Unit V
Caring Throughout the Lifespan

Unit VI
Psychosocial Considerations

Unit VII
Scientific Basis for Nursing Practice

Unit VIII
Basic Physiological Needs

Unit IX
Clients with Special Needs

ELSEVIER

evolve

To access your Student Resources, visit the Web address below:

http://evolve.elsevier.com/Canada/Potter/fundamentals/

- **Student Learning Activities**
  Include crosswords, hangman puzzles, matching games, case studies, and short answer questions.
- **Review Questions**
  Include answers and rationales.
- **Concept Map Exercises**
  Challenge you to work with multiple nursing diagnoses and recognize their relationship to medical diagnoses.
- **Animations**
  Include exciting images related to various chapters in the textbook.
- **Critical Thinking Exercises**
  Challenge you to recognize how nursing process and critical thinking come together so that you can provide the best care for your clients.
- **Video Clips**
  Demonstrate important steps in a variety of nursing skills throughout the textbook.
- **WebLinks**
  Take you to hundreds of exciting websites carefully chosen to supplement the content of the textbook.
- **Content Updates**
  Include the latest information from the authors of the textbook to keep you current with recent developments in this area of study.

With over 1100 illustrations

Canadian Fundamentals of Nursing

Patricia A. Potter, RN, MSN, PhD, CMAC, FAAN
Research Scientist
Barnes-Jewish Hospital
St. Louis, Missouri

Anne Griffin Perry, RN, MSN, EdD, FAAN
Professor and Interim Director of Research
Saint Louis University School of Nursing
Saint Louis University Health Sciences Center
St. Louis, Missouri

Janet C. Ross-Kerr, RN, BScN, MS, PhD
Professor, Faculty of Nursing
University of Alberta
Edmonton, Alberta

Marilynn J. Wood, RN, BSN, MSN, DrPH
Professor, Faculty of Nursing
University of Alberta
Edmonton, Alberta

ELSEVIER
MOSBY

3rd Edition

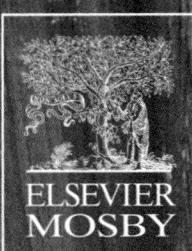

NOTICE

Neither the Publisher not the Editors assume any responsibility for any loss or injury and/or damage to persons or property arising out of or related to any use of the material contained in this book. It is the responsibility of the treating practitioner, relying on independent expertise and knowledge of the patient, to determine the best treatment and method of application for the patient.

Library and Archives Canada Cataloguing in Publication

Potter, Patricia Ann
Canadian fundamentals of nursing / Patricia A. Potter, Anne Griffin Perry; Canadian editors, Janet C. Ross-Kerr, Marilynn J. Wood—3rd ed.
Includes bibliographical references and index.
ISBN-13: 978-0-7796-9961-2 ISBN-10: 0-7796-9961-0
1. Nursing—Textbooks. 2. Nursing—Canada—Textbooks.
I. Perry, Anne Griffin II. Kerr, Janet C., 1940- III. Wood, Marilynn J. IV. Title.
RT41.P68 2005 610.73 C2004-907453-9

Publisher: Ann Millar
Developmental Editors: Heather McWhinney and Joanne Sanche
Managing Developmental Editor: Martina van de Velde
Projects Manager: Liz Radojkovic
Production Editor: Marcel Chiera
Copy Editor: Barb Every
Cover and Interior Design: Kathi Gosche
Typesetting and Assembly: Graphic World
Printing and Binding: Transcontinental

Elsevier Canada
1 Goldthorne Ave., Toronto, ON, Canada M8Z 5S7
Phone: 1-866-896-3331
Fax: 1-866-359-9534

ISBN-13: 978-0-7796-9961-2
ISBN-10: 0-7796-9961-0

Printed in Canada

2 3 4 5 10 09 08 07 06 05

Canadian Fundamentals of Nursing

Canadian Contributors

Canadian Editors

Janet C. Ross-Kerr, RN, BScN, MS, PhD
Professor, Faculty of Nursing, University of Alberta
Edmonton, Alberta

Marilynn J. Wood, RN, BSN, MSN, DrPH
Professor, Faculty of Nursing, University of Alberta
Edmonton, Alberta

Canadian Contributors

Marion Allen, RN, PhD
Associate Dean; Professor, Faculty of Nursing,
University of Alberta
Edmonton, Alberta

Marjorie C. Anderson, RN, PhD
Associate Professor, Retired
Faculty of Nursing
University of Alberta
Edmonton Alberta

Debbie Fraser Askin, RNC, MN
Assistant Professor, Faculty of Nursing
University of Manitoba
Winnipeg, Manitoba

Barbara J. Astle, RN, BScN, MN, PhD (candidate)
Doctoral Candidate, Faculty of Nursing
University of Alberta
Edmonton, Alberta
Formerly Nursing Instructor, Faculty of Nursing
University of Calgary
Calgary, Alberta

Maureen Barry, BScN, MScN
Senior Lecturer, Faculty of Nursing
University of Toronto
Toronto, Ontario

Zoraida DeCastro Beekhoo, RN, MA
Lecturer, Faculty of Nursing
University of Toronto
Toronto, Ontario

Donna Best, RN, BN, MN, ACNP
Associate Professor, School of Nursing
Memorial University of Newfoundland
St. John's, Newfoundland

Judee E. Onyskiw, RN, PhD
Canada Research Chair in Family Violence and Health
Associate Professor, Faculty of Nursing
University of New Brunswick
Fredericton, New Brunswick

Shelley Raffin Bouchal, RN, BScN, MN, PhD
Assistant Professor, Faculty of Nursing
University of Calgary
Calgary, Alberta

Ann Brokenshire, RN, BScN, MEd
Instructor, School of Nursing
Ryerson University
Toronto, Ontario

Barbara Brown, RN, BA, BScN, MScN
Associate Professor, School of Nursing
McMaster University
Hamilton, Ontario

Marion Clauson, RN, MSN, PNC(C)
Senior Instructor; Associate Director, Undergraduate Programs
School of Nursing
University of British Columbia
Vancouver, British Columbia

Rene A. Day, RN, PhD
Professor and Associate Dean, Executive and Partnership Development
Faculty of Nursing
University of Alberta
Edmonton, Alberta

Jan Park Dorsay, RN, MN, ACPN(D)
Assistant Clinical Professor, Faculty of Health Sciences
McMaster University
Hamilton, Ontario

Jane Drummond, RN, PhD
Professor, Faculty of Nursing
University of Alberta
Edmonton, Alberta

Wendy Duggleby, DSN, RN, AOCN
Associate Professor, College of Nursing
University of Saskatchewan
Saskatoon, Saskatchewan

Susanna Edwards, RN, BScN, MSc, PhD(pc)
Assistant Professor, School of Nursing
Ryerson University
Toronto, Ontario

Frances Fothergill-Bourbonnais, RN, BScN, MN, PhD
Professor, School of Nursing
University of Ottawa
Ottawa, Ontario

Jo-Ann E.T. Fox-Threlkeld, RN, BN, MSc, PhD
Professor Emeritus, School of Nursing
McMaster University
Hamilton, Ontario

Julie A. Gilbert, RN, BScN, MN
Sessional Instructor, Faculty of Nursing
University of Alberta
Edmonton, Alberta

Nancy C. Goddard, RN, BScN, MN, PhD
Adjunct Assistant Professor, University of Alberta
Edmonton, Alberta
Nursing Instructor, Red Deer College
Red Deer, Alberta

Sonya Grypma, RN, PhD
Assistant Professor, School of Health Sciences
University of Lethbridge
Lethbridge, Alberta

Kathryn A. Smith Higuchi, RN, BScN, MEd, PhD
Assistant Professor, School of Nursing
University of Ottawa
Ottawa, Ontario

Kaysi Eastlick Kushner, RN, PhD
Assistant Professor, Faculty of Nursing
University of Alberta
Edmonton, Alberta

Maureen Leahey, RN, PhD
Manager, Outpatient Mental Health Program
Director, Family Therapy Training Program
Calgary Health Region
Adjunct Associate Professor, Faculties of Nursing and Medicine (Psychiatry)
University of Calgary
Calgary, Alberta

Lenora Marcellus, RN, PhD (candidate)
Instructor, School of Nursing
University of Victoria
Victoria, British Columbia
Doctoral Candidate
University of Alberta
Edmonton, Alberta

Jean McClennon-Leong, RN, MN, APNP
Professor, Faculty of Nursing
Northeast Wisconsin Technical College
Green Bay, Wisconsin
Master's Student
University of Alberta
Edmonton, Alberta

Maureen McQueen, RN, MN
Coordinator, Undergraduate Programs
Centre for Nursing and Health Studies
Athabasca University
Athabasca, Alberta

Jennifer Medves, RN, PhD
Assistant Professor
School of Nursing
Queen's University
Kingston, Ontario

Jill Milne, RN, MN, PhD
Postdoctoral Fellow, Faculty of Nursing
University of Alberta
Edmonton, Alberta

Deborah Mings, RN, MHSc, ACNP, GNC(C)
Clinical Nurse Specialist, Rehabilitation and Complex Continuing Care
St. Peter's Hospital
Hamilton Ontario

Anita Molzahn, RN, BScN, MN, PhD
Professor, School of Nursing
University of Victoria
Victoria, British Columbia

Katherine N. Moore, RN, PhD
Associate Professor, Faculty of Nursing
University of Alberta
Edmonton, Alberta

Linda Reutter, RN, PhD
Professor, Faculty of Nursing
University of Alberta
Edmonton, Alberta

Ginette Lemire Rodger, RN, BScN, MAdmN, PhD
Vice President, Professional Practice; Chief Nursing Executive
The Ottawa Hospital
Ottawa, Ontario

Daria Romaniuk, RN, BN, MN
Assistant Professor, School of Nursing
Ryerson University
Toronto, Ontario

Donna M. Romyn, RN, PhD
Associate Professor; Director, Centre for Nursing and Health Studies
Athabasca University
Athabasca, Alberta

Cheryl Sams, RN, BScN, MSN
School of Nursing
York University and Seneca College
Toronto, Ontario

Carla Shapiro, RN, MN
Instructor II, Faculty of Nursing
University of Manitoba
Winnipeg, Manitoba

D. Lynn Skillen, PhD, RN
Professor, Faculty of Nursing
University of Alberta
Edmonton, Alberta

Marlene Smadu, RN, BScN, MAdEd, ED
Associate Dean, Regina Site
College of Nursing
University of Saskatchewan
Regina, Saskatchewan

Shirley Solberg, BN, MN, PhD
Associate Professor, School of Nursing
Memorial University of Newfoundland
St. John's, Newfoundland

T.C. Stephen, RN, BScN, MN
Sessional Instructor, Faculty of Nursing
University of Alberta
Edmonton, Alberta

Sally Thorne, RN, PhD
Professor and Director, School of Nursing
University of British Columbia
Vancouver, British Columbia

Ardene Robinson Vollman, RN, BScN, MA, PhD
Adjunct Associate Professor
Faculties of Nursing, Medicine (Community Health Sciences), and Kinesiology
University of Calgary
Calgary, Alberta

Fay F. Warnock, RN, PhD
Assistant Professor, School of Nursing
University of British Columbia
Vancouver, British Columbia

Lorraine M. Wright, RN, PhD
Professor Emeritus, School of Nursing
University of Calgary
Calgary, Alberta

Contributors

Jeanette Adams, PhD, MSN, APRN, CRNI
Nursing Consultant
Coconut Grove, Florida

Myra. A. Aud, PhD, RN
Assistant Professor
Sinclair School of Nursing, University of Missouri–Columbia
Columbia, Missouri

Marjorie Baier, RN, PhD, APRN, BC
Associate Professor
School of Nursing, Southern Illinois University Edwardsville
Edwardsville, Illinois

Janice Boundy, RN, PhD
Professor, Director of Graduate Program
Saint Francis College of Nursing
Peoria, Illinois

Anna Brock, PhD, MSN, MEd, BSN
Professor
University of Southern Mississippi College of Nursing
Hattiesburg, Mississippi

Pamela L. Cherry, RN, BSN, MSN, DNSc
Associate Professor of Nursing
Humboldt State University
Arcata, California

Janice C. Colwell, RN, MS, CWOCN
Clinical Nurse Specialist, Wound, Ostomy & Skin Care
University of Chicago Hospitals
Chicago, Illinois

Eileen Costantinou, RN, MSN
Professional Practice Consultant
Barnes-Jewish Hospital
St. Louis, Missouri

Christine Durbin, RN, MSN, JD, PhDc
Instructor, School of Nursing
Southern Illinois University–Edwardsville
Edwardsville, Illinois

Margaret Ecker, RN, MS, PNP
Director of Education
Saint John's Health Center
Santa Monica, California

Martha Keene Elkin, RN, MS, IBCLC
Nursing Educator for Associate Degree Nursing
Private Practice Lactation Consultant
Mother Care of Maine
Sumner, Maine

Susan Jane Fetzer, RN, BA, BSN, MSN, MBA, PhD
Associate Professor
University of New Hampshire
Durham, New Hampshire

Victoria N. Folse, PhD, APRN, CS, LCPC
Assistant Professor
Illinois Wesleyan University
Bloomington, Illinois

Leah W. Frederick, MS, RN CIC
Infection Control Consultant
Infection Control Consultants
Scottsdale, Arizona

Amy Hall, RN, BSN, MS, PhD
Associate Professor
Saint Francis Medical Center College of Nursing
Peoria, Illinois

Mimi Hirshberg, RN, MSN
Clinical Assistant Professor
Barnes College of Nursing and Health Studies
University of Missouri–St. Louis
St. Louis, Missouri
IV Therapist
Vascular Access Service
Barnes-Jewish Hospital
St. Louis, Missouri

Steve Kilkus, RN, MSN
Nursing Faculty
Edgewood College
Madison, Wisconsin

Judith Ann Kilpatrick, RN, DNSc
Assistant Professor
Widener University School of Nursing
Chester, Pennsylvania

Kristine M. L'Ecuyer, RN, MSN, CCNS
Adjunct Assistant Professor
Saint Louis University School of Nursing
St. Louis, Missouri

Joyce Larson, PhD, MS, RN
President, Founder Culture and Counts
Adjunct Hillsborough Community College
Tampa, Florida

Ruth Ludwick, BSN, MSN, PhD, RNC
Professor
Kent State University, College of Nursing
Kent, Ohio

Annette G. Lueckenotte, MS, RN, BC, GNP GCNS
Gerontologic Nurse Practitioner and Educator
Barnes-Jewish West County Hospital
St. Louis, Missouri

Elaine K. Neel, BSN, MSN
Nursing Instructor
Graham Hospital School of Nursing
Canton, Illinois

Dula Pacquiao, BSN, MA, EdD
Professor, Director of Transcultural Nursing Institute and Coordinator of Graduate Program
Kean University
Union, New Jersey

Nancy C. Panthofer, RN, MSN
Lecturer
Kent State University College of Nursing
Kent, Ohio

Elaine U. Polan, RNC, BSN, MS
Nursing Program Supervisor
Vocational Education and Extension Board Practical Nursing Program
Uniondale, New York

Patsy L. Ruchala, DNSc, RN
Director and Professor
Orvis School of Nursing
University of Nevada–Reno
Reno, Nevada

Debbie Sanazaro, RN, MSN, GNP
Assistant Professor
Saint Louis University School of Nursing
St. Louis, Missouri

Marilyn Schallom, RN, MSN, CCRN, CCNS
Surgical Critical Care Clinical Nurse Specialist
Barnes-Jewish Hospital
St. Louis, Missouri

Patricia A. Stockert, RN, BSN, MS PhD
Associate Professor, Coordinator
Saint Francis Medical Center College of Nursing
Peoria, Illinois

Marshelle Thobaben, RN, MS, PHN, APNP, FNP
Chair and Professor
Humboldt State University
Arcata, California

Pamela Becker Weilitz, RN, MSN(R), BC, ANP, M-SCNS
Adult Nurse Practitioner
Private Practice
St. Louis, Missouri

Joan Domigan Wentz, BSN, MSN
Assistant Professor
Jewish Hospital College of Nursing and Allied Health
St. Louis, Missouri

Rita Wunderlich, BSN, MSN(r), PhD
Assistant Professor
Saint Louis University
School of Nursing
St. Louis, Missouri

Reviewers

Phil Bourget, RN, MN
Nursing Faculty
Georgian College
Barrie, ON

Christine Boyle, RN, BScN, MA
Nursing Instructor
Mount Royal College
Calgary, AB

Ethel Bratt
Faculty, Nursing Division
Nursing Education Program of Saskatchewan
Saskatchewan Institute of Applied Science and Technology (Wascana Campus)
Regina, SK

Madeleine Buck, BSc(N), MSc
Assistant Director, School of Nursing
McGill University
Montreal, QC

Carol Butler RN, BScN, MScN
Program Coordinator Practical Nursing
Fanshawe College
London Ontario

Lorna Butler, RN, BScN, MN, PhD
Professor, School of Nursing
Dalhousie University
Halifax, Nova Scotia

Michelle Connell, BScN, MEd
Years 1 & 4 Collaborative Nursing Degree Coordinator
Centennial College
Scarborough, ON

Kathryn Crooks RN, Ph.D (candidate)
Coordinator, Undergraduate Nursing Program
Medicine Hat College
Medicine Hat, AB

Katherine Cummings, RN BScN MHSc
Professor of Nursing
University of Ontario/Durham College
Oshawa, ON

Elizabeth Domm, RN, MSN
Assistant Professor, College of Nursing
University of Saskatchewan
Regina, SK

Rebecca Dyck, RN, BScN, MA
Nursing Instructor
Dawson College
Montreal, Quebec

Susan Eldred, RN, BScN, MBA, PHN
Coordinator, Year One Generic Program
Faculty of Health Sciences, School of Nursing
University of Ottawa
Ottawa, ON

Ann Fisk, RN, MEd
Instructor, Nursing Department
Red Deer College
Red Deer, AB

Kerri L. Honeychurch, RN, BScN, MEd
Professor of Nursing
Seneca College of Applied Arts and Technology
Toronto, ON

Nina Hrycak, RN, BScN, MEd, PhD
Associate Professor of Nursing
University of Calgary
Calgary, AB

Jean Jackson, RN, BScN, MAEd
Coordinator PN and PSW Programs
Durham College
Oshawa, ON

Kathy King, RN, CCRN, BScN, MA, PhD (candidate)
Professor, Nipissing University/Canadore College BScN Program
North Bay, ON

Ola Lunyk-Child, BScN, MScN, RN, PhD (candidate)
Assistant Professor of Nursing & Level 1 Chair, BScN Program
McMaster University
Hamilton, ON

Lesley MacMaster, RN, MSc
Nursing Faculty
Georgian College
Barrie, ON

Jeanne Molnar, RN, BN, MEd
Professor/Co-ordinator, BScN Program
Algonquin College
Ottawa, Ontario

Wendy Motley, RN, BScN, MN
Nursing Instructor
Red Deer College,
Red Deer, Alberta

Barbara Reid, RN(EC), BScN, MHSc
Professor of Nursing
Northern College of Applied Arts and Technology
Timmins, ON

Frances Ross, RN, MScN
Professor of Nursing
George Brown College
Toronto, ON

Stephen Sanche, MD, FRCPS
Assistant Professor, Division of Infectious Diseases
Royal University Hospital
Saskatoon, SK

Carol Ann Sherman, RN, MSN, CPCN
Faculty Lecturer, School of Nursing
McGill University
Montreal, QC

Susan Sproul RN, BScN, MScN
Professor of Nursing, Collaborative Nursing Program
University of Ontario Institute of Technology/Durham College
Oshawa, ON

Jean Stevens, RN, MA
Curriculum Coordinator, Nursing Programs
Georgian College
Barrie, ON

Beth Swart, RN, BScN, MES
Professor, School of Nursing
Ryerson University
Toronto, ON

Sylvia van der Weg, RN, BSCN, MA(Ed)
Professor of Nursing
Georgian College
Barrie, ON

Mireille Walsh, BScN, RN, ENC(C), MScN (candidate)
Professor, Northeastern Ontario Collaborative Nursing Program
Northern College
Timmins, ON

Kathryn Weatherall, RN, MEd
Nursing Faculty
Georgian College
Barrie, ON

Sandy Wiesenthal, RN, MN
Professor, Centre for Nursing
George Brown College
Toronto, ON

Karen Wilson, BScN, MSc
Level 1 Coordinator, Collaborative BScN Program
Conestoga College
Kitchener, ON

Leanne J. Wyrostok RN, MN
Senior Instructor/Nursing Skills Clinician, Faculty of Nursing
University of Calgary
Calgary, AB

Student Preface

Learning Objectives begin each chapter to help you focus on the key information that follows.

Chapters end with **Key Concepts** to help you review.

Critical Thinking Exercises help you apply essential content.

Review Questions at the end of each chapter help you review and evaluate what you have learned. Answers and rationales are provided at the back of the book.

Key Terms are listed at the end of each chapter and are boldfaced and defined in the text. Page numbers help you quickly find where each term is defined.

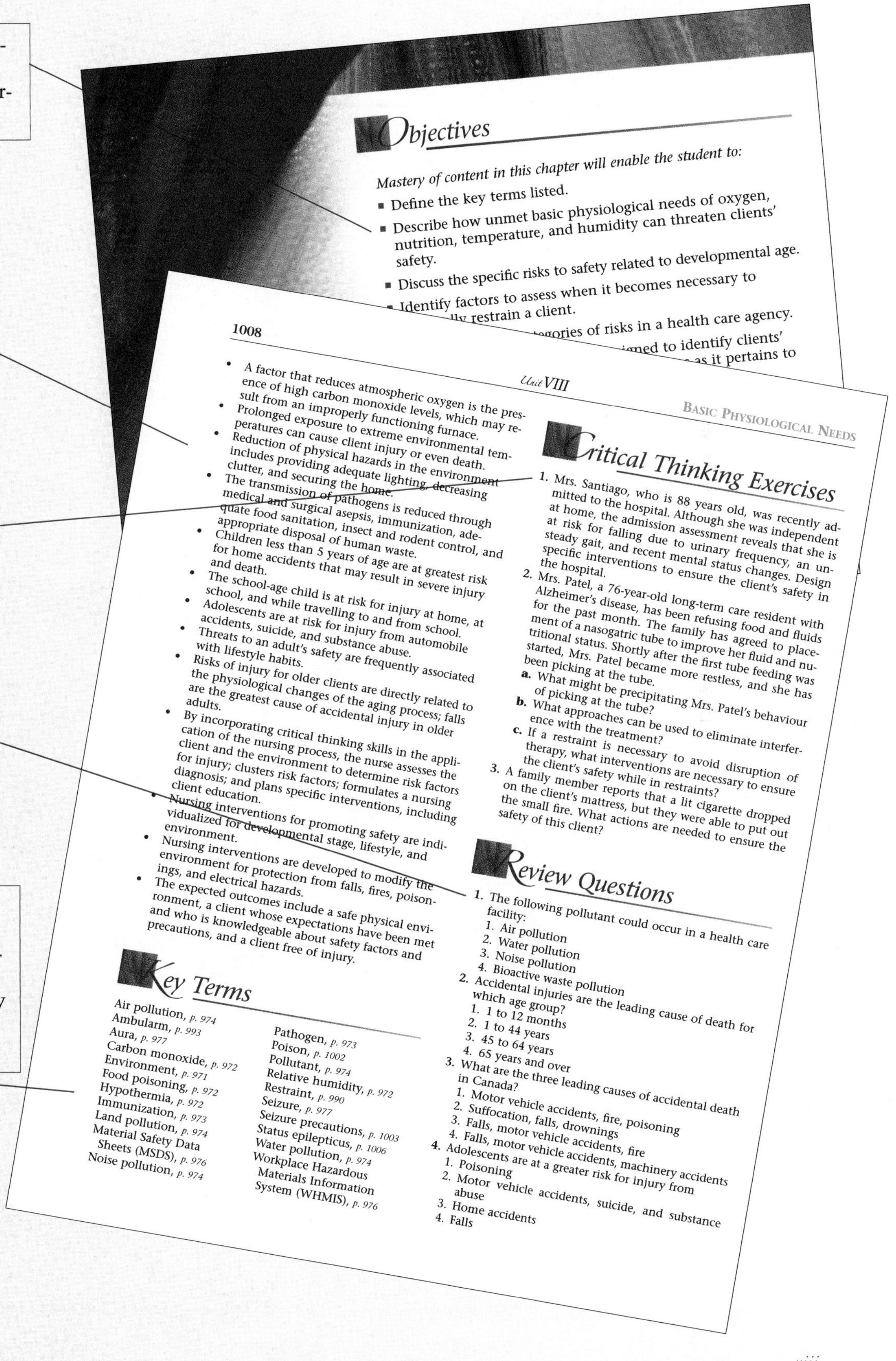
Objectives

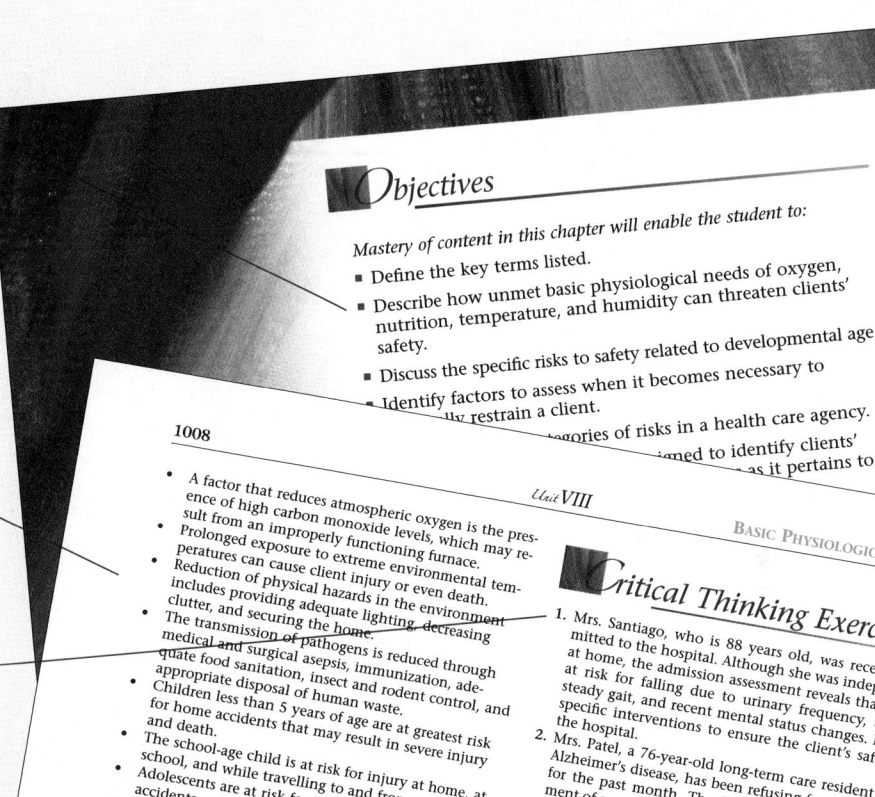

Mastery of content in this chapter will enable the student to:

- Define the key terms listed.
- Describe how unmet basic physiological needs of oxygen, nutrition, temperature, and humidity can threaten clients' safety.
- Discuss the specific risks to safety related to developmental age.
- Identify factors to assess when it becomes necessary to ...lly restrain a client.
- ...egories of risks in a health care agency.
- ...gned to identify clients' ... as it pertains to

1008 *Unit* VIII BASIC PHYSIOLOGICAL NEEDS

- A factor that reduces atmospheric oxygen is the presence of high carbon monoxide levels, which may result from an improperly functioning furnace.
- Prolonged exposure to extreme environmental temperatures can cause client injury or even death.
- Reduction of physical hazards in the environment includes providing adequate lighting, decreasing clutter, and securing the home.
- The transmission of pathogens is reduced through medical and surgical asepsis, immunization, adequate food sanitation, insect and rodent control, and appropriate disposal of human waste.
- Children less than 5 years of age are at greatest risk for home accidents that may result in severe injury and death.
- The school-age child is at risk for injury at home, at school, and while travelling to and from school.
- Adolescents are at risk for injury from automobile accidents, suicide, and substance abuse.
- Threats to an adult's safety are frequently associated with lifestyle habits.
- Risks of injury for older clients are directly related to the physiological changes of the aging process; falls are the greatest cause of accidental injury in older adults.
- By incorporating critical thinking skills in the application of the nursing process, the nurse assesses the client and the environment to determine risk factors for injury; clusters risk factors; formulates a nursing diagnosis; and plans specific interventions, including client education.
- Nursing interventions for promoting safety are individualized for developmental stage, lifestyle, and environment.
- Nursing interventions are developed to modify the environment for protection from falls, fires, poisonings, and electrical hazards.
- The expected outcomes include a safe physical environment, a client whose expectations have been met and who is knowledgeable about safety factors and precautions, and a client free of injury.

Key Terms

Air pollution, *p. 974*
Ambularm, *p. 993*
Aura, *p. 977*
Carbon monoxide, *p. 972*
Environment, *p. 971*
Food poisoning, *p. 972*
Hypothermia, *p. 972*
Immunization, *p. 973*
Land pollution, *p. 974*
Material Safety Data Sheets (MSDS), *p. 976*
Noise pollution, *p. 974*
Pathogen, *p. 973*
Poison, *p. 1002*
Pollutant, *p. 974*
Relative humidity, *p. 972*
Restraint, *p. 990*
Seizure, *p. 977*
Seizure precautions, *p. 1003*
Status epilepticus, *p. 1006*
Water pollution, *p. 974*
Workplace Hazardous Materials Information System (WHMIS), *p. 976*

Critical Thinking Exercises

1. Mrs. Santiago, who is 88 years old, was recently admitted to the hospital. Although she was independent at home, the admission assessment reveals that she is at risk for falling due to urinary frequency, an unsteady gait, and recent mental status changes. Design specific interventions to ensure the client's safety in the hospital.
2. Mrs. Patel, a 76-year-old long-term care resident with Alzheimer's disease, has been refusing food and fluids for the past month. The family has agreed to placement of a nasogatric tube to improve her fluid and nutritional status. Shortly after the first tube feeding was started, Mrs. Patel became more restless, and she has been picking at the tube.
   a. What might be precipitating Mrs. Patel's behaviour of picking at the tube?
   b. What approaches can be used to eliminate interference with the treatment?
   c. If a restraint is necessary to avoid disruption of therapy, what interventions are necessary to ensure the client's safety while in restraints?
3. A family member reports that a lit cigarette dropped on the client's mattress, but they were able to put out the small fire. What actions are needed to ensure the safety of this client?

Review Questions

1. The following pollutant could occur in a health care facility:
   1. Air pollution
   2. Water pollution
   3. Noise pollution
   4. Bioactive waste pollution
2. Accidental injuries are the leading cause of death for which age group?
   1. 1 to 12 months
   2. 1 to 44 years
   3. 45 to 64 years
   4. 65 years and over
3. What are the three leading causes of accidental death in Canada?
   1. Motor vehicle accidents, fire, poisoning
   2. Suffocation, falls, drownings
   3. Falls, motor vehicle accidents, fire
   4. Falls, motor vehicle accidents, machinery accidents
4. Adolescents are at a greater risk for injury from
   1. Poisoning
   2. Motor vehicle accidents, suicide, and substance abuse
   3. Home accidents
   4. Falls

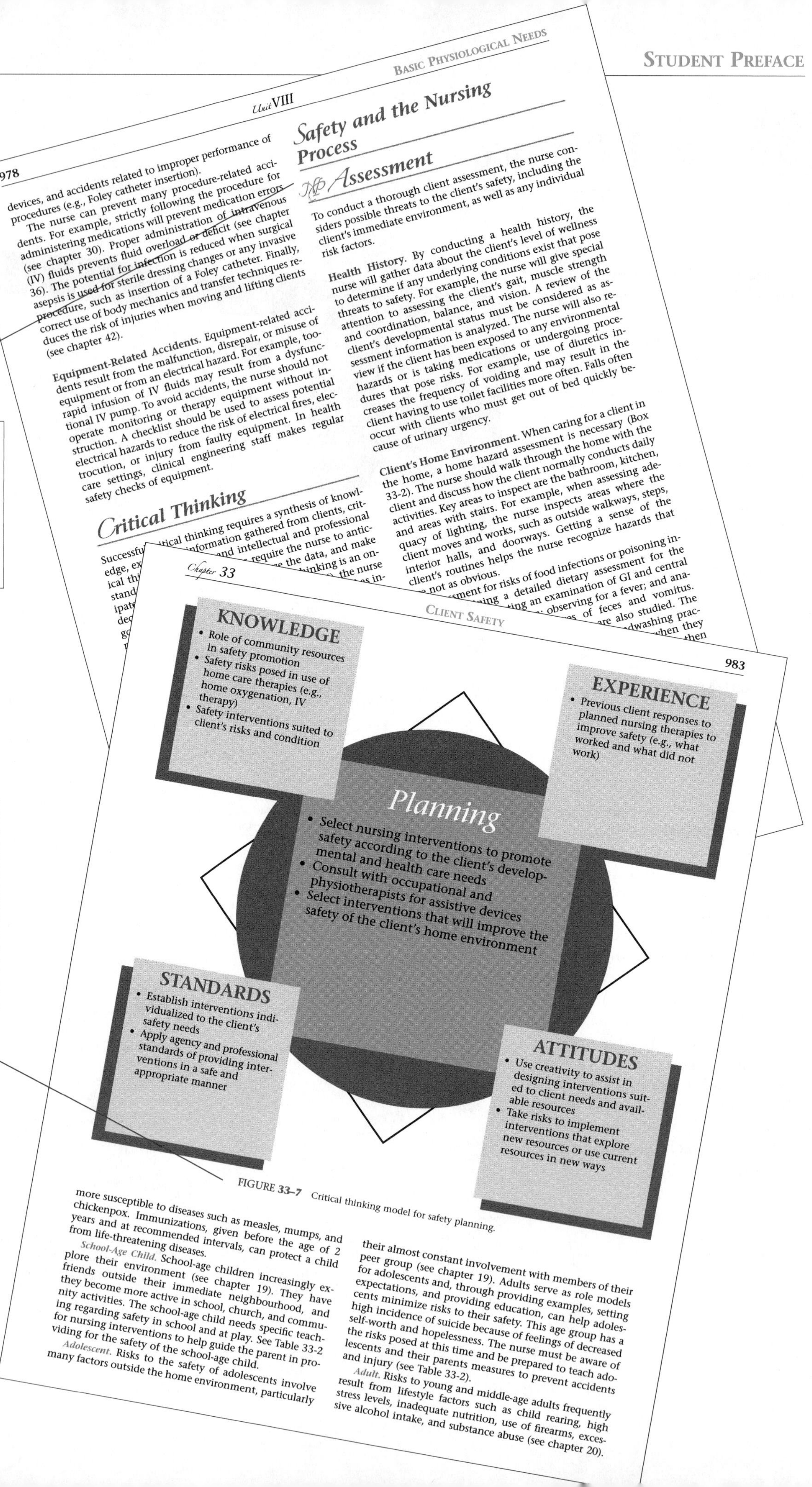
978
Unit VIII
BASIC PHYSIOLOGICAL NEEDS
devices, and accidents related to improper performance of procedures (e.g., Foley catheter insertion).
The nurse can prevent many procedure-related accidents. For example, strictly following the procedure for administering medications will prevent medication errors (see chapter 30). Proper administration of intravenous (IV) fluids prevents fluid overload or deficit (see chapter 36). The potential for infection is reduced when surgical asepsis is used for sterile dressing changes or any invasive procedure, such as insertion of a Foley catheter. Finally, correct use of body mechanics and transfer techniques reduces the risk of injuries when moving and lifting clients (see chapter 42).
Equipment-Related Accidents. Equipment-related accidents result from the malfunction, disrepair, or misuse of equipment or from an electrical hazard. For example, too-rapid infusion of IV fluids may result from a dysfunctional IV pump. To avoid accidents, the nurse should not operate monitoring or therapy equipment without instruction. A checklist should be used to assess potential electrical hazards to reduce the risk of electrical fires, electrocution, or injury from faulty equipment. In health care settings, clinical engineering staff makes regular safety checks of equipment.
Critical Thinking
Safety and the Nursing Process
Assessment
To conduct a thorough client assessment, the nurse considers possible threats to the client's safety, including the client's immediate environment, as well as any individual risk factors.
Health History. By conducting a health history, the nurse will gather data about the client's level of wellness to determine if any underlying conditions exist that pose threats to safety. For example, the nurse will give special attention to assessing the client's gait, muscle strength and coordination, balance, and vision. A review of the client's developmental status must be considered as assessment information is analyzed. The nurse will also review if the client has been exposed to any environmental hazards or is taking medications or undergoing procedures that pose risks. For example, use of diuretics increases the frequency of voiding and may result in the client having to use toilet facilities more often. Falls often occur with clients who must get out of bed quickly because of urinary urgency.
Client's Home Environment. When caring for a client in the home, a home hazard assessment is necessary (Box 33-2). The nurse should walk through the home with the client and discuss how the client normally conducts daily activities. Key areas to inspect are the bathroom, kitchen, and areas with stairs. For example, when assessing adequacy of lighting, the nurse inspects areas where the client moves and works, such as outside walkways, steps, interior halls, and doorways. Getting a sense of the client's routines helps the nurse recognize hazards that are not as obvious.
Chapter 33
CLIENT SAFETY
983
KNOWLEDGE
• Role of community resources in safety promotion
• Safety risks posed in use of home care therapies (e.g., home oxygenation, IV therapy)
• Safety interventions suited to client's risks and condition
EXPERIENCE
• Previous client responses to planned nursing therapies to improve safety (e.g., what worked and what did not work)
Planning
• Select nursing interventions to promote safety according to the client's developmental and health care needs
• Consult with occupational and physiotherapists for assistive devices
• Select interventions that will improve the safety of the client's home environment
STANDARDS
• Establish interventions individualized to the client's safety needs
• Apply agency and professional standards of providing interventions in a safe and appropriate manner
ATTITUDES
• Use creativity to assist in designing interventions suited to client needs and available resources
• Take risks to implement interventions that explore new resources or use current resources in new ways
FIGURE 33–7 Critical thinking model for safety planning.
more susceptible to diseases such as measles, mumps, and chickenpox. Immunizations, given before the age of 2 years and at recommended intervals, can protect a child from life-threatening diseases.
School-Age Child. School-age children increasingly explore their environment (see chapter 19). They have friends outside their immediate neighbourhood, and they become more active in school, church, and community activities. The school-age child needs specific teaching regarding safety in school and at play. See Table 33-2 for nursing interventions to help guide the parent in providing for the safety of the school-age child.
Adolescent. Risks to the safety of adolescents involve many factors outside the home environment, particularly their almost constant involvement with members of their peer group (see chapter 19). Adults serve as role models for adolescents and, through providing examples, setting expectations, and providing education, can help adolescents minimize risks to their safety. This age group has a high incidence of suicide because of feelings of decreased self-worth and hopelessness. The nurse must be aware of the risks posed at this time and be prepared to teach adolescents and their parents measures to prevent accidents and injury (see Table 33-2).
Adult. Risks to young and middle-age adults frequently result from lifestyle factors such as child rearing, high stress levels, inadequate nutrition, use of firearms, excessive alcohol intake, and substance abuse (see chapter 20).

The five-step **Nursing Process** provides a consistent framework for presentation of content in clinical chapters.

The unique **Critical Thinking Model** clearly shows how nursing process and critical thinking come together to help you provide the best care for your clients.

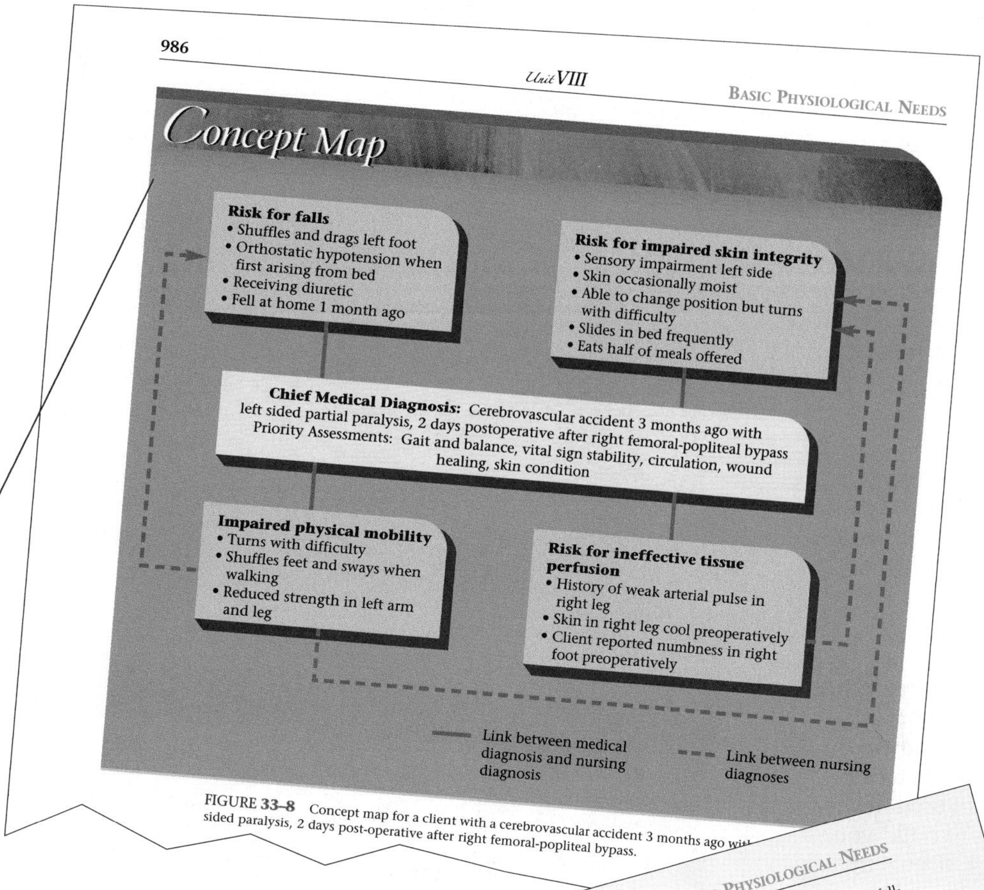

986
Unit VIII
BASIC PHYSIOLOGICAL NEEDS
Concept Map
Risk for falls
• Shuffles and drags left foot
• Orthostatic hypotension when first arising from bed
• Receiving diuretic
• Fell at home 1 month ago
Risk for impaired skin integrity
• Sensory impairment left side
• Skin occasionally moist
• Able to change position but turns with difficulty
• Slides in bed frequently
• Eats half of meals offered
Chief Medical Diagnosis: Cerebrovascular accident 3 months ago with left sided partial paralysis, 2 days postoperative after right femoral-popliteal bypass
Priority Assessments: Gait and balance, vital sign stability, circulation, wound healing, skin condition
Impaired physical mobility
• Turns with difficulty
• Shuffles feet and sways when walking
• Reduced strength in left arm and leg
Risk for ineffective tissue perfusion
• History of weak arterial pulse in right leg
• Skin in right leg cool preoperatively
• Client reported numbness in right foot preoperatively
Link between medical diagnosis and nursing diagnosis
Link between nursing diagnoses
FIGURE 33–8 Concept map for a client with a cerebrovascular accident 3 months ago wi... sided paralysis, 2 days post-operative after right femoral-popliteal bypass.

Concept Maps show you the association among multiple nursing diagnoses and their relationship to medical diagnoses.

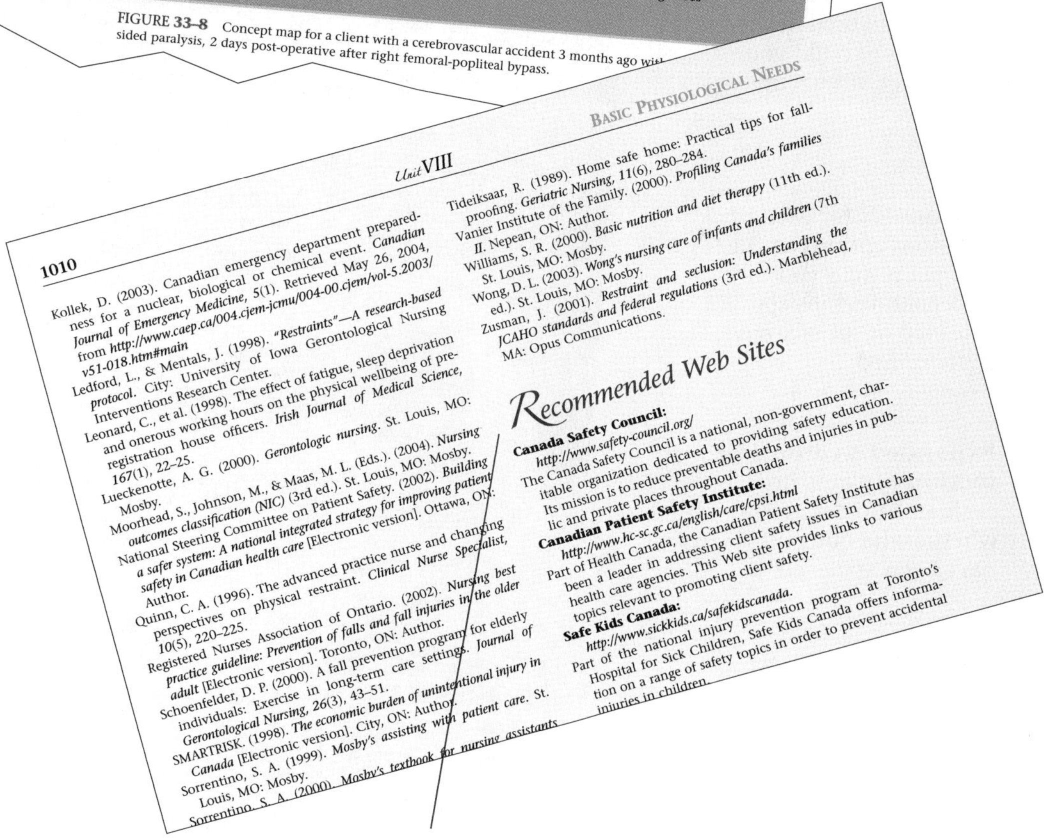

1010 Unit VIII BASIC PHYSIOLOGICAL NEEDS

Kollek, D. (2003). Canadian emergency department preparedness for a nuclear, biological or chemical event. *Canadian Journal of Emergency Medicine, 5*(1). Retrieved May 26, 2004, from http://www.caep.ca/004.cjem-jcmu/004-00.cjem/vol-5.2003/v51-018.htm#main

Ledford, L., & Mentals, J. (1998). *"Restraints"—A research-based protocol*. City: University of Iowa Gerontological Nursing Interventions Research Center.

Leonard, C., et al. (1998). The effect of fatigue, sleep deprivation and onerous working hours on the physical wellbeing of pre-registration house officers. *Irish Journal of Medical Science, 167*(1), 22–25.

Lueckenotte, A. G. (2000). *Gerontologic nursing*. St. Louis, MO: Mosby.

Moorhead, S., Johnson, M., & Maas, M. L. (Eds.). (2004). *Nursing outcomes classification (NIC)* (3rd ed.). St. Louis, MO: Mosby.

National Steering Committee on Patient Safety. (2002). *Building a safer system: A national integrated strategy for improving patient safety in Canadian health care* [Electronic version]. Ottawa, ON: Author.

Quinn, C. A. (1996). The advanced practice nurse and changing perspectives on physical restraint. *Clinical Nurse Specialist, 10*(5), 220–225.

Registered Nurses Association of Ontario. (2002). *Nursing best practice guideline: Prevention of falls and fall injuries in the older adult* [Electronic version]. Toronto, ON: Author.

Schoenfelder, D. P. (2000). A fall prevention program for elderly individuals: Exercise in long-term care settings. *Journal of Gerontological Nursing, 26*(3), 43–51.

SMARTRISK. (1998). *The economic burden of unintentional injury in Canada* [Electronic version]. City, ON: Author.

Sorrentino, S. A. (1999). *Mosby's assisting with patient care*. St. Louis, MO: Mosby.

Sorrentino, S. A. (2000). *Mosby's textbook for nursing assistants*

Tideiksaar, R. (1989). Home safe home: Practical tips for fall-proofing. *Geriatric Nursing, 11*(6), 280–284.

Vanier Institute of the Family. (2000). *Profiling Canada's families II*. Nepean, ON: Author.

Williams, S. R. (2000). *Basic nutrition and diet therapy* (11th ed.). St. Louis, MO: Mosby.

Wong, D. L. (2003). *Wong's nursing care of infants and children* (7th ed.). St. Louis, MO: Mosby.

Zusman, J. (2001). *Restraint and seclusion: Understanding the JCAHO standards and federal regulations* (3rd ed.). Marblehead, MA: Opus Communications.

Recommended Web Sites

Canada Safety Council:
http://www.safety-council.org/
The Canada Safety Council is a national, non-government, charitable organization dedicated to providing safety education. Its mission is to reduce preventable deaths and injuries in public and private places throughout Canada.

Canadian Patient Safety Institute:
http://www.hc-sc.gc.ca/english/care/cpsi.html
Part of Health Canada, the Canadian Patient Safety Institute has been a leader in addressing client safety issues in Canadian health care agencies. This Web site provides links to various topics relevant to promoting client safety.

Safe Kids Canada:
http://www.sickkids.ca/safekidscanada.
Part of the national injury prevention program at Toronto's Hospital for Sick Children, Safe Kids Canada offers information on a range of safety topics in order to prevent accidental injuries in children.

Recommended Web Sites list up-to-date online resources

Nursing Care Plans feature a revised format that helps you understand the process of assessment, the association of assessment findings with defining characteristics of nursing diagnoses, the identification of goals and outcomes, selection of interventions, and the process for evaluating care.

Assessment section tells you how to gather data instead of just listing findings.

Nursing Intervention Classification and **Nursing Outcome Classification** terminologies are used in the care plans to build your knowledge of nursing concepts.

Rationales for each of the interventions in the care plans help you to understand why a specific step or set of steps is performed.

Expanded Evaluation section explains how to evaluate and determine whether the outcomes have been achieved.

Research Highlight boxes provide abstracts of current nursing research studies and explain the implications for your daily practice.

Safety Alerts indicate techniques you can use to ensure client and nurse safety.

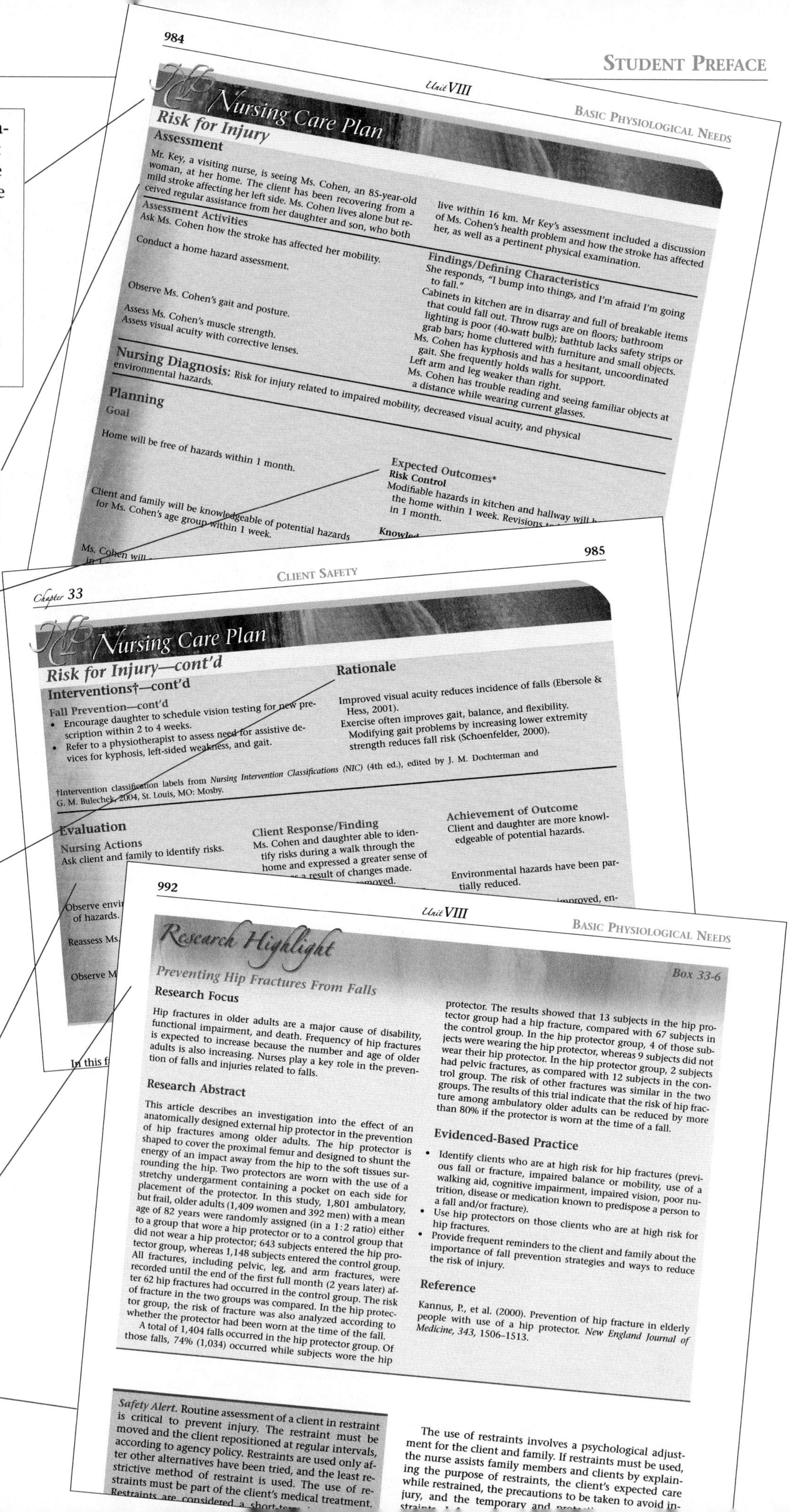
984

Unit VIII

BASIC PHYSIOLOGICAL NEEDS

Nursing Care Plan

Risk for Injury

Assessment

Mr. Key, a visiting nurse, is seeing Ms. Cohen, an 85-year-old woman, at her home. The client has been recovering from a mild stroke affecting her left side. Ms. Cohen lives alone but received regular assistance from her daughter and son, who both live within 16 km. Mr Key's assessment included a discussion of Ms. Cohen's health problem and how the stroke has affected her, as well as a pertinent physical examination.

Assessment Activities	Findings/Defining Characteristics
Ask Ms. Cohen how the stroke has affected her mobility.	She responds, "I bump into things, and I'm afraid I'm going to fall."
Conduct a home hazard assessment.	Cabinets in kitchen are in disarray and full of breakable items that could fall out. Throw rugs are on floors; bathroom lighting is poor (40-watt bulb); bathtub lacks safety strips or grab bars; home cluttered with furniture and small objects.
Observe Ms. Cohen's gait and posture.	Ms. Cohen has kyphosis and has a hesitant, uncoordinated gait. She frequently holds walls for support.
Assess Ms. Cohen's muscle strength.	Left arm and leg weaker than right.
Assess visual acuity with corrective lenses.	Ms. Cohen has trouble reading and seeing familiar objects at a distance while wearing current glasses.

Nursing Diagnosis: Risk for injury related to impaired mobility, decreased visual acuity, and physical environmental hazards.

Planning

Goal	Expected Outcomes*
Home will be free of hazards within 1 month.	Risk Control Modifiable hazards in kitchen and hallway will b... the home within 1 week. Revisions t... in 1 month.
Client and family will be knowledgeable of potential hazards for Ms. Cohen's age group within 1 week.	Knowl...
Ms. Cohen will ...	

985

CLIENT SAFETY

Chapter 33

Nursing Care Plan

Risk for Injury—cont'd

Interventions†—cont'd	Rationale
Fall Prevention—cont'd • Encourage daughter to schedule vision testing for new prescription within 2 to 4 weeks. • Refer to a physiotherapist to assess need for assistive devices for kyphosis, left-sided weakness, and gait.	Improved visual acuity reduces incidence of falls (Ebersole & Hess, 2001). Exercise often improves gait, balance, and flexibility. Modifying gait problems by increasing lower extremity strength reduces fall risk (Schoenfelder, 2000).

†Intervention classification labels from *Nursing Intervention Classifications (NIC)* (4th ed.), edited by J. M. Dochterman and G. M. Bulechek, 2004, St. Louis, MO: Mosby.

Evaluation

Nursing Actions	Client Response/Finding	Achievement of Outcome
Ask client and family to identify risks.	Ms. Cohen and daughter able to identify risks during a walk through the home and expressed a greater sense of ... a result of changes made.	Client and daughter are more knowledgeable of potential hazards.
Observe envi... of hazards.	...moved.	Environmental hazards have been partially reduced.
Reassess Ms. ...		...improved, en...
Observe M...		

In this f...

992

Unit VIII

BASIC PHYSIOLOGICAL NEEDS

Research Highlight

Preventing Hip Fractures From Falls

Box 33-6

Research Focus

Hip fractures in older adults are a major cause of disability, functional impairment, and death. Frequency of hip fractures is expected to increase because the number and age of older adults is also increasing. Nurses play a key role in the prevention of falls and injuries related to falls.

Research Abstract

This article describes an investigation into the effect of an anatomically designed external hip protector in the prevention of hip fractures among older adults. The hip protector is shaped to cover the proximal femur and designed to shunt the energy of an impact away from the hip to the soft tissues surrounding the hip. Two protectors are worn with the use of a stretchy undergarment containing a pocket on each side for placement of the protector. In this study, 1,801 ambulatory, but frail, older adults (1,409 women and 392 men) with a mean age of 82 years were randomly assigned (in a 1:2 ratio) either to a group that wore a hip protector or to a control group that did not wear a hip protector; 643 subjects entered the hip protector group, whereas 1,148 subjects entered the control group. All fractures, including pelvic, leg, and arm fractures, were recorded until the end of the first full month (2 years later) after 62 hip fractures had occurred in the control group. The risk of fracture in the two groups was compared. In the hip protector group, the risk of fracture was also analyzed according to whether the protector had been worn at the time of the fall.

A total of 1,404 falls occurred in the hip protector group. Of those falls, 74% (1,034) occurred while subjects wore the hip protector. The results showed that 13 subjects in the hip protector group had a hip fracture, compared with 67 subjects in the control group. In the hip protector group, 4 of those subjects were wearing the hip protector, whereas 9 subjects did not wear their hip protector. In the hip protector group, 2 subjects had pelvic fractures, as compared with 12 subjects in the control group. The risk of other fractures was similar in the two groups. The results of this trial indicate that the risk of hip fracture among ambulatory older adults can be reduced by more than 80% if the protector is worn at the time of a fall.

Evidenced-Based Practice

- Identify clients who are at high risk for hip fractures (previous fall or fracture, impaired balance or mobility, use of a walking aid, cognitive impairment, impaired vision, poor nutrition, disease or medication known to predispose a person to a fall and/or fracture).
- Use hip protectors on those clients who are at high risk for hip fractures.
- Provide frequent reminders to the client and family about the importance of fall prevention strategies and ways to reduce the risk of injury.

Reference

Kannus, P., et al. (2000). Prevention of hip fracture in elderly people with use of a hip protector. *New England Journal of Medicine, 343*, 1506–1513.

Safety Alert. Routine assessment of a client in restraint is critical to prevent injury. The restraint must be moved and the client repositioned at regular intervals, according to agency policy. Restraints are used only after other alternatives have been tried, and the least restrictive method of restraint is used. The use of restraints must be part of the client's medical treatment. Restraints are considered a short-te...

The use of restraints involves a psychological adjustment for the client and family. If restraints must be used, the nurse assists family members and clients by explaining the purpose of restraints, the client's expected care while restrained, the precautions to be taken to avoid injury, and the temporary and protec... straints...

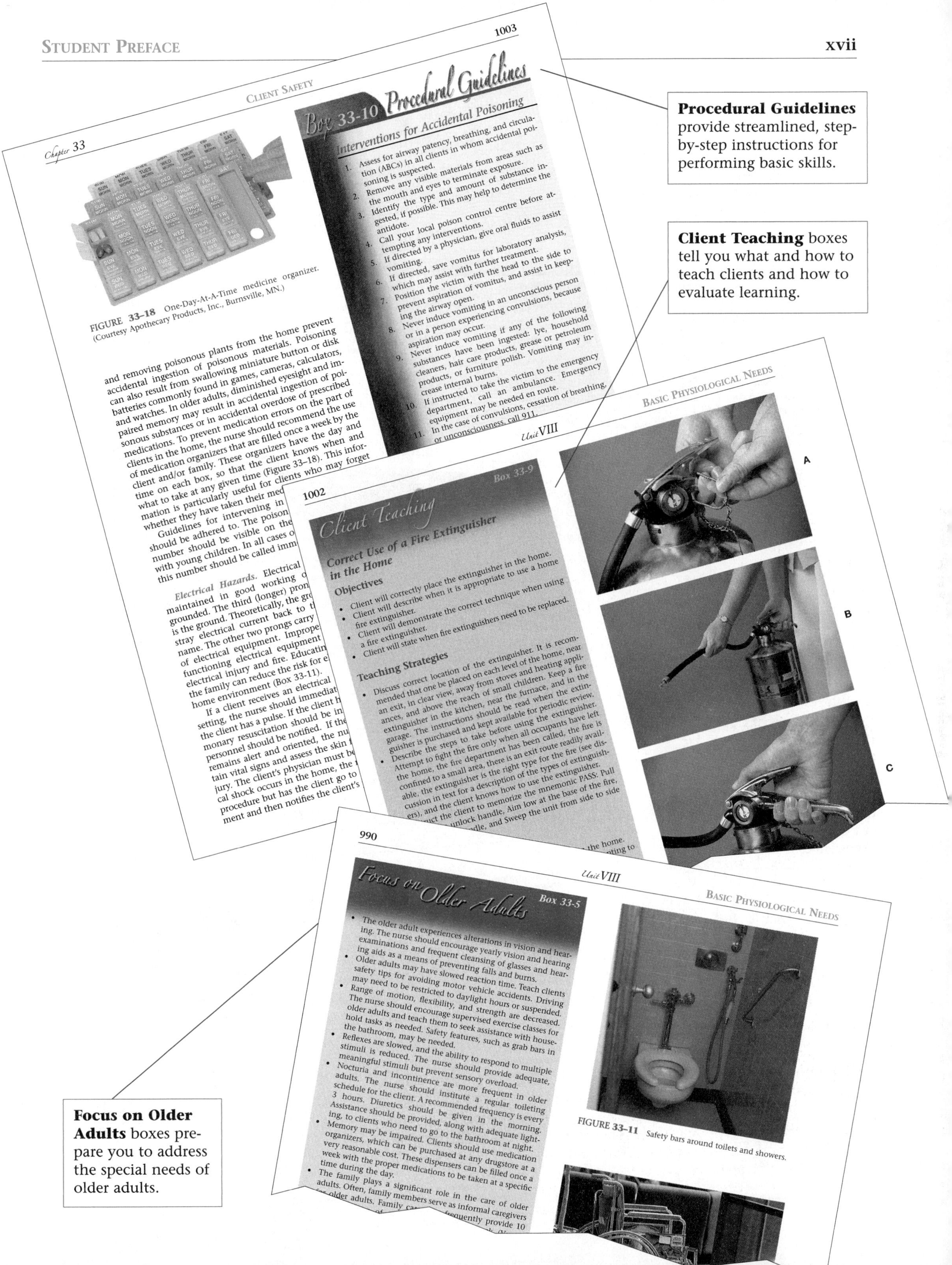

Procedural Guidelines provide streamlined, step-by-step instructions for performing basic skills.

Client Teaching boxes tell you what and how to teach clients and how to evaluate learning.

Focus on Older Adults boxes prepare you to address the special needs of older adults.

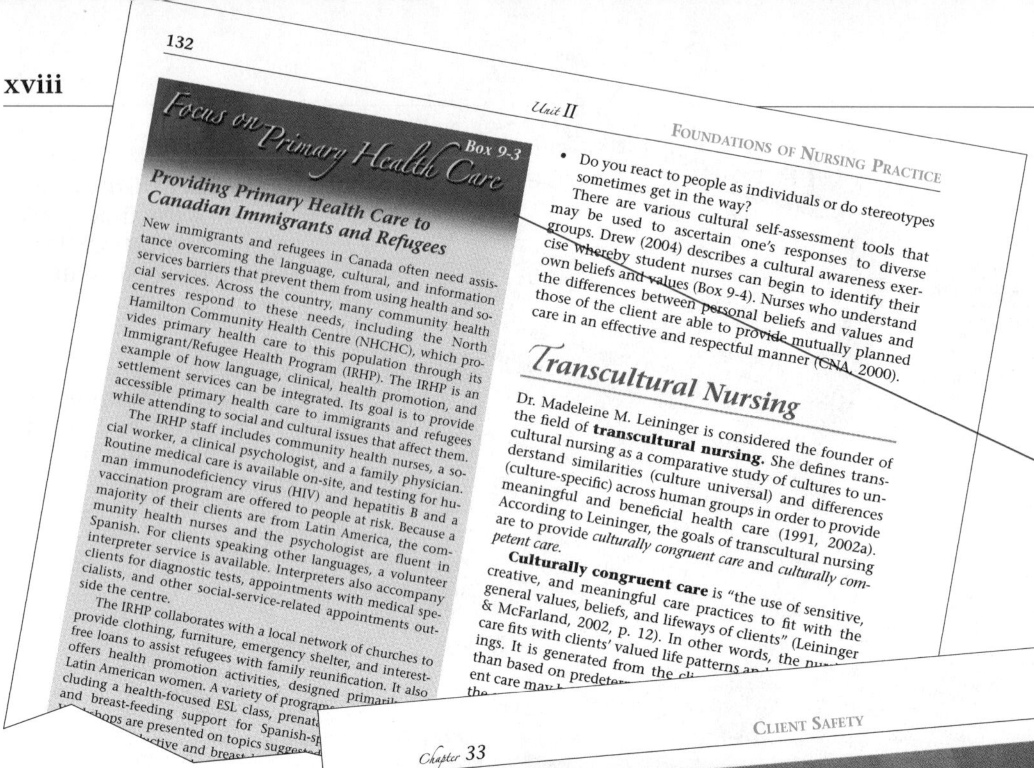

132 *Unit II* FOUNDATIONS OF NURSING PRACTICE

Focus on Primary Health Care Box 9-3

Providing Primary Health Care to Canadian Immigrants and Refugees

New immigrants and refugees in Canada often need assistance overcoming the language, cultural, and information services barriers that prevent them from using health and social services. Across the country, many community health centres respond to these needs, including the North Hamilton Community Health Centre (NHCHC), which provides primary health care to this population through its Immigrant/Refugee Health Program (IRHP). The IRHP is an example of how language, clinical, health promotion, and settlement services can be integrated. Its goal is to provide accessible primary health care to immigrants and refugees while attending to social and cultural issues that affect them.

The IRHP staff includes community health nurses, a social worker, a clinical psychologist, and a family physician. Routine medical care is available on-site, and testing for human immunodeficiency virus (HIV) and hepatitis B and a vaccination program are offered to people at risk. Because a majority of their clients are from Latin America, the community health nurses and the psychologist are fluent in Spanish. For clients speaking other languages, a volunteer interpreter service is available. Interpreters also accompany clients for diagnostic tests, appointments with medical specialists, and other social-service-related appointments outside the centre.

The IRHP collaborates with a local network of churches to provide clothing, furniture, emergency shelter, and interest-free loans to assist refugees with family reunification. It also offers health promotion activities, designed primarily ... Latin American women. A variety of program... cluding a health-focused ESL class, prenat... and breast-feeding support for Spanish-sp... ...hops are presented on topics sugges... ...ctive and breast...

- Do you react to people as individuals or do stereotypes sometimes get in the way?

There are various cultural self-assessment tools that may be used to ascertain one's responses to diverse groups. Drew (2004) describes a cultural awareness exercise whereby student nurses can begin to identify their own beliefs and values (Box 9-4). Nurses who understand the differences between personal beliefs and values and those of the client are able to provide mutually planned care in an effective and respectful manner (CNA, 2000).

Transcultural Nursing

Dr. Madeleine M. Leininger is considered the founder of the field of **transcultural nursing.** She defines transcultural nursing as a comparative study of cultures to understand similarities (culture universal) and differences (culture-specific) across human groups in order to provide meaningful and beneficial health care (1991, 2002a). According to Leininger, the goals of transcultural nursing are to provide *culturally congruent care* and *culturally competent care.*

Culturally congruent care is "the use of sensitive, creative, and meaningful care practices to fit with the general values, beliefs, and lifeways of clients" (Leininger & McFarland, 2002, p. 12). In other words, the nur... care fits with clients' valued life patterns an... ings. It is generated from the cli... than based on predeter... ent care may...

Focus on Primary Health Care boxes highlight how the principles of primary health care can be applied to the topic of the chapter.

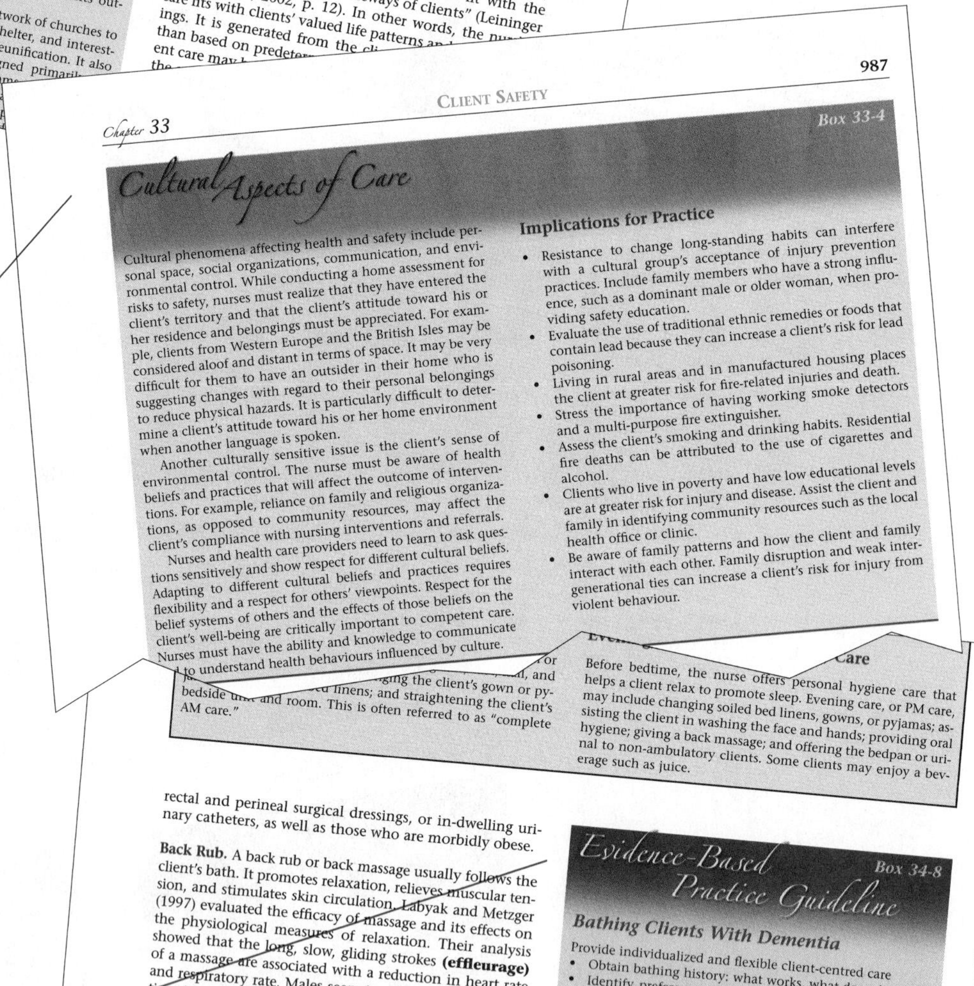

987

Chapter 33 CLIENT SAFETY

Cultural Aspects of Care Box 33-4

Cultural phenomena affecting health and safety include personal space, social organizations, communication, and environmental control. While conducting a home assessment for risks to safety, nurses must realize that they have entered the client's territory and that the client's attitude toward his or her residence and belongings must be appreciated. For example, clients from Western Europe and the British Isles may be considered aloof and distant in terms of space. It may be very difficult for them to have an outsider in their home who is suggesting changes with regard to their personal belongings to reduce physical hazards. It is particularly difficult to determine a client's attitude toward his or her home environment when another language is spoken.

Another culturally sensitive issue is the client's sense of environmental control. The nurse must be aware of health beliefs and practices that will affect the outcome of interventions. For example, reliance on family and religious organizations, as opposed to community resources, may affect the client's compliance with nursing interventions and referrals.

Nurses and health care providers need to learn to ask questions sensitively and show respect for different cultural beliefs. Adapting to different cultural beliefs and practices requires flexibility and a respect for others' viewpoints. Respect for the belief systems of others and the effects of those beliefs on the client's well-being are critically important to competent care. Nurses must have the ability and knowledge to communicate ...d to understand health behaviours influenced by culture.

Implications for Practice

- Resistance to change long-standing habits can interfere with a cultural group's acceptance of injury prevention practices. Include family members who have a strong influence, such as a dominant male or older woman, when providing safety education.
- Evaluate the use of traditional ethnic remedies or foods that contain lead because they can increase a client's risk for lead poisoning.
- Living in rural areas and in manufactured housing places the client at greater risk for fire-related injuries and death.
- Stress the importance of having working smoke detectors and a multi-purpose fire extinguisher.
- Assess the client's smoking and drinking habits. Residential fire deaths can be attributed to the use of cigarettes and alcohol.
- Clients who live in poverty and have low educational levels are at greater risk for injury and disease. Assist the client and family in identifying community resources such as the local health office or clinic.
- Be aware of family patterns and how the client and family interact with each other. Family disruption and weak intergenerational ties can increase a client's risk for injury from violent behaviour.

...ging the client's gown or py... ...d linens; and straightening the client's bedside u... and room. This is often referred to as "complete AM care."

...Care

Before bedtime, the nurse offers personal hygiene care that helps a client relax to promote sleep. Evening care, or PM care, may include changing soiled bed linens, gowns, or pyjamas; assisting the client in washing the face and hands; providing oral hygiene; giving a back massage; and offering the bedpan or urinal to non-ambulatory clients. Some clients may enjoy a beverage such as juice.

Cultural Aspects of Care boxes prepare you to care for clients of diverse populations by identifying actions needed to meet different cultural needs and preferences.

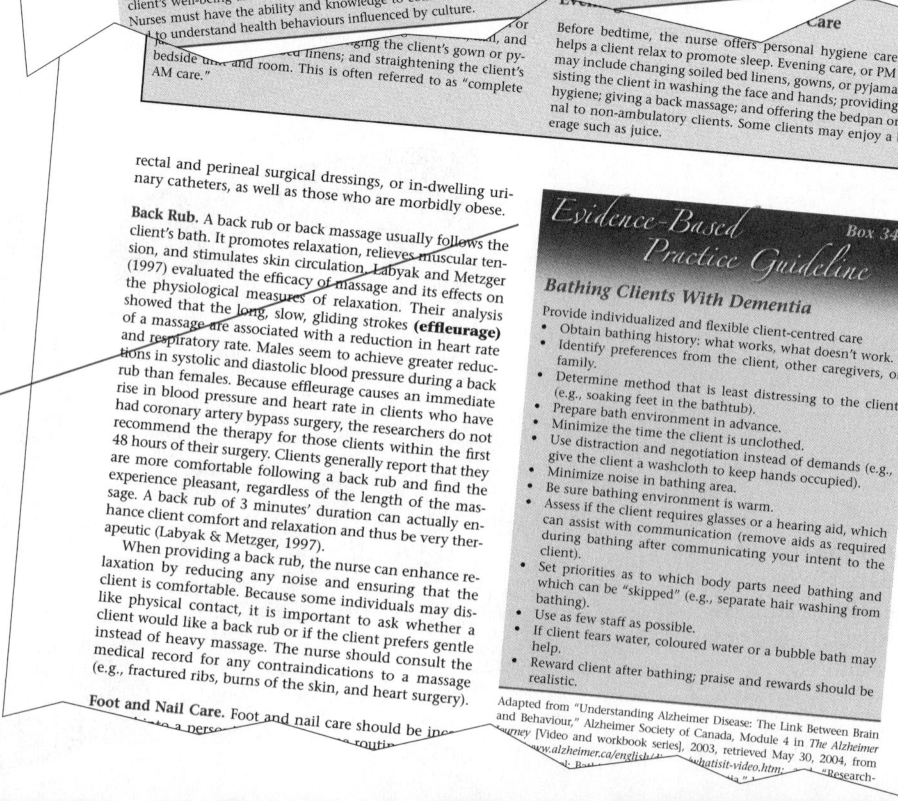

rectal and perineal surgical dressings, or in-dwelling urinary catheters, as well as those who are morbidly obese.

Back Rub. A back rub or back massage usually follows the client's bath. It promotes relaxation, relieves muscular tension, and stimulates skin circulation. Labyak and Metzger (1997) evaluated the efficacy of massage and its effects on the physiological measures of relaxation. Their analysis showed that the long, slow, gliding strokes **(effleurage)** of a massage are associated with a reduction in heart rate and respiratory rate. Males seem to achieve greater reductions in systolic and diastolic blood pressure during a back rub than females. Because effleurage causes an immediate rise in blood pressure and heart rate in clients who have had coronary artery bypass surgery, the researchers do not recommend the therapy for those clients within the first 48 hours of their surgery. Clients generally report that they are more comfortable following a back rub and find the experience pleasant, regardless of the length of the massage. A back rub of 3 minutes' duration can actually enhance client comfort and relaxation and thus be very therapeutic (Labyak & Metzger, 1997).

When providing a back rub, the nurse can enhance relaxation by reducing any noise and ensuring that the client is comfortable. Because some individuals may dislike physical contact, it is important to ask whether a client would like a back rub or if the client prefers gentle instead of heavy massage. The nurse should consult the medical record for any contraindications to a massage (e.g., fractured ribs, burns of the skin, and heart surgery).

Foot and Nail Care. Foot and nail care should be inc... ...to a perso... ...routi...

Evidence-Based Practice Guideline Box 34-8

Bathing Clients With Dementia

Provide individualized and flexible client-centred care

- Obtain bathing history: what works, what doesn't work.
- Identify preferences from the client, other caregivers, or family.
- Determine method that is least distressing to the client (e.g., soaking feet in the bathtub).
- Prepare bath environment in advance.
- Minimize the time the client is unclothed.
- Use distraction and negotiation instead of demands (e.g., give the client a washcloth to keep hands occupied).
- Minimize noise in bathing area.
- Be sure bathing environment is warm.
- Assess if the client requires glasses or a hearing aid, which can assist with communication (remove aids as required during bathing after communicating your intent to the client).
- Set priorities as to which body parts need bathing and which can be "skipped" (e.g., separate hair washing from bathing).
- Use as few staff as possible.
- If client fears water, coloured water or a bubble bath may help.
- Reward client after bathing; praise and rewards should be realistic.

Adapted from "Understanding Alzheimer Disease: The Link Between Brain and Behaviour," Alzheimer Society of Canada, Module 4 in *The Alzheimer Journey* [Video and workbook series], 2003, retrieved May 30, 2004, from www.alzheimer.ca/english/... ...whatisit-video.htm; ... "Research-...

Evidence-Based Practice Guideline boxes provide examples of recent state-of-the-science guidelines for nursing practice.

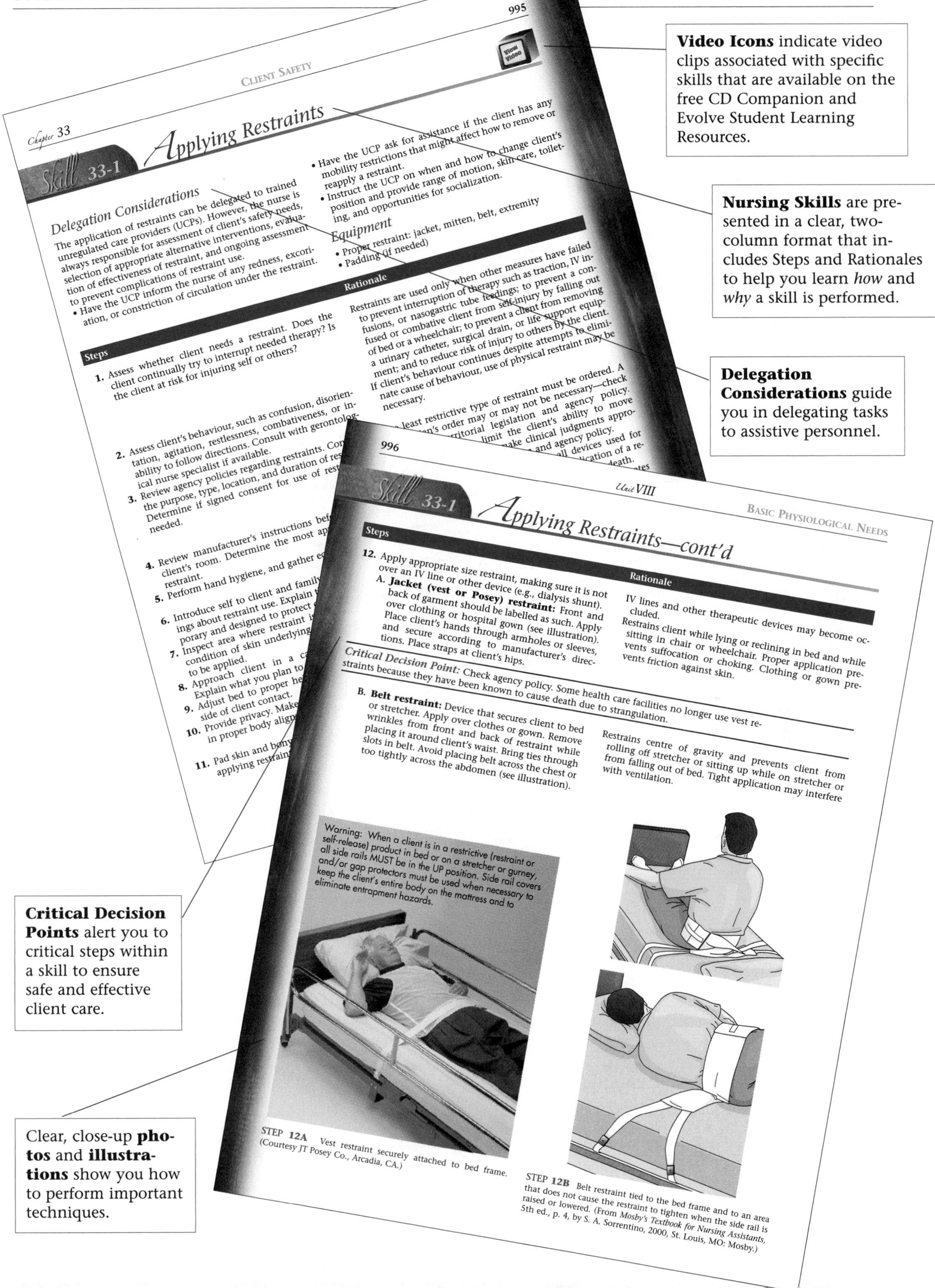
995

CLIENT SAFETY

View Video

Chapter 33

Skill 33-1 Applying Restraints

Delegation Considerations

The application of restraints can be delegated to trained unregulated care providers (UCPs). However, the nurse is always responsible for assessment of client's safety needs, selection of appropriate alternative interventions, evaluation of effectiveness of restraint, and ongoing assessment to prevent complications of restraint use.

- Have the UCP inform the nurse of any redness, excoriation, or constriction of circulation under the restraint.
- Have the UCP ask for assistance if the client has any mobility restrictions that might affect how to remove or reapply a restraint.
- Instruct the UCP on when and how to change client's position and provide range of motion, skin care, toileting, and opportunities for socialization.

Equipment

- Proper restraint: jacket, mitten, belt, extremity
- Padding (if needed)

Steps	Rationale
1. Assess whether client needs a restraint. Does the client continually try to interrupt needed therapy? Is the client at risk for injuring self or others?	Restraints are used only when other measures have failed to prevent interruption of therapy such as traction, IV infusions, or nasogastric tube feedings; to prevent a confused or combative client from self-injury by falling out of bed or a wheelchair; to prevent a client from removing a urinary catheter, surgical drain, or life support equipment; and to reduce risk of injury to others by the client. If client's behaviour continues despite attempts to eliminate cause of behaviour, use of physical restraint may be necessary.
2. Assess client's behaviour, such as confusion, disorientation, agitation, restlessness, combativeness, or inability to follow directions. Consult with gerontological nurse specialist if available.	
3. Review agency policies regarding restraints. ... the purpose, type, location, and duration of ... Determine if signed consent for use of ... needed.	...least restrictive type of restraint must be ordered. A ...'s order may or may not be necessary—check ...ritorial legislation and agency policy. ...limit the client's ability to move ...ake clinical judgments appro... and agency policy. ...ll devices used for ...ication of a re... death.
4. Review manufacturer's instructions ... client's room. Determine the most ... restraint.	
5. Perform hand hygiene, and gather ...	
6. Introduce self to client and family ... ings about restraint use. Explain ... porary and designed to protect ...	
7. Inspect area where restraint ... condition of skin underlying ... to be applied.	
8. Approach client in a ... Explain what you plan to ...	
9. Adjust bed to proper he... side of client contact.	
10. Provide privacy. Make ... in proper body align...	
11. Pad skin and bony ... applying restrain...	

996

Unit VIII BASIC PHYSIOLOGICAL NEEDS

Skill 33-1 Applying Restraints—cont'd

Steps	Rationale
12. Apply appropriate size restraint, making sure it is not over an IV line or other device (e.g., dialysis shunt).	IV lines and other therapeutic devices may become occluded.
A. **Jacket (vest or Posey) restraint:** Front and back of garment should be labelled as such. Apply over clothing or hospital gown (see illustration). Place client's hands through armholes or sleeves, and secure according to manufacturer's directions. Place straps at client's hips.	Restrains client while lying or reclining in bed and while sitting in chair or wheelchair. Proper application prevents suffocation or choking. Clothing or gown prevents friction against skin.

Critical Decision Point: Check agency policy. Some health care facilities no longer use vest restraints because they have been known to cause death due to strangulation.

Steps	Rationale
B. **Belt restraint:** Device that secures client to bed or stretcher. Apply over clothes or gown. Remove wrinkles from front and back of restraint while placing it around client's waist. Bring ties through slots in belt. Avoid placing belt across the chest or too tightly across the abdomen (see illustration).	Restrains centre of gravity and prevents client from rolling off stretcher or sitting up while on stretcher or from falling out of bed. Tight application may interfere with ventilation.

Warning: When a client is in a restrictive (restraint or self-release) product in bed or on a stretcher or gurney, all side rails MUST be in the UP position. Side rail covers and/or gap protectors must be used when necessary to keep the client's entire body on the mattress and to eliminate entrapment hazards.

STEP 12A Vest restraint securely attached to bed frame. (Courtesy JT Posey Co., Arcadia, CA.)

STEP 12B Belt restraint tied to the bed frame and to an area that does not cause the restraint to tighten when the side rail is raised or lowered. (From *Mosby's Textbook for Nursing Assistants,* 5th ed., p. 4, by S. A. Sorrentino, 2000, St. Louis, MO: Mosby.)

Video Icons indicate video clips associated with specific skills that are available on the free CD Companion and Evolve Student Learning Resources.

Nursing Skills are presented in a clear, two-column format that includes Steps and Rationales to help you learn *how* and *why* a skill is performed.

Delegation Considerations guide you in delegating tasks to assistive personnel.

Critical Decision Points alert you to critical steps within a skill to ensure safe and effective client care.

Clear, close-up **photos** and **illustrations** show you how to perform important techniques.

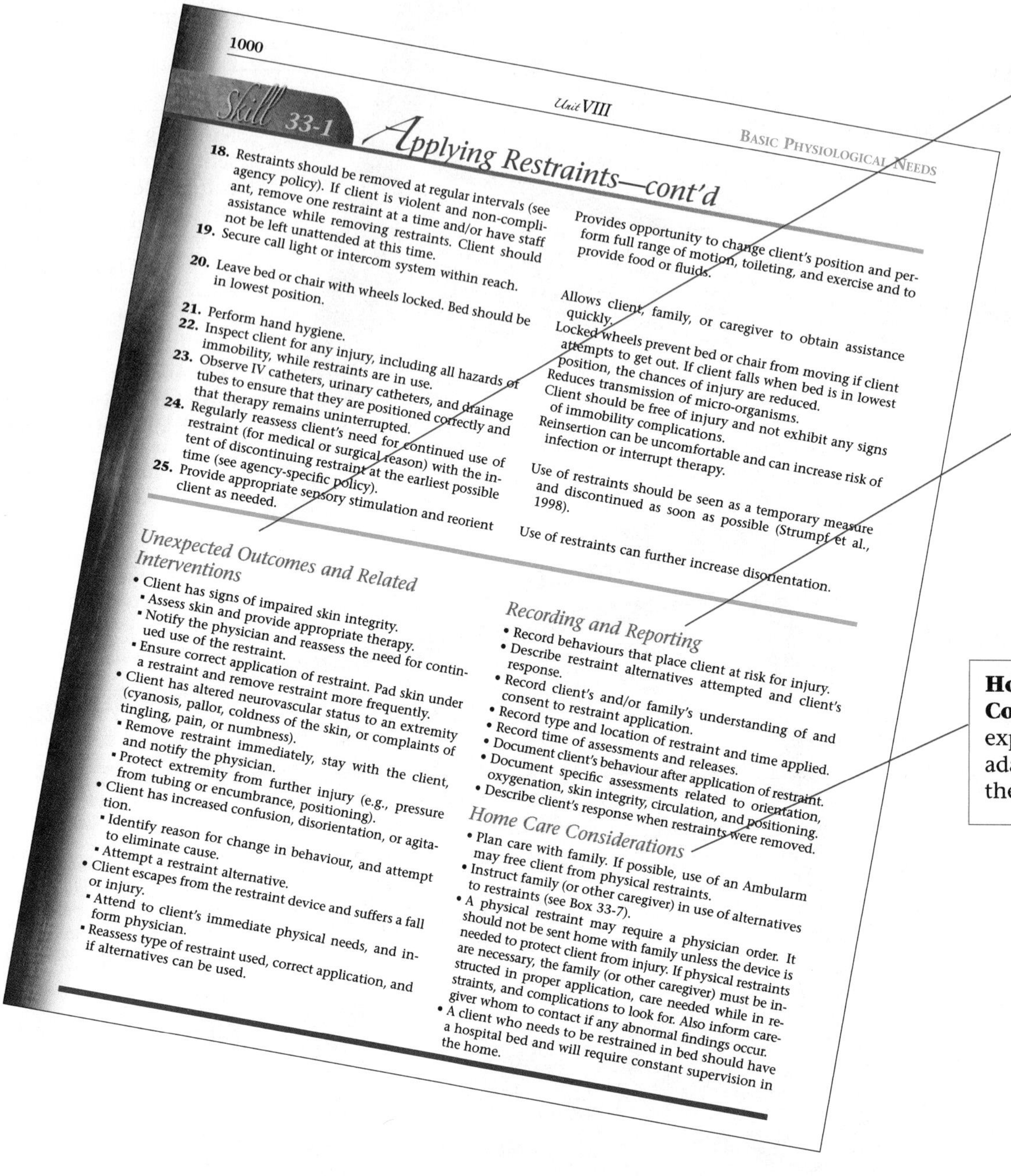

1000 *Unit* VIII BASIC PHYSIOLOGICAL NEEDS

Skill 33-1 *Applying Restraints—cont'd*

18. Restraints should be removed at regular intervals (see agency policy). If client is violent and non-compliant, remove one restraint at a time and/or have staff assistance while removing restraints. Client should not be left unattended at this time.	Provides opportunity to change client's position and perform full range of motion, toileting, and exercise and to provide food or fluids.
19. Secure call light or intercom system within reach.	Allows client, family, or caregiver to obtain assistance quickly.
20. Leave bed or chair with wheels locked. Bed should be in lowest position.	Locked wheels prevent bed or chair from moving if client attempts to get out. If client falls when bed is in lowest position, the chances of injury are reduced.
21. Perform hand hygiene.	Reduces transmission of micro-organisms.
22. Inspect client for any injury, including all hazards of immobility, while restraints are in use.	Client should be free of injury and not exhibit any signs of immobility complications.
23. Observe IV catheters, urinary catheters, and drainage tubes to ensure that they are positioned correctly and that therapy remains uninterrupted.	Reinsertion can be uncomfortable and can increase risk of infection or interrupt therapy.
24. Regularly reassess client's need for continued use of restraint (for medical or surgical reason) with the intent of discontinuing restraint at the earliest possible time (see agency-specific policy).	Use of restraints should be seen as a temporary measure and discontinued as soon as possible (Strumpf et al., 1998).
25. Provide appropriate sensory stimulation and reorient client as needed.	Use of restraints can further increase disorientation.

Unexpected Outcomes and Related Interventions

- Client has signs of impaired skin integrity.
  - Assess skin and provide appropriate therapy.
  - Notify the physician and reassess the need for continued use of the restraint.
  - Ensure correct application of restraint. Pad skin under a restraint and remove restraint more frequently.
- Client has altered neurovascular status to an extremity (cyanosis, pallor, coldness of the skin, or complaints of tingling, pain, or numbness).
  - Remove restraint immediately, stay with the client, and notify the physician.
  - Protect extremity from further injury (e.g., pressure from tubing or encumbrance, positioning).
- Client has increased confusion, disorientation, or agitation.
  - Identify reason for change in behaviour, and attempt to eliminate cause.
  - Attempt a restraint alternative.
- Client escapes from the restraint device and suffers a fall or injury.
  - Attend to client's immediate physical needs, and inform physician.
  - Reassess type of restraint used, correct application, and if alternatives can be used.

Recording and Reporting

- Record behaviours that place client at risk for injury.
- Describe restraint alternatives attempted and client's response.
- Record client's and/or family's understanding of and consent to restraint application.
- Record type and location of restraint and time applied.
- Record time of assessments and releases.
- Document client's behaviour after application of restraint.
- Document specific assessments related to orientation, oxygenation, skin integrity, circulation, and positioning.
- Describe client's response when restraints were removed.

Home Care Considerations

- Plan care with family. If possible, use of an Ambularm may free client from physical restraints.
- Instruct family (or other caregiver) in use of alternatives to restraints (see Box 33-7).
- A physical restraint may require a physician order. It should not be sent home with family unless the device is needed to protect client from injury. If physical restraints are necessary, the family (or other caregiver) must be instructed in proper application, care needed while in restraints, and complications to look for. Also inform caregiver whom to contact if any abnormal findings occur.
- A client who needs to be restrained in bed should have a hospital bed and will require constant supervision in the home.

Unexpected Outcomes and Related Interventions alert you to what might go wrong and provide guidelines for appropriate responses.

Recording and Reporting provides guidelines for what to chart and report with each skill.

Home Care Considerations explain how to adapt skills for the home setting.

Preface to the Instructor

The future of nursing both in Canada and around the world promises dynamic change and continual challenges. Canadian nurses of tomorrow need a broad knowledge base from which to provide care. They will assume the lead in preserving nursing practice and demonstrate its importance in maintaining and improving the health of Canadians. Nurses of tomorrow need to become critical thinkers, client advocates, clinical decision makers, and client educators within a broad spectrum of care services.

Canadian Fundamentals of Nursing is designed for beginning students in all types of professional nursing programs. The comprehensive coverage provides fundamental nursing concepts, skills, and techniques of nursing practice and a firm foundation for more advanced areas of study.

The third edition of ***Canadian Fundamentals of Nursing*** has been extensively revised and thoroughly edited so that it is easier to read and comprehend. At 45 chapters, the text is more concise than the previous edition. All chapters have been adapted or rewritten so that they are placed clearly in a context that reflects Canadian standards, traditions, research, and practice. The text has also been reorganized to reflect the order in which topics are usually taught. For example, foundational chapters such as The Development of Nursing Practice in Canada and Research as a Basis for Practice now appear in Part One.

Canadian Fundamentals of Nursing discusses the entire scope of primary, acute, and restorative care. This revision emphasizes the central role of primary health care in all areas of nursing practice. It also focuses on evidence-based practice in skills and care plans to help students understand how the latest research findings should guide their clinical decision-making. The text includes 22 Concept Maps that visually demonstrate the relationship between multiple nursing diagnoses for associated medical diagnoses. Nursing Skills and Nursing Care Plans have been expanded.

This textbook has resulted from the combined efforts of many talented professionals committed to excellence. Contributors from across Canada worked with general editors to ensure that the entire text reflects the Canadian health care system, Canadian health and social organizations, and issues about health care that are uniquely Canadian. Reviewers scrutinized the chapters and made many helpful suggestions for revision. We appreciate the dedication and enthusiasm of all these dedicated professional nurse colleagues. Throughout the text we have attempted to acknowledge the contributions of nurses, both past and present, who have made a difference in the lives of Canadians. We are very proud to be associated with such fine individuals.

Features

Key features of the text include the following:

Classic Features

- **Comprehensive** coverage and readability of all fundamental nursing content.
- **Full-colour** text to enhance visual appeal and instructional value.
- **Nursing process** provides a consistent organizational framework.
- **Primary health care and health promotion** discussed throughout the text.
- Important nursing **skills** are presented in a clear, two-column format with rationales for all steps; rationales are based on research.
- Covers **health promotion, acute and tertiary care,** and **restorative care** to address today's practice in various settings.
- **Cultural diversity** is presented in Chapter 9, stressed in clinical examples throughout the text, and highlighted in special boxes.
- **Research Highlight** boxes integrated throughout the text provide current nursing research studies and explain the implications for daily practice. Many of these present Canadian research.
- **Client education** is stressed in boxes that list teaching objectives, strategies, and evaluation for clinical topics throughout the text.
- **Gerontological nursing** principles are addressed in **Focus on Older Adults** boxes throughout the text.
- **Diverse clinical settings** are discussed, including clinics, long-term care facilities, and the home, as well as acute care settings.
- Historical boxes entitled **Milestones in Canadian History** provide information about nursing leaders and critical events in Canadian nursing history.
- Critical thinking in clinical chapters is presented through a dimensional **critical thinking model** that visually demonstrates the ongoing assimilation of knowledge, critical thinking attitudes, intellectual and professional standards, and experience in relationship to clinical decision making and the nursing process.
- **NIC** and **NOC classifications** are included in sample nursing care plans.
- Real **Critical pathways** from progressive health care agencies address collaborative care in the home and acute care settings.
- **Procedural Guidelines** boxes provide streamlined, step-by-step instructions for performing very basic skills.

New and Revised Features

- **Focus on Primary Health Care boxes** highlight how the principles of primary health care can be applied to the topic of the chapter; all these boxes are Canadian
- **Nursing process** chapters have been condensed and consolidated into one chapter, making key concepts clearer for students
- References updated throughout to include **Canadian research and practice standards,** e.g., Health Canada, Statistics Canada, the CNA, and RNAO Best Nursing Practice Guidelines
- New comprehensive and Canadian chapter on **health assessment and physical examination**
- **New and expanded information** on home care, culture, hand hygiene, Calgary Family Assessment Model, complementary and alternative therapies, and palliative care.
- **Concept maps** added, to show the association between multiple nursing diagnoses and their relationship to medical diagnoses
- **Nursing Care Plans** feature a revised format that offers more detail on how to conduct an assessment and consider the defining characteristics that indicate nursing diagnoses. The plans incorporate NIC and NOC classifications to familiarize students with this nomenclature. The evaluation section describes how to evaluate outcomes of care
- **Unexpected Outcomes and Related Interventions** highlighted within nursing skills
- **Evidence-Based Practice Guidelines** boxes provide examples of recent state-of-the-science guidelines for nursing practice
- **Safety Alerts** indicate techniques students can use to ensure client and nurse safety
- **End-of-chapter review questions** help students review and evaluate what they have learned. Answers and rationales are provided at the back of the book
- **Planning discussions** include sections on *Goals and Outcomes, Setting Priorities,* and *Continuity of Care* to help beginning students plan and prioritize comprehensive client care
- **Annotated "Recommended Web sites"** section at the end of each chapter direct the student to current Web-based resources, most of which are Canadian
- **Free CD Companion** in each text has been enhanced to include **Test-Taking Skills** in addition to Butterfield's **Fluids and Electrolytes** program, and **Glossary**
- **Practical Nursing in Canada** appendix provides important information on this nursing role in Canada

Canadian Ancillaries

- Canadian **Study Guide** provides an ideal supplement to help students understand and apply the content of the text. Each chapter includes multiple sections:
  - Preliminary reading includes a chapter assignment from the text
  - Comprehensive Understanding identifies topics and main ideas from the text in outline format. By completing the outline, students learn to extract key information from the chapter. Once completed, these outlines serve as ideal review tools for exams.
  - Review Questions are exam-style multiple-choice questions that require students to provide a rationale for their answers.
  - Clinical chapters include an Application of Critical Thinking Synthesis Model that expands the case study from the chapter's sample care plan and asks students to develop a step in the synthesis model based on the nurse and client in the scenario. This helps students learn to apply both content learned and the critical thinking synthesis model.
  - Skills Performance Checklists are included so that students can evaluate skill competency.
- Canadian **Instructor's Manual with Test Bank.**
- evolve **Online Courseware** includes Canadian WebLinks, Canadian Instructor's Manual, Computerized Test Bank, Electronic Image Collection, PowerPoint Slides, and Procedure Checklists.

Acknowledgments

Adapting a nursing text for the Canadian market is an enormous undertaking, and in this third Canadian edition, every chapter has been written for Canadian readers. We would like to acknowledge the contributions of each of our Canadian authors, who developed and wrote outstanding material in a short time frame. Their dedication and content expertise is evident throughout and we thank them for the extraordinary effort put forward to make this book a success. We would also like to thank:

- Ann Millar, Publisher of Elsevier Canada, for her support and encouragement throughout the development and production of this text.
- Heather McWhinney, Developmental Editor, for her dedication to the quality of this text
- Joanne Sanche, Developmental Editor, for her meticulous work in reading and editing the text
- Marcel Chiera, Production Editor, for his unrelenting attention to ensuring that the text was ready for production
- Barbara Every, Copy Editor, for her thorough reading and editing of the manuscript

Contents

Unit I Health and Health Care in Canada

1 Health and Wellness, 1

Linda Reutter, RN, PhD (Canadian author)

2 The Canadian Health Care Delivery System, 18

Ardene Robinson Vollman, RN, BScN, MA, PhD (Canadian author)

Patricia A. Potter, RN, MSN, PhD, CMAC, FAAN

3 The Development of Nursing Practice in Canada, 34

Janet C. Ross-Kerr, RN, BScN, MS, PhD (Canadian author)

Unit V Caring Throughout the Lifespan

18 Developmental Theories, 336

Jane Drummond, RN, PhD (Canadian author)

Lenora Marcellus, RN, PhD (candidate) (Canadian author)

Elaine U. Polan, RNC, BSN, MS

19 Conception Through Adolescence, 356

Elaine U. Polan, RNC, BSN, MS

Shirley Solberg, BN, MN, PhD (Canadian author)

20 Young to Middle Adult, 397

Patsy L. Ruchala, DNSc, RN

Marion Clauson, RN, MSN, PNC(C) (Canadian author)

21 Older Adult, 413

Myra A. Aud, PhD, RN

Wendy Duggleby, DSN, RN, AOCN (Canadian author)

Unit VI Psychosocial Considerations

26 Stress and Adaptation, 539

Marjorie Baier, RN, PhD, APRN, BC

Ginette Lemire Rodger, RN, BScN, MAdmN, PhD (Canadian author)

Unit VII Scientific Basis for Nursing Practice

27 Vital Signs, 561

Susan Jane Fetzer, RN, BA, BSN, MSN, MBA, PhD

Maureen McQueen, RN, MN (Canadian author)

28 Health Assessment and Physical Examination, 616

D. Lynn Skillen, PhD, RN (Canadian author)

Rene A. Day, RN, PhD (Canadian author)

Marjorie C. Anderson, RN, PhD (Canadian author)

Tracey Stephen, RN, BScN, MN (Canadian author)

Julie A. Gilbert, RN, BScN, MN (Canadian author)

30 Medication Administration, 832

Amy Hall, RN, BSN, MS, PhD

Debbie Fraser Askin, RNC, MN (Canadian author)

31 Complementary and Alternative Therapies, 920

Steve Kilkus, RN, MSN

Jean McClennon-Leong, RN, MN, APNP (Canadian author)

Unit VIII Basic Physiological Needs

32 Activity and Exercise, 940

Rita Wunderlich, BSN, MSN(r), PhD

Ann Brokenshire, RN, BScN, MEd (Canadian author)

45 Care of Surgical Clients, *1600*

Marilyn Schallom, RN, MSN, CCRN, CCNS

Frances Fothergill-Bourbonnais, RN, BScN, MN, PhD (Canadian author)

Appendix Practical Nursing in Canada, *1653*

Vivian Lucas, RN, MEd

Review Question Answers, *1672*

Review Question Rationales, *1675*

Index, *1701*

1

Health and Wellness

Linda Reutter, RN, PhD (Canadian author)

Objectives

Mastery of content in this chapter will enable the student to:

- Define the key terms listed.
- Discuss ways that definitions of health have been conceptualized.
- Describe key characteristics of medical, behavioural, and socio-environmental approaches to health.
- Identify factors that have led to each approach to health.
- Discuss contributions of the following Canadian documents to conceptualizations of health and health determinants: Lalonde Report, Ottawa Charter, Epp Report, Strategies for Population Health, Toronto Charter.
- Discuss key health determinants and their interrelationships in influencing health.
- Contrast distinguishing features of health promotion and disease prevention.
- Describe the three levels of disease prevention.
- Identify the five health promotion strategies discussed in the Ottawa Charter.
- Analyze how the nature and scope of nursing practice are influenced by different conceptualizations of health and health determinants.

Just what is health? The answer is that there is no single definition: The term is used in many different contexts to refer to many different aspects of life (Naidoo & Wills, 1994). Health concepts and determinants have changed significantly in the past 30 years. This change has major implications for Canadian nursing in the 21st century. Nurses' perceptions of health—and what determines it—influence how and with whom they conduct their practice. The importance of health as a concept that influences nursing is reflected in nursing models and frameworks, where *health* appears alongside *person, environment,* and *nursing* (see chapter 5). In each framework, health concepts are congruent with the assumptions and focus of the model. Most important, the nature and scope of nursing depend on a nurse's definition of health and its determinants.

Conceptualizations of Health

Discussion about the nature of health revolves around its relationship to *disease, illness,* and *wellness*. Often, debates focus on negative or positive terms. When health is negatively defined as the absence of disease, health and illness are represented on a continuum, with maximum health at one end and death at the other. When health is positively defined, however, health and illness are viewed as distinct but interrelated concepts. Therefore, one can have disease, such as a chronic illness, and have healthy characteristics as well.

How should one define disease and illness, then? Many people use the words *illness* and *disease* interchangeably. Others suggest that **disease** is an objective state of ill health, the pathology of which can be detected by medical

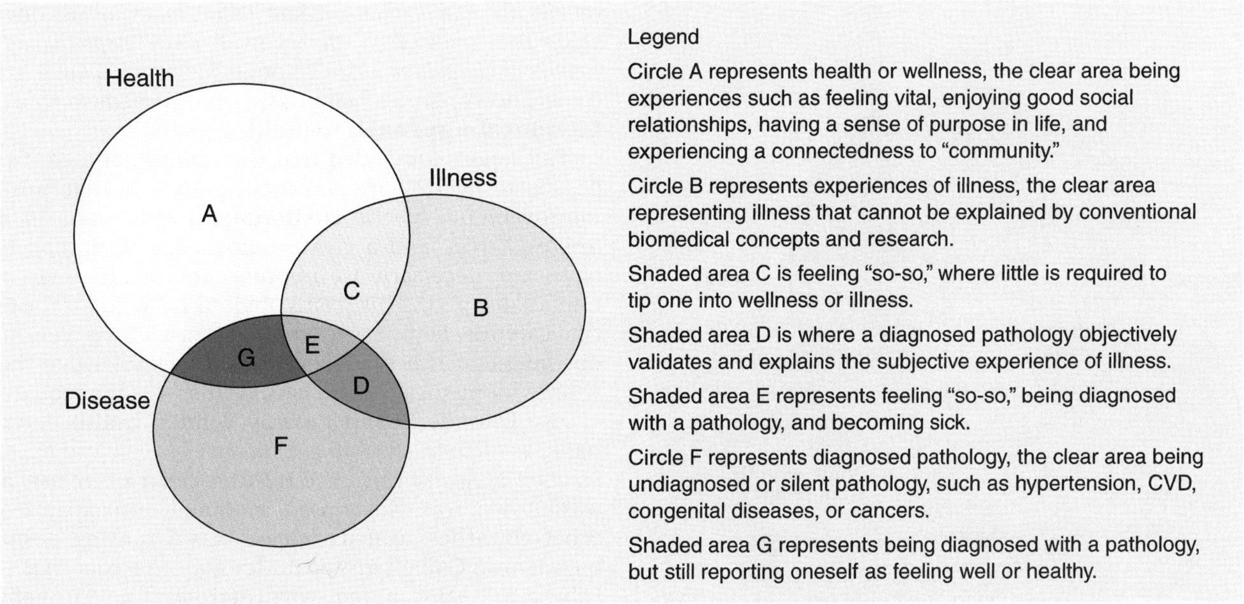
Health
Illness
Disease
A
B
C
D
E
F
G
Legend
Circle A represents health or wellness, the clear area being experiences such as feeling vital, enjoying good social relationships, having a sense of purpose in life, and experiencing a connectedness to "community."
Circle B represents experiences of illness, the clear area representing illness that cannot be explained by conventional biomedical concepts and research.
Shaded area C is feeling "so-so," where little is required to tip one into wellness or illness.
Shaded area D is where a diagnosed pathology objectively validates and explains the subjective experience of illness.
Shaded area E represents feeling "so-so," being diagnosed with a pathology, and becoming sick.
Circle F represents diagnosed pathology, the clear area being undiagnosed or silent pathology, such as hypertension, CVD, congenital diseases, or cancers.
Shaded area G represents being diagnosed with a pathology, but still reporting oneself as feeling well or healthy.

FIGURE **1–1** Health, illness, and disease. (From *Issues in Health Promotion Series. 3. Health Promotion and Empowerment: Practice Frameworks* by R. Labonte, 1993, Toronto, ON: Centre for Health Promotion, University of Toronto, & ParticipACTION.)

science, whereas **illness** is a subjective experience of loss of health (Jensen & Allen, 1993; Labonte, 1993; Naidoo & Wills, 1994). Figure 1–1 shows the relationship among health, illness, and disease.

Definitions beyond the absence of disease usually have multi-dimensional components, including physical, mental, social, and spiritual health. Although some consider this broad definition of health to be synonymous with wellness (Labonte, 1993; Pender, Murdaugh, & Parsons, 2002), others argue that health and wellness are different concepts: **Health** is an objective process characterized by functional stability, balance, and integrity, whereas **wellness** is a subjective experience (Jensen & Allen, 1993; Orem, 1995).

The word *health* is derived from the Old English word *hoelth,* meaning whole of body. Historically, physical wholeness was important for social acceptance, and people with contagious or disfiguring diseases were often ostracized. Good health was considered natural, whereas disease was unnatural. As science progressed, illness was regarded less negatively because it could be countered by scientific medicine. In 1947, after World War II, the World Health Organization (WHO) defined health as "a state of complete physical, mental and social well-being, and not merely the absence of disease and infirmity." This is still the most commonly cited definition of health.

Classifications of Health Conceptualizations

Pender (2002) classified health in three ways:

- **Stability-oriented definition.** Health was defined as the maintenance of physiological, functional, and social norms.
- **Actualization-oriented definition.** Health was defined as the actualization of human potential. Those who adhere to this definition often use the terms health and wellness interchangeably.
- **Combined actualization and stability definition.** Pender (1996) incorporated both actualization and stabilization concepts in her definition of health: "Health is the actualization of inherent and acquired human potential through goal-directed behaviour, competent self-care and satisfying relationships with others, while adjustments are made as needed to maintain structural integrity and harmony with relevant environments" (p. 22).

The Canadian health scholar Labonte (1993) developed a multi-dimensional conceptualization of health that reflects both actualization and stability perspectives. Aspects include:

- Feeling vital and full of energy.
- Having good social relationships.
- Having a feeling of control over one's life and living conditions.
- Being able to do things one enjoys.
- Having a sense of purpose.
- Feeling connected to community.

Labonte categorized these characteristics using the WHO dimensions of physical, mental, and social well-being (Figure 1–2).

Historical Approaches to Health in Canada

Definitions of health come from different contexts. How then has health been viewed in Canada and what has influenced our thinking about it? In recent years, the three major approaches to health have been medical, behavioural, and socio-environmental (Labonte, 1993). These

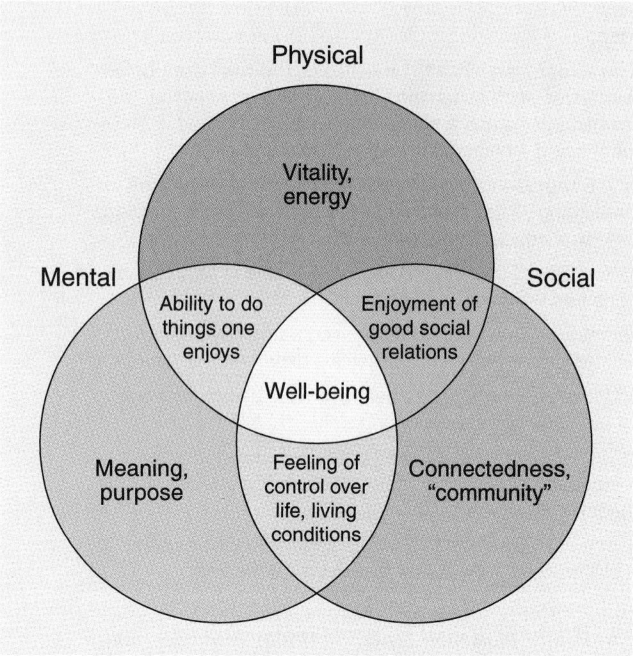

FIGURE 1–2 Dimensions of health and well-being. (From *Issues in Health Promotion Series. 3. Health Promotion and Empowerment: Practice Frameworks,* by R. Labonte, 1993, Toronto, ON: Centre for Health Promotion, University of Toronto, & ParticipACTION.)

approaches are a useful framework to examine the evolution of health orientations in Canada.

Medical Approach

The **medical approach,** which represents a stability orientation to health (Pender et al., 2002), has dominated Western thinking for most of the 20th century. It emphasizes that medical intervention restores health. Health problems are defined as **physiological risk factors**—those physiologically defined characteristics that are precursors to, or risk factors for disease. Examples include hypertension, hypercholesterolemia, genetic predispositions, and obesity. In the medical approach, an adequate health care system is paramount to ensuring healthy populations.

Focusing on treatment of disease and infirmity was strongly supported after World War II, when new technological and scientific medical advances facilitated the medical approach. In Canada, post-war economic growth increased funding to build new hospitals. National health insurance was also created to remove financial barriers to care. Many believed that scientific medicine could solve most health problems and that accessible and quality health care (or, more correctly, illness care) would improve the health of Canadians. Within this approach, less emphasis was given to health promotion and disease prevention.

Behavioural Approach

By the early 1970s, increasingly large amounts of money were spent on health care, but the health status of the population did not improve proportionately. To better understand what contributed to illness and death, the Minister of Health and Welfare, Marc Lalonde, commissioned a study that resulted in the report, *A New Perspective on the Health of Canadians.* The Lalonde Report (1974), as it became known, shifted emphasis from a medical to a **behavioural approach** to health.

The report concluded that the traditional medical approach to health care was inadequate and that "further improvements in the environment, reductions in self-imposed risks, and a greater knowledge of human biology" are necessary to improve the health status of Canadians (p. 6). This seems obvious now, but at the time the Lalonde Report was the first modern government document in the Western world to acknowledge that a strictly biomedical health care system was inadequate.

The Lalonde Report broadly defined health determinants as *lifestyle, environment, human biology,* and *the organization of health care.* The **health field concept,** as it was known, was widely used, modified, and expanded by other countries, and its release was a turning point in broadening Canadians' attitudes about factors that contribute to health, along with the role of government in promoting health (Health Canada, 1998).

Of the four elements in the health field concept, lifestyle received the most attention. In 1978, the Canadian government established the Health Promotion Directorate in the Department of National Health and Welfare, the first official health promotion undertaking of its kind. Its aim was to decrease **behavioural risk factors** such as smoking, substance abuse, lack of exercise, and an unhealthy diet. Public health programs such as Operation Lifestyle and ParticipACTION were developed through this department.

Why did lifestyle, rather than environment, become the focus of health promotion efforts? Some suggested that lifestyle behaviours contributed to chronic diseases such as cancer, heart disease, and injuries—the leading causes of morbidity and mortality in Canada (Labonte, 1993; Rootman & Raeburn, 1994). Better understanding of behavioural social psychology revealed what motivated individuals to engage in healthy or unhealthy behaviours.

The behavioural approach influences how health professionals, including nurses, promote and maintain health. It places responsibility for health on the individual, thereby favouring health promotion strategies such as education and social marketing. Strategies are often based on the assumption that if people know the risk factors for disease they will engage in healthy behaviours. Indeed, positive health practices among Canadians increased during this time. With the ParticipACTION initiative, for instance, many people increased their exercise. Anti-smoking campaigns led to a substantial decrease in smoking.

Socio-Environmental Approach

By the mid-1980s, however, the behavioural approach to health and illness prevention fell into disfavour. Labonte (1993) cited several possible reasons. First, studies showed that lifestyle improvements were made primarily by well-educated, well-employed, and higher income Canadians. Public health professionals said that the Lalonde Report deflected attention from one's environment. The report was criticized for how environment and lifestyle were defined. Lifestyle, according to the report, was within an individual's control. Health risks were "self-imposed" behaviours. This led to "victim-blaming" and views that health was largely an individual responsibility. Critics of the report suggested that health-related behaviours could not be separated from the social contexts in which they occurred. Some wondered if individuals chose poor health or if their living and working conditions were barriers that affected their ability to engage in healthy behaviours.

In the **socio-environmental approach,** health is closely tied to the social structure. For example, poverty and unhealthy physical and social environments, such as air pollution, water quality, and work hazards, can influence health directly. Thus, Canadian public health professionals expanded Lalonde's health field concept to emphasize the social context of health and the relationship between personal health behaviours and social and physical environments (Hancock & Perkins, 1985).

Internationally, more attention was also given to the social context of health. The WHO Regional Conference in Europe in 1984 produced a discussion paper identifying the social conditions that influence health (WHO, 1984). Just as Canada led the behavioural approach to health with the Lalonde Report, it was now instrumental in focusing on social and environmental conditions. In 1986, the First International Conference on Health Promotion was held in Ottawa. The conference was sponsored by the WHO, the Canadian Public Health Association (CPHA), and Health and Welfare Canada. It produced a watershed document called the *Ottawa Charter for Health Promotion,* which supported a socio-environmental approach. This document has since been translated into more than 40 languages.

Ottawa Charter for Health Promotion. The Ottawa Charter (WHO, 1986) identified **prerequisites for health** as peace, shelter, education, food, income, a stable ecosystem, sustainable resources, social justice, and equity. These prerequisites clearly go beyond lifestyles or personal health practices to include social, environmental, and political contexts. Attention to these prerequisites places responsibility for health on society rather than only on individuals. Focus on social justice and equity also incorporated the concept of empowerment—one's ability to define, analyze, and solve problems—as an important goal for health professionals (Registered Nurses Association of British Columbia, 1994). Indeed, Wallerstein (1992) contended that powerlessness could be the health determinant influencing other risk factors. Consequently, health promotion literature emphasizes the concept of empowerment.

An understanding of the determinants of health is continually evolving. For instance, four additional prerequisites for health were identified at the International Health Promotion Conference in Jakarta, Indonesia, and were subsequently incorporated into the Jakarta Declaration (WHO, 1997). These were *human rights, social security, social relations,* and *empowerment of women.*

The Ottawa Charter incorporated the new 1984 WHO definition of health as follows: Health is viewed as the extent to which an individual or group is able, on the one hand, to realize aspirations and satisfy needs; and on the other hand, to change or cope with the environment. Health is seen as a resource for everyday living; not the object of living. Health is a positive concept emphasizing social and personal resources as well as physical capacities.

Rather than defining health as an ideal state of well-being (as in the 1947 WHO definition), the 1984 definition suggested that people in a variety of situations—even those with physical disease or nearing death—could be considered healthy. Note that the WHO 1984 definition includes both actualization and stability orientations (Pender et al., 2002). This definition identified health as a social and individual concept. It emphasized health's dynamic and positive nature and viewed it as a fundamental human right (Naidoo & Wills, 1994).

The Ottawa Charter outlined five major strategies to promote health:

- Building healthy public policy.
- Creating supportive environments.
- Strengthening community action.
- Developing personal skills.
- Reorienting health services.

These strategies are detailed later in the chapter.

Achieving Health for All. Concepts from the Ottawa Charter were incorporated into another important Canadian document called *Achieving Health for All: A Framework for Health Promotion.* This report, developed under the leadership of Jake Epp, Minister of National Health and Welfare from 1984 to 1989, became Canada's blueprint for achieving the WHO goal of Health for All 2000. The Epp Report (1986), as it has come to be known, also inspired health promotion around the world (Figure 1-3).

The Epp Report identified three major health challenges influencing Canadians: reducing inequities, improving prevention, and enhancing coping. It acknowledged disparities in health, particularly between low- and high-income people, and that living and working conditions were critical determinants of health. It stated that effective ways to prevent injuries, illnesses, chronic conditions, and disabilities needed to be identified. Enhancing a client's capacity to cope acknowledged the belief that the dominant diseases in Canada—unlike infectious diseases of earlier times—were chronic conditions that could not be cured. Therefore, the challenge became one of assisting people to manage and cope with chronic conditions to enable them to live meaningful and productive lives. The Epp Report emphasized society's responsibility to ensure that supports are available for people experiencing chronic medical conditions, stress, mental illness, and problems associated with aging. It also recognized the need for supports for caregivers. The report identified self-care, mutual aid, and healthy environments as ways that these challenges could be addressed, emphasizing both personal and social responsibility. Specific strategies to address the challenges included fostering public participation, strengthening community health services, and coordinating healthy public policy.

The Ottawa Charter and the Epp Report each reflect a socio-environmental approach in which health is seen as more than just the absence of disease and engaging in healthy behaviours; rather, this approach emphasizes

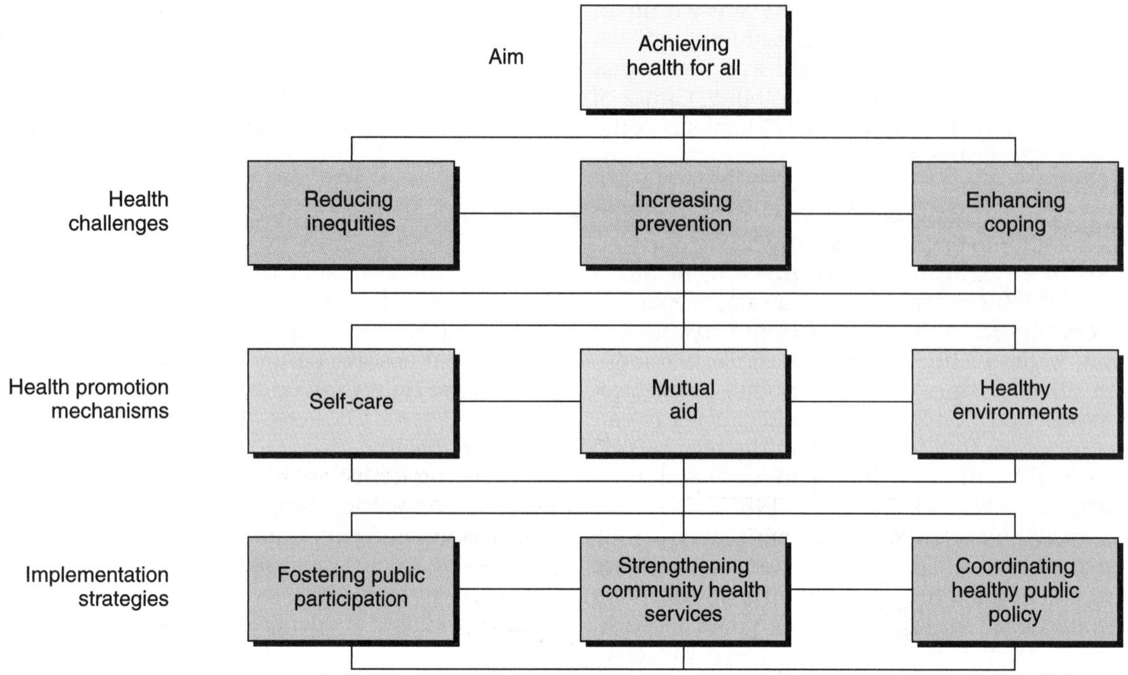

FIGURE **1–3** Achieving health for all: A framework for health promotion. (From *Achieving Health for All: A Framework for Health Promotion* by J. Epp, 1986, Ottawa, ON: Health and Welfare Canada.)

connectedness, self-efficacy, and capacity to engage in meaningful activities (see Figure 1–2).

Risk Factors and Risk Conditions. Labonte (1993) categorized the major determinants of health in a socio-environmental approach as psychosocial risk factors and socio-environmental risk conditions:

- **Psychosocial risk factors** are complex psychological experiences resulting from social circumstances that include isolation, lack of social support, limited social networks, low self-esteem, self-blame, and low perceived power.
- **Socio-environmental risk conditions** are social and environmental living conditions that include poverty, low educational or occupational status, dangerous or stressful work, dangerous physical environments, pollution, discrimination, relative political or economic powerlessness, and inequalities of income or power.

A socio-environmental approach to health suggests that political, social, and cultural forces affect health and well-being directly and indirectly through their influence on personal health behaviours. Socio-environmental risk conditions can lead to psychosocial risk factors, which then result in unhealthy behaviours (Figure 1–4). This means that health professionals should recognize the influence of one's environment on personal behaviours. This perspective suggests that "health-inhibiting" behaviours could be coping strategies to manage the stress created by living and working conditions that decrease access to resources. Nurses should consider the *context* of health behaviours, rather than focusing only on the behaviour itself. In other words, "to change behaviour it may be necessary to change more than behaviour" (Wilkinson, 1996, p. 64). For example, rather than working "downstream" to assist people who are experiencing the negative health effects of socio-environmental conditions, nurses can work with others to advocate for policies that ensure affordable housing, financial support to those with low incomes, and safe, fulfilling work environments.

Strategies for Population Health. In Canada, there has been further emphasis on the determinants of health through the **population health approach** (Figure 1–5). This approach, initiated by the Canadian Institute of Advanced Research, was officially endorsed by the federal, provincial, and territorial ministers of health in the report titled *Strategies for Population Health: Investing in the Health of Canadians* (Federal, Provincial, and Territorial Advisory Committee on Population Health [ACPH], 1994). In a population health approach, "the entire range of known individual and collective factors and conditions that determine population health status, and the interactions among them, are taken into account in planning action to improve health" (Health Canada, 1998). The population health approach emphasizes the use of epidemiological data to determine the etiology of health and disease. Much like the Lalonde Report, it moved away from a clinical focus, which emphasized treatment of individuals with disease, and instead emphasized social and individual factors that influence a population's health.

The key **health determinants** identified in this document are:

- Income and social status.
- Social support networks.
- Education.
- Employment and working conditions.
- Physical environments.

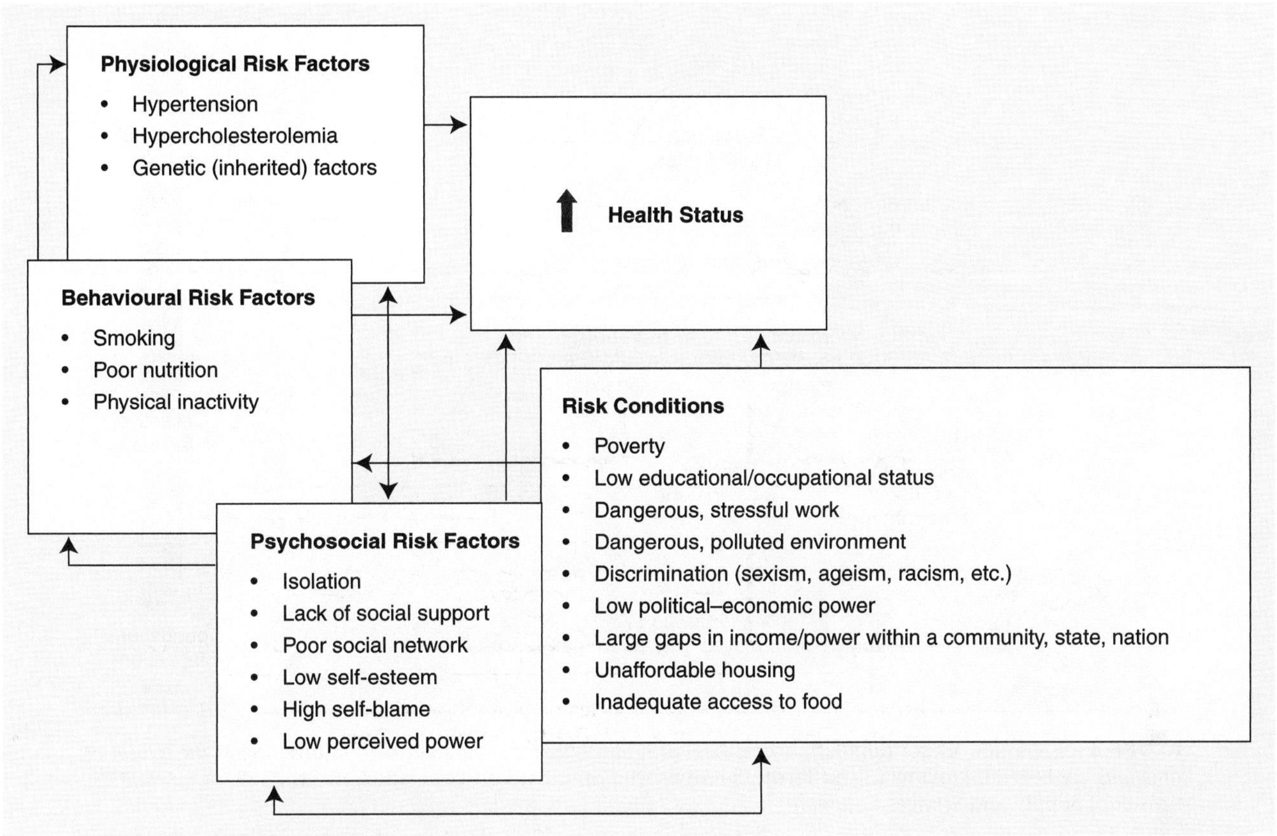

FIGURE **1–4** Socio-environmental approach to health. (From *Issues in Health Promotion Series. 3. Health Promotion and Empowerment: Practice Frameworks,* by R. Labonte, 1993, Toronto, ON: Centre for Health Promotion, University of Toronto, & ParticipACTION.)

- Biology and genetic endowment.
- Personal health practices and coping skills.
- Healthy child development.
- Health services.

In 1996, Health Canada added *gender, culture,* and *social environments* to this list. Note that the list includes individual level (personal health practices and coping skills, biology and genetic endowment) and at the population level (education, employment, and income distribution).

Toronto Charter on the Social Determinants of Health. In the early to middle 1990s, Canadian social and health policies changed significantly with political, economic, and social conditions (Bryant, 2002). The decade witnessed increasing social and economic inequalities (Raphael, Bryant, & Curry-Stevens, 2004). In 2002, a conference was held in Toronto on the state of 10 social determinants of health to explore the implications of these conditions for the health of Canadians and to outline policy directions to strengthen these determinants (Raphael et al., 2004). The conference resulted in the *Toronto Charter on the Social Determinants of Health* (*http://www.atkinson.yorku.ca/SHPM/torontoCharter1.pdf*), which outlined action for governments, media, and public health agencies and associations. The determinants identified as particularly important to the health of Canadians and relevant to policy were *early childhood development, education, employment and working conditions, food security, health care services, housing shortages, income and its equitable distribution, social safety nets, social exclusion,* and *unemployment and employment security.* These determinants reflected growing concern that social safety nets were eroding.

Determinants of Health

The following are some of the major determinants of health affecting Canadians (Health Canada, 1996). Each determinant influences the others. This is only an introduction to the determinants; There are many excellent sources of information about each of them.

Income and Social Status (Income Distribution)

Income and social status is the greatest determinant of health (ACPH, 1994; Canadian Institute for Health Information [CIHI], 2004; Raphael et al., 2004; WHO, 1997). Canadians who live in poverty have poorer health. Low-income Canadians are more likely to die earlier and to suffer more illnesses than those with higher incomes, regardless of age, sex, race, culture, and place of residence. Mortality rates are highest in poor neighbourhoods (Wilkins, Berthelot, & Ng, 2002), and it is estimated that 23% of Canadians' premature loss of

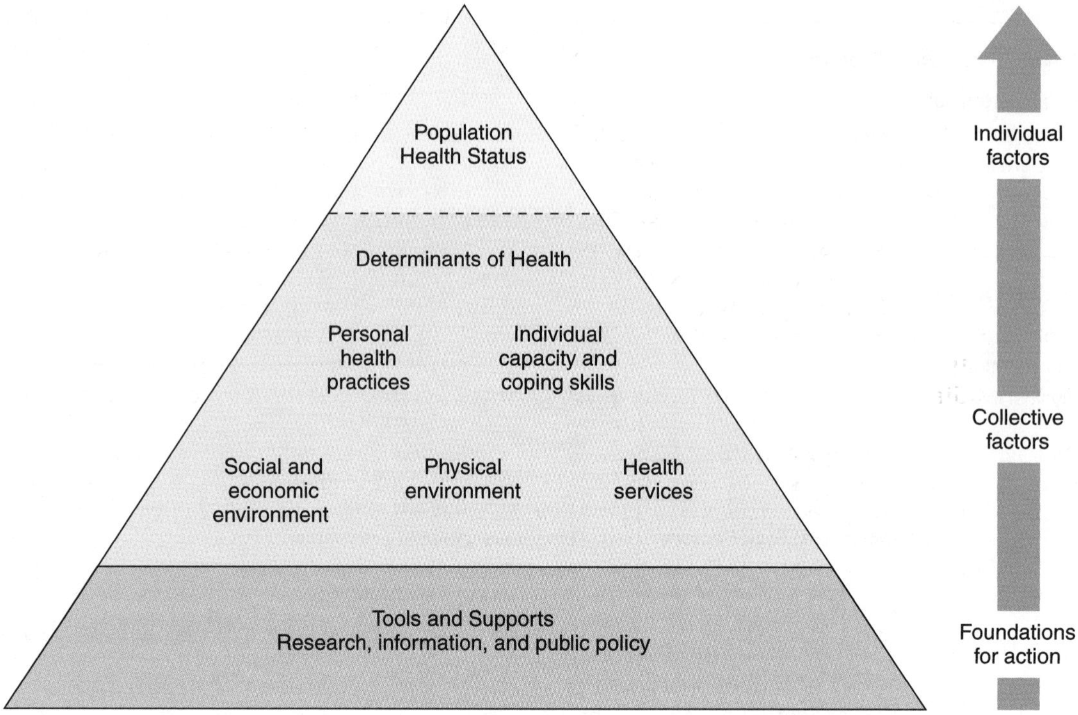

FIGURE **1–5** Framework for population health. (From *Strategies for Population Health: Investing in the Health of Canadians,* by Federal, Provincial, and Territorial Advisory Committee on Population Health, 1994, Ottawa, ON: Minister of Supply and Services Canada.)

life can be accounted for by income differences (Raphael, 2004).

From Statistics Canada's low-income cut-offs (National Council of Welfare, 2002), in 1999, 16% of Canadians lived in low-income households, with much higher rates for single mothers (52%), single older women (49%), people with disabilities in urban areas (36%), off-reserve Aboriginal peoples (56%), and recent urban immigrants (52%) (Lee, 2000). Less than half of Canadians (47%) in the lowest income group rate their health as very good or excellent, compared with 73% in the highest group (ACPH, 1999). People with lower incomes are also more likely to have chronic health problems (Roberge, Berthelot, & Wolfson, 1995); lower levels of self-esteem, sense of mastery, and coherence; and higher levels of depression (ACPH, 1999). Children living in poverty are more likely to have chronic medical problems such as asthma and psychiatric disorders (Canadian Council on Social Development, 1997) and are at greater risk for poor school performance (Lipps & Frank, 1997; Ross & Roberts, 1999). A study by the Canadian Council on Social Development found that family income is crucial to child development. The risks for negative child outcomes in a family with two children are noticeably higher for families with incomes below $30,000 (Ross & Roberts, 1999).

With each step up the economic ladder, Canadians' health status improves. This suggests that ill health is related to more than absolute material deprivation. Social deprivation may also influence health, perhaps through its effects on personal control and uncertainty (Wilkinson & Marmot, 1998).

Income inequality, the increasing gap between the rich and the poor (Dunn, 2002; Phipps, 2003), is also reflected in the concentration of poverty in certain urban neighbourhoods (Federation of Canadian Municipalities, 2003). Societies with greater gaps between rich and poor may have lower overall health (Dunn, 2002; Wilkinson, 1996). For example, countries with longer life expectancies such as Sweden and Japan also have smaller differences in income (Wilkinson, 1996). Some investigators suggest that economic inequality is the single greatest threat to the well-being of Western societies (Kawachi & Kennedy, 1997). Why is this so? Although ways that income inequality influences health are still being debated, some investigators speculate that people with different economic resources are socially distanced from one another, thereby losing commitment to public institutions that influence the cohesiveness of communities (Raphael, 1999; Wilkinson, 1996). Countries with economic inequality have higher levels of poverty, fewer public services, and weaker social safety nets (Raphael, 1999). Interestingly, income inequality has affected the United States more than it has affected Canada, which is attributed to Canada's progressive tax system, more public goods, and less geographic segregation by income (Dunn, 2002).

Social Support Networks

Social support affects health, health behaviours, and health care utilization (Stewart, 2000) through practical, emotional, informational, and affirmational support (House, 1981). Indeed, some experts believe that relationships may be as important to health as established risk factors such as smoking and high blood pressure

(ACPH, 1999). A strong body of research links social support with positive health outcomes (Berkman, 1995; Cohen, 1992).

In general, Canadians have reported high levels of support. In the National Population Health Survey in 1996/1997, four of five Canadians reported they had someone to confide in, whom they could count on in a crisis or for advice, and who made them feel loved and cared for. Nevertheless, there were variations: Women generally reported higher levels of support than did men, and single parents reported lower levels of support than did other household types. Lower income Canadians also reported less support (ACPH, 1999).

Support from families and friends and from informal and formal groups can provide practical aid during times of crisis and emotional support in times of distress and change. Social support also assists coping and behavioural changes and can help individuals solve problems and maintain a sense of mastery and control over their lives. For instance, Stewart, Hart, and Mann (2000) found that telephone support groups for people with both hemophilia and AIDS and for their caregivers improved psychological health. A survey of young parents in Alberta identified that spouses, family, and friends were major sources of support in encouraging healthy behaviours (exercise, diet) by providing emotional, affirmational, and practical support, including child care and financial assistance (Reutter, Dennis, & Wilson, 2001). In another study, a peer-visiting support program for new family caregivers of stroke survivors lowered both inpatient and outpatient hospital use for stroke survivors (Hart et al., 2000).

Education

Some investigators suggest that literacy and education are important influences of health status because they affect many other health determinants (Perrin, 1998). Education increases job opportunities and income security, giving one the knowledge and skills to solve problems and gain a sense of control over one's life. It also increases one's access to health information and services (ACPH, 1994).

Canadians with low literacy skills are more likely to be unemployed and to live in poverty, suffer poorer health, and die earlier than Canadians with high literacy skills (ACPH, 1999). As well, people with higher education levels tend to smoke less, be more physically active, and have access to healthier foods and physical environments (ACPH, 1999). These findings suggest that education can influence many other health determinants such as income, physical environment, and health practices.

Employment and Working Conditions

Employment and working conditions significantly affect physical, mental, and social health. Paid work provides financial resources, a sense of identity and purpose, social contacts, and opportunities for personal growth (CPHA, 1996a). Unemployed people have reduced life expectancy and experience significantly more health problems than do employed people (Bartley, Ferrie, & Montgomery, 1999). However, working conditions can also pose significant hazards. Temporary employees, part-time workers, and people working in low-wage jobs have high levels of job insecurity and, frequently, periods of unemployment. Often such jobs do not provide benefits or pensions, which can lead to uncertainty and stress.

Work pace and time are also key health influences, especially among professionals and managers (Canadian Policy Research Networks, 2002). In 2000, one third of Canadian workers experienced stress at work from "too many demands or too many hours." More than one third of 25- to 44-year-old women who worked full time and have children reported stress, and the same is true of about one in four men (Statistics Canada, 1999). Workplace stress is linked to increased risk of physical injuries at work, high blood pressure, cardiovascular disease, depression, and increases in smoking and drinking (Jackson, 2004).

Although injuries are often only associated with physical jobs such as manufacturing and construction, injury rates are also high in retail and in health and social services sectors (Jackson, 2004).

Physical Environments

Housing, indoor air quality, and community planning are important determinants of health. Contaminants in air, water, food, and soil also adversely affect health, sometimes contributing to cancer, birth defects, respiratory illness, and gastrointestinal ailments. Children from low-income families, who often live in substandard housing and in neighbourhoods near highways and industrial areas, are particularly likely to be exposed to these contaminants (ACPH, 1999). Childhood asthma, which is highly sensitive to airborne contaminants, has increased significantly in the last two decades.

Recently, environmental tobacco smoke (ETS, or second-hand smoke) has received considerable attention in Canada. Pregnant women, fetuses, and young children are especially susceptible to the effects of ETS, which include complications during pregnancy, low birth weight, increased risk of sudden infant death syndrome and ear infections, reduced lung development, and increased risk of respiratory illnesses (U.S. Department of Health and Human Services, 1994). In 1996 and 1997, an estimated 33% of children in Canada under the age of 12 years were regularly exposed to ETS in the home (de Groh & Morrison, 2002).

Another important aspect of the environment, which is closely related to income, is affordable and adequate housing. The number of homeless people in Canada is increasing, in part because of reduced government funding of social housing and lack of affordable rental accommodation (Bryant, 2004). Homeless Canadians include increasing numbers of women and children, adolescents, people with mental illness, and Aboriginal people (ACPH, 1999). Many studies have shown that homeless populations have more health problems such as respiratory conditions, epilepsy, arthritis, and poor oral and dental health. They are also more likely to die an early death (Hwang, 2001).

Poor housing conditions can affect health directly, but a lack of affordable housing can also *indirectly* affect health through its influence on other determinants (Bryant, 2004). Spending a disproportionate amount of income on rent, for example, reduces the amount of money that families can spend on food, clothing, and medical care.

Biology and Genetic Endowment

Heredity—an important health determinant—is strongly influenced by social and physical environments, and considerable effort has been expended to prevent congenital defects through monitoring and improved pre-conception and prenatal care (ACPH, 1999). This effort has led to substantial decreases in anomalies at birth.

Age is also a strong determinant of health, although there may be differences related to different aspects of health. For example, both physical health and levels of stress decrease with increasing age (Denton & Walters, 1999). With aging, there is a normal decline in vision, nerve conduction velocity, muscular strength, bone mass, and kidney function. Many older people develop chronic diseases (ACPH, 1999). However, one should ask how much of this decline is related to biological aging and how much is the result of other determinants such as socio-economic status, social support, and personal health practices.

Personal Health Practices and Coping Skills

Recall that personal health practices are the primary focus of the behavioural approach to health. Effective coping skills help people to face challenges without resorting to risk behaviours such as substance abuse. Remember, too, that many so-called risk behaviours may, in fact, be coping strategies for stress and strain due to living circumstances. For example, considerable evidence shows that low-income women use smoking as a coping strategy (Stewart et al., 1996).

Although many Canadians are making changes in their personal health practices, there is considerable room for improvement. Adolescents and young adults are particularly vulnerable to negative health practices (ACPH, 1999).

Three lifestyle practices with major detrimental health consequences are physical inactivity, poor nutrition, and smoking.

- *Physical inactivity* promotes weight gain and obesity (CIHI, 2004). It is a major risk factor for a number of diseases. Active living benefits include a reduced risk for cancer, diabetes, heart disease, and osteoporosis and an enhanced feeling of well-being (Bouchard, Shephard, & Stephens, 1994).
- *Poor nutrition,* in particular overconsumption of fats, sugars, and starches, is linked to major causes of disease including some cancers, cardiovascular diseases, Type 2 diabetes, hypertension, osteoarthritis, strokes, and gallbladder disease (CIHI, 2004). Obesity is now considered a major public health problem. In 2001, 56% of men and 39% of women were overweight or obese. In 2000 to 2001, more than one third (36%) of children aged 2 to 11 years were overweight or obese. Although Canadians have decreased total fat consumption, only about one in three reported eating the recommended number of fruits and vegetables daily (CIHI, 2004). Several factors influence food consumption patterns, including household income, food advertising, and availability of nutritious choices. In Canada, those on social assistance are at greater risk of experiencing food insecurity, the limited or uncertain availability of nutritious foods. Food insecurity is significantly associated with poor and fair health, multiple chronic conditions, obesity, distress, and depression (Che & Chen, 2001).
- *Smoking* is the single most important preventable cause of death (Shields & Tremblay, 2002). In 1996, one fifth of all deaths from the three leading causes—cancer, heart disease, and stroke—were attributed to cigarette smoking (Makomaski Illing & Kaiserman, 1999). Smoking is also the single largest modifiable risk factor contributing to low birth weight and infant mortality (Steinhauer, 1998).

Although smoking rates have dropped dramatically in Canada in the past three decades, groups that are particularly at risk for increased smoking are young women generally and young women and men with low-income status (ACPH, 1999). Forty-four per cent of men and 36% of women in the lowest income bracket reported smoking, whereas only 24% of men and 22% of women in the highest income bracket were smokers (Health Canada, 2003). Aboriginal people are another group at greater risk for the ill effects of smoking, about 63% of whom smoke (Health Canada, 1995).

Many factors influence personal health behaviours: income, education, gender, culture, and social support. Therefore, although health education helps to influence behaviours, it is clearly not sufficient. Individuals need access to resources to develop and maintain health-enhancing behaviours. Social policies such as income security and non-smoking legislation will make "healthy choices the easy choices."

Healthy Child Development

All determinants influence child development, especially the negative effects of poverty, but healthy child development is a separate determinant because of its importance to lifelong health. In the past decade, increasing evidence suggests that events during conception and before the age of 6 years influence children's health for the rest of their lives (CIHI, 2004). Three conditions for healthy child development are adequate and equitable income, effective parenting, and supportive environments (CIHI, 2004; Stroick & Jenson, 1999).

From conception to birth, two significant health risks are low birth weight and effects of maternal tobacco, alcohol, and drug use (Steinhauer, 1998). A baby with low birth weight is almost twice as likely to die at birth or during its first year and has almost twice the risk of lifelong diseases and disabilities, including cerebral palsy, visual problems, attention deficit hyperactivity disorder, learning disabilities, and respiratory problems (McCormick, Gortmaker, & Sobol, 1990). Other factors that contribute to low birth weight include a mother's isolation, lack of psychosocial supports, chronic high stress, and abuse during pregnancy (Garmezy, 1991; Goodyer, 1990).

From birth through the toddler years, the family environment is important, particularly to establish attachment to a primary caregiver during the first 2 years of life (Steinhauer, 1998). Throughout the toddler, preschool, and school-aged years, meeting a child's development needs is crucial. Family conflict, violence, and poverty threaten healthy child development. Schools in which students feel secure, respected, challenged, and cared for are important factors to ensure that children succeed in school. Community support is also important (Steinhauer, 1998).

Health Services

Approximately 25% of a population's health status is attributed to the quality of its health care services (Saskatchewan Public Health Association, 1994). Quality, accessible acute care treatment, long-term care, home care, and preventive services are therefore important. More funding is given to acute-care services than to health promotion and disease prevention—services that contribute even more to population health. Prenatal care, well-child and immunization clinics, education services about healthy lifestyles, and services that maintain older adults' health and independence are important examples of preventive and primary health care services that Canadians should continue to develop. Canada's national health insurance scheme is considered a hallmark of society (National Forum on Health, 1997). Principles of the *Canada Health Act*—universality, portability, accessibility, comprehensiveness, and public administration—apply to the provision of medically insured services. Increasingly, the trend in health care service provision is from institutionalized care to community-based care, decision making based on the best available evidence, and more regional administration. In the 1990s, all Canadian provinces and territories restructured their health care services, and most areas have undergone major cutbacks in services. Concern about the sustainability of Canada's health care system is discussed in chapter 2.

Gender

Gender is "the array of society-determined roles, personality traits, attitudes, behaviours, values, relative power and influence that society ascribes to the two sexes on a differential basis" (Health Canada, 1996). Many health issues are a function of gender-based social roles, and gender can influence health status, behaviours, and care. In Canada, men are more likely than women to die prematurely, largely as a result of heart disease, unintentional fatal injuries, cancer, and suicide. Women, however, are more likely to suffer from depression, stress (often due to efforts to balance work and family life), chronic conditions such as arthritis and allergies, and injuries and death from family violence (ACPH, 1999). The negative effects of lower levels of income, education, and social support on health are greater for women than for men (Denton & Walters, 1999). Indeed, when considering the determinants of health discussed in this section, think about how gender may affect each determinant. For example, why are women more likely to live in poverty? How and why do smoking rates differ by gender? The recently created Institute for Gender and Health at the Canadian Institutes of Health Research (*www.cihr.ca*) explores gender effects on health.

Culture

Cultural and ethnic factors influence how people interact with a health care system, their participation in programs of prevention and health promotion, their access to health information, their health-related lifestyle choices, and their understanding of health and illness (Health Canada, 1996). Cultural factors also influence whether and how determinants are met (see chapter 9). For example, health and social well-being are affected by racially motivated harassment in schools and workplaces. Language differences can lead to isolation and decreased social support networks. Prejudice can deny individuals opportunities for education, employment, and access to housing (Health Canada, 1996).

Social Environments

Social environments are defined as "the array of values and norms of a society [that] influence in varying ways the health and well-being of populations. In addition, social stability, recognition of diversity, safety, good working relationships and cohesive communities provide [support] that reduces or avoids many potential risks to good health" (Health Canada, 1996). This determinant is clearly related to other factors and expands on the social support determinant by incorporating broader community characteristics, norms, and values. Healthy social environments include freedom from discrimination and prejudice—particularly for people marginalized by income, age, gender, activity limitations, ethnicity, and sexual orientation. Reducing income inequalities increases community cohesiveness. The determinant of social environment is also evident in the Jakarta Declaration prerequisites of human rights, social security, and social relations (WHO, 1997).

One important aspect of the social environment that affects nurses' roles is violence—both in the home and in the community. Violence takes many forms, all of which may have damaging short- and long-term effects on mental, physical, and spiritual well-being (ACPH, 1999). Women, children, youth, and older adults are particularly at risk for domestic violence (CPHA, 1997). Although the Canadian national crime rate has decreased for more than a decade, it is still much higher than it was three decades ago (Statistics Canada, 2003). Recently, greater attention has been directed to violence experienced by nurses in the workplace (Duncan et al., 2001).

Strategies to Influence Health Determinants

All health determinants influence each other. For example, all determinants influence healthy child development, and poverty influences all other determinants. Personal health practices and coping skills are influenced by income, education, culture, gender, social support, and other factors. What, then, does an understanding of these determinants and their interrelationships mean for nurses? To assist clients and communities, nurses should:

- Understand the myriad and complex factors influencing health situations.
- Consider root causes of health situations and strive to influence them (see Figure 1–4).
- Consider multiple strategies to enhance a population's health status.
- Co-operate with other sectors and the public to enhance health.

Health Promotion and Disease Prevention

Recall that health is often viewed as qualitatively different from disease. This understanding has led to a differentiation of the concepts of health promotion and disease prevention, even though they are interrelated. Health promotion is defined in the Ottawa Charter as "the process of enabling people to increase control over, and improve, their health" (WHO, 1986). Health promotion is therefore much broader than disease prevention. Pender (1996) differentiated between health promotion and disease prevention as follows: **health promotion** is "directed toward increasing the level of well-being and self-actualization" (p. 34); **disease prevention** "is directed toward decreasing the probability of experiencing health problems" (p. 34).

Some authors consider health promotion as one aspect of primary prevention (Leavell & Clark, 1965; Neuman, 1995). For example, in the initial formulations of the levels of prevention, health promotion was viewed as one component of primary prevention, and it was not necessarily disease specific—it included diet and exercise, for instance (Leavell & Clark, 1965).

There are three levels of disease prevention:

- *Primary prevention* includes activities that protect against a disease *before* signs and symptoms occur. Examples include immunization to prevent infectious diseases and reduction of risk factors such as inactivity, smoking, and air pollution.
- *Secondary prevention* includes activities that promote *early detection* of disease so that prompt treatment can be initiated to halt disease and limit disability. Examples include preventive screening for cancer, such as breast self-examination, mammography, or testicular self-examination; blood pressure screening to detect hypertension; and blood sugar screening to detect diabetes.
- *Tertiary prevention* includes activities that *minimize residual disability* from disease and help the client learn to live productively with limitations. An example is a cardiac rehabilitation program entered after a myocardial infarction.

In a prevention paradigm, the nurse assesses risk factors for disease and works to alleviate them. Health promotion, however, does not necessarily focus on a specific disease (Laffrey & Craig, 2000). Health promotion focuses on enhancing a person's competencies and capacities and is committed to empowerment and community-based health planning (Robertson, 1998). Health promotion is often political because it is associated with structural and systemic inequities and has a strong social justice philosophy. Health promotion is guided by the following principles (CPHA, 1996b):

- *Health promotion addresses health issues in context.* It recognizes relationships among individual, social, and environmental factors.
- *Health promotion supports a holistic approach* that recognizes physical, mental, social, ecological, cultural, and spiritual aspects of health.
- *Health promotion requires a long-term perspective.*
- *Health promotion is multi-sectoral.* Because most health determinants lie outside health care, sectors other than health must be involved to change unhealthy living and working conditions.
- *Health promotion draws on knowledge from a variety of sources.* It uses knowledge from disciplines such as social, economic, political, environmental, medical, and nursing sciences, as well as from first-hand experiences.

Health Promotion Strategies

The Ottawa Charter identified five broad strategies to enhance health. The following is a brief introduction to each of these **health promotion strategies.**

1. Build Healthy Public Policy. Advocating healthy public policies is a priority strategy for health promotion in Canada. Indeed, some suggest that this strategy is the foundation of all others because policies shape how money, power, and material resources are distributed to society (CPHA, 1996b). Advocating healthy public policy is a collaborative effort to identify the most important areas where policy can make a difference. Nurses should work with others to develop policy options, encourage public dialogue, persuade decision makers to adopt the healthiest option, and follow up to make sure the policy is implemented (CPHA, 1996b). Cathy Crowe, a Toronto nurse and co-founder of the Toronto Disaster Relief Committee (*http://www.tdrc.net*), is an excellent example of a nurse advocating for healthy public policy both locally and nationally.

The CPHA recommends that more emphasis be given to policies that create healthy living conditions and enable those who are least powerful to express their concerns. This priority is also reflected in the *Toronto Charter on the Social Determinants of Health*, discussed earlier.

Given that the determinants of health are broad, healthy public policy necessarily extends beyond traditional health agencies and government health departments to other sectors such as agriculture, education, transportation, labour, social services, energy, and housing. Therefore, policy-makers in all government sectors and organizations should know the health consequences of their policies.

Increasingly, policy advocacy is incorporated into nursing role statements (e.g., Community Health Nurses Association of Canada, 2003; International Council of Nurses, 2001) and nursing education curricula (Rains & Barton-Kriese, 2001; Reutter & Duncan, 2002; Reutter & Williamson, 2000).

Nurses should think about what policies have contributed to health problems, what policies would help alleviate the problem, and how they can champion public policies. For example, how do current welfare incomes—which are lower than the national poverty line (National Council of Welfare, 2004)—influence the ability of welfare recipients to obtain adequate food and shelter and participate meaningfully in Canadian society?

2. Create Supportive Environments. The Ottawa Charter (WHO, 1986) states that "the overall guiding principle . . . is the need to encourage reciprocal maintenance, to take care of each other, our communities and our natural environment." This strategy helps ensure that physical environments are healthy and safe and that living and working conditions are stimulating and satisfying. Creating supportive environments also means protecting the natural environment and conserving natural resources (WHO, 1986).

An excellent example of an initiative that helps create supportive environments is the Comprehensive School Health Program, which focuses on improving school environments by providing health instruction, social support, support services, and positive physical environments (Mitchell & Laforet-Fliesser, 2003).

3. Strengthen Community Action. Strengthening communities is a requisite for successful health promotion and for community health nursing practices in Canada (Community Health Nurses Association of Canada, 2003; CPHA, 1996b). This strategy is often referred to as community development, and it implies that communities identify issues and work together to make changes that will enhance health. In a community development approach, health professionals help community groups identify important issues and organize and implement plans and strategies to resolve these issues. Public participation in all phases of community programming is key to community development (Labonte, 1993).

4. Develop Personal Skills. This strategy, which is probably most familiar to nurses, helps clients develop personal skills, enhance coping, and gain control over their health and environments so that they can make healthy lifestyle choices. Personal skills development includes health education, but it also emphasizes adequate support and resources.

5. Reorient Health Services. Health system reform has two objectives: to shift emphasis from treating disease to improving health and to make the health care system more efficient and effective (CPHA, 1996b). A proactive approach to health requires improved access to primary health care services, increased community development, improved community-based care services, increased family-based care, and public participation. In Canada, there is considerable emphasis on developing the primary health care model, which nursing associations in Canada have advocated for many years (Ogilvie & Reutter, 2002; see chapter 2).

Population Health Promotion Model: Putting It All Together

This chapter has presented the two major approaches to health in the 1990s: health promotion and population health. Hamilton and Bhatti (1996) integrated these two concepts into one model that shows their relationship (Figure 1–6). Aimed at developing actions to improve health, the model explores four major questions: "On *what* can we take action?" "*How* can we take action?" "*With whom* can we act?" and "*Why* take action?" (Saskatchewan Health, Population Health Branch, 2002).

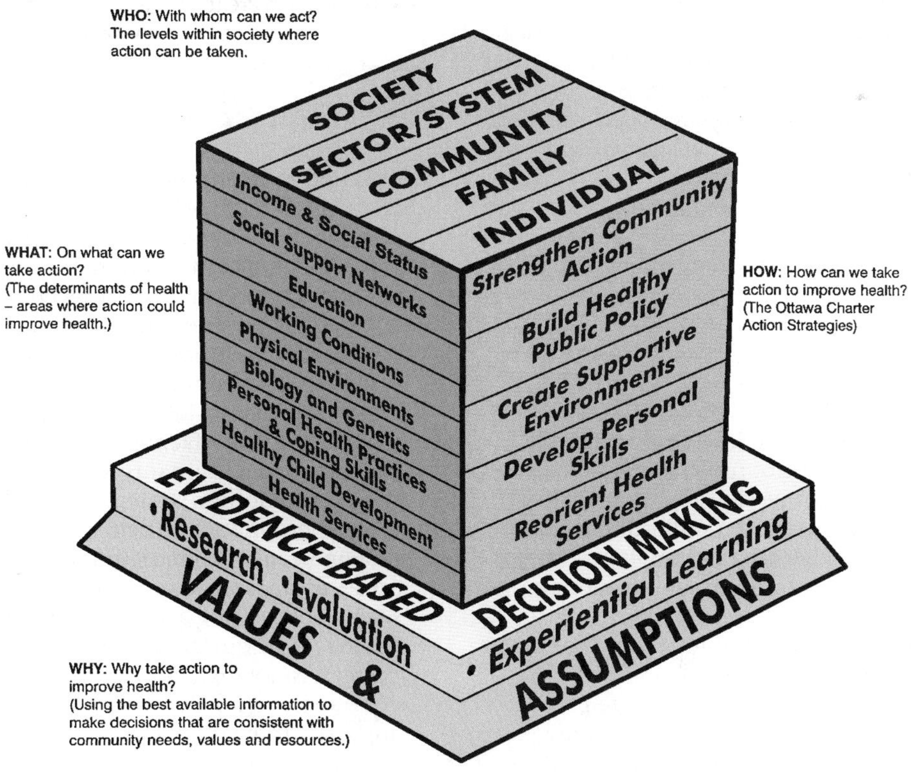

FIGURE **1–6** Population Health Promotion Model. (From *Population Health Promotion: An Integrated Model of Population Health and Health Promotion,* by N. Hamilton and T. Bhatti, 1996, Ottawa, ON: Health Promotion Development Division, Health Canada. Copyright 1996 by Minister of Public Works and Government Services Canada, 2000.)

The document *Strategies for Population Health* (ACPH, 1994) indicates what health determinants action could be taken (the *what*). The Ottawa Charter provides a comprehensive set of five strategies to enhance health (the *how*). Together, these documents suggest that to enhance population health, action must be taken on a variety of levels (the *who*). Clearly, nurses must direct these strategies toward individuals and families, communities, individual sectors of society (such as health or environmental sectors), and society as a whole. For example, to promote the health of lower income clients, nurses can help them access resources and support that will enhance their personal skills. Community programs such as school lunch programs, recreational activities, collective kitchens, and support groups can be provided. Nurses can lobby government sectors responsible for housing and employment to implement healthy public policies about affordable housing, job creation, income security, and financially accessible health services. On a societal level, nurses can raise awareness about the negative effects of poverty on health and well-being and can advocate policies that will decrease poverty. The population health promotion model shows how evidence-based decision making is a foundation to ensure that policies and programs focus on the right issues, take effective action, and produce successful results (Hamilton & Bhatti, 1996), the why of action (Saskatchewan Health, Population Health Branch, 2002). Evidence is based on research, experiential learning, and evaluation of programs, policies, and projects. Values and assumptions that are the foundation of the model include:

- Stakeholders representing the various determinants must collaborate to address health determinants.
- Society is responsible for its members' health status.
- Health status is a result of people's health practices and their social and physical environments.
- Opportunities for healthy living are based on social justice, equity, and relationships of mutual trust and caring, rather than power and status.
- Health care, health protection, and disease prevention complement health promotion.
- Active participation in policies and programs is essential.

Key Concepts

- Health conceptualizations and determinants influence the nature and scope of professional practice.
- Definitions of health can be classified in several ways; recent definitions reflect a multi-dimensional perspective and a positive orientation.
- Three recent approaches to health are medical, behavioural, and socio-environmental.
- Behavioural approaches focus primarily on health practices.
- Socio-environmental approaches emphasize psychosocial factors and socio-environmental conditions.
- Health determinants are interrelated.
- Canada is a leader in shifting views on health and health determinants.
- Health promotion differs from disease prevention.
- Three levels of disease prevention are primary (protection against disease), secondary (activities that promote early detection), and tertiary (activities directed toward minimizing disability from disease and helping clients learn to live productively with their limitations).
- The Ottawa Charter identifies five major categories of health promotion strategies.

Key Terms

Actualization-oriented definition, *p. 3*
Behavioural approach, *p. 4*
Behavioural risk factors, *p. 4*
Combined actualization and stability definition, *p. 3*
Determinants of health, *p. 6*
Disease, *p. 2*
Disease prevention, *p. 12*
Health, *p. 3*
Health field concept, *p. 4*
Health promotion, *p. 12*
Health promotion strategies, *p. 12*
Illness, *p. 3*
Medical approach, *p. 4*
Physiological risk factors, *p. 4*
Population health approach, *p. 6*
Prerequisites for health, *p. 5*
Psychosocial risk factors, *p. 6*
Socio-environmental approach, *p. 5*
Socio-environmental risk conditions, *p. 6*
Stability-oriented definition of health, *p. 3*
Wellness, *p. 3*

Critical Thinking Exercises

1. Describe your current level of health. What criteria did you use? Which definition of health discussed in this chapter best matches your understanding of health? Consider another definition of health discussed in this chapter. Does your current level of health change on the basis of this definition? How might your nursing practice differ depending on which conceptualization of health you choose to guide your practice?
2. What do you consider to be the three most important health problems facing Canadians today? What are the major determinants of these problems? Which health promotion strategies would you consider the most appropriate for them?
3. Imagine you are a community health nurse working in an area where there are many low-income women who smoke. Using a socio-environmental approach to health, what questions would you need to address to decrease smoking behaviour in your area? How would your approach differ if you were using a behavioural approach to health?

Review Questions

1. The Lalonde Report is significant in that it was the first to emphasize
   1. A behavioural approach to health
   2. A medical approach to health
   3. A socio-environmental approach to health
   4. Physiological risk factors

2. The "watershed" document that marked the shift from a lifestyle to a social approach to health was the
   1. Lalonde Report
   2. National Forum on Health
   3. Toronto Charter
   4. Ottawa Charter

3. The major determinants of health in a socio-environmental view of health are
   1. Psychosocial risk factors and socio-environmental risk conditions
   2. Physiological risk factors and behavioural risk factors
   3. Behavioural and psychosocial risk factors
   4. Behavioural and socio-environmental risk factors

4. The main reason that intersectoral collaboration is a necessary strategy to reach the goal of Health for All is
   1. The determinants of health are broad
   2. Intersectoral collaboration is cost-effective
   3. Intersectoral collaboration encourages problem solving at a local level
   4. Intersectoral collaboration is less likely to result in conflict

5. Providing immunizations against measles is an example of
   1. Health promotion
   2. Primary prevention
   3. Secondary prevention
   4. Tertiary prevention

6. Which one of the following statements does NOT accurately characterize health promotion?
   1. Health promotion addresses health issues within the context of the social, economic, and political environment.
   2. Health promotion emphasizes empowerment.
   3. Health promotion strategies focus primarily on helping people to develop healthy behaviours.
   4. Health promotion is political.

7. The belief that health is primarily an *individual* responsibility is most congruent with the ___________ approach to health.
   1. Medical
   2. Behavioural
   3. Socio-environmental
   4. Public health

8. All of the following statements accurately describe the Population Health Promotion Model, EXCEPT
   1. The model suggests that action can address the full range of health determinants.
   2. The model incorporates the health promotion strategies of the Ottawa Charter.
   3. The model focuses primarily on interventions at the society level.
   4. The model attempts to integrate the concepts of population health and health promotion.

9. Which of the following is the most influential health determinant?
   1. Personal health practices
   2. Income and social status
   3. Health care services
   4. Physical environment

10. Health promotion activities are aimed at
    1. Providing protection against disease
    2. Increasing the level of well-being
    3. Avoiding injury or illness
    4. Teaching clients to learn to live with their limitations

References

Bartley, M., Ferrie, J., & Montgomery, S. (1999). *Living in a high-unemployment economy: Understanding the health consequences.* In M. Marmot & R.Wilkinson (Eds.), *Social determinants of health* (pp. 81–104). Oxford, England: Oxford University Press.

Berkman, L. (1995). The role of social relations in health promotion. *Psychosomatic Medicine, 57,* 245–254.

Bouchard, C., Shephard, R., & Stephens, T. (Eds.). (1994). *Physical activity, fitness, and health: International proceedings and consensus statement.* Champaign, IL: Human Kinetics.

Bryant, T. (2002). The role of knowledge in public health and health promotion policy change. *Health Promotion International, 17,* 89–98.

Bryant, T. (2004). Housing and health in Canada. In D. Raphael (Ed.), *Social determinants of health: Canadian perspectives* (pp. 217–232). Toronto, ON: Canadian Scholars Press.

Canadian Council on Social Development. (1997). *The progress of Canada's children 1997.* Ottawa, ON: Author.

Canadian Institute for Health Information. (2004). *Improving the health of Canadians.* Ottawa, ON: Author.

Canadian Policy Research Networks. (2002). *Long hours of work and stress.* Retrieved May 11, 2004, from *www.jobquality. ca/indicator%5Fe/phy005.stm*

Canadian Public Health Association. (1996a). *The health impacts of unemployment: A position paper.* Ottawa, ON: Author.

Canadian Public Health Association. (1996b). *Action statement for health promotion in Canada.* Ottawa, ON: Author.

Canadian Public Health Association. (1997). *Health impacts of social and economic conditions: Implications for public policy.* Ottawa, ON: Author.

Che, J., & Chen, J. (2001). Food insecurity in Canadian households [Electronic version]. *Health Reports, 12*(4), 11–22.

Cohen, S. (1992). Stress, social support, and disorder. In H. Veiel & U. Baumann (Eds.), *The meaning and measurement of social support* (pp. 109–124). New York: Hemisphere.

Community Health Nurses Association of Canada. (2003). *Community health nursing standards of practice.* Retrieved May 12, 2004, from *http://www.communityhealthnursescanada.org/Standards%20of%20Practice.pdf*

de Groh, M., & Morrison, H. (2002). Environmental tobacco smoke and deaths from coronary heart disease in Canada. *Chronic Diseases in Canada, 23*(1), 13–16.

Denton, M., & Walters, V. (1999). Gender differences in structural and behavioral determinants of health: An analysis of the social production of health. *Social Science and Medicine, 48,* 1221–1235.

Duncan, S., et al. (2001). Nurses' experience of violence in Alberta and British Columbia hospitals. *Canadian Journal of Nursing Research, 32*(4), 57–78.

Dunn, J. R. (2002). *Are widening income inequalities making Canada less healthy?* Retrieved May 20, 2004, from Ontario Public Health Association Web site: *http://www.opha.on.ca/resources/incomeinequalities/incomeinequalities.pdf*

Epp, J. (1986). *Achieving health for all: A framework for health promotion.* Ottawa, ON: Health and Welfare Canada.

Federal, Provincial, and Territorial Advisory Committee on Population Health. (1994). *Strategies for population health: Investing in the health of Canadians.* Ottawa, ON: Minister of Supply and Services Canada.

Federal, Provincial, and Territorial Advisory Committee on Population Health. (1999). *Toward a healthy future: Second report on the health of Canadians.* Ottawa, ON: Minister of Public Works and Government Services Canada.

Federation of Canadian Municipalities. (2003). *Falling behind: Our growing income gap.* Prepared by Caryl Arundel and Associates in association with Henson Consulting Ltd. Retrieved May 13, 2004, from *http://www.fcm.ca/english/communications/igover.pdf*

Garmezy, N. (1991). Resiliency and vulnerability to adverse developmental outcomes associated with poverty. *The American Behavioral Scientist, 34,* 416–430.

Goodyer, I. (1990). Family relationships, life events and childhood psychopathology. *Journal of Child Psychology and Psychiatry, and Allied Disciplines, 31,* 161–192.

Hamilton, N., & Bhatti, T. (1996). *Population health promotion: An integrated model of population health and health promotion.* Ottawa, ON: Health Promotion Development Division, Health Canada.

Hancock, T., & Perkins, F. (1985). The mandala of health: A conceptual model and teaching tool. *Health Education, 24*(1), 8–10.

Hart, G., et al. (2000). Stroke and heart failure in seniors: Dyadic peer support for family caregivers. In M. J. Stewart (Ed.), *Chronic conditions and caregiving in Canada: Social support strategies* (pp. 146–171). Toronto, ON: University of Toronto Press.

Health Canada. (1995). Tobacco use among high priority groups. *Fact Sheets: Tobacco use among Aboriginal peoples.* Ottawa, ON: Author.

Health Canada. (1996). *Towards a common understanding: Clarifying the concepts of population health.* Ottawa, ON: Author.

Health Canada. (1998). *Taking action on population health: A position paper for health promotion and programs branch staff.* Ottawa, ON: Author.

Health Canada. (2003). *Smoking behaviour of Canadians.* Retrieved May 12, 2004, from *http://www.hc-sc. gc.ca/pphb-dgspsp/ ccdpc-cpcmc/cancer/publications/nphs-sboc/nphs12_e.html*

House, J. (1981). *Work, stress, and social support.* Menlo Park, CA: Addison-Wesley.

Hwang, S. (2001). Homelessness and health. *Canadian Medical Association Journal, 164*(2), 229–233.

International Council of Nurses. (2001). *Guidelines on shaping effective health policy.* Geneva, Switzerland: Author.

Jackson, A. (2004). The unhealthy Canadian workplace. In D. Raphael (Ed.), *Social determinants of health: Canadian perspectives* (pp. 79–94). Toronto, ON: Canadian Scholars Press.

Jensen, L., & Allen, M. (1993). Wellness: The dialectic of illness. *Image—The Journal of Nursing Scholarship, 25,* 220–224.

Kawachi, I., & Kennedy, B. (1997). The relationship of income inequality to mortality: Does the choice of indicator matter? *Social Science and Medicine, 45,* 1121–1127.

Labonte, R. (1993). *Health promotion and empowerment: Practice frameworks. Issues in Health Promotion Series #3.* Toronto, ON: Centre for Health Promotion, University of Toronto, & ParticipACTION.

Laffrey, S., & Craig, D. (2000). Health promotion for communities and aggregates: An integrated model. In M. J. Stewart (Ed.), *Community nursing: Promoting Canadians' health* (2nd ed., pp. 105–125). Toronto, ON: W. B. Saunders.

Lalonde, M. (1974). *A new perspective on the health of Canadians.* Ottawa, ON: Government of Canada.

Leavell, H., & Clark, A. (1965). *Preventive medicine for doctors in the community* (3rd ed.). New York: McGraw-Hill.

Lee, K. (2000). *Urban poverty in Canada. A statistical profile.* Ottawa, ON: Canadian Council on Social Development.

Lipps, G., & Frank, J. (1997). The social context of school for young children. *Canadian Social Trends, 47,* 22–26.

Makomaski Illing, E., & Kaiserman, M. (1999). Mortality attributable to tobacco use in Canada and its regions, 1994 and 1996. *Chronic Diseases in Canada, 20*(3), 111–117.

McCormick, M., Gortmaker, S., & Sobol, A. (1990). Very low birthweight children: Behavior problems and school difficulties in a national sample. *Journal of Pediatrics, 117,* 687–693.

Mitchell, I., & Laforet-Fliesser, Y. (2003). Promoting healthy school communities. *Canadian Nurse, 99*(8), 21–24.

Naidoo, J., & Wills, J. (1994). *Health promotion: Foundations for practice.* London: Bailliere Tindall.

National Council of Welfare. (2002). *Poverty profile 1999.* Ottawa, ON: Minister of Public Works and Government Services Canada.

National Council of Welfare. (2004). *Income for living?* Ottawa, ON: Minister of Public Works and Government Services Canada.

National Forum on Health. (1997). *Canada health action: Building on the legacy. Synthesis reports and issues papers* (Vol. 2). Ottawa, ON: Author.

Neuman, B. (1995). *The Neuman systems model: Applications to nursing education and practice* (2nd ed.). Norwalk, CT: Appleton & Lange.

Ogilvie, L., & Reutter, L. (2002). Primary health care: Complexities and possibilities from a nursing perspective. In J. Ross-Kerr and M. Wood (Eds.), *Canadian nursing: Issues and perspectives* (4th ed., pp. 441–465). Toronto, ON: Harcourt Canada.

Orem, D. (1995). *Nursing: Concepts of practice* (5th ed.). New York: McGraw-Hill.

Pender, N. (1996). *Health promotion in nursing practice* (3rd ed.). Stamford, CT: Appleton & Lange.

Pender, N., Murdaugh, C., & Parsons, M. (2002). *Health promotion in nursing practice* (4th ed.). Upper Saddle River, NJ: Prentice Hall.

Perrin, B. (1998). *How does literacy affect the health of Canadians? A profile paper.* Ottawa, ON: Minister of Public Works and Government Services Canada. Retrieved November 26, 2004, from *http://www.phac-aspc.gc.ca/ph-sp/phdd/literacy/literacy. html*

Phipps, S. (2003). *The impact of poverty on health: A scan of the research literature.* Canadian Institute for Health Information and Canadian Population Health Initiative. Retrieved November 26, 2004, from *http://secure. cihi.ca/cihiweb/products/CPHIImpactonPoverty_e. pdf*

Rains, J., & Barton-Kriese, P. (2001). Developing political competence: A comparative study across disciplines. *Public Health Nursing 18,* 219–224.

Raphael, D. (1999). Health effects of economic inequality. *Canadian Review of Social Policy, 44,* 25–40.

Raphael, D. (2004). Introduction to the social determinants of health. In D. Raphael (Ed.), *Social determinants of health: Canadian perspectives* (pp. 1–18). Toronto, ON: Canadian Scholars Press.

Raphael, D., Bryant, T., & Curry-Stevens, A. (2004). Toronto charter outlines future health policy directions for Canada and elsewhere [Electronic version]. *Health Promotion International, 19,* 269–273.

Registered Nurses Association of British Columbia. (1994). *Creating the new health care: A nursing perspective.* Vancouver, BC: Author.

Reutter, L., Dennis, D., & Wilson, D. (2001). Young parents' understanding and actions related to the determinants of health. *Canadian Journal of Public Health, 92,* 335–339.

Reutter, L., & Duncan, S. (2002). Preparing nurses to promote health-enhancing public policies. *Policy, Politics, and Nursing Practice 3,* 294–305.

Reutter, L., & Williamson, D. (2000). Advocating healthy public policy: Implications for baccalaureate nursing education. *The Journal of Nursing Education, 39*(1), 21–26.

Roberge, R., Berthelot, J., & Wolfson, M. (1995). Health and socio-economic inequalities. *Canadian Social Trends 37,* 15–19.

Robertson, A. (1998). Shifting discourses on health in Canada: From health promotion to population health. *Health Promotion International, 13,* 155–166.

Rootman, I., & Raeburn, J. (1994). The concept of health. In A., Pederson, M. O'Neill, & I. Rootman (Eds.), *Health promotion in Canada* (pp. 56–71). Toronto, ON: W.B. Saunders.

Ross, D., & Roberts, P. (1999). *Income and child well-being: A new perspective on the poverty debate.* Ottawa, ON: Canadian Council on Social Development.

Saskatchewan Health, Population Health Branch. (2002) *A Population health promotion framework for Saskatchewan Regional Health Authorities.* Retrieved February 17, 2005, from *http://www.health.gov.sk.ca/ic_pub_3793_skhlthframewk.pdf*

Saskatchewan Public Health Association. (1994). *The determinants of health: Position paper.* Regina, SK: Author.

Shields, M., & Tremblay, S. (2002). The health of Canada's communities [Electronic version]. *Supplement to Health Reports, 13,* 1–24.

Statistics Canada. (1999, November 9). General social survey: Time use. *The Daily.* Retrieved May 11, 2004, from *www.statcan.ca*

Statistics Canada (2003, July 24). Crime statistics 2002. *The Daily.* Retrieved May 25, 2004, from *www.statcan.ca*

Steinhauer, P. (1998). Developing resiliency in children from disadvantaged populations. In *Determinants of health: Children and youth: Vol. 1. Canada health action: Building on the legacy.* Papers commissioned by the National Forum on Health. Sainte-Foy, QC: MultiMondes.

Stewart, M. (2000). Social support, coping, and self-care as public participation mechanisms. In M. J. Stewart (Ed.), *Community nursing: Promoting Canadians' health* (2nd ed.). Toronto, ON: W.B. Saunders.

Stewart, M., et al. (1996). Smoking among disadvantaged women: Causes and cessation. *Canadian Journal of Nursing Research, 28*(1):41.

Stewart, M., Hart, G., & Mann, K. (2000). Overcoming the loneliness of hemophiliacs with AIDS and their caregivers through telephone support. In M. J. Stewart (Ed.), *Chronic conditions and caregiving in Canada: Social support strategies* (pp. 117–145). Toronto, ON: University of Toronto Press.

Stroick, S., & Jenson, J. (1999). *What is the best policy mix for Canada's young children?* (CPRN Study No. F/09). Ottawa, ON: Canadian Policy Research Networks.

U.S. Department of Health and Human Services. (1994). *Preventing tobacco use among young people: A report of the surgeon general.* Atlanta, GA:U.S. Public Health Service, Centers for Disease Control and Prevention.

Wallerstein, N. (1992). Powerlessness, empowerment, and health: Implications for health promotion programs. *American Journal of Health Promotion, 6*(3), 197–205.

Wilkins, R., Berthelot, J., & Ng, E. (2002). Trends in mortality by neighbourhood income in urban Canada from 1971 to 1996. *Health Reports, 13*(Suppl.), 1–28.

Wilkinson, R. (1996). *Unhealthy societies: The afflictions of inequality.* London: Routledge.

Wilkinson, R., & Marmot, M. (1998). *Social determinants of health: The solid facts.* Copenhagen, Denmark: World Health Organization. Retrieved November 26, 2004, from *http://www.euro.who.int/document/e81384.pdf*

World Health Organization. (1984). *A discussion document on the concept and principles of health promotion.* Copenhagen, Denmark: European Office of the World Health Organization.

World Health Organization. (1986). *Ottawa charter for health promotion.* Ottawa, ON: Canadian Public Health Association.

World Health Organization. (1997). *The Jakarta Declaration on health promotion into the 21st century.* Retrieved November 26, 2004, from *http://www. who.int/hpr/NPH/docs/jakarta_declaration_en.pdf*

Recommended Web Sites

Canadian Health Network:
www.canadian-health-network.ca

The Canadian Health Network Web site is offered by Health Canada and major Canadian health organizations. It offers many links to numerous sources of health information on key health topics and population groups. It includes resources on how to stay healthy and prevent disease and injury.

Canadian Institute for Health Information (CIHI):
www.cihi.ca

The CIHI is a not-for-profit Canadian organization working to improve the health of Canadians and the health care system. One of its goals is to generate public awareness about factors affecting good health. This Web site offers current information and numerous links to government health reports.

National Literacy and Health Program:
http://www.nlhp.cpha.ca

The Canadian Public Health Association's National Literacy and Health Program (NLHP) promotes awareness among health professionals of the association between literacy and health. This Web site provides links to services, projects, and publications of the NLHP.

Population Health:
http://www.hc-sc.gc.ca/hppb/phdd/approach/index.html

This Health Canada Web site addresses the population health approach and the determinants of health. It provides links to health promotion research and documents.

World Health Organization publications:
http://www.who.int/pub/en/

This Web site provides links to the publications of the World Health Organization, including the World Health Report.

2

The Canadian Health Care Delivery System

Ardene Robinson Vollman, RN, BScN, MA, PhD (Canadian author)
Patricia A. Potter, RN, MSN, PhD, CMAC, FAAN

Objectives

Mastery of content in this chapter will enable the student to:

- Define the key terms listed.
- Discuss the evolution of Canada's social safety net and medicare program.
- Identify and define the principles of the *Canada Health Act.*
- Discuss clients' rights to health care.
- Discuss the role of nurses in different health care delivery settings.
- Describe the five levels of health care.
- Describe the types of services found within each level of health care.
- Discuss principal factors influencing health care reform.
- Explain the roles of primary health care and home care in health care reform.

Nurses are an essential part of the Canadian health care system. They make up the largest employment group within the system and are recognized as invaluable to the health of Canadians. Nursing services are necessary for virtually every client seeking care of any type. However, nursing finds itself in the middle of a health care dilemma. Fewer nurses provide care to greater numbers of clients. Registered nurses form the largest occupational group in Canada, with a membership of 230,957. Coupled with 60,123 registered (licensed) practical nurses, and some 5,000 registered psychiatric nurses, the profession contributes a formidable workforce to the health care system (Canadian Institute for Health Information [CIHI], 2003a, 2003b; Box 2-1). However, there are not enough nursing graduates to meet demands. Over the past decade, the size of the Canadian nursing workforce has remained relatively stable, but the size of the Canadian population has increased by 9.1%, leading to a decrease in the number of nurses per capita (CIHI, 2004a, 2004b). This shortage of nurses has been aggravated by an aging workforce, a high retirement rate, and a lack of full-time positions.

Because nursing is such an important part of the health care delivery system, nurses must understand the health care system and the issues that affect how care is provided to clients and their families. Every nurse practising today needs to appreciate that the health care system is a business whose central issues are rising costs and availability of quality services. Financial pressures have forced hospitals and other institutions to shift priorities. Some institutions have attempted to control costs by cutting the workforce and support services, and some institutions have made financial incentives a priority over quality care. Nursing professionals can help restructure delivery systems and maintain a level of excellence in health care. More than ever, a nurse's role in client advocacy will be critical to ensure that everyone's health care needs are served. The success of any health care business depends on nursing's participation to create systems to deliver quality, cost-effective care. In the face of rapid change and staff shortages, nursing must lead the way and retain its values for client care.

Box 2-1 Facts About Nursing in Canada, 2003

- In 2003, there were 258, 393 nurses (RNs) in Canada, constituting 78% of the total nursing workforce; this was an increase of 1.4% from 2002.
- Licensed practical nurses (LPNs) numbered 63,138 or 20.4% of the total nursing workforce; and there were 5,107 registered psychiatric nurses (RPNs) (1.6% of the total nursing workforce).
- There was a ratio of 131 RNs per 10,000 population in 2003.
- 40% of new RN graduates (those graduating in the last 5 years) earned a baccalaureate degree prior to entering practice.
- 7.3% of the RN workforce are foreign graduates while 1.7% of LPNs employed in Canada received their education in a foreign country.
- 62.4% of RNs practice in the hospital sector; 10.5% in long-term care facilities; 12.6% in community health and home care; 2.7% in educational institutions; 2.1% in offices and clinics; and 10.8% in other settings.
- 46.8% of LPNs are employed in hospitals, while 36.9% practice in long-term care settings.
- 94.7% of RNs are female and 5.3% are male; 93.2% of LPNs are female, while 6.8% are male.
- The average age of RNs is 44.5, of LPNs is 44.4, and of RPNs is 46.2.
- There are more RNs aged 55-59 in the Canadian nursing workforce than those aged 25-29. Of the LPN workforce, 15.1% are 55 or more years old.

Source: CIHI, Workforce Trends of Registered Nurses in Canada, 2003, Author, 2004; CIHI, Workforce Trends of Licensed Practical Nurses in Canada, 2003, Author, 2004; CIHI, Workforce Trends of Registered Psychiatric Nurses in Canada, 2003, Author, 2004.

Box 2-2 Milestones in Canadian Nursing History

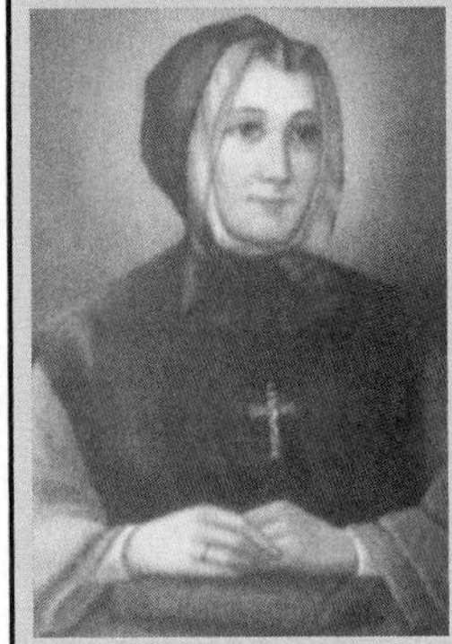

Marguerite d'Youville, 1701–1771

Born near Montreal in 1701, Marguerite d'Youville defied social conventions and fought for the rights of the poor (Mitchell, 1958). The niece of an explorer, she married fur trader François d'Youville—a notorious bootlegger and gambler (McGuire, 1982). After François' death in 1730, d'Youville and a band of like-minded women founded the Sisters of Charity. To support their work among the sick and the poor, they established farms, a mill, a bakery, a brewery, and a tobacco factory. After their refuge was destroyed by fire in 1745, the order moved to Montreal's General Hospital, of which d'Youville became director. Initially, the sisters were derided as "les grises," meaning tipsy women—a snide reference to Marguerite's late husband, a bootlegger. They wore a grey habit: hence their nickname the Grey Nuns.

During English-French hostilities from 1756 to 1760, the Grey Nuns cared for sick and wounded soldiers, including British prisoners of war. The order was known for its excellent hospitals, in which they cared for anyone, regardless of race, colour, creed, or financial status. As the first non-cloistered order of nuns in New France, the sisters visited the sick in their homes, becoming the first visiting nurses. They established hospitals in Quebec, Manitoba, Saskatchewan, and Alberta, and in remote northern communities.

In 1959, the Roman Catholic Church beatified Marguerite d'Youville. She was canonized in 1990, and is the only Canadian saint.

Sources: *Three Centuries of Canadian Nursing,* by J. Gibbon and M. Mathewson, 1947, Toronto, ON: Macmillan; *Marguerite d'Youville: A Pioneer for Our Times,* by S. R. McGuire, 1982, Ottawa, ON: Novalis; and *Marguerite d'Youville,* by E. Mitchell, 1958, Montreal, QC: Palm. Painting by Flore Barrette, s.g.m., 1959.

Evolution of the Canadian Health Care Delivery System

Canada has a range of social programs that protects the interests of all Canadians. Known as the **social safety net,** this network of programs reflects Canadians' basic values and wishes to promote human rights and social justice. It includes programs such as family allowance, welfare, and unemployment insurance. **Medicare** is also a key element of Canada's social safety net. Medicare is Canada's national health insurance system, which uses taxes to finance medically necessary services for all citizens, thus providing "free" health care to all. It has been a source of national pride and fierce debate. Indeed, few issues are as important to Canadians as health care.

Early Health Care in Canada

Europeans who came to Canada in the 15th century brought infectious diseases that flourished under poor sanitary conditions. Settlements enacted public health laws to control the spread of diseases. For years, government care was limited to essential services (such as care of the insane and impromptu measures for dealing with epidemics). There were no permanent boards of health; families, churches, and local communities were expected to be self-reliant in handling all other medical and social problems. The first Canadian nurses were nuns from religious orders, such as the legendary Marguerite d'Youville (Box 2-2).

Canada was founded in 1867 (Confederation) with the *British North America Act,* which determined federal and provincial jurisdictions. Responsibility for health, education, and social services was delegated to the provinces. However, the provinces did not have the tax base necessary to support the extensive services required to meet the needs of the public. After Confederation, the country became increasingly urban and industrial. Immigration, crowded living conditions, and poor housing and sanita-

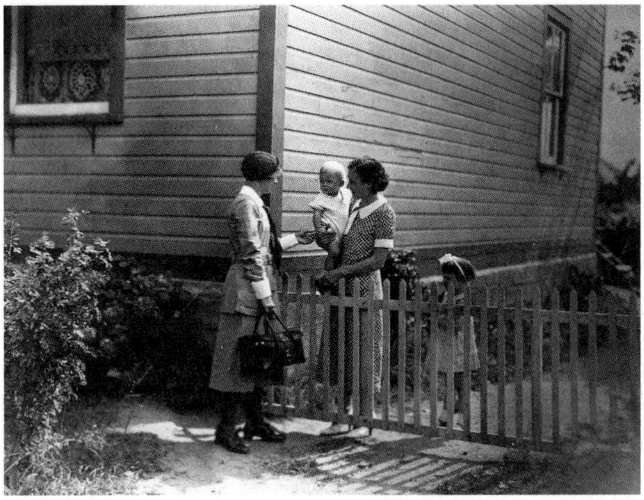

FIGURE 2–1 In the early 1900s, charitable medical services were provided by community agencies such as the Victorian Order of Nurses.

tion led to more disease. Provinces enacted public health acts to establish local boards of health to hire medical health officers and sanitary inspectors. Those working in the community with the poor were the first public health nurses. Churches and charities continued to provide hospital care.

By 1920, many health and social programs had expanded, and voluntary, charitable organizations formed, including the Children's Aid Society (1891), the Red Cross (1896), the Victorian Order of Nurses (1897), and the Canadian Mental Health Association (1918). Municipalities organized services for the poor and established hospitals. Those who could not pay still depended on charity (Figure 2–1). Fraternal societies (such as the Knights of Columbus) and unions created trusts that members could access when ill, injured at work, or unemployed. Such programs were precursors of modern unemployment insurance.

With World War I, citizens demanded support for widows, children, and elder family members who lost sons in the war. Manitoba passed *Mothers' Pension Act* in 1916 for women and older adults who could demonstrate financial need.

As urbanization continued, rural communities had difficulty attracting and paying physicians. The federal *Municipality Act* in 1916 gave communities the power to levy taxes to pay for physicians. The spread of the Great Depression across Canada during the 1930s had a dramatic effect on the health care system. Many families could not pay their medical bills, and a hospital stay caused financial ruin for many. These hardships inspired Canadians to create a prepaid medical and hospitalization insurance plan. In 1947, Premier Tommy Douglas of Saskatchewan was the first to introduce a public insurance plan that covered the costs of hospital services. By 1961, all provinces and territories had agreed to provide coverage for inpatient hospital care, with the federal and provincial/territorial governments each roughly paying half the costs of hospital and diagnostic services.

The next step was to ensure medical services outside hospitals. Once again, Saskatchewan took the lead. In 1962, it unilaterally instituted its *Medical Care Insurance Act* against the wishes of physicians, prompting a 23-day doctors' strike. In 1964, the Hall Commission recommended "strong federal government leadership and financial support for medical care" (Wilson, 1995). Based on these recommendations, the *Medical Care Act* was passed in 1966. Federal grants were awarded on a cost-sharing basis with the provinces if programs provided universal, comprehensive, portable, and publicly administered coverage of health care. Again, the federal and provincial/territorial governments agreed to equally share health care expenses. By 1972, all provincial and territorial insurance plans extended their coverage to include medical services provided outside hospitals. Modern medicare began that year because all Canadian citizens now had free access to hospital and medical care, regardless of their personal wealth.

Although programs prospered, cost sharing did not last. The Canadian government enacted the *Federal Provincial Fiscal Arrangements and Established Programs Financing Act* (1977) to replace cost sharing with block transfers of funds. These block transfers led the way to decreased federal contributions. Soon, extra billing of clients by hospitals and provider groups over what the universal insurance program covered became an issue. Universal medicare was threatened.

The *Canada Health Act* of 1984 amalgamated the previous acts of 1957 and 1966: It reaffirmed the insurance method of health care funding and effectively outlawed extra billing and user fees. It added the principle of accessibility to the principles of universality, portability, comprehensiveness, and public administration (Table 2-1). Under previous acts, access to services was through physician gatekeepers. Revisions in the act now allowed multiple points of access and insurance for care providers other than physicians. Although there was opposition to the act, by 1987 all provinces followed its principles (Health Canada, 1992).

The Evolution of Other Social Programs

Just as the health care system evolved to meet the needs of all Canadians, so, too, did other social programs. After World War II, Canada created many federal social programs that offered support to all Canadians, including those most in need. For example, the first universal social program in Canada was family allowance. The *Family Allowance Act* (1945) gave every family a monthly allowance, regardless of means. Social programs expanded to include universal old age security (1951), programs for the disabled, and revisions to the unemployment insurance system. In 1966, the *Canada Pension Plan* was introduced, and the *Canada Assistance Plan Act* was passed to subsidize social assistance and other welfare programs. The *Guaranteed Income Supplement* for low-income recipients of old age security was introduced in 1967, with a spousal allowance added in 1975.

Table 2-1 Canada Health Act (1984)

1. **Public administration**	The plan must be administered and operated on a nonprofit basis by a public authority, responsible to the provincial/territorial government and subject to audits of its accounts and financing transactions.
2. **Comprehensiveness**	The plan must cover all medically necessary hospital and physician services and, when the province or territory permits, services rendered by other health care practitioners.
3. **Universality**	Every permanent resident of a province or territory is entitled to receive the insured health care services provided by the plan on uniform terms and conditions.
4. **Portability**	Coverage for insured services must be maintained when an insured person moves or travels within Canada or travels outside of Canada.
5. **Accessibility**	Insured residents must have reasonable access to medically necessary hospital and physician services, regardless of their income, age, health status, gender, or geographical location. Additional charges for insured services are not permitted.

Adapted from *Canada Health Act: Introduction.* Accessed February 8, 2005, from *http://www.hc-sc.gc.ca/medicare/home.htm*

The Organization of Health Care

Under the Canadian constitution, the administration and delivery of health care services is a provincial and territorial responsibility. Medicare is often described as an interlocking set of 10 provincial and 3 territorial health care plans (Health Canada, 2004). However, the federal government also has a role in health care administration.

Federal Jurisdiction

The federal government is responsible for:

- Setting and administering national principles for the health care system through the *Canada Health Act.*
- Assisting in the financing of provincial/territorial health care services through fiscal transfers. The federal government transfers tax money to provinces and territories to share the cost of health care services. Provinces and territories must adhere to the principles outlined in the *Canada Health Act* as a prerequisite for obtaining their transfer shares.
- Delivering health services for certain groups (e.g., First Nations and Inuit, veterans, and inmates of federal penitentiaries).
- Providing government policy and programs that promote health and prevent disease; for example, the federal government approves drugs, assesses environmental risks, and provides grant money for public health programs like prenatal education.

Provincial and Territorial Jurisdiction

Each province and territory develops and administers its own health care insurance plan. The provincial/territorial government role is to finance and plan its health care services, following the five principles outlined in the *Canada Health Act* (see Table 2-1). For example, the province or territory decides where hospitals or long-term care facilities will be located and organized; how many physicians, nurses, and other care providers will be needed; and how much money to spend on health care services.

The provincial and territorial health insurance plans pay for physician and hospital costs. They also pay for some of the costs of rehabilitation and long-term care services. However, each provincial and territorial plan is unique, and details of what is covered and by how much varies across the country. For example, coverage for drugs, ambulance services, and home care varies by province. To help pay for services not covered by provincial or territorial insurance, Canadians can buy private health insurance policies. Employers often offer individual or group insurance plans.

Right to Health Care

Canadians believe that everyone has a right to health care. After one enters the health care system, one becomes a client and thus has certain rights. Generally, consumers have a right to determine what kind of health care should be available to them. However, the *Canadian Charter of Rights and Freedoms* (1982) does not explicitly include health care as a right. As a result, one must look to federal and provincial legislation to prove legal entitlement. (Quebec is the only province that has included health care rights within its legislation.) The *Canada Health Act* influences rights by setting conditions for federal funding (see Table 2-1). These provisions ensure that Canadians have access to "medically required services and hospital services without financial or other barriers; that these services will be administered on a public, not-for-profit basis, and that [consumers] be compensated for health care services inside or outside Canada at the same rate as if the service had been provided in their province of residence" (Wilson, 1995, pp. 29–30). Note that the right to have health care costs *covered* is guaranteed, not the right to health care itself.

Rights Within the System

In the midst of this debate, the Consumers' Association of Canada developed a list of Consumers' Rights to Health Care (1989, as cited in Wilson, 1995; Table 2-2). Sutherland and Fulton (1992) articulated a number of rights that Canadian health care workers expect, namely, the right to reasonable working conditions, including

Table 2-2 Consumer Rights for Health Care

1. Right to be informed	(a) about preventive health care including education on nutrition, birth control, drug use, appropriate exercise (b) about the health care systems including the extent of government insurance coverage for services, supplementary insurance plans, the referral system to auxiliary health, and social facilities and services in the community (c) about the individual's own diagnosis and specific treatment program including prescribed surgery and medication, options, effects, and side effects (d) about the specific costs of procedures, services, and professional fees undertaken on behalf of the individual consumer (e) about the policies and procedures of the health care facility or program
2. Right to be respected as the individual with a major responsibility for his or her own health care.	(a) right that confidentiality of his or her own health records be maintained (b) right to refuse experimentation or undue painful prolongation of his or her life, and restrict participation in teaching programs (c) right of adult to refuse treatment; right to die with dignity (d) right to considerate and respectful care
3. Right to participate in decision making affecting his or her own health.	(a) through consumer representation at each level of government in planning and evaluating the system of health services, the types and qualities of service, and the conditions under which health services are delivered (b) with the health professionals and personnel involved in his or her direct health care
4. Right to equal access to health care regardless of the individual's economic status, sex, age, creed, ethnic origin, and location.	(a) right to access to adequately qualified health personnel (b) right to a second medical opinion (c) right to prompt response in emergencies (d) right to expect continuity of care

From *Policy Statement on Consumers and Health Care,* by Consumers' Association of Canada, 1972, 1989, Ottawa, ON: Author. The complete *Policy Statement on Consumers and Health Care* is available at the Consumers' Association Web site at *www.consumer.ca*

safety and absence of discrimination. Workplace hazards for which workers need protection include exposure to infectious organisms, noise, radiation, back injury, burnout, toxic fumes, and injury. Nurses should assure workers that employee health records are kept confidential.

Settings for Health Care Delivery

Although service organization and delivery varies across Canada, the types of agencies delivering those services are comparable. There are institutional agencies; formal community agencies; agencies that cover hospitals, homes and communities; and agencies run by volunteers or the private sector.

Institutional Sector

This sector includes hospitals, long-term care facilities, psychiatric facilities, and rehabilitation centres. All offer health care services to **inpatients** (clients who stay at an institution for diagnosis, treatment, or rehabilitation). Most also offer services to **outpatients** (clients who visit an institution for these services).

Hospitals. Hospitals have traditionally been major health care agencies. Publicly funded acute care hospitals are the most common site of health employment in Canada. **Acute care** is health care delivered for a short time (usually days to weeks) that diagnoses and/or treats an immediate health problem. An acute illness appears suddenly and lasts a short time, typically less than 3 months. Most hospitals specialize in acute care.

Hospital services vary and may include emergency and diagnostic services, general inpatient services, surgical intervention, intensive care units, outpatient services, and rehabilitation facilities. The goal of hospitals is to provide the highest quality of care possible so that clients can be discharged early but safely to the home or to a facility that can adequately manage remaining health care needs.

There are five types of hospitals: community hospitals, regional or general hospitals, teaching hospitals, university health science centres, and specialized hospital treatment centres. These hospitals are distinguished by their size, the types of service provided, and their connection to academic institutions. Hospitals are public or private. Public hospitals are financed and operated by a government agency at the local, provincial, or national level and provide services at a not-for-profit rate. Private hospitals are owned and operated by groups such as churches, corporations, businesses, and charitable organizations.

Although few in number, military hospitals in Canada provide medical care for members of the military and their families. There are also veterans' hospitals that provide residential and extended care and rehabilitation to aging, injured, and disabled veterans.

Hospital nurses perform a variety of roles. They provide nursing care to clients, including teaching about their conditions and how to care for themselves following discharge. They also coordinate the care provided by members of the health care team. Many nurses specialize, for example, in caring for clients with cancer or cardiac problems. Other hospital roles include nurse manager, clinical nurse specialist, infection control coordinator, clinical educator, and clinical nurse researcher.

Long-Term Care Facilities. A **long-term care (extended care) facility** provides accommodations and 24-hour intermediate and custodial care (e.g., nursing, rehabilitation, dietary, recreational, social, and religious services) for residents of any age with chronic or debilitating illnesses or disabilities. Most residents are frail, older adults with multiple health issues. Some are younger adults with severe, chronic health conditions. A long-term care facility is the resident's temporary or permanent home; therefore, the surroundings should be as homelike as possible. The philosophy of care is to provide a planned, systematic, and interdisciplinary approach that helps residents reach and maintain their highest level of function. In these settings, nurses plan and coordinate resident care, manage chronic illnesses, and conduct rehabilitation programs. Nursing roles for education, management, and family-related interventions abound.

Psychiatric Facilities. Located in hospitals, independent outpatient clinics, or mental health clinics, these facilities offer inpatient and outpatient services. Nurses collaborate with doctors, psychologists, social workers, and therapists to make plans that enable a client to return to the community. At discharge from inpatient facilities, clients are usually referred for follow-up through community-based agencies.

Rehabilitation Centres. A **rehabilitation centre** is a residential institution that provides therapy and training, the goal being to decrease clients' dependence on care. Many centres offer programs that teach the client or family to achieve maximum function after a stroke, head or spinal cord injury, or other impairment. Drug rehabilitation centres help clients withdraw from dependence and return to the community. Nurses in rehabilitation centres collaborate closely with physical and occupational therapists.

Community Sector

Community services are directed at primary and secondary care and should be easily accessible to clients in locations where they live, work, play, and attend school. Outreach programs provide services and locate clients who might not show up at traditional health care centres. Community health care agencies include physicians' offices, clinics, community health centres, home health care agencies, and crisis intervention centres.

Public Health. The public health sector monitors environmental and biological hazards and disease transmission. Nurses are the primary professionals in public health clinics and offer well-baby clinics, school health programs, and screening programs of various types, as well as geriatric surveillance, health promotion, and disease prevention programs. For example, during an outbreak of a communicable disease such as meningitis, the public health system mobilizes to detect cases early and prevent transmission to others, often through mass vaccination and public education. The public health sector also offers a range of services within schools and communities.

Physician Offices. Physician offices offer primary care and tend to focus on the diagnosis and treatment of specific illnesses rather than on health promotion. In this setting, nurses take vital signs, prepare clients for examination, and collaborate with physicians to conduct physical examinations and histories, offer health education, and recommend therapies.

Community Health Centres and Clinics. Staff at these centres plan, manage, and deliver comprehensive services to designated geographic areas or specific at-risk populations. Community health centres typically offer a variety of health and social services, including family medicine, social work, counseling, and health promotion and community development programs. Many are staffed by a multidisciplinary team of professionals working in close association with hospitals and other health and social services. They focus on primary health care and direct their programs and services to the individual, family, group, and community (Wilson, 1995). Primary care services delivered by nurses are different from those delivered by physicians. Nursing stresses education and self-care, not diagnosis and treatment. A nurse-managed clinic helps clients to assume more responsibility for their health. Long-term advanced practice nurses improve client outcomes by enabling clients to remain functional within their homes and communities.

Assisted Living. **Assisted-living facilities** are community-based residential facilities where adults live in their own apartments and are provided with a range of support services, such as meals, social and recreational programs, laundry, housekeeping, transportation, and health checks (Sorrentino, 2004). Facilities range from apartment-like buildings with hundreds of units to small group homes that house three to four residents. Partial funding for assisted living may be provided by medicare.

Home Care. **Home care** is the provision of health care services and equipment to clients and families in their homes. Home care primarily involves nursing care but also includes other professional and non-professional services that clients may need to stay in their homes. Services are offered through the respective health regions by community health nurses and other health professionals employed by a variety of agencies.

Home care was originally created to provide care for people following hospital discharge. However, all levels of care can occur within the home setting (see Levels of Care). Clients include older adults; families with children; people with mental, physical, or developmental disabilities; people with acute or chronic medical conditions; and people in the recovery, rehabilitative, or life-ending stages of disease. Most Canadian cities have large and growing palliative home care programs that are operated separately from the regular home care programs. These palliative care services allow people to have care at home during a terminal illness.

Home care includes a range of professional and support services. Professional services including nursing care; physiotherapy and occupational, respiratory, and speech therapy; nutrition counseling; and social work. Support services are non-medical services and include personal care, assistance with activities of daily living, and assistance with home management.

Adult Daycare Centres. **Adult daycare centres** may be associated with a hospital or long-term care facility or exist as independent centres. Frequently, clients do not require hospitalization but need continuous health care services. These clients include, for example, clients with dementia, older adults needing physical rehabilitation, individuals needing counseling, and individuals with chemical dependency. Nurses in daycare centres provide continuity between the care delivered at home and care delivered in the centre. For instance, nurses can ensure that the client continues to take prescribed medications and can administer specific treatments; the nurse can also assist the client through counselling sessions. Knowledge of community needs and resources is essential in providing adequate support to clients who often spend only a few hours a week in the daycare setting (Ebersole & Hess, 1994).

Community and Voluntary Agencies. National, provincial, and regional **voluntary agencies** meet specific needs. Examples include the Canadian Heart and Stroke Foundation and the Canadian Diabetes Association. Most voluntary agencies do not provide treatment but have programs to prevent and detect specific illnesses. Public education is a major focus. Some voluntary agencies provide financial support for the training of physicians and nurses. Voluntary agencies depend on the help of professional and lay volunteers; financial support is often from fundraising and donations. Canadian examples include the Victorian Order of Nurses, Canadian Red Cross, and Meals on Wheels.

Occupational Health. Occupational health refers to health services offered to clients within their place of work. The primary health professionals are community health nurses with special preparation in workplace health and knowledge of workplace hazards. Large corporations often monitor and assist the health and safety of employees through individual and group health activities. Such services may employ occupational health nurses, physiotherapists, and occupational therapists.

Hospice/Palliative Care. A **hospice** is a family-centred care system that enables a person to live in comfort, with independence and dignity while relieving strains caused by a life-threatening illness. Hospice care is palliative, not curative (see chapter 25). Its multidisciplinary approach involving physicians, nurses, social workers, pharmacists, and pastoral care staff is critical. Hospice nurses work in hospitals, free-standing structures called hospices, or the client's home, caring for the client and family during the terminal phase of illness and at the time of death. They may continue to offer bereavement counselling to the family following the client's death.

Parish Nursing. **Parish nursing** is becoming more popular as faith communities promote and maintain members' health. In some cases, this care fills the gap in public health services; in others, it is a preference or a convenience. Parish and public systems often collaborate to provide interventions that integrate clients' values, faith, beliefs, and practices (Krasnansky, 1999).

Levels of Care

There are five **levels of health care:** promotive, preventive, curative (diagnosis and treatment), rehabilitative, and supportive (including home care, long-term care, and palliative care) (Canadian Nurses Association, [CNA] 2003).

Level 1: Health Promotion

The first level of health care, **health promotion,** includes services and activities designed to improve or maintain health status. Examples include the provision of wellness services, anti-smoking education, promotion of self-esteem in children and adolescents, and advocacy for healthy public policy.

Health promotion takes place in many settings. For example, community clinics offer programs such as prenatal nutrition classes that promote the health of the woman, fetus, and infant. The *Ottawa Charter for Health Promotion* (World Health Organization [WHO], 1986) details five action strategies for health promotion: building healthy public policy, creating supportive environments, strengthening community action, developing personal skills, and reorienting health services. The Ottawa Charter details how health professionals can enable clients to make decisions that affect their health. Further, it states, "The fundamental conditions and resources for health are peace, shelter, food, income, a stable ecosystem, sustainable resources, social justice, and equity." This is the foundation of health promotion (see chapter 1).

Level 2: Disease and Injury Prevention

The second level of health care delivery includes illness prevention services to help clients, families, and communities reduce risk factors for disease and injury (see chapter 4). Prevention strategies include clinical (screening, immunizing), behavioural (lifestyle change, support groups), or environmental (societal pressure for a healthy environment; see chapter 1).

Level 3: Diagnosis and Treatment

The focus of diagnosis and treatment is on recognizing and treating clients' existing health problems. These are the most used services of the health care delivery system. Within this level of care are three sublevels: primary, secondary, and tertiary care. These typically refer to health care activities aimed at individuals, rather than families or communities.

- **Primary care** is the first contact a client makes with the health care system that leads to a decision regarding a course of action to resolve any actual or potential health problem. The providers of primary care are often physicians and nurse practitioners. Settings for primary care include physicians' offices, nurse-managed clinics, schools, and occupational settings. The focus is on early detection and routine care, with emphasis on education to prevent recurrences. (Do not confuse primary care with **primary health care;** they are different concepts. Primary health care focuses on the community and population health and uses a particular philosophy of service delivery that is founded upon social justice and equity as described in the WHO [1978] Alma Ata Declaration.) See Primary Health Care.

- **Secondary care** involves provision of a specialized medical service by a physician specialist or a hospital on referral from a primary care practitioner. A client has developed recognizable signs and symptoms that are either definitively diagnosed or require further diagnostic review. Secondary settings include hospitals and the home.
- **Tertiary care** is specialized and highly technical care in diagnosing and treating complicated or unusual health problems. Clients who require tertiary care present with an extensive, often complicated, pathological condition. Tertiary settings are usually regional hospitals or provincial health science centres that house sophisticated diagnostic equipment and perform complex therapeutic procedures that require advanced expertise by medical and nursing specialists.

Level 4: Rehabilitation

Rehabilitation is the restoration of a person to the fullest physical, mental, social, and vocational functioning possible (Clemen-Stone, McGuire, & Eigsti, 1998). Clients require rehabilitation after a physical or mental illness, injury, or chemical addiction. Initially, rehabilitation may focus on preventing complications from the illness or injury. As a condition stabilizes, rehabilitation is necessary until clients return to their previous level of function or they reach a new level of function limited by their illness or disease. The goal is to assist a client in regaining maximal functional status, thereby enhancing quality of life while promoting independence and self-care.

Rehabilitation services include physiotherapy, occupational and speech therapy, and social services. Ideally, rehabilitation begins the moment a client enters a health care setting for treatment. For example, some orthopaedic programs now have clients undergo physiotherapy exercises before major joint repair so as to enhance their recovery. With the emphasis on early discharge from hospitals, most clients require some level of rehabilitative care. Rehabilitation occurs in many health care settings, including rehabilitation institutions, outpatient settings, and the home.

Level 5: Supportive Care

Clients of all ages with chronic (i.e., long-term) or progressive (i.e., worsens over time) illnesses or disabilities may require supportive care. Supportive care describes a collection of health, personal, and social services provided over a prolonged period to people who are disabled, who never were functioning independently, or who have a terminal disease. The need for supportive health care services is growing. People are living longer, and many of those with chronic health care needs have no immediate family members to care for them. Supportive care is available within institutional settings (e.g., long-term care facilities, assisted-living settings), communities (e.g., adult day care centres), or the home (e.g., home care, home-delivered meals; Lueckenotte, 2000).

Palliative care is part of supportive care. Palliative care is services for people living with progressive, life-threatening illnesses or conditions. It aims to reduce discomfort but not produce a cure. Palliate means to soothe or relieve. The goal of palliative care is to meet the physical, emotional, social, and spiritual needs of the client and family. Palliative care can be provided in hospitals, hospices, or homes.

Respite care is another component of supportive care. Respite care is a service that provides short-term relief or time off for family caregivers. Adult day care is one form of respite care. However, respite care can also be provided within the home by health professionals and trained volunteers. The caregiver is able to leave the home for errands or just take a break from caregiving responsibilities.

Health Care Spending

Health care expenditures aim to maintain and improve the health status of Canadians (Federal, Provincial, and Territorial Advisory Committee on Population Health, 1999). Public funds are spent on health services used by individuals, on services that benefit society, and on the administration of the system. Expenditures reflect the volume of use and the costs of health goods and services. Except for a few years in the mid-1990s, when health budgets were cut to fight mounting deficits, spending has increased dramatically, particularly in the last 7 years. In September 2004, the federal government committed to providing an extra $41.2 billion in extra federal funding to the health care system over the next 10 years.

Total Health Care Expenditures

In 2003, Canada's total health expenditures were predicted to be $121.4 billion (Conference Board of Canada, 2004). Hospitals and other institutions account for the largest share of total expenditures (39.4%), followed by drugs (16.2%) and remuneration for physicians (12.9%). This total health care expenditure represents an average of $3,839 per capita (i.e., per person) per year. Per capita spending is higher for children and older adults. Although older adults comprise 12.6% of the population, they account for approximately 50% of hospital costs (CIHI, 2004b).

Canada contributes 9.7% of its gross domestic product to health care; comparatively, the United States contributes 13.9%; Sweden 8.7%, and the United Kingdom and Japan 7.6%—all of which have equally good or better population health statistics (Organization for Economic Co-operation and Development, 2004).

A 2004 Conference Board of Canada study compared Canada and 23 Organisation for Economic Co-operation and Development (OECD) industrialized countries. Canada is the third-highest spender on health care and the sixth-highest public spender. Yet, in terms of health status, Canada ranks at number 13. Although Canada's life expectancy and self-reported health ranks at number 5, the country ranks poorly in factors such as the incidence of traffic accidents and obesity, air pollution, and health outcome indicators. The study shows that despite Canada's high and escalating health care expenditures, a corresponding improvement in health care is not evident.

Challenges to the Health Care System

Canada's health care system is faced with many issues and challenges, including the rising costs of care and problems with equality and access.

Cost Accelerators

Cost accelerators include new technology, new pharmaceuticals, an increase in chronic and new diseases, and changing demographics and expectations (CIHI, 2004b). Large salary settlements for health care providers also push up health care costs.

- New technologies are now available such as new-generation antibiotics, diagnostic imaging equipment, and specialized beds or support surfaces. Drugs and technologies are treating diseases and disabilities more successfully than ever. Mortality rates are declining due to effective (and expensive) drugs and treatments However, most new drugs and technologies are very expensive because of high development costs.
- Demographics affect costs. As the population ages, chronic and age-related diseases are increasing, largely because older people are more likely to become ill and disabled. They require more treatment and drugs, resulting in higher costs to the system. Another demographic that has resulted in higher health care costs is maternal age, which has risen steadily in the past 15 years. It costs more to provide prenatal care for an older woman than for a younger woman.
- Canadians are better informed than ever about their health care options. They demand high quality care for their tax dollars. For example, clients might ask a physician to order an expensive diagnostic test such as magnetic resonance imaging (MRI), whereas 15 years ago they would have been satisfied with a simple X-ray.
- Large salary increases for unionized health care providers (including nurses) have increased costs for health care.

Equality and Access

A key principle of the *Canada Health Act* is universality. This means that the Canadian health care system must strive to provide equal care and access to care for all.

Income assistance programs for older adults and welfare recipients cover some health care expenses not covered by medicare, such as optometric, dental, and pharmaceutical care. However, Canadians with low wages may experience unequal access and consequently, lower health status. Lower-income Canadians visit dentists less often than middle- or upper-income Canadians and also are less likely to seek preventive eye care. Although Aboriginal Canadians are fully insured for dental care, they report visiting dentists less often than other Canadians.

Privatization of Services. Governments are struggling to maintain the principle of universality against the benefits and problems of privatization. At present, not all health services are available and accessible to all Canadians. For example, some infertility treatments and laser eye surgeries are private and are, therefore, available to only to those who can pay. Discussions continue about what constitutes "medically necessary services" and what core services should be available and accessible to everyone. Many experts contend that medicare can only be saved by privatizing more parts of the system.

Shortages of Health Care Professionals. Accessibility is compromised by shortages of physicians, nurses, and technicians, particularly in rural areas, but increasingly in cities as well. People are waiting months for treatment or travelling to other cities for procedures that they once could have had in their hometowns. Waiting times in Canada are among the highest in OECD countries (Conference Board of Canada, 2004).

Health services are scarce resources in Canada. The shortage of family physicians and nurses is impacting health care services at all levels. Two studies by the CNA (1997, 2002) have confirmed that the shortage is projected to continue. Factors contributing to the shortage include a sharp decline in nursing graduates in the 1990s, the trend toward entry to practice at a later age, insufficient capacity in nursing education programs, a large percentage of nurses retiring in the next two decades, and the aging population creating a greater demand for nursing services (CNA, 2002).

Trends and Reforms in Canada's Health Care System

Health care in Canada has been undergoing restructuring and reform since the early 1980s. The Canadian health care system has been scrutinized and compared with other systems. One of the main reforms has been the shift to community care from acute and institutional care (Attenborough, 1997).

Numerous recent federally and provincially sponsored reports have made recommendations for reforming the system. Two influential national reports on Canada's health care system include the Kirby Report (*The Health of Canadians,* 2002) and the Romanow Commission (2002; Box 2-3).

There is a new urgency to health care reform because many experts claim that our current rate of health care expenditures is unsustainable. Studies show that that the aging population and the rising costs associated with it will result in total health care spending jumping from $89.5 billion in 2000 to $243.8 billion in 2020 (Conference Board of Canada, 2001). When these fig-

Box 2-3 Influential Health Care Reports

The Romanow Commission

Romanow concluded that medicare is sustainable and must be preserved because it represents the core values of Canadians. His top priority was to modernize the *Canada Health Act* by providing funds and making specific recommendations in these key areas:

- Creating a new diagnostic service fund
- Building information technology infrastructure
- Improving access (i.e., for rural and remote areas and Aboriginal peoples)
- Ensuring and measuring quality
- Improving and expanding primary health care
- Strengthening and expanding home care
- Offering catastrophic drug coverage

Romanow did not attach a specific cost to any of his recommendations, but he did stress accountability for funding and services provided. He promoted the concept of a National Health Council with wide responsibility for indicators, benchmarks, and performance measurement.

The Kirby Report

Kirby concluded that the present medicare system is not sustainable. He believed that the private sector should have a stronger role in health care delivery. He pointed out the impact of spiralling health care costs on other social programs. He did not address the core values underlying the health care system or recommend changes to the *Canada Health Act.* He identified as priorities the need for:

- Moving funding for hospitals to a service-based model
- Granting more responsibility to regional health authorities for delivering and/or contracting out publicly insured health services
- Reforming primary health care
- Offering a health care guarantee to Canadians (e.g., a time limit for wait times; if the wait time is exceeded, the government will pay for care done elsewhere)

Like Romanow, Kirby emphasized the importance of accountability for services and funding. Instead of a National Health Council (as recommended by Romanow), he suggested an appointed council of fewer members with limited advisory functions.

Sources: *Building on Values: The Future of Health Care in Canada—Final Report,* by R. Romanow, Commissioner, 2002, Ottawa, ON: Commission on the Future of Health Care in Canada; and *The Health of Canadians—The Federal Role,* by M. Kirby, 2002, Ottawa, ON, available from *http://www.parl.gc.ca/37/2/parlbus/commbus/senate/com-e/soci-e/rep-e/repoct02vol6-e.htm*

ures are adjusted for inflation, spending goes from $80.7 billion in 2000 to $147 billion in 2020. In other words, it almost doubles. The proportion of provincial and territorial revenues devoted to health will grow from about 32% in 2001 to 44% in 2020 (Conference Board of Canada, 2001, 2004).

Because health care costs are rising faster than government revenues, some Canadians and decision makers believe that spending on health care will eventually crowd out spending on other programs in the social safety net and will consume 100% of all monies (MacKinnon, 2004). This will create a huge social problem. If health care spending absorbs all available monies, what will happen to programs such as education, social services, transportation safety, and environmental protection, all of which have a profound impact on health?

Many recommendations have been put forth. The next section explores two key recommendations that have been made to improve our health care system.

Primary Health Care

According to the CNA, primary health care (PHC) is a philosophy and a model for improving health that focuses on promoting health and preventing illness. Although treating existing illness is part of PHC, attention is primarily on aspects of peoples' lives that make them sick (CNA, 2002). PHC addresses issues such as diet, lifestyle choices, income, housing, education, relationships, and environmental toxins.

The CNA has been actively promoting PHC in Canada and around the world since the early 1980s, shortly after the publication of the World Health Organization's 1978 document Alma-Ata Declaration: Health for All by Year 2000. Based on a philosophy of social justice and equality, this document called for countries to provide essential health services to everyone. Services included health education, adequate food, safe water and adequate sanitation, maternal and child health care, and immunization. There was an emphasis on the prevention and control of endemic diseases, appropriate treatment of common diseases and injuries, and provision of essential drugs.

PHC has been the focus of almost all Canadian health reports of the last 15 years and has been cited as the key to reform and sustainability. Speaking at the CNA convention in June 2002, Roy Romanow stated, "Primary health care is the single most important basis from which to renew the health care system" (CNA, 2002).

PHC is committed to promoting essential health care services (promotive, preventive, curative, rehabilitative, and supportive), with a strong emphasis on the principles of health promotion and disease prevention.

PHC builds interventions that lead to improved health outcomes for an entire population (Shoultz & Hatcher, 1997). The PHC model (Figure 2–2) focuses on collaboration among health professionals, community members, and others working in multiple sectors, emphasizing health promotion, development of health policies, and prevention of diseases for all individuals. A closer look at each sector shows that they are all linked and that events within each sector have an impact, either positive or negative, on each other and on the outcome of the popula-

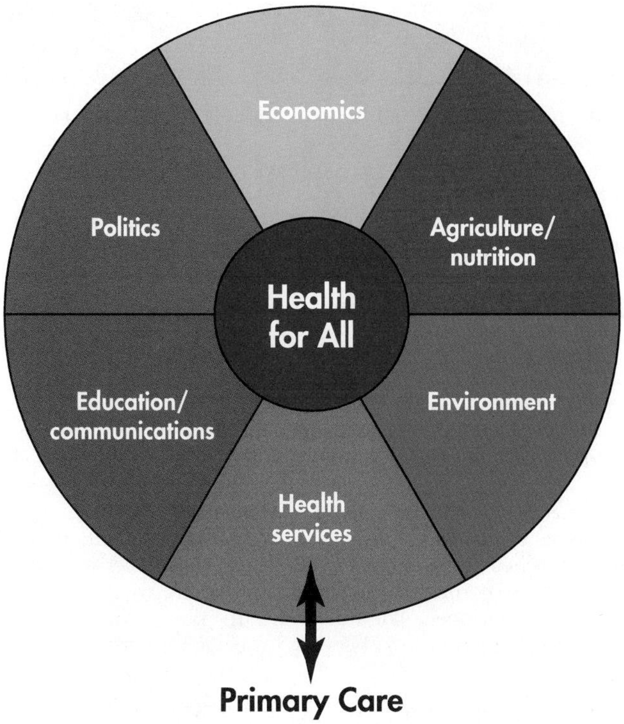

FIGURE 2–2 Primary health care model: A multi-sectoral or intersectoral approach. (From "Looking beyond primary health care: an approach to community-based action," by P. Hatcher, J. Shoultz, and W. Patrick, 1996, *Nursing Outlook, 45,* p. 24.)

tion's health (Hatcher, Patrick, & Shoultz, 1994). For example, the health problems that commonly affect members of a lower socio-economic level can often be traced to poor community services (e.g., water treatment, waste disposal, air quality, and transportation services). A PHC approach requires a multi-sectoral approach by addressing many of the determinants of health (Shoultz & Hatcher, 1997).

PHC is usually associated with the following five principles, all of which emphasize prevention and promotion, as well as investment in sustainability (CNA, 2003):

- Public participation
- Health promotion and disease prevention
- Use of appropriate skills and technology
- Accessibility (an equal distribution of care)
- Intersectoral collaboration (e.g., the integration of health, social services, and education; links between hospitals and community services)

Throughout this book, Focus on Primary Health Care boxes highlight the vital role nurses play in providing primary health care. Box 2-4 links real health care situations to PHC principles.

Many Canadians do not understand the concept of primary health care. They confuse it with related approaches to health care such as primary care, health promotion, and population health. Even health care leaders and providers use the term *primary health care* to mean different things. For many people, the distinction between primary health care and primary care is difficult to understand. Access to primary care is a key element of primary health care, but it is only one component. Primary care focuses on personal health services, whereas primary health care looks beyond primary care, with essential elements that include health education, proper nutrition, maternal/child health care, family planning, immunizations, and control of locally endemic diseases.

Even those Canadians who understand primary health care may not support it. Members of the public think of health care as an "illness based system that will be there when they need it" (CNA, 2003). Money spent on the primary health care priorities of promotion and prevention may not appear to benefit them. Some professionals do not support a primary health care model, which requires interdisciplinary collaboration and flexible boundaries between health care professions.

PHC is a sensible approach to health care that is cost-effective and benefits those most in need. It offers vulnerable people the chance for a healthy life. For example, by attending a community health program on infant and child care, parents will learn the importance of recognizing signs and symptoms of urinary tract infection (UTI) in children and understand that they must seek medical treatment if they suspect their child has a UTI. With this knowledge, parents may prevent long-term serious complications of untreated UTIs, such as kidney damage. This will save the child and family distress and will ultimately significantly reduce health care costs.

In a restructured health system that emphasizes primary health care, programs will cross sectors. For example, trauma programs will have health promotion activities (bicycle helmets, road safety education), preventive programming (helmet legislation), secondary and tertiary care (emergency transportation and care for accident-related trauma), and rehabilitation (head injury recovery programs). Programs may cover multiple sites, may be defined by a particular disease or population group (e.g., children), and will comprise multiple disciplines and sectors of society (e.g., health, education, justice systems). Nursing will have a significant role in every aspect of a PHC integrated program.

Because of its integrated approach, primary health care may hold the key to our looming health care crisis. If Canadians stay healthier because more money is spent on primary health care, they will need less medical care and the proportion of money going to medical care will decline. If health care, education, social services, and the voluntary sector have integrated programs, competition among the various sectors for government monies may decline. This integration requires all sectors to think beyond its own boundaries (Box 2-5).

Home Care

Canadian health care is shifting from an institutional-based system to one in which community care is playing a greater role (see chapter 4). Home care is an increasingly important part of community health care. According to the Romanow Commission, it is one of the fastest growing components of the health care system (2002). Services that used to be provided exclusively in hospitals, doctors' offices, clinics, or long-term

Box 2-4 Focus on Primary Health Care

The Five Principles of Primary Health Care

The five principles of primary health care (PHC) are health promotion and disease prevention, accessibility, intersectoral collaboration, public participation, and use of appropriate skills and technology.

Accessibility

In most large Canadian cities, teams of nurses, physicians, social workers, counsellors, nutritionists, and other professionals bring primary health care to the streets. They seek out street people to assess and monitor their health. Many of these people are in poor health, with inadequate shelter, poor hygiene, poor diet, and lack of support. Many are addicted to drugs or alcohol. Diseases such as HIV/AIDS and hepatitis C are common. Most street people are not comfortable seeking out or accessing care, so they stay away from doctor's offices or hospitals. Nurses on "street teams" care for individuals who are in need; they also address the needs of entire populations. For example, a nurse cares for a 17-year-old prostitute who is 8 months pregnant and addicted to crack. The nurse also runs a community program called "Having Healthy Babies" for young, vulnerable women.

Intersectoral Collaboration

A PHC model at work can be seen at the Northeast Community Health Centre (NCHC) in Edmonton. Located on a major bus route close to schools, the centre addresses the health care needs of new immigrants, older adults, women, adolescents, and children. Intersectoral collaboration is thriving at the centre, which provides a full range of services, including health promotion, chronic disease management, emergency services, laboratory services, and diagnostic imaging. The staff include nutritionists, audiologists, social workers, public health nurses, emergency nurses, nurse practitioners, cultural workers, and physicians. A community advisory committee provides direction for the centre by planning services.

Public Participation

An innovative model of PHC delivery is taking place in James Bay, British Columbia, a small community of largely low-income, single-parent families and older adults. Public participation is vital to the success of the James Bay Community Project (JBCP); it features a volunteer program (with 200 volunteers), a youth clinic that does outreach for youths at risk, a women's clinic, and a men's health project. JBCP is known for its integrated multidisciplinary practice, particularly the blend of nursing and physician services and health care and social services.

Health Promotion

A public health nurse in southern Ontario was running an educational program for low-income mothers about nutrition, child development, and community action. The group shared their ideas about how to meet their family's nutritional requirements on tight budgets. They were alarmed to learn that a national bakery was closing its local day-old bread outlet. The nurse coached the women to call a local newspaper reporter, who, in turn, contacted the bakery's president, who agreed to keep the outlet open. The nurse's health promotion activities resulted in a decision that benefited the community.

Appropriate Skills and Technology

The skills of nurse, nurse practitioners, emergency nurses, and other health care professionals can be put to excellent use in collaborative PHC settings. Both the NCHC and JBCP make appropriate use of all staff skills to provide health care to their respective communities.

These centres are also making excellent use of technology to improve communication and health care. For example, the Edmonton NCHC has an integrated information system that enables the various professionals to share files and information.

An appropriate technology is the telephone triage systems **(telehealth)** now used in many provinces and territories. Individuals may dial a toll free number and are immediately connected to a qualified nurse who can answer their health questions. These systems have been a success. For example, the nurses in the New Brunswick program have been able to respond to the questions and concerns of almost 75% of callers. This technology has provided better access to health care for many Canadians, particularly for those in rural and remote areas.

Source: Canadian Nurses Association (2003, September). Primary Health Care—the time has come. *Nursing Now, 16,* 1–4.

care facilities now can be provided in people's homes. Clients are now sent home sooner after hospital procedures. Despite the spending increases, home care accounts for only 2% to 6% of provincial health budgets (Health Canada, 1999).

Home care is not considered medically necessary and therefore is not covered under the *Canada Health Act.* Every province and territory has a publicly funded home care program, but the services offered and how they are delivered vary widely across the county. All provinces and territories fund assessment and case management, nursing care, and support services for eligible clients. Clients may pay for extra professional or support services through insurance or out of pocket.

The CNA advocates for an effective and equitable home care system (1998), and calls for:

- Accessible, publicly funded and publicly administered home care services coast to coast
- The application of the *Canada Health Act* principles to home care programs
- The rooting of a national initiative in the principles of PHC
- The granting of priority status to the needs of family caregivers
- The integration of a health care provider human resource plan

In his commission, Roy Romanow recommends making home care an essential service for post-acute clients,

Case Study — Box 2-5

Primary Health Care

During a community meeting in a core area of a small city, parents, educators, health care providers, and volunteers agreed to pilot an integrated program to prevent obesity in children. Social services and volunteers run a breakfast program, fruits and vegetables for twice-daily snacks are donated by a local grocery store, and nutritionists and kinesiologists educate the teachers and help them to integrate nutrition and physical fitness into the curriculum. The schools commit to having students and teachers walk outside for at least 15 minutes every day and establish rules for school lunches (e.g., children are not allowed to bring pop). Nurse practitioners set up visits with the parents of children identified as being overweight or at risk. A follow-up high school program is being developed for the children who remain overweight or at risk. If only 10% of the children in the program develop a healthier lifestyle, the savings to the health care system in future years would pay for the cost of the program.

palliative care clients, and mentally ill clients. If these recommendations were implemented, home care for some would become a publicly funded health care right, just like a hospital stay or a doctor's visit.

Romanow points out two main reasons to increase funding for home care:

- People will maintain their independence and their health for longer.
- The program would be cost-effective. A national home care study found that home care and home support save money be preventing accidents and keeping people out of expensive acute care beds (Hollander & Chappell, 2001).

Some believe that Romanow's recommendations for home care do not go far enough. The focus for change is on short-term care but leaves out the ongoing care needs of the frail and elderly, people with disabilities, those with chronic mental health problems, and families with children with special needs. Many of these individuals do not require expensive nursing care, but rather need support services that enable them to function independently (Hollander, 2002). Studies have shown that public home care and other community services provided to frail older adults cost less than institutional care (Hébert et al., 2001; Hollander & Chappell, 2001).

The Role of Nurses in Health Care Reform

Nurses play a key role in health care reform, both as leaders at the political and community level and in their everyday work life. To keep health care reforms front and centre as nurses practise, they need to stay current with the issues and debates of the day. Plans for the future should not be left only to nurse administers and nursing associations. Every nurse should read the Romanow and Kirby Reports and understand the concepts discussed in them.

Key Concepts

- Medicare is a key part of Canada's social safety net.
- Government plays a major role in the Canadian health care system by funding national health insurance and by setting health care policy according to the principles of the *Canada Health Act (1984).*
- The *Canada Health Act* outlaws extra billing and user fees and upholds health care delivery must be universal, portable, comprehensive, accessible, and publicly administered.
- Health care services are provided in a variety of institutional and community settings, across all age groups, and for individual, family, group, community, and population clients.
- There are five levels of health care: promotive, preventive, curative, rehabilitative, and supportive.
- Escalating costs are driving health care reform efforts, challenging health care institutions to deliver care more efficiently without sacrificing quality.
- Issues of equality, access, and continuity of care also challenge the health care system.
- To achieve continuity of care when a client is discharged from a hospital, the staff nurse must anticipate and identify the client's continuing needs and then work with all members of the multidisciplinary team to develop a plan that transfers the client's care from the hospital to another environment.
- The rise of primary health care and home care is a result of reforms to the health care system.
- Successful health promotion and disease prevention programs, such as those found in community health centres, schools, and community clinics, are designed to help clients acquire healthier lifestyles and achieve a decent standard of living.
- Home care is one of the fastest growing components of the health care system, partly because clients are sent home from hospital sooner.

Key Terms

Accessibility, *p. 22*
Acute care, *p. 23*
Adult daycare centres, *p. 25*
Assisted-living facilities, *p. 24*
Comprehensiveness, *p. 22*
Extended care facility, *p. 24*
Health promotion, *p. 25*
Home care, *p. 24*
Hospice, *p. 25*
Inpatients, *p. 23*
Levels of health care, *p. 25*
Long-Term care facility, *p. 24*
Medicare, *p. 20*
Outpatients, *p. 23*
Palliative care, *p. 26*
Parish nursing, *p. 25*
Portability, *p. 22*
Primary care, *p. 25*
Primary health care, *p. 26*
Public administration, *p. 22*
Quality improvement, *p. 31*
Rehabilitation, *p. 26*
Rehabilitation centre, *p. 24*
Respite care, *p. 26*
Secondary care, *p. 26*
Social safety net, *p. 20*
Telehealth, *p. 30*
Tertiary care, *p. 26*
Universality, *p. 22*
Voluntary agencies, *p. 25*

Critical Thinking Exercises

1. Debate the following issues in relation to the future of the Canadian health care system: escalating costs, privatization, continuity of care, accessibility.
2. Consider and describe how the national economy, changes in the population, and technology have changed the Canadian health care system. Identify what implications these changes have for nursing practice.
3. Consider Mr. Wilson, a 68-year-old client who will have major surgery to replace the joint in his hip. Afterward, extensive therapy will be needed for him to walk normally again. Describe the type of health care services that might become involved in his care.

Review Questions

1. Canada contributes 9.7% of its gross domestic product (GDP) to health care. Which one of the following countries contributes a greater percentage of their GDP to their health care system?
   1. The United Kingdom
   2. The United States
   3. Japan
   4. Sweden
2. Canada's social safety net does NOT include
   1. Legal aid
   2. Medicare
   3. Family allowance
   4. Welfare
3. The first universal social program in Canada was
   1. Medicare
   2. Canada Pension Plan
   3. Family Allowance
   4. War Widows' Assistance
4. The *Canada Health Act (1984)* has the following five principles
   1. Public administration, comprehensiveness, universality, portability, accessibility
   2. Social justice, equity, acceptability, efficiency, effectiveness
   3. Accountability, equality, economy, collaboration, coordination
   4. Insured health services, compensation for providers, hospital services, community care, and prescription drugs
5. An adult daycare centre is an example of a(n)
   1. Home care organization
   2. Institutional agency
   3. Community agency
   4. Ambulatory care centre
6. What are the five levels of health care services?
   1. Promotive, preventive, curative, rehabilitative, supportive
   2. Prevention, protection, diagnosis, treatment, palliative care
   3. Promotion, prevention, treatment, primary health care, diagnosis
   4. Assessment, diagnosis, planning, implementation, evaluation
7. The largest share of health expenditures go to
   1. Prescription drugs
   2. Home care
   3. Physicians
   4. Hospitals
8. Which is NOT a cause of Canada's increasing health care costs?
   1. Workplace injuries
   2. The aging of the population
   3. New technologies and drugs
   4. An increase in chronic and new diseases
9. A nurse organizes a blood pressure screening program. This is an example of which health care service?
   1. Health promotion
   2. Illness prevention
   3. Continuing care
   4. Rehabilitation
10. The provision of specialized medical services by a physician specialist or a hospital is known as
    1. Primary care
    2. Primary health care
    3. Secondary care
    4. Tertiary care

References

Attenborough, R. (1997). The Canadian health care system: Development, reform and opportunities for nurses. *Journal of Obstetric, Gynecologic, and Neonatal Nursing, 26*(2), 229–234.

Canadian Institute for Health Information. (2003a). *Workforce trends of licensed practical nurses in Canada, 2002.* Ottawa, ON: Author. Available from LPN database.

Canadian Institute for Health Information. (2003b). *Workforce trends of registered nurses in Canada, 2002.* Ottawa, ON: Author. Available from LPN database.

Canadian Institute for Health Information. (2004a). *Health personnel trends in Canada, 1993–2002* (pp. 190–201). Ottawa, ON: Author.

Canadian Institute for Health Information. (2004b). *Health spending in Canada, 1993–2003.* Ottawa, ON: Author.

Canadian Nurses Association. (1997, January). Out in Front—Advanced Nursing Practice. *Nursing Now, 2,* 1–4.

Canadian Nurses Association. (2002). *Planning for the future: Nursing human resource projections.* Ottawa, ON: Author.

Canadian Nurses Association. (2003, September). Primary health care—The time has come. *Nursing Now, 16,* 1–4.

Clemen-Stone, S., McGuire, S. L., & Eigsti, D. G. (1998). *Comprehensive community health nursing* (5th ed.). St. Louis, MO: Mosby.

Conference Board of Canada. (2001). *The future cost of health care in Canada, 2000 to 2020: Balancing affordability and sustainability.* Ottawa ON: Author.

Conference Board of Canada. (2004). *Understanding health care cost drivers and escalators.* Ottawa ON: Author.

Consumers' Association of Canada. (1972, 1989). *Policy statement on consumers and health care.* Ottawa, ON: Author.

Ebersole, P., & Hess, P. (1994). *Toward healthy aging: Human needs and nursing response* (4th ed.). St. Louis, MO: Mosby.

Federal, Provincial, and Territorial Advisory Committee on Population Health. (1999). *Toward a healthy future. Second report on the health of Canadians.* Ottawa, ON: Author.

Gibbon, J., & Mathewson, M. (1947). *Three centuries of Canadian nursing*. Toronto, ON: Macmillan.

Hatcher, P. A., Patrick, W., & Shoultz, J.. (1994). Impacts: A primary health care game to develop global health consciousness. *Journal of Family and Community Health, 17*(2):74–77.

Health Canada. (1992). *Canada Health Act annual report.* Ottawa, ON: Author.

Health Canada. (2004). *Canada's health care system.* Retrieved October 4, 2004, from: *http://www.hc-sc.gc.ca/english/care/index.html*

Hébert, R., et al. (2001). Resources and costs associated with disabilities of elderly people living at home and in institutions. *Canadian Journal on Aging, 20*(1), 1–22.

Hollander, M. J. (2002). *Unfinished business: The case for chronic home care services: A policy paper.* Victoria, BC: Hollander Analytical Services, Ltd..

Hollander, M. J., & Chappell, N. L. (2001). *Final report of the study on the comparative cost analysis of home care and residential care services.* Victoria, BC: National Evaluation of the Cost-Effectiveness of Home Care.

Kirby, M. (Chair). (2002). *The health of Canadians—The federal role.* Ottawa: Standing Senate Committee on Social Affairs, Science and Technology.

Krasnansky, S. (1999, Spring). Parish nursing—Who are parish nurses? APHA Section Newsletter: *Public Health Nursing,* 4, 1999.

Lueckenotte, A. (2000). *Gerontologic nursing* (2nd ed.). St. Louis, MO: Mosby.

MacKinnon, J. (2004). *The arithmetic of health care.* CMAJ. 2004 September 14; 171(6): 603–604.

McGuire, S. R. (1982). *Marguerite d'Youville: A pioneer for our times.* Ottawa, ON: Novalis.

Mitchell, E. (1958). *Marguerite d'Youville.* Montreal, QC: Palm.

Organisation for Economic Co-operation and Development. (2004). *OECD Health Data 2003: A comparative analysis of 30 countries.* France: Author. Retrieved May 31, 2004, from *http://www.oecd.org/dataoecd/10/20/2789777.pdf*

Romanow, R. J. (2002). *Building on values: The future of health care in Canada—Final report.* Ottawa, ON: Commission on the Future of Health Care in Canada.

Shoultz, J., & Hatcher, P. A. (1997). Looking beyond primary care to primary health care: An approach to community-based action. *Nursing Outlook, 45*(1), 23–26.

Sorrentino, S.A. (2004). *Mosby's Canadian textbook for the support worker.* Toronto: Elsevier Canada.

Sutherland, R. W., & Fulton, M. J. (1992). *Health care in Canada.* Ottawa, ON: The Health Group.

Wilson, D. M. (1995). *The Canadian health care system.* Edmonton, AB: Health Canada.

World Health Organization. (1978). *Alma-Ata Declaration: Health for all by year 2000.* Geneva, Switzerland: Author.

World Health Organization. (1986). *The Ottawa Charter for health promotion.* Geneva, Switzerland: Author.

Recommended Web Sites

Canadian Institute of Health Information:
http://www.cihi.ca

The Canadian Institute of Health Information (CIHI) is a not-for-profit organization that seeks to improve the health of Canadians and the health care system by providing health information.

Canadian Public Health Association:
http://www.cpha.ca

The Canadian Public Health Association (CPHA) is a national, not-for-profit association representing public health in Canada with links to the international public health community.

Commission on the Future of Health Care in Canada:
http://www.hc-sc.gc.ca/english/care/romanow/index1.html

This Health Canada Web site provides an overview of the Romanow Commission and access to the 2002 Commission report.

Health Canada:
http://www.hc-sc.gc.ca

This Government of Canada Web site provides numerous links to information about the Canadian health care system, including links to the *Canada Health Act* and other legislation, federal reports, and related publications.

3

The Development of Nursing Practice in Canada

Janet C. Ross-Kerr, RN, BScN, MS, PhD (Canadian author)

Objectives

Mastery of content in this chapter will enable the student to:

- Define the key terms listed.
- Discuss the historical development of professional nursing.
- Discuss the historical development of nursing education in Canada.
- Describe educational programs available for professional nurses.
- List the roles and career opportunities for nurses.
- Discuss the role of nursing organizations and practice acts.
- Describe trends affecting nurses' roles and responsibilities.

Over the centuries, the goals of nursing have been to help people maintain their health and to provide comfort and care to the sick. Modern nursing is a professional discipline with a unique body of knowledge applied to the needs of individuals and families. The foundations of professional practice emerge from historical and philosophical traditions in nursing and health, social policy and practice, and ongoing research in nursing. It is interesting to explore the origins of nursing, as these have contributed in large measure to the knowledge and skills used in practice today. The evolution of nursing has brought the profession to a challenging and exciting time in its history (Box 3-1). There are tremendous opportunities to improve the health and quality of life of clients and communities with advances in professional knowledge and practice.

The philosophical and theoretical basis of the profession provides the necessary foundation for practice (see chapter 5). Virginia Henderson's definition of nursing (1966) was adopted by the **International Council of Nurses (ICN)** in 1973, and it applies well to current nursing:

> The unique function of the nurse is to assist the individual, sick or well, in the performance of those activities contributing to health [and] its recovery, or to a peaceful death that the client would perform unaided if he had the necessary strength, will, or knowledge. And to do this in such a way as to help the client gain independence as rapidly as possible. (p. 15)

As a profession, nursing is committed to public service. The practice of nursing requires specialized knowledge that must be learned and carries a high degree of responsibility. Nursing is practical in nature, motivated by altruism and based on ethical standards.

The profession of nursing evolves as society, health care needs, and social policies change. Nursing responds and adapts to change. This chapter traces the roots of the nursing profession over many centuries to its establishment and development in Canada. Although there has been a dramatic increase in the nature and extent of knowledge and skills required for nursing, the professional mandate has remained relatively constant over time and continues to be an inspiring force for the profession. The transformation of the profession to the modern era is highlighted.

Box 3-1 Milestones in Nursing History

1639	Three nuns from France establish the Hôtel Dieu at Quebec.
1641	Jeanne Mance arrives at Quebec with Maisonneuve and his men to found a settlement at Montreal.
1642	After overwintering at Quebec, they establish Ville Marie on the Island of Montreal, where Jeanne Mance cares for the sick and founds the Hôtel-Dieu.
1737	The Grey Nuns or Sisters of Charity of Montreal is formed by Marguerite d'Youville as the first non-cloistered order of nuns in New France; they visit the sick in their homes.
1855	Florence Nightingale takes command of nursing sick and wounded British soldiers during the Crimean War.
1859	Nightingale's *Notes on Nursing: What It Is and What It Is Not* is published.
1896	The Nurses' Associated Alumni of the United States and Canada is formed with Isabel Hampton as its first president.
1897	The Victorian Order of Nurses is created under the sponsorship of Lady Aberdeen to undertake visiting nursing.
1902	Sigma Theta Tau, Nursing Honor Society, is established by six student nurses from Indiana University.
1905	The first issue of *The Canadian Nurse* is published with Dr. Helen McMurchy as editor.
1908	The Canadian National Association of Trained Nurses (later changed to the Canadian Nurses Association) is founded with Mary Agnes Snively as president.
1968	*Nursing Papers* is published by McGill University under the editorship of Dr. Moyra Allen; it is subsequently renamed the *Canadian Journal of Nursing Research.*
1971	The first national Nursing Research Conference is held in Ottawa, sponsored by the University of British Columbia School of Nursing and supported by the Department of National Health and Welfare.
1982	The Medical Research Council establishes a working group on Nursing Research and this group recommends the establishment of doctoral programs for nurses in Canada and the need for funds designated specifically for nursing research.
1988	The first Nursing Research development grants are given by the Medical Research Council/National Health Research Development Program joint initiative to five Canadian universities (British Columbia, Alberta, Manitoba, Toronto, Dalhousie).
2000	The federal government commits $2.5 billion in the Canada Health and Social Transfer for health and education.
2005	Province of Ontario adopts the baccalaureate degree as entry to practice.

Highlights of World Nursing History

Nursing's historical roots are deep and honourable and can be traced over many centuries. In the 16th century BC, the ancient Egyptians recognized the importance of preventing illness and maintaining health. They understood that diet was important for maintaining good health, and consumed a reasonably well-balanced diet of fruits, vegetables, fish, milk, legumes, seeds, and oil. Priest-physicians ministered to the people, using herbs to relieve pain and using a variety of treatments based on spiritual/mythological beliefs in the causation of illness. The *Papyrus Ebers* and the *Edwin Smith Papyrus,* discovered in Thebes in 1862, document the Egyptians' knowledge of disease and treatment and have helped us understand how they dealt with health and illness as far back as the old empire (3300–1500 BC).

The theories of health and illness of the ancient Egyptians provided a framework for the development of medicine in ancient Greece. Although the early Greeks believed in the spiritual causes of disease, Hippocrates (circa 460–370 BC) was the first to make observations of patients and develop treatments on the basis of symptoms. He founded a school of medicine on the island of Cos and produced numerous books on disease and illness. Hippocrates is considered the father of scientific medicine and Western medical ethics, developing methods of treating disease and establishing ethical principles upon which practice was based. Through his influence, medicine developed into a science. Galen (AD 130–303), another Greek physician-scientist, made important contributions to physiology through research on animals and wrote a number of books, eventually moving to Rome and becoming physician to the gladiators. Through Galen and other Greek physicians, this knowledge had an influence upon the Romans.

The Romans recognized the importance of fresh water and hygiene for public health. As the cities grew and water supplies became inadequate, Roman engineers developed aqueducts to carry fresh water from distant springs. They also developed public baths and constructed public toilets and sewers, greatly improving the health of the population.

The Hebrews believed in a spiritual basis of illness. They believed that following the Ten Commandments promoted health. They also recognized the importance of nutrition in maintaining health. They developed dietary laws that protected the public by prescribing what foods could or could not be eaten together and guidelines for safely eating the meat of slaughtered animals. Nurses cared for the sick in the home and community and served as midwives during childbirth.

During the early Christian period with its emphasis on love for others, nursing became a caring service undertaken by women. Around AD 400, Fabiola, a well-to-do Christian woman in Rome, offered respite to ill and fatigued pilgrims travelling to the holy land. Later, during the Middle Ages (AD 1100–1300), hospitals were built to provide care for the sick. The Benedictine Order originated with St. Benedict of Nursia in AD 529 and is the oldest of the Catholic nursing orders. The Knights Hospitallers of the Order of St. John of Jerusalem emerged from the Benedictine nursing tradition to become one of a number of religious orders formed during the Crusades (11th to 13th centuries) committed to caring for and defending pilgrims. Hospices were constructed for pilgrims. When the Protestant Reformation took hold in Europe following the Crusades, monasteries were disbanded and the hospitals and other institutions where monks and nuns cared for the sick and weary were closed. When new hospitals were built, untrained and unsuitable individuals were responsible for nursing patients. Conditions deteriorated as lack of sanitation prevailed and disease spread rapidly.

During the 17th century, conditions began to improve as greater emphasis was placed on nursing. St. Vincent de Paul founded The Sisters of Charity in 1633 to care for the sick, poor, and orphaned. Because this was the first non-cloistered order, the nuns went into the community to care for people for the first time. For the most part, women who entered the convents to become nurses came from the upper classes and were well educated. In Germany, Pastor Theodore Fliedner established an Institute of Deaconesses at Kaiserwerth in 1836 in order to prepare women to serve as nurses.

Nineteenth Century and Florence Nightingale

The movement to improve standards of nursing care in the mid-19th century was spearheaded by Florence Nightingale, who is considered the founder of modern nursing. Brought up in a wealthy family, Florence Nightingale railed against the customs of her time that did not allow middle and upper class women to work outside the home: "Why have women passion, intellect, moral activity—these three—and a place in society where no one of the three can be exercised?" (Nightingale, 1872/1979). She was well educated and, against the wishes of her family, sought to prepare herself for nursing by travelling to Kaiserwerth, Germany, where she worked with the German deaconesses under Pastor Fliedner. She later worked in France with nuns in the French nursing orders. Her initial nursing experience was developing the nursing services at Harley Street Hospital in London. She saw an opportunity to introduce nursing to the British army and subsequently was asked to organize a group of nurses to go to the Crimea.

Nightingale and her staff of nurses made every possible attempt to care for the wounded and make them comfortable in ways that would foster their recovery. They were able to achieve dramatic reductions in morbidity and mortality rates, indeed saving thousands of wounded British soldiers, by applying principles of cleanliness and comfort to nursing care. Accounts of Nightingale's work were distributed to the British press by a reporter covering the war. Nightingale's successful nursing care of wounded soldiers soon became widely known and had a remarkable impact on attitudes toward nursing. Nightingale helped to elevate the status of nursing so that it became accepted as a suitable field of work for women outside the home. At the same time, remarkable advances in health care and the rise of hospitals created a need for nurses, and the nursing profession became one of the most significant avenues of work for women in this century. Nursing thus became an instrument of women's emancipation against the prevailing middle-class restrictions on women working outside the home.

Early History of Nursing in Canada

The roots of nursing and health care in North America may be found in the values and ideals of the European settlers in New France. At a time when knowledge of disease was primitive, technology was virtually non-existent, and a few herbal remedies were the only medicines available, the practice of nursing developed as an integral part of the emerging health care system. Nursing care was often the sole weapon in fighting infectious disease. Its importance is underscored in accounts of the devastating epidemics of smallpox, diphtheria, cholera, and other infectious diseases that continually ravaged the population (Ross-Kerr, 2003).

A long-established indigenous society existed in North America prior to the arrival of the first settlers. As early as Columbus' voyage, there were anywhere from 1 to 10 million people living in North America (Reich, 1984). The Native peoples also had health knowledge of their own, including the use of herbal remedies.

The First Nurses and Hospitals in New France

In 1608, Champlain selected Quebec as the site for a colony of settlers to support the growing fur trade. For the next two decades, the first colonists to New France provided their own health care. The first laywoman to provide nursing care in New France was Marie Rollet Hébert. She and her husband Louis Hébert, who was a surgeon-apothecary, emigrated with their three children at the request of Champlain in 1617. Mme Hébert became the first woman to emigrate to the new world from France and cared for Native people and settlers alike. Her husband's apothecary and agricultural skills helped prevent starvation and mitigate illness (Brown, 1966). Although she was a layperson, Mme Hébert extended care to Natives and settlers who were ill just as she would for ill family members, the latter being a customary role for women at the time.

The first nurses to tend the sick in a type of health centre were male attendants at a "sick bay" established at the French garrison in Port Royal in Acadia in 1629 (Gibbon & Mathewson, 1947). The Jesuit priests, who were missionary immigrants to New France, also served as types of nurses. They found that in order to carry out their mission to convert the Natives to Christianity, they had to minister to the sick. Many religious orders and laypersons came to New France voluntarily to assist the Jesuits. Most of the women who came to New France were motivated by Christian ideals of educating Native children and caring for the sick. Although small in number, these women led the young colony's efforts in health care and teaching. They proved remarkably resilient as they battled small pox epidemics and tended to those injured in the Iroquois wars.

The first nursing mission was established in 1639 at Sillery, outside the citadel of Quebec, by three nuns from the Hospitalières de la Miséricorde. As a result of the Iroquois wars, the nuns abandoned this mission in 1644 and opened another mission inside the citadel, where they nursed French settlers. This mission later became known as Hôtel-Dieu, Quebec's first hospital. In 1641, Jeanne Mance came to New France to found a hospital of the yet unsettled region of Ville Marie (later Montreal); Mance and her fellow travellers were not warmly received. Their intentions to care for the sick were viewed with suspicion by the settlers. When she arrived at Ville Marie in 1642, Mance was the only person with health care knowledge in the new settlement. She was a leader in the community and became an inspiration for later generations of nurses (Box 3-2).

A Canadian order of nuns, the Sisters of Charity of Montreal, formed in 1737 by Marguerite d'Youville (see chapter 2), became the first visiting nurses in Canada. They began as a small group of women who pooled their possessions to form a refuge for the poor and needy (Gibbon & Mathewson, 1947). Because some colonists doubted their charitable intentions, the women were called "les soeurs grises," a derogatory term meaning both the "Grey Nuns" and the "tipsy nuns." However, the goodness of their intentions was clear and they were respected for their work. They proudly referred to themselves as the "Grey Nuns" from then on, and were given a charter to take over the General Hospital of Montreal. To meet their hospital expenses, these resourceful women made military garments and tents, started a brewery and a tobacco plant, and operated a freight and cartage business (Ross-Kerr, 2003).

Box 3-2 Milestones in Canadian Nursing History

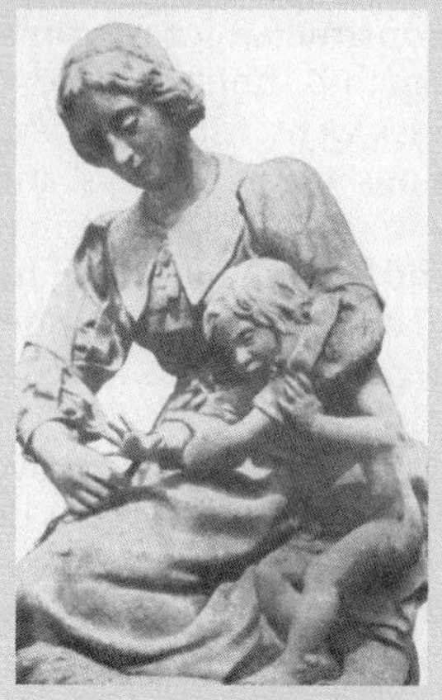

Jeanne Mance, 1606–1673

Born to a wealthy family in France in 1606, Jeanne Mance became known as co-founder of the city of Montreal and Canada's first lay nurse. In 1641, she sailed to New France with Paul de Chomédey, Sieur de Maisonneve, and 40 others. The group was charged with establishing a hospital in what would later become Montreal.

However, arriving in Quebec after a difficult 2-month voyage, the settlers learned that the governor of New France would not support their mission. As winter approached, the party settled in Quebec City. Mance spent the winter learning about nursing and health care in New France from local Augustinian nuns.

In the spring, the settlers travelled to Montreal and began building houses and a hospital named Hôtel-Dieu. The next year, during an attack by the Iroquois, several settlers were killed and others were taken hostage. The remaining settlers, however, were able to finish the hospital and build a stockade around their colony.

By 1649, the settlers' funds were low and the colony was close to disbanding. Mance sailed to Paris to raise money and recruit more settlers. Over the next few years, relations with the Iroquois were poor. A guard was placed at the hospital and Mance slept within the fort, with good reason: In 1650, the Iroquois killed 30 settlers. The French and Iroquois reached a truce in 1654, and Mance was able to move back to her home at the Hôtel-Dieu.

Mance and her nurses worked amid grim conditions. Nevertheless, her Catholic faith sustained her. Although conditions were poor and finances precarious at best, Jeanne Mance succeeded in establishing the first hospital in Montreal. Today, the Canadian Nurses Association awards its highest honour in the name of this courageous pioneer.

Nursing During the British Regime

During the war between the British and the French in 1756, the Grey Nuns designated a ward of the General Hospital of Montreal for the care of English soldiers, thus caring for soldiers on both sides of the conflict. There was a marked contrast between Canada and Britain in the status of nursing and the quality of care provided at this time. Nursing in Britain had fallen into disrepute following Henry VIII's renunciation of the Catholic Church. The nursing orders of nuns, which had previously provided the nursing services in the large London hospitals, were replaced by women of questionable morals and little knowledge. However, nursing remained strong in early Canada because of France's influence, where nursing was more highly regarded.

Infectious diseases carried by immigrants and travellers spread rapidly in the British colonies. The increasing populace and continuing epidemics created a need for more health care facilities. In areas not served by the French-Canadian nursing orders, institutions were established with standards similar to those in Britain at the time (Canadian Nurses Association [CNA], 1968). Laywomen offered their services and organized groups to provide proper care, but because they lacked knowledge and skill, these efforts were largely unsuccessful. The established French-Canadian orders expanded their services and new English-speaking orders were founded to help the sick and the poor.

Opening of the West and the Grey Nuns

In 1844, four Grey Nuns embarked on a perilous canoe journey from Montreal to St. Boniface, Manitoba, where their mission was to care for the sick. Soon after their arrival, a series of epidemics began. The nuns visited the sick at home, where they cared for people with measles, dysentery, and smallpox, and treated them with medicines and local herbs.

The Grey Nuns travelled west by ox cart over rough terrain to arrive in what is now Alberta in 1859 to establish their first mission in Lac Ste. Anne, where they saw clients in their homes and cared for them in the convent. Later they established small missions in what is now northern Saskatchewan and the Northwest Territories to provide health care in Native settlements. In 1895, they constructed the Edmonton General Hospital because settlement was burgeoning there. Arriving before most of the settlers, the sisters established systems of health care to care for the sick.

Nursing Education in Canada

In 1860, Florence Nightingale established a financially independent School of Nursing in association with St. Thomas's Hospital in London, England. Interest in the new school was high. Soon hospital training schools for nurses based on this model were established throughout Europe and North America.

Unfortunately, the educational programs of the Nightingale school were missing from the new hospital schools. This was largely because the new schools had no financing and required students to provide nursing service to the hospital in return for their education and living expenses, enabling hospitals to provide nursing services at minimal cost. The race to establish hospitals in the early 1890s was undoubtedly spurred on by the financial benefits of establishing associated schools of nursing. The early hospitals were stretched financially because they did not charge the poor. Services thus had to be of high enough quality to attract paying clients. Because trained nurses were more effective than untrained aides, paying clients were more likely to enter a hospital that employed trained nurses. However, trained nurses were in limited supply and one way to guarantee a supply of nurses was to operate a training school (Young, 1994).

The First Canadian Nursing Schools

The first hospital diploma school in Canada, the St. Catharines Training School, opened in 1874 at the St. Catharines General and Marine Hospital. Admission standards were "plain English education, good character, and Christian motives" (*St. Catharines Annual Report,* as cited in Healey, 1990). At the time, nursing was still considered an undesirable vocation for a refined lady in Canada, the only acceptable profession being teaching (Healey, 1990). Students learned chemistry, sanitary science, physiology, anatomy, and hygiene. They were taught to observe patients for changes in temperature, skin condition, pulse, respirations, and functions of organs and to report "faithfully" to the attending physician (Healey, 1990).

The School for Nurses at the Toronto General Hospital was established in 1881, with Mary Agnes Snively being superintendent in 1884 (Box 3-3). Although work and living conditions were poor, Miss Snively worked hard to improve the program. In 1896, she introduced a 3-year course with 84 hours of practical nursing and 119 hours of instruction by the medical staff (Gibbon & Mathewson, 1947).

Box 3-3 Milestones in Canadian Nursing History

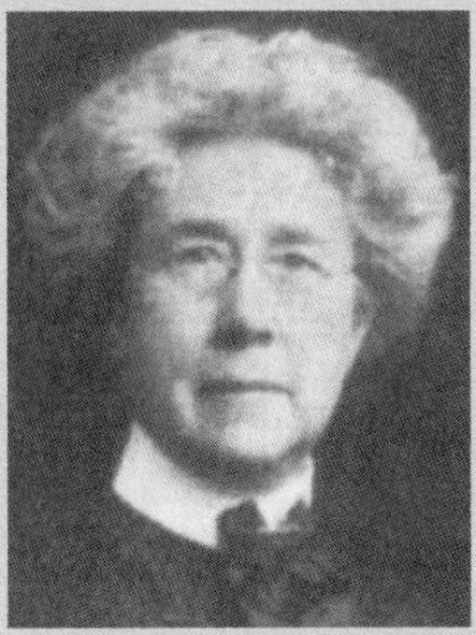

Mary Agnes Snively, 1847–1933

Born in St. Catharines, Ontario, Mary Agnes Snively was a teacher before she was a nurse. Upon graduation from the school of nursing at Bellevue Hospital, New York, in 1894, she became Lady Superintendent of Nurses at Toronto General Hospital (TGH).

Students provided most of the nursing care at TGH, at little cost to the hospital. Snively found no organized plan for classes or clinical experience, nor was there a residence (students were housed in various locations in the hospital). Written records of nursing care, medical orders, and client histories were also lacking. There were problems recruiting desirable applicants because the school had so many hardships.

Snively rectified all these deficiencies. A residence was soon built, she developed a curriculum plan including nursing theory and practice, and she lengthened the education period to 3 years. By the end of her tenure in 1910, TGH was the largest school of nursing in Canada and served as a model for others.

Snively achieved acclaim for her organizational work. She attended the 1899 founding meeting of the International Council of Nurses (ICN) in London, England, and was elected first honorary treasurer of the ICN, becoming vice president a few years later. In 1908, she was elected first president of the Provisional Organization of the Canadian National Association of Trained Nurses (later the CNA).

From *Three Centuries of Canadian Nursing,* by J. Gibbon and M. Mathewson, 1947, Toronto, ON: Macmillan; and *Jean I. Gunn, Nursing Leader,* by N. Riegler, 1997, Markham, ON: Associated Medical Services with Fitzhenry and Whiteside.

In Montreal, after several unsuccessful attempts, The School for Nurses at the Montreal General Hospital was established in 1890 under the direction of Nora Livingston. Conditions were deplorable, but Miss Livingston quickly made improvements. The popularity of the school increased rapidly. Miss Livingston reported 169 applications in the first year, from which 80 students were accepted (Gibbon & Mathewson, 1947).

The move to establish hospital schools of nursing swept the country. The Winnipeg General Hospital initiated the first Training School for Nurses in 1887 to serve the entire West. A measure of its success was that 134 of its graduates served as nurses in World War I (Gibbon & Mathewson, 1947). By 1890, hospitals in Fredericton, Saint John, Halifax, and Charlottetown had opened schools. Vancouver General Hospital began a school in 1891, and in Alberta, a school was opened in Medicine Hat in 1894. By 1930, there were approximately 330 schools of nursing in Canada (CNA, 1968; Box 3-4).

Box 3-4 Milestones in Canadian Nursing History

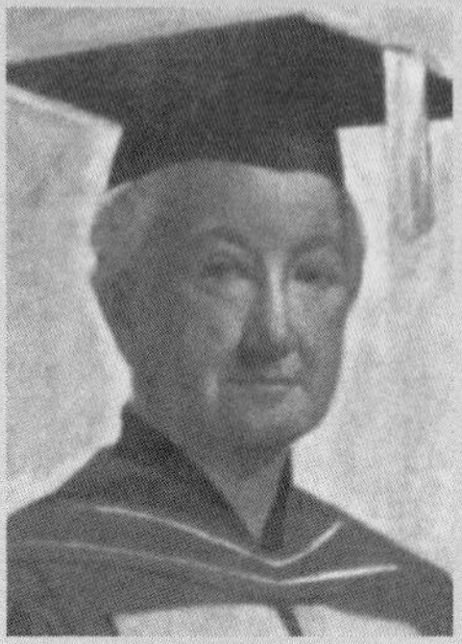

Jean I. Gunn, 1882–1941

Born in 1882 in Belleville, Ontario, Jean Gunn was superintendent of nurses at the Toronto General Hospital in 1913, a role that included directing the School of Nursing.

Shortly after Gunn took up the position, she recruited several outstanding nursing administrators. With strong leadership to assist her, she became involved in provincial, national, and international health and nursing organizations, eventually chairing the Red Cross's committee on surgical dressings during World War II. In this role, she oversaw production of millions of dressings by female civilian volunteers.

Nurses were in short supply during this time. With most men in the armed forces, many industrial jobs were now open to women and at wages far surpassing those of nurses. In 1917, Gunn pressed for the establishment of a permanent cadre of trained nurses for national service. She also worked tirelessly for the registration of nurses.

Jean Gunn advocated for nursing and nurses on many fronts. She castigated hospital boards for reviewing costs of hospital services while ignoring the savings that accrued from educating a nurse. She decried the exploitation of nurses in schools of nursing and envisioned university degree programs in nursing.

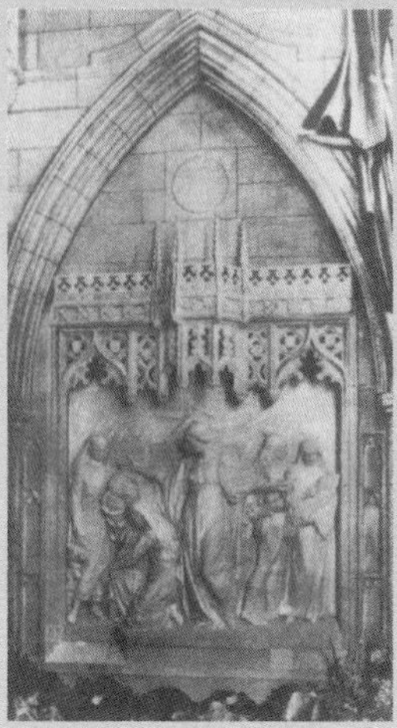

Gunn is perhaps best remembered for her work toward the Nurses' War Memorial, which recognized the service of military nurses during World War I through a bas-relief sculpture in white marble. The memorial was unveiled on Parliament Hill in 1924. In 1932, the Canadian Nurses Association's crest was added to the sculpture.

In recognition of her outstanding service to nursing and health throughout her life, Gunn received a number of honours in her final years, including a King's Jubilee Medal in 1935 and a Doctor of Laws degree from the University of Toronto. Jean Gunn was a leader among leaders in nursing.

Source: *Jean I. Gunn, Nursing Leader,* by N. Riegler, 1997, Markham, ON: Associated Medical Services with Fitzhenry and Whiteside.

The Impact of Nursing Organizations on Nursing Education

At the same time that hospital training schools for nurses were being established, nurses began to organize themselves to advocate for educational standards and legislation in their profession. Women's associations were key to the public health crusade in Canada and to the rise of nursing organizations. The National Council of Women under the presidency of Lady Ishbel Aberdeen, wife of the governor general of Canada, approved the formation of the Victorian Order of Nurses (VON) in 1898. Lady Aberdeen had persevered with her idea of establishing the VON after she was struck by the plight of women in Western Canada who had to give birth in remote locations with no assistance. The formation of the VON signified a professional standard of education for Canadian nurses that recognized the need not only for altruism and compassion but also for nursing knowledge.

Nurses from around the world were beginning to organize themselves, inspired by the leadership of women like Ethel Gordon Bedford Fenwick. Editor of the *British Journal of Nursing,* she attended the 1893 Congress of Charities, Corrections and Philanthropy in Chicago, where she spoke of British struggles to achieve registration for nurses. Her North American colleagues had similar concerns. After the congress, they formed the American Society of Superintendents of Training Schools for Nurses of the United States and Canada, later to become the National League for Nursing Education, whose goal was to raise standards of nursing education. Soon afterward in 1896, the Nurses' Associated Alumnae of the United States and Canada was formed, becoming the American Nurses Association in 1911. A major goal was to secure legislation to differentiate between trained and untrained nurses (CNA, 1968).

In 1899, Bedford Fenwick founded the ICN, with Britain, Germany, and the United States as member organizations. Nations without national nursing organizations could not become members. Although Canada did not yet have a national nursing organization, Mary Agnes Snively, Superintendent of Nurses at Toronto General Hospital, was elected the first honourary treasurer of the ICN in 1899 (CNA, 1968).

The Origins of the Canadian Nurses Association and Provincial Nursing Associations. The Canadian Society of Superintendents of Training Schools for Nurses was formed in 1907. The next year, the Provisional Society of the Canadian National Association of Trained Nurses (CNATN) was formed with Mary Agnes Snively as president (CNA, 1968). Membership in this new national organization was through affiliated societies in the provinces. At the ICN meeting in 1909, Canada became a full-fledged member of the organization. Later, the CNATN streamlined its organization when registration of nurses was established through legislation in each province. Its name was changed to the Canadian Nurses Association (CNA) in 1924 and it became a federation of provincial associations in 1930.

The struggle for women's rights helped nurses to secure laws to regulate their profession. Nurses formed provincial nurses' associations and sought legislation that would set educational standards and improve nursing care. The first province to gain legislation was Nova Scotia, where a voluntary registration act was passed in 1910. It also allowed non-graduate nurses to register. Initial acts passed in other provinces contained more restrictive standards. Admission criteria and curricula were set for nursing schools, as were rules governing registration and discipline of practising nurses.

All provinces and two territories eventually secured mandatory registration, requiring that all practising nurses register with the regulatory body approved by the provincial nursing act. The distinguishing feature of mandatory rather than permissive legislation is a statute containing a definition of the scope of nursing practice. Nurses' functions are outlined more explicitly under mandatory registration (Wood, 2003). Licensure laws are designed to protect the public against unqualified and incompetent practitioners.

The First University Programs

The devastating consequences of World War I and the influenza pandemic of 1918 led to support for public health programs and new patterns of health care delivery. Community health was promoted, and nurses were seen as central players who needed university-level education. To this end, the Canadian Red Cross Society awarded grants to a number of Canadian universities to develop post-graduate courses in public health nursing: Toronto, McGill, British Columbia, Alberta, Dalhousie, and Western Ontario.

The first Canadian undergraduate nursing degree program was established at the University of British Columbia in 1919, with Ethel Johns as director. The operating costs of the new department were to be borne by the hospital, an incentive for the university to support the program. The program was non-integrated, in that "the university assumed no responsibility for the two or three years of nursing preparation in a hospital school of nursing" (Bonin, 1976, p. 7).

Several new 5-year, non-integrated degree programs began at Canadian universities in the 1920s and 1930s: the University of Western Ontario, the University of Alberta and l'Institut Marguerite d'Youville, the University of Ottawa, and St Francis Xavier University. The religious order associated with the University of Ottawa launched what was essentially a hospital diploma program in 1933.

From the Depression to the Post World War II Years

When nursing schools were established, women's education was a low priority. Nursing students were exploited in the hospital-based programs, effectively subsidizing hospital operations. Nursing leaders fought to improve education at nursing schools and limit service, developing a standard curriculum that they urged schools to use. To eliminate weak programs, they encouraged the closure of hospital schools with insufficient beds. In 1932, the first national study of nursing education in Canada was conducted by Dr. George Weir. His report confirmed what nurses already knew about nursing schools: The conditions were deplorable, the health of students was in jeopardy, and education was secondary to hospital service (Weir, 1932).

The Depression "brought unemployment and hardship to nurses" (Allemang, 1974, p. 172). Clients could no longer afford to employ private-duty nurses, which had been the most promising area of employment for graduate nurses (Gunn, 1933). During the Depression, Canadian universities faced reduced revenues, staff layoffs, and difficult working conditions. The Depression was especially hard on McGill University, which depended on funds from private sources. During the Depression, raising private funds became next to impossible. Leaders of McGill's nursing school had fought unsuccessfully for years for a degree program. Once the university's finances began to deteriorate, the Board of Governors threatened to close the school altogether. The school's director, Bertha Harmer, gave up her salary, the faculty bought books for the library, and nursing alumnae groups all over the country raised funds to ensure the survival of the McGill School (Tunis, 1966).

During World War II, health education became a priority as doctors and nurses were needed to care for military personnel as well as civilians. Nurses who held critical positions as administrators, supervisors, teachers, and public health nurses were recruited for military service and left their positions. There soon occurred a shortage of nurses.

During and after the war, a new interest in nursing education led to increased external university funding, more scholarships and bursaries from private foundations, the growth of existing schools, and the founding of new programs. Queens and McMaster Universities initiated programs in 1941, followed by the University of Manitoba in 1943, Mount St. Vincent University in 1947, and Dalhousie University in 1949. At McGill, new funds flowed in, and in 1944, supporters of the school were rewarded with a 5-year non-integrated degree program.

Most non-integrated programs offered a 2- to 3-year apprenticeship-based hospital diploma program "sandwiched" between 2 years of university study. The non-integrated degree pattern with its stepladder approach to nursing education was well established, and the hospital programs on which this approach depended had been entrenched for many years. However, the new interest in nursing education led to exciting innovations. In 1942, the University of Toronto introduced an integrated basic degree program. Under the leadership of Edith Kathleen Russell (see chapter 4), courses in arts and sciences were combined with nursing courses and planned to enhance student development. Unlike the instructors of non-integrated programs, university instructors supervised student clinical practice in the hospitals. Four years after the introduction of the University of Toronto basic degree program, a second basic degree program was developed at McMaster University under Gladys Sharpe's direction. As they evolved over the years, these programs had tremendous influence across Canada, and the University of Toronto model became the dominant model for university nursing education in Canada.

Expansion in the 1950s and 1960s

In the 1960s, existing nursing degree programs expanded, and new programs emerged in other universities. The first master's degree program in nursing was established at the University of Western Ontario in 1959, followed in the 1960s and 1970s by universities across the country. In 1962, the Canadian Nurses Foundation was established as a separate entity from the CNA, to provide scholarships, bursaries, and fellowships for graduate study in nursing.

Nursing schools' financial dependence left them at the mercy of hospital administrators. "The lack of nursing instructors and of other graduate nurses on patient care units meant that there were few role models for students for observation, questions and general discussion. In most cases senior students were left in charge of teaching junior students, and this with very limited supervision" (Paul, 1998, pp. 133–134). Many have suggested that this was not a true apprenticeship model because there were few masters to guide the students (Chapman, 1969).

Nursing leaders called for better faculty preparation, more integrated programs, and more university-based opportunities for students, such as student placements and increased enrolments. The movement to separate nursing education programs from the authority of hospitals began in earnest. Studies of nursing education identified persistent problems. A study by Mussallem found that hours on duty for students in hospital schools of nursing were too long, there were too few nursing instructors, and the instructors were not qualified (CNA, 1965). In a 1965 survey, 65% of hospital schools reported that clinical assignments were based on the service needs of the patient care units, not on the students' educational needs (CNA, 1965).

Universities resisted introducing basic integrated degree programs because of the costs associated with low student-teacher ratios required for clinical nursing. It was cheaper for universities to let hospitals finance clinical education, but this meant that universities granted degrees for work over which they had no control. In 1964, the Royal Commission on Health Services castigated universities for this practice. By the late 1960s, the basic integrated degree program finally became the program of choice.

From the 1970s to 2000

In 1975, the Alberta Task Force on Nursing Education proposed their entry to practice position, which was that all new nursing graduates be qualified at the baccalaureate level. Over the past 25 years, provincial governments have been increasing the capacity of their provincial degree-granting nursing education programs to accommodate all students studying nursing at the undergraduate level (CNA, 1991). Most provincial and regulatory bodies have made the baccalaureate degree an entry to the practice of nursing (CNA, 2004).

Throughout the 1970s and 1980s, university faculties and schools of nursing developed research resources so they could offer doctoral programs. The first doctoral nursing program was established at the University of Alberta Faculty of Nursing in 1991 and others quickly followed. Today there are 12 doctoral nursing programs in Canada.

Nursing Education Today

With the increased complexities of health care and the expansion of knowledge about care, beginning practitioners require a broad education base. New curricula and collaborative baccalaureate programs across the country attest to the profession's commitment to maintaining high standards of health care and responding to society's changing health needs. The Internet, computerized learning programs, shared faculty via teleconferencing, and weekend and evening courses provide practising nurses with many options to complete degrees. Some universities have innovative programs at the baccalaureate level in an accelerated 12-month program when the candidate holds a baccalaureate degree in science. Baccalaureate and master's degree programs are also offered through distance education.

Standards for nursing education are monitored by each province to ensure that educational programs are of appropriate quality and respond to changes in health care. As professionals, nurses must acquire, maintain, and continuously enhance the knowledge, skills, attitudes, and judgment required to meet client needs in an evolving health care system. The responsibility for educational support for competent nursing practice is shared among individual nurses, professional nursing organizations, educational institutions, and governments (Wood, 2003).

Post-Graduate Degrees

The need for nurses with post-graduate degrees is rising, along with the need for research. A master's degree in nursing is necessary for nurses seeking the role of advanced practice nurse, clinical nurse specialist, nurse practitioner, nurse administrator, or nurse educator. (These roles are described later in this chapter.) Most master's programs in Canada focus on advanced nursing practice. This provides the nurse with advanced preparation in nursing science, theory, and practice, with emphasis on research-based clinical practice.

Nurses with doctorates can undertake research that advances knowledge and evidence-based practice in clinical settings (see chapter 6). This research enhances the quality of nursing care and improves Canadians' health outcomes.

Continuing and In-Service Education

Nurses need skills and knowledge to practise in a constantly changing health care environment. Today's continuing education programs help nurses learn current nursing skills, knowledge, and theory. **Continuing education** includes formal, organized, and educational programs offered by provincial associations and educational and health care institutions.

As well, health care agencies and institutions offer **in-service education** programs, designed to increase the knowledge, skills, and competencies of nurses and other health care professionals employed by the institution. For example, a hospital might offer an in-service program to teach nurses about primary nursing before it is implemented at the hospital.

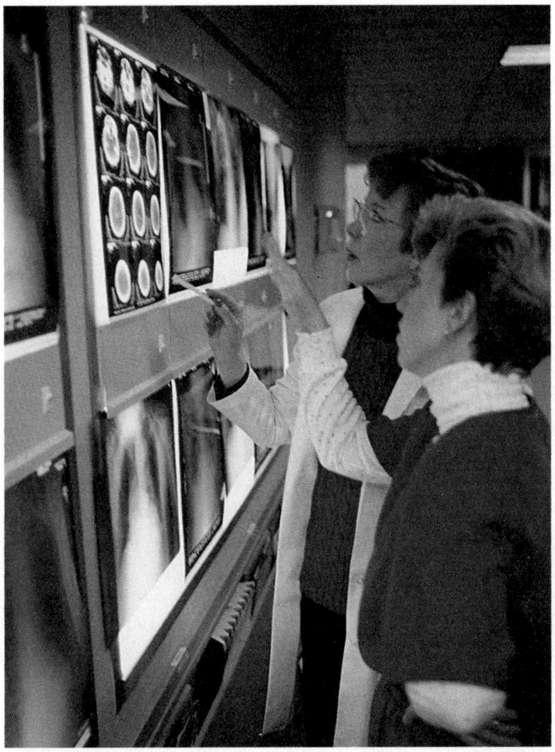

FIGURE **3–1** Nurse specialist consults on a difficult client case.

Professional Roles and Responsibilities

Contemporary nursing requires that the nurse possess knowledge and skills for a variety of professional roles and responsibilities. In the past, the principal role of nurses was to provide care and comfort as they carried out specific nursing functions. Today the nursing role has expanded to include increased emphasis on health promotion as well as concern for the client as a whole.

Nurses fulfill a variety of functions within many settings. The positions in which nurses work are evolving as health care agencies and the health care system address advancing technology and knowledge in medicine, nursing, and health in general. Career roles are specific employment positions or paths. Because of increasing educational opportunities for nurses, the growth of nursing as a profession, and a greater concern for job enrichment, the nursing profession offers expanded roles and different kinds of career opportunities (Figure 3–1). Examples of career roles include nurse educators, advanced practice nurses, nurse managers and administrators, quality improvement nurses, consultants, and even business owners. Box 3-5 describes some of the many nursing roles.

Professional Nursing Organizations

A **professional organization** is the voice of a profession and deals with issues of concern to those practising in the profession. Professional nursing organizations establish educational and practice standards for nurses, carry out the regulatory functions of registration and licensure, and discipline members who do not meet the standards. The terms *registration* and *licensure* have different meanings, although they are often used interchangeably. Registration refers to the listing of a member in good standing on the membership roster of an organization, whereas licensure refers to the granting by a government body of the exclusive right to practise a profession to a member in good standing. In most provinces and territories (except Ontario and the Yukon), governments entrust administration of the legislation to the professional nursing association.

Nursing associations in each province/territory are the voice for registered nurses in those regions of the country. These organizations are the official representatives of the nursing profession and interact with provincial/territorial government officials on issues concerning the health of the populace and the role of the nursing profession. They also collaborate with other health professions' organizations on matters of mutual interest and help their members maintain competence through continuing education. Nursing organizations aim to increase public understanding of nursing and its impact on the health of individuals, families, and communities.

Some professional organizations and special interest groups focus on specific areas such as critical care, nursing administration, or research. Examples include the Canadian Gerontological Nursing Association, the Canadian Association of Neuroscience Nurses, and the Aboriginal Nurses Association of Canada. These organizations seek to improve the standards of practice, expand nursing roles, and foster the welfare of nurses within the specialty areas. In addition, professional organizations present education programs and publish journals.

Nurses form a large and very powerful group and have made important gains on health care issues through the leadership provided by their professional organizations. As the national voice of professional nurses, the CNA is the representative of nurses across the country to the federal government and national organizations (Box 3-6). The CNA collaborates with other national nursing and health organizations on issues related to practice, education, and research. The organization holds regular meetings and discussions with government officials to ensure that the federal government is aware of nursing's positions on health issues, including its national agenda for health care reform.

The CNA works for the improvement of health standards and the availability of health care services for all people, fosters high standards of nursing, stimulates and promotes the professional development of nurses, and advances their economic and general welfare. It gives individual nurses a collective means to influence health policy at the national level. It regularly presents briefs to the House of Commons on areas such as taxation, poverty, health, unemployment insurance, employment opportunities, part-time work, economic and social affairs, science and technology, and federal-provincial fiscal arrangements, including funding for health care. For example, following extensive lobbying by the CNA, in February 2000, the federal government committed $2.5 billion to the Canada Health and Social Transfer, with a substantial portion of

Box 3-5 Categories of Nursing Roles

Nurse clinician	A nurse who provides direct client care.
Advanced practice nurse	A clinical nurse with graduate preparation in nursing who provides primary care, usually in partnership with a physician or group of physicians. The advanced practice nurse has authority to prescribe medications (with the exception of narcotics) and treat health problems within the scope of nursing practice.
Clinical nurse specialist	An advanced practice nurse with preparation in a specialized area of nursing practice; may specialize in a specific disease, such as cancer or AIDS, or in a specific field, such as pediatrics or gerontology.
Nurse practitioner	A nurse with advanced preparation in nursing who works usually in outpatient, ambulatory care, or community-based setting. Provides care for clients with complex problems using a holistic approach.
Nursing educator	A nurse with graduate preparation who works primarily in schools of nursing, staff development departments of health care agencies, and client education departments. Educators in schools of nursing teach students to become professional nurses. Educators in staff development departments provide programs for nurses within their institution, such as safety training and instruction about new equipment or procedures. Educators in client education departments teach ill or disabled clients and their families how to provide care in the home.
Nursing administrator	A nurse prepared at the graduate level, who manages client care and the delivery of specific nursing services in a health care agency. Needs to be skilled in business and management, as well as to understand all aspects of nursing and client care. Functions may include budgeting, staffing, strategic planning of programs and services, employee evaluation, and employee development.
Nursing researcher	A nurse prepared at the doctoral level, who investigates problems to improve nursing care and to further define and expand the scope of nursing practice (see chapter 6). May be employed in an academic setting, hospital, or independent professional or community service agency.

Box 3-6 Canadian Nurses Association Vision Statement

- A commitment to the public interest where excellence in client centred care drives the nursing agenda.
- Nursing services form the core of the health care delivery system.
- Registered nurses are a provider of choice for primary, holistic health care services for Canadians.
- As an access point to the health care system, registered nurses assess, admit, and discharge clients from health services, provide a wide range of nursing interventions, and support clients along a continuum of care.
- Registered nurses, as expert health educators and counsellors, are sought to help people change their health behaviours and to help families and communities stay healthy.
- From hospital to clinic, from home to main street, registered nurses are highly accessible, visible health care providers.
- Independent professionals, registered nurses practice autonomously but also bring their expertise to interdisciplinary teams.
- As dynamic managers, nurses lead nursing teams, coordinate a broad range of services, and are equal partners on health care teams.
- Powerful leadership is fostered through advanced practice, certification, baccalaureate, master's, and doctoral nursing programs.
- Recognized nationally and internationally, nurses are leaders who influence health care policies at all levels and act as public authorities on health care issues.
- Accomplished and educated, nurses continually expand their expertise and knowledge through formal and informal professional development.
- Funded nursing research ensures a research-based norm for practise, and supports the rich body of nursing knowledge.

Adapted from *CNA's Vision Statement,* by the Canadian Nurses Association, 1998, Ottawa, ON: Author.

that amount being earmarked for nursing. After the 2004 federal election, the CNA lobbied federally for its Common Vision Statement on health care in order to develop an agreement with the provinces to ensure "an adequate supply of health providers, pan-Canadian benchmarks and real targets for timely access to care, the expansion of the continuum of care and sufficient, on-going and predictable federal long-term funding" (Media Statement, 2004).

Unions

In Canada, professional associations and unions operate separately. Professional organizations initially were responsible for collective bargaining. However, the 1973 Supreme Court decision in the appeal of the Saskatchewan case *Service Employees International Union* [SEIU] *v Nipiwan District Staff Nurses Association* (where the Staff Nurses Association was a unit of the Saskatchewan Registered Nurses Association) led to the separation of professional associations across the country (S.E.I.U. Local 333, 1973). The Staff Nurses Association had applied to be certified as a bargaining unit, but this was denied on the basis of the potential conflict of interest in determining salaries of registered nurses because the Staff Nurses Association's Board of Directors could include nurse managers. Within a decade, every province had both a separate nursing association and a union. Some nursing unions represent both registered nurses and registered practical nurses (licensed practical nurses).

A movement to establish a national voice for unionized nurses began in the late 1960s, and the CNA established a labour relations department in 1977 to disseminate information about collective bargaining and to provide educational assistance to members. In 1981, the National Federation of Nurses' Unions was formed to represent the interests of nurses in both watchdog and lobbying activities. This organization became the Canadian Confederation of Nurses' Unions and by 2004 all provinces except Quebec were members (*www.cnfu.ca*, 2004). When nursing positions were cut dramatically in the mid-1990s, unions represented nurses on an institution-by-institution basis. Nursing unions have lobbied for professional responsibility clauses in union contracts and are primary participants as the representatives of nurses in particular provinces/territories at the bargaining table when new contracts are negotiated.

Standards of Nursing Practice

As a self-regulating profession, nursing sets its own standards of practice, which serve as objective guidelines for nurses to provide and evaluate care. Such standards are developed and established based on research and clinical evidence. They help assure clients that they are receiving high-quality care. Quality assurance programs use measures to ensure that standards of practice are high. Because health is a provincial responsibility, each professional nursing organization is responsible for developing the standards for nursing practice in its particular province. In Table 3-1, the standards developed for the province of Ontario by the College of Nurses of Ontario (CNO) are outlined to serve as an example of nursing practice standards.

Nursing Best Practice Guidelines

Recently, there has been a focus in all professions on ensuring that those professionals providing service understand practice guidelines. "Best practices" are guiding principles leading to the most appropriate courses of action in certain standard practice situations. They are different from the much more general nursing practice standards in that they apply to specific clinical practice situations. Since 1999, the Ontario Ministry of Health and Long-Term Care has given annual funding of $1.5 million to the Registered Nurses Association of Ontario (RNAO) to develop, pilot implement, evaluate, and disseminate "best practice guidelines" or statements of what nurses would be expected to do in particular client situations. This is a multi-year project to assist nurses in Ontario to provide informed and high-quality care.

The five broad clinical topics designated as primary centres of focus were gerontology, primary health care, home health care, mental health care, and emergency care. The RNAO has held numerous conferences for Ontario nurses to familiarize them with the guidelines as well as a national conference and two international conferences in 2001 and 2003 (Box 3-7).

Other provinces and territories are interested in these guidelines because they can be applied in other areas of Canada. Health Canada has provided funding for national dissemination of the materials and translation in French. This is a project of great interest to nurses across the country.

Ethical Standards of Practice

Fundamental to all professions are ethical standards that guide practice. Normally these standards are expressed as "codes" of ethics and have emerged in the modern era from the Nuremberg Code, developed in 1947 as a result of the post-World War II war crimes investigation of experimentation on human beings. The first **code of ethics** for nursing was developed by the ICN in 1953. This provided a model for member countries to develop their own codes of ethics. A code of ethics defines the principles by which nurses function (see chapter 7).

In 1954, the CNA adopted the code of ethics developed by the ICN (1953). This was followed by the development of the CNA *Code of Ethics: An Ethical Basis for Nursing in Canada*, which was most recently updated in 2002. The *Code of Ethics* provides nurses with direction for ethical decision making and practice in everyday situations. Because nursing in Canada is a provincial responsibility, by law, each province and territory has to specify a code of ethics for nurses. Therefore, each provincial statute regulating nursing incorporates a code of ethics; many provinces use the CNA *Code of Ethics* in their statutes.

Registration/Licensure

In all provinces and territories, nursing practice acts regulate the licensure and practice of nursing. Each province or territory defines for itself the scope of nursing practice because constitutional responsibility for education and health care rests with individual provinces (i.e., the legal limits of nurses' professional role). Many provincial nursing practice acts have been revised to reflect nursing's growing autonomy and expanding roles. In all provinces except Ontario and Quebec, provincial nursing associations assume responsibility for defining and monitoring standards. Legislation in each province outlines nursing scope of practice. In addition, nurses working in hospitals and other health agencies also practice according to the policies of the organizations. These policies are more detailed and are specific to the nature of the care provided within the particular health agency. In most provinces and territories, nursing registration requires that the student complete a prescribed course of study from an approved program.

Certification

As nursing education has developed, the practice has expanded. The CNA, spurred on by the need to certify nursing specialties, passed a resolution at its convention in 1980 to develop certification examinations, which are voluntary. The CNA identified the following purposes of certification: "to provide an opportunity for practitioners to validate their expertise in a specialty; to promote high standards of nursing practice in order to provide quality nursing care to the people of Canada; and to identify through a recognized credential those nurses who have met the specialty standard" (1986). There were 17 specialties for which nurses could apply for certification in 2004, including critical care, nephrology, occupational health, perioperative, gerontological, emergency, neuroscience, oncology, perinatal nursing, and psychiatric/

Table 3-1 Standards of Professional Practice

The following are broad descriptions of the expectations of nurses and apply to all nurses in every area of practice. Although written by the CNO for nurses in Ontario, the general themes are relevant for nurses across the country.

Accountability

Each nurse is accountable to the public and responsible for ensuring that her or his practice and conduct meets legislative requirements and the standards of the profession.
Nurses are responsible for their actions and the consequences of those actions. Part of this accountability includes conducting themselves in ways that promote respect for the profession.
Nurses demonstrate this standard by:

- advocating for clients, the profession, and the health care system
- ensuring practice is consistent with standards of practice, guidelines, and legislation
- taking responsibility for errors when they occur and taking appropriate action to maintain client safety
- refraining from performing activities for which they are not competent

Continuing Competence

Each nurse maintains and continually improves her/his competence by participating in the College of Nurses of Ontario's Quality Assurance (QA) Program.
Competence is the nurse's ability to use knowledge and skill in a given role, situation, and practice setting. Continuing competence ensures the nurse is able to perform in a changing health environment. It also contributes to quality nursing practice and increases the public's confidence in the nursing profession.
Nurses demonstrate this standard by:

- assuming responsibility for their own professional development and for sharing knowledge with others
- engaging in a learning process to enhance their practice
- advocating for quality practice improvements in the workplace

Ethics

Each nurse understands, upholds, and promotes the values and beliefs described in the CNO standard entitled Ethics.
Ethical nursing care means promoting the values of client well-being, respecting client choice, assuring privacy and confidentiality, respecting sanctity and quality of life, maintaining commitments, respecting truthfulness, and ensuring fairness in the use of resources. It also includes acting with integrity, honesty, and professionalism.
Nurses demonstrate this standard by:

- identifying ethical issues and communicating these to the health team
- identifying options to resolve ethical issues
- identifying personal values and ensuring they do not conflict with professional practice

Knowledge

Each nurse possesses, through basic education and continuing learning, knowledge relevant to her or his professional practice.
RNs and RPNs study from the same body of nursing knowledge. RPNs study for a shorter period of time resulting in a more focused or basic foundation of knowledge. RNs study for a longer period of time for a greater breadth and depth of knowledge. All nurses add to their basic education and foundational knowledge throughout their careers by pursuing ongoing learning.
Nurses demonstrate this standard by:

- providing an evidence-based rationale for all decisions
- being informed about the various nursing roles and their relationship to one another
- understanding the legislation and standards relevant to nursing and the practice area
- knowing how cultural background relates to health needs

Knowledge Application

Each nurse continually improves the application of professional knowledge.
The quality of professional nursing practice reflects nurses' application of knowledge. Nurses apply knowledge to practice using nursing frameworks, theories, and/or processes.
Nurses demonstrate this standard by:

- identifying and recognizing abnormal or unexpected client responses and taking action
- planning care approaches with the client
- managing multiple nursing interventions simultaneously
- evaluating the outcome of interventions and modifying the care plan
- integrating research findings into professional service and practice

Leadership

Nurses demonstrate leadership by providing, facilitating and promoting the best possible care or service to the public.
Leadership requires self-knowledge (understanding one's beliefs and values and being aware of how one's behaviour affects others), respect, trust, integrity, shared vision, learning, participation, good communication techniques, and the ability to be a change facilitator. All nurses have opportunities for leadership.
Nurses demonstrate this standard by:

- role-modelling professional values, beliefs, and attributes
- collaborating with clients and the health team to provide professional practice that respects client rights
- providing direction to, collaborating with, and sharing knowledge and expertise with novices, students, and unregulated care providers
- participating in nursing associations, committees, or interest groups

From *Professional Standards (Revised 2002),* by College of Nurses of Ontario, 2004, Toronto, ON: Author.

Table 3-1 Standards of Professional Practice—cont'd

Relationships

Each nurse establishes and maintains respectful, collaborative, therapeutic and professional relationships.
Relationships include therapeutic nurse-client relationships and professional relationships with colleagues, health team members, and employers.

- **Therapeutic Nurse-Client Relationships**

The clients' needs are the focus of the therapeutic relationship, which is based on trust, respect, intimacy, and the appropriate use of power. It is the nurse's responsibility to establish and maintain the therapeutic relationship.
Nurses demonstrate this standard by:

- demonstrating respect, empathy, and interest for clients
- maintaining boundaries between professional, therapeutic relationships and non-professional, personal relationships
- ensuring that their personal needs are met outside of the therapeutic nurse-client relationship
- ensuring clients' needs remain the focus of the nurse-client relationship
- **Professional Relationships**

Professional relationships are based on trust and respect, and result in improved client care
Nurses demonstrate this standard by:

- role-modelling positive collegial relationship
- using communication and interpersonal skills to establish and maintain collegial relationships
- demonstrating knowledge of, and respect for, each other's roles, knowledge, expertise and unique contribution to the team
- demonstrating effective conflict-resolution skills

Box 3-7 RNAO Nursing Best Practice Guidelines

Caregiving Strategies for Older Adults with Delirium, Dementia and Depression
Best Practice Guideline for the Subcutaneous Administration of Insulin in Adults with Type 2 Diabetes
Promoting Asthma Control in Children
Assessment and Device Selection for Vascular Access
Adult Asthma Care Guidelines for Nurses: Promoting Control of Asthma
Assessment and Management of Pain
Assessment and Management of Stage I to IV Pressure Ulcers
Assessment and Management of Venous Leg Ulcers
Breastfeeding Best Practice Guidelines for Nurses
Client Centred Care
Crisis Intervention
Enhancing Healthy Adolescent Development
Establishing Therapeutic Relationships
Integrating Smoking Cessation into Daily Nursing Practice
Prevention of Constipation in the Older Adult Population
Prevention of Falls and Fall Injuries in the Older Adult
Promoting Continence Using Prompted Voiding
Reducing Foot Complications for People with Diabetes
Risk Assessment and Prevention of Pressure Ulcers
Screening for Delirium, Dementia and Depression in Older Adults
Supporting and Strengthening Families Through Expected and Unexpected Life Events
(See *http://www.rnao.org/bestpractices/completed_guidelines/bestPractice_ firstCycle.asp* for links to these guidelines.)

mental health. The certification program offered under the auspices of the CNA has been highly successful, for it has provided a means of recognizing the specialized knowledge and skills necessary in a great number of areas of practice. It is likely that even more specialty groups will apply to be part of the certification program in the future.

Conclusion

We have seen in this chapter that organized nursing has been a part of the social setting in Canada since the early days of the European settlement at Quebec, a period of more than three and a half centuries. The first nurses who came to found hospitals and to provide care for Natives and settlers were motivated by altruism and serve as excellent role models for nurses today. Altruism, a hallmark of any profession, remains an important characteristic of the nursing profession despite the vast difference in the health care settings of yesterday and today.

A fundamental and guiding principle of the French-Canadian hospitals that survived largely intact into the 20th century was that care was available to all regardless of their background, status in life, or ability to pay. This continues to be a principle for which nurses, through their professional organizations, have argued for determinedly in national debates on the nature and continuing direction of Canada's national health insurance program. In the face of pressure to reshape medicare, nurses have continued to strongly resist calls for privatization of more aspects of the health system. They have also repeatedly called for all health professionals to be remunerated on a salary or contract basis (Ross-Kerr, 2003).

Although the nature of nursing practice is changing rapidly in the light of restructuring and regionalization of health care services, there are certain fundamental characteristics of nursing that continue to be held in high regard by professional nurses. A time-honoured value in nursing is that the client is the central focus of care and that it is important to take the whole person into account when planning care. In the past, the hospital has served as the primary environment of care. However, changes in the organization and financing of health care have fuelled a movement to shift a great deal of care away from the hospital to settings in the community such as community health centres and homes of clients.

Multidisciplinary teams are an integral component of the health care organization in the community. However, nurses are the primary health care professionals in community settings both in home care and in community health settings. Thus, expanded and enhanced educational systems for nurses that incorporate knowledge and skills for community health and home care nursing are essential to meet the health needs of the populace in the health settings of today.

Nursing today requires a vast range of knowledge and skills, and thus educational programs to prepare nurses for the health systems of today and tomorrow are demanding. Nurses have unlimited opportunities for fulfilling careers in a vast array of general and specialty areas. There is a tremendous range of educational opportunities open to nurses throughout their careers to enhance knowledge and skills and to move into new areas if desired. In nursing practice, nurses carry more responsibility for care than ever before. Nursing educators have challenging opportunities in practice, education, and research. Nursing scientists are on the cutting edge of health research and the results of their investigations have changed health practices around the world.

The transformation of the nursing profession and the educational programs that support it in the past century has been truly remarkable. Despite monumental obstacles, nurses have demonstrated the value of their service, the integrity of their goals, the quality of their educational programs, and the strength of their commitment. Although we do not know what will unfold as we move through the 21st century, it is certain that the nursing profession will continue to evolve in the interest of providing a high quality of nursing care to the populace.

Key Concepts

- Nursing has responded to the health care needs of society, which were influenced by economic, social, and cultural variables of a specific era.
- Nursing in Canada is rooted in the traditions of good nursing that developed in New France.
- Florence Nightingale revolutionized nursing as an acceptable profession for lay nurses in the late 1800s and early 1900s.
- The development of a system of nursing education in Canada emerged from the early nursing sisterhoods and from schools of nursing based on the Nightingale model.
- Baccalaureate entry to practice is well on its way to full implementation in Canada.
- Basic nursing education is acquired in collaborative college-university or university programs.
- Nurses have a variety of career opportunities and roles, including nurse clinician, advanced practice nurse, clinical nurse specialist, nurse practitioner, educator, administrator, and researcher.
- Professional nursing organizations establish standards of education and practice for nurses, carry out the regulatory functions of registration and professional conduct, deal with issues of concern to specialist groups within the nursing profession, and empower nurses to influence health care policy and practice.
- Nursing sets its own standards of practice—from scientific research and the work of nurse clinical experts—to ensure high-quality care.

Key Terms

Advanced practice nurse, *p. 44*
Clinical nurse specialist, *p. 44*
Code of ethics, *p. 45*
Continuing education, *p. 42*
In-Service Education, *p. 42*
International Council of Nurses (ICN), *p. 35*
Nurse clinician, *p. 44*
Nurse practitioner, *p. 44*
Nursing administrator, *p. 44*
Nursing educator, *p. 44*
Nursing researcher, *p. 44*
Professional organization, *p. 43*

Critical Thinking Exercises

1. Explain the importance of Florence Nightingale's work on the establishment of nursing as a profession.
2. Observe various levels of nursing practice, such as a staff nurse, advanced practice nurse, and nurse educator. Identify similarities and differences in their roles and educational preparation.
3. Outline some career objectives for yourself after completing your nursing program. Think about what you want to do as a professional nurse and then outline strategies for achieving these goals.

Review Questions

1. The founder of modern nursing is
   1. Hippocrates
   2. Florence Nightingale
   3. Jeanne Mance
   4. Mary Agnes Snively
2. The founder of the Sisters of Charity of Montreal, which later became known as the Grey Nuns, is
   1. Marie Hébert
   2. St. Vincent de Paul
   3. Marguerite d'Youville
   4. Lady Ishbel Aberdeen
3. The first doctoral nursing program in Canada was established in
   1. 1890
   2. 1933
   3. 1975
   4. 1991

4. Advanced practice nurses generally
   1. Work in the university setting
   2. Function independently
   3. Work in partnership with a physician or group of physicians
   4. Function as unit directors
5. Nursing has a code of ethics that professional registered nurses follow, which
   1. Defines the principles by which nurses' provide care to their clients
   2. Ensures identical care to all clients
   3. Protects the client from harm
   4. Improves self-health care
6. Which of the following is NOT a function of a professional nursing organization?
   1. Regulates registration and professional conduct
   2. Monitors unregulated care providers
   3. Collaborates with other health care organizations on matters of mutual interest
   4. Establishes standards of education and professional practice
7. The practice of nursing is regulated by
   1. The CNA
   2. Nursing practice acts
   3. Best practice guidelines
   4. Hospital administrators and taxpayers
8. Some of the professional standards outlined by the College of Nurses of Ontario include
   1. Accountability, ethics, leadership
   2. Administration of medications, personal hygiene, and grooming
   3. Care of vulnerable populations
   4. Care of people in financial crises
9. Except for Ontario and Quebec, minimum standards for nursing education are set by
   1. The nursing school
   2. The provincial/territorial nursing association
   3. The Canadian Nurses Association (CNA)
   4. The Canadian Nurses Federation (CNF)
10. A role of a nursing union is to
    1. Devise ethical standards to guide practice
    2. Set standards of practice
    3. Represent nurses at the bargaining table when new contracts are negotiated
    4. Carry out the regulatory functions of registration and licensure

References

Allemang, M. M. (1974). *Nursing education in the United States and Canada, 1873–1950: Leading figures, forces, views on education.* Ph.D. dissertation, University of Washington, Seattle.

Bonin, M. A. (1976). *Trends in integrated basic degree nursing programs in Canada: 1942–1972.* Unpublished Ph.D. dissertation, University of Ottawa, Ottawa, ON.

Brown, G. (Ed.). (1966). *Dictionary of Canadian biography: 1000 to 1790* (Vol. 1). Toronto, ON: University of Toronto Press.

Canadian Nurses Association. (1965). *Report on the Canadian Nurses Association School Improvement Program.* Ottawa, ON: Author.

Canadian Nurses Association. (1968). *The leaf and the lamp.* Ottawa, ON: Author.

Canadian Nurses Association. (1986). CNA's Certification Program: An Information Booklet. Ottawa, ON: Author.

Canadian Nurses Association. (1991). NB for BN: Province joins nurses' call for degree. *Edufacts, 1*(2), 1.

Canadian Nurses Association. (1998). *CNA's vision statement.* Ottawa, ON: Author.

Canadian Nurses Association and Canadian Association of Schools of Nursing. (2004). *Joint Position Statement: Educational Preparation for Entry to the Practice of Nursing.* Ottawa, ON: Author.

Chapman, M. E. (1969). *Nursing education and the movement for higher education for women: A study of interrelationship, 1870–1900.* Doctor of Education thesis, Columbia University, New York.

College of Nurses of Ontario. (1996). *Professional standards for registered nurses and registered practical nurses in Ontario.* Toronto, ON: Author.

Gibbon, J. M., & Mathewson, M. S. (1947). *Three centuries of Canadian nursing.* Toronto, ON: Macmillan.

Gunn, J. I. (1933, March). Educational adjustments recommended by the survey. *Canadian Nurse, 29,* 139–145.

Healey, P. (1990). *The Mack training school for nurses.* Doctoral dissertation, University of Texas, Austin.

Henderson, V. (1966). *The nature of nursing.* New York: Macmillan.

Nightingale, F. (1979). *Cassandra.* New York: The Feminist Press of the City University of New York. (Original work published 1872)

Media Statement by the Canadian Medical Association, Canadian Nurses Association, Canadian Pharmacists Association, and Canadian Healthcare Association. Retrieved September 15, 2004, from *http://www.cna-nurses.ca/_frames/search/searchframe.htm*

Paul, P. (1998). Nursing education becomes synonymous with nursing service: The development of training schools. In J. C. Ross-Kerr (Ed.), *Prepared to care: Nurses and nursing in Alberta.* Edmonton: The University of Alberta Press.

Reich, J. R. (1984). *Colonial America.* Englewood Cliffs, NJ: Prentice-Hall.

Riegler, N. (1997). *Jean I. Gunn, nursing leader.* Markham, ON: Associated Medical Services with Fitzhenry and Whiteside.

Ross-Kerr, J. (2003). Early nursing in Canada, 1600–1760: A legacy for the future. In J. C. Ross-Kerr & M. J. Wood (Eds.), *Canadian nursing: Issues and perspectives* (pp. 3–13). Toronto, ON: Elsevier Science.

Ross-Kerr, J. (2003). Issues in the organization and financing of health care. In J. C. Ross-Kerr & M. J. Wood (Eds.), *Canadian nursing: Issues and perspectives* (pp. 3–13). Toronto, ON: Elsevier Science.

Royal Commission on Health Services. (1964). *Report.* Ottawa, ON: Queen's Printer.

S.E.I.U. Local 333 v Nipawin District Staff Nurses Association et al. (1973) Carswell, SK 120[1974] 1 W.W.R. 653, 41 D.L.R. (3d) 6, 73 C.L.L.C. 14,193, [1975] 1 S.C.R. 382.

Tunis, B. L. (1966). *In caps and gowns.* Montreal, QC: McGill University Press.

Weir, G. M. (1932). *Survey of nursing education in Canada.* Toronto, ON: University of Toronto Press.

Wood, M. J. (2003). Monitoring standards in nursing education. In J. C. Ross-Kerr & M. J. Wood (Eds.), *Canadian nursing: Issues and perspectives.* Toronto, ON: Elsevier Science.

Young, S. L. (1994) *Standards in diploma nursing education: The involvement of the University of Alberta, 1920–1970.* Master of Nursing thesis, University of Alberta, Edmonton.

Recommended Web Sites

Canadian Association for the History of Nursing (CAHN):
http://www.ualberta.ca/~jhibberd/CAHN_ACHN/
An affiliate group of the Canadian Nurses Association, the CAHN offers information about Canadian nursing history and promotes historical research.

Canadian nursing organizations:
http://www.nurses.info/ organizations_canada.htm
This site offers a list of current Canadian nursing organizations, including contact information.

Registered Nurses Association of Ontario (RNAO) Best Practice Guidelines:
http://www.rnao.org/bestpractices/
The RNAO launched the Nursing Best Practice Guidelines Project in November 1999 with funding from the Ontario Ministry of Health and Long Term Care. This Web site directs users to all completed Best Practice Guidelines and in-progress guidelines. All guidelines may be downloaded free of charge.

4

Community-Based Nursing Practice

Kaysi Eastlick Kushner, RN, PhD (Canadian author)

Objectives

Mastery of content in this chapter will enable the student to:

- Define the key terms listed.
- Explain the relationship between public health nursing and community health nursing.
- Differentiate between community health nursing and community-based nursing.
- Discuss the role of the community health nurse.
- Discuss the role of the nurse in community-based practice.
- Explain the characteristics of clients from vulnerable populations that influence a nurse's approach to care.
- Describe the roles and competencies important for success in community health nursing practice.
- Describe elements of a community assessment.

Today's health care climate is rapidly changing in response to economic pressures, technological and medical advances, and client participation in health care. As a result, many clients are receiving care in the community rather than in hospital. There is a growing need to deliver health care where people live, work, and learn through a community nursing model. Community care focuses on health promotion, disease prevention, and restorative and palliative care. The goals of community nursing are to keep individuals healthy, provide in-home care for ill or disabled clients, encourage client participation and choice in care, and contain costs.

Promoting individual and community health has always been key to the holistic practice of nursing. In the 1730s, the Grey Nuns were established as Canada's first community nursing order. More than a century later in England, Florence Nightingale articulated a nursing philosophy grounded in knowledge of environmental conditions. By the end of the century, the Victorian Order of Nurses was providing in-home nursing, often in outpost and remote regions. After World War I, community nursing responsibilities "extended to screening programs to detect disease at early stages, to helping to maintain a healthy environment, and to providing nursing care" (Ross-Kerr, 1996, p. 11).

Canadians such as Kate Brighty (Box 4-1) and Edith Kathleen Russell (see Box 4-5) pioneered community health nursing and public health nursing in Canada. Today nursing is leading the way in assessing, implementing, and evaluating all types of public and community health services needed by clients. Community health nursing and community-based nursing are needed to improve the health of the general public.

Achieving Healthy Populations and Communities

Nurses practising in the community face many challenges in promoting the health of populations and community groups. A **population** is a collection of individuals who have in common one or more personal or environmental characteristics (Stanhope & Lancaster, 2004). Examples of populations include

Box 4-1 Milestones in Canadian Nursing History

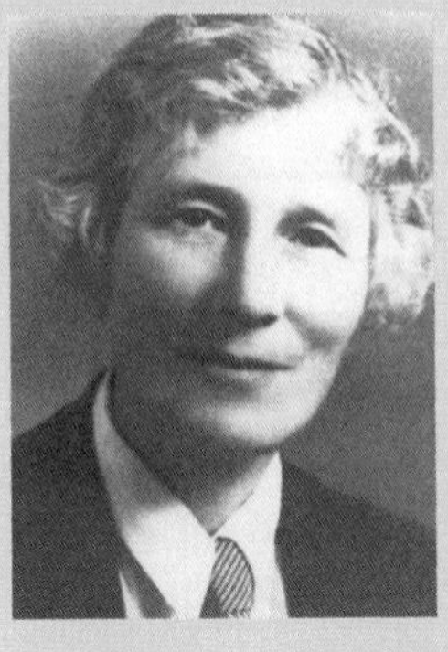

Kate Brighty Colley, 1883–1985

Born in England in 1883, Kate Brighty immigrated with her parents to Nova Scotia at the age of 3 years. She graduated from the Royal Alexandra Hospital School of Nursing in Edmonton in 1917, after which she enlisted with the Canadian Army Medical Corps in Calgary.

After completing a course in public health nursing at the University of Alberta in 1919, Brighty was one of the first nurses to be appointed to the staff of the new Alberta Department of Public Health. Soon afterward, the Alberta Department of Agriculture engaged her to teach home nursing, bedside care, and hygiene in Grande Prairie.

In the same year, Brighty was appointed matron of the second municipal hospital in Alberta, the Mission Hospital at Onoway. Because there were no physicians in the region, she and her two employees staffed the hospital and visited rural patients on horseback. In 1923, she returned to the Department of Public Health to establish a district nursing centre at Buck Lake near Pendryl, southwest of Edmonton—an area that had no roads at the time—and then another centre, farther north at Wanham, near the Peace River. Here she travelled by cutter to assist women in labour and those who were ill.

In 1925, Brighty took a post-graduate course in public health nursing at Columbia University, New York. Upon her return to Alberta in 1928, she was appointed director of public health nurses and, a year later, inspector of hospitals.

In her new post, Brighty established a number of new district nursing centres. As a former district nurse, she understood the problems these nurses faced, and she travelled widely to visit staff. She expanded the health education program and gave talks on the radio on health, hygiene, nutrition, and child welfare. These broadcasts were important to residents of remote areas, where little formal health care was available.

Brighty was active in the Alberta Association of Registered Nurses and, in 1936, was elected president of the organization. She wrote the first history of nursing in Alberta, the *AARN Blue Book*.

Brighty retired in 1943 to Vancouver, where she contributed regularly to the *Halifax Chronicle, Atlantic Monthly,* and other magazines. In 1970, she published *While Rivers Flow: Stories of Early Alberta,* experiences and short stories based on her public health nursing practice.

Sources: AARN Museum and Archives 91.41-P24; *While Rivers Flow: Stories of Early Alberta,* by K. Brighty Colley, 1970, Saskatoon, SK: The Western Producer; *These Were Our Yesterdays: A History of District Nursing in Alberta,* by I. Stewart, 1979, Altona, MB: Friesen Printers.

Canadians inclusively, or more specifically, high-risk infants, older adults, or a cultural group such as Aboriginals. A healthy population is composed of healthy individuals, and the health of individuals is considered an overall aggregate that reflects an average or general healthiness or health status. In determining a population's health status, individual characteristics are considered, such as occurrence of illness, disability, and death; lifespan; education; and living conditions.

A **community** is a group of people that share a geographic (locational) dimension and a social (relational) dimension (Edwards & Moyer, 2000). The social dimension—which comprises individual relationships, interactions among groups, and shared characteristics among members—distinguishes a community from a population. Examples of communities include geographic groupings (e.g., neighbourhoods) and shared interest groups (e.g., women's health networks). A healthy community consists of healthy individuals engaged in collective relationships that create a supportive living environment. Both individual and community characteristics are used to determine community health status. Key characteristics of a healthy community include a collective capacity to solve problems; adequate living conditions; environmental safety; and sustainable resources such as employment, health and educational facilities.

To understand community health nursing, one first needs to know how public health works. The emphasis in **public health** is on the health of the entire population. Historically, government-funded agencies have supported public health programs that improve food and water safety and provide adequate sewage disposal. Public health policy has largely been responsible for the dramatic gain in life expectancy for North Americans during the last century (McKay, 2005; Shah, 1994; Stanhope & Lancaster, 2004).

The goal of public health is to achieve a healthy environment for all. Principles of public health can be applied to individuals, families, groups, or communities. By using public health principles, the nurse is better able to understand the environments in which clients live, the factors that influence client health, and the types of interventions supportive of client health. Figure 4–1 illustrates a framework for public health programs that provides a means of organizing program development in public health practice (Edwards & Moyer, 2000).

As discussed in chapter 1, **population health** emerged in Canada in the 1990s as an approach to public health. The overall goals of a population health approach are to maintain and improve the health of the entire population and to eliminate health disparities (Health Canada, 1998).

The population health approach provides a framework for thinking about health and for taking action to improve the health of populations. Action is primarily directed at community levels. Strategies address the determinants of health in order to improve population health and reduce risks (see chapter 1). Most health determinants involve other sectors of society such as education, agriculture, business, and government. Therefore, multisectoral collaboration between health and other sectors is essential in a population health approach. This approach

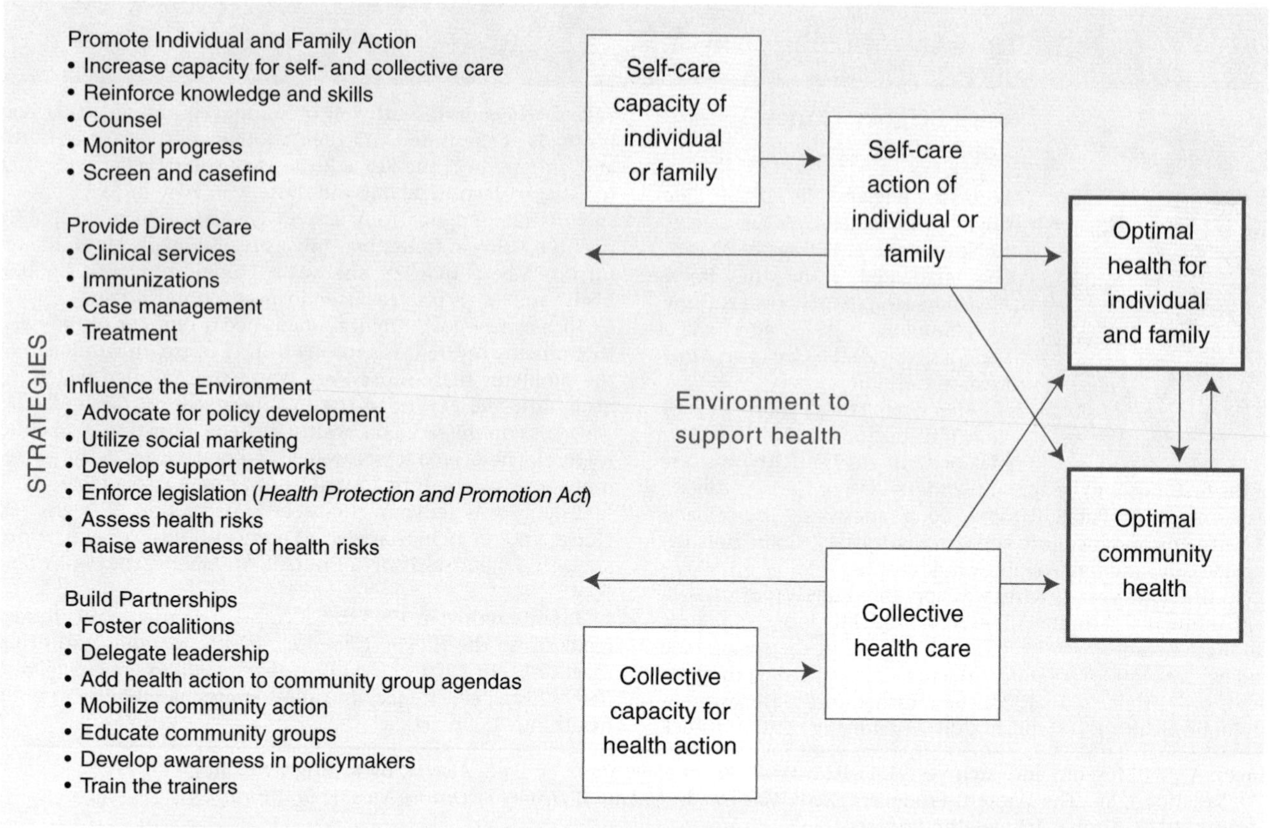

FIGURE 4–1 Framework for public health programs. (From *Building and Sustaining Collective Health Action: A Framework for Community Health Practitioners,* by N. Edwards et al., 1995, Ottawa ON: Community Health Research Unit, Pub. No. DP95-1, as cited in "Community Needs and Capacity Assessment: Critical Component of Program Planning," by N. Edwards and A. Moyer, in *Community Nursing: Promoting Canadian's Health,* 2nd ed., M. Stewart, Ed., 2000, Toronto, ON: W. B. Saunders.)

further broadens the scope of nursing practice in the community. Population-based public health programs focus on disease prevention, health protection, and health promotion, which provide the foundation for health care services at all levels (see chapter 2).

Community Nursing Practice

The scope of **community nursing practice** includes population-focused health promotion, protection, maintenance, and restoration; community-, family-, and individual-focused health promotion; and individual-focused rehabilitation or palliative care at the end of life. The term is broad, encompassing public health nursing, community health nursing, and community-based nursing.

Public Health Nursing and Community Health Nursing

The terms *community health nursing* and *public health nursing* are sometimes used interchangeably. There are similarities. **Public health nursing** merges knowledge from the public health sciences with professional nursing theories to safeguard and improve the health of populations in the community (Canadian Public Health Association [CPHA], 1990). A public health focus requires understanding the needs of a population. Focus may be narrowed to vulnerable populations, such as older adults, low-income families, or recent immigrants. Public health professionals must understand factors that influence the health promotion and health maintenance of groups, trends and patterns influencing the occurrence of disease or risks within populations, environmental factors contributing to health and illness, and political processes used to influence public policy. A public health nurse requires preparation at the basic entry level and may require a baccalaureate degree in nursing that includes preparation for public health nursing. A public health specialist has a graduate degree with a focus in the public health.

Community health nursing promotes and protects the health of individuals, families, groups, communities, and populations (Community Health Nurses Association of Canada [CHNAC], 2003). It involves coordinating care and planning services, programs, and policies by collaborating with individuals, caregivers, families, other disciplines, communities, and governments (CHNAC, 2003). It combines knowledge of nursing theory, social sciences, and public health sciences.

Community health nursing includes public health nursing, home health nursing, community mental health nursing, and occupational health nursing (CHNAC, 2003; McKay, 2005). The focus is broader than that of public health, emphasizing both the community's health and direct care to subpopulations within that community. Nurses use their clinical expertise to provide direct care (e.g., a case manager follows clients recovering from stroke and provides rehabilitation services). By focusing on subpopulations, the community health nurse cares for the whole community and considers the individual to be one member of a group. The practice focus of various specialties within community health nursing can be compared to the shifting perspective of a camera lens: for example, home health nurses zoom in to focus on individual clients, then wide angle their view to consider family and community, whereas public health nurses more often shift from a wide angle view of populations to a close-up on specific risk groups or families (CHNAC, 2003).

An advanced degree may not be required for community health nursing. However, nurses with a graduate degree in nursing who practise in community settings are considered community health nurse specialists, regardless of their public health experience (Stanhope & Lancaster, 2004).

Both public health nursing and community health nursing provide primary health care. **Primary health care** focuses on education, rehabilitation, support services, and health promotion and disease prevention. It involves multidisciplinary teams and collaboration with other sectors as well as with secondary and tertiary care facilities (see chapter 2). Primary health care principles guide community health nurses to use empowerment-based models of community practice (Chalmers & Bramadat, 1996). **Empowerment** may be most simply described as a means by which people, individually and collectively in organizations and communities, exercise their ability to effect change.

Public and community health nursing practice require a distinct set of skills and knowledge. Expert community health nurses understand the needs of a population or community through experiences with families and groups. They think critically in applying a wide range of knowledge to find the best approaches for partnering with their clients. Public health nurses perceive value in their distinctive practice, which enables them to see "the big picture" owing to their "broad health knowledge base, in-depth understanding of the community and community resources, and . . . appreciation of individual–family–community inter-relationships" (Reutter & Ford, 1996, p. 8).

A successful community health nursing practice involves building relationships with the community and being responsive to changes within it (CPHA, 1990; Diekemper, SmithBattle, & Drake, 1999). For example, when a community experiences an increased incidence of grandparents caring for their grandchildren, a nurse can provide support by creating an educational program with local schools. The community health nurse is responsive by being active in the community; knowing its members, needs, and resources; and establishing health promotion and disease prevention programs. This often means working with other professional systems and individuals and encouraging them to respond to a population's needs. Empowerment-based skills of client advocacy, communication, and the design of new systems in co-operation with existing systems help make community nursing practice effective. Figure 4–2 depicts an integrated model of community health promotion. The model shows how community nursing care encompasses action aimed at illness care; prevention of illness, disease, or injury; and health promotion. These three actions complement one another, even as their underlying aims, approaches to care, and perceptions of clients differ.

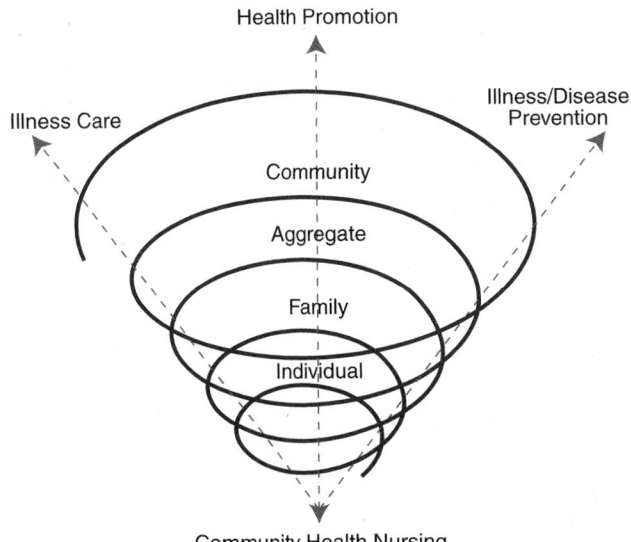

FIGURE 4–2 Integrated model of community health promotion. (From "Health Promotion for Communities and Aggregates: An Integrated Model," by S. C. Laffrey and D. M. Craig, in *Community Nursing: Promoting Canadians' Health,* 2nd ed., pp. 105–125, M. J. Stewart, Ed., 2000, Toronto, ON: W. B. Saunders.)

Community-Based Nursing

Community-based nursing involves acute, chronic, and palliative care of clients and families that enhances their capacity for self-care and promotes autonomy in decision making (Ayers, Bruno, & Langford, 1999). Nursing takes place in community settings such as the home, long-term care facility, or clinic, but the focus is care of the individual or family. The nurse's competence is based on critical thinking and decision making at the level of the individual client—assessing health status, selecting nursing interventions, and evaluating care outcomes. Because they provide care where clients live, work, and play, community-based nurses need to be individual and family oriented while appreciating a community's values (Zotti, Brown, & Stotts, 1996).

Components of community-based nursing practice include self-care as a client and family responsibility; preventive care; care within the community context; continuity of care between home and health system services; and collaborative client care among health practitioners (Hunt & Zurek, 1997). Nursing supports and improves clients' quality of life. Illness is seen as one aspect of clients' everyday lives. Nursing tends to be problem focused, addressing client needs for primary, secondary, and tertiary prevention (Hunt, 1998).

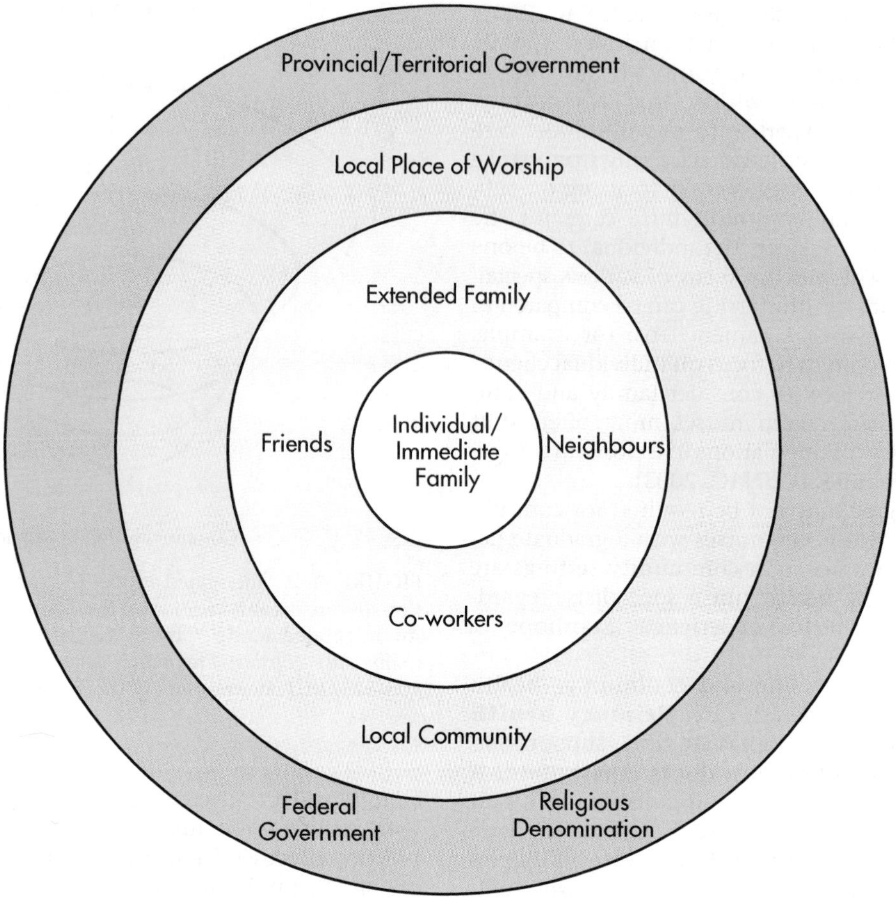

FIGURE **4–3** These concentric circles represent the social interaction units of the human ecology model. (Adapted from *Community-Based Nursing Care: Making the Transition,* by M. Ayers, A. A. Bruno, and R. W. Langford, 1999, St. Louis, MO: Mosby.)

The philosophical foundation for community-based nursing is the human ecological model, which conceptualizes human systems as open and interactive with the environment (Chalmers, Bramadat, & Andrusyszyn, 1998). In an ecological model, the individual is viewed within the larger systems of family, community, culture, and society. The social interaction units seen in Figure 4–3 depict four circles: the inner circle of the client and the immediate family, the second circle of people and settings that have frequent contact with the client and family, the third circle of the local community and its values and policies, and the outer circle of larger social systems such as government and church (Ayers et al., 1999). A community-based nurse must understand the interaction of all units while caring for clients and families in their natural environment. Nurses typically become involved in the domain of the first three circles. For example, a home health nurse with a client recently diagnosed with diabetes works closely with the client and family on establishing a care plan. The nurse uses his or her observations of the client's lifestyle when planning an exercise schedule and meal routines. Knowing community resources (e.g., shops with glucose monitoring supplies and local diabetes support groups) enables the nurse to provide comprehensive support.

Community-based nursing is family-centred care (Ayers et al., 1999). This care requires knowledge of family theory (see chapter 16), communication (see chapter 14), group dynamics, and cultural diversity (see chapter 9). The nurse collaborates with clients and families to help them assume responsibility for their health care decisions. The family is involved in planning, decision making, implementation, and evaluation of health care approaches. Community-based health professionals, together with members of the community, define the problem and develop strategies to remedy the problem. Eventually, local community members or groups assume the responsibility for running programs, which is consistent with a commitment to empowerment (Labonte, 1993).

The Changing Focus of Community Nursing Practice

Community nursing practice has changed in recent decades in response to social, economic, and political influences. Changes were documented by Chalmers et al. (1998), who interviewed community health nurse educators, administrators, and staff nurses who worked in public

Box 4-2 Trends in Community Health Nursing

- Increasing focus on at-risk, high-acuity, and high-needs populations
- Decreasing services to low-risk and well families
- Community development/community mobilization
- Closer links with institutions for discharge planning
- More acute care in the community
- More care of young disabled individuals at home
- Change in nurses' working conditions (e.g., evening practice)
- Little case-finding in the community
- Closer contact within primary care team
- Greater specialization
- Increasing skills mix in the community
- Increasing first-contact primary care role/nurse-management clinics

From "The Changing Environment of Community Health Practice and Education: Perceptions of Staff Nurses, Administrators, and Educators," by K. I. Chalmers, I. J. Bramadat, and M. A. Andrusyszyn, 1998, *Journal of Nursing Education, 37,* p. 109.

health agencies, home care and home health services, and community health centres in Manitoba. The nurses noted a shift in practice focus from universal programs to programs directed to high-risk or vulnerable groups. This shift has resulted in increasing demands placed on community health nurses who are faced with more complex care situations. Box 4-2 summarizes trends predicted by these community health workers. The identified trends, many of which have already influenced nursing practice, remain relevant as they reflect ongoing shifts in practice.

From interviews with public health nurses in Alberta, Reutter and Ford (1998) concluded that nursing roles and activities are also changing, particularly in response to economic policies and program decisions. Although many changes are consistent with the principles of primary health care and health promotion, there is concern that some changes put universal accessibility of services at risk.

Vulnerable Populations

Community health nurses care for clients from diverse cultures and backgrounds and with various health conditions. However, changes in the health care delivery system have made high-risk groups the nurse's principal clients. Community health nurses, for example, may not visit low-risk mothers and babies. Instead, adolescent mothers or mothers with drug addiction are more likely to receive home care services.

Vulnerable populations of clients are those who are likely to develop health problems as a result of excess risks, who have barriers to access to health care services, or who are dependent on others for care. Individuals living in poverty, older adults, homeless people, individuals in abusive relationships, substance abusers, severely mentally ill people, and new immigrants are examples of vulnerable populations (Hwang, 2000). Vulnerable individuals and their families often belong to more than one of these groups. In addition, health care vulnerability affects all age groups (Corrarino et al., 2000). Vulnerable individuals may also be a specific population with a distinct health care problem. For example, the older adult who has had a heart transplant presents specific health care needs (Baas et al., 2002).

Frequently, vulnerable clients come from a variety of cultures, have beliefs and values different from the mainstream culture, face language barriers, and have few sources of social support (Chalmers et al., 1998). Their special needs form the backdrop for the challenges nurses face in caring for increasingly complex acute and chronic health conditions.

To provide competent care to vulnerable populations, nurses in community health practice must be comfortable with diversity. Culture, race, ability, economic status, gender, and sexual orientation are all aspects of diversity in Canadian society. Sensitivity to diversity requires more than tolerance of difference, a phrase that implies that the dominant culture is the reference point. Rather, community nursing practice that is sensitive to diversity embraces diversity as valuable to individual and social well-being.

Chapter 9 addresses factors influencing individual differences within cultural groups and the nurse's role in providing culturally competent care. To be culturally competent, the nurse must be more than just sensitive to a client's cultural uniqueness. The nurse must be able to appraise and understand clients' cultural beliefs, values, and practices to work with them to determine their needs and the interventions most likely to improve their health. The nurse cannot judge or evaluate a client's beliefs and values about health in terms of the nurse's own culture. Communication and caring practices are critical to understanding clients' perceptions of their problems and to planning effective, culturally competent health care. The nurse needs to be aware of cultural and ethnic determinants of health, differing beliefs about health and medicine among ethnic communities, and barriers to accessing care for members of ethnic minorities (Shah, 1994).

Vulnerable populations typically experience poorer health outcomes than those clients with ready access to resources and health care services. Higher morbidity and mortality rates pose real threats to members of ethnically and racially diverse minority groups (Barr et al., 2002; Hwang, 2000). Members of vulnerable groups frequently have cumulative risks or combinations of risk conditions that make them more sensitive to the adverse effects of individual risk factors that others might overcome (Rew et al., 2001). Community nurses must assess clients from vulnerable populations by considering multiple risks and the clients' ability to cope with stressors. Box 4-3 summarizes guidelines for assessing clients from vulnerable population groups.

Poor and Homeless Clients. Low-income Canadians are less likely to rate their health as very good or excellent, and are more likely to suffer chronic illness and die earlier than Canadians with higher incomes, regardless of age, sex, race, and place of residence (Canadian Population Health Initiative, 2004). People who live in

Box 4-3 Guidelines for Assessing Members of Vulnerable Population Groups

Setting the Stage

Create a comfortable, non-threatening environment.
Learn about the culture of your clients so you understand cultural practices and values that may influence their health care practices.
Provide a culturally competent assessment by understanding the meaning of language and nonverbal behaviour in the client's culture.
Be sensitive to the fact that the individual or family may have priorities other than health, including financial or legal problems. You may need to help with their concerns before you can address health concerns.
Collaborate with others as appropriate; you should not provide financial or legal advice. However, do connect your client with someone who can help.

Nursing History of an Individual or Family

You may have only one opportunity to work with a vulnerable person or family. Try to complete a history that provides information needed to help on that day. Organize what you need to ask, and understand why the data are necessary.
Use a comprehensive assessment form that has been modified to focus on the special needs of the vulnerable group, but remain flexible. With some clients, it is both impractical and unethical to ask all the questions on the form. If you are likely to see the client again, ask the less pressing questions at the next visit.
Be sure to include questions about social support, economic status, resources for health care, developmental issues, current health problems, medication, and how the person or family manages their health status. Your goal is to obtain information that will enable you to provide family-centred care.
Does the individual have any condition that compromises his or her immune status, such as AIDS, or is the individual undergoing therapy that would result in immunodeficiency, such as cancer chemotherapy?

Physical Examination or Home Assessment

Complete as thorough a physical examination (on an individual) or home assessment as you can. Collect only data for which you have a use.
Be alert for signs of physical abuse or substance use (e.g., bruises, being underweight).
Assess a family's home using observation skills. Does the family live in an insect- or rat-infested environment? Do they have running water, functioning plumbing, electricity, and a telephone? Is perishable food left on tables and countertops? Are bed linens reasonably clean? Is paint peeling on the walls and ceilings? Is ventilation and the temperature adequate? Is the family exposed to raw sewage or animal waste? Is the home adjacent to a busy highway, exposing the family to high noise levels and automobile exhaust?

From *Community Health Nursing: Process and Practice for Promoting Health,* (6th ed.), by M. Stanhope and J. Lancaster, 2004, St. Louis, MO: Mosby.

poverty are more likely to live in hazardous environments, work at high-risk jobs, eat less nutritious foods, and experience multiple stressors. Clients with low incomes face practical problems such as limited access to transportation, quality child care to support employment, and medication or dental coverage from supplementary health benefits. Low-income status is prevalent among lone-parent families, unattached older adults (mostly women), and Aboriginal families (Canadian Population Health Initiative, 2004).

Homeless people have even fewer resources than the poor (Box 4-4). Their vulnerability lies in their social condition, lifestyle, and environment, which diminish their ability to maintain or improve their health or access health care. Homeless people live on the streets or in temporary accommodation such as shelters and boarding houses. They tend to distrust health and social services as bureaucratic and normative, using them only when their health has deteriorated (Thibaudeau & Denoncourt, 2000). Chronic health problems worsen because of barriers to supportive self-care and medical care. The homeless have a high incidence of mental illness and substance abuse. The nurse must help homeless people identify their capacities and resources, their eligibility for assistance, and interventions to help improve their health.

Abused Clients. Physical, emotional, and sexual abuse, as well as neglect, are major public health problems, particularly affecting older adults, women, and children (CPHA, 1994; Sebastian, 2004). "All forms of violence have damaging short- and long-term effects on mental, physical and spiritual well-being" (CPHA, 1994, p. 1). Risk factors for abusive relationships include mental health problems, substance abuse, socio-economic stressors, and dysfunctional family relationships. There may not be any risk factors present. Abuse occurs in many settings, including the home, workplace, school, health care facility, and public areas, and is most often committed by an acquaintance of the victim (CPHA, 1994). When dealing with clients at risk for or who may have suffered abuse, the nurse must provide protection. Interviews with clients should occur in private when the individual suspected of being the abuser is not present. Clients who have been abused fear retribution if they discuss their problems with a health care provider. Most regions have reporting agencies or "hot lines" for notification when an individual has been identified as being at risk.

Clients Who Engage in Risk Behaviours. Risk behaviours include tobacco use, substance abuse, and unsafe sex. Tobacco use continues to be a public health issue, accounting for at least one quarter of all deaths in adults

Research Highlight

Box 4-4

AIDS Prevention Street Nurse Program

Research Focus

The AIDS Prevention Street Nurse Program in Vancouver, BC, provides outreach HIV and sexually transmitted infection prevention for vulnerable, high-risk clients. Community health nurses with the program use harm reduction and health promotion approaches in their work. Harm reduction includes needle exchange for injection drug use, education to promote safer drug use and sexual behaviour, and support to clients in addiction treatment programs. Nurses go where the clients are: clinics, drop-in centres, detoxification centres, jails, door-to-door in hotels, or on the street.

Research Abstract

The purpose of the program evaluation study was to describe the nurses' work and its impact on clients, the challenges nurses faced, and the program fit with other services. Program nurses were interviewed, as were clients of the program including street youth, sex trade workers, and injection drug users. Challenges facing nurses include building trust with clients, providing needed care or resources, and involving other health care providers. Clients reported gaining knowledge, feeling better about themselves, being supported, and changing their behaviours to help themselves and others.

Evidence-Based Practice

- Key strategies to reaching vulnerable populations include working with clients "at their location, on their own terms, and according to their own agenda" and encouraging and facilitating client participation and choice.
- Client empowerment can be promoted through nurses' non-judgmental care, trust, and respect.
- Educating marginalized clients about health promotion and harm prevention increases their self-concept and encourages them to change their behaviour.

References

Hilton, A. B., Thompson, R., & Moore-Dempsey. L. (2000). Evaluation of the AIDS Prevention Street Nurse Program: One step at a time. *Canadian Journal of Nursing Research, 32*(1), 17–38.

Hilton, A. B., Thompson, R., Moore-Dempsey, L., & Hutchinson, K. (2001). Urban outpost nursing: The nature of the nurses' work in the AIDS prevention street nurse program. *Public Health Nursing, 18*(4), 273–280.

aged 35 to 84 years (Health Canada, 1999). Tobacco use among Aboriginal people, youth, and particularly young women is a concern (Health Canada, 2003). Understanding what tobacco means for clients is an important first step in working with them to address related issues and change risk behaviours.

Substance abuse is a general term that describes the use of illegal drugs and the abuse of alcohol and prescribed medications such as anti-anxiety agents and narcotic analgesics. Clients who abuse substances frequently also have health and socio-economic problems. For example, health problems for cocaine users can include nasal and sinus disorders and cardiac alterations that can be fatal (Sebastian, 2004). A substantial proportion of adult AIDS cases have been attributed to injection drug use (Geduld et al., 2003). Substance abuse, particularly alcohol abuse, remains a serious problem among Canadian adolescents (Gillis, 2000). Socio-economic problems often result from financial strain, employment loss, and family breakdown. Health care providers can help clients by assessing substance use for amount, frequency, and use. Often these clients avoid health care for fear of being judged by health care providers and concern over being turned in to the police.

Unsafe sexual practices and multiple risk-taking behaviours remain high among young people, particularly among young men (Health Canada, 1999). Unsafe sex creates serious health and social risks, including the risks of unplanned pregnancy and acquiring sexually transmitted infections (e.g., HIV/AIDS). Unplanned adolescent pregnancy creates risks for both mothers and infants, including pregnancy complications (DiCenso & Van Dover, 2000), low income, low academic achievement, unemployment, and violence (Gillis, 2000).

Clients With Chronic Conditions. "Chronic conditions are impairments in function, development, or disease states that are irreversible or have a cumulative effect" (Ogden Burke et al., 2000, p. 211). There are physical and emotional aspects of living with chronic conditions. Societal trends toward greater family mobility, maternal employment, smaller families, and female-headed low-income families are challenges for families caring for children with chronic conditions (Ogden Burke et al., 2000). Older adults experience more chronic conditions as they age (Health Canada, 1999). The shift in health care service delivery from institutional to community-based care places demands on families, particularly women, to provide caregiving in the community. Community health nurses work with clients, families, and communities to ensure adequate support for family caregivers and to promote access to resources and services.

When a client has a severe mental illness, multiple health and socio-economic problems must be explored. Many such clients are homeless or marginally housed. Others are unable to work or provide self-care. They require medication therapy, counselling, housing, and vocational assistance. No longer hospitalized in long-term psychiatric institutions, clients with mental illness are offered resources within their community. However, many communities face continuing difficulties in the establishment of comprehensive, coordinated, and accessible community-based service networks (Health Canada, 2002; Shah, 1994). Many clients who lack functional skills are left with fewer and more fragmented services. An increasing number of young mentally ill people have only episodic hospital care. Collaboration among community resources is key to helping mentally ill people obtain health care.

Women and Girls. Health is considered a gendered experience. Men are more likely to die prematurely than women, but women are more likely to experience depression, chronic illness, and family violence (Health Canada, 1999). As noted, women are at greater risk for problems related to low income, violence, selected risk behaviours, and the stressors associated with unpaid caregiving. Such risks are further complicated for some by geographically isolated settings (Leipert & Reutter, 1998). Community health nurses recognize the need to listen to, respect, and communicate with women in their communities (Leipert, 1999).

Youth and Older Adults. Unintentional injuries, unemployment, depression, and suicide are a concern among youth, particularly among young men and in Aboriginal communities. "Community health nurses who are concerned with adolescent health promotion must consider the broad range of factors that affect adolescent health decisions and behaviours. Individual, family and environmental factors must be considered, together with many structural and societal factors" (Gillis, 2000, p. 257).

With the increasing numbers of older adults, there is a corresponding increase in the number of clients with chronic disease and a greater demand for health care (Craig, 2000). Nurses must view health promotion from a broad perspective, by understanding what health means to older adults and ways they can maintain their own health. When individuals feel empowered to control their own health, they have less incidence of disability from chronic disease (Baas et al., 2002). Nurses can help improve the quality of life for older adults.

Competencies, Roles, and Activities in Community Health Nursing

A nurse in community practice must have a broad base of knowledge and skills to work with clients to meet their health care needs and develop community relationships. Primary health care and health promotion approaches help the nurse recognize the interplay between individual experience and social conditions, the value of diversity, and the importance of building capacity to promote health-enhancing change. In community health nursing practice, "nurses are responsible for the maintenance of professional nursing standards and of public health standards by being accountable for the quality of their own practice, striving for excellence, ensuring that their knowledge is current and taking advantage of opportunities for life long learning" (CPHA, 1990, p. 5). Cradduck (2000) concludes that the "legacy of community health nursing is its multidimensional role, community orientation, and advocacy" (p. 367). The CHNAC (2003) identifies five standards of practice for community health nurses: promoting health, building individual/community capacity, building relationships, facilitating access and equity, and demonstrating professional responsibility and accountability. These standards reflect a community health nursing process that enacts values and beliefs in caring, primary health care principles, multiple ways of knowing, individual/community partnerships, and empowerment. A summary of key roles and practice dimensions is presented below.

Direct Care/Service Provider. Community health nurses act as direct care and service providers when they work with clients to promote and protect health and to prevent injury and illness. In many communities, home visiting remains integral to community health nursing practice, as do services like health assessment and immunization clinics. Care may involve treating illness, monitoring risk conditions, educating or guiding informed decision making, and supporting client self-care.

Educator. Community health nurses must demonstrate competency in client education. They work with individuals and groups. Perinatal classes, infant care, child safety, and cancer screening are just some of the health education programs in which a nurse in community practice may participate (Corrarino et al., 2000).

As an educator, the nurse draws on a broad knowledge base as well as communication and learning process theory. The nurse provides information to support community, family, and individual decision making. The nurse may participate in formal education sessions such as prenatal classes, or in informal sessions such as discussions with families during home visits. Nurses guide and support client decision making during life transitions such as new parenthood, school entry, adolescence, and death. Clients need information to make decisions about health issues, but this is not enough to produce behavioural change. The nurse supports clients in applying information in their everyday lives.

Consultant. The nurse as consultant applies a broad knowledge base to provide information and support participation in health activities. In this role, the nurse involves not only clients, but also community members, care providers, professionals from other disciplines, members of other sectors, policy-makers, and government. The nurse responds to inquiries about and makes referrals to community resources. The nurse also develops collaborative relationships to support client access to these resources.

Facilitator. To facilitate is to promote. As a facilitator, the community health nurse works within a participatory process to identify issues, develop goals for change, and implement strategies for action and evaluation of results. Leadership, enabling, and advocacy skills are key to these activities. Leadership focuses on supporting processes that build capacity among participants, rather than on directing or controlling decision making. Enabling encourages client participation and experiential learning.

Box 4-5 Milestones in Canadian Nursing History

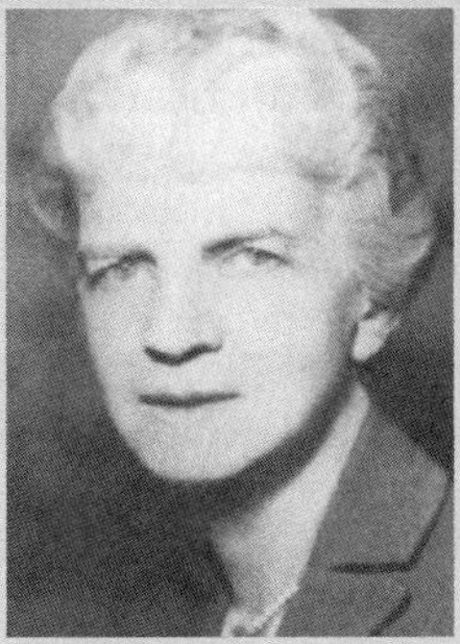

Edith Kathleen Russell, 1886–1964

Kathleen Russell was born in Windsor, Nova Scotia, in 1886. She entered the Toronto General Hospital School of Nursing in 1915, and after graduating, worked with the Department of Public Health in Toronto. In 1920, the Department of Public Health Nursing at the University of Toronto was established, and Russell was appointed its first director.

Russell recognized the great need for improved nursing education. At the time, an apprenticeship system in hospital schools was the norm, in which students, rather than graduate nurses, fulfilled nursing tasks. The primary focus of the hospital school system was not education but hospital service; the incentive was mainly financial. Although public health nursing was her department's original focus, Russell turned her attention to hospital nursing. She gained the support of the University of Toronto and the Rockefeller Foundation for an experiment in basic nursing education and obtained a grant of more than a quarter of a million dollars. Notably, this was at the height of the Depression, when other university schools were fighting for their very existence.

Russell's diploma program, begun in 1933, prepared nurses for hospital and public health nursing. In 1942, her program evolved into an integrated basic degree program controlled by the university, in which clinical practice was obtained at affiliated hospitals under supervision of university instructors. This program was the first of its kind in Canada, and was hailed throughout the world as an important new system of nursing education. Today, hospital-based schools of nursing have largely given way to schools in the general educational system, either in community colleges or universities, and most provinces are moving to the degree as the basic credential for nursing practice. Kathleen Russell is widely recognized as the architect of the integrated degree nursing program.

Source: *A Divine Discontent: Edith Kathleen Russell, Reforming Educator,* by H. Carpenter, 1982, Toronto, ON: University of Toronto Faculty of Nursing.

Advocacy fosters equity and accessibility, especially among vulnerable populations.

Communicator. Communication is fundamental to community health nursing. Skill as an effective communicator is closely related to the leadership, enabling, and advocacy skills of the facilitator. As a communicator, the nurse may use negotiation and mediation to foster collaboration. Communication skills support all other activities in community health nursing practice.

Collaborator. Collaboration is a way of working together that is characterized by recognition of interdependence, collective responsibility, and negotiated equity in relationships (Gray, 1989; Labonte, 1993). Collaboration involves more than linking or networking with others. The community health nurse participates in a collective process as a collaborator with clients, community members, agencies, and sectors. This process is supported by developing honest relationships and mutual respect, recognizing many forms of expertise, valuing diversity, and being organized and committed.

Coordinator. The coordinator's role has long been associated with nursing practice. Community health nurses work with clients and diverse agencies to coordinate or organize activities, resources, access, and care to promote client health. Coordinator activities complement activities as direct care/service provider, educator, social marketer, and community developer.

Researcher. Research is used to generate information, identify issues, determine directions for action, consider strategies to promote change, and evaluate results. The nurse must learn to review research and apply knowledge to practice. Community health nurses also engage in research projects as participants or investigators.

Social Marketer. Social marketing is an approach to social change, typically focused on behavioural change, that uses marketing and change theory in the design, implementation, and management of programs aimed at promoting awareness and acceptability of a social idea or practice in a specified subpopulation (Kotler & Roberto, 1989). Development of successful social marketing programs is supported by interdisciplinary and intersectoral environments that provide a broad base of knowledge, skill, and expertise in community health promotion. Community health nurses may act as social marketers to promote public awareness of issues and available programs and to build support for social action initiatives.

Community Developer. As a community developer, the community health nurse must support community participation. Participation encourages open identification of issues, shared decision making, egalitarian relationships, and collective ownership of action (Labonte, 1993). Participation and empowerment are closely linked.

Policy Formulator. Activities as a policy formulator include identifying the need for policy and program development; participating in program development, implementation, and evaluation; and helping to establish policies.

Community Assessment

A nurse needs to assess the community—the environment in which clients live and work. Without an understanding of that environment, any effort to promote the client's health and to support change is unlikely to succeed.

The community can be seen as having three components: structure or locale, the people, and the social systems. A complete assessment, such as the framework presented by Vollman, Anderson, and McFarlane (2004) involves studying each component to begin to identify needs for health policy, health program development, and service provision. When assessing the locale or structure, the nurse should travel around the community and observe its design, the location of services, and the locations where residents congregate. Information about social systems, such as schools or health care facilities, may be acquired by visiting various sites and learning about their services. Community statistics from a local library or health department can help assess a population's demographics. Discussion with community members is also helpful. It is essential to identify community resources and capacities as well as issues and problems (Edwards & Moyer, 2000).

Once the nurse has a good understanding of the community, individual or family client assessment may then be performed against that background. For example, consider the situation of the nurse assessing a client's home for safety. Does the client have secure locks on doors? Are windows secure and intact? Is lighting along walkways and entryways operational? The nurse conducts the assessment, with full knowledge of the level of community violence and the resources that are available to the client when help is necessary. No individual or family assessment should occur in isolation from the environment and conditions of the client's community.

Promoting Clients' Health

The challenge for nurses in community health practice is how to promote and protect the health of clients, whether within the context of their community or with the community as the focus. The nurse may bring together the resources necessary to improve the continuity of care of clients. In collaboration with clients, health and social service providers, and other community members, the nurse coordinates health care services, locates appropriate services, and develops innovative approaches to address clients' health issues.

Perhaps the key to being an effective community health nurse is the ability to understand clients' everyday lives. The foundation for this understanding is the establishment of strong, caring relationships with clients (see chapters 15 and 16) that support empowerment as an active growth process rooted in cultural, religious, and personal belief systems (Falk-Rafael, 2001). The "quasi-insider" status of nurses in a community often leads to the identification of local patterns and needs that can be addressed through programs, policies, and advocacy (SmithBattle, Diekemper, & Leander, 2004) that are responsive, supportive, and effective. This is difficult because the time that nurses have to spend with clients continues to decline. However, the expert nurse is able to advise, counsel, and teach after being accepted into the client's family or the community and by understanding what makes clients unique. The day-to-day activities of family and community life, and the cultural, economic, and political environment influence how the nurse adapts nursing interventions. The time of day an individual client goes to work, the availability of the spouse and client's parents to provide child care, and the family values that shape views about health are just a few examples of the many factors nurses must consider in community health practice. Once the nurse acquires a picture of a client's life, interventions designed to promote health and prevent disease can be introduced. Similarly, understanding the relationships, activities, and concerns of client groups and communities is central to health promotion practice.

Community health nursing practice is influenced by trends that focus attention on consumer participation, aggregates and communities, independent and interdependent practice, health promotion (Stewart & Leipert, 2000), population health, and health and social system reform that emphasizes community-based service delivery. The "continuing challenge will be to translate all these trends into the everyday practice of community health nurses in Canada" (Stewart & Leipert, 2000, p. 609) in ways that respect and promote collective as well as individual and family responsibility for health in everyday life.

Key Concepts

- The principles of public health nursing practice aim at assisting individuals in acquiring a healthy environment in which to live.
- The community health nurse cares for the community as a whole and considers the individual or family to be one member of a group at risk.
- A successful community health nursing practice involves building relationships with the community and being responsive to changes within it.
- The community-based nurse's competence is based on decision making at the level of the individual client.
- Within the ecological model of community-based nursing, the individual is viewed within the larger systems of family, community, culture, and society.
- Vulnerable individuals and their families often belong to more than one vulnerable group.
- The special needs of vulnerable populations form the backdrop for the challenges nurses face in caring for these clients' increasingly complex acute and chronic health conditions.
- Exacerbations of chronic health problems among the homeless are common because they have few resources.
- An important principle in dealing with clients at risk for or who may have suffered abuse is protection of the client.
- Clients who are substance abusers may often avoid health care for fear of being turned in to authorities.
- In community health practice, it is important to understand what health means to older adults and the steps they can take to maintain their own health.
- A community health nurse must be competent in fulfilling a multidimensional role, including activities as care or service provider, educator, consultant, facilitator, communicator, collaborator, coordinator, researcher, social marketer, community developer, and policy formulator.

- Assessment of a community includes assessing three elements: structure or locale, the people, and the social systems.
- An important consideration in becoming an effective community health nurse is to strive to understand clients' lives.

Key Terms

Community, *p. 53*
Community-based nursing, *p. 55*
Community health nursing, *p. 54*
Community nursing practice, *p. 54*
Empowerment, *p. 55*
Population, *p. 52*
Population health, *p. 53*
Primary health care, *p. 55*
Public health, *p. 53*
Public health nursing, *p. 54*
Vulnerable populations, *p. 57*

Critical Thinking Exercises

1. As a nurse working with the family of a severely disabled child, you learn that there is an absence of respite services to provide parental support and limited educational resources in your community. What activities or roles of the community health nurse would be important to establish a special-education daycare service, operated by volunteer educators?
2. Mr. Crowder is a 42-year-old man with diabetes mellitus and visual impairment. Your assessment reveals that he is homeless and that he currently spends nights in a shelter two blocks away. He has been unable to acquire medications or proper diet to control his blood sugar. What factors might you consider in attempting to support Mr. Crowder's adherence to medication administration?
3. Conduct a community assessment of an area that you have visited infrequently. Observe the community locale by driving or walking through the more populated area. Look for the following services: hospital, clinic, pharmacy, grocery store, schools, park or playground, and police and fire departments.

Review Questions

1. The overall goals of a population health approach are to
   1. Maintain and improve the health of the entire population and to eliminate health disparities
   2. Gather information on incident rates of certain diseases and social problems
   3. Assess the health care needs of individuals, families, or communities
   4. Develop and implement public health policies and improve access to care
2. Public health nursing is a nursing approach that merges knowledge from professional nursing theories and the
   1. Population sciences
   2. Public health sciences
   3. Environmental sciences
   4. Mental health sciences
3. Community-based nursing involves the acute, chronic, and palliative care of clients and families that enhances their capacity for
   1. Nursing care that promotes autonomy in decision making
   2. Improving their health care and self-care
   3. Self-care and promotes autonomy in decision making
   4. Learning about their illnesses
4. Vulnerable populations of clients are those who are more likely to develop health problems as a result of
   1. Chronic diseases, homelessness, and poverty
   2. Lack of transportation, dependence on others for care, and lack of initiative
   3. Poverty, unlimited access to health care services, and mental illness
   4. Excess risks, barriers to health care services, and dependence on others for care
5. Which is NOT an aspect of competent care of vulnerable populations?
   1. Providing culturally appropriate care
   2. Creating a comfortable, non-threatening environment
   3. Assessing living conditions
   4. Offering financial or legal advice
6. Major public health problems affecting older adults, women, and children are
   1. Prescribed medication abuse, poverty, sexual abuse
   2. Physical, emotional, and sexual abuse, as well as neglect
   3. Acute illnesses, neglect, abandonment
   4. Financial strain, poverty, physical abuse
7. A successful community health nursing practice requires
   1. A PhD
   2. An ability to build relationships with the community and be responsive to changes within the community
   3. Taking a passive role in the community
   4. Subspecialty training in an acute-care area
8. Teaching classes about infant care, child safety, and cancer screening are examples of a nurse in the role of a(n)
   1. Consultant
   2. Collaborator
   3. Educator
   4. Facilitator
9. A community health nurse who is directing a client to community resources is an example of a nurse in the role of a
   1. Consultant
   2. Collaborator
   3. Coordinator
   4. Researcher

10. A community includes the following three elements, each of which must be assessed:
    1. Structure or locale, people, and social systems
    2. People, neighbourhoods, and social systems
    3. Health care systems, geographic boundaries, and people
    4. Environment, families, and social systems

References

Ayers, M., Bruno, A. A., & Langford, R. W. (1999). *Community-based nursing care: Making the transition*. St. Louis, MO: Mosby.

Baas, L. S., Bell, B., Stuebbe, S. D., Giesting, R., & Wagoner, L. E. (2002). The challenge of managing the care of older heart transplant recipients. *AACN Clinical Issues, 13,* 114–131.

Barr, R. G., Somers, S., Speizer, F. E., Camargo, C. A. (2002). Patient factors and medication guidline adherence among older women with asthma. *Archives of Internal Medicine, 162,* 1761–1768.

Brighty Colley, K. (1970). *While rivers flow: Stories of early Alberta.* Saskatoon, SK: The Western Producer.

Canadian Population Health Initiative. (2004). *Summary report: Improving the health of Canadians.* Ottawa, ON: Canadian Institute for Health Information.

Canadian Public Health Association. (1990, November). *Community health–public health nursing in Canada: Preparation and practice.* Ottawa, ON: Author.

Canadian Public Health Association (1994). *Violence in society: A public health perspective.* Ottawa, ON: Author.

Chalmers, K. I., & Bramadat, I. J. (1996). Community development: Theoretical and practical issues for community health nursing in Canada. *Journal of Advanced Nursing, 24,* 719–726.

Chalmers, K. I., Bramadat, I. J., & Andrusyszyn, M. A. (1998). The changing environment of community health practice and education: Perceptions of staff nurses, administrators, and educators. *Journal of Nursing Education, 37,* 109–117.

Community Health Nurses Association of Canada. (2003, May). *Canadian community health nursing standards of practice.* Retrieved from *www.communityhealthnursescanada.org*

Corrairino, J. E., Walsh, P. J., Boyle, M. L., & Anselmo, D. (2000). The cool kids coalition: A community effort to reduce scald burn risk in children. *MCN The American Journal of Maternal/Child Nursing, 25,* 10–17.

Cradduck, G. R. (2000). Primary health care practice. In M. J. Stewart (Ed.), *Community nursing: Promoting Canadians' health* (2nd ed.). Toronto, ON: W. B. Saunders.

Craig, D. M. (2000). Health promotion with older adults. In M. J. Stewart (Ed.), *Community nursing: Promoting Canadians' health* (2nd ed.). Toronto, ON: W. B. Saunders.

DiCenso, A., & Van Dover, L. (2000). Prevention of adolescent pregnancy. In M. J. Stewart (Ed.), *Community nursing: Promoting Canadians' health* (2nd ed.). Toronto, ON: W. B. Saunders.

Diekemper, M., SmithBattle, L., & Drake, M. A. (1999). Bringing the population into focus: A natural development in community health nursing practice. Part I. *Public Health Nursing, 16,* 3–10.

Edwards, N. C., & Moyer, A. (2000). Community needs and capacity assessment: Critical component of program planning. In M. J. Stewart (Ed.), *Community nursing: Promoting Canadians' health* (2nd ed.). Toronto, ON: W. B. Saunders.

Falk-Rafael, A. (2001). Empowerment as a process of evolving consciousness: A model of empowering care [Electronic version]. *Advances in Nursing Science, 24*(1), 1–16.

Geduld, J., & Gatali, M. (2003). Estimates of HIV prevalence and incidence in Canada, 2002 [Electronic version]. *Canada Communicable Disease Report, 29,* 197–207.

Gillis, A. J. (2000). Adolescent health promotion: An evolving opportunity for community health nurses. In M. J. Stewart (Ed.), *Community nursing: Promoting Canadians' health* (2nd ed.). Toronto, ON: W. B. Saunders.

Gray, B. (1989). *Collaborating: Finding common ground for multiparty problems.* San Francisco: Jossey-Bass.

Health Canada. (1998). *Taking action on population health.* Ottawa, ON: Author.

Health Canada. (1999). *Toward a healthy future.* Ottawa, ON: Author.

Health Canada. (2002). *A report on mental illnesses in Canada.* Ottawa, ON: Author.

Health Canada. (2003). *Canadian tobacco use monitoring survey (CTUMS).* Ottawa, ON: Author.

Hunt, R. (1998). Community-based nursing: Philosophy or setting? *American Journal of Nursing, 98*(10), 44–47.

Hunt, R., & Zurek, E. L. (1997). *Introduction to community based nursing.* Philadelphia: Lippincott.

Hwang, S. (2000). Mortality among men using homeless shelters in Toronto, Ontario. *The Journal of the American Medical Association 283*(16), 2152–2157.

Kotler, P., & Roberto, E. (1989). *Social marketing.* New York: Free Press.

Labonte, R. (1993). *Health promotion and empowerment: Practice frameworks.* Toronto, ON: Centre for Health Promotion, University of Toronto, & ParticipACTION.

Laffrey, S. C., & Craig, D. (2000). Health promotion for communities and aggregates: An integrated model. In M. J. Stewart (Ed.), *Community nursing: Promoting Canadians' health* (2nd ed.). Toronto, ON: W. B. Saunders.

Leipert, B. (1999). Women's health and the practice of public health nurses in Northern British Columbia. *Public Health Nursing 16*(4), 280–289.

Leipert, B., & Reutter, L. I. (1998). Women's health and community health nursing practice in geographically isolated settings: A Canadian perspective. *Health Care for Women International, 19,* 575–588.

McKay, M. (2005). Community health nursing in Canada. In L. L. Stamler & L. Yiu (Eds.), *Community health nursing: A Canadian perspective.* Toronto, ON: Pearson Prentice Hall.

Ogden Burke, S, Kauffmann, E., Wiskin, N. M. W., & Harrison, M. B. (2000). Children with chronic conditions and their families in the community. In M. J. Stewart (Ed.), *Community nursing: Promoting Canadians' health* (2nd ed.). Toronto, ON: W. B. Saunders.

Reutter, L. I., & Ford, J. S. (1996). Perceptions of public health nursing: Views from the field. *Journal of Advanced Nursing, 24,* 7–15.

Reutter, L. I., & Ford, J. S. (1998). Perceptions of changes in public health nursing practice: A Canadian perspective. *International Journal of Nursing Studies, 35,* 85–94.

Rew, L., et al. (2001). Correlates of resilience in homeless adolescents. *Journal of Nursing Scholorship, 33*(1), 33–40.

Ross-Kerr, J. C. (1996). The growth of community health nursing in Canada. In J. Ross-Kerr & J. MacPhail (Eds.), *An introduction to issues in community health nursing in Canada.* Toronto, ON: Mosby.

Sebastian, J. G. (2004). Vulnerability and vulnerable populations: An introduction. In M. Stanhope & J. Lancaster (Eds.), *Community health nursing: Process and practice for promoting health* (6th ed.). St. Louis, MO: Mosby.

Shah, C. P. (1994). *Public health and preventive medicine in Canada* (3rd ed). Toronto, ON: University of Toronto Press.

SmithBattle, L., Diekemper, M., & Leander, S. (2004). Moving upstream: Becoming a public health nurse, part 2. *Public Health Nursing, 21*(2), 95–102.

Stanhope, M., & Lancaster, J. (2004). *Community health nursing: Process and practice for promoting health* (6th ed.). St. Louis, MO: Mosby.

Stewart, I. (1979). *These were our yesterdays: A history of district nursing in Alberta.* Altona, MB: Friesen Printers.

Stewart, M. J., & Leipert, B. (2000). Community health nursing in the future. In M. J. Stewart (Ed.), *Community nursing: Promoting Canadians' health* (2nd ed). Toronto, ON: W. B. Saunders.

Thibaudeau, M. F., & Denoncourt, H. (2000). Nursing practice in outreach clinics for the homeless in Montreal. In M. J. Stewart (Ed.), *Community nursing: Promoting Canadians' health* (2nd ed.). Toronto, ON: W. B. Saunders.

Vollman, A. R., Anderson, E. T., & McFarlane, J. (2004). *Canadian community as partner.* Toronto: Lippincott Williams & Wilkins.

Zotti, M. E., Brown, P., & Stotts, R. C. (1996). Community-based nursing versus community health nursing: What does it all mean? *Nursing Outlook, 44*(5), 211–217.

Recommended Web Sites

Canadian Public Health Association:
http://www.cpha.ca
The Canadian Public Health Association (CPHA) is a national, independent, not-for-profit, voluntary association representing public health in Canada.

Community Health Nurses Association of Canada:
http://www.communityhealthnursescanada.org
The Community Health Nurses Association of Canada is a national-level organization. It provides standards and information on community health nursing.

Fact Sheet—Primary Health Care Approach:
http://www.cna-nurses.ca/pages/fact_sheets/primary_ health_care _approach.htm
This Canadian Nurses Association publication defines and describes primary health care in Canada.

Health Canada: Health Promotion Online:
http://www.hc-gc.gc.ca/english/for_you/hpo/index.html
This federal Web site provides links to many useful health promotion resources and guides that will aid health professionals and community leaders.

Victorian Order of Nurses:
http://www.von.ca/
The Victorian Order of Nurses (VON) is Canada's leading charitable organization addressing community health and social needs.

5

Theoretical Foundations of Nursing Practice

Sally Thorne, RN, PhD (Canadian author)
Anne Griffin Perry, RN, MSN, EdD, FAAN

Objectives

Mastery of content in this chapter will enable the student to:

- Define the key terms listed.
- Appreciate the role of theorizing in the development of nursing knowledge.
- Differentiate between various nursing theories.
- Describe challenges associated with theorizing about nursing.
- Appreciate the historical development of nursing theory.
- Recognize selected conceptual frameworks for nursing.
- Interpret current debates within nursing theory.
- Describe the relationship between theorizing and other forms of knowledge development in nursing.

Modern nursing is guided by a knowledge base and set of principles for systematically applying that knowledge in an expanding array of contexts. Although certain nursing tasks can be mastered by most people trained to do them, the hallmark of nursing practice is this knowledge and its application across a range of unique circumstances. The purpose of nursing theory is to make sense of nursing knowledge, so that nurses can use it in a professional and accountable manner (Beckstrand, 1978).

A **theory** is a purposeful set of assumptions or propositions that show relationships between concepts. Theories are useful because they provide a systematic view of explaining, predicting, and prescribing phenomena. A **nursing theory** is a conceptualization of some aspect of nursing communicated for the purpose of describing, explaining, predicting, and/or prescribing nursing care (Meleis, 2005). Theories constitute much of the knowledge of a discipline, and theory and inquiry are vital linkages to each other (Fawcett et al., 2001). Nursing theories provide nurses with a perspective to view client situations, a way to organize data, and a method to analyze and interpret information.

Early Nursing Practice and the Emergence of Theory

Excellent nursing practices have been documented throughout history (Yura & Walsh, 1983). However, modern nursing, in which the knowledge and practice of nursing were formalized into a professional context, started with the work of Florence Nightingale. Nightingale was a visionary leader in Victorian England, who created systems for nursing education and practice (see chapter 3). Contemporary authors are beginning to explore Nightingale's work as a potential theoretical and conceptual model for nursing. Her "descriptive theory" provided nurses with a way to think about nursing with a frame of reference that focuses on clients and the environment.

Since Nightingale's era, nursing's status and authority have parallelled the authority of women in society. Following World War II, major developments in science and technology powerfully influenced health care, including nursing. Nursing science came into its own. No longer simply an application of the knowledge of other disciplines, nursing now had its own unique body of knowledge.

Since the 1960s, scientific knowledge has exploded in all disciplines, including health sciences, basic physical sciences, social and biobehavioural sciences, social theory, ethical theory, and the philosophy of science. Nursing knowledge both draws from and contributes to all these disciplines. It interprets and systematizes relevant facts and theories for use in nursing practice.

Major developments in nursing theory occurred in the late 1960s (Meleis, 2005). The health care system was expanding and changing, influenced by scientific discoveries and technological applications. Disease intervention was now more sophisticated and scientifically driven. The focus of health care had shifted from attending to the sick and injured to curing and eradicating disease. Physicians increasingly influenced the structure of health care. For the first time, nurses realized that they needed to articulate exactly how their role differs from those in other disciplines (Chinn & Kramer, 2004; Engebretson, 1997; Fawcett, 2005; Newman, 1972).

The drive for early nursing theorizing came from nursing educators, who noted that traditional ways of preparing professional nurses were becoming outdated. Until the 1960s, a nursing apprenticeship model, augmented by lectures by physicians, had seemed sufficient. Nursing educational leaders of this era were inspired to theorize about nursing as a way to structure and define what a curriculum oriented to nursing knowledge might look like (Dean, 1995; Orem & Parker, 1964; Torres, 1974). This meant grappling with large theoretical and philosophical questions, such as:

- What is the focus and scope of nursing?
- How is nursing unique and different from other health care professions?
- What should be the proper knowledge base for professional practice in nursing?

To answer these questions, early theorists developed conceptual frameworks, which organized core nursing concepts and the relationships among these concepts. These conceptual frameworks were "mental maps" whose purpose was to make sense of the information and decisional processes nurses needed to apply knowledge in nursing practice (Ellis, 1968; D. E. Johnson, 1974a; McKay, 1969; Wald & Leonard, 1964). Expressing nursing knowledge in scientific language created a context in which **nursing science** could be accepted and could flourish (Cull-Wilby & Peppin, 1987; Jones, 1997). However, these nursing theories were not the kind of scientific theories that one sets out to prove or disprove with empirical evidence (Levine, 1995); rather, they represented mental structures intended for the purpose of organizing knowledge nurses would need and the processes by which they would access and apply it to unique practice situations. Table 5-1 defines some basic terms that underpin the structure of scientific theorizing.

Nursing Process

Early nursing theories organized knowledge that a nurse would use in any clinical encounter. However, they did not involve a way to systematically apply that knowledge in each new situation (Field, 1987). Nursing knowledge was first systematically applied by Orlando in 1961. She conceived of a problem-solving approach that came to be known as the **nursing process** (Yura & Walsh, 1998). The nursing process originally involved four steps: assessment, planning, intervention, and evaluation. Each step

Table 5-1 **The Structure of Scientific Theorizing**

Term	Description
Concept	A mental formulation of objects or events. Concepts represent the basic way in which ideas are organized and communicated.
Operational definition	Description of concepts articulated in such a way that they can be applied to decision making in practice. It links concepts with other concepts and with theories and often includes the essential properties and distinguishing features of a concept.
Theory	Purposeful set of assumptions or propositions about concepts. A theory shows relationships between concepts and thereby provides a systematic view of phenomena so that they may be explained, predicted, or prescribed.
Assumption	Statement describing concepts or connecting two concepts that are accepted as factual or true. Assumptions include the "taken for granted" ideas about the nature and purpose of concepts as well as the structure of theory.
Phenomena	Aspects of reality that can be consciously sensed or experienced (Meleis, 1997). Nursing concepts and theory are often understood as the theoretical approach to making sense of the phenomena of nursing.
Theoretical model	Mental representation of how things work. An architect's plan for a house, for example, is not the house, but contains an extensive amount of information about how all of the building elements will be brought together to create the house.
Conceptual framework	The theoretical structure that links concepts together for a specific purpose. When its purpose is to show how something works, it can also be described as theoretical models. Conceptual frameworks that link the major nursing concepts and phenomena direct nursing decisions (e.g., what to assess, how to make sense of data, how to plan, how to enact a plan, and how to evaluate whether the plan has had the intended outcome). Frameworks are variously called nursing models, conceptual frameworks, or nursing theories (Meleis, 1997).

represented a distinct way in which general nursing knowledge could be applied to unique and individual nurse-client situations (Carnevali and Thomas, 1993; Henderson, 1966; Meleis, 2005; Torres, 1986).

- Assessment phase. Nurses would gather information to help them understand the client as a unique case, including biological, socio-cultural, environmental, spiritual, and psychological data related to the client's health or illness experience. They would then organize the data and interpret major issues and concerns (Barnum, 1998). This culminated in the nursing diagnosis—nursing's perspective on the appropriate focus for the client (Durand & Prince, 1966).
- Planning phase. Nurses would prioritize the issues raised during assessment in relation to the nursing diagnoses, identify which issues could be supported or assisted by nursing intervention, and create a plan of care.
- Intervention phase. During this phase, the plan would be carried out.
- Evaluation phases. The plan's success or failure would be judged both against the plan itself and against the client's overall health status. The goal of evaluation was to determine whether the intended outcomes had been achieved or if the nursing strategies needed to be revised.

The nursing process was intended as a cycle in which thoughtful interpretation preceded action, and the effects of action were evaluated in relation to the original situation.

The nursing process was widely accepted because it was a logical way to describe basic problem-solving processes and it used knowledge effectively to guide nursing decisions (Henderson, 1982). Nurses soon adapted the nursing process to represent a continuous rapid cycling of information through the phases. Although it was generally accepted as a useful way to organize and explain knowledge use in clinical practice (Meleis, 2005), some later theorists deemed the nursing process too linear and rigid for nursing's purposes (Varcoe, 1996).

In current practice, terms like *clinical judgment* are used to refer to reasoning processes that rely upon *critical thinking* and multiple *ways of knowing;* clinical judgment implies the systematic use of the nursing process to invoke the complex intuitive and conscious thinking strategies that are part of all clinical decision making in nursing (Alfaro-LeFevre, 2004; Benner & Tanner, 1987; Tanner, 1993).

Conceptual Frameworks

The conceptual framework builders of the late 1960s and beyond are usually referred to as *the nursing theorists.* All were fascinated with how excellent nurses systematically organize general knowledge in order to understand an individual client's situation and determine which of numerous strategies would work best to restore health and ameliorate or prevent disease (Orem & Parker, 1964). This reasoning process was different from linear, cause-and-effect reasoning, and it was what the nursing theorists understood to be the hallmark of nursing excellence (Barnum, 1998; Meleis, 2005). Indeed, when excellent nurses made brilliant clinical decisions, it was often difficult to determine how they used knowledge in making these decisions (Benner, Tanner, & Chesla, 1996).

The building of **models for nursing** was an attempt to theorize how all nurses might be taught to organize and synthesize knowledge so that they develop excellent reasoning skills (Raudonis & Acton, 1997). These theorists worked out frameworks and models to depict theoretical structures that would enable a nurse to grasp all aspects of a clinical situation and the larger implications of options for nursing care. Table 5-2 lists four types of theory.

Table 5-2 Types of Theory

Type of Theory	Description
Grand theory	Global, conceptual framework that provides insight into abstract phenomena, such as human behaviour or nursing science. Grand theories are broad in scope and therefore require further specification through research before they can be fully tested (Chinn and Kramer, 2004). A grand theory is not intended to provide guidance for specific nursing interventions, but to provide the structural framework for broad, abstract ideas about nursing. They are sometimes called paradigms because they come to represent distinct world views about those phenomena and provide the structural framework within which smaller-range theories are developed and tested.
Middle-range theory	Encompasses a more limited scope and is less abstract. Middle range theories address specific phenomena or concepts and reflects practice (administration, clinical, or teaching) The phenonoma or concepts tend to cross different nursing fields and reflect a variety of nursing care situations.
Descriptive theory	Describes phenomena (e.g., responses to illness of patterns of coping), speculates on why phenomena occur, and describes the consequences of phenomena. Descriptive theories have to ability to explain, relate, and in some situations predict nursing phenomena (Meleis, 2005). Descriptive nursing theories do not direct specific nursing activities, but they may help to explain client assessments and possibly guide future nursing research.
Prescriptive theory	Addresses nursing interventions and predicts the consequences of a specific intervention. In nursing, a prescriptive theory should designate the prescription (i.e., nursing interventions), the conditions under which the prescription should occur, and the consequences (Meleis, 2005). Prescriptive theories are action oriented, which tests the validity and predictability of a nursing intervention. These theories guide nursing research to develop and test specific nursing interventions (Fawcett, 2005).

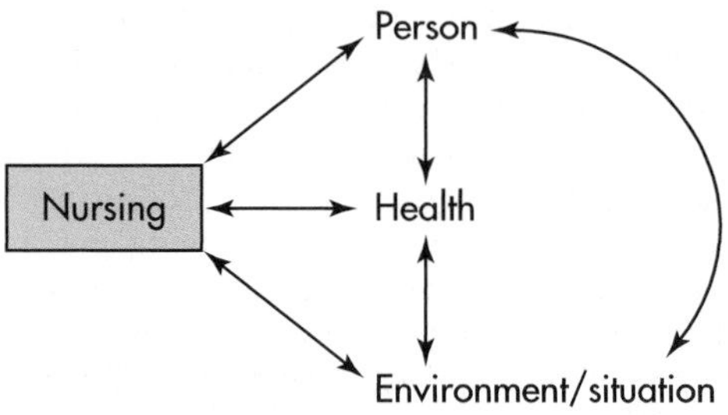

FIGURE **5–1** Nursing's metaparadigm concepts.

Metaparadigm Concepts

Each conceptual framework attempted to define nursing by creating a theoretical definition for the substance and structure of the key bodies of knowledge needed to understand clinical situations (Figure 5–1). This knowledge was called the **metaparadigm concepts** and included person, environment, health, and nursing (Fawcett, 1992).

Client and Person

By the 1960s, it was recognized that nurses did much more than simply care for hospitalized patients. Because of this, theorists used the term *client* to refer to the person at the centre of any nursing process. The term signified a range of health states, including both sick and well people, and a more negotiated relationship between the nurse and the individual toward whom the nurse's action was directed. At the same time, nursing was becoming aware of its potential to deliver care beyond the individual—to families, groups, and communities. However, although theoretical work to articulate the role of nursing in families and communities began around this time, most early conceptual models focused on the individual.

To help nurses systematically organize and make sense of vast information that could be relevant to any client, most early models clearly defined the concept of *the person.* Some understood the person as a system of interacting parts, others as a system of competing human needs. Some recognized that humans had biological, psychological, social, and spiritual dimensions. Each framework drew attention to multiple human domains so that the nurse could understand each experience of health and illness for its uniqueness in the context of an individual's body, feelings, and situation. Each model provided a whole picture of the individual so that the implications of any action or intervention could be thoroughly understood and nursing care could be systematically individualized.

Environment

Each conceptual framework understood that the person is embedded in and interacts with a complex environmental system. This environment might involve the person's family and social ties, the community, the health care system, and geographical and political issues that affect health. The early conceptual frameworks helped nurses understand the larger context of every experience of health and illness. The frameworks anticipated a future in which nurses would lead advances in social and health policy, health promotion, and community development.

Health

Because nursing has a social mandate to do good for both the individual and society, the early theorists struggled to articulate a goal for nursing. They defined health as more than the absence of disease or injury, but as an ideal state of optimal health or total well being to which all individuals can aspire (see chapter 1). This definition reflects a vision that nursing applies to both the individual and society, to all clients, sick or well. People with chronic illness can aspire to health just like others. Physically healthy clients with psychological or spiritual challenges are included in this ideal vision. Although perfect health might not always be achievable, nurses can help clients reach a state of health that is whole, productive, and satisfying.

Nursing

Each conceptual framework included a unique definition of nursing that linked a view of the client with an understanding of the person's environment and life and health goals.

Built on a distinct subset of knowledge, each conceptual framework presented a coherent and complete belief system about nursing practice, although they used different terms and aligned ideas differently. Nursing scholars assumed that one model would eventually become dominant (Alligood and Choi, 1998). This led to competition among the frameworks, and their application in practice became rigid and codified. The focus shifted from guiding nurses to think systematically, to using language in particular ways and filling out assessment forms correctly. Many nurses found these frameworks actually inhibited their systematic thinking. Much debate followed about the utility of the models.

Philosophy of Nursing Science

When nursing theorists began developing frameworks and models, nurses understood knowledge development as a matter of science and discovery. Theories were considered to be logical propositions that could be rigorously tested and proven to answer (or not answer) the hypothetical questions posed by a discipline. The early theorists created frameworks for the complex reasoning in nursing practice. However, they were working toward a vision without the tools needed to enact that vision. They were using the traditional scientific way of understanding how knowledge works without appreciating the limitations of science, especially in relation to complex problems. As well, they lacked the other kinds of knowledge that would become more obvious as thinkers in all disciplines moved beyond their traditional boundaries.

Scientific Revolutions

Thomas Kuhn, a philosopher of science, created a way of thinking about science and knowledge that led to many more options. First published in the early 1960s, his work was popular in the 1970s and 1980s as scholars realized how his ideas could develop knowledge. Kuhn challenged the traditional notion of science as a logical progression of discoveries. He argued that major scientific developments occurred when scientists thought about problems in radically new and different ways. These ways of thinking were so different from the traditional that an entirely different world view or "paradigm shift" developed. According to Kuhn, scientific advances happen when people think creatively and look beyond the norm. With creative thinking, they can understand problems that were once considered irresolvable (e.g., quantum physics introduced the idea that the behaviour of very small particles could explain atomic behaviour in ways that defied explanation using conventional Newtonian physics). This new way of thinking about the **philosophy of science** led nurses to consider their theoretical frameworks as more than theoretical propositions about logical relationships among concepts, but as actual world views, or **paradigms,** that would help them grasp the complexities of nursing (Fry, 1995).

Complexity Science

A second major shift in scientific thinking occurred with chaos theory (Gleick, 1987). This theory originated from observations of physics in which predictable patterns were found among factors that could not be predicted scientifically. This theory created a new way of approaching complex situations. Rejecting the simple cause-and-effect relationships used in traditional science, chaos theory led to what has been termed *complexity science.* In this kind of science, dynamic and interactive phenomena are interpreted within their natural context rather than by isolating their parts. They are reduced to the smallest properties that can be observed, and their actions are studied with little interference from real-life influences. For example, chaos theory helps us understand that, in sensitive systems, minor variations in initial conditions (e.g., barometric pressure) can explain such large-scale physical patterns over time (e.g., hurricanes). These ideas created a new language to apply to nursing. Nurses' experiences of health and illness are difficult to understand out of their individual context. Chaos theory gave them a new way to think about nursing (Coppa, 1993; Ray, 1998).

Nursing's Ways of Knowing

As ideas shifted, nursing theorists realized that science was just one of several knowledge forms necessary for their practice discipline. In 1978, Carper published an influential paper on patterns of knowing in nursing. The paper articulated a critical role not only for empirical science, but also for ethical, personal, and esthetic knowledge. Later, theorists added socio-political knowledge (White, 1995) to the list of central **ways of knowing** essential to excellent clinical nursing practice. These ideas contributed to discussions emerging in other social and life sciences around *how* we know what we know (Chinn & Kramer, 2004; Kikuchi & Simmons, 1999).

Paradigm Debates Within Nursing

With the new philosophical approach to scientific knowledge, nursing struggled with how to define itself as both an art and a science, as both an applied and a practical science (Donaldson, 1995; J. L. Johnson, 1991; Rodgers, 1991; Sarter, 1990). Its ideas about its theoretical foundations shifted. Some scholars began to question conceptual models as a valid form of theorizing (Holden, 1990). The frustration resulting from overly formal and rigid application of many of these models led to a period of what has been called *model bashing* (Engebretson, 1997). However, the problem confronting the early theorists remained: How does one organize and make sense of all possible bodies of knowledge that nursing might draw from and apply them intelligently to the challenges that arise in an individual clinical case?

In this context, many nurse scholars began to appreciate the original theories as being philosophical statements rather than scientific prescriptions. However, one group of theorists, considering some of the original theories to be overly simplistic and insufficiently holistic, began to categorize nursing models as belonging to entirely different paradigms of thinking (Parse, 1987). They depicted the majority of nursing's models and frameworks as old-fashioned and outdated, claiming that they reduced an understanding of the human person to fragmented parts out of context, and they coined the term *totality paradigm* frameworks to discredit these models. In contrast, they distinguished one particular set of conceptual frameworks as radically different in that they were both holistic and philosophically sophisticated, calling them *simultaneity paradigm frameworks* (Parse, 1987). Advocates of these simultaneity theories continue to represent them as philosophically and morally superior to the traditional ways of thinking that they believe were embedded in the collection of diverse theories that they refer to as the totality paradigm models (Cody, 1995; Nagle & Mitchell, 1991; Newman, 1992).

Nursing Diagnosis

Another discussion about nursing theory centred on nursing diagnosis. The conceptual framework builders focused on models to assess and interpret data about individual client situations. They were less explicit about planning, implementing, and evaluating nursing care. To fill this gap, **nursing diagnosis** emerged as an additional phase in that process. It became a discrete focus of nursing theorizing.

In the 1970s, scholars noted a need for a precise language to categorize and document nursing diagnoses into a taxonomy (Warren & Hoskins, 1990). This resulted in the formation of the North American Nursing Diagnoses Association, known as NANDA (see chapter 12), which held a series of consensus conferences to agree upon a list of the common client problems addressed by practicing nurses. This movement attracted debate on the merits of a fixed list of nursing diagnoses (as in NANDA) in contrast to the theoretically infinite options for nursing care that were the objective of the conceptual model builders (Fitzpatrick, 1990; Roy, 1982). Although it has been recognized as practical rather than theoretical (Fitzpatrick, 1990), the NANDA listing has become popular as a device to organize nursing care because it allows for efficient categorization into computer databases and the subsequent articulation of standardized nursing care plans. (Warren & Hoskins, 1990). However, despite its popularity with health care administrators, NANDA is commonly recognized by nurses as a system that relies entirely upon an agreement about what constitutes average health and illness experiences. It can therefore create worrisome barriers to nurses committed to the individualized care of clients who are understood as unique human beings.

Reflections on Conceptualizing Nursing

The scientific and philosophical work of nursing today is built on the foundation of early nursing theories. Nursing's theoretical history can be seen as an enlightened attempt to articulate excellent clinical reasoning in nursing. However, the discipline has yet to capture the mystery of how excellent nurses use knowledge. Theorizing in nursing is perhaps best understood as an extended philosophical struggle to understand how excellent nurses think. The excitement is best seen in the struggle, not in specific answers. When reflecting on nursing's theoretical history, it is best not to favour one theory over another. Rather, appreciate the creativity of our predecessors as they tried to make sense of our complex discipline.

Table 5-3 Milestones in Nursing Theory Development

1859	Florence Nightingale's *Notes on Nursing: What It Is and What It Is Not* published
1952	*Nursing Research,* nursing's first peer-reviewed scientific journal, established
1952	Hildegard Peplau's text on *Interpersonal Relations in Nursing* published
1955	Virginia Henderson's definition of nursing first published in the 5th edition of Harmer & Henderson's basic nursing text.
1961	Ida Orlando introduces nursing process
1970	Martha Rogers' model first published
1970	Callista Roy's model first published
1971	Dorothea Orem's model first published
1976	First North American Nursing Diagnoses Association (NANDA) on nursing diagnosis
1976	University of British Columbia model for nursing first published
1978	Barbara Carper's paper on fundamental patterns of knowing in nursing published
1979	Evelyn Adam's model first published (English version 1980)
1981	Rosemary Parse's model first published
1987	McGill model of nursing first published

Major Theoretical Models

This section is a brief capsule summary of some of the major theoretical models. It illustrates a variety of approaches as well as similarities and differences among theories. It may be helpful to view the conceptual frameworks in terms of larger theories on which they have drawn, such as adaptation theory, systems theory, or human needs theory. However, because many nursing theorists based their models on complex combinations of theories from many disciplines, the categorization used here may seem overly simplified (Table 5-3).

Practice-Based Theories

All nursing conceptual models were designed to guide and shape practice. However, few derived their theoretical inspiration directly from the practice setting. If this direction had been vigorously pursued, current nursing theories might effectively reflect societal and demographic changes, current health belief models and therapeutic strategies, and political struggles occurring in health care delivery. The early practice theories similarly reflected the issues that were shaping the role and context of nursing in their time.

Florence Nightingale. Whereas most later theorists drew on social and psychological theories, Nightingale was inspired by nursing practice. When she wrote *Notes on Nursing* (1859/1946), she described conditions needed to promote health and healing. Her observations during the Crimean War provided the first set of principles for nursing practice. Nightingale recognized the importance of the environment, including the need for clean patient areas and fresh air and light. She ensured that the wounded were warm, comfortable, and adequately fed. Torres (1986) notes that Nightingale gave nurses a way to think about their clients and the environment. By focusing care on an environment conducive to healing instead of on disease processes, Nightingale's conceptualization clearly differentiated the role of nursing from that of medicine.

The McGill Model. This Canadian nursing model was conceived by Dr. Moyra Allen (Box 5-1) and developed by her and her colleagues (Gottleib & Rowat, 1987). Systematically studying actual nursing situations, the model developers created a way of thinking about nursing that focused on promoting health. They recognized that many clients' health concerns were best approached through changes in lifestyle. They focused on the individual in the context of the family and, like Nightingale, viewed nursing as complementary to medicine. The main features of the McGill model include "a focus on health rather than illness and treatment, on all family members rather than the patient alone, on family goals, rather than on the nurse's, and on family strengths rather than their deficits" (Gottlieb & Feeley, 1999, p. 194). Over time, the model has been developed to demonstrate its application within a range of clinical contexts and settings (e.g., Feeley & Gerez-Lirette, 1992; Feeley & Gottlieb, 1998).

Needs Theories

Many early theorists organized their thinking by conceptualizing the client as representing a collection of needs. This reflected a common orientation to studying the nature of people made popular in the 1960s when needs, drives, and competencies were thought to hold potential for understanding human behaviour. Of these theories, Maslow's (1954) hierarchy of needs was one of the best known and most influential (see chapter 15). The idea that human behaviour can be explained by the competing demands of various basic human needs features prominently in many nursing models.

Virginia Henderson. Henderson conceptualized the person as a compilation of 14 basic human needs: to breathe, eat and drink, eliminate, move and maintain posture, rest and sleep, dress and undress, maintain body temperature, be clean, avoid danger, communicate, worship, work, play, and learn. Viewing the client like this helped Henderson define a nurse's role. Accordingly, she defined nursing practice as assisting the individual, sick or well, in the performance of those activities that will contribute to health, recovery, or a peaceful death. Henderson's model has remained popular in practice because its language is familiar and easy to comprehend. As well, it shows the nurse how a person's biological, psychological, social, and spiritual components combine to influence the way illness is experienced and health can be regained.

Dorothea Orem. Orem's self-care theory, which has its origins in Henderson's work, is used widely in both nursing practice and research. Orem's theory is actually three distinct, though related, theories that show how people are responsible for meeting universal self-care requisites, which are:

- maintaining sufficient intake of air, water, and food;
- maintaining a balance between activity and rest, and between solitude and interaction;
- providing for elimination processes;
- preventing hazards to life, functioning, and well-being;
- promoting functioning and growth in social groups in accordance with human potential (Orem, 2001).

Recognizing human needs and drawing on developmental theory, Orem's theory focused on the individual's role in maintaining health. This theory emerged when the passive role of the client was being questioned, and the health care system was less likely to take full charge of people's health. With increased understanding of illness patterns, it acknowledged the impact of multiple lifestyle factors such as smoking, diet, and exercise. Orem's theory reminded nurses that people can look after their own health and that they must learn to care for themselves within their families and communities. Thus, the role of the nurse, according to Orem, is to act temporarily for the client until he or she can resume a more independent role in self-care.

Interactionist Theories

Interactionist theories focused on the relationships between nurses and their clients. These theorists defined more clearly the specific human communicative and behavioural patterns by which practitioners met their clients' needs. They drew from the work of psychologists and psychoanalysts who shaped their thinking as they reframed definitions of the nursing profession.

Hildegard Peplau. Peplau, a psychiatric specialist, defined the core of nursing as the interpersonal relationship between the nurse and the client. Drawing from the work of psychoanalyst Harry Stack Sullivan, Peplau viewed this relationship as interactive and therapeutic, with a goal of having the client live independently away from the hospital. In Peplau's time, long-term stays in large inpatient psychiatric hospitals were common; her vision of nursing challenged this practice. Peplau articulated her view with the following words: "The kind of person each nurse becomes makes a substantial difference in what each patient will learn as he is nursed through his experience with illness" (1952, p. vii). Peplau's nurse was "an investigator, prober, interpreter, and reporter, using the rich data she extracts from the patient concerning his life. She

Box 5-1 Milestones in Canadian Nursing History

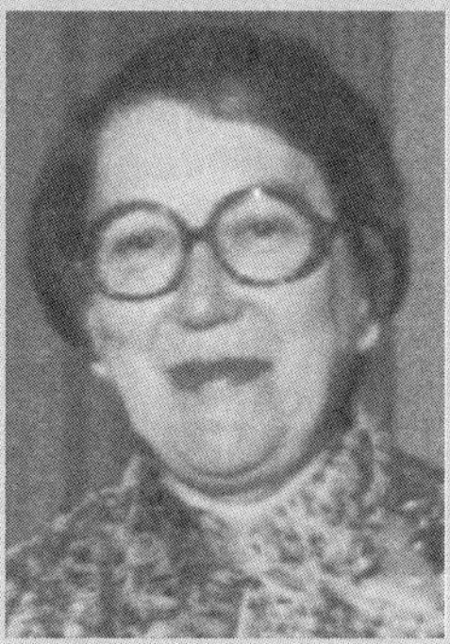

Moyra Allen, 1921–1998

A creative and independent thinker, Moyra Allen was one of the first Canadian nurses to earn a doctoral degree. She lobbied for collective bargaining rights for nurses and was the founding president of the United Nurses of Montreal. She was also the founder of *Nursing Papers,* renamed the *Canadian Journal of Nursing Research.*

Dr. Allen was a founding member of the committee that developed the criteria for accreditation of nursing schools. She designed an evaluation model for nursing schools and evaluated schools in South America, India, and Ghana. She joined the faculty of the School of Nursing at McGill in 1954 and became professor emeritus in 1985 upon her retirement.

In demonstrating her model of nursing, now known as the McGill model Dr. Allen established The Health Workshop in 1977, a community health facility where she put into practice a developmental concept of health and nursing as a prototype of primary health care. The workshop, viewed as complementary to existing services, was staffed with nurses, a community development officer, and a health librarian. The workshop's purpose was to demonstrate the validity of a local health resource managed by nurses that focused on long-term family health. It was an innovative way to improve the health status of families coping with illness and problems.

Dr. Allen received numerous awards, including the Jeanne Mance Medal. In 1987, she became a member of the Order of Canada for her outstanding contributions to nursing.

develops insights, his and hers, into the meaning of a patient's behaviour and helps the patient recognize and change patterns that obstruct achievement of his goals" (Barnum, 1994, p. 217). An early advocate of an orderly and systematic approach to care, Peplau created a way of thinking about nursing that directed nurses toward preventing illness and maintaining health.

Joyce Travelbee. Writing in the late 1960s and early 1970s, Travelbee also viewed nursing as an interpersonal process. In contrast to Peplau's psychoanalytic orientation, she drew from abstract ideas deriving from a form of thinking known as existential philosophy to operationalize this directive. Travelbee viewed nursing's client as including not only the individual but also the family and the community. In her definition of nursing, Travelbee articulated that the role of the nurse was to assist clients to "prevent or cope with the experience of illness and suffering and, if necessary, to find meaning in these experiences" (1971, p. 7). Travelbee emphasized that nurses should recognize the humanity of their clients and suggested that even the term "patient" should be regarded as a stereotypic categorization. Recognizing the reciprocity of human interaction, Travelbee focused nursing's attention on the communication that occurs between nurses and their clients as an important vehicle toward finding meaning in illness.

Evelyn Adam. Influenced by Dorothy Johnson, as well as the earlier interactionist theorists (Creekmur et al., 1986), Canadian theorist Evelyn Adam articulated the essence of nursing as a helping process (1979, 1991). From her perspective, the nurse played a complementary-supplementary role in supporting the client's strength, knowledge, and will. Adam's model drew on Henderson's framework of basic human needs and extended it into a model that would explain not only how nurses conceptualized the person, but also how they applied that knowledge in the context of a helping relationship characterized by empathy, caring, and mutual respect.

Systems Theories

In the 1970s and 1980s, when conceptual models for nursing were becoming more sophisticated and structured, several drew upon general systems theory (von Bertalanffy, 1968) for guidance in conceptualizing the complexity of human health. The main appeal of systems theory was that it accounted for the whole of an entity (the system) and its component parts (subsystems) as well as the interactions between the parts and the whole. In this way, systems theory allowed nursing theorists to expand the conceptualization of nursing through both structure and process, viewing the individual as an open system in constant interaction with its environment. Being outside the system, the nurse became one of the many forces that would have an impact on the system. Using a systems theory approach, nurses would understand that there are interactions between a system, its component parts, and its environment. They would recognize that to intervene in any one part of a system would produce reactions and consequences in other parts of the system and in the system as a whole. These general principles, considered common to all living systems, featured in all the systems models of nursing, regardless of how each theorist depicted the nature of the system.

Dorothy Johnson. Johnson's theoretical work was popularized in the early 1960s through class notes and speeches, but remained unpublished until much later (D. E. Johnson, 1974b). In her nursing model, Johnson identified the individual as a behavioural system with seven subsystems, each of which has a goal, a set, and a choice. The goals of the subsystems are based on the notion of drives, which are considered universal and applicable to all clients. However, the meanings attributed to each goal and the set of behaviours by which goals were achieved were seen as highly individual and therefore unique to each client. Together with the choices made by the client in relation to meeting his or her behavioural system goals, each subsystem also had a function that could be considered analogous to the physiological function of a biological system (Meleis, 2005).

The UBC Model. The behavioural systems model developed at the University of British Columbia School of Nursing was inspired by Johnson's model and was developed by a team led by Margaret Campbell that included several of Johnson's former students. Broadening the view of human experience based on behavioural drives, the UBC model considered the behavioural system to be composed of nine basic human needs, each of which is shaped by the psychological and socio-cultural environment in which it is expressed (M. A. Campbell, Cruise, & Murakami, 1976). Needs are universal and therefore fundamental to human experience. However, the specific goals toward which needs-related human behaviour are directed and the strategies for achieving those goals are unique to individuals and their particular physiological, psychological, or social circumstances (Thorne et al., 1993). Thus, the UBC model provided a structure by which general knowledge about human health and illness could be combined with particular knowledge about each individual client. In accordance with the tenets of general systems theory, the goal of nursing was balance of the behavioural system. The nurse's role is to foster, protect, sustain, and teach (M. A. Campbell, 1987) and thereby bring about not only system balance but also stability and optimal health.

Betty Neuman. Neuman's approach to theorizing nursing differed from that of other systems theorists in that she did not rely on concepts concerning needs and drives, nor did she break the system into any component parts. Neuman understood the person to be a physiological, psychological, socio-cultural, developmental, and spiritual being (Meleis, 2005). She oriented the attention of the nurse to the client system in a health-oriented and holistic manner (Neuman, 1982). Neuman considered the client system to have innate factors consistent with being human, as well as unique factors that characterized each individual person. She considered each client to have a unique set of response patterns determined and regulated by this core structure. Because the person is considered vulnerable to environmental stressors, Neuman conceptualized the role of the nurse as focusing on actual and potential stressors. Therefore, her model focused on prevention.

Sr. Callista Roy. In contrast to many other systems approaches, Roy did not consider the client to be a behavioural system, but rather an adaptive system. She viewed the person as a biopsychosocial being in constant interaction with a changing environment (Roy, 1984). Roy understood the person to have four modes of adaptation: physiological needs, self-concept, role function, and interdependence (Roy, 1974). As an adaptive system, the person has two major internal processes by which to adapt, and these represented the cognator and the regulator subsystems (Roy & Andrews, 1999). Using these mechanisms, Roy's model described and explained the interconnectedness of all aspects of human adaptation and conceptualized the role of the nurse in managing the stimuli that influence that adaptation (Meleis, 2005).

Simultaneity Theories

The theorists who identify their work as belonging to the simultaneity paradigm consider their theories to be radically different from the practice, needs, interactionist, and systems theories. Although these theories were first articulated long before the paradigm debate took hold, and before the terms simultaneity and totality were used to categorize the various theories, the language of simultaneity has become prominent in distinguishing this group of nursing theories from others. A characteristic feature of these theories is what Rogers (1970) called the "unitary human being." Previous theories sought to identify aspects of the individual that could represent an abstract conceptualization of the whole, but that also provided some access to the person and his or her problems, needs, or goals. In contrast, the simultaneity theorists view the individual as an entirely irreducible whole. Further, simultaneity theorists consider this holistic individual to be inherently and holographically connected with the universal environment. Thus, they represent a distinct way of articulating an understanding of the client of nursing and of nursing's role in relation to that client.

Martha Rogers. Martha Rogers's model (1970) was considered revolutionary in presenting the individual as an energy field in constant interaction with the environment, which itself was also an irreducible energy field, coextensive with the universe (Bultmeier, 2000). Nursing's role according to Rogers was to focus upon the life process of a human being along a time-space continuum (Rogers, 1970). An early proponent of pattern recognition, Rogers believed that pattern gave the energy field its identity and its distinguishing characteristics (Bultmeier, 2000). The object of nursing was to help the client reach maximum health potential in the context of change and development from a lower to a higher level of diversity.

Rosemary Parse. Parse's theory of "man–living–health" (1981), later termed "human becoming" (1999), also viewed the individual as a unitary and holistic being who is "continuously coconstituting patterns of relating" (Parse, 1997, p. 171) in mutual process with the universe. Nurses facilitate this process through their presence; their caring and their own patterns of relating support assist the individual in the human becoming process. Parse's nursing model does not articulate goals for nursing in the traditional sense of defining health; instead, it relies on the notion of people in a continuous process of making choices and changing health priorities. According to Parse's theory, nurses engage with people in their process of becoming through the application of three core processes: explicating, dwelling with, and moving beyond (Parse, 1999).

Jean Watson. Watson (1979) considered the individual to be a totality who can be viewed as a transpersonal self. According to Watson, the individual is much more than simply a body and an ego and can be more usefully understood as "an embodied spirit; a transpersonal transcendent evolving consciousness; unity of mindbody-spirit; person–nature–universe as oneness, connected" (Watson, 1999, p. 129). Watson intended that nurses do far more than deal with physical illness and attend to their primary function, which is caring. From Watson's perspective, caring infuses all aspects a nurse's role and draws attention to nursing acts as containing an esthetic that facilitates healing and growth (see chapter 15).

Theorizing the Future

Theoretical knowledge leads us to reflect on "the basic values, guiding principles, elements, and phases of a conception of nursing" (Meleis, 2005). The goals of theoretical knowledge are to stimulate thinking and create a broad understanding of the science and practice of the nursing discipline (King & Fawcett, 1997). Although our current vantage point helps us appreciate the inherent complexity of these objectives, the creativity and vision modeled by these early theorists continue to inspire nursing theorizing.

Nursing is solidly established as a distinct health discipline with its own unique science; however, current theorists draw heavily from philosophy to work out some of nursing's theoretical challenges. As June Kikuchi (1999) pointed out, much nursing theorizing of the past several decades has confused rather than clarified our thinking. As nursing scholarship includes stronger philosophical as well as scientific inquiry, nursing will be conceptualized with increasing clarity (Silva, Sorrell, & Sorrell, 1995).

Many nurse philosophers and scientists are using new ways of tackling the main problem in nursing theory—applying expanding, dynamic, and multiple sources of knowledge to a diverse range of client situations. The problem of understanding the general and applying it to the particular appears in the work of many scholars.

Afaf Meleis, a scholar of nursing theory, challenged nurses to direct their theorizing away from the processes by which nurses use knowledge and toward the equally challenging issues associated with the substance of that knowledge (1987). Accepting this challenge, many nursing scholars have shifted their theorizing to include both theoretical and substantive knowledge. Liaschenko (1997; Liaschenko & Fisher, 1999) has oriented our theorizing toward three levels of abstraction: knowing the case, the client, and the person. Engebretson (1997) positioned nursing theory in relation not only to biomedicine but also to Eastern and holistic understandings of health and illness. Starzomski and Rodney (1997) worked toward articulating the link between our definitions of health and more philosophical notions of the greater social good. J. C. Campbell and Bunting (1991) explored the possibilities of critical social and feminist theories for emancipatory theorizing in nursing. Watson (1990; Brenwick & Webster, 2000) developed the idea of embedding caring as a moral component of nursing theory. And Yeo (1989) considered the implications of ethical reasoning for nursing theory.

The interrelationships between practice and theorizing are of increasing interest to nursing scholars. A dialogue in which the dynamic interaction between clinical practice and theorizing (termed **praxis**) has started to emerge (Clarke, James, & Kelly, 1996; Mitchell, 1995; P. G. Reed, 1995; J. Reed & Ground, 1997; Thorne, 1997). This newer theorizing does not seek static truths about nursing; rather, it creates a foundation upon which we can build, challenge, and integrate an infinite range of new knowledge and new ideas. As nursing theorist Myra Levine once wrote, "theory is the poetry of science" (1995, p. 14). Theorizing brings familiar concepts of nursing together into bold new configurations, making disconnected aspects of human experience part of a greater whole. In so doing, it makes the discipline come alive for us all.

Key Concepts

- The hallmark of nursing is knowledge and the way nurses use it.
- Nursing science has evolved in a historical and social context.
- Nursing theory represents the attempts by nursing scholars to articulate ways in which knowledge from various sources can be used systematically to guide professional, accountable, and defensible nursing practice.
- Much of the early theorizing in nursing was specifically designed to guide nursing curriculum development so that nursing education would be focused on the knowledge unique to nursing.
- Nursing process is nursing's fundamental problem-solving process by which new situations are assessed, plans are developed, and interventions carried out and evaluated.
- Nursing requires application of bodies of general knowledge to an infinite range of unique situations. Nursing process and nursing theory represent strategies to guide the process of such application.
- The major components of nursing theory, sometimes called the metaparadigm concepts, are person, environment, health, and nursing.
- Nursing's understanding of the role of science has shifted as more complex forms of science have been articulated by philosophers of science; science is no longer limited to simple relationships like cause and effect but provides us with strategies for understanding much more complex kinds of relationships and phenomena.
- Nursing knowledge derives from various sources in addition to science, including esthetics, personal knowing, socio-cultural knowing, and ethics.
- Nursing theorists based their conceptual frameworks on a variety of ways of thinking about human behaviour and experience; some drew their ideas from what they saw happening in excellent nursing practice, whereas others drew from theories of human behaviour, such as needs, interaction, or systems.
- Nursing conceptual frameworks include those for understanding both the person as nursing's client and the nurse's role in relation to that person.
- Although each framework may have attempted to organize nursing knowledge and systematic reasoning processes in a different way, each was aiming for a very similar ideal of excellent decision making in nursing practice.
- Although nursing theoretical frameworks are no longer considered useful as prescriptive models for practice, they provide a way of conceptualizing nursing's interests and of identifying researchable nursing problems.
- As nursing theorizing evolves, the role of philosophy in helping nurses understand their relationship to knowledge has become increasingly relevant.

Key Terms

Assumption, *p. 68*
Concept, *p. 68*
Conceptual framework, *p. 68*
Descriptive theory, *p. 69*
Grand theory, *p. 69*
Metaparadigm concepts, *p. 70*
Middle-range theory, *p. 69*
Models for nursing, *p. 69*
Nursing diagnosis, *p. 71*
Nursing process, *p. 68*
Nursing science, *p. 68*
Nursing theory, *p. 67*
Operational definition, *p. 68*
Paradigms, *p. 71*
Phenomena, *p. 68*
Philosophy of science, *p. 71*
Praxis, *p. 76*
Prescriptive theory, *p. 69*
Theoretical model, *p. 68*
Theory, *p. 67*
Ways of knowing, *p. 71*

Critical Thinking Exercises

1. How do you think that different ways of conceptualizing the human person/client might influence the kinds of decisions nurses might make in their practice? Consider how understanding the person in terms of needs, system theory, or interaction might lead you to notice certain things and not others.
2. What sorts of gaps in information or misunderstandings might occur if nurses failed to use a systematic way of thinking about each individual client in their care?
3. How do you think that conceptual frameworks and nursing theories might be used to generate research questions for developing knowledge for evidence-based practice?
4. Why is it useful for nurses to question how they know what they know?

Review Questions

1. A theory is a set of assumptions or propositions that is useful because it
   1. Helps people meet their self care needs
   2. Isolates concepts
   3. Helps the nurse implement care
   4. Provides a systematic view of explaining, predicting, and prescribing phenomena
2. The drive for early nursing theorizing came from
   1. Physicians
   2. Political leaders
   3. Nursing educators
   4. Policy-makers
3. The nursing process originally involved which four basic steps?
   1. Assessment, planning, intervention, evaluation
   2. Assessment, nursing diagnosis, planning, intervention
   3. Nursing diagnosis, planning, intervention, evaluation
   4. Planning, assessment, intervention, evaluation
4. The metaparadigm concepts included
   1. The person, environment, health, and nursing
   2. The theories of Thomas Kuhn
   3. Chaos theory and games theory
   4. The grounded theory approach
5. The main problem confronting early nursing theorists was
   1. How to differentiate between nursing theories and medical theories
   2. How to reconcile the generalizations of the North American Nursing Diagnoses Association with the unique situations of each client
   3. How to organize and make sense of general nursing knowledge and apply this knowledge to an individual clinical case
   4. Whether to use theories from other disciplines such as philosophy and to apply them to nursing
6. According to Kuhn, scientific advances happen when creative individuals
   1. Approach a problem in a new way
   2. Use the cause-and-effect model to solve problems
   3. Use the work of other scientists to solve problems
   4. Use empirical evidence to solve problems
7. The McGill Model
   1. Focuses on health rather than on illness or treatment
   2. Accounts for holistic aspects of the individual, rather than component parts
   3. Views the person as an energy field in constant interaction with the environment
   4. Considers the human experience to be based on behavioural drives
8. Hildegard Peplau considered the core of nursing to be
   1. The role of the individual in health maintenance
   2. The relationship between the nurse and client
   3. Advancing nursing theories
   4. Caring
9. Theorist Evelyn Adam articulated the essence of nursing as
   1. A collaboration with health care professionals
   2. A helping process
   3. The management of clients and health care systems
   4. All of the above
10. Systems theorists considered the human being to be
    1. An irreducible whole
    2. A whole and component parts
    3. An embodiment of mind, body, and spirit
    4. All of the above
11. Parse's theory relies on
    1. A traditional definition of illness and health
    2. The idea of people engaging in a continuing process of making choices
    3. The notion of nursing as a caring profession
    4. All of the above

References

Adam, E. (1979). *Être infirmière.* Montréal, QC: Editions HRW Ltée.

Adam, E. (1991). *To be a nurse* (2nd ed.). Philadelphia: W. B. Saunders.

Alfaro-LeFevre, R. (2004). *Critical thinking in nursing: A practical approach* (3rd ed.). Philadelphia: W. B. Saunders.

Alligood, M. R. and Choi, E. C. (1998). Evolution of nursing theory development. In A. M. Tomey and M. R. Alligood (Eds.), *Nursing theorists and their work* (4th ed.). St. Louis, MO: Mosby.

Barnum, B. J. S. (1998). *Nursing theory: Analysis, application, evaluation* (5th ed.). Philadelphia: J. B. Lippincott.

Beckstrand, J. (1978). The notion of a practice theory and the relationship of scientific and ethical knowledge to practice. *Research in Nursing & Health, 1,* 131–136.

Benner, P., & Tanner, C. (1987). Clinical judgement: How expert nurses use intuition. *American Journal of Nursing, 87*(1), 23–31.

Benner, P., Tanner, C. A., & Chesla, C. A. (1996). *Expertise in nursing practice: Caring, clinical judgement, and ethics.* New York: Springer.

Brenwick, J. M., & Webster, G. A. (2000). *Philosophy of nursing: A new vision for health care.* Albany, NY: SUNY Press.

Bultmeier, K. (2000). Roger's science of unitary human beings in nursing practice. In M R. Alligood & A. Marriner-Tomey (Eds.), *Nursing theory: Utilization and application* (2nd ed.). St. Louis, MO: Mosby.

Campbell, J. C., & Bunting, S. (1991). Voices and paradigms: Perspectives on critical and feminist theory in nursing. *Advances in Nursing Science, 13*(3), 1–15.

Campbell, M. A. (1987). *The UBC model for nursing: Directions for practice.* Vancouver: The University of British Columbia School of Nursing.

Campbell, M. A., Cruise, M. J., & Murakami, T.R. (1976). A model for nursing: University of British Columbia School of Nursing. *Nursing Papers, 8*(2), 5–9.

Carnevali, D. L., & Thomas, M. D. (1993). *Diagnostic reasoning and treatment decision making in nursing.* Philadelphia: Lippincott.

Carper, B.A. (1978). Fundamental patterns of knowing in nursing. *Advances in Nursing Science,* 1, 13–23.

Chinn, P. L., & Kramer, M. K. (2004). *Integrated knowledge development* in nursing (6th ed.). St. Louis, MO: Mosby.

Clarke, B., James, C., & Kelly, J. (1996). Reflective practice: Reviewing the issues and refocussing the debate. *International Journal of Nursing Studies, 33,* 171–180.

Cody, W. K. (1995). About all those paradigms: Many in the universe, two in nursing. *Nursing Science Quarterly, 8,* 144–147.

Coppa, D. F. (1993). Chaos theory suggests a new paradigm for nursing science. *Journal of Advanced Nursing, 18,* 985–991.

Creekmur, T., DeFelice, J., Hodel, A., & Petty, C.Y.et al. (1986). Evelyn Adam: Conceptual model for nursing. In A. Marriner (Ed.), *Nursing theorists and their work* (pp. 131–143). St. Louis, MO: Mosby.

Cull-Wilby, B. L., & Peppin, J. I. (1987). Towards a coexistence of paradigms in nursing knowledge development. *Journal of Advanced Nursing, 12,* 515–521.

Dean, H. (1995). Science and practice: The nature of knowledge. In A. Omery, C. E. Kasper, & G. G. Page (Eds.), *In search of nursing science.* Thousand Oaks, CA: Sage.

Donaldson, S. K. (1995). Nursing science for nursing practice. In A. Omery, C. E. Kasper, & G. G. Page (Eds.), *In search of nursing science.* Thousand Oaks, CA: Sage.

Durand, M., & Prince, R. (1966). Nursing diagnosis: Process and decision. *Nursing Forum, 4,* 50–64.

Ellis, R. (1968). Characteristics of significant theories. *Nursing Research, 17,* 217–222.

Engebretson, J. (1997). A multiparadigm approach to nursing. *Advances in Nursing Science, 20*(1), 21–33.

Fawcett, J. (1992). Contemporary conceptualizations of nursing: Philosophy or science. In J. F. Kikuchi & H. Simmons (Eds.), *Philosophic inquiry in nursing.* Newbury Park, CA: Sage.

Fawcett, J. (2005). *Contemporary nursing knowledge: Analysis and evaluation of nursing models and theories* (2nd ed.). Philadelphia: F. A. Davis.

Fawcett, J (2001). On Nursing Theories and Evidence, *Journal of Nursing Scholarship 33*(2): 115.

Feeley, N., & Gerez-Lirette, T. (1992). Development of professional practice based on the McGill model of nursing in an ambulatory care setting. *Journal of Advanced Nursing, 17,* 801–808.

Feeley, N., & Gottlieb, L. N. (1998). Classification systems for health concerns, nursing strategies, and client outcomes: Nursing practice with families who have a child with a chronic illness. *The Canadian Journal of Nursing Research, 30,* 45–49.

Field, P. A. (1987). The impact of nursing theory on the clinical decision making process. *Journal of Advanced Nursing, 12,* 563–571.

Fitzpatrick, J. J. (1990). Conceptual basis for the organization and advancement of nursing knowledge: Nursing diagnosis/taxonomy. *Nursing Diagnosis, 1,* 102–106.

Fry, S. T. (1995). Science as problem solving. In A. Omery, C. E. Kasper, & G. G. Page (Eds.), *In search of nursing science.* Thousand Oaks, CA: Sage.

Gleick, J. (1987). *Chaos: Making a new science.* New York: Penguin.

Gottlieb, L. N., & Feeley, N. (1999). Nursing intervention studies: Issues related to change and timing in children and families. *The Canadian Journal of Nursing Research, 30,* 193–212.

Gottlieb, L. N., & Rowat, K. (1987). The McGill model of nursing: A practice-derived model. *Advances in Nursing Science, 9,* 51–61.

Henderson, V. (1966). *The nature of nursing.* New York: Macmillan.

Henderson, V. (1982). The nursing process: Is the title right? *Journal of Advanced Nursing, 7,* 103–109.

Holden, R. J. (1990). Models, muddles and medicine. *International Journal of Nursing Studies, 27,* 223–234.

Johnson, D. E. (1974a). Development of theory: A requisite for nursing as a primary health profession. *Nursing Research, 23,* 372–377.

Johnson, D. E. (1974b). The behavioral system model for nursing. In J. P. Riehl & C. Roy (Eds.), *Conceptual models for nursing practice.* New York: Appleton-Century-Crofts.

Johnson, J. L. (1991). Nursing science: Basic, applied, or practical? Implications for the art of nursing. *Advances in Nursing Science, 14*(1), 7–16.

Jones, M. (1997). Thinking nursing. In S. E. Thorne & V. E. Hayes (Eds.), *Nursing praxis: Knowledge and action.* Thousand Oaks, CA: Sage.

Kikuchi, J. F. (1999). Clarifying the nature of conceptualizations about nursing. *The Canadian Journal of Nursing Research, 30*(4), 115–128.

Kikuchi, J. F., & Simmons, H. (1999). Practical nursing judgment: A moderate realist conception. *Scholarly Inquiry for Nursing Practice, 13,* 43–55.

King, I. M., & Fawcett, J. (1997). *The language of nursing theory and metatheory.* Indianapolis, IN: Sigma Theta Tau International Center Nursing Press.

Kuhn, T. S. (1962). *The structure of scientific revolutions.* Chicago: University of Chicago Press.

Levine, M. E. (1995). The rhetoric of nursing theory. *Image—The Journal of Nursing Scholarship, 27,* 11–14.

Liaschenko, J. (1997). Knowing the patient? In S. E. Thorne & V. E. Hayes (Eds.), *Nursing praxis: Knowledge and action.* Thousand Oaks, CA: Sage.

Liaschenko, J., & Fisher, A. (1999). Theorizing the knowledge that nurses use in the conduct of their work. *Scholarly Inquiry for Nursing Practice, 13,* 29–41.

Maslow, A. H. (1954). *Motivation and personality.* New York: Harper & Row.

McKay, R. (1969). Theories, models, and systems for nursing. *Nursing Research, 18,* 393–400.

Meleis, A. I. (1987). ReVisions in knowledge development: A passion for substance. *Scholarly Inquiry for Nursing Practice, 1,* 5–19.

Meleis, A. I. (2005). *Theoretical nursing: Development and progress* (3rd ed. revised reprint). Philadelphia: Lippincott.

Mitchell, G. J. (1995). Reflection: The key to breaking with tradition. *Nursing Science Quarterly, 8,* 57.

Nagle, L. M., & Mitchell, G. J. (1991). Theoretic diversity: Evolving paradigmatic issues in research and practice. *Advances in Nursing Science, 14,* 17–25.

Neuman, B. M. (1982). *The Neuman systems model: Application to nursing education and practice.* Norwalk, CT: Appleton-Century-Crofts.

Newman, M. A. (1972). Nursing's theoretical evolution. *American Journal of Nursing, 20,* 449–453.

Newman, M. A. (1992). Prevailing paradigms in nursing. *Nursing Outlook,* 40, 10–13, 32.

Nightingale, F. (1859/1946). *Notes on nursing: What it is and what it is not.* Philadelphia: Lippincott.

Orem, D. E. (2001). *Nursing: Concepts of practice* (6th ed.). New York: McGraw Hill.

Orem, D. E., & Parker, K. S. (1964). *Nursing content in preservice nursing curriculums.* Washington, DC: Catholic University of America Press.

Orlando, I. J. (1961). *The dynamic nurse–patient relationship: Function, process, and principles.* New York: GP Putnam's Sons.

Parse, R. R. (1981). *Man–living–health: A theory of nursing.* New York: Wiley.

Parse, R. R. (1987). *Nursing science: Major paradigms, theories, and critiques.* Philadelphia: W. B. Saunders.

Parse, R. R. (1997). Transforming research and practice with the human becoming theory. *Nursing Science Quarterly, 10*(4) 171.

Parse, R. R. (1999). Nursing science: The transforming of practice. *Journal of Advanced Nursing, 30,* 1383–1387.

Peplau, H. E. (1952). *Interpersonal relations in nursing.* New York: G. P. Putnam's Sons.

Raudonis, B. M., & Acton, G. J. (1997). Theory-based nursing practice. *Journal of Advanced Nursing, 26,* 138–145.

Ray, M. A. (1998). Complexity and nursing science. *Nursing Science Quarterly, 11,* 91–93.

Reed, J., & Ground, I. (1997). *Philosophy for nursing.* London: Arnold.

Reed, P. G. (1995). A treatise on nursing knowledge development for the 21st century: Beyond postmodernism. *Advances in Nursing Science, 17*(3), 70–84.

Rodgers, B. L. (1991). Deconstructing the dogma in nursing knowledge and practice. *Image—The Journal of Nursing Scholarship, 23,* 177–181.

Rogers, M. E. (1970). *An introduction to the theoretical basis of nursing.* Philadelphia: F. A. Davis.

Roy, C. (1974). The Roy adaptation model. In J. P. Riehl & C. Roy (Eds.), *Conceptual models for nursing practice.* New York: Appleton-Century-Crofts.

Roy, C. (1984). *Introduction to nursing: An adaptation model* (2nd ed.). Englewood Cliffs, NJ: Prentice-Hall.

Roy, C. (1982). Historical perspective of the theoretical framework for the classification of nursing diagnosis. In M. J. Kim & D.A. Moritz (Eds.), *Classification of nursing diagnoses: Proceedings of the third and fourth national conferences held in St. Louis, MO, in 1978 and 1980* (pp. 235–246). New York: McGraw-Hill.

Roy, C., & Andrews, H. A. (1999). *The Roy adaptation model: The definitive statement* (2nd ed.). East Norwalk, CT: Appleton & Lange.

Sarter, B. J. (1990). Philosophical foundations of nursing theory: A discipline emerges. In N. L. Chaska (Ed.), *The nursing profession: Turning points* (pp. 223–229). St. Louis, MO: Mosby.

Silva, M. C., Sorrell, J. M., & Sorrell, S. C. (1995). From Carper's patterns of knowing to ways of being: An ontological philosophical shift in nursing. *Advances in Nursing Science, 18*(1), 1–13.

Starzomski, R., & Rodney, P. (1997). Nursing inquiry for the common good. In S. E. Thorne & V. E. Hayes (Eds.), *Nursing praxis: Knowledge and action* (pp. 219–236). Thousand Oaks, CA: Sage.

Tanner, C. A. (1993). Rethinking clinical judgement. In N. L. Diekelman & M. L. Notter (Eds.), *Transforming RN education: Dialogue and debate* (2nd ed., pp. 15–41). New York: NLN Press (14-2511).

Thorne, S. E. (1997). Introduction: Praxis in the context of nursing's developing inquiry. In S. E. Thorne & V. E. Hayes (Ed.), *Nursing praxis: Knowledge and action* (pp. xi–xxiii). Thousand Oaks, CA: Sage.

Thorne, S., et al. (1993). A nursing model in action: The University of British Columbia experience. *Journal of Advanced Nursing, 18,* 1259–1266.

Torres, G. (1974). Curriculum process and the integrated curriculum. In National League for Nursing (Eds.), *Unifying the curriculum: The integrated approach* (pp. 15–31). New York: National League for Nursing (15-1522).

Torres, G. (1986). *Theoretical foundations of nursing.* Norwalk, CT: Appleton-Century-Crofts.

Travelbee, J. (1971). *Interpersonal aspects of nursing.* Philadelphia: F. A. Davis.

Varcoe, C. (1996). Disparagement of the nursing process: The new dogma? *Journal Advanced Nursing,* 23,120–125.

von Bertalanffy, L. (1968). *General systems theory: Foundations, development, application.* New York: George Braziller.

Wald, F. S., & Leonard, R. C. (1964). Toward development of nursing practice theory. *American Journal of Nursing, 13,* 309–313.

Warren, J. J., & Hoskins, L. M. (1990). The development of NANDA's nursing diagnosis taxonomy. *Nursing Diagnosis, 1,* 162–168.

Watson, J. (1979). *Nursing: The philosophy and science of caring.* Boston: Little, Brown & Co.

Watson, J. (1990). Caring knowledge and informed moral passion. *Advances in Nursing Science, 13*(1), 15–24.

Watson, J. (1999). *Postmodern nursing and beyond.* Edinburgh, Scotland: Churchill Livingstone.

White, J. (1995). Patterns of knowing: Review, critique, and update. *Advances in Nursing Science, 17*(4), 73–86.

Yeo, M. (1989). Integration of nursing theory and nursing ethics. *Advances in Nursing Science, 11*(3), 33–42.

Yura, H., & Walsh, M. B. (1988). *The nursing process: Assessing, planning, implementing, evaluating* (5th ed.). Norwalk, CT: Appleton-Century-Crofts.

Recommended Web Sites

Department of Nursing, Clayton College and State University Nursing "Theory Link Page":
http://healthsci.clayton.edu/eichelberger/nursing.htm

This collection offers links to a wide range of nursing theories, including theories of nursing in general and theories about substantive fields within nursing.

Hahn School of Nursing, University of San Diego "The Nursing Theory Page":
http://www.sandiego.edu/nursing/theory/

This site orients the student to most of the major nursing theorists and resources to expand an understanding of their contributions.

6

Research as a Basis for Practice

Marilynn J. Wood, RN, BSN, MSN, DrPH (Canadian author)
Anne Griffin Perry, RN, MSN, EdD, FAAN

Objectives

Mastery of content in this chapter will enable the student to:

- Define the key terms listed.
- Identify the various ways to acquire knowledge.
- Discuss methods for developing new nursing knowledge.
- Define nursing research.
- Discuss Canadian nursing research priorities.
- Identify ethical principles important in undertaking research.
- Explain how the rights of human research subjects are protected.
- Discuss methods of locating research reports in nursing and related areas.
- Explain how to organize information from a research report.
- Discuss the process of research utilization.

Nursing knowledge must continuously expand to keep approaches to nursing care relevant and current. Without new knowledge, nursing cannot improve therapies such as infant care, pain management, grief counseling, or client education. The major source of new knowledge is research, which provides a solid foundation for nursing practice. Nurses need a sound knowledge base to support practice, and research is essential to build that knowledge. Nursing practice is based on theory, values, and evidence.

Nurses base decisions on these as well on other influences such as ethics, the law, working conditions, and work environments. Evidence-based practice is nursing's goal, yet it raises issues, such as the need for targeted research in specific practice areas and the need for better dissemination of research findings (CNA, 1998).

The scientific knowledge needed for nursing practice is discovered, tested, and enhanced through nursing research. The multidisciplinary nature of nursing challenges nurses not only to keep up with nursing research, but also to know the status of research in other disciplines such as the behavioural and physical sciences.

Nursing research is a systematic examination of phenomena important to the nursing discipline, as well as to nurses, their clients, and families. Its purpose is to expand the knowledge base for practice by answering nurses' questions. Nursing research addresses a range of issues related to actual and potential client populations and to individual and family responses to health problems. Some research tests nursing theories; other research generates theory from findings. This "back-and-forth" relationship between theory and research is the way knowledge develops in any discipline (Brink & Wood, 2001).

The International Council of Nurses (ICN, 1986) supports nursing research as a means to improve people's health and welfare. Research identifies new knowledge, improves education and practice, and uses resources effectively. In 1983, the National Center for Nursing Research (NCNR) in the United States and the ICN established priorities for nursing research. These priorities were to promote the in-depth knowledge base for nursing practice, to recognize nursing research as an integral part of nursing practice and education, to facilitate cross-cultural research, to ensure adequate preparation of nurse researchers, and to encourage all national nursing associations to establish ethical research standards (NCNR/ICN, 1990).

In 1995, the Canadian Nurses Association (CNA), the Canadian Association of University Schools of Nursing, and the Canadian Association for Nursing Research developed research priorities. These priorities identify the need to expand the knowledge base for nursing practice in Canada, including the study of contextual issues such as the social, political, and environmental predictors of health, specific clinical populations, and a range of interventions from health promotion strategies to specific clinical measures (Canadian Association of University Schools of Nursing, 1997).

Nursing research improves nursing practice, raising the profession's standards. Involvement in research takes many forms: designing studies, being on a research team, collecting data, using research findings to change clinical practice, improving client outcomes, and maintaining health care costs (Titler et al., 1994). Promoting research and using it in practice increases the scientific knowledge base for nursing practice. Clients benefit from these improvements to practice.

The History of Nursing Research

Nursing research provides a strong foundation for practice (Box 6-1). During the Crimean War, Florence Nightingale's detailed and systematic observation of nursing actions and outcomes resulted in major changes in nursing practice (see chapter 3). Her work demonstrated the importance of systemic observational research to nursing practice.

In Canada, the establishment of university nursing courses in the 1920s, followed by master's degree programs in the 1950s and 60s, was key to the development of nursing research (see chapter 3). The first master's degree program, established at the University of Western Ontario in 1959, highlighted the need for Canadian research capacity in nursing.

The first nursing research journal, *Nursing Research,* was launched in the United States in 1952. The first nursing research journal published in Canada, *Nursing Papers* (later the *Canadian Journal of Nursing Research*), was established at McGill University in 1969. Other journals slowly followed. Today, nurses publish their research in a variety of nursing journals (Box 6-2) as well as other disciplines' journals.

In 1971, McGill University established the Centre for Nursing Research in Canada. The same year, the first National Conference on Nursing Research in Canada was held in Ottawa. These conferences were held annually or biennially for several years. Papers of the early conferences were published as monographs. Nursing research conferences increased and began to be sponsored by professional, research, and academic organizations. As well, nurses began to participate in the research conferences of interdisciplinary groups such as the Canadian Association on Gerontology.

Box 6-1 Historical Milestones in the Development of Canadian Nursing Research

1858	Florence Nightingale publishes *Notes on Matters Affecting the Health, Efficiency and Hospital Administration of the British Army* and *Notes on Hospitals.*
1920	Public health courses offered at the universities of British Columbia (UBC), Alberta (U of A), Toronto (U of T), McGill, Dalhousie, and Western Ontario (UWO).
1923	Goldmark report on U.S. nursing education identifies deficiencies in the system.
1932	Weir report, sponsored by the Canadian Nurses Association and Canadian Medical Association calls for better nursing education and service.
1952	The American Nurses Association first publishes *Nursing Research.*
1959	First Canadian Nursing master's degree program launched at UWO.
1964–1965	First nursing research project funded by a Canadian federal granting agency; *International Journal of Nursing Studies* and *International Nursing Index* launched.
1969–1970	*Nursing Papers,* forerunner of the *Canadian Journal of Nursing Research,* published at McGill; Lysaught report, *An Abstract for Action,* published.
1971	McGill launches Centre for Nursing Research; first national Canadian conference held on nursing research; both financed by The Department of National Health and Welfare.
1978	Heads of university nursing schools and deans of graduate studies attend The Kellogg National Seminar on Doctoral Education in Nursing.
1982	The Alberta Foundation for Nursing Research, first funding agency for nursing research, established; the Working Group on Nursing Research established by the Medical Research Council (MRC).
1985	Report of the Working Group on Nursing Research is released by MRC.
1988	MRC and the National Health Research and Development Program establish joint initiative to structure nursing research grants.
1992	First fully funded Canadian Nursing PhD programs launched first at U of A, followed by UBC, McGill, and U of T.
1994	McMaster University launches nursing PhD; MRC's mandate now includes health research.
1999	The Nursing Research Fund launched with a $25 million grant over 10 years; the Canadian Health Services Research Foundation administers the funds. PhD nursing program launched at the University of Calgary.
2004	PhD in Nursing program initiated at Dalhousie University.
	Forum on doctoral education held in Toronto under the auspices of CASN to develop a national position paper on the PhD in Nursing for Canada.

Throughout the 1970s and 1980s, university faculties and schools of nursing built their research resources so that they could mount doctoral programs. The first provincially approved doctoral nursing program was established at the University of Alberta Faculty of Nursing in 1991. The University of British Columbia School of Nursing followed later that year with programs at McGill University and the University of Toronto following in 1993. In the late 1990s and early 2000s, other programs were launched, bringing the total to 12.

Growing awareness of the importance of nursing research gradually led to research funds becoming available. The year 1964 marked the first time that a federal granting agency funded nursing research in Canada (Good, 1969). For the next few decades, the primary source of federal funds for nursing research was the National Health Research and Development Program. In 1982, the Alberta government responded to requests for funding and established the Alberta Foundation for Nursing Research with $1,000,000 to be distributed over the first 5 years. This was the first research-granting agency in Canada to fund nursing research exclusively. The Foundation did excellent work for 12 years before tight budgets and downsizing led to the government's decision not to award further funds.

Also in 1982, the Medical Research Council (MRC) established the Working Group on Nursing Research, which recommended the establishment of doctoral nursing programs and the mandatory funding of nursing research by the MRC (1985). In 1988, the MRC and the National Health Research and Development Program launched a joint initiative to provide support for nursing researchers. Several key Canadian researchers received funding under this venture. In 1994, the MRC broadened its mandate from exclusively biomedical research to health research. Under the new guidelines, most nursing research was now eligible for funding.

Meanwhile, in the United States, a study of nursing by the Institute of Medicine (1983) recommended that the federal government increase funds for scientific research in nursing and that a national organization be established to place nursing research "in the mainstream of scientific investigation." Acting on this recommendation in the U.S. Congress established the NCNR in 1985 and the National Institute of Nursing Research (NINR) in 1993. The NINR (2000) supports:

> Clinical and basic research to establish a scientific basis for the care of individuals across the life span—from management of patients during illness and recovery to the reduction of risks for disease and disability and the promotion of healthy life styles. According to its mandate the Institute seeks to understand and ease the symptoms of acute and chronic illness, to prevent or delay the onset of disease or disability or slow its progression, and to improve the clinical settings in which care is provided. . . . Research extends to problems encountered by patients, families, and caregivers. It also emphasizes the special needs of at-risk and underserved populations.

Insufficient and inconsistent funding for Canadian nursing research indicated a need for a Canadian national funding body similar to the NINR. Nurses had long been asking for such assistance. There were adequate numbers of doctorally prepared nursing researchers, and their research priorities were clear (Box 6-3). In 1999, in response to intensive lobbying by the CNA, the federal government established the Nursing Research Fund, budgeting $25,000,000 for nursing research ($2,500,000 over each of the following 10 years), with the funds to be administered by the Canadian Health Services Research Foundation. The research areas targeted for support included nursing policies, management, human resources, and nursing care. A total of $500,000 each year is designated for the Open Grants Competition, $500,000 to the Canadian Nurses Foundation for research on nursing care, $750,000 for training (post-doctoral fellowships and student grants), and $250,000 for knowledge networks and dissemination activities. To date, five Chairs in Nursing Research have been funded by this initiative, representing excellence in nursing research across Canada. The incumbents are to develop research capacity in a particular area of nursing:

- Dr. Lesley Degner, University of Manitoba: Development of Innovative Nursing Interventions to Influence Practice and Policy in Cancer Care, Palliative Care, and Cancer Prevention
- Dr. Alba Dicenso, McMaster University: Evaluation of Nurse Practitioner/Advanced Practice Nurse Roles and Interventions
- Dr. Nancy Edwards, University of Ottawa: Multiple Interventions in Community Health Nursing Care
- Dr. Janice Lander, University of Alberta: Evaluating Innovative Approaches to Nursing Care
- Dr. Linda O'Brien-Pallas, University of Toronto: Nursing Human Resources for the New Millennium (*www.chsrf.ca/nursing_research_fund/action_e.php*)

Early nursing research focused on the roles and characteristics of nurses rather than on client care. The Lysaught (1970) report in the United States recommended increased research in nursing practice and education. By the mid-1970s, more nurses were receiving doctoral preparation and initiating research in both the United States and

Box 6-2 Nursing Research Journals (Non-Specialty Based)

Decade	Journal Title
1950s	*Nursing Research*
1960s	*Image—The Journal of Nursing Scholarship*
	Canadian Journal of Nursing Research (originally *Nursing Papers*)
	International Journal of Nursing Studies
1970s	*Advances in Nursing Science*
	Research in Nursing and Health
	Western Journal of Nursing Research
1980s	*Applied Nursing Research*
	Journal of Nursing Measurement
	Nursing Science Quarterly
	Scholarly Inquiry for Nursing Practice
1990s	*Clinical Nursing Research*
	Qualitative Health Research
	Measurement of Nursing Outcomes
	Canadian Nursing Research Priorities

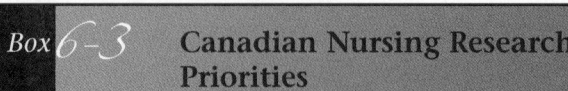

Box 6-3 Canadian Nursing Research Priorities

Priority 1: Nursing Practice

- Context (including determinants of health, health reform, and ethical issues)
- Populations (vulnerable groups as well as specific clinical populations)
- Interventions (wide range, from health promotion to comfort measures)

Priority 2: Outcomes

- Development of valid measures for multiple dimensions
- Links with clinical judgement

Priority 3: Enhanced Links Between Research and Practice

- Development of body of nursing knowledge

Data from *Canadian Nursing Research Priorities, Results of Phase III of National Nursing Research Symposium,* by Canadian Association of University Schools of Nursing, 1997, Ottawa ON: Author, available from *http://www.CAUSN.org/English/ Research/research.htm*

Canada. In the Report of the Commission on Canadian Studies, Professor Thomas Symons (1975) noted that the slow start of graduate programs and inadequate support had resulted in few nursing research projects, publications, and investigations into Canadian health care.

Nursing research has focused progressively on evidence-based practice in response to demands to justify care practices and systems by improving client outcomes and controlling costs. **Evidence-based practice** is the integration of the best research evidence with evidence from expert clinical practice and other sources to produce the best possible care for clients. The scope of nursing research has also broadened to include historical and philosophical inquiry. The establishment of a Centre for Philosophical Nursing Research at the University of Alberta exemplifies this new direction.

Three new training centres funded by the Nursing Research Fund at the Canadian Health Services Research Foundation are mandated to increase research capacity in nursing and related disciplines:

- The Centre for Knowledge Transfer is a national training centre at the University of Alberta that provides funding for students and offers courses in knowledge utilization and transfer (*www.ckt-ctc.ca*).
- The FERASI Centre in Quebec is a joint initiative among l'Université de Montréal, McGill University, and l'Université Laval to build research capacity in the administration of nursing services. It focuses on developing partnerships with health care decision makers in order to provide training opportunities and insights into the decision- making environment. Funding is provided for student scholarships (*www.ferasi.umontreal.ca*).
- The Ontario Training Centre in Health Services and Policy Research involves six Ontario universities for the purpose of enhancing health services and policy research. The centre is located at McMaster University and involves collaboration with Toronto, York, Ottawa, Laurentian, and Lakehead (*www.otc-hsr.ca*).

Knowledge Development in Nursing

Knowledge that provides the rationale for nursing practice is organized in a variety of ways. In her classic article on patterns of knowing in nursing, Carper (1978) identified four patterns: empirics or the science of nursing, esthetics or the art of nursing, personal knowing, and ethics or the moral component (Table 6-1). These different types of knowledge focus on the meaning and value of nursing knowledge. With evidence-based practice, the evidence can be derived from any of these sources of knowledge.

Empirics: The Science of Nursing

Carper (1978) described empirics as "knowledge that is systematically organized into general laws and theories for the purpose of describing, explaining and predicting phenomena of special concern to the discipline of nursing" (p. 14). This pattern of knowing implies an objective reality, from the study of which one can interpret the meaning of particular phenomena and develop understandings of other similar phenomena. Fundamental to this model is the rational stance in which one can generalize from a sample to a population. The theoretical or conceptual models and frameworks help to explain particular phenomena in health and illness and to identify important questions for nursing research. The goal of scientific research is to produce this type of knowledge.

Esthetics: The Art of Nursing

Nursing incorporates an artistic, expressive component, which involves knowledge and understanding. As Carper (1978) noted, "The art of nursing involves the active transformation of the patient's behavior into a perception of what is significant in it—that is, what need is being expressed by the behavior" (p. 17). She further stated that perception is beyond mere recognition and, as such, moves nursing activities into the esthetic realm.

Personal Knowledge

This pattern of knowing can be the most difficult to understand and to teach. The nature of the relationship formed with the client and the depth and quality of the interpersonal experience are fundamental to the realm of personal knowledge. As Carper (1978) stated, "Personal knowledge is concerned with the knowing, encountering and actualizing of the concrete, individual self" (p. 18). Many have attempted to understand the nature of therapeutic relationships. How is a nurse successful in assisting a client to reach health goals through the rapport established with the individual? Perhaps "the nurse in the therapeutic use of self rejects approaching the patient-client as an object and strives instead to actualize an authentic personal relationship between two persons" (Carper, 1978, p. 19).

Table 6-1 Fundamental Patterns of Knowing in Nursing

I. Empirics: The Science of Nursing	Knowledge developed through systematic research to describe and explain phenomena.
II. Esthetics: The Art of Nursing	Creativity, with an artistic or expressive component.
III. Personal Knowledge	Knowledge derived from the depth and power of the interpersonal relationship with the client.
IV. Ethics: The Moral Component	Knowledge that emerges from ethical dilemmas practice and based on what ought to be done in particular situations.

From Fundamental Patterns of Knowing in Nursing, by B. A. Carper, *Advances in Nursing Science, 1*(1), p. 13.

Ethics: The Moral Component

Nurses are faced with ethical questions that centre on what ought to be done in particular situations. Ethics goes beyond ethical theories, principles, and codes of professional conduct to dilemmas such as choosing the best of two or more actions, none of which are totally desirable. Now that technology can prolong life, ethical dilemmas have become more frequent and complex. As Carper (1978) stated, "The ethical pattern of knowing in nursing requires an understanding of different philosophical positions regarding what is good, what ought to be desired, and what is right; of different ethical frameworks devised for dealing with the complexities of moral judgments; and of various orientations to the notion of obligation" (p. 21).

The Development of Research in Nursing

A mature discipline uses multiple research methods to develop a unique knowledge base (Barrett, 1998). A person continuously acquires knowledge, using critical thinking to interpret and evaluate complex information.

The Scientific Paradigm

The term *paradigm* was introduced by Kuhn (1970) and can be loosely defined as a way of thinking (see chapter 5). According to Kuhn, a dominant research paradigm can be identified during any one era. Eventually this paradigm will no longer provide solutions to research problems and will be challenged by new ideas. It will then be replaced by a new paradigm, and the process continues. The dominant paradigm for most of the 19th and 20th centuries has been positivism. Positivism emphasizes tested and systematized experience, rather than speculation, and focuses on the search for cause-and-effect relationships to explain phenomena. In this paradigm, the scientific method arose as the major research approach.

Researchers using the **scientific method** pose research questions and collect and analyze data to find answers to the questions. The process is rigorous and systematic and is guided by scientific principles, the most important of which is empiricism, meaning that only things that can be observed by the human senses can be called facts. Positivists also use deductive reasoning, in which a **hypothesis** (hypothetical proposition) is tested experimentally to confirm or reject theoretical explanations of phenomena.

The scientific method is an objective means of acquiring and testing knowledge by which researchers try to understand, explain, predict, or control nursing phenomena. The method is characterized by systematic, orderly procedures that, although not without fault, seek to limit the possibility for error and minimize the likelihood that any bias or opinion by the researcher might influence the results of research and, thus, the knowledge gained. Brink and Wood (2001) described the **research process** as follows: The process begins with a researchable question. If properly stated, the question will guide the rest of the process; thus, asking the question is a crucial step. There are three levels of questions, and the appropriate level is chosen based on how much is known about the research topic. Once an initial question has been formulated, the literature is searched to discover what is already known about the topic and to determine if the question needs to be revised in light of prior knowledge. The level of the question determines the research design needed to answer it. Table 6-2 describes the basic steps in planning nursing research.

The research design provides the ground rules for data collection and analysis, ensuring that the research question will have a valid answer. The design steps are systematic and precise to control unwanted influences that might affect the answer. For example, in a study of the relationship between diet and heart disease, influences such as stress or smoking must be controlled, as they are known to influence heart disease. The design also specifies the type of sample and sample selection techniques that will provide the best data for the study.

Evidence that is part of experience **(empirical data)** is gathered from the sample through measurement techniques that quantify the variables in the research question. Techniques include interviews, tests of knowledge, physiological measures such as heart rate and blood pressure, and so forth. When the evidence is analyzed, the result answers the original question and becomes the basis for discovering new knowledge.

A goal of scientific research is to understand phenomena so that the knowledge gained can be applied generally, not just to isolated cases. This goal is achieved by studying a sample that represents a larger population, thus increasing the likelihood that the results will apply across that population.

In the scientific paradigm, researchers conduct studies that contribute to the testing or development of theories, thereby advancing knowledge that can be applied in nursing practice.

The Qualitative Paradigm

Positivism has been criticized by those who believe that reality and our perception of reality are so intertwined that we cannot separate them. Interpretivism is an alternative to

Table 6-2 Basic Steps in Planning Nursing Research

Steps	Levels I	Levels II	Levels III
Question	What?	What is the relationship?	Why?
Problem	Little known about topic	Conceptual base; variables have been studied before	Theoretical base
Purpose	Declarative statement	Question or hypothesis	Hypothesis
Design	Exploratory descriptive	Descriptive survey, correlational or comparative	Experiment
Sample	Convenience sample or total population	Probability sample	Random assignment to treatment and control groups
Methods	Qualitative, unstructured data; some quantitative descriptive data	Quantitative data collected by all methods	Quantitative data
Analysis	Content analysis; descriptive statistic	Correlation or tests of association; regression	Differences between means: *t*-test, ANOVA
Answer	Description of processes, concepts, or population	Explanation of relationship among variables	Test of theory

Modified from *Basic Steps in Planning Nursing Research* (inside cover), by P. Brink and M. Wood, 2001, Sudbury, MA: Jones & Bartlett.

positivism, representing the view that we construct our own world as we strive to make sense of our social environments (Milburn et al., 1995). The research that flows from interpretivism can be broadly designated as qualitative research. Qualitative research avoids the empirical notion of the study of people as objects and strives instead to understand human behaviour in the context of those being studied. A qualitative researcher studies the behaviours, experiences, perceptions, and motives of individuals in social and cultural settings (Parahoo, 1997).

There are several approaches to qualitative research, each very different from the others. Unlike the scientific approach, qualitative approaches often have their own unique philosophic base, making comparisons difficult. Streubert and Carpenter (1999, p. 10) identified the following six characteristics common to all qualitative research:

- belief in multiple realities
- commitment to identifying an approach to understanding that will support the phenomenon studied
- commitment to the participant's point of view
- conduct of inquiry in a way that does not disturb the natural context of the phenomena of interest
- acknowledged participation of the researcher in the research
- conveyance of the understanding of phenomena by reporting in a literary style rich with participants' commentary

The idea of multiple realities is a challenge to positivist thinking, which proposes that researchers are searching for one reality or truth. Interpretivists say that because the experience of individuals is unique, each one can come to know the world differently, leading to many truths rather than one. This belief leads qualitative researchers to seek multiple ways of understanding the world, and to change methods and data collection strategies as needed, rather than following a single prescribed set of strategies. It follows that the participant's point of view would be the focus of the research and would guide the process. The researcher becomes a co-participant in the process of understanding the participant's point of view.

Qualitative research is carried out in the participants' natural setting to maintain a natural context. The researcher is a participant, and it is acknowledged that this will affect the participants and the setting. Objectivity is not a goal in qualitative research; rather, subjectivity from the participants' perspective is sought. Because of the nature of the data, rich with personal experience and example, the research is usually reported in a literary style, similar to storytelling. Liberal quotation from the participants adds to the richness of the report.

Research Designs

Nursing research approaches vary depending upon the specific problem to be studied. The paradigms of positivism and interpretivism lead to two different research approaches, often categorized as quantitative (scientific method) and qualitative (interpretive). Neither is used exclusively in nursing research, although positivism and the scientific method are dominant. Nonetheless, interpretivism and qualitative methods have much to offer nursing research. The next section describes some common research designs in these two categories.

Nursing Research in the Scientific Paradigm

Scientific nursing research (quantitative nursing research) is the investigation of nursing phenomena that can be precisely measured and quantified. Examples are pain severity, rates of wound healing, and body temperature changes. These designs fall within the scientific paradigm and provide rigorous, systematic, objective examination of specific concepts and their relationships. The goal is to test theory using numerical data, statistical analysis, and controls to eliminate bias (Brink & Wood, 2001; Knapp, 1998; Polit & Beck, 2004).

Experimental Research. Experimental design is the hallmark of scientific research. Experiments are appropriate designs for questions at Level III (see Table 6-2), which ask why one variable causes a predictable change in another variable. In a **true experiment,** the conditions under which the variables are studied are tightly controlled to provide objective testing of hypotheses, which predict cause-and-effect relationships. Experimental research requires that the data be collected and quantified in a prescribed manner.

The requirements of a true experiment are as follows:

- The study usually includes at least one control or comparison group, which does not receive the nursing measure being investigated. The results for this group are compared with those of the experimental group—the group that receives a treatment or intervention. The **subjects**—people selected for the comparison and experimental groups—are randomly assigned to these groups, so that the groups are as similar as possible to each other prior to the intervention. Random assignment of subjects ensures that all subjects have the same chance to be in the control or experimental (treatment) group and that variables that could affect the outcome of the study are randomly distributed between the groups and therefore are no more likely to affect experimental subjects than control subjects.
- There must be an experimental variable that is manipulated by the researcher. For example, in a study of the effect of preoperative teaching on post-operative anxiety, the researcher manipulates preoperative teaching by providing it for the experimental group but not for the control group. The expectation is that the differences in post-operative anxiety measures between the two groups can be attributed to the effect of preoperative teaching because all other factors are under control. However, the researcher cannot control clients' prior experiences, such as hearing others' stories about surgery. Psychological factors, which cannot be controlled, may influence the subject's level of anxiety. If clients are randomly assigned to the two groups, however, those with negative prior experiences should be distributed equally between the two groups, and these experiences would affect both groups equally. Thus, differences between the groups in post-operative anxiety can still be attributed to the preoperative teaching intervention.
- The researcher proposes theory-based and statistically tested hypotheses about the action of the variables to answer the research question. For example, in a study of preoperative teaching, the hypothesis might be, "Clients who receive structured preoperative teaching will have significantly lower postoperative anxiety levels than clients who do not receive structured preoperative teaching." The researcher must explain why lower anxiety is expected in a discussion of the theory behind the study.

A **quasi-experimental research design** is one in which groups are formed and the conditions are controlled, but the subjects are not randomly assigned to a control group or treatment conditions. These designs also answer questions at Level III (Brink & Wood, 2001). In many health care settings, assigning subjects randomly to experimental and control groups is not feasible. Quasi-experimental research is often carried out for practical reasons related to the subjects themselves. For example, to test the effect of a new intervention in Alzheimer care, carrying out two treatments on the unit at the same time might confuse the clients. A quasi-experiment could use two Alzheimer care units: one as the experimental unit, where all clients would receive the new intervention, and the second as the control group, in which clients would receive the usual care but not the new intervention. The two groups would be compared before and after the intervention on the outcome variable. The weakness in a quasi-experiment is the researcher does not know if the two groups were equivalent prior to the intervention. Unrecognized differences between the two units might exist that could influence the outcome of the study. For instance, clients on one unit might have more cognitive impairment than those on the other unit, and thus could influence the outcome.

Descriptive Survey Designs. Surveys are designed to answer Level II questions about relationships among variables. The research question that leads to a survey design will begin with "What is the relationship between . . . ?" and will address two or more variables (Brink & Wood, 2001). For example, what is the relationship between ethnicity and suicide among university students?

Many types of research use surveys in which a group of people is compared on two or more variables. The purpose is to discover relationships among variables in the population. In a survey design, the sample makes the difference between a good survey and a poor one. The sample should be representative of the population so that generalizations can be made on the basis of the sample data. There are three key elements in a survey. First, a random sample of the population must be drawn, from which inferences can be made about the population. Second, the population sampled should be large enough to keep sampling error to a minimum. Third, the measurement tools (e.g., questionnaires, interviews) must be accurate measures of the study variables.

Exploratory Descriptive Designs. Exploratory descriptive designs provide in-depth descriptions of populations or variables not previously studied. Level I (basic) questions are asked because not much is known about the topic. They typically begin with "what"; for example, "What are the health-promoting behaviours of older adults living in subsidized housing?" The results provide a detailed description of the variable or population. No relationships among variables are posited at this stage, although the results might indicate that relationships should be examined in subsequent research.

Data Analysis. Except for some exploratory descriptive studies in which the outcome is a verbal description, all quantitative studies use statistical analysis. In experimental designs, one must discover if the experimental and control groups are significantly different from each other after the intervention has been applied. Statistical tests that provide a test of group means are generally used for experiments.

Descriptive survey designs use statistical techniques to test for significant relationships among the variables. Generally these are correlational tests that indicate whether the subject's score on one variable (e.g., blood pressure) is related to that same subject's score on another variable (e.g., weight). The results of a correlational analysis of these two variables would indicate how much influence increased body weight has on blood pressure.

Exploratory descriptive studies use several techniques to analyze data, depending upon the type collected. Unstructured data that do not lend themselves to numerical form are summarized verbally. If quantitative measures are used to collect the data, they can be described numerically as well as verbally. Descriptions usually include measures of central tendency (mean, median, or mode) and dispersion (range, standard deviation).

Nursing Research in the Qualitative Paradigm

Qualitative nursing research poses questions about nursing phenomena that cannot be quantified and measured. Examples are the study of the experience of pregnancy and the culture of a long-term care facility. To answer questions about these phenomena, researchers must understand the perspective of the person in the situation. Researchers using qualitative methods can choose one of many design strategies, including ethnography, phenomenology, and grounded theory. As with scientific research, the research question is the basis for the choice of design. Ethnography is chosen if the research question leads to the study of behaviour within a specific group or culture, phenomenology if the question relates to the experience of the participants, and grounded theory if the researcher is interested in studying a social process.

Ethnography. **Ethnography** involves the observation and description of behaviour in social settings. It comes from anthropology, where it provides the means to study the culture of groups of people. Anthropologists use participant observation as the major source of data collection, together with other sources such as artifacts and photographs. Nurse researchers use ethnography to study the behaviour of nurses and their clients in a variety of settings. The goal of ethnography is to understand the culture of the study population as the culture is practised in its own setting. The focus is on the cultural norms and social forces that shape behaviour in a given setting. The researcher becomes an accepted member of the community under study and collects data through repeated interviews of informants from the community. Data collection continues until understanding has been reached about why the members of the community behave as they do. Interview data are supplemented by other forms, such as artifacts and historical documents; the result is a rich description of the culture.

Phenomenology. The focus of **phenomenology** is on the lived experience of a specific phenomenon from the perspective of the people who are in the situation. Phenomenology has its roots in German philosophy of the early 20th century, stemming from the philosopher, Husserl (1962), who posited that only those who experience phenomena are capable of communicating them to the outside world. The researcher must learn to understand a phenomenon from the viewpoint of those experiencing it. For example, an investigator may want to study the impact of surrogate decision making regarding end-of-life decisions (Jeffers, 1998). The goal of this research is to describe fully the lived experience of surrogate decision makers, their perceptions of the surrogate role, the decision-making process, and the meaning of the decisions. The data's source is the subject, and the data are the result of in-depth conversations. The units of analysis are the conversations, which are coded and analyzed to extract the meaning to the subjects of the phenomenon.

Grounded Theory. **Grounded theory** as a research method was developed by Glaser and Strauss (1967) as a means of generating hypotheses and theories about social processes inductively from the data. The grounded theory is "discovered," developed, and verified through a rigorous process of data collection and analysis. Glaser and Strauss advocated that researchers not review the literature prior to carrying out the study, as they might be influenced by what others have found. The strength of the grounded theory approach comes from examining the situation afresh and opening up the possibility of a new perspective on an old problem (Parahoo, 1997).

For example, in studying the process of weaning from mechanical ventilation, Wunderlich and Perry (1999) interviewed clients who were successfully weaned from mechanical ventilation. The interview data prompted the investigators to suggest that social support was the most important factor in the clients' success. This information, along with findings from another study, has begun to define some theoretical concepts for preparing clients to be weaned from mechanical ventilation (Ketchum & Perry, 1999).

Conducting Nursing Research

Nurses conduct research in a variety of settings. Student nurses and practitioners participate in investigations of client outcomes and nursing care, commonly called quality assurance or improvement studies (see chapter 10). Data are collected to determine the influence of nurses on achievement of client care objectives in a particular clinical setting. Because the results usually apply only to one facility, this research is not scientific. However, it is important to the facility involved because it can demonstrate the contributions made by nurses to client care and improve processes if necessary.

Clinical nursing research should be undertaken by nurses educated to conduct scientific investigations (Figure 6–1). An experienced researcher is usually more qualified than a beginner to undertake a complex, long-term project. Nurses new to research may, however, assist with data collection, conduct replication studies (studies

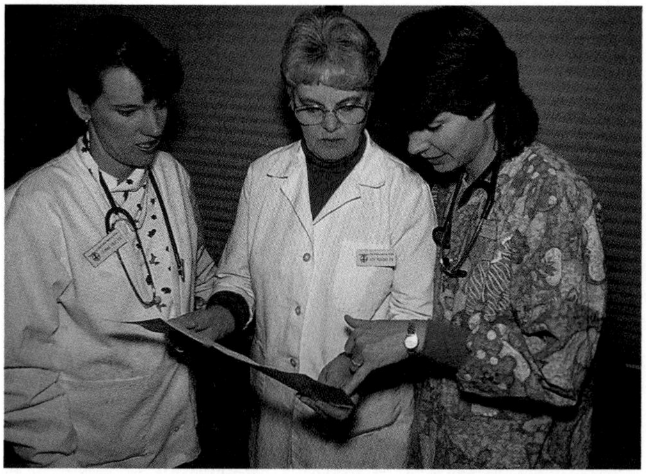

FIGURE **6–1** Nurses collaborating on research.

previously performed elsewhere), or conduct less complex studies.

Research Mindedness and Roles of Nurses in Research

Research mindedness means "awareness of, and openness to, nursing research" (Ross-Kerr & MacPhail, 1996, p. 118). Every nurse needs to be research minded by keeping up with current research, contributing to the development of research questions, conducting research, or incorporating findings into practice.

Nurses are expected to participate in research by identifying clinical problems in practice, assisting with data collection, and using research findings in clinical practice. Nurses should read research critically, use standards to assess the readiness of the findings for clinical practice, identify clinical problems in nursing practice, and help investigators gain access to clinical sites.

Research requires advanced preparation, usually obtained in graduate programs. Nurses with a master's degree are active members of a research team, assuming the role of clinical expert and creating an environment that supports nursing research and the integration of research findings into practice.

Doctorally prepared nurses are expected to design studies independently, as well as collaborate with other clinicians and researchers in conducting studies. Nurses serving as principal investigators are responsible for acquiring funding for research from public and private sources.

Ethical Issues in Research

Research must meet ethical standards in ways that respect the dignity and preserve the well-being of human research participants. In Canada, every health care facility and university receiving public funds for research must meet federal standards for protecting human research participants. The most recent standard is the Tri-Council Policy Statement (Medical Research Council et al, 2002), which requires that the institution have in place a Research Ethics Board (REB) to review all research proposals to determine if ethical principles are being upheld (Box 6-4). The REB focuses on informed consent and weighs benefits versus harms from the research. No research may be carried out in a university or health care facility without the approval of the REB. All proposals are subject to review. However, if data collection processes (such as quality assurance studies) are a normal part of institutional business, performance reviews, or testing within normal educational requirements and are not for research purposes, they are exempt from REB review.

To refine existing knowledge and develop new knowledge, clinical research sometimes uses new procedures whose outcome is doubtful or unknown. This research may seem to conflict with the purpose of nursing practice, which is to meet specific clients' needs. In such cases, the researcher must structure the investigation to avoid or minimize harm to the subjects. Although not all undesirable effects can be anticipated, researchers are obligated to inform everyone involved about the known potential risks. Other basic human rights must also be observed. These principles are set forth by the CNA (1983, 1991). Procedures for obtaining **informed consent** must be outlined in the study protocol. The consent form must describe in lay language the purpose of the study, the role of the subjects, types of data that are to be obtained, how the data are obtained, the duration of the study, subject selection, procedures, risks to the subject (including financial risks), potential benefits (including the possibility of no benefit), alternatives to participation, and contact information concerning the principal investigator and local REB. The consent process gives subjects complete information regarding the study's risks, benefits, and costs so that they can make an informed decision.

The REB also determines if the researcher has the necessary knowledge and skills to undertake the research, including familiarity with the clinical area in which the data will be collected and sufficient research training and experience. For example, a nurse planning a study of psychiatric clients should be familiar with psychiatric nursing principles and theory, as well as research procedures for data collection and analysis.

Rights of Other Research Participants

Student nurses and practising nurses may be asked to participate in research as data collectors or may be involved in the care of clients participating in a study. All participants, including health care professionals, have the right to be fully informed about the study, its procedures (including the consent process and risk factors), and physical or emotional injuries that clients could experience as a result of participation. Often, the physical risks are more obvious than the emotional risks. For example, clients may be asked to give highly personal, intrusive information, which some may find stressful. The researcher should prepare all participants, including nurses delivering care, for this possibility and assist them in coping with the effects. Participants also have the right to see

Box 6-4 Guiding Ethical Principles for Research in Canada

1. *Respect for Human Dignity:* This principle aspires to protect the multiple and interdependent interests of the person—bodily, psychological, and cultural integrity.
2. *Respect for Free and Informed Consent:* Presumes that individuals have the capacity and right to make free and informed decisions.
3. *Respect for Vulnerable Persons:* Children, institutionalized people, or others who are vulnerable are entitled, on grounds of human dignity, caring, solidarity, and fairness, to special protection against abuse, exploitation, or discrimination.
4. *Respect for Privacy and Confidentiality:* Standards of privacy and confidentiality protect the access, control, and dissemination of personal information and thus help to protect mental or psychological integrity. These standards are consonant with values underlying privacy, confidentiality, and anonymity.
5. *Respect for Justice and Inclusiveness:* The ethics review process should be independent and use fair methods, standards, and procedures. No segment of the population should be unfairly burdened with the harms of research. There are particular obligations to protect vulnerable individuals unable to protect their own interests. Individuals and groups who may benefit from advances in research must neither be discriminated against nor neglected.
6. *Balancing Harms and Benefits:* Research ethics require a favourable harms-benefit balance so that the foreseeable harms should not outweigh anticipated benefits.
7. *Minimizing Harm:* Non-maleficence, the duty to avoid, prevent, or minimize harms to others, is considered essential in research. No research subjects should be subjected to unnecessary risks of harm, and their participation in research must be essential to achieving important aims for science and for society.
8. *Maximizing Benefit:* Beneficence, the duty to benefit others, in research ethics means a duty to maximize net benefits. In most research, the primary benefits produced are for society and for the advancement of knowledge, rather than for the individual research participant.

Adapted from Tri-Council Policy on Research Ethics: *Context of an Ethics Framework,* available from *http://www.nserc.ca/programs/ethics/english/intro01.htm*

review forms from the REB that certify approval of the study. Participants can refuse to carry out research procedures if they are concerned about ethical aspects.

Applying Research Findings to Nursing Practice

Research evidence as a basis for scholarly, professional decision making in clinical practice is essential for providing competent, efficient, and state-of-the art nursing care (McCaughan et al., 2002). Advances in care through research are meaningless unless they reach nurses at the point of care. Nurses make links between research findings and nursing care by reading relevant literature, identifying appropriate clinical problems, and incorporating **research utilization** activities into the nursing practice of a specific nursing unit or agency.

Nurses must read journals that contain research reports, as well as textbooks and other journals in nursing and related fields. Findings from research may be suitable for use in nursing practice. This book uses Research Highlight boxes to illustrate how research can progress from clinical problem investigation to application in day-to-day client care (Box 6-5). To use findings in clinical practice, nurses must know the problems already studied, understand relevant research studies, and determine which findings apply to their client's needs.

Research Report Versus Clinical Article

Nurses must distinguish research reports or articles from other literature. The article may not report results from a study even if the title contains the word *research.* The only way to determine if an article reports research results is to examine its contents. Sometimes, however, an article's title can give a clue to its contents. Phrases such as "a study of" or "comparison of" suggest a research report. The abstract and the introductory paragraphs of an article can also indicate whether the article is based on research. A typical research report includes the following:

- An introductory section that presents the purpose, a summary of literature used to formulate the study, the hypotheses tested, or the research questions posed.
- A methods section that describes the methods used to conduct the study, including the sample, type of data collected, and the device or instrument used to measure empirical information.
- A results section that describes the results of the study, including statistical tests used to analyze data.
- A discussion section that presents the author's interpretation of the results, including conclusions and implications that can be drawn from the study.
- References that list articles and other research used to support the study.

If the report is written by a researcher who conducted the study, it is a **primary source.** Any other article about the study is considered a **secondary source** (e.g., an article by an author not involved in the study who collected the information from another source). Most nursing textbooks are secondary sources. Their authors incorporate knowledge and information gathered from nursing and related literature, including research written by original investigators.

Locating Research Studies

In the health care field, several resources can help nurses find research articles. To locate primary research sources, nurses should go to the journals where original research reports are published. The most efficient way to locate

Research Highlight

Box 6-5

A Comparison of Three Anaesthetics for Infant Circumcision

Research Focus

This study addressed misconceptions about infant pain and infants' responses to anaesthetics.

In the past, beliefs about the safety and effectiveness of current anesthetics have resulted in many newborns being circumcised without anesthesia. Clinical practice was changed as a result of this research, involving both nursing and medicine.

Research Abstract

The objective of this study was to compare ring block, dorsal penile nerve block, a topical eutectic mixture of local anesthetics (EMLA), and topical placebo when used for neonatal circumcision. The placebo represented current practice, with no anesthetic for neonatal circumcision. The design was a randomized controlled trial set in antenatal units in two tertiary care hospitals in Edmonton, Alberta. A consecutive sample of 52 healthy, full-term, male newborns, aged 1 to 3 days, was admitted to the study. Physiological and behavioural monitoring occurred in a series of trials: baseline, drug application, preparation, circumcision, and post-circumcision. Surgical procedures defined the following four stages of the circumcision: cleansing, separation, clamp on, and clamp off. Methemoglobin level was assessed 6 hours after surgery. The main outcome measures were heart rate, cry, and methemoglobin level. Newborns in the untreated placebo group exhibited homogeneous responses that consisted of sustained elevation of heart rate and high-pitched cry throughout the circumcision and following. Two newborns in the placebo group became ill following circumcision (choking and apnea). The three treatment groups all had significantly less crying and lower heart rates during and following circumcision compared with the untreated group. The ring block was equally effective through all stages of the circumcision, whereas the dorsal penile nerve block and EMLA were not effective during foreskin separation and incision. Methemoglobin levels were highest in the EMLA group, although no newborn required treatment. It was concluded that the most effective anesthetic is the ring block; EMLA is the least effective. It is our recommendation that an anesthetic should be administered to newborns prior to undergoing circumcision.

Implications for Practice

- The effects of pain in infants are significant, and measures to reduce or eliminate severe pain experienced during circumcision should be taken.
- Measures to be taken to reduce pain should be discussed with parents before the procedure.
- The effects of pain on neonates in other invasive procedures should be considered.

Reference

Lander, J., et al. (1997). Comparison of ring block, dorsal penile nerve block and topical anesthesia for neonatal circumcision: A randomized controlled trial. *Journal of the American Medical Association*, 278, 2157–2162.

research articles is to consult a computerized database or an index of journal articles, such as the *Cumulative Index to Nursing and Allied Health Literature (CINAHL), International Nursing Index, MEDLINE,* and *PubMed.*

Major nursing journals publish research studies or research reports. Some journals, such as *Nursing Research,* are devoted solely to research; other nursing journals, such as the *American Journal of Critical Care,* publish both original research reports and clinical reports. Most specialty practice journals publish research articles devoted to the particular specialty.

Research Utilization

Usually the results of one study, no matter how convincing, do not provide sufficient evidence to change policy and practice. Multiple studies with similar findings must be assessed before the findings can be applied. Beginners should look for articles that provide a systematic review, an examination of all the research on a given topic that critically evaluates the methods used, and a summary of the findings. A good systematic review can provide the basis for changing policy and practice.

Even the evidence provided by good systematic reviews is often not sufficient to change practice. Ehrenberg and Estabrooks (2004) report that a survey of 5,947 clients in European hospitals revealed that less than 4.6% of those who were at risk for or already had pressure ulcers were given adequate prevention measures. This is despite research evidence showing that at least 50% of pressure ulcers are preventable and despite clinical guidelines developed from the research and distributed widely in several countries. This survey clearly illustrates the research/practice gap in nursing and the consequences for clients when the latest research is not used.

Much current research focuses on ways to improve the utilization of new knowledge in practice. A summary of steps to foster success is found in Box 6-6.

Evidence-Based Practice and Research

Evidence-based practice incorporates critical thinking and research utilization competencies (Stetler et al., 1998). The research utilization skills enable the nurse to systematically transfer or translate research-based knowledge into the clinical practice setting (Kajermo et al., 2001). Evidence-based practice recognizes that the best evidence may not be research based but, in fact, may be the evidence of clinical experts in the field. Integration of evidence-based practice is essential for competent, safe nursing care.

Evidence-based practice and research-based practice are terms often used interchangeably. However, research-based practice refers to the use of knowledge based on

Box 6-6 Steps for Successful Research Utilization

1. Relevance—Topic/problem needs to be relevant to the nursing and administration staff participating in the utilization project.
   a. Identify and gather research studies appropriate to the clinical problem.
   b. Critique the research studies.
   c. Determine the merit of each study in terms of applicability to clinical practice.
   d. Develop a specific practice innovation based on researching findings of studies critiqued.
   e. Apply the practice innovation based on research findings of studies critiqued.
   f. Determine outcomes of the innovation.
   g. Evaluate outcomes of the innovation for widespread use.
2. Education—Prepare method to educate and inform staff about the research utilization process.
3. Support—Determine necessary support resources (e.g., librarian, university faculty, doctorally prepared researchers) to streamline and assist in the process.
4. Expectation—Create a climate where utilization of research findings in a practice setting is expected.
5. Alignment—Set goals for research utilization, implemenation of change, and the educational process.
6. Reward—Acknowledge the work of others in utilizing research findings; build activities into career building.
7. Caring—Emphasize state-of-the-art nursing care and the impact on the client and family, and acknowledge impact on the total care provided by the staff, not just the people active in the research utilization project.
8. Continue to incorporate the innovation into daily client care routine.

Data from "Supporting Nurses in Their Quest for Evidence-Based Practice: Research Utilization and Conduct," by R. Maljanian, 2000, *Outcomes Management for Nursing Practice, 4*(4), p. 144; and "Strategies for Teaching Nursing Research: Teaching Baccalaureate Nursing Students," by H. R. Feldman, 1996, *Western Journal of Nursing Research, 18,* p. 479.

systematic research studies, whereas evidence-based practice also takes into account a nurse's clinical experience, practice trends, and even individual client preferences (Barnsteiner & Prevost, 2002; Stevens, 2001).

In a policy statement released in 1998, the CNA stated that evidence-based decision-making by registered nurses "is key to quality nursing practice" (CNA, 1998, p. 1). Nurses need not only skills to access and appraise existing research, but also scientific knowledge and skills to change practice settings and to promote evidence-based decisions about client care.

Evidence-based nursing practice deemphasizes ritual, isolated, and unsystematic clinical experiences; ungrounded opinion; and tradition as a basis for nursing practice. It stresses the use of research findings, and as appropriate, quality improvement data, other evaluation data, and the consensus of recognized experts and affirmed experience to support a specific practice (Stetler, et al. 1998). Evidence-based practice is nursing's goal, yet it raises issues, such as the need for targeted research in specific practice areas and the need for better dissemination of research findings (CNA, 1998). Many aspects of health care are not justly served by one discipline's research. The expertise of several disciplines must be brought to bear on complex health issues. Just as nurses play a vital role on the health care team, so they are crucial to multidisciplinary health research. Policy-makers in the broader arena of health must hear the voice of nursing, which is so essential to client care. Nurses need a sound knowledge base to support practice, and research is essential to build that knowledge.

Key Concepts

- There are four patterns of nursing knowledge: empirics, esthetics, personal knowledge, and ethics.
- A scientific investigation is an orderly, planned, and controlled study of reality that can be applied to general situations and that tests theories.
- Nursing research looks at physical or psychosocial responses of people of all ages in various states of health and illness.
- An experimental research study controls factors that could influence the results, includes comparison and experimental treatment groups of subjects, and uses random means for selecting study subjects.
- A qualitative research study organizes information in narrative format so that phenomena can be described and patterns of relationships can be discovered.
- Participation of human subjects in research requires the researcher to obtain informed consent of study subjects, to maintain the confidentiality of subjects, and to protect subjects from undue risk or injury.
- When summarizing data reported in a research study, the nurse should note when, how, where, and by whom the investigation was conducted and who and what were studied.
- A researchable clinical nursing problem is one that is not satisfactorily resolved by present nursing interventions, occurs frequently in a particular group, can be measured or observed, and has a possible solution within the realm of nursing practice.
- To determine if research findings can be used in nursing practice, the nurse considers the scientific worth of the study, substantiating evidence from other studies, the similarity of the research setting to the nurse's own clinical practice setting, the status of current nursing theory, and factors affecting the feasibility of application.

Key Terms

Empirical data, *p. 85*
Ethnography, *p. 88*
Evidence-based practice, *p. 84*
Grounded theory, *p. 88*
Hypothesis, *p. 85*
Informed consent, *p. 89*
Nursing research, *p. 81*
Phenomenology, *p. 88*
Primary source, *p. 90*
Qualitative nursing research, *p. 88*

Quantitative nursing research, *p. 86*
Quasi-experimental research design, *p. 87*
Research mindedness, *p. 89*
Research process, *p. 85*
Research utilization, *p. 90*
Scientific method, *p. 85*
Scientific nursing research, *p. 86*
Secondary source, *p. 90*
Subjects, *p. 87*
Surveys, *p. 87*
True experiment, *p. 87*

Critical Thinking Exercises

1. The nurse is concerned about learning to properly treat a pressure ulcer. Explain the benefits to the client if the nurse learns how to treat the sore by drawing from information in the research literature rather than using the scientific method.
2. The research literature reflects many different methods for treating pressure ulcers. If you wished to determine the best method for doing this, what type of research design would you use?
3. The nurses working on an orthopedic unit decide to study the factors that commonly result in client falls on their unit. How could they design a study to answer their questions?

Review Questions

1. The first provincially approved doctoral program was established in
   1. 1969
   2. 1974
   3. 1982
   4. 1991
2. Empirics is described by Carper (1978) as
   1. The artistic expression of knowledge
   2. Knowledge derived from the interpersonal relationship with the client
   3. Knowledge derived from ethical dilemmas
   4. Knowledge systematically organized into general laws and theories
3. The scientific method is characterized by
   1. Systematic procedures that seek to limit error and eliminate bias
   2. Studies of behaviours, experiences, perceptions, and motives
   3. A commitment to the participants's point of view
   4. The use of the participants' natural setting
4. If the research question leads to the study of behaviour within a specific culture, the design chosen is
   1. Phenomenology
   2. Grounded theory
   3. Ethnography
   4. Quantitative research
5. Subjectivity is the goal of
   1. Positivism
   2. Qualitative research
   3. True experiments
   4. The scientific method
6. Which research method is quantitative?
   1. Grounded theory
   2. Phenomenology
   3. Ethnography
   4. Quasi-experimental research
7. A sample in a survey design
   1. Is the main component of qualitative research
   2. Should be representative of the population surveyed
   3. Should be small enough to keep sampling error to a minimum
   4. Should be no different from the control group
8. Procedures for obtaining informed consent do NOT include
   1. Describing the purpose of the study
   2. Describing the role of the subjects
   3. Giving the names of other participants in the study
   4. Describing the risks of the subject
9. In a quasi-experimental research design, subjects are assigned to
   1. An empirical group
   2. An ethnographic group
   3. A control group or treatment condition
   4. An experimental group
10. Evidence-based practice
    1. Enables the transfer of clinical practice techniques into a positivist paradigm
    2. Requires that evidence be always research based
    3. Is synonymous with research-based practice
    4. Uses knowledge based on research studies and takes into account a nurse's clinical experience and client preferences.

References

Barnsteiner, J., & Prevost, S. (2002). How to interpret evidence-based practice: Some tried and true pointers. *Reflections on Nursing Leadership, 28*(2), 18–21.
Barrett, E. A. M. (1998). Unique nursing research methods: The diversity chant of pioneers. *Nursing Science Quarterly, 11*(3), 94–96.
Brink, P., & Wood, M. (2001). *Basic steps in planning nursing research* (inside cover). Sudbury, MA: Jones & Bartlett.
Canadian Association of University Schools of Nursing. (1997). *Canadian nursing research priorities: Results of Phase III of National Nursing Research Symposium*. Ottawa, ON: Author.
Canadian Nurses Association. (1983). *Ethical guidelines for nursing research involving human subjects*. Ottawa, ON: Author.
Canadian Nurses Association. (1991). *Code of ethics for registered nurses*. Ottawa, ON: Author.
Canadian Nurses Association. (1998). *Policy statement: Evidence-based decision-making and nursing practice*. Ottawa, ON: Author.
Carper, B. A. (1978). Fundamental patterns of knowing in nursing. *Advances in Nursing Science, 1*(1),13–23.
Carroll, D. L., et al. (1997). Barriers and facilitators to the utilization of nursing research. *Clinical Nurse Specialist CNS, 11*(5), 207–212.
Ehrenberg A., & Estabrooks, C. (2004). Why using research matters. *Journal of Wound, Ostomy, and Continence Nursing, 32*(2), 62–66.

Feldman, H. R. (1996). Strategies for teaching nursing research: teaching baccalaureate nursing students. *Western Journal of Nursing Research, 18,* 479–481.

Glaser, B., & Strauss, A. (1969). *The discovery of grounded theory.* Chicago: Aldine.

Good, S.R. (1969). *Submission to the study of support of research in universities for the Science Secretariat of the Privy Council.* Ottawa, ON: Canadian Nurses Association and Canadian Nurses Foundation.

Husserl, E. (1962). *Ideas: General introduction to pure phenomenology.* New York: Collier.

Institute of Medicine, Division of Health Care Services. (1983). *Nursing and nursing education: Public policies and private actions.* Washington, DC: National Academy.

International Council of Nurses. (1986). *Nursing research: ICN position statement.* Geneva: Author.

Jeffers, B. R. (1998). The surrogate's experience during treatment decision making. *Medsurg Nursing, 7*(6), 357–363.

Kajermo K.N., et al. (2001). Nurses' experiences of research utilization within the framework of an educational programme, *Journal of Clinical Nursing. 10*(5):671.

Ketchum, K., & Perry, A. C. (1999). *Patients' perceptions in weaning from mechanical ventilation.* Manuscript submitted for publication.

Knapp, T. R. (1998). *Quantitative nursing research.* Thousand Oaks, CA: Sage Publications.

Kuhn, T. (1970). *The structure of scientific revolutions* (2nd ed.). Chicago: University of Chicago Press.

Lysaught, J. P. (1970). *An abstract for action.* New York: McGraw-Hill.

Maljanian, R. (2000). Supporting nurses in their quest for evidence-based practice: Research utilization and conduct. *Outcomes Management for Nursing Practice, 4*(4),155–158.

McCaughan, D., et al. (2002). Acute care nurses' perceptions of barriers to using research information in clinical decision-making. *Journal of Advanced Nursing, 39*(1), 46–60.

Medical Research Council of Canada. (1985). *Report to the Medical Research Council of Canada by the Working Group on Nursing Research.* Ottawa, ON:Author.

Medical Research Council of Canada, the Natural Sciences and Engineering Research Council of Canada, & the Social Sciences and Humanities Research Council of Canada. (2003). *Tri-Council Policy Statement: Ethical conduct for research involving humans, 1998 (with 2000, 2002 updates).* Retrieved November 25, 2004, from *www.pre.ethics.gc.ca/english/pdf/TCPS June2003_E.pdf*

Milburn, K., et al. (1995). Combining methods in health promotion research: Some considerations about appropriate use. *Health Education Journal,* 54, 347–356.

National Center for Nursing Research/International Council of Nurses. (1990). *Nursing research worldwide: Report of the Task Force on International Nursing Research.* Geneva, Switzerland: Author.

National Institute of Nursing Research. (1997). *National Institute of Nursing Research mission statement.* Bethesda, MD: National Institutes of Health. Retrieved August 15, 2004, from *http://www.nih.gov/ninr/ NINR2000A.RO.html*

Parahoo, K. (1997). *Nursing research: Principles, process and issues.* London: MacMillan Press.

Polit, D. F., & Beck, C. T. (2004). *Nursing research: Principles and methods* (7th ed.). Philadelphia: Lippincott.

Polit, D. F., & Hungler, B. P. (1999). *Nursing research: Principles and methods* (6th ed.). Philadelphia: Lippincott.

Ross-Kerr, J. C., & MacPhail, J. (1996). *Canadian nursing: Issues and perspectives.* Toronto, ON: Mosby-Year Book.

Stetler, C. B., et al. (1998). Evidence-based practice and the role of nursing leadership. *Journal of Nursing Administration, 28*(7), 45–53.

Stevens, K. (2001). Systematic reviews: The heart of evidence-based practice. *AACN Clinical Issues, 12*(4), 529–538.

Streubert, H. J., & Carpenter, D. R. (1999). *Qualitative research in nursing: Advancing the humanistic imperative* (p. 10). Philadelphia: Lippincott.

Symons, T. H. B. (1975). *To know ourselves: The report of the Commission of Canadian Studies* (p. 212). Ottawa, ON: Association of Universities and Colleges of Canada.

Titler, M. G., et al. (1994). Infusing research into practice to promote quality care. *Nursing Research, 43*(50), 307–313.

Walsh, M. (1997). Barriers to research utilization and evidence based practice in A & E nursing. *Emergency Nurse, 5*(2), 24–27.

Recommended Web Sites

Canadian Nurses Association:
http://www.can-nurses.ca
Contains information about policies and position statements for nursing research in Canada, as well as information on research funding.

Canadian Nurses Foundation:
http://www.canadiannursesfoundation.com
This site provides information on available research funding as well as scholarships for students.

The Canadian Health Services Research Foundation:
http://www.chsrf.ca
Contains information about funding for health services research, as well as the Nursing Research Fund.

Canadian Institutes of Health Research:
http://www.cihr.ca
Web pages for all 13 Institutes for Health Research in Canada.

7

Nursing Values and Ethics

Shelley Raffin Bouchal, RN, BScN, MN, PhD (Canadian author)
Margaret Ecker, RN, MS, PNP

Objectives

Mastery of content in this chapter will enable the student to:

- Define the key terms listed.
- Discuss the role of values in the study of ethics.
- Examine and clarify personal values.
- Discuss how values influence client care.
- Explain the relationship between ethics and professional practice.
- Describe some basic ethical philosophies relevant to health care.
- Apply a method of ethical analysis to a clinical situation.
- Identify contemporary ethical issues in nursing practice.

Values and ethics are inherent in all nursing acts. A **value** is a strong personal belief. It is an ideal that a person or group (such as nurses) strives to uphold. **Ethics** refers to the study of the philosophical ideals of right and wrong behaviour. It also commonly refers to the values and standards to which individuals and professions strive (e.g., health care ethics, nursing ethics). In other words, ethics are a reflection of what matters most to people or professions. Nurses and other health care professionals agree to national codes of ethics that offer a guideline for difficult questions that occur in practice and demonstrate to the public an overview of professional practice standards. For example, the Canadian Nurses Association (CNA) publishes a **code of ethics** (2002) that outlines nurses' professional values and ethical commitments to their clients.

Because of their prominent and intimate role in the provision of health care, nurses continually make decisions about the right thing to do in different circumstances. Often, there is no best answer or course of action. To manage these difficult situations, nurses need a keen awareness of their values and those of their clients, a good understanding of ethics, and a sound approach to ethical decision making. They also must be guided by a broader understanding of ethics through the application of theories and sets of principles (Yeo & Moorehouse, 1996).

Values

Values are at the heart of ethics. A value is a personal belief about the worth of a given idea, attitude, custom, or object that sets standards that influence behaviour (Maslow, 1959; Rokeach, 1973). An individual's values reflect cultural and social influences, relationships, and personal needs. Values vary among people and develop and change over time.

The CNA *Code of Ethics* (2002) is organized around eight values that are central to ethical nursing practice. Providing safe, competent, and ethical care and promoting health and well-being, choice, and dignity are some of the values in the code. Each provincial nursing association also has shared values, such as those held in position statements and practice standards. These standards reflect the values of the profession and clarify what is expected of each practising nurse.

Because of the intimacy of the nurse-client relationship, nurses must be aware of their personal values as well as the values of clients, physicians, employers, or other groups. To understand the values of others, it is important to understand one's own values: what they are, where they came from, and how they relate to others' values.

Value Formation

People acquire values in many ways, beginning in early childhood. Throughout childhood and adolescence, people learn to distinguish right from wrong and to form values on which to base their actions. This is known as moral development (see chapter 18). Family experiences strongly influence value formation. In some families, children are strictly disciplined and expected to conform to the parents' standards of right and wrong. In others, children receive little discipline or limitations. These variations in child rearing create variations in values and in adult behaviour.

Values are also learned outside the family. People's culture, ethnic, and religious communities strongly influence their values, as do schools, peer groups, and work environments. **Cultural values** are those adopted as a result of a person's social setting. A basic task of the young adult is to identify personal values within the context of the community. Over time, an individual acquires values by choosing some that are strongly held in the community and discarding or transforming others.

Individual experience also influences one's values. For example, a person who suffers much in life may have very different values from someone whose life has been free of suffering. Nurses and other care providers must respect the wide variety of values that clients may hold.

Values Clarification

Clarifying one's values helps to articulate one's point of view. Values are key to the way an individual sees the world. They influence how a person interprets confusing or conflicting information. As people mature and experience new situations, their values change. They may reorder their values or replace old values with new ones. As a result, the person may modify attitudes and behaviour. The willingness to change shows a healthy attitude and an ability to adapt to new experiences.

To adopt new values, a person must be aware of his or her existing values and how they affect behaviour. **Values clarification** is the process of appraising one's personal values (Box 7-1). It is not a set of rules, nor does it suggest that certain values should be accepted by all people. Rather, it is a process of personal reflection. People who clarify their values make careful choices. The result of values clarification is greater self-awareness and personal insight.

By understanding their personal values, nurses better understand their clients' and colleagues' values. "Value conflict" is when personal values are at odds with those of a client, colleague, or institution. Values clarification plays a major role in resolving these dilemmas. As well, nurses can better advocate for a client when they can identify personal values and the values of the client.

Once the skill of clarifying personal values is mastered, the nurse can help clients identify their personal priorities, values, and emotions. This may help clients resolve conflicts between values and behaviours. The goal of values clarification with clients is effective nurse-client communication. As the client becomes more willing to express problems and feelings, the nurse can better establish an individualized care plan.

Structured communication is a useful way to clarify values with a client. Simple strategies that promote the process of sharing feelings can be effective. For example, responding to a client by repeating the client's sentence as a question ("You wish you could be at home?") will encourage the client to elaborate. Avoiding questions that can be answered with a yes or no encourages the client to answer in greater detail. Rather than asking, "Do you want to live at home with your daughter?" the nurse might say, "Tell me how you feel about living at home with your daughter."

How the nurse responds can motivate the client to examine personal thoughts and actions. When the nurse makes a clarifying response, it should be brief and nonjudgmental. For example, when talking with a client who exercises rarely, the nurse might ask, "What is your understanding of the purpose of exercise?" An effective clarifying response encourages the client to think about personal values after the exchange is over without imposing the nurse's own values onto the client's. In this

Box 7-1 Three Steps of Values Clarification

Choosing One's Beliefs and Behaviours

Choosing from alternatives
Choosing freely
Considering all consequences

Prizing One's Beliefs and Behaviours

Prizing and cherishing the choice
Publicly affirming the choice

Acting on One's Beliefs

Making the choice part of one's behaviour
Acting with a pattern of consistency and repetition

A Values Clarification Exercise

1. Consider a choice that you make about a fundamental value. For example, how do you feel about abortion? Or what do you consider your obligations to society? Think through all the possible choices and the consequences of each choice.
2. Describe how you might make your choice clear to friends, family, colleagues. How would they know that you cherish this particular value?
3. List three or four activities in which you might participate where your behaviour reflects consistent commitment to this specific value.

Adapted from *Values and Teaching* (2nd ed.), by L. E. Raths, M. Harmin, and S. B. Simon, 1979, Columbus, OH: Merrill Publishing.

Box 7-2 Canadian Nurses Association Code of Ethics

The following is the CNA's statement of the eight values that must be upheld in nursing practice. The complete code of ethics also includes responsibility statements outlining how nurses can incorporate these values into their practice; it can be found on the CNA Web site (see Recommended Web Sites at the end of this chapter).

Values

Safe, Competent, and Ethical Care

Nurses value the ability to provide safe, competent, and ethical care that allows them to fulfill their ethical and professional obligations to the people they serve.

Health and Well-Being

Nurses value health promotion and well-being and assisting persons to achieve their optimum level of health in situations of normal health, illness, injury, and disability, or at the end of life.

Choice

Nurses respect and promote the autonomy of persons and help them to express their health needs and values and also to obtain desired information and services so that they can make informed decisions.

Dignity

Nurses recognize and respect the inherent worth of each person and advocate for respectful treatment of all persons.

Confidentiality

Nurses safeguard information learned in the context of a professional relationship and ensure it is shared outside the health care team only with the person's informed consent, or as may be legally required, or where the failure to disclose would cause significant harm.

Justice

Nurses uphold principles of equity and fairness to assist persons in receiving a share of health services and resources proportionate to their needs and promoting social justice.

Accountability

Nurses are answerable for their practice, and they act in a manner consistent with their professional responsibilities and standards of practice.

Quality Practice Environments

Nurses value and advocate for quality practice environments that have the organizational structures and resources necessary to ensure safety, support, and respect for all persons in the work setting.

Source: *Code of Ethics for Registered Nurses,* by Canadian Nurses Association, August 2002, Ottawa, ON: Author.

way, the nurse respects the client's self-direction and avoids inappropriately introducing personal values into the conversation.

Values clarification plays a key role in communication. Especially when the topic concerns issues of personal health, private habits, and quality of life, participants in a discussion will benefit from clarity of values. The nurse who appreciates values can identify differences between personal opinion and the values that others embrace. Through values clarification, the nurse better serves the needs of clients, especially when values differ. By demonstrating respect for the client's differences and helping the client to clarify values, the nurse is better able to teach and to heal.

Ethics

Ethics is the study of good conduct, character, and motives. It is concerned with determining what is good or valuable for all people. Often the terms *ethics* and *morals* or ***morality*** are used interchangeably (Johnstone, 1999). Morals or morality is often stated as private, personal standards of what is right and wrong based on social mores or customs. Ethics, on the other hand, is a dynamic process of dialogue and action. Acts that are ethical often reflect a commitment to standards beyond personal preferences—standards on which individuals, professions, and societies agree.

Professional Nursing and Ethics

Codes of Ethics. A code of ethics is a set of ethical principles that are accepted by all members of a profession. A profession's ethical code is a collective statement about the group's expectations and standards of behaviour. Codes serve as guidelines to assist nurses and other professionals when questions arise about correct practice or behaviour. The nursing code of ethics, as in other professions, sets forth ideals of conduct.

A code serves only as a guideline for ethical practice. It does not provide rules of behaviour for every circumstance. Situations are unique to the context in which they occur. The environment or institution can greatly influence the values that nurses are encouraged to uphold. Further, a code does not offer guidance as to which values should take priority or how to balance them in practice. A code must also be adopted in relation to the law, professional standards, and ethical principles (CNA, 2002).

The CNA and the International Council of Nurses have established widely accepted codes for nurses that re-

Box 7-3 International Council of Nurses Code of Ethics

Nurses have four fundamental responsibilities: to promote health, to prevent illness, to restore health, and to alleviate suffering. The need for nursing is universal. Inherent in nursing is respect for human rights, including the right to life, to dignity, and to be treated with respect. Nursing care is unrestricted by considerations of age, colour, creed, culture, disability or illness, gender, nationality, politics, or social status. Nurses render health services to the individual, the family, and the community and coordinate their services with those of related groups.

Nurses and People

The nurse's primary responsibility is to people requiring nursing care.

In providing care, the nurse respects human rights, values, customs, and spiritual beliefs of the individual, family, and community. The nurse provides the individual with sufficient information on which to base consent for care and related information.

The nurse holds personal information in confidence and uses judgment in sharing it.

The nurse shares with society the responsibility for initiating and supporting action to meet the health and social needs of the public, particularly those of vulnerable populations.

The nurse also shares responsibility to sustain and protect the natural environment from depletion, pollution, degradation, and destruction.

Nurses and Practice

The nurse carries personal responsibility and accountability for nursing practice and for maintaining competence by continual learning.

The nurse maintains a standard of personal health such that the ability to provide care is not compromised.

The nurse uses judgment regarding individual competence when accepting and delegating responsibility.

The nurse at all times maintains standards of personal conduct that reflect well on the profession and enhance public confidence.

Nurses and the Profession

The nurse assumes the major role in determining and implementing acceptable standards of critical nursing practice, management, research, and education.

The nurse is active in developing a core of research-based professional knowledge.

The nurse, acting through the professional organization, participates in creating and maintaining equitable social and economic working conditions in nursing.

Nurses and Co-Workers

The nurse sustains a cooperative relationship with co-workers in nursing and other fields.

The nurse takes appropriate action to safeguard individuals when their care is endangered by a co-worker or any other person.

From *ICN Code of Ethics for Nurses* by International Council of Nurses, 2000, Geneva, Switzerland, The Council.

flect the principles of responsibility, accountability, and advocacy (Boxes 7-2 and 7-3). Nurses agree to be responsible for specific actions and accountable for the consequences. They also agree to maintain competence in their practice and to use competence in the application of judgment. To act as an advocate, the nurse must promote and protect clients' rights.

Responsibility. **Responsibility** refers to the characteristics of reliability and dependability. It implies an ability to distinguish between right and wrong. In professional nursing, responsibility includes a duty to perform actions well and thoughtfully. When administering a medication, for example, a nurse is responsible for assessing the client's need for the drug, for giving it safely and correctly, and for evaluating the response to it. By agreeing to act responsibly, the nurse gains trust from clients, colleagues, and society.

Nurses are responsible for ensuring safe and competent care for clients and respecting their fundamental rights to dignity, privacy, and information. For example, nurses are to treat all clients as people worthy of respect, provide care in a discreet manner that respects the client's physical privacy and minimizes unwanted intrusions, and be truthful when providing information (CNA, 2002).

Accountability. **Accountability** means being able to answer for one's actions. The nurse balances accountability to the client, the profession, the employer, and society. For example, a nurse may know that a client who will be discharged soon is confused about how to administer insulin. The action that a nurse takes in response to this situation will be guided by the sense of accountability. The client, the institution, and society rely on the good judgment of the nurse and trust that the nurse will take action in response to this situation. The nurse may request more hospitalization to provide further teaching or arrange home care to continue teaching at home. The goal is the prevention of injury to the client. The nurse's sense of accountability guides actions that achieve this goal

According to the CNA (2002), nurses who are enacting professional accountability are (a) evaluating new professional practices and reassessing existing ones, (b) ensuring they have the skill to provide these practices, (c) safeguarding the quality of nursing care that clients receive, and (d) sharing their knowledge with others through mentorship and giving feedback to others when appropriate.

Professional accountability is also the mandate of professional associations. Professional associations both check unethical practice in a profession and support conscientious professionals who may be under pressure to act unethically or to overlook unethical activity by colleagues. They have the authority to register and discipline nurses. They also set and maintain professional standards of practice and communicate them to the public. These standards, developed by nursing clinical experts, provide a basic structure against which nursing care is objectively measured. They do not eliminate the need for individualized care plans; rather, the nurse incorporates the standards into each client's care plan.

Advocacy. The ethical responsibility of being an advocate is to "see that the [client's] rights and interests are protected in health care settings" (Davis et al., 1997, p. 76). The CNA advises nurses to advocate for all persons in their care (2002). This includes protecting the client's right to choice by providing information, obtaining informed consent for all nursing care, and respecting clients' decisions. Nurses should protect clients' right to dignity by advocating for appropriate use of interventions in order to minimize suffering, intervening if others fail to respect the dignity of the client, and working to promote health and social conditions that allow people to live and die with dignity. Nurses should protect the clients' right to confidentiality by helping them access their health records (subject to legal requirements), intervening if other members of the health care team fail to respect their confidentiality, and following policies that protect their privacy. The *Code of Ethics* also states that nurses should advocate for the discussion of ethical issues among team members, clients, and families, and nurses should advocate for health policies that enable fair and inclusive allocation of resources.

Advocacy is sometimes controversial in the nursing literature because it is at times associated with informing on wrongdoers, or "whistle-blowing" (Tschudin, 1995). However, advocacy should be seen as essential to nursing because of the holistic nurse-client relationship. Nurses usually interact with clients over longer time intervals than do other professionals. Clients and families may reveal information not generally shared with physicians or others. Details about family life, information about coping styles, personal preferences, and fears and insecurities are likely to come out during nursing interventions (Shannon, 1997). Therefore, nurses are in an ideal position to act as advocates. However, nurses should remember that they are not the only advocates. The nursing point of view is part of the larger picture that is best built by all members of the health care team. Physicians, other health care professionals, professional organizations, and the client's family also act as the client's advocates.

Ethical Theory

An understanding of ethics provides a foundation for logical and consistent decision making. Ethics have to do with examining the moral basis for judgments, actions, duties, and obligations. For centuries, moral philosophers have tried to answer two questions: What is the meaning of right and good? What is the morally right thing to do in this situation? Nurses are mainly concerned with the second question because they are often in situations where they must make decisions that affect client well-being.

Philosophical discussion about health care issues has progressed over time, just as developments in health care and society itself have progressed. The philosophical constructions that shape the discussions have also changed. Ethics began as a standard reference point for the determination of right action. It has grown into a field of study filled with differences of opinion, competing systems of values, and deeply meaningful efforts to understand human interaction with new technologies. Some knowledge of ethical theories that have shaped our thinking is necessary to understand the development of nursing ethics. The following section introduces a variety of contemporary ethical theories. It is neither exclusive nor comprehensive.

Deontology. A traditional ethical theory, **deontology** proposes a system of ethics that is perhaps most familiar to practitioners in health care. Its foundations are often associated with the work of the 18th century philosopher Immanuel Kant (1724–1804). Deontology defines actions as right or wrong based on their "right-making characteristics such as fidelity to promises, truthfulness, and justice" (Beauchamp & Childress, 2001). It locates the essence of right or wrong within these principles. Deontology specifically does not look to consequences of actions to determine rightness or wrongness. Instead, it critically examines a situation for the existence of essential rightness or wrongness. Ethical principles such as justice, allowing free choice (autonomy), and doing the greatest good (beneficence) serve to define right or wrong. If an act is just, respects autonomy, and provides good, then the act will be ethical. The process depends on a mutual understanding and acceptance of these principles.

Difficulty arises when a person must choose among conflicting principles, which is often the case in health care ethical dilemmas. For example, applying the principle of respect for autonomy can be confusing when dealing with the health care of children. The health care team may recommend a treatment, but the parent may disagree or refuse the recommendation. In discussion of the dilemma, participants may refer to a guiding principle such as respect for autonomy. But questions will remain. Whose autonomy should receive the respect? The parent's? Who should speak for the child's best interest? Society often struggles to understand who should be ultimately responsible for the well-being of children. A commitment to respect autonomy does not guarantee that controversy can be avoided.

Utilitarianism. A utilitarian system of ethics proposes that the value of something is determined by its usefulness. This philosophy may also be known as **consequentialism** because its main emphasis is on the outcome or consequence of action. A third term associated with this philosophy is **teleology,** from the Greek word *telos,* meaning "end," or the study of ends or final causes. Its philosophical foundations were first proposed by John

Stuart Mill (1806–1873), a British philosopher and social commentator. The greatest good for the greatest number of people is the guiding principle for determining right action in this system. As with deontology, this theory relies on the application of a certain principle, namely, measures of "good" and "greatest" (Beauchamp & Childress, 2001). The difference between utilitarianism and deontology is in the focus on consequences or outcomes. Utilitarianism measures the effect that an act will have; deontology looks to the presence of principle regardless of outcome.

Individuals or groups may have conflicting definitions of "greatest good." For example, research suggests that education regarding safer sex practices may reduce the spread of human immunodeficiency virus. But some argue that education about sex should be provided in the family and that sex education in public schools diminishes the role and the value of family. For some, the greater good is defined as educating the greatest number of people in the most effective way possible. For others, the greater good is the preservation of family values and the protection of individual choices regarding sex education of children. The concepts of utilitarianism provide guidance, but they do not invariably provide for universal agreement.

Bioethics. In the 1970s, a group of ethics scholars concluded that current ethical theories were not sufficient for the health care field because they did not give specific guidance for important moral questions that arise in the context of medicine. A new theory called **bioethics** was developed, which specifically addressed issues relevant to health care. The central idea of bioethics is that moral decision making in health care should be guided by four principles: autonomy, beneficence, non-maleficence, and justice. According to this theory, health care providers should examine each situation, determine which of the principles has priority, and use that principle to guide action.

Autonomy. **Autonomy** refers to a person's independence. As a standard in ethics, autonomy represents an agreement to respect another's right to determine a course of action. Respect for another's autonomy is fundamental to the practice of health care. It is why clients are included in all aspects of decision making regarding their care. The agreement to respect autonomy involves the recognition that clients have the right to be respected and supported by the nurse regarding their health care decisions. For example, the purpose of the preoperative consent that clients must read and sign before surgery is the assurance in writing that the health care team respects the client's independence by obtaining permission to proceed. The consent process implies that a client may refuse treatment, and in most cases the health care team must agree to follow the client's wishes. Health care professionals agree to abide by a standard of respect for the client's autonomy.

Beneficence. **Beneficence** means doing or promoting good for others. It involves taking positive actions to help others. Commitment to beneficence helps to guide difficult decisions wherein the benefits of a treatment may be challenged by risks to the client's well-being or dignity. A child's immunization may cause temporary discomfort, but the benefits of protection from disease, both for the individual and for society, outweigh the discomfort. The agreement to act with beneficence also requires that the best interests of the client remain more important than self-interest. For example, a nurse does not simply follow medical orders but acts thoughtfully to understand client needs and then works actively to meet those needs.

Non-maleficence. Maleficence refers to harm or hurt; thus **non-maleficence** is the avoidance of harm or hurt. In health care ethics, ethical practice involves not only the will to do good, but also the equal commitment to do no harm. The health care professional tries to balance the risks and benefits of a plan of care while striving to do the least harm possible. This principle is often helpful in guiding discussions about new or controversial technologies. For example, a new bone marrow transplant procedure may promise a chance at cure. The procedure, however, may require long periods of pain and suffering. These discomforts should be considered in light of the suffering that the disease itself might cause, and in light of the suffering that other treatments might cause. The commitment to provide least harmful interventions illustrates the term *non-maleficence.* The standard of non-maleficence promotes a continuing effort to consider the potential for harm even when it may be necessary to promote health.

Justice. **Justice** refers to fairness. The term often is used during discussions about resources. What constitutes a fair distribution of resources may not always be clear. In these cases, national discussion about just distribution of resources often helps to clarify methods for achieving fairness. In Canada, nurses confront issues of justice at the governmental and institutional levels (Ross-Kerr & MacPhail, 1996), which affects the care that nurses are able to provide to their clients. Questions that will continue to intensify include, Which people in need of treatment should be given priority? How much money should go to services in acute care facilities? Should resources be reallocated to disease prevention or to health promotion? Should private fee-for-service health care be encouraged or even tolerated? (Yeo & Moorehouse, 1996) These are ethical questions that require further exploration of values, principles, and priorities to guide decisions in resource allocation.

Feminist Ethics. A newer philosophy focuses on feminism and ethics. Feminist ethicists consider their work a critique of conventional ethics, as well as a critique of social values. Their work focuses on continuing inequalities between people (Holmes & Purdy, 1992; Wolf, 1996). They look to the nature of relationships between people for guidance in working out ethical dilemmas. Writers with a feminist perspective concentrate more on practical solutions than on ethical theory.

Changes in the regard of women reflect new perspectives in women's relationship to family, to work, to science, and to society (Sherwin, 1992). For example, until the early 1980s, moral development was thought to reach the highest stages more often in men than in women. According to this theory, moral development occurred in predictable stages. The most complex stage involved a sense of justice, and young girls did not reach this stage as often as young boys (Kohlberg, 1981). Research from the early 1980s disputed these findings. Carol Gilligan (1982) proposed that Kohlberg's tools to measure moral development were gender biased. Gilligan went on to build a revised theory of moral development from her findings. She attempted to accommodate gender differences. Specifically, she concluded that young girls tend to pay attention to community and to individual circumstances and that young boys tend to process dilemmas through ideals or principles determined abstractly.

Feminist ethics philosophy builds on the idea that principles may distract participants from dealing with larger issues of community. Feminist ethicists value the role of relationships and stories about relationships. They emphasize the importance of stories and the role of community over an attention to universal principles. In fact, they argue that it is impossible to be unbiased or not influenced by relationships to people. They propose that the natural human urge to be influenced by relationships is a positive value (Wolf, 1996).

This system of ethics also addresses issues of gender inequality. Feminists propose that an inequality of attention to women can be remedied by routinely asking, in the midst of any ethical dilemma, how bioethical decisions will affect women (Sherwin, 1992). For example, in a discussion regarding the ethics of fetal surgery (surgical intervention before birth of the child), feminist ethics would propose that questions about the effects of the intervention on the mother are at least as important as questions about the effects on the fetus. In a discussion about a proposal to ration services to the very old so that younger people would have better resources, feminists might ask how such a proposal would affect women. In our society, there are more older women than older men. Bell (1992) concludes, "If age becomes a standard for limiting the provision of health care, the limits that will be set will affect women more drastically than they affect men." Gender-based investigations in ethical discussion would ensure that social facts about women, and men, are addressed.

Critics of feminist ethics argue that feminist ethics favours social relevance at the sacrifice of moral content. In this argument, the critics agree that feminists are concerned about inequities that occur in society, but they argue that a feminist reluctance to endorse universal principles decreases their moral strength.

Ethic of Care. The ethic of care and feminist ethics are closely related. Many theorists who developed ideas about the ethic of care are nurses. The ethic of care explores the notion of care as a central activity of human behaviour. Those who write about **ethic of care** maintain that ethical theory based on principles is a male-biased theory. They advocate a more female-biased theory that is based on understanding relationships, especially personal narratives.

Nel Noddings (1984), an early proponent of the ethic of care, used the term "the one-caring" to identify the individual who provides care, and "the cared-for" to refer to the client. In adopting this language, Noddings hoped to emphasize the role of feelings but not at the expense of conventional principles such as autonomy and beneficence. Edmund Pellegrino (1985), a physician, wrote about the moral obligation of physicians and nurses to incorporate notions of care into a definition of professional behaviour. His definition of care included the obligation to appreciate, understand, and even share the pain or condition of a client.

Some nurse authors propose a nursing ethics that distinguishes the work of nurses from that of physicians (Boyer and Nelson, 1990; Fry, 1989; Leininger, 1988; Watson, 1994). As Leininger (1988) wrote, care has been the "central and unifying domain for the body of knowledge and practices in nursing." These writers propose that dilemmas can be solved by attention to relationships and by attention to clients' stories. A focus on the individual client narratives will lead to clarity about decisions, because individual values and moral preferences are often revealed within clients' personal histories.

If the term *care* is used too loosely, however, it can become sentimental and ineffective. Critics of ethics of care warn that sentimentalizing nursing belittles it—that the nursing point of view may be seen as less strong or less important than the facts associated with medical findings (Boyer & Nelson, 1990). Nonetheless, restating common ethical dilemmas in the language of care provides new and refreshing access to discussion and, it is to be hoped, solution. Is it caring to place a disabled relative in a long-term care facility? Is a shortened hospital stay an expression of caring? How, and for whom? The ethic of care philosophy tries to locate ethical discourse at the level where these activities of relationship are located, rather than in an intellectual discussion.

Relational Ethics. Like feminist ethics and ethics of care, **relational ethics** attempts to go beyond bioethics to explain some of the complexities of the nurse's moral obligation to the client; it focuses on how we treat others. Relational ethics theory proposes that our ethical understandings are formed in, and emerge from, our relationships with others. Nurse ethicists have suggested that "being in relationship" with others is the essence of nursing practice; therefore, nursing ethics must be relational (Bergum, 1992, 2002; Bishop & Scudder, 1999; Cameron, 2004; Gadow, 1999; Hartrick Doane, 2002). In other words, nursing ethics exists in the relationship between nurse and the "other," whether that other be client, family, community, or colleague. They suggest that ethical behaviour is displayed in the daily interactions, the way in which nurses relate to others. According to Bergum (1998), relational ethics "is a way of being rather than a mode of decision making. It is how we insert a needle, how we enter into conversation, how we show respect, or how we are with each other."

Within the relationship, the nurse uses nursing knowledge and acts with intent to work toward enhancing health and well-being. The nurse always considers the unique needs of the client as an individual. Mutual respect is created, with attention to the needs, wishes, expertise, or experience of both nurse and client (Bergum & Dosseter, in press).

How to Process an Ethical Dilemma

An **ethical dilemma** is a conflict between two sets of human values, both of which are judged to be good but which cannot both be fully served. Ethical dilemmas can cause distress and confusion for clients and caregivers. The nurse may well be faced with ethical questions that have not previously been examined and for which no practical wisdom exists. The nurse must be able to examine issues and apply experience and wisdom in each situation. Storch (1999) defined the notion of being "ethically fit" as being "mentally engaged in the human activity of ethical reflection and justification" (p. 353). Such fitness requires nurses to be knowledgeable and skillful as they engage in problem solving. Ethical issues must be processed carefully and deliberately. An ethical decision is not based solely on emotions or on what people want and feel; however, the process promotes the free expression of feelings.

Wherever an ethical dilemma is resolved—in a committee setting, at the bedside, or in a family conference—the nurse applies a careful, critical processing of the dilemma. Resolving an ethical dilemma requires deliberate, systematic thinking (Miller & Babcock, 1996). It also requires negotiation of differences, incorporation of conflicting ideas, and an effort to respect differences of opinion. The process of negotiating ethical dilemmas may in part be the process of understanding ambiguities. Nurses need to be knowledgeable and adept in making logical, fair, and consistent decisions. Ethical decision-making models offer a variety of methods for coming to informed conclusions (Box 7-4).

Each step in the processing of an ethical dilemma resembles steps in critical thinking. The nurse begins by gathering information and moves through assessment, identification of the problem, planning, implementation, and evaluation. The first step guides the nurse in determining whether the problem is an ethical one. Not all problems are ethical in nature. The nurse learns to distinguish ethical problems from questions of procedure, legality, or medical diagnosis. To distinguish an ethical problem from other problems, Curtin and Flaherty (1982) recommended that the nurse decide whether the problem has one or more of the following characteristics:

- It cannot be resolved solely through a review of scientific data. To make this determination, it will be necessary to gather detailed information about the situation. This information may come from medical records, health care literature, or consultation with colleagues or the client and the client's family. What at first appears to be a dilemma may resolve on the nurse's learning, for example, that a review of a diagnostic procedure reveals a different prognosis.
- It is perplexing. One cannot easily think logically or make a decision about the problem. Or, the nurse may disagree with a decision that others are making, and the difference of opinion is perplexing.
- The answer to the problem will have a profound relevance for several areas of human concern.

A part of gathering information includes an examination of one's own values as they relate to the issues. The distinction between personal opinion and the facts of the case, or the opinions of others, is essential for resolution to proceed. To clarify the true ethical issues in any situation, a nurse needs to be aware of personal responses. People come to different conclusions about the same situation with no malice intended toward other people. Remembering this will help the nurse arbitrate conversations.

After reviewing relevant information and personal values, a clear statement of the ethical problem becomes the groundwork to begin negotiation. Discussions are more likely to remain focused and constructive when all parties agree on the statement of the dilemma. The group then lists possible courses of action. Possibilities may occur at any time during deliberations. After alternatives are considered, people in an ethical conflict come to a point of resolution or agreement, and action is taken. Decisions are made that can be evaluated in an ongoing manner (Box 7-5).

Documentation of the ethical process can take a variety of forms. Whenever the process involves a family conference or results in a change in the plan of care, the process should be documented in the medical record. Some institutions may use a formal consultation format whenever a request for discussion comes to the ethics committee. If the ethical dilemma does not directly affect client care, however, documentation may occur by means of minutes from a meeting or in a memorandum to affected parties. In the following case study, the nursing concerns and the family conferences would be recorded in the medical record and in nursing flow sheets.

> On your unit, a 35-year-old woman has been hospitalized in the final stages of brain cancer. She is a single mother with two young children. Although she has been treated by both conventional and experimental treatments, the tumour continues to grow, and the medical team has agreed that further treatment would be futile. You have cared for this client during past admissions, and during an especially open discussion, she expressed wishes to explore "do not resuscitate" (DNR) orders. During the current admission, her primary physician is out of town. The attending physician does not know the client personally, but he has spent time with her. He has reviewed the clinical data and agrees that the client is entering the terminal stage of her disease. In his opinion, however, the client is not ready to discuss end-of-life issues. He states that the client has declined to discuss DNR orders with him. You ask the physician to convene a family conference about the issues. He refuses, stating that he believes the client is not ready to participate.

Step 1. Is this an ethical dilemma? What may at first appear to be a question of ethics may be resolved by clarifying one's knowledge base about clinical facts. A review of policy and procedure, or of standards of care, may explain legal obligations that determine a course of action, regardless of personal opinion. If the question remains

Box 7-4 Two Ethical Decision-Making Frameworks

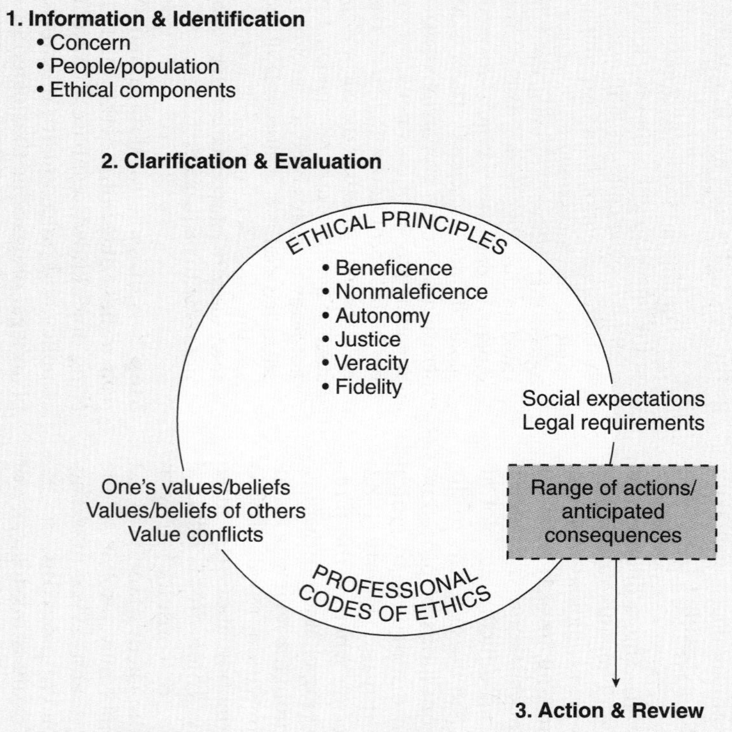

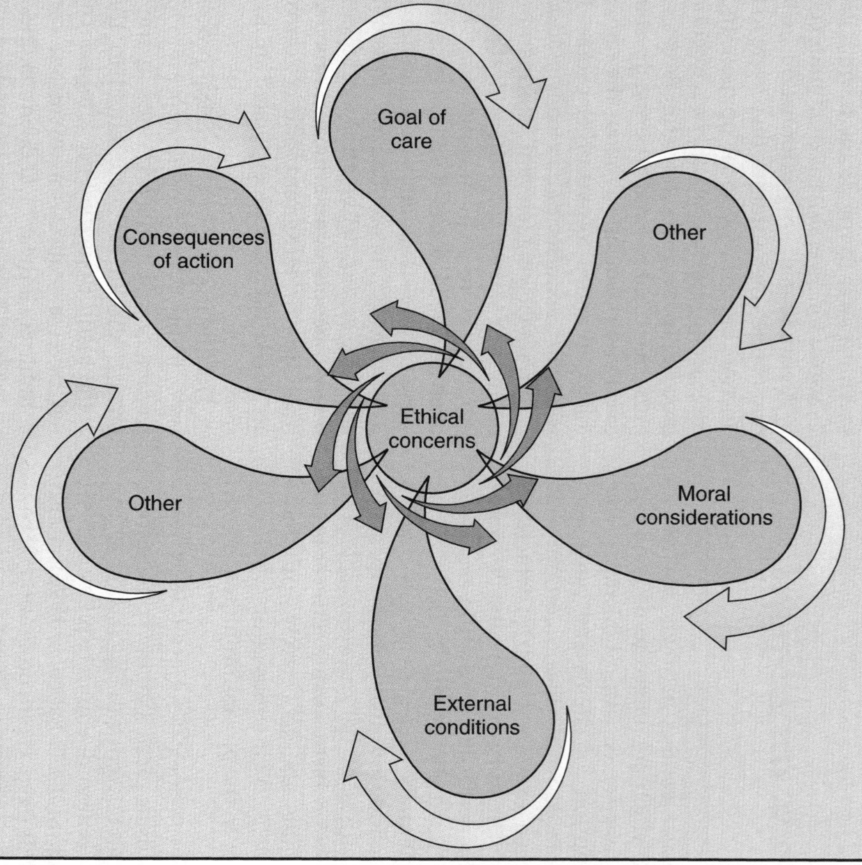

Sources: "Model for Ethical Decision Making for Policy and Practice," by J. L. Storch, in *Toward a Moral Horizon: Nursing Ethics for Leadership and Practice* (p. 515), J. Storch, P. Rodney, and R. Starzomski, Eds., 2004, Toronto, ON: Pearson Education. Reprinted with permission; and "A Model for Questioning," in *Ethical Decision-Making For Registered Nurses in Alberta: Guidelines and Recommendations* (p. 15), by Alberta Association of Registered Nurses, February 1996, Edmonton, AB: Author.

Box 7-5 How to Process an Ethical Dilemma

Step 1. Is this an ethical dilemma? If a review of scientific data does not resolve the question, the question is perplexing, and the answer will have profound relevance for several areas of human concern, then an ethical dilemma may exist.
Step 2. Gather all of the information relevant to the case. To be sure it is a true dilemma, it will be important to review all pertinent information. Occasionally an overlooked fact may provide quick resolution. At this point, client, family, institutional, and social perspectives are important sources of relevant information.
Step 3. Examine and determine your own values on the issues. Values clarification provides a foundation for clarity and for confidence during discussions that will be necessary for resolution of a dilemma.
Step 4. Verbalize the problem. A clear, simple statement of the dilemma may not always be easy, but it is essential for the next step to take place.
Step 5. Consider possible courses of action. To respect all sides of an issue, it is helpful to list potential actions, especially when the list will reflect opinions that conflict.
Step 6. Negotiate the outcome. Sometimes courses of action that seem unlikely at the beginning of the process take on new possibility as they are put to rational and respectful consideration. Negotiation requires a confidence in one's own point of view and a deep respect for the opinions of others.
Step 7. Evaluate the action.

perplexing, and the answer will have profound relevance for several areas of human concern, then an ethical dilemma may exist.

The single mother's situation meets the criteria for an ethical dilemma. Further review of scientific data will probably not contribute to a resolution of the dilemma, but it is important to review the data carefully to make this determination. The disagreement does not revolve around whether the client is in a terminally ill state, so further clinical information will not change the basic question: Should the client have an opportunity to discuss DNR orders at this time? The question is perplexing. Two professional team members disagree on an assessment of a client's readiness to confront the difficult issues related to dying. The answer to the question, "Is this client ready to discuss end of life?" has important implications. If she is not ready, then raising the issue may cause anguish and fear in the client and her family. If she is ready and the team avoids discussion, she may suffer unnecessarily in silence. If she is very close to death, then the lack of a DNR order will necessitate cardiopulmonary resuscitation (CPR) in a futile situation. You know that CPR can cause pain. If applied in a situation where further life is unlikely, then CPR could prolong suffering and reduce dignity.

Step 2. Gather as much information as possible that is relevant to the case. Because resolution to dilemmas may arise from unlikely sources, incorporate as much knowledge as possible at every step of the process. At this point, the information could include laboratory and test results, the clinical state of the client, and current literature about the diagnosis or condition of the client. It may include investigation of the psychosocial concerns of the client, as well as those of her significant others. The client's religious, cultural, and family orientations are part of the nurse's assessment.

You obtain all the clinical information that is pertinent to the question. It may be helpful to determine if the client retains most cognitive functions, even though her tumour is aggressive. You review the chart and discuss this aspect with the physician, and you agree that the client is fully competent, but afraid and overwhelmed by the prognosis. Because two professionals disagree on a client's state of mind, it may be helpful to reassess the client or request that an independent person assess the client's readiness to discuss end-of-life issues. Sometimes family members or significant others hold important clues to a client's state of mind.

Step 3. Examine and determine your own values on the issues. This step is important for all participants in the discussion. At this stage, the nurse and others will practice values clarification and differentiate between their own values and the values of the client and other team members. Essential parts of the goal are the forming one's own opinion and the respecting others' opinions.

At this point, you stop to reflect on your own values. You realize that your own religious practices would not prohibit you from deciding to forgo further treatment if you were in the client's condition. You also realize that you do not yet have family members who rely on you, such as children or elderly parents. This client's religious practices are perhaps more strictly constructed than your own. Her religion discourages actions that diminish life in any way, and you realize that she may have come to see a DNR order as giving up, or as "acting like God." In addition, you understand that the attending physician has not had time to know this client as her own physician has or as you have. You continue to believe that the client would be capable of a discussion, despite her statements to the physician. In fact, you believe that she would benefit from a discussion, because perhaps the combination of an unfamiliar caretaker and declining physical health have silenced her, even though her fears and concerns persist.

Step 4. Verbalize the problem. Once all relevant information has been gathered, then accurate definition of the problem may proceed. It is helpful to state the problem in a few sentences. By agreeing to a statement of the problem, the group can proceed with discussion in a focused way.

Here, the problem seems to be this: Should this client discuss DNR at this time? What are the benefits and risks of a DNR order at this time? Another important question relates to the client's current state of mind: Is she afraid to speak? Is she feeling cut off from her normal network (a primary physician)? Are these feelings contributing to confusion about DNR decisions?

Step 5. Consider possible courses of action. What options are available within the context of the situation and the client's values?

Once you have asked the basic question, other questions and possible courses of action arise. Should you initiate a discussion with the client independently of the physician? Would you be outside your professional role if you facilitated a DNR order? What if your assessment were incorrect? Would you contribute not to the dignity but to the distress of the client? The answers to these questions may be elusive, because they depend on an understanding of client feelings and values that are not necessarily obvious. Even if the nurse cannot legally write a DNR order, the nurse can influence a physician's or client's decision regarding DNR; therefore, troubling questions remain.

Step 6. Negotiate the outcome. This step represents the most important and delicate part of the process. These negotiations may happen informally at the bedside or in the charting room. Or a formal ethics meeting may be necessary. The nurse's point of view represents a unique contribution to the discussion.

If an ethics committee meeting is convened, then the discussion will usually be multidisciplinary. A facilitator or chairperson will ensure that all points of view are examined and that all pertinent issues are identified. A decision or recommendation is the usual outcome of discussion. In the best of circumstances, participants discover a course of action that meets criteria for acceptance by all. Occasionally, however, participants may leave the discussion disappointed or even opposed to the decision. But in a successful discussion, all members will have agreed on an action or decision that can be implemented.

The discussion focuses on the disagreement between your assessment and the physician's regarding the client's readiness to discuss end-of-life issues. The principles involved during the discussion include beneficence and non-maleficence: Which plan would provide the most good for this client, a DNR order or no order? A separate question addresses the client's point of view: Would a discussion with the client promote well-being or promote anguish? The principle of autonomy reveals that a troublesome question remains: Does the client want something different from what she is expressing?

With several members of the health care team present, the discussion proceeds. You present your point of view. You continue to sense that the client is ready to discuss DNR orders but that she may be reluctant to trust the circumstances of this admission. But you also respect the attending physician and his analysis and continue to be concerned that the client may have experienced a change of mind between the last admission and this one. In the end, the team proposes the following: a formal meeting with the client, where you, the attending physician, and a supportive family member are all present. You support this proposal because you sense that it will maximize the support of the client's existing network. In addition, you recognize that in a trusting environment, the client is more likely to express her fears, insecurities, and wishes. Team members agree to keep the discussion open ended and exploratory. You suggest that rather than asking if the client wants a DNR order, perhaps the team could wait for her to bring up the issue. In this way, the team could be assured of her consent and willingness to participate in the discussion.

Step 7. Evaluate the action.

At the meeting, the client in fact opens up. She expresses relief at the chance to explore her options and feelings. Pain management issues are clarified. She wants to discuss a DNR order but requests a visit from her priest before making a final decision.

Institutional Ethics Committees

Most health care institutions have established ethics committees to support the processing of ethical dilemmas. Ethics committees are usually multidisciplinary. They can be a valuable resource for the nurse who identifies an ethical conflict or dilemma.

Ethics committees serve several purposes: education, policy recommendation, and case consultation or review. Unfortunately, not all health care professionals are aware of the ethics committee available in their institution (Storch & Griener, 1992). Further, some nurses who are aware resist submitting a case or issue to such a committee (Storch, 1994). Nevertheless, any involved person, including nurses, physicians, clients, and families of clients may request access to an ethics committee.

Ethical issues may also be processed in settings other than in a committee. Nurses provide insight about ethical problems at family conferences, staff meetings, or in one-to-one meetings. Many ethical problems begin when people feel misled or are not aware of their options and do not know when to speak up about their concerns. Such concerns may be addressed in a variety of constructive settings. Formal help from an ethics committee may be sought after other avenues of communication have been pursued. Ethics committees do not replace important relationships; however, they complement relationships and offer a valuable resource for strengthening them.

Ethical Issues in Nursing Practice

With increased professional responsibility and accountability, and with changes in the workplace and the health care system, nurses are increasingly facing a myriad of ethical issues. Ethical issues are faced daily while providing client care (e.g., ensuring consent is informed, following advance directives, and withdrawing food and nutrition) and while relating with other health care providers. Nurses also must be aware of ethical implications of emerging societal issues involving health care, such as health care funding and delivery.

Client Care Issues

Informed Consent. The intimacy and integrity of the nurse-client relationship demand that nurses protect the rights of their clients. This is achieved as nurses follow standards, policies, guidelines, and legislation regarding consent to treatment. **Informed consent** is consent based on accurate and complete information (see chapter 8). The goal of informed consent is to protect the client's right to autonomy. The CNA *Code of Ethics* (2002) states that to promote autonomy, some of the nurse's ethical responsibilities include:

- building trusting relationships to ensure that the client's choice is understood, expressed, and advocated

- providing the desired information and support required so that clients can act on their own behalf
- assisting clients in obtaining the best current knowledge about their health condition
- being sensitive to the timing of the information and how the information is presented
- ensuring that nursing care is always provided with the client's informed consent, recognizing that the client has the right to refuse or withdraw consent
- respecting the informed choices of competent clients (except if these are contrary to the law)

There can be many unethical scenarios involving consent: clients signing consent forms without understanding what they are consenting to; a nurse mistakenly assuming that a doctor has explained a medical procedure to a client before obtaining the client's consent; a consent being obtained from a client who does not speak English without the assistance of an interpreter; a client consenting to a procedure without knowing about associated risks or potential adverse side effects.

Although obtaining informed consent for medical procedures is not a nursing duty, the nurse may witness the client's signature on the consent form. When nurses provide consent forms for clients to sign, their main responsibility lies with ensuring the client fully understands the nature of the treatment or procedure. If not, notification of the physician must occur so that the physician can clarify or provide additional information.

Advance Directives. People receiving health care often worry, in the event of their becoming incapacitated and unable to express their wishes, that they will be "hooked up to machines" and receive treatment that they do not wish (Figure 7–1). Advance directives have been suggested as one way to address this problem (see chapter 8). **Advance directives** are "the means used to document and communicate a person's preferences regarding life-sustaining treatment in the event that they become incapable of expressing those wishes for themselves" (CNA, 1998b, p. 1). Advance directives are commonly expressed in two ways: (a) an instruction directive, or living will, identifies *what* life-sustaining treatment a person wishes in certain situations, and (b) a proxy directive, or power or attorney for personal care, explains *who* is to make health care decisions if the person becomes incompetent (CNA, 1998b). A routine part of any admission to a hospital now usually includes inquiry about the client's advance directives; if they exist, they are included as part of the medical record. It has become necessary for nurses to be aware of the legal status of all types of advance directives in their province or territory.

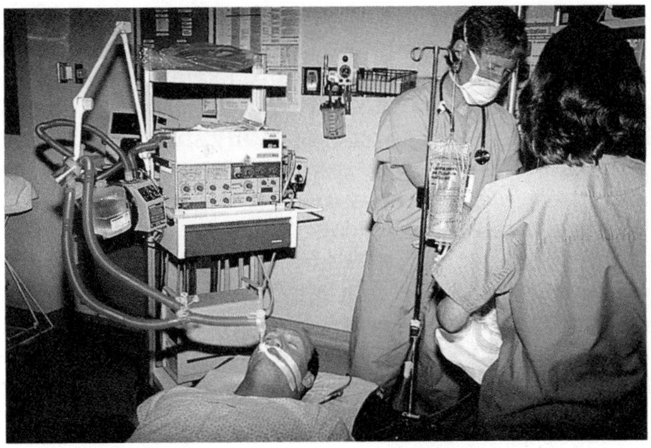

FIGURE **7–1** Advance directives communicate a person's wishes if the person becomes unable to express them.

The nurse has several roles regarding advance directives. A nurse may be involved in helping clients plan an advance directive by discussing its uses and helping clients clarify their values and wishes for end-of-life treatment. The nurse's role also includes following the advance directive, alerting others to changes in the client's wishes, and advocating on behalf of the client or substitute decision maker if the client's wishes or advance directive are not being followed.

Withdrawal of Food and Hydration. Maintaining nutrition is a natural life-sustaining measure and common part of the nursing role. A change in the client's ability to drink and eat raises many issues. When food and hydration is administered for a prolonged period to a client who is not expected to improve, then some nurses may view this care as extraordinary or heroic, whereas others see this as humane.

Current literature suggests fluids should not be routinely administered to dying individuals or automatically withheld from them, but rather given based on the goals of care and a careful assessment of the client's comfort. A position statement by the CNA on end-of-life care (1994) stresses the importance of the health care team to determine whether food and fluid are most beneficial or harmful to a client. The following questions may aid health care professionals in reflecting on the goals of care: Will the client's well-being be enhanced by artificial nutrition? Are there symptoms that could be relieved or aggravated? Could hydration enhance the client's mental status or level of consciousness? Will it temporarily prolong the client's life? Is that the wish of the client and family? (Zerwekh, 1997).

Using artificial hydration may present dilemmas when it is merely maintaining physical life (e.g., when the person is in a vegetative state or is near death). Nurses should know that withholding food will eventually lead to starvation and death and under most circumstances is not considered an ethical action. However, it is considered appropriate to withhold or discontinue life-sustaining medical interventions if they are not benefiting the client or are contrary to the client's wishes.

Issues in the Work Environment

Ethical issues in the workplace are problematic when they compromise practice by preventing nurses from making effective decisions. Inter-professional issues can include inequalities/power differentials, particularly when physicians devalue nursing knowledge or when communication between physicians and nurses is limited.

Most institutions require nurses to function interdependently; that is, to trust in the professional expertise of nurse colleagues. Inter-professional issues between nurse colleagues presents challenges to safe ethical care. The devotion between members of the same profession, and

Research Highlight — Box 7-6

Ethics in Nursing Practice

Research Focus

Researchers were interested in exploring ethical issues in Canadian public health and identifying strategies to support ethical practice.

Research Abstract

In this qualitative study, 22 public health nurses (11 in rural and 11 in urban settings) were asked to describe ethical problems they had experienced in their work. Situations described stemmed from a relational nature as opposed to an active choice between options. Data analysis revealed that ethical issues can be organized into five interrelated themes: relationships with health care professionals, systems issues, character of relationships, respect for people, and putting self at risk.

Evidence-Based Practice

- All aspects of public health nursing have ethical components.
- Nurses must strive to optimize the "good" while maintaining supportive relationships with others.

Reference

Oberle, K., & Tenove, S. (2000). Ethical issues in public health nursing. *Nursing Ethics, 7*(5), 425–438.

Focus on Primary Health Care — Box 7-7

Encouraging Public Participation in Policies Related to Funding of Health Services

- Ensure that consumers have adequate information on the issue (what is currently privately and publicly funded).
- In public forums, ensure that there is a strong mandate from consumers, and that these consumers are connected with formal and informal access to constituents.
- In choosing consumer representatives, select individuals who have strong personalities so as not to be intimated by the so-called experts during group discussion.

their obligation to collectively promote the public's welfare, underlies their professional relationship. In their role of caregiver, nurses inherit clear expectations of how they should behave within their role as professionals.

Reporting the wrongdoing of a colleague can be distressful. Nurses worry about how to report or deal with unacceptable practice and still maintain healthy relationships with other colleagues. They need to examine relative risks and benefits and decide on appropriate action. For example, a nurse might ponder the risks to clients of not reporting poor practice, compared with the benefits of maintaining collegial relationships (Box 7-6). Nurses need to be prepared to struggle with difficult questions and reflect on the facts and their internal values and perspectives. Such concerns, although having elements of a classic dilemma, reveal the complexity and impact of relational issues within the workplace. When positive professional relationships are absent, both the profession and the professionals suffer.

Emerging Societal Issues

Emerging societal issues such as funding and delivery of health care are important to all heath care providers. Changes and pressures are altering the Canadian health care system. Closing hospital beds, deciding how to allocate resources, and deciding what to publicly fund are all ethical issues. Issues related to health care costs and funding also raise ethical questions for health care providers and consumers.

To control these costs, strict attention is paid to **resource allocation.** If the percentage of Canada's revenues required to support health care continue to increase, health could take up all government resources within the next 20 years (Commission on the Future of Health Care in Canada, 2002). Some governments are examining methods (e.g., user fees and privatization) that threaten to change the foundation of the Canadian health care system—equal access to and public funding of all medically necessary services to all Canadians, regardless of their ability to pay (National Forum on Health, 1997).

Recently there has been much debate in Canada on the relationship between public and private funding of health care. Nurses play a key role in fostering public participation so that consumers are involved in public discussions of the issue (Box 7-7). A question often pondered in the media is "Do we want a two-tiered system?"

The private sector is already part of our public system. People against privatization speak of risks to the integrity and viability of our public health care system that may result from an expanded role for private providers. A prime example is the rapid growth of magnetic resonance imaging clinics, which permit individuals to purchase faster service and use test results to "jump the queue" into the public system for treatment. Difficult ethical questions are raised when considering the delivery of "core" medical services through private means. Examples such as the above speak to the tension of "individual liberty" versus the "common good." Some ask, Why should those who can afford it be prevented from insuring privately just because there is public insurance for the same procedure? Others advocate for the "collective," believing the benefits private care might offer such as reduced waiting times would be overshadowed by the threat to the whole system. The ethical basis for the concept is a presumed overriding Canadian societal value of social solidarity. Private versus public health care is an issue that causes much ethical tension.

Key Concepts

- Values clarification helps nurses explore personal values and feelings and to decide how to act on personal beliefs. It also facilitates nurse-client communication.
- Ethics refers to the study of philosophical ideals of right and wrong behaviour.
- A code of ethics provides a foundation for professional nursing. Professional nursing promotes accountability, responsibility, and advocacy.
- Theories of bioethics refers to ethical issues specific to the health care delivery. They are based on the principles of autonomy, beneficence, nonmaleficence, and justice.
- The relational theory goes beyond bioethics by addressing the role of relationship in the ethical delivery of health care. It maintains that the client-nurse relationship is the foundation of nursing ethics.
- Professional nurses maintain competence in practice and assume responsibility for nursing judgments.
- Ethical problems arise from differences in values, changing professional roles, technological advances, and social issues.
- A standard process for thinking through ethical dilemmas helps providers resolve conflict or uncertainty about right actions.
- Critical thinking is an important part of processing ethical dilemmas.
- The nurse's point of view provides a unique and valuable voice in the resolution of ethical dilemmas.

Key Terms

Accountability, *p. 99*
Advance directives, *p. 107*
Autonomy, *p. 101*
Beneficence, *p. 101*
Bioethics, *p. 101*
Code of ethics, *p. 96*
Consequentialism, *p. 100*
Cultural values, *p. 97*
Deontology, *p. 100*
Ethic of care, *p. 102*
Ethical dilemma, *p. 102*
Ethics, *p. 96*
Informed consent, *p. 106*
Justice, *p. 101*
Morality, *p. 98*
Non-maleficence, *p. 101*
Relational ethics, *p. 102*
Resource Allocation, *p. 108*
Responsibility, *p. 99*
Teleology, *p. 100*
Value, *p. 96*
Values clarification, *p. 97*

Critical Thinking Exercises

1. Complete the values clarification exercise (Box 7-1) with your classmates or others. Compare the answers and discuss the differences.
2. You are a clinic nurse in a small community clinic. A 45-year-old male client has been coming to the clinic for several years for treatment and support of his acquired immunodeficiency syndrome (AIDS). During recent months, he has lost his long-term companion to AIDS. In addition, both his parents died many years ago. His clinical condition has deteriorated. His vision is failing, his nutritional status is difficult to maintain, and he has been hospitalized three times in the past 3 months for pneumonia. He asks for your help in planning his suicide. Discuss your response to his request. Begin by acknowledging that assisted suicide and euthanasia are illegal in Canada. Examine your personal feelings about suicide. Include a discussion about your understanding of AIDS: Where does it come from? Who gets the disease? Why? What are your feelings and opinions about people with AIDS? Construct your response, keeping in mind the ethical principles of justice, autonomy, beneficence, and nonmaleficence. Because all of these principles conflict in this example, it will be important to identify each and to recognize personal responses to the role that each plays in this narrative. Just as important is the role that one imagines they play for the client, especially as they differ from one's own. What are your possible courses of action?
3. You have been assigned the care of a 98-year-old woman who was recently admitted with a diagnosis of pneumonia. She has a history of cardiac disease and takes a number of medications. She had been fairly active until the past few days, when her cough worsened and she developed a fever. You note that her pulse has become weak and thready and that her respirations are increasingly laboured. The client is now too weak to respond to you. When you mention to the family that you may need to call the physician and even "call a code," the son and the daughter become distraught, saying that they do not want their mother to be kept alive on "machines." They report that they have discussed this situation with their mother. You find that documentation of these wishes is not in the chart. The family members have not discussed this situation with their doctor. What actions would you consider taking at this moment? Take into account the ethical principles of autonomy and beneficence. What are your personal values about interventions at the end of life?

Review Questions

1. Values clarification plays a major role in:
   1. Creating a set of rules for conduct
   2. Identifying values that should be accepted by all
   3. Resolving issues of "value conflict"
   4. Developing a code of ethics
2. In Canada, access to health care means that all citizens have equal access to medically necessary services. Many jurisdictions have implemented private magnetic resonance imaging clinics. A discussion about the ethics of this situation would involve predominately the principle of
   1. Accountability
   2. Autonomy
   3. Relational ethics
   4. Justice, because the question in this situation is how to determine the just distribution of resources
3. It may seem redundant when health care providers, including professional nurses, agree to "do no harm" to

their clients. The point of this agreement is to reassure the public that in all ways the health care team will not only work to heal clients, but that they agree to do this in the least painful and harmful way possible. The principle that describes this agreement is called
   1. Beneficence
   2. Accountability
   3. Non-maleficence
   4. Respect for autonomy

4. A child's immunization may cause discomfort during administration, but the benefits of protection from disease, both for the individual and for society, outweigh the temporary discomforts. This involves the principle of
   1. Beneficence
   2. Fidelity
   3. Non-maleficence
   4. Respect for autonomy

5. If a nurse assesses a client for pain and then offers a plan to manage the pain, the principle that encourages the nurse to monitor the client's response to the plan is
   1. Beneficence
   2. Justice
   3. Non-maleficence
   4. Respect for autonomy

6. Including clients in decision making regarding their care and respecting their choices of treatment demonstrate the principle of:
   1. The National League for Nursing
   2. The Canadian Nurses Association
   3. The Canadian Medical Association
   4. The National Institutes of Health, Nursing Division

7. Nurses agree to be advocates for their clients. Practice of advocacy calls for the nurse to
   1. Seek out nursing supervisor in conflicting situations
   2. Work to understand the law as it applies to the client's clinical condition
   3. Assess the client's point of view and prepare to articulate this point of view
   4. Document all clinical changes in the medical record in a timely manner

8. Which of the following is NOT part of the nurse's role as client advocate?
   1. Intervening if others fail to respect the client's dignity
   2. Protecting the client's right to confidentiality and privacy
   3. Making nursing care decisions for the client
   4. Advocating for appropriate use of interventions to minimize suffering

9. The philosophy sometimes called the ethics of care suggests that ethical dilemmas can best be solved by attention to
   1. Relationships
   2. Ethical principles
   3. Clients
   4. Code of ethics for nurses

10. Ethical dilemmas often arise over a conflict of opinion. Once the nurse has determined that the dilemma is ethical, a critical first step in negotiating the difference of opinion would be to
   1. Consult a professional ethicist to ensure that the steps of the process occur in full
   2. Gather all relevant information regarding the clinical, social, and spiritual aspects of the dilemma
   3. List the ethical principles that inform the dilemma so that negotiations agree on the language of the discussion
   4. Ensure that the attending physician has written an order for an ethics consultation to support the ethics process

References

Alberta Association of Registered Nurses. (1996). *Ethical decision-making for registered nurses in Alberta: Guidelines and recommendations.* Edmonton, AB: Author.

Beauchamp, T., & Childress, J. (2001). *Principles of biomedical ethics* (4th ed.). New York: Oxford University Press.

Bell, N. K. (1992). If age becomes a standard for rationing health care. In H. B. Holmes & L. M. Purdy (Eds.), *Feminist perspectives in medical ethics.* Bloomington: Indiana University Press.

Bergum, V. (1992). Beyond rights: The ethical challenge. *Phenomenology & Pedagogy, 10,* 75–84.

Bergum, V. (2002). Ethical challenges of the 21st century: Attending to relations. *Canadian Journal of Nursing Research, 34*(2), 9–15.

Bergum, V., & Dossetter, J. (in press). *Relational ethics: The full meaning of respect.* Hagerstown, MD: University Publishing Group.

Bergum V. (1998). *Relational Ethics. What is it?* Retrieved August 10, 2004 from *http://www.phen.ab.ca/materials/intouch/vol1/intouch1-02.html*

Bishop, A. H., & Scudder, J. R. (1999). A philosophical interpretation of nursing. *Scholarly Inquiry for Nursing Practice: An International Journal, 13*(1), 17–27.

Boyer, J. R., & Nelson, J. L. (1990). A comment on Fry's "The Role of Caring in a Theory of Nursing Ethics." *Hypatia, 5,* 153–158.

Cameron, B. (2004). Ethical moments in practice: The nursing "how are you" revisited. *Nursing Ethics, 11*(1), 53–62.

Canadian Nurses Association. (1994). *A question of respect: Nurses and end of life treatment dilemmas.* Ottawa, ON: Author.

Canadian Nurses Association: *Advance Directives: The Nurses Role.* Ottawa, 1998b : Author.

Canadian Nurses Association. (2002). *Code of ethics for registered nurses.* Ottawa, ON: Author.

Commission on the Future of Health Care in Canada. (2002). *Building on values: The future of health care in Canada: Final report.* Ottawa, ON: Author.

Curtin, L., & Flaherty, M. J. (1982). *Nursing ethics: Theories and pragmatic.* Bowie, MD: Brady.

Davis, A. J., et al. (1997). *Ethical dilemmas and nursing practice* (4th ed.). Stamford, CT: Appleton and Lange.

Fry, S. T. (1989). The role of caring in a theory of nursing ethics. *Hypatia, 4*(2), 88–103.

Gadow, S. (1999). Relational narrative: The postmodern turn in nursing ethics. *Scholarly Inquiry for Nursing Practice, 13,* 57–70.

Gilligan, C. (1982). *In a different voice.* Cambridge, MA: Harvard University Press.

Hartrick Doane, G. (2002). Am I still ethical? The socially-mediated process of nurses' moral identity. *Nursing Ethics, 9*(6), 623–635.

Holmes, H. B., & Purdy, L. M. (Eds.). (1992). *Feminist perspectives in medical ethics.* Bloomington: Indiana University Press.

International Council of Nurses. (2000). *ICN code of ethics for nurses.* Geneva, Switzerland: Author.

Johnstone, M. J. (1999). *Bioethics: A nursing perspective.* Harcourt, Australia: Harcourt/Saunders.

Kohlberg, L. (1981). *Essays on moral development* (Vols. 1–3). San Francisco: Harper & Row.

Leininger, M. (1988). *Caring: An essential human need.* Detroit, MI: Wayne State University Press.

Maslow, A. (1959). *New knowledge in human values.* New York: Harper & Row.

Miller, M. A., & Babcock, D. E. (1996). *Critical thinking applied to nursing.* St. Louis, MO: Mosby.

National Forum on Health. (1997). *Canada health action: Building on the legacy* (Vols. 1–2). Ottawa, ON: Author.

Noddings, N. (1984). *Caring: A feminist approach to ethics and moral education.* Berkeley: University of California Press.

Pellegrino, E. D. (1985). The caring ethic: The relation of physician to patient. In A. H. Bishop & J. R. Scudder (Eds.), *Caring, curing, coping: Nurse, physician, and patient relations* (pp. 8–30). Birmingham: University of Alabama Press.

Raths, L. E., Harmin, M., & Simon, S. B. (1979). *Values and teaching* (2nd ed.). Columbus, OH: Merrill Publishing.

Rokeach, M. (1973). *The nature of human values.* New York: Free Press.

Ross-Kerr, J., & MacPhail, J. (1996). *Concepts in Canadian nursing.* St. Louis, MO: Mosby.

Shannon, S. E. (1997). The roots of interdisciplinary conflict around ethical issues. *Critical Care Nursing Clinics of North America, 9*(1), 13–28.

Sherwin, S. (1992). *No longer patient: Feminist ethics and health care.* Philadelphia: Temple University Press.

Storch, J. L. (1994). Ethics in health care in Canada. In B. Bolaria & H. Dickenson (Eds.), *Health and illness and health care in Canada.* Toronto, ON: Harcourt Brace.

Storch, J. L. (1999). Ethical dimensions of leadership. In J. Hibberd & D. Smith (Eds.), *Nursing management in Canada* (2nd ed.). Toronto, ON: W. B. Saunders.

Storch, J. L., & Griener, G. G. (1992). Ethics committees in Canadian hospitals: Report of the 1990 pilot study. *Health Care Manage Forum, 5*(1), 19–26.

Storch, J., Rodney, P., & Starzomski, R. (Eds.). (2004). *Toward a moral horizon: Nursing ethics for leadership and practice.* Toronto, ON: Pearson Education.

Tschudin, V. (1995). Editorial. Advocacy in Nursing. *Nursing Ethics, 2*(1), 1.

Watson, J. (Ed.). (1994). *Applying art and science of human caring.* New York: National League of Nursing Press.

Wolf, S. M. (Ed.). (1996). *Feminism and bioethics.* New York: Oxford University Press.

Yeo, M., & Moorehouse, A. (1996). *Concepts and cases in nursing ethics* (2nd ed.). Toronto, ON: Broadview Press.

Zerwekh, J. (1997). Do dying patients need IV fluids? *American Journal of Nursing, 97*(3), 26–31.

Recommended Web Sites

Canadian Bioethics Society:
http://www.bioethics.ca

The Canadian Bioethics Society (CBS) was founded in 1988 by the amalgamation of the Canadian Society of Bioethics and the Canadian Society for Medical Bioethics. Members of the society include health care administrators, lawyers, nurses, philosophers, physicians, theologians, and others concerned with the ethical and humane dimensions of health care. The Web site offers information about the annual CBS conference, national and international ethics organization links, and relevant ethics journals from a variety of disciplines.

Canadian Nurses Association–Code of Ethics:
http://www.cna-nurses.ca/_frames/ethics/ethicsframe.htm

Provides a link to the Canadian Nurses Association and the *Code of Ethics for Registered Nurses.*

Centre for Applied Ethics:
http://www.ethics.ubc.ca

The University of British Columbia established this centre in 1993. It is primarily an interdisciplinary research centre that studies a variety of ethics topics. The Web site has links to other ethics organizations and ethics resources. The centre's newsletter is also available on the Web site.

Nursing Ethics.ca:
http://www.nursingethics.ca/

This Web site has Canadian resources that support ethical nursing practice.

Provincial Health Ethics Network (Alberta):
http://www.phen.ab.ca/

The Provincial Health Ethics Network (PHEN) was established as a society in Alberta in 1995. It provides information for all Albertans about ethics and access to health ethics resources. Its mission is to facilitate examination, discussion, and decision making with respect to ethical issues in health and health care.

8

Legal Implications in Nursing Practice

Carla Shapiro, RN, MN (Canadian author)
Christine Durbin, RN, MSN, JD, PhDc

Objectives

Mastery of content in this chapter will enable the student to:

- Define the key terms listed.
- Explain legal concepts that apply to nurses.
- Describe the legal responsibilities and obligations of nurses.
- List sources for standards of care for nurses.
- Define legal aspects of nurse-client, nurse-physician, nurse-nurse, and nurse-employer relationships.
- List the elements needed to prove negligence.
- Give examples of legal issues that arise in nursing practice.

Safe nursing practice includes knowing the legal boundaries within which nurses must function. Nurses must understand the law to protect themselves from liability and to protect their clients' rights. Nurses need not fear the law but rather should view it as representing what society expects from them. Laws are continually changing to meet the needs of the people they are intended to protect. As technology has expanded the role of the nurse, the ethical dilemmas associated with client care have increased and often become legal issues as well. As health care evolves in our society, so do the legal implications for health care. Although federal laws apply to all provinces and territories, nurses must also be aware that laws do vary across the country. It is important for nurses to know the laws in their province or territory that affect their practice. Being familiar with the law enhances nurses' ability to be client advocates.

Legal Limits of Nursing

Nurses have a fiduciary relationship with their clients. A fiduciary relationship is one in which a professional, the nurse, provides services that by their nature cause the recipient, the client, to trust in the specialized knowledge and integrity of the professional. Nurses are obligated in the fiduciary relationship to provide knowledgeable, competent, and safe care.

Although legal challenges to nurses were once rare, the situation is changing. The public is better informed than in the past about their rights to health care and are more likely to seek damages for professional negligence. The courts have upheld the concept that nurses must provide a reasonable standard of care. Thus, it is essential that nurses understand the legal limits influencing their daily practice.

Sources of Law

The Canadian legal system can be divided into two main categories: public law and private law. Public law is chiefly concerned with relations between individuals and the state or society in general and includes constitutional, taxation, administrative, human rights, and criminal law. Private law involves disputes between individuals and covers areas such as wills, contracts, marriage and divorce, and civil wrongs (e.g., negligence). Whereas public law is addressed in the same manner across the country, two systems deal with private law issues—**civil law** (based on Roman law) in Quebec, and **common law** (based on British common law) throughout the rest of the country. These two systems differ primarily in their legal processes. In each system, courts interpret the rules made by the legislature in the context of specific disputes.

When either a civil or a criminal case goes to court, decisions are based on previous case rulings. How courts rule on the circumstances and facts surrounding the case is called a *precedent*. If a case has been previously decided on similar facts, the court is bound to follow that decision. Not every jurisdiction will have case law on a given issue. For example, cases regarding a client's right to refuse treatment are not found in every province. In such situations, other jurisdictions are consulted for guidance. Generally, breaches of private law result in the payment of money to compensate the aggrieved party for damages incurred. Violations of public law may result in a range of remedies, including fines or imprisonment.

Statute law is created by elective legislative bodies such as Parliament and provincial or territorial legislatures. Federal statues apply throughout the country, and provincial and territorial statues apply only in the province or territory in which they were created. Examples of provincial statutes are the *Regulated Health Professions Act* in Ontario and nursing practice acts throughout the country, which describe and define nursing practice within each province. Examples of federal statutes are the new *Assisted Human Reproduction Act* (2004), the *Controlled Drugs and Substances Act* (1996), and the *Food and Drugs Act* (1985).

Professional Regulation

Like all self-governing professions in Canada, nursing is regulated at the provincial or territorial level. Each province and territory has legislation that grants authority to a nursing regulatory body. These regulatory bodies are accountable to the public for ensuring safe, competent, and ethical nursing care. Regulatory bodies are responsible for granting certificates of registration, offering practice support, ensuring continuing competence of its members, investigating complaints against members' conduct, and disciplining members when necessary. Regulatory bodies are also responsible for developing codes of ethics, setting standards of practice, and approving nursing education programs (McIntyre & Thomlinson, 2003).

There are separate regulatory bodies for registered nurses and practical nurses. Some provinces also have regulatory bodies for registered psychiatric nurses. These regulatory bodies are called either the provincial association or the college of nursing (e.g., the Alberta Association of Registered Nurses, the College of Licensed Practical Nurses of Alberta, the College of Nurses of Ontario). The trend appears to be a move to the college model, with a stronger focus on regulation of practice and accountability to the public.

Nurses must be registered by the professional nursing association or college of the province or territory in which they practise. The requirements for registration (or licensure, where applicable) varies across the country, but most provinces and territories have minimum education requirements and require the person to pass an examination. All provinces and territories (except Quebec) use the Canadian Registered Nurse Examination. Quebec has created its own examination. Registration (or licensure) permits people to practise nursing and use the applicable nursing title and initials: registered nurse and RN or registered practical nurse and RPN. All nurses require verification of their credentials either by having their name appear on a register or by holding a valid license to practise.

Registration can be suspended or revoked by the regulatory body if a nurse's conduct violates provisions in the registration statute. For example, nurses who perform illegal acts such as selling controlled substances jeopardize their registration status. Due process must be followed before registration can be suspended or revoked. Due process means that nurses must be notified of the charges brought against them and have an opportunity to defend themselves against the charges in a hearing. Hearings do not occur in courts but are usually conducted by the regulatory body. If a nurse loses the professional license or is removed from the provincial or territorial register and the case involves civil or criminal wrongs, then further legal consequences may follow.

Standards of Care

Standards of care are legal guidelines for nursing practice. Standards establish an expectation for nurses to provide safe and appropriate client care. If nurses do not perform duties within accepted standards of care, they may place themselves in jeopardy of legal action and, more important, place their clients at risk for harm and injury. Nursing standards of care arise from a variety of sources. These include statutes and laws of broad application, such as the statutes and common law relating to human rights, privacy, and negligence; provincial statutes that specifically apply to health care professionals or nurses only; and the detailed regulations, practice standards, and codes of ethics that are generated by the professional associations. Nursing standards are also outlined in the written policies and procedures of employing institutions.

All provincial and territorial legislatures have passed health professions and/or **nursing practice acts** that define the scope of nursing practice. These acts set educational requirements for nurses, distinguish between nursing and medical practice, and generally define nursing practice. The rules and regulations enacted by the provincial or territorial regulatory body help to define the practice of nursing more specifically. For example, a nursing association may develop a rule regarding intravenous therapy. All nurses are responsible for knowing the provisions of the nursing practice act for the province or territory in which they work, as well as the rules and regulations enacted by the provincial or territorial regulatory administrative bodies.

Professional organizations are another source for defining standards of care. The Canadian Nurses Association has developed standards for nursing practice, policy statements, and similar resolutions. The standards delineate the scope, function, and role of the nurse in practice. Nursing specialty organizations also have standards of practice defined for certification of nurses who work in specific specialty areas such as the operating room or critical care. These same standards also serve as practice guidelines for defining safe and appropriate nursing care in specialty areas.

The Canadian Council on Health Services Accreditation requires that accredited health care institutions have written nursing policies and procedures that detail how nurses are to perform their duties. These internal standards of care are usually quite specific and are found in procedural manuals on most nursing units. For example, a procedure or policy outlining the steps that should be taken when changing a dressing or administering medication gives specific information about how nurses are to perform these tasks. Nurses must know the policies and procedures of their employing institution because they must all follow the same standard of care. Institutional policies and procedures must conform to laws and cannot conflict with legal guidelines that define acceptable standards of care.

In a negligence lawsuit, these standards are used to determine whether the nurse has acted as any reasonably prudent nurse in a similar setting with the same credentials would act. A nursing expert is called to testify about the standards of nursing care as applied to the facts of the case (Box 8-1). The expert may be called to define and explain to the court what a reasonably prudent nurse would have been expected to do under the facts of the case from any similar setting around the country. It is recognized and understood that nursing practice differs based on the rural or urban nature of the institutional setting. Additionally, home health care, occupational health nursing, and other community-based clinical settings require that the expert be familiar with the standards of care in these settings versus the traditional hospital or institutional setting. The expert must have the credentials, experience, and understanding of what the standard of care should have been in the case at hand. The expert witness is distinguished from the fact witness. Staff nurses may testify in a court proceeding as fact witnesses if they have first-hand personal experience with the facts of the case. The expert witness evaluates the defendant's professional judgments and behaviour under the circumstances being reviewed.

Usually, general duty nurses are legally responsible for meeting the same standards as other general duty nurses in similar settings. However, specialized nurses, such as critical care or dialysis nurses, are held to standards of care and skill exercised by those in the same specialty as defined by applicable standards. All nurses must know the standards of care they are expected to meet within their specific specialty and work setting. Ignorance of the law or of standards of care is not a defence against negligence. Nor is being asked to perform an out-of-scope procedure by an employer. The law as written will overrule any agency policy or procedure.

Legal Liability Issues in Nursing Practice

Torts

A **tort** is a civil wrong made against a person or property. Torts may be classified as intentional or unintentional. **Intentional torts** are willful acts that violate another's rights (Keatings & Smith, 2000). Examples are assault,

Box 8-1 Anatomy of a Lawsuit

Pleadings—Statements of Claim and Defence

- The plaintiff outlines what the defendant(s) did wrong and how that caused injury.
- The statement of claim is then issued by the court and served upon the defendants.
- Statements of claim are often very broad and may be served upon the employer, institution, and all members of the health care team involved in the client's care at the relevant time.
- The defendant must deliver a statement of defence to the allegations. The defendant(s) can admit or deny each allegation in the petition.

Procedures of Discovery

Pretrial proceedings permit each side to gather legally relevant information from the other and usually lead to a settlement between the parties before a trial.

(1) *Examination for discovery*—plaintiff's lawyer is permitted to question each defendant under oath. Examination for discovery usually takes place in private offices, with only the parties, their lawyers, and a reporter present to record a transcript of the testimony. Questioning can be wide-ranging and detailed in order to discover useful information. Answers given to questions will be available for trial.

(2) *Discovery of documents*—each side can be forced to produce all documents relevant to the litigation. Medical records and nurses' notes may be of particular value.

(3) *Independent medical examination of the plaintiff*—to determine the extent of the plaintiff's injuries. Negligence is not actionable without proof of damage.

(4) *Discovery by interrogatories*—similar to the examination for discovery but involves a series of written questions, which must be answered under oath.

Expert Witnesses

Each side usually selects experts to help explain and interpret the evidence as it emerges. A nursing expert may be called upon to establish the appropriateness of nursing care provided.

Pretrial Conference

The purpose of the pretrial conference is to identify points of contention, narrow down the issues, and encourage settlement out of court.

- In some jurisdictions, the pretrial conference may be mandatory.
- A pretrial conference is presided over by a judge and attended by counsel for the various parties. Most settlements take place without any admission of liability.

Trial

Usually takes place several years after filing of the initial statement of claim. Most nursing negligence cases are heard and decided by a judge alone. Usually, damages are assessed at trial.

battery, invasion of privacy, and false imprisonment. Negligence is example of an unintentional tort.

Intentional Torts

Assault. Assault is conduct (such as a physical or verbal threat) that creates in another person apprehension or fear of imminent harmful or offensive contact. No actual contact is necessary in order for damages for assault to be awarded (Fridman, 2003; Osborne, 2003). It is an assault for a nurse to threaten to give a client an injection or to threaten to restrain a client for an X-ray procedure when the client has refused consent. The key issues are whether the client was afraid of being harmed in the situation and the client's consent. In a lawsuit wherein assault is alleged, the client's consent would bar the claim of assault against a nurse.

Battery. Battery is any intentional physical contact with a person without consent. The contact can be harmful to the client and cause an injury, or it can be merely offensive to the client's personal dignity (Sneiderman, Irvine, & Osborne, 2003). In the example of a nurse threatening to give a client an injection without the client's consent, if the nurse actually gives the injection, it is considered battery. Battery could even be life-saving, as in the Ontario case of *Malette v. Shulman* (1990). In that case, the plaintiff was unconscious and bleeding profusely. The physician determined that she needed a life-saving blood transfusion. Prior to the transfusion, a nurse found a signed card in the plaintiff's purse that identified her as a Jehovah's Witness and stated that under no circumstances was she to receive blood. Despite this, the physician chose to administer the blood to preserve the client's life. The plaintiff survived, recovered from her injuries, and successfully sued the physician for battery (Sneiderman et al., 2003).

In some situations, consent is implied. For example, if a client gets into a wheelchair or transfers to a stretcher after being advised that it is time to be taken for an X-ray procedure, the client has given implied consent to the procedure. A client has the right to revoke or withdraw consent at any time.

Invasion of Privacy. The tort of invasion of privacy protects the client's right to be free from unwanted intrusion into his or her private affairs. Clients are entitled to confidential health care. Nursing standards for what constitutes confidential information are based on professional ethics and the common law. The ideals of privacy and sensitivity to the needs and rights of clients who may not choose to have nurses intrude on their lives, but who depend on nurses for their care, guide the nurse's judgment. The nurse's fiduciary duty requires that confidential information not be shared with others except on a need-to-know basis.

One form of invasion of privacy is the release of a client's medical information to an unauthorized person, such as a member of the press or the client's employer. The information that is contained in a client's medical record is a confidential communication. It should be shared with health care providers for the purpose of medical treatment only.

A client's medical record is confidential. The nurse should not disclose the client's confidential medical information without the client's consent. For example, a nurse should respect a wish not to inform the client's family of a terminal illness. Similarly, a nurse should not assume that a client's spouse or family members know all of the client's history, particularly with respect to private issues such as mental illness, medications, pregnancy, abortion, birth control, or sexually transmitted infections.

However, confidentiality is not an absolute value, and in certain circumstances, breaching confidentiality is justifiable. There are times when a nurse may be required by law (statutory duty) to breach confidentiality and disclose information to a third party. For example, each province and territory has laws that require health care workers to report suspected child abuse to a local child-protection agency. Or nurses may be required to release information about a client when they are subpoenaed (given a legal order) to testify in court.

Nurses are under no legal obligation to release confidential information to the police except in rare cases in which the life, safety, or health of the client or an innocent third party is in jeopardy (such as when a client tells a nurse that he or she intends to hurt or kill someone; Tapp, 1996). Such a statement should be reported to the authorities of the institution and to the police. Other admissions made by a client to a nurse about past or future criminal activity may not have to be disclosed unless the nurse is compelled to do so by a court of law. The conflict between confidentiality and risk of public harm is not always clear. In cases where a nurse has serious concerns about the welfare of others (e.g., a client who has human immunodeficiency virus [HIV] and admits to having unsafe sex or donating blood), the nurse should first suggest and strongly encourage the client to disclose this information. If the client refuses, then the nurse should seek consultation with professional colleagues and supervisors. A careful balancing of the need for privacy and confidentiality of privileged communication would need to be weighed carefully.

Computers and Confidentiality. Most health care facilities use computer systems to maintain client records. Access to confidential client information is generally controlled by means of a variety of technological safeguards, including magnetized cards and passwords. It is important that these security devices not be shared with others and that access cards be used to retrieve files only when warranted. The improper use of one's magnetized card and password to seek out confidential information could lead to legal repercussions or disciplinary action.

Likewise, the use of e-mail messages carries a potential legal risk because they are susceptible to unauthorized access by third parties. E-mail messages may also be introduced as evidence in any court or legal proceedings (Tapp, 2001).

False Imprisonment. The tort of false imprisonment serves to protect a person's individual liberty and basic rights. Preventing a client from leaving a health care facility voluntarily may constitute the tort of false imprisonment. The inappropriate or unjustified use of restraints (e.g., by confining a person to an area, using physical or chemical restraints) may also be viewed as false imprisonment. Nurses must be aware of their facility's policies and specific legislation in their jurisdiction (e.g., under the *Mental Health Act*) relating to when and how restraints can be used (Canadian Nurses Protective Society [CNPS], 2004).

Unintentional Torts

Negligence. When nurses are sued, most often the proceedings against them are for the tort of negligence, also referred to as malpractice (Sneiderman et al., 2003). **Negligence** in nursing is conduct that falls below a standard of care established by law. No intent is needed for negligence to occur. It is characterized chiefly by inadvertence, thoughtlessness, or inattention. Negligence may involve carelessness, such as not checking an ID bracelet, resulting in administration of the wrong medication. However, carelessness is not always the cause. If nurses perform a procedure for which they have not been educated and do it carefully, but still harm the client, a claim of negligence could be made. In general, courts define nursing negligence as the failure to use that degree of skill or learning ordinarily used under the same or similar circumstances by members of the nursing profession (Box 8-2).

Nurses can be found liable for negligence if the following criteria are established: (a) the nurse (defendant) owed a duty to the client (plaintiff); (b) the nurse did not carry out that duty; (c) the client was injured; and (d) the nurse's failure to carry out the duty caused the injury.

The ability to predict harm (i.e., the foreseeability of risk) is evaluated in negligence cases. The circumstances surrounding the injury are evaluated to determine if it was likely that the injury or harm to the client could have been expected from the care that was or was not provided. The cause of the injury is also investigated through the evaluation of the actual and the nearest causes of the injury. Had it not been for what the nurse did or did not do, could an injury have been prevented?

The case of *Downey v. Rothwell* (1974) is a good example of nursing negligence. This case involved a plaintiff who suffered a severe arm injury when she fell off an examining table while under the care of a nurse. The client, who had a history of epilepsy, informed the nurse that she was about to have a seizure. The nurse left the client unattended on an examining table while she left the room for a few moments. During this time, the client had a seizure, fell onto the floor, and broke her arm. The nurse should have anticipated the client was about to have a seizure and ensured her safety either by moving her to the floor or by putting up guard rails on the examining table. In this case, there was an undertaking by the nurse to provide care, a reliance on this nurse by the client, and a foreseeable risk. The nurse was found negligent in this case and her employers were held vicariously liable.

In the case of *Granger v. Ottawa General Hospital* (1996), two nurses (a staff nurse and her team leader) were found negligent in the care they provided to a woman in labour. During labour, the plaintiff's fetal heart monitor strip showed deep, persistent, variable decelerations. The staff nurse did not appreciate that these were a sign of fetal distress and did not immediately report these findings to others on the obstetrical team. This resulted in severe and permanent brain injury to the baby, leaving her severely disabled. In this case, the nurse breached her duty to exercise appropriate skill in making an assessment and to communicate the information to the physicians.

Preventing Negligence. The best way for nurses to avoid being negligent is to follow standards of care; give competent health care; insist on appropriate orientation, continuing education, and adequate staffing; communicate with other health care providers; develop a caring rapport with the client; and document assessments, interventions, and evaluations fully.

The health care record is a permanent record of the nursing process. Careful, complete, and thorough documentation is one of the best defences against allegations of negligence or violations of nursing standards. An institution has a legal duty to maintain nursing records. Nursing notes contain substantial evidence needed to understand the care received by a client. If records are lost or incomplete, there is a presumption that the care was negligent and therefore the cause of the client's injuries. In addition, incomplete or illegible records undermine the credibility of the health care provider.

In the case of *Kolesar v. Jeffries* (1976), the Supreme Court of Canada addressed the issue of poor record keeping. In that case, a client underwent major spinal surgery and was transferred to a surgical unit, where he was nursed on a Stryker frame. The client was found dead the following morning. There were no nursing notes recorded from 2200 hours the previous evening until 0500, when he was found dead. Although at trial several nurses and nursing assistants testified that they had tended to the client multiple times throughout the night, the court inferred that "nothing was charted because nothing was done." One of the nurses was held negligent for this client's death.

It is very important for documentation to be done in a timely manner. Any significant changes in the client's condition must be reported to the physician and documented in the chart (see chapter 13). Recording nursing care notes in a notebook and then transferring them to the chart at the end of the shift can be a dangerous

Box 8-2 Common Negligent Acts

- Medication errors that result in injury to clients
- Intravenous therapy errors resulting in infiltrations or phlebitis
- Burns to clients caused by equipment, bathing, or spills of hot liquids and foods
- Falls resulting in injury to clients
- Failure to use aseptic technique where required
- Errors in sponge, instrument, or needle counts in surgical cases
- Failure to give a report, or giving an incomplete report, to an oncoming shift
- Failure to adequately monitor a client's condition
- Failure to notify a physician of a significant change in a client's status

practice. If this practice is followed, other care providers may administer medications or provide care to the client without up-to-date information. Harm may come to a client whose record is not accurate and current. Nurses must always follow the particular style of charting adopted by their employer (Phillips, 1999a).

Truthful documentation is also essential. If an error is made in the documentation, it is important to follow the policies and procedures of the institution to correct it. Obliterating or erasing errors may appear to be a cover-up and lead to charges of fraud. The credibility of a nurse who goes to court will be negatively affected if it appears that the nurse's initial charting has been changed after an injury has occurred to a client. This scenario is exemplified in the case of *Meyer v. Gordon* (1981). Nurses did not adequately monitor a woman in labour, and their notes were sloppy and vague. The fetus experienced severe distress, required resuscitation upon delivery, and was transferred to another hospital. When a nurse realized that the documentation was deficient, she altered it. However, the original chart had already been photocopied and sent to the second hospital. At trial, it was obvious that the original document had been tampered with. The court held that the nursing staff had been negligent in several respects, and the judge severely condemned the nurse's tampering with the evidence.

Nurses should also know the current nursing literature in their areas of practice. They should know and follow the policies and procedures of the institution in which they work. Nurses should be sensitive to common sources of client injury, such as falls and medication errors. Finally, nurses must communicate with the client, explain the tests and treatment to be performed, document that specific explanations were provided to the client, and listen to the client's concerns about the treatment.

Nurse-client relationships are very important, not only in ensuring quality care but also in minimizing legal risks. Trust develops between a nurse and client. Clients who believe that the nurses performed their duties correctly and were concerned with their welfare are less likely to initiate a lawsuit against the nurse. Sincere caring for clients is an essential role of the nurse and is an effective risk-management tool. However, caring will not totally protect the nurse if negligent practice occurs. When a client is injured, the investigation into the incident may implicate the nurses even if the client feels kindly toward them.

Criminal Liability

Although the vast majority of nursing liability issues involve private law matters (e.g., torts), the criminal law is also relevant. Canadian nurses have been charged with criminal offences such as assault, administering a noxious substance, and criminal negligence causing death (a category of manslaughter). The difference between the tort of negligence and criminal negligence charges is the degree to which the act deviated from the standard of a reasonably competent practitioner. For example, in the case of criminal negligence, the Crown must prove that there was *extreme* carelessness on the part of the nurse, indicating "wanton or reckless disregard for the lives or safety of other persons" (*Criminal Code,* 1985, 219 [1]).

Consent

A signed consent form is required for all routine treatment, procedures such as surgery, some treatment programs such as chemotherapy, and research involving clients. A client signs general consent forms when admitted to the hospital or other health care facility. The client or representative must sign a special consent or treatment form before each specialized procedure or treatment.

Provincial and territorial laws detail individuals who are legally able to give consent to medical treatment. Nurses should know the law in their own jurisdiction and be familiar with the policies and procedures of their employing institution regarding consent.

Generally the following factors must be verified for consent to be legally valid:

- The person must have the legal and mental capacity to make a treatment decision.
- The consent must be given voluntarily without coercion.
- The person must understand the risks and benefits of the procedure or treatment, the risks of not undergoing the procedure or treatment, and any available alternatives.

If a client is deaf, illiterate, or speaks a foreign language, an official interpreter must be available to explain the terms of consent. A family member or acquaintance who is able to speak a client's language should not be used to interpret health information except as a last resort. A client under the effects of a sedative is not able to clearly understand the implications of an invasive procedure. Every effort should be made to assist the client in making an informed choice.

Nurses must be sensitive to the cultural issues of consent. The nurse must understand the way in which clients and their families communicate and make important decisions. It is essential for nurses to understand the various cultures with which they interact. The cultural beliefs and values of the client may be very different from those of the nurse. It is important for nurses not to impose their own cultural values on the client (see chapter 9).

Informed Consent. **Informed consent** is a person's agreement to allow something to happen, such as surgery or an invasive procedure, based on a full disclosure of the likely risks, benefits, alternatives, and consequences of refusal (Black, 1999). Informed consent creates a legal duty for the physician and/or health care provider to disclose material facts in terms the client can reasonably understand to make an informed choice (Sneiderman et al., 2003). The explanation should also describe treatment alternatives, as well as the risks involved in all treatment options. Failure to obtain consent in situations other than emergencies may result in a claim of battery. Without informed consent, a client may bring a lawsuit against the health care provider for negligence, even if the procedure had been done in a competent manner. Informed consent requires providing adequate information for the client to form a decision and documenting that decision.

The following factors are required for informed consent (Sneiderman et al., 2003):

- A brief, complete explanation of the procedure or treatment.

- Names and qualifications of people performing and assisting in the procedure.
- A description of any possible harm, including permanent damage or death, that may occur as a result of the procedure.
- An explanation of alternative therapies to the proposed procedure/treatment, as well as the risks of doing nothing. Clients also need to be informed of their right to refuse the procedure/treatment without discontinuing other supportive care and their right to withdraw their consent even after the procedure has begun.

Informed consent is part of the physician-client relationship. Because nurses do not perform surgery or direct medical procedures, obtaining clients' informed consent does not usually fall within the nursing duty. Even though the nurse assumes the responsibility for witnessing the client's signature on the consent form, the nurse does not legally assume the duty of obtaining informed consent. The nurse's signature witnessing the consent means that the client voluntarily gave consent, that the client's signature is authentic, and that the client appears to be competent to give consent (Sneiderman et al., 2003). When nurses provide consent forms for clients to sign, the clients should be asked if they understand the procedures for which consent is being given. If they deny understanding or the nurse suspects they do not understand, the nurse must notify the physician or nursing supervisor. Some consent forms also have a line for the physician to sign after explaining the risks and alternatives to a client. Such a form is helpful in a court case when a client alleges that consent was not informed. If a client refuses treatment, this rejection should also be written, signed, and witnessed.

If a client participates in an experimental treatment program or submits to use of experimental drugs or treatments, an even more detailed and stringently regulated informed consent form is used. An organization's institutional review board should review the information in the consent form for research involving human subjects. The client may withdraw from the experiment at any time (see chapter 6).

Many procedures that nurses perform (e.g., insertion of intravenous [IV] or nasogastric tubes) do not require a formal written consent, yet clients still deserve the protection of their right to give or refuse consent to treatment. Implied consent to treatment is very often involved in nursing procedures. For example, when the nurse approaches the client with a syringe in hand and the client rolls over to expose the injection site, consent is implied. If the client resists the injection either verbally or through actions, the nurse must not proceed with the procedure. Forcing or otherwise treating a client without consent could result in criminal or civil charges of assault and battery. Many advanced practice nurses are now autonomously treating clients. It is therefore likely that formal written consent for nursing procedures will also be expected for the treatment received from advance practice nurse specialists.

Parents are usually the legal guardians of pediatric clients, and therefore they must sign consent forms for treatment. If the parents are divorced, the parent with legal custody must give consent. Occasionally a parent or guardian refuses treatment for a child. In those cases, the court may intervene on the child's behalf. The practice of making the child a ward of the court and administering necessary treatment is relatively common in such cases.

The example of 13-year-old Tyrell Dueck from Saskatchewan illustrates such a case. The teen was diagnosed with cancer in the fall of 1998. He completed part of his chemotherapy when he decided that he did not want more treatment or the recommended amputation of his leg, believing that he had been "cured by God" and further treatment was unnecessary. His statements were consistent with his family's Christian value system. Following his parents' advice, the boy wished to undergo alternative therapy at a clinic in Mexico. The treating physicians maintained that without further conventional treatment, Tyrell would die within a year. A judge concluded that Tyrell had been given inaccurate information by his father about the benefits and risks of the proposed alternative therapy and therefore was unable to make an informed consent or refusal. Thus, the family's wishes to forgo conventional treatment were legally overruled, and the boy's grandparents were to take him for treatments. Before the enforced treatment could be started, however, tests revealed that the cancer had already spread and the treatment would no longer be helpful. The teen was returned to the care of his parents and he died a short time later.

In some instances, obtaining informed consent is difficult or simply not possible. If, for example, the client is unconscious, consent must be obtained from a person legally authorized to give consent on the client's behalf. Other surrogate decision makers may have legally been delegated this authority through proxy directives or court guardianship procedures. In emergency situations, if it is impossible to obtain consent from the client or an authorized person, the procedure required to benefit the client or save a life may be undertaken without liability for failure to obtain consent. In such cases, the law assumes that the client would wish to be treated. This is referred to as the *emergency doctrine*.

Clients with mental health problems and frail, older adults must also be given the opportunity to give consent. They retain the right to refuse treatment unless a court has legally determined that they are incompetent to decide for themselves.

Nursing Students and Legal Liability

Nursing students are liable if their actions cause harm to clients. If a client is harmed as a direct result of a nursing student's actions or lack of action, the liability is generally shared by the student, instructor, hospital or health care facility, and university or educational institution. Nursing students should never be assigned to perform tasks for which they are unprepared, and they should be carefully supervised by instructors as they learn new skills. Although nursing students are not considered employees of the hospital, the institution has a responsibility to monitor their acts. Nursing students are expected to perform as professional nurses would in providing safe client care. Faculty members are usually responsible for instructing and observing students, but in some situations, staff nurses serving as preceptors may share these responsibilities. Every nursing school should provide clear definitions of student, preceptor, and faculty responsibility (Phillips, 2002).

When students are employed as nursing assistants or nurses' aides when not attending classes, they should not perform tasks that do not appear in a job description for a nurses' aide or assistant. For example, even if a student has learned to administer intramuscular medications in class, this task may not be performed by a nurses' aide. If a staff nurse overseeing the nursing assistant or aide knowingly assigns work without regard for the person's ability to safely conduct the task as defined in the job description, the staff nurse would also be liable. If students employed as nurse's aides are requested to perform tasks that they are not prepared to safely complete, this information should be brought to the supervisor's attention so that the needed help can be obtained.

Professional Liability Protection

Most nurses in Canada are employed by publicly funded health care facilities that carry malpractice insurance. These facilities are considered employers and therefore are vicariously liable for negligent acts of their employees as long as the employees were working within the normal scope and course of practice (Keatings & Smith, 2000). Because of this legal principle, if an employee is found liable in a civil lawsuit, the employer is generally ordered to pay the damages (CNPS, 1998). A nurse who exceeds the bounds of acceptable practice or is self-employed would be fully liable for his or her own negligence. All nurses should be aware of their employment status and professional liability coverage.

The CNPS is a non-profit society established in 1988 to provide legal support and liability protection to nurses. The services of CNPS are available free as a benefit of membership in a subscribing provincial or territorial professional association or college. The only two jurisdictions in Canada not included in CNPS are British Columbia and Quebec. Registered nurses in British Columbia are covered by their own insurance corporation, and those in Quebec have commercial insurance available through the Order of Nurses of Quebec. CNPS services are available to nurses in a variety of work settings, including independent practice and volunteer settings. Nurses can obtain confidential assistance from a nurse lawyer by contacting the CNPS toll-free by telephone, Monday to Friday from 0845 to 1630 hours EST at 1-800-267-3390.

A nurse providing emergency assistance at an accident scene would not be covered by an employer's insurance policy because the care given would not be the responsibility of the employer. However, some provinces have passed "Good Samaritan" laws (e.g., Alberta's *Emergency Medical Aid Act*) that prevent voluntary rescuers from being sued for wrongdoing unless it can be proven that they displayed gross negligence. Nurses must be familiar with these laws in their own province or territory (Phillips, 1999b).

Abandonment, Assignment, and Contract Issues

Short Staffing. During nursing shortages or periods of staff downsizing, the issue of inadequate staffing may arise. Legal problems may result if there are not enough nurses or an appropriate mix of staff to provide competent care. If assigned to care for more clients than is reasonable, nurses should bring this information to the attention of the nursing supervisor. In addition, a written protest such as a workload or staffing report form should be completed to document the nurse's concerns about client safety. Most provinces and territories have some reporting mechanism in place to document heavy workload or staffing situations. Although such a protest may not relieve nurses of responsibility if a client suffers injury because of inattention, it would show that they were attempting to act reasonably. Whenever a written protest is made, nurses should keep a copy of this document in their personal file. Most administrators recognize that knowledge of a potential problem shifts some of the responsibility to the institution.

Nurses should not walk out when staffing is inadequate, because charges of abandonment could be made. A nurse who refuses to accept an assignment may be considered insubordinate, and clients would not benefit from having even fewer staff available. It is important to know the institution's policies and procedures and the nursing union's collective agreement on how to handle such circumstances before they arise.

Floating. Nurses are sometimes required to "float" from the area in which they normally practise to other nursing units. In one case, a nurse in obstetrics was assigned to an emergency room. A client entered the emergency room and complained of chest pain. The client was given too great a dosage of lidocaine by the obstetrical nurse and died after suffering irreversible brain damage and cardiac arrest. The nurse lost the negligence lawsuit. Nurses must practice within their level of competence. Nurses should not be floated to areas where they have not been adequately cross-trained. Nurses who float should inform the supervisor of any lack of experience in caring for the type of clients on the nursing unit. They should also request and be given orientation to the unit. A supervisor can be held liable if a staff nurse is given an assignment he or she cannot safely perform.

Physicians' Orders. The physician is responsible for directing medical treatment. Nurses are obligated to follow physicians' orders unless they believe the orders are in error, violate hospital policy, or would harm clients. Therefore, all orders must be assessed, and if one is found to be erroneous or harmful, further clarification from the physician is necessary. If the physician confirms the order and the nurse still believes it is inappropriate, the supervising nurse should be informed. A nurse should not proceed to perform a physician's order if it is foreseeable that harm will come to the client. The nursing supervisor should be informed and given a written memorandum detailing the events in chronological order; the reasons for refusing to carry out the order should also be written to protect the nurse from disciplinary action. The supervising nurse should help resolve the questionable order. A medical or pharmacy consultant may be called in to help clarify the appropriateness or inappropriateness of the order. A nurse carrying out an inaccurate or inappropriate order may be legally responsible for any harm suffered by the client.

In a negligence lawsuit against a physician and a hospital, one of the most frequently litigated issues is whether the nurse kept the physician informed of the client's condition. To inform a physician properly, nurses must perform a competent nursing assessment of the client to determine the signs and symptoms that are significant in relation to the attending physician's tasks of diagnosis and treatment. Nurses must be certain to document that the physician was notified and to document his or her response, the nurse's follow-up, and the client's response. For example, nurses noticed that a client with a cast on his leg was experiencing poor circulation to his foot. The nurses recorded these changes, but did not notify the doctor. The client subsequently developed gangrene and required an amputation. The hospital, physician, and nursing staff were all charged with negligence.

The physician should write all orders, including "do not attempt resuscitation" (DNR) orders, which many physicians are reluctant to write out because they fear legal repercussions for criminal neglect or failure to act. The nurse must make sure that orders are transcribed correctly. Verbal orders are not recommended because they increase the possibilities for error. If a verbal order is necessary (e.g., during an emergency), it should be written and signed by the physician as soon as possible, usually within 24 hours. The nurse should be familiar with the institution's policy and procedures regarding verbal orders.

Dispensing Advice Over the Phone. Providing advice over the telephone is a high-risk activity because diagnosing over the phone is extremely difficult. The nurse is legally accountable for advice given over the phone. The most common allegations of negligence in this area are providing inadequate advice, improper referrals, and failure to refer (CNPS, 1997). It is essential that nurses precisely follow institutional guidelines and policies and thoroughly document each call to avoid serious repercussions for all parties.

Contracts and Employment Agreements. In Canada, most nurses belong to unions or associations that engage in collective bargaining on behalf of a group. The collective agreements between employers and union members are written contracts that set out the conditions of employment (e.g., salary, hours of work, benefits, layoffs, and termination). Many laws, including labour laws, apply to nurses. For example, laws outline eligibility for and details of workers' compensation or maternity benefits. It is important for nurses to understand the employment laws in the province or territory where they work.

By accepting a job, a nurse enters into an agreement with an employer. The nurse will perform professional duties competently, adhering to the policies and procedures of the institution. In return, the employer pays for the nursing services and ensures facilities and equipment are adequate for safe care.

Legal Issues in Nursing Practice

Abortion

The Supreme Court of Canada handed down a ruling in the 1988 case of *R. v. Morgentaler* stating that the *Criminal Code* regulations on legal access to abortion were unconstitutional. The *Criminal Code* had required a woman seeking abortion to secure the approval of a hospital-based committee before the procedure could be performed. By rejecting the *Criminal Code* provisions, the Supreme Court in effect tossed the abortion issue back to Parliament, but Parliament has not rewritten a criminal law policy on abortion. Abortion is thus unregulated by law, which is tantamount to its legalization. However, the legal entitlement to abortion does not mean abortion services are readily available. Because health care facilities are not obliged to offer abortions, many do not do so. Thus, access remains a continuing issue.

Drug Regulations and Nurses

Canadian law closely regulates the administration of drugs. Two federal acts control the manufacture, distribution, and sale of food, drugs, cosmetics, and therapeutic devices in Canada: the *Food and Drugs Act* and the *Controlled Drugs and Substances Act*. The *Food and Drugs Act* lists the drugs that can be sold only by prescription (e.g., antibiotics) and drugs that are subject to stringent controls (e.g., barbiturates, amphetamines). These drugs require specific handling and record keeping. The *Controlled Drugs and Substances Act* controls the manufacture, distribution, and sale of narcotics (e.g., morphine, codeine). However, it also regulates other drugs that are controlled in the same manner as narcotics, such as cocaine and marijuana. Most institutions have policies about medication administration and record keeping, especially for controlled drugs and narcotics. Nurses must be aware of their employer's policies.

Nurses are not legally entitled to prescribe drugs. However, in several jurisdictions, nurse practitioners may prescribe certain non-narcotic drugs specific to their area of practice.

The administration of medications following a physician's prescription is a basic nursing responsibility. A competent nurse is expected to know the purpose and effect of any drug administered, as well as potential side effects and contraindications. It is also a nurse's responsibility to question any doctor's orders that may be incorrect or unsafe. A nurse who follows a doctor's order that is unclear or incorrect may be found negligent.

Communicable Diseases

The care of people with communicable diseases such as HIV, acquired immunodeficiency syndrome (AIDS), hepatitis, and severe acute respiratory syndrome (SARS) has legal implications for nurses. Health care workers are at risk for exposure to communicable diseases due to the nature of their work. Despite the best attempts to protect oneself against communicable diseases through the proper and consistent use of protective gear (e.g., latex gloves or masks), accidental needle-stick injuries or life-threatening illnesses such as SARS can still occur. Nurses have an ethical and legal obligation to provide care to all assigned clients, and employers have an obligation to provide their employees with necessary protective gear.

In all cases involving privacy, confidentiality, and disclosure, there is the need to balance the rights of the people infected with a communicable disease with those of the public or health care workers. Both civil and criminal liability can result if private information is disclosed without authorization. Nurses must understand the reporting laws in the province or territory in which they practise. Courts can order disclosure of AIDS clients' records in situations that are not addressed by a statute, even without the client's consent. Whenever information is requested on a client by any third parties, including insurance companies or employers, nurses must obtain a signed release from the client before releasing confidential information. Not every health care worker who comes in contact with a client has a need to know the client's HIV status. Confidential information must be protected.

The courts have upheld the employer's right to fire a nurse who refuses to care for an AIDS client. Nurses who flatly refuse to care for HIV-infected clients or possibly a client with SARS may be reprimanded or fired for insubordination. The Canadian Nurses Association *Code of Ethics for Registered Nurses* (2002) states that nurses must not discriminate in the provision of nursing care on the basis of factors such as a person's sexual orientation, health status, or lifestyle (p. 15). One limitation outlined in the code regarding a nurse's right to refuse care to a client is that nurses are not obligated to comply with a person's wishes when this is contrary to the law (e.g., assisting suicide). If the care requested is contrary to the nurse's personal values, such as assisting with an abortion, the nurse must provide appropriate care until alternative care arrangements are arranged.

Nurses must be concerned with balancing the rights of protecting themselves with protecting the client's rights. Both are afforded protection against discrimination and protection of privacy by human rights legislation. Most legal cases involving nurses and communicable diseases currently relate to the protection needed for nurses as employees. Strict compliance with standard precautions/routine practices and the use of transmission-based precautions (e.g., airborne or droplet) for clients known or suspected of having other serious illnesses is the nurse's wisest strategy (see chapter 29).

Death and Dying

Many legal issues surround the event of death, including a basic definition as to when a person is considered dead. The only province that has a statutory definition of death is Manitoba, which defines it as "the irreversible cessation of all brain function" (*Vital Statistics Act,* 1987). However, this "brain death" definition has become standard medical practice across Canada. Until the 1960s, death was defined as the irreversible cessation of cardiopulmonary functioning. However, two developments beginning around that time necessitated a shift to the brain: (a) the emergence of artificial life-support devices that could maintain cardiopulmonary functioning in a brain-dead person, and (b) the emergence of organ transplants—death had to be redefined so that organs could be donated.

Ethical and legal questions are raised by the related issues of euthanasia and assisted suicide. **Euthanasia** is an act undertaken by one person with the motive of relieving another person's suffering and the knowledge that the act will end the life of that person (Downie, 2004). In Canada, euthanasia is illegal. It is legally irrelevant whether the client has consented to the act because section 14 of the *Criminal Code* states, "no person can consent to have death inflicted on him." And according to section 241 of the *Criminal Code,* it is an offence to "aid a person to commit suicide, whether suicide ensues or not" (1985).

On the other hand, the law draws a distinction between "killing" and "letting die." Euthanasia and assisted suicide are considered killing. Withholding or withdrawing life-prolonging treatment is considered "letting die." The disease process causes the client to die a natural death. Thus, a mentally competent client has the legal right to refuse life-prolonging treatment. If, for example, such a client requests that her ventilator be disconnected, understanding that she will die as a result, her wishes must be honoured in accordance with the principle of "no treatment without consent."

In the case of *Nancy B. v. Hôtel-Dieu de Québec* (1992), a young, mentally competent client who was totally and permanently paralyzed by a neurological disease twice asked that her ventilator be disconnected. After the second refusal, she sought a court order to enforce her will. The order was granted by the Quebec Superior Court, which ruled that as a mentally competent client, she could not be treated without consent. It should also be noted that even if a client has not asked for the termination of life-prolonging treatment (either directly or by way of an advance directive), physicians are still allowed, after consultation with family members, to terminate such treatment when it no longer offers any reasonable hope of benefit to the person.

When clients reject life-prolonging treatment, the nurse focuses on the goal of caring versus curing. Nurses have a legal obligation to treat the deceased person's remains with dignity (see chapter 25). Wrongful handling of a deceased person's remains could cause emotional harm to the surviving family.

Advance Directives and Health Care Surrogates

The **advance directive** is a mechanism enabling a mentally competent person to plan for a time when he or she may lack the mental capacity to make medical treatment decisions. It comes into effect only when the person becomes incompetent to speak for himself or herself. The advance directive is a more sophisticated concept than that of the living will, although the two terms are often confused. A **living will** is a document in which the person makes an anticipatory refusal of life-prolonging measures during a future state of mental incompetence. On the other hand, an advance directive is not restricted to the rejection of life-support measures; its focus is on treatment preferences, which may include both requests and refusals of treatment. The advance directive assumes two forms: the instructional directive (in which the maker of the document spells out specific directions to govern care in more detail than is generally found in the living will); and the proxy directive (in which the person appoints someone as a health care agent to make treatment decisions on his or her behalf). Legislation in British Columbia, Alberta, Saskatchewan, Manitoba, Ontario, Prince Edward Island, Newfoundland and Labrador, and the Yukon gives full legal effect to both kinds of directives; the proxy directive is also recognized in Quebec and Nova Scotia. Even in provinces and territories that do not recognize an instructional directive, there is nothing prohibiting a physician from following a directive.

If nurses know about the existence of a health care directive, they are required to follow it. Nurses are also required to follow the wishes of a validly appointed proxy (assuming these instructions are legal). A proxy has the right to receive all medical information concerning the client's condition and proposed plan of care. Failure to comply with a proxy's directions could result in charges of battery being laid.

If a physician ignores the advance directive, the nurse must bring the advance directive to the physician's attention, and document that he or she did so along with the physician's response to this information. The nurse should also notify the supervisor, who can then give direction regarding institutional policies and guidelines for such circumstances.

The psychiatric advance directive is a new type of advance directive. Individuals with mental health problems complete these directives during periods of mental stability and competence. It outlines how the person wishes to be treated in the future should their underlying mental illness causes them to lose decision-making capacity. For example, it may specify preferences for and against certain interventions (e.g., electroconvulsive therapy) or medications. The psychiatric advance directive can also designate a surrogate decision maker to act on the person's behalf in the event of an incapacitating mental health crisis.

Organ Donation

Legally competent people are free to donate their bodies or organs for medical use. Every province and territory has human tissue legislation that provides for both the *inter vivos* (live donor) and *post-mortem* (cadaveric) donation of tissues and organs. For example, a mentally competent adult is allowed to donate a kidney, a lobe of the liver, or bone marrow. Regarding cadaveric donation, statutes provide that adults may consent to organ donation after death. If the deceased had left no direction for post-mortem donation, then consent may be obtained from the person's family. In two provinces—Manitoba and Nova Scotia—the statutes contain "required request" provisions that come into effect when a deceased person had not consented to organ removal but is considered a good donor candidate. In such an event, the physician is legally obliged to seek permission from the family. In many hospitals, a nurse transplant coordinator performs this function.

Mental Health Issues

Treating clients with mental health problems raises legal and ethical issues. Provincial mental health legislation such as the *Mental Health and Consequential Amendments Act* (S.M. 1998) provides direction for health care professionals, protects client autonomy, and recognizes that some individuals with severe mental health problems may lack the ability to appreciate the consequences of their health condition.

A client can be admitted to a psychiatric unit involuntarily or on a voluntary basis. Clients admitted on a voluntary basis should be treated no differently than any other client. They have the right to refuse treatment and the right to discharge themselves from hospital. However, if the client may cause harm to self or others, provincial mental health legislation permits police officers (or other authorized parties) to bring the person for examination and treatment without the person's consent (Morris, Ferguson, & Dykeman, 1999).

Potentially suicidal clients may be admitted to psychiatric units. If the client's history and medical records indicate suicidal tendencies, the client must be kept under supervision. A lawsuit may result if a client attempts suicide within the hospital. The allegations in the lawsuits would be that the institution failed to provide adequate supervision or safeguard the facilities. Documentation of precautions against suicide is essential.

Public Health Issues

It is important that nurses, especially those employed in community health settings, understand the public health laws. Public health acts, which have been enacted in all provinces and territories, are directed toward the prevention, treatment, and suppression of communicable disease (Sneiderman et al., 2003). Community health nurses have the legal responsibility to follow the laws enacted to protect the public health. These laws may include reporting suspected abuse and neglect, such as child abuse, elder abuse, or domestic violence; reporting communicable diseases; and reporting of other health-related issues enacted to protect the public's health.

Some provinces (e.g., Ontario) have legislation under their health protection acts that require proof of immunization for school entry. In these provinces, however, exceptions are permitted for medical or religious grounds and reasons of conscience (Health Canada, 1997). Although a signed consent is not required for an immunization, nurses are advised to obtain some documentation (evidence) that they discussed the risks and benefits with the parent or legal guardian. Nurses should be aware of their employer guidelines for documentation.

Every province and territory has child abuse legislation that requires health care professionals, such as nurses, to report witnessed or suspected child abuse or neglect directly to child protection agencies. To encourage reports of suspected cases, the laws offer legal immunity for the reporter if the report is made in good faith.

Health care professionals who do not report suspected child abuse or neglect maybe held liable for civil or criminal action. Several provinces and territories also have laws that require health care workers to report witnessed or suspected abuse of clients within facilities (e.g., *The Protection of Persons in Care Act* in Manitoba). These reports must be made directly to a public authority. Even if public reporting is not required, nurses should report all suspicions of client abuse to their supervisors. It is essential for nurses to know their provincial or territorial laws and employer policies regarding the reporting of abuse.

Risk Management

Risk management is a system of ensuring appropriate nursing care by identifying potential hazards and eliminating them before harm occurs (Guido, 2001). The steps involved in risk management include identifying possible risks, analyzing them, acting to reduce them, and evaluating the steps taken.

One tool used in risk management is the **incident report** or **adverse occurrence report.** When a client is harmed or endangered by incorrect care, such as a drug error, a nurse completes an incident report (see chapter 13). These reports are analyzed to determine how future problems can be avoided. For example, if incident reports show that drug errors commonly involve a new IV pump, the risk manager will ensure staff has been properly trained on its use. In-service education may be all that is necessary to prevent future errors.

The underlying rationale for quality assurance in risk-management programs is the highest possible quality of care. Some insurance companies and medical and nursing organizations require the use of quality-assurance and risk-management procedures. Quality care is the responsibility of both the employer and the individual provider.

Risk management requires good documentation. The nurse's documentation can be the evidence of what actually was done for a client and can serve as proof that the nurse acted reasonably and safely. Documentation should be thorough, accurate, and performed in a timely manner. When a lawsuit is being evaluated, the nurse's notes are very often the first record to be reviewed by the plaintiff's counsel. If the nurse's credibility is questioned because of these documents, the risk of greater liability exists for the nurse. The nurse's notes are risk-management and quality-assurance tools for the employer and the individual nurse.

Professional Involvement

Nurses must be involved in their professional organizations and on committees that define the standards of care for nursing practice. If current laws, rules and regulations, or policies under which nurses must practise do not reflect reality, nurses must become involved as advocates to see that the scope of nursing practice is accurately defined. Nurses must be willing to represent nursing and the client's perspective in the community as well. The voice of nursing can be powerful and effective when the organizing focus is the protection and welfare of the public entrusted to their care.

Key Concepts

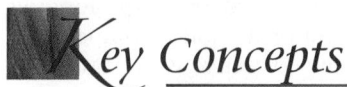

- With increased emphasis on client rights, nurses in practice today must understand their legal obligations and responsibilities to clients.
- The civil law system is concerned with the protection of a person's private rights, and the criminal law system deals with the rights of individuals and society.
- A nurse can be found liable for negligence if the following criteria are established: the nurse (defendant) owed a duty of care to the client (plaintiff), the nurse did not carry out that duty, the client was injured, and the nurse's failure to carry out the duty caused the client's injury.
- Clients are entitled to confidential health care and freedom from unauthorized release of information.
- Under the law, practising nurses must follow standards of care, which originate in nursing practice acts and regulations, the guidelines of professional organizations, and the written policies and procedures of employing institutions.
- Nurses are responsible for confirming that informed consent has been given for any surgery or other medical procedure before the procedure is performed.
- Nurses are responsible for performing all procedures correctly and exercising professional judgment as they carry out physicians' orders.
- Nurses are obligated to follow physicians' orders unless they believe the orders are in error or could be detrimental to clients.
- Staffing standards determine the ratio of nurses to clients, and if the nurse is required to care for more clients than is reasonable, a formal protest should be made to the nursing administration.
- Legal issues involving death include documenting all events surrounding the death and treating the deceased person with dignity.
- A competent adult can legally give consent to donate specific organs, and nurses may serve as witnesses to this decision.
- All nurses should know the laws that apply to their area of practice.
- Depending on provincial statutes, nurses are required to report suspected child abuse and certain communicable diseases.
- Nurses are client advocates and ensure quality of care through risk management and lobbying for safe nursing practice standards.
- Nurses must file incident reports in all situations when someone could or did get hurt.

Key Terms

Advance directive, *p. 122*
Adverse occurrence report, *p. 124*
Assault, *p. 116*
Battery, *p. 116*
Civil law, *p. 113*
Common law, *p. 113*
Euthanasia, *p. 122*
Incident reports, *p. 124*
Informed consent, *p. 118*
Intentional torts, *p. 115*
Living will, *p. 122*
Negligence, *p. 117*
Nursing practice acts, *p. 114*
Risk management, *p. 124*
Standards of care, *p. 114*
Statute law, *p. 114*
Tort, *p. 115*

Critical Thinking Exercises

1. Nurse Rossi and Nurse Kao are getting on an elevator to go down to the cafeteria. There are several visitors present in the elevator, as well as hospital personnel. Nurse Rossi and Nurse Kao are talking about a client who is in the intensive care unit who has just tested positive for HIV. They identify the client as the man in Room 14B. One of the visitors on the elevator who overhears this information is a woman who is engaged to the client in Room 14B.
   a. Have Nurse Rossi and Nurse Kao breached a client's right to confidential health care?
   b. Would the client in Room 14B have any legal cause of action against the nurses?
   c. Even though the client's fiancée may have a right to know the HIV status of her future husband, is there any duty on the part of the nurses to disclose confidential information to the fiancée?
2. While transporting a client down the hall on a stretcher, Nurse Reyes stops to chat with an orderly. The side rails on the stretcher are down, and while Nurse Reyes has her back to the stretcher, the client rolls over, falls off the stretcher, and fractures his hip. In a lawsuit by the client against Nurse Reyes, what must the client establish to prove negligence against the nurse?

Review Questions

1. The *Nursing Practice Acts* are an example of
   1. Statute law
   2. Common law
   3. Public law
   4. Criminal law
2. Treating a client without the person's consent is considered
   1. Battery
   2. Negligence
   3. Implied consent
   4. Expressed consent
3. The nurse restrains a client without the client's permission and without a physician's order. The nurse may be guilty of
   1. Assault
   2. False imprisonment
   3. Invasion of privacy
   4. Neglect
4. A confused client who fell out of bed because side rails were not used when they were ordered is an example of which type of liability?
   1. False imprisonment
   2. Assault
   3. Battery
   4. Negligence
5. Even though the nurse may obtain the client's signature on a form, obtaining informed consent is the responsibility of the
   1. Student
   2. Student's instructor and the hospital or health care facility
   3. University or educational institution
   4. Supervising nurse
6. What should you do if you think the client does not understand the procedure for which he or she is being asked to give consent?
   1. Do not be concerned if the consent is already signed.
   2. Notify the physician or nursing supervisor.
   3. Send the client for the procedure and discuss it afterward.
   4. Ask a family member to give consent.
7. When a client is harmed as a result of a nursing student's actions or lack of action, the liability if generally held by
   1. The student alone
   2. The student's instructor or preceptor
   3. The hospital or health care facility
   4. All of the above
8. When the nurse stops to help in an emergency at the scene of an accident, if the injured party files suit and the nurse's employing institution's insurance does not cover the nurse, the nurse would probably be covered by
   1. The nurse's automobile insurance
   2. The nurse's homeowner's insurance
   3. The Patient Care Partnership, which may grant immunity from suit if the injured party consents
   4. The Good Samaritan laws, which grant immunity from suit if there is no gross negligence
9. The nurse is obligated to follow a physician's order unless
   1. The order is a verbal order.
   2. The physician's order is illegible.
   3. The order has not been transcribed.
   4. The order is in error, violates hospital policy, or would be detrimental to the client.

10. If a third party (e.g., insurance company of employer) requests health information on a client, the nurse must
1. Provide the information
2. Refuse to provide the information
3. Obtain a signed release by the client before releasing the information
4. Contact the client's family or lawyer

References

Black, H. C. (1999). *Black's law dictionary* (7th ed.). St. Paul, MN: West Publishing.

Canadian National Report on Immunization. May 1997. CCDR Supplement Volume 24 S4. Available from *http://www.phac-aspc.gc.ca/publicat/ccdr-rmtc/97vol23/23s4/index. html*

Canadian Nurses Association. (2002). *Code of ethics for registered nurses.* Ottawa, ON: Author.

Canadian Nurses Protective Society. (1997, September). Telephone advice. *infoLAW Bulletin, 6*(1).

Canadian Nurses Protective Society. (1998, April). Vicarious liability. *infoLAW bulletin, 7*(1).

Canadian Nurses Protective Society. (2004, May). Patient restraints. *infoLAW bulletin, 13*(2).

Controlled Drugs and Substances Act, S.C., c. 19 (1996).

Criminal Code, R.S.C. 1985, c. C-46.

Downey v. Rothwell, 5 W.W.R. 311, 49 D.L.R. (3d) 82 (Alta. S.C. 1974).

Downie, J. (2004). *Dying justice: A case for decriminalizing euthanasia and assisted suicide in Canada.* Toronto, ON: University of Toronto Press.

Food and Drugs Act, R.S.C., c. F-27 (1985).

Fridman, G. H. L. (2003). *Introduction to the Canadian law of torts* (2nd ed.). Markham, ON: LexisNexis Canada.

Granger v. Ottawa General Hospital, O.J. No. 2129 (Gen. Div. 1976).

Guido, G. (2001). *Legal and ethical issues in nursing* (3rd ed.). Upper Saddle River, NJ: Prentice Hall.

Health Canada. (1997, May). *Canada communicable disease report* (Suppl., Vol. 23 S4). Ottawa, ON: Public Health Agency of Canada.

Keatings, M., & Smith, O. (2000). Ethical and legal issues in Canadian nursing (2nd ed.). Toronto, ON: W. B. Saunders Canada.

Kolesar v. Jeffries, 9 O.R. (2d) 41, 59 D.L.R. (3d) 367 (S.C.C. 1976).

Malette v. Shulman, (1990), CarswellOnt 642, 2 C.C.L.T. (2d), 1, 72 O.R. (2d).

McIntyre, M., & Thomlinson, E. (2003). Realities of Canadian nursing: Professional, practice, and power issues. Philadelphia: Lippincott Williams & Wilkins.

Mental Health and Consequential Amendments Act, S.M., c. 36 (1998).

Meyer v. Gordon, 17 C.C.L.T. 1 (B.C. S.C. 1981).

Morris, J. J., Ferguson, M., & Dykeman, M. J. (1999). *Canadian nurses and the law* (2nd ed.). Toronto, ON: Butterworths.

Nancy B. v. Hôtel-Dieu de Québec, R.J.Q. 361, 86 D.L.R. (4th) 385, 69 C.C.C. (3d) 450 (S.C. 1992).

Osborne, P. H. (2003). *Essentials of Canadian law: The law of torts* (2nd ed.). Toronto, ON: Irwin Law.

Phillips, E. (1999a). The author responds to: If it's not charted it's not done? *The Canadian Nurse, 95*(5), 12.

Phillips, E. (1999b). Is there a risk in being a Good Samaritan? *The Canadian Nurse, 95*(8):43–44.

Phillips, E. (2002). Managing Legal Risks in Preceptorships. *The Canadian Nurse, 98*(9) 25–26.

R. V. Morgentaler, 37 C.C.C. (3d) 449 (S.C.C. 1988).

Sneiderman, B., Irvine, J., & Osborne, P. (2003). *Canadian medical law* (3rd ed.). Scarborough, ON: Thompson Canada.

Tapp, A. (1996). Release of confidential information to the police. *The Canadian Nurse, 92*(3), 49–50.

Tapp, A. (2001). The legal risks of e-mail. *The Canadian Nurse, 97*(3), 35–36.

Vital Statistics Act, R.S.M., c. V60, s. 2 (1987).

Recommended Web Sites

Canadian Nurses Association—Provincial/Territorial Organizations:
http://www.cna-nurses.ca/pages/nursing_links/ nurselinkframe.htm
This Canadian Nurses Association (CNA) site offers up-to-date Web links and contact information for all provincial and territorial nursing colleges and associations.

The Canadian Nurses Protective Society:
http://www.cnps.ca
The Canadian Nurses Protective Society (CNPS) helps nurses manage their professional legal risks by offering legal support and liability protection. The members-only section of the Web site (the user name is the acronym of your professional association or college, and the password is "assist") provides information on a variety of legal topics affecting Canadian nursing practice.

The College of Licensed Practical Nurses of Nova Scotia:
http://www.clpnns.ca/outofprovlinks.htm
This site provides links to all provincial licensing authorities.

Department of Justice Canada:
http://laws.justice.gc.ca/en/
This site provides links to consolidated statutes, including the Criminal Code of Canada.

The Health Law Institute of Dalhousie University: The End of Life Project:
http://as01.ucis.dal.ca/dhli/cmp_advdirectives_faq/default.cfm
This site contains information about the Canadian law pertaining to various aspects of end of life care, including advance directives and withholding of life-sustaining treatment.

9

Culture and Ethnicity

Barbara J. Astle, RN, BScN, MN, PhD (candidate) (Canadian author)
Dula Pacquiao, BSN, MA, EdD

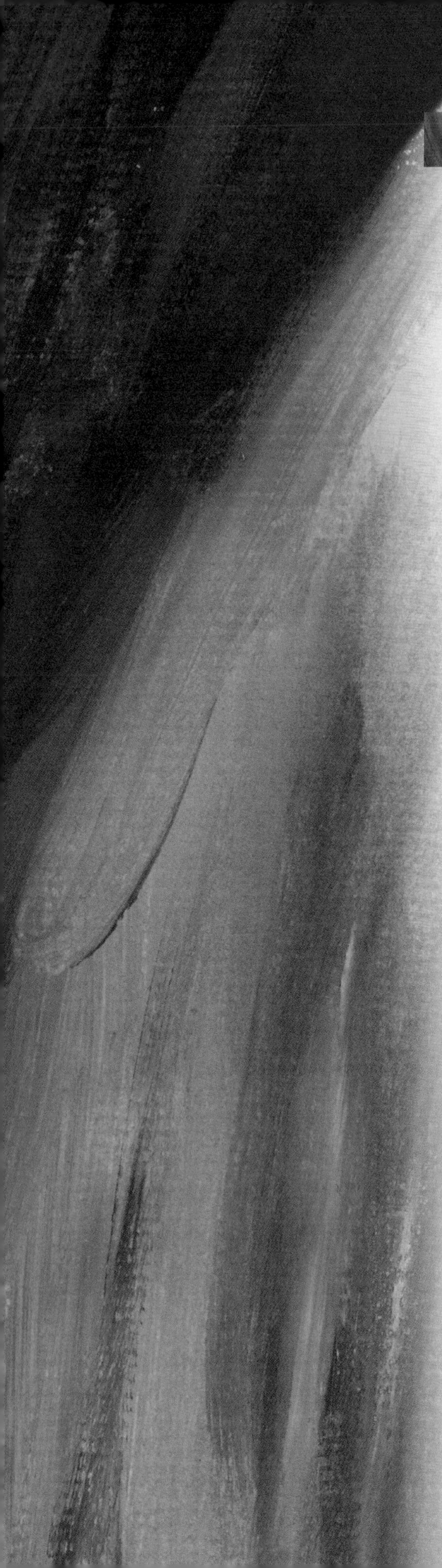

Objectives

Mastery of content in this chapter will enable the student to:

- Define the key terms listed.
- Describe how cultural awareness influences nursing care.
- Describe social and cultural influences in health, illness, and caring patterns.
- Differentiate culturally congruent care from culturally competent care.
- Use cultural assessment to identify significant values, beliefs, and practices critical to nursing care.
- Identify major components of cultural assessment.
- Apply research findings in culturally competent care.

Canada has always been a multicultural nation. At the time of Confederation, there were more than 50 different Aboriginal groups—each with their own language and culture—as well as settlers from England, France, and other European countries. Eventually, people from around the world immigrated to Canada.

The ethnocultural profile of Canada is continually evolving. According to the 2001 Census, there has been a three-fold increase in the numbers of visible minorities since 1981. (For the purposes of the Census, a *visible minority* is a person who is neither Aboriginal nor white-skinned Caucasian.) In 2001, almost 4 million individuals identified themselves as visible minorities, representing about 13% of the total population. Just 20 years ago, visible minorities comprised only 4.7% of the population. In fact, the visible minority population is growing much faster than the total population. Between 1996 and 2001, the visible minority population increased 27%, and the total population increased only 6%. If recent immigration trends continue, the visible minority population is expected to account for 20% of Canada's population by 2016 (Statistics Canada, 2003; Figure 9–1).

Figure 9–2 shows the most common visible minority groups in Canada. The three largest groups are Chinese, South Asians, and Blacks. In 2001, there were over a million Chinese people in Canada, representing 3.5% of the national population and 26% of the visible minority population. South Asians (i.e., people from the Indian subcontinent, which includes India, Pakistan, and Bangladesh, among other countries) are the fastest growing minority group, representing 3.1% of Canada's total population and 23% of all visible minorities. Blacks represent 2.2% of Canada's total population and 17% of the visible minority population.

Many people from these visible minority groups (about 30%) were born and raised in Canada (Statistics Canada, 2003). Indeed, some minority groups such as the Japanese and Blacks have been in Canada for hundreds of years. Nevertheless, the increased numbers of visible minorities is largely due to immigration patterns. Approximately 18% of Canada's total population has been born outside of the country (Statistics Canada, 2003). Canada ranks second only to Australia as the country with the highest proportion of foreign-born citizens. However, per capita, Canada receives more immigrants than any other country, including Australia and the United States (Statistics Canada, 2003). Increasingly, immigrants to Canada are from Asian countries, including the Middle East. In 1961, only 3% of immigrants to Canada were Asian and 90%

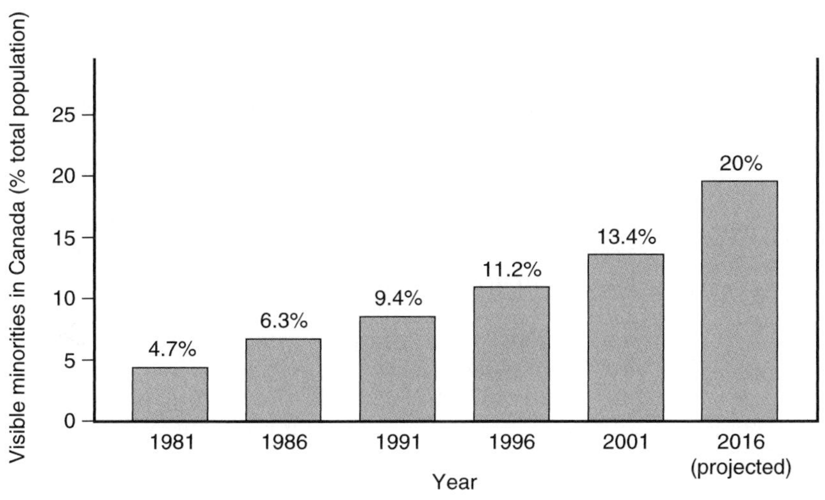

FIGURE **9–1** Visible minorities as a percentage of the total population in Canada, 1981 to 2001 and beyond. (Adapted from *Canada's Ethnocultural Portrait: The Changing Mosaic,* by Statistics Canada, 2003, accessed October 1, 2004, from *http://www12.statcan.ca/english/census01/products/analytic/companion/etoimm/canada.cfm#immigrants_ increasingly_asia)*

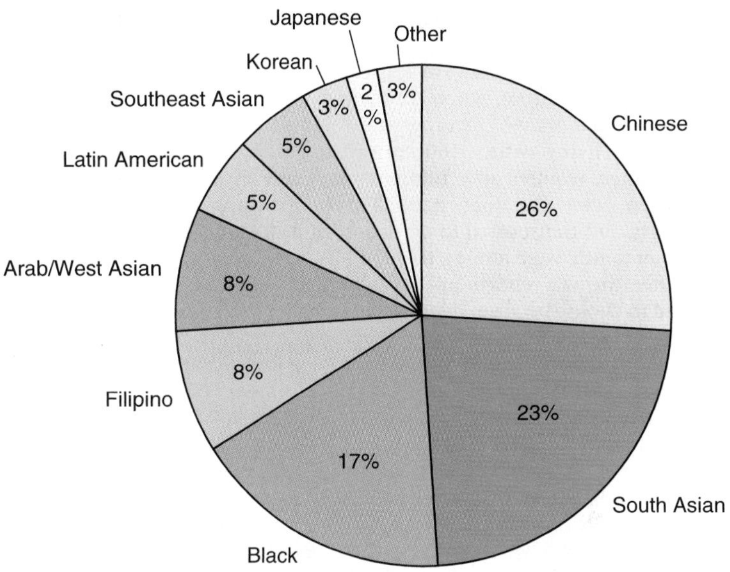

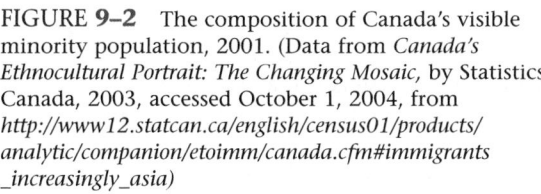

FIGURE **9–2** The composition of Canada's visible minority population, 2001. (Data from *Canada's Ethnocultural Portrait: The Changing Mosaic,* by Statistics Canada, 2003, accessed October 1, 2004, from *http://www12.statcan.ca/english/census01/products/analytic/companion/etoimm/canada.cfm#immigrants _increasingly_asia)*

were European; by 2001, 58% of immigrants were Asian and only 19% were European. Immigration has now outpaced the natural birth rate, accounting for 53% of overall population growth (Canadian Heritage, 2004). Immigrants and refugees come to Canada from around the world, creating over 200 ethnic groups in Canada (Statistics Canada, 2003).

Of course, another significant part of Canada's cultural mosaic is the Aboriginal population. In the 2001 Census, over 1.3 million people reported having at least some Aboriginal ancestry, representing 4.4% of the total population. Further details of the Aboriginal population are given later in this chapter.

In response to this diversity, Canadian nurses must understand cultural influences in health, illness, and caring patterns (Galanti, 2000, 2004). A nurse who appreciates the significance of culture will approach clients confidently and provide care in a sensitive, holistic manner (Box 9-1). Nurses should also recognize that they bring their own cultural values and beliefs to the client-nurse relationship. Nurses must not impose these on clients, but must respect the differences that each client brings to the care environment. With this understanding between nurses and clients, care can become mutually effective and respectful (Canadian Nurses Association [CNA], 2000). With the ever-changing demographics of a multicultural population, nurses must be prepared to adapt to these changes to provide effective care to all Canadians.

Cultural Concepts

Culture consists of the totality of socially transmitted knowledge of values, beliefs, norms, and lifeways of a particular group that guides their thoughts and behaviours (Leininger, 2002a; Purnell & Paulanka, 1998). Culture evolves as a way of life by a group of people who deal with similar issues over a period of time in their environment. It is passed from one person to the next, and from one generation to the next, often through social and religious customs and intellectual and artistic activities. It is a dynamic, ever-changing process.

Box 9-1 Milestones in Canadian Nursing History

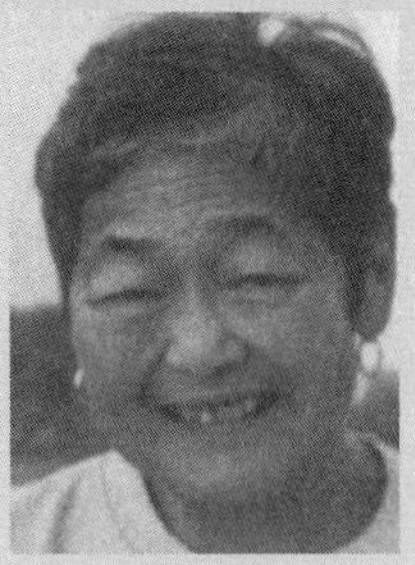

May Aiko Watanabe Yoshida, 1930–2000

Born in Vancouver, British Columbia, May Watanabe Yoshida was a clinical nurse, teacher, and researcher. She focused her professional life on the need to understand clients and their families in the light of their cultural heritage. Not surprisingly, her respect for the cultures and traditions of others grew out of her personal experiences of discrimination growing up as a Japanese Canadian.

Racist attitudes toward Japanese were rampant in Canada from the time the first immigrants arrived in the late 19th century. Laws excluded Asians from most professions, the civil service, and teaching. All Japanese Canadians—including the Canadian-born children of immigrants—were denied the right to vote. Anti-Japanese feeling came to a head after Japan attacked Pearl Harbor, when the Canadian government used the *War Measures Act* to order the removal of all Japanese Canadians living within 160 km of the Pacific Coast. Some 21,000 men, women, and children of Japanese ancestry—75% of whom were Canadian nationals—were stripped of their property and transported to detention camps. May Watanabe and her family were among them.

After the war ended in 1945, Japanese Canadians were forced to choose between deportation to Japan or dispersal east of the Rocky Mountains. The Watanabes chose to relocate in southern Ontario. A brilliant student, May entered the nursing program at McMaster University in Hamilton and graduated in 1953. She went on to earn a master's degree in 1959.

As a clinician, May Yoshida was well known for her work with immigrant families. Specializing in parent-child nursing, she focused on child-bearing and child-rearing practices of various ethnic groups. She came to believe that people's cultural traditions were central to their health and well-being. Professor Yoshida's many research projects on a range of cultural issues, together with her compelling lecturing style, made her a popular speaker internationally. Her work on caring for diverse culture was groundbreaking and her influence considerable.

Culture has both **visible** (easily seen) and **invisible** (less observable) components. The invisible value-belief system of a particular culture is the major driving force behind visible practices. For example, although a Sikh man can be easily identified by the visible artifacts that he wears (uncut hair with wooden comb, beard, turban, steel bracelet, and short sword), the meanings and beliefs associated with these artifacts are not readily apparent. These artifacts symbolize a devotee's allegiance to the pillars of Sikhism, and removal of these artifacts without expressed consent of the individual or his family is considered sacrilegious and violates the ethnoreligious identity of the person (Singh, 2000).

In any society, there is a dominant culture that exists along with other variant cultural patterns (Kluckholn, 1976). These variant patterns may be referred to as *diverse cultures, subcultures,* or *minority cultures.* Although subcultures may have similarities with the dominant culture, they maintain their unique life patterns, values, and norms. In Canada, the dominant culture is Anglo-Canadian with origins from Western Europe. **Subcultures** such as the Ukrainian and Acadian cultures represent various ethnic, religious, and other groups with distinct characteristics from the dominant culture. **Ethnicity** refers to groups whose members share a social and cultural heritage. For example, ethnic groups may share common values, language, history, physical characteristics, and geographical space. The most important characteristic of an ethnic group is that its members feel a sense of common identity. Individuals may declare their ethnic identity as, for example, Scottish, Vietnamese, or Colombian. A term that is usually contrasted with ethnicity is **race,** which is limited to the common biological attributes shared by a group, such as skin colour (Leininger & McFarland, 2002; Spector, 2000). Examples of racial classifications include Blacks and Caucasians.

In any intercultural encounter, there is an insider or native perspective **(emic world view)** and an outsider's perspective **(etic world view).** A nurse is baffled by a Korean female's request for seaweed soup for her first meal after giving birth. The nurse has an emic view of professional postpartum care, and as an outsider to the Korean culture, the nurse is not aware of the significance of the practice to the client. Conversely, the Korean client who has an etic view of Canadian professional care assumes that seaweed soup should be available in the hospital because it cleanses the blood and promotes healing and lactation (*Korean Health Beliefs,* 2003). Unless the nurse seeks the client's emic view, he or she is likely to suggest other varieties of soups available, disregarding the cultural meaning of the practice to the client.

The processes of enculturation and acculturation facilitate cultural learning. Socialization into one's primary culture as a child is known as **enculturation.** The process of adapting to and adopting characteristics of a new culture is **acculturation** (Leininger & McFarland, 2002). Acculturation outcomes may result in varying degrees of affiliation with the dominant culture. **Assimilation** results when people give up their ethnic identity in favour of the dominant culture (Spector, 2000).

In Canada, rather than assimilation, the preferred outcome is **multiculturalism,** where immigrants and others maintain their culture and different cultures interact peacefully within the nation. In 1971, Canada became the first country in the world to officially adopt a multiculturalism policy. Over the years, various laws have been passed to protect and promote the rights of minorities in Canada (Box 9-2). Canadians believe, as enshrined in the multiculturalism policy, that citizens should be able to retain their unique ethnic cultures and traditions within a Canadian context.

Ethnic Heritage and Ethnohistory

Knowledge of a client's country of origin and its history and ecological contexts are significant to health care. For example, Haitian immigrants have linguistic and

Box 9-2 Legislation Recognizing Diversity in Canada

Significant Legislative Events for Diversity in Canada

Official Languages Act (1969)—
(Updated September 15, 1988)
This act recognizes English and French equally as Canada's official languages. The 1988 amendment to this act outlines the obligations of Canadian federal institutions to be committed to promoting full recognition and use of both English and French in Canadian society, as well as supporting the development of the Anglophone and Francophone communities across the country.

Canadian Constitution Act (1982)
This act replaced the *British North America Act* as Canada's Constitution, outlining how Canada governs and structures its society. It also recognizes three main groups of Aboriginal peoples in Canada: Indians, Inuit, and Métis.

Canadian Charter of Rights and Freedoms (1982)
Written into the Canadian Constitution in 1982, the Charter is a statement of the basic human rights and freedoms of all Canadians.

Canadian Multiculturalism Act (1988)
In recognition of Canada's cultural diversity, this act enshrines the enhancement and preservation of multiculturalism in Canada.

communication patterns distinct from those of Jamaicans, even though they both come from the Caribbean and have a common history of slavery. Differences can be traced to their colonial history and intermingling with the local indigenous people. Hindu immigrants from Jamaica have different cultural characteristics from those originating from India because of the cultural contexts of the different regions. Their nutritional, communication, and health patterns may be more similar to African Jamaicans than South Asian Hindus. In giving care for an Indian Hindu who grew up in Jamaica, the nurse can expect that the client will interact more like a Jamaican although he or she looks south Indian.

People immigrate to another country for various reasons and have different motivations for acculturating to the new country. Refugees may be relocated without any choice in their initial residence, in contrast to immigrants, who have options as to where they go. Refugees experience greater dislocation and deprivation than immigrants who enter Canada with specialized skills and education and have the option to return to their homeland. Age of immigration may determine the level of acculturation, with younger immigrants acculturating faster than their older counterparts. Similarities shared by an immigrant group with the dominant culture in society are strong predictors of how easily the person will adjust. Although acculturation and length of residence in the new culture are related, the outcome may be affected by other factors such as education, racial characteristics, and familiarity with the language and religion. A nurse may ask clients what the condition or situation was that brought them to Canada and how they feel they are adjusting.

The nurse should also be aware that newly arrived immigrants and refugees, especially from developing countries, are vulnerable to a variety of health conditions, including tuberculosis, hepatitis B, anemia, dental caries, intestinal parasites, nutritional deficiencies, immunization deficiencies, and mental and emotional problems like depression and post-traumatic stress disorder (Fowler, 1998; Kemp, 2004). New immigrants and refugees also frequently experience language barriers, social isolation, separation from family, and lack of information about available resources (Fowler, 1998). Therefore, nurses should be aware of and advocate for primary health care programs in the community for these vulnerable clients (Box 9-3).

Cultural Conflicts

Culture provides the context for valuing, evaluating, and categorizing our life experiences. Because values, morals, and norms are transmitted from one generation to another, members of ethnic groups may display **ethnocentrism,** a tendency to hold one's own way of life as superior to others. Health care practitioners who do not understand cultural differences often resort to **cultural imposition,** when they use their own values and lifeways as the absolute guide in dealing with clients and interpreting their behaviours. Hence, a nurse who believes that pain is to be borne quietly as a demonstration of strong moral character will be annoyed by a client's insistence on having pain medication and may try to deny the client's discomfort.

Ethnocentrism is the root of stereotypes, biases, and prejudices against others perceived to be different from the valued group. Nurses must avoid **stereotypes,** which are generalizations about any particular group that prevent further assessment of unique characteristics. When action is taken on one's prejudices, **discrimination** occurs, which is treating people unfairly based on their group membership. Often people do not realize that they are displaying prejudice or discrimination, but simply react negatively or fearfully to cultural differences.

Cultural Awareness

Nurses must be tolerant and non-judgmental about clients' beliefs and practices. Nurses also must acknowledge that they bring their own personal cultural perspectives to the client-nurse relationship. Nurses must not impose their cultural values on clients and must respect the uniqueness and differences that each will bring to the care environment (CNA, 2000). To do so, nurses must be aware of how their own culture may influence how they provide client care (Andrews & Boyle, 2003; Drew, 2004). One strategy for nurses to become culturally self-aware is to conduct a self-assessment to examine their biases and feelings. Nurses must critically examine their own beliefs, which can have a direct impact upon the care that they provide to their clients. For example, Sorrentino (2004) recommends reflecting on the following questions:

- How have people in your social network influenced and shaped you?

Focus on Primary Health Care Box 9-3

Providing Primary Health Care to Canadian Immigrants and Refugees

New immigrants and refugees in Canada often need assistance overcoming the language, cultural, and information services barriers that prevent them from using health and social services. Across the country, many community health centres respond to these needs, including the North Hamilton Community Health Centre (NHCHC), which provides primary health care to this population through its Immigrant/Refugee Health Program (IRHP). The IRHP is an example of how language, clinical, health promotion, and settlement services can be integrated. Its goal is to provide accessible primary health care to immigrants and refugees while attending to social and cultural issues that affect them.

The IRHP staff includes community health nurses, a social worker, a clinical psychologist, and a family physician. Routine medical care is available on-site, and testing for human immunodeficiency virus (HIV) and hepatitis B and a vaccination program are offered to people at risk. Because a majority of their clients are from Latin America, the community health nurses and the psychologist are fluent in Spanish. For clients speaking other languages, a volunteer interpreter service is available. Interpreters also accompany clients for diagnostic tests, appointments with medical specialists, and other social-service-related appointments outside the centre.

The IRHP collaborates with a local network of churches to provide clothing, furniture, emergency shelter, and interest-free loans to assist refugees with family reunification. It also offers health promotion activities, designed primarily for Latin American women. A variety of programs are offered, including a health-focused ESL class, prenatal drop-in centre, and breast-feeding support for Spanish-speaking women. Workshops are presented on topics suggested by participants, such as reproductive and breast health, cervical cancer prevention, parenting, and family communication. People find out about these sessions by word of mouth or are personally invited, in keeping with the Latin American cultural preference for "personalismo"—a personal approach.

From "Providing Primary Health Care to Immigrants and Refugees: The North Hamilton Experience," by N. Fowler, 1998, *Canadian Medical Association Journal, 159,* pp. 388–391, available at *http://collection.nlc-bnc.ca/100/201/300/cdn_medical_association/cmaj/vol-159/issue-4/0388.htm.* Reprinted with permission.

- Do you assume if something works for you, it must work for others?
- Do you think there are "right" and "wrong" ways of doing things?
- Are you ever critical of another person's lifestyle because it is different than your own?
- Do you sometimes consider that other people's lifestyles, religious beliefs, superstitions, and attitudes are silly or odd?
- Do you try to convert others to your religion or way of thinking and doing things?
- Do you react to people as individuals or do stereotypes sometimes get in the way?

There are various cultural self-assessment tools that may be used to ascertain one's responses to diverse groups. Drew (2004) describes a cultural awareness exercise whereby student nurses can begin to identify their own beliefs and values (Box 9-4). Nurses who understand the differences between personal beliefs and values and those of the client are able to provide mutually planned care in an effective and respectful manner (CNA, 2000).

Transcultural Nursing

Dr. Madeleine M. Leininger is considered the founder of the field of **transcultural nursing.** She defines transcultural nursing as a comparative study of cultures to understand similarities (culture universal) and differences (culture-specific) across human groups in order to provide meaningful and beneficial health care (1991, 2002a). According to Leininger, the goals of transcultural nursing are to provide *culturally congruent care* and *culturally competent care.*

Culturally congruent care is "the use of sensitive, creative, and meaningful care practices to fit with the general values, beliefs, and lifeways of clients" (Leininger & McFarland, 2002, p. 12). In other words, the nursing care fits with clients' valued life patterns and set of meanings. It is generated from the clients themselves, rather than based on predetermined criteria. Culturally congruent care may be distinct from the values and meanings of the professional health care system. Discovering clients' culture care values, meanings, beliefs, and practices as they relate to nursing and health care requires nurses to be learners of clients' culture and to partner with clients and families in defining the characteristics of meaningful and beneficial care (Leininger, 2002b).

Leininger and McFarland (2002) define **culturally competent care** as "the explicit use of culturally based care and health knowledge in sensitive, creative, and meaningful ways to fit the general lifeways and needs of individuals or groups for beneficial and meaningful health and well-being or to help them face illness, disabilities, or death" (p. 84). Culturally competent care, therefore, is a process whereby nursing care is delivered based on knowledge of the clients' cultural heritage, beliefs, and attitudes (Giger & Davidhizer, 1999). It requires the practitioner to bridge cultural gaps in caring, work with cultural differences, and enable clients and families to receive meaningful care. To provide culturally competent care, the nurse must have specific ability, knowledge, sensitivity, openness, and flexibility to adjust to cultural differences (Suh, 2004). The nurse then is able to develop meaningful interventions to promote optimal health among individuals.

Campinha-Bacote (2002) further defines cultural competence as an ongoing process, where the nurse continuously strives to work within the client's cultural context. Therefore, health care providers develop cultural competence rather than possess it. This ongoing process involves assimilating the following: cultural awareness,

Box 9-4 Cultural Awareness Exercise

- Consider where and how knowledge about your heritage was passed on to you.
- Who are the people in your social network responsible for influencing and shaping the lives of the young people?
- Seek out someone who has a background, heritage, or ethnicity different from your own.
- Ask that person's permission for an interview and ask where and how the person's cultural heritage was passed on to him or her. Ask the person the same questions you asked yourself in identifying your basic cultural richness.
- Analyze the sociocultural similarities and differences each of you have.
- Try to predict potential areas of conflict between the two views as well as the positive and congruent strengths.
- Ask yourself, "What potential strengths in similarities between us should I build on to begin interactions with this person?"

Adapted from "Cultural Competence in Partnerships With Communities" by J. C. Drew, in *Canadian Community as Partner: Theory and Practice in Nursing* (p. 183), A. R. Vollman, E. T. Anderson, & J. McFarlane, Eds., 2004, Philadelphia, PA: Lippincott Williams & Wilkins.

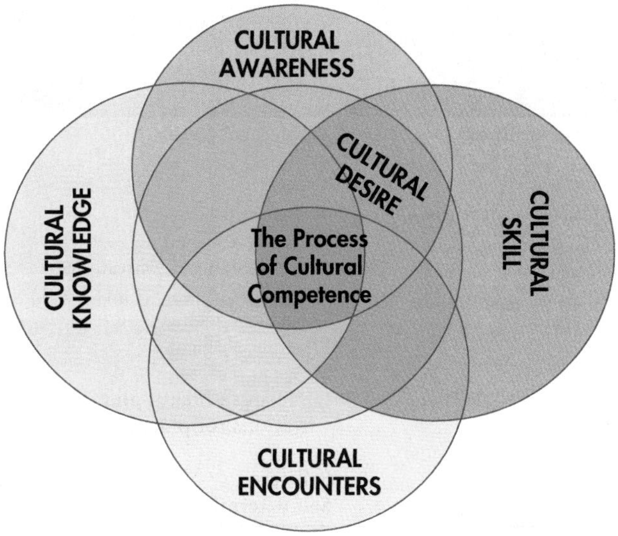

FIGURE **9–3** The process of cultural competence. (From "The Process of Cultural Competence in the Delivery of Health Care Services: A Model of Care," by J. Campinha-Bacote, 1999, *Journal of Transcultural Nursing, 13*(3), p. 181. Printed with permission from Transcultural C.A.R.E. Associates, Cincinnati, Ohio.)

knowledge, skill, encounters, and desire, as shown in Figure 9-3. ***Cultural awareness*** is being aware of one's own background, and involves an in-depth self-examination to recognize biases, prejudices, and assumptions (see Box 9-4). *Cultural knowledge* is knowing about the client's culture. It involves learning about diverse groups, including their values, health beliefs, care practices, and world view. Knowledge of culturally relevant information will assist the nurse in planning and implementing a treatment regimen that meets the unique needs of each client (Bhimani & Acorn, 1998; CNA, 2004). For example, a nurse assigned to a female Egyptian-Canadian client decides to seek information about the Egyptian culture. Upon learning that female modesty and gender-congruent care are valued in the culture, the nurse encourages female relatives to assist with the client's hygiene needs. *Cultural skills* include assessment of social, cultural, and biophysical factors influencing client care. *Cultural encounters* involve engaging in cross-cultural interactions that can teach about other cultures. *Cultural desire* is the motivation and commitment to learn from others, accept the role as learner, be accepting of cultural differences, and build upon cultural similarities.

Culturally competent care can and should be practiced in all clinical settings. Although nurses are responsible for providing culturally competent care, nursing regulatory bodies, professional associations, educational institutions, governments, and health services delivery and accreditation organizations share the responsibility of supporting culturally competent care (CNA, 2004). Nurses must form partnerships among other health care providers, clients, and funding agencies to facilitate culturally diverse practices in health services and to optimize clients' health outcomes.

Cultural Context of Health and Caring

Health, illness, and caring are phenomena embedded in a culture (Kleinman, 1979; Leininger, 2002a). Culture is the context in which groups of people interpret and define their experiences relevant to life transitions such as birthing, illness, and dying. It is the system of meanings by which people make sense of their experiences. Culture is the framework used in defining social phenomena such as when a person is healthy or requires intervention. For example, in most African groups, a robust body is considered a sign of health in the same way that a plump baby is viewed as healthy in some Hispanic cultures (Higgins, 2000; Loustaunau & Sobo, 1997). In Jamaican culture, pregnancy is not viewed as a medical condition but rather as a normal life transition; hence, a pregnant woman need not go to a doctor unless she has a problem (Sobo, 1993).

Table 9-1 provides a comparison of cultural contexts of health and illness in Western and non-Western cultures. Attributed causes of illness are highly influenced by cultural beliefs. For example, among the Hmong refugees (a group of people who originated from the mountainous regions of Laos), epilepsy is believed to be caused by wandering of the soul; hence, treatment includes intervention by a shaman who can perform the ritual to retrieve the client's soul (Fadiman, 1997). Their belief is distinct from the scientifically determined neurological abnormality causing seizures.

The biomedical orientation of Western cultures emphasizing scientific investigation and reducing the human body into distinct parts is in conflict with the holistic conceptualization of health and illness in non-Western

Table 9-1 Comparative Cultural Contexts of Health and Illness

	Western Cultures	Non-Western Cultures
Cause of illness	Biomedical causes	Imbalance between humans and nature Supernatural Magico-religious
Method of diagnosis	Scientific, high-tech Specialty focused Organ-specific manifestations	Naturalistic, magico-religious Holistic Mixed Global, non-specific symptomatology
Treatment	Specialty specific Pharmacological Surgery	Holistic Mixed (magico-religious, supernatural herbal, biomedical, etc.)
Practitioners/Healers	Uniform standards and qualifications for practice	May be learned through apprenticeship Criteria for practice not uniform Reputation established in community
Caring pattern	Self-care Self-determination	Caring provided by others Group reliance and interdependence

Data from "Disease Etiologies in Non-Western Medical Systems," by G. Foster, 1976, *American Anthropology, 78,* p. 773; *Patients and Healers in the Context of Culture,* by A. Kleinman, 1979, Berkeley: University of California Press; and *Transcultural Nursing: Concepts, Theories, Research and Practice* (3rd ed.), by M. Leininger and M. McFarland, 2002, New York: McGraw-Hill.

cultures. Holism (see chapters 1 and 15) is evident in the belief in continuity between humans and nature, and between human events and metaphysical and magico-religious phenomena. Hence, epilepsy as conceived by the Hmong people is caused by loss of one's spirit to the magical and supernatural forces in nature. Establishing a diagnosis of epilepsy in Western cultures requires scientifically proven techniques and confirmed criteria for the abnormality. Such medical criteria are meaningless to the Hmong, who believe in the global causation of the illness that goes beyond the mind and body of the person to forces in nature. The choice of healers or health care practitioners is conditioned by the attributed cause. Whereas a Hmong will seek a shaman, a Westerner will seek a qualified neurologist. A shaman, on the other hand, has an established reputation in the Hmong community, and the shaman's qualifications are neither determined by standardized criteria nor confined to specific bodily systems. A shaman uses rituals symbolizing the supernatural, spiritual, and naturalistic modalities of prayers, herbs, and incense burning.

The dominant value orientation in North American society is individualism and self-reliance in achieving and maintaining health. Caring approaches generally promote the client's independence and ability for self-care. In collectivistic cultures that value group reliance and interdependence such as traditional South Asians, caring behaviours are manifested by actively providing physical and psychosocial support for kin members. Adult clients are not expected to be solely responsible for their care and well-being; rather, family members and kin are relied upon to make decisions and provide for their care (Pacquiao, 2001). An older Chinese woman's refusal to independently perform rehabilitation exercises after hip surgery until her daughter is present to assist her may be misconstrued by nurses as lack of self-responsibility and motivation for her care. In contrast, the client may interpret the nurse's insistence on self-reliance as uncaring behaviour.

Cultural Healing Modalities and Healers

Health care systems have evolved into externalizing or internalizing systems (Young, 1976). **Externalizing systems** connect health and illness to social and cosmological factors. For instance, acquired immunodeficiency syndrome (AIDS) may be seen as punishment from God for one's evil deeds (cosmological) or transgression of social taboos (dishonouring one's elders). **Internalizing systems** are observed in modern societies with highly scientific and technological capacity to examine internal structural and biological causes of health and illness. An example is the Western biomedical system, which has been criticized for being specialty driven and having a tendency to minimize effects of social and cultural factors on health and illness.

Disparities in health outcomes between the rich and poor illustrate the influence of socio-economic factors in morbidity and mortality. Social factors such as poverty and lack of access to health resources compromise the health status of the poor and unemployed. Cultural practices may pose advantages or health risks to members of a particular society. Sedentary lifestyle and high caloric intake have increased risks to cardiovascular disorders among Canadians who value a convenient and efficient way of life. This value is translated into fast foods, driving instead of walking, and using technology to perform many of the physical tasks of daily life.

Foster (1976) has identified two distinct categories of healers cross-culturally. **Naturalistic practitioners** attribute illness to natural, impersonal, and biological forces that cause alteration in the equilibrium of the human body. Healing emphasizes naturalistic modalities using herbs, chemicals, heat, cold, massage, and surgery. In contrast, **personalistic practitioners** believe that health and illness can be caused by active influence of an external agent, which can be human (i.e., sorcerer) or nonhuman (e.g., ghosts, evil, or deity). Personalistic beliefs emphasize the importance of humans' relationship with

Research Highlight

Box 9-5

The Desi Ways: Traditional Health Practices of South Asian Women in Canada

Research Focus

It is unclear how traditional practices are used in the South Asian population in Canada and what challenges women confront in using them. Cultural knowledge of the health behaviours and traditional practices of South Asian immigrant women in Canada enables nurses to be culturally sensitive in providing care.

Abstract

In Canada, South Asian women have stated that they have felt humiliated by Western health care providers for using traditional healing and health practice. Using critical enthnographic methods, this study conducted 50 interviews, 12 focus group discussions, and community meetings with South Asian women in Canada. The interviews were conducted in the participant's language of choice. Thematic analysis was completed on the transcribed interviews. *Health* for South Asian women is understood in terms of well-being and mental and physical happiness. It is viewed holistically as part of everyday life and being in balance. The women reported that they included many traditional health practices or *desi ways* in their everyday lives. *Desi* is a Punjabi term for traditional health practices. The study findings revealed the women practiced a variety of traditional health practices, including dietary regimens, prayers, home remedies, consultations, and rituals with hakims, updits, badjis, homeopaths, veds, and jyotshis. Participants stated diverse reasons for using traditional health practices, including beliefs and prior experiences, the nature and severity of problems, family members, and the feasibility of using these practices. However, traditional health practices were rarely used exclusively by these women; rather, they were used only on an episodic or daily basis.

Evidence-Based Practice

- Clients may have difficulty communicating their cultural values and practices to outsiders such as nurses. South Asian women often do not report that they use traditional approaches because they fear ridicule and want to maintain their relationship with the Western health care provider.
- Clients want choices when accessing health care and want to be supported in using traditional practices.
- Nurses need to be sensitive and open to the diversity of health practices among various cultures. This entails understanding the meaning traditional practice holds for the clients and respecting their choices.

Reference

Hilton, B. A., et al. (2001). Being strong: The desi ways: Traditional health practices of South Asian women in Canada. *Health Care for Women International, 22,* 553–567.

others, both living and deceased, and with their deities. For example, a voodoo priest uses modalities that combine supernatural, magical, and religious beliefs through the active facilitation of an external agent or personalistic practitioner. A Haitian woman who believes in voodoo attributes her illness to a curse placed by someone and seeks the services of a voodoo priest to remove the cause. Personalistic approaches also include naturalistic modalities such as massage, aromatherapy, and herbs (see chapter 31). Some clients seek both types of practitioners to achieve health and treat illness.

Because of coexisting and simultaneous use of both healing systems, nurses must avoid making rash judgments about clients' practices. Nurses need to gain knowledge and understanding of folk remedies used by clients to prevent cultural imposition (Box 9-5). For example, many Southeast Asian cultures practice folk remedies such as coining, cupping, pinching, and burning to relieve aches and pains and remove bad wind or noxious elements that cause illness. It should be noted that other groups, including Eastern Europeans, also use cupping to treat respiratory ailments. These remedies leave peculiar visible markings on the skin in the form of ecchymosis, superficial burns, strap marks, or local tenderness. Cultural ignorance may lead a practitioner to call authorities for suspicion of abuse. Different groups commonly use herbal therapy with some distinct differences from each other. Instead of dismissing the practice as dangerous and incompatible with Western medicine, practitioners need to investigate further whether the practice needs changing. Consultation and collaboration with herbalists and other naturalistic practitioners can prevent unwarranted distress for the client.

Culture and the Experience of Grief and Loss

Dying and death bring a resurgence of traditions that have been meaningful to groups of people most of their lives (see chapter 25). Societies assign different meanings to death of a child, a young person, and an older adult. In Western cultures with strong future time orientation and where children are expected to survive their parents, death of a young person is devastating. In cultures where infant mortality rates are high, however, the emotional distress over a child's death is tempered by the reality of the commonly observed risks of growing up. Hence, untimely death of an adult may be mourned more deeply.

Societies that believe in the concept of reincarnation, such as devout Hindus and Buddhists, may view death as a step toward rebirth. Care of the dying is focused in supporting the client's preparation for a good death. The family will pray and read religious scriptures to the client to improve his or her chances in the next cycle. Buddhists generally believe that life is suffering and suffering is mitigated when a person moves beyond the earthly desires and atones for past misdeeds. A dying Hindu male prepares for a good death by refusing nourishment and medications, concentrating all his energies on the spiritual aspects of the journey to the next cycle (Pacquiao, 2002).

Culture strongly influences pain expression and need for pain medication. Whereas most people in the dominant Western culture desire freedom from pain and suffering, other groups accept suffering. Nurses need not assume that pain relief is equally valued across groups. For example, many Filipino mothers tolerate the pain of childbirth without complaining or asking for medication because they believe that pain is a form of spiritual atonement for one's past deeds (Pacquiao, 2001).

Clients may suffer *cultural pain* when their valued way of life is disregarded by practitioners (Leininger & McFarland, 2002). Inability of Orthodox Jews to pray in groups at the bedside with the dying client because of limitations in the number of visitors allowed can cause cultural pain in the client and family. Working with the family and their religious/spiritual leader will facilitate culturally congruent care (Pacquiao, 2003).

Regulatory mandates and organizational policies intended to benefit clients should be implemented with sensitivity and understanding of their cultural life patterns. The high value that Western society places on individual autonomy and self-determination may be in direct conflict with diverse groups. Advance directives, informed consent, and consent for hospice are examples of mandates that may violate clients' values. Informed consent and advance directives protect the right of the individual to know and make decisions, ensuring continuity of these rights even to the time when the individual is incapacitated. However, other cultures are organized so that the group assumes decision making for a family member in these situations and is trusted to make the right decision for the individual. Indeed, some groups such as Asian Canadians and South Asian Canadians may expect their family to make decisions for them, and family members may prefer to protect the individual from unnecessary suffering by knowing the reality of imminent death. These cultures value group interdependence and view individual autonomy as an unnecessary burden for a loved one who is ill (Pacquiao, 2002, 2003).

In the case of cultures that share the religious belief that events in their life are God's will, prognostication is not an acceptable human act. Hence, devout Muslims may object to a diagnosis of terminal illness or cancer. Cultural knowledge and skills are needed to enable nurses to provide culturally congruent care for dying clients and work with their families and religious leaders. Rituals associated with death and dying are highly conditioned by culture. Orthodox Jews rally behind members of their congregation and provide care for the dying as well as assistance to the family. They may visit the client in groups of about 10 and pray together at the bedside (Bonura et al., 2001). Among Orthodox Jews and Muslims, a special group knowledgeable in the religious rituals is called to perform post-mortem care. Gender congruent care and provision of privacy are strictly observed as a show of respect for the dead person. Immediate burial is generally scheduled; hence, preparations should be planned with the family beforehand. Among Orthodox Jews, the dead person is generally buried before sundown (Bonura et al., 2001). Some Buddhists may refuse to move the dead body after death because of their belief that the spirit of the dead takes some time to leave the body. They define death as the absence of consciousness and loss of body warmth. Indeed, many other groups do not agree with using brain death as a criterion of death (Lin, 2002).

The dominant practice of bringing a stillborn fetus to the mother immediately after birth to promote healthy grieving is not viewed as positive in some cultures. Some Asian Indians regard this practice as adding to the mother's and family's suffering. Hindus and Buddhists believe that it is the soul that lives on and the body is only a shell. A dead body without the soul is but an empty shell (Vatuk, 1996).

The meaning and expressions of grief are culturally constituted. Among the usually stoic East Asians, the social position and status of the deceased reflects the extent to which mourners publicly express grief. Korean families may hire people to lead the open grieving. Loud crying and screaming is to be expected.

Religious beliefs also affect attitudes toward cremation, organ donation, and the treatment of body parts. Devout Muslims may refuse an autopsy or organ donation for fear of desecrating the dead and because of their belief that one has to be whole to appear in front of the creator. Burial is preferred over cremation (Geissler, 1998). A Muslim client who is having a leg amputated may request a blessing of the leg from a priest (Imam) before surgery (Pacquiao, 2003).

Cultural Assessment

A comprehensive cultural assessment is the basis for providing culturally competent care. Combined with critical thinking skills, a cultural assessment provides the knowledge necessary for transcultural nursing care (Andrews & Boyle, 2003). Cultural assessment is a systematic and comprehensive examination of the cultural care values, beliefs, and practices of individuals, families, and communities. The goal of cultural assessment is to generate from the clients themselves significant information that will enable culturally congruent care (Leininger & McFarland, 2002). There are several models for cultural assessment, each involving different levels of skill and knowledge. Leininger's Sunrise Model (Leininger & McFarland, 2002) in Figure 9–4 demonstrates the inclusiveness of culture in everyday life and helps to explain why cultural assessment must be comprehensive. The model assumes that cultural care values, beliefs, and practices are embedded in the cultural and social structural dimensions of society, which include environmental contexts, language, and ethnohistory (i.e., significant historical experiences of a particular group). For example, the experience with the Great Depression of older adults has sometimes resulted in their tendency to be frugal. A nurse needs to have clients share stories about their lives that will reveal the broad picture of who they are and the cultural lifestyle they embrace. Leininger's model differentiates folk care, which is caring as defined by the people, from the health care professions, which is based on the scientific, biomedical caring system.

Davidhizar and Giger (1998) and Giger and Davidhizar (2004) also developed a **transcultural assessment model,** which builds upon Leininger's work.

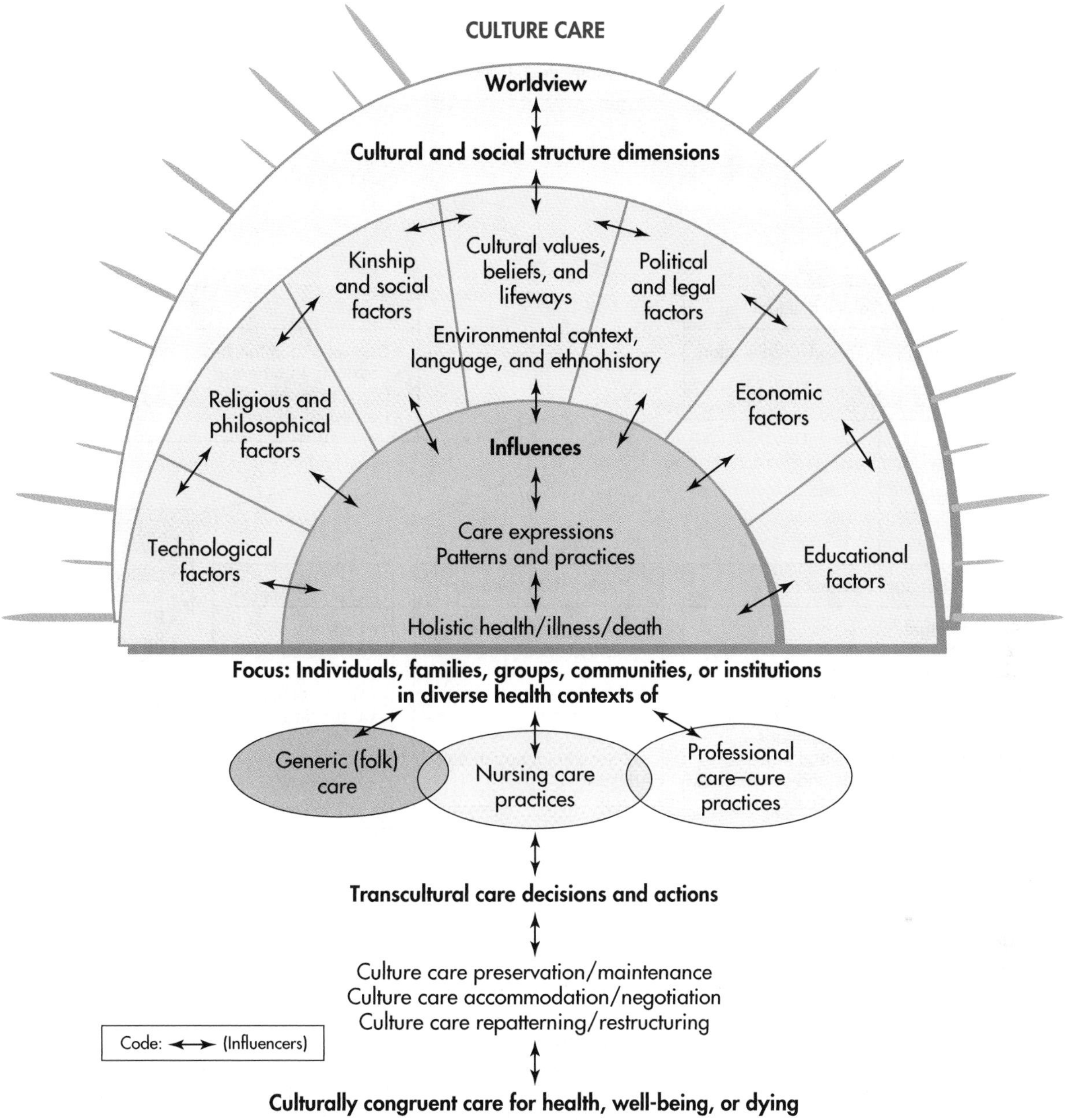

FIGURE **9–4** Leininger's culture care theory and Sunrise Model. (From *Transcultural Nursing: Concepts, Theories, Research and Practice,* 3rd ed, p. 80, by M. M. Leininger and M. R. McFarland, 2002, New York: McGraw-Hill.)

The underlying premise of their model is that each person is culturally unique and should be assessed according to six cultural phenomena: communication, space, social organization, time, environmental control, and biological variations (Figure 9–5). These phenomena are apparent in all cultural groups, but their application in the practice setting will be variable. Giger and Davidhizar's transcultural assessment model offers a means for nurses to assess clients' unique health care needs, including cultural health practices. This model has been specifically developed for use in nursing practice.

Whichever assessment model is used, a nurse begins cultural assessment by knowing population demographic changes in the community setting of practice. Nurses should anticipate the client populations that use their services and gain some knowledge about their cultures before they come to the setting. Having background knowledge about a culture assists the nurse in conducting a focused assessment when time is limited. Demographics can be gathered from the local and regional census data, as well as from the demographic breakdown of clients who come to the setting. Population demographics might include the distribution of ethnic groups, education, occupations, and incidence of the most common illnesses. Comprehensive cultural assessment requires skill and time; hence, preparation and anticipation of need are important.

One problem in cultural assessment is the lack of ability to assess the insider or emic perspective of the clients

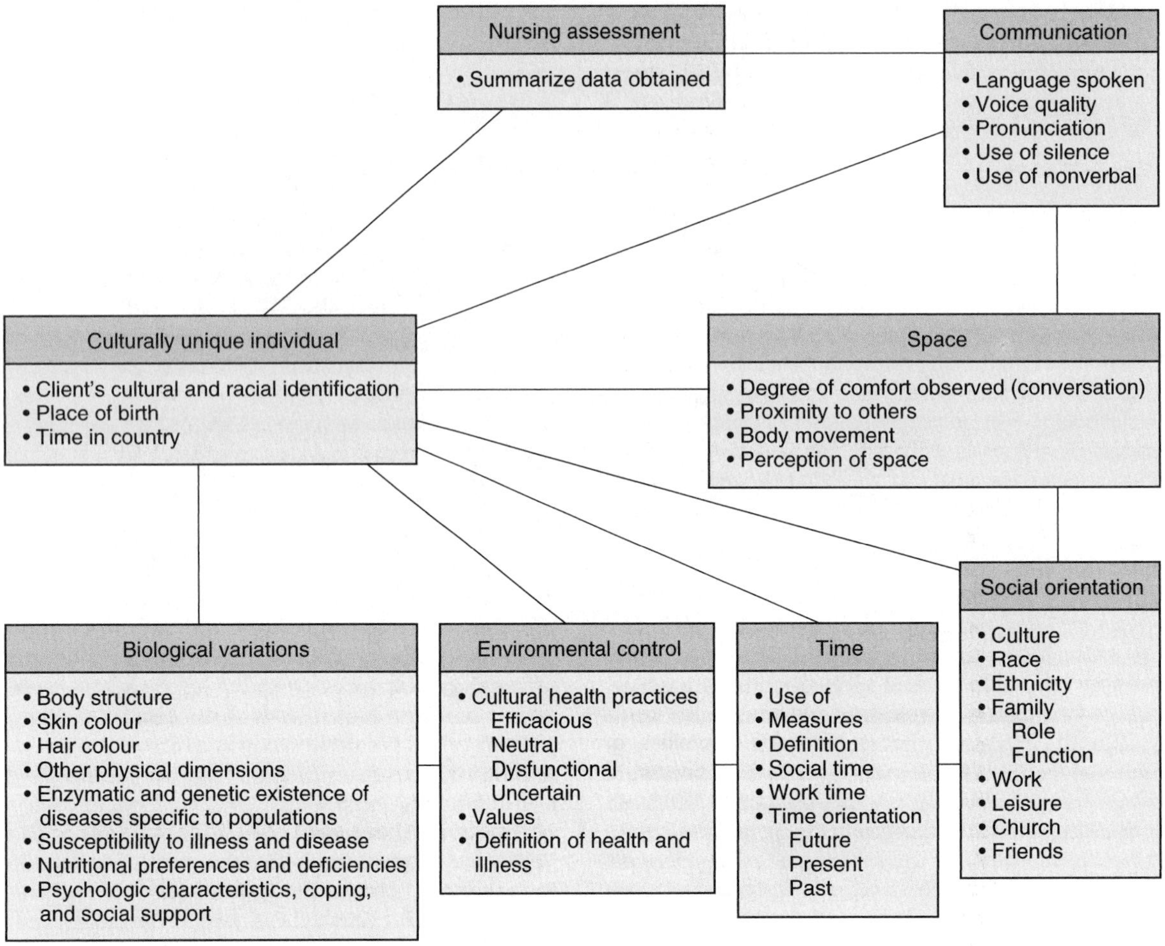

FIGURE **9–5** Giger and Davidhizar's Transcultural Assessment Model. (From *Transcultural Nursing: Assessment and Intervention,* 4th ed., p. 8, by J. N. Giger and R. E. Davidhizar, 2004, New York: McGraw-Hill.)

and interpret the information during the assessment. It helps to use open-ended questions (e.g., What do you think caused your illness?), focused questions (e.g., Did you have this problem before?), and contrast questions (e.g., How different is this problem from the one you had previously?). The aim is to encourage clients to describe values, beliefs, and practices that are significant to their care that may be taken for granted unless otherwise uncovered. Culturally oriented questions are by nature broad and require a lot of descriptions. Nurses need to have a set of questions to elicit the clients' descriptions. Table 9-2 provides a list of guiding questions relevant to various social and cultural dimensions.

Selected Components of Cultural Assessment

Cultural assessment is important to the total care of any client. A nurse will learn over time various skills needed to gather an accurate and comprehensive assessment. The following sections list certain components of cultural assessment that provide information useful in planning and delivering nursing care. Nurses should use the following information as a starting point to assess the similarities and differences of clients and families. However, nurses must not assume that just because clients come from the same region or country they share similar values, beliefs, attitudes, and experiences and their response to illness and treatment will be the same. Other experiences to consider are socio-economic class, educational background, family heritage, work/occupation, length of time in Canada, urban/rural origin, and other individual characteristics, such as disability, sexual orientation, and strength of ethnic identity (St. Hill, Lipson, & Meleis, 2003).

Communication Patterns

Distinct linguistic and communication patterns are associated with different cultural groups. These patterns reflect core cultural values of a society. In the dominant Western culture, which upholds individualism, assertive communication is valued because it shows autonomy and self-determination. People are expected to say what they mean and mean what they say. In collectivistic cultures, communication is shaped by the context of relationships among participants. Promoting group harmony is given priority, so participants interact based on their expected positions and relationships within the social hierarchy. Individuals are more likely to remain respectful

Table 9-2 Cultural Assessment Guide

	Suggested Questions
Cultural identity/ancestry/heritage	Where were you born?
	Where were your parents born?
Ethnohistory	How long have you/your parents resided in this country?
	What is your ethnic background or ancestry?
	How strongly are you influenced by your culture?
	Why did you leave your homeland?
Social organization	Who lives with you?
	Who do you consider members of your family?
	Where do you live?
	Where do other members of your family live?
	How do you contact them?
	How often do you have contact with your family members?
	Who makes the decisions for you or your family?
	Who do you go to outside of your family for support?
	What do you expect your family members to do for you?
	How different are your expectations of them from other times?
	What expectations do you have of your family members who are males, females, old, or young?
Socio-economic status	What do you do for a living?
	What did you do back in your homeland?
	Where did you go to school?
	What did you finish in school?
	How different is your life here from back home?
	Do you have a primary care provider?
	What other care providers have you seen?
Biocultural ecology and health risks	What is your purpose for coming here?
	What caused your problem?
	Have you had this problem before?
	Does this problem affect your life and your family? How?
	Are there other members of your family with this kind of problem?
	How do you treat this problem at home?
	Who do you go to for this kind of problem?
	What other plans do you have for dealing with this problem?
	What do you think we should do for you?
	What other problems do you have?
	Have these problems occurred to any other member of your family?
Language and communication	What language(s) do you speak at home?
	What language(s) are you most comfortable speaking?
	In what language(s) can you read and write?
	How do you want us to talk to you?
	How should we address or call you?
	What kinds of communication upset or offend you?
	What words would you use to describe how you feel?
	Do you need an interpreter?
	Would you prefer a female or male interpreter?
Religion/spirituality	What is your religion?
	Who is your religious or spiritual leader?
	Do you want to be in touch with your religious leader?
	How do we contact your spiritual leader?
	What are some of the things we need to do within your religion?
	How do you practice your religion?
	Are there specific dietary practices you follow?
Caring beliefs and practices	What do you do to keep yourself well?
	What do you do to show someone you care?
	How does your family or you take care of sick family members?
	Which caregivers do you seek when you are sick?
	How do you decide when to go and which one to go to?
	How different is what we do from what your family does for you when you are sick?
	Are we doing what you think we should be doing for you?
	How should we give you care?
Experience with professional health care	Since you came to this country, have you had contact with doctors or hospitals?
	How do you compare your past experience with now?
	What were some of the problems that you encountered?
	How were they resolved?
	What were the positive experiences you had?
	What type of care provider do you prefer? Why?
	If you have a choice, what changes do you wish to see?

and show deference to older adults or family leaders, even though they may disagree on an issue. Differences in status and position, age, gender, and outsider versus insider determine the content and process of communication. Among Asian cultures, for example, face-saving communication promotes harmony by indirect, ambiguous communication and conflict avoidance. Messages spoken may have little to do with their meanings. Saying "no" to a superior or older person may not be permitted; hence, a subordinate's affirmative response may only mean "I heard you" rather than full agreement.

In cultural groups with distinct linear hierarchy, negotiation of conflict occurs between people within the same level of position or authority. Identifying and working with established family hierarchy can prevent miscommunication. In cultures with highly differentiated gender roles, some clients may place more value on the advice of a male nurse than a female nurse. By recognizing and working within this cultural context, the nurse can become more effective in achieving outcomes.

Non-verbal communication patterns include the use of touch and silence, eye contact, and facial expressions. For example, the high value that the traditional Chinese culture places on emotional self-control and correct behaviour has limited the use of touch. Physical contact beyond a handshake is uncommon among many Chinese people; touch, such as hugging and kissing, is generally reserved for loved ones and then is used only in moderation. Open expression of emotions is considered bad taste except in very private circumstances. Emotions are thought to interfere with self-control and may be construed as weakness.

Social Organization

Cultural groups consist of units of organization delineated by kinship, status hierarchy, and appropriate roles for their members. In the dominant Western society, the most common unit of social organization is the nuclear family where adult children are expected to establish separate residences from their parents. In collectivistic cultures, family composition may be extended to distant blood relatives across generations and non-blood kin. Kinship may be extended to both the father's and mother's side of the family (bilineal) or limited to the side of either father (patrilineal) or mother (matrilineal). Patrilineally extended families are observed among Chinese and Hindus, where a woman is expected to move into her husband's clan after marriage and kinship ties with her family of orientation (her own parents and siblings) are minimized. The nurse must consider all options when determining a client's next of kin. This is especially relevant to new immigrants and refugees, who may not have relocated with intact families. Collectivistic groups may regard members of their ethnic group as closest kin and would want to consult them for health care decisions, as well as permit them to speak on their behalf.

A client's status within the social hierarchy is generally linked with qualities such as age and gender, as well as achieved status such as education and position. The dominant culture in Canada emphasizes achievement as the determinant of status, whereas most collectivistic cultures give higher priority to age and gender. The eldest male is next to his father in terms of authority in many Asian and African cultures. A Korean mother is subject to the authority of her oldest son in the absence of her husband. Older adults generally occupy higher status in some societies such that grandparents may impose their decisions over their married children regarding the care of the grandchildren. Nurses determine who has authority for making decisions within the family and how to communicate with the proper individuals.

Expected roles of members are defined by culture and may be differentiated by gender. In Islamic and Arabic cultures, usually females are the caregivers and males are the providers and major decision makers. Thus, a woman from these cultures may insist on staying at the bedside of her child, in-laws, or husband. To assume, however, that as the primary caregiver she can be relied upon to make decisions independently is unrealistic. An Orthodox Jewish husband may respond to questions posed to his wife, which can annoy nurses operating from a context of individual autonomy. The family social hierarchy needs to be determined as soon as possible to prevent offending clients and their families. Working with established family hierarchy prevents delays and achieves outcomes in nursing care.

Religious and Spiritual Beliefs

Religious and spiritual beliefs are major influences in the person's attitudes toward health and illness, pain and suffering, and life and death. The distinction between religion and spirituality is often blurred. It is advisable for a nurse to understand the emic perspective of the client. Many cultures do not separate religion and spirituality, whereas many have a totally distinct concept of spirituality. To a Hmong animist, spirits could be those of dead ancestors or forces external to the person. To an Anglo-Canadian, spirituality may mean an inner, personal relationship with God. Although discussion of religious and spiritual philosophies is difficult in a hospital setting, nurses must assess what is important to the spiritual well-being of clients and learn as much as possible about clients' spiritual and religious practices (see chapter 24).

Devout Muslims pray five times daily and undergo an obligatory ritual cleansing of some parts of their body before praying. Nurses need to anticipate the ritual cleansing needs of the client and provide privacy for praying. Diagnostic procedures may be rescheduled so that Buddhist clients can participate in the festivities of their New Year. Anticipating the needs of Jewish clients during Sabbath, when they refrain from using electrical appliances, requires creative accommodations by the staff such as placing articles of care near the client so he or she need not use the call light or telephone to get assistance. Consent for emergency surgeries can be sent by facsimile to the rabbi, who can contact the client's next of kin unreachable by telephone during Sabbath.

Religious beliefs are evident in clients' dietary practices. Devout Hindus avoid beef, and many are vegetarians. Many Buddhists are vegetarians. *Halal* foods, which include meat, fish, fresh fruit, vegetables, eggs, milk, and cheese, are permissible for Muslims. Halal meat comes from animals that have been slaughtered during a prayer ritual. Prohibited, or *Haram,* foods include non-Halal meat, animals with fangs, pork products, gelatin products, and alcohol (Akhtar, 2002). Fasting during daylight is required during the 28 days of Ramadan, observed during the ninth lunar month. Although children and sick and frail individuals are exempt from fasting, nurses must not assume that these individuals will eat regular meals during Ramadan. Rescheduling of treatments and medications may be required to prevent complications such as hypoglycemia.

Jewish clients who follow a Kosher diet will avoid meat from carnivores, pork products, and fish without scales or fins. Kosher meat comes from permissible animals that are slaughtered with the least amount of suffering. Kosher foods must not be contaminated by non-Kosher foods. Hence meat is served separately from dairy, and dishes used for serving and eating these products are also kept separate among strict adherents (Selekman, 2003).

Background information should be available to the nursing staff about major holy days and practices for commonly encountered religions. Such information prevents scheduling non-emergency treatments and procedures on major holy days such as the Jewish Yom Kippur, Rosh Hashanah, or Passover. Religious mandates followed by Jehovah's Witnesses require followers to have bloodless surgery and to avoid blood transfusions. Nurses should identify and contact clients' religious and spiritual leaders before problems arise. These leaders can be called upon to act as cultural brokers in times of crises. On admission, nurses should obtain this information from clients or their family.

Time Orientation

All cultures have past, present, and future time dimensions. It is important for a nurse to understand a client's time orientation. This information can be useful in planning a day of care, setting up appointments for procedures, and helping a client plan self-care activities in the home. Differences exist in the dimensions of time that cultures emphasize and the manner of expressing time. Time orientation is reflected in communication patterns. Future time orientation minimizes present time, so that communication tends to be direct and focused on task achievement. Business time is separate and distinct from social time. This is the norm in the dominant Canadian culture. In contrast, collectivistic cultures emphasize past and present times to preserve social hierarchy and promote group harmony. Social time is often emphasized and mixed with business time. Rushed, hurried, and businesslike communication may be perceived as uncaring or disrespectful.

Present time orientation is in conflict with the dominant organizational norm in health care that emphasizes punctuality and adherence to appointments. This should be expected, and adjustments need to be made when dealing with ethnic groups. Improving clients' access to health services mandates culturally congruent time schedules that accommodate their cultural patterns. When making appointments and referrals, anticipated barriers to time adherence should be explored and managed with the client.

Environmental Control

Environmental control refers to the individual's perception of his or her ability to control factors in the environment. Specifically, it refers to the individual's perception of causes of illness and how their behaviour can prevent or treat illness. It also refers to the person's use of cultural healing modalities and healers (see "Cultural Healing Modalities and Healers"). During cultural assessment, the nurse should identify the client's health practices and respect them (Box 9-6). Information about folk remedies and cultural healers used by the client should be obtained. Unless these practices are harmful, they should be incorporated into the client's care plan. If the practice may be harmful (e.g., the client uses an herbal remedy that interferes with a prescribed drug), the nurse immediately notifies the physician and educates the client about the potential harm.

Biological Variations and Socio-Cultural Health Risks

Identification of clients' health risks related to sociocultural and biological history can be assessed on admission. Distinct health risks can be attributed to the ecological context of the culture. For example, immigrants

Case Study — Box 9-6

A recent Chinese immigrant to Canada has given birth to her first child. Once the newborn has been cared for and is resting, the nurse asks the new mother if she would like to take a shower. The mother refuses but appears complacent. The Chinese mother's belief is that if she takes a shower she could get rheumatism in old age. Then the mother's food tray arrives and she does not touch or eat anything. For this newcomer to Canada, the hospital food may seem different and served in an unfamiliar manner. Her family brings food into the hospital, which consists of a diet of plain rice and salted pork. As well, two different soups are brought in, which are thought to bring heat, "the yang," into her body, thereby removing the impurities from her system.

In the traditional Chinese culture, good health means to have a balance between yin and yang. There is the belief that all body systems interact with one another and the environment to produce a balanced state of wellness. In consultation with the mother, the nurse is able to assess and understand why she is refusing to shower and eat the hospital food. With this increased understanding, the nurse is able to mutually negotiate with the mother some alternatives to her care to accommodate her needs, without jeopardizing her care or making her feel stressed. The nurse appropriately assesses that rather than showering, the mother would prefer a basin of water and a cloth that she could use to clean herself. In terms of her dietary requests, it was determined that she could have the food from home, as long as they did not interfere or jeopardize her health status. As a result, the nurse's sensitivity and respect for the new mother's cultural beliefs enables the mother to relax and restore her health in a culturally appropriate manner. The nurse was open to learning the cultural beliefs of the new mother and then collaborating with the mother on decisions about her care.

originating from the region near the Nile River are generally predisposed to parasitic infestations endemic to the region. Immigrants from developing countries with poor sanitary conditions and water supply may present infections such as hepatitis. In addition, biological variations exist between people in different ethnic groups. As a result, some ethnic groups have greater risk of developing certain health conditions. For example, certain genetic disorders are linked with specific ethnic groups, such as Tay-Sachs among Ashkenazi Jews and malignant hypertension among Black Canadians.

Application of Cultural Assessment Components to Canadian Aboriginals

Aboriginal people represent an important and increasingly growing group within Canada. Within the past century, the Aboriginal population increased 10-fold, whereas the overall population of Canada increased by only a factor of six (Statistics Canada, 2001a). The Canadian constitution recognizes three groups of Aboriginal peoples: Indians, Métis, and Inuit. The North American Indian has the largest population with 608,850 people, followed by the Métis with 292,310, and lastly the Inuit with 45,070 people (Statistics Canada, 2001b, 2001c). These three groups have their own unique languages, heritages, cultural practices, and spiritual beliefs. Within each group, there are many subgroups, each with their own unique culture. The term *Indian* describes all the Aboriginal peoples in Canada who are not Métis or Inuit. These include the nations or groups of people who were originally living in Canada before the European explorers began to arrive about 500 years ago (Canadian Health Network, 2004). There are three legal definitions used to describe Indians in Canada: Status, Non-Status, and Treaty Indians. *Status Indians* refer to an Indian person who is registered under the *Indian Act* (Indian and Northern Affairs Canada, 2004), which is an act that regulates the management of reservations and sets out certain federal obligations. *Non-Status Indians* refers to Indian persons who are not registered under the *Indian Act* (Indian and Northern Affairs Canada, 2004). A *Treaty Indian* is a status Indian who belongs to a First Nation that signed a treaty with the Crown (Indian and Northern Affairs Canada, 2004).

Many Aboriginal people find the term *Indian* offensive and outdated, so in the 1970s the term "First Nation" became a preferred replacement for Treaty Indians. In addition, many Indian people adopted the term "First Nations" to replace the word "band" in the name of their community (Indian and Northern Affairs Canada, 2004; Wasekeesikaw, 2003). Some Aboriginal people prefer the more inclusive term *First Peoples* rather than the word *nation* because in English this word does not fit with the Aboriginal social structure (Canadian Health Network, 2004). The first explorers to North America originally used the term *Indian,* as they thought they had discovered India (Canadian Health Network, 2004). First Nations people claim that the roots of the term *Indian* reflect a history of colonialism and therefore the term is inappropriate (Wasekeesikaw, 2003).

The following sections describe how variations from the dominant culture may be seen among Canadian Aboriginals. It should be kept in mind that these discussions are general in nature and that each client must be assessed as an individual.

Communication Patterns

There are approximately 53 Aboriginal languages, with Algonquian being the largest and most widespread language family in Canada (Reimer & Redskye, 1998). Many of these languages may have other dialects. For example, the Cree language has identified nine dialects related to certain areas of Canada (McMillan, 1988). However, many Aboriginal people living in urban areas, like the Cree, speak English or are bilingual (Yonge & Bernard, 1998). However, because some Aboriginals do not speak any English, the nurse may need to find a translator familiar with the specific language or dialect. Translating is often difficult, because many Aboriginal languages do not have one single word that is similar to an English word. When an interpreter is used, this person must be knowledgeable about medical terminology, as well as the cultural aspects of the Aboriginal lifestyle (Lutumba Ntetu & D'arc Fortin, 1996).

There may be some variation in non-verbal communication among Aboriginal people. Some believe that it is disrespectful to engage in direct eye contact and others do not, depending upon the situation. For example, the Cree view direct eye contact as controlling, whereas the Ojibwa view brief eye contact as acceptable when greeting a person and occasionally throughout an interview (Reimer & Redskye, 1998). On the other hand, people of the Kwa-Kwa'ka-wakw First Nation believe it is disrespectful not to look at the speaker (Voyageur, 1998). Many Aboriginal people are very comfortable with silence. The Kwa-Kwa'ka-wakw First Nation people consider silence a virtue and do not speak just for the sake of speaking (Voyageur, 1998). Speaking is reserved for matters of extreme importance.

Instead of using the handshake on meeting another person, some Aboriginal people extend the hand and lightly touch the hand of the person they are greeting. The Kwa-Kwa'ka-wakw First Nation people use handshakes and verbal greetings with non-family members, reserving hugs and embraces for family.

Social Organization

Traditionally, for many Aboriginal people the biological family is the centre of social organization and includes all members of the extended family. However, over time with the migration of Aboriginal people to urban centres, the closeness of the extended family has given way to the nuclear family. In some bands, such as the Cree, elders are so highly respected for their vast experience and knowledge that aunts and uncles are often called mother and father, respectively. Younger Cree who move to urban centres may be deprived of the guidance and support of their elders and other members of the extended family, and thus may experience confusion and feelings of isolation.

Religious and Spiritual Practices

Spirituality, rather than religion, is the core meaning for such people as the Cree (Yonge & Bernard, 1998). The circle is the common symbol of spirituality that illustrates harmony of body, mind, and spirit. The circle has four aspects or directions: spiritual, physical, mental, and emotional. All directions must be present for a person to acquire health. Health and religion cannot be separated in the Aboriginal world view. Indeed, there is a link between traditional religion and healing ceremonies. Other Aboriginal people have been influenced by Christianity, and so have become baptized, confirmed, and married according to European ways.

Time Orientation

Aboriginal people can be oriented either to the present or to both the past and present. For example, the Ojibwa people's time orientation to the past is apparent by showing their respect for traditions, elders, and harmony with nature. Their time orientation to the present is revealed by showing concern for what is happening now, which should be enjoyed and attended to. The Cree people have mainly a present time orientation: Traditionally, they based their timing on the seasons, which met all present needs. For people with a present time orientation, conceptualizing the future may be difficult.

The nurse may need to acknowledge that a present-oriented Aboriginal person has difficulty adhering to scheduled clinic appointments. Services to this group may need to be flexible and accessible. Also, some present-oriented Aboriginal people believe it is very important to establish a relationship before discussing a personal health concern. For example, an Ojibwa client may be quick to notice if the health care professional is impatient or hurried and does not take time to establish a rapport. Because certain tasks are associated with present needs, it may be difficult for the nurse to counsel and advise an Aboriginal client about crucial future events, such as taking medications. The present-oriented Aboriginal client may eat two meals today, four meals tomorrow, no meals the next day, and three meals the day after. This becomes an important nursing consideration if a medication must be taken three times a day with meals. The nurse must devise a plan of care that considers the client's life situation. Of course, as Aboriginal people leave the reserves for larger urban centres, they often become more future-oriented as they adopt the habits and values of the society around them.

Environmental Control

In general, Aboriginal people subscribe to a holistic concept of health. Traditionally, Aboriginal people have linked health to spiritual beliefs and living in harmony with the environment. For example, the natural environment for the Kwa-kwa'ka-wakw people is thought to be a source of great wisdom and power (Voyageur, 1998). Explanations of various diseases and illnesses can vary from group to group. For example, the Cree thought that breaking a taboo resulted in an illness. The principle for prevention of illness is the maintenance of harmony in the mind, body, and spirit and the avoidance of factors that may lead to disharmony. Some Aboriginal groups have merged traditional and modern methods to improve health.

Aboriginal groups recognize a variety of healers, including herbalists, diagnosticians, and shamans. The Cree believe that healers or shamans possess specialized knowledge that allows them to understand the earth and the spirit world. The Cree healer uses rituals and herbs to promote healing.

Biological Variations and Aboriginal Health Issues

Over the past 50 years, dramatic changes in lifestyle have affected the social, environmental, and health status of Aboriginal people (Harris et al., 1997; Shestowsky, 1995). The disease patterns in many First Nations and Inuit communities continue to resemble those found in developing countries, despite gains in recent years (Health Canada, 2003). In addition, the prevalence of major chronic diseases including diabetes, cardiovascular disease (Healthy Ontario, 2004), cancer, and arthritis/rheumatis appears to be increasing in this population (Vollman, Anderson, & McFarlane, 2004). High rates of unintentional injuries, deaths from drowning, and other accidents are also affecting children in Aborginal families (Vollman et al., 2004).

Tuberculosis. Although the incidence of tuberculosis has dropped steadily over the past several decades, First Nations and Inuit people have a rate almost seven times higher than the national rate based upon 1998 figures (Health Canada, 2004a; Hoeppner & Marciniuk, 2000). Factors contributing to such a high rate include overcrowding and safe or unreliable water supplies in these communities. As well, many older people still carry the bacteria in their bodies; if not treated, they may relapse and infect others.

Hepatitis A. The rate of hepatitis A infection among First Nations and Inuit people tends to be significantly higher than the Canadian average (Minuk & Uhanova, 2003). The major factors believed to contribute to these periodic outbreaks are poor housing, poor water supplies, and lack of sewage treatment.

Diabetes Mellitus. Diabetes is a major health problem for Aboriginal peoples in Canada. The prevalence of diabetes among Aboriginal people is three to five times times the national average (Health Canada, 2003b). The factors contributing to this rate appear to be a combination of genetic susceptibility, a change from a physically active lifestyle to a sedentary lifestyle, and a diet high in sugar, fats, and salt. Aboriginal people with diabetes are usually less than 45 years old, but in the general Canadian population most are over 60 years old. Increasingly, however, Type 2 diabetes is being diagnosed in Aboriginal children (Health Canada, 2003b). The earlier onset of the disease leads to an earlier onset of complications, as well as excessive mortality rates in the early and middle adult years. In Inuit communities, the rate of diabetes is still relatively low, but there are concerns that this may change if people alter their traditional eating patterns and lifestyle (Health Canada, 2003b).

HIV/AIDS. HIV/AIDS cases among Aboriginal peoples have increased steadily over the past decade, whereas the annual number of AIDS cases has levelled off in the rest of the population (Health Canada, 2001). Aboriginal people represent 16% of all new HIV infections cases in Canada. Of these cases, 40% are under the age of 30 and 45% are women (Health Canada, 2001). This increase may be because Aboriginal people are overrepresented in high-risk groups, such as prison inmates and intravenous drug users. In addition, because of the high mobility of many Aboriginal people, the HIV risk found in the inner urban areas could be transferred to remote Aboriginal communities (Laboratory Centre for Disease Control, 1998). Currently, research is limited in the area of HIV prevention efforts targeted at Canadian Aboriginal youth. Mujumdar, Chambers, and Roberts (2004) emphasize the importance of researching HIV and AIDS among the Aboriginal youths so that culture-sensitive education can be provided, as well as appropriate prevention interventions for this group.

Alcohol and Substance Abuse. It is difficult to collect accurate figures, but the abuse of alcohol and other substances is perceived to be common in some First Nations communities (Health Canada, 2004b). Alcohol and substance abuse can be viewed as part of a set of complex issues affecting the social and physical well-being of the individual, family, and community. The First Nations and Inuit Health Programs has established the National Native Alcohol and Drug Abuse Program, which assists First Nations and Inuit communities to institute and operate programs aimed at reducing the level of alcohol, drug, and solvent abuse among their target populations on reserves. The National Native Alcohol and Drug Abuse Program emphasizes training, prevention, treatment, research, and development.

Suicide. The suicide rates in Inuit and First Nations communities are three to five times greater than the rates found in the Canadian population (Health Canada, 2003a). Possible factors contributing to the suicide rate include poor living conditions and lack of economic opportunity.

Implications for Nursing Practice

Canada's Aboriginal peoples have a rich heritage; the nurse should be aware of and appreciate their unique cultural values and traditions. Aboriginal culture includes a variety of traditional approaches to promoting health and preventing illness. Whenever possible, incorporating these approaches into a plan of care can benefit the client. Such nursing practice demonstrates respect both for the client's culture and for standard Western medical practice.

The importance of cultural competence when providing nursing care to Aboriginal people has been recognized by the Royal Commission on Aboriginal Peoples, the Canadian Medical Association, the Inuit Regional Health Survey, and the Aboriginal Women's Health Report (Dokis, 2001–2002). Dokis recognizes that for nurses to achieve cultural competence, they must understand the disparities between Aboriginal and non-Aboriginal health beliefs. Dokis is studying cultural competency to gain a better understanding of non-Aboriginals' and Aboriginals' ideas about health and community. Increasingly, nurse scholars are investigating the health problems of the Aboriginal peoples to provide culturally competent care (Browne & Fiske, 2001; Gregory et al., 1999; Majumdar et al., 2004; Smith, 2003).

Key Concepts

- Culture is the context for interpreting human experiences such as health and illness and provides direction to decisions and actions.
- Transcultural nursing is a comparative study and understanding of cultures to identify culture-specific and culture-universal caring constructs across cultures.
- Culturally congruent care is meaningful, supportive, and facilitative because it fits valued life patterns of clients; it is achieved through cultural assessment.
- Culturally competent care requires knowledge, attitudes, and skills supportive of implementation of culturally congruent care.
- Cultural assessment requires a comprehensive and thorough investigation of a client's cultural values, beliefs, and practices; it may involve assessing communication patterns, social organization, religious and spiritual beliefs, time orientation, environmental control, and biological and socio-cultural health risks.

Key Terms

Acculturation, *p. 130*
Assimilation, *p. 130*
Cultural awareness, *p. 133*
Cultural imposition, *p. 131*
Culturally competent care, *p. 132*
Culturally congruent care, *p. 132*
Culture, *p. 129*
Discrimination, *p. 131*
Emic world view, *p. 130*
Enculturation, *p. 130*
Ethnicity, *p. 130*
Ethnocentrism, *p. 131*
Etic world view, *p. 130*
Externalizing systems, *p. 134*
Internalizing systems, *p. 134*
Invisible culture, *p. 130*
Multiculturalism, *p. 130*
Naturalistic practitioner, *p. 134*
Personalistic practitioner, *p. 134*
Race, *p. 130*
Stereotypes, *p. 131*
Subcultures, *p. 130*
Transcultural assessment model, *p. 136*
Transcultural nursing, *p. 132*
Visible culture, *p. 130*

Critical Thinking Exercises

1. You were about to begin giving a male Arabic Muslim his morning care when he stated, "I don't want a bath now." He got annoyed when you tried explaining that you have to do it at this time. Before you left the

room, he asked you to leave a basin of water and towel by his bedside. He also asked you to get his prayer rug from his closet.
   a. How would you respond to the client?
   b. What might be the reasons for his refusal and annoyance?
2. A 50-year-old Chinese woman is hospitalized with a respiratory condition. She insisted that you give her warm water and rub her back with Tiger balm liniment. When her lunch came, consisting of a turkey sandwich, tossed salad, and milk, she asked that you take it back.
   a. How would you respond to the client's requests?
   b. What is the significance of her requests?
   c. Why did she refuse her lunch?
3. You are assigned to a 60-year-old South Asian Hindu widow who is admitted with chest pain and shortness of breath. The client recently arrived from India to visit her son and pregnant daughter-in-law. She can speak only Gujarati and understands very little English. She is accompanied by her son.
   a. What areas would you include in your focused cultural assessment?
   b. How would you communicate with the client?
   c. Identify ways to preserve and/or accommodate the client's culture.
   d. What aspects of the client's lifeway may need repatterning?

Review Questions

1. Socialization into one's primary culture as a child is known as
   1. Enculturation
   2. Acculturation
   3. Assimilation
   4. Multiculturalism
2. Multiculturalism results when an individual
   1. Has an experience with a new or different culture that is extremely negative
   2. Maintains his or her culture and interacts peacefully with other peoples of other cultures
   3. Gives up his/her ethnic identity in favour of the dominant culture
   4. Adapts to and adopts a new culture
3. Cultural self-awareness is an in-depth self-examination of one's
   1. Background, recognizing biases and prejudices
   2. Social, cultural, and biophysical factors
   3. Engagement in cross-cultural interactions
   4. Motivation and commitment to caring
4. Culturally competent care is the process of
   1. Learning about vast cultures
   2. Delivering care based on knowledge of the client's cultural heritage, beliefs, and attitudes
   3. Influencing treatment and care of clients
   4. Motivation and commitment to caring
5. Ethnocentrism is the root of
   1. Stereotypes, biases, and prejudices
   2. Meanings by which people make sense of their experiences
   3. Cultural beliefs
   4. Individualism and self-reliance in achieving and maintaining health
6. When action is taken on one's prejudices
   1. Discrimination occurs
   2. Sufficient comparative knowledge of diverse groups is obtained
   3. Delivery of culturally congruent care is ensured
   4. Effective intercultural communication develops
7. The dominant value orientation in Western society is
   1. Use of rituals symbolizing the supernatural
   2. Group reliance and interdependence
   3. Healing emphasizing naturalistic modalities
   4. Individualism and self-reliance in achieving and maintaining health
8. Disparities in health outcomes between the rich and poor illustrates a(n)
   1. Illness attributed to natural, impersonal, and biological forces.
   2. Biological and socio-cultural health risks.
   3. Influence of socio-economic factors in morbidity and mortality.
   4. Combination of naturalistic, religious, and supernatural modalities.
9. Culture strongly influences pain expression and need for pain medication. However, cultural pain
   1. May be suffered by a client whose valued way of life is disregarded by practitioners
   2. Is more intense, thus necessitating more mediation
   3. Is not expressed verbally or physically
   4. Is expressed only to others of like culture
10. The dominant values in Western society on individual autonomy and self-determination
   1. Rarely have an effect on other cultures
   2. Do not have an effect on health care
   3. May hinder ability to get into hospice programs
   4. May be in direct conflict with diverse groups

References

Akhtar, S. (2002). Nursing with dignity. VII. Islam. Nursing Times, 98(16), 40.

Andrews, M. M., & Boyle, J. S. (2003). *Transcultural concepts in nursing care* (4th ed.). Philadelphia: Lippincott Williams & Wilkins.

Bhimani, R., & Acorn, S. (1998). Managing within a culturally diverse environment. *Canadian Nurse, 94*(8), 32–36.

Bonura, D., et al. (2001). Culturally congruent end-of-life care for Jewish patients and their families. *Journal of Transcultural Nursing, 12*(3), 211–220.

Browne, A. J., & Fiske, J. (2001). First Nations women's encounters with mainstream health care services. *Western Journal of Nursing Research, 23*(2), 126–147.

Campinha-Bacote, J. (2002). The process of cultural competence in the delivery of healthcare services: A model of care. *Journal of Transcultural Nursing, 13*(3), 181–184.

Canadian Health Network. (2004). Glossary. Retrieved July 18, 2004, from *http://www.candadian-health-network.ca/servlet/ContentServer?pagename=pagename=CHN-RCS/CH*

Canadian Heritage. (2004). *Multiculturalism. Message from the Honourable Jean Augustine.* Retrieved September 20, 2004, from *http://www.canadianheritage.gc.ca/progs/multi/reports/ann2002-2003/message_e.cfm*

Canadian Nurses Association. (2000, February). Cultural diversity: Challenges and changes. *Nursing NOW, 3,* 1–4.

Canadian Nurses Association. (2004). *Promoting culturally competent care.* Ottawa, ON: Author.

Davidhizar, R. E., & Giger, J. N. (Eds.). (1998). *Canadian transcultural nursing: Assessment and intervention.* St. Louis, MO: Mosby.

Dokis, L. (2001–2002). Cultural competence for registered nurses. *Canadian Women's Health Network, 4/5*(5/1), 17–18.

Drew, J. D. (2004). Cultural competence in partnership with communities. In A. R. Vollman, E. T. Anderson, & J. McFarlane (Eds.), *Canadian community as partner: Theory and practice in nursing* (pp. 157–186). Philadelphia: Lippincott Williams & Wilkins.

Fadiman, A. (1997). *The spirit catches you and you fall down.* New York: Farrar, Straus & Giroux.

Foster, G. (1976). Disease etiologies in non-Western medical systems. *American Anthropologist, 78,* 773–782.

Fowler, N. (1998). Providing primary health care to immigrants and refugees: The North Hamilton experience. *Canadian Medical Association Journal, 159,* 388–391.

Galanti, G. A. (2000). An introduction to cultural differences. *Western Journal of Medicine, 172,* 335–336.

Galanti, G. A. (2004). *Caring for patients from different cultures* (3rd ed.). Philadelphia: University of Pennsylvania Press.

Geissler, E. (1998). *Mosby's pocket guide series of cultural assessment* (2nd ed.). St. Louis, MO: Mosby.

Giger, J. N., & Davidhizar, R. E. (Eds.). (2004). *Transcultural nursing: Assessment and intervention* (4th ed.). St. Louis, MO: Mosby.

Gregory, D., Whalley, W., Olson, J., Bain, M., Harper, G. G., Roberts, L., & Russell, C. (1999). Exploring the experience of Type 2 Diabetes in urban aboriginal people. *Canadian Journal of Nursing Research,* 31(1), 101–115.

Harris, S. B., et al. (1997). The prevalence of NIDDM and associated risk factors in native Canadians. *Diabetes Care, 20,* 185–187.

Health Canada. (2001). *1999–2000 Annual review, August 2000—HIV/AIDS.* Retrieved July 18, 2004, from *http://www.hc-sc.gc.ca/fnihb/cp/annualreview/hiv_aids.htm*

Health Canada. (2003a). *Just for you: Aboriginal people.* Retrieved July 12, 2004, from *http://www.hc-sc.gc.ca/english/for_you/aboriginals.html*

Health Canada. (2003b). *Aboriginal diabetes initiative.* Retrieved July 18, 2004, from *http://www.hc-sc.gc.ca/fnihb/cp/adi/introduction.htm*

Health Canada. (2004a). *Why do Native people have such a high rate of tuberculosis (TB)?* Retrieved December 1, 2004, from *http://www.canadian-health-network.ca/servlet/ContentServer?cid=1007039&pagename=CHN-RCS%2FCHNResource%2FFAQCHNResourceTemplate&c=CHNResource&lang=En&repGroupTopic=Aboriginal+Peoples+KS*

Health Canada. (2004b). *Aboriginal peoples.* Retrieved December 1, 2004, from *http://www.canadian-health-network.ca/servlet/ContentServer?cid=1044475860190&pagename=CHN-RCS%2FPage%2FGTPageTemplate&c=Page&lang=En*

Healthy Ontario (2004). *Senior's health features: Different strokes.* Retrieved July 18, 2004, from *http://www.healthyontario.ca/english/features_details.asp?channel_id-4&aggregate_id*

Higgins, B. (2000). Puerto Rican cultural beliefs: Influence on infant feeding practices. *Journal of Transcultural Nursing, 11*(1), 12.

Hoeppner, V. H., & Marciniuk, D. D. (2000). Tuberculosis in aboriginal Canadians. *Canadian Respiratory Journal, 7*(2), 141–146.

Indian and Northern Affairs Canada. (2004) Status—most often asked questions. Retrieved December 1, 2004, from *http://www.ainc-inac.gc.ca/pr/pub/ywtk/index_e.html*

Kemp, C. (2004). Promoting healthy partnerships with refugees and immigrants. In A. R. Vollman, E. T. Anderson & J. McFarlane (Eds.). *Canadian community as partner: Theory and practice in nursing* (pp. 407–430). Philadelphia: Lippincott Williams & Wilkins.

Kleinman, A. (1979). *Patients and healers in the context of culture.* Berkeley: University of California Press.

Kluckholn, F. (1976). Dominant and variant value orientations. In P. Brink (Ed.), *Transcultural nursing: A book of readings* (pp. 63–81). Englewood Cliffs, NJ: Prentice Hall.

Korean health beliefs. (2003). Retrieved December 1, 2004, from *http://www.hawcc.hawaii.edu/nursing/RNKorean00.htm*

Leininger, M. M. (Ed.). (1991). *Culture care diversity and universality: A theory of nursing.* New York: NLN Press.

Leininger, M. (2002a). Essential transcultural nursing care concepts, principles, examples and policy statements. In M. Leininger & M. R. McFarland (Eds.), *Transcultural nursing: Concepts, theories, research and practice* (3rd ed., pp. 45–69). New York: McGraw-Hill.

Leininger, M. (2002b). Culture care theory: A major contribution to advance transcultural nursing knowledge and practices. *Journal of Transcultural Nursing, 13*(3), 189–192.

Leininger, M., & McFarland, M. R. (2002). *Transcultural nursing: Concepts, theories, research and practice* (3rd ed.). New York: McGraw-Hill.

Lin, Y. (2002). Crossing the gate of death in Chinese Buddhist culture. Retrieved December 1, 2004, from Buddhist Yogi C. M. Chen's Web site: *http://www.yogichen.org/efiles/mbk16.html*

Loustaunau, M. O., & Sobo, E. J. (1997). *The cultural context of health, illness and medicine.* Westport, CT: Bergin & Garvey.

Lutumba Ntetu, A., & D'arc Fortin, J. (1996). Pour un reajustement des approaches aupres des autochtones. *Canadian Nurse, 92*(3), 42–46.

Majumdar, B. B., Chambers, T. L., & Roberts, J. (2004). Community-based, culturally sensitive HIV/AIDS education for Aboriginal adolescents: Implications for nursing practice. *Journal of Transcultural Nursing, 15*(1), 69–73.

McMillan, A. D. (1988). *Native peoples and cultures of Canada.* Vancouver, BC: Douglas & McIntyre.

Minuk, G. Y., & Uhanova, J. (2003). Viral hepatitis in the Canadian Inuit and First Nations populations. *Canadian Journal of Gastroenterology, 17*(12), 707–712.

Pacquiao, D. F. (2001). Cultural incongruities of advance directives. *Bioethics Forum, 17*(1), 27–31.

Pacquiao, D. F. (2002). Ethics and cultural diversity: A framework for decision-making. *Bioethics Forum, 17*(3–4), 12–17.

Pacquiao, D. F. (2003). Cultural competence in ethical-decision-making. In M. M. Andrews & J. S. Boyle. (2003). *Transcultural concepts in nursing care.* Philadelphia: Lippincott Williams & Wilkins.

Purnell, L. D., & Paulanka, B. J. (1998). *Transcultural healthcare: A culturally competent approach.* Philadelphia: F. A. Davis.

Reimer, J. J., & Redskye, C. (1998). The Canadian Ojibwa. In R. E. Davidhizar & J. N. Giger (Eds.), *Canadian transcultural nursing: Assessment and intervention* (pp. 197–213). St. Louis, MO: Mosby.

Selekman, J. (2003). People of Jewish Heritage. In L. D. Purnell & B. J. Paulanka (Eds.), *Transcultural healthcare: a culturally competent approach* (pp. 234–248). Philadelphia: F. A. Davis.

Shestowsky, B. (1995). Health-related concerns of Canadian Aboriginal people residing in urban areas. *International Nursing Review, 42*(1), 23–26.

Singh, P. (2000). *The Sikhs.* New York: Random House.

Smith, D. (2003). Maternal-child health care in Aboriginal communities. *Canadian Journal of Nursing Research, 35*(2), 143–152.

Sobo, E. (1993). *One blood: The Jamaican body.* Albany, NY: SUNY Press.

Sorrentino, S. A. (2004). *Mosby's Canadian textbook for the support worker.* Toronto, ON: Elsevier Canada.

Spector, R. E. (2000). *Cultural diversity in health & illness* (5th ed.). Upper Saddle River, NJ: Prentice Hall Health.

Statistics Canada. (2001a). *Aboriginal peoples of Canada.* Retrieved December 1, 2004, from *http://www.statcan.ca:8096/bsolc/english/bsolc?catno=97F0011X*

Statistics Canada. (2001b). *Aboriginal peoples of Canada: Metis.* Retrieved December 1, 2004, from *http://www12.statcan.ca/english/census01/Products/Analytic/companion/abor/groups2.cfm*

Statistics Canada. (2001c.). *Aboriginal peoples of Canada:North American Indians.* Retrieved December 1, 2004, from *http://www12.statcan.ca/english/census01/Products/Analytic/companion/abor/groups1.cfm*

Statistics Canada. (2003). *Census: Canada's Ethnocultural portrait: The changing mosaic.* Retrieved October 2, 2004, from *http://www12.statcan.ca/english/census01/products/analytic/companion/etoimm/canada.cfm#immigrants_increasingly_asia*

St. Hill, P., Lipson, J. G., & Meleis, A. I. (2003). *Caring for women cross-culturally.* Philadelphia: F. A. Davis.

Suh, E. E. (2004). The model of cultural competence through an evolutionary concept analysis. *Journal of Transcultural Nursing, 15*(2), 93–102.

Vatuk, S. (1996). The art of dying in Hindu India. In H. M. Spiro, M. G. McCrea Curnen, & I. P. Wandel (Eds.), *Facing death* (pp. 121–128). New Haven, CT: Yale University Press.

Vollman, A. R., Anderson, E. T., & McFarlane, J. (2004). *Canadian community as partner: Theory and practice in nursing.* Philadelphia: Lippincott Williams & Wilkins.

Voyageur, E. (1998). Kwa-kwa'ka-wakw First Nation. In R. E. Davidhizar & J. N, Giger (Eds.), *Canadian transcultural nursing: Assessment and intervention* (pp. 214–229). St. Louis, MO: Mosby.

Wasekeesikaw, F. H. (2003). Challenges for the new millennium: Nursing in First Nations communities. In M. McIntyre & E. Thomlinson (Eds.), *Realities of Canadian nursing: Professional, practice, and power issues* (pp. 447–469). Philadelphia: Lippincott Williams & Wilkins.

Yonge, O., & Bernard, M. (1998). The Cree living in urban settings. In R. E. Davidhizar & J. N. Giger (Eds.), *Canadian transcultural nursing: Assessment and intervention* (pp. 179–196). St. Louis, MO: Mosby.

Young, A. (1976). Internalizing and externalizing medical systems: An Ethiopian example. In C. Currer & M. Stacey (Eds.), *Concepts of health, illness and disease: A comparative perspective.* Oxford, England: Berg.

Recommended Web Sites

Canadian Ethnocultural Council:
http://www.ethnocultural.ca/

This Web site explains the purposes of the Canadian Ethnocultural Council (CEC), which is a non-profit, non-partisan coalition of national ethnocultural organizations representing ethnocultural groups across Canada. Links to other related publications and sites related to ethnocultural groups are included.

Citizen and Immigration Canada—Cultural Profiles Project:
http://www.settlement.org/cp/

This Web site provides an overview of the life and customs of immigrants to Canada. Each profile includes a summary fact sheet and information about their culture, food, health, landscape, climate, arts, holidays, and literature.

Cultures Canada:
http://www.culturescanada.ca

This Web site is sponsored by Canadian Heritage and provides a current directory listings to multiculturalism, cultural communities, organizations, and other links to information related to and celebrating Canada's cultural diversity.

10

Client Care: Leadership, Delegation, and Quality Management

Patricia A. Stockert, RN, BSN, MS, PhD
Marlene Smadu, RN, BScN, MAdEd, ED (Canadian author)

Box 10-3

Focus on Primary Health Care

Nursing Leadership in Primary Health Care

Nursing as a profession has taken a strong leadership role in implementing primary health care (PHC) throughout the world. Since 1978, the International Council of Nurses, the Canadian Nurses Association (CNA), and other national and provincial/territorial nursing associations have been instrumental in lobbying for inclusion of PHC principles and programs in health provider education, in service planning and delivery, and in research and evaluation. The CNA actively promotes initiatives to incorporate PHC into nursing practice and policy.

Nurses continue to have a leadership role in primary health care. As Deborah Tamlyn, the president of the CNA, stated in her inaugural speech in June, 2004, "More and more, nurses have legitimate power and believe in their ability to re-generate and renew the health care system. Across Canada and around the globe we are seeing examples of how nurses can lead initiatives in reshaping the health system to one that addresses the social determinants of health and is based on principles of primary health care."

Nurses provide primary health care at all levels and maintain links between individuals, families, communities, and the rest of the health care system. Working with other members of the health care team and other sectors or on their own, nurses explore new and better ways of keeping well, improving health, and preventing disease and disability. Nurses improve equity and access to health care and add quality to the outcome of care.

Sources: *International Council of Nurses Position Statement: Nurses and Primary Health Care; Annual Report,* by Canadian Nurses Association, 2003. Accessed August 24, 2004, from *http://www.newswire.ca/en/releases/archive/June2004/23/c7832.html*

Box 10-4 Developing a Vision for a Nursing Unit

What Is the Nursing Unit's Purpose or Mission?

Articulating why we exist
Knowing our clients (internal and external)
Demonstrating our uniqueness
Understanding the uniqueness of our clients
Demonstrating how we accomplish organizational goals or vision

How Will Staff Work With Clients and Families?

Placing client and family needs first with a client-focused approach
Involving clients and families in all aspects of care
Making communication a priority

What Are the Standards of the Work Unit?

All staff will be competent.
Each staff member is accountable for the care delivered to clients.
Staff will work collaboratively with all members of the health care team.

Key Values

Creating an environment of caring
Being self-motivated and self-managed
Supporting a learning environment

Team Nursing. **Team nursing** developed in response to the nursing shortage following World War II (Ritter-Teitel, 2002). It involves the delivery of nursing care by various staff members. A registered nurse (RN) leads a team of other RNs, registered practical nurses/licensed practical nurses (RPNs/LPNs), and/or unregulated care providers (UCPs). The team members provide client care under the direction of the team leader. The team leader coordinates overall care, develops care plans, provides care requiring complex nursing skills, problem solves with physicians and other professionals, and helps the team evaluate their care (Wywialowski, 1997). UCPs are often given client assignments instead of being assigned particular tasks. A disadvantage of this model is that the client may see an RN infrequently. Risks exist if an RN is unable to make necessary client assessment and clinical decisions. Also, continuity of care may suffer because of the task orientation and if nurses are not assigned the same clients daily. Advantages are the collaborative working style, the autonomy of the team leader, and the decision making that occurs at a clinical level (Ritter-Teitel, 2002).

Total Patient Care. **Total patient care** delivery was the original care model developed during Florence Nightingale's time. It became popular in the 1970s and 1980s, when the numbers of RNs were increasing. In this model, an RN is responsible for all aspects of care for one or more clients. The RN may assign or delegate aspects of care to an RPN/LPN or UCP but remains accountable for care of all assigned clients. The nurse works directly with the client, family, physician, and health care team members. The model typically has a shift-based focus. The same nurse does not necessarily care for the same client over time. Continuity of care from shift to shift or day to day is compromised if staff members do not clearly communicate client needs to one another.

Primary Nursing. The **primary nursing** model aimed to place RNs at the bedside and improve nursing accountability for client outcomes and relationships among staff (Ritter-Teitel, 2002). The model was popular in the 1970s and early 1980s when hospitals employed more RNs. Primary nursing supports a philosophy of strong nurse-client relationships. An RN assumes responsibility for a caseload of clients. Typically, the RN selects the clients and cares for the same clients during their stay in the health care setting. The RN assesses client needs, develops care plans, and ensures that appropriate nursing care is delivered. Primary nursing maintains continuity of care across shifts, days, or visits. It can be applied in any

Table 10-1 Examples of Management Structures

Structural Approach	Characteristics
Centralized management	Single administrator leads organization, with directors overseeing departments. Decisions are made from top down, with little staff input. Managers have minimal responsibility or accountability for 24-hour operation of nursing unit.
Decentralized management	Structure may be similar to centralized management. Often there are fewer directors. Staff members with the most knowledge about an issue make decisions. Managers often have 24-hour accountability and responsibility for staff, budget, and day-to-day management of work unit.
Matrix	Traditional hospital departments are reorganized into business units. Staff may report to more than one manager.

health care setting. When a primary nurse is off-duty, associate nurses, including RPNs/LPNs or other RNs, follow the care plan. If differences in opinion occur, associates and primary nurses collaborate to redefine the plan as needed. Although primary nursing requires more RNs, the model is not necessarily more costly than others. Ritter-Teitel (2002) contends that care consistently managed by one RN can minimize delays in therapies, improve collaboration with other professionals, and enhance the client-nurse relationship. The RN has a high level of clinical autonomy and authority that enhances collaboration with physicians (Ritter-Teitel, 2002).

Case Management. Case management coordinates and links health care services to clients and their families while streamlining costs and maintaining quality (Dadich, 2003). Case management is "a collaborative process which assesses, plans, implements, coordinates, monitors, and evaluates the options and services required to meet an individual's health needs, using communications and available resources to promote quality, cost-effective outcomes" (Case Management Society of America, 2003). Clinicians, as individuals or in teams, manage clients with specific case types (e.g., clients presenting complex nursing and medical problems) and are usually held accountable for quality and cost management.

Case managers coordinate clients' acute care in hospital, supervise care delivered by staff members, coordinate discharge planning, and follow-up with clients after discharge. Some case managers work exclusively in the community. Case managers often oversee a caseload of clients with complex nursing and medical problems. Many case managers use critical pathways or CareMaps—multidisciplinary treatment plans for clients of a specific case type (see chapter 12). The plans help in the delivery of timely, coordinated care. Guesswork is eliminated because all members of the health care team work from the same plan.

Box 10-5 Responsibilities of the Nurse Manager

- Assist staff in establishing annual goals for the unit and systems needed to accomplish goals.
- Monitor professional nursing standards of practice on the unit.
- Develop an ongoing staff development plan, including one for new employees.
- Recruit new employees (interview and hire).
- Conduct routine staff evaluations.
- Establish self as a role model for positive customer service (customers include clients, families, and other health care team members).
- Submit staffing schedules for the unit.
- Conduct regular client rounds and problem solve client or family complaints.
- Establish and implement a unit quality improvement plan.
- Review and recommend new equipment for the unit.
- Conduct regular staff meetings.
- Conduct rounds with physicians.
- Establish and support staff and interdisciplinary committees.

Decentralized Decision Making

The nurse executive supports managers by creating a management structure that will help achieve organizational goals and provide support to care delivery staff (Table 10-1). With a vision for nursing established, the manager directs and supports staff to realize that vision.

Decentralized management, in which decision making occurs at the staff level, is common in health care organizations. The advantage of this structure is that managers and staff are actively involved in shaping an organization's identity and determining success. Decentralized management requires workers to be empowered to accept greater responsibility for the quality of client care (Ellis & Hartley, 2005; Lilley, 2002). A decentralized structure leads to increased collaboration, staff competency, and satisfaction.

The nurse manager is critical to successful nursing units or groups. Box 10-5 illustrates the diverse responsibilities of nurse managers. For decentralized decision making to work, managers must move decisions down to the lowest level. All staff (RNs, RPNs/LPNs, UCPs, and secretaries) need to be actively involved. They must be well informed, asked to join committees, and encouraged to participate in problem-solving activities.

Key elements in decision making are responsibility, autonomy, authority, and accountability (Cox, 1995; Ritter-Teitel, 2002). The CNA (2003b) outlines principles and criteria for decentralized decision making (Box 10-6).

Responsibility refers to the duties and activities that an individual is employed to perform. Responsibility reflects ownership. The individual who oversees the employee must allocate responsibility and the employee must accept it. Managers must be sure that staff understand

Box 10-6 Principles for Decentralized Decision Making

- Decision making is based on having the appropriate number of positions and the competencies required to ensure safe, competent, and ethical care.
- Nurse administrators and managers (including supervisors, middle, and senior managers) are responsible for ensuring the appropriate staff mix.
- Legislative, professional, and organizational parameters are respected.
- The safety of clients must never be compromised by substituting less qualified workers when the competencies of a registered nurse (RN) are required.
- The staffing decision-making process recognizes the unique and shared competencies of each care provider group.
- Responsibility and accountability of care providers are clear.
- RNs at all levels in the organization are involved in decision making that affects nursing practice, client care, and the work environment.
- Staffing decisions are evidence-based.
- Organizations and other stakeholders, including RNs, ensure that the elements necessary for a quality professional practice environment are in place.
- RNs are leaders in implementing collaborative practice and promoting effective communication among all members of the health care team.

their responsibilities, particularly during change. For example, when hospitals restructure and client care delivery models change, the manager must clearly define the RN's role within the new care delivery model. If decentralized decision making is in place, professional staff can help shape the new RN role. All RNs are responsible for knowing their role on the unit. For example, a primary nurse is responsible for assessing all assigned clients, developing care plans, and evaluating the success of the plans.

Autonomy is the freedom to decide and act (Hicks, 2003). Autonomy, consistent with the scope of professional nursing practice, maximizes the effectiveness of the nurse (Hicks, 2003). With autonomy, a nurse can make independent decisions about client care. The nurse plans care for the client within the scope of nursing practice and provides nursing interventions without seeking physician permission (Ritter-Teitel, 2002). For example, a nurse has the autonomy to design a discharge teaching plan based on specific client needs. Innovation by nurses, increased productivity, higher nurse retention, and greater client satisfaction are results of autonomy in nursing practice (Hicks, 2003).

Authority is the right to act in areas where an individual has been given and accepts responsibility (Cox, 1995). For example, a primary nurse who finds that the nursing team did not follow a discharge teaching plan for an assigned client has the authority to consult with other nurses to learn why the plan was not followed. The primary nurse has the final authority in selecting the best course of action for the client's care.

Accountability means being answerable for one's actions. It involves follow-up and reflection on one's decisions to evaluate effectiveness (Cox, 1995). A primary nurse is accountable for clients' outcomes. In the example about the discharge teaching plan, the primary nurse is accountable for ensuring that the client learns to do self-care at home.

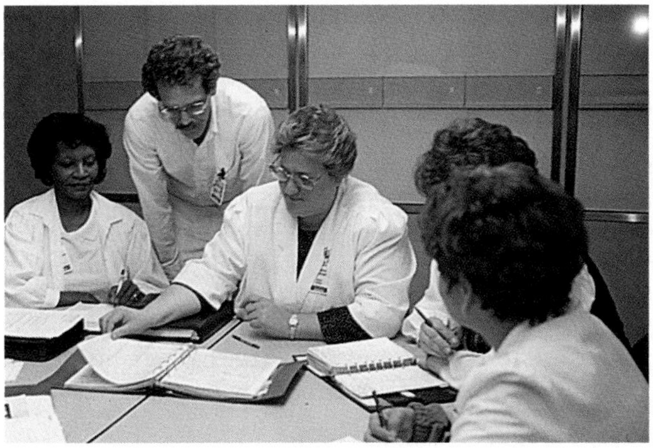

FIGURE **10–1** Staff collaborating on practice issues.

A successful decentralized nursing unit exercises the four elements of decision making: responsibility, autonomy, authority, and accountability. The staff must meet routinely to discuss how to maintain an equality and balance in these elements. Individuals should be comfortable in expressing differences in opinion and in challenging the status quo, while understanding their own responsibility, autonomy, authority, and accountability.

Supporting Staff Involvement. In decentralized decision-making structures, all staff members actively participate in unit activities (Figure 10–1). Staff members benefit from the knowledge and skills of the entire work group. If the staff values knowledge and their colleagues' contributions, client care improves. The nursing manager supports staff involvement through the following approaches.

Establishment of Nursing Practice Problem-Solving Committees or Professional Shared Governance Councils. Chaired by senior clinical staff, these groups are empowered to maintain care standards for nursing practice on their work unit. The committees review and establish standards of care, develop policy and procedures, resolve client satisfaction issues, or develop new documentation tools. To ensure the delivery of quality care, the committees should focus on client outcomes rather than only on work issues (Hansten & Washburn, 1999). Mechanisms are established so that all staff have input on practice issues. Managers might not sit on the committee, but they receive progress reports. The types of work on the nursing unit determines committee membership. Professionals from other disciplines (e.g., pharmacy, respiratory therapy, or clinical nutrition) might participate in practice committees or shared governance councils.

Nurse-Physician Collaborative Practice. A nursing unit's care delivery model influences nurse and physician collaboration. If the unit practises team nursing, team leaders should participate in physician rounds. If the unit practises primary nursing, the physician should communicate either with each primary nurse or with the associate nurse who is assuming care for the client on that day. In a home care or other community care setting, the staff should be able to reach physicians easily and work together on decisions regarding client care. The manager should avoid taking care of problems for the staff. Instead, staff members should keep physicians informed about important client issues. Physicians are invited to attend practice committees when clinical problems are addressed and to present timely in-service programs on new medical procedures or research findings.

Interdisciplinary Collaboration. The emphasis on efficiency in health care delivery brings all members of the health care team together. Whenever systems or programs are redesigned, interdisciplinary involvement is crucial because most health care processes involve more than one discipline (CNA, 2003a). Nursing staff must recognize the importance of prompt referrals and timely communication with other health professionals. Including professionals from various disciplines in practice projects, in-service programs, conferences, and staff meetings fosters interdisciplinary collaboration.

Staff Communication. Communication with staff is one of the manager's greatest challenges, especially in a large work group. It is difficult to ensure that all staff receive the correct message. In the present health care environment, staff quickly become uneasy and distrusting if they fail to hear about planned changes on their work unit. A manager cannot be responsible for all communication but can use several approaches to communicate quickly and accurately with all staff. Examples are circulating newsletters, posting minutes of committee meetings, and using list servers and e-mail. Meetings should be held to discuss vital issues. Members of practice or quality improvement committees should communicate with selected staff so that everyone is contacted and asked for input.

Staff Education. Nursing staff should grow in knowledge. Ongoing education helps staff learn medical and nursing practice trends. The nurse manager facilitates learning by planning in-service programs, sending staff to classes and conferences, and having staff present case studies or practice issues at meetings. Staff members are responsible for upgrading skills and knowledge when their competencies are lacking.

Leadership Skills for Nursing Students

Nursing students must prepare for leadership roles. This does not mean they have to quickly learn how to lead a nursing team; rather, they first learn to become dependable and competent care providers. Nursing students are responsible and accountable for the care they provide. Although their authority is limited and they must consult with instructors and staff, the students must not avoid making decisions in client care. Students can learn to become leaders by making good clinical decisions, learning from mistakes, seeking guidance, collaborating with nurses, and striving to improve during each client interaction. Leadership skills that nursing students can learn to use include clinical care coordination, team communication, delegation, and knowledge building.

Clinical Care Coordination

A student must acquire the skills necessary to ensure timely and effective client care. At first, students might have only one client, but eventually they will coordinate the care of groups of clients. Clinical care coordination includes clinical decision making, priority setting, use of organizational skills and resources, time management, and evaluation.

Clinical Decisions. When a nurse assesses a client, the first activity is to assess the client's condition in order to determine the client's needs and required nursing therapies. Decision making is a fundamental element of nursing work (Boblin-Cummings, Baumann, & Deber, 1999). Leadership and decision-making skills are required as the nurse engages in the complex interactions—collaboration, negotiation, and delegation—required to elicit the involvement of others. The initial contact is important to developing a caring relationship with a client. The nurse takes a critical thinking approach, applying previous knowledge and experience to the decision-making process (see chapter 11).

The nursing process is the framework nurses use to determine the level of care required, implement the care plan, and evaluate the results (see chapter 12). If the nurse fails to make accurate clinical judgments, undesirable outcomes may result. The client's condition might worsen or remain the same when it might have improved. Accurate clinical decision making keeps the nurse focused on the proper course of action.

Priority Setting. The nurse must decide which client's needs or problems to address first. Wywialowski (1997) describes categories of priority nursing needs of individual clients:

- *First-order priority needs*—An immediate threat to a client's survival or safety, such as an obstructed airway, loss of consciousness, or an anxiety attack.
- *Second-order priority needs*—Actual problems for which the client or family has requested immediate help, such as comfort measures, nausea, or a full bladder or bowel.
- *Third-order priority needs*—Relatively urgent actual or potential problems that the client or family does not recognize, such as monitoring for post-operative complications or anticipating teaching needs of a client who may be unaware of side effects of a drug.
- *Fourth-order priority needs*—Actual or potential problems with which the client or family may need help in the future, such as teaching for self-care in the home.

Many clients can have all four types of priorities, requiring a nurse to make careful judgments in choosing a course of action. First-order priority needs demand a nurse's immediate attention. When a client has diverse priority needs, it helps to focus on basic needs. For example, a client in traction who is about to eat says he is uncomfortable from being in one position. Before helping the client to eat, the nurse repositions him and offers basic hygiene measures. The client is more interested in eating now that he is comfortable. He is also more receptive to instructions from the nurse.

Nurses must meet the priority needs of groups of clients. This requires knowing the priority needs of each client, assessing each client's needs as soon as possible, and addressing first- and second-priority needs in a timely manner (Wywialowski, 1997). To identify which clients require assessment first, the nurse uses the change-of-shift report, the agency's classification system that identifies client acuity, and the client record. The nurse considers resources, recognizes that priority needs can change, and uses time wisely. With time, nurses learn to spontaneously rank clients' needs by priority or urgency.

Priorities are also made based on client expectations. If a client is resistant to a therapy or disagrees with the approach, a care plan will be ineffective. Working closely with the client and showing a caring attitude is important. A nurse should discuss priorities with the client to establish co-operation.

Organizational Skills. A nurse learns to become efficient by combining various nursing activities—in other words, doing more than one thing at a time. For example, while obtaining a specimen, the nurse combines therapeutic communication skills, teaching interventions, and assessment and evaluation. Nurses continually strengthen relationships with clients. Each time they are with a client they convey a caring attitude and share necessary information. They observe the client's behaviours and responses to therapies and evaluate responses to interventions.

Events may occur that interfere with plans. For example, as a nurse begins an education session with a client and family, an X-ray technician arrives to take a chest film. The nurse's priorities conflict with those of the technician. Both must focus on the client's needs. The client may have experienced symptoms earlier that require a chest film. In this case, the X-ray must be completed. However, if the chest film is a routine order from 2 days ago and the client's condition is stable, the technician may be willing to return later because the education session is a priority at this time.

Use of Resources. Effective use of resources, including members of the health care team, is key to clinical care coordination. Students should never hesitate to ask staff for assistance, especially when it would make a client safer or more comfortable. For example, help with turning, positioning, and ambulating clients is needed for clients with impaired mobility. Complicated procedures, such as dressing changes, can be more efficient with help with equipment and supplies. This is an excellent way for students to learn to work with UCPs. Students must recognize their limitations. For example, a student may assess a client and find clinical signs and symptoms but be unfamiliar with the underlying condition. Consultation with an RN leads to confirmation of findings and assurance that the proper care is delivered. Throughout their professional careers, nurses are always facing new situations. Leaders know their limitations and seek guidance from colleagues.

Time Management. Nurses can experience stress on a clinical unit while trying to meet the multiple needs of clients. Time management skills can help manage stress. These skills involve learning how, where, and when to use your time. Client goals should direct priorities. For example, a nurse is caring for two clients on a surgical nursing unit: One had surgery the day before, and the other is anticipating discharge the next day. The first client's goals centre on restoring physiological function, the second client's, on preparation for self-care at home. The nurse, in reviewing the therapies required for both clients, organizes his or her time to deliver care and achieve client goals. The nurse must anticipate when medication administration and diagnostic testing will occur and plan the best time for therapies such as dressing changes and client ambulation.

A worksheet can help nurses manage time. With each client, it helps to make a list that sequences the nursing activities to be performed. The change-of-shift report may help with sequencing because it details the client's condition and care provided. Consider activities that have specific time limits, such as administering a pain medication before a procedure or instructing clients before discharge. The nurse also analyzes activities scheduled by agency policies or routines (e.g., medications or intravenous [IV] tubing changes). A nurse notes which activities need to be done at a certain time and which activities can be done on discretion (Wywialowski, 1997). Medications must be administered within a specific schedule, but a nurse can also perform other activities while in the client's room. Estimate the time needed for all activities. Activities requiring assistance of colleagues take longer because the nurse must plan around their schedule.

It is best to complete one task before starting another and to complete activities started with one client before moving on to the next. If the nurse focuses on each client, errors will be fewer and care will be less fragmented. To manage time well, the nurse must anticipate the day's activities, combine activities when possible, and avoid non-essential interruptions.

Evaluation. Evaluation is a critical part of clinical care coordination. Evaluation is an ongoing process. Once nurses begin a therapy, they should immediately evaluate its effectiveness and the client's response. The evaluation process compares expected client outcomes with actual outcomes. For example, a clinic nurse assesses a diabetic client's foot ulcer to determine if healing is progressing and expected outcomes are met. Evaluation reveals the need to revise approaches to care and introduce new therapies. A nurse cannot always evaluate care immediately. For example, she or he must anticipate when to return to a client's bedside to evaluate care, 30 minutes after a medication was administered, 15 minutes after an IV line has begun infusing, or 60 minutes after discussing discharge instructions with the client and family.

Focusing on evaluation of a client's progress and outcomes, rather than tasks, lessens the chance of distraction. The nurse must constantly inquire about the client's condition and healing progress.

Team Communication. As part of a team, each nurse must communicate openly and professionally. In an enriching work environment, staff members are honest and direct, listen to and respect each other, and share ideas and information. On a hospital unit, nurses tell colleagues about clients with emerging problems, physicians who have been called for consultation, and solutions to complex nursing problems. In a clinic, they share unusual diagnostic findings or convey information about a client's family support. An efficient team knows it can count on all members. Sharing expectations of what, when, and how to communicate helps establishes a strong team.

Delegation. Changes in staff mix have resulted in UCPs now delivering care to clients (Boblin-Cummings et al., 1999; McGillis Hall, 1997). In the new working environment, a nurse must understand the evolving role of nursing and delegated care responsibilities.

Delegation refers to the transferring of responsibility for the performance of an activity or task while retaining accountability for the outcome (American Nurses Association, 1995). The CNA (1995) states that because nursing practice is knowledge-based and not task-based, the responsibility for nursing cannot be delegated even when specific tasks or procedures are delegated. One purpose of delegation is to improve efficiency. Asking a staff member to obtain an ordered specimen while the nurse attends to a client's pain medication request prevents a delay in the client's pain relief. Delegation can also provide job enrichment. A nurse shows trust in colleagues by delegating tasks to them and showing staff members that they are integral to the delivery of care. A nurse never delegates a task that he or she dislikes doing or would not do independently because this can create negative feelings and poor working relationships. For example, if a nurse is in the room when a client asks to be placed on a bedpan, the nurse should assist the client rather than leave the room to find the UCP. Remember that although the delegation of a task transfers the responsibility and authority to another person, the nurse who is delegating retains accountability for the delegated task.

It is important to recognize that *tasks* are delegated, not clients (CNA, 1995). Leah Curtin (1994), a distinguished nursing leader and editor of the journal *Nursing Management,* wrote that unregulated personnel should not be at the bedside, but at the nurse's side. This means that a UCP should not be assigned sole responsibility for client care. The nurse in charge of client care decides which activities the UCP can perform independently and which activities must be performed by the nurse and UCP in partnership. One way to accomplish this is to have the nurse and UCP conduct rounds together. The nurse can assess each client as the UCP attends to basic client needs. The nurse then delegates care based upon assessment findings and priorities.

An RN is always responsible for assessing a client's ongoing status, but if a client is stable, the RN may delegate an activity such as vital sign monitoring to the UCP. In most settings, the RN makes judgments about when to delegate. However, an RPN/LPN may direct care in many long-term care facilities. Box 10-7 lists some guidelines for delegation of tasks in accordance with the RN's legal scopes of practice. As the leader of the health care team, the RN must know how to give clear instructions, effectively prioritize client needs and therapies, and give staff members timely and meaningful feedback

Effective delegation is a skill nursing students need to observe and practice to improve clinical management skills. When nurses delegate, they give someone else the authority to carry out a care task, but they remain accountable for the overall nursing care of the client (CNA, 1995; Parkman, 1996). A nurse cannot simply assign an UCP to tasks without considering the implications. The nurse assesses a client and determines a plan of care before identifying which tasks someone else can perform. When directing a UCP, the RN must decide the degree of supervision that is required. Is this the first time a staff member has performed the task? Does the client present

Box 10-7 The Five Rights of Delegation

Right Task

The right task is one that can be delegated for a specific client, such as tasks that are repetitive, require little supervision, and are relatively noninvasive.

Right Circumstances

The appropriate client setting, available resources, and other relevant factors are considered. In an acute care setting, clients' conditions can change quickly. Good clinical decision-making is needed to determine what to delegate.

Right Person

The right person is delegating the right tasks to the right person to be performed on the right person.

Right Direction/Communication

A clear, concise description of the task, including its objective, limits, and expectations, is given. Communication must be ongoing between RN and unregulated care providers during a shift of care.

Right Supervision

Appropriate monitoring, evaluation, intervention as needed, and feedback are provided. Unregulated care providers should feel comfortable to ask questions and seek assistance.

Modified from *Delegation: Concepts and Decision-Making Process,* by National Council of State Boards of Nursing, 1995, Chicago, IL: Author.

a complicating factor necessitating the RN's assistance? Does the staff member have prior experience with a particular type of client in addition to having received training on skill performance? The RN's final responsibility is to evaluate if the UCP performed a task properly and if desired outcomes were realized.

Appropriate delegation begins with knowing which tasks can be delegated. This requires the RN to be familiar with the provincial or territorial nursing practice act, institutional policies and procedures, and the institution's job description for UCPs. These standards help to define the necessary level of competency of UCPs.

Provincial regulations define the scope of an RN's practice, including those activities that only RNs can perform (e.g., client assessment and planning care). Although most provinces identify the delegation and supervision of work as an RN's responsibility, each province addresses the specifics of delegation differently. In Ontario, British Columbia, and Alberta, for example, legislation that applies to all regulated health professions identifies specific tasks or activities that can be performed by only certain professions. In British Columbia, these authorized tasks are known as *reserved acts,* in Ontario they are called *controlled acts,* and in Alberta they are known as *restricted activities*. UCPs are not allowed to perform acts authorized for RNs unless they have been properly delegated by an RN, and only if they are within the UCP's job description and employer policy (Sorrentino, 2004).

An institution's policies, procedures, and job descriptions for UCPs provide specific guidelines regarding which tasks or activities can be delegated. The job description should specify any required education and the types of tasks UCPs can perform, either independently or with an RN's direct supervision. Institutional policy helps in defining the amount of training required of UCPs while employed. Procedures specify who is qualified to perform a given nursing procedure, whether supervision is necessary, and the type of reporting required. Job descriptions, policies, and procedures should comply with provincial laws and regulations. Nurses should have a means to access policies easily or have supervisory staff who can inform them as to the UCP's job duties.

Competency of UCPs is important because there may be no consistent standard for training across institutions or jurisdictions. To delegate, the RN must know that the UCP is competent to perform the procedure. This means that the RN should be familiar with the worker's training program. Frequently, RNs become preceptors in a UCP's training. The RN is assigned for a limited time to supervise a staff member directly and to observe his or her skill performance. Participating in UCP training and the refining of their skills can build trust and facilitate communication within the health care team (Parkman, 1996).

Effective delegation requires trust between the RN and UCPs. It also requires constant communication—sending clear messages and listening so that all participants understand expectations regarding client care. An RN should provide clear instructions when delegating tasks. These instructions may initially focus on the procedure itself as well as on the unique needs of the client. As the RN becomes more familiar with a staff member's scope of practice, trust builds and fewer instructions may be needed, but clarification of clients' specific needs will always be necessary.

A key step in delegation is evaluation of the staff member's performance and the client's outcomes. When UCPs do a good job, it is important to provide praise and recognition. If the staff member's performance is unsatisfactory, the RN must give constructive feedback, specifically discussing mistakes and how they could have been avoided. Giving feedback in private in a professional manner preserves the staff member's dignity. A UCP may fail to meet expectations because of inadequate training or assignment of too many tasks. The RN may need to review or demonstrate a procedure with staff or schedule additional training with the education department. The delegation of too many tasks might be a nursing practice issue. All staff should discuss delegation on their unit because UCPs may need help in learning how to prioritize and RNs may need to ensure that they are not overdelegating.

A few tips for nurses on appropriate delegation (Keeling et al., 2000) are as follows:

- *Assess the knowledge and skills of the delegate.* Nurses should determine what the UCP knows and what he or she can do by asking open-ended questions that will elicit conversation and details; for example, "How do you prepare the tubing before giving an enema?"
- *Match tasks to the delegate's skills.* Nurses need to know what skills are included in the UCP training program at their facility and to determine if personnel have learned critical thinking skills, such as knowing the difference between normal clinical findings and changes to report.
- *Communicate clearly.* Nurses should provide unambiguous directions by describing a task, the desired outcome, and the time period for completion of the task. Rather than giving instructions through another staff member, nurses should make the person feel part of the team. For example, "I'd like you to help me by getting Mr. Floyd up to ambulate before lunch. Be sure to check his blood pressure before he stands and write your finding on the graphic sheet. OK?"
- *Listen attentively.* Nurses should listen to the UCP's responses as they give directions. Is the person comfortable asking questions or requesting clarification? Nurses need to be especially attentive if the person has a deadline from another nurse and to help sort out priorities.
- *Provide feedback.* Nurses should give feedback about performance, regardless of outcome. They must tell the person about a job well done, or, if an outcome is undesirable, find a private place to discuss what occurred, any miscommunication, and how to achieve a better outcome in the future.

Knowledge Building. All nurses recognize that ongoing learning is key to competence. A leader values knowledge. Opportunities for learning occur with each interaction with client and colleagues and at every meeting where clinical care issues are discussed. In-service programs, workshops, and courses offer current information on health care. To become a leader, a nurse actively pursues learning opportunities, both formal and informal, and learns to share knowledge with colleagues.

Quality Improvement

For nursing care to be effective, management and organizational structures must support it. Management and staff need a common understanding of the organization's goals and vision. Studies reveal that quality practice environments produce better client outcomes and more satisfied clients and staff. These workplaces have lower rates of infection, shorter lengths of stay, and higher staff retention (Aiken et al., 2002; Aiken, Havens, & Sloane, 2000; Scott, Sochalski, & Aiken, 1999). Initiatives such as the College of Nurses of Ontario's Quality Assurance Practice Consultation Program (2004) and the Registered Nurses Association of British Columbia's Quality Practice Environment Program (2003) assess organizational attributes that enhance practice. The assessment is voluntary, but response by hospitals is encouraging. This review activity helps create and support a magnet workplace, which includes a flexible work environment, investment in education, professional autonomy, and flat management structures (Buchan, 1999).

In an intense and demanding workplace, finding the time to reflect on work processes can be a challenge. Quality and value in health care emerged as key issues in the 1990s.

Organizational programs such as **total quality management (TQM)** and **continuous quality improvement (CQI)** were developed to encourage staff to reflect on how to improve work. Quality management recognizes that the client or customer defines quality (Wendt & Vale, 2003). Value is a function of balance between excellent care and services, good outcomes, and cost (Joint Commission on Accreditation of Healthcare Organizations [JCAHO], 2002). Most organizations have moved away from programs identified as TQM or CQI, and instead focus on the more generic and pervasive concept of **quality improvement (QI).** The Canadian Council on Health Services Accreditation (CCHSA) defines QI as "an organizational philosophy that seeks to meet clients' needs and exceed their expectations by using a structured process that selectively identifies and improves all aspects of service" (2003, p. 1). The CCHSA (2003) describes quality as responsiveness, system competency, client/community focus, and work life. QI focuses on improving organization performance related to processes.

To improve client outcomes, organizations must systematically monitor, analyze, and improve processes (JCAHO, 2002). Typically, many individuals are involved in a single process. Take medication delivery, for example: Physicians prescribe the medications, pharmacists prepare them, secretaries communicate orders and changes, transporters deliver them, and nurses administer them. With so many individuals involved in most work processes, strong leadership, employee empowerment, good collaboration, effective communication, and support of staff's ideas are essential for successful QI.

Box 10-8 Dimensions of Performance

Doing the Right Thing

The *efficacy* of the procedure or treatment in relation to the client's condition
The *appropriateness* of a specific test, procedure, or service to meet the client's clinical needs

Doing the Right Thing Well

The *availability* of a test, procedure, treatment, or service to the client who needs it
The *timeliness* with which a test, procedure, treatment, or service is provided
The *effectiveness* of tests, procedures, treatments, and services
The *continuity* of services provided to the client with respect to other services, practitioners, and providers over time
The *safety* of the client and others to whom the services are provided
The *efficiency* with which care and services are provided
The *respect and caring* with which care and services are provided

Modified from *Comprehensive Accreditation Manual for Hospitals: The Official Handbook,* by Joint Commission on Accreditation of Healthcare Organizations, 2002, Chicago, IL: Author.

Quality in Nursing Practice

JCAHO (2002) identifies performance as what is done and how well it is done to provide health care (Box 10-8). Nursing processes directly influence clients. Nursing practice is a priority for nursing managers and staff. Nurses must evaluate their success in delivering client care. Is care appropriate and competent? What outcomes does the client experience? These questions drive any QI effort.

The outcomes of care are a measure of the health care team's performance. With all disciplines contributing to client care, managing quality is a multidisciplinary effort. The nurse manager and staff play a critical role in recognizing trends in nursing practice, identifying recurrent problems, and initiating improvements to the quality of care. A nurse manager should enforce a work ethic that encourages staff to continually improve care. The first step is to define quality of nursing practice.

Quality Defined. Standards or guidelines define the meaning of quality. For example, to judge if rehabilitation has been delayed, there must be a standard indicating when rehabilitation should begin. Quality of care in nursing practice is not arbitrarily defined. A definition of quality begins with the mission, vision, philosophy, and values of the nursing department. These statements define how all nurses within an organization are to perform and which services must be provided. Written values give direction for professional standards and care guidelines that lead to positive client outcomes. Figure 10–2 provides a framework for quality nursing care.

Professional Standards. Professional standards are authoritative statements used by the profession in describ-

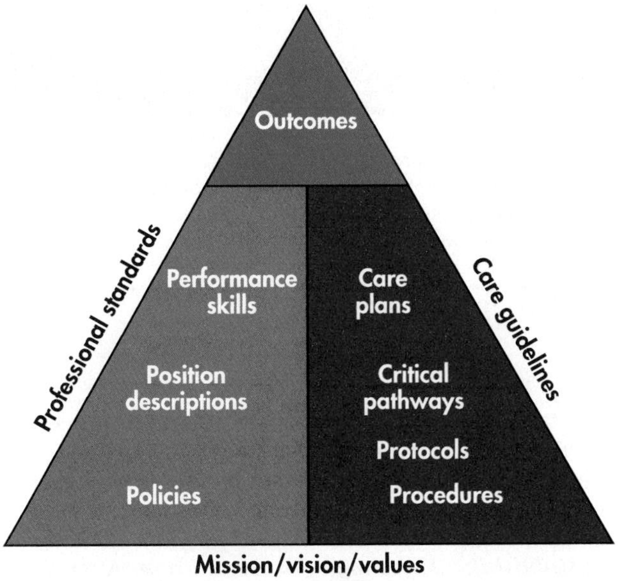

FIGURE **10–2** Framework for quality. (Data from "Outcomes: The Mainstay of a Framework for Quality Care," by D. A. Peters, 1995, *Journal of Nursing Care Quality, 10*(1), p. 61.)

ing the responsibilities for which its practitioners are accountable (Peters, 1995). Included are the policies and position descriptions that identify performance expectations within an organization. Standards are an organization's interpretation of the professional's competency. The adherence to professional standards is measured through professional outcomes.

Care Guidelines. Care guidelines are statements to assist in determining the most effective preventative methods, diagnoses, treatments, and management of diseases and other health conditions. Guidelines can be developed by single disciplines (Registered Nurses Association of Ontario, 2003) or be multidisciplinary in focus. An example of a nursing clinical protocol is one used for instructing clients newly diagnosed with diabetes. The effectiveness of clinical guidelines is measured through client outcomes.

Care guidelines include procedures, care plans, protocols, and critical pathways. Procedures are step-by-step descriptions of how to perform a skill. An example is the nursing skill for changing a sterile dressing. Most skills require cognitive abilities and manual dexterity. Clinical protocols outline steps for treating certain conditions (Peters, 1995). A course of action is usually prescribed in specific terms under specific conditions. For example, a protocol establishes actions in the treatment of a pressure ulcer.

Outcomes. Outcomes are conditions to be achieved as a result of care. Analysis of outcomes is key to QI (Johnson, Mass, & Moorhead, 2000; Titler, 2001). An **outcome** reveals if interventions are effective, if clients progress, how well standards are being met, and if changes are necessary. Outcomes are the backbone for organizing and managing care and quality (Peters, 1995). When nurses think about outcomes, their actions are purposeful and focused on improving clients' health. There are two types of outcomes (Peters, 1995).

1. *Professional outcomes.* These measure a nurse's performance. Professional standards of care, institutional policies, and job descriptions set expectations for the delivery of care and the nurse's responsibility for care. These discipline-specific outcomes are key to evaluating practice quality (Johnson et al., 2000). For example, the RN is responsible for the ongoing assessment of clients' status and communicating status changes to appropriate staff.
2. *Client outcomes.* These measure the client's status after receiving care. Client outcomes are defined in care plans and clinical guidelines, such as critical pathways and clinical protocols. Outcomes are generally organization specific and are stated as expected goals (Johnson et al., 2000). For example, a goal states that following reminiscent therapy, a client will be able to discuss concerns regarding the client's life-threatening illness.

Developing QI Teams. Health care providers collaborate on teams for QI efforts. A team with the goal of improving the admission process might include nursing staff, admissions staff, transporters, physicians, and pharmacists. In organization-wide teams, staff from all departments focus on a process that affects the entire organization. For example, such a team might focus on the medical record that is used by all departments. Unit-based QI teams identify clinical priorities for a work unit. Client understanding of discharge instructions and the associated education process is an example of a unit-based QI project for a nursing unit.

Components of a QI Program. QI programs focus on processes or systems that significantly contribute to outcomes. To identify areas for improvement, an organization considers those activities that are high volume, high risk, and/or problem areas (CCHSA, 2003). A systematic approach is required to ensure that all staff support the QI goals. Many Canadian health care organizations use the CCHSA's standards and criteria for QI, as well as one or more of the available process-improvement models. The models have similar elements, such as process or problem identification, establishment of a target to guide the process, collection and analysis of data, interpretation of results, and implementation of the improvements followed by evaluation of the improvements (Wendt & Vale, 2003). An organization may use the CCHSA standards to organize its QI program, but use a QI model such as FOCUS-PDCA (Table 10-2) to structure problem analysis and resolution.

Responsibility for a QI Program. Leadership and planning are essential to creating a work culture that supports QI. The work environment should be a non-threatening place that promotes teamwork; treats people with respect, dignity, and trust; encourages open communication; and benefits everyone involved in QI (Wendt & Vale, 2003). Most organizations have a director responsible for QI activities. Individual staff members are responsible for

Table 10-2 Models for Process Improvement

Pride	Focus-PDCA	Fade
Process—select one to improve	**F**ind process to improve	**F**ocus on a problem
Relevant dimensions of performance measurement	**O**rganize team that knows process	**A**nalyze the problem
Interpret data and evaluate variance	**C**larify current knowledge of process	**D**evelop a plan
Design or redesign the process	**U**nderstand causes of process variation	**E**xecute the plan
Execute the plan	**S**elect process improvement	
Improve—validate by remeasuring	**PDCA: P**lan, **D**o, **C**heck, **A**ct	

Modified from "Optimizing Performance Through Process Improvement," by P. Keill and T. Johnson, 1994, *Journal of Nursing Care Quality, 9*(1), p. 1.

monitoring practice, making decisions about ways to improve practice, and evaluating results.

Scope of Service. Each nursing care area involved in the care of a select group of clients provides a well-defined set of services. A unit's scope of service includes the types of clients and the types of processes used to deliver care. An example is a general medicine unit in a hospital that cares for middle-aged and older clients with diabetes, heart disease, and gastrointestinal disorders. The unit's processes include IV administration, diabetes education, referrals for cardiac diagnostic testing, and endoscopy. Understanding the scope of service allows staff to focus on quality. Unit-based committees review services that are considered a priority for clients. This helps prioritize activities within the unit's scope of service.

Developing Quality Indicators. A **quality indicator** is a quantitative measure that helps determine if a service conforms to established standards or requirements. The quality indicator is the focus for a QI project, with the staff monitoring criteria that will show whether indicator standards have been met. There are three types of indicators: structure, process, and outcome.

Structure indicators evaluate the structure or systems for delivering care; an example is adherence in checking whether forms documenting restraint use are completed correctly. Process indicators evaluate the manner in which care is delivered (e.g., the process of pain assessment and clients' referral to community services). Outcome indicators, as described earlier, evaluate the end result of care (e.g., incidence of nosocomial infection and adherence to medication therapy). Outcomes are the most important indicators in any QI program, but structural and process indicators cannot be ignored.

Processes of care are closely related to outcomes and the structure in which a process of care occurs, enhances, or hinders the effectiveness of care (Titler, 2001). To judge whether standards of care are met, processes and outcomes are measured. For example, a staff measures its success in implementing a new process of diabetes instruction and also measures the outcome: can clients administer insulin correctly? When selecting quality indicators, teams should consider processes and related outcomes that are most likely to improve nursing practice. Processes to improve may include the following:

- A weak process that is causing problems (e.g., poor pain management for clients with cancer)
- A stable process that is adequate but can improve (e.g., waiting time for ambulatory surgery clients)
- A process linked to negative outcomes (e.g., care of IV access sites with the occurrence of phlebitis).

Establishing Thresholds for Evaluation. After selecting a quality indicator, the staff chooses quantitative measures for the indicator. The occurrence of an indicator, or the percentage of times the indicator is observed (e.g., the number of surgical clients who can explain their discharge instructions), is a common measure. A threshold is a standard for determining if a problem exists. A measurement that falls below the threshold indicates a problem. For example, a staff may set a threshold that 95% of clinic clients over the age of 65 years will receive flu shots. If only 90% had flu shots, the threshold is not being met, and staff must review factors interfering with client education and adherence. When QI is ongoing, staff continuously improve outcomes or performance by raising thresholds.

Data Collection and Analysis. Data collection and analysis can be simple or complex. The key is to obtain accurate results that guide decisions about quality care. Many organizations that value QI conduct formal research (see chapter 6). When formal research is not done, staff may collect data on frequencies or percentages for a predetermined number of clients. Such data provide information on practice trends and problems. Sufficient data should be collected on the right criteria. QI teams usually can access resources that help determine how much information in needed for QI analysis. If a team is evaluating diabetic instruction and insulin administration, they might monitor the use of teaching materials, staff's compliance with teaching standards, and each client's score on a return demonstration test. When sufficient data are collected, the team can determine if problems exist and analyze possible causes.

Evaluation of Care. Monitoring of quality indicators helps to evaluate whether a specifically defined process reaches desired outcomes. If results meet or exceed a threshold, or if performance is within controls set for a process, the process is effective. When thresholds are not met or when performance is below the control limits set, staff must look for the cause of problems. For example, staff must discover why diabetic clients score an average of only 70% on a return demonstration test. Staff review practice activities and look for ways to reinforce nursing care standards or improve practice.

When a process is not effective, the staff may use a QI model (e.g., FOCUS-PDCA). A model helps staff to isolate the aspect of the process to improve, organize an expert team that knows the process, clarify knowledge about the process, understand sources of variation, and select an improvement. In the diabetes example, staff nurses, dietitians, diabetes nurse specialists, and pharmacists should be on the QI team. The team determines factors associated with a practice problem and recommends ways to improve the process and achieve desired outcomes.

Resolution of Problems. Staff develop action plans to improve the process and outcomes. Actions should be achievable. Merely notifying staff of a problem is unlikely to improve outcomes. In FOCUS-PDCA, staff *P*lan the action or improvement to make, *D*o or implement the change, *C*heck or analyze results of the change, and then *A*ct on the findings. For example, the QI team discovers that clients are not administering insulin correctly due to insufficient information. Clients lack information because staff do not start teaching early enough (as soon as clients learn that they require insulin). Also, the staff lack teaching materials. The team recommends that the pharmacy includes instructional materials when insulin is sent to the unit and that a clinical pharmacist assist with insulin therapy instruction. The staff nurses and nurse specialist develop a practice protocol that outlines specific content to teach the client how to administer injections.

Evaluation of Improvement. The staff evaluate the success of the action plan. In the example, they monitor the new teaching process and the results of client testing. If test scores improve, outcomes have improved; if they do not improve, a new action plan is needed. When desired outcomes are not met, the staff reinstitutes the QI process.

Communication of Results. The results of QI activities must be communicated to staff in appropriate departments. If they are not communicated, practice changes will likely not occur. Regular discussions of QI activities through staff meetings, newsletters, and memos are examples of communication strategies. Often, a QI study reveals information requiring organization-wide change. The organization must respond to the problem with the resources needed for change. For example, organizations may respond by revising policies and procedures, modifying standards of care, or implementing system changes.

Key Concepts

- A manager must set a vision or philosophy for a work unit, ensure appropriate staffing, mobilize staff and institutional resources to achieve objectives, motivate staff members to carry out their work, set standards of performance, and make the right decisions to achieve objectives.
- An empowered nursing staff has decision-making authority to change how they practise.
- Nursing care delivery models vary by the responsibility of the RN in coordinating care delivery and the roles other staff members play in assisting with care.
- Continuity of nursing care can be compromised in total patient care delivery, functional nursing, and team nursing.
- Critical to the success of decentralized decision making is making staff members aware that they have the responsibility, authority, autonomy, and accountability for the care they give and the decisions they make.
- A nurse manager can foster decentralized decision making by establishing nursing practice committees, supporting nurse-physician and interdisciplinary collaboration, setting and implementing quality improvement plans, and maintaining timely staff communication.
- Clinical care coordination involves accurate clinical decision making, establishing priorities, efficient organizational skills, appropriate use of resources and time management skills, and an ongoing evaluation of care activities.
- To promote an enriching professional environment, each member of a nursing work team is responsible for open, professional communication.
- Delegation involves transferring responsibility for performing an activity while retaining accountability for the outcome.
- When done correctly, delegation can improve job efficiency and job enrichment.
- An important responsibility for the nurse who delegates nursing care is evaluation of the staff member's performance and client outcomes.
- In a quality improvement environment, every staff member becomes involved in finding ways to improve or change work processes so as to promote client or customer satisfaction.
- A well-organized quality improvement program focuses on processes or systems that significantly contribute to improvement of outcomes.

Key Terms

Accountability, *p. 153*
Authority, *p. 153*
Autonomy, *p. 153*
Case management, *p. 152*
Continuous quality improvement (CQI), *p. 158*
Decentralized management, *p. 152*
Delegation, *p. 156*
Functional nursing, *p. 150*
Outcome, *p. 159*
Primary nursing, *p. 151*
Quality improvement (QI), *p. 158*
Quality indicator, *p. 160*
Responsibility, *p. 152*
Team nursing, *p. 151*
Total patient care, *p. 151*
Total quality management (TQM), *p. 158*

Critical Thinking Exercises

1. John, an RN, is working with Tammy, an unregulated care provider, to manage care for five clients. John has completed morning assessments and rounds on the assigned clients and is giving Tammy directions for what she needs to do in the next hour. John says to Tammy, "Why don't you go to Room 415 and see what Mr. Thomas needs and go to Room 418 to check if Mrs. Landry is doing all right." Based on what you know about delegation, were these appropriate or inappropriate directions for Tammy? Provide a rationale for your answer.
2. The unit in which you are working has identified a problem: Clients are receiving initial doses of newly ordered medications 6 to 8 hours after the order is written. Your manager asks you to be the head of a quality improvement team to investigate this problem. Who would you want to be on your team? What would your first priority be? What data would you want to collect related to this problem?
3. You have just received morning shift report on your clients. You have been assigned the following clients:
   - A 52-year-old man who was admitted yesterday with a diagnosis of angina. He is scheduled for a cardiac stress test at 0900.
   - A 60-year-old woman who was transferred out of intensive care at 0630 today. She had uncomplicated coronary bypass surgery yesterday.
   - A 45-year-old man who experienced a myocardial infarction 3 days ago and is complaining of pain rated as 5 on a scale of 0 to 10.
   - A 76-year-old woman who had a permanent pacemaker inserted yesterday and is complaining of incision pain rated as a 7 on a scale of 0 to 10.

   Which one of these clients do you need to see first? Explain your answer.

Review Questions

1. The nursing model of client care in which tasks are divided, with one nurse assuming responsibility for specific tasks, for example, hygiene and dressing changes, and another nurse assuming responsibility for medication administration, is
   1. Team nursing
   2. Total patient care
   3. Functional nursing
   4. Primary nursing
2. The model of nursing care delivery that was developed with the aim of placing RNs at the bedside and improving nursing's accountability for client outcomes and the professional relationships among staff members is
   1. Team nursing
   2. Total patient care
   3. Functional nursing
   4. Primary nursing
3. The type of care management approach that coordinates and links health care services to clients and their families while streamlining costs and maintaining quality is
   1. Case management
   2. Total patient care
   3. Functional nursing
   4. Primary nursing
4. The type of management structure in which there is the potential for greater collaborative effort, increased competency of staff, and ultimately a greater sense of professional accomplishment and satisfaction is
   1. Case management
   2. Primary nursing
   3. Total patient care
   4. Decentralized
5. While administering medications, the nurse realizes she has given the wrong dose of medication to a client. The nurse acts by completing an incident report and notifying the client's physician. The nurse is exercising
   1. Authority
   2. Responsibility
   3. Accountability
   4. Decision making
6. Many managers distribute biweekly newsletters of ongoing unit or health care agency activities and post minutes of committee meetings in an accessible location for all staff to read. This is an example of
   1. Problem-solving committees
   2. Nurse/physician collaborative practice
   3. Interdisciplinary collaboration
   4. Staff communication
7. During the morning rounds, a nurse assesses the client's condition. He had major heart surgery 2 days ago. His vital signs are stable and his incision is clean and healing well. He complains of pain in his lower leg where the vein graft was removed. The nurse finds that the IV infusion is running on time but only 100 mL remains before the infusion runs out. An order exists for the IV infusion to continue. A second order of priority is
   1. The need to replace the IV bag with a new one
   2. The need to have an analgesic administered to the client for his leg pain
   3. The need to instruct the client on complications of wound health
   4. The need for the nurse to determine if the pharmacy has delivered IV solutions ordered for the day
8. A client is experiencing an anxiety attack. This is which priority nursing need for this client?
   1. First-order priority
   2. Second-order priority
   3. Third-order priority
   4. Fourth-order priority
9. The nurse checks on her client who was admitted to the hospital with pneumonia. He has been coughing profusely and has required nasotracheal suctioning. He has an IV infusion of antibiotics. He is febrile. The client asks the nurse if he can have a bath because he has been perspiring profusely. The nurse may dele-

gate to the unregulated care provider working with her today the task of
1. Assessing vital signs
2. Changing IV dressing
3. Nasotracheal suctioning
4. Administering a bed bath

10. An example of a quality improvement outcome indicator is the
1. Rate of post-operative wound infection
2. Percentage of time it takes to count narcotics by nursing staff every shift
3. Number of clients receiving post-operative education on possible surgical complications
4. Time it takes for a client to be transported from the emergency department to an inpatient nursing unit

References

Aiken, L. H., et al. (2002). Hospital nurse staffing and patient mortality, nurse burnout, and job dissatisfaction. *The Journal of the American Medical Association, 288*(16), 1987–1993.

Aiken, L. H., Havens, D. S., & Sloane, D. M. (2000). The Magnet Nursing Services Recognition Programme: A Comparison of Two Groups of Magnet Hospitals. *American Journal of Nursing, 100*(3), 26–35.

American Nurses Association. (1997). Position statement on registered nurse utilization of unlicensed assistive personnel. Retrieved November 24, 2004, from *http://www.nursingworld.org/readroom/position/uap/uapuse.htm.*

Boblin-Cummings, S., Baumann, A., & Deber, R. (1999). Critical elements in the process of decision making: A nursing perspective. *Canadian Journal of Nursing Leadership, 12*(1), 6–13.

Buchan, J. (1999). Still attractive after all these years? Magnet hospitals in a changing health care environment. *Journal of Advanced Nursing, 30*(1), 100–108.

Canadian Council on Health Services Accreditation. (2003). *2003 Accreditation recognition guidelines.* Ottawa, ON: Author.

Canadian Nurses Association. (1995). *Unregulated health care workers supporting nursing care delivery—Position statement.* Ottawa, ON: Author.

Canadian Nurses Association. (2002). *Nursing leadership—Position statement.* Ottawa, ON: Author.

Canadian Nurses Association. (2003a). *Scopes of practice—Joint position statement.* Ottawa, ON: Author.

Canadian Nurses Association. (2003b). *Staffing decisions for the delivery of safe nursing care—Position statement.* Ottawa, ON: Author.

Case Management Society of America. (2003). Membership information. Retrieved November 24, 2004, from *http: http://www.cmsa.org/Membership/*

College of Nurses of Ontario. (2004). *Quality assurance practice consultation program.* Toronto, ON: Author.

Cortes, T., Noyes, B., & Brennan, E (2000). Is now the time to design new care delivery models? *Journal of Nursing Administration, 30*(9), 403–404.

Cox, S. (1995, Fall). *Managing the workplace 2000.* Seminar conducted at Barnes-Jewish Hospital, St. Louis, MO.

Curtin, L. (1994). The heart of patient care. *Nursing Management, 25*(5), 7–8.

Dadich, K. A. (2003). Care delivery strategies. In P. S. Yoder-Wise (Ed.), *Leading and managing in nursing* (3rd ed., pp. 253–274). St. Louis, MO: Mosby.

Ellis, J.R., & Hartley, C.L. (2005). *Managing and coordinating nursing care* (4th ed). Philadelphia, PA: Lippincott Williams & Wilkins.

Hansten, R., & Washburn, M. (1999). Seven steps to shift from tasks to outcomes. *Nursing Management, 30*(7), 24–27.

Hicks, F. (2003). Collective action. In P. S. Yoder-Wise (Ed.), *Leading and managing in nursing* (3rd ed., pp. 155–171). St. Louis, MO: Mosby.

Johnson, M., Mass, M. L., & Moorhead, S. (2000). *Nursing outcomes classification (NOC)* (2nd ed.). St. Louis, MO: Mosby.

Joint Commission on Accreditation of Healthcare Organizations. (2002). *Comprehensive accreditation manual for hospitals: The official handbook.* Oakbrook Terrace, IL: Author.

Keeling, B., et al. (2000). Appropriate delegation. *American Journal of Nursing, 100*(12): 24A–24D.

Keill, P., & Johnson, T. (1994). Optimizing performance through process improvement. *Journal of Nursing Care Quality, 9*(1), 1–9.

Lilley, L. (2002). Shared governance: Turning decisions over to staff. In E. Howkins & C. Thornton (eds.), *Managing and leading innovation in health care* (pp 211–219). London: Bailliere Tindall.

Maddox, P. J. (1999). Quality management in nursing practice. In J. Lancaster (Ed.), *Nursing issues in leading and managing change.* St. Louis, MO: Mosby.

McGillis Hall, L. (1997). Staff mix models: Complementary or substitution roles for nurses. *Nursing Administration Quarterly, 21*(2), 31–39.

National Council of State Boards of Nursing. (1995). *Delegation: Concepts and decision-making process.* Chicago, IL: Author.

Parkman, C. A. (1996). Delegation: Are you doing it right? *American Journal of Nursing, 96*(9), 42–47.

Peters, D. A. (1995). Outcomes: The mainstay of a framework for quality care. *Journal of Nursing Care Quality, 10*(1), 61–69.

Pinkerton, S. E. (2001). Nurses executives: Who are they; what do they do; and what challenges do they face? In J. C. McCloskey & H. K. Grace (Eds.), *Current issues in nursing* (6th ed., pp. 26–29). St. Louis, MO: Mosby.

Registered Nurses Association of British Columbia. (2003). Quality practice environment program. Vancouver, BC: Author.

Registered Nurses Association of Ontario. (2003). *A phenomenal journey: The Nursing Best Practice Guidelines Project: Shaping the future of nursing.* Toronto, ON: Author.

Ritter-Teitel, J. (2002). The impact of restructuring on professional nursing practice. *Journal of Nursing Administration, 32*(1), 31–41.

Scott, J. G., Sochalski, J., & Aiken, L. (1999). Review of magnet hospital research: Findings and implications for professional nursing practice. *The Journal of Nursing Administration, 29*(1), 9–19.

Sorrentino, S. (2004). *Mosby's Canadian textbook for the support worker.* Toronto, ON: Elsevier.

Street, M. M. (1973). *Watch-Fires on the mountains: The life and writing of Ethel Johns.* Toronto, ON: University of Toronto Press.

Tebbitt, B. V. (1997). Nurse executives: Who are they, what do they do, and what challenges do they face? In J. C. McCloskey & H. K. Grace (Eds.), *Current issues in nursing* (5th ed., pp. 26–31. St. Louis, MO: Mosby.

Titler, M. G. (2001). Outcomes management for quality improvement. In J. C. McCloskey & H. K. Grace (Eds.), *Current issues in nursing* (6th ed., pp. 246–254). St. Louis, MO: Mosby.

Wendt, D. A., & Vale, D. J. (2003). Managing quality and risk. In P. S. Yoder-Wise (Ed.), *Leading and managing in nursing* (3rd ed., pp. 173–189). St. Louis, MO: Mosby.

Werner, K. M. (1999). Nursing's role in improving the quality of health care. In B. Chery & S. R. Jacob (Eds.), *Contemporary nursing: Issues, trends and management.* St. Louis, MO: Mosby.

Wywialowski, E. (1997). *Managing client care* (2nd ed.). St. Louis, MO: Mosby.

Recommended Web Sites

Canadian Council of Health Services Accreditation:
http//www.cchsa.ca
The Canadian Council on Health Services Accreditation (CCHSA) is a national, non-profit, independent organization whose role is to help health services organizations, across Canada and internationally, examine and improve the quality of care and service they provide to their clients.

Canadian Nurses Association:
http//www.cna-nurses.ca
The Canadian Nurses Association (CNA) is a federation of 11 provincial and territorial nursing associations representing more than 120,000 registered nurses. CNA's mission is to advance the quality of nursing in the interest of the public.

Canadian Nursing Students Association:
http//www.aeic.ca
The Canadian Nursing Students' Association (CNSA) is the national voice of Canadian nursing students in diploma and baccalaureate registered nursing programs. Its aim is to increase the legal, ethical, professional, and educational aspects of nursing. CNSA is dedicated to an active and positive promotion of nurses and the nursing profession as a whole.

Institute for Healthcare Improvement:
http://www.ihi.org/ihi
The Institute for Healthcare Improvement (IHI) is a not-for-profit organization driving the improvement of health by advancing the quality and value of health care.

International Council of Nurses:
http://www.icn.ch/
The International Council of Nurses (ICN) is a federation of national nurses' associations, representing nurses in more than 120 countries. Operated by nurses for nurses, ICN works to ensure quality nursing care for all, sound health policies globally, and the advancement of nursing knowledge.

11

Critical Thinking in Nursing Practice

Patricia A. Potter, RN, MSN, PhD, CMAC, FAAN
Donna M. Romyn, RN, PhD (Canadian author)

Objectives

Mastery of content in this chapter will enable the student to:

- Define the key terms listed.
- Discuss the nurse's responsibility in making clinical decisions.
- Discuss how reflection can improve a nurse's practice.
- Describe how intuition affects clinical decisions.
- Compare and contrast critical thinking competencies.
- Describe the components of a critical thinking model for clinical decision making.
- Discuss critical thinking skills used in nursing practice.
- Explain the relationship between clinical experience and critical thinking.
- Discuss the critical thinking attitudes used in clinical decision making.
- Explain how professional standards influence a nurse's clinical decisions.
- Discuss the relationship of the nursing process to critical thinking.

Nurses face an endless variety of situations involving clients, family members, health care staff, and peers. In every clinical situation, nurses must think critically and make sound judgments so that clients receive the very best nursing care. Critical thinking is not a simple, step-by-step, linear process that can be learned overnight; it is acquired through hard work, commitment, and curiosity. Ideally, critical thinking becomes a habit of mind, a part of each nurse's character (N. Facione & P. Facione, 1996).

Clinical Decisions in Nursing Practice

Nurses are responsible for making accurate clinical decisions. Clinical decision making separates professional nurses from technical or ancillary personnel. Nurses, for example, act immediately when a client's clinical condition deteriorates, decide if a client is experiencing complications that warrant notification of the physician, and determine whether a teaching plan for a client is ineffective and must be revised. A nurse must think critically, solve problems, and find the best solution for clients' needs in order to assist clients in maintaining, regaining, or improving their health. However, most clients have health care problems for which there are no clear solutions. Each client's problem is unique, a product of many factors, including the client's physical health, lifestyle, culture, relationship with family and friends, living environment, and experiences. Thus, a nurse does not always have a clear picture of the client's needs and the appropriate actions to take when first meeting a client. Instead, the nurse must learn to question and explore different perspectives in order to find the best solution to help the client (Whiteside, 1997).

Because no two clients have identical health problems, a nurse is always challenged to observe each client closely, search for and examine ideas and inferences about client problems, consider scientific principles relating to the problems, recognize the problems, and develop an approach to nursing care. A nurse learns to creatively seek new knowledge as needed, act quickly when events change, and make sound decisions that promote the client's well-being. The challenges of clinical decision making are part of what makes nursing fulfilling. Over time, a nurse gains the expertise to test and refine nursing approaches, learn from successes and failures, and apply new knowledge. Critical thinking, problem solving, and decision making are central to nursing practice.

Critical Thinking Defined

Thinking and learning are interrelated, lifelong processes (Chaffee, 1994). Over time, knowledge and experience in clinical practice help broaden the nurse's ability to make thoughtful observations, judgments, and choices. **Critical thinking** is an active, organized, cognitive process used to carefully examine one's thinking and the thinking of others (Chaffee, 1994). It involves forming conclusions, making decisions, drawing inferences, and reflecting (Gordon, 1995). It means taking nothing for granted. A critical thinker identifies and challenges assumptions, considers key aspects of a situation, imagines and explores alternatives, considers ethical principles, applies reason and logic, and thus makes informed decisions. Critical thinking begins by asking these questions: What do I really know about this nursing care situation? How do I know it? What options are available to me? (Paul & Heaslip, 1995). For example, What do I really know about a client's pain? How do I know the client is in pain? What options are available to relieve the pain? Unless such questions are asked, a nurse can easily form inaccurate conclusions and take inappropriate actions.

Critical thinking requires a certain basic level of intellectual humility (i.e., acknowledging one's own ignorance) and a commitment to thinking and reasoning. It leads to a precise and accurate assessment of a situation and enables the nurse to act on the basis of knowledge gained from the situation and from nursing science. Critical thinking also requires one to ask questions, be well informed, face and reconsider personal biases, and think clearly about issues (P. Facione, 1990). Core critical thinking skills, when applied to nursing, are useful in showing the complex nature of clinical decision making (Table 11-1). Being able to apply these skills takes practice, a sound knowledge base, and thoughtful consideration of the knowledge gained in the clinical care of clients.

Nurses who apply critical thinking in their work focus on options for solving problems and making decisions, rather than hastily and carelessly forming quick, simple solutions (Kataoka-Yahiro & Saylor, 1994). Indeed, nurses who work in crisis situations such as those that occur in the emergency department or the intensive care unit must often act quickly when client problems develop. However, even these nurses exercise discipline in decision making so as to avoid premature and inappropriate decisions. Thinking critically helps a nurse advocate for clients and make better-informed choices about their care. Critical thinking is more than just problem solving—it is an attempt to continually improve how one addresses problems in client care. Each clinical experience helps a nurse pursue learning opportunities that are focused on excellence in practice. There are three important aspects of critical thinking: reflection, language, and intuition.

Table 11-1 Critical Thinking Skills

Skill	Description	Nursing Practice Applications
Interpretation	Categorization Clarifying meaning	Be systematic in data collection. Look for patterns to categorize data (e.g., nursing diagnoses [see chapter 12]). Clarify any data you are uncertain about.
Analysis	Examining ideas Analyzing arguments	Be open-minded as you look at information about a client. Do not make careless assumptions. Do the data reveal what you believe is true, or are there other options?
Evaluation	Assessing results Assessing arguments	Look at all situations objectively. Use criteria (e.g., expected outcomes, pain characteristics, learning objectives) to determine results of nursing actions. Reflect on your own behaviour.
Inference	Examining evidence Speculating or conjecturing alternatives Drawing conclusions	Look at the meaning and significance of findings. Are there relationships between findings? Does the data about the client help you determine that a problem exists?
Explanation	Stating results Justifying procedures Presenting arguments	Support your findings and conclusions. Use knowledge to select strategies you use in the care of clients.
Self-regulation	Self-examination Self-correction	Reflect on your experiences. Identify in what way you can improve your own performance. What will make you feel that you have been successful?

Adapted from *Critical Thinking: A statement of Expert Consensus for Purposes of Educational Assessment and Instruction. The Delphi Report: Research Findings and Recommendations Prepared for the American Philosophical Association,* by P. Facione, 1990, Washington, DC: American Philosophical Association (ERIC Document Reproduction Services No. ED 315-423).

Reflection

An important aspect of critical thinking is **reflection,** the process of purposefully thinking back or recalling a situation to discover its purpose or meaning (Miller & Babcock, 1996). Nurses should think back on a client situation, make sense of the experience, and thus gain insight into the meaning of the situation. For example, after caring for a client who is recovering from heart surgery, one might reflect on how the client reacted when discussing diet restrictions and exercise guidelines. What did it mean when the client said, "I don't know what my family will think about this new diet," or "Exercise has never been something I enjoyed doing"? Such reflection provides new insight (Smith & Johnston, 2002). It involves taking time to honestly review everything one can remember about a situation. Reflection requires adequate knowledge and is necessary for self-evaluation when reviewing one's successes or opportunities for improvement. However, O'Neill and Dluhy (1997) caution new clinicians not to question every judgment they make. Emphasizing reflection can deter thinking in a clinical situation because of the second-guessing it can create.

With reflection, a nurse seeks to understand the relationships between concepts learned in the classroom and real-life clinical situations. In the earlier example, the client's response to new diet and exercise guidelines may result from fear, denial, or concern over family support. Reflection allows the nurse to consider all possibilities, refer to knowledge learned previously, and then return to assess the client, identify relevant problems, and clarify any concerns. Reflection allows a nurse to judge personal performance while also judging whether standards of nursing practice were followed. It is a process that helps make sense of an experience so that the next time a similar situation arises, the nurse can use approaches that were successful or revise a previous approach to achieve better client outcomes. For example, a nurse considers the client's comments and his or her responses to the client's comments. Did I respond so the client could express his views openly? Did I listen? Did I form unfounded conclusions without sufficient information?

Engaging in reflection is an individualized process (Miller & Babcock, 1996), and learning to be reflective takes practice (Box 11-1). When reflecting on a clinical experience, a nurse should be open to new information and consider the perspective of both the client and nurse. Paget (2001) suggested that reflective practice has the potential for improving nurses' clinical practice and for influencing their self-awareness and the manner in which they interact with clients (Box 11-2). Paget also argued that the routine use of reflective practice can positively affect client outcomes.

Because nursing is a self-governing profession, each professional organization and nursing regulatory body has developed tools to help nurses systematically reflect on their practice and assess their competency (e.g., Alberta Association of Registered Nurses *Continuing Competency Program* and the College of Nurses of Ontario *Self-Assessment Tool*). Although the format of these tools varies somewhat, they all reflect the knowledge, skills, attitudes, and judgments expected of the nurse. Students may also find these tools useful in assessing their progress in acquiring the competencies required of graduate nurses. The Web site of each provincial or territorial professional nursing association contains the tools currently in use in its jurisdiction (see Recommended Web Sites).

Box 11-1 Tips on Facilitating Reflection

- As you care for a client, consider your client's situation and what your assessment findings mean. What physical or psychological changes are occurring? How does this compare to normal functioning?
- When you chart or report on your client, consider the meaning of his or her symptoms and associated treatment. Always ask what could be happening (Fowler, 1998).
- Reflect carefully on any critical incidents (e.g., safety episodes, cardiac arrests, pivotal events in the progression of a client's disease; Bittner & Tobin, 1998). What occurred? What actions were taken? How did the client respond? Were there other actions you might have taken?
- At the end of each working day, take time to reflect. Ask yourself whether you achieved your original plan of care. If you did, what made it successful? If you did not, what were the barriers or factors requiring changes? What would you do differently or the same?
- Keep a journal or summative description of your experiences with clients. Be sure to include the following elements: identification, description, significance, and implications (Baker, 1996). Telling a story and drawing a picture are two ways to identify the situation or experience. Describe what you felt, thought, and did. Analyze the significance of the experience by considering feelings, thoughts, and possible meanings. Describe the implications of the experience in terms of your own clinical practice or self-perceptions as a learner. Refer to the journal often when you care for clients in similar situations. The journal can become a rich resource for you to revisit important experiences and gain insight into the thoughts and actions that make up clinical practice.
- Talk with a colleague who works with you and has observed your clinical work. Ask if his or her observations are the same as yours.
- Keep all written care plans or clinical papers. Use them as a resource for future clients. Maintain a logical filing system.
- Make time for reflection, both after having cared for a client and before caring for new clients with similar conditions. How is your current client similar to or different from previous clients?

Language

Another important aspect of critical thinking is the use of language. The ability to use language is closely associated with the ability to think meaningfully (Miller & Babcock, 1996). To think critically, a nurse must be able to use language precisely and clearly. Vague and inaccurate language reflects sloppy thinking.

Clear communication with clients, families, and health care professionals is crucial. When a nurse uses incorrect terminology, jargon, or vague descriptions, communication is ineffective. This deficiency may become obvious if the client is unable to co-operate with nursing therapies or if members of the nursing team do not follow through

Research Highlight — Box 11-2

Reflective Practice Improves Nursing Practice

Research Focus

Reflective practice, the use of reflection to help nurses expand and develop their clinical knowledge, is considered a useful method for developing nurses' practice. Techniques for developing reflective practice are being used in academic settings. The question is, does reflective practice influence a nurse's practice and client outcomes?

Research Abstract

This was an evaluative study to determine whether student nurses who had participated in a reflective practice course or course module perceived any change in their clinical practice. The study involved both undergraduate and graduate nurses. The research used a combination of focus groups (small groups of students sharing views together), questionnaires, and individual phone interviews. The majority of students found reflective practice useful, particularly when a group approach was used. In groups, students are able to discuss clinical events with individuals from similar backgrounds and experiences. The process of learning to reflect was perceived to improve students' self-awareness, their attitudes toward clients, and their insight into the clinical environment. Most students also felt that reflective practice changed their clinical practice in a way that benefited clients. Once learned, the skill of reflecting can be a medium for constant reviewing of professional practice. For a few students, reflective practice helped them learn to apply research findings to a specific area of clinical practice.

Evidence-Based Practice

The benefits of reflective practice should be considered for any student wishing to use reflection on a regular basis. Reflective practice was found to:

- Provide students with new insight
- Enhance communication skills
- Encourage use of research findings
- Increase a student's ability to reflect in actual practice
- Improve students' ability to deal with others more honestly and openly

Reference

Paget, T. (2001). Reflective practice and clinical outcomes: Practitioners' views on how reflective practice has influenced their clinical practice. *Journal of Clinical Nursing, 10*(2), 204–214.

on the nurse's recommendations. Critical thinking requires a framing of one's thoughts so that the focus and message are clear. It helps to reflect on one's language and to consider whether one communicates and expresses an idea, position, or judgment precisely and clearly.

Intuition

Intuition is the direct understanding of particulars in a situation without conscious deliberation (Benner, Hooper-Kyriakidis, & Stannard, 1999). It is an inner sense that something is so. In other words, intuition occurs when an experienced nurse walks into a client's room, looks at the client's appearance without the benefit of a thorough assessment, and senses that the client is about to deteriorate physically. Intuition in nursing develops as one's clinical experience increases. Intuition appears to act as a trigger, sparking an analytical process that leads nurses in a conscious search to acquire data that confirm their sense of change in a client's status (King & Clark, 2002). For example, when first entering the room to check on a client, an experienced surgical nurse may suspect that something is wrong. The nurse senses by looking at the client that something is out of place and the client is likely experiencing a surgical complication. The nurse then acts on intuition by gathering information to determine whether a problem really exists. For example, the nurse will ask how the client feels and will assess vital signs, the client's wound, and the intravenous line status.

It is important to remember, however, that nurses cannot safely act on intuition alone. They must use various cognitive and emotional cues to trigger critical thinking and then to select nursing interventions. It is critical to know what knowledge one has, but it is even more critical to know what one does not know. Nurses should trust their intuition as a "red flag" or signal that something is not quite right, but they should not take intuition as an automatic truth. As soon as intuition strikes, a nurse should probe further to assess a client's situation (Fowler, 1998). If nurses do not recognize what they do not know about their clients, there is a risk that clients will receive improper care. Each clinical situation requires careful and thoughtful analysis for accurate and sound clinical decisions to be made.

Thinking and Learning

Learning is a lifelong process. Intellectual and emotional growth involves acquiring new knowledge and refining the ability to think, solve problems, and make judgments. To learn, one must be flexible and open to new information. The science of nursing is growing rapidly, and there will always be new information to apply in practice. Over time, as nurses have new experiences and apply the knowledge gained, they become better able to form hypotheses, present ideas, and make valid conclusions.

A nurse must learn to think about a client's status and to anticipate nursing needs. Anticipation involves looking ahead and asking, What is the client's status? How might it change? How can nursing knowledge be applied to improve the client's condition? Thinking cannot become routine or standardized. Instead, the nurse should look beyond the obvious in any clinical situation, explore the client's unique responses to health alterations, and recognize what actions are necessary to benefit the client's well-being. This process does not mean that the nurse knows nothing about a client until they meet: A nurse's experience with other clients aids in recognizing patterns of behaviour, seeing commonalities in signs and symptoms, and anticipating reactions to therapies. Thinking about those experiences enables the nurse to better anticipate client needs and recognize problems when they develop.

Nursing practice is always changing. As new knowledge becomes available, nurses must challenge traditional ways of doing things and discover those interventions that are most effective, have scientific relevance, and result in better client outcomes. For example, for many years, nurses were taught to massage a client's reddened skin to improve circulation. Nursing research has shown that massaging a reddened pressure area causes capillary injury and promotes skin breakdown. Massage of reddened skin is no longer practised, and the use of alternating airflow mattresses is the new, accepted therapy for pressure ulcer care. By applying current knowledge, a nurse is able to think critically and to positively influence nursing practice.

Levels of Critical Thinking in Nursing

The ability to think critically expands as a nurse gains new knowledge and experience and matures into a competent professional. Kataoka-Yahiro and Saylor (1994) developed a critical thinking model that incorporates three levels of critical thinking in nursing: basic, complex, and commitment.

Basic Critical Thinking

At the basic level of critical thinking, a learner trusts that experts have the right answers for every problem. Thinking is concrete and based on a set of rules or principles. For example, a nurse uses an institution's procedure manual to confirm how to insert a Foley catheter. The nurse follows the procedure step by step without adjusting it to meet a client's unique needs (e.g., positioning to accommodate the client's pain or mobility restrictions). For basic critical thinkers, answers to complex problems are either right or wrong (e.g., there is too much or insufficient air in the Foley catheter balloon), and one right answer usually exists for each problem. Basic critical thinking is an early step in the development of reasoning ability (Kataoka-Yahiro & Saylor, 1994), revealing that the individual has had limited critical thinking experience. Despite the tendency to be governed by others, a person gradually learns to accept the diverse opinions and values of experts (e.g., instructors and staff nurse role models). However, inexperience, weak competencies, and inflexible attitudes can restrict a person's ability to move to the next level of critical thinking.

Complex Critical Thinking

A person begins to detach from authorities and analyze and examine alternatives more independently at the complex level of critical thinking. Kataoka-Yahiro and Saylor (1994) noted that the nurse's best answer to a problem at this level is, "It depends." The person's thinking abilities and initiative to look beyond expert opinion begin to develop. A nurse realizes that alternative, and perhaps conflicting, solutions exist. Consider the case of Mr. Rosen, a 36-year-old man who underwent hip surgery. He is having pain but refuses his prescribed analgesic. His physician is concerned that the client will not progress as planned, delaying rehabilitation. While discussing the importance of rehabilitation with Mr. Rosen, the nurse respects the client's decision to avoid taking pain medication. The nurse learns that the client practices meditation at home and decides to discuss this with the client as a pain control option.

In complex critical thinking, each solution has benefits and risks that the nurse weighs before making a final decision. Options are acknowledged and thinking becomes more creative and innovative. There is a willingness to consider deviations from standard protocols or policies when complex situations develop. Nurses learn a variety of different approaches for the same therapy.

Commitment

The third level of critical thinking is commitment (Kataoka-Yahiro & Saylor, 1994). The individual anticipates the need to make choices without assistance from others and then assumes accountability for them. At this level, the nurse does more than just consider the complex alternatives that a problem poses. At the commitment level, the nurse chooses an action or belief based on the alternatives available and stands by it. Sometimes an action may be no action, or the nurse may choose to delay an action until a later time but does so as a result of experience and knowledge. Because the nurse assumes accountability for the decision, attention is given to the results of the decision and a determination of whether it was appropriate.

Critical Thinking Competencies

Critical thinking competencies are the cognitive processes a nurse uses to make judgments. These competencies include (a) general critical thinking, (b) specific critical thinking in clinical situations, and (c) specific critical thinking in nursing (Kataoka-Yahiro & Saylor, 1994).

General critical thinking competencies are not unique to nursing. They are used in other disciplines and in nonclinical, everyday situations. General critical thinking competencies include applying the scientific method, problem solving, and decision making. Specific critical thinking competencies are applied by physicians, nurses, and other health care professionals when making clinical care decisions. These specific competencies include diagnostic reasoning/inference and clinical decision making. Finally, the critical thinking competency specific to nursing practice is the application of the nursing process.

General Critical Thinking Competencies

Applying the Scientific Method. The scientific method is an approach to reasoning that is used in nursing, medicine, and other disciplines. Using this approach, one seeks the truth or verifies that a set of facts agrees with reality. Nurse researchers use the **scientific method** when testing hypotheses or research questions in nurs-

Table 11-2 Steps of the Scientific Method

Step	Example in Practice
Identify the problem to be investigated.	Family members have difficulty communicating with a dying loved one.
Collect data about the problem.	Review previous studies about grieving families. Review literature on methods for improving communication. Talk with dying clients about the kinds of feelings they think are important to communicate.
Formulate a hypothesis or research question to examine or explain the problem.	Family members who receive instruction on ways to communicate with dying loved ones will be perceived as more supportive by the dying family member.
Test the hypothesis or answer the research question.	Include family members in a group session on communication approaches. Have the family members use the new approaches when communicating with their dying loved ones.
Evaluate the results of the study to determine if the hypothesis was supported or refuted or the research question was answered.	Interview the clients to determine if they perceive family members to be more supportive.

ing practice situations (Table 11-2). For example, a nurse researcher might observe that clients in a hospice program often have difficulty communicating their feelings to family members. The nurse learns more about what causes this problem and considers the possibility that family members might have ineffective communication skills. The nurse asks the question, "Can family members who receive instruction in communication principles provide support to loved ones with a life-threatening illness?" The nurse might design a study that involves formal instruction in communication skills and uses a support group to help family members practise and apply the skills. Once the instruction and application are complete, the nurse might ask clients to evaluate their feelings about their communication with loved ones. The nurse hopes that results from the study will give other nurses working in hospice settings useful approaches for improving family communication. The scientific method is one formal way to approach a problem, plan a solution, test the solution, and come to a conclusion (see chapter 6).

Problem Solving. We all face problems every day, such as a computer program that does not function properly or a kitchen cabinet that fails to close completely. When a problem arises, we obtain information and then use the information in addition to what we already know to find a solution. Clients routinely present problems in nursing practice. For example, a nurse visits a home care client and learns that she has had difficulty taking her medications regularly. The nurse knows the client was discharged from the hospital and had five medications prescribed. The nurse sits down with the client and finds out that she has two over-the-counter medications that she takes regularly as well. When the nurse asks the client to show the medications that she takes in the morning, the nurse notices that the client has difficulty reading the medication labels. The client is able to describe the medications she is to take but is uncertain about the times of administration. The nurse recommends having the client's pharmacy relabel the medications in larger lettering. In addition, the nurse shows her examples of pill organizers that can allow her to sort her medications by time of day for 7 days.

Effective **problem solving** also involves evaluating the solution over time to be sure that it is still effective. If a problem recurs, it may become necessary to try different options. From the earlier example, during a follow-up visit, the nurse finds that the client has organized her medications correctly and can read the labels without difficulty. The nurse obtained information that correctly clarified the cause of the client's problem and tested a solution that proved successful. Having solved a problem in one situation adds to the nurse's practice experience and allows the nurse to apply that knowledge in future client situations.

Decision Making. When a person faces a problem or situation and must choose a course of action from several options, the person is engaged in decision making. **Decision making** is an end point of critical thinking that one hopes will lead to problem resolution. The decision-making process involves a series of steps: (a) recognizing and defining the problem, (b) assessing options, (c) weighing each option against a set of criteria, (d) testing possible options, (e) considering the consequences of the decision, and (f) making a final decision. For example, decision making occurs when a person chooses a family physician. The individual defines the problem (needs a physician), assesses all options (considers recommended physicians or looks for one whose office is close to home), considers each physician according to a set of criteria (experience, friendliness, reputation), tests possible options (talks directly with the physicians), considers the consequences of the decision (examines the pros and cons of selecting one physician over another), and then makes a final decision.

Although there is a sequence of steps, decision making also involves moving back and forth between steps. Using such a process leads to a conclusion that is informed and supported by evidence and reason (Bandman & Bandman, 1995). Examples of decision making in the clinical area include deciding on a choice of dressings for a wound or selecting the best approach for teaching a family how to assist a stroke client who is returning home. The nurse learns to make sound decisions by approaching each clinical situation thoughtfully and by applying each component of the decision-making process.

Specific Critical Thinking Competencies

Diagnostic Reasoning and Inference. As soon as a nurse receives information about a client in a particular clinical situation, **diagnostic reasoning** begins. In this process, the nurse gathers data by assigning meaning to the behaviours, physical signs, and symptoms presented by the client to logically determine the client's health status (O'Neill & Dluhy, 1997). Part of diagnostic reasoning is **inference,** which is the process of drawing conclusions from related pieces of evidence (Smith Higuchi & Donald, 2002). Forming a nursing diagnosis is a type of diagnostic reasoning (see chapter 12). For example, when a client presents symptoms of restlessness, guarded posturing, moaning, and abdominal discomfort, the nurse must retrieve knowledge regarding pain in the abdomen and then reason in a direct and precise way to determine the specific nature of the client's pain. The nurse collects as much information as possible to be sure a nursing diagnosis is accurate. Nurses do not make medical diagnoses, but they do assess and monitor clients closely and compare the client's signs and symptoms with those that are common to a medical diagnosis. This type of diagnostic reasoning assists in making clinical inferences or judgments about a client's progress. When certain symptoms present themselves, the nurse considers all variables influencing the client, including what is known about the client's pathological condition, to infer if the client is doing better or worse.

Consider this clinical example. Mrs. Spellman had a myocardial infarction (heart attack) 10 months ago. She must periodically be monitored for signs and symptoms of recurrent cardiac problems, such as chest pain, shortness of breath, and/or irregularity of vital signs. If Mrs. Spellman has a regular heart rate, denies discomfort, and is breathing without difficulty, the nurse may infer that the client's cardiac status is stable. The nurse must critically analyze changing clinical situations in order to immediately determine a client's status. Analysis of the client's condition allows the nurse to initiate appropriate therapies (e.g., activity restriction) so that the client's condition does not worsen. In addition, diagnostic conclusions made by the nurse will help the physician understand a problem more quickly and select proper medical therapies.

Clinical Decision Making. When approaching a clinical problem such as a client who has developed a pressure ulcer, the nurse collaborates with the client to identify the problem and choose nursing interventions that will meet mutually established goals of care. Nurses make clinical decisions all the time to improve a client's health or maintain wellness, either by minimizing the severity of the problem or by resolving it completely. The **clinical decision-making process** requires careful reasoning so that the options for the best client outcomes are chosen on the basis of the client's condition and the priority of the problem.

When making clinical decisions, the nurse first asks why a decision is necessary. For example, Mrs. Witowski is an 87-year-old client who lives alone. Her daughter, Marie, who lives nearby, is Mrs. Witowski primary caregiver. During a recent clinic visit, the nurse, Ruth, observes a bruised area of the skin over Mrs. Little's right hip. Mrs. Little says that she bruised herself when she slipped and fell on the edge of her bathtub. Knowing the client's age and the physiological changes that occur with aging, Ruth knows a decision is needed about whether Mrs. Little is living in a safe environment. To make a decision about actions to take to promote healing and prevent further injury, Ruth must collect facts and then select the information that is relevant to confirm the client's problems (Smith Higuchi & Donald, 2002). Ruth must consider Mrs. Little's physical condition (e.g., strengths and limitations), her home environment, and whether repeated injuries have been part of the client's history.

Strader (1992) identified decision-making criteria to assist nurses in making appropriate choices:

- What needs to be achieved? (healing of the skin, a safe home environment)
- What needs to be preserved? (mobility, nutrition, comfort, and safety)
- What needs to be avoided? (further tissue injury or infection and further falls)

The answers to these questions help the nurse make clinical decisions and then set priorities as they relate to the client's situation. Because each client brings different variables to a situation, an activity may be more of a priority in one situation and less of a priority in another. For example, if a client is immobile and incontinent of urine, the nurse recognizes skin integrity as a greater priority than if the client were mobile and incontinent of urine. The nurse must not assume that certain health situations produce automatic priorities. For example, a surgical client is expected to experience some post-operative pain, which often becomes a nursing priority. However, if the client has severe anxiety that heightens pain perception, the nurse may have to focus on anxiety relief before pain relief measures can be effective.

After determining a client's nursing care priorities, the nurse selects therapies most likely to relieve each problem. A range of choices may be available, from nurse-administered to client self-care strategies. The nurse collaborates with the client and then selects, tests, and evaluates the chosen approaches. The nurse anticipates what might go wrong and considers ways to minimize or prevent problems. For example, Ruth talks with Marie, about the need to check her mother's bathroom for obstacles that could create a risk for falls. She also recommends a complete home safety assessment. From the findings, Ruth can suggest ways to minimize hazards and prevent further injury.

Nurses make decisions about individual clients and about groups of clients. A nurse in a hospital unit usually cares for several clients. The nurse uses criteria such as the clients' clinical condition, Maslow's hierarchy of needs (see chapter 15), risks involved in treatment delays, and clients' expectations of care to determine which clients have the greatest priorities for care. For example, a client who has a sudden drop in blood pressure along with a change in consciousness requires the nurse's attention immediately as opposed to the client who needs assistance with a walk down the hallway. The nurse visits the client who has had no visitors and has recently been given a diagnosis of cancer before checking on the recovering surgical client who is with family. For nurses to be able to manage the wide variety of problems associated with groups of clients, skilful, prioritized decision making is critical (Box 11-3).

Specific Clinical Thinking in Nursing

Applying the Nursing Process. Nurses apply the **nursing process** as a competency when delivering client care (Kataoka-Yahiro & Saylor, 1994). The nursing process consists of five steps: assessment, nursing diagnosis, planning, implementation, and evaluation (see chapter 12). Its purpose is to assist nurses to identify and treat clients' health concerns. Use of the nursing process allows nurses to help clients meet agreed-upon outcomes for better health (Figure 11–1). The process provides a systematic approach for gathering client data, critically examining and analyzing the data, identifying the client's response to a health problem, determining priorities, establishing goals and expected outcomes of care, taking appropriate action, and evaluating whether the action is effective. The process incorporates general and specific critical thinking competencies, described earlier, in a manner that focuses on a client's unique needs. The format for the nursing process is unique to the nursing discipline and provides a common language and process for nurses to "think through" clients' clinical problems (Kataoka-Yahiro & Saylor, 1994).

Creativity, or the use of innovation, characterizes the nursing process, which responds to the ever-changing needs of a client. For example, after evaluating the results of nursing care and finding that the client has not improved, the nurse can reassess a client's condition to update data, redefine problems, and select new interventions. The nursing process is not linear. In clinical practice, a nurse will move back and forth, using steps of the nursing process that are most appropriate to a client's presenting situation.

The nursing process is a blueprint for care. It provides a creative, organized framework for the delivery of nursing care, yet it is flexible enough to be used in all settings. At any time in the care of a client, a nurse may move back and forth from one step of the process to another should new data emerge. The nurse must always be critically thinking and recognizing which step of the process is being used. Throughout the clinical chapters of this text, the relationship of critical thinking to the nursing process will be emphasized.

Box 11-3 Clinical Decision Making for Groups of Clients

Identify each client's nursing problems and decide which are the most urgent based on basic needs, the clients' changing or unstable status, and problem complexity.

Consider the time it will take to care for clients whose problems are of high priority.

Consider the resources you have to manage each problem, other staff willing to assist, and clients' family members.

Consider how to involve the clients as decision makers and participants in care.

Decide how to combine activities to resolve more than one client problem at a time.

Decide what, if any, nursing care procedures can be delegated to unregulated care providers so that you can devote your time to activities requiring professional nursing knowledge.

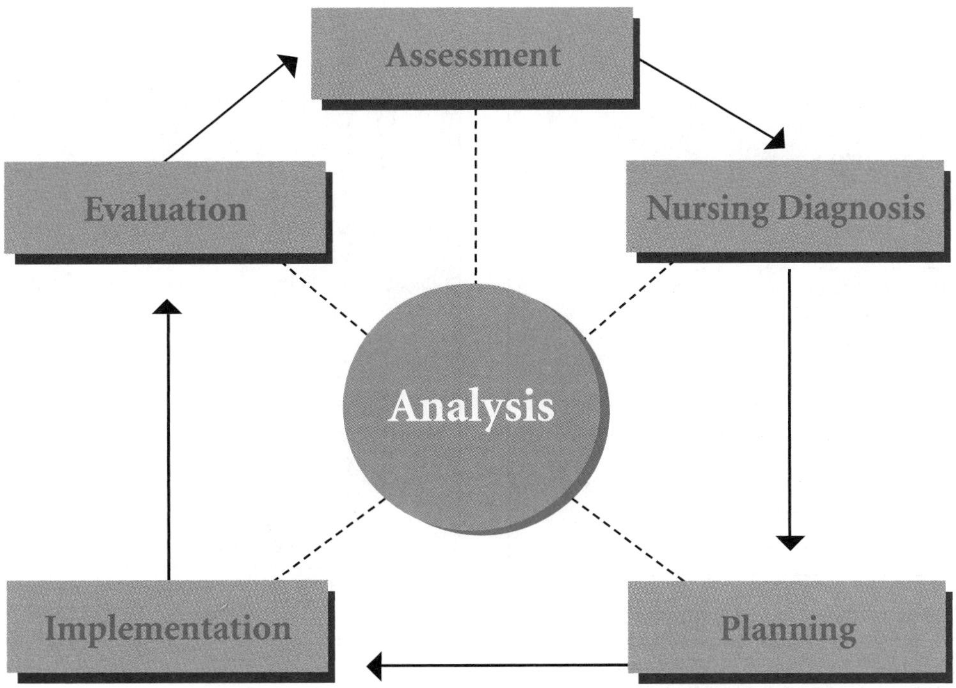

FIGURE **11–1** Five-step nursing process model.

Critical Thinking Model

Models help to explain concepts. Because critical thinking in nursing is complex, a model can help to explain the factors involved in making decisions and judgments about clients. Kataoka-Yahiro and Saylor (1994) developed a model of critical thinking for nursing judgment based in part on previous work by Paul (1993), Glaser (1941), Perry (1979), and Miller and Malcolm (1990; Figure 11–2). The model defines the outcome of critical thinking as nursing judgment that is relevant to nursing problems in a variety of settings. According to this model, there are five components of critical thinking:—(a) knowledge base, (b) experience, (c) competencies, (d) attitudes, and (e) standards. The elements of the model combine to explain how nurses make clinical judgments that are necessary for safe, effective nursing care (Box 11-4). The following sections describe knowledge base, experience, attitudes, and standards. Critical thinking competencies, the third component of critical thinking, are described in the previous section. The critical thinking competency specific to nursing is the use of the nursing process.

Specific Knowledge Base

The first component of critical thinking is a nurse's knowledge base. This varies according to a nurse's educational experience, including basic nursing education, continuing education courses, and additional university degrees. In addition, it includes the initiative a nurse shows in reading the nursing literature to remain current in nursing science. A nurse's specific knowledge base includes information and theory from the basic sciences, humanities, behavioural sciences, and nursing. Nurses use their knowledge base in a different way from other health care disciplines in how they think about client problems. For example, a nurse's broad knowledge base gives the nurse a holistic view of clients and their health care needs. The depth and extent of knowledge influence the nurse's ability to think critically about nursing problems. Consider this scenario:

Robert Perez previously earned a bachelor's degree in education and taught high school for 1 year. He is starting his third year of study in his nursing program. He has successfully completed his required courses in the sciences, health ethics, introduction to nursing concepts, and communication principles. His first clinical course focuses on health promotion with a clinical assignment on a general medicine clinic. Although he is still a novice nurse, his experiences as a teacher and his preparation and knowledge base in nursing will help him know how to interview clients and begin to make clinical decisions about clients' health promotion practices.

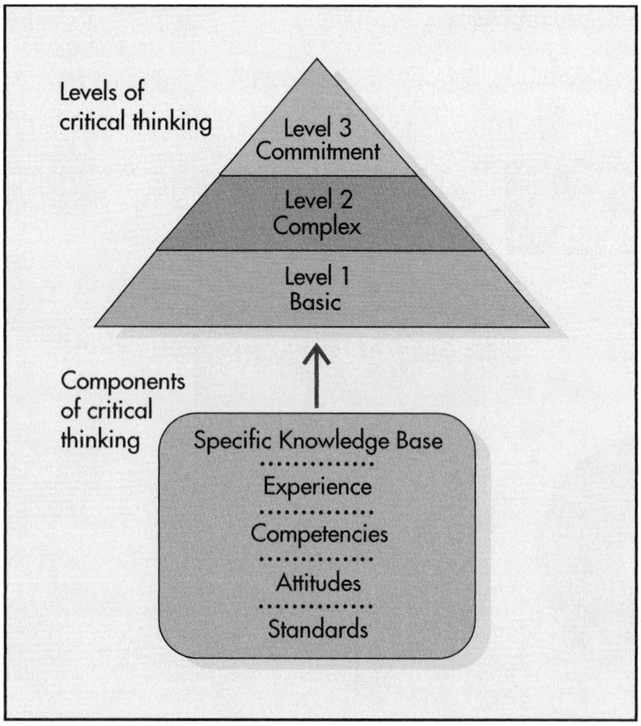

FIGURE **11–2** Critical thinking model for nursing judgment. (Redrawn from "A Critical Thinking Model for Nursing Judgment," by M. Kataoka-Yahiro and C. Saylor, 1994, *Journal of Nursing Education, 33*(8), p. 351. Adapted from Glaser, 1941; Miller & Malcolm, 1990; Paul, 1993; and Perry, 1979.)

Box 11-4 Components of Critical Thinking in Nursing

I. Specific knowledge base in learning.
II. Experience in nursing.
III. Critical thinking competencies.
  A. General critical thinking competencies
  B. Specific critical thinking competencies in clinical situations
  C. Specific critical thinking competency in nursing
IV. Attitudes for critical thinking
  A. Confidence
  B. Independence
  C. Fairness
  D. Responsibility
  E. Risk taking
  F. Discipline
  G. Perseverance
  H. Creativity
  I. Curiosity
  J. Integrity
  K. Humility
V. Standards for critical thinking
  A. Intellectual standards
    1. Clear
    2. Precise
    3. Specific
    4. Accurate
    5. Relevant
    6. Plausible
    7. Consistent
    8. Logical
    9. Deep
    10. Broad
    11. Complete
    12. Significant
    13. Adequate (for purpose)
    14. Fair
  B. Professional standards
    1. Ethical criteria for nursing judgement
    2. Criteria for evaluation
    3. Professional responsibility

Adapted from "A Critical Thinking Model for Nursing Judgment," by M. Kataoka-Yahir and C. Saylor, 1994, *Journal of Nursing Education, 33,* p. 351. Data from "The Art of Redesigning Instruction," by R. W. Paul, in *Critical Thinking: How to Prepare Students for a Rapidly Changing World,* edited by J. Willsen and A. J. A. Blinker, 1993, Santa Rosa, CA: Foundation for Critical Thinking.

Experience

The second component of the critical thinking model is nursing experience. Unless a nurse practices and make decisions about client care, critical thinking in clinical decision making will not develop. In clinical situations, the nurse learns from observing, sensing, talking with clients and families, and then reflecting actively on all experiences. Clinical experience is the laboratory for testing nursing knowledge. The nurse will learn that "textbook" approaches lay important groundwork for practice, but safe adaptations or revisions in approaches must often be made to accommodate the setting, the unique qualities of the client, and the experience the nurse has gained from using the approaches with previous clients. With experience, the nurse begins to understand clinical situations, recognize cues of clients' health patterns, and interpret cues as relevant or irrelevant. Perhaps the best lesson to be learned by a new nursing student is to value all client experiences, because they become stepping stones for building new knowledge and stimulating innovative thinking.

During the previous summer, Robert worked as a nurse assistant in a long-term care facility. This experience gave him the opportunity to interact with older adults and provide basic nursing care. As Robert thinks about his clinical experience at the clinic, he recognizes he still has a lot to learn. However, each client has provided him valuable learning experiences. Specifically, he has been able to develop good interviewing skills and understand the importance of the family in an individual's health, and he has learned the role nurses play as client advocates. His time in the physical assessment laboratory and the long-term care facility have helped him begin to be a watchful observer. Robert also knows that his previous experience as a teacher will help him apply educational principles in his nursing role.

Attitudes for Critical Thinking

The fourth component of the critical thinking model is attitudes. Paul (1993) identified 11 attitudes that are central features of a critical thinker (see Box 11-4). These attitudes define how a successful critical thinker approaches a problem. For example, when a client complains of anxiety before undergoing a diagnostic procedure, the nurse will be curious and explore possible reasons for the client's concerns. The nurse will also show discipline in completing a thorough assessment. Attitudes of inquiry involve an ability to recognize that problems exist and to accept the general need for evidence in support of what is asserted to be true (Watson & Glaser, 1980). Critical thinking attitudes offer guidelines for how to approach a problem or decision-making situation. An important part of critical thinking is interpreting, evaluating, and making judgments about the adequacy of various arguments and available data. Knowing when more information is needed, knowing when information is misleading, and recognizing one's own knowledge limits are examples of how critical thinking attitudes play a key role in decision making. Table 11-3 summarizes how critical thinking attitudes apply to nursing practice.

Table 11-3 Critical Thinking Attitudes and Applications in Nursing Practice

Critical Thinking Attitude	Application in Practice
Confidence	Learn how to introduce yourself to a client. Speak with conviction when you begin a treatment or procedure. Do not lead a client to think that you are uncertain of being able to perform care safely. Always be prepared before performing a nursing activity.
Thinking independently	Read the nursing literature, especially when there are different views on the same subject. Talk with colleagues and share ideas about nursing interventions.
Fairness	Listen to both sides in any discussion. If a client or family member complains about a colleague, listen to the story and then speak with the colleague as well. Weigh all facts.
Responsibility and accountability	Ask for help if you are uncertain about an aspect of client care. Report any problems immediately. Follow standards of practice in your care.
Risk taking	If your knowledge causes you to question a physician's order, do so. Be willing to recommend alternative approaches to nursing care when colleagues are having little success with clients.
Discipline	Be thorough and manage your time effectively. Use known scientific and practice-based criteria for activities such as assessment and evaluation.
Perseverance	Be wary of an easy answer. If colleagues give you information about a client and some facts seem to be missing, clarify the information or talk to the client directly. If problems of the same type continue to occur on a nursing unit, bring colleagues together, look for a pattern, and find a solution.
Creativity	Look for different approaches if interventions are not working. A client may need a different positioning technique or a different instructional approach.
Curiosity	Always ask why. A clinical sign or symptom can indicate a variety of problems. Explore and learn more about the client so as to make appropriate clinical judgments.
Integrity	Recognize when your opinions may conflict with those of a client; review your position, and decide how best to proceed to reach mutually beneficial outcomes. Do not compromise nursing standards or honesty in delivering nursing care.
Humility	Recognize when you need more information to make a decision. When you are newly assigned to a clinical unit and you are unfamiliar with the clients, ask to be oriented to the area. Ask RNs regularly assigned to the area for assistance. Read the professional journals regularly to keep updated on new approaches to care.

Confidence. To be confident is to feel certain in one's ability to accomplish a task or goal. Confidence grows with experience and the maturity to recognize one's strengths and limitations. Confidence is not arrogance or the feeling of superiority. Confident critical thinkers are aware of the balance between what they know and what they do not know. When a nurse shows confidence, clients recognize it in the manner in which the nurse communicates and performs nursing care. Confidence builds trust between the nurse and client and is often instrumental in achieving client outcomes.

Thinking Independently. As people mature and gain new knowledge, they learn to consider a wide range of ideas and concepts before forming an opinion or making a judgment. This does not mean they ignore other people's ideas. All sides of a given situation should be considered. However, a critical thinker does not usually accept or reject another person's ideas without question. To think independently, one questions others' ways of interpreting knowledge and looks for rational and logical answers to problems. Independent thinking and reasoning are essential to the improvement and expansion of nursing practice.

Fairness. Critical thinkers are just. They recognize their own biases and prejudices and do not allow them to affect their decisions. Fairness helps one to look at a situation objectively and completely, analyzing all viewpoints, before making a decision. Imagination and compassion helps one to be fair. Imagining what clients are experiencing can help a nurse see situations with new perspective and appreciate their complexity.

Responsibility and Accountability. A nurse is responsible for correctly performing nursing care activities based on standards of practice. Standards of practice are the minimum level of performance expected of nurses to provide safe, competent, and ethical care (Canadian Nurses Association, 2002). For example, the nurse does not take shortcuts (e.g., failing to identify a client) when administering medications. The nurse who intervenes for a client must be answerable or accountable for the outcomes of any nursing actions. A nurse who is accountable is reliable and willing to recognize when nursing care is ineffective. Ultimately, the nurse assumes accountability for whatever decisions and resultant actions are made on the client's behalf.

Risk Taking. Risk-taking is often perceived as dangerous. Driving too fast is a risk that might result in injury to the driver and others. But risk taking does not have to cause injury. Without intellectual risk taking, knowledge cannot advance. A critical thinker is willing to take risks in trying different approaches to solving problems. Being willing to be wrong, willing to take a stance on an issue, and willing to form close therapeutic relationships with clients help nurses discover new ideas. The willingness to take risks often comes from experience with similar problems. Nurses in the past have taken risks in trying different approaches to skin and wound care, pulmonary hygiene, and pain management, to name a few. When taking a risk, the nurse considers all options, analyzes and minimizes danger to a client, and acts in a well-reasoned, logical, and thoughtful manner.

Discipline. A disciplined thinker misses few details and follows an orderly approach when making decisions or taking action. Disciplined thinking ensures that decisions are made systematically and in a comprehensive manner. For example, assessment of a client's pain includes more than just noting the location. The nurse also assesses the severity of pain, its duration, factors that aggravate or relieve the pain, and the effect of the pain on the client's lifestyle (see chapter 38). An in-depth, disciplined assessment of the client's pain ensures correct identification of the nature of pain and the selection of the most appropriate nursing interventions.

Perseverance. A critical thinker takes on a problem with determination and diligence despite opposition. Perseverance helps critical thinkers find solutions to client care problems. This attitude is especially important when problems remain unresolved or when they reoccur. The nurse learns as much as possible about a problem, tries various approaches to care, and continues to seek additional resources until a successful approach is found. For example, a client who is unable to speak following throat surgery often poses communication challenges for the nurse. Perseverance leads the nurse to try different communication approaches (e.g., message boards or alarm bells) until a method is found that the client can easily use. A critical thinker who perseveres is not satisfied with minimal effort, but works to achieve the highest level of quality care.

Creativity. Creativity involves using imaginative and innovative skills in problem solving. This means finding new or innovative solutions to client problems while upholding standards of practice. Creativity is a great motivator that enables one to generate options and alternative approaches (Miller & Babcock, 1996). Often clients pose problems that require unique approaches. A client's clinical problems, social support systems, and living environment are just some factors that can make even simple nursing procedures complicated without a creative approach. For example, a home health nurse is helping an older client with arthritis gain greater mobility. The client has difficulty lowering and raising herself in a chair because of pain and limited range of motion in her knees. The nurse solves the problem by using wooden blocks to elevate the chair legs so that the client can easily sit and stand with minimal discomfort.

Curiosity. A critical thinker seeks knowledge. Curiosity drives a critical thinker to ask the question, Why? In any clinical situation, a nurse learns a great deal about a client. As the nurse analyzes client information, data patterns emerge that are not always clear. Curiosity motivates the nurse to inquire further and to investigate a clinical situation so that all the information needed to make a decision is obtained.

Integrity. A person of integrity acts according to a sound moral and ethical position. Integrity builds trust from peers and subordinates. Nurses face many dilemmas in clinical practice, and few avoid making mistakes. Nurses with integrity are honest and willing to admit to mistakes or inconsistencies in their behaviour, ideas, and beliefs. They strive to achieve high standards of practice even in the face of adversity. Critical thinkers question and test personal knowledge and beliefs as rigorously as they test the knowledge and beliefs of others.

Humility. It is important to be humble and admit to one's own limitations in knowledge and skills. Critical thinkers admit what they do not know and try to acquire the knowledge needed to make proper decisions. Clients' safety and welfare may be at risk if nurses do not acknowledge when they are unable to deal with a practice problem. The nurse must rethink a situation, acquire additional knowledge, and then use the new information to form opinions, draw conclusions, and take action.

Standards for Critical Thinking

The fifth component of the critical thinking model includes intellectual and professional standards (Kataoka-Yahiro & Saylor, 1994).

Intellectual Standards. Paul (1993) identified 14 intellectual standards universal for critical thinking (see Box 11-4). These standards are commonly applied when a nurse conducts the nursing process. When considering a client problem, the nurse must apply intellectual standards such as preciseness, accuracy, and consistency to ensure that all data are available for making sound clinical decisions. For example:

Mrs. Lamar is an 82-year-old client who is transferred from intensive care to a general medicine nursing unit. During his assessment, the nurse, Robert, finds an ulcer on Mrs. Lamar's left foot. A quick check of the client's medical record reveals a description of the ulcer by one of the intensive care unit nurses from 2 days earlier. The client is receiving a topical medication for the ulcer. To be consistent in his assessment, Robert uses the same assessment criteria applied during the last examination. He methodically inspects the affected area of the skin, asks if the client is experiencing discomfort, measures the size of the ulcer, and notes the appearance of any drainage. The wound location and appearance are described in Mrs. Lamar's medical record using specific anatomical terms. Robert examines Mrs. Lamar further to ensure that his findings are accurate and to determine if any other ulcers are present. He also assesses the client's ability to ambulate, knowing that the ulcer could impair function. By applying appropriate intellectual standards, Robert is able to determine that the ulcer is healing and has improved since the last assessment.

A rigorous use of intellectual standards in clinical practice ensures that critical thinking is not haphazard.

Professional Standards. Professional standards for critical thinking refer to ethical criteria for nursing judgments, scientific and practice-based criteria used for evaluation, and criteria for professional responsibility (Paul, 1993). Application of professional standards requires that nurses use critical thinking for the good of individuals or groups (Kataoka-Yahiro & Saylor, 1994). Professional standards promote the highest level of quality nursing care.

Excellent nursing practice reflects sound ethical standards. In Canada, ethical nursing standards are guided by the Canadian Nurses Association *Code of Ethics for Registered Nurses* (2002). Client care requires more than just the application of scientific knowledge. Focussing on a client's values and beliefs helps a nurse to make clinical decisions that are just, faithful to the client's choices, and beneficial to the client's health and well-being. Critical thinkers maintain a sense of self-awareness through conscious awareness of their beliefs, values, feelings, and the multiple perspectives that clients, family members, staff, and peers present in clinical situations (Ludwick & Sedlak, 1998). Chapter 7 summarizes how to process ethical dilemmas.

Critical thinking also requires the use of scientifically based and practice-based criteria for making clinical judgments. These criteria may be scientifically based on research findings (see chapter 6) or practice based on standards developed by clinical experts and quality improvement initiatives. An example is the *Best Practice Guidelines* developed by the Registered Nurses Association of Ontario (*http://www.rnao.org/bestpractices/*), which include standards for the treatment of select clinical conditions. Another example is clinical criteria used to categorize clinical phenomena, such as categorizing (staging) pressure ulcers by assessing skin temperature, tissue consistency, and depth of wound (see chapter 43). Scientific and practice-based evaluation criteria set the minimum requirements necessary to ensure appropriate and high-quality care.

Nurses routinely use scientific and practice-based criteria to assess clients' conditions and to determine the efficacy of nursing interventions. For example, accurate assessment of symptoms such as pain or shortness of breath includes use of assessment criteria such as the duration, severity, location, aggravating or relieving factors, and effects on daily lifestyle (see chapter 28). Assessment criteria allow a nurse to accurately determine the nature of a client's symptom, select appropriate therapies, and then evaluate if the therapies are effective.

Standards of professional responsibility are cited in institutional practice guidelines, professional organizations' standards of practice, and nursing practice acts. These standards outline the responsibilities and accountabilities that a nurse must assume in guaranteeing quality health care to the public.

Critical Thinking Synthesis

By placing the nursing process within the context of the critical thinking model, one is able to see two processes occur together (Figure 11–3). As nurses engage in the nursing process, they are also synthesizing critical thinking knowledge, experience, competencies, standards, and attitudes. The nurse who assesses a client's pain does not focus only on what the client reports about the pain and what the nurse is able to observe and measure. The nurse also reflects on prior experience with clients who have had similar pain to compare it with the new client's

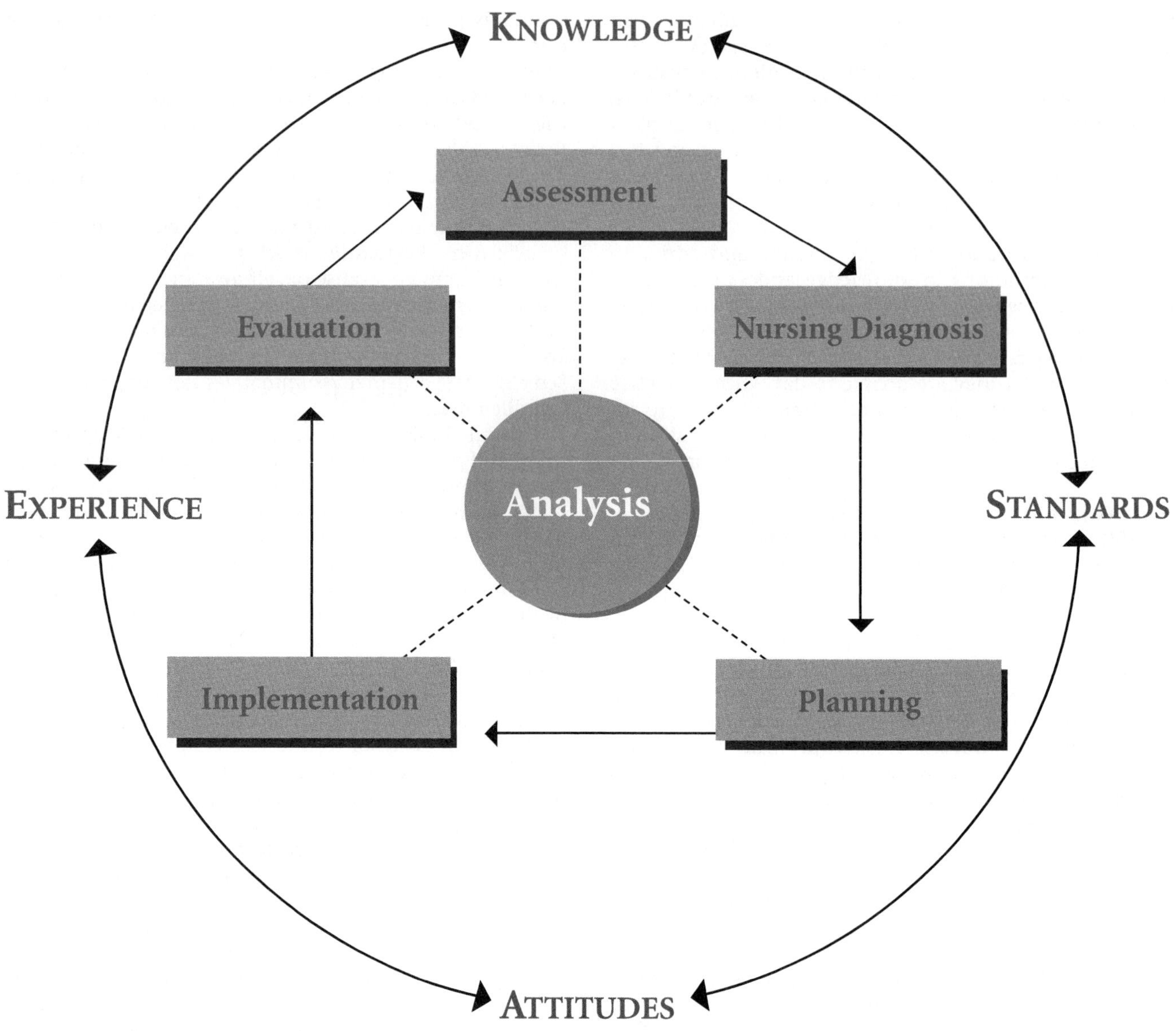

FIGURE **11–3** Synthesis of critical thinking with the nursing process competency.

response. The nurse refers to scientific texts to see how the pain might be relieved. The nurse also displays intellectual standards in being sure the pain assessment is accurate and objective. Finally, the nurse exercises the attitudes necessary for the client to be cared for fairly and responsibly.

The nursing process and critical thinking are synthesized, meaning the two come together in a manner that allows a student to become a competent. This text provides a model that reinforces the importance of critical thinking in practice. Throughout the clinical chapters of this text, the components of critical thinking are summarized to help readers better understand its relationship to the nursing process.

Key Concepts

- To assist clients in maintaining, regaining, or improving their health, a nurse must be able to think critically, solve problems, and find the best solution for a client's problems.
- The nurse who is a good critical thinker faces problems without forming a quick, simple solution, but rather considers the value of all available options.
- By reflecting on a client situation and making sense of the experience, the nurse gains insight into the meaning of the situation.

- Reflection is a form of self-evaluation that helps the nurse judge personal performance.
- To become a critical thinker, the nurse must be able to use language precisely and clearly.
- Intuition acts as a trigger, sparking an analytical process that leads nurses in a conscious search to acquire data that confirm their sense of change in a client's status.
- The three levels of critical thinking in nursing are basic, complex, and commitment.
- To make a decision, a person must recognize and define the problem or situation, assess all options, weigh each option against a set of criteria, test possible options, consider the consequences of the decision, and then make a final decision.
- Diagnostic reasoning occurs when a nurse assigns meaning to the behaviours, physical signs, and reported client symptoms that arise in a clinical situation.
- A nurse makes clinical decisions by identifying client problems and then choosing the best nursing interventions that will reach mutually established goals.
- The model of critical thinking for nursing judgment consists of five elements: knowledge, experience, critical thinking competencies (e.g., nursing process), attitudes, and standards.
- With experience, a nurse learns to understand clinical situations, recognize cues of clients' health patterns, and interpret cues as relevant or irrelevant.
- Critical thinking attitudes help a nurse to know when more information is needed and when information is misleading and to recognize personal knowledge limits.
- The nurse's use of intellectual standards during assessment ensures a complete database of information.
- Professional standards for critical thinking refer to ethical criteria for nursing judgments, scientific and practice criteria to be used for evaluation, and criteria for professional responsibility.
- As the nurse engages in the nursing process, the nurse is also synthesizing critical thinking knowledge, experience, standards, and attitudes.

Key Terms

Clinical decision-making process, *p. 172*
Critical thinking, *p. 167*
Decision making, *p. 171*
Diagnostic reasoning, *p. 172*
Inference, *p. 172*
Intuition, *p. 169*
Nursing process, *p. 173*
Problem solving, *p. 171*
Reflection, *p. 168*
Scientific method, *p. 170*

Critical Thinking Exercises

1. Select a day and write a journal entry describing any one of the following experiences that stimulated your thinking: an interaction you had with a client, an interaction you had with a family member, or an interaction you had with someone you were trying to help. In the entry, do each of the following:
   a. Describe, as thoroughly as you can, your thoughts, feelings, and actions.
   b. Describe your decision-making process.
   c. Describe what you would do differently if a similar incident were to occur.
   d. Describe your strengths and weaknesses in dealing with the situation.
2. The following nurse's note was entered for Mrs. Simmons, a client who visited the general medicine clinic.

   Mrs. Simmons visited the general medicine clinic presenting with a 7-day bout of blurred vision and dizziness. Client reports vision is blurred or distorted, preventing her from performing routine activities such as preparing meals, writing cheques, and, some mornings, performing her own hygiene and grooming. She has the most difficulty seeing close objects, although her distance vision is also blurred. Blurring is present with and without use of glasses. On examination, pupils are equal and reactive to light and accommodation. Visual fields are normal. She was unable to read newsprint in the newspaper or read the instructions on the nutrition information chart on the wall. She is active in her local church activities, but this has declined recently. Mrs. Simmons denies having a headache but has also noticed some dizziness. She is currently taking estrogen, a calcium supplement, and Inderal.

Evaluate the nurse's note for the use of intellectual standards. What is complete and significant in the note versus superficial or trivial? What is relevant versus irrelevant? What is clear versus unclear?

3. Consider the following statements and describe which is an example of inference, problem solving, or clinical decision making. Support your answer with a rationale.
   a. As the nurse enters a client's room, she observes that the intravenous (IV) line is not infusing at the ordered rate. The nurse checks the flow regulator on the tubing, looks to see if the client is lying on the tubing, checks the point of connection between the tubing and the IV catheter, and then checks the condition of the site where the IV catheter enters the client's skin.
   b. The client is turning frequently in bed, holds his abdomen with his left hand, and tells the nurse, "My stomach is killing me." The nurse examines the client's abdomen, inspects the incision made during surgery 24 hours ago, and asks the client to rate the discomfort on a scale of 0 to 10. The client rates the pain a 9, compared with a 4 just 3 hours ago. The nurse concludes the pain is related to incisional trauma and administers a prescribed analgesic. The nurse checks the client 30 minutes later and finds that the client is more relaxed and the pain is at a 5.
   c. The nurse reviews a client's medical record and finds that the client has ingested only 600 mL of fluids over the last 24 hours. The client also has a low urinary output. The nurse conducts an assessment and finds the client to have poor skin turgor and difficulty concentrating when asked questions

about his medical history. The nurse exits the client's room and tells the physician that the client is likely becoming dehydrated.

4. Mr. Yousif is a terminally ill client. His wife and son are asking you about the type of pain control he is receiving. Mrs. Yousif is requesting that the physician increase her husband's medication, even if it means he will not be responsive. She does not want her husband to suffer. The son is vehemently opposed to too much narcotic and believes that his father is still able to make decisions for himself. Mr. Yousif remains alert much of the time and is able to talk with you about his feelings regarding death. He seems to appreciate your talking with him. How might you apply the critical thinking attitudes of fairness, responsibility, and creativity in this case?

Review Questions

1. The following process involves forming conclusions, making decisions, drawing inferences, and reflecting:
   1. Assessment
   2. Critical thinking
   3. Thinking independently
   4. Intellectual humility
2. The nurse identifies ways he can improve his own performance. He reflects on his nursing experiences. This is an example of the core critical thinking skill
   1. Inference
   2. Explanation
   3. Analysis
   4. Self-regulation
3. During the day, the nurse spends time instructing a client in how to self-administer insulin. After discussing the techniques and demonstrating an injection, the nurse has the client try it. After two attempts, it is obvious that the client does not understand how to prepare the correct dose. When the nurse returns to the medication room, he discusses the situation with the charge nurse, reviewing his approach with the client and asking for her suggestions on his technique. This is an example of
   1. Reflection
   2. Risk taking
   3. Client assessment
   4. Care plan evaluation
4. An experienced surgical nurse enters a client's room and suspects that the client is experiencing a surgical complication. The nurse begins an assessment of vital signs, the client's wound, the intravenous line status, and an analysis of how the client feels to gather information and verify whether the nurse's_____ was correct and a problem really exists.
   1. Knowledge
   2. Intuition
   3. Reflection
   4. Risk taking
5. A nurse uses an institution's procedure manual to confirm how to insert a Foley catheter. The level of critical thinking the nurse is using is
   1. Commitment
   2. Complex critical thinking
   3. Scientific method
   4. Basic critical thinking
6. A client has nursing diagnoses of anxiety and deficient knowledge concerning his impending surgery. The nurse decides that the client's anxiety must be addressed first in order for the client to be receptive to any formal instruction about surgery. This decision is considered a part of
   1. Assessment
   2. Planning
   3. Intervention
   4. Evaluation
7. A client had hip surgery 24 hours ago. When beginning the nursing shift, the nurse refers to the written plan of care, noting that the client has a drainage device collecting wound drainage. The physician's order requires that the physician be notified when drainage in the device exceeds 100 mL for the day. When the nurse enters the room, the nurse looks at the device and carefully notes the amount of drainage currently in the device. This is an example of
   1. Assessment
   2. Planning
   3. Intervention
   4. Evaluation
8. The nurse asks a client how she feels about her impending surgery for breast cancer. Before the discussion, the nurse reviewed the description in his textbook of loss and grief in addition to therapeutic communication principles. The critical thinking component involved in the nurse's review of the literature is
   1. Experience
   2. Problem solving
   3. Knowledge application
   4. Clinical decision making
9. A 72-year-old woman has been a client on the medical unit for about 4 days. When she was first admitted, she was alert and oriented. In the last 24 hours, she has become acutely confused and has repeatedly attempted to get out of bed. The nursing staff has discussed the possibility of using restraints; however, one nurse insists that use of orientation and meaningful diversion should be tried. This is an example of the critical thinking attitude
   1. Integrity
   2. Risk taking
   3. Thinking independently
   4. Responsibility and accountability
10. The nurse does not take shortcuts (e.g., failing to identify a client) when administering medications. This is an example of the critical thinking attitude
    1. Responsibility and accountability
    2. Thinking independently
    3. Fairness
    4. Discipline

References

Baker, C. R. (1996). Reflective learning: A teaching strategy for critical thinking. *Journal of Nursing Education, 35*(1), 19–22.

Bandman, E. L., & Bandman, B. (1995). *Critical thinking in nursing* (2nd ed.). Norwalk, CT: Appleton & Lange.

Benner, P., Hooper-Kyriakidis, P., & Stannard, D. (1999). *Clinical wisdom and interventions in critical care.* Philadelphia: W. B. Saunders.

Bittner, N. P., & Tobin, E. (1998). Critical thinking: Strategies for clinical practice. *Journal for Nurses in Staff Development, 14,* 267–272.

Canadian Nurses Association. (2002). *Code of Ethics for Registered Nurses.* Ottawa, ON: Author.

Chaffee, J. (1994). *Thinking critically* (3rd ed.). Boston: Houghton Mifflin.

Facione, N., & Facione, P. (1996). Externalizing the critical thinking in knowledge development and clinical judgement. *Nursing Outlook, 44,* 129–136.

Facione, P. (1990). *Critical thinking: A statement of expert consensus for purposes of educational assessment and instruction. The Delphi report: Research findings and recommendations prepared for the American Philosophical Association.* Milbrae, CA: California Academic Press. (ERIC Document Reproduction Service No. ED 315-423)

Fowler, L. P. (1998). Improving critical thinking in nursing practice. *Journal for Nurses in Staff Development, 14,* 183–187.

Glaser, E. (1941). *An experiment in the development of critical thinking.* New York: Bureau of Publications, Teachers College, Columbia University.

Gordon, M. (1995). *Nursing diagnosis: Process and application* (3rd ed.). St. Louis, MO: Mosby.

Kataoka-Yahiro, M., & Saylor, C. (1994). A critical thinking model for nursing judgment. *Journal of Nursing Education, 33,* 351–356.

King, L., & Clark, J. M. (2002). Intuition and the development of expertise in surgical ward and intensive care nurses. *Journal of Advanced Nursing, 37,* 322–329.

Ludwick, R., & Sedlak, C. A. (1998). Ethical issues and critical thinking: Students' stories. *NursingConnections, 11*(3), 12–18.

Miller, M. A., & Babcock, D. E. (1996). *Critical thinking applied to nursing.* St. Louis, MO: Mosby.

Miller, M. A., & Malcolm, N. S. (1990). Critical thinking in the nursing curriculum. *Nursing & Health Care, 11,* 67–73.

O'Neill, E. S., & Dluhy, N. M. (1997). A longitudinal framework for fostering critical thinking and diagnostic reasoning. *Journal of Advanced Nursing, 26,* 825–832.

Paget, T. (2001). Reflective practice and clinical outcomes: Practitioners' views on how reflective practice has influenced their clinical practice. *Journal of Clinical Nursing, 10,* 204–214.

Paul, R. W. (1993). The art of redesigning instruction. In J. Willsen & A. J. A. Blinker (Eds.), *Critical thinking: How to prepare students for a rapidly changing world.* Santa Rosa, CA: Foundation for Critical Thinking.

Paul, R. W., & Heaslip, P. (1995). Critical thinking and intuitive nursing practice. *Journal of Advanced Nursing, 22,* 40–47.

Perry, W. (1979). *Forms of intellectual and ethical development in the college years: A scheme.* New York: Holt, Rinehart, & Winston.

Smith, B., & Johnston, Y. (2002). Using structured clinical preparation to stimulate reflection and foster critical thinking. *Journal of Nursing Education, 41,* 182–185.

Smith Higuchi, K. A., & Donald, J. G. (2002). Thinking processes used by nurses in clinical decision making. *Journal of Nursing Education, 41,* 145–153.

Strader, M. (1992). Critical thinking. In E. J. Sullivan & P. J. Decker (Eds.), *Effective management in nursing* (3rd ed.). Redwood City, CA: Addison Wesley Nursing.

Watson, G., & Glaser, E. (1980). *Watson-Glaser critical thinking appraisal manual.* New York: MacMillan.

Whiteside, C. (1997). A model for teaching critical thinking in the clinical setting. *Dimensions of Critical Care Nursing, 16,* 152–165.

Recommended Web Sites

Canadian Nurses Association:
http://www.cna-nurses.ca
The Canadian Nurses Association Web site provides links to the provincial and territorial professional nursing associations. Access the link to your provincial or territorial association to view the self-assessment tool currently in use in your jurisdiction.

Critical Thinking: To Think Like a Nurse:
http://www.cariboo.bc.ca/nursing/faculty/heaslip/nrsct.htm
The author of this Web site discusses the intellectual capacities and skills nurses need to acquire to become disciplined, self-directed, critical thinkers.

Critical Thinking in Nursing:
http://hsc.unm.edu/consg/conct/
This site provides a definition of critical thinking, an overview of critical thinking research, strategies for teaching, learning and evaluating critical thinking skills, and links to other information and resources related to critical thinking.

Critical Thinking in Nursing: Web Resources:
http://hsc.unm.edu/consg/conct/resources.shtml#Web
This Web site includes links to a wide range of Web-based resources related to critical thinking. In addition, it includes a link to a bibliography of print-based articles related to critical thinking in nursing.

Tim van Gelder's Critical Thinking on the Web: Nursing:
http://www.austhink.org/critical/pages/nursing.html
Included on this Web site are links to a number of articles that explore a variety of issues related to continuing competency in nursing.

12

The Nursing Process

Patricia A. Potter, RN, MSN, PhD, CMAC, FAAN
Marilynn J. Wood, RN, BSN, MSN, DrPH (Canadian author)
Janet C. Ross-Kerr, RN, BScN, MS, PhD (Canadian author)
Julie A. Gilbert, RN, BScN, MN (Canadian author)
Tracey Stephen, RN, BScN, MN (Canadian author)
Rene A. Day, RN, PhD (Canadian author)

Objectives

Mastery of content in this chapter will enable the student to:

- Define the key terms listed.
- Discuss and use the steps of the nursing process.
- Discuss the relationship of critical thinking to the steps of the nursing process.
- Discuss the steps that constitute nursing assessment.
- Explain why client expectations are important to include in assessment.
- State the sources of data for a nursing assessment.
- State the purpose of a nursing health history.
- List and discuss the steps of forming a nursing diagnosis.
- Formulate nursing diagnoses from a nursing assessment.
- Explain the relationship of planning to assessment and nursing diagnosis.
- Discuss the process of priority setting.
- Discuss the difference between a goal and an expected outcome.
- Discuss the process of selecting nursing interventions.
- Describe the purposes of a written nursing care plan.
- Explain the relationship of implementation to the diagnostic process.
- Identify preparatory activities that the nurse uses before implementation.
- Identify the five elements of the evaluation process.
- Describe how evaluation leads to discontinuation, revision, or modification of a care plan.

A nurse follows the **nursing process** to organize and deliver nursing care. The nursing process is a systematic approach that applies knowledge from the biological, physical, and social sciences to unique client situations. It is used to identify, diagnose, and treat human responses to health and illness. The nursing process involves five steps: assessment, nursing diagnosis, planning, implementation, and evaluation (Figure 12–1):

- *Assessment.* The nurse gathers information in order to understand the client's unique situation.
- *Nursing diagnosis.* The nurse organizes and interprets the data and makes a nursing diagnosis, which is nursing's perspective on the appropriate focus for the client.
- *Planning.* The nurse prioritizes proposed strategies and interventions and creates a care plan.

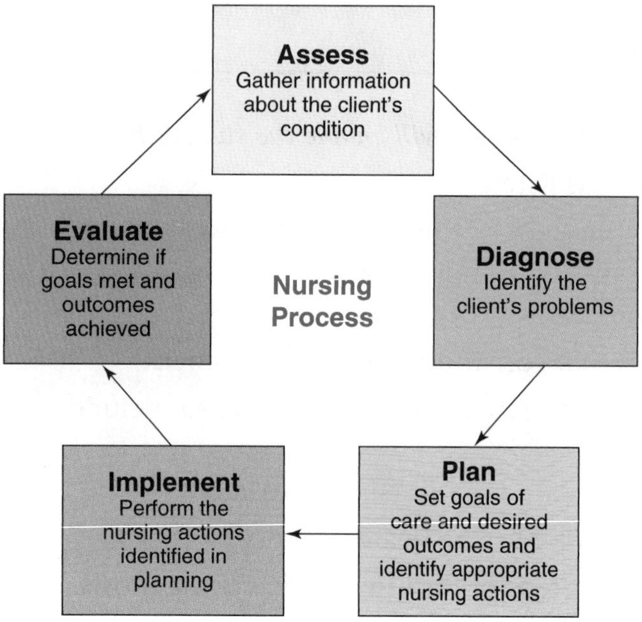

FIGURE **12–1** The five-step nursing process.

- *Implementation.* The nurse carries out the care plan.
- *Evaluation.* The nurse determines if intended outcomes have been achieved or if the nursing strategies needed to be revised.

The nursing process enables nurses to organize and systematize nursing practice. Using this process, the nurse makes inferences about the meaning of a client's response to health problems or generalizes about the client's functional states of health. A pattern then begins to form. For example, if a client is having acute back pain, a nurse may infer that the client's mobility will be limited. The nurse applies the nursing process in gathering information (e.g., noting whether the client is able to walk, stand, and sit normally) until an accurate nursing diagnosis is determined, such as the following: *impaired physical mobility related to acute back pain.* The clear definition of the client's problem provides the basis for nursing interventions (i.e., nursing treatment to enhance client outcomes) and evaluation of outcomes.

The nursing process provides a framework for nurses to think critically and make sound and reasonable decisions. Rather than being linear, the nursing process is dynamic and continuous, enabling nurses to modify care as clients' needs change. Clients often have multiple needs; thus, the nurse will simultaneously apply the process to each of those needs. When nurses think critically, the client becomes an active participant and the outcome is a comprehensive, individualized approach to care.

The nursing process applies to the care of all client systems, including individuals, families, groups, and communities. It differentiates nursing practice from that of physicians and other health care professionals. Use of the nursing process alone does not ensure excellent nursing care, however. The process is a tool or system that must be approached with confidence, responsibility, integrity, fairness, creativity, discipline, and perseverance. Nurses who successfully use the nursing process to improve the care of their clients are independent thinkers, astute observers, empathetic listeners, and clear communicators.

Step 1: Nursing Assessment

During a nursing **assessment,** the nurse applies the nursing process to systematically collect, verify, analyze, and communicate data about a client. Data are collected from both primary (the client) and secondary sources (e.g., family, health professionals, and medical records). The purpose of the assessment is to establish a **database** about the client's needs, health problems, and responses to these problems. The data contain information about health practices, family and social support, goals, values, and expectations about the health care system.

An assessment must be relevant to a particular health problem. For example, in an emergency setting, with a client who has a possible ruptured disk, the nurse must gather information about the injury; intensity, type, and location of pain; initial first aid measures; and medication allergies. These data are relevant for eventual analysis of the type of pain, its possible source, and pain relief approaches.

In facilities, nurses collect assessment data on standardized nursing assessment forms designed to collect targeted relevant data quickly and efficiently. In community settings, where clients often present with less acute problems, the assessment focuses on the client's condition, circle of family and friends, and resources within the community (Bryans & McIntosh, 1996). Nurses apply principles of critical thinking when conducting an assessment (see chapter 11). Critical thinking is the active, organized, cognitive process used to carefully examine one's thinking. By thinking critically, a nurse can see the big picture while forming conclusions or making decisions about a client's condition. When gathering data about a client, the nurse simultaneously synthesizes relevant knowledge, clinical experiences, critical thinking standards and attitudes, and standards of practice (Figure 12–2). Critical thinking thus helps the nurse to direct a meaningful and purposeful assessment.

Knowledge about the physical, biological, and social sciences enables the nurse to ask the right questions, collect relevant history, and gather physical assessment data related to the client's health care needs. For example, if a client has a ruptured lumbar disk, the nurse with sufficient knowledge knows to ask if the client has pain radiating from the buttocks down the leg and whether the pain affects mobility. Nurses also apply standards of practice and accepted standards for physical assessment data when assessing clients. They also apply knowledge gained though prior clinical experience. For example, a nurse who has cared for other clients with back pain knows that the pain can be disabling by limiting normal motion. Thus, the nurse assesses how much the pain affects the client's ability to walk and perform daily living activities. New nurses can sharpen assessment skills by validating unexpected assessment findings with more experienced nurses and observing assessments performed by skilled professionals.

Nurses think critically when applying clinical knowledge and experience and when deciding on which

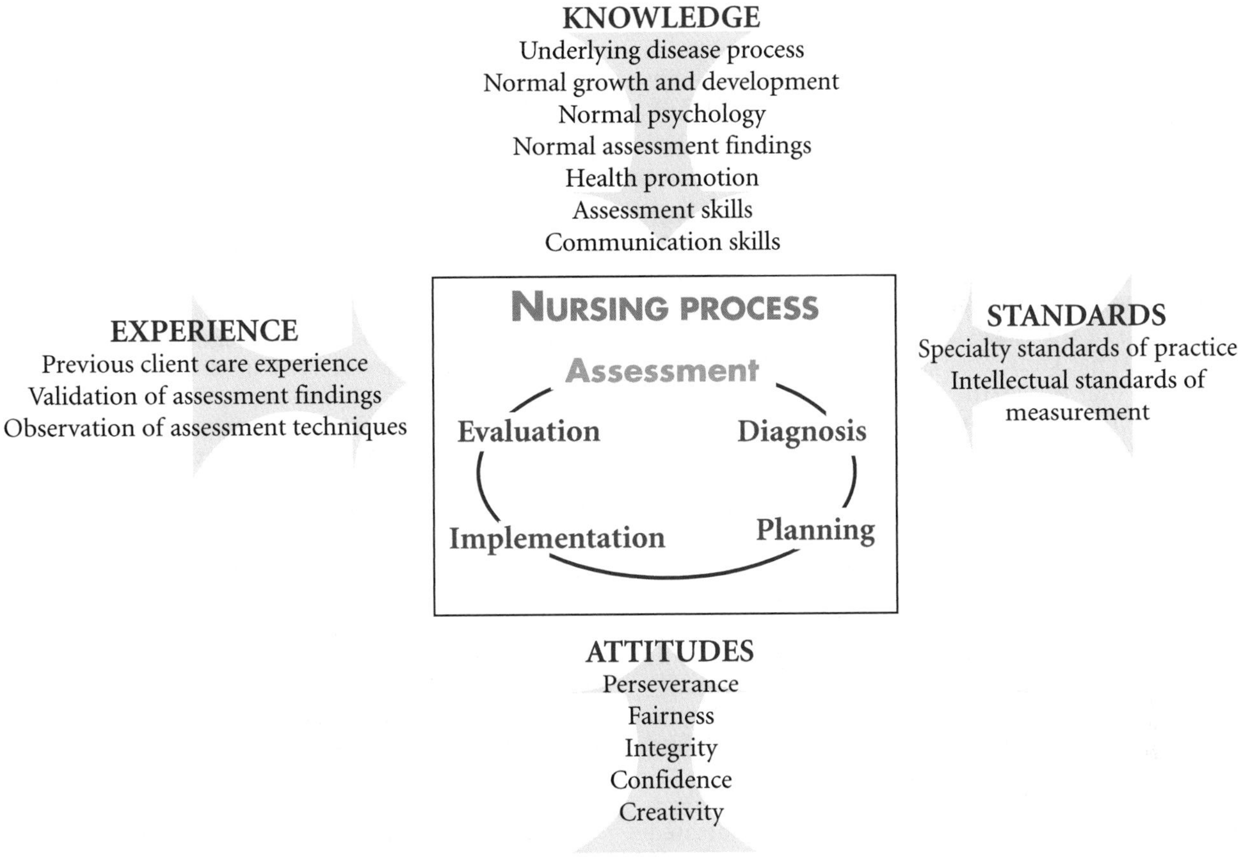

FIGURE **12–2** Critical thinking and the assessment process.

questions to ask or measurements to make in an assessment. Judgment develops and matures over time. During a first client meeting, the nurse must decide if an assessment can be a quick overview or a detailed examination of the client's case. An overview is usually based on the client's presenting priorities, the nurse's specialty area of practice, or the treatment situation. For example, an emergency department nurse uses the A-B-C (airway-breathing-circulation) approach with clients who have acute injuries or life-threatening conditions. In contrast, a psychiatric nurse may have more time to gather data and may choose to focus on the client's reality, anxiety level, and potential for violence (Carnevali & Thomas, 1993).

Nurses must be able to differentiate key data from the data mass. A **cue** is information that nurses acquire through their five senses. If the nurse uses an intensely focused assessment, important cues may be missed. Rather, the nurse should interpret cues from the client to determine how in-depth an assessment should be. Assessment is dynamic; it should allow the nurse to freely explore relevant problems as they appear.

After an initial assessment, a nurse focuses on the client's potential problems by conducting a more comprehensive assessment. Two approaches may be used: theory based or problem oriented. The theory-based approach involves the use of a structured database format, based upon an accepted theoretical framework or practice standard. Using this approach, the nurse identifies the categories of information needed to make a comprehensive assessment of the client's condition and problems. Using the problem-oriented approach, the nurse focuses on the client's presenting situation. For example, the nurse's assessment might begin with a problem area such as grieving and spread out to other relevant areas of the client's life. The nurse reviews with the client the nature of the loss and then broadens to categories such as the influence of loss on lifestyle, family relationships, and work habits (see chapter 25). The nurse thoroughly analyzes the problems of loss and grief before planning interventions that will help the client cope with the grief.

Nurses always try to stay a step ahead of the assessment. Once a question is asked or an observation is made, the information often branches to an additional series of questions or observations. Nurses who do not anticipate assessment questions may not recognize problems. Knowing how to frame questions is a basic skill, refined over time. Nurses decide which questions are relevant to the situation and necessary for a complete assessment. The nurse's thoughts about the client develop from ideas gleaned from cues or data. A nurse's ability to assign meaning to the data that are collected and analyzed largely depends on knowledge and experience.

Assessment is part of a nurse's collaborative role. The nurse makes clinical observations about a client, reports the client's situation relative to a medical problem, and then follows delegated medical activities prescribed by the physician. In the independent role of a health care provider, the nurse assesses a client's response to health problems and institutes nursing interventions to maintain or improve the client's health. Accurate assessment is crucial to ensure client needs are properly identified and the right course of action is implemented. Nurses also assess clients' responses to nursing interventions.

Organization of Data Gathering

Before beginning an assessment, a nurse should organize the assessment process and decide which data to collect. Nurses must have a focus when initiating the nurse-client interaction. Why has the client sought health care? What is the purpose of the nurse-client interaction? Who will be involved? What knowledge does the nurse have about the situation that brings the nurse and client together? These factors influence the nurse's success in developing a relationship with the client that leads to a directed, purposeful, and comprehensive assessment.

During an assessment, many interactions (verbal and non-verbal) occur between the nurse and client. Verbal data include information that is communicated through words that are spoken, written, or signed (i.e., sign language) and their meaning (Stephen, 1997). Clues about a client's overall state may be revealed in choice of words, vocabulary level, volume, and speed of speech. For example, clients who speak loudly, respond inappropriately to questions, and have difficulty focusing and completing sentences reveal clues about their intellectual and emotional health.

Non-verbal data include information communicated through body language. Clients present physiological responses that relay information, such as posturing, breathing patterns, and body movement. Body language tends to be involuntary; therefore, it may be a more accurate expression of feelings and emotions than verbal language. Sometimes, non-verbal communication is purposeful and voluntary. For example, clients may point to the location where they are feeling pain or they may use their hands to describe the amount or type of pain they are experiencing. Other examples of purposeful body language include massaging an area, supporting an injured limb, and protecting a tender area (Stephen, 1997).

Nurses use the five senses to accurately assess a client's behaviour. The senses collect experiences that the nurse can classify and judge (Bandman & Bandman, 1995). For example, when a nurse observes a client having difficulty breathing, sense impressions are formed that the client is in trouble. These sense impressions are sources of knowledge and often are reliable clues that lead the nurse to a more deliberate assessment. The skills of physical examination (see chapter 28) enable the nurse to explore physical findings accurately and in detail, such as measurement of respiratory rate, rhythm, and depth. When making judgments, nurses connect sense experiences to nursing knowledge to ensure accurate reasoning.

As a client and nurse interact, the nurse asks relevant questions to gather more data. If the nurse does not ask the right questions, the database may be incomplete and the conclusions (i.e., the nursing diagnoses), inaccurate. Any inferences about the client are separated from actual data.

Data Collection

Assessment data must be descriptive, concise, and complete. An assessment should not include inferences or interpretative statements that are not supported with data. Nurses apply intellectual standards of critical thinking (see chapter 11) to collect the details necessary to understand clients' problems or needs. For example, when a client tells a nurse about difficulty sleeping, the nurse will ask relevant questions, such as, "Do you have trouble falling asleep?" or "Do you have trouble staying asleep?" The nurse may also ask a specific question, such as, "How many hours of sleep do you average each night?" Note that the nurse asks only one question at a time. Nurses should avoid asking questions in the negative, such as, "You don't take sleeping pills, do you?" These questions can put clients in an awkward position. In this example, if the client answers in the affirmative, he or she is admitting to doing something of which the nurse disapproves. These kinds of questions do not encourage openness, and may even lead to incorrect information being recorded.

A client's database begins with the client's perception of a symptom or health problem; additional data are obtained from the perceptions and observations of the family, the nurse's observations, or reports from other members of the health care team. A nurse might begin an assessment by saying, "Tell me what brings you to the clinic" or "How has your fatigue affected your daily way of life?" Open-ended questions allow clients to tell their stories in detail and to relate what is important. In this way, the nurse can quickly focus on the client's priorities.

As a client begins to reveal information, the nurse immediately begins to anticipate the need for other questions and considers what the existing data means. For example, a client may describe pain as a "sharp, throbbing pain in the back." The nurse's observation may be as follows: "The client lies on the right side with knees flexed. Facial grimacing is present. The client is unable to turn without assistance." The nurse then conducts a focused examination and records only observations (e.g., tenderness over the fourth and fifth lumbar vertebrae) and avoids interpreting behaviour (e.g., "The client tolerates pain poorly"). The information obtained is summarized in a short, concise format using correct medical terms (e.g., "Client describes a constant, sharp, throbbing pain in the lower lumbar area of the back. Turning is limited. Pain began 48 hours ago after the client fell off a ladder"). Complete data collection results from obtaining all information relevant to the actual or potential health problem. The nursing requires information that answers the questions, When, where, and what are the duration and influencing factors for the client's problems?

Collecting inaccurate or incomplete data may lead to incorrect identification of the client's health care needs and subsequent inappropriate nursing diagnoses. Inaccurate data result if a nurse fails to collect information relevant to a specific area or if a nurse is disorganized or unskilled in assessment techniques. The assessment will be incomplete if a nurse neglects to obtain all information about a specific area or make unwarranted assumptions.

Types of Data

Data collection involves the gathering of subjective and objective data from or about a client. **Subjective data** are clients' perceptions about their health problems. Only clients can provide this kind of information. For example, a client's report of feeling fearful about impending surgery is a subjective finding. Other examples of subjective data include feelings of anxiety, pain, or mental stress. Although only clients can provide subjective data relevant to their feelings, nurses need to be aware that these problems can result in physiological changes, which are identified through objective data collection.

Objective data are observations or measurements made by the data collector. Assessment of a client's wound and a description of client behaviour are examples of observed objective data. The measurement of objective data is based on an accepted **standard,** such as the centimetres on a measuring tape or known definitions of behaviours. Body temperature and blood pressure are other examples of measured objective data.

Sources of Data

Data are obtained from the client, family, significant others, health care team members, and health records. Data are also obtained though physical examination, results of diagnostic and laboratory tests, and pertinent nursing and medical literature. The nurse's own past experiences with similar types of clients help validate data accuracy. Each source of data provides information about the client's level of wellness, anticipated prognosis, risk factors, health practices and goals, and patterns of health and illness, as well as information relevant to the client's health care needs.

Client. A client is usually the best source of information. The client who is oriented and answers questions appropriately can provide the most accurate information about health care needs, lifestyle patterns, present and past illnesses, perception of symptoms, and changes in ability to perform **activities of daily living (ADLs;** i.e., daily self-care activities necessary for independence, including ambulating, eating, dressing, bathing, brushing the teeth, and grooming). It is necessary, however, for nurses to consider the setting where they interact with the client. A client experiencing acute symptoms in an emergency department will not be able to offer the same depth of information as one who comes to a primary care clinic for a routine checkup. In order to gather a detailed database, it is important for nurses to always pay attention to their clients. Clients are less likely to fully reveal the nature of their health care problems when health care providers show little interest.

Family and Significant Others. Family members and significant others can be interviewed as primary sources of information about infants, children, and critically ill, intellectually disabled, disoriented, or unconscious clients. In cases of severe illness or emergency situations, families may be the only available sources of data about a client's health-illness patterns, current medications, allergies, onset of illness, and other needed information.

The family and significant others are also important secondary sources of information. They can confirm findings provided by a client. It is important to include them in assessment of the client when appropriate and when desired by the client. Often spouses or close friends will attend an assessment and provide their view of the client's health problems or needs. They may supply information about the client's current health status, when changes in the client's status occurred, and how the client's functioning has been affected. Family members are a valuable source of information about a client because they observe how health problems affect the client's daily activities. Their knowledge about the client's needs can affect the way care is delivered (e.g., how a client swallows or eats a meal, how a client makes choices, or how a client reacts to pain).

Health Care Team Members. For a comprehensive assessment, nurses must communicate with other health care team members, such as physicians, other nurses, physiotherapists, and others. In the acute care setting, the change of shift report is often the vehicle for nurses from one shift to convey information to nurses on the oncoming shift (see chapter 13). The health care team provides information about the client's interactions within the health care environment; the client's reaction to information, diagnostic procedures, and nursing and medical therapies; and the client's response to visitors. Every member of the health care team is a potential source of information, and the team can identify and communicate data and verify information from other sources.

Medical Records. The medical record contains data about the client's medical history, laboratory tests, and diagnostic study results. By reviewing past and present medical records, nurses can identify patterns of illness, previous responses to treatment, and past methods of coping. Information in a client's record is confidential and health care agencies have policies governing how the information can be shared among health care providers.

Other Records. Other records such as educational, military, and employment records may contain pertinent health care information (e.g., immunizations and prior illnesses). If the client received services at a community health centre or day care clinic, the nurse should obtain data from these records but must first secure written permission from the client or guardian. All information is confidential and is treated as part of the client's legal medical record (see chapter 8).

Literature Review. Reviewing nursing, medical, and pharmacological literature about a client's illness helps the nurse complete the assessment database. The review increases the nurse's knowledge about the expected symptoms, treatment, and prognosis of specific illnesses, as well as established standards of therapeutic practice.

Nurse's Experience. Through experience, a nurse learns to ask questions that yield the most useful information. A nurse's expertise develops after testing and refining propositions, questions, and principle- or standard-based expectations. For example, while caring for a client with back pain, the nurse learns many lessons: The nurse recognizes behaviours demonstrated by clients in acute pain. The nurse also notes how positioning techniques comfort the client. The nurse sees first-hand how administering a pain medication regularly achieves better pain control than waiting for the client to request it. Critical thinking is strengthened by practical experience and the opportunity to make decisions. A nurse's ability to assess clients improves from applying past experience, relevant knowledge, and focusing on data collection that avoids unnecessary information.

Methods of Data Collection

The nurse uses the interview, the nursing health history, the physical examination, and results of laboratory and diagnostic tests to establish the assessment database.

Interview. The first step in establishing the database is to collect subjective information by interviewing the client. An **interview** is an organized conversation with the client to obtain the client's health history and information about the current illness. During an interview, nurses have the opportunity to do the following:

- Introduce themselves to the client and explain their role and that of other health care professionals
- Establish a sense of caring for the client as an individual
- Establish a therapeutic relationship with the client
- Gain insight about the client's concerns and worries
- Determine the client's goals and expectations of the health care system
- Obtain cues about which parts of the data collection phase require further in-depth investigation

The interview should help clients relate their own interpretation and understanding of their condition. The nurse and client must be partners during the interview, rather than the nurse controlling the interview. A therapeutic relationship with the client is essential (see chapter 15).

An interview includes three phases: orientation, working, and termination.

Case Study — Box 12-1

Daniel Shea is the registered nurse assigned to Mr. Brown. Daniel is preparing an admission history on Mr. Brown, a 51-year-old man hospitalized for the first time. Mr. Brown is presenting with a history of diarrhea for 3 weeks. He also has a number of other physical problems including a history of emphysema, which requires a complete nursing assessment. Mr. Brown is married and has a 30-year-old son who has two children of his own.

Daniel: Good afternoon, Mr. Brown. I'm Daniel. I'll be doing the initial assessment of your situation to help us plan your nursing care. We call this a health interview. Any information you give me is confidential. The total interview should take about 20 to 30 minutes. Is it okay if I begin the interview in a few minutes?

Mr. Brown: How about giving me a half-hour? My wife is about to leave. She needs to go pick up the grandkids at day care. That way we can have some time together. I'll be ready after that.

Daniel: That's fine. Because you're in a private room, I will do the health interview here. (Mr. Brown nods.) Thirty minutes later, Daniel returns to the room.

Daniel: Okay. Before I get started, do you have any questions for me?

Mr. Brown: Yes. Why is there an outlet for oxygen on the wall above my bed? Does that mean that I'm really sick—did they put me in a special room?

Daniel: No, that's not it. Every bed in this hospital has an oxygen outlet located on the wall above the head of the bed. The reason is that this hospital has a central oxygen delivery system, and when a client needs oxygen, we're able to supply it quickly, easily, and safely.

Mr. Brown: Okay. I wasn't actually worried. I was basically just curious. That was the only piece of equipment I couldn't explain.

Daniel: (pause) Mr. Brown, you mentioned that you and your wife have a son and grandchildren. Tell me a bit about your family.

Orientation Phase. The orientation phase begins with the nurse's introduction to the client and an explanation of the interview's purpose. The nurse must explain why the data are being collected (e.g., a nursing health history) and assure the client that information obtained will remain confidential and will be used by health care professionals for the client's care. This phase is important in establishing trust with the client.

Box 12-1 is an introduction to a case study that will be used throughout this chapter to demonstrate the nursing process. To begin, the nurse, Daniel, spends a few minutes becoming acquainted with the client, Mr. Brown. After introducing his role to Mr. Brown, Daniel reviews the interview process and its objectives, confidentiality, and length. Before beginning the interview, Daniel asks his client if he has any questions and answers his client's question. Daniel's open-ended question encourages Mr. Brown to begin the interview in a direction in which he feels comfortable.

Working Phase. During this phase of the interview, the nurse gathers information about the client's health status. The nurse may choose to use a health history form or instead use an open-ended interview technique that allows the client to direct the conversation based upon the problems identified. The nurse uses a variety of communication strategies such as listening, paraphrasing, focusing, summarizing, and clarifying (see chapter 14). The nurse's critical thinking directs the interview so that sufficient detail can be gathered about the client's condition. The following is an example of Daniel's interview:

Daniel: Tell me, Mr. Brown, about your difficulty breathing.

Mr. Brown: I can't get my breath after I do even the simplest activities.

Daniel: Can you give me an example?

Mr. Brown: After I get up in the morning, shower, and dress myself, I just can't catch my breath. I already feel worn out before I even start my day. I am beginning to feel helpless.

Daniel: (silence to encourage Mr. Brown to say more)

Mr. Brown: This problem with my heart is not something I ever expected.

The initial interview is normally the most extensive interview. Major topics covered include biographical data, the progress of the current illness, the client's perceptions and beliefs about the illness, and the health history. Ongoing interviews, which occur each time a nurse interacts with a client, do not need to be as extensive. They update the client's status and are more focused on changes in previously identified ongoing and new problems.

Termination Phase. When concluding an interview, the nurse summarizes the important points and asks the client whether the summary was accurate. The interview is terminated in a friendly manner, with the nurse indicating specifically when there will be additional contact. For example, an appropriate way for Daniel to end his interview would be, "Thank you for your help, Mr. Brown. You have given me a good picture of your health and how you have been affected. You have indicated that you would like to know more about the procedures scheduled for your treatment. You also hope to be able to breathe more easily with less discomfort. Is that correct? This information will be helpful in planning your care. Another nurse will be caring for you this evening, but I'll be back on duty tomorrow morning. Do you have any other questions? Is there anything I can do for you now?"

Interview strategies should be adapted on the basis of the client's responses. Pertinent health data are obtained when the nurse is prepared for the interview and is able to carry it out with minimal interruption.

Interview Techniques. The manner in which the interview is conducted is just as important as the questions asked. Attention to the environment, client comfort, and good communication techniques usually ensures a successful interview. During the interview, the nurse directs the flow of the discussion so that adequate information is obtained and the client has the opportunity to contribute freely.

An interview may be focused or comprehensive. As the nurse listens and considers the information shared, the client may be directed to give more detail or discuss a topic that seems to reveal a possible problem. Because the client's report will include subjective information, the nurse uses data from the interview to later validate with objective data. For example, if the client reports difficulty breathing, the nurse will later assess the client's respiratory rate and listen to (auscultate) lung sounds.

During the interview, the nurse obtains information about a client's physical, developmental, emotional, intellectual, social, and spiritual dimensions. Physical and developmental information reflects expected functioning and reveals any pathological changes induced by illness, trauma, or developmental crisis. Emotional information includes the client's behavioural responses to changes in health and pattern of living. Relevant emotional information includes mood, perceptions, body image, self-concept, and attitudes about sexuality. Intellectual information includes intellectual performance, problem-solving ability, educational level, communication patterns, and attention span. Social information involves environmental, cultural, ethnic, or social patterns that can affect the present or future level of wellness (e.g., values about health care and attitudes about family support). Nurses also collect information about life goals, values, and religious practices, which are part of the spiritual dimension (see chapter 24).

The interview is an opportunity for the nurse to observe the client's appearance, behaviour, and interactions within the health care environment. If family members are present at the interview, the nurse observes interactions between the client and family. Nurses determine whether the data obtained by observation are consistent with those obtained by verbal communication. For example, if the client states no concern about an upcoming diagnostic test but appears anxious and irritable, the data conflict. Observations during an interview lead nurses to gather additional objective information to form accurate conclusions.

Clients also obtain information during the interview. If a positive nurse-client relationship has been established, the client will feel comfortable asking the nurse questions to help make decisions about goals and the plan of care. In addition, the interview is a first step toward helping a client obtain education or counselling. For example, the interview allows a nurse to determine a client's readiness and ability to learn so that appropriate educational interventions can be used. It is also important for nurses to ask clients about their expectations of health care providers.

Nursing Health History. The **nursing health history** is data collected about the client's current level of wellness, including a **review of systems (ROS),** family and health history, socio-cultural history, spiritual health, and mental and emotional reactions to illness. The history is obtained during an interview and is a major component of assessment in the nursing process.

The client's health history provides subjective data on the client's health care experiences and current health and lifestyle habits. The information is entirely from the client's point of view. The goal is to identify patterns of health and illness, risk factors for physical and behavioural health problems, deviations from the expected, and available resources for adaptation. Although many health history forms are structured, the nurse learns to use the questions as starting points. A good assessor learns to refine and broaden questions as needed so that the client's unique needs are correctly assessed. Client priorities, time available for data collection, and duration the client will remain in a particular setting determine how complete a history will be. For example, a client arrives at an emergency department with a fractured wrist and will be discharged home in a few hours. The health history will focus on the fracture and what assistance the client will require to cope with it. In contrast, nurses admitting a client to a long-term care facility need to collect a detailed history as a baseline. Baseline data are used to plan future interactions and as a reference point for identifying changes in a client's health status over time. Although there are many formats for the nursing health history, all contain similar basic components (Box 12-2).

Recording Nursing Health History Findings. There are two points of view about recording history findings. One is that nurses should record data on standardized forms as the client responds to questions. The other view is that

Box 12-2 Guidelines for a Comprehensive Nursing Health History

A. ***Identifying Data.*** Name, age, sex, date and place of birth.
B. ***Reason for Health History Interview.***
C. ***Present State of Health.*** General state of health, health goals. If an illness is present, gather data about the nature of the illness by conducting a symptom analysis (see chapter 28).
D. ***Developmental Variables.***
- Marital status: single, married, separated, widowed, divorced.
- Number of children.
- Developmental stage (see chapter 18).
- Current occupation.
- Significant life experiences (e.g., education, previous occupations, financial situations, retirement, coping-stress-tolerance, and measures normally used to reduce stress).
- Safety hazards (e.g., biological, chemical, ergonomic, physical, psychosocial, reproductive).
- Housing, environmental hazards (e.g, type of housing, location, living arrangements; specific hazards in the home or community).
- Safety measures (e.g., use of seat belts, presence of smoke detectors and fire extinguishers, and other measures related to specific hazards of work, community, and home).

E. ***Psychological Variables.*** Mental processes, relationships, support systems, statements about client's feelings about self.
F. ***Spiritual Variables.*** Rituals, religious practices, beliefs about life, clients' source for guidance in acting on beliefs, and the relationship with family in exercising faith.
G. ***Socio-cultural Variables.***
- Culture—beliefs and practices related to health and illness (see chapter 9).
- Primary language and other languages spoken.
- Recreation (exercise, hobbies, socializing, use of leisure time).
- Family/significant others. Include family composition, relationships, special problems experienced by family, client and family response to stress, roles, and support systems. The family history provides information about family structure, interaction, and function that may be useful in planning care. For example, a cohesive, supportive family can help a client adjust to an illness or disability and should be incorporated into the plan of care. However, if the client's family is not supportive, it may be better to not involve them in care. Outline a family tree (genogram, see chapter 16) to determine whether the client is at risk for genetic illnesses and to identify areas of health promotion and illness prevention.

H. ***Physiological Variables*** (body structure and function).
- Past history of illnesses and injuries, including dates.
- Current medications: Prescribed, over-the-counter, and/or illicit drugs. Include name, dose, schedule, duration and reason for use, expected effects and side effects; if illicit drug, include type, amount, response, adverse reaction, drug-related accidents/arrests, attempts to quit.
- Review of Systems (ROS). The ROS is a systematic method for collecting data on all body systems. It is likely that not all questions in each system will be covered in every history. Nevertheless, some questions about each system are included, particularly when a client mentions a symptom or sign. The nurse begins with open-ended questions about the usual functioning of each body system and any noted changes, and follows with specific questions such as the ones noted under each system. Nurses also focus on measures taken by the client to promote and maintain health, and prevent illness or injury. The following are included in the ROS:
- **General presentation of symptoms:** Fever, chills, malaise, pain, sleep patterns and disturbances, fatigue, recent alterations in weight.
- **Integumentary:** Itching, colour or texture change, lesions, dryness and use of creams/lotions, changes in hair or nails.
- **Ocular:** Visual acuity, blurring, pain, recent change in vision, discharge, excessive tearing, date of last examination.
- **Auditory:** Hearing loss, pain, discharge, dizziness, ringing in ears, wax.
- **Upper Respiratory:** Nosebleeds, discharge from nose, nasal allergies, sinus problems, frequency of colds and usual method of treatment, sore throat and usual type of home remedy, hoarseness or voice changes.
- **Lower Respiratory:** Use of tobacco (amount and number of years smoking; exposure to others smoking; if smoker, attempts to stop smoking), exposure to airborne pollutants, cough, sputum, wheezing, shortness of breath, tuberculosis test and results, date of last chest X-ray.
- **Breasts and Axillae:** Rashes, lumps, discharge, pain; breast self-examination practices.
- **Lymphatic:** Pain; swelling.
- **Cardiovascular:** Chest pain or distress, precipitating causes, timing and duration, relieving factors, dyspnea, orthopnea, edema, hypertension, exercise tolerance circulatory problems, varicose veins.
- **Gastrointestinal:** Appetite, digestion, food intolerance, dysphagia, heartburn, abdominal pain, nausea or vomiting, bowel regularity, use of laxatives, change in stool colour or contents, constipation or diarrhea, flatulence, hemorrhoids, rectal examinations.
  a. Dietary Pattern: Number of servings per day of each of the food groups, using Canada's Food Guide to Healthy Eating for serving size (see chapter 39); restrictions to food choice; special diets; use of salt; calculate adequacy of fluid intake (should be 30 to 40 mL of fluid/kg of body weight); indicate sources of calcium and amounts per day, alcohol use (average number of ounces/week, recent changes in pattern of consumption).

Adapted from *A Syllabus for Adult Health Assessment,* edited by D. L. Skillen and R. A. Day, 2004, Edmonton, AB: Faculty of Nursing, University of Alberta.

Box 12-2 Guidelines for a Comprehensive Nursing Health History—cont'd

- **Urinary:** Painful urination; blood, stones, or pus in urine; bladder or kidney infections; difficulty stopping urinary stream; dribbling or hesitancy; sudden feeling of need to pass urine; frequent urination; nocturia (having to get up to void during the night); incontinence (see chapter 41).
- **Genital/Reproductive:**
  a. Male: Puberty onset, difficulty with erections, emissions, testicular pain, libido, infertility, urethral discharge, genital lesions, exposure to and history of STIs, self-testicular examinations, testicular lump or pain, hernias, sexual preference, birth control and safer sex practices used.
  b. Female: Menses (onset, duration, regularity, flow, discomfort, date of last menstrual period), age at menopause (occurrence of hot flashes, night sweats, vaginal discharge), date of last PAP smear, pregnancies (number, miscarriages, abortions), exposure to and history of STIs, sexual preference, birth control and safer sex practices used.
- **Musculoskeletal:** Pain, joint stiffness or swelling, restricted motion, muscle wasting, weakness, general mobility.
- **Neurological:** Injury, headaches, dizziness, fainting, abnormalities of sensation or coordination, tremors, seizures.
- **Endocrine:** Excessive sweating, thirst, hunger or urination; intolerance to heat or cold; changes in distribution of facial hair; thyroid enlargement or tenderness; unexplained weight change; change to glove, shoe size.
- **Hematologic:** Anemia; bruise or bleed easily; transfusions.
- **Psychiatric:** Depression, mood changes, difficulty concentrating, nervousness, anxiety, suicidal thoughts, irritability.
- **Immunologic:** Communicable diseases (indicate disease and age or year), immunization status (indicate year of most recent immunization), allergies (known allergens and reactions; medic-alert identification worn).

nurses should jot down key points during the interview but wait until the interview is complete to write up the detailed information. The latter approach allows nurses to focus their attention on the client during the interview, rather than on writing.

Physical Examination. During the **physical examination,** vital signs and other objective measurements are taken and all body systems are examined. The purpose is to objectively validate information obtained from the nursing health history. New information can also be identified. See chapter 28 for complete details about the physical examination.

Diagnostic and Laboratory Data. Diagnostic and laboratory data are an important part of the nursing assessment because they can identify or verify alterations noted during the nursing health history and physical examination. For example, during the history, the client indicates recurrent upper respiratory tract infections and presently has a productive cough with brown sputum. The nurse notes during the physical examination that the client has an elevated body temperature, increased respirations, and decreased breath sounds in the right lower lobe. The nurse reviews results of a complete blood count (CBC) to look for an elevated white blood cell (WBC) count, indicative of an infection. In addition, the nurse checks the results of a chest X-ray examination to determine if there is right lung congestion. Together, the findings suggest the client may have pneumonia. Laboratory data are compared with the established **norms** for a particular test, age group, and gender. Nurses identify variations from the usual and interpret findings according to the disease process and treatments. In addition, nurses use laboratory data to evaluate the success or failure of nursing and medical interventions.

Formulating Nursing Judgments

The successful interpretation of assessment data requires critical thinking. When nurses correctly collect and analyze data, they are able to make necessary clinical decisions for their clients' care. Useful and appropriate assessment data must refer to the intended purpose of nursing and relate to the client's health problems (Bandman & Bandman, 1995). These interrelated concepts are the basis for nursing judgments. Critical thinking in client assessment enables nurses to fully understand clients' problems, judge the extent of the problems more carefully, and discover possible relationships between or among problems.

Data Clustering. After validating and interpreting assessment data, nurses organize the information into meaningful clusters, keeping in mind the client's response to illness. A cluster is a set of signs or symptoms that are grouped together in a logical order. During data clustering, nurses organize data and focus on client functions needing support and assistance for recovery. Focused data clustering using a systems approach or another health patterns approach assists the nurse to correctly classify and organize data. For example, a client who has recently been diagnosed with diabetes, has had no opportunity to talk with a physician, and is asking questions about insulin obviously has a problem related to inadequate knowledge. As the nurse clusters cues, such as the client asking questions and reporting no previous experience with insulin use, a pattern of meaning forms. Clustering of data helps the nurse to focus on identification of the problem.

During data clustering, certain cues alert the nurse's thinking processes and help generate nursing diagnoses. Nurses become experienced in recognizing features of health problems such as pain, anxiety, or immobility. Over time, the nurse stores knowledge from previous experiences so that more complicated clustering becomes possible. This knowledge explains the difference in the skill of a beginning nurse and a more expert nurse.

Data Documentation

Documentation is the last part of a complete assessment. The nursing process requires thorough, concise, and accurate documentation. If an item is not recorded, it is lost and unavailable. When recording data, nurses should pay attention to facts and be as descriptive as possible. Anything heard, seen, felt, or smelled should be reported exactly. Objective information must be recorded using accurate terminology (e.g., weighs 170 kg, abdomen is soft and non-tender to palpation). Subjective information from a client is recorded in quotation marks. When entering data, nurses should avoid generalizing or forming judgments through written communication. Collecting concise and accurate information through the health history interview provides the basis for the physical examination and ongoing care of the client. Thorough documentation ensures that information is available to those caring for the client's needs.

Step 2: Nursing Diagnosis

Nursing diagnosis, the second step of the nursing process, is a term used to classify health problems within the domain of nursing. A **nursing diagnosis** is a clinical judgment about individual, family, or community responses to actual and potential health problems or life processes (NANDA International, 2003). It is a statement that describes the client's actual or potential response to a health problem that the nurse is licensed and competent to treat. *Impaired skin integrity, risk for infection,* and *deficient knowledge* are examples of nursing diagnoses. Just as a **medical diagnosis** (physician's clinical judgment of disease) of diabetes mellitus provides the basis for selection of medical therapies (e.g., insulin, an 1,800-calorie diet, and moderate exercise), the nursing diagnosis of *impaired skin integrity* provides the basis for selection of nursing therapies (e.g., application of pressure relief devices, regular turning schedules, and skin care). The accurate selection of nursing diagnoses requires a nurse to use critical thinking and good clinical judgment.

Evolution of Nursing Diagnosis

Nursing diagnosis was first introduced in the nursing literature in 1950 (McFarland & McFarlane, 1989). Fry (1953) proposed that nursing could be more creative by the formulation of nursing diagnoses and an individualized nursing care plan. This proposal emphasized the nurse's independent practice (e.g., education and symptom relief) compared with the dependent practice driven by physicians' orders (e.g., medication administration and wound treatment). Initially, professional nursing did not support nursing diagnoses, and most provincial and territorial nursing legislation prior to the 1970s excluded references to diagnosis or prescriptive therapies. As a result, nurses hesitated to use nursing diagnoses in their practice.

However, nursing theorists encouraged defining nursing in terms of client problems and were partly responsible for the interest and eventual use of nursing diagnosis in contemporary nursing education, practice, administration, and research.

In 1973, the first U.S. national conference for the classification of nursing diagnosis was held to identify nursing functions and establish a classification system. "A classification system for nursing defines the body of knowledge for which nursing is held accountable" (Carpenito, 1995). Over the years, participants of these conferences have developed the accepted nursing diagnoses (Box 12-3). In 1982, a professional association, the North American Nursing Diagnosis Association (NANDA), was established. The purpose of NANDA was "to develop, refine, and promote a taxonomy of nursing diagnostic terminology of general use for professional nurses" (Kim, McFarland, & McLean, 1984). Recently, NANDA changed its name to **NANDA International** (NANDA International, 2003) to better reflect the international utility of nursing diagnosis. NANDA International's work provides a common language for the health problems that nurses deal with. The organization is the leader in nursing diagnosis classification and is widely recognized by members of the nursing profession as having the responsibility to do so.

Nursing diagnosis is recognized in Canada and the United States as an innovative means of translating nursing observations and assessments into standard conclusions using a common nomenclature. Although nursing diagnosis is part of basic nursing preparation in Canada, it has not yet been incorporated into provincial and territorial nursing practice standards or legislation. The exception is in Ontario, where practice standards require the formulation and documentation of nursing diagnoses. The Canadian Nurses Association defines nursing as a "dynamic, caring, helping relationship in which the nurse assists the client to achieve and maintain optimal health. The nurse fulfills this purpose by applying knowledge and skills from nursing and related fields using the nursing process" (1986). Although this definition does not specifically mention diagnosis, it promotes the nursing process and therefore gives support to diagnosis along with the other steps of the process. It may be that the introduction of new health profession legislation, which defines controlled acts that nurses are permitted to perform, may lead to the more widespread application of nursing diagnosis in Canadian nursing legislation and standards. In the meantime, Higuchi et al. (1999) reported that Canadian nurses are more likely to document nursing diagnoses when institutions have formal educational programs and computer-generated care plans.

Critical Thinking and the Nursing Diagnostic Process

A nurse integrates what is known from previous experience and scientific and practical knowledge bases, applies critical thinking attitudes and intellectual standards, and refers to standards of practice in making well-reasoned, accurate, and relevant nursing diagnoses (Figure 12–3). The critical thinking process (see chapter 11) is required in diagnostic reasoning and judgment.

Diagnostic Process. Diagnostic reasoning is a process of using the data gathered about a client to logically explain a clinical judgment, in this case making a nursing

Box 12-3 NANDA Nursing Diagnoses

Activity intolerance
Risk for **Activity** intolerance
Impaired **Adjustment**
Ineffective **Airway** clearance
Latex **Allergy** response
Risk for latex **Allergy** response
Anxiety
Death **Anxiety**
Risk for **Aspiration**
Risk for impaired parent/infant/child **Attachment**
Autonomic dysreflexia
Risk for **Autonomic** dysreflexia
Disturbed **Body** image
Risk for imbalanced **Body** temperature
Bowel incontinence
Effective **Breast-feeding**
Ineffective **Breast-feeding**
Interrupted **Breast-feeding**
Ineffective **Breathing** pattern
Decreased **Cardiac** output
Caregiver role strain
Risk for **Caregiver** role strain
Impaired **Comfort**
Impaired verbal **Communication**
Readiness for enhanced **Communication**
Decisional **Conflict**
Parental role **Conflict**
Acute **Confusion**
Chronic **Confusion**
Constipation
Perceived **Constipation**
Risk for **Constipation**
Coping
Ineffective **Coping**
Ineffective community **Coping**
Readiness for enhanced community **Coping**
Defensive **Coping**
Compromised family **Coping**
Disabled family **Coping**
Readiness for enhanced family **Coping**
Ineffective **Denial**
Impaired **Dentition**
Risk for delayed **Development**
Diarrhea
Risk for **Disuse** syndrome
Deficient **Diversional** activity
Disturbed **Energy** field
Impaired **Environmental** interpretation syndrome
Adult **Failure** to thrive
Risk for **Falls**
Dysfunctional **Family** processes: alcoholism
Family processes
Interrupted **Family** processes
Fatigue
Fear
Fluid balance
Deficient **Fluid** volume
Excess **Fluid** volume
Risk for deficient **Fluid** volume
Risk for imbalanced **Fluid** volume
Impaired **Gas** exchange
Grieving
Anticipatory **Grieving**
Dysfunctional **Grieving**
Delayed **Growth** and development
Risk for disproportionate **Growth**
Ineffective **Health** maintenance
Health-seeking behaviours
Impaired **Home** maintenance
Hopelessness
Hyperthermia
Hypothermia
Disturbed personal **Identity**
Functional urinary **Incontinence**
Reflex urinary **Incontinence**
Stress urinary **Incontinence**
Total urinary **Incontinence**
Urge urinary **Incontinence**
Risk for urge urinary **Incontinence**
Disorganized **Infant** behaviour
Risk for disorganized **Infant** behaviour
Readiness for enhanced organized **Infant** behaviour
Ineffective **Infant** feeding pattern
Risk for **Infection**
Risk for **Injury**
Risk for perioperative-positioning **Injury**
Decreased **Intracranial** adaptive capacity
Deficient **Knowledge**
Knowledge (specify)
Risk for **Loneliness**
Impaired **Memory**
Impaired bed **Mobility**
Impaired physical **Mobility**
Impaired wheelchair **Mobility**
Nausea
Unilateral **Neglect**
Noncompliance
Imbalanced **Nutrition:** less than body requirements
Imbalanced **Nutrition:** more than body requirements
Nutrition
Risk for imbalanced **Nutrition:** more than body requirements
Impaired **Oral** mucous membrane
Acute **Pain**
Chronic **Pain**
Impaired **Parenting**
Parenting
Risk for impaired **Parenting**
Risk for **Peripheral** neurovascular dysfunction
Risk for **Poisoning**
Post-trauma syndrome
Risk for **Post-trauma** syndrome
Powerlessness
Risk for **Powerlessness**
Ineffective **Protection**
Rape-trauma syndrome
Rape-trauma syndrome: compound reaction
Rape-trauma syndrome: silent reaction
Relocation stress syndrome

From *NANDA Nursing Diagnoses: Definitions and Classification 2003–2004,* by NANDA International, 2003, Philadelphia: Author. Adapted with permission.

Continued

Box 12-3 NANDA Nursing Diagnoses—cont'd

Risk for **Relocation** stress syndrome
Ineffective **Role** performance
Bathing/hygiene **Self-care** deficit
Dressing/grooming **Self-care** deficit
Feeding **Self-care** deficit
Toileting **Self-care** deficit
Self-concept
Chronic low **Self-esteem**
Situational low **Self-esteem**
Risk for situational low **Self-esteem**
Self-mutilation
Risk for **Self-mutilation**
Disturbed **Sensory** perception
Sexual dysfunction
Ineffective **Sexuality** patterns
Impaired **Skin** integrity
Risk for impaired **Skin** integrity
Sleep
Sleep deprivation
Disturbed **Sleep** pattern
Impaired **Social** interaction
Social isolation
Chronic **Sorrow**
Spiritual distress
Risk for **Spiritual** distress
Readiness for enhanced **Spiritual** well-being
Risk for **Sudden Infant Death Syndrome**
Risk for **Suffocation**
Risk for **Suicide**
Delayed **Surgical** recovery
Impaired **Swallowing**
Effective **Therapeutic** regimen management
Ineffective **Therapeutic** regimen management
Ineffective community **Therapeutic** regimen management
Ineffective family **Therapeutic** regimen management
Management of **Therapeutic** regimen
Ineffective **Thermoregulation**
Disturbed **Thought** processes
Impaired **Tissue** integrity
Ineffective **Tissue** perfusion
Impaired **Transfer** ability
Risk for **Trauma**
Impaired **Urinary** elimination
Urinary elimination
Urinary retention
Impaired spontaneous **Ventilation**
Dysfunctional **Ventilatory** weaning response
Risk for other-directed **Violence**
Risk for self-directed **Violence**
Impaired **Walking**
Wandering

From *NANDA Nursing Diagnoses: Definitions and Classification 2003–2004,* by NANDA International, 2003, Philadelphia: Author. Adapted with permission.

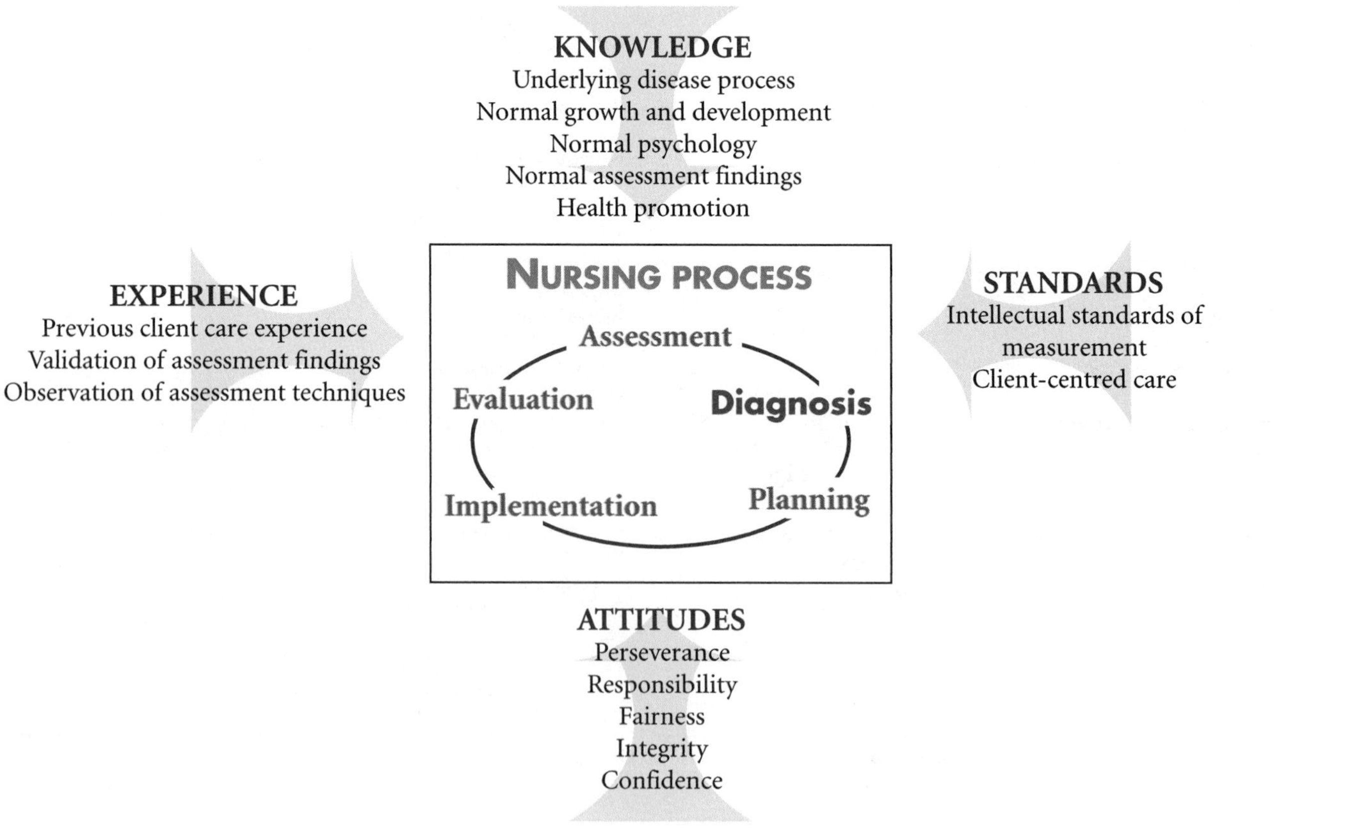

FIGURE **12–3** Critical thinking and the nursing diagnostic process.

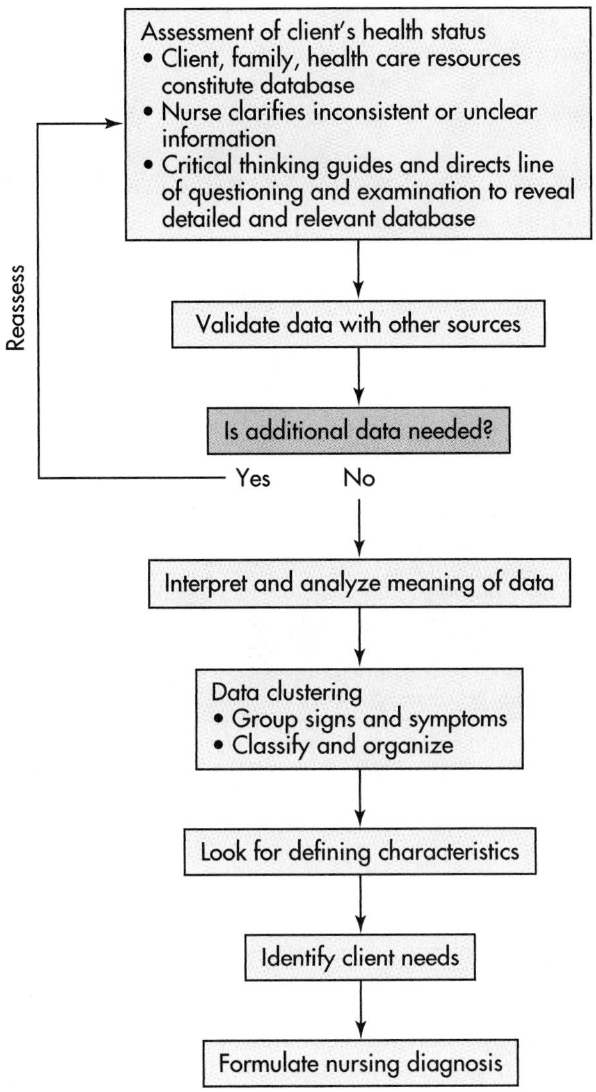

FIGURE **12–4** The nursing diagnostic process.

Box 12-4 Summary of Relevant Data From Mr. Brown's Complete Assessment

Physical and Developmental

Diarrhea for 3 weeks
Productive cough upon rising each morning
Occasional rales in lung bases
7-kg weight loss 3 weeks before hospitalization
Hemoglobin 120 g/L
Slight change of emphysema shown on chest roentgenogram
Distended abdomen
Squamous cell cancer
Biopsy obtained during outpatient colonoscopy June 24
Smoked for 15 years, 2 packs a day (30 pack-years)
Family history of stomach cancer
Family history of heart attack
Married 30 years
Self-employed for 20 years
One adult son, 30 years old
Two grandchildren
Two sisters, 50 and 48, with no major health problems
Anemia
Crackles auscultated in lung fields

Intellectual

Talkative
Frequently asks nurses if he has cancer and "Can it be treated?"
Good attention span

Emotional

Anxious
Withdrawn after biopsy report of squamous cell cancer
Awaiting colon resection and temporary colostomy

Social

Walks with neighbour
Active in his neighbourhood
Visits regularly with his son and grandchildren

Spiritual

Methodist
Attends church weekly
Reads Bible daily

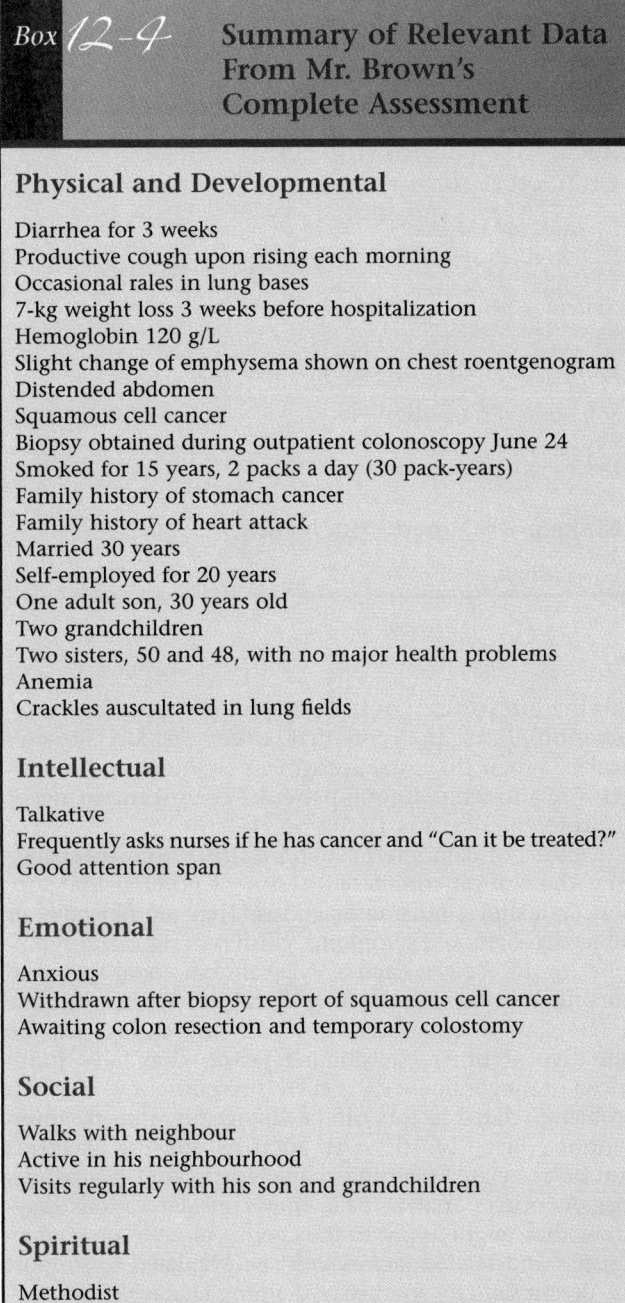

diagnosis. The **diagnostic process** includes decision-making steps, including gathering the assessment database, validating data, analyzing and interpreting data, identifying client needs, and formulating nursing diagnoses (Figure 12–4). The diagnostic process is dynamic and requires the nurse to reflect on existing assessment data and health care needs of the client (Da Cruz & Acuri, 1998). The nurse uses scientific knowledge and experience to analyze and interpret data collected about the client. The nurse then identifies the client's health care problems and writes nursing diagnoses, which form the basis for a plan of care. Clinical situations demand that diagnostic reasoning be thorough and rigorous in order for data to support a nursing diagnosis.

Analysis and Interpretation of Data. Data analysis involves (a) recognizing patterns or trends, (b) comparing them with widely accepted standards for normal, such as professional standards and knowledge and normal diagnostic test values, and (c) making a reasoned conclusion. As mentioned in the assessment section, the nurse organizes information into meaningful clusters, a set of signs or symptoms grouped together in a logical order. Alone, these signs or symptoms cannot be the basis of a nursing diagnosis. However, when clustered together as a group, the nurse sees a relationship between and among these assessment findings. Consider the case of Mr. Brown introduced earlier. Box 12-4 is a summary of relevant data collected by Daniel Shea (the registered nurse) from Mr. Brown's assessment. Singly, these symptoms could be related to multiple nursing diagnoses, but by analyzing these symptoms together, the nurse begins to think about functional health patterns (e.g., client's

Box 12-5 Example of Data Analysis: Mr. Brown

Recognize Pattern (Cluster of Defining Characteristics)

Diarrhea for 3 weeks
Ribbon-shaped or watery stools
Distended abdomen
Cramping before and during each bowel movement

Compare With Normal Standards

Soft, formed stool daily
Abdomen soft, non-distended
Defecation non-painful

Make a Reasoned Conclusion

Bowel elimination problem

Box 12-6 Sample Nursing Diagnosis With Defining Characteristics and Related Factors

Diagnosis: Diarrhea
Definition: Passage of loose, unformed stool

Defining Characteristics:

- At least three loose, liquid stools a day
- Hyperactive bowel sounds
- Urgency
- Abdominal pain
- Cramping

Related Factors:

- *Psychological:* High stress and anxiety
- *Situational:* Alcohol abuse, toxins, laxative abuse, travel, radiation, tube feedings, adverse medication effects, contaminants
- *Physiological:* Inflammation, malabsorption, irritation, infectious processes, parasites

Adapted from *NANDA Nursing Diagnoses: Definitions and Classification 2003–2004,* by NANDA International, 2003, Philadelphia: Author.

elimination pattern) or body system function (e.g., oxygenation), and the potential effect on Mr. Brown's health. When the nurse recognizes a pattern and identifies a relationship among patterns, client-centred needs begin to emerge (Box 12-5).

Clusters of data often contain **defining characteristics,** the clinical criteria or assessment findings that support (validate) a nursing diagnosis. They are objective or subjective signs and symptoms, clusters of signs and symptoms, or risk factors. Each NANDA International-approved nursing diagnosis has defining characteristics that validate it (NANDA International, 2003). **Related factors** are causative or other contributing factors that have influenced or may influence the client's response to the health problem; related factors can be changed by nursing interventions. Box 12-6 shows an approved nursing diagnosis and its associated defining characteristics and related factors. As nurses analyze data, they consider various diagnoses that might apply to the client. All defining characteristics and related factors must be evaluated to support the diagnosis. The absence of defining characteristics suggests that a proposed diagnosis should be rejected.

Identification of Client Needs. Before finalizing a nursing diagnosis, the nurse identifies the client's general health care needs or problems. For example, after reviewing clusters of data, such as dyspnea, increased respiratory rate, and cough, the nurse recognizes that the client has a general respiratory problem. However, before a nurse can effectively give care, the problem must be more specifically defined. NANDA International has a variety of nursing diagnoses that can apply to a respiratory problem (e.g., *ineffective breathing pattern, impaired gas exchange,* or *ineffective airway clearance*). It is critical for the nurse to eventually arrive at the correct diagnostic label for the client's need (Collier, McCash, & Bartram, 1996). When identifying the client's general problem, the nurse considers all assessment data and focuses on pertinent, relevant, and abnormal data (Gordon, 1994). It may help the inexperienced nurse to think of the problem identification phase as the general health care problem and the formulation of the nursing diagnosis as the specific health care problem. The nurse moves from general to specific.

It is important for the nurse to review the assessment data to identify client needs and not focus solely on the client's illness or medical diagnosis. For example, a client has a nursing diagnosis of *social isolation related to relocation into extended care.* Although this client has Parkinson's disease, his greatest need is to increase social supports and familiarity with his new surroundings.

Formulation of the Nursing Diagnosis. Once patterns and clusters of data containing defining characteristics are sorted and client needs or problems are identified, the nurse is ready to formulate nursing diagnoses. NANDA International (2003) has identified three types of nursing diagnoses: actual diagnoses, risk diagnoses, and wellness diagnoses.

- An **actual nursing diagnosis** describes a client's responses to health conditions/life processes. It is based on assessment data and supported by defining characteristics.
- A **risk nursing diagnosis** describes responses to health conditions/life processes that may develop in a vulnerable client. For example, a client with a spinal cord injury that limits mobility is at *risk for impaired skin integrity.* This diagnosis is based on data revealing risk factors (e.g., physiological, psychosocial factors) that increase the client's vulnerability to developing the condition.
- A **wellness nursing diagnosis** describes responses to levels of wellness in a client that has a readiness for

Table 12-1 Formulation of Nursing Diagnoses for Mr. Brown

Clustering Data	Identification of Client Need	Nursing Diagnosis
Diarrhea for 3 weeks Distended abdomen Family history of stomach cancer	Alteration of elimination patterns	Diarrhea related to irritation
Weight loss: 7 kg	Excessive weight loss	Altered nutrition: less than body requirements related to inability to absorb nutrients because of chronic diarrhea for 3 weeks
Anemia 30 pack-year history of smoking Slight change of emphysema shown on chest X-ray film Crackles auscultated in lung fields Productive cough on rising each morning	Risk for post-operative respiratory complications	Risk for ineffective airway clearance after surgery related to incisional pain
Temporary colostomy	Possible change in body image	Risk for situational low self-esteem related to change in body image
Scheduled surgery: Abdominal incision Client verbalization of fear of stomach cancer Client withdrawal after biopsy report Anxiety	Changes in interpersonal interactions	Ineffective individual coping related to fear about unknown prognosis

Box 12-7 Sources of Diagnostic Error

Collecting

Lack of knowledge or skill
Inaccurate data
Missing data
Disorganization

Interpreting

Inaccurate interpretation of cues
Failure to consider conflicting cues
Using an insufficient number of cues
Using unreliable or invalid cues
Failure to consider cultural influences or developmental stage

Clustering

Insufficient cluster of cues
Premature or early closure
Incorrect clustering

Labelling

Wrong diagnostic label selected
Evidence exists that another diagnosis is more likely
Condition is a collaborative problem
Failure to validate nursing diagnosis with client
Failure to seek guidance

enhancement. This diagnosis is used when the client wishes to achieve a higher level of wellness; for example, *family coping: potential for growth related to unexpected birth of twins*. The nurse and the family work together to adapt to the stressors associated with twins, with the outcome directed at an enhanced level of coping.

Review Box 12-4, which summarizes data from Mr. Brown's preoperative assessment. Table 12-1 demonstrates data clustering, identification of Mr. Brown's needs, and formulation of nursing diagnoses for Mr. Brown.

Diagnostic Errors

Errors can occur in the nursing diagnostic process during data collection, clustering, interpretation, and statement of the diagnosis (Box 12-7). These sources of error demonstrate the level of critical thinking required for an accurate nursing diagnostic process.

To avoid the most common errors in formulating nursing diagnoses, the nurse should do the following:

- Identify the client's response, not the medical diagnosis (Carpenito, 2000).
- Identify a NANDA International diagnostic statement rather than the symptom. Nursing diagnoses are derived from a cluster of defining characteristics; one symptom is insufficient for problem identification. For example, shortness of breath, pain on inspiration, and productive cough with thick secretions should cue the nurse to *ineffective breathing pattern related to increased airway secretions.*
- Identify a treatable etiology (i.e., the cause of the nursing diagnosis) rather than a clinical sign or chronic problem. Nursing interventions are directed toward correcting the etiology of the problem. A diagnostic test or a chronic dysfunction is not an etiology that can be

treated by a nursing intervention. A client with pneumonia may present restlessness, hypoxia, abnormal blood gas levels, and dyspnea. "Impaired gas exchange related to altered blood gases" is an incorrect diagnostic statement. *Impaired gas exchange related to alveolar capillary membrane changes* is a correct statement.

- Identify the problem caused by the treatment or diagnostic study rather than the treatment or study itself. Clients experience many responses to diagnostic tests and medical treatment. These responses are the area of nursing concern. The diagnosis "cardiac catheterization related to angina" should be restated to read *anxiety related to lack of knowledge about cardiac catheterization.*
- Identify the client response to the equipment rather than the equipment itself. Clients are often unfamiliar with medical technology. The diagnosis "anxiety related to cardiac monitor" can be changed to *deficient knowledge regarding the need for cardiac monitoring.*
- Identify the client's problems rather than the nurse's problems. Nursing diagnoses are always client centred and form the basis for goal-directed care. "Potential complications related to poor vascular access" indicates a nursing problem in initiating and maintaining intravenous (IV) therapy. The diagnosis *risk for infection related to presence of invasive lines* properly focuses on client needs.
- Identify the client problem rather than the nursing intervention. Nursing interventions are planned to alleviate client problems and are not part of the diagnostic statement. Failure to state a diagnostic label results in an inability to evaluate problem resolution. The statement "offer bedpan frequently because of altered elimination patterns" should be changed to identify the problem and etiology. *Diarrhea related to food intolerance* corrects the misstatement and allows proper implementation of the nursing process.
- Identify the client problem rather than the goal. Goals are based upon accurate identification of a client's problems. The goals then serve as a basis to determine if problem resolution is achieved. If the problem is not first identified, goal selection and evaluation of problem resolution is difficult. "Client needs high-protein diet related to potential alteration in nutrition" should be changed to *imbalanced nutrition: less than body requirements related to inadequate protein intake* to allow for planning to correct the etiology.
- Make professional rather than prejudicial judgments. Nursing diagnoses data and should not include the nurse's personal beliefs. The nurse's judgment can be removed from "risk for impaired skin integrity related to poor hygiene habits" by changing the diagnosis to read *risk for impaired skin integrity related to knowledge about perineal care.*
- Identify the problem and etiology. Be careful to avoid a circular statement. Such statements are vague and give no direction to nursing care. "Alteration in comfort related to pain" can be changed to identify the client problem and the cause: *ineffective breathing pattern related to incisional pain.*
- Identify only one client problem in the diagnostic statement. Every problem has different specific expected outcomes. Confusion during the planning step occurs when multiple problems are included in a nursing diagnosis. "Pain and anxiety related to difficulty in ambulating" should be restated as two nursing diagnoses, such as *impaired physical mobility related to pain in right knee* and *anxiety related to difficulty in ambulating.* It is permissible to include multiple etiologies contributing to one client problem, for example, *dysfunctional grieving related to diagnosed terminal illness and change in family role* would be an acceptable diagnostic statement.

Step 3: Planning Nursing Care

Once a nurse assesses a client's condition and identifies appropriate nursing diagnoses, a plan is developed for the client's nursing care. **Planning** involves establishing client goals and expected outcomes and selecting nursing interventions. The interventions are chosen to resolve the client's problem and achieve the goals and outcomes. Planning requires decision-making and problem-solving skills (Liukkonen, 1992). During planning, priorities are set because a client often has more than one nursing diagnosis and a variety of proposed interventions. During the planning process, the nurse reviews pertinent literature and collaborates with the client, family, and other members of the health care team. A plan of care is dynamic and will change as the client's needs are met or as new needs are identified.

Establishing Priorities

Priority setting involves ranking nursing diagnoses in order of importance. Priorities are established to help the nurse anticipate and sequence nursing interventions when a client has multiple problems or alterations (Carpenito, 1997). Because clients have multiple nursing diagnoses, the nurse and client select mutually agreed-on priorities based on the urgency of the problem, the client's safety and desires, the nature of the treatment indicated, and the relationship among the diagnoses.

Priorities are classified as high, intermediate, or low (Table 12-2). High-priority nursing diagnoses are those that, if untreated, could result in harm to the client. For example, *risk for other-directed violence, impaired gas exchange,* and *acute pain* are high-priority nursing diagnoses because they involve safety, maintaining adequate oxygenation, and providing comfort, which are always considered high priorities. However, it is always important to consider each client's unique case. Consider Mr. Brown, who was introduced earlier. He has now successfully undergone surgery for a colon resection. Among Mr. Brown's nursing diagnoses are *acute pain, risk for ineffective airway clearance, deficient knowledge,* and *ineffective peripheral tissue perfusion.* Mr. Brown's high priorities are pain control post-operatively and maintaining a patent airway. Pain control is the highest priority because unless it is managed, Mr. Brown will be unable to cough effectively to remove secretions for a clear airway. High priorities can occur in both the psychological and physiological dimensions, and the nurse should avoid classifying only physiological nursing diagnoses as high priority. For example, lowering anxiety may become a priority over teaching information about impending surgery. If the client is too anxious to learn, then the nurse is unable to

Table 12-2 Priority Setting for Mr. Brown

Mr. Brown has returned to the post-operative nursing unit following surgery for a colon resection. His condition presents numerous nursing diagnoses. The nurse sets priorities as follows:

Nursing Diagnoses	Rationale
High Priority	
Risk for ineffective airway clearance related to abdominal incisional pain	Client is at risk for post-operative pulmonary complications such as atelectasis and pneumonia, unless he is able to cough and deep breathe. Nurse will institute aggressive pulmonary hygiene.
Acute pain related to tissue trauma of surgical incision	Client is experiencing typical acute incisional pain. If the pain is not controlled or managed to a level the client can tolerate, it will be difficult for the client to participate in pulmonary hygiene.
Intermediate Priority	
Ineffective peripheral tissue perfusion related to post-operative venous status and risk for thrombophlebitis	All clients are at risk for altered peripheral tissue perfusion following major abdominal surgery. Mr. Brown does not currently show signs of thrombophlebitis; however, preventive measures such as frequent turning, leg exercises, and early ambulation will be essential.
Low Priority	
Deficient knowledge regarding post-operative home care related to inexperience	Mr. Brown will require instruction on wound care, infection prevention, and nutrition. The nurse will plan to begin teaching once pain control is achieved and the client is receptive to learning.
Risk for infection related to 15-year-history of smoking	This diagnosis reflects the client's long-term needs. The client will have to have a desire and willingness to change behaviour and stop smoking. Post-discharge referral to a smoking cessation class may be appropriate.

address a knowledge deficit at that time. Anxiety becomes the initial priority.

Intermediate priority nursing diagnoses involve the non-emergent, non-life-threatening needs of the client. In Mr. Brown's case, the intermediate priority pertains to the nursing diagnosis of *ineffective peripheral tissue perfusion*. Mr. Brown has no immediate impairment in circulation but is at risk for post-operative venous stasis. Aggressive preventive care is a part of Mr. Brown's routine post-operative care. Thus, maintaining normal circulation to the lower extremities becomes the nurse's immediate priority.

Low-priority nursing diagnoses are client needs that may not be directly related to a specific illness or prognosis but may affect the client's future well-being. Many low-priority diagnoses focus on the client's long-term health care needs. For example, Mr. Brown eventually will be discharged following surgery and will be required to manage his wound and nutritional needs in the home. *Deficient knowledge* is an important diagnosis that the nurse must attend to, but teaching the client is a low priority, especially if pain management and a patent airway have not been achieved. The nurse will begin teaching Mr. Brown as soon as the client becomes receptive and able to learn.

The order of priorities changes as a client's condition changes, sometimes within a matter of minutes. Each time a nurse begins a sequence of care such as at the beginning of a hospital shift or a client's clinic visit, it is important to reorder priorities. Thus, the nurse must monitor assessment data to be sure that nursing diagnoses have been identified or that existing diagnoses have been resolved.

Whenever possible, the client should be involved in priority setting. In some situations, the client and the nurse assign different priority rankings to nursing diagnoses. If both place different values on health care needs and treatments, these differences can be resolved through open communication. However, when the client's physiological and emotional needs are at stake, the nurse needs to assume primary responsibility for setting priorities.

Critical Thinking in Establishing Goals and Expected Outcomes

Once a nursing diagnosis is identified for a client, the nursing process consists of finding the best approach to address and resolve the problem. Goals and expected outcomes are specific statements of client behaviour or physiological responses that a nurse sets to achieve problem resolution. The goals and outcomes provide a clear focus for the type of interventions necessary to care for the client. When goals and outcomes are met, a client's health problems are resolved. For example, when a client has a diagnosis of *impaired physical mobility related to acute pain,* there are two associated health problems: reduced mobility and pain. Appropriate goals would include, "Client will achieve normal mobility" and "Client will achieve pain control." Both goals are necessary because the nurse must attend to both the client's mobility and comfort needs. In order for the nurse to monitor progress toward the ultimate goals, outcomes or measurable criteria to evaluate goal achievement are necessary. Outcomes for the goal of "Client will achieve normal mobility" include "Client will initiate turning and repositioning in bed" and

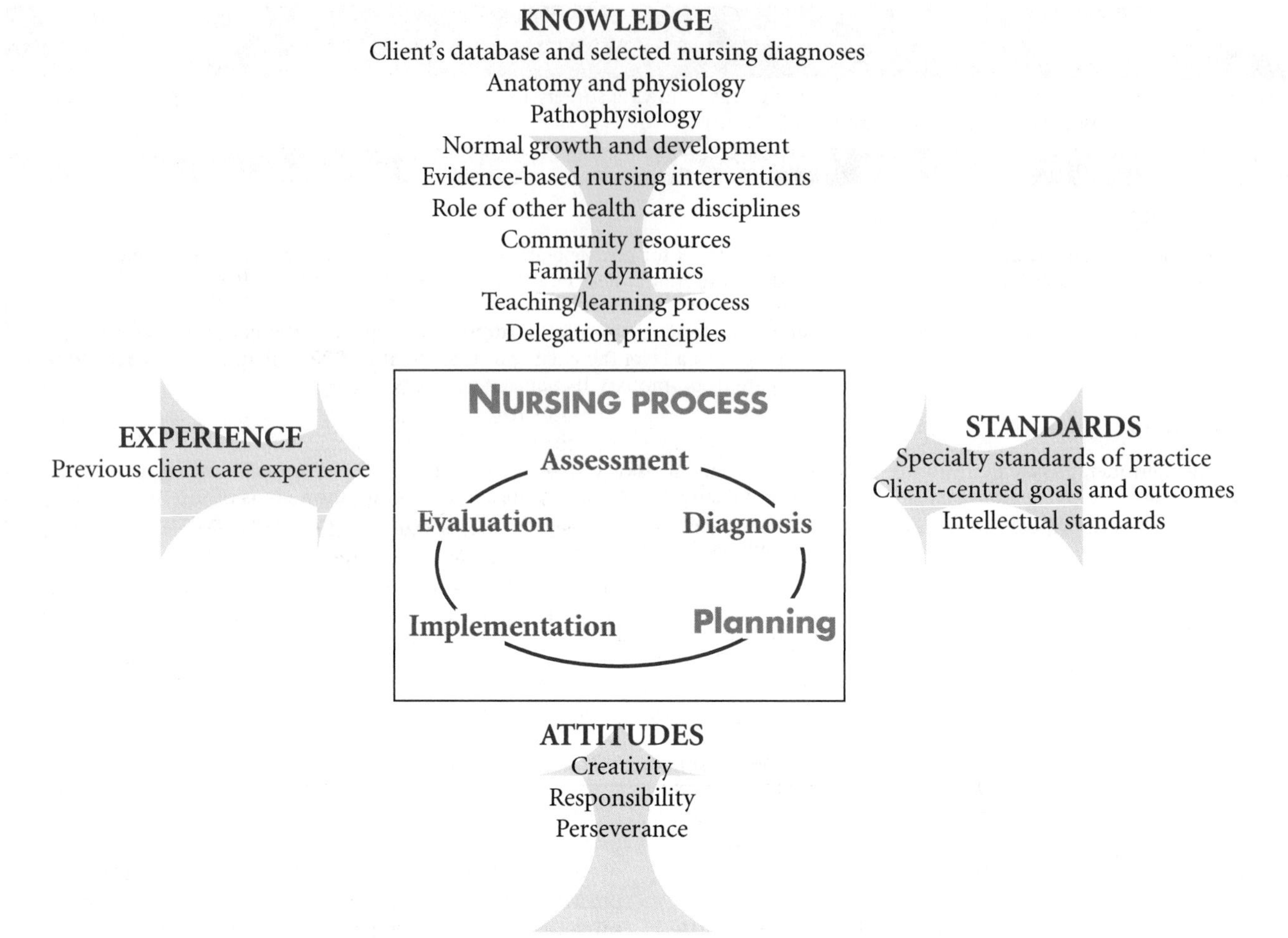

FIGURE **12–5** Critical thinking and the process of planning care.

"Client will sit and stand by first post-operative evening." Outcomes for the goal of "Client will achieve pain control" include "Client will report pain severity below 4 on a scale of 0 to 10" and "Client will report ability to sleep during the night without discomfort." The nurse's interventions will include exercise therapy (ambulation and turning), analgesic administration, and non-pharmacological pain management (relaxation exercises). The purposes for writing goals and expected outcomes are to (a) direct the selection and use of nursing interventions and (b) provide focus for evaluation of the interventions.

Planning nursing care requires critical thinking (Figure 12–5). The nurse evaluates the nursing diagnoses, the urgency of the problems, and the resources of the client and the health care delivery system (Bandman & Bandman, 1995). The nurse applies knowledge from the medical, socio-behavioural, and nursing sciences to plan care. Goals, expected outcomes, and interventions are selected by considering previous experience with similar client problems and established professional standards. The goals and outcomes must meet intellectual standards by being relevant to client needs, specific, singular, observable, measurable, and time limited. The nurse uses critical thinking attitudes in selecting interventions with the greatest likelihood of success. For example, the nurse creatively selects comfort measures that the client practises at home in choosing a plan for managing the client's chronic pain. Figure 12–6 illustrates the relationships among nursing diagnoses, goals, expected outcomes, and nursing interventions within the nursing process.

Goals of Care. A **client-centred goal** is a specific and measurable behaviour or response that reflects a client's highest possible level of wellness and independence in function. Examples include, "Client will perform self-care hygiene independently," "Client will remain free of infection," and "Client will accept body image alteration." A goal contains singular behaviours or responses. For example, "Client will communicate needs and adhere to treatment plan" is written incorrectly because the statement includes two different behaviours: communicate and adhere. A goal must also be observable and measurable. A nurse is able to observe the condition of a surgical wound and measure the amount of drainage or appearance of the incision for the goal, "Client will remain free of infection." The specific criteria used to measure success of a goal are written in the form of outcome statements (see Expected Outcomes). Each goal and outcome must be time limited so that the health care team has a common time frame for problem resolution. The time frame

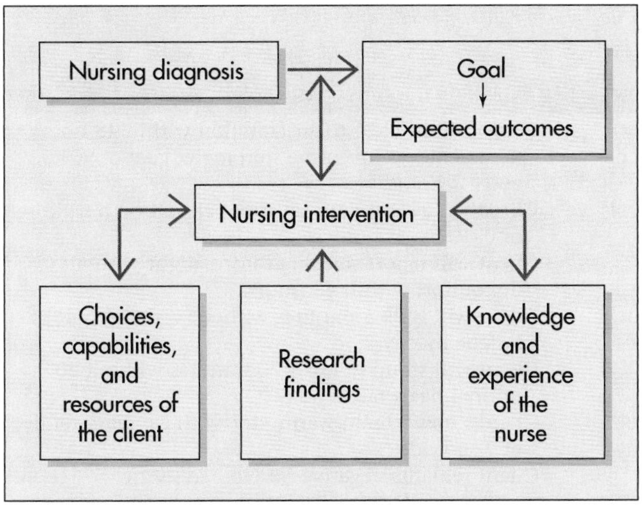

FIGURE **12–6** From diagnosis to outcome. (Revised and redrawn from *Nursing Diagnosis: Process and Application,* 3rd ed., by M. Gordon, 1994, St. Louis, MO: Mosby.)

depends on the nature of the problem, etiology, overall condition of the client, and treatment setting. For example, a client with acute pain following surgery will likely have a shorter time frame for achievement of goals than a client with chronic recurrent pain. The statements, "Client will achieve pain control within 48 hours" and "Client will remain free of infection by discharge home" are correctly written goals.

Role of the Client in Goal Setting. The nurse should involve the client and family (when appropriate) in prioritizing the goals of care and developing a plan to achieve those goals (McCloskey & Bulechek, 1994). Clients should also understand and see the value of nursing therapies. When clients share the nurse's goals, they are more likely to participate in the plan of care.

Goals should be realistic and based on client needs and resources. For clients to participate in goal setting, they should be alert and have some degree of independence in ADLs, problem solving, and decision making. This is important because the nurse and client partner together in the client's care. If clients' cognitive and physical impairments are so severe that they cannot actively participate in goal setting, the nursing team acts on their behalf to develop client-centred goals. When developing goals, the nurse acts as an advocate for the client to develop nursing interventions to promote the client's return to health or to prevent further deterioration (Carpenito, 1997).

Goals should not only meet the immediate needs of the client, but should also strive toward prevention and rehabilitation. Two types of goals, short-term goals and long-term goals, are developed for the client, depending upon the nature of the client's need or problems and the nature of the nursing services provided.

Short-Term Goals. A **short-term goal** is an objective that can be achieved within a short time frame, usually less than a week (Carpenito, 1997). With the present health care system and shorter hospital stays, short-term goals are the direction for the immediate care plan. In the case of Mr. Brown, the client has the nursing diagnosis of *acute pain related to the tissue trauma of a surgical incision.* A short-term goal for Mr. Brown would be, "Client will achieve comfort within 24 hours post-operatively." The goal is realistic because of the importance placed on managing post-operative pain.

Long-Term Goals. A **long-term goal** is an objective that can be achieved over a longer time frame, usually over weeks or months. Long-term goals may be appropriate for problem resolution after discharge, especially from acute care settings (Carpenito, 1997). Long-term goals are appropriate for clients in home care settings, those adapting to chronic illnesses who reside in long-term care facilities, and for some clients in rehabilitation, mental health, ambulatory care, and community nursing settings (Carpenito, 1997). For example, Mr. Brown has the nursing diagnosis of *deficient knowledge regarding post-operative home care related to inexperience.* A long-term goal for Mr. Brown may be, "Client will adhere to post-operative activity restrictions for 1 month." Long-term goals focus on prevention, rehabilitation, discharge, and health education. Failure to set long-term goals may prevent continuity of care.

Expected Outcomes. An **expected outcome** is a specific measurable change in a client's status that is expected to occur in response to nursing care. An outcome is an objective criterion for measuring goal achievement. Client outcomes identify and measure the desired results of nursing interventions and practice (Deaton, 1998). Outcomes provide a focus for nursing care because they are the desired responses of a client's condition in the physiological, social, emotional, developmental, or spiritual dimensions. The expected outcomes determine when a specific, client-centred goal has been met and evaluate the response to nursing care and the resolution of the etiology of a nursing diagnosis.

Several expected outcomes are usually developed for each nursing diagnosis and goal. The rationale for the multiple expected outcomes is that few client problems can be resolved by one nursing action. In addition, the listing of the step-by-step expected outcomes guides the nurse in planning interventions. Expected outcome statements should be written sequentially, with time frames. Time frames give nurses progressive steps in which to move a client toward recovery and offer an order for nursing interventions. Time frames also set limits for problem resolution. For example, if Mr. Brown has the goal, "Client will adhere to post-operative activity restrictions from 1 month," appropriate outcome statements will include, "Client will describe activity restrictions imposed post-operatively within 2 days post-op" and "Client will explain reasons for activity restrictions by day of discharge."

Once a nurse develops goals and expected outcomes for a client's diagnosis, the interventions in the plan of care are selected. Developing a plan of care must incorporate the contributions of evidence-based research (see chapter 6), other health care disciplines, the family, and community resources. The nurse also applies previous experiences to determine what has worked or not worked in similar situations. This clinical testing of interventions

Table 12-3 Mr. Brown's Nursing Diagnoses, Goals, and Expected Outcomes

Nursing Diagnoses	Goals	Expected Outcomes
Risk for ineffective airway clearance related to abdominal incisional pain	Client will maintain patent airway through post-operative period to discharge.	Lungs will be clear to auscultation within 48 hours. Client achieves incentive spirometer goal of 90% every 2 hours.
Acute pain related to tissue trauma of surgical incision	Client will achieve pain control within 48 hours.	Client will report pain severity below 4 on a scale of 0–10 by 24 hours. Client will report sleeping during night without discomfort within 48 hours.
Activity intolerance related to reduced oxygenation from blood loss	Client will increase ambulation progressively during post-operative period.	Client will walk 5 minutes without verbal report of fatigue by day 2. Client will sit up in chair 20 minutes without abnormal heart rate by day 2.
Ineffective peripheral tissue perfusion related to post-operative venous stasis	Client will maintain adequate peripheral tissue perfusion by discharge.	Client's toes remain warm, dry, with capillary refill of 2 seconds. Client remains negative for Homan's sign.

helps the nurse to choose therapeutic interventions for each new client. As goals, outcomes, and interventions are developed, the nurse must be committed to accepted standards of practice from nursing and other disciplines. The nurse displays attributes such as creativity, perseverance, and humility when developing a plan of care.

Consider, again, the case of Mr. Brown. It is now 1 day after Mr. Brown's bowel resection surgery. He was found to have colon cancer. His operative course has some complications. His blood loss has been greater than anticipated, and his hemoglobin level is now 85 g/L. He is fatigued, and his tolerance of routine post-operative leg exercises and ambulation is poor. He therefore has a new nursing diagnosis of *activity intolerance.* Although he is receiving around-the-clock pain medications, he still periodically reports pain at a level above 5 on the pain scale. It is important for the nurse to continue to emphasize the need for pulmonary hygiene. Because of his current fatigue and level of pain, teaching Mr. Brown is not a priority at this time. Table 12-3 shows the relationship between nursing diagnoses, goals, and expected outcomes for Mr. Brown.

Guidelines for Writing Goals and Expected Outcomes. It is important to write goals and outcomes clearly so that all members of the nursing team understand a client's plan of care and are able to collaborate on achieving the same goals and outcomes. Written goals and expected outcomes must be client centred, singular, observable, measurable, time limited, mutual, and realistic.

Client Centred. Outcomes and goals should reflect the client behaviour and responses expected as a result of nursing interventions. A common error occurs when the goals are written to reflect the nurse's goals or outcomes. A correct outcome statement is, "Client will ambulate in the hall three times a day." A common error is to write, "Ambulate client in the hall three times a day."

Singular Goal or Outcome. Each goal and expected outcome statement should address only one behaviour or response. This limitation ensures a precise method to evaluate the client's response to a nursing intervention. If an outcome statement reads, "Client's lungs will be clear to auscultation, and respiratory rate will be 20 breaths per minute by 8/22," but the nurse evaluates the client after suctioning and finds the lungs to be clear with the respiratory rate at 28 per minute, it would be difficult to determine whether the expected outcome was achieved. By splitting the outcome into two parts, "Lungs will be clear to auscultation by 8/22" and "Respiratory rate will be 20 breaths per minute by 8/22," the nurse can determine specifically the outcome that has been achieved. In addition, singularity assists the nurse in determining if modifying the care plan is necessary.

Observable. The nurse must be able to observe whether change has taken place. Observable changes can occur in physiological findings, the client's level of knowledge, perceptions or expressed feelings, and behaviour. The results can be obtained by directly asking the client about the condition or can be observed by using assessment skills. For example, the goal, "Client will be able to self-administer insulin" is observed through the outcomes, "Client prepares insulin dosage correctly by 8/30" and "Client performs subcutaneous injection correctly by 8/31." The outcome statement, "Client will appear less anxious" is not a correct statement because there is no specific behaviour observable for "will appear."

Measurable. Goals and expected outcomes are written to give the nurse a standard against which to measure the client's response to nursing care. Examples are, "Body temperature will remain 37.0," and "Apical pulse will remain between 60 and 100 beats per minute." A goal or an outcome that is stated in measurable terms allows the nurse to objectively quantify changes in the client's status. A common mistake is to use vague qualifiers such as *normal, stable, acceptable,* or *sufficient* in the expected outcome statement. Vague terms result in guesswork in determining the client's response to care. Terms specifically describing quality, quantity, frequency, length, or weight allow the nurse to evaluate whether outcomes are achieved.

Time Limited. The time frame for each goal and expected outcome indicates when the expected response should occur. Time frames help determine that progress is being made at a reasonable rate. When the date of evaluation arrives, the nurse assesses the client to determine whether that particular expected outcome has been reached. If the outcome is unmet, but it is still appropriate for the client's care, another future evaluation date is set. Time frames promote accountability in the delivery of nursing care.

Mutual Factors. Mutually set goals and expected outcomes ensure that the client and nurse agree on the direction and time limits of care. Mutual goal setting can increase the client's motivation and co-operation. The nurse does not impose personal values on the client. However, the nurse must be aware of standards of practice, client safety, and basic human needs. The nurse may need to direct some of the goals and expected outcomes to keep the client physically and emotionally stable and safe.

Realistic. The nurse sets goals and expected outcomes that can be achieved. This approach provides clients with a sense of accomplishment and can increase the client's motivation and co-operation. When establishing realistic goals, the nurse assesses the available resources, the client's potential, and the economic costs to reach expected outcomes.

Critical Thinking in Planning Nursing Interventions

Nursing interventions are any treatment or action, based upon clinical judgment and knowledge, that nurses perform to enhance clients' outcomes (McCloskey & Bulechek, 2000). Nursing interventions are designed to assist the client in moving from the present level of health to that which is described in the goal and measured by the expected outcomes (Gordon et al., 1994). Implementation of these interventions occurs during the implementation phase of the nursing process (see Step 4: Implementing Nursing Care).

Choosing suitable nursing interventions involves decision making. The nurse uses critical thinking by applying knowledge of the client's situation, experience from caring for similar clients, critical thinking attitudes, and standards to select interventions that will successfully meet established goals and expected outcomes for each diagnostic statement. In addition, to initiate the intervention, the nurse must (a) know the **scientific rationale** for the intervention, (b) have the necessary psychomotor and interpersonal skills, and (c) be able to function within a particular setting to use the available resources effectively (McCloskey & Bulechek, 2000).

Types of Interventions. Nursing interventions can be grouped into three categories according to how they are initiated: nurse initiated or independent, physician initiated or dependent, and collaborative. One client may require all three categories, whereas another client may need only nurse- and physician-initiated interventions.

Nurse-Initiated Interventions. Nurses can act within their scope of practice to intervene on a client's behalf. **Nurse-initiated interventions** are the independent response of the nurse to the client's health care needs and nursing diagnoses. Nurse-initiated interventions are autonomous actions based on scientific rationale that are expected to benefit the client in a predictable way (McCloskey & Bulechek, 2000). They involve aspects of professional nursing practice encompassed by licensure and law. These interventions require no supervision or direction from others. For example, independent nursing actions include instructing clients in ways to manage their nutrition and positioning clients to minimize pressure on bony prominences.

Nurse-initiated interventions do not require an order from a physician, independent care provider (e.g., nurse practitioner), or other health professional. Physicians frequently include in their written orders the specifics of independent nursing interventions. However, according to most nursing practice acts, nursing actions pertaining to ADLs, health education, health promotion, and counselling are in the domain of nursing practice.

Physician-Initiated Interventions. **Physician-initiated interventions** are based on a physician's response to treat or manage a medical diagnosis. They are included in the physicians' orders written in the client's medical record. Nurse practitioners who are licensed provincially are also able to write orders for such interventions. The nurse intervenes by carrying out the independent provider's written orders. This may be in the form of an individual written order, a signed treatment protocol, or standing orders. Administering medications, implementing an invasive procedure, changing a dressing, and preparing a client for diagnostic tests are examples of physician-initiated interventions. It is not always within the legal scope of practice for the nurse to prescribe and order these treatments independently, but nurses can complete such orders and individualize approaches to their administration. For example, a physician may order a dressing change twice a day and a bone scan for a client. The nurse incorporates both of these orders into the client's plan of care so that they are safely and efficiently completed.

Each physician-initiated intervention requires specific nursing responsibilities and technical nursing knowledge. For example, when administering medications, the nurse is responsible for knowing the classification of the drug, its physiological action, normal dosage, side effects, and nursing interventions related to its action or side effects (see chapter 30). When a specific diagnostic or laboratory test is ordered by a physician or nurse practitioner, the nurse is responsible for scheduling the test, preparing the client, and knowing the normal findings and nursing implications associated with it.

Collaborative Interventions. **Collaborative interventions** are therapies that require the knowledge, skill, and expertise of multiple health care professionals. For example, Mr. Joseph is a 68-year-old man with a history of dementia who also has hemiplegia from a recent cerebrovascular accident (stroke). His cognitive functions are limited, he is at risk for problems related to impaired sensation and mobility, and he is unable to independently complete ADLs. In order for Mr. Joseph to maintain his present level of health, he requires multiple interventions, including nursing interventions to prevent pressure ulcers, physiotherapy interventions to prevent musculoskeletal changes from immobility, and occupational therapy interventions for eating and hygiene needs. The care for this client requires the coordination of interventions from multiple health care professionals, all with the goal of maintaining Mr. Joseph's present level of health.

Preventing Intervention Errors. Nurse-initiated, physician-initiated, and collaborative interventions require critical thinking and decision making. The nurse does not automatically implement physician-initiated or collaborative interventions but must determine whether they are appropriate for the client. Every nurse faces an inappropriate or incorrect order at some time. The nurse with a strong knowledge base recognizes the error and seeks to correct it. Recognizing incorrect therapies is particularly important when administering medications or implementing procedures. An error can occur in writing the order or transcribing it to a documentation form or computer screen. Clarifying an order is competent nursing practice, and it protects the client and members of the health care team. The nurse carrying out an incorrect or inappropriate intervention is as much in error as the person who wrote or transcribed the original order and is liable for any complications resulting from the error.

Selection of Interventions. A nurse does not select interventions haphazardly. All clients who have the diagnosis of *Anxiety,* for example, do not have the same interventions. Anxiety related to the uncertainty of an impending diagnostic test will be treated differently than anxiety related to a threat to loss of family role function. When choosing interventions, nurses consider the following six factors: (a) characteristics of the nursing diagnosis, (b) expected outcomes, (c) research base (nursing knowledge) for the interventions, (d) feasibility of the intervention, (e) acceptability to the client, and (f) their nursing competencies (McCloskey & Bulechek, 1998, 2000; Box 12-8). The nurse may review standardized care plans, the Nursing Interventions Classification (NIC), critical pathways, policy or procedure manuals, textbooks, and nursing literature. **Collaboration** with the client, family, and other members of the health team is

Box 12-8 Choosing Nursing Interventions

Characteristics of the Nursing Diagnosis

- Interventions must be directed toward altering the etiological (causative) factors associated with the diagnosis.
- When an etiological factor cannot change, the interventions must be directed toward treating the signs and symptoms (e.g., NANDA defining characteristics).
- For potential or high-risk diagnoses, interventions must be aimed at altering or eliminating the risk factors for the diagnosis.

Expected Outcomes

- Client outcomes must be specified before selecting an intervention.
- Because an outcome is stated in terms used to evaluate the effectiveness of an intervention, this language can assist in selecting the intervention.
- Nursing Interventions Classification (NIC) is designed to show the link to Nursing Outcomes Classification (NOC) (Johnson, Maas, & Moorehead, 2000).

Research Base

- Research in support of a nursing intervention will indicate the effectiveness of the intervention.
- Refer to research articles or evidence-based practice protocols that describe the use of research findings in similar clinical situations and settings.
- When research is not available, the nurse uses scientific principles (e.g., infection control) or consults a clinical expert.

Feasibility

- A specific intervention may have the potential for interacting with other interventions chosen by the nurse or other health care providers.
- The nurse must be knowledgeable of the total plan of care.
- Consider cost: Is the intervention clinically effective and cost efficient?
- Consider time: Are time and personnel resources available?

Acceptability to the Client

- An intervention must be acceptable to the client and family and congruent with the client's goals, health care values, and culture.
- To facilitate informed choice, clients must know how they are expected to participate and the anticipated effect of the intervention.

Capability of the Nurse

- The nurse must be able to carry out the intervention.
- The nurse must be knowledgeable of the scientific rationale for the intervention.
- The nurse must possess the necessary psychosocial and psychomotor skills to complete the intervention.
- The nurse must be able to function within the particular setting to effectively use health care resources.

Adapted from *Nursing Interventions Classification (NIC),* (4th ed.) edited by J. M. Dochterman and G. M. Bulechek, 2004, St. Louis, MO: Mosby.

also useful for individualizing nursing interventions. In addition, the nurse also reviews previous clinical experiences and priorities to select the nursing interventions with the best potential for success. With experience, the deliberation process becomes more efficient and experience based (Benner, 1984).

Nursing Interventions Classification. The Iowa Intervention Project has developed a taxonomy of nursing interventions that provides a level of standardization to enhance communication of nursing care across settings and to compare outcomes (Dochterman & Bulechek, 2004; Iowa Intervention Project, 1993). Extensive nursing research, expert review, and clinical judgment have merged to form the NIC taxonomy: 486 interventions are grouped into 30 classes and 7 domains for ease of use (Table 12-4). Each class includes interventions that will enhance the condition of a client who has an alteration within the class (Box 12-9). Each intervention then has a variety of nursing activities from which the nurse chooses to perform (Box 12-10). In addition, NIC interventions have been linked with NANDA International nursing diagnoses (Dochterman & Jones, 2003; NANDA International, 2003). For example, if a client has a problem with activity and exercise management, specifically the diagnosis of *activity intolerance,* there are a variety of interventions from which to choose (e.g., body mechanics promotion or exercise promotion). NIC is a valuable resource when selecting appropriate interventions. NIC is evolving and is practice oriented; it is designed to enable nurses in all practice settings to have a standard classification system for documenting nursing care. The classification is designed to be comprehensive, including independent and collaborative interventions that cover all specialty areas (Carter et al., 1995). However, it still remains the nurse's decision to determine which interventions are most appropriate for each client's needs and situation.

Developing a Plan of Care

When planning care, a nurse will usually have more interventions than are necessary to meet a client's expected outcomes. Some are discarded as inappropriate, and others are adapted to the client's needs and abilities. As a result, the list of possible interventions is narrowed down to those suitable to the client (Redman, 2001). These interventions are then written on the nursing care plan.

A **nursing care plan** is a guide for clinical care. It also serves as a document that communicates a client's nursing care to all members of the health care team. It is made available to the team as a ready reference for nursing care interventions.

Purpose of Care Plans. A written care plan is designed to direct clinical care and to decrease the risk of incomplete, incorrect, or inaccurate care. The plan is organized so that any nurse can quickly identify the client's nursing diagnoses, goals, outcomes, and required nursing interventions. In hospitals, outpatient settings, and community-based settings, the client often receives care from more

Box 12-9 Example of Level 3 Interventions for Activity and Exercise Management

A. Activity and Exercise Management

Interventions to organize or assist with physical activity and energy conservation and expenditure.

Level 3 Interventions

Body Mechanics Promotion
Energy Management
Exercise Promotion
Exercise Promotion: Strength Training
Exercise Promotion: Stretching
Exercise Therapy: Ambulation
Exercise Therapy: Balance
Exercise Therapy: Joint Mobility
Exercise Therapy: Muscle Control
Teaching Prescribed Activity/Exercise

Examples of Linked Nursing Diagnoses:
Activity Intolerance
Fatigue
Mobility, Impaired Physical

From *Nursing Interventions Classification (NIC),* (4th ed.), edited by J. M. Dochterman and G. M. Bulechek, 2004, St. Louis, MO: Mosby.

Box 12-10 Example of Level 3 Interventions and Associated Nursing Activities

Body Mechanics Promotion

Examples of Activities:

- Determine client's commitment to learning and using correct posture
- Collaborate with physiotherapy in developing a body mechanics promotion plan
- Determine client's understanding of body mechanics and exercises
- Instruct client on structure and function of spine and optimal posture for moving and using the body
- Instruct client need for correct posture to prevent fatigue, strain, or injury
- Instruct client how to use posture and body mechanics while performing any physical activities
- Determine client awareness of own musculoskeletal abnormalities and potential effects of posture and muscle tissue
- Instruct to use firm mattress, chair, or pillow as appropriate
- Instruct to avoid sleeping prone
- Assist to demonstrate appropriate sleeping positions
- Assist to avoid sitting in the same position for prolonged periods
- Demonstrate how to shift weight from one foot to another while standing

From *Nursing Interventions Classification (NIC),* (4th ed.), edited by J. M. Dochterman and G. M. Bulechek, 2004, St. Louis, MO: Mosby.

Table 12-4 Nursing Interventions Classification (NIC) Taxonomy

Domain 1	Domain 2	Domain 3
Level 1 Domains		
1. **Physiological: Basic** Care that supports physical functioning	2. **Physiological: Complex** Care that supports homeostatic regulation	3. **Behavioral** Care that supports psychosocial functioning and facilitates life-style changes
Level 2 Classes		
A *Activity and Exercise Management:* Interventions to organize or assist with physical activity and energy conservation and expenditure	G *Electrolyte and Acid-Base Management:* Interventions to regulate electrolyte/acid-base balance and prevent complications	O *Behavior Therapy:* Interventions to reinforce or promote desirable behaviors or alter undesirable behaviors
B *Elimination Management:* Interventions to establish and maintain regular bowel and urinary elimination patterns and manage complications due to altered patterns	H *Drug Management:* Interventions to facilitate desired effects of pharmacological agents	P *Cognitive Therapy:* Interventions to reinforce or promote desirable cognitive functioning or alter undesirable cognitive functioning
C *Immobility Management:* Interventions to manage restricted body movement and the sequelae	I *Neurologic Management:* Interventions to optimize neurologic functions	Q *Communication Enhancement:* Interventions to facilitate delivering and receiving verbal and nonverbal messages
D *Nutrition Support:* Interventions to modify or maintain nutritional status	J *Perioperative Care:* Interventions to provide care before, during, and immediately after surgery	R *Coping Assistance:* Interventions to assist another to build on own strengths, to adapt to a change in function, or to achieve a higher level of function
E *Physical Comfort Promotion:* Interventions to promote comfort using physical techniques	K *Respiratory Management:* Interventions to promote airway patency and gas exchange	S *Patient Education:* Interventions to facilitate learning
F *Self-Care Facilitation:* Interventions to provide or assist with routine activities of daily living	L *Skin/Wound Management:* Interventions to maintain or restore tissue integrity	T *Psychological Comfort Promotion:* Interventions to promote comfort using psychological techniques
	M *Thermoregulation:* Interventions to maintain body temperature within a normal range	
	N *Tissue Perfusion Management:* Interventions to optimize circulation of blood and fluids to the tissue	

From *Nursing Interventions Classification (NIC),* (4th ed.), edited by J. M. Dochterman and G. M. Bulechek, 2004, St. Louis, MO: Mosby.

than one nurse, physician, or other health professional. A written nursing care plan makes possible the coordination of nursing care, subspecialty consultations, and diagnostic test scheduling.

The care plan can identify and coordinate resources used to deliver nursing care. The listing of specific equipment and supplies necessary for nursing actions is an economically efficient mechanism for selecting equipment. If all equipment and supplies are included in the care plan, the nurse's time is used effectively.

The nursing care plan enhances the continuity of nursing care by listing specific nursing actions necessary to achieve the goals and outcomes of care. These nursing actions can be carried out daily. A correctly formulated written care plan facilitates the continuity of care from one nurse to another. As a result, all nurses have the opportunity to deliver high-quality, consistent care.

Written nursing care plans organize information exchanged by nurses in change-of-shift reports (see chapter 13). Nurses focus their reports on nursing care and treatments and client outcomes as delineated in care plans. At the end of shifts, nurses discuss care plans and the client's overall progress with the next caregivers. Thus, all nurses are able to discuss current and pertinent information about the client's plan of care.

The written care plan also includes the long-term needs of the client. Incorporating the goals of the care plan into discharge planning is particularly important for a client who will be undergoing long-term rehabilitation in the community or who will require ongoing home care. A complete care plan enhances the continuity of nursing care between nurses in the hospital and community.

When developing an individualized care plan, the nurse involves the family and client. The family is a resource to help the client meet health goals. In addition, meeting some of the family's needs can improve the client's level of wellness.

Most written plans include expected outcome criteria used in the evaluation of care. Proper listing of the criteria provides the nurse with objective statements that help

Table 12-4 Nursing Interventions Classification (NIC) Taxonomy—cont'd

Domain 4	Domain 5	Domain 6	Domain 7
4. Safety Care that supports protection against harm	**5. Family** Care that supports the family unit	**6. Health System** Care that supports effective use of the health care delivery system	**7. Community** Care that supports the health of the community
U *Crisis Management:* Interventions to provide immediate short-term help in both psychological and physiological crises V *Risk Management:* Interventions to initiate risk-reduction activities and continue monitoring risks over time	W *Childbearing Care:* Interventions to assist in understanding and coping with the psychological and physiological changes during the childbearing period Z *Childrearing Care:* Interventions to assist in rearing children X *Lifespan Care:* Interventions to facilitate family unit functioning and promote the health and welfare of family members throughout the lifespan	Y *Health System Mediation:* Interventions to facilitate the interface between patient/family and the health care system a *Health System Management:* Interventions to provide and enhance support services for the delivery of care b *Information Management:* Interventions to facilitate communication among health care providers	c *Community Health Promotion:* Interventions that promote the health of the whole community d *Community Risk Management:* Interventions that assist in detecting or preventing health risks to the whole community

From *Nursing Interventions Classification (NIC),* (4th ed.), edited by J. M. Dochterman and G. M. Bulechek, 2004, St. Louis, MO: Mosby.

determine whether the goals of care have been achieved. The complete care plan is the blueprint for nursing action. It provides direction for implementation of the plan and a framework for evaluation of the client's response to nursing actions.

Institutional Care Plans. Institutional care plans are concise documents that become part of the client's medical record. Many hospitals use the Kardex nursing care plan. **Kardex** is a trade name for a card-filing system that allows quick reference to the particular needs of the client for certain aspects of nursing care. Information about medications, activity levels, level of self-care, diet, treatments, and procedures is usually included on the outside of the card. The nursing care plan is commonly placed on the inside (Figure 12–7). Each institution has its own format for the Kardex, but the basic information contained on it is universal. The care plan section of the Kardex also has institutional variations. One institution might use a three-column nursing care plan, which includes the problem, goal or outcome, and nursing action. Another institution may incorporate a four-column nursing care plan, which includes the nursing diagnosis, goal or outcome, nursing action, and evaluation. Although the format of the care plan varies from setting to setting, its overall purpose is to provide a written guideline for care so that the health care needs of the client and subsequent therapies are communicated among the health care team.

The focus of a nursing care plan will differ by setting and the evolving client situation. For example, the nursing care plan developed for the client returning home is usually based solely on long-term health needs. The plan includes interventions to involve the client, family, and significant others in assuming more responsibility for care because the client is to receive nursing care in the home. Same-day surgeries usually have plans focused on clients' short-term needs (e.g., immediate recovery from surgery and instructions for assuming self-care following discharge). A long-term care facility will have a plan of care focused on the client's long-term needs.

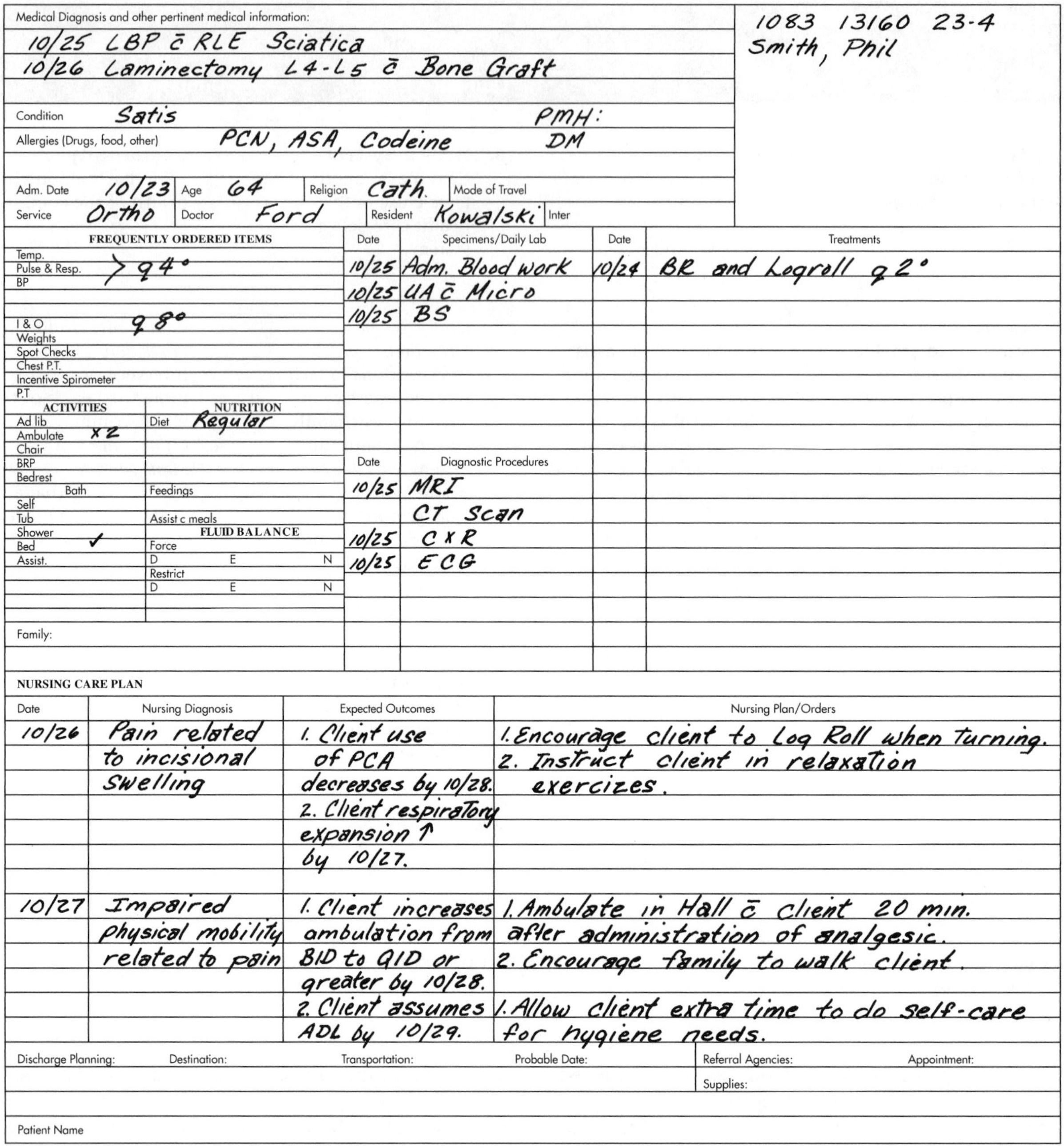

Medical Diagnosis and other pertinent medical information:
10/25 LBP c̄ RLE Sciatica
10/26 Laminectomy L4-L5 c̄ Bone Graft

1083 13160 23-4
Smith, Phil

Condition: Satis
PMH: DM
Allergies (Drugs, food, other): PCN, ASA, Codeine

Adm. Date	10/23	Age	64	Religion	Cath.	Mode of Travel	
Service	Ortho	Doctor	Ford	Resident	Kowalski	Inter	

FREQUENTLY ORDERED ITEMS
Temp. / Pulse & Resp. / BP: q 4°
I & O: q 8°
Weights
Spot Checks
Chest P.T.
Incentive Spirometer
P.T

Date	Specimens/Daily Lab
10/25	Adm. Blood work
10/25	UA c̄ Micro
10/25	BS

Date	Treatments
10/24	BR and Logroll q 2°

ACTIVITIES
Ad lib
Ambulate x 2
Chair
BRP
Bedrest

NUTRITION
Diet: Regular

Bath: Self / Tub / Shower / Bed ✓ / Assist.
Feedings: Assist c meals

FLUID BALANCE
Force: D E N
Restrict: D E N

Date	Diagnostic Procedures
10/25	MRI
	CT Scan
10/25	CXR
10/25	ECG

Family:

NURSING CARE PLAN

Date	Nursing Diagnosis	Expected Outcomes	Nursing Plan/Orders
10/26	Pain related to incisional swelling	1. Client use of PCA decreases by 10/28. 2. Client respiratory expansion ↑ by 10/27.	1. Encourage client to Log Roll when turning. 2. Instruct client in relaxation exercizes.
10/27	Impaired physical mobility related to pain	1. Client increases ambulation from BID to QID or greater by 10/28. 2. Client assumes ADL by 10/29.	1. Ambulate in Hall c̄ client 20 min. after administration of analgesic. 2. Encourage family to walk client. 1. Allow client extra time to do self-care for hygiene needs.

Discharge Planning: Destination: Transportation: Probable Date: Referral Agencies: Appointment:
Supplies:
Patient Name

FIGURE 12–7 Nursing care plan on a nursing Kardex.

Standardized Care Plans. The use of computers and the need to efficiently organize the nurse's time have resulted in standardized care plans, which are pre-written plans created for a specific nursing diagnosis or clinical problem (e.g., immobility, abdominal surgery, or postpartum care). After completing a nursing assessment, the nurse determines whether a standardized care plan should be used for that particular client. Even if the care plan is generally appropriate for a client, the nurse must add or delete information on the standardized form to individualize it for the client's needs. Failure to do so can result in incomplete and inaccurate care. For example, the nurse selects a nursing diagnosis and then individualizes the standard care plan by making selections from menus. Each care plan lists generalized nursing diagnoses, goals, outcome criteria, and interventions for specific clients (Figure 12–8).

Computerized/standardized nursing care plans streamline and augment care planning. They are designed to incorporate current evidence-based practice guidelines to achieve the desired client outcomes for a specific group of clients. These plans also encourage the nurse to incorporate individual client care needs into the plan of care.

Care Plans for Community-Based Settings. Planning care for clients in community-based settings, for example, clinics, community centres, or client's homes, involves using the same principles of nursing practice. However, in these settings, the nurse must complete a more

NURSING STANDARD CARE PLAN

Nursing Diagnosis: INEFFECTIVE BREATHING PATTERN

Related to: ______
(respiratory muscle fatigue, anxiety, pain, impaired respiratory mechanics such as chest tubes, incisions, anatomy)

Date Initiated/ Initials	Expected Outcomes	Date to be Met/Initials	Date Met/ Initials
______	Patient will verbalize understanding of ______ .	______	______
______	Patient will demonstrate ability to perform ______ .	______	______
______	Patient will pace and schedule activities.	______	______
______	Patient will use relaxation techniques for breathing control.	______	______
______	Patient will maintain respiratory rate of ______ with PaC02 of ______ .	______	______
______	Other: ______	______	______

Relevant baseline data: ______

Referrals: (date contacted)

☐ Nurse Specialist: ______ ☐ Home Care: ______ ☐ Social Work: ______
☐ Other: ______ ☐ Other: ______

Date Initiated/ Initials	Nursing Interventions	Date Inactivated/ Initials
	1. Assess respiratory function for rapid, shallow, irregular, or slow breathing, dyspnea, use of accessory muscles, breath sounds, restlessness, confusion, and cyanosis every ______ .	
	2. Monitor patient's mental status/LOC every ______ .	
______ ______ ______	3. Maintain adequate airway by: ☐ a. cough/splinting every ______ ☐ b. suction every ______ ☐ c. incentive spirometry every ______	______ ______ ______
	4. Pace and schedule activity to avoid dyspnea resulting from fatigue. Schedule is ______	
	5. Provide physical and emotional support during episodes of respiratory distress by: ______	
______ ______ ______ ______ ______	6. Provide teaching specific to patient or support person's needs. Initiate individual plan: ☐ a. pursed lip breathing ☐ b. coughing/splinting techniques (specify) ______ ☐ c. relaxation techniques (specify) ______ ☐ d. diaphragmatic breathing ______ ☐ e. other: ______	______ ______ ______ ______ ______
______ ______ ______ ______	7. Other interventionsl specific to patient: a. ______ b. ______ c. ______ d. ______	______ ______ ______ ______
	Signature/Initials: ______	

☐ **PLAN OF CARE MUTUALLY SET WITH PATIENT AND/OR FAMILY**

FIGURE **12–8** Standardized nursing care plan. (Courtesy Barnes-Jewish Hospital, St. Louis, MO.)

comprehensive community, home, and family assessment. In this setting, the client/family unit is in equal partnership with health care professionals. Ultimately, the client/family must be able to independently provide the majority of health care. The nurse designs a plan to (a) educate the client/family about the necessary care techniques, (b) teach the client/family how to integrate care within family activities, and (c) allow the client/family to assume a greater percentage of care in graduated increments. Last, the plan is designed to include nurses' and the client's/ family's evaluation of expected outcomes.

Critical Pathways or CareMaps. **Critical pathways** or **CareMaps** may also be used to direct client care. A critical pathway or CareMap is a document that includes the client's expected outcomes predicted by members of the health care team (see chapter 13). It enables staff from all disciplines, such as medicine, nursing, pharmacy, and social work, to develop integrated care plans for a projected length of stay or number of visits for clients with a specific case type. For example, a pathway for a surgical procedure such as a colon resection will recommend daily activities, consults, procedures, discharge planning activities, and educational topics expected for the client's progression to discharge. A critical pathway ensures better continuity of care because it clearly details the responsibility of each health care discipline. When well developed, pathways incorporate evidence-based protocols typically used in the care of the specific case type. The nurse and other health team members use the pathway as a documentation tool to monitor a client's progress and ensure continuity of care.

Initially, critical pathways were developed to manage clients in acute care settings. However, these pathways are now integrated into community-based settings (Leininger & Laux, 1998). When using critical pathways to plan care, many other forms (e.g., the nursing care plan, flow sheets, and nurses' notes) are eliminated because all of the pertinent components are included on the pathway format.

Concept Maps. Students care for clients who present with multiple health problems and related nursing diagnoses. It is often not realistic to have a written columnar plan developed for each nursing diagnosis. Plus, the columnar plans do not contain a means to show the association between different nursing diagnoses and nursing interventions. A **concept map** is a tool that assists students in appraising their thinking processes (Daley et al., 1999). It is a diagram of client problems and interventions that shows their relationships to one another (Schuster 2002). When used as a plan of care, a concept map fosters a careful consideration of evidence from clinical practice. Students learn to consider the context of nursing practice in their conceptualization of nursing problems (Daley et al., 1999). The use of a concept map promotes critical thinking and helps student nurses to organize complex client data, process complex relationships, and achieve a holistic view of a client's situation (Baugh & Mellott, 1998).

There are different approaches to writing concept maps. Schuster (2000) suggested some simple steps in preparing for concept mapping and in developing a clinical plan of care:

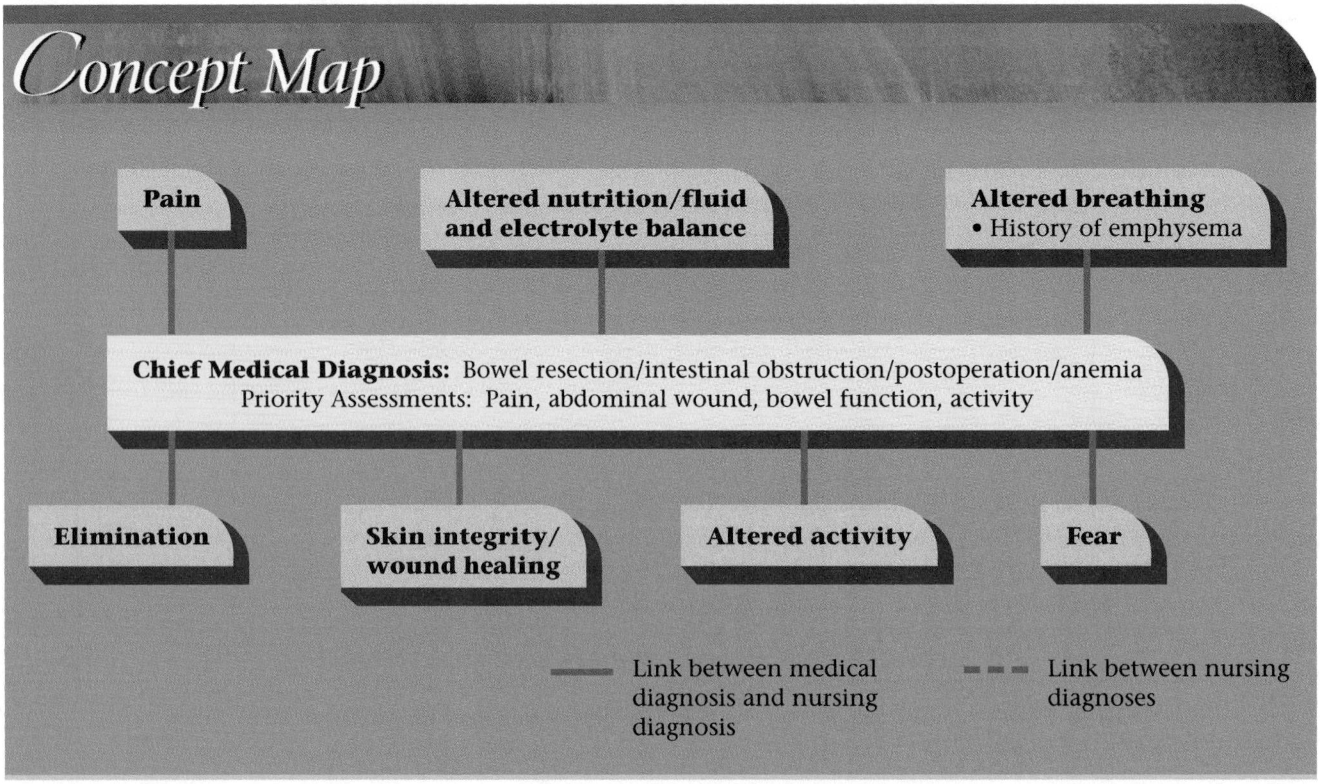

FIGURE 12–9 Concept map with nursing and medical diagnoses.

1. Before caring for an assigned client, gather the clinical assessment database from the client's medical record, including health history, physical assessment data, laboratory and diagnostic data, medication history, and treatment plan.
2. Review information on the client's health problems, treatments, and medications in course textbooks, pharmacology texts, and other related resources.
3. Review on the nursing unit any standardized nursing care plans, clinical pathways, clinical protocols, or client education materials appropriate for client care preparation.
4. Prepare the map by first developing a skeleton diagram of the client's health problems. Write the client's major medical diagnoses in the middle of the map, then add associated nursing care needs like spokes on a wheel (Figure 12–9). Often students initially have difficulty labelling nursing diagnoses correctly. It is important for the student to recognize the major nursing care focus for the client. Later, appropriate diagnostic labels can be added to the map.
5. Identify and group clinical assessment data, treatments, medications, and medical history data related to the nursing diagnoses (Figure 12–10). These include assessments the students must complete during their first contact with their client. Remember, sometimes symptoms apply to more than one nursing diagnosis. Repeat symptoms under different categories when appropriate; for example, lethargy and fatigue would be appropriate under "decreased cardiac output," "altered nutrition," and "impaired gas exchange."

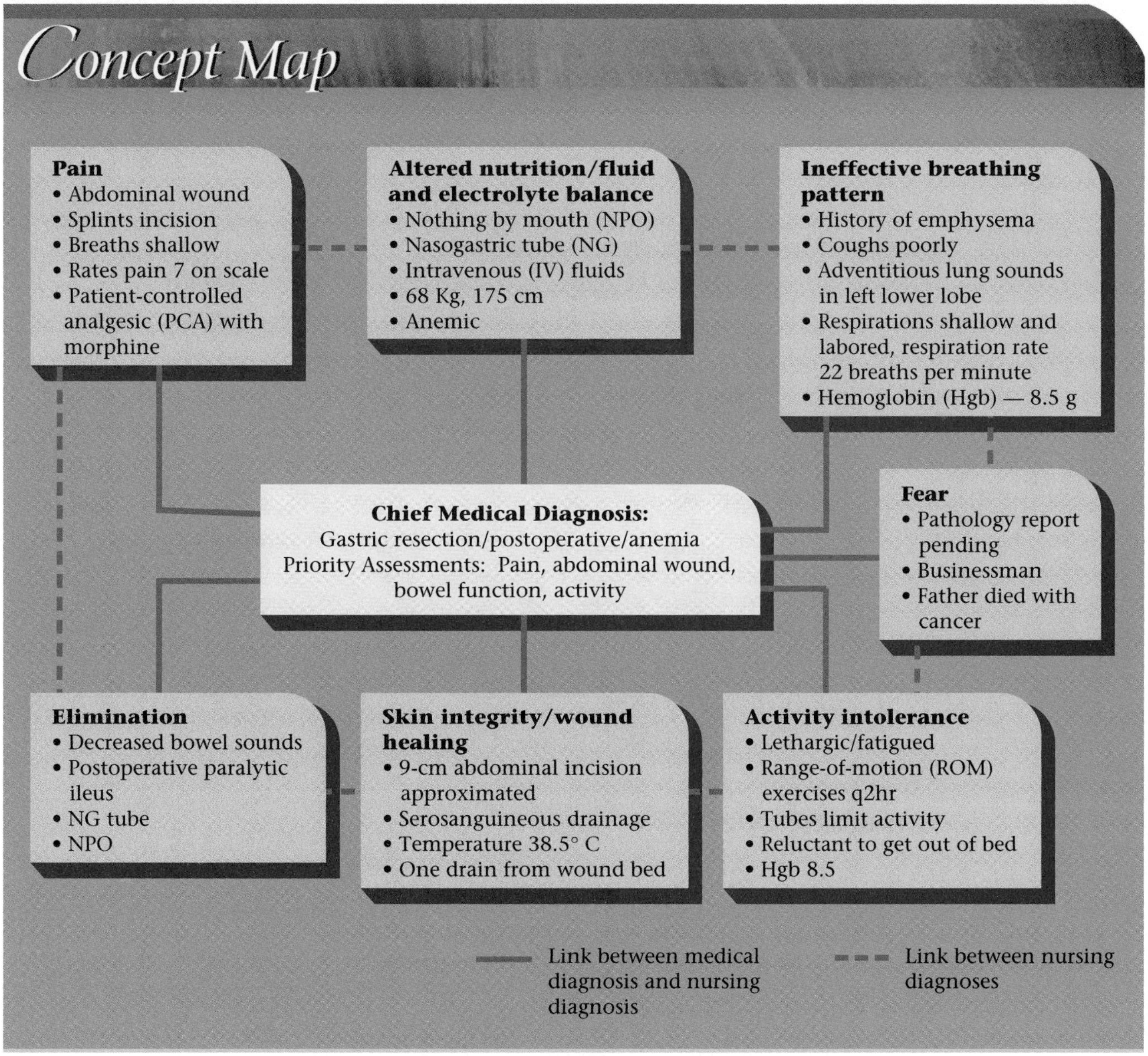

FIGURE **12–10** Concept map data to support nursing diagnoses.

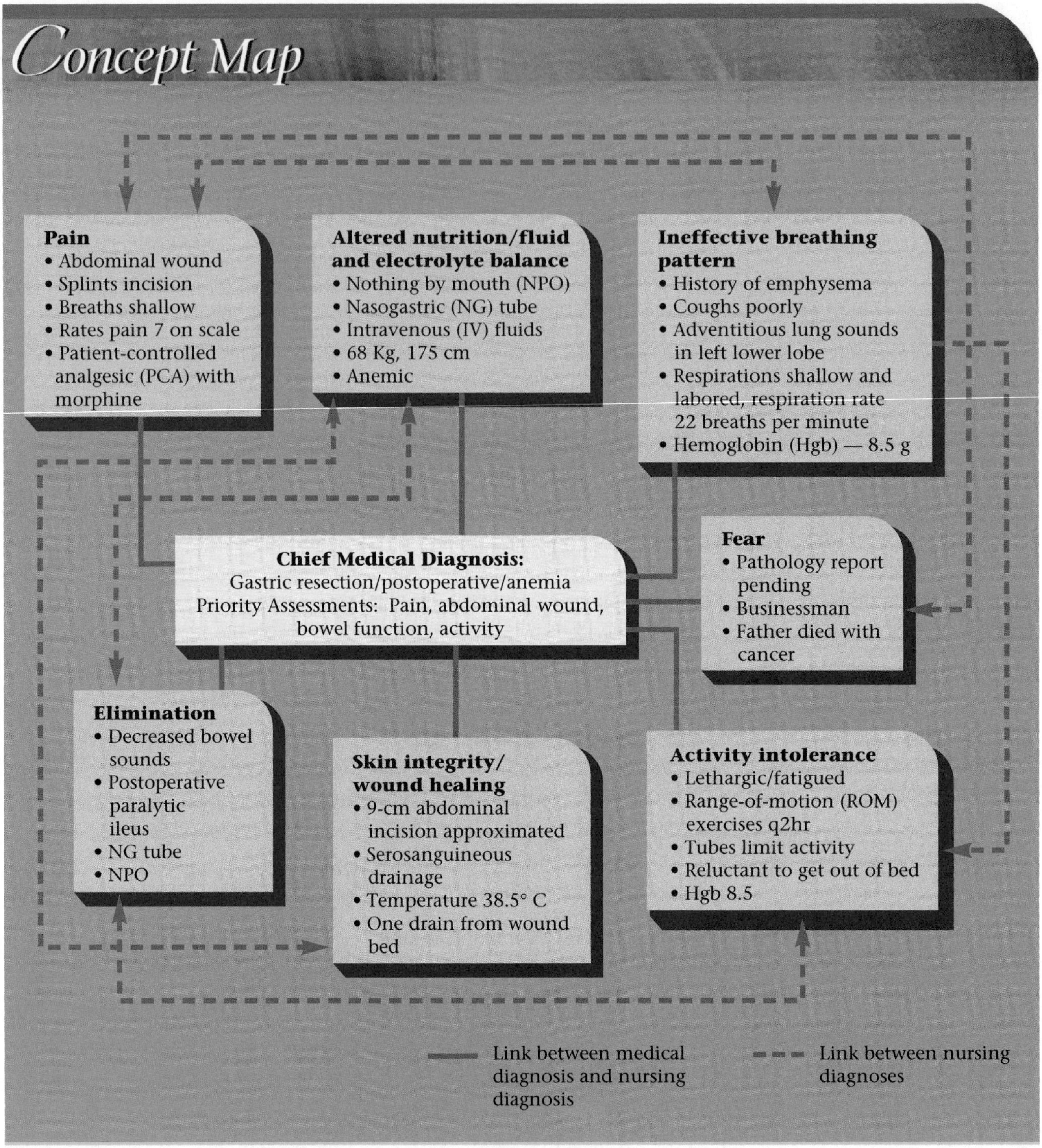

FIGURE **12–11** Concept map relationships between nursing diagnoses.

6. Next, analyze relationships among the nursing diagnoses. Draw lines between nursing diagnoses to indicate relationships (Figure 12–11). It is important to make accurate, meaningful, and complete associations between concepts. A student must be able to explain why nursing diagnoses are related.
7. Finally, on a separate sheet of paper or on the map itself, list nursing interventions to attain the outcomes for each nursing diagnosis (Box 12-11). This step corresponds to the planning phase of the nursing process.
8. While caring for the client, write down the client's responses to each nursing activity. Also write your clinical impressions and inferences regarding the client's progress toward expected outcomes and the effectiveness of interventions.

Box 12-11 Example of Nursing Interventions for Nursing Diagnoses on Concept Map

Pain

Reinforce appropriate use of patient-controlled analgesia (PCA) device.
Splint abdomen.
Position for comfort.
Use distraction or guided imagery.

Ineffective Breathing Pattern

Support incisional area during cough/deep breathing exercises.
Administer incentive spirometer every 2 hours.
Turn every 2 hours.
Monitor respiratory rate, chest excursion.
Auscultate breath sounds.
Monitor hemoglobin level.
Position semi-Fowler's, Fowler's if tolerated.

9. Keep the care map with you throughout the clinical day. As the plan is revised, take notes and add or delete nursing interventions. Use the information recorded on the map for your documentation of client care.

Critical thinkers learn by organizing and relating cognitive concepts. Concept maps help students to link concepts such as nursing diagnoses and to assimilate the interrelationships so as to create a unique meaning and organization of information. A concept map will help students link important ideas between client problems and treatments for those problems. A map helps to build the structure of what a student knows, as well as reveal what a student does not understand, so that the student can learn to ask the right questions.

Consulting Other Health Care Professionals

Planning nursing care involves consultation with other members of the health care team. **Consultation** is a process in which the expertise of a specialist is sought to identify ways to handle problems in client management or the planning and implementation of therapies. Although it may occur at any step in the nursing process, consultation is most often needed during planning and implementation, when the nurse is more likely to identify a problem requiring additional knowledge, skills, or resources. Consultation is based on the problem-solving approach, and the consultant is the stimulus for change.

Step 4: Implementing Nursing Care

Implementation, the fourth step of the nursing process, begins after the care plan has been developed. With the care plan based on clear and relevant nursing diagnoses, the nurse then initiates interventions that are most likely to support or improve the client's health status. In theory, implementation of the nursing care plan follows the planning component of the nursing process. However, in many health care settings, implementation may begin directly after assessment. For example, immediate implementation is necessary when the nurse identifies urgent needs of the client in situations such as cardiac arrest or sudden death of a loved one.

Implementation is the step of the nursing process in which nurses provide care to clients. The nurse initiates and completes actions or interventions necessary for achieving the goals and expected outcomes of nursing care. A **nursing intervention** is any treatment, based upon clinical judgment and knowledge, that a nurse performs to enhance client outcomes (Dochterman & Bulechek, 2004). Interventions include direct and indirect care and may be aimed at individuals, families, or the community. **Direct care** interventions are treatments performed through interaction with the client. For example, a client may require direct intervention in the form of medication administration, intravenous (IV) infusion, or grief counselling. **Indirect care** interventions are treatments performed away from the client but on behalf of the client or group of clients (Dochterman & Bulechek, 2004). Examples of indirect care include actions aimed at managing the client's environment (e.g., safety and infection control), documentation, and interdisciplinary collaboration.

Implementation is a continuous process that interacts with all steps of the nursing process. As the nurse carries out interventions, the client's condition can change, requiring further assessment, or the client may respond to the interventions as expected, based on evaluation (Table 12-5). For implementation to be effective, the nurse must be knowledgeable about the implementation process, implementation skills, and specific direct and indirect care interventions.

Protocols and Standing Orders

At times, nursing interventions are developed, communicated, and organized on the basis of protocols or standing orders. A **protocol** provides a standard of care or clinical guideline that can be individualized for each client depending on how an institution recommends protocol implementation. Nurses who provide primary care for clients in an outpatient setting frequently follow diagnostic and treatment protocols. In such a setting, nurses assess the client and identify abnormalities. The protocol delineates the conditions that nurses are permitted to treat, such as controlled hypertension, and the types of treatment they are permitted to administer, such as antihypertensive medications. A protocol can also be strictly within the framework of independent nursing interventions, such as a protocol for admission and discharge, pain management, or initiating cardiopulmonary resuscitation (CPR). Protocols are also used in interdisciplinary settings for diagnostic testing and physical, occupational, and speech therapies.

A **standing order** is a pre-printed document containing orders for the conduct of routine therapies, monitoring guidelines, and/or diagnostic procedures for specific clients with identified clinical problems. The orders

Table 12-5 Sample Nursing Care Plan

CASE STUDY: A nursing care plan has been developed for Mrs. Coyle, a 32-year-old woman who had a normal vaginal delivery of a 3,700-gm newborn. The nursing diagnosis of *impaired urinary elimination related to perineal swelling after vaginal delivery* provides the focus for the plan. Just before inserting the straight catheter, the nurses reassesses Mrs. Coyle to determine if she has voided spontaneously. Spontaneous voiding of 150 mL of urine would indicate that the straight catheterization procedure would no longer be appropriate. However, Mrs. Coyle has not voided and the straight catheterization is still indicated.
NURSING DIAGNOSIS: Impaired urinary elimination related to perineal swelling after vaginal delivery.
DEFINITION: Impaired urinary elimination is the state in which an individual experiences a disturbance in urine elimination.*

Assessment	Goals/*Outcomes*	Implementation	Evaluation (Outcomes)
Client has not voided in 8 hours.	Achieve emptying of bladder (8/17) as evidenced by: *Urine output greater than 240 mL during single voiding.*	Insert straight catheter, using sterile technique, if client has not voided in 8 hours and bladder is palpable.	1000 mL of clear yellow urine is returned via straight catheter (8/16).
Fluid intake for last 8 hours is 2400 mL.			Bladder is not palpable (8/16).
Client states that she "feels the urge" to void and experiences bladder discomfort.	*Verbalizes no urge to void and no bladder discomfort.*		Client no longer has urge to void (8/17).
Bladder is palpable to 2 cm below umbilicus.	*Bladder is not palpable.*		Client no longer complains of bladder discomfort (8/17).

*Data from *NANDA Nursing Diagnoses: Definitions and Classification 2003–2004,* by NANDA International, 2003, Philadelphia: Author.

direct the conduct of client care in various clinical settings. Standing orders must be approved and signed by the licensed, prescribing physician or health care provider in charge of care before their implementation. Often they are implemented at the time a client is admitted to a health care setting. Standing orders are commonly found in critical care settings, where client's needs can change rapidly and require immediate attention. Such a standing order might specify certain medications, such as lidocaine for an irregular heart rhythm. After assessing the client and identifying the irregular rhythm, the critical care nurse gives the specified medication without first notifying the physician. The physician's initial order covers the nurse's action. Standing orders are also common in the community health setting, in which the nurse encounters situations that do not permit immediate contact with a physician. Thus, standing orders and protocols give the nurse legal protection to intervene appropriately in the client's best interest.

Before implementing any intervention, the nurse must use sound judgment in determining whether the intervention is correct and appropriate. The nurse is responsible for having correct theoretical knowledge and developing the clinical competency necessary to perform the intervention. Nursing responsibility is equally great for all types of interventions.

Critical Thinking in Implementation

When nurses use the nursing process, they make two types of decisions. During the diagnostic process, nurses form conclusions, make decisions, and draw inferences about the client's assessment data and health care needs (Miller & Babcock, 1996). Next, nurses use a methodical, systematic, research-based approach to plan and select appropriate nursing interventions (Gordon, 1994). The selection of nursing interventions for a specific client is part of the clinical decision making of the nurse (Dochterman & Bulechek, 2004). Six factors should be considered when choosing interventions:

1. *Desired or expected client outcome*—Outcomes are the criteria against which to judge the success of a nursing intervention. The nurse identifies for each client the outcomes that can be reasonably expected and attained as a result of nursing intervention (see Step 3: Planning Nursing Care).
2. *Characteristics of the nursing diagnosis*—An intervention should be directed toward altering the etiological or related factor of a client's nursing diagnosis. An intervention will alter the related factor or treat the client's signs and symptoms. For a risk nursing diagnosis, interventions are aimed at altering or eliminating risk factors for the diagnosis.
3. *Evidence base for the intervention*—A nurse should know the evidence base for an intervention. An evidence base includes the research or proven practice guidelines that indicate the effectiveness of using an intervention with certain types of clients (Dochterman & Bulechek, 2004). Sometimes choosing among nurse-initiated interventions can be difficult because research is not available to support all nursing interventions (Snyder, Egan, & Nojima, 1996). Some interventions have been widely tested for specific populations. Examples are interventions in client education and pain management. Other interventions are still in the development phase, with scant evidence of their efficacy. When evidence is not

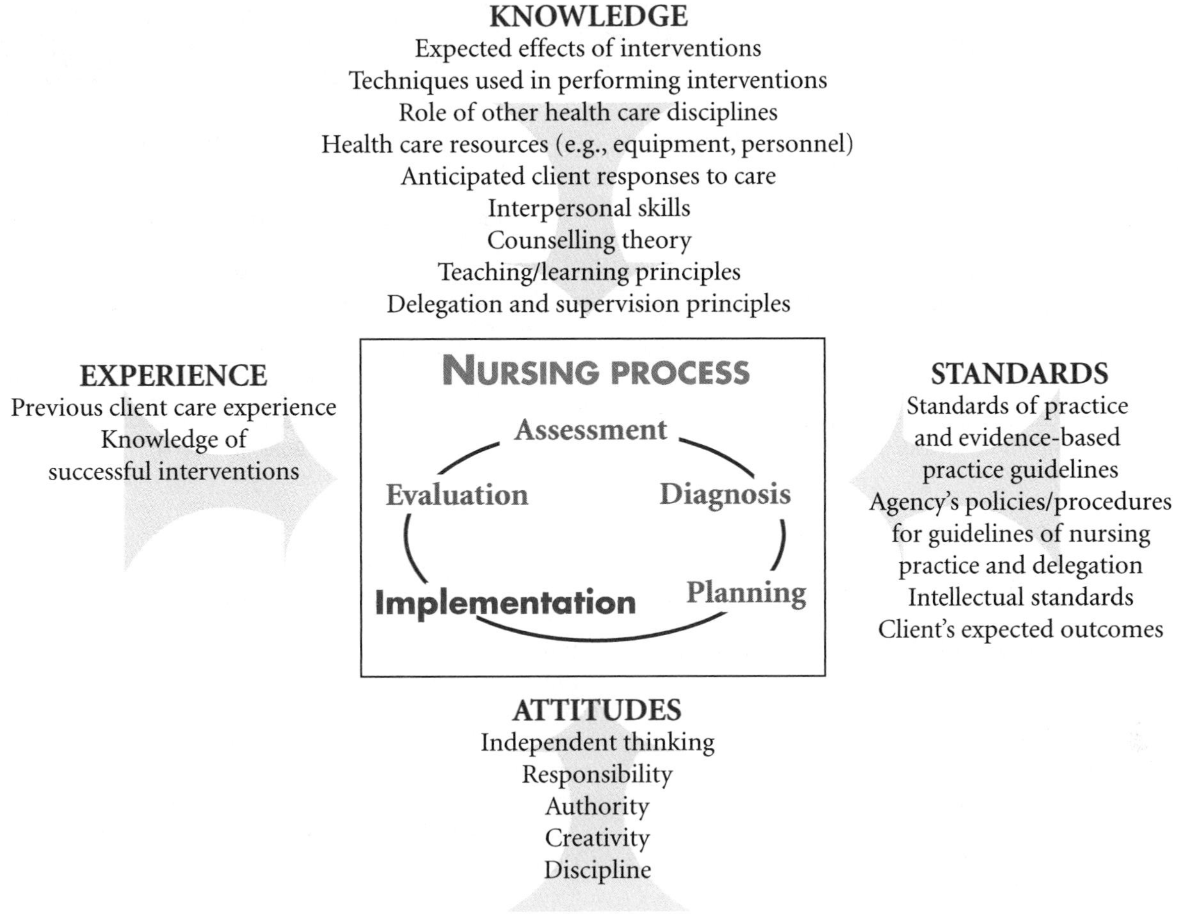

FIGURE **12–12** Critical thinking and the process of implementing care.

available, the nurse uses scientific principles and/or consults with clinical experts.

4. *Feasibility for performing an intervention*—The nurse must consider how a proposed intervention will affect other interventions delivered by the nurse or other members of the health care team. For example, a nurse should consider how educating a client about lifestyle changes would affect the information a dietician covers during diet instruction. The cost and time it takes to deliver an intervention must also be considered when determining if an intervention is feasible.
5. *Acceptability to the client*—An intervention must be acceptable to a client and family (Dochterman & Bulechek, 2004). When choosing interventions, the nurse explains how the client is to participate, what the intervention involves, and how the client might be affected. This type of summary is necessary for clients to make informed decisions about their care. It is also important to consider the client's values, beliefs, and culture when selecting interventions.
6. *Capability of the nurse*—A nurse must be competent to perform the intervention. The nurse must have knowledge of the scientific rationale for the intervention, possess necessary psychomotor and interpersonal skills, and function within the setting to effectively use all resources. No one nurse is expert in all interventions. Consultation with other nurses and disciplines is critical.

The critical thinking model discussed in chapter 11 provides a framework for how to make decisions for implementing nursing care (Figure 12–12). The nurse implements the care plan using the knowledge bases necessary for care planning and implementation. An important knowledge base is the NIC taxonomy developed by the University of Iowa. The interventions help to differentiate nursing practice from the practice of other health care professionals (Box 12-12).

Prior clinical experiences are important to consider. What interventions have worked and what have not worked in previous situations? The nurse learns to adapt interventions according to different client needs and situations. To intervene effectively, the professional and agency standards of practice must be followed. The standards of practice offer guidelines for the selection of interventions, their frequency, and whether the procedures may be delegated. Intellectual standards are also applied when performing interventions. For example, any client instruction should be relevant, clear, logical, and complete to promote client learning. All critical thinking attitudes apply to implementation. For example, being confident when performing a procedure builds trust with a client. Creativity and self-discipline will guide the nurse in reviewing, modifying, and

Box 12-12 Purposes of the Nursing Interventions Classification (NIC) Project

1. Standardization of the nomenclature (e.g., labelling, describing) of nursing interventions. Needed to standardize the language nurses use to describe specific actions used to deliver nursing care.
2. Expansion of nursing knowledge about connections between nursing diagnoses, treatments, and outcomes. These connections will be determined through the study of actual client care using a database that the classification will generate.
3. Development of nursing and health care information systems. Information systems will standardize a system for describing the interventions that nurses perform.
4. Teaching decision making to nursing students. Defining and classifying nursing interventions will help in teaching beginning nurses how to determine a client's need for care and respond appropriately. In addition, a classification of nursing interventions will make it easier to identify nursing interventions requiring higher knowledge and skill levels.
5. Determination of the cost of services provided by nurses.
6. Planning for resources needed in all types of nursing practice settings.
7. Language to communicate the unique functions of nursing.
8. Articulate with the classification systems of other health care providers.

From *Nursing Interventions Classification (NIC),* (4th ed.), edited by J. M. Dochterman and G. M. Bulechek, 2004, St. Louis, MO: Mosby.

implementing interventions. A critical thinker shows integrity by questioning personal knowledge. A beginning student or practitioner still needs supervision from an instructor or experienced nurse to guide the decision-making process for implementation.

When making decisions about implementing care, the nurse should do the following:

- Consider all possible nursing actions (e.g., pain-control measures, including analgesia, relaxation, and positioning).
- List all possible consequences associated with each possible nursing action (e.g., relief of pain, no relief of pain, and an adverse reaction to analgesia).
- Determine the probability that each of the consequences will occur (e.g., the client's pain decreased with previous analgesia and positioning; therefore adverse reactions are unlikely).
- Judge the value of that consequence to the client (e.g., the client's pain will most likely be decreased with analgesia and positioning).

Implementation Process

Preparation for implementation ensures efficient, safe, and effective nursing care. Preparatory activities include reassessing the client, reviewing and revising the existing nursing care plan, organizing resources and care delivery, and anticipating and preventing complications.

Reassessing the Client. Assessment is a continuous process that occurs each time a nurse interacts with a client. When new data are gathered and a new client need is identified, the nurse modifies the care plan. During the initial phase of implementation, the nurse reassesses the client. This is a partial assessment that may focus on one dimension of the client, such as level of comfort, or on one system, such as the cardiovascular system. The reassessment provides a way to determine whether the proposed nursing action is still appropriate for the client's level of wellness. For example, the nurse plans to ambulate a client following lunch; however, a reassessment reveals shortness of breath and increased fatigue, which requires the nurse to return the client to bed. When new data are obtained and a new client need is identified, the nurse modifies the nursing care plan.

Reviewing and Revising the Existing Nursing Care Plan. After reassessing a client, the nurse reviews the care plan, compares assessment data to validate the stated nursing diagnoses, and determines whether the nursing interventions remain the most appropriate for the clinical situation. If the client's status has changed and the nursing diagnosis and related nursing interventions are no longer appropriate, the nursing care plan needs to be modified. An out-of-date or incorrect care plan compromises the quality of nursing care, whereas review and modification enable the nurse to provide timely nursing interventions to best meet the client's needs. A nurse modifies the written care plan as follows:

1. Revises data in the assessment column to reflect the client's current status. Dates new data to inform other members of the health care team of the time that the change occurred.
2. Revises nursing diagnoses. Deletes nursing diagnoses that are no longer relevant, revises related factors, and adds and dates new nursing diagnoses. In addition, revises and dates the client's priorities, goals, and expected outcomes.
3. Revises specific interventions to correspond to the new nursing diagnoses and client goals. This revision reflects the client's present status.
4. Decides what methods of evaluation will be used to determine if outcomes are achieved.

The following example shows how a nurse reviews and revises a plan. A care plan was developed preoperatively for Mr. Brown. As he progressed through the post-operative period, his nursing needs changed. The nurse made modifications in the care plan for one nursing diagnosis: *risk for ineffective airway clearance related to abdominal incisional pain* (Table 12-6). On the second post-operative day, the nurse assessed the client and noted decreased chest wall movements, crackles that were auscultated in the right lower lobes, and an elevated temperature (39° C). Mr. Brown also reported increased abdominal pain. Mr. Brown had a standing order for a chest X-ray examination, which

Table 12-6 Modified Nursing Care Plan for Mr. Brown

NURSING DIAGNOSIS: Risk for ineffective airway clearance related to abdominal incisional pain.
Modified Nursing Diagnosis: Ineffective airway clearance related to decreased inspiratory effort secondary to abdominal incisional pain.
DEFINITION: Ineffective airway clearance is the state in which an individual is unable to clear secretions or obstructions from the respiratory tract to maintain a clear airway.*

Assessment	Goals/*Outcomes*	Implementation	Evaluation
Smoked two packs/day for 15 years; chest X-ray film showing slight change of emphysema; crackles auscultated in RLL; scheduled for abdominal surgery	Airway will remain clear (11/8) as evidenced by: *Lungs clear to auscultation* *Client coughs productively*	**Airway management†** Demonstrate turn, cough, and deep breathing exercise to client. Have client perform exercises every 2 hours while awake.	Productive cough produced. Airway clear to auscultation.
Modified 24 Hours After Surgery			
Decreased chest wall movements; crackles bilaterally in base that do not clear with coughing; elevated temperature (39° C); reports incisional pain 6 on scale of 0 to 10	Airway will remain clear (11/8) as evidenced by: *Lungs clear to auscultation* *Temperature <37.8° C* *Pain intensity will be less than client's baseline*	**Airway management†** Administer chest physiotherapy to all lobes of the lung: 8-12-4-8-12-4. Have Mr. Brown perform incentive spirometry every 2 hours around the clock. Teach client to splint incision with pillow before and during coughing. Administer analgesics as ordered for incisional pain. **Airway suctioning** Suction nasotracheally every 2 hours if client is unable to cough productively.	Lung fields are clear on auscultation. Client becomes afebrile. Chest X-ray film demonstrates atelectasis resolving. Client does not report increased pain during coughing.

*Data from *NANDA Nursing Diagnoses: Definitions and Classification 2003–2004,* by NANDA International, 2003, Philadelphia: Author.
†Intervention categories supported by NIC. From *Nursing Interventions Classification (NIC),* (4th ed.), edited by J. M. Dochterman and G. M. Bulechek, 2004, St. Louis, MO: Mosby.

was taken immediately and revealed the collapse of alveoli in the right lower lobe. The nursing diagnosis was revised to an actual diagnosis with a different etiology, *ineffective airway clearance related to decreased inspiratory effort secondary to abdominal incisional pain.* The nursing diagnostic label was revised because of the presence of right lower lobe crackles and decreased chest wall movement. The goal of Mr. Brown's airway becoming clear was still appropriate. Specific new nursing interventions such as the use of incentive spirometry and the optional use of suctioning were developed to assist in preventing further alveolar collapse. Finally, the nurse determined the method of evaluation for the new clinical problem.

Organizing Resources and Care Delivery. Before delivering an intervention, the nurse prepares the necessary supplies and decides on the time and provider of care. All supplies should be gathered and put in a convenient location, usually where they will be used. Extra supplies should be available in case of mishaps. It is the nurse's responsibility to determine whether to perform an intervention or to delegate it to another member of the nursing team. The nurse's assessment of the client should direct the decision about delegation, not the intervention alone. For example, unregulated care providers (UCPs) are trained to ambulate clients. However, if a nurse learns that a client recently experienced cardiac irregularities, the nurse may decide to personally assist the client with ambulation and evaluate the client's cardiac status.

Preparation for care delivery also involves preparing the client for nursing interventions. Controlling environmental factors, positioning, and taking care of other physical needs (e.g., elimination) should precede initiation of interventions. The nurse should also consider the client's level of endurance and plan only the amount of activity that the client can comfortably endure.

The client benefits most from nursing interventions when surroundings are compatible with activities. Privacy promotes relaxation when body parts are exposed. Reducing distractions enhances a client's learning opportunities. Provision of adequate space and lighting provides for efficiency when procedures are performed. Before beginning to perform interventions, the nurse should make the client as physically and psychologically comfortable as possible. Symptoms such as nausea, dizziness, or pain, for example, frequently interfere with a client's full concentration and co-operation. Administering comfort measures before initiating interventions enables the client to participate more fully. In the case of analgesic administration, for example, if client alertness is needed, the dose of pain medication should be sufficient to relieve discomfort but not impair mental faculties.

Anticipating and Preventing Complications. Risks to the client arise from illness, conditions, and treatment. The nurse must identify these risks, evaluate the relative benefit of the treatment versus the risk, and initiate risk prevention measures. For example, the client with pre-existing left-sided paralysis following a stroke 2 years earlier is at risk for developing a pressure ulcer following orthopedic surgery, which requires traction and bed rest. The nurse's knowledge of pathophysiology helps in identifying the risk of complications that can occur. Scientific rationales for how certain interventions (e.g., pressure relief devices and turning and repositioning) can prevent or minimize complications help the nurse to evaluate the usefulness of preventive measures. If the client's post-operative pain is not controlled, the risk for pressure ulcer development increases because pain may limit the client's ability to change position frequently. The nurse anticipates when the client's pain will be aggravated, administers ordered analgesics, and then positions the client to remove pressure on the skin and underlying tissues.

Identifying Areas of Assistance. Some nursing situations require the nurse to seek additional assistance, knowledge, and/or nursing skills. Before implementing care, the nurse reviews the plan to determine the need for assistance and the type required. Situations requiring additional personnel vary. Assistance may be needed in performing a procedure, comforting a client, or preparing the client for a procedure. For example, a nurse assigned to care for an immobilized client will need additional personnel to help turn, transfer, and position the client. The nurse needs to determine the number of additional personnel and when they are needed. The nurse then explains the type of assistance needed, when it is needed, and how the client has responded in the past when more than one caregiver is involved.

Some nursing situations require additional knowledge and skills, such as when administering a new medication or implementing a new procedure. Such information can be obtained from the agency's procedure manual and the literature. If the nurse is still uncertain about the new medication or procedure, the nurse can consult other members of the health care team. Assistance can come from another staff nurse, a supervisor, an educator, or a nurse specialist.

Box 12-13

Focus on Primary Health Care

Implementing Preventive Measures

Preventive nursing actions promote health and prevent illness. Prevention includes assessment and promotion of the client's health potential, application of prescribed measures (e.g., immunizations), health teaching, and identification of risk factors for illness and/or trauma.

Consider, for example, the case of Mrs. Schmidt, who is providing in-home care to her elderly mother, maintaining a career, and caring for two school-age children as a single parent. Mrs. Schmidt tells the nurse that she is experiencing a great deal of stress. The nurse can implement preventive measures to assist Mrs. Schmidt in controlling some of the stress. The nurse initiates stress-reducing interventions, such as relaxation therapy, for Mrs. Schmidt. In addition, the nurse assists Mrs. Schmidt in identifying community agencies and resources, such as respite care. The nurse teaches Mrs. Schmidt how to provide hygiene, nutrition, and medications for her mother. Together, the nurse and Mrs. Schmidt identify signs and symptoms that indicate whether her mother's health status is changing and what actions should be taken.

Preventive nursing interventions are a fundamental aspect of primary health care and are needed in all types of care settings and with all age groups.

Direct Care

Nurses provide a variety of direct care measures. Because interaction with the client is involved, the nurse must always be sensitive to the client's clinical condition, values and beliefs, expectations, and cultural views. This sensitivity ensures an individualized approach. All direct care measures require competent, safe practice. When administering direct care, the nurse learns to avoid or compensate for clients' adverse reactions to therapy and ensures preventive care (Box 12-13).

Activities of Daily Living. Acute and chronic conditions and diseases can disrupt a client's ability to perform ADLs. An acute condition or disease is characterized by symptoms that are usually severe and present for a relatively short time, usually less than 6 months. An episode of acute disease results in recovery to a state of health and activity comparable to the state before the disease, passage into a chronic phase of the disease, or death. An example is the post-operative client who because of lingering sedation and pain is often unable to independently complete all ADLs. While progressing through the post-operative period, the client gradually depends less on nurses for completing ADLs.

A chronic disease or condition persists longer. Although the symptoms are usually less severe than those of the acute phase of the same disease, chronic disease may result in complete or partial disability. An example is a client with partial paralysis after a cerebrovascular accident (stroke). The client will be unable to use the affected extremity or extremities and generally will require long-term assistance with ADLs.

The client's need for assistance with ADLs may be temporary, permanent, or rehabilitative. In the case of temporary assistance with ADLs, the client needs assistance for a limited period of time. A client with impaired mobility because of bilateral arm casts has a temporary need for assistance. After the casts are removed, the client will gradually regain the strength and range of motion needed to perform ADLs. However, a client with a total self-care deficit related to an irreversible injury high in the cervical spinal cord has a permanent need for assistance. It is unrealistic for the nurse to plan a rehabilitation program with the goal that this client will be able to independently complete all ADLs. However, through restorative care, the client will learn new ways to perform ADLs, thus becoming more independent.

As is the case with any intervention, assessment verifies a client's need for assistance with ADLs. Clients whose assessment data reveal fatigue, limitations in mobility, confusion, and pain, for example, often need assistance with ADLs. A client who experiences severe shortness of breath may avoid eating because of the associated fatigue. The nurse will assist the client with feeding and plan for more frequent, small meals to maintain the client's nutrition. Assistance with ADLs can range from partial assistance to complete care. In clients with chronic conditions, assistance with ADLs can change from day to day.

When assisting with ADLs, the nurse must also assess client preferences. For example, a client whose activities are limited because of mobility restrictions may prefer to have assistance with partial hygiene but maintain independence in feeding and grooming activities. Involving the client in planning the timing and types of interventions with ADLs can boost the client's self-esteem and willingness to become more independent.

Instrumental Activities of Daily Living. Illness or disability can alter clients' ability to be independent in society. **Instrumental activities of daily living (IADLs)** include such skills as shopping, preparing meals, writing checks, and taking medications. Nurses within the home care and community health setting have an excellent opportunity to assist clients in adapting to perform IADLs. Often family and friends can assist clients. In the acute care setting, it is important for a nurse to anticipate how a client's illness might affect the ability to perform IADLs so that appropriate referrals can be made to support the client following discharge.

Physical Care Techniques. Nurses deliver an array of physical care techniques. Examples include turning and positioning clients, performing invasive procedures, administering medications, and providing comfort measures. Physical techniques involve the safe and competent administration of nursing skills or procedures (e.g., urinary catheter insertion, range-of-motion exercises, and administration of injections). The specific knowledge and skills needed to carry out these nursing procedures are detailed in subsequent clinical chapters in this text. However, there are common methods in all procedures that must be used, including promoting safety, following infection-control practices, using an organized approach, and positioning clients correctly. When these methods are integrated within a procedure, the ultimate outcome is safe and effective nursing care.

To carry out a procedure, the nurse must be knowledgeable about the procedure itself, the standard frequency, the steps, and the expected outcomes. In a hospital, the nurse completes many procedures each day. Before conducting a new procedure, the nurse assesses personal competencies and determines the need for assistance, new knowledge, or new skills.

Lifesaving Measures. A **lifesaving measure** is implemented when a client's physiological or psychological state is threatened. The purpose of the lifesaving measure is to restore physiological or psychological equilibrium. Such measures include administering emergency medications, instituting CPR, intervening to protect a confused or violent client, and obtaining immediate counselling from a crisis centre for a severely anxious client. As with any procedure, the nurse must be knowledgeable about the lifesaving procedure and expected outcomes. If an inexperienced nurse faces a situation requiring emergency measures, the proper nursing action may be to get an experienced professional.

Counselling. Counselling is a direct care method that helps the client use a problem-solving process to recognize and manage stress and to facilitate interpersonal relationships among the client, family, and health care team. Nurses provide counselling to help the client accept actual or impending changes resulting from stress. Counselling involves emotional, intellectual, spiritual, and psychological support. A client and family who need nursing counselling have normal adjustment difficulties and are upset or frustrated, but they are not necessarily psychologically disabled. For example, more families are now taking care of their relatives who have physical disabilities following surgery, stroke, or chronic illnesses. These families need assistance in adjusting to the demands placed on the caregiver. Likewise, the recipient of care also needs assistance in adjusting to the disability. Clients with psychiatric diagnoses require therapy by nurses specializing in psychiatric nursing or by social workers, psychiatrists, or psychologists.

Many counselling techniques are used to foster cognitive, behavioural, developmental, experiential, and emotional growth. Most of the techniques listed in Box 12-14 require additional knowledge beyond the scope of this text. Counselling encourages individuals to examine available alternatives and decide which choices are useful and appropriate. When clients are able to examine alternatives, they can develop a sense of control and are able to better manage stress. To assist clients in need of counselling, the nurse must be able to identify the need for counselling and possess communication skills to develop a therapeutic relationship (Sundeen et al., 1998).

Clients needing counselling include those who must adjust lifestyle patterns, as in smoking cessation, weight reduction, or increasing activity. Clients coping with chronic or disabling diseases require counselling to help them adapt to changes in lifestyle or body image as the disease progresses. During life-threatening illnesses, clients and families need counselling to cope with the possibility of death.

Teaching. Counselling is closely aligned with teaching. Both involve using communication skills to effect a change in the client. However, with counselling, the change results in the development of new attitudes and feelings, whereas in teaching the focus of change is intellectual growth or the acquisition of new knowledge or psychomotor skills (Redman, 2001).

Teaching is an implementation method used to present correct principles, procedures, and techniques of health care to clients and to inform clients about their health

Box 12-14 Counselling Strategies and Selected Examples Used by Nurses

Behaviour Modification

Client changes from smoking to meditating to cope with stress
Client uses exercise as a health promotion activity

Bereavement Counselling

Nurse assists client in productive reminiscing of loved one
Nurse supports client in removing loved one's belongings from home

Biofeedback

Regulation of stress
Meditation

Relaxation Exercises

Progressive muscle relaxation exercises
Meditation

Crisis Intervention

Therapy designed to assist in coping with crisis
Anticipatory guidance to recognize and avoid modifiable crises

Play Therapy

Assist children through play to cope with loss and grief
Assist children in coping with chronic illness
Assist children in becoming competent in self-care activities

status (see chapter 17). As a nursing responsibility, teaching is implemented in all health care settings (Figure 12–13). The nurse is responsible for assessing the learning needs and readiness of clients and is accountable for the quality of education delivered. The teaching-learning process is an interaction between the teacher and the learner in which specific learning objectives are presented (Redman, 2001). This process provides the organizational structure and framework for client education. The teaching-learning process is much like the basic nursing process.

During assessment, the nurse determines the client's learning needs and readiness to learn. The nurse then interprets the data to formulate nursing diagnoses that reflect the identified needs. During planning, the nurse and client establish goals and outcomes for learning, with consideration of the skills and knowledge clients will require in their self-care. Implementation is the initiation of the teaching strategies designed to achieve the learning goals. Finally, evaluation measures the learning that has occurred. The purpose of the teaching-learning process is to develop and implement a teaching plan individualized for the client's needs, level of knowledge, and learning resources. The goal is to give clients the knowledge and skills necessary to assume health-related behaviours.

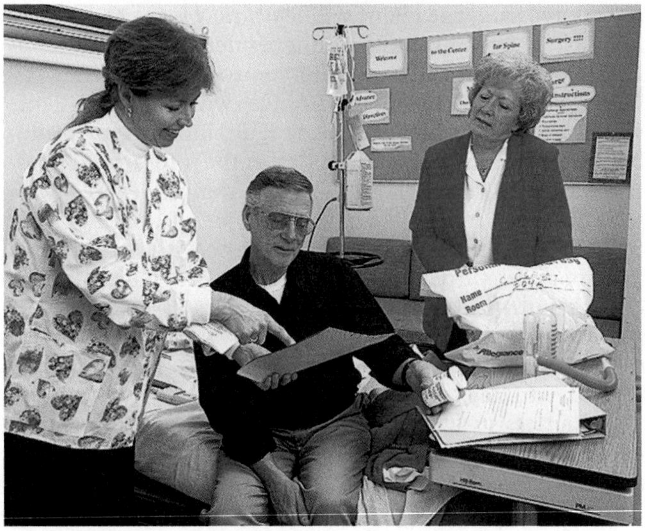

FIGURE **12–13** A nurse teaching a client about his discharge instructions.

Observing for Adverse Reactions. An **adverse reaction** is a harmful or unintended effect of a medication, diagnostic test, or therapeutic intervention. Adverse reactions can follow any nursing interventions; therefore, the nurse learns to anticipate and know the adverse reactions to expect. For instance, the client receiving feedings through a nasogastric tube is at risk for aspiration. The nurse should elevate the head of the bed and have pharyngeal suction equipment at the bedside before initiating the feedings.

Nursing actions that control for adverse reactions reduce or counteract the reaction. For example, when applying a moist heat compress, the nurse assesses the area requiring the compress. Following application of the compress, the nurse evaluates the area every 5 minutes for any adverse reaction, such as excessive reddening of the skin from the heat or skin maceration from the moisture of the compress. When completing a physician-directed intervention, such as medication administration, the nurse understands the known and potential side effects of the drug. After administration of the medication, the nurse evaluates the client for any adverse effects. The nurse should be aware of drugs that can counteract the side effects. For example, a client may have an unknown hypersensitivity to penicillin and may develop hives after three doses. The nurse records the reaction and stops further administration of the drug. The nurse also consults the physician's orders and, for example, may administer diphenhydramine (Benadryl), an antihistamine and antipruritic medication, to reduce the allergic response and to relieve the itching.

When caring for a client who is undergoing a diagnostic test, the nurse must understand the test and any potential adverse effects. For example, a client has not had a bowel movement in 24 hours after a barium enema. Because bowel impaction is a potential side effect of a barium enema, the nurse increases fluid intake and instructs the client to let the nursing personnel know when a bowel movement occurs.

Although adverse effects are not common, they do occur. Ultimately, the nurse wants to prevent any adverse effects. It is imperative that the nurse recognizes the signs and symptoms of an adverse reaction and intervenes in a timely manner.

Indirect Care

Indirect care measures are actions that support the effectiveness of direct care interventions (McCloskey & Bulechek, 2000). Indirect care often involves managerial measures, such as emergency cart checking, environmental management (i.e., making client rooms safe, assigning client rooms), and supply management. Other examples of indirect care include documentation, order transcription, computer entry, telephone consultation, and specimen management and transport. A good percentage of a nurse's time is spent in indirect and unit management activities. Communication of information about clients (e.g., change-of-shift report and consultation) is critical to ensuring that direct care activities are planned, coordinated, and ultimately performed with the proper resources. Delegation of care to UCPs is another indirect care activity. When performed correctly, delegation ensures that the right care providers perform the right tasks so that the nurse and UCP work most efficiently for the client's benefit.

Communicating Nursing Interventions. Nursing interventions are written and/or communicated orally. Written interventions are part of the nursing care plan and client's permanent medical record. In many institutions, **interdisciplinary care plans** are developed. These plans represent the contributions of all disciplines caring for a client. For example, a client recovering from total hip surgery will have a care plan for the problem of impaired mobility that includes interventions from nursing, the surgeon, and physiotherapy. Any client care plan reflects proposed nursing interventions. After the interventions are completed, the client's response to the treatment is recorded on the appropriate record (see chapter 13). The record entry usually includes a brief description of pertinent assessment findings, the specific procedure, and the client's response. This information validates the need for the specific nursing intervention. Writing the time and the details of the intervention documents that the procedure was completed.

Nursing interventions are also communicated orally between nurses and other health care professionals. Unless communication is timely and accurate, caregivers may be uninformed, interventions may be needlessly duplicated, procedures may be delayed, or tasks may be left undone (Gerteis et al., 1993). Clients can quickly tell when the health care team communicates poorly, indicating that no one is in charge. Nurses commonly communicate orally when conferring with colleagues, changing shifts, transferring a client to another unit, or discharging a client to another health care agency. Whether the nursing intervention is written or communicated orally, the language should be clear and concise.

Delegating, Supervising, and Evaluating Others' Work. Depending on the system of health care delivery, the nurse who develops the care plan frequently does not perform all of the nursing interventions. Some activities may be delegated to other members of the health care team and coordinated by the nurse. Repetitive, non-invasive interventions such as range-of-motion exercises, ambulation, grooming, and hygiene measures are typically delegated to UCPs such as support workers. A licensed practical nurse/registered practical nurse can perform these measures in addition to medication administration and certain invasive tasks (e.g., catheterization, dressing care, and suctioning). The delegating nurse is responsible for ensuring that the person who is assigned the task is competent to perform the task and that the task is completed according to the standard of care (McCloskey et al., 1996). Chapter 10 covers guidelines for effective delegation.

Step 5: Evaluating Nursing Care

The nursing process is a series of nursing actions based on and supported by clinical judgments. The previous sections of this chapter describe how the nurse uses critical thinking skills to gather client data, form nursing diagnoses, and develop and implement a plan of care. **Evaluation,** the final step of the nursing process, is crucial to determine whether the client's condition or well-being improves. Evaluation involves two components: examining a condition or situation and judging whether change has occurred. Ideally, after an intervention takes place, evaluation should reveal an improvement.

The nurse applies all that is known about a client and the client's condition, as well as experience with previous clients, to evaluate whether nursing care was effective. The nurse conducts evaluation measures to determine if expected outcomes are met, not the nursing interventions. The expected outcomes are the standards against which the nurse judges if goals have been met and thus if care is successful.

Critical Thinking and Evaluation

Evaluation is one of the most critical phases of the nursing process because it determines the usefulness and effectiveness of nursing practice (Lin, 1996). During evaluation, the nurse decides if the previous steps of the nursing process were effective by examining the client's responses and comparing them with the behaviours or physical indicators stated in the expected outcomes. For example, a client may have a diagnosis of *impaired oral mucous membrane related to effects of chemotherapy.* The nurse administers oral care and adjusts the client's food intake with the intent of meeting the outcome of, "Client's mucosa will be well hydrated and client will deny oral pain." Evaluation will involve inspection of the oral mucosa and questioning the client about pain. Evaluation is not simply recording that oral care was performed. Evaluation informs the nurse of the need to change or revise the care plan when interventions are ineffective or less effective than anticipated. Effective evaluation requires the use of critical thinking skills (Figure 12–14).

Evaluation is ongoing whenever the nurse has contact with the client. Once an intervention has been delivered, the nurse gathers objective and subjective data from the

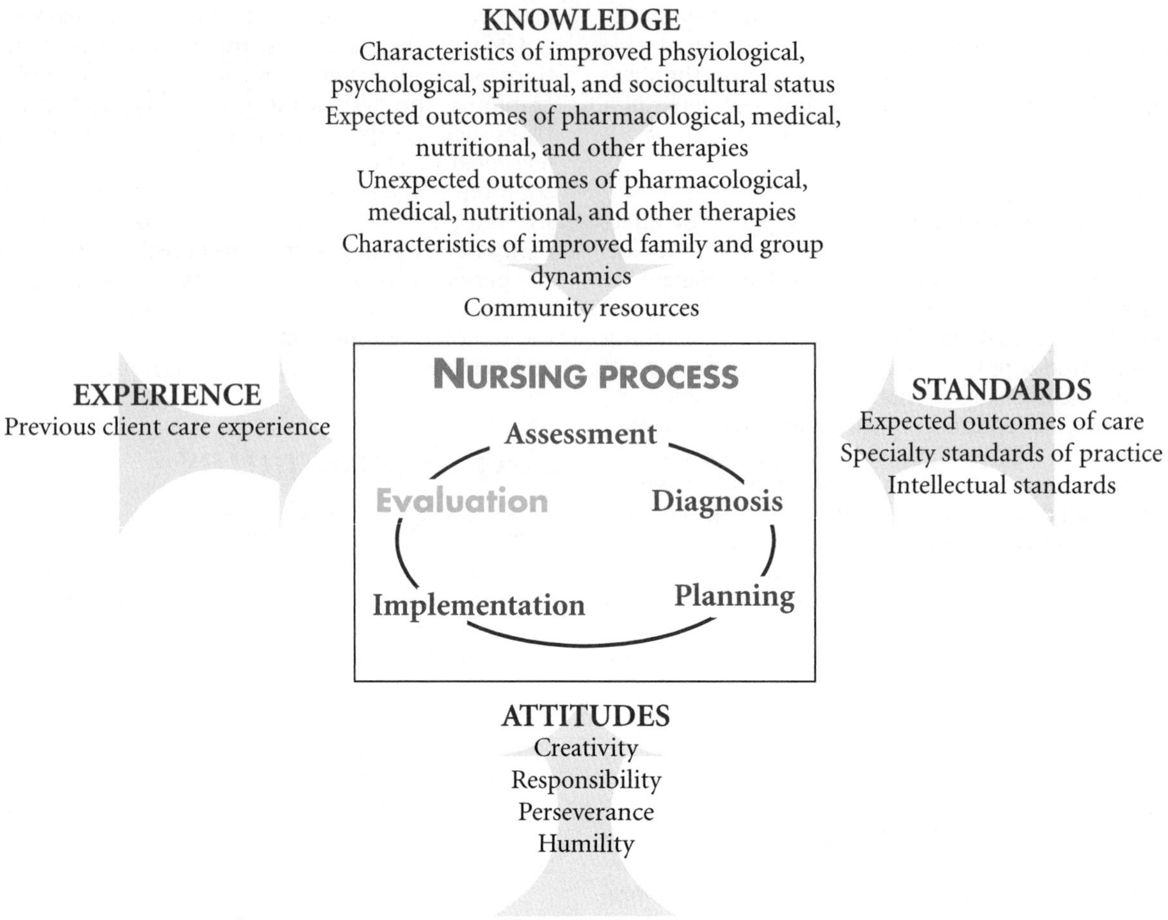

FIGURE **12–14** Critical thinking and evaluation.

client, family, and health care team members. The nurse also reviews knowledge regarding the client's current condition, treatment, resources available for recovery, and the anticipated outcomes. By referring to previous experiences when caring for similar clients, the nurse is in a better position to know how to evaluate the client. Finally, the nurse applies critical thinking attitudes and standards to determine whether outcomes of care are achieved. If outcomes are met, the overall goals for the client are also met. The nurse compares client behaviour and responses assessed before and after nursing intervention. Critical thinking directs the nurse to analyze evaluation findings. What do I know about the client's health problem, and has it improved? For example, has the skin's appearance returned to normal after administering pressure relief therapies? Is pain relieved following the use of guided imagery and distraction? Is the client expressing less anxiety following instruction and the opportunity to ask questions about his diagnosis?

During evaluation, the nurse makes clinical decisions and redirects nursing care to best meet client needs. For example, when evaluating a client for a change in vital signs, the nurse applies knowledge of the disease process, physiological responses to interventions, and the correct procedure for vital sign measurement to interpret whether a change has occurred and whether the change is desirable. A client experiencing deficient fluid volume following blood loss from surgery may have an increased heart rate and reduced blood pressure. The nurse knows that these signs represent the expected physiological response to an isotonic fluid loss (see chapter 36). The nurse knows the client has a history free of complications and rules out other factors that may cause an increased heart rate or drop in blood pressure. After administering IV fluids and making the client comfortable so as to reduce stressors, the nurse returns to evaluate if vital signs have returned to an acceptable level or to the client's baseline before surgery. Evaluative findings determine the nurse's next course of action.

Positive evaluations occur when desired results are met and lead the nurse to conclude that nursing interventions are effective. In the example above, a return to normal vital signs indicates that the client achieves the goal of a normal fluid balance. Negative evaluations or undesired results, such as the continuation of an elevated or irregular heart rate, indicate that interventions are not effective in minimizing or resolving the actual problem or avoiding an at-risk problem. A negative evaluation reveals that the client has not met the expected outcomes. As a result, the nurse changes the plan of care by trying different therapies or changing the frequency or approach of existing therapies.

This sequence of critically evaluating and revising therapies continues until clients' problems, as defined by

Table 12-7 Evaluation of Mr. Brown's Plan of Care

Assessment	Goals	Expected Outcomes	Evaluative Measures	Evaluation Statement
Decreased chest wall movements	Airway will become clear in 48 hours.	Chest excursion will increase by 2.5 cm.	Auscultate lung fields bilaterally.	Lung sounds reveal crackles in bases with clearing on left during coughing.
Crackles bilaterally in bases do not clear with coughing		Lungs will be clear to auscultation within 48 hours.	Observe and record volume of air inspired by client using spirometry.	Client is achieving 60% of incentive spirometry goal.
Chest X-ray film reveals right lower lobe infiltrate present		Client will achieve 90% of incentive spirometry goal in 24 hours.		
Elevated temperature (39° C)		Temperature will be 37.8° C in 48 hours.	Measure client's oral temperature.	Temperature is 38.3° C.
Reports incisional pain 5–6 on scale of 0–10		Pain intensity will be less than client's baseline in 24 hours.	Administer pain scale.	Client rates pain at level of 6. Client continues to have difficulty clearing airway due to ongoing abdominal pain.

nursing diagnoses, are appropriately resolved. Evaluation is dynamic and ever changing, depending on the client's nursing diagnoses and condition. As problems change, so too may expected outcomes. A client whose health status continuously changes requires more frequent evaluation. In addition, priority diagnoses are usually evaluated first. For example, a nurse evaluates a client's *acute pain* before evaluating the status of *deficient knowledge.*

The Evaluation Process

The purpose of nursing care is to assist the client in resolving health problems, preventing potential problems, and maintaining health. The evaluation process, which determines the effectiveness of nursing care, includes five elements: (a) identifying evaluative criteria and standards, (b) collecting data to determine whether the criteria or standards are met, (c) interpreting and summarizing findings, (d) documenting findings and any clinical judgment, and (e) terminating, continuing, or revising the care plan.

Identifying Criteria and Standards. A nurse evaluates care by knowing what to look for. With clearly defined goals and expected outcomes, the nurse has objective criteria from which to judge the client's response to care.

Goals. A goal specifies the expected behaviour or response that indicates resolution of a nursing diagnosis or maintenance of health. It is a summary statement of what is to be accomplished when all expected outcomes have been met. In the case of Mr. Brown, who is 2 days post-operative, the nursing diagnosis of *ineffective airway clearance related to decreased inspiratory effort secondary to abdominal incisional pain* remains his primary health problem. The nurse selected the goal of, "Client's airway will become clear in 48 hours." Successful achievement of this goal depends on the success of rigorous pulmonary hygiene (Table 12-7). The nurse compares evaluative findings with all expected outcomes to determine if the goal is achieved. For example, the nurse auscultates the client's lungs to determine if crackles have decreased and lung sounds are clear. When a goal has been accomplished, the nurse knows that interventions were successful. If a goal remains unmet, either the plan must continue or revisions may be necessary. In Mr. Brown's case, revisions are likely needed.

Goals often are based on standards of care or guidelines established for minimal safe practice. For example, the Infusion Nurses Society (INS) has standards of care for prevention of the IV complication phlebitis. When a nurse cares for a client with a peripheral intravenous line, the goal of, "The IV site will remain free of phlebitis" is established on the basis of sound practice standards. The INS has developed a scale containing physical criteria for determining phlebitis (chapter 36).

Expected Outcomes. Expected outcomes are the expected measurable results of the goal-oriented nursing process. A nurse-sensitive client outcome is a measurable client or family state, behaviour, or perception, largely influenced by and sensitive to nursing interventions (Moorhead, Johnson, & Mass, 2004). Outcomes are statements of progressive, step-by-step responses or behaviours that the client must accomplish to achieve the goals of care. An outcome defines the effectiveness, efficiency, and measurement of the results of nursing interventions (Deaton, 1998). When outcomes are achieved, the related factors for a nursing diagnosis no longer exist. For example, for Mr. Brown's nursing diagnosis of *ineffective airway clearance related to decreased inspiratory effort secondary to abdominal incisional pain,* the client must achieve the goal of the airway remaining clear. This goal will be accomplished by meeting the outcomes of, "The client's lungs will become clear to auscultation within 48 hours," "Client will achieve 90% of incentive spirometry goal," and "Oral temperature will return to normal within 48 hours." If the outcomes are met, the nurse has successfully promoted mucus clearance and the maintenance of a patent airway.

It is important to understand that evaluation is not a description of the achievement of an intervention. Evaluation of Mr. Brown *does not* involve observing his ability to use the incentive spirometer. Evaluation *does* involve the actual incentive spirometry volume achieved by the client compared with the desired outcome of 90%.

During the planning phase of the nursing process, nurses must select an observable client state, behaviour, or self-reported perception that will reflect goal achievement. One valuable resource is the Nursing Outcomes Classification (NOC), which provides a classification system of nurse-sensitive outcomes. NOC is designed to provide the language for the evaluation step of the nursing process. The purposes of NOC are to (a) identify, label, validate, and classify nursing-sensitive client outcomes; (b) field test and validate the classification; and (c) define and test measurement procedures for the outcomes and indicators using clinical data (Moorhead et al., 2004). The NOC project complements the work of NANDA International and the NIC project. The NOC classification offers nurse-sensitive outcomes for NANDA nursing diagnoses (Table 12-8). For each outcome, there are specific recommended evaluation indicators.

If a critical pathway or CareMap is used to direct client care, the nurse and team members clearly know what client outcomes are to be met for a given day. If there is variance (unexpected outcomes or outcomes occurring at a different time than expected), the nurse reports these responses and revises the plan of care as needed. By having outcomes clearly documented on either a CareMap or other documentation form, the nurse and other health care providers clearly know what to evaluate. All members of the health care team should monitor a client's progress. Each nurse summarizes data on an ongoing basis to ensure that the client is progressing to an optimal level of health.

Collecting Evaluative Data. When nurses provide care to clients, two aspects of care must be evaluated. First, what is the client's response to nursing care? Was the therapy effective in improving the client's physical or emotional heath? Did the client benefit? It is important to evaluate whether each client reaches a level of wellness or recovery that the health care team and client established in the goals of care. Second, have the client's expectations of care been met? The nurse asks clients about their perceptions of care, such as, "Did you receive the type of pain relief you expected?" "Did you receive enough information to care for your baby at home?" This level of evaluation is important to determine the client's satisfaction with care and to strengthen the partnering between nurse and client. The nurse selects appropriate evaluative measures to evaluate client response and expectations.

Evaluating a client's response to nursing care requires the use of evaluative measures, which are the assessment skills and techniques used to collect data for evaluation (e.g., auscultation of lung sounds, observation of a client's skill performance, discussion of the client's feelings, and inspection of the skin). In fact, evaluative measures are the same as assessment measures but are performed at the point of care when decisions are made about the client's status and progress. The intent of assessment is to identify what problems exist, if any. The intent of evaluation is to determine if the known problems have remained the same, improved, worsened, or otherwise changed. In Mr. Brown's situation, the nurse uses evaluative measures that include auscultation of lung sounds, measurement of the inhaled volume on the incentive spirometer, and measurement of the client's oral temperature (see Table 12-7).

In many clinical situations, it is important to collect evaluative measures over a period of time to determine if a pattern of improvement or change exists. A one-time observation of a pressure ulcer is insufficient to determine that the ulcer is healing. It is important to note a

Table 12-8 Linkages Between Nursing Outcomes Classification and Nursing Diagnoses

Nursing Diagnosis	Suggested Outcomes	Indicators (examples)
Pain	Comfort level	Reported physical well-being Reported satisfaction with symptom control Expressed satisfaction with pain control
	Pain control	Recognizes pain onset Uses analgesics appropriately Reports pain controlled
	Pain: disruptive effects	Difficulty eating Impaired mood
	Pain level	Reported pain level Frequency of pain Muscle tension
Ineffective airway clearance	Aspiration control	Avoids risk factors Positions self upright for eating
	Respiratory status: airway patency	Moves sputum out of airway Free of adventitious lung sounds
	Respiratory status: gas exchange	Ease of breathing PaO_2 and $PaCO_2$ within normal limits (WNL)
	Respiratory status: ventilation	Respiratory rate in expected range Chest expansion symmetrical Shortness of breath not present

Adapted from *Nursing Outcomes Classification (NOC)* (3rd ed.), edited by S. Moorhead, M. Johnson, and M. Maas, 2004, St. Louis, MO: Mosby.

consistency in change. For example, over a period of 2 days, is the pressure ulcer gradually decreasing in size, is the amount of drainage declining, is the redness of inflammation resolving? Recognizing a pattern of improvement or deterioration allows the nurse to reason and decide whether the client's problems are resolved.

The primary source of data for evaluation is the client. However, the nurse also uses the family and other caregivers as data sources. For example, the nurse might ask a family member to report on the amount of food the client eats during a meal. A nurse might consult with a colleague about how the client responded to pain medication on a previous shift.

Interpreting and Summarizing Findings. Expert nurses engage in an ongoing dialogue with a situation (Benner, Hooper-Kyriakidis, & Stannard, 1999). They are able to read a clinical situation and then provide an appropriate response. An expert nurse recognizes relevant evidence, even evidence that sometimes does not match clinical expectations, and makes judgments about a client's condition. To develop clinical judgment, a novice nurse learns to match a clinical situation with expected outcomes and clinical goals to determine if a client's status is improving or not. When interpreting findings, the nurse compares expected responses and physiological signs and symptoms with those actually seen from the evaluative database. Comparing expected and actual findings allows the nurse to interpret and judge the client's condition and whether predicted changes have occurred (Table 12-9). To objectively evaluate whether a goal has been achieved, the nurse should use the following steps:

1. Examine the goal statement to identify the desired client behaviour or response.
2. Assess the client for the presence of that behaviour or response.
3. Compare the established outcome criteria with the behaviour or response.
4. Judge the degree of agreement between outcome criteria and the behaviour or response.
5. If there is no agreement (or only partial agreement) between the outcome criteria and the behaviour or response, consider what is/are the barriers. Why did they not agree?

Evaluation of each expected outcome and its place in the sequence of care is essential. Failure to evaluate each expected outcome results in an inability to determine the place in which the sequence faltered. In other words, the nurse is not able to revise and redirect the care plan at the most appropriate time. If the client achieves the expected outcomes, the nurse either continues the care plan or discontinues interventions because the goal of care is met. If evaluation determines that the expected outcomes were not met or only partially met, the nurse begins reassessment and revision of the care plan.

There are different degrees of goal achievement. If the client's response matches or exceeds the outcome criteria, the goal is met. If the client's behaviour begins to show changes but does not yet meet criteria set, the goal is partially met. If there is no progress, the goal is not met (Table 12-10). A clearly defined goal with specific outcomes is easily measured (see Guidelines for Writing Goals and Expected Outcomes).

Documenting Findings. Documentation and reporting are an important part of the evaluation process. A client's medical record must be accurate in order for nurses to make ongoing evaluations. When documenting the client's response to interventions, the nurse always includes the same evaluative measures gathered during assessment. The nurse presents a clear argument from the data about whether a client is progressing or not. All objective data should be documented using precise measurements and thorough detail (see chapter 13). The nurse's documentation must record subjective data appropriately, for example, "Client reports that nausea has

Table 12-9 Evaluation Measures to Determine the Success of Goals and Expected Outcomes

Goals	Evaluative Measures	Expected Outcomes
Client's pressure ulcer will heal within 7 days.	Inspect colour, condition, and location of pressure ulcer. Measure diameter of ulcer daily. Note odour and colour of drainage from ulcer.	Erythema will be reduced in 2 days. Diameter of ulcer will decrease in 5 days. Ulcer will have no drainage in 2 days. Skin overlying ulcer will be closed in 7 days.
Client will tolerate ambulation to end of hall by 11/20.	Palpate client's radial pulse before exercise. Palpate client's radial pulse 10 minutes after exercise. Assess respiratory rate during exercise. Observe client for dyspnea or breathlessness during exercise.	Pulse will remain below 110 beats per minute during exercise. Pulse rate will return to resting baseline within 10 minutes after exercise. Respiratory rate will remain within two breaths of client's baseline rate. Client will deny feeling of breathlessness.
Client will have improved grief resolution by 1/15.	Ask client about frequency of periods of crying, sadness. Review client's sleeping log. Review client's dietary intake.	Client reports decreased frequency of crying, sadness in 2 months. Client has periods of 6-7 hours of sleep without interruption within 10 days. Client has no weight loss in 1 month.

Table 12-10 Examples of Objective Evaluation of Goal Achievement

Goals	Outcome Criteria	Client Response	Evaluation Findings
Client will self-administer insulin by 12/18.	Client prepares insulin dosage in syringe by 12/17. Client demonstrates self-injection by 12/18.	Client prepared accurate dosage in syringe on 12/17. Client administered morning insulin dosage; self-injection was correctly performed on 12/18.	Client has progressed and achieved desired behaviour.
Client's lungs will be free of secretions by 11/30.	Coughing will be nonproductive by 11/29. Lungs will be clear to auscultation by 11/30. Respirations will be 20 per minute by 11/30.	Client coughed frequently and productively on 11/29. Lungs were clear to auscultation on 11/30. Respirations were 18 per minute on 11/29.	Client will require continued therapy. Condition is improving.
Client will be able to perform self-care measures without discomfort in 2 days.	Client will rate pain as 3 on a scale of 0-10 within 2 days. Client will initiate bathing within 2 days.	Client rates severe right-sided abdominal pain as 5 on a scale of 0-10 while attempting bathing on day 2.	Client's condition still indicates a problem. Continued therapy with possibly new care measures is required.

subsided." Written nursing progress notes, assessment flow sheets, and information shared among nurses during change-of-shift reports should communicate a client's progress toward meeting expected outcomes and goals for the nursing plan of care.

Care Plan Revision and Critical Thinking

As goals are evaluated, the nurse makes adjustments to the care plan as indicated. If a goal was successfully met, that portion of the care plan is discontinued. Unmet and partially met goals require the nurse to continue intervention. After a nurse reassesses a client, nursing diagnoses may be modified or added with appropriate goals and expected outcomes, and interventions are established. The nurse also redefines priorities. This is an important step in critical thinking—knowing how the client is progressing and how problems either resolve or worsen.

In the case of Mr. Brown, his pain continues to be a problem. The nurse on days recognized that Mr. Brown was not using his PCA device routinely. Mr. Brown consistently was reporting pain at a level of 6 on a scale of 0 to 10. The nurse revises the plan of care to place more emphasis on pain control (Box 12-15). The nurse reviews the care plan developed immediately following surgery for the nursing diagnosis of *acute pain*. In addition, the nursing diagnosis of *ineffective airway clearance* has already been revised to include poor pain control as the related factor. The nurse revises the *acute pain* care plan's expected outcomes and interventions for managing Mr. Brown's abdominal pain. The nurse's logic in revising the plan is to focus attention on pain management and to administer pain relief therapies so that Mr. Brown can then breathe deeper, cough with minimal discomfort, and eventually achieve airway clearance.

The nurse's careful monitoring and early detection of problems are a client's first line of defence. Nurses must learn to anticipate the client's future course (Benner, Stannard, & Hooper, 1996). Clinical judgments are based on the nurse's observations of what is occurring with a specific client and not merely what may happen to clients in general. Frequently, changes are very subtle. Evaluation must be client specific, based on a close familiarity with each client's behaviour, physical status, and reaction to caregivers. Critical thinking skills promote accurate evaluation, which leads to the appropriate revision of ineffective care plans and discontinuation of unsuccessful therapy.

Discontinuing a Care Plan. After determining that expected outcomes and goals have been achieved, the nurse confirms this evaluation with the client when possible. If the nurse and client agree that the expected outcomes have been met, the nurse discontinues that care plan. For example, a client has the nursing diagnosis of *deficient knowledge regarding self-administration of insulin related to inexperience.* To achieve the goal of accurate client administration of insulin, the nurse establishes outcomes including, "Client will describe the purpose of insulin by 9/20," "Client will correctly prepare insulin in syringe by 9/20," and "Client will administer insulin injection independently by 9/22." The nurse asks the client to describe the purpose of insulin and observes as the client prepares the dosage and administers the injection. When outcomes are met successfully, it is not necessary to teach additional information about insulin administration. The care plan can be documented as discontinued. Continuity of care assumes that care provided is relevant to client needs. Significant time is wasted when achieved goals are not communicated.

Modifying a Care Plan. When goals are not met, the nurse identifies the variables or factors that interfere with goal achievement. Usually a change in the client's condition, needs, or abilities makes alteration of the care plan necessary. For example, when teaching self-administration of insulin, the nurse discovers that the client has developed a new problem, a tremor associated with a side effect

Box 12-15 Modification of Nursing Care Plan for Mr. Brown

Mr. Brown is continuing to have difficulty with abdominal incision pain. As a result, Mr. Brown has resisted pulmonary hygiene implemented by the nursing staff. The nurse on the evening shift returns to Mr. Brown's room to reassess the client's condition.

Assessment Activities	Findings/Defining Characteristics
Auscultate client's lung sounds.	Crackles present in both lower lobes
Observe client use incentive spirometer and observe volume of air inspired.	Achieves only 60% to 70% of incentive spirometry goal
Observe client's ability to turn, cough, and deep breathe.	Reluctant to turn, cough, and deep breathe; states that pain is "too much"
Observe client's technique with splinting incision during coughing.	Does not splint abdominal incision
Measure oral temperature.	Oral temperature of 39.8° C
Monitor use of patient-controlled analgesia (PCA) device and ask client to rate pain on a scale of 0 to 10.	Infrequent, irregular use of PCA Rates incisional pain as 6 on a scale of 0 to 10

Nursing Diagnosis: Acute Pain Related to Surgical Trauma of Incision

Planning

Goal	Expected Outcomes*
Client's pain will be reduced in 24 hours.	***Pain Control*** Client will use PCA more frequently, receiving 6 mg morphine every hour for next 24 hours. Client's level of pain decreases to level below baseline within 36 hours. Client will splint incision before each cough and deep breathing exercise.

Interventions†	Rationale
Pain Management	
Instruct client in proper use of PCA and rationale for regular use of medication.	PCA is a drug delivery system that allows clients to self-administer opioids with minimal risk of overdose. On-demand doses typically add 1 mg morphine every 6 minutes, with a total hourly limit of 6 mg.
Have client administer a single PCA dose 10 minutes before performing incentive spirometry.	Provides level of pain relief before incentive spirometer exercise that will cause expansion of thoracic and abdominal muscles.
Demonstrate correct splinting procedure. Allow for return demonstration by client.	Splinting provides support to underlying tissues disrupted by surgical incision, preventing stimulation of pain fibres.
Assist client in performing splinting during coughing and deep breathing and during turning and repositioning.	
When pain is under control, instruct client in relaxation exercises.	Relaxation techniques provide individuals with self-control when discomfort or pain occurs, reversing the physical and emotional stress of pain.

Evaluation

Nursing Actions	Client Response/Finding	Achievement of Outcome
Ask client to rate severity of pain on scale of 0 to 10 after coughing or activities such as routine hygiene.	Client rates pain at level of 5 after coughing. Is able to perform hygiene activities with pain at level of 3 to 4.	Pain control is improving. Continue reinforcement of splinting and use of PCA.
Observe regularity of client splinting incision during turning, coughing and deep breathing.	Client uses splinting technique about 75% of the time. May forget to splint when coughing develops without warning. Turns without splinting.	Reinforce use of splinting during turning.
Check dosage delivered on PCA pump for 24-hour period.	Client receiving average of 4 to 6 mg morphine per hour.	Client using PCA more regularly, receiving safe dosage of medication.

†Intervention classification label from *Nursing Interventions Classification (NIC),* (4th ed.), edited by J. M. Dochterman and G. M. Bulechek, 2004, St. Louis, MO: Mosby.
*Outcome label from *Nursing Outcomes Classification (NOC)* (3rd ed.), edited by S. Moorhead, M. Johnson, and M. Maas, 2004, St. Louis, MO: Mosby.

of a medication. The client is unable to draw medication from a syringe or inject the needle safely. As a result, the original outcome of, "Client will administer insulin injection independently" cannot be met. The nurse introduces new interventions (instructing wife in insulin administration) and revises outcomes to meet the goal of care.

Lack of goal achievement may also result from an error in nursing judgment or failure to follow each step of the nursing process. Clients frequently have multiple and complex problems. The nurse should always remember the possibility of overlooking or misjudging something. When there is failure to achieve a goal, no matter what the reason, the entire nursing process sequence for that nursing diagnosis is repeated to discover changes that need to be made to promote, maintain, or restore the client's health.

Reassessment. A complete reassessment of all client factors relating to the nursing diagnosis and etiology is necessary when modifying a plan. Reassessment requires critical thinking when the nurse compares new data about the client's condition with previously assessed information. Often a nurse applies knowledge from experiences with other clients to direct the reassessment process. Encounters over time with clients and families who have similar health problems give nurses a strong background of knowledge to use for anticipating client needs and planning care. For example, consider Mr. Brown, who has the nursing diagnosis of *acute pain related to surgical trauma of incision.* Two days following surgery, Mr. Brown continues to have a poor appetite despite no obvious surgical complications. If the client continues to have pain, the nurse may automatically associate loss of appetite with discomfort. However, the nurse may recall a previous client who became depressed following surgery. After exploring the problem further, the nurse learns that Mr. Brown's family has not been visiting, the client is fearful of his cancer diagnosis, he has loss of appetite, and he is not sleeping well. Although the client continues to have pain, a new priority diagnosis may be *anticipatory grieving related to losses associated with illness.* Focusing on this diagnosis may improve the client's appetite more than the original plan. As in the original assessment, data are collected from all sources. Depending on the nurse's findings, assessing variables that were not covered on the initial assessment may be necessary.

Reassessment ensures that the database is accurate and current. It may also reveal the missing link (i.e., a critical piece of new information that was overlooked and thus interfered with goal achievement). All new data are sorted, validated, and clustered to analyze and interpret differences from the original database. The nurse documents reassessment data to alert other nursing staff to the client's status.

Nursing Diagnoses. After reassessment, the nurse determines accurate nursing diagnoses for the situation. The nurse asks whether the correct diagnosis was selected and whether it and the etiological factor are current. The problem list should then be revised to reflect the client's changed status. A new diagnosis may be made. If a previous diagnosis no longer accurately reflects the problem, it should be discontinued. For example, after finding that the client with diabetes is unable to self-administer insulin, the nurse finds a family member who is available as a resource. To develop a plan designed to educate an alternate caregiver about the administration of insulin, the nurse then establishes a new diagnosis: *ineffective health maintenance related to impaired dexterity.*

A nurse's care is based on an accurate list of nursing diagnoses. Accuracy is more important than the number of diagnoses selected. As the client's condition changes, the diagnoses do as well.

Goals and Expected Outcomes. When care plans are revised, the nurse reviews goals and expected outcomes for needed changes. Even the goals for unchanged nursing diagnoses should be examined for appropriateness because a change in one problem may affect others. Determining that each goal and expected outcome is realistic for the problem, etiology, and time frame is particularly important. Unrealistic expected outcomes and time frames make goal achievement difficult.

The nurse clearly documents goals and expected outcomes for new or revised nursing diagnoses so that all team members are aware of the revised care plan. When the goal is still appropriate but has not yet been met, the nurse may change the evaluation date to allow more time. All goals and expected outcomes should be client centred, with realistic expectations for client achievement.

Interventions. Evaluating interventions requires examining two factors: the appropriateness of the interventions selected and the correct application of the intervention. The appropriateness of an intervention may be based on the standard of care for a client's health problem. A **standard of care** is the minimum level of care accepted to ensure high quality of care to clients. Standards of care define the types of therapies typically administered to clients with defined problems or needs. If the client who is post-operative for abdominal surgery has a specific nursing diagnosis, such as *ineffective airway clearance,* the standard of care established by a nursing department for this problem may include pain-control measures with coughing or deep breathing exercises to help the client breathe more easily with a clear airway. The nurse reviews the standard of care to determine whether the right interventions have been chosen or whether additional interventions are required.

Increasing or decreasing the frequency of interventions is one approach to ensure appropriate application of the intervention. The nurse adjusts interventions according to the client's response to therapy and previous experience with similar clients. For example, if a client continues to have congested lung sounds, the nurse increases the frequency of coughing and deep breathing exercises to remove secretions.

During evaluation, the nurse may find that some planned interventions are designed for an inappropriate level of nursing care. If the level of care needs to be changed, a different action verb, such as *assist* in place of *provide,* may be substituted. Sometimes the level of care is appropriate but the interventions are unsuitable because of a change in the expected outcome. In this case, the interventions should be discontinued and new interventions planned.

Changes in implementation should be guided by the nature of the client's unfavourable response. Consulting with other nurses may yield suggestions for improving the approach to care delivery. Senior nurses are often excellent resources because of their experience. Simply changing the care plan is not enough. The nurse must implement the new plan and re-evaluate the client's response to the nursing actions.

Occasionally during evaluation, the nurse may discover unmet client needs. This possibility should be anticipated. The nursing process is designed to be a systematic, problem-solving approach to individualized client care, but there is an array of variables for each client with a health care problem. Clients with the same health care problem are not treated the same way. As a result, the nurse sometimes makes errors in judgment. The systematic use of evaluation provides a way for nurses to catch these errors in judgment. The nurse consistently incorporates evaluation into practice to minimize errors and ensure that the client's plan of care is appropriate and relevant.

Key Concepts

- All steps of the nursing process involve critical thinking skills to identify, diagnose, and treat human responses to health and illness.
- Nursing assessment involves the collection, verification, and analysis of data to establish a database about a client's needs, health problems, and responses to those problems.
- Subjective data are the client's perceptions; objective data are observations or measurements made by the data collector.
- The client, family members, and members of the health care team are important sources of information about the client's health status.
- During an interview, the nurse and the client both obtain information.
- To form a nursing judgment, the nurse critically assesses a client, validates the data, interprets the information gathered, looks for diagnostic cues, and identifies the client's problems.
- Nursing diagnoses state the actual or potential problems of the client's health status.
- Nursing diagnoses are necessary to develop a plan of care that will help the client and family adapt to changes resulting from an illness or change in lifestyle.
- Planning nursing care involves determining and prioritizing client goals, identifying expected outcomes, and a developing a written nursing care plan.
- A nurse writes goals and expected outcomes to direct selection and use of nursing interventions and to provide focus for evaluation of client care.
- A client-centred goal is specific, measurable, time limited, and mutually set with a client when possible.
- An expected outcome is an objective criterion for goal achievement.
- The Nursing Interventions Classification (NIC) taxonomy provides a standardization to assist nurses in selecting suitable interventions for clients' problems.
- Implementation is the step of the nursing process in which nurses provide direct and indirect nursing care interventions to clients.
- During the initial phase of implementation, the nurse reassesses the client to determine whether the proposed nursing action is still appropriate for the client's level of wellness.
- Counselling is a direct care method that helps the client use a problem-solving process to recognize and manage stress and to facilitate interpersonal relationships among the client, family, and health care team.
- Preventive nursing actions include assessment and promotion of the client's health potential, application of prescribed measures (e.g., immunizations), health teaching, and identification of risk factors for illness and/or trauma.
- Evaluation is a step of the nursing process that allows a nurse to determine whether nursing interventions are successful in improving a client's condition or well-being.
- A nurse interprets evaluative findings to judge the client's condition and to know whether predicted changes have occurred.
- Documentation of evaluative findings allows all members of the health team to know a client's progress.

Key Terms

Activities of daily living (ADLs), *p. 187*
Actual nursing diagnosis, *p. 196*
Adverse reaction, *p. 219*
Assessment, *p. 184*
Client-centred goal, *p. 200*
Collaboration, *p. 204*
Collaborative interventions, *p. 203*
Concept map, *p. 210*
Consultation, *p. 213*
Counselling, *p. 219*
Critical pathways (CareMaps), *p. 210*
Cue, *p. 185*
Database, *p. 184*
Defining characteristics, *p. 196*
Diagnostic process, *p. 195*
Direct care, *p. 213*
Evaluation, *p. 221*
Expected outcome, *p. 201*
Goals, *p. 201*
Implementation, *p. 213*
Indirect care, *p. 213*
Instrumental activities of daily living (IADLs), *p. 219*
Interdisciplinary care plans, *p. 221*
Interview, *p. 188*
Kardex, *p. 207*
Lifesaving measure, *p. 219*
Long-term goal, *p. 201*
Medical diagnosis, *p. 192*
NANDA International, *p. 192*
Norms, *p. 191*
Nurse-initiated interventions, *p. 203*
Nursing care plan, *p. 205*
Nursing diagnosis, *p. 192*
Nursing health history, *p. 189*
Nursing intervention, *p. 213*
Nursing process, *p. 183*
Objective data, *p. 187*
Physical examination, *p. 191*
Physician-initiated interventions, *p. 203*
Planning, *p. 198*
Protocol, *p. 213*
Preventive nursing actions, *p. 218*
Related factors, *p. 196*
Risk nursing diagnosis, *p. 196*
Scientific rationale, *p. 203*
Short-term goal, *p. 201*
Standard, *p. 187*
Standard of care, *p. 228*
Standing order, *p. 213*
Subjective data, *p. 187*
Wellness nursing diagnosis, *p. 196*

Critical Thinking Exercises

1. Mrs. Lewis comes to the well-baby clinic for her infant's 1-month examination. She tells her nurse, Ethan, that the baby has not been sleeping well during the night. In addition, Mrs. Lewis has noted a rash on the baby's abdomen. Write three questions that Ethan might ask to assess the two potential problems Mrs. Lewis has presented. What assessment technique might the nurse apply to assess the rash that would not be used to assess the baby's sleep pattern?
2. Mrs. Spezio has a pressure ulcer over the coccyx that is 5 cm in diameter and approximately 1 cm deep. The tissue surrounding the ulcer is inflamed and tender to touch. Mrs. Spezio is transferring from a long-term care facility where she had resided for 6 months following a massive stroke. She is unable to move independently in bed and does not sense pressure or discomfort over her coccyx or hips. Given this clinical situation, identify the defining characteristics and related factors for the nursing diagnosis *impaired skin integrity.*
3. Write a goal and expected outcome for each of the following clinical scenarios:
   a. Mr. Jacko has recently been diagnosed with asthma and is to be discharged tomorrow. His physician has ordered a metred dose inhaler for Mr. Jacko to use daily. The client has not used an inhaler before. He asks the nurse, "What do I do at home if I have trouble using this thing?" The nursing diagnosis for Mr. Jacko is *deficient knowledge regarding use of a metred dose inhaler related to inexperience.*
   b. Ms. Kapoor has been suffering from a high fever for several days. She is diaphoretic and very fatigued. She has difficulty turning herself in bed because she has little energy and she is overweight. The skin over her bony prominences is intact at this time, with some redness appearing over the coccyx area. Reddened area blanches with fingertip pressure. The nursing diagnosis for Ms. Kapoor is *risk for impaired skin integrity related to moisture and impaired mobility.*
4. Sunjita is assigned to care for Ms. Reznick, who has been diagnosed with Crohn's disease, an inflammatory bowel condition. Ms. Reznick has had considerable abdominal pain, accompanied by cramping and frequent diarrhea. Her nursing history shows that she has lost 7 kg over the last 2 months. Her appetite has been poor. One of the many nursing diagnoses for Ms. Reznick is *imbalanced nutrition: less than body requirements related to decreased nutrient intake and increased nutrient loss through diarrhea.* What factors should Sunjita consider in selecting interventions for Ms. Reznick?
5. Mr. Vicar has been visiting the clinic for more than a month. He visits weekly for follow-up care for a chronic venous stasis ulcer of the left leg. The nurse's note at the time of his first visit contained the following information: "Ulcer with irregular margins, 4 cm wide by 5 cm long, approximately 0.5 cm deep, draining foul-smelling purulent yellowish drainage. Subcutaneous tissue visible. Skin around ulcer, brownish rust in colour. Zinc oxide and calamine gauze applied to ulcer; elastic wrap bandage applied to gauze. Client instructed to return in 1 week." As the nurse who is caring for the client on the follow-up visit, what expected outcomes would you anticipate for the goal of, "Wound will demonstrate healing within 4 weeks"? What evaluative measures would you use to determine if the wound is healing?

Review Questions

1. The purpose of assessment is to
   1. Establish a database concerning the client
   2. Teach the client about his or her health
   3. Implement nursing care
   4. Delegate nursing responsibility
2. During data clustering, the nurse
   1. Implements the nursing process
   2. Provides documentation of nursing care
   3. Organizes data and focuses attention on client functions
   4. Reviews the data with other health care providers
3. A nursing diagnosis is
   1. A clinical judgment about individual, family, or community responses to actual and potential health problems or life processes
   2. The identification of a disease condition based on a specific evaluation of physical signs, symptoms, the client's medical history, and the results of diagnostic tests and procedures
   3. The diagnosis and treatment of human responses to health and illness
   4. The advancement of the development, testing, and refinement of a common nursing language
4. The nursing diagnosis, *Family coping: potential for growth related to unexpected birth of twins,* is an example of a
   1. Wellness nursing diagnosis
   2. Risk nursing diagnosis
   3. Potential nursing diagnosis
   4. Diagnostic nursing diagnosis
5. Once a nurse assesses a client's condition and identifies appropriate nursing diagnoses a
   1. Plan is developed for nursing care
   2. Physical assessment begins
   3. List of priorities is determined
   4. Review of the assessment is conducted with other team members
6. Priorities are established to help the nurse anticipate and sequence nursing interventions when a client has multiple problems or alterations. Priorities are determined by the client's
   1. Physician
   2. Non-emergent, non–life-threatening needs
   3. Future well-being
   4. Urgency of problems

7. Which of the following is an example of indirect care?
   1. Actions are aimed at managing environment and documentation
   2. Medication administration is performed
   3. Psychological counselling is provided
   4. Intravenous infusion is begun
8. An out-of-date care plan
   1. Means the client was discharged
   2. Compromises the quality of care
   3. Ensures that the nursing care was delivered
   4. Identifies that the client response was successful
9. The evaluation process, which determines the effectiveness of nursing care, includes
   1. Implementing, evaluating, documenting, revising, and continuing
   2. Planning, diagnosing, interpreting, evaluating, and revising
   3. Identifying, collecting, interpreting, documenting, and terminating, continuing, or revising the care plan
   4. Assessing, diagnosing, planning, implementing, and evaluating
10. Unmet and partially met goals require the nurse to
   1. Compare the client's response with that of another client
   2. Relinquish care of the client to another nurse
   3. Continue intervention
   4. Begin new interventions

References

Bandman, E. L., & Bandman, B. (1995). *Critical thinking in nursing* (2nd ed.). Norwalk, CT: Appleton & Lange.

Baugh, N. G., & Mellott, K. G. (1998). Clinical concept mapping as preparation for student nurses' clinical experiences. *Journal of Nursing Education, 37*(6), 253–256.

Benner, P. (1984). *From novice to expert: Excellence and power in clinical nursing practice.* Menlo Park, CA: Addison-Wesley.

Benner, P., Hooper-Kyriakidis, P., & Stannard, D. (1999). *Clinical wisdom and interventions in critical care.* Philadelphia: W. B. Saunders.

Benner, P., Stannard, D., & Hooper, P. L. (1996). A "thinking-in-action" approach to teaching clinical judgment: A classroom innovation for acute care advanced practice nurses. *Advanced Practice Nursing Quarterly, 1*(4), 70–77.

Bryans, A., & McIntosh, J. (1996). Decision making in community nursing: An analysis of the stages of decision making as they relate to community nursing. *Journal of Advanced Nursing, 24*(1), 24–30.

Canadian Nurses Association. (1986). *Definition of nursing practice and standards for nursing practice.* Ottawa, ON: Author.

Carnevali, D. L., & Thomas, M. D. (1993). *Diagnostic reasoning and treatment decision making in nursing.* Philadelphia: J. B. Lippincott.

Carpenito, L. J. (1995). *Nursing diagnoses: Application to clinical practice* (6th ed.). Philadelphia: J. B. Lippincott.

Carpenito, L. J. (1997). *Nursing diagnoses: Application to clinical practice* (7th ed.). Philadelphia: J. B. Lippincott.

Carpenito, L. J. (2000). *Nursing diagnoses: Application to clinical practice* (8th ed.). Philadelphia: J. B. Lippincott.

Carter, J., et al. (1995). Using the Nursing Interventions Classification to implement Agency for Health Care Policy and Research guidelines. *Journal of Nursing Care Quality, 9*(2), 76–86.

Collier, I. C., McCash, K. E., & Bartram, J. M. (1996). *Writing nursing diagnoses: A critical thinking approach.* St. Louis, MO: Mosby.

Da Cruz, D. A. L. M, & Acuri, E. A. M. (1998). The influence of nursing diagnosis on information processing on undergraduate students. *Nursing Diagnosis, 9*(3), 93–100.

Daley, B. J., et al. (1999). Concept maps: A strategy to teach and evaluate critical thinking. *Journal of Nursing Education, 38*(1), 42–47.

Deaton, C. (1998). Outcomes measurement. *Journal of Cardiovascular Nursing, 12*(4), 49–51.

Dochterman, J. M., & Jones, D. A. (Eds.). (2003). *Unifying nursing languages: The harmonization of NANDA, NIC, and NOC.* Washington, DC: American Nurses Association.

Dochterman, J. M., & Bulechek, G. M. (Eds.). (2004). *Nursing interventions classification (NIC)* (4th ed.). St. Louis, MO: Mosby.

Fry, V. S. (1953). The creative approach to nursing. *American Journal of Nursing, 53,* 301–302.

Gerteis, M., et al. (Eds.). (1993). *Through the patient's eyes.* San Francisco: Jossey-Bass Health Series.

Gordon, M. (1994). *Nursing diagnosis: Process and application* (3rd ed.). St. Louis, MO: Mosby.

Gordon, M., et al. (1994). Clinical judgment: An integrated model. *Advances in Nursing Science, 16,* 55–70.

Higuchi, K.A., Smith Dulberg, C., and Duff, V. (1999). Factors Associated with Nursing Diagnosis Utilization in Canada. *Nursing Diagnosis, 10*(4) 137–147.

Iowa Intervention Project. (1993). The NIC taxonomy structure. *Image—The Journal of Nursing Scholarship, 25,* 187–192.

Johnson, M., Maas, M., & Moorhead, S. (2000). *Nursing outcomes classification (NOC)* (2nd ed.). St. Louis, MO: Mosby.

Kim, M. J., McFarland, G. K., & McLean, A. M. (Eds.). (1984). *Classification of nursing diagnoses: Proceedings of the fifth conference (NANDA).* St. Louis, MO: Mosby.

Leininger, S. M., & Laux, L. H. (1998). The continuum of health care: Highlights of orthopaedic and general medical pathways. *Home Health Care Management and Practice, 10*(4), 1–10.

Lin, C. (1996). Patient satisfaction with nursing care as an outcome variable: Dilemmas for nursing evaluation researchers. *Journal of Professional Nursing, 1294,* 207–216.

Liukkonen, A. (1992). The nurse's decision-making process and the implementation of psychogeriatric nursing in a mental hospital. *Journal of Advanced Nursing, 17*(3), 356–361.

McCloskey, J. C., & Bulechek, G. M. (1994). Standardizing the language for nursing treatments: An overview of the issues. *Nursing Outlook, 42,* 56–63.

McCloskey, J. C., & Bulechek, G. M. (1998). Nursing interventions core to specialty practice. *Nursing Outlook, 46*(2), 67–76.

McCloskey, J. C., & Bulechek, G. M. (2000). *Nursing interventions classification (NIC)* (3rd ed.). St. Louis, MO: Mosby.

McCloskey, J. C., et al. (1996). Nurses' use and delegation of indirect care interventions. *Nursing Economic$, 14*(1), 22–33.

McFarland, G. K., & McFarlane, E. A. (1989). *Nursing diagnosis and intervention: Planning for patient care.* St. Louis, MO: Mosby.

Miller, M. A., & Babcock, D. E. (1996). *Critical thinking applied to nursing.* St. Louis, MO: Mosby.

Moorhead, S., Johnson, M., & Maas, M. (Eds.). (2004). *Nursing outcomes classification (NOC)* (3rd ed.). St. Louis, MO: Mosby.

NANDA International. (2003). *NANDA nursing diagnoses: Definitions and classifications, 2003–2004.* Philadelphia: Author.

Redman, B. K. (2001). *The practice of patient education* (9th ed.). St. Louis, MO: Mosby.

Schuster, P. M. (2000). Concept mapping: Reducing clinical care plan paperwork and increasing learning. *Nurse Educator, 25*(2), 76–81.

Schuster, P. M. (2002). *Concept mapping: A critical-thinking approach to care planning.* St. Louis, MO: Mosby.

Skillen, D. L., & Day, R. A. (Eds.). (2004). *A syllabus for adult health assessment.* Edmonton, AB: Faculty of Nursing, University of Alberta.

Snyder, M., Egan, E. C., & Nojima, Y. (1996). Defining nursing interventions. *Image—Journal of Nursing Scholarship, 28*(2), 137–141.

Stephen, T. (1997). Symptom analysis. In *Adult health assessment series* [CD-ROM]. Edmonton, AB: DataStar Education Systems and Services (Producer and Distributor).

Sundeen, S. J., et al. (1998). *Nurse-client interaction: Implementing the nursing process* (6th ed.). St. Louis, MO: Mosby.

Recommended Web Sites

Center for Nursing Classification and Clinical Effectiveness:
http://www.nursing.uiowa.edu/centers/cncce

The University of Iowa's Center for Nursing Classification and Clinical Effectiveness was established to facilitate ongoing research of the Nursing Interventions Classification (NIC) and Nursing Outcomes Classification (NOC). This site provides an overview of the NIC and NOC and offers information about publications.

NANDA International:
http://www.nanda.org

NANDA (North American Nursing Diagnosis Association) International maintains this Web site. It provides current information on nursing diagnosis research, publications, links, and Internet resources.

13

Documenting and Reporting

Martha Keene Elkin, RN, MS, IBCLC
Maureen Barry, BScN, MScN (Canadian author)

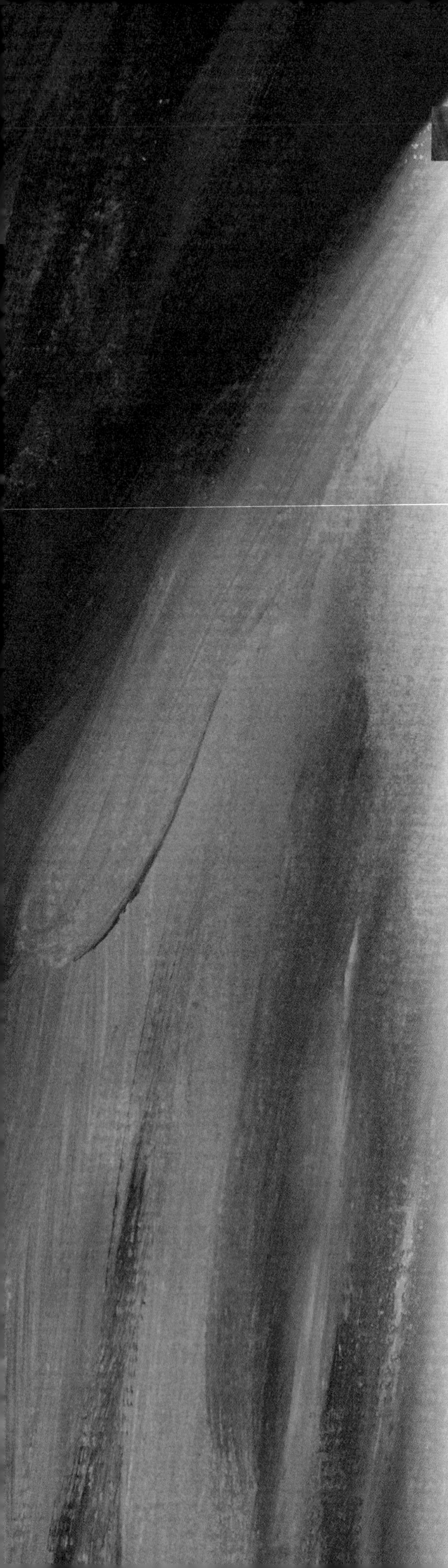

Objectives

Mastery of content in this chapter will enable the student to:

- Define the key terms listed.
- Describe multidisciplinary communication within the health care team.
- Identify purposes of a health care record.
- Discuss legal guidelines for documentation.
- Maintain confidentiality of records and reports.
- Describe five quality guidelines for documentation and reporting.
- Describe the different methods used in record keeping.
- Discuss the advantages of standardized documentation forms.
- Identify elements to include when documenting a client's discharge plan.
- Describe the role of critical pathways in multidisciplinary documentation.
- Identify the important aspects of home care and long-term care documentation.
- Discuss issues related to computerization in documentation.
- Describe the purpose and content of a change-of-shift report.
- Explain how to verify telephone orders.

Documentation is anything written or printed that is relied on as record or proof for authorized persons. Documentation within a client medical record is a vital aspect of nursing practice. Nursing documentation must be accurate, comprehensive, and flexible enough to retrieve critical data, maintain continuity of care, track client outcomes, and reflect current standards of nursing practice. Information in the client record provides a detailed account of the quality of care delivered to clients. Effective documentation ensures continuity of care, saves time, and minimizes the risk of errors (Yocum, 2002).

Effective documentation can positively affect the quality of life and health outcomes for clients. Accrediting agencies such as the Canadian Council on Health Services Accreditation (CCHSA) offer guidelines for documentation. However, documentation and reporting practices differ among institutions and jurisdictions and are influenced by ethical, legal, medical, and agency guidelines.

As members of the health care team, nurses need to communicate information about clients accurately and in a timely, effective manner. The quality of client care depends on caregivers' ability to communicate with one another. All health care providers require accurate information about clients in order to devise an organized, comprehensive care plan. If the care plan is not communicated to all members of the health care team, care can be fragmented, tasks repeated, and therapies delayed or omitted. Data recorded, reported, or communicated to other health care professionals are confidential and must be protected.

The health care environment creates many challenges for accurately documenting and reporting client care. The quality of care, the standards of regulatory agencies and nursing practice, and the legal guidelines for nursing practice make documentation and reporting a critical responsibility of a nurse. Whether the transfer of client information occurs through verbal reports, written documents, or electronic transfer, there are principles that the nurse must follow to maintain confidentiality of information.

Confidentiality

Nurses are legally and ethically obligated to keep information about clients confidential. Nurses may not discuss a client's examination, observation, conversation, or treatment with other clients or staff not involved in the client's care. Only staff directly involved in a specific client's care have legitimate access to the records. Clients frequently request copies of their health records, and they have the right to do so. Knowing that clients may read their own record should influence the choice of language used in documentation. Each institution has policies for controlling the manner in which records are shared. In most situations, clients are required to give written permission for release of medical information.

Nurses are responsible for protecting records from all unauthorized readers. When nurses and other health care professionals have a legitimate reason to use records for data gathering, research, or continuing education, appropriate authorization must be obtained according to agency policy. Student nurses and faculty may be required to present identification indicating they have authorized access to the record. The nurse should know the location of the record at all times. The record is stored by the health care agency after the treatment ends.

Multidisciplinary Communication Within the Health Care Team

Client care requires effective communication among members of the health care team. Communication takes place through the client's record or chart, reports, and consultations.

A client's **record** or chart is a confidential, permanent legal documentation of information relevant to a client's health care. Information about the client's health care is recorded after each client contact. The record is a continuing account of the client's health care status and is available to all members of the health care team. All records contain the following information:

- Client identification and demographic data
- Informed consent for treatment and procedures
- Advance directives
- Admission nursing history
- Nursing diagnoses or problems
- Nursing or multidisciplinary care plan
- Record of nursing care treatment and evaluation
- Medical history
- Medical diagnosis
- Therapeutic orders
- Medical and health discipline's progress notes
- Reports of physical examinations
- Reports of diagnostic studies
- Client education
- Summary of operative procedures
- Discharge plan and summary

Reports are oral, written, or audiotaped exchanges of information between caregivers (Figure 13–1). Common reports given by nurses include change-of-shift reports, telephone reports, transfer reports, and incident reports (see Reporting). A physician may call a nursing unit to receive a verbal report on a client's condition and progress. The laboratory submits a written report providing the results of diagnostic tests. Incident reports are documented on a record that is not part of the client's medical record (see chapter 8).

Information is also communicated through discussions or conferences among team members. For example, a discharge planning conference often involves members of all disciplines (e.g., nursing, social work, dietary, medicine, and physiotherapy), who meet to discuss the client's progress toward established discharge goals. **Consultations** are another form of discussion whereby one professional caregiver gives formal advice about the care of a client to another caregiver. For example, a nurse caring for a client with a chronic wound may need a consultation with a wound care specialist. **Referrals** (an arrangement for services by another care provider), consultations, and conferences must be documented in a client's permanent record so that all caregivers can plan care accordingly.

Purposes of Records

A record is a valuable source of data that is used by all members of the health care team. Its purposes include communication and care planning, legal documentation,

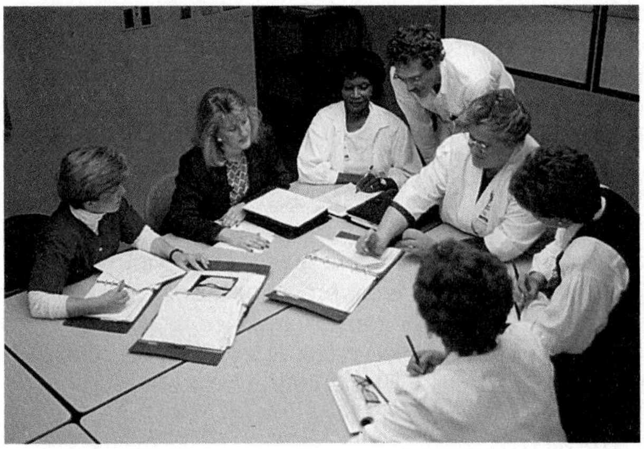

FIGURE **13–1** Staff communicate information about their clients during a change-of-shift report.

education, funding and resource management, research, and quality review.

Communication and Care Planning

The record is a means by which health care team members communicate client needs and progress, individual therapies, content of conferences, client education, and discharge planning. The care plan needs to be clear to anyone reading the chart. The record should be the most current and accurate source of information about a client's health care status.

The manner in which the nursing process is conducted with a client is communicated in the record. The admitting nursing history and physical assessment is comprehensive and provides a baseline of the client's health status on admission to the facility. These data usually contain biographical information (e.g., age and marital status), method of admission, reason for admission, a brief medical-surgical history (e.g., previous surgeries or illnesses), allergies, current medication (prescribed and over-the-counter), the client's perceptions about illness or hospitalization, and a review of health risk factors. A physical assessment of all body systems is either incorporated into the nursing history or included on a separate form (see chapter 28).

The medical progress notes should complement nursing process information. The notes detail the physician's findings at the time of assessment. Nurses first refer to the client's medical record for relevant assessment findings so that they can anticipate the client's status and then conduct an individualized assessment.

The record provides data that nurses use to identify and support nursing diagnoses, establish expected outcomes of care, and plan and evaluate interventions. Information from the record adds to the nurse's observations and assessment. The nurse does not need to collect information that is already available. If there is reason to believe that the information is inaccurate, information should be verified and appropriate changes made to the client's record.

Legal Documentation

Accurate documentation is one of the best defences against allegations of nursing negligence (see chapter 8). To limit nursing liability, nurses must clearly document the individualized, goal-directed nursing care that was provided to a client. The record must describe exactly what happened to a client. Charting should be done immediately after providing care. Even though nursing care may have been excellent, in a court of law "care not documented is care not provided." Nurses need to indicate all assessments, interventions, client responses, instructions, and referrals in the medical record.

Common negligent errors in documentation include (a) not charting the correct time when events occurred, (b) failing to record verbal orders or failing to have them signed, (c) charting actions in advance to save time, and (d) documenting incorrect data (Martin, 1994). Table 13-1 provides guidelines for legally sound documentation.

Education

A client's record contains a variety of information, including diagnoses, signs and symptoms of disease, successful and unsuccessful therapies, diagnostic findings, and client behaviours. By reading the client care record, the nurse can learn the nature of an illness and the client's response to the illness. No two clients have identical records, but patterns of information can be identified in records of clients with similar health problems. By studying records, students identify patterns for various health problems and begin to anticipate the type of care required for a client.

Funding and Resource Management

The client care record shows how health care agencies have used their financial resources. Various tools help monitor the timing and reasons for health team-client interactions. These data are then compared with documented entries on the chart to demonstrate the need for and efficacy of health care resources. Health care interactions and tasks are assigned specified points in relation to time spent with each client in some form of workload assignment system.

Research

Statistical data relating to the frequency of clinical disorders, complications, use of specific medical and nursing therapies, recovery from illness, and deaths can be gathered from client records. For example, as part of a quality improvement program for clients receiving intravenous (IV) therapy, a nurse manager reviews clients' records to investigate the incidence of infection in clients with a specific type of IV catheter. The client record review indicates that the infection rate is increased, and the nurse manager and staff nurses design a new specific method for IV catheter care. Once this new intervention is implemented, the manager again reviews clients' records to determine if the infection rate decreases.

A nurse may use clients' records during a clinical research study to investigate a new nursing intervention. For example, a nurse wants to compare a new method of pain control with a standard pain protocol using two groups of clients. The client records provide data on the two types of interventions: the new method and the standard pain control. The nurse researcher collects data from the clients' records that describe the type and dose of analgesic medications used, objective assessment data, and clients' subjective reports of pain relief. The researcher then compares the findings to determine if the new method was more effective that the standard pain control protocol.

Some data collection activities may be part of the quality improvement practices at an agency, whereas other activities may be actual clinical research studies. Different types of permission must be secured before reviewing client records for any type of research study or data analysis. The researcher must be sure the data collection and analysis adhere to provincial and agency policies.

Quality Review

A regular review of information in client records gives a basis for evaluation of the quality and appropriateness of care. This audit may be either a review of care received by discharged clients or an evaluation of care currently being given. Nurses or cross-discipline members of a committee monitor records throughout the year to determine if quality improvement standards are met, comparing each to a predetermined set of criteria (see chapter 10). Deficiencies are shared with the nursing staff so that corrections in policy or practice can be made.

Table 13-1 Legal Guidelines for Recording

Guidelines	Rationale	Correct Action
Do not erase, apply correction fluid, or scratch out errors made while recording.	Charting becomes illegible: It may appear as if you were attempting to hide information or deface record.	Draw single line through error, write word *error* above it and sign your name or initials and date. Then record note correctly.
Do not write retaliatory or critical comments about client or care by other health care professionals.	Statements can be used as evidence for non-professional behaviour or poor quality of care.	Enter only objective descriptions of client's behaviour; client comments should be quoted.
Correct all errors promptly.	Errors in recording can lead to errors in treatment.	Avoid rushing to complete charting; be sure information is accurate.
Record all facts.	Record must be accurate and reliable.	Be certain entry is factual; do not speculate or guess.
Do not leave blank spaces in nurse's notes.	Another person can add incorrect information in space.	Chart consecutively, line by line; if space is left, draw line horizontally through it and sign your name at end.
Record all entries legibly and in black ink.	Illegible entries can be misinterpreted, causing errors and lawsuits; ink cannot be erased; black ink is more legible when records are photocopied or transferred to microfilm.	Never erase entries or use correction fluid, and never use pencil.
If an order is questioned, record that clarification was sought.	If you perform an order known to be incorrect, you are just as liable for prosecution as the physician is.	Do not record, "physician made error." Instead, chart that "Dr. Wong was called to clarify order for analgesic."
Chart only for yourself.	You are accountable for information you enter into chart.	Never chart for someone else (exception: if caregiver has left unit for day and calls with information that needs to be documented, include the name of the source of information in the entry and include that the information was provided via telephone).
Avoid using generalized, empty phrases such as "status unchanged" or "had good day."	Specific information about client's condition is missing—information is too generalized and has no meaning.	Use complete, concise descriptions of care.
Begin each entry with time, and end with your signature and title.	This guideline ensures that correct sequence of events is recorded; signature indicates who is accountable for care delivered.	Do not wait until end of shift to record important changes that occurred several hours earlier; be sure to sign each entry.
Do not "pre-chart" (documenting an entry prior to performing a treatment or an assessment or prior to giving a medication)	Pre-charting invites error and thus endangers the health and safety of the client; it is also illegal and can constitute falsification of medical records.	Document during or immediately after giving care or administering a medication.
For computer documentation keep your password to yourself.	Maintains security and confidentiality.	Once logged into the computer, do not leave the computer screen unattended.

Guidelines for Quality Documentation and Reporting

High-quality documentation and reporting enhance efficient, individualized client care. Quality documentation and reporting have six important characteristics: they are factual, accurate, complete, current, and organized, and they comply with standards set by the CCHSA and provincial or territorial regulatory bodies.

Factual

A record must contain descriptive, objective information about what a nurse sees, hears, feels, and smells. An objective description is the result of direct observation and measurement. Inferences without supporting factual data are unacceptable because they can be misunderstood. Words such as *appears, seems,* or *apparently* are also not acceptable because they suggest that the nurse is stating an opinion. For example, the description "the client seems anxious" does not accurately communicate facts and does not inform another caregiver of the details regarding the behaviours exhibited by the client that led to the use of the word *anxious*. The phrase *seems anxious* is a conclusion without supported facts. It is best to describe the client's behaviours (for example, increased pulse rate, increased respirations, and increased restlessness) and to document the client's exact words within quotation marks (e.g., "Client states, 'I feel very nervous and out of control.'").

Accurate

The use of exact measurements establishes accuracy. For example, a description such as "Intake, 360 mL of water" is more accurate than "Client drank an adequate amount of fluid." These measurements can later be used as a means to determine whether a client's condition has changed. Charting that an abdominal wound is "5 cm in length without redness, drainage, or edema" is more descriptive than "large wound healing well."

Documentation of concise data should be clear and easy to understand, with unnecessary words and irrelevant details left out. For example, the fact that the client is watching TV is only relevant when this activity is significant to the client's status and plan of care.

Use of an institution's accepted abbreviations, symbols, and system of measures (e.g., metric) ensures that all staff members use the same language in their reports and records. A nurse should use abbreviations carefully to avoid misinterpretation. For example, od (every day) can be misinterpreted to mean O.D. (right eye). To minimize errors, if abbreviations are confusing, a nurse should spell them out in their entirety. The Joint Commission on Accreditation of Healthcare Institutions published a list of abbreviations in January 2004 that should no longer be used in written medical documents (Karch, 2004). Suggestions include the following: write "unit" instead of "U"; always use a zero before a decimal point (e.g., 0.25 mg); and do not write a zero alone after a decimal point (e.g., write 5 mg—not 5.0 mg).

Correct spelling demonstrates a level of competency and attention to detail. Many terms can easily be misinterpreted (e.g., *dysphagia* or *dysphasia* and *dram* or *gram*). Some spelling errors can also result in serious treatment errors; for example, the names of certain medications such as digitoxin and digoxin or morphine and Numorphan are similar and must be transcribed carefully to ensure that the client receives the correct medication.

Record entries must be dated and a method used to identify the authors of entries. Therefore, each entry in a client's record ends with the caregiver's full name or initials and status, such as "Holly Lee, RN." Each time initials are used, the full name and status must previously appear on the same page so that the individual entering initials can be readily identified. A nursing student enters full name, student nurse abbreviation (e.g., SN or NS), and educational institution, such as "Henri Gauthier, SN 1 (student nurse—year one), U of S (University of Saskatchewan)."

Records need to reflect accountability during the time frame of the entry, which is best accomplished when nurses chart only their own observations and actions. The signature holds that nurse accountable for information recorded. If information was inadvertently omitted from the record, it is acceptable for nurses to ask colleagues to chart information after they leave work. The entry needs to clearly show what was done and by whom (e.g., "At 1100 hrs Sam Roustas, RN, called and reported that at 0800 hrs morphine sulfate 5 mg subcutaneously was administered to client for abdominal pain").

Nurses should refer to agency policy before making late entries, correcting errors, or completing an omission. Late entries are often documented by writing the current date and time in the next available space and writing "late entry for (date and shift)" (Sullivan, 2000). For adding information to an existing entry, Sullivan also suggests using the current date and time in the next space and adding "addendum to note of (date and time of prior note)."

Complete

The information within a recorded entry or a report needs to be complete, containing appropriate and essential information. Criteria for thorough communication exist for certain health problems or nursing activities (Table 13-2). The nurse makes written entries in the client's medical record, describing the administered nursing care and the client's response. An example of a thorough nurse's note follows:

> 1915 Client verbalizes sharp, throbbing pain localized along lateral side of right ankle, beginning approximately 15 minutes ago after twisting his foot on the stairs. Client rates pain as 8 on a scale of 0-10. Pain increased with movement, slightly relieved with elevation. Pedal pulses equal bilaterally. Right ankle circumference 1 cm larger than left. Ice applied. Percocet 2 tabs given for pain. Client states pain somewhat relieved with ice, rates pain as 6 on a scale of 0-10. Physician notified. Lee Turno, RN.

Current

Timely entries are essential in the client's ongoing care. Documentation should occur during or as soon as possible after the incident or intervention and events should be presented chronologically to reflect a clear record of events (College of Nurses of Ontario, 2004). To increase accuracy and decrease unnecessary duplication, many health care agencies use bedside records, which facilitate immediate documentation of information as it is collected from a client. The following activities and findings should be communicated at the time of occurrence:

- Vital signs
- Administration of medications and treatments
- Preparation for diagnostic tests or surgery
- Change in client's status and who was notified (e.g., physician, manager, client's family)
- Admission, transfer, discharge, or death of a client
- Treatment for a sudden change in status

This information is usually included in flow sheets kept at the bedside. Nurses usually keep notes on a worksheet when caring for several clients, making notes as the care occurs to ensure that entries recorded later in the record are accurate.

Health care agencies use military time, a 24-hour system that avoids misinterpretation of AM and PM times (Figure 13–2). Instead of two 12-hour cycles in standard time, the military clock is one 24-hour time cycle. The military clock ends with midnight at 2400 and begins with 1 minute after midnight at 0001. For example, 10:22 AM is 1022 military time; 1:00 PM is 1300 military time.

Organized

The nurse communicates information in a logical order. For example, an organized note describes the client's pain, nurse's assessment and interventions, and the client's response. To write notes about complex situations in an organized fashion, the nurse thinks about the situation and often makes notes of what is to be included before beginning to write in the permanent legal record.

Complies With Standards

Documentation needs to follow standards set by the CCHSA and provincial or territorial regulatory bodies in order to maintain institutional accreditation and decrease

Table 13-2 Examples of Criteria for Reporting and Recording

Topic	Criteria to Report or Record
Assessment	
Subjective data	Description of episode in quotation marks Onset, location, description of condition (severity, duration, frequency; precipitating, aggravating, and relieving factors)
Client behaviour (e.g., anxiety, confusion, hostility)	Onset, behaviours exhibited, precipitating factors
Objective data (e.g., rash, tenderness, breath sounds)	Onset, location, description of condition
Nursing Interventions and Evaluation	
Treatments (e.g., enema, bath, dressing change)	Time administered, equipment used (if appropriate), client's response (objective and subjective changes) compared with previous treatment; for example, "client denied pain during dressing change" or "client reported severe abdominal cramping during enema"
Medication administration	Immediately after administration, document time medication given, preliminary assessment (e.g., pain level, vital signs), client response or effect of medication; for example, "1500 Pain reported at 6 (scale 0–10). Tylenol 500 mg given PO 1530: Client reports pain level 2 (scale 0–10)" or "Pruritus and hives developed over lower abdomen 1 hour after penicillin was given"
Client teaching	Information presented, method of instruction (e.g., discussion, demonstration, videotape, booklet), client response, including questions and evidence of understanding such as return demonstration or change in behaviour
Discharge planning	Measurable client goals or expected outcomes, progress toward goals, need for referrals

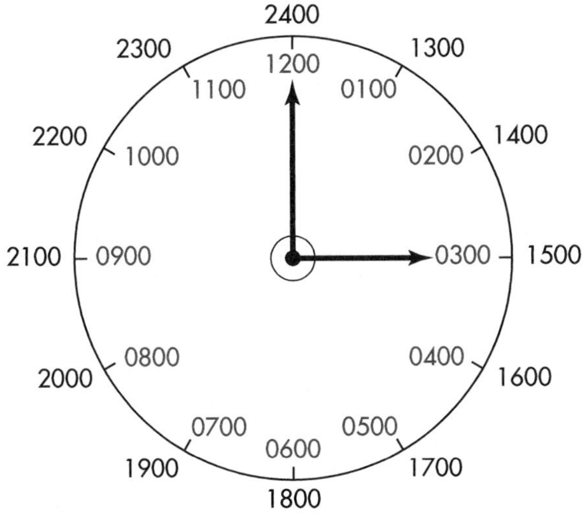

FIGURE **13–2** Military time clock.

the risk of liability. Current standards require that all clients who are admitted to a health care institution have an assessment of physical, psychosocial, environmental, self-care, client education, and discharge planning. In addition, criteria for standards stress the importance of evaluating client outcomes, including the client's response to treatments, teaching, or preventive care.

Common Documentation Systems

There are several documentation systems for recording client data. These systems are selected by the nursing service and reflect the philosophy of the department. The same documentation system is used throughout a specific agency and may also be used throughout a health care system.

Narrative Documentation

Narrative documentation is the traditional method for recording nursing care. It is simply the use of a story-like format to document information specific to client conditions and nursing care. Narrative charting, however, has many disadvantages, including the tendency to repeat information, to be time consuming, and to require the reader to sort through much information to locate desired data.

Problem-Oriented Medical Records

The **problem-oriented medical record (POMR)** is a method of documentation that emphasizes the client's problems. Data are organized by problem or diagnosis. Ideally, each member of the health care team contributes to a single list of identified client problems. This assists in coordinating a common plan of care. The POMR has the following major sections: database, problem list, care plan, and progress notes.

Database. The database section contains all available assessment information pertaining to the client (e.g., history and physical examination, the nurse's admission history and ongoing assessment, the dietitian's assessment, laboratory reports, and radiological test results). The database is the foundation for identifying client problems and planning care. The database is revised as new data become available. It accompanies clients through successive hospitalizations or clinic visits.

Problem List. After data are analyzed, problems are identified and a single list is made. The problems include the client's physiological, psychological, social, cultural, spiritual, developmental, and environmental needs. The problems are listed in chronological order and filed in the front of the client's record to serve as an organizing guide for the client's care. New problems are added as they are identified. When a problem has been resolved, the date is recorded and it is highlighted, or a line is drawn through the problem and its number.

Care Plan. A care plan is developed for each problem by the disciplines involved in the client's care (see chapter 12). Nurses may document the plan of care in a variety of formats. Generally, these plans of care include nursing diagnoses, expected outcomes, and interventions.

Progress Notes. Health care team members monitor and record the progress of a client's problems (Box 13-1). The information can be expressed in various formats of structured notes. One method is the SOAP charting. **SOAP:** S—subjective data (verbalizations of the client), O—objective data (that which is measured and observed), A—assessment (diagnosis based on the data), P—plan (what the caregiver plans to do). Some institutions add an I and E (i.e., **SOAPIE**). The I stands for intervention, and the E represents evaluation. The logic for SOAPIE notes is similar to that of the nursing process: Collect data about the client's problems, draw conclusions, and develop a plan of care. The nurse numbers each SOAP note and titles it according to the problem on the list.

A second progress note method is the **PIE** format. It is similar to SOAP charting in its problem-oriented nature. However, it differs from the SOAP method in that PIE charting has a nursing origin, whereas SOAP originated from medical records. The format simplifies documentation by unifying the care plan and progress notes. PIE differs from SOAP notes because the narrative does not include assessment information. A nurse's daily assessment data appear on flow sheets, preventing duplication of data. The narrative note includes P—problem, I—intervention, and E—evaluation. The PIE notes are numbered or labelled according to the client's problems. Resolved problems are dropped from daily documentation after the nurse's review. Continuing problems are documented daily.

A third progress note format is **focus charting.** It involves use of **DAR** notes, which include D—data (both subjective and objective), A—action or nursing intervention, and R—response of the client (i.e., evaluation of effectiveness). One distinction of focus charting is its movement away from charting only problems, which has a negative connotation. Instead, the notes are structured according to client concerns: a sign or symptom, a condition, a nursing diagnosis, a behaviour, a significant event, or a change in a client's condition. Documentation is written in accordance with the nursing process, nurses are encouraged to broaden their thinking to include any client concerns, not just problem areas, and critical thinking is encouraged. Focus charting is easily understood by caregivers and adaptable to most health care settings. Focus charting helps track the client's condition and progress (Smith, 2000).

Box 13-1 Examples of Progress Notes Written in Different Formats

SOAP (Subjective—Objective—Assessment—Plan)

1/19/05 Knowledge deficit related to inexperience regarding surgery
1630
S—"I'm worried about what it will be like after surgery."
O—Client asking frequent questions about surgery. Has had no previous experience with surgery. Wife present, acts as a support person.
A—Knowledge deficit regarding surgery related to inexperience. Client also expressing anxiety.
P—Explain routine preoperative preparation. Demonstrate and explain rationale for turning, coughing, and deep breathing (TCDB) exercises. Provide explanation and teaching booklet on post-operative nursing care. S. Lazarus, RPN

PIE (Problem—Intervention—Evaluation)

P—Knowledge deficit regarding surgery related to inexperience.
I—Explained to client normal preoperative preparations for surgery. Demonstrated TCDB exercises. Provided booklet to client on post-operative nursing care.
E—Client demonstrates TCDB exercises correctly. Needs review of post-operative nursing care. S. Lazarus, RPN

Focus Charting (Data—Action—Response)

D—Client stating, "I'm worried about what it will be like after surgery." Client asking frequent questions about surgery. Has had no previous experience with surgery. Wife present; acts as a support person.
A—Explained to client normal preoperative preparations for surgery. Demonstrated TCDB exercises. Provided booklet to client on post-operative nursing care.
R—Client demonstrates TCDB exercises correctly. Needs review of post-operative nursing care. S. Lazarus, RPN
NOTE: Some agencies also add P (Plan).

Source Records

In a **source record,** the client's chart is organized so that each discipline (e.g., nursing, medicine, social work, respiratory therapy) has a separate section in which to record data. One advantage of a source record is that caregivers can easily locate the proper section of the record in which to make entries. Table 13-3 lists the components of a source record.

A disadvantage of the source record is that details about a specific problem may be distributed throughout

Table 13-3 Organization of Traditional Source Record

Sections	Contents
Admission sheet	Specific demographic data about client: legal name, identification number, sex, age, birth date, marital status, occupation and employer, health card number, nearest relative to notify in an emergency, religious preference, name of attending physician, date and time of admission
Physician's order sheet	Record of physician's orders for treatment and medications, with date, time, and physician's signature
Nurse's admission assessment	Summary of nursing history and physical examination
Graphic sheet and flow sheet	Record of repeated observations and measurements such as vital signs, daily weights, and intake and output
Medical history and examination	Results of initial examination performed by physician, including findings, family history, confirmed diagnoses, and medical plan of care
Nurses' notes	Narrative record of nursing process: assessment, nursing diagnosis, planning, implementation, and evaluation of care
Medication records	Accurate documentation of all medications administered to client: date, time, dose, route, and nurse's signature
Physician's progress notes	Ongoing record of client's progress and response to medical therapy and review of disease process
Health care disciplines' records	Entries made into record by all health-related disciplines: radiology, social work, and laboratories
Discharge summary	Summary of client's condition, progress, prognosis, rehabilitation, and teaching needs at time of dismissal from hospital or health care agency

Box 13-2 Sample Narrative Note

8/6/05 1100
Client states, "I'm having a hard time catching my breath." Respirations, laboured at 32/min; P 120; BP 112/70. Client using intercostal muscles during inhalation. Breath sounds auscultated, crackles and wheezes over both lower lobes. Chest excursion equal bilaterally. Head of bed elevated to Fowler's position. Arterial blood gas (ABG) sample obtained at 1045 and O_2 started at 2 L/min per nasal prongs as ordered. Remained at bedside to calm client. P. Haske, RN
1130 Results of ABGs reported to Dr Stein are pH 7.34; Pco_2 44 mm Hg; Po_2 80 mm Hg. Client breathing less laboured now R 28/min; P 96; BP 110/72. Crackles and wheezing still audible on auscultation. Client resting quietly. P. Haske, RN

the record. For example, the nurse describes the character of abdominal pain and use of relaxation therapy and analgesic medication in the nurses' notes. The physician's notes describe the progress of the client's bowel obstruction and the plan for surgery in a separate section of the record. The results of X-ray examinations that show the location of the bowel obstruction are in the test results section of the record. The method by which source records are organized does not show how information from the disciplines is related or how care is coordinated to meet all of the client's needs.

The notes section is where nurses enter a narrative description of nursing care and the client's response (Box 13-2). It is also a section for documenting care that is provided by the physician in the nurse's presence. The nurse may record key diagnostic test results from other sections of the record in the nurses' notes if they are of major importance in the care of the client.

Charting by Exception

Charting by exception (CBE) is an approach that is used to eliminate redundancy, ensure concise documentation of routine care, emphasize abnormal findings, and identify trends in clinical care. While making documentation more effective, it can significantly reduce time spent in charting (Cummins & Hill, 1999). It is a shorthand method for documenting normal findings and routine care based on clearly defined standards of practice and predetermined criteria for nursing assessments and interventions. Clearly defined standards of practice that specify nurses' responsibilities to clients provide the framework for routine care of all clients. With standards integrated into documentation forms, such as predefined normal assessment findings or predetermined interventions, a nurse need only document significant findings or exceptions to the predefined norms. In other words, the nurse writes a progress note only when the standardized statement on the form is not met. Assessments are standardized on flow sheets or other forms so that all caregivers evaluate and document findings consistently (Figure 13–3).

Because the standard assessments are located in the chart, client data are already present on the permanent record, so nurses do not have to keep temporary notes for later transcription and caregivers have easy access to current data. The assumption with CBE is that all standards are met unless otherwise documented. When nurses see entries in the chart, they know that something out of the ordinary has been observed or has occurred. For that reason, when changes in a client's condition have developed, it is easy to track them.

When clients' conditions change, thorough and precise descriptions of what happens to clients and the actions taken are essential. CBE can pose legal risks if nurses are not disciplined in documenting exceptions. CBE can also be problematic when related documentation forms

Ottawa–Carleton Hospital
Medical–Surgical Interdisciplinary Patient Care Flow Sheet

Initials in Box = Assessment findings meet standards and procedures. Interventions tolerated well.
∗ in Box = Significant finding(s) **not normal or changed.** See Progress Notes.
➔ in Box = Significant finding(s) has NOT CHANGED.

Complete and initial all relevant items. Leave others blank.

CAREMAP NAME:

YEAR ____	DAY
MONTH _____	TIME

NEUROLOGICAL	Alert & oriented to person, place, time. Behaviour appropriate to situation. Pupils equal & reactive to light. Purposeful movement of all extremities and symmetry of strength. Sensation intact. Gag & cough reflex intact.
Assessment ☐ Pre-existing Impairment	
CARDIOVASCULAR	Regular radial pulse. No edema, no chest pain, no diaphoresis.
Assessment ☐ Pre-existing Impairment	
RESPIRATORY	Respirations, quiet, regular, unlaboured. Sputum absent or clear. Nail beds and lips within patient's normal colour. Breath sounds clear & audible both lung fields. Oximetry as per patient's parameters.
Assessment ☐ Pre-existing Impairment	
Auscultation	
Chest Care (e.g., DB & C)	
GASTROINTESTINAL	No nausea, vomiting, or pain. Bowel movements within patient's own normal.
Assessment ☐ Pre-existing Impairment	
Bowel Sounds Present	
Incontinent Stool (follow skin care protocol)	
GENITOURINARY	GENITALIA: normal. VAGINAL FLOW: Scant to moderate, light pink to serosanguinous to brownish drainage. No foul odours or bright red bleeding. Few clots may be present. BLADDER: Urine clear, yellow to amber. Urinary drainage system patent, if present. No pain or burning on voiding. FOLEY: cleansed with Savlon q shift.
Assessment Genitalia ☐ Pre-existing Impairment	
Vaginal Flow	
Assessment Bladder ☐ Foley	
Incontinent Urine (follow skin care protocol)	

CAREMAP NAME:

YEAR ____	DAY
MONTH _____	TIME

PERIPHERAL VASCULAR	Extremities pink, warm. Sensation intact. Peripheral pulses palpable. No limb edema, no calf tenderness.
Assessment ☐ Pre-existing Impairment	
MUSCULOSKELETAL/ADL	No swelling, tenderness, or muscle spasms. Functional ROM for all joints. MOBILITY/ADL: Able to ambulate; steady balance; purposeful gait. Progressing toward goals as per CareMap.
Assessment ☐ Pre-existing Impairment	
Mobility	
ADL	
SKIN INTEGRITY	Skin colour within patient's norm; skin warm & intact; mucous membranes moist.
Assessment ☐ Pre-existing Impairment	
Hygiene needs met per CareMap (A.M. & hs care)	
Skin care protocol in use	
PAIN/COMFORT	Patient describes pain as nil, mild, or moderate & is satisfied with management. PAIN SCALE: 1–10
Location #1	
Location #2	
Pain Score #1 / #2	
PSYCHOSOCIAL DISCHARGE PLANNING	ADAPTATION: Patient is adapting to hospitalization & illness. DISCHARGE PLANNING: Plans progressing according to CareMap.
Assessment: Adaptation	
Assessment: Discharge	
NUTRITION	Maintaining healthy body weight. ORAL: Consuming & tolerating at least 3/4 of prescribed diet. No nausea or vomiting. No dehydration. SWALLOWING: No coughing/choking on liquids/solids. TUBE FEED: Tolerating prescribed type, rate, & amount of enteral feeding.
Assessment:	
Assessment: Oral Feeding	
Assessment: Swallowing	
Assessment: Tube Feeding	
SLEEP	1 = Slept Well 2 = Slept at Intervals 3 = Slept Poorly
Assessment	

FIGURE 13–3 Example of a standardized form (in this case, a client care flow-sheet) that can be used when charting by exception; predefined normal assessment findings are listed on the form and the nurse notes when assessment findings are not normal or have changed. (Adapted from Ottawa-Carleton Hospital: Queensway-Carleton Campus, Nepean, ON.)

Ottawa–Carleton Hospital
Medical–Surgical Interdisciplinary Patient Care Flow Sheet

Initials in Box = Assessment findings meet standards and procedures. Interventions tolerated well.
⁎ in Box = Significant finding(s) **not normal or changed.** See Progress Notes.
→ in Box = Significant finding(s) has NOT CHANGED.

Complete and initial all relevant items. Leave others blank.

CAREMAP NAME:

YEAR ____ DAY
MONTH _____ TIME

SAFETY — Low risk for falls or wandering. Basic safety precautions in place.
Assessment

TEACHING/LEARNING — Receptive to & understands treatment goals & care needs. Educational goals met as per CareMap.
Assessment

PERIPHERAL/CENTRAL LINES/ SALINE LOCK — Absence of redness, swelling, or tenderness at site. IV infusing at prescribed rate. Saline lock patent. IV site checked q 2 h. △ = dressing change. D/C = IV discontinued.

Site 1: _____ Site Assessment
☐ Lock
☐ Peripheral Tubing/Dressing △
☐ Central Discontinued D/C
☐ Other ____

Site 2: ____ Site Assessment
☐ Lock
☐ Peripheral Tubing/Dressing △
☐ Central Discontinued D/C
☐ Other ____

WOUND — No redness, inflammation. Incision well approximated. Sutures, SteriStrips, staples intact. R = staples, sutures removed. △ = dressing change. DRAINAGE: S = serous, SS = serosanguinous, SG = sanguinous, P = purulent. AMOUNT: 1 = nil, 2 = small, 3 = moderate, 4 = copious.

Site 1: ____ Site Assessment
Dressing dry & intact
Drainage/Dressing △

Site 2: ____ Site Assessment
Dressing dry & intact
Drainage/Dressing △

CAREMAP NAME:

YEAR ____ DAY
MONTH _____ TIME

DRAINS — Patent & draining as expected. DRAINAGE: S = serous, SS = serosanguinous, P = purulent. AMOUNT: 1 = nil, 2 = small, 3 = moderate, 4 = copious. SH = shortened. R = removed.
Location #1
Location #2

TRANSURETHRAL PROCEDURES — URINE: C = clear, P = pink, T = tea-coloured, M = moderate sanguinous, SC = sanguinous with clots. R = catheter removed. HNV = has not voided.
Foley catheter patent & draining
Bladder irrigation Continuous
Manual
Type of urine drainage
Voiding satisfactory post removal

FIGURE **13–3, cont'd** Example of a standardized form (in this case, a client care flow-sheet) that can be used when charting by exception; predefined normal assessment findings are listed on the form and the nurse notes when assessment findings are not normal or have changed. (Adapted from Ottawa-Carleton Hospital: Queensway-Carleton Campus, Nepean, ON.)

do not have space allotted for documenting client and family perspectives.

Critical Pathways or CareMaps

In many organizations, the standardized plan of care is summarized into critical pathways for a specific disease or condition. The **critical pathways** or **CareMaps** are multidisciplinary care plans that include client health concerns, key interventions, and expected outcomes within an established time frame. The use of a computerized charting system allows many disciplines to access the chart, and this integration of information from the different disciplines can be accessed easily from every computer terminal at any time. The nurse and other team members such as physicians, dietitians, social workers, physiotherapists, and respiratory therapists use the same critical pathway to monitor the client's progress during each shift or, in the case of home care, every visit. In general, the critical pathway or CareMap identifies the expected outcomes for each day of care (Figure 13–4). Individual client values and preferences must be considered at every point of the critical pathway so that care remains individualized.

Critical pathways promote integration of information so that each discipline has access to notes written by others. It also reduces duplication and the amount of charting (Brugh, 1998). Unexpected occurrences, unmet goals, and interventions not specified within the clinical pathway time frame are called **variances.** A variance occurs when the activities on the clinical pathway are not completed as predicted or the client does not meet the expected outcomes. An example of a negative variance is when a post-operative client develops pulmonary complications requiring oxygen therapy and monitoring with pulse oximetry. A positive variance occurs when a client progresses more rapidly than expected (e.g., use of a Foley catheter may be discontinued a day early). A variance analysis is necessary to review the data for trends and for developing and implementing an action plan to respond to the identified client problems (Box 13-3). In addition, variances may result from changes in the client's health or may occur as a result of other health complications not associated with the primary reason for which the client requires care. The nurse's responsibility is to address the variance and to justify the actions taken to manage the critical pathway deviation (Iyer & Camp, 1999). Over time, the reoccurrence of similar variances may lead the health care team to revise a critical pathway.

Box 13-3 Example of Variance Documentation

A 56-year-old client is on a surgical unit one day after cholecystectomy. His temperature is slightly elevated, his breath sounds are decreased bilaterally at the bases of both lobes of the lungs, and he is slightly confused. Ordinarily, at 1 day post-operatively, the client should be afebrile with clear lungs. The following is an example of the variance documentation for this client.

9/23/05 1000

Breath sounds diminished bilaterally at the bases. T 37.8; P 92; R 28/min; oxygen saturation 84%. Daughter states he is "confused" and did not recognize her when she arrived a few minutes ago. Oxygen started at 2 L/min via nasal prongs as per standing orders. Will monitor pulse oximetry and vital signs every 15 minutes. Physician notified of change in status. Daughter at bedside.

Common Record-Keeping Forms

A variety of forms are available that are specially designed for the type of information nurses routinely document. The categories within a form are usually derived from institutional standards of practice or guidelines established by accrediting agencies.

Admission Nursing History Forms

A nursing history form is completed when a client is admitted to a nursing care unit. The history form guides the nurse through a complete assessment to identify relevant nursing diagnoses or problems (see chapter 12). Data on history forms provide baselines that can be compared with changes in the client's condition. Each institution designs a nursing history form that is consistent with professional standards of practice. This form may be incorporated into discharge summary forms as the initial data.

Flow Sheets and Graphic Records

Flow sheets are forms that allow nurses to quickly and easily enter assessment data about the client, including vital signs and routine repetitive care, such as hygiene measures, ambulation, meals, weights, and safety and restraint checks. The format of the flow sheet varies depending on the agency and the data being recorded. For example, some flow sheets may be used only to record vital signs; others may be more comprehensive (Figure 13–5; note that Figure 13–3 shows a flow sheet that is used for CBE). Flow sheets use a coding system for data entry. It is important to fill out all spaces on the flow sheet even if it is only "N/A" for items that are "not applicable." If a space is blank, it can raise doubts about whether an intervention was or was not done (Sullivan, 2000). If an occurrence on the flow sheet is unusual or changes significantly, a focus note is needed. For example, if a client's blood pressure becomes dangerously high, the nurse completes a focus assessment and records this, as well as action taken, in the progress notes. Flow sheets provide a quick, easy reference for the health care team members in assessing a client's status. Critical care and acute care units commonly use flow sheets for all types of physiological data (Box 13-4).

Box 13-4 Benefits of Using a Flow Sheet

- Information is accessible to all members of the health care team.
- Time spent on writing a narrative note is decreased.
- Information is current.
- Errors resulting from transfer of information are decreased.
- Team members can quickly see trends over time.

Client Care Summary or Kardex

Many hospitals now have computerized systems that provide basic, summative information in the form of a client care summary. This is printed out for each client during each shift. This summary is continually updated and provides the nurse with a current detailed list of orders, treatment, and diagnostic testing. In some settings, a **Kardex,** which is a portable "flip-over" file or notebook, is kept at the nurses' station. Most Kardex forms have an activity and treatment section and a nursing care plan section that organize information for quick reference as nurses give change-of-shift reports or make walking rounds. An updated Kardex eliminates the need for repeated referral to the chart for routine information throughout the day. In many institutions, Kardex entries are done in pencil because of the need for frequent revisions as the client's needs change. In settings in which the Kardex is a permanent part of the client's record, entries are made in ink.

Information commonly found on the client care summary or Kardex includes the following:

- Basic demographic data (e.g., age, religion)
- Physician's name
- Primary medical diagnosis
- Current physician's treatment orders to be carried out by the nurse (e.g., dressing changes, ambulation, glucose monitoring)
- Nursing care plan
- Nursing orders (e.g., education sessions, symptom relief measures, counselling)
- Scheduled tests and procedures
- Safety precautions to be used in the client's care
- Factors related to activities of daily living
- Nearest relative/guardian or person to contact in an emergency
- Emergency code status
- Allergies

Acuity Records or Workload Measurement Systems

Acuity records (also known as **workload measurement systems**) provide a method of determining the hours of care and staff required for a given group of clients. A client's acuity level is based on the type and number of nursing interventions required for providing care in a 24-hour period. The acuity level determined by the nursing care allows clients to be rated in comparison with one another. For example, an acuity system might rate bathing clients from 1 to 5 (1 is totally dependent, 5 is independent). A client returning from surgery requiring frequent monitoring and extensive care may be listed with an acuity level of 1. On the same continuum, another client awaiting discharge after a successful recovery from surgery has an acuity level of 5. Accurate acuity ratings may also be used to justify overtime and the number and qualifications of staff needed to safely care for clients. The client-to-staff ratios established for a unit depend on a composite gathering of data for the 24-hour interventions that are necessary for each client receiving care.

Standardized Care Plans

Many institutions have attempted to make documentation easier for nurses with **standardized care plans.** The plans, based on the institution's standards of nursing practice, are preprinted, established guidelines that are used to care for clients who have similar health problems. After a nursing assessment is completed, the staff nurse identifies the standard care plans that are appropriate for the client. The care plans are placed in the client's medical record. Modifications can be made in ink to the standardized plans to individualize the therapies. Most standardized care plans also allow the nurse to write in specific goals or desired outcomes of care and the dates by which these outcomes should be achieved.

One advantage of standardized care plans is establishment of clinically sound standards of care for similar groups of clients. These standards can be useful when quality improvement audits are conducted. Another advantage is education. Nurses learn to recognize the accepted requirements of care for clients. The standardized care plans can also improve continuity of care among professional nurses.

The use of standardized care plans is controversial. The major disadvantage is the risk that the standardized plans prevent nurses from providing unique, individualized therapies for clients. When standardized care plans are used, the nurse remains responsible for an individualized approach to care. Standardized care plans cannot replace the nurse's professional judgment and decision making. In addition, care plans need to be updated on a regular basis to ensure that content is current and appropriate. Many hospitals are computerizing care plans. Daily computer-generated care plans are printed and incorporate several nursing diagnoses or problems in a single care plan. Such a system facilitates the process of revision and individualization of plans.

Discharge Summary Forms

Much emphasis is placed on preparing a client for an efficient, timely discharge from a health care facility. A client's discharge should also result in desirable outcomes. Multidisciplinary involvement in discharge planning helps to ensure that a client leaves the hospital in a timely manner with the necessary resources in place (Box 13-5).

Ideally, discharge planning begins at admission. Nurses revise the care plan as the client's condition changes. The client and family members are involved in the discharge planning process so that they have the information needed to return home. Discharge information and instructions should include data such as the following:

- Instruction in potential food-drug interactions, nutrition intervention, and modified diets
- Rehabilitation techniques to support adaptation to and/or functional independence in the environment
- Access to available community resources
- Circumstances in which clients should obtain further treatment or follow-up care
- Methods of obtaining follow-up care
- The client's and family's responsibilities in the client's care

DATE:				
CRITICAL PATH	ADMISSION	OR DAY	POST-OP DAY 1	DAY 2
CONSULTS	– Discharge planner/ Social work PRN – Medical, Anesthesia	– Physiotherapist	– Clinical nurse specialist refers to Geriatrician PRN – Dietitian PRN – OT. referral	
TESTS			See Standing Orders: – CBC	
TEACHING	REVIEW: – Pre-op teaching, client & family – CareMap – Pain control – Diet: ↑ protein, ↑ fibre	REINFORCE: – Pain control – DB & C* – Quad, ankle pumps	PHYSIO REVIEWS: – Bed exercises	PHYSIO REVIEWS: – exercises REVIEW: – CareMap PRN
MEDICATIONS	REVIEW: – Client-specific meds – Analgesic PRN – Anesthetist pre-op orders	– Client-specific meds – IM analgesic – Anti-emetic	– Client-specific med – IM analgesic – Anti-emetic	– Client-specific meds – Oral analgesic – Anti-emetic – Bowel routine
TREATMENTS/ ASSESSMENT	– V/S /shift & PRN – Mental status PRN* – CSM* /shift – Measure for TED stocking – Foam, air mattress monkey bar, fracture pan – IV as ordered – Foley PRN if ordered – Intake & output/shift – 5-lb skin traction if ordered	– V/S OR routine – CSM/shift – TED stocking to unaffected leg – DB & C – IV as ordered – Foley PRN if ordered – Intake & output/shift – Monitor hemovac – Monitor dressing	– V/S /shift – Mental status PRN – CSM/shift – TED stocking to unaffected leg – DB & C – IV as ordered – Foley PRN if ordered – Intake & output/shift – Monitor hemovac – Monitor dressing – Physio assists to chair — weight bearing as ordered	– V/S /shift – Mental status PRN – CSM/shift – TED stocking to both legs – DB & C – D/C IV if drinking well – D/C Foley – D/C Intake & output – D/C hemovac, apply pressure drsg. to drain – dry dressing to incision – Ambulate with Physio weight-bearing orders
HYGIENE/ACTIVITY	Bed bath – Bedrest	Post-op bath – Bedrest for 24 h, pillow under affected leg PRN – Head of bed 30° for short periods only – Position for comfort, unaffected side – Pillow between legs for turns on side	Bed bath – Bedrest or up in chair if able – Encourage physio exercises – Up in chair	Bed bath/sink with help – May be up for meals – Encourage physio exercises – Up with walker assist × 2 – Physio assists to chair
DIET	– DAT, NPO as ordered – Screen food allergy, nutrition risk – Special diet PRN	– NPO – full fluids, soft, light to DAT – Special diet PRN	– DAT – Special diet PRN	– DAT + ↑ protein drink TID – Special diet PRN
DISCHARGE PLANS	– Complete Client History & initiate consults PRN – *Notify CNS/Discharge Planner if: 1.>70 yr lives alone or with minimal home support. 2. From home, retirement facility + confusion		Assessment/referral: – If sent from Acute Care facility plan return on day 4 – GAU* – Rehab – Convalescence – Home – Other facility	ASSESS: – Need for home care – Physio assessment for discharge or transfer – Rehab forms completed PRN
PATIENT OUTCOMES Activity achieved (✓)	– Adequate pain control – Verbalizes understanding of condition, treatment & hospitalization, if able – Maintain present skin integrity & ROM in unaffected limbs	– Adequate pain control – Demonstrates DB & C and leg exercises, if able	– Demonstrates & participates in physio bed exercises, as able – Verbalizes adequate pain control with analgesia, as able. – Chair	– Verbalizes/understands plans for mobilization, if able. – Verbalizes adequate pain control with po analgesia, as able ___FWB ___PWB ___NWB ___walker or ___________ distance _____ assist of _____ ____ chair
	Variance [✓] if not met			
* Key *CNS complete F.I.M. PRN * DB & C = Deep breathing & coughing * CSM = circulation, movement, warmth, sensation *CNS = Clinical Nurse Specialist				

FIGURE **13–4** Example of a critical pathway (CareMap) for a fractured hip. (Adapted from Ottawa-Carleton Hospital, 2000, Queensway-Carleton Campus, Nepean, ON: Author.)

DAY 3	DAY 4	DAY 5	DAY 6	(Initial) DAY 7 – DISCHARGE INDICATORS
– Home Care Physio Referral Form PRN – Pastoral Care PRN	– Dietitian PRN – Notify if protein drink not taken			____ – Consults/reassessment completed
– CBC, lytes, INR – Confusion Scale (OT)			– Confusion Scale (OT)	____ – Laboratory/X-ray results within acceptable range
REVIEW: – Nutrition, bowel routine	REVIEW: – Application & care of TED stockings (client & family)	ENCOURAGE: – Application of TED stocking PHYSIO REVIEWS: – Home exercises – Adoptive equipment rental/ purchase and use (OT)	REVIEW: – Discharge plan – Incision care – Signs of infection – Home medications	Client Verbalizes Understanding of: ____ – Anticoagulant Tx ____ – Discharge medication ____ – *S/S of infection & incision care
– Client-specific meds – Oral analgesic – Bowel routine	– Client-specific meds – Oral analgesic – Bowel routine	– Client-specific meds – Oral analgesic – Bowel routine	– Client-specific meds – Oral analgesic – Bowel routine	____ – Bowels functioning ____ – Response to client-specific medication acceptable ____ – Pain controlled/ manageable
– V/S BID – Mental status PRN – CSM/shift – TED stocking to both legs – DB & C – Reassess IV if still in – Assess level of hydration – Incision care PRN – Physiotherapy weight bearing as ordered	– V/S daily – CSM BID – TED stockings to both legs – Incision care PRN – Physiotherapy weight bearing as ordered	– V/S daily – CSM BID – TED stockings to both legs – Assess tub transfers, toilet transfers (OT) – Teach lower body self-care (OT) – Incision care PRN – Physiotherapy weight bearing as ordered	– V/S daily – CSM BID – TED stockings to both legs – Incision care PRN – Demonstrates home exercises to Physio – Physiotherapy weight bearing as ordered	____ – V/S within normal limits × 8 h ____ – CSM to legs same as prior to surgery ____ – TED stocking applied to both legs ____ – Incision care done — abnormality on Progress Notes ____ – Clips left in (send clip remover if necessary) OR ____ – Clip removed ____ – SteriStrips applied
Sink, if able – Up for meals – Encourage physio exercises – Up with walker ☐ Day/evening walk if able	Self-care, if able – Activity as tolerated (some assistance) – Up with walker/crutches ☐ Day/evening walk if able	Shower with assistance – Self ADL dress in own clothes as able – Up with walker/crutches ☐ Day/evening walk	Self-care, assist – Self ADL dress in own clothes as able – Up with walker/ crutches ☐ Day/evening walk	____ – Self-care ____ – Assistance required ____ – Self ADL dress in own clothes ____ – Assistance required (Progress Notes) ____ – Up with walker/crutches independently ____ – Limited mobility (Progress Notes)
– DAT + ↑ protein drink TID – Request extra fluids for meals – Special diet PRN	– DAT + ↑ protein drink TID – Request extra fluids for meals – Special diet PRN	– DAT + ↑ protein drink TID – Request extra fluids for meals – Special diet PRN	– DAT + ↑ protein drink TID – Request extra fluids for meals – Special diet PRN	____ – DAT OR ____ – Special diet tolerated
– Client, family are aware of discharge plans	– Physio initiates outpatient referral PRN – Transfer to/meet RN from GAU – If sent from acute care hospital return if bed available	– Physio/Home care arranges services arranges services/ equipment – Evaluate discharge readiness: V/S stable, mobility, ADL at pre-hospital status – OT assessment done	– Physio arranges outpatient appt. PRN – Confirm discharge plans with family	____ Discharge at 10:00 h
– No evidence of infection – Client & family understand discharge plan and are aware of planned date of discharge/transfer – PO fluids 1500 mL daily ___FWB ___PWB ___NWB ___walker or __________ distance _____ assist of ___ ____ chair	– Demonstrates increasing independent activity, if able – Understands purpose of TED stockings, if able – PO fluids 1500 mL daily ___FWB ___PWB ___NWB ___walker or __________ distance _____ assist of ____ ____ chair	– No signs of wound infection, normal temperature, increasing mobility with/without assistance, if able – PO fluids 1500 mL daily – Bowel routine effective ___FWB ___PWB ___NWB ___walker or __________ distance _____ assist of _____ ____ chair	– Increasing independence with mobility, if able – Recognizes signs of infection to report to doctor, if able – PO fluids 1500 mL daily – Bowel routine effective ___FWB ___PWB ___NWB ___walker or __________ distance ____ assist of ____ ____ chair	____ Client discharged with ability to manage at home ___FWB ___PWB ___NWB ___walker or __________ distance _____ assist of _____ ____ chair
[ ] Discharge Plan (650) not documented	[ ] GAU N/A (801)	[ ] Unable to return (800) to Valley Hospital (Progress Notes)		☐ Discharge delayed (Progress Notes) (999)

*GAU = Geriatric Assessment Unit *S/S = signs and symptoms

Ottawa–Carleton Hospital Post-Op Flow Sheet

Key to Amount	Key to Colour	Key to Urine Colour
– – Nil	br – Bright Red	c – clear
S – Small	dr – Dark Red	tc – tea colour
M – Moderate	b – Brown	p – pink
L – Large	dg – Dark Green	br – bright red
Sc – Scant	lg – Light Green	dr – dark red
	y – yellow	rc – red with clots
	p – pink	b – brown

DATE	MONTH YEAR													
PAIN	TIME													
	– absent/comfortable													
	– relieved with meds													
	– meds not effective													
CHEST														
	– clear													
	– congested													
	– D B & C													
	– D B & C with encouragement													
ABDOMEN														
	– soft													
	– distended													
BOWEL SOUNDS														
	– absent													
	– sluggish													
	– normal													
	– passing flatus													
DRESSING														
	– dry, intact													
	– reinforced													
	– amount of drainage (key)													
	– colour of drainage (key)													
DIET														
	NPO													
	– sips/ice chips													
	– fluids													
	– diet tolerated													
	– diet not tolerated													

Ottawa–Carleton Hospital Post-Op Flow Sheet

Key to Amount	Key to Colour	Key to Urine Colour
– – Nil	br – Bright Red	c – clear
S – Small	dr – Dark Red	tc – tea colour
M – Moderate	b – Brown	p – pink
L – Large	dg – Dark Green	br – bright red
Sc – Scant	lg – Light Green	dr – dark red
	y – yellow	rc – red with clots
	p – pink	b – brown

DATE	MONTH YEAR													
AMBULATION	TIME													
	– active exercise in bed													
	– dangles													
	– up as ordered													
	– up and about													
	– not tolerating activity													
URINE														
	– colour (key)													
P.V. LOSS														
	– colour (key)													
	– amount (key)													
CIRCULATION														
	– temp. satis.													
	– temp. unsatis.													
	– pulses – present													
	– absent													
	– edema – absent													
	– present													
	– cyanosis/pallor													
	– sensation – absent													
	– present													
DRAINAGE														
	– N.G. tube													
	– colour (key)													

FIGURE **13–5** Example of a client care flow sheet. (Adapted from Ottawa-Carleton Hospital, 2000, Queensway-Carleton Campus, Nepean, ON: Author.)

Box 13-5 Discharge Summary Information

- Use clear, concise descriptions in client's own language.
- Provide step-by-step description of how to perform a procedure (e.g., home medication administration). Reinforce explanation with printed instructions.
- Identify precautions to follow when performing self-care or administering medications.
- Review signs and symptoms of complications that should be reported to a physician.
- List names and phone numbers of health care providers and community resources that the client can contact.
- Identify any unresolved problem, including plans for follow-up and continuous treatment.
- List actual time of discharge, mode of transportation, and who accompanied the client.

Box 13-6 Home Care Forms for Documentation

The usual forms used to document home care include:

- Client assessment
- Referral source information/intake form
- Discipline-specific care plans
- Physician's plan of treatment
- Medication sheet
- Clinical progress notes
- Miscellaneous (conference notes, verbal order forms, telephone calls)
- Discharge summary
- Reports to third-party payers

Modified from Iyer PW, Camp NH: *Nursing documentation: a nursing process approach,* St. Louis, 1999, Mosby.

- Medication instructions, including when to take each medication and why, the dose, the route, precautions, possible adverse reactions, and when and how to get prescriptions refilled.

Further, a common standard in nursing practice is to educate clients about the nature of their disease process, its likely progress, and the signs and symptoms of complications.

When a client is discharged from inpatient care, a discharge summary is prepared that includes information from members of the health care team. The summary is given to the client or family or to the home care, rehabilitation, or long-term care agency. Discharge summary forms make the summary concise and instructive (Figure 13–6). A summary form emphasizes previous learning by the client and family and care that should be continued in any restorative care setting. When given directly to clients, the form may be attached to pamphlets or teaching brochures.

Home Health Care Documentation

Home health care continues to grow with shorter hospitalizations and larger numbers of older adults requiring home care services. Documentation in the home health care system has different implications than in other areas of nursing. One primary difference is that the majority of care is witnessed by the client and family rather than by the nurse. Nurses must have astute assessment skills to gather the needed information about changes in the client's health care status. In addition, documentation systems need to provide the entire health care team with information needed to work together effectively (Box 13-6).

Some parts of the record are needed in the home with the client; other information is needed in an office setting. Thus, duplication of documentation is necessary unless agency policies specify which forms are to be left at the office and which are to be left in the clients' homes. Computerized client records may address these different needs. With the use of modems and laptop computers, records can be available in multiple locations, allowing greater access to the multidisciplinary needs that are often present in home care.

Long-Term Health Care Documentation

An increasing number of older adults require care in long-term care facilities. Because many individuals will live in this setting for the rest of their lives, they are referred to as **residents** rather than clients. In the long-term care setting, nursing personnel face challenges much different from those in the acute care setting (Iyer & Camp, 1999). Because residents are often stable, daily documentation is done using flow sheets. Assessment done several times a day in the acute care setting may be required only weekly or monthly in the long-term care setting.

In long-term care, governmental agencies and provincial and territorial laws are instrumental in determining the standards and policies for documentation. Documentation is used to review the levels of care given to and needed by residents in long-term care facilities.

Long-term care agencies also may have skilled care units where clients require increased levels of care in response to mandates for shorter hospital stays. Multidisciplinary communication among such health care providers is essential.

Computerized Documentation and the Electronic Health Record

Nurses have been using computerized systems for supplies, equipment, stock medications, and diagnostic testing for some time. However, increasingly hospitals are using computerized documentation systems. Many systems

Ottawa–Carleton Hospital
Discharge Protocol

ADMITTING INFORMATION
(Completed by Nurse on Admission)

Admission Date: ________ Doctor: ________
Diagnosis: ________

Support Systems: ☐ Spouse ☐ Children ☐ Friend/Neighbour ☐ None
☐ Other: ________

Community Services: CCAC: ☐ Nursing ☐ OT ☐ PT ☐ Homemaking
☐ GAOT ☐ Helpline ☐ Day Hospital ☐ Meals on Wheels
☐ Seniors Support ☐ Other (describe): ________

If not admitted from home, name of facility: ________

DISCHARGE SUMMARY (Completed on Discharge)
Discharge Date: ________ Time: ________ Level: ________ Quad: ________

Discharge Destination: ☐ Home alone ☐ Home with other: ________
☐ Facility: ________ ☐ Informed of DC Date: ________
☐ Transfer & Referral Form ☐ Transportation arranged: ________

Accompanied By: ☐ Spouse ☐ Relative/friend ☐ Alone ☐ Other: ________

Appliances/Aids: ☐ None ☐ Crutches ☐ Cane ☐ Walker ☐ Other: ________

Community Referrals Arranged: CCAC: ☐ Nursing ☐ OT ☐ PT ☐ Homemaking
☐ GAOT ☐ Helpline ☐ Day Hospital ☐ Meals on Wheels
☐ Seniors Support ☐ Other (describe): ________

Outpatient Follow-Up: ☐ None ☐ Clinic ☐ Physician's office ☐ Other: ________
☐ Tests ________

Discharge Medications: ☐ None Prescription ☐ Yes ☐ No Teaching ☐ Yes ☐ No

Discharge Teaching Completed: ☐ Yes ☐ No Comments: ________

Incision Assessed: ☐ Yes ☐ No ☐ Not applicable Comments: ________

Patient's Condition on Discharge:
Bladder Function: ☐ Good ☐ Fair ☐ Poor Independence: ☐ Good ☐ Fair ☐ Poor
Bowel Function: ☐ Good ☐ Fair ☐ Poor Nutrition: ☐ Good ☐ Fair ☐ Poor
Emotional Status: ☐ Good ☐ Fair ☐ Poor Skin: ☐ Good ☐ Fair ☐ Poor

Date: ________ Nurse's Signature: ________

KEY:
ADL = Activities of Daily Living
CNS = Clinical Nurse Specialist
GAOT = Geriatric Assessment Outreach Team
N/A = Not Applicable
RRT = Registered Respiratory Therapist
ARDU = Alzheimer & Related Disorder Unit
DC = Discharge
LTC = Long-Term Care
OT = Occupational Therapy
Rx = Treatment
CCAC = Community Care Access Centre
Dx = Diagnosis
MRSA = Methicillin-Resistant *Staphylococcus Aureus*
PT = Physiotherapy
SOB = Short of Breath

FIGURE **13–6** Example of a discharge summary form. (Adapted from Ottawa-Carleton Hospital, 2000, Queensway-Carleton Campus, Nepean, ON: Author.)

CLIENT PROBLEMS (Referral Criteria):
Multidisciplinary Team members to ✓ and date problems applicable to client. All referrals to be written in the Client's Orders and processed through the ACC.

MEDICAL HISTORY

- ☐ _____ Many chronic medical problems **Refer: Social Worker** **Refer: CNS** (if patient >75 yrs)
- ☐ _____ Many ER visits or hospital admissions **Refer: Social Worker**
- ☐ _____ Cancer, AIDS/HIV, or terminal illness & client/family needing support **Dr. to consider Palliative Care**
- ☐ _____ Behavioural or psychological problems **Dr. to consider Geriatrician, Psychogeriatric/Psychiatry, ARDU**
- ☐ _____ Other (describe)

HEALTH MANAGEMENT

- ☐ _____ Positive MRSA screen **Refer: Infection Control**
- ☐ _____ Needs stress management training **Refer: OT**

MEDICATIONS

- ☐ _____ Noncompliant or needs education
- ☐ _____ Uncertain of drug allergy reaction
- ☐ _____ DC medications differ from admission & is taking >6 schedule medications
- ☐ _____ Frequent medication changes or multiple generic brands, numerous herbal preparation **Refer: Pharmacist**
- ☐ _____ Taking multiple medications (>75 yr) **Refer: CNS**
- ☐ _____ Other (describe)

RESPIRATORY

- ☐ _____ O_2 titration, spirometry
- ☐ _____ Home O_2 or home O_2 candidate
- ☐ _____ Needs education: disease, devices
- ☐ _____ Candidate for Asthma Clinic **Refer: RRT**
- ☐ _____ Respiratory problem with mobility restrictions & safety issues
- ☐ _____ Respiratory deficiency, SOB, difficulty clearing secretions **Refer: PT**
- ☐ _____ Pneumonia **Refer: PT Refer: RRT**
- ☐ _____ Needs energy conservation, work simplication, & relaxation training **Refer: OT**
- ☐ _____ Other (describe)

SKIN

- ☐ _____ Delayed wound healing
- ☐ _____ Decubitus ulcer, exudating open wound, large burn, nutritional edema
- ☐ _____ Positioning & pressure relief **Refer: Dietitian Refer: CNS Refer: OT**
- ☐ _____ Limited mobility due to wound on joint **Refer: PT Refer: CNS**
- ☐ _____ Lymphedema, skin care problem **Refer: CNS**
- ☐ _____ Other (describe)

PAIN

- ☐ _____ Needs pain/symptom management **Dr. to consider Palliative Care**
- ☐ _____ Origin is musculoskeletal, articular, neural, gross edema
- ☐ _____ Palliative patient with pain **Refer: PT Refer: OT**

NUTRITION

- ☐ _____ Dysphagia **Refer: Speech Therapy** **Refer: Dietitian**
- ☐ _____ Malnutrition or weight loss
- ☐ _____ Inadequate food intake (prolonged)
- ☐ _____ Special diet
- ☐ _____ Enteral/parenteral nutrition
- ☐ _____ Needs diet intervention/teaching
- ☐ _____ Diabetic — new or uncontrolled
- ☐ _____ Candidate for Diabetes Info. Program
- ☐ _____ Candidate for Lipid Clinic **Refer: Dietitian**
- ☐ _____ Other (describe)

ELIMINATION

- ☐ _____ Stoma care problem (any age)
- ☐ _____ Altered bowel function
- ☐ _____ Altered urinary function **Refer: CNS**
- ☐ _____ Other (describe)

COGNITIVE & SENSORY

- ☐ _____ Cognitive impairment **Refer: OT Refer: CNS (if patient >75 yr)**
- ☐ _____ Motivational problems **Refer: CNS (if patient >75 yr)** **Refer: OT**

- ☐ _____ Communication difficulty (recent) **Refer: Speech Therapy**
- ☐ _____ Other (describe)

MOBILITY

- ☐ _____ Concern for ADL safety/independence
- ☐ _____ Need for wheelchair
- ☐ _____ Meal preparation **Refer: OT Refer: Dietitian**
- ☐ _____ Restricted/unsafe mobility
- ☐ _____ Severe general weakness/balance difficulties
- ☐ _____ Recent inability to do stairs at home
- ☐ _____ Problem moving in bed or transferring **Refer: PT Refer: CNS (if patient >75 yr)**
- ☐ _____ Other (describe)

PSYCHOSOCIAL

- ☐ _____ Lives alone and at risk
- ☐ _____ Unable to return to previous living situation
- ☐ _____ Financial concerns for living needs
- ☐ _____ Indications of abuse
- ☐ _____ Needs 24-h supervision
- ☐ _____ Anticipated DC to a facility
- ☐ _____ Sole caregiver for dependent person
- ☐ _____ Caregiver unable to manage **Refer: Social Worker Refer: CNS (if patient >75 yr) Refer: OT** **Refer: Geriatric Day Hospital**
- ☐ _____ Other (describe)

SPIRITUAL

- ☐ _____ Fear or anxiety related to Dx or Rx
- ☐ _____ Questioning meaning or purpose of life, self or situation, values & beliefs
- ☐ _____ Non-urgent sacramental care needed **Refer: Hospital Chaplain**
- ☐ _____ Acute fear or anxiety or grief
- ☐ _____ Urgent sacramental care needed **Notify on-call chaplain**
- ☐ _____ Other (describe)

FIGURE **13–6, cont'd** Example of a discharge summary form. (Adapted from Ottawa-Carleton Hospital, 2000, Queensway-Carleton Campus, Nepean, ON: Author.)

Box 13-7 Benefits of Automated Speech-Recognition (ASR) Technology

- Comprehensive nursing documentation with minimal nursing effort
- Decreased charting errors and omissions
- Consistent documentation patterns
- Increased interdisciplinary communication
- Considerable time savings for the nurse
- Clear, concise, legible documentation
- Increased compliance with accreditation standards

Box 13-8 Objectives of Computer-Based Patient Care Record (CPCR)

- Improved uniformity, accuracy, and retrievability of data about client care
- Confidentiality of health care information ensured in the system
- Access for authorized health care providers from any department
- Ability to retrieve information selectively and choose various formats for examining it
- Assistance with clinical application, including analysis tools, risk assessment, and clinical reminders
- Support for data collection in a manner that adequately supports health care providers' direct entry and stores information according to a defined vocabulary
- Easy access to client data, fast retrieval, and versatile data display that facilitates improved health care delivery
- Availability of a lifelong record of health-related events incorporating records from various settings and time periods

Adapted from *High Performance Computing and Communications FY 1997 Implementation Plan,* by National Coordination Office for Computing, Information, and Communications, 1996, Washington, DC: U.S. Government Printing Office.

give access to data across the continuum (regardless of setting) and capture useful information from both individual clients and population groups.

Current software programs allow nurses to quickly enter specific assessment data, fill in forms with typical entry choices, allow narrative for unique situations, have adequate computer memory for large amounts of data, and automatically transfer information to different reports. Computers also help generate nursing care plans and document all facets of client care.

Typical user interfaces (e.g., keyboard and monitor) require typing skills and can result in data entry errors. **Graphic user interfaces** (e.g., touch pads, mouse, and icons) are not well suited for nursing. Pen-based handwriting recognition or **automated speech-recognition** or voice-recognition technology may eventually become extremely effective for nursing documentation (Box 13-7). Handhelds or **personal digital assistants (PDAs)** have the potential to increase nursing productivity by providing access to clinical and reference material, providing a means to decrease medication errors, and reducing documentation time (Scordo, Yeager, & Young, 2003). Nurses can document at the bedside—at the point of care. **Point-of-care information systems** consist of PDAs that nurses carry to the bedside and a server computer located in the nursing station.

A complete **computer-based patient care record (CPCR)** is a comprehensive system that uses many components of data collection (Box 13-8). The CPCR permits the nurse to have an instrumental role in development of this form of documentation.

A number of **electronic health record (EHR)** initiatives are underway in Canada to support effective health care delivery (Canadian Nurses Association [CNA], 2002). An EHR is accessible online from many separate, interoperable automated systems within an electronic network (Health Canada, 2003). The distinguishing features of the EHR are that it is electronic, longitudinal, accessible, available to the client, and comprehensive (CNA, 2002).

There are legal risks associated with computerized documentation and initiatives like the EHR. Anyone could access a computer station within a hospital and gain information on any client. Confidentiality of access to computerized records is a major issue. Security requires the use of a password to enter and sign off computer files. The computer password must never be shared with anyone other than the person to whom it was assigned. A good system requires periodic changes in passwords to prevent unauthorized persons from tampering with records. In addition, most staff have access only to clients in their work area. Select staff may be given authority to access all client records.

Nurses need to know how to correct charting errors on a computer. As with any documentation method, data that have been part of the record are not deleted. Incorrect entries must be corrected, indicating who made the correction and when.

One of the challenges of computerized documentation is inclusion of the nursing process (Ammenwerth et al., 2001). There are important preconditions for the success of computer-based nursing process documentation, including a high acceptance of the nursing process, careful preparation of predefined care plans, organizational preparation, and inclusion of future users in the development process. It is also essential to have sufficient technical equipment with integration into the hospital information system.

The transition to computerized documentation presents both opportunities and challenges to nurses and nurse managers (Figure 13–7). The successful implementation of a computerized documentation system requires preparation, involvement, and commitment of the entire nursing staff. Tools for transforming existing documents into interactive interdisciplinary computerized forms have been developed. Some studies, however, have shown that during the transition when charting must be done on both paper and the computer, the time spent on documentation was not excessive (Korst, 2003).

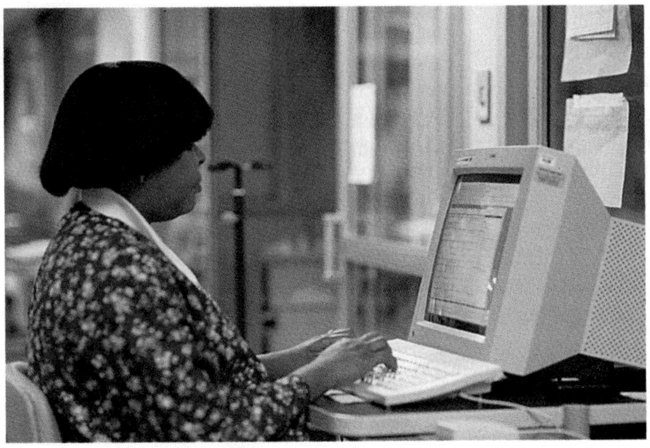

FIGURE **13–7** Computerized documentation systems can improve uniformity, accuracy, and retrievability of data.

Reporting

Nurses communicate information about clients so that all team members can make appropriate decisions about their care. Any verbal report must be timely, accurate, and relevant. Nurses make four types of reports—change-of-shift reports, telephone reports, transfer reports, and incident reports. Under certain circumstances, RNs can also receive telephone orders or verbal orders.

Change-of-Shift Reports

At the end of each shift, nurses report information about their assigned clients to the nurses working on the next shift. The purpose of the report is to provide continuity of care among nurses who are caring for a client. For example, if one nurse finds a certain pain-relief measure effective for a client, this information must be relayed to the next nurse caring for that client so that pain-control interventions can be continued.

A **change-of-shift report** may be given orally in person, by audiotape recording, by writing information on a summary report sheet, or during "walking-planning" rounds at each client's bedside. Oral reports can be given in conference rooms, with staff members from both shifts participating. Oral reports can also take the form of one-to-one reports given by the night nurse to the day nurse, for example. An advantage of oral reports is that they allow staff members to ask questions or clarify explanations. When nurses make rounds, the client and family members also have the opportunity to participate in any decisions. The nurses can see the client together to perform needed assessments, evaluate progress, and discuss the interventions best suited to the client's needs. An audiotape report is given by the nurse who has completed care for the client and is left for the nurse on the next shift to review. Taped reports can improve efficiency by being recorded before the end of the shift when time is available and by avoiding social conversations between peers. However, it is essential to schedule an opportunity for the oncoming nurses to ask questions for clarification after listening to the taped report.

Because of the many responsibilities nurses have to assume, change-of-shift reports must be conducted quickly and efficiently (Table 13-4). An effective report describes clients' health status and tells staff on the next shift exactly what kind of care they require. A change-of-shift report should *not* simply be a reading of documented information. Instead, significant facts about clients are reviewed (e.g., condition of wounds, episodes of chest pain) to provide a baseline for comparison during the next shift. Data about clients need to be objective, current, and concise.

An organized report follows a logical sequence. To prepare for the report, the nurse gathers information from work sheets, the client's records, and the care plan. A systematic approach, such as the nursing process, can provide staff with critical information. The following is an example of a change-of-shift report:

Background information: *Cy Tolan in bed 4, a 32-year-old client of Dr. Lang, is scheduled for a colon resection this morning. He has had ulcerative colitis for 2 years. He was admitted last night with slight abdominal discomfort. This is his first surgery. He knows he may require a colostomy.*

Assessment: *Mr. Tolan expressed difficulty falling asleep last night. He had several questions about surgery. Early in the night he called for assistance several times.*

Nursing diagnosis: *His chief nursing care problems are anxiety related to inexperience with surgery and risk for body image disturbance.*

Teaching plan: *He asks appropriate questions about surgery. Staff on evenings explained post-operative routines. I reinforced information with him early in the night. He stated that he felt less anxious.*

Treatments: *Cleansing enemas till clear were administered at 2100; no blood was noted in the return. He complained of some abdominal cramping immediately afterward, but that subsided. He received flurazepam 15 mg PO at 2330, and I gave him a back rub. He was awake at 0630 and stated he slept OK.*

Family information: *His wife remained with him last evening until the end of visiting hours. She has returned and is in the room this morning.*

Discharge plan: *Mr. Tolan is a very active person at home. He plays tennis and basketball and swims. Mrs. Tolan is concerned about how he might react to a colostomy. I suggest making a referral to the enterostomal therapist early, if the colostomy is performed.*

Priority needs: *Right now, Mr. Tolan is relaxing in his room. The operative consent has been signed. All preoperative procedures have been completed except for his preop medications, due on call to the operating room.*

When giving a report, nurses should use a professional demeanour. Since they often have to discuss clients, nurses, and family members in behavioural terms, they must avoid using judgmental language such as *unco-operative, difficult,* or *bad* when describing such behaviours.

In many settings, unregulated care providers (UCPs) are involved in the change-of-shift report. UCPs are part of the team and can contribute more when they also know a client's condition and the nursing team's priorities in care. The nurse can use the report to emphasize to UCPs the tasks to be done.

Table 13-4 Comparison of Do's and Don'ts of Change-of-Shift Report

Dos	Don'ts
Provide only essential background information about client (i.e., name, sex, age, physician's diagnosis, and medical history).	Don't review all routine care procedures or tasks (e.g., bathing, scheduled changes).
Identify client's nursing diagnoses or health care problems and their related causes.	Don't review all biographical information already available in written form.
Describe objective measurements or observations about client's condition and response to health problem, emphasize recent changes.	Don't use critical comments about client's behaviour, such as "Mrs. Wills is so demanding."
Share significant information about family members as it relates to client's problems.	Don't make assumptions about relationships between family members.
Continuously review ongoing discharge plan (e.g., need for resources, client's level of preparation to go home).	Don't engage in idle gossip.
Relay to staff significant changes in the way therapies are given (e.g., different position for pain relief, new medication).	Don't describe basic steps of a procedure.
Describe instructions given in teaching plan and client's response.	Don't explain detailed content unless staff members ask for clarification.
Evaluate results of nursing or medical care measures (e.g., effect of back rub or analgesic administration).	Don't simply describe results as "good" or "poor." Be specific.
Be clear about priorities to which oncoming staff must attend.	Don't force oncoming staff to guess what to do first

Telephone Reports

Nurses inform physicians of changes in a client's condition and communicate information to nurses on other units about client transfer. The laboratory staff or a radiologist may phone to report results of diagnostic tests. Telephone reports should provide clear, accurate, and concise information. Information in a telephone report is documented when significant events or changes in a client's condition have occurred. To document a phone call, the nurse includes when the call was made, who made it (if other than the writer of the information), who was called, to whom information was given, what information was given, and what information was received. For example, "At 1005 called Dr. Morgan's office; S. Thomas, RN, was informed that Mr. Rush's stat potassium level drawn at 0800 was 3.2. C. Skala, RN."

Transfer Reports

Clients may transfer from one unit to another to receive different levels of care. For example, clients transfer from an intensive care unit or the recovery room to general nursing units when they no longer require intense monitoring. To promote continuity of care, nurses may give **transfer reports** by phone or in person. When giving a transfer report, nurses include the following information:

- Client's name, age, primary physician, and medical diagnosis
- Summary of progress up to the time of transfer
- Current health status (physical and psychosocial)
- Allergies
- Emergency code status
- Family support
- Current nursing diagnoses or problem and care plan
- Any critical assessments or interventions to be completed shortly after transfer (helps receiving nurse to establish priorities of care)
- Need for any special equipment, such as isolation equipment, suction equipment, or traction

After completion of the transfer report, the receiving nurse needs an opportunity to ask questions about the client's status. In some cases, written documentation must include a record of information reported.

Incident Reports

An incident is any event that is not consistent with the routine operation of a health care unit or routine care of a client. Examples of incidents include client falls, needlestick injuries, a visitor having symptoms of illness, medication administration errors, accidental omission of ordered therapies, and circumstances that led to injury or risk for client injury. Analysis of **incident reports** (also known as adverse occurrence reports) helps with the identification of trends in systems and unit operations that justify changes in policies and procedures or the scheduling of in-service seminars. Incident reports are an important part of a unit's quality improvement program (see chapter 8).

Telephone or Verbal Orders

A telephone order (TO) involves a physician stating a prescribed therapy over the phone to an RN. A verbal order (VO) may be accepted when there is no opportunity for a physician to write the order, as in emergency situations. Clarifying for accuracy is important when an RN accepts physician's orders over the telephone or verbally. The order needs to be verified by repeating it clearly and precisely. The RN is responsible for writing the order on the physician's order sheet in the client's permanent record and signing it. An example follows: "1/16/2005 1920 acetaminophen 325 mg PO 2 tabs now and q4h prn. TO Dr. Reiss/Carol Skala, RN." The physician later verifies the TO legally by signing it within a set time period (e.g.,

Box 13-9 Guidelines for Telephone Orders and Verbal Orders

- Clearly determine the client's name, room number, and diagnosis.
- Repeat any prescribed orders back to the physician.
- Use clarification questions to avoid misunderstandings.
- Write telephone order (TO) or verbal order (VO), including date and time, name of client, the complete order; and sign the name of the physician and nurse.
- Follow agency policies; some institutions require telephone (and verbal) orders to be reviewed and signed by two nurses.
- The physician must co-sign the order within the time frame required by the institution (usually 24 hours).

24 hours). TOs are frequently given at night or during an emergency and need to be used only when absolutely necessary. In some situations, it may be prudent to have a second person listen to TOs. Box 13-9 provides guidelines that can be used to prevent errors in receiving telephone orders and verbal orders.

Key Concepts

- The medical record is a legal document and requires information describing the care that is delivered to a client.
- All information pertaining to a client's health care management that is gathered by examination, observation, conversation, or treatment is confidential.
- Multidisciplinary communication is essential within the health care team.
- Accurate record keeping requires an objective interpretation of data with precise measurements, correct spelling, and proper use of abbreviations.
- A nurse's signature on an entry in a record designates accountability for the contents of that entry.
- Any change in a client's condition warrants immediate documentation to keep a record accurate.
- Problem-oriented medical records are organized by the client's health care problems.
- The intent of SOAP, SOAPIE, PIE, or DAR charting is to organize entries in the progress notes according to the nursing process.
- Critical pathways or CareMaps provide members of the health care team with a way to document their contributions to the client's total plan of care.
- Home care documentation is accessible to a variety of caregivers in the home.
- Long-term care documentation is multidisciplinary and closely linked with fiscal requirements of governmental review.
- Computerized information systems provide information about clients in an organized and easily accessible fashion.
- The major purpose of the change-of-shift report is to maintain continuity of care.
- When information pertinent to care is communicated by telephone or verbally, the information needs to be verified.
- Incident reports objectively describe any event that is not consistent with the routine care of a client.

Key Terms

Acuity records, *p. 248*
Automated speech recognition, *p. 252*
CareMaps, *p. 244*
Change-of-shift report, *p. 253*
Charting by exception (CBE), *p. 241*
Computer-based patient care record (CPCR), *p. 252*
Consultations, *p. 235*
Critical pathways, *p. 244*
DAR, *p. 240*
Documentation, *p. 234*
Electronic health record (EHR), *p. 252*
Flow sheets, *p. 244*
Focus charting, *p. 240*
Graphic user interfaces, *p. 252*
Incident reports, *p. 254*
Kardex, *p. 248*
Personal digital assistants (PDAs), *p. 252*
PIE, *p. 240*
Point-of-care information systems, *p. 252*
Problem-oriented medical record (POMR), *p. 239*
Record, *p. 235*
Referrals, *p. 235*
Reports, *p. 235*
Residents, *p. 249*
SOAP, *p. 240*
SOAPIE, *p. 240*
Source record, *p. 240*
Standardized care plans, *p. 248*
Transfer report, *p. 254*
Variances, *p. 244*
Workload measurement systems, *p. 248*

Critical Thinking Exercises

1. Joseph Vojnovic is an 80-year-old man admitted with a diagnosis of possible pneumonia. He complains of general malaise and a frequent productive cough, worse at night. Vital signs are as follows: blood pressure 150/90 mm Hg; pulse rate 92 beats per minute; respirations 22 breaths per minute; and temperature 38.5° C. During your initial assessment, he coughs violently for 40 to 45 seconds without expectorating. His lungs have wheezes and coarse crackles at both bases. He states, "It hurts in my chest when I cough." Differentiate between objective and subjective data in this case example.
2. The nurse positions Mr. Vojnovic in a semi-Fowler's position, encourages increased fluid intake, and gives Tylenol 650 mg PO as ordered for fever. One hour later, the client is resting in bed. Vital signs are as follows: blood pressure 130/86 mm Hg; pulse 86 beats per minute; respirations 22 breaths per minute; and temperature 37.7° C. He states he has been able to sleep. His fluid intake has been 200 mL of water. Use the given information to write a nurse's progress note, using the PIE format.
3. Near the end of your shift, you have identified *fluid volume deficit* as a nursing diagnosis for Mr. Vojnovic. Since his admission he has had fluid intake of about 600 mL, and his urine output was 300 mL of dark, con-

centrated urine. His temperature is back up to 38.4° C, his mucous membranes are dry, and he states he feels very weak. List what should be included in the change-of-shift report.

4. Several days later, following treatment with intravenous antibiotics, Mr. Vojnovic is feeling much better and preparations are being made for discharge. He is to take Keflex 500 mg q6h for the next 10 days, continue to drink extra fluids, and get extra rest. He lives alone. Although he is generally co-operative, he does not like drinking water or taking pills. He is to make an appointment with his physician for 1 week from today and should call the physician if he develops symptoms of recurrence. Write a discharge summary that is concise and instructive.

Review Questions

1. Which of the following agencies or associations specify accreditation guidelines for documentation?
   1. Canadian Council on Health Services Accreditation (CCHSA)
   2. Canadian Nurses Association
   3. Canadian Provincial and Territorial Professional Associations
   4. Canadian Nurses Foundation
2. Which of the following statements is true about the use of abbreviations and documentation?
   1. Check the agency policy to see its approved list of abbreviations.
   2. Abbreviations save time for the reader.
   3. Abbreviations are not allowed in client records.
   4. Abbreviating as much as possible saves time for nurses.
3. Which of the following is the best example of effective documentation?
   1. Client's condition much improved from previous day
   2. Lesion on lower leg is red and weeping
   3. Codeine 30 mg po given for incisional pain (6/10) left hand
   4. No complaints of shortness of breath
4. Data recorded, reported, or communicated to other health care professionals are
   1. Public knowledge
   2. Available to all ancillary agencies
   3. Confidential and must be protected
   4. Available to all interested parties
5. Clients frequently request copies of their medical records. The nurse understands that
   1. Clients have the right to read those records
   2. Clients are not allowed to read those records
   3. Only the health care workers have access to the records
   4. Only the families may read the records
6. Critical pathways, or CareMaps, are care plans that
   1. Guide nursing care for all diseases
   2. Are used only by nurses
   3. Include key interventions and expected outcomes
   4. Are written by the physician
7. Acuity records are designed to
   1. Guide all nursing care
   2. Document the client admission
   3. Determine hours of care needed
   4. Establish guidelines for client care
8. Ideally, discharge planning begins
   1. At the time clients are preparing for discharge
   2. At admission
   3. After a diagnosis is made
   4. After acuity has been determined
9. In long-term care facilities, the client is referred to as a(n)
   1. Resident
   2. Occupant
   3. Patient
   4. Client
10. A telephone order involves
    1. A physician giving any health care worker an order via the phone
    2. No liability on the part of the nurse taking of a phone order
    3. Taking a physician's order only in an acute emergency
    4. Clarification, accuracy, and verification

References

Ammenwerth, E., et al. (2001). Nursing process documentation systems in clinical routine—Prerequisites and experiences. *International Journal of Medical Informatics, 64*(2–3), 187–200.

Brugh, L. A. (1998). Automated clinical pathways in the patient record: Legal implications. *Nursing Case Management, 3*(3), 131–137.

Canadian Nurses Association. (2002, April). Demystifying the electronic health record. *Nursing Now, 13*. Retrieved August 21, 2004 from *http://www.cna-urses.ca/_frames/issuestrends/issuestrendsframe.htm*

College of Nurses of Ontario. (2004). *Documentation*. Toronto, ON: Author.

Cummins, K. M, & Hill, M. T. (1999). Charting by exception, a timely format for you? *American Journal of Nursing, 99*(3), 24G–24J.

Health Canada. (2003). *Electronic health record*. Retrieved August 21, 2004, from *www.hc-sc.gc.ca/ohih-bsi/theme/ehr_dse/index_e .html*

Iyer, P. W., & Camp, N. H. (1999). *Nursing documentation: A nursing process approach*. St. Louis, MO: Mosby.

Karch, A. M. (2004). What's wrong with U? JCAHO places limits on abbreviations used in practice. *American Journal of Nursing, 104*(6), 65–66.

Korst, L. M. (2003). Nursing documentation time during implementation of an electronic medical record. *Journal of Nursing Administration, 33*(1), 24–30.

Martin, F. (1994). Documentation tips to help you stay out of court. *Nursing, 24*(6), 63–64.

National Coordination Office for Computing, Information, and Communications. (1996). *High performance computing and communications FY 1997 implementation plan*. Washington, DC: U.S. Government Printing Office.

Ottawa-Carleton Hospital. (2000). [Ottawa-Carleton Hospital patient care flow sheets and summaries]. Queensway-Carleton Campus, Nepean, ON: Author.

Scordo, K. A., Yeager, S., & Young, L. (2003). Use of personal digital assistants with acute care nurse practitioner students. *AACN Clinical Issues, 14*(3), 350–362.

Smith, L. S. (2000). How to use FOCUS charting. *Nursing, 30*(5), 76.

Sullivan, G. H. (2000). Keeping your charting on course. *RN, 63*(5), 75–80.

Yocum, R. F. (2002). Documenting for quality patient care. *Nursing, 32*(8), 58–63.

Recommended Web Sites

Canadian Council on Health Services Accreditation:
http://www.cchsa.ca

The Canadian Council on Health Services Accreditation (CCHSA) is a national, non-profit, independent organization whose role is to help health services organizations, across Canada and internationally, examine and improve the quality of care and service they provide to their clients.

Canadian Nurses Association: Provincial/Territorial Organizations:
http://www.cna-nurses.ca/_frames/aboutcna/ aboutusframe.html

This part of the Canadian Nurses Association Web site provides links to each provincial and territorial nursing association. Most associations provide information about documentation standards and requirements in their province or territory.

Canadian Nursing Informatics Association:
http://www .cnia.ca

The Canadian Nursing Informatics Association (CNIA) is an affiliate group of the Canadian Nurses Association and has been established to be the voice for health informatics in Canada. Nursing informatics refers to the integration of nursing science, computer science, and information science to document and communicate data and knowledge in nursing practice. This Web site provides links to sites featuring current research and educational initiatives in nursing informatics.

College of Nurses of Ontario (CNO):
http://www.cno.org/pubs/ compendium.html#comp

This site provides a link to the CNO publication, *Practice Standards: Documentation* (2004). Although written specifically for nurses in Ontario, many aspects of these practice standards are relevant to all Canadian nurses.

14

Communication

Joyce Larson, PhD, MS, RN
Nancy C. Goddard, RN, BScN, MN, PhD (Canadian author)

Objectives

Mastery of content in this chapter will enable the student to:

- Define the key terms listed.
- Describe aspects of critical thinking that are important to the communication process.
- Describe the five levels of communication and their uses in nursing.
- Describe the basic elements of the communication process.
- Identify significant features and therapeutic outcomes of nurse-client helping relationships.
- List nursing focus areas within the four phases of a nurse-client helping relationship.
- Identify significant features and desired outcomes of nurse-health team member relationships.
- Describe qualities, behaviours, and communication techniques that affect professional communication.
- Discuss effective communication techniques for clients at various developmental levels.
- Identify client health states that contribute to impaired communication.
- Discuss nursing care measures for clients with special communication needs.

Communication is a lifelong learning process for the nurse. Nurses make the intimate journey with clients and their families from the miracle of birth to the mystery of death. It is important to build therapeutic communications for this journey. Nurses must communicate effectively with people under stress. They must function as client advocates and as members of interdisciplinary teams who often have different priorities for client care. Nurses must also be able to communicate their own needs to avoid burnout and remain effective care providers (Balzer Riley, 2004). In the midst of competing demands and technological complexity, it is the intimate moment of connection that makes the difference in the quality of care and meaning of the illness experience for both the client and the nurse (Balzer Riley, 2004). Therefore, nurses must become competent in a variety of communication techniques in order to develop and maintain effective relationships. The Conference Board of Canada considers communication and interpersonal relationship skills to be critical factors for successful employment (Devito, Shimoni, & Clark, 2005). Failure to effectively communicate may lead to poor client outcomes such as increased pain and suffering and may increase liability and decrease professional credibility.

The qualities, behaviours, and therapeutic communication techniques described in this chapter characterize professionalism in helping relationships. Although the term *client* is often used, the same principles can be applied when communicating with any person, in any nursing situation.

Communication and Interpersonal Relationships

At the core of nursing are therapeutic interpersonal relationships based on caring, mutual respect, and dignity. Communication is the means to establish these helping-healing relationships. Because all behaviour communicates, and all communication influences behaviour, nurses must become experts in communication if they are to be effective care providers.

The nurse's ability to relate to others—establishing and maintaining a relationship, being authentic, and responding appropriately—is a crucial aspect of interpersonal communication. Good interpersonal communication also requires the nurse to develop a sense of mutuality, a belief that the nurse-client relationship is a partnership and that both are equal participants. Nurses must honour the fact that people are complex and ambiguous beings. Often, more is communicated than at first apparent, and client responses are not always what the nurse might expect. It is helpful for the nurse to purposefully focus on positive intentions for the other person and to use the technique of re-imagining a possible future (Hartrick, 1997) so that a vision of hope and better health can be shared. For example, a client who has had a heart attack can be provided with an opportunity to develop an intention to improve health by choosing healthy behaviours like stress-reducing activities, an exercise regimen, and improved dietary habits.

A new perspective of human relationships suggests that energy fields permeate and connect all beings. Although the idea of using energy to heal has recently re-emerged in the West, it has long been present in Eastern cultures. Healers in Eastern and primitive cultures often focused on the concept of balancing energy within each human being to maintain health (Minor, 2001). Therefore, it is not surprising that nurses often perceive a strong sense of connection to others within helping relationships. Nurses know that attitudes and emotions are easily transmitted. Every nuance of posture, every small expression and gesture, every word chosen, every attitude held—all have the potential to hurt or heal through the exchange of human energy. Knowing that intention and behaviour directly influence human energy fields, and therefore health, gives nurses tremendous ethical responsibility to do no harm to those entrusted to their care. Communication must be respected for its potential power and not carelessly misused to hurt, manipulate, or coerce others. Good communication empowers others and enables people to know themselves and make their own choices, an essential aspect of the healing process. Nurses have tremendous opportunity to bring about good things for themselves, their clients, and their colleagues through this kind of therapeutic communication.

Developing Communication Skills

Gaining expertise in communication requires an understanding of the communication process and reflection about one's personal communication experiences. Nurses who have developed good critical thinking skills are the best communicators. They can draw from theoretical knowledge about communication and integrate this knowledge with what has been learned through personal experience. They can interpret messages received from others, analyze their content, make inferences about their meaning, evaluate their effect, explain rationale for communication techniques used, and self-examine personal communication skills (Creasia & Parker, 2001).

Other qualities of critical thinking also matter to the communication process. Critical thinking characteristics provide guidelines for how to approach a problem. These characteristics include curiosity, perseverance, creativity, self-confidence, independence, fairness, integrity, and humility. Curiosity motivates the nurse to learn more about a person, and clients are more likely to communicate with nurses who express an interest in them. Perseverance and creativity are also conducive to communication because they help the nurse identify innovative solutions. Self-confidence is important because the nurse who demonstrates confidence can more readily establish interpersonal helping-trust relationships and convey competence in the professional role. A sense of independence permits the nurse to communicate with colleagues and share ideas about nursing interventions. Such an attitude sometimes involves risk taking because colleagues may question the suggested nursing interventions. At the same time, an attitude of fairness enables the nurse to listen to both sides in any discussion. Nurses with integrity are able to recognize when their opinions conflict with those of the client, review positions objectively, and decide how to communicate to reach mutually beneficial decisions. Furthermore, humility is necessary to recognize and communicate the need for more information before a decision can be made (Paul, 1993).

Interpersonal communication may be challenging because it is based on an individual's **perception** of received information and is therefore subject to misinterpretation. Perception is based on information acquired through the five senses of sight, hearing, taste, touch, and smell (Stuart & Laraia, 2001). It is a function of the mind, a process of organizing and interpreting sensory information to arrive at a meaningful conclusion. An individual's culture, education, and personal background also influence perception. Critical thinking can help the nurse overcome **perceptual biases,** human tendencies that interfere with accurately perceiving and interpreting messages from others. People often assume that others would think, feel, act, react, and behave as they would in similar circumstances. They tend to distort or ignore information that goes against their expectations, preconceptions, or stereotypes (Beebe et al., 2004). By thinking critically about personal communication habits, the nurse can learn to control these tendencies and become more effective in interpersonal relationships.

As communication skills develop, the nurse's competence in the nursing process also grows. Communication skills must be integrated throughout the nursing process as nurses collaborate with clients and health team members to achieve goals (Box 14-1). Nurses use communication skills to gather, analyze, and transmit information and to accomplish the work of each step of the process. Assessment, diagnosis, planning, implementation, and

Box 14-1 Communication Throughout the Nursing Process

Assessment

Verbal interviewing and history taking
Visual and intuitive observation of non-verbal behaviour
Visual, tactile, and auditory data gathering during physical examination
Written medial records, diagnostic tests, and literature review

Nursing Diagnosis

Intrapersonal analysis of assessment findings
Validation of health care needs and priorities via verbal discussion with client
Handwritten or computer-mediated documentation of nursing diagnosis

Planning

Interpersonal or small-group health team planning sessions
Interpersonal collaboration with client and family to determine implementation methods
Written documentation of expected outcomes
Written or verbal referral to health team members

Implementation

Delegation and verbal discussion with health care team
Verbal, visual, auditory, and tactile health teaching activities
Provision of support via therapeutic communication techniques
Contact with other health resources
Written documentation of client's progress in medical record

Evaluation

Acquisition of verbal and non-verbal feedback
Comparison of actual and expected outcomes
Identification of factors affecting outcomes
Modification and update of care plan
Verbal and/or written explanation of revisions of care plan to client

evaluation all depend on effective communication among nurse, client, family, and others on the health care team. Although the nursing process is a reliable framework for client care, it will not work well unless the nurse masters the art of effective interpersonal communication.

The nature of the communication process requires nurses to constantly make decisions about what, when, where, why, and how to convey messages to others. The nurse's decision making is always contextual—the unique features of any situation influence the nature of the decisions made. For example, the explanation of the importance of following a prescribed diet to a client with a newly diagnosed medical condition will differ from the explanation to a client who has repeatedly chosen not to follow diet restrictions.

Throughout this chapter, brief clinical examples guide students in the use of effective communication techniques. Many situations present communication challenges. For example, some clients may not express their feelings or needs, others may have cognitive or physical disabilities that impair speech, and some may speak very little English. Because the best way to acquire skill is through practice, it is useful for students to discuss and role-play these scenarios before experiencing them in the clinical setting. Consider that clients, family, nurse colleagues, unregulated care providers, physicians, or other health team members might be involved and decide which communication techniques might be most effective.

Levels of Communication

Nurses use different levels of communication in their professional role. The nurse's communication skills need to include techniques that reflect competence in each level.

Interpersonal Communication

Interpersonal communication is one-to-one interaction between the nurse and another person that often occurs face to face. It is the level most frequently used in nursing situations and lies at the heart of nursing practice. It takes place within a social context and includes all the symbols and cues used to give and receive meaning.

Because meaning resides in people and not in words, messages received may be different from messages intended. Nurses work with people who have different opinions, experiences, values, and belief systems, so meaning must be validated or mutually negotiated between participants. Meaningful interpersonal communication results in exchange of ideas, problem solving, expression of feelings, decision making, goal accomplishment, team building, and personal growth.

Transpersonal Communication

Transpersonal communication is interaction that occurs within a person's spiritual domain. Many people use prayer, meditation, guided reflection, religious rituals, or other means to communicate with their "higher power." Nurses who value the importance of human spirituality often use this form of communication with clients and for themselves.

Small-Group Communication

Small-group communication is interaction that occurs when a small number of people meet together and share a common purpose. This type of communication is usually goal directed and requires an understanding of group dynamics. When nurses work on committees, lead client support groups, form research teams, or participate in client care conferences, a small-group communication process is used. Darley (2002) suggested two principles to ensure effective communication and working relationships between people in any group: respecting people as partners and listening actively to the other people in the group.

Intrapersonal Communication

Intrapersonal communication is a powerful form of communication that occurs within an individual. It is communication with oneself, also known as self-talk, and is exemplified in one's thinking (Beebe et al., 2004).

People's thoughts strongly influence perceptions, feelings, behaviour, and self-concept. Intrapersonal communication creates a set of conditions through which life is experienced. Nurses should be aware of the nature and content of their own thinking and try to replace negative, self-defeating thoughts with positive assertions. Positive self-talk can be used as a tool to improve health and self-esteem, both for the nurse and the client. For example, guided imagery can be used to enhance coping and reduce stress (see chapter 26). Self-instruction can provide a mental rehearsal for difficult tasks or situations. Nurses and clients can use intrapersonal communication to develop self-awareness and a positive self-concept that will enhance appropriate self-expression.

Public Communication

Public communication is interaction with an audience. Nurses have opportunities to speak with groups of consumers about health-related topics, present scholarly work to colleagues at conferences, or lead classroom discussions with peers or students. Public communication requires special adaptations in eye contact, gestures, voice inflection, and use of media materials to communicate messages effectively. Effective public communication increases audience knowledge about health-related topics, health issues, and other issues important to the nursing profession.

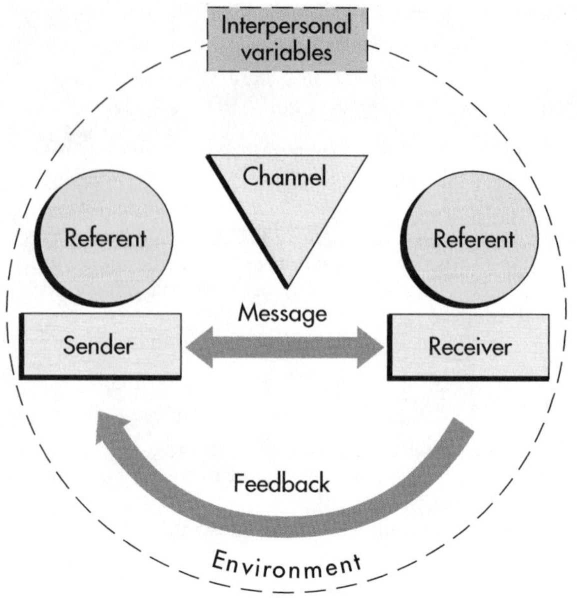

FIGURE **14–1** Communication is an active process between sender and receiver.

Basic Elements of the Communication Process

Communication is an ongoing, dynamic, and multidimensional process. Its basic elements are shown in Figure 14–1 and described in the following paragraphs. Nursing situations have many unique aspects that influence the nature of communication and interpersonal relationships. Nurses must use critical thinking to focus on each aspect of communication so that interactions can be purposeful and effective.

Referent

The **referent** motivates one person to communicate with another. In a health care setting, sights, sounds, odours, time schedules, messages, objects, emotions, sensations, perceptions, ideas, and other cues initiate communication. The nurse who knows the stimulus that initiated communication is able to develop and organize messages more efficiently and better perceive meaning in another's message. A client request for help prompted by difficulty breathing brings a different nursing response than a request prompted by boredom.

Sender and Receiver

The **sender** is the person who encodes and delivers the message, and the **receiver** is the person who receives and decodes the message. The sender puts ideas or feelings into a form that can be transmitted and is responsible for accuracy and emotional tone. The sender's message acts as a referent for the receiver, who is responsible for attending to, translating, and responding to the sender's message. Sender and receiver roles change back and forth as people interact; sending and receiving may even occur simultaneously. The more the sender and receiver have in common and the closer the relationship, the more likely they will accurately perceive one another's meaning and respond accordingly.

Messages

The **message** is the content of the communication. It may contain verbal, non-verbal, and symbolic language. Messages are interpreted by those who receive them through personal perceptions that may or may not distort the meaning intended by the sender. Two nurses can provide the same information yet convey very different messages according to their personal communication styles. One nurse can send the same message to two people and be understood differently by each. Nurses can send effective messages by expressing themselves clearly, directly, and in a manner familiar to the receiver. Watching the listener for non-verbal cues that suggest confusion or misunderstanding helps the nurse know whether the message needs to be clarified. Communication can be difficult when participants have different levels of education and experience. "Your incision is well approximated without purulent drainage," means the same as "Your wound edges are together, and there are no signs of infection," but clients better understand the latter message. The nurse must be sure clients can read before sending messages in writing.

Channels

Channels are means of conveying and receiving messages through visual, auditory, and tactile senses. Facial expressions send visual messages, spoken words travel through auditory channels, and touch uses tactile channels. The more channels the sender uses to convey a message, the more clearly it is usually understood. For example, when teaching about insulin self-injection, the nurse talks about and demonstrates the technique, gives the client printed information, and encourages hands-on practice with the vial and syringe. Nurses use verbal, non-verbal, and mediated (technological) communication channels. They send and receive information in person, by informal or formal writing, over the telephone or pager, by audiotape and videotape, through fax and electronic mail, and through computer-interactive and information sites.

Feedback

Feedback is the message returned by the receiver. It indicates whether the meaning of the sender's message was understood. Senders need to seek verbal and non-verbal feedback to ensure that good communication has occurred. To be effective, the sender and receiver must be sensitive and open to each other's messages, clarify the messages, and modify behaviour accordingly. In a social relationship, both people assume equal responsibility for seeking openness and clarification, but the nurse assumes primary responsibility in the nurse-client relationship.

Interpersonal Variables

Interpersonal variables are factors within both the sender and receiver that influence communication. Perception is one such variable; each person's view of reality is unique and formed by his or her expectations and experiences. People sense, interpret, and understand events differently. A nurse might say, "You have been very quiet since your family left. Is there something on your mind?" One client might perceive the nurse's question as showing caring and concern; another might perceive the nurse as being intrusive. Other interpersonal variables include educational and developmental levels, socio-cultural backgrounds, values and beliefs, emotions, gender, physical health status, and roles and relationships. Variables associated with illness, such as pain, anxiety, and medication effects, can also affect nurse-client communication.

Environment

The **environment** is the setting for sender-receiver interaction. For effective communication, the environment should meet participant needs for physical and emotional comfort and safety. Noise, temperature extremes, distractions, and lack of privacy or space may create confusion, tension, and discomfort. Environmental distractions are common in health care settings and can interfere with messages sent between people; therefore, nurses must try to control the environment as much as possible to create favourable conditions for effective communication.

Forms of Communication

Messages are conveyed verbally, non-verbally, and symbolically. As people communicate, they express themselves through words, movements, voice inflection, facial expressions, and use of space. These elements can work in harmony to enhance a message or conflict with one another to contradict and confuse it.

Verbal Communication

Verbal communication uses spoken or written words. Verbal language is a code that conveys specific meaning as words are combined. The most important aspects of verbal communication are discussed below.

Vocabulary. Communication is unsuccessful if senders and receivers cannot translate each other's words and phrases. When a nurse cares for a client who speaks another language, an interpreter may be necessary. Even those who speak the same language use subcultural variations of certain words: *dinner* may mean a noon meal to one person and the last meal of the day to another. Medical jargon (technical terminology used by health care providers) may sound like a foreign language to clients and should be used only with other health team members. Children may use special words to describe bodily functions or a favourite blanket or toy. Teenagers often use words in unique ways that are unfamiliar to adults.

Denotative and Connotative Meaning. A single word can have several meanings. Individuals who use a common language share the denotative meaning: *baseball* has the same meaning for everyone who speaks English, but *code* denotes cardiac arrest primarily to health care providers. The connotative meaning is the shade or interpretation of a word's meaning influenced by the thoughts, feelings, or ideas people have about the word. Families who are told a loved one is in serious condition may believe that death is near, but to nurses *serious* may simply describe the nature of the illness. Nurses should carefully select words that cannot be easily misinterpreted, especially when explaining a client's medical condition or therapy. Even a much-used phrase such as "I'm going to take your vital signs" can be unfamiliar to an adult or frightening to a child.

Pacing. Conversation is more successful at an appropriate speed or pace. Nurses should speak slowly enough to enunciate clearly. Talking rapidly, using awkward pauses, or speaking slowly and deliberately can convey an unintended message. Long pauses and rapid shifts to another subject may give the impression that the nurse is hiding the truth. Pacing is improved by thinking before speaking and by developing awareness of the cadence of one's speech.

Intonation. Tone of voice dramatically affects a message's meaning. Depending on intonation, even a simple question or statement can express enthusiasm, anger, concern, or indifference. The nurse must be aware of voice tone to avoid sending unintended messages. For example, clients may interpret a nurse's tone of voice as condescending, and further communication may be inhibited. A client's voice tone often provides information about his or her emotional state or energy level.

Clarity and Brevity. Effective communication is simple, brief, and direct. Fewer words result in less confusion. Clarity is achieved by speaking slowly, enunciating clearly, and using examples to make explanations easier to understand. Repeating important parts of a message also clarifies communication. Phrases such as "you know" or "OK?" at the end of every sentence detract from clarity. Brevity is achieved by using short sentences and words that express an idea simply and directly. "Where is your pain?" is much better than "I would like you to describe for me the location of your discomfort."

Timing and Relevance. Timing is critical in communication. Even though a message is clear, poor timing can limit its effectiveness. For example, the nurse should not begin routine teaching when a client is in severe pain, emotional distress, or distracted by pressing matters. Often the best time for interaction is when a client expresses an interest in communicating. If messages are relevant or important to the situation at hand, they are more effective. When a client is facing emergency surgery, discussing the risks of smoking is less relevant than explaining perioperative procedures.

Non-Verbal Communication

Non-verbal communication includes all five senses and everything that does not involve the spoken or written word. It has been estimated that approximately 7% of meaning is transmitted by words, 38% is transmitted by vocal cues, and 55% is transmitted by body cues. Non-verbal communication serves a variety of purposes. It can be used to accent, complement, contradict, regulate, repeat, or substitute for verbal messages (Devito et al., 2005). Non-verbal messages may be sent intentionally or unintentionally and are multi-channelled (Falikowski, 1996). Non-verbal communication is often subconsciously motivated and therefore may express intended meaning more accurately than spoken words (Stuart & Laraia, 2001). When there is incongruity between verbal and non-verbal communication, the receiver usually "hears" the non-verbal message as the true message.

All kinds of non-verbal communication are important, but interpreting them can be difficult. Sociocultural background is a major influence on the meaning of non-verbal behaviour. Non-verbal messages between people of different cultures can easily be misinterpreted. Because the interpretation of non-verbal behaviour is subjective, it is important to check its perceived meaning (Adler, Towne, & Rolls, 2001). There are many kinds of non-verbal behaviour.

Personal Appearance. Personal appearance includes physical characteristics, facial expression, manner of dress and grooming, and adornments. These factors help communicate physical well-being, personality, social status, occupation, religion, culture, and self-concept. First impressions are largely based on appearance. Nurses learn to develop a general impression of client health and emotional status through appearance, and clients develop a general impression of the nurse's professionalism and caring in the same way.

Posture and Gait. Posture and gait are forms of self-expression. The way people sit, stand, and move reflects attitudes, emotions, self-concept, and health status. For example, an erect posture and a quick, purposeful gait communicate a sense of well-being and confidence. Leaning forward conveys attention. A slumped posture and slow shuffling gait may indicate depression, illness, discomfort, or fatigue.

Facial Expression. The face is the most expressive part of the body. Facial expressions convey emotions such as surprise, fear, anger, happiness, and sadness. Some people have an expressionless face, or flat affect, which reveals little about what they are thinking or feeling. An inappropriate affect is a facial expression that does not match the content of a verbal message, for example, smiling when describing a sad situation. People can be unaware of the messages their expressions convey. For example, a nurse may frown in concentration while doing a procedure and the client may interpret this as anger or disapproval. Clients often closely observe nurses. Consider the impact a nurse's facial expression might have on a person who asks, "Am I going to die?" The slightest change in the eyes, lips, or facial muscles can reveal the nurse's feelings. Although it is hard to control all facial expression, the nurse should try to avoid showing shock, disgust, dismay, or other distressing reactions in the client's presence.

Eye Contact. People signal readiness to communicate through eye contact. Maintaining eye contact during conversation shows respect and willingness to listen. Eye contact also allows people to closely observe one another. Lack of eye contact may indicate anxiety, defensiveness, discomfort, or lack of confidence in communicating. However, people from Asian or some Aboriginal cultures may consider eye contact intrusive, threatening, or harmful and minimize or avoid its use. Looking down on a person establishes authority, whereas interacting at the same eye level indicates equality in the relationship. Rising to the same eye level of an angry person helps establish one's autonomy.

Gestures. Gestures emphasize, punctuate, and clarify the spoken word. Gestures alone carry specific meanings, or they may create messages with other communication cues. A finger pointed toward a person may communicate several meanings, but when accompanied by a frown and stern voice, the gesture becomes an accusation or threat. Pointing to an area of pain may be more accurate than describing the pain's location.

Sounds. Sounds such as sighs, moans, groans, or sobs also communicate feelings and thoughts. Combined with other non-verbal communication, sounds help send clear messages. Sounds can be interpreted in several ways: Moaning can convey pleasure or suffering, and crying can communicate happiness, sadness, or anger. The nurse must validate such non-verbal messages with the client to interpret them accurately.

Territoriality and Personal Space. Territoriality is the need to gain, maintain, and defend one's right to space. Territory is important because it provides people with a sense of identity, security, and control. Territory can be separated and made visible to others, such as a fence around a yard or a bed in a hospital room. Personal space

Box 14-2 Zones of Personal Space and Touch

Zones of Personal Space

Intimate zone (0 to 45 cm)
Holding a crying infant
Performing physical assessment
Bathing, grooming, dressing, feeding, and toileting a client
Changing a client's dressing
Personal zone (45 cm to 1 metre)
Sitting at a client's bedside
Taking the client's nursing history
Teaching an individual client
Exchanging information at change of shift
Social zone (1 to 4 metres)
Participating in client care rounds
Sitting at the head of a conference table
Teaching a class for clients with diabetes
Conducting a family support group
Public zone (4 metres and greater)
Speaking at a community forum
Testifying at a legislative hearing
Lecturing to a class of students

Zones of Touch

Social zone (permission not needed)
Hands, arms, shoulders, back
Consent zone (permission needed)
Mouth, wrists, feet
Vulnerable zone (special care needed)
Face, neck, front of body
Intimate zone (great sensitivity needed)
Genitalia, rectum

is invisible, individual, and travels with the person. During interpersonal interaction, people maintain varying distances between each other depending on their culture, the nature of their relationship, and the situation. When personal space becomes threatened, people respond defensively and communicate less effectively. Situations dictate whether the interpersonal distance between nurse and client is appropriate. Examples of nursing actions within zones of personal space are listed in Box 14-2, along with zones of touch. Nurses frequently move into clients' territory and personal space because of the nature of caregiving. The nurse must convey confidence, gentleness, and respect for privacy, especially when actions require intimate contacts or involve a client's vulnerable zone.

Symbolic Communication

Good communication requires awareness of **symbolic communication,** the verbal and non-verbal symbolism used by others to convey meaning. Art and music are forms of symbolic communication that nurse can use to enhance understanding and promote healing. Dreams, drawings, metaphorical language, a child's play, and even the symptoms of illness are all symbolic forms of self-expression that have rich messages for health care providers (Seigel, 1989).

Metacommunication

Metacommunication is an essential ingredient of effective interpersonal interaction. It is communication *about* communication and includes all of the factors that contribute to how a message is perceived by others (Arnold & Boggs, 2003). Metacommunication reflects the relational aspects of communication (Adler et al., 2001) and can help people better understand what they have communicated. For example, the nurse observes a young client holding his body rigidly erect and his voice is sharp as he says, "Going to surgery is no big deal." The nurse replies, "You say having surgery doesn't bother you, but you look and sound tense. I'd like to help." This is metacommunication, and it may result in further exploration of the client's feelings and concerns.

Professional Nursing Relationships

Professional relationships are created through the nurse's application of knowledge, understanding of human behaviour and communication, and commitment to ethical behaviour. Having a philosophy based on caring and respect for others will help the nurse be more successful in establishing relationships of this nature.

Nurse-Client Helping Relationships

Helping relationships are the foundations of clinical nursing practice. In such relationships, the nurse assumes the role of professional helper and comes to know the client as an individual who has unique health needs, human responses, and patterns of living. The relationship is therapeutic, promoting a psychological climate that facilitates positive change and growth. The nurse's therapeutic use of communication is the mechanism by which clients can achieve successful outcomes for the problems currently preventing them from achieving optimum health (Fortinash & Holoday-Worret, 2000). There is an explicit time frame, a goal-directed approach, and a high expectation of confidentiality. The nurse establishes, directs, and takes responsibility for the interaction, and the client's needs take priority over the nurse's needs. The relationship is also characterized by the nurse's non-judgmental acceptance of the client. Acceptance conveys a willingness to hear a message or to acknowledge feelings. It does not mean the nurse must always agree with the client or approve of the client's decisions or actions. A helping relationship between nurse and client does not just happen—it is created with care and skill and is built on the client's trust in the nurse.

The nurse-client relationship is characterized by a natural progression of four goal-directed phases: pre-interaction, orientation, working, and termination phases (Box 14-3). These phases may begin before the nurse meets the client and continue until the caregiving relationship ends. Even a brief interaction displays an abbreviated version of these phases. For example, the student nurse may gather client information to prepare in advance for caregiving, meet the client and establish trust, accomplish health-related goals through use of the nursing process, and say goodbye at the end of the day.

Socializing is an important initial component of interpersonal communication. It helps people get to know one another and relax. It is easy, superficial, and not deeply personal, whereas therapeutic interactions are often more intense, difficult, and uncomfortable. A nurse often uses social conversation to lay a foundation for a closer relationship: "Hi, Mr. Simpson. I hear it's your birthday today. Happy birthday!" A friendly, informal, and warm communication style helps establish trust, but nurses must get beyond social conversation to talk about issues or concerns affecting the client's health. During social conversation, clients may ask personal questions about the nurse's family, place of residence, and so forth. Students often wonder whether it is appropriate to reveal such information. The skilful nurse uses judgment about what to share and provides minimal information or deflects such questions with gentle humour and refocuses conversation back to the client.

Creating a therapeutic environment depends on the nurse's ability to communicate, comfort, and help clients meet their needs. Comfort has been acknowledged as a critical value inherent in the practice of nursing. Hawley (2000) identified comforting strategies from the perspective of emergency department clients. Participants described nurses' comforting strategies under the following categories: competent and immediate technical/physical care, positive talk, vigilance, attention to physical discomforts, and attending to family. The comforting strategies used by nurses resulted in the clients feeling safe, secure, cared about, more relaxed, and better able to cope with pain and the unknown.

In a therapeutic relationship, nurses often encourage clients to share personal stories, which are called narrative interactions. Through narrative interactions, nurses begin to understand the context of others' lives and learn what is meaningful for them from their perspective (Canales, 1997). For example, a nurse asked a client to tell about a time in his life when he had to make a hard decision. The client related the following story:

> *When I was a young man, I worked on the family farm. An uncle died and left me some money. All of a sudden, I could afford to go to college, but Dad didn't want me to go because he needed me there. I had to decide whether to stay or go, and it was real hard, because at first I just wanted to get away. I talked to our preacher, and he said it was up to me, to pray about it and do what my heart told me to. So I stayed. Oh, I've thought from time to time what I might have made of myself, but I never regretted it. I had a good life in farming.*

From this brief story, the nurse understood that it was important to the client to put his family's needs above his personal desires and that seeking spiritual guidance was an important component of his decision making. This same information may not have been revealed had the

Box 14-3 Phases of the Helping Relationship

Pre-interaction Phase

Before meeting the client, the nurse:
- Reviews available data, including the medical and nursing history
- Talks to other caregivers who may have information about the client
- Anticipates health concerns or issues that may arise
- Identifies a location and setting that will foster comfortable, private interaction
- Plans enough time for the initial interaction

Orientation Phase

When the nurse and client meet and get to know one another, the nurse:
- Sets the tone for the relationship by adopting a warm, empathetic, caring manner
- Recognizes that the initial relationship may be superficial, uncertain, and tentative
- Expects the client to test the nurse's competence and commitment
- Closely observes the client and expects to be closely observed by the client
- Begins to make inferences and form judgments about client messages and behaviours
- Assesses the client's health status
- Prioritizes the client's problems and identifies the client's goals
- Clarifies the client's and nurse's roles
- Forms contracts with the client that specify who will do what
- Lets the client know when to expect the relationship to be terminated

Working Phase

When the nurse and client work together to solve problems and accomplish goals, the nurse:
- Encourages and helps the client to express feelings about his or her health
- Encourages and helps the client with self-exploration
- Provides information needed to understand and change behaviour
- Encourages and helps the client to set goals
- Takes actions to meet the goals set with the client
- Uses therapeutic communication skills to facilitate successful interactions
- Uses appropriate self-disclosure and confrontation

Termination Phase

During the ending of the relationship, the nurse:
- Reminds the client that termination is near
- Evaluates goal achievement with the client
- Reminisces about the relationship with the client
- Separates from the client by relinquishing responsibility for his or her care
- Achieves a smooth transition for the client to other caregivers as needed

nurse used a standard history form that usually only elicits short answers.

The nurse and client work as a team in a helping relationship. The nurse offers clients the opportunity to make choices, even as simple as choosing a bath time or whether to take a pain medication (as needed). The nurse also acts as an advocate to keep the client informed of health care alternatives and give support in decision making.

A good way to encourage client autonomy is to collaborate with others. For example, the nurse can ask clients and family members for input and suggestions about goals, interventions, and evaluation of the plan of care. Collaboration builds relationships and is based on principles of mutual gain and respect. It reflects a desire to satisfy the needs of both parties (Dubrin & Geerinck, 2002). Collaborative communication promotes personal responsibility, permits self-expression, and strengthens the client's problem-solving ability. Research has shown that successful collaboration requires an active and committed involvement by both client and nurse and a joint effort toward problem solving. Such a relationship will enhance the client's well-being and the nurse's feeling of success (Paavilainen & Astedt-Kurki, 1997).

Nurse-Family Relationships

Many nursing situations, especially those in community and home care settings, require the nurse to form helping relationships with entire families. The same principles that guide one-to-one helping relationships also apply when the client is a family unit—although communication within families requires additional understanding of the complexities of family dynamics, needs, and relationships (see chapter 16).

Nurse-Health Team Relationships

Nurses function in roles that require interaction with multiple health team members. Many elements of the nurse-client helping relationship are also applied in these collegial relationships, which are focused on accomplishing the work and goals of the clinical setting. Communication in such relationships may be geared toward team building, facilitating group process, collaboration, consultation, delegation, supervision, leadership, and management (see chapter 10). A variety of communication skills are needed, including presentational speaking, persuasion, group problem solving, providing performance reviews, and writing business reports.

Social and therapeutic interactions are needed between the nurse and health team members to build morale and strengthen relationships within the work setting. Everyone has interpersonal needs for acceptance, inclusion, identity, privacy, power and control, and affection (Stewart & Logan, 1998). Nurses need friendship, support, guidance, and encouragement from one another to cope with the many stressors imposed by the nursing role and must extend the same caring communication used with clients to build positive relationships with colleagues and co-workers.

Nurse-Community Relationships

Many nurses form relationships with community groups by participating in local organizations, volunteering for community service, or becoming politically active. Nurses in a community-based practice must be able to establish relationships with their community to be effective change agents (see chapter 4). Communication within the community occurs through channels such as neighbourhood newsletters, public bulletin boards, newspapers, radio, television, and electronic information sites. Nurses can use these forms of communication to share information and discuss issues important to community health.

Elements of Professional Communication

Professional appearance, demeanour, and behaviour are important in establishing the nurse's trustworthiness and competence. They communicate that the nurse has assumed the professional helping role, is clinically skilled, and is focused on the client. Inappropriate appearance or behaviour harms one's professional image.

A professional is expected to be clean, neat, well-groomed, conservatively dressed, and scent and odour free. Professional behaviour should reflect warmth, friendliness, confidence, and competence. Professionals speak in a clear well-modulated voice, use good grammar, listen to others, help and support colleagues, and communicate effectively. Being on time, organized, well-prepared, and equipped for the responsibilities of the nursing role also communicate one's professionalism.

Courtesy

Common courtesy is part of professional communication. To practice courtesy, the nurse says hello and goodbye, knocks on doors before entering, and uses self-introduction. Nurses also state their purpose, address people by name, say please and thank you to team members, and apologize for inadvertently making an error or causing someone distress. Being discourteous is rude and insensitive. It sets up barriers between nurse and client and causes friction among team members.

Use of Names

Self-introduction is important. The nurse's failure to give a name, indicate status (e.g., registered nurse or licensed practical nurse), or acknowledge the client can create uncertainty about the interaction and convey lack of commitment or caring. Making eye contact and smiling at others gives them recognition. Addressing others by name conveys respect for human dignity and uniqueness. Because using last names is respectful in most cultures, nurses should use the client's last name in the initial interaction, but may later use the first name if requested to do so by the client. The nurse should ask others how they would like to be addressed. Using first names is appropriate for infants, young children, and close team members. Do not use terms of endearment such as "honey," "dear," "Grandma," or "sweetheart." Do not refer to clients by diagnosis, room number, or other attribute (e.g., "the cancer client in Room 118"). Not using proper names is demeaning and sends the message that the nurse does not care enough to know the person as an individual.

Privacy and Confidentiality

Maintaining confidentiality is an important aspect of professional behaviour. The nurse must safeguard the client's right to privacy by carefully protecting information of a sensitive, private nature (see chapter 8). Sharing personal information or gossiping about others violates nursing ethical codes and practice standards. It sends the message that the nurse cannot be trusted and damages interpersonal relationships. Team members directly involved in the client's care should be given only relevant information about the client's status. Respect for clients is demonstrated when the nurse treats them with dignity and maintains their physical and emotional privacy.

Trustworthiness

Trust is relying on someone without doubt or question. Being trustworthy means helping others without hesitation when needed. To foster trust, the nurse communicates warmth and demonstrates consistency, reliability, honesty, integrity, and competence. Sometimes it is not easy for a client to ask for help. Trusting another person involves risk and vulnerability, but it also fosters open, therapeutic communication and enhances the expression of feelings, thoughts, and needs. Without trust, a nurse-client relationship rarely progresses beyond social interaction and superficial care. Avoid dishonesty at all costs. Knowingly withholding key information, lying, or distorting the truth violates both legal and ethical standards of practice.

Autonomy and Responsibility

Autonomy is the ability to be self-directed and independent in accomplishing goals and advocating for others. Professional nurses make choices and accept responsibility for the outcomes of their actions (Townsend, 2003). They take initiative in problem solving and communicate in a manner that reflects what they really need and want (Burden, 1997). Autonomy can be beneficial to the client because people who seek health care are often concerned about losing control of decisions that influence how they live.

Assertiveness

Assertive behaviour allows individuals to act in their own best interests without infringing on or denying the rights of others (Devito et al., 2005). It is characterized by openness, confidence, self-awareness, respect for others, and independence.

Nurses can teach assertiveness skills to others as a means for promoting health. Assertive people express feelings and emotions confidently, spontaneously, and honestly. They make decisions and control their lives more effectively than do non-assertive individuals. They can better deal with criticism and manipulation by others and learn to say no, set limits, and resist intentionally imposed guilt.

Assertive responses are characterized by feelings of security, competence, power, optimism, and professionalism. They are good tools for dealing with criticism, change, negative conditions in personal or professional life, and conflict or stress in relationships. Assertive responses often contain "I" messages, such as "I want," "I need," "I think," or "I feel."

Communication Within the Nursing Process

In the following section, the focus of the nursing process is on providing care for clients who need special assistance with communication. However, the implementation section contains examples of therapeutic communication techniques that are appropriate strategies for use in any interpersonal nursing situation.

NP Assessment

Assessment of a client's ability to communicate includes gathering data about the many contextual factors that influence communication. The word *context* refers to all of the parts of something that help determine its meaning. A context for communication includes physical and psychological elements, including participants' internal factors and characteristics, the nature of their relationship, the situation prompting communication, the environment, and the socio-cultural elements present (Beebe et al., 2004). Box 14-4 lists the contextual factors that influence communication. Assessing these contextual factors helps the nurse make sound decisions during the communication process.

Physical and Emotional Factors. Assessing the psychophysiological factors that influence communication is especially important. There are many altered health states and human responses that limit communication. People with hearing or visual impairments have fewer channels through which to receive messages (see chapter 44). Facial trauma, laryngeal cancer, or endotracheal intubation may prevent movement of air past vocal cords or mobility of the tongue, resulting in inability to articulate words. An extremely breathless person must use oxygen to breathe rather than speak. People with aphasia after a stroke or in late-stage Alzheimer's disease often cannot understand or form words. Certain mental illnesses such as psychoses or depression may cause clients to demonstrate flight of ideas, constant verbalization of the same words or phrases, a loose association of ideas, or slowed speech pattern. People with high anxiety may be unable to perceive environmental stimuli or hear explanations. Finally, unresponsive or heavily sedated people cannot send or respond to verbal messages.

Review of the client's medical record helps provide relevant information about the client's ability to communicate. The health history and physical examination may document physical barriers to speech, neurological deficits, and pathophysiology affecting hearing or vision. Reviewing the client's medication record is also important. For example, opiates, antidepressants, neuroleptics, hypnotics, or sedatives may cause a client to slur words or use incomplete sentences. The nursing progress notes may reveal other factors that contribute to communication difficulties, such as the absence of family members who could provide more information about a confused client.

Box 14-4 Contextual Factors Influencing Communication

Psychophysiological Context

The internal factors influencing communication:
Physiological status (e.g., pain, hunger, weakness, dyspnea)
Emotional status (e.g., anxiety, anger, hopelessness, euphoria)
Growth and development status (e.g., age, developmental tasks)
Unmet needs (e.g., safety/security, love/belonging)
Attitudes, values, and beliefs (e.g., meaning of illness experience)
Perceptions and personality (e.g., optimist/pessimist, introvert/extrovert)
Self-concept and self-esteem (e.g., positive or negative)

Relational Context

The nature of the relationship between the participants:
Social, helping, or working relationship
Level of trust between participants
Level of caring expressed
Level of self-disclosure between participants
Shared history of participants
Balance of power and control

Situational Context

The reason for the communication:
Information exchange
Goal achievement
Problem resolution
Expression of feelings

Environmental Context

The physical surroundings in which communication takes place:
Privacy level
Noise level
Comfort and safety level
Distraction level

Cultural Context

The socio-cultural elements that affect the interaction:
Educational level of participants
Language and self-expression patterns
Customs and expectations

Assessment should include communicating directly with clients to provide information about their ability to attend to, interpret, and respond to stimuli. If clients have difficulty communicating, it is important to assess how they are affected by the problem. The client who cannot communicate effectively will often have difficulty expressing needs and responding appropriately to the environment. A client who is unable to speak can be at risk for injury unless an alternate communication method can be found. If there are barriers to communicating directly with the client, then family or friends can be important resources about the client's communication patterns and abilities.

Developmental Factors. Aspects of a client's growth and development also influence nurse-client interaction. For example, an infant's self-expression is limited to crying, body movement, and facial expression, whereas older children can express their needs more directly. The nurse adapts communication techniques to the special needs of infants and children. Communication with children and their parents requires special considerations. The nurse can include the parents, child, or both as sources of information about the child's health, depending on the child's age. A young child can be given toys or other distractions so that the parent can give full attention to the nurse. Children are especially responsive to non-verbal messages, and sudden movements, loud noises, or threatening gestures can be frightening. Children often prefer to make the first move in interpersonal contacts and do not like adults to stare or look down at them. A child who has received little environmental stimulation may be behind in language development, thus making communication more challenging.

Age also influences communication. Age alone does not determine an adult's capacity for communication. However, approximately 12% of Canadians who are age 65 and older have a speech disorder that limits self-expression or their ability to understand others (The Canadian Association of Speech-Language Pathologists, n.d.). Box 14-5 highlights tips for communicating with older adults who have communication needs and barriers. These tips can also be applied to all clients with communication problems.

Socio-cultural Factors. Culture is a blueprint for thinking, feeling, behaving, and communicating. Nurses need to be aware of the typical patterns of interaction that characterize various cultures. For example, Inuit and First Nations peoples often value privacy, respect, and silence. Whereas European Canadians are more open and willing to discuss private family matters, Aboriginal Canadians may be reluctant to reveal personal or family information to strangers. Personal information is often conveyed indirectly through storytelling. Across the Canadian prairies, Hutterite colonies form a large portion of the rural population. These communities have a hierarchical social order, and elders make decisions that affect all community members. For the Hutterites, teaching individual responsibility for health-related choices would not be consistent with communalism and their culture (Brunt, Lindsey, & Hopkinson, 1997). Awareness of such cultural values will facilitate communication between the nurse and the client (see chapter 9).

Foreign-born people may not speak or understand English or French. Those who speak a second language often experience difficulty with self-expression or language comprehension. To practice cultural sensitivity in

Focus on Older Adults Box 14-5

Tips for Improved Communication With Older Adults Who Have Communication Needs/Barriers

- Always start the communication process by checking for a hearing aid.
- Amplify your voice if necessary.
- Get the clients' attention before speaking. Face them so they can see your mouth.
- Structure the environment so it is conducive to good communication. Minimize visual and auditory distractions.
- Make sure there is adequate lighting.
- When caring for clients with communication disorders, remember their deficit. Do not assume a communication breakdown is the result of the client being uncooperative.
- Do not expect to communicate the same way as you would with a non-impaired person. Instead, act as a communication partner whose job is to facilitate the clients' self-expression and comprehension.
- Speak slowly and clearly while maintaining eye contact. Use short sentences with simple words.
- Supplement your words with visual gestures.
- Match your body language to your speech. For example, when reporting favourable test results, the message that the news is good should be evident in your expressions, posture, and tone of voice.
- Summarize the most important points of the conversation.
- Give clients plenty of time to ask and answer questions.
- Allow them to make errors. Do not constantly correct them. Suppress the desire to finish sentences.
- Be a good listener despite time constraints that make listening difficult.
- Stick to one topic at a time.
- Whenever possible have a family member or caregiver in the room with you. This person will usually be most familiar with the client's communication patterns and can assist in the communication process.

From "Overcoming communication disorders in the elderly," by E. Mandel, M. Shulman, and T. Begany, 1997, *Patient Care, 31*(2), pp. 55–58. Copyright 1997 by Medical Economics, Thomas Health Care. Adapted with permission.

communication, the nurse must understand that people of different cultures use different degrees of eye contact, personal space, gestures, voice modulation, pace of speech, touch, silence, and meaning of language. Nurses must avoid interpreting messages from their cultural perspective, but rather consider communication in the context of the client's background. Nurses must never stereotype, patronize, or make fun of other cultures.

Gender. Gender is another factor that influences how we think, act, feel, and communicate. Male and female communication patterns tend to differ, which can sometimes create barriers to effective communication (Beebe et al., 2004).

Males communicate to achieve goals, establish individual status and authority, and compete for attention and power. They typically prefer to talk about topics that do not expose personal feelings. Men tend to speak directly when giving criticism or orders. They use more banter, teasing, and playful put-downs. Men usually want others to know of their accomplishments.

Females communicate to build connections with others, include others, and co-operate with, respond to, show interest in, and support others. Women enjoy discussing feelings and personal issues and find closeness in dialogue. They tend to downplay their achievements. Women speak indirectly, couching criticism and commands in praise or vagueness to avoid causing offence or hurt feelings. A male nurse might say to his colleague, "Help me turn Jeremy." A female nurse might say, "Jeremy needs to be turned," expecting her colleague to understand the implied request for help. Research has shown there are differences in the way male and female nurses use silence, touch, and humour in their practice (Perry, 1996).

To practice gender sensitivity in communication, the nurse must recognize the differences in male and female patterns to avoid misinterpreting messages sent by someone of the opposite gender. The nurse must also be careful to avoid conversations with sexual overtones, gender-denigrating jokes, and male-female stereotyping.

Nursing Diagnosis

Most individuals experience difficulty with some aspect of communication. People who are free of illness or disability may lack skills in attending, listening, responding, and self-expression. Most often, the nurse's care is directed toward those individuals who experience serious communication impairments.

The primary nursing diagnostic label used to describe the client who has limited or no ability to communicate verbally is *impaired verbal communication.* This is the state in which an individual experiences a decreased or absent ability to receive, process, transmit, and use symbols (Johnson et al., 2001). A client will have defining characteristics such as the inability to articulate words, inappropriate verbalization, difficulty forming words, and difficulty in comprehending, which the nurse clusters together to form the diagnosis. This diagnosis is useful for a wide variety of clients with special problems and needs related to communication, such as impaired perception, reception, and articulation. Although a client's primary problem may be impaired verbal communication, the associated difficulty in self-expression or altered communication patterns may also contribute to other nursing diagnoses:

- Anxiety
- Social isolation
- Ineffective coping
- Compromised family coping
- Powerlessness
- Impaired social interaction

The related (contributing) factors for a nursing diagnosis focus on the causes of the communication disorder. In the case of impaired verbal communication, these can be physiological, mechanical, anatomical, psychological, cultural, or developmental in nature. Accuracy in the identification of related factors is necessary so that the nurse selects interventions that can effectively resolve the diagnostic problem. For example, the diagnosis of *impaired verbal communication related to cultural difference (immigrant from China learning English)* would be managed very differently than the diagnosis of *impaired verbal communication related to deafness*.

Planning

Once the nurse has identified the nature of the client's communication dysfunction, several factors must be considered as the care plan is designed. Motivation is a factor in improving communication, and clients often require encouragement to try different approaches. It is especially important to involve the client and family in decisions about the plan of care to determine whether suggested methods are acceptable. The nurse needs to make sure basic comfort and safety needs are met before introducing new communication methods and techniques. When the focus is on practising communication, the nurse should allow adequate time for practice and arrange for a quiet, private place that is free of distractions such as television or visitors. Communication aids may be needed, such as a writing board for a client with a tracheostomy or a special call system for a client who is paralyzed.

Goals and Outcomes. The primary goal of nursing interventions is to facilitate the development of a sense of trust between the client and the nurse or other health care providers. It is important to identify expected outcomes for all clients, particularly when impaired communication is a concern. Outcomes are very specific and measurable and provide the means to determine if the broader goal is met. For example, outcomes for the client might include the following:

- Client initiates conversation about diagnosis or health care problem.
- Client is able to attend to appropriate stimuli.
- Client conveys clear and understandable messages with family members and health care team.
- Client expresses increased satisfaction with the communication process.

At times, nurses care for well clients whose difficulty in sending, receiving, and interpreting messages interferes with healthy interpersonal relationships. In this case, impaired communication may be a contributing factor to other nursing diagnoses such as *impaired social interaction* or *ineffective coping*. Nurses can plan interventions to help such clients improve their communication skills. For example, the nurse can model effective communication techniques and provide feedback regarding the client's communication. Role play can help clients rehearse situations in which they have difficulty communicating. Expected outcomes for a client in this situation might include demonstrating the ability to appropriately express needs, feelings, and concerns; communicating thoughts and feelings more clearly; engaging in appropriate social conversation with peers and staff; and increasing feelings of autonomy and assertiveness.

Setting of Priorities. Nurses must always maintain an open line of communication so that the client can express any emergent needs or problems. This openness may involve an intervention as simple as keeping a call light in reach for a client restricted to bed, or providing communication augmentative devices (e.g., message board, Braille computer). When the nurse plans to have lengthy interactions with a client, physical care priorities should be addressed, so that the discussion can be uninterrupted. The nurse should make the client comfortable by ensuring that symptoms are under control and that elimination needs have been met.

Continuity of Care. To ensure an effective care plan, the nurse may need to collaborate with other health team members who have expertise in communication strategies. Speech therapists can help clients with aphasia, interpreters may be needed for clients who speak a foreign language, and psychiatric nurse specialists might help angry or highly anxious clients to communicate more effectively.

Implementation

In carrying out any care plan, nurses need to use communication techniques that are appropriate for the client's individual needs. Before learning how to adapt communication methods to help clients with serious communication impairments, it is necessary to learn the communication techniques that serve as the foundation for professional communication. It is also important to understand those communication techniques that create barriers to effective interaction.

Therapeutic Communication Techniques. **Therapeutic communication techniques** are specific responses that encourage the expression of feelings and ideas and convey the nurse's acceptance and respect. Learning these techniques helps the student develop awareness of the variety of nursing responses available for use in different situations. Although some of the techniques may seem artificial at first, skill and comfort will increase with practice. Tremendous satisfaction will result as therapeutic relationships and outcomes are achieved.

Active Listening. **Active listening** means to be attentive to what the client is saying both verbally and non-verbally. Active listening facilitates client communication. With active listening, trust is enhanced because the nurse communicates acceptance and respect for the client. Several non-verbal skills have been identified as facilitative skills for attentive listening. They can be identified by the acronym SOLER (Townsend, 2003):

S—Sit facing the client. This posture gives the message that the nurse is there to listen and is interested in what the client is saying.

O—Observe an open posture (i.e., keep arms and legs uncrossed). This posture suggests that the nurse is "open" to what the client says. A "closed" position may convey a defensive stance, possibly invoking a similar response in the client.

L—Lean toward the client. This posture conveys that the nurse is involved and interested in the interaction.

E—Establish and maintain intermittent eye contact. This behaviour conveys involvement in and willingness to listen to what the client is saying. Absence of eye contact or shifting of the eyes gives the message that the nurse is not interested in what is being said.

R—Relax. It is important to communicate a sense of being relaxed and comfortable with the client. Restlessness communicates a lack of interest and may also convey a feeling of discomfort that may be transferred to the client.

Sharing Observations. Nurses make observations by commenting on how the other person looks, sounds, or acts. Stating observations often helps the client communicate without the need for extensive questioning, focusing, or clarification. This technique can help start a conversation with quiet or withdrawn people. The nurse does not state observations that might anger, embarrass, or upset the client, such as telling someone "You look a mess!" Even if such an observation is made with humour, the client can become resentful.

Sharing observations differs from making assumptions, which means drawing unwarranted conclusions about the other person without validating them. Making assumptions puts the client in the position of having to contradict the nurse. Examples might include the nurse interpreting fatigue as depression or assuming that untouched food indicates lack of interest in meeting nutritional goals. Making observations is a gentler and safer technique: "You look tired," "You seem different today," or "I see you haven't eaten anything."

Sharing Empathy. **Empathy** is the ability to understand another person's reality, to accurately perceive unspoken feelings, and to communicate this understanding to the other. To express empathy, the nurse must understand the other person's feelings. Such empathic understanding requires the nurse to be both sensitive and imaginative, especially if the nurse has not had similar experiences. Showing empathy is an important goal to work for, essential for showing concern and communicating support for others. Statements reflecting empathy are highly effective because they tell the person that the nurse heard the feeling content, as well as the factual content, of the communication. Empathy statements are neutral and non-judgmental. They can be used to establish trust in difficult situations. For example, the nurse might say to an angry client who has limited mobility after a stroke: "It must be very frustrating to know what you want and not be able to do it."

Sharing Hope. Nurses recognize that hope is essential for healing and learn to communicate a "sense of possibility" to others. Appropriate encouragement and positive feedback are important in fostering hope and self-confidence and for helping people achieve their potential and reach their goals. The nurse can instill hope by commenting on the positive aspects of the other person's behaviour, performance, or response. Sharing a vision of the future and reminding others of their internal resources and coping abilities can also strengthen hope. Clients can be reassured that there are many kinds of hope and that meaning and personal growth can come from illness experiences. For example, the nurse might say to a client discouraged about a poor prognosis: "I believe you will find a way to face your situation, because I have seen your courage and creativity in the past."

Sharing Humour. Humour is an important but underused resource in nursing interactions. According to Astedt-Kurki and Isola (2001), humour has positive effects on both a person's psyche and physiology. Laughter signifies positive events to people and may contribute to feelings of togetherness, closeness, and friendliness (Balzer Riley, 2004). Shulman and Haugo (2003) noted that humour positively influences the immune system by decreasing levels of stress related hormones that suppress immune function, such as catecholamines and cortisol, and increasing the number and activity level of defensive immune cells, such as activated T cells. Furthermore, they add that humour is a social lubricant that enhances interpersonal communication in several additional ways: It releases emotional tension; permits cognitive reframing; fosters feelings of power and security; creates a nurturing atmosphere; proves a means for expressing empathy; and facilitates social bonding, intimacy, and conflict resolution.

Today it is common for nurses to care for clients from different cultures. When the nurse interacts with clients who do not have a full grasp of the language, it is important to realize the jokes and statements meant to be humorous may not be understood or may be misinterpreted. It is also important to recognize that when either a nurse or client tries to speak in another language, mistakes may occur. The ability to laugh at oneself and with others serves to ease the anxiety that may be present in an intercultural situation (Geiger & Davidhizar, 1999).

A kind of dark, negative humour is sometimes used after difficult or traumatic situations as a way to deal with unbearable tension and stress. This coping humour has a high potential for being misinterpreted as uncaring by people not involved in the situation. For example, student nurses are sometimes offended and wonder how staff can laugh and joke after unsuccessful resuscitation efforts. When nurses use coping humour within earshot of clients or their loved ones, great emotional distress can result.

Sharing Feelings. Emotions are subjective feelings that result from one's thoughts and perceptions. Feelings are not right, wrong, good, or bad, although they may be pleasant or unpleasant. If feelings are not expressed, stress and illness can worsen. Nurses can help clients express emotions by making observations, acknowledging feelings, encouraging communication, giving permission to express "negative" feelings, and modelling healthy emotional self-expression. At times, clients may direct anger or frustration prompted by their illness toward the nurse, who should not take such expressions personally. Acknowledging clients' feelings communicates that the nurse listened to and understood the emotional aspects of their illness situation.

When nurses care for clients, they must be aware of their own emotions because feelings are difficult to hide.

Students may wonder whether it is helpful for the nurse to share feelings with clients. Sharing emotion makes nurses seem more human and can bring people closer. It is appropriate to share feelings of caring, or even cry with others, as long as the nurse is in control of how those feelings are expressed and does so in a way that does not burden the client or break confidentiality. Clients are perceptive and can sense a nurse's emotions. It is usually inappropriate to discuss negative personal emotions such as anger or sadness with clients. A social support system of colleagues is helpful, and employee assistance programs, peer group meetings, and the use of interdisciplinary teams such as social work and pastoral care provide other means for nurses to safely express feelings away from clients.

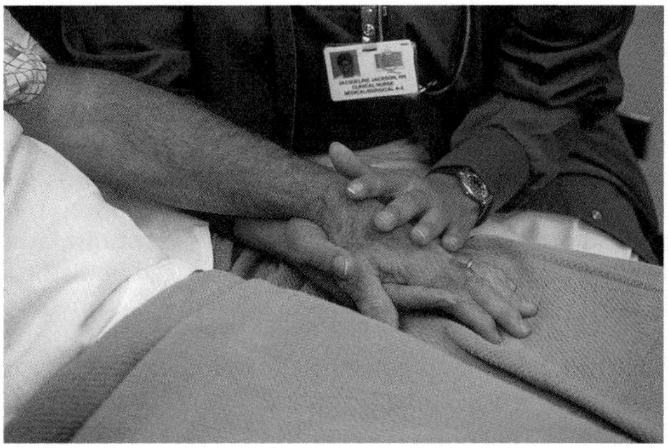

FIGURE **14–2** The nurse uses touch to communicate.

Using Touch. In today's fast-paced technical environments, nurses are required to bring the sense of caring and human connection to their clients (see chapter 15). Touch is one of the nurse's most potent forms of communication. Many messages, such as affection, emotional support, encouragement, tenderness, and personal attention, are conveyed through touch. Comfort touch, such as holding a hand, is especially important for severely ill clients, who are facing physical and emotional losses. Nurses use touch not connected with procedures to get a client's attention, arouse them from sleep, begin a nursing intervention, add emphasis to explanations, make requests, bring comfort, emphasize or point things out, and thank clients (Routasalo, 1996; Figure 14–2).

Seed (1995) found that students may initially find giving intimate care to be stressful, especially when caring for clients of the opposite gender, and that students learn to cope with intimate contact by changing their perception of the situation. Because much of what nurses do involves touching, nurses must learn to be sensitive to other's reactions to touch and use it wisely. Touch should be as gentle or as firm as needed and delivered in a comforting, non-threatening manner. There are times when touch should be withheld; for example, highly suspicious or angry people may respond negatively or even violently to the nurse's touch.

Using Silence. It takes time and experience to become comfortable with silence. Most people have a natural tendency to fill empty spaces with words, but sometimes what those spaces really need is time for the nurse and client to observe one another, sort out feelings, think how to say things, and consider what has been communicated. Silence can prompt people to talk. Silence allows the client to think and gain insight. In general, the nurse should allow the client to break the silence, particularly when the client has initiated it (Stuart & Laraia, 2001).

Silence is particularly useful when people are confronted with decisions that require much thought. For example, silence may help a client gain confidence needed to share the decision to refuse medical treatment. Silence also allows the nurse to pay particular attention to non-verbal messages such as worried expressions or loss of eye contact. Remaining silent demonstrates the nurse's patience and willingness to wait for a response when the other person is unable to reply quickly. Silence may be especially therapeutic during times of profound sadness or grief.

Providing Information. Providing information that the client needs or wants to know empowers the client to make informed decisions, experience less anxiety, and feel safe and secure. It is also an integral aspect of health teaching. Hiding information from clients is not usually helpful, particularly when they seek it. If a physician withholds information, the nurse needs to clarify the reason with the physician. Clients have a right to know about their health status and what is happening in their environment. Information of a distressing nature needs to be communicated with sensitivity, at a pace appropriate to what the client can absorb, and in general terms at first: "John, your heart sounds have changed from earlier today, and so has your blood pressure. I'll let your doctor know." The nurse provides information that enables others to understand what is happening and what to expect: "Mrs. Evans, John is getting an echocardiogram right now. This test uses painless sound waves to create a moving picture of his heart structures and valves and should tell us what is causing his murmur."

Clarifying. To check whether understanding is accurate, the nurse can restate an unclear or ambiguous message to clarify the sender's meaning. Instead of restating the message, the nurse can also ask the other person to rephrase it, explain further, or give an example of what the person means. Without clarification, the nurse may make invalid assumptions and miss valuable information. Despite efforts at paraphrasing, the nurse may not understand the client's message and should let the client know if this is the case: "I'm not sure I understand what you mean by 'sicker than usual.' What is different now?"

Focusing. Focusing is used to centre on key elements or concepts of a message. If conversation is vague or rambling or clients begin to repeat themselves, focusing is a useful technique. The nurse does not use focusing if it interrupts clients while discussing an important issue. Rather, the nurse uses focusing to guide the direction of conversation to important areas: "We've talked a lot about your medications, but let's look more closely at the trouble you're having in taking them on time."

Paraphrasing. Paraphrasing is restating another's message more briefly using one's own words. Through paraphrasing, the nurse sends feedback that lets the client know that the nurse is actively involved in the search for understanding. Practice is required to paraphrase accurately. If the meaning of a message is changed or distorted through paraphrasing, communication may become ineffective. For example, a client may say, "I've been overweight all my life and never had any problems. I can't understand why I need to be on a diet." Paraphrasing this statement by saying, "You don't care if you're overweight or not," is incorrect. It would be more accurate to say, "You're not convinced you need a diet because you've stayed healthy."

Asking Relevant Questions. Nurses ask relevant questions to seek information needed for decision making. Nurses should ask only one question at a time and fully explore one topic before moving to another area. During client assessment, questions follow a logical sequence and usually proceed from general to more specific. Open-ended questions allow the client to take the conversational lead and introduce pertinent information about a topic. For example, "What's your biggest concern at the moment?" Focused questions are used when specific information is needed in an area: "How has your pain affected your life at home?" The nurse should allow clients to fully respond to an open-ended question before asking more focused questions. Closed-ended questions elicit a yes, no, or one-word response: "How many times a day are you taking pain medication?" They are generally less useful during therapeutic exchanges, although they may be needed during assessment.

Asking too many questions can be dehumanizing, because seeking factual information does not allow the nurse or client to establish a more meaningful relationship or deal with important emotional issues. It may be a way for the nurse to ignore uncomfortable areas in favour of more comfortable, neutral topics. A useful exercise is to try conversing without asking the other person a single question. By giving general leads ("Tell me about it."), making observations, paraphrasing, focusing, providing information, and so forth, nurses can discover much of importance that would have remained hidden if questions alone were used during the communication process.

Summarizing. Summarizing is a concise review of key aspects of an interaction. Summarizing brings a sense of satisfaction and closure to an individual conversation and is especially helpful during the termination phase of a nurse-client relationship. By reviewing a conversation, participants focus on key issues and can add additional relevant information as needed. Beginning a new interaction by summarizing a previous one helps the client recall topics discussed and shows the client that the nurse has analyzed communication. Summarizing also clarifies expectations, as in this example of a nurse manager who has been working with a dissatisfied employee: "You've told me a lot of reasons about why you don't like this job and how unhappy you've been. We've also come up with some possible ways to make the situation better, and you've agreed to try some and let me know if any of them help."

Self-Disclosure. Self-disclosures are subjectively true, personal experiences about the self and are intentionally revealed to another person. This is not therapy for the nurse; rather, it shows clients that their experiences can be understood and are not unique. The nurse may choose to share experiences or feelings that are similar to those of the client and may emphasize both the similarities and differences. This kind of self-disclosure is indicative of the closeness of the nurse-client relationship and involves a particular kind of respect for the client. It is offered as an expression of genuineness and honesty by the nurse and is an aspect of empathy (Stuart & Laraia, 2001). Self-disclosures should be relevant and appropriate and made to benefit the client rather than the nurse. They are used sparingly so that the client is the focus of the interaction: "That happened to me once, too. It was devastating, and I had to face some things about myself that I didn't like. I went for counselling, and it really helped. What are your thoughts about seeing a counsellor?"

Confrontation. To confront someone in a therapeutic way, the nurse helps the other person become more aware of inconsistencies in his or her feelings, attitudes, beliefs, and behaviours (Stuart & Laraia, 2001). This technique improves client self-awareness and helps the client recognize growth and deal with important issues. Confrontation should be used only after trust has been established, and it should be done gently, with sensitivity: "You say you've already decided what to do, yet you're still talking a lot about your options."

Non-Therapeutic Communication Techniques. Certain communication techniques can hinder or damage professional relationships. These specific techniques are referred to as non-therapeutic or blocking and will often cause recipients to activate defences to avoid being hurt or negatively affected. Non-therapeutic techniques tend to discourage further expression of feelings and ideas and may engender negative responses or behaviours in others.

Asking Personal Questions. "Why don't you and Sandeep get married?" Asking personal questions that are not relevant to the situation, simply to satisfy the nurse's curiosity, is not appropriate professional communication. Such questions are nosy, invasive, and unnecessary. If clients wish to share private information, they will. If the nurse needs to know more about the client's interpersonal roles and relationships, a question such as "How would you describe your relationship with Sandeep?" can be asked.

Giving Personal Opinions. "If I were you, I'd put your mother in a long-term care facility." When the nurse gives a personal opinion, it takes decision making away from the client. It inhibits spontaneity, stalls problem solving, and creates doubt. Personal opinions differ from professional advice. At times, clients need suggestions and help to make choices. Suggestions are presented to clients as options because the final decision rests with the client. Remember, the problem and its solution belong to the other person and not the nurse. A much better response would be, "Let's talk about what options are available for your mother's care."

Changing the Subject. "Let's not talk about your problems with the insurance company. It's time for your walk." Changing the subject when another person is trying to communicate something important is rude and shows a lack of empathy. It tends to block further communication, and the sender may then withhold important messages or fail to openly express feelings. Thoughts and spontaneity are interrupted, ideas become tangled, and information provided may be inadequate. In some instances, changing the subject can serve as a face-saving manoeuvre. If this happens, reassure the client you will return to his concerns: "After your walk, let's talk some more about what's going on with your insurance company.

Automatic Responses. "Older adults are always confused." "Administration doesn't care about the staff." Stereotypes are generalized beliefs held about people. Making stereotyped remarks about others reflects poor nursing judgment and can threaten nurse-client or team relationships. A cliché is a stereotyped comment such as "You can't win them all" that tends to belittle the other person's feelings and minimize the importance of his or her message. These automatic phrases communicate that the nurse is not taking concerns seriously or responding thoughtfully. Another kind of automatic response is parroting, repeating what the other person has said, word for word. Parroting is easily overused and is not as effective as paraphrasing. A simple "oh?" can give the nurse time to think if the other person says something that takes one by surprise.

A nurse who is task oriented automatically makes the task or procedure the entire focus of interaction with clients, missing opportunities to communicate with them as individuals and meet their needs. Task-oriented nurses are often perceived as cold, uncaring, and unapproachable. When students first perform technical skills, it is difficult to integrate therapeutic communication because of the need to focus on the procedure. In time, the nurse can learn to integrate communication with high-visibility tasks and accomplish several goals simultaneously.

False Reassurance. "Don't worry, everything will be all right." When a client is seriously ill or distressed, the nurse may be tempted to offer hope to the client with statements such as "You'll be fine" or "There's nothing to worry about." When a client is reaching for understanding, false reassurance from the nurse may discourage open communication. Offering reassurance not supported by facts or based in reality can do more harm than good. Although it might be intended kindly and have the secondary effect of helping the nurse avoid the other person's distress, it tends to block conversation and discourage further expression of feelings. A more facilitative nursing response would be "It must be difficult not to know what the surgeon will find. What might be helpful to you at this time?"

Sympathy. "I'm so sorry about your mastectomy, it must be terrible to lose a breast." **Sympathy** is concern, sorrow, or pity felt for the client generated by the nurse's personal identification with the client's needs. Sympathy is a subjective look at another person's world that prevents a clear perspective of the issues confronting that person. Sympathy focuses on the nurse's feelings rather than the client's (Balzer Riley, 2004). Although sympathy is a compassionate response to another's situation, it is not as therapeutic as empathy. The nurse's own emotional issues can prevent effective problem solving and impair good judgment. A more empathetic approach would be "The loss of a breast is a major change. How do you think it will affect your life?"

Asking for Explanations. "Why are you so anxious?" A nurse may be tempted to ask the other person to explain why the person believes, feels, or has acted in a certain way. Clients frequently interpret "why" questions as accusations or think the nurse knows the reason and is simply testing them. Regardless of motivation, "why" questions can cause resentment, insecurity, and mistrust. If additional information is needed, it is best to phrase a question to avoid using the word "why." "You seem upset. What's on your mind?" is more likely to help the anxious client to communicate.

Approval or Disapproval. "You shouldn't even think about abortion, it's not right." Nurses must not impose their own attitudes, values, beliefs, and moral standards on others while in the professional helping role. Other people have the right to be themselves and make their own decisions. Judgmental responses by the nurse often contain terms such as *should, ought, good, bad, right,* or *wrong.* Agreeing or disagreeing sends the subtle message that nurses have the right to make value judgments about client decisions. Approving implies that the behaviour being praised is the only acceptable one. Often the client shares a decision with the nurse, not in an effort to seek approval but to provide a means to discuss feelings. On the other hand, disapproving implies that the client must meet the nurse's expectations or standards. Instead, the nurse should help clients explore their own beliefs and decisions. The nursing response, "Tell me why you are considering abortion," gives the client a chance to express ideas or feelings without fear of being judged.

Defensive Responses. "No one here would intentionally lie to you." Becoming defensive in the face of criticism implies the other person has no right to an opinion. The sender's concerns may be ignored when the nurse focuses on the need for self-defence, defence of the health care team, or defence of others. When clients express criticism, nurses should listen to what they have to say. Listening does not imply agreement. To discover reasons for the client's anger or dissatisfaction, the nurse must listen uncritically. By avoiding defensiveness, the nurse can defuse anger and uncover deeper concerns: "You believe people have been dishonest with you. That must make it difficult to trust anyone. What would you like to happen from this point on?"

Passive or Aggressive Responses. "Things are bad, and there's nothing I can do about it." "Things are bad, and it's all your fault." Passive responses serve to avoid conflict or sidestep issues. They reflect feelings of sadness, depression, anxiety, powerlessness, and hopelessness. Aggressive responses provoke confrontation at the other person's expense. They reflect feelings of anger, frustration, resentment, and stress. Nurses who lack assertive skills may also use triangulation, complaining to a third party rather than confronting the problem or expressing concerns directly to the source. This lowers team morale and draws others into the conflict situation. Assertive communication is a far more professional approach for the nurse to take.

Arguing. "How can you say you didn't sleep a wink, when I heard you snoring all night long?" Challenging or arguing against perceptions denies that they are real and valid to the other person. They imply that the other person is lying, misinformed, or uneducated. The skilful nurse can give information or present reality in a way that avoids argument: "You say you feel like you didn't get any rest at all last night. What do you think might help you to sleep better?"

Adapting Communication Techniques for the Client With Special Needs. Interacting with those who have conditions that impair communication requires special thought and sensitivity. Such clients benefit greatly when the nurse adapts communication techniques to their unique circumstances or developmental level. For example, the nurse caring for a client with impaired verbal communication related to cultural differences may provide a table of simple words in the client's language. The nurse and client use the table to help communicate about basic needs such as food, water, toileting, pain relief, sleep, and so forth. Research findings suggest that many of the difficulties in communicating with clients with severe communication impairment can be viewed as a breakdown in understanding, arising from the lack of an understandable communication system that could be used by nurse and client (Box 14-6; Hemsley et al., 2001).

The nurse's actions are directed at meeting the goals and expected outcomes identified in the plan of care, addressing both the communication impairment and its contributing factors. Box 14-7 lists many methods available to encourage, enhance, restore, or substitute for verbal communication. The nurse must be sure that the client is physically able to use the chosen method and that it does not cause frustration by being too complicated or difficult.

Box 14-8 provides general guidelines for communicating with children and adolescents. Students may consult pediatric nursing textbooks for more detailed information about communication and establishing nurse-client relationships with children and their parents.

In helping older adults with impaired communication, the primary goal is to establish a reliable communication system that is easily understood by all health care team members. Effective communication involves adapting to any special needs resulting from sensory, motor, or cognitive impairments that may be present. Nurses can also encourage older adults to share life stories and reminisce about the past, which has a therapeutic effect and increases their sense of well-being. The nurse should avoid sudden shifts from subject to subject. It is helpful to include the client's family and friends and to become familiar with the client's favourite topics for conversation.

Research Highlight — Box 14-6

Difficulty in Communicating With Clients Unable to Speak

Research Focus

Effective communication with clients is critical to effective nursing practice. The focus of this descriptive study was to provide information about nurses' experiences in communicating with clients who have severe communication impairment.

Research Abstract

The study was designed to include interviews with 20 nurses who cared for clients with severe communication impairment. The interview protocol explored positive and negative experiences of providing nursing care to clients with severe communication impairments as a result of cerebral palsy or traumatic brain injury. Frequency counts and descriptive analyses were conducted to identify the major themes emerging from the interviews.

The results suggest that nurse-client communication is difficult when the client has severe communication impairment, although some nurses discovered effective strategies to facilitate communication with such clients. Many of the difficulties result from misunderstandings between nurse and client caused by ineffective communication.

Evidence-Based Practice

The results suggest a need for nurses to have the following:

- Education in the use of alternative modes of communication
- Access to a variety of simple augmentative communication devices for use with clients who are unable to speak
- Collaboration with speech pathologists on the development of preadmission information and bedside training for people who are admitted to the hospital with severe communication impairment

Reference

Hemsley, B., et al. (2001). Nursing the patient with severe communication impairment. *Journal of Advanced Nursing, 35*(6), 827–835.

NP Evaluation

The nurse and client determine whether the plan of care has been successful by evaluating the client communication outcomes. The nurse evaluates nursing interventions to determine what strategies or interventions were effective and what client changes resulted because of the

Box 14-7 Communicating With Clients Who Have Special Needs

Clients Who Cannot Speak Clearly (e.g., Aphasia, Dysarthria, Deafness)

Listen attentively, be patient, and do not interrupt. Ask simple questions that require "yes" or "no" answers. Allow time for understanding and response. Use visual cues (e.g., words, pictures, and objects) when possible. Allow only one person to speak at a time.

Do not shout or speak too loudly.

Encourage the client to converse.

Let clients know if you have not understood them. Collaborate with speech therapist as needed. Use communication aids:

- Pad and felt-tipped pen or Magic Slate
- Communication board with commonly used words, letters, or pictures denoting basic needs
- Call bells or alarms
- Sign language
- Use of eye blinks or movement of fingers for simple responses ("yes" or "no")

Clients Who Are Cognitively Impaired

Reduce environmental distractions while conversing. Get client's attention prior to speaking.

Use simple sentences and avoid long explanations. Ask one question at a time.

Allow time for client to respond.

Be an attentive listener.

Include family and friends in conversations, especially in subjects known to client.

Clients Who Are Unresponsive (e.g., unconscious or in a coma)

Call client by name during interactions.

Communicate both verbally and by touch.

Speak to client as though he or she can hear. Explain all procedures and sensations.

Provide orientation to person, place, and time. Avoid talking about client to others in his or her presence. Avoid saying things client should not hear.

Always assume that clients can hear and understand everything said at their bedside.

Clients Who Do Not Speak English

Speak to client in normal tone of voice (shouting may be interpreted as anger).

Establish method for client to signal desire to communicate (call light or bell).

Provide an interpreter (translator) as needed. Avoid using family members, especially children, as interpreters. Develop communication board, pictures, or cards. Translate words from native language into English list for client to make basic requests.

Have dictionary (English/French, English/Cree, and so forth) available if client can read.

Box 14-8 Developmental Aspects of Communication

Communicating With Infants

Use firm touch and gentle physical contact such as cuddling, patting, or rocking.

Hold infant so he or she can see the parents.

Talk softly to the infant.

Communicating With Toddlers and Preschoolers

Interact with parents before communicating with child. Assume a position that is at the child's eye level. Allow children to touch and examine objects that will come in contact with them.

Offer a choice only if one exists.

Focus communication on the child, not on the experience of others.

Use simple words and short sentences.

Keep unfamiliar equipment out of view until it is needed. Communicate through transition objects such as dolls, puppets, or stuffed animals before questioning a young child directly.

Communicating With Children

Allow time for the child to feel comfortable. Avoid sudden or rapid advances, broad smiles, staring, or other threatening gestures.

Talk to the parent if the child is initially shy. Give older children the opportunity to talk without the parents present.

Speak in a quiet, unhurried, and confident voice. Give correct reason for why something is done or how equipment works.

State directions and suggestions specifically and positively. Be honest and let the child know what to expect and how to participate.

Allow the child to express concerns and fears; allow time for questions.

Use a variety of communication techniques such as drawing or play.

Communicating With Adolescents

Give undivided attention.

Listen, listen, listen.

Be courteous, calm, and open-minded.

Avoid judging or criticizing.

Choose important issues when taking a stand.

Make expectations clear.

Respect their privacy and views.

Praise good points and tolerate differences.

Encourage expressions of ideas and feelings.

Adapted from *Whaley and Wong's Nursing Care of Infants and Children* (6th ed., pp. 519–541), by D. Wong et al., 1999, St. Louis, MO: Mosby.

Box 14-9 Sample Communication Analysis

Nurse: "Good morning, Mr. Simpson."
(Smiles, approaches bed holding clipboard)
Acknowledging by name, social greeting to begin conversation
Client: "What's good about it?"
(Arms crossed over chest, frowning, direct stare)
Non-verbal signs of anger
Nurse: "You sound unhappy."
(Pulls up chair and sits at bedside)
Sharing observation, non-verbal communication of availability
Client: "You'd be unhappy, too, if nobody would answer your questions."
(Angry voice tone, challenging expression)
Further expression of feelings facilitated by nurse making accurate observation
Nurse: "Are you saying that you need some information you haven't been able to get?"
Clarifying what has been implied
Client: "Oh, I've tried to get it, all right. But nothing does any good."
Feeling powerless
Nurse: "I'd like to hear more about it."
(Leans forward slightly, lays clipboard in lap)
Offering self, removing barriers to active listening
Client: "You're probably just like all the rest of the incompetents in this hospital. Why should I talk to you?"
Testing and challenging nurse
Nurse: "This hospital has a fine staff, Mr. Simpson. I'm sure no one would intentionally keep information from you."
Feeling threatened and being defensive, a non-therapeutic technique
Client: "All right then: Why wouldn't that girl tell me what my blood sugar was?"
Nurse: "I'm not sure. If I were you, I'd forget about it and get a fresh start."
Giving advice and using cliché, which was non-therapeutic; would have been better to acknowledge that client had a right to know the information
Nurse: "I'm going to test your glucose in a minute, and I'll tell you the results." (does test) "Your blood sugar was 20."
Providing information, demonstrating trustworthiness
Client: "That's up pretty high, isn't it?"
(Worried facial expression)
Feeling very concerned about test results
Nurse: (Nods) . . . long pause . . .
Non-verbal affirmation, use of silence to allow client time to absorb information and gather thoughts
Client: "I'll never be normal again."
(Tears in eyes and voice)
Expressing feelings, which is therapeutic
Nurse: "This illness has changed a lot of things for you, hasn't it?"
Empathy statement, acknowledging implied feelings
Client: "I'm sorry, I shouldn't cry. I'm acting like a baby."
Embarrassed about showing his emotions
Nurse: "I don't think you're acting like a baby. I think being able to express your feelings is important and healthy."
(Hands him tissue box)
Sharing perception, giving professional opinion, meeting comfort needs
Client: "I'm so afraid complications will set in since my blood sugar is high."
(Stares out window)
Feels free to express deeper concerns, but they are hard to face
Nurse: "What kinds of things are you worried about?"
Open-ended question to seek information
Client: "I could lose a leg, like my mother did. Or go blind. Or have to live hooked up to a kidney machine for the rest of my life. I could go crazy!"
Nurse: "Go crazy? I'm not sure what you mean."
(Puzzled and faintly alarmed facial expression)
Concerned about meaning, trying to clarify
Client: "Go crazy from worrying, I guess."
(Both laugh)
Use of humour defuses tension
Nurse: "You've been thinking about all kinds of things that could go wrong, and it adds to your worry not to be told what your blood sugar is."
Summarizing to let client "hear" what he has communicated
Client: "I always think the worst."
(Shakes head in exasperation)
Expressing insight into his "inner dialogue"
Nurse: "I'll pass along to the tech that it's OK to tell you your glucose levels. And later this afternoon, I'd like us to talk more about some things you can do to help avoid these complications and set some goals for controlling your glucose."
(Stands up, keeps looking at client)
Providing information, encouraging collaboration and goal setting
Giving non-verbal cue that conversation is nearing end
Client: "OK, if you can stand an old pessimist like me."
(Smiles, appears relaxed)
Trust established, willing to work with nurse; anxiety lessened
Nurse: "Old pessimists are my favourite challenge! Seriously, I'm glad you let me know what was going on, and I'd like to help."
(Humour, positive reinforcement for client's willingness to communicate)

interventions. For example, if using a pen and paper proves frustrating for a non-verbal client whose handwriting is shaky, the care plan can be revised to include use of a picture board instead. If expected outcomes are not met or progress is not satisfactory, the nurse needs to determine what factors influenced the outcomes and then modify the plan of care.

Nurses can evaluate the effectiveness of their own communication by making process recordings, written records of their verbal and non-verbal interactions with clients. Process recording analysis reveals how the nurse can improve personal communication techniques to make them more effective. Box 14-9 contains a sample communication analysis of such a record. Analyzing a process recording enables the nurse to do the following:

- Determine whether he or she encouraged openness and allowed the client to "tell his or her story," expressing both thoughts and feelings
- Identify any missed verbal or non-verbal cues or conversational themes
- Examine whether nursing responses blocked or facilitated the client's efforts to communicate

- Determine whether nursing responses were positive and supportive or superficial and judgmental
- Examine the type and number of questions that were asked
- Determine the type and number of therapeutic communication techniques used
- Discover any missed opportunities to use humour, silence, or touch

Evaluation of the communication process will help nurses gain confidence and competence in interpersonal skills. Becoming an effective communicator greatly increases the nurse's professional satisfaction and success. There is no skill more basic, no tool more powerful.

Key Concepts

- Communication is a powerful therapeutic tool and an essential nursing skill used to influence others and achieve positive health outcomes.
- Communication involves the entire human being, including body, mind, emotions, and spirit.
- Critical thinking facilitates communication through creative inquiry, focused self-awareness and awareness of others, purposeful analysis, and control of perceptual biases.
- Nurses consider many contexts and factors influencing communication when making decisions about what, when, where, how, why, and with whom to communicate.
- Nurses use intrapersonal, interpersonal, transpersonal, small-group, and public interaction to achieve positive change and health goals.
- Communication is most effective when the receiver and sender accurately perceive the meaning of one another's messages.
- Message transmission is influenced by the sender's and receiver's physical and developmental status, perceptions, values, emotions, knowledge, sociocultural background, roles, and environment.
- Effective verbal communication requires appropriate vocabulary, intonation, clear and concise phrasing, proper pacing of statements, and proper timing and relevance of a message.
- Non-verbal communication may convey the true meaning of a message more accurately than verbal communication, and it includes personal appearance, posture, facial expressions, eye contact, sounds, and personal space.
- Helping relationships are strengthened when the nurse demonstrates caring by establishing trust, empathy, autonomy, confidentiality, and professional competence.
- Effective communication techniques are facilitative and tend to encourage the other person to openly express ideas, feelings, or concerns.
- Ineffective communication techniques are inhibiting and tend to block the other person's willingness to openly express ideas, feelings, or concerns.
- The nurse must blend social and informational interactions with therapeutic communication techniques so that others can explore feelings and manage health issues.
- Methods that facilitate communication with children include sitting at eye level; interacting with parents; using simple, direct language; and incorporating play activities.
- Older-adult clients with sensory, motor, or cognitive impairments require the adaptation of communication techniques to compensate for their loss of function and special needs.
- Clients with impaired verbal communication require special consideration and alterations in communication techniques to facilitate the sending, receiving, and interpreting of messages.
- Desired outcomes for clients with impaired verbal communication include increased satisfaction with interpersonal interactions, the ability to send and receive clear messages, and attending to and accurately interpreting verbal and non-verbal cues.

Key Terms

Active listening, *p. 271*
Assertive, *p. 268*
Autonomy, *p. 268*
Channels, *p. 262*
Communication, *p. 259*
Empathy, *p. 271*
Environment, *p. 263*
Feedback, *p. 263*
Interpersonal communication, *p. 261*
Interpersonal variables, *p. 263*
Intrapersonal communication, *p. 261*
Message, *p. 262*
Metacommunication, *p. 265*
Non-verbal communication, *p. 264*
Perception, *p. 260*
Perceptual biases, *p. 260*
Public communication, *p. 262*
Receiver, *p. 262*
Referent, *p. 262*
Sender, *p. 262*
Small-group communication, *p. 261*
Symbolic communication, *p. 265*
Sympathy, *p. 275*
Therapeutic communication techniques, *p. 271*
Transpersonal communication, *p. 261*
Verbal communication, *p. 263*

Critical Thinking Exercises

1. Mrs. Mary Goodrunning, an Aboriginal Canadian of Chipewyan descent, must learn how to manage her diabetes mellitus and self-administer insulin injections. What communication techniques could the nurse use to help her?
2. Jan, a nurse colleague of Mary Ellen, is having difficulty standing up to Dr. Fielding, a physician who has an abrupt, intimidating communication style. Jan frequently complains of tension headaches, pent up anger, and crying easily. What could Mary Ellen do to help Jan?
3. Mr. Hess, a client with Parkinson's disease living at a long-term care facility, has a stiff, expressionless face, a result of his disease. He sits slumped in a recliner chair all day and seems lost in his own world, rarely

looking at or interacting with anyone. When he does talk, he mumbles in a soft voice and his words are difficult to understand. What nursing interventions might establish a helping-healing relationship with Mr. Hess?

4. Mrs. Velma Eberhard, a member of a Hutterite colony in western Canada, is considering whether or not she should have her two young children immunized before they begin attending school. What communication techniques could the nurse use to help her decide, and what traps must the nurse avoid in such a situation?
5. Mrs. Esther Larson, a client who is receiving palliative care, confides in the nurse that she feels overwhelmed with the number of issues she must attend to now that she's facing the possibility of death. She says, "My thoughts are all over the place. I don't know where to start." What communication techniques, based on the critical thinking model, could the nurse use to help her at this point?

Review Questions

1. Communication is not the message that was intended but rather the message that was received. The statement that best helps explain this is as follows:
   1. Clear communication can ensure the client will receive the message intended.
   2. Sincerity in communication is the responsibility of the sender and the receiver.
   3. Attention to personal space can minimize misinterpretation of communication.
   4. Contextual factors, such as attitudes, values, beliefs, and self-concept, influence communication.
2. The nurse demonstrates active listening by
   1. Agreeing with the client
   2. Repeating everything the client says to clarify
   3. Assuming a relaxed posture and leaning toward the client
   4. Smiling and nodding continuously throughout the interview
3. The nurse builds helping, caring relationships by
   1. Asking the client personal questions
   2. Establishing trust and demonstrating empathy
   3. Not asking the client to do anything painful
   4. Being sympathetic and protective of the client
4. Gender influences how a person thinks, acts, feels, and communicates. In Western culture, it is important for the nurse to remember that
   1. Males communicate to achieve goals, establish individual status and authority, and compete for attention and power; females communicate to build connections with others
   2. Males use indirect communication to meet their needs, whereas females communicate directly
   3. Males grow up using aggressive communication, whereas females use passive communication
   4. Males and females should be treated equally; therefore it serves no purpose to distinguish between genders in communication
5. The statement that best explains the role of collaboration with others for the client's plan of care is that the professional nurse
   1. Collaborates with colleagues and the client's family to provide combined expertise in planning care
   2. Consults the physician for direction in establishing goals for clients
   3. Depends on the latest literature to complete an excellent plan of care for clients
   4. Works independently to plan and deliver care and does not depend on other staff for assistance
6. "I'm not sure I understand what you mean by 'sicker than usual.' What is different now?" The nurse is using the therapeutic technique of
   1. Paraphrasing
   2. Providing information
   3. Clarifying
   4. Focusing
7. "We've talked a lot about your medications, but let's look more closely at the trouble you're having in taking them on time." The nurse is using the therapeutic technique of
   1. Paraphrasing
   2. Providing information
   3. Clarifying
   4. Focusing
8. "If I were you, I'd put your mother in a long-term care facility." The nurse is using the non-therapeutic technique of
   1. Asking personal questions
   2. Changing the subject
   3. Giving personal opinions
   4. Automatic responses
9. When working with an older adult, the nurse should remember to avoid
   1. Touching the client
   2. Shifting from subject to subject
   3. Allowing the client to reminisce
   4. Asking the client how he or she feels
10. A nurse should consider zones of personal space and touch when caring for clients. If the nurse is taking the client's nursing history, he or she should be
    1. 0 to 45 cm from the client
    2. 45 cm to 1 m from the client
    3. 1 to 4 m from the client
    4. 4 m or farther from the client

References

Adler, B., Towne, N., & Rolls, J. (2001). *Looking out: Looking in* (1st Canadian ed.). Toronto, ON: Harcourt.

Arnold, E., & Boggs, K. (2003). *Interpersonal relationships: Professional communication skills for nurses* (4th ed.). St. Louis, MO: Saunders.

Astedt-Kurki, P., & Isola, A. (2001). Humour between nurse and patient, and among staff. *Journal of Advanced Nursing, 35,* 452–458.

Balzer Riley, J. (2004). *Communication in nursing* (5th ed.). St. Louis, MO: Mosby.

Beebe, S., et al. (2004). *Interpersonal communication: Relating to others* (3rd Canadian ed.). Toronto, ON: Prentice Hall.

Brunt, J., Lindsey, E., & Hopkinson, J. (1997). Health promotion in the Hutterite community and the ethnocentricity of empowerment. *Canadian Journal of Nursing Research, 29*(1), 17–28.

Burden, N. (1997). Using self-responsibility to improve communication: One nurse's perspective. *Journal of Perianesthesia Nursing, 12*(1):25–31.

Canadian Association of Speech Language Pathologists and Audiologists. (n.d.). *Speech and Hearing Fact Sheet.* Retrieved December 21, 2004, from *www.caslpa.ca/PDF/fact%20sheets/speechhearingfactsheet.pdf*

Canales, M. (1997). Narrative interaction: Creating a space for therapeutic communication. *Issues in Mental Health Nursing, 18,* 477–494.

Creasia, J., & Parker, P. (2001). *Conceptual foundations of professional nursing practice.* St. Louis, MO: Mosby.

Darley, M. (Ed.). (2002). *Managing communication in health care.* New York: Baillere Tindall/Harcourt.

Devito, J., Shimoni, R., & Clark, D. (2005). *Messages: Building interpersonal communication skills.* Toronto, ON: Pearson.

Dubrin, J., & Geerinck, T. (2002). *Human relations: Interpersonal, job-oriented skills* (Canadian ed.). Toronto, ON: Prentice Hall.

Falikowski, A. (1996). *Mastering human relations* (3rd Canadian ed.). Scarborough, ON: Prentice Hall.

Fortinash, K., & Holoday-Worret, P. (2000). *Psychiatric mental health nursing* (2nd ed.). St. Louis, MO: Mosby.

Geiger, J., & Davidhizar, R. (1999). *Transcultural nursing: Assessment and intervention* (3rd ed.). St. Louis, MO: Mosby.

Hartrick, G. (1997). Relational capacity: The foundation for interpersonal nursing practice. *Journal of Advanced Nursing, 26,* 523–528.

Hawley, M. (2000). Nurse comforting strategies. *Clin Nursing Research, 9,* 441–459.

Hemsley, B., et al. (2001). Nursing the patient with severe communication impairment. *Journal of Advanced Nursing, 35,* 827–835.

Johnson, M., et al. (Eds.). (2001). *Nursing diagnoses, outcomes, and interventions: NANDA, NOC, and NIC linkages.* St. Louis, MO: Mosby.

Minor, A. (2001). Therapeutic touch. *Healthcare Review, 14*(3), 4.

Paavilainen, E., & Astedt-Kurki, P. (1997). The client-nurse relationship as experienced by public health nurses: Toward better collaboration. *Public Health Nursing, 14*(3), 137–142.

Paul, R. (1993). The art of redesigning instruction. In J. Willsen & A. J. A. Binker (Eds.), *Critical thinking: How to prepare students for a rapidly changing world.* Santa Rosa, CA: Foundation for Critical Thinking.

Perry, B. (1996). Influence of nurse gender on the use of silence, touch, and humor. *International Journal of Palliative Nursing, 2*(1), 7–14.

Routasalo, P. (1996). Non-necessary touch in the nursing care of elderly people. *Journal of Advanced Nursing, 23,* 904–911.

Seed, A. (1995). Crossing the boundaries: Experiences of neophyte nurses. *Journal of Advanced Nursing, 1,* 1136–1143.

Seigel, B. (1989). *Peace, love and healing.* New York: Harper & Row.

Shulman, N., & Haugo, Z. (2003). An overview of the science and practice of humor–HA! *Primary Care Reports, 9*(1), 1–7.

Stewart, J., & Logan, C. (1998). *Together: Communicating interpersonally* (5th ed.). Boston: McGraw-Hill.

Stuart, G., & Laraia, M. (2001). *Principles and practice of psychiatric nursing* (7th ed.). St. Louis, MO: Mosby.

Townsend, M. (2003). *Psychiatric mental health nursing: Concepts of care* (4th ed.). Philadelphia: F. A. Davis.

Wong, D., et al. (1999). *Whaley and Wong's nursing care of infants and children* (6th ed.). St. Louis, MO: Mosby.

Recommended Web Sites

American Sign Language Dictionary:
http://commtechlab .msu.edu/sites/aslweb/browser.htm
This site provides an English and manual alphabet/dictionary, a brief history of sign language, and links to other sites.

Communicative Disorders Assistant Association of Canada:
http://www.cdaac.ca/links.html
This site provides links to various Canadian and international resources for people with conditions that affect communication.

Guidelines for Good Communication with Children:
http://childdevelopmentinfo.com/parenting/communication.shtml
This Web site by the Child Development Institute offers tips on positive communication with children.

Jest of the Health of It!:
http://www.jesthealth.com
This site provides links to articles and resources about using therapeutic humour in nursing practice.

Medscape:
http://www.medscape.com/px/urlinfo
Medscape is a resource for physicians and nurses that requires a one-time registration (free of charge) and offers links to current literature on numerous health care topics. Enter "Communication" in the search frame, and the site will list current articles on communication in health care.

National Institute on Deafness and Other Communication Disorders:
http://www.nidcd.nih.gov/
Part of the National Institutes of Health (NIH), the National Institute on Deafness and Other Communication Disorders (NIDCD) is mandated to conduct and support biomedical and behavioural research and research training in the normal and disordered processes of hearing, balance, smell, taste, voice, speech, and language.

15

Caring in Nursing Practice

Patricia A. Potter, RN, MSN, PhD, CMAC, FAAN
Cheryl Sams, RN, BScN, MSN (Canadian author)

Objectives

Mastery of content in this chapter will enable the student to:

- Define the key terms listed.
- Discuss the role that caring plays in building a nurse-client relationship.
- Compare and contrast theories on the concept of caring.
- Discuss the potential implications when nurses' and clients' perceptions of caring differ.
- Explain how an ethic of care influences nurses' decision making.
- Describe ways to convey caring through presence and touch.
- Describe the therapeutic benefit of listening to clients.
- Explain the relationship between knowing a client and clinical decision making.

Caring is central to nursing practice, but perhaps it has never been more important because of today's hectic health care environment. The pressure and time constraints on health care workers in most health care settings can result in nurses and other health professionals becoming cold and indifferent to client needs. Canadian author Chantal Cara (2003) believes that the current health care climate and emphasis on restructuring threatens to dehumanize client care. She stressed that the nursing profession must ensure that caring continues to be a strong force within all areas of nursing—in the clinical, administrative, educational, and research fields. Technological advances must be provided within a context of skilful and compassionate care. Empathy and compassion should be a natural part of every client encounter. A caring attitude helps a nurse to focus on the client—to know the person, to explore the person's problems, and to find solutions. A nurse who is able to engage clients in a caring and compassionate manner and who recognizes the therapeutic value of caring will make enormous contributions to the health and well-being of those clients.

Think about an experience you have had with the health care system. Then read the scenarios in Box 15-1. Select the one that most successfully conveys a sense of caring.

There is little doubt that the first scenario depicts a nurse who cares. The nurse's calm presence, parallel eye contact, attention to the client's concerns, and physical closeness all convey a person-centred, compassionate approach. The second scenario conveys indifference and interest only in nursing tasks. During times of illness or when a person seeks the professional guidance of a nurse, caring is essential in helping the individual reach positive outcomes.

Learning about caring in nursing practice enables students to better understand their clients and to improve their approaches to care delivery (Box 15-2).

Theoretical Views on Caring

Caring in nursing has been studied from a variety of philosophical and ethical perspectives since the time of Florence Nightingale. A number of nursing scholars have developed theories on caring because of its importance in nursing and

Case Study Box 15-1

A 42-year-old woman is recovering from a mastectomy. A nurse enters her hospital room and gives a warm greeting while touching her lightly on the shoulder. The nurse sits down, makes eye contact with the woman, and asks how she is feeling. The woman tells the nurse that she is anxious about the pathology report, which she has not yet received. While listening to the woman's story, the nurse gently takes her hand. She sits for a minute after the woman has stopped talking. She then looks at the intravenous (IV) solution, briefly examines the woman, and checks the vital sign summary on the bedside computer screen. As she leaves, she tells the woman to be sure to call if she wishes to talk.

A second nurse enters the room, looks at the IV solution, checks the vital sign summary, quickly says hello to the client but does not sit down or touch the person. Eye contact is from the nurse's lofty vertical position to the client's vulnerable horizontal position. The nurse asks a few brief questions about the client's symptoms and then leaves.

in human relationships in general. This chapter does not detail every theoretical position on caring, but it should help beginning nurses understand that caring is at the heart of a nurse's ability to work with people in a respectful and therapeutic way.

Caring Is Primary

A caring approach requires more than knowledge of a client's health issues, disease, and illness; it requires an understanding of the whole person. (*Holism* is a concept meaning wholeness.) Nurses care for a whole person, who has physical, developmental, emotional, social, intellectual, and spiritual dimensions (Figure 15–1).

The classic works of Patricia Benner (1984) and Benner and Wrubel (1989) offer nurses a hallmark theory that provides a rich, holistic understanding of nursing practice and caring through the interpretation of expert nurses' stories. After listening to nurses' stories and analyzing their meaning, Benner described caring as the essence of excellent nursing practice. The stories revealed to Benner nursing behaviours and decisions that express caring. **Caring** means that people, events, projects, and things matter to people (Benner & Wrubel, 1989). It is a word for being connected. Because caring determines what matters to a person, it describes a wide range of involvements, from parental love to friendship, from caring for one's work to caring for and about one's clients. Personal concern for another person, event, or thing provides motivation and direction for people to care. Caring is an inherent feature of nursing practice, whereby nurses help clients to recover from illness, give meaning to that illness, and maintain or re-establish connection. Nurses who care pay attention; they notice which interventions are successful, and this concern then guides future caregiving.

Each individual is unique, bringing different experiences, values, and cultural perspectives to a health care encounter. Caring is always specific and relational for each nurse-client encounter. Caring facilitates a nurse's ability to know a client, allowing the nurse to recognize a client's problems and to find and implement individualized solutions.

In addition to their work in understanding caring, Benner and Wrubel (1989) described the relationship between health, illness, and disease. Health is not the absence of illness, nor is illness identical to disease (see chapter 1). Health is a state of being that people define in relation to their own values, personality, and lifestyle.

Research Highlight Box 15-2

Enhancing Caring Practices

Research Focus

Caring has been shown to facilitate healing in clients and to improve client satisfaction with nursing care. A question to ask is, can human caring be taught? Can nursing educators present instructional methods that will improve students' caring practices?

Research Abstract

Hoover implemented an innovative 15-week module on nursing as human caring for a group of undergraduate nurses. The aim of the study was to improve students' understanding of caring practices and to thus make them more caring practitioners. The researcher interviewed students before and after completing the module to understand the impact of this module on their caring practices. For example, to gain a fuller understanding of the students' practices, they were asked what factors facilitated and impeded their caring in practice.

The students reported an increased self-awareness in regard to (a) connecting in relationships with self and others, (b) finding purpose and meaning in life, and (c) clarifying values. Several students spoke of becoming more tolerant of others, recognizing the uniqueness of people and appreciating their perspectives. By recognizing themselves as caring people, the students gained meaning in their lives. Many were able to relate a great deal of satisfaction in recognizing that they were caring people and nursing allowed them to express that. Finally, students also expressed an enhanced appreciation of what they valued.

Evidence-Based Practice

- Students who use caring in their practice also use a more holistic approach to care delivery. They recognize the importance of getting to know clients in order to elicit and therefore better meet their needs.
- The caring model involves a closeness, commitment, and involvement in the nurse-client relationship. This can be stressful for both nurse and client. The students who participated in the caring module were able to work through the emotional issues and practical constraints, which allowed them to grow spiritually and connect with clients at a deeper level.

Reference

Hoover, J. (2002). The personal and professional impact of undertaking an educational module on human caring. *Journal of Advanced Nursing, 37*(1), 79–86.

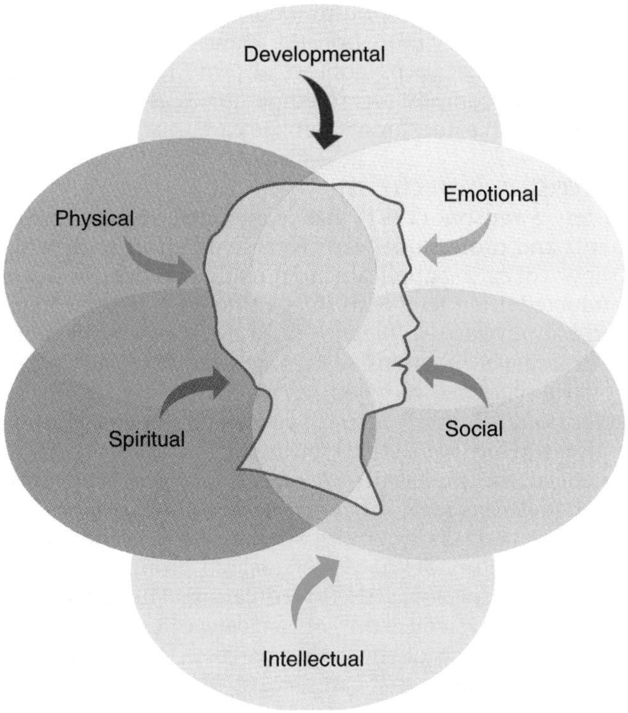

FIGURE **15–1** A whole person has physical, developmental, emotional, social, intellectual, and spiritual dimensions. (Adapted from *Mosby's Canadian Textbook for the Support Worker,* 1st Canadian ed., p. 33, by S. A. Sorrentino, 2004, Toronto: ON: Elsevier Canada.)

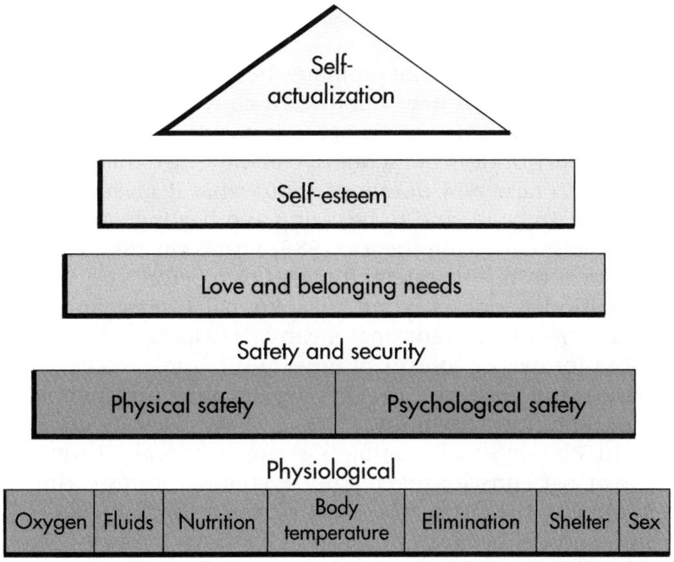

FIGURE **15–2** Maslow's hierarchy of needs. (Redrawn from *Motivation and Personality,* by A. H. Maslow, 1970, Upper Saddle River, NJ: Prentice Hall.)

Health exists along a continuum. Illness is the experience of loss or dysfunction, whereas disease is the manifestation of an abnormality at the cellular, tissue, or organ level. Belle Brown, Weston, and Stewart (2003) described disease as "the thing that is wrong with the body-as-machine" and illness as "the patient's personal experience of sickness—the thoughts, feelings, and behaviour of someone who feels sick" (p. 35). They also pointed out that "a disease is what everyone with that disease has in common, but the illness of each person is unique" (p. 36). Disease and illness do not necessarily coexist. A person may have a disease but not experience the sense of being ill or a decrease in function. For example, a client may have had diabetes for many years but not sense being ill until the disease begins to impair his vision. Illness therefore only has meaning within the context of a person's life. Because illness is the human experience of loss or dysfunction, any treatment or intervention given without consideration of its meaning to an individual is likely to be worthless. Expert nurses understand the difference between health, illness, and disease. They listen to their clients' stories about their illness so that they can understand the meaning of the illness and provide therapeutic, client-centred care (Registered Nurses Association of Ontario, 2002a).

Caring Is Universal

Caring is universal. To be cared for is a basic human need (Leininger, 1978). Basic human needs must be met for survival and health (e.g., food, water, safety, and love). The extent to which basic needs are met is a major factor in a person's level of health. Maslow's hierarchy of needs (1970) is a model that nurses can use to understand the interrelationships of basic human needs (Figure 15–2). According to this model, certain human needs are more basic than others; that is, some needs must be met before others. The need to feel cared for is akin to the need for love and belonging, which is a mid-level human need that is essential for overall wellness.

From a **transcultural** perspective, Madeleine Leininger (1978) described the concept of care as the essence and central, unifying, and dominant domain that distinguishes nursing from other health disciplines. Care, unlike cure, is oriented to assisting an individual or group in improving a human condition. Acts of caring refer to the nurturing and skilful activities, processes, and decisions that assist people in ways that are empathetic, compassionate, and supportive. Leininger's studies of numerous world cultures have found that care helps protect, develop, nurture, and provide survival to people. Care is vital to recovery from illness and to the maintenance of healthy life practices in all cultures.

Leininger (1988) stressed nurses' understanding of both universal and non-universal folk and professional caring behaviours as crucial to the care of clients. Although caring is a universal phenomenon, the expressions, processes, and patterns of caring vary among cultures. Caring is personal, and thus expressions of caring differ for each client. To meet the needs of all clients, nurses must learn specific behaviours and words that reflect human caring in different cultures (see chapter 9).

Caring Is Transformative

Clients and their families should expect a high quality of human interaction from nurses. Unfortunately, many conversations between clients and their nurses are brief and disconnected. Jean Watson's theory of caring (1979, 1988) is a holistic nursing model that suggests that a conscious intention to care promotes healing and wholeness (Hoover, 2002). It does not discard conventional science or modern nursing practices, but is complementary to it. The theory of caring describes a consciousness that allows nurses to raise new questions about what it means to be a nurse, to be ill, and to be caring and healing. Watson's transpersonal caring theory (1988) rejects the disease orientation to health care and places care before cure. The practitioner looks beyond the external disease and its treatment by conventional means. Transpersonal caring looks for deeper sources of inner healing to protect, enhance, and preserve a person's dignity, humanity, wholeness, and inner harmony.

In Watson's view, caring is almost spiritual. Through his or her consciousness, a nurse communicates caring-healing to the client. This takes place during a single caring moment between nurse and client. An interconnectedness forms between the one cared for and the one caring. The model is **transformative,** as both the nurse and the client are influenced by the relationship, for better or for worse (Hoover, 2002). The caring-healing consciousness can promote healing (Cara, 2003). Application of Watson's caring model in practice can enhance nurses' caring practices.

Canadian theorist Sister Simone Roach (1997) also focused on the integration of caring and spirituality. Her caring theory comprises five concepts: compassion, competence, confidence, conscience, and commitment. Pusari (1998) applied Roach's theory in work with people with life-threatening illness. She proposed that Sister Roach's caring elements be extended to also include the concepts of courage, culture, and communication, thus making the theory more holistic. These eight concepts incorporate physical, psychological, emotional, spiritual, and cultural components to guide nurses as they provide comprehensive and individualistic care.

Caring is Nurturing

Kristen Swanson (1991) has conducted research with clients and professional caregivers in an effort to develop a theory of caring applicable to nursing practice. Swanson conducted interviews with three different groups: women who had miscarried, parents and health care professionals in a newborn intensive care unit, and socially at-risk mothers who had received long-term, public health intervention. All groups were in a perinatal (before, during, or after the birth of a child) setting or context and had experienced the phenomenon of caring. Each group was asked questions regarding how caring was experienced or expressed in their situation. After analyzing the stories and descriptions of the three research groups, Swanson was able to develop a theory of caring. The theory describes caring as consisting of five categories or processes (Table 15-1). Each of the caring processes has definitions and subdimensions that can serve as the basis for nursing interventions. Swanson (1991) defined caring as a nurturing way of relating to a valued other, toward whom one feels a personal sense of commitment and responsibility. This theory supports the claim that caring is a central nursing phenomenon but not necessarily unique to nursing practice.

The contributions by Swanson (1991) are valuable in providing direction for how to develop useful and effective caring strategies. Thus, the research findings used to

Table 15-1 **Swanson's Theory of Caring**

Caring Process	Definitions	Subdimensions
Knowing	Striving to understand an event as it has meaning in the life of the other	Avoiding assumptions about the life of the other Centring on the one cared for Seeking cues
Being with	Being emotionally present to the other	Engaging the self or both Being there Conveying ability Sharing feelings
Doing for	Doing for the other as he or she would do for the self if it were at all possible	Not burdening Comforting Anticipating Performing skilfully Protecting
Enabling	Facilitating the other's passage through life transitions (e.g., birth, death) and unfamiliar events	Preserving dignity Informing/explaining Supporting/allowing Focusing Generating alternatives
Maintaining belief	Sustaining faith in the other's capacity to get through an event or transition and face a future with meaning	Validating/giving feedback Believing in/holding in esteem Maintaining a hope-filled attitude Offering realistic optimism "Going the distance"

From "Empirical Development of a Middle-Range Theory of Caring," by K. M. Swanson, 1991, *Nursing Research, 40*(3), p. 161.

develop the theory can be used in clinical nursing practice. For example, Swanson (1999) tested the effects of caring-based counselling on women's emotional well-being in the first year after miscarrying. Results from the study showed that caring-based counselling had significant benefit in reducing women's depression and anger, particularly for women in the first 4 months following miscarriage. Future research is needed to determine if Swanson's caring theory applies to other populations of clients.

Summary of Theoretical Views

There are common themes in nursing caring theories. Caring is highly relational. The nurse and the client enter into a relationship that is much more than one person simply "doing tasks for" another. There is a mutual give-and-take that develops as nurse and client begin to know and care for one another. Sociologist Arthur Frank (1998) has written about his experiences after being diagnosed with advanced testicular cancer at the age of 40: "What I wanted when I was ill, was a mutual relationship of *persons* who were also clinician and client" It was important for Frank to be seen as one of two fellow human beings, not the dependent client being cared for by the expert technical clinician.

Clients sense when a nurse does not care. Failing to show interest in a client or ignoring a request immediately conveys an uncaring attitude. In contrast, clients know when a nurse cares. They are then more willing to disclose details that enable the nurse to understand their particular experience of illness. Benner and Wrubel (1989) related the story of a clinical nurse specialist who learned from a client what caring is all about: "I felt that I was teaching him a lot, but actually he taught me. One day he said to me (probably after I had delivered some well-meaning technical information about his disease), 'You are doing an OK job, but I can tell that every time you walk in that door you are walking out.'" The client perceived that the nurse was simply going through the motion of teaching and showed little caring toward the client. In a study of oncology clients, one client described a nurse's caring as "putting the heart in it" and "having an investment" that makes clients feel that you are with them (Radwin, 2000). This allows the nurse to become a coach and partner rather than a detached provider of care.

Another theme is the importance of understanding the context of the person's life and illness, including his or her physical and social environment, family, friends, and the community. For some, the context may be a comfortable home, a loving family, a fulfilling career, close friends, and community support. For others, it may be poverty, family strife, alcoholism, and unemployment. Another factor that influences context is stage of personal development (see chapter 18). The concept of illness for a child, adolescent, middle age adult, or older adult largely depends on the individual's developmental stage. For example, fear and anxiety are common among ill children, especially if thoughts about illness, hospitalization, or procedures are based on incomplete or unclear information. Emotional development may also influence beliefs about health-related matters. Thus a nurse uses different techniques for teaching about contraception to an adolescent than would be used for an adult.

To feel valued and cared for, most people need to be involved with making sense of their illness or situation. Through careful questioning, the nurse can explore a client's thoughts, feelings, experiences, and ideas. Exploring the following questions with a client can help the nurse to understand a client's perception of illness: How was the illness first recognized? How does the client feel? What does the client think is the cause? How does the illness affect the client's daily life practices? Knowing the context of a client's illness helps the nurse to choose and individualize interventions that will actually help the client. This approach is more successful than simply selecting interventions based on the client's symptoms or disease process.

Clients' Perceptions of Caring

Swanson's theory of caring (1991) provides an excellent beginning to understanding the behaviours and processes that characterize caring. Other researchers have also studied caring from clients' perceptions (Table 15-2). Knowing the behaviours that clients perceive as caring helps nurses to understand what clients expect of them as caregivers. Clients have always valued nurses' effectiveness in performing tasks, but, clearly, they also value the affective dimension of nursing care (Williams, 1997). Establishing a reassuring presence, recognizing an individual as unique, and being attentive to the client are recurrent caring behaviours identified by researchers. All clients are unique; however, understanding common behaviours that clients associate with caring will help the beginning student learn to express caring in practice.

Clients' experiences with and views of health care services and providers affect how they use the health care system and how they can benefit from it (Gerteis et al., 1993). When clients sense that health care providers are interested in them as people, they are more willing to follow recommendations and therapeutic plans. Williams (1997) studied the relationship between clients' perceptions of four dimensions of caring and their satisfaction with nursing care. Clients in the study indicated higher levels of satisfaction when they perceived nurses to be caring. Radwin (2000) found that oncology clients associated excellent nursing care with attentiveness, partnership, individualization, rapport, and caring. As institutions look for ways to improve client satisfaction, creating a caring environment is a crucial and worthwhile goal.

Nurses new to clinical practice must consider clients' perception of caring and the best approaches to providing care. The behaviours that researchers have associated with caring offer an excellent starting point. Beginning nurses also must determine individual clients' perceptions and unique expectations. Researchers have learned that frequently clients and nurses differ in their perceptions of caring (Mayer, 1987). For this reason, nurses should focus on relationship building so that they learn what matters to their clients. Knowing who clients are helps the nurse to select those caring approaches that are most appropriate to the clients' needs.

Table 15-2 A Comparison of Research Studies Exploring Nurse Caring Behaviour (as Perceived by Clients)

Riemen (1986)		Attree (2001)	Mayer (1986)
Perceptions of Female Clients	Perceptions of Male Clients	General Medical Clients' and Families' Perceptions	Perceptions of Cancer Clients
Responding to client's uniqueness	Being physically present so client feels valued	Checking up on clients	Knowing how to give injections and manage equipment
Being perceptive and supportive of client's concerns	Returning voluntarily without being called	Being compassionate and patient	Being cheerful
Being physically present	Making client feel comfortable, relaxed, and secure	Demonstrating sensitivity and sympathy	Encouraging clients to call if they have problems
Having attitudes and displaying behaviours that make client feel valued as a human being	Attending to comfort and needs of client before doing tasks	Using a calm, gentle, and kind approach	Putting clients first
Returning to client voluntarily without being asked	Using a kind, soft, pleasant, gentle voice and attitude		Anticipating that first experiences are the hardest
Showing concern that is comforting and relaxing			
Using a soft, gentle voice			
Invoking feelings of security			
Invoking feelings in client of wanting to reciprocate			

Ethic of Care

Caring is considered by many to be a moral imperative. Through caring for others, human dignity is protected, enhanced, and preserved. Watson (1988) suggested that caring, as a moral ideal, provides the stance from which a nurse intervenes. This stance ensures the practice of ethical standards for good conduct, character, and motives (see chapter 7). The term *ethics* refers to the ideals of right and wrong behaviour. In any client encounter, a nurse must know what behaviour is ethically appropriate. An ethic of care ensures that nurses do not make decisions based solely on intellectual or analytical principles. Instead, an ethic of care places caring at the centre of decision making. Is it caring to provide clean needles to drug addicts? Should pregnant adolescents be advised about abortion?

An **ethic of care** is concerned with relationships between people and with a nurse's character and attitude toward others. Nurses who function from an ethic of care are sensitive to unequal relationships that can lead to an abuse of one person's power over another—intentional or otherwise. Clients and families can feel intimidated by professionals; illness, suffering, lack of information, and unfamiliar circumstances can lead to feelings of vulnerability. An ethic of care ensures the nurse is the client's advocate, solving ethical dilemmas by attending to relationships and by considering each client's unique situation.

Caring is an integral element of the ethical framework of the Canadian Nurses Association (CNA) professional standards (1997). The standards appear in the CNA's *Code of Ethics for Registered Nurses* (see chapter 7). They are incorporated into most provincial nursing standards except for Quebec, which include caring as an element in their document, *Outlook of Practice Nursing*. The College of Nurses of Ontario's 1999 publication, *The Therapeutic Nurse-Patient Relationship* states that the caring attitudes and behaviours as well as knowledge and skill are necessary to deliver optimum nursing care. As well, the RNAO (2002b) best practice guideline, *Establishing Therapeutic Relationships,* includes caring as a core element of nursing.

Caring in Nursing Practice

Scholars disagree as to whether caring can be taught or is more fundamentally a way of being. When caring is a normal part of a person's life, it is a product of the person's culture, values, experiences, and relationships. People who have not been cared for often find it difficult to act in caring ways. As nurses deal with health and illness in their practice, they grow in the ability to care. Nursing behaviours that show caring include providing presence, a caring touch, and listening. Nurses make an effort to know the client, provide spiritual care, and include the family.

Providing Presence

To provide **presence** is to have a person-to-person encounter that conveys closeness and a sense of caring. Fredriksson (1999) explained that presence involves "being there" and "being with." "Being there" is not only a physical presence, but also communication and understanding. The interpersonal relationship of "being there" seems to depend on the fact that a nurse is attentive to the client (Cohen, Hausner, & Johnson, 1994). This type of presence is something the nurse offers to the client to achieve a goal, such as support, comfort, or encouragement, to diminish the intensity of unwanted feelings or for reassurance (Fareed, 1996; Pederson, 1993).

"Being with" is also interpersonal. Nurses give of themselves: They are available and at their clients' disposal (Pederson, 1993). If clients accept the nurse, they will invite him or her to see, share, and touch their vulnerability and suffering. The nurse then enters the client's world. In this presence, clients are able to put words to feelings and to understand themselves in ways that lead to identifying solutions, seeing new directions, and making choices (Gilje, 1997).

When a nurse establishes presence, then eye contact, body language, voice tone, listening, and having a positive and encouraging attitude act together to create an openness and understanding. The message conveyed is that the other's experience matters to the one caring (Swanson, 1991). Establishing presence with a client enhances a nurse's ability to learn from the client, leading to more appropriate nursing care.

Establishing presence is especially important with clients who are under stress. Waiting for test results and preparing for an unfamiliar procedure are just two examples of stressful events. The nurse's presence can help to allay anxiety and fear related to stress. Giving reassurance and thorough explanations about a procedure, remaining at the client's side, and coaching the client through the experience all convey a presence that is invaluable to the client's well-being.

Touch

Clients face situations that can be embarrassing, frightening, and painful. Whatever the feeling or symptom, clients look to nurses for comfort. Touch is one way to offer **comfort** and communicate concern and support.

Touch leads to a connection between nurse and client. It involves contact and non-contact touch (Fredriksson, 1999). Contact touch involves obvious skin-to-skin contact, whereas non-contact touch refers to eye contact. It is difficult to separate the two. Both are described within three categories: task-orientated touch, caring touch, and protective touch (Fredriksson, 1999).

A nurse uses task-orientated touch when performing a task or procedure. The skilful and gentle performance of a nursing procedure conveys competence and makes the client feel secure. Procedures are more effective when administered carefully and with consideration for client concerns. For example, if a client is anxious about having a nasogastric tube inserted, the nurse provides comfort by explaining how the procedure will be done and what the client will feel. Throughout the procedure, the nurse talks quietly with the client to provide reassurance and support.

Caring touch is a form of non-verbal communication that can increase a client's comfort and security, enhance self-esteem, and improve reality orientation (Boyek & Watson, 1994). It may be expressed in the way a nurse holds a client's hand, gives a back massage, gently positions a client, or converses. A caring touch helps the nurse connect with the client and shows acceptance of the individual (Tommasini, 1990).

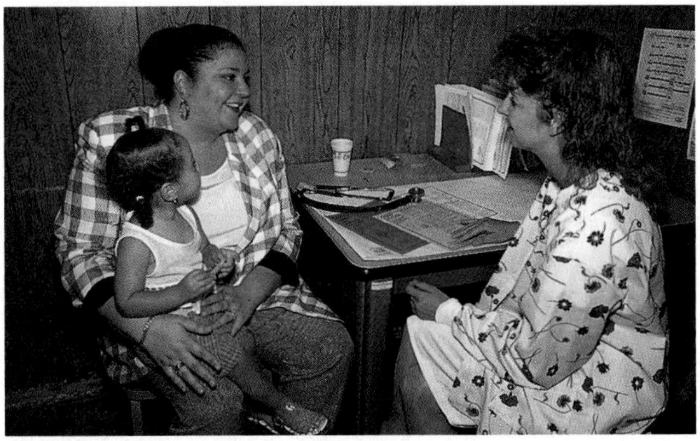

FIGURE **15–3** Nurse listening to a client.

Protective touch is a form of touch that protects the nurse and/or client (Fredriksson, 1999). The client may view it either positively or negatively. The most obvious form of protective touch is used to prevent an accident, for example, holding and bracing the client to avoid a fall. Protective touch can also protect the nurse emotionally. A nurse might withdraw from a client when the nurse cannot tolerate suffering or needs to escape from a tense situation. When used in this way, protective touch can elicit negative feelings in a client (Fredriksson, 1999).

Because touch conveys many messages, it must be used with discretion. Clients generally sanction task-orientated touch, as most individuals give nurses and doctors a license to enter their personal space to provide care. However, exceptions can exist because of clients' cultural backgrounds. A nurse should understand if clients are accepting of touch and how they interpret the nurse's intentions.

Listening

Caring involves an interpersonal interaction that is much more than two people simply talking back and forth. In a caring relationship, the nurse establishes trust, opens lines of communication, and listens to the client (Figure 15–3). Listening is crucial, because it conveys the nurse's full attention and interest. Listening includes not only "taking in" what a client says, but also interpreting and understanding what is said and reflecting that understanding to the person talking (Kemper, 1992). Listening to the meaning of what a client says helps create a mutual relationship.

When individuals become ill, they usually have a story to tell about the meaning of their illness. Any critical or chronic illness affects all of a client's life choices and decisions, sometimes affecting the individual's identity. Being able to tell that story helps the client break the distress of illness. Thus, a story needs a listener. Frank (1998) described his own feelings during his experience with cancer: "I needed a [health care professional's] gift of listening in order to make my suffering a relationship between *us,* instead of an iron cage around *me.*" He needed to be able to express what he needed when he was ill. The personal concerns that are part of a client's illness story determine what is at stake for the client. Caring through listening enables the nurse to be a participant in the client's life.

Listeners need to silence themselves to listen with openness (Fredriksson, 1999). Fredriksson described silencing one's mouth and also the mind. It is important to remain intentionally silent and to concentrate on what the client has to say. Nurses must be able to give clients their full, focused attention as their stories are told.

When ill people tell their stories, they reach out to others. Telling the story implies a relationship that can develop only if the clinician exchanges his or her stories as well. Frank (1998) argued that professionals do not routinely take seriously their own need to be known as part of a clinical relationship. Yet, unless the professional acknowledges this need, there is no reciprocal relationship, only an interaction (Campo, 1997). There is pressure on the clinician to know as much as possible about the client, but it isolates the clinician from the client. In contrast, knowing and being known each supports the other (Frank, 1998).

Learning to listen to a client can be difficult. It is easy to become distracted by tasks, colleagues, or other clients waiting to have their needs attended to. However, the time one takes to listen (and listen effectively) is worthwhile both in the information gained and in the strengthening of the nurse-client relationship. Listening involves paying attention to the individual's words and tone of voice and entering his or her frame of reference. By observing the expressions and body language of the client, the nurse can find cues to help assist the client in exploring ways to achieve greater peace, take action, or do whatever a situation requires (Hungelmann et al., 1996). Chapter 14 discusses additional listening techniques.

Knowing the Client

One of the five caring processes described by Swanson (1991) is knowing the client. This concept comprises both the nurse's understanding of a specific client and the nurse's subsequent selection of interventions (Radwin, 1995). Knowing develops over time as a nurse learns the array of clinical conditions within a specialty and the behaviours and physiological responses of clients. To know a client means that the nurse avoids assumptions, focuses on the client, and engages in a caring relationship with the client that reveals information and cues that facilitate critical thinking and clinical judgments. Knowing the client is at the core of the process by which nurses make clinical decisions. By establishing a caring relationship, the nurse, through the mutuality that develops, comes to better know the client as a unique individual and to then choose the most appropriate and helpful nursing therapies.

The caring relationships that a nurse develops over time, coupled with the nurse's growing knowledge and experience, provide a rich source of meaning when changes in a client's clinical status occur. Expert nurses develop the ability to detect changes in clients' conditions almost effortlessly. Clinical decision making, perhaps the most important nursing responsibility, involves various aspects of knowing the client: responses to therapies, routines, and habits; coping resources; physical capacities and endurance; and body typology and characteristics (Tanner et al., 1993). Experienced nurses know additional facts about their clients, such as their experiences, behaviours, feelings, and perceptions (Radwin, 1995). When clinical decisions are made accurately in the context of knowing a client well, improved client outcomes will result. Swanson-Kauffman (1986) noted that when care is based on knowing the client, it is perceived by clients as personalized, comforting, supportive, and healing.

Knowing a client is much more than simply gathering data about the client's clinical signs and condition. Of course, this information must be gathered. But success in knowing the client lies in the relationship that is established. To know a client is to enter into a caring, social process that results in "bonding," whereby the client comes to feel known by the nurse (Lamb & Stempel, 1994). The bonding then sets the stage for the relationship to evolve into "working" and "changing" phases so that the nurse can help the client become involved in his or her care and accept help when needed.

Spiritual Caring

Spiritual health is achieved when people find a balance between their own life values, goals, and belief systems and those of others. Research has shown a link between spirit, mind, and body. An individual's beliefs and expectations can and do have effects on the person's physical well-being (Coe, 1997).

Establishing a caring relationship with a client involves an interconnectedness between the nurse and the client. This interconnectedness is why Watson (1979) described the caring relationship in a spiritual sense. Spirituality offers a sense of connectedness as well, intrapersonally (connected with oneself), interpersonally (connected with others and the environment), and transpersonally (connected with the unseen, God, or a higher power). When a caring relationship is established, the client and the nurse come to know one another so that both move toward a healing relationship. Establishing a caring relationship requires the nurse to do the following:

- Mobilizing hope for the client and for the nurse
- Finding an interpretation or understanding of illness, symptoms, or emotions that is acceptable to the client
- Assisting the client in using social, emotional, or spiritual resources

Chapter 24 describes in detail the significance that spirituality plays in an individual's health.

Family Care

Caring for an individual does not occur in isolation from the person's family. Nurses need to know the family almost as thoroughly as they know the client (Figure 15–4). The family is an important resource. Success with

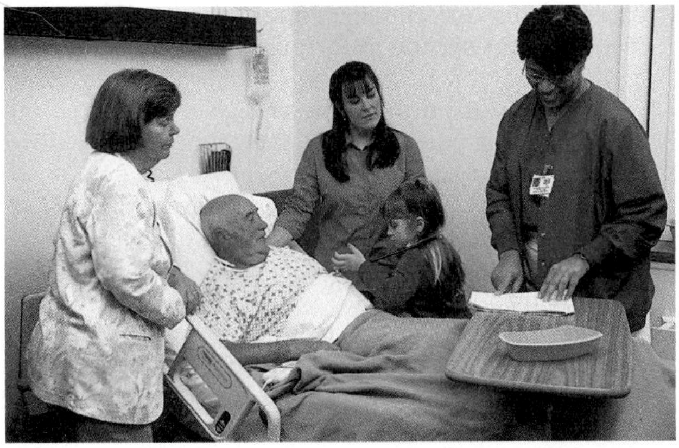

FIGURE **15-4** The nurse discusses the client's health care needs with the family.

Box 15-3 Nurse Caring Behaviours as Perceived by Families

- Being honest
- Giving clear explanations
- Keeping family members informed
- Trying to make the client comfortable
- Showing interest in answering questions
- Providing necessary emergency care
- Assuring the client that nursing services will be available
- Answering family members' questions honestly, openly, and willingly
- Allowing clients to do as much for themselves as possible
- Teaching the family how to keep the relative physically comfortable

Data from "Cancer Patients' and Families' Perceptions of Nurse Caring Behaviors," by D. K. Mayer, *Topics in Clinical Nursing, 8*(2), p. 63.

nursing interventions often depends on the family's willingness to share information about the client, their acceptance and understanding of therapies, whether the interventions fit with the family's daily practices, and whether the family can support and deliver the therapies recommended.

Mayer (1986) identified 10 nurse caring behaviours that were perceived as most helpful by families of clients with cancer (Box 15-3). These helpful behaviours can also be implemented to develop a caring relationship with all families. Ensuring the client's well-being and helping the family to become active participants are critical for family members. The nurse begins a relationship by learning who makes up the client's family and what their roles are in the client's life. Showing the family care and concern for the client creates an openness that then enables a relationship to form with the family. Caring for the family takes into consideration the context of the client's illness and the stress it imposes on all members (see chapter 16).

The Challenge of Caring

Many nurses enter the profession because they want to help people. Hoover (2002) found that when nurses affirm themselves as caring individuals, they achieve a meaning and purpose to their lives. The profession of nursing, unlike medicine, can care for and assist people without medical diagnoses or new technologies and treatments. Caring is a motivating force for people to become nurses and it becomes the source of satisfaction when nurses know they have made a difference in their clients' lives.

It is a challenge to care in today's health care system. Being a part of the helping professions is difficult and demanding. Nurses have less time to spend with clients, making getting to know them more difficult. A reliance on technology and cost-effective health care strategies and efforts to standardize and refine work processes undermine the nature of caring. Too often clients become just a number, with their real needs either overlooked or ignored.

In 1993, Oberle and Davies identified that a major cause of nursing disillusionment is when nurses' personal values, which are entrenched in an ethic of caring, are in conflict with their agencies' emphasis on technological proficiency. Nurses often oppose the current biomedical and corporate ethos. However, researchers have found that supportive colleagues, professional standards, and ethics education help nurses to practice ethical care (Rodney et al., 2002). Other strategies to enable nurses to demonstrate more caring behaviours include introducing greater flexibility into the work environment structure, rewarding experienced nurse mentors, improving nurse staffing, and providing nurses with autonomy over their practice.

Nurses should be aware that the need to build caring relationships with clients must be balanced with the need to maintain scientific objectivity (Hawthorne & Yurkovich, 2002). However, clients cannot be treated like machines if health care is to make a positive difference in their lives. Instead, health care must become more humanizing. As professionals, nurses play an important role in making care an integral part of health care delivery. This role begins by nurses' making caring a part of the philosophy and environment in the workplace. Incorporating care concepts into standards of nursing care establishes the guidelines for professional conduct. Finally, during the day to-day practice with clients and families, nurses must be committed to caring and establishing the relationships necessary for the delivery of personal, compassionate, and meaningful nursing care.

Key Concepts

- Caring is at the heart of a nurse's ability to work with people in a respectful and therapeutic way.
- Caring is always specific and relational for each nurse-client encounter.

- For caring to achieve cure, nurses must learn those culturally specific behaviours and words that reflect human caring in different cultures.
- Because illness is the human experience of loss or dysfunction, any treatment or intervention given without consideration of its meaning to the individual is likely to be worthless.
- Swanson's theory of caring includes five caring processes: knowing, being with, doing for, enabling, and maintaining belief.
- Caring involves a mutual give and take that develops as nurse and client begin to know and care for one another.
- It is difficult to show caring to clients without gaining an understanding of who they are and their perception of their illness.
- Presence involves a person-to-person encounter that conveys closeness and a sense of caring that involves "being there" and "being with" clients.
- Research has shown that touch, both contact and non-contact, includes task-orientated touch, caring touch, and protective touch.
- The skilful and gentle performance of a nursing procedure conveys security and a sense of competence in the nurse.
- Listening includes interpreting and understanding what is said.
- Knowing the client is at the core of the process by which nurses make clinical decisions.
- A nurse demonstrates caring by helping family members become active participants in a client's care.

Key Terms

Caring, *p. 284*
Comfort, *p. 289*
Ethic of care, *p. 288*
Presence, *p. 288*
Transcultural, *p. 285*
Transformative, *p. 286*

Critical Thinking Exercises

1. Lindsey is a senior nursing student assigned to care for Mrs. Lowe, a 62-year-old client being treated for lymphoma (cancer of the lymph nodes). Mrs. Lowe is to receive an injection for her pain. In what way can Lindsay show caring in the way she administers the injection to Mrs. Lowe?
2. Mr. Leonard is a 42-year-old man who is married and has two teenage daughters. He underwent surgery this morning for an angioplasty to correct obstruction of his coronary arteries. The recovery room nurse calls the nursing division and tells you that Mr. Leonard has arrived, is stable, and will likely be there for 2 to 3 hours. His doctor will be up to the division shortly. What can you do to demonstrate caring for Mr. Leonard?
3. During your next clinical practicum, select a client to talk with for at least 15 to 20 minutes. Ask the client to tell you about his or her illness. Review the skills of listening in this chapter and in chapter 14. Immediately after your discussion, reflect on the discussion with the client and answer the following questions:
   a. What do you believe the client was trying to tell you about his or her illness?
   b. Why was it important for the client to share his or her story?
   c. What did you do that made it easy or difficult for the client to talk with you?
   d. Would you rate yourself a good listener? If not, why? If so, explain.
   e. The next time you are assigned to a clinical agency, ask to read their philosophy and standards of care documents. Does the language in the documents represent a caring ethic?

Review Questions

1. A nurse hears a colleague tell a student nurse that she never touches the clients unless she is performing a procedure or doing an assessment. The nurse should inform the colleague that
   1. She does not touch the clients either
   2. Touch is a verbal communication
   3. Touch is one way to offer comfort and communicate concern and support
   4. There is never a problem with using touch
2. One of the five caring processes is "knowing" the client. This concept is best described as
   1. Gathering task-oriented information
   2. Knowing reasons for the client's physician preference
   3. Knowing the client's personal business information
   4. Avoiding assumptions and focussing on the client.
3. A nurse is overheard saying that there is no place in nursing for spiritual caring. An appropriate retort would be,
   1. "You are correct. Religion is a personal decision."
   2. "Nurses should not teach their religious beliefs to their clients."
   3. "Spiritual care should be left to a professional."
   4. "There is a link between spirit, mind, and body that can have a direct effect on a client's health."
4. A nurse is overheard complaining about a client's family being "too involved" in the client's care. An appropriate response would be,
   1. "The family is an important resource."
   2. "You are right, the family should just stay out of nursing matters!"
   3. "The client doesn't like her family anyway."
   4. "The family will not follow through with care when she goes home."
5. To enable nurses to demonstrate more caring behaviours, nurse managers should
   1. Increase nurses' wages
   2. Increase working hours
   3. Introduce greater flexibility in the work environment
   4. Increase physican's input concerning nursing functions

6. As professionals, nurses play an important role in making care an integral part of health care delivery. This begins by nurses
   1. Making caring a part of the philosophy and environment in the workplace
   2. Incorporating personal views in the workplace
   3. Disregarding the family's views of care
   4. Making all decisions in the care of the clients
7. A nurse can demonstrate caring by helping family members to
   1. Make health care decisions for the client
   2. Provide activities of daily living (ADLs)
   3. Become active participants in care
   4. Remove themselves from any form of personal care
8. Listening is not only "taking in" what a client says; it also includes
   1. Interpreting and understanding of what is said and reflecting that understanding to the person talking
   2. Injecting the nurse's personal views and statements
   3. Correcting any errors in the client's understanding
   4. Incorporating the views of the physician
9. Presence involves a person-to-person encounter that
   1. Provides personal care to a client
   2. Conveys a closeness and a sense of caring
   3. Describes being in close contact with a client
   4. Enables clients to care for self
10. By considering the clients' perceptions of caring, nurses are better able to
    1. Understand what clients expect of them as caregivers
    2. Be more efficient in performing tasks
    3. Provide continuity of care
    4. Establish nursing priorities

References

Attree, M. (2001). Patients' and relatives' experiences and perspectives of "good" and "not so good" quality care. *Journal of Advanced Nursing, 33*(4), 456–466.

Benner, P. (1984). *From novice to expert.* Menlo Park, CA: Addison-Wesley.

Benner, P., & Wrubel, J. (1989). *The primacy of caring: Stress and coping in health and illness.* Menlo Park, CA: Addison Wesley.

Boyek, K., & Watson, R. (1994). A touching story. *Elderly Care, 3,* 20–21.

Campo, R. (1997). *The poetry of healing: A doctor's education in empathy, identification, and desire.* New York: W. W. Norton.

Canadian Nurses Association. (1997). *The code of ethics for registered nurses.* Ottawa, ON: Author.

Cara, C. (2003). A pragmatic view of Jean Watson's caring theory. *International Journal for Human Caring, 7*(3), 51–61.

Coe, R. M. (1997). The magic of science and the science of magic: An essay on the process of healing. *Journal of Health and Social Behavior, 38*(3), 1–8.

Cohen, M. Z., Hausner, J., & Johnson, M. (1994). Knowledge and presence: Accountability as described by nurses and surgical patients. *Journal of Professional Nursing, 3,* 177–185.

College of Nurses of Ontario. (1999). *The therapeutic nurse-patient relationship.* Toronto, ON: Author.

Fareed, A. (1996). The experience of reassurance: Patients' perspectives. *Journal of Advanced Nursing, 23,* 272–279.

Frank, A. W. (1998). Just listening: Narrative and deep illness. *Family, Systems and Health, 16*(3), 197–212.

Fredriksson, L. (1999). Modes of relating in a caring conversation: A research synthesis on presence, touch, and listening. *Journal of Advanced Nursing, 30*(5), 1167–1176.

Gerteis, M., et al. (1993). What patients really want. *Health Management Quarterly, 15,* 2–6.

Gilje, F. (1997). Presence: US-Norway nursing research perspectives. In J. K. Hummelvoll & U. A. Lindstrom (Eds.), *Nordiska Perspektiv Psykiatrisk Omvudnad.* Lund, Sweden: Studentlitteratur.

Hawthorne, D., & Yurkovich, N. (2002). Nursing as science: A critical question. *The Canadian Journal of Nursing Research, 34*(2), 53–64.

Hoover, J. (2002). The personal and professional impact of undertaking an educational module on human caring. *Journal of Advanced Nursing, 37*(1), 79–86.

Hungelmann, J., et al. (1996). Focus on spiritual well-being: Harmonious interconnectedness of mind-body-spirit—Use of the JAREL spiritual well-being scale. *Geriatric Nursing, 17*(6), 262–266.

Kemper, B. J. (1992). Therapeutic listening: Developing the concept. *Journal of Psychosocial Nursing and Mental Health Services, 7,* 21–23.

Lamb, G.S, & Stempel, J.E. (1994). Nurse case management from the client's view: Growing as insider-expert. *Nursing Outlook, 42*(7), 7–13.

Leininger, M. (1978). *Transcultural nursing: Concepts, theories and practices.* New York: John Wiley & Sons.

Leininger, M. (1988). *Care: The essence of nursing and health.* Detroit, MI: Wayne State University Press.

Maslow, A. H. (1970). *Motivation and personality.* Upper Saddle River, NJ: Prentice Hall.

Mayer, D. K. (1986). Cancer patients' and families' perceptions of nurse caring behaviors. *Topics in Clinical Nursing, 8*(2), 63–69.

Mayer, D. K. (1987). Oncology nurses' versus cancer patients' perceptions of nurse caring behaviors: A replication study. *Oncology Nursing Forum, 14*(3), 48–52.

Pederson, C. (1993). Presence as a nursing intervention with hospitalized children. *Maternal-Child Nursing Journal, 3,* 75–81.

Pusari, N. D. (1998). Eight 'Cs' of caring: A holistic framework for nursing terminally ill patients. *Contemporary Nurse, 7*(3), 156–160.

Radwin, L. (1995). Knowing the patient: A process model for individualized interventions. *Nursing Research, 44,* 364–370.

Radwin, L. (2000). Oncology patients' perceptions of quality nursing care. *Research in Nursing & Health, 23*(3), 179–190.

Registered Nurses Association of Ontario. (2002a). Client Centred Care. Retrieved January 5, 2005, from *http://www.rnao.org/bestpractices/completed_guidelines/BPG_Guide_C2_CCC.asp*

Registered Nurses Association of Ontario. (2002b). *Establishing therapeutic relationships.* Retrieved January 5, 2005, from *http://www.rnao.org/bestpractices/completed_guidelines/bestPractice_firstCycle.*

Riemen, D. J. (1986). The essential structure of a caring interaction: Doing phenomenology. In P. L. Munhall, & C. J. Oiler (Eds.), *Nursing research: A qualitative perspective* (pp. 85–108). Norwalk, CT: Appleton-Century-Crofts.

Roach, S. (1997). *Caring from the heart: The convergence of caring and spirituality.* Mahwah, NJ: Paulist Press.

Rodney, P., et al. (2002). Navigating toward a moral horizon: A multisite qualitative study of ethical practice in nursing. *The Canadian Journal of Nursing Research, 34*(3), 75–102.

Sorrentino, S. A. (2004). *Mosby's Canadian textbook for the support worker* (1st Canadian ed.). Toronto, ON: Elsevier Canada.

Swanson, K. M. (1991). Empirical development of a middle-range theory of caring. *Nursing Research, 40*(3), 161–166.

Swanson, K. M. (1999). Effects of caring, measurement, and time on miscarriage impact and women's well-being. *Nursing Research, 48*(6), 288–298.

Swanson-Kauffman, K. (1986). Caring in the instance of unexpected early pregnancy loss. *Topics in Clinical Nursing, 8*(2), 37–46.

Tanner, C., et al. (1993). The phenomenology of knowing the patient. *Image—The Journal of Nursing Scholarship, 25,* 273–280.

Tommasini, N. R. (1990). The use of touch with the hospitalized psychiatric patient. *Archives of Psychiatric Nursing, 4,* 213–220.

Watson, M. J. (1979). *Nursing: The philosophy and science of caring.* Boston: Little, Brown.

Watson, M. J. (1988). New dimensions of human caring theory. *Nursing Science Quarterly, 1,* 175–181.

Williams, S. A. (1997). The relationship of patients' perceptions of holistic nurse caring to satisfaction with nursing care. *Journal of Nursing Care Quality, 11*(5), 15–29.

Recommended Web Sites

International Association for Human Caring:
www.humancaring.org/journal/index.htm

The focus of the Web site is to advance nursing and other related disciplines in the knowledge of caring and caring theory. This site provides access to the *International Journal for Human Caring,* which is a well-recognized journal that details research on caring.

Nursing as Caring:
http://www.nursingascaring.com/index.html

This Web site is dedicated to describing current research, development, practice, and education projects related to the theory of Nursing As Caring. It also lists a bibliography of publications on the subject of caring.

16

Family Nursing

Lorraine M. Wright, RN, PhD (Canadian author)
Maureen Leahey, RN, PhD (Canadian author)
Anne Griffin Perry, RN, MSN, EdD, FAAN

Objectives

Mastery of content in this chapter will enable the student to:

- Define the key terms listed.
- Discuss how the term *family* can be defined.
- Examine current trends in the Canadian family.
- Discuss the way family members influence one another's health.
- Compare family as context to family as client and explain the way that these perspectives influence nursing practice.
- State the three major categories of the Calgary Family Assessment Model (CFAM) and understand subcategories important to consider in a family assessment.
- Describe key concepts of the Calgary Family Intervention Model (CFIM).
- Ask assessment questions to learn relevant information about family functioning in the context of health or illness.
- Discuss family nursing skills needed to conduct a family interview.

The family continues to be a central institution in Canadian society. Over the decades, the role of the family in health care has been evolving. In the early 20th century, visiting public health nurses and private duty nurses worked closely with family members while providing nursing care in the client's home. After World War II and the implementation of Medicare, most nursing services were delivered in hospitals, rather than homes. As a result, families were generally excluded from their relatives' nursing care, and doctors and nurses were considered to be the final authority to determine what was best for the client (Canadian Nurses Association [CNA], 1997). Over the last 20 to 30 years, however, families and health care professionals have been forging more collaborative relationships, where families' needs and contributions are taken into consideration.

Today, nurses strive to provide *family-centred care,* also known as *family nursing.* **Family nursing** is based on the assumption that all people, regardless of age, are a member of some type of family form, and individuals are best understood within the context of the family. A change in one family member, such as an illness or health condition, affects the other family members. Family nursing promotes, supports, and provides for the well-being and health of the family and individual family members (Astedt-Kurki et al., 2002). Nurses are responsible for first understanding the makeup (configuration), structure, and coping capacity of the family and then building on the family's relative strengths and resources (Feeley & Gottleib, 2000). Studies have shown that when nurses and families establish meaningful relationships, families are better able to manage the illness and nurses gain greater clinical confidence and job satisfaction (Leahey et al., 1995). The goal of family nursing is to help the family and its individual members reach and maintain maximum health throughout and beyond the illness experience. Family nursing is the focus of the future across all practice settings and is emphasized in all health care environments.

What Is a Family?

Defining *family* may initially appear to be a simple undertaking. However, different definitions have resulted in heated debates among social scientists and legislators. The family can be defined biologically, legally, or as a social network with personally constructed ties and ideologies. To some clients, family may include only people who are related by marriage, birth, or adoption. To others, aunts, uncles, close friends, cohabiting people, and even pets are considered family. Families are as diverse as the individuals that compose them, and clients may have deeply ingrained values about their families that deserve respect. Thus, the nurse must think of family as defined by each individual. In other words, the nurse can think of the **family** as a set of relationships that the client identifies as family or as a network of individuals who influence each other's lives, whether or not there are actual biological or legal ties.

The nurse's personal beliefs do not have to coincide with those of the client. To provide individualized care, the nurse understands that families take many forms and have diverse cultural and ethnic orientations. In addition, no two families are alike; each has its own strengths, weaknesses, resources, and challenges (Bell et al., 2001). However, some general characteristics of a family include future obligations and caregiving functions, such as protection, nourishment, and socialization of its members (Stuart, 1991).

Current Trends in the Canadian Family

Although the institution of the family remains strong, the family itself is changing. Nurses should be aware of current trends and social factors that impact the structure and function of the family. The following information about current family trends is based on data from Statistics Canada's 2001 Census.

Family Forms

Family forms are patterns of people considered by family members to be included in the family (Box 16-1). Although all families have some common characteristics, each family form has unique problems and strengths. The nurse needs to have an open mind about what constitutes a family so that potential resources and concerns are not overlooked.

The proportion of "traditional" families (married parents and biological children) has been declining over the decades, whereas the proportion of common-law and lone-parent families has been increasing (Figure 16–1). The number of couples without children at home is also increasing: In 1981, 32% of married and common-law couples had no children living at home; by 2001, this number had risen to 37%. This increase in couples without children at home is partly due to lower fertility rates, couples delaying having children, and increased life expectancy, which is resulting in greater numbers of older couples with independent adult children (Statistics Canada, 2002a). Figure 16–2 shows the proportions of families with and without children at home.

Divorce rates have increased dramatically since the 1950s, and although the rate seems to be dropping, it is now estimated that 38% of Canadian marriages will end in divorce (Statistics Canada, 2004). Most divorced people eventually remarry, resulting in blended families with complex sets of relationships among step-parents, stepchildren, half-brothers and half-sisters, and extended family members. In 2001, step families and blended families accounted for 12% of all couples with children. When transitioning to a blended family, parents must deal with sometimes hostile or upset reactions of the children, the extended families, and ex-spouse. Parents also must address the new family organization, including roles and relationships.

Although able to marry by law in only certain parts of the country, homosexual couples define their relationships in family terms. According to the 2001 Census, homosexual couples accounted for 0.5% of all couples. Some homosexual families include children, either through adoption, artificial insemination, or from prior

Box 16-1 Family Forms

Nuclear Family

Consists of two parents (married or common-law) and their children

Extended Family

Includes the nuclear family and other relatives (perhaps grandparents, aunts, uncles, cousins)

Step Family

Formed when at least one child in a household is from a previous relationship of one of the parents

Blended Family

Formed when both patients bring children from previous relationships into a new, joint living situation, or when there are children from the current union and children from previous unions living together

Lone-Parent Family

Consists of one parent (either father or mother) and one or more children. The lone-parent family is formed when one parent leaves the nuclear family because of death, divorce, or desertion, or when a single person decides to have or adopt a child.

Other Family Forms

These relationships include married and common-law couples without children, "skip-generation" families (grandparents caring for grandchildren), "non-families" (adults living alone), and homosexual couples (with or without children).

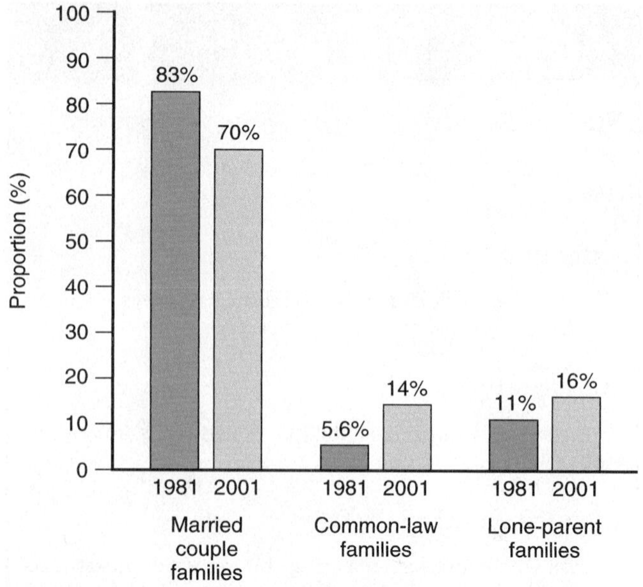

FIGURE **16–1** Proportion of married, common-law, and lone-parent families, 1981 and 2001. (Adapted from *Profile of Canadian Families and Households: Diversification Continues,* Statistics Canada, 2002. Retrieved October 12, 2004, from *http://www12.statcan.ca/english/census01/Products/Analytic/companion/fam/canada.cfm*)

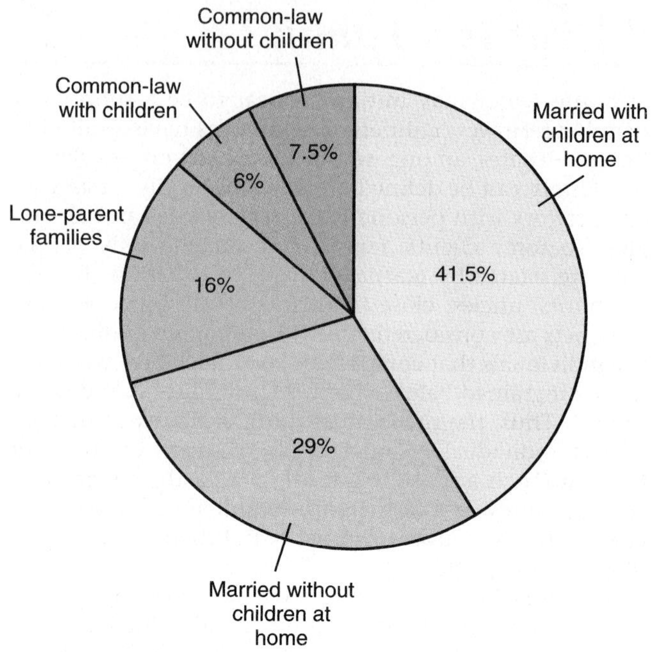

FIGURE **16–2** Proportion of families with and without children at home, 2001. (Adapted from *Canadian Families and Households,* Statistics Canada, 2002. Retrieved October 12, 2004, from *http://www12.statcan.ca/english/census01/Products/Analytic/companion/fam/canada.cfm*)

relationships. About 15% of female couples and 3% of male couples have children.

Grandparents are also increasingly being called on to raise their grandchildren. In 2001, about 1% of all grandparents were living with their grandchildren without either of the childrens' parents involved (Statistics Canada, 2003a). This parenting responsibility is most often a consequence of legal intervention when parents are deemed unfit or renounce their parental obligations.

The rate of teenagers giving birth declined steadily over the last 25 years, probably due to increased sexual education, the availability of contraceptives, and the use of abortion (Statistics Canada, 2000). Nevertheless, adolescents who give birth are now more likely to raise the child themselves rather than placing the child for adoption (The Vanier Institute of the Family, 2000). A teenage pregnancy tends to have health and social consequences for the baby and mother and often severely stresses family relationships and resources. In addition, there is an increased risk for continued poverty for these families. Child-bearing often interferes with education, thereby limiting the mother's employment opportunities. Adolescent parents are often already struggling with the normal tasks of development and identity but now must also accept a responsibility that they may not be ready for physically, emotionally, socially, and/or financially.

Marital Roles

Marital roles are also more complex as families increasingly comprise two wage earners. The majority of mothers—both wives and lone mothers—work outside the home; over 75% of mothers with children over 6 years old are in the workforce (The Vanier Institute of the Family, 2000). Balancing employment and family life creates a variety of challenges in terms of child care and household work. Concerns that maternal employment is detrimental for children are unsubstantiated (Harvey, 1999). However, finding quality substitute child care is a major issue for parents. Managing household tasks can also be a major challenge. Research demonstrates that although equal division of labour receives verbal approval, the majority of household tasks remain "women's work." There is some evidence that the fathering role is changing. Fathers are now expected to participate more fully in day-to-day parenting responsibilities.

Economic Status

In 2000, the median income of Canadian families was about $55,000. However, about 18% of all Canadian children and 17% of older adults lived below Health Canada's low-income cut-off (Statistics Canada, 2003b). In fact, in 2000, about 13% of all families were living in low-income households, and almost half (46%) of all lone-parent families with children under 18 years old were living in low-income households (Statistics Canada, 2003b). Distribution of wealth greatly affects the capacity to maintain health. Low educational preparation, poverty, and decreased amounts of support compound one another, magnifying each other's impact *on* sickness in the family, and magnifying the amount of sickness *in* the family.

Family Caregivers

The fastest-growing age group in Canada is 80 years of age and over. This aging of the population has affected family life cycle, especially the middle generation. Often,

Box 16-2

Focus on Older Adults

- The nurse must consider caregiver strain; caregivers are usually either spouses, who may also be an older adult and may have declining physical stamina, or middle-age children, who often have other responsibilities.
- Later-life families have a different social network than younger families because friends and same-generation family members may have died or been ill themselves. The nurse may need to look for social support within the community and religious affiliation.
- Greater physical health impairment increases the risk of depression in the older adult.
- As in the other stages of life, members of later-life families need to be working on developmental tasks (see chapter 21).
- Abuse of older adults in families occurs across all social classes. Family members and family caregivers are the most frequent abusers. Unexplained bruises and skin trauma should not be ignored.

family members serve as informal caregivers for older adults and others with disabilities. The majority of these caregivers are women, and they frequently provide 10 hours or more of unpaid assistance per week (The Vanier Institute of the Family, 2000). Family caregiving involves the routine provision of services and personal care activities for a family member by spouses, siblings, or parents. Caregiving activities might include personal care (bathing, feeding, or grooming), monitoring for complications or side effects of medications, instrumental activities of daily living (shopping or housekeeping), and ongoing emotional support.

Whenever an individual becomes dependent on another family member for care and assistance, significant stress affects both the caregiver and the care recipient. The caregiver must continue to meet the demands of his or her normal lifestyle (e.g., raising children, working full time, or dealing with personal problems or illness). In many cases, older adult children care for their parents or older relatives. Although family caregivers often find that providing care has many rewards, they usually also have to balance caregiving with career and other family responsibilities. To provide care for a family member, this group frequently must make major adjustments to integrate the challenges and time commitments of caring for a family member with their own lives (Hunt, 2003). Caregivers' physical and emotional health may suffer, as may their careers and family relationships (The Vanier Institute of the Family, 2000).

Box 16-2 provides a list of family nursing gerontological concerns.

The Family and Health

The family is the primary social context in which health promotion and disease prevention take place (Box 16-3). The health of the family is influenced by many factors (e.g., its relative position in society, economic resources, and geographical boundaries). The family's beliefs, values, and practices also strongly influence health-promoting behaviours of its members (Hartrick, 2000). In turn, the health status of each individual influences how the family unit functions and its ability to achieve goals. When the family satisfactorily functions to meet its goals, its members tend to feel positive about themselves and their family. Conversely, when they do not meet goals, families view themselves as ineffective.

Good health may not be highly valued in some families; in fact, detrimental practices may be accepted. In some cases, a family member may provide mixed messages about health. For example, a parent may continue to smoke while telling children that smoking is bad for them. Family environment is crucial because health behaviour reinforced in early life has a strong influence on later health practices. In addition, the family environment can be a crucial factor in an individual's adjustment to a crisis. Although illness can strain relationships, research indicates that family members have the potential to be a primary force for coping.

Box 16-3

Focus on Primary Health Care

Community health nurses meet families in a wide variety of settings and have tremendous opportunities to use holistic family nursing practices. Nursing duties in health promotion include newborn assessments, bereavement visits, school health, occupational health, substance abuse programs, palliative care, infusion clinics, home care, and numerous other clinical encounters.

When implementing family nursing, health promotion interventions are needed to improve or maintain the physical, social, emotional, and spiritual well-being of the family and its members (Ford-Gilboe, 2002). Individual members and the total family are encouraged to reach their optimal levels of wellness. Identifying attributes that contribute to healthy, resilient families has been a focus of ongoing research for at least three decades. "Strong" families that adapt to expected transitions and unexpected crises and change tend to be characterized by clear communication among members, good problem-solving skills, a commitment to each other and to the family unit, and a sense of cohesiveness and spirituality (Svavarsdottir, McCubbin, & Kane, 2000). Health promotion programs aimed at enhancing these attributes are available for families and children in many communities. The nurse must be aware of family-oriented offerings so that families can be referred as needed. Health promotion behaviours that the nurse needs to encourage are often tied to the developmental stage of the family, such as programs for the child-bearing family about adequate prenatal care.

Attributes of Healthy Families

Ruebin Hill's classic work (1958) noted that it is possible to explain the reactions of crisis-proof and crisis-prone families. The crisis-proof, or effective, family is able to integrate the need for stability with the need for growth and change. This family has a flexible structure that allows adaptable performance of tasks and acceptance of help from outside the family system. The structure is flexible enough to allow adaptability but not so flexible that the family lacks cohesiveness and a sense of stability. The effective family has control over the environment and exerts influence on the immediate environment of home, neighbourhood, and school. The ineffective, or crisis-prone, family may lack or believe it lacks control over these environments.

Recently, health promotion research has started to focus on the stress-moderating effect of **hardiness** and **resiliency** as factors that contribute to long-term health. *Family hardiness* has been defined as the internal strengths and durability of the family unit and is characterized by a sense of control over the outcome of life, a view of change as beneficial and growth producing, and an active rather than passive orientation in adapting to stressful events (McCubbin, McCubbin, & Thompson, 1996). A hardy family can transcend long periods and inevitable lifestyle changes. *Family resiliency* is the ability to cope with expected and unexpected stressors. The family's ability to adapt to role changes, developmental milestones, and crises shows resilience. The goal of the family is not only to survive the challenge, but also to thrive and grow as a result of the newly gained knowledge. Resources and techniques that a family or individuals within the family use to maintain health can show a family's level of resiliency (Svavarsdottir et al., 2000).

Family Nursing

Nursing practice is enhanced by a family-centred approach. Nurses should examine family patterns, relationships, and interactions when they consider how a health problem or illness affects a family and how a family affects a health problem or illness. A nurse's relationship with the family has a significant influence on client and family functioning (Leahey & Harper-Jaques, 1996). A positive collaborative relationship with family members that is based on mutual respect and trust is essential (Figure 16–3).

To begin working with families, nurses must have a scientific knowledge base in family theory and an adequate knowledge base in family nursing. Although the past and present health care systems tend to emphasize the individual, family focus is now needed in order to be able to safely discharge clients back to the family or community settings.

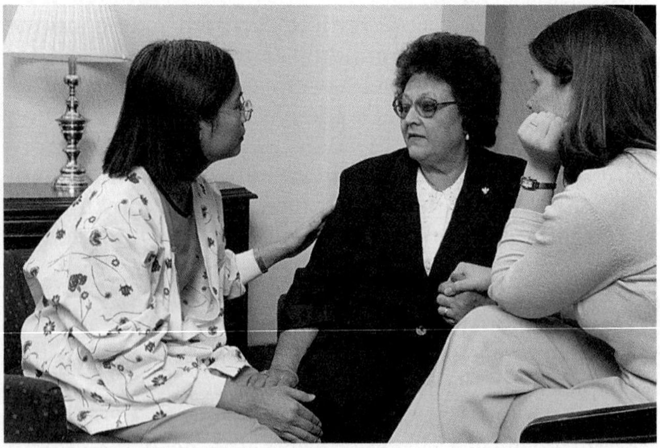

FIGURE **16–3** Nurse and family members.

Family nursing can be described as focusing on either family as context or family as client. The choice of approach used depends on the situation and the abilities of the nurse.

Family as Context

When considering the family as context, the nurse focuses either on the individual client within the context of his or her family or on the family with the individual as context (CNA, 1997). The approach that a nurse uses is related to the clinical setting, the clinical problem, and realistic and practical considerations. An example of the first approach is a nurse interviewing a man with heart disease asking the man's wife about the family's diet and possible family stressors. The wife's abilities to support her husband's efforts at changing eating patterns and use of stress management techniques are also assessed. The main focus is on the health of the client within the environment of the family. An example of the second approach is a community health nurse interviewing the adult daughter of a woman with multiple sclerosis to discuss how the daughter is coping with her mother at home. Family members may need direct interventions themselves.

With both approaches, the nurse assesses the extent to which the family provides the individual's basic needs. Family members should be considered as valuable resources. They can provide the nurse with information about how they have been helping the client maintain health and manage health problems. When clients are unable to communicate, families can provide important information about the client and indicate the client's wishes. All nurses should be competent at considering the family as context. Even if the nurse does not have an opportunity to involve the family directly, the nurse should still consider the client as a member of a family (CNA, 1997).

Family as Client

When the family as client is the approach, the nurse focuses on the entire family—its processes and relationships (e.g., parenting or family caregiving). The focus of nursing assessment is usually on family patterns and interactions among family members rather than on individual characteristics. The nursing process concentrates on the extent to which these patterns and processes are consistent with reaching and maintaining family and individual health. Nursing practice that focuses on family as client is also known as *family systems nursing,* and it usually requires an in-depth knowledge of family dynamics and family systems theory. Therefore, nurses who practice family systems nursing usually have extensive clinical practice skills and a post-graduate degree. Dealing with complex family system problems often requires an interdisciplinary approach. The nurse must always be aware of the limits of nursing practice and make referrals when appropriate. When the family is viewed as the client, the nurse will aim to support communication among all family members. This support ensures that the family remains informed as to the nurse's intent and progress in providing health care. Often the nurse must support conflict resolution between family members so that each member can confront and resolve problems in a healthy way. The nurse also helps family members use the external and internal resources that are necessary. Ultimately, the nurse's aim is to help the family reach a point of optimal function.

Assessing the Needs of the Family: The Calgary Family Assessment Model

Family assessment is essential to providing adequate family care and support. To help families adjust to acute and chronic illness, nurses need to understand the family unit, what the illness means to the family members, what the illness means to family functioning, how the family has been affected by the illness, and the support the family requires (Neabel, Fothergill-Bourbonnais, & Dunning, 2000). Box 16-4 lists families who should especially be considered for a family assessment. During an assessment, the nurse, client, and family collaboratively engage in conversation to systematically collect information and reflect on issues important to the client's well-being at this particular time.

The **Calgary Family Assessment Model (CFAM)** is a framework nurses may follow to do a thorough family assessment (Wright & Leahey, 2000). It has received wide recognition and faculties and schools of nursing around the world have adopted it. The International Council of Nurses recognizes it as one of the four leading family assessment models in the world (Schober & Affara, 2001). The CFAM focuses on three major categories of family life: the structural dimension, the developmental dimension, and the functional dimension. Each category has several subcategories; however, not all subcategories are relevant to all families (Figure 16–4). The nurse must decide, on a family-by-family basis, which subcategories are relevant at *each* point in time. Using too many subcategories may overwhelm a nurse with data; using too few may distort a family's strengths and/or problems. The model provides a framework to draw from during discussions about family issues.

Box 16-4 Families Who Should Be Considered for a Family Assessment

Families who may benefit most from a family assessment include those who:

- Are experiencing emotional, physical, and/or spiritual suffering or disruption caused by a family crisis (e.g., acute illness, injury, or death)
- Are experiencing emotional, physical, and/or spiritual suffering or disruption caused by a developmental milestone (e.g., birth, marriage, or child leaving home)
- Define a problem as a family issue (e.g., the impact of chronic illness on the family)
- Have a child or adolescent whom they identify as having difficulties (e.g., school phobia or fear of cancer treatment)
- Are experiencing issues that are serious enough to jeopardize family relationships (e.g., terminal illness or abuse)
- Have a family member who is about to be admitted to the hospital for psychiatric treatment
- Have a child who is about to be admitted to the hospital

From *Nurses and Families: A Guide to Family Assessment and Intervention* (3rd ed., p. 17), by L. M. Wright and M. Leahey, 2000, Philadelphia: F. A. Davis.

Structural Assessment

The structural dimension of the family includes the following:

- *Internal structure*—The people who are included in the family and how they are connected to each other
- *External structure*—The relationships the family has with people and institutions outside the family
- *Context*—The whole situation or background relevant to the family

Internal Structure. The internal structure of the family—its composition and connections among family members—can be further divided into six subcategories: composition, gender, sexual orientation, rank order, subsystems, and boundaries.

Composition. Composition refers to the individual members who form the family. The family composition is not limited to the traditional, nuclear family, but may include any of the various family forms discussed earlier (see Box 16-1). It is important to note whether there have been any recent additions or losses to the family composition.

Questions to Ask the Family: *Who is in your family? Does anyone else live with you, for example, grandparents, boarders? Has anyone recently moved out, married, or died? Is there anyone else you think of as a family member who is not biologically related?*

Gender. Gender is the set of beliefs about or expectations of male and female behaviour and experiences. These beliefs are fundamental to male and female relationships and are influenced by culture, religion, and family. It is useful to understand how males and females in a particular family may view the world differently.

Questions to Ask the Family: *How have your parents' ideas about masculinity and femininity affected your own? Do you have expectations of your children based on their gender? Is the division of labour in your family based on gender roles?*

Sexual Orientation. Included here are heterosexual, homosexual, bisexual, and transgendered orientations (see chapter 23). Heterosexism, a belief that privileges male-female bonding over other types of bonding, is a

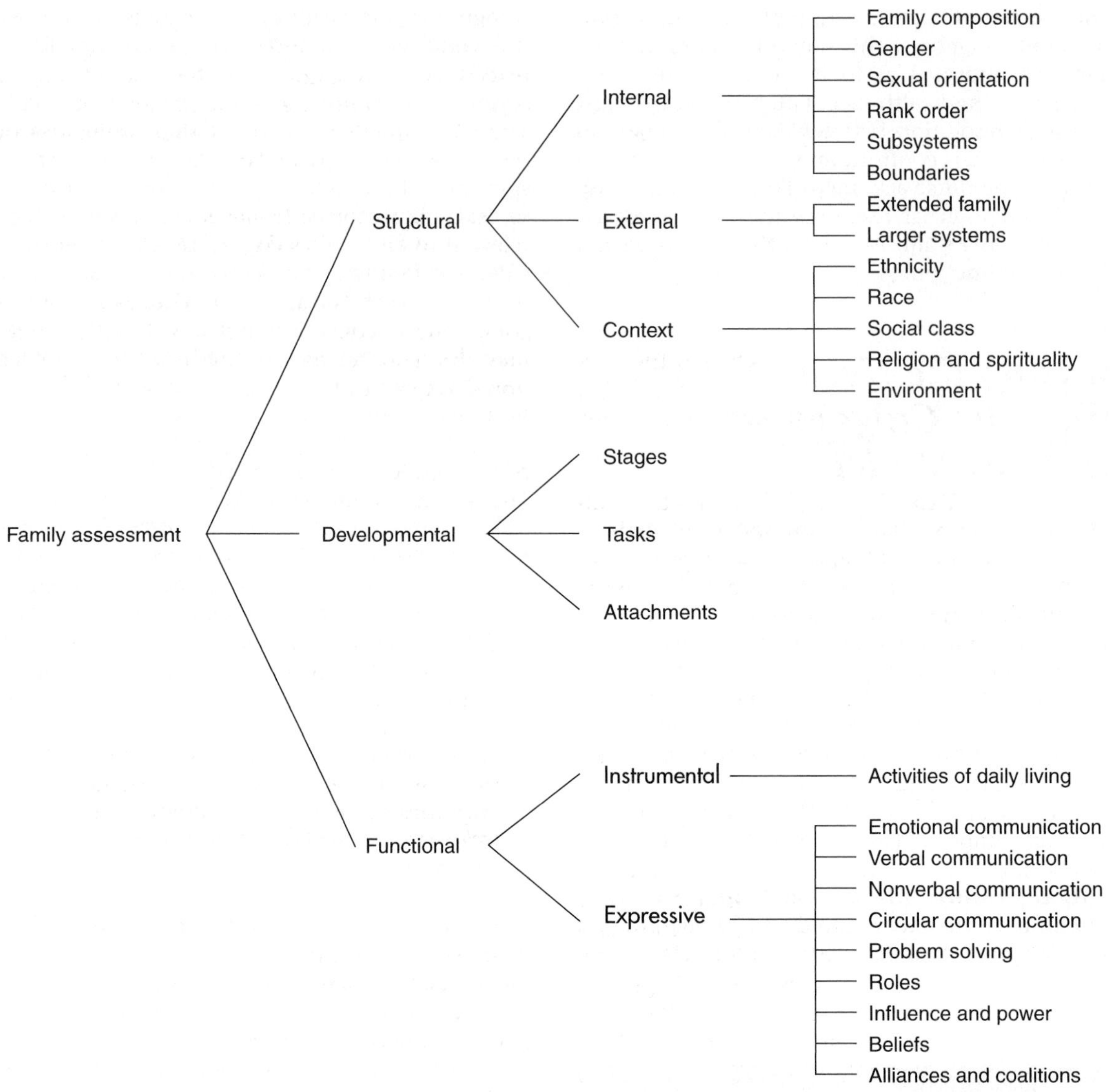

FIGURE **16–4** Branching diagram of the CFAM. (From *Nurses and Families: A Guide to Family Assessment and Intervention,* 3rd ed., p. 68, by L. M. Wright and M. Leahey, 2000, Philadelphia: F. A. Davis.)

form of bias that can affect families and health care providers. Discrimination of sexual orientation continues to be an issue in North American society. Unless it is particularly relevant to the client or family's presenting concern, the nurse does not usually ask questions about sexual orientation but is careful when asking general questions to avoid stereotyping or making assumptions.

Rank Order. The order of children by age and gender is called rank order. The birth order, gender, and distance in age between siblings are important factors to consider because they may influence roles and behaviours. Also important is the child's characteristics and the family's idealized "program" for the child (going to school, college, university, work, getting married, etc.).

Questions to Ask the Family: *How many children are in your family? What are the ages of the children? Do you have expectations of the eldest that are different than for the younger children?*

Subsystems. Subsystems are smaller groups of relationships within a family. Subsystems can be created based on generation, interests, skills, or gender. For example, a family could have a sibling subsystem, a husband-wife subsystem, and a parent-child subsystem. Each family member usually belongs to several subsystems, and in each subsystem, they play a different role, use different skills, and have a different level of power. For example, a teenager behaves differently with her younger sister than she does with her father. Adapting to the demands of different subsystems is a necessary skill for each family member.

Questions to Ask the Family: *What are your family's subgroups? Are there frequent disagreements among and between subgroups? If your family had more or fewer subgroups, what effect do you think that might have?*

Boundaries. Boundaries define family subsystems and distinguish one subsystem from another. They define how members participate in each subsystem. For example, a child in a parent-child subsystem may be given certain responsibilities and power but not be expected to be involved with family decision making. Boundaries can be weak, rigid, or flexible and they change over time as family members age or are gained or lost.

Questions to Ask the Family: *Whom do you talk with if you feel happy? Whom do you talk with if you feel sad? Are there any "unwritten" rules in the family about topics that are never to be discussed with someone outside of the family?*

External Structure. External structure refers to the connections that family members have to those outside the family. There are two subcategories to external structure: extended family and larger systems.

Extended Family. Extended family includes the family of origin and present generation and step-relatives. How each member sees self as an individual, yet also as part of the family, is a critical structural area for assessment. The nurse should note whether family members make many references to the extended family during the interview.

Questions to Ask the Family: *Where do your parents live? How often do you have contact with them and/or your brothers and sisters? Which family members do see or speak with regularly? To which relatives are you closest?*

Larger Systems. Larger systems are groups with whom the family has meaningful contact. Groups include health care providers, work, church, school, friends, and social agencies such as public welfare, child welfare, foster care, and courts. Usually, contact with such larger systems is helpful. However, some families have difficult relationships with individuals from these groups, which can create stress for the family.

Questions to Ask the Family: *What agency professionals are involved with your family? How many agencies regularly interact with you? How is this involvement helpful or unhelpful?*

Context. Context refers to the situation or background relevant to the family. A family can be viewed in the context of ethnicity, race, social class, spirituality and/or religion, and environment.

Ethnicity. Ethnicity, which is the concept of a family's "peoplehood," is an important influence on family interaction. Ethnicity often influences a family's function, structure, perspectives, values, health beliefs, and philosophies (see chapter 9). Cultural and ethnic heritage can affect, for example, religious practices, child-rearing practices, recreational activities, and nutrition. Members may subscribe to differing beliefs, traditions, and restrictions, even within the same generation.

Questions to Ask the Family: *Do you think of your family has having a strong ethnic identity? Has your ethnic background influenced your health care? Could you tell me about ethnic traditions you practice? How are your practices similar or different from those suggested by our health clinic?*

Race. Race influences individual and group identification and is closely connected to ethnicity. Family members' interactions among themselves and with health care providers are influenced by racial attitudes, stereotypes, and discrimination. If ignored, these influences can harm the nurse and family's relationship.

Questions to Ask the Family: *If you and I were of the same race, would our conversation be different? If so, how?*

Social Class. Social class is shaped by education, income, and occupation. Each class has its own values, lifestyles, and behaviours that influence family interaction and health care practices.

Questions to Ask the Family: *What is your job, and how many hours a week do you work? Does anyone in the family work shifts? How does that influence your family functioning? What level of education have you completed? Does your family have economic problems at this time?*

Spirituality and/or Religion. Family members' spiritual or religious beliefs, rituals, and practices can influence their ability to cope with or manage an illness or health concern (Wright, 2004). Spirituality is often an underused resource in family work (see chapter 24).

Questions to Ask the Family: *Are you involved with a church, temple, mosque, or synagogue? Would you discuss a family problem with anyone from your place of worship? Are your spiritual beliefs a resource to you?*

Environment. The family environment refers to the larger community, neighbourhood, and home. Environmental factors that my affect family functioning include adequate space and access to schools, day care, recreation, and public transportation.

Questions to Ask the Family: *What are the advantages and disadvantages of living in your neighbourhood? What community services do your family use? What community services would you like to learn about?*

Structural Assessment Tools. The CFAM encourages nurses to create genograms and ecomaps to help document and understand the structure of a family and its contact with outside individuals and organizations. A **genogram** is a sketch of the family structure and relevant information about family members (Figure 16–5). Some agencies have genogram forms, but genograms can also be sketched on other forms, such as admission forms or Kardex cards. The genogram becomes part of the documentation about the client and family. In some facilities, the information is collected on admission and then hung at the client's bedside, serving as a visual reminder to all health care professionals involved with the client to think about the family. An **ecomap** is a sketch of the family's contact with those outside the family (Figure 16–6). The family members who share the household are depicted in the centre of the ecomap, and various important extended family members or larger systems are sketched in to show their relationship to the family.

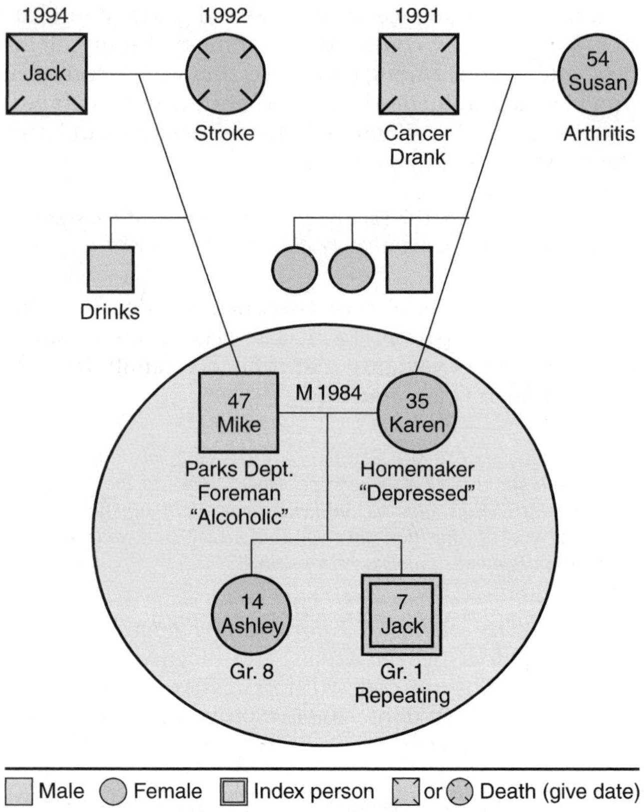

FIGURE **16–5** Sample family genogram. (Adapted from *Nurses and Families: A Guide to Family Assessment and Intervention,* 3rd ed., p. 90, by L. M. Wright and M. Leahey, 2000, Philadelphia: F. A. Davis.)

Nurses should draw genograms and ecomaps for families with whom they will be involved for more than 1 day. Information for brief genograms and ecograms can be gleaned from family members during the structural assessment. The most essential information for genograms includes data about ages, occupation or school grade, religion, ethnicity, and current health status of each family member. For a brief genogram, the nurse focuses only on information that is relevant to the family and health problem.

Developmental Assessment

Families, like individuals, change and grow over time. Although families are all unique, they tend to go through certain stages that require the family to adjust, adapt, and change roles. Each developmental stage presents challenges and includes tasks that need to be completed before the family can successfully move on to the next stage. Family development is more than the concurrent development of children and adults. It is the interaction between an individual's development and the phase of the family developmental life cycle that can be significant for family functioning. Therefore, in addition to understanding family structure, nurses should understand the developmental life cycle of each family.

Carter and McGoldrick's model of family life stages (1982, 1999) describes the emotional aspects of lifestyle transition and the changes and tasks necessary for the family to proceed developmentally (Table 16-1). The nurse can use this model to promote behaviours to achieve essential tasks and help families prepare for transitions. It should be noted that the model presented in Table 16-1 does not address diverse family forms, such as blended families, lone-parent families, families without children, or common-law partners.

Functional Assessment

A functional assessment focuses mainly on how family members interact and behave toward each other. The nurse assesses how family members function by closely observing their interactions. There are two subcategories of family functioning: instrumental and expressive functioning.

Instrumental Functioning. Instrumental functions are the normal activities of daily living such as preparing meals, eating, sleeping, and attending to health needs. For families with health problems, these activities often become a challenge. Roles often change as family members cope with illness and disability in the family.

> Questions to Ask the Family: *Who is usually responsible for housekeeping and child care? Do other family members help with these tasks? Does anyone in the family require help with activities of daily living? Who usually provides this help?*

Expressive Functioning. Expressive functions are the ways in which people communicate. Illness and disability often alter expressive functioning within the family. A diagnosis may cause intense feelings of anxiety or grief, both within the person being diagnosed and within other family members. Nurses should encourage families to explore their understanding of illness and how it impacts their lives. There are 10 subcategories of expressive functioning: emotional, verbal, non-verbal, and circular communication; problem solving; roles; influence; beliefs; and alliances and coalitions.

Emotional Communication. Emotional communication refers to the range and types of feelings that are expressed by the family. Most families express a wide range of feelings. However, families with problems often have rigid patterns with a narrow range of emotional expression. For example, a family coping with a father's diagnosis of cancer may be consumed with anxiety and not express optimism or hope for the future. Family roles and gender may affect emotional expression.

> Questions to Ask the Family: *How can you tell when each member of your family is happy, sad, or under stress? How do you express happiness, sadness, or stress?*

Verbal Communication. The nurse should observe a family's verbal communication, focusing on the meaning of the words in terms of the relationship. Is communication among family members clear and direct or is it vague

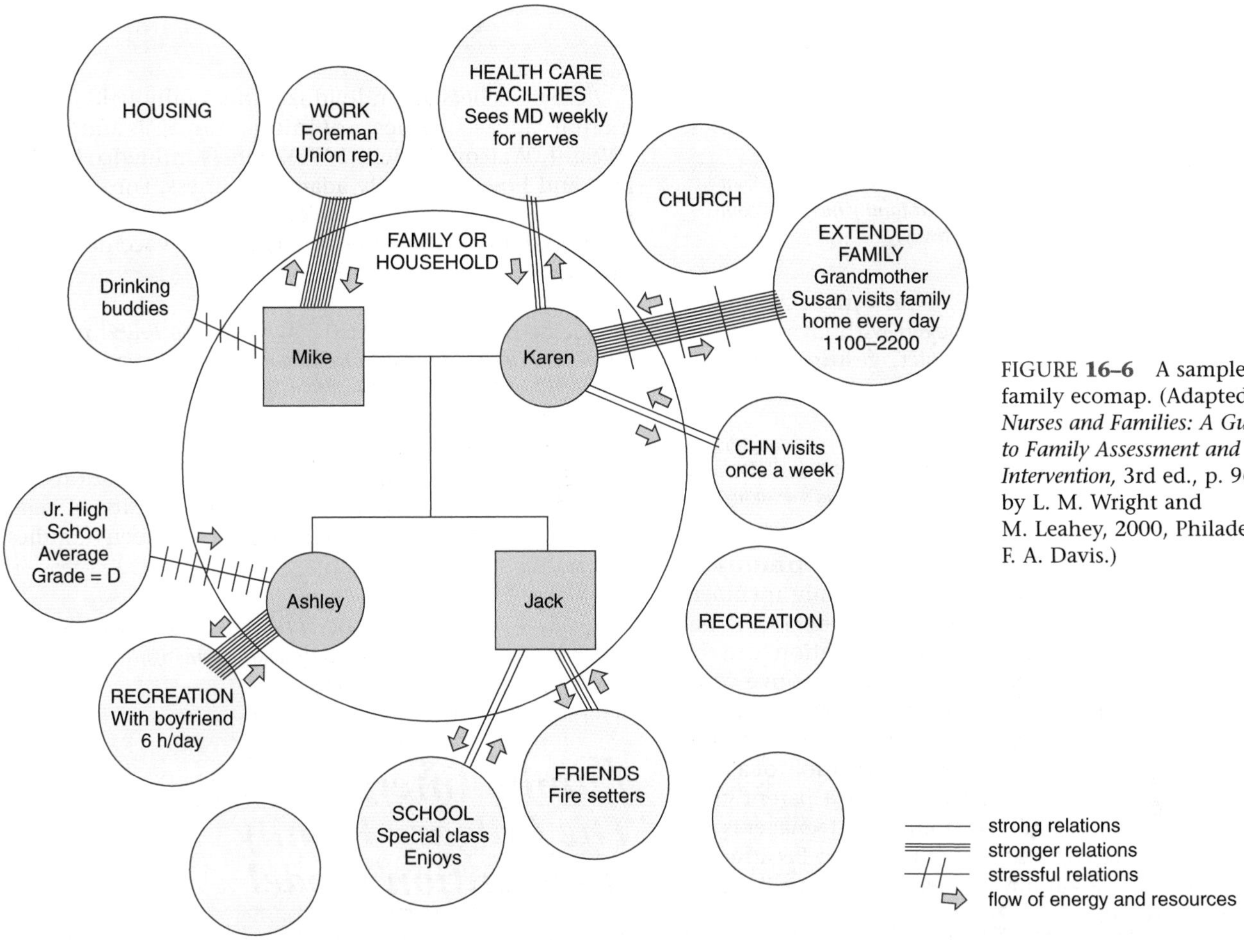

FIGURE **16–6** A sample family ecomap. (Adapted from *Nurses and Families: A Guide to Family Assessment and Intervention,* 3rd ed., p. 96, by L. M. Wright and M. Leahey, 2000, Philadelphia: F. A. Davis.)

Table 16-1 Stages of the Family Life Cycle

Family Life Cycle Stage	Emotional Process of Transition: Key Principles	Changes in Family Status Required to Proceed Developmentally
Between families: unattached young adult	Accepting parent-offspring separation	a. Differentiation of self in relation to family of origin b. Development of intimate peer relationships c. Establishment of self in work
Joining of families through marriage: newly married couple	Commitment to new system	a. Formation of marital system b. Realignment of relationships with extended families and friends to include spouse
Family with young children	Accepting new generation of members into system	a. Adjusting marital system to make space for children b. Taking on parental roles c. Realignment of relationships with extended family to include parenting and grandparenting roles
Family with adolescents	Increasing flexibility of family boundaries to include children's independence	a. Shifting of parent-child relationships to permit adolescents to move into and out of system b. Refocus on midlife material and career issues c. Beginning shift toward concerns for older generation
Launching children and moving on	Accepting multitude of exits from and entries into family system	a. Renegotiation of marital system as dyad b. Development of adult-to-adult relationships between grown children and their parents c. Realignment of relationships to include in-laws and grandchildren d. Dealing with disabilities and death of parents (grandparents)
Family in later life	Accepting shifting of generational roles	a. Maintaining own or couple functioning and interests in the face of physiological decline; exploration of new familial and social role options b. Support for more central role for middle generation c. Making room in system for wisdom and experience of older adults; supporting older generations without overfunctioning for them d. Dealing with loss of spouse, siblings, and other peers, and preparation for own death; life review and integration

Reprinted from McGoldrick M, Carter E: The stages of the family life cycle. In Walsh F: *Normal family processes,* 1982, Guilford Press.

and indirect? The nurse should also ask family members their opinions about how well the family communicates.

Questions to Ask the Family: *Which family member communicates most clearly? How might your family members communicate with each other more effectively?*

Non-Verbal Communication. Non-verbal communication consists of messages conveyed without words, including body language, eye contact, gesturing, crying, and tone of voice.

Questions to Ask the Family: *How do you think your daughter feels when your son rolls his eyes while she's talking? Who shows the most distress when talking about your dad's drinking?*

Circular Communication. **Circular communication** refers to communication between family members that is reciprocal; that is, each person influences the behaviour of the other. Circular communication can be adaptive or maladaptive. For example, an adaptive communication pattern is when a parent comforts a child because the child cries. Because the parent responds to the child, the child feels safe and secure. An example of a maladaptive communication pattern is when a parent criticizes a teenager for not phoning home. The teenager is angry for being criticized and avoids the parent. Because the teenager avoids the parent, the parent becomes angrier and criticizes more.

Questions to Ask the Family: *You mentioned that your wife frequently makes demands of you. What do you do then? How do you think that impacts her?*

Problem Solving. Problem solving refers to how a family solves its own problems.

Questions to Ask the Family: *Who first notices problems? How does your family tend to deal with problems? Is one member more proactive than others about solving problems?*

Roles. Roles are established patterns of behaviour for family members, often developed through interactions with others. Formal roles include those of mother, husband, friend, and so forth. Informal roles can include, for example, those of the "softy," "angel," or "scapegoat."

Questions to Ask the Family: *Who is the "good listener" in your family? Who is "the angel"?*

Influence. Influence refers to methods of affecting or controlling another's behaviour. Influence may be instrumental (the use of privileges as reward for behaviour; e.g., the promise of candy, computer time), psychological (the use of communication to influence behaviour; e.g., praise, admonishment), or corporal (the use of body contact; e.g., hugging, hitting).

Questions to Ask the Family: *What method does your mom use to get Noreen to go to bed at the right time? How does your grandma get Luis to attend school when he refuses?*

Beliefs. Beliefs are individual- and family-held fundamental ideas, values, opinions, and assumptions (Wright, Watson, & Bell, 1996). Beliefs influence behaviour and how the family adapts to illness. For example, if a family believes that vaccinations may cause long-term disabilities, the parents may decline vaccinating an infant.

Questions to Ask the Family: *What do you believe is the cause of your husband's depression? What do you believe would be the effect on your chronic pain if you choose to participate in that treatment?*

Alliances and Coalitions. Alliances and coalitions involve the directionality, balance, and intensity of relationships among family members or between families and nurses.

Questions to Ask the Family: *If the children are playing well together, who would most likely start them fighting? Who would stop them from fighting?*

Family Intervention: The Calgary Family Intervention Model

After the assessment, the nurse needs to intervene to help families meet their needs. A range of family nursing interventions can be offered to families. Some, such as parent education and caregiver support, are general; others are specific and require therapeutic communication and family interviewing skills. The ultimate goal is to help family members discover solutions that reduce or alleviate emotional, physical, and spiritual suffering. Whether caring for a client with the family as context or directing care to the family as client, nursing interventions aim to increase family members' abilities in certain areas, to remove barriers to health care, and to do things that the family cannot do for itself. The nurse guides the family in problem solving, provides practical services, and conveys a sense of acceptance and caring by listening carefully to family members' concerns and suggestions.

Nurses must tailor their interventions to each family and the chosen domain of family functioning. The nurse must remember that each family is unique. As well, nurses can only offer interventions to the family. They should not instruct or insist on a particular kind of change or way of family functioning.

The **Calgary Family Intervention Model (CFIM)** is a companion model to the CFAM and can be used as a guide for family interventions (Wright & Leahey, 2000). The CFIM focuses on promoting and improving family functioning in three domains: cognitive (thinking), affective (feeling), and behavioural (doing). Interventions may affect functioning in any or all of the three domains. For example, the clinic nurse informs a wife that her husband who has amyotrophic lateral sclerosis is still capable of large gross motor movement and suggests that he could help with chores in the house, such as bringing the laundry upstairs. This intervention challenges the wife's thinking that her husband was incapable of work, influences the wife to feel less depressed over her husband's declining physical capacity, and leads to the wife changing her behaviour by including her husband when doing other household chores.

The CFIM recommends many nursing practices that promote family functioning, including asking interventive questions, offering commendations, providing information, validating emotional responses, encouraging illness narratives, supporting family caregivers, and encouraging respite.

Asking Interventive Questions

One of the simplest but most effective ways that nurses can help families is by engaging in a conversation with families and asking them questions. The practice of asking questions leads the family to reflect on their situation, clarify their opinions and ideas, and understand how they are affected by their family member's illness or condition. By hearing their own responses to questions, family members can better understand themselves and each other, and perhaps discover new solutions. Interventive questions also provide important information to the nurse.

There are two types of interventive questions: linear and circular questions (Tomm, 1987, 1988). **Linear questions** provide the nurse with information about a client or family. They explore a family member's descriptions or perceptions of a problem. For example, when exploring a couple's perceptions of their daughter's anorexia nervosa, the nurse could begin with linear questions: "When did you notice that your daughter had changed her eating habits?" "Why do you think she stopped eating normally?" These questions inform the nurse of the woman's eating patterns and illuminate family perceptions or beliefs about eating patterns.

Circular questions help determine changes that could be made in a client's or family's life. They help explain a problem. For example, with the same family, the nurse could ask, "Who is most worried about Cheyenne's anorexia?" "How does Mother show that she's worrying the most?" Circular questions help the nurse understand relationships between individuals, beliefs, and events, and provide valuable information to help create change. In this way, circular questions often make new cognitive connections, paving the way for different family behaviours. Whereas linear questions may imply that the nurse knows what is best for the family, circular questions facilitate change by inviting the family to discover their own answers. Linear questions tend to target specific yes or no answers, thereby limiting the options for the family. For example, "Have you tried time-out to discipline your 3 year old?" An alternative circular question might be, "Which type of discipline seems to work best for your 3 year old?" There are several types of circular questions, and each can affect the cognitive, affective, and behavioural domains. These types include difference questions, behavioural effect questions, hypothetical/future-oriented questions, and triadic questions (Wright & Leahey, 2000; Table 16-2).

Offering Commendations

Families do not always look at their own system as one that has inherently positive components. The nurse can help the family become aware of its own unique strengths, thereby increasing its potential and capabilities. A **commendation** is a statement that emphasizes the strengths or abilities of the family. While spending time with the family, the nurse may observe many instances in which the family displays positive attributes. It is important to acknowledge these to the family so that they can appreciate their own resiliency. By commending a family's strengths and competencies, nurses can offer family members a new view of themselves. The nurse should look for patterns of behaviour to commend, rather than a single occurrence. For example, the nurse may say, "Your family is showing much courage in living with your wife's cancer for 5 years," or "I'm very impressed with how the family worked together during the crisis." Families coping with chronic, life-threatening, or psychosocial problems frequently feel hopeless in their efforts to overcome or live with the illness. Therefore, nurses can never offer too many truthful commendations. In a study of families experiencing chronic illness, families reported that the nursing team's commendations were "an extremely important facet of the process" (Robinson, 1998).

Family strengths include clear communication, adaptability, healthy child-rearing practices, support and nurturing among family members, and the use of crisis for growth. The nurse can help the family focus on these strengths instead of its problems and weaknesses.

Providing Information

Families need information from health care professionals about developmental issues, health promotion, and illness management, especially if the illness is complex (Levac, Wright, & Leahey, 2002; Robinson, 1998). Accurate and timely information is essential for the family to make decisions and cope with difficult situations. One of the roles the nurse will need to adopt is that of educator. Health education is a process by which information is shared by nurse and client in a two-way fashion. Family and client needs for information may be recognized through direct questioning, but they are generally far more subtle. The nurse may recognize that the father is fearful of cleaning the newborn's umbilical cord or that an older adult woman is not using her cane safely. Respectful communication is required. Often the subtle needs for information can be approached by saying, "I notice you are trying to not touch the umbilical cord; I see that a lot." Or, "You use the cane the way I did before I was shown a way to keep from falling or tripping over it; do you mind if I show you?" When the nurse assumes a humble position instead of coming across as an authority on the subject, this attitude often decreases the client's defences and invites the client to listen without feeling embarrassed.

Table 16-2 Types of Circular Questions

Type of Question	Examples to Elicit Change in the Following Domains: Cognitive Domain	Affective Domain	Behavioural Domain
Difference question			
Explores differences between people, relationships, time, ideas, or beliefs.	What is the best advice given you about supporting your son with AIDS? What is the worst advice?	Who in the family is most worried about how AIDS is transmitted?	Which family member is best at getting your son to take his medication on time?
Behavioural Effect Question			
Explores connections between how one family member's behaviour affects other members	What do you know about the affect of life-threatening illness on children?	How does your son show that he is afraid of dying?	What could you do to show your son that you understand his fears?
Hypothetical/Future-oriented Question			
Explores family options and alternative actions or meanings in the future	What do you think will happen if these skin grafts continue to be painful for your son?	If your son's skin grafts are not successful, what do you think his mood will be? Angry? Resigned?	When will your son engage in treatment for his contractures?
Triadic Question			
Question posed to a third person about the relationship between two other people	If your father were not drinking daily, what would your mother think about his receiving treatment for alcoholism?	What does your father do that makes your mother less anxious about his condition?	If your father were willing to talk with your mother about solutions to his addiction, what could he say?

Adapted from *Nurses and Families: A Guide to Family Assessment and Intervention* (3rd ed., pp. 162–163), by L. M. Wright and M. Leahey, 2000, Philadelphia: F. A. Davis.

Validating or Normalizing Emotional Responses

Validation of intense emotions can alleviate feelings of isolation and loneliness and help family members make the connection between a family member's illness and the family's emotional response. For example, after a diagnosis of a life-shortening illness, families frequently feel out of control or frightened. It is important for nurses to validate these strong emotions and to reassure families that they will adjust and learn new ways to cope.

Encouraging Illness Narratives

Too often, clients and family members are encouraged to talk only about medical aspects of their illness rather than emotional aspects. An **illness narrative** is the person's story of how the illness affects their whole being, including their emotional, intellectual, social, and spiritual dimensions. Hearing the person's illness narrative helps the nurse understand the person's strengths and challenges. This information enables the nurse to offer commendations acknowledging the client's abilities. Many people also find that the telling of their story helps them better understand themselves, their experience, and their family's experience.

The need to communicate what it is like to live in our individual, separate worlds of experience, particularly within the world of illness, is powerful in human relationships (Nichols, 1995; Wright, 2004). Frequently, nurses believe that listening entails on obligation to "fix" whatever concerns or problems are raised. However, showing compassion and offering commendations is usually more therapeutic or helpful than offering solutions to problems (Bohn, Wright, & Moules, 2003; Hougher Limacher, 2003; Hougher Limacher & Wright, 2003; Moules, 2002).

Encouraging Family Support

Nurses can enhance family functioning by encouraging and assisting family members to listen to each other's concerns and feelings. This assistance can be particularly useful if a family member is embracing some constraining beliefs when a loved one is dying or has died (Wright & Nagy, 1993). For example, a family may believe that to talk with the ill person about death and dying would hasten the person's death.

Supporting Family Caregivers

Family members are often afraid of becoming involved in the care of an ill member without a nurse's support. One way the nurse can best provide family care is through supporting family caregivers. Without adequate preparation or support, caregiving can be stressful, causing a decline in the health of the caregiver and the care receiver or even the development of abusive relationships.

Despite its demands, caregiving can be a positive and rewarding experience (Picot, Youngblut, & Zeller, 1997). Whether it is a wife caring for a husband or a daughter caring for a mother, caregiving is an interactional process. The interpersonal dynamics between family members influence the ultimate quality of caregiving. Thus the nurse can play a key role in helping family members develop better communication and problem-solving skills to build the relationships needed for successful caregiving.

Researchers have identified variables, such as caregiver and care recipient expectations of one another, that influence caregiving quality. Carruth (1996) has studied the concept of **reciprocity,** acknowledging the importance of the capability of care recipients to share exchanges that contribute to a caregiver's perception of self-worth. When the caregiver knows that the care recipient appreciates his or her efforts and values the assistance provided, a healthier and more satisfying caregiving relationship will exist. When caregiver and client solve problems together, overprotection or oversolicitous behaviour can be avoided. Clients feel in control of their care and responsible for care decisions. The caregiver also feels very positive and enjoys the caregiving experience (Isaksen, Thuen, & Hanestad, 2003).

Encouraging Respite

Nurses should encourage respite for caregivers, who may feel guilty about needing or wanting to withdraw from the caregiving role. Caregivers may not recognize their needs for respite. Sometimes an ill person may be encouraged to accept another person's temporary assistance so that family members can take a break. Whatever the situation, the nurse should remember that each family's need for respite varies.

Providing care and support for family caregivers often involves using available family and community resources for respite. A useful caregiving schedule is one where all family members participate, extended family members share any financial burdens posed by caregiving, and distant relatives send cards and letters communicating their support. However, it is imperative for the nurse to understand the relationship between potential caregivers and care recipients. If the relationship is not a supportive one, community services may be a resource for both the client and family.

Use of community resources might include locating a service required by the family or providing respite care so that the family caregiver has time away from the care recipient. Examples of services that may be beneficial to families include caregiver support groups, housing and transportation services, food and nutrition services, housecleaning, legal and financial services, home care, hospice, and mental health resources. Before referring a family to a community resource, it is critical that the nurse understands the family's dynamics and knows whether support is desired or welcomed. Often a family caregiver will resist help, feeling obligated to be the sole source of support to the care recipient. The nurse must be sensitive to family relationships and help caregivers understand the normalcy of caregiving demands.

Interviewing the Family

Once nurses have a clear conceptual framework for assessment and intervention, they can begin to learn the competencies and skills needed to conduct family interviews. Family interviews follow the same basic principles as any client interview (see chapter 12). However, family interviews can be more complex because there are more people involved. The nurse must develop keen perceptual, conceptual, and executive skills. *Perceptual skills* refer to the ability to make relevant observations. In family interviewing, the nurse must observe multiple interactions and relationships simultaneously. *Conceptual skills* are the ability to formulate observations of the entire family and give meaning to those observations. Remember, however, that observations and subsequent judgments are subjective and not conclusive. *Executive skills* are the actual therapeutic interventions that the nurse carries out in an interview. These therapeutic interventions elicit responses from family members and are the basis for further observations and conceptualizations. During an interview, the nurse monitors responses from a client and family to form opinions and concepts about therapeutic interventions. The type of therapeutic intervention that the nurse gives depends on the nurse's clinical expertise and experience in working with families.

Table 16-3 lists various stages of a family interview and the executive skills that might be used during each stage. By using the skills presented in Table 16-3, nurses can engage a family to assess, explore, and identify strengths and problems. The nurse can also decide to intervene or refer the family to another health professional. Note that these skills should not necessarily be applied to all families. The nurse should tailor the interview to each family's individual context.

It is important to realize that not all family interviews are formal, lengthy processes. Even if a nurse does not have the time to organize a formal family interview, the nurse can still engage the family in productive, therapeutic conversation. Every conversation between the nurse, client, and/or family members improves communication and understanding, and no conversation is trivial. Therapeutic conversations can be as short as one sentence or as long as time allows. All conversations, regardless of time, have the potential to bring the family together (Hougher Limacher & Wright, 2003; McLeod, 2003). Even brief interviews, or conversations, have tremendous healing potential because they offer families the opportunity to acknowledge and affirm their problems and seek solutions (Hougher Limacher, 2003; Moules, 2002; Tapp, 2001).

The integration of task-oriented client care with interactive, purposeful conversation distinguishes a time-effective interview (taking less than 15 minutes). Providing information and involving the family in decision making are integral parts of the process. The nurse searches for opportunities to engage in purposeful conversations with families, which may include the following:

- Routinely inviting families to accompany the client to the unit, clinic, or hospital
- Routinely including families in the admission procedure
- Routinely inviting families to ask questions
- Acknowledging the client and family's expertise in managing the health problem at home
- Routinely consulting clients and families about their ideas for treatment and discharge

Table 16-3 Family Interviewing Skills for Nurses Using the CFAM and CFIM

Perceptual/Conceptual Skills	Executive Skills
The nurse understands the following:	The nurse might do the following:
Stage 1: Engagement	
1. An individual family member is best understood in the context of the family.	1. Invite all family members who are concerned about or involved with the problem to attend the first interview.
2. Initial efforts to involve both partners and/or parents provide a broad view of the family and increases engagement among its members.	2. Try to involve both partners and/or parents in initial sessions.
3. Providing structure to the interview reduces anxiety and increases engagement, especially during times of crisis.	3. Explain the purpose, length, and structure of the interview to family members and ask if they have any questions about the interview.
4. Family members are most comfortable talking about the structural aspects of the family.	4. Introduce yourself, and ask family members to share their names, ages, work or school, years married, and so forth.
Stage 2: Assessment	
1. The CFAM is an important tool that can be used to understand family dynamics.	1. Explore the components of the structural, developmental, and functional aspects of the CFAM to assess strengths and problem areas. Not all components of the CFAM need to be explored if they are not relevant to the situation.
2. Obtaining a detailed description and history of the presenting problem is important.	2. Ask family members, including children, to explain their understanding of the presenting problem: "How do you see the problem?"
3. The presenting problem is often related to other concerns in the family. For example, a child's outbursts may be related to a family conflict.	3. Explore with the family if there are other problems or concerns connected to the presenting problem.
4. Noting differences generates more specific information. • That is: (a) Clarifying *differences between individuals* reveals information about family functioning. (b) Clarifying *differences between relationships* reveals information about family structure. (c) Clarifying differences *between family members or in relationships at various points in time* reveals information about family development.	4. Inquire about differences between individuals, relationships, and points in time. • For example: (a) Ask the child, "Who is better at getting you to do those things in the evening, Mother or Father?" (b) "Do Father and Ingo fight more or less than Father and Hannah?" (c) "Do you worry more, less, or the same about your husband's health since his heart attack?"
5. The information obtained from the family assessment is used to create a strengths/problems list. Strengths/problems may be present in the structural, functional, or developmental dimensions of family life. For example: (a) Structural: Adjusting to lone-parenthood (b) Developmental: Adjusting to children leaving home (c) Functional: Reacting to a family-held belief, such as, "Father would be displeased with us for still crying about his death."	5. State to the family your understanding of their strengths/problems and ask if you are correct. After verifying them with the family, record your conclusions. • E.g., "We've identified that being a new single parent and also having to cope with your children leaving home are your two major concerns. Have I understood this correctly?"
6. Some problems are beyond the scope of the nurse's competence. Referral is necessary when medical symptoms have not been fully assessed or long-standing emotional or behavioural problems exist.	6. Tell the family whether you will continue to work with them on problems or will refer them to another professional. (If referring, proceed to Stage 4, Termination.) • E.g., "Now that I have a more complete understanding of your concerns, I think it is necessary to have your son examined by a pediatrician."
7. An extensive inquiry into the most pressing problems is necessary before intervening.	7. Ask the family which issue they think is most important and then explore it in depth. If the family cannot agree, discuss the lack of consensus. • E.g., "About which of the problems we have discussed today are you most concerned?"
8. Assessment is complete when sufficient information has been obtained to clearly understand the presenting problem.	8. State your understanding of the problem(s) to the family and obtain their commitment to work on a specific problem.

Adapted from *Nurses and Families: A Guide to Family Assessment and Intervention* (3rd ed., pp. 195–202), by L. M. Wright and M. Leahey, 2000, Philadelphia: F. A. Davis.

Table 16-3 Family Interviewing Skills for Nurses Using the CFAM and CFIM—cont'd

Perceptual/Conceptual Skills	Executive Skills
Stage 3: Intervention	
1. Families have problem-solving abilities. Families not only possess the capability to change, but also to identify and implement solutions.	1. Encourage family members to explore possible solutions to problems. • E.g., "You've mentioned that your mother is critical of herself. What do you think she could do to feel more positive?"
2. Interventions are focused on the cognitive, affective, and/or behavioural domains of functioning, as described in the CFIM. It is not always necessary to design interventions for all domains simultaneously.	2. Plan interventions to influence one or all of the domains of functioning described in the CFIM. • For example: (a) Cognitive: Invite family to think differently. (b) Affective: Encourage different affective expressions. (c) Behavioural: Ask family to perform new tasks.
3. Lack of information can inhibit the family's problem-solving abilities. Often, with additional information, families can provide their own creative and unique solutions to problems.	3. Provide information to the family that will support further problem solving. • E.g., ask the family if they would like to hear about some typical reactions a three-year-old has to a new baby. This intervention targets cognitive functioning.
4. Persistent, intense emotions can often block the family's problem-solving abilities. • Families who predominantly experience emotions such as sadness or anger are often unable to deal with problems until the emotional constraint is removed.	4. When appropriate, validate family members' emotional responses. • E.g., a son who is suppressing grief may need confirmation of the normal grieving process. This intervention targets the affective functioning.
5. Suggesting specific tasks can often provide a new way for family members to behave in relation to one another.	5. Assign tasks aimed at improving family functioning. • E.g., suggest that the father and son spend one evening a week together in a common activity. This intervention influences behavioural functioning.
Stage 4: Termination	
A. If consultation or referral is necessary: 1. Families appreciate additional professional resources when problems are complex.	1. Refer individuals and/or family members for consultation or ongoing treatment. • E.g., "I think that your family needs professional input beyond what I can offer. Therefore, I would like to refer you to the learning centre."
B. If family interviewing with nurse continues: 1. Evaluating the family interviews at regular intervals is important.	1. Collaborate with family members about the present status of problems and initiate termination when sufficient progress is made.
2. Interviews over a prolonged period can foster excessive dependency. The nurse must be careful to not inadvertently encourage dependency.	2. If necessary, mobilize other supports for the family and begin to initiate termination by decreasing the frequency of sessions. Nurses can inadvertently provide "paid friendship" unless they mobilize other supports such as partner, friends, or relatives.
3. Recognizing family members' constructive efforts to solve problems is helpful.	3. Commend family members' positive efforts to resolve problems, regardless of whether you think significant improvement has occurred. • E.g., "Your family has made tremendous efforts to find ways to care for your elderly father at home and still attend to your children's needs."
4. Individuals and families appreciate backup support in times of stress.	4. If appropriate, extend an invitation for further meetings should problems recur or if the family wants consultation.

Key Concepts

- Family members influence one another's health beliefs, practices, and status.
- The concept of family is highly individual; thus the nurse should base care on the client's definition of family rather than on an inflexible definition of family.
- Family nursing requires that nurses continually examine the current trends in the Canadian family and its health care implications.
- A healthy, resilient family is able to integrate the need for stability with the need for growth and change. The family can be viewed as context—where the nurse focuses either on the individual client within the context of his or her family or on the family with the individual as context, or the family can be viewed as client (family systems nursing)—where the nurse focuses on family interactions.
- The Calgary Family Assessment Model (CFAM) provides a conceptual framework to guide nurses in assessing the structural, developmental, and functional aspects of the family.
- Genograms and ecomaps are structural assessment tools that provide the nurse with a pictorial image of the family's structure and relation to outside influences.
- Family members as caregivers are often spouses who may be either older adults themselves or adult children trying to work full time, care for aging parents, and launch teenagers successfully.
- Illness and disability often alter expressive functioning and communication within the family.
- The Calgary Family Intervention Model (CFIM) is a companion model to the CFAM and guides nurses in implementing family interventions; it is focused on improving family functioning in three domains: cognitive (thinking), affective (feeling), and behavioural (doing).
- One of the simplest and most effective ways that nurses can help families is by asking them interventive questions.
- Offering commendations is important because they encourage the family to recognize their strengths and competencies.
- Other nursing interventions to help the family include providing information, validating emotional responses, encouraging illness narratives, supporting family caregivers, and encouraging respite for family caregivers.
- Family caregiving is an interactional process that occurs within the context of the relationships among its members.
- Family interviews require the nurse to have perceptual, conceptual, and executive skills; interviews may be formal and lengthy or casual and brief.

Key Terms

Calgary Family Assessment Model (CFAM), *p. 301*
Calgary Family Intervention Model (CFIM), *p. 306*
Circular communication, *p. 306*
Circular questions, *p. 307*
Commendation, *p. 307*
Ecomap, *p. 303*
Family, *p. 297*
Family forms, *p. 297*
Family nursing, *p. 296*
Genogram, *p. 303*
Hardiness, *p. 300*
Illness narrative, *p. 308*
Linear questions, *p. 307*
Reciprocity, *p. 309*
Resiliency, *p. 300*

Critical Thinking Exercises

1. Kathy Mendolson is a palliative care nurse working with a family of four: Wai-Ling, a 45-year-old single mother; her adolescent sons, Chun and Wang; and Heng, her 76-year-old mother, who is in the last stages of terminal breast cancer. The family has lived together for 10 years, ever since they immigrated to Canada from Hong Kong. Heng helped Wai-Ling parent Chun and Wang and supported Wai-Ling when her husband died five years ago. Wai-Ling has decided to care for Heng in the family's home until the elderly mother dies. Kathy will assist this family to achieve their goal.
   a. What parts of the CFAM should Kathy use when assessing the family's needs?
   b. How can Kathy help the family achieve their goal of caring for their elderly family member at home?
   c. How can Kathy determine this family's strengths, suffering, and resources?
   d. What cultural aspects are important to consider with a family who has immigrated to Canada and is now facing the death of another loved one in the family?
2. Dan and Kim divorced seven years ago and neither has remarried. They have three daughters: Annie, Angela and Abby, ages 10, 12, and 14. At the time of the divorce, Dan was HIV positive and the disease has been active for five years. Kim has had repeated tests and remains HIV negative. Dan is responding to therapy slowly. Kim and Dan share parenting responsibilities and have a friendly relationship. They have decided it would be easier for the family to live together again so that Dan can be active in his children's lives without placing caregiver demands on Kim when the extended family visits overnight. Kim also wants to care for her former husband.
   a. What family development tasks are important to assess with this family as they attempt to reunite?
   b. How should the nurse determine what support services the family needs?
   c. What assessment questions would be useful to ask to assess how the illness is affecting this family and if there are any signs of emotional, physical, or spiritual suffering?

3. Mr. and Mrs. Baillargeron, both in their early 50s, are the youngest members of large French-Canadian Catholic families. They work full time and have two teenage children. Both sets of their parents are in their 80s and have chronic health problems. All of their siblings live farther away.
   a. How can the nurse help Mr. and Mrs. Baillargeron access resources to aid in caring for their parents and maintain the responsibilities of their own family unit?
   b. What developmental tasks does this family have?
   c. What kinds of questions could the nurse ask to assess the family's emotional and verbal communication (found in CFAM's functional assessment category)?

Review Questions

1. The nurse must think of family as:
   1. Parents and their children
   2. People related by marriage, birth, or adoption
   3. The nuclear family and aunts, uncles, grandparents, and cousins
   4. A set of relationships that the client identifies as family
2. The client is remarried, and her two children from a previous marriage live in the same household. Her husband's children visit on the weekend. This is an example of a(n)
   1. Nuclear family
   2. Blended family
   3. Extended family
   4. Alternative family
3. Which of the following is NOT a current trend?
   1. The proportion of couples without children at home is increasing.
   2. The proportion of "traditional" families is declining.
   3. The proportions of common-law and lone-parent families are increasing.
   4. The rate of teenagers giving birth has increased steadily.
4. The primary social context in which health promotion and disease prevention take place is
   1. At educational institutions
   2. From friends and colleagues
   3. From doctors and nurses
   4. The family
5. Two factors that contribute to the long-term health of a family are
   1. Structure and function
   2. Caregiving and reciprocity
   3. Hardiness and resiliency
   4. Context and system
6. When nurses view the family as client, their primary focus is on the
   1. Health and development of an individual member existing within a specific environment
   2. Family process and relationships
   3. Family relational and transactional concepts
   4. Family within a system
7. Asking a client "Who is in your family?" helps to assess
   1. Internal structure
   2. External structure
   3. Context
   4. Instrumental functioning
8. According to the CFAM, emotional communication is a subcategory of
   1. Instrumental functioning
   2. Development
   3. Internal structure
   4. Expressive functioning
9. "What do you think when your husband won't visit your son in the hospital?" is an example of a circular question. Asking the family circular questions is an effective way to
   1. Facilitate change by inviting the family to discover their own answers
   2. Encourage family members to be caregivers
   3. Validate their emotional responses
   4. Target specific yes or no answers
10. During a family interview, the nurse can
    1. Educate the family
    2. Enforce change
    3. Engage a family to assess, explore, and identify strengths and problems
    4. Establish roles

References

Astedt-Kurki, P., et al. (2002). Development and testing of a family nursing scale. *Western Journal of Nursing Research, 24*(5), 567–579.

Bell, J. M., et al. (2001). Learning to nurse the family [Editorial]. *Journal of Family Nursing, 7*(2), 117–126.

Bohn, U., Wright, L. M., & Moules, N. J. (2003). A family systems nursing interview following a myocardial infarction: The power of commendations. *Journal of Family Nursing, 9*(2), 151–165.

Canadian Nurses Association. (1997, September). The family connection. *Nursing Now, 3*. Retrieved December 15, 2004, from *http://www.cna-nurses.ca/_frames/issuestrends/issuestrendsframe.htm*

Carruth, A. K. (1996). Development and testing of the caregiver reciprocity scale. *Nursing Research, 45*, 92–97.

Carter, B., & McGoldrick, M. (Eds.). (1999). *The expanded family life cycle: Individual, family and social perspectives* (3rd ed.). Boston: Allyn and Bacon.

Feeley, N., & Gottlieb, L. N. (2000). Nursing approaches for working with family strengths and resources. *Journal of Family Nursing, 6*(1), 9–24.

Ford-Gilboe, M. (2002). Developing knowledge about family health promotion by testing the developmental model of health and nursing. *Journal of Family Nursing, 8*, 140–156.

Frank, A. W. (1995). *The wounded storyteller: Body, illness, and ethics*. Chicago: University of Chicago Press.

Hartrick, G. (2000). Developing health-promoting practice with families: One pedagogical experience. *Journal of Advanced Nursing, 3*, 27–34.

Harvey, E. (1999). Short-term and long-term effects of early parental employment on children: The National Longitudinal Survey of Youth. *Developmental Psychology, 35*(2), 445–459.

Hill, R. (1958). Generic features of families under stress. *Social Casework, 39*, 139–158.

Hougher Limacher, L. (2003). *Commendations: The healing potential of one family systems nursing intervention.* Unpublished doctoral thesis, University of Calgary, Calgary, Alberta.

Hougher Limacher, L., & Wright, L. M. (2003). Commendations: Listening to the silent side of a family intervention. *Journal of Family Nursing, 9*(2), 130–135.

Hunt, C. K. (2003). Concepts in caregiver research. *Journal of Nursing Scholarship, 35,* 27–32.

Isaksen, A. S., Thuen, F., & Hanestad, B. (2003). Patients with cancer and their close relatives: Experiences with treatment, care, and support. *Cancer Nursing, 26*(1), 68–74.

Leahey, M., & Harper-Jaques, S. (1996). Family-nurse relationships: Core assumptions and clinical implications. *Journal of Family Nursing, 2*(2), 133–151.

Leahey, M., et al. (1995). The impact of a family systems nursing approach: Nurses' perceptions. *Journal of Continuing Education in Nursing, 26,* 219–225.

Levac, A. M. C., Wright, L. M., & Leahey, M. (2002). Children and families: Models for assessment and intervention. In J. Fox (Ed.), *Primary health care of infants, children, and adolescents* (2nd ed., pp. 10–19). St. Louis, MO: Mosby.

McCubbin, M. A., McCubbin, H. I., & Thompson, A. I. (1996). Family Hardiness Index (FHI). In H. I. McCubbin, A. I. Thompson, & M. S. McCubbin (Eds.), *Family assessment: Resiliency, coping, and adaptation, inventories for research and practice.* Madison: University of Wisconsin Press.

McLeod, D. L. (2003). *Opening space for the spiritual: Therapeutic conversations with families living with serious illness.* Unpublished doctoral dissertation, University of Calgary, Alberta.

Moules, N. J. (2002). Nursing on paper: Therapeutic letters in nursing practice. *Nursing Inquiry, 9*(2), 104–113.

Neabel, B., Fothergill-Bourbonnais, F., & Dunning, J. (2000). Family assessment tools: A review of the literature from 1978–1997. *Heart & Lung, 29,* 196–209.

Nichols, M. P. (1995). *The lost art of listening.* New York: Guilford Press.

Picot, S. J. F., Youngblut, J., & Zeller, R. (1997). Development and testing of a measure of perceived caregiver rewards in adults. *Journal of Nursing Measurement, 5,* 33–52.

Robinson, C. A. (1998). Women, families, chronic illness, and nursing interventions: From burden to balance. *Journal of Family Nursing, 4*(3), 271–290.

Schober, M., & Affara, F. (2001). *The family nurse: Frameworks for practice.* Geneva, Switzerland: International Council of Nurses.

Statistics Canada. (n.d.). *Teenage pregnacy.* Retrieved December 15, 2004, from *http://www.statcan.ca/english/kits/preg/preg3.htm*

Statistics Canada. (2001). *Census families in private households, by family structure and presence of children, by provinces and territories (2001 Census).* Retrieved October 12, 2004, from *www.statcan.ca/english/Pgdb/famil54a.htm*

Statistics Canada. (2002a). *Canadian families and households.* Retrieved October 12, 2004, from *http://www12.statcan.ca/english/census01/Products/Analytic/companion/fam/canada.cfm*

Statistics Canada. (2002b). *Profile of Canadian families and households: Diversification continues.* Retrieved December 15, 2004, from *http://www12.statcan.ca/english/census01/Products/Analytic/companion/fam/contents.cfm*

Statistics Canada. (2003a, December 9). Grandparents and grandchildren. *The Daily.* Catalogue number 11-001-XIE. Retrieved October 12, 2004, from *http://www.statcan.ca/Daily/English/031209/d031209b.htm*

Statistics Canada. (2003b). *Income of Canadian families.* Retrieved December 15, 2004, from *http://www12.statcan.ca/english/census01/Products/Analytic/companion/inc/canada.cfm*

Statistics Canada. (2004, May 4). *Divorces: 2001 and 2002. The Daily.* Catalogue number 11-001-XIE. Retrieved December 15, 2004, from *http://www.statcan.ca/Daily/English/040504/d040504a.htm*

Stuart, M. (1991). An analysis of the concept of family. In A. Whall & J. Fawcett (Eds.), *Family theory development in nursing: State of the science and art* (pp. 31–42). Philadelphia: F. A. Davis.

Svavarsdottir, E. K., McCubbin, M. A., & Kane, J. H. (2000). Well-being of parents of young children with asthma. *Research in Nursing & Health, 23,* 346–358.

Tapp, D. M. (2001). Conserving the vitality of suffering: Addressing family constraints to illness conversations. *Nursing Inquiry, 8*(4), 254–263.

Tomm, K. (1987). Interventive interviewing: Part II. Reflexive questioning as a means to enable self-healing. *Family Process, 26,* 167–183.

Tomm, K. (1988). Interventive interviewing: Part III. Intending to ask lineal, circular, strategic or reflexive questions? *Family Process, 27,* 1–15.

The Vanier Institute of the Family. (2000). *Profiling Canada's families II.* Nepean, ON: Author.

Wright, L. M. (2004). *Spirituality, suffering, and illness: Ideas for healing.* Philadelphia: F. A. Davis.

Wright, L. M., & Leahey, M. (2000). Nurses and families: A guide to family assessment and intervention. Philadelphia: F. A. Davis.

Wright, L.M., & Nagy, J. (1993). Death: The most troublesome family secret of all. In E. Imber Black (Ed.), *Secrets in families and family therapy* (pp. 121–137). New York: W. W. Norton.

Wright, L. M., Watson, W. L., & Bell, J. M. (1996). *Beliefs: The heart of healing in families and illness.* New York: Basic Books.

Recommended Web Sites

Child & Family Canada:
http://www.cfc-efc.ca

Fifty Canadian non-profit organizations have come together under the banner of Child & Family Canada to provide relevant information to families and those who work with children and families. The Canadian Child Care Federation maintains this public education Web site.

The Vanier Institute of the Family:
http://www.vifamily.ca

The Vanier Institute of the Family was established in 1965 under the patronage of Governor General Georges P. Vanier and Madame Pauline Vanier. It is a national voluntary organization dedicated to promoting the well-being of Canadian families through research, publications, education, and advocacy. This Web site provides links to numerous publications related to important trends and issues affecting Canadian families, including a link to an online publication of *Profiling Canada's Families.*

17

Client Education

Amy Hall, RN, BSN, MS, PhD
Janet C. Ross-Kerr, RN, BScN, MS, PhD (Canadian author)

Objectives

Mastery of content in this chapter will enable the student to:

- Define the key terms listed.
- Identify three main goals of client education.
- Identify the nurse's role in client education.
- Identify the purposes of client education.
- Describe learning domains and basic learning principles.
- Differentiate factors that determine motivation to learn and ability to learn.
- Compare and contrast the nursing and teaching processes.
- Write learning objectives for a teaching plan.
- Describe characteristics of a good learning environment.
- Describe ways to incorporate teaching and routine nursing care.
- Identify methods for evaluating learning.

Educating clients is a role for nurses in all health care settings. Clients and family members have the right to health education so that they can make informed decisions about their health and lifestyle. Thus, nurses have an ethical responsibility to teach their clients about health care practices. The nurse often clarifies information provided by physicians and other health care providers and may become the primary source of information needed for people adjusting to health problems (Oermann, Harris, & Dammeyer, 2001). In primary health care settings, the nurse is often the main source of information about health promotion and illness prevention (Box 17-1).

Shorter hospital stays, increased demands on nurses' time, more chronically ill clients—all make education especially important. Client education helps ensure continuity of care as clients move from one health care setting to another. A well-designed, comprehensive teaching plan that meets a learner's needs can reduce health care costs, improve quality of care, help clients gain optimal wellness, and increase independence (Cooper et al., 2001).

Goals of Client Education

The goal of client education is to assist individuals, families, or communities in achieving optimal levels of health (Edelman & Mandle, 2002). A main tool of primary health care, education helps individuals, families, and communities to maintain and improve their health, reduce hardship, and contain health care costs. Client education has three main goals (Box 17-2):

- Maintaining and promoting health and preventing illness
- Restoring health
- Coping with impaired functioning

Box 17-1

Focus on Primary Health Care

Educating Clients in order to Promote Health and Prevent Disease

Promotion of health through prevention of disease is an important goal of primary health care. Nurses are essential in preventing many diseases (e.g., cardiovascular disease) by teaching clients about evidence supporting preventive actions and lifestyle change. Clients need to know about risk factors and how they can avoid or reduce their risk of developing the disease. In order to teach clients effective health practices, nurses need to be aware of the evidence in the literature and to apply this to counselling clients. They can also help clients make lifestyle changes by helping interpret the meaning of the evidence.

In order to communicate information successfully, nurses need to use simple, clear and non-technical language that clients can understand and to develop rapport with clients so that they are able to receive and act on the information. Characteristics of a positive relationship with the client include empathic understanding, genuineness, unconditional regard, intimacy and reciprocity, respect for the client's right to control lifestyle, and mutual trust.

Because clients may face serious barriers to making lifestyle changes, nurses need to carry out an assessment to determine the readiness for behaviour change and the feasibility of carrying out the change. Nurses must understand principles of learning and behaviour change theories in order to set the stage for determining how meaningful lifestyle change might be possible for the client.

Clients need to develop an awareness of their own behaviour, a process that can by enhanced by self-monitoring. When clients can identify areas of difficulty and how they can be addressed, goals can be set collaboratively to ensure that clients are able to change their behaviour. Breaking long term goals into shorter term goals tends to enhance self-efficacy and client satisfaction. Focusing on behaviour change rather than physiological outcomes is recommended because the former is within the control of the client. Once the goal is set, feedback on its attainment is important to support the client's efforts. The use of social support from family or friends can be a positive influence in terms of helping clients achieve their goals.

From "Promoting Prevention: Skill Sets and Attributes of Health Care Providers Who Deliver Behavioural Interventions," L. E. Burke and J. Fair, 2003, *Journal of Cardiovascular Nursing, 18*(4), pp. 256–266.

Box 17-2 Topics for Health Education

Health Maintenance and Promotion and Illness Prevention

First aid
Avoidance of risk factors (e.g., smoking, alcohol)
Stress management
Growth and development
Hygiene
Immunizations
Prenatal care and normal child-bearing
Nutrition
Exercise
Safety (in home and health care setting)
Screening (e.g., blood pressure, vision, cholesterol level)
Behaviour modification to change risk behaviours (e.g., quitting smoking, treatment for substance abuse treatment)

Restoration of Health

Client's disease or condition
Anatomy and physiology of body system affected
Cause of disease
Origin of symptoms
Expected effects on other body systems
Prognosis
Limitations on function
Rationale for treatment
Medications
Tests and therapies
Nursing measures
Surgical intervention
Expected duration of care
Hospital or clinic environment
Hospital or clinic staff
Long-term care
Methods for client participation in care
Limitations posed by disease or surgery

Coping With Impaired Functions

Home care
Medications
Intravenous therapy
Diet
Activity
Self-help devices
Rehabilitation of remaining function
Physiotherapy
Occupational therapy
Speech therapy
Prevention of complications
Knowledge of risk factors
Implications of non-compliance with therapy
Environmental alterations

Maintaining and Promoting Health and Illness Prevention

In the home, clinic, or other community setting, the nurse provides information and skills that people need to maintain and improve their health (see Box 17-2). For example, in prenatal classes, nurses teach expectant parents about fetal development and physical and psychological changes during pregnancy. They also teach about the importance of healthy food choices, exercise, and avoiding substances that might harm the fetus. Greater knowledge can result in better health. When clients become more health conscious, they are more likely to seek early diagnosis of health problems (Redman, 2001).

Restoring Health

Many clients seek information and skills that will help them regain or maintain their health (see Box 17-2). However, clients who find it difficult to adapt to illness may be more passive. The nurse learns to identify clients' willingness to learn and to help motivate interest in learning (Assessment, the Foundation of Good Teaching, 2002).

The family can be a vital part of a client's return to health and may need to know as much as the client. If the nurse excludes the family from a teaching plan, conflicts may arise. For example, if the family does not understand a client's need to regain independent function, their efforts may encourage dependency and slow recovery. Nurses should assess the client-family relationship before involving the family in a teaching plan (see Chapter 16).

Coping With Impaired Functioning

Some clients must learn to cope with permanent health alterations. For example, a client whose ability to speak is lost after surgery of the larynx must learn new ways to communicate. A client with severe heart disease must learn to modify risk factors that might cause further heart damage. After the client's needs are identified and the family has displayed willingness to help, the nurse teaches family members to assist the client with health care management (e.g., giving medications through gastric tubes and doing passive range-of-motion exercises).

Teaching and Learning

Teaching is an interactive process that promotes learning. Generally, teaching and learning begin when a person identifies a need for knowing or acquiring an ability to do something. A nurse-teacher provides information that prompts the client to engage in activities that lead to a desired change. Teaching is most effective when it responds to the learner's needs. The teacher assesses these needs by asking questions, observing the client, and determining the client's interests. With successful teaching, clients can learn new skills or change existing attitudes (Redman, 2001; Box 17-3).

Role of the Nurse in Teaching and Learning

Nurses have an ethical responsibility to teach their clients. The Canadian Nursing Association's code of ethics (2002) indicates that clients have the right to make informed decisions about their care. The information clients need to make such decisions must be accurate, complete, and relevant to their needs. The nurse should anticipate clients' needs for information based on their physical condition and treatment plans. The nurse often clarifies information provided by physicians and other health care providers and may become the primary source of information for adjusting to health problems (Oermann, Harris, and Dammeyer, 2001).

Clients and their families often ask nurses for health information. However, in some cases, the need for information may be less apparent. The nurse needs to observe and listen carefully to determine clients' information and learning needs. When nurses value education and ensure their clients' learn necessary information, clients are better prepared to assume health care responsibilities.

Research Highlight — Box 17-3

Learning Preferences of Clients with Cancer

Research Focus

Adult clients living with cancer have unique learning needs. This study aimed to identify the best methods to meet these needs.

Research Abstract

This study had three phases. In the first phase, a multidisciplinary team identified key categories of information that should be included in an educational program. The key categories included topics such as cancer diagnosis and treatment, coping, medication side effect management, sexuality, and pain control. The second phase included 100 structured interviews. The third phase of the study included a 37-item survey based on information obtained during the interviews.

The survey asked 1,310 clients with cancer to recall what they were taught about their treatment and their educational preferences. Results: Discussions with physicians were the most favoured learning method, followed by personal communication with nurses. Women were more likely to prefer speaking with a nurse for all content areas, whereas men were more likely to discuss sexuality with their physicians. The majority of respondents did not attend support groups, and interest in computer-assisted learning (e.g., the Internet) was low. However, respondents expressed interest in using a toll-free number to access information and support.

Evidence-Based Practice

- Clients with cancer want clear, accurate information about their diagnosis and related treatment options.
- Adult clients with cancer prefer interactive, personal communication with physicians or nurses.
- Printed material is preferred to computer-assisted learning.
- Assessing and adapting educational information and approaches to clients' needs and preferences enhances the success of educational efforts.
- Nurses must remain creative and responsive to their clients when providing client education.

Reference

Chelf, J., et al. (2002). Learning and support preferences of adult patients with cancer at a comprehensive cancer center. *Oncology Nursing Forum, 29*(5), 863–867.

Teaching as Communication

Effective teaching depends on effective communication (see chapter 14). To be a good teacher, a nurse must listen empathetically, observe astutely, and speak clearly. Many intrapersonal variables influence both the nurse and client's style and approach, including attitudes, values, culture and emotions, and knowledge. Both the client and the nurse are also affected by the client's motivation and ability to learn, which depends on physical and psy-

Box 17-4 Appropriate Teaching Methods Based on Domains of Learning

Cognitive

Discussion (one-on-one or group)
May involve nurse and one client or nurse with several clients.
Promotes active participation and focuses on topics of interest to client.
Allows peer support.
Enhances application and analysis of new information.

Lecture

Is more formal method of instruction because it is teacher controlled.
Helps learner acquire new knowledge and gain comprehension.
Includes question-and-answer session.
Designed specifically to address client's concerns.
Assists client in applying knowledge.

Role Play, Discovery

Allows client to actively apply knowledge in controlled situation.
Promotes synthesis of information and problem solving.

Independent Projects (e.g., Computer-assisted Instruction), Field Experience

Allows client to assume responsibility for learning at own pace.
Promotes analysis, synthesis, and evaluation of new information and skills.

Affective

Role play
Allows expression of values, feelings, and attitudes.
Discussion (group)
Allows client to acquire support from others in group.
Permits client to learn from others' experiences.
Promotes responding, valuing, and organizing.
Discussion (one-on-one)
Allows discussion of personal, sensitive topics of interest or concern.

Psychomotor

Demonstration
Provides presentation of procedures or skills by nurse.
Permits client to incorporate modelling of nurse's behaviour.
Allows nurse to control questioning during demonstration.

Practise

Enables client to perform skills using equipment in a controlled setting.
Provides repetition.
Return demonstration.
Permits client to perform skill as nurse observes.
Provides excellent source of feedback and reinforcement.

Independent Projects, Games

Require teaching method that promotes adaptation and origination of psychomotor learning.
Permit learner to use new skills.

chological health, education, developmental stage, and previous knowledge.

Domains of Learning

Learning occurs in three domains: cognitive (understanding), affective (attitudes), and psychomotor (motor skills; Bloom, 1956). Any topic to be learned may involve one domain, all domains, or any combination of the three. For example, clients with diabetes must learn how diabetes affects the body and how to control blood glucose levels for better health (cognitive domain). They must also learn to accept the chronic nature of diabetes by learning positive coping mechanisms (affective domain). Finally, many clients with diabetes must learn to test their blood glucose levels at home. This requires learning how to use a glucose meter (psychomotor domain). Understanding each learning domain prepares the nurse to select appropriate teaching methods (Box 17-4).

Cognitive Learning

Cognitive learning includes all intellectual behaviours and requires thinking (Bastable, 2003). In the hierarchy of cognitive behaviours, the simplest behaviour is acquiring knowledge and the most complex is evaluation.

Knowledge. Using knowledge involves acquiring new facts or information and being able to recall them. For example, the client learns about a prescribed medication and is able to describe its purpose and potential side effects.

Comprehension. Comprehension is the ability to understand the meaning of learned material. For example, the client is able to explain how a new medication will improve a physical condition.

Application. Application uses abstract, newly learned ideas in a practical situation. For example, the client develops a medication schedule according to normal mealtimes to ensure optimal desired effects of the medication.

Analysis. Analysis involves breaking down information into organized parts, allowing a client to discriminate important from unimportant information. For example, the client is able to distinguish which medication side effects are most common and which are least common.

Synthesis. Synthesis is the ability to apply knowledge and skills to produce a new whole. For example, the client experiences side effects from a medication and takes steps to prevent them.

Evaluation. Evaluation is a judgment of the worth of information given for a specific purpose. For example, the client recognizes the need for more information about insulin to plan a safe exercise program.

Affective Learning

Affective learning concerns expressions of feelings and acceptance of attitudes, opinions, or values. Values clarification (see chapter 7) is an example of affective learning. The simplest behaviour in the affective learning hierarchy is receiving, and the most complex is characterizing (Krathwohl, Bloom, & Masia, 1964).

Receiving. Receiving is receptivity to another person's words. For example, a woman shows a willingness to listen to a nurse explain the surgical procedure for removal of a breast by maintaining eye contact while the nurse is talking.

Responding. Responding means participating through listening and reacting verbally and non-verbally. The person reveals that he or she is engaged in the exchange. For example, the client responds verbally by asking the nurse about the appearance of the incision following surgery.

Valuing. Valuing means attaching worth to an object, concept, or behaviour. Learners demonstrate valuing through their behaviour. For example, a client reveals the value she places on her body image by refusing to look at her incision following breast surgery.

Organizing. Organizing refers to the development of a value system that identifies and organizes or reorganizes values and resolves conflicts. For example, the client reorganizes her value system and resolves conflict by accepting changes created by surgery and planning for a prosthesis fitting.

Characterizing. Characterizing involves acting and responding with a consistent value system. The person behaves consistently when values are tested or challenged. For example, the client who accepted a diagnosis of breast cancer and did not fear losing a breast assumes her regular routine after surgery and is able to discuss positive self-feelings with others.

Psychomotor Learning

Psychomotor learning involves acquiring skills that require the integration of mental and muscular activity, such as the ability to walk or to use an eating utensil. The simplest behaviour in the hierarchy is perception and the most complex is origination (Rankin & Stallings, 2001; Redman, 2001).

Perception. Perception is being aware of objects or qualities through the use of sensory organs, which give cues to performing a task. For example, a client who has had a stroke needs to learn to use a walker. While learning this skill, the client begins to recognize that different walking surfaces require adjustments in placing the walker.

Set. A set is a readiness to take a particular action. There are three sets: mental, physical, and emotional. For example, a young man injured in a car accident uses judgment to determine the best way to get out of a wheelchair (mental readiness). The man aligns and postures properly (physical readiness). He also commits (emotional readiness) to do strengthening exercises regularly to aid in his recovery.

Guided Response. A guided response is the performance of an act under an instructor's supervision. For example, a client prepares an insulin injection after watching a nurse's demonstration. The nurse provides immediate reinforcement after the client correctly performs the self-injection.

Mechanism. A mechanism is a higher level of behaviour from which a person gains confidence and skill. Usually the skill is more complex or involves several more steps than a guided response. For example, a client learns to fill the insulin syringe for different insulin doses.

Complex Overt Response. A complex overt response involves performing a complex motor skill smoothly and accurately without hesitation. For example, a client who is recently paralyzed from a spinal injury learns to perform self-catheterization.

Adaptation. Adaptation occurs when a person learns to change a motor response to solve problems. For example, a new mother returning to work learns how to collect breast milk, store it, and coordinate pumping times with her baby's feeding demands and her work schedule.

Origination. Origination is a highly complex motor skill that involves creating new movement patterns. A person acts on the basis of existing psychomotor skills and abilities. For example, a client who has left-sided paralysis learns to eat, dress, and walk.

Basic Learning Principles

Before nurses can teach, they must understand how people learn. Learning depends on the learning environment and on the individual's ability to learn, learning style, and motivation.

Learning Environment

The ideal environment for learning is a well-lit, well-ventilated room with appropriate furniture and a comfortable temperature. A quiet setting with few distractions and interruptions helps concentration. A nurse can provide privacy even in a busy hospital by closing cubicle curtains or taking the client to a quiet spot. In the home, a bedroom might separate the client from household activities. If the client desires, family members or significant others may share in discussions. However, some clients may be reluctant to discuss their illness when others, even close family members, are in the room.

Ability to Learn

The ability to learn depends on emotional, intellectual, and physical capabilities and on developmental stage. If a client's learning ability is impaired, the nurse should modify or postpone teaching activities.

Emotional Capability. Emotions can aid or prevent a person from learning. Mild anxiety may help a person focus. However, stronger levels of anxiety can be incapacitating, creating an inability to attend to anything other than to relieve the anxiety. The prospect of change makes many people anxious. Seriously ill people, who are faced with multiple losses, may be extremely anxious and distressed. Nurses must be sensitive to a client's level of anxiety. If a person is incapacitated with anxiety, the nurse needs to find a way to alleviate the anxiety. This may mean teaching relaxation techniques before attempting to teach a task or a procedure.

Intellectual Capability. Clients have different levels of intellectual ability. The nurse must assess the client's knowledge and intellectual level before beginning a teaching plan. For example, measuring liquid or solid food portions requires the ability to perform mathematical calculations. Reading a medication label or discharge instructions requires reading and comprehension skills. Following directions when performing self-care in accordance with limitations requires comprehension and application skills.

Physical Capability. The ability to learn often depends on physical health. To learn psychomotor skills, a client must possess the necessary strength, coordination, and sensory acuity. The nurse should not overestimate the client's physical ability. The following physical attributes are required to learn psychomotor skills:

- Size (height and weight match the task to perform or the equipment to use [e.g., crutch walking])
- Strength (ability of the client to follow a strenuous exercise program)
- Coordination (dexterity needed for complicated motor skills, such as using utensils or changing a bandage)
- Sensory acuity (visual, auditory, tactile, gustatory, and olfactory; sensory resources needed to receive and respond to messages taught)

Any physical condition (e.g. pain, fatigue, or hunger) that depletes energy also impairs the ability to learn. For example, a client in a weakened state who has just spent hours undergoing diagnostic tests is likely to be too fatigued to learn. Nurses must assesses the client's energy level by noting the client's willingness to communicate, the degree of activity initiated, and the client's responsiveness to questions. The nurse may halt teaching if the client needs rest.

Developmental Stage. Age and stage of development affects the ability to learn (Box 17-5). Without proper biological, motor, language, and personal-social development, many types of learning cannot take place.

Learning in Children. As a child matures, intellectual growth moves from concrete to abstract. Therefore, information should be understandable, and the expected outcomes realistic and based on the child's developmental stage. Developmentally appropriate teaching aids should also be used (Figure 17–1).

Adult Learning. Many adults are independent, self-directed learners. However, they may become dependent in new learning situations. Adults typically learn more successfully when they are encouraged to use past experiences to solve problems. Adult clients and nurses should collaborate on educational topics and goals. Needs or issues that are important to the adult should be addressed early in the teaching-learning process. Ultimately, adults must accept responsibility for changing their own behaviours. Assessing what the adult client currently knows, teaching what the client wants to know, and setting mutual goals will improve the outcomes of care and education (Bastable, 2003).

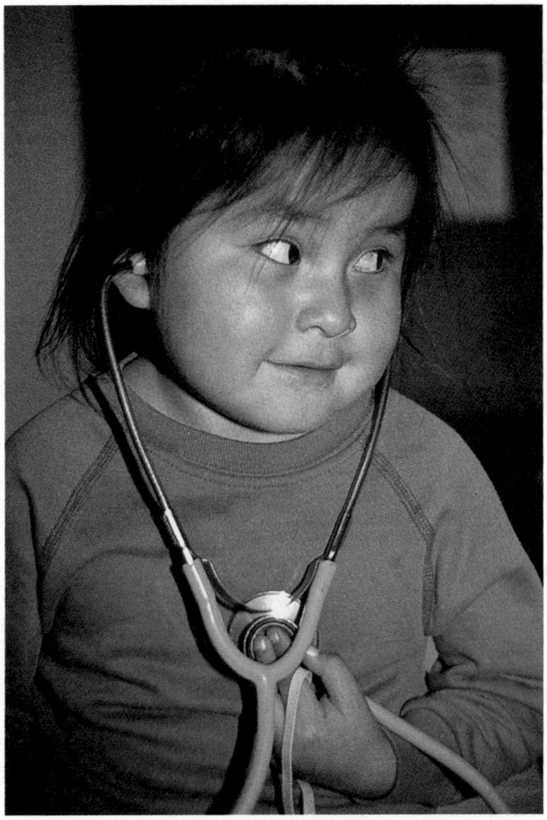

FIGURE **17–1** The preschool child learns not to be afraid of medical equipment by being allowed to handle the stethoscope and imitating its use.

Learning Style and Preference

People have different learning styles and preferences. Everyone processes information differently by seeing and hearing, reflecting and acting, reasoning logically and intuitively, and analyzing and visualizing. Some people are visual learners. They learn best by watching. Audiovisual presentations and visual demonstrations often work best for this type of learner. Other people learn best when they are able to manipulate tools and find out how they work. Some people learn by taking detailed notes; others prefer to only listen. Some people need to be engaged in activities and discussion to learn effectively. Others may be too shy to enjoy this type of learning and prefer to learn from an orderly, structured presentation.

When developing teaching plans, the nurse should ask clients how they like to learn. With groups, it may not be possible to address every client's preferences. However,

Box 17-5 Teaching Methods Based on Client's Development Capacity

Infant

Keep routines (e.g., feeding, bathing) consistent.
Hold infant firmly while smiling and speaking softly to convey sense of trust.
Have infant touch different textures (e.g., soft fabric, hard plastic).

Toddler

Use play to teach procedure or activity (e.g., handling examination equipment, applying bandage to doll).
Offer picture books that describe story of children in hospital or clinic.
Use simple words such as cut instead of laceration to promote understanding.

Preschooler

Use role-playing, imitation, and play to make it fun for preschoolers to learn.
Encourage questions and offer explanations. Use simple explanations and demonstrations.
Encourage children to learn together through pictures and short stories about how to perform hygiene.

School-Age Child

Teach necessary psychomotor skills. (Complicated skills, such as learning to use a syringe, may take considerable practice.)
Offer opportunities to discuss health problems and answer questions.

Adolescent

Help adolescent learn about feelings and need for self-expression.
Collaborate on teaching activities.
Let adolescents make decisions about health and health promotion (safety, sex education, substance abuse).
Use problem solving to help adolescents make choices.

Young or Middle Adult

Encourage participation in teaching plan by setting mutual goals.
Encourage independent learning.
Offer information so that adult can understand effects of health problem.

Older Adult

Teach when client is alert and rested.
Involve adult in discussion or activity.
Focus on wellness and the person's strength.
Use approaches that enhance sensorially impaired client's reception of stimuli (see chapter 44).
Keep teaching sessions short.

including a combination of approaches to meet multiple learning styles can ensure that most people's learning preferences are met (Felder, 2002).

Motivation to Learn

Motivation is a person's desire or willingness to learn; it may result from a social, task mastery, or physical motive and it influences a person's behaviour (Redman, 2001). Thus, if one does not want to learn, learning is unlikely to occur.

Social Motives. Social motives demonstrate a need for connection, social approval, or self-esteem. For example, new parents demonstrate a need for connection and social approval when they validate ideas about parenting with friends or with health care workers with whom they have rapport.

Task Mastery Motives. Task mastery motives are driven by desire for achievement. For example, a high school student with diabetes begins to test blood glucose levels and determine insulin dosages before leaving home and establishing independence. The desire to live independently and manage the disease provides the motivation to master the task or skill. After succeeding at a task, a person is usually motivated to achieve more.

Physical Motives. Physical motives come from a desire to maintain and improve health. Those motivated by the need to survive or overcome hardship are often more motivated than those who wish merely to improve their health (Rankin & Stallings, 2001). For example, a client who has had a leg amputated may be extremely motivated to learn to use assistive devices, whereas a client who is overweight but otherwise healthy may not be motivated to exercise.

Many people will not adopt new health behaviours or change unhealthy behaviours unless they perceive a disease as a threat, overcome barriers to changing health practices, and see the benefits of such changes. Thus, a client with lung disease may continue to smoke. An obese client may worsen a heart condition by refusing to follow a low-fat diet.

Motivation and Social Learning Theory. Health education often involves changing people's attitudes and values. Change can only occur when education plans and interventions are based on sound learning theories. A number of theories address the complex client education process (Bastable, 2003; Redman, 2001). One of these is **social learning theory,** which helps educators understand learners and develop interventions that enhance motivation and learning (Bandura, 2001; Bastable, 2003; Saarmann, Daugherty, & Riegel, 2002).

Table 17-1 Comparison of the Nursing and Teaching Processes

Basic Steps	Nursing Process	Teaching Process
Assessment	Collect data about client's physical, psychological, social, cultural, developmental, and spiritual needs from client, family, diagnostic tests, medical record, health history, and literature.	Gather data about client's learning needs, motivation, ability to learn, and teaching resources from client, family, learning environment, medical record, health history, and literature.
Nursing diagnosis	Identify appropriate nursing diagnoses based on assessment findings.	Identify client's learning needs on basis of three domains of learning.
Planning	Develop individualized care plan. Set diagnosis priorities based on client's immediate needs. Collaborate with client on care plan.	Establish learning objectives, stated in behavioural terms. Identify priorities regarding learning needs. Collaborate with client on teaching plan. Identify type of teaching method to use.
Implementation	Perform nursing care therapies. Include client as active participant in care. Involve family/significant other in care as appropriate.	Implement teaching methods. Actively involve client in learning activities. Include family/significant other participation as appropriate.
Evaluation	Identify success in meeting desired outcomes and goals of nursing care. Alter interventions as indicated when goals are not met.	Determine outcomes of teaching-learning process. Measure client's ability to achieve learning objectives. Reinforce information as needed.

When people believe that they can execute a particular behaviour, they are more likely to perform the behaviour consistently and correctly (Bandura, 1997). *Self-efficacy,* a social learning theory concept, refers to a person's perceived ability to successfully complete a task. Beliefs about self-efficacy arise from four sources: enactive mastery experiences, vicarious experiences, verbal persuasion, and physiological and affective states (Bandura, 1997). Understanding these sources lets nurses develop appropriate interventions. For example, a nurse teaching a boy with asthma to use an inhaler expresses positive reinforcement (verbal persuasion). The nurse then demonstrates how to use the inhaler (vicarious experience). The boy uses the inhaler (enactive mastery experience). As the boy's wheezing and anxiety decrease from using the inhaler, he experiences positive feedback, further enhancing his confidence to use the inhaler (physiological and affective states). Interventions such as these enhance perceived self-efficacy, which in turn improves the achievement of desired outcomes.

Integrating the Nursing and Teaching Processes

The nursing and teaching processes are related (Redman, 2001) and usually take place concurrently. Like the nursing process, the teaching process requires assessment, nursing diagnosis, planning, implementation, and evaluation. However, the processes are not exactly the same. The nursing process is broader. For example, determining a client's health needs requires assessing all data sources. The teaching process is focused on data sources that reveal the client's learning needs, willingness and ability to learn, and available teaching resources. Table 17-1 compares the teaching and nursing processes.

The teaching process requires assessment. The client's ability to learn, motivation, and needs should be assessed and analyzed. A diagnostic statement specifies the information or skills that the client requires. The nurse sets specific **learning objectives** (i.e., what the learner will be able to do after successful instruction) and implements the teaching plan using teaching and learning principles to ensure that the client acquires knowledge and skills. Finally, the teaching process requires an evaluation of learning based on learning objectives.

NP Assessment

During assessment, the nurse determines the client's health care needs (see chapter 12). The client may reveal a need for health care information or the nurse may identify a need for education. Learning needs identified by both the client and the nurse determine the content to be learned. An effective assessment forms the basis on which instruction can be individualized for each client (Redman, 2001).

Learning Needs. Most clients can identify at least some of their own learning needs. Effective questioning and assessment tools help a nurse to determine a client's perceived learning needs. By listening carefully and using open-ended and closed questions (see chapter 14), nurses can often find out what a client wants to know. Assessment tools can help clients to determine their learning needs. For example, a short educational needs checklist was developed for clients with coronary artery disease (Martinali et al., 2001). Clients who used this checklist to prepare for visits to a cardiology clinic were better able to identify their educational needs and experienced less anxiety before their appointments.

The nurse also determines what information is critical to teach. Because a client's health status is dynamic, learning needs change constantly and assessment should be ongoing. The nurse assesses the following:

- Client's understanding of health status, implications and threat of illness, types of therapy, and prognosis.

For example, the nurse asks a client newly diagnosed with Type 1 diabetes, "Tell me what you know about diabetes and why you need to take insulin."
- Information or skills needed by the client to perform self-care and to understand the implications of a health problem. Health care team members anticipate learning needs related to specific health problems. For example, the nurse teaches an adolescent boy to perform testicular self-examination.
- Client's experiences that influence the need to learn. For example, a woman having her second child is more likely to be familiar with the implications of pregnancy than a woman who is pregnant for the first time.

Ability to Learn. Many factors can impair the ability to learn, including body temperature, electrolyte levels, oxygenation status, and blood glucose level. Several factors may influence a client at one time. The nurse assesses the client's ability to learn by considering the following:
- Physical strength, movement, dexterity, and coordination. The nurse determines the client's ability to perform skills.
- Sensory deficits that may affect the ability to understand or follow instruction (see chapter 44).
- Reading level. Reading level can be difficult to assess because functional illiteracy is often easy to conceal. One way to assess a client's reading level and level of understanding is to ask the client to read instructions from a teaching brochure and then explain its meaning.
- Developmental level. Developmental level influences teaching approaches (see Box 17-5).
- Cognitive function. Cognitive function includes memory, knowledge, association, and judgment.

Motivation to Learn. The nurse asks questions that identify a client's motivation level, which help to determine whether the client is prepared and willing to learn. The nurse assesses the client's motivation by studying the following:
- Behaviour (e.g., attention span, tendency to ask questions, memory, and ability to concentrate during the teaching session).
- Health beliefs and perception of a health problem and the benefits and barriers to treatment. For example, a nurse asks a client with coronary artery disease, "Explain how heart disease will affect you over time. What value is there in eating a low-fat diet?"
- Perceived ability to complete a required health behaviour.
- Desire to learn.
- Attitudes about health care providers (e.g., role of client and nurse in making decisions). For example, a nurse asks, "In what way can I best help you?"
- Knowledge of information to be learned. The client must play an active role in seeking health-based information.
- Pain, fatigue, anxiety, or other physical symptoms that can interfere with the ability to maintain attention and participate. In acute care settings, a client's physical condition can easily detract from learning.
- Socio-cultural background. A client's beliefs and values about health and various therapies may be influenced by socio-cultural norms or tradition (see chapter 9). Educational efforts can be especially challenging when clients and educators do not speak the same language.
- Learning style preference. Clients who learn better by seeing and hearing may benefit from a video. Clients who learn best by reasoning logically and intuitively may learn better if presented with written material that they can analyze and discuss with others.

Teaching Environment. The nurse assesses the following factors when choosing a teaching environment:
- Distractions or persistent noise. A quiet area should be set aside for teaching.
- Comfort of the room, including ventilation, temperature, lighting, and furniture.
- Room facilities and available equipment.

Resources for Learning. Assessment of resources includes a review of available teaching tools. If a client requires family support, the nurse assesses the readiness and ability of family and friends to learn to care for the client and reviews resources in the home. The nurse assesses the following:
- Client's willingness to have family members involved in the teaching plan and care. (Information about the client's health care is confidential unless the client chooses to share it.)
- Family members' perceptions and understanding of the client's illness and its implications. Family members and clients' perceptions should match; otherwise, conflicts may arise in the teaching plan.
- Family's willingness and ability to participate in care. Family members must be responsible, willing, and able to assist in care activities, such as bathing or administering medications.
- Resources in the home. These resources include health care equipment and a suitable rearrangement of rooms.
- Teaching tools, including brochures, audiovisual materials, or posters. Printed material should present current and easy-to-understand information that matches the client's reading level.

Nursing Diagnosis

After assessing the client's ability and need to learn, the nurse interprets data to form an accurate diagnosis (Box 17-6). This diagnosis ensures that teaching will be goal directed and individualized. If a client has several learning needs, the nursing diagnoses will guide priority setting. Classifying diagnoses by the three learning domains helps the nurse to focus on subject matter and teaching methods. Examples of nursing diagnoses that indicate a need for education include the following:
- Ineffective health maintenance
- Health-seeking behaviours
- Impaired home maintenance
- Deficient knowledge
- Ineffective therapeutic regimen management
- Ineffective community therapeutic regimen management
- Ineffective family therapeutic regimen management
- Non-compliance

Nursing Diagnostic Process — Box 17-6

Risk for Injury

Assessment Activities	Defining Characteristics	Nursing Diagnosis
Have client describe how to walk with crutches. Have client demonstrate three-point crutch walking on level surfaces and up stairs.	States has not received information about use of crutches. Asks questions about how to use crutches. Uses crutches inappropriately. Cannot go up or down stairs on crutches.	Deficient knowledge (psychomotor) regarding use of crutches related to lack of exposure.

When health care problems can be managed through education, the diagnostic statement is *deficient knowledge.* For example, an older adult may be unable to manage a medication regimen because of the number of medications that must be taken at different times of the day. Education may improve the client's ability to schedule and take the medications.

Some nursing diagnoses also indicate that teaching is inappropriate. The nurse may identify conditions that hinder learning (e.g., nursing diagnosis of pain or activity intolerance). In these cases, the nurse delays teaching until the nursing diagnosis is resolved or the health problem is controlled.

Planning

After identifying a client's learning needs and making a nursing diagnosis, the nurse develops a teaching plan, sets goals and expected outcomes, and works with the client to select a teaching method (see Care Plan). Expected outcomes or learning objectives determine which teaching strategies and approaches are appropriate. Client participation is essential.

Developing Learning Objectives. Learning objectives identify the expected outcome of instruction and establish learning priorities. Objectives help a nurse to manage time and resources.

Objectives are either for a short term or a long term. Short-term objectives meet the client's immediate learning needs, such as needing knowledge about an upcoming test. Long-term objectives, which are often broader, help a client adapt to a long-term challenge. Learning objectives, which will guide the teaching plan, include the same criteria as outcomes in a nursing care plan:

- Singular behaviours
- Observable or measurable content
- Timing or conditions under which the objective is measured
- Goals mutually set by the nurse and client

Each objective focuses on a single behaviour that will determine the client's ability to meet health care outcomes. A behavioural objective contains an active verb, describing what the learner will do after the objective is met, such as *will administer* an injection. Behavioural objectives are measurable and observable and indicate how learning will be evidenced (e.g., "will perform *three-point crutch gait*"). The objective describes precise behaviours and content. Nurses should avoid vague or non-specific objectives that do not explain what the learner is to do.

An objective is more precise when it describes the conditions or timing under which the behaviour occurs. Conditions and time frames should be realistic and designed for the learner's needs (e.g., "will identify the side effects of medication by discharge"). It also helps to consider conditions under which the client or family will perform the behaviour (e.g., "will walk from bedroom to bathroom using crutches"). A nurse sets criteria for acceptable performance on the basis of the desired level of accuracy, success, or satisfaction. For example, "a client undergoing therapy for a fractured leg will walk on crutches to the end of the hall within 3 days." Criteria are more acceptable when the teacher and learner establish them mutually. However, the nurse serves as a resource in setting the minimum criteria for success.

After formulating objectives, the nurse and client establish a teaching plan. The nurse integrates basic teaching principles and develops a well-timed, organized teaching plan.

Setting Priorities. Teaching priorities are based on the client's immediate needs, nursing diagnoses, and learning objectives. They are also based on the client's main concerns, anxiety level, and the time available to teach.

Timing. When is the right time to teach? Before a client is hospitalized? When a client enters a clinic or a long-term care facility? At discharge? At home? The answer is all of them, because clients continue to have learning needs and opportunities as long as they stay in the health care system. The nurse should plan to teach when the client is most attentive, receptive, and alert.

However, timing can be difficult, particularly in an acute care setting, because the focus is on an early discharge. By the time the client is ready to learn, discharge may already be scheduled. Therefore, nurses need to anticipate a client's educational needs. Donovan and Ward (2001) found that clients were better able to manage pain after receiving structured education at an oncology clinic. In this case, the nurses had anticipated their client's needs.

The length of teaching sessions also influences learning. Concentration decreases with prolonged sessions. Frequent sessions of about 20 minutes are more easily tolerated. The nurse should assess a client's level of concentration by observing non-verbal cues such as poor eye contact or slumped posture. Teaching sessions should be held often enough to document the client's learning progress.

Nursing Care Plan

Learning Needs

Assessment

Connie, a nurse in a surgeon's office, is preparing Mr. Holland for a colon resection, which is scheduled in 1 week. Mr. Holland, age 75, has recently been diagnosed with colorectal cancer. Connie's assessment focuses on Mr. Holland's readiness to learn and factors that might affect his ability to understand the procedure and related post-operative care.

Assessment Activities	Findings/Defining Characteristics
Assess Mr. Holland's readiness to learn, and ask what the surgeon has already told him about the surgery.	Mr. Holland responds, "I can't remember what the doctor told me at my last appointment. My surgery is scheduled for next week."
Ask Mr. Holland to explain post-operative care, including performing a return demonstration of deep breathing and coughing.	Mr. Holland is unable to describe post-operative care or provide a return demonstration of deep breathing and coughing.
Assess Mr. Holland's visual acuity.	Mr. Holland says he has difficulty reading small print.

Nursing Diagnosis: Deficient knowledge related to lack of recall and exposure to information.

Planning

Goal	Expected Outcomes* **Knowledge: Treatment Procedure**
Client will describe preoperative and post-operative care to nurse before surgery.	Mr. Holland will verbalize understanding of surgical procedure and related care on the day of surgery.
Client will participate in post-operative care during hospitalization.	Mr. Holland will demonstrate deep breathing and coughing; he will advance his level of activity after his surgery.

*Outcome labels from *Nursing Outcomes Classification (NOC)* (3rd ed.), edited by S. Moorhead, M. Johnson, and M. L. Maas, 2004, St. Louis, MO: Mosby.

Interventions†	Rationale
Learning Readiness Enhancement	
Determine readiness to learn and what the client perceives as important to know.	The adult client's learning is enhanced when the client is ready to learn and the information is perceived as important (Bastable, 2003).
Learning Facilitation	
Give client large-print brochure describing preoperative and post-operative care during educational session.	Providing clients with educational methods that use multiple senses is effective in educating older adults. Large fonts with contrasting colours are easier to visualize for the older adult (Maas et al., 2001).
Explain post-operative care, demonstrate deep breathing and coughing, and have client perform return demonstration.	Improving self-efficacy by using role modelling and having the client perform behaviours enhances the successful adoption of healthy behaviours (Bandura, 1997).

†Intervention classification labels from *Nursing Interventions Classification (NIC)* (4th ed.), edited by J. M. Dochterman and G. M. Bulecheck, 2004, St. Louis, MO: Mosby.

Evaluation

Nursing Actions	Client Response/Finding	Achievement of Outcome
Ask Mr. Holland what he can expect before and after surgery.	Mr. Holland is able to state understanding of preoperative and post-operative care.	Mr. Holland's anxiety level has decreased, and he reports he is ready for surgery.
Observe client as he demonstrates deep breathing and coughing and advances his activity post-operatively.	Mr. Holland is able to cough and breathe deeply post-operatively, but he is hesitant to advance his activity level after surgery.	Outcome of advancing activity postoperatively has not been totally achieved. Address and manage barriers inhibiting attainment of this outcome (e.g., pain), and continue to encourage and educate client.

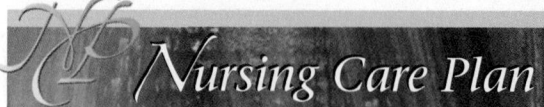

The frequency of sessions depends on the learner's abilities and the complexity of the material. For example, a child newly diagnosed with diabetes will require more visits to an outpatient centre than will an older adult who has had diabetes for 15 years and who lives in a long-term care facility. Intervals between teaching sessions should not be so long that the client might forget information.

Organizing Teaching Material. An outline helps organize information into a logical sequence. Material should progress from simple to complex. A person must learn simple facts and concepts before learning associations or complex concepts.

Essential content should come first because people are more likely to remember information that is taught early. Repetition reinforces learning. Summarizing key points helps the learner remember important information (Bastable, 2003).

Maintaining Learning Attention and Participation. Active participation is key to learning. People learn better when more than one of the body's senses is stimulated. Nurses should engage the clients' interest by changing the tone and intensity of their voice, making eye contact, using gestures, asking questions, and encouraging participation with activities such as role-playing.

Building on Existing Knowledge. An effective teacher presents information that builds on a learner's existing knowledge. For example, a client who has had multiple sclerosis must begin a new medication that is given subcutaneously. On assessment, the nurse asks the client about experience with injections. The client explains that she gave her father insulin injections for many years. The nurse individualizes the teaching plan by building on the client's previous knowledge and experience with insulin injections.

Selecting Teaching Methods. A teaching method is the way that the teacher delivers information. It is based on the client's learning needs. More than one method may be used for instruction. For example, a client who learns best in the psychomotor domain will benefit from demonstrations and supervised practice. The client masters skills by manipulating equipment and practising manual skills. Discussions, question-and-answer sessions, and formal lectures can all be effective methods, depending on the client's needs and learning style. When choosing appropriate teaching methods, the nurse encourages the client to offer suggestions.

Selecting Resources. The nurse is responsible for ensuring that clients' educational needs are met. Sometimes client needs are highly complex. In these cases, the nurse identifies appropriate health education resources within the health care system or the community. Examples of resources for client education include diabetes education clinics, cardiac rehabilitation programs, prenatal classes, and support groups. The nurse obtains a referral if necessary, encourages clients to attend these sessions, and reinforces information taught.

Writing Teaching Plans. In all health care settings, nurses develop written teaching plans for use by colleagues. The nurse responsible for developing the teaching plan incorporates all pertinent information into the plan, including topics for instruction, resources (e.g., equipment, teaching booklets, and referrals to education programs), recommendations for involving family, and objectives of the teaching plan. A plan may be lengthy or in outline form.

In an acute care setting, plans are concise and focused on the primary learning needs of the client because there is limited time for teaching. A home care teaching plan or outpatient clinic plan may be more comprehensive because nurses may have more time to instruct clients and clients are often less anxious in outpatient settings.

A plan should provide continuity of instruction, particularly when several nurses are involved in a client's care. The more specific the plan, the easier it is to follow.

NP Implementation

Implementing a teaching plan depends on the nurse's ability to analyze assessment data when identifying learning needs and developing the teaching plan (see Care Plan). The nurse evaluates the learning objectives and determines the best teaching and learning methods to help the client to meet expected goals and outcomes. The nurse uses a diversified approach to create an active learning environment (Box 17-7).

Teaching Approaches. A teaching approach is different from a method. Because a a learner's needs and motives can change over time, the nurse must be ready to modify teaching approaches.

Telling. The telling approach is useful when limited information must be taught (e.g., preparing a client for an emergency diagnostic procedure). The nurse outlines the task to be done by the client and gives instructions. This method provides no opportunity for feedback.

Selling. The selling approach uses two-way communication. The nurse paces instruction according to the client's response. Specific feedback is given to the client who learns successfully. For example, the client learns a step-by-step procedure for changing a dressing.

Participating. Participating involves setting objectives and becoming involved in the learning process together. The client helps decide content, and the nurse guides and counsels the client with pertinent information. There is opportunity for discussion, feedback, mutual goal setting, and revision of the teaching plan.

Entrusting. The entrusting approach provides the client with the opportunity to manage self-care. The nurse observes the client's progress and remains available to assist without introducing more new information.

Reinforcing. **Reinforcement** is using a stimulus that increases the probability of a response. A person who receives reinforcement before or after learning a desired behaviour is likely to repeat the behaviour. People usually

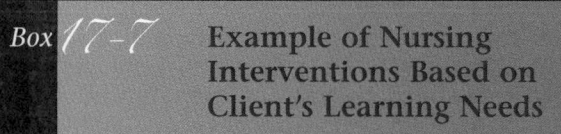

Box 17-7 Example of Nursing Interventions Based on Client's Learning Needs

Assessment Data

Mr. Kennedy, age 67, has a 15-year history of Type 2 diabetes. He is in the hospital because of an infected foot ulcer that requires frequent dressing changes. Mr. Kennedy used to take oral hypoglycemic agents to control his blood sugar levels. However, he now needs to start home insulin injections because of the infection and wound. He must also learn how to change his dressings. Mr. Kennedy is anxious about his discharge and requests information about a local diabetes support group. The case manager indicates that Mr. Kennedy will be discharged soon.

Cognitive Interventions

- Ask Mr. Kennedy about what he believes he needs to know before his discharge.
- Encourage Mr. Kennedy to help establish learning outcomes and goals.
- Provide Mr. Kennedy with teaching materials regarding insulin preparation, administration, and how to recognize and manage hypoglycemia and hyperglycemia.
- During teaching sessions, give Mr. Kennedy examples of what problems he might experience at home and ask him how he would respond to the situations (e.g., if the wound's drainage increased and became purulent, what would he do?).

Affective Interventions

- Encourage Mr. Kennedy to attend a support group meeting if possible to allow learning from others' experiences.
- Encourage Mr. Kennedy to verbalize his feelings and fears about this change in his health status.
- Have Mr. Kennedy role-play how he will respond to his friends when they ask him about his health status.
- As he acquires new skills and behaviours, provide Mr. Kennedy with feedback and positive reinforcement.

Psychomotor Interventions

- Demonstrate insulin preparation and injection techniques.
- Demonstrate use of blood sugar metre and recording of blood sugar measurement results.
- Demonstrate dressing changes.
- Have Mr. Kennedy perform return demonstrations of insulin preparation and injection, blood sugar testing, and dressing changes.

respond better to positive reinforcement (Bastable, 2003). The effects of negative reinforcement, such as criticizing, can decrease an undesired response, but are less predictable and often undesirable. Feedback is a common form of reinforcement.

Three types of reinforcers are social, material, and activity. Most nurses use social reinforcers (e.g., encouraging words) to acknowledge a learned behaviour. Examples of material reinforcers are food, toys, and music. These reinforcers work best with young children. Activity reinforcers are based on the principle that people are motivated to engage in an activity if after its completion they are able to engage in a more desirable activity. For example, clients with dementia may be more willing to bathe if they can go for a walk with the nurse afterward. Activity reinforcers work when a client is self-motivated. Choosing an appropriate reinforcer requires attention to individual preferences. Observing behaviour often helps reveal the best reinforcer to use. Reinforcers should never be used as threats and are not effective with every client.

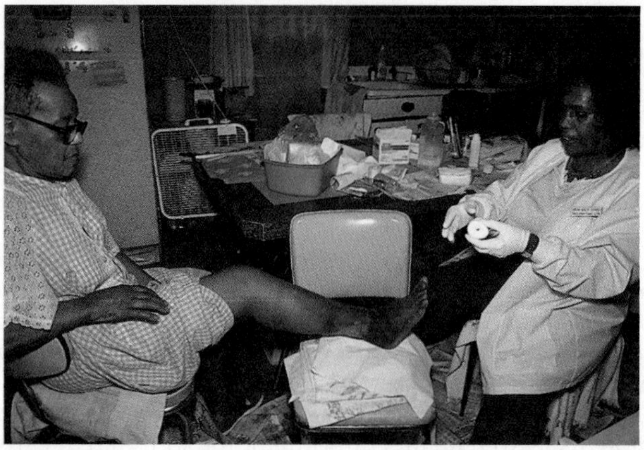

FIGURE **17–2** The nurse incorporates teaching about wound care during a home visit.

Incorporating Teaching With Nursing Care. Many nurses teach effectively while delivering nursing care. This ability becomes easier as a nurse gains confidence in clinical skills. For example, while hanging blood, the nurse explains why the blood is needed and the symptoms indicated with transfusion reactions that should be reported immediately. When the nurse follows a teaching plan informally, the client feels less pressure to perform and learning becomes more of a shared activity. Teaching during routine care is efficient and cost-effective (Figure 17–2).

Implementing Teaching Methods. A nurse's choice of teaching methods depends on the client's learning needs, the time available for teaching, the environment, the resources, and the nurse's own comfort level with teaching. Skilled teachers are flexible in altering teaching methods according to the learner's responses and in using teaching tools that work best with a particular method (Table 17-2). The following are a variety of teaching methods.

One-on-One Discussion. In one-on-one discussion, the nurse presents information informally, allowing the client to ask questions or share concerns. Various teaching aids such as models or diagrams can be used during the discussion, depending on the client's learning needs.

Group Instruction. Groups are an economical way to teach several clients at once. Clients interact and learn from others' experiences. Groups can also foster positive attitudes that help clients meet learning objectives (Rankin & Stallings, 2001).

Table 17-2 Teaching Tools for Instruction

Description	Learning Implications
Printed Material	
Written teaching tools available as pamphlets, booklets, brochures	Material must be easily readable for learner. Information must be accurate and current. Method is ideal for understanding complex concepts and relationships.
Programmed Instruction	
Written sequential presentation of learning steps requiring that learners answer questions and that teachers tell them whether they are right or wrong	Instruction is primarily verbal, but teacher may use pictures or diagrams. Method requires active learning, giving immediate feedback, correcting wrong answers, and reinforcing right answers. Learner works at own pace.
Computer Instruction	
Use of programmed instruction format in which computers store response patterns for learners and select further lessons on basis of these patterns (programs can be individualized)	Method requires reading comprehension, psychomotor skills, and familiarity with computer.
Nonprint Materials	
Diagrams	
Illustrations that show interrelationships by means of lines and symbols	Method demonstrates key ideas, summarizes, and clarifies key concept.
Graphs (Bar, Circle, or Line)	
Visual presentations of numerical data	Graphs help learner to grasp information quickly about single concept.
Charts	
Highly condensed visual summary of ideas and facts that may highlight series of ideas, steps, or events	Charts demonstrate relationship of several ideas or concepts. Method helps learners know what to do.
Pictures	
Photographs or drawings used to teach concepts in which the third dimension of shape and space is not important	Photographs are more desirable than diagrams because they more accurately portray the details of the real item. Drawings are pertinent for removing the superfluous detail present in real objects.
Physical Objects	
Use of actual equipment, objects, or models to teach concepts or skills	Models are useful when real objects are too small, large, or complicated or are unavailable. Learners can manipulate objects that are to be used later in skill.
Other Audiovisual Materials	
Slides, audiotapes, television, and videotapes used with printed material or discussion	Materials are useful for clients with reading comprehension problems and visual deficits.

Group instruction often involves both lecture and discussion. Lectures are highly structured and help clients learn standard content. However, they do not encourage active thinking; thus, discussion and practice sessions are essential (Rankin & Stallings, 2001).

Preparatory Instruction. Clients are often anxious about unfamiliar tests or procedures. Providing information about procedures helps clients to anticipate what will happen. Here are guidelines for giving preparatory explanations:

- Describe physical sensations during the procedure, but do not evaluate them. For example, when drawing a blood specimen, explain that the client will feel a sticking sensation as the needle punctures the skin.
- Describe the cause of the sensation to prevent misinterpretation of the experience. For example, explain that a needle stick burns because the alcohol used to cleanse the skin enters the puncture site.
- Prepare clients only for aspects of the experience that are common to other clients. For example, explain that it is normal for a tight tourniquet to cause a person's hand to tingle and feel numb.

Demonstrations. Demonstrations help teach psychomotor skills such as preparing a syringe, bathing an infant, walking with a crutch, or measuring a pulse. Clients are able to observe a skill before practising it. They are most effective when clients first observe the nurse and then perform a **return demonstration** to practice the skill. A demonstration should be combined with discussion to clarify concepts and feelings. An effective demonstration requires advanced planning:

- Position the client to provide a clear view of demonstration.
- Review the rationale and steps of the procedure.
- Assemble and organize equipment. Make sure it works.
- Perform each step in sequence while analyzing the knowledge and skills involved.
- Determine when to give explanations, considering the client's learning needs.
- Adjust speed and timing of the demonstration according to the client's abilities and anxiety level.

The nurse demonstrates a skill in the same order in which the client will perform it. The demonstration involves the following:

- Performing each step slowly and accurately
- Encouraging the client to ask questions so that each step is understood
- Explaining the rationale for each step
- Allowing the client to observe each step
- Allowing the client to handle equipment and practice the skill under supervision

The client demonstrates the procedure to ensure that learning has occurred. The demonstration should occur under the same conditions that will be experienced at home or in the place where the skill is to be performed. For example, for a client learning to walk with crutches, the nurse simulates the home environment. If short, narrow steps lead to the client's bedroom, the client should learn to climb similar stairs in the hospital.

Analogies. Learning occurs when a teacher translates complex language or ideas into words or concepts that the client understands. **Analogies** aid learning by supplementing verbal instruction with familiar images that make complex information more real and understandable. For example, when explaining arterial blood pressure, an analogy is the flow of water through a hose. To use analogies, follow these general principles:

- Be familiar with the concept.
- Know the client's background, experience, and culture.
- Keep the analogy simple and clear.

Role Playing. Role-play helps teach new ideas and attitudes. During role-play, clients play themselves or someone else and rehearse a desired behaviour. For example, a nurse teaches a parent to respond to a child's behaviour by pretending to be a child having a temper tantrum. This role-playing allows the parent to practice responding in this situation. The nurse evaluates the parent's response and determines whether an alternative approach would be more appropriate. Role-play helps clients learn skills and feel confident in their ability to perform them independently.

Simulation. Simulation helps teach problem solving, application, and independent thinking. During individual or group discussion, a nurse poses a problem or situation for clients to solve. For example, clients with heart disease are asked to plan a low-fat meal. The nurse asks the clients to present their diet, providing an opportunity to identify mistakes and reinforce correct information.

Paying Attention to Barriers to Learning. Many situations or conditions present a barrier to learning. For example, the client may have a low reading level (functionally illiterate), learning disability, sensory alteration, or poor memory. Nursing interventions that can be used when caring for clients who are illiterate or who have learning disabilities are summarized in Box 17-8. Clients understand fewer medical words than health care professionals predict. Researchers have found that printed educational material is consistently written above most clients' reading level. Unfortunately, the gap between a client's reading level and educational materials is often undetected by health care professionals (Winslow, 2001). Nurses must use words that clients understand. They should pay special attention to the learning needs of those clients who have reading problems, learning disabilities, sensory alterations, and to those whose first language is not English or French.

Illiteracy and Learning Disabilities. The most recent survey on literacy rates in Canada found that about 22% of Canadian adults fall into the lowest level of literacy. These people have only rudimentary reading and writing skills. For example, they are not able to read and understand a label on a medicine container. A further 26% of Canadians can only read material that is simple and familiar. Therefore, almost half of Canadians have problems with reading materials encountered in everyday life (Perrin, 1998).

Some people have learning disabilities, which are disorders that may impair ability to acquire, organize, remember, understand, or apply information (Learning Disabilities Association of Canada, 2002). Learning disabilities may interfere with the person's ability to learn or use oral or written language and/or mathematics. If a client's learning disability impairs mathematical ability, teaching can be challenging, especially if complex medication dosages and frequencies must be learned. Some clients have ADHD (attention deficit and hyperactivity disorder). These people may have difficulty recalling information and staying focused during educational sessions; they may also have a low threshold of frustration (Mennies, 2001).

Sensory Alteration and Other Barriers. Some clients, including many older adults, have sensory deficits (see chapter 44). Sensory changes such as visual and hearing changes require teaching methods that enhance functioning. For example, the nurse faces the client with hearing problems and speaks in a low tone of voice during discussions (lower tones are easier to hear than higher tones). Clear, written materials should be provided. Clients with visual problems can benefit from large print materials. Clients with slower cognitive function and reduced short-term memory (which may include some older adults or clients who have had strokes) learn and remember effectively if the learning is paced properly and the material is relevant to the learner's needs and abilities.

Language. The diverse backgrounds of Canadians can challenge a nurse to provide culturally sensitive care (see chapter 9). Clients may not understand instructions that are not in their native language (see Chapter 14). The nurse needs to ascertain a client's level of English (or French) before choosing teaching methods or tools.

Client Teaching

Box 17-8

Clients With Barriers to Learning

Objectives

- Client will understand information presented.
- Client will perform desired behaviours accurately.

Teaching Strategies

- Establish trust with the client before beginning the teaching learning session.
- Limit teaching objectives; present only crucial information to avoid overwhelming the learner.
- Use simple terminology to enhance the client's understanding.
- Avoid medical jargon. If necessary, explain medical terms using basic one- or two-syllable words.
- Schedule short teaching sessions at frequent intervals; minimize distractions during teaching sessions.
- Begin and end each teaching session with the most important information.
- Present information slowly; allow ample time for understanding of the material.
- Repeat important information.
- Give many examples that have meaning to the client (e.g., relate new material to previous life experience).
- Build on existing knowledge.
- Use visual cues and simple analogies when appropriate.
- Frequently ask the client for feedback to determine if the client comprehends information.
- Demonstrate procedures such as measuring dosages; ask for return demonstrations (provides opportunity to clarify instructions and time to review procedures).
- Provide teaching materials that reflect the reading level of the client; use material that is written with short words and sentences, large type, and simple format (generally, information written on a fifth-grade reading level is recommended for adult learners).
- Model appropriate behaviour and use role-playing to help client learn how to ask questions and ask for help effectively.
- Allow clients to progress at their own pace.
- Include family members or other caregivers in the education process.

Evaluation

- Ask the client to verbalize understanding of information taught.
- Observe and evaluate the client's ability to perform desired behaviours.

Data from *Nurse as Educator: Principles of Teaching and Learning for Nursing Practice,* by S. Bastable, 2003, Sudbury, MA: Jones & Bartlett; "Teaching Adult Patients With Learning Disabilities," by J. Mennies, 2001, *Nursing Spectrum, 14*(21), p. 20; *In Other Words . . . Can They Understand? Testing Patient Education Materials With Intended Readers,* by H. Osborne, 2001, Retrieved November 1, 2001, from *http://www.healthliteracy.com/oncallnov2001.htm;* and *Literacy, ESL, and Health Care,* by C. Meyers, 2002, Retrieved December 22, 2004, from *http://www.caslpa.ca/english/resources/literacy.asp*

Needs of Clients With Severe Illness. Adapting to serious illness or disability is difficult for most people. They need to grieve. This process gives them time to adapt psychologically to the emotional and physical implications of illness. People experience the stages of grieving as theorized by Kübler-Ross (see chapter 25) at different rates and sequences, depending on their self-concept before illness, the severity of the illness, and the changes and losses caused by the illness. Not everyone experiences every stage. Sensitivity is required to educate clients while they are grieving and adjusting to their illness.

Readiness to learn is related to the grieving stage (Table 17-3). Clients cannot learn when they are unwilling or unable to accept the reality of illness. However, properly timed teaching can help a client to adjust to illness or disability. The nurse identifies the client's stage of grieving on the basis of the client's behaviours. When the client enters the stage of acceptance, the stage compatible with learning, the nurse introduces a teaching plan. Continuous assessment of the client's behaviours determines the stages of grieving.

NP Evaluation

Client education is not complete until the nurse evaluates outcomes of the teaching-learning process (see Care Plan). The nurse determines whether clients have learned the material. Evaluation reinforces correct behaviour, helps learners realize how they should change incorrect behaviour, and helps the teacher determine adequacy of teaching (Cronbach, 1977; Redman, 2001). Success depends on the client's ability to meet the established outcome and goals by which the nurse can evaluate success. The following checklist helps evaluate client education (Rankin & Stallings, 2001):

- Were the objectives clearly stated in a way that allowed client behaviours to be observed?
- Were the client's goals or outcomes realistic?
- Were the learner's needs assessed thoroughly?
- Did the client perceive the education as important, and did the client state a willingness to change behaviour?
- What obstacles or problems were encountered that provided barriers to change?
- Were educational goals set mutually between the nurse and the client?
- Were the interventions individualized to help the client meet the learning objectives?
- Was the client's behavioural change measured and documented accurately?
- Does the client continue to have a skill deficiency? If so, what changes in interventions should be made to enhance skill attainment?

Measurement Methods. In direct observation, the nurse has the client demonstrate the behaviours described in the learning objectives. If the evaluation process indicates

Table 17-3 Relationship Between Learning and Psychosocial Adaptation to Illness

Stage	Client's Behaviour	Learning Implications	Rationale
Denial or disbelief	Client avoids discussion of illness ("There's nothing wrong with me"), withdraws from others, and disregards physical restrictions. Client suppresses and distorts information that has not been presented clearly.	Provide support, empathy, and careful explanations of all procedures while they are being done. Let client know you are available for conversation. Explain situation to family or significant other if appropriate. Teach in present tense (e.g., explain what client needs to know to be discharged).	Client is not prepared to deal with problem. Attempts to teach client will result in further anger or withdrawal. Provide only information client pursues or requires.
Anger	Client blames, complains, and often directs anger toward nurse or others.	Do not argue with client, but listen to concerns. Teach in present tense. Reassure family of client's normalcy.	Client needs opportunity to express feelings and anger. Client is still not prepared to face future.
Bargaining	Client offers to live better life in exchange for promise of better health ("If God lets me live, I promise to manage my disease better").	Continue to introduce only reality and teaching in present tense.	Client is still unwilling to accept limitations.
Resolution	Client begins to express emotions openly, realizes that illness has created changes, and begins to ask questions.	Encourage expression of feelings. Begin to share information needed for future, and set aside formal times for discussion.	Client begins to perceive need for assistance and is ready to accept responsibility for learning.
Acceptance	Client recognizes reality of condition, actively pursues information, and strives for independence.	Focus on future skills and knowledge required. Continue to teach in present tense. Involve family in planning and teaching for discharge.	Client is more easily motivated to learn. Acceptance of illness reflects willingness to deal with its implications.

a knowledge or skill deficit, the nurse repeats or modifies the teaching plan. Watching clients demonstrate behaviours shows the nurse if correct techniques are used. However, a client may behave differently later. Therefore, observation works best in real-life situations.

Oral and written questioning are other useful evaluation methods. Questions are best used for behaviours that are not easily demonstrated. The nurse should phrase questions to ensure that the learner understands them and that objectives are truly measured.

Another form of evaluation includes self-reports (oral and written) and self-monitoring (written). An example is a client's written log of the foods eaten in a specific time period, matched against a new diet. The nurse relies on the client's honesty and memory in self-reporting.

Client Expectations. Evaluations of nursing care and teaching sessions help determine if a client's needs and expectations have been met. At the end of the session, the nurse asks clients to identify information that was missing and should have been covered. Clients may also fill out written evaluations of a teaching session or course. Anonymous written evaluations may be more truthful than face-to-face evaluations.

Evaluation may reveal new learning needs or new factors that are interfering with learning, enabling a nurse to try alternative teaching methods. When a client has difficulty in an acute care setting, the nurse may make a referral to resources, such as home care or an outpatient clinic, for further education and evaluation.

Documentation of Client Teaching. Because client teaching often occurs informally between nurse and client, it is difficult to document it consistently. A nurse is legally responsible for providing accurate, timely client information that promotes continuity of care; therefore, it is essential to document the outcomes of teaching. Rankin and Stallings (2001) suggested documenting the following regarding client education:

- *Assessment data and reassessment of learning needs.* Provides important information needed when developing the teaching plan.
- *Nursing diagnoses, client needs, and educational priorities.* Provides support for goals and outcomes that are established.
- *Interventions planned.* A specific plan, including the methods to be used in instruction, enhances continuity of care. When viewing the planned interventions, nurses can determine what information needs to be provided to the client.
- *Interventions provided.* Specifically describing the subject matter enables other nurses to follow up and reinforce teaching (e.g., "Explained side effects of Inderal" or "Demonstrated umbilical cord care"). Note the date, time, and specific client or clients taught. Avoid generalizations (e.g., "medications taught"). When resources such as pamphlets or audiovisual materials are used, the nurse documents this in the client's record.
- *Client's response and outcomes of care.* Documenting evidence of learning (e.g., a return demonstration or the

ability to verbalize the purpose and side effects of a medication) informs staff about the client's progress and determines information that must still be taught.

- *Ability of client and/or family to manage needs after discharge.* An evaluation of remaining educational needs on discharge helps identify the need for outpatient or home health follow-up. If referrals are appropriate, the client and/or family are often able to meet their needs.

Key Concepts

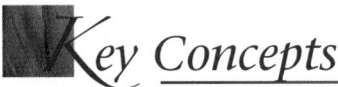

- The nurse ensures that clients, families, and communities receive information needed to maintain optimal health.
- Health education is aimed at the promotion, restoration, and maintenance of health.
- Teaching is most effective when it is responsive to the learner's needs.
- Teaching is a form of interpersonal communication, with the teacher and student actively involved in a process that increases the student's knowledge and skills.
- The ability to learn depends on a person's physical and cognitive attributes.
- The ability to attend to the learning process depends on physical comfort and anxiety levels and the presence of environmental distraction.
- A person's health beliefs influence the willingness to gain knowledge and skills necessary to maintain health.
- Teaching must be timed to coincide with the client's readiness to learn.
- Clients of different age groups require different teaching strategies as a result of developmental capabilities.
- The client should be an active participant in a teaching plan, agreeing to the plan, helping choose instructional methods, and recommending times for instruction.
- Learning objectives describe what a person is to learn in behavioural terms.
- A combination of teaching methods improves the learner's attentiveness and involvement.
- A teacher is more effective when presenting information that builds on a learner's existing knowledge.
- Nurses should assess which learning materials, methods, and approaches will be most effective for each client, based on that client's individual abilities and challenges.
- A nurse evaluates a client's learning by observing performance of expected learning behaviours under desired conditions.
- Effective documentation describes the entire process of client education, promotes continuity of care, and demonstrates that educational standards have been met.

Key Terms

Affective learning, *p. 320*
Analogies, *p. 330*
Cognitive learning, *p. 319*
Learning, *p. 319*
Learning objectives, *p. 323*
Motivation, *p. 322*
Psychomotor learning, *p. 320*
Reinforcement, *p. 327*
Return demonstration, *p. 330*
Social learning theory, *p. 322*
Teaching, *p. 318*

Critical Thinking Exercises

1. Mrs. S. has a 10-year history of hypertension and a 5-year history of diabetes. Recently her hypertension has worsened and she has been diagnosed with depression. Her medications, which have recently been changed, include 25 mg captopril (Capoten) three times a day, 240 mg diltiazem (Cardizem CD) every morning, 1,500 mg metformin (Glucophage XR) before the evening meal, and 100 mg sertraline (Zoloft) by mouth at bed time.

   The nurse identifies the priority nursing diagnosis as deficient knowledge related to change in medications. The nurse wants to develop a plan of care that uses the three domains of learning. What are the client's teaching priorities? Which learning needs would require a cognitive method? Which needs would be more appropriate to satisfy through affective or psychomotor methods?
2. The nurse is caring for a client who is being discharged after an appendectomy. He takes medication to treat attention deficit and hyperactivity disorder. Which teaching strategies should the nurse use when providing discharge information to this client?
3. A 23-year-old man has recently sustained a spinal cord injury after being involved in a diving accident that has left him paralyzed from the waist down. He verbally abuses the staff and expresses anger toward his family and friends when they come to visit. He needs to begin learning transfer techniques. Which stage of grieving is this client experiencing? What approach should the nurse take in planning education for this client?
4. A 65-year-old woman is taking her 72-year-old husband home after surgery. Which interventions should the nurse use in helping this couple make the transition to home smoothly?

Review Questions

1. A client must learn to use a walker. Acquisition of this skill will require learning in the
   1. Cognitive domain
   2. Affective domain
   3. Psychomotor domain
   4. Attentional domain

2. The nurse should plan to teach a client about the importance of exercise
   1. When there are visitors in the room
   2. When the client's pain medications are working
   3. Just before lunch, when the client is most awake and alert
   4. When the client is talking about current stressors in his or her life
3. A client newly diagnosed with cervical cancer is going home. The client is avoiding discussion of her illness and post-operative orders. In teaching the client about discharge instructions, the nurse should
   1. Teach the client's spouse
   2. Focus on knowledge the client will need in a few weeks
   3. Provide only the information the client needs to go home
   4. Convince the client that learning about her health is necessary
4. A community health nurse is about to teach a Grade 12 health class about nutrition. To achieve the best learning outcomes, the nurse should
   1. Provide information using a lecture
   2. Use simple words to promote understanding
   3. Complete an extensive literature search focusing on eating disorders
   4. Develop topics for discussion that require problem solving
5. A nurse is going to teach a client how to perform a breast self-examination. The behavioural objective that would best measure the client's ability to perform the examination is as follows:
   1. The client will verbalize the steps involved in breast self-examination within 1 week.
   2. The nurse will explain the importance of performing breast self-examination once a month.
   3. The client will perform breast self-examination correctly before the end of the teaching session.
   4. The nurse will demonstrate breast self-examination on a breast model provided by the Canadian Cancer Society.
6. A client who is having chest pain is going for an emergency cardiac catheterization. The most appropriate teaching approach in this situation is the
   1. Telling approach
   2. Selling approach
   3. Entrusting approach
   4. Participating approach
7. The nurse is teaching a parenting class to a group of pregnant adolescents and has given the adolescents baby dolls to bathe and talk to. This is an example of
   1. Discovery
   2. An analogy
   3. Role-playing
   4. A demonstration
8. A client with a learning disability is being started on a new antihypertensive medication. In teaching the client about the medication, the nurse should
   1. Demonstrate measuring dosages and ask for return demonstration
   2. Provide only written material
   3. Present the information once
   4. Expect the client to understand the information quickly
9. A client must learn how to administer a subcutaneous injection. The nurse knows the client is ready to learn when the client
   1. Has been given written instructions
   2. Expresses the importance of learning the skill
   3. Can see and understand the markings on the syringe
   4. Has the dexterity needed to prepare and inject the medication
10. A client who is hospitalized has just been diagnosed with diabetes. He is going to need to learn how to give himself injections. The best teaching method would be
    1. Demonstration
    2. Group instruction
    3. One-on-one discussion
    4. Simulation

References

Assessment, the foundation of good teaching. (2002). *Patient education management, 9*(4), 40–65.

Bandura, A. (1997). *Self-efficacy: The exercise of control.* New York: W. H. Freeman.

Bandura, A. (2001). Social cognitive theory: An agentic perspective. *Annual Review of Psychology, 52,* 1–26.

Bastable, S. (2003). *Nurse as educator: Principles of teaching and learning for nursing practice.* Sudbury, MA: Jones & Bartlett.

Bloom, B. S. (Ed.). (1956). *Taxonomy of educational objectives: The classification of educational goals: Vol. 1. Cognitive domain.* New York: Longman.

Burke, L. E., & Fair, J. (2003). Promoting prevention: Skill sets and attributes of health care providers who deliver behavioural interventions. *Journal of Cardiovascular Nursing, 18*(4), 256–266.

Canadian Nurses Association. (2002). *Code of ethics for registered nurses.* Ottawa, ON: Author.

Chelf, J., et al. (2002). Learning and support preferences of adult patients with cancer at a comprehensive cancer center. *Oncology Nursing Forum, 29*(5), 863–867.

Cooper, H., et al. (2001). Chronic disease patient education: Lessons from meta-analyses. *Patient Education and Counseling, 44,* 107–117.

Cronbach, L. J. (1977). *Educational psychology* (3rd ed.). New York: Harcourt Brace Jovanovich.

Dochterman, J. M., & Bulecheck, G. M. (Eds.). (2004). *Nursing interventions classification (NIC)* (4th ed.). St. Louis, MO: Mosby.

Donovan, H., & Ward, S. (2001). A representational approach to patient education. *Journal of Nursing Scholarship, 33*(3), 211–216.

Edelman, C. L., & Mandle, C. L. (2002). *Health promotion throughout the life-span* (5th ed.). St. Louis, MO: Mosby.

Felder, R. (2002). *Learning styles.* Accessed January 6, 2005, from *http://www.ncsu.edu/felder-public/Learning_Styles.html*

Krathwohl, D. R., Bloom, B. S., & Masia, B. B. (1964). *Taxonomy of educational objectives: The classification of educational goals: Handbook 2. Affective domain.* New York: David McKay.

Learning Disabilities Association of Canada. (2002). *Official definition of learning disabilities.* Accessed January 7, 2005, from *http://www.ldac-taac.ca/english/defined/definew.htm*

Maas, M., et al. (Eds.). (2001). *Nursing care of older adults: Diagnoses, outcomes, and interventions.* St. Louis, MO: Mosby.

Martinali, J., et al. (2001). A checklist to improve patient education in a cardiology outpatient setting. *Patient Education and Counseling, 42,* 231–238.

Mennies, J. (2001). Teaching adult patients with learning disabilities. *Nursing Spectrum, 14*(21), 20.

Moorhead, S., Johnson, M., & Maas, M. L. (Eds.). (2004). *Nursing outcomes classification (NOC)* (3rd ed.). St. Louis, MO: Mosby.

Oermann, M., Harris, C., & Dammeyer, J. (2001). Teaching by the nurse: How important is it to patients? *Applied Nursing Research, 14*(1), 11–17.

Osborne, H. (2001). *In other words . . . can they understand? Testing patient education materials with intended readers.* In Rankin, S. H., & Stallings, K. D. (2001). *Patient education: Issues, principles, practices* (4th ed.). Philadelphia: Lippincott.

Perrin, B. (1998). *How does literacy affect the health of Canadians?* Minister of Public Works and Government Services, Canada. Accessed December 22, 2004, from *http://www.phac-aspc.gc.ca/ph-sp/phdd/literacy/literacy2.html#situation*

Redman, B. K. (2001). *The practice of patient education* (9th ed.). St. Louis, MO: Mosby.

Saarmann, L., Daugherty, J., & Riegel, B. (2002). Teaching staff a brief cognitive-behavioral intervention. *Medsurg Nursing, 11*(3), 144–151.

Winslow, E. (2001). Patient education materials: Can patients read them, or are they ending up in the trash? *American Journal of Nursing, 101*(10), 33–38.

Recommended Web Sites

University Health Network Patient Education Program

http://www.uhn.ca/patient/pen/tgh_twh_pen.asp?nav=2;5.5—18k—5Nov 2004 –

This Web site is sponsored by the University Health Network in Toronto under the auspices of the Toronto General and Toronto Western sites. It contains a wealth of information on a variety of topics to assist in teaching clients.

Health Canada

http://www.hc-sc.gc.ca/

Health Canada's Web site provides many resources on a variety of health issues and topics to assist in client education.

National Institutes of Health

http://health.nih.gov/

This Web site provides a great many resources for client education prepared by the National Institutes of Health in the U.S.

18

Developmental Theories

Jane Drummond, RN, PhD (Canadian author)
Lenora Marcellus, RN, PhD (candidate) (Canadian author)
Elaine U. Polan, RNC, BSN, MS

Objectives

Mastery of content in this chapter will enable the student to:

- Define the key terms listed.
- Identify basic principles of growth and development.
- Discuss factors influencing growth and development.
- Identify five major traditions that underlie modern developmental theories.
- Name and describe the major developmental theories associated with each tradition.
- Describe and compare the mechanisms that underlie the major developmental theories.
- Discuss nursing implications for the application of developmental principles to client care.

All people progress through phases of growth and development, from the simple to the complex, and at a highly individualized rate. Understanding typical growth and development helps nurses predict, prevent, and detect any changes from clients' expected patterns. Using theory to understand growth and development provides a useful framework within which nurses can develop approaches and programs that can further enhance the developmental well-being of individuals (Berk, 2003; Bukatko & Daehler, 2001; Edelman & Mandle, 2002). Developmental theories are also important in helping nurses assess and treat a client's response to an illness. Understanding the process of human development guides caregivers in planning appropriate individualized care for clients.

For many years, human growth and development have been described as orderly, predictable processes beginning with conception and continuing until death. However, it is no longer assumed that all people progress through universal linear phases of growth and development. This view is increasingly being recognized as not inclusive of differences in gender, culture, and sexuality. Human growth and development is now seen as a process in which socio-cultural, biological, and psychological forces interact with the individual over time (Elder, 1998). As a result, theorists have been moving away from description and toward explanation. How do humans develop? What are the mechanisms, or explanatory components, that underlie human growth and development?

In this chapter, five broad traditions of human development are introduced and the mechanisms of development espoused by key theorists are outlined. Examples of implications for the nursing process that follow from the mechanisms are offered. Detailed descriptions of human development are found in the following three chapters of this text.

Growth and Development

Growth and development are synchronous processes that are interdependent in the healthy individual. Growth and development depend on a sequence of endocrine, genetic, constitutional, environmental, and nutritional influences (Edelman & Mandle, 2002).

Physical Growth

Growth is the quantitative, or measurable, aspect of an individual's increase in physical measurements. Measurable growth indicators include changes in height, weight, teeth, skeletal structures, and sexual characteristics. For example, children generally double their birth weight by 5 months of age and their birth height by 36 months. Physical growth is not just genetic but is also affected by other contextual factors such as socio-economic status.

Development

Development implies a progressive and continuous process of change leading to increased skill and capacity to function. Development is the result of complex interactions between biological and environmental influences (Salkind, 2004). These changes are qualitative in nature and difficult to measure in exact units. Developmental changes have certain predictable characteristics: They proceed from simple to complex, from general to specific, from head to toe (cephalocaudal), and from the trunk to the extremities (proximodistal). For example, a child's progressions from rolling over to crawling to walking are developmental changes.

Factors Influencing Growth and Development

There are three major categories of factors that influence human growth and development: (a) genetic or natural forces within the person, (b) the environment in which the person lives, and (c) the interaction that takes place between these two (Table 18-1).

The nurse applies knowledge of these factors in selecting approaches to promote typical growth and developmental progression. It is important, for example, that as part of planning for a client's pregnancy, the nurse considers the client's genetic endowment, age, socio-economic status, culture (Box 18-1), available support system, and preconception state of health.

Traditions of Developmental Theories

A theory is an organized, often observable, logical set of statements about a subject. Human developmental theories are models intended to account for how and why people become as they are (Thomas, 1997). All of the theories of development discussed in this chapter make different contributions to our understanding of the developmental process.

To help the reader understand the number of developmental theories, this chapter has been grouped into five traditions of (or ways of thinking about) theory development: organicism, psychoanalytic/psychosocial, mechanistic, contextualism, and dialecticism. The areas of learning and spiritual development are covered in chapters 17 and 24, respectively.

Each tradition emphasizes different underlying developmental mechanisms. **Mechanisms** of development are the explanatory components of each theory, or the means by which the developmental tasks are achieved. They are the processes or factors that underlie the developmental process within each theory and they enable developmental progression. These underlying mechanisms are proposed to be universal and act across the lifespan, not just in childhood. Although developmental theories are often presented within a framework of stage-like progressions, what the stages actually represent are the outcomes produced by these mechanisms at each specific age.

Organicism

Organicism refers to a theoretical focus on the organism itself. Theories in this tradition hold that development is a result of biologically driven behaviour and the person's adaptation to the environment. Biophysical and cognitive/moral theories of development are included in this tradition.

Biophysical Developmental Theories

Biophysical developmental theories describe and explain how our physical bodies grow and change. The changes that occur as a newborn infant grows into adulthood can be quantified and compared against established norms, keeping in mind that there may be regional and cultural differences and differences related to the availability of resources in the environment for adequate growth.

How does the physical body age? What are the triggers that move the body from the physical characteristics of childhood, through adolescence, to the physical changes of adulthood? Biological influences on development include many factors such as genetics and exposure to teratogens (e.g., maternal diseases, drugs, X-rays, or other hazardous substances that interfere with the normal development of the fetus). All biophysical theories give some credence to the roles of nature and nurture. However, the theories differ sharply on how much influence individual and environmental forces have on development (Berk, 2003).

Gesell's Theory of Maturational Development. Arnold Gesell (1880–1961) was a psychologist who obtained his medical degree to help him explain the physiological processes he was observing in the behaviour of children. Through extensive observations in the 1940s, he developed behavioural norms that serve as a primary source of information for childhood development today.

Fundamental to Gesell's theory of development is the notion that the pattern of growth and development is directed by the activity of the genes, although at that time the genetic mechanism was unknown to him. He believed that environmental factors can support, change, and modify the pattern, but that they do not generate the progressions of development (Gesell, 1948). Gesell proposed that the pattern of maturation follows a fixed developmental sequence in all humans and that *critical periods* exist, which are times when the presence or absence of particular experiences makes a biological system functional or non-functional (Keating & Hertzman, 1999). For example, if a child's visual defect is not identified until the start of school, usual message pathways in the brain may not become fully developed and long-term vision may be impaired (Cynader & Frost, 1999).

Sequential development is seen in fetuses, where there is a specified order of development of the various organ systems (Crain, 1992). After birth, children grow according to their genetic blueprint and gain skills in an orderly fashion, but at each individual's own pace. For example, most children will learn first how to hold a cup with digital grasp at around 15 months of age and will handle a cup well, lifting, drinking, and replacing, at 21 months of age. Gesell was clear that not every child develops those skills at exactly the same time. He pointed out that the environment does play a part in the development of the child, but that it does not have any part in the sequence of development. Gesell believed that children could not be pushed to develop faster than their own unique timetable permitted. He also went as far as to propose that it is our biological body that determines our behavioural development.

Table 18-1 Major Factors Influencing Growth and Development

Categories	Implications
Genetic or Natural Factors	
Heredity	Genetic endowment determines sex, race, hair and eye colour, physical growth, stature, and to some extent psychological uniqueness.
Temperament	Temperament is the characteristic psychological mood with which the child is born. It influences interactions between an individual and the environment.
Environmental Factors	
Family	Family purposes are to protect, teach, and nurture its members. Family functions include means for survival, security, assistance with emotional and social development, assistance with maintenance of relationships, instruction about society and world, and assistance in learning roles and behaviours. Family influences through its values, beliefs, customs, and specific patterns of interaction and communication.
Peer group	Peer group provides new and different learning environment. Peer group provides different patterns and structures of interaction and communication, necessitating different style of behaviour. Functions of peer group include allowing individual to learn about success and failure; to validate and challenge thoughts, feelings, and concepts; to receive acceptance, support, and rejection as unique people apart from family; and to achieve group purposes by meeting demands, pressures, and expectations.
Health environment	Level of health affects an individual's responsiveness to environment and responsiveness of others to the individual. Availability and accessibility of resources to support health.
Nutrition	Growth is regulated by dietary factors. Adequacy of nutrients influences whether and how physiological needs, as well as subsequent growth and development needs, are met. The availability of quality nutrients also affects growth.
Rest, sleep, and exercise	Balance between rest, sleep, and exercise is essential to rejuvenating body. Disturbances diminish growth, whereas equilibrium reinforces physiological and psychological health.
Living environment	Factors affecting growth and development include season, climate, community life, socioeconomic status, and quality of the physical environment (air, water, land). Developing embryo may be exposed to teratogenic substances (e.g., alcohol, chemicals, or radiation) that cause abnormal development.
Political and policy environment	Municipal, provincial, and federal policies directly affect the health and well-being of individuals, families, and communities.
Interacting Factors	
Life experiences	Individuals develop by applying what has been learned through experience to their current situation. Experiences emerge from both biological and environmental sources. The individual creates meaning from these experiences and builds on them.
Prenatal health	Biological and maturational factors (genetics, maternal age, medical problems) and environmental factors (maternal health, nutrition, use of tobacco and alcohol, use of prenatal services) together affect fetal growth and development.
State of health	Health is a product of both intrinsic (biology) and extrinsic (quality of environment, availability of resources for health) factors. Changes to health status such as illness or injury may cause inability to cope and respond to underlying processes and demands of development.

Cultural Aspects of Care — Box 18-1

Nurses need to assess the cultural background of their clients and be prepared to change their practice so that it is congruent with each client's beliefs and values concerning growth and development. For example, within many Aboriginal cultures, the concept of a circle or cycle is a fundamental theme (Smylie, 2001) and can be applied to human development. Human states and concepts are considered to be part of the life cycle of the earth, which also includes plants, animals, and seasons (Smylie, 2000). For people, this life cycle may be described as a continuum of age-related roles and qualities of being, including physical, mental, emotional, and spiritual well-being. All aspects of human development are viewed as being in harmony with the cycle of life in nature. As in nature, each part of the cycle needs to be balanced with the other parts. Roles and expectations related to developmental age reflect traditional values of respect, honour, balance, and harmony. Figure 18–1 represents the circle of life or the medicine wheel as applied to the human life cycle.

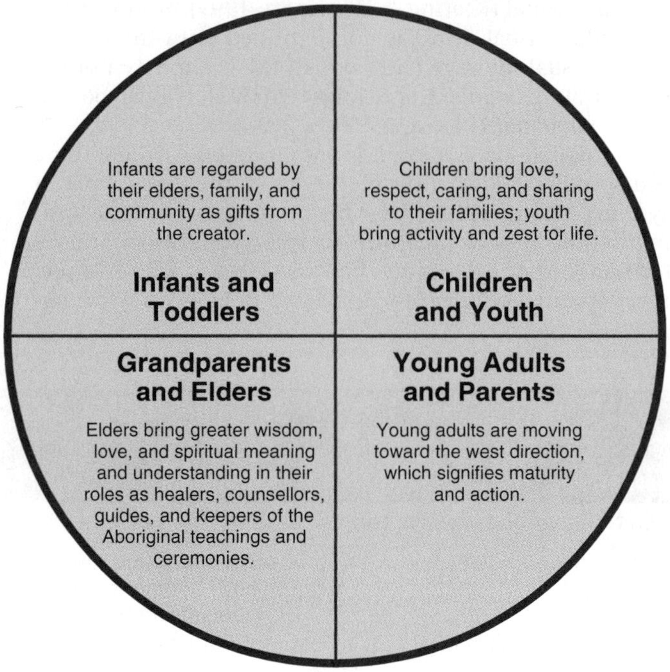

FIGURE **18–1** An Aboriginal perspective on human development: The circle of life (or the medicine wheel) as applied to the human life cycle. (Redrawn from "A Guide for Health Professionals Working with Aboriginal Peoples," by J. Smylie, 2001, *Journal SOGC, 100,* p. 55.)

Mechanisms of Maturational Development. **Maturation** is the biological internal regulatory mechanism that governs the emergence of all new skills and abilities that appear with advancing age (Kuhn, 1984). Maturation involves an individual's biological ability, physiological condition, and desire to learn more mature behaviour. To mature, the individual may have to relinquish previous behaviour and learning, integrate new patterns into existing behaviour, or both. Maturation influences the sequence and timing of the changes associated with growth and development. For example, the infant relinquishes crawling for walking because walking permits greater investigation of the environment and more learning. However, the infant cannot walk until the biological ability and structures to perform the action (i.e., increased muscle cells and tone) have developed.

Differentiation is the process by which cells and structures become modified and refine their characteristics. It is a simple-to-complex development of activities and functions. Embryonic cells begin as vague and undifferentiated and develop into complex, highly diversified cells, tissues, and organs.

Nursing Implications. Nurses consider maturational development in their care planning when they help mothers sequence play activities appropriate for learning of sitting, rolling, creeping, crawling, and walking. Nurses consider sequential development of fetuses and critical periods when they counsel expectant mothers about environmental teratogens during the first trimester of pregnancy. Nurses also support development during critical periods when they develop early intervention programs for parents.

Chess and Thomas's Theory of Temperament Development. **Temperament** is a physical and emotional response style that affects a child's interactions with others (Hockenberry et al., 2003). It is the way a person adjusts to life experiences and is thought to originate within the person's genetic makeup. A child's temperament influences how others respond to the child and his or her needs. Knowledge of temperament helps parents to have a clearer perspective of their child and enables health care providers to guide them appropriately (Hockenberry et al., 2003).

Psychiatrists Stella Chess and Alexander Thomas conducted a landmark 20-year longitudinal study of development that included children from a range of populations, including children of middle-class parents and intellectually disabled children of working-class parents. The breadth of the data allowed them to look at the behaviour of people from childhood to early adulthood as they interacted with their environment. Their work defined the concept of temperament (Chess & Thomas, 1986). They proposed that temperament is biologically derived.

Chess and Thomas described three common categories of temperament but explained that there are wide ranges of the behaviour and approximately 30% of children do not appear in any of these groups:

- *The easy child*—Easygoing and even-tempered. Regular and predictable in his or her habits. Is open and adaptable to change and displays a mild to moderately intense mood that is typically positive.
- *The difficult child*—Highly active, irritable, and irregular in habits. Negative withdrawal toward others is typical, and the child requires a more structured environment. Adapts slowly to new routines, people, or

situations. Mood expressions are usually intense and primarily negative.

- *The slow-to-warm-up child*—Typically reacts negatively and with mild intensity to new stimuli. Adapts slowly with repeated contact unless pressured and responds with mild but passive resistance to novelty or changes in routine.

Mechanisms of Temperament Development. Temperament theory proposes that biologically derived temperament characteristics drive children's interaction with the environment. Chess and Thomas (1986) proposed that it is through "goodness of fit" between the individual and the immediate environment that human development is modulated. This proposal places significant responsibility for child development outcomes within the family. For instance, the difficult child who has trouble making the transition from one activity or environment to a new one will function best in a family that maintains routine and has a slow easy attitude toward the introduction of change. The same child in a family that has few routines will have much more difficulty moving from one activity (like play) to the next activity (like sleep). In the first example, there is "goodness of fit" between the temperament of the child and the family environment.

Nursing Implications. Nurses can help families identify the unique characteristics of their infants and children. For instance, Kathryn Barnard and her research team have developed an approach called Keys to Caregiving (Sumner, 1995), which assists nurses to help new parents identify their infants' usual behaviour and communication styles. Nurses can help families adapt their habits and routines to match their children's temperaments. Nurses can also consider temperament styles when working with adults and families in teaching or support situations.

Cognitive Developmental Theories

Cognitive developmental theories focus on reasoning and thinking processes, including the changes in how people come to perform intellectual operations. These operations are related to the ways people learn to understand the world in which they live. Mental processes, including perceiving, reasoning, remembering, and believing, permit certain types of emotional behaviour. For example, a child will have a different emotional reaction to the death of a grandparent compared with the death of an older sibling or parent.

Unlike biophysical theories, cognitive developmental theories emphasize that although the developmental process originates with the person, it is greatly influenced by interactions between the person and the environment. Therefore, theories of cognitive development emphasize the active role that the individual plays in the developmental process. Cognitive theories are considered to be within the organicism tradition because development is still seen as originating within the organism.

Jean Piaget's Theory of Cognitive Development. Jean Piaget (1896–1980), a Swiss biologist and philosopher, studied how people come to know their world. **Piaget's theory of cognitive development** addresses the development of children's intellectual organization and how they think, reason, perceive, and make meaning of the physical world. His theory includes four periods with a number of stages within each (Table 18-2). It recognizes that people move through these specific periods at different rates but in the same sequence or order (Berk, 2003; Crain, 1992; Maier, 1965). He also theorized that this would be true in all cultures. He acknowledged that biological maturation plays a role in this developmental theory but believed that rates of development depend on the intellectual stimulation and challenge in the environment of the person. Piaget found that children acquire knowledge through acting on the environment. In other words, the individual plays an active role in his or her development.

Mechanisms of Cognitive Development. Although it is helpful to be aware of the stages, what is most important to learn from Piaget's theory is that he considered development to be a spontaneous process in which individuals play an active role in their own development. That is, biological maturation plays a role but the rates of development depend upon the intellectual stimulation and challenge in the environment of the child. These environmental challenges are internalized through the mechanisms of **assimilation** and **accommodation.** Assimilation is the process of making sense of new information in comparison with what is already known. Accommodation occurs when the individual adapts ways of thinking to a new experience or new information. Taken together, these processes reflect adaptation to new information or experience. In a health care situation, a person who has a headache can evaluate it as an everyday or usual experience. In this process, they are assimilating it to what they know already as their experience of their body. That is, they have occasional headaches and this is usual. When headaches become extreme or constant, then the same person will need to accommodate the headache pain to a different understanding of their experience of their body. For instance, they may learn to see themselves as a person who has migraines or as a person with a brain tumour who requires surgery.

The mechanisms of cognitive development apply across the lifespan and to all client situations. As such, they also apply to the moral theories and theories of adult development that are described in the following pages.

Nursing Implications. Most clients need to know about new ways of adjusting or behaving with respect to their health. Assimilation and accommodation represent adaptation of the client to new health challenges. Nurses need to support this process through providing information and support as clients come to terms with new health situations. Nurses must also offer positive feedback when clients successfully adapt to their challenges.

Moral Developmental Theories

Moral developmental theories are a subset of cognitive theory and describe the development of moral reasoning. Moral reasoning is how people think about the rules of ethical or moral conduct but it does not predict what a person would actually do in a given situation.

Table 18-2 Piaget's Theory of Cognitive Development

Stage and Age	Description	Nursing Interventions
Period 1: Sensorimotor (birth to 2 years)	The infant develops the schema or action pattern for dealing with the environment (Berk, 2003; Singer & Revenson, 1996). These schemas may include hitting, looking, grasping, or kicking (Figure 18–2). Schemas become self-initiated activities; for example, the infant learning that sucking achieves a pleasing result generalizes the action to suck fingers, blanket, or clothing. Successful achievement leads to greater exploration. In the second year, infants are able to form primitive mental images as they acquire object permanence. Before this, they do not realize that objects out of sight exist. When a 6-month-old is shown a toy before it is hidden, he or she will not search for it. At 18 months, the child can understand that even if it cannot be seen it still exists and will search for it.	Educating parents about the need to promote infants' exploration of the environment will support development of action patterns that develop motor and cognitive skills.
Period II: Preoperational (2 to 7 years of age)	Children learn to think with the use of symbols and mental images. Still egocentric, the child sees objects and people from only one point of view: the child's own. Play is the initial method of non-language use of symbols. This is a time of parallel play. Parallel play can be observed as children engage in activities side by side without a common goal. Imitation and make-believe play are ways to represent experience (Berk, 2003; Singer & Revenson, 1996). Later, language develops and broadens possibilities for thinking about the past or the future. Children can now communicate about events with others. As the language fits into a logical form, it mirrors the thinking process at the time.	Recognize the use of play as the way the child understands the events taking place. Parents can be assisted in the use of play materials such as toy thermometers and stethoscopes to encourage children to communicate feelings about health care procedures.
Period III: Concrete operations (7 to 11 years of age)	Children now achieve the ability to perform mental operations. For example, the child can now think about an action that before was performed physically. At the earlier stage, the child could count to 10 but now he or she can count and understand what each number represents. Children can now describe a process without actually performing it. At this time, they are able to coordinate two perspectives. In other words, they can appreciate the difference between their perspective and that of a friend. Reversibility is the primary characteristic of concrete operational thought. Children can mentally reverse the direction of their thoughts. Children can now mentally classify objects according to their quantitative dimensions, known as seriation. Another major accomplishment of this stage is conservation, or the ability to see objects or quantities as remaining the same despite a change in their physical appearance (Berk, 2003; Singer & Revenson, 1996). Children can begin to co-operate and share with new information about the acts they perform.	Encourage parents to guide the child to perform helpful activities within the home, such as doing chores in exchange for privileges (TV time, play with friends).
Period IV: Formal operations (11 years to adulthood)	The individual's thinking moves to abstract and theoretical subjects. Thinking can venture into such subjects as achieving world peace, finding justice, and seeking meaning in life. Adolescents can organize their thoughts in their minds. They have the capacity to reason with respect to possibilities. New cognitive powers allow the adolescent to do more far-reaching problem solving. This thinking matures, and the depth of understanding increases with experience.	The ability to think abstractly and theoretically enables adolescents to participate more fully in their own health care decisions.

Moral development is the ability of an individual to distinguish right from wrong and to develop ethical values on which to base his or her actions (Berk, 2003). Although various theorists have addressed moral development within their respective theories, Piaget and Kohlberg are the two who have done the most to propose a theory of moral development. These theories are within the organicism tradition because they are grounded in cognitive development theory and seen as originating from within the individual. The mechanisms of cognitive development and the general nursing interventions also apply to the moral development theories because they emerged from the original work of Piaget.

Jean Piaget. Piaget believed that moral development goes through a series of successive stages just as cognition and learning do. **Piaget's theory of moral development** presents three stages of morality: the **premoral stage,** the **conventional stage,** and the **autonomous stage.** In the premoral stage, the child has no obligation to rules. In

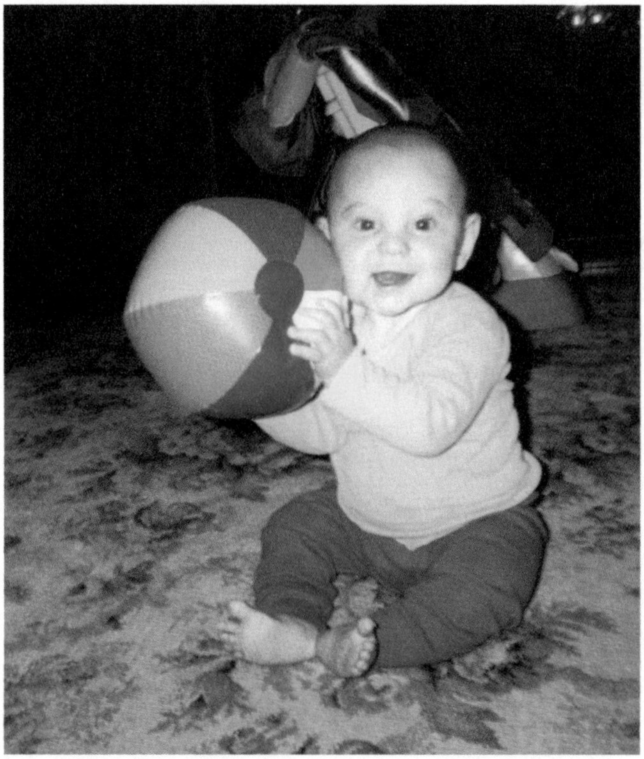

FIGURE **18–2** Successfully achieving action patterns such as grasping leads to learning and more exploration.

the conventional stage, children follow the rules set up by those in authority, such as their parents, teachers, clergy, or police. When a person reaches the stage of autonomous morality, moral judgments are based on mutual respect for the rules. A person also considers the consequences of a moral decision. In making moral judgments that involve others, the person at this stage starts to consider information related to the subjective intent (Berk, 2003).

Piaget believed children initially follow the rules without understanding them. Children see these rules as fixed and handed down by adults or by God and therefore think they cannot change them. Young children base their moral decisions on the extent of the consequences to the action, not necessarily on the action itself. For example, a young child will not eat a cookie before supper, not because the mother said not to, but because the child is afraid of the punishment that would result if he or she did. Around 10 or 11 years of age, children's cognitive ability matures and the rules children follow are understood within the context of community life. Children understand that the rules can be modified "by legal channels" if everyone agrees to change the rules (Singer & Revenson, 1996). Moral maturity is the internalization of the principles, the desire to weigh all of the relationships and circumstances before making a decision.

Lawrence Kohlberg. Lawrence Kohlberg (1927–1987) expanded on Piaget's moral developmental theory. From a series of moral dilemmas presented to boys aged 10, 13, and 16 years, he identified six stages of moral development under three levels (Kohlberg, 1981; Table 18-3). Kohlberg found a link between moral development and Piaget's cognitive development theory. He theorized that a child's moral development does not advance if the child's cognitive development does not also mature. In this way, **Kohlberg's theory of moral development** follows Piaget's cognitive developmental theory. According to Kohlberg, levels and stages do not occur at specific ages, and people develop to different levels of moral development.

Kohlberg's Critics. Although Kohlberg is recognized as a leader in moral developmental theory, critics have questioned the applicability of his study beyond the study population of young males of the Western philosophical tradition. Research attempting to support Kohlberg's theory with people raised in the Eastern philosophies found that those study participants never rose above Stages 3 or 4 of Kohlberg's model. Does that mean that they have not reached as high a level of moral development as most of the adults raised in the Western traditions? Or is it that Kohlberg's research design did not allow a way to measure those raised within a different culture?

Kohlberg has also been criticized for age and gender bias. Carol Gilligan, an associate, has criticized Kohlberg for his gender biases (Berk, 2003). Gilligan's research looked at moral development and concentrated on the differences that may be related to gender. According to Gilligan, all developmental theories are subject to gender bias, and only recently has our society researched and recognized the differences between men and women in the way they think and how they have been raised to make decisions (Kail, 2002).

Carol Gilligan. Gilligan (1936–present) proposed that Kohlberg's theory is biased in favour of men. She believes there may be parallel ways that men and women develop, with one not being superior to the other. Basic to Gilligan's argument is the developmental difference in relationships and issues of dependency between women and men (Berk, 2003; Crain, 1992; Gilligan, 1982; Schroeder, 1992). **Separation** and **individuation** are critically tied to male development. Separation refers to the child's recognition of biological distinctness and is based on his emergence from a dependent relationship with his mother. This separation from the mother is essential for the boy in his development of masculinity. Girls do not need to separate from their mothers to achieve feminine identity; it is through this attachment to their mother that their identity is formed. Most developmental theories use achievement of increasing separation as a developmental norm. When women are measured against this norm as it relates to their need to maintain relationships, they are seen as failures or less evolved developmentally. Individuation is based on the child's awareness of differences in will, viewpoint, and needs. This process permits the individual to gradually assume a more independent role and identity.

Male moral development may focus on logic, justice, and social organization, whereas female moral development focuses on interpersonal relationships. Interestingly, studies using Gilligan's critique as the research design have been inconclusive. As a result, Gilligan's position remains controversial (Cavanaugh, 1993).

Table 18-3 Kohlberg's Moral Development Theory

Level and Stage	Description	Nursing Implications
Level I: Preconventional Level	The person reflects on moral reasoning based on personal gain. The person's moral reason for acting, the "why," relates to the consequences the person believes will occur. These consequences can come in the form of punishment or reward. Therefore, children may view illness as a punishment for fighting with their siblings or disobeying their parents.	The nurse must be aware of this thinking and reinforce teaching that the child cannot become ill because of wrongdoing.
Stage 1: Punishment and obedience orientation	Response to a moral dilemma is in terms of absolute obedience to authority and rules. Avoidance of punishment or the unquestioning deference to authority is characteristic motivation to behave. The child will do something because an authority figure tells him or her to do it.	
Stage 2: Instrumental relativist orientation	The person recognizes there is more than one right view. The decision to do something morally right is based on satisfying one's own needs and occasionally the needs of others.	
Level II: Conventional Level	The person sees moral reasoning based on his or her own personal internalization of societal and others' expectations. A person wants to fulfill the expectations of the family, group, or nation and also develop a loyalty to and actively maintain, support, and justify the order. Moral decision making at this level moves from "What's in it for me?" to "How will it affect my relationships with others?"	Nurses may observe this level of moral development when family members make end-of-life decisions for their loved ones. Grief support will involve an understanding of the level of moral decision making of each family member (see chapter 25).
Stage 3: Good boy-nice girl orientation	The individual wants to please others and win approval by "being nice," meaning having good motives, showing concern for others, and keeping mutual relationships through trust, loyalty, respect, and gratitude.	
Stage 4: Society-maintaining orientation	Expands focus from relationships with others to societal concerns. Right behaviour is doing one's duty, showing respect for authority, and maintaining the social order. Adolescents in this stage may choose not to attend a party where drugs will be used, not because they are afraid of getting caught, but because they know that it is not right.	
Level III: Post-conventional Level	The person finds a balance between basic human rights and obligations and societal rules and regulations. Individuals move away from moral decisions based on authority or conformity to groups to define their own moral values and principles. Individuals at this stage start to look at what an ideal society would be like.	Nurses focus not only on their individual practice, but also on social determinants that affect the well-being of a community, such as poverty and homelessness.
Stage 5: Social contract orientation	An individual follows the laws but recognizes the possibility of changing the law to improve society. The individual also recognizes that different social groups may have different values but believe in basic rights, such as liberty and life.	
Stage 6: Universal ethical principle orientation	"Right" is defined by the decision of conscience in accord with self-chosen ethical principles. These principles are abstract, like the Golden Rule, and appeal to logical comprehensiveness, universality, and consistency (Kohlberg, 1981). Stage 5 emphasizes the basic rights and the democratic process, whereas Stage 6 defines the principles by which agreements will be most just.	

Psychoanalytic/Psychosocial Tradition

Theories in the **psychoanalytic/psychosocial tradition** describe the development of personality, thinking, behaviour, and emotions. This development is thought to occur with varying degrees of influence from internal biological forces and external societal/cultural forces.

Sigmund Freud

The first person to provide a formal, structured theory of personality development was Sigmund Freud (1856–1939). His goal was to promote successful participation in society through the development of balance between pleasure-seeking drives and societal pressures. In **Freud's psychoanalytic model of personality development,** he asserted that mature adults should have a strong sense of conscience that allows for the experience of pleasure within the boundaries of society. He believed that two

Table 18-4 **Freud's Five Stages of Psychosexual Development**

Level and Stage	Description	Nursing Implications
Stage 1: Oral (birth to 12 to 18 months)	Initially, sucking and oral satisfaction is not only vital to life, but also extremely pleasurable in its own right. Late in this stage, the infant begins to realize that the mother/parent is something separate from self. Disruption in the physical or emotional availability of the parent (e.g., inadequate bonding or chronic illness) could have an impact on the infant's development.	For an infant, feeding and sucking produces pleasure and comfort. Feedings should be offered whenever the infant requires them.
Stage 2: Anal (12 to 18 months to 3 years)	The focus of pleasure changes to the anal zone. Children become increasingly aware of the pleasurable sensations of this body region with interest in the products of their effort. Through the toilet-training process, the child is asked to delay gratification in order to meet parental and societal expectations.	The nurse should teach the parents that toilet training should be as positive an experience as possible. Offering praise gives the child a sense of control.
Stage 3: Phallic or oedipal (3 to 6 years)	The genital organs become the focus of pleasure. The boy becomes interested in the penis; the girl becomes aware of the absence of the penis, known as penis envy. This is the time of exploration and imagination as the child fantasizes about the parent of the opposite sex as his or her first love interest, known as the Oedipal or Electra complex. By the end of this stage, the child attempts to reduce this conflict by identifying with the parent of the same sex in a way to win recognition and acceptance.	Assure parents that a child's identifying with the parent of the same sex is a normal developmental phase.
Stage 4: Latency (6 to 12 years)	Sexual urges from the earlier Oedipal stage are repressed and channelled into productive activities that are socially acceptable. Within the educational and social worlds of the child, there is much to learn and accomplish. This is where the child places energy and effort.	Encourage the child to pursue physical and intellectual challenges.
Stage 5: Genital (puberty through adulthood)	This is a time of turbulence when earlier sexual urges reawaken and are directed to an individual outside the family circle. Unresolved prior conflicts surface during adolescence. Once conflicts are resolved, the individual is then capable of having a mature adult sexual relationship.	Educate parents that the child needs to be encouraged to be independent and make his or her own decisions, within safe limits.

internal biological forces essentially drive psychological change in the child: sexual **(libido)** and aggressive energies. Motivation for behaviour is to achieve pleasure and avoid pain created by these forces. These forces come into conflict with the reality of the world as maturational changes occur.

Freud's theory has five psychosexual developmental stages, each associated with different pleasurable zones serving as the focus for gratification and bodily pleasure (Behrman & Kliegman, 2000; Berk, 2003; Table 18-4). Freud's theory has been soundly criticized for gender and cultural biases. Some of Freud's critics contend that people are more influenced by their life experiences than by their sexual energies. Despite these criticisms, it is clear that Freud gave other theorists a basis for observation of emotion and behaviour. Many other psychoanalytic theories maintain the idea that development is an ongoing process of resolving conflict between issues of biological maturation and societal expectations.

Mechanisms of Freud's Theory. Components of personality emerge through Freud's developmental stages. The mechanisms of Freud's personality development theory are the id, the ego, and the superego. Freud believed that the functions of these mechanisms regulate behaviour. The id, basic instinctual impulses driven to achieve pleasure, is the most primitive part of the personality and originates in the infant. The ego represents the reality mechanism mediating conflicts between the environment and the forces of the id. The ego helps us judge reality accurately, regulate impulses, and make good decisions. The third mechanism, the **superego,** performs regulating, restraining, and prohibiting actions. Often referred to as the conscience, the superego is influenced by the standards of outside social forces (parent, teacher).

Nursing Implications. The functions of the id, ego, and superego form the historical basis of many, if not all, subsequent theories of personality and social emotional development. Nurses need to remember that according to Freudian theory, mature human personality is the product of conflict between instinctual drives that seek pleasure and the restraints of adaptive human society. When activities associated with basic pleasure (e.g., eating, sexual activity, and elimination) are altered by illness or disability, knowledgeable and empathetic nursing care is required.

Erik Erikson

Erik Erikson (1902–1994) expanded Freud's psychoanalytic stages into a psychosocial model that covered the whole lifespan, not just childhood and adolescence (Behrman & Kliegman 2000; Berk, 2003; Erikson, 1963, 1997). He broadened the factors responsible for influencing development to include socialization.

According to **Erikson's eight stages of life theory,** each person goes through eight stages of development (Table 18-5). In each stage, the person needs to accomplish a particular task before moving on to the next stage. Each task is framed with opposing conflicts that the person must balance. For example, an adolescent needs to develop a sense of personal identity despite many conflicting societal choices (Stage 5, identity versus role confusion). Each stage builds upon the successful resolution of the previous developmental conflict. Readiness for the task is necessary for success. Once mastered, tasks are challenged and tested during new situations or at times of conflict (Hockenberry et al., 2003). For example, the infant's trust is built through consistent, reliable caregiving, and the concept of trust is tested when an infant is hospitalized or after the birth of a new baby sibling.

Mechanisms of Erikson's Theory. *Maturation* and *ego* activity are the primary mechanisms of development in Erikson's eight stages of life. The ego mediates the conflicts between the biological needs and societal norms, and maturation establishes the timeline. The developmental result of these mechanisms is described as an **epigenesis** (successive gradual change). If the process is adaptive, then a person has successive positive outcomes.

Nursing Implications. The theory of the eight stages of life implies that the quality of early developmental work is important. For instance, children living in environments where violence is common and trust has not been attained are at greater risk of experiencing poor intimate relationships. The mechanism of epigenesis implies that the original required trust elements cannot be retrieved; at best such a person can only learn to live with the fear and anger associated with this mistrust. Nurses therefore need to practice within the health promotion model in order to build the familial, community, and societal supports to the early stages of life (trust, autonomy, and initiative).

John Bowlby

John Bowlby (1907–1990) was a child psychiatrist interested in children's mental health. **Bowlby's attachment and separation theory** proposes that the conflict between attachment and separation needs to be resolved in order to produce healthy social and emotional developmental outcomes across the lifespan. A basic premise of the theory is that the quality of attachment relationships stems from interactions between infants and their caregivers. These interactions reflect the degree to which infants can rely on their caregivers to provide proximity and companionship, a safe haven in the face of threat or anxiety, and a secure base from which to explore. Failure to achieve secure attachment results in an inability throughout the lifespan to separate from caregivers and reconnect to new relationships (including work, friendship, and intimate relationships) in a healthy way.

Mechanisms of Bowlby's Theory. Early in life, two complementary behavioural systems, attachment and caregiving, combine into a self-regulating system that supports people in their healthy attachments to and separations from others. The child's experiences within this self-regulating system cause the child to develop a cognitive working model (or "map") of self, other, and the relationship between them. The ability to regulate emotion and behaviour are influenced by this working model at each developmental stage throughout life.

Nursing Implications. Nurses need to design approaches that address both the quality of the attachment system and the caregiving system. For instance, in the situation in which a young child is hospitalized, the nurse would need to consider the security of the child and to provide high-quality substitute care, including making developmentally appropriate efforts to keep the child attached to his or her primary caregiver (e.g., using pictures, phone calls, liberal visiting hours, parent sleepovers). Alternatively, in a situation in which nurses work with parents in impoverished environments, the nurse needs to support the caregivers through provision of material, social, and educational resources.

Robert Havighurt

Robert Havighurst (1900–1991) was influenced by Erikson's work and observations of the developmental tasks critical to healthy development. Havighurst defined a series of essential tasks that arise from predictable internal and external pressures (Ashburn, 1978). These pressures include increasing physical maturity, cultural pressure of society, and the individual's personal goals and aspirations.

According to **Havighurst's developmental tasks,** several sources of pressure may be present at the same time. Increasing physical maturity is associated with the development of skills such as walking, talking, or eating. Cultural pressure creates the conditions necessary to learn social behaviours and ethical norms. Although the adolescent girl may be physically able to bear a child, the preparation and timing for the onset of parenthood can also be considered from a perspective of cultural pressure from both the youth and adult cultures.

Havighurst believed that there are critical periods when the individual is most receptive to the learning necessary to achieve success in performing these tasks. Effective learning and achievement of tasks during one period lead to happiness and success with later tasks. Failure leads to unhappiness, disapproval by society, and difficulty with later tasks. An example is the struggle that adolescents might experience in preparing for a work career after having failed to develop fundamental skills in reading and math.

Havighurst's theory is limited in its cultural application according to critics who believe that it describes developmental milestones from the perspective of middle-class norms within the American culture. It would be difficult to fit all cultural or ethnic mores within this theoretical framework.

Mechanisms and Nursing Implications. Havighurst's work builds on that of Freud and Erikson. Therefore, the mechanisms and nursing implications from Freud and Erikson also apply to Havighurst's developmental tasks.

Table 18-5 Erikson's Eight Stages of Life

Stage and Developmental Period/Age	Description	Nursing Implications
1. **Trust versus mistrust** (infancy: birth to 1 year)	The infant learns to trust others. Trust is achieved when the infant will let the caregiver out of sight without undo distress. Key to this stage is consistent caregiving. The question answered at this stage is "Can I trust the world?"	The parent's struggle with building competence can be assisted by the nurse's use of anticipatory guidance and other educative interventions. The parent may need guidance to understand the importance of a safe, nurturing environment when meeting the child's needs.
2. **Autonomy versus sense of shame and doubt** (toddler years: 1 to 3 years)	The toddler learns to be independent and develops self-confidence. Not learning independence creates feelings of shame and doubt. Independence is accomplished by accomplishing self-care activities, including walking, feeding, and toileting. Toddlers also develop autonomy by making choices. The question answered at this stage is "Can I control my own behaviour?"	The nurse can model empathetic guidance that offers support for and understanding of the challenges of this stage. Harsh punishment and never offering choices are not appropriate.
3. **Initiative versus guilt** (preschool years: 3 to 6 years)	The child learns to initiate his or her activities. Accomplishing this task teaches the child to seek challenges in later life. Children use fantasy and imagination to explore their environment. Conflicts often arise between the child's desire to explore and the limits placed on his or her behaviour. These conflicts may lead to feelings of frustration and guilt. The questioned answered during this stage is "Can I become independent of my parents and explore my limits?"	Teaching impulse control and co-operative behaviours to the child are necessary for this stage.
4. **Industry versus inferiority** (middle childhood: 6 to 11 years)	The child develops a sense of competence in physical, cognitive, and social areas. Not learning new skills may lead to a sense of inadequacy and inferiority. Successfully achieving this task leads to positive attitudes toward work in adulthood (Erikson, 1963). The question answered at this stage is "Can I master the skills necessary to survive and adapt?"	The nurse can encourage parents to offer the child many opportunities to pursue new interests and challenges.
5. **Identity versus role confusion** (adolescence: 12 to 18 years)	The task of adolescence is to try out several roles and form a unique identity. Dramatic physiological changes associated with sexual maturation also mark this stage. Acquiring a sense of identity is essential for making later adult decisions such as vocation or marriage partner. There are also new social demands, opportunities, and conflicts that relate to the emergent identity and separation from family. The question answered at this stage is "Who am I, and what are my beliefs, feelings, and attitudes?"	The nurse can provide education and anticipatory guidance for the parent about the changes and challenges to the adolescent. Nurses can also assist hospitalized adolescents in dealing with their illness by giving them enough information to allow them to make decisions about their treatment plan.
6. **Intimacy versus isolation** (young adulthood: 18 to 35 years)	The primary task of young adulthood is to form close, personal relationships. This is the time to become fully active in the community. If young people have not achieved a sense of personal identity, they may be unable to form meaningful attachments and experience feelings of isolation. The question answered during this stage is "Can I give of myself fully to another?"	The nurse should understand that during hospitalization young adults may benefit from the support of their partner or significant other because this strengthens their need for intimacy.
7. **Generativity versus self-absorption and stagnation** (middle age: 35 to 65 years)	The task of middle adulthood is to help younger people. The ability to expand one's personal and social involvement is critical to this stage of development. Middle-age adults should be able to see beyond their needs and accomplishments to the needs of society. Dissatisfaction with one's achievements often leads to self-absorption and stagnation. The question answered during this stage is "What can I offer succeeding generations?"	Nurses can assist adults in choosing creative ways to foster social development. Middle-age people may find a sense of fulfillment by volunteering some time in a local school, hospital, or place of worship.
8. **Integrity versus despair** (old age: 65 years and over)	Older adults reflect on their life and feel satisfaction or disappointment. By suffering physical and social losses, the adult may also suffer loss of status and function, such as through retirement or illness. The person may also have internal struggles, such as the search for meaning in life. Meeting these challenges creates the potential for growth and wisdom (Figure 18–3). The question answered during this stage is "Has my life been worthwhile?"	Nurses are in positions of influence within their communities and can contribute to the valuing of people at all ages and stages. People at all ages and stages need to feel valued, appreciated, and needed.

Adapted from *An Introduction to Theories of Human Development,* by N. Salkind, 2004, Thousand Oaks, CA: Sage.

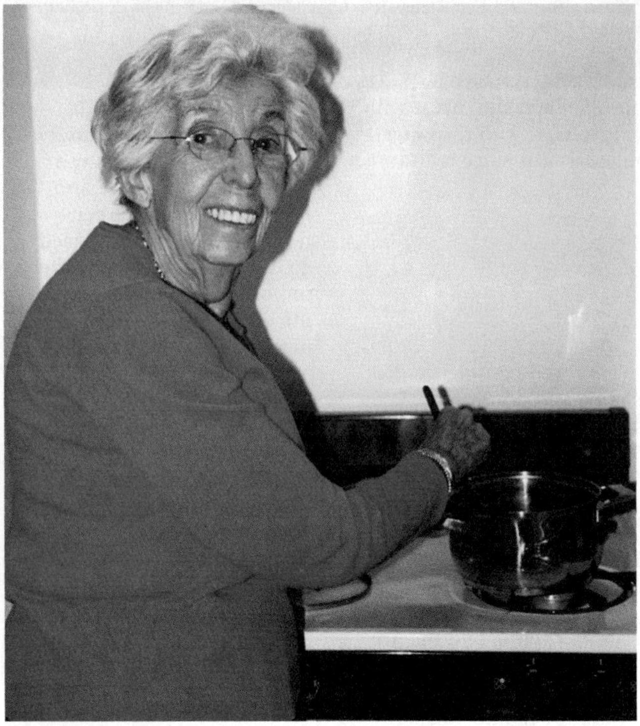

FIGURE **18–3** Maintaining independence is important to one's self-esteem.

Roger Gould

Psychiatrist Roger Gould reviewed the work of other theorists and found that a lack of understanding of the adult years contributed to the maturing and changing of personality (Gould, 1972). (Table 18-6 compares the major themes of the three most prominent adult theorists.) Gould conducted extensive research that supported a set of development themes within stages of adult development. Gould found that over the adult years, people dismantle the protective thinking developed during childhood. Over a period of years, beliefs are shed, marking a shift from childhood into adult consciousness.

Gould's development themes start when individuals are in their 20s with the theme, "I have to get away from my parents." This theme is challenged in minor ways before the end of high school but culminates as young people begin to live away from home. The move away from parental influence is gradual as young adults establish themselves as adults.

The second theme occurs when individuals reach their early 30s and ask, "Is what I am the only way for me to be?" This question occurs when young adults experience the consequences of the decisions of their independence. Everything does not work out magically as might have been expected. There are failures to be overcome. Acceptance for who they are is essential. So, too, is acceptance of their own growing children as being unique and separate.

The third theme occurs when individuals reach their mid- to late 30s and asks, "Have I done the right thing? Is there time to change?" These questions recognize the complexities of adult decisions. The impact of a growing family and aging parents influences this theme. There is the beginning of a sense of how much time is left to meet desired goals.

The fourth theme, identified in individuals in their 40s, "The die is cast," is indicative of resignation and the belief that possibilities are limited. The personality is set. Changes in career are believed to be less likely to be successful. Parents are blamed for their lack of choices. Regret is faced for mistakes made with children.

During the period when individuals are in their 50s a decrease in negativism occurs. Gould finds people generally realize their mortality and are concerned for their state of health. There is less responsibility for the welfare of the children and more attachment to the spouse, as might be expected.

Gould believes his research describes a sequential process that takes place between the internal life (personality) of adults and their outer world (culture, lifestyle). For example, Gould looked at the timing and sequencing of an event, as well as the individual's adjustment and transition into a particular stage. It seemed clear to Gould that events of adulthood may be similar in adults; however, the timing and sequencing affects the adjustment and consequences in different individuals. Marriage, for example, may occur before or after pregnancy, the time between the birth of the first and second child may differ, and retirement may occur in one's 50s or 60s.

Mechanisms and Nursing Implications. As with Havighurst, Gould's work builds on that of Freud and Erikson. Therefore, the mechanisms and nursing implications from Freud and Erikson also apply to Gould's theory of development.

Mechanistic Tradition

The **mechanistic tradition** presents the organism as similar to a machine. Development depends on the level of stimulation, the kind of stimulation, and the history of stimulation from the environment. The environment is considered to activate (Dixon & Lerner, 1984) human development, and behaviour is seen as responsive to environmental forces rather than driven only by internal causes like maturation. Social learning theories follow from this tradition and are presented in chapter 17.

Contextualism

The way that we describe and explain human development is increasingly tied to our understanding of environment and context. Developmental theories within the **contextual tradition** focus on the relationship between the individual and his or her social context. Within this tradition, the individual and the environment are viewed as mutually influential, acting on one another in dynamic interaction (Dixon & Lerner, 1984). Human development is therefore seen as the process of continuously adapting to changing environments.

Table 18-6 Adult Developmental Theorists

Adult Stages (Approximate Ages)	Erikson	Havighurst	Gould
Early-early adult (16–22 years)	Intimacy versus isolation	Early adulthood stage	Theme: "I have to get away from my parents."
Middle-early adult (22–28 years)	Ability to form intimate relationships	Selecting a mate Learning to live with a marriage partner Starting a family Rearing children Getting started in an occupation Taking on civic responsibilities Finding a congenial social group	Gradually establishing control of self as an adult
Late-early adult (28–35 years)			Theme: "Is what I am the only way for me to be?" Demonstrating independent competence while overcoming failures
Middle adult (35–45 years)	Generativity versus self-absorption and stagnation Ability to expand personal and social involvement	Middle age Assisting teenage children to become responsible adults Achieving adult social and civic responsibility Reaching and maintaining satisfactory performance in one's occupation Developing adult leisure-time activities Relating to one's spouse as a person Accepting and adjusting to the physiological changes of middle age Adjusting to aging of parents	Theme: "Have I done the right thing?" Learning to live with ambivalence without need to prove self Beginning sense of time to effect wanted results
Middle adult (continued) (40–50 years) Middle adult (continued) (50–65 years)			Theme: "The die is cast." Believing that possibilities are limited Seeing time as having an end point Decreased negativism Increased feelings of self-satisfaction Realizing mortality and concern for health
Late adult/old age (65 years and over)	Integrity versus despair, disgust Ability to adapt to changes in lifestyle, functional level, and family structure	Later maturity Adjusting to decreasing physical strength and health Adjusting to retirement and reduced income Adjusting to death of a spouse Establishing an affiliation with one's age group Adopting and adapting social roles in a flexible way Satisfactory physical living space	

Urie Bronfenbrenner

Urie Bronfenbrenner (1917–present), a developmental psychologist at Cornell University, has developed a theory that stresses the importance of the interaction between the developing individual and his or her surrounding social environments. **Bronfenbrenner's bioecological theory** involves considering multiple "layers" of the environment:

- The **microsystem** consists of the immediate settings, activities, and personal relationships of the individual. Examples of microsystems include family, classroom, workplace, or recreation group.
- The **mesosystem** is made up of the relationships between the different settings in which the person spends time. Examples of mesosystems include relationships between families and schools, workplaces and schools, families and spiritual organizations (church parish, mosque, temple), and spiritual organizations and schools.
- The **exosystem** is a set of specific social structures that do not directly contain the individual but exert direct and indirect influence on individual development. Examples of exosystems include the health care

system, the education system, the justice system, and religious institutions.
- The **macrosystem** consists of all of the elements contained in the individual's micro-, meso-, and exosystems plus the general underlying philosophy, cultural orientation, and values within which the person lives (Salkind, 2004). The macrosystem includes overarching dimensions such as political orientation, economic model, and cultural values.

Mechanisms of the Bioecological Theory. Lev Semenovich Vygotsky (1896–1934) introduced a concept called the **zone of proximal development,** which is the key developmental mechanism of ecological theories. This zone is the space between the individual's potential and his or her actual developmental status. For instance, a toddler may have a 10-word vocabulary, but potentially could have a repertoire of hundreds of words. Activity that links those two states promotes development. For instance, parents who use joint referencing (looking at things that their toddlers are looking at and naming them) will promote toddler vocabulary development within the zone of proximal development.

Bronfenbrenner's modern conception of developmental processes follows directly from Vygotsky's idea of the zone of proximal development but expands upon it. In the case of language acquisition, developmental support processes occur in all levels of the system. At the macrosystem level, a support process that would be supportive of language development in young children would be the adoption of a national child care policy to support working parents. Such a policy would inform regulations around issues like education level of child care workers, ratio of child to worker in child care centres, space requirements per child, and so on.

Nursing Implications. An appropriate goal of nursing practice is to influence wellness by promoting health in all layers of the bioecological system. The ecological model applies to nursing practice beyond the individual level of health promotion to higher levels of the social context. Therefore, Bronfenbrenner's theory fits well with current emphasis on primary health care (Box 18-2).

Focus on Primary Health Care — Box 18-2

Bronfenbrenner's Ecological Theory and Primary Health Care

Three principles of primary health care are to (a) foster public participation, (b) educate the client in order to promote health and prevent illness, and (c) foster intersectoral collaboration. Bronfenbrenner's ecological model of human development fits well with these principles. At each environmental layer (as described by Bronfenbrenner), nurses can initiate actions to promote health:

- Microsystem—includes the individual and his or her immediate setting (family, school, workplace, neighbourhood, etc.). The nurse can help the individual develop personal skills, healthy lifestyles and activities, and supportive environments. For example, a nurse can help teach family members caring for an elderly parent how to balance family care and self-care to keep themselves healthy.
- Mesosystem—relations among the individual's various immediate settings. To strengthen the mesosystem, the nurse can work toward strengthening community action. The nurse can link the family to community supports such as adult respite services and older adults' activities groups.
- Exosystem—relations among structures, sectors, services, and policies. The exosystem is strengthened when nurses promote healthy public policy. Nurses are practising at this level when they participate in ways to develop links between typically separate services such as the health care system and the social service system. For example, a nurse can volunteer to be on planning committees and other decision-making bodies.
- Macrosystem—societal values. To promote optimum health at the macrosystem level, the nurse can be an advocate for social change. For example, a nurse who believes that more value should be placed on older adults in our society might advocate for higher standards and staff-resident ratios in long-term care facilities. This might include writing letters to the editor, joining community or national advocacy groups, and lobbying politicians.

Dialecticism

In the **dialectic tradition,** all developmental theories are considered mutually interactive. Developmental theorists are increasingly proposing that change or development can occur within the framework of multiple theories. A key element of the dialectic tradition is the ability to incorporate multiple contexts. An example of a dialectic approach from the biomedical sciences is the theory of gene expression. The theory of gene expression links genetics, the environment, and their influences on human behaviour and disease. In the human development disciplines, examples of dialectical thinking include the growing awareness of the effect of the economic environment on human development at the population level. Resilience is also a new theoretical approach in which the interaction between two processes, previously studied separately, is examined.

Keating and Hertzman's Population Health Theory

Human development has historically been considered an individual characteristic. Daniel Keating and Clyde Hertzman's **population health approach** (1999) maintains that human development is a population phenomenon. These Canadian developmental theorists refer to the strong association between the health of a population, developmental outcomes, and the social and economic forces affecting the larger society. They base their developmental theory on epidemiological data that suggest that improved literacy (one marker of human development) is related to improvements in the following socio-economic conditions: family economic

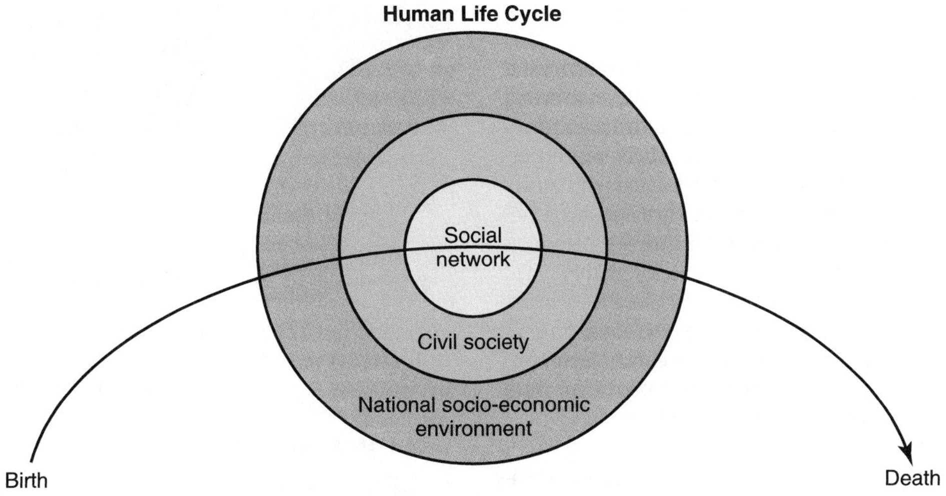

FIGURE **18–4** Framework for human development and the social determinants of health. (Redrawn from *Developmental Health and the Wealth of Nations: Social, Biological and Educational Dynamics,* p. 30, edited by D. P. Keating and C. Hertzman, 1999, New York: Guilford.)

status, school community economic status, and national economic status.

They proposed that health, behaviour, and cognitive functions are largely set in early life and are then influenced further by succeeding events that flow from the socio-economic environment. Keating and Hertzman define **developmental health** as the physical and mental health, well-being, coping, and competence of human populations. Developmental health arises primarily as a function of the overall quality of the social environment, including the national socio-economic environment, civil society, and social network. Their population approach to human development is outlined in Figure 18–4.

Mechanisms of the Population Health Theory. Keating and Herzman (1999) proposed three interrelated regulatory systems as the mechanisms for human population development. Each regulatory system develops in interaction between the individual's biological processes and his or her multiple social-economic environments.

- Emotional regulation involves the modulation of emotional reactions. Emotional regulation plays an important role in competent social functioning.
- Attention regulation involves regulation of the arousal and reactivity of the brain. Attainment of attention regulation contributes to the individual being able to pursue goals and respond to challenges to those goals.
- Social regulation involves regulation of social interaction, including aspects such as mutual affection and warmth, particularly in nurturing relationships.

Together, these three regulatory systems are thought to influence later competence as individuals interact reciprocally with their socio-economic environments.

Nursing Implications. Nurses have typically practised in a way that focuses on the health and well-being of individuals. Evidence shows that to promote well-being, health professionals need to implement practices that take into account the impact of the socio-economic context on the health of the individual. The ecological levels of health promotion activities are directly applicable to the population health approach (see Box 18-2). A population health approach helps identify these socio-economic factors and provides direction for designing nursing interventions that address them.

Resilience Theory

Resilience is defined as the maintenance of positive adjustment under challenging life conditions (Luthar, Cocchetti, & Becker, 2000). The notion of resilience alerts us to the possibility that positive adjustment processes may differ by environment (Luthar, 1999) and that positive adjustments can and do occur in less than optimal situations. This approach arose in child psychiatry when clinicians observed that some children and adolescents were able to thrive in severely adverse conditions (e.g., poverty, maternal depression, and paternal criminality), whereas others faltered (Rutter, 1979).

Mechanisms of Resilience. Resilience theory focuses on the interaction between protective processes and vulnerability processes. **Vulnerability processes** (physical illness, psychological stresses, social risk) and **protective processes** (self-efficacy, good parenting and problem solving, good social support acquisition and maintenance) are examined together to understand and explain human growth and development. Individual factors found to promote resilience include self-efficacy, positive attitude, literacy, social competence, and a history of success. Family-level processes that protect from adversity include coherent response to crisis, social supports, stability, flexibility, effective parenting, and responsibilities outside the home (Drummond et al., 1996–1997). Community-level processes that promote resilience include control over policy, collaborative and co-operative organization, widespread citizen participation in community, and volunteerism.

Resilience and family adaptation theory has been used to design interventions to support children and families at risk (Drummond et al., 2002). The current emphasis in resilience research is on protective processes (a positive perspective) within the context of key risk situations, usually defined by factors like poverty, chronic illness, and civil conflict. This emphasis is a progression from the previous emphasis on pathological processes only, but it does not yet capture the richness of the dynamic between vulnerability processes and protective processes (Drummond et al., 2002). The challenge is to design research that can study both resilience processes (protective processes and vulnerability processes) as they occur together.

Nursing Implications. The focus of nursing practice is directly on the individual, family, and community factors that will promote health. Nursing practice is usually focused on situations that are stressful and challenging for individuals and families, such as illness and loss. Resilience acknowledges the complexity of these moments and asks what it is about these challenging situations that nurses can use to help the family succeed (Box 18-3). For example, a young single woman dealing with the birth of her first child will benefit from nursing interventions that focus on both protective processes (linking to support group, learning parenting skills) and vulnerability processes (ensuring adequate health care, arranging for financial support).

Research Highlight — Box 18-3

Supporting Parents: Can Intervention Improve Parent-child Relationships?

Research Focus

Healthy child development has been identified as one of the key determinants of health and resiliency in adulthood. Two studies examined interventions aimed at improving the parent-child relationship and enhancing resiliency among children considered at risk due to poverty and/or parents' young age, inexperience, or lack of education.

Research Abstract

These two pilot studies were randomized control trials designed to test the effects of two support interventions. The first intervention, Keys to Caregiving, used a family-centred approach to provide parents with tools necessary for high-quality interactions with their infants. A post-test only experimental design was used to study 16 adolescent mothers and their infants. The second intervention, Natural Teaching Strategies, focused on developing mutually satisfying methods for parents to communicate with their preschoolers. A pretest–post-test design was used to study 29 families of children enrolled in Head Start programs. In both groups, parent-child interactions were enhanced in the treatment groups. Both interventions pointed to the potential effect of supportive intervention on parent-child interactions over time.

Evidence-Based Practice

- Helping parents develop realistic expectations of their child's development and improving the quality of parent-child relationships are important support mechanisms for families at risk.
- Parent training and support has the potential to positively alter the style of interactions between parents and children.

Reference

Letourneau, N., et al. (2001). Supporting parents: Can intervention improve parent-child relationships? *Journal of Family Nursing, 7*(2), 159–187.

Developmental Theories and Nursing

From the diverse set of theories included in this chapter, it is clear that human behaviour is truly complex. No one theory successfully describes human growth and development in all of its complexity. Theorists demonstrate their own values and beliefs in their focus and the subjects chosen for their work, and they work within a cultural and historical perspective. The theories included here are meant to provide the basis for meaningful thought and observation of an individual's pattern of growth and development and the role of environments in it. This observation and reflection provides nurses with a framework within which to predict human responses to health and illness and to recognize deviations from the norm.

Accurate assessment of patterns of growth and development helps to set the stage for future patterns of adjustment to life (Edelman & Mandle, 2002). A clear understanding of these patterns and the contexts within which they occur assists the nurse in planning questions for health screening and health history and in health teaching for clients of all ages. Nurses need to consider an individual's development within the context of their families, social relationships, communities, and the larger society.

Developmental theories help nurses to use critical thinking skills when asking how and why people respond as they do. A nurse's assessment of a client requires a thorough analysis and interpretation of data to form accurate conclusions about a client's developmental needs. Accurate identification of client need relies on the nurse's ability to consider developmental theory in data analysis. A nurse compares typical developmental behaviours with those projected by the developmental theory. Examples of nursing diagnoses applicable to clients with developmental issues include: *risk for delayed development, delayed growth and development, risk for disproportionate growth, presence of adversity severe enough to compromise typical growth and development,* and *insufficient stimulation from key environmental supports to development.* Further detail regarding these diagnoses can be found in chapter 12.

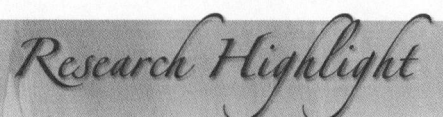

Key Concepts

- Nurses provide care for individuals and families throughout their lives. Developmental theories provide a basis for nurses to assess, interpret, and understand the responses seen in their clients.
- People continue to develop throughout their lives.
- Individuals have unique patterns of growth and development within broad limits.
- Development is not just a series of distinct linear tasks, but it is a process that varies across and within individuals (Hartup, 2002).
- There are three major categories of factors that influence human growth and development: (a) genetic or natural forces within the person, (b) the environment in which the person lives, and (c) the interaction that takes place between these two.
- Theories within the organic tradition explore how individuals develop when mostly biological components are believed to stimulate developmental progress.
- Theories in the psychoanalytic/psychosocial tradition describe development of the human personality from the point of view of conflict resolution between the internal biological forces and the external societal/cultural forces.
- The mechanistic approach positions human development and behaviour as responses to environmental forces rather than driven by internal causes like maturation.
- Within the contextual tradition, the individual and the environment are viewed as mutually influential, acting on one another in dynamic interaction.
- In the dialectical tradition, the complete complexity of development is acknowledged. Theorists who work in this tradition strive to combine divergent ways of viewing human development.

Key Terms

Accommodation, *p. 342*
Assimilation, *p. 342*
Autonomous stage, *p. 343*
Biophysical development theories, *p. 338*
Bowlby's attachment and separation theory, *p. 346*
Bronfenbrenner's bioecological theory, *p. 350*
Cognitive development theories, *p. 341*
Contextual tradition, *p. 350*
Conventional stage, *p. 343*
Developmental health, *p. 351*
Dialectic tradition, *p. 350*
Differentiation, *p. 340*
Epigenesis, *p. 346*
Erikson's eight stages of life theory, *p. 345*
Exosystem, *p. 350*
Freud's psychoanalytic model of personality development, *p. 345*
Gould's development themes, *p. 348*
Havighurst's developmental tasks, *p. 348*
Individuation, *p. 345*
Kohlberg's theory of moral development, *p. 343*
Libido, *p. 345*
Macrosystem, *p. 350*
Maturation, *p. 340*
Mechanisms, *p. 338*
Mechanistic tradition, *p. 350*
Mesosystem, *p. 350*
Microsystem, *p. 350*
Moral developmental theories, *p. 343*
Organicism, *p. 338*
Piaget's theory of cognitive development, *p. 341*
Piaget's theory of moral development, *p. 341*
Population health approach, *p. 350*
Premoral stage, *p. 343*
Protective process, *p. 351*
Psychoanalytic/psychosocial tradition, *p. 345*
Resilience, *p. 351*
Separation, *p. 345*
Superego, *p. 345*
Temperament, *p. 341*
Vulnerability processes, *p. 351*
Zone of proximal development, *p. 350*

Critical Thinking Exercises

1. A 76-year-old woman has just been diagnosed with breast cancer. She also has severe cardiovascular disease that limits her choices of treatment. Her oncologist has recommended a series of chemotherapy treatments that her cardiologist believes would be fatal. Her family is urging her to do all that is recommended. The client, who is in good spirits despite her prognosis, chooses palliative care. Interpret the responses of this family using attachment and separation perspectives.
2. A 50-year-old woman is anxious because her children, 20 and 23 years of age, are no longer living at home. Her husband is still working full time but planning to retire in 2 years. She is concerned that she is not needed and is bored with her life. Identify the developmental task of Erickson's theory that best fits this woman's situation. How will the nurse assist this client in changing her lifestyle while understanding her developmental tasks?
3. A public health nurse conducting a routine assessment of an 18-month-old toddler is concerned about the child being underweight for his age. Upon further discussion, the father reveals that he is not working at present and the family is having financial troubles. Using your knowledge of Bronfenbrenner's bioecological theory, what approach and subsequent strategies would be helpful for these parents?
4. Two 11-year-old girls are spending the day together at the mall. They exit one store, and one of the girls shows her friend a small purse that she stole from the store. Her friend is upset and wonders how she should respond. Use moral development theory to discuss this issue.

Review Questions

1. Children generally double their birth weight by 5 months of age. This is an example of
   1. Development
   2. Heredity
   3. State of health
   4. Physical growth

2. ________ development is the ability of an individual to distinguish right from wrong and to develop ethical values on which to base his or her actions.
   1. Moral
   2. Cognitive
   3. Psychosocial
   4. Psychoanalytic
3. Theories in this tradition hold that development is a result of biology and adaptation.
   1. Organicism
   2. Psychoanalytic/psychosocial
   3. Contexualism
   4. Dialecticism
4. Which of the following factors is considered an environmental factor that affects human development:
   1. Family
   2. Heredity
   3. State of health
   4. Genetics
5. The developmental theorist who believed his research described a sequential process that resolved conflict between the internal life (personality) of adults and their outer world (culture) was
   1. Erickson
   2. Bronfenbrenner
   3. Freud
   4. Gould
6. "The die is cast" is consistent with Gould's theme for the
   1. 30s
   2. 40s
   3. 50s
   4. 70s
7. According to Piaget's theory of cognitive development, during this stage, the individual's moral thinking moves to abstract and theoretical subjects. Thinking can venture into such subjects as achieving world peace, finding justice, and seeking meaning in life.
   1. Formal operations
   2. Concrete operations
   3. Sensorimotor
   4. Preoperational
8. The nurse who is working with a school committee to develop playground safety guidelines is focusing on which level of the bioecological model?
   1. Mesosystem
   2. Microsystem
   3. Exosystem
   4. Macrosystem
9. Which of the following nursing interventions is representative of a population health approach?
   1. Parent teaching
   2. Developing a clinical practice guideline
   3. Participating in a community coalition to improve community housing
   4. Assisting an individual in obtaining funding support for home care
10. A resilient individual is able to experience positive development despite challenging life circumstances. For a young single mother with two young children, access to quality daycare represents the following:
   1. A vulnerability process
   2. A critical period
   3. Attachment
   4. A protective process

References

Behrman, R., & Kliegman, R. (2000). *Nelson textbook of pediatrics* (16th ed.). Philadelphia: W. B. Saunders.

Berk, L. (2003). *Child development* (6th ed.). Boston: Allyn & Bacon.

Bukatko, D., & Daehler, M. (2001). *Child development: A thematic approach* (4th ed.). Boston: Houghton Mifflin.

Cavanaugh, J. C. (1993). *Adult development and aging* (2nd ed.). Pacific Grove, CA: Brooks/Cole.

Chess, S., & Thomas, A. (1986). *Temperament in clinical practice.* New York: Guilford Press.

Crain, W. (1992). *Theories of development: Concepts and applications* (3rd ed.). Englewood Cliffs, NJ: Prentice Hall.

Cynader, M., & Frost, B. (1999). Mechanisms of brain development: Neuronal sculpting by the physical and social environment. In D. Keating D & C. Hertzman (Eds.), *Developmental health and the wealth of nations: Social, biological, and educational dynamics* (pp. 153–185). New York: Guilford.

Dixon, R., & Lerner, R. (1984). A history of systems in developmental psychology. In M. Bornstein and M. Lamb (Eds.), *Developmental psychology: An advanced textbook* Hillsdale, NJ: Lawrence Erlbaum.

Drummond, J., et al. (1996–1997). Risk and resiliency in two samples of Canadian families. *Health and Canadian Society, 4*(1), 117–152.

Drummond, J., et al. (2002). The Family Adaptation Model: Examination of dimensions and relations. *Canadian Journal of Nursing Research, 34*(1), 29–46.

Edelman, C., & Mandle, C. (2002). *Health promotion throughout the lifespan.* St. Louis, MO: Mosby.

Elder, G. (1998). The life course and human development. In W. Damon (Ed.), *Handbook of child psychology* (5th ed., Vol. 1, pp. 939–1028). New York: John Wiley & Sons.

Erikson, E. (1963). *Childhood and society.* New York: Norton.

Erikson, E. (1997). *The lifecycle completed.* New York: Norton.

Gesell, A. (1948). *Studies in child development.* New York: Harper.

Gilligan, C. (1982). *In a different voice: Psychological theory and women's development.* Cambridge, MA: Harvard University Press.

Gould, R. L. (1972). The phases of adult life: A study in developmental psychology. *The American Journal of Psychiatry, 129,* 521–531.

Hartup, W. (2002). *Growing points in developmental science: An introduction.* New York: Psychology Press.

Hockenberry, M. J., et al. (2003). *Wong's nursing care of infants and children* (7th ed.). St. Louis, MO: Mosby.

Kail, R. (2002). *Advances in child development and behaviour* (Vol. 32). Burlington, MA: Elsevier.

Keating, D., & Hertzman, C. (1999). *Developmental health and the wealth of nations: Social, biological, and educational dynamics.* New York: Guilford.

Kohlberg, L. (1981). *The philosophy of moral development: Moral stages and the idea of justice.* San Francisco: Harper & Row.

Kuhn, D. (1984). Cognitive Development. In Bornstein, M.H. & Lamb, M.E (Eds.). *Developmental Psychology: An advanced textbook.* Hillsdale NJ: Lawrence Erlbaum Assoc. (pp. 133–180).

Letourneau, N., et al. (2001). Supporting parents: Can intervention improve parent-child relationships? *Journal of Family Nursing, 7*(2), 159–187.

Luthar, S. S. (1999). *Poverty and children's adjustment.* New York: Sage.

Luthar, S. S., Cocchetti, D., & Becker, B. (2000). The construct of resilience: A critical evaluation and guidelines for future work. *Child Development, 71*(3), 543–562.

Maier, H. W. (1965). *Three stories of child development.* New York: Harper & Row.

Rutter, M. (1979). Protective factors in children's responses to stress and disadvantage. In M. W. Kent & J. E. Rolf (Eds.), *Primary prevention of psychopathology* (Vol. 3, pp. 49–74). Hanover, NH: University Press of New England.

Salkind, N. (2004). *An introduction to theories of human development.* Thousand Oaks, CA: Sage.

Schroeder, B. A. (1992). *Human growth and development.* St. Paul, MN: West Publishing.

Schuster, C.S. (1992). Selected theories of developoment. In Schuster, C.S. & Ashburn, S.S. (Eds.), *The process of human development: A holistic life-span approach.* (pp. 893–896). New York: J.B. Lippincott

Singer, D. G., & Revenson, T. A. (1996). *A Piaget primer: How a child thinks.* New York: Penguin Books.

Smylie, J. (2000). A guide for health professionals working with Aboriginal Peoples: The sociocultural context of Aboriginal Peoples in Canada. *Journal SOGC, 100,* 1–12.

Smylie, J. (2001). A guide for health professionals working with Aboriginal Peoples: Health issues affecting Aboriginal Peoples. *Journal SOGC, 100,* 1–15.

Sumner, G. (1995). Keys to caregiving: A new NCAST program for health care providers and parents of newborns. *Zero to Three, 5,* 33–35.

Thomas, R. M. (1997). *Moral development theories: Secular and religious—A comparative study.* Westport, CT: Greenwood Press.

Recommended Web Sites

Canadian Institute of Child Health:
http://www.cich.ca

The Canadian Institute of Child Health (CICH) is dedicated to improving the health of children and youth in Canada. Activities range from research and policy recommendations to community development and resource building. The four key areas of activity focused on by the CIHR include supporting healthy pregnancy and childbirth, fostering healthy child development, ensuring the environment is safe for children, and monitoring the state of children's health.

Centre of Excellence for Early Childhood Development:
http://www.excellence-earlychildhood.ca/encyclopedia

The mandate of the Centre of Excellence for Early Childhood Development (CEECD) is to foster the dissemination of scientific knowledge on the social and emotional development of young children and on the policies and services that influence this development. The CEECD also formulates recommendations on the services needed to ensure optimum early childhood development. This page of the CEECD Web site lists a variety of issues and behaviours common to children under 5 years old, with links to articles on the subjects written by leading researchers in the field.

Health Canada Centre for Healthy Human Development (CHHD):
http://www.hc-sc.gc.ca/pphb-dgspsp/chhd-sdsh/index.html

The CHHD uses a life stages approach and is responsible for implementing policies and programs that enhance the conditions within which healthy development takes place. The Centre addresses the determinants of health and facilitates successful movement through the life stages. The Centre acts through programs addressing healthy child development, families, aging and lifestyles, public information, and education (Canadian Health Network), as well as issues related to rural health and support of the voluntary sector.

Nursing Child Assessment Satellite Training (NCAST):
http://www.ncast.org/

Based out of the University of Washington, this organization aims to give professionals, parents, and other caregivers the knowledge and skills to provide nurturing environments for young children. NCAST disseminates and develops research-based products and training programs for practitioners and researchers in many disciplines and settings, which can be used with typically developing children, those at risk for developmental delays, and those diagnosed with special health care needs.

19

Conception Through Adolescence

Elaine U. Polan, RNC, BSN, MS
Shirley Solberg, BN, MN, PhD (Canadian author)

Objectives

Mastery of content in this chapter will enable the student to:

- Define the key terms listed.
- Discuss physiological and psychosocial health concerns during the transition of the child from intrauterine to extrauterine life.
- Describe characteristics of physical growth of the unborn child and from birth to adolescence.
- Describe cognitive and psychosocial development from birth to adolescence.
- Describe the interactions that occur between parent and child.
- Explain the role of play in the development of the child.
- Identify factors that contribute to self-esteem in youth.
- Describe the influence of the school environment on the development of the child.
- Plan culturally appropriate health promotion activities for children of all backgrounds.
- Discuss ways in which the nurse can help parents meet their children's developmental needs.

Human growth and development are continuous, intricate, complex processes that are often divided into stages organized by age groups. This arbitrary, chronological division is used because it coincides with the timing and sequence of maturational changes that allows the child to progress through a series of developmental stages and associated tasks (Box 19-1). Major developmental theories can be found in chapter 18. This chapter focuses on the various physical, psychosocial, and cognitive changes. It also focuses on health risks and concerns during the various stages of growth and development.

Selecting a Developmental Framework for Nursing

Providing developmentally appropriate nursing care is easier when planning is based on a theoretical framework (see chapter 18). An organized, systematic approach ensures that the child's needs are assessed and met by the care plan. If nursing care is delivered only as a series of isolated actions, some of the child's developmental needs may be overlooked. A developmental approach encourages organized care directed at the child's current level of functioning to motivate self-direction and health promotion. For example, nurses might instruct parents to encourage toddlers to feed themselves to advance their developing independence and thus promote their sense of autonomy. Understanding an adolescent's need to be independent should prompt the nurse to negotiate with the adolescent to establish a contract about the care plan and its implementation.

Box 19-1 Developmental Age Periods

Prenatal Period: Conception to Birth

Germinal: Conception to approximately 2 weeks
Embryonic: 2 to 8 weeks
Fetal: 8 to 40 weeks (birth)

A rapid growth rate and total dependency make this one of the most crucial periods in the developmental process. The relationship between maternal health and certain manifestations in the newborn emphasizes the importance of adequate prenatal care to the health and well-being of the infant.

Infancy Period: Birth to 12 or 18 Months

Neonatal: Birth to 28 days
Infancy: 1 to approximately 12 months

The infancy period is one of rapid motor, cognitive, and social development. Through bonding with the caregiver (parent), the infant establishes a basic trust in the world and the foundation for future interpersonal relationships. The critical first month of life, termed the neonatal period, although part of infancy, is often differentiated from the remainder because of the major physical adjustments to extrauterine existence and the psychosocial adjustment of the parents to their new roles.

Early Childhood: 1 to 6 Years

Toddler: 1 to 3 years
Preschooler: 3 to 6 years

This period, which extends from the time the child begins walking until school entry, is characterized by intense activity and discovery. It is a time of marked physical and psychosocial development. Motor development advances steadily. Children at this age acquire language and wider social relationships, learn role standards, gain self-control and mastery, develop increasing awareness of dependence and independence, and begin to develop a self-concept.

Middle Childhood: 6 to 12 Years

Frequently referred to as the *school age,* this period of development is one in which the child expands relationships outside the family group and activities are centred around peer relationships. There is steady advancement in physical, cognitive, and psychosocial development with emphasis on developing skill competencies. Social co-operation and early moral development take on more importance with relevance for later life stages. This is a critical period in the development of a self-concept.

Adolescence: 12 to approximately 19

The period of rapid maturation and change known as adolescence is considered to be a transitional period that begins at the onset of puberty and extends to the point of entry into the adult world—usually high school graduation. Biologic and psychological maturation are accompanied by physical and emotional turmoil, and there is redefining of the self-concept. In the late adolescent period, the child begins to internalize all previously learned values and to focus on an individual, rather than a group, identity.

Adapted from *Wong's Nursing Care of Infants and Children* (7th ed.), by M. J. Hockenberry et al., 2003, St. Louis, MO: Mosby.

Conception

From the moment of conception, human growth proceeds at a predictable and rapid rate. During gestation or the prenatal period, the embryo grows from a single cell to a complex, physiological being. All major organ systems develop in utero, with most functioning before birth.

Intrauterine Life

Intrauterine life that reaches full term usually lasts approximately 9 calendar months, or 40 weeks. The length of pregnancy is computed using **Nagele's rule,** which counts back 3 months from the first day of the last menstrual period and then adds 7 days. **Fertilization** occurs when a sperm penetrates the ovum and the material from both cell nuclei unites. The newly formed organism, known as a **zygote,** has its full genetic complement (1 pair of sex chromosomes and 22 pairs of autosomal chromosomes). The ovum and the sperm each contribute one chromosome to each pair. It is through this mechanism that genetically programmed conditions (such as Down syndrome) and genetically determined characteristics (such as eye colour) are transmitted from parent to child.

The zygote moves through the fallopian tube to the uterus within 3 to 4 days. During this time, the zygote continues to divide. Within 3 days, a solid ball of cells, the **morula,** has formed. The morula continues to develop and forms a central cavity, or **blastocyst.** Even at this early stage of development, cells begin to differentiate in structure and function. Cells at one end of the blastocyst develop into the **embryo,** and those at the opposite end form the **placenta.** Between days 6 and 10, enzymes are secreted that allow the blastocyst to burrow into the endometrium and become completely covered, a process known as **implantation.** Chorionic villi, fingerlike projections that emerge from the outer sac surrounding the embryo, obtain oxygen and nutrition from the maternal blood supply and dispose of carbon dioxide and waste products.

The placenta produces essential hormones that maintain the pregnancy. Because the placenta is porous, noxious materials such as viruses and drugs can pass from mother to child. The effect of noxious agents on the unborn child depends on the developmental stage in which exposure takes place, with the embryonic stage (2 to 8 weeks after conception) being the most crucial because the organ systems and the main external features are developing. The period of gestation is divided equally into three periods called trimesters.

First Trimester. During the first trimester, the first 3 calendar months, fetal cells continue to differentiate and develop into essential organ systems. As cellular change (differentiation) and rapid organ growth **(organogenesis)** occur, each organ is vulnerable to conditions in the environment. Interference with growth can cause the congenital absence of an organ system or extensive structural or functional alterations. Because several organ systems develop at the same time, disruption of one system often occurs with disruption of others. Toward the end of the first trimester, it is possible to detect fetal heart tones by fetoscope or ultrasound.

Second Trimester. During the second trimester, the end of month 3 through month 6, the height of the uterus above the symphysis pubis is an indicator of fetal growth and approximate gestational age. Between 16 and 20 weeks, the mother begins to feel fetal movement. This feeling of life is referred to as **quickening.**

By the end of the sixth month, most organ systems are complete and can function. The **fetus** is therefore considered viable, or capable of life outside the uterus, if given intensive environmental support. Fingers and toes are differentiated, rudimentary kidneys function, and the sex of the fetus can be determined. The fetus is covered with **vernix caseosa,** a cheese-like substance coating the skin. **Lanugo,** or fine hair, covers most of the body. These substances protect the thin, fragile skin and decrease in amount as the pregnancy nears its completion; thus infants born before 38 weeks' gestation have more of these protective coverings than do full-term infants.

Third Trimester. During the last 3 months of intrauterine life, the fetus grows to approximately 50 cm in length. Subcutaneous fat is stored, and weight increases to between 3.2 and 3.4 kg. The skin thickens, lanugo begins to disappear, and the fetal body becomes rounder and fuller.

A tremendous spurt in brain growth begins during this trimester and lasts well into the first few years of life. The central nervous system has established its total number of neurons and connections between neurons, and myelination of nerve fibres progresses at a rapid rate.

At the end of the third trimester, the normal fetus is physically able to make the transition from intrauterine to extrauterine life. The cardiac system can change its circulation to end bypassing of the lungs. The lungs are capable of maintaining the inflated state for gas exchange. The primitive temperature maintenance systems, reflexes, and sensory organs are ready for use.

Health Promotion. There are many topics that nurses can address with pregnant clients in order to protect the health of the fetus and mother. Topics may vary depending on the stage of pregnancy. For example, during the first trimester of pregnancy, women should be educated about nutrition and exposure to **teratogens,** two factors known to affect prenatal development. During the second trimester, the nurse can help the client plan for the impending birth. This is often a good time for education about gestational rest, nutrition, dental care, physical activity, and infant feeding options. It is also a good time to discuss the risks of **preterm labour** and actions that can be taken to prevent it. During the third trimester, parents often seek information regarding the childbirth process and birth-setting options. Box 19-2 lists some of the many topics that nurses can address with pregnant women and their partners. Nurses can make a significant difference in supporting the functions of young families. Following an assessment of the couple's strengths and weaknesses, nurses can direct parents to available services to enhance their coping skills (Knauth, 2001).

Transition From Intrauterine to Extrauterine Life

The transition from intrauterine to extrauterine life requires rapid changes in the newborn. The nurse assesses the newborn's ability to make these changes and plans for appropriate nursing interventions (Askin, 2002). Circulatory, pulmonary, and thermal changes all contribute to the infant's adaptation to neonatal life. Gestational age and development, exposure to depressant drugs before or during labour, and the newborn's own behavioural style also influence the adjustment to the external environment. Therefore, initial assessment encompasses a variety of physical and psychosocial elements. The nurse also provides early opportunities for the parents and infant to develop close emotional bonds.

Physical Changes

An immediate assessment of the newborn's condition is performed to determine the physiological functioning of the major organ systems. The most extreme physiological change occurs when the newborn leaves the in utero circulation and develops independent respiratory functioning. Nursing care is directed at maintaining an open airway, stabilizing and maintaining body temperature, and protecting the newborn from infection. The most widely used assessment tool is the **Apgar score.** Heart rate, respiratory effort, muscle tone, reflex irritability, and colour are rated to determine overall status. The Apgar assessment is generally conducted at 1 and 5 minutes after birth and may be repeated until the newborn's condition stabilizes. Table 19-1 outlines the scoring criteria of physiological functioning. A total score of 0 to 3 signifies severe distress, a score of 4 to 6 represents moderate difficulty, and a score of 7 to 10 indicates little difficulty in adjusting to extrauterine life. The nurse can use the Apgar score to determine areas requiring further assessment and careful observation. In addition, the nurse monitors and records the newborn's early elimination patterns (i.e., voiding and passage of meconium) as well as body temperature and other vital signs.

Psychosocial Changes

After conducting a physical evaluation and applying identification bracelets, the nurse promotes the parents' and newborn's need for close physical contact. Early parent-child interaction encourages parent-child attachment. Physical factors (e.g., fatigue, hunger, and health) and emotional factors (e.g., needs for affection and touch) are assessed.

Focus on Primary Health Care

Box 19-2

Health Promotion Topics for the Pregnant Client

First Trimester Health Concerns

Nutrition. Mothers who eat well have fewer complications of pregnancy and childbirth and bear healthier babies than those with poor nutritional intake (Hilton, 2002; Kail, 2001). Inadequate prenatal nutrition has been associated with lower birth weight (Behrman, Kliegman, & Jenson, 2000), and low-birth-weight infants have an increased risk for learning disorders, temperament problems, neurological and motor impairment, and developmental delays. The importance of adequate folic acid intake before and during pregnancy should be stressed (Box 19-3). Folic acid intake is believed to be responsible for decreasing the incidence of neural tube defects (Hilton, 2002). See chapter 39 for a description of the nutritional needs of the pregnant woman.

Teratogens. Agents capable of producing functional or structural damage to the developing fetus are called teratogens. The nurse educates the mother about avoiding exposure to teratogenic agents. One such teratogen is the rubella virus, which can cause stillbirth or congenital anomalies, primarily when exposure is in the first trimester. Many drugs are teratogenic during the first trimester. Past and present use of home remedies, medications (prescription and over-the-counter), and illegal drugs must be carefully assessed. Benefits of any drug needed to maintain the mother's health must be weighed against potential harm to the fetus.

Cigarette smoke and alcohol are also teratogens. Smoking during pregnancy has been shown to reduce birth weight and increase the incidence of premature birth and fetal and neonatal death (Kail, 2001; Pletsch & Morgan, 2002). It is also considered a risk factor for impaired growth and development among young children (Health Canada, 1999a). Alcohol consumed during pregnancy is known to cause fetal alcohol syndrome, fetal alcohol effect, and alcohol-related birth defects (Kail, 2001). Pregnant women must be educated about the risks of cigarette smoke and alcohol on the unborn.

Second Trimester Health Concerns

Preterm Labour. Preterm labour is labour that begins before the 37th week of pregnancy. With technological advances, it is possible for 500-g babies of 24 to 26 weeks' gestation to survive; however, there may be significant risk of morbidity and disability. Causes of preterm labour are poorly understood and may be the result of maternal or fetal problems. Maternal risk factors include physiological stresses such as renal and cardiovascular disease, diabetes mellitus, or uterine and cervical abnormalities. Urinary tract infections greatly increase the risk of preterm labour. Because of dramatic changes occurring in the renal system, it is possible for a mother to have an asymptomatic urinary tract infection. Voiding habits should be discussed with the mother during this time. Research has also demonstrated an increased risk for preterm labour among mothers living in poverty, smokers, and mothers receiving poor prenatal care (Berk, 2003). Multiple pregnancies and fetal infections are two of the potential fetal factors for preterm labour. Interventions to prevent preterm labour can include medications, intravenous fluids, and bed rest.

Third Trimester Health Concerns

Birth-setting choices. Hospitals have been the traditional setting for childbirth for the past 60 years because emergency backup is available in case of birth complications. Many hospitals have taken a family-centred approach to childbirth.

In some areas of the country, birthing centres are available for those who prefer a more home-like setting. Women delivering in this setting are required to attend childbirth classes, and the pregnancy must be considered low risk. Physicians and midwives with hospital privileges may attend births in these facilities. Mothers must understand that there is always a possibility of transfer to a hospital if the conditions warrant.

A growing number of mothers choose to deliver at home when professional midwifery services are available. Control over the birth process and the desire for a more natural birth are common reasons why some mothers choose home births. Another reason is so that the entire family or other people close to the family can be part of the birth. Nurses can support the mother by offering information and resources to help her choose the birth setting.

Client Teaching

Box 19-3

Folic Acid for Women Contemplating Pregnancy

Objective

- Client will consume 0.4 mg of folic acid (vitamin B_9) every day.

Teaching Strategies

- Educate females of child-bearing age about the benefits of folic acid to a developing fetus.
- Discuss the need for women to have an adequate daily intake of folic acid before pregnancy because the moment of conception is not always known. Folic acid is a water-soluble vitamin and is readily excreted in the urine.
- Encourage consumption of 0.4 mg of folic acid daily. This amount may be consumed in food sources; however, adolescents are usually deficient. Deficiency is not related to socio-economic status.
- Discuss foods rich in folic acid, such as green leafy vegetables, liver, kidney, and asparagus. Limited amounts may be found in milk, poultry, and eggs.
- Assist clients in developing menus with folic acid-rich foods. Teach women to read the labels of breakfast cereals to determine if they are fortified with folic acid.
- Encourage clients to take a daily prenatal multivitamin to supplement dietary intake.

Evaluation

- Have client identify dietary sources of folic acid.
- Review client's 3-day diet intake diary.

Table 19-1 Apgar Scoring

Sign	Score 0	Score 1	Score 2
Heart rate	Absent	Slow (below 100)	Over 100
Respiratory effort	Absent	Slow, irregular, hypoventilation	Good, crying lustily
Muscle tone	Flaccid	Some flexion of extremities	Active motion, well flexed
Reflex irritability	No response	Crying, some motion	Vigorous cry
Colour	Blue, pale	Pink body, blue hands and feet	Completely pink

Adapted from *Wong's Nursing Care of Infants and Children* (7th ed.), by M. J. Hockenberry et al., 2003, St. Louis, MO: Mosby.

Merely placing the family together does not promote closeness. The parents and newborn must be willing and able to respond to each other. Most healthy newborns are awake and alert for the first half-hour after birth. This is a good time for parent-child interaction to begin. Close body contact, often including skin-to-skin contact and breast-feeding, is a satisfying way for most families to start. If immediate contact is not possible, the nurse incorporates it into the care plan as early as possible, which may mean bringing the newborn to an ill parent or bringing the parents to an ill or premature child.

Bonding occurs when parents and newborn elicit reciprocal and complementary behaviour. Parental bonding behaviours include attentiveness and physical contact. Newborn bonding behaviour involves maintenance of contact with the parent. Preterm newborns, ill newborns, and ill mothers may have difficulty forming this bond if separation is prolonged; they need to be carefully assessed for any problems with attachment. The bonding process is further complicated if parents are unable to care for the infant. The nurse should give the parents support throughout the early bonding process, particularly if the newborn or mother is ill or if the newborn is separated from the parents.

Health Risks

The removal of nasopharyngeal and oropharyngeal secretions with suction or a bulb syringe ensures airway patency. Newborns are susceptible to heat loss and cold stress (Askin, 2002). Because hypothermia increases oxygen needs, the newborn's body temperature must be stabilized and maintained. The newborn may be placed directly on the mother's abdomen and covered in warm blankets; dried and wrapped in warm blankets, with the head well covered; or placed unclothed in an infant warmer with a temperature probe in place. For newborns unable to sustain adequate body temperature, isolettes and incubators, which supply radiant heat, are preferred. Box 19-4 outlines measures to prevent cold stress.

Prevention of infection is a major concern in the care of the newborn, whose immune system is immature. Good hand-washing technique is the most important factor in protecting the newborn and nurse from infection. Cover gowns do not need to be worn while providing care for the healthy newborn once the blood and amniotic fluid have been removed from the infant's skin (Hockenberry et al., 2003). Other precautions include wearing gloves when touching mucous membranes or non-intact skin (e.g., caused by surgery or injury) and when drawing blood (e.g., heel stick; Garner, 1996).

Box 19-4 Measures to Prevent Cold Stress

Mechanism of Heat Loss	Nursing Intervention
Evaporation	Immediately dry newborn after delivery. Wrap in blanket. Delay first bath until temperature and other vital signs are stable.
Conduction	Warm objects that have direct contact with newborn. Cover newborn's head.
Convection	Prevent unnecessary exposure to cold.
Radiation	Use radiant warmer until temperature stabilizes. Avoid cold drafts.

The most commonly used prophylactic treatment against ophthalmic conjunctivitis is erythromycin (0.5%) because it prevents *Neisseria gonorrhoeae* and other infections, which can be transmitted during passage through an infected vaginal canal. Application should occur during the newborn's initial assessment.

Vitamin K is administered as a single intramuscular injection shortly after birth. Vitamin K is important for the synthesis of prothrombin necessary for clotting. Normally, the intestinal flora synthesizes vitamin K, and by about the third day the infant should have enough intestinal flora to start to synthesize its vitamin K.

The stump of the moist umbilical cord is an excellent medium for bacterial growth. The cord should be cleansed with soap and water and dried at each diaper change. Until the cord dries and falls off, the diaper should be folded below the umbilicus to prevent accumulation of moisture.

Newborn

The **neonatal period** is the first month of life. During this stage, the newborn's physical functioning is mostly reflexive, and stabilization of major organ systems is the body's primary task. Behaviour greatly influences interaction between the newborn and the environment and caregivers. For example, the average 2-week-old newborn smiles spontaneously and is able to regard the mother's face. The impact of these reflexive behaviours is generally a surge of feelings of love that prompt the mother to cuddle the baby.

Nurses can apply their knowledge of this stage of growth and development to promote newborn and parental health. If the nurse understands, for example, that the newborn's cry is usually a response to an unmet need (such as hunger), parents can be assisted in identifying ways to meet those needs, such as counselling the parents to feed their baby on demand rather than on a rigid schedule.

Physical Changes

A comprehensive nursing assessment is usually performed as soon as the newborn's physiological functioning is stable, generally within a few hours after birth. The nurse measures height, weight, head circumference, temperature, pulse, and respirations and observes general appearance, body functions, sensory capabilities, reflexes, and responsiveness.

The average newborn weighs 3,400 g, is 50 cm in length, and has a head circumference of 35 cm. Up to 10% of birth weight is lost in the first few days of life, primarily through fluid losses by respiration, urination, defecation, and low fluid intake. Birth weight is usually regained by the second week of life, and a gradual pattern of increase in weight, height, and head circumference is evident. During the first month, these increases average 226 to 455 g in weight per week, 0.6 to 2.5 cm in length, and 2 cm in head circumference.

The newborn's heart rate ranges from 120 to 160 beats per minute. The average blood pressure is 85/54 mm Hg. The newborn's respiratory movements are primarily abdominal and vary in rate and rhythm, with an average rate of 30 to 60 breaths per minute. The axillary temperature ranges from 36° to 37.5° C and generally stabilizes within 24 hours after birth.

Normal physical characteristics include the continued presence of lanugo on the skin of the back; cyanosis of the hands and feet for the first 24 hours; and a soft, protuberant abdomen. Skin colour varies according to racial and genetic heritage and gradually changes during infancy. **Molding,** or overlapping of the soft skull bones, allows the fetal head to adjust to various diameters of the maternal pelvis and is a common occurrence with vaginal births. The bones readjust within a few days, producing a rounded appearance. The sutures and **fontanels** are usually palpable at birth. The diamond shape of the anterior fontanel and the triangular shape of the posterior fontanel between the unfused bones of the skull are shown in Figure 19–1.

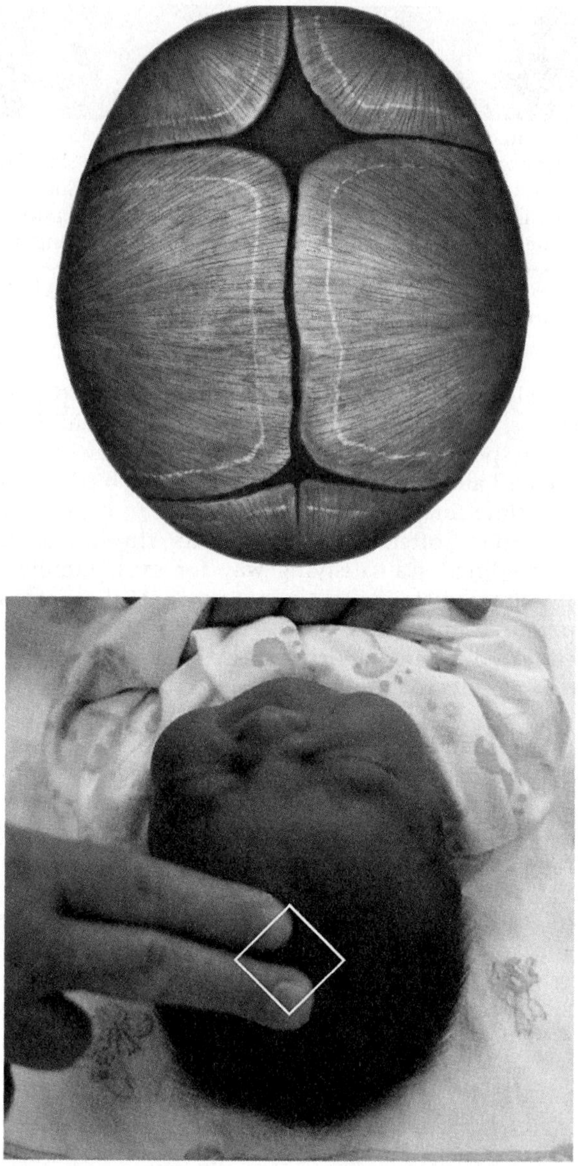

FIGURE **19–1** Fontanels and suture lines. (From *Wong's Nursing Care of Infants and Children* (7th ed.), by M. J. Hockenberry et al., 2003, St. Louis, MO: Mosby.)

Neurological function is assessed by observing the newborn's level of activity, alertness, irritability, responsiveness to stimuli, and reflexes. Normal reflexes include sucking, rooting, grasping, yawning, coughing, sneezing, hiccoughing, blinking in response to bright lights, and startling (pulling arms and legs inward) in response to sudden, loud noises. An absence of any of these or other reflexes indicates **prematurity,** possible trauma, or central nervous system complications. Assessment of these reflexes is vital because the newborn depends largely on reflexes for survival and in response to its environment. Figure 19–2 shows the tonic neck reflex: When newborns are lying supine, they reflexively turn the head to one side, extend the arm on the side to which the head is turned, and flex the other arm.

Normal newborn behaviours include periods of sucking, crying, sleeping, and wakefulness. Movements are generally sporadic, but they are symmetrical and involve all four extremities. The relatively flexed fetal position of intrauterine life continues as the newborn attempts to maintain an enclosed, secure feeling. Newborns respond to sensory stimuli, particularly the primary caregiver's face, voice, and touch.

Except for the first hour after birth, when they are in a quietly alert state, newborns sleep almost continuously for first 2 to 3 days to recover from the exhausting birth process. Thereafter, sleep periods vary from 20 minutes to 6 hours with little day-night differentiation.

Cognitive Changes

Early cognitive development begins with innate behaviour, reflexes, and sensory functions. Newborns initiate reflex activities, learn behaviours, and learn their desires. For example, newborns reflexively turn to the nipple

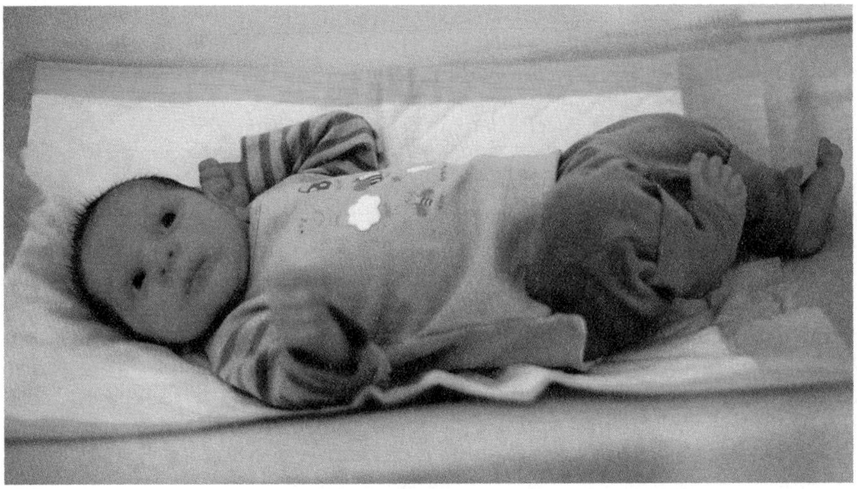

FIGURE **19–2** Tonic neck reflex. Newborns assume this position while supine. (Courtesy Elaine Polan, RNC, BSN, MS.)

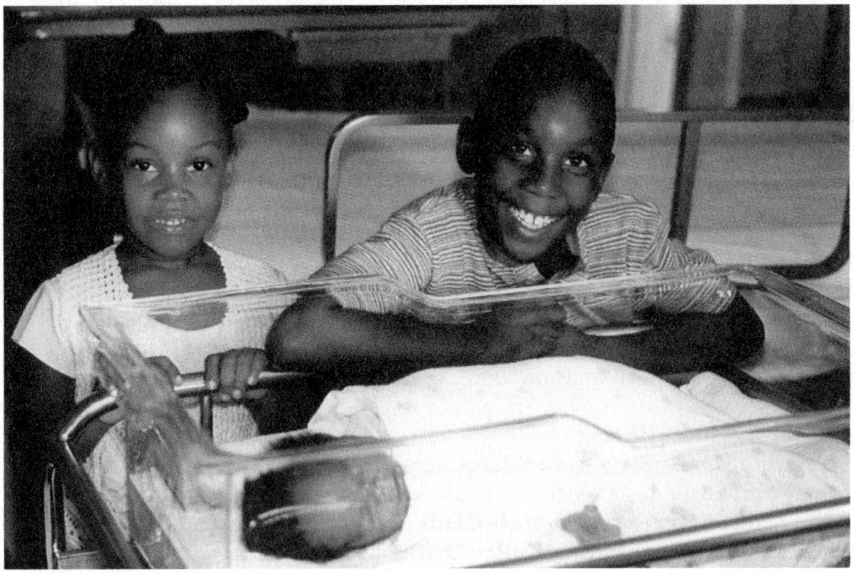

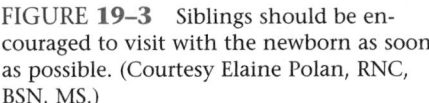

FIGURE **19–3** Siblings should be encouraged to visit with the newborn as soon as possible. (Courtesy Elaine Polan, RNC, BSN, MS.)

(rooting) and learn that crying results in parent response of feeding, diapering, and cuddling.

Sensory functions contribute to cognitive development in the newborn. At birth, children can focus on objects about 3 to 4 cm from their faces and can perceive forms. A preference for the human face is apparent. Auditory and vestibular (i.e., equilibrium) systems function from birth. These sensory capabilities allow newborns to elicit stimuli rather than simply receive them. Parents should be taught the importance of providing sensory stimulation, such as talking to their newborns and holding them to see their faces. This allows infants to seek or take in stimuli, thereby enhancing learning and promoting cognitive development.

Psychosocial Changes

During the first month of life, parents and newborns normally develop a strong bond that grows into a deep attachment. Interactions during routine care enhance or detract from the attachment process. The processes of feeding, changing, bathing, and comforting an infant promote interaction and provide a foundation for deep attachments. Early on, older siblings should have the opportunity to be involved with the newborn. Family involvement helps support growth and development and promotes nurturing (Figure 19–3).

If parents or newborns experience health complications after birth, bonding may be compromised. Infants' behavioural cues may be weak or absent, and caregiving may be less mutually satisfying. Tired, ill parents have difficulty interpreting and responding to their infants. Children who have congenital anomalies are often too weak to be responsive to parental cues and require special supportive nursing care. For example, infants born with heart defects may tire easily during feedings. They may rest frequently after several bursts of sucking. They may awaken frequently, crying because they are hungry again. Mothers may think that the infants are being fussy or that they are inadequate as mothers. Both infants and mothers may feel frustrated. In this case, bonding is not enhanced and may even be reduced unless nursing intervention breaks the sequence of events.

Research on the frequency of crying in infants shows that although there is individual variation, the newborn cries more just after birth and again 4 to 6 weeks after birth than at other times (Barr, Hopkins, & Green, 2000). Rather than being a sign of distress in infants, crying may be an adaptive response to extrauterine life. For newborns, crying is a means of communication to provide cues to parents. Babies may cry because their diapers are wet, they are hungry, they want to be held, or they need a change in position or activity. Their crying may frustrate the parents if they cannot see an apparent cause. With the nurse's help, parents can learn to recognize infants' cry patterns and take appropriate action when necessary.

Health Risks

Hyperbilirubinemia refers to an excessive amount of accumulated bilirubin in the blood and is characterized by a yellow colouring of the skin, or jaundice. The accumulation occurs when the infant's body is unable to balance the destruction of red blood cells and the use or excretion of by-products. The balance can be upset by prematurity, inadequate intake during breast-feeding, excess production of bilirubin, certain disease states, or a disturbance in the liver. Bilirubin at high levels is highly toxic to neurons and places newborns at risk for brain injury. Phototherapy is used to help break down the bilirubin for easier excretion. During phototherapy, the infant's eyes must be shielded to protect them from exposure to the light. Because excretion of the extra bilirubin can cause watery stools, adequate fluid balance in the infant must be maintained.

Health Concerns

Screening. The nurse coordinates screening tests and other laboratory tests as needed. Blood tests can determine **inborn errors of metabolism** (IEMs). This term applies to genetic disorders caused by the absence or deficiency of a substance, usually an enzyme, essential to cellular metabolism that results in abnormal protein, carbohydrate, or fat metabolism. Although IEMs are rare, they account for a significant proportion of health problems in children. Neonatal screening can detect phenylketonuria (PKU), hypothyroidism, and galactosemia and thus allow appropriate treatment that can prevent permanent intellectual disability and other health problems. Routine screening of newborns for PKU is recommended (Feldman, 1994). Other screening may be necessary depending on the family history (e.g., cystic fibrosis or hemophilia).

Circumcision. Circumcision is controversial in this country and is not recommended as a routine procedure by the Canadian Paediatric Society (1996). The controversy surrounds the risks and benefits, especially with respect to pain control. Risks have been identified as hemorrhage, infection, adhesions, and meatal stenosis. Benefits include prevention of penile cancer and urinary tract infections, and preservation of male body image to be consistent with peers (Hockenberry et al., 2003). Parents must give informed consent before the procedure. Care of the site depends on the type of method used for the procedure. The newborn should be checked frequently for evidence of swelling or oozing and the ability to void.

Infant

Infancy, the period from 1 month to 1 year of age, is characterized by dramatic physical growth and change. Psychosocial development advances and interaction between infants and the environment is greater and more meaningful. Infants who giggle and roll over in response to tickling are interacting more with their social environments and are displaying a greater response than when they merely smile in response to a hug.

Physical Changes

Steady and proportional growth of the infant is more important than absolute growth values. The infant's growth can be compared with charts of normal age- and gender-related growth measurements. Using growth charts, the nurse can also evaluate an infant's growth patterns by recording weight, length, and head circumference at selected intervals. Measurements recorded over time are the best way to monitor growth and identify problems. An infant with a growth problem may be generally below the expected norms at all intervals or may experience an acute, brief interference with growth. An infant with a feeding problem or a genetic condition such as cystic fibrosis may be below the expected norm for weight.

Size increases rapidly during the first year; birth weight doubles in approximately 5 months and triples by 12 months. An average weight gain is 680 g during the first 5 months and 340 g for months 7 to 12. Height increases an average of 2.5 cm during each of the first 6 months and 3.8 cm for the next 6 months. This 50% increase in birth height occurs primarily in the trunk, with the chest diameter approximating that of the head by the first birthday (Hockenberry et al., 2003). The fontanels become smaller: the posterior fontanel closes at about 2 months and the anterior at about 12 to 18 months.

Physiological functioning stabilizes, and by the end of the first year the heart rate is 90 to 140 beats per minute, the blood pressure averages 95/65 mm Hg, and the respiratory rate is 30 to 35 breaths per minute. Patterns of body function also stabilize, as evidenced by predictable sleep, elimination, and feeding routines. Motor development proceeds steadily in a cephalocaudal (from the head toward the feet) direction. Table 19-2 identifies milestones in motor development.

Cognitive Changes

The infant learns by experiencing and manipulating the environment. Developing motor skills and increasing mobility expand an infant's environment and, with developing visual and auditory skills, enhance cognitive development. For these reasons, Piaget (1952) named his first stage of cognitive development, which extends until around the third birthday, the sensorimotor period (see chapter 18). Before the acquisition of language, the extraordinary development of the mind occurs through the

Table 19-2 Milestones in Infant Motor Development

Month 3	Month 6	Month 9	Month 12	Month 15
Gross Motor				
Lifts head 90 degrees when prone Sits with support	Sits without support Crawls on abdomen with arms	Attains sitting position independently Pulls self to standing position	Walks holding onto walls and furniture (cruising) Stands alone Takes 1 to 2 steps	Walks alone
Fine Motor				
Grasps and briefly holds objects and takes them to mouth	Uses palm grasp with fingers encircling object Transfers cube from hand to hand	Crude thumb-finger pincer grasp Bangs hand-held cubes together	Places tiny object, such as raisin, into container Makes marks with crayon	Scribbles with crayon Builds tower of two cubes

Adapted from "The Denver II: A Major Revision and Restandardization of the Denver Developmental Screening Test," by W. K. Frankenburg et al., 1992, *Pediatrics, 89*(1), p. 93.

child's developing senses and motor abilities. For example, a 1-month-old infant can follow the path of a moving object. Improved visual acuity and eye-hand coordination allow grasping and exploration of objects. In addition, rudimentary colour vision begins by 2 months and improves throughout the first year, making the environment more interesting to see and explore. The infant's hearing also improves, allowing localization and discrimination of sounds.

Infants need opportunities to develop and use their senses. Nurses must evaluate the appropriateness and adequacy of these opportunities. For example, ill or hospitalized infants may lack the energy to interact with their environments, thereby slowing their cognitive development. Infants need to be stimulated according to their temperament, energy, and age. The nurse uses stimulation strategies that maximize the development of infants while conserving their energy and orientation. An example of this approach is the nurse talking to and encouraging an infant to suck on a pacifier while administering the infant's tube feeding.

Language. Speech is an important aspect of cognition that develops during the first year. Infants proceed from crying, cooing, and laughing to imitating sounds, comprehending the meaning of simple commands, and repeating words with knowledge of their meaning. By 1 year, infants recognize their own names and have two- or three-word vocabularies, usually including *Da-Da, Ma-Ma,* and *no.* The nurse can promote language development by encouraging mothers to name objects on which their infants' attention is focused.

Psychosocial Changes

Separation. During their first year, infants begin to differentiate themselves from others as separate beings capable of acting on their own. Initially, infants are unaware of the boundaries of self, but through repeated experiences with the environment, they learn where the self ends and the external world begins. As infants determine their physical boundaries, they begin to respond to others.

Two- and 3-month-old infants begin to smile responsively rather than reflexively. Similarly, they can recognize differences in people when their sensory and cognitive capabilities improve. By 8 months, most infants can differentiate a stranger from a familiar person and respond differently to the two. Close attachment to the primary caregivers, most often parents, is usually established by this age. Infants seek out these people for support and comfort during times of stress. The ability to distinguish self from others allows infants to interact and socialize within their environments. By 9 months, for example, infants play simple social games such as patty-cake and peekaboo. More complex interactive games such as hide-and-seek involving objects are possible by the age of 1 year. Erikson (1963) described the psychosocial developmental crisis for the infant as trust versus mistrust. If the infant's physical and emotional needs are met, then the infant begins to develop a sense of security (see chapter 18).

The nurse assesses the availability and appropriateness of experiences contributing to psychosocial development. Hospitalized infants may have difficulty establishing physical boundaries because of repeated bodily intrusions and painful sensations. Limiting these negative experiences and providing pleasurable sensations are interventions that support early psychosocial development. Extended separations from parents complicate the bonding process and increase the number of caregivers with whom the infant must interact. Ideally, the parents should provide the majority of care during hospitalization. When parents are not present, an attempt should be made to limit the number of caregivers who have contact with the infant and to follow the parents' directions for care. These interventions will foster the infant's continuing development of trust.

Play. Play is a meaningful set of activities through which individuals interact with their environment and relate to others. Play provides opportunities for the infant to develop many motor skills. Much of infant play is exploratory as they use their senses to observe and examine their own bodies and objects of interest in their surroundings. For example, placing their toes in their mouths provides infants with pleasure and information about their own body and helps form their early self-concept. Play becomes manipulative as the child learns control of the hands. Adults can facilitate infant learning by planning activities that promote the development of milestones and by providing toys that are safe for the infant to explore with the mouth and manipulate with the hands, such as rattles, blocks, stacking rings, and stuffed animals. Infants most frequently engage in solitary (one-sided) play but do enjoy watching others, particularly siblings. Infants need to be played with and stimulated through interactions with others.

Health Risks

Sudden Infant Death Syndrome. Sudden Infant Death Syndrome (SIDS) is the sudden and unexpected death of an apparently healthy infant. SIDS is rare before 1 month of age, and peaks between 2 and 4 months of age. However, it can occur in infants up to a year old. Three babies die of SIDS every week in Canada (Canadian Foundation for the Study of Infant Deaths, 2004). The cause of SIDS is not understood, but Health Canada (1999b) recommends the following precautions:

- Infants should sleep on their back on a firm, flat surface.
- Provide a smoke-free environment before and after birth.
- Keep a baby's crib free of such clutter as pillows, pillow-like items, comforters, or duvets.
- Dress and cover the infant lightly to avoid overheating.
- Mothers should breast-feed if possible.

Accidental Injury. Injury is a major cause of death in children 6 to 12 months old. An understanding of the major developmental accomplishments during this time period will allow for injury prevention planning. Box 19-5 lists the main types of injuries occurring in this age group and possible prevention strategies.

Child Abuse. Nurses need to be aware that child abuse can occur during any stage of a child's life, beginning in infancy. Child abuse refers to violence, emotional or sexual mistreatment, or neglect of a child or adolescent. More children suffer from neglect than any other type of abuse. Many suffer from more than one type of abuse. The *Canadian Incidence Study of Reported Abuse and Neglect* (Trocmé et al., 2001) confirmed there were four cases of neglect, two cases of physical abuse, two cases of emotional maltreatment, and one case of sexual abuse for every 1,000 children in Canada. Protection of children from abuse comes under the jurisdiction of a province or territory. All provinces and territories include a mandatory reporting law for health professionals to report suspected abuse. Box 19-6 includes possible signs and symptoms of child abuse. These indications are relevant for children from infancy through adolescence.

A combination of signs and symptoms or a pattern of injury should arouse suspicion. It is important for the health care provider to be aware of certain disease processes (e.g., mongolian spots, which are flat, dark birthmarks that may look like bruises) and cultural practices (e.g., coining, in which the skin is rubbed or scratched with a coin to improve circulation or restore balance) that may mimic signs of abuse.

Health Concerns

Nutrition. The quality and quantity of nutrition influence the infant's growth and development. The nurse helps parents select a nutritionally adequate diet for their infant. The nurse must understand that nutrition is influenced by many variables (e.g., culture, food preferences, slow eating, or food allergies) and that no diet is effective for all children or for one age group.

Feeding Alternatives. Supplying essential nutrients to the infant is both the nurse's and parents' goal. The nurse should support the parents' choice of feeding methods and facilitate a successful feeding process (Gill, 2001). Breast-feeding is considered the most complete nutritional source until 6 months of age. Breast milk contains protein, fats, carbohydrates, and immunoglobulins that bolster the infant's ability to resist infection (Box 19-7). Breast-feeding has been associated with a decreased frequency of gastroenteritis, otitis media, and food allergies (Behrman et al., 2000; Health Canada, 1998; Hockenberry et al., 2003).

If breast-feeding is not possible or not desired by the parent, an acceptable alternative is iron-fortified commercially prepared formula. Formulas are convenient, contain standard ingredients, and are fortified with vitamins and minerals. Cow's milk and imitation milks are not recommended in the first year because infants are not able to properly digest the contained fat. Cow's milk also contains more sodium and protein and less iron than formula (Hockenberry et al., 2003). Because cow's milk is low in iron and high in calcium and phosphorus, absorption of iron may be decreased, causing anemia.

The average 1-month-old infant takes approximately 540 to 630 mL of breast milk or formula per day. This amount increases slightly during the first 6 months and decreases when solid foods are introduced. The amount of formula per feeding and the number of feedings vary among infants.

Developmentally, infants are not ready for solid food until 6 months of age. Before 6 months, the infant's gastrointestinal tract cannot handle the complex nutrients in solid food, and the extrusion reflex causes food to be pushed out of the mouth. Also, early introduction to solid foods may cause allergies.

Cereals and well-cooked and pureed fruits, vegetables, and meats eaten during the second 6 months of life provide iron and additional sources of vitamins. These nutrients become especially important when infants are taken off breast milk or formula and begun on whole cow's milk after the first birthday. Because the amount and frequency of feedings vary among infants, the nurse should discuss differing feeding patterns with parents.

Honey has been used to sweeten water and coat pacifiers. Honey should not be used in infants less than 1 year old because of the potential for infant botulism poisoning (Behrman et al., 2000).

Box 19-5 Injury Prevention During Infancy

Age: Birth–4 Months

Major Developmental Accomplishments

Involuntary reflexes, such as the crawling reflex, may propel infant forward or backward, and the startle reflex may cause the body to jerk
May roll over
Increasing eye-hand coordination and voluntary grasp reflex

Injury Prevention

Aspiration

Not as great a danger to this age-group, but should begin practising safeguarding early (see under Age: 4–7 Months)
Never shake baby powder directly on infant; place powder in hand and then on infant's skin; store container closed and out of infant's reach
Hold infant for feeding; do not prop bottle
Know emergency procedures for choking*
Use pacifier with one-piece construction and loop handle

Suffocation/Drowning

Keep all plastic bags stored out of infant's reach; discard large plastic garment bags after tying in a knot
Do not cover mattress with plastic
Use a firm mattress and loose blankets; no pillows
Make sure crib design follows federal regulations and mattress fits snugly—crib slats no further than 6 cm apart
Position crib away from other furniture and away from radiators
Do not tie pacifier on a string around infant's neck
Remove bibs at bedtime
Never leave infant alone in bath
Do not leave infant under 12 months alone on adult or youth mattress

Falls

Always raise crib rails
Never leave infant on a raised, unguarded surface
When in doubt as to where to place child, use the floor

Injury Prevention—cont'd

Falls—cont'd

Restrain child in infant seat and never leave child unattended while the seat is resting on a raised surface
Avoid using a high chair until child can sit well with support

Poisoning

Not as great a danger to this age-group, but should begin practicing safeguards early (see under Age: 4–7 Months)

Burns

Install smoke detectors in home
Use caution when warming formula in microwave oven; always shake the bottle and check temperature of liquid before feeding
Check bathwater temperature
Do not pour hot liquids when infant is close by, such as sitting on lap
Do not leave infant in the sun for more than a few minutes; keep exposed areas covered
Wash flame-retardant clothes according to label directions
Use cool-mist (rather than hot-mist) vaporizers
Do not leave child in parked car
Check surface heat of car restraint before placing child in seat

Motor Vehicles

Transport infant in federally approved, rear-facing infant seat, preferably in backseat (Figure 19–4)
Never place infant seat in front passenger seat with an air bag
Do not place child in a carriage or stroller behind a parked car

Bodily Damage

Avoid sharp, jagged objects
Keep diaper pins closed and away from infant
Never shake a baby (can cause shaken baby syndrome); advise caregivers to seek help if they feel irritated or overwhelmed by a baby's crying

Age: 4–7 Months

Major Developmental Accomplishments

Rolls over
Sits momentarily
Grasps and manipulates small objects
Picks up a dropped object
Has well-developed eye-hand coordination
Can focus on and locate very small objects
Mouthing is very prominent
Can push up on hands and knees
Crawls backward

Injury Prevention

Aspiration

Keep buttons, beads, syringe caps, and other small objects out of infant's reach
Keep floor free of any small objects

Injury Prevention—cont'd

Aspiration—cont'd

Do not feed infant hard candy, nuts, food with pits or seeds, or whole or circular pieces of hot dog
Exercise caution when giving teething biscuits, because large chunks may be broken off and aspirated
Do not feed infant while child is lying down
Inspect toys for removable parts

Suffocation

Keep all latex balloons out of reach
Remove all crib toys that are strung across crib or playpen when child begins to push up on hands or knees or is 5 months old
Keep baby powder and baby oil, if used, out of reach

Adapted from *Wong's Nursing Care of Infants and Children* (7th ed.), by M. J. Hockenberry et al., 2003, St. Louis, MO: Mosby.
*Further information available from *Keep Kids Safe 1-2-3-4,* Transport Canada (2001).

Continued

Box 19-5 Injury Prevention During Infancy—cont'd

Age: 4–7 Months—cont'd

Injury Prevention—cont'd

Falls

Restrain in a high chair
Keep crib rails raised to full height
Do not use baby walkers; baby walkers are no longer sold or imported into Canada because of their high rate of injuries they cause

Poisoning

Make sure that paint for furniture or toys does not contain lead
Hang plants or place on high surface rather than on floor
Store any toxic substances, such as cleaning fluid, paints, pesticides out of the reach of babies on a high shelf or in locked cabinet
Discard used containers of poisonous substances
Do not store toxic substances in food containers
Know telephone number of local poison control center (usually listed in front of telephone directory)

Burns

Keep faucets out of reach
Place hot objects (candles, incense) on high surface
Limit exposure to sun; apply sunscreen

Motor Vehicles

See under Age: Birth–4 Months

Bodily Damage

Give toys that are smooth and rounded, preferably made of wood or plastic
Avoid long, pointed objects as toys
Avoid toys that are excessively loud
Keep sharp objects out of infant's reach
See also Age: Birth—4 Months

Age: 8–12 Months

Major Developmental Accomplishments

Crawls/creeps
Stands, holding onto furniture
Stands alone
Cruises around furniture
Walks
Climbs
Pulls on objects
Throws objects
Is able to pick up small objects; has pincer grasp
Explores by putting objects in mouth
Dislikes being restrained
Explores away from parent

Injury Prevention

Aspiration

Keep small objects out of reach of children
Take care in feeding solid table food to ensure that very small pieces are given
Do not use beanbag toys or allow child to play with dried beans
See also under Age: 4–7 Months

Suffocation/Drowning

Keep doors of ovens, dishwashers, refrigerators, coolers, and front-loading clothes washers and dryers closed at all times
If storing an unused appliance, such as a refrigerator, remove the door
Supervise contact with inflated balloons; immediately discard popped balloons and keep uninflated balloons out of reach
Fence swimming pools
Always supervise when near any source of water, such as baths, cleaning buckets, drainage areas, toilets
Keep bathroom doors closed
Eliminate unnecessary pools of water
Keep one hand on child at all times when in tub

Injury Prevention—cont'd

Falls

Fence stairways at top and bottom if child has access to either end
Dress infant in safe shoes and clothing (soles that do not "catch" on floor, tied shoelaces, pant legs that do not touch floor)
Ensure that furniture is sturdy enough for child to pull self to standing position and cruise

Poisoning

Never call medications candy
Do not administer medications unless so prescribed by a practitioner
Replace medications and poisons immediately after use; replace caps properly if a child-protector cap is used

Burns

Place guards in front of or around any heating appliance, fireplace, or furnace
Keep electrical wires hidden or out of reach
Place plastic guards over electrical outlets; place furniture in front of outlets
Keep hanging tablecloths out of reach (child may pull down hot liquids or heavy or sharp objects)

Adapted from *Wong's Nursing Care of Infants and Children* (7th ed.), by M. J. Hockenberry et al., 2003, St. Louis, MO: Mosby.

Box 19-6 Clinical Manifestations of Potential Child Abuse and Neglect

Physical Neglect

Suggestive Physical Findings

- Failure to thrive (infants), signs of malnutrition (e.g., unhealthy looking skin and hair, sunken eyes or cheeks), evidence of poor health care
- Poor personal hygiene, especially of teeth, unclean and/or inappropriate dress
- Frequent injuries from lack of supervision

Suggestive Behaviours

- Dull and inactive (infants)
- Self-stimulatory behaviours, such as finger-sucking or rocking
- Begging or stealing food, vandalism, or shoplifting
- Absenteeism from school
- Drug or alcohol addiction

Emotional Abuse and Neglect

Suggestive Physical Findings

- Failure to thrive
- Feeding disorders, such as rumination
- Enuresis (bed wetting after toilet training has been established)
- Sleep disorders

Suggestive Behaviours

- Self-stimulatory behaviours such as biting, rocking, sucking
- Stranger anxiety and lack of social smile (infants)
- Withdrawal, unusual fearfulness
- Antisocial behaviour, such as destructiveness, stealing, cruelty
- Extremes of behaviour, such as overcompliant, passive, aggressive, or demanding
- Lags in emotional and intellectual development, especially language
- Suicide attempts

Physical Abuse

Suggestive Physical Findings

- Bruises and welts on face, lips, mouth, back, buttocks, thighs, or areas of torso
- Regular patterns descriptive of object used, such as belt buckle, hand, wire hanger, chain, wooden spoon, squeeze or pinch marks, round cigar or cigarette burns, burns in the shape of an iron, radiator, or electric stove burner
- Burns, injuries, fractures, lacerations or bruises in various stages of healing on soles of feet, palms of hands, back, or buttocks
- Absence of "splash" marks and presence of symmetric burns
- Unusual symptoms, such as abdominal swelling, pain, and vomiting from punching
- Descriptive marks such as from human bites or pulling out of hair
- Unexplained repeated poisoning or unexplained sudden illness

Physical Abuse—cont'd

Suggestive Behaviours

- Wariness of physical contact with adults
- Apparent fear of parents or of going home
- Lying very still while surveying environment, lack of reaction to frightening events
- Inappropriate reaction to injury, such as failure to cry from pain
- Apprehensiveness when hearing other children cry
- Indiscriminate friendliness and displays of affection, superficial relationships
- Acting-out behaviour, attention-seeking behaviours
- Withdrawn behaviour

Sexual Abuse

Suggestive Physical Findings

- Bruises, bleeding, lacerations or irritation of external genitalia, anus, mouth, or throat
- Torn, stained, or bloody underclothing
- Pain on urination or pain, swelling, and itching of genital area, penile discharge, unusual odour in the genital area
- Sexually transmitted infection, non-specific vaginitis, venereal warts, or presence of sperm
- Difficulty in walking or sitting
- Recurrent urinary tract infections
- Pregnancy in young adolescent

Suggestive Behaviours

- Sudden emergence of sexually related problems, including excessive or public masturbation, age-inappropriate sexual play, promiscuity, or overtly seductive behaviour
- Withdrawn behaviour, excessive daydreaming, preoccupation with fantasies, especially in play
- Poor relationships with peers
- Sudden changes, such as anxiety, loss or gain of weight, clinging behaviour
- In incestuous relationships, excessive anger at mother for not protecting child
- Regressive behaviour, such as bed-wetting or thumb-sucking
- Sudden onset of phobias or fears, particularly fears of the dark, men, strangers, or particular settings or situations (e.g., undue fear of leaving the house or staying at the day care centre or the babysitter's house)
- Running away from home
- Substance abuse, particularly of alcohol or mood-elevating drugs
- Profound and rapid personality changes, especially extreme depression, hostility, and aggression (often accompanied by social withdrawal)
- Rapidly declining school performance
- Suicidal attempts or ideation

From *Wong's Nursing Care of Infants and Children* (7th ed.), by M. J. Hockenberry et al., 2003, St. Louis, MO: Mosby.

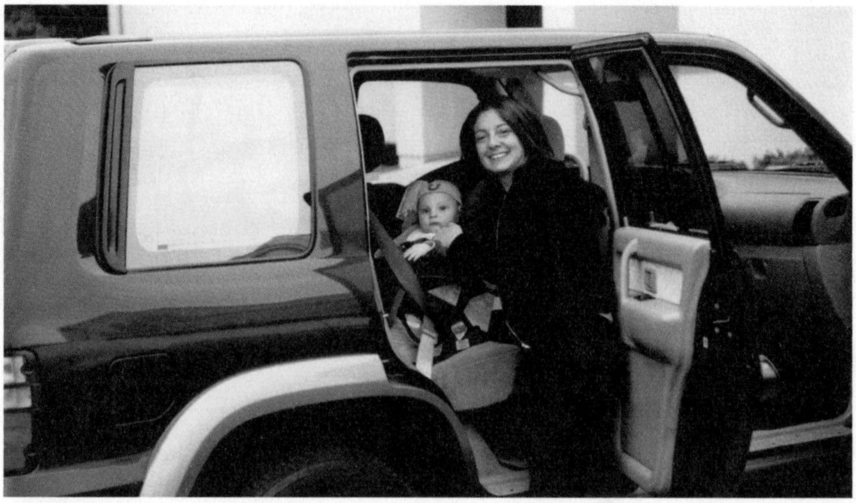

FIGURE **19–4** Federally approved infant car restraint. Note that the seat is rear facing in the back seat. (Courtesy Elaine Polan, RNC, BSN, MS.)

Research Highlight

Box 19-7

Breast-Feeding

Research Focus

Success in breast-feeding largely depends on the information and support a woman receives during the postpartum period. Nurses can play an important role in assisting mothers in their attempts to breast-feed.

Research Abstract

The purpose of this study was to describe how nurses facilitated mothers' breast-feeding attempts during their hospital stay. Also investigated were the mother's perceptions of support by their nurses. Earlier research indicated that a mother's choice to breast-feed is influenced by several factors, including age, education, ethnicity, and income. Those who have difficulties initiating or continuing breast-feeding often have feelings of failing, which may further undermine their confidence in parenting. Different forms of support include informational support, tangible support, emotional or interpersonal support, and appraisal support. Informational support provides the mother with information verbally, non-verbally, or in writing. Tangible support uses physical assistance and/or money. Appraisal support encourages and evaluates the mother's progress. Using a research approach known as ethnography, information was obtained from the subjects by interview and observation. Some of the nurses were reported to be well informed and knowledgeable about breast-feeding and willing to offer support. However, the mothers interviewed reported that they were disappointed and did not feel supported. They felt frustrated and discouraged. Mothers wanted the nurses to stay with them during their feeding attempts. They thought the written instructions were not supportive enough for them to feel satisfied.

Evidence-Based Practice

- Nurses must provide education and support to breast-feeding mothers.
- Nurses must try to anticipate mother's needs rather than wait to be told.
- All nurses should use consistent approaches to best facilitate breast-feeding.
- Nurses should provide breast-feeding mothers with verbal support and written information.
- Nurses should assess mothers' support system's knowledge of breast-feeding.

Reference

Gill, S. (2001). The little things: Perceptions of breastfeeding support. *Journal of Obstetric, Gynecologic, and Neonatal Nursing, 30*(4), 401–409.

Supplementation. The need for dietary vitamin and mineral supplements depends on the infant's diet. Full-term infants are born with some iron stores. The breast-fed infant absorbs adequate iron from breast milk during the first 4 to 6 months of life. After 6 months, iron-fortified cereal is generally considered an adequate supplemental source. Because iron in formula is less readily absorbed than that in breast milk, formula-fed infants should receive iron-fortified formula throughout the first year. Infants who are breast-fed, especially those in more northerly areas, need to receive a vitamin D supplement to prevent rickets (Ward et al., 2003).

Adequate concentrations of fluoride to protect against dental caries are not available in human milk, and therefore fluoridated water or supplemental fluoride is generally recommended. The presence of fluoride in formula depends on the type of formula and the source of water used in preparing the concentrated forms. Fluoride supplementation may be necessary.

Overfeeding. The association between overfeeding, infant obesity, and later adult obesity is still controversial. However, early feeding experiences can influence later eating habits. The nurse should therefore emphasize bal-

Cultural Aspects of Care — Box 19-8

Cultural practices and beliefs have a significant influence on the choice of infant feeding methods. Although cultural norms exist, application of the norms may not be appropriate for all individuals.

Implications for Practice

- Immigrants to Canada from poorer countries may choose to bottle-feed their infants because it is believed to be better and more modern. Others may choose bottle-feeding because of a desire to adapt to the North American culture.
- Many cultures choose not to give the infants colostrum (the antibody-rich secretion produced in the first hours of lactation, before the milk comes in). Filipinos, Vietnamese, Koreans, Nigerians, and East Indians are a few of the 50 known cultures that delay breast-feeding until the milk has come in.
- Other cultures may begin breast-feeding immediately after delivery and offer the breast each time the infant cries.
- Cultural attitudes regarding breast-feeding, modesty, and dietary beliefs are important considerations for the nurse.

Data from *A Multicultural Perspective of Breastfeeding in Canada,* by T. Agnew, J. Gilmore, and P. Sullivan, 1997, Ottawa, ON: Health Canada; *Health Promotion Throughout the Life Span* (5th ed.), by C. Edelman and C. Mandle, 2002, St. Louis, MO: Mosby; and "The Little Things: Perceptions of Breastfeeding Support," by S. Gill, 2001, *Journal of Obstetric, Gynecologic, and Neonatal Nursing, 30*(4), p. 401.

anced nutrition and good dietary habits through feeding experiences mutually satisfying for the parents and infant. Eating habits are frequently affected by the family's socio-cultural background. Certain cultures regard "a fat baby as a healthy baby." Because some cultures consider a fat baby to be a sign of good mothering, any suggestion to limit intake or slow weight gain may be seen as a threat. It is important for the nurse to develop an understanding of the cultural influences to develop effective nursing interventions (Box 19-8).

Dentition. The average age that the first tooth erupts is 7 months, but there is considerable variation among infants because of their genetic endowment. An occasional infant is born with a tooth, whereas others remain toothless at 1 year. The order of tooth eruption is fairly predictable with the lower central incisors being first to appear, closely followed by the upper central incisors. Most 1-year-olds have six teeth.

Teething may result in considerable discomfort for some infants and little or none for others. The inflammation of the gums before the tooth emerges may result in a low-grade fever and irritability. Some infants have increased drooling, biting, or finger sucking. Biting on a frozen teething ring or ice cube wrapped in a washcloth may be soothing. Over-the-counter teething medications to rub on the inflamed gums and appropriate doses of acetaminophen are helpful when the infant is irritable and has difficulty eating or sleeping.

Most dentists recommend that parents cleanse their infant's teeth after each feeding. The parent can place a clean, wet washcloth or piece of gauze over a finger and use it to wipe the infant's teeth. Because of the risk of developing dental caries, discourage prolonged breast- or bottle-feeding, especially after the infant is asleep and is likely to leave milk in the mouth and around the teeth. The infant should never go to bed with a bottle of juice or milk (Behrman et al., 2000).

Immunizations. The widespread use of immunizations has resulted in the dramatic decline of infectious diseases over the past 50 years and is therefore a most important factor in health promotion during childhood. Although most immunizations can be given to people of any age, it is recommended that the administration of the primary series begin soon after birth and be completed during early childhood. The Canadian Paediatric Society (2004) has added flu vaccine to the list of recommended immunizations for children between the ages of 6 months and 2 years of age. Vaccines are among the safest and most reliable drugs used. Minor side effects may occur, and serious reactions are rare. Parents must receive instructions regarding the potential side effects of immunizations. High fever and extreme irritability should be reported to their health care provider.

Complacency and fear regarding the side effects of certain vaccines, especially diphtheria and tetanus toxoids and pertussis vaccine (DTP), have resulted in large numbers of children not receiving appropriate immunizations during recent years. An important role for the nurse is to discuss the importance of vaccination for infants and children, provide up-to-date information to parents, and encourage them to make an informed decision for their child. General contraindications to vaccination include moderate illness, allergic response to a previous dose of a particular vaccine, immunosuppression, and people receiving high doses of corticosteroids. Live virus vaccines are generally not recommended for pregnant women (Behrman et al., 2000).

Sleep. Sleep patterns vary among infants, with many having their days and nights mixed up until 3 to 4 months of age. By this time, most infants sleep between 9 and 11 hours a night. Total daily sleep averages 15 hours. Most infants take one or two naps a day by the end of the first year. Sleep disturbances with a physiological basis are rare, with the possible exception of colic. Common sleep disturbances are described in Table 19-3.

Toddler

Toddlerhood ranges from 12 to 36 months. The toddler has increasing independence, physical mobility, and cognitive abilities. Toddlers are increasingly aware of their

Table 19-3 Selected Sleep Disturbances During Infancy and Early Childhood

Disorder/Description	Management
Nighttime Feeding	
Colic, irritability Prolonged need for night bottle or breast-feeding Child goes to sleep at the breast or with a bottle Irregular sleep patterns Child returns to sleep after feeding; other comfort measures (e.g., rocking or holding) are usually ineffective	Soothe, rock for brief periods, offer pacifier Gradually increase daytime feeding intervals to 4 hours or more Offer last feeding as late as possible at night Gradually increase amount of fluid during day Offer no bottles in bed Put to bed *awake* When child is crying, check at progressively longer intervals each night; reassure child but do not hold, rock, take to parent's bed, or give bottle or pacifier
Developmental Night Crying	
Child age 6–12 months with undisturbed nighttime sleep now awakes abruptly; may be accompanied by nightmares	Reassure parents that this phase is temporary Enter room immediately to check on child but keep reassurances *brief* Avoid feeding, rocking, taking to parent's bed, or any other routine that may initiate trained night crying
Trained Night Crying (Inappropriate Sleep Associations)	
Child typically falls asleep in place other than own bed (e.g., rocking chair or parent's bed) and is brought to own bed while asleep; on awakening, cries until usual routine is instituted (e.g., rocking)	Put child in own bed when *awake* If possible, arrange sleeping area separate from other family members Check crying child at progressively longer intervals each night; reassure child but do not resume usual routine
Refusal to Go to Sleep	
Child resists bedtime and comes out of room repeatedly Nighttime sleep may be continuous, but frequent awakenings and refusal to return to sleep may occur and become a problem if parent allows child to deviate from usual sleep pattern	Evaluate if hour of sleep is too early (child may resist sleep if not tired) Assist parents with consistent bedtime routine If child persists in leaving bedroom, close door for progressively longer periods Reinforce positive behaviour
Nighttime Fears	
Child resists going to bed or wakes during the night because of fears Child seeks parent's physical presence and falls asleep easily with parent nearby.	Evaluate if hour of sleep is too early (child may fantasize when nothing to do but think in dark room) Calmly reassure the frightened child; keeping a night-light on may be helpful Use reward system with child to provide motivation to deal with fears Avoid patterns that can lead to additional problems (e.g., sleeping with child or taking child to parent's room)
Overwhelming fears	If child's fear is overwhelming, consider desensitization (e.g., progressively spending longer periods of time alone; consult professional help for protracted fears) Distinguish between nightmares and sleep terrors (confused partial arousals)

abilities to control and are pleased with successful efforts. This success leads them to continue attempting to control their environments. Unsuccessful attempts at control may result in negative behaviour and temper tantrums.

Physical Changes

The rapid development of motor skills allows the child to participate in self-care activities such as feeding, dressing, and toileting. Initially, the toddler walks with a broad stance and gait, protuberant abdomen, and arms out to the sides for balance. Soon the child begins to navigate stairs, using a rail or the wall to maintain balance. Locomotion skills eventually include running, jumping, standing on one foot for several seconds, and kicking a ball. Most toddlers can ride tricycles, climb ladders, and run well by their third birthday.

Fine motor capabilities move from scribbling spontaneously to drawing circles and crosses accurately. By 3 years, the child draws simple stick people and can usually stack a tower of small blocks. Increased locomotion skills, the ability to undress, and development of sphincter control allow toilet training if the toddler has developed the necessary language and cognitive abilities. Parents often consult nurses for an assessment of readiness for toilet training. Recognition by the child of the urge to urinate and defecate is a crucial component in the child's mental readiness. At this stage, children usually show a willingness to please parents and take pride in their accomplishments (Kinservik & Friedhoff, 2000). The nurse needs to remind parents that patience, consistency, and a nonjudgmental attitude, in addition to the child's readiness, are essential to successful toilet training.

The cardiopulmonary system becomes stable in the toddler years. The heart and respiratory rates slow to an average of 110 beats and 25 breaths per minute, respectively, and the blood pressure varies slightly from infancy. The average blood pressure for a toddler is 90/50 mm Hg.

The anterior fontanel closes between 12 and 18 months of age, ending the period of most rapid growth of the skull and brain. Routine measurement of head circumference should be done until 3 years of age.

The rate of increase in weight and length slows. By 2½ years, the child weighs four times the birth weight. Height during the toddler years increases by approximately 7.5 cm a year, mainly as a result of increases in leg length. The average height of 2-year-olds is 85 cm. Slowed growth rates are accompanied by decreased caloric need, and smaller food intake leads some parents to worry about the adequacy of dietary intake. Parents need encouragement to offer appropriate servings of food from Canada' Food Guide and to avoid force feeding or allowing the child to fill up on foods that are high in fat and sugar. The nurse can reassure parents that the child's nutrition is adequate by demonstrating the child's satisfactory status on a growth chart.

Cognitive Changes

Toddlers' completion of the development of **object permanence,** their ability to remember events, and their beginning ability to put thoughts into words at about 2 years of age signal their transition to Piaget's (1952) **preoperational thought** stage of cognitive development (see chapter 18). Toddlers recognize that they are separate beings from their mothers, but they are unable to assume the view of another. They use symbols to represent objects, places, and people. This function is demonstrated when children imitate the behaviour of another that they viewed earlier (e.g., pretend to shave like daddy), pretend one object is another (e.g., a doll is a baby), and use language to stand for absent objects (e.g., request bottle).

Language. The 18-month-old child uses approximately 10 words. The 24-month-old child has a vocabulary of up to 300 words and is generally able to speak in two-word sentences (Deering & Cody, 2002). "Who's that?" and "What's that?" typify questions asked during this period. Expressions such as "me do it" and "that's mine" demonstrate the 2-year-old child's use of pronouns and desire for independence and control. Despite the expanded vocabulary of an older toddler, many toddlers' favourite word is *no* until well into the third year. Offering choices to the toddler helps reduce their sense of frustration and builds their sense of independence (Deering & Cody, 2002).

Because children's moral development is closely associated with their cognitive abilities, the moral development of toddlers is only beginning and is also egocentric. Toddlers do not understand concepts of right and wrong. However, they understand that some behaviours bring pleasant results and others elicit unpleasant results. Therefore, until toddlers achieve a higher level of cognitive function, they behave simply to avoid the unpleasant and seek out the pleasant (Hockenberry et al., 2003).

Psychosocial Changes

According to Erikson (1963), a sense of autonomy emerges during the toddler years (see chapter 18). Children strive for independence by using their developing muscles to do everything for themselves and control their bodily functions. Their strong wills are frequently exhibited in negative behaviour when caregivers attempt to direct their actions. Temper tantrums may result when toddlers are frustrated by parental restrictions. Parents need to provide toddlers with graded independence, allowing them to do things that do not result in harm to themselves or others. This strategy prevents them from doubting their abilities or feeling a sense of shame for what they have done. Firm consistent limits, patience, and support allow toddlers to develop socially acceptable behaviour and cope with the frustration of learning self-control (Kinservik & Friedhoff, 2000).

Socially, toddlers remain strongly attached to their parents and fear separation from them. In their parents' presence, toddlers feel safe and their curiosity is evident in their exploration of the environment. The child continues to engage in solitary play during toddlerhood but also begins to participate in parallel play, which is playing beside rather than with another child. Toddlers who are just learning what belongs to them are often possessive of their toys. They learn the joy of sharing when they offer parents toys to hold and the parents express pleasure.

Health Risks

The newly developed locomotion abilities and insatiable curiosity of toddlers put them at risk for injury. Toddlers need close supervision at all times, particularly when in environments that have not been childproofed (Figure 19–5). Creating a safe, childproof environment in the home is essential to helping prevent accidental injuries.

Poisonings occur frequently because children near 2 years of age are interested in placing any object or substance in their mouths to learn about it. Parents must remove or lock up all possible poisons, including plants, cleaning materials, and medications. Lead poisoning can pose a health hazard for younger children (Health Canada, 1997). Health care providers need to educate families living in older homes about the risks, screening, and treatment of lead poisoning. The toddlers' lack of awareness regarding the danger of water and their newly developed walking skills make drowning a major cause of accidental death in this age group. Toddlers can easily get separated from a parent because they will often wander away. It is important to closely supervise a toddler, especially if in an open public space. Limit setting is extremely important for toddlers' safety. Toddlers must remain in car seats (Kamerling, 2002). Children often learn

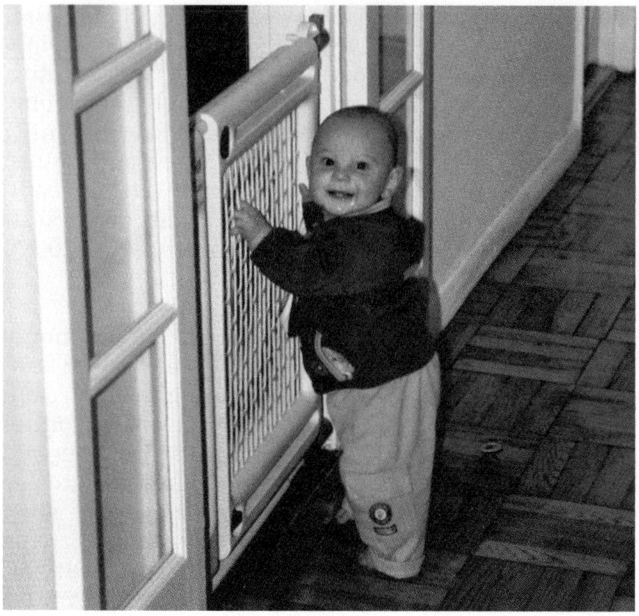

FIGURE **19–5** Safety precautions should be provided for toddlers. (Courtesy Elaine Polan, RNC, BSN, MS.)

to release the car restraints, and parents must be firm in their resolve not to drive unless the children are securely restrained. Toddlers completely depend on their parents for physical safety. Health care workers must educate parents on the proper use of child passenger restraint use. Table 19-4 identifies developmental abilities acquired during this age period and injury prevention strategies.

Health Concerns

Nutrition. Most toddlers change from breast milk or formula to cow's milk. Nutritional requirements are increasingly met by solid foods. Because the consumption of more than 1 L of milk per day usually decreases the child's appetite for these essential solid foods and results in inadequate iron intake, the nurse should advise parents to limit milk intake to between 500 and 750 mL (2 to 3 servings) per day. Children should not drink low fat or skim milk until 2 years of age because they need the fat in whole milk for physical and intellectual growth. The healthy toddler requires a balanced daily intake of bread and grains, vegetables, fruit, dairy products, and proteins (see chapter 39). Because parents frequently overestimate the size of a normal serving for their child, the nurse should discuss normal serving sizes.

Special dietary considerations are required for children who are ill, are undergoing surgery, or have conditions involving ingestion, absorption, or use of nutrients. Alterations in the type of foods and caloric requirements may be necessary. Strict vegetarian diets for children also require careful planning to ensure adequate, balanced protein intake. Regardless of children's health status, several basic principles of nutrition apply. Mealtime has psychosocial and physical significance. If the parents struggle to control toddlers' dietary intake, problem behaviour and conflicts may result. Toddlers often develop "food jags," or the desire to eat one food repeatedly. Rather than becoming disturbed by this behaviour, parents should be encouraged to offer a variety of nutritious foods at meals and to provide only nutritious snacks between meals. Serving finger foods to toddlers allows them to eat by themselves and to satisfy their need for independence and control. Small, reasonable servings allow toddlers to eat all of their meals.

Preschooler

The **preschool period** refers to the years between 3 and 5 years of age. Children refine the mastery of their bodies and often are eager to begin school. Many people consider these the most intriguing years of parenting because children are less negative and can more effectively share their thoughts, interact, and communicate. Physical development occurs at a slower pace than cognitive and psychosocial development.

Physical Changes

Physical development continues in the preschool years. Heart and respiratory rates range from 60 to 100 beats and 23 to 25 breaths per minute, respectively. Blood pressure rises slightly to an average of 92/56 mm Hg. Children gain about 2.27 kg per year; the average weight at 3 years is 14.5 kg, at 4 years is 16.8 kg, and at 5 years is about 18.6 kg. Preschoolers grow 6 to 7.5 cm per year, double their birth length around 4 years, and stand an average of 1-m tall by their fifth birthday. The elongation of the legs results in a more slender appearance. Little difference exists between the sexes, although boys are slightly larger with more muscle and less fatty tissue.

Large and fine muscle coordination improves. Preschoolers run well, walk up and down steps with ease, and learn to hop. By 5 years, they can usually skip on alternate feet, jump rope, and begin to skate and swim. Improving fine motor skills allows intricate manipulations. They learn to copy crosses and squares. Triangles and diamonds are usually mastered between 5 and 6 years. Scribbling and drawing help to develop fine muscle skills and eye-hand coordination needed for the printing of letters and numbers.

Children need opportunities to learn and practice new physical skills. Early intervention programs are important to help children develop these skills, especially among disadvantaged children. Nursing care of healthy and ill children includes an assessment of the availability of these opportunities. Although children with acute illnesses benefit from rest and exclusion from usual daily activities, children who have chronic conditions or who have been hospitalized for long periods need ongoing exposure to developmental opportunities. The parents and nurse weave these opportunities into the children's daily experiences, depending on their abilities, needs, and energy level.

Cognitive Changes

Preschoolers continue to master the preoperational stage of cognition. The first phase of this period, known as preconceptual thought (2 to 4 years), is characterized by perceptual-bound thinking, in that children judge people, objects, and events by their outward appearance or what seems to be (Piaget, 1952). For example, a child

Table 19-4 Injury Prevention for Toddlers and Preschoolers

Developmental Abilities Related to Risk of Injury	Injury Prevention
	Motor Vehicles
Walks, runs, and climbs Able to open doors and gates Can ride tricycle Can throw ball and other objects	Continue to use federally approved car restraint. Toddlers weighing 10 to 18 kg should be placed in a forward-facing child seat that is anchored to the vehicle frame with a tether strap. Children weighing 18 to 36 kg should use a booster seat. Supervise child while playing outside to avoid entering street Do not allow child to play on curb or behind a parked car Do not permit child to play in pile of leaves, snow, or anywhere they are not visible Supervise tricycle riding Children playing outside must be properly supervised Teach child to obey pedestrian safety rules Supervise children when near traffic
	Drowning
Has great curiosity Helpless in water, unaware of its danger; depth of water has no significance	Supervise closely when near any source of water, including buckets Keep bathroom doors and lid on toilet closed Have fence around swimming pool and lock gate Teach swimming and water safety (not a substitute for protection)
	Burns
Able to reach heights by climbing, stretching, standing on toes, and using objects as a ladder Pulls objects Explores any holes or opening Can open drawers and closets Unaware of potential sources of heat or fire Plays with mechanical objects	Turn pot handles toward back of stove Place electric appliances, such as coffeemaker or frying pan, toward back of counter Place guardrails in front of radiators, fireplaces, and other heating elements Store matches and cigarette lighters in locked or inaccessible area; discard carefully Place burning candles, incense, hot foods, ashes, embers, and cigarettes out of reach Do not let tablecloth hang within child's reach Do not let electric cord from iron or other appliance hang within child's reach Cover electrical outlets with protective devices Keep electrical wires hidden or out of reach Do not allow child to play with electrical appliance, wires, or lighters Stress danger of open flames; teach what "hot" means Always check bathwater temperature; adjust hot-water heater temperature to 49° C or lower; do not allow children to play with faucets Apply a sunscreen with SPF 15 or higher when child is exposed to sunlight
	Poisoning
Explores by putting objects in mouth Can open drawers, closets, and most containers Climbs Cannot understand warning labels	Place all potentially toxic agents (including plants) in a locked cabinet or out of reach Replace medications and poisons immediately; replace child-resistant caps properly Refer to medications as drugs, not as candy Do not store large surplus of toxic agents Promptly discard empty poison containers; never reuse to store a food item or other poison Teach child not to play in trash containers Never remove labels from containers of toxic substances Know number and location of nearest poison control centre (usually listed in front of telephone directory)

From *Wong's Nursing Care of Infants and Children* (7th ed.), by M. J. Hockenberry et al., 2003, St. Louis, MO: Mosby.

Continued

Table 19-4 Injury Prevention for Toddlers and Preschoolers—cont'd

Developmental Abilities Related to Risk of Injury	Injury Prevention
	Falls
Able to open doors and some windows Goes up and down stairs Depth perception unrefined	Keep screen in window, nail securely, and use guardrail Place gates at top and bottom of stairs Keep doors locked or use child-resistant doorknob covers at entry to stairs, high porch, or other elevated area, such as laundry chute Remove unsecured or scatter rugs Apply non-skid mat in bathtub or shower Keep crib rails fully raised and mattress at lowest level Place carpeting under crib and in bathroom Keep large toys and bumper pads out of crib or playpen (child can use these as "stairs" to climb out) Move to youth bed when child is able to crawl out of crib Dress in safe clothing (soles that do not "catch" on floor, tied shoelaces, pant legs that do not hang on floor) Never leave unattended in shopping cart or stroller Supervise at playgrounds; select play areas with soft ground cover and safe equipment
	Choking and Suffocation
Puts things in mouth May swallow hard or non-edible pieces of food	Avoid large, round chunks of meat, such as whole hot dogs (slice lengthwise into thin pieces) Avoid fruit with pits, fish with bones, dried beans, hard candy, chewing gum, nuts, popcorn, grapes, marshmallows Choose large, sturdy toys without sharp edges or small removable parts Discard old refrigerators, ovens, and so on; if storing old appliance, remove doors Keep automatic garage door opener in inaccessible place Select safe toy boxes or chests without heavy, hinged lids Keep window blind strings out of child's reach Remove drawstrings from clothing
	Bodily Damage
Still clumsy in many skills Easily distracted from tasks Unaware of potential danger from strangers or other people	Avoid giving child sharp or pointed objects—such as knives, scissors, or toothpicks—especially when child is walking or running Do not allow lollipops or similar objects in mouth when walking or running Teach safety precautions (e.g., to carry fork or scissors with pointed end away from face) Store all dangerous tools, garden equipment, and firearms in locked cabinet Be alert to danger of animals, including household pets Use safety glass and decals on large glassed areas, such as sliding glass doors Teach personal safety Teach name, address, and phone number and to ask for help from appropriate people (cashier, security guard, police officer) if lost; have identification on child (sewn in clothes, inside shoe) Avoid personalized clothing in public places Teach child to never go with a stranger Teach child to tell parents if anyone makes child feel uncomfortable in any way Always listen to child's concerns regarding others' behaviour Teach child to say "no" when confronted with uncomfortable situations

From *Wong's Nursing Care of Infants and Children* (7th ed.), by M. J. Hockenberry et al., 2003, St. Louis, MO: Mosby.

may think that a 240-mL glass full of fluid contains more than a 300-mL glass that also contains 240 mL of fluid because the smaller glass appears fuller. Even if they watch the fluid from the smaller glass being poured into the larger glass and the smaller glass refilled, they will still assert that the full, smaller glass contains more.

Thinking is hindered by their limited attention and attending skills. **Artificialism,** the misconception that everything in the world has been created by humanity, may result in children asking questions such as who built the mountains. Another misconception of preschool thinking, **animism,** the attribution of animal life to inanimate objects, often results in statements such as "Trees cry when their branches are broken." A third misconception is a type of reasoning called **immanent justice,** the notion that the world has a built-in code of law and order and therefore the natural world punishes bad behaviour. For example, a child might think that he became sick because he lied to his mother.

Around the age of 4 years, the intuitive phase of preoperational thought develops. Children's ability to think more complexly is demonstrated by their ability to classify objects according to size or colour and by questions such as, "Why do they call it the 31st day of the month instead of the 30 last?" Egocentricity persists, but during these 3 years, it begins to be replaced with social interaction, as is illustrated by the 5-year-old child who offers a bandage to a child with a cut finger. Children become aware of cause-and-effect relationships, as illustrated by the statement, "The sun sets because people want to go to bed." Early causal thinking is also evident in preschoolers' transductive thoughts (reasoning occurs from one particular to another). If two events are related in time or space, children link them in a causal fashion. The hospitalized child, for example, may reason, "I cried last night, and that's why the nurse gave me the shot." As children near the age of 5 years, they begin to use or can be taught to use rules to understand causation. They then begin to reason from the general to the particular. This development forms the basis for more formal logical thought. The child now reasons, "I get a shot twice a day, and that's why I got one last night."

Preschoolers' knowledge of the world remains closely linked to concrete (perceived by the senses) experiences. Even their rich fantasy life is grounded in the perception of reality. The mixing of the two aspects can lead to many childhood fears and may be misinterpreted by adults as lying when children are actually presenting reality from their perspective.

The greatest fear of this age group appears to be that of bodily harm, and it can be seen in children's fear of the dark, thunderstorms, and medical personnel. This fear often makes children unwilling to allow nursing interventions such as measurement of vital signs. Preschoolers may co-operate if they are allowed to help the nurse measure the blood pressure of a parent or if they are allowed to manipulate the nurse's equipment.

The preschooler's moral development expands to include a beginning understanding of behaviours considered socially right or wrong. The child continues to be motivated, however, by the wish to avoid punishment and the desire to obtain a reward. The primary difference between this stage of moral development and that of a toddler is that a preschooler is better able to identify behaviours that elicit rewards or punishment and begins to label these behaviours as right or wrong.

Language. Preschoolers' vocabularies continue to increase rapidly, and by the age of 6 years, children know more than 10,000 words (Deering & Cody, 2002). Language is more social, and questions expand to "Why?" and "How come?" Phonetically similar words such as *die* and *dye* or *wood* and *would* might cause confusion in preschool children. The nurse avoids such words when preparing children for procedures and assesses comprehension of explanations.

Psychosocial Changes

The world of preschoolers expands beyond the family into the neighbourhood where children meet other children and adults. Their curiosity and developing initiative lead to the active exploration of the environment, the development of new skills, and the making of new friends. Preschoolers have a surplus of energy that permits them to plan and attempt many activities that may be beyond their capabilities, such as pouring milk into their cereal bowls. Guilt arises within children when they overstep the limits of their abilities and feel they have not behaved correctly. Children who in anger have wished their sibling were dead experience guilt if that sibling becomes ill. Children need to be taught that "wishing" for something to happen does not make it occur. Parents should allow preschoolers to do tasks on their own but set firm limits and provide guidance.

During times of stress or illness, preschoolers may revert to bedwetting or thumb sucking and want the parents to feed, dress, and hold them. These dependent behaviours are often confusing and embarrassing to parents, who can benefit from the nurse's reassurance that they are the child's normal coping behaviours. The nurse should provide experiences that these children can master. Such successes help children return to their prior level of independent functioning. As language skills develop, children should be encouraged to talk about their feelings. Play is also an excellent way for preschoolers to vent frustration or anger and is a socially acceptable way to deal with stress.

Play. Children become more social after the third birthday as they shift from parallel to associative play. Children playing together engage in similar if not identical activity; however, there is no division of labour or rigid organization or rules. Most 3-year-old children are able to play with one other child in a co-operative manner in which they make something or play designated roles such as mother and baby. By the age of 4 years, children play in groups of two or three, and by 5 years, the group has a temporary leader for each activity.

In many play activities, preschoolers display awareness of social context. Sex-role identification is strengthening, and children most often assume roles of people of their own sex. Children frequently mimic or repeat social experiences. This tendency is especially significant for the nurse working with hospitalized children. Through play, children may express questions, fears, anger, and misunderstanding about their illnesses and care. The nurse should be alert to such clues and ensure that children can play within energy limits. Play can provide a healthy outlet for frustration, especially when children have been subjected to painful or restrictive experiences against their will.

Imaginary play depends on children's memory of things they have seen or heard. This socio-dramatic play involving other children occupies about a third of 5-year-old children's playtime. Pretending allows children to learn to understand other's points of view, develop skills in solving social problems, and become more creative. Some children have imaginary playmates, which are a sign of creativity and healthy development.

Health Risks

As fine and gross motor skills develop, the child becomes more coordinated with better balance; nevertheless, falls and other accidents remain a leading cause of injury. Guidelines for injury prevention in the toddler also apply to the preschooler (see Table 19-4). The nurse should alert parents of children in this age group to the risks of poisoning and pedestrian-motor vehicle accidents. Children up to 18 kg must be in forward-facing child seats, and children weighing 18 to 36 kg must use a booster seat. The leading cause of death in Canadian children is unintentional injury (Canadian Institute of Child Health

[CICH], 2000). All of these injuries are preventable. Children should be taught about safety in the home and reinforced early in elementary school.

Health Concerns

Nutrition. Nutrition requirements for the preschooler vary little from those of the toddler. The average daily intake is 1,800 calories. Parents may still worry about the amount of food their child is consuming. However, the quality of the food is more important than quantity in most situations. Preschoolers consume about half of the average adult portions. Finicky eating habits are characteristic of the 4-year-old; the 5-year-old is more interested in trying new foods.

Sleep. Preschoolers average 12 hours of sleep a night and take infrequent naps. Sleep disturbances are common during these years. Disturbances may range from trouble getting to sleep to nightmares to prolonging bedtime with extensive rituals. Frequently, the child has had an overabundance of activity and stimulation. Having children follow a set routine before bedtime helps them prepare for sleep.

Vision. Preschoolers should routinely be screened for vision problems. One of the common problems in the preschool period is amblyopia. Early detection and treatment can improve vision for most children (Berry et al., 2001).

School-Age Children and Adolescents

School-age children and adolescents lead demanding, challenging lives. The developmental changes between ages 6 and 19 years are diverse and span all areas of growth and development. Physical, psychosocial, cognitive, and moral skills are developed, expanded, refined, and synchronized. The environment in which the individual develops skills also expands and diversifies. Instead of the boundaries of family and close friends, the environment now may include the school, community, and church. Because of expectations for development, increasing skill and knowledge base, and environmental expansion, the individual experiences new difficulties and dilemmas. With age-specific assessment, the nurse must review the appropriate developmental expectations for each age group. For example, before assessing risk-taking behaviours, the nurse recognizes that adolescents normally strive to achieve a sense of identity while developing a moral code compatible with society.

The nurse needs to direct school-age children and adolescents toward normal developmental behaviours, assisting them in improving their abilities and using them to cope. Table 19-5 provides an overview of developmental behaviour typical of school-age children and adolescents.

Table 19-5 Developmental Behaviours of School-Age Children and Adolescents

School-Age Children	Adolescents
Relationships with Parents	
Children gradually learn that parents are less than perfect; children can be disillusioned with parents and wish that friends' parents were their own. They still rely on parents for unconditional love, security, guidance, and nurturing.	Adolescents' desire for increasing independence and autonomy yet continuing need for some dependence and limit setting by parents place strain on their relationship. Effective communication and democratic parenting are best tools for meeting this challenge.
Relationships with Siblings	
Siblings seem to be at odds with one another at home, yet they are each other's best defenders away from home. Younger children often idolize older siblings, and this frequently leads to competition. Older children may envy attention that younger siblings require and be quite bossy and somewhat abusive.	Younger siblings rarely understand their adolescent siblings' need for privacy. Adolescents often enjoy interacting with and guiding younger brothers and sisters when timing is convenient for them and they can remain in control.
Relationships with Peers	
During primary grades (6–7 years), children of both sexes play together, depending on who is available and interested. Around age 8, social groupings of same-sex peers form. These "gangs" allow children to declare their independence from parental rules and establish their own rules of membership and behaviour. This period is often referred to as *secret society* of childhood. Preadolescent (10–12 years) friendships are characterized by having best friend of same sex. These relationships may be transient, but they are intense and allow discussion of all areas of life. Childhood "crushes" are common.	Peer group is factor of critical influence to adolescents, who have increasing need for recognition and acceptance. Companionship offered by peer groups provides secure environment for individuals to try out new ideas and share similar feelings and attitudes. Adolescents often form cliques with peers from same socio-economic group with similar interests. Cliques, which are highly exclusive, help their members develop their identities.

Table 19-5 Developmental Behaviours of School-Age Children and Adolescents—cont'd

School-Age Children	Adolescents
Self-concept	
Children's feelings of competence regarding mastery of tasks are key elements in forming self-esteem. Children need to receive positive feedback regarding their efforts. It is important for children to develop skills in at least one area such as reading, music, or swimming.	Formal and informal peer groups are primary force in shaping self-concept of group members. Popularity and recognition within peer group enhance self-esteem and reinforce self-concept. Total immersion in peer group may make it appear that adolescents have no original thoughts and are incapable of making decisions. Adolescents who withdraw from peers into isolation struggle with developing identity.
Fears	
There is decline in fears related to body safety. Fears of supernatural such as ghosts and witches persist and decline slowly. New fears related to school and family occur. They fear ridicule from teachers and friends and disapproval and rejection of parents. They also become frightened about death and items that they hear on news such as war and destruction of environment.	Fears in this age group centre around peer group acceptance, body changes, loss of self-control, and emerging sexual urges. Adolescents constantly examine their bodies for changes and signs of imperfection. Any defect, real or imagined, is cause of endless worry.
Coping Patterns	
To deal with stress, school-agers use problem solving and defence mechanisms such as denial and aggression. Several categories of coping behaviours of hospitalized school-agers include inactivity (total silence, lack of activity, and apathy), orientation or precoping (looking and listening, walking around and exploring, and asking questions), co-operation (compliance with care), resistance (attempt to get away from the situation by turning away or making physical or verbal attacks), and controlling (assuming responsibility for self-care and suggesting how things could be done).	Coping behaviours expand with experiences adolescents have gained from life and from developing cognitive maturity. By age 15, most use full range of defence mechanisms, including rationalization and intellectualization. Adolescents' problem-solving abilities have matured, and they can reason through philosophical discussions and complex situations that require abstract thinking and proposition of hypotheses. Some adolescents use avoidance coping strategies in which the problem is denied or repressed and an attempt is made to reduce tension by engaging in substance abuse or avoiding people.
Morals	
Children learn rules from parents, but their understanding of rules or reasons for them is limited until about 10 years. Before that, they are concerned with own needs first and may cheat to win. After 10 years of age, justice is based on "eye for an eye," and punishment should correct situation (e.g., if children break something, they should pay to have it fixed).	According to Kohlberg (1964), as youths approach adolescence, they reach conventional level, where internalization of expectations of their family and society begins. Initially there is considerable conformity to rules to win praise or approval from others and to avoid social disapproval or rejection; later, they seek to avoid criticism from people of authority in institutions.
Diversional Activity	
School-agers play co-operatively in group activities such as sports and jumping rope. Play becomes competitive, and children often have difficulty learning to lose. Teasing, insults, dares, superstitions, and increased sensitivity are characteristics of this age.	Many teenagers develop special interests in certain sports and concentrate on developing maximal skills therein. Recreational activities are often determined by what is popular with peers and what can provide independence from parents (e.g., computers, cars).
Nutrition	
Children have definite likes and dislikes. Few nutritional deficiencies occur in this age group. Children have voracious appetites after school and need quality snacks such as fruit and sandwiches to avoid empty calorie foods such as chips and candy.	Total nutritional needs become greater during adolescence. Girls' caloric needs decrease, and their need for protein increases slightly. Adolescents need to increase their consumption of iron-rich foods, and growth spurts increase calcium demand.

The nurse must also increasingly involve the child or adolescent in charting a developmental course. Not only can they describe their feelings about the changes, but they can also think through these changes. Problem solving becomes more purposeful and sophisticated and results in the achievement of the outcomes that they desire. This paced, active participation may initiate a style of involvement in lifelong self-care.

School-age children and adolescents must cope with many changes. For example, 6-year-old children beginning school are confronted with new authority figures, teachers, and new rules and restrictions. They need to cooperatively work and play with a large group of children of various cultural backgrounds. School-age children must meet the challenge of developing cognitive skills that enhance their reasoning and allow them to learn to read, write, and manipulate numbers. Because of the stress of these changes, a child may develop physical and psychosocial health problems (e.g., increased susceptibility to upper respiratory infections, school maladjustment, inadequate peer relationships, or poor performance in school). The nurse designs health promotion interventions that are based on the child's developmental stage.

School-Age Child

During these "middle years" of childhood, the foundation for adult roles in work, recreation, and social interaction is laid. In industrialized countries, this school-age period begins when the child starts formal schooling around the age of 6 years. **Puberty,** around 12 years of age, signals the end of middle childhood. Great developmental strides are made during these years as children develop competencies in physical, cognitive, and psychosocial skills.

The school or educational experience expands the child's world and is a transition from a life of relatively free play to a life of structured play, learning, and work. The school and home influence growth and development, requiring adjustment by the parents and child. The child must learn to cope with rules and expectations presented by the school and peers. Parents must learn to allow their child to make decisions, accept responsibility, and learn from life's experiences.

Physical Changes

The rate of growth during these early school years is slower than any time since birth but continues steadily. A particular child may not follow the pattern precisely. The school-age child appears slimmer than the preschooler as a result of changes in fat distribution and thickness (Edelman & Mandle, 2002). Growth accelerates at different times for different children. The average increase in height is 5 cm per year, and weight, which is more variable, increases by 1.8 to 3.2 kg per year. An average 6-year-old is 112.5-cm tall and weighs 20.9 kg; the average 12-year-old is 147.5-cm tall and weighs 40 kg. Many children double their weight during these middle childhood years (Hockenberry et al., 2003).

School provides children with the opportunity to compare themselves with children of the same age. The physical examination is an excellent opportunity for the nurse to discuss with the child and parents the influences of genetic endowment, nutrition, and exercise on height and weight. Annual measurement of height and weight may reveal alterations in growth that are symptoms of the onset of a variety of childhood diseases.

Boys are slightly taller and heavier than girls during these early school years. Approximately 2 years before puberty, children experience a rapid acceleration in skeletal growth. Girls, who reach puberty first, begin to surpass boys in height and weight, which causes embarrassment to both sexes. Puberty occurs in North American girls between the ages of 9 and 13 years, and in boys, between the ages of 11 and 14 years.

Cardiovascular functioning is refined and stabilized during the school-age years. The heart rate averages 75 to 100 beats per minute, the blood pressure normalizes to approximately 110/65 mm Hg, and the respiratory rate stabilizes to 20 to 30 breaths per minute. Lung growth is minimal, and respirations become slower, deeper, and more regular. However, by the end of this period the heart is six times the size it was at birth and has generally reached its adult size.

School-age children become more graceful during the school years because their large-muscle coordination improves and their strength doubles. Most children practise the basic gross motor skills of running, jumping, balancing, throwing, and catching during play, resulting in refinement of neuromuscular function and skills. Fine motor skills improve and as control is gained over fingers and wrists, children become proficient in a wide range of activities, although there is much individual difference in the rate and degree of proficiency.

Most 6-year-olds can hold a pencil adeptly and print letters and words. By 12 years, the child can make detailed drawings and write sentences in script. Activities such as painting, drawing, playing computer games, and making models allow children to practise and improve newly refined skills. Parents should encourage children to pursue these activities. Table 19-6 describes specific gross motor and fine motor skills and their use in self-care activities.

The improved fine motor capabilities of school-age children allow them to become very independent in bathing, dressing, and taking care of other personal needs. They develop strong personal preferences in the way these needs are met. Illness and hospitalization threaten children's control in these areas; therefore, it is important to allow them to participate in care and maintain as much independence as possible. For example, children whose care demands restriction of fluids cannot be allowed to decide the amount of fluids they will drink in 24 hours, but they can help decide the type of fluids and can help keep a record of intake.

Assessment of neurological development is often based on fine motor coordination. This assessment may include penmanship, stacking ability, and performance of sequential, rapid, alternating movements such as touching the finger to the nose and then to the examiner's finger (smooth movement without tremors is the normal response). Fine motor coordination is critical to success in the typical school, where children must be able to hold pencils and crayons, use scissors and rulers, and develop computer skills. The opportunity to practise

Table 19-6 Motor Development in the School-Age Child

6–7 Years	8–10 Years	11–12 Years
Fine Motor Skills		
Uses knife to butter bread and learns to cut tender meat Cuts, folds, and pastes paper Prints with pencil Draws person with 12–16 details Copies triangle at 6 years and diamond by 7 years Colours within lines of picture Needs assistance to clean teeth thoroughly	Uses knife and fork simultaneously Learns to thread needle and tie knot Uses hammer, saw, and screwdriver Becomes proficient at writing cursive Uses symbols in drawing (e.g., bird, star) Builds simple models of cars and planes and does simple handcrafts Can learn to floss teeth effectively and be independent in tooth care	Learns to peel apples and potatoes Sews simple garments on machine Builds simple objects like birdhouse Enjoys using decorative script Begins to use creative and artistic talents Builds complex models of cars and planes and does complex handcrafts Learns to play musical instrument Becomes proficient in caring for teeth with braces and other appliances
Gross Motor Skills		
Remains in constant motion Moves more cautiously at 7 years than at 6 years Hops and jumps into small squares Learns to roller skate, skip rope, ride bicycle, and swim	Can catch, throw, and hit baseball Engages in alternate rhythmic hopping Engages in complex styles of skipping rope accompanied by verbal jingles	Can do standing broad jump of 1.5 m Can do standing high jump of 1 m Plays games involving simultaneous use of two or more complex motor skills such as rollerblading, skateboarding, or hockey
Self-care		
Takes bath without supervision Often returns to finger feeding Learns to brush and comb hair in acceptable fashion without help Puts on most clothes but may need assistance with final adjustments	Learns to clean bathroom after bath Enjoys fixing own snacks and sack lunch Learns to part hair and insert barrettes Dresses self completely and can help younger siblings with clothes Can make own bed	Dusts, vacuums, and straightens own room Learns to cook simply prepared foods Washes, dries, and fixes own hair Learns to sort, wash, dry, and press own clothing Learns to care for fingernails and toenails

these skills through schoolwork and play is essential to the acquisition of coordinated, complex behaviours.

Other physical changes take place during the school-age years. Steady skeletal growth in the trunk and extremities occurs, and small- and long-bone ossification is present but not complete by 12 years. Dental growth is prominent during the school-age years. The first permanent or secondary teeth erupt at approximately 6 years of age. Development of the permanent teeth has been occurring for some time prior to eruption. The root is absorbed, leaving the crown, which causes the tooth to become loose and fall out. This event makes room for the new permanent tooth. Eruption usually begins with the 6-year molar and follows the same order as with the primary teeth. By 12 years, all primary teeth have been shed, and the majority of permanent teeth have erupted. Infrequent or inadequate dental care remains a persistent problem for many children.

As skeletal growth progresses, body appearance and posture change. Earlier posture, which was characterized by a stoop-shouldered, slight lordosis and prominent abdomen, changes to a more erect posture. It is essential that children, especially girls after the age of 12 years, be evaluated for scoliosis, the lateral curvature of the spine.

Eye shape alters because of skeletal growth. This improves visual acuity, and normal adult 20/20 vision is achievable. Screening for vision and hearing problems is easier, and results are more reliable because school-age children can more fully understand and co-operate with the test directions. The public health nurse typically assesses the dental, visual, and auditory status of school-age children and refers those with possible deviations to their family practitioner or pediatrician.

Cognitive Changes

Cognitive changes provide the school-age child with the ability to think in a logical manner about the here and now and to understand the relationship between things and ideas (Hockenberry et al., 2003). The thoughts of school-age children are no longer dominated by their perceptions, and thus their ability to understand the world greatly expands. Around 7 years of age, children enter Piaget's third stage of cognitive development, known as **concrete operations,** in which they are able to use symbols to carry out operations (mental activities) in thought rather than in action. They begin to use logical thought processes with concrete materials (objects, people, and events they can touch and see).

Children in the concrete operational stage are considerably less egocentric than younger children and develop the ability to concentrate on more than one aspect of a situation. School-age children now have the ability to recognize that the amount or quantity of a substance remains the same even when its shape or appearance changes. For instance, two balls of clay of equal size retain the same amount of clay even when one is flattened and the other remains in ball shape.

The mental process of **classification** becomes more complex during the school years. The young child can separate objects into groups according to shape or colour, whereas the school-age child understands that the same element can exist in two classes at the same time. The school-age child is becoming a "thinker" and is less egocentric and more capable of understanding another's views and feelings (Bukatko & Daehler, 2001).

Middle childhood youngsters can use their newly developed cognitive skills to solve problems. Some individuals are better than others at problem solving because of intelligence, education, and experience, but all children can improve these skills. Children who are good problem solvers demonstrate the following characteristics: a positive attitude that the problem can be solved with persistence, a concern for accuracy, the ability to divide the problem into parts for study, and the ability to avoid guessing while searching for facts. Adults can help children improve their problem-solving strategies by helping them define the problem, plan a solution, and then evaluate their solution. Nurses can use these strategies to help school-age children understand their illness and assume responsibility for their general health.

Language Development. Language growth is so rapid during middle childhood that it is no longer possible to match age with language achievements. Children improve their use of language and expand their structural knowledge. They become more aware of the rules for linking words into phrases and sentences. They can also identify generalizations and exceptions to rules. They accept language as a means for representing the world in a subjective manner and realize that words have arbitrary, rather than absolute, meanings. They can use different words for the same object or concept, and they understand that a single word may have many meanings. Similar to younger children, school-age children watch parents and other adults to gain clues about how to understand events (Deering & Cody, 2002). Many school-age children use "bad language" to gain peer status and to shock adults. It often begins with bathroom language and progresses to sexual or genital words. Children begin to think about language, which enables them to appreciate jokes and riddles. Language acquisition is nurtured by social interactions with their parents and caretakers (Bukatko & Daehler, 2001).

Psychosocial Changes

Erikson (1963) identified the developmental task for school-age children as industry versus inferiority (see chapter 18). During this time, children strive to acquire competence and skills necessary for them to function as adults. School-age children who are positively recognized for success feel a sense of worth. Those faced with failure can feel a sense of unworthiness, which may result in withdrawal from school and peers.

Moral Development. The need for a moral code and social rules becomes more evident as school-age children's cognitive abilities and social experiences increase. For example, 12-year-old children are able to consider what society would be like without rules because of their ability to reason logically and their experiences with group play. They view rules as necessary principles of life, not just dictates from authorities. In the early school years, children strictly interpret and adhere to rules. As they develop, their judgments are more flexible and they can evaluate rules for applicability to a given situation. School-age children consider motivations and behaviour when making judgments about the way their behaviours affect themselves and others. The ability to be flexible when applying rules and to take the perspective of others is essential in developing moral judgments. These abilities are present at times in earlier years but are more consistently displayed in later school years.

Peer Relationships. Group and personal achievements are important to the school-age child. Success is important in physical and cognitive activities. Play involves peers and the pursuit of group goals. Although solitary activities are not eliminated, they are overshadowed by group play. Learning to contribute, collaborate, and work co-operatively toward a common goal becomes a measure of success (Figure 19–6).

The school-age child prefers same-sex peers to opposite-sex peers. In general, girls and boys view the opposite sex negatively. Peer influence becomes diverse during this stage of development. Conformity is evidenced in mannerisms, clothing styles, and speech patterns, which are reinforced and influenced by contact with peers. During this period, clubs and peer groups become prominent. Group identity increases as the school-age child approaches adolescence.

Sexual Identity. Freud described middle childhood as the latency period because he felt that children of this period had little interest in their sexuality. Today, many researchers believe that school-age children have a great deal of curiosity about their sexuality. Some may experiment, but this play is usually transitory. Children's curiosity about adult magazines or meanings of sexually explicit words is also an example of their sexual interest. This is the time for children to have exposure to sex education, including information on sexual maturation, reproduction, and relationships (Edelman & Mandle, 2002).

Health Risks

Accidents and injuries are a major health problem affecting school-age children. Motor vehicle accidents and accidents related to recreational activities or equipment are the leading causes of death or injury from the age of 1 year to adult-

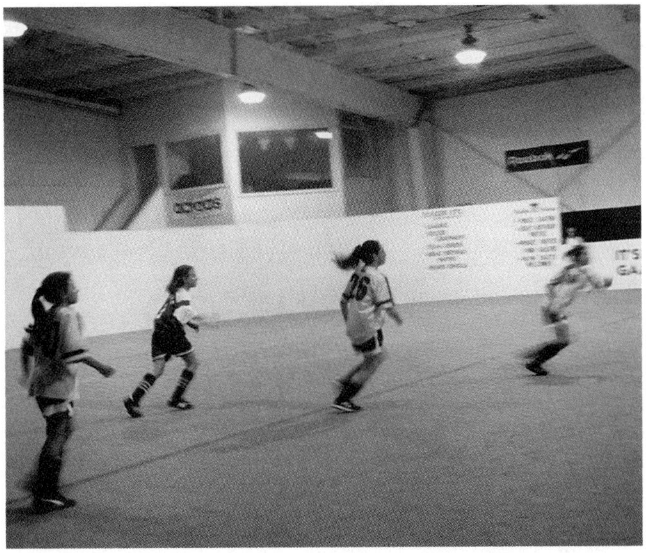

FIGURE **19–6** School-age children gain a sense of achievement by working and playing with peers. (Courtesy Elaine Polan, RNC, BSN, MS.)

hood (Edelman & Mandle, 2002). Unintentional injuries account for nearly half of all childhood deaths (Table 19-7).

Although falls account for a major portion of pediatric hospital admissions, they account for less than 5% of pediatric deaths resulting from injury. However, even though an accident may not result in death, it still can be a major cause of disability in children. More children die from automobile accidents than from all major preventable childhood diseases. The rates of injury and death have begun to decrease with the institution of automobile child restraint laws.

School-age children are also significantly affected by respiratory illnesses, especially asthma, cancer (CICH, 2000), and heart disease (Hockenberry et al., 2003). In this age group, these problems have a relatively low mortality rate but a high morbidity rate compared with accidents. Cancers are the second leading cause of death in children 1 to 14 years of age (Hockenberry et al.). Leukemia is the most frequent type, with brain tumours and lymphoma second and third, respectively.

Infections account for the majority of all childhood illnesses; respiratory infections are the most prevalent. The common cold remains the chief illness of childhood. Children living in poverty are more prone to disease and disability. Intellectual disabilities, learning disorders, sensory impairments, and malnutrition are far more prevalent among children living in poverty (Health Canada, 1999a).

Poverty and the prevalence of illness are highly correlated, probably because access to health promotion and preventative health care activities are minimal for children living in poverty. Poor nutrition and access to early intervention programs continue to be major health concerns for impoverished families. Education, social and health care reform, and environmental change are necessary if the nurse wants to positively influence the health of children. Children's developing cognitive and psychomotor skills make it possible for them to become more involved in health promotion and the management of chronic illness.

Health Concerns

During the school-age years, identity and self-concept become stronger and more individualized. School-age children are aware of their body and are sensitive about being exposed. Nurses should provide for privacy and offer explanations of common procedures. This approach helps foster children's self-esteem and lessens their fear of pain and intrusion (Popovich, 2000).

Health Education. The school-age period is crucial for the acquisition of behaviours and health practices for a healthy adult life. Because cognition is advancing during the period, effective health education must be developmentally appropriate. Promotion of good health practices is a nursing responsibility. A comprehensive school health approach includes programs, activities, and services that take place in schools and their surrounding communities in order to enable children and youth to improve their health and develop to their fullest potential (Canadian Association for School Health, 2003; Box 19-9).

School-age children should receive age-appropriate sexual health education that begins before the onset of sexual activity (Behrman et al., 2000). Other topic areas for elementary health education curricula include the promotion of adequate nutrition, oral hygiene, and regular health supervision. School-age children should also be exposed to programs that highlight tobacco, drug, and alcohol use prevention (Health Canada, 1999a).

Nurses also instruct parents regarding health promotion appropriate for the school-age child. Parents need to recognize the importance of annual checkups for immunizations, screenings, and dental care. When their school-age child reaches 10 years of age, parents need to talk with the child about upcoming pubertal changes. Topics should include introductory information regarding menstruation, sexual intercourse, and reproduction. Nurses should provide age-appropriate written materials to aid parents in their efforts. The settings where health promotion activities can occur are varied, including the classroom, school-based clinic, community-based clinic, or in the community itself.

Table 19-8 presents a list of possible health promotion topics for school-age children.

Safety. Because accidents are the leading cause of death and injury in the school-age period, safety is a priority health teaching consideration. Nurses can contribute to the general health of children by educating them about safety measures to prevent accidents. At this age, children should be encouraged to take responsibility for their own safety.

Nutrition. Nurses can contribute to the promotion of healthy lifestyle habits, including nutrition. School-age children should participate in educational programs that enable them to plan, select, and prepare healthy meals

Table 19-7 Injury Prevention During School-Age Years

Developmental Abilities Related to Risk of Injury	Injury Prevention
	Motor Vehicles
Is increasingly involved in activities away from home Is excited by speed and motion Can be reasoned with Does not always perceive injury risk Is easily distracted by environment	Educate child regarding proper use of seat belts while a passenger in a vehicle Maintain discipline while a passenger in a vehicle (e.g., keep arms inside, do not lean against doors or interfere with driver) Remind parents and children that no one should ride in the bed of a pickup truck Emphasize safe pedestrian behaviour Insist child wears safety apparel (e.g., helmet) where applicable, such as when riding a bicycle or using a skateboard
	Drowning
Is apt to overdo May work hard to perfect a skill Is cautious, but not fearful	Teach child to swim Teach basic rules of water safety Select safe and supervised places to swim Check sufficient water depth for diving Insist child swims with a companion Use an approved flotation device in water or boat Learn CPR
	Burns
Has increasing independence Enjoys trying new things	Make sure smoke detectors are in homes Set hot water temperatures (49° C–54° C) to avoid scald burns Instruct child in behaviour in areas involving contact with potential burn hazards (e.g., gasoline, matches, bonfires or barbecues, lighter fluid, firecrackers, cigarette lighters, cooking utensils, chemistry sets) Instruct child to avoid climbing or flying kites around high-tension wires Instruct child in proper behaviour in the event of fire (e.g., fire drills at home and school) Teach child safe cooking (use low heat, avoid any frying, be careful of steam burns, scalds, or exploding foods, especially from microwaving)
	Substance Abuse and Poisoning
May be easily influenced by peers Has strong allegiance to friends	Educate child regarding hazards of taking non-prescription drugs and chemicals, including tobacco and alcohol Teach child to say "no" if offered illegal or dangerous drugs or alcohol Keep potentially dangerous products in properly labeled receptacles—preferably locked and out of reach
	Bodily Damage
Has increased physical skills Needs strenuous physical activity Is interested in acquiring new skills and perfecting attained skills Is daring and adventurous, especially with peers Frequently plays in hazardous places Confidence often exceeds physical capacity Desires group loyalty and has strong need for friends' approval Attempts hazardous feats Delights in physical activity Is likely to overdo Growth in height exceeds muscular growth and coordination	Help provide facilities for supervised activities Encourage playing in safe places Keep firearms safely locked up Teach proper care of, use of, and respect for devices with potential danger (e.g., power tools) Teach children not to tease or surprise dogs, invade their territory, take dogs' toys, or interfere with dogs' feeding Teach safety regarding use of corrective devices (glasses); if child wears contact lenses, monitor duration of wear to prevent corneal damage Stress careful selection, use, and maintenance of sports and recreation equipment such as skateboards and in-line skates Emphasize proper conditioning, safe practices, and use of safety equipment for sports or recreational activities Caution against engaging in hazardous sports, such as those involving trampolines Use safety glass and decals on large glassed areas, such as sliding glass doors Use window guards to prevent falls Teach stranger safety Avoid personalized clothing in public places Caution child to never go with a stranger Have child tell parents if anyone makes child feel uncomfortable in any way Always listen to child's concerns regarding others' behaviour Teach child to say "no" when confronted with uncomfortable situations

From *Wong's Nursing Care of Infants and Children* (7th ed.), by M. J. Hockenberry et al., 2003, St. Louis, MO: Mosby.

and snacks. These foods should be consistent with *Canada's Food Guide for Healthy Eating* guidelines, which include limiting intake of fats and increasing intake of complex carbohydrates, fruits, and vegetables. Box 19-10 outlines several learning activities appropriate for this age group. In addition, nurses need to encourage daily physical activity for all children.

Growth may slow down during the school-age period compared with infancy and adolescence. Obesity is believed to begin during infancy and childhood (Edelman & Mandle, 2002). Obesity places the child at increased risk for hypertension, diabetes, and coronary heart disease. Emotionally, the obese child is at risk for problems caused by low self-esteem (Jerum & Melnyk, 2001). Obesity may occur because children often rush into the home after school or play and eat the most easily obtainable and appealing foods. Unfortunately, these foods are often high in calories and low in nutrition. Providing nutritious snacks is often the best way for a parent to ensure good nutritional intake. Caregivers should provide ready access to fresh fruit, raw vegetables, cheese, popcorn, and high-protein snacks such as skim-milk pudding and hot chocolate. Children should be praised when making healthy food choices (Jerum & Melnyk, 2001). Nurses must consider cultural, economic, and social issues when planning successful interventions (Edelman & Mandle, 2002).

Nurses can help families and children prevent obesity through proper nutrition and exercise. Today's families may often eat in fast-food restaurants where the food is high in fat, calories, and salt. Nurses need to encourage healthy food choices in these situations. Selections should include meats that are not breaded and are broiled, shakes that are made with low-fat yogurt or skim milk, and fruits and vegetables that are fresh or prepared in a low-calorie manner.

Box 19-9 Critical Functions of Comprehensive School Health

- Promote health promotion and illness prevention measures, with attention to multicultural, linguistic, physical, cognitive, and emotional factors.
- Intervene to assist children and youth who are in need or at risk.
- Help support those who are already experiencing poor health.
- Foster parental education on health issues.
- Identify learning disabilities early and begin appropriate interventions to foster learning and self-esteem.
- Facilitate growth and self-actualization.
- Emphasize positive health attitudes.
- Foster positive life skills that enhance successful coping.
- Encourage involvement of individuals, families and communities as active partners in their health care.

Adapted from *Consensus statement on comprehensive school health,* Canadian Association for School Health, 2003. Retrieved November 3, 2004, from *http://www.schoolfile.com/cash/consensus.htm*

Adolescent

Adolescence is the period of development between childhood and adulthood, usually between 12 and 19 years of age. The term *adolescent* usually refers to psychological maturation of the individual, whereas *puberty* refers to the point at which reproduction becomes possible. The hormonal changes of puberty result in changes in the appearance of the young person (i.e., the primary sexual characteristic involving the reproductive organs mature and the secondary sexual characteristic changes such as the development of pubic hair and female breasts begin). Mental development during puberty results in the ability to hypothesize and deal with abstractions. In addition, adolescents become much more social, and their behavioural patterns become much less predictable. Adjustments and adaptations are needed to cope with these simultaneous changes and the attempt to establish a mature sense of identity. In the past, many have re-

Table 19-8 Health Promotion for the School-Age Child

School-Age Health Concerns	Health Promotion Interventions
Nutrition	Provide nutrition education that promotes healthy lifestyle; e.g., limiting fat intake to 30% of calories, saturated fat to 10% of calories.
Oral hygiene	Provide examples of low cariogenic snacks. Review mechanics of dental hygiene: brushing, flossing. Stress importance of biannual dental checkups.
Infections	Provide immunization information and follow-up. Teach infection prevention practices (hand washing, care of minor skin injuries). Teach concepts of viral and bacterial illness.
Tobacco, alcohol, and drug use	Provide tobacco use prevention programs. Provide information regarding the hazards of drug use.
Human sexuality	Provide information about sexual maturation and reproduction in age-appropriate manner. Encourage parents to view their child's sexual curiosity as part of the developmental process. Discuss with parents the learning needs of their child regarding sexuality. Provide age-appropriate sexual health education.

Box 19-10 Interventions to Promote Nutrition Education

Make healthy foods (fruits, vegetables, whole grains, low-fat snacks) available in school vending machines and at school sporting events.
Discourage the use of high-fat foods (chocolate bars) as part of school fund-raising projects.
Avoid the use of food as rewards for behaviour; use verbal praise and token gifts to reinforce healthy eating and physical activity.
Have teachers and school personnel model healthy eating habits.
Ask children to select foods from a fast-food restaurant menu and to identify those foods high in fat, cholesterol, and sodium.
Ask each child to keep a diary of foods eaten in 1 day; using *Canada's Food Guide for Healthy Eating,* evaluate these foods.
Have students keep a diary to identify cues for their eating behaviour (e.g., hunger, stress, other people, social situations).
Teach students how to read and discuss the nutrition labels on foods.
Ask students to examine television commercials, magazine advertisements, and billboards to identify social influences on eating and physical activities.
Use role-playing to help students learn to cope with social and peer pressures to eat specific foods.
Have students identify environmental barriers to healthy eating.
Have students prepare nutritious foods, plan menus, and develop a recipe book of healthy foods.
Involve parents in nutrition education through homework assignments or by inviting parents to attend student-led nutrition fairs.

Modified from "Guidelines for School Programs to Promote Lifelong Healthy Eating," by Center for Communicable Diseases, 1997 *Journal of School Health, 67,* pp. 9–26 .

ferred to adolescence as a stormy and stressful period filled with inner turmoil, but today it is recognized that most teenagers successfully meet the challenges of this period. These challenges may cause the adolescent to be moody and difficult. Within adolescence, three subphases exist: early adolescence, including puberty (12 to 14 years), middle adolescence (14 to 17 years), and late adolescence (17 to 19 years). Opportunities, challenges, changes, skills, pressures, and physical, cognitive, and psychosocial development vary widely between the subphases (Table 19-9).

The nurse's understanding of development provides a unique perspective for helping teenagers and parents anticipate and cope with the stresses of adolescence. Primary health care activities, particularly education, can promote healthy development. These activities occur in a variety of settings and can be directed at the adolescent, parents, or both. For example, the nurse can conduct seminars in a high school to provide practical suggestions for solving problems of concern to a large group of students, such as treating acne or making responsible decisions about drugs or alcohol use. Similarly, a group education program for parents about how to cope with teenagers would promote parental understanding of adolescent development. These programs can be held in the school, clinic, private office, or community centre. To learn more about specific topics or problems, the nurse must identify teenagers' needs and desires. Involvement produces more active, interested learners.

Physical Changes

Physical changes occur rapidly in adolescence. Sexual maturation occurs with the development of primary and secondary sexual characteristics. Four main focuses of the physical changes are as follows:

- Increased growth rate of skeleton, muscle, and viscera
- Sex-specific changes, such as changes in shoulder and hip width
- Alteration in distribution of muscle and fat
- Development of the reproductive system and secondary sex characteristics

Wide variation exists in the timing of physical changes associated with puberty between sexes and within the same sex. Girls tend to begin their physical changes earlier than boys. Variations are more pronounced in boys (Behrman et al., 2000). The sequence of pubertal growth changes is the same in most individuals (Table 19-10).

Changes are created by hormonal fluctuations within the body when the hypothalamus begins to produce gonadotropin-releasing hormones. This change sends the pituitary a signal to secrete gonadotropic hormones. Gonadotropic hormones stimulate ovarian cells to produce **estrogen** and testicular cells to produce **testosterone.** These hormones contribute to the development of secondary sex characteristics such as hair growth and voice changes and play an essential role in reproduction. The changing concentrations of these hormones are also linked to acne and body odour. Understanding these hormonal changes enables the nurse to reassure adolescents and educate them about body care needs.

Boys who mature early have been shown by some researchers to be more poised, relaxed, good-natured, skilled in athletic activities, and more likely to be school leaders than boys who mature late. In contrast, girls who mature early have been found to be less sociable and more shy and introverted, perhaps from feeling so conspicuous (Edelman & Mandle, 2002).

Being like their peers is extremely important for adolescents. Nurses need to stress that there are ranges of normal for sexual changes. As with increases in height and weight, the pattern of sexual changes is more significant than their time of onset. Large deviations from normal frames require investigation.

Any deviation in the timing of the physical changes can be extremely difficult for adolescents to accept. The nurse should therefore provide emotional support for those undergoing early or delayed puberty. Even adoles-

Table 19-9 Growth and Development During Adolescence

Early Adolescence (11–14 years)	Middle Adolescence (14–17 years)	Late Adolescence (17–20 years)
Growth		
Rapidly accelerating growth reaches peak velocity Secondary sex characteristics appear	Growth decelerating in girls Stature reaches 95% of adult height Secondary sex characteristics well-advanced	Physically mature Structure and reproductive growth almost complete
Cognition		
Explores newfound ability for limited abstract thought Experience uncertainty as they are confronted with new values Comparison of "normality" with peers of same sex	Developing capacity for abstract thinking Enjoys intellectual powers, often in idealistic terms Concern with philosophic, political, and social problems	Establishes abstract thought Can perceive and act on long-range operations Able to view problems comprehensively Intellectual and functional identity established
Identity		
Preoccupied with rapid body changes Tries out various roles Measurement of attractiveness by acceptance or rejection of peers Conformity to group norms	Modifies body image Very self-centred; increased narcissism Tendency toward inner experience and self-discovery Has a rich fantasy life Idealistic Able to perceive future implications of current behaviour and decisions; variable application	Body image and gender-role definition nearly secured Mature sexual identity Phase of consolidation of identity Stability of self-esteem Comfortable with physical growth Social roles defined and articulated
Relationships With Parents		
Defining independence-dependence boundaries Strong desire to remain dependent on parents while trying to detach No major conflicts over parental control	Major conflicts over independence and control Low point in parent-child relationship Greatest push for emancipation; disengagement Final and irreversible emotional detachment from parents; mourning	Emotional and physical separation from parents completed Independence from family with less conflict Emancipation nearly secured
Relationships With Peers		
Seeks peer affiliations to counter instability generated by rapid change Upsurge of close, idealized friendships with members of the same sex Struggle for mastery takes place within peer group	Strong need for identity to affirm self-image Behavioural standards set by peer group Acceptance by peers extremely important—fear of rejection Exploration of ability to attract the opposite sex	Peer group recedes in importance in favour of individual friendship Testing of male-female relationships against possibility of permanent alliance Relationships characterized by giving and sharing
Sexuality		
Self-exploration and evaluation Limited dating, usually socializes with a group Limited intimacy	Multiple plural relationships Decisive turn toward heterosexuality (if is homosexual, knows by this time) Exploration of "self-appeal" Feeling of "being in love" Tentative establishment of relationships	Forms stable relationships and attachment to another Growing capacity for mutuality and reciprocity Dating Intimacy involves commitment rather than exploration and romanticism
Psychological Health		
Wide mood swings Intense daydreaming Anger outwardly expressed with moodiness, temper outbursts, and verbal insults and name-calling	Tendency toward inner experiences; more introspective Tendency to withdraw when upset or feelings are hurt Vacillation of emotions in time and range Feelings of inadequacy common; difficulty in asking for help	More constancy of emotion Anger more apt to be concealed

From *Wong's Nursing Care of Infants and Children* (7th ed.), by M. J. Hockenberry et al., 2003, St. Louis, MO: Mosby.

Table 19-10 Average Sequences of Physiological Changes in Adolescence

Characteristics	Girls*	Boys*
Beginning of skeletal growth spurt	8–14½ (peak: 12)	10½–16 (peak: 14)
Beginning of breast development	8–13	
Enlargement of testes and scrotal sac		10–13½
Appearance of straight, pigmented pubic hair, which gradually becomes curly	8–14	10–15
Early voice changes (cracks)		11–14½
Enlargement of penis and prostate gland		11–14½
Menarche	10–18 (average: 12¼)	
Spermatogenesis (ejaculation of sperm)		11–17 (average: 13½)
Ovulation and completion of breast development	14–18 (average: 15½)	
Appearance of downy facial hair		12–17
Appearance of axillary (underarm) hair and increased output of oil and sweat-producing glands, which may lead to acne	10–16	12–17
Widening and deepening of female pelvis, with deposition of subcutaneous fat that gives rounded appearance to body	10–18	
Increase in shoulder width		11–21
Deepening of voice in males, with appearance of coarse and pigmented facial hair and appearance of chest hair		16–21

*Age range is in years.

cents whose physical changes are occurring at the normal times may seek reassurance about their normalcy.

Height and weight increases usually occur during the prepubertal growth spurt. The growth spurt for girls generally begins between 8 and 14 years of age. Height increases 5 to 20 cm, and weight increases by 7 to 25 kg. The male growth spurt usually takes place between 10 and 16 years of age. Height increases approximately 10 to 30 cm, and weight increases by 7 to 30 kg. The final 20% to 25% of adult height and 50% of adult weight is gained during this time (Hockenberry et al., 2003).

Girls attain 90% to 95% of their adult height by **menarche** (the onset of menstruation) and reach their full height by 16 to 17 years of age, whereas boys continue to grow taller until 18 to 20 years of age. Fat is redistributed into adult proportions as height and weight increase, and gradually the adolescent torso takes on an adult appearance. Although there are individual and sex differences, growth follows a similar pattern for both sexes. Growth in the length of the extremities occurs earliest, making the hands and feet appear very large and the legs very long; the individual often appears awkward and clumsy. At the same time, the lower jaw and nose become longer and the forehead higher and wider as the baby face of childhood disappears. Next, the thighs widen; then the shoulders broaden, and growth of the trunk proceeds. Widening of the female hips and broadening of the male shoulders continue throughout adolescence.

Personal growth curves help the nurse assess physical development. The individual's sustained progression along the curve, however, is more important than a comparison with the norm. The nurse charts growth measurements during routine health assessments to evaluate changes.

Adolescents are sensitive about physical changes that make them different from peers. For this reason, they are generally interested in the normal pattern of growth and their personal growth curves. Consequently, the nurse should share this information to reassure adolescents that their own patterns are normal.

Cognitive Changes

According to Piaget, the changes that occur within the mind and the widening social environment of the adolescent result in the highest level of intellectual development, known as formal operations (see chapter 18). However, without an appropriate educational environment, some people may not attain this stage. Those who are guided toward rational thinking may reach this stage early.

The adolescent develops the ability to determine possibilities, rank possibilities, solve problems, and make decisions through logical operations. The teenager can think abstractly and deal effectively with hypothetical problems. When confronted with a problem, the teenager can consider an infinite variety of causes and solutions. The adolescent can move beyond the physical or concrete properties of a situation and use reasoning powers to understand the abstract. School-age children think about what is, whereas adolescents can imagine what might be. These newly developed abilities allow the individual to have more insight and skill in playing video games, computer games, and board games that require abstract thinking and deductive reasoning about many possible strategies. A teenager can solve problems requiring simultaneous manipulation of several abstract concepts.

Development of this ability to reason abstractly is important in the pursuit of an identity. For example, newly acquired cognitive skills allow the teenager to define appropriate, effective, and comfortable sex-role behaviours and to consider their impact on peers, family, and society. The ability to think logically about these behaviours and their outcomes encourages the adolescent to develop personal thoughts and means of expressing sexual identity. In addition, a higher level of cognitive functioning makes the adolescent receptive to more detailed and diverse information about sexuality and sexual behaviours. For example, sex education can include an explanation of physiological sexual changes and birth control measures.

By middle adolescence, an introspective quality emerges. At this time, adolescents believe that they are unique, giving rise to their risk-taking behaviours. They often express that they "can drive fast and not get into an accident." Other typical adolescent behaviours include self-consciousness and the desire for privacy.

The complex development of thought during this period leads adolescents to question society and its values. Although adolescents have the capability to think as well as an adult, they do not have experiences on which to build. It is common for teenagers to consider their parents too narrow-minded or too materialistic. This perception can result in conflicts between teens and their parents. Cognitive abilities and performance vary greatly among adolescents. In fact, an adolescent may perform at different levels in different situations on the basis of past experiences, formal education, and motivation in the use of logic and effective deductive reasoning.

Language Skills. Language development is fairly complete by adolescence, although vocabulary continues to expand. The primary focus becomes communication skills that can be used effectively in various situations. Adolescents need to communicate thoughts, feelings, and facts to others. The skills used in communication situations are varied. Adolescents must select the person with whom to communicate, decide on the message, and choose the way to transmit the message. For example, the way teenagers tell parents about failing grades is not the same as the way that they tell friends. Adolescents develop different skills and styles of communication and learn how and when to use them most effectively. These diverse communication skills are used and refined throughout life (Deering & Cody, 2002). Good communication skills are critical for overcoming peer pressure and unhealthy behaviours. The following are some hints for communicating with adolescents:

- Do not avoid discussing sensitive issues. Asking questions about sex, drugs, and school opens the channels for further discussion.
- Ask open-ended questions.
- Look for the meaning behind their words or actions.
- Be alert to clues to their emotional state.
- Involve other individuals and resources when necessary.

Psychosocial Changes

The search for personal identity is the major task of adolescent psychosocial development. Teenagers must establish close peer relationships or remain socially isolated. Erikson (1963) viewed identity (or role) confusion as the prime danger of this stage and suggested that the cliquishness and intolerance of differences seen in adolescent behaviour are defences against identity confusion (Erikson, 1968). Adolescents work at becoming emotionally independent from their parents, while retaining family ties. In addition, they need to develop their own ethical systems based on personal values. Choices about vocation, future education, and lifestyle must be made. The various components of total identity evolve from these tasks and compose adult personal identity that is unique to the individual. Indecisiveness and the inability to make an occupational choice are behaviours indicating negative resolution of the developmental task.

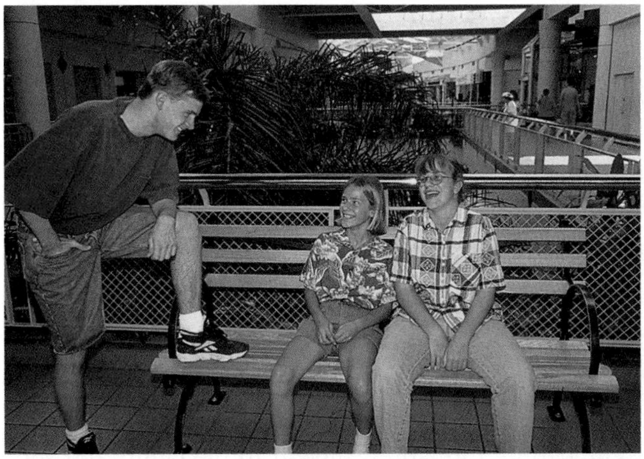

FIGURE **19–7** Social interactions strengthen a teen's identity.

Gender Identity. Achievement of gender identity is enhanced by the physical changes of puberty. According to Freud, these physiological changes of puberty stimulate the libido, the energy source that fuels the sex drive (see chapter 18). This change is evidenced by the teenager's interest in romantic relationships, as well as by their practice of masturbation. The physical evidence of maturity encourages the development of masculine and feminine behaviours. If these physical changes involve deviations, the person has more difficulty developing a comfortable sexual identity. Adolescents depend on these physical clues because they want assurance of maleness or femaleness and because they do not wish to be different from peers.

Other influences on gender identity are cultural attitudes and expectations of sex-role behaviour and available role models (Katz, 2003). The masculine and feminine behaviours that teenagers see affect the way that they express sexuality.

Group Identity. Adolescents seek a group identity because they need esteem and acceptance (Figure 19–7). Similarity in dress or speech is common in teenage groups. Popularity is a major concern for teens. Peer groups provide the adolescent with a sense of belonging, approval, and the opportunity to learn acceptable behaviour. Popularity with opposite-sex and same-sex peers is important. The strong need for group identity seems to conflict at times with the search for personal identity. It is as though adolescents require close bonds with peers so that they can later achieve a sense of individuality.

Family Identity. The movement toward stronger peer relationships contrasts with adolescents' movements away from parents. Although financial independence for adolescents is not the norm in Canadian society, many adolescents work part time, using their income to bolster independence. When adolescents cannot have a part-time job because of studies, school-related activities, and other factors, parents can provide allowances for clothing and incidentals, which encourage adolescents to develop decision-making and budgeting skills.

Some adolescents and families have more difficulty during these years than others. Adolescents need to make choices, act independently, and experience the consequences of actions. This testing, however, is best done against a firm, supportive, family foundation. The family needs to allow independence while providing a haven in which adolescents can contemplate actions. Families unable to provide this support complicate movement toward identity formation. Support to the family and adolescent may be essential to their success.

Nurses can assist families in considering ways that are appropriate for them to foster the independence of their adolescent while maintaining family structure. Many of these discussions often involve curfews, jobs, and participation in family chores. Emancipation from the immediate family is most successful when accomplished gradually and results in a balance between independence and family ties.

Vocational Identity. Selecting an occupation or a vocational direction in life is a goal for adolescents. Because of society's changing needs, adolescents must be future oriented when making these choices. However, adolescents do not know which jobs will be available and rewarding 10 or 20 years in the future, and thus selecting a career is a complicated task. The nurse should provide emotional support during this process and help adolescents select courses of action that promote self-satisfaction, identity, and continued opportunity for growth.

Moral Identity. The development of moral judgment depends heavily on cognitive and communication skills and peer interaction. Although moral development begins in early childhood, it is consolidated in adolescence because of the presence of certain skills. Adolescents learn that rules are co-operative agreements that can be modified to fit the situation, rather than absolutes. Regarding rules, adolescents learn to use their own judgment rather than to use the rules to avoid punishment as in earlier years. Kohlberg (1964) explained moral development in terms of stages (see chapter 18). At the highest level, morality is derived from individual principles of conscience. Adolescents judge themselves by internalized ideals, which often leads to conflict between personal and group values. Group values become less significant in later adolescence.

Not all adolescents attain the same level of moral development. There is, however, a general forward movement through the stages of moral development, and the sequence of the stages is similar for all individuals, even when their time of achievement varies. Kohlberg's moral development theory (1964) focuses on justice based on reciprocity and equal respect. Females have been found to be more likely to give caring responses to moral problems. Males have been found to give more justice-oriented responses.

Health Identity. Healthy adolescents evaluate their own health according to feelings of well-being, ability to function normally, and absence of symptoms (CICH, 2000; Hockenberry et al., 2003).

Interventions to improve health perception might, therefore, concentrate on the adolescent period. The rapid changes during this period make primary health care programs especially crucial. Adolescents try new roles, begin to stabilize their identity, and acquire values and behaviours from which their adult lifestyle will evolve.

Health Risks

Injuries. Injuries, including self-inflicted injuries and injuries caused by motor vehicle accidents and poisoning, are the leading cause of death in adolescents (CICH, 2000). Feelings of being indestructible lead to risk-taking behaviour. Many injuries are preceded by the use of alcohol (Health Canada, 1999a). Youths continue to be both the victims and perpetrators of violence.

Suicide. Suicide is increasing as a cause of death in adolescents between 15 and 19 years of age, particularly among Aboriginal youth (CIHI, 2000). Depression and social isolation commonly precede a suicide attempt, but suicide probably results from a combination of several factors (Box 19-11).

The nurse must be able to identify the factors associated with adolescent suicide risk and precipitating events. In addition, the nurse should be alert to the following warning signs, which often occur for at least a month before suicide is attempted:

- Decrease in school performance
- Withdrawal
- Loss of initiative
- Loneliness, sadness, and crying
- Appetite and sleep disturbances
- Verbalization of suicidal thought

Immediate referrals to mental health professionals need to be made when assessment suggests that adolescents may be considering suicide. Guidance can help them focus on the positive aspects of life and strengthen coping abilities.

Substance Abuse. Adolescents may believe that mood-altering substances create a sense of well-being or improve level of performance. All adolescents are at risk for experimental or recreational substance use, but those who have dysfunctional families are more at risk for chronic use and physical dependency. Some adolescents believe that substance use makes them more mature. They further believe that they will look and feel better with drug usage. The majority of adolescents experiment with marijuana. Other substances frequently abused by teens include steroids, which are used to enhance their athletic performances. It is believed that the use of these products may increase the likelihood of using other illicit drugs (Health Canada, 1999a).

Tobacco use continues to be a problem among adolescents and is carefully monitored within Canada (Canadian

Box 19-11 Suicide Risk Assessment

History

Previous suicide attempt
Family member or friend has attempted suicide
History of child abuse or neglect
Past psychiatric hospitalization
Death of a parent when child was young

Individual Factors

Hopelessness
Marked, persistent depression
Alcohol or drug abuse
Impulsive
Difficulty tolerating frustration
Feelings of self-hatred or excessive guilt, feelings of humiliation
Thinking disorder (wishes to join a deceased person, hears voices telling to kill self)
Physical/body image problems (delayed puberty, chronic illness, disability, attention deficit hyperactivity disorder, learning disorders)
Gender identity concerns; gay or lesbian in an unsupportive environment
Sees self as totally helpless—a victim of fate
A need to do things perfectly

Family Factors

Difficult home situation—long, bitter parent-child conflict
Hostile parents
Overt rejection by one or both parents
Divorce or separation of parents
Recent or impending move
Family breakup or parental loss
Exposure to unrealistically high parental expectations
Parental indifference with very low expectations

Social/Environmental Factors

Firearms in the home
Incarceration
Lack of effective social support system
Isolation
Exposure to suicide of another
Few social, vocational, educational opportunities

From *Wong's Nursing Care of Infants and Children* (7th ed.), by M. J. Hockenberry et al., 2003, St. Louis, MO: Mosby.

Tobacco Use Monitoring Survey, 2001). In 2001, 22.5% of 15- to 19-year-olds in Canada smoked cigarettes. The federal *Tobacco Act* passed in 1997 prohibits the sale of tobacco products to those under the age of 18 years. However, the federal government depends on the provinces to enforce this act and compliance of retailers varies (Canadian Cancer Society, 2002).

Eating Disorders. The number of eating disorders is on the rise in adolescent girls, and knowledge of growth progression may be a way to discourage radical weight reduction activities. If an adolescent deviates radically from the usual pattern, further assessment is necessary to identify the cause. Areas to include in the assessment are past and present diet history, food records, eating habits, attitudes, health beliefs, and socio-economic and psychosocial factors (Hockenberry et al., 2003; Kail, 2001). Weight extremes resulting from excessive or inadequate caloric intake are common during the adolescent years. Allowing the adolescent to see when and how the weight curve changed can be a first step in identifying the problem and implementing dietary changes.

Although anorexia nervosa and bulimia are classified as separate eating disorders, there is significant overlap between the two (Kail, 2001). Anorexia nervosa is considered a clinical syndrome with both physical and psychosocial components. The majority of clients are adolescents and young women. Attending a highly competitive high school and being from a professional, upper-middle-class family increases the risk for this disorder. People with anorexia nervosa have an intense fear of gaining weight and refuse to maintain body weight at the minimal normal weight for their age and height.

Bulimia nervosa is most identified with binge eating and behaviours to prevent weight gain, including self-induced vomiting, misuse of laxatives and other medications, and excessive exercise (Kail, 2001). Because adolescents rarely volunteer information about behaviours to prevent weight gain, it is important to take a thorough dietary history. Bulimia is considered a biopsychosocial illness. Society's expectations for thinness may have a strong influence on the development of these eating disorders. Eating disorders are thought to be more common among females, but it is important to note that males may suffer from these disorders as well. Causes of eating disorders are the same for both females and males.

Sexual Experimentation. Sexual experimentation is common among adolescents. Peer pressure, physiological and emotional changes, and societal expectations contribute to early heterosexual and homosexual relations. Two prominent consequences of adolescent sexual activity are sexually transmitted infections and pregnancy (Bukatko & Daehler, 2001).

Sexually Transmitted Infections. The incidence of **sexually transmitted infections (STIs)** is increasing in adolescents (CICH, 2000). Therefore, sexually active adolescents must be screened for STIs, even when they have no symptoms. The annual physical examination of a sexually active adolescent should include a thorough sexual history and a careful examination of the genitalia so that genital warts, herpes, and other STIs are not missed. Recommended tests for women include Papanicolaou (Pap) smears, cervical cultures for gonorrhea and *Chlamydia* species, and syphilis tests; for men, urethral cultures for gonorrhea and *Chlamydia* species and syphilis tests are recommended. If men have participated in homosexual activities, rectal and pharyngeal cultures also need to be taken to check for gonorrhea. The health care provider can be proactive by using the interview process to identify risk factors in the adolescent (Berk, 2003). Once identified, the risk factors should lead to strategies for prevention.

Human immunodeficiency virus (HIV), which causes acquired immunodeficiency syndrome (AIDS), is transmitted through unprotected sexual intercourse, the use of shared needles, and infected blood products (see chapter 23). Therefore, the risk-taking behaviours of adolescent sexual activity and drug use make adolescents vulnerable to the threat of AIDS and other STIs. Adolescents who have placed themselves at risk for AIDS should be tested for HIV. Knowledge of HIV/AIDS needed to be improved among adolescents (Council of Ministers of Education, 2003).

Pregnancy. In a national survey, 7% of the sexually active girls in grades 9 and 11 reported they became pregnant and 6% of the sexually active boys reported getting a partner pregnant (Council of Ministers of Education, 2003). Adolescent pregnancy occurs across socio-economic classes, in public and private schools, among all ethnic and religious backgrounds, and in all parts of the country. Teenage pregnancy with early prenatal supervision is considered less harmful to both mother and child than earlier believed. Pregnant teens need special attention to nutrition, as well as health supervision and psychological support.

Health Concerns

Adolescents must form healthy habits of daily living. The nurse needs to emphasize the importance of exercise, sleep, nutrition, and stress reduction habits and to identify ways to adapt them to each adolescent. To do this, the nurse must assess the individual's positive and negative habits and attitudes about health. Extensive and long-term follow-up is required if individualized interventions are to succeed. The nurse needs to be aware of the prevalence of health problems and to make assessments accordingly.

Health Education. Community and school-based health programs for adolescents focus on health promotion and illness prevention. Nurses are involved in community health through screening and teaching programs (Table 19-11).

Through their primary health care efforts in the school and community, nurses can make a contribution in improving the health of adolescents (Health Canada, 1999a). Discussions with adolescents must be private and confidential. Deering and Cody (2002) found that for adolescents to reveal intimate information about their risk-taking behaviours, they must first feel comfortable and respected as individuals. Developing and implementing programs to respond to adolescents' needs are an important strategy. Helping adolescents make decisions about their health care strengthens their autonomy and promotes healthy behaviours (Dickey & Deatrick, 2000; McGahee, Kemp, & Tingen, 2000).

Nurses can play an important role in preventing injuries and accidental deaths. Injury prevention activities; support of organizations that promote responsible behaviour, including Mothers Against Drunk Driving (MADD) and Drug Abuse Resistance Education (DARE); and encouragement of students to participate in organizations such as Students Against Drunk Driving (SADD) are types of important activities. Stimulating adolescents to discuss alternatives to driving when under the influence of drugs or alcohol prepares them to consider alternatives when such an occasion arises. The nurse must identify those adolescents at risk for abuse, provide education to prevent accidents related to substance abuse, and provide counselling to those in rehabilitation.

Nurses can play a strategic role in an anti-smoking movement. Smoke prevention programs can be initiated

Table 19-11 Health Promotion for the Adolescent

Adolescent Health Concerns	Health Promotion Intervention
Unintentional injuries	Advise adolescent to take driver's education course and to wear seat belts. Inform the adolescent of risk associated with drinking and driving, use of drugs. Promote helmet use by adolescent bicyclists and motorcyclists. Ensure adolescent receives proper orientation to the use of all sports equipment. Encourage adolescent to swim with a "buddy."
Firearm use and violence	Teach conflict resolution skills.
Tobacco, alcohol, and drug use	Screen for tobacco (including smokeless), alcohol, and drug use and inform of the risks of use.
Suicide	Offer suicide prevention information. Teach methods to deal with a suicidal peer. Promote suicide alternatives.
Sexually transmitted infections	Provide adolescent with information regarding disease, mode of transmission, and related symptoms. Encourage safer sex; including abstinence from sexual activity or the use of condoms. Provide accurate information about the consequences of sexual activity.

in schools. Peer-support programs have been found to be a good means of preventing smoking. Communities can also play a role in creating tobacco control policies at the local level (Dickey & Deatrick, 2000).

The nurse must provide sex education and counselling. Nurses play a key role in counselling teenagers on ways to avoid pregnancies. The nurse can also assist adolescents in making decisions about the pregnancy (e.g., becoming a parent, adoption, or abortion). Some schools have instituted day-care programs so that the adolescent mother can continue her schooling after the baby is born. Whatever choice the adolescent makes, it is important that she receive appropriate health care including counselling.

Extensive educational efforts to prevent the spread of AIDS and other STIs in this age group are a nursing responsibility. Formal or informal education, in a one-on-one or group setting, may occur in the school or community. Speakers and organizations can be used to help in the educational process.

Rural Adolescents. Approximately 22% of Canadians live in rural areas; however, this percentage varies by province and territory. Areas of concern for adolescents living in rural areas are limited privacy, recreational facilities, and access to specialized services.

Nurses can play an important role in improving the health of the adolescent living in rural areas. Decreasing barriers to care, health promotion education, development of coping strategies, and assessment of health beliefs are important areas for the nurse to address.

Minority Adolescents. By the next century, it is expected that minorities as a group will become the majority. Minority adolescents have been identified as experiencing a greater percentage of health problems and barriers to health care.

Issues of concern for these adolescents living in a high-risk environment include learning or emotional difficulties, death related to violence, unintentional injuries, and increased rate for adolescent pregnancy and STIs, including AIDS. Poverty is a major factor negatively affecting the lives of minority adolescents. Limited access to culturally appropriate health services is common. Nurses can make a significant contribution to improving access to appropriate health care for adolescents. Health promotion initiatives must be based on topics of concern for these adolescents.

Nurses working in the community must adopt culturally sensitive interventions to meet the needs of minority adolescents and their families (Hockenberry et al., 2003). They must be able to communicate in another language by speaking it or using an interpreter. Teaching materials need to be written in the appropriate language. Information regarding health beliefs and healing practices must be assessed. With knowledge about various cultures and the means to care for minority adolescents, the nurse acts as an advocate to ensure accessibility of appropriate services.

Aboriginal Adolescents. Health status and factors affecting it are worse for Canadian Aboriginal adolescents than any other adolescent population. Suicide is a greater problem among Aboriginal youth than other youth in Canada, especially among young males (CICH, 2000). Aboriginal adolescents are more likely to have crowded living conditions and live in communities where alcohol and substance abuse is high. Likewise, the incidence of unemployment and reported sexual and physical abuse is higher than in non-Aboriginal communities (Health Canada, 1999a). Some problems persist for Aboriginal peoples, such as overcrowded living conditions and high rates of employment when they live in urban areas of Canada.

Nurses working with Aboriginal adolescents need to be aware of the unique factors that may affect these young people's health. They need to be sensitive to culturally appropriate interventions. Many Aboriginal communities are taking responsibility for their own health and well-being, developing their own health services, and including traditional methods of healing to improve well-being.

Key Concepts

- A developmental perspective helps the nurse understand commonalities and variations in each stage and the impact they have on the client's health.
- During the intrauterine period, while embryo and fetus grow and develop, genetic factors and environmental factors (teratogens) may cause impairments in any body system.
- Physiological, cognitive, and psychosocial development continue from conception through adolescence, and the nurse must be familiar with normal parameters to determine potential problems and promote normal development.
- Physical growth during the school years is slow and steady until the skeletal growth spurt just before puberty.
- The major psychosocial developmental task of the school-age child is the development of a sense of competence.
- Cognitively, the young school-age child develops the ability to think in a logical manner.
- The prepubertal growth spurt usually occurs 2 years earlier in girls than in boys.
- Adolescents move forward to the last stage of cognitive development, formal operations, in which they begin to think in an abstract manner, reflect on thought processes, and plan for the future.
- Adolescence begins with puberty, when the primary sexual characteristic involving the reproductive organs mature and the secondary sexual characteristic changes such as the development of pubic hair and female breasts begin.
- Adolescents are able to solve complex mental problems by using deductive reasoning.
- The adolescent's rapid change in physical appearance heightens self-consciousness and concerns regarding body image.
- Accidents are the major cause of death in all age groups.

- Motor vehicle accidents are the major cause of accidental death in adolescence.
- Adolescents begin the long process of emancipation from their parents and need parental support to accomplish this in a timely manner.

Key Terms

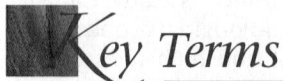

Adolescence, *p. 385*
Animism, *p. 376*
Apgar score, *p. 359*
Artificialism, *p. 376*
Blastocyst, *p. 358*
Bonding, *p. 361*
Classification, *p. 381*
Concrete operations, *p. 381*
Embryo, *p. 358*
Estrogen, *p. 386*
Fertilization, *p. 358*
Fetus, *p. 359*
Fontanels, *p. 362*
Hyperbilirubinemia, *p. 364*
Immanent justice, *p. 376*
Implantation, *p. 358*
Inborn errors of metabolism, *p. 364*
Infancy, *p. 364*
Lanugo, *p. 359*
Menarche, *p. 388*
Molding, *p. 362*
Morula, *p. 358*
Nagele's rule, *p. 358*
Neonatal period, *p. 361*
Object permanence, *p. 373*
Organogenesis, *p. 359*
Placenta, *p. 358*
Prematurity, *p. 362*
Preoperational thought, *p. 373*
Preschool period, *p. 374*
Preterm labour, *p. 359*
Puberty, *p. 380*
Quickening, *p. 359*
School-age, *p. 378*
Sexually transmitted infections (STIs), *p. 392*
Teratogens, *p. 389*
Testosterone, *p. 386*
Toddlerhood, *p. 371*
Vernix caseosa, *p. 359*
Zygote, *p. 358*

Critical Thinking Exercises

1. Mrs. Yeigh is attending the antepartum clinic for the first visit. A major area for focus is health promotion. What other topics should the nurse present at this time? Mrs. Yeigh asks whether it is better to breast-feed or bottle-feed.
2. The parents of 2-year-old Tyrese are concerned because he cries and fusses when they leave him at the day care centre and go to work. Identify nursing measures that will minimize separation anxiety for Tyrese.
3. What measure can parents and teacher use to help the school-age child accomplish Erikson's task for this stage of development?
4. Twelve-year-old Maya is brought to the pediatric clinic for a physical examination. She is concerned about her lack of physical development compared with her peers. Discuss ways to educate Maya about puberty and the variations that occur.
5. Fifteen-year-old Ricardo wants very much to belong and be accepted by his peers. He expresses concern when his peers begin to plan a party with alcohol and drugs. What should be discussed to help support his feelings and need to belong?

Review Questions

1. Maternal risk factors associated with preterm labour include
   1. Physiological stresses, e.g., renal disease
   2. Ethnicity
   3. Fetal infections
   4. Nutrition
2. The most extreme physiological change occurs when the newborn leaves the in utero circulation and develops
   1. Respiratory functioning
   2. Cardiac functioning
   3. Reflex irritability
   4. Temperature control
3. Breast-fed infants require supplemental
   1. Vitamin C
   2. Calcium
   3. Vitamin D
   4. Zinc
4. A toddler pretends to shave after watching his father shave. This is an example of Piaget's
   1. Sensorimotor stage
   2. Intuitive phase of preoperational thought stage
   3. Autonomy stage
   4. Preoperative thought stage
5. By this age, children are able to play with others in a co-operative manner and have a temporary leader for each activity.
   1. 3 years of age
   2. 4 years of age
   3. 5 years of age
   4. 6 years of age
6. Preschoolers sleep an average of
   1. 8 hours a night and takes frequent naps
   2. 12 hours a night and takes infrequent naps
   3. 10 hours a night and takes frequent naps
   4. 6 hours a night and takes frequent naps
7. The nurse can counsel a parent that her child can floss his teeth effectively and be independent in tooth care by the age of
   1. 8 to 10 years
   2. 6 to 7 years
   3. 11 to 12 years
   4. 7 to 8 years
8. The chief illness of childhood is
   1. Flu
   2. Common cold
   3. Measles
   4. Ear infections
9. When nurses are communicating with adolescents, they should
   1. Avoid discussing sensitive issues, such as asking questions about sex and drugs
   2. Ask closed-ended questions to get straight answers
   3. Be alert to clues to their emotional state
   4. Avoid looking for meaning behind adolescents' words or actions

10. The leading cause of death in adolescence is
    1. Homicide
    2. Substance abuse
    3. Injuries
    4. Eating disorders

References

Agnew, T., Gilmore, J., & Sullivan, P. (1997). *A multicultural perspective of breastfeeding in Canada* (Catalogue No. H39-386/1997E). Ottawa, ON: Health Canada.

Askin, D. (2002). Complications in the transition from fetal to neonatal life. *Journal of Obstetric, Gynecologic, and Neonatal Nursing, 31*(3), 318–327.

Barr, R., Hopkins, B., & Green, J. (Eds.). (2000). *Crying as a sign, a symptom and a signal: Clinical, emotional and developmental aspects of infant and toddler crying.* London: MacKeith Press.

Behrman, R., Kliegman, R., & Jenson, H. (2000). *Nelson textbook of pediatrics.* Philadelphia: W. B. Saunders.

Berk, L. (2003). *Child development* (6th ed.). Boston: Allyn & Bacon.

Berry, B., et al. (2001). Preschool vision screening using the MTI-Photo screener. *Pediatric Nursing, 27*(1), 27–34.

Bukatko, D., & Daehler, M. (2001). *Child development: A thematic approach* (4th ed.). Boston: Houghton Mifflin.

Canadian Association for School Health. (2003). *Consensus statement on comprehensive school health.* Retrieved November 3, 2004, from *http://www.schoolfile.com/cash/consensus.htm*

Canadian Cancer Society. (2002). *A critical analysis of youth access laws.* Ottawa, ON: Author.

Canadian Foundation for the Study of Infant Deaths. (2004). *Information about sudden infant death syndrome (SIDS).* Retrieved December 19, 2004, from *http://www.sidscanada.org*

Canadian Institute of Child Health. (2000). *The health of Canada's children: A CIHI profile* (3rd ed.). Ottawa, ON: Author.

Canadian Paediatric Society (1996). Clinical practice Guidelines. Neonatal circumcision revisited. Ref. No. FN96-01. Retrieved December 19, 2004, from *http://www.cps.ca/english/statements/FN/fn96-01.htm*

Canadian Paediatric Society (2004). Recommendations for the use of influenza vaccines for children. Ref. No. ID04-01. Retrieved December 19, 2004, from *http://www.cps.ca/english/ca/statements/ID/ID04-01.htm*

Canadian Tobacco Use Monitoring Survey (CTUMS), (2001). Retrieved December 19, 2004, from *www.hc-sc.ca/hecs-sesc/tobacco/ctums.htm*

Center for Communicable Diseases. (1996). Guidelines for school programs to promote lifelong healthy eating. *Journal of School Health, 67,* 9–26.

Council of Ministers of Education, Canada (2003). Canadian youth, sexual health and HIV/AIDs study: Factors influencing knowledge, attitudes and behaviours. Toronto, ON: Authors.

Deering, C., & Cody, D. (2002). Communicating with children and adolescents. *American Journal of Nursing, 102*(3), 34–41.

Dickey, S., & Deatrick, J. (2000). Autonomy and decision making for health promotions in adolescence. *Pediatric Nursing, 26*(5), 461–467.

Edelman, C., & Mandle, C. (2002). *Health promotion throughout the life span* (5th ed.). St. Louis, MO: Mosby.

Erikson, E. H. (1963). *Childhood and society* (2nd ed.). New York: Norton.

Erikson, E. H. (1968). *Identity: Youth and crises.* New York: Norton.

Feldman, W. (1994). Screening for phenylketonuria. In the Canadian Task Force on the Periodic Health Examination. *Canadian Guide to Clinical Preventative Health Care,* 180–188. Ottawa, ON: Health Canada. Retrieved December 19, 2004, from *http://www.ctfphc.org/Full_Text_printable/ ch17full.htm*

Frankenburg, W. K., et al. (1992). The Denver II: A major revision and restandardization of the Denver Development Screening Test. *Pediatrics, 89*(1), 91–97.

Garner, J. (1996). Guidelines for isolation precautions in hospitals. *Infection Control and Hospital Epidemiology, 17*(1), 53–80.

Gill, S. (2001). The little things: Perceptions of breastfeeding support. *Journal of Obstetric, Gynecologic, and Neonatal Nursing, 30*(4), 401–409.

Health Canada. (1997). *Health and environment: Partners for life* (Catalogue No. H49-112/1997E). Ottawa, ON: Author.

Health Canada. (1998). *Nutrition for healthy term infants. Joint statement of Health Canada, the Paediatric Society, and the Dieticians of Canada* (Catalogue No. H39-153/1-1998E). Ottawa, ON: Author.

Health Canada. (1999a). *Healthy development of children and youth: The role of the determinants of health* (Catalogue No. H39-501/1999E). Ottawa, ON: Author.

Health Canada. (1999b). *Joint statement: Reducing the risk of sudden infant death syndrome in Canada* (Catalogue No. H39-466/2/1999) [Brochure]. Ottawa, ON: Author.

Hilton, J. (2002). Folic acid intake of young women. *Journal of Obstetric, Gynecologic, and Neonatal Nursing, 31*(2), 172–177.

Hockenberry, M. J., et al. (2003). *Wong's nursing care of infants and children* (7th ed.). St. Louis, MO: Mosby.

Jerum, A., & Melnyk, B. (2001). Effectiveness of intervention to prevent obesity and obesity-related complications in children, adolescents. *Pediatric Nursing, 27*(6), 606–610.

Kail, R. (2001). *Children and their development* (2nd ed.). Upper Saddle River, NJ: Prentice Hall.

Kamerling, S. (2002). Airbags and children: Making correct choices in child passenger restraints. *MCN. The American Journal of Maternal Child Nursing, 27*(5), 264–273.

Katz, A. (2003). "Where I come from we don't talk about that": Exploring sexuality and culture among Blacks, Asians and Hispanics. *AWHONN Lifelines, 6*(6), 533–536.

Kinservik, M., & Friedhoff, M. (2000). Control issues in toilet training. *Pediatric Nursing, 26*(3), 267–272.

Knauth, D. (2001). Marital change during the transition to parenthood. *Pediatric Nursing, 27*(2), 169–172.

Kohlberg, L. (1964). Development of moral character and moral ideology. In M. L. Hoffman & L. N. W. Hoffman (Eds.), *Review of child development research* (Vol. 1). New York: Russell Sage Foundation.

McGahee, T., Kemp, V., & Tingen, M. (2000). A theoretical model for smoking prevention studies in preteen children. *Pediatric Nursing, 26*(2), 135–138, 141.

Piaget, J. (1952). *The origins of intelligence in children.* New York: International Universities Press.

Pletsch, P., & Morgan, S. (2002). Smoke-free families: A tobacco control program for pregnant women and their families. *Journal of Obstetric, Gynecologic, and Neonatal Nursing, 31*(1), 39–47.

Popovich, D. (2000). Sexuality in early childhood: Pediatric nurses' attitudes, knowledge, and clinical practice. *Pediatric Nursing, 26*(5), 484–492.

Transport Canada (2001). Keep kids safe 1-2-3-4. Ottawa, ON: Minister of Public Works and Government Services, [Brochure] Catalogue No. T46-27/2001E. Retrieved December 19, 2004, from *http://www-tc.gc/roadsafety/tp/tp13511/menu.htm*

Trocmé, N., et al. (2001). *Canadian incidence study of reported child abuse and neglect: Final report.* Ottawa, ON: Minister of Public Works and Government Services Canada.

Ward, L., et al. (2003). *Risk factors for Vitamin D deficiency rickets among children living in Canada: Results of an incidence study through the Canadian Paediatric Surveillance Program.* Presented at the Canadian Society of Endocrinology and Metabolism Annual Meeting, Ottawa, ON.

Recommended Web Sites

Canadian Adolescents at Risk Research Network:
http://educ.queensu.ca/~caarrn/pub.htm
The Canadian Adolescents at Risk Research Network (CAARRN) is a Queen's University research program funded by the Canadian Population Health Initiative (CPHI) to study adolescent health. This Web site offers links to a number of reports and publications on adolescent health topics.

Canadian Institute of Child Health:
http://www.cich.ca/
The Canadian Institute of Child Health (CIHI) is a national, charitable organization dedicated to promoting the health of children and youth in Canada. The CIHI works with government and industry to address children's safety and health care issues and develop appropriate policies. This Web site offers evidence-based resources of interest to health care professionals, teachers, and parents.

Canadian Paediatric Society: Position Statements:
http://www.cps.ca/english/publications/statementsalphabetical.htm
This Web site includes the Canadian Paediatric Society's position statements on a variety of child health issues. It has updates as they are developed.

20

Young to Middle Adult

Patsy L. Ruchala, DNSc, RN
Marion Clauson, RN, MSN, PNC(C) (Canadian author)

Objectives

Mastery of content in this chapter will enable the student to:

- Define the key terms listed.
- List and discuss major life events and developmental tasks of young and middle adults.
- Discuss the significance of family in the life of the adult.
- Describe normal physiological changes in young and middle adulthood and in pregnancy.
- Discuss cognitive and psychosocial changes occurring during the adult years.
- Describe health concerns of young and middle adults.
- Apply clinical decision making to administer care to young and middle adults.

Young and middle adulthood is a period of challenges, rewards, and crises. Challenges may include the demands of working and raising families; rewards may include career, family, and personal successes; crises may include job loss and caring for aging parents.

Adult developmental changes are based on earlier characteristics that help shape subsequent behaviour and characteristics. Each person's development, however, is a unique process (Stuart & Laraia, 2001). Young adulthood is the period between the late teens and the mid- to late 30s (Edelman & Mandle, 2002). Young adults constitute approximately 20% of the population (Statistics Canada, 2001). During young adulthood, individuals move away from their families of origin, establish career goals, and decide to marry and begin families or remain single. Young adults must adapt to new experiences and newly acquired independence.

Middle age occurs between the mid- to late 30s and the mid-60s, when people become aware of changes in reproductive and physical abilities. This is a time when individuals may reassess life goals. In 2001, about 41% of the Canadian population were middle-age adults (Statistics Canada, 2001). The population aged 45 to 64 years increased by 36% between 1991 and 2001 and is expected to increase a further 30% during the next decade.

Developmental theories provide nurses with a basis for understanding the life events and developmental tasks of the young and middle adult. Developmental theorists Erikson (1963, 1982), Gould (1972), Havighurst (1972), and Gilligan (1993) have described the phases of adulthood and related developmental tasks (see chapter 18).

Nurses may themselves be young or middle adults coping with the demands of their respective developmental period. They must be careful to recognize the needs of their clients even if they are not experiencing the same challenges and events. Nurses can help young and middle adults achieve their potential by offering support and providing information and appropriate referrals.

Young Adult

Physical Changes

The young adult has usually completed physical growth by the age of 20 years. Young adults are usually quite active, experience fewer severe illnesses than older age groups, tend to ignore physical symptoms, and often postpone seeking health care. Physical characteristics of young adults begin to change as middle age approaches.

Clients in this developmental stage may benefit from a personal lifestyle assessment to identify habits that increase the risk for cardiac, malignant, pulmonary, renal, or other chronic diseases. A personal lifestyle assessment of the young adult includes assessment of general life satisfaction; hobbies and interests; habits such as diet, sleeping, exercise, sexual habits, and use of caffeine, alcohol, and illicit drugs; home conditions, including housing and finances; and occupational environment, including type of work, exposure to hazardous substances, and physical or mental strain.

Cognitive Changes

Cognitive changes refer to variations in reasoning and thinking. Critical thinking habits increase steadily through the young and middle adult years. Formal and informal education, life experiences, and work opportunities increase the individual's conceptual and problem-solving skills. Because young adults are continually evolving and adjusting to changes in the home, workplace, and personal lives, their decision-making processes should be flexible.

Choosing an occupation is a major task of young adults and involves knowing their skills, talents, and personality characteristics. Many young adults, however, lack the resources or the support systems to pursue higher education or develop work skills. As a result, some young adults may have limited occupational choices.

Understanding how adults learn helps the nurse to develop teaching plans (see chapter 17). Adults enter the learning situation with a background of unique life experiences, including illness. Therefore, the nurse should always view adults as individuals. When determining what amount of information the individual needs to make decisions about the prescribed course of therapy, the nurse should consider those factors that may affect the individual's compliance with the regimen, including educational level, socio-economic factors, motivation, and desire to learn.

Psychosocial Changes

The emotional health of the young adult is related to the individual's ability to address and resolve personal and social tasks. The young adult often wants to prolong adolescence yet assume adult commitments. Between the ages of 23 and 28 years, people usually refine self-perception and ability for intimacy. From ages 29 to 34 years, people usually focus on achieving personal and occupational goals and improving their socio-economic status. For many young adults, a dual-income family is needed to achieve and maintain middle-class status. Career and personal counselling can help individuals identify career choices and set realistic goals.

Ethnicity and gender issues influence an adult's life and can pose challenges for nursing care. Each person holds culture-bound definitions of health and illness. An understanding of ethnicity, race, and gender differences enables the nurse to provide individualized care (see chapter 9). Men and women have experienced changes in their traditional gender roles. In many cultures, the man has traditionally assumed familial authority. However, in the last 30 years, women have been entering the workforce and pursuing careers. About 57% of Canadian women age 15 years and over are in the labour force (Career Statistics, 2004). Women contribute significantly to their families' incomes. As a result, many women deal with the stresses of being wife, mother, and employee. Likewise, men are more aware of parental and household responsibilities (Stuart & Laraia, 2001). Some men choose to put careers on hold to be stay-at-home dads.

Career. Young men and women hope to have fulfilling careers. They may formulate short- and long-term career goals. Successful employment ensures economic security and promotes friendships, social activities, support, and self-respect.

Two-career marriages are increasing. Although there are many benefits to both partners working (e.g., improved finances), there are also many potential stressors (e.g., child-care demands, household needs, increased physical, mental, or emotional demands). To reduce stress in a two-career family, neither partner should assume all household responsibilities. For some families, a solution is to hire a housekeeper. Others may set up an equal division of household and child-care duties.

Sexuality. The young adult usually has the emotional maturity necessary to develop mature sexual relationships and establish intimacy. Young adults who have failed to achieve the developmental tasks of adolescence may develop relationships that are superficial (Stuart & Laraia, 2001).

For most young adults, the emotional aspect of sexual activity is as important as its type or frequency. Adults should be encouraged to explore various aspects of their sexuality and be aware that their sexual needs and concerns evolve (see chapter 23).

Singlehood. Social pressure to get married is not as great as it once was. The average age for first marriage for women is 27 years and for men is 30 years (Statistics Canada, 1999). For young adults who remain single, parents and siblings become the nucleus for a family, although the single young adult usually maintains independence. Close friends and associates of the single young adult may also be viewed as the individual's "family." Some singles choose to become parents, either biologically or through adoption.

The single population is increasing partly because women have greater career opportunities than before and partly because single individuals often choose to live together rather than marry. As well, many adults become single again after an unsuccessful marriage.

Marriage. Every married couple's relationship is unique. Although no rules guarantee a successful marriage, some guidelines are useful for building a happy marriage. Before marriage the couple ideally should (a) ensure that their emotions are based on love rather than physical attraction, (b) explore their motivations for marriage, (c) develop clear communication, (d) accept that behaviour and habits are unlikely to change after marriage, and (e) determine their compatibility in important beliefs and values.

When establishing a household and family, the married couple must work as a team. Individuals require maturity and self-esteem to accomplish the following major tasks of marriage: establishing an intimate relationship; deciding on and working toward mutual goals; establishing guidelines for decision-making issues; setting standards for social interactions; and choosing morals, values, and ideologies acceptable to both. Accomplishing these tasks provides the foundation for a stable relationship.

Marriage also requires the couple to learn patterns of sexual expression, establish roles, and practise effective conflict resolution and decision-making skills. Each partner may experience a sense of loss of individuality in the transition from *me* to *we*.

Child-bearing Cycle. Conception, pregnancy, birth, and the puerperium (postpartum) period are phases of the child-bearing cycle. The changes during these phases are complex (Box 20-1). Childbirth education classes can prepare the pregnant woman, her partner, and other support people to participate in the birthing process. Social support has a positive impact on pregnant women and their families (Box 20-2). A current trend is to have a lay **doula** or support person in addition to the woman's partner present during labour to offer physical, emotional, and informational support.

Breast-feeding offers many advantages to both the new mother and baby (see chapter 43). However, for the inexperienced mother, breast-feeding may cause anxiety and frustration. Women who have had no contact with newborns or other mothers who breast-feed may require assistance to breast-feed successfully. The nurse must be alert for signs that the mother needs information and assistance. By observing the mother while she breast-feeds, the nurse may catch problems such as improper positioning or ineffective sucking by the infant (Registered Nurses Association of Ontario, 2003).

The personal and social changes occurring in the lives of a couple after the birth of a baby cannot be underestimated (Figure 20–2). The nursing assessment of the couple's response to the birthing experience and parent-child attachment are discussed later in this chapter.

Parenthood. Contraception allows couples to decide when and if to start a family. One factor influencing this decision is the reason for wanting a child. Social pressures may encourage a couple to have a child or may influence them to limit the number of children they have. Economic considerations frequently enter into the decision because raising children is expensive. Because couples are getting married later and are postponing pregnancies, general health status and age are also factors in whether the couple decides to have children.

Parenting roles must be defined and practised. Nurturing and socialization needs of the children can put pressure on the couple's intimate relationship. In addition, parents' images of the "perfect parent" may conflict with reality.

Alternative Family Structures and Parenting. The norms and values about family life in Canada continuously evolve, as demonstrated by recent judicial rulings on same-sex marriage. Greater numbers of infants are born to cohabiting (common-law) couples (see chapter 16). Parents may also be single or homosexual couples. Often parents from alternative family structures feel a lack of support and bias from the health care system (Coll, Surrey, & Weingarten, 1998). The needs of same-sex parents and their children may include support for the adoption of children and the parenting role.

Focus on Primary Health Care — Box 20-1

Preparation for Parenthood

Preparing for child-bearing and parenthood involves many decisions and choices for the child-bearing family. These include the decision to have a baby, the choice of care provider and place of birth, how to obtain information and prepare for childbirth, and how to feed and care for the newborn.

The nurse in a hospital or community prenatal clinic has many opportunities to assist the child-bearing family by providing information that enables informed decision making. Nurses help families to seek preconceptual counselling for known or suspected health risks that might affect the mother or fetus during pregnancy. They also refer families to other health care professionals for unique concerns. By providing a list of questions that could be asked of a care provider on a first visit, the nurse encourages expectant parents to select a care provider they will be comfortable with and who will meet their needs.

Prenatal education programs offered by hospital and community nurses provide information about coping strategies and support during pregnancy, labour, and the early postpartum period (Figure 20–1). Classes specifically for preparation for Cesarean birth or for siblings and grandparents may also be available. All classes are structured to meet the unique needs, goals, and learning styles of the expectant family.

Adapted from *Maternal-Newborn Nursing and Women's Health Care* (7th ed., pp. 285–293), by S. B. Olds et al., 2004, Upper Saddle River, NJ: Pearson Prentice Hall.

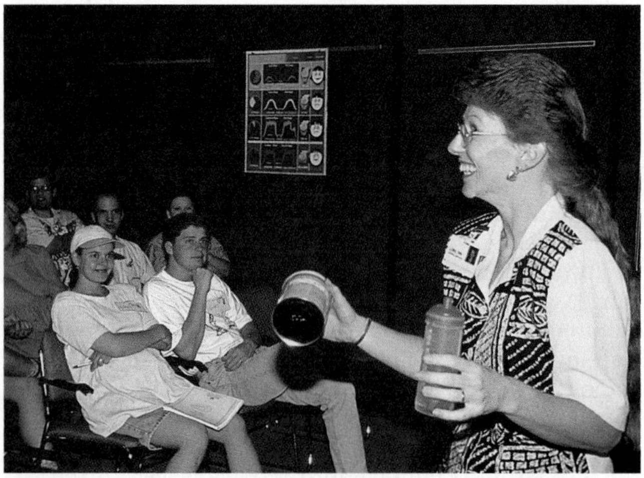

FIGURE **20–1** Nurse-instructor and expectant parents share information about pregnancy and childbirth.

Hallmarks of Emotional Health. Most young adults have the physical and emotional resources and support systems to meet their many challenges, tasks, and responsibilities. During psychosocial assessment of young adults, the nurse can assess for 10 hallmarks of emotional health that indicate successful maturation in this developmental stage (Box 20-3).

Health Risks

Health risk factors for a young adult originate in the community, lifestyle patterns, and family history.

Lifestyle. Lifestyle habits such as poor food choices, smoking, stress, substance abuse, and inactivity increase the risk of illness. For example, prolonged stress can cause ulcers, emotional disorders, and infections (see chapter 26). Smoking and second-hand smoke can cause lung cancer and pulmonary, cardiac, and vascular diseases. The nurse's role in health promotion is to identify lifestyle risk factors and provide education and support to reduce unhealthy behaviours.

Family History. A family history of a disease may put a young adult at risk for developing it in the middle or older adult years. For example, a family history of certain cancers or cardiovascular, renal, endocrine, or neoplastic disease increases the family member's risk of developing the disease.

Accidental Death and Injury. Accidents are the leading cause of injury and death in young adults (Lemone & Burke, 2004). Death and injury can occur from motor vehicle or other accidents, physical assaults, and suicide attempts. Motor vehicle accidents causing injuries and fatalities are double the rate in 20- to 24-year-olds than for the population as a whole (Statistics Canada, 1999). They are the leading cause of accidental injury for young and middle adults (Canadian Institute for Health Information, 2003). They also may cause permanent disability.

Physical assault and violence also may cause injury or death. Factors that may predispose to violence include poverty, family breakdown, child abuse and neglect, and access to firearms. It is important that the nurse perform

Research Highlight — Box 20-2

Culture and Social Support in Pregnancy

Research Focus

Although Mexican-Americans have lower levels of prenatal care and socio-economic status than other Americans, they have relatively the same or better infant mortality rates and favourable birth-weight distributions. This study looked into the reasons why, and its conclusions about the value of social support during pregnancy can also apply to Canadian settings.

Research Abstract

The purpose of this study was to describe the role of social supports to American Hispanic families during pregnancy. Hispanic mothers, family members, and health care providers were interviewed, and regional data and demographics were analyzed. Findings indicated that pregnancy outcomes were positive because of a socialization process that helped pregnant Hispanic women and family members adapt and change to support the pregnancy. The aspects of mutual adaptation helped reinforce the family structure, integrate cultural beliefs, define roles for both mother and family members, define the nature of mother-child and family-child relationships, and facilitate a positive process through a supportive orientation.

Evidence-Based Practice

- Recognizing the importance of cultural and social contexts in which pregnancies occur is an important aspect of nursing care and intervention.
- Family support of pregnant women is a major factor in the well-being of pregnant women and their unborn children.
- Health care practices and policy focused on increasing social support of pregnant women could improve birth outcomes.

Reference

Domian, E. (2001). Cultural practices and social support of pregnant women in a northern New Mexico community. *Journal of Nursing Scholarship, 33*(4), 331–336.

Box 20-3 Ten Hallmarks of Emotional Health

A sense of meaning and direction in life
Successful negotiation through transitions
Absence of feelings of being cheated or disappointed by life
Attainment of several long-term goals
Satisfaction with personal growth and development
When married, feelings of love for partner; when single, satisfaction with social interactions
Satisfaction with friendships
Generally cheerful attitude
Acceptance of constructive criticism
No unrealistic fears

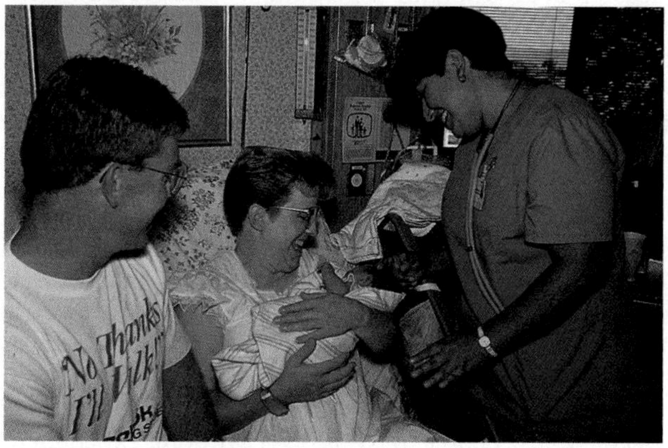

FIGURE **20–2** The birth of a newborn causes many personal and social changes in the parents' lives. (From Stanhope, M., & Lancaster, J. (2001). *Community and public health nursing,* 5th ed. St. Louis: Mosby.)

a thorough psychosocial assessment, including such factors as behaviour patterns, history of physical abuse and substance abuse, education, work history, and social support systems, to detect personal and environmental risk factors for violence.

Substance Abuse. Substance abuse directly or indirectly contributes to mortality and morbidity in young adults. Regular heavy drinking (five or more drinks on one occasion) is most common among youth aged 20–24 (Statistics Canada, 2002). Intoxication is often a factor in motor vehicle accidents.

Dependence on stimulant or depressant drugs can result in death. Overdose of a stimulant drug ("upper") can stress the cardiovascular and nervous systems and lead to death. The use of depressants ("downers") can lead to an accidental or intentional overdose and death. The nurse can provide counselling and support for clients seeking treatment for substance abuse.

Substance abuse can not always be diagnosed, particularly in its early stages. Non-judgmental questions about use of legal drugs (prescribed drugs, over-the-counter drugs, tobacco, and alcohol), soft drugs (marijuana), and illegal drugs (cocaine or heroin) should be a routine part of any physical assessment. Important information may be obtained by making specific inquiries about past medical problems, changes in food intake or sleep patterns, or problems of emotional lability. Reports of arrests because of driving while intoxicated, domestic or child abuse, or disorderly conduct should alert the health care provider to probe the possibility of drug abuse.

Unplanned Pregnancies. Unplanned pregnancies, although more common among adolescents, account for over 40% of pregnancies in young and middle adult Canadian women (Childbirth by Choice Trust, n.d.). Unplanned pregnancies are a source of stress that can result in adverse health outcomes for the mother, infant, and family. Often young adults have educational and career goals that take precedence over family development. Interference with these goals can affect future relationships and later parent-child relationships.

Determining situational factors that may affect the outcome of an unplanned pregnancy is important. When assessing the woman with an unplanned pregnancy, it is important for the nurse to explore issues such as family support systems; potential parenting disorders; depression; coping mechanisms; and possible financial, career, or housing problems.

Sexually Transmitted Infections. Sexually transmitted infections (STIs) are a major health problem in young adults. STIs include syphilis, chlamydia, gonorrhea, genital herpes, and acquired immunodeficiency syndrome (AIDS) (see chapter 23). STIs have immediate physical effects such as discharge and discomfort. They also can lead to chronic disorders (genital herpes), infertility (gonorrhea), or death (AIDS). Many people have an STI without experiencing symptoms. Young adults need information about transmission, prevention, symptoms, and management of STIs.

Many young adults have misconceptions regarding transmission and treatment of STIs. Partners are encouraged to know one another's sexual history and sexual practices. The nurse should be alert for STIs when clients come to clinics with complaints of urological or gynecological problems (see chapter 28). Young adults should be assessed for their knowledge and use of safer sex practices and genital self-examinations.

Environmental or Occupational Factors. A common environmental or occupational risk factor is exposure to work-related hazards or agents, which may cause diseases and cancer (Table 20-1). Such diseases include silicosis from inhalation of talcum and silicon dust and emphysema from inhalation of smoke. Cancers resulting from occupational exposures may involve the lung, liver, brain, blood, or skin. Questions regarding occupational exposure to hazardous materials should be a routine part of the nurse's assessment.

Health Concerns

Infertility. Infertility refers to a prolonged time to conceive, usually more than 1 full year. An estimated 7% to 8% of reproductive couples are infertile, and many are young adults (Dodds & Armson, 1997). However, about half of the couples evaluated and treated in infertility clinics become pregnant. In about 20% of infertile couples, the cause is unknown. Female factors such as ovulatory dysfunction or a pelvic factor and male factors such as sperm and semen abnormalities are responsible for about 80% of infertility (Breslin & Lucas, 2003). Couples who delay conception until their mid-30s may also experience fertility problems. For some infertile couples, the nurse may be the first resource identified. Nursing assessment of the infertile couple should include comprehensive histories of both the male and female partners to determine factors that may have affected fertility as well as pertinent physical findings (Lowdermilk & Perry, 2003).

Exercise. Exercise patterns can affect health status. Exercise that produces a sustained increase in the pulse rate for 15 to 20 minutes three times a week improves cardiopulmonary function by decreasing blood pressure and heart rate. In addition, exercise decreases fatigue, insomnia, tension, and irritability. The nurse should conduct a thorough musculoskeletal assessment, including joint mobility and muscle tone, and a psychosocial assessment for improved tolerance to stress to determine the effects of exercise.

Routine Health Screening. Poor adherence to routine screening examinations can put the client at risk for severe illnesses because of failed early detection. Clients should be encouraged to perform monthly skin, breast, or male genital self-examination (see chapter 28). In 2003, the most frequently diagnosed cancers were breast cancer in women and prostate cancer in men (Canadian Cancer Society, 2004). The incidence of beast cancer is steadily increasing. Therefore, the nurse's role is extremely important in educating female clients about breast self-examination and the current breast screening recommendations. The nurse must also include information about testicular self-examination in health teaching with young male adults. Prolonged exposure to ultraviolet rays of the sun or in

Table 20-1 Occupational Hazards/Exposures Associated With Diseases and Cancers

Job Category	Occupational Hazard/Exposure	Work-related Condition
Agricultural workers	Pesticides, infectious agents, gases, sunlight	Pesticide poisoning, "farmer's lung," skin cancer
Automobile workers	Asbestos, plastics, lead, solvents	Asbestosis, dermatitis
Carpenters	Wood dust, wood preservatives, adhesives	Nasopharyngeal cancer, dermatitis
Cement workers	Cement dust, metals	Dermatitis, bronchitis
Dry cleaners	Solvents	Liver disease, dermatitis
Glass workers	Heat, solvents, metal powders	Cataracts
Hospital workers	Infectious agents, cleansers, latex gloves, radiation	Infections, latex allergies, unintentional injuries, back injuries
Insulators	Asbestos, fibrous glass	Asbestosis, lung cancer, mesothelioma
Office computer workers	Repetitive wrist motion on computers and eye strain	Tendonitis, carpal tunnel syndrome, tenosynovitis

From *Community and Public Health Nursing* (6th ed.), by M. Stanhope and J. Lancaster, 2004, St. Louis, MO: Mosby.

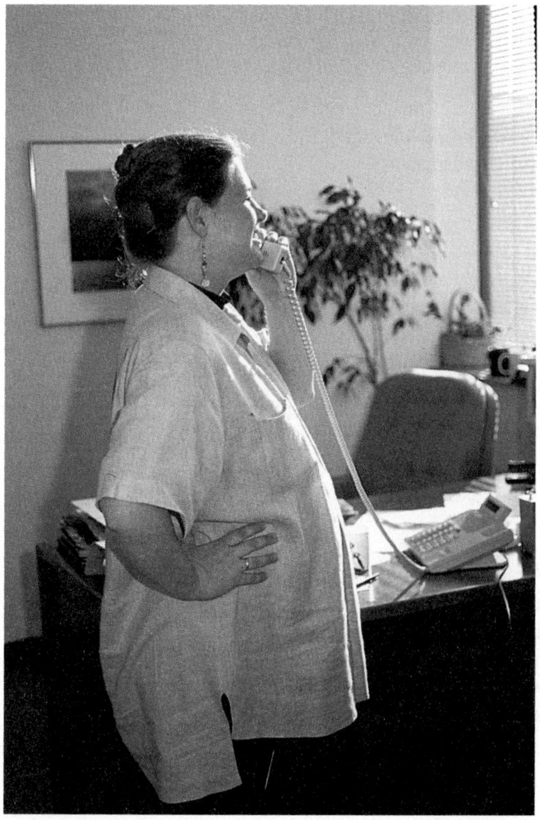

FIGURE **20–3** The ability to handle day-to-day challenges at work minimizes stress.

tanning salons by the adolescent and young adult can increase the risk for development of skin cancer later in life. Routine assessment of the skin for recent changes in colour or presence of lesions and changes in their appearance should be encouraged.

Job Stress. Job stress can occur every day or from time to time. Most young adults are able to handle day-to-day crises (Figure 20–3). Situational job stress may occur when a new boss enters the workplace, a deadline is approaching, or the worker is given new responsibilities. A recent trend in today's business world (and major source of job stress) is corporate downsizing, which leads to layoffs and increased responsibilities for remaining employees. Job stress also occurs when a person becomes dissatisfied with a job. Because individuals perceive jobs differently, the types of job stressors vary from person to person. The nurse's assessment of the young adult should include a description of the adult's work, including conditions and hours, duration of employment, changes in sleep or eating habits, and evidence of increased irritability or nervousness.

Family Stress. Family stressors can occur at any time in family life. Family life has peaks, when everyone in the family works together, and valleys, when everyone appears to pull apart. Situational stressors occur during events such as births, deaths, illnesses, marriages, and job losses. Because of changing relationships and structures in the emerging young adult family, stress is frequently high. Stress may be related to a number of variables and may lead to dysfunction in the young adult family. Stress and the possible resulting family dysfunction may account for the high divorce rate during the first 3 to 5 years of marriage for young adults under the age of 30 years. When a client seeks health care and presents stress-related symptoms, the nurse should ask if the person has recently experienced a life-changing event.

Each family has certain predictable roles or jobs for members. These roles enable the family to function and be an effective part of society. One necessary role is the family leader. In most families, one parent is the leader or both parents act as co-leaders. In single-parent families, the parent or occasionally a member of the extended family is the family leader. When this role changes as a result of illness, a situational crisis may occur. The nurse should assess environmental and familial factors, including support systems and coping mechanisms commonly used by family members.

Pregnancy. Although the physiological changes of pregnancy and childbirth occur only in the woman, cognitive and psychosocial changes and health concerns affect the

Table 20-2 Major Physiological Changes During Pregnancy

Signs and Symptoms	Causes
First trimester	
Amenorrhea	Fertilization and implantation of egg Increases in hormone levels
Morning sickness	Increased serum hormone levels
Breast changes Enlargement Tenderness Darkened and enlarged nipples	Increased estrogen levels
Urinary frequency	Pressure of uterus on bladder
Fatigue	Increases in hormone levels Increased nutritional demands Decreased nutritional intake resulting from morning sickness
Second trimester	
Integumentary changes Pigmented nipple and breast Hyperpigmentation of abdominal line (linea nigra) Mottling of cheeks or forehead (chloasma or "mask of pregnancy") Localized or generalized pruritis	Increased levels of melanocyte-stimulating hormone
Hypertrophy of gums causing gingival swelling and bleeding	Proliferation of interdental papillary blood vessels, resulting in local inflammation and hyperplasia
Increasing size of uterine fundus	Growth of fetus
Sensation of movement or gaslike movements (quickening)	Fetal movement
Braxton Hicks contractions	Expanding uterus and preparation of uterus for labour
Third trimester	
Increased colostrum	Hormonal influence; preparation of breasts for lactation
Increased urinary frequency	Pressure on bladder from enlarged fetus

Data from *Maternity Nursing* (6th ed.), by D. Lowdermilk and S. Perry, 2003, St. Louis, MO: Mosby; and *Maternal-Infant Nursing Care,* by E. Dickason, B. Silverman, and J. Kaplan, 1998, St. Louis, MO: Mosby.

entire child-bearing family (Diemer, 1997). The entire family, therefore, needs education about pregnancy, labour, delivery, breast-feeding, and integration of the newborn into the family structure.

Women who are anticipating pregnancy benefit from good health practices before conception, including eating a balanced diet, exercising, attending regular dental checkups, and avoiding alcohol, drugs, and smoking. Women trying to become pregnant should not try weight-reduction diets.

Prenatal Care. **Prenatal care** is the routine examination of the pregnant woman by a family physician, obstetrician, nurse practitioner, or midwife. Health promotion interventions are important during the prenatal period and can improve the well-being of the woman and fetus. Prenatal care includes a thorough physical assessment of the pregnant woman during regularly scheduled intervals; provision of information regarding STIs, vaginal infections, and urinary infections that could adversely affect the fetus; and counselling about exercise patterns, diet, and child care. Regular prenatal care can address health concerns that arise during the pregnancy.

Physiological Changes. The physiological changes and needs of the pregnant woman vary with each trimester (Table 20-2). Temporary changes also occur in visual and hearing acuity, taste, and smell. The nurse must be familiar with these physiological changes, their causes, and helpful interventions. All women experience some physiological changes in the first trimester, but some changes affect only certain women. During the second trimester, growth of the uterus and fetus results in some of the physical signs of pregnancy, and the woman will be able to see her growing abdomen and feel the fetal movements. During the third trimester, irregular, short contractions **(Braxton-Hicks contractions),** fatigue, and urinary frequency may occur. Close to the onset of labour, the woman may experience a burst of energy during which she prepares for the baby's arrival, a period called **nesting.**

The **puerperium** is a period of approximately 6 weeks after delivery. During this time, the woman's body reverts to its pre-pregnant physical status. The nurse should assess the woman's knowledge of and ability to care for both herself and for her newborn baby. Assistance with infant feeding and care and assessment of parenting skills and maternal-infant interactions are particularly important.

Table 20-3 Major Psychosocial Changes During Pregnancy

Category	Implications for Nursing
Body image	Morning sickness and fatigue may contribute to poor body image. Increase in breast size may make the woman feel more feminine and sexually appealing but may also be uncomfortable. Begins to "show" during the second trimester. General feeling of well-being when woman can feel the baby move and hear the heartbeat.
Role changes	Both partners think about and can have feelings of uncertainty about impending role changes. May have feelings of ambivalence about becoming parents and concern about ability to be parents.
Sexuality	Need reassurance that sexual activity will not harm fetus. Desire for sexual activity may be influenced by body image. May desire cuddling and holding rather than sexual intercourse.
Coping mechanisms	Need reassurance that childbirth and child rearing are natural and positive experiences, but can also be stressful. Provide guidance with preparation for childbirth and encourage participating in childbirth classes.
Stresses during puerperium	May return home from hospital fatigued and unfamiliar with infant care. May experience physical discomfort or feelings of anxiety. May be necessary for woman to return to work soon after delivery with subsequent feelings of guilt, anxiety, or, possibly, sense of freedom or relief.
Postpartum blues and depression	Postpartum blues symptoms include transient emotional or mood disturbances such as weepiness, insomnia, anxiety and poor concentration about 3 to 6 days after birth. Postpartum depression symptoms include extreme anxiety, sense of failure, feelings of guilt, sleep disturbances, appetite disorders, excessive concerns about the baby, and suicide ideation. Interventions include medication, therapy, counselling and support.

Psychosocial Changes. Like the physiological changes of pregnancy, psychosocial changes may occur at various times during the 9 months of pregnancy and in the puerperium. Table 20-3 summarizes the major categories of psychosocial changes and implications for nursing intervention.

Acute Care. The young adult years are generally a time of good physical and emotional health. Potential health hazards may be related to lifestyle. Acute care for young adults is frequently related to accidents, substance abuse, exposure to environmental and occupational hazards, stress-related illnesses, respiratory infections, gastroenteritis, influenza, urinary tract infections, and minor surgery.

Although cancer is relatively infrequent in young adults, more females are diagnosed with cancer than males because of the frequency of breast and reproductive system cancers (Marrett et al. & the Cancer in Young Adults in Canada [CYAC] Working Group, 2002).

An acute, minor illness can cause a disruption in the life activities of the young adult and increase stress in an already hectic lifestyle. Dependency and limitations posed by treatment regimens can also increase frustration for the young adult. To give young adults control of their health care choices, it is important for the nurse to keep them informed about their health status and involve them in health care decisions.

Restorative and Continuing Care. Chronic conditions are not common in young adulthood, but they can occur. Chronic illnesses such as hypertension, coronary artery disease, and diabetes may have their onset in young adulthood without being known to the young adult until later in life. Causes of chronic illness and disability in the young adult can include accidents, multiple sclerosis, rheumatoid arthritis, AIDS, and cancer. Chronic illness and disability can affect the accomplishment of important developmental tasks in young adulthood. They can reduce a young adult's independence and require the person to change personal, family, and career goals. The young adult with chronic illness or disability may experience developmental problems related to sense of identity. The person needs support in the establishment of independence, reorganization of intimate relationships and family structure, and launching of a chosen career (Lemone & Burke, 2004).

Middle Adult

The middle adult years begin around the early to mid 30s and last through the late 60s. Personal and career achievements have often already been experienced. Many middle adults enjoy assisting their children and other young people to become productive and responsible adults. They may also begin to help aging parents. Using leisure time in satisfying and creative ways is a challenge that, if met satisfactorily, enables middle adults to prepare for retirement.

Although most middle adults have achieved socioeconomic stability, recent trends in corporate downsizing have left many middle adults either jobless or forced to accept lower-paying jobs.

Men and women must adjust to inevitable biological changes. Middle adults adapt self-concept and body image to physiological realities and changes in physical appearance. Exercising, eating well, getting enough sleep, and practising good hygiene promote healthy bodies and a positive attitude toward physiological changes.

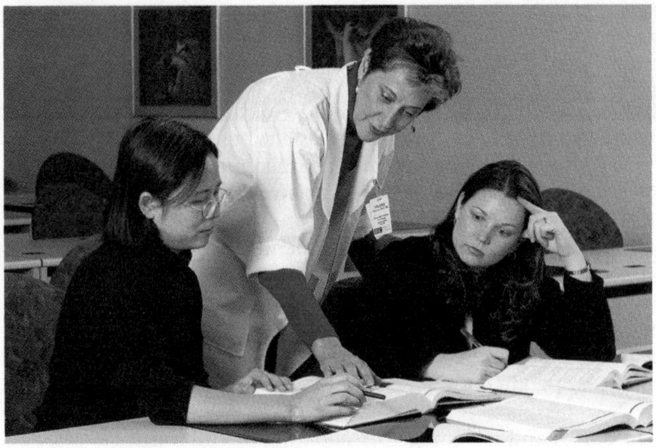

FIGURE **20–4** Mentoring younger people is important to many middle adults.

Physical Changes

Major physiological changes occur between 40 and 65 years of age. Table 20-4 summarizes these normal developmental changes that the nurse considers when conducting a physical examination. The most visible changes are greying of the hair, wrinkling of the skin, and thickening of the waist. Decreases in hearing and visual acuity are often noted during this period. Often these physiological changes have an impact on self-concept and body image. For women, the most significant physiological change during middle age is menopause. Men may also notice several sexual changes as androgen levels decrease, such as less firm erections and less frequent ejaculation (see chapter 23). However, many middle-aged men are still capable of producing fertile sperm and fathering a child.

Perimenopause and Menopause. Menstruation and ovulation occur in a cyclical rhythm in the woman from adolescence into middle adulthood. Perimenopause is the period during which ovarian function declines, resulting in a diminishing number of ova and irregular menstrual cycles. During this perimenopause time, however, women can still become pregnant. **Menopause** is the permanent cessation of menstruation. It occurs primarily because the ovaries stop producing the hormones estrogen and progesterone. Menopause typically occurs between 45 and 60 years of age. Approximately 10% of women have no symptoms of menopause other than cessation of menstruation, 70% to 80% are aware of other changes but have no problems, and approximately 10% experience changes severe enough to interfere with activities of daily living.

Cognitive Changes

Changes in the cognitive function of middle adults are rare except with illness or trauma. The middle adult can learn new skills and information. Some middle adults enter educational or vocational programs to prepare themselves for entering the job market or changing jobs.

Psychosocial Changes

The psychosocial changes in the middle adult may involve expected events, such as children moving away from home, or unexpected events, such as a marital separation or the death of loved one. Many middle adults may find themselves in the **"sandwich generation,"** having the responsibility of raising their own children while caring for aging parents. These changes may result in stress that can affect the middle adult's overall level of health. During middle age, the person examines life goals and relationships. Often a "mid-life crisis" results, in which the person feels turmoil or anxiety about the course of his or her life and desires change. As a result, the person may change relationships, lifestyle, or occupation.

Nurses should assess the major life changes occurring in the middle adult and the impact that the changes have on that person's state of health. Nursing assessment should also include individual psychosocial factors such as coping mechanisms and sources of social support.

In the middle adult years, as children depart from the household, the family enters the post-parental family stage. Time and financial demands on the parents decrease, and the couple faces the task of redefining their relationship. If grandchildren arrive, grandparenting styles must be chosen. It is during this period that many middle adults begin to take on a healthier lifestyle. Assessment of health promotion needs for the middle adult include adequate rest, leisure activities, regular exercise, good nutrition, reduction or cessation in the use of tobacco or alcohol, and regular screening examinations. Assessment of the middle adult's social environment is also important, including relationship concerns; communication and relationships with children, grandchildren, and aging parents; and caregiver concerns with their own aging or disabled parents.

According to Erikson's developmental theory (1968, 1982), the primary developmental task of the middle years is to achieve generativity (see chapter 18). Generativity is the willingness to care for and guide others. Middle adults can achieve generativity with their own children or other younger people (Figure 20–4). If middle adults fail to achieve generativity, stagnation occurs. This state is shown by excessive concern with themselves or destructive behaviour toward their children and the community.

Career Transition. Career changes may occur by choice or as a result of changes in the workplace or society. In recent decades, middle adults more often change occupations for a variety of reasons, including limited upward mobility, decreasing availability of jobs, and seeking an occupation that is more challenging to the individual. In some cases, technological advances or other changes force middle adults to seek new jobs. Such changes, particularly when unanticipated, may result in stress that can affect health, family relationships, self-concept, and other dimensions.

Sexuality. After the departure of their last child from the home, many couples rejuvenate their relationships and find increased marital and sexual satisfaction during middle age. The onset of menopause can affect the sexual health of the middle adult woman. A woman may desire increased sexual activity because pregnancy is no longer possible. Menopausal women may also experience vaginal dryness and dyspareunia or pain during sexual intercourse (see chapter 23). During middle age, a man may notice changes in the strength of his erection and a

Table 20-4 Physical Assessment Findings in the Middle Adult

Body System	Expected Findings
Integument	Intact condition Appropriate distribution of pigmentation Slow, progressive decrease in skin turgor Graying and loss of hair (baldness patterns in males are established by age 55; hair loss after this time might have other causes.)
Head and neck	Symmetry of scalp, skull, and face Normal accessory organs of vision
Eyes	Visual acuity by Snellen chart that is less than 20/50 Pupillary reaction to light and accommodation Normal visual fields and extraocular movements Normal retinal structures
Ears	Normal auditory structures and acuity
Nose, sinuses, and throat	Patent nares and intact sinuses, mouth, and pharynx Location of trachea at midline Non-palpable lateral thyroid lobes
Thorax and lungs	Increased anteroposterior diameter Respiratory rate 12–20 breaths per minute and regular Ratio of respiratory rate to heart rate: 1:4 Normal tactile fremitus, resonance, and breath sounds
Heart and vascular system	Normal heart sounds Systole: S_1 less than S_2 at base Diastole: S_1 greater than S_2 at apex Point of maximal impulse: at fifth intercostal space in midclavicular line and 2 cm or less in diameter Temperature: 36.1°–37.6° C Pulse: 60–100 bpm (conditioned athlete 50) Blood pressure: 130 mm Hg systolic 85 mm Hg diastolic All pulses palpable
Breasts	Decreased size resulting from decreased muscle mass Normal nipples
Abdomen	No tenderness or organomegaly Decreased strength of abdominal muscles
Female reproductive system	Change in menstrual cycle and in duration and quality of menstrual flow to cessation of menses "Hot flashes" Change in cervical mucosa
Male reproductive system	Normal penis and scrotum Prostatic enlargement in some individuals
Musculoskeletal system	Decreased muscle mass Decreased range of joint motion
Neurological system	Appropriate affect, appearance, and behaviour Lucidity and appropriate level of cognitive ability Intact cranial nerves Adequate motor responses Responsive sensory system

decrease in his ability to experience repeated orgasm. Other factors influencing sexuality during this period include work stress; diminished health of one or both partners; and the use of prescription medications with side effects that may influence sexual desire or functioning (e.g., anti-hypertensive agents). Both partners may experience stresses related to sexual changes or a conflict between their sexual needs and self-perceptions and social attitudes or expectations.

Family Types. Psychosocial factors involving the family may include the stresses of singlehood, marital changes, transition of the family as children leave home, and the care of aging parents.

Singlehood. Many adults over 35 years of age have never been married. Many of them have chosen to delay marriage and parenthood. Some single middle adults, however, have chosen to become parents, either biologically or through adoption. Many single middle adults may have no relatives but share a family type of relationship with close friends or work associates. Consequently, some single middle adults may feel isolated during traditional "family" holidays such as Thanksgiving or Christmas. In times of illness, single adults may have to rely on relatives or friends. Nursing assessment of single middle adults should include a thorough assessment of psychosocial factors, including the individual's definition of family and available support systems.

Marital Changes. Marital changes that may occur during middle age include death of a spouse, separation, divorce, and the choice of remarrying or remaining single. A widowed, separated, or divorced client goes through a period of grief and loss in which it is necessary to adapt to the change in marital status. Normal grieving progresses through a series of phases, and resolution of grief may take a year or more. The nurse should assess effective coping of the middle adult to the grief and loss associated with certain life changes (chapter 25).

If a single middle adult decides to marry, the stressors of marriage are similar to those for the young adult.

Family Transitions. The departure of the last child from the home may be a stressor. Many parents welcome freedom from child-rearing responsibilities, whereas others feel lonely or without direction because of this change (known as "empty-nest" syndrome). Eventually parents must reassess their marriage, resolve conflicts, and plan for the future. Occasionally this readjustment phase may lead to marital conflicts, separation, and divorce.

Care of Aging Parents. Increasing lifespans have led to increased numbers of older adults in the population. Therefore, greater numbers of middle adults must address the personal and social issues confronting their aging parents. Many become caregivers for their older parents.

Housing, employment, health, and economic realities have changed the traditional social expectations between generations in families. The middle adult and the older adult parent may have conflicting priorities related to their relationship while the older adult strives to remain independent. Negotiations and compromises help in defining and resolving problems. Nurses deal with middle and older adults in the community, long-term care facilities, and hospitals. The nurse can help identify the health needs of both groups and can assist the multigenerational family in determining the health and community resources available to them as they make decisions and plans. The nurse should also assess family relationships to determine family members' perceptions of responsibility and loyalty in relation to caring for older adult members. It is also important for the nurse to assess environmental resources (e.g., number of rooms in the house, stair rails, or handrails in bathrooms) needed for adults to care for their older parents.

Health Concerns

Physiological concerns for the middle adult include stress, level of wellness, obesity, and the formation of positive health habits. When adults seek health care, the nurse's focus on the goal of wellness can guide clients to evaluate health behaviours, lifestyle, and environment. Attention to risk factors that can be altered to improve the client's health, such as stress, obesity, use of tobacco, excessive alcohol consumption, poor nutrition, and unsafe sexual practices, can increase the quality of life and add years to it.

Stress and Stress Reduction. Middle adults' perceptions of health and health behaviours are often important factors in maintaining health. Today's complex world makes individuals prone to stress-related illnesses such as heart attacks, hypertension, migraine headaches, ulcers, colitis, autoimmune disease, backache, arthritis, and cancer. Stress levels may also increase as the middle adult tries to balance responsibilities related to employment, family life, care of children, and care of aging parents.

Throughout life, people are exposed to many stressors (see chapter 26). After these stressors are identified, the client and nurse can work together to intervene and modify the stress response. Specific interventions for stress reduction falls into three categories. First, the frequency of stress-producing situations can be minimized. Together the nurse and client identify approaches to prevent stressful situations, such as habituation, change avoidance, time blocking, time management, and environmental modification. The second category is psychophysiological preparation to increase stress resistance, such as increasing self-esteem, improving assertiveness, redirecting goal alternatives, and reorienting cognitive appraisal. Last, the physiological response to stress can be avoided. The nurse uses relaxation techniques, imagery, and biofeedback to recondition the client's response to stress. Chapter 31 explains these general interventions in greater detail.

Levels of Wellness. The nurse must be able to assess the health status of the middle adult client. Such assessment offers direction for planning nursing care and is useful in evaluating the effectiveness of nursing interventions. Table 20-4, which shows the expected physical assessment findings of the middle adult, can be used with other standard assessment techniques as a guide for physical assessment (see chapter 28).

Obesity. Obesity, defined as having a body mass index of 30 or more, is a growing health concern for middle adults. The prevalence of obesity among Canadian adults almost tripled from 5.6% in 1985 to 14.8% in 1998 (Canadian Institutes of Health Research, 2003). Health consequences of obesity include such conditions as high blood pressure, high blood cholesterol, Type 2 (non-insulin dependent) diabetes, coronary heart disease, osteoarthritis, and obstructive sleep apnea. Continued focus on the goal of wellness can assist clients in evaluating health behaviours and lifestyle that contribute to obesity during the middle adult years. Counselling related to physical activity and nutrition is an important component of the plan of care for overweight and obese clients.

Forming Positive Health Habits. A habit is a person's usual practice or manner of behaviour. This behaviour pattern is reinforced by frequent repetition until it becomes the individual's customary way of behaving. Some habits support health, such as exercise, eating a balanced diet, participating in routine screening and diagnostic tests (e.g., laboratory work for cholesterol, mammography), reducing stress, and daily brushing and flossing of teeth. Other habits involve risk factors to health, such as smoking, consuming excessive alcohol, using drugs, or eating foods with little or no nutritional value.

During assessment, the nurse frequently obtains data indicating clients' positive and negative health behaviours. In the planning, implementation, and evaluation phases, the nurse helps the client maintain habits that protect health and offers healthier alternatives to poor habits.

Health teaching and health counselling are often directed at improving health habits (Box 20-4). The more fully the nurse understands the dynamics of behaviour and habits, the more likely interventions will help the client to achieve or reinforce health-promoting behaviours.

To help clients form positive health habits, the nurse becomes a teacher and facilitator. By providing information about how the body functions and how habits are formed and changed, the nurse raises clients' understanding of the impact of behaviour on health. A nurse cannot change clients' habits. Clients have control of and are responsible for their own behaviours. The nurse can explain psychological principles of changing habits and offer information about health risks. Ultimately, however, the client decides which behaviours will become habits of daily living. Barriers to change exist (Box 20-5). Unless these barriers are minimized or eliminated, it is futile to encourage the client to take actions that are going to be blocked.

As they do with adolescents and young adults, nurses continue educating middle adults about STIs, substance abuse, and accident prevention.

Client Teaching Box 20-4

Positive Health Habits

Objective

- Client will increase exercise patterns to include three 2-km walks per week to assist in weight loss and improve cardiopulmonary functions.

Teaching Strategies

- Review with client the daily work schedule and identify potential times for exercise.
- Inform client about the effect of exercise on weight control and improved cardiac function.
- Demonstrate how to calculate target heart rate and assess pulse correctly.
- Provide warm-up and cool-down exercises and demonstrate how to do them.
- Instruct client about support shoes for walking exercises.

Evaluation

- Have client keep log of exercise periods.
- Have client demonstrate pulse measurement.
- Have client demonstrate warm-up and cool-down exercises.
- Inspect client's feet for blisters or sores.

Anxiety. Anxiety is a common response to change, conflict, and perceived control of the environment (Stuart & Laraia, 2001). Adults often experience anxiety in response to the physiological and psychosocial changes of middle age. Such anxiety can motivate the adult to rethink life goals and can stimulate productivity. For some adults, however, this anxiety precipitates psychosomatic illness and preoccupation with death. In this case, the middle adult views life as being half or more over and thinks in terms of the time left to live.

Clearly, a life-threatening illness, marital transition, or job stressor increases the anxiety of the client and family. The nurse may need to use crisis intervention or stress management techniques to help the client adapt to the changes of the middle adult years (see chapter 26).

Depression. Depression is a mood disorder that manifests itself in many ways. Although the most frequent age of onset is between the ages of 25 and 44 years, it is common among adults in the middle years and may have many causes (Stuart & Laraia, 2001). The risk factors for depression include being female; disappointments or losses at work, school, or in family relationships; departure of the last child from the home; and family history. The incidence of depression in women is twice that of men.

People experiencing mild depression describe feeling sad, blue, downcast, down in the dumps, and tearful. Other symptoms include difficulty in sleeping (insomnia) or sleeping too much (hypersomnia), irritability, feelings of social disinterest, and decreased alertness. Physical changes such as weight loss or weight gain, headaches, or feelings of fatigue regardless of the amount of rest may also be depressive symptoms. Depression that occurs during the middle years is commonly characterized by moderate to high anxiety and physical complaints. Mood changes and depression are common phenomena during menopause. Depression may be worsened by the abuse of alcohol or other substances. Nursing assessment of the depressed middle adult includes focused data collection regarding individual and family history of depression, mood changes, cognitive changes, behavioural and social changes, and physical changes. Assessment data should be collected from both the client and the client's family. Family data may be particularly important, depending on the level of depression being experienced by the middle adult.

Primary Health Care Programs. Primary health care programs for young and middle adults are designed to

Box 20-5 Barriers to Change

External Barriers	Internal Barriers
Lack of facilities	Lack of knowledge
Lack of materials	Lack of motivation
Lack of social supports	Insufficient skills to effect change in health habits
	Undefined short- and long-term goals

prevent illness, promote health, and detect disease in the early stages. Nurses can make valuable contributions to the community's health by taking an active part in the planning of screening and teaching programs and support groups for young and middle adults.

Family planning, birthing, and parenting skills are program topics in which adults might be interested. Health screening for diabetes, hypertension, eye disease, and cancer is a good opportunity for the nurse to perform assessment and provide health teaching and health counselling.

Health education programs can promote changes in behaviour and lifestyle. The nurse as health teacher offers information that enables the client to make decisions about health practices within the context of health promotion for young to middle adults. The nurse must be sure that educational programs are culturally appropriate (Box 20-6). Changes to more positive health practices during young and middle adulthood may lead to fewer or less complicated health problems during older adulthood. During health counselling, the nurse and client design a plan of action that addresses the client's health and well-being. Through objective problem solving, the nurse helps the client grow and change.

Acute Care. Acute illnesses and conditions experienced in middle adulthood may be similar to those of young adulthood. Injuries and acute illnesses in middle adulthood, however, may take a longer recovery period because of the slowing of recuperative processes. In addition, acute illnesses and injuries experienced in middle adulthood are more likely to become chronic conditions.

Restorative and Continuing Care. Chronic illnesses such as diabetes mellitus, hypertension, rheumatoid arthritis, chronic obstructive pulmonary disease, or multiple sclerosis may affect the roles and responsibilities assumed by the middle adult. Strained family relationships, modifications in family activities, increased health care tasks, increased financial stress, the need for housing adaptation, social isolation, medical concerns, and grieving may all result from chronic illness. The degree of disability and the client's perception of both the illness and the disability determine the extent to which lifestyle changes will occur. A few examples of the problems experienced by clients who develop debilitating chronic illness during adulthood include role reversal, changes in sexual behaviour, and alterations in self-image. Along with the current health status of the chronically ill middle adult, the nurse must assess the knowledge base of both the client and family. This assessment should include the medical course of the illness and the prognosis for the client. In addition, the nurse determines the coping mechanisms of the client and family, adherence to treatment and rehabilitation regimens, and the need for community and social services, along with appropriate referrals.

Cultural Aspects of Care — Box 20-6

All women experience menopause but the process of menopause is unique for every woman. The culture in which women participate, beginning in early childhood contributes to how women learn to respond. The experience of menopause for Korean women in Canada has been studied. Findings reveal that although menopause symptoms required management, the women considered menopause to be a natural process. They used herbs and maintained health diets as well Western medicine to deal with menopause.

Implications for Practice

- Be aware of cultural influences that may affect the experience of menopause, and how women seek assistance from health care providers.
- Educational materials that combine Western remedies with traditional approaches may be more easily accepted and utilized.
- Cultural norms and taboos may influence women's willingness to discuss personal issues such as menopause. Information sessions on the topic, or more broadly related to women and aging, should be held in community settings where women might gather and feel comfortable.

From "A Critical Ethnography of Korean Canadian Women's Menopause Experience," by J. Elliott, H. Berman, and S. Kim, 2002, *Health Care for Women International, 23*(4), pp. 377–388.

Key Concepts

- Adult development involves orderly and sequential changes that adults experience over time.
- Young adults are in a stable period of physical development, except for changes related to pregnancy.
- Cognitive development continues throughout the young and middle adult years.
- Emotional health of young adults is correlated with the ability to address and resolve personal and social problems.
- Young adults must choose a career and decide whether to remain single or marry and begin a family.
- Pregnant women need to understand physiological changes occurring in each trimester.
- Psychosocial changes and health concerns during pregnancy and the puerperium period affect the mother and the rest of the family.
- Health promotion interventions are important during the prenatal period and can improve the well-being of the woman and fetus.
- Mid-life transition begins when a person becomes aware that physiological and psychosocial changes signify passage to another stage in life.
- Two significant physiological changes of the middle years are menopause in women and changes in sexual response in men.
- Cognitive changes are rare in middle age except in cases of illness or physical trauma.
- Psychosocial changes for middle adults may be related to career transition, sexuality, marital changes, family transition, and care of aging parents.

- Health goals of middle adults commonly involve preventing stress-related illnesses, participating in health assessments, and adopting positive health habits.

Key Terms

Braxton-Hicks contractions, *p. 404*
Breast-feeding, *p. 400*
Doula, *p. 400*
Infertility, *p. 402*
Menopause, *p. 406*
Nesting, *p. 404*
Prenatal care, *p. 404*
Puerperium, *p. 404*
Sandwich generation, *p. 406*

Critical Thinking Exercises

1. Katya K. is a 24-year-old woman who smokes two packs of cigarettes per day. She began smoking when she was 14 years old. Katya complains to the nurse at the clinic, "I just can't seem to kick the habit no matter how hard I try." What information does the nurse need to know to assist Katya in quitting smoking?
2. Rohan D., 48 years old, married, and the father of 13- and 16-year-old sons, has recently had to assume the responsibility of caring for his 78-year-old mother after she suffered a stroke. Describe the nurse's role in assisting Rohan in caring for his mother.

Review Questions

1. The young adult has usually completed physical growth by the age of
   1. 18 years
   2. 20 years
   3. 25 years
   4. 30 years
2. When assessing young adults, the nurse will find this population usually has a high level of wellness. However, it is important to direct health care education toward activities related to
   1. Health promotion
   2. Primary prevention
   3. Secondary prevention
   4. Tertiary prevention
3. When determining what amount of information the individual needs to make decisions about the prescribed course of therapy, the nurse should consider those factors that may affect the individual's compliance with the regimen, including educational level, socio-economic factors, and
   1. Sexuality
   2. Lifestyle
   3. Gender
   4. Motivation and desire to learn
4. A common physiological change in the second trimester of pregnancy is
   1. Morning sickness
   2. Amenorrhea
   3. Increased colostrum
   4. Braxton-Hicks contractions
5. The most common cause of injury in young adults is
   1. Suicide
   2. Motor vehicle accidents
   3. Substance use
   4. Cancer
6. Close friends and associates of the single young adult may also be viewed as the individual's
   1. Siblings
   2. "Family"
   3. Alternative family structure
   4. Substitute parents
7. A young man's father and paternal grandfather had myocardial infarctions (heart attacks) in their 50s. He has a risk for a future myocardial infarction. The young man faces what type of health risk?
   1. Lifestyle
   2. Poor personal hygiene
   3. Family history
   4. Hereditary disease
8. In the middle adult years, the family enters which stage?
   1. Generative stage
   2. Independence stage
   3. Post-parental family stage
   4. Family orientation stage
9. To improve an adult's health habits, the nurse often uses health counselling and
   1. Medications
   2. Referrals
   3. Health teaching
   4. Stress management techniques
10. To help recondition the client's response to stress, the nurse can use biofeedback, imagery, and
    1. Medication
    2. Time management strategies
    3. Relaxation techniques
    4. Assertiveness training

References

Breslin, E. T., & Lucas, V. A. (2003). *Women's health nursing: Toward evidence-based practice.* St. Louis, MO: Saunders.

Canadian Cancer Society. (2004). *Media backgrounder: Canadian Cancer Statistics 2004.* Retrieved May 29, 2004, from *http://www.cancer.ca/ccs/internet/mediareleaselist/0,3208,3172_210504871_1angld-en,00.html*

Canadian Institute for Health Information. (2003). *National Trauma Registry: 2003 Report: Major injury in Canada.* Ottawa, ON: Author.

Canadian Institutes of Health Research. (2003, April 28). *News release: Backgrounder.* Retrieved December 8, 2004, from *http://www.cihr-irsc.gc.ca/e/7972.html*

Career statistics: Women in the workforce. (2004, March 15). *Macleans.* Retrieved May 24, 2004, from *http://www.macleans.ca/topstories/life/article.jsp?content=20040315_77252_77252*

Childbirth by Choice Trust. (n.d.). *Contraceptive use in Canada.* Retrieved May 24, 2004, from *http://www.cbctrust.com/contraceptive.html*

Coll, C., Surrey, J., & Weingarten, K. (1998). *Mothering against the odds.* New York: The Guilford Press.

Dickason, E., Silverman, B., & Kaplan, J. (1998). *Maternal-infant nursing care.* St. Louis, MO: Mosby.

Diemer, G. (1997). Expectant fathers: Influence of perinatal education on stress, coping, and spousal relations. *Research in Nursing & Health, 20*(4), 281–293.

Dodds, L., & Armson, B. A. (1997). Is Canada's sex ratio in decline? *Canadian Medical Association Journal, 157*(1), 46–48.

Edelman, C., & Mandle, C. (2002). *Health promotion throughout the lifespan* (5th ed.). St. Louis, MO: Mosby.

Elliott, J., Berman, H., & Kim, S. (2002). A critical ethnography of Korean Canadian women's menopause experience. *Health Care for Women International, 23*(4), 377–388.

Erikson, E. (1963). *Childhood and society* (2nd ed.). New York: W. W. Norton.

Erikson, E. (1968). *Identity: Youth and crisis.* New York: W. W. Norton.

Erikson, E. (1982). *The life cycle completed: A review.* New York: W. W. Norton.

Gilligan, C. (1993). *In a different voice.* Cambridge, MA: Harvard University Press.

Gould, R.L. (November, 1972). The phases of adult life: A study in developmental psychology. *Am J Psychiatry, 129*(5).

Havighurst, R. (1972). Successful aging. In R. H. Williams, C. Tibbits, & W. Donahue (Eds.), *Process of aging* (Vol. 1). New York: Atherton.

Health Canada. (2000). *1998/1999 Canadian sexually transmitted diseases (STD) surveillance report.* Retrieved May 29, 2004, from *http://www.hc-sc.gc.ca/pphb-dgspsp/publicat/ccdr-rmtc/00vol26/26s6/index.html*

Lemone, P., & Burke, K. (2004). *Medical surgical nursing: Critical thinking in client care* (3rd ed.). Upper Saddle River, NJ: Pearson Prentice Hall

Lowdermilk, D., & Perry, S. (2003). *Maternity nursing* (6th ed.). St. Louis, MO: Mosby.

Marrett, L. D., et al., & the Cancer in Young Adults in Canada (CYAC) Working Group. (2002). Cancer incidence in young adults in Canada: Preliminary results of a cancer surveillance project. *Chronic Diseases in Canada, 23*(2), 58–64.

Olds, S. B., et al. (2004). *Maternal-newborn nursing and women's health care* (7th ed.). Upper Saddle River, NJ: Pearson Prentice Hall.

Registered Nurses Association of Ontario (RNAO). (2003). *Breastfeeding Best Practice Guidelines for nurses.* Toronto, ON: Author.

Stanhope, M., & Lancaster, J. (2004). *Community and public health nursing* (6th ed.). St. Louis, MO: Mosby.

Statistics Canada. (1999). *Statistical report on the health of Canadians.* Catalogue No. 82-570XIE. Retrieved December 8, 2004, from *http://www.statcan.ca/english/freepub/82-570-XIE/intro.htm*

Statistics Canada. (2001). *Shifts in the population size of various age groups.* Retrieved December 8, 2004, from *http://www12.statcan.ca/english/census01/Products/standard/themes/RetrieveProductTable.cfm*

Stuart, G., & Laraia, M. (2001). *Principles and practice of psychiatric nursing* (7th ed.). St. Louis, MO: Mosby.

Recommended Web Sites

Breastfeeding Committee for Canada:
http://www.breastfeedingcanada.ca
The Breastfeeding Committee for Canada was established in 1991 as a Health Canada initiative. This Web site addresses Canadian breast-feeding issues.

Canadian Cancer Society:
http://www.cancer.ca
This site provides information on specific cancers, clinical trials, support services, and how to get involved.

Canadian Women's Health Network:
http://www.cwhn.ca
The goal of the Canadian Women's Health network is to share information, resources, and strategies to improve women's health.

Population and Public Health Branch: Adult Health:
http://www.phac-aspc.gc.ca/ah-sa_e.html
This Web site links to the Public Health Agency of Canada: Adult Health and links to topics concerning Canadian adult health issues, including information on chronic diseases, infectious diseases, and healthy living.

21

Older Adult

Myra A. Aud, PhD, RN
Wendy Duggleby, DSN, RN, AOCN (Canadian author)

Objectives

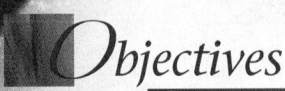

Mastery of content in this chapter will enable the student to:

- Define the key terms listed.
- Discuss demographic trends related to older adults in Canada.
- Identify common myths and stereotypes about older adults.
- List the types of community-based and institutional health care services available to older adults.
- Identify selected biological and psychosocial theories of aging.
- Discuss common developmental tasks of older adults.
- Describe common physiological changes of aging.
- Differentiate among delirium, dementia, and depression.
- Discuss issues related to psychosocial changes of aging.
- Describe selected health concerns of older adults.
- Identify nursing interventions related to the physiological, cognitive, and psychosocial changes of aging.

The identification of 65 years of age as the start of older adulthood dates back to social reform in Germany in the 19th century. The age of 65 years continues to be used as the lower boundary for "old age" in demographics and social policy, although many older adults consider themselves to be "middle-aged" well into their seventh decade. Chronological age may have little relation to the reality of aging for an older adult. Each of us ages in our own ways according to our own schedules and life histories. Even though in this chapter generalizations will be made about the aging process and its effect on individuals, every older adult is unique and must be approached as a unique individual by the nurse.

The number of older adults in Canada is growing, both absolutely and as a proportion of the total population. In 2001, there were 3.7 million adults over 65 years in Canada, representing 12% of the population (National Advisory Council on Aging [NACA], 2003). This number represented an increase of 3.7% since 1997. Geographic variations in the aging population exists across Canada, with the lowest proportion of older adults in Nunavut (2.6%) and the highest in Saskatchewan (14.6%; Health Canada, 2002). The number of older adults is expected to increase to 6.9 million (18% of the population) by 2021 (Health Canada, 2004). Part of that increase is due to extension of the average lifespan. A 65-year-old woman in 2001 could expect to live another 13 years, a 65-year-old man, another 7 years (Health Canada, 2004).

Two other factors that contribute to the projected increase in the number of older adults are aging of the baby boom generation and the growth of the population segment over 85 years. The baby boomers are the large cohort of adults born between 1946 and 1964. The first baby boomers will reach the age of 65 years in 2011. As baby boomers age, social and health care programs will need to expand to meet their needs as well as the needs of the fastest-growing group of adults, those who are 85 years and older. The numbers in this group have doubled since 1981 to 430,000 in 2001 and are expected to grow to 1.6 million in 2031 (4% of the population).

The diversity of the over 65 years group is also projected to increase (Health Canada, 2002). Approximately 25% of Canadian older adults were born outside of Canada. Most immigrated when they were young. In 1997, 3% of immigrants arriving each year were older adults. This number is expected to increase as immigration patterns change. Most immigrant older adults can speak one or both of Canada's official languages; however, 4% cannot. In the over 65 years group, women are more likely than men to be unable to speak either French or English. In 1996, 5.2% of older women and 3.5% of older men were unable to speak either official language. Currently, older adults make up a small proportion of Canada's Aboriginal population (3.5%; Health Canada, 2002). However, the number of older Aboriginals is expected to triple by 2016 as their population ages and lives longer. Nurses must take the cultural, ethnic, and racial diversity represented by these numbers into account as they care for older adults from these groups. Examples of culturally sensitive nursing approaches to older adults include respect for preferences in food, music, and religion; attentive listening; use of physical assessment norms appropriate for the ethnic group; and asking about personal health practices, family customs, lifestyle preferences, and spiritual resources (Ebersole & Hess, 2001). Chapter 9 provides further information on culturally competent care.

Variability Among Older Adults

The nursing care of older adults poses special challenges because of great variation in their physiological, cognitive, and psychosocial health. Older adults also vary widely in their levels of functional ability. The majority of older adults are active and involved members of their communities. A smaller number have lost the ability to care for themselves, are confused or withdrawn, and/or are unable to make decisions concerning their needs. Most older adults live in non-institutional settings, either with family members or alone (29% of older adults live alone; NACA, 2002). Only 7% of all older adults resided in institutions such as long-term care facilities (Health Canada, 2004). Age influences living arrangements: The proportion of older adults living with a spouse decreases with age, the proportion living alone increases with age, and the proportion living in an institution increases with age.

Aging does not inevitably lead to disability and dependence. Most older people remain functionally independent despite the increasing prevalence of chronic disease. Nursing assessment, a complex and challenging process, can provide valuable clues to the effect of a disease or illness on a client's functional status. Chronic conditions add to the complexity of assessment and care of the older adult. Approximately 80% of older adults have multiple chronic conditions, with arthritis, hypertension, heart disease, vision impairment, and diabetes mellitus being the most common in non-institutionalized older adults (NACA, 2002). These chronic conditions impose limitations on activities: Slightly more than 20% of adults 65 to 74 years of age and nearly 50% of adults 85 years or over report some limitations on activities (Health Canada, 2004).

The physical, cognitive, and psychosocial aspects of aging are closely related. For the older person, a reduced ability to respond to stress, the experience of multiple losses, and the physical changes associated with normal aging may combine to place the person at high risk for illness and functional deterioration. Although the interaction of these physical and psychosocial factors can be serious, the nurse should not assume that all older adults have signs, symptoms, or behaviours representing disease and decline or that these are the only items to be assessed. The older adult's strengths and abilities must also be identified during the assessment.

Terminology

As the number of older adults increases, the specialty of gerontological nursing is gaining in importance. Several terms are used, at times interchangeably, to describe this specialty (Lueckenotte, 2000).

- **Geriatrics** is the branch of medicine that deals with the physiological and psychological aspects of aging and with the diagnosis and treatment of diseases affecting older adults.
- **Gerontology** is the study of all aspects of the aging process and its consequences.
- **Gerontological nursing** is concerned with assessment of the health and functional status of older adults; diagnosis, planning, and implementing health care and services to meet the identified needs; and evaluating the effectiveness of such care. This is the term most often used by nurses specializing in this field.
- **Gerontic nursing,** a seldom-used term that is gaining use, considers the nursing care of older adults to be the art and practice of nurturing, caring, and comforting rather than merely the treatment of disease.

Myths and Stereotypes

Despite ongoing research in the field of gerontology, false beliefs, or myths, about older adults persist. These stereotypes include beliefs about the physical and psychosocial characteristics and the lifestyles of older adults. Stereotypes, both positive and negative, may be held by younger and older adults but do not automatically imply age-based prejudice (Chasteen, Schwarz, & Park, 2002). However, when health care providers holding negative stereotypes care for older adults, those stereotypes may adversely affect the quality of the care provided. Nurses, although personally susceptible to the myths and stereotypes held by society, have the responsibility to dispel the myths and replace the stereotypes with accurate information.

Older adults are sometimes stereotyped as ill and disabled. However, although many experience chronic conditions or have at least one disability that limits their performance of activities of daily living (ADLs), only 6% of older adults describe their health as poor or fair (Health Canada, 2002). Other common misconceptions hold that older adults are not interested in sex and that any interest in sexual activities is abnormal and should be discouraged. Yet older adults report continued enjoyment of sexual relationships.

Some people believe that older adults are forgetful, confused, rigid, bored, and unfriendly and that they are unable to understand and learn new information. Yet centenarians, the oldest of the old, are described as having an optimistic outlook on life, good memories, broad social contacts and interests, and tolerance for others (Ebersole & Hess, 1998). Although the process of learning may be affected by age-related changes in vision or hearing or by reduced energy and endurance, older adults are lifelong learners. The nurse should use teaching techniques that compensate for sensory changes, provide additional time for remembering and responding, and present concrete rather than abstract material to facilitate learning by older adults. Other effective teaching techniques draw from the older adult's past experiences and correspond to the identified interests of the older adult rather than to the content areas believed important by the health care professional. Box 21-1 presents additional teaching strategies that the nurse can use to address the special learning needs of older adults.

Box 21-1 Older Adult Client's Special Learning Needs

Teaching Strategies

- Make sure the client is ready to learn before trying to teach. Watch for clues that would indicate that the client is preoccupied or too anxious to comprehend the material.
- Sit facing the client so that he or she can watch your lip movements and facial expressions.
- Speak slowly.
- Keep your tone of voice low; older adults can hear low sounds better than high-frequency sounds.
- Present one idea at a time.
- Emphasize concrete rather than abstract material.
- Give the client enough time in which to respond because older adults' reaction times are longer than those of younger people.
- Focus on a single topic to help the client concentrate.
- Keep environmental distractions to a minimum.
- Defer teaching if the client becomes distracted or tired or cannot concentrate for other reasons.
- With permission of the older adult, invite another member of the household to join the discussion.
- Use audio, visual, and tactile cues to enhance learning and help the client remember information.
- Ask for feedback to ensure that the information has been understood.
- Use past experience; connect new learning to that already learned.
- Compensate for physical discomfort and sensory alterations.
- Support a positive self-image in the learner.
- Use creative teaching strategies.
- Respond to identified interests of learners.
- Emphasize and integrate emotional and personal values in the acquisition of skills and ideas.

Adapted from *Geriatric Nursing and Healthy Aging,* by P. Ebersole and P. Hess, 2001, St. Louis, MO: Mosby. (Original source: "Handle With Caring: Meeting Elderly Clients' Special Learning Needs," by S. Fielo and M. Rizzolo, 1988, *Nursing & Health Care, 9*[4], p. 193.)

Stereotypes about lifestyles include mistaken notions about living arrangements and finances. Most older adults live in non-institutional settings, either with family members or alone. Misconceptions about the financial status of older adults range from beliefs that many are affluent to beliefs that many are poor. In 2000, about 17% of non-institutionalized Canadian older adults were living in low-income households (Statistics Canada, 2003). Low-income rates among Canadian older adults are among the lowest in countries of the Organisation for Economic Co-operation and Development. However, unattached older adults, particularly women, are more likely to have low incomes. This statistic is expected to change because of women's increased workforce participation. In a society that values attractiveness, energy, and youth, these myths and stereotypes lead to the undervaluing of older adults. Some people believe that older adults are unattractive and become worthless after they leave the workforce. Others consider the knowledge and experience of older adults to be too old-fashioned to have any current value. These notions underlie the concept of **ageism,** which is discrimination against people because of increasing age, just as racism and sexism are discrimination based on skin colour and gender, respectively. Ageism has the potential to undermine the self-confidence of older adults, limit their access to care, and distort caregivers' understanding of the uniqueness of each older adult (Cutillo-Schmitter, 1996).

Today there are laws banning discrimination on the grounds of age. The economic and political power of older adults also acts against ageism. Older adults are a significant proportion of the consumer economy. As voters and activists in various issues, they influence the formation of public policy. Their participation adds a unique perspective to social, economic, and technological issues because they have experienced almost 100 years of developments. In the past 100 years, we have gone from riding in horse-drawn carriages to observing space shuttle flights. Gaslights and steam power have given way to electricity and nuclear power. Typewriters and carbon paper have been replaced by computers and copier machines. Older adults have lived through the Great Depression. They have also experienced two world wars and the Korean conflict. Older adults have seen changes in health care as the era of the family doctor gave way to the age of specialization. After witnessing the government initiatives that established the Old Age Security Program, Canada Pension Plan, and National Health Insurance System (Medicare), older adults are currently living with the changes imposed by health care reform. Having lived through all of these events and changes, older adults have stories and examples of coping with change to share with others.

Nurses' Attitudes Toward Older Adults

It is important for nurses to assess their attitudes toward older adults, their own aging, and the aging of their family, friends, and clients. The attitudes of the nurse toward older adults result partly from personal experiences with older adults, education, employment experiences, attitudes of co-workers and employers, and the nurse's own age. Given the increasing number of older adults in health care settings, cultivation of positive attitudes toward older adults and specialized knowledge about aging and the health care needs of older adults are priorities for nurses.

Positive attitudes are based in part on a realistic portrayal of the characteristics and health care needs of older adults. In the past, negative attitudes about aging and older adults have contributed to the persistence of stereotypes of older adults as dependent and less attractive than younger clients. Nursing care, under the influence of these attitudes, has often ignored the opportunity to respect older adults and actively involve them in care decisions and activities. At times, hospitals and long-term care facilities have treated older adults as objects to be acted upon rather than as independent, dignified adults. What older adults perceive as important in promoting their independence may differ from what nurses and other caregivers may assume to be important. For example, a research study found that older adults selected balance as the most important skill for staying independent, but nurses selected managing medications (Mastrian, 2001).

Theories of Aging

Various theorists have attempted to describe the complex biopsychosocial process of aging. Although many theories have been developed, there is no single universally accepted theory that predicts and explains the complexities of the aging process. The nurse must be aware of the scientific attempts to explain the aging process and the concepts included in the theories. Although the theories are in various stages of development and have limitations, nurses can use them to increase their understanding of the phenomena affecting the health and well-being of older adults.

The biological theories of aging are categorized as either **stochastic theories** or **non-stochastic theories** (Ebersole & Hess, 2004). Stochastic theories view aging as the result of random cellular damage that occurs over time. The accumulated damage leads to the physical changes characteristic of the aging process. According to the non-stochastic theories, genetically programmed physiological mechanisms within the body control the process of aging. In another approach to the explanation of the biological changes of the aging process, Sloane (1992) suggested a "rule of thirds" in which functional decline from disease, aging itself, and inactivity or disuse each contribute equally to the aging process.

The psychosocial theories of aging attempt to explain changes in behaviour, roles, and relationships that come with aging. As with biological theories of aging, no single theory is universally accepted. The theories also reflect the values held by the theorist and society at the time the theory was first articulated. The three classic psychosocial theories of aging are disengagement theory, activity theory, and continuity theory (Ebersole & Hess, 1998). Disengagement theory, the oldest psychosocial theory, states that aging individuals withdraw from customary roles and engage in more introspective, self-focused activities as society disengages from them (Cummings & Henry, 1961). The activity theory, unlike the disengagement theory, considers the continuation of activities performed during middle age as necessary for successful aging (Lemon, Bengston, & Peterson, 1972). Continuity theory or developmental theory (Neugarten, 1964) states that personality remains the same and behaviour becomes more predictable as people age. The personality and behaviour patterns developed during a lifetime determine the degree of engagement and activity in older adulthood.

Critics suggest, however, that all three psychosocial theories either fail in some measure to consider the many factors that affect an individual's response to the aging process or address those factors in a simplistic fashion.

Developmental Tasks for Older Adults

Theories of aging are closely linked to the concept of developmental tasks appropriate for distinct stages of life. Although no two individuals age in the same way, either biologically or psychosocially, frameworks outlining developmentally appropriate tasks for older adults have been developed. Seven developmental tasks for older adults are listed in Box 21-2.

These developmental tasks are common to many older adults and are associated with varying degrees of change and loss. The more common losses are health, significant others, a sense of being useful, socialization, income, and independent living. The ways that older adults adjust to the changes of aging are highly individualized. For some, adaptation and adjustment are relatively easy. For others, coping with the changes caused by aging may require the assistance of family, friends, and health care professionals. The nurse must be sensitive to the effect of such losses on older adults and their families and be prepared to offer support.

Older adults must adjust to the physical changes that accompany aging. The extent and timing of these changes vary from individual to individual, but as body systems age, changes in appearance and functioning occur. These changes are not associated with a disease but are normal changes. The presence of disease may alter the timing of the changes or their impact on daily life. Structural and

Box 21-2 Developmental Tasks of the Older Adult

- Adjusting to decreasing health and physical strength
- Adjusting to retirement and reduced or fixed income
- Adjusting to death of a spouse
- Accepting self as aging person
- Maintaining satisfactory living arrangements
- Redefining relationships with adult children
- Finding ways to maintain quality of life

functional changes associated with aging are described in the section on physiological development.

Although a great majority of Canadian older adults are retired, 6% of them are employed outside the home (NACA, 2003). A large number of employed older adults work on a part-time basis (41%). Many return to paid work following initial retirement. In 1994, 13% of Canadian retirees reported they had returned to paid work following initial retirement. Older adults retired from employment outside the home are challenged to cope with the loss of that work role. Older adults who worked at home and the spouses of those who worked outside the home also face role changes as they retire.

Because retirement is usually anticipated, people can make financial plans and plan replacement activities. Many older adults welcome retirement as a time to pursue new interests and hobbies, to participate in volunteer activities, to continue their education, or to start a new business career. Retirement plans for some older adults include changes of residence such as moving to a different city or province or moving to a different type of housing.

Reasons other than retirement may also lead to changes of residence. For example, physical impairments may require relocation to a smaller, single-level home. Health problems may require the older adult to live with relatives or friends or move to an assisted-living or long-term care facility. A change in living arrangements for the older adult may require an extended period of adjustment during which assistance and support from health care professionals, friends, and family members are needed. However, although changes in residence occur, the majority of Canadian older adults report that they enjoy good housing (NACA, 2003).

The majority of older adults are faced with the death of a spouse. In 1996, almost half (46%) of all older women were widows, and 12.7% of older men were widowers (NACA, 2002). Some older adults must cope with the death of adult children and grandchildren. All experience the deaths of friends. These deaths represent both losses and reminders of personal mortality. Coming to terms with these deaths is often difficult. By assisting older adults through the grieving process, the nurse can help them resolve the issues posed by these deaths.

The redefining of relationships with children that occurred as those children grew up and left home continues as older adults experience the challenges of aging. A variety of issues may arise, including, but not limited to, role reversal, control of decision making, dependence, conflict, guilt, and loss. How these issues surface in situations and how they are resolved depends in part on the past relationship between the older adult and the adult children. All of the involved parties bring past experiences and powerful emotions with them. When adult children assist the older adults of their family, they must find ways to balance the demands of their own children and their careers. Adult children also determine how much assistance to provide and how much decision-making authority to assume. As adult children and aging parents negotiate the parameters of the changed roles, nurses may act as counsellors to both the parents and the children. Nurses can assist adult children by listening and by helping them distinguish between changes and behaviours related to illness, normal aging changes, and their parents' lifelong preferences and patterns of behaviour.

In the face of the changes that come with aging, older adults must find ways to maintain their quality of life. What defines quality of life varies from person to person. Nurses must listen to what the older adult considers to be most important rather than making assumptions about that individual's priorities. Together the nurse and the older adult may set objectives that lead to the maintenance of quality of life, whether quality of life is defined as maintenance of social relationships, continuing to live alone, or continuing activities such as driving or gardening.

Community-Based and Institutional Health Care Services

Nurses encounter older adult clients in a wide variety of community-based and institutional health care settings. Outside of the acute care hospital setting, nurses care for older adults in private homes and apartments, adult day care centres, assisted-living facilities (also known as supportive housing), and long-term care facilities. Long-term care facilities provide accommodations, 24-hour nursing care, and support services for people who cannot care for themselves at home but do not need hospital care. Assisted-living facilities are designed for residents who need only minimal to moderate care. Residents live independently in their own apartments and are provided with support services such as homemaking or personal care. Some assisted-living facilities are small group homes where residents share common eating and living areas. In some provinces, personal care homes are offered as a type of assisted-living facility. A **personal care home** is a private business that provides accommodation, meals, and supervision or assistance with personal care in family-like atmosphere. Nursing services are not usually included in assisted-living facilities.

Nurses can also assist older adults and their families by providing information and answering questions as they make choices among care options. During the decision-making period, the actual move from a private home to an assisted-living or long-term care facility, and the time after the move, the nurse's role is to support the older adult and the family. The nurse can provide information about the selection of a good assisted-living or long-term care facility (Box 21-3). The best way to evaluate quality is to visit that facility and inspect it personally (Rantz, Popejoy, & Zwygart-Stauffacher, 2001).

Assessing the Needs of Older Adults

Gerontological nursing offers creative approaches for maximizing the potential of older adults. The Canadian Gerontological Nursing Association (1996) standards of practice were developed to define the uniqueness and

Focus on Older Adults Box 21-3

Selecting a Personal Care Home

A personal care home, like all assisted-living facilities, is for adults who need minimal to moderate assistance. It provides an adult with accommodation, meals, and supervision or assistance with personal care. Advise clients that an important step in the selection process is to visit the facility. Clients should select a home that offers the features that are most important to them. Suggest clients to do the following when visiting a personal care home:

- Notice the atmosphere. The facility should feel like a home. Residents should be able to personalize their rooms and have privacy. There should be enough space to meet residents' requirements.
- Ask to see the license.
- Talk to the staff and residents about the care services provided, recreation activities, and transportation.
- Ask about the experience and training of staff.
- Ask if residents are encouraged to do things they like to do around the home such as tidying their room.
- Talk about how much money you will pay to live in the home and what you will receive in return.
- Ask to see the menu plan.
- Ask to see a copy of the residents' rights and privileges.
- Ask about the rules of the home.

Adapted from *Selecting a Personal Care Home,* Saskatchewan Health, 2000. Retrieved August 18, 2004, from *http://www.health.gov.sk.ca/rr_selecting_prsnl_care.html*

scope of gerontological nursing practice, which includes functions such as assessment. With comprehensive assessment information regarding the older adult's strengths, resources, and limitations, the nurse and the older adult identify needs and problems and select interventions that maintain the older adult's physical abilities and create an environment for psychosocial and spiritual well-being. A thorough assessment requires the nurse to actively engage older adults and provide them with enough time to share important information about their health. The nurse assesses for changes in physiology, cognition, and psychosocial behaviour.

Nursing assessment must take into account five key points to ensure an age-specific approach: (a) the interrelation between physical and psychosocial aspects of aging, (b) the effects of disease and disability on functional status, (c) the decreased efficiency of homeostatic mechanisms, (d) the lack of standards for health and illness norms, and (e) altered presentation and response to specific disease (Lueckenotte, 2000). Obtaining a comprehensive assessment of an older adult often takes more time than an assessment of a younger adult because of the longer life and medical history and the potential complexity of that history. By planning to spend extra time with the assessment, the nurse and the older adult are less likely to feel rushed. During the physical examination, the nurse may find it necessary to allow rest periods or to conduct the assessment in several sessions because of the reduced energy and limited endurance experienced by some frail older adults.

Sensory changes may also affect data gathering. The nurse's choices of communication techniques will be influenced by any visual or hearing impairments experienced by the older adult. If older adults are unable to understand the nurse's visual or auditory cues, assessment data may be inaccurate or misleading. For example, if a client has difficulty hearing the nurse's questions, his or her responses may be inappropriate and the nurse may wrongly believe the client is confused. Communication techniques for the nurse to use when older adults have visual impairments include the following:

- Sit or stand in front of the client in full view.
- Face the older adult while speaking; do not cover your mouth.
- Provide diffuse, bright, non-glare lighting.
- Encourage clients with assistive devices such as glasses or magnifiers to use them.

Techniques for the nurse to use when older adults are hearing-impaired include the following:

- Speak directly to the client; do not cover your mouth.
- Speak in clear, low-pitched tones at a moderate rate and volume.
- Reduce background noises; move to a quiet, private room.
- Ask if there is a "good ear," and speak toward that ear.
- Encourage clients with assistive devices such as hearing aids or "microphone plus earphones" to use them.
- Make sure the hearing aid is working properly (check the battery, check that the hearing aid is turned on, adjust volume controls).
- Check the ear canal for cerumen impaction.

Memory deficits, if present, will affect the accuracy and completeness of the data collected. Information contributed by a family member or other caregiver may be necessary to supplement the older adult's recollection of past medical events and information such as allergies and immunizations. Tact must be used when involving another person in the assessment interview with the older adult. The additional person supplements the answers of the older adult with the consent of the older adult, but the older adult remains the focus of the interview.

With older clients, signs and symptoms of diseases and laboratory values may be different than those for younger clients. For example, the classic signs and symptoms of diseases may be absent, blunted, or atypical in older adults (Lueckenotte, 2000). These differences may be due to age-related changes in organ systems and homeostatic mechanisms, progressive loss of physiological and functional reserves, or coexisting acute or chronic conditions (Emmett, 1998). As a result, the older adult with a urinary tract infection may present with confusion, loss of appetite, weakness, dizziness, or fatigue instead of fever, dysuria, frequency, or urgency. The older adult with pneumonia may have tachycardia, tachypnea, and confusion without the more common symptoms of fever and productive cough. Instead of substernal chest pain and diaphoresis, the older adult with a myocardial infarction may experience no pain, epigastric discomfort, referred pain, restlessness, hypotension, or confusion. Variations from the usual norms for laboratory values may be due to age-related changes in cardiac, pulmonary, renal, and metabolic function (Beers & Berkow, 2000). Examples of laboratory values that may be increased by the aging process include, but are not limited to, alkaline phosphatase, serum cholesterol, triglycerides, serum glucose (postprandial), and serum uric acid. Examples of laboratory values that may be decreased by the aging process include, but are not limited to, serum calcium, serum creatine kinase, and creatinine clearance.

Physiological Changes

Perception of well-being can define quality of life. Understanding the older adult's perceptions about health status is essential for accurate assessment and development of clinically relevant interventions. Older adults' concepts of health generally depend on personal perceptions of functional ability. Therefore, older adults engaged in ADLs usually consider themselves healthy, whereas those whose activities are limited by physical, emotional, or social impairments may perceive themselves as ill.

There are frequently observed physiological changes in older adults that are called normal. Finding these "normal" changes during an assessment is not unexpected. These physiological changes are not always pathological processes in themselves, but they may make older adults more vulnerable to some common clinical conditions and diseases. Some older adults experience all of these physiological changes, and others experience only a few. The body changes continuously with age, and specific effects on particular older adults depend on health, lifestyle, stressors, and environmental conditions. The nurse should know about these normal, or more commonly experienced, changes in order to provide appropriate care for older adults and to assist with adaptation to the changes. Common physiological changes are summarized in Table 21-1.

General Survey. The general survey occurs during the initial nurse-client encounter and includes a quick, but careful, head-to-toe scan of the older adult that the nurse documents in a concise description. An initial inspection of an older adult might reveal eye contact and facial expression appropriate to the situation, as well as common aging changes such as facial wrinkles, grey hair, loss of body mass in the extremities, and an increase of body mass in the trunk.

Integumentary System. With aging, the skin loses resilience and moisture. The epithelial layer thins, and elastic collagen fibres shrink and become rigid. Wrinkles of the face and neck reflect lifelong patterns of muscle activity and facial expressions, the pull of gravity on tissue, and diminished elasticity.

Spots and lesions may also be present on the skin. Smooth, brown, irregularly shaped spots (age spots, or senile lentigo) initially appear on the backs of the hands and on forearms. Small, round, red or brown cherry angiomas may be found on the trunk. Seborrheic lesions or keratoses may appear as irregular, round or oval, brown watery lesions. Years of sun exposure contribute to the aging of the skin and may lead to premalignant and malignant lesions. Examination of skin lesions must rule out three malignancies related to sun exposure: melanoma, basal cell carcinoma, and squamous cell carcinoma (Beers & Berkow, 2000; see chapter 28).

Head and Neck. The facial features of the older adult become more pronounced from loss of subcutaneous fat and skin elasticity. Facial features may appear asymmetrical because of missing teeth or improperly fitting dentures. In addition, common vocal changes include a rise in pitch and a loss of power and range.

Visual acuity declines with age. This decline may be the result of retinal damage, reduced pupil size, development of opacities in the lens, or loss of lens elasticity. Presbyopia is common in older adults and is the gradual decline in the ability to focus on close objects. There is a reduced ability to see in darkness and to adapt to abrupt changes from dark areas to light areas (and the reverse). Ambient lighting (soft, indirect light that usually lights up the entire room) is generally the best type of lighting for older adults. However, older adults also have increased sensitivity to the effects of glare, and interventions to increase ambient light should not increase glare. Changes in colour vision and discolouration of the lens make it difficult to distinguish between blues and greens and among pastel shades.

Auditory changes are often subtle. The earliest losses of hearing acuity may be ignored until friends and family members comment on it. A common age-related change in auditory acuity is called presbycusis. Presbycusis affects the ability to hear high-pitched sounds and sibilant consonants such as *s, sh,* and *ch.* Before the nurse assumes presbycusis, it is necessary to inspect the external auditory canal for the presence of cerumen (ear wax). Impacted cerumen is an easily treated cause of diminished hearing acuity.

Taste buds atrophy and lose sensitivity. The older adult is less able to discern among salty, sweet, sour, and bitter tastes. The sense of smell is also decreased, further reducing taste. Salivary secretion is reduced.

Thorax and Lungs. Because of changes in the musculoskeletal system, the configuration of the thorax sometimes changes. After the age of 55 years, respiratory muscle strength begins to decrease (Beers & Berkow, 2000). The antero-posterior diameter of the thorax increases. Because of the increased incidence of osteoporosis in older adults, vertebral changes due to osteoporosis lead to dorsal kyphosis, the curvature of the thoracic spine sometimes called "dowager's hump." Calcification of the costal cartilage can cause decreased mobility of the ribs. The chest wall gradually becomes stiffer. Lung expansion decreases. If kyphosis or chronic obstructive lung disease is present, breath sounds are distant.

Heart and Vascular System. Decreased contractile strength of the myocardium results in a decreased cardiac output. The decrease is significant when the older adult is stressed by anxiety, excitement, illness, or strenuous activity. The body tries to compensate for decreased cardiac output by increasing the heart rate during exercise. However, after exercise, it takes longer for the older adult's rate to return to baseline.

Table 21-1 Common Physiological Changes With Aging

System	Common Changes
Integument	loss of skin elasticity (wrinkles, sagging, dryness, easily tears)
	pigmentation changes, glandular atrophy (oil, moisture, sweat glands)
	thinning hair (facial hair: decreased in men, increased in women)
	slower nail growth, atrophy of epidermal arterioles
Respiratory	decreased cough reflex
	decreased removal of mucus, dust, irritants from airways (decreased cilia)
	decreased vital capacity (increased anterior-posterior chest diameter)
	increased chest wall rigidity
	fewer alveoli, increased airway resistance
	increased risk of respiratory infections
Cardiovascular	thickening of blood vessel walls
	narrowing of vessel lumen
	loss of vessel elasticity
	lower cardiac output
	decreased number of heart muscle fibres
	decreased elasticity and calcification of heart valves
	decreased baroreceptor sensitivity
	decreased efficiency of venous valves
	increased pulmonary vascular tension
	increased systolic blood pressure
	decreased peripheral circulation
Gastrointestinal	periodontal disease
	loss of teeth
	decrease in saliva, gastric secretions, and pancreatic enzymes
	smooth muscle changes with decreased esophageal peristalsis and small intestinal motility
Musculoskeletal	decreased muscle mass and strength, decalcification of bones, degenerative joint changes, dehydration of intervertebral disks (decreased height)
Neurological	degeneration of nerve cells, decrease in neurotransmitters, decrease in rate of conduction of impulses
Sensory	
Eyes	decreased ability to focus on near objects (presbyopia)
	difficulty adjusting to changes from light to dark
	yellowing of the lens
	altered colour perception
	increased sensitivity to glare
	smaller pupils
Ears	loss of acuity for high-frequency tones (presbycusis)
	thickening of tympanic membrane
	sclerosis of inner ear
	may have buildup of earwax (cerumen)
Taste	often diminished, may have fewer taste buds
Smell	often diminished
Touch	decreased skin receptors
Proprioception	decreased awareness of body positioning in space
Genitourinary	fewer nephrons
	decreased renal blood flow
	decreased bladder capacity
Men	enlargement of prostate
Women	reduced sphincter tone
Reproductive	
Female	decreased estrogen production
	degeneration of ovaries
	atrophy of vagina, uterus, breasts
Male	sperm count diminishes
	smaller testes
	erections less firm and slow to develop
Endocrine	
General	alteration in hormone production with decreased ability to respond to stress
Thyroid	decreased secretion
Thymus	involution of thymus gland
Cortisols, glucocorticoids	increased anti-inflammatory hormone
Pancreas	increased fibrosis, decreased secretion of enzymes and hormones

Adapted from *Geriatric Nursing and Healthy Aging,* by P. Ebersole and P. Hess, 2001, St. Louis, MO: Mosby.

Systolic and/or diastolic blood pressures may be abnormally elevated. More than 50% of older adults have systolic or diastolic hypertension (systolic pressure >140 mm Hg, diastolic pressure >90 mm Hg; Beers & Berkow, 2000). Although a common chronic condition, hypertension is not a normal aging change; it predisposes older adults to heart failure, stroke, renal failure, coronary heart disease, and peripheral vascular disease.

Peripheral pulses are frequently weaker in the lower extremities, although still palpable. Older adults may report that their lower extremities are cold, particularly at night. Changes in the peripheral pulses in the upper extremities are less common.

Breasts. In older women, the breasts sag due to decreased muscle mass, tone, and elasticity. Atrophy of glandular tissue, coupled with more fat deposits, results in a slightly smaller, less dense, and less nodular breast. Gynecomastia, enlarged breasts in men, may be due to medication side effects, hormonal changes, or obesity. Although usually occurring in women, breast cancer can also occur in older men.

Gastrointestinal System and Abdomen. Aging leads to an increase in the amount of fatty tissue in the trunk. As a result, the abdomen increases in size. Because muscle tone and elasticity decrease, it also becomes more protuberant. Gastrointestinal function changes include a slowing of peristalsis and alterations in secretions. The older adult may experience these changes as the development of intolerance to certain foods and discomfort due to delayed gastric emptying. Alterations in the lower gastrointestinal tract may lead to constipation, flatulence, or diarrhea.

Reproductive System. Changes in the structure and function of the reproductive system occur as the result of hormonal alterations. Female menopause is related to a reduced responsiveness of the ovaries to pituitary hormones and a resultant decrease in estrogen and progesterone levels. In men, there is no definite cessation of fertility associated with aging. Spermatogenesis begins to decline during the fourth decade but continues into the ninth. The changes in reproductive structure and function, however, do not affect libido. Less frequent sexual activity can result from illness, death of a sexual partner, decreased socialization, or loss of sexual interest.

Urinary System. Hypertrophy of the prostate gland may develop in older men. This hypertrophy enlarges the gland, and pressure is displaced to the neck of the bladder. As a result, urinary retention, frequency, incontinence, and urinary tract infections may occur. In addition, prostatic hypertrophy can result in difficulty initiating voiding and maintaining a urinary stream. Benign prostatic hypertrophy must be distinguished from cancer of the prostate. Cancer of the prostate is the most frequently diagnosed cancer in men over the age of 70, resulting in the death of 1 of 26 men who are diagnosed (Canadian Cancer Society, 2004).

Urinary incontinence is an abnormal condition for older women, although it is experienced by 25% of middle-aged and older women (Canadian Continence Foundation, 2004). Older women, particularly those who have had children, can experience stress incontinence, an involuntary release of urine that occurs when they cough, sneeze, or lift an object. This type of incontinence is a result of a weakening of the perineal and bladder muscles. Other types of urinary incontinence are transient, urge, overflow, functional, reflex, and mixed incontinence (see chapter 40). The Registered Nurses Association of Ontario [RNAO] (2002b) recommends assessing risk factors for urinary incontinence, which include individual factors (fluid intake, medications, functional ability, and medical history) and environmental factors.

Musculoskeletal System. With aging, muscle fibres are reduced in size. Muscle strength diminishes in proportion to the decline in muscle mass. Bone mass also declines. Older adults who exercise regularly do not lose as much bone and muscle mass or muscle tone as those who are inactive. Twenty-five percent of Canadian women over the age of 50 years have osteoporosis (Osteoporosis Society of Canada, 2004). Women who maintain calcium intake throughout life and into menopause have less bone demineralization than women with low calcium intake. Older men with poor nutrition and decreased mobility are also at risk for bone demineralization. One of eight men in Canada has osteoporosis.

Neurological System. The decrease in the number of neurons in the nervous system that begins in the middle of the second decade can lead to changes such as those affecting the senses described earlier. In addition, the older adult may experience a decreased sense of balance or uncoordinated motor responses. Older adults frequently report alterations in the quality and the quantity of sleep, including difficulty falling asleep, difficulty staying asleep, difficulty falling asleep again after waking during the night, waking too early in the morning, and excessive daytime napping (see chapter 37).

Cognitive Changes

A common misconception about aging is that cognitive impairments are widespread among older adults. Younger adults often assume that older adults are confused and no longer able to handle their affairs. Structural and physiological changes within the brain, such as reduction in the number of cells, deposition of lipofuscin and amyloid in cells, and change in neurotransmitter levels, are a normal part of aging and are seen in older adults with and without cognitive impairment. Symptoms of cognitive impairment such as disorientation, loss of language skills, loss of the ability to calculate, and poor judgment are not normal aging changes. When the nurse identifies these changes during the assessment, further investigation of the underlying causes is indicated.

The three common conditions affecting cognition are **delirium, dementia,** and **depression** (Table 21-2). The nurse may find that distinguishing among these three conditions is challenging but essential for selecting appropriate nursing interventions. The RNAO published best practice guidelines to screen for delirium, dementia, and depression in older adults (2003). Appropriate nursing interventions

Table 21-2 A Comparison of the Clinical Features of Delirium, Dementia, and Depression

Clinical Feature	Delirium	Dementia	Depression
Onset	Acute/subacute, depends on cause, often at twilight or in darkness	Chronic, generally insidious, depends on cause	Chronic, generally insidious, depends on cause
Course	Short, diurnal fluctuations in symptoms, worse at night, in darkness, and on awakening	Long, no diurnal effects, symptoms progressive yet relatively stable over time	Diurnal effects, typically worse in the morning, situational fluctuations, but less than with delirium
Progression	Abrupt	Slow but uneven	Variable, rapid, or slow but even
Duration	Hours to less than 1 month, seldom longer	Months to years	At least 6 weeks, can be several months to years

Data from "Assessing Cognitive Function," by M. Foreman et al., 1996, *Geriatric Nursing, 17*(5), p. 228.

are specific to the cause of the cognitive impairment. The use of techniques such as reality orientation, validation therapy, and reminiscence also depends on the nature of the cognitive impairment.

Delirium. Delirium, or acute confusional state, is a potentially reversible cognitive impairment that often has a physiological cause. Physiological causes of delirium include, but are not limited to, electrolyte imbalances, cerebral anoxia, hypoglycemia, medications, drug effects, tumours, subdural hematomas, and cerebrovascular infection, infarction, or hemorrhage. Delirium in older adults sometimes accompanies systemic infections and may be the presenting symptom for pneumonia or urinary tract infection. Delirium may also be due to environmental factors such as sensory deprivation or unfamiliar surroundings or to psychosocial factors such as emotional distress or pain. Although delirium may occur in any setting, an older adult in the acute care setting is especially at risk because of predisposing factors (physiological, psychosocial, and environmental) in combination with the medical condition that led to the hospital admission.

Delirium is characterized by fluctuations in cognition, mood, attention, arousal, and self-awareness. Other signs may be hallucinations, occasional incoherent speech, disturbed sleep-wake cycle, and disorientation. The onset of delirium is typically sudden, and there are rapid fluctuations in symptoms and severity. The presence of delirium requires prompt assessment and intervention. The cognitive impairment secondary to delirium is usually reversed once the cause of delirium is identified and treatment started unless there has been permanent brain injury.

Dementia. Dementia is a generalized impairment of intellectual functioning that interferes with social and occupational functioning. Cognitive function deterioration leads to a decline in the ability to perform basic and instrumental ADLs. Unlike delirium, dementia is characterized by a gradual, progressive, irreversible cerebral dysfunction. Because of the close resemblance of delirium and dementia, the presence of delirium must be ruled out whenever dementia is suspected. Bolla, Filley, and Palmer (2000) described four major types of dementia: Alzheimer's disease (50%), diffuse Lewy body disease (DLBD) (15%), frontal-temporal dementia (15%), and vascular dementia (10%). Other causes of dementia, such as infection or trauma, account for another 10% of cases. In Canada, approximately 34.5% of adults over the age of 85 years have dementia, compared with 2.4% of those aged 65 to 74 years (Alzheimer Society, 2004).

The most common form of dementia is **Alzheimer's disease.** The cause of the disease is not known, and although several theories are being studied, none are definitive. Cholinesterase-inhibiting medications (donepezil, rivastigmine, galantamine) are currently prescribed to slow the progression of symptoms. These medications prevent the breakdown of the neurotransmitter acetylcholine by the enzyme cholinesterase (Conn, 2001). It is hypothesized that by increasing the amount of acetylcholine available to transmit impulses among neurons, cognition in some older adults with Alzheimer's disease will improve. The characteristic progressive symptoms of Alzheimer's disease are loss of memory (amnesia), loss of the ability to recognize objects and people (agnosia), loss of the ability to perform familiar tasks (apraxia), and loss of language skills (aphasia). As Alzheimer's disease progresses, the older adult becomes more dependent on caregivers for assistance with ADLs. Safety issues must be addressed as the disease progresses and the ability to judge risks diminishes.

Like Alzheimer's disease, DLBD is progressive. The features of DLBD include dementia, fluctuating cognition, visual and/or auditory hallucinations, and the motor features of Parkinsonism.

Frontal-temporal dementia has an insidious onset and progresses slowly. Early symptoms include poor hygiene, lack of social tact, hyper-orality, and sexual disinhibition. Incontinence is an early symptom in frontal-temporal dementia, although it is a late symptom in the more common Alzheimer's disease. Repetitive behaviours (wandering, clapping, singing, picking up objects) are frequently observed. Safety and behaviour managements are major concerns for caregivers.

The cause of vascular dementia is interruption of blood supply to areas of the brain by thromboembolism, hemorrhage, or ischemia (Bolla et al., 2000). Symptoms of vascular dementia vary with the areas of the brain affected. Progression of vascular dementia may be either stepwise with repeated episodes of damage to the brain over time or steadily progressive. Management of vascular dementia parallels the recommendations for cerebrovascular disease (i.e., reduction of risk factors by treatment of hypertension, hyperlipidemia, carotid disease, arrhythmias, diabetes mellitus, and polycythemia vera). Because the use of nicotine has been linked with vascular disease, older adults with vascular dementia should stop or reduce their use of tobacco products. If the older adult has a cardiac arrhythmia such as atrial fibrillation, anticoagulant therapy may be indicated to reduce the risk of thromboembolism.

Nursing management of older adults with any form of dementia must consider the needs of the older adult with dementia and the needs of the family. Those needs change as the progressive nature of dementia leads to increased cognitive deterioration. In addition to the physical needs of the older adult, safety needs and psychosocial needs must be considered. The older adult's family needs information and support. Nursing care objectives are individualized and promote the use of the remaining functional abilities.

Depression. Late-life depression may be experienced by 15% to 20% of community-based older adults (RNAO, 2003). Depression reduces happiness and well-being, contributes to physical and social limitations, complicates the treatment of concomitant medical conditions, and increases the risk of suicide. The presentation of depression in older adults differs from that of younger adults. Older adults are more likely to talk about being "blue" or "down in the dumps" and may express feelings of diminished life satisfaction (Miller, 2004).

Delirium and depression, both reversible disorders, are often mistaken for irreversible dementia in the older adult because cerebral dysfunction and cognitive impairment occur with these conditions as well as with dementia. Careful and thorough assessment of older adults with cognitive impairment is essential in order to distinguish among delirium, dementia, and depression. The beginning nurse may choose to consult with a clinical nurse specialist in gerontology. Accurate assessment is necessary to select appropriate nursing interventions.

Psychosocial Changes

The psychosocial changes that occur with aging involve changes in roles and relationships. Roles and relationships within the family change as parents become grandparents, adult children become caregivers for aging parents, or spouses become widows or widowers. Group membership roles and relationships change as the older adult retires from work, moves from a familiar neighbourhood, or stops attending social activities because of declining health status.

The nurse assesses both the nature of the psychosocial changes facing an older adult and the adaptation of the older adult to those changes. In the assessment, the nurse asks how the older adult feels about self, self in relation to others, and self as aging. Areas to be addressed during the assessment include the family, intimate relationships, past and present occupation, finances, housing, social networks, activities, and spirituality. Specific topics related to these areas include retirement, housing and environment, social isolation, sexuality, and death.

Retirement. Retirement is often mistakenly associated with passivity and seclusion. In actuality, it is a stage of life characterized by transitions and role changes. The psychosocial stresses of retirement may be related to role changes with the spouse or within the family and to loss of role. There may also be problems related to social isolation and finances. The age of retirement varies. Retirement, which may be mandatory or voluntary, occurs at a variety of ages. But whether it occurs at the age of 55, 65, or 75 years, retirement is one of the major turning points in life.

Pre-retirement planning is an important advisable task for middle-age individuals. People who plan in advance for retirement generally have a smoother transition into retirement. Pre-retirement planning is more than financial planning, although financial planning is important. Planning begins with consideration of the "style" of retirement desired and includes an inventory of interests, current skills, and general health. Meaningful retirement planning is critical because retirement can last for 30 or more years.

Retirement has an impact on more individuals than the retired person. Spouses, adult children, and grandchildren are all affected. When the spouse is still working, the retired person faces time alone. For example, the working spouse may have new ideas about the amount of participation in housework expected of the retired person. Friction may develop when the plans of the retired person conflict with the work responsibilities of the working spouse. The working spouse may also have expectations of the retired person that need clarification. For couples, the adjustment to retirement is affected by the quality of their communication with each other, their process of decision making about issues such as money or activities, their adherence to either traditional or shared role orientations, and their level of affection and intimacy (Ebersole & Hess, 2004). Adult children may expect the retired person to become an automatic babysitter for the grandchildren.

Loss of the work role has a major impact on some retired people. When so much of life has revolved around work and the personal relationships at work, the loss of the work role may be devastating. Personal identity may be rooted in the work role, and with retirement a new identity must be constructed. The structure imposed on daily life by a work schedule is also lost with retirement, as are the social exchanges and interpersonal support that occur in the workplace. In the adjustment to retirement, the older adult is challenged to develop a personally meaningful schedule and a supportive social network.

The most powerful factors that influence the retired person's satisfaction with life are health status, the option to continue working, and sufficient income (Ebersole & Hess, 2004). Positive pre-retirement expectations also contribute to satisfaction in retirement. The nurse can help the older adult and family prepare for retirement by discussing with them several key areas, including relations with spouse and children, meaningful activities to replace the work role, adjusting or rebuilding social networks, issues related to income and health promotion and maintenance, and long-range planning, including wills and advance directives.

Social Isolation. Social isolation and loneliness are significant issues for older adults regardless of gender and geographic location (Havens et al., 2004). Social isolation is an objective measure of contacts with other people. Loneliness is the dissatisfaction with the level of social contact. There are two forms of isolation: Isolation may be a choice to interact with others, or it may be a response to conditions that inhibit the ability or the opportunity to interact with others (Ebersole & Hess, 2004). Whether or not isolation is a choice for older adults, they are vulnerable to its consequences.

Living alone and having multiple chronic illnesses are factors contributing to social isolation and loneliness (Havens et al., 2004). Some older adults see themselves as unattractive and rejected because of changes in their personal appearance due to normal aging or because of body image changes following illness or surgery (Ebersole & Hess, 2004). Older adults who are confused or incontinent, who are unable to communicate, who are institutionalized, or who are poor or homeless may feel isolated. The societal trend toward the geographic dispersion of families leads to decreased opportunities for interaction among family members.

The nurse can assist lonely older adults to rebuild social networks and reverse patterns of isolation (Ebersole & Hess, 2004). Many communities have outreach programs designed to make contact with isolated older adults. Outreach programs may meet nutritional needs, such as Meals on Wheels; socialization needs, such as daily telephone calls by volunteers; or needs for activities, such as outings. Social service agencies in most communities welcome older adults as volunteers and provide them with the opportunity to serve and to be served. Other organizations within communities such as churches, colleges, and libraries offer a variety of programs for older adults that increase the opportunity to meet people with similar activities, interests, and needs.

Sexuality. Sexuality is increasingly recognized as an important factor in the care of older adults. All older adults, whether healthy or frail, need to express sexual feelings. Sexuality involves love, warmth, sharing, and touching, not just the act of intercourse. Sexuality is linked with identity and validates the belief that people can give to others and have the gift appreciated.

Maintaining sexual health requires integration of somatic, emotional, intellectual, and social aspects of the sexual being. To help the older adult achieve or maintain sexual health, the nurse needs to understand the physical changes in sexual response (see chapter 23). The nurse should provide privacy for any discussion of sexuality and should maintain a non-judgmental attitude. Open-ended questions inviting the older adult to explain sexual activities or concerns may elicit more information than a list of closed-ended questions about specific activities or symptoms. Older adults may appreciate information about the typical age-related changes in sexuality. Information about the prevention of sexually transmitted infections should be included when appropriate.

The older adult's libido does not decrease, although frequency of sexual activity may decline. An older woman who does not understand physical changes affecting sexual activity may be concerned that her sex life is nearly over with the onset of menopause. The older man may feel the same when he discovers a change in the firmness of his erection, a decreased need for ejaculation with each orgasm, or a longer recovery period between episodes of intercourse.

In addition to the physical changes that affect sexual functioning, many older adults use prescription medications that depress sexual activity as a side effect, such as antihypertensives, antidepressants, sedatives, and hypnotics. Some drugs increase libido in older adults. For example, phenothiazines increase sexual desire in women, and levodopa has a similar effect in men.

While considering the older adult's need for sexual expression, the nurse must not ignore the important need to touch and be touched. Touch is an overt expression with many meanings and is an important part of sexuality. Touch can complement traditional sexual methods or serve as an alternative sexual expression when physical intercourse is not desired or possible and thus can serve as an important method of achieving intimacy (Wallace, 1996). The nursing student needs to recognize that knowledge of older adults' sexual and intimacy needs will increase with professional growth. Experience in caring for older adults combined with the ability to establish therapeutic connection allows the nurse to learn how to explore clients' sexual concerns. Knowing an older adult's sexual needs allows the nurse to incorporate this information into the nursing care plan.

The sexual preferences of older adults are as diverse as those of the younger population. Not all older adults are heterosexual. Little information is available regarding older adult homosexuals and their health care needs, although Wojciechowski (1998) described the health care needs of older lesbian women and older heterosexual women as similar. To be effective caregivers for older homosexuals, nurses need to be aware of their own beliefs about sexuality and the potential impact of those beliefs on their ability to provide care.

Nurses may find that they are called on to advise older adults and help other health care professionals understand the sexual needs of older adults. Not all nurses feel comfortable counselling older adults about sexual health and need not feel obligated to do so. But all nurses should be prepared to refer older adults to appropriate professional counsellors.

Housing and Environment. The extent of the older adult's ability to live independently strongly determines housing choices. Changes in social roles, family responsibilities, and health status influence older adults' living arrangements. Some choose to live with family members. Others prefer their own homes or apartments near their families. Leisure or retirement communities provide older people with living and social opportunities in a one-generation setting. Federally subsidized housing, where available, offers apartments with communal, social, and, in some cases, food service arrangements.

When assisting older adults with housing needs, the nurse should assess their activity level, financial status, access to public transportation and community activities, environmental hazards, and support systems. Housing choices should also look to the future needs of the older adults in so far as these can be anticipated. A housing unit with only one floor and without exterior steps may be a prudent choice for the older adult with severe arthritis who has already had some lower extremity joint replacement surgeries and anticipates the need for future surgeries.

Housing and environment have a major impact on the health of older adults. The environment can support or hinder physical and social functioning, enhance or drain energy, and complement or tax existing physical changes such as vision and hearing. For example, the colours red, orange, and yellow are easiest for older adults to see. In contrast, older adults have difficulty distinguishing between green and blue and among pastel shades. To help older adults in health care settings find their rooms, pictures or other decorations near their doors can be used as landmarks. Door frames and baseboards in a colour that contrasts with the colour of the wall improve perception of the boundaries of halls and rooms. Glare from highly polished floors, metallic fixtures, and windows is poorly tolerated.

Furniture should be comfortable and designed for the musculoskeletal changes of older adults. Older adults should examine furniture carefully for size, comfort, and function before purchasing it. Furniture should be easy to get into and out of and should provide back support. Dining room chairs should be tested for comfort during meals and for height in relation to the table. Older adults may prefer transferring out of a wheelchair to another chair for meals because some styles of wheelchairs do not let older adults sit close enough to the table to eat comfortably. Raising the table to clear the wheelchair arms may bring the table closer to the older adult but may make it too high for comfortable use. To make getting out of bed easier and safer, the height of the bed should allow the older adult's feet to be flat on the floor when the older adult is sitting on the side of the bed.

The goal of nursing assessment of the environment is the promotion of independence and functional ability (Fielo & Warren, 2001). Assessment of safety, a major component of the older adult's environment, includes risks within the environment and the older adult's ability to recognize and respond to the risks. Risks include factors leading to injury within the home, such as water heaters set at excessively hot temperatures or throw rugs that could cause a fall, and factors outside of the home, such as deteriorating sidewalks and steps or a high incidence of street crime.

Death. Part of the life history of an older adult is the experience of the death of family members and friends (see chapter 25). This experience includes the loss of the older generations of their families and sometimes the loss of a child or grandchild. One third of Canadian older adults have experienced the death of a spouse (Health Canada, 2002). As the older adult ages, friends gradually die. Despite these experiences, it would be wrong to assume that the older adult is comfortable with the idea of death.

Fear of death in old age is a multi-dimensional concept. Religiosity and external locus of control have a direct impact on fear of death (Cicirelli, 1999). Ethnicity and gender indirectly affect fear of death by influencing religiosity. Age and socio-economic status affect fear of death by influencing a person's external locus of control. The stereotype that the death of an older adult is a blessing and the culmination of a full life will not apply to every older adult. Even as death approaches, many older adults still have unfinished business and are not prepared to die. Families and friends may not be ready to let go of the older adult. The nurse may be the person to whom the older adult and family members or friends turn to for assistance in coping with death and loss.

Addressing the Health Concerns of Older Adults

The three most common causes of death in Canadian older adults are heart disease, cancer, and stroke. Other frequently reported causes of death are respiratory disease, accidents/falls, diabetes, kidney disease, and liver disease (Health Canada, 2002). All of these causes of death have preventive measures that could potentially reduce the frequency of these conditions and delay disability and/or death (Rubenstein & Nahas, 1998).

Health Canada's NACA (2003) has identified the following areas that require action to improve the health of older adults:

- Injury prevention
- Promotion of physical activity
- Suicide prevention
- Reducing the cost of prescription drugs
- Improving the quality of home and institutionalized care
- Addressing the shortage of geriatricians
- Increasing incomes of older adults
- Increasing affordable rental housing
- Reducing the rate of economic crime victimization
- Abolishing mandatory retirement at the age of 65 years

Nurses participate in activities such as health screenings and fairs that can identify older adults at risk and advise them about disease prevention and health promotion measures (Davidhizar, Eshleman, & Moody, 2002). Many communities offer wellness programs where older adults can access information about health promotion and disease prevention (Box 21-4). Nurses in acute care and long-term care settings also assess the health status of older adults, intervene in acute situations, and, with the older adults, plan strategies to reduce risk and manage chronic conditions. Each contact with an older adult, regardless of setting, offers opportunities to teach and counsel.

Nursing interventions for older adults are directed toward improving or maintaining the older adult's health needs and concerns. Although various interventions cross all three levels of care—health promotion, acute care, and restorative care—there are approaches unique

Focus on Primary Health Care — Box 21-4

Older Adult Wellness Programs

Focusing on self-care abilities and practices that foster health while aging are important nursing interventions (Pender, Murdaugh, & Parsons, 2002). Factors that have been reported to affect older adults' willingness to engage in health promotion activities include socio-economic factors, beliefs and attitudes, encouragement by a health care professional, access to resources, age, number of chronic illnesses, and mental and physical health (Resnick, 2003). Generally, older adults seem to be less interested in engaging in health promotion activities for the purpose of lengthening their lives but may have greater interest in these activities if they improve quality of life (Resnick, 2003).

In order to help older adults maintain function and improve quality of life, the Saskatoon Health Region, in conjunction with several other community agencies, has established an Older Adult Wellness Program. The program goals are to

1. Encourage older adults to adopt lifestyle choices and practices that preserve their health.
2. Promote the concept of mutual aide and social support among older adults in the community (capacity building).
3. Alter or adapt social economic or physical surroundings to preserve and enhance the health of older adults.

The program is housed in a public health centre and employs two full-time registered nurses. As part of this program, the nurses provide educational programs on promoting older adults' health to the community, health care professionals, and older adults. They also organize and provide a program to increase physical activity and decrease falls. Preventive services such as health screening and immunizations are also offered to older adults. A community resource directory has been published and is used by older adults and nurses to access services for program participants.

From *Older Adult Wellness Program Annual Report* by Saskatoon Health Region, 2003, Saskatoon, SK: Author, p. 1–23.

Research Highlight — Box 21-5

Benefits of a Health Promotion Program

Research Focus

The purpose of this study was to evaluate participation, processes, and impact of the Seniors Active Living in Vulnerable Elders (ALIVE) program. ALIVE was a 10-month health promotion program for low-income older adults in Alberta.

Research Abstract

The ALIVE program consisted of exercise classes, health information sessions (i.e., health concerns), and newsletters delivered in older adults' apartment buildings for 10 months. At the end of 10 months, 34 of the older adults who participated and 3 of the program staff were asked to answer the following questions:

1. What factors influenced older adults' participation in the program?
2. How did the program impact those who attended?
3. How did the program work?

The most frequent reason for joining the program was because the person recognized the benefits of exercise; and the most frequent reason for not attending the program was having other priorities. The main participant impact was "feeling better." Participants described feeling physically and mentally better and reported enjoying the social interaction. Fun, program delivery adaptations, autonomy, social interactions, and staff-participant relationships were discovered to be important program processes.

Evidence-Based Practice

- Health promotion programs need to be fun and flexible and to encourage social interactions.
- Program delivery adaptations reduce barriers to participation by being offered in the daytime in a familiar location, requiring no cost, and requiring no transportation.
- Nurses play a key role in planning, implementing, and evaluating health promotion programs for older adults.

Reference

Buijs, R., et al. (2003). Promoting participation: Evaluation of a health promotion program for low income seniors. *Journal of Community Health Nursing, 20*(2), 93–107.

to each level. When planning interventions, it is important for the nurse to incorporate the older adult's routines or rituals when possible because the older adult feels more secure when routines are continued. The interventions generally are aimed at promoting independence and supporting self-care abilities.

Health Promotion and Maintenance: Physiological Concerns

Older adults believe that activity is important for staying fit and remaining independent and that their own positive actions contribute to wellness and quality of life (Clark, 1998). The factors that lead to wellness in advanced age have not been fully identified, but four important factors seem to be genetics, good luck, good health habits, and preventive measures (Rubenstein & Nahas, 1998). The nurse is unable to do anything about an older adult's genetic heritage or luck, but the nurse is in a unique position to establish health maintenance programs that promote older adults' wellness and to recommend preventive measures. Such programs have been found to have a positive impact on the physical, mental, and social health of older adults (Buijs et al., 2003; Box 21-5). Senior citizens' centres, churches, schools, shopping malls, libraries, and hospital lobbies can be used as settings to conduct screening tests and present information on health topics. Using creative approaches, the nurse can include health promotion activities for older adults in all health care settings.

Approximately 80% of older adults living at home have at least one chronic health condition. The most common conditions are arthritis, high blood pressure, back problems, chronic heart problems, cataracts, and diabetes (Health Canada, 2002). The effect of chronic conditions on the lives of older adults varies widely, but, in general, chronic conditions diminish well-being and threaten the independence of older adults. Nursing interventions are often directed at the management of these conditions, but interventions can also focus on prevention (Rubenstein & Nahas, 1998). General preventive measures that nurses can recommend to older adults include the following:

- Regular exercise
- Weight reduction if overweight
- Management of hypertension
- Smoking cessation
- Immunization for influenza, pneumococcal pneumonia, and tetanus

Approximately 70,000 to 75,000 hospitalizations and 6,700 deaths each year are attributed to influenza (Menec et al., 2003). Annual immunization for influenza of all older adults is strongly recommended, with special emphasis on the immunization for influenza of residents of long-term care facilities and clients of any age with chronic cardiovascular, pulmonary, and metabolic disorders (Gomolin & Kathpalia, 2002). Receipt of the pneumococcal pneumonia vaccine is recommended for all adults over 65 years of age. Unlike influenza vaccine, pneumococcal pneumonia vaccine is given only once, although revaccination 6 to 8 years after the initial vaccination is recommended by some authorities (Beers & Berkow, 2000). For tetanus immunization, booster injections every 10 years are recommended for adults who have had the primary series for tetanus immunization. However, not all older adults are current with their booster injections and some never received the primary series of injections. Nurses should ask older adults about the current status of all three types of immunizations, provide information about the immunizations, and make arrangements for the older adult to receive the immunizations as needed. Nurses should also refer older adults for screening for the early detection of cancer and depression.

Most older adults are interested in their health and are capable of taking charge of their lives. They want to remain independent and to prevent disability (Figure 21–1). Initial screenings establish baseline data that can be used to determine wellness, identify health needs, and design health maintenance programs. Following initial screening sessions, nurses can share information on nutrition, exercise, medications, and safety precautions with older adults. Information on specific conditions such as hypertension or arthritis or on self-care procedures such as foot and skin care may also be provided. By providing information about health promotion and self-care, nurses can significantly improve the health and well-being of older adults.

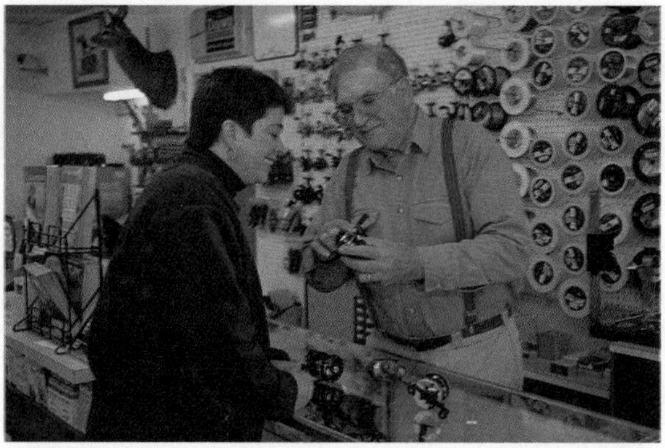

FIGURE 21–1 This older adult works part-time at a sporting goods store.

Heart Disease. Heart disease is the leading cause of death in older adults. Common cardiovascular disorders are hypertension and coronary artery disease. Hypertension is diagnosed when repeated blood pressure measurements of 90 mm Hg or greater diastolic and 140 mm Hg or greater systolic are present. Although over 30% of Canadians have elevated diastolic and/or systolic pressures (Health Canada, 2002), the fact that hypertension is common does not make it normal or harmless. Systolic pressures higher than 160 mm Hg are associated with increased risk of stroke, increased risk of cardiovascular mortality, and increased risk of overall mortality (Beers & Berkow, 2000). In coronary artery disease, partial or complete blockage of one or more coronary arteries leads to myocardial ischemia and myocardial infarction. The risk factors for both hypertension and coronary artery disease include smoking, obesity, lack of exercise, and stress. Additional risk factors for coronary artery disease include hypertension, hyperlipidemia, and diabetes mellitus. Nursing interventions for hypertension and coronary artery disease address weight reduction, exercise, dietary changes limiting salt and fat, stress management, and smoking cessation. Client teaching includes information about medications, blood pressure monitoring, nutrition, stress reduction techniques, and the symptoms indicating the need for emergency care.

Cancer. Malignant neoplasms are the second most common cause of death among older adults. Nurses participate in programs to educate older adults about early detection, treatment, and risk factors. Examples include smoking cessation, teaching breast self-examination (see chapter 28), and encouraging all older adults to have annual screening for fecal occult blood. It is also important to educate older adults about the signs of cancer and encourage prompt reporting of non-healing skin lesions, unexpected bleeding, change in bowel habits, and unexplained weight loss (Rubenstein & Nahas, 1998). Detection is complicated when cancer symptoms are mistakenly identified as part of the normal aging process, and the nurse must carefully distinguish between normal aging and pathological conditions.

Stroke (Cerebrovascular Accident). Cerebrovascular accidents, the third leading cause of death in Canada, occur as brain ischemia or brain hemorrhage (Health Canada, 2002). In brain ischemia, there is an inadequate supply of blood to areas of the brain due to blockage of blood vessels or general circulatory failure. Brain hemorrhage, either subarachnoid hemorrhage or intracerebral hemorrhage, is less common than brain ischemia. Risk factors for cerebrovascular accidents include hypertension, hyperlipidemia, diabetes mellitus, history of transient ischemic attacks, and family history of cardiovascular disease.

Treatment usually includes hospitalization for days or months, depending on the degree of brain injury. Cerebrovascular accidents may impair the functional abilities of older adults and limit their ability to live independently. The scope of nursing interventions ranges from teaching older adults about risk reduction strategies to care of the older adult after a cerebrovascular accident and during recovery and rehabilitation.

Smoking. Cigarette smoking has been recognized as the major preventable cause of death and disease in Canada (Health Canada, 2004). Smoking cessation is a health promotion strategy for older adults just as it is for younger adults. Older smokers can still benefit from smoking cessation (Boyd, 1996). In addition to reducing risk, smoking cessation may stabilize existing conditions such as chronic obstructive pulmonary disease. Smoking cessation may even contribute to the extension of life or of independent functioning.

There are four sequential approaches that nurses may use to encourage smoking cessation (Boyd, 1996). First, the nurse asks the older adult about smoking, including the type of tobacco product used, the frequency of smoking, and the number of years smoking. The nurse then provides information about the ill effects of smoking and recommends quitting. If the client does not choose to quit smoking, the nurse should suggest a reduction in smoking. The nurse offers to help develop a plan for quitting (e.g., discusses the use of nicotine gum or patches and asking family members to reduce smoking). Lastly, the nurse, on subsequent visits with the older adult, offers encouragement and assistance in modifying the plan as necessary. Although some mistakenly believe that older adults do not want to quit smoking or are unable to quit, some older adults do choose to quit smoking and do succeed.

Alcohol Abuse. It is estimated that up to 12% of older adults consume 14 or more drinks a week (Statistics Canada, 2004). Studies of alcohol abuse in older adults report two patterns: a lifelong pattern of heavy drinking that continues and a late-onset pattern when heavy drinking begins late in life. Frequently cited causes of excessive alcohol use are depression, loneliness, and lack of social support.

Abuse of alcohol may be under-identified in older adults. Signs of alcohol abuse are subtle, and the assessment may be complicated by coexisting dementia or depression. Suspicion of alcohol abuse increases when there is a history of repeated falls and accidents, a change in behaviour or personality, social isolation, recurring episodes of memory loss and confusion, a history of skipping meals or medications, and difficulty managing household tasks and finances (Peterson & Zimberg, 1996). When abuse of alcohol is suspected, treatment includes age-specific approaches that acknowledge the stresses experienced by the older adult and encourage involvement in activities that match the older adult's interests and boost feelings of self-worth. The identification and treatment of coexisting depression is also important.

Nutrition. How older adults meet their needs for good nutrition is influenced by lifelong eating habits and situational factors. Lifelong eating habits based in tradition, ethnicity, and religion influence choices of what foods are eaten and how those foods are prepared. Situational factors affecting nutrition include access to food stores, adequate finances, the physical and cognitive capability for food preparation, and a place to store food and prepare meals.

The nutritional needs of older adults are affected by their levels of activity and by clinical conditions. Level of activity has implications for the total amount of calories, with more sedentary older adults usually needing fewer calories than more active older adults. However, caloric requirements are not determined solely by activity. Additional calories may be required in clinical situations such as recovery from surgery, whereas calories may be restricted when the older adult is diabetic or overweight. Beyond caloric requirements, therapeutic diets may restrict fat, sodium, or simple sugars or may increase fibre or foods high in calcium, iron, vitamin A, or vitamin C.

Good nutrition for older adults includes appropriate caloric intake and limited intake of fat, salt, refined sugars, and alcohol. Although the nutritional guidelines displayed in Canada's Food Guide are the basic recommendations for older adult nutrition (see chapter 39), some older adults do not follow these guidelines. Protein intake may be lower than recommended if older adults have reduced financial resources or limited access to grocery stores. Difficulty chewing meat may also limit protein intake. Fat intake may be higher than recommended because of the substitution of fast-food restaurant meals for meals prepared at home or because of methods of cooking featuring fried foods and sauces using butter and cream. Extra salt and sugar may be used while cooking or at the table to compensate for a diminished sense of taste. Vitamin intake may be reduced if shopping for fresh fruits and vegetables is difficult.

Older adults with dementia have special nutritional needs. As their memory and their functional skills decline with the progression of dementia, they lose the ability to remember when to eat, how to prepare food, and, eventually, how to feed themselves. At the same time, their caloric needs may increase because of the energy expended in pacing and wandering activities. Nurses and other caregivers of older adults with dementia should routinely monitor weight and food intake, serve food that is easy to eat, provide assistance with eating, and offer food supplements as needed to maintain weight (Yen, 1997). Mealtime interventions for older adults with dementia also provide opportunities for socialization and practise with functional skills.

Dental Problems. Dental problems are common in older adults and include problems with natural teeth and dentures. Dental caries, gingivitis, broken or missing teeth, and ill-fitting or missing dentures may affect nutritional adequacy, cause pain, and lead to infection. The nurse can help prevent dental and gum disease through education about routine dental care (see chapter 34). The nurse can also help older adults find dental services that offer reduced rates and that are accessible to those with impaired mobility.

Exercise. Older adults should be encouraged to maintain physical exercise and activity. The primary benefits of exercise include maintaining and strengthening functional ability and promoting a sense of enhanced well-being. An exercise such as walking builds endurance, increases muscle tone, improves joint flexibility, strengthens bones, reduces stress, and contributes to weight loss (Butler, 1998). Other benefits of a program of exercise include improvement of cardiovascular function, improved plasma lipoprotein profiles, increased metabolic rate, increased gastrointestinal transit time, and improved sleep quality (Butler et al., 1998). Frail older adults who exercise may experience improved mobility, gait, and balance as well as less difficulty getting up from a chair or climbing stairs. Exercise may also have a positive effect on anxiety and depression (Gunnarsson & Judge, 1997).

The nurse should plan an exercise program that meets physical needs while allowing for physical impairments and encourage the older adult to persevere with the exercise program. Willingness to participate in and persevere with an exercise program is influenced by general beliefs about exercise, specific benefits from exercise, past experiences with exercise, personal goals, personality, and any unpleasant sensations associated with exercise (Resnick & Spellbring, 2000). Walking is the preferred exercise of many older adults (Figure 21–2). Walking and other low-impact exercises such as riding an exercise (stationary) bicycle or exercises in a swimming pool protect the musculoskeletal system and joints (Ellingson & Conn, 2000). Other exercises can be incorporated into the older adult's activities of daily living. For example, arm and leg circles can be performed while watching television. However, before beginning an exercise program, the older adult should have a physical examination. Exercise programs for sedentary older adults who have not been exercising regularly should begin conservatively and progress slowly. Safety considerations include wearing shoes and clothing appropriate to the exercise, drinking water before and after exercising, avoiding outdoor exercise when the weather is very warm or very cold, and exercising with a partner. Nurses should instruct the older adult to stop exercising and seek help if chest pain or tightness, shortness of breath, dizziness or light-headedness, or palpitations are experienced during exercise (Gunnarsson & Judge, 1997).

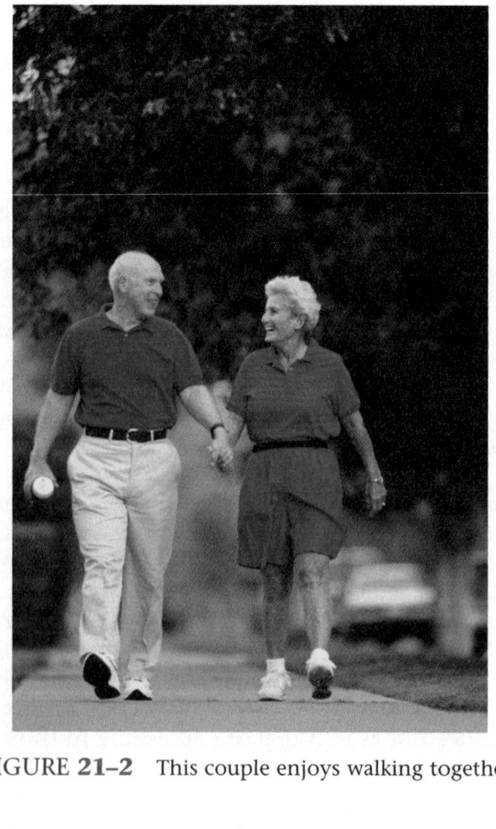

FIGURE **21–2** This couple enjoys walking together.

Arthritis. Arthritis is a common condition in older adults, especially in women. The degree to which the mobility of older adults is impaired depends on the extent of the disease and joints affected. The impact of arthritis on the lives of older adults is a combination of the changes in joint range of motion and stability and the amount of pain experienced. Arthritis has no cure, but recently developed pharmacological agents can decrease pain and swelling and therefore increase joint motion. Nursing interventions are aimed at promoting comfort, functional ability, and safety. Education about self-care techniques, joint protection, and exercises for flexibility and strength is also important.

Falls. Falls are a safety concern of many older adults. Falls may lead to fear of additional falls, withdrawal from usual activities, and loss of independence (see chapter 33). Hospitalization and placement in a long-term care facility may be required. Falls account for 87% of unintentional injuries resulting in hospitalization for adults aged 71 years and over and 75% of the deaths from injury (Health Canada, 2002). A fracture will be sustained in 5% of those falls. Falls are more frequent and more serious for older adults over the age of 85 years.

Causes of falls are a combination of individual and environmental factors (RNAO, 2002a). Individual factors include impaired vision; cardiovascular conditions such as postural hypotension or syncope; conditions affecting mobility such as arthritis, muscle weakness, and foot problems; conditions affecting balance; alterations in bladder function such as frequency or incontinence; cognitive impairment; and adverse medication reactions. Environmental factors include, but are not limited to, poor lighting, slippery or wet floors, stairs or sidewalks in poor repair, shoes in poor repair or with slippery soles, and household items that could be tripped over, such as throw rugs, foot stools, and electric extension cords.

Nursing interventions are directed toward the management of health-related conditions and the reduction of environmental hazards. Older adults taking medications that may have adverse effects such as postural hypotension, dizziness, or sedation, can be instructed to be aware of these potential effects and to take precautions such as changing position slowly or holding onto sturdy furniture if unsteady. Encouraging older adults to perform exercises aimed at increasing leg strength and balance also reduce the risk of falls (Robson et al., 2003). Simple interventions in the home such as rearranging furniture to provide a clear pathway to the bathroom and providing a night light in the bathroom can reduce falls related to nighttime trips to the toilet. Picking up throw rugs and other items on the floor reduces slipping and tripping. Nurses can also instruct older adults in the safe use of assistive devices such as canes, walkers, and wheelchairs.

Sensory Impairments. The older adult usually has changes in vision, hearing, taste, and smell that are a result of normal aging. Chapter 44 describes in detail the nursing interventions used to maintain and improve sensory function.

Pain. Between 25% and 50% of older adults living in the community (Gloth, 2000) and between 56% and 77% of older adults in long-term care facilities experience pain (Kaasalainen & Crook, 2003). The causes of pain in older adults include acute and chronic conditions (e.g., trauma, infection, and neuropathies). Many factors influence the management of pain, including cultural influences on the meaning and expression of pain for older adults, fears related to the use of analgesic medications, and the problem of pain assessment with cognitively impaired older adults. Nurses caring for older adults are challenged to advocate for appropriate and effective pain management and to use standardized pain tools in their assessments (see chapter 38).

Medication Use. Older adults take more prescription and over-the-counter drugs than any other age group. They account for 12% of the population, but use as much as 40% of prescription medications (NACA, 2002). In 1997, 56% of Canadian older adults reported taking two or more medications a day (Health Canada, 2002). The most commonly used medications are cardiovascular drugs, antihypertensives, analgesics, antiarthritic agents, sedatives, tranquilizers, laxatives, and antacids (Eliopoulos, 1999). **Polypharmacy,** the concurrent use of many medications, increases the risk for adverse reactions. Although polypharmacy may reflect inappropriate prescribing, the concurrent use of multiple medications may be necessary if the older adult has multiple acute and chronic conditions. However, periodic and thorough review of all medications being used is important to restrict the number of medications used to the fewest necessary. The nurse's role with an older adult undergoing drug therapy is to ensure the greatest therapeutic benefit with the least amount of harm.

Older adults are at risk for adverse reactions because of age-related changes in the absorption, distribution, metabolism, and excretion of drugs (Table 21-3). Medications may interact with one another, adding or negating the effect of another drug. Medications may also cause confusion; affect balance and mobility; cause dizziness, nausea, and vomiting; or lead to constipation, urinary frequency, or incontinence. Because of these effects, some older adults are unwilling to take medications.

Managing medications is a very important component of maintaining and promoting good health in old age. For some older adults on large numbers of medications, safely managing medications can be a complex activity that can easily become overwhelming. Up to 50% of older adults take their medications incorrectly because they do not understand the instructions about their medications, further complicating medication assessment (Hayes, 1998). Nurses can provide valuable assistance to their older adult clients as they carry out this important self-care activity.

The nurse works collaboratively with the older adult to ensure safe and appropriate use of prescribed and over-the-counter medications. The older adult should be taught the names of all drugs being taken, when and how to take them, and the desirable and undesirable effects of the drugs. The nurse also teaches how to avoid adverse effects and/or interactions of drugs and how to establish and follow an appropriate self-administration pattern. Strategies for reducing the risk for an adverse medication reaction in the older adult include reviewing the medications with the older adult at each visit, examining for potential interactions with food or other drugs, simplifying and individualizing the drug regimen, taking every opportunity to inform the older adult and family about all aspects of medication use, and encouraging the older adult to question the physician, advanced practice nurse, and/or pharmacist about all prescribed and over-the-counter drugs.

When drugs are used in the management of confusion, special care is necessary. The sedatives and tranquilizers sometimes prescribed for acutely confused older adults may themselves cause or exacerbate confusion. These drugs should be carefully administered, taking into account age-related changes in body systems that can affect the pharmacokinetic activity. When confusion has a physiological cause (such as an infection), the cause, rather than the confused behaviour, should be specifically treated. When confusion varies by time of day or is related to environmental factors, the nurse can use creative, non-pharmacological measures such as making the environment more meaningful, providing adequate light, encouraging use of assistive devices (glasses, hearing aids), or even encourage the client to make telephone calls to friends or family members to hear reassuring voices.

Health Promotion and Maintenance: Psychosocial Health Concerns

Interventions supporting the psychosocial health of older adults resemble those for other age groups. However, some interventions are more crucial for older adults experiencing social isolation, cognitive impairment, or stresses related to retirement, relocation, or approaching death. These interventions include therapeutic communication, touch, reality orientation, validation therapy, reminiscence, and interventions to improve body image.

Therapeutic Communication. With therapeutic communication, the nurse perceives and respects the older adult's uniqueness and meets the older adult's expectations. Older adults expect nurses to be attentive, caring, and knowledgeable (Santo-Novak, 1997). Attentive nurses provide care in a timely fashion, meeting client's expressed or unexpressed needs. A caring nurse expresses attitudes of concern, kindness, and compassion. Knowledgeable nurses not only demonstrate procedural competence, but they are also adept at recognizing needs

Table 21-3 Age-Related Changes Affecting Drug Therapy in Older Adults

Change	Effect	Nursing Measures
Drier mucous membrane of oral cavity	Tablets and capsules may stick to roof or sides of mouth and not be swallowed, or dissolve in and irritate mouth.	Offer fluids before drug administration to moisten mouth and ample fluids during administration. Inspect client's mouth or advise client to inspect mouth for any tablet or capsule that may not have been swallowed (dentures and reduced oral sensations may cause client to be unaware of presence of medication). Unless contraindicated, break large tablets to facilitate swallowing.
Decreased circulation to lower bowel and vagina; lower body temperatures	Suppositories require more time to melt and can be expelled undissolved.	Explore possibility of using alternative route. Allow more time for suppository to melt. Check client or advise to check that the suppository has melted before getting out of bed to resume activities.
Decreased tissue elasticity; reduced muscle mass and activity	Poor seal of tissues after injection and oozing or poor absorption may result.	Use Z-track injection technique for injections to facilitate sealing (see chapter 30).
Decreased pain sensation	Infection or other problem at injection site may not be detected.	Cleanse any medication that has oozed onto skin. Check injection sites regularly.
Decreased cardiac efficiency	Greater risk exists for circulatory overload during intravenous administration of medications.	Monitor intravenous drip closely. Observe for signs of circulatory overload, such as rise in blood pressure, rapid respirations, coughing, or shortness of breath.
Less gastric acid	Slower absorption of drugs that require low gastric pH may result.	Ensure that gastric acid is not further reduced by other drugs such as antacids.
Increase in adipose tissue compared with lean body mass; decreased cardiac output	Drugs stored in adipose tissue (lipid-soluble drugs) have increased tissue concentrations and decreased plasma concentrations and accumulate and remain in body longer. Plasma levels of drugs can increase while less is deposited in reservoirs (particularly true of water-soluble drugs).	Ensure that dosages are adjusted for age. Become familiar with adverse effects of drugs being administered and observe for these effects.
Reduced serum albumin levels	The administration of protein-bound drugs together can result in drugs competing for the same protein molecules. Some drugs may not effectively bind and may be less effective.	Advise physician of other protein-bound drugs client is taking when new protein-bound drug is prescribed. Highly protein-bound drugs include acetazolamide, amitriptyline, cefazolin, chlordiazepoxide, chlorpromazine, cloxacillin, digitoxin, furosemide, hydralazine, nortriptyline, phenylbutazone, phenytoin, propranolol, rifampin, salicylates, spironolactone, sulfisoxazole, and warfarin. Ensure that serum albumin level is evaluated along with blood level of drug. (If serum albumin level is low, client is at greater risk for toxicity despite normal or low blood levels of drug.)
Reduced number of functioning nephrons; decreased glomerular filtration rate; reduced blood flow	Biological half-life is extended, and drugs take longer to be filtered from body; risk of adverse reactions is increased.	Ensure that age-adjusted dosages are prescribed for drugs excreted through renal system.

From *Manual of Gerontologic Nursing* (2nd ed.), by C. Eliopoulos, 1999, St. Louis, MO: Mosby.

and relaying information. Older adult clients also expect nurses to respect their individuality (Marini, 1999). The nurse who meets these expectations and communicates effectively will be accepted as one who has a genuine concern for the older adult's welfare. However, the nurse cannot simply enter an older adult's environment and immediately establish a therapeutic relationship; the nurse first must be knowledgeable and skilled in communication techniques (see chapter 14).

Touch. Throughout life, touch tells us about our environment and the people around us. Gentle touch conveys affection and friendliness. A firm handclasp may convey security. Touch is a therapeutic tool that nurses can use to help comfort older adults. It can provide sensory stimulation, induce relaxation, provide physical and emotional comfort, orient the person to reality, convey warmth, and communicate interest. It is a powerful physical expression of a relationship.

Older adults may be deprived of touching when separated from family or friends. An older adult who is isolated, dependent, or ill; who fears death; or who lacks self-esteem has a greater need for touch. The nurse may recognize touch deprivation by behaviours as simple as an older adult reaching for the nurse's hand or standing close to the nurse. When nurses use touch, they must be aware of cultural variations as well as individual preferences (see chapter 9). Touch should convey respect and sensitivity. Touch should not be used in a condescending way such as patting an older adult on the head.

Reality Orientation. **Reality orientation** is a communication technique used to make an older adult more aware of time, place, and person. The purposes of reality orientation include restoring a sense of reality, improving the level of awareness, promoting socialization, elevating independent functioning, and minimizing confusion, disorientation, and physical regression.

Although the nurse can use reality orientation techniques in any health care setting, they may be especially useful in the acute care setting. The older adult experiencing a change in environment, surgery, illness, or emotional stress is at risk for becoming disoriented. Environmental changes, such as the bright lights, unfamiliar noises, and lack of windows in specialized units of a hospital, often lead to disorientation and confusion. Absence of familiar caregivers is also disorienting. When anesthesia, sedatives, tranquilizers, analgesics, and physical restraints are used, disorientation is increased. The nurse should anticipate and monitor for disorientation and confusion as possible consequences of hospitalization, relocation, surgery, loss, or illness and should incorporate interventions based on reality orientation into the care plan.

The key elements of reality orientation include frequent reminders of person, time, and place; the use of environmental aids such as clocks, calendars, and personal belongings; and stability of environment, routine, and staff (Eliopoulos, 1999). For individuals with dementia, reality orientation should only be used for information needed for safe function (Miller, 2004). Communication is always respectful, patient, and calm. The nurse answers questions from the older adult simply and honestly with sensitivity and a caring attitude.

Validation Therapy. **Validation therapy** is an alternative approach to communication with a confused older adult. Whereas reality orientation insists that the confused older adult agree with our statements of time, place, and person, validation therapy accepts the description of time and place as stated by the confused older adult. Older adults with dementia are less likely to benefit and more likely to become agitated by the caregiver's insistence on the "correct" time, place, and person.

In validation therapy, statements and behaviours of the confused older adult are not challenged or disputed. The statements and behaviours are believed to represent an inner need or feeling. The appropriate nursing intervention is to recognize and address that inner need or feeling. Validation does not involve reinforcing the confused older adult's misperceptions, but reflects sensitivity to hidden meanings in statements and behaviours. By listening with sensitivity and validating what is expressed, the nurse conveys respect, reassurance, and understanding. Validating or respecting confused older adults' feelings in the time and place that is real to them is more important than insisting on the literally correct time and place (Day, 1997).

Reminiscence. **Reminiscence** is recalling the past. Many older adults find enjoyment in sharing past experiences. As therapy, reminiscence uses the recollection of the past to bring meaning and understanding to the present and to resolve current conflicts (Eliopoulos, 1999). Looking back to positive resolutions to problems reminds the older adult of coping strategies used successfully in the past. Reminiscing is also a way to express personal identity. Reflection on past achievements supports self-esteem. For some older adults, the process of looking back on past events uncovers new meanings for those events.

During the assessment process, the nurse may use reminiscence to assess self-esteem, cognitive function, emotional stability, unresolved conflicts, coping ability, and expectations for the future (Eliopoulos, 1999). Reminiscence also occurs during direct care activities. Taking time to ask questions about past experiences and listening attentively conveys to an older adult the nurse's attitudes of respect and concern (Puentes, 1998). Although reminiscence is often used in a one-on-one situation of nurse and older adult, reminiscence can also be a group therapy for cognitively impaired or depressed older adults. The nurse organizes the group and selects strategies to start a conversation. For example, the nurse might ask the group to discuss families or childhood memories. The group's size, structure, process, goals, and activities are adapted to meet its members' needs.

Body-Image Interventions. The way that older adults present themselves influences body image and feelings of isolation. Some physical characteristics of older adulthood are socially desirable, such as distinguished-looking gray hair. Other features are also impressive, such as a lined face that displays character or wrinkled hands that convey a lifetime of hard work. Consequences of illness and aging that threaten the older adult's body image include invasive diagnostic procedures, pain, surgery, loss of sensation in a body part, skin changes, loss of scalp hair, and incontinence. Body image is also affected by the use of devices such as dentures, hearing aids, artificial limbs, in-dwelling catheters, ostomy devices, and enteral feeding tubes.

The importance to the older adult of presenting a socially acceptable image must be considered. When older adults have acute or chronic illnesses, the related physical dependence makes it difficult for them to maintain body image. The nurse influences the older adult's appearance by assisting with grooming and hygiene. It takes little effort to assist the older adult with combing hair, cleaning dentures, shaving, or changing clothing. The nurse should also be sensitive to odours in the environment. Odours created by urine and some illnesses are often present. By controlling odours, the nurse may encourage visitors to stay longer or visit more often.

Older Adults and the Acute Care Setting

Older adults in the acute care setting need special attention to help them adjust to the acute care environment and to meet their basic needs for comfort, safety, nutrition, hydration, and skin integrity. The acute care setting poses increased risk for adverse events such as delirium, dehydration, malnutrition, nosocomial infections, urinary incontinence, and falls.

The risk for delirium is increased when hospitalized older adults experience immobilization, infection, dehydration, pain, and hypoxia. Multiple medications and multiple medical diagnoses are also risk factors for delirium (Simon, Jewell, & Brokel, 1997). Non-medical causes of delirium include placement in unfamiliar surroundings, separation from supportive family members, and stress. Impaired vision or hearing contributes to confusion and interferes with attempts to reorient the older adult. When the prevention of delirium fails, interventions begin with treatment of the cause. Supportive interventions include encouraging family visits, providing memory cues (clocks, calendars, name tags), and compensating for sensory deficits. Reality orientation techniques may be useful.

Older adults are at greater risk for dehydration and malnutrition during hospitalization because of standard procedures such as limiting food and fluids in preparation for diagnostic tests (Sullivan, Sun, & Walls, 1999). The risk for dehydration and malnutrition is also increased when older adults are unable to reach beverages or to feed themselves while in bed or connected to medical equipment. Interventions include getting the client out of bed, providing beverages and snacks frequently, and including favourite foods and beverages in the diet plan.

The increased risk for nosocomial infections in older adults is related to age-related reductions in immune system response. The use of in-dwelling urinary catheters accounts for 80% of nosocomial urinary tract infections (Lee & Burnett, 1998). Other nosocomial infections include surgical site infection, pneumonia, and bloodstream infections (Russell, 1999). Prevention begins with hand hygiene and measures to minimize the risk of infection from procedures (see chapter 29). Prevention also includes measures to increase the older adult's resistance to infection.

Older adults in acute care settings are also at risk for becoming incontinent of urine (transient incontinence). Causes of transient urinary incontinence include delirium, untreated urinary tract infection, excessive urine production, medications, restricted mobility, and constipation or impaction (Bradway, Hernly, & the NICHE faculty, 1998). Interventions for transient urinary incontinence are geared to correcting contributing factors. The interventions may include an individualized plan to provide voiding opportunities and modification of the environment to improve access to the toilet. In-dwelling urinary catheters should be avoided if possible. Measures to prevent skin breakdown should be used.

The increased risk for skin breakdown and the development of pressure ulcers is related to changes in aging skin and to situations that arise in the acute care setting such as immobility, incontinence, and malnutrition. The key points in the prevention of skin breakdown are avoiding pressure, reducing shear forces and friction, providing skin care and moisture management, and providing nutritional support (Maklebust, 1997; see chapter 43).

Older adults in the acute care setting are at risk for falling and sustaining injuries. Many of the falls occur as the older adult gets out of bed without assistance. Sedating medications may increase unsteadiness. Medications causing orthostatic hypotension may also increase the risk for falls because of the blood pressure drop when the older adult gets out of a bed or chair. Diuretics increase the risk for falling because the person must get out of bed often to void. Attempts to get out of bed when physically restrained may lead to injury when the older adult becomes entangled in the restraint. Equipment such as wires from monitors, intravenous tubing, urinary catheters, and other medical devices become obstacles to safe ambulation. Impaired vision may prevent the older adult from seeing tripping hazards such as garbage cans. Confused older adults who may try to get out of bed although weak, unsteady, or drowsy may benefit from reality orientation or the presence of family members and friends. Interventions to reduce the risk for falling include assistance with ambulation, strengthening exercises, medication monitoring, assistance with toileting, and removal of tripping hazards (see chapter 33).

Older Adults and Restorative Care

Restorative care refers to two types of ongoing care. The first type of restorative care continues the convalescence from acute illness or surgery that began in the acute care setting. The second type of restorative care addresses chronic conditions that affect day-to-day functioning. Both types of restorative care take place in private homes and in long-term care settings.

Interventions during convalescence from acute illness or surgery are directed toward regaining or improving the prior level of independence in ADLs. Interventions that began in the acute care setting should be continued and later modified as convalescence progresses. To achieve this continuation, the acute care setting's discharge information should include information on the ongoing interventions (e.g., exercise routines, wound care routines, medication schedules, vital sign monitoring, and blood glucose monitoring). Interventions should also address the restoration of interpersonal relationships and activities either at their previous level or at the level desired by the older adult.

When restorative care addresses chronic conditions, the goals of care include stabilizing the chronic condition, promoting health, and promoting independence in ADLs. Interventions to stabilize the chronic condition may focus on regulation or prevention. An example of a regulatory intervention is the monitoring of blood glucose levels in diabetes. An example of prevention is a smoking cessation program for the older adult with chronic obstructive pulmonary disease.

Health promotion interventions for older adults, as addressed in this chapter, should occur in all health care settings. For example, nurse-directed programs in long-term care settings improve ambulation, reverse urinary incontinence, and reduce confusion.

Interventions to promote independence in ADLs address physical ability, cognitive ability, and safety. The physical ability to perform ADLs requires strength, flexibility, and balance. Accommodation must be made for impairments of vision, hearing, and touch. The cognitive ability to perform ADLs requires the ability to recognize, judge, and remember. Cognitive impairments, such as Alzheimer's disease, may interfere with the safe performance of ADLs, although the older adult is still physically capable of the activities. Interventions to promote independence in ADLs adapt these requirements to the needs and lifestyle of the older adult. Safety is always an important consideration. The older adult should be able to perform the ADLs with the least amount of risk that is acceptable to the older adult.

Beyond the basic ADLs, the older adult's ability to perform instrumental activities of daily living (IADLs) must be assessed and appropriate interventions implemented. IADLs are tasks such as using a telephone, preparing meals, shopping, doing laundry, cleaning the home, and driving an automobile. To remain independent at home or in assisted-living residences, older adults must be able to perform IADLs, be able to purchase services by outside workers, or have a supportive network of family and friends who assist with these tasks.

Restorative care measures focus on activities to prevent, improve, reduce, or eliminate problems. Priorities of care are established, client goals and expected outcomes are determined, and appropriate interventions are selected. These are done with the older adult's participation so that the interventions are understood and conflicts in approaches or priorities can be avoided. The older adult's lifetime experiences, values, and socio-cultural patterns are the basis for planning individual care. When the older adult's cognitive status prevents participation in health care decisions, the family or significant others must be included. Family and friends are rich sources of data because they knew the older adult before the impairment. Frequently, they can provide explanations for the older adult's behaviours and suggest methods of management. Thoughtful assessment and planning leads to goals of care that consider the influence of normal aging changes, facilitate an optimal level of comfort and coping, and promote independence in self-care activities.

Key Concepts

- The number of older adults, especially the number of older adults over the age of 85 years, is increasing.
- Because nurses' attitudes toward older adults influence the quality of care, those attitudes should be based on accurate information about older adults, rather than myths and stereotypes.
- Biological and psychosocial theories of aging offer possible explanations for the changes seen in aging, but every older adult is a unique individual who ages in a unique way.
- The physical changes that accompany aging are considered to be normal, not pathological, although they may predispose the older adult to disease.
- Cognitive impairment is not normal in older adults and requires assessment and intervention.
- Cognitive impairment includes acute, potentially reversible disorders and chronic, irreversible, progressive disorders.
- Areas affected by psychosocial changes of aging include retirement, social isolation, change in housing, death, and sexuality.
- Nursing interventions for psychosocial concerns include therapeutic communication, touch, reality orientation, validation therapy, reminiscence, and interventions to improve body image.
- The leading causes of death in the older population are heart disease, cancer, stroke, lung disease, accidents/falls, diabetes, kidney disease, and liver disease.
- Health promotion recommendations for older adults include good nutrition, regular exercise, smoking cessation, measures to reduce the risk for falls, and measures to reduce adverse medication reactions.
- Acute care settings place older adults at risk for delirium, dehydration, malnutrition, nosocomial infections, urinary incontinence, and falls.
- Restorative nursing interventions, whether accomplished in the older adult's home or in long-term care institutions, stabilize chronic conditions, promote health, and promote independence in basic and instrumental activities of daily living.

Key Terms

Ageism, *p. 416*
Alzheimer's disease, *p. 423*
Delirium, *p. 422*
Dementia, *p. 422*
Depression, *p. 422*
Geriatrics, *p. 415*
Gerontic nursing, *p. 415*
Gerontological nursing, *p. 415*
Gerontology, *p. 415*
Non-stochastic theories, *p. 417*
Personal care home, *p. 418*
Polypharmacy, *p. 431*
Reality orientation, *p. 433*
Reminiscence, *p. 433*
Stochastic theories, *p. 417*
Validation therapy, *p. 433*

Critical Thinking Exercises

1. Mr. Wong, 73 years old, has come to the clinic for a routine check of his blood pressure. It is normal (130/80 mm Hg). He tells you that he wants to do everything he can to stay healthy. What advice can you give him on health promotion and disease prevention?
2. Mrs. Doshi's daughter has come with her to the clinic. She is concerned about her mother's memory. She tells you that her mother's memory has been excellent but has suddenly become poor. Two days ago Mrs. Doshi phoned her daughter six times in 2 hours asking where her husband (the late Mr. Doshi) was, and when told of his death 4 years ago, denied this fact. When her daughter arrived at her house to check on her, she found that Mrs. Doshi had emptied the contents of all the closets onto the floor and accused her daughter of theft. Mrs. Doshi has spent the last two nights at her daughter's house because her daughter is concerned about her safety. From Mrs. Doshi's daughter's report, you suspect delirium (acute confusional state). What questions should you ask and what areas should you assess to identify the possible causes of Mrs. Doshi's confusion?
3. A nursing colleague tells you that she does not know very much about assessing older adults and asks for some pointers on how to do a good, thorough assessment. What advice can you give her on the process of geriatric assessment?

Review Questions

1. Two factors contribute to the projected increase in the number of older adults:
   1. Financial success and improved environment
   2. Fewer medical problems associated with aging
   3. Improved medication plan and increase in federal health care funding
   4. The aging of the "baby boom" generation and the growth of the population segment over the age of 85 years
2. Which of the following is true about the theories of aging?
   1. Genetic changes are solely responsible.
   2. Environment is the main factor.
   3. There is no single theory that explains aging.
   4. Disease causes a decline in function.
3. The three common conditions affecting cognition in older adults are
   1. Stroke, heart attack, and cancer of the brain
   2. Cancer, Alzheimer's disease, stroke
   3. Delirium, depression, and dementia
   4. Blindness, hearing loss, and stroke
4. Sexuality is recognized as a factor in the care of older adults; thus
   1. Any expression of sexuality should be discouraged
   2. All older adults, whether healthy or frail, need to express sexual feelings
   3. A decrease in an older adult's need for sexual expression occurs
   4. The need to touch and be touched is decreased
5. The older adult's libido does not decrease; however
   1. Frequency of sexual activity may decline
   2. Physical changes usually will not affect sexual functioning
   3. The need to touch and be touched is decreased
   4. The sexual preferences of older adults are not as diverse
6. Visual acuity declines with age. Presbyopia is a progressive decline in
   1. Distinguishing between blues and greens and among pastel shades
   2. The ability to see in darkness
   3. The ability to focus on near objects
   4. Adaptation to abrupt changes from dark areas to light areas
7. A common age-related change in auditory acuity is called
   1. Presbycusis
   2. Presbyopia
   3. Calcification
   4. Hypertrophy
8. Taste buds atrophy and lose sensitivity. The older adult is less able to discern
   1. Salty, sweet, sour, and bitter tastes
   2. Hot and cold temperatures
   3. Moistness and dryness
   4. Spicy and bland tastes
9. Changes in the musculoskeletal system lead to changes in the configuration of the thorax. This is known as
   1. Hypertrophy
   2. Calcification
   3. Presbycusis
   4. Kyphosis
10. Frontal-temporal dementia has an insidious onset and progresses slowly. Early symptoms include
    1. Poor hygiene, lack of social tact, and sexual disinhibition
    2. More involvement in surroundings and social situations
    3. Fluctuating cognition, and visual and/or auditory hallucinations
    4. Motor features of parkinsonism

References

Alzheimer Society. (2004). *Alzheimer disease statistics.* Retrieved December 6, 2004, from *http://www.alzheimer.ca/english/disease/stats-intro.htm*

Beers, M., & Berkow, R. (2000). *The Merck manual of geriatrics* (3rd ed.). Whitehouse Station, NJ: Merck.

Bolla, L., Filley, C., & Palmer, R. (2000). Dementia DDx: Office diagnosis of the four major types of dementia. *Geriatrics, 55*(1), 34–37, 41–42, 45–46.

Boyd, N. (1996). Smoking cessation: A four-step plan to help older patients quit. *Geriatrics, 51*(11), 52–57.

Bradway, C., Hernly, S., & the NICHE faculty. (1998). Urinary incontinence in older adults admitted to acute care. *Geriatric Nursing, 19,* 98–102.

Buijs, R., et al. (2003). Promoting participation: Evaluation of a health promotion program for low income seniors. *Journal of Community Health Nursing, 20*(2), 93–107.

Butler, R. (1998). Tell your patients to take a walk. *Geriatrics, 53*(5), 15, 19.

Butler, R., et al. (1998). Physical fitness: Benefits of exercise for the older patient. *Geriatrics, 53*(10), 46, 49–52, 61–62.

Canadian Cancer Society. (2004). *Prostrate cancer statistics.* Retrieved December 8, 2004, from *http://www.cancer.ca/ccs/internet/standard/0,3182,3172_14471__langId-en,00.html*

Canadian Continence Foundation. (2004). *Facts on incontinence.* Retrieved December 8, 2004, from *http://www.continence-fdn.ca/indexeng.htm*

Canadian Gerontological Nursing Association. (1996). *Canadian Gerontological Nursing Association Standards of Nursing Practice.* Retrieved December 8, 2004, from *http://www.cgna.net/standards.htm*

Chasteen, A., Schwarz N., & Park D. (2002). The activation of aging stereotypes in younger and older adults, *Journal of Gerontological & Psychological Science, Soc Sci* 57B:P540.

Ciricelli, V. (1999). Personality and demographic factors in older adults' fear of death, *Gerontologist, 39*:569.

Clark, C. (1998). Wellness self-care by healthy older adults. *Image Journal of Nursing Scholarship,* 30, 351.

Conn, D. (2001). Cholinesterase inhibitors: Comparing the options for mild-to-moderate dementia. *Geriatrics, 56*(9), 56–57.

Cummings, E., & Henry, W. (1961). *Growing old: The process of disengagement.* New York: Basic Books.

Cutillo-Schmitter, T. (1996). Aging: Broaden our view for improved nursing care. *Journal of Gerontological Nursing, 22*(7), 31–42.

Davidhizar, R., Eshleman, J., & Moody, M. (2002). Health promotion for aging adults. *Geriatric Nursing, 23*(1), 28–34.

Day, C. (1997). Validation therapy: A review of the literature. *Journal of Gerontological Nursing, 23*(4), 29–34.

Ebersole, P., & Hess, P. (1998). *Toward healthy aging: Human needs and nursing response* (5th ed.). St. Louis, MO: Mosby.

Ebersole, P., & Hess, P. (2001). *Geriatric nursing and healthy aging.* St. Louis, MO: Mosby.

Ebersole, P., & Hess, P. (2004). *Toward healthy aging: Human needs and nursing response* (6th ed.). St. Louis, MO: Mosby.

Eliopoulos, C. (1999). *Manual of gerontologic nursing* (2nd ed.). St. Louis, MO: Mosby.

Ellingson, T. & Conn, V (2000) Exercise and quality of life in elderly individuals. *Journal of Gerontological Nursing, 26*(3), 17.

Emmett, K. (1998). Nonspecific and atypical presentation of disease in the older patient. *Geriatrics, 53*(2), 50–52, 58–60.

Fielo, S., & Rizzolo, M. (1988). Handle with caring: Meeting elderly clients' special learning needs. *Nursing & Health Care, 9*(4), 193–195.

Fielo, S., & Warren, S. (2001). Home adaptation: Helping older people age in place. *Geriatric Nursing, 22*(5), 239–246.

Foreman, M., et al. (1996). Assessing cognitive function. *Geriatric Nursing, 17*(5), 228–232.

Gloth, F. M., III. (2000). Factors that limit pain relief and increase complications. *Geriatrics, 55*(10), 46–48, 51–54.

Gomolin, I., & Kathpalia, R. (2002). Influenza: How to prevent and control nursing home outbreaks. *Geriatrics, 57*(1), 28–30, 33–34.

Gunnarsson, O., & Judge, J. (1997). Exercise at midlife: How and why to prescribe it for sedentary patients. *Geriatrics, 52*(5), 71–72, 77–80.

Havens, B., et al. (2004). Social isolation and loneliness: Differences between older rural and urban Manitobans. *Canadian Journal of Aging, 23,* 129–140.

Hayes, K. (1998). Randomized trial of geragogy-based medication instruction in the emergency department. *Nursing Research, 47,* 211.

Health Canada. (2002). *Canada's aging population.* Retrieved April 10, 2004, from *www.hc-sc.gc/ca/seniors/pub*

Health Canada. (2004). *Canada's seniors at a glance.* Retrieved April 10, 2004, from *www.hc-sc.gc/ca/seniors/pub*

Kaasalainen, S., & Crook, J. (2003). A comparison of pain-assessment tools for use with elderly long term care residents. *Canadian Journal of Nursing Research, 35*(4), 58–71.

Lee, V., & Burnett, E. (1998). A case report: Special needs of hospitalized elders. *Geriatric Nursing, 19,* 185–191.

Lemon, B., Bengston, V., & Peterson, J. (1972). An exploration of the activity theory of aging: Activity types and life satisfaction among in-movers to a retirement community. *Journal of Gerontology, 27* 511–523.

Lueckenotte, A. (2000). Gerontologic assessment. In A. Lueckenotte (Ed.), *Gerontologic nursing* (2nd ed.). St. Louis, MO: Mosby.

Maklebust, J. (1997). Pressure ulcers: Decreasing the risk for older adults. *Geriatric Nursing, 18*(6), 250–254.

Marini, B. (1999). Institutionalized older adults' perceptions of nurse caring behaviours. *Journal of Gerontological Nursing, 25*(5):11.

Mastrian, K. (2001). Differing perceptions in defining safe independent living for elders. *Nursing Outlook, 49,* 213.

Menec, V., et al. (2003). The impact of influenza-associated respiratory illnesses on hospitalizations, physicians visits, emergency room visits and mortality. *Canadian Journal of Public Health, 94*(1), 59–64.

Miller, C. (2004). *Nursing for wellness in older adults. Theory and practice* (4th ed.). Philadelphia: Lippincott.

National Advisory Council on Aging. (2002). Cautions Medications. *Expressions, 15*(1), 1–8.

National Advisory Council on Aging. (2003). *Interim report card: Seniors in Canada.* Retrieved December 8, 2004, from *http://www.phac-aspc.gc.ca/seniors-aines/naca/report_card2003/rptcard2003_toc_e.htm*

Neugarten, B. (1964). *Personality in middle and late life.* New York: Atherton.

Osteoporosis Society of Canada. (2004). *About osteoporosis.* Retrieved December 8, 2004, from *http://www.osteoporosis.ca http://www.osteoporosis.ca/english/about%20osteoporosis/default.asp?s=1*

Pender, N. J., Murdaugh, C. L., & Parsons, M. A. (2002). *Health promotion in nursing practice* (4th ed.). Upper Saddle River, NJ: Prentice Hall.

Peterson, M., & Zimberg, S. (1996). Treating alcoholism: An age-specific intervention that works for older patients. *Geriatrics, 51*(10), 45–49.

Puentes, W. (1998). Incorporating simple reminiscence techniques into acute care nursing practice. *Journal of Gerontological Nursing, 24*(2), 14–20.

Rantz, M., Popejoy, L., & Zwygart-Stauffacher, M. (2001). *The new nursing homes: A 20-minute way to find great long-term care.* Minneapolis, MN: Fairview Press.

Registered Nurses Association of Ontario. (2002a). *Prevention of fall injuries in the older adult.* Retrieved April 10, 2004, from *http://www.rnao.org/bestpractices/completed_guidelines/BPG_Guide_C1_Prevent_Falls.asp*

Registered Nurses Association of Ontario. (2002b). *Promoting continence using prompted voiding.* Retrieved April 10, 2004, from *http://www.rnao.org/bestpractices/completed_guidelines/BPG_Guide_C1_Promote_Continence.asp*

Registered Nurses Association of Ontario. (2003). *Screening for delirium, dementia and depression in older adults.* Retrieved April 10, 2004, from *http://www.rnao.org/ bestpractices/completed_guidelines/BPG_Guide_C3_ddd.asp*

Resnick, B. (2003). Health promotion practices of older adults: Testing an individualized approach. *Journal of Clinical Nursing, 12*(1), 46–55.

Resnick, B. & Spellbring, A (2000) Understanding what motivates older adults to exercise. *Journal of Gerontological Nursing, 26*(3), 34.

Robson, S., et al. (2003). Steady as you go (SAYGO): A falls-prevention program for seniors living in the community. *Canadian Journal on Aging, 22*(2), 207–216.

Rubenstein, I., & Nahas, R. (1998). Primary and secondary prevention strategies in the older adult. *Geriatric Nursing, 19*(1), 11–17.

Russell, B. (1999). Nosocomial infections. *American Journal of Nursing, 99*(6), 24J–24P.

Santo-Novak, D. (1997). Older adults' descriptions of their role expectations of nursing. *Journal of Gerontological Nursing 23*(1):32

Saskatchewan Health. (2000). *Selecting a personal care home.* Retrieved December 8 , 2004, from *http://www.health.gov.sk.ca/rr_selecting_prsnl_care.html*

Saskatoon Health Region. (2003). *Older adult wellness program annual report.* Saskatoon, SK: Author.

Statistics Canada. (2003). *Income of Canadian families.* Retrieved December 15, 2004, from *http://www12.statcan.ca/english/census01/Products/Analytic/companion/inc/canada.cfm*

Simon, L., Jewell, N., & Brokel, J. (1997). Management of acute delirium in hospitalized elderly: A process improvement project. *Geriatric Nursing, 18,* 150–154.

Sloane, P. (1992). Normal aging. In R. Ham & P. Sloane (Eds.), *Primary care geriatrics: A case based approach* (2nd ed.). St. Louis, MO: Mosby.

Statistics Canada. (2004). *Basic statistics on older adults and drinking.* Retrieved December, 8, 2004, from *http://www.statcan.ca/english/freepub/82-221-XIE/00601/high/drink.htm*

Sullivan, D., Sun, S., & Walls, R. (1999). Protein-energy undernutrition among elderly hospitalized patients. *The Journal of the American Medical Association, 281,* 2013–2019.

Wallace, M. (1996). Touch and intimacy. In A. Lueckenotte (Ed.), *Gerontologic nursing* (pp. 217–231). St. Louis, MO: Mosby.

Wojciechowski, C. (1998). Issues in caring for older lesbians. *Journal of Gerontological Nursing, 24*(7), 28–33.

Yen, P. (1997). Weight loss resulting from Alzheimer's disease. *Geriatric Nursing, 18*(3), 132–133.

Recommended Web Sites

Alzheimer Society of Canada:
http://www.Alzheimer.ca

The Alzheimer Society of Canada provides current information on Alzheimer's disease, related dementias, caregiving, support, research, treatment, and programs and services.

Canadian Gerontological Nursing Association:
http://www.cgna.net

This Web site provides information on gerontological nursing in Canada, including current standards of practice.

Health Canada Division of Aging and Seniors:
http://www.hc-sc.gc.ca/seniors-aines

This federal Web site provides links to new services, publications, and news releases on issues relevant to aging.

22

Self-Concept

Victoria N. Folse, PhD, APRN, CS, LCPC
Judee E. Onyskiw, RN, PhD (Canadian author)

Objectives

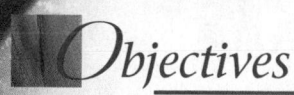

Mastery of content in this chapter will enable the student to:

- Define the key terms listed.
- Discuss factors that influence the following components of self-concept: identity, body image, and role performance.
- Identify stressors that affect self-concept and self-esteem.
- Describe the components of self-concept as related to psychosocial and cognitive developmental stages.
- Explore ways in which the nurse's self-concept and nursing actions can affect the client's self-concept and self-esteem.
- Incorporate research findings to promote evidence-based practice for identity confusion, disturbed body image, low self-esteem, and role conflict.
- Examine cultural considerations that affect self-concept.
- Apply the nursing process to promote a client's self-concept.

Self-concept is how one thinks about oneself. It is a subjective sense of the self and a complex mixture of unconscious and conscious thoughts, attitudes, and perceptions. It affects how a person manages situations and relationships. Self-concept also affects one's self-esteem, or how one feels about oneself. Self-concept and self-esteem are often used interchangeably, but it is important to understand the distinction. Self-esteem stems from self-concept, and self-esteem influences self-concept. Self-concept is a descriptive term, whereas self-esteem is an evaluative term. Appropriate use of these terms facilitates communication among health care providers and ensures that the care plan is individualized to meet each client's needs.

Nurses care for clients who face health problems that can threaten their self-concept and self-esteem (e.g., loss of bodily function, decline in activity tolerance, and difficulty in managing a chronic illness). Nurses play a key role in helping clients adjust to alterations in self-concept and in supporting components of self-concept that enable clients to cope with difficulties.

Scientific Knowledge Base

Developing and maintaining self-concept and self-esteem begin at a young age and continue across the lifespan. Parents and other primary caregivers, as well as culture and environment, influence the development of a child's self-concept and self-esteem. In general, young children tend to rate themselves higher than they rate other children, perhaps a reflection of their egocentric view of the world. Adolescence is a particularly critical time when many variables affect self-concept and self-esteem (Figure 22–1). The adolescent experience appears to adversely affect self-esteem, more so for girls than for boys. Maturational changes are generally regarded as positive for boys: there is no sudden physical change in boys to indicate puberty. For girls, adolescence brings menarche, its associated symptoms, the development of breasts, and a gain in body fat. As a result, adolescent girls may be more sensitive to their appearance and how others view them (Park, 2003).

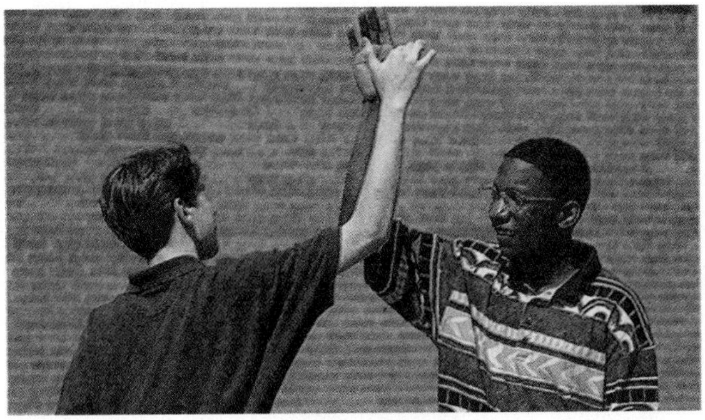

FIGURE 22–1 Participating in group activities can foster adolescents' self-esteem. (From *Mosby's Textbook for the Home Care Aide,* 2nd ed., by J. Birchenall and E. Streight, 2003, St. Louis, MO: Mosby.)

In adulthood, men tend to report higher levels of self-esteem than do women. However, the exact magnitude of this gender difference and the way it varies across the lifespan remain unclear. Job satisfaction and job performance are linked to self-esteem. When individuals are terminated or laid off from a job, they lose their job identity and their self-perceptions may be altered or diminished. They may not be motivated to be active socially or may even become depressed. A developmental goal of adulthood is to establish a sense of self that is stable and transcends relationships and situations.

In older adults, the sense of self may be negatively affected by the emotional and physical changes associated with aging (Robins et al., 2002). When older adults lose a partner or develop health problems, for example, they may experience negative changes in independence or social interaction. These changes may alter their self-concept and self-esteem.

Ethnic and cultural differences in self-concept and self-esteem have also been demonstrated across the lifespan, and recent findings suggest that differences in the development of self-concept may exist (Twenge & Crocker, 2002). Sensitivity to factors that affect self-concept and self-esteem in diverse cultures is essential to ensure an individualized approach to health care.

How individuals view themselves and how they perceive their health are closely related. Clients' beliefs in personal health can enhance their self-concept. Statements such as "I can get through anything" or "I've never been sick a day in my life" indicate that a person's thoughts about personal health are positive. Illness, hospitalization, and surgery can also affect self-concept. Chronic illness may affect the ability to provide financial support, thereby affecting an individual's self-esteem and perceived roles within the family. Negative perceptions regarding health status may be reflected in such statements as "It's not worth it anymore" or "I'm a burden to my family." Further, chronic illness can affect identity and body image, as reflected in statements such as "I'll never get any better" or "I can't stand to look at this disfigurement."

What individuals think and how they feel about themselves affect the way they care for themselves physically and emotionally and the way they care for others. How one behaves is generally consistent with both self-concept and self-esteem. Individuals who have poor self-concepts often do not feel in control of situations and may not feel worthy of care, which can influence decisions regarding health care. Knowledge of variables that affect self-concept and self-esteem is critical for nurses to provide effective treatment.

Nursing Knowledge Base

Development of Self-Concept

The development of self-concept is a complex lifelong process that involves many factors. Erikson's psychosocial theory of development (1963) remains helpful in understanding key tasks that individuals face at various stages of development. Successful mastery of each stage can translate to a positive sense of self (Box 22-1).

A nurse learns to recognize an individual's failure to achieve an age-appropriate developmental stage or an individual's regression to an earlier stage in a period of crisis. This understanding allows a nurse to individualize care and determine appropriate nursing interventions. Self-concept is always changing and is based on the following:

- Sense of competency
- Perceived reactions of others to one's body
- Ongoing perceptions and interpretations of other people's thoughts and feelings
- Personal and professional relationships
- Racial identity
- Academic and employment-related identity
- Spiritual identity
- Personality structure
- Perceptions of events that have an impact on the self
- Mastery of prior and new experiences
- Current feelings about the physical, emotional, and social self
- Self-expectations

Components and Interrelated Terms of Self-Concept

A positive self-concept gives a sense of meaning, wholeness, and consistency to a person. A healthy self-concept has a high degree of stability and generates positive feelings toward the self. The components of self-concept frequently considered by nurses are identity, body image, and role performance. Self-esteem is traditionally viewed as a closely related concept.

Identity. **Identity** involves the internal sense of individuality, wholeness, and consistency of a person over time and in various circumstances. Identity implies being distinct and separate from others. Identity develops over time and ends in being a whole and unique self. The core of identity is being "oneself." A child learns culturally and socially accepted values, behaviours, and roles through observing others and modelling their behaviour. Identity is often gained from self-observation and from what individuals are told about themselves (Stuart & Laraia, 2001). An individual first identifies with parenting

Box 22-1 Self-Concept: Developmental Tasks

0 to 1 Year

Develops trust from consistency in caregiving and nurturing interactions of parents and others
Distinguishes self from environment

1 to 3 Years

Begins to communicate likes and dislikes
Increasingly autonomous in thoughts and actions
Appreciates body appearance and function
Develops self through modelling, imitation, and socialization

3 to 6 Years

Takes initiative
Identifies with a gender
Gains an enhanced self-awareness
Increases language skills, including identification of feelings
Sensitive to family feedback

6 to 12 Years

Incorporates feedback from peers and teachers
Increases self-esteem with new skill mastery (e.g., reading, math, sports, music)
Sexual identity strengthens
Aware of strengths and limitations

12 to 20 Years

Accepts body changes/maturation
Examines attitudes, values, and beliefs; establishes goals for the future
Feels positive about expanded sense of self
Interacts with those whom he or she finds sexually attractive or intellectually stimulating

Mid-20s to Mid-40s

Has intimate relationships with family and significant others
Has stable, positive feelings about self
Experiences successful role transitions and increased responsibilities

Mid-40s to Mid-60s

Accepts changes in appearance and physical endurance
Reassesses life goals
Shows contentment with aging

Late 60s On

Feels positive about own life and its meaning
Interested in providing a legacy for the next generation

figures and later with teachers, peers, and role models. To form an identity, a child must be able to bring together learned behaviours and expectations into a coherent, consistent, and unique whole (Erikson, 1963).

Achieving one's identity is necessary for the development of intimate relationships because one's identity is expressed in relationships with others. Sexuality is a part of one's identity. Gender identity is a person's conceptualization of the self as a man or as a woman and includes one's sexual orientation. This image and its meaning depend on culturally determined values that are affected by socialization (see chapter 23).

Racial or cultural identity develops from identification and socialization within an established group, as well as through the experience of integrating the response of individuals outside the cultural or racial group into one's sense of self. Self-concept may be most influenced by political, social, and cultural influences during childhood. In general, a positive relationship exists between identification with social groups and personal self-esteem. In addition, when racial identity is central to self-concept and is positive, self-esteem tends to be high (Twenge & Crocker, 2002). People who experience discrimination, prejudice, or environmental stressors such as poverty or living in high-crime neighbourhoods may conceptualize themselves differently from those who have not had the same stressors (Ruiz, Roosa, & Gonzales, 2002). Further, the opinion or approval of others may not constitute the basis for self-esteem in the same way for all racial and cultural groups. Cultural differences in self-concept exist and may also demonstrate some age-specific trends (Box 22-2).

Body Image. **Body image** involves attitudes related to the body, including physical appearance, structure, or function. Feelings about body image include those related to sexuality, femininity and masculinity, youthfulness, health, and strength. These mental images are not always consistent with a person's actual physical structure or appearance. Some body image distortions have deep psychological origins such as those that occur in an eating disorder like anorexia nervosa. Other alterations occur as a result of situational events such as the loss or change in a body part. The majority of men and women experience some degree of body dissatisfaction, which can affect body image and overall self-concept. Disturbances in body image can be exaggerated when a change in health status occurs. The way others view a person's body and the feedback offered is also influential. For example, a controlling, violent husband might tell his wife that she is ugly and that no one else would want her. Over time, with repeated humiliation and degradation, she may incorporate this image into her self-concept.

Body image is affected by cognitive growth and physical development. Normal developmental changes such as puberty, menopause, and aging have an effect on body image. Body image is influenced by hormonal changes during adolescence. The development of secondary sex characteristics and changes in body fat distribution affect an adolescent's self-concept. In the older adult, changes associated with

Cultural Aspects of Care — Box 22-2

Racial and cultural identity are important components of a person's self-concept. Early in growth and development, an individual develops this identity within the family context. As people grow, the cultural aspects of their self-concept may be reinforced through family, social, or cultural experiences. A person's self-concept may be strengthened or challenged through political, social, or cultural influences experienced in school or work environments.

Implications for Practice

- Recognize that positive or negative cultural role modelling and past experiences can influence self-concept.
- Develop an open, non-restrictive attitude when assessing for and encouraging cultural practices to improve a client's self-concept.
- Ask clients what they think is important to help them feel better or gain a stronger sense of self.
- Encourage cultural identity by individualizing hygiene practices, dietary choices, and clothing to meet each client's self-concept needs.

Data from "Global Self-Esteem Across the Life Span," by R. W. Robins et al., 2002, *Psychology and Aging, 17*(3), p. 423; "Predictors of Self-Esteem for Mexican American and European American Youths: A Reexamination of the Influence of Parenting," by S. Y. Ruiz, M. W. Roosa, and N. A. Gonzales, 2002, *Journal of Family Psychology, 16*(1), p. 70; and "Race and Self-Esteem: Meta-Analyses Comparing Whites, Blacks, Hispanics, Asians, and American Indians," by J. M. Twenge and J. Crocker, 2002, *Psychology Bulletin, 128*(3), p. 371.

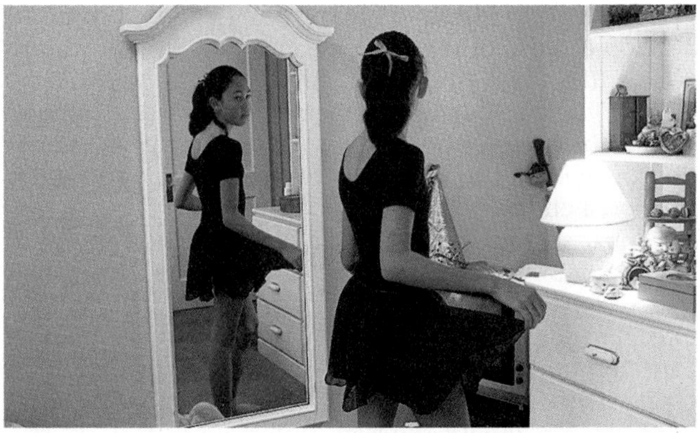

FIGURE 22–2 An individual's appearance influences self-concept. (From *Mosby's Textbook for Nursing Assistants*, 6th ed., by S. A. Sorrentino, 2004, St. Louis, MO: Mosby.)

aging (i.e., wrinkles, greying hair, and decreasing visual acuity, hearing, and mobility) can also affect body image.

Cultural and societal attitudes and values also influence body image. Culture and society dictate accepted norms of body image and can influence one's attitudes (Figure 22–2). Values such as ideal body weight and shape, as well as attitudes toward body markings, piercing, and tattoos, are culturally based. In North American society, youth, beauty, and wholeness are emphasized, as apparent in television programs, movies, and advertisements. People in Western cultures have been socialized to dread the normal aging process, whereas people in Eastern cultures view aging more positively and have great respect for older adults.

Body image depends only partly on the reality of the body. When physical changes occur, individuals may or may not incorporate these changes into their body image. For example, people who have experienced significant weight loss may not perceive themselves as thin and thus may present with a distorted body image. Body image issues are often associated with impaired self-concept and self-esteem and frequently focus on thinness for females and muscularity for males (Cohane & Pope, 2001).

Role Performance. **Role performance** is the way in which an individual perceives his or her ability to carry out significant roles. Common roles include mother or father, wife or husband, daughter or son, sister or brother, employee or employer, and friend. An individual's perception of competency in a role may or may not match other people's evaluation. Roles that individuals follow in given situations involve socialization to expectations or standards of behaviour. Patterns are stable and change only minimally during adulthood. Individuals learn behaviours that are approved by society through the following processes:

- *Reinforcement-extinction:* Certain behaviours become common or are avoided, depending on whether they are approved and reinforced or discouraged and punished.
- *Inhibition:* An individual learns to refrain from behaviours, even when tempted to engage in them.
- *Substitution:* An individual replaces one behaviour with another, which provides the same personal gratification.
- *Imitation:* An individual acquires knowledge, skills, or behaviours from other members of the social or cultural group.
- *Identification:* An individual internalizes the beliefs, behaviour, and values of role models into a personal, unique expression of self.

Ideal societal role behaviours are often hard to achieve in real life. Individuals have multiple roles and individual needs that often conflict. For example, an individual may be a mother of three children, a child of elderly parents, and an employee. Each role involves meeting certain expectations. To function effectively in multiple roles, a person must know the expected behaviour and values, desire to conform to them, and be able to meet the role requirements. Successful adults learn to distinguish between ideal role expectations and realistic possibilities. Fulfillment of these expectations leads to an enhanced sense of self. Difficulty or failure in meeting role expectations leads to deficits and often contributes to decreased self-esteem or altered self-concept.

Self-Esteem. **Self-esteem** is an individual's overall sense of self-worth or the emotional appraisal of the self. It represents the overall judgment of personal worth or value (Judge & Bono, 2001). Self-esteem is positive when one feels capable, worthwhile, and competent (Rosenberg, 1965).

According to Erikson (1963), young children begin to develop a sense of usefulness or industry by learning to act on their own initiative. Children's self-esteem is related to their evaluation of their effectiveness at school, within the family, and in social settings. Others' evaluation of the child is also likely to have a profound influence on a child's self-esteem.

Global self-esteem levels tend to be highest in childhood, possibly because children's sense of self is inflated by a variety of positive sources (Robins et al., 2002). Self-esteem tends to decline in adolescence, which may be partially understood in the context of maturational changes associated with puberty and increased expectations associated with the transition from primary to secondary school. This decline may also be associated with a shift to more realistic information about the self. Social and emotional support has been shown to be positively related to self-esteem and well-being in early adolescence (Park, 2003; Yarcheski, Mahon, & Yarcheski, 2001).

> ***Safety Alert.*** Individuals with low self-esteem are more likely to engage in practices harmful to their health. A decline in self-esteem in adolescence is often associated with an increased need for attention. This need for attention may be demonstrated in unsafe behaviours, such as premature sexual activity, unprotected sex, or substance abuse. In addition, adolescents may take more risks when they begin to drive. These risks threaten the adolescent's health and have implications for health care interventions.

Self-esteem levels rise gradually during adulthood and decline sharply in old age (Robins et al., 2002). In general, this pattern holds true across gender, socio-economic status, and ethnicity. Erikson's emphasis on the generativity stage (1963; see chapter 18) may explain the rise in self-esteem and self-concept in adulthood. The individual is focused on being increasingly productive and creative at work, while at the same time promoting and guiding the next generation. Other than childhood, the mid-60s represents the highest level of self-esteem across the lifespan. At around the age of 70 years, self-esteem declines sharply, which, according to Erikson's stages of development, reflects a diminished need for self-promotion and a shift in self-concept to a more modest and balanced view of the self (Robins et al., 2002).

A consideration of the relationship between a person's self-concept and his or her ideal self can enhance understanding of self-esteem. The ideal self consists of the aspirations, goals, values, and standards of behaviour that a person considers ideal and strives to attain. The ideal self originates in the preschool years and develops throughout life; it is influenced by societal norms and the expectations and demands of parents and significant others. In general, a person whose self-concept comes close to matching the ideal self has high self-esteem, whereas a person whose self-concept varies widely from the ideal self suffers from low self-esteem. A child who excels in school and who is liked by peers is more likely to have high self-esteem than is a child who has difficulty in school and is not liked by peers.

Self-evaluation is an ongoing mental process. A positive sense of self-esteem is an important variable in determining how an individual functions in the world. A person's ability to contribute to society in a meaningful way often affects self-concept and self-esteem. Once established, basic feelings about the self tend to be constant, although there may be some fluctuation. A situational crisis may temporarily affect one's self-esteem. Individuals who are sick and unable to be involved in society may feel worthless. The nurse's acceptance of a client as an individual with worth and dignity can help maintain and improve the client's self-esteem.

Stressors Affecting Self-Concept

A self-concept stressor is any real or perceived change that threatens identity, body image, or role performance (Figure 22–3). A stressor challenges a person's adaptive capacities. The most important factor in determining an individual's response is the individual's perception of the stressor. The ability to re-establish balance is related to numerous factors, including the number of stressors, duration of the stressors, and health status (see chapter 26). The normal process of maturation and development itself is a stressor. Changes that occur in physical, spiritual, emotional, sexual, familial, and socio-cultural health can affect self-concept. Being able to adapt to stressors is likely to lead to a positive sense of self, whereas failure to adapt often leads to a negative sense of self.

Any change in health can be a stressor that potentially affects self-concept. A physical change in the body can lead to an altered body image affecting identity and self-esteem. Chronic illnesses often alter role performance, which may alter one's identity and self-esteem. Loss of a partner can lead to loss of identity and lower self-esteem (Van Baarsen, 2002). An essential process in adjusting to loss is the development of a new self-concept. The case study in Box 22-3 illustrates the interrelationships among the components of self-concept.

Crisis occurs when a person cannot overcome obstacles with the usual methods of problem solving and adaptation. Any crisis potentially threatens self-concept and self-esteem. Some crises, such as the one presented in Box 22-3, directly affect all components of self-concept. The stressors created as a result of a crisis can also affect health status if the person is unable to adapt. If the resulting identity confusion, disturbed body image, low self-esteem, role conflict, role strain, role ambiguity, or role overload are not relieved, illness may result. For example, a diagnosis of cancer places additional demands on a person's established living pattern. It changes the person's appraisal of and satisfaction with the current level of physical, emotional, and social functioning. Self-esteem, learned resourcefulness, and social support have been shown to predict health-related quality of life for long-term survivors of cancer, with self-esteem being the strongest predictor (Pedro, 2001). Health-related quality of life may increase with interventions such as nurse-led support groups aimed at supporting and improving self-esteem. During self-concept crises, supportive and educative resources can help a person learn new ways of coping and responding to the stressful event or situation to maintain or enhance self-concept.

Identity Stressors. Developmental markers such as puberty, menopause, retirement, and decreasing physical

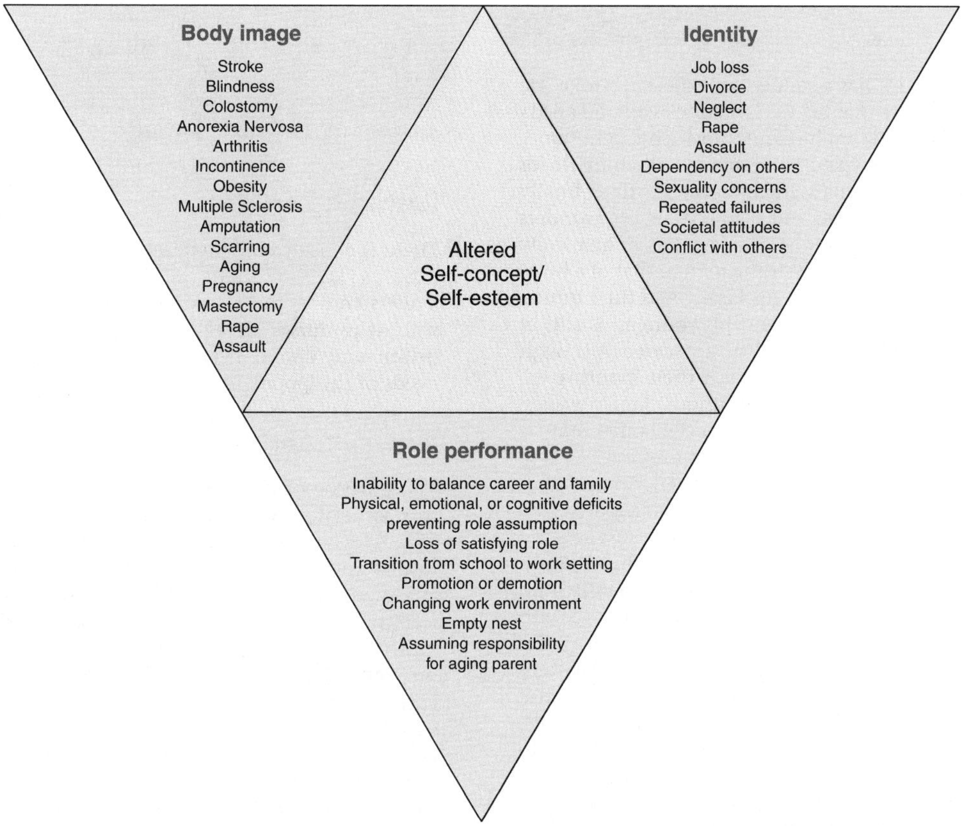

FIGURE **22–3** Common stressors that influence self-concept. (From *Wong's Nursing Care of Infants and Children*, 7th ed., edited by M. Hockenberry et al., 2003, St. Louis, MO: Mosby.)

abilities may affect identity. Identity, like body image, is closely related to appearance and abilities. An individual's identity is affected by stressors throughout life but is particularly vulnerable during adolescence, a time marked by great change. Adolescents are trying to adjust to the physical, emotional, and mental changes of increasing maturity, which can result in insecurity and anxiety. It is also a time when the adolescent is developing psychosocial competence, including coping strategies (see chapter 26). A positive self-concept in adolescence impacts psychological and physical health in young adulthood (Box 22-4).

An adult generally has a more stable identity and thus a more firmly developed self-concept. Cultural and social stressors, rather than personal stressors, may have more impact on an adult's identity. For example, an adult may have to balance career and family, or make choices regarding honouring religious or cultural traditions. Retirement may mean the loss of an important means of achievement and continued success. People at retirement may begin to re-evaluate their identities and accomplishments. Loss of a significant other can lead the surviving individual to re-examine aspects of his or her identity.

Identity confusion results when people do not maintain a clear, consistent, and continuous consciousness of personal identity. It may occur at any stage of life if a person is unable to adapt to identity stressors. Under extreme stress, an individual may experience disturbed personal identity, a state in which the differences between the self and others cannot be determined.

Body Image Stressors. Changes in the appearance, structure, or function of a body part requires an adjustment in body image. An individual's perception of the change and the relative importance placed on body image will affect the significance of a loss of function or change in appearance. For example, if a woman's body image incorporates reproductive functions as the ideal, a hysterectomy secondary to uterine cancer may be a very significant alteration and may result in a perceived loss of femininity or wholeness. Changes in body appearance, such as an amputation, facial disfigurement, or burns, are obvious stressors affecting body image. Mastectomy and colostomy are surgical procedures that alter body appearance and function. Even though these changes may be undetected by others, they can have a significant impact on the individual. Even some elective changes such as breast augmentation or reduction can affect body image. Chronic illnesses such as heart and renal disease decrease function. Anticipated body changes resulting from the developmental process can also affect body image. In addition, the effects of pregnancy, significant weight gain or loss, pharmacological management of illness, or radiation therapy change body image. Negative body image can lead to adverse health outcomes.

Many people associate success with a specific body part or function. For example, athletes may consider their

Case Study Box 22-3

Amil, a 48-year-old man, has a sudden, unexpected stroke. He had not even been aware that he was hypertensive. Amil awakens in the hospital to find that he cannot move his right hand. He cannot care for himself and is unable to turn himself for days. With the nurse's constant encouragement, he is finally able to pull himself out of bed and into a chair. He wonders what lies ahead for him. Amil's body image has dramatically changed from that of a physically strong man to that of a helpless individual. Amil worries about his family and their future. His oldest child is away at college, and his youngest is still in high school. Amil and his wife, Meredith, are scared. Although Meredith works, they are not able to meet their monthly expenses or to educate their children without Amil's wages. Amil's role as primary financial provider for the family may be drastically changed if his condition does not improve.

Amil's self-esteem diminishes as his recovery and rehabilitation progress slowly. His self-concept has changed from a person who is self-sufficient to someone who must rely on others. Although he is now at home in the rehabilitation process, Amil is not able to perform tasks for the family and must wait until his wife and son get home to help him with activities that require strength. Amil's adaptation capabilities are stretched to the maximum, although his physician tells him that he is very fortunate to be alive. Amil's identity is not clear to him anymore. He has no clear role within the family, his body image has been drastically altered, and his self-esteem is spiralling lower and lower.

Amil continues in outpatient physiotherapy. He requires significant time and energy even for simple tasks. Nevertheless, he slowly begins to gain some strength. After several months, he is able to return to work, with a few modifications to ensure his safety. He has some diminished mental agility and muscle weakening, but he is able to perform most aspects of his job. His self-esteem improves, and his body image is enhanced. Although he still feels somewhat altered, his physical capabilities closely resemble those he had before the stroke.

bodies and physical activities to be the focus of personal success. Adaptation and rehabilitation may be affected if they can never again participate in athletics because of an accident or injury. To surgeons, an amputation of a finger would significantly alter their ability to perform surgery. This change may affect their perception of worth as individuals. Body image changes necessitate the revision of long-accepted self-perceptions, as well as alterations in lifestyle. To regain a positive self-concept and self-esteem, each person must adapt to his or her body image stressors.

Society's response to an individual's physical changes may be affected by the conditions surrounding the alteration. For example, paralysis resulting from an act of war may result in the individual being treated as a hero and being praised for self-sacrifice. However, paralysis resulting from a car accident in which the person was intoxicated would likely result in a very different response from society.

Role Performance Stressors. Throughout life a person undergoes numerous role changes. Normal changes associated with growth and maturation result in developmental transitions. Situational transitions occur when parents, spouses, children, or close friends die or people move, marry, divorce, or change jobs. A health-illness transition is a movement from a state of health or well-being to one of illness. A shift along the continuum from illness to wellness is as stressful as a shift from wellness to illness. Any of these transitions may lead to role conflict, role ambiguity, role strain, or role overload.

Role conflict results when a person simultaneously assumes two or more roles that are inconsistent, contradictory, or mutually exclusive. For example, when a middle-age woman with teenage children assumes responsibility for caring for her older parents, conflicts may arise in relation to being both the adult child and the caregiver of her parents. Negotiating a balance of time and energy between her

Research Highlight Box 22-4

Adolescent Self-Concept and Health

Research Focus

There is considerable literature on adolescent self-concept but little is known about its long-term impact on health. Understanding the role of self-concept in adolescent health will help nurses develop strategies to promote adolescent health and design health education programs to meet the needs of this population.

Research Abstract

The purpose of this longitudinal study was to examine factors associated with adolescent self-concept and the impact of adolescent self-concept on psychological and physical health and health behaviour in later adulthood. The study analyzed data from two cycles of the National Population Health Survey, a general health survey of a representative sample of Canadians aged 12 years or older in the 10 provinces. Findings showed that girls tend to have lower self-concept in adolescence than do boys of the same age. Self-concept was associated with household income and with adolescents' perceived level of emotional support. A weak self-concept was predictive of depression six years later among girls, physical inactivity among boys, and obesity among adolescents of both sexes. A strong self-concept had a positive long-term effect on girls' (but not boys') self-perceived health.

Evidenced-Based Practice

- Adolescent self-concept and self-esteem are important issues to be addressed when promoting adolescent health in a variety of settings.
- Nurses should provide emotional support to adolescents and assist them to access emotional support from significant others in their lives.
- Health promotion policies and health education programs would benefit from including strategies to enhance adolescents' self-concept and self-esteem.

Reference

Park, J. (2003). Adolescent self-concept and health into adulthood [Catalogue 82-003]. *Health Reports, 14,* 41–52.

children and parents may also create role conflicts. The perceived importance of each conflicting role influences the degree of conflict experienced. The **sick role** involves the expectations of others and society regarding how one should behave when sick. Role conflict may occur when general societal expectations (take care of yourself and you will get better) and the expectations of co-workers (need to get the job done) collide. The conflict of taking care of oneself while getting everything done can be a major challenge.

Role ambiguity involves unclear role expectations. When there are unclear expectations, people may be unsure about what to do or how to do it. Such a situation is often stressful and confusing. Role ambiguity is common in adolescence. Adolescents are pressured by parents, peers, and the media to assume adult-like roles, but many adolescents lack the resources to move beyond the role of dependent children. Role ambiguity is also common in employment situations. In complex, rapidly changing, or highly specialized organizations, employees often become unsure about job expectations.

Role strain blends role conflict and role ambiguity. Role strain may be expressed as a feeling of frustration when a person feels inadequate or unsuited to a role. Role strain is often associated with gender role stereotypes (Stuart & Laraia, 2001). Others may perceive women in positions traditionally held by men as less competent, less objective, or less knowledgeable than their male counterparts. Women may feel that they must work harder and be better to compete. Men in traditionally female roles may also encounter gender bias.

Role overload involves having more roles or responsibilities within a role than are manageable. It is frequently reflected in an individual who unsuccessfully attempts to meet the demands of work and family while carving out some personal time. Often during periods of illness or change, those involved, either as the one who is ill or as a significant other, find themselves in role overload.

Self-Esteem Stressors. Individuals with high self-esteem are generally more resilient and are better able to cope with demands and stressors than those with low self-esteem. Low self-worth can contribute to feeling unfulfilled and misunderstood and can result in depression and unremitting uneasiness or anxiety. Illness, surgery, or accidents that change life patterns may also influence feelings of self-worth. Chronic illnesses such as diabetes, arthritis, and cardiac dysfunction require changes in accepted and long-assumed behavioural patterns. The more the chronic illness interferes with the ability to engage in activities contributing to feelings of worth or success, the more it affects self-esteem.

Self-esteem stressors vary with developmental stages. Perceived inability to meet parental expectations, harsh criticism, inconsistent discipline, and unresolved sibling rivalry may reduce children's level of self-worth. Some data suggest that the maximum difference in self-esteem between boys and girls occurs in junior high school and also indicate that a gender difference exists in early adolescent coping strategies (Byrne, 2000).

Negative thinking and low self-esteem in college-age women have been shown to be potential predictors for later development of depression (Pedan et al., 2000).

Focus on Older Adults — Box 22-5

- Promoting a positive self-concept in all older adults is essential, but it is especially important for those experiencing disability or frailty.
- Conducting a life review or participating in a reminiscence group, recording an oral history, or arranging a photo scrapbook of meaningful life events are examples of activities to help older adults feel a sense of self-worth about their life while providing a legacy for younger family members (Eliopoulos, 2001).
- Potential threats to the self-esteem of older adults may arise from the institutional environments where they receive care. These threats can include dependence, devaluation, depersonalization, functional impairments, and lack of control over one's environment. Nursing interventions directed toward reducing or eliminating these threats result in improved quality of life for the older adult (Miller, 1999).
- Self-concept may be negatively affected in older adulthood secondary to a number of life changes, including health problems, declining socio-economic status, spousal loss or bereavement, loss of social support, and decline in achievement experiences following retirement (Stuart & Laraia, 2001).
- Be alert to older adults' preoccupation with physical complaints; conduct a comprehensive assessment and encourage clients to verbalize needs, feelings, and emotions such as fear, insecurity, and loneliness (Robins et al., 2002).
- By actively listening and accepting the person's feelings, being respectful, and praising health-seeking behaviours, the nurse will convey that the older adult is worthwhile.

Stressors affecting self-esteem include failures in work and relationships. Pregnancy also introduces unique self-concept stressors. Low self-esteem is one of the strongest predictors of postpartum depression (Beck, 2001). In older adults, self-concept stressors include health problems, declining socio-economic status, spousal loss or bereavement, loss of social support, and decline in achievement experiences following retirement (Box 22-5).

Family Effect on Self-Concept Development

The family plays a key role in creating and maintaining the self-concepts of its members. Children develop a basic sense of who they are from family members. Children learn from family members accepted norms for how one should think, feel, and behave. Some scholars suggest that parents are the most important influence on children's development. Specifically, a relationship exists between parents who respond in a firm, consistent, and warm manner and children's positive self-esteem and school achievement (Ruiz et al., 2002). Parents who are harsh, inconsistent, or have low self-esteem themselves may behave in ways that foster negative self-concepts in their children. Even well-meaning parents can cultivate negative self-concepts in children. To assist clients in developing a positive self-concept, the nurse may first need to assess the family's style of relating (see chapter 16).

The Nurse's Effect on the Client's Self-Concept

A nurse's acceptance of a client with an altered self-concept helps promote positive change. When a client's physical appearance has changed, likely both the client and the family will observe the nurse's verbal and non-verbal responses and reactions. Nurses need to be aware of their own feelings, ideas, values, expectations, and judgments. Self-awareness is critical in initially understanding and accepting others. Nurses who are secure in their own identities more readily accept and thus reinforce clients' identities. It is important for nurses to assess and clarify the following self-concept issues about themselves:

- Own thoughts and feelings about lifestyle, health, and illness
- Awareness of how one's non-verbal communication may affect clients and families
- Personal values and expectations and how they affect clients
- Ability to convey a non-judgmental attitude toward clients
- Preconceived attitudes toward cultural differences in self-concept and self-esteem

The client with a change in body appearance or function can be extremely sensitive to verbal and non-verbal responses of the health care team. A positive and matter-of-fact approach to care can provide a model for the client and family to follow. By conveying genuine interest and acceptance, nurses can have a positive effect on clients. Recognizing and including self-concept issues in planning and delivering care can positively influence client outcomes. Building a trusting nurse-client relationship and appropriately involving the client and family in decision making can enhance self-concept. An individualized approach may highlight a client's unique needs, including incorporating alternative health care practices or methods of spiritual expression.

Nurses can also have a significant impact on their client's body image. For example, a nurse can facilitate a woman's acceptance of her mastectomy by showing acceptance of the mastectomy scar. Clients closely watch other people's reactions to their wounds and scars. A facial expression showing shock or disgust can contribute to the woman developing a negative body image. It is critical for nurses to monitor their responses toward the client. Statements such as "This wound is healing nicely" or "This looks healthy" can be very affirming to the client.

Inadvertently frowning or grimacing when performing procedures can profoundly affect the client. The nurse's non-verbal behaviours help to convey the level of caring that exists for a client and can affect self-esteem (Figure 22–4). For example, the self-concept of an incontinent client can be threatened by the perception that the caregivers find the situation unpleasant. Nurses should anticipate their own reactions, acknowledge them, and focus on the client instead of on the unpleasant task or situation. If nurses can put themselves in the client's position, they can envision measures to ease embarrassment, frustration, and anger.

Preventative measures, early identification, and appropriate treatment can minimize the intensity of self-esteem stressors and the potential effects for the client and family. The nurse learns to design specific self-concept interventions to fit a client's profile of risk factors. It is essential to assess the client's perception of a problem and to work collaboratively to resolve self-concept issues. For example, low-income women defined different barriers to returning to work than those that had been traditionally identified by professionals (Box 22-6). Thus, the nurse must use a different set of interventions for this group of clients.

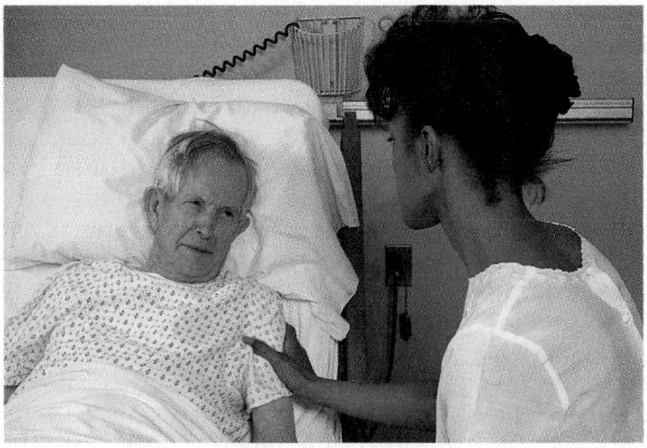

FIGURE **22–4** Nurses can use touch and eye contact to enhance a client's self-esteem.

Critical Thinking

Self-concept profoundly influences a person's response to illness. A critical thinking approach to care is essential. This approach requires synthesis of knowledge, experience, information gathered from clients and families, critical thinking attitudes, and intellectual and professional standards. The nurse needs to use solid clinical judgment, anticipate the required information, collect and analyze the data, and make appropriate decisions regarding client care.

In the case of self-concept, the nurse must integrate knowledge from nursing and other disciplines, including self-concept theory and communication principles, and consider cultural and developmental factors. Previous experience in caring for clients with alterations in self-concept assists the nurse in individualizing care for each client. The nursing process is continuous until the client's self-concept is improved, restored, or maintained.

Self-Concept and the Nursing Process

NP Assessment

In assessing self-concept and self-esteem, the nurse first focuses on the various components of self-concept (identity, body image, and role performance). Assessment should also include behaviours suggestive of an altered self-concept (Box 22-7), actual and potential self-concept

Research Highlight

Box 22-6

Promoting Self-Esteem and Self-Sufficiency

Research Focus

Low-income women encounter many barriers as they struggle to enter the workforce and become self-sufficient. Understanding the barriers that women face from the women's perspective is important so that nurses can develop interventions specifically targeted to assist these women in achieving self-sufficiency and health.

Research Abstract

A group of low-income women participated in a qualitative study to identify barriers to achieving self-sufficiency. The women were attending an occupational skills training centre designed to assist low-income, unemployed, or underemployed women in their transition to the workforce. The women identified eight obstacles to self-sufficiency, including lack of self-esteem, especially about returning to school; having "bad" relationships with men; lack of support from family and friends; limited life options; lack of training; lack of quality programs; criminal histories; and fear of success. Inadequate child care and transportation were not identified as barriers by the women themselves but were viewed as socially acceptable reasons for not working.

Evidence-Based Practice

Promoting empowerment, building self-esteem, and developing self-efficacy in women living in low income are important means of promoting behavioural change.

- Nursing resources should be aimed at addressing fundamental self-concept deficits.
- Modifying the nursing approach to match identified client needs is needed to ensure client and family health.
- Follow-up services, including home care and community health, are needed to promote family health.

Reference

Brown, S. G., & Barbosa, G. (2001). Nothing is going to stop me now: Low-income women as they become self-sufficient. *Public Health Nursing, 18*(5), 364–372.

stressors (see Figure 22–3), and coping patterns. Gathering comprehensive assessment data requires the nurse to critically synthesize information from multiple sources (Figure 22–5).

In addition to direct questioning, much of the data regarding self-concept are effectively gathered through observing the client's non-verbal behaviour and by paying attention to the content of the client's conversation. The nurse should take note of the manner in which clients talk about significant people in their lives, because this observation can provide clues to both stressful and supportive relationships, as well as to key roles that the client assumes. Using knowledge of developmental stages to determine what areas are likely to be important to the client, the nurse should inquire about these aspects of the person's life. For example, the nurse might ask a 65-year-old client about his or her life and what has been important to him or her. At this stage of development, individuals are examining their lives and considering the impact they have had in the world. The individual's conversation will likely provide data relating to role performance, identity, self-esteem, stressors, and coping patterns. At appropriate times, it may be useful to ask specific questions (Table 22-1).

Box 22-7 Behaviours Suggestive of Altered Self-Concept

Avoidance of eye contact
Slumped posture
Unkempt appearance
Overly apologetic
Hesitant speech
Overly critical or angry
Frequent or inappropriate crying
Negative self-evaluation
Excessively dependent
Hesitant to express views or opinions
Lack of interest in what is happening
Passive attitude
Difficulty in making decisions

Coping Behaviours. The nursing assessment should also include considering previous coping behaviours; the nature, number, and intensity of the stressors; and the client's internal and external resources. Knowledge of how a client has dealt with stressors in the past can provide insight into the client's style of coping. People do not address all issues in the same way, but often use a familiar coping pattern for newly encountered stressors. As the nurse identifies previous coping patterns, it is useful to determine whether these patterns have contributed to healthy functioning or created more problems. For example, the use of drugs or alcohol during times of stress often creates additional stressors (see chapter 26).

Exploring resources and strengths, such as the availability of significant others or prior use of community resources, can be important in formulating a realistic and effective plan. It is also critical to understand how the client views the situation. For example, it may be that older women are more accustomed to changes in their health status because of the aging process in general, and experiencing heart disease may be one more aspect of growing older. On the other hand, a cardiac event occurring in

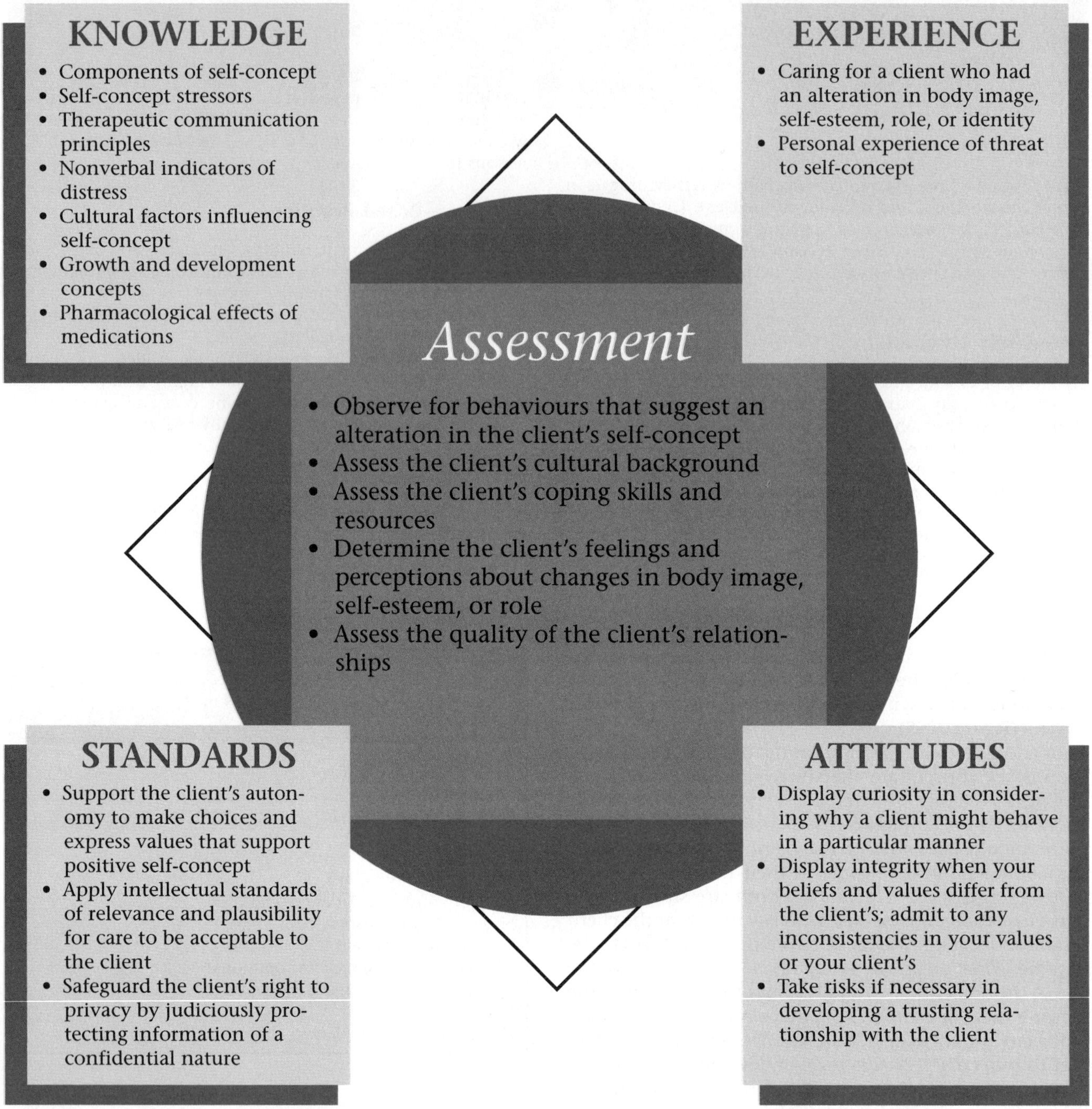
KNOWLEDGE
• Components of self-concept
• Self-concept stressors
• Therapeutic communication principles
• Nonverbal indicators of distress
• Cultural factors influencing self-concept
• Growth and development concepts
• Pharmacological effects of medications
EXPERIENCE
• Caring for a client who had an alteration in body image, self-esteem, role, or identity
• Personal experience of threat to self-concept
Assessment
• Observe for behaviours that suggest an alteration in the client's self-concept
• Assess the client's cultural background
• Assess the client's coping skills and resources
• Determine the client's feelings and perceptions about changes in body image, self-esteem, or role
• Assess the quality of the client's relationships
STANDARDS
• Support the client's autonomy to make choices and express values that support positive self-concept
• Apply intellectual standards of relevance and plausibility for care to be acceptable to the client
• Safeguard the client's right to privacy by judiciously protecting information of a confidential nature
ATTITUDES
• Display curiosity in considering why a client might behave in a particular manner
• Display integrity when your beliefs and values differ from the client's; admit to any inconsistencies in your values or your client's
• Take risks if necessary in developing a trusting relationship with the client

FIGURE **22–5** Critical thinking model for self-concept assessment.

middle age may be less expected and more problematic for women in terms of family and career responsibilities and thus elicit a more dramatic change in anxiety (Plach, Napholz, & Kelber, 2001).

Significant Others. Valuable data may also evolve out of conversations with family and significant others. These individuals may have insights into the person's way of dealing with stressors or knowledge about what is important to the person's self-concept. The way the person talks about the client and the significant others' non-verbal behaviours may provide information about what kind of support is available for the client.

Client Expectations. Also important in assessing self-concept is the person's expectations. Asking clients how they believe interventions will make a difference can indicate their expectations and provide an opportunity to discuss their goals. For example, a nurse working with a client who is experiencing anxiety related to an upcoming diagnostic test might ask about the relaxation exercise that they have been practising together. The client's

Table 22-1 Nursing Assessment of Client's Self-Concept

Assessment Questions*	Responses Reflecting Difficulties With Self-Concept
Identity	
"How would you describe yourself?"	Derogatory answers (e.g., "I don't know; there's not too much worth mentioning") should raise concern.
Body Image	
"What aspects of your appearance do you like?" "Are there any aspects of your appearance that you would like to change? If yes, describe the changes you would make."	Most people can identify something about their appearance that they like (e.g., "I have nice eyes"). If a person cannot identify any positive characteristic, this is suggestive of a negative body image and poor self-esteem. Most people have something that they would like to change (e.g., "My nose is too big" or "My hips are too large"), but a long list of problem areas may suggest difficulties with self-concept.
Self-esteem	
"Tell me about the things you do that make you feel good about yourself." "How do you feel about yourself?"	Statements about not having any strengths or being able to do anything well should raise concern.
Role Performance	
"Tell me about your primary roles (e.g., partner, parent, friend, sister, professional role, volunteer). How effective are you at carrying out each of these roles?"	The nurse should listen for the number of primary roles identified. A large number of primary roles will put the client at risk for role conflict and role overload. As with questions above, if the client indicates that he or she does not feel that these roles are adequately covered, the person may be experiencing alterations in self-concept. Although most people carry out many roles and often feel as though some of them are not adequately addressed, listen for the person's perception about his or her overall role competency.

*In addition to the client's verbal response, the nurse should note non-verbal behaviours. Hesitant speech, poor eye contact, and hunched posture suggest alterations in self-concept.

response will provide the nurse with valuable information about the client's beliefs and attitudes regarding the efficacy of the intervention as well as the potential need to modify the nursing approach.

Nursing Diagnosis

The nurse has to carefully consider assessment data to identify a client's actual or potential problem areas. The nurse relies on knowledge and experience, applies appropriate professional standards, and looks for clusters of defining characteristics that indicate a nursing diagnosis. Although there are multiple nursing diagnostic labels for altered self-concept, the following list provides examples of self-concept-related nursing diagnoses:

- Impaired adjustment
- Anxiety
- Disturbed body image
- Caregiver role strain
- Decisional conflict
- Ineffective coping
- Ineffective denial
- Fear
- Hopelessness
- Disturbed personal identity
- Risk for loneliness
- Ineffective role performance
- Chronic low self-esteem
- Situational low self-esteem
- Ineffective sexuality patterns
- Impaired social interaction
- Spiritual distress
- Risk for self-directed violence

Making nursing diagnoses about self-concept is complex. Often, isolated data could be the defining characteristics for more than one nursing diagnosis (Box 22-8). For example, a client might express feelings of uncertainty and inadequacy. These are defining characteristics for both *anxiety* and *situational low self-esteem.* Awareness that the client is demonstrating defining characteristics for more than one nursing diagnosis can guide the nurse to gather specific data to validate and differentiate the underlying problem. To further assess the possibility of *anxiety* as the nursing diagnosis, the nurse might consider whether the person has any of the following defining characteristics: Is the person experiencing increased muscle tension, shakiness, a sense of being "rattled," or restlessness? These symptoms would suggest *anxiety* as the more appropriate diagnosis. On the other hand, if the person expresses a predominantly negative self-appraisal, including inability to handle situations or events and difficulty making decisions, these characteristics would suggest that *situational low self-esteem* may be the more appropriate nursing diagnosis. To further aid the nurse in differentiating between the two diagnoses, information regarding recent events in the person's life and how the person has viewed himself or herself in the past would

Nursing Diagnostic Process — Box 22-8

Assessment Activities	Defining Characteristics	Nursing Diagnosis
Observe client's behaviour during conversation.	Client demonstrates restlessness, inability to maintain eye contact, facial tension, increased perspiration, and self-preoccupation.	Anxiety related to accidental injury, pain, uncertainty of outcome of upcoming surgery
Empathically communicate, "Tell me how you are coping" or "Let's talk about what you are thinking and feeling about tomorrow's procedure."	Client replies, "I'm scared. They may amputate my leg tomorrow. I just don't know how I'll manage. I couldn't sleep last night. On top of the pain, I just kept thinking about everything."	

provide insight into the most appropriate nursing diagnosis. As additional data are gathered, usually the priority nursing diagnosis becomes evident.

To validate critical thinking regarding a nursing diagnosis, the nurse can share observations with the client and allow the client to verify the nurse's perception. This approach often results in the client providing additional data, which further clarifies the situation. In the above example, if the nurse said, "I notice you haven't eaten much breakfast or lunch today," the response to this statement coupled with the client's non-verbal communication could facilitate further discussion. An alternative approach may be to state, "I notice you jumped when I came up behind you. Are you feeling uneasy today?" This statement could allow the client to verify whether he or she is in fact anxious and to tell the nurse about any concerns.

Planning

During planning, the nurse again synthesizes knowledge, experience, critical thinking attitudes, and standards (Figure 22–6). Critical thinking ensures that the client's care plan integrates all that the nurse knows about the individual, as well as key critical thinking elements (see Care Plan). Professional standards are especially important to consider when the nurse develops a plan of care. These standards often establish ethical or evidence-based practice guidelines for selecting effective nursing interventions.

Another method to assist in planning care is a concept map (Figure 22–7). This concept map shows the relationship between a medical diagnosis, post-operative reconstruction of severe facial scars, and the four nursing diagnoses. The concept map also links the nursing diagnoses and shows how they are interrelated. In this example, there is a relationship between disturbed body image and situational low self-esteem. As the client's facial scars improve, she should begin to feel better about her appearance.

Goals and Outcomes. The nurse develops an individualized plan of care for each nursing diagnosis. The nurse and client set realistic expectations for care. Goals should be individualized and realistic with measurable outcomes. In establishing goals, the nurse should consult with the client about whether the goals are perceived as realistic. Consultation with significant others, mental health clinicians, and community resources can result in a more comprehensive and workable plan. Once a goal has been formulated, the nurse should consider how the data that illustrated the problem would change if the problem were diminished. These changes should be reflected in the outcome criteria. For example, a client is diagnosed with *situational low self-esteem related to a recent job layoff*. The nurse and client establish a goal: "Client's self-esteem and self-concept should begin to improve in 2 weeks." Examples of expected outcomes directed toward that goal include the following:

- The client will discuss a minimum of three areas of her life where she is functioning well.
- The client will be able to voice the recognition that losing her job is not reflective of her worth as a person.
- The client attends a support group for out-of-work professionals.

Setting Priorities. The care plan presents the goals, expected outcomes, and interventions for a client with an alteration in self-concept. Interventions focus on helping the client adapt to the stressors that led to the self-concept disturbance and on supporting and reinforcing methods of coping.

Often a client perceives a situation as overwhelming and may feel hopeless about returning to the previous level of functioning. The client may need time to adapt to physical changes.

Establishing priorities may include therapeutic communication to address self-concept issues to ensure that the client's ability to address physical needs is maximized. The nurse should look for strengths in both the individual and the family and provide resources and education to assist the client to change limitations into strengths. Client teaching creates understanding of the normalcy of certain situations (e.g., nature of a chronic disease, change in a relationship, or effect of a loss). Often, once this is understood, the sense of hopelessness and helplessness decreases.

Continuity of Care. The perceptions of significant others are important to incorporate into the plan of care. Individuals who have experienced deficits in self-concept before the current episode of treatment may have

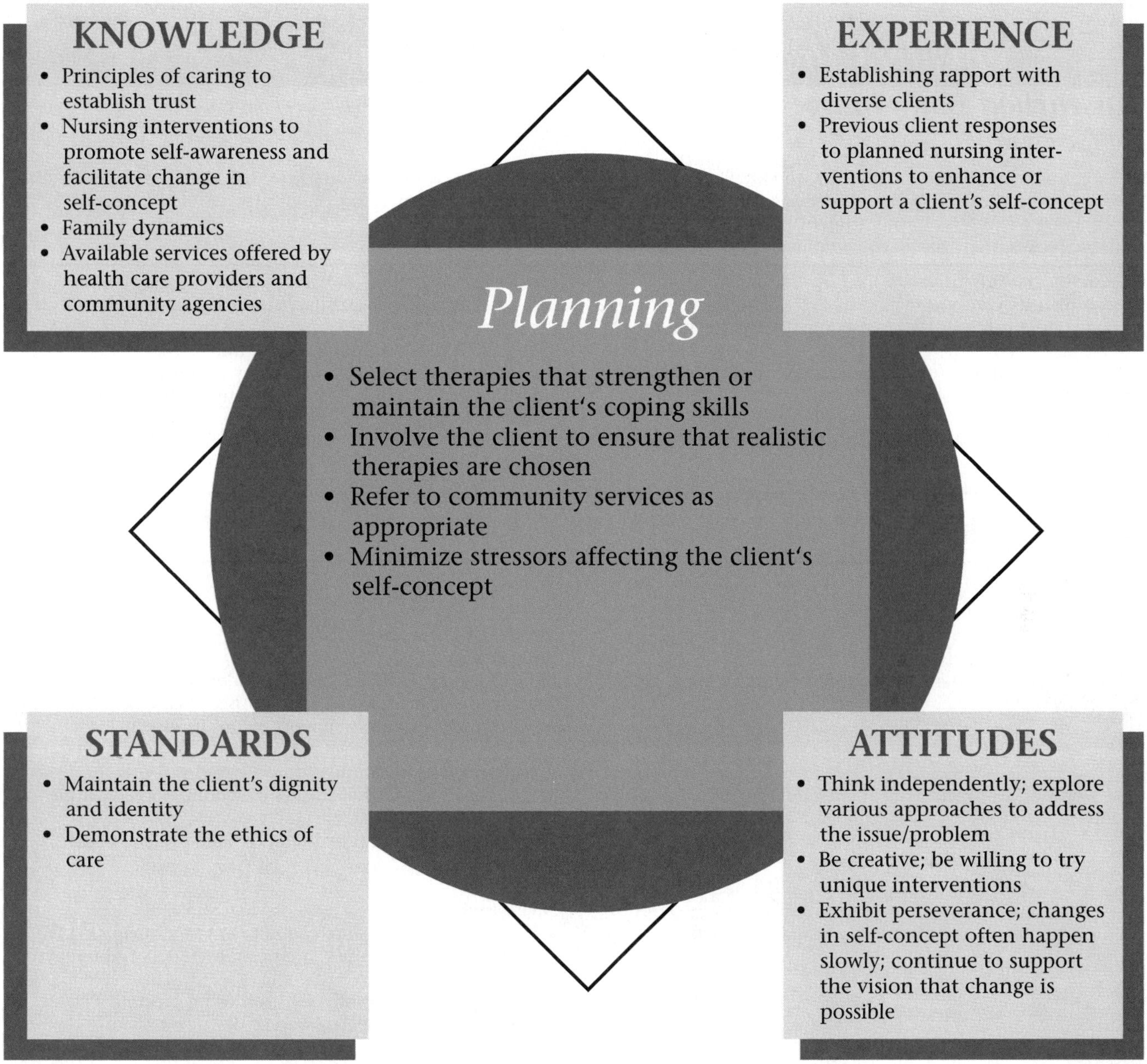
KNOWLEDGE
• Principles of caring to establish trust
• Nursing interventions to promote self-awareness and facilitate change in self-concept
• Family dynamics
• Available services offered by health care providers and community agencies
EXPERIENCE
• Establishing rapport with diverse clients
• Previous client responses to planned nursing interventions to enhance or support a client's self-concept
Planning
• Select therapies that strengthen or maintain the client's coping skills
• Involve the client to ensure that realistic therapies are chosen
• Refer to community services as appropriate
• Minimize stressors affecting the client's self-concept
STANDARDS
• Maintain the client's dignity and identity
• Demonstrate the ethics of care
ATTITUDES
• Think independently; explore various approaches to address the issue/problem
• Be creative; be willing to try unique interventions
• Exhibit perseverance; changes in self-concept often happen slowly; continue to support the vision that change is possible

FIGURE **22–6** Critical thinking model for self-concept planning.

established a system of support including mental health clinicians, clergy, and other community resources. Before involving the family, the nurse needs to consider the client's desires for their involvement and cultural norms regarding who most frequently makes decisions in the family.

Implementation

As with all the steps of the nursing process, a therapeutic nurse-client relationship is central to the implementation phase. Once the goals and outcome criteria have been developed, the nurse considers nursing interventions for promoting a healthy self-concept and helping the client move toward the goals. To develop effective nursing interventions, the nurse should consider the nursing diagnosis and broad interventions that address the diagnosis. These broad, standard interventions should be tailored to the individual client. Regardless of the health care setting, it is important that nurses work with clients and their families or significant others to promote a healthy self-concept. For example, nursing interventions may include strategies to help clients regain or restore the elements that contribute to a strong and secure sense of self. The approaches that nurses choose will vary according to the level of care required.

Health Promotion. The nurse may work with clients to help them develop healthy lifestyle behaviours that contribute to a positive self-concept (Box 22-9).

Nursing Care Plan

Disturbed Body Image

Assessment

Mrs. Johnson, a 45-year-old married woman who underwent a unilateral radical mastectomy because of malignancy, has been assigned to Miss Carr, a student nurse. Mrs. Johnson's physical assessment has been completed, and she has been adequately medicated for pain. Miss Carr sits down to discuss how the mastectomy has affected Mrs. Johnson's self-concept.

Assessment Activities	Findings/Defining Characteristics
Assess identity concerns (e.g., sexual role, femininity). Ask Mrs. Johnson how the mastectomy is affecting her sense of self.	Mrs. Johnson looks away, shakes her head, and states, "I don't feel feminine. My husband says it doesn't affect how he feels about me, but I don't believe him."
Observe Mrs. Johnson's mood and interactions with others, including family members.	Intermittent eye contact, frequent crying when alone, pulling hospital gown tightly across chest, superficial conversations with family members.
Determine Mrs. Johnson's participation in self-care activities.	Avoids looking in mirror; refuses to bathe, comb hair, or brush her teeth.

Nursing Diagnosis: Disturbed body image related to negative thoughts and feelings to actual change in body.

Planning

Goal	Expected Outcomes*
Mrs. Johnson will identify and express feelings verbally and non-verbally.	**Body Image** Mrs. Johnson will discuss disturbed body image with staff members and significant others within 3 days. Mrs. Johnson will consider exploring support groups by discharge.
Mrs. Johnson will participate in self-care related to mastectomy.	**Acceptance/Health Status** Mrs. Johnson will look at tissue surrounding surgery within 2 days. Mrs. Johnson will begin to attend to basic hygiene needs within 2 days.
Mrs. Johnson will identify and use resources outside the hospital.	**Social Involvement** Mrs. Johnson will verbalize commitment to participating in community resources (e.g., mastectomy support group) by discharge. By post-operative visit, Mrs. Johnson will determine if she wishes to attend support group.

*Outcome classification labels from *Nursing Outcomes Classification (NOC)* (3rd ed.), edited by S. Moorhead, M. Johnson, and M. Maas, 2004, St. Louis, MO: Mosby.

Interventions†	Rationale
Coping Enhancement	
Initially assign the same staff members to work with Mrs. Johnson.	Continuity in care will facilitate the establishment of a therapeutic relationship; familiarity and trust will enhance communication.
Approach Mrs. Johnson and initiate conversation; use silence and active listening to promote communication.	Mrs. Johnson's ability to initially find the words for what she is experiencing may be limited.
Remain aware of your own feelings regarding Mrs. Johnson's bodily changes and physical appearance.	Inadvertently communicating discomfort or negativity will interfere with Mrs. Johnson's ability to openly communicate her feelings.
Have Mrs. Johnson spend time alone and with supportive family members for crying, recording in her journal, reflection, or prayer.	Encourages expression of thoughts and feelings including depression, grief, resentment, and fear of rejection.
Facilitate evaluation of overall self-concept.	The impact on body image may influence other aspects of self-concept and self-esteem, including perception of identity and role performance.

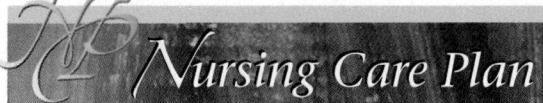

Nursing Care Plan

Disturbed Body Image—cont'd

Interventions†—cont'd	Rationale
Coping Enhancement—cont'd	
Involve Mrs. Johnson's husband in discussion of uncomfortable issues such as areas of sexual concerns.	Family involvement is an essential element of comprehensive care. Sexuality is a basic need and concern for both men and women, yet can be one of the most difficult discussions for clients to initiate.
Assist Mrs. Johnson to identify and use appropriate support systems outside the hospital including home health care.	Support can assist the client in feeling normal again and in integrating a new body image into her self-concept.

†Intervention classification labels from *Nursing Interventions Classification (NIC)* (4th ed.), edited by J. M. Dochterman and G. M. Bulechek, 2004, St. Louis, MO: Mosby.

Evaluation

Nursing Actions	Client Response/Finding	Achievement of Outcome
Ask Mrs. Johnson how effective she feels in her ability to identify and express feelings verbally and nonverbally.	Mrs. Johnson responds, "It's hard for me to talk about myself, but I have really made an effort to talk about what the loss of my breast means to me."	Mrs. Johnson reports improvement in communication skills and success with discussing disturbed body image with primary nurse and husband.
Observe Mrs. Johnson's participation in self-care related to mastectomy.	Mrs. Johnson assumed responsibility for basic hygiene immediately after establishing the goal and has used a mirror to examine her mastectomy scar.	Mrs. Johnson has increased her independence and has begun to integrate body image change into her self-concept.
Assist Mrs. Johnson to identify resources outside the hospital; secure a commitment to use resources.	Mrs. Johnson will verbalize commitment to participating in community resources (e.g., mastectomy support group).	Outcome has not been completely achieved; Mrs. Johnson has expressed hesitancy in attending a support group, but is receptive to home care. Home care nurse to ensure goal is re-evaluated and addressed as appropriate.

Acute Care. In the acute care setting, the nurse is likely to care for clients who are experiencing potential threats to their self-concept because of the nature of the treatment and diagnostic procedures. Threats to a person's self-concept can result in anxiety or fear. Numerous stressors, including unknown diagnoses, the need to make changes in lifestyle, and change in functioning, may be present and need to be addressed. In the acute care setting, there is often more than one stressor, thus increasing the overall stress level for the client and family.

Nurses in the acute care setting also encounter clients who are faced with the need to adapt to an altered body image as a result of surgery or other physical changes. Often a visit by someone who has experienced similar changes and adapted to them (e.g., someone who has had a laryngectomy) may be helpful. The timing of such a visit is important. Because addressing these needs may be difficult while in an acute care setting, appropriate follow-up and referrals, including home care, are essential. The nurse needs to be sensitive to the client's level of acceptance of the change. Forcing confrontation with the change before the client is ready could delay the person's acceptance. Signs that a person may be receptive to such a visit would include the client's asking questions related to how to manage a particular aspect of what has happened or looking at the changed area. As the client expresses readiness to integrate the body change into his or her self-concept, the nurse can either let the client know about groups that are available or ask the client if he or she would like the nurse to make the contact. Another way in which nurses can facilitate adjustment to a change in physical appearance is through their own response to the change. As the nurse responds with acceptance, this models acceptance for both the client and the family.

Restorative Care. Often in a long-term nurse-client relationship in a home care environment, nurses have the opportunity to work with clients to attain a more positive self-concept (Box 22-10). Interventions designed to help a client attain a positive self-concept are based on the premise that the client first develops insight and self-awareness concerning problems and stressors and then acts to solve the problems and cope with the stressors. This approach, outlined by Stuart and Laraia (2001), can

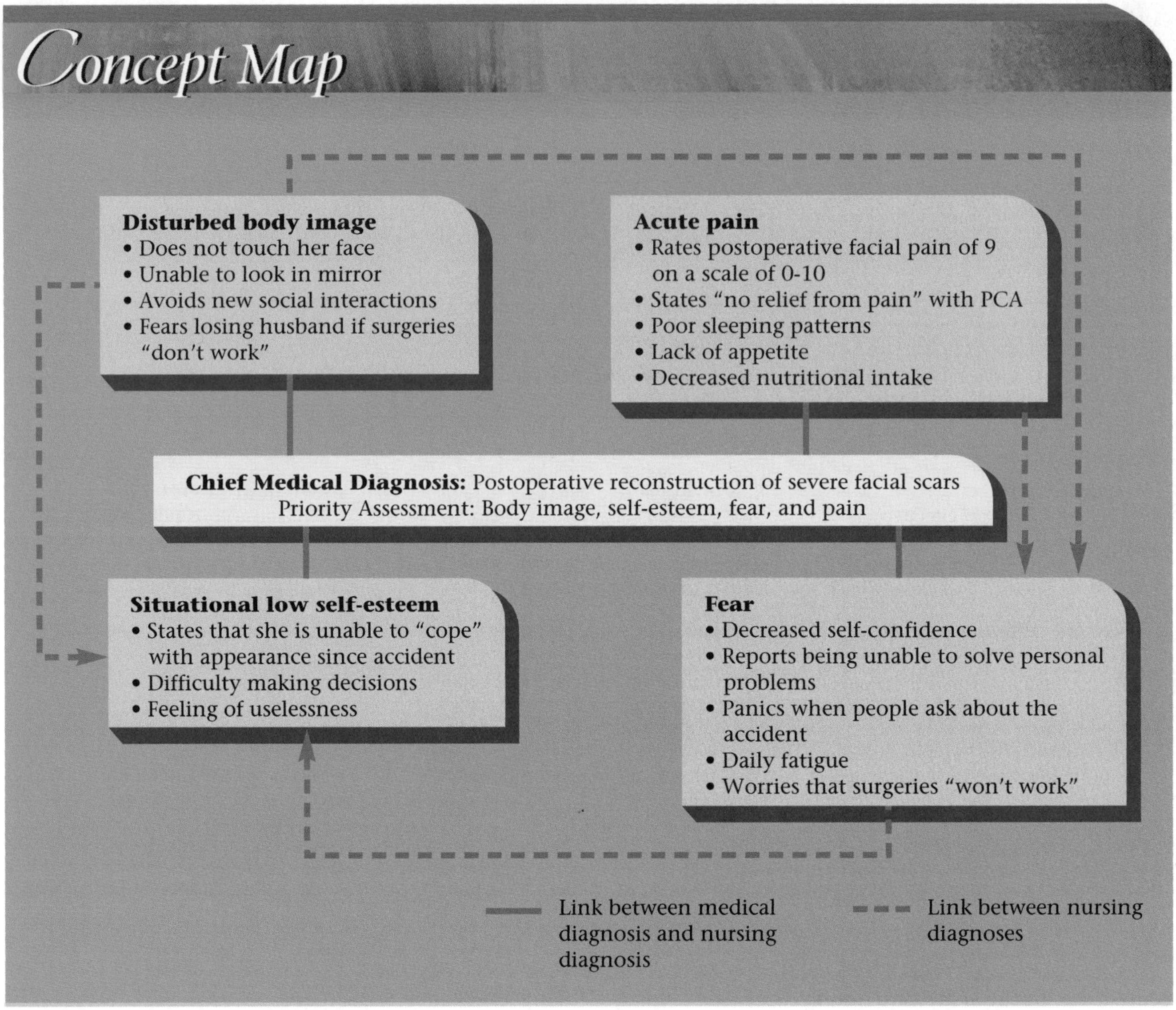
Concept Map
Disturbed body image
• Does not touch her face
• Unable to look in mirror
• Avoids new social interactions
• Fears losing husband if surgeries "don't work"
Acute pain
• Rates postoperative facial pain of 9 on a scale of 0-10
• States "no relief from pain" with PCA
• Poor sleeping patterns
• Lack of appetite
• Decreased nutritional intake
Chief Medical Diagnosis: Postoperative reconstruction of severe facial scars
Priority Assessment: Body image, self-esteem, fear, and pain
Situational low self-esteem
• States that she is unable to "cope" with appearance since accident
• Difficulty making decisions
• Feeling of uselessness
Fear
• Decreased self-confidence
• Reports being unable to solve personal problems
• Panics when people ask about the accident
• Daily fatigue
• Worries that surgeries "won't work"
Link between medical diagnosis and nursing diagnosis
Link between nursing diagnoses

FIGURE **22–7** Concept map for client who is post-operative for reconstruction of severe facial scars.

be incorporated into client teaching for alterations in self-concept, including situational low self-esteem, which might present in the home care setting.

Increasing the client's self-awareness is achieved through establishing a trusting relationship that allows the client to openly explore thoughts and feelings. A priority nursing intervention continues to be the expert use of communication skills to clarify client and family expectations. Open exploration can make the situation less threatening for the client and encourages behaviours that expand self-awareness. Encouraging the client's self-exploration is achieved by accepting the client's thoughts and feelings, by helping the client to clarify interactions with others, and by being empathetic. The nurse encourages self-expression and stresses the client's self-responsibility. Promoting the client's self-evaluation involves helping the client to define problems clearly and to identify positive and negative coping mechanisms. The nurse works closely with the client to help analyze adaptive and maladaptive responses, contrast different alternatives, and discuss outcomes.

Collaborating with the client in establishing realistic goals involves helping the client identify alternative solutions and develop realistic goals based on them. This collaboration facilitates real change and encourages further goal-setting behaviours. The nurse designs opportunities that result in success, reinforces the client's skills and strengths, and assists the client in getting needed assistance. Assisting the client in becoming committed to decisions and actions to achieve goals involves teaching the client to move away from ineffective coping mechanisms and to develop successful coping strategies. Supporting attempts that are health promoting is essential, because with each success another attempt can be

Focus on Primary Health Care Box 22-9

Promoting Client Self-Concept

The focus of primary health care is to promote health and prevent illness by stressing client education and self-care. Measures that support adaptation to stress, such as proper nutrition, regular exercise within the client's capabilities, measures that facilitate adequate sleep and rest, and stress-reducing practices may contribute to a healthy self-concept and therefore promote health and well-being.

Nurses are in a unique position to identify lifestyle practices that put a person's self-concept at risk or are suggestive of an altered self-concept. For example, a young teacher visits a clinic with complaints of being unable to sleep and experiencing anxiety attacks. In gathering the nursing health history, the nurse may learn of lifestyle practices such as excessive use of alcohol or non-prescription drugs, too little rest, or a large number of life changes occurring simultaneously. These data, when taken together, may suggest actual or potential self-concept disturbances. The nurse in this situation determines how the client views the various lifestyle elements to facilitate the client's insight into behaviours. If necessary, the nurse provides needed health teaching or makes appropriate referrals to other community services. Clients who are experiencing threats to or alterations in self-concept often benefit from mental health and community resources to promote increased awareness. Knowledge of available community resources allows the nurse to make appropriate referrals.

made. Supporting adaptive, flexible coping is critical to intervening in self-concept alterations.

Establishing a therapeutic environment and a therapeutic relationship (see chapter 14) and increasing self-awareness are critical to successfully intervening with clients who have alterations in self-concept, whether care is focused on health promotion, dealing with an acute process, or addressing restorative care. To support a client in developing a positive self-concept, the nurse must convey genuine caring (see chapter 15). The nurse can then establish a partnership with the client to address underlying problems.

Client Teaching Box 22-10

Alterations in Self-Concept

Objective

- Risks for situational low self-esteem will be reduced in the home care setting.

Teaching Strategies

- Reinforce client's expression of thoughts and feelings; clarify meaning of verbal and non-verbal communication.
- Encourage opportunities for self-care.
- Elicit client's perceptions of strengths and weaknesses.
- Convey verbally and behaviourally that client is responsible for behaviour.
- Identify relevant stressors with client and ask for appraisal of them.
- Explore client's adaptive and maladaptive coping responses to problems.
- Collaboratively identify alternative solutions; encourage alternatives not previously tried.
- Continue to reinforce strengths and successes.

Evaluation

- Confirm perception of and actual use of improved communication skills.
- Observe level of participation in decisions that affect care.
- Confirm with client and family that the increase in activities and tasks has been a positive experience.
- Observe the client's establishment of a simple routine.
- Observe the client take necessary action to change maladaptive coping responses and maintain adaptive responses.
- Confirm with client and family how new coping resources can be applied to continued change.

Modified from *Principles and Practice of Psychiatric Nursing* (7th ed.), by G. W. Stuart and M. T. Laraia, 2001, St. Louis, MO: Mosby.

NP Evaluation

Client Care. Evaluating success in meeting each client's goal and the established expected outcomes requires critical thinking (Figure 22–8). Frequent evaluation of client progress is recommended so that changes can be instituted if necessary. The nurse uses knowledge of behaviours and characteristics of a healthy self-concept when reviewing the client's behaviours. This method determines whether outcomes have been met.

Expected outcomes for a client with a self-concept disturbance may include non-verbal behaviours indicating a positive self-concept, statements of self-acceptance, and acceptance of change in appearance or function. Key indicators of clients' self-concept can be their non-verbal behaviours. For example, a client who has had difficulty making eye contact may demonstrate a more positive self-concept by making more frequent eye contact. Social interaction, adequate self-care, acceptance of the use of prosthetic devices, and statements indicating understanding of teaching all indicate progress. A positive attitude toward rehabilitation and increased movement toward independence facilitate a return to pre-existing roles at work or at home. Patterns of interacting can also reflect changes in self-concept. For example, a client who has been hesitant to express his or her views may more readily offer opinions and ideas as self-esteem increases. The goals of care may be unrealistic or inappropriate as the client's condition changes. The nurse may need to revise the plan, reflecting on successful experiences with other clients. Client adaptation to major changes may take a year or longer, but the fact that this period is long does not suggest problems with adaptation. The nurse should look for signs that the client has reduced some stressors

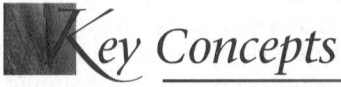

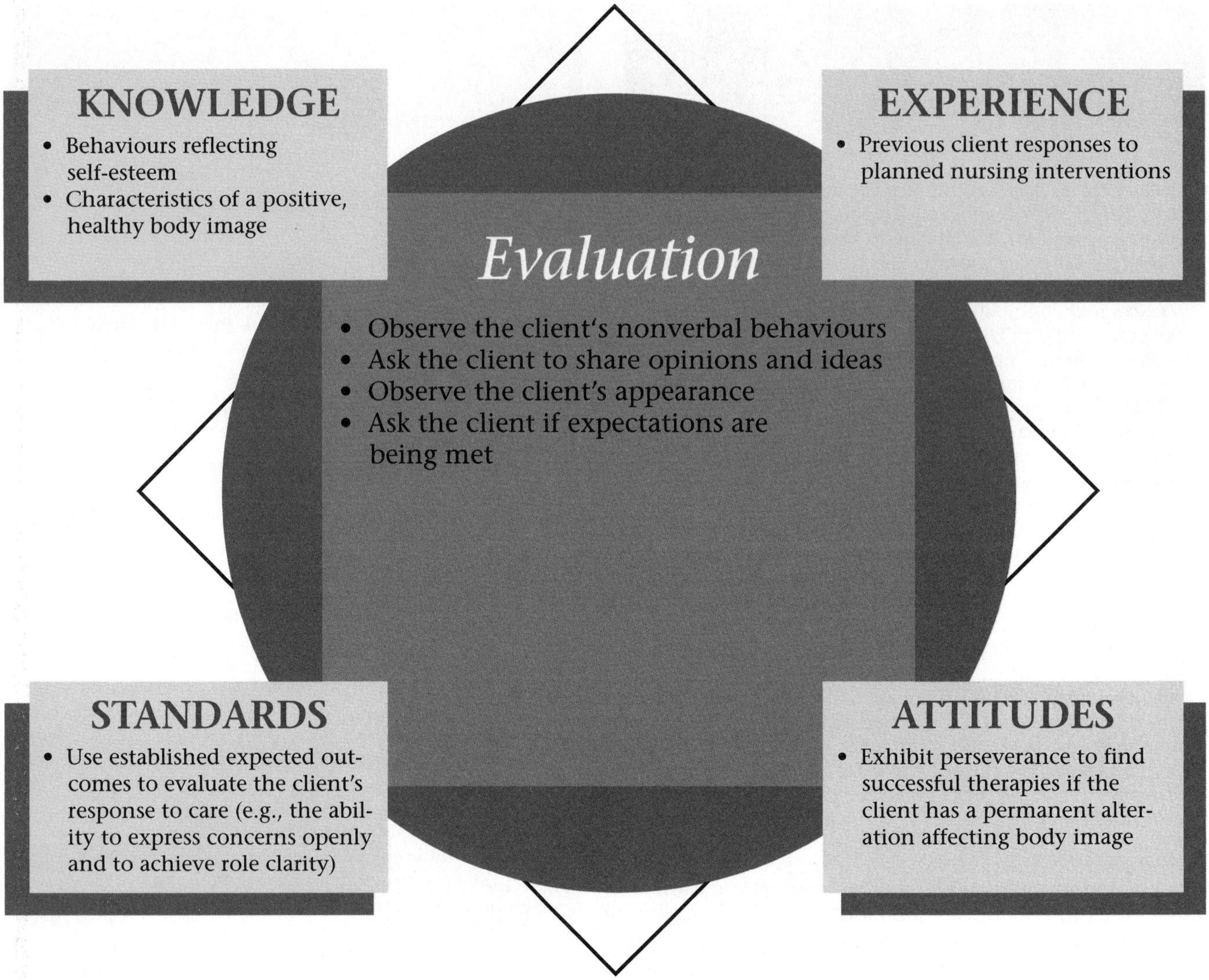
KNOWLEDGE
• Behaviours reflecting self-esteem
• Characteristics of a positive, healthy body image
EXPERIENCE
• Previous client responses to planned nursing interventions
Evaluation
• Observe the client's nonverbal behaviours
• Ask the client to share opinions and ideas
• Observe the client's appearance
• Ask the client if expectations are being met
STANDARDS
• Use established expected outcomes to evaluate the client's response to care (e.g., the ability to express concerns openly and to achieve role clarity)
ATTITUDES
• Exhibit perseverance to find successful therapies if the client has a permanent alteration affecting body image

FIGURE **22–8** Critical thinking model for self-concept evaluation.

and that some behaviours have become more adaptive. Changes in self-concept take time. Although change may be slow, care of the client with a self-concept disturbance can be rewarding.

Client Expectations. If the nurse has developed a good rapport with the client, the client may be able to share how things are going from his or her perspective. The nurse may be able to facilitate this sharing by initiating a review of what has happened over time. This review offers the nurse the opportunity to share perceptions and encourages clients to consider and voice how they have conceptualized any changes.

Key Concepts

- Self-concept is an integrated set of conscious and unconscious attitudes and perceptions about the self.
- Components of self-concept are identity, body image, and role performance.
- Each developmental stage involves factors that are important to developing a healthy, positive self-concept.
- Identity is particularly vulnerable during adolescence.
- Body image is the mental picture of one's body and is not necessarily consistent with a person's actual body structure or appearance.
- Body image stressors include changes in physical appearance, structure, or functioning caused by normal developmental changes or illness.
- Self-esteem is the emotional appraisal of self-concept and reflects the overall sense of being capable, worthwhile, and competent.
- Self-esteem stressors include developmental and relationship changes, illness (particularly chronic illness involving changes in what were normal activities), surgery, accidents, and the responses of other individuals to changes resulting from these events.

- Role stressors, including role conflict, role ambiguity, and role strain, may originate in unclear or conflicting role expectations and may be aggravated by illness.
- The nurse's self-concept and nursing actions can have an effect on a client's self-concept.
- Planning and implementing nursing interventions for self-concept disturbance involve increasing the client's self-awareness, encouraging self-exploration, aiding in self-evaluation, helping formulate goals for adaptation, and assisting the client in achieving those goals.

Key Terms

Body image, *p. 442*
Identity, *p. 441*
Identity confusion, *p. 445*
Role ambiguity, *p. 447*
Role conflict, *p. 446*
Role overload, *p. 447*
Role performance, *p. 443*
Role strain, *p. 447*
Self-concept, *p. 440*
Self-esteem, *p. 443*
Sick role, *p. 447*

Critical Thinking Exercises

1. You are assigned to care for a 23-year-old Chinese-Canadian client who sustained multiple fractures to his face and femur 4 days ago in a motor vehicle accident. He had surgery the evening of admission to repair his femur but was admitted to wait for surgery to his face. The client lives with his girlfriend and their 7-month-old daughter and works as a janitor in the local university. He left China with his mother when he was a young child and has grown up in Canada. You have been with him for most of the morning. He was in moderate pain, which was treated with morphine. His pain rating decreased from 6 to 3 on a scale of 0 to 10 but the morphine left him drowsy. During the morning, he shared with you some of his concerns about when he will be able to return to work. You are in the room when the surgeon tells him about his upcoming surgery. A temporary tracheotomy is planned because of the extensive surgery needed in the nasal and throat area. After the surgeon leaves, the client tells you that he does not want the tracheotomy. He indicates that he is unclear about what it actually entails, even though the surgeon explained it in fairly simple terms. He states, "I just want to get back to normal." How would you address his comment regarding "get back to normal" and his lack of understanding regarding the tracheotomy?
2. A 16-year-old girl is preparing for discharge from the hospital after giving birth 2 days earlier. She is unmarried, uninvolved with the baby's father, and has minimal familial support to assist her in caring for her newborn. Before admission, she arranged to give the baby up for adoption. She reaffirms this as a good decision because she will be able to return to school immediately and still graduate with her peers. The client confides in you that her biggest concerns right now are how she feels about herself and how she looks. Taking into account the developmental needs of this adolescent, how will you collaborate with her to establish priority interventions to address her self-concept deficits?
3. As a part of your community health experience, you are assigned to visit a 75-year-old woman who has gone to live with her daughter after being hospitalized for agitation and aggression secondary to Alzheimer's disease. When you go to their home, you find the 55-year-old daughter tearful. She says, "I just don't know if I can do this. She is so confused. She calls me two or three times a night to sit with her; sometimes she doesn't even recognize me. I've been missing a lot of work. Even when I'm there, I'm not as productive as I was before she came to live with us." What additional assessment data would be important to gather? What provisional nursing diagnosis could be made for the daughter?

Review Questions

1. When a nurse is caring for a client after mastectomy, interventions to promote physiological stability and pain control are necessary. In addition, the nurse also needs to design nursing interventions directed toward improving her
   1. Mobility
   2. Self-concept
   3. Activity tolerance
   4. Self-care activities
2. Developing self through modelling, imitation, and socialization is a self-concept developmental task during the ages of
   1. 0 to 1 year
   2. 1 to 3 years
   3. 3 to 6 years
   4. 6 to 12 years
3. The following involves the internal sense of individuality, wholeness, and consistency of a person over time and in various circumstances:
   1. Body image
   2. Self-concept
   3. Role performance
   4. Identity
4. Adolescents are at risk for body image disturbance. An accurate statement about body image is that
   1. Body image is not influenced by the opinions of others
   2. Body image refers to the external features of a person
   3. Body image includes actual and perceived perceptions of one's body
   4. Physical changes during adolescence are quickly incorporated into the person's body image
5. Certain behaviours become common or are avoided, depending on whether they are approved and reinforced or discouraged and punished. This process is called
   1. Reinforcement-extinction
   2. Inhibition
   3. Substitution
   4. Identification

6. When an individual internalizes the beliefs, behaviour, and values of role models into a personal, unique expression of self, the process is called
   1. Reinforcement-extinction
   2. Inhibition
   3. Substitution
   4. Identification
7. An individual's identity is affected by stressors throughout life, but the group that is particularly vulnerable to stressors because of it being a time of great change is
   1. Infants
   2. Children
   3. Adolescents
   4. Adults
8. When a person does not maintain a clear, consistent, and continuous consciousness of personal identity, it results in
   1. Identify confusion
   2. Low self-esteem
   3. Low self-concept
   4. Body image difficulties
9. The nurse asks the client, "How do you feel about yourself?" The nurse is assessing the client's
   1. Identity
   2. Body image
   3. Self-esteem
   4. Role performance
10. Increasing a client's self-awareness is achieved
    1. By establishing a trusting relationship that allows the client to explore his or her thoughts and feelings
    2. By accepting the client's thoughts and feelings
    3. By helping the client to define his or her problems clearly
    4. Through having the client identify his or her positive and negative coping mechanisms

References

Beck, C. T. (2001). Predictors of postpartum depression: An update. *Nursing Research, 50*(5), 275–285.

Birchenall, J., & Streight, E. (2003). *Mosby's textbook for the home care aide* (2nd ed.). St. Louis, MO: Mosby.

Byrne, B. (2000). Relationships between anxiety, fear, self-esteem, and coping strategies in adolescence. *Adolescence, 35*(137), 201–215.

Cohane, G. H., & Pope, H. G., Jr. (2001). Body image in boys: A review of the literature. *International Journal of Eating Disorders, 29,* 373–379.

Dochterman, J. M., & Bulechek, G. M. (Eds.). (2004). *Nursing interventions classification (NIC)* (4th ed.). St. Louis, MO: Mosby.

Eliopoulos, C. (2001). *Gerontologic nursing* (5th ed.). Philadelphia: Lippincott.

Erikson, E. (1963). *Childhood and society* (2nd ed.). New York: W. W. Norton.

Hockenberry, M., et al. (Eds.). (2003). *Wong's nursing care of infants and children* (7th ed.). St. Louis, MO: Mosby.

Judge, T. A., & Bono, J. E. (2001). Relationship of core self-evaluations traits—self-esteem, generalized self-efficacy, locus of control, and emotional stability—with job satisfaction and job performance: A meta-analysis. *Journal of Applied Psychology, 86*(1), 80–92.

Miller, C. A. (1999). *Nursing care of older adults: Theory and practice* (3rd ed.). Philadelphia: Lippincott.

Moorhead, S., Johnson, M., & Maas, M. (Eds.). (2004). *Nursing outcomes classification (NOC)* (3rd ed.). St. Louis, MO: Mosby.

Park, J. (2003). Adolescent self-concept and health into adulthood [Catalogue 82-003]. *Health Reports, 14,* 41–52.

Peden, A.R., et al. (2000). Negative thinking mediates the effect of self-esteem on depressive symptoms in college women. *Nursing Research, 49*(4), 201–207.

Pedro, L. W. (2001). Quality of life for long-term survivors of cancer: Influencing variables. *Cancer Nursing, 24*(1), 1–11.

Plach, S. K., Napholz, L., & Kelber, S. T. (2001). Differences in anxiety and role experiences between three age groups of women with heart disease, *Archives of Psychiatric Nursing, 15*(4), 195–199.

Robins, R. W., et al. (2002). Global self-esteem across the life span. *Psychology and Aging, 17*(3), 423–434.

Rosenberg, M. (1965). *Society and the adolescent self-image.* Princeton, NJ: Princeton University Press.

Ruiz, S. Y., Roosa, M. W., & Gonzales, N. A. (2002). Predictors of self-esteem for Mexican American and European American youths: A reexamination of the influence of parenting. *Journal of Family Psychology, 16*(1), 70–80.

Sorrentino, S. A. (2004). *Mosby's textbook for nursing assistants* (6th ed.). St. Louis, MO: Mosby.

Stuart, G. W., & Laraia, M. T. (2001). *Principles and practice of psychiatric nursing* (7th ed.). St. Louis, MO: Mosby.

Twenge, J. M., & Crocker, J. (2002). Race and self-esteem: Meta-analyses comparing whites, blacks, Hispanics, Asians, and American Indians. *Psychology Bulletin, 128*(3), 371–408.

Van Baarsen, B. (2002). Theories on coping with loss: The impact of social support and self-esteem on adjustment to emotional and social loneliness following a partner's death in later life. *The Journals of Gerontology. Series B, Psychological Sciences and Social Sciences, 57*(1), S33–S42.

Yarcheski, A., Mahon, N. E., & Yarcheski, T. J. (2001). Social support and well-being in early adolescents: The role of mediating variables. *Clinical Nursing Research, 10*(2), 163–181.

Recommended Web Sites

Fact Sheet: Managing Self-Esteem in Adolescence
http://www.calgaryhealthregion.ca/hecomm/mental/Adolescence/ManagingSelf-Esteem.pdf
Discusses the importance of self-esteem throughout the lifespan and provides suggestions to improve self-esteem.

My Body, My Self:
http://www.enablelink.org/disability/ disab_articles.html?showdisability=1&id=1308
This article describes self-esteem and body acceptance for people with disabilities and suggests ideas or strategies to help individuals adjust to and accept a disability. The author recommends changing priorities and taking better care of one's health.

Children and Self-Esteem:
http://www.cmha.ca/english/info_centre/mh_pamphlets/mh_pamphlet_21.htm
This electronic pamphlet published by the Canadian Mental Health Association offers advice on how to promote positive self-esteem in children.

Adolescent Self-Concept and Health into Adulthood:
http://www.statcan.ca/english/freepub/82-003-SIE/2003000/pdf/82-003-SIE2003005.pdf
This Statistics Canada report examines factors associated with adolescent self-concept and the impact of adolescent self-concept on later health and health behaviour in young adulthood.

Mental Health Promotion Among Newcomer Female Youth: Post-Migration Experiences and Self-Esteem
http://www.swc-cfc.gc.ca/pubs/ 0662320840/index_e.html
This site presents the findings of a research project on newcomer Canadian female adolescents, examines mental health promotion issues for this group, and makes recommendations.

University of Alberta, University Health Centre: Food, Weight & Body Image:
http://www.uofaweb.ualberta.ca/healthinfo/nav02.cfm?nav02=27622&nav01=27614
This site addresses body image and healthy weight, including discussions on standards of beauty, food and dieting, and eating disorders. It includes a table of healthy weights, based on body mass index, and a directory of contacts at the University of Alberta.

23

Sexuality

Anna Brock, PhD, MSN, MEd, BSN
Marilynn J. Wood, RN, BSN, MSN, DrPH (Canadian author)
Janet C. Ross-Kerr, RN, BScN, MS, PhD (Canadian author)

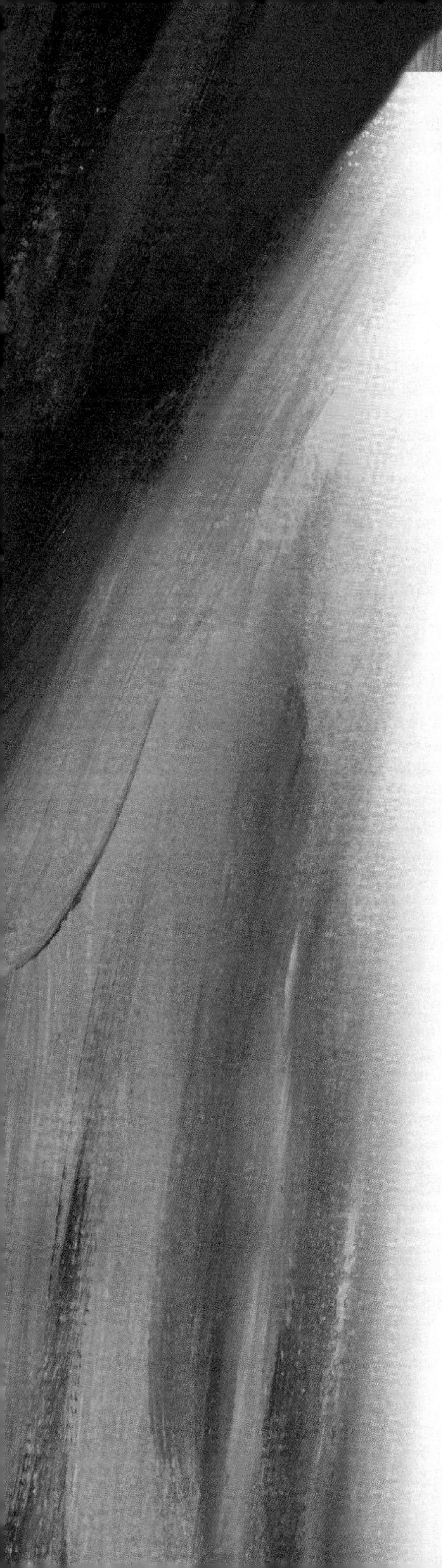

Objectives

Mastery of content in this chapter will enable the student to:

- Define the key terms listed.
- Discuss the nurse's role in maintaining or enhancing a client's sexual health.
- Discuss the complexities of sexual and gender identity and sexual orientation.
- Describe key concepts of sexual development across the lifespan.
- Describe the sexual response cycle.
- Identify high-risk and safer sex behaviours.
- Identify common sexually transmitted infections (STIs).
- Identify major types of sexual dysfunction and potential causes.
- Assess a client's sexuality.
- Define appropriate nursing diagnoses for clients with alterations in sexuality.
- Identify and describe nursing interventions to promote sexual health.
- Evaluate a client's sexual health.
- Identify potential referral resources for clients' sexual concerns outside the nurse's level of expertise.
- Use critical thinking skills in assisting clients in meeting their sexual needs.

Sexuality and its expression are vital elements in the wholeness of human beings. The powerful force of sexuality creates the capacity for physical closeness, pleasure, and emotional intimacy. It is central to our sense of self-esteem and our body image (Pangman & Seguire, 2000). Sexuality includes biological, sociological, psychological, spiritual, and cultural dimensions of each person's being. In addition, it is influenced by values, attitudes, behaviours, relationships with others, and the need to establish emotional closeness with others (MacLaren, 1995).

Sexual health means a person has freedom from physical and psychological impairment, awareness of and positive attitudes toward sexual functioning, and accurate knowledge about sexuality (Heath & White, 2001). Sexual health is an important aspect of one's overall health. Consequently, sexual health care throughout the lifespan is an essential component of comprehensive health care and health promotion (Pangman & Seguire, 2000). Nurses have an important role in the development of positive, healthful sexuality for youth, adolescents, adults, and older adults. Nurses can educate clients to achieve positive outcomes such as improved self-esteem, respect for others, non-exploitive sexual relationships, and rewarding sexual relations. Nurses can also educate clients to help prevent adverse outcomes such as unwanted pregnancy, **sexually transmitted infections (STIs;** also known as sexually transmitted diseases, or STDs), or sexual dysfunction (Health Canada, 2003).

Religious teachings, culturally prescribed gender roles, beliefs about sexual orientation, and social and environmental climates influence both the client's and the health care provider's value systems. Nurses need to explore their own beliefs and prejudices and strive to develop a non-judgmental and caring approach that integrates sexual health care into everyday practice.

Scientific Knowledge Base

To assist clients in meeting their sexual needs, a nurse must have a sound scientific knowledge base about sexual and gender identity, sexual orientation, sexual development, the sexual response cycle, high-risk and safer sex behaviours, STIs, contraception, and abortion.

Sexual and Gender Identity

Sexual identity is the objective labelling of a person as male or female. Most people would probably say that there are two sexes and that sexual identification is fairly straightforward. Conventional wisdom would say that simply examining a person's genitalia will determine whether the person is male or female (Vilain, 2004). According to the XY sex-determination system, females have two of the same kind of sex chromosomes (XX), and males have two distinct sex chromosomes (XY). However, people do not always fit neatly within this system of sexual identification. Variations in genitalia, gonads, chromosomes, or hormones occur in an estimated 17 of 1,000 births in Canada (Johnson, 2004). For example, some people are born with ambiguous genitalia, which makes determining the sex of the infant difficult. Several genetic conditions can disrupt the development of the fetus such that the baby is neither fully male nor fully female (Liao, 2003). A child with an androgen disorder may have male-like genitalia and might genetically be a girl; another child might have male hormones and may have the external appearance of a girl.

Gender identity refers to the degree to which a person identifies as male, female, or some combination. It begins in infancy as the child becomes aware of the differences of the sexes and perceives that he or she is male or female. People's gender identity is usually consistent with their sex at birth; however, this is not always the case. For example, **transsexuality** occurs when people have physical bodies that are "at odds" with their gender identity. Transsexuals may have female bodies but feel like men, or male bodies but feel like women (Johnson, 2004). Current research indicates that gender identity disorder is caused by hormonal fluctuations at a crucial time in fetal development (Society for Human Sexuality, 2004). Many people with transsexuality choose to undergo sex reassignment so that their physical sex is congruent with their gender identity, a process involving surgery and the administration of hormones.

Sexual Orientation

Sexual orientation describes the predominant gender preference of a person's sexual attraction over time. **Heterosexuality** is sexual preference for members of the opposite sex. **Homosexuality** is sexual preference for members of the same sex. **Bisexuality** is an equal or almost equal preference for either sex. In a recent Statistics Canada survey, 1% of the respondents identified themselves as homosexual (gay men and lesbian women) and about 0.7% of respondents identified themselves as bisexual (Canadian Community Health Survey, 2004). Nurses must not assume that they know their clients' gender identity or sexual orientation. Anyone could be lesbian, gay, bisexual, transsexual, or heterosexual. If nurses learn of their clients' sexual orientation, they should not assume that they may tell anyone else or include it in the medical record without the client's knowledge. Some people might want to keep their sexual orientation private.

Earlier thinking about sexual orientation led many to believe that heterosexuals were normal and mentally healthy and everyone else was abnormal or psychologically disordered. Today, this theory is summarily rejected; scientists agree that homosexuality, transsexuality, and bisexuality are not disorders and are not associated with mental illness or abnormal psychological functioning. Nevertheless, many people still display **homophobia,** which is the prejudicial treatment of, or negative attitudes about, lesbian, gay, bisexual, or transsexual people and those who are perceived to be of these gender or sexual identities. Homophobia can include a range of emotions and behaviour from discomfort, fear, and disgust to hatred and violence. The nurse who is non-judgmental and equipped with an appropriate knowledge base can help to address the problems of homophobia and provide nursing care that that does not discriminate against the client's sexual orientation.

Sexual Development

As a person grows and develops, so does his or her sexuality. Each stage of development brings changes in sexual functioning and the role of sexuality in relationships.

Infancy and Childhood. The awareness of one's sexual identity and sexual development begins in infancy with the attitudes about the physical body communicated by the caregivers (Haroian, 2000). From birth on, children are treated differently according to their gender. The differential treatment results in shaping the behaviour of the child. During the school years, children expand their horizons from parents and family. Parents, teachers, and the child's peer group serve as role models and teach about how men and women act and relate with each other. School-age children generally have questions regarding the physical and emotional aspects of sex (Finan, 1997). They need accurate information from home and school about body and emotional changes during this period and what to expect as they move into puberty. Knowledge about normal emotional and physical changes associated with puberty may decrease the anxieties as these changes begin to happen. An uninformed child may be frightened by menstruation or nocturnal emission and view them as evidence of a dreadful disease.

Puberty/Adolescence. The emotional changes during puberty and adolescence are as dramatic as the physical changes. The adolescent functions within a powerful peer group, with the almost constant anxiety of "Am I nor-

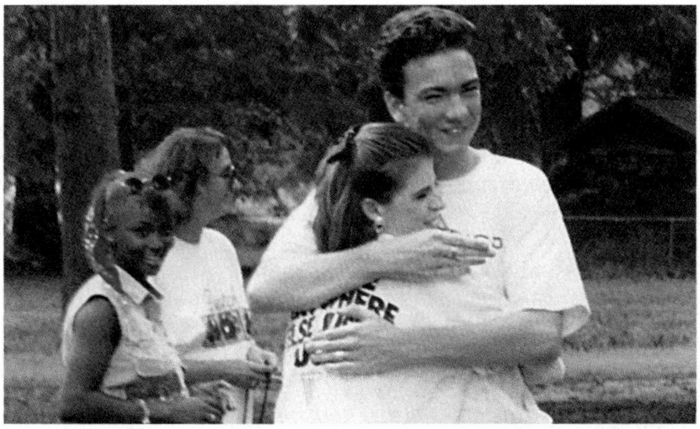

FIGURE **23–1** Adolescents function within a powerful network of peers as they explore their sexual and gender identity.

mal?" and "Will I be accepted?" Same-sex peers or friends remain influential in defining appropriate behaviour, but the task of establishing a romantic relationship begins (Figure 23–1).

During adolescence, teenagers usually begin to explore their sexual identity and ability to attract sexual partners (Beausang, 2000). It is the norm for youth, rather than the exception, to experiment sexually and often with multiple partners (Beitz, 1998); thus it is essential that youth have access to sexual health services, including information on topics such as body changes, sexual health promotion, STIs, contraception, and pregnancy. Such services are designed to promote sexual health and to encourage responsible decision making regarding sexual choices.

Public health professionals have been alarmed by the trend toward greater sexual activity at increasingly younger ages, particularly because of the adverse consequences. In 1998 in Canada, 21,000 girls between 15 and 19 years of age had abortions, and almost 20,000 girls of that age group gave birth, translating into a rate of 19.8 births for every 1,000 girls (Canadian Institute of Health Information, 2004). Following teenage pregnancy, mothers and their children often experience health, financial, and social problems (Jewell, Tacchi, & Donovan, 2000). Similarly, exposure to STIs and unwanted sexual activity can lead to psychological disturbances, impairments in the development of healthy social and interpersonal relationships, and long-term physical health problems.

Nurses may be most effective in their goals to support teenagers by helping parents develop confidence in educating their children about sexuality. Factual information regarding sexuality and sexual activity is important, but equally or perhaps more important is guidance in establishing a personal value or belief system to use as a framework for decision making. In healthy family networks, much of this guidance will have been conveyed in the course of child rearing. Parents need to understand the importance of providing information, sharing their values, and promoting sound decision-making skills. Parents and significant others need to be counselled that even with the best guidance and information, adolescents will make their own decisions and must be held accountable for those decisions.

Adolescence is often a time when individuals explore their primary sexual orientation. Some teenagers may recognize their preference as distinctly homosexual, which can be frightening and confusing for an adolescent. Support for the adolescent's sexual identity is important during this time and can come from a variety of sources, such as school counsellors, clergy, family, or health professionals.

Adulthood. The adult has gained physical maturation but is continuing to explore and define emotional maturation in relationships. Intimacy and sexuality are issues for all adults of all sexual orientations, whether they are in a sexual relationship, choose to abstain from sex, are single, widowed, divorced—whatever circumstances arise. People can be sexually healthy in numerous ways. Sexual activity is often defined as a basic need, but sexual desire can be channelled healthily into other forms of intimacy throughout a lifetime.

As sexually active adults develop intimate relationships, they need to learn techniques of stimulation that are satisfying to both themselves and their sexual partners. Some adults may need confirmation that alternative ways of sexual expression other than penile-vaginal intercourse are normal. Other individuals may require significant education or therapy to achieve mutually satisfying sexual relationships.

Through middle adulthood, physical changes can affect sexual functioning. Decreasing levels of estrogen in **perimenopausal** and menopausal women may lead to diminished vaginal lubrication and decreased vaginal elasticity. Both of these changes may lead to **dyspareunia,** which is painful intercourse. Declining levels of testosterone result in decreased desire for sexual activity. Suggestions such as using vaginal lubrication and creating time for caressing and tenderness can help clients adjust to normal changes related to aging.

As men age, they are likely to experience an increase in the post-ejaculatory refractory period, delayed ejaculation, and other changes. Advising clients of these normal changes related to aging can ease concerns regarding functioning. Aging adults may also need to adjust to the impact of chronic illness, medications, aches, pains, and other health concerns that affect sexuality.

Older Adulthood. As people age, some shift their priority from genital sex to other means to express sexual desire. Activity that includes affection, romance, intimacy, and companionship may be enough to satisfy the sexual needs of some older adults (Figure 23–2). However, not all older adults have a declining interest in sex. The majority of people have the capacity to stay sexually active into very late life and regard sexual activity as important to their overall well-being and quality of life (Gott, 2001). Aging does, however, affect sexual functioning (Box 23-1). The accompanying psychological and physical transitions require flexibility in thinking and adjustment to the changes; those who manage the transition are poised for emotional and sexual satisfaction (Palacios, Tobar, & Menendez, 2002). The nurse's approach to the care of older clients must include sexual

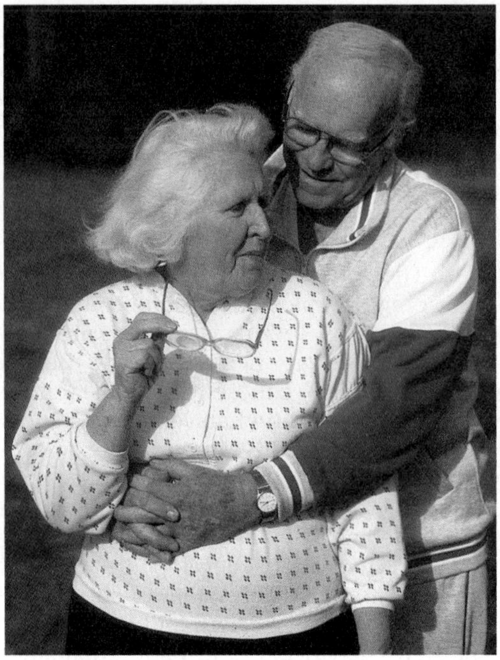

FIGURE 23–2 Intimacy and affection are important to older adults.

health education about and for older adults (Pangman & Seguire, 2000).

Focus on Older Adults — Box 23-1

Changes Affecting Sexuality in Older Adults

- Sexuality and continued interest in sex throughout late life generally reflects life patterns (Lueckenotte, 2000).
- Pathological problems with the aging sexual response are often related to illnesses and medications. For example, impotence is often due to the use of tranquilizers, antidepressants, antihypertensives, or phenothiazines. Removal of causative agent generally results in resolution of the problem (Lueckenotte, 2000).
- In women, vaginal tissue atrophies and lubrication is diminished or delayed over time.

Strategies to Deal With Sexual Issues in Older Adults

- Acknowledge that sexual impulses are normal and do not disappear as people age; sex and love are not just for the young.
- Demonstrate recognition, acceptance, and respect for an older adult's sexuality by displaying a willingness to openly discuss sex and sexuality-related concerns.
- Keep abreast of current research in the field of sexuality and aging and communicate these findings to nursing colleagues and older adult clients to promote a more realistic understanding of aging and sexuality (Eliopoulos, 2001).

Sexual Response Cycle

The **sexual response cycle** is the sequence of physiological events that occur when a person becomes sexually aroused and participates in sexually stimulating activities. The cycle is characterized by four phases: appetitive (sexual desire or libido), arousal, orgasm, and resolution. Both men and women experience the phases, albeit with different timing, and there is considerable variability from person to person in duration and response in each phase.

In the appetitive phase, a person begins to want sexual intimacy or gratification. It occurs before sexual arousal and activity, and occurs mainly in the mind, rather than the body. This phase may be triggered by a variety of stimuli, including sight, sound, smell, touch, taste, fantasy, and memory. The arousal and orgasm phases are a result of **vasocongestion** and **myotonia,** the basic physiological responses of sexual arousal. In women, this reaction leads to vaginal lubrication, swelling of the clitoris and the labia minora and majora, and engorgement of the outer third of the vagina (orgasmic platform). In men, vasocongestion leads to erection of the penis. Both men and women also experience increased breathing, heart rate, and blood pressure. Myotonia, or neuromuscular tension, gradually increases throughout the body during the excitement and plateau phases. Myotonia peaks during orgasm, resulting in involuntary contractions of the woman's vagina and the man's vas deferens and urethra. In men, contractions of the ejaculatory duct in the prostate gland cause semen to be ejected through the urethra and penis. Women and men may experience contractions of the arm and leg muscles, facial muscles, and gluteal muscles. During the resolution phase, vasocongestion and myotonia return to pre-arousal levels.

Sexual Behaviour

Sexual behaviour typically comprises the broad array of sexual activities people participate in, such as masturbation, hugging, kissing, manual stimulation of a partner, vaginal or anal penetration, oral-genital stimulation, oral-anal stimulation, sexual excitement while looking at erotica, and telephone or "cyber" sex (Bernhard, 2002; Engender Health, 2004). It is difficult to say what is "normal" and what is "abnormal" because "what is unusual or atypical varies between cultures and from one period to another. Defining normality is extremely difficult (and arbitrary), because the definition involves making a value judgement and therefore labelling how we view other people" (de Silva, 1999, p. 654). What is acceptable for some people is unthinkable for others.

How do we draw the line? Whatever people find pleasurable is "normal" as long as it occurs between *consenting adults* who are having sexual experiences through choice, in a safe environment where rules and boundaries are negotiated and respected.

High-Risk Sexual Behaviour. Because semen, vaginal fluids, and other body fluids can be transferred between partners, unprotected sex can result in pregnancy or the transmission of STIs. ***Safer sex*** refers to those activities that present minimal or reduced risk for disease transmission or unintended pregnancy. *Unsafe sex* refers to activities that present a high risk for infection, unintended pregnancy, or injury. Unsafe sex includes anal-penile or vaginal-penile intercourse without a condom (Society for Human Sexuality, 2004). Having sex with multiple partners also is unsafe sexual behaviour. When barriers such as condoms are not used, penile-anal intercourse is likely the riskiest activity, followed by penile-vaginal intercourse, oral-anal sex, and oral-genital sex.

The dynamics of sexual risk taking are not fully understood, but numerous studies have found correlations between drug/alcohol use, sexual abuse, and unsafe sex (Keller et al., 1996; Kenney, Reinholtz & Angelini, 1998). Adolescents, especially, tend to have a sense of being invincible, believing that unwanted pregnancy, STIs, and other negative outcomes of sexual behaviour are not likely to happen to them (Ross, Channon-Little, & Rosser, 2000).

Safety Alert. Increasingly, adolescents engage in oral sex, thinking there is less risk for acquiring STIs. However, herpes can be transmitted from genitals to mouth or mouth to genitals during unprotected oral sex, and it is possible to acquire a bacterial infection of the mouth or throat from someone with a bacterial STI such as gonorrhea, syphilis, or chlamydia. Education about the risk must include parents and teachers as well as adolescents.

Sexually Transmitted Infections

There are more than 20 STIs that concern public health officials and health care providers (McIlhaney, 2000). In Canada, health officials are beginning to see increases in all of the infections that, by law, must be reported, including genital chlamydia, gonorrhea, and infectious syphilis (Division of STD Prevention and Control [DSTDP&C], 2000).

A major problem in dealing with STIs is finding and treating the people who have them. Some people may not even know that they are infected because symptoms are absent or go unnoticed. Because sexual behaviour may include the whole body rather than just the genitalia, many parts of the body are potential sites for an STI. The ears, mouth, throat, tongue, nose, and eyelids can be used for sexual pleasure. The perineum, anus, and rectum are also frequently included in sexual activity. Furthermore, any contact with another person's body fluids around the head or an open lesion on the skin, anus, or genitalia can transmit an STI.

Sometimes people do not seek treatment because they are embarrassed to discuss sexual symptoms or concerns (Box 23-2). They may also hesitate to talk about their sexual behaviour if they believe that it is not "normal." This hesitation to seek help often hinders the detection of an STI.

Infectious Syphilis. Syphilis, a bacterial infection, can be transmitted through oral, vaginal-penile, or anal sex with an infected person. A pregnant woman with syphilis can pass it on to her baby, leading to birth defects or death. Although not common, syphilis also can be transmitted via injection drug use or through broken skin or sores. Syphilis can be diagnosed with a simple blood test and is easily treated with antibiotics. If it is not treated, syphilis can affect the brain, blood vessels, heart, and bones. It can also cause death.

Genital Chlamydia. Genital chlamydia affects both men and women. The most common of all bacterial STIs, chlamydial infection may cause an abnormal genital discharge and burning with urination. Once diagnosed with chlamydial infection, a person can be treated with an antibiotic.

There are many serious complications of genital chlamydia in women, including chronic pelvic pain, infertility, and ectopic pregnancy. If undetected and thus untreated, it can progress to pelvic inflammatory disease (PID) in women, a very painful and sometimes debilitating disease. It is estimated that as many as 20% to 40% of chlamydia cases develop into PID (DSTDP&C, 2000). Recent research findings suggest that genital chlamydial infection is also a risk factor for the transmission of HIV infection and it could be a risk factor for cervical cancer (Anttila et al., 2003). However, as many as 85% of chlamydia infections in women and 40% of infections in men do not cause symptoms and so people are unaware that they are infected (McIlhaney, 2000). In men, the group with the highest prevalence rate is the 20- to 24-year-old age group. In women, the group with the highest rate is the 15- to 19-year-old age group (DSTDP&C, 2000).

Gonorrhea. Gonorrhea is easily transmitted during vaginal-penile and anal-penile intercourse and during oral sex (Birley et al., 2002). It can affect the penis, cervix, rectum or anus, throat, and eyes. Pain during sex or during urination, or unusual discharge, may be indications of a gonorrheal infection. Gonorrhea must be treated with antibiotics. If left untreated, it may cause serious health problems, including infertility. It can also cause blindness in a baby born to an infected woman (DSTDP&C, 2000; Planned Parenthood Federation of Canada, 2004b). Gonorrhea is the second most commonly reported bacterial STI in Canada, and it is also increasing in prevalence. This infection is found most often in young adults: 15- to 19-year-old women and 20- to 24-year-old men (DSTDP&C, 2000).

Human Papillomavirus. Human papillomavirus (HPV) is not reportable, although it is a very serious STI. It is strongly linked with cervical cancer (DSTDP&C, 2000). External genital warts are a manifestation of HPV and can occur on the penis, scrotum, perineum, vulva, and perianal area. The HPV virus that produces these warts can also lead to warts in the vagina, on the cervix, and inside the urethra and anus (Beutner et al., 1998); they usually appear as small, hard painless bumps. If untreated, they may grow and develop a fleshy, cauliflower-like appearance. Because they are caused by a virus, genital warts cannot be cured. They are treated with a topical drug (applied to the skin), by freezing, or if they recur, with injections. If the warts are very large, they can be removed surgically.

Genital Herpes. Genital herpes is the most common cause of genital ulceration and is often transmitted by people who have no visible or symptomatic lesions

Research Highlight — Box 23-2

The Effect of Social Stigma and Shame on STI-Isolated Care

Research Focus

At-risk clients who perceive that they will be judged adversely because of sexually transmitted infections (STIs) are less likely to seek appropriate care.

Research Abstract

The purpose of this study was to assess the relationship between social stigma and shame associated with seeking treatment for STIs. Participants included 847 males and 1,126 females (mean age was 24.9 years) recruited from clinics and community-based organizations and through street intercept in seven cities. The STI-related stigma and STI-related shame scales were administered during face-to-face interviews. The findings revealed that males were more likely than females to have suspected gonorrhea in the past, but females were more likely than males to have received a gonorrhea or human immunodeficiency virus (HIV) test in the past year. A significantly higher proportion of males were classified in the "high shame" group. Gonorrhea testing was related to female gender, younger age, enrolment in a health facility, health service use in the past year, suspicion of gonorrhea, and low levels of STI-related stigma. HIV testing was related to older age, health service use, gonorrhea testing, and low levels of STI-related stigma. STI-related shame was not related to gonorrhea testing or HIV testing.

Evidence-Based Practice

- STI-related stigma, rather than shame, decreases the likelihood of a person being tested for gonorrhea or HIV.
- Nurses have the potential through education to promote community norms of healthy sexuality and STI-related care. They can act as advocates for STI-related care and prevention programs in high schools and colleges, organizing opportunities to discuss the issues of sexual at-risk behaviours.
- Nurses' awareness of their own and others' feelings and attitudes about STIs will enable them to respond more effectively to the needs of the client.
- Use of a caring, open, non-judgmental manner with clients with STIs will increase the likelihood of a person seeking treatment.

Reference

Fortenberry, J. D., et al. (2002). Relationships of stigma and shame to gonorrhea and HIV screening. *American Journal of Public Health, 92*(3), 378–381.

(Mindel, 1998). Genital herpes can cause extensive ulceration (painful blisters or open sores), with severe pain. Without treatment, episodes can last for 3 or more weeks, and many people with herpes have recurrent episodes. At present, the viral infection is incurable; antiviral drugs can only control the symptoms.

Human Immunodeficiency Virus (HIV) Infection. The human immunodeficiency virus (HIV) is the virus that causes AIDS (acquired immunodeficiency syndrome). Essentially, HIV destroys the body's ability to defend against infection. Many people do not have symptoms when they first are infected with HIV, although some may have a flu-like illness within 1 to 2 months following exposure. More persistent or severe symptoms may not appear for 10 years or more following infection. During the asymptomatic period, however, the virus is actively multiplying, infecting, and killing cells of the immune system. As the immune system weakens, a variety of complications occur (National Institute of Allergy and Infectious Diseases [NIAID], 2003).

AIDS is the term applied to the most advanced stages of HIV infection. The syndrome can result in many infections that do not usually affect healthy people. In people with AIDS, these infections are often severe and sometimes fatal. People with AIDS are particularly prone to developing cancers, especially those caused by viruses such as Kaposi's sarcoma or cervical cancer, or cancers of the immune system such as lymphomas.

HIV is present in the majority of body fluids. For transmission to occur, therefore, some exchange of body fluid, particularly blood, must occur. Primary routes of transmission include contaminated intravenous needles, unprotected sexual activity (anal intercourse, vaginal intercourse, and oral-genital sex), and transfusion of blood and blood products. HIV can also be spread from infected mothers to their babies at birth or during breastfeeding. There is no evidence that HIV is spread through sweat, tears, saliva, or urine.

In Canada, by the end of 2002, an estimated 56,000 people were living with HIV infection (including AIDS), which was an increase of about 12% from the estimate at the end of 1999. Rates of infection are highest in men who have sex with men, Aboriginal people, injection drug users, and immigrants from countries where HIV is endemic (Centre for Infectious Disease Prevention and Control [CIDPC], 2003). Many Canadians who are currently infected with HIV do not know it.

Although there are medications that permit individuals with HIV to be healthy longer and help to prevent the transmission of HIV from a pregnant woman to her newborn, medications cannot cure the disease (McIlhaney, 2000).

Prevention of Sexually Transmitted Infections. People most likely to be infected with an STI are those who have unprotected sex with multiple partners or unprotected sex with someone who has had many partners. Injection drug users are also a high-risk group. Primary prevention of STIs starts with changing the sexual behaviour that places people at risk for infection. Targeted health promotion to high-risk groups that emphasizes education and counselling regarding safer sexual behaviour is essential.

Safer Sex. Safer sex refers to the sexual practices and behaviour that reduce the risk of contracting and transmitting STIs, especially HIV. When a partner is infected or the status of a partner is not known, it is critical to practise safer sex. For penile-vaginal and penile-anal penetration, partners should use condoms. Oral sex also requires safer sex practices; if a woman is the recipient, a thin piece of rubber, a latex dental dam, a female condom, or a cut-open, unlubricated male condom should be placed between the mouth and the vulva before any oral contact is made. With male partners, the penis should be covered with an unlubricated condom before any oral contact is made (Engender Health, 2004).

Using Condoms. Condoms were originally sold to promote birth control. However, when used correctly, they also provide protection against STIs. A condom acts as a barrier to keep blood, semen, or vaginal fluids from passing from one person to another. In Canada, condoms are free at many public health clinics and are readily available from drugstores and supermarkets. The condom can be made from latex, polyurethane, or natural membranes such as sheepskin or lambskin. Latex and polyurethane condoms reduce the risk of most STIs (including HIV) and help to protect against pregnancy. Natural membrane condoms do not protect against STIs because some bacteria and viruses can pass through the small pores in the material (CIDPC, 2002).

A female condom is a strong, soft, clear sheath made of polyurethane. It is placed inside the vagina before sex and protects against pregnancy and STIs (including HIV). When placed correctly, one end covers the cervix and the other end covers the external genitalia (Planned Parenthood Federation of Canada, 2004a).

Contraception

Contraception is a crucial facet of sexual health to avoid unwanted pregnancies. Some forms of contraception require a health care provider's intervention: hormonal contraception (e.g., birth control pills or patch, injectable contraceptives), IUDs (intrauterine devices), the diaphragm, the vaginal contraceptive ring, and the cervical cap. Permanent, surgical procedures are available to men (vasectomy) and women (tubal ligation). Other forms of contraception do not require a prescription or intervention from a health care provider: condoms, contraceptive sponges, vaginal spermicides, and fertility awareness methods (i.e., timing of intercourse in relation to the menstrual cycle). Table 23-1 summarizes some of the contraception choices available.

Effective contraception involves factors relating to the sexually active couple, the method of contraception, the couple's understanding of the contraceptive method, the consistency of use, and the compliance with the requirements of the chosen method. Personal characteristics that have been identified as positively influencing contraceptive use include motivation to avoid unplanned pregnancy, ability to plan, comfort with sexuality, and previous contraceptive use (Running & Berndt, 2003). Cultural and religious background may permit certain practices and prohibit others. For example, the teachings of the Roman Catholic Church prohibit the use of artificial contraception.

Emergency Contraception. Emergency contraception pills (ECPs or "morning after" pills) are available and can prevent a woman from becoming pregnant after unprotected vaginal-penile sex. ECPs are most effective up to 3 days following intercourse and are recommended to women when contraception was not used, a condom broke, a diaphragm slipped, a birth control shot was given over 1 week late, or two or more birth control pills were missed. Women can obtain ECPs from family physicians, hospital emergency rooms, or walk-in clinics. In Quebec and British Columbia, pharmacists may dispense ECPs without a physician's prescription. ECPs are available for free or at minimum cost at many university health services, sexual health clinics, birth control clinics, Planned Parenthood clinics, and women's health clinics. Adolescent girls do not require parental consent to obtain ECPs and no medical examination is required. In 2004, Health Canada proposed to amend the Food and Drug Regulations and allow ECPs to be available without a prescription from a physician (Government of Canada, 2004). The amendment requires public consultation, which is currently in process. If approved, all Canadian women and girls will be able to obtain ECPs from their local pharmacists.

Abortion

Since 1988, Canada has been one of the few countries without any criminal law restricting abortion. There are no requirements for waiting periods, parental or spousal consent, gestational limits, or restrictions on types of abortion. Abortion is also a safe procedure, especially if done within the first trimester of pregnancy. Some provinces fully fund all abortions; others only fund abortions performed in hospitals. However, access to abortion services is often a problem for women living outside major centres. Two thirds of abortions are done in hospitals; the remaining are done in abortion clinics and health centres. However, only 18% of hospitals across the nation provide abortions (Canadian Abortion Rights Action League, 2003). In Prince Edward Island and Nunavut, no hospitals perform abortions.

Abortion continues to be a hotly debated issue. Women and their partners who are faced with an unwanted pregnancy often consider abortion. The nurse can provide an environment in which the issue of abortion can be openly discussed, allowing exploration of various options with an unwanted pregnancy. The nurse should discuss religious, social, and personal issues in a non-judgmental manner with clients. Reasons for choosing an abortion vary and may include terminating an unwanted pregnancy or aborting a fetus known to have birth defects. When abortion is chosen as a way of dealing with an unwanted pregnancy, the woman, and often her partner, may experience a sense of loss, grief, and/or guilt. Guilt may surface immediately or may be more covert and manifest as sexual dysfunction or altered perceptions.

Health care providers must reflect on personal values related to abortion. The health care provider is entitled to personal views and should not be forced to participate in counselling or procedures contrary to beliefs and values. Nurses should choose specialties or places of employment where their personal values are not compromised and the care of a client in need of health care is not jeopardized.

Table 23-1 Available Contraception

Type	Effectiveness	Description
Male condom	86% to 97%	A thin, skin-tight sheath placed on an erect penis to stop sperm from entering a partner's body. Water-based lubricants can make them more comfortable, increase sensation, and reduce the risk of breakage.
Female condom	79% to 85%	A lubricated pouch that is placed in the vagina before penile insertion; it stops sperm from entering the woman's body. It may break or slip and some women may have difficulty placing it correctly.
Birth control pills	98% to 99%	Pills taken every day that contain a low dose of hormones (estrogen and progestin or progestin alone). The ovaries are prevented from releasing an egg for fertilization, eggs are prevented from implanting, and the mucus around the cervix is thickened, which makes entry of the sperm more difficult. Requires a prescription.
Cervical cap	80% to 91%	A small flexible cup that is inserted into the vagina before penile insertion. It covers the cervix and prevents sperm from entering the uterus. The caps are available in different sizes; proper fitting by a trained health professional is required.
Intrauterine device (IUD)	99%	A small piece of plastic or copper that is inserted into the uterus by a physician. Sperm is prevented from fertilizing an egg, or, if an egg is fertilized, it cannot implant in the uterus. Some also release hormones to prevent pregnancy. IUDs can stay in place for 1 to 8 years.
Birth control patch	99.2% to 99.4%	A thin, 2-cm × 2-cm patch that can be worn on the lower abdomen, buttock, upper arm, or upper torso. The patch is applied once a week for 3 consecutive weeks; the fourth week is patch free. The mechanism of action is the same as that of oral contraceptives.
Injectable contraception	99.7%	Progestin is injected into a woman's arm or buttocks once every 12 weeks. The hormone prevents the ovaries from releasing eggs. A physician or nurse administers the injections.
Vaginal contraceptive ring	98.3% to 99.4%	A soft, flexible, transparent ring that is self-inserted into the vagina and delivers hormones over 3 weeks, after which time the ring is removed for 1 week. A new ring is then inserted.
Contraceptive sponge	80% to 91%	A soft sponge that is filled with spermicide and placed in the vagina before vaginal-penile intercourse. It is effective for 24 hours following placement. The sponge must be kept in place for 6 hours after intercourse.
Vaginal spermicides	78% to 90%	Gels, films and suppositories, which contain a spermicidal agent, are inserted into the vagina before vaginal-penile intercourse. The agent kills sperm and acts as a physical barrier to prevent any surviving sperm cells from entering the cervix. This approach may be used by women who are at low risk for STIs and whose partners are at low risk.
Fertility Awareness	90% to 98%	A woman can monitor her fertility patterns and know when she is most likely and least likely to conceive on the basis of daily observations of body temperature and cervical mucous. She must abstain from vaginal-penile intercourse when she is fertile. It can also be used to achieve pregnancy.
Tubal ligation	99.5%	A surgical procedure in which a woman's fallopian tubes are tied into a loop and then cut. This is done under general anaesthetic and should be considered a permanent procedure.
Vasectomy	99.9%	A minor surgical procedure for men in which the vas deferens that carry the sperm are cut, "tied," cauterized, or otherwise interrupted. The semen no longer contains sperm after the tubes are cut, and conception cannot occur. The procedure can be done in a physician's office under local anaesthetic. This should be considered a permanent procedure.

Adapted from *Contraception,* Planned Parenthood Federation of Canada, 2004, retrieved June 25, 2004, from *http://www.ppfc.ca/ppfc/content.asp?articleid=248;* and "New Contraceptive Methods: Update 2003," by A. Pettinato and S. J. Emans, 2003, *Current Opinion in Pediatrics, 15,* pp. 362–369.

Nursing Knowledge Base

In planning to assist clients in addressing their sexual needs, the nurse uses critical thinking skills and basic nursing knowledge. Nurses may draw from the following areas of nursing knowledge: socio-cultural dimensions of sexuality, how to discuss sexual issues, infertility, sexual abuse, sexual dysfunction, and conditions that create sexual health concerns.

Socio-cultural Dimensions of Sexuality

Sexuality is influenced by cultural rules and norms that determine what is acceptable behaviour within the culture (Box 23-3). Society plays a powerful role in shaping

Cultural Aspects of Care — Box 23-3

Female Genital Cutting

The cultural genesis of female circumcision or female genital cutting (FGC) is no longer known, but approximately 2 million girls and women around the world are subjected to FCG each year, despite laws that ban the practice in many countries (Cook, Dickens, & Fathalla, 2002). The practice occurs mainly in Africa (e.g., Gambia, Guinea, Kenya, Mali, Mauritania, Nigeria, Senegal, Somalia, Sudan, Uganda, and Yemen; United Nations Population Fund and Population Reference Bureau, 2003) and is observed in some immigrants from these regions to Canada.

The World Health Organization (WHO) has distinguished various types of FGC; in the majority of cases, it involves the excision of the clitoris and the labia minora. In extreme cases, almost all of the external genitalia are excised and then the vulva is stitched so that only a tiny opening is present. Typically, unqualified personnel perform these procedures, often with crude instruments and without anaesthesia (Department of Gender and Women's Health [DGWH], 2001). FGC occurs at various ages: it may be undertaken when girls are newborns, during childhood, adolescence, at marriage, or during the first pregnancy. In some cultures, a woman is re-infibulated (re-stitched) following labour and delivery. FGC is strongly condemned by the WHO, the International Council of Nurses, the International Confederation of Midwives, and others.

Implications for Practice

- With the large numbers of ethnic groups immigrating to Canada (e.g., Somalis), FGC is a real issue that Canadian nurses are facing.
- FGC can result in problems with urination, menstruation, and sexual intercourse, as well as difficulties with childbirth.
- During delivery, the vulva must be opened to allow for the delivery of the baby and to prevent the formation of fistulae (i.e., abnormal passages or sinuses). Following delivery, health professionals may be requested by a woman, her partner, or her family to re-stitch the opened vulva.
- Because of the wide-ranging physical, psychological, and sexual risks associated with such procedures, health professionals should not re-infibulate an opened vulva (DGWH, 2001).

sexual values and attitudes and in supporting specific expression of sexuality in its members. Each cultural and social group has its own set of rules and norms that guide the behaviour of its members. These rules become an integral part of an individual's thinking and underlie sexual behaviour, including, for example, how people find partners, whom they choose as partners, how they relate to one another, how often they have sex, and what they do when they have sex.

Many factors affect people's sexual health and their willingness to discuss this private part of life. Some clients tend to be hesitant to talk about sexual matters. They may talk more freely to a nurse or other health care provider of the same sex (Iannotta, 2002).

Discussing Sexual Issues

Sexuality is a significant part of each person's being, yet sexual assessment and interventions are not always included in health care. The area of sexuality can be emotionally charged for nurses as well as for clients. Discomfort with talking about sexual issues, lack of information, and differences in values between the client and the nurse may prevent the nurse from discussing issues regarding sexuality with clients. The most valuable tool that the nurse can develop for providing care in areas of sexuality is effective, non-judgmental communication. Nurses who have difficulty discussing topics related to sexuality should explore their discomfort and develop a plan for addressing their discomfort.

Discussing matters of a sexual nature can also be extremely embarrassing for clients. Often, clients will not bring up sexual health issues. They may worry about looking stupid, using incorrect words, or being offensive, or they may simply have no way of describing their concerns. It is critical to be comfortable in asking questions about sexuality and in responding to issues that arise from such questioning. A perceptive and educated approach to talking about sexuality can offer the support that many clients require.

Effective communication about sexuality requires caring, sensitivity, tact, compassion, the use of appropriate language, and non-discriminatory attitudes. Paying attention to pertinent non-verbal cues can aid effective communication (Pangman & Seguire, 2000). When talking with people about sexuality, it is important not to have preconceived notions about their sexual identity or activity. Homosexual and bisexual people may be invisible within health care settings if health professionals assume heterosexual sexual orientation and fail to obtain complete sexual histories. Older adults' sexual health may also be overlooked if health care professionals stereotype them as asexual.

Alterations in Sexual Health

Infertility. **Infertility** is the inability to conceive after 1 year of unprotected intercourse. A couple who wants to conceive and cannot may experience a sense of failure and may feel that their bodies are somehow defective. Infertility may become an emotionally draining facet of their lives. With advances in reproductive technology, infertile couples face many choices that involve religious and ethical values and financial constraints.

Choices for the infertile couple include medical assistance with fertilization, adoption, or adapting to the possibility of remaining childless. Organizations such as infertility support groups or international adoption groups can provide couples with support. For example, the Infertility Awareness Association of Canada, a national support group for couples with infertility, can be helpful in offering educational resources and support for a couple.

Sexual Abuse. Sexual abuse is a widespread health problem in our society. Abuse crosses all gender, socio-economic, age, and ethnic groups. Most often, this abuse is at the hands of a former intimate partner or family member.

Sexual abuse has far-ranging effects on physical and psychological functioning (Dickinson et al., 1999).

Evidence of sexual abuse in children may be uncovered during history taking or physical examination (see chapter 28). Symptoms that should raise suspicion of the possibility of sexual abuse include a child showing an early, exaggerated awareness of sex or exhibiting seductive behaviour toward adults; swelling or bruising of the external genitalia, anus, breasts, or buttocks; lacerations of or a foreign substance in the vagina or anus; and an STI in a child under 15 years of age. In Canada, nurses are required by law to report suspected child abuse to child protection authorities. Signs and symptoms of abuse in adults are listed in Box 23-4.

When sexual abuse is recognized, support needs to be mobilized for the person and the family. All family members may require therapy in situations of incest to promote healthy interactions and relationships. Rape victims may need to work through the crisis before feeling comfortable with intimate expressions of affection. The partner may need support in understanding this process and ways to assist the victim. Children who have been sexually abused need to understand that they are not at fault for the incident. The parents must understand that their response is critical to how the child reacts and adapts. The nurse may come in contact with clients confronting these stressors. Nurses are in an ideal position to assess occurrences of sexual violence and to educate individuals regarding community services. Nurses should be aware of resources for referral and support in the community.

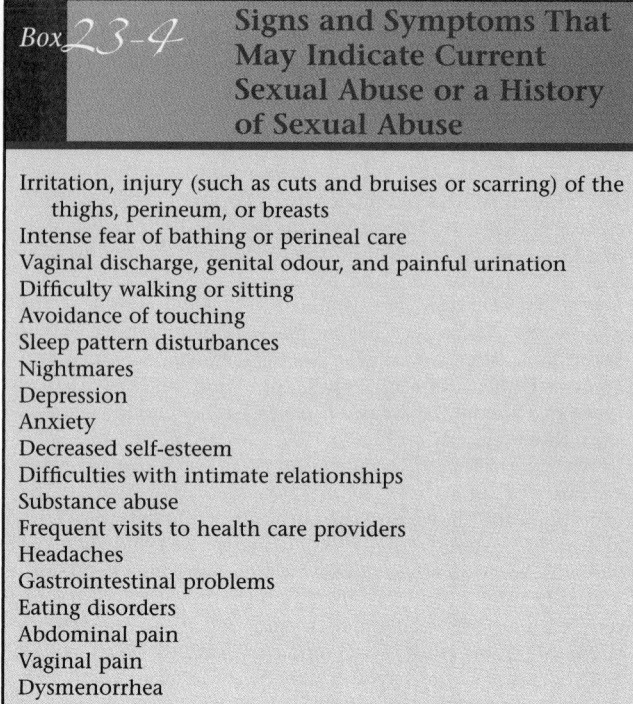

Box 23-4 Signs and Symptoms That May Indicate Current Sexual Abuse or a History of Sexual Abuse

Irritation, injury (such as cuts and bruises or scarring) of the thighs, perineum, or breasts
Intense fear of bathing or perineal care
Vaginal discharge, genital odour, and painful urination
Difficulty walking or sitting
Avoidance of touching
Sleep pattern disturbances
Nightmares
Depression
Anxiety
Decreased self-esteem
Difficulties with intimate relationships
Substance abuse
Frequent visits to health care providers
Headaches
Gastrointestinal problems
Eating disorders
Abdominal pain
Vaginal pain
Dysmenorrhea

Adapted from "Sequelae of Abuse: Health Effects of Childhood Sexual Abuse, Domestic Battering, and Rape," by D. Bohn and K. Holz, 1996, *Journal of Nurse-Midwifery, 41*(6), p. 442.

Sexual Dysfunction. **Sexual dysfunction** is the absence of complete sexual functioning (Tables 23-2 and 23-3). Sexual dysfunction is a common, complex problem that arises because of biological, psychological, and interpersonal factors. Sexual problems and dysfunction are often associated with health problems such as heart disease, diabetes, and mental illness. It is not known how many people experience sexual dysfunction, and it is most likely a minority who seek help. Researchers estimate that between 10% and 52% of men and 25% and 63% of women have sexual problems, although the prevalence of sexual dysfunctions that meet the diagnostic criteria is lower (Heiman, 2002). For most people, sexual dysfunction is perplexing, emotionally disturbing, and socially troubling.

Sexual dysfunction can usually be treated with either medical (mostly pharmacological) or psychological interventions (e.g., cognitive and behavioural methods). The aim is typically to achieve changes in physical (genital response, orgasms) or subjective (greater desire, ease of orgasm) responses (Heiman, 2002).

Sexual Dysfunction in Women. Loss of sexual desire is the most common reason that women seek help for sexual dysfunction (Butcher, 1999a). Despite considerable research, sexual desire is poorly understood. Some medical conditions (including depression) and stress and fatigue affect sexual desire. Painful intercourse is another common sexual dysfunction in women. Recurring sexual pain can produce a cycle in which trepidation because of previous pain leads to avoidance of the sexual activity that produced it, which in turn leads to lack of arousal, failure to achieve orgasm, and loss of sexual desire (Butcher, 1999b). This cycle can evolve to avoidance of sexual activity altogether.

Sexual Dysfunction in Men. One of the most common types of sexual dysfunction for men is erectile dysfunction (ED). It is estimated that about 27% of sexually active Canadian men experience ED, which is the repeated inability to achieve or maintain an erection (Auld & Brock, 2002). There are many health problems that can lead to ED, including heart disease, hypertension (or its treatment), diseases of the prostate, diabetes mellitus, multiple sclerosis, and depression. Indeed, ED might be a warning sign of an undiagnosed health problem.

Clients With Particular Sexual Health Concerns

Pregnant and Postpartum Women. Female sexual interest tends to fluctuate during pregnancy, with increased interest during the second trimester and often decreased interest during the first and third trimesters. There is often a decrease in libido during the first trimester because of nausea, fatigue, and breast tenderness. During the second trimester, there is an increased blood flow to the pelvic area to supply the placenta and sexual enjoyment and libido increases. During the third trimester, the increased abdominal size may make finding a comfortable position difficult.

The most prevalent sexual problem during pregnancy is fear of harming the fetus. However, there is no associa-

Table 23-2 Types of Sexual Dysfunction

Category	Type	Define
Sexual desire disorders	Hypoactive sexual desire disorder	Persistent or recurrent deficiency or absence of sexual fantasies and desire for sexual activity.
	Sexual aversion disorder	Persistent or recurrent extreme aversion to, and avoidance of, all or almost all genital sexual contact with a sexual partner.
Sexual arousal disorders	Female sexual arousal disorder	Failure to attain or maintain the lubrication-swelling response or experience a subjective sense of sexual excitement and pleasure in a female during sexual activity.
	Male erectile dysfunction	Persistent or recurrent inability to attain, or maintain until completion of the sexual activity, an adequate erection.
Orgasmic disorders	Female orgasmic disorder (anorgasmia)	The recurrent and persistent inhibition of the female orgasm, as manifested by the absence or delay of orgasm following a period of sexual excitement judged adequate in intensity and duration to produce such a response.
	Male orgasmic disorder (retarded ejaculation)	Persistent or recurrent delay in, or absence of, orgasm following a normal sexual excitement phase during sexual activity that the clinician, taking into account the person's age, judges to be adequate in focus, intensity, and duration.
	Premature ejaculation	Persistent or recurrent ejaculation with minimal sexual stimulation before, upon, or shortly after penetration and before the person wishes it.
Sexual pain disorders	Dyspareunia	Recurrent or persistent genital pain in either a male or female before, during, or after sexual intercourse that is not associated with vaginismus or with lack of lubrication.
	Vaginismus	An involuntary constriction of the outer one third of the vagina that prevents penile insertion and intercourse.
Sexual dysfunction due to drugs/diseases		With these disorders, the sexual dysfunction is judged to be caused by the direct physiological effects of a general medical condition or use of a substance.

Table 23-3 Predisposing Factors to Sexual Dysfunction

Category	Predisposing Factor
Biological factors	Suggestive evidence exists of a relationship between serum testosterone and hypoactive sexual desire in men and increased libido in women. Certain medications, such as antihypertensives, antipsychotics, antidepressants, anxiolytics, and anticonvulsants may be linked to hypoactive sexual desire disorder. Erectile disorders in men may be affected by arteriosclerosis and diabetes. In women, consumption of alcohol, as well as certain medications, have been shown to affect ability to have orgasms. Various organic factors have also been associated with painful intercourse in both men and women.
Psychological factors	A number of psychological factors have also been associated with sexual desire disorders, as well as with virtually all sexual disorders. A few of these factors include religious orthodoxy, secret sexual deviations, fear of pregnancy, childhood sexual abuse, rape, fears, anxiety, and depression.
Transactional model of stress/adaptation	The etiology of sexual disorders is most likely influenced by multiple factors.

tion between birth complications and sexual intercourse (von Sydow, 1999). If women have a history of miscarriages or premature labour, they may be advised to avoid sexual intercourse during the early months of pregnancy. Other restrictions such as no orgasms or no sexual arousal may be required to protect high-risk pregnancies (Mayo Foundation for Medical Education and Research, 2004).

Clients Recovering From Surgery. Surgeries that result in disfigurement, especially of the face, breasts, genitalia, and reproductive organs, frequently have harmful effects on a client's self-image and sexuality (de Marquiegui & Huish, 1999). The effects of surgery, whether temporary or permanent, are often not fully anticipated and may not have their full impact until after discharge from the hospital. Clients' partners might also have adjustments to make and may find it difficult to resume sexual activity. Coping with their anxiety, fear, or depression about the surgery is essential. Nurses ought to support clients to discuss their concerns, especially sexual anxieties, because problems can become deep-rooted and more complicated to resolve over time (de Marquiegui & Huish, 1999). Clients who have had ileostomies, colostomies, or urostomies will be particularly concerned about possible loss of control, unpleasant smells or sounds, seepage or broken bags, and their partners' responses (see chapters 40 and 41). Perioperative counselling and support is essential for these clients.

Clients With Illness or Disabilities. Illness and disability often affect sexual health. During periods of illness, individuals may experience major physical changes, the effects of drugs or treatments, the emotional stress of a prognosis, concern about future functioning, and separation from significant others. Situational stressors could include survival of a heart attack (myocardial infarction); cancer diagnosis and treatment; or chronic disease such as diabetes, multiple sclerosis, or Parkinson's disease. The nurse should not assume that sexual functioning is not a concern because of a client's age or severity of prognosis. In some instances, clients may wrongly believe that their condition prohibits sexual activity, or they may need some guidance to promote satisfactory sexual functioning (Nusbaum, Hamilton, & Lenahan, 2003).

Many myths are prevalent about people with disability, including that they are asexual or somehow different. Without doubt, long-term disability can have profound effects on a person's sense of sexuality and sexual function. Congenital or birth impairments commonly affect a person's sexual development; for example, the resulting lack of privacy and independence may mean that people with disabilities miss out on typical sexual experiences (Glass & Soni, 1999). Acquired disabilities may have different implications: Impairments sustained in one's youth may bring about low social and sexual confidence, and people who sustain disabilities as adults may be far more aware of what they have lost. It is important that health professionals validate a disabled person's sexuality. Nurses can do this by sensitively initiating conversations about sexual function and safer sex practices.

Critical Thinking

Successful critical thinking requires synthesis of knowledge, experience, information gathered from clients, critical thinking attitudes, and intellectual and professional standards. Clinical judgment requires the nurse to anticipate the information necessary, analyze the data, and make appropriate decisions regarding client care. Figure 23–3 demonstrates that the nurse must consider numerous critical thinking elements, as well as client assessment data, that contribute to appropriate nursing diagnoses.

In the case of sexuality, the nurse integrates knowledge from nursing and other disciplines. The nurse must have a good understanding, for example, of the human sexual response, safer sex practices, and the risks and behaviours associated with sexual problems to anticipate how to assess a client and then how to interpret findings. Previous experience in caring for clients whose sexuality becomes threatened helps the nurse approach the next client in a more reflective and helpful way. Clients will have different customs and values from those of the nurse. Professional standards call for the nurse to respect each client as an individual.

Sexuality and the Nursing Process

A person's sexuality has physical, psychological, social, and cultural elements. The nurse must assess all relevant elements to determine a client's sexual well-being. The nurse should build a sound knowledge base and be willing to explore personal issues regarding sexuality. The nursing role in addressing sexual concerns can range from ongoing assessment to providing information to counselling to referral.

NP Assessment

Factors Affecting Sexuality. In gathering a sexual history, the nurse should consider physical, functional, relationship, lifestyle, and self-esteem factors that may influence sexual functioning. Sexual desire varies among individuals; some people want and enjoy sexual activity every day, whereas others only want it once a month, and still others have no sexual desire and are quite comfortable with that fact. Sexual desire becomes an issue if the person wants to feel sexual desire more often, if the person believes it is necessary to measure up to some cultural norm, or if there is a discrepancy between the sexual desires of the partners in a relationship.

The nurse assesses for factors that typically can influence sexual desire. A person may experience a decrease in sexual desire for physical reasons, such as pain or discomfort during sexual activity. Minor illness, medications, and fatigue can also decrease sexual desire. Lifestyle factors, such as poor communication between sexual partners, the use or abuse of alcohol, lack of sleep, lack of time, or the demands of caring for a new baby can also be influencing factors. After identifying factors that can potentially affect sexual desire, the nurse confirms them with the client and then determines the extent to which sexual function is impaired.

Sexual Health History. When taking a health history, the nurse should include a few questions related to sexual functioning to determine whether the client has any sexual concerns. These questions can be incorporated in the review of systems and addressed in a routine, matter-of-fact manner. The nurse needs to understand the reasons for the question and be able to provide them to the client on request. An opening statement such as "Sex is an important part of life and can be affected by our health status. To better understand your health, it is useful to know . . ." is a possible introduction to these questions. Other questions for adults might include the following:

- How do you feel about the sexual aspects of your life?
- Have you noticed any changes in the way you feel about yourself (as a man, woman, husband, or wife)?

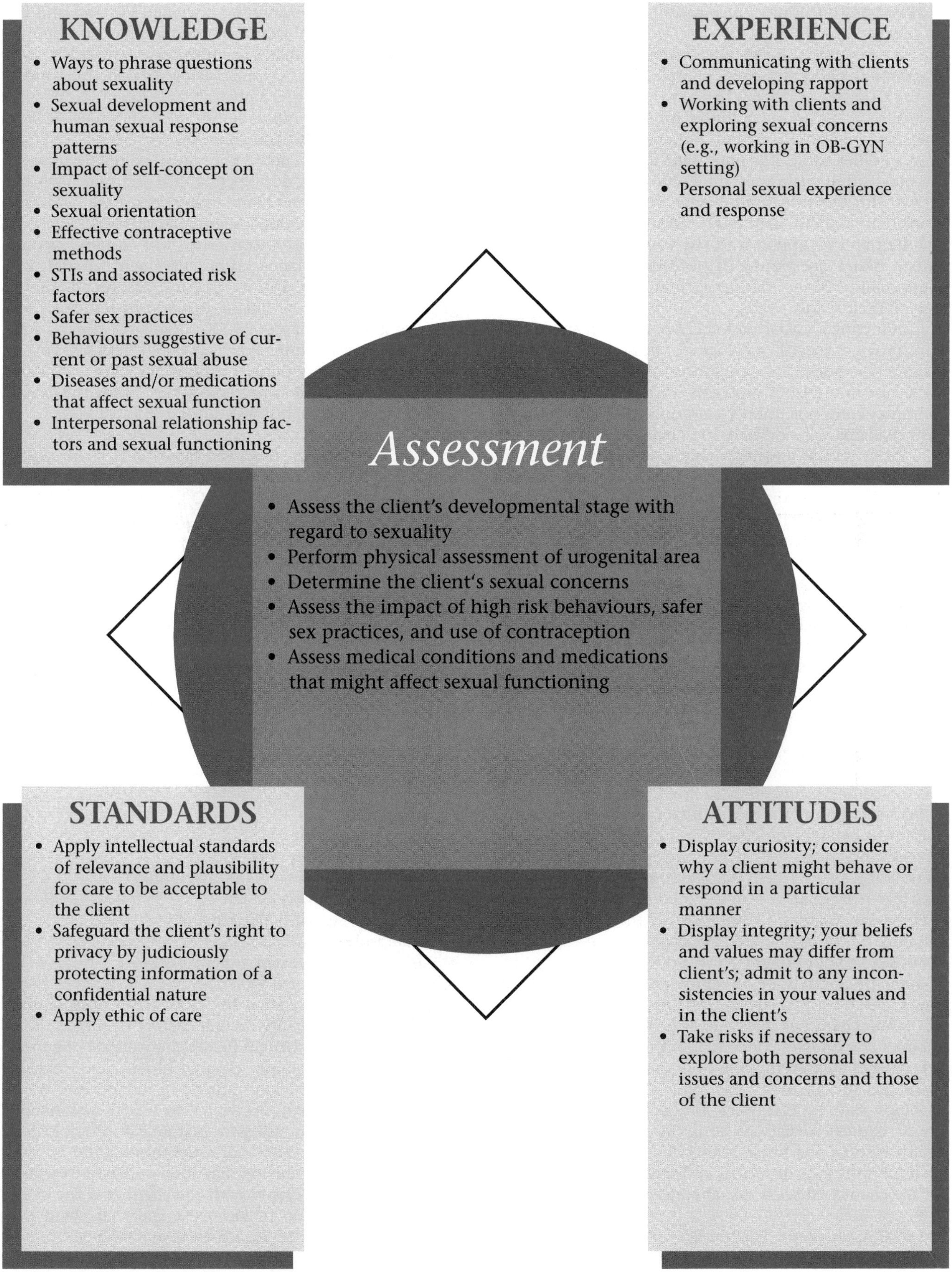
KNOWLEDGE
• Ways to phrase questions about sexuality
• Sexual development and human sexual response patterns
• Impact of self-concept on sexuality
• Sexual orientation
• Effective contraceptive methods
• STIs and associated risk factors
• Safer sex practices
• Behaviours suggestive of current or past sexual abuse
• Diseases and/or medications that affect sexual function
• Interpersonal relationship factors and sexual functioning
EXPERIENCE
• Communicating with clients and developing rapport
• Working with clients and exploring sexual concerns (e.g., working in OB-GYN setting)
• Personal sexual experience and response
Assessment
• Assess the client's developmental stage with regard to sexuality
• Perform physical assessment of urogenital area
• Determine the client's sexual concerns
• Assess the impact of high risk behaviours, safer sex practices, and use of contraception
• Assess medical conditions and medications that might affect sexual functioning
STANDARDS
• Apply intellectual standards of relevance and plausibility for care to be acceptable to the client
• Safeguard the client's right to privacy by judiciously protecting information of a confidential nature
• Apply ethic of care
ATTITUDES
• Display curiosity; consider why a client might behave or respond in a particular manner
• Display integrity; your beliefs and values may differ from client's; admit to any inconsistencies in your values and in the client's
• Take risks if necessary to explore both personal sexual issues and concerns and those of the client

FIGURE **23–3** Critical thinking model for sexuality assessment.

- How has your illness, medication, or surgery affected your sex life?
- It is not unusual for people with your condition to be experiencing some sexual changes. Have you noticed any changes, or do you have any concerns?

When caring for older adults, nurses may adjust their assessment approach. When gathering a sexual history from an older adult, it is important to keep in mind that the older adult may have difficulty discussing intimate details with health care providers. The nurse has the responsibility to help maintain the sexuality of older adults by offering the opportunity to discuss any concerns. Often, asking questions on the topic of sexuality in a comfortable, relaxed manner facilitates older adults' discussing their sexual needs.

Conducting a sexual assessment of children and adolescents provides special challenges for health care providers. Issues of language, of promoting normal development while not minimizing problems, of screening for sexual concerns while not unduly alarming them, are all common challenges. In addition, the sexual counselling of minors raises ethical and legal issues regarding the client's rights to health care and education on the one hand, and the parents' or guardian's right to supervise information on the other. Use of an open, positive, interested disposition when introducing sexual questions is helpful.

Because of the prevalence of domestic violence and sexual abuse, questions relating to abusive relationships can be important. Questions that address domestic violence or abuse should be addressed to the client in private. A question such as "Are you in a relationship in which someone is hurting you?" may compel a client to reveal present or previous abuse. An additional question such as "Has anyone ever forced you to have sex you did not wish to participate in?" may more specifically encourage the client to discuss concerns. Recognizing both subjective and objective signs and symptoms of abuse can aid in recognition of this too-common problem (see Box 23-4).

While gathering the sexual history of clients, it is also helpful to explore the client's use of contraception and safer sex practices. Adolescents may respond to a comment that reassures them that having questions related to sexuality is normal. A lead-in could be "Many teenagers have questions about STIs or whether their bodies are developing at the right rate. Do you have any questions about sex or your body?"

Some individuals are too embarrassed or do not know how to ask questions about sexuality. The nurse may detect that a client has questions if he or she makes a sexual joke or expresses concern about relations with his or her partner. Observing for and listening to concerns about sexuality takes practise. With experience, the nurse develops skill in clarifying and paraphrasing to help clients express sexual concerns. By including it in the health history, the nurse acknowledges that sexuality is an important part of health and creates an opportunity for the client to discuss sexual concerns.

Physical Assessment. The physical examination is important in evaluating the cause of sexual concerns or problems and may be the best opportunity to teach a client about sexuality. In examining a woman's breasts and the external and internal genitalia, the nurse has the opportunity to assess the woman's reaction, answer questions, and provide information. A woman can learn to perform breast self-examination during a physical assessment (see chapter 28). In addition, the nurse may choose to teach pelvic floor muscle exercises (also known as Kegel exercises; see chapter 40). Toning of the pelvic floor muscle often decreases as a result of stretching during childbirth and loss of general elasticity during aging. Maintaining good tone helps prevent bladder or rectal prolapse into the vagina (cystocele or rectocele), reduces problems with later urinary incontinence, and can enhance sexual enjoyment through and beyond menopause. During physical assessment of the genitalia, men can be taught to perform testicular self-examination (see chapter 28). Knowledge of normal scrotal anatomical structures aids men in detecting signs of testicular cancer. The nurse can instruct both men and women on signs and symptoms of STIs during the examination when clients' histories suggest risks for STIs.

Client Expectations. As in the case of any client assessment, it is important to understand the client's expectations regarding his or her care. Questions such as "What would you like to have happen in regard to [expressed concern]?" and "What initial steps might you take?" can help the person identify desired outcomes. It is important for the nurse to set aside personal views and not assume what a client's expectations might be.

NP Nursing Diagnosis

After completing an assessment and applying critical thought to the diagnostic process (Box 23-5), the nurse selects diagnoses applicable to the client's needs. Possible nursing diagnoses related to sexual functioning are listed below:

- Anxiety
- Ineffective coping
- Interrupted family processes
- Deficient knowledge (contraception/STIs)
- Sexual dysfunction
- Ineffective sexuality patterns
- Social isolation
- Risk for other-directed violence
- Risk for self-directed violence

Clues that may signal at-risk or an actual nursing diagnosis related to sexuality include history of surgery of reproductive organs, changes in appearance, past or current physical or sexual abuse, chronic illness, and developmental milestones such as puberty or menopause. When making nursing diagnoses related to sexual dysfunction, the nurse must have assessed anatomical, physiological, socio-cultural, and situational issues thoroughly.

When making a nursing diagnosis in regard to sexuality, the nurse must clarify with the client that the defining characteristics do in fact exist and that client perceives a problem with regard to sexuality. Determining the etiological or contributing factors is important to focus effective planning and to select appropriate nursing

Nursing Diagnostic Process — Box 23-5

Assessment Activities	Defining Characteristics	Nursing Diagnosis
Observe readiness to discuss sexual concerns through verbalization (e.g., "When can I return to life as normal?" or "There goes my love life") or behaviour (e.g., exhibitionism)	Client verbalizes concern that sexual activity may cause another myocardial infarction or death.	Ineffective sexuality patterns related to fear of recurrent myocardial infarction or death during intercourse.
Ask client and spouse about previous level and method of sexual expression (e.g., frequency, initiator).		
Observe for affectionate behaviour (e.g., touching, hand holding, kissing).	Client's spouse exhibits reluctance to touch client.	
In privacy, ask spouse about perceptions of recovery and return to full functioning.	Spouse verbalizes concern that client will need continuous care, attention, and protection.	
Observe for anxiety (e.g., hand wringing)	Client maintains eye contact, shifts position frequently.	

interventions. For example, the nursing interventions appropriate for the nursing diagnosis of *chronic low self-esteem* would be different for other etiological factors. *Self-esteem disturbance related to chronic, recurring herpes infection* would lead to counselling and education on how to maintain safer sexual practices. In contrast, *self-esteem disturbance related to sexual abuse* would require counselling and referral to community resources (e.g., crisis services or sexual abuse support group).

Planning

Goals and Outcomes. During planning, the nurse again synthesizes information from multiple resources (Figure 23–4). The nurse uses critical thinking skills to integrate professional standards and knowledge about the client's sexuality into the care plan. It is especially important to maintain a client's dignity and identity when developing the care plan. For example, conveying respect for a client's gender preferences by including a lesbian or gay partner in the plan to the degree that the client wishes can assist the client in maintaining his or her identity and dignity.

The nurse develops an individualized care plan for each nursing diagnosis (see Care Plan). The nurse and client together set realistic goals for care. Expected outcomes need to be individualized and realistic. For example, for a client with a nursing diagnosis of *sexual dysfunction related to dyspareunia or hypoactive sexual desire,* the nurse and client develop a goal to be free from pain or discomfort during sexual intercourse. Expected outcomes for this goal may include that the client will do the following:

- Report decreased anxiety and greater satisfaction with sexual activity
- Consistently use a water-soluble lubricant before sexual intercourse
- Avoid the use of feminine hygiene products that destroy the natural flora and secretions of the vaginal walls

A concept map is useful for organizing client care (Figure 23–5). This concept map shows the relationship of a medical diagnosis (e.g., decreased libido and depression) with the four nursing diagnoses identified from the client assessment data. The map also shows the links and relationship with the nursing diagnosis. For example, ineffective coping affects and contributes to social isolation; as long as the client has ineffective coping, the social isolation continues or perhaps worsens.

Setting Priorities. A useful framework to guide planning is the PLISSIT model developed by Annon (1976). In this model, there are progressively more involved levels of intervention. The *P* stands for permission giving. During assessment, the nurse's questions can bring up the topic of sexuality and can give the individual permission to talk about sexual concerns. *LI* stands for limited information, which involves providing basic information regarding sexuality and sexual functioning. An example would be discussing nocturnal emissions with a prepubescent boy to minimize fear that might develop if the boy did not know this was a normal part of development. *SS* stands for specific suggestions, whereby the nurse provides specific suggestions regarding a sexual concern or issue. For example, a post-menopausal woman might be concerned about her lack of vaginal lubrication, and the nurse might suggest use of a water-based lubricant during sexual intercourse. The concern expressed might be one that the nurse is not equipped to address. In this case, the nurse should refer to another health care provider. The *IT* stands for intensive therapy. At this level of intervention, the nurse's role would be to refer the client to a qualified practitioner, such as a social worker or sex counsellor for individualized therapy. The level of intervention nurses plan depends in part on their own experience and knowledge. When a client requires specific suggestions or intensive therapy, the nurse may recommend referral to a specialist.

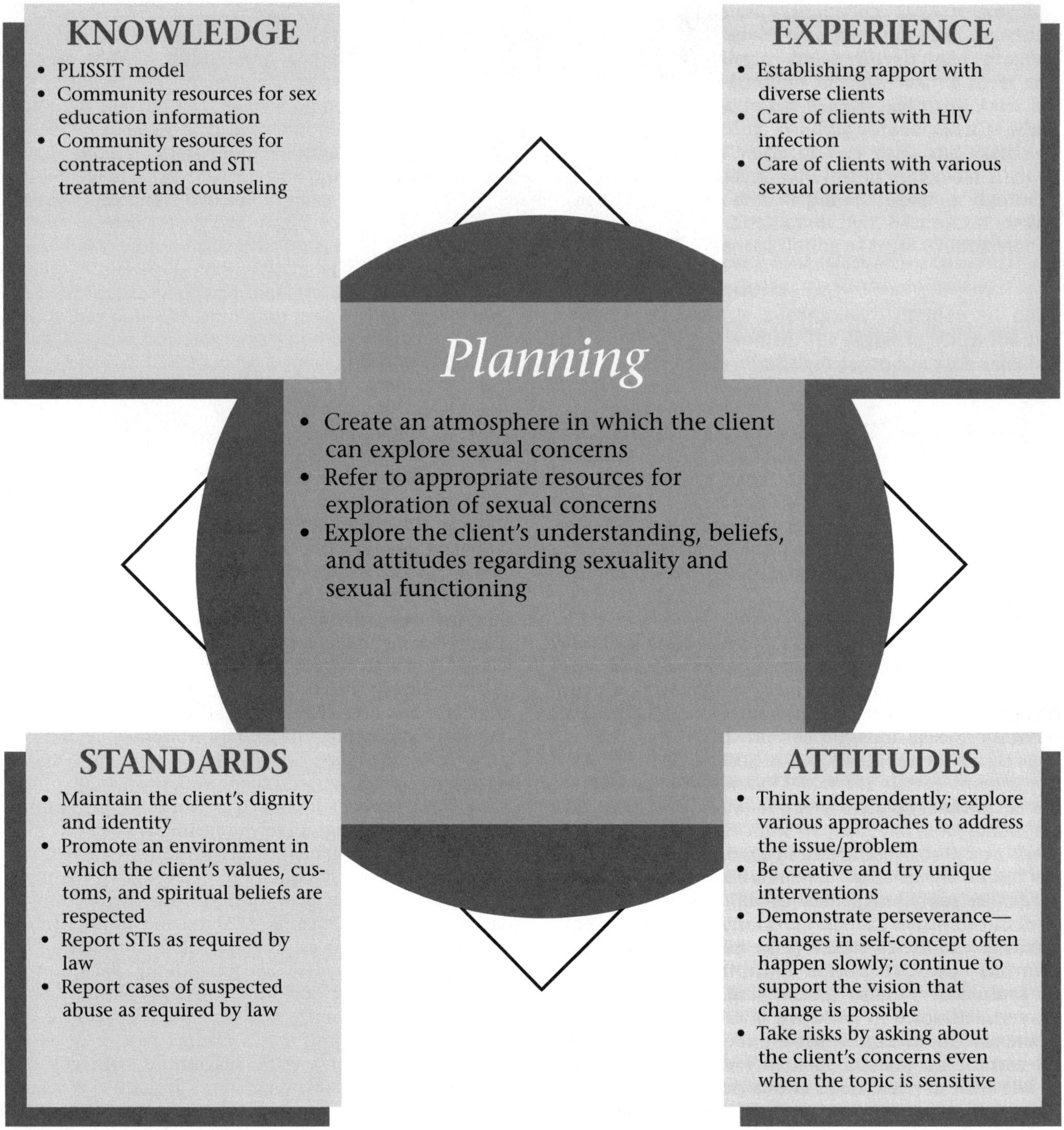
KNOWLEDGE
• PLISSIT model
• Community resources for sex education information
• Community resources for contraception and STI treatment and counseling
EXPERIENCE
• Establishing rapport with diverse clients
• Care of clients with HIV infection
• Care of clients with various sexual orientations
Planning
• Create an atmosphere in which the client can explore sexual concerns
• Refer to appropriate resources for exploration of sexual concerns
• Explore the client's understanding, beliefs, and attitudes regarding sexuality and sexual functioning
STANDARDS
• Maintain the client's dignity and identity
• Promote an environment in which the client's values, customs, and spiritual beliefs are respected
• Report STIs as required by law
• Report cases of suspected abuse as required by law
ATTITUDES
• Think independently; explore various approaches to address the issue/problem
• Be creative and try unique interventions
• Demonstrate perseverance—changes in self-concept often happen slowly; continue to support the vision that change is possible
• Take risks by asking about the client's concerns even when the topic is sensitive

FIGURE **23–4** Critical thinking model for sexuality planning.

Continuity of Care. Planning in the area of sexuality may include referrals to community resources (Box 23-6). Sexual conflicts in marriage or trauma related to sexual abuse or incest may require intensive treatment with a mental health professional or certified sex therapist. For women in abusive relationships, most communities have battered women's shelters that provide counselling and serve as a safe haven for them while they make further plans.

NP Implementation

Health Promotion. Because of their education, clinical expertise, and wellness orientation, nurses are among the best-situated professionals to develop and deliver sexual health initiatives. The nurse can promote sexual health by identifying clients at increased risk, providing appropriate information, helping individuals gain insight into

Nursing Care Plan

Sexual Dysfunction

Assessment

Mr. Clements is a 46-year-old client who was last seen in the office 2 months ago, when he was found to have mild hypertension and was given a prescription for propranolol (Inderal). His blood pressure today is 122/82 mm Hg.

Jack Constant, a nursing student, talks with Mr. Clements after reading his records, which include the recent diagnosis of mild hypertension, the order for propranolol, and the current blood pressure reading of 122/82 mm Hg. The record also indicates that Mr. Clements is married and living with his wife.

Jack tells Mr. Clements of the improvement in his blood pressure since his last visit. He inquires if Mr. Clements is taking his medication regularly. Mr. Clements reports that he has been taking his medication regularly. He relates that it scared him when his blood pressure was up because both his parents had died of strokes. Jack then inquires if he has noted any side effects from the medicine. Mr. Clements says not really, except he is maybe a little more tired than he used to be. Jack then asks, "Some people find that certain blood pressure medications affect their sexual performance. Have you noticed any changes in sexual functioning since you began your medication?" Mr. Clements replies that he finds he just is not very interested in sex any more and that this is becoming somewhat of a problem between him and his wife. Her interest does not seem to have waned at all, he tells Jack.

Assessment Activities	Findings/Defining Characteristics
Ascertain when Mr. Clements began noticing his decreased interest in sex.	He responds that it was at about the same time he started taking propranolol.
Ask Mr. Clements about his sexual relationship with his wife before taking propranolol.	He states they used to have intercourse 1 to 3 times per week.
Ask Mr. Clements if he has noticed any changes in his erect penis.	He states he sometimes has trouble having an erection.
Ask Mr. Clements if there have there been any changes to his lifestyle since the first of the year.	He denies any changes.

Nursing Diagnosis: Sexual dysfunction related to side effects of antihypertensive medication.

Planning

Goal	Expected Outcomes*
	Sexual Functioning
Client will express satisfaction with sexual relationship with wife within 1 month.	Client will report a renewed interest in sex within 1 month. Client will report resolution of problem with impotence.

*Outcome classification labels from *Nursing Outcomes Classification (NOC)* (3rd ed.), edited by S. Moorhead, M. Johnson, and M. Maas, 2004, St. Louis, MO: Mosby.

Interventions†	Rationale
Sexual Counseling	
• Establish trust and respect with client. Offer privacy during conversations.	Conveys sense of caring, increasing likelihood of client's ability to express concerns fully (Ross et al., 2000).
• Discuss possible effects of antihypertensive on sexual functioning, and encourage client to discuss sexual concerns with physician.	Helps client to understand possible cause for sexual difficulties. Gives client important option to review with physician (Riley, 1999).
• Encourage client to discuss concerns with his wife. Role play so that client can practise ways to approach concerns.	Many of the sexual problems in relationships involve poor communication (Finan, 1997).
Anxiety Reduction	
• Assure client that there are other blood pressure medications available that can maintain blood pressure control and that do not negatively affect sexual function.	Gives client sense of control knowing that there are options and that blood pressure can continue to be safely managed (Running & Berndt, 2003).

†Intervention classification labels from *Nursing Interventions Classification (NIC)* (4th ed.), edited by J. M. Dochterman and G. M. Bulechek, 2004, St. Louis, MO: Mosby.

Evaluation

Nursing Actions	Client Response/Finding	Achievement of Outcome
Ask Mr. Clements if his sexual relations with his wife has increased during return office visit.	He responds that since he has been on new medication his interest in sex is back to normal and he has no trouble now having an erection.	Mr. Clements reports sexual interest and function with the new medication.

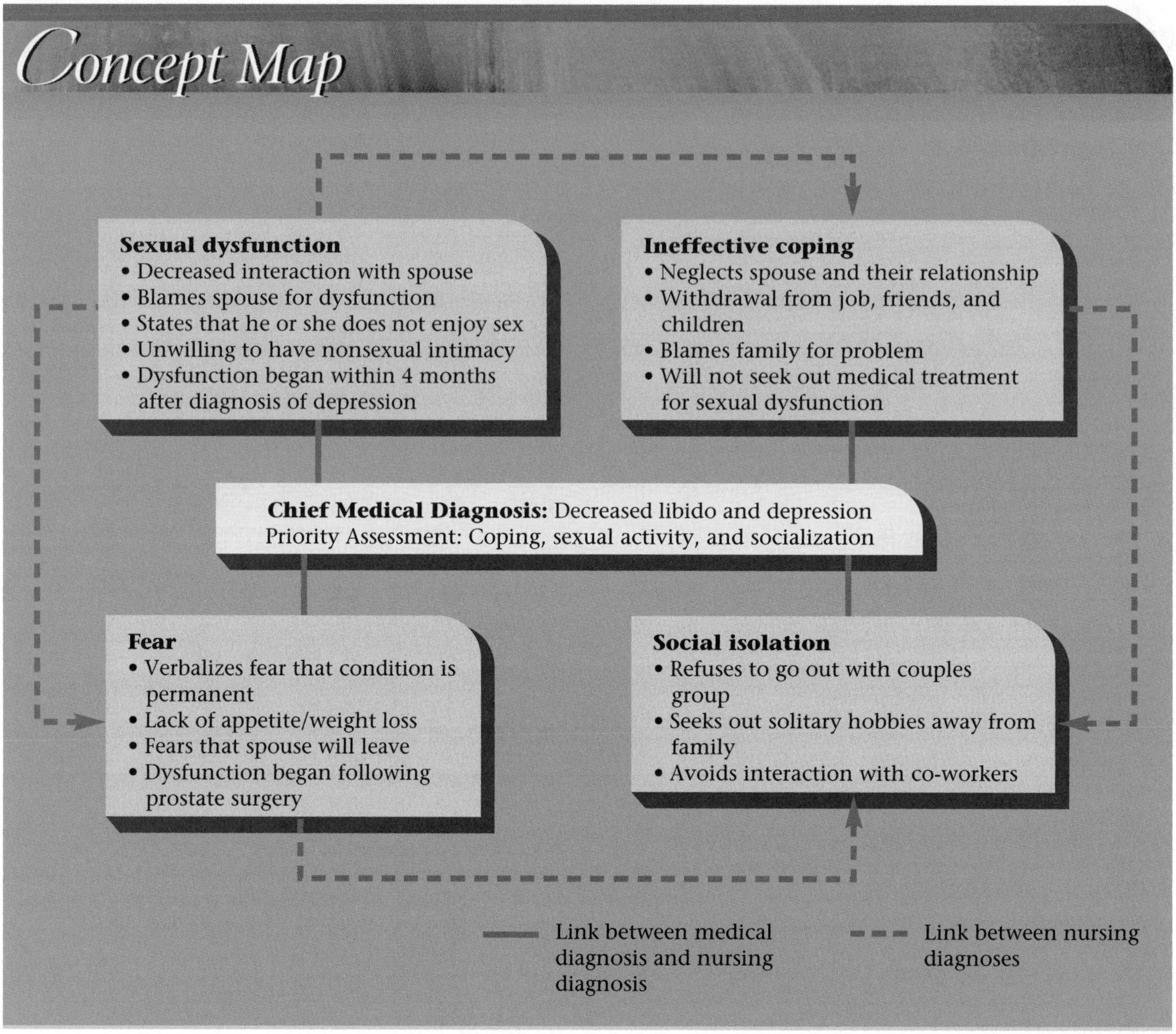
Concept Map
Sexual dysfunction
• Decreased interaction with spouse
• Blames spouse for dysfunction
• States that he or she does not enjoy sex
• Unwilling to have nonsexual intimacy
• Dysfunction began within 4 months after diagnosis of depression
Ineffective coping
• Neglects spouse and their relationship
• Withdrawal from job, friends, and children
• Blames family for problem
• Will not seek out medical treatment for sexual dysfunction
Chief Medical Diagnosis: Decreased libido and depression
Priority Assessment: Coping, sexual activity, and socialization
Fear
• Verbalizes fear that condition is permanent
• Lack of appetite/weight loss
• Fears that spouse will leave
• Dysfunction began following prostate surgery
Social isolation
• Refuses to go out with couples group
• Seeks out solitary hobbies away from family
• Avoids interaction with co-workers
Link between medical diagnosis and nursing diagnosis
Link between nursing diagnoses

FIGURE **23–5** Concept map for client with decreased libido and depression.

their problems, and exploring methods to deal with them effectively. A health promotion perspective ought to guide nurses in designing informal educational opportunities, continuing education, peer learning activities for adolescents, community and political initiatives, and health care professional education (Beitz, 1998). Topics for education vary, depending on the nursing diagnosis (Box 23-7).

Acute Care. Nursing interventions that address alterations in sexuality generally are aimed at raising awareness, assisting in clarification of issues or concerns, and/or providing information. Nurses who have pursued specialized education in sexual functioning and counselling may provide more intensive sex therapy. Nurses should recognize when an individual's needs exceed their expertise and provide appropriate referral.

The initial intervention often includes exploring present sexual practices with the individual. The individual should be encouraged to investigate and acknowledge social and ethical values and consider the role of sexuality in his or her self-concept. When there is significant discrepancy between values and past or present practices, the person may need referral for more intensive counselling.

Major developmental milestones (e.g., puberty or menopause) should prompt education about effects on sexuality. Situational crises such as a life change with pregnancy, illness, extreme financial stress, placement of a spouse in a long-term care facility, or loss and grief affect sexuality. Effects may last for days, months, or years and can generate performance anxieties that lead to continued sexual dysfunction. If an individual is prepared for possible changes in sexual functioning, performance anxieties may be minimized.

Box 23-6 Community Resources Relating to Sexuality

Planned Parenthood
Sex therapists
Clinical psychologists
Social workers
Health department (often for both family planning and STIs)
Groups that provide education/services for those with particular conditions include the following:
 Canadian Diabetes Association
 Heart and Stroke Foundation of Canada
 Muscular Dystrophy Canada
Sexual abuse support groups
Women's shelters (for those who have been physically and/or sexually abused)
Hotlines for help (will have lists of community support resources)

When concerns are assessed and identified, they can be addressed in the context of the client's value system. In response to identified concerns, the nurse may initiate discussion in pertinent areas. It may be appropriate to discuss sexual practices such as oral-genital sex or mutual masturbation as methods of expressing intimate affection when penile-vaginal intercourse is contraindicated. A partner experiencing musculoskeletal problems that cause joint pain, muscle spasms, stiffness, or problems with flexibility or mobility may appreciate a discussion of various positions for intercourse. Pillows placed about the body or under joints may reduce pain during sexual activity. Additional relief may be obtained by taking a warm shower or bath before sexual activity or using a waterbed to minimize pressure on painful joints (Nusbaum et al., 2003). Use of fantasy or a sense of playfulness may add new romance or stimulation to a long-term relationship. A couple may need confirmation or assurance that the acting out of non-harmful fantasy is normal and healthy.

Restorative Care. In the home, the nurse can help to create an environment that is comfortable for sexual activity. This may involve recommending ways to arrange the bedroom to accommodate an individual's limitations. For example, wheelchair-bound individuals may prefer to move the chair close to the side of the bed at an angle that allows for more ease in touching and caressing. Suggestions regarding how to accommodate barriers such as Foley catheters or drainage tubes can contribute to enhanced sexual activity.

In the long-term care setting, facilities should make proper arrangements for privacy during residents' sexual experiences (Lueckenotte, 2000). The ideal situation is to set up a pleasant room that can be used for a variety of activities but may also be reserved for private visits with a spouse or partner. If this is not feasible, making arrangements for the roommate of a client to have another place to be can allow a couple time alone.

Focus on Primary Health Care — Box 23-7

Sexual Health Education Topics

- Guidelines for normal development. For example, the nurse might talk to a toddler's mother regarding a new baby, to a school-age child regarding the appearance of pubic hair, or to a 60-year-old man regarding delayed ejaculation. Details of physiological changes should be provided as a part of general health care. Providing client education gives permission for clients to raise questions or concerns regarding personal functioning.
- Contraception, when talking with clients of child-bearing age. The discussion should include desire for children, usual sexual practices, acceptable methods of contraception, frequency of sexual activity, comfort with genital touching, comfort with sharing contraceptive responsibility with the partner, and comfort with interruption of sexual acts. The nurse might ask, "Are you using contraception with your partner now?" and then follow up, based on the client's answer. For clients who do not have a regular contraceptive method, who do not have a reliable contraceptive method, or who are not satisfied with their current method, the various methods of contraception should be reviewed to provide necessary information for an informed choice. The best method is the one that the person will use consistently.
- Safer sex practices, when talking with sexually active adolescents and clients having more than one sex partner or whose partner has other sexual experiences. Information should be provided regarding sexually transmitted infection symptoms and transmission, use of condoms, and risky sexual activities (e.g., trauma from penile-anal sex). An area to consider in discussing sexual relating is the emotional risks within a relationship. Role play can be a useful educational tool in helping a person learn to say no or negotiate with a partner to use a condom.
- The need for regular health examinations. Regular health examinations are important for maintaining sexual health. The annual health examination also provides an easy opportunity to discuss contraception and safer sex practices. Regular breast self-examinations, mammograms, and Papanicolaou (Pap) smear are important for women, as are testicular self-examinations for men.

NP Evaluation

Client Care. The nurse reviews client responses to interventions to determine if goals and outcome criteria have been met (Figure 23–6). Critical thinking ensures that the nurse applies what is known about sexuality and the client's unique situation.

Having follow-up discussions with the client or spouse will determine whether goals and outcomes have been achieved. Sexuality is felt more than observed, and sexual expression requires an intimacy that is not amenable to observation. Clients can be asked to relate risk factors, verbalize concerns, and share experiences and their level of satisfaction. The nurse can also observe behavioural

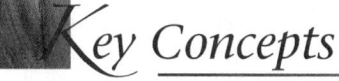

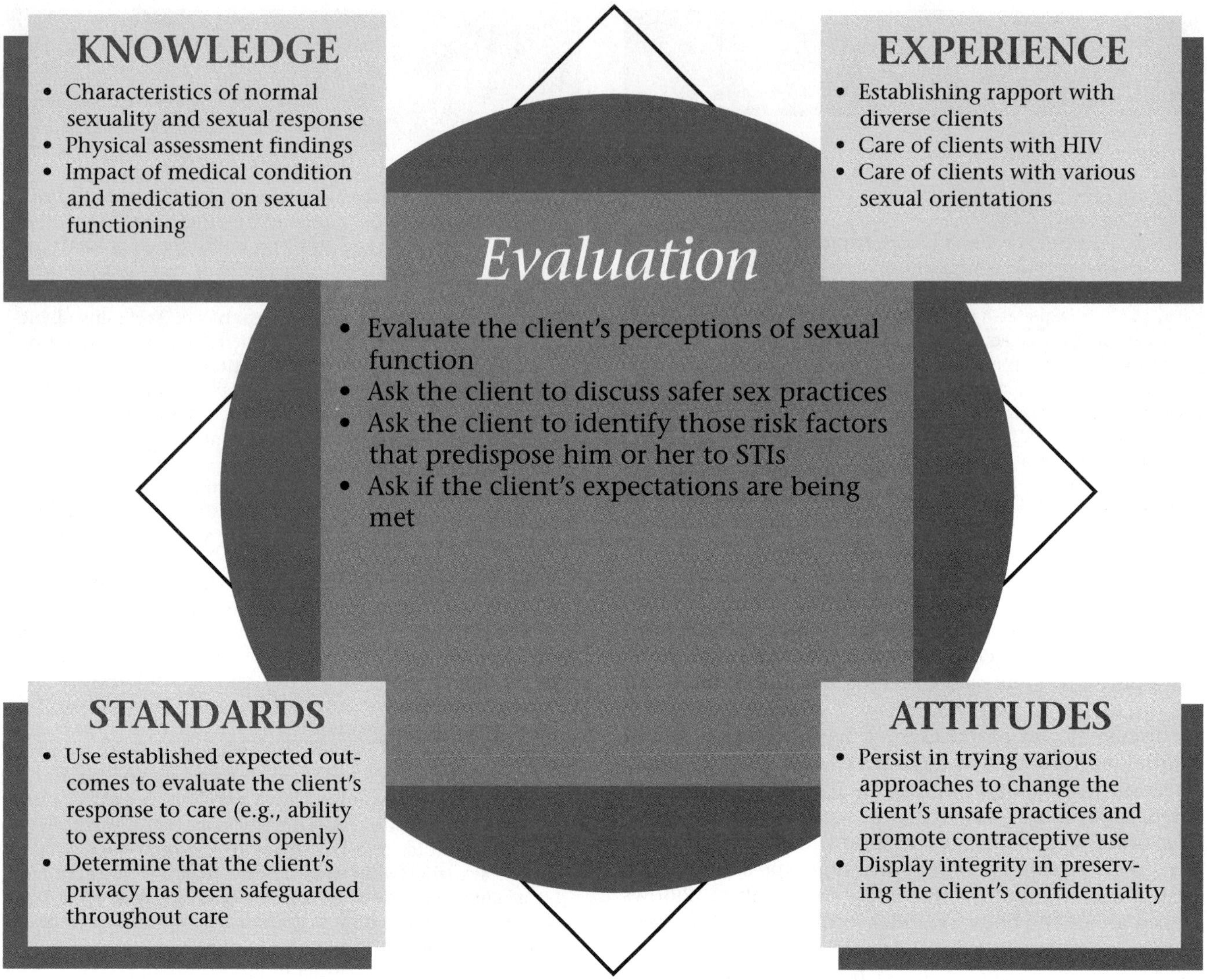
KNOWLEDGE
• Characteristics of normal sexuality and sexual response
• Physical assessment findings
• Impact of medical condition and medication on sexual functioning
EXPERIENCE
• Establishing rapport with diverse clients
• Care of clients with HIV
• Care of clients with various sexual orientations
Evaluation
• Evaluate the client's perceptions of sexual function
• Ask the client to discuss safer sex practices
• Ask the client to identify those risk factors that predispose him or her to STIs
• Ask if the client's expectations are being met
STANDARDS
• Use established expected outcomes to evaluate the client's response to care (e.g., ability to express concerns openly)
• Determine that the client's privacy has been safeguarded throughout care
ATTITUDES
• Persist in trying various approaches to change the client's unsafe practices and promote contraceptive use
• Display integrity in preserving the client's confidentiality

FIGURE **23–6** Critical thinking model for sexuality evaluation.

cues, such as eye contact, posture, and extraneous hand movements that indicate comfort or suggest continued anxiety or concern as topics are addressed. As outcomes are evaluated, the individual, spouse, and nurse may need to modify expectations or establish time frames in which to achieve the target goals. All involved may need to be reminded of the individual nature of sexual expression and the multiple factors that affect perceptions and responses. Sexual wellness is not an absolute. An individual must define what is acceptable and satisfying. The partner's level of sexual satisfaction must also be considered. Sexual performance is seldom the exclusive focus of sexual satisfaction. Open communication and positive self-esteem are essential factors in effectively resolving concerns.

Client Expectations. In evaluating the outcomes of interventions related to sexuality, the nurse must consult with the client. Resolution of sexual concerns must meet the client's perceptions of improvement. An individual must define what is acceptable and satisfying. In considering the status of sexual health, the client's partner's perceptions of sexual satisfaction are also significant.

Key Concepts

- Sexuality is related to all dimensions of health; therefore, sexual concerns or problems should be addressed as a part of nursing care.
- Sexuality is a part of each individual's identity and includes sexual identity, gender identity, and sexual orientation.
- Attitudes toward sexuality vary widely and are influenced by religious beliefs, society's values, the family, and other factors.
- Nurses' attitudes toward sexuality also vary and may differ from those of clients; nurses should be sensitive to clients' sexual preferences and needs.
- The sexual response cycle includes four phases: appetitive, arousal, orgasm, and resolution.

- Sexual development is a process beginning in infancy and involves some level of sexual behaviour or growth in all developmental stages.
- The physiological sexual response changes with aging, but aging does not lead to diminished sexuality.
- Sexual health involves physical and psychosocial aspects and contributes to an individual's sense of self-worth and positive interpersonal relationships.
- Sexual dysfunction can result from an easily identified etiology or varied and complex etiologies.
- Interventions for sexual dysfunctions depend on the condition and the client; interventions may include giving information, teaching specific exercises, improving communication between partners, and referral to a knowledgeable professional.
- Choice and use of contraceptive methods are affected by desire for children, usual sexual practices, acceptable methods of contraception, frequency of sexual activity, comfort with genital touching, comfort with sharing contraceptive responsibility with the partner, and comfort with interruption of sexual acts.
- A brief review of sexuality should be included in every nursing assessment of a client's level of wellness.
- Most nursing interventions to enhance a client's sexual health involve providing information and education.

Key Terms

Bisexuality, *p. 464*
Contraception, *p. 469*
Dyspareunia, *p. 465*
Gender identity, *p. 464*
Heterosexuality, *p. 464*
Homophobia, *p. 464*
Homosexuality, *p. 464*
Infertility, *p. 471*
Myotonia, *p. 466*
Perimenopausal, *p. 465*
Safer sex, *p. 466*
Sexual dysfunction, *p. 466*
Sexual health, *p. 472*
Sexual identity, *p. 463*
Sexual orientation, *p. 464*
Sexual response cycle, *p. 466*
Sexuality, *p. 463*
Sexually transmitted infections (STIs), *p. 463*
Transsexuality, *p. 464*
Vasocongestion, *p. 466*

Critical Thinking Exercises

1. Your current clinical experience is in a community health care setting. You are conducting the initial interview with a 48-year-old man who started taking antihypertensives 2 weeks ago. You take his blood pressure and find it to be 136/74 mm Hg. You ask him how he has been doing since his last visit. He looks down at the floor and says, "Oh, OK I guess. Seems like I'm just getting old now." What kind of follow-up would be indicated based on this information?
2. You are assigned to care for a 15-year-old girl who was admitted after a motor vehicle accident. Yesterday she had an internal fixation of a fractured ankle. In gathering her nursing history, you explore sexuality and learn that she has just recently become sexually active with her boyfriend of 3 months. When you ask about safer sex and the use of birth control, she tells you that she knows she does not have to worry about STIs with him because he is just not one of those kinds of boys. In regard to birth control, she says that her boyfriend has reassured her that because he is pulling out before ejaculation, there is no risk of her becoming pregnant. How would you proceed?
3. You are working on a rehabilitation unit and caring for a 67-year-old man who had a stroke 3 weeks ago. He shares a room with another man who is recovering from a stroke. He has been progressing in his self-care skills and is now able to get around with a cane, feed himself, and do most of his bath. His wife is in fairly good health, and the plan is for him to return home within the next 1 to 2 weeks. As you work with him one morning, he says to you, "You know, one of the things that is hardest about being here is not being able to sleep in the same bed as Greta. I miss her so much. Even though she visits every day, it is just not the same." How would you explore his comment, and what planning would you consider?

Review Questions

1. Gender identity is the individual's
   1. Sexual behaviour
   2. Sexual orientation
   3. Sense of being male, female, or some combination
   4. Sense of preferring one sex over the other
2. Sexual health refers to
   1. Having no sexually transmitted infections
   2. Awareness of and positive attitudes toward sexual functioning
   3. Using contraception consistently
   4. Sexual activity with multiple partners
3. Inability or difficulty in sexual functioning caused by numerous factors is called
   1. Sexual behaviour
   2. Sexual response
   3. Sexual orientation
   4. Sexual dysfunction
4. A major problem in dealing with sexually transmitted infections (STIs) is that
   1. Symptoms are often absent or go unnoticed
   2. Most STIs cannot be treated with antibiotics
   3. Little is known about how they are transmitted
   4. Little can be done to help
5. The most common bacterial STI is
   1. Syphilis
   2. Genital chlamydia
   3. Gonorrhea
   4. HIV/AIDS
6. Which of the following methods of contraception BOTH require a health care provider's intervention?
   1. Diaphragm and intrauterine device (IUD)
   2. Condoms and hormones
   3. Cervical caps and condoms
   4. Sterilization and vaginal spermicidals

7. Which of the following is the most effective contraception method for women?
   1. Female condom
   2. Birth control pill
   3. Contraceptive sponge
   4. Vaginal spermicide
8. The most valuable tool the nurse can develop when providing sexual health care is
   1. Knowledge of right and wrong sexual behaviours
   2. Effective, non-judgmental communication
   3. Nursing diagnoses
   4. Firm personal convictions about what constitutes normal sexual behaviour
9. When the nurse is gathering a sexual history from an older adult, the nurse must keep in mind that
   1. Older adults do not usually participate in sexual activity
   2. Older men always lose fertility
   3. Older adults may have difficulty discussing intimate matters
   4. Both older men and women are sexually dysfunctional
10. A useful framework for the nurse to guide planning and set priorities about sexual activity for a client is the
   1. PLISSIT model
   2. NANDA International guidelines
   3. NIC and NOC guidelines
   4. Nurse's own theory of sexual behaviour

References

Annon, J. S. (1976). The PLISSIT model: A proposed conceptual scheme for the behavioral treatment of sexual problems. *Journal of Sex Education and Therapy, 2,* 1–15.

Anttila, T., et al. (2003). Serotypes of *Chlamydia trachomatis* and risk for development of cervical squamous cell carcinoma. *Journal of the American Medical Association, 285,* 47–51.

Auld, R. B., & Brock, G. (2002). Sexuality and erectile dysfunction: Results of a national survey. *Journal of Sexual & Reproductive Medicine, 2,* 50–54.

Beausang, C. C. (2000). Personal stories of growing up sexually. *Issues in Comprehensive Pediatric Nursing, 23,* 175–192.

Beitz, J. M. (1998). Sexual health promotion in adolescents and young adults: Primary prevention strategies. *Holistic Nursing Practice, 12,* 27–37.

Bernhard, L. A. (2002). Sexuality and sexual health care for women. *Clinical Obstetrics and Gynecology, 45,* 1089–1098.

Beutner, K. R., et al. (1998). External genital warts: Report of the American Medical Association Consensus Conference. AMA Expert Panel on External Genital Warts. *Clinical Infectious Diseases, 27,* 796–806.

Birley, H., et al. (2002). Sexually transmitted diseases: Microbiology and management. *Journal of Medical Microbiology, 51,* 793–807.

Bohn, D., & Holz, K. (1996). Sequelae of abuse: Health effects of childhood sexual abuse, domestic battering, and rape. *Journal of Nurse-Midwifery, 41*(6), 442–456.

Butcher, J. (1999a). ABC of sexual health: Female sexual problems. I: Loss of desire—What about the fun? *British Medical Journal, 318,* 41–43.

Butcher, J. (1999b). ABC of sexual health: Female sexual problems. II: Sexual pain and sexual fears. *British Medical Journal, 318,* 110–112.

Canadian Abortion Rights Action League. (2003). *Protecting abortion rights in Canada.* Ottawa, ON: Author.

Canadian Community Health Survey. (2004, June). Retrieved July 7, 2004, from *http://www.statcan.ca/Daily/English/040615/d040615b.htm*

Canadian Institute of Health Information. (2004). *Teen pregnancy, by outcome of pregnancy and age group, count and rate per 1,000 women aged 15 to 19, Canada, provinces and territories, 1998.* Retrieved June 22, 2004, from *http://www.statcan.ca/english/freepub/82-221-XIE/01201/tables/html/P411.htm*

Centre for Infectious Disease Prevention and Control, Population and Public Health Branch, Health Canada. (2002). *Condoms, sexually transmitted infections, safe sex and you.* Ottawa, ON: Health Canada.

Centre for Infectious Disease Prevention and Control, Population and Public Health Branch, Health Canada. (2003). Estimates of HIV prevalence and incidence in Canada, 2002. *Canada Communicable Disease Report, 29,* 197–206.

Cook, R. J., Dickens, B. M., & Fathalla, M. F. (2002). Female genital cutting (mutilation/circumcision): Ethical and legal dimensions. *International Journal of Gynecology & Obstetrics, 79,* 281–287.

de Marquiegui, A., & Huish, M. (1999). ABC of sexual health: A woman's sexual life after an operation. *British Medical Journal, 318,* 178–181.

de Silva, W. P. (1999). ABC of sexual health. Sexual variations. *British Medical Journal, 318,* 654–656.

Department of Gender and Women's Health, Department of Reproductive Health and Research, Family and Community Health, World Health Organization. (2001). *Female genital mutilation: The prevention and the management of the health complications. Policy guidelines for nurses and midwives.* Geneva, Switzerland: World Health Organization.

Dickinson, L. M., et al. (1999). Health-related quality of life and symptom profiles of female survivors of sexual abuse. *Archives of Family Medicine, 8*(1), 35–43.

Division of STD Prevention and Control, Bureau of HIV/AIDS, STI and TB, Centre for Infectious Disease Prevention, Health Canada. (2000). 1998/1999 Canadian sexually transmitted diseases (STD) surveillance report. *Canada Communicable Disease Report, 26*(S6), 1–36.

Dochterman, J. M., & Bulechek, G. M. (Eds.). (2004). *Nursing interventions classification (NIC)* (4th ed.). St. Louis, MO: Mosby.

Eliopoulos, C. (2001). *Gerontological nursing* (5th ed.). Philadelphia: Lippincott Williams & Wilkins.

Engender Health. (2004). *Sexuality and sexual health: Online minicourse.* Retrieved June 25, 2004, from *http://www.engenderhealth.org/res/onc/sexuality/index.html*

Finan, S. F. (1997). Promoting healthy sexuality: Guidelines for the school-age child and adolescent. *The Nurse Practitioner, 22*(11), 62, 65–67, 71–72.

Glass, C., & Soni, B. (1999). ABC of sexual health: Sexual problems of disabled patients. *British Medical Journal, 318,* 518–521.

Gott, C. M. (2001). Sexual activity and risk-taking in later life. *Health & Social Care in the Community, 9,* 72–78.

Government of Canada. (2004, May 18). *Government of Canada proposes access to "morning after pill" without a prescription.* Retrieved June 25, 2004, from *http://www.news.gc.ca/cfmx/CCP/view/en/index.cfm?articleid=86279*

Haroian, L. (2000). Child sexual development. *Electronic Journal of Human Sexuality, 3.* Retrieved August 15, 2004, from *www.ejhs.org*

Health Canada. (2003). *Canadian guidelines for sexual health education* (Cat. No. H39-300/2003E). Ottawa, ON: Community Acquired Infections Division, Centre for Infectious Disease Prevention and Control, Author.

Heath, H., & White, I. (2001). *Challenging sexuality in health care.* Oxford: Blackwell Science.

Heiman, J. R. (2002). Sexual dysfunction: Overview of prevalence, etiological factors, and treatments. *Journal of Sex Research, 39,* 73–78.

Iannotta, J. G. (Ed.). (2002). *Emerging issues in Hispanic health: Summary of a workshop.* Washington, DC: The National Academies Press.

Jewell, D., Tacchi, J., & Donovan, J. (2000). Teenage pregnancy: Whose problem is it? *Family Practice, 17,* 522–528.

Johnson, O. S. (2004). *The sexual spectrum: Exploring human diversity.* Vancouver, BC: Raincoast Books.

Keller M., et al. (1996). Adolescents' views of sexual decision-making, *Image: The Journal of Nursing Scholarship, 28*(2), 125.

Kenney J.W, Reinholtz C.O,, & Angelini P.O. (1998). Sexual abuse, sex before age 16, and high-risk behaviors of young females with sexually transmitted diseases, *Journal of Obstetric, Gynecologic, and Neonatal Nursing, 27*(1), 54.

Liao, L. M. (2003). Learning to assist women born with atypical genitalia: Journey through ignorance, taboo and dilemma. *Journal of Reproductive and Infant Psychology, 21,* 229–238.

Lueckenotte, A. G. (2000). *Gerontologic nursing* (2nd ed.). St. Louis, MO: Mosby.

MacLaren, A. (1995). Primary care for women: Comprehensive sexual health assessment. *Journal of Nurse-Midwifery, 40*(2), 104–119.

Mayo Foundation for Medical Education and Research. (2004). *Sex during pregnancy.* Retrieved June 25, 2004, from *http://www.mayoclinic.com/invoke.cfm?id=HO00140*

McIlhaney, J. S. (2000). Sexually transmitted infection and teenage sexuality. *American Journal of Obstetrics and Gynecology, 183,* 334–338.

Mindel, A. (1998). Genital herpes—How much of a public-health problem? *Lancet, 351*(Suppl. 3), 16–18.

Moorhead, S., Johnson, M., & Maas, M. (Eds.). (2004). *Nursing outcomes classification (NOC)* (3rd ed.). St. Louis, MO: Mosby.

National Institute of Allergy and Infectious Diseases, National Institutes of Health, U.S. Department of Health and Human Services. (2003). *An introduction to sexually transmitted infections.* Retrieved January 12, 2005, from *http://www.niaid.nih.gov/factsheets/stdinfo.htm*

Nusbaum, M. R., Hamilton, C., & Lenahan, P. (2003). Chronic illness and sexual functioning. *American Family Physician, 67,* 347–354.

Palacios, S., Tobar, A. C., & Menendez, C. (2002). Sexuality in the climacteric years. *Maturitas, 43*(Suppl. 1), S69–S77.

Pangman, V. C., & Seguire, M. (2000). Sexuality and the chronically ill older adult: A social justice issue. *Sexuality and Disability, 18,* 49–59.

Pettinato, A., & Emans, S. J. (2003). New contraceptive methods: Update 2003. *Current Opinion in Pediatrics, 15,* 362–369.

Planned Parenthood Federation of Canada. (2004a). *Contraception.* Retrieved June 25, 2004, from *http://www.ppfc.ca/ppfc/content.asp?articleid=248*

Planned Parenthood Federation of Canada. (2004b). *Sexually transmitted infections (STIs).* Retrieved June 25, 2004, from *http://www.ppfc.ca/ppfc/content.asp?articleid=70*

Riley A. (1999). Sex in old age: continuing pleasure or inevitable decline? *Geriatric Medicine, 29*(3), 25.

Ross, M. W., Channon-Little, L. D., & Rosser, B. R. (2000). *Sexual health concerns: Interviewing and history taking for health practitioners* (2nd ed.). Philadelphia: F. A. Davis.

Running, A., & Berndt, A. (2003). *Management guidelines for nurse practitioners working in family practice.* Philadelphia: F. A. Davis.

Society for Human Sexuality. (2004). *Guide to safe sex.* Retrieved June 25, 2004, from *http://www.sexuality.org/safesex.html*

United Nations Population Fund and Population Reference Bureau. (2003). *Country profiles for population and reproductive health: Policy developments and indicators 2003.* New York, NY: Author.

Vilain, E. (2004, April 19). Commentary: Gender blender: Intersexual? Transsexual? Male, female aren't so easy to define. *Los Angeles Times.*

von Sydow, K. (1999). Sexuality during pregnancy and after childbirth: A metacontent analysis of 59 studies. *Journal of Psychosomatic Research, 47,* 27–49.

Recommended Web Sites

Public Health Agency of Canada:
http://www.phac-aspc.gc.ca/publicat/cgshe-ldnemss/

Canadian Guidelines for Sexual Health Education, a publication developed by Health Canada in collaboration with sexual health experts, provides information for health care professionals and others to develop and improve sexual health education policies and programs that address the diverse needs of Canadians.

Public Health Agency of Canada:
http://www.phac-aspc.gc.ca/std-mts/

Sexual Health and Sexually Transmitted Infections works with provinces, non-governmental organizations, and health care providers to improve and maintain the sexual health and well-being of Canadians. The site offers links to sexual health and sexually transmitted infection information, publications, and resources.

Sunnybrook and Women's College Health Sciences Centre:
http://www.womenshealthmatters.ca/centres/sex/index.html

Developed by Sunnybrook and Women's College Health Sciences Centre and the Centre for Research in Women's Health, this site provides information about women's sexual matters, including sexual expression, how female bodies work, pregnancy, birth control, abortion, and safer sex.

24

Spiritual Health

Patricia A. Potter, RN, MSN, PhD, CMAC, FAAN
Sonya Grypma, RN, PhD (Canadian author)

Objectives

Mastery of content in this chapter will enable the student to:

- Define the key terms listed.
- Discuss research findings that suggest spiritual practices influence clients' health status.
- Describe the relationship between faith, hope, and spiritual well-being.
- Discuss theoretical foundations for spiritual care.
- Compare and contrast the concepts of religion and spirituality.
- Perform an assessment of a client's spirituality.
- Explain how a nurse's caring relationship with clients affects their ability to gain spiritual insight.
- Discuss barriers and bridges to spiritual intervention in nursing care.
- Discuss nursing interventions designed to promote spiritual health.
- Evaluate attainment of spiritual health.

The word **spirituality** derives from the Latin word *spiritus,* which refers to breath or wind. The spirit gives life to, or animates, a person. It signifies whatever is at the centre of all aspects of a person's life (Dombeck, 1995). A person's health depends on a balance of physical, psychological, sociological, cultural, developmental, and spiritual factors. Friedemann, Mouch, and Racey (2002) defined spirituality as the act of connecting to systems such as God, nature, or other people to find meaning through relationships. Spirituality can be the important factor that helps individuals achieve the balance needed to maintain health and well-being and to cope with illness.

Spirituality is a highly personal matter. Caring for a client's spiritual needs means caring for the whole person, accepting his or her beliefs and experiences, and helping the client with issues surrounding meaning and hope (Childe, 2002). Being able to determine the importance spirituality holds for clients depends on a nurse's ability to develop a caring relationship (see chapter 15).

Nurses must recognize spirituality in their clients and be aware of their own spirituality in order to provide appropriate spiritual care. Expert nurses help clients use their spiritual resources as they identify what is meaningful in their lives and cope with the impact of illness and life stressors.

Scientific Knowledge Base

Research shows an association between spirituality and health. There may be beneficial health outcomes when individuals engage their beliefs in a higher power and sense a source of strength or support. The healing power of prayer may lower blood pressure (Koenig et al., 1997), reduce stress before surgery (Saudia et al., 1991), enhance cancer treatment (Lambe et al., 1996), or relieve depression and improve the immune status of clients with AIDS (Adair et al., 1991; Carson and Green, 1992). Prayer and meditation are frequently used as methods for coping and minimizing physical stressors. For example, meditation is successful in treating chronic pain, insomnia, anxiety, and depression (Culligan, 1996). Prayer is beneficial for clients and has also been found to be beneficial for nurses. A study of 1,000 nurses found that nurses used prayer to enhance their professional performance (Cavenish et al., 2004).

There is a link between mind, body, and spirit; however, the relationship is not clearly understood. Nevertheless, studies show that an individual's beliefs and expectations can and do have effects on the person's physical well-being (Coe, 1997). For example, recent Canadian studies showed that spirituality influences health for Orthodox Jewish women during child-bearing years (Semenic, Callister, & Feldman, 2004), mental health inpatients (Baetz et al., 2002), and informal caregivers of elderly and disabled clients (Sawatzky & Fowler-Kerry, 2003). A nurse will be more successful in helping clients achieve desirable health outcomes after learning to support clients and families spiritually as well as mentally and physically.

Nursing Knowledge Base

Historical Perspectives

Nursing has a rich spiritual heritage. Spirituality was at the core of early nursing philosophies and practice until the 19th century (McSherry, 2001). Organized nursing grew out of religious orders, where nuns were primarily responsible for providing nursing care. In Canada, the earliest nurses belonged to Roman Catholic orders devoted to care of the sick—most notably the Sisters of Charity of Montreal (Grey Nuns) founded by Marie Marguerite d'Youville in 1737 (Paul, 2000). This non-cloistered order was responsible for bringing a Judeo-Christian model of nursing to the most remote areas of western and northern Canada. Religion provided a lens through which to acknowledge spiritual needs, express spiritual care, and pursue spiritual health.

Florence Nightingale's ideas of modern nursing were first taught in London in 1860. Her model of Western nursing, rooted in Christianity, was spread around the world during the colonial era (Paul, 2000). Canadian missionary nurses were among those British subjects who brought modern nursing to India, Japan, Korea, and China at the turn of the 20th century (Grypma, 2004). For many people, the concepts of spirituality and religion were linked, and until the 1970s, nurses used the terms interchangeably (Taylor, 2002).

In the 20th century, confidence in religion was replaced by confidence in medical science. By the 1970s, nursing had evolved from a religious vocation to an increasingly secular profession. Spirituality, associated with religion, was devalued. Over time, the general public became dissatisfied with a purely medical approach to care, partly because there was a growing realization that science does not possess all the answers to existential questions raised by clients (McSherry, 2001). Nurses felt a spiritual gap in the profession and began to find ways to articulate and incorporate spirituality into practice and research. Spirituality was conceptualized as broader and more encompassing than any particular religion or culture. Between 1980 and 2000, renewed interest in spirituality was reflected by an increase in related literature in nursing, as well as a growing interest in parish nursing as a way for faith communities in Canada to reclaim their healing mission (Olson, Simington & Clark, 1998). At present, clients and caregivers are looking to nurses as leaders in spiritual care because of nursing's unique spiritual heritage and continual presence at the centre of health care delivery (McSherry, 2001).

Theoretical Perspectives

Many nursing theorists describe clients as bio-psycho-social-spiritual beings, and most advocate holistic care (Barnum, 2003; Taylor, 2002). Those who advocate holistic care typically identify spirituality as an aspect of nursing care. The concept that humans are multi-dimensional beings is still used as a basis for nursing models today (Figure 24–1).

Several theoretical nursing models have identified spirituality as an aspect of nursing practice (Taylor, 2002):

- Virginia Henderson (*The Nature of Nursing,* 1966) identified three nursing abilities that are related to spirituality: ability to express feelings and thoughts, ability to play and recreate, ability to learn and satisfy curiosity. *Spiritual care could entail assisting clients to worship or pursue recreational activities.*
- Joyce Travelbee (Human-to-human relationship model, 1971) portrayed nursing as an interpersonal process involving preventing, alleviating, or helping individuals/families/communities find meaning in illness or suffering. Witnessing or assisting clients through experiences like illness give nurses opportunities to create meaning. *Spiritual care could entail instilling meaning and hope through verbal communication.*
- Jean Watson (Theory of human caring, 1999) recognized a societal need for the universal, mysterious, and powerful forces of love and care. Human caring is a spiritual act that assists clients to achieve a greater sense of self as well as harmony with body, mind, and soul. *Spiritual care could entail connecting with a client through therapeutic presence, communication, silence, or movement.*
- Betty Neuman (Systems model, 1995) maintained that each person or group constitutes a system of physiological, psychological, sociological, cultural, developmental, and spiritual variables that exist along a developmental continuum. The spiritual continuum can range from lack of awareness or denial to a highly developed spiritual consciousness. *Spiritual care could entail assisting clients to identify goals, increase spiritual awareness, and access spiritual resources.*

Nursing theories are broad and encompassing, and are meant to be adapted for use in a variety of areas of nursing practice. *Nursing frameworks* are more specific, describing ways in which spirituality can be incorporated into care of culturally diverse clients (Andrews & Boyle, 1999) or families (Friedemann, 1995). *Nursing models* may be expressly geared to spiritual caregiving, providing guidelines to a particular group of nurses (such as Christian or parish nurses) or a particular practice setting (such as a faith community; M. B. Clark & Olson, 2000; O'Brien, 2003; Shelly, 2000). Nursing theories are not meant to address practical specifics about spiritual caregiving. Rather, they serve to establish a system of assumptions and principles that nurses can use to guide their practice. Nurses may draw from more than one theory to develop effective approaches to client care (Taylor, 2002).

Traditional Concepts in Spiritual Health

A variety of concepts are used to describe spiritual health. To provide meaningful and supportive spiritual care, a nurse must understand the concepts of spirituality, faith,

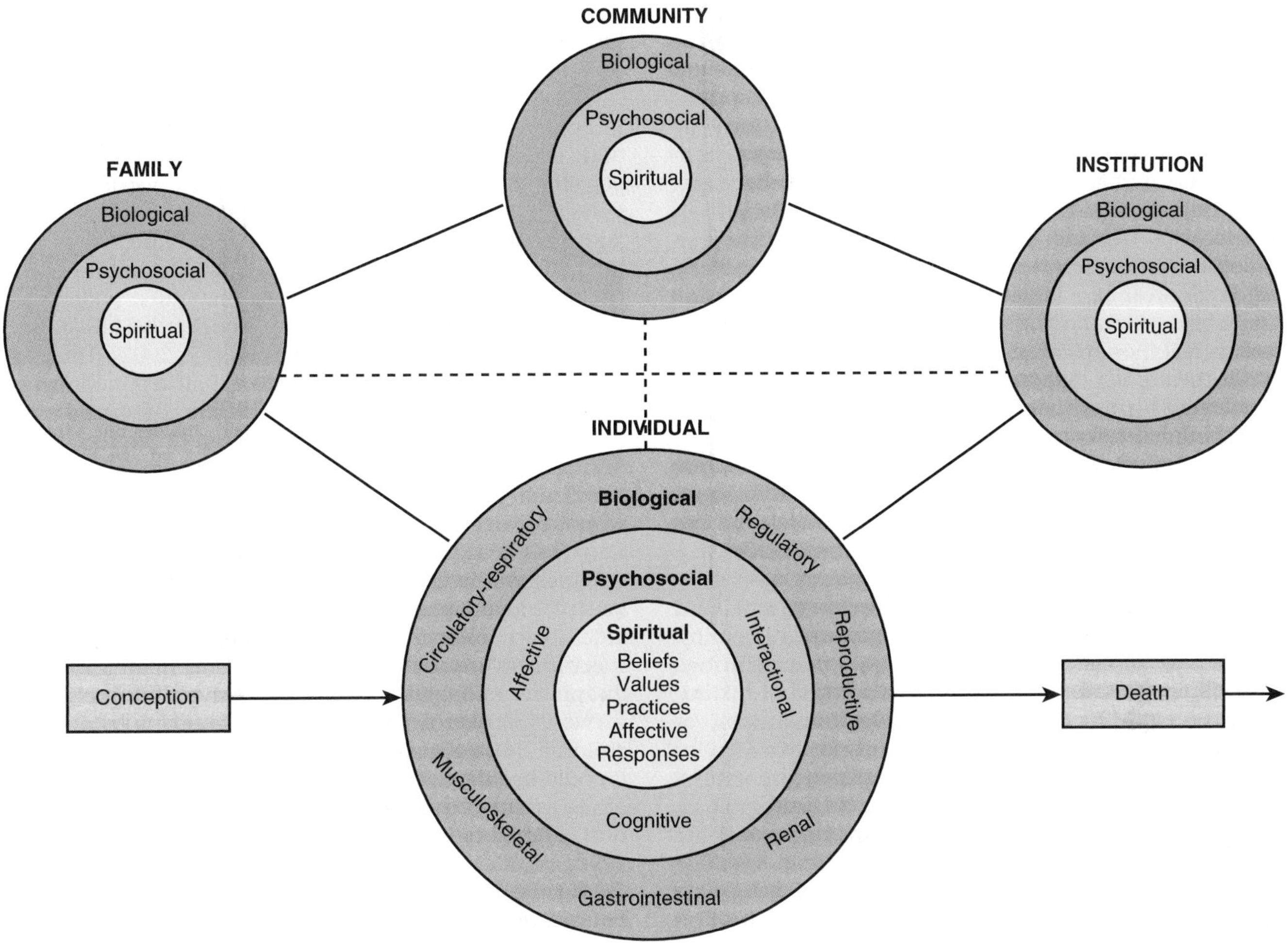

FIGURE **24–1** Model of spiritual relationships. (Adapted from Stallwood & Stoll, in *The Intersystem Model,* p. 5, by B. M. Artinian and M. M. Conger, 1997, Thousand Oaks, CA: Sage.)

religion, and hope. Each concept offers direction in understanding the views that individuals have of life and its value.

Spirituality. Spirituality is a concept that is unique to each individual and dependent on a person's culture, development, life experiences, beliefs, and ideas about life. An individual's spirituality enables the person to love, have faith and hope, seek meaning in life, and nurture relationships with others. Spirituality offers a sense of connectedness intrapersonally (connected within oneself), interpersonally (connected with others and the environment), and transpersonally (connected with the unseen, God, or a higher power). The notion of "relationship" is central to the concept of spirituality in nursing.

Spiritual well-being is a state of wholeness or health in which a person has a sense of connection with others and dwells in peace in relationships. Spiritual health is achieved when people find a balance between their life values, goals, and belief systems and their relationship within themselves and with others. **Spiritual care** involves facilitating relationships, assisting clients to transcend the current situation for higher meaning and purpose, providing hope, and allowing individuals to experience connectedness with others (McEwen, 2004).

Spirituality begins as children learn about themselves and their relationships with others. Children's ideas of a higher power or supreme being are often based on what is presented to them in their homes or religious community. Adolescents may reconsider their child-like concept of a spiritual power and, in the search for an identity, may question values and practices. Canadian teens and young adults who have been reared in a religious tradition frequently "drop out" of their religious system as they search for a personalized belief system and seek a clearer meaning to life (Bibby, 2002).

Many adults experience spiritual growth by entering into lifelong relationships. An ability to care meaningfully for others and the self is evidence of a healthy spirituality. Older adults often turn to important relationships and the giving of themselves to others as spiritual tasks. As people mature, they often turn inward to enduring values and to a concept of a supreme being or a higher meaning that has been sustaining and meaningful. A healthy spirituality in older adults is one that gives peace and acceptance of the self and that is often based on a lifelong relationship with a supreme being. Illness and loss can threaten and challenge the spiritual developmental process or can precipitate a spiritual crisis. Nurses can help clients cope with the spiritual health concerns triggered by critical events (Meyerhoff et al., 2002). It thus becomes important for the nurse to understand the nature and status of a client's belief system and spiritual health.

There are individuals who either do not believe in the existence of God **(atheist)** or who believe that any ultimate reality is unknown **(agnostic).** Agnostics believe that the existence of a God or higher power cannot be proven or disproved. This does not mean that spirituality is not an important concept for the atheist or agnostic. Atheists search for meaning in life through their work and their relationships with other individuals (Burnard, 1988). Because atheists feel they are alone, they sense a strong responsibility for themselves. They also tend to believe in a joint responsibility for others. In acting for themselves, they feel they should also act for all of humankind (Burnard, 1988). It is important for agnostics to discover meaning in what they do or how they live. Because agnostics find no ultimate meaning for the way things are, they believe that we as people bring meaning to what we do (Burnard, 1988).

Faith. Spirituality enables one to love, have faith and hope, seek meaning in life, and nurture relationships. The concept of faith is described in the literature in two ways. In the first, faith is defined as a cultural or institutional religion, such as Judaism, Buddhism, Islam, or Christianity. Second, **faith** is a relationship with a divinity, higher power, authority, or spirit that incorporates a reasoning faith (belief) and a trusting faith (action; D. G. Benner, 1985). Reasoning faith is an individual's belief and confidence in something for which there is no proof. Sometimes that involves a belief in a higher power, spirit guide, God, or Allah (Fryback, 1993). However, faith also might be the manner in which a person chooses to live life. Faith in this sense enables action. For example, a person might believe that having a positive outlook on life is the best way to achieve life's goals.

The belief that comes with faith involves **transcendence,** or an awareness of that which one cannot see or know in ordinary physical ways (Reed, 1987). It gives purpose and meaning to an individual's life, allowing for action. For example, clients with cancer who have faith in a positive outlook on life might pursue more knowledge about their disease and continue to pursue daily activities rather than resign themselves to the disease's symptoms. Hall (1998) studied clients diagnosed with human immunodeficiency virus (HIV) and found that spirituality frames individuals' lives. Individuals become open to discover their unique spiritual meaning after a crisis that threatens health. Their faith becomes strengthened, and they are better able to go on with life and engage in activities that fit the new definition of their selves.

Religion. Many people use the terms *religion* and *spirituality* interchangeably. Although closely associated, these terms are not synonymous. **Religion** is an organized system of beliefs concerning the cause, nature, and purpose of the universe, especially belief in or the worship of God or gods (Andrews & Boyle, 1999). It is a structured search for the spiritual and an outward expression of spirituality (Emblen, 1992). Religious practice encompasses spirituality, but spirituality need not include religious practice. Whereas the aim of religious care is to help clients maintain their belief systems and worship practices, the aim of spiritual care is to facilitate spiritual health (Taylor, 2002).

Spirituality is informed by, and expressed through, both culture and religion. **Culture** represents a way of perceiving, behaving, and evaluating the world. It provides a blueprint or guide for determining values, beliefs, and practices (Andrews & Boyle, 1999). A person's spiritual nature may be expressed in religious and philosophical beliefs and practices, and these may differ widely depending on the person's race, gender, social status, religion, ethnicity, and experience (Taylor, 2002). Thus, although nurses may make an intellectual distinction between spirituality and religion or culture, the boundaries are much less distinct in actual experience (Macrae, 2001).

Organized religion can provide a framework for understanding the meaning of existence and a structure for worship. According to a national survey, 88% of Canadian adults and 80% of teens describe themselves as religious (Bibby, 2002). There is considerable religious diversity and there are many geographic regions that provide health care to multi-faith users. Pluralism and respect for diversity is highly valued. Canadians generally disapprove of religious groups aggressively attempting to convert others, particularly vulnerable people such as children, immigrants, and the elderly (Bibby, 2002), and, it could be added, the sick. In nursing, it is never appropriate to proselytize, impose one's own religious orientation, or discriminate based on religion (Shelly & Miller, 1999; W. R. Miller & Thoresen, 2003). Confusion over the difference between proselytizing and spiritual care is one reason nurses give for hesitating to discuss spiritual concerns with their clients (Vance, 2001). The Canadian Nurses Association code of ethics and an ethic of caring (see chapter 7) provide guidelines for nurses. Generally, it is important to ensure that client's choices are honoured and their vulnerabilities are not exploited.

Hope. Spirituality is a key element in hope. When a person has the attitude of something to live for and look forward to, hope is present. **Hope** is a multi-dimensional concept that provides comfort while enduring life threats and personal challenges (Morse & Doberneck, 1995). Hope is also closely associated with faith. It is energizing, giving individuals a motivation to achieve and the resources to use toward that achievement. People express hope in all aspects of their lives to help them deal with life stressors. Hope is an invaluable personal resource whenever someone is faced with a loss (see chapter 25) or a challenge that seems difficult to achieve. Morse and Doberneck (1995) conducted research with four groups of clients: heart transplant recipients, spinal cord injured clients, breast cancer survivors, and breast-feeding mothers intending to continue nursing while employed. Their research identified seven concepts of hope: an initial assessment of threat, envisioning of options and setting goals, preparing for negative outcomes, assessing for resources, seeking out supportive relationships, evaluating signs that reinforce goals, and determining to endure. Thus, hope can be a complex and unique concept for each individual.

Spiritual Challenges

When illness, loss, grief, or a major life change affects a person, either spiritual resources help a person move to recovery or spiritual needs and concerns develop. **Spiritual distress** is the disruption of an individual's "life principle," which fills the person's entire being and transcends or exceeds one's biological and psychosocial nature (North American Nursing Diagnosis Association [NANDA], 2003). A catastrophic illness, for example, can upset a person's spiritual well-being sufficiently to cause doubt and loss of faith. Spiritual distress may cause the person to feel alone or even abandoned. Individuals may question their spiritual values, raising questions about their way of life and purpose for living. Spiritual distress also occurs when a person's beliefs conflict with prescribed treatment or when the person is unable to practice rituals.

Acute Illness. Sudden, unexpected illness can create significant spiritual distress. For example, both the 50-year-old man who has a heart attack and the 20-year-old who is a victim of a motor vehicle accident face crises that may threaten their spiritual health. The illness or injury creates an unanticipated scramble to integrate and cope with new realities (e.g., disability). People look for ways to remain faithful to their beliefs and value systems. They may pray, attend religious services, or reflect on the positive aspects of their lives. Often conflicts can develop around a person's beliefs and the meaning of life. Anger is not uncommon, and clients may express it against God, their families, themselves, or the nurse.

The strength of clients' spirituality influences how they cope with sudden illness and how quickly they recover. Yim and Vande Creek (1996) developed a spiritual healing critical pathway for coronary artery bypass clients. Their research has shown that knowledge of clients' spiritual well-being can be used to maximize their recovery. Hope and the ability to speak about life values help the individual gain meaning from illness and influence recovery from heart surgery. The pathway identifies clients' spiritual recovery and recommends interventions that help clients find purpose and worth to recover.

Chronic Illness. People with chronic illness often suffer debilitating symptoms that change their lifestyles. A symptom is more than a signal for a persistent health problem or a clue for diagnosing a disease. A symptom can give a person permission to take needed rest, be a sign of impending disruption, or even raise feelings about the person's self-worth and strength (P. Benner and Wrubel, 1989). Symptoms are meaningful to the individual, and that meaning is shaped by the person's history and the current context of the illness.

With chronic illness, independence can be threatened, causing fear, anxiety, and dispiritedness. Dependence on others can create a feeling of powerlessness. A person may feel a loss of a sense of purpose in life that affects the inner strength needed to deal with alterations in functioning. A person's spirituality can influence how he or she adapts to changes resulting from chronic illness. Successful adaptation can strengthen a person spiritually. A re-evaluation of life may occur. Those who use their spiritual resources are better able to re-establish a self-identity and live to their potential.

Terminal Illness. Terminal illness commonly causes fears of physical pain, isolation, the unknown, and dying (Turner et al., 1995). However, when people experience periods of disease remission, they may become asymptomatic for long periods of time and put off the idea of illness and death. Terminal illness creates an uncertainty about what death means and thus may cause spiritual distress. However, some clients have a spiritual peace that enables them to face death without fear. Hall (1998) interviewed 10 men and women in advanced-stage HIV disease who reported having spiritual or religious experiences that had helped them cope. These individuals discovered a unique spiritual meaning after a health crisis. Living with HIV required clearing one's life of the stressful existence, problematic relationships, and social memberships that did not work. Spirituality helped them find peace in themselves and their death.

Individuals experiencing a terminal illness examine their life and question its meaning. Common questions asked include "Why is this happening to me?" or "What have I done?" Family and friends can be affected just as much as the client. Terminal illness causes family members to ask important questions about its meaning and how it will affect their relationship with the client (see chapter 25).

Fryback (1993) conducted a study to learn how people with a terminal illness describe health. Clients in the study identified the following three domains of health: mental/emotional, spiritual, and physical (Figure 24–2).

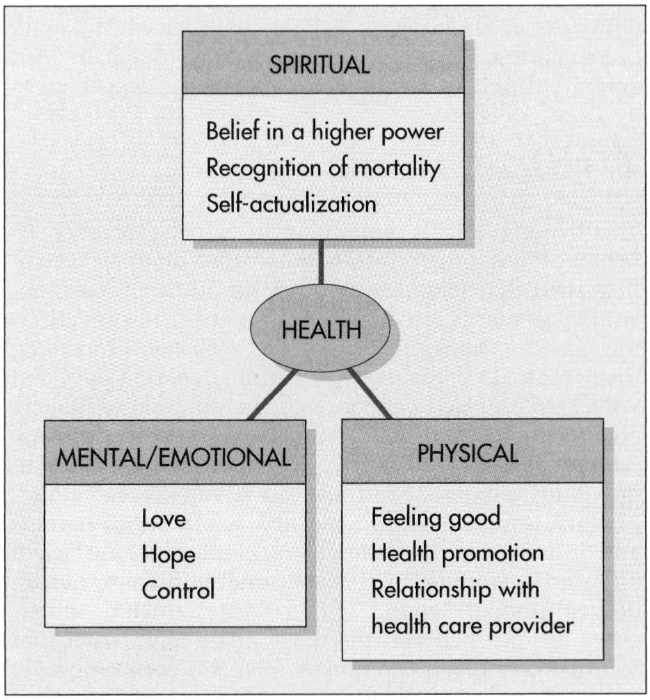

FIGURE 24–2 Domains of health based on perceptions of terminally ill clients. (Adapted from "Health for People With a Terminal Diagnosis," by P. B. Fryback, 1993, *Nursing Science Quarterly, 6*[3], p. 147.)

The spiritual domain was seen as being essential for health and included having a relationship with a higher power, recognizing mortality, and striving for self-actualization. Although many of the participants in the study either attended church or stated a desire to do so, others found that spirituality was not dependent on a religion or church. They associated health with belief in a higher power that gave them faith and the ability to love (Fryback, 1993). The study revealed that when terminally ill clients have a perception of being unhealthy, it is not due to the disease but to being unable to live their lives fully and do the things they desire.

Near-Death Experience. Nurses may care for clients who have had a near-death experience (NDE). An NDE is a psychological phenomenon of people who either have been close to clinical death or may have recovered after being declared dead. It is not associated with a mental disorder (Basford, 1990). People who experience an NDE after cardiopulmonary arrest, for example, often tell the same story of feeling themselves rising above their bodies and watching caregivers initiate lifesaving measures. Most individuals describe passing through a tunnel to a bright light, encountering loved ones who had died, and feeling an inner tranquility and peace. Instead of moving toward the light, they learn it is not time for them to die and they return to life.

Clients who have an NDE are often reluctant to discuss it, thinking family or caregivers will not understand. Isolation and depression can occur. However, individuals experiencing an NDE who can discuss it with family or caregivers find acceptance and meaning from this powerful experience. They consistently report positive after-effects, including a positive attitude and spiritual development (Turner et al., 1995). After a client has survived cardiopulmonary arrest, it is important for the nurse to remain open and give the client a chance to explore what happened.

Critical Thinking

The helping role is important in nursing practice (P. Benner, 1984). Clients look to nurses for a different kind of help than that sought from other health care professionals. Expert nurses can anticipate the personal issues affecting clients' abilities to receive and seek help, including their spiritual well-being. Critical thinking knowledge and skills help a nurse to enhance clients' spiritual well-being and health. While using the nursing process, the nurse applies knowledge, experience, attitudes, and standards in providing appropriate spiritual care (Figure 24–3).

Nursing research has identified a number of barriers and bridges to spiritual caregiving. Barriers include lack of knowledge, confidence, time, personal spiritual resources, or institutional support. Other barriers include differences of faith between the nurse and client, belief that spiritual care is not the nurse's role, and confusion over proselytizing versus spiritual care (Grant, 2004; Louis and Alpert, 2000; McSherry, 1998; Vance, 2001). Key elements acting as bridges include nurses' readiness and preparation, recognition of client/family cues of spiritual concerns, experience in spiritual intervention, and ability to pray (Van Dover & Bacon, 2001).

Knowledge about spirituality begins with nurses' insight about their own spirituality. Friedemann et al. (2002) believe it is important that nurses experience a self-exploration through reading, religious involvement, or activities such as meditation to understand their own beliefs and values. Applying knowledge of spiritual concepts, principles of caring (see chapter 15), and therapeutic communication skills (see chapter 14) enables a nurse to recognize and understand a client's spiritual needs. Personal experience in caring for clients in spiritual distress can be invaluable in helping each new client to examine coping options, test values, and try out new behaviours.

A client's spirituality is unique, and thus a nurse must apply critical thinking in order to determine whether intervention is necessary and how to sensitively provide spiritual care. Applying intellectual standards enables the nurse to help clients acquire spiritual healing. It is particularly important in giving spiritual care to apply sound ethical standards. For example, interventions such as relaxation exercises or meditation can be coercive and/or unethical if they are routinely prescribed without considering the clients' individual needs and interests (Friedemann et al., 2002). An ethic of caring (see chapter 7) provides nurses with a framework for decision making. A client's spiritual beliefs may influence choice of therapy and cause conflict with professionals. An ethic of care places the nurse as the client's advocate, working through ethical dilemmas by attending to relationships and honouring the client's personal choices.

Spiritual Health and the Nursing Process

At the core of nursing is a commitment to caring and respect for an individual's uniqueness. In the case of spirituality, it is even more important for the nurse to respect each client's personal beliefs. Fundamental differences exist in the ways in which people experience the world and find meaning in that experience (Martsolf & Mickley, 1998). There is a danger that any blanket application of a concept of spirituality will be equally disrespectful to the views of clients who embrace a broadly religious view of the world and of those who adopt a more secular (nonreligious) orientation.

Application of the nursing process from the perspective of a client's spiritual needs is not simple. It goes beyond assessing a client's religious practices. Understanding a client's spirituality and then appropriately identifying the level of support and resources needed requires a new, broader perspective. Heliker (1992) described the importance of shared compassion and community. *Compassion* comes from the Latin words *pati* and *cum,* meaning "to suffer with." *Community* is derived from the Latin word meaning "fellowship." To be compassionate is to "enter into places of pain, to share in brokenness with other human beings" (Heliker, 1992). To practise compassion as a nurse requires awareness of the very human tie between clients and a healing community. This kind of work will generally consist of quiet conversations, effective listening, and communication through presence and touch (Draper & McSherry, 2002).

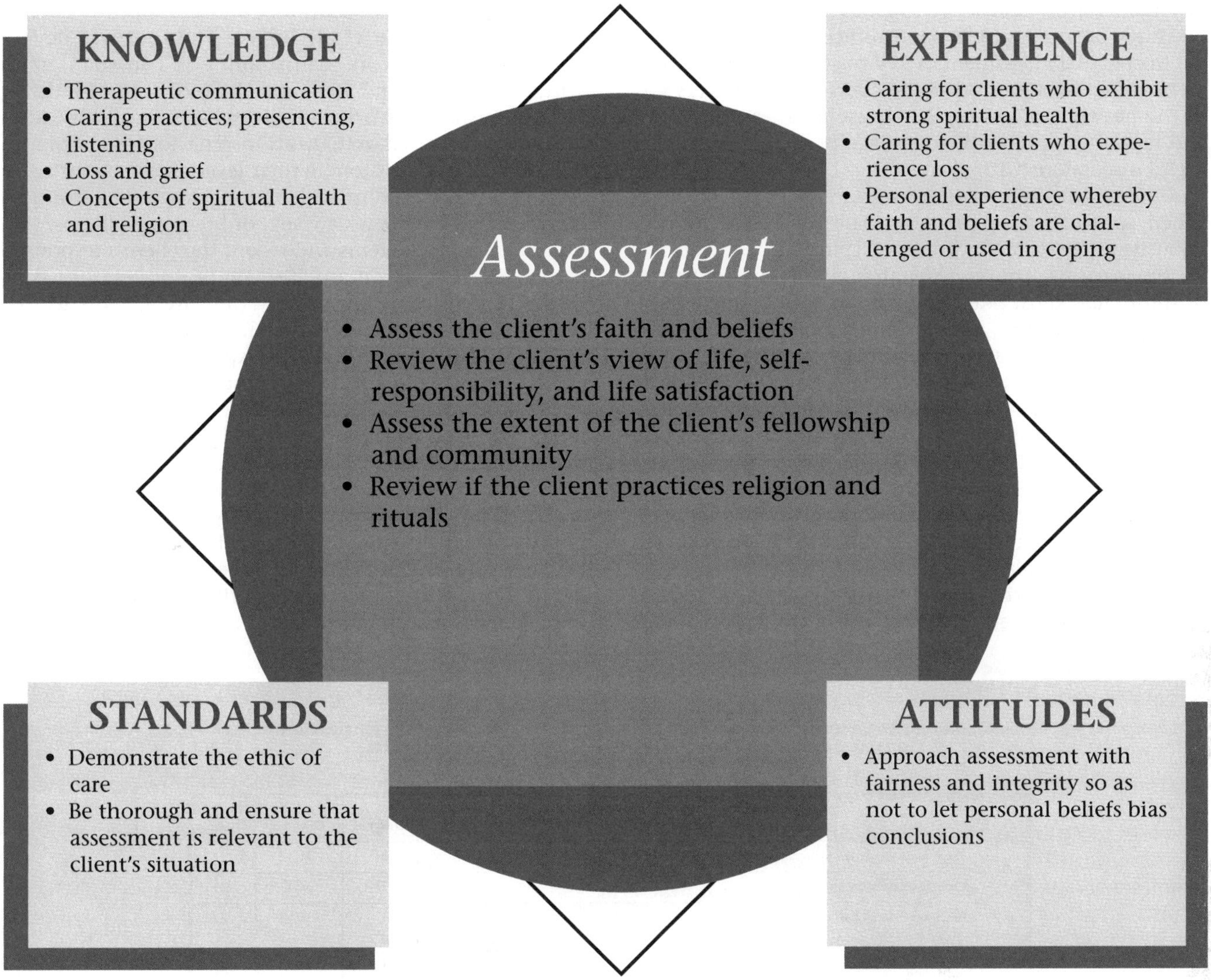

KNOWLEDGE
• Therapeutic communication
• Caring practices; presencing, listening
• Loss and grief
• Concepts of spiritual health and religion
EXPERIENCE
• Caring for clients who exhibit strong spiritual health
• Caring for clients who experience loss
• Personal experience whereby faith and beliefs are challenged or used in coping
Assessment
• Assess the client's faith and beliefs
• Review the client's view of life, self-responsibility, and life satisfaction
• Assess the extent of the client's fellowship and community
• Review if the client practices religion and rituals
STANDARDS
• Demonstrate the ethic of care
• Be thorough and ensure that assessment is relevant to the client's situation
ATTITUDES
• Approach assessment with fairness and integrity so as not to let personal beliefs bias conclusions

FIGURE **24–3** Critical thinking model for spiritual health assessment.

The nurse must remove from the assessment any personal biases or misconceptions and be willing to share and discover a client's meaning and purpose in life, sickness, and health. One question usually asked on an admission form is the client's "religion." Such a question leaves little doubt that the accepted position is that of a "believer" (Burnard, 1988). It is important for nurses to sort out value judgments about other people's belief systems. Working through values clarification exercises can be helpful (see chapter 7). If nurses are believers, do they judge harshly the unbeliever? If nurses are agnostic or atheist, do they dismiss the believer? Nurses must accept and acknowledge others' beliefs and not try to convert them. A nurse learns to look beyond a personal view when establishing a client relationship. This approach means identifying the common values that make us human and respecting the commitments and values that make humans unique. Love, trust, hope, forgiveness, meaning, and community are spiritual needs we all have. Learning to share these needs helps the nurse find a way to give clients spiritual care and support.

Another important aspect of spiritual care is recognizing that a client may not have a spiritual problem. Clients bring certain spiritual resources that the nurse can engage as resources to help them assume healthier lives, recover from illness, or face impending death. Supporting and recognizing the positive side of a client's spirituality will ensure effective, individualized nursing care.

NP Assessment

The purpose behind a spiritual assessment determines how such assessments are constructed and used. Catterall et al. (1998) suggested a two-stage approach to assessment. The first stage is commonly found in acute care settings, where an initial assessment identifies a client's religious beliefs, affiliations, and practices. This information is important for making referrals to appropriate clergy and attempting to adapt clients' practices (e.g., diet preferences or rituals) into their care. The second stage is a more in-depth assessment for clients who the nurse feels are experiencing or at risk for spiritual distress. With time pressures on nurses, it is often difficult to obtain an in-depth spiritual assessment. A key to success is to conduct an ongoing assessment over the course of the client's stay in the health care setting. The nurse must establish trust and rapport and have the opportunity to conduct meaningful discussions with clients.

Once a trusting relationship with a client is established, spiritual caring can occur. The nurse learns to consciously integrate an attitude of spiritual care into the nursing process. The assessment should focus on aspects of spirituality most likely to be influenced by life experiences, events, illness, and hospitalization. Even conducting an assessment can be therapeutic because it conveys a level of caring and support. Friedemann et al. (2002) noted, "An assessment done well is not simply a collection of data but becomes an intervention." The nurse who understands the overall approach to spiritual assessment can enter into thoughtful discussions with the client and gain a greater awareness of the individual's personal resources. These resources ought to be incorporated into an effective plan of care.

The JAREL spiritual well-being scale (Figure 24–4) provides nurses and other health care professionals with a simple tool for assessing a client's spiritual well-being (Hungelmann et al., 1996). The tool was developed for clients from Christian, non-Christian, and atheist belief systems. Items on the tool comprise three key dimensions: faith/belief, life/self-responsibility, and life satisfaction/self-actualization. The tool is simple to use, requiring clients to rate their level of agreement with each item on a 5-point scale (strongly agree to strongly disagree). For clients with visual or literacy problems, the nurse can read the items and record the client's response. If the client's score on any item, group of items, or particular dimension is low, it may indicate an area to explore further (Hungelmann et al., 1996).

The tool helps the nurse to explore with clients any perceptions or concerns they might have. For example, if a client disagrees about accepting life situations, the nurse will need to learn how the client is accepting and managing an illness. Whether a nurse uses a tool like the JAREL scale or directs an assessment with questions that are based on principles of spirituality, the nurse must not impose personal value systems on the client. This is particularly true when the client's values and beliefs are similar to those of the nurse, as it can then become very easy to make false assumptions.

DIRECTIONS: PLEASE CIRCLE THE CHOICE THAT **BEST** DESCRIBES HOW MUCH YOU AGREE WITH EACH STATEMENT. CIRCLE ONLY **ONE** ANSWER FOR EACH STATEMENT. THERE IS NO RIGHT OR WRONG ANSWER.

		Strongly Agree	Moderately Agree	Agree	Disagree	Moderately Disagree	Strongly Disagree
1.	Prayer is an important part of my life.	SA	MA	A	D	MD	SD
2.	I believe I have spiritual well-being.	SA	MA	A	D	MD	SD
3.	As I grow older, I find myself more tolerant of others' beliefs.	SA	MA	A	D	MD	SD
4.	I find meaning and purpose in my life.	SA	MA	A	D	MD	SD
5.	I feel there is a close relationship between my spiritual beliefs and what I do.	SA	MA	A	D	MD	SD
6.	I believe in an afterlife.	SA	MA	A	D	MD	SD
7.	When I am sick I have less spiritual well-being.	SA	MA	A	D	MD	SD
8.	I believe in a supreme power.	SA	MA	A	D	MD	SD
9.	I am able to receive and give love to others.	SA	MA	A	D	MD	SD
10.	I am satisfied with my life.	SA	MA	A	D	MD	SD
11.	I set goals for myself.	SA	MA	A	D	MD	SD
12.	God has little meaning in my life.	SA	MA	A	D	MD	SD
13.	I am satisfied with the way I am using my abilities.	SA	MA	A	D	MD	SD
14.	Prayer does not help me in making decisions.	SA	MA	A	D	MD	SD
15.	I am able to appreciate differences in others.	SA	MA	A	D	MD	SD
16.	I am pretty well put together.	SA	MA	A	D	MD	SD
17.	I prefer that others make decisions for me.	SA	MA	A	D	MD	SD
18.	I find it hard to forgive others.	SA	MA	A	D	MD	SD
19.	I accept my life situations.	SA	MA	A	D	MD	SD
20.	Belief in a supreme being has no part in my life.	SA	MA	A	D	MD	SD
21.	I cannot accept change in my life.	SA	MA	A	D	MD	SD

FIGURE **24–4** JAREL spiritual well-being scale. (From "Focus on Spiritual Well-Being: Harmonious Interconnectedness of Mind-Body-Spirit—Use of the JAREL Spiritual Well-Being Scale," by J. Hungelmann et al., 1996, *Geriatric Nursing, 17*[6]. Copyright 1987 by J Hungelmann, E Kenkel-Rossi, L Klassen, R Stollenwerk, Marquette University College of Nursing, Milwaukee, WI.)

Faith/Belief. Each individual has some source of authority and guidance in his or her life. It is that inner voice or outer authority that leads people to choose and act on their beliefs. The authority can be a supreme being, a code of conduct, a specific religious leader, family or friends, oneself, or a combination of sources. Faith in an authority provides a sense of confidence that guides a person in exercising beliefs and experiencing growth. Knowing a client's sources of strength and faith can direct interactions with them. The nurse can assess a person's faith in an authority by asking, "To what or whom do you look as a source of strength or faith in life?" or "What is your personal source of strength or hope?"

The nurse determines if the client has a religious source of guidance that conflicts with medical treatment plans. This conflict can seriously affect the options that nurses and other health care providers can offer clients. For example, if a client looks to the Jehovah's Witnesses as a source of authority, blood products cannot be accepted as a form of treatment. Christian Scientists often refuse any medical intervention because they believe that their faith will heal them.

It is also important to understand a client's philosophy of life (Semenic et al., 2004; Box 24-1). Asking the client, "Tell me what is most important in your life" or "Tell me what gives your life meaning," may help to assess what is the basis of the client's belief system regarding meaning and purpose in life. This information reveals the client's spiritual focus and may help to reflect the impact that illness, loss, or disability has on the person's life. Depending on a client's religious practices, views about health and the response to illness may influence how nurses provide support (Table 24-1).

Life and Self-Responsibility. Spiritual well-being includes life and self-responsibility (Hungelmann et al., 1996). Individuals who can accept change in life, make decisions about their lives, and forgive others in times of difficulty have a higher level of spiritual well-being. During illness, clients often are unable to accept limitations or know what to do to regain a functional and meaningful life. Their sense of helplessness may reflect spiritual distress. However, if clients are able to adapt to changes and seek solutions for how to deal with any limitations, spiritual well-being reflects an important coping resource. The nurse assesses whether clients understand the limitations or threats posed by an illness and the manner in which they have chosen to adjust to them. In addition, questions to ask might include "Tell me how you feel about the changes caused by this illness" and "How do these changes affect what you now need to do?"

Life Satisfaction. Spiritual well-being seems to be tied to satisfaction with life and what one has accomplished

Research Highlight

Box 24-1

Spiritual/Cultural Dimensions of Childbirth for Canadian Orthodox Jewish Women

Research Focus

Giving birth is a pivotal and life-changing event. A woman's perception of her childbirth experience is influenced by culture. Religious faith or spiritual belief lends perspective to the meaning of significant life experiences. Little is known about the spiritual/cultural meanings of giving birth.

Research Abstract

The purpose of this study was to describe the meaning of the childbirth experience among Canadian Orthodox Jewish women. Interviews were conducted with 30 Orthodox Jewish women who had given birth within 2 weeks to healthy full-term newborns at a Montreal Jewish hospital. Five themes reflecting spiritual/cultural dimensions of childbirth were identified: (1) birth as a significant life event, (2) birth as a bittersweet paradox, (3) the spiritual dimensions of giving birth, (4) the importance of obedience to rabbinical law, and (5) a sense of support and affirmation.

When speaking of their childbirth experiences, these women spoke of awe, reverence, purpose in the creation of a new life, and the meaning of birth as an integral part of the spiritual dimension of their lives. Meaning was created as women obeyed rabbinical law when bearing a child. Obedience to the laws of purity and modesty were foundational to family life. It was important to observe the Sabbath and other religious holidays even while hospitalized, as was keeping ancient rituals of naming and circumcision.

Evidence-Based Practice

- Appreciate the central role of motherhood to the Orthodox Jewish woman.
- Within the framework of rabbinical law, spirituality is infused into every aspect of daily lives.
- Women may request head cover or extra gowns to preserve modesty.
- Visits from extended family are considered *mitzvah,* or good deed.
- Sabbath observance might include having the nurse diaper or bathe newborns.
- Amulet or prayer card might be used to keep the newborn safe from harm.
- Commercial cow milk-based formula is not kosher; ensure availability of soy formula if the mother chooses not to breastfeed.
- A newborn boy will be circumcised in an important religious ceremony on the 8th day.
- Family may be reluctant to reveal the newborn's intended name (e.g., for birth certificate) until after the naming ceremony.

Reference

Semenic, S. E., Callister, L. C., and Feldman, P. (2004). Giving birth: The voices of Orthodox Jewish women living in Canada. *Journal of Obstetric, Gynecologic, and Neonatal Nursing, 33*(1), 80–87.

Table 24-1 **Religious Beliefs About Health**

Religious/Cultural Group	Health Care Beliefs	Response to Illness
Hinduism	Accepts modern medical science.	Illness is caused by past sins. Prolonging life is discouraged.
Sikhism	Accepts modern medical science.	Females to be examined by females. Removing undergarments causes great distress.
Buddhism	Accepts modern medical science. Believes in the Four Noble Truths taught by Buddha: Life is suffering, suffering is caused by desire, suffering can be eliminated by eliminating desire, and to eliminate desire, one must follow an eightfold path of understanding, purpose, speech, conduct, vocation, effort, thinking, and meditation.	May refuse treatment on Holy Days. Dharma, the law of nature, teaches that life is impermanent and all people have to age and die. May want a Buddhist priest. Usually accept death as last stage of life and may permit withdrawal of life support. Does not practise euthanasia.
Islam	Must be able to practise the Five Pillars of Islam. May have a fatalistic view of health.	Uses faith healing. Family members are a comfort. Group prayer is strengthening. May permit withdrawal of life support. Does not practise euthanasia.
Judaism	Believes in the sanctity of life. God and medicine must have a balance. Observance of the Sabbath is important. May refuse treatments on the Sabbath.	Visiting the sick is an obligation. The sick are obligated to seek care. Euthanasia is forbidden.
Christianity	Accepts modern medical science. Many follow complementary alternative medicine (see chapter 31).	Life supports are discouraged. Uses prayer, faith healing. Appreciates visits from clergy. Some will use laying on of hands. Sacraments of Holy Communion and the Anointing of the Sick may be practised.
Canadian Hutterites	Accept modern science. About 80% seek out alternative therapies. Live on colonies to help remove from earthly distractions that impede spiritual practice and devotion. Not appropriate to pray for good health, but rather wisdom to live a healthy life or bear suffering without complaint.	Appreciate receiving education about their health. Prefer straightforward discussions. Respect health professionals. Families expect to be involved in health care discussions (Davidhizar & Giger, 1998).
Canadian Ojibwa *(Anishanaabe)*	Central value is that everything belongs to everyone in extended family. Health is spiritual experience. Disease and illness may be caused by soul loss or spiritual intrusion (Davidhizar & Giger, 1998).	Families generally want to be involved in health care decisions. Desire to get to know nurse before sharing problems. May use Western medicine blended with traditional healing practices (Davidhizar & Giger, 1998).

(Hungelmann et al., 1996). When people are satisfied with life and how they are using their abilities, more energy is available to deal with difficulties and resolve problems. Haase et al. (1992) proposed that satisfaction is associated with acceptance. Acceptance is the process of resolving issues within oneself or dealing with life experiences and is closely tied to hope and spirituality. A nurse can assess a client's life satisfaction by asking, "How happy or satisfied are you with your life?" or "Tell me to what extent you feel satisfied with what you have accomplished in life."

Culture. Spirituality is a personal experience within a cultural context (Pincharoen & Congdon, 2003). It is important to know clients' culture and values. It is common in many cultures for individuals to feel that they have led a worthwhile and purposeful life (Box 24-2). Remaining connected with their cultural heritage often helps clients define their place in the world and express their spirituality. Asking clients about their faith and belief systems is a good beginning for understanding the relationship between culture and spirituality.

Fellowship and Community. Fellowship is one kind of relationship an individual can have with other people (Farran et al., 1989), including immediate family, close friends, associates at work or school, fellow members of a church, and neighbours. More specifically, fellowship includes the community of shared faith between clients and their support networks. The nurse can ask, "With whom do you find the greatest source of support in times of difficulty?" or "When you have faced difficult times in the past, how has that resource been helpful?" The nurse explores a client's support networks and their relationship

Cultural Aspects of Care — Box 24-2

Spirituality should not be limited to a client's religious perspective, but rather should include all of life. In caring for clients from different cultures, the nurse must determine what is important in their lives and what provides them with inner strength and meaning. Clients are usually attempting to find meaning in the changing circumstances of their health and illness. Often spirituality and health are closely associated. For example, Chiu (2001) found that Chinese immigrant women with breast cancer used the following as spiritual resources: family; traditional Chinese values; art, prose and literature; alternative therapy; Chinese support groups; and religion. Pincharoen and Congdon (2003) investigated how spirituality helped Thai older adults maintain health and found that finding harmony through a healthy mind and body was critical.

Implications for Practice

- Explore spirituality of clients from different cultures by assessing the meaning of health and how clients achieve balance, stability, peace, or comfort in their lives.
- Offer a universal and holistic approach to assessing clients' needs by demonstrating caring and using therapeutic communication techniques.
- Promote an environment during assessment in which human rights, values, customs, and spiritual beliefs are respected.
- Include appropriate pastoral care professionals in the assessment process.
- Avoid use of language that alienates or discriminates between different religions.

with the client. It is unwise to assume that a given network offers the kind of support a client desires. For example, calling the client's clergy to request a visit might be inappropriate if the client finds little fellowship with that individual or community. Does the client have one significant fellowship or several?

Ritual and Practice. One of the easiest areas to assess about a client's spirituality is the use of rituals and practices. Rituals include participation in a religious group or private worship, prayer, sacraments such as baptism or communion, fasting, singing, meditating, scripture reading, and making offerings or sacrifices. Different religions have established various rituals for certain life events. For example, Buddhists practise baptism later in life and find burial or cremation acceptable at death. Muslims wash the body of a dead family member and wrap it in white cloth with the head turned toward the right shoulder. Orthodox and Conservative Jews circumcise their newborn sons 8 days after birth. The nurse assesses whether a client's usual rituals or practices have been interrupted as a result of illness or hospitalization. A ritual can provide the client with structure and support during difficult times. If rituals are important to the client, the nurse uses them as part of nursing intervention.

Vocation. Individuals express their spirituality on a daily basis in life routines, work, play, and relationships (Farran et al., 1989). Spirituality can be used in their vocation in life and be part of their identity. The nurse determines if illness or hospitalization has altered the clients' ability to express their spirituality. Expression of spirituality may include showing an appreciation for life, living in the moment and not worrying about tomorrow, appreciating nature, expressing love toward others, and being productive. Questions might include "Has your illness affected the way you live your life spiritually?" or "Has your illness affected your ability to express what's important in life for you?" When illness or loss prevents clients from expressing their spirituality, the nurse must understand the implications psychologically, socially, and spiritually and provide appropriate guidance and support.

Client Expectations. It is important to include in any client assessment a review of the clients' expectations for their health care. The nurse and the client explore what the client expects of caregivers and what he or she hopes to gain. The nurse should not anticipate a client's expectations. What a nurse assumes a client needs may have nothing to do with what the client actually expects or wants. Assessing client expectations requires the nurse to ask questions such as "What do you hope we will be able to do for you?" or "Your expectations are important to us; how can we make your care most satisfactory?" During times of loss or crisis, the client might simply desire a trusting and open relationship with the nurse. It might also be important that the client perceive caregivers to be accepting of his or her religious rituals. Asking clients what they expect of caregivers and then meeting those expectations can help to establish a strong relationship.

Nursing Diagnosis

A spiritual assessment allows a nurse to learn a great deal about a client and the extent that spirituality plays in the client's life. Exploring the client's spirituality may reveal responses to health problems that require nursing intervention, or it may reveal the existence of a strong set of resources that enable the client to cope effectively. As nurses analyze data to find patterns of defining characteristics, they select appropriate nursing diagnoses (Box 24-3). When identifying diagnoses, the nurse must recognize the significance that spirituality has for all types of health problems. Pain, fear, anxiety, and self-care deficit are just some examples of common nursing diagnoses that will require the nurse to incorporate spiritual care principles.

Two nursing diagnoses pertain to spirituality: *readiness for enhanced spiritual well-being* and *spiritual distress* (NANDA, 2003). *Readiness for enhanced spiritual well-being* means the client is able to experience meaning and purpose in life through connectedness with self and others. A client with this nursing diagnosis has potential resources to draw from when faced with illness or a threat to well-being. If the client does not know how to engage personal resources to cope with health problems, the nurse offers support in exploring options. The nursing

Nursing Diagnostic Process — Box 24-3

Assessment Activities	Defining Characteristics	Nursing Diagnosis
Ask client to describe his or her source of faith.	Client expresses an inner strength and source of guidance.	Readiness for enhanced spiritual well-being
Have client describe level of satisfaction with life.	Life has purpose and meaning, provides community service as a volunteer.	
Determine who provides the greatest source of strength and support to the client during times of difficulty.	Person pursues interactions with friends and family.	

diagnosis of *spiritual distress* creates a different clinical picture. Defining characteristics from a nurse's assessment may find patterns that reflect a person's dispiritedness (e.g., expressing lack of hope, meaning, or purpose in life; refusing interaction with spiritual leaders, friends, or family; inability to express previous creativity; or inability to pray). A client with *spiritual distress* requires care that focuses on establishing or renewing faith and hope and offering resources that the client accepts.

Accurate selection of diagnoses requires critical thinking. The nurse reviews concrete data (e.g., religious rituals and sources of fellowship), an assessment of previous client experiences, the nurse's own spirituality, and the appraisal of the client's spiritual well-being. Defining characteristics must be validated and clarified with the client before a diagnosis and plan of care are made. Commonly, clients will have multiple nursing diagnoses. The concept map in Figure 24–5 provides an example of how multiple diagnoses can be interrelated.

Each diagnosis must have an accurate related factor so that resulting interventions can be purposeful and goal directed. The following nursing diagnoses may apply to clients in need of spiritual care:

- Anxiety
- Compromised family coping
- Disabled family coping
- Readiness for enhanced family coping
- Ineffective coping
- Interrupted family processes
- Fear
- Dysfunctional grieving
- Hopelessness
- Powerlessness
- Chronic low self-esteem
- Readiness for enhanced spiritual well-being
- Spiritual distress
- Risk for spiritual distress

Planning

During the planning step of the nursing process, the nurse develops a plan of care for each of the client's nursing diagnoses. Critical thinking is again important because the nurse must reflect on previous experience and apply knowledge and critical thinking when selecting the most appropriate nursing interventions (Figure 24–6). Prior experience in selecting interventions that support clients' spiritual well-being is invaluable when the nurse considers the best options for clients with similar types of situations or problems. The nurse also integrates the knowledge gathered from assessment and knowledge of resources and therapies available for spiritual care to develop an individualized plan of care (see Care Plan). The nurse matches the client's needs with those interventions that are supported and recommended in the clinical and research literature.

Confidence becomes an important critical thinking attitude as the nurse attempts to build a caring relationship with the client. Confidence works to build trust, enabling nurse and client to enter into a healing relationship together. Attempting to meet or support clients' spiritual needs is not simple, and often the new nurse will require humility in recognizing that additional resources may be needed. The nurse's skills in helping clients interpret and understand the meaning of illness and loss, for example, may be limited. Because spiritual care is so personal, standards of autonomy and self-determination are critical in supporting the client's decisions about the plan of care.

Goals and Outcomes. A spiritual care plan must include realistic and individualized goals along with relevant outcomes. It is important for both nurse and client to collaborate closely in setting goals and choosing related interventions. Setting realistic goals will require the nurse to know the client well. In cases in which spiritual care requires helping clients adjust to loss or stressful life situations, goals may be long-term oriented. However, short-term outcomes can be established so that the client progressively reaches a more spiritually healthy situation. The following is an example of a goal and associated outcomes:

- The client will improve personal harmony and connections with members of his or her support system.
- The client will be able to express acceptance of his or her illness.
- The client reports the ability to rely on family members for support.
- The client initiates social interactions with family and friends.

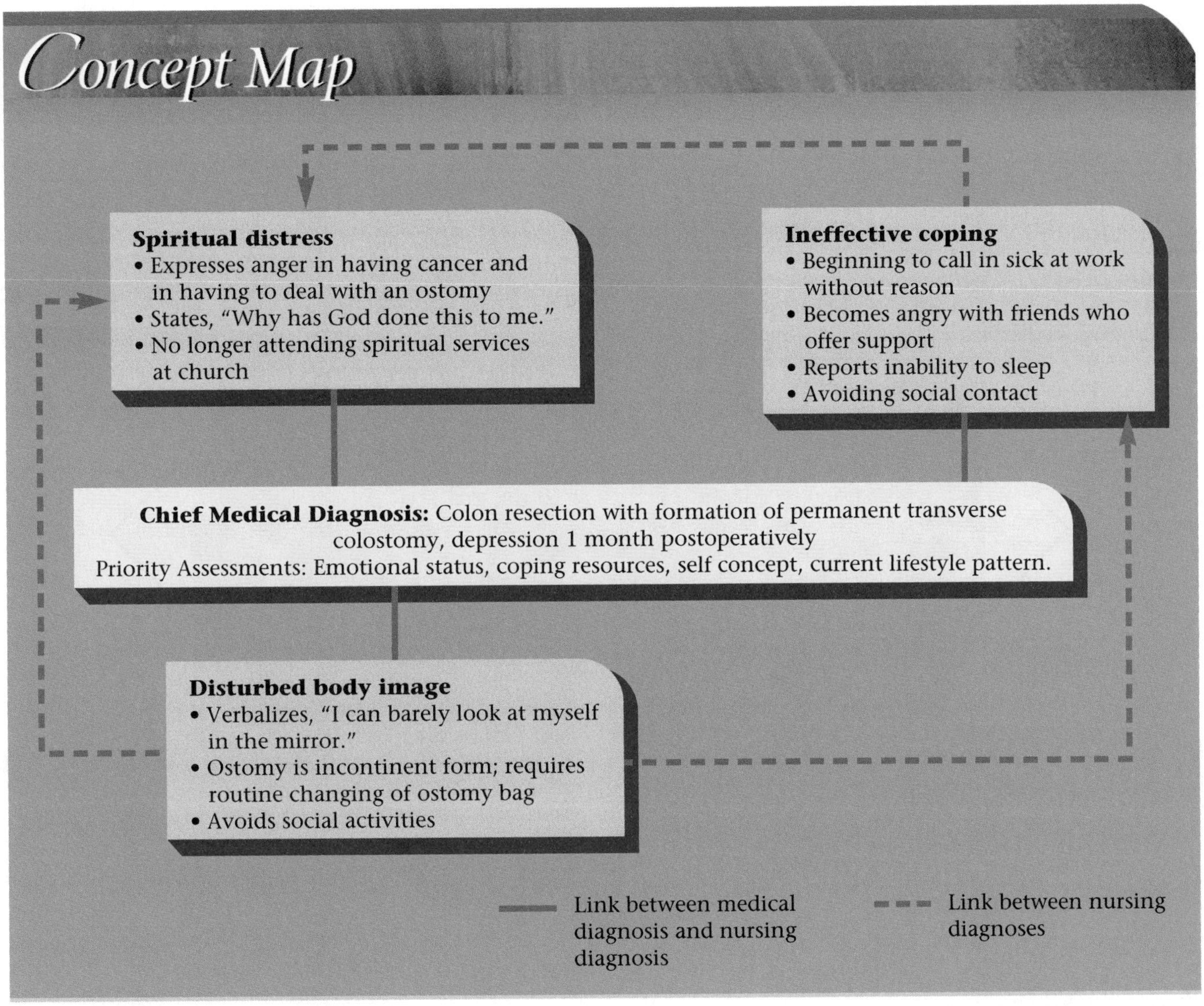
Concept Map
Spiritual distress
• Expresses anger in having cancer and in having to deal with an ostomy
• States, "Why has God done this to me."
• No longer attending spiritual services at church
Ineffective coping
• Beginning to call in sick at work without reason
• Becomes angry with friends who offer support
• Reports inability to sleep
• Avoiding social contact
Chief Medical Diagnosis: Colon resection with formation of permanent transverse colostomy, depression 1 month postoperatively
Priority Assessments: Emotional status, coping resources, self concept, current lifestyle pattern.
Disturbed body image
• Verbalizes, "I can barely look at myself in the mirror."
• Ostomy is incontinent form; requires routine changing of ostomy bag
• Avoids social activities
Link between medical diagnosis and nursing diagnosis
Link between nursing diagnoses

FIGURE **24–5** Concept map for client with colon resection with formation of permanent transverse colostomy and depression 1 month post-operatively.

Setting Priorities. Spiritual health is closely tied to physical and psychological well-being. When a client is in acute distress, the nurse focuses care on the relief of symptoms to provide the client with a sense of control. Then the nurse supports the client's efforts to express the emotional and intellectual aspects of his or her spirituality. When a client has a chronic or terminal condition, the nurse's priorities may shift to helping the client deal with unresolved losses and to connect with the spiritual resources available. The nurse needs to reinforce the everyday life patterns that the client uses to maintain coherence and practise individuation.

Continuity of Care. Significant others, such as spouses, siblings, parents, and friends, need to be involved in the client's care, as appropriate. The nurse learns from the assessment which individuals or groups have formed a relationship with the client. These individuals may become involved in all levels of the nurse's plan. The client's support network may assist in giving physical care, providing emotional comfort, and sharing spiritual support. In a hospital setting, one of the best resources to use in planning a client's spiritual care is the hospital's pastoral care department. A health care chaplain has special expertise in dealing with the spiritual problems confronted by clients. These professionals should be part of the health care team, lending insight about how and when to best support clients and families.

If the client participates in a formal religion, members of the clergy, parish nurses, or members of the church, temple, mosque, or synagogue may need to be involved in the plan of care. Depending on the client's health status and needs, part of the plan will involve a continuation of appropriate religious rituals. The nurse must make sure that any icons or religious materials such as scriptures or a prayer book are made available.

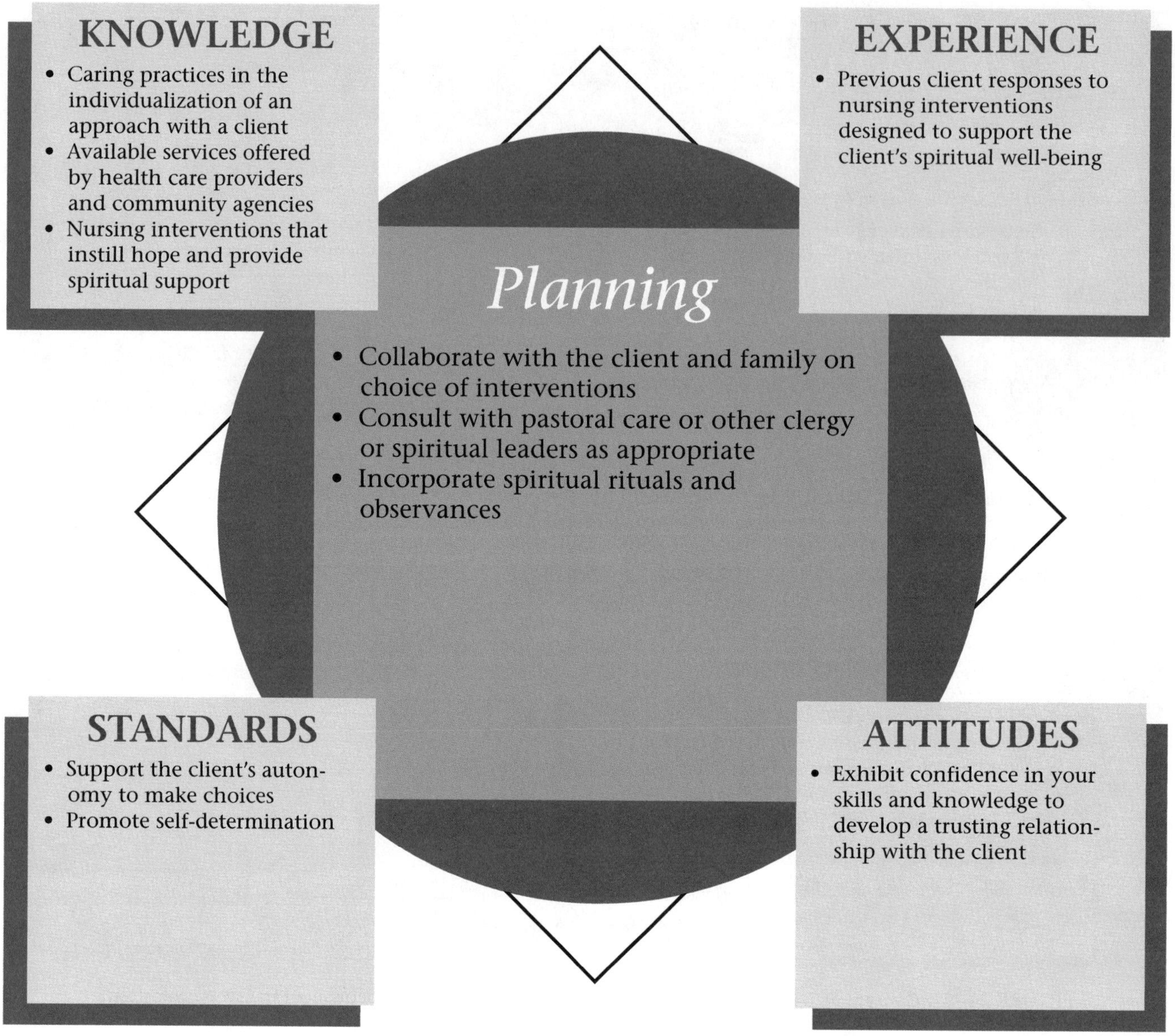
KNOWLEDGE
• Caring practices in the individualization of an approach with a client
• Available services offered by health care providers and community agencies
• Nursing interventions that instill hope and provide spiritual support
EXPERIENCE
• Previous client responses to nursing interventions designed to support the client's spiritual well-being
Planning
• Collaborate with the client and family on choice of interventions
• Consult with pastoral care or other clergy or spiritual leaders as appropriate
• Incorporate spiritual rituals and observances
STANDARDS
• Support the client's autonomy to make choices
• Promote self-determination
ATTITUDES
• Exhibit confidence in your skills and knowledge to develop a trusting relationship with the client

FIGURE **24–6** Critical thinking model for spiritual health planning.

Implementation

Whether a nurse can provide spiritual care depends on the nurse's ability to establish a caring relationship with a client. Spiritual care interventions need not be time-consuming. Partnering with clients helps nurses to determine the most appropriate and effective interventions, which may include touch, rest, nature, reminiscence, imagery, and humour (Meyerhoff et al., 2002). The client and nurse discover together the meaning that illness or loss poses for the client and the impact that it has on the meaning and purpose of life. Achieving this level of understanding with a client enables the nurse to deliver care in a sensitive, creative, and appropriate manner (Box 24-4).

Health Promotion. Spiritual care should be a central theme in promoting an individual's overall well-being. In settings where health promotion activities occur, clients are often in need of information, counselling, and guidance to make the necessary choices to remain healthy. Nurses providing primary health care can contribute to clients' spiritual well-being partly by establishing a positive presence (Box 24-5). They can also support a healing relationship through a variety of methods.

Supporting a Healing Relationship. A nurse looks beyond health problems and recognizes a client's broader needs. For example, the nurse does not just treat a client's back pain, but rather considers how the pain influences ability to function and achieve goals. A **holistic** view

Nursing Care Plan

Spiritual Distress

Assessment

James is a 24-year-old who has recently been diagnosed with AIDS. The clinic nurse, Leah, has been talking with James during his last three visits. During that time, James expresses a fear of dying. His partner, Will, visits James at home periodically but much less often than before the diagnosis. Leah now talks with James in a private conference area.

Assessment Activities	Findings/Defining Characteristics
Leah asks James, "How has your illness affected your own source of strength or hope?"	James responds, "I don't believe this is happening to me. How can God do this to me? There are moments when I just feel so angry. What is going to happen to me?"
Leah responds, "This is obviously a very difficult time. Who in your life provides you the greatest source of support?"	James begins to cry and admits, "I feel so alone. Will has just not been there when I need him. My family wants to help but they live out of town."
Leah clarifies, "You sound as though it would help to have someone to talk to."	James responds, "It would, but it is so hard to find someone I can trust and who will listen."
Leah questions, "You mentioned you could not understand why God has done this to you. How has this experience affected your faith and beliefs?"	James responds, "It has been hard. I have never been a religious person. My church does not accept homosexuality, but I always have had a faith in God. Will and I have attended a new ecumenical service at the local college. I have not been attending lately."

Nursing Diagnosis: Spiritual distress related to fear and uncertainty of terminal illness.

Planning

Goal	Expected Outcomes*
	Hope
Client will express a sense of purpose.	Client will discuss how the experience of having AIDS may have a positive influence in life within 1 month. Client expresses a sense of confidence in treatments available for AIDS in 2 weeks.
	Spiritual Well-being
Client establishes connection with significant others.	Client reports having more visits with partner and family members in next 2 weeks (e.g., telephone and e-mail to out-of-town relatives).
Client establishes connection with spiritual advisor and/or member of faith community	Client reports having been in contact with member/s of faith community (e.g., clergy, parish nurse, leader of ecumenical service he had been attending at local college). Client schedules attendance at AIDS support group in 1 month.

*Outcome labels from *Nursing Outcomes Classification (NOC)* (3rd ed.), edited by S. Moorhead, M. Johnson, and M. L. Maas, 2004, St. Louis, MO: Mosby.

Interventions†	Rationale
Hope Instillation	
• Plan instructional session to discuss typical course of AIDS, emphasizing the typical pattern of remissions with drug therapy. Review therapies available for treatment.	Knowledge about disease will help client think as a person living with AIDS rather than dying with AIDS (Hall, 1998). Reality of disease course will help instill hope.
Spiritual Support	
• Encourage client's expression of loneliness through establishing a caring presence.	Presencing reflects being in tune with the client and displays caring. It is an effective technique that makes a topic of discussion more approachable (P. Benner & Wrubel, 1989).
• Listen to client's feelings and concerns. • Plan discussion session with client that includes his partner. Have client discuss his ability to cope with AIDS and its spiritual meaning .	People question and become open to discover their unique spiritual meaning after a crisis that threatens health (Hall, 1998). Provides client a resource from client's community of faith to share concerns.
• Encourage contact with family members. • Recommend contact with spiritual resources (e.g., clergy, parish nurse, spiritual advisor from faith community). • Recommend client consider attending AIDS support group sponsored by local college.	Connections with a support system can provide meaning to illness and offer sources of hope.

†Intervention classification labels from *Nursing Interventions Classification (NIC)* (4th ed.), edited by J. M. Dochterman and G. M. Bulecheck, 2004, St. Louis, MO: Mosby.

Continued

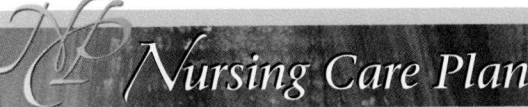

Nursing Care Plan

Spiritual Distress—cont'd

Evaluation

Nursing Actions	Client Response/Finding	Achievement of Outcome
Ask client how he currently feels about having AIDS.	"I am not quite as frightened as I was a few weeks ago. I believe the treatments will help me. I have been on the combination therapy for 2 weeks. I just hope it works."	James reports an improved outlook and confidence in treatment. May continue to have doubt about outcome.
Have client describe the session that included Will.	"It meant a great deal to tell Will how I feel. I know now he wants to help, but did not know how. Since then, we have talked on the phone almost every day."	Successfully increased connection with significant other. May require support or guidance on how to discuss sensitive feelings with partner.
Have client describe contact with family members.	"My sister has been great. She has been sending me lengthy e-mails and has pointed out some helpful Web sites. My mother and father are short on the phone; I think they are struggling with this diagnosis, too."	Successfully increased connection with sister. May require information on various ways that family members deal with a diagnosis of AIDS. Encourage keeping lines of communication open with family.
Have client describe contact with member/s of faith community.	"Will and I attended the ecumenical service again. A bulletin announcement invited newcomers to join small fellowship groups. We are planning to call the small group leader to get more information."	Successfully initiated contact with faith community. May require ongoing encouragement as seeks a place of belonging and fellowship.
Ask client if he scheduled attendance at the support group.	"I have called the college. The support group meets next Tuesday evening. I plan to be there."	Client schedules attendance at support group.

enables the nurse to establish a helping role and a healing relationship. Three factors are evident when a healing relationship develops between nurse and client:

- Mobilizing hope for the nurse, as well as for the client
- Finding an interpretation or understanding of the illness, pain, anxiety, or other stressful emotion that is acceptable to the client
- Assisting the client in using social, emotional, and spiritual resources (P. Benner, 1984)

Hope motivates people with strategies to face challenges in life. The nurse can help a client find things to hope for. For example, a client who has been newly diagnosed with diabetes might hope to learn how to manage the disease so as to continue a productive and satisfying way of life. Hope helps a client work toward recovery. To help clients achieve hope, the nurse and client work together to find an explanation of the situation that is acceptable to both. Then the nurse helps the client realistically exercise hope. This help might include supporting a client's positive attitude toward life or a desire to be informed and to make decisions.

To further support a healing relationship, the nurse must remain aware of the client's spiritual resources and needs. It is always important for clients to express their beliefs and find spiritual comfort. When life stressors or illness create confusion or uncertainty for the client, the nurse must recognize the possible effect on a client's well-being. How can spiritual resources be used and strengthened? The nurse may begin by encouraging a client to discuss the effect that illness has had on personal beliefs and faith. This discussion gives the nurse the chance to clarify any misconceptions or inaccuracies in information. Having a clear sense of what illness may hold for an individual helps the person to apply all resources toward recovery.

Acute Care. Within acute care settings, clients experience multiple stressors that threaten their sense of control. Support and enhancement of a client's spiritual well-being can be a challenge when the focus of health care seems to be one of treatment and cure rather than care. The nurse works closely with clients and their support networks in finding ways to make spiritual resources part of the plan of care.

Support Systems. Use of support systems is important in any health care setting. Support systems provide clients with the greatest sense of well-being during hospitalization and serve as a human link connecting the client, the nurse, and the client's lifestyle before an illness (C. C. Clark et al., 1991). Part of the client's caregiving environment is the regular presence of supportive family and friends. The nurse plans care with the client and the client's support network to promote the interpersonal bonding that is needed for recovery. The support system is a source of faith and hope, and it can be an important

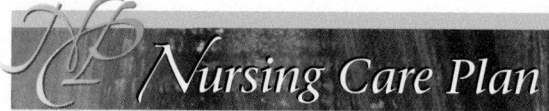

Case Study Box 24-4

Spiritual Nursing Interventions

Case Study Focus

This case study describes spiritual health interventions used by Canadian public health nurses to help a family confronted with a loss of meaning precipitated by the diagnosis of a child's chronic condition. These health interventions continued through the boy's childhood and adolescence.

The Perez Family

After their son Michael's lack of language development, unpredictability, erratic behaviour, and repetitive rocking movements were diagnosed as autism, Marie and Edwin felt overwhelmed by emotional stress. They struggled to find meaning in their lives and the life of their son, while experiencing a loss of hopes and dreams for a "normal" son.

Spiritual Interventions

Communication. When Michael's diagnosis was confirmed, the public health nurse focused on establishing a relationship with the family. Communication facilitated the processing of feelings and responses to the loss of hopes and dreams as the family struggled to find meaning in the face of unwelcome challenges. Marie needed to express how tired she felt and occasionally questioned why this load had been given to her family. Edwin needed solitude to cope with intense feelings, but this made Marie feel that he was withdrawing. The nurse suggested Edwin journal his feelings, which he found helpful.

Connectedness. The nurse helped the family identify and nurture significant relationships. The family identified significant family members, close friends, and members of their faith community, and asked them to meet as a group. At the first meeting, Marie and Edwin asked if the group would be willing to meet to provide support and counselling. Everyone agreed, and the group met weekly for 15 years. Marie and Edwin also nurtured connectedness with God by attending spiritual retreats, practising prayer, and partnering with a spiritual director.

Bibliotherapy. Bibliotherapy is the use of books to provide healing, enhance the expression of feelings, and gain insight. Through reading, the Perez family gained new information about families who cope with illness. The nurse encouraged Edwin, Marie, and Mary (Michael's sister) to compare their situation with those in the books and to write out a new ending for one of the experiences. This exercise allowed the Perez family to reflect on changes they could make to have a better experience of living with a child with a developmental disability.

Music Therapy. Music's healing power has long been established, even though music therapy as a spiritual intervention is new to nurses. The nurse suggested a referral to a music therapist, who used and taught a variety of music styles to engage and calm Michael. Edwin and Marie also listened to tranquil music to relieve their own spiritual distress.

Prayer. Marie and Edwin prayed for their son's health and for strength for themselves. Other family and friends prayed for ongoing support. The Perez family said they could "feel" the prayers of others. They felt that God heard their prayers of petition and trusted God with Michael's future.

Reference

Meyerhoff, H., et al. (2002). Spiritual nursing interventions. *Canadian Nurse, 98*(3), 21–24.

Focus on Primary Health Care Box 24-5

Establishing Presence

Clients have reported that the presence of nurses and their caregiving activities contribute to a sense of well-being and provide hope for recovery (C. C. Clark et al., 1991). Behaviours that establish the nurse's presence include giving attention, answering questions, listening, and having a positive and encouraging (but realistic) attitude. The ability to establish presence is part of the art of nursing. It is not simply being in the same room with a client while performing procedures or sharing information. Presencing involves "being with" a client versus "doing for" a client (P. Benner, 1984). Presencing involves offering a closeness with the client, physically, psychologically, and spiritually.

When health promotion is the focus of care, the nurse's presence becomes important in instilling confidence in clients' abilities to take the steps necessary to remain healthy. Research shows that the best way to convey a caring presence is to listen to the client (Emblen & Halstead, 1993). Other ways include involving family in discussions about clients' health, displaying self-confidence when providing health instruction, and supporting clients' faith in the choices they make. The client who seeks health care may be fearful of experiencing an illness that would threaten loss of control and looks for someone to offer competent direction. The nurse's encouraging words of support and the nurse's calm and decisive approach establish a presence that builds trust and well-being (see chapter 15).

resource in conducting the religious rituals on which some clients rely.

When it is known that clients depend on family and friends for support, the nurse encourages them to visit the client regularly. Often illness and the treatment environment intimidate family members and friends. The nurse helps family members to feel welcome and encourages them to be themselves during visits. Their support and presence can be used to promote healing. Encouraging the family to bring meaningful religious symbols to the client's bedside can offer significant spiritual support.

Another important resource to clients is spiritual advisors and members of the clergy. Many hospitals have pastoral care departments that assist in notifying community clergy of their congregants' admission or who can provide trained clergy for support. In addition, some congregations have parish nurses who provide hospitalized congregants with spiritual support. Pastoral care professionals are expert at giving attention to how an illness influences a person's beliefs and how beliefs can influence illness and recovery. The nurse should ask if clients desire to have a member of the clergy or parish nurse visit during their hospitalization. All pastoral care professionals should be made welcome on nursing units. When requested by clients or families, the nurse should keep pastoral care professionals informed of any physical, psychosocial, or spiritual concerns affecting the client. The nurse shows respect for clients' spiritual values and

Table 24-2 Religious Dietary Regulations Affecting Health Care

Religion	Dietary Practices
Hinduism	Some sects are vegetarians. The belief is not to kill *any* living creature.
Buddhism	Some are vegetarians, and many will not use alcohol or tobacco and may hesitate to use drugs. Many will fast on Holy Days.
Islam	Prohibits consumption of pork and alcohol. Fasting is done during the month of Ramadan.
Judaism	Some observe the kosher dietary restrictions of avoiding pork and shellfish and not preparing and eating milk and meat at the same time.
Christianity	Some Baptists, Evangelicals, and Pentecostals discourage the use of alcohol, caffeine, and tobacco. Some Roman Catholics may fast during Lent, Ash Wednesday, Good Friday, and 1 hour before receiving Communion.
Jehovah's Witnesses	Members may avoid food prepared with or containing blood.
Mormonism	Members abstain from alcohol, caffeine, and tobacco.
Russian Orthodox Church	Followers must observe fast days as well as a "no meat" rule on Wednesdays and Fridays. During Lent, all animal products, including dairy products and butter, are forbidden.
First Nations	Food practices influenced by individual nations' beliefs.

needs by willingly co-operating with others giving spiritual care and by facilitating the administration of sacraments, rites, and rituals.

Providing privacy for the client, family, and pastoral care professionals is a thoughtful and sensitive gesture. The nurse determines the proper routine in a client's religion by asking the clergy, family, or client. Often a client within the hospital may want to discuss spiritual concerns in the evening or late at night, when support services such as clergy and social services are unavailable. The nurse can help to meet the client's needs through careful, skilled, and active listening.

Diet Therapies. Food and nutrition are important aspects of client care and often an important component of some religious observances (Table 24-2). Food and the rituals surrounding the preparation and serving of food can be important to a person's spirituality. The nurse can consult with the dietitian to integrate the client's dietary preferences into daily care. In the event that an agency cannot prepare food in the preferred way, the family may be asked to bring meals that accommodate dietary restrictions.

Supporting Rituals. Nurses provide spiritual care by supporting clients' participation in spiritual rituals and activities. This support is especially important for older adults, who typically perceive themselves as highly spiritual (Isaia, Parker, & Murrow, 1999; Box 24-6). Personal care of the client should be planned to allow time for religious readings, spiritual visitations, or attendance at religious services. Some churches and synagogues offer audio tapes of their services for those members who cannot attend in person. Family members can plan a prayer session or an organized reading of scriptures on a regular basis. Arrangements may need to be made with pastoral care staff for the client and family to receive the sacraments. Clergy will routinely offer to make home visits for people unable to attend religious services. Taped meditations, classical or religious music, and televised religious services provide other effective options. The nurse should be respectful of icons, medals, prayer rugs, or crosses that clients bring to a health setting to be sure they are not accidentally lost, damaged, or misplaced.

Focus on Older Adults — Box 24-6

- There is an association between an older adult's spirituality and ability to adjust or cope with real or anticipated losses (Simington, 1996).
- The very old are more likely to be interested in the non-organizational aspects of religion than in active participation (Courtney et al., 1992).
- Belief in the afterlife increases as adults grow older. Visits from clergy, social workers, lawyers, and even financial advisors can be made available so that clients feel prepared. Leaving a legacy to loved ones (e.g., oral histories, works of art, photographs) provides a sense of meaning (Ebersole & Hess, 1998).
- Higher levels of religiosity in older women may be related to the social structure in which women typically participate, including church activities, caregiving, and nurturing (Levin, Taylor, & Chatters, 1994).
- Older adult caregivers, such as those caring for another with Alzheimer's disease, often have a need to express spiritual needs. Feelings of guilt, hopelessness, fear, and the distresss of "playing God" are just some of the feelings that caregivers might express that could reflect spiritual distress (C. A. Miller, 1999).
- Spiritual beliefs and practices may also help caregivers cope and find a sense of peace (Sawatzky & Fowler-Kerry, 2003).

Restorative and Continuing Care. For clients who are recovering from a long-term illness or disability or who suffer chronic or terminal disease, spiritual care becomes especially important. Many of the nursing interventions applicable in health promotion and acute care apply to this level of health care as well.

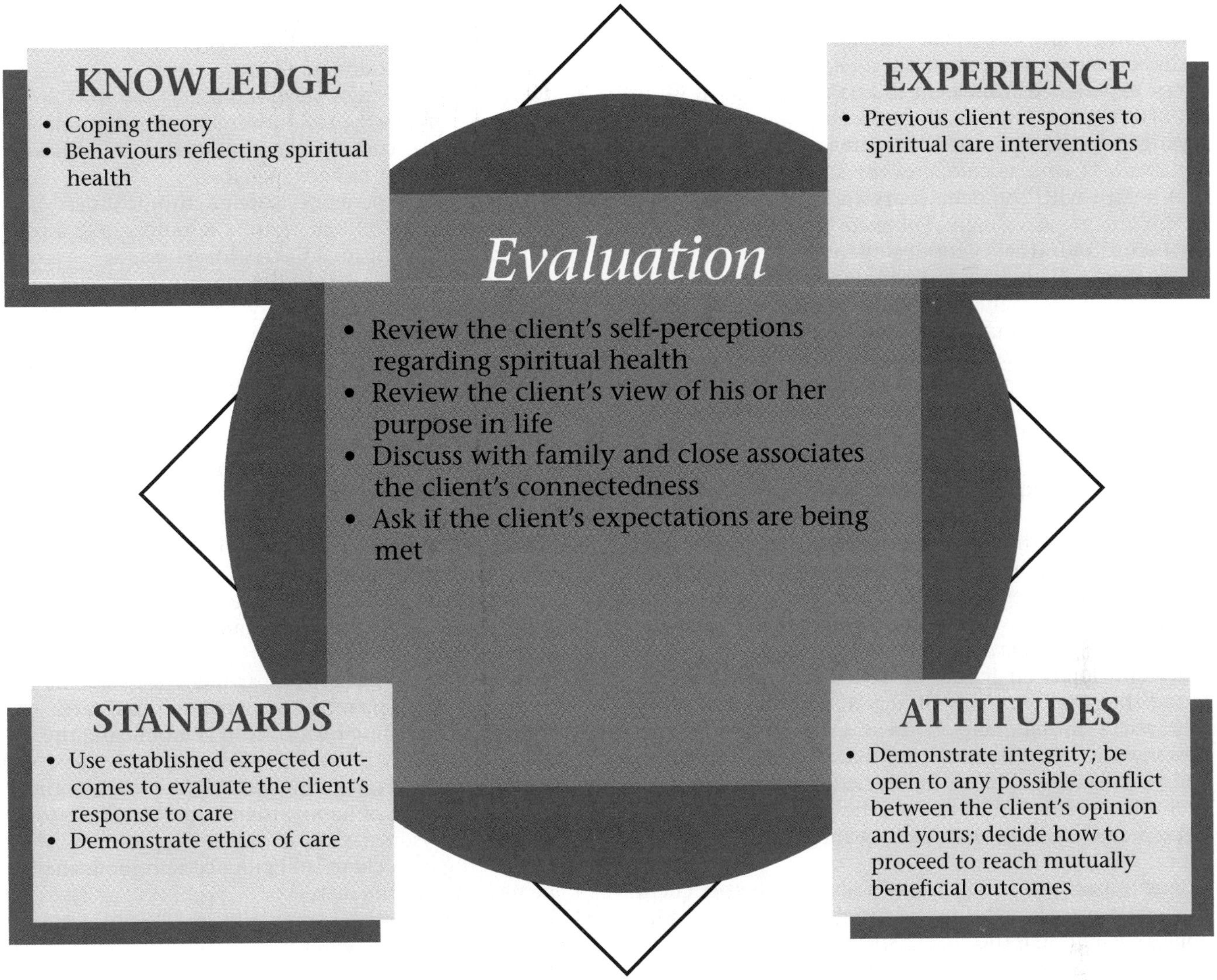
KNOWLEDGE
• Coping theory
• Behaviours reflecting spiritual health
EXPERIENCE
• Previous client responses to spiritual care interventions
Evaluation
• Review the client's self-perceptions regarding spiritual health
• Review the client's view of his or her purpose in life
• Discuss with family and close associates the client's connectedness
• Ask if the client's expectations are being met
STANDARDS
• Use established expected outcomes to evaluate the client's response to care
• Demonstrate ethics of care
ATTITUDES
• Demonstrate integrity; be open to any possible conflict between the client's opinion and yours; decide how to proceed to reach mutually beneficial outcomes

FIGURE **24–7** Critical thinking model for spiritual health evaluation.

Prayer. The act of prayer gives an individual the opportunity to renew personal faith and belief in a higher being in a specific, focused way that may be highly ritualized and formal or quite spontaneous and informal. Prayer has been shown to be an effective coping resource for physical as well as psychological symptoms. Clients may pray in private or pursue opportunities for group prayer with family, friends, or clergy. The nurse can be supportive of prayer by giving the client privacy if desired, learning if the client wishes to have the nurse participate, and by suggesting prayer when it is known to be a coping resource for the client. If prayer is not suitable for a client, an alternative may be to read from a book (e.g., the Bible or the Koran) selected by the client or from poetry or other inspirational texts.

Supporting Grief Work. Clients who experience terminal illness or who have been recently disabled by disease or injury will require the nurse's support in grieving over and coping with their loss (see chapter 25). Supporting a client during times of grief can be enhanced by a spiritual relationship with the client.

NP Evaluation

The evaluation of a client's spiritual care requires the nurse to think critically to determine if efforts at restoring or maintaining the client's spiritual health were successful (Figure 24–7). The nurse will consider spiritual concepts and coping theory (see chapter 26) in evaluating whether the client has been able to adjust to those factors that threaten spiritual well-being. Outcomes established during the planning phase will serve as the standards to evaluate the client's progress. In addition, an ethic of caring ensures that the nurse evaluates any ethical concerns that may arise in the course of the client's spiritual care and support. The nurse's evaluation includes a review of the client's response to care and whether the client's expectations were achieved.

Client Care. Attainment of spiritual health is a lifelong goal. Clients will experience the need to clarify values, reshape philosophies, strengthen relationships, and live those experiences that help to shape one's purpose in life. The nurse provides spiritual care while always evaluating whether planned outcomes and goals were achieved. The nurse compares the client's level of spiritual health with the behaviours and perceptions noted in the nursing assessment. For example, if the nurse's assessment finds the client losing hope, the follow-up evaluation will involve a discussion with the client to determine if the client has regained a purpose for living. Family and friends can be a useful source of evaluative information. Successful outcomes should reveal the client developing an increased or restored sense of connectedness with significant others, family, and/or faith community; maintaining, renewing, or reforming a sense of purpose in life; and, for some, establishing or renewing a confidence and trust in God, a supreme being or power.

For clients with a serious or terminal illness, evaluation focuses on the goal of helping the client retain faith and hope or expressing openly life's uncertainties. The nurse evaluates how clients are accepting their illness and whether hope has enabled them to recognize their mortality and focus on living for each day. Fryback (1993) found that the terminally ill, regardless of whether they followed a formal religion, held a belief in a higher power, which gave them a sense that God was with them and they were not alone. The nurse must not assume all clients have such faith. However, the nurse's support aims to help clients accept their destiny and to be at peace.

Client Expectations. The nurse evaluates whether client expectations were met. In regard to spiritual care, this involves evaluating if the client's spiritual practices were respected and if the nurse-client relationship was one of caring and support. Both the client and family should be able to relate whether opportunities were offered for religious rituals. With respect to the nurse-client relationship, does the client express trust and confidence in the nurse? Is the client able to discuss important issues or topics? Is the client comfortable in expressing spiritual needs with the nurse? Ask the client to reflect on the quality of the nurse-client relationship. Asking, "Do you feel your expectations of me in supporting your spiritual needs were met?" will determine whether an effective healing relationship was developed.

Key Concepts

- Nurses must develop a caring relationship in order to understand clients' spirituality.
- There may be beneficial health outcomes of spirituality.
- Canadian nursing has a rich spiritual heritage that has influenced contemporary practice.
- Nursing theories provide principles that nurses can use to guide spiritual care practice.
- Spirituality is highly personal and unique to each individual.
- Faith is a relationship with God or a higher power or authority that enables action and gives purpose and meaning to an individual's life.
- Religion is a system of organized beliefs and worship that a person practises to outwardly express spirituality.
- Hope provides comfort and a motivation to achieve when a person is faced with a loss.
- When clients experience acute or chronic illness or a terminal disease, either spiritual resources help a person recover or spiritual distress develops.
- Common religious rituals include private worship, prayer, singing, use of a rosary, and scripture reading.
- A spiritual assessment is most successful when the nurse applies knowledge that pertains to therapeutic communication, principles of loss and grief, and knowledge of caring practices.
- The personal nature of spirituality requires open communication and the establishment of trust between nurse and client.
- If a client's religious beliefs conflict with medical treatment, options to nurses and other health care providers can be limited.
- An important part of spiritual assessment is learning who of the client's friends or family share a community of faith.
- A hospital's pastoral care department is a valuable resource to use in planning a client's spiritual care.
- Central to a healing relationship is mobilizing the client's hope.
- Part of a client's caregiving environment can be the regular presence of family, friends, parish nurses, or spiritual advisors.
- Depending on a client's religion, certain foods may be restricted in the diet.
- Prayer is an effective coping resource for physical and psychological symptoms.
- When evaluating spiritual care, successful outcomes should reveal the client developing an increased or restored sense of connectedness with significant others and maintaining, renewing, or reforming a sense of purpose in life.

Key Terms

Agnostic, *p. 490*
Atheist, *p. 490*
Culture, *p. 490*
Faith, *p. 490*
Holistic, *p. 500*
Hope, *p. 490*
Religion, *p. 490*
Spiritual care, *p. 489*
Spiritual distress, *p. 491*
Spiritual well-being, *p. 489*
Spirituality, *p. 487*
Transcendence, *p. 490*

Critical Thinking Exercises

1. Mr. Gadacz is a 40-year-old businessman with over 100 employees. A 12-hour workday is not unusual for him. Last evening, he was admitted to the cardiac care unit with severe chest pain resulting from a myocardial infarction (heart attack). He is now stabilized but fre-

quently asks about his diagnostic tests and what he needs to do to be able to go home. He tells his nurse, "My doctor tells me I will need surgery once I am more stable. I hope he can do that soon. I just can't believe this is happening. I worry about what will happen to my business while I am gone." Identify three approaches you might use as his nurse to conduct a spiritual assessment with Mr. Gadacz.

2. Tejal is a new graduate nurse caring for Ms. Rosenbaum for the first time. Ms. Rosenbaum has been diagnosed with uterine cancer. Tejal is helping Ms. Rosenbaum with her meal tray when she says, "I noticed that the information in your chart says you are Jewish. Would you like me to call a rabbi to visit? Are there any diet considerations we should be making for you?" Are Tejal's assessment and resultant interventions appropriate for this situation?
3. Critical thinking is an ongoing process. When you learn that you are assigned to Fangzhou Lin, you note that the Kardex information includes his religion, Buddhist, and his place of birth, Hong Kong. A colleague tells you he can speak some English. The client is 80 years old and reportedly has a hearing deficit. What knowledge might you wish to reflect on critically before beginning a spiritual assessment of this client?

Review Questions

1. Caring for a client's spiritual needs means
   1. The nurse must have the same beliefs as the client
   2. Praying for the client
   3. Accepting the client's beliefs and experiences
   4. Calling for a religious leader if the nurse determines a need
2. An individual who does not believe in the existence of God is an
   1. Agnostic
   2. Atheist
   3. Anarchist
   4. Agenic
3. Hope is a concept related to spirituality that can be best described as:
   1. Satisfaction with someone or something
   2. Having a bond with another person for ongoing support
   3. Having confidence in something for which there is no proof
   4. Having something to live for and look forward to
4. Canadian Hutterites believe that suffering
   1. May be prevented through prayer
   2. May be caused by soul loss
   3. Is a public matter
   4. Is a burden to be borne without complaint
5. Client's rituals and practice
   1. Have no place in modern medicine
   2. Have no place in the hospital
   3. Can get in the way of nursing care
   4. Provide structure and support for the client
6. Establishing presence is not simply being in the same room with a client but also
   1. Involves offering a closeness with the client, physically, psychologically, and spiritually
   2. Involves performing procedures
   3. Involves sharing technical information with the client
   4. Involves all team members
7. For Hindus it is important to consider that
   1. Some sects are vegetarian
   2. Followers must observe fast days
   3. Many individuals avoid meats containing blood
   4. Members abstain from alcohol and caffeine
8. Jehovah Witnesses may avoid
   1. Caffeine and chocolate
   2. Pork and shellfish
   3. Dairy products and caffeine
   4. Food prepared with or containing blood
9. Members of the Mormon faith
   1. Avoid pork and shellfish
   2. Avoid alcohol, caffeine, and tobacco
   3. Practise vegetarianism
   4. Do not eat milk and meat at the same time
10. Clients who experience terminal illness or who have suffered recent disability because of a disease or injury can benefit from
    1. Grief work
    2. Diet therapy
    3. Acupuncture
    4. Values clarification

References

Adair, M. N., et al. (1991). New behavioral strategies for enhancing immune function. *AIDS Patient Care, 5,* 297–300.

Andrews, M. M., & Boyle, J. S. (1999). *Transcultural concepts in nursing care* (3rd ed.), Philadelphia: Lippincott.

Artinian, B. M., & Conger, M. M. (1997). *The intersystem model: Integrating theory and practice.* Thousand Oaks, CA: Sage.

Baetz, M., et al. (2002). Canadian psychiatric inpatient religious commitment: An association with mental health. *Canadian Journal of Psychiatry, 47,* 159–165.

Barnum, B. S. (2003). *Spirituality in nursing: From traditional to new age* (2nd ed.). New York: Springer.

Basford, T. K. (1990). *Near death experience: An annotated bibliography.* New York: Garland.

Benner, D. G. (1985). *Baker encyclopedia of psychology.* Grand Rapids, MI: Baker Book House.

Benner, P. (1984). *From novice to expert.* Menlo Park, CA: Addison-Wesley.

Benner, P., & Wrubel, J. (1989). *The primacy of caring.* Menlo Park, CA: Addison-Wesley.

Bibby, R. (2002). *Restless gods: The renaissance of religion in Canada.* Toronto, ON: Stoddart.

Burnard, P. (1988). The spiritual needs of atheists and agnostics. *Professional Nurse, 4*(3), 130–132.

Carson, V. B., & Green, H. (1992). Spiritual well-being: A predictor of hardiness in patients with acquired immunodeficiency syndrome. *Journal of Professional Nursing, 8,* 209–220.

Catterall, R. A., et al. (1998). The assessment and audit of spiritual care. *International Journal of Palliative Nursing, 4,* 162–168.

Cavendish, R., et al. (2004). Nurses enhance performance through prayer [Electronic version]. *Holistic Nursing Practice, 18,* 26–31.

Childe, G. (2002). Spiritual healing. *Nursing Standard, 16*(44), 27–.

Chiu, L. (2001). Spiritual resources of Chinese immigrants with breast cancer in the USA. *International Journal of Nursing Studies, 38,* 175–184.

Clark, C. C., et al. (1991). Spirituality: Integral to quality care. *Holistic Nursing Practice, 5*(3), 67–76.

Clark, M. B., & Olson, J. K. (2000). *Nursing within a faith community: Promoting health in times of transition.* Thousand Oaks, CA: Sage.

Coe, R. M. (1997). The magic of science and the science of magic: An essay on the process of healing. *Journal of Health and Social Behavior, 38*(3), 1–8.

Courtney, B. C., et al. (1992). Religiosity and adaptation in the oldest-old. In L. W. Poon (Ed.), *The Georgia centenarian study* Amityville, NY: Baywood.

Culligan, K. (1996, August 31). Spirituality and healing in medicine. *America,* p. 17.

Davidhizer, R. E., & Giger, J. N. (1998). *Canadian transcultural nursing.* Toronto, ON: Mosby.

Dochterman, J. M., & Bulechek, G. M. (2004). *Nursing interventions classification (NIC)* (4th ed.). St. Louis, MO: Mosby.

Dombeck, M. B. (1995). Dream-telling: A means of spiritual awareness. *Holistic Nursing Practice, 9*(2), 37–47.

Draper, P., & McSherry, W. (2002). A critical view of spirituality and spiritual assessment. *Journal of Advanced Nursing, 39*(1), 1–2.

Ebersole, P., & Hess, P. (1998). *Toward healthy aging* (5th ed.). St. Louis, MO: Mosby.

Emblen, J. D. (1992). Religion and spirituality defined according to current use in nursing literature. *Journal of Professional Nursing, 8*(1), 41–47.

Emblen, J. D., & Halstead, L. (1993). Spiritual needs and interventions: Comparing the views of patients, nurses, and chaplains. *Clinical Nursing Specialist, 7*(4), 175–182.

Farran, C. J., et al. (1989). Development of a model for spiritual assessment and intervention. *Journal of Religion Health, 28*(3),185–194.

Friedemann, M. L. (1995). *The framework of systemic organization: A conceptual approach to families and nursing.* Thousand Oaks, CA: Sage.

Friedemann, M. L., Mouch, J., & Racey, T. (2002). Nursing the spirit: The Framework of Systemic Organization. *Journal of Advanced Nursing, 39*(4), 325–332.

Fryback, P. B. (1993). Health for people with a terminal diagnosis. *Nursing Science Quarterly, 6*(3), 147–149.

Grant, D. (2004). Spiritual interventions: How, when and why nurses use them [Electronic version]. *Holistic Nursing Practice, 18*(1), 36–41.

Grypma, S. (2004). Neither angels of mercy nor foreign devils: Revisioning Canadian missionary nurses in China, 1935–1947. *Nursing History Review, 12,* 97–119.

Haase, J. E., et al. (1992). Simultaneous concept analysis of spiritual perspective, hope, acceptance, and self-transcendence. *Image—The Journal of Nursing Scholarship, 24*(4), 141–147.

Hall, B. A. (1998). Patterns of spirituality in persons with advanced HIV disease. *Research in Nursing & Health, 21,* 143–153.

Heliker, D. (1992). Reevaluation of a nursing diagnosis: Spiritual distress. *Nursing Forum, 27*(4), 15–20.

Hungelmann, J., et al. (1996). Focus on spiritual well-being: Harmonious interconnectedness of mind-body-spirit—Use of the JAREL spiritual well-being scale. *Geriatric Nursing, 17*(6), 262–266.

Isaia, D., Parker, V., & Murrow, E. (1999). Spiritual well-being among older adults. *Journal of Gerontological Nursing, 26*(8),15–21.

Koenig, H. G., et al. (1997). Attendance at religious services, interleukin-6, and other biological parameters of immune function in older adults. *International Journal of Psychiatry in Medicine, 27,* 233–250.

Lambe, M., et al. (1996). Malignant melanoma: Reduced risk associated with early childbearing and multiparity. *Melanoma Research, 6,* 147–153.

Levin, J. S., Taylor, R. J., & Chatters, L. M. (1994). Race and gender differences in religiosity among older adults: Findings from four national surveys. *Journal of Gerontology, 49,* S137–S145.

Louis, A., & Alpert, P. (2000). Spirituality for nurses and their practice. *Nursing Leadership Forum, 5,* 43–51.

Macrae, J. A. (2001). *Nursing as a spiritual practice: A contemporary application of Florence Nightingale's views.* New York: Springer.

Martsolf, D. S., & Mickley, J. R. (1998). The concept of spirituality in nursing theories: Differing world-views and extent of focus. *Journal of Advanced Nursing, 27,* 294–303.

McEwen, M. (2004). Analysis of spirituality content in nursing textbooks. *Journal of Nursing Education, 43,* 20–30.

McSherry, W. (1998). Nurses' perceptions of spirituality and spiritual care. *Nursing Standard 13*(4):36–40

McSherry, W. (2001). Spiritual crisis? Call a nurse. In H. Orchard (Ed.), *Spirituality in health care contexts* (pp. 107–117). London: Jessica Kingsley.

Meyerhoff, H., et al. (2002). Spiritual nursing interventions. *Canadian Nurse, 98,* 21–24.

Miller, C. A. (1999). *Nursing care of older adults: Theory and practice* (3rd ed.). Philadelphia: Lippincott.

Miller, W. R., & Thoresen, C. E. (2003). Spirituality, religion and health: An emerging research field [Electronic version]. *The American Psychologist, 58*(1), 24–35.

Moorhead, S., Johnson, M., & Maas, M. (Eds.). (2004). *Nursing outcomes classification (NOC)* (3rd ed.). St. Louis, MO: Mosby.

Morse, J. M., & Doberneck, B. (1995). Delineating the concept of hope. *Image: The Journal of Nursing Scholarship, 27*(4), 277–285.

North American Nursing Diagnosis Association. (2003). *NANDA nursing diagnoses: Definitions and classifications 2003—2004.* Philadelphia: Author.

O'Brien, M. E. (2003). *Parish nursing: Healthcare ministry within the church.* Sudbury, MA: Jones & Bartlett.

Olson, J., Simington, J. A., & Clark, M. B. (1998). Educating parish nurses. *Canadian Nurse,* 9440–9444.

Paul, P. (2000). The history of the relationship between nursing and faith traditions. In M. B. Clark and J. K. Olson (Eds.), *Nursing within a faith community: Promoting health in times of transition* (pp. 147–159). Thousand Oaks, CA: Sage.

Pincharoen, S., & Congdon, J. G. (2003). Spirituality and health in older Thai persons in the United States. *Western Journal of Nursing Research, 25*(1), 93–108.

Reed, P. G. (1987). Spirituality and well-being in terminally ill hospitalized adults. *Research in Nursing & Health, 10,* 335–344.

Saudia, T. L., et al. (1991). Health locus of control and helpfulness of prayer. *Heart & Lung, 20,* 60–65.

Sawatzky, J. E., & Fowler-Kerry, S. (2003). Impact of caregiving: Listening to the voice of informal caregivers. *Journal of Psychiatric and Mental Health Nursing, 10,* 277–286.

Semenic, S. E., Callister, L. C., & Feldman, P. (2004). Giving birth: The voices of Orthodox Jewish women living in Canada. *Journal of Obstetric, Gynecologic and Neonatal Nursing, 33,* 80–87.

Shelly, J. A. (2000). *Spiritual care: A guide for caregivers.* Downers Grove, IL: Intervarsity Press.

Shelly, J. A., & Miller, A. (1999). *Called to care: A Christian theology of nursing.* Downers Grove, IL: Intervarsity Press.

Simington, J. (1996). Attitudes toward the old and death, and spiritual well-being. *Journal of Religion and Health, 35,* 21–32.

Taylor, E. J. (2002). *Spiritual care: Nursing theory, research, and practice.* Upper Saddle River, NJ: Prentice Hall.

Turner, R. P., et al. (1995). Religious or spiritual problem: A culturally sensitive diagnostic category in the DSM-IV. *The Journal of Nervous and Mental Disease, 183*(7), 435–444.

Vance, D. L. (2001). Nurses' attitudes towards spirituality and spiritual care. *MEDSURG Nursing, 10,* 264–268.

Van Dover, L. J., & Bacon, J. M. (2001). Spiritual care in nursing practice: A close-up view. *Nursing Forum, 36,* 18–30.

Yim, R. J. R., & Vande Creek, L. (1996). Unbinding grief and life's losses for thriving recovery after open heart surgery. *Caregiver Journal, 12*(2), 8–20.

Recommended Web Sites

Canadian Association for Parish Nursing Ministry: *http://www.capnm.ca*

The Canadian Association for Parish Nursing Ministry is committed to the development of the resource of parish nursing within Canada.

Center for Spirituality and Healing: *http://www.csh.umn.edu*

Established in 1995 at the University of Minnesota, the Center for Spirituality and Healing provides education about integrative medicine, combining biomedical, complementary, cross-cultural, and spiritual care.

Center for Spirituality, Theology and Health: *http://www.dukespiritualityandhealth.org*

The purpose of the Center is to conduct research on the effects of spirituality on physical and mental health.

Nurses Christian Fellowship: *http://www.intervarsity.org/ncf/facgrad/scr.html*

Nurses Christian Fellowship is a Christian organization with the goal of integrating Christianity into nursing care. This link examines the scope and trend of research related to spiritual care.

25

The Experience of Loss, Death, and Grief

Debbie Sanazaro, RN, MSN, GNP
Barbara Brown, RN, BA, BScN, MScN (Canadian author)

Objectives

Mastery of content in this chapter will enable the student to:

- Define the key terms listed.
- Identify the nurse's role in assisting clients who have experienced loss, death, and grief.
- Describe and compare the phases of grieving from Kübler-Ross, Bowlby, and Worden.
- List and discuss the five categories of loss.
- Describe the types of grief.
- Describe characteristics of a person experiencing grief.
- Discuss variables that influence a person's response to grief.
- Develop a nursing care plan for a client or family experiencing loss and grief.
- Explain reasons for the need for improved end-of-life care for clients.
- Discuss principles of palliative care.
- Describe how to involve family members in palliative care.
- Describe the procedure for care of the body after death.
- Discuss the nurse's own loss experience when caring for dying clients.

Loss and grief are experiences that affect not only clients and their families, but the nurses who care for them as well. Canada and other Western societies present a death-denying culture (Northcott & Wilson, 2001). This means that Canadians often deny the need to express grief and to feel the pain associated with a loss, both of which are beneficial to healing. Grief affects survivors physically, psychologically, socially, and spiritually as a result of very real, concrete losses. Death of a client, for example, leaves family, friends, and caregivers feeling powerless. Most nurses enter the profession with the intent of helping clients recover from illness, adjust to illness-related changes in lifestyle, and move toward health restoration. It is frightening to learn that knowledge, skill, and technology cannot always come together to result in cure.

The nurse's role in facilitating the grief process includes assisting survivors to feel the loss, express the loss, and complete the tasks of the grief process (End-of-Life Nursing Education Consortium [ELNEC], 2000). To be effective, the nurse must have a thorough understanding of a client's loss, its significance and meaning to the client and family, and how it affects the client and family's ability to carry on. Providing care for clients in crisis from loss or at the end of life requires knowledge and caring to help bring comfort to clients and families, even when a hope for cure is gone. Helping clients to a peaceful, dignified death is an important aspect of nursing care. Although working with dying clients is difficult, nurses also find it to be a rewarding and often life-changing experience, both professionally and personally (Perry, 1998).

Table 25-1 Types of Loss

Definition	Implications of Loss
Loss of external objects (e.g., loss, misplacement, deterioration, theft, destruction by natural causes)	Extent of grieving depends on object's value, sentiment attached to it, and its usefulness.
Loss of known environment (e.g., moving from a neighbourhood, hospitalization, a new job, moving out of intensive care unit)	Loss occurs through maturational or situational events and through injury or illness. Loneliness or newness of unfamiliar setting threatens self-esteem and makes grieving difficult.
Loss of a significant other (e.g., being promoted, moving, or running away; loss of a family member, friend, trusted nurse, acquaintance, or animal companion)	Significant other typically fulfills another person's need for psychological safety, love and belonging, and self-esteem.
Loss of an aspect of self (e.g., body part, psychological or physiological function)	Illness, injury, or developmental changes result in loss of aspect of self that causes grief and permanent changes in body image and self-concept.
Loss of life (e.g., death of family members, friend, or acquaintance; own death)	Loss of life creates grief for those left behind. Person facing death often fears pain, loss of control, and dependency on others.

Scientific Knowledge Base

Loss

Throughout our lives, we form attachments and suffer losses. We develop independence from our parents, start and leave school, change friends, begin careers, and form relationships. The growing-up process is natural and positive, yet as we move our lives forward, we suffer necessary losses (Hasler, 1996). **Necessary losses** are an integral part of each person's life. We expect our losses to be recovered and replaced by something different or better, but there are other losses that cause us to suffer an unbearable change in our safety and security (Hasler, 1996). Losses such as death of a loved one, divorce, or loss of independence are significant and can have long-term effects on physical and psychological health.

Loss comes in many forms depending on the values and priorities learned within a person's sphere of influence, including family, friends, society, and culture. A person experiences loss in the absence of an object, person, body part or function, emotion, or idea that was formerly present (Table 25-1). Losses may be actual or perceived. An **actual loss** is any loss of a person or object that can no longer be felt, heard, known, or experienced by the individual. Examples could include the loss of a body part, child, relationship, or role at work. Lost objects that have been valued by a client include any possession that is worn out, misplaced, stolen, or ruined by disaster. For example, a child may grieve over the loss of a favourite toy. A **perceived loss** is any loss that is uniquely defined by the grieving client. It may be less obvious to others. An example is the loss of confidence or prestige. Perceived losses are easily overlooked or misunderstood, yet the process of grief follows the same sequencing and progression as actual losses. Individual interpretation makes a difference in how the perceived loss is uniquely valued and the response that one will have during grieving.

Losses may also be maturational, situational, or both. A **maturational loss** includes any change in the developmental process that is normally expected during a lifetime. One example would be a mother's feeling of loss as a child goes to school for the first time. Events associated with maturational loss are part of normal life transitions, but the feelings of loss persist as grieving helps a person cope with the change. **Situational loss** includes any sudden, unpredictable external event. Often this type of loss includes multiple losses rather than a single loss, such as an automobile accident that leaves a driver paralyzed, unable to return to work, and grieving over the loss of the passenger in the accident.

The type of loss and the perception of the loss influence the depth and duration of grief that a person experiences. Each individual responds to loss differently. It is incorrect to assume that the loss of an object does not generate the same level of stress as loss of a loved one. The value an individual places on the lost object (e.g., a family pet) determines the emotional response to the separation. A nurse must assess the special meaning that a loss has for a client and its effect on the client's health and well-being.

Hospitalization and chronic illness or disability are special circumstances that have multiple associated losses. When clients enter a hospital, they lose their privacy, control over body functions and their daily routines, their modesty, and any illusions that they may have about their personal indestructibility. A chronic illness or disability adds concern over financial security. Furthermore, long-term illness may require a job change, threaten independence, and force alterations in lifestyle. Even a brief illness or hospitalization requires temporary shifts in family role functioning. Chronic or debilitating illness may pose a major threat to the stability of relationships.

Death is the ultimate loss. Although death is part of the continuum of life and a universal and inevitable part of being human, it is also a mystical event that generates anxiety and fear. Death ends relationships and separates people. Even with a strong spiritual grounding, facing death is often difficult for the dying person, as well as for the person's family, friends, and caregivers. A person's terminal illness reminds close friends and associates of their own mortality. A person with an advanced, progressive, ultimately fatal illness, such as chronic renal failure, end-stage heart failure, amyotrophic lateral sclerosis, or metastatic cancer, faces many levels of suffering. It is difficult to be sick, and many people dislike seeking help from others, yet nearly all want companionship in the face of death (Finucane, 2002).

Callahan (1995) suggested that talking about death has been banished from our society, our everyday lives, our language, and even our thinking. Feelings of guilt, anger, and fear arise when death must finally be faced. It may cause family members and caregivers to withdraw at a time when the dying person needs a trusted, unhurried companion, acting with gentle advocacy and humility. Moreover, as professional caregivers increasingly assist the dying, families have become less involved in the care of their loved ones (Northcott & Wilson, 2001). The way a person approaches dying will be influenced by personal fundamental beliefs and values, past experiences with death, culture, spirituality, and the quality of the human emotional support available.

Table 25-2 The Grief Process

Kübler-Ross's Five Stages of Dying	Bowlby's Four Phases of Mourning	Worden's Four Tasks of Mourning
Denial	Numbing	Accepting the reality of loss
Anger	Yearning and searching	Working through the pain of grief
Bargaining	Disorganization and despair	Adjusting to the environment without the deceased
Depression	Reorganization	Emotionally relocating the deceased and moving on with life
Acceptance		

Grief

Grief is the emotional response to a loss. It is manifested in a variety of ways that are unique to an individual and based on personal experiences, cultural expectations, and spiritual beliefs (Farber, Egnew, & Herman-Bertsch, 1999; see chapters 9 and 24). Coping with grief after a loss involves the process of mourning, the outward social expression of a loss (ELNEC, 2000). It involves working through the grief until an individual accepts and adapts to his or her expectations to go on in life without that which was lost.

Bereavement includes grief and mourning—the inner feelings and outward reactions of the survivor (ELNEC, 2000). Survivors go through a bereavement period that is not linear. It does not proceed in sequential stages that can be precisely predicted, which may imply passivity on the part of the bereaved. Rather, an individual will move back and forth through a series of stages and/or tasks many times, possibly extending over a period of several years, before the process is completed. Although no one really "gets over" a loss, the individual can heal and learn to live with a loss (ELNEC, 2000). There are several theorists who have developed stages of the grieving process and a series of tasks for survivors to work through their bereavement and adapt to life with a loss.

Theories of Grief

Kübler-Ross's Stages of Dying. The framework for Kübler-Ross's theory (1969) is behaviour oriented and includes five stages (Table 25-2). During **denial,** an individual acts as though nothing has happened and may refuse to believe or understand that a loss has occurred. In the **anger** stage, the individual resists the loss and may strike out at everyone and everything. During **bargaining,** the individual postpones awareness of the reality of the loss and may try to deal in a subtle or overt way as though the loss can be prevented. A person finally realizes the full impact and significance of the loss during the stage of **depression,** when the individual may feel overwhelmingly lonely and withdraw from interpersonal interaction. Finally, during the **acceptance** stage, the individual accepts the loss and begins to look to the future.

Bowlby's Phases of Mourning. Bowlby's attachment theory (1980) is the foundation for his theory on mourning. Attachment is described as an instinctive behaviour that leads to the development of affectionate bonds between children and their primary caregiver. These bonds are present and active throughout the life cycle. Later the bonds are generalized to other people with whom individuals form close relationships. Attachment behaviour ensures our survival because it keeps us in close contact with people who can offer us protection and support.

Bowlby described four phases of mourning (see Table 25-2). As in the case of the other grief theories, a person can move back and forth between any two of the phases while responding to the loss. The **numbing** phase may last from a few hours to a week or more and may be interrupted by periods of extremely intense emotion. It is the briefest phase of mourning. The grieving person may describe this phase as feeling "stunned" or "unreal." Numbing may serve to protect the body from the onslaught or consequence of the loss. The second phase of **yearning and searching** arouses emotional outbursts of tearful sobbing and acute distress in most people. The phase is painful, but must be endured (Hasler, 1996). Parkes (1972) has explained that it is necessary for the bereaved person to experience the pain of grief in order to get the grief work done. Then, anything that continually allows the person to avoid or suppress the pain can be expected to prolong the course of mourning. Common physical symptoms include tightness in the chest and throat, a shortness of breath, feelings of weakness and lethargy, insomnia, and loss of appetite. A person may also experience an intense yearning for the object or individual who is lost. This phase may last for months or years. During the phase of **disorganization and despair,** an individual may endlessly examine how and why the loss occurred. It is common for the person to express anger at anyone who might be responsible. Gradually, this examination gives way to an acceptance that the loss is permanent. During the final phase of **reorganization,** which may require as much as a year or more, the person begins to accept unaccustomed roles, acquire new skills, and build new relationships. People experiencing this phase must be encouraged to untie themselves from their old relationship, while not devaluing it or feeling that in so doing they are lessening its importance (Hasler, 1996).

Worden's Four Tasks of Mourning. Worden's four tasks of mourning (1991) imply that people who mourn can be actively involved in helping themselves and can be assisted by outside intervention. Although time varies greatly in individuals, the tasks typically require a minimum of a full year to work through.

- *Task I: To accept the reality of the loss.* Even when a death has been expected, there is always some period of disbelief and surprise that the event has really happened. This task involves the processes required to accept that the person or object is gone and will not return.
- *Task II: To work through the pain of grief.* Even though people respond to loss differently, it is impossible to experience a loss and work through grief without emotional pain. Individuals who deny or shut off the pain prolong their grief.
- *Task III: To adjust to the environment in which the deceased is missing.* According to Worden, a person does not realize the full impact of a loss for at least 3 months. At this point, many friends and associates stop calling and the person is left to ponder the full impact of loneliness. People completing this task must take on roles formerly filled by the deceased, including some tasks that they never fully appreciated.
- *Task IV: To emotionally relocate the deceased and move on with life.* The goal of this task is not to forget the deceased or give up the relationship with the deceased but to have the deceased take a new, less prominent place in a person's emotional life. This is often the most difficult task to complete because people fear that if they make other attachments, they will forget their loved one or be disloyal. A person completes this stage after realizing that it is possible to love other people without loving the deceased person less.

Types of Grief. Knowledge of types of grief, which are based on characteristics or signs and symptoms of grief, enables a nurse to implement appropriate bereavement therapies.

Normal Grief. Normal or uncomplicated grief consists of the normal feelings, behaviours, and reactions to a loss, including resentment, sorrow, anger, crying, loneliness, and temporary withdrawal from activities. Often the normal grief response to a loss can prove positive, helping one to mature and develop as a person. As people mature, they develop ways of dealing with losses and learn to maintain and enhance their feelings of safety and security (Hasler, 1996).

Anticipatory Grief. The process of disengaging or "letting go" that occurs before an actual loss or death has occurred is called **anticipatory grief.** For example, once a person or family receives a terminal diagnosis, they begin the process of saying goodbye and completing life affairs. The process becomes more stressful when the client is unable to make decisions as a result of deterioration in health. Unless guided by a client's explicit decisions regarding end-of-life care, the family assumes the responsibility of deciding whether to continue life-sustaining measures. The family must weigh factors such as the client's values and choices, the medical facts and probabilities, the burden of treatment, the expected future quality of life for the client, and the limitations of their own emotional resources (Tilden et al., 2001).

When dying takes a long time, the client's loved ones may have few symptoms of grief once the death occurs. This seeming absence of grief symptoms may result because the family has engaged in the grief process over time. By the time the moment of death arrives, much of the shock, denial, and tearfulness have already been experienced.

There are risks in anticipatory grieving. Family members may withdraw emotionally from the client too soon, leaving the client with no emotional support as death approaches. There may also be complications if a person who was thought to be near death survives. Family members may then have difficulty reconnecting and may even be resentful that the person has lived past life expectancy.

Complicated Grief. When a person has difficulty progressing through the normal phases or stages of grieving, bereavement becomes complicated. In these cases, bereavement appears to "go wrong" and loss never resolves. This can threaten a person's relationships with others. Complicated grief includes four types:

- *Chronic grief:* Active acute mourning that is characterized by normal grief reactions that do not subside and continue over very long periods of time (ELNEC, 2000). People verbalize an inability to "get past" the grief.
- *Delayed grief:* Characterized by normal grief reactions that are suppressed or postponed and the survivor consciously or unconsciously avoids the pain of the loss (ELNEC, 2000). Active grieving is held back, only to resurface later, usually in response to a trivial loss or upset. For example, a wife may appear to grieve for only a few weeks after the death of her spouse, but then become distraught and sad a year later when she attends a family gathering. The extreme sadness is a delayed response to the death of her husband.
- *Exaggerated grief:* People become overwhelmed by grief, and they cannot function. This may be reflected in the form of severe phobias or self-destructive behaviour such as alcoholism, substance abuse, or suicide.
- *Masked grief:* Survivors are not aware that behaviours that interfere with normal functioning are a result of their loss (ELNEC, 2000). For example, a person who is grieving may develop alterations in eating or sleeping patterns.

Disenfranchised Grief. People experience grief when a loss is experienced and cannot be openly acknowledged, socially sanctioned, or publicly shared (ELNEC, 2000). Examples include the loss of a partner from acquired immunodeficiency syndrome (AIDS), or the loss of a child in utero or at birth.

Application of Grief Theory to Other Types of Loss. Although grief theories apply mainly to the way that individuals cope with the death of a loved one, they also apply to other losses. The theories are relevant when describing the way people respond to a loss of body function, as in the case of organ transplantation or heart attack, and disability such as amputation of a limb or paralysis. Grief theory applies to individuals who progress through stages of mourning for lost independence, body integrity, and a change in body image. These individuals experience emotional pain that is very real as they progress through the stages of grieving.

Nursing Knowledge Base

Nursing knowledge has traditionally focused on the acute care setting, where losses are more physical in nature. As nurses enter the home and community setting, the definitions of loss are more comprehensive and in many ways different. Nurses must develop interventions for each unique client situation.

Factors Influencing Loss and Grief

The way that an individual perceives a loss and responds to it during bereavement is influenced by many factors.

Human Development. People of differing ages and stages of development will display different and unique symptoms of grief. For example, toddlers are unable to understand loss or death, but they feel great anxiety over loss of objects and separation from parents. School-age children experience grief over the loss of a body part or function. They often associate misdeeds with causing death. Middle-age adults usually begin to re-examine life and are sensitive to their own physical changes. Older adults often experience anticipatory grief because of aging and the possible loss of self-care abilities. Aging is frequently associated with losses such as physical changes, loss of employment, loss of social respect, loss of relationships, and threat to a sense of fulfillment and contributions made in life. However, Lund (1989) found that older adults are often resilient in responding to grief, despite it being a highly stressful process (Box 25-1).

Psychosocial Perspectives of Loss and Grief. Loss and death are life experiences that each person faces. Death is an overwhelming experience that affects everyone involved in the loss situation or in the death of the individual. According to psychologists, the valuing of individuals is a unique, learned response of a specific culture and society (Binstock & Spector, 1997). Concepts, perspectives, and definitions of loss are described within a cultural bias of a specific society (Witoszek, 1998). Age, gender, status, race, spirituality, religious beliefs, intellect, achievement, self-expression, and cultural opportunity are the basis for an individual to define and qualify the definition of life or death (Cressy, 1997). The nurse is part of that same psychosocial environment and shares many of the biases or perspectives gained during sociological development. Norms for psychosocial patterns of loss and grief are reflected in caregivers as well as in clients.

An individual's expression of grief evolves as the person matures. Personal experiences shape the coping mechanisms that the individual uses to deal with stressors. As psychologists explain, the coping mechanisms that were effective in the past are repeated as a first response to the pain of a loss. When older coping strategies are unsuccessful, new coping mechanisms are attempted (see chapter 26). When faced with a loss, a client learns what is needed for his or her own coping through repetition that is based on the successes and failures of different coping mechanisms. Sometimes the number or depths of losses become overwhelming, and familiar coping styles are not successful. For example, in the case of disenfranchised grief, society has different expectations than the person experiencing the loss, and routine coping strategies become ineffective or unavailable. Professional assistance is often required to help the client and family understand and deal realistically with losses.

Socio-economic Status. Socio-economic status influences a person's ability to obtain options and use support mechanisms when coping with loss. Generally, an individual feels greater burden from a loss when there is a lack of financial, educational, or occupational resources. For example, a client with limited finances may not be able to replace a home lost in a fire or may not be able to purchase necessary medications to manage a newly diagnosed disease. These clients require referral to community social service agencies that can provide needed resources.

Personal Relationships. When loss involves a loved one, the quality and meaning of the relationship are critical in understanding a person's grief experience. It has been said that to lose your parents is to lose your past, to lose your spouse is to lose your present, and to lose your child is to lose your future. When a relationship between two individuals has been very close, the one left behind can have great difficulty coping. Support from family and friends is based in part on the person's relationships with members of a social network and the manner and circumstances of the loss. People who do not receive support and compassion from others may have difficulty grieving.

Nature of the Loss. The ability to resolve grief depends on the meaning of the loss and the situation surrounding the loss. The ability to accept help from others influences

Focus on Older Adults — Box 25-1

- Bereavement adjustments are multi-dimensional in that nearly every aspect of a person's life can be affected by a loss.
- The overall effect of bereavement on the physical and mental health of many older spouses is not as devastating as expected.
- Older bereaved spouses commonly experience both positive and negative feelings simultaneously.
- Loneliness and problems associated with completing the tasks of daily living are two of the most common and difficult adjustments for older bereaved spouses.
- There is a great deal of diversity in how older bereaved adults adjust to the deaths of spouses.

Data from "Conclusions About Bereavement in Later Life and Implications for Interventions and Future Research," by D. A. Lund, in *Older Bereaved Spouses: Research With Practical Application*, edited by D. A. Lund, 1989, New York: Hemisphere.

whether the bereaved will be able to cope. The visibility of a loss influences the support a person receives. For example, the loss of one's home from a fire will bring support from the community, whereas a private loss of an important possession may bring less support from others. Some losses are not highly visible, such as reproductive loss (e.g., miscarriage, stillbirth, abortion, giving up a child for adoption, infertility). The Centre for Reproductive Loss was founded in Montreal to help those who have suffered such a loss to acknowledge and deal with their unspoken grief (Gray & Lassance, 2003).

The suddenness of a loss can often cause slower resolution from grief. For example, a sudden and unexpected death is generally more difficult for a family to accept than one following a long-term chronic disease.

Culture and Ethnicity. A person's cultural background strongly influences attitudes toward life-sustaining treatments during terminal illness (Blackhall et al., 1999). Cultural background and family practices also influence people's interpretation of a loss and the expression of grief (Box 25-2). When individuals lose control over aspects of their life due to illness, their basic core belief systems are critical components of culture that they can and often do hold on to (Thomas, 2001). Culture affects how clients and their support systems or families respond to loss (see chapter 9). For example, in the Western hemisphere, the grieving process is usually personal and private, with individuals showing restrained emotion. However, the ceremonies surrounding a person's death offer time for grief resolution and reminiscing. In Eastern nations, such as the Philippines or China, respect for the dead is shown by wailing and physically demonstrating grief for a specified period of time. Despite these trends, members of the same ethnocultural background may respond to loss and death differently. Nurses must acquire an understanding and appreciation of each client's cultural values as they apply to the experience of loss, death, and grieving.

Canada is a multicultural society and, as such, there are many cultural contexts and responses to dying, death, and bereavement (Northcott & Wilson, 2001). Nurses must be able to support and guide clients and families along the final life journey in a culturally informed and acceptable manner. Culturally sensitive practices are needed to guide the development of effective nursing interventions. Latimer (2000) suggested that "sincere interest, respect, flexibility and knowledge are the keys to meeting the needs of patients and families in a culturally sensitive way" (p. 93).

Spiritual Beliefs. Individuals' spirituality significantly influences their ability to cope with loss. Some of the spiritual resources that clients may depend upon during a loss include faith in a higher power or influence, their community of fellowship with friends, their sources of hope and meaning in life, and their use of religious rituals and practices. Loss can sometimes cause internal conflicts about spiritual values and the meaning of life. Clients who have a strong interconnectedness with a higher power or others are often very resilient and able to face death with relatively minimal discomfort (see chapter 24).

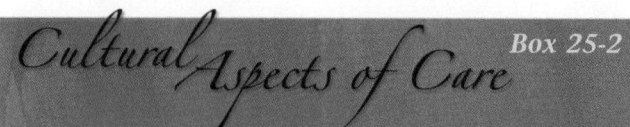

Cultural Aspects of Care — Box 25-2

At the end of life, rituals, mourning practices, and specific expressions of grief of all cultures are necessary for participants to have a sense of acceptance and inner peace. There is controversy as to whether appropriate care at the end of life achieves a "good death" or an "acceptable death" for clients. Do clients achieve a sense of comfort and peace during the death experience? Most hospital policies and procedures support an "acceptable death" for the client who is dying. This means providing basic standard levels of care and support, which may or may not take into account a client's cultural beliefs and practices. The expectation is that death be non-theatrical, disciplined, and with minimal exchange of emotions. In contrast, Kagawa-Singer (1998) described a "good death" as one that allows social adjustments and personal preparations for the transition that will occur. A good death allows time for the client and family to make both the private and public preparations that are needed to help the family begin the adjustment to a world without their loved one, and for the client to complete unfinished tasks. The disengagement that occurs between the person who is dying and loved ones takes many forms because of cultural differences:

- Hindus envision a circular pattern of life and death with multiple deaths and rebirths.
- Christians believe in a more linear trajectory as expressed in the construct of a heaven where all good people will gather after death and a hell where lost souls will go for eternity.
- Some Aboriginal cultures envision the land of the dead as a parallel world, where the spirits of the dead can directly affect the lives of the living.
- For other cultures, the disengagement can be abrupt and final, even to the point of sanctions against speaking names of the deceased to avoid keeping them from leaving earth and gaining peace.

Implications for Practice

- A nurse's concept of social support must be broadened to include greater variation in the timing, form, and mode of support provided to grieving clients and families.
- Cultural beliefs influence who makes up a client's support network and what support is acceptable to both give and receive during death.
- Care provided at the end of life within the client and family's cultural context draws from the resources of their whole lives.

Data from "The Cultural Context of Death Rituals and Mourning Practices," by M. Kagawa-Singer, 1998, *Oncology Nursing Forum, 25*(10), p. 1752.

Coping With Grief and Loss

In order to support clients and families during loss, nurses must understand how people normally cope with grief and loss. Nursing interventions involve reinforcing the client's successful coping mechanisms and introducing new coping approaches. Chapter 26 summarizes the nursing care principles for assisting clients in coping with stressful situations.

Hope. **Hope** is the anticipation of a continued good, an improvement or lessening of something unpleasant. It is a multi-dimensional concept that is energizing and provides comfort while one endures life threats and personal challenges (Bierman et al., 1998; Morse & Doberneck, 1995). Hope enhances coping skills and even influences a person's survival (Doka, 1993). A person often reveals hope through an expression of expectations for life, the present, and the future. Often in terminal illness, a client focuses hope on milestones (e.g., a child's high school graduation or the completion of a project at work), significant events (e.g., an upcoming anniversary), or the relief of pain or other disabling symptoms (Weissman and Matson, 1999). Spiritual distress is often based on the person's definition of hope or lack of hope. People may view hope as encouragement to work toward recovery. Others may view hope more negatively by not being able to see any future favourable outcomes.

Hope can be found in all aspects of life as a force that helps one cope with life stressors. It has purpose and direction and gives reason for being (Post-White et al., 1996). The existence and maintenance of hope depend on a person having strong relationships and a sense of emotional connectedness to others. Nurses and other health care professionals may provide that personal connectedness essential to hope. Hope is often the basis from which clients find meaning in their illness. Hopefulness enables one to see life as enduring or having sustained meaning or purpose (Chochinov, 2002). Nurses have reported that they feel they make the greatest difference in clients' lives by helping them keep hope alive (Perry, 2002). Chapter 24 discusses the conceptual components of hope and related nursing care implications.

Critical Thinking

When nurses care for clients who have experienced losses, successful critical thinking requires a synthesis of knowledge, previous experience with loss and grief, and information gathered from clients and families. The nurse must apply both critical thinking attitudes and intellectual and professional standards to provide appropriate and responsive nursing care.

During assessment, the nurse must analyze all sources of information that lead to the selection of appropriate nursing diagnoses (Figure 25–1). To understand the process of grief and its effect on the client and family, the nurse integrates knowledge from nursing and other disciplines and previous experiences in caring for clients suffering loss. Knowledge of the stages of grief, for example, enables a nurse to better empathize with a client and family and to understand the client's behaviours. Through identification of the stages of grief, the nurse is able to direct assessment questions. The application of critical thinking attitudes and standards then helps the nurse to apply this information in a relevant and therapeutic way for the client's benefit. For example, the critical thinking attitude of perseverance is needed to learn as much as possible about the type of grief a client is experiencing to ultimately select the most appropriate nursing interventions. The use of intellectual standards such as significance and relevance help to ensure that the information gathered is pertinent to the client's unique situation. Professional standards include those of bioethics, the dying person's bill of rights (Box 25-3), and clinical standards such as guidelines for managing cancer pain. All provide evidence-based guidelines for a thorough assessment and humane, compassionate nursing care.

The Nursing Process and Grief

NP Assessment

When a nurse cares for a client who has experienced or is facing a loss, assessment includes the client, family, and significant others. Grief assessment is ongoing throughout the course of an illness for the client and family and for the bereavement period after the death for the survivors (ELNEC, 2000). The nurse should not assume how or if the client or family experiences grief. The nurse should also avoid assuming that a particular behaviour indicates grief; rather, the nurse should allow clients to share what is happening in their own way. An effective nurse encourages clients to tell their stories. This requires the nurse to establish trust with clients and to evoke a caring presence. It is helpful to have clients and families find a time and place to express their grief and describe their experiences (Figure 25–2). The nurse interviews clients and families separately unless a client requests having family members present. A thorough and comprehensive approach to the assessment of grief will result in a well-designed plan of care that will facilitate clients' abilities to work through grief.

A nurse begins by interviewing the client and family, using honest and open communication. Listening carefully and observing the client's responses and behaviours are important. The nurse assumes a neutral perspective and remains alert for non-verbal cues such as facial expressions, voice tones, and topics that are avoided. While gathering data, the nurse summarizes and validates any impressions formed with the client and family so that appropriate nursing diagnoses can be made. Information from other health care workers, such as physicians, social workers, and members of pastoral care will contribute to the database.

Type and Stage of Grief. It is important for the nurse to assess how a client is reacting rather than how the client *should be* reacting. The sequencing of stages or behaviours of grief may occur in order, they may be skipped, or they may reoccur. A single behaviour can be representative of any number of types of grief. Therefore, the identification of the type and stage of grief should be used only to guide the nurse's assessment and not to judge the outcomes of the grieving process. The application of a theorist's phase of grief aids the nurse in the accurate assessment of a situation. For example, if a client is complaining of loneliness and difficulty falling asleep, the nurse considers all factors surrounding the loss. When did the loss occur? What type of loss occurred? The client may be experiencing a normal grief reaction, or if the loss occurred 2 years previously, the client may be experiencing chronic grief.

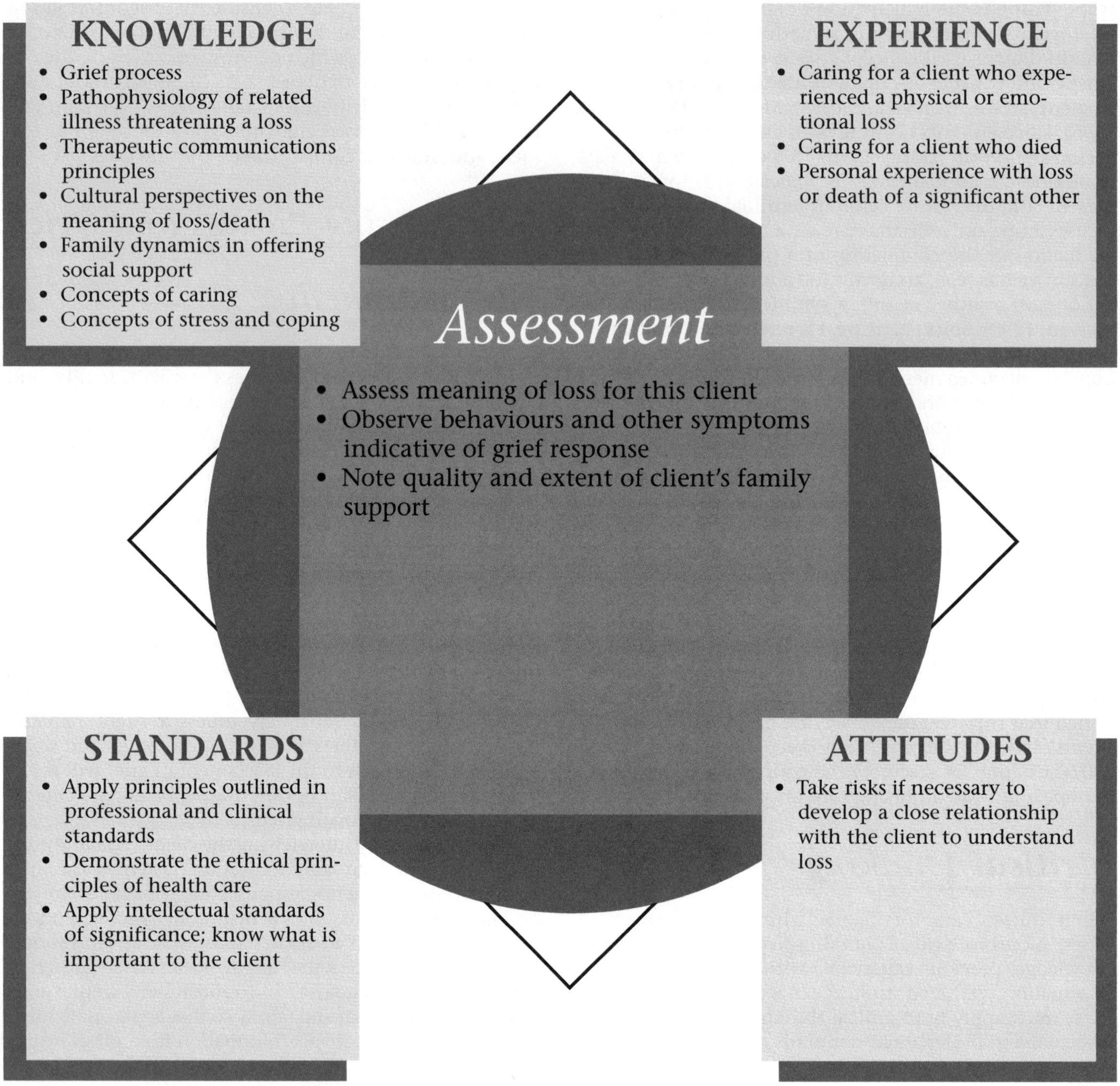
KNOWLEDGE
• Grief process
• Pathophysiology of related illness threatening a loss
• Therapeutic communications principles
• Cultural perspectives on the meaning of loss/death
• Family dynamics in offering social support
• Concepts of caring
• Concepts of stress and coping
EXPERIENCE
• Caring for a client who experienced a physical or emotional loss
• Caring for a client who died
• Personal experience with loss or death of a significant other
Assessment
• Assess meaning of loss for this client
• Observe behaviours and other symptoms indicative of grief response
• Note quality and extent of client's family support
STANDARDS
• Apply principles outlined in professional and clinical standards
• Demonstrate the ethical principles of health care
• Apply intellectual standards of significance; know what is important to the client
ATTITUDES
• Take risks if necessary to develop a close relationship with the client to understand loss

FIGURE **25–1** Critical thinking model for loss, death, and grieving assessment.

The nurse asks clients to describe their loss and how it has affected them. "Tell me how your diagnosis of heart disease makes you feel." The nurse can anticipate characteristics or responses during a phase of grieving but should allow clients to describe their feelings as thoroughly as possible. "How has this change in your life affected you today?" "Tell me more." The nurse probes and validates feelings expressed in the client's emotions: "You seem angry, tell me more . . . ," "You seem sad, tell me . . . ," "What are your feelings about. . . ." The nurse avoids premature assumptions about the phase of grief a client might be experiencing so as to avoiding terminating assessment too early.

Grief Reactions. The nurse uses psychological and physical assessment skills to gather a complete database about the client, family, or both. Although no two people grieve exactly the same way, most people who grieve have at least some outward signs and symptoms (Box 25-4). Clinical reasoning is needed to analyze the data cues and to determine the appropriate related cause. For example, a client who is experiencing dysfunctional grieving may have a changing affect, withdrawn activity level, somatic complaints such as headache, upset stomach, and alterations in concentration. The nurse might associate these symptoms with any number of problems such as anxiety, gastrointestinal disturbances, or even impaired memory.

Box 25-3 A Dying Person's Bill of Rights

I have the right to be in control.
I have the right to be treated as a living human being until I die. I have the right to have a sense of purpose.
I have the right to be cared for by those who can maintain a sense of hopefulness.
I have the right to express my feelings and emotions about my approaching death in my own way.
I have the right to have a respected spirituality. I have the right to participate in decisions about my care. I have the right to expect continuing medical and nursing attention even though "cure" goals must be changed to "comfort" goals.
I have the right not to die alone.
I have the right to be comfortable.
I have the right to have my questions answered honestly. I have the right not to be deceived.
I have the right to have help from and for my family in accepting my death.
I have the right to die in peace and dignity.
I have the right to laugh and to be angry and sad. I have the right to retain my individuality and not be judged for my decisions that may be contrary to beliefs of others. I have the right to be cared for by caring, sensitive, knowledgeable people who will try to understand my needs and will be able to gain some satisfaction in helping me face my death.

Adapted from "The Dying Person's Bill of Rights," by A. J. Barbus, 1975, *American Journal of Nursing, 75,* p. 99; and *Hospice RN: Patient's Bill of Rights,* 2003, *http://www.geocities.com/HotSprings/5120/bill.htm*

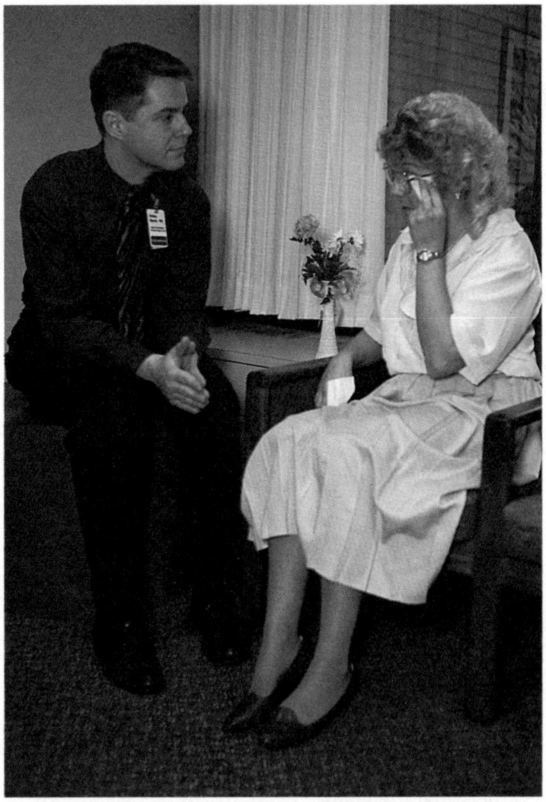

FIGURE **25–2** Nurses find a private place to listen to clients express their grief.

However, the focus is to assess the client's symptoms in context. What is the meaning and significance of loss, and how is it affecting the client in physical and psychological ways? What does the client associate the symptoms with? In what way are the symptoms related to one another when they occur? What symptoms are observed when the client openly expresses grief? Over what time period have the symptoms been present: before the loss, during the loss? Careful analysis refines the nurse's ability to make judgments about the client's condition.

A loss takes place in a social context. When the primary provider in a family has a terminal illness, the family begins to reorganize itself as soon as the client is no longer able to fulfill the same number and types of roles. When a person is disabled, the client and family undergo similar reorganization, realigning roles and responsibilities to meet the demands. During this time, clients and families can experience a variety of physical and psychological symptoms. The nurse assesses the entire family's response to loss, recognizing that family members may be dealing with different aspects of grief than the client. Good interviewing and physical assessment skills guide the nurse as caregiver and as an advocate of the client in planning appropriate nursing care.

Factors That Affect Grief. Because a number of factors influence loss and the grief response, it helps to discuss the meaning of loss to the client and family. This usually

Box 25-4 Symptoms of Normal Grief Feelings

Feelings

Sadness
Anger
Guilt or self-reproach
Anxiety
Loneliness
Fatigue
Helplessness
Shock/numbness (lack of feeling)
Yearning
Emancipation/relief

Cognitions (Thought Patterns)

Disbelief
Confusion
Preoccupation about the deceased
Sense of the presence of the deceased
Hallucinations
Hopelessness ("I'll never be OK again")

Physical Sensations

Hollowness in the stomach
Tightness in the chest
Tightness in the throat
Oversensitivity to noise
Sense of depersonalization ("Nothing seems real")
Feeling short of breath
Muscle weakness
Lack of energy
Dry mouth

Behaviours

Sleep disturbances
Appetite disturbances
Absentminded behaviour
Dreams of the deceased
Sighing
Crying
Carrying objects that belonged to the deceased

Table 25-3 Assessment of Factors Influencing Grieving

Factor	Areas/Suggestions/Questions to Explore
Nature of relationships	Functions of the family, community, and society *Examples:* How long have you known your friend? What role has your mother played in your family? What is your relationship? Will it change? How will family relationships change as a result of the loss?
Social support system	Availability of family, friends, health care workers *Examples:* Who is present? Absent? Supportive? Non-supportive? What do family/friends do that is most meaningful? Are family/friends available when needed? Are health care workers accepting and exploring ways to preserve the client's dignity and lifestyle?
Nature of loss	Actual versus perceived; death issues; impact on roles *Examples:* Tell me what the loss means to you. What factors help you to grieve? What factors interfere with grieving? What past experiences or outcomes have you had with loss?
Cultural and spiritual beliefs	Values, cultural norms, spirituality, customs, attitudes *Examples:* What is your belief about death? Meaning of life? What customs do you value at the time of death? How is this loss viewed by others of your culture or religious group? Do religious practices interfere with medical treatments? Who has the right to say "yes" or "no" to life-sustaining measures?
Loss of personal life goals	Actual or perceived individual losses affecting future decisions and options *Examples:* What is your goal in life for . . .? How has this changed as a result of your diagnosis? How will your role change your personal goals? What planning have you and your family made for your own life?
Family's grief	Relationships, involvement with the dying process *Examples:* Observe client and family's level of grief, patterns of behaviour, rank of leadership or power. What has helped family members deal with problems in the past? What was not helpful? What are the family's strengths and weaknesses?
Survivor risk factors	High risk, such as sudden death, violent death, loss of a child *Examples:* Describe your feelings at this time. Let's talk about why you think you could have prevented this. Are you feeling guilty because . . .? What are unresolved issues or perceptions toward others?
Hope	Goals, worth, adaptation to future changes *Examples:* Tell me what you think about your treatment plan. What do you expect will happen to you? How does this illness affect your goals in life? What are you hoping for following your surgery?

provides information that allows the nurse to explore a number of topics in detail, such as personal characteristics of the person experiencing loss, the nature of family relationships, support systems, and cultural and spiritual beliefs (Table 25-3). The nurse must then apply assessment skills from appropriate specialty areas (e.g., spiritual or family assessment; see chapters 24 and 16, respectively) to acquire a thorough understanding of the client's loss.

End-of-Life Decisions. Although living wills or advanced directives are not recognized legally in all provinces (Keatings & Smith, 2000), the Canadian Nurses Association (CNA), along with other national health organizations, developed the *Joint Statement on Advance Directives* (1994). In this document, the CNA states that "all persons have the right to make decisions regarding their health care and treatment, including the right to request or refuse life-sustaining treatment" (p. 1). An advance directive documents a person's preferences regarding life-sustaining treatment and communicates these preferences if the person becomes incapable of doing so for himself or herself (CNA, 1998). Nurses must be aware of the legal status of advance directives in their province or territory and the laws regarding a person's competence to consent to treatment (see Chapter 8).

When a person has a terminal illness, family members must face end-of-life decisions that have ethical, legal, and practical implications. Families experience a very high level of stress when deciding whether to withdraw life-sustaining treatments (Tilden et al., 2001). Although some clients may have advance directives, it is important for family members to know a client's wishes in regard to life-sustaining measures.

The *Code of Ethics for Registered Nurses* (CNA, 2002) identifies three values that are pertinent to nurses assisting individuals in end-of-life decision making: (a) health and well-being—nurses must ensure that an individual's wishes as stated in an advance directive are respected and continuing care and support are provided, (b) choice—nurses must respect and promote the autonomy of individuals and help clients to express their needs and values and obtain appropriate care, and (c) dignity—nurses must advocate on the client's behalf and examine biological, psychological, social, cultural, and spiritual factors that affect end-of-life treatment decisions (CNA, 1998).

Benner et al. (2003) articulated a set of core nursing principles regarding end-of-life care, in which "attending to death as a human passage" is central. A nurse must assess the client's and family's wishes for end-of-life care, including the preferred place for death, the use of and the level of life-sustaining measures, and expectations regarding pain control and symptom management (Box 25-5). Does the client want to try all available treatments? Does the family or client insist on use of a feeding tube for continued nutritional support after the client stops eating? When life support requires use of a mechanical ventilator, is this something the client wants? Does the family feel comfortable in administering analgesics? Family members face complex decisions with unresolved burdens and guilt, limited knowledge, and an inability to conceptualize the dying trajectory or how a person's final days or weeks will be experienced (Forbes, Bern-Klug, & Gessert, 2000). The nurse must give the client and family time to discuss their preferences. Often it is necessary to return to a conversation on a subsequent day or visit. If the nurse feels uncomfortable in assessing a client's wishes, it is important to find a health care provider who is experienced with discussing end-of-life issues and can assist in communicating a client's preferences to the health care team.

End-of-life care is one of the more significant topics a nurse will discuss with clients. A nurse cannot keep what is learned about a client's preferences private. Good interdisciplinary teamwork is essential to provide quality end-of-life care. Thus, the nurse must communicate what is known about client preferences and decisions in change-of-shift reports, health team conferences, written care plans, and ongoing consultation with physicians and other health team members.

Research Highlight — Box 25-5

Family Perception of End-of-Life Care

Research Focus

Family members are often involved in providing care during a dying person's last month of life. Their perspectives of how the person's last days of life are spent provide valuable insight in the quality of end-of-life care.

Research Abstract

This is a retrospective study of decedents and their families. Data about family views of health services and clinicians' care during the last month of life were collected. Researchers also conducted telephone surveys of family members using a 58-item survey. The survey obtained information about family members' perceptions of end-of-life care.

Findings suggest that a high rate of advance planning and a high level of clinician respect for client-family preferences existed. There was a low use of aggressive, life-sustaining treatments and greater frequency of decisions to forego aggressive treatments rather than to discontinue them once started. All clients who died at home preferred that location. However, almost half of clients who received care in a hospital preferred that setting. One third of the families indicated their family member experienced moderate to severe pain in the final week of life. Families had more complaints about the management of pain for decedents who died at home, even though they did not report higher levels of pain. Generally, there was a high level of satisfaction with clinicians' efforts to manage pain.

Evidence-Based Practice

- It is important to learn directly from clients and families their wishes regarding preferred location of the client's death.
- Families of dying clients may have low expectations of pain management; nevertheless, aggressive therapies are needed to help comfort dying clients.
- Nurses should recognize that family members are more aware of pain management problems and bear more responsibility for direct care of such needs.
- Nurses should provide guidance and support to help families administer necessary pain therapies.

Reference

Tolle, S., et al. (2000). Family reports of barriers to optimal care of the dying. *Nursing Research, 49*(6), 310–317.

Nurses' Experience With Grief. When caring for grieving clients, nurses must assess their own emotional well-being. Self-reflection, which is a part of critical thinking, is a valuable tool in assessing whether one's sadness is related to the client, to unresolved personal experiences from the past, or to a combination of both. It is normal to have personal feelings and emotions about certain illnesses and death. However, it is inappropriate to place personal family situations and values before those of the client. Talking with friends and professional colleagues may help the nurse resolve conflicts about caring for dying clients. Some nurses choose to work in a specialty area where there are few deaths. Part of being a professional involves knowing oneself and when to move away from a situation.

Client Expectations. The nurse must assess the client's and family's expectations for nursing care. The client's perceptions and expectations can influence how the nurse prioritizes nursing diagnoses. For example, if clients perceive that their level of pain and discomfort is severe, they will be less attentive to the nurse's attempts to discuss the significance and meaning of their loss. Before the nurse can begin meaningful discussion or counselling, the client must be comfortable. The nurse should assess the client's expectations within the context of the loss by asking questions such as, "How can we help you cope with your loss?" "What do you feel is necessary from us for you to be able to resolve the grief you feel?" "What is most important that we do for you while you are under our care?"

It is important to give family members the chance to explain how they perceive the nurse's role and what their goals are for the health care team. This helps the nurse to clarify any misunderstandings that might exist. For example, the family may have unrealistic expectations regarding the treatment available to the client and the anticipated effects.

Nursing Diagnosis

From data collected during assessment, the nurse identifies a nursing diagnosis that accurately reflects the needs of the client or family experiencing the loss. Critical thinking skills are the tools used to apply concepts of assessment, clustering of cues, and drawing a conclusion of the actual or perceived needs of the client. The nurse will cluster defining characteristics and identify the nursing diagnosis applicable to the client's situation (Box 25-6). Clustering of client or family behaviours, actual or potential losses, the client's attempts at coping, and data involving the nature and meaning of the loss will lead to individualized nursing diagnoses, such as the following:

- Anxiety
- Caregiver role strain
- Compromised family coping
- Ineffective coping
- Ineffective denial
- Fear
- Anticipatory grieving
- Dysfunctional grieving
- Hopelessness
- Powerlessness
- Social isolation
- Spiritual distress
- Readiness for enhanced spiritual well-being

The presence of one or two defining characteristics is usually insufficient to make an accurate diagnosis. The nurse must carefully review the data to consider if competing diagnoses exist. For example, if a dying person cries, displays anger, and reports nightmares, this could signal several possible nursing diagnoses because these characteristics are common to more than one diagnosis. Possibilities include *pain, ineffective coping,* and *spiritual distress.* The nurse examines all available data and inquires about the presence of other behaviours and symptoms until an accurate diagnosis can be identified.

Part of the diagnostic process is to identify the appropriate related factor for each diagnosis. For example, *dysfunctional grieving related to the loss of the ability to walk from paralysis* will require different interventions than *dysfunctional grieving related to the loss of a job.*

In order to promote a holistic approach to care, wellness-oriented diagnoses need to be included such as *readiness for enhanced spiritual well-being.* These diagnoses allow for recognizing and drawing from client strengths. As well, the nursing diagnostic process is continual because the client situation will change.

When identifying nursing diagnoses for the dying client, other problems are identified separately according to specific standards of care. Other nursing diagnoses can include *disturbed body image, impaired physical mobility,* or *ineffective role performance.* More physical nursing diagnoses are identified when the client begins to experience the physical changes accompanying death, including *impaired urinary elimination* and/or *bowel incontinence, acute pain, nausea, disturbed sensory perception,* and *ineffective breathing pattern.* The comfort of the dying, including pain control and the acceptance of the dying process by the family, are realistic expectations for the nurse to deal with in the dying situation. With terminal illness, physical assessment of the dying process is ongoing so that the nurse can adapt or validate the actual nursing diagnoses with the changing condition of the client.

Nursing Diagnostic Process — Box 25-6

Assessment Activities	Defining Characteristics	Nursing Diagnosis
Ask client to discuss future goals and plans.	Client sighs and says, "I have no future."	Hopelessness related to failing physical condition
Observe client's non-verbal behaviour.	Client becomes passive with little affect and turns away from speaker.	
Offer client choices and observe responses.	Client shrugs and says, "What does it matter?"	
Assess activity level.	Client refuses to eat. Client sleeps all the time, keeping blinds closed and lights out. Client refuses to participate in care.	

Planning

Grieving is the natural response to loss and thus has a therapeutic value. The focus in planning nursing care is to support the client physically, emotionally, developmentally, and spiritually in the expression of grief. Figure 25–3 illustrates the interrelatedness of critical thinking factors during the planning phase of the nursing process. Application of critical thinking ensures a well-designed plan in which the nurse supports the client's personhood, self-esteem, and autonomy by including the client in decisions about the plan of care. When caring for the dying client, it is important to devise a plan that helps a client to die with dignity and offers family members the assurance that their loved one is cared for with care and compassion (see Care Plan).

Goals and Outcomes. The nurse establishes realistic goals and expected outcomes based on the client's nursing

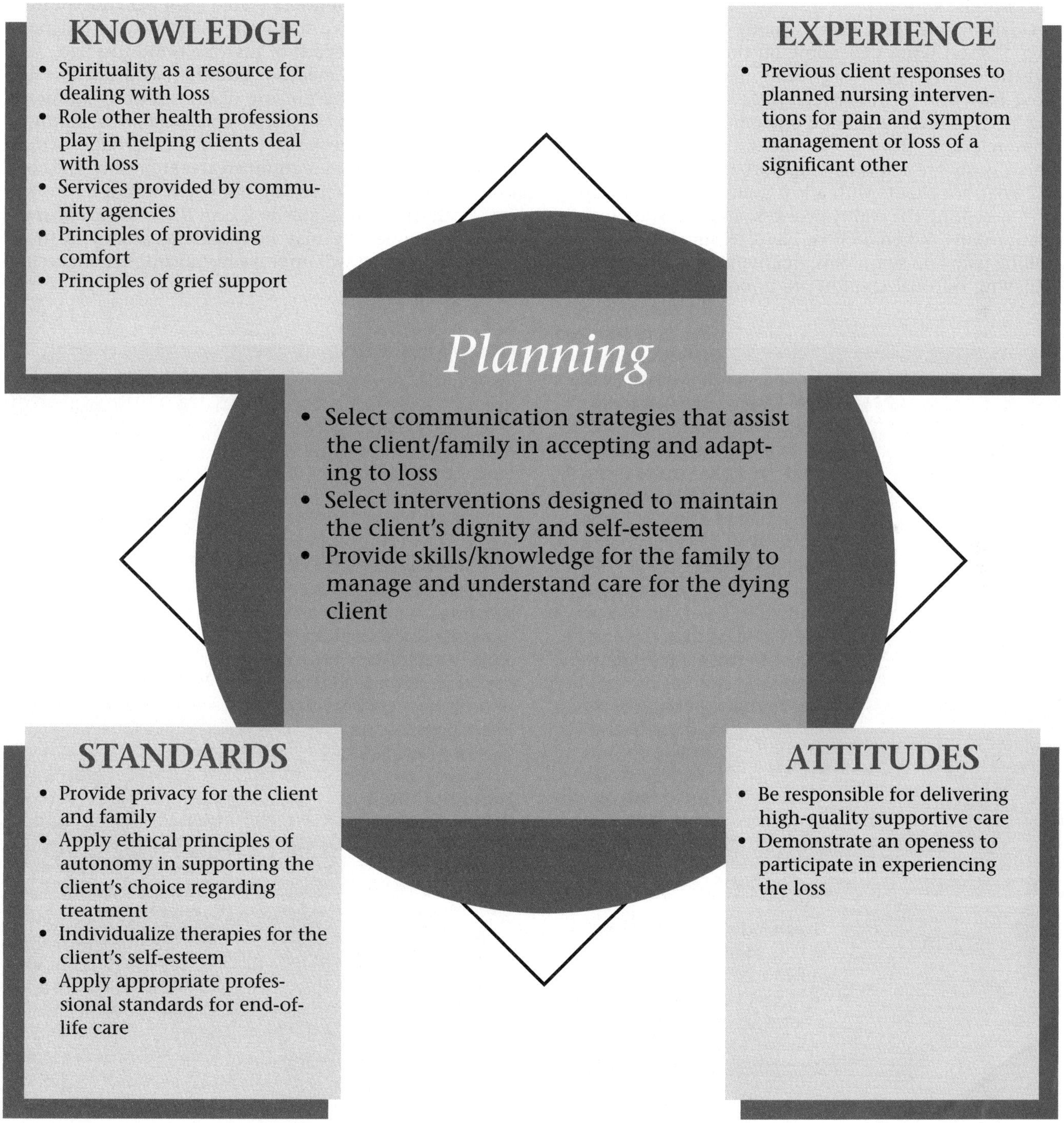
KNOWLEDGE
• Spirituality as a resource for dealing with loss
• Role other health professions play in helping clients deal with loss
• Services provided by community agencies
• Principles of providing comfort
• Principles of grief support
EXPERIENCE
• Previous client responses to planned nursing interventions for pain and symptom management or loss of a significant other
Planning
• Select communication strategies that assist the client/family in accepting and adapting to loss
• Select interventions designed to maintain the client's dignity and self-esteem
• Provide skills/knowledge for the family to manage and understand care for the dying client
STANDARDS
• Provide privacy for the client and family
• Apply ethical principles of autonomy in supporting the client's choice regarding treatment
• Individualize therapies for the client's self-esteem
• Apply appropriate professional standards for end-of-life care
ATTITUDES
• Be responsible for delivering high-quality supportive care
• Demonstrate an openess to participate in experiencing the loss

FIGURE **25–3** Critical thinking model for loss, death, and grieving planning.

diagnoses. Client resources such as physical energy and activity tolerance, supportive family members, spiritual faith, and methods for coping are integrated into the plan of care. For example, if a terminally ill client has the diagnosis of *powerlessness related to planned cancer therapy,* a goal of "Client will be able to discuss expected course of disease" will be realistic if the client is able to remain attentive and participate in educational discussions without becoming fatigued. In contrast, an expected outcome of "Client will participate in series of short planned teaching discussions about disease" accounts for the client's need to have short teaching sessions so as to avoid exhaustion.

Goals of care for a client dealing with loss might be long or short term, depending on the nature of the loss and the client's phase of grieving. Because a client may move back and forth between phases of grief, the nurse may need to revise goals and outcomes to ensure they remain relevant. Having the client partner in deciding which goals are relevant is important. General nursing care goals for clients with a loss include accommodating grief, accepting the reality of a loss, and renewing regular relationships. When a client has a terminal illness, controlling pain and symptoms, maintaining autonomy, and achieving spiritual comfort are important goals. For the goal of "achieving a sense of dignity," expected outcomes might include the following:

- Client will be able to continue parental responsibilities in care of toddler.
- Client will express hopefulness that cancer treatment will control symptoms.
- Client will engage in playing chess with friends on a weekly basis.

Setting Priorities. When a client has multiple nursing diagnoses, the problems cannot be addressed simultaneously. At any given time, two or three problems will demand the nurse's attention. Figure 25–4 is a concept map developed for a client medically diagnosed with depression following the death of his wife 6 months ago. As a result of the client's medical condition, associated health problems include the nursing diagnoses of *dysfunctional grieving, disturbed sleep pattern,* and *imbalanced nutrition: less than body requirements.* The nurse determines which of the three diagnoses requires greater attention. The continuing grief experienced by the client might be the focus. Until the client is able to accept his loss and begin resolving his grief, he may be unable to attend to those interventions that will improve his nutritional intake and sleep status.

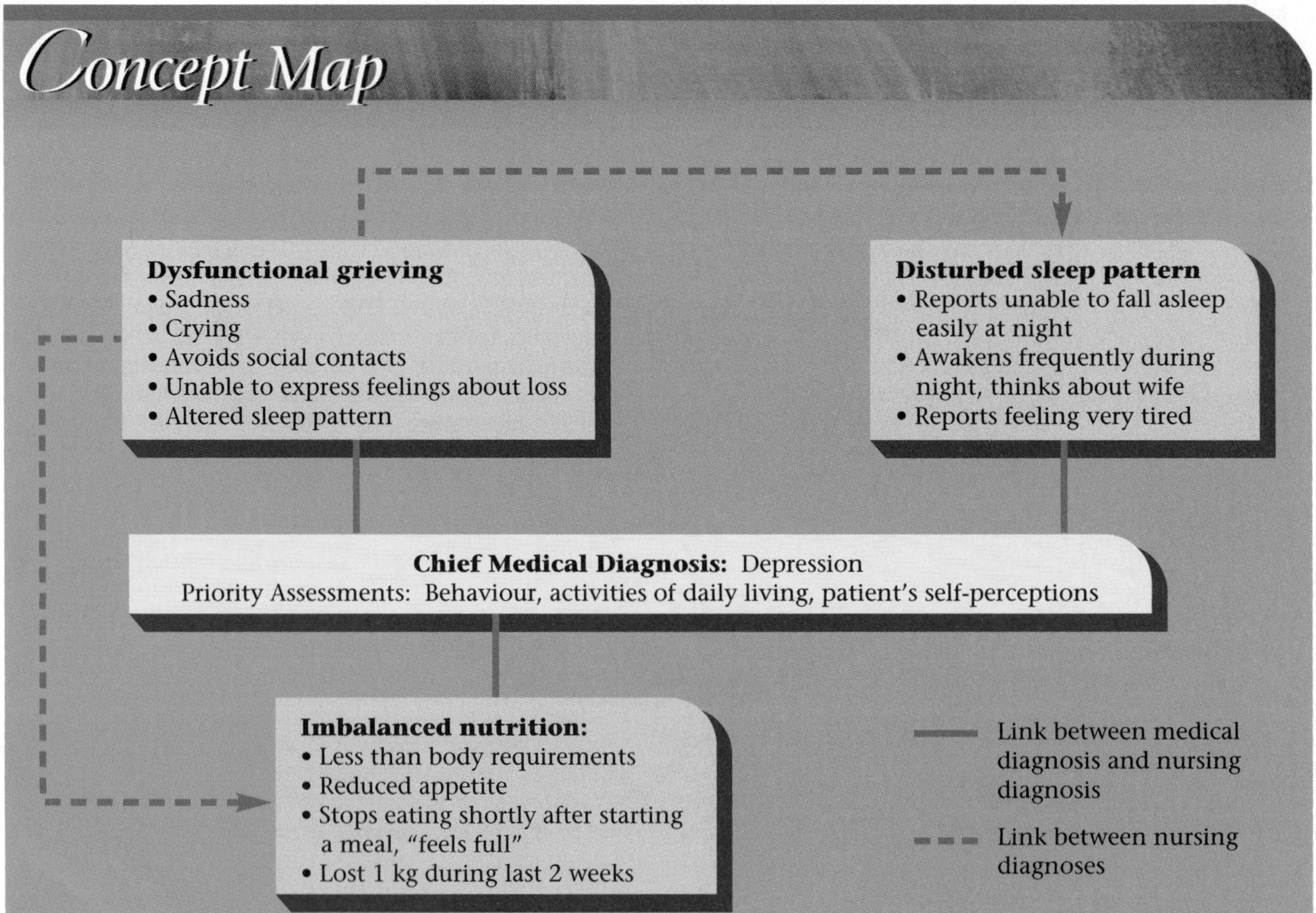

FIGURE **25–4** Concept map for a client with depression following death of wife.

Clients' conditions always change. Ongoing assessment of a client's condition can quickly focus the nurse's attention on a new problem. The nurse must always consider what are the client's most urgent physical or psychological needs requiring immediate intervention. The nurse considers the client's expectations and preferences in regard to the priorities of care. If the terminally ill client's priorities include controlling pain and maintaining self-esteem, pain control will be the priority when analgesics become ineffective and the client experiences

Nursing Care Plan

Ineffective Coping

Assessment

Jan Runyon is the nurse who admits Mr. Miller, a 48-year-old man, from the emergency department to the intensive care unit (ICU) following massive head trauma incurred in a motor vehicle accident. Mr. Miller is a successful business executive who has a wife and two sons. The physician has explained to the family that Mr. Miller's prognosis is poor. Tests are under way to determine the extent of brain injury. Mrs. Miller and the children are in the ICU waiting area, waiting on word about Mr. Miller.

Assessment Activities	Findings/Defining Characteristics
Jan asks Mrs. Miller, "Tell me how you are feeling about your discussion with the physician."	"I know they are doing everything they can. He is going to be OK, I just know he is. He has never been sick a day in his life."
Jan observes Mrs. Miller's interaction with her children.	Mrs. Miller has difficulty problem solving. The family has posed several questions to her as to what she plans to say to the insurance company and Mr. Miller's employees. Mrs. Miller is unable to decide what to say at this time.
Jan overhears Mrs. Miller on the phone in the waiting area.	Mrs. Miller states over the phone, "Don't worry, he's having some tests right now. I know, Bill, he will be back in the office before you know it. Tell the staff everything will be OK."
Jan accompanies the transplant coordinator, who asks Mrs. Miller if the family has ever discussed organ donation.	Mrs. Miller responds, "Bill will be fine, that's not important right now!"

Nursing Diagnosis: Ineffective coping related to husband's traumatic injury and uncertainty of prognosis.

Planning

Goal	Expected Outcomes*
	Grief Resolution
Wife will accept client's impending death within 48 hours.	Wife will verbalize to caregiver within the next 6 hours that husband's death is actually impending. Wife will inform children of their father's likely death within 24 hours. Wife will make a decision about organ donation within the next 12 hours. Wife will discuss immediate lifestyle changes that will occur as a result of husband's death over next 48 hours.
Wife will demonstrate effective expression of grief within next 48 hours.	Wife will discuss with children their concerns about what they need to do as a family to prepare for father's impending death within next 48 hours. Wife will discuss effects loss has on her personally with caregiver within next 48 hours.

*Outcome classification label from *Nursing Outcomes Classification (NOC)* (3rd ed.), edited by S. Moorhead, M. Johnson M, and M. L. Maas, 2004, St. Louis, MO: Mosby.

Interventions†	Rationale
Presence	
• Display interest in wife's situation and accept her behaviours of denial.	Recognizing denial (based on Kübler-Ross's theory) gives the staff direction for planning unique interventions based on grief theory (Cressy, 1997).
• Establish trust and a positive regard by creating an atmosphere of sharing. Offer privacy and security.	Privacy offers a place of security to exhibit personal needs and to work through feelings (McLean, 1999). Anxiety about losing dignity when expressing grief will hinder an honest expression of feelings.

Continued

Nursing Care Plan

Ineffective Coping—cont'd

Interventions†—cont'd	Rationale
Grief Work Facilitation	
• Offer wife encouragement to explore and verbalize feelings of grief.	Encouragement refocuses on current needs and minimizes dysfunctional adaptation behaviours by facilitating resolution of grief through problem-solving skills (Braza, 1993).
• Identify personal coping strategies used in the past; assess effectiveness and promote when appropriate.	Previously successful coping strategies are the first to be used when one is under stress (Cressy, 1997). Discouraging maladaptive behaviours will minimize dysfunctional grieving (Lenhardt, 1997).
• Determine wife's acceptance of available community resources and initiate as appropriate: significant other (business partner), children, clergy (family is Methodist), or other health care workers.	Professionals can use their expertise to direct the grieving process (Catalano, 1995). Trust in relationships already formed will speed the therapeutic communication process (Stocker, 1994).

†Intervention classification labels from *Nursing Interventions Classification (NIC)* (4th ed.), edited by J. M. Dochterman and G. M. Bulechek, 2004, St. Louis, MO: Mosby.

Evaluation

Nursing Actions	Client Response/Finding	Achievement of Outcome
Say to client, "This has been a difficult time. Your husband's injury has been so sudden."	Wife responds, "I still cannot believe it. The doctors do not believe he will live through the night."	Shows beginning acknowledgement of client's impending death.
Ask, "Tell me how you are feeling now."	Wife explains, "I am worried about my kids. The boys are both close to their dad. I feel this unbelievable sadness."	Able to express normal grieving behaviours.
Observe wife's behaviour when with children.	Wife discusses decisions that must be made because of impending death of husband. Allows children to express their sadness.	Wife is able to express grief with family; maintains role as supportive mother.

acute distress. If the client is progressing as desired, the nurse may refocus priorities to address unmet needs. For example, the client suffering depression caused by his wife's death also has problems of imbalanced nutrition and a disturbed sleep pattern. If the client reports an improved appetite and has shown weight stabilization since the last clinic visit, the nurse can focus more attention on the sleep pattern disturbance. The nurse must remember that the client's expectations, clinical condition, and preferences influence priorities. If a terminally ill client places more emphasis on spiritual support versus other priorities such learning about planned treatments, the nurse must attend to the client's priorities. Meeting client priorities may allow the nurse to then address other needs more effectively with less effort.

Continuity of Care. Interdisciplinary teams help to identify and meet the needs of those who experience losses. Dieticians, clergy, physicians, social workers, physiotherapists, psychologists, and other specialty health care workers can assist a client and family in their grief. A coordinated team approach to managing a client's needs results in a well managed care plan. When a client dies, the loss experienced by the nurse and colleagues can be shared within the professional group. Support is needed to promote healing for all who worked with the dying client. Conflicts and differences can be openly discussed and solutions found in a healthy manner with the client as the primary focus. By working together, the sharing of experiences, feelings, alternatives, and solutions become the basis for dealing with future losses.

Often, terminally ill clients return home and require continued intense nursing care. Home care nurses collaborate closely with family members to meet the client's ongoing needs. Important interventions to include in planning are arranging for main-floor access, arranging appropriate medical equipment, and providing sufficient family respite. When it is realistic for the client to remain independent, therapeutic strategies should bolster the client's sense of autonomy and the ability to function as independently as possible (Chochinov, 2002). For example, judicious application of orthotic devices, along with physiotherapy and occupational therapy, can often bolster a client's functional capacity.

Implementation

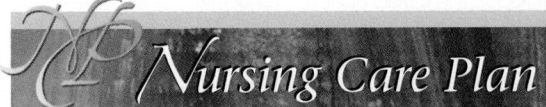

Health Promotion. Although a return to full function is not an expected outcome for a terminally ill client or even for a client who has significant disability, the goal should be to enable the client to return to optimal physical and emotional functioning. The goal of nursing care is to help clients and families cope with the stressors in their lives and to move toward healthy grief resolution. Nurses help clients and families to deal with loss, make decisions about the client's health care, and adjust to any disappointment, frustration, and anxiety created by their loss.

Therapeutic Communication. Nursing care of the grieving client and family begins with establishing a caring presence and determining the significance of their loss. This is difficult if the client is unwilling or unable to express feelings or is experiencing numbing or denial. The nurse must use therapeutic communication strategies that enable clients to discuss their loss and find ways to work through it. The nurse's presence, attentive listening, and use of open-ended questions allow clients to freely share their thoughts and concerns. The use of closed-ended questions often results in the client discussing only what the nurse presumes is the problem. For example, asking the client, "Does knowing you have cancer make you fearful?" will not likely reveal as much as, "Tell me how your diagnosis of cancer is making you feel." The nurse should acknowledge the client's grief and show support by demonstrating caring behaviours throughout the discussion (see chapter 15). The nurse will gain the client's trust by showing a desire to enter into a caring, therapeutic relationship with the client. Listening attentively to the client can be very therapeutic for the client and will reveal details that will help plan effective care.

If a client chooses not to share feelings or concerns, the nurse should convey a willingness to be available when needed. If the nurse is reassuring and respectful of the client's need for dignity and privacy, a therapeutic relationship will likely develop. Sometimes clients need to begin resolving their grief before they can discuss their loss.

Some clients will not discuss feelings about their loss. The nurse must observe for expressions of anger, denial, depression, or guilt. Nurses must also know their own feelings before encouraging clients to express their anger. Individuals may retaliate against family, staff, or physicians. Clients can also become demanding and accusing. The nurse must remain supportive by letting clients and family members know that feelings such as anger are normal. For example, the nurse might say, "You are obviously upset. I just want you to know I am here to talk with you if you want." The nurse must avoid barriers to communication such as denying the client's grief, providing false reassurance, or avoiding discussion of sensitive issues (see chapter 14).

No topic that a dying client wishes to discuss should be avoided. When the client wants to talk, it is important for the nurse to find time to do so. This can be challenging for a nurse with limited experience with dying clients or who works in a busy acute care setting. The nurse should respond to questions openly and honestly and provide information that helps clients and their families to understand their condition, the trajectory or future course of their disease, the benefits and burdens of treatment, and values and goals (Forbes et al., 2000). In some cases, the nurse may recognize the need for the client to consult with pastoral care or counselling services.

Promoting Hope. Hope can be an energizing resource for clients experiencing loss. For each dimension of hope, there are nursing strategies that promote hope.

- *Affective dimension.* Show empathic understanding of the client's strengths. Reinforce expressions of courage, positive thinking, and realistic goal setting. Encourage expression of both positive and negative feelings.
- *Cognitive dimension.* Offer information about the illness and correct any misunderstanding or misinformation. Clarify or modify the client's perceptions.
- *Behavioural dimension.* Assist the client in using personal resources and making use of external supports to balance the need for independence with healthy interdependence and dependence.
- *Affiliative dimension.* Encourage clients to foster supportive relationships with others.
- *Temporal dimension.* Focus on short-term goals as life expectancy diminishes.
- *Contextual dimension.* Encourage development of achievable goals. Reminisce about achievements or positive moments in time so that the client can derive meaning from suffering.

Facilitating Mourning. Nursing care strategies can help clients move through uncomplicated grief (Worden, 1991). The following guidelines are helpful for people who are mourning a death, facing death, and grieving over an actual loss:

- *Help the client accept that loss is real.* Discuss how the loss or illness occurred or was discovered, when, under what circumstances, who told them about it, and other similar topics to help make the event real and to place it in perspective.
- *Support efforts to live without the deceased person or in the face of disability.* A problem-solving approach is often helpful. Have clients or family make a list of their problems, help them prioritize them, and then lead them step-by-step through a discussion of how they might tackle each one. Encourage them to make use of family members, community resources, or others who can help.
- *Encourage establishment of new relationships.* Many people fear that establishing new relationships would be disloyal. They need reassurance that new relationships do not mean that they are replacing the person who has died. Encourage the client to become involved in social relationships that are non-threatening (e.g., religious gatherings or volunteer activities).
- *Allow time to grieve.* It is common to have "anniversary reactions" around the time of the loss in subsequent years. Some people worry that they are going crazy when sadness or other signs of grief recur after a period of relative calm. Encourage the client to reminisce.
- *Interpret "normal" behaviour.* Being distractible, having difficulty sleeping or eating, and thinking they have heard the deceased's voice are common following loss. These symptoms do not mean an individual has an emotional problem or is becoming ill in some way. Reinforce that these occurrences are normal and will resolve over time.

- *Provide continuing support.* Clients and their families may need to talk and may look to the nurse for support for many months or years following a loss. If the nurse has occasion to see the client or family after an extended time, it is appropriate to ask about how they are coping or adjusting. This gives them the opportunity to talk if needed.
- *Be alert for signs of ineffective coping.* Be aware of coping mechanisms that may be harmful, such as alcohol or substance abuse, which can include excessive use of over-the-counter pain medications or sleep aids.

Acute Care

Palliative Care. People who face life-threatening illnesses have many medical and technological advances available to reverse the course of their disease or to prolong their lives. For clients with serious life-limiting illness, it becomes important for health care providers to find ways to help clients approach their end of life. Such is the aim of **palliative care,** to relieve suffering and improve the quality of living and dying (Ferris et al., 2002). More than 220,000 Canadians die each year, with approximately 160,000 needing palliative care. However, only an estimated 5% of dying Canadians and their families receive palliative care services (Senate of Canada, 2000).

Palliative care is for any age, any diagnosis, at any time, and not just during the last few months of life. Chochinov (2002) explained that when the preservation of dignity becomes the goal of palliation, care options encompass the physical, psychological, social, spiritual, and existential aspects of the client's illness. Palliative care thus allows clients to make more informed choices, achieve better alleviation of symptoms, and have more opportunity to work on issues of life closure. Ferris et al. (2002) have designed the *Model to Guide Patient and Family Care,* which provides a comprehensive approach for palliative caregivers using nationally accepted principles and norms of practice.

According to the World Health Organization (2003), when health care providers deliver palliative care, they do the following:

- Provide relief from pain and other distressing symptoms
- Affirm life and regard dying as a normal process
- Neither hasten nor postpone death
- Integrate psychological and spiritual aspects of client care
- Offer a support system to help clients live as actively as possible until death.
- Offer a support system to help families cope during the client's illness and their own bereavement
- Enhance the quality of life

Ferris et al. (2002) add that palliative care also helps clients and families "prepare for and manage self-determined life closure and the dying process" and promotes opportunities for meaningful and valuable experiences, personal and spiritual growth, and self-actualization" (p. 114).

Palliative care is a philosophy of total care. A palliative care approach ensures that a client experiences a "good death," free of avoidable pain and suffering, in accord with the client's and family's wishes, and reasonably consistent with clinical, cultural, and ethical standards (Tolle et al., 2000). Palliative care is one of the most interdisciplinary and team-based approaches (Northcott & Wilson, 2001) and includes physicians, nurses, social workers, pastoral care professionals, physiotherapists, occupational therapists, and pharmacists. Massage therapists or music/art therapists who provide alternative therapies might also be a part of the team (see chapter 31).

The Canadian Hospice Palliative Care Association Nursing Standards Committee (2002) has developed nursing standards of practice for hospice palliative care. These nursing standards reflect the six dimensions of the supportive care model: valuing, connecting, empowering, doing for, finding meaning, and preserving integrity (Davies & Oberle, 1990).

Palliative care is compassionate and supportive of dying people and their families. Nurses play a key role in providing care to the dying and are "often the most intimate contact and constant presence" (CNA, 2000). Thus, one of the most important skills a nurse provides in palliative care is establishing a caring relationship with both client and family. It also becomes very important for the nurse to provide appropriate symptom-control measures to maintain the client's dignity and self-esteem, to prevent feelings of abandonment or isolation, and to provide a comfortable and peaceful environment at the time of death.

Symptom Control. Comfort for a dying client requires management of symptoms of disease and therapies. For many clients, symptom distress is characteristic of the dying experience (Chochinov, 2002). Symptom distress is the experience of discomfort or anguish related to the progression of a disease. Clients experience anguish from not knowing or being unaware of aspects of their health status or treatment. Worry or fear are common in many clients and may heighten their perception of discomfort. The nurse assesses the character of the client's symptoms carefully in order to select appropriate therapies. Chapter 38 details the assessment of pain. Providing information about treatment options or the anticipated unfolding of an illness helps to preserve the dignity of clients and families plagued by not knowing what the future holds (Hinton, 1999). Complementary therapies are sometimes used for symptom management; these include, for example, therapeutic touch, aromatherapy, biofeedback, homeopathy, acupuncture, and relaxation therapy (Fisher, Ross, & MacLean, 2000).

One symptom common among the terminally ill is dyspnea, or air hunger. The sense of suffocation can cause great panic in the client and significant stress in the caregiver (Tarzian, 2000). As the client panics, unable to get a breath, the dyspnea worsens. Tarzian interviewed nurses who cared for the terminally ill and found that surrendering and sharing control help reduce pain and anxiety in these clients. For example, a client may choose to switch oxygen devices, even though they deliver the same concentration of oxygen. However, if the client believes there is a difference, it might be enough to relieve the dyspnea at least briefly. When there are options in respiratory therapy, it helps to give the client a choice.

Management of air hunger also involves the judicious administration of morphine and anxiolytics for relief of respiratory distress. Table 25-4 summarizes nursing care measures for additional symptoms of terminal disease.

Table 25-4 **Promoting Comfort in the Terminally Ill Client**

Symptoms	Characteristics or Causes	Nursing Implications
Discomfort	Any source of physical irritation may worsen pain.	Provide thorough skin care including daily baths, lubrication of skin, and dry, clean bed linens to reduce irritants.
	As client approaches death, mouth remains open, tongue becomes dry and edematous, and lips become dry and cracked.	Provide oral care at least every 2 to 4 hours. Use soft toothbrushes or foam swabs for frequent mouth care. Apply a light film of petroleum jelly to lips and tongue (chapter 34).
	Blinking reflexes diminish near death, causing drying of cornea.	Eye care removes crusts from eyelid margins. Artificial tears reduce corneal drying.
Fatigue	Metabolic demands of a cancerous tumour cause weakness and fatigue.	Help client to identify values or desired tasks; then help client to conserve energy for only those tasks. Promote frequent rest periods in a quiet environment.
	Exhaustion phase of the general adaptation syndrome causes energy depletion.	Time and pace nursing care activities.
Nausea	Nausea may occur as a side effect of medications and as a result of severe pain.	Administer antiemetics: provide oral care at least every 2 to 4 hours; offer clear liquid diet and ice chips; avoid liquids that increase stomach acidity such as coffee, milk, and citric acid juices.
Constipation	Narcotic medications and immobility slow peristalsis. Lack of bulk in diet or reduced fluid intake may occur with appetite changes. Constipation can add to discomfort.	Give preventive care, which is most effective: increase fluid intake; include bran, whole grain products, and fresh vegetables in diet; encourage exercise (chapter 39). Administer prophylactic stool softeners.
Diarrhea	Diarrhea results from disease process (e.g., colon cancer) and complications of treatment or medications.	Assess for fecal impaction. Confer with physician to change medication if possible. Provide low-residue diet.
Urinary incontinence	Incontinence results from progressive disease (e.g., involvement of spinal cord, reduced level of consciousness.)	Protect skin from irritation or breakdown. Indwelling urinary catheter or condom catheters may be used (chapter 40).
Inadequate nutrition	Nausea and vomiting can decrease appetite.	Serve smaller portions and bland foods, which may be more palatable.
	Depression from grieving may cause anorexia.	Allow home-cooked meals, which may be preferred by client and gives the family a chance to participate.
Dehydration	As disease progresses, client is less willing or able to maintain oral fluid intake.	Remove factors causing decreased intake; give antiemetics, apply topical analgesics to oral lesions. Reduce discomfort from dehydration; give mouth care at least every 4 hours; offer ice chips or moist cloth to lips.
Ineffective breathing patterns, e.g., dyspnea, shortness of breath	Disease progression that involves lung tissue, e.g., progression of cancer, pneumonia, pulmonary edema, may affect breathing.	Treat or control underlying cause.
	Anemia reduces oxygen-carrying capacity.	Maximize client's oxygenation, e.g., position client upright, provide supplemental oxygen, maintain a patent airway, reduce anxiety or fever.
	Anxiety, which increases oxygen demand. Fever, which increases oxygen demand.	Administer medications such as bronchodilators, inhaled steroids, or narcotics to suppress cough and ease breathing and apprehension.

Because therapies and clinical recommendations in palliative care are constantly evolving, nurses must stay current (Fisher et al., 2000).

Maintaining Dignity and Self-Esteem. The notion of dignity varies from client to client, and between one circumstance and the next (Chochinov, 2002). Dignity may revolve around a person's positive sense of self-regard, a feeling that the essence of who one is remains intact, along with an ability to invest in and gain strength from a rich spiritual life (Daaleman & VandeCreek, 2000). Dignity may also revolve around the extent to which clients feel valued and how they are treated by caregivers.

A nurse can promote a client's self-esteem and dignity by taking a therapeutic stance that conveys respect for the client as a whole person with feelings, accomplishments, and passions independent of the illness experience (Chochinov, 2002). Giving importance to what a client holds dear acknowledges individual personhood, while also strengthening the empathic, therapeutic communication between the client, the client's family, and the nurse. Spending time to let clients share their life experiences, particularly about what has been meaningful, enables the nurse to know clients better. Knowing clients then facilitates choice of therapies that promote client decision making and autonomy.

For many clients, receiving spiritual comfort helps to preserve dignity and self-esteem. Facilitating connections to a spiritual practice or community and supporting the expression of culturally held beliefs is very important. Clients may also benefit by being assured that some aspect of their lives may transcend death. In other words, the client gains comfort from knowing that something of one's life will continue after death. Participating in a life project such as making an audio tape or videotape for the family, writing letters, or keeping a journal can offer clients the comfort of knowing that something of their essence will survive beyond (Chochinov, 2002). Chapter 24 further discusses some of the spiritual practices and religious rituals that can support people in need of spiritual comfort.

Basic to promoting self-esteem and dignity is attending to the client's appearance and surroundings. Cleanliness, absence of body odours, attractive clothing, and personal grooming all contribute to a sense of worth. When helping a client tend to bodily functions, the nurse always shows respect, even when the client becomes dependent. It is important to keep the client's immediate surroundings pleasant by opening curtains and letting light change from the bright of day to the dark of night. The quick removal of liquid stool or vomitus will remove unpleasant odours.

Disabilities experienced by the client may threaten dignity, especially when caregivers take control of the client's life. The nurse allows the client to make nursing care decisions (e.g., how and when to administer personal hygiene, diet preferences, and timing of nursing therapies). The nurse keeps the client and family well informed about planned therapies, their purpose, and anticipated effects. It is also important to provide the client with privacy during nursing care procedures and when the client and family need time together.

Preventing Abandonment and Isolation. A terminally ill client is often fearful of dying alone. Therefore it is important for the nurse to answer the call light quickly and to explain when staff will be giving care and performing assessments throughout the day and night. The nurse should establish presence and use appropriate touch when performing care measures. The nurse must be available to answer questions, even if there is no need for data, no further decisions to make, or no further curative interventions to offer (Finucane, 2002). Clients may feel a sense of involvement when sharing a room and interacting with staff. Clients can share conversation and companionship with roommates and visitors. The choice of private or shared room should be discussed with the client and family whenever possible.

Family is always considered as the unit of care in palliative care. If family members have difficulty accepting the client's impending death, they may avoid visitation. When family members do visit, it is important for the nurse to talk with them and keep them informed of the client's progress. It may be useful to give family members helpful hints about what to discuss with clients. For example, the nurse can help improve the family member's communication skills by role modeling attentive listening and offering reassurance. The nurse should encourage the family to discuss activities other family members are involved in, to reminisce about enjoyable times, and to inquire about the client's concerns. It is also helpful to find simple and appropriate care activities for the family to perform, such as feeding the client, washing the client's face, combing hair, and filling out the client's menu. Older adults often become particularly lonely at night and may feel more secure if a family member stays at the bedside during the night. The nurse should allow visitors to remain with dying clients at any time if the client wants them. Also, the nurse must know how to contact family members at any time if the client requests a visit or if the client's condition worsens.

Providing a Comfortable and Peaceful Environment. The nurse keeps a client comfortable through frequent repositioning, keeping bed linens dry, and controlling extraneous environmental noise. Pictures, cherished objects, cards or letters from family members and friends, and plants and flowers create an environment that is more familiar and comforting. The nurse offers the client frequent back massage or guided imagery exercises and allows the client time to listen to preferred types of music. A comfortable, pleasant environment helps clients to relax, which promotes their ability to sleep and minimizes severity of symptoms.

Fear of Dying and Death. People are afraid of dying and death for many different reasons. The process of dying with its associated pain and loss of dignity, not knowing what will happen after death, or dying before accomplishing dreams and goals are all possible reasons. The intensity of the fear varies with each person and his or her circumstances, including age, culture, sex, personal experiences, family situation, social supports, and religious beliefs. Lugton and Kindlen (1999) pointed out that nurses need to help clients realistically appraise these threats. They also need to listen and understand as clients express their emotions.

Support for the Grieving Family. The family may be the primary caregivers when the client chooses to die at home. Family members need the nurse's support, and they benefit from being taught ways to care for their loved one (Box 25-7). Caring for a family member can be emotionally stressful and physically exhausting for the family caregiver. Not all families can manage care on their own. In the home setting, the nurse provides the opportunity for the family to be temporarily relieved of their duties so that they can rest. Respite care is a resource available through hospice programs.

Families also need to be informed of home care, hospice, and community service options so that they can choose among the resources available. The Saint Elizabeth Health Care Foundation in Canada has sponsored a free-of-charge publication called *Family Hospice Care.* This is a practical and informative resource written to help families meet the needs of their terminally ill loved ones (van Bommel, 1999). In some cases, families may need assistance and support in making the decision about placement in a health care facility.

The nurse keeps the family informed so that they can anticipate the type of symptoms the client will likely experience and the implications for care. The nurse encourages family members to express their grief openly with the client and to give the client the opportunity to

Client Teaching Box 25-7

Preparing the Dying Client's Family

Objectives

- Family will be able to provide appropriate physical care for the dying client in the home.
- Family will be able to provide appropriate psychological support to the dying client.

Teaching Strategies

- Describe and demonstrate feeding techniques and selection of foods to facilitate ease of chewing and swallowing.
- Demonstrate bathing, mouth care, and other hygiene measures, and allow family to perform return demonstration.
- Show a video on simple transfer techniques to prevent injury to themselves and the client; help family to practise.
- Instruct family on need to enforce rest periods.
- Teach family to recognize signs and symptoms to expect as the client's condition worsens and provide information on whom to call in an emergency.
- Discuss ways to support the dying person and listen to needs and fears.
- Solicit questions from family and provide information as needed.

Evaluation

- Have the family members demonstrate physical care techniques (e.g., turning, feeding, mouth care).
- Ask the family members to describe how they vary approaches to care when the client has symptoms such as pain or fatigue.
- Ask the family to discuss how they feel about their ability to support the client.

discuss any remaining concerns or requests. The family also needs personal time to share their concerns with the nurse and to ask questions about treatment options, course of the client's disease, and the meaning of the client's behaviours. It is wise for the nurse to communicate news of the client's impending death when the family is together, if possible. Family members can provide support for one another. The nurse conveys the news in a private area and remains willing to stay with the family as needed.

In the hospital setting, the nurse assists in planning a visitation schedule for family members to prevent the client and family from excessive fatigue. Young children should visit dying parents. At the time of the client's death, the nurse helps the family to stay in communication with the client through frequent visits, caring silence, attentive listening, touch, and telling the client of their love. After the client's death, the nurse assists the family with decision making such as notification of a mortician, transportation of family members, and collection of the client's belongings.

Hospice Care. **Hospice** care is an alternative care delivery model for the terminally ill. It is one phase of palliative care. Hospice is not a facility but a concept for family-centred care designed to assist the client in being comfortable and maintaining a satisfactory lifestyle until death. Hospice services are available in the home, hospital, stand-alone facilities, and long-term care settings. Availability and accessibility vary across Canada. Components of hospice care programs include the following:

- Client and family as the unit of care
- Coordinated home care with access to available inpatient and long-term care facility beds
- Control of symptoms (physical, sociological, psychological, and spiritual)
- Physician-directed services
- Provision of an interdisciplinary care team of physicians, nurses, spiritual advisors, social worker, and counsellors
- Medical and nursing services available at all times
- Bereavement follow-up after a client's death
- Use of trained volunteers for frequent visitation and respite support

Canada's first hospice was established in Toronto in 1979. Casey House in Toronto and the John Gordon home in London, Ontario, provide hospice care for people dying from AIDS. Canuck Place in Vancouver is the only children's hospice in North America. Canuck Place provides a continuum of care that comprises three components, including respite, palliative, and bereavement (Davies et al., 2003). Generally, clients accepted into a hospice program have less than 6 months to live, although this criterion is being challenged across Canada.

The nurse's role in hospice is to meet the primary wishes of the dying client and to be open to individual desires of each client. The nurse supports a client's choice in maintaining comfort and dignity. Whether the client ultimately dies at home or in a health care facility, the client's wishes are followed with the understanding that whatever their choice, it is made "for the good of all who are involved." When options are complicated by family needs, hospice will try to work with the clients' wishes. A hospice program emphasizes palliative care with the client and family as active participants. Client care goals are mutually set, and all participants fully understand the options and desires of the client. Efforts by the hospice team are made to meet the client's desires and to encourage the family to stay within those guidelines. Often a bereavement visit or visits will be made by the staff of the hospice team to the family even after the death of the client to help the family move through the grieving process successfully.

Many clients prefer to die at home in a familiar setting, whereas others choose not to burden their families and so prefer die in a hospital or long-term care facility. It is important that the hospice team know the client's preference. Many clients suffer physical ailments that prevent them from being cared for at home despite the willingness of family and friends to care for the client. The health and welfare issues are viewed from a broader perspective than just the client's desires. The concern for family needs is also taken into consideration by the hospice team.

A client in hospice may become hospitalized, and the health care team will coordinate care between the home and inpatient setting. There is always the effort to keep clients at home for as long as possible. The family provides basic supportive care. However, if the family cannot meet all of the client's needs, a nurse is available to coordinate and administer symptom management therapies. The interdisciplinary team has the goal of 24-hour accessibility as needed. As a client's death becomes imminent, members of the hospice team are there to give support to the client and family.

Care After Death. When a client dies in a hospital setting, the nurse provides **post-mortem care.** It is important to care for the client's body with dignity and sensitivity and in a manner consistent with the client's religious or cultural beliefs. After death, the body undergoes many physical changes. For that reason, care must be provided as soon as possible to prevent tissue damage or disfigurement of body parts.

Provincial and territorial legislation require hospitals to formulate policies and procedures based on current laws to validate death, identify potential organ or tissue donors, and to provide post-mortem care. For transplantation of organs, the client must be maintained on ventilatory and circulatory support until vital organs are harvested. The family must clearly understand that the client is "brain dead," that the equipment (i.e., ventilator and vasopressor medications) is not keeping the client alive but keeping the physical body in a state so that the organs will not be damaged before harvesting.

The nurse can be very helpful in supporting families through the organ and tissue request process. It is important to provide a private area to discuss all issues with the family. The staff member designated to make a request, such as a formal transplant coordinator, a social worker, chaplain, or the nurse, must offer the family clarification of what defines brain death because support systems must remain in place even after the client is pronounced "dead" for vital organ retrieval (i.e., heart, lungs, kidneys, and liver). The nurse reinforces explanations throughout the organ retrieval process. The family must know who legally can give final consent, what options there are for organ or tissue donation, whether there are associated costs, and how donation will affect burial or cremation. Non-vital tissues such as corneas, skin, long bones, and middle ear bones can be harvested when the client is proclaimed dead without artificially maintaining vital functions. If the client did not make specific documented requests before death, the family must agree on organ and tissue donation. Nurses should review their provincial or territorial organ retrieval laws and institutional policy and procedure regarding the formal consent process.

Another area that is difficult for the nurse and family concerns autopsy. According to Dracup and Bryan-Brown (1998), getting permission through delicate questioning is difficult at best. The doctor usually asks for permission for an autopsy, but it is often the nurse who answers questions and supports the family's choices. It is very difficult to approach a grieving family with such a request. Dracup and Bryan-Brown (1998) suggested showing the value that an autopsy can have by improving knowledge in the field of medicine. To help the living, the autopsy can lead to new therapies or new understanding of diseases. The more reasons the nurse can think of to support organ donation or autopsy, the more the family will be helped to realize the good that can be accomplished by either donation or research autopsy.

Clients' and families' cultural beliefs are very important in post-mortem care (see chapter 9). Maintaining the integrity of rituals and mourning practices gives families a sense of acceptance of the client's death and an inner peace. The ethical decisions that surround a client's death are based on the values of a culture. Health care providers must determine the makeup of a family network and which members should be involved about decisions such as organ donation and end-of-life care.

The nurse is responsible for coordination of all aspects of care surrounding a client's death. Box 25-8 summarizes the nurse's and physician's responsibilities for care of the body after death. It is important for the nurse to be familiar with institutional policies and procedures that are established for post-mortem care. Many of these practices also depend on the individuals' unique experiences and preferences.

The family becomes the primary client when the actual death has occurred, and the shift of concern moves from the deceased client to the living family. At this time, it becomes important to appropriately use the resources that are available. For example, pastoral care staff can be a helpful resource to assist the family even before the actual death, if no bereavement team is available. However, it is important to know whether the family chooses to have spiritual counsellors present. Some families prefer to grieve alone, whereas others may desire the support of others. Social workers and counsellors can also offer assistance. If the family's expectations for support are unknown, the simple questions and suggestions for assistance can be offered by anyone who assists the family.

Documentation of all of the events surrounding a client's death is important to avoid misunderstandings and to clarify final events in a client's life. There are legal guidelines supported by each facility's policies and procedures that must be followed and accurately documented. Box 25-9 lists the content to be documented about end-of-life care. Documentation will validate the success of meeting the goals identified for the client or provide a justification for the failure to meet any goals. Complete and accurate documentation offers a summary of activities that can become the focus for risk management or legal investigations.

A doctor or coroner must sign some of the medical forms, but the registered nurse must record most of the forms. Gathering of information for the forms may be delegated to unregulated care providers, but the nurse must chart the data on the nurse's notes. A licensed professional should witness the signing of forms.

In cases of legal matters, the family expects a clear, concise description of what occurred in the care of the client at the time of death. Opinions must be avoided, and facts are stated in a non-judgmental, objective fashion. Provincial and territorial guidelines will direct what type of information is charted and when it is to be charted. The Supreme Court of Canada has enshrined the

Box 25-8 Procedural Guidelines

Care of the Body After Death

Equipment: Bath towels, washcloths, wash basin, scissors, shroud kit with name tags, bed linen, room deodorizer, documentation forms.

Delegation: Care of the body after death can be delegated to unregulated care providers except for requests of organ/tissue donation. Check agency policy for which staff member is to remove any invasive tubes or lines.

1. Physicians must certify the death—time pronounced, therapy used, and actions taken. (This may not be the policy in all agencies. Follow agency policy.)
2. Physicians may request an autopsy, especially for unusual circumstances.
3. Trained staff member provides an option for donation of organs or tissue—personal, religious, and cultural needs should be included during this process.
4. Nurses work with sensitivity to preserve the client's and family's dignity.
   a. Check orders for any specimens or special orders needed by the physician.
   b. Make arrangements for staff, spiritual advisor, or others to stay with the family while preparing the body for viewing; ask for special requests for viewing (e.g., shaving, a special gown, Bible in hand, rosary at the bedside).
   c. Before shaving of male client: Determine if the family wishes client to remain unshaven if it was his custom to wear a beard. Determine if client's religion or culture has a preference to facial hair.
   d. Remove all equipment, tubes, supplies, and dirty linens according to protocol (unless organ donation is to take place; in that case, leave support systems in place).
   e. Cleanse the body thoroughly, apply clean sheets, and remove all trash from the room.
   f. Brush and comb client's hair. Apply any personal hairpiece.
   g. Position according to protocol—the eyes should be closed by gently holding them down a few minutes; dentures should be in the mouth to maintain facial alignment; packing should not be visible during viewing.
   h. Cover with a clean sheet up to the chin with arms outside covers if possible.
   i. Lower the lighting, and spray a deodorizer if possible to remove unpleasant odours.
   j. Give the family the option to view or not to view and go with them.
   k. Clarify that either option is acceptable.
   l. Encourage the family to say goodbye through both touch and talk.
   m. Do not rush this process. Once the family is more comfortable, ask if they would like to be left alone. Remind them that they can call you if needed.
   n. Clarify personal belongings that are to stay with the body or who has taken personal items; documentation will require both a descriptor of the objects and the name of who received them, with the time and date.
   o. Do not discard items found after the family is gone—call the family and tell them what was found and ask who might pick it up—describing the articles will be helpful in the decision-making process for the client's family.
   p. Apply name tags according to protocol—such as at the wrist, right big toe, or outside a shroud.
   q. Complete documentation in the nursing notes. This will vary depending on the agency (see Box 25-9).
   r. Remain sensitive to other hospitalized clients or visitors when transporting the body, such as covering the body with a clean sheet and watching to avoid visitors when moving the body to another part of the hospital or to the exit for the funeral home.
   s. Follow all protocol and policies to meet all legal requirements in caring for the body.

Box 25-9 Documentation of End-of-Life Care

Time of death and actions taken to prevent the death if applicable
Who pronounced the client's death
Any special preparation and type of donation, including time, staff, and company
Who was called and who came to the hospital—donor organization, morgue, funeral home, chaplain, and individual family members making any decisions
Personal articles left on the body and taped to skin or tubes left in
Personal items given to the family—specific names and descriptors of items
Time of discharge and destination of the body
Location of name tags on the body
Special requests by the family
Any other personal statements that might be needed to clarify the situation

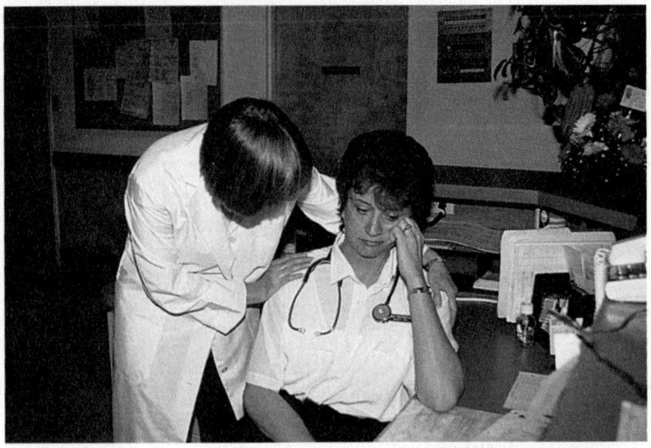

FIGURE **25–5** Nurses benefit from support of colleagues during their time of loss.

right of clients to access their health records. Copies of parts of the chart can be given to family members with a written request and the approval of the physician and hospital (see agency guidelines). The nurse must understand and uphold the legal guidelines of documentation at all times (see chapter 13).

The Grieving Nurse. When a nurse has cared for a client for a period of time, it is possible to have deep personal feelings of loss and sadness when the client dies. McPhee and Markowitz (2002) described an almost universal desire to hold on to the person who is dying, with the ability to "let go" becoming a fundamental challenge. When a nurse is able to "let go," there are four fundamental things to hold on to: faith, memory, love, and one another.

There are many ways in which a nurse can attempt to cope with the loss of a dying client. Attending the viewing at the mortuary or funeral is one way to say goodbye. Writing a letter of sympathy to the family can prove helpful. It is natural for a nurse to go through the grieving process. When a nurse works in an area where there are multiple losses, it is easy for bereavement overload to develop unless there are ways to process grief. The nurse might feel frustration, anger, guilt, sadness, or anxiety. Often nurses seek out other nurses or health care workers to discuss their own grief (Figure 25–5). It is important for nurses to develop their own support systems that allow time away from the care setting and opportunities to share personal feelings. Stress management techniques (see chapter 26) can help to restore a nurse's energy and continued enjoyment in caring for clients. The nurse's self-care is critical to survival and recovery from loss, not only for the nurse's sake, but also for the sake of future clients.

NP Evaluation

Client Care. A nurse will care for clients and families at every phase of the grief process. This requires the nurse to remain aware of signs and symptoms of grief, even when clients are not specifically seeking care directly related to a loss. These same signs and symptoms offer criteria to evaluate whether a client is able to deal with a loss and progress through the grief process. Critical thinking ensures that the evaluation process is thorough and relevant to the client's situation (Figure 25–6).

The nurse refers to the goals and expected outcomes established in the plan of care to determine the effectiveness of nursing interventions. By comparing actual client behaviours with expected outcomes, the nurse evaluates the client's health status and whether there is a need to revise the plan of care. For example, if the goal is to have the client communicate a sense of hope with family members, the nurse evaluates the verbal and non-verbal communication process for cues related to hope. The client's responses will determine if new therapies are needed or if existing therapies should be revised. The nurse continues to evaluate the progress of the client, the effectiveness of the interventions, and the interactions between the family and client. It is important for the client and family to share experiences and be active participants in the evaluation process.

Client Expectations. The client expects individualized care, including relief of symptoms, preservation of dignity, and support of the family to maximize quality of life. The success of the evaluation depends partially on the bond formed with the client. Unless the client trusts the nurse, the sharing of personal expectations or desires is not likely to occur. It becomes important for the nurse to take the time to talk with the client and learn if expectations are being met. The following are examples of questions that will validate the achievement of client expectations:

- Am I helping you in the way you have hoped?
- Would you like me to assist you in a different way?
- Do you have a specific request that I have not been able to meet?
- What is most important for us to do for you at this time?
- Are we dealing with your problems in a timely manner?

Through communication and evaluation, the nurse will continue to determine if outcome criteria were met to support the goals of care. Often the evaluation of the client's needs is easy, but the process is more complex as it relates to the family. Once rapport is established, the nurse must be vigilant to avoid problems that threaten that rapport.

Key Concepts

- When caring for clients who have experienced a loss, the nurse facilitates the grief process by assisting survivors in feeling the loss, expressing the loss, and moving through the tasks of the grief process.
- Loss comes in many forms depending on the values and priorities learned within a person's sphere of influence, including family, friends, society, and culture.
- The type of loss and the perception of the loss influence the degree of grief a person experiences.

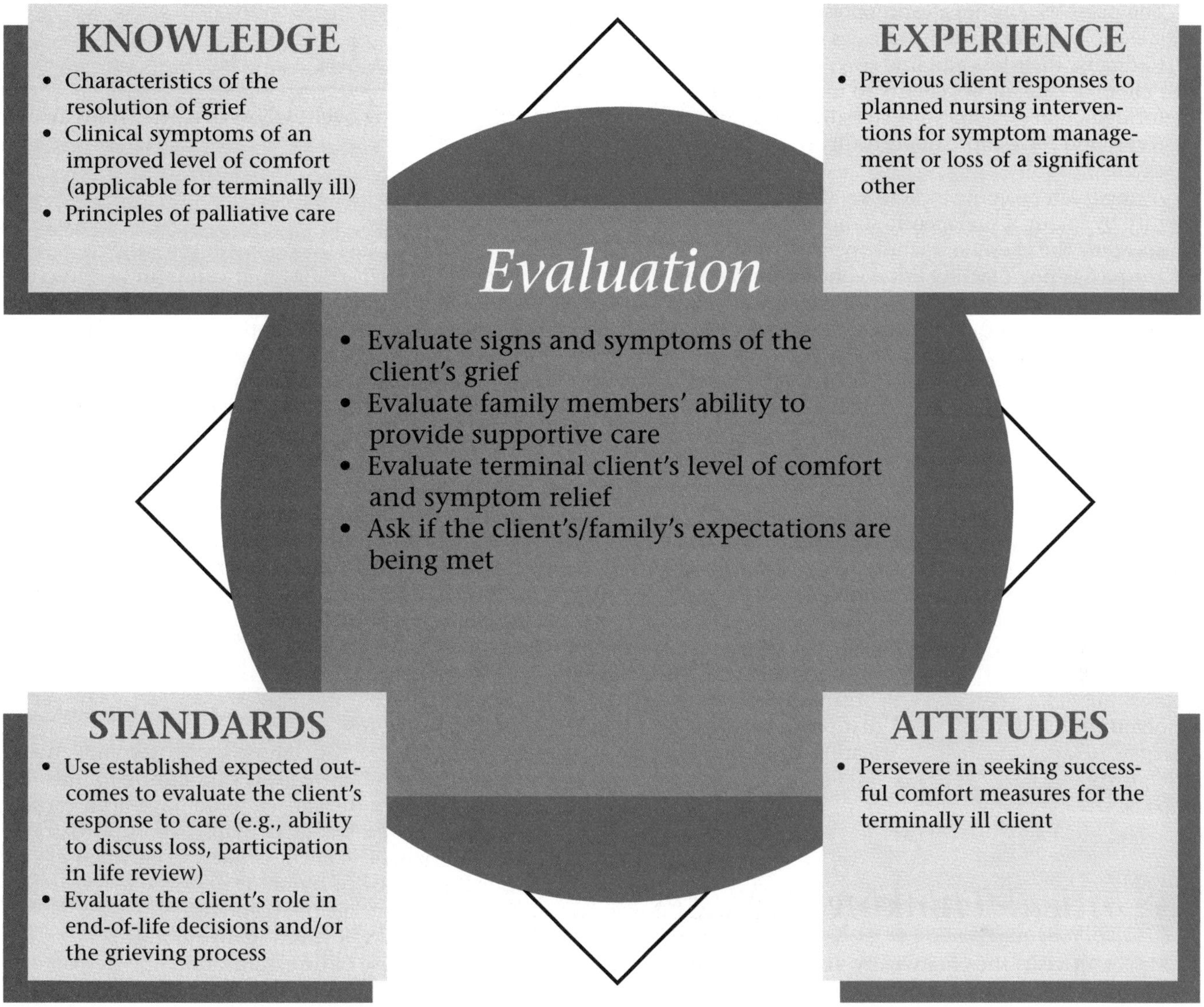
KNOWLEDGE
• Characteristics of the resolution of grief
• Clinical symptoms of an improved level of comfort (applicable for terminally ill)
• Principles of palliative care
EXPERIENCE
• Previous client responses to planned nursing interventions for symptom management or loss of a significant other
Evaluation
• Evaluate signs and symptoms of the client's grief
• Evaluate family members' ability to provide supportive care
• Evaluate terminal client's level of comfort and symptom relief
• Ask if the client's/family's expectations are being met
STANDARDS
• Use established expected outcomes to evaluate the client's response to care (e.g., ability to discuss loss, participation in life review)
• Evaluate the client's role in end-of-life decisions and/or the grieving process
ATTITUDES
• Persevere in seeking successful comfort measures for the terminally ill client

FIGURE **25–6** Critical thinking model for loss, death, and grieving evaluation.

- Death is difficult for the dying person, as well as for the person's family, friends, and caregivers.
- Survivors go through a bereavement period that is not linear; rather, an individual will move back and forth through a series of stages and/or tasks many times, possibly extending over a period of several years.
- Several theorists have developed stages of the grieving process and a series of tasks for survivors to successfully complete their bereavement and adapt to life with a loss.
- A nurse's knowledge of the types of grief allows for the implementation of appropriate bereavement interventions.
- The way an individual perceives and responds to a loss is influenced by development, psychosocial perspectives, socio-economic status, personal relationships, nature of loss, culture, and spiritual beliefs.
- Nursing interventions involve reinforcing clients' successful coping mechanisms and introducing new coping approaches such as the promotion of hope.
- When assessing clients in grief, the nurse does not assume how or if clients experience grief or whether a particular behaviour indicates grief; rather, the nurse allows clients to share what is happening in their own way.
- A nurse must assess the terminally ill client's and family's wishes for end-of-life care, including the preferred place for death, the level of life-sustaining measures to use, and expectations regarding pain and symptom management.
- The nurse develops a plan of care by integrating clients' resources such as physical energy and activity tolerance, supportive family members, spiritual faith, and methods for coping.

- The nurse establishes a caring presence and uses therapeutic communication strategies that enable clients to discuss their loss and find ways to resolve it.
- Palliative care allows clients to make more informed choices, achieve better alleviation of symptoms, and have more opportunity to work on issues of life closure.
- A nurse can promote a client's self-esteem and dignity by taking a therapeutic stance that conveys respect for the client as a whole person.
- Hospice is not a facility but a concept for family-centred care designed to assist the client in being comfortable and maintaining a satisfactory lifestyle until death.

Key Terms

Acceptance, *p. 513*
Actual loss, *p. 512*
Anger, *p. 513*
Anticipatory grief, *p. 514*
Bargaining, *p. 513*
Bereavement, *p. 513*
Denial, *p. 513*
Depression, *p. 513*
Disorganization and despair, *p. 513*
Grief, *p. 513*
Hope, *p. 517*
Hospice, *p. 531*
Maturational loss, *p. 512*
Necessary losses, *p. 512*
Numbing, *p. 513*
Palliative care, *p. 528*
Perceived loss, *p. 512*
Post-mortem care, *p. 531*
Reorganization, *p. 513*
Situational loss, *p. 512*
Yearning and searching, *p. 513*

Critical Thinking Exercises

1. Mr. Singh visits the community health clinic and tells the nurse, "I don't know what's wrong with me. I lost my wife 6 months ago and I still get angry that God let her die. I still miss her so much. I have been going out with friends, but I just don't enjoy it that much. There are times when I wake up at night and I think my wife is still here. What is wrong with me? I thought I would be feeling better by now." How could the nurse respond to Mr. Singh?
2. You are assigned to care for two clients. Mrs. Rossi has rheumatoid arthritis and is experiencing severe joint pain in both hands. Mrs. Nester has bone cancer and has experienced ongoing deep pain in the back and hips, with some discomfort also in the lower extremities. Refer to chapter 38 on content about pain. Then discuss in what way management of pain will differ between the two clients.
3. A nursing colleague is discussing her client with you. She says, "My client is a 48-year-old man with a degenerative neurological disease. The disease is progressive. He is having trouble walking and taking care of his daily needs. The only thing I can do is assist him with bathing, feeding, and walking. He really is not a candidate yet for palliative care." What would be your response to your colleague?

Review Questions

1. A child is grieving over the loss of a pet. This is an example of a(n)
   1. Actual loss
   2. Perceived loss
   3. Situational loss
   4. Maturational loss
2. A middle-age man comes to a community clinic for his annual flu shot. In the discussion with the nurse, she learns that he still works at a local law firm. However, he has recently lost two important cases and his boss has been applying pressure on him "to turn it around." The client may be experiencing a(n)
   1. Actual loss
   2. Perceived loss
   3. Situational loss
   4. Maturational loss
3. The community health nurse's job is to provide grief counselling for the community residents where a major flood has occurred. The loss associated with flooding is best described as a(n)
   1. Actual loss
   2. Perceived loss
   3. Situational loss
   4. Maturational loss
4. The client has been diagnosed with terminal brain cancer. When the nurse visits him during rounds, he asks her whether the cancer could have been caused by something he ate or perhaps exposure to some chemical toxin. The client is likely experiencing
   1. Bowlby's phase of numbing
   2. Kübler-Ross's stage of acceptance
   3. Worden's tasks of emotionally relocating
   4. Bowlby's phase of disorganization and despair
5. According to Kübler-Ross's *Stages of Dying,* during this phase, the client may feel overwhelmingly lonely and withdraw from interpersonal interaction:
   1. Denial
   2. Anger
   3. Bargaining
   4. Depression
6. Since the death of his wife, the client has assumed full responsibility for the care of his children. He has noticed over the last few weeks that friends are calling less often. He is most likely in the following phase of mourning:
   1. Anticipatory grieving
   2. Worden's task III of mourning
   3. Kübler Ross's phase of bargaining
   4. Bowlby's phase of disorganization and despair
7. Which of the following is one of the most common and difficult issue faced by older bereaved spouses?
   1. Adjusting to physical problems
   2. Overcoming mental health problems
   3. Completing the tasks of daily living
   4. Managing finances

8. "Client will express hopefulness that cancer treatment will control symptoms." is an example of a(n)
   1. Goal
   2. Intervention
   3. Plan
   4. Expected outcome
9. A 16-year-old client has been admitted to the intensive care unit after suffering a closed head injury. The client is soon declared brain dead. The physician and nurse are preparing to approach the family to consider donation of the heart and lungs. When working with families in this situation, it is important to explain that
   1. The ventilator is being used to prevent brain death
   2. The ventilator maintains organ perfusion until time for harvesting
   3. Tissues such as corneas can be harvested only if the client remains ventilated
   4. Organ donation can occur only if the client has made a request to donate organs in the past
10. This type of care allows clients to make more informed choices, achieve better alleviation of symptoms, and have more opportunity to work on issues of life closure:
   1. Acute care
   2. Mourning care
   3. Palliative care
   4. Terminal care

References

Barbus, A. J. (1975). The dying person's bill of rights. *American Journal of Nursing, 75,* 99.

Benner, P., et al. (2003). Attending death as a human passage: Core nursing principles for end-of-life care. *American Journal of Critical Care, 12*(6), 558–561.

Bierman, A. S., et al. (1998). Assessing access as a first step towards improving the quality of care for very old adults. *The Journal of Ambulatory Care Management, 21*(3), 17–26.

Binstock, R. H., & Spector, W. D. (1997). Five priority areas for research on long-term care. *Health Services Research, 32*(5), 715–730.

Blackhall, L. J., et al. (1999). Ethnicity and attitudes towards life-sustaining technology. *Social Service in Medicine, 48,* 1779–1789.

Bowlby, J. (1980). *Attachment and loss: Vol. 3. Loss, sadness, and depression.* New York: Basic Books.

Braza, K. (1993, March). Families and the grief process. *ARCH Factsheet, 21.* Retrieved December 12, 2004, from *http://www.archrespite.org/archfs21.htm*

Callahan, D. (1995). Terminating life-sustaining treatment of the demented. *The Hastings Center Report, 25,* 25–31.

Canadian Hospice Palliative Care Association Nursing Standards Committee. (2002). *Hospice palliative care nursing standards of practice.* Ottawa, ON: Canadian Hospice Palliative Care Association.

Canadian Nurses Association, et al. (1994). *Joint statement on advance directives.* Ottawa, ON: Author.

Canadian Nurses Association. (1998). *Advance directives: The nurse's role, ethics in practice.* Ottawa, ON: Author.

Canadian Nurses Association. (2000). *Fact sheet: Palliative care.* Ottawa, ON: Author.

Canadian Nurses Association. (2002). *Code of ethics for registered nurses.* Ottawa, ON: Author.

Catalano, J. T. (1995). *Ethical and legal aspects of nursing* (2nd ed.). Springhouse, PA: Springhouse.

Chochinov, H. M. (2002). Dignity-conserving care—A new model for palliative care: Helping the patient feel valued. *Journal of the American Medical Association, 287*(17), 2253–2260.

Cressy, D. (1997). *Birth, marriage, and death: Ritual, religion, and the life- cycle in Tudor and Stuart England.* New York: Oxford University Press.

Daaleman, T. P., & VandeCreek, L. (2000). Placing religion and spirituality in end-of-life care. *Journal of the American Medical Association, 284,* 2514–2517.

Davies, B., et al. (2003). The impact on families of a children's hospice program. *Journal of Palliative Care, 19*(1), 15–26.

Davies, B., & Oberle, K. (1990). Dimensions of the supportive role of the nurse in palliative care. *Oncology Nursing Forum, 17*(1), 87–94.

Dochterman, J. M., & Bulechek, G. M. (Eds.). (2004). *Nursing interventions classification (NIC)* (4th ed.). St. Louis, MO: Mosby.

Doka, K. J. (1993). *Living with life-threatening illness: A guide for patients, their families, and caregivers.* New York: Lexington.

Dracup, K., & Bryan-Brown, C. W. (1998). Asking difficult questions. *American Journal of Critical Care, 7*(6), 399–401.

End-of-Life Nursing Education Consortium. (2000). American Association of Colleges of Nursing and City of Hope National Medical Center.

Farber, S. J., Egnew, T. R., & Herman-Bertsch, J. L. (1999). Issues in end-of-life care: Family practice faculty perceptions. *The Journal of Family Practice, 48*(7), 525–530.

Ferris, F. D., et al. (2002). A model to guide patient and family care: Based on nationally accepted principles and norms of practice. *Journal of Pain and Symptom Management, 24*(2), 106–123.

Finucane, T. E. (2002). Care of patients nearing death: Another view. *Journal of the American Geriatrics Society, 50*(3), 551–553.

Fisher, R., Ross, M. M., & MacLean, M. J. (Eds.). (2000). *A guide to end-of-life care for seniors.* Ottawa, ON: Health Canada.

Forbes, S., Bern-Klug, M., & Gessert, C. (2000). End-of-life decision making for nursing home residents with dementia. *Journal of Nursing Scholarship, 32*(3), 251–258.

Gray, K., & Lassance, A. (2003). *Grieving reproductive loss: The healing process.* Amityville, NY: Baywood.

Hasler, K. (1996). Understanding and managing bereavement. *Nursing Standard, 10*(24), 51–54.

Hinton, J. (1999). The progress of awareness and acceptance of dying assessed in cancer patients and their caring relatives. *Palliative Medicine, 13,* 19–35.

The Hospice RN. (2003). Patients bill of rights. Retrieved January 18, 2005, from *http://www.geocities.com/hotsprings/5120/bill.htm*

Kagawa-Singer, M. (1998). The cultural context of death rituals and mourning practices. *Oncology Nursing Forum, 25*(10), 1752–1756.

Keatings, M., & Smith, O. B. (2000). *Ethical and legal issues in Canadian nursing* (2nd ed.). Toronto, ON: W. B. Saunders.

Kübler-Ross, E. (1969). *In death and dying.* New York: MacMillan.

Latimer, E. J. (2000). Cultural diversity in palliative care: Celebrating uniqueness. *The Canadian Journal of Continuing Medical Education, 12*(11), 93–110.

Lenhardt, A. M. C. (1997). Grieving disenfranchised losses: Background and strategies for counselors. *The Journal of Humanistic Education and Development, 35*(4), 208.

Lugton, J., & Kindlen, M. (1999). *Palliative care: The nursing role.* Edinburgh, Scotland: Churchill Livingston.

Lund, D. A. (1989). Conclusions about bereavement in later life and implications for interventions and future research. In D. A. Lund (Ed.), *Older bereaved spouses: Research with practical application.* New York: Hemisphere.

McLean, S. (1999). The definition of death: Contemporary controversies. *BMJ, 319*(7207), 458A.

McPhee, S. J., & Markowitz, A. J. (2002). Reflections at a palliative care unit. *Journal of the American Medical Association, 288*(10), 1279.

Moorhead, S., Johnson, M., & Maas, M. (Eds.). (2004). *Nursing outcomes classification (NOC)* (3rd ed.). St. Louis, MO: Mosby.

Morse, J. M., & Doberneck, B. (1995). Delineating the concept of hope. *Image—The Journal of Nursing Scholarship, 27*(4), 277–285.

Northcott, H. C., & Wilson, D. M. (2001). *Dying and death in Canada*. Aurora, ON: Garamond Press.

Parkes, C. M. (1972). *Bereavement: Studies of grief in adult life*. London: Tavistock.

Perry, B. (1998). *Moments in time: Images of exemplary nursing care*. Ottawa, ON: Canadian Nurses Association.

Perry, B. (2002). Nurses' work: Growth and satisfaction. *Canadian Nurse, 98*(10), 19–22.

Post-White, J., et al. (1996). Hope, spirituality, sense of coherence, and quality of life in patients with cancer. *Oncology Nursing Forum, 23*(10), 1571–1579.

Senate of Canada. (2000). *Quality end-of-life care: The right of every Canadian: Final report of the Standing Senate Committee on Social Affairs, Science and Technology*. Retrieved May 18, 2004, from *http://www.parl.gc.ca/36/2/parlbus/commbus/senate/com-e/upda-e/rep-e/repfinjun00-e.htm*

Stocker, S. (1994). Beyond grief: A guide to reconciling life after loss. *Prevention, 46*(8), 88–96.

Tarzian, A. J. (2000). Caring for dying patients who have air hunger. *Image—The Journal of Nursing Scholarship, 32,*137–143.

Thomas, N. D. (2001). The importance of culture throughout all of life and beyond. *Holistic Nursing Practice, 15*(2), 40–46.

Tilden, V. P., et al. (2001). Family decision-making to withdraw life-sustaining treatments from hospitalized patients. *Nursing Research, 50*(2), 105–115.

Tolle, S., et al. (2000). Family reports of barriers to optimal care of the dying. *Nursing Research, 49*(6), 310–317.

van Bommel, H. (1999). *Family hospice care: Pre-planning and care guide*. Scarborough, ON: Resources Supporting Family and Community Legacies.

Weissman, D. E., & Matson, S. (1999). Pain assessment and management in the long-term care setting. *Theoretical Medicine and Bioethics, 20*(1), 31–43.

Witoszek, N. (1998). *Talking to the dead: A study of Irish funerary traditions*. Atlanta, GA: Rodopi.

Worden, J. W. (1991). *Grief counseling and grief therapy: A handbook for the mental health practitioner* (2nd ed.). New York: Springer.

World Health Organization. (2003). *Palliative care*. Retrieved December 12, 2004, from *http://www.who.int/hiv/topics/palliative/PalliativeCare/en*

Recommended Web Sites

Bereaved Families of Ontario:
http://www.bereavedfamilies.net

This site provides support programs and resources for people of all ages who have lost a family member.

Canadian Hospice Palliative Care Association:
http://www.chpca.net/home.htm

The Canadian Hospice Palliative Care Association (CHPCA) is a national association that offers leadership in the pursuit of excellence in care for people approaching death. One of its goals is to advocate for improved hospice palliative care policy, resource allocation, and supports for caregivers.

Regional Palliative Care Program in Edmonton Alberta:
http://www.palliative.org

The objective this Web site is to provide information to health care professionals that will help them to reflect on their practice with the terminally ill. This site offers palliative care tips, nursing notes, a caregiver guide, and links to publications and other resources.

26

Stress and Adaptation

Marjorie Baier, RN, PhD, APRN, BC
Ginette Lemire Rodger, RN, BScN, MAdmN, PhD (Canadian author)

Objectives

Mastery of content in this chapter will enable the student to:

- Define the key terms listed.
- Describe the three stages of the general adaptation syndrome.
- Differentiate acute stress disorder and post-traumatic stress disorder.
- Discuss the integration of stress theory with nursing theories.
- Formulate nursing diagnoses from assessment data.
- Describe stress management techniques beneficial for coping with stress.
- Discuss the process of crisis intervention.
- Develop a care plan for clients experiencing stress.
- Discuss how stress in the workplace can affect the nurse.

Stress is universal and necessary for survival, affecting every person regardless of age, gender, race, economic condition, or educational level. Knowledge about stress is important because health care professionals must recognize stress in clients and families and intervene effectively. In addition, health care professionals are affected by stressful events. Nurses must recognize the signs and symptoms of stress and be knowledgeable about stress management techniques to design stress management interventions for their clients and families, as well as to aid personal coping.

People use the term ***stress*** in many ways. First, stress is an experience a person is exposed to through a stimulus or stressor. **Stressors** are disruptive forces operating within or on any system (Neuman, 1995). Stress is also the appraisal, or perception, of a stressor. **Appraisal** is how people interpret what is happening , the impact of the stressor on themselves, and what they can do about it (Lazarus, 1999). Finally, stress is a general term that links environmental demands and the person's capacity to meet those demands (Kasl, 1992). Stress in this context refers to the consequences of the stressor, as well as to the person's appraisal of the stressor.

People experience stress as a consequence of daily life events and experiences. Stress can result in personal growth and facilitate development (Aguilera, 1998). It is a motivating force that stimulates thought processes and helps people stay alert to their environment. However, stress also causes discomfort and retreat. When stress overwhelms a person's coping mechanisms, disequilibrium occurs, and a **crisis** results (Aguilera, 1998). If symptoms of stress persist beyond the duration of the stressor, a person has experienced a **trauma** (Hyer & Sohnle, 2001). How people react to stress depends on how they view and evaluate the impact of the stressor, its effect on their situation, their available supports, and their usual coping mechanisms.

Scientific Knowledge Base

Over 60 years ago, Walter Cannon proposed the **fight-or-flight response** to stress, which is arousal of the sympathetic nervous system (Aldwin, 2000). This reaction prepares a person for action by increasing heart rate; diverting blood from the intestines to the brain and striated muscles; and increasing

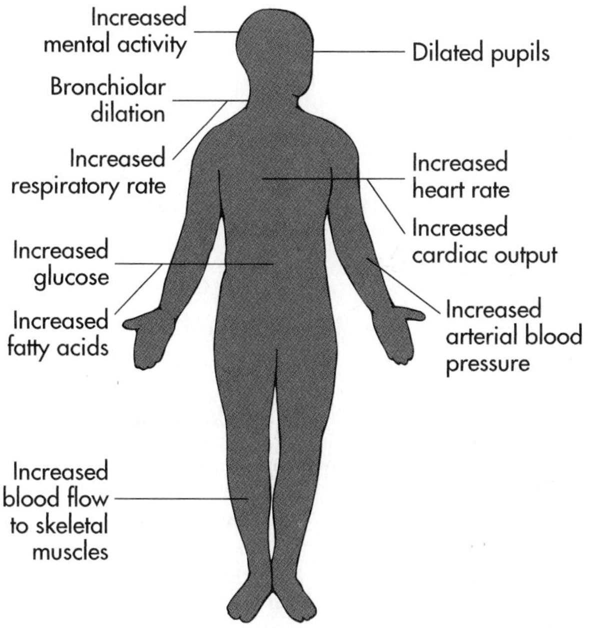

FIGURE **26–1** Fight-or-flight response.

blood pressure, respiratory rate, and blood sugar levels (Figure 26–1).

Neurophysiological responses to stress function through negative feedback. This is a process by which the controlling mechanism senses an abnormal state, such as lowered body temperature, and makes an adaptive response, such as initiating shivering to generate body heat. Cannon coined the term ***homeostasis*** to describe the phenomenon of establishing and maintaining internal physio-chemical equilibrium (Chrousos, Loriaux, & Gold, 1988). Stress is associated with the activation of the hypothalamus-pituitary-adrenal axis. The link between the stressor and the hypothalamus gland is still unknown, but the presence of corticotropin-releasing hormone (CRH) in the brain is sufficient to initiate the stress response (Dunn, 1989). CRH elicits changes in both the nervous and the endocrine pathway. The major mechanisms of neuroresponse to a stressor are controlled by the reticular formation, the limbic system, the midbrain, the pons, and the medulla oblongata, whereas the endocrine response is controlled mainly by the pituitary gland.

- *Reticular Formation.* The reticular formation is a small integrative cluster of neurons in the brain stem and spinal cord. It continuously monitors the physiological status of the body through connections with sensory and motor tracts. For example, certain cells within the reticular formation can cause a sleeping person to regain consciousness or increase the level of consciousness when a need arises.
- *Limbic System.* The limbic system is another integrative cluster of neurons that interconnect several parts of the brain. It is involved in emotional experience and can modify the way a person acts. Stress will cause increased activities of this system.
- *Midbrain and the Pons.* The midbrain joins the lower part of the brain stem and the spinal cord with the higher part of the brain and acts as a reflex centre for certain auditory, visual, and posture reflexes. The pons mainly relays impulses to and from the medulla oblongata to other parts of the brain and the peripheral nervous system, and it also controls the rate and depth of breathing.
- *Medulla Oblongata.* The medulla oblongata controls vital functions necessary for survival, including heart rate, blood pressure, and respiration. Impulses travelling to and from the medulla oblongata can increase or decrease these vital functions. For example, regulation of the heartbeat is the result of sympathetic or parasympathetic nervous system impulses travelling from the medulla oblongata to the heart. The heart rate increases in response to pulses from sympathetic fibres and decreases with impulses from parasympathetic fibres.
- *Pituitary Gland.* The pituitary gland, a small gland attached to the hypothalamus, supplies hormones that control vital functions. The role of this gland is central to the endocrine pathway of stress response. The pituitary gland produces hormones necessary for adaptation to stress, such as the adrenocorticotropic hormone, which in turn produces cortisol. In addition, the pituitary gland regulates the secretion of thyroid, gonadal, and parathyroid hormones. Hormone secretion, like other homeostatic mechanisms, is normally regulated by a feedback mechanism that continuously monitors hormone levels in the blood. When hormone levels drop, the pituitary gland receives a message to increase hormone secretion. When hormone levels rise, the pituitary gland decreases hormone production.

General Adaptation Syndrome

In the 1930s, 1940s, and 1950s, Hans Selye, a Canadian Nobel Prize winner, expanded on Cannon's fight-or-flight hypothesis to describe the **general adaptation syndrome (GAS),** a three-stage reaction to stress (Selye, 1991). The GAS describes how the body responds to stressors through the alarm reaction, the adaptation (or resistance) stage, and the exhaustion stage. The GAS can be triggered either directly by a physical event or indirectly by a psychological event (Lazarus, 1999).

The GAS is an immediate physiological response of the body to stress and involves several body systems, especially the autonomic nervous system and the endocrine system (Figure 26–2). When a demand is made on the body, such as an injury or fear, the GAS is initiated by the pituitary gland. The pituitary gland is closely linked to the hypothalamus, which secretes **endorphins.** Endorphins are hormones that act on the mind like morphine and opiates, producing a sense of well-being and reducing pain (Lazarus, 1999). In this way, the GAS defends against stress both by activating the neuroendocrine system and by providing endorphins that decrease awareness of the pain.

During the **alarm reaction,** rising hormone levels result in increased blood volume, blood glucose levels, epinephrine and norepinephrine amounts, heart rate, blood flow to muscles, oxygen intake, and mental alertness

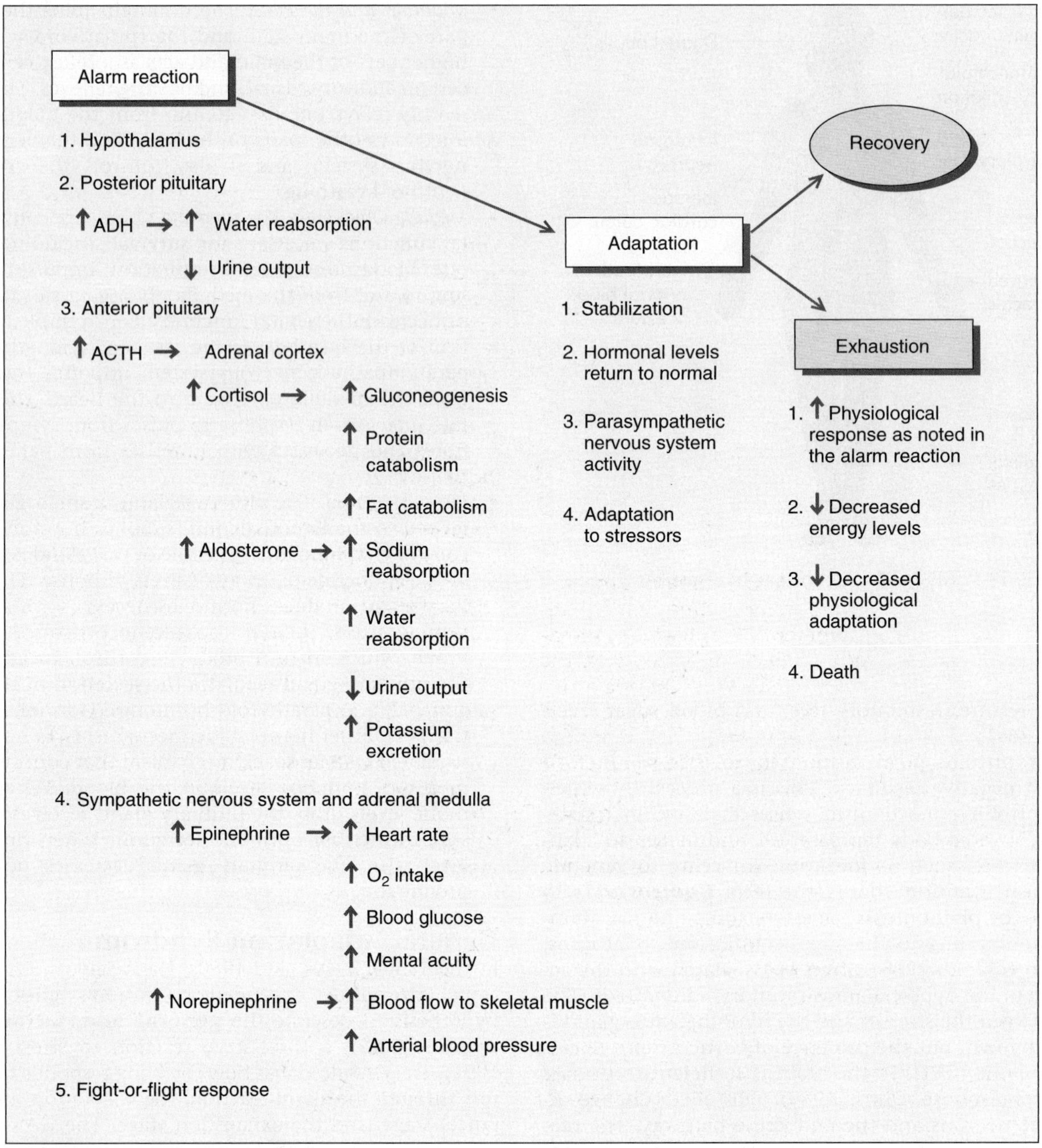

FIGURE **26–2** General adaptation syndrome (GAS).

(Selye, 1991). In addition, the pupils of the eyes dilate to produce a greater visual field. This change in body systems prepares an individual for fight or flight and may last from 1 minute to many hours. If the stressor poses an extreme threat to life or remains for a long time, the person progresses to the second stage, adaptation.

During the **adaptation stage,** the body stabilizes and responds in an opposite manner to the alarm reaction. Hormone levels, heart rate, blood pressure, and cardiac output return to normal, and the body repairs any damage that may have occurred. However, if the stressor remains, and there is no adaptation, the person enters the third stage, exhaustion.

The **exhaustion stage** occurs when the body can no longer resist the effects of the stressor and when the energy necessary to maintain adaptation is depleted. The physiological response is intensified, but the person's energy level is compromised, and adaptation to the stressor diminishes. The body is unable to defend itself against the impact of the event, physiological regulation diminishes, and, if the stress continues, death may result.

Physiological responses to stress also include immunological responses, although the mechanisms through which stress affects the immune system are unclear (Aldwin, 2000). The immune system differentiates between self and non-self, so that, under normal condi-

Box 26-1 Factors Influencing the Response to Stressors

Aspects of a Stressor That Would Influence the Stress Response

Intensity
Scope
Duration
Number and nature of other stressors
Predictability

Characteristics of the Individual That Would Influence the Stress Response

Level of personal control
Availability of social supports
Feelings of competence
Cognitive appraisal

tions, one's own cells are not treated as threats in the way that bacteria, viruses, parasites, or toxins are treated. Typically, the immune system recognizes bacteria, for example, as a threat and attacks them. An antigen on the surface of the bacteria cells identifies the bacteria as invaders. After being exposed to a particular antigen, the immune system remembers how to respond to that antigen and is prepared to respond with antibodies when the same antigen appears at a later time. However, a virus might create an antigen that is very similar to a naturally occurring protein and the immune system would attack it as if it were a threat. Problems occur when the immune system misinterprets antigens and responds too vigorously, leading to an autoimmune illness.

Selye (1991) noted that a prolonged state of stress could cause disease. Stress can make people ill as a result of (a) increased levels of powerful hormones that change our bodily processes; (b) coping choices that are unhealthy, such as not getting enough rest or a proper diet or use of tobacco, alcohol, caffeine, or other substances; and (c) neglect of warning signs of illness or failure to adhere to prescribed medicines or treatments (Monat & Lazarus, 1991).

Reaction to Psychological Stress

The GAS is activated for both physical and psychological threats. Psychological threats are different for each person and produce differing reactions (Box 26-1). Lazarus (1999) maintained that a person is under stress only if the person evaluates the event or circumstance as personally significant. Evaluating an event for its personal meaning is called **primary appraisal.** Appraisal of an event or circumstance is an ongoing perceptual process (Aguilera, 1998). If primary appraisal results in the person identifying the event or circumstance as a harm, loss, threat, or challenge, the person experiences stress. If stress is present, **secondary appraisal** focuses on possible coping strategies. Balancing factors contribute to restoring equilibrium. According to crisis theory (Aguilera, 1998), feedback cues lead to reappraisals of the original perception. Therefore, coping behaviours constantly change as new information is perceived.

Coping is the person's effort to manage psychological stress (Lazarus, 1999). Effectiveness of coping strategies depends on the individual's needs. For this reason, no single coping strategy works for everyone or for every stress. The same person may cope differently from one time to another. In stressful situations, people may use a combination of problem-focused coping and emotion-focused coping strategies. In other words, when under stress, a person obtains information and takes action to change the situation, as well as regulating emotions tied to the stress. In some cases, a person avoids thinking about the situation or changes the way he or she thinks about it, without changing the actual situation itself (Lazarus, 1999).

Lazarus suggested that not only does the type of stress make a difference, but also people's goals, their beliefs about themselves and the world, and personal resources determine how they cope with stress. "Resources include intelligence, money, social skills, supportive family and friends, physical attractiveness, health and energy, and ways of thinking, such as optimism" (Lazarus, 1999).

Psychological adaptive behaviours are also referred to as coping mechanisms. Such mechanisms can be task oriented, involving the use of direct problem-solving techniques to cope with the threats. They can also be **ego-defence mechanisms,** the purpose of which is to regulate emotional distress and thus give a person protection from anxiety and stress. Ego-defence mechanisms are indirect methods of coping with stress.

Ego-defence mechanisms, first described by Sigmund Freud, are unconscious behaviours that offer psychological protection from a stressful event. Everyone uses them to help protect against feelings of worthlessness and anxiety. Occasionally a defence mechanism can become distorted and is no longer able to assist the person in adapting to a stressor. There are many ego-defence mechanisms (Box 26-2). They are frequently activated by short-term stressors and usually do not result in psychiatric disorders.

Types of Stress

Selye identified two types of stress: **distress,** or damaging stress, and **eustress,** stress that protects health. Eustress is motivating energy, such as happiness, hopefulness, and purposeful movement (Varcarolis, 2002). Eustress is a positive, healthy adaptation to stressors in daily life. It is within this context that Selye (1974) wrote his book *Stress Without Distress*. However, Aldwin in 2000 wrote that the idea of healthy stress is controversial because it is difficult to tell whether a person has benefited from stress or is coping by denying the stress in some way. There are several types of stress, including work stress, family stress, chronic stress, acute stress, daily hassles, trauma, and crisis. "Work and family stress interact, family being the background for work stress, and work the background for family stress" (Lazarus, 1999). One person may see a stimulus as a challenge, leading to mastery and growth. Another sees the same stimulus as a threat, leading to stagnation and loss. Lazarus suggests a spillover of stresses

Box 26-2 Examples of Ego-Defence Mechanisms

- Compensation is making up for a perceived deficiency in one aspect of self-image by exaggerating a feature considered an asset. (Example: A poor communicator becomes an elite athlete.)
- Conversion is unconsciously repressing an anxiety-producing emotional conflict and changing it into physical symptoms. (Example: A person who is waiting for test results may appear calm but experience difficulty sleeping, loss of appetite).
- Denial is avoiding emotional conflicts by refusing to consciously acknowledge anything that might cause intolerable emotional pain. (Example: An adolescent with diabetes does not alter her diet, saying "a few treats aren't going to hurt me.")
- Displacement is transferring emotions, ideas, or wishes from a stressful situation to a less anxiety-producing substitute. (Example: A person is angry with his boss but yells at his child.)
- Projection is assigning one's feelings to someone or something else. (Example: A child says she needs a night-light because her doll is afraid of the dark.)
- Rationalization is making excuses for one's behaviour or a situation while ignoring the real reason. (Example: An older man experiences hearing loss, but says he cannot understand others because they are mumbling.)
- Regression is coping with a stressor through actions and behaviours associated with an earlier developmental period. (Example: A 3-year-old wants a bottle when a new baby comes into the family.)

between work and home. The individual with family responsibilities and a full-time job outside the home may experience chronic stress. Chronic stress occurs in stable conditions and from stressful roles. Another example of chronic stress is living with a long-term illness. Conversely, acute stress is provoked by time-limited events that are threatening for a relatively brief period. Further complicating chronic or acute stress are daily hassles that are recurrent, such as commuting to work, maintaining a house, dealing with difficult people, and managing money.

When a trauma occurs, its effects may last well after the traumatizing event ends (Hyer & Sohnle, 2001). **Post-traumatic stress disorder (PTSD)** begins with an **acute stress disorder** (ASD; Hyer & Sohnle, 2001). An ASD begins with the person experiencing, witnessing, or being confronted with a traumatic event and responding with intense fear, helplessness, or horror (American Psychiatric Association [APA], 2000). Other criteria of the ASD are that the person displays at least three acute dissociative symptoms, has at least one re-experiencing symptom, displays marked avoidance of stimuli that arouse memories of the trauma, shows marked hyperarousal, and has these symptoms between 2 days and 4 weeks after the trauma (Hyer & Sohnle, 2001). Examples of traumatic events that lead to ASD are motor vehicle crashes, natural disasters, violent personal assault, and military combat. Symptoms of PTSD may have a delayed onset longer than 4 weeks and persists longer than 1 month (APA, 2000). People with PTSD may experience **flashbacks,** or recurrent and intrusive recollections of the event. Traumatic events that can lead to PTSD include the same events that lead to ASD (Box 26-3).

Conversely, research is beginning to show that trauma can have positive effects. It can lead to greater self-knowledge, improved coping skills, stronger social ties, and changes in values and perspectives (Hyer & Sohnle, 2001).

A crisis implies that a person is facing a turning point in life. That is, previous ways of coping are not effective and the person must change. Gerald Caplan, in 1964, described crisis intervention. Caplan distinguished two types of crises, those associated with changing developmental levels, or **developmental crises,** and **situational crises.** The frame of reference for a crisis is from the view of the person experiencing the crisis. Aguilera's crisis theory (1998) maintains that the vital question for a person in crisis is, "What does this mean to you; how is it going to affect your life?" What is extremely stressful for one person might not be stressful to another. The factors influencing the return of equilibrium or homeostasis are the perception of the event, situational supports, and coping mechanisms. A basic assumption of crisis theory is that a person can either advance or regress as a result of a crisis, depending upon how the crisis is managed (Lazarus, 1999).

Nursing Knowledge Base

Nurses have proposed theories related to stress and coping. Because stress plays a role in vulnerability to disease, symptoms of stress often require nursing intervention.

Nursing Theory and the Role of Stress

Neuman Systems Model is based on the concepts of stress and reaction to stress. This nursing theory views nursing as being responsible for developing interventions to prevent or reduce stressors on the client or to make them more bearable for the client (Neuman, 1995). Because the Neuman model is a systems model, it is applied to not only understand clients' individual responses to stressors, but families' and communities' responses as well. All systems experience multiple stressors, each of which has a differing potential to disturb the person's, family's, or community's balance. Examples of stress may include intrapersonal stressors, such as an illness or injury; interpersonal stressors, such as an argument or misunderstanding; or extrapersonal stressors that arise because of life circumstances, such as financial problems. Every person has developed a set of responses to stress that constitute the "normal line of defence" (Neuman, 1995). This line of defence helps to maintain health and wellness. However, when "physiological, psychological, sociocultural, developmental, or spiritual influences" are unable to buffer stress, the normal line of defence is broken, and disease can result. In this belief, Neuman Systems Model coincides with Selye's general adaptation syndrome.

Neuman Systems Model (1995) stresses the importance of accuracy in assessment and interventions that

Research Highlight

Box 26-3

Understanding Risks for Developing Psychological Distress

Research Focus

When caring for clients who have experienced trauma such as motor vehicle crashes, assaults, and industrial accidents, nurses focus first on life-threatening effects of the trauma. However, other consequences of trauma, such as psychological distress, may be unnoticed. Nurses need to be aware of risk factors for anxiety, depression, and post-traumatic stress disorder following trauma.

Research Abstract

The purpose of this study was to describe the pre-trauma characteristics of 152 people (87 women and 65 men) who experienced significant psychological distress shortly after physical injury. Individuals who had received treatment in the emergency department were contacted and asked to complete three questionnaires: the Posttraumatic Stress Disorder Scale, the Impact of Event Scale (IES), and the Hospital Anxiety and Depression Scale. A fourth questionnaire, the Abbreviated Injury Scale, was completed based upon a medical record review by the researchers. The presence of significant psychological distress among the 152 people identified from all of the people receiving emergency treatment was documented. Overall, the people identified with distress reported very little functional impairment and a high level of contentment before the traumatic event. Most of their injuries were relatively minor and not life-threatening. However, 141 (93%) of the subjects met the diagnostic criteria for post-traumatic stress disorder (PTSD). The IES revealed that the subjects were experiencing high levels of trauma-related distress. The researchers examined the relationship between pre-trauma variables and the total score on the IES. The pre-trauma factors of being unemployed and having experienced previous trauma accounted for 10% of the variance in the total IES score. The researchers concluded that (a) trauma perceived as mild by medical personnel can result in severe stress, anxiety, and depression for the client; (b) high functioning before a traumatic event does not protect the client from developing PTSD; and (c) pre-trauma unemployment can contribute to psychological distress after a traumatic injury.

Evidence-Based Practice

- Regardless of the severity of trauma or previous level of functioning, clients who have experienced a traumatic injury are at risk for developing PTSD.
- Nurses must monitor the client's perception of the meaning and impact of a traumatic injury, regardless of the apparent severity of the trauma.
- Two risk factors for developing PTSD after a traumatic injury are unemployment before the trauma and previous trauma.

Reference

Joy, D., et al. (2000). Post-traumatic stress reactions after injury. *The Journal of Trauma, 48*(3), 490–494.

promote optimal wellness using primary, secondary, and tertiary prevention strategies. According to Neuman's theory, the goal of primary prevention is to promote client wellness by stress prevention and reduction of risk factors. Secondary prevention occurs after symptoms appear. The nurse determines the meaning of the illness and stress to the client and the client's needs and resources for meeting them. Tertiary prevention begins when the client system is becoming more stable and recovering. At the tertiary level of prevention, the nurse supports rehabilitation processes involved in healing, moving the client back to wellness and the primary level of disease prevention. Neuman's model of nursing views the person, family, or community as constantly changing in response to the environment and stressors.

Pender's health promotion model proposes that health promotion is directed toward increasing the level of well-being of an individual or group (Pender, Murdaugh, & Parsons, 2002). Conversely, primary, secondary, and tertiary prevention (health protection) focus on avoiding negative events. Pender considered stress reduction strategies important to reduce threats to well-being, to help people fulfill their potential, and to shape and maintain health behaviours. To change behaviour, the client must initiate the change and behave differently in interactions. People want to live in ways that enable them to be as healthy as possible and to be capable of assessing their own abilities and assets. Based on these assumptions of the capability and desire of people to be healthy, Pender suggested strategies for prevention and health promotion related to stress management.

Situational, Maturational, and Socio-cultural Factors

Potential stressors and coping mechanisms vary across the lifespan. For example, adolescence, adulthood, and old age bring different stressors. Appraisal of stressors, amount and type of social support, and coping strategies are balancing factors when assessing stress, and all depend on previous life experiences (Aguilera, 1998). Furthermore, situational and socio-cultural stressors place people who are vulnerable at higher risk for prolonged stress.

Situational Factors. Situational stress can arise from the person's current circumstances, such as moving, changing jobs (stressful job changes can include promotions, transfers, downsizing, restructuring, changes in supervisors, and additional responsibilities), and adjusting to a chronic illness or condition. Common diseases and conditions that provoke stress are obesity, hypertension, diabetes, depression, asthma, and coronary artery disease. Being a family caregiver may also cause situational stress,

Research Highlight

Box 26-4

Spousal Support for Psychological Distress

Research Focus

Holistic nursing care includes the client's family. Family members, especially the spouse, have an impact on the client's recovery from cardiac disease and surgery. More information is needed about stress experienced by spouses of clients in cardiac rehabilitation and interventions to help spouses cope with stress.

Research Abstract

The purposes of this study were (a) to describe the distress experienced by 213 spouses of men in cardiac rehabilitation, (b) to identify the most common heart disease stressors experienced by the women, (c) to compare distressed and non-distressed spouses in terms of demographic variables and coping strategies, and (d) to identify specific intervention needs for spouses of clients undergoing cardiac rehabilitation. Spouses were recruited by telephone at the time of the admission of the spouse into the cardiac rehabilitation program. Subjects agreed to participate in five spousal support group sessions and to complete five questionnaires that assessed psychological distress, coping, marital intimacy, family functioning, and heart disease hassles. The Brief Symptom Inventory measured psychological distress. Based upon this scale, 66 subjects were categorized as being psychologically distressed. Symptoms of distress were feeling tense, having trouble falling asleep, and feeling easily hurt. The group of spouses who were distressed was significantly younger than the group who were not distressed. The distressed spouses coped with the stress by disengagement strategies, such as avoidance, wishful thinking, self-criticism, and withdrawal. The Heart Disease Hassles Scale is a 75-item scale that identified common heart disease-related stressors. The five highest ranked stressors identified by spouses in this study were (a) worries about treatment, recovery, and prognosis; (b) moodiness of the client; (c) worries about the client returning to work and about money; (d) sexual concerns; and (e) helplessness or apathy on the part of the client and increased spousal responsibility.

Evidence-Based Practice

- Spouses of clients in cardiac rehabilitation could benefit from the following:
  - Stress-management techniques, such as relaxation training, assertiveness training, and self-care techniques
  - Training in problem-solving and cognitive-based coping strategies
  - Support groups for spouses
- Younger women need to be especially identified for supportive interventions when their husbands are in cardiac rehabilitation

Reference

O'Farrell, P., Murray, J., & Hotz, S. B. (2000). Psychologic distress among spouses of patients undergoing cardiac rehabilitation. *Heart & Lung, 29*(2), 97–104.

although the source of stress may not necessarily be the caregiving, but other factors in the caregiver's life such as work or finances (Chiriboga 1992). Spouses and other family members also experience stress when a loved one is ill (Box 26-4).

Maturational Factors. Stressors vary with life stage. Preadolescents experience stress related to self-esteem issues, changing family structure due to divorce or death of a parent, or hospitalizations. As adolescents search for their identity with peer groups and separate from their families, they undergo stress. In addition, they face questions about using mind-altering substances, sexuality, jobs, school, and career choices that cause stress. Stress for adults centre around major changes in life circumstances (Aguilera, 1998). These changes include the many milestones of beginning a family and a career, losing parents, seeing children leave home, and accepting physical aging. In old age, stressors include the loss of autonomy and mastery due to general frailty or health problems that limit stamina and strength (Pearlin & Mullan, 1992; Box 26-5).

Socio-cultural Factors. Environmental and social stressors can lead to developmental problems. Potential stressors in any age group, but especially stressful for young people, include prolonged poverty and physical disability. Children are vulnerable when relationships with parents and caregivers are lost through divorce, imprisonment, or death or when parents have mental illness or substance abuse disorders. Furthermore, living under conditions of continuing violence, disintegrated neighbourhoods, or homelessness is damaging for people of any age, but especially for young people (Pender et al., 2002).

A person's cultural background also greatly influences the perception of and reaction to stress. A client's culture defines what is stressful to the person and ways of coping with stress (Aldwin, 2000). For example, cultural background may determine whether or not a person stoically accepts pain without complaint (Box 26-6).

Critical Thinking

When caring for a client experiencing stress, the nurse uses critical thinking skills to understand the stressor and the client's stress response. The nurse integrates knowledge from nursing and other disciplines, previous experiences, and information gathered from clients to understand stress and its impact on the client and family. The nurse must know the neurophysiological changes that occur with stages of the general adaptation syndrome. She or he must also be able to determine the client's perception of the situation and assess client behaviours and coping abilities. If the client's usual coping skills are unsuccessful or support systems are inadequate, the nurse

Focus on Older Adults

Box 26-5

- There are very few age-related differences in coping strategies, and older adults are just as effective at coping as younger adults (Aldwin, 1992).
- Older adults are incorrectly presumed to be unique and more vulnerable to the effect of stressors; however, the effect of psychosocial factors on health status is not altered by age (Kasl, 1992).
- Losses in later life may be less stress provoking than generally assumed, partly because certain life transitions are anticipated and people prepare by coping in advance (Pearlin & Mullan, 1992).
- A study of stress and coping in old-old clients (ages 75 to 91 years) found them to be least likely to view their lives as having problems, and they expended less effort in coping (Aldwin et al., 1996). This may be because the life experiences and perspectives of older adults may make most problems seem insignificant, older adults have acquired appropriate stress management techniques, or both.
- The timing of stress-inducing events can significantly influence older adults' ability to cope. Many older adults experience several stressful events (e.g., loss of a spouse and new medical diagnosis) within a brief time frame, which may result in reduced coping ability.
- In people 85 years and older, there is a clear connection among age, loss, and stress (Pearlin & Mullan, 1992). Stresses in this age group are related to confronting one's own diminished autonomy and mastery (Pearlin & Mullan, 1992).
- Older adults effectively use religious coping in response to medical illness and disasters (Foster, 1997).
- Anxiety disorders are the most prevalent disorders in later life and are continuations of lifelong illnesses (Hyer & Sohnle, 2001).

will need to use crisis intervention counselling (see Crisis Intervention).

With experience, the nurse learns to understand the client's unique perspective and to recognize responses to stress. In addition, personal experiences with stress and coping help the nurse to empathize with clients who are experiencing stress.

The nurse should be confident in the belief that stress can be effectively managed by the nurse, if necessary, and by the client. Clients who are overwhelmed and perceive events as being beyond their capacity to cope will rely on the nurse as an expert and may require either direct intervention or guidance. Through a nurse's expert advice and counsel, many clients gain confidence in their ability to move past the stressful event or illness. The nurse must always respect the client's perception of or perspective about the stressor. Effort must be made to have clients explain their unique viewpoint and situation. Standards of practice can help a nurse make an accurate assessment of a client's stress, coping mechanisms, and support system before intervening.

Nursing Process

NP Assessment

When assessing a client's stress level and coping resources, the nurse must ask the client to share personal and sensitive information. Therefore, the nurse must first establish a trusting nurse-client relationship. By asking questions, listening carefully, observing non-verbal behaviour and the client's environment, the nurse learns about the client's stress. The nurse uses critical thinking skills to synthesize and analyze information

Cultural Aspects of Care

Box 26-6

Cultural context shapes the types of environmental stimuli that produce stress. For example, diverse cultures address developmental transitions and life's turning points differently. How a person leaves the parental home, experiences health crises or chronic illness, cares for the family, or becomes disabled or dependent are all culturally bound. Furthermore, how a person appraises stress is also dependent upon the person's culture. What is perceived as a stressor in one culture might be viewed as a minor problem in another. Coping strategies are also influenced by culture. According to Aldwin, cultures vary in their emotion-focused and problem-focused coping strategies. Some cultures stress that emotions should be controlled, others that they should be expressed. Problem-focused coping refers to controlling or managing stress. Different cultures control stress in different ways. Finally, cultures provide different institutions for coping with stress. These include the legal system for conflict resolution, advice givers or support groups, and rituals.

Implications for Practice

- Realize that stressors and coping styles vary with different cultures.
- Use introspection to examine one's own perceptions of stress and coping in a cultural context.
- Assess the influence of culture on a client's appraisal of stress.
- Determine the institutions within a client's culture that may facilitate coping.

From *Stress, Coping and Development: An Integrative Perspective,* by C. M. Aldwin, 2000, New York: Guilford Press.

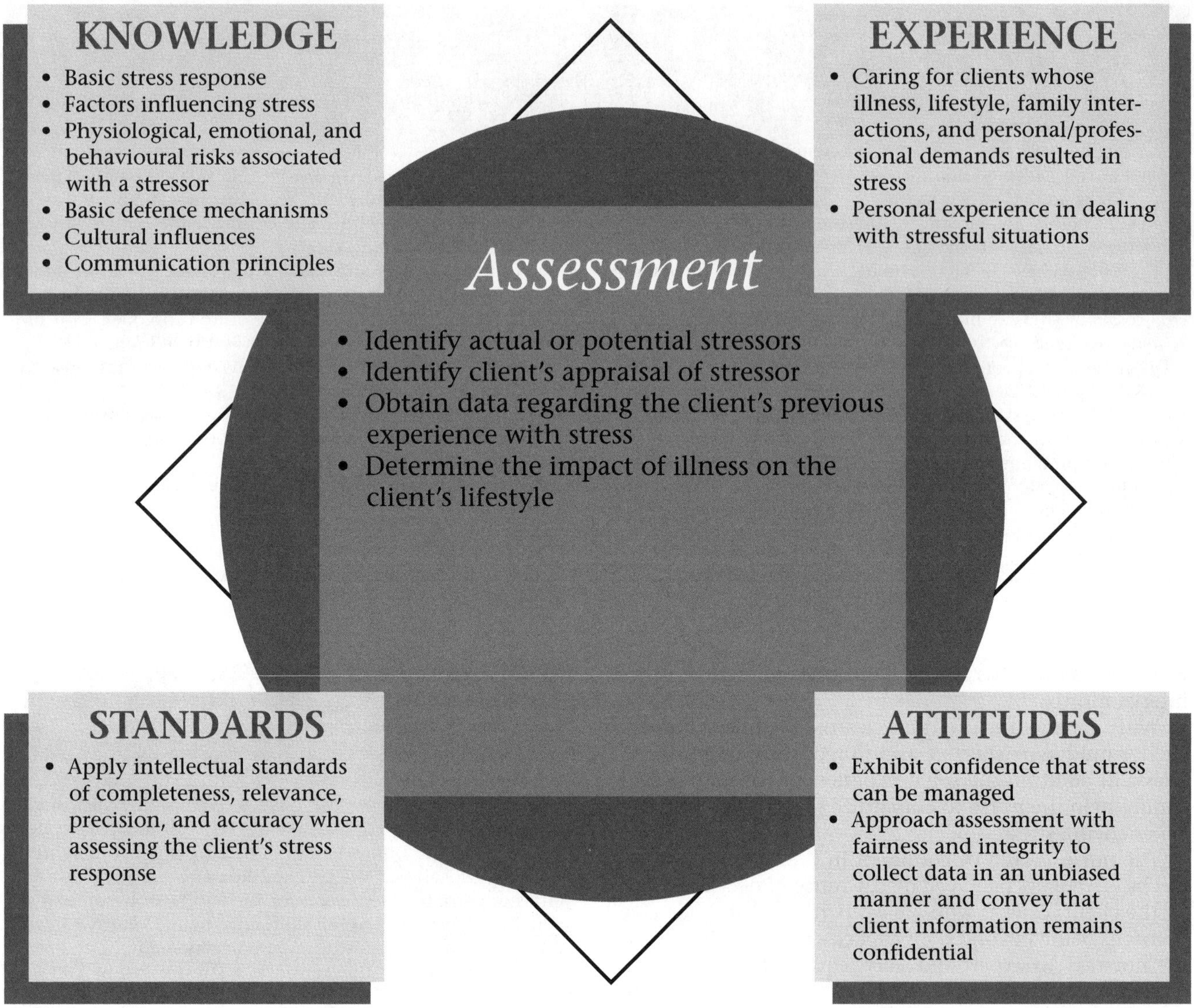
KNOWLEDGE
• Basic stress response
• Factors influencing stress
• Physiological, emotional, and behavioural risks associated with a stressor
• Basic defence mechanisms
• Cultural influences
• Communication principles
EXPERIENCE
• Caring for clients whose illness, lifestyle, family interactions, and personal/professional demands resulted in stress
• Personal experience in dealing with stressful situations
Assessment
• Identify actual or potential stressors
• Identify client's appraisal of stressor
• Obtain data regarding the client's previous experience with stress
• Determine the impact of illness on the client's lifestyle
STANDARDS
• Apply intellectual standards of completeness, relevance, precision, and accuracy when assessing the client's stress response
ATTITUDES
• Exhibit confidence that stress can be managed
• Approach assessment with fairness and integrity to collect data in an unbiased manner and convey that client information remains confidential

FIGURE **26–3** Critical thinking model for stress and coping assessment.

(Figure 26–3). Often clients have difficulty expressing what is troubling them until they have the opportunity to talk with someone who has time to listen.

Stress can affect an individual, family, or community. Stress in a family might be from critical illness, job loss, or a move. Stress in a community might be a natural disaster such as a major flood or the unexpected death of a beloved teacher or teenager.

Subjective Findings. When assessing a client's level of stress and coping resources, the nurse arranges a non-threatening physical environment, without a desk as a barrier, for the interaction (Varcarolis, 2002). The nurse assumes the same height as the client, arranging the interview environment so that eye contact can be comfortably maintained or avoided. This can be accomplished by placing chairs at a 90-degree angle or side by side to reduce the intensity of the interaction (Varcarolis, 2002). The nurse gathers information about the health status of the client from the client's perspective and begins the process of developing a trusting relationship with the client. The nurse uses the interview to determine the client's view of the stress, coping resources, any possible maladaptive coping, and adherence to prescribed medical recommendations, such as medication or diet (Monat & Lazarus, 1991; Table 26-1). If the client is using denial as a coping mechanism, the nurse must be alert to whether the person is overlooking necessary information. As in all interactions with the client, the nurse must respect the confidentiality and sensitivity of the information shared.

Objective Findings. The nurse obtains objective findings about stress and coping by observing the client's appearance and non-verbal behaviour during the interview, including grooming and hygiene, handshake and gait, body language, speech quality, eye contact, and attitude. Before or at the end of the interview, depending upon the client's

Table 26-1 Focused Assessment Interview

Factors to Assess	Questions and Approaches	Physical Assessment Strategies
Perception of stressor	Ask the client what is of most concern at this time. Ask the client about problems sleeping, eating, working, and concentrating. Ask whether the client has had accidents in the home, in the car, or on the job.	Observe non-verbal behaviour and expressions of feelings that indicate anxiety, fear, anger, irritability, or tension.
Available coping resources	Ask the client about current friendships and contacts with family members. Ask what the client has done in the past to cope with similar problems or stress. Ask how the client spends leisure time.	Observe whether the person is alone or with others. Observe grooming and hygiene. Observe the person's communication skills. Observe if the person is able to ask for help. Observe developmental level and socio-cultural circumstances.
Maladaptive coping used	Ask about use of tobacco, alcohol, drugs, medications, and caffeine.	Observe for effects of smoking, alcohol, drugs, and caffeine.
Adherence to healthy practices	Ask if the client sees a physician or nurse practitioner regularly for checkups. Ask about nutritional habits, exercise, use of seat belts, helmets (if applicable), and safer sex.	Monitor pulse, blood pressure, weight. Observe non-verbal behaviour.

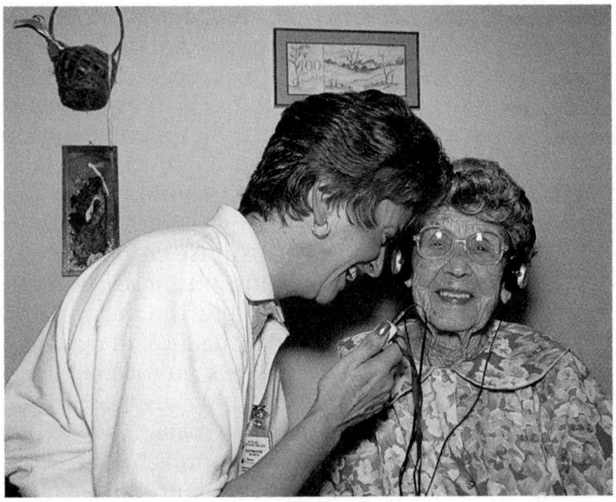

FIGURE 26–4 Sharing a joke or laughing with clients can reduce stress and support a therapeutic relationship.

anxiety level, the nurse takes basic vital signs to assess for physiological signs of stress such as elevated blood pressure, heart rate, or respiratory rate (Figure 26–4).

> ***Safety Alert.*** Medical conditions such as hypoxia and thyroid dysfunction that are common in older adults can initially present symptoms that mimic the consequences of stress and anxiety. For this reason, a thorough physical assessment of an older adult appearing stressed or anxious is necessary to rule out potentially serious medical disorders. In addition, it is critical to differentiate signs of stress and crisis in older adults from dementia and from acute confusion, a condition that can be life threatening.

Client Expectations. It is crucial that the nurse understands the meaning of the precipitating event to the client and how stress is affecting the client's life. The nurse must allow the client time to express priorities for coping. For example, if a woman has just been told that a breast mass was identified on a routine mammogram, the nurse must discern what the client wants and needs most from the nurse. Some clients identify an immediate need for information about biopsy or mastectomy; others need guidance and support on how to share the news with family members. In some cases, when nothing can be done to change or improve the situation, allowing the client to use denial as a coping mechanism can be helpful. Gaining an understanding of client expectations does not mean excluding important aspects of care simply because a client does not identify them as needs. However, by inquiring about client expectations and priorities, the nurse will be better able to ensure that *all* of the client's needs will be addressed in some way.

ND Nursing Diagnosis

The nurse clusters data that indicate a potential or actual stressor and the client's response. Keeping in mind previous knowledge and experiences with clients under stress, the nurse then makes individualized nursing diagnoses (Box 26-7).

Nursing diagnoses for people experiencing stress generally focus on coping. Major defining characteristics of *ineffective coping* include verbalization of an inability to cope and an inability to ask for help. The nurse identifies defining characteristics by asking clients what currently concerns them most and allowing them sufficient time to answer. The nurse observes for non-verbal signs of anxiety,

Nursing Diagnostic Process — Box 26-7

Assessment Activities	Defining Characteristics	Nursing Diagnosis
Ask client about change in sleeping patterns.	Sleep disturbance; difficulty falling asleep at night	Ineffective coping
	Sighing	
Ask client to complete a sleep diary for 2 weeks.	Excessive sleeping	
Observe client's behaviour and response to questions during assessment.	Fatigue	
	Inability to concentrate	
	Inaccurate response to questions	
	Inappropriate laughing or crying	
Observe client's appearance.	Poor grooming	
	Self-harm	
Ask client about changes in eating patterns.	Weight gain or loss	
	Lack of interest in food	

fear, anger, irritability, and tension. Other defining characteristics include the presence of life stress, an inability to meet role expectations and basic needs, alteration in societal participation, self-destructive behaviour, change in usual communication patterns, high rate of accidents, excessive food intake, drinking, smoking, and sleep disturbances. The nurse identifies these behaviours as part of the subjective and objective data collection. Stress can result in multiple nursing diagnoses, such as the following:

- Anxiety
- Caregiver role strain
- Chronic pain
- Post-traumatic stress syndrome
- Powerlessness

Crises differ from stress in the degree of severity, although there are many similarities between stress and crises. A client who perceives a situation as stressful, who is unable to cope in ways that have worked before, and who has insufficient supports is experiencing a crisis. A crisis is devastating and requires use of all resources available (Aguilera, 1998). Unlike stress, which ends when the stressor is gone, the effects of a trauma can last for years (Hyer & Sohnle, 2001).

Planning

Goals and Outcomes. Desirable outcomes for people experiencing stress are (a) effective coping, (b) family coping, (c) caregiver emotional health, and (d) psychosocial adjustment: life change (Moorhead, Johnson, & Maas, 2004). The nurse may select interventions for stress and improved coping such as coping enhancement or crisis intervention, which are in the *Nursing Interventions Classification (NIC)* (Dochterman & Bulechek, 2004). In addition, the nurse selects individualized interventions after considering the nursing diagnosis, the resources available to the client, and the goals identified by the client and nurse (Figure 26–5).

Nursing interventions may be designed within the framework of primary, secondary, and tertiary prevention. At the primary level of prevention, nursing activities are directed to identifying individuals and populations who may be at risk for stress (Stuart & Wright, 1995). Nursing interventions at the secondary level include actions directed at symptoms, such as protecting the client from self-harm. Tertiary-level interventions assist the client in readapting and might include relaxation training and time management training (see Care Plan). Another method of planning care involves using a concept map (Figure 26–6). The nurse creates the map after identifying relevant nursing diagnoses from the assessment database. In this example, the nursing diagnoses are linked to the client's medical diagnosis of post-traumatic stress response. The concept map shows the relationships with the nursing diagnoses: *post-traumatic stress syndrome, ineffective coping, anxiety,* and *risk for other directed violence.* This approach uses critical thinking skills to organize client data and plan for client-centred care.

Just as the nursing assessment of stress and coping depends on the client's perception of the problem and coping resources, the interventions focus on a partnership with the client and support system, usually the family. In the case of a family or community stressor and impaired family or community coping, the view of the situation and resources is broader.

Setting Priorities. When prioritizing needs for a person experiencing stress or a crisis, the first question to be answered is, "What is happening in your life that you needed to come today?" or "What happened in your life that is *different?*" This question requires the client to focus. The nurse should then assess the client's perception of the event, situational supports, and what the client usually does when faced with a problem (Aguilera, 1998). As in all areas of nursing, safety of the client and family is the first priority.

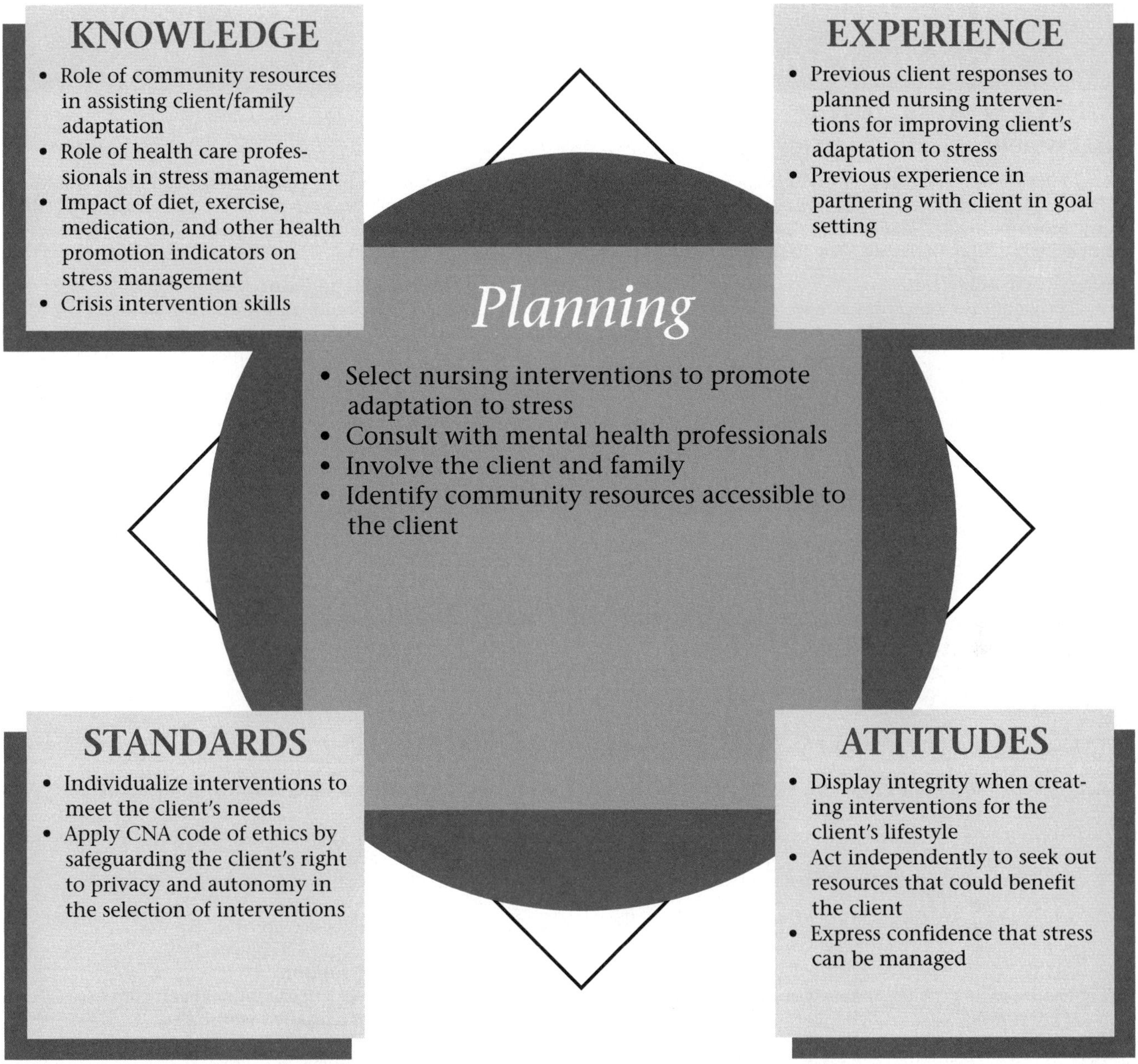
KNOWLEDGE
• Role of community resources in assisting client/family adaptation
• Role of health care professionals in stress management
• Impact of diet, exercise, medication, and other health promotion indicators on stress management
• Crisis intervention skills
EXPERIENCE
• Previous client responses to planned nursing interventions for improving client's adaptation to stress
• Previous experience in partnering with client in goal setting
Planning
• Select nursing interventions to promote adaptation to stress
• Consult with mental health professionals
• Involve the client and family
• Identify community resources accessible to the client
STANDARDS
• Individualize interventions to meet the client's needs
• Apply CNA code of ethics by safeguarding the client's right to privacy and autonomy in the selection of interventions
ATTITUDES
• Display integrity when creating interventions for the client's lifestyle
• Act independently to seek out resources that could benefit the client
• Express confidence that stress can be managed

FIGURE **26–5** Critical thinking model for stress and coping planning.

Safety Alert. Direct questions help to determine if the person is suicidal or homicidal. The nurse might ask, "Are you thinking of killing yourself or someone else?" If so, the nurse should calmly determine if the person has a plan and determine how lethal the means are. If suicide or homicide is not an issue, the nurse should consider other threats to the safety of people who are under client's care and provide for their temporary care or supervision if necessary. When immediate assessment is completed and safety is ensured, the problem-solving process should begin (Aguilera, 1998).

Continuity of Care. There are times when the scope of nursing practice is insufficient to meet all of the client's needs. Clients experiencing stress from medical conditions or psychiatric disorders present needs that require the nurse to consult with advanced practice mental health nurses, psychiatrists, psychologists, psychiatric social workers, or others. Such a multidisciplinary approach to care is often most effective in addressing the holistic needs of the client and should be included in the planning of care. The nurse's role is to recognize the need for collaboration and consultation, inform the client about potential resources, and make arrangements for interventions, such as consultations, group sessions, or therapy as needed.

Nursing Care Plan

Caregiver Role Strain

Assessment

When Maya Bhatt, RN, first goes to Carl's house, she finds the home to be in slight disarray. The lawn is overgrown, there are dirty dishes in the sink, and an empty can of soup is sitting on the kitchen counter. Carl is standing in the living room folding clothes from a laundry basket, and Evelyn, Carl's wife, is sitting in a chair watching TV. Evelyn was recently diagnosed with Alzheimer's disease.

Assessment Activities	Findings/Defining Characteristics
Ask Carl about his recent stressors and coping strategies.	He continues to fold clothes during the visit, stating, "There's so much to do that I don't even know where to begin." Carl describes being awakened 3 to 4 times per night to find Evelyn wandering in the house. He states that he has no outside activities and his children live in other provinces. He does have several close friends who live nearby but does not know of community resources.
Observe Carl's grooming and hygiene.	Carl is unshaven and appears dishevelled.
Ask Carl about his sleep and nutrition patterns.	Carl states that he has lost 9 kg in the past 6 months and that his appetite has been poor.
Assess Carl's mood and affect by asking how he is feeling.	Carl states, "I feel very tired. Everything feels overwhelming."
Assess Carl's suicide potential.	Carl denies being suicidal.
Assess health status and health care status.	Carl has not seen a nurse practitioner or physician for his own health in over a year.

Nursing Diagnosis: Caregiver role strain related to recent diagnosis of wife's Alzheimer's disease.

Planning

Goal	Expected Outcomes*
	Caregiver Physical Health
Client will appear rested in 1 month.	• Client will report waking up less frequently during the night within 1 week. • Client will verbalize approaches used to involve others in wife's caregiving activities within 2 weeks.
Client will maintain a stable weight over next 4 weeks.	• Client will re-establish normal eating pattern within 1 week. • Client will report improved appetite.
	Caregiver Lifestyle Disruption
Client will state that he has resumed one outside activity within 1 month.	• Client will report a balanced routine that incorporates time for own rest or relaxation with 1 week.

*Outcome classification labels from *Nursing Outcomes Classification (NOC)* (3rd ed.), edited by S. Moorhead, M. Johnson, and M. L. Maas, 2004, St. Louis, MO: Mosby.

Interventions†	Rationale
Caregiver Support	
• Assist client in establishing a consistent care routine.	Routines can help tasks be simplified and more time efficient.
• Discuss ways that client agrees will simplify care routine such as hiring a teenage neighbour to mow the lawn, buying frozen meals, having groceries delivered, having a cleaning service twice a month.	Caregivers experience stress outside of their caregiving roles. Frequently, providing ways to assist the caregiver with home maintenance, meal planning, and shopping assists caregivers with stress management.
• Identify sources of respite care by encouraging client to identify available friends who can assist with caregiving.	Successful caregiving cannot normally occur with only one caregiver. Caregiver may be hesitant to ask for help because of past family conflict (Gulanick, Klopp, & Galanes, 2003).
• Explore community resources such as home care, adult day care, and Meals on Wheels with client.	Feelings of burden have been found to be lower among caregivers with social supports (Solomon & Draine, 1995).
• Teach client stress-management techniques.	Stress, especially long-term stress, can precipitate physical illness.
• Set up monthly health checks for client that include vital sign and weight checks.	Teaching the caregiver health maintenance strategies is important to sustain his own physical and mental health (Dochterman & Bulechek, 2004).

†Intervention classification labels from *Nursing Interventions Classification (NIC)* (4th ed.), edited by J. M. Dochterman and G. M. Bulechek, 2004, St. Louis, MO: Mosby.

Continued

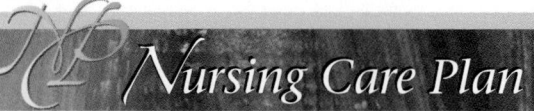

Nursing Care Plan

Caregiver Role Strain—cont'd

Evaluation

Nursing Actions	Client Response/Finding	Achievement of Outcome
Observe for signs of fatigue.	Carl states he feels more rested and less depressed.	Carl is able to sleep for 6 hours during night and takes a 30-minute nap in the afternoon.
Review new care routines. Ask client what other modifications may need to be made.	Carl buys frozen meals to use when he is busy with other caregiving.	Carl has reduced his personal expectation that he must cook every meal himself.
Ask client about how community and additional family support is helping to relieve stress.	Meals on Wheels delivers lunch 5 days per week. A neighbour mows the lawn for Carl.	Carl is mobilizing community resources.
Ask client to compare past and present energy levels.	Carl reports having more energy and smiles spontaneously.	Carl has improved balance in routine between Evelyn's and his own.
Weigh client regularly.	Carl reports gaining 2 kg in 1 month.	Carl has resumed a normal eating pattern.
Ask client about recent food intake.	Carl reports having eaten lunch with Evelyn on the day of the visit.	

Concept Map

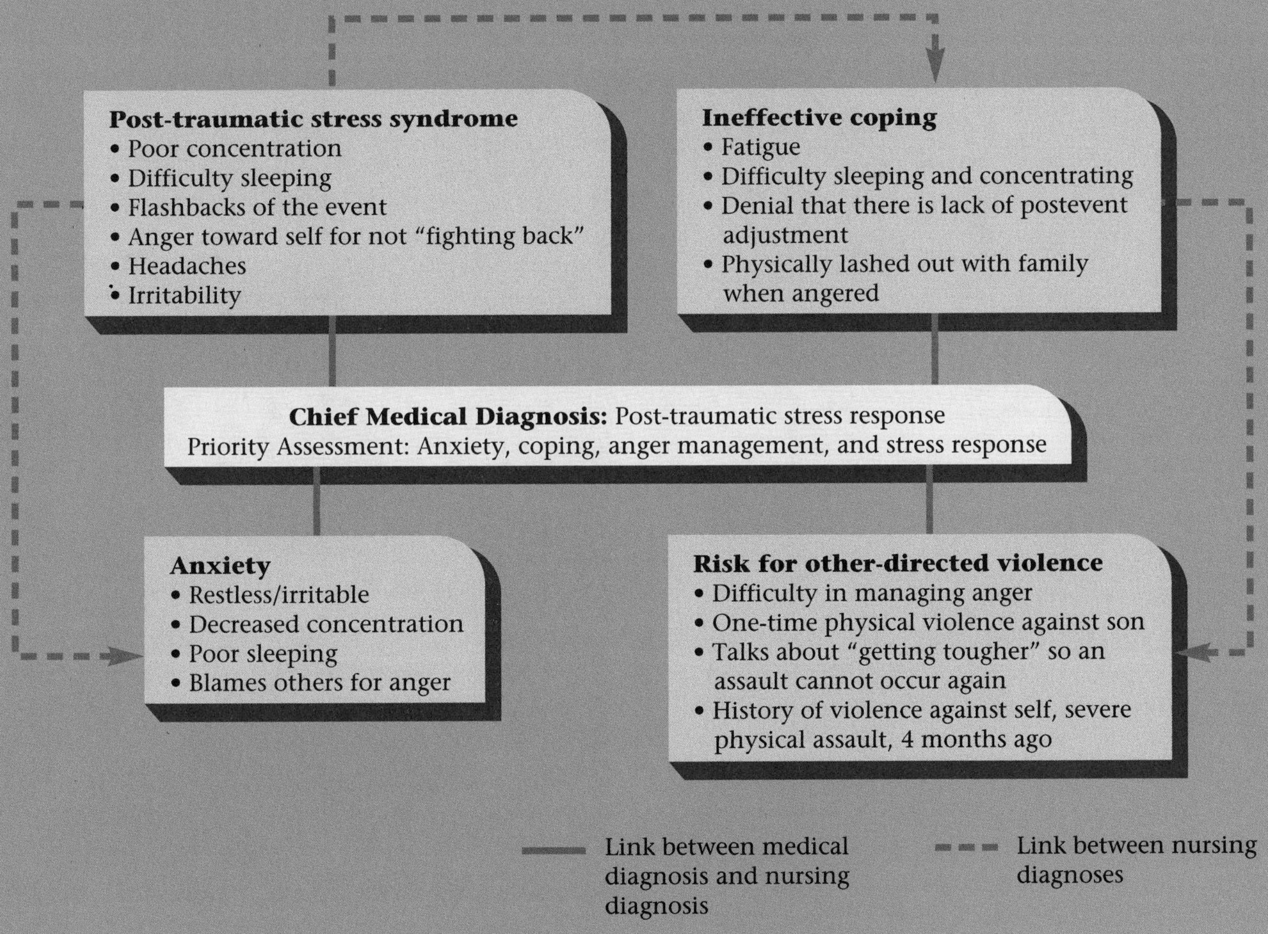
Post-traumatic stress syndrome
• Poor concentration
• Difficulty sleeping
• Flashbacks of the event
• Anger toward self for not "fighting back"
• Headaches
• Irritability
Ineffective coping
• Fatigue
• Difficulty sleeping and concentrating
• Denial that there is lack of postevent adjustment
• Physically lashed out with family when angered
Chief Medical Diagnosis: Post-traumatic stress response
Priority Assessment: Anxiety, coping, anger management, and stress response
Anxiety
• Restless/irritable
• Decreased concentration
• Poor sleeping
• Blames others for anger
Risk for other-directed violence
• Difficulty in managing anger
• One-time physical violence against son
• Talks about "getting tougher" so an assault cannot occur again
• History of violence against self, severe physical assault, 4 months ago
Link between medical diagnosis and nursing diagnosis
Link between nursing diagnoses

FIGURE 26–6 Concept map for client with post-traumatic stress response 4 months after a severe assault.

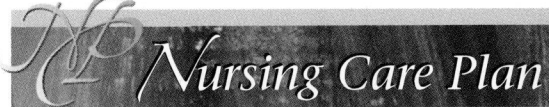

NP Implementation

Health Promotion. Three primary modes of intervention for stress are to decrease stress-producing situations, increase resistance to stress, and learn skills that reduce physiological response to stress (Pender et al., 2002). The nurse is in a position to educate clients and families about the importance of health promotion (Box 26-8; Box 26-9). Several strategies help increase resistance to stress and reduce response to stress.

Focus on Primary Health Care — Box 26-8

Nurses address their client's stress or potential stress in many different primary health care situations. They consider the stress in the lives of communities, families, and individuals. In a community setting, a nurse might instruct a group of teenage mothers on how to care for their newborns and themselves. The goal of the instruction is to improve the health and safety of the babies and to prevent stress, health breakdown, and crises in the lives of these vulnerable women. In a home setting, a nurse might help the family of a woman who has cancer to recognize and deal with symptoms of stress in their lives. In an interview at a community clinic, a nurse might assess the stress in the life of a client with sleep problems and plan interventions to help the client sleep.

Client Teaching — Box 26-9

Stress Management Strategies

Objective

- Coping with daily hassles in the workplace will improve.

Teaching Strategies

- Assist the client in analyzing new job possibilities if necessary.
- Instruct the client to avoid excessive change in lifestyle when other stress is present.
- Instruct the client in time management skills to become more organized and set priorities.
- Assist the client in creating a daily exercise plan.
- Assist the client in developing a well-balanced diet that avoids excessive caffeine intake (i.e., coffee, tea, chocolate).
- Assist the client in building a network of social support.
- Train the client in progressive muscle relaxation or other relaxation techniques.

Evaluation

- Observe client for signs of stress.
- Ask client to keep a record of hours of sleep.
- Ask client to list participation in activities that are soothing or enjoyable.

Data from *Health Promotion in Nursing Practice* (4th ed.), by N. J. Pender, C. Murdaugh, and M. A. Parsons, 2002, Upper Saddle River, NJ: Howorth Press.

Regular Exercise. A regular exercise program improves muscle tone and posture, controls weight, reduces tension, and promotes relaxation. In addition, exercise reduces the risk of cardiovascular disease and improves cardiopulmonary functioning. Clients who have a history of a chronic illness, who are at risk for developing an illness, or who are older than 35 years of age should begin a physical exercise program only after discussing the plan with a physician. In general, for a fitness program to have positive physical effects, a person should exercise daily for an hour (Figure 26–7).

Support Systems. A support system of family, friends, and colleagues who listen, offer advice, and provide emotional support benefits a client experiencing stress. There are many support groups available to individuals, such as those sponsored by the Heart and Stroke Foundation of Canada, the Canadian Cancer Society, local hospitals and churches, and mental health organizations.

Time Management. Time management techniques include developing lists of tasks to be performed in order of priority; for example, those tasks that require im-

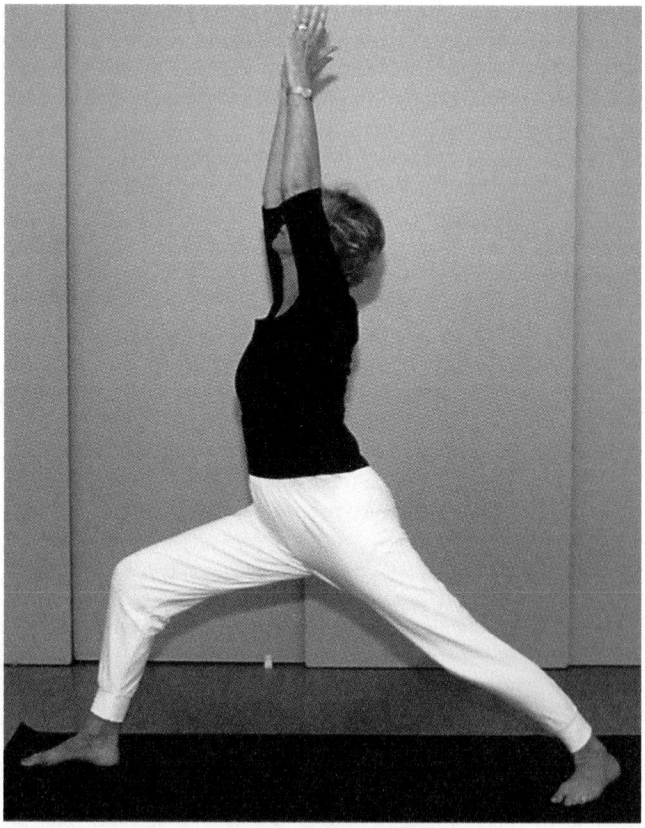

FIGURE **26–7** Regular exercise assists in coping with stress.

mediate attention, those that are important and can be delayed, and those tasks that are routine and can be accomplished when time becomes available. In many cases, setting priorities helps individuals identify tasks that are not necessary or perhaps can even be delegated to someone else.

Guided Imagery and Visualization. Guided imagery is based on the belief that a person can significantly reduce stress with imagination (see chapter 31). Guided imagery is a relaxed state in which a person actively uses imagination in a way that allows visualization of a soothing, peaceful setting. Typically the image created or suggested uses many sensory words to engage the mind and offer distraction and relaxation.

Progressive Muscle Relaxation. In the presence of anxiety-provoking thoughts and events, a common physiological symptom is muscle tension. Physiological tension will be diminished through a systematic approach to releasing tension in major muscle groups. Typically, a relaxed state is achieved through deep chest breathing, and then the client is directed to alternately tighten and relax muscles in specific groupings (see chapter 31).

Assertiveness Training. Assertiveness comprises skills for helping individuals communicate effectively regarding their needs and desires. The ability to resolve conflict with others through assertiveness training is important for reducing stress. When assertiveness is taught in a group setting, benefits of the experience are increased.

Journal Writing. For many people, keeping a private, personal journal provides a therapeutic outlet for stress, and it is well within the realm of nursing to suggest journal keeping to clients experiencing difficult situations. In a private journal, clients can express a full range of emotion and vent their honest feelings without hurting anyone's feelings and without concern for how they might appear to others.

Stress Management in the Nurse's Workplace. Rapid changes in health care technology, diversity in the workforce, organizational restructuring, and changing work systems can place stress on nurses (Bauman et al, 2001; Manning, Curtis, & McMillen, 1999). Additional causes of job stress include particular job assignments, difficult schedules, shift work, fear of failure, and inadequate support services (Manning et al., 1999). **Burnout** occurs as a result of chronic stress. Burnout is "a syndrome of emotional exhaustion, depersonalization of others, and perceptions of reduced personal accomplishment, resulting from intense involvement with people in a care-giving environment" (Aguilera, 1998).

If nurses recognize feelings of burnout, they can make changes in their behaviour to cope with workplace stress. An important step is identifying the limits and scope of responsibilities at work (Aguilera, 1998). Recognizing the areas over which one has control and can change and those that one does not have responsibility for is a vital insight. Making a clear separation between work and home life is crucial as well. Strengthening friendships outside of the workplace, arranging for temporary social isolation for personal "recharging" of emotional energy, and spending off-duty hours in interesting activities all help reduce burnout.

Acute Care

Crisis Intervention. When stress overwhelms a person's usual coping mechanisms and demands mobilization of all available resources, it becomes a crisis (Aguilera, 1998). A crisis creates a turning point in a person's life because it changes the direction of a person's life in some way. According to Aguilera (1998), the precipitating event usually occurs from 1 to 2 weeks before the individual seeks help, but it may have occurred within the past 24 hours. Generally, a crisis is resolved in some way within approximately 6 weeks. Crisis intervention aims to return the person to a pre-crisis level of functioning and to promote growth (Figure 26–8).

Because usual coping strategies are ineffective in managing the stress of the precipitating event, the person or family must use new coping mechanisms to manage a crisis. The use of unfamiliar strategies can result either in a heightened awareness of previously unrecognized strengths and resources or in deterioration in functioning. Thus, a crisis is often referred to as a situation of both danger and opportunity. Some people or families emerge from a crisis state functioning more effectively, whereas others are weakened, and still others completely dysfunctional.

Crisis intervention is a specific type of brief psychotherapy with prescribed steps (Aguilera, 1998). Crisis intervention is more directive than traditional psychotherapy or counselling and can be used by any member of the health care team who has been trained in its techniques. The basic approach is problem solving and focuses only on the problem presented by the crisis.

When using a crisis intervention approach, the nurse helps the client make the mental connection between the stressful event and the client's reaction to it. This is crucial because the person may be unable to see the whole situation clearly. The nurse also helps the person become aware of present feelings, such as anger, grief, or guilt, to help the individual reduce tension. In addition, the nurse helps the client explore coping mechanisms, perhaps identifying ways of coping that the client had not thought of. Finally, the nurse may help increase the person's social contacts if the person has been internally focused and isolated (Aguilera, 1998).

Restorative and Continuing Care. A person under stress recovers when the stress is removed or coping strategies are successful; however, a person who has experienced a crisis has changed, and the effects may last for years or for the rest of the person's life (Shontz, 1975). The final stage of adapting to a crisis is acknowledgement of the long-term implications of the crisis (Shontz, 1975). If a person has successfully coped with a crisis and its consequences, he or she becomes a more mature and healthy person. When a person has recovered from a stressful situation, the time is right for introducing stress management skills

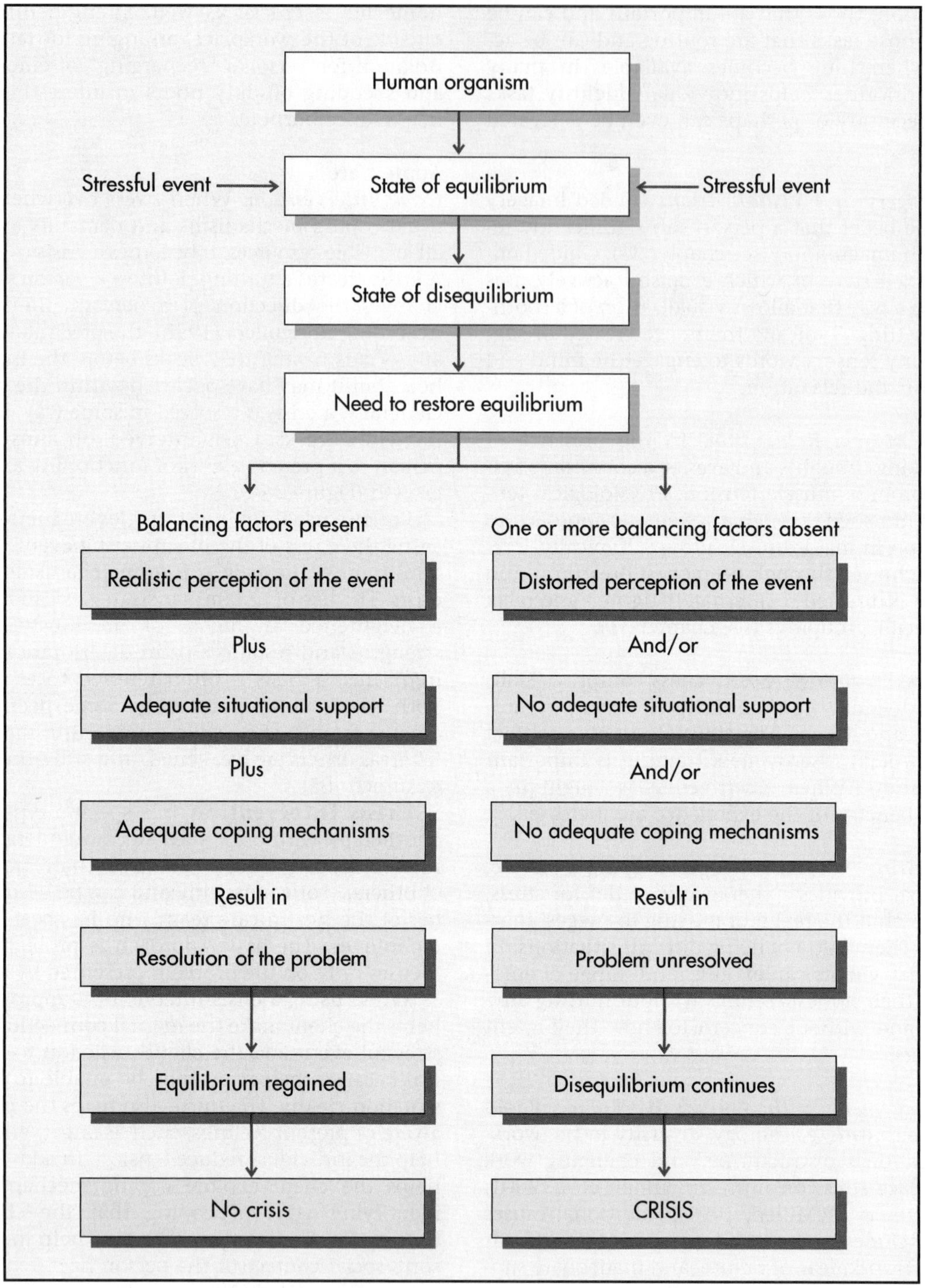

FIGURE **26–8** Crisis intervention model. (Redrawn from *Crisis Intervention: Theory and Methodology,* 8th ed., by D. C. Aguilera, 1998, St. Louis, MO: Mosby.)

to reduce the number and intensity of stressful situations in the future.

Evaluation

Client Care. By evaluating the goals and expected outcomes of care, the nurse knows if the nursing interventions were effective and if the client is coping with the identified stress. The nurse reviews the measurable goals and assesses whether or not the client has met the criteria for success as stated in the outcomes. If the nursing interventions have not been effective in helping the client achieve targeted goals, the nurse must re-evaluate the strategies implemented and revise the care plan in light of the client's current health status (Figure 26–9).

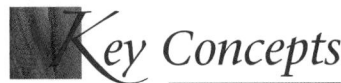

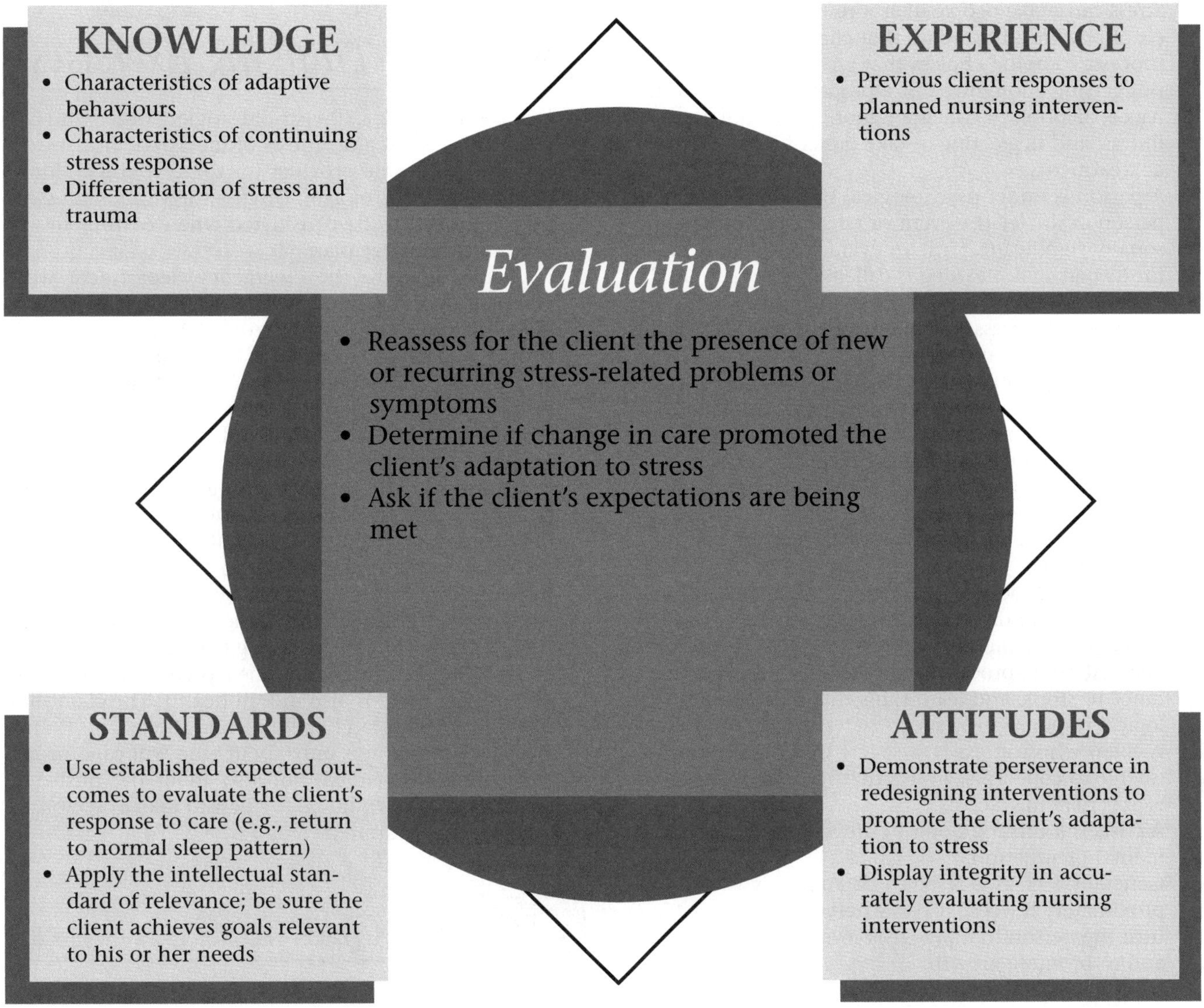
KNOWLEDGE
• Characteristics of adaptive behaviours
• Characteristics of continuing stress response
• Differentiation of stress and trauma
EXPERIENCE
• Previous client responses to planned nursing interventions
Evaluation
• Reassess for the client the presence of new or recurring stress-related problems or symptoms
• Determine if change in care promoted the client's adaptation to stress
• Ask if the client's expectations are being met
STANDARDS
• Use established expected outcomes to evaluate the client's response to care (e.g., return to normal sleep pattern)
• Apply the intellectual standard of relevance; be sure the client achieves goals relevant to his or her needs
ATTITUDES
• Demonstrate perseverance in redesigning interventions to promote the client's adaptation to stress
• Display integrity in accurately evaluating nursing interventions

FIGURE **26–9** Critical thinking model for stress and coping evaluation.

To evaluate whether goals and outcomes of care have been achieved, the nurse observes client behaviours and talks with the client and family, if appropriate. If contact with a client ends before goals have been achieved, the client should be referred to appropriate resources so that progress is not delayed or interrupted.

Client Expectations. It is crucial to maintain ongoing communication with clients regarding the care plan. Clients under severe stress or trauma often feel powerless and vulnerable. The nurse can help to reduce these feelings by actively involving clients and families in assessment, prioritizing, goal setting, and evaluation. Involving clients enables them to direct their energy positively and encourages them to take responsibility for their health. It also sets the stage for open communication, which makes it easier for the client to report on interventions that are successful and helps the nurse better understand why some interventions fail to meet their goals.

An essential part of the evaluation process is collaborating with clients to determine if their own expectations from nursing have been met. Revisions to the care plan must then include steps to address client expectations.

Key Concepts

- The general adaptation syndrome is an immediate physiological response of the whole body to stress and involves several body systems, especially the autonomic nervous system and the endocrine system. Physiological responses to stress also include immunological changes.

- Stress can make people ill as a result of increased levels of powerful hormones that change our bodily processes; coping choices that are unhealthy, such as not getting enough rest or a proper diet or use of tobacco, alcohol, or caffeine; ignoring warning signs of illness; and neglecting to take prescribed medicines or treatments.
- A person is under psychological stress only if the person evaluates the event or circumstance as personally significant. Such an evaluation of an event for its personal meaning is called primary appraisal.
- There are several types of stress, including work stress, family stress, chronic stress, acute stress, daily hassles, trauma, and crisis.
- Rapid changes in health care technology, diversity in the workforce, organizational redesign, and changing work systems can place stress on nurses.
- Potential stressors and coping mechanisms vary across the lifespan, from childhood through adolescence, adulthood, and old age.
- Coping means making an effort to manage psychological stress.
- Coping is a process that is constantly changing to manage demands on a person's resources.
- Three primary modes for stress intervention are to decrease stress-producing situations, increase resistance to stress, and learn skills that reduce physiological response to stress.
- A client whose stress is so severe that the person is unable to cope in any ways that have worked before is experiencing a crisis.
- A crisis is a turning point in life and can be developmental or situational.
- Generally a crisis is resolved in some way within approximately 6 weeks. Crisis intervention aims to return the person to a pre-crisis level of functioning and to promote growth.

Key Terms

Critical Thinking Exercises

1. You are caring for a 30-year-old single mother who has recently received a diagnosis of metastatic breast cancer. She is the sole provider for three young children (all under 7 years of age). Discuss the various stressors that will need to be considered when writing an appropriate discharge plan.
2. A client comes to the emergency department with complaints of dizziness, which are not related to any physical finding on examination. During the health history, the client reports that her life is very stressful and she is barely coping. She finalized her divorce 3 months ago, is working 32 hours per week, and is attending college. Her ex-husband recently lost his job and can no longer pay child support. She tearfully confesses that she thinks she might be pregnant but does not want her ex-husband to know. Develop nursing diagnoses related to this situation.
3. An older woman is admitted to the hospital with a fractured hip. Before her injury, she lived with her husband, who has advancing Alzheimer's disease. While she is hospitalized, he is staying with a niece who lives 50 km away, but this cannot be a permanent situation because her niece is also in frail health. The client has no children who can help her when she returns home. She is concerned not only about who will care for her after she is discharged, but also about her husband. What approach would be the best to take in establishing goals for treatment?

Review Questions

1. The vital functions necessary for survival, which include heart rate, blood pressure, and respiration, are controlled by the
   1. Medulla oblongata
   2. Reticular formation
   3. Pituitary gland
   4. Limbic system
2. While assessing a person for effects of the general adaptation syndrome, the nurse should be aware that
   1. Heart rate increases in the adaptation state
   2. Blood volume increases in the exhaustion stage
   3. Vital signs return to normal in the exhaustion stage
   4. Blood glucose level increases during the alarm reaction stage
3. A client avoids emotional conflict by refusing to consciously acknowledge anything that might cause intolerable emotional pain. The client is using the defence mechanism
   1. Conversion
   2. Denial
   3. Dissociation
   4. Displacement

4. When doing an assessment of a young woman who was in an automobile accident 6 months before, the nurse learns that the woman has vivid images of the crash whenever she hears a loud, sudden noise. The nurse recognizes this as
   1. Social phobia
   2. Acute anxiety
   3. Post-traumatic stress disorder
   4. Borderline personality disorder
5. A man is adjusting to a chronic illness; the chronic illness can be considered a(n)
   1. Socio-cultural stress
   2. Maturational stress
   3. Situational stress
   4. Environmental stress
6. A child who has been in a house fire comes to the emergency department with her parents. The child and parents are upset and tearful. During the nurse's first assessment for stress, the nurse should say,
   1. "Tell me whom I can call to help you."
   2. "Tell me what upsets you the most about this experience."
   3. "I will contact someone who can help get you temporary housing."
   4. "I will sit with you until other family members can come help you get settled."
7. The nurse is evaluating the coping success of a client experiencing stress from being newly diagnosed with multiple sclerosis and psychomotor impairment. The nurse realized that the client is coping successfully when the client says,
   1. "I am going to learn to drive a car so I can be more independent."
   2. "My sister says she feels better when she goes shopping, so I will go shopping."
   3. "I have always felt better when I go for a long walk. I will do that when I get home."
   4. "I am going to attend a support group to learn more about multiple sclerosis and what I will be able to do."
8. The nurse knows that the client is recovering from the stress of an emergency surgery when the client says,
   1. "I am going to change jobs."
   2. "I am learning progressive relaxation training."
   3. "I plan to have plastic surgery while I am here in the hospital."
   4. "I am planning to sell my house and move within the next 6 weeks."
9. A staff nurse is talking with her nursing supervisor about the stress she feels on the job. The supervising nurse recognizes that
   1. Nurses who feel stress usually pass the stress along to their clients
   2. A nurse who feels stress is ineffective as a nurse and should not be working
   3. Nurses who talk about feeling stress are unprofessional and should calm down
   4. Nurses frequently experience stress with the rapid changes in health care technology and organizational restructuring
10. Generally, a person's crisis is resolved in some way within approximately
   1. 6 weeks
   2. 1 month
   3. 6 months
   4. 2 weeks

References

Aguilera, D. C. (1998). *Crisis intervention: Theory and methodology* (8th ed.). St. Louis, MO: Mosby.

Aldwin, C. (1992). Aging, coping, and efficacy: Theoretical framework for examining coping in life-span developmental context. In M. Wykle, E. Kahava, & J. Kowal (Eds.), *Stress and health among the elderly* (pp. 96–115). New York: Springer.

Aldwin, C. M. (2000). *Stress, coping, and development: An integrative perspective.* New York: Guilford.

Aldwin, C. M., et al. (1996). Age differences in stress, coping, and appraisal: Findings from the Normative Aging Study. *Journal of Gerontology. Series B, Psychological Sciences and Social Sciences, 51*(4), P179–P188.

American Psychiatric Association. (2000). *Diagnostic and statistical manual of mental disorders* (4th ed.). Washington, DC: Author.

Bauman, A., et al. (2001). *Commitment and care: The benefits of a healthy workplace for nurses, their patients and the system. A policy synthesis.* Ottawa, ON: Canadian Health Research Foundation.

Chiriboga, D. A. (1992). Paradise lost: Stress in the modern age. In M. Wykle, E. Kahava, & J. Kowal (Eds.), *Stress and health among the elderly* (pp. 35–72). New York: Springer.

Chrousos, G. P., Loriaux, L., & Gold, P. W. (1988). The concept of stress and its historical development. In G. P. Chrousos, L. Loriaux, & P. W. Gold (Eds.), *Mechanisms of physical and emotional stress* (pp. 3–10). New York: Plenum Press.

Dochterman, J. M., & Bulechek, G. M. (Eds.). (2004). *Nursing interventions classification (NIC)* (4th ed.). St. Louis, MO: Mosby.

Dunn, A. J. (1989). CRF as mediator of stress responses neurochemical and behavioral aspects. In L. Bueno, S. Collins, & J.-L. Junien (Eds.), *Stress and digestive mobility* (pp. 13–22). London: John Libbey.

Foster, J. (1997). Successful coping, adaptation and resilience in the elderly: An interpretation of epidemiological data. *The Psychiatric Quarterly, 68*(3), 189–219.

Gulanick, M., Klopp, A., & Galanes, S. (2003). *Nursing care plans: Nursing diagnosis and intervention* (5th ed.). St. Louis, MO: Mosby.

Hyer, L. A., & Sohnle, S. J. (2001). *Trauma among older people.* Ann Arbor, MI: Taylor & Francis.

Kasl, S. V. (1992). Stress and health among the elderly: An overview of issues. In M. Wykle, E. Kahava, & J. Kowal (Eds.), *Stress and health among the elderly* (pp. 5–35). New York: Springer.

Lazarus, R. (1999). *Stress and emotion: A new synthesis.* New York: Springer.

Manning, G., Curtis, K., & McMillen, S. (1999). *Stress: Living and working in a changing world.* Duluth, MN: Whole Person Associates.

Monat, A., & Lazarus, R. (1991). *Stress and coping: An anthology.* New York: Columbia University Press.

Moorhead, S., Johnson, M., & Maas, M. (Eds.). (2004). *Nursing outcomes classification (NOC)* (3rd ed.). St. Louis, MO: Mosby.

Neuman, B. (1995). *The Neuman systems model* (3rd ed.). Stamford, CT: Appleton & Lange.

Pearlin, L. I., & Mullan, J. T. (1992). Loss and stress in aging. In M. Wykle (Ed.), *Stress and health among the elderly.* New York: Springer.

Pender, N. J., Murdaugh, C., & Parsons, M. A. (2002). *Health promotion in nursing practice* (4th ed.). Upper Saddle River, NJ: Howorth Press.

Selye, H. (1974). *Stress without distress*. New York: J. B. Lippincott.

Selye, H. (1991). History and present status of the stress concept. In A. Monat & R. Lazarus (Eds.), *Stress and coping: An anthology* (pp. 21–35). New York: Columbia University Press.

Shontz, F. (1975). *The psychological aspects of physical illness and disability*. New York: Macmillan.

Solomon, P., & Draine, J. (1995). Subjective burden among family members of mentally ill adults: Relation to stress, coping, and adaptation. *The American Journal of Orthopsychiatry, 65*(3), 419–427.

Stuart, G., & Wright, L. (1995). Applying the Neuman systems model to psychiatric nursing practice. In B. Neuman (Ed.), *The Neuman systems model* (3rd ed.). Stamford, CT: Appleton & Lange.

Varcarolis, E. M. (2002). *Foundations of psychiatric mental health nursing: A clinical approach* (4th ed.). St. Louis, MO: Saunders.

Recommended Web Sites

Health Care Information Resources: Stress Links:
http://hsl.mcmaster.ca/tomflem/stress.html
This Web site provides links to health care information for clients, their families, and health care workers.

Heart & Stroke Foundation of Canada: Manage your Stress–Resources:
http://ww1.heartandstroke.ca/Page.asp?PageID=33&ArticleID=484&Src=living&From=SubCategory
This page of the Heart & Stroke Foundation's Web site provides information and resources related to coping with stress.

Stress WWW virtual library:
http://www.clas.ufl.edu/users/gthursby/stress/
This site provides links to online information on the topic of stress, including books, journals, organizations, and Web links.

Yale New Haven Health System: Stress Management:
http://yalenewhavenhealth.org/library/healthguide/en-us/illnessconditions/ topic.asp?hwid=rlxsk
This site provides information on diseases, health concerns, treatment options, and prevention regarding stress management.

27

Vital Signs

Susan Jane Fetzer, RN, BA, BSN, MSN, MBA, PhD
Maureen McQueen, RN, MN (Canadian author)

Objectives

Mastery of content in this chapter will enable the student to:

- Define the key terms listed.
- Explain the principles and mechanisms of thermoregulation.
- Describe nursing measures that promote heat loss and heat conservation.
- Discuss physiological changes associated with fever.
- Accurately assess tympanic, oral, rectal, and axillary temperatures.
- Accurately assess pulse, respirations, oxygen saturation, and blood pressure.
- Explain the physiology of normal regulation of blood pressure, pulse, oxygen saturation, and respirations.
- Describe factors that cause variations in body temperature, pulse, oxygen saturation, respirations, and blood pressure.
- Describe cultural and ethnic variations with blood pressure assessment.
- Identify ranges of acceptable vital sign values for an infant, a child, and an adult.
- Explain variations in technique used to assess an infant's, a child's, and an adult's vital signs.
- Describe the benefits and precautions involving self-measurement of blood pressure.
- Identify when vital signs should be taken.
- Accurately record and report vital sign measurements.
- Appropriately delegate vital sign measurement to unregulated care providers.

The most frequent measurements obtained by health practitioners are those of temperature, pulse, blood pressure, respiratory rate, and oxygen saturation. As indicators of health status, these measures indicate the effectiveness of circulatory, respiratory, neural, and endocrine body functions. Because of their importance, they are referred to as **vital signs.** Many factors—such as the temperature of the environment, the client's physical state, and illness—cause vital signs to change, sometimes to outside an acceptable range. Pain can also profoundly affect vital signs. A thorough discussion of pain and pain assessment is found in chapter 38.

Measurement of vital signs provides data to determine a client's usual state of health (baseline data). A change in vital signs can indicate a change in physiological function. Assessment of vital signs allows the nurse to identify nursing diagnoses, implement planned interventions, and evaluate success when vital signs have returned to acceptable values. An alteration in vital signs may signal the need for medical or nursing intervention.

Vital signs are a quick and efficient way of monitoring a client's condition, identifying problems, or evaluating the client's response to intervention. When the nurse learns the physiological variables influencing vital signs and recognizes the relationship of vital sign changes to other physical assessment findings, precise determinations of the client's health problems can be made. The basic techniques of inspection, palpation, and auscultation are used to determine vital signs. These skills are simple but should not be taken for granted. Careful measurement techniques ensure accurate findings. Vital signs and other physiological measurements are the basis for clinical problem solving. Vital sign assessment is an essential function when nurses and physicians collaborate to determine the client's health status.

Guidelines for Measuring Vital Signs

Vital signs are a part of the database that a nurse collects during assessment. Box 27-1 provides a reference for acceptable values in the adult client. Vital signs are obtained during a complete physical assessment (see chapter 28) or as needed to assess a client's condition. Establishing a database of vital signs during a routine physical examination serves as a baseline for future assessments. The client's needs and condition determine when, where, how, and by whom vital signs are measured. The nurse must be able to measure vital signs correctly or delegate the measurement of vital signs appropriately to unregulated care providers. When vital signs are obtained, the nurse must understand and interpret the values, communicate findings appropriately, and begin interventions as needed. The following guidelines assist the nurse in incorporating vital sign measurement into nursing practice:

- The nurse caring for the client is responsible for vital sign measurement. Measurement of selected vital signs (i.e., in stable clients) may be delegated to unregulated care providers.
- Equipment should be functional and appropriate for the size and the age of the client. Equipment used to measure vital signs (e.g., a thermometer) must work properly to ensure accurate findings.
- Equipment should be selected on the basis of the client's condition and characteristics (e.g., an adult-size blood pressure cuff should not be used for a child).
- The nurse knows the client's usual range of vital signs. A client's usual values may differ from the acceptable range for that age or physical state. The client's usual values serve as a baseline for comparison with later findings. Thus, a nurse can detect a change in condition over time.
- The nurse knows the client's medical history, therapies, and prescribed medications. Some illnesses or treatments cause predictable vital sign changes. Some medications affect one or more of the vital signs.
- The nurse controls or minimizes environmental factors that may affect vital signs. For example, assessing the client's temperature in a warm, humid room may yield a value that is not a true indicator of the client's condition.
- The nurse uses an organized, systematic approach when taking vital signs. Each procedure requires a step-by-step approach to ensure accuracy.
- The manner of approach to the client can alter the vital signs. The nurse approaches the client in a calm, caring manner while demonstrating proficiency in handling the supplies needed for vital sign measurement.
- The nurse collaborates with the physician to decide the frequency of vital sign assessment (Box 27-2).
- The nurse uses vital sign measurements to determine indications for medication administration. For example, the physician may order certain cardiac drugs to be given only within a range of pulse or blood pressure values. Antipyretics are often administered when

Box 27-1 Vital Signs: Acceptable Ranges for Adults

Temperature Range: 36° to 38° C

Average oral/tympanic: 37° C
Average rectal: 37.5° C
Average axillary: 36.5° C

Pulse

60 to 100 beats per minute

Respirations

12 to 20 breaths per minute

Blood Pressure

Average: 120/80 mm Hg
Pulse pressure: 30 to 50 mm Hg

Box 27-2 When to Take Vital Signs

When the client is admitted to a health care facility
In a hospital or care facility on a routine schedule according to the physician's order or the institution's standards of practice
Before and after a surgical procedure
Before and after an invasive diagnostic procedure
Before, during, and after the administration of medications that affect cardiovascular, respiratory, and temperature-control function
When the client's general physical condition changes (as with loss of consciousness or increased intensity of pain)
As a client's physical condition worsens (it may be necessary to monitor vital signs as often as every 5 to 15 minutes)
Before and after nursing interventions influencing a vital sign (e.g., before a client previously on bed rest ambulates or before a client performs range-of-motion exercises)
When the client reports non-specific symptoms of physical distress (e.g., feeling "funny" or "different")

temperature is elevated outside of the acceptable range for the client. Therefore, the nurse does not administer these drugs if the vital sign assessment indicates the measurements are within the specified acceptable range.
- The nurse analyzes the results of vital sign measurement. The nurse is often in the best position to assess all clinical findings about a client. Vital signs are not interpreted in isolation. The nurse must also know related physical signs or symptoms and be aware of the client's ongoing health status.
- The nurse verifies, documents, and communicates significant changes in vital signs. Baseline measurements allow a nurse to identify changes in vital signs. When vital signs appear abnormal, it may help to have another nurse or a physician repeat the measurement. The nurse informs the physician or nurse in charge of abnormal vital signs.
- The nurse develops a teaching plan to instruct the client or caregiver in vital sign assessment and the significance of findings.

Body Temperature

Physiology

The body temperature is the difference between the amount of heat produced by body processes and the amount of heat lost to the external environment.

Heat produced − Heat lost = Body temperature

Despite extremes in environmental conditions and physical activity, temperature-control mechanisms keep the body's **core temperature** (temperature of the deep tissues) relatively constant (Figure 27–1). However, surface temperature fluctuates depending on blood flow to the skin and the amount of heat lost to the external environment. Because of these surface temperature fluctuations, acceptable body temperature ranges from 36° to 38° C. The body's tissues and cells function best within the relatively narrow temperature range.

The site of temperature measurement (oral, rectal, axillary, tympanic membrane, esophageal, pulmonary artery, or even urinary bladder) is one factor that determines the client's temperature. For healthy young adults, the average oral temperature is 37° C. In clinical practice, nurses learn the temperature range of individual clients. No single temperature is normal for all people.

The measurement of body temperature is aimed at obtaining a representative average temperature of core body tissues. Sites reflecting core temperatures are more reliable indicators of body temperature than sites reflecting surface temperatures (Box 27-3). In addition, the temperature value obtained may differ depending on the measurement site.

Regulation. The balance between heat lost and heat produced, or **thermoregulation,** is precisely regulated by physiological and behavioural mechanisms. For the body temperature to stay constant and within an acceptable range, the relationship between heat production and heat loss must be maintained. This relationship is regulated by neurological and cardiovascular mechanisms. The nurse applies knowledge of temperature-control mechanisms to promote temperature regulation.

Neural and Vascular Control. The **hypothalamus,** located between the cerebral hemispheres, controls body temperature the same way that a thermostat works in the home. A comfortable temperature is the "set point" at which a heating system operates. In the home, a decrease in environmental temperature activates the furnace, whereas a rise in temperature shuts the system down. The hypothalamus is like the home's furnace; it senses minor changes in body temperature. The anterior hypothalamus controls heat loss, and the posterior hypothalamus controls heat production.

When nerve cells in the anterior hypothalamus become heated beyond the set point, impulses are sent out to reduce body temperature. Mechanisms of heat loss include sweating, vasodilation (widening) of blood vessels, and in-

Box 27-3 Core and Surface Temperature Measurement Sites

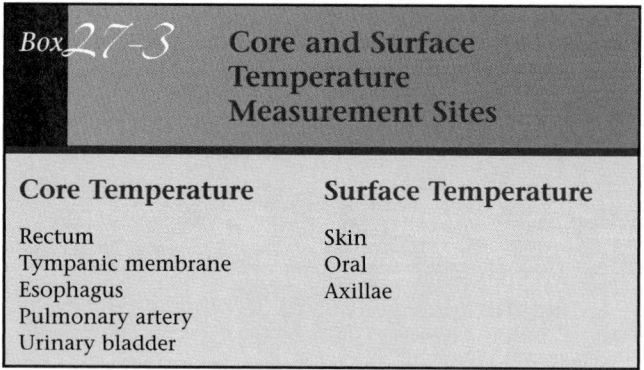

Core Temperature	Surface Temperature
Rectum	Skin
Tympanic membrane	Oral
Esophagus	Axillae
Pulmonary artery	
Urinary bladder	

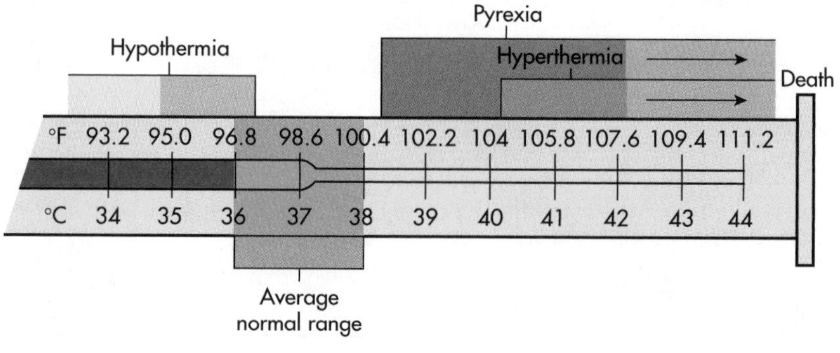

FIGURE **27–1** Ranges of normal temperature values and physiological consequences of abnormal body temperature.

hibition of heat production. Blood is redistributed to surface vessels to promote heat loss. If the posterior hypothalamus senses the body's temperature is lower than the set point, heat conservation mechanisms are instituted. Vasoconstriction (narrowing) of blood vessels reduces blood flow to the skin and extremities. Compensatory heat production is stimulated through voluntary muscle contraction and muscle shivering. When vasoconstriction is ineffective in preventing additional heat loss, shivering begins. Disease or trauma to the hypothalamus or to the spinal cord, which carries hypothalamic messages, can cause serious alterations in temperature control.

Heat Production. Thermoregulation depends on the normal function of heat production processes. Heat is produced in the body as a by-product of metabolism, which is the chemical reaction in all body cells. Food is the primary fuel source for metabolism. Activities requiring additional chemical reactions increase the metabolic rate. As metabolism increases, additional heat is produced. When metabolism decreases, less heat is produced. Heat production occurs during rest, voluntary movements, involuntary shivering, and non-shivering thermogenesis.

- Basal metabolism accounts for the heat produced by the body at absolute rest. The average **basal metabolic rate (BMR)** depends on the body surface area. Thyroid hormones also affect the BMR. By promoting the breakdown of body glucose and fat, thyroid hormones increase the rate of chemical reactions in almost all cells of the body. When large amounts of thyroid hormones are secreted, the BMR can increase 100% above normal. Absence of thyroid hormones can cut the BMR in half, causing a decrease in heat production. The male sex hormone testosterone increases BMR. Men have a higher BMR than women.
- Voluntary movements such as muscular activity during exercise require additional energy. The metabolic rate can increase up to 2,000 times normal during exercise. Heat production can increase up to 50 times normal.
- **Shivering** is an involuntary body response to temperature differences in the body. The skeletal muscle movement during shivering requires significant energy. In vulnerable clients, shivering can seriously deplete energy sources, resulting in further physiological deterioration. Shivering can increase heat production four to five times greater than normal. The heat that is produced assists in equalizing the body temperature, and the shivering ceases.
- **Non-shivering thermogenesis** occurs primarily in neonates. Because neonates cannot shiver, they rely on vasoconstriction via an increase in norepinephrine. As well, a limited amount of vascular brown tissue (fat) is metabolized for heat production.

Heat Loss. Heat loss and heat production occur simultaneously. The skin's structure and exposure to the environment result in constant, normal heat loss through radiation, conduction, convection, and evaporation.

Radiation is the transfer of heat from the surface of one object to the surface of another without direct contact between the two. Up to 85% of the human body's surface area radiates heat to the environment. Peripheral vasodilation increases blood flow from the internal organs to the skin to increase radiant heat loss. Peripheral vasoconstriction minimizes radiant heat loss. Radiation increases as the temperature difference between the objects increases. However, if the environment is warmer than the skin, the body absorbs heat through radiation.

The nurse increases heat loss through radiation by removing clothing or blankets. The client's position enhances radiation heat loss (e.g., standing exposes a greater radiating surface area and lying in a fetal position minimizes heat radiation). Covering the body with dark, closely woven clothing also reduces the amount of heat lost from radiation.

Conduction is the transfer of heat from one object to another with direct contact. Heat conducts through contact with solids, liquids, and gases. When the warm skin touches a cooler object, heat is lost. Conduction normally accounts for a small amount of heat loss. The nurse increases conductive heat loss when applying an ice pack or bathing a client with a cool cloth. Applying several layers of clothing reduces conductive loss. The body gains heat by conduction when contact is made with materials warmer than skin temperature (e.g., application of an aquathermia pad).

Convection is the transfer of heat away by air movement. A fan promotes heat loss through convection. Convective heat loss increases when moistened skin comes into contact with slightly moving air.

Evaporation is the transfer of heat energy when a liquid is changed to a gas. The body continuously loses heat by evaporation. About 600 to 900 mL a day evaporates from the skin and lungs, resulting in water and heat loss. By regulating perspiration or sweating, the body promotes additional evaporative heat loss. Millions of sweat glands located in the dermis of the skin secrete sweat through tiny ducts on the skin's surface. When body temperature rises, the anterior hypothalamus signals the sweat glands to release sweat. Sweat evaporates from the skin surface, resulting in heat loss. During exercise and emotional or mental stress, sweating is one way to lose excessive heat produced by the increased metabolic rate. **Diaphoresis** is visible perspiration primarily occurring on the forehead and upper thorax, though it can also be seen elsewhere on the body. Excessive evaporation can cause skin scaling and itching, as well as drying of the nares and pharynx.

A lowered body temperature inhibits sweat gland secretion. People who have a congenital absence of sweat glands or a serious skin disease that impairs sweating are unable to tolerate warm temperatures because they cannot cool themselves adequately.

Skin in Temperature Regulation. The skin regulates temperature through insulation of the body, vasoconstriction (which affects the amount of blood flow and heat loss to the skin), and temperature sensation. The skin, subcutaneous tissue, and fat keep heat inside the body. When blood flow between skin layers is reduced, the skin alone is an excellent insulator. People with more body fat have more natural insulation than do slim and muscular people.

In the human body, the internal organs produce heat. During exercise or increased sympathetic stimulation, the amount of heat produced is greater than the usual core temperature. Blood flows from the internal organs, carrying heat to the body surface. The skin is well supplied with blood vessels, especially the areas of the hands, feet, and ears. Blood flow through these vascular areas of the skin may vary from minimal flow to as much as 30% of the blood ejected from the heart. Heat transfers from the blood, through vessel walls, to the skin's surface and is lost to the environment through the heat-loss mechanisms. The body's core temperature remains within safe limits.

The degree of vasoconstriction determines the amount of blood flow and heat loss to the skin. If the core temperature is too high, the hypothalamus inhibits vasoconstriction. As a result, blood vessels dilate, and more blood reaches the skin's surface. On a hot, humid day, the blood vessels in the hands are dilated and easily visible. In contrast, if the core temperature becomes too low, the hypothalamus initiates vasoconstriction and blood flow to the skin lessens, thus conserving body heat.

Behavioural Control. Humans voluntarily act to maintain comfortable body temperature when exposed to temperature extremes. The ability of a person to control body temperature depends on (a) the degree of temperature extreme, (b) the person's ability to sense feeling comfortable or uncomfortable, (c) thought processes or emotions, and (d) the person's mobility or ability to remove or add clothes. Body temperature control is difficult if any of these abilities are absent or lost. Infants can sense uncomfortably warm conditions but need assistance in changing their environment. Older adults may need help in detecting cold environments and minimizing heat loss. Illness, a decreased level of consciousness, or impaired thought processes results in an inability to recognize the need to change behaviour for temperature control. When temperatures become extremely hot or cold, health-promoting behaviours, such as removing or adding clothing, have a limited effect on controlling temperature. The nurse assesses for variables that place clients at high risk for ineffective thermoregulation.

Factors Affecting Body Temperature

Many factors affect body temperature. Changes in body temperature within an acceptable range occur when the relationship between heat production and heat loss is altered by physiological or behavioural variables. The nurse must be aware of these factors when assessing temperature variations and evaluating deviations from normal.

Age. At birth, the newborn leaves a warm, relatively constant environment and enters one in which temperatures fluctuate widely. Temperature-control mechanisms are immature. An infant's temperature may respond drastically to changes in the environment. Extra care is needed to protect the newborn from environmental temperatures. Clothing must be adequate, and exposure to temperature extremes must be avoided. A newborn loses up to 30% of body heat through the head and therefore needs to wear a cap to prevent heat loss. When protected from environmental extremes, the newborn's body temperature is maintained between 35.5° and 37.5° C.

Temperature regulation is unstable until children reach puberty. The normal temperature range gradually drops as individuals approach older adulthood. The older adult has a narrower range of body temperatures than the younger adult. Oral temperatures of 35° C are not unusual for older adults in cold weather. However, the average body temperature of older adults is approximately 36° C. Older adults are particularly sensitive to temperature extremes because of deterioration in control mechanisms, particularly poor vasomotor control (control of vasoconstriction and vasodilation), reduced amounts of subcutaneous tissue, reduced sweat gland activity, and reduced metabolism.

Exercise. Muscle activity requires an increased blood supply and an increased carbohydrate and fat breakdown. This increased metabolism causes an increase in heat production. Any form of exercise can increase heat production and thus body temperature. Prolonged strenuous exercise, such as long-distance running, can temporarily raise body temperatures up to 41° C.

Hormone Level. Women generally experience greater fluctuations in body temperature than men. Hormonal variations during the menstrual cycle cause body temperature fluctuations. Progesterone levels rise and fall cyclically during the menstrual cycle. When progesterone levels are low, the body temperature is a few tenths of a degree below the baseline level. The lower temperature persists until ovulation occurs. During ovulation, greater amounts of progesterone enter the circulatory system and raise the body temperature to previous baseline levels or higher. These temperature variations can be used to predict a woman's most fertile time to achieve pregnancy.

Body temperature changes also occur in women during menopause (cessation of menstruation). Women who have stopped menstruating may experience periods of intense body heat and sweating lasting from 30 seconds to 5 minutes. There may be intermittent increases in skin temperature of up to 4° C during these periods, referred to as *hot flashes*. This is due to the instability of the vasomotor controls for vasodilation and vasoconstriction.

Circadian Rhythm. Body temperature normally changes 0.5° to 1° C during a 24-hour period. However, temperature is one of the most stable rhythms. The temperature is usually lowest between 1:00 AM and 4:00 AM (Figure 27–2). During the day, body temperature rises steadily, until a maximum temperature value at about 6:00 PM, and then declines to early morning levels. Temperature patterns are not automatically reversed in people who work at night and sleep during the day. It takes 1 to 3 weeks for the cycle to reverse. In general, the circadian temperature rhythm does not change with age.

Stress. Physical and emotional stress increase body temperature through hormonal and neural stimulation. These physiological changes increase metabolism, which increases heat production. The client who is anxious about entering a hospital or a physician's office may register a higher normal temperature (see chapter 26).

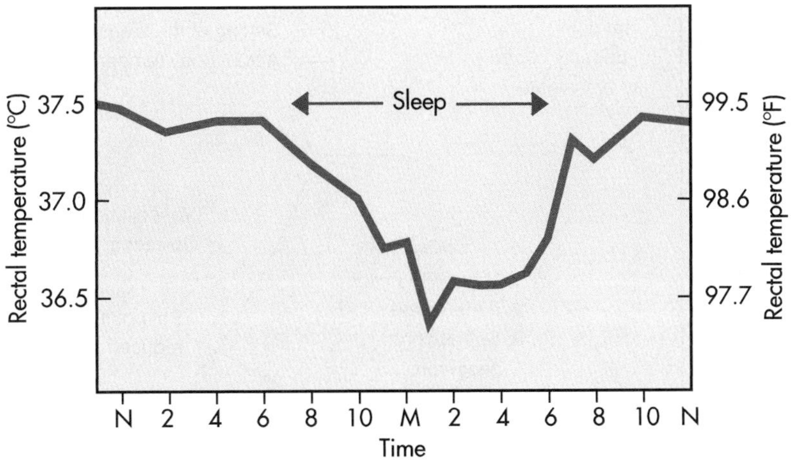

FIGURE **27–2** Temperature cycle for 24 hours.

Environment. Environment influences body temperature. If body temperature is measured in a very warm room, a client may be unable to regulate body temperature by heat-loss mechanisms, and the body temperature will be elevated. If the client has just been outside in the cold without warm clothing, body temperature may be low because of extensive radiant and conductive heat loss. Infants and older adults are most likely to be affected by environmental temperatures because their temperature-regulating mechanisms are less efficient.

Temperature Alterations. Changes in body temperature outside the usual range affect the hypothalamic set point. These changes can be related to excess heat production, excessive heat loss, minimal heat production, minimal heat loss, or any combination of these alterations. The nature of the change affects the type of clinical problems that a client experiences.

Fever. **Pyrexia,** or **fever,** occurs because heat-loss mechanisms are unable to keep pace with excess heat production, resulting in an abnormal rise in body temperature. A fever is usually not harmful if it stays below 39° C, and a single temperature reading may not indicate a fever. In addition to physical signs and symptoms of infection, a fever determination is based on several temperature readings at different times of the day compared with the usual value for that person at that time.

A true fever results from an alteration in the hypothalamic set point. **Pyrogens** such as bacteria and viruses cause a rise in body temperature. Pyrogens act as antigens, triggering immune system responses. The hypothalamus reacts to raise the set point, and the body responds by producing and conserving heat. Several hours may pass before the body temperature reaches the new set point. During this period, the person experiences chills, shivers, and feels cold, even though the body temperature is rising (Figure 27–3). The chill phase resolves when the new set point, a higher temperature, is achieved. During the next phase, the plateau, the chills subside and the person feels warm and dry. If the new set point is "overshot" or the pyrogens are removed (e.g., destruction of bacteria by antibiotics), the third phase of a febrile episode occurs. The hypothalamus set point drops, initiating heat loss responses. The skin becomes warm and flushed because of vasodilation. Diaphoresis assists in evaporative heat loss. When the fever "breaks," the person becomes **afebrile.**

Fever is an important defence mechanism. Temperature elevations up to 39° C enhance the body's immune system. During a **febrile** episode, white blood cell production is stimulated. Increased temperature reduces the concentration of iron in the blood plasma, suppressing the growth of bacteria. Fever also fights viral infections by stimulating interferon, the body's natural virus-fighting substance.

Analyzing a fever pattern can help health care professionals make diagnoses. Fever patterns differ depending on the causative pyrogen (Box 27-4). The increase or decrease in pyrogen activity results in fever spikes and declines at different times of the day. The duration and degree of fever depend on the pyrogen's strength and the ability of the individual to respond. The term **fever of unknown origin (FUO)** refers to a fever that does not have a determined etiology (cause).

During a fever, cellular metabolism increases and oxygen consumption rises. The body's metabolism increases 13% for every degree Celsius of temperature elevation. Heart and respiratory rates increase to meet the metabolic needs of the body for nutrients. The increased metabolism uses energy that produces additional heat. If the client has a cardiac or respiratory problem, the stress of a fever can be great. A prolonged fever can weaken a person by exhausting energy stores. Increased metabolism requires additional oxygen. If the demand for additional oxygen cannot be met, cellular hypoxia (inadequate oxygen) occurs. Myocardial hypoxia produces angina (chest pain). Cerebral hypoxia produces confusion. Interventions during a fever may include oxygen therapy. Water loss through increased respiration and diaphoresis can be excessive, placing a client at risk for fluid volume deficit. Dehydration can be a serious problem for older adults and children with low body weight. Maintaining optimum fluid volume status is an important nursing intervention (see chapter 36).

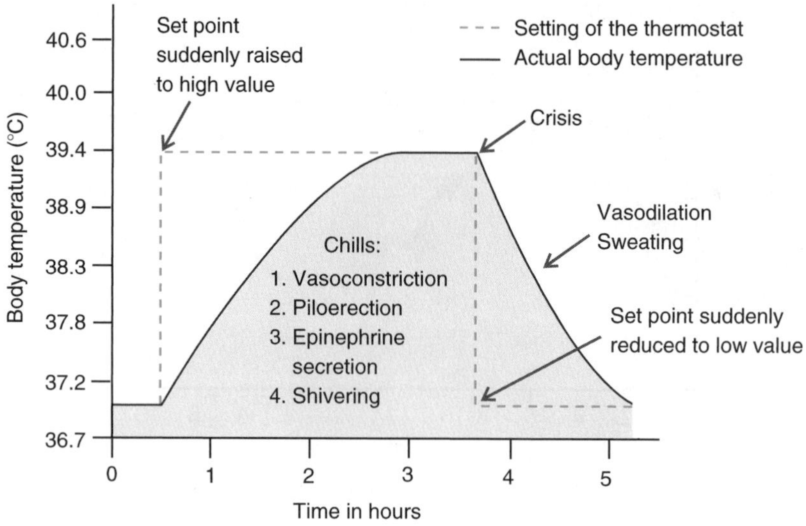

FIGURE **27–3** Effect of changing the set point of the hypothalamic temperature control during a fever. (Adapted from *Textbook of Medical Physiology,* 10th ed., by A. C. Guyton and J. E. Hall, 2002, Philadelphia: W. B. Saunders.)

Box 27-4 Patterns of Fever

Sustained—A constant body temperature continuously above 38° C that demonstrates little fluctuation.

Intermittent—Fever spikes interspersed with usual temperature levels. Temperature returns to acceptable value at least once in 24 hours.

Remittent—Fever spikes and falls without a return to normal temperature levels.

Relapsing—Periods of febrile episodes interspersed with acceptable temperature values. Febrile episodes and periods of normothermia may be longer than 24 hours.

Hyperthermia. **Hyperthermia** is an elevated body temperature due to the body's inability to promote heat loss or reduce heat production. Whereas fever is an upward shift in the set point, hyperthermia results from an overload of the body's thermoregulatory mechanisms. Any disease or trauma to the hypothalamus can impair heat-loss mechanisms. **Malignant hyperthermia** is a hereditary condition of uncontrolled heat production, occurring when susceptible people receive certain anaesthetic drugs.

Heatstroke. Prolonged exposure to the sun or high environmental temperatures can overwhelm the body's heat-loss mechanisms. Heat also depresses hypothalamic function. These conditions cause **heatstroke,** a dangerous heat emergency with a high mortality rate. Clients at risk include those who are very young or very old and those who have cardiovascular disease, hypothyroidism, diabetes, or alcoholism. Also at risk are those who take medications that decrease the body's ability to lose heat (e.g., phenothiazines, anticholinergics, diuretics, amphetamines, and beta-adrenergic receptor antagonists) and those who exercise or work strenuously (e.g., athletes, construction workers, and farmers).

Signs and symptoms of heatstroke include confusion, delirium, excess thirst, nausea, muscle cramps, visual disturbances, giddiness, and incontinence. The most important sign is hot, dry skin. Victims of heatstroke do not sweat because of severe electrolyte loss and hypothalamic malfunction. Vital signs reveal a body temperature sometimes as high as 45° C, with an increase in heart rate and lowering of blood pressure. If the condition progresses, the person becomes unconscious with fixed, unreactive pupils. Permanent neurological damage occurs unless cooling measures are rapidly started.

Heat Exhaustion. **Heat exhaustion** occurs when profuse diaphoresis results in excess water and electrolyte loss. The client exhibits signs and symptoms of fluid volume deficit (see chapter 36). First aid includes transporting the client to a cooler environment and restoring fluid and electrolyte balance.

Hypothermia. Heat loss during prolonged exposure to cold overwhelms the body's ability to produce heat, causing hypothermia. **Hypothermia** is classified by core temperature measurements:

- Mild hypothermia occurs when body temperature is between 34° C and 36° C.
- Moderate hypothermia occurs when body temperature is between 30° C and 34° C.
- Severe hypothermia occurs when body temperature is less than 30° C.

Hypothermia can be unintentionally induced, such as falling through the ice of a frozen lake. During surgical procedures, it may be intentionally induced to reduce metabolic demand and the body's need for oxygen. Accidental hypothermia usually develops gradually and may go unnoticed for several hours. When body temperature drops to 35° C, uncontrolled shivering, loss of memory, depression, and poor judgment occur. As the body temperature falls below 34.4° C, heart rate, respiratory rate, and blood pressure fall. The skin becomes cyanotic. If hypothermia progresses, a person experiences cardiac dysrhythmia, loss of consciousness, and unresponsiveness to painful stimuli. In cases of severe hypothermia, a person may demonstrate clinical signs similar to death (e.g., lack of response to stimuli and extremely slow respirations and pulse). The assessment of core temperature is critical when hypothermia is suspected. A special low reading thermometer may be required because standard devices do not register below 35° C.

Frostbite occurs when the body is exposed to subnormal temperatures. Ice crystals forming inside the cell can result in permanent circulatory and tissue damage. Areas particularly susceptible to frostbite are the earlobes, tip of the nose, and fingers and toes. The injured area becomes white, waxy, and firm to the touch. The client loses sensation in the affected area. Intervention includes gradual warming measures, analgesia, and protection of the injured tissue.

Nursing Process and Thermoregulation

Knowledge of the physiology of body temperature regulation helps the nurse to assess the client's response to temperature alterations and to intervene safely. Independent measures can be implemented to increase or minimize heat loss, promote heat conservation, and increase comfort. These measures complement the effects of medically ordered therapies during illness. Many measures can also be taught to family members, parents of children, or other caregivers.

NP Assessment

Sites. There are several sites for measuring core and surface body temperature. The core temperatures of the pulmonary artery, esophagus, and urinary bladder are used in intensive care settings. These measurements require the use of continuous invasive devices placed in body cavities or organs and continually display readings on an electronic monitor.

Intermittent temperature measurements are obtained from the routinely used invasive sites of the mouth, rectum, tympanic membrane, and axilla. Non-invasive chemically prepared thermometer patches can also be applied to the skin. Oral, rectal, axillary, and skin temperature sites rely on effective blood circulation at the measurement site. The heat of the blood is conducted to the thermometer probe. Tympanic temperature relies on the radiation of body heat to an infrared sensor. Because the tympanic membrane shares the same arterial blood supply as the hypothalamus, tympanic temperature is considered a core temperature.

Each site must be measured correctly (Skill 27-1) to ensure accurate temperature readings. The temperature obtained varies depending on the site used, but should be between 36.0° C and 38.0° C. Rectal temperatures are usually 0.5° C higher than oral temperatures, and axillary temperatures are usually 0.5° C lower than oral temperatures. Each of the common temperature measurement sites has advantages and disadvantages (Box 27-5). The nurse chooses the safest and most accurate site for the client. When possible, the same site should be used when repeated measurements are necessary.

Thermometers. Two types of thermometers are commonly available for measuring body temperature: electronic and disposable. A third type, the mercury-in-glass thermometer, was once the standard device for the clinical setting. However, most municipalities have prohibited the sale or use of mercury-containing medical devices because of the potential hazards.

Each device measures temperature using the **Celsius** or **Fahrenheit** scale. Electronic thermometers allow the nurse to convert scales by activating a switch. When it is necessary to convert temperature readings, the following formulas can be used:

1. To convert Fahrenheit to Celsius, subtract 32 from the Fahrenheit reading and multiply the result by 5/9

$$C = (F - 32°) \times 5/9$$
$$\text{Example: } 40° \text{ C} = (104° \text{ F} - 32° \text{ F}) \times 5/9$$

2. To convert Celsius to Fahrenheit, multiply the centigrade reading by 9/5 and add 32 to the product.

$$F = (9/5 \times C) + 32°$$
$$\text{Example: } 104° \text{ F} = (9/5 \times 40° \text{ C}) + 32°$$

Electronic Thermometer. The electronic thermometer consists of a rechargeable battery-powered display unit, a thin wire cord, and a temperature-processing probe covered by a disposable plastic sheath (Figure 27–4). Separate unbreakable probes are available for oral and rectal use. The oral probe can also be used for axillary temperature measurement. Within 20 to 50 seconds of insertion, a reading appears on the display unit. A sound signals when the peak temperature reading has been measured.

Another form of electronic thermometer is used exclusively for tympanic temperature. An otoscope-like speculum with an infrared sensor tip detects heat radiated from the tympanic membrane. Within 2 to 5 seconds of placement in the auditory canal, a reading appears on the dis-

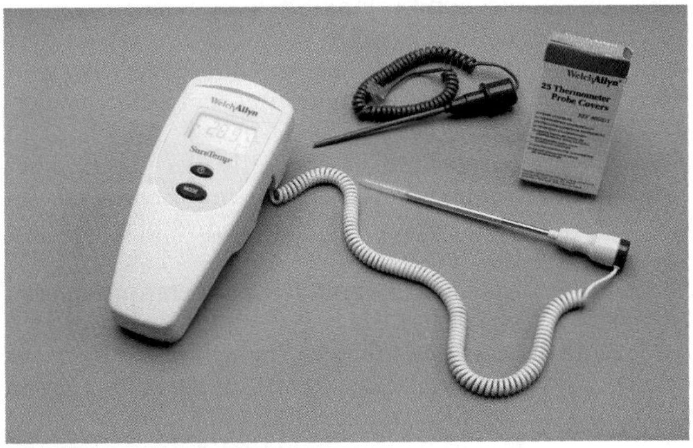

FIGURE 27–4 Electronic thermometer. Blue probe is for oral or axillary use. Red probe is for rectal use.

Text continued on p. 576

Skill 27-1 Measuring Body Temperature

Delegation Considerations

The skill of temperature measurement can be delegated to unregulated care providers (UCPs). The nurse is responsible for assessing the impact of changes in body temperature. It is important for the nurse to do the following:

- Inform the UCP of appropriate route and device to measure temperature.
- Inform the UCP of specific factors related to client that can falsely raise or lower temperature.
- Inform the UCP of the frequency of temperature measurement for select client.
- Determine that the UCP is aware of the usual values for client.
- Inform the UCP of the abnormalities that should be reported to the nurse.

Equipment

- Appropriate thermometer
- Soft tissue or wipe
- Lubricant (for rectal measurements only)
- Pen, vital sign flow sheet or record form
- Disposable gloves, plastic thermometer sleeve or disposable probe cover

Steps	Rationale
1. Assess for signs and symptoms of temperature alterations and for factors that influence body temperature.	Physical signs and symptoms may indicate abnormal temperature. Nurse can accurately assess nature of variations.
2. Determine any previous activity that would interfere with accuracy of temperature measurement. When taking oral temperature, wait 20 to 30 minutes before measuring temperature if client has smoked or ingested hot or cold liquids or foods.	Smoking or oral intake of food or fluids can cause false oral temperature readings.
3. Determine appropriate temperature site and device for client.	Chosen based on advantages and disadvantages of each site (see Box 27-5). Disposable single-use thermometer is used for client who is on isolation precautions.
4. Explain route by which temperature will be taken and importance of maintaining proper position until reading is complete.	Clients are often curious about such measurements and should be cautioned against prematurely removing thermometer to read results.
5. Perform hand hygiene.	Reduces transmission of microorganisms.
6. Obtain temperature reading.	
A. Oral temperature measurement with electronic thermometer	
(1) Apply disposable gloves (optional).	Use of oral probe cover, which can be removed without physical contact, minimizes need to wear gloves.
(2) Remove thermometer pack from charging unit. Attach oral probe (blue tip) to thermometer unit. Grasp top of probe stem, being careful not to apply pressure on the ejection button.	Charging provides battery power. Ejection button releases plastic probe cover from tip.
(3) Slide disposable plastic probe cover over thermometer probe until cover locks in place (see illustration).	Soft plastic cover will not break in client's mouth and prevents transmission of microorganisms between clients.
(4) Have client sit or lie in bed. Ask client to open mouth; then gently place thermometer probe under tongue in posterior sublingual pocket lateral to centre of lower jaw (see illustration).	Heat from superficial blood vessels in sublingual pocket produces temperature reading. With electronic thermometer, temperatures in right and left posterior sublingual pocket are significantly higher than in area under front of tongue.
(5) Ask client to hold thermometer probe with lips closed.	Maintains proper position of thermometer during recording.
(6) Leave thermometer probe in place until audible signal occurs and client's temperature appears on digital display; remove thermometer probe from under client's tongue.	Probe must stay in place until signal occurs to ensure accurate reading.
(7) Push ejection button on thermometer stem to discard plastic probe cover into appropriate receptacle.	Reduces transmission of microorganisms.

Steps	Rationale

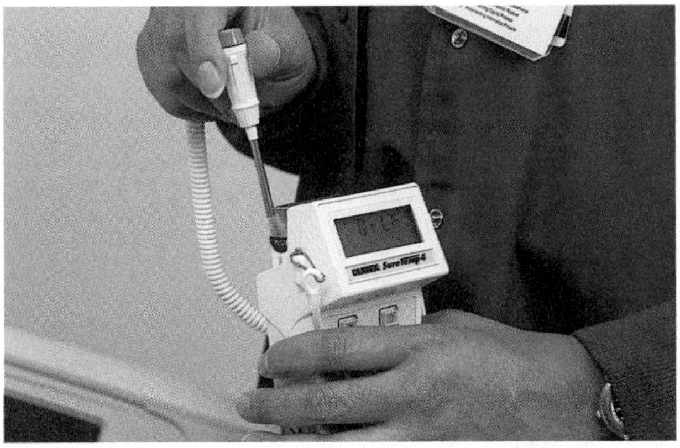

STEP **6A(3)** Inserting thermometer stem into plastic probe cover.

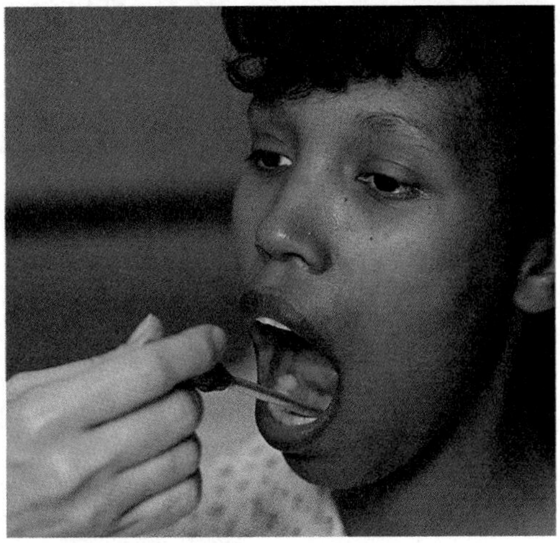

STEP **6A(4)** Probe under tongue in posterior sublingual pocket.

Steps	Rationale
(8) Return thermometer stem to storage well of recording unit.	Protects probe from damage. Returning probe automatically causes digital reading to disappear.
(9) If gloves worn, remove and dispose in appropriate receptacle. Perform hand hygiene.	Reduces transmission of microorganisms.
(10) Return thermometer to charger.	Maintains battery charge.
B. Rectal temperature measurement with electronic thermometer	
(1) Draw curtain around bed and/or close room door. Assist client to Sims' position with upper leg flexed. Move aside bed linen to expose only anal area. Keep client's upper body and lower extremities covered with sheet or blanket. Remind client to remain in Sims' position until procedure is complete.	Maintains client's privacy, minimizes embarrassment, and promotes comfort. Exposes anal area for correct thermometer placement.
(2) Apply disposable gloves.	Maintains standard precautions/routine practices when exposed to items soiled with body fluids (e.g., feces).
(3) Remove thermometer pack from charging unit. Attach rectal probe (red tip) to thermometer unit. Grasp top of probe stem, being careful not to apply pressure on the ejection button.	Charging provides battery power. Ejection button releases plastic probe cover from tip.
(4) Slide disposable plastic probe cover over thermometer probe until cover locks in place.	Probe cover prevents transmission of microorganisms between clients.
(5) Squeeze liberal portion of lubricant on tissue. Dip thermometer's blunt end into lubricant, covering 2.5 to 3.5 cm for adult.	Lubrication minimizes trauma to rectal mucosa during insertion. Tissue avoids contamination of remaining lubricant in container.
(6) With nondominant hand, separate client's buttocks to expose anus. Ask client to breathe slowly and relax.	Fully exposes anus for thermometer insertion. Relaxes anal sphincter for easier thermometer insertion.
(7) Gently insert thermometer into anus in direction of umbilicus, 3.5 cm for adult. Do not force thermometer.	Ensures adequate exposure against blood vessels in rectal wall.
(8) If resistance is felt during insertion, withdraw thermometer immediately. Never force thermometer.	Prevents trauma to mucosa.

Critical Decision Point: If thermometer cannot be adequately inserted into rectum, remove thermometer and consider alternative method for obtaining temperature.

Skill 27-1 Measuring Body Temperature—cont'd

Steps	Rationale

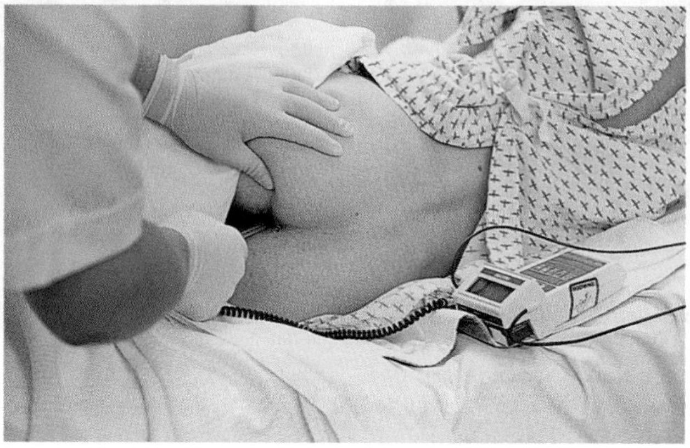

STEP **6B(9)** Probe positioned in anus.

Steps	Rationale
(9) Once positioned, leave thermometer probe in place (see illustration) until audible signal occurs and client's temperature appears on digital display; remove thermometer probe from anus.	Probe must stay in place until signal occurs to ensure accurate reading.
(10) Push ejection button on thermometer stem to discard plastic probe cover into appropriate receptacle. Wipe probe with alcohol swab, paying particular attention to ridges where probe cover connects to probe.	Reduces transmission of microorganisms.
(11) Return thermometer stem to storage well of recording unit.	Protects probe from damage. Returning probe automatically causes digital reading to disappear.
(12) Wipe client's anal area with soft tissue to remove lubricant or feces and discard tissue. Assist client in assuming a comfortable position.	Provides for comfort and hygiene.
(13) Remove and dispose of gloves in appropriate receptacle. Perform hand hygiene.	Reduces transmission of microorganisms.
(14) Return thermometer to charger. Verify that charger and probes are wiped with alcohol daily.	Maintains battery charge. Reduces transmission of microorganisms.
C. Axillary temperature measurement with electronic thermometer	
(1) Draw curtain around bed and/or close door.	Maintains client's privacy, minimizes embarrassment.
(2) Assist client to a supine or sitting position.	Provides easy access to axilla.
(3) Move clothing or gown away from shoulder and arm.	Exposes axilla for correct thermometer probe placement.
(4) Remove thermometer pack from charging unit. Be sure oral probe (blue tip) is attached to thermometer unit. Grasp top of probe stem, being careful not to apply pressure on the ejection button.	Charging provides battery power. Ejection button releases plastic cover from probe.
(5) Slide disposable plastic probe cover over thermometer probe until cover locks in place.	Soft plastic cover prevents transmission of microorganisms between clients.

Steps	Rationale

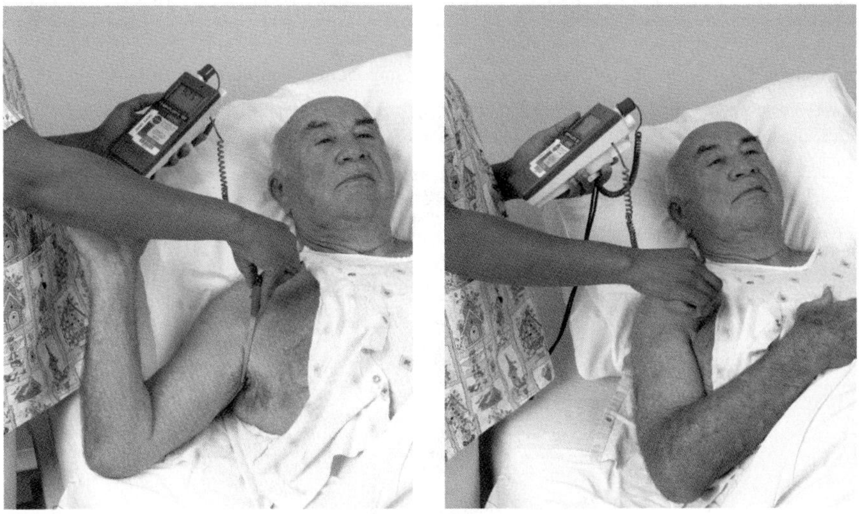

STEP **6C(7)** Thermometer tip in axilla.

Steps	Rationale
(6) Raise client's arm away from torso; inspect for skin lesion and excessive perspiration. Insert probe into centre of axilla, lower arm over probe, and place arm across client's chest (see illustration).	Maintains proper position of probe against blood vessels in axilla.

Critical Decision Point: Do not use axilla if skin lesions are present because local temperature may be altered and area may be painful to touch.

Steps	Rationale
(7) Hold probe in place until audible signal occurs and temperature appears on digital display.	Probe must stay in place until signal occurs to ensure accurate reading.
(8) Remove probe from axilla.	
(9) Push ejection button on thermometer stem to discard plastic probe cover into appropriate receptacle.	Reduces transmission of microorganisms.
(10) Return thermometer stem to storage well of recording unit.	Protects probe from damage. Returning probe automatically causes digital reading to disappear.
(11) Assist client in assuming a comfortable position, replacing linen or gown.	Restores comfort and promotes privacy.
(12) Perform hand hygiene.	Reduces transmission of microorganisms.
(13) Return thermometer unit to charger.	Maintains battery charge.
D. Tympanic membrane temperature with electronic thermometer	
(1) Assist client in assuming comfortable position with head turned toward side, away from nurse. Right-handed caregivers should obtain temperature from client's right ear. Left-handed caregivers should obtain temperature from client's left ear.	Ensures comfort and exposes auditory canal for accurate temperature measurement. The less acute the angle of approach, the better the probe seal.
(2) Note if there is obvious earwax in the client's ear canal.	To ensure clear optical pathway, lens cover of speculum must not be impeded by earwax. Switch to other ear or select alternative measurement site if needed.
(3) Remove thermometer handheld unit from charging base, being careful not to apply pressure on the ejection button.	Base provides battery power. Removal of handheld unit from base prepares it to measure temperature. Ejection button releases plastic probe cover from tip.

Skill 27-1 *Measuring Body Temperature—cont'd*

Steps	Rationale

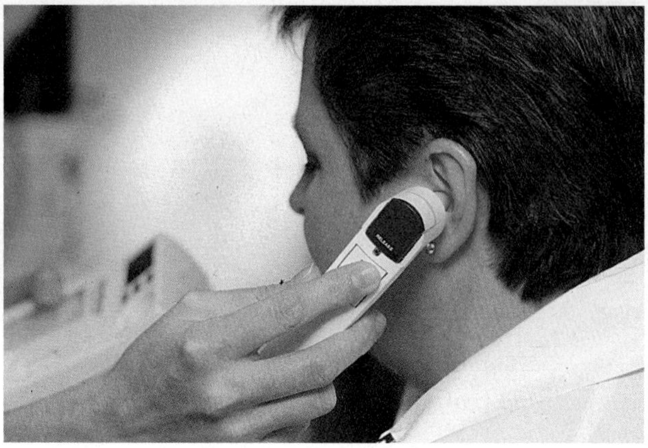

STEP **6D(5)c** Tympanic thermometer with probe cover inserted into auditory canal.

Steps	Rationale
(4) Slide clean disposable speculum cover over otoscope-like lens tip until it locks into place, being careful not to touch lens cover.	Lens cover must be unimpeded by dust, fingerprints, or earwax to ensure clear optical pathway.
(5) Insert speculum into ear canal following manufacturer's instructions for tympanic probe positioning:	Correct positioning of the probe with respect to ear canal ensures accurate readings.
a. Pull ear pinna backward, up, and out for an adult.	The ear tug straightens the external auditory canal, allowing maximum exposure of the tympanic membrane.
b. Move thermometer in a figure-eight pattern.	Some manufacturers recommend movement of the speculum tip in a figure-eight pattern, which allows the sensor to detect maximum tympanic membrane heat radiation.
c. Fit otoscope probe snugly into canal and do not move (see illustration).	Gentle pressure seals ear canal from ambient temperature, which can alter readings as much as 2.7° C.
d. Point speculum tip toward nose.	
(6) As soon as probe is in place, depress scan button on handheld unit. Leave thermometer probe in place until audible signal occurs and client's temperature appears on digital display.	Depression of scan button causes infrared energy to be detected. Otoscope tip must stay in place until signal occurs to ensure accurate reading.
(7) Carefully remove speculum from auditory meatus.	
(8) Push ejection button on handheld unit to discard plastic probe cover into appropriate receptacle.	Reduces transmission of microorganisms. Automatically causes digital reading to disappear.
(9) If a second reading is necessary, replace probe lens cover and wait 2 to 3 minutes before inserting the probe tip.	Lens cover must be free of cerumen to maintain optical path. Time allows ear canal to regain usual temperature (Giuliano et al., 2000).
(10) Return handheld unit to charging base.	Protects sensory tip from damage.
(11) Assist client in assuming a comfortable position.	Restores comfort and sense of well-being.
7. Perform hand hygiene.	Reduces transmission of microorganisms.
8. Discuss findings with client as needed.	Promotes participation in care and understanding of health status.
9. If temperature is assessed for the first time, establish temperature as baseline if it is within normal range.	Used to compare future temperature measurements.

Steps	Rationale
10. Compare temperature reading with client's previous baseline and acceptable temperature range for client's age group.	Normal body temperature fluctuates within narrow range; comparison reveals presence of abnormality. Improper placement or movement of thermometer can cause inaccuracies. Second measurement confirms initial findings of abnormal body temperature.

Unexpected Outcomes and Related Interventions

- Temperature 1° C above usual range
  - Assess possible sites (e.g., central line catheter, wounds, etc.) for localized infection and for related data suggesting a systemic infection.
  - Implement appropriate nursing measures (see Box 27-9).
- Persistent fever
  - Notify physician and administer antipyretic and antibiotics as ordered.
- Temperature 1° C below usual range
  - Remove any drafts, wet clothing, or linen.
  - Apply extra blankets, and, unless contraindicated, offer warm liquids.

Recording and Reporting

- Record temperature in nurses' notes or vital sign flow sheet. Measurement of temperature after administration of specific therapies should be documented in narrative form in nurses' notes.
- Report abnormal findings to nurse in charge or physician.

Home Care Considerations

- Assess temperature and ventilation of client's environment to determine existence of any environmental condition that may influence outcome of client's temperature.
- In the home, clients may continue to use mercury-in-glass thermometers (see Box 27-6). Assess safe storage of mercury-in-glass thermometers to protect from breakage and mercury spills. Educate client and caregiver about mercury hazards.

Box 27-5 Advantages and Disadvantages of Select Temperature Measurement Sites

Tympanic Membrane

Advantages

Easily accessible site
Minimal client repositioning required
Provides core reading
Very rapid measurement (2 to 5 seconds)
Can be obtained without disturbing or waking client
Eardrum close to hypothalamus; sensitive to core
Unaffected by oral intake of food, fluids, smoking
Can be used for tachypneic clients
Can be used in newborns to reduce infant handling and heat loss (Bailey & Rose, 2001)

Disadvantages

More variability of measurement than with other core temperature devices
Requires removal of hearing aids before measurement
Should not be used with clients who have had surgery of the ear or tympanic membrane
Requires disposable probe cover
Expensive
Does not accurately measure core temperature changes during and after exercise
Possible distortion of temperature readings for clients with otitis media
Cerumen impaction can lower readings (Giuliano et al., 2000)
Questions about measurement accuracy in newborns
Cannot obtain continuous measurement
Affected by ambient temperature devices such as incubators, radiant warmers, and facial fans (Giuliano et al., 2000)

Rectum

Advantages

Argued to be more reliable when oral temperature cannot be obtained

Disadvantages

May lag behind core temperature during rapid temperature changes (Giuliano et al., 2000)
Should not be used for children with diarrhea or clients who have had rectal surgery, a rectal disorder, or decreased platelets
Should not be used for routine vital signs in newborns
Requires positioning and may be source of client embarrassment and anxiety
Risk of body fluid exposure
Requires lubrication

Mouth

Advantages

Accessible; requires no position change
Comfortable for client
Provides accurate surface temperature reading
Reflects rapid change in core temperature
Acceptable route for clients with endotracheal tube in place (Fallis, 2000)

Continued

Box 27-5 Advantages and Disadvantages of Select Temperature Measurement Sites—cont'd

Mouth—cont'd

Disadvantages

Affected by ingestion of fluids or foods, smoke, and oxygen delivery
Should not be used with clients who have had oral surgery, trauma, history of epilepsy, or shaking chills
Should not be used with infants, small children, or confused, unconscious, or uncooperative clients
Risk of body fluid exposure

Axilla

Advantages

Safe and non-invasive
Can be used with newborns and unco-operative clients

Disadvantages

Long measurement time
Requires continuous positioning by nurse
Lags behind core temperature during rapid temperature changes
Requires exposure of thorax
Not recommended for detecting fever in infants and young children

Skin

Advantages

Inexpensive
Provides continuous reading
Safe and non-invasive
Does not require disturbing client
Can be used for neonates
Easy to read

Disadvantages

Lags behind other sites during temperature changes, especially during hyperthermia
Adhesion can be impaired by diaphoresis or sweat
Can be affected by environmental temperature
Unreliable during chill phase of fever

play unit. A sound signals when the peak temperature reading has been measured.

The greatest advantages of electronic thermometers are that they can be inserted immediately, their readings appear within seconds, and they are easy to read. The plastic sheath is unbreakable and ideal for children. Their expense is a major disadvantage. Maintaining cleanliness of the probes is an important consideration. If not properly cleaned between clients, gastrointestinal contamination of the rectal probe can be a vector of disease transmission. The thermometer must be wiped daily with alcohol, and the thermometer probe must be wiped with an alcohol swab after each client. Particular attention must be paid to the probe hub, which has ridges, where the probe cover is secured to the probe.

Disposable Thermometers. Disposable single-use thermometers are thin strips of plastic with a temperature sensor at one end. They are used for oral or axillary temperatures, particularly with children (Figure 27–5). They are useful when caring for clients on isolation precautions (see chapter 29) to avoid the need to take electronic instruments into client rooms. They are inserted the same way as an oral or axillary thermometer and used only once. Chemical dots on the thermometer change colour to reflect the temperature reading. The thermometer is removed after 60 seconds and read after waiting about 10 seconds to ensure the temperature reading has stabilized. Research has shown that disposable single-use thermometers tend to overestimate or underestimate true temperature readings (Erickson, Meyer, & Woo, 1996). As a result, the device is only recommended for screening purposes in adults. When an abnormal temperature is suspected, the temperature should be confirmed with an electronic thermometer.

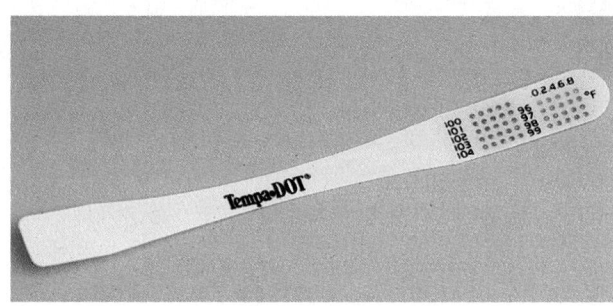

FIGURE **27–5** Disposable, single-use thermometer strip.

Another form of disposable thermometer is a temperature-sensitive patch or tape. Applied to the forehead or abdomen, the patch changes colour at different temperatures. These thermometers are also useful for screening clients, especially infants, for altered temperature. If an abnormal temperature is suspected, the temperature must be confirmed with an electronic temperature device. Disposable thermometers are not appropriate for monitoring temperature therapies.

Glass Thermometers. The mercury-in-glass thermometer is a glass tube sealed at one end with a mercury-filled bulb at the other. Exposure of the bulb to heat causes the mercury to expand and rise in the enclosed tube. The length of the thermometer is marked with Centigrade or Fahrenheit calibrations. Obtaining a temperature with a

Box 27-6 Procedural Guidelines

Use of a Mercury-in-Glass Thermometer

Equipment: Mercury-in-glass thermometer (rectal or oral), plastic sleeve, lubricating jelly (rectal only), disposable gloves.

Delegation Considerations: The skill of measuring body temperature can be delegated to unregulated care providers (see Skill 27-1).

1. Perform hand hygiene. Apply disposable gloves to avoid contact with body fluids (e.g., saliva, stool).
2. Hold end (if colour-coded, tip will be blue or red) of glass thermometer with fingertips to reduce contamination of bulb.
3. Read mercury level while gently rotating thermometer at eye level. If mercury is above desired level, grasp tip of thermometer securely, stand away from solid objects, and sharply flick wrist downward. Briskly shaking lowers mercury level in glass tube. Continue shaking until reading is below 35.6° C. Thermometer reading must be below client's actual temperature before use.
4. Insert thermometer into plastic sleeve cover to protect from body secretions (e.g., saliva, stool). Apply lubricant to cover 2.5 to 3.5 cm on rectal thermometer.
5. Place thermometer using technique appropriate to oral, rectal, or axillary site (see Skill 27-1).
6. Leave thermometer in place 3 minutes for oral or rectal temperature, 2 minutes for axillary temperature, or according to agency policy.
7. Remove the thermometer. Carefully discard the plastic sleeve. Wipe off secretions with clean tissue, moving toward the bulb.
8. Read thermometer at eye level, findings, store thermometer in storage container. Remove gloves and perform hand hygiene.

mercury-in-glass thermometer requires careful preparation of the device (Box 27-6). In addition to proper positioning of the thermometer using the oral, rectal, or axillary site, the nurse must maintain this position for the appropriate length of time to obtain an accurate reading. In addition to the time delay, the mercury-in-glass device is easily breakable and when broken, releases hazardous mercury. Although health care agencies no longer use glass thermometers, many clients may have mercury-in-glass thermometers in their homes. If a thermometer is broken or a mercury spill is suspected, the nurse is required to take immediate action (Box 27-7). It is also important to teach clients and their families what to do in the event of breakage of a mercury-in-glass thermometer.

NP Nursing Diagnosis

The nurse identifies assessment findings and clusters defining characteristics to form a nursing diagnosis. Nursing diagnoses for clients with body temperature alterations include the following:

Box 27-7 Steps to Take in the Event of a Mercury Spill

1. Do NOT touch spilled mercury droplets. If skin contact has occurred, immediately flush area with water for 15 minutes.
2. If possible, remove client from immediate contaminated environment.
3. Change any clothing or linen that has been contaminated with mercury. Perform hand hygiene thoroughly after changing. Wash clothing before reuse.
4. Notify the environmental services department or obtain a mercury spill kit if available.
5. Follow procedures for mercury removal as directed by Material Safety Data Sheet (MSDS). Spills are removed using special absorbent materials, filtered vacuum equipment, and protective clothing.
6. Promote exhaust ventilation to reduce concentration of mercury vapours.
7. Follow agency guideline for laundering clothing.
8. Complete incident report as directed by institution procedure.

- Risk for imbalanced body temperature
- Hyperthermia
- Hypothermia
- Ineffective thermoregulation

For example, an increase in body temperature, flushed skin, skin warm to touch, and tachycardia indicate the diagnosis *hyperthermia*. The nursing diagnosis will be stated as either an at-risk or actual temperature alteration. If the client possesses risk factors for temperature alterations, the nurse minimizes or eliminates them.

Once a diagnosis is determined, the nurse must accurately select the related factor or etiology (Box 27-8). The related factor allows the nurse to select appropriate nursing interventions. In the example of hyperthermia, a related factor of vigorous activity will result in much different interventions than a related factor of decreased ability to perspire.

NP Planning

During planning, the nurse integrates the knowledge gathered from assessment and the client history to develop an individualized care plan (see Care Plan). The nurse matches the client's needs with those interventions that are supported and recommended in the clinical research literature.

Goals and Outcomes. The care plan for a client with alteration in temperature must include realistic and individualized goals along with relevant outcomes. The nurse must collaborate closely with the client in setting goals and outcomes and choosing nursing interventions. Expected outcomes are established to gauge progress toward returning the body temperature to an acceptable range. If the temperature alteration requires the nurse to help the client modify the environment, goals may be long term (e.g., obtaining appropriate clothing to wear in cold weather). Short-term goals, such as regaining normal

Nursing Diagnostic Process Box 27-8

Activities	Defining Characteristics Assessment	Nursing Diagnosis
Obtain vital signs, including temperature, pulse, respirations, SpO_2.	Increased body temperature above usual range Tachycardia Tachypnea Hypoxemia	Ineffective thermoregulation related to aging and inability to adapt to environmental temperature
Palpate skin.	Warm, dry skin	
Observe client's appearance and behaviour while talking and resting.	Restlessness Confusion Flushed appearance	
Review medical history.	Found in unventilated apartment during heat wave; 85 years old with history of dementia	

range of body temperature, may be helpful in improving client health. Outcomes must relate to what the nurse learns about the client. For example, if a client has had excessive diaphoresis during a fever episode, an outcome for the goal of attaining fluid and electrolyte balance might be stated, "Client intake and output will be equal for the next 24 hours."

Setting Priorities. The severity of a temperature alteration and its effects, together with the client's general health status, influence the nurse's care priorities. Safety is a top priority. Often, other medical problems complicate the care plan. For instance, alterations in body temperature affect the body's requirements for fluids. Clients with heart problems may have difficulty tolerating required fluid replacement therapy.

Continuity of Care. Clients at high risk for alterations in body temperature require an individualized care plan directed at maintaining normothermia (normal body temperature) and reducing risk factors. For example, the outcome of care may be that the client can explain actions to take during a heat wave. The nurse teaches the client and caregiver the importance of thermoregulation and actions to take during very hot weather. Education is particularly important for parents, who need to know how to take action at home when an infant or child develops a temperature alteration.

Implementation

Health Promotion. Health promotion for clients at risk for altered body temperature is directed toward promoting balance between heat production and heat loss. Client activity, temperature of the environment, and clothing are all considered. The nurse teaches clients to avoid strenuous exercise in hot, humid weather; to drink fluids such as water or clear fruity juices before, during, and after exercise; to wear light, loose-fitting, light-coloured clothes; to avoid exercising in areas with poor ventilation; to wear a protective covering over the head when outdoors; and to expose themselves to hot climates gradually.

Prevention is the key for clients at risk for hypothermia. Prevention involves educating clients, family members, and friends. Clients most at risk include the very young and the very old and people debilitated by trauma, stroke, diabetes, drug or alcohol intoxication, sepsis, and Raynaud's disease. Mentally ill or disabled clients may acquire hypothermia because they are unaware of the dangers of cold conditions. People without adequate home heating, shelter, diet, or clothing are also at risk. Fatigue, skin colour (Black Canadians are more susceptible), malnutrition, hypoxemia, and body piercing also contribute to the risk of frostbite.

Acute Care

Fever. When an elevated body temperature develops, the nurse initiates interventions to treat fever. The objective of therapy is to increase heat loss, reduce heat production, and prevent complications.

The procedures used to intervene and treat the temperature depend on the cause, any adverse effects, and the strength, intensity, and duration of the elevation. The nurse plays a key role in assessing and implementing temperature-reducing strategies (Box 27-9). The physician may try to determine the cause of the elevated temperature by isolating the causative pyrogen. The nurse may be asked to obtain necessary culture specimens for laboratory analysis such as urine, blood, sputum, and wound sites (see chapter 29). The physician will order antibiotic medications to be given after the cultures have been obtained. Administering antibiotics destroys pyrogenic bacteria and eliminates the body's stimulus for the elevated temperature.

Most fevers in children are viral, last only briefly, and have limited effects. However, children still have immature temperature-control mechanisms and temperatures can rise rapidly. Dehydration and febrile seizures can occur during rising temperatures of children between 6 months and 3 years of age. Febrile seizures are unusual in children over 5 years of age. The extent of the temperature, often exceeding 38.8° C, seems to be more important than the rapidity of the temperature increase. Children are at particular risk for fluid volume deficit because they can quickly lose large amounts of fluids in

Nursing Care Plan

Hyperthermia

Assessment

Mr. Coburn is a 45-year-old teacher who arrives at the outpatient clinic with the complaint of malaise.

Assessment Activities	Findings/Defining Characteristics
Palpate skin.	Mr. Coburn's skin is warm and dry to touch.
Observe client's behaviour while talking and resting.	Mr. Coburn appears to have laboured breathing. His face is flushed.
Obtain vital signs.	Blood pressure right arm 116/62, left arm 114/64; right radial pulse 128, regular and bounding; respiratory rate 26; SpO_2 98% on room air; oral temperature 39.2° C.
Review medical history.	He reports smoking one pack of cigarettes per day and recently began expectorating yellow-green sputum. He has been tired for the past 3 days and upon rising in the morning has been dizzy.

Nursing Diagnosis: Hyperthermia related to infectious process.

Planning

Goals	Expected Outcomes*
	Thermoregulation
Client will regain normal range of body temperature within next 24 hours.	Body temperature will decline at least 1° C within next 8 hours.
Client will attain sense of comfort and rest within next 48 hours.	Client will verbalize increased satisfaction with rest and sleep pattern.
	Client will report increase in energy level within next 3 days.
	Vital Signs
Fluid and electrolyte balance will be maintained during next 3 days.	Intake will equal output within next 24 hours. No evidence of postural hypotension during ambulation.

*Outcome classification labels from *Nursing Outcomes Classification (NOC)* (3rd ed.), edited by S. Moorhead, M. Johnson, and M. L. Maas, 2004, St. Louis, MO: Mosby.

Interventions†	Rationale
Fever Treatment	
• Instruct client to reduce external coverings and keep clothing and bed linen dry.	Promotes heat loss through conduction and convection.
• Instruct client to monitor temperature at home and administer acetaminophen every 4 hours as ordered for temperature over 39° C.	Antipyretics reduce set point.
• Instruct client to limit physical activity and increase frequency of rest periods over next 2 days.	Activity and stress increase metabolic rate, contributing to heat production.
• Instruct client to increase oral fluids of choice.	Fluids lost through insensible water loss require replacement.

†Intervention classification labels from *Nursing Interventions Classification (NIC)* (4th ed.), edited by J. M. Dochterman and G. M. Bulechek, 2004, St. Louis, MO: Mosby.

Evaluation

Nursing Actions	Client Response/Finding	Achievement of Outcome
Obtain orthostatic blood pressure measurements.	Blood pressure measurements lying, sitting, and standing are within 5 mm Hg of each other.	Fluid volume status adequate.
Ask Mr. Coburn if he has had any episodes of dizziness.	Mr. Coburn denies dizziness.	
Review Mr. Coburn's fluid record.	Increased consumption of oral fluids.	Fluid volume status adequate.
Ask Mr. Coburn if his energy level has changed since the last visit.	He responds, "I am sleeping much better and have returned to work with a lot more energy."	Improved rest and sleep pattern and increased energy level.

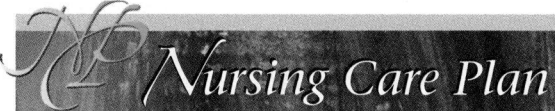

Box 27-9 Nursing Measures for Clients with a Fever

Assessment

- Obtain core temperature during each phase of febrile episode.
- Assess for contributing factors such as dehydration, infection, or environmental temperature.
- Identify physiological response to temperature.
  - Obtain all vital signs.
  - Observe skin colour.
  - Assess skin temperature.
  - Observe for shivering and diaphoresis.
  - Assess client comfort and well-being.
- Determine phase of fever: chill, plateau, fever break.

Intervention (Unless Contraindicated)

- Obtain blood cultures when ordered. Blood specimens are obtained to coincide with temperature spikes when the antigen-producing organism is most prevalent.
- Initiate therapies to minimize heat production.
  - Reduce the frequency of activities that increase oxygen demand such as excessive turning and ambulation.
  - Allow rest periods.
  - Limit physical activity.
- Initiate therapies to maximize heat loss.
  - Reduce external covering on client's body to promote heat loss through radiation and conduction. Do not induce shivering.
  - Keep clothing and bed linen dry to increase heat loss through conduction and convection.
- Initiate therapies to meet requirements for increased metabolic rate.
  - Provide supplemental oxygen therapy as ordered to improve oxygen delivery to body cells.
  - Provide measures to stimulate appetite and offer well-balanced meals.
  - Provide fluids (at least 3 L per day for client with normal cardiac and renal function) to replace fluids lost through insensible water loss and sweating.
- Initiate therapies to promote client comfort.
  - Encourage oral hygiene because oral mucous membranes dry easily from dehydration.
  - Control temperature of the environment without inducing shivering.
- Identify onset and duration of febrile episode phases.
- Examine previous temperature measurements for trends.
- Initiate health teaching as indicated.

proportion to their body weight. The nurse maintains accurate intake and output records and encourages fluids.

A fever may be a hypersensitivity response to a drug. Drug fevers can be accompanied by other allergy symptoms such as rash or pruritus (itching). Treatment involves withdrawing the medication.

Antipyretics are drugs that reduce fever. Nonsteroidal drugs such as acetaminophen, salicylates, indomethacin, and ketorolac reduce fever by increasing heat loss. Corticosteroids reduce heat production by interfering with the immune system and can mask signs of infection. Corticosteroids are not used to treat a fever. However, the nurse must be aware of their effect on suppressing the client's ability to develop a fever in response to a pyrogen.

Non-pharmacological therapy for fever involves methods that increase heat loss by evaporation, conduction, convection, or radiation. Traditionally, nurses have used tepid sponge baths, bathing with alcohol water solutions, applying ice packs to axillae and groin areas, and cooling fans. These therapies should be avoided because they lead to shivering. There is no demonstrated advantage of these methods over antipyretic medications. Blankets cooled by circulating water delivered by motorized units increase conductive heat loss. The nurse must follow manufacturer's instructions for applying these hypothermia blankets because of the risk for skin breakdown and "freeze burns." Placing a bath blanket between the client and the hypothermia blanket and wrapping distal extremities (fingers, toes, and genitalia) is recommended to reduce the risk of injury to the skin and tissue from hypothermia therapy.

Nursing measures to enhance body cooling must avoid stimulating shivering. Shivering is counterproductive and can increase energy expenditure up to 400%. Wrapping the client's extremities has been recommended to reduce the incidence and intensity of shivering. A dependent nursing intervention for shivering may involve giving medications (e.g., meperidine or butorphanol) that can reduce shivering.

Heatstroke. Heatstroke is an emergency. First aid treatment for heatstroke includes moving the client to a cooler environment, reducing clothing covering the body, placing cool wet towels over the skin, and using oscillating fans to increase convective heat loss. Emergency medical treatment may include intravenous (IV) fluids, irrigating the stomach and lower bowel with cool solutions, and hypothermia blankets.

Hypothermia. The priority treatment for hypothermia is to prevent a further decrease in body temperature. Removing wet clothes, replacing them with dry clothes, and wrapping the client in blankets is a key nursing intervention. In emergencies away from a health care setting, the client lies under blankets next to a warm person. A conscious person benefits from drinking hot liquids such as soup, while avoiding alcohol and caffeinated fluids. Other measures include keeping the head covered, placing the client near a fire or in a warm room, or placing heating pads next to areas of the body (head and neck) that lose heat the quickest.

Restorative and Continuing Care

The nurse educates the client who has been febrile about the importance of taking and continuing any antibiotics as directed until the course of treatment is completed. Children and older adults are at risk for fluid volume deficit because they can quickly lose large amounts of fluids in proportion to their body weight. Identifying preferred fluids and encouraging oral fluid intake is an important ongoing nursing intervention.

Evaluation

All nursing interventions are evaluated by comparing the client's actual response to the expected outcomes of the care plan. This reveals whether goals of care have been met or if a revision to the plan is needed. After any intervention, the nurse measures the client's temperature to evaluate for change. In addition, the nurse uses other evaluative measures such as palpation of the skin and assessment of pulse and respirations. If therapies are effective, body temperature will return to an acceptable range, other vital signs will stabilize, and the client will report a sense of comfort.

Pulse

The pulse is the palpable bounding of blood flow noted at various points on the body. Blood flows through the body in a continuous circuit. The pulse is an indicator of circulatory status.

Physiology and Regulation

Electrical impulses originating from the sinoatrial node travel through heart muscle to stimulate cardiac contraction. Approximately 60 to 70 mL of blood enters the aorta with each ventricular contraction **(stroke volume).** With each stroke volume ejection, the walls of the aorta distend, creating a pulse wave that travels rapidly toward the distal ends of the arteries. The pulse wave moves 15 times faster through the aorta and 100 times faster through the small arteries than the ejected volume of blood. When a pulse wave reaches a peripheral artery, it can be felt by palpating the artery lightly against underlying bone or muscle. The pulse is the palpable bounding of the blood flow in the peripheral artery. The number of pulsing sensations occurring in 1 minute is the pulse rate.

The volume of blood pumped by the heart during 1 minute is the **cardiac output,** the product of heart rate and the ventricle's stroke volume. In an adult, the heart normally pumps 5,000 mL of blood per minute. A change in heart rate or stroke volume does not always change the heart's output or the amount of blood in the arteries. For example, if a person's heart rate is 70 beats per minute and the stroke volume is 70 mL, the cardiac output is 4,900 mL per minute. What happens if the heart rate drops to 60 beats per minute and the stroke volume rises to 85 mL (Box 27-10)?

Mechanical, neural, and chemical factors regulate the strength of heart contractions and its stroke volume. However, when mechanical, neural, or chemical factors are unable to alter stroke volume, a change in heart rate will result in a change in blood pressure. As heart rate increases, there is less time for the heart to fill. As heart rate increases without a change in stroke volume, blood pressure will decrease. As the heart rate slows, filling time is

Box 27-10 Cardiac Output Determination

Pulse rate × Stroke volume = Cardiac output
70 beats per minute × 70 mL/beat = 4.9 L/minute
60 beats per minute × 85 mL/beat = 5.1 L/minute

increased and blood pressure increases. The inability of blood pressure to respond to increases or decreases in heart rate may indicate a health deviation and must be reported to the physician.

The cause of an abnormally slow, rapid, or irregular pulse may alter cardiac output. The nurse assesses the heart's ability to meet the demands of the body's tissue for nutrients by palpating a peripheral pulse or by using a stethoscope to listen to heart sounds (apical rate).

Assessment of Pulse

Any artery can be assessed for pulse rate, but the radial and carotid arteries are commonly used because they are easily palpated. When a client's condition suddenly worsens, the carotid site is recommended for quickly finding a pulse. The heart will continue delivering blood through the carotid artery to the brain as long as possible. When cardiac output declines significantly, peripheral pulses weaken and are difficult to palpate.

The radial and apical locations are the most common sites for pulse rate assessment. People who are learning to monitor their own heart rates use the radial pulse (e.g., athletes, people taking heart medications, and clients starting a prescribed exercise regimen). If the **radial pulse** at the wrist is abnormal or intermittent resulting from dysrhythmias, or if it is inaccessible because of a dressing or cast, the apical pulse is assessed. When a client takes medication that affects the heart rate, the apical pulse may provide a more accurate assessment of heart function. The brachial or apical pulse is the best site for assessing an infant's or young child's pulse because other peripheral pulses are deep and difficult to palpate accurately.

Assessment of other peripheral pulse sites such as the brachial or femoral artery is unnecessary when routinely obtaining vital signs. Other peripheral pulses are assessed when a complete physical is conducted, when surgery or treatment has impaired blood flow to a body part, or when there are clinical indications of impaired peripheral blood flow (see chapter 28). Table 27-1 summarizes pulse sites and criteria for measurement. Skill 27-2 outlines pulse rate assessment.

Use of a Stethoscope. When assessing the apical rate, the nurse uses a stethoscope (Figure 27–6). The five major parts of the stethoscope are the earpieces, binaurals, tubing, bell chestpiece, and diaphragm chestpiece.

The plastic or rubber earpieces should fit snugly and comfortably in the nurse's ears. The binaurals should be angled and strong enough so that the earpieces stay firmly in the ears without causing discomfort. To ensure the best reception of sound, the earpieces follow the con-

Table 27-1 Pulse Sites

Site	Location	Assessment Criteria
Temporal	Over temporal bone of head, above and lateral to eye	Easily accessible site used to assess pulse in children
Carotid	Along medial edge of sternocleidomastoid muscle in neck	Easily accessible site used during physiological shock or cardiac arrest when other sites are not palpable
Apical	Fourth to fifth intercostal space at left midclavicular line	Site used to auscultate for apical pulse
Brachial	Groove between biceps and triceps muscles at antecubital fossa	Site used to assess status of circulation to lower arm Site used to auscultate blood pressure
Radial	Radial or thumb side of forearm at wrist	Common site used to assess character of pulse peripherally and assess status of circulation to hand
Ulnar	Ulnar side of forearm at wrist	Site used to assess status of circulation to hand; also used to perform an Allen's test
Femoral	Below inguinal ligament, midway between symphysis pubis and anterior superior iliac spine	Site used to assess character of pulse during physiological shock or cardiac arrest when other pulses are not palpable; used to assess status of circulation to leg
Popliteal	Behind knee in popliteal fossa	Site used to assess status of circulation to lower leg
Posterior tibial	Inner side of ankle, below medial malleolus	Site used to assess status of circulation to foot
Dorsalis pedis	Along top of foot, between extension tendons of great and first toe	Site used to assess status of circulation to foot

tour of the ear canal pointing toward the face when the stethoscope is in place.

The polyvinyl tubing should be flexible and 30 to 40 cm long. Longer tubing decreases the transmission of sound waves. The tubing should be thick walled and moderately rigid to eliminate transmission of environmental noise and to prevent the tubing from kinking, which distorts sound wave transmission. Stethoscopes can have single or dual tubes.

The chestpiece consists of a bell and a diaphragm that are rotated into position. The diaphragm or bell must be in proper position during use to hear sounds through the stethoscope. The nurse can test the position of the chestpiece by tapping lightly on the diaphragm to determine which side is functioning. The diaphragm is the circular, flat portion of the chestpiece covered with a thin plastic disk. It transmits high-pitched sounds created by the high-velocity movement of air and blood. Bowel, lung, and heart sounds are auscultated using the diaphragm. The nurse positions the diaphragm to make a tight seal against the client's skin (Figure 27–7). Enough pressure is exerted to leave a temporary red ring on the client's skin when the diaphragm is removed.

The bell is the bowl-shaped chestpiece usually surrounded by a rubber ring. The ring avoids chilling the client with cold metal when placed on the skin. The bell transmits low-pitched sounds created by the low-velocity movement of blood. Heart and vascular sounds are auscultated using the bell. The nurse applies the bell lightly, resting the chestpiece on the skin (Figure 27–8). Compressing the bell against the skin reduces low-pitched sound amplification and creates a "diaphragm of skin." Some stethoscopes have one chestpiece that combines the features of the bell and diaphragm. When the nurse uses light pressure, the chestpiece is a bell, whereas exerting more pressure converts the bell into a diaphragm.

The stethoscope is a delicate instrument and requires proper care for optimal function. The earpieces should be removed regularly and cleaned of cerumen (earwax). The bell and diaphragm are cleaned of dust, lint, and body oils. The tubing is cleaned with mild soap and water. Nurses are encouraged to have their own stethoscope. However, if several nurses use the same stethoscope, the earpieces should be cleansed with an antiseptic before use.

Character of the Pulse

Assessment of the radial pulse includes measurement of the rate, rhythm, strength, and equality. When auscultating an apical pulse, the nurse assesses rate and rhythm only.

Rate. Before measuring a pulse, the nurse reviews the client's baseline rate for comparison (Table 27-2). Some practitioners prefer to make baseline measurements of the pulse rate as the client assumes a sitting, standing, and lying position. Postural changes cause changes in pulse rate because of alterations in blood volume and sympathetic activity. The heart rate temporarily increases when a person changes from a lying to a sitting or standing position.

When assessing the pulse, the nurse must consider the variety of factors influencing the pulse rate (Table 27-3). A single factor or a combination of these factors may cause significant changes. If the nurse detects an abnormal rate while palpating a peripheral pulse, the next step is to assess the apical rate. The apical rate requires auscultation of heart sounds, which provides a more accurate assessment of cardiac contraction.

The nurse assesses the apical rate by listening for heart sounds (see chapter 28). The nurse tries to identify the first and second heart sounds (S_1 and S_2). At normal slow rates, S_1 is low pitched and dull, sounding like a "lub." S_2 is higher pitched and shorter, creating the sound "dub." Each set of "lub-dub" is counted as one heartbeat. Using the diaphragm or bell of the stethoscope, the nurse counts the number of lub-dubs occurring in 1 minute.

Text continued on p. 588

Skill 27-2 Assessing the Radial and Apical Pulses

View Video

Delegation Considerations

The skill of pulse measurement can be delegated to unregulated care providers (UCPs). The nurse is responsible for assessing changes in pulse. It is important for the nurse to do the following:

- Inform the UCP of client history or risk for irregular pulse.
- Inform the UCP of frequency of pulse measurement for select client.
- Determine that the UCP is aware of the usual values for the client.
- Inform the UCP of the abnormalities that should be reported to the nurse.

Equipment

- Stethoscope (apical pulse only)
- Wristwatch with second hand or digital display
- Pen, vital sign flow sheet or record form
- Alcohol swab

Steps	Rationale
1. Determine need to assess radial or apical pulse:	Nurse uses clinical judgment to determine need for assessment.
a. Note risk factors for alterations in apical pulse.	Certain conditions place clients at risk for pulse alterations. Heart rhythm can be affected by heart disease, cardiac dysrhythmias, onset of sudden chest pain or acute pain from any site, invasive cardiovascular diagnostic tests, surgery, sudden infusion of large volume of IV fluid, internal or external hemorrhage, and administration of medications that alter heart function.
b. Assess for signs and symptoms of altered stroke volume and cardiac output, such as dyspnea, fatigue, chest pain, orthopnea, syncope, palpitations (person's unpleasant awareness of heartbeat), jugular venous distension, edema of dependent body parts, cyanosis or pallor of skin.	Physical signs and symptoms may indicate alteration in cardiac function.
2. Assess for factors that normally influence pulse rate and rhythm: age, exercise, position changes, fluid balance, medications, temperature, sympathetic stimulation.	Allows nurse to accurately assess presence and significance of pulse alterations.
3. Determine previous baseline apical rate (if available) from client's record. Otherwise, note baseline radial rate.	Allows nurse to assess for change in condition. Provides comparison with future apical pulse measurements.
4. Explain that pulse or heart rate is to be assessed. Encourage client to relax and not speak.	Activity and anxiety can elevate heart rate. Client's voice interferes with nurse's ability to hear sound when apical pulse is measured.
5. Perform hand hygiene.	Reduces transmission of microorganisms.
6. If necessary, draw curtain around bed and/or close door.	Maintains privacy.
7. Obtain pulse measurement.	
A. Radial pulse	
(1) Assist client in assuming a supine or sitting position.	Provides easy access to pulse sites.
(2) If supine, place client's forearm straight alongside body or across lower chest or upper abdomen with wrist extended straight (see illustration). If sitting, bend client's elbow 90 degrees and support lower arm on chair or on nurse's arm. Slightly flex the wrist with palm down (see illustration).	Relaxed position of lower arm and slight flexion of wrist promotes exposure of artery to palpation without restriction.
(3) Place tips of first two fingers of hand over groove along radial or thumb side of client's inner wrist (see illustration).	Fingertips are most sensitive parts of hand to palpate arterial pulsation. Nurse's thumb has pulsation that may interfere with accuracy.
(4) Lightly compress against radius, obliterate pulse initially, and then relax pressure so that pulse becomes easily palpable.	Pulse is more accurately assessed with moderate pressure. Too much pressure occludes pulse and impairs blood flow.

Skill 27-2 Assessing the Radial and Apical Pulses—cont'd

Steps	Rationale

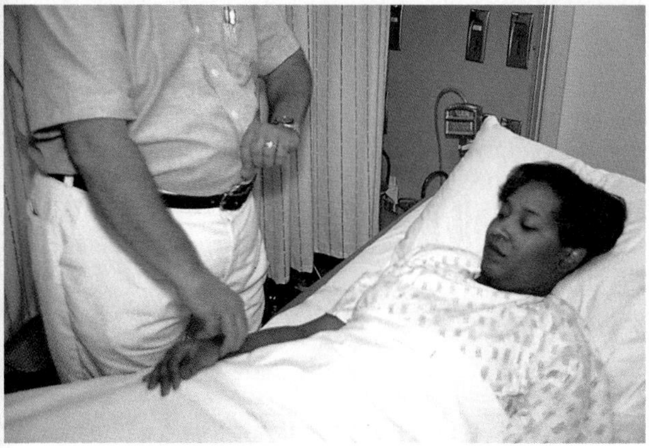

STEP **7A(2)** Pulse check with client's forearm at side with wrist extended.

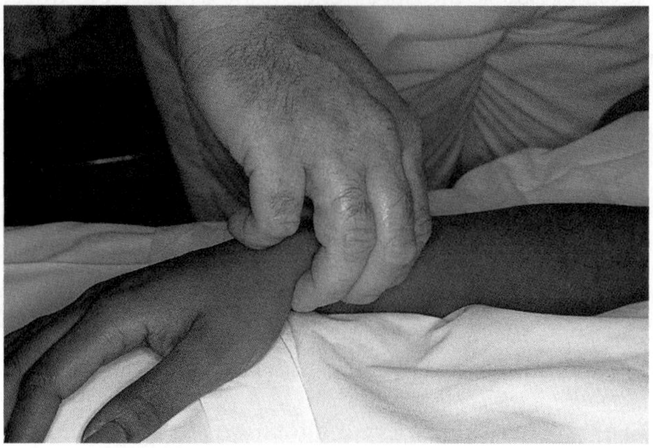

STEP **7A(3)** Hand placement for pulse checks.

Steps	Rationale
(5) Determine strength of pulse. Note whether thrust of vessel against fingertips is bounding, strong, weak, or thready.	Strength reflects volume of blood ejected against arterial wall with each heart contraction.
(6) After pulse can be felt regularly, look at watch's second hand and begin to count rate: When sweep hand hits number on dial, start counting with zero, then one, two, and so on.	Rate is determined accurately only after nurse is assured pulse can be palpated. Timing begins with zero. Count of one is first beat palpated after timing begins.
(7) If pulse is regular, count rate for 30 seconds and multiply total by 2.	A 30-second count is accurate for rapid, slow, or regular pulse rates.
(8) If pulse is irregular, count rate for 1 minute (60 seconds). Assess frequency and pattern of irregularity.	Inefficient contraction of heart fails to transmit pulse wave, interfering with cardiac output and resulting in irregular pulse. Longer time ensures accurate count.

Critical Decision Point: If pulse is irregular, do an apical/radial pulse assessment to detect a pulse deficit. Count apical pulse while colleague counts radial pulse. Begin apical pulse count out loud to simultaneously assess pulses. If pulse count differs by more than 2, a pulse deficit exists.

B. Apical pulse

Steps	Rationale
(1) Assist client to supine or sitting position. Move aside bed linen and gown to expose sternum and left side of chest.	Exposes portion of chest wall for selection of auscultatory site.
(2) Locate anatomical landmarks to identify the point of maximal impulse (PMI), also called the apical impulse (see illustrations a–d). Heart is located behind and to left of sternum with base at top and apex at bottom. Find angle of Louis just below suprasternal notch between sternal body and manubrium; can be felt as a bony prominence (illustration a). Slip fingers down each side of angle to find second intercostal space (ICS; illustration b). Carefully move fingers down left side of sternum to fifth ICS (illustration c) and laterally to the left midclavicular line (MCL; illustration d). A light tap felt within an area 1 to 2 cm of the PMI is reflected from the apex of the heart.	Use of anatomical landmarks allows correct placement of stethoscope over apex of heart, enhancing ability to hear heart sounds clearly. If unable to palpate the PMI, reposition client on left side. In the presence of serious heart disease, the PMI may be located to the left of the MCL or at the sixth ICS.

Steps	Rationale

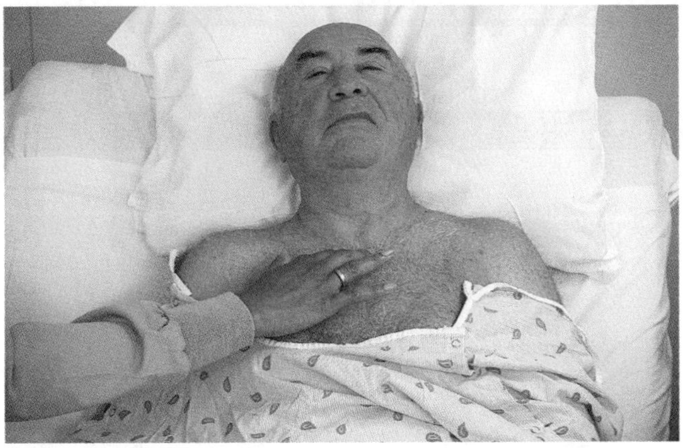

STEP **7B(2)a** Locating the angle of Louis.

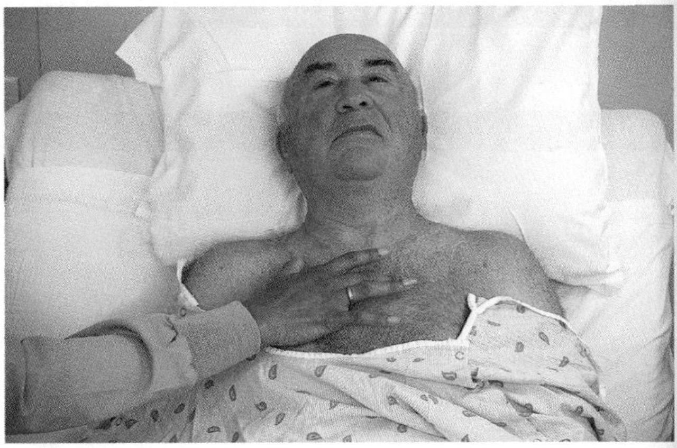

STEP **7B(2)b** Locating the second intercostal space (ICS).

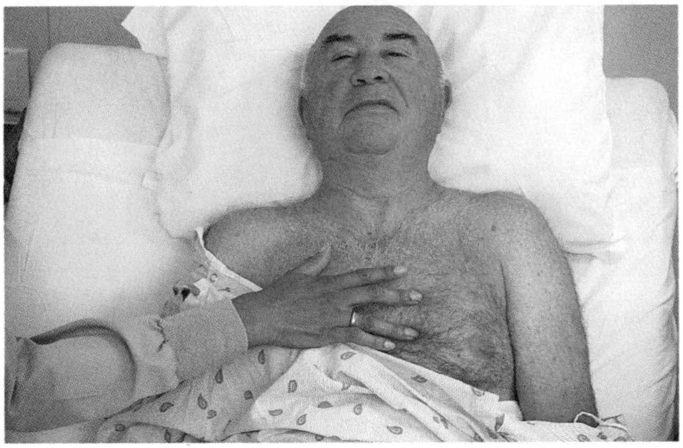

STEP **7B(2)c** Locating the fifth ICS.

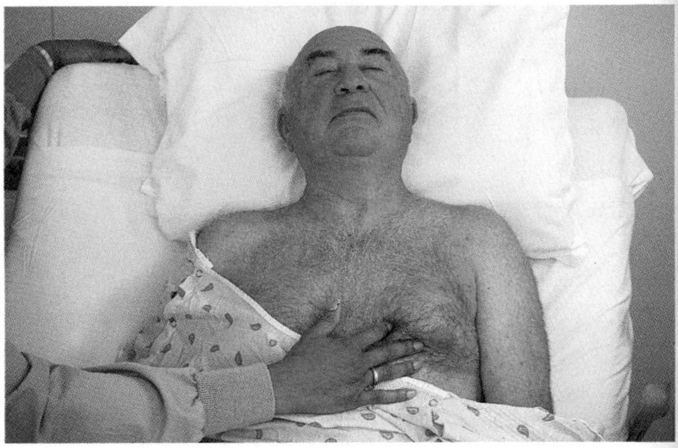

STEP **7B(2)d** Identifying the midclavicular line (MCL).

Steps	Rationale
(3) Place diaphragm of stethoscope in palm of hand for 5 to 10 seconds.	Warming of metal or plastic diaphragm prevents client from being startled and promotes comfort.
(4) Place diaphragm of stethoscope over PMI at the fifth ICS, at left MCL, and auscultate for normal S_1 and S_2 heart sounds (heard as "lub-dub"; see illustrations).	Allow stethoscope tubing to extend straight without kinks that would distort sound transmission. Normal sounds S_1 and S_2 are high pitched and best heard with the diaphragm.
(5) When S_1 and S_2 are heard with regularity, use watch's second hand and begin to count rate: When sweep hand hits number on dial, start counting with zero, then one, two, and so on.	Apical rate is determined accurately only after nurse is able to auscultate sounds clearly. Timing begins with zero. Count of one is first sound auscultated after timing begins.
(6) If apical rate is regular, count for 30 seconds and multiply by 2.	Regular apical rate can be assessed within 30 seconds.
(7) If heart rate is irregular or client is receiving cardiovascular medication, count for 1 minute (60 seconds).	Irregular rate is more accurately assessed when measured over longer interval.
(8) Note regularity of any dysrhythmia (S_1 and S_2 occurring early or later after previous sequence of sounds; for example, every third or every fourth beat is skipped).	Regular occurrence of dysrhythmia within 1 minute may indicate inefficient contraction of heart and alteration in cardiac output.
(9) Replace client's gown and bed linen; assist client in returning to comfortable position.	Restores comfort and promotes sense of well-being.

Skill 27-2 *Assessing the Radial and Apical Pulses—cont'd*

Steps	Rationale

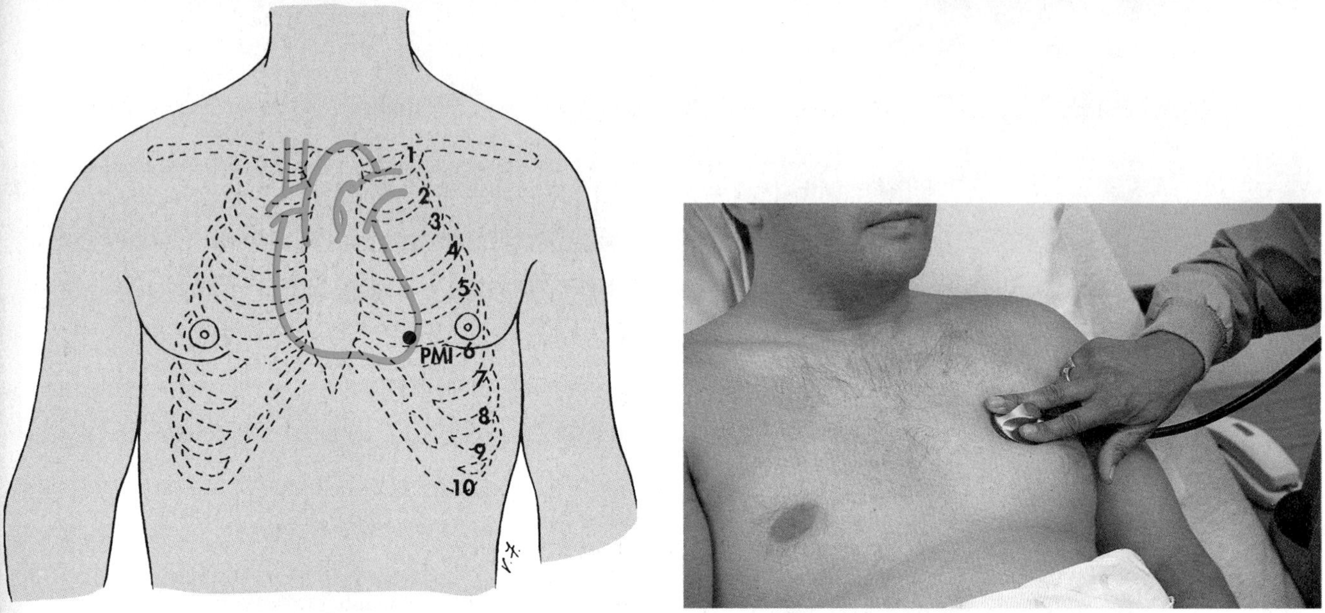

A B

STEP **7B(4)** **A,** Location of PMI in adult. **B,** Stethoscope over PMI.

Steps	Rationale
(10) Clean earpieces and diaphragm of stethoscope with alcohol swab as needed.	Controls transmission of microorganisms when nurses share stethoscope.
8. Perform hand hygiene.	Reduces transmission of microorganisms.
9. Discuss findings with client as needed.	Promotes participation in care and understanding of health status.
10. Compare readings with previous baseline and/or acceptable range of heart rate for client's age (see Table 27-2).	Evaluates for change in condition and alterations.
11. Compare peripheral pulse rate with apical rate and note discrepancy.	Differences between measurements indicate pulse deficit and may warn of cardiovascular compromise. Abnormalities may require therapy.
12. Compare radial pulse equality and note discrepancy.	Differences between radial arteries indicate compromised peripheral vascular system.
13. Correlate pulse rate with data obtained from blood pressure and related signs and symptoms (palpitations, dizziness).	Pulse rate and blood pressure are interrelated.

Unexpected Outcomes and Related Interventions

- Radial pulse is weak and thready.
  - Assess both radial pulses and compare findings. Local obstruction to one extremity (e.g., clot, edema) may decrease peripheral blood flow.
  - Perform complete assessment of all pulses (see chapter 28).
  - Observe for symptoms associated with decreased tissue perfusion (e.g., pallor and cool skin temperature of tissue distal to the weak pulse).
  - Measure apical and radial pulse simultaneously to determine presence of pulse deficit.
- Apical pulse is greater than 100 beats/minute (tachycardia).
  - Assess for presence of fever, anxiety, pain, recent exercise, hypotension, decreased oxygenation, or dehydration, all of which can elevate pulse.

- Obtain complete vital signs.
- Assess for factors associated with decreased cardiac output (e.g., chest pain, dyspnea, dizziness).

• Apical pulse is less than 60 beats/minute (bradycardia).
  - Assess for the presence of factors that may alter heart rate (e.g., digoxin or other cardiac medications). It may be necessary to withhold prescribed medications until the physician can evaluate the need to adjust dosage.
  - Assess for factors associated with decreased cardiac output.

Recording and Reporting

• Record pulse rate with assessment site in nurses' notes or vital signs flow sheet. Measurement of pulse rate after administration of specific therapies should be documented in narrative form in nurses' notes.
• Report abnormal findings to nurse in charge or physician.

Home Care Considerations

• Assess home environment to determine room that will afford quiet environment for auscultating apical rate.

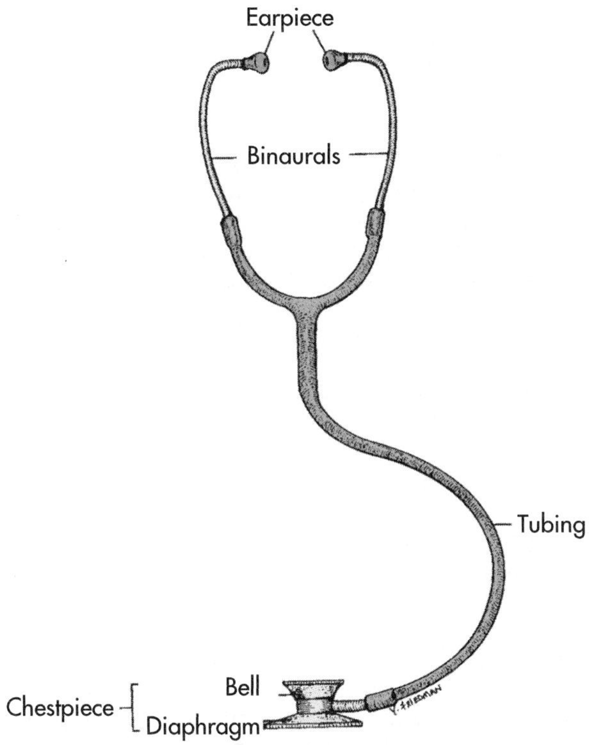

FIGURE **27–6** Parts of a stethoscope.

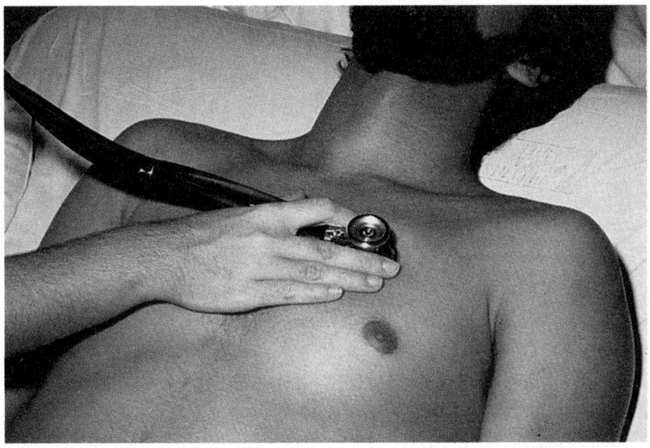

FIGURE **27–7** Positioning the diaphragm of the stethoscope firmly and securely when auscultating high-pitched heart sounds.

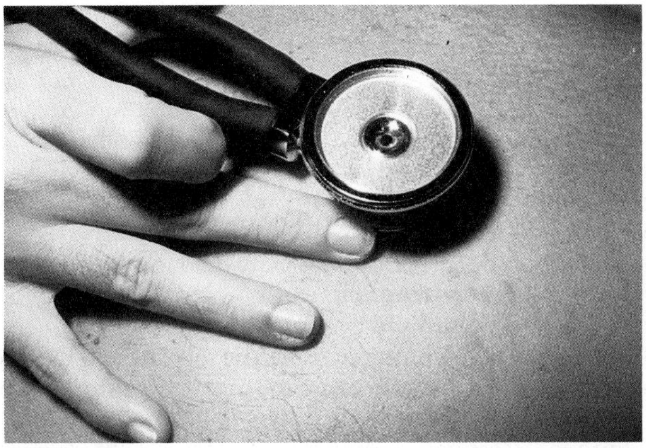

FIGURE **27–8** Positioning the bell of the stethoscope lightly on the skin to hear low-pitched heart sounds.

Table 27-2 Acceptable Ranges of Heart Rate

Age	Heart Rate (Beats per Minute)
Infant	120–160
Toddler	90–140
Preschooler	80–110
School-age child	75–100
Adolescent	60–90
Adult	60–100

Data from *AACN's Clinical Reference for Critical Care Nursing* (4th ed.), by M. R. Kinney et al., 1998, St. Louis, MO: Mosby.

Table 27-3 Factors Influencing Pulse Rates

Factor	Increases Pulse Rate	Decreases Pulse Rate
Exercise	Short-term exercise.	A conditioned athlete will have a lower heart rate at rest.
Temperature	Fever and heat.	Hypothermia.
Emotions	Acute pain and anxiety increase sympathetic stimulation, affecting heart rate.	Unrelieved severe pain increases parasympathetic stimulation, affecting heart rate; relaxation.
Drugs	Positive chronotropic drugs such as epinephrine.	Negative chronotropic drugs such as digitalis; beta and calcium blockers.
Hemorrhage	Loss of blood increases sympathetic stimulation.	
Postural changes	Standing or sitting.	
Pulmonary conditions	Diseases causing poor oxygenation such as asthma, chronic obstructive pulmonary disease (COPD).	Lying down.

Peripheral and apical pulse rate assessment may reveal variations in heart rate. Two common abnormalities in pulse rate are tachycardia and bradycardia. **Tachycardia** is an abnormally elevated heart rate, above 100 beats per minute in adults. **Bradycardia** is a slow heart rate, below 60 beats per minute in adults.

An inefficient contraction of the heart that fails to transmit a pulse wave to the peripheral pulse site creates a **pulse deficit.** To assess a pulse deficit, the nurse and a colleague assess radial and apical rates simultaneously and then compare rates. The difference between the apical and radial pulse rates is the pulse deficit. For example, an apical rate of 92 beats per minute with a radial rate of 78 beats per minute leaves a pulse deficit of 14 beats per minute. Pulse deficits are frequently associated with abnormal rhythms.

Rhythm. Normally, a regular interval occurs between each pulse or heartbeat. An interval interrupted by an early or late beat or a missed beat indicates an abnormal rhythm or **dysrhythmia.** A dysrhythmia threatens the heart's ability to provide adequate cardiac output, particularly if it occurs repetitively. The nurse identifies a dysrhythmia by palpating an interruption in successive pulse waves or auscultating an interruption between heart sounds. If a dysrhythmia is present, the regularity of its occurrence should be assessed and the apical rate is auscultated (see chapter 28). Dysrhythmias may be described as regularly irregular or irregularly irregular.

To document a dysrhythmia, a physician may order an electrocardiogram, Holter monitor, or telemetry. An electrocardiogram records the electrical activity of the heart for a 12-second interval. This test requires placement of electrodes across the client's chest followed by recording of the heart rhythm. The Holter monitor records 24 hours of electrical activity in a small tape recorder that the client wears. Access to the information recorded is not available until after the 24 hours have passed and the data are printed for review. Cardiac telemetry provides continuous monitoring of the heart's electrical activity transmitted to a stationary monitor. Telemetry permits observation of heart rhythm during all of the client's daily activities and thus allows for immediate treatment if the rhythm becomes erratic or unstable.

Children often have a sinus dysrhythmia, which is an irregular heartbeat that speeds up with inspiration and slows down with expiration. This is a normal finding and can be verified by having the child hold his or her breath; the heart rate should then become regular.

Strength. The strength or amplitude of a pulse reflects the volume of blood ejected against the arterial wall with each heart contraction and the condition of the arterial vascular system leading to the pulse site. Normally, the pulse strength remains the same with each heartbeat. Pulse strength may be graded or described as strong, weak, thready, or bounding. It is included during assessment of the vascular system (see chapter 28).

Equality. Pulses on both sides of the peripheral vascular system should be assessed. The nurse assesses both radial pulses to compare the characteristics of each. A pulse in one extremity may be unequal in strength or absent in many disease states (e.g., thrombus [clot] formation, aberrant blood vessels, cervical rib syndrome, or aortic dissection). All symmetrical pulses can be assessed simultaneously except for the carotid pulse. The carotid pulse should never be measured simultaneously because excessive pressure may occlude blood supply to the brain or trigger carotid reflexes that may result in alterations in blood pressure.

Nursing Process and Pulse Determination

Pulse assessment determines the general state of cardiovascular health and the response to other system imbalances. Tachycardia, bradycardia, and dysrhythmias are defining characteristics of many nursing diagnoses, including the following:

- Activity intolerance
- Anxiety
- Decreased cardiac output
- Fear

- Deficient/excess fluid volume
- Impaired gas exchange
- Hyperthermia
- Hypothermia
- Acute pain
- Ineffective tissue perfusion

The nursing care plan includes interventions based on the nursing diagnosis identified and the related factor. For example, the defining characteristics of an abnormal heart rate, exertional dyspnea, and a client's verbal report of fatigue lead to a diagnosis of *activity intolerance.* The nurse evaluates client outcomes by assessing the pulse rate, rhythm, strength, and equality following each intervention.

Respiration

Human survival depends on the ability of oxygen (O_2) to reach body cells and carbon dioxide (CO_2) to be removed from the cells. Respiration is the mechanism that the body uses to exchange gases between the atmosphere and the blood and between the blood and the cells. Respiration involves **ventilation** (the movement of gases in and out of the lungs), **diffusion** (the movement of oxygen and carbon dioxide between the alveoli and the red blood cells), and **perfusion** (the distribution of red blood cells to and from the pulmonary capillaries). Analyzing respiratory efficiency requires integrating assessment data from all three processes. Ventilation is assessed by determining respiratory rate, respiratory depth, and respiratory rhythm. Diffusion and perfusion can be assessed by determining oxygen saturation.

Physiological Control

Breathing is generally a passive process. Normally, a person thinks little about it. The respiratory centre in the brain stem regulates the involuntary control of respirations. Adults normally breathe in a smooth, uninterrupted pattern, 12 to 20 times a minute.

Ventilation is regulated by levels of CO_2, O_2, and hydrogen ion concentration (pH) in the arterial blood. The most important factor in the control of ventilation is the level of CO_2 in the arterial blood. An elevation in the CO_2 level causes the respiratory control system in the brain to increase the rate and depth of breathing. The increased ventilatory effort removes excess CO_2 (hypercarbia) by increasing exhalation. However, clients with chronic lung disease have ongoing hypercarbia. For these clients, chemoreceptors in the carotid artery and aorta become sensitive to **hypoxemia,** or low levels of arterial O_2. If arterial oxygen levels fall, these receptors signal the brain to increase the rate and depth of ventilation. Hypoxemia helps to control ventilation in clients with chronic lung disease. Because low levels of arterial O_2 provide the stimulus that allows the client to breathe, administration of high oxygen levels can be fatal for clients with chronic lung disease.

Mechanics of Breathing

Although breathing is normally passive, muscular work is involved in moving the lungs and chest wall. Inspiration is an active process. During inspiration, the respiratory centre sends impulses along the phrenic nerve, causing the diaphragm to contract. Abdominal organs move downward and forward, increasing the length of the chest cavity to move air into the lungs. The diaphragm moves approximately 1 cm, and the ribs retract upward from the body's midline approximately 1.2 to 2.5 cm. During a normal, relaxed breath, a person inhales 500 mL of air. This amount is referred to as the **tidal volume.** During expiration, the diaphragm relaxes and the abdominal organs return to their original positions. The lung and chest wall return to a relaxed position (Figure 27–9). Expiration is a passive process. The normal rate and depth of ventilation, **eupnea,** is interrupted by sighing. The sigh, a prolonged deeper breath, is a protective physiological mechanism for expanding small airways and alveoli not ventilated during a normal breath.

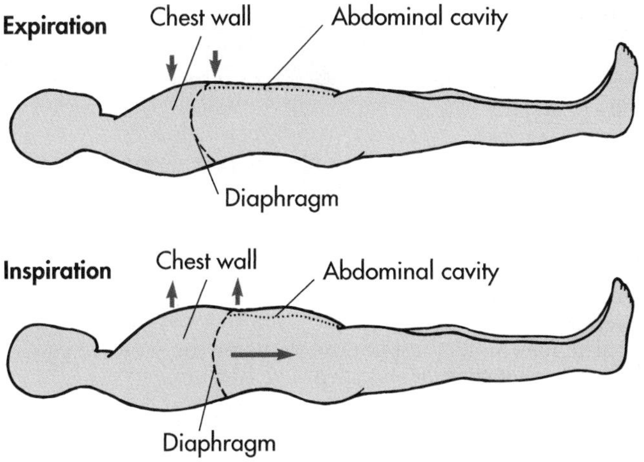

FIGURE **27–9** Illustration of diaphragmatic and chest wall movement during inspiration and expiration.

The accurate assessment of respirations depends on the nurse's recognition of normal thoracic and abdominal movements. During quiet breathing, the chest wall gently rises and falls. Contraction of the accessory muscles of breathing (i.e., the intercostal muscles between the ribs and the muscles in the neck and shoulders) is not visible. During normal quiet breathing, diaphragmatic movement causes the abdominal cavity to rise and fall slowly.

Assessment of Ventilation

The nurse does not require any special equipment to measure respirations; however, respirations are often haphazardly measured. A nurse must not estimate respirations. Accurate measurement requires observation and palpation of chest wall movement.

A sudden change in the character of respirations may be important. Because respiration is tied to the function of numerous body systems, the nurse must consider all variables when changes occur (Box 27-11). For example, abdominal trauma may injure the phrenic nerve, which is responsible for diaphragmatic contraction. The nurse must understand the extent of the injury and the implications for the respiratory system.

Box 27-11 Factors Influencing Character of Respirations

Exercise

Exercise increases rate and depth to meet the body's need for additional oxygen and to rid the body of CO_2.

Acute Pain

Pain alters rate and rhythm of respirations; breathing becomes shallow.
Client may inhibit or splint chest wall movement when pain is in area of chest or abdomen.

Anxiety

Anxiety increases rate and depth as a result of sympathetic stimulation.

Smoking

Chronic smoking changes the lung's airways, resulting in increased rate of respirations at rest when not smoking.

Body Position

A straight, erect posture promotes full chest expansion.
A stooped or slumped position impairs ventilatory movement.
Lying flat prevents full chest expansion.

Medications

Narcotic analgesics, general anaesthetics, and sedative hypnotics depress rate and depth.
Amphetamines and cocaine may increase rate and depth.
Bronchodilators slow rate by causing airway dilation.

Neurological Injury

Injury to the brain stem impairs the respiratory centre and inhibits respiratory rate and rhythm.

Hemoglobin Function

Decreased hemoglobin levels (anemia) reduce oxygen-carrying capacity of the blood, which increases respiratory rate.
Increased altitude lowers the amount of saturated hemoglobin, which increases respiratory rate and depth.
Abnormal blood cell function (e.g., sickle cell disease) reduces ability of hemoglobin to carry oxygen, which increases respiratory rate and depth.

A skillful nurse does not let a client know that respirations are being assessed. A client aware of the nurse's intentions may consciously alter the rate and depth of breathing. Measurement can best be done immediately after measuring pulse rate, with the nurse's hand still on the client's wrist as it rests over the chest or abdomen. When assessing a client's respirations, the nurse should keep in mind the client's usual ventilatory rate and pattern, the influence any disease or illness has on respiratory function, the relationship between respiratory and cardiovascular function, and the influence of therapies on respirations. The objective measurements of an assessment of respiratory status include the rate and depth of breathing and the rhythm of ventilatory movements (Skill 27-3).

Respiratory Rate. The nurse observes a full inspiration and expiration when counting ventilation or respiration rate. The respiratory rate varies with age (Table 27-4).

An apnea monitor is a respiratory monitoring device that aids the nurse's assessment. This device uses leads attached to the client's chest wall that sense movement. The absence of chest wall movement triggers the apnea alarm. Apnea monitoring is used frequently with infants in the hospital and at home to observe for prolonged apneic events.

Table 27-4 Acceptable Range of Respiratory Rates for Age

Age	Rate (Breaths per Minute)
Newborn	30–60
Infant (6 months)	30–50
Toddler (2 years)	25–32
Child	20–30
Adolescent	16–19
Adult	12–20
Older Adult	16–25

Ventilatory Depth. The depth of respirations is assessed by observing the degree of excursion or movement in the chest wall. The nurse subjectively describes ventilatory movements as deep, normal, or shallow. A deep respiration involves a full expansion of the lungs with full exhalation. Respirations are shallow when only a small quantity of air passes through the lungs and ventilatory movement is difficult to see. Objective techniques are used if the nurse observes that chest excursion is unusually shallow (see chapter 28). Table 27-5 summarizes alterations of breathing patterns.

Ventilatory Rhythm. Breathing pattern can be determined by observing the chest or the abdomen. Diaphragmatic breathing results from the contraction and relaxation of the diaphragm and is best observed by watching abdominal movements. Healthy men and children usually demonstrate diaphragmatic breathing. Women tend to use thoracic muscles to breathe; movements are observed in

Skill 27-3 Assessing Respirations

View Video

Delegation Considerations

The skill of respiration measurement can be delegated to unregulated care providers (UCPs). The nurse is responsible for assessing for change in respiration rate, rhythm, and depth. It is important for the nurse to do the following:

- Inform the UCP of client history or risk for increased or decreased respiratory rate or irregular respirations.
- Inform the UCP of frequency of respirations measurement for specific client.
- Determine that the UCP is aware of the usual values for the client.
- Inform the UCP of the abnormalities that should be reported to the nurse.

Equipment

- Wristwatch with second hand or digital display
- Pen, vital sign flow sheet or record form

Steps	Rationale
1. Determine need to assess client's respirations:	Nurse uses clinical judgment to determine need for assessment.
a. Note risk factors for respiratory alterations.	Certain conditions place client at risk for alterations in ventilation detected by changes in respiratory rate, depth, and rhythm. The following conditions can result in respiratory alteration: fever, pain, anxiety, diseases of chest wall or muscles, constrictive chest or abdominal dressings, gastric distension, chronic pulmonary disease (emphysema, bronchitis, asthma), traumatic injury to chest wall with or without collapse of underlying lung tissue, presence of a chest tube, respiratory infection (pneumonia, acute bronchitis), pulmonary edema and emboli, head injury with damage to brain stem, and anemia.
b. Assess for signs and symptoms of respiratory alterations such as bluish or cyanotic appearance of nail beds, lips, mucous membranes, and skin; restlessness, irritability, confusion, reduced level of consciousness; pain during inspiration; laboured or difficult breathing; adventitious breath sounds (see chapter 28), inability to breathe spontaneously; thick, frothy, blood-tinged, or copious sputum produced on coughing.	Physical signs and symptoms may indicate alterations in respiratory status related to ventilation.
2. Assess pertinent laboratory values:	
A. Arterial blood gases (ABGs): Normal ABGs (values may vary slightly within institutions): pH 7.35–7.45 $PaCO_2$ 35–45 PaO_2 80–100 SaO_2 95%–100%	Arterial blood gases measure arterial blood pH, partial pressure of O_2 and CO_2, and arterial O_2 saturation, which reflects client's oxygenation status.
B. Pulse oximetry (SpO_2): Acceptable SpO_2 90%–100%; 85%–89% may be acceptable for certain chronic disease conditions; less than 85% is abnormal (see Skill 27-4).	SpO_2 less than 85% is often accompanied by changes in respiratory rate, depth, and rhythm.
C. Complete blood count (CBC): Normal CBC for adults (values may vary within institutions and references consulted): *Hemoglobin:* 132 to 173 g/L, males; 117 to 155 g/L, females *Hematocrit:* 0.43 to 0.49, males; 0.38 to 0.44, females *Red blood cell count:* 4.7 to 5.74 × 10^{12}/L, males; 4.2 to 4.87 × 10^{12}/L, females.	CBC measures red blood cell count, volume of red blood cells, and concentration of hemoglobin, which reflects client's capacity to carry O_2.
3. Determine previous baseline respiratory rate (if available) from client's record.	Allows nurse to assess for change in condition. Provides comparison with future respiratory measurements.

Skill 27-3 Assessing Respirations—cont'd

Steps	Rationale
4. Perform hand hygiene. Draw curtain around bed and/or close door.	Prevents transmission of microorganisms. Maintains privacy.

Critical Decision Point: Clients with difficulty breathing (dyspnea), such as those with congestive heart failure, abdominal ascites, or in late stages of pregnancy, should be assessed in the position of greatest comfort. Repositioning may increase the work of breathing, which will increase respiratory rate.

Steps	Rationale
5. Be sure client is in comfortable position, preferably sitting or lying with the head of the bed elevated 45 to 60 degrees. Be sure client's chest is visible. If necessary, move bed linen or gown.	Sitting erect promotes full ventilatory movement. Ensures clear view of chest wall and abdominal movements.
6. Place client's arm in relaxed position across the abdomen or lower chest, or place nurse's hand directly over client's upper abdomen (see illustration).	A similar position used during pulse assessment allows respiratory rate assessment to be inconspicuous. Client's hand or your hand rises and falls during respiratory cycle.
7. Observe complete respiratory cycle (one inspiration and one expiration).	Rate is accurately determined only after nurse has viewed respiratory cycle.
8. After cycle is observed, look at watch's second hand and begin to count rate: When sweep hand hits number on dial, begin time frame, counting one with first full respiratory cycle.	Timing begins with count of one. Respirations occur more slowly than pulse; thus timing does not begin with zero.
9. If rhythm is regular, count number of respirations in 30 seconds and multiply by 2. If rhythm is irregular, less than 12, or greater than 20, count for 1 full minute.	Respiratory rate is equivalent to number of respirations per minute. Suspected irregularities require assessment for at least 1 minute.

Critical Decision Point: Respiratory rate less than 12 or greater than 20 requires further assessment (see chapter 28) and may require immediate intervention.

Steps	Rationale
10. Note depth of respirations, subjectively assessed by observing degree of chest wall movement while counting rate. Nurse can also objectively assess depth by palpating chest wall excursion or auscultating the posterior thorax after rate has been counted (see chapter 28). Depth is described as shallow, normal, or deep.	Character of ventilatory movement may reveal specific disease state restricting volume of air from moving into and out of the lungs.

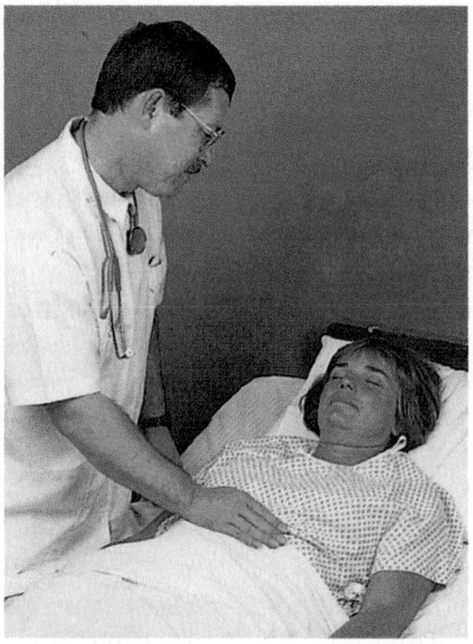

STEP **6** Nurse's hand over client's abdomen to check respiration.

Steps	Rationale
11. Note rhythm of ventilatory cycle. Normal breathing is regular and uninterrupted. Sighing should not be confused with abnormal rhythm.	Character of ventilations can reveal specific types of alterations.

Critical Decision Point: Any irregular respiratory pattern or periods of apnea (the cessation of respiration for several seconds) are symptoms of underlying disease in the adult and must be reported to the physician or nurse in charge. Further assessment may be required (see chapter 28) and immediate intervention may be needed. An irregular respiratory rate and short apneic spells are normal for newborns.

Steps	Rationale
12. Replace bed linen and client's gown.	Restores comfort and promotes sense of well-being.
13. Perform hand hygiene.	Reduces transmission of microorganisms.
14. Discuss findings with client as needed.	Promotes participation in care and understanding of health status.
15. If respirations are assessed for the first time, establish rate, rhythm, and depth as baseline if within normal range.	Used to compare future respiratory assessment.
16. Compare respirations with client's previous baseline and normal rate, rhythm, and depth.	Allows nurse to assess for changes in client's condition and for presence of respiratory alterations.

Unexpected Outcomes and Related Interventions

- Client has abnormal respiratory rate, depth, or states a feeling of being short of breath.
  - Observe for related factors, including obstructed airway, abnormal breath sounds, productive cough, restlessness, irritability, anxiety, confusion.
  - Position client to improve ventilation such as in a sitting position (semi- or high-Fowler's), unless contraindicated.
  - When possible, remove respiratory irritants from the environment, such as second-hand smoke, perfumes, and so forth.

Recording and Reporting

- Record respiratory rate and character in nurses' notes or vital sign flow sheet. Indicate type and amount of oxygen therapy if used by client during assessment. Measurement of respiratory rate after administration of specific therapies should be documented in narrative form in nurses' notes.
- Report abnormal findings to nurse in charge or physician.

Home Care Considerations

- Assess for environmental factors in the home that may influence client's respiratory rate such as second-hand smoke, poor ventilation, or gas fumes.

the upper chest. Laboured respirations usually involve the accessory muscles of respiration visible in the neck. When something such as a foreign body interferes with the movement of air in and out of the lungs, the intercostal spaces retract during inspiration. A longer expiration phase is evident when the outward flow of air is obstructed (e.g., asthma).

With normal breathing, a regular interval occurs after each respiratory cycle. Infants tend to breathe less regularly. The young child may breathe slowly for a few seconds and then suddenly breathe more rapidly. While assessing respirations, the nurse estimates the time interval after each respiratory cycle. Respiration is regular or irregular in rhythm.

Assessment of Diffusion and Perfusion

The respiratory processes of diffusion and perfusion can be evaluated by measuring the oxygen saturation of the blood. Blood flow through the pulmonary capillaries provides red blood cells for oxygen attachment. After oxygen diffuses from the alveoli into the pulmonary blood, most of the oxygen attaches to hemoglobin molecules in red blood cells. Red blood cells carry the oxygenated hemoglobin molecules through the left side of the heart and out to the peripheral capillaries, where the oxygen detaches, depending on the needs of the tissues.

The percent of hemoglobin that is bound with oxygen in the arteries is the percent of saturation of hemoglobin (or SaO_2). It is usually between 95% and 100%. SaO_2 is affected by factors that interfere with ventilation, perfusion, or diffusion (see chapter 35). The saturation of venous blood (SvO_2) is lower because the tissues have removed some of the oxygen from the hemoglobin molecules. A normal value for SvO_2 is 70%. SvO_2 is affected by factors that interfere with or increase the tissue's need for oxygen.

Measurement of Arterial Oxygen Saturation. A pulse oximeter permits the indirect measurement of oxygen saturation (Skill 27-4). The pulse oximeter is a probe with

Table 27-5 Alterations in Breathing Pattern

Alteration	Description
Bradypnea	Rate of breathing is regular but abnormally slow (less than 12 breaths per minute).
Tachypnea	Rate of breathing is regular but abnormally rapid (greater than 20 breaths per minute).
Hyperpnea	Respirations are laboured, increased in depth, and increased in rate (greater than 20 breaths per minute). Occurs normally during exercise.
Apnea	Respirations cease for several seconds. Persistent cessation results in respiratory arrest.
Hyperventilation	Rate and depth of respirations increase. Hypocarbia may occur.
Hypoventilation	Respiratory rate is abnormally low, and depth of ventilation may be depressed. Hypercarbia may occur.
Cheyne-Stokes respiration	Respiratory rate and depth are irregular, characterized by alternating periods of apnea and hyperventilation. Respiratory cycle begins with slow, shallow breaths that gradually increase to abnormal rate and depth. The pattern reverses, breathing slows and becomes shallow, climaxing in apnea before respiration resumes.
Kussmaul's respiration	Respirations are abnormally deep, regular, and increased in rate.
Biot's respiration	Respirations are abnormally shallow for two to three breaths followed by irregular period of apnea.

a light-emitting diode (LED) and photo detector connected by cable to an oximeter (Figure 27–10). The LED emits light wavelengths that are absorbed differently by the oxygenated and deoxygenated hemoglobin molecules. The photo detector detects the light-absorbing differences, and the oximeter calculates the pulse saturation (SpO_2). SpO_2 is a reliable estimate of SaO_2 when the SaO_2 is over 70%. Values obtained with pulse oximetry are less accurate at saturations less than 70% (Grap, 2002).

The photo detector is contained within the oximeter probe. Selecting the appropriate probe is important to reduce measurement error. Digit probes are spring-loaded and conform to various sizes. Earlobe probes have greater accuracy at lower saturations and are least affected by peripheral vasoconstriction (Grap, 2002). Disposable sensor pads can be applied to a variety of sites, even the bridge of an adult's nose or the sole of an infant's foot. The ability of the photo detector to measure SpO_2 is affected by factors that affect light transmission or peripheral arterial pulsations (Box 27-12). An awareness of these factors allows accurate interpretation of abnormal SpO_2 measurements.

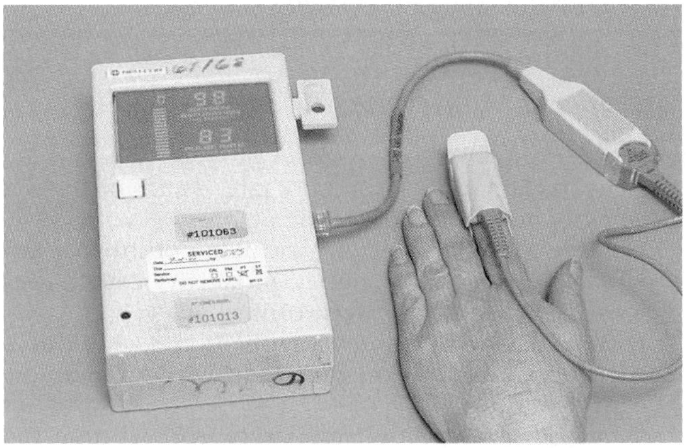

FIGURE **27–10** Portable pulse oximeter with digit probe.

Nursing Process and Respiratory Vital Signs

Vital sign measurement of respiratory rate, pattern, and depth, along with SpO_2, allows the nurse to assess ventilation, diffusion, and perfusion. The nurse may also conduct other assessments to measure respiratory status (see chapter 28). Each measurement can provide clues in determining the nature of a client's problem. Respiratory assessment data are defining characteristics of many nursing diagnoses, including the following:

- Activity intolerance
- Ineffective airway clearance
- Anxiety
- Ineffective breathing pattern
- Impaired gas exchange
- Acute pain
- Ineffective tissue perfusion
- Dysfunctional ventilatory weaning response

The nursing care plan includes interventions based on the nursing diagnosis identified and the related factor. For example, the defining characteristics of tachypnea, changes in depth of respirations, use of accessory muscles, cyanosis, and a decline in SpO_2, lead to a diagnosis of *impaired gas exchange*. Related factors may include postoperative lobectomy with chest tube placement, a history of chronic obstructive lung disease, and history of heavy smoking. The nurse evaluates client outcomes by assessing the respiratory rate, ventilatory depth, rhythm, and SpO_2 following each intervention.

Blood Pressure

Blood pressure is the force exerted on the walls of an artery by the pulsing blood under pressure from the heart. Blood flows throughout the circulatory system because of pressure changes. It moves from an area of high pressure to an area of low pressure. Systemic or arterial blood pressure, the blood pressure in the system of arteries in the body, is a good indicator of cardiovascular

Skill 27-4 Measuring Oxygen Saturation (Pulse Oximetry)

Delegation Considerations

The skill of oxygen saturation measurement can be delegated to unregulated care providers (UCPs). The nurse is responsible for assessing the impact of changes in oxygen saturation. It is important for the nurse to do the following:

- Inform the UCP to notify nurse immediately of any reading lower than SpO_2 of 90%.
- Inform the UCP of appropriate sensor site and probe for measurement of oxygen saturation.
- Inform the UCP of frequency of oxygen saturation measurements for specific client.
- Determine that the UCP is aware of factors that can falsely lower SpO_2 (see Box 27-11).

Equipment

- Oximeter
- Oximeter probe appropriate for client and recommended by manufacturer
- Acetone or nail polish remover
- Pen, vital sign flow sheet or record form

Steps	Rationale
1. Determine need to measure client's oxygen saturation:	Nurse uses clinical judgment to determine need for assessment.
a. Note risk factors for alteration of oxygen saturation	Certain conditions place clients at risk for decreased oxygen saturation: acute or chronic compromised respiratory function; recovery from general anaesthesia or conscious sedation; traumatic injury to chest wall with or without collapse of underlying lung tissue; ventilator dependence; changes in supplemental oxygen therapy.
b. Assess for signs and symptoms of alterations in oxygen saturation such as altered respiratory rate, depth, or rhythm; adventitious breath sounds (see chapter 28); cyanotic appearance of nail beds, lips, mucous membranes, and skin; restlessness, irritability, confusion; reduced level of consciousness; laboured or difficult breathing.	Physical signs and symptoms may indicate abnormal oxygen saturation.
2. Assess for factors that normally influence measurement of SpO_2 such as oxygen therapy, hemoglobin level, and temperature.	Allows nurse to accurately assess oxygen saturation variations. Peripheral vasoconstriction related to hypothermia can interfere with SpO_2 determination.
3. Review client's medical record for physician's order or consult agency policy or procedure manual for standard of care.	Medical order may be required to assess oxygen saturation.
4. Determine previous baseline SpO_2 (if available) from client's record.	Baseline information provides basis for comparison and assists in assessment of current status and evaluation of interventions.
5. Perform hand hygiene.	Reduces transmission of microorganisms.
6. Explain purpose of procedure to client and how oxygen saturation will be measured. Instruct client to breathe normally.	Promotes client cooperation and increases compliance. Prevents large fluctuations in minute ventilation and possible error in SpO_2 readings.
7. Assess site most appropriate for sensor probe placement (e.g., digit, earlobe). Site must have adequate local circulation and be free of moisture.	Peripheral vasoconstriction can interfere with SpO_2 determination. Dark nail polish and acrylic nails impede sensor detection of emitted light and produce falsely elevated SpO_2. Moisture impedes ability of sensor to detect SpO_2 levels.
8. Position client comfortably. If finger is chosen as monitoring site, support lower arm.	Ensures probe positioning and decreases motion artifact that interferes with SpO_2 determination.
9. Instruct client to breathe normally.	Prevents large fluctuations in respiratory rate and depth and possible changes in SpO_2.
10. If finger is to be used, remove any fingernail polish with acetone from digit to be assessed.	Ensures accurate readings. Opaque coatings decrease light transmission; nail polish containing blue pigment can absorb light emissions and falsely alter saturation.
11. Attach sensor probe to monitoring site. Instruct client that clip-on probe feels like a clothespin on the finger but will not hurt.	Pressure of sensor probe's spring tension on a peripheral digit or earlobe may be unexpected.

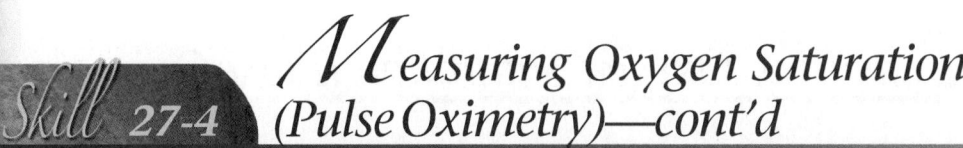

Skill 27-4 Measuring Oxygen Saturation (Pulse Oximetry)—cont'd

Steps	Rationale
Critical Decision Point: Do not attach probe to finger, ear, or bridge of nose if area is edematous or skin integrity is compromised. Do not attach probe to fingers that are hypothermic. Select ear or bridge of nose if adult client has history of peripheral vascular disease. Earlobe and bridge of nose sensors are not used for infants and toddlers because of skin fragility. Disposable adhesive probes contain latex and should not be used if client has latex allergy.	
12. Turn on oximeter by activating power. Observe pulse waveform/intensity display and audible beep. Correlate oximeter pulse rate with client's radial pulse. Differences require reevaluation of oximeter probe placement and may require reassessment of pulse rates.	Pulse waveform/intensity display enables detection of valid pulse or presence of interfering signal. Pitch of audible beep is proportional to SpO_2 value. Double-checking pulse rate ensures oximeter accuracy. Oximeter pulse rate, client's radial pulse, and apical pulse rate should be the same. Any difference requires reevaluation of oximeter sensor probe placement and reassessment of pulse rates.
13. Leave probe in place until oximeter readout reaches constant value and pulse display reaches full strength during each cardiac cycle. Inform client that oximeter will alarm if the probe falls off or if client moves the probe. Read SpO_2 on digital display.	Reading may take 10 to 30 seconds, depending on site selected.
14. If continuous SpO_2 monitoring is planned, verify SpO_2 alarm limits and alarm volume, which are preset by the manufacturer at a low of 85% and a high of 100%. You must determine limits for SpO_2 and pulse rate alarms based on each client's condition. Verify that alarms are on. Assess skin integrity under sensor probe and relocate sensor probe at least every 4 hours.	Alarms must be set at appropriate limits and volumes to avoid frightening clients and visitors. Spring tension of sensor probe or sensitivity to disposable sensor probe adhesive can cause skin irritation and lead to disruption of skin integrity.
15. Assist client in returning to comfortable position.	Restores comfort and promotes sense of well-being.
16. Perform hand hygiene.	Reduces transmission of microorganisms.
17. Discuss findings with client as needed.	Promotes participation in care and understanding of health status.
18. If intermittent or spot-checking SpO_2 measurements are planned, remove probe and turn oximeter power off. Store probe in appropriate location.	Batteries can be depleted if oximeter is left on. Sensor probes are expensive and vulnerable to damage.
19. Compare SpO_2 readings with client baseline and acceptable values.	Comparison reveals presence of abnormality.
20. Correlate SpO_2 with SaO_2 obtained from arterial blood gas measurements (see chapter 36) if available.	Documents reliability of noninvasive assessment.
21. Correlate SpO_2 reading with data obtained from respiratory rate, depth, and rhythm assessment (see Skill 27-3).	Measurements assessing ventilation, perfusion, and diffusion are interrelated.

Unexpected Outcomes and Related Interventions

- SpO_2 is less than 90%.
  - Verify that oximeter probe is intact and correctly positioned.
  - Obtain vital signs and notify physician if indicated.
  - Observe for signs associated with decreased oxygenation (e.g., anxiety, restlessness, tachycardia, cyanosis).
  - Verify that supplemental oxygen delivery system is delivered as ordered and is functioning properly.
  - Position client to promote optimal ventilation.
- Pulse rate indicated on the oximeter is less than client's radial or apical pulse
  - Reposition sensor probe to an alternative site with increased blood flow.
  - Assess client for signs of altered cardiac output (e.g., decreased blood pressure, cool skin, confusion).

Recording and Reporting

- Record SpO_2 value on nurses' notes or vital sign flow sheet, indicating type and amount of oxygen therapy used by client during assessment. Also record any signs and symptoms of oxygen desaturation in narrative form in nurses' notes. Report abnormal findings to nurse in charge or physician.

Recording and Reporting—cont'd

- Assessment of oxygen saturation after administration of specific therapies should be documented in narrative form in nurses' notes.
- Record in nurses' notes client's use of continuous or intermittent pulse oximetry.

Home Care Considerations

- Pulse oximetry is used in home care to noninvasively monitor oxygen therapy or changes in oxygen therapy.
- Instruct caregivers to examine oximeter site prior to applying sensor.
- Instruct caregivers on procedure to implement when oxygen saturation not within acceptable values.

Box 27-12 Factors Affecting Determination of Pulse Oxygen Saturation (SpO_2)

Interference With Light Transmission

Outside light sources can interfere with the oximeter's ability to process reflected light.

Carbon monoxide (caused by smoke inhalation or poisoning) artificially elevates SpO_2 by absorbing light similar to oxygen.

Client motion can interfere with the oximeter's ability to process reflected light.

Jaundice may interfere with the oximeter's ability to process reflected light.

Intravascular dyes (methylene blue) absorb light similar to deoxyhemoglobin and artificially lower saturation.

Reduction of Arterial Pulsations

Peripheral vascular disease (atherosclerosis) can reduce pulse volume.

Hypothermia at assessment site decreases peripheral blood flow.

Pharmacological vasoconstrictors (epinephrine, phenylephrine, dopamine) decrease peripheral pulse volume.

Low cardiac output and hypotension decrease blood flow to peripheral arteries.

Peripheral edema can obscure arterial pulsation.

Tight probe records venous pulsations in the finger that compete with arterial pulsations.

health. The heart's contraction forces blood under high pressure into the aorta. The peak of maximum pressure when ejection occurs is the **systolic** blood pressure. When the ventricles relax, the blood remaining in the arteries exerts a minimum or **diastolic** pressure. Diastolic pressure is the minimal pressure exerted against the arterial walls at all times.

The standard unit for measuring blood pressure is millimeters of mercury (mm Hg). The measurement indicates the height to which the blood pressure can raise a column of mercury. Blood pressure is recorded with the systolic reading before the diastolic (e.g., 120/80). The difference between systolic and diastolic pressure is the **pulse pressure.** For a blood pressure of 120/80, the pulse pressure is 40.

Physiology of Arterial Blood Pressure

Blood pressure reflects the interrelationships of cardiac output, peripheral vascular resistance, blood volume, blood viscosity, and artery elasticity. A nurse's knowledge of these hemodynamic variables helps in the assessment of blood pressure alterations.

Cardiac Output. A person's cardiac output (CO) is the volume of blood pumped by the heart (stroke volume [SV]) during 1 minute (heart rate [HR]):

$$CO = HR \times SV$$

The blood pressure (BP) depends on the cardiac output and peripheral vascular resistance (R):

$$BP = CO \times R$$

When volume increases in an enclosed space, such as a blood vessel, the pressure in that space rises. Thus, as cardiac output increases, more blood is pumped against arterial walls, causing the blood pressure to rise. Cardiac output can increase as a result of an increase in heart rate, greater heart muscle contractility, or an increase in blood volume. Changes in heart rate can occur faster than changes in heart muscle contractility or blood volume. An increase in heart rate may decrease the heart's filling time. As a result, there is a decrease in blood pressure.

Peripheral Resistance. Blood circulates through a network of arteries, arterioles, capillaries, venules, and veins. Arteries and arterioles are surrounded by smooth muscle that contracts or relaxes to change the size of the lumen. The size of arteries and arterioles changes to adjust blood flow to the needs of local tissues. For example, when more blood is needed by a major organ, the peripheral arteries constrict, decreasing their supply of blood. More blood becomes available to the major organ because of the resistance change in the periphery. Normally, arteries and arterioles remain partially constricted to maintain a constant flow of blood. Peripheral vascular resistance is the resistance to blood flow determined by the tone of vascular musculature and diameter of blood vessels. The smaller the lumen of a vessel, the greater peripheral vascular resistance to blood flow. As resistance rises, arterial blood pressure rises. As vessels dilate and resistance falls, blood pressure drops.

Blood Volume. The volume of blood circulating within the vascular system affects blood pressure. Most adults have a circulating blood volume of 5,000 mL. Normally,

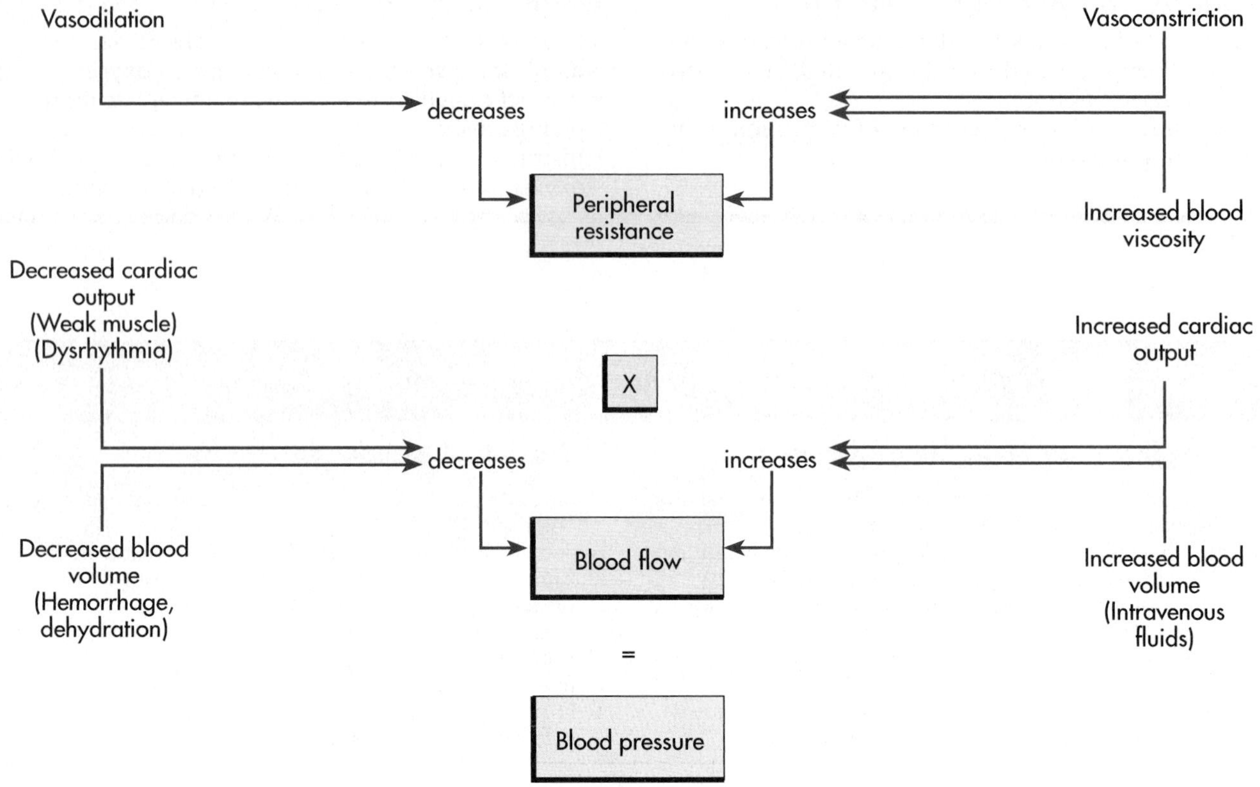

FIGURE **27–11** Hemodynamic factors that affect blood pressure.

the blood volume remains constant. However, if volume increases, more pressure is exerted against arterial walls. For example, the rapid, uncontrolled infusion of IV fluids elevates blood pressure. When circulating blood volume falls, as in the case of hemorrhage or dehydration, blood pressure falls.

Viscosity. The thickness or viscosity of blood affects the ease with which blood flows through small vessels. The **hematocrit,** or percentage of red blood cells in the blood, determines blood viscosity. When the hematocrit rises and blood flow slows, arterial blood pressure increases. The heart must contract more forcefully to move the viscous blood through the circulatory system.

Elasticity. Normally, the walls of an artery are elastic and easily distensible. As pressure within the arteries increases, the diameter of vessel walls increases to accommodate the pressure change. Arterial distensibility prevents wide fluctuations in blood pressure. However, in certain diseases, such as arteriosclerosis, the vessel walls lose their elasticity and are replaced by fibrous tissue that cannot stretch well. With reduced elasticity, there is greater resistance to blood flow. As a result, when the left ventricle ejects its stroke volume, the vessels no longer yield to pressure. Instead, a given volume of blood is forced through the rigid arterial walls, and the systemic pressure rises. Systolic pressure is more significantly elevated than diastolic pressure as a result of reduced arterial elasticity.

Each hemodynamic factor significantly affects the others. For example, as arterial elasticity declines, peripheral vascular resistance increases. The complex control of the cardiovascular system normally prevents any single factor from permanently changing the blood pressure. For example, if the blood volume falls, the body compensates with an increased vascular resistance. Figure 27–11 illustrates how hemodynamic variables can affect blood pressure.

Factors Influencing Blood Pressure

Blood pressure is not constant but is continually influenced by many factors. One blood pressure measurement cannot adequately reflect a client's blood pressure. Even under the best conditions, blood pressure changes from heartbeat to heartbeat. Blood pressure trends, not individual measurements, guide nursing interventions. Understanding these factors ensures a more accurate interpretation of blood pressure readings.

Age. Normal blood pressure levels vary throughout life (Table 27-6). They increase during childhood. The level of a child's or adolescent's blood pressure is assessed with respect to body size and age. An infant's blood pressure ranges from 65–115/42–80. The normal blood pressure for a 7-year-old is 87–117/48–64. Larger children (heavier and/or taller) have higher blood pressures than smaller children of the same age. During adolescence, blood pressure continues to vary according to body size.

An adult's blood pressure tends to increase with advancing age. The optimal blood pressure for a healthy, middle-

Table 27-6 Average Optimal Blood Pressure for Age

Age	Blood Pressure (mm Hg)
Newborn (3000 g)	40 (mean)
1 month	85/54
1 year	95/65
6 years*	105/65
10–13 years*	110/65
14–17 years*	120/75
>18	<120/80

From "The Seventh Report of the Joint National Committee on Detection, Evaluation, and Treatment of High Blood Pressure," by A. V. Chobanian et al., 2003, *JAMA, 289*(19), p. 2560.
*In children and adolescents, hypertension is defined as blood pressure that is, on repeated measurement, at the 95th percentile or greater adjusted for age, height, and gender (NHBPEP, 1997).

Table 27-7 Classification of Blood Pressure for Adults Ages 18 and Older

Category	Systolic (mm Hg)	Diastolic (mm Hg)
Optimal	<120	<80
Normal	<130	<85
High normal	130–139	85–89
Grade 1 hypertension	140–159	90–99
Grade 2 hypertension	160–179	100–109
Grade 3 hypertension	≥180	≥110

Adapted from *Recommendations for the Management of Hypertension. Part 1: Hypertension as a Public Health Risk—The Canadian Response,* Canadian Hypertension Education Program, 2004, Retrieved May 27, 2004, from *http://www.chs.md/index2.html (Introduction Slide 8).*

age adult is less than 120/80. Values of 130–139/85–89 are considered high normal (Canadian Hypertension Education Program [CHEP], 2004; Table 27-7). Older adults may have a rise in systolic pressure related to decreased vessel elasticity; however, blood pressure greater than 140/90 increases an older adult's risk for hypertension and other related illness.

Stress. Anxiety, fear, pain, and emotional stress result in sympathetic stimulation, which increases heart rate, cardiac output, and peripheral vascular resistance. The effects of sympathetic stimulation increase blood pressure.

Ethnicity. The incidence of hypertension (high blood pressure) is higher among ethnic groups such as South Asians, Aboriginals, and Black Canadians. Genetic and environmental factors are believed to be contributing factors.

Gender. There is no clinically significant difference in blood pressure levels between boys and girls. After puberty, males tend to have higher blood pressure readings. After menopause, women tend to have higher levels of blood pressure than men of similar age.

Diurnal Variation. Blood pressure levels vary over the course of a day. Blood pressure is typically lowest in the early morning, gradually rises during the morning and afternoon, and peaks in late afternoon or evening. No two people have the same pattern or degree of variation. Students may find it interesting to have their blood pressure checked by a friend at intervals during 24 hours.

Medications. Some medications can directly or indirectly affect blood pressure. During blood pressure assessment, the nurse asks whether the client is receiving antihypertensive or other cardiac medications, which lower blood pressure (Table 27-8). Another class of medications affecting blood pressure is opioid analgesics, which can lower blood pressure.

Other. Blood pressure can be reduced for several hours after a period of exercise. Older adults often experience a 5- to 10-mm fall in blood pressure about 1 hour after eating.

Hypertension

The most common alteration in blood pressure is **hypertension.** Hypertension is an often asymptomatic disorder characterized by persistently elevated blood pressure. The diagnosis of high normal in adults is made when an average of two or more diastolic readings on at least two subsequent visits is between 85 and 89 mm Hg or when the average of multiple systolic blood pressures on two or more subsequent visits is between 130 and 139 mm Hg. Hypertension is noted with diastolic readings greater than 90 mm Hg and systolic readings greater than 140 mm Hg (CHEP, 2004). Categories of hypertension have been developed and determine medical intervention (see Table 27-7). One elevated blood pressure measurement does not qualify as a diagnosis of hypertension. However, if the nurse assesses a high reading during the first blood pressure measurement (e.g., 150/90 mm Hg), the client is encouraged to return for another checkup within 2 months.

Hypertension is associated with the thickening and loss of elasticity in the arterial walls. Peripheral vascular resistance increases within thick and inelastic vessels. The heart must continually pump against greater resistance. As a result, blood flow to vital organs such as the heart, brain, and kidney decreases.

People with a family history of hypertension are at significant risk. Obesity, cigarette smoking, heavy alcohol consumption, high sodium (salt) intake, sedentary lifestyle, and continued exposure to stress are also linked to hypertension. The incidence of hypertension is greater in people with diabetes, older adults, and some ethnic groups. It is a major factor underlying deaths from strokes and is a contributing factor to myocardial infarctions (heart attacks). When clients are diagnosed with hypertension, the nurse helps to educate them about blood pressure values, long-term follow-up care and therapy, the usual lack of symptoms (the fact that it may not be

Table 27-8 Antihypertension Medications

Medication Type	Names	Action
Diuretics	Furosemide (Lasix), spironolactone (Aldactone), metolazone, polythiazide, benzthiazide	Lower blood pressure by reducing reabsorption of sodium and water by the kidneys, thus lowering circulating fluid volume
Beta-adrenergic blockers	Atenolol (Tenormin), nadolol (Corgard), timolol maleate (Blocadren), propranolol (Inderal)	Combine with beta-adrenergic receptors in the heart, arteries, and arterioles to block response to sympathetic nerve impulses; reduce heart rate and thus cardiac output
Vasodilators	Hydralazine hydrochloride (Apresoline), minoxidil (Loniten)	Act on arteriolar smooth muscle to cause relaxation and reduce peripheral vascular resistance
Calcium channel blockers	Diltiazem (Cardizem, Dilacor XR), verapamil hydrochloride (Calan SR), nifedipine (Procardia), nicardipine (Cardene)	Reduce peripheral vascular resistance by systemic vasodilation
Angiotensin-converting enzyme (ACE) inhibitors	Captopril (Capoten), enalapril (Vasotec), lisinopril (Prinivil, Zestril), benazepril (Lotensin)	Lower blood pressure by blocking the conversion of angiotensin I to angiotensin II, preventing vasoconstriction; reduce aldosterone production and fluid retention, lowering circulating fluid volume

"felt"), therapy's ability to control but not cure hypertension, and a consistently followed treatment plan that can ensure a relatively normal lifestyle (CHEP, 2004).

Hypotension

Hypotension is considered present when the systolic blood pressure falls to 90 mm Hg or below. Although some adults have a low blood pressure normally, for the majority of people, low blood pressure is an abnormal finding associated with illness.

Hypotension occurs because of the dilation of the arteries in the vascular bed, the loss of a substantial amount of blood volume (e.g., hemorrhage), or the failure of the heart muscle to pump adequately (e.g., myocardial infarction). Hypotension associated with pallor, skin mottling, clamminess, confusion, increased heart rate, or decreased urine output is life threatening and should be reported to a physician immediately.

Orthostatic hypotension, also referred to as **postural hypotension,** occurs when a normotensive person (a person having normal blood pressure) develops symptoms and low blood pressure when rising to an upright position. When a healthy individual changes from a lying, to sitting, to standing position, the peripheral blood vessels in the legs constrict. Constriction of the lower extremity vessels when standing prevents the pooling of blood in the legs due to gravity. Thus, no symptoms are normally felt in standing. In contrast, when clients have a decreased blood volume, their blood vessels are already constricted. When a volume-depleted client stands, there is a significant drop in blood pressure with an increase in heart rate to compensate for the drop in cardiac output. Clients who are dehydrated, anemic, or have experienced prolonged bed rest or recent blood loss are at risk for orthostatic hypotension. Some medications can cause orthostatic hypotension if misused, especially in older adults or young clients. Blood pressure should always be measured before administering such medications.

The nurse assesses for orthostatic hypotension during vital sign measurements by obtaining blood pressure and pulse with the client supine, sitting, and standing. When recording orthostatic blood pressure measurements, the nurse records the client's position in addition to the blood pressure measurement. For example: 140/80 supine, 132/72 sitting, 108/60 standing. The readings are obtained 1 to 3 minutes after the client changes position. In most cases, orthostatic hypotension is detected within a minute of standing. If orthostatic hypotension is assessed, the client is assisted to a lying position and the physician or nurse in charge is notified. While obtaining orthostatic measurements, the nurse observes for other symptoms of hypotension such as fainting, weakness, or light-headedness. Because the skill of orthostatic measurements requires critical thinking and ongoing nursing judgment, this procedure is not delegated to unregulated care providers.

Measurement of Blood Pressure

Arterial blood pressure may be measured either directly (invasively) or indirectly (non-invasively). The direct method requires the insertion of a thin catheter into an artery. Tubing connects the catheter to electronic monitoring equipment. The monitor displays a constant arterial pressure waveform and reading. Because of the risk of sudden blood loss from an artery, invasive blood pressure monitoring is used only in intensive care settings. The more common non-invasive method requires use of the sphygmomanometer and stethoscope. The nurse measures blood pressure indirectly by auscultation or palpation. Auscultation is the most widely used technique (Skill 27-5).

Blood Pressure Equipment. In order to assess blood pressure, the nurse must know how to use a sphygmomanometer and stethoscope. A **sphygmomanometer** includes a pressure manometer, an occlusive cloth or vinyl cuff that encloses an inflatable rubber bladder, and a pressure bulb with a release valve that inflates the bladder. The two types of manometers are the aneroid and the mercury (Figure 27–12). Aneroid manometers have the advantages of being safe, lightweight, portable, and compact. The

Text continued on p. 605

Skill 27-5 Measuring Blood Pressure

View Video

Delegation Considerations

In most provinces and territories, the skill of blood pressure measurement can be delegated to unregulated care providers (UCPs). The nurse is responsible for assessing changes in blood pressure. It is important for the nurse to do the following:

- Inform the UCP if client has alterations affecting the appropriate limb for blood pressure measurement.
- Inform the UCP of appropriate-size blood pressure cuff for designated extremity.
- Inform the UCP if client is at risk for orthostatic hypotension.
- Inform the UCP of frequency of blood pressure measurement for select client.
- Determine that the UCP is aware of the usual values for the client.
- Inform the UCP of the abnormalities that should be reported to the nurse.

Equipment

- Aneroid sphygmomanometer
- Cloth or disposable vinyl pressure cuff of appropriate size for client's extremity
- Stethoscope
- Alcohol swab
- Pen, vital sign flow sheet or record form

Steps	Rationale
1. Determine need to assess client's blood pressure (BP):	Nurse uses clinical judgment to determine need for assessment.
a. Note risk factors for alteration in BP.	Certain conditions place clients at risk for BP alteration: history of cardiovascular disease, renal disease, diabetes, circulatory shock (hypovolemic, septic, cardiogenic, or neurogenic), acute or chronic pain, rapid IV infusion of fluids or blood products, increased intracranial pressure, postoperative conditions, toxemia of pregnancy.
b. Observe for signs and symptoms of BP alterations:	Physical signs and symptoms may indicate alterations in BP.
(1) Assess for symptoms of high BP: headache (usually occipital), flushing of face, nosebleed, and fatigue in older adults.	High BP (hypertension) is often asymptomatic until pressure is very high.
(2) Assess for symptoms associated with low BP: dizziness, mental confusion; restlessness; pale, dusky, or cyanotic skin and mucous membranes; cool, mottled skin over extremities.	
2. Determine best site for BP assessment. Avoid applying cuff to extremity when IV fluids are infusing; an arteriovenous shunt or fistula is present; breast or axillary surgery has been performed on that side; extremity has been traumatized, diseased, or requires a cast or bulky bandage. The lower extremities may be used when the brachial arteries are inaccessible.	Inappropriate site selection may result in poor amplification of sounds, causing inaccurate readings. Application of pressure from inflated bladder temporarily impairs blood flow and can further compromise circulation in extremity that already has impaired blood flow.
3. Select appropriate cuff size.	Improper cuff size results in inaccurate readings (see Table 27-9). If cuff is too small, it tends to come loose as inflated and results in false high readings. If the cuff is too large, false low readings may be recorded. For the adult client, the bladder, enclosed by the cuff, should encircle 80% of the arm.
4. Determine previous baseline BP (if available) from client's record.	Allows nurse to assess for change in condition. Provides comparison with future BP measurements.
5. Identify factors likely to interfere with accuracy of BP measurement: exercise, coffee (i.e., caffeine), smoking. Encourage client to avoid exercise and smoking for 15–30 minutes, and ingestion of caffeine for 60 minutes before assessment of BP (CHEP, 2004).	Exercise and smoking can cause false elevations in BP. Smoking increases BP immediately and lasts up to 15 minutes. The effects of coffee or caffeine increases BP for up to 3 hours (Pickering, 2001).

Skill 27-5 Measuring Blood Pressure—cont'd

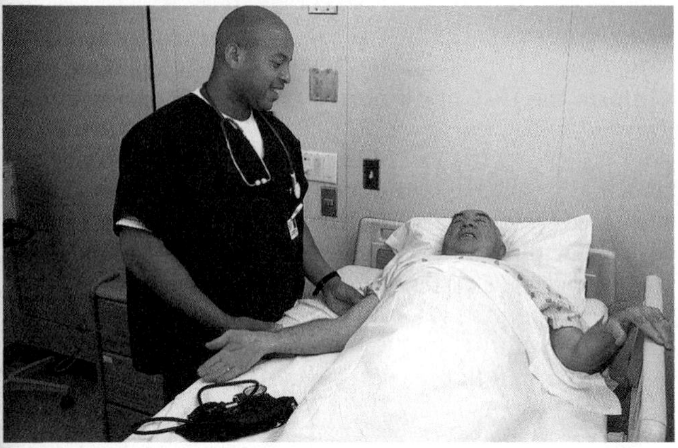

STEP **8** Client's forearm supported in bed.

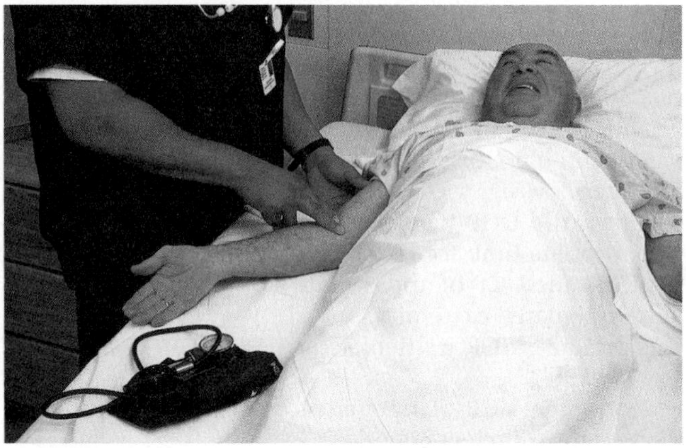

STEP **10** Nurse palpating client's brachial artery.

6. Perform hand hygiene. Have client assume sitting or lying position. Be sure room is warm, quiet, and relaxing.

Reduces transmission of microorganisms. Maintains client's comfort during measurement. The client's perceptions that the physical or interpersonal environment is stressful affect the BP measurement.

7. Explain to client that BP is to be assessed and have client rest at least 5 minutes before measurement. When possible, client should be sitting in a chair with feet touching floor (CHEP, 2004). Ask client not to speak when BP is being measured.

Allows client to relax and helps to avoid falsely elevated readings. Blood pressure readings taken at different times can be objectively compared when assessed with client at rest. Talking to a client when the BP is being assessed may increase readings.

8. With client sitting or lying, position client's forearm at heart level; position thigh flat (provide support as needed). For arm, turn palm up (see illustration); for thigh, position with knee slightly flexed.

If extremity is unsupported, client may perform isometric exercise that can increase diastolic blood pressure.

9. Expose extremity (arm or leg) fully by removing constricting clothing.

Ensures proper cuff application.

Critical Decision Point: Do not place blood pressure cuff over clothing.

10. Palpate brachial artery (arm; see illustration) or popliteal artery (leg). Position cuff 2.5 cm above site of pulsation (antecubital or popliteal space).

Inflating bladder directly over artery ensures proper pressure is applied during inflation.

11. Apply bladder of cuff above artery by centring arrows marked on cuff over artery. If no centre arrows on cuff, estimate the centre of the bladder and place this centre over artery. With cuff fully deflated, wrap cuff evenly and snugly around extremity (see illustrations).

Loose-fitting cuff causes false high readings.

12. Measure blood pressure.

A. Two-step method

(1) Relocate brachial pulse. Palpate the artery distal to the cuff with fingertips of nondominant hand while inflating cuff rapidly to pressure 30 mm Hg above point at which pulse disappears. Slowly deflate cuff and note point when pulse reappears. Deflate cuff fully and wait 30 seconds.

Estimating prevents false low readings, which may result in the presence of an auscultatory gap. Maximal inflation point for accurate reading can be determined by palpation. If unable to palpate artery because of weakened pulse, an ultrasonic stethoscope can be used (see chapter 28). Deflating cuff prevents venous congestion and false high readings.

(2) Place stethoscope earpieces in ears and be sure sounds are clear, not muffled.

Each earpiece should follow angle of ear canal to facilitate hearing.

(3) Relocate brachial or popliteal artery and place bell or diaphragm chestpiece of stethoscope over it. Do not allow chestpiece to touch cuff or clothing (see illustration).

Proper stethoscope placement ensures optimal sound reception. Stethoscope improperly positioned causes muffled sounds that often result in false low systolic and false high diastolic readings.

Steps	Rationale

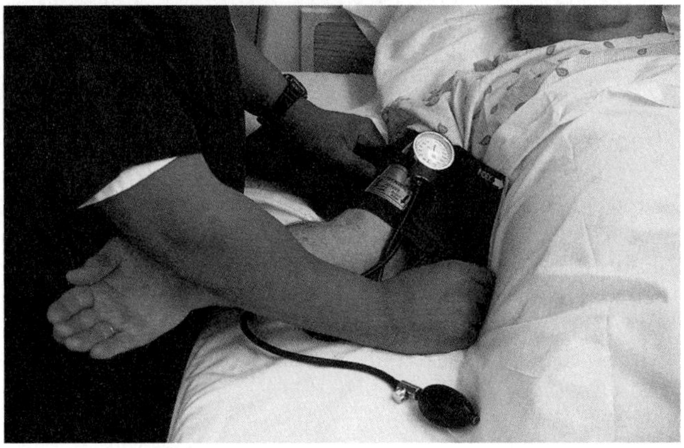

A

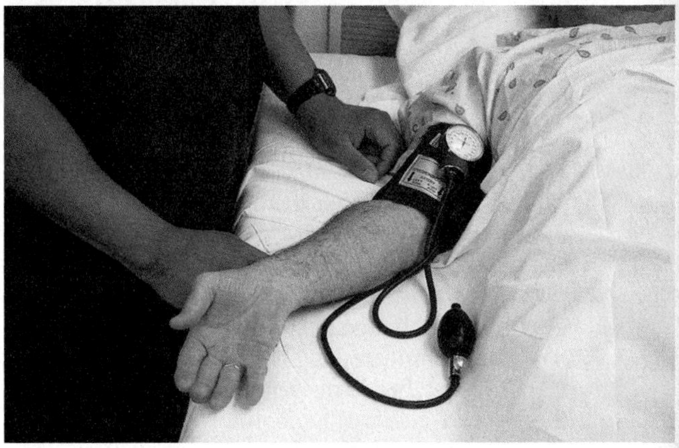

B

STEP **11** **A,** Centre bladder of cuff above artery. **B,** Blood pressure cuff wrapped around upper arm.

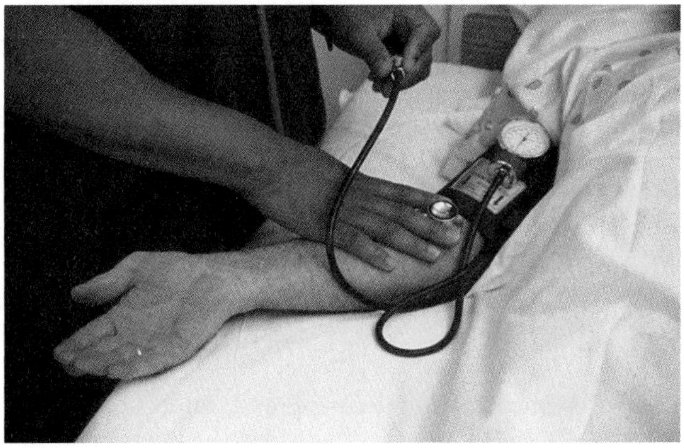

STEP **12A(3)** Stethoscope over brachial artery to measure BP.

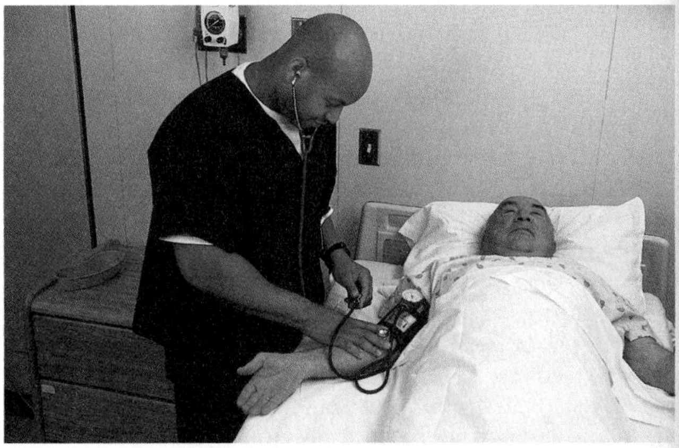

STEP **12A(4)** Inflating BP cuff.

Steps	Rationale
(4) Close valve of pressure bulb clockwise until tight. Quickly inflate cuff to 30 mm Hg above palpated systolic pressure (client's estimated systolic pressure; see illustration).	Tightening of valve prevents air leak during inflation. Inflation ensures accurate measurement of systolic pressure.
(5) Slowly release pressure bulb valve and allow needle of manometer gauge to fall at rate of 2 mm Hg/second.	Too rapid or slow a decline in pressure can cause inaccurate readings.
(6) Note point on manometer when first clear sound is heard. The sound will slowly increase in intensity.	First Korotkoff sound indicates systolic pressure (see Figure 27–14).
(7) Continue to deflate cuff, noting point at which muffled or dampened sound appears.	Fourth Korotkoff sound involves distinct muffling of sounds and is recommended as indication of diastolic pressure in children.
(8) Continue to deflate cuff gradually, noting point at which sound disappears in adults. Listen for 10 to 20 mm Hg after the last sound, and then allow remaining air to escape quickly.	Beginning of the fifth Korotkoff sound is recommended as indication of diastolic pressure in adults. Continuous cuff inflation causes arterial occlusion, resulting in numbness and tingling of client's arm.
B. One-step method	
(1) Place stethoscope earpieces in ears and be sure sounds are clear, not muffled.	Each earpiece should follow angle of ear canal to facilitate hearing.

Skill 27-5 *Measuring Blood Pressure—cont'd*

Steps	Rationale
(2) Relocate brachial or popliteal artery and place bell or diaphragm chestpiece of stethoscope over it. Do not allow chestpiece to touch cuff or clothing.	Proper stethoscope placement ensures optimal sound reception. Stethoscope improperly positioned causes muffled sounds that often result in false low systolic and false high diastolic readings.
(3) Close valve of pressure bulb clockwise until tight. Quickly inflate cuff to 30 mm Hg above palpated systolic pressure.	Tightening of valve prevents air leak during inflation. Inflation ensures accurate measurement of systolic pressure.
(4) Slowly release pressure bulb valve and allow needle of manometer gauge to fall at rate of 2 mm Hg/second.	Too rapid or slow a decline in pressure can cause inaccurate readings.
(5) Note point on manometer when first clear sound is heard. The sound will slowly increase in intensity.	First Korotkoff sound indicates systolic pressure.
(6) Continue to deflate cuff, noting point at which muffled or dampened sound appears.	Fourth Korotkoff sound involves distinct muffling of sounds and is recommended as indication of diastolic pressure in children.
(7) Continue to deflate cuff gradually, noting point at which sound disappears in adults. Listen for 10 to 20 mm Hg after the last sound, and then allow remaining air to escape quickly.	Beginning of the fifth Korotkoff sound is recommended as indication of diastolic pressure in adults. Continuous cuff inflation causes arterial occlusion, resulting in numbness and tingling of client's arm.
13. Remove cuff from extremity unless measurement must be repeated. Two readings separated by 1 minute should be taken (CHEP, 2004). If readings are different by more than 5 mm Hg, additional readings are necessary. If this is the first assessment of client, repeat blood pressure assessment on other extremity.	Comparison of BP in both extremities detects circulation problems. (Normal difference of 5 to 10 mm Hg exists between extremities.)
14. Assist client in returning to comfortable position and cover upper arm if previously clothed.	Promotes participation in care and understanding of health status.
15. Perform hand hygiene.	Reduces transmission of microorganisms.
16. Discuss findings with client as needed.	Restores comfort and promotes sense of well-being.
17. Compare reading with previous baseline and/or acceptable value of blood pressure for client's age.	Evaluates for change in condition and alterations.
18. Compare blood pressure in both arms or both legs.	If using upper extremities, the arm with the higher pressure should be used for subsequent assessments unless contraindicated.
19. Correlate blood pressure with data obtained from pulse assessment and related cardiovascular signs and symptoms.	Blood pressure and heart rate are interrelated.

Unexpected Outcomes and Related Interventions

- Unable to obtain BP reading
  - Assess for signs of decreased cardiac output (e.g., weak thready pulse, confusion, pallor, or cyanosis).
  - Palpate radial artery if strong, reposition BP cuff, and repeat measurement.
  - Use palpation method to obtain BP.
  - If BP is low or obtainable, place client in supine position.
  - Notify physician.
- BP is less than 90 mm Hg, systolic
  - Repeat BP measurement
  - If using automatic BP device, switch and use auscultation or palpation method to obtain client's BP.
  - Notify physician.
- BP is elevated above client's usual value
  - Repeat measurement in other arm.
  - Assess client for headache, confusion, fatigue.
  - Report elevated BP to physician.

Recording and Reporting

- Inform client of value and need for periodic reassessment.
- Record blood pressure in nurses' notes or vital sign flow sheet. Measurement of blood pressure after administration of specific therapies should be documented in narrative form in nurses' notes.
- Report abnormal findings to nurse in charge or physician.

Home Care Considerations

- Assess home noise level to determine room that will provide quietest environment for assessing BP.
- Consider electronic blood pressure cuff for home if client has hearing difficulties and adequate dexterity.

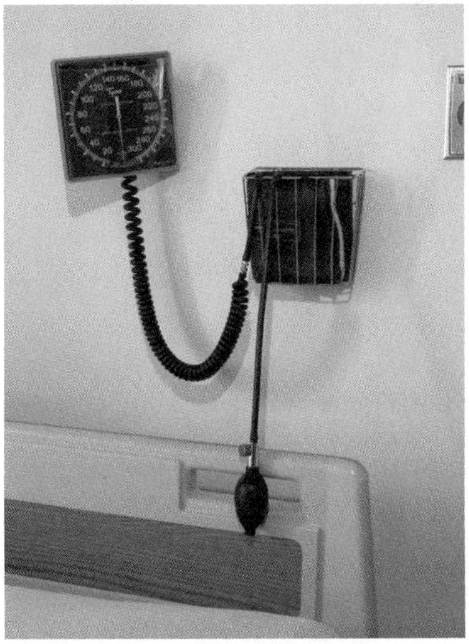

FIGURE **27–12** Wall-mounted aneroid sphygmomanometer.

aneroid manometer has a glass-enclosed circular gauge containing a needle that registers millimeter calibrations. Before using the aneroid model, the nurse makes sure that the needle is pointing to zero and that the manometer is correctly calibrated. Aneroid sphygmomanometers require biomedical calibration at routine intervals to verify their accuracy.

Mercury manometers, once the gold standard, are less common because they contain mercury, a hazardous substance. However, some agencies or specific units, for example, operating rooms or intensive care units, may still use the mercury manometer. Pressure created by the inflation of the compression cuff moves the column of mercury upward against the force of gravity. Millimeter calibrations mark the height of the mercury column. To ensure accurate readings, the mercury column should fall freely as pressure is released and should always be at zero when the cuff is deflated. Accurate readings are obtained by looking at the meniscus of the mercury at eye level. Looking up or down at the mercury results in distorted readings. Because most municipalities have prohibited the sale or use of mercury-containing devices because of the potential hazards, fewer mercury manometers are available, but they still exist.

Cloth or disposable vinyl compression cuffs contain the inflatable bladder and come in several sizes. The size selected is proportional to the circumference of the limb being assessed (Figure 27–13). Ideally, the width of the cuff should be 40% of the circumference (or 20% wider than the diameter) of the midpoint of the limb on which the cuff is to be used. The bladder, enclosed by the cuff, should encircle at least 80% of the arm of an adult and the entire arm of a child. In children, the lower edge of the cuff should be above the antecubital fossa, allowing room for placement of the stethoscope bell or diaphragm. Blood pressure measurements will not be accurate unless the correct size blood pressure cuff is applied appropriately.

Before using a sphygmomanometer, the nurse should inspect the parts of the release valve and the pressure bulb. The valve should be clean and freely moveable in either direction. If it sticks or becomes too tightly closed, the deflation of the pressure cuff will be hard to regulate. The pressure bulb is made of tough rubber and should be free of leaks.

Auscultation. The best environment for blood pressure measurement by auscultation is a quiet room at a comfortable temperature. Although the client may lie or stand, sitting is the preferred position. In most cases, blood pressure readings obtained with the client in the supine, sitting, and standing positions are similar.

The client's position during routine blood pressure determination should be the same during each measurement to permit a meaningful comparison of values. Before assessment, the nurse should attempt to control factors responsible for artificially high readings, such as pain, anxiety, or exertion. The client's perceptions that the physical or interpersonal environment is more or less stressful will affect the blood pressure measurement. Blood pressure measurements taken at the client's place of employment or in a physician's office are higher than those taken at the client's home.

During the initial assessment, the nurse should obtain and record the blood pressure in both arms. Normally, there is a difference of 5 to 10 mm Hg between the arms. In subsequent assessments, the blood pressure should be measured in the arm with the higher pressure. Pressure differences greater than 10 mm Hg indicate vascular problems and are reported to the physician or nurse in charge.

The nurse asks the client to state his or her usual blood pressure. If the client does not know, the nurse informs the client after measuring and recording the blood pressure. This is a good opportunity to educate the client about optimal values of blood pressure, the risk factors for developing hypertension, and dangers of hypertension.

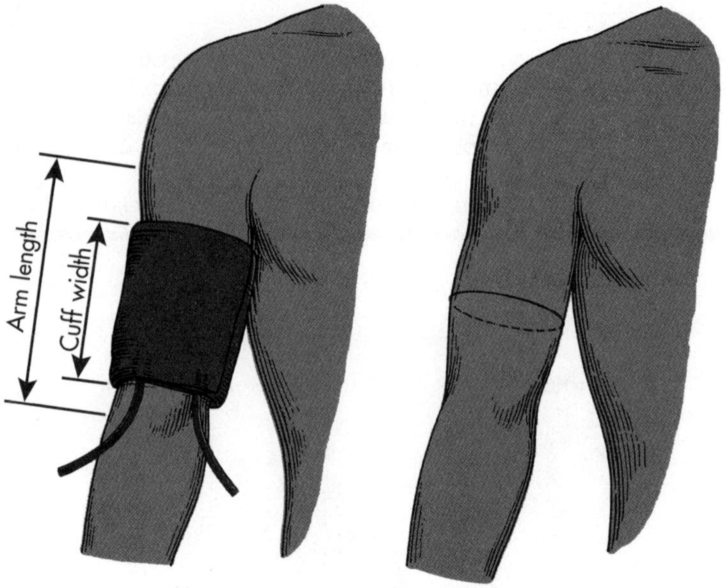

FIGURE **27–13** Guidelines for proper blood pressure cuff size: Cuff width 20% more than upper arm diameter, or 40% of circumference and two thirds of arm length.

Research Highlight *Box 27-13*

Effect of Crossing Legs on Blood Pressure Measurement

Research Focus

Blood pressure measurement is an important factor when determining the diagnosis of hypertension. Because hypertension can lead to serious complications, eliminating errors in measuring blood pressure is important.

Research Abstract

The purpose of this study was to determine if the client's position affects the measurement of blood pressure. One hundred and three older adults participated in a study to determine the influence of leg crossing. The blood pressure of male and female older adults with and without a diagnosis of hypertension was measured twice. Blood pressure was measured after 3 minutes of rest while sitting with feet flat on the floor. A second blood pressure was measured after the subjects had crossed one leg over the knee for 3 minutes. Results indicate that systolic and diastolic blood pressure were greater when legs were crossed for both groups of subjects.

Evidence-Based Practice

- Clients should be instructed to keep their feet flat on the floor during blood pressure measurement.
- A client's positions should be considered when comparing two different blood pressure measurements.

Reference

Keele-Smith, R., & Price-Daniel, C. (2001). Effects of crossing legs on blood pressure measurement. *Clinical Nursing Research, 10*(2), 202–213.

Indirect measurement of arterial blood pressure works on a basic principle of pressure. Blood flows freely through an artery until an inflated cuff applies pressure to tissues and causes the artery to collapse. After the cuff pressure is released, the point at which blood flow returns and sound appears through auscultation is the systolic pressure.

In 1905, Korotkoff, a Russian surgeon, first described the sounds heard over an artery distal to the blood pressure cuff. The first Korotkoff sound is a clear rhythmical tapping corresponding to the pulse rate that gradually increases in intensity. *Onset of the sound corresponds to the systolic pressure.* A murmur or swishing sound occurs as the cuff continues to deflate, resulting in the second Korotkoff sound. As the artery distends, there is turbulence in blood flow. The third Korotkoff sound is a crisper and more intense tapping. The fourth Korotkoff sound becomes muffled and low-pitched as the cuff is further deflated. At this point, the cuff pressure has fallen below the pressure within the vessel walls; *this sound is the diastolic pressure in infants and children.* The fifth Korotkoff sound marks the disappearance of sound. *In adolescents and adults, the fifth sound corresponds with the diastolic pressure* (Figure 27–14). In some clients, the sounds are clear and distinct. In other clients, only the beginning and ending sounds are clear.

The Canadian Hypertension Education Program (2004) recommends recording two numbers for a blood pressure measurement: the point on the manometer when the first sound is heard for systolic and the point on the manometer when the fifth sound is heard for diastolic. Some institutions recommend recording the point when the fourth sound is heard as well, especially for clients with hypertension. The numbers are divided by slashed lines (e.g., 120/80 or 120/100/80), the arm used to measure the blood pressure is noted (e.g., right arm [RA] 130/70), and the client's position when the pressure is assessed (e.g., sitting); Box 27-13.

Many medical decisions and nursing interventions about a client's health care are made based on blood pressure findings. The importance of obtaining an accurate

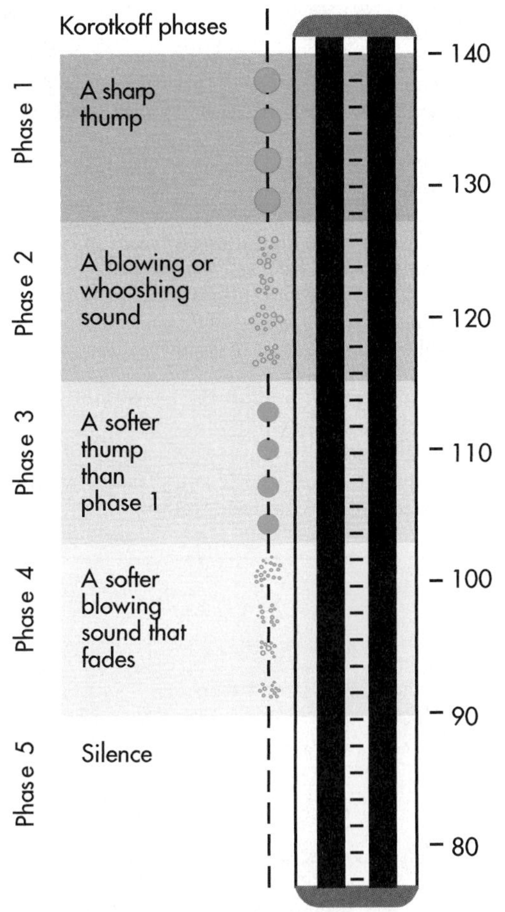

FIGURE **27–14** The sounds auscultated during blood pressure measurement can be differentiated into five Korotkoff phases. In this example, blood pressure is 140/90.

blood pressure cannot be overemphasized. There are several sources for error. Table 27-9 summarizes common mistakes in measurement. When a nurse is unsure of a reading, a colleague should reassess the blood pressure.

Assessment in Children. All children 3 years of age through adolescence should have blood pressure checked at least yearly. Blood pressure in children changes with growth and development. The nurse can help parents to understand the importance of this routine screening to detect children who may be at risk for hypertension. The measurement of blood pressure in infants and children is difficult for several reasons:

- Different arm size requires careful and appropriate cuff size selection. Do not choose a cuff based on the name of the cuff. An "infant" cuff may be too small for some infants.
- Readings are difficult to obtain in restless or anxious infants and children. A delay of at least 15 minutes to allow children to recover from recent activities and apprehension is recommended. Preparing the child for the blood pressure cuff's unusual sensation can increase co-operation. Most children will understand the analogy of a "tight hug on your arm."
- Placing the stethoscope too firmly on the antecubital fossa can cause errors in auscultation.
- Korotkoff sounds are difficult to hear in children because of low frequency and amplitude. A pediatric stethoscope bell can be helpful.

Ultrasonic Stethoscope. If a nurse is unable to auscultate sounds because of a weakened arterial pulse, an ultrasonic stethoscope can be used (see chapter 28). This stethoscope allows the nurse to hear low-frequency systolic sounds and is commonly used when measuring the blood pressure of infants, children, and low blood pressure in adults.

Palpation. The indirect palpation technique is useful for clients whose arterial pulsations are too weak to create Korotkoff sounds. Severe blood loss and decreased heart contractility are examples of conditions that result in blood pressures too low to auscultate accurately. Only the systolic blood pressure can be assessed by palpation because the diastolic pressure is difficult to appreciate (Box 27-14). When the palpation technique is used, the systolic value and the manner in which it was measured are recorded (e.g., RA 90/—, palpated, supine).

The palpation technique is used along with auscultation in some instances. In some hypertensive clients, the sounds usually heard over the brachial artery when the cuff pressure is high disappear as pressure is reduced and then reappear at a lower level. This temporary disappearance of sound is the **auscultatory gap.** It typically occurs between the first and second Korotkoff sounds. The gap in sound may cover a range of 40 mm Hg and thus may cause an underestimation of systolic pressure or overestimation of diastolic pressure. The examiner must be certain to inflate the cuff high enough to hear the true systolic pressure before the auscultatory gap. Palpation of the radial artery helps to determine how high to inflate the cuff. The examiner inflates the cuff 30 mm Hg above the pressure at which the radial pulse was palpated. The range of pressures in which the auscultatory gap occurs is recorded (e.g., BP RA 180/94 with an auscultatory gap from 180 to 160, sitting).

Lower Extremity Blood Pressure. Dressings, casts, IV catheters, or arteriovenous fistulas or shunts can make the upper extremities inaccessible for blood pressure measurement. Blood pressure must then be measured in the lower extremities. Comparing upper extremity blood pressure with that in the legs is also necessary for clients with certain peripheral vascular abnormalities. The popliteal artery, palpable behind the knee in the popliteal space, is the site for auscultation. The cuff must be wide and long enough to allow for the larger girth of the thigh. Placing the client in a prone position is best. If such a position is impossible, the client should be asked to flex the knee slightly for easier access to the artery. The cuff is positioned 2.5 cm above the popliteal artery with the bladder over the posterior aspect of the midthigh (Figure 27–15). The procedure is identical to brachial artery auscultation. Systolic pressure in the legs is usually higher by 10 to 40 mm Hg than in the brachial artery, but the diastolic pressure is the same.

Table 27-9 Common Mistakes in Blood Pressure Assessment

Error	Effect
Bladder or cuff too wide	False low reading
Bladder or cuff too narrow	False high reading
Cuff wrapped too loosely or unevenly	False high reading
Deflating cuff too slowly	False high diastolic reading
Deflating cuff too quickly	False low systolic and false high diastolic reading
Arm below heart level	False high reading
Arm above heart level	False low reading
Arm not supported	False high reading
Stethoscope that fits poorly or impairment of the examiner's hearing, causing sounds to be muffled	False low systolic and false high diastolic reading
Stethoscope applied too firmly against antecubital fossa	False low diastolic reading
Inflating too slowly	False high diastolic reading
Repeating assessments too quickly	False high systolic reading
Inaccurate inflation level	Inaccurate interpretation of systolic and diastolic readings
Multiple examiners using different Korotkoff sounds for diastolic readings	False high systolic and low diastolic reading

Box 27-14 Palpating the Systolic Blood Pressure

1. Apply blood pressure cuff to the upper arm in the same manner as the auscultation method.
2. Continually palpate the pulse of the brachial, radial, or popliteal artery with fingertips of one hand.
3. Inflate blood pressure cuff 30 mm Hg above the point at which the radial pulse is palpated.
4. Release valve and allow manometer needle mercury to fall 2 mm Hg per second.
5. As soon as the pulse is palpable, note the manometer reading, which will be the systolic blood pressure.
6. Deflate cuff rapidly and completely.
7. Remove cuff from extremity and discuss findings with client as needed. Record pressures systolic/—, palpated (e.g., BP 108/—, palpated).

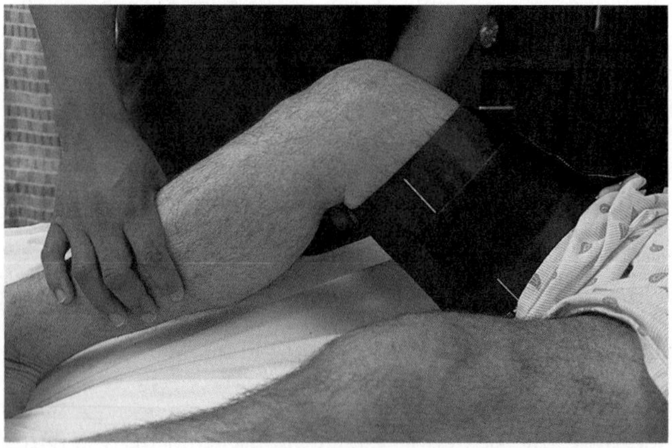

FIGURE **27–15** Lower extremity blood pressure cuff positioned above the popliteal artery at midthigh with knee flexed.

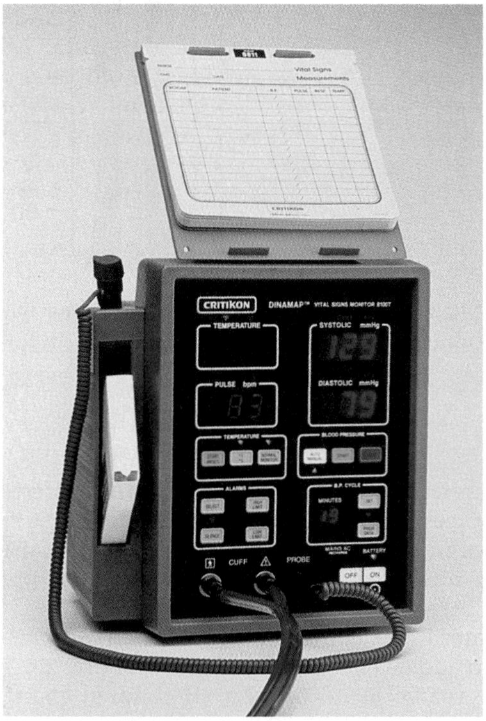

FIGURE **27–16** Automatic blood pressure monitor. (Dinamap Vital Signs Monitor is a trademark of Critikon, Inc. Photo courtesy Critikon, Inc., Tampa, FL.)

Automatic Blood Pressure Devices. Many electronic devices can determine blood pressure automatically (Figure 27–16). These devices are applied when frequent blood pressure assessment is required such as in the critically ill or potentially unstable client, during or after invasive procedures, or when therapies require frequent monitoring (e.g., IV heart and blood pressure medications). However, some client conditions are not appropriate for automatic blood pressure devices (Box 27-15).

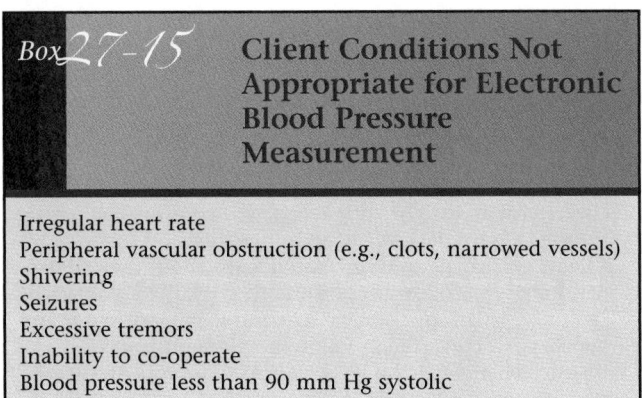

Box 27-15 Client Conditions Not Appropriate for Electronic Blood Pressure Measurement

Irregular heart rate
Peripheral vascular obstruction (e.g., clots, narrowed vessels)
Shivering
Seizures
Excessive tremors
Inability to co-operate
Blood pressure less than 90 mm Hg systolic

Whereas the auscultatory technique relies on the detection of Korotkoff sounds, some electronic devices rely on the principle of oscillometry. The system includes either a microphone or a pressure sensor built into the inflatable cuff. The microphone or acoustic system hears Korotkoff sounds and registers diastolic and systolic readings. The pressure sensor or ultrasonic system responds to the pressure waves generated by the movement of blood through the artery. The sensor determines the initial burst of oscillations and translates the information into a systolic pressure reading. The diastolic pressure is measured when the oscillations are lowest, just before they stop.

A baseline blood pressure should be obtained using the auscultatory method before applying automatic devices. A comparison assists in evaluation of a client's status and allows proper programming of the device. Once the blood pressure cuff is applied, the nurse can program the device to obtain and record blood pressure readings at preset intervals. Alarm limits can be programmed to alert the nurse if the blood pressure measurement is outside desired parameters.

Automatic devices are easy to use and efficient when repeated or when frequent measurements are indicated. The ability to use a stethoscope is not required. However, automatic devices are more sensitive to outside interference and are susceptible to error. The microphone or pressure sensor must be positioned directly over the artery for proper function. Client movements, vibration, or outside noise can interfere with the microphone or sensor signal. Most automatic blood pressure devices are unable to process sounds or vibrations of low blood pressure. The range of device sophistication also can make blood pressure measurement comparisons difficult.

The use of automatic blood pressure devices permits assessment of blood pressure during interpersonal interactions. However, the nurse should avoid speaking to the client for at least a minute before initiating a blood pressure recording. Talking to a client when the blood pressure is being assessed can increase readings 10% to 40% (Pickering, 2001).

Self-Measurement of Blood Pressure. More people measure their own blood pressures because of improved technology in home monitoring devices and a greater interest in health promotion. Two of the more common devices used by the general public include portable home sphygmomanometers and stationary automatic blood pressure machines.

The portable home devices include the aneroid sphygmomanometer and electronic digital readout devices that do not require use of a stethoscope. The electronic devices inflate and deflate cuffs with the push of a button. The electronic devices may be easier to manipulate but can easily become inaccurate and require recalibration more than once a year. Because of their sensitivity, improper cuff placement or movement of the arm can cause electronic devices to give incorrect readings.

Stationary automatic blood pressure devices can be found in public places such as drug stores, fitness clubs, banks, airports, or work sites. Users simply rest their arms within the machine's inflatable cuff, which contains a pressure sensor. The cuff fits over clothing. A visual display tells users their blood pressure within 60 to 90 seconds. The reliability of the stationary machines is limited. Blood pressure values may vary by 5 to 10 mm Hg or more (for both systolic and diastolic values) compared with pressures taken with a manual sphygmomanometer.

Self-measurement of blood pressure has several benefits. Elevated blood pressure may be detected in people previously unaware of a problem. People with high normal blood pressure can provide information about the pattern of blood pressure values. Clients with hypertension can benefit from participating actively in their treatment through self-monitoring, which may help compliance with treatment. The disadvantages of self-measurement include improper use of the device and inaccurate readings. A client may be needlessly alarmed with one elevated reading. Clients with hypertension may become overly conscious of their blood pressures and make inappropriate self-adjustment of medications.

Consumers can learn to use self-measurement devices if they have the information needed to perform the procedure correctly and if they know when to seek medical attention. The nurse can advise clients of possible inaccuracies in the blood pressure devices, help clients understand the meaning and implications of readings, and teach them proper measurement techniques.

Nursing Process and Blood Pressure Determination

The assessment of blood pressure and pulse is used to evaluate the general state of cardiovascular health and responses to other system imbalances. Hypotension, hypertension, orthostatic hypotension, and narrow or wide pulse pressures are defining characteristics of certain nursing diagnoses, including the following:

- Activity intolerance
- Anxiety
- Decreased cardiac output
- Deficient/excess fluid volume
- Risk for injury
- Acute pain
- Ineffective tissue perfusion

The nursing care plan includes interventions based on the nursing diagnosis identified and the related factor.

Focus on Primary Health Care **Box 27-16**

Health Promotion and Vital Signs

Temperature

- Identify client's ability to initiate preventive health measures and recognize alteration in body temperature. Educate client and caregiver about measures to prevent body temperature alterations.
- Teach clients at risk for hypothermia and frostbite (older adults, homeless people, etc.) about risk factors: fatigue; malnutrition; hypoxemia; cold, wet clothing; alcohol intoxication.
- Teach clients at risk for heat stroke (older adults, athletes, travellers, people who work outside, etc.) about risk factors: strenuous exercise in hot, humid weather; sudden exposure to hot climates; insufficient fluid intake.
- Teach clients the importance of taking and continuing antibiotics as directed until course of treatment is completed.

Pulse Rate

- Clients taking certain prescribed cardiac medications should learn to assess their own pulse rates to detect side effects of medications.
- Clients undergoing cardiac rehabilitation should learn to assess their own pulse rates to determine their response to exercise.

Blood Pressure (BP)

- Teach client risk factors for hypertension. People with family history of hypertension are at significant risk. Obesity, cigarette smoking, heavy alcohol consumption, high blood cholesterol and triglyceride levels, and continued exposure to stress are risk factors linked to hypertension.
- Clients with hypertension should learn about their BP values, long-term follow-up care and therapy, the usual lack of symptoms, therapy's ability to control but not cure, and benefits of a consistently followed treatment plan.
- Instruct clients on the importance of appropriate-size BP cuff for home use.
- Instruct client or primary caregiver to take BP at same time each day and after client has had a brief rest. Take BP sitting or lying down, and use the same position and arm each time pressure is taken.
- Instruct client or primary caregiver that if it is difficult to hear the pressure, it may be that the cuff is too loose, not big enough, or too narrow; the stethoscope is not over arterial pulse; the cuff was deflated too quickly or too slowly; or the cuff was not pumped high enough for systolic readings.

Respirations

- Clients who demonstrate decreased ventilation may benefit from being taught deep breathing and coughing exercises (see chapter 45).
- Instruct caregiver to contact home care nurse or physician if unusual fluctuations in respiratory rate occur.
- Teach client signs and symptoms of hypoxemia: headache, somnolence, confusion, dusky colour, shortness of breath, dyspnea.
- Teach client effect of high-risk behaviours such as cigarette smoking on oxygen saturation.

For example, the defining characteristics of hypotension, dizziness, pulse deficit, and dysrhythmia lead to a diagnosis of *decreased cardiac output*. Related factors may include poor oral intake, excessive heat exposure, and a history of valvular heart disease. The related factor guides the choice of nursing interventions. The nurse evaluates client outcomes by assessing the blood pressure following each intervention.

Health Promotion and Vital Signs

The emphasis on health promotion and health maintenance, as well as early discharge from hospital settings, has resulted in an increase in the need for clients and their families to monitor vital signs in the home. Teaching considerations affect all vital sign measurements and should be incorporated within the client's plan of care (Box 27-16).

When considering how to teach clients and their families about vital sign measurements and their importance and significance, the client's age is an important factor. With the increased older adult population, there is a need for caregivers to be aware of changes that are unique to older adults (Box 27-17).

Recording Vital Signs

Special graphic flow sheets exist for recording vital signs (Figure 27–17). The nurse identifies the institution's procedure for documenting on the graphic or vital sign flow sheet. In addition to the vital sign values, the nurse records in the nurses' notes any accompanying or precipitating symptoms such as chest pain and dizziness with abnormal blood pressure, shortness of breath with abnormal respirations, cyanosis with hypoxemia, or flushing and diaphoresis with elevated temperature. The nurse documents any interventions initiated as a result of vital sign measurement such as administration of oxygen therapy or an antihypertensive medication.

Clients being managed on critical paths or CareMaps may have vital sign values listed as outcomes (see chap-

Focus on Older Adults

Box 27-17

Temperature

- Normal body temperatures are lower in later life; mean body temperature ranges from 36° to 36.8° C orally and 36.6° to 37.2° C rectally (Eliopoulos, 2001).
- Know the older adult's baseline body temperature when making a determination about febrile status. Document the actual temperature and its deviation from baseline, rather than using terminology such as "febrile" or "afebrile" (Miller, 1999).
- Manifestations of delayed or diminished febrile response to infection are subtle, variable in presentation, and very difficult to assess. Do not assume that an infection in an older adult will cause an elevated temperature (Miller, 1999).
- The nurse needs to be especially attentive to subtle temperature changes and other manifestations of fever in this population, such as tachypnea, anorexia, falls, delirium, and overall functional decline (Lueckenotte, 1998).
- Increased age is associated with a reduced ability to respond to cold environments due to inefficient vasoconstriction, decreased cardiac output, diminished shivering, and reduced muscle mass and subcutaneous tissue.
- A reduced ability to respond to hot environments is due to impaired sweating mechanisms and decreased cardiac output (Eliopoulos, 2001).

Pulse Rate

- If it is difficult to palpate the pulse of an older adult or obese client, a Doppler device will provide a more accurate reading.
- The older adult has a decreased heart rate at rest (Ebersole & Hess, 2001).
- Once elevated, the pulse rate of an older adult takes longer to return to normal resting rate (Lueckenotte, 2000).
- When assessing older women with sagging breasts, the breast tissue should be gently lifted and the stethoscope placed at the fifth intercostal space or the lower edge of the breast.
- Heart sounds may be muffled or difficult to hear in older adults because of an increase in air space in the lungs.

Blood Pressure (BP)

- Older adults, especially those who are frail, have lost upper arm mass, requiring special attention to selection of BP cuff size.
- An older adult's BP may elevate with age. However, such elevations should not be considered a normal aspect of aging and older adults need to have minor elevations monitored (Chobanian et al., 2003).
- Older adults have an increase in systolic pressure related to decreased vessel elasticity. The diastolic pressure remains the same, resulting in a wider pulse pressure (Lueckenotte, 2000).
- Older adults are instructed to change position slowly and wait after each change to avoid postural hypotension and prevent injuries.

Respirations

- Aging causes ossification of costal cartilage and downward slant of ribs, resulting in a more rigid rib cage, which reduces chest wall expansion. Kyphosis and scoliosis that can occur in older adults may also restrict chest expansion and decrease tidal volume (Sheahan & Musialowski, 2001).
- Older adults may depend more on diaphragmatic and accessory abdominal muscles during respiration than on weakened thoracic muscles (Sheahan & Musialowski, 2001).
- Decreased efficiency of respiratory muscles results in breathlessness at low exercise levels.
- A change in lung function with aging results in respiratory rates that are generally higher in older adults, with a normal of 16 to 25 breaths per minute (Lueckenotte, 2000).
- Responses to hypercapnia and hypoxia are reduced 50% in older adults as compared with the young, limiting the ability of older adults to respond to hypoxia with respiratory changes (Ebersole & Hess, 2001).
- Identifying an acceptable pulse oximeter probe site may be difficult on older adults because of the likelihood of peripheral vascular disease, decreased cardiac output, cold-induced vasoconstriction, and anemia.

ter 12). If a vital sign value is above or below the anticipated outcomes, a variance note is written to explain the nature of the variance and the nurse's course of action. For example, a CareMap for a client who has undergone a thoracotomy may have an outcome during the postoperative period of "afebrile." If the client has a fever, the nurse's variance note may address possible sources of fever (e.g., retained pulmonary secretions) and nursing interventions (e.g., increased suctioning, postural drainage, or hydration).

Key Concepts

- Vital signs include the physiological measurement of temperature, pulse, blood pressure, respirations, and oxygen saturation.
- Vital signs are measured as part of a complete physical examination or in a review of a client's condition.
- The nurse assesses vital sign changes with other physical assessment findings, using clinical judgment to determine measurement frequency.
- Knowledge of the factors influencing vital signs assists the nurse in determining and evaluating abnormal values.
- Vital signs provide a basis for evaluating response to nursing interventions.
- Vital signs are best measured when the client is inactive and the environment is controlled for comfort.
- The nurse assists the client in maintaining body temperature by initiating interventions that promote heat loss, production, or conservation.
- A fever is one of the body's normal defence mechanisms.

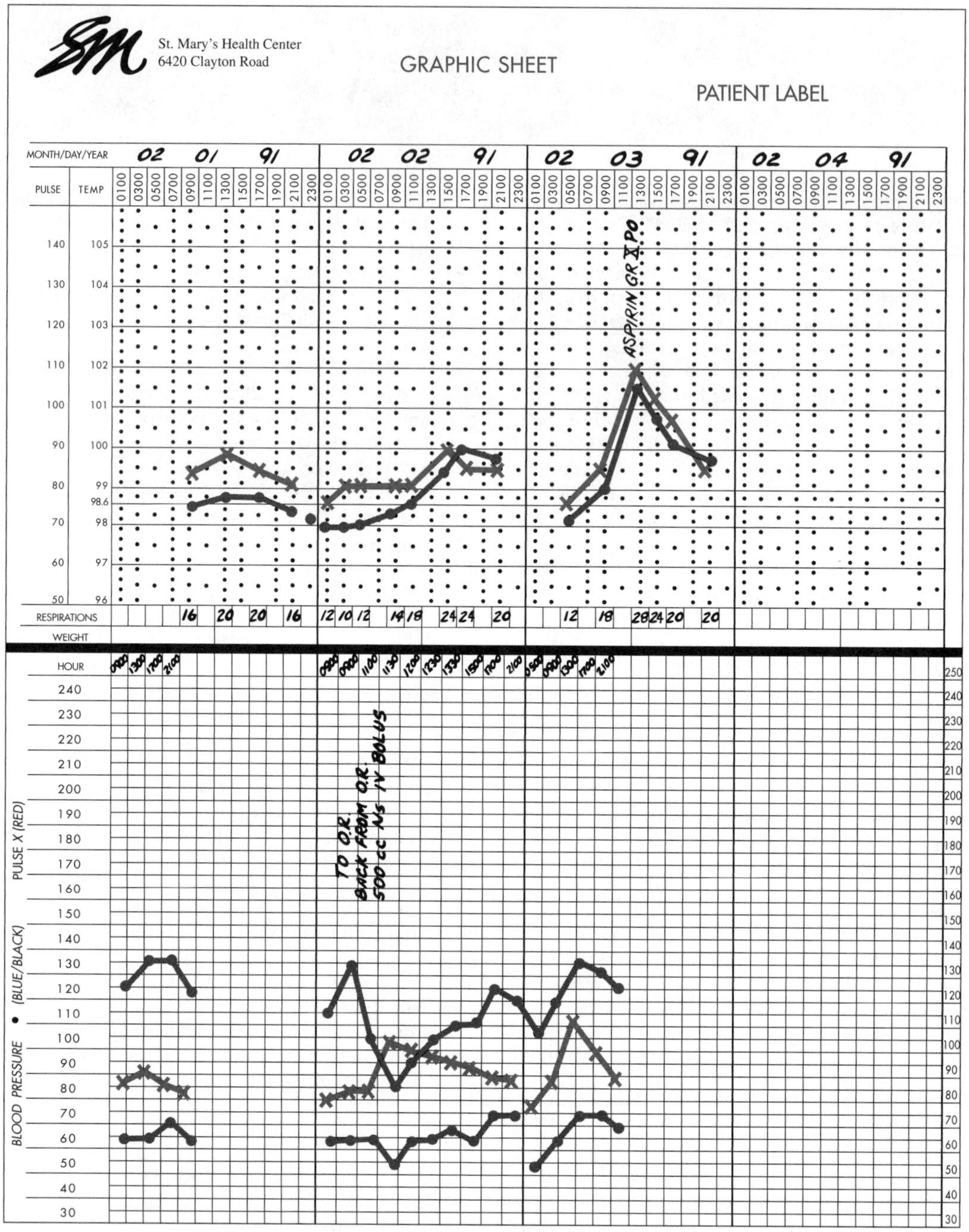

FIGURE **27–17** Vital signs graphic flow sheet. (Courtesy St. Mary's Health Center, St. Louis, MO.)

- Rectal temperature measurements should not be performed on newborn infants or adults with rectal alterations.
- Respiratory assessment includes measurement to determine the effectiveness of ventilation, perfusion, and diffusion.
- Several hemodynamic variables contribute to blood pressure determination.
- Hypertension is diagnosed only after an average of readings made during two or more subsequent visits reveals an elevated blood pressure.
- Errors in blood pressure measurement can be made by selecting and applying the cuff improperly.
- Changes in one vital sign can influence characteristics of the other vital signs.

Key Terms

Afebrile, *p. 567*
Antipyretics, *p. 579*
Auscultatory gap, *p. 607*
Basal metabolic rate (BMR), *p. 565*
Blood pressure, *p. 594*
Bradycardia, *p. 588*
Cardiac output, *p. 581*
Celsius, *p. 569*
Conduction, *p. 565*
Convection, *p. 565*
Core temperature, *p. 564*
Diaphoresis, *p. 565*
Diastolic, *p. 579*
Diffusion, *p. 589*
Dysrhythmia, *p. 588*
Eupnea, *p. 589*
Evaporation, *p. 565*
Fahrenheit, *p. 569*
Febrile, *p. 567*
Fever, *p. 567*
Fever of unknown origin (FUO), *p. 567*
Frostbite, *p. 569*
Heat exhaustion, *p. 568*
Heatstroke, *p. 568*
Hematocrit, *p. 598*
Hypertension, *p. 599*
Hyperthermia, *p. 568*
Hypotension, *p. 600*
Hypothalamus, *p. 564*
Hypothermia, *p. 568*
Hypoxemia, *p. 589*
Malignant hyperthermia, *p. 568*
Non-shivering thermogenesis, *p. 565*
Orthostatic hypotension, *p. 600*
Perfusion, *p. 589*
Postural hypotension, *p. 600*
Pulse deficit, *p. 588*
Pulse pressure, *p. 597*
Pyrexia, *p. 567*
Pyrogens, *p. 567*
Radial pulse, *p. 581*
Radiation, *p. 565*
Shivering, *p. 565*
Sphygmomanometer, *p. 600*
Stroke volume, *p. 581*
Systolic, *p. 597*
Tachycardia, *p. 588*
Thermoregulation, *p. 564*
Tidal volume, *p. 589*
Ventilation, *p. 589*
Vital signs, *p. 562*

Critical Thinking Exercises

1. A 47-year-old Aboriginal man is coming to the health clinic for a routine physical examination by the nurse practitioner. The unregulated care provider (UCP) obtains the following vital signs: tympanic temperature, 36.9° C; right radial pulse rate of 96 beats per minute and irregular; BP, sitting, right arm 162/82 mm Hg, left arm 150/70 mm Hg; SpO_2, 95% on room air; respiratory rate, 22 breaths per minute.
   a. As the admitting nurse, what questions would you ask this client to evaluate his risk for hypertension?
   b. Based on these vital signs, what actions should you take?
2. A teenage mother brings her 3-year-old child to the walk-in health centre. She notes that he has been fussy, has not had much of an appetite, and is not his active self. The boy is crying and struggling to get out of his mother's lap during the interview. You note that he is small for his age, but otherwise well-developed.
   a. Describe the sequence you would use for obtaining vital signs.
   b. When selecting the appropriate equipment for obtaining the vital signs, what, if any, special considerations are needed?
   c. The UCP reports she has obtained a temperature of 37.7° C. What additional information do you request from the UCP?
3. A 52-year-old woman is admitted to the medical unit for chronic dyspnea and discomfort in her left chest with deep breathing and coughing. She has been smoking for 35 years and has a 20-year history of emphysema. Over the past 4 months, she has lost 4.5 kg and currently weighs 50 kg.
   a. When delegating the vital signs to UCPs, what information and directions should you provide?
   b. The blood pressure and heart rate are within acceptable ranges. The temperature is 37.5° C, obtained with an oral electronic thermometer; the respiratory rate 32 breaths per minute and shallow; and the SpO_2 is 89%. Based on these results, list your actions in priority.
4. An 82-year-old resident in a subacute extended care facility is being treated for pneumonia with antibiotics. She has been on bed rest for the past 2 days. She has a history of hypertension, treated with diuretics, but is otherwise healthy. She has been afebrile for the past 24 hours and is eager to walk to the activity room. She has activity orders "up ad lib."
   a. Should a UCP be delegated to assist with ambulation?
   b. What places this client at risk for fainting?
   c. Why should the nurse obtain orthostatic measurements?
5. A 25-year-old Asian woman arrives at the prenatal clinic for her first visit. She is 8 months pregnant. The UCP checks her vital signs, height, and weight. The client weighs 104 kg and is 160 cm tall; BP in right arm is 210/92 mm Hg; HR, 104 beats per minute; respiratory rate, 24 breaths per minute; tympanic temperature, 37.1° C. You are concerned with the client's blood pressure and repeat the measurement. You obtain 148/86 mm Hg in the right arm and 144/84 mm Hg in the left arm.
   a. What blood pressure measurement should be recorded? Provide some possible explanations for the difference between your measurements and the UCP's.
   b. How might you explain the abnormal vital signs to the client?
   c. What will be included in your discharge teaching?

Review Questions

1. During a nursing assessment, an adult client is noted to have shallow respirations at a rate of 8 beats per minute. His heart rate is 46 beats per minute. His vital signs would be described as
   1. Bradycardia and apnea
   2. Tachycardia and apnea
   3. Bradycardia and bradypnea
   4. Tachycardia and bradypnea

2. A pulse deficit provides information about the heart's ability to adequately perfuse the body. A pulse deficit is
   1. The difference between the radial and apical pulse rates
   2. The digital pressure felt when taking radial and ulnar pulses
   3. The amount of pressure felt when taking radial and ulnar pulses
   4. The difference between the systolic and diastolic blood pressure readings
3. As individuals approach older adulthood, body temperature tends to
   1. Gradually drop
   2. Gradually rise
   3. Fluctuate
   4. Remain the same
4. If a blood pressure cuff is too small, the blood pressure reading will be
   1. Falsely low
   2. Falsely high
   3. Difficult to hear because sounds will be muffled
   4. Dependent on the examiner's hearing acuity
5. Clients with apnea experience
   1. Difficult respirations requiring more effort
   2. Slowness of breathing followed by rapid breathing
   3. Cessation of breathing that may be temporary
   4. Lack of oxygen to body tissues and organs
6. An older adult recently on bed rest is assisted out of bed. The nurse measures his blood pressure as the client changes position and the results are as follows: 140/80 supine, 132/72 sitting, 108/60 standing. The client also mentions he feels light-headed. The nurse should immediately
   1. Assist the client to return to a supine position
   2. Obtain a blood pressure in the other arm
   3. Report the findings to the nurse in charge
   4. Help the client to walk
7. A nurse is taking vital signs and notes that the client has a strong radial pulse that diminishes in intensity and has an interruption in rhythm about every four to six beats. The nurse should immediately
   1. Report the findings to a physician
   2. Measure a 60-second apical pulse
   3. Connect the client to a cardiac monitor
   4. Obtain a 60-second apical-radial pulse
8. Nursing interventions such as applying an ice pack or cool cloths act to decrease body temperature through
   1. Conduction
   2. Convection
   3. Evaporation
   4. Radiation
9. Poor oxygenation of the blood ordinarily will affect the pulse rate and cause it to become
   1. Bounding
   2. Irregular
   3. Faster than normal
   4. Slower than normal
10. The basic techniques of which of the following are used to determine vital signs?
    1. Inspection, palpation, and auscultation
    2. Inspection, blood work, and X-rays
    3. Rhythm, rate, and open communication
    4. Psychology, physiology, and nursing skills

References

Bailey, J., & Rose, P. (2001). Axillary and tympanic membrane temperature recording in the preterm neonate: A comparative study. *Journal of Advanced Nursing, 34*(4), 465–474.

Canadian Hypertension Education Program. (2004). *Recommendations for the management of hypertension. Part 1: Hypertension as a public health risk—The Canadian response.* Retrieved May 27, 2004, from *http://www.chs.md/index2.html* (Introduction at *http://www.chs.md/Documentation/CHEP2004_Intro_Feb16.ppt*, slide 8.)

Chobanian, A. V., et al.. (2003). The seventh report of the Joint National Committee on Prevention, Detection, Evaluation, and Treatment of High Blood Pressure. *Journal of the American Medical Association, 289*(19), 2560–2572.

Dochterman, J. M., & Bulechek, G. M. (Eds.). (2004). *Nursing interventions classification (NIC)* (4th ed.). St. Louis, MO: Mosby.

Ebersole, P., & Hess, P. (2001). *Geriatric nursing and healthy aging.* St. Louis, MO: Mosby.

Eliopoulos, C. (2001). *Gerontologic nursing* (5th ed.). Philadelphia: Lippincott.

Erickson, R. S., Meyer, L. T., & Woo, T. M. (1996). Accuracy of chemical dot thermometers in critically ill adults and young children. *Image—The Journal of Nursing Scholarship, 28,* 23–28.

Fallis, W. M. (2000). Oral measurement of temperature in orally intubated critical care patients: State of the science review. *American Journal of Critical Care, 9*(5), 334–343.

Giuliano, K. K., et al. (2000). Temperature measurement in critically ill adults: A comparison of tympanic and oral methods. *American Journal of Critical Care, 9*(4), 254–261.

Grap, M. J. (2002). Applying research at the bedside: Pulse oximetry and update 2002. *Critical Care Nurse, 22*(3), 69–76.

Guyton, A. C., & Hall, J. (1995). *Textbook of medical physiology* (9th ed.). Philadelphia: W. B. Saunders.

Kinney, M. R., et al. (1998). *AACN's clinical reference for critical care nursing* (4th ed.). St. Louis, MO: Mosby.

Lueckenotte, A. G. (1998). *Pocket guide to gerontologic assessment* (3rd ed.). St. Louis, MO: Mosby.

Lueckenotte, A. G. (2000). *Gerontologic nursing* (3rd ed.). St. Louis, MO: Mosby.

Maas, M. L., et al. (Eds.). (2001). *Nursing care of older adults: Diagnoses, outcomes, and interventions.* St. Louis, MO: Mosby.

Miller, C. A. (1999). *Nursing care of older adults: Theory and practice* (3rd ed.). Philadelphia: Lippincott.

Moorhead, S., Johnson, M., & Maas, M. (Eds.). (2004). *Nursing outcomes classification (NOC)* (3rd ed.). St. Louis, MO: Mosby.

National High Blood Pressure Education Program (NHBPEP) (1997). National Heart, Lung, and Blood Institute; National Institutes of Health: The sixth report of the Joint National Committee on Detection, Evaluation, and Treatment of High Blood Pressure. *Archives of Internal Medicine, 157,* 2413.

Pickering, T. G. (2001). Self-monitoring of blood pressure. In W. B. White (Ed.), *Blood pressure monitoring in cardiovascular medicine and therapeutics.* Totowa, NJ: Humana Press.

Sheahan, S. L., & Musialowski, R. (2001). Clinical implications of respiratory system changes in aging. *Journal of Gerontological Nursing, 27*(5), 26–34.

Recommended Web Sites

Canadian Hypertension Society:
http://www.chs.md/index2.html
The Canadian Hypertension Society's mission is to promote the prevention of hypertension through research and education. This site offers information on hypertension to health professionals and the public.

Centre for Chronic Disease Prevention and Control: Cardiovascular Disease:
http://www.phac-aspc.gc.ca/ccdpc-cpcmc/cvd-mcv/links_e.html
This Public Health Agency of Canada Web site provides links to a variety of Canadian resources on cardiovascular health, including the Heart and Stroke Foundation of Canada and the Canadian Stroke Network.

Guidelines and Protocols Advisory Committee, Detection and Diagnosis of Hypertension:
http://www.healthservices.gov.bc.ca/msp/protoguides/gps/hypertension/hyperdiag.pdf
Part of BC Health Services, the Guidelines and Protocols Advisory Committee developed this document to recommend proper blood pressure measurement technique and equipment.

Public Health Agency of Canada: The Healthy Heart Kit:
http://www.phac-aspc.gc.ca/ccdpc-cpcmc/hhk-tcs/index.html
Sponsored by Health Canada and the Heart and Stroke Foundation of Canada, this Web site provides information on several issues related to cardiovascular health, including high blood pressure and heart disease.

28

Health Assessment and Physical Examination

D. Lynn Skillen, PhD, RN (Canadian author)
Rene A. Day, RN, PhD (Canadian author)
Marjorie C. Anderson, RN, PhD (Canadian author)
Tracey Stephen, RN, BScN, MN (Canadian author)
Julie A. Gilbert, RN, BScN, MN (Canadian author)

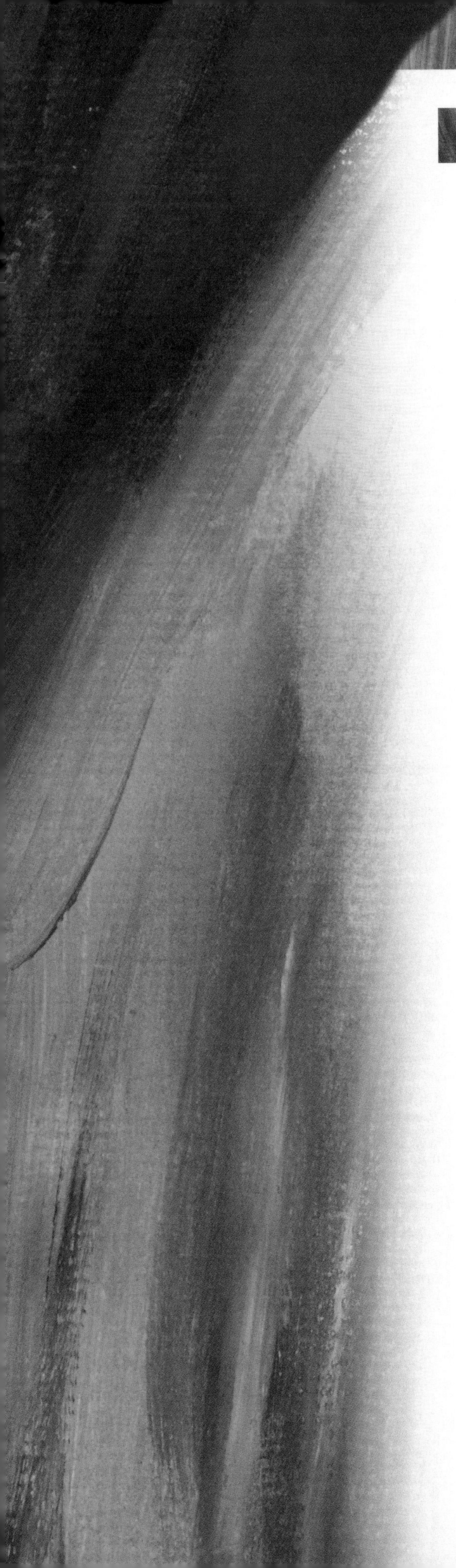

Objectives

Mastery of content in this chapter will enable the student to:

- Define the key terms listed.
- Conduct a symptom/sign analysis as the basis for a focused physical examination.
- Describe the basic physical examination techniques.
- Describe preparation of the nurse, client, and environment for the physical examination.
- Describe the essential techniques to be used during physical examination of body systems and regions.
- Explain the rationale underlying techniques and procedures used during the physical examination.
- Describe the specific characteristics to be assessed during the physical examination of body systems and regions.
- Describe the expected findings during the physical examination of the adult.
- Identify expected age-related changes during physical examination of the adult.
- Apply the database collected during a health history interview to a focused physical examination, considering developmental, physical, psychological, physiological, socio-cultural, and spiritual aspects of health.
- Integrate data on preventive screening examinations and client self-examinations in the physical examination.
- Relate knowledge of principles of communication to the physical examination.
- Discuss topics to assess for determining client learning needs.
- Identify teaching and learning opportunities for client health promotion.
- Document physical findings using standard format, appropriate terminology, physical examination criteria, and principles of recording.

Whether employed in urban, rural, remote, or international health care settings, Canadian nurses must have a foundation in physical examination knowledge and skills. Nurses in inner city clinics, tertiary level hospitals, northern health centres, industry, rural hospitals, home care services, mental health services, continuing care institutions, military clinics, and international volunteer organizations all require **physical assessment** skills (Boxes 28-1 and 28-2). Nurses promoting health in health fairs, physicians' offices/medicentres, public health screening clinics, primary health care facilities, remote nursing stations, international projects with vulnerable populations, or with Canadian workers offshore must also be prepared to conduct focused client assessments.

Research Highlight

Box 28-1

Physical Examination Use by Continuing Care Nurses

Research Focus

Maximizing health and confronting functional impairments are goals of gerontological nursing. The health of older adults is often fragile because of age-related change complicated by chronic illnesses. Nurses need physical assessment skills in order to identify changes in older adults' health status and to provide these clients with appropriate care. This study examined what factors hinder assessment and what factors help assessment.

Research Abstract

In 1995, research was conducted in Alberta on registered nurse case managers' reported use of assessment skills with older clients. Nineteen continuing care facilities in a provincial health region participated. After expert review and pilot testing, questionnaires were distributed to two independent groups: nurse administrators/staff development coordinators and case managers (response rate = 73%). Qualitative data were analyzed using descriptive, interpretive, and pattern coding. Factors that constrained or facilitated physical assessment in continuing care were identified. Time constraints, characteristics of clients and their families, colleagues, the organizations, and case managers themselves deterred physical assessment However, clients' age-related changes and diverse disease processes required ongoing monitoring by nurses using physical examination skills. When administrators and colleagues expected case managers to perform physical examinations, physical assessment was facilitated. Use of physical assessment skills was critical for the multi-faceted roles of the case manager.

Evidence-Based Practice

- Nurse case managers need to be prepared to conduct physical assessment of their gerontological clients.
- Health care administrators need to actively support physical assessments by nurse case managers by making assessment an expectation for the position, putting into place relevant in-service programs and audiovisual learning resources, and providing the time by establishing manageable staff:client ratios.
- Nurse change agents in education, administration, and practice need to address the constraining factors among gerontological nurse case managers themselves and to emphasize the facilitating factors that were identified in older clients, health care colleagues, and continuing care organizations for physical assessments.

Reference

Adapted from Skillen, D. L., Anderson, M. C., & Knight, C. L. (2001). The created environment for physical assessment by case managers. *Western Journal of Nursing Research, 32*, 72–89.

Research Highlight

Box 28-2

Physical Examination Use by Occupational Health Nurses (OHNs)

Research Focus

The focus of this research was to determine the following:

- The use of assessment skills by nurses in occupational health settings
- The importance that OHNs assign to physical assessment skills
- OHNs' assessment of their own physical assessment skills

Research Abstract

In 1997, all nurses in Alberta who reported employment in occupational health when renewing their registration were mailed a questionnaire to be answered anonymously. The questionnaire had been subjected to expert review and pilot testing. One hundred and thirty-seven completed questionnaires were returned (response rate = 39%); 103 OHNs reported using physical assessment skills with workers. The most frequent physical conditions and problems for which they used these skills were sprains and strains; ear, eye, nose, and throat problems; cardiac conditions; respiratory problems; and post-injury assessments. For their nursing specialty, they indicated that the priority physical examination skills were assessment of the musculoskeletal system, peripheral vascular and cardiovascular systems, head and neck region, thorax and lungs, and neurological system. Competence in physical assessment was very important to 96 OHNs; 56 rated their level of competence in performing physical assessment as strong, 57 rated their level between strong and weak, and 23 rated their level as weak. At least 90 OHNs believed that competence in physical assessment was necessary for effectiveness in occupational health nursing practice.

Evidence-Based Practice

- OHNs need to be competent in performing physical assessment.
- OHNs need opportunities to strengthen physical assessment skills.
- Competent physical assessment contributes to OHN effectiveness in workplaces.

Reference

Adapted from Skillen, D. L., Seglie, J., & Anderson, M. (1998). Beyond bandaids: Are OHNs using physical assessment skills? *AOHNA Newsletter, 19*(1): 5, 10.

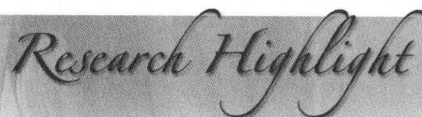

Nurses use four basic examination modes: **inspection, palpation, percussion,** and **auscultation** to conduct client assessments. Using these modes, nurses do the following:

- Obtain baseline client data as comparison for future assessment findings
- Refute, confirm, or supplement an existing client database
- Use knowledge gained during symptom/sign analysis to focus physical examination
- Detect client response to treatment
- Identify changes in client condition or function
- Determine indications for client referral to other members of the interdisciplinary health care team
- Identify learning needs and opportunities for clients
- Identify high-risk clients by screening, for example, for high blood pressure, tuberculosis exposure, and sexually transmitted infections (STIs)
- Detect treatable client conditions early
- Think critically about examination focus and findings
- Interpret patterns in examination findings and make clinical nursing judgments
- Determine when more comprehensive examinations, including diagnostic tests, are indicated
- Individualize client care
- Practise primary, secondary, and tertiary prevention
- Document physical examination findings for communication to other members of the interdisciplinary health care team
- Promote continuity of client care by making ongoing, objective, and focused or comprehensive examinations.

After collecting **subjective data** in the **health history** (see chapter 12) and conducting a symptom/sign analysis, nurses collect **objective data** about clients during a physical examination. By obtaining the client history first, nurses initiate a relationship with clients that promotes trust and sharing of key information relevant to the physical assessment. Subjective client data about levels of wellness, presenting concern, family history, changes in life patterns, socio-cultural history, spiritual health, and mental or emotional reactions to illness or body changes determine the areas requiring attention in the physical examination. The **symptom/sign analysis** assists nurses to plan a focused physical examination and address the client's presenting complaint or concern. Comprehensive head-to-toe examinations that review all client body systems and regions may be required and are preferred for baseline data. Canadian research compared two strategies for teaching nursing students how to conduct complete physical examinations (Box 28-3).

Box 28-3 Research on Lecture Versus Computer to Teach Health Assessment

Computer-managed instruction (CMI) is an instructional strategy using the computer to provide learning objectives and learning resources and to assess learner performance. The main objective of this study was to compare the outcomes of two teaching strategies for health assessment: CMI versus the traditional lecture method. The study was quasi-experimental and incorporated two experimental treatments applied on two occasions with first-year undergraduate baccalaureate nursing students in Alberta. The variables examined were cognitive performance of learners, learner attitude toward the instructional strategy, learner retention of knowledge, time to master the learning objectives, and relationship between learner characteristics and effectiveness of the instructional strategy. No significant difference was found between groups on cognitive performance as measured by written and practical examination scores. There was no significant difference between groups in the time spent meeting the learning objectives by either instructional strategy. The majority of students preferred a combination of instructional methods for learning health assessment content.

Adapted from "Computer-Managed Instruction: An Alternative Teaching Strategy," by R. Day and L. Payne, 1987, *Journal of Nursing Education, 26,* pp. 30–36.

Purposes of Physical Examination

Nurses plan the physical examination based on clients' stated needs, the subjective information obtained in the health history, and the symptom/sign analysis. Ideally, nurses obtain baseline data for every client by completing a comprehensive health history and physical examination. Subjective information helps nurses to understand the life context of their clients, identify health needs in dialogue with them, and focus on their primary concern. Objective information permits nurses to make clinical judgments, seize teaching and learning opportunities, and document clients' health status for continuity in health care based on standardized assessment techniques. The accuracy of nurses' assessments influences the management of clients' health problems (Box 28-4).

Comprehensive client histories and examinations enable nurses to identify clients' strengths and resources; promote wellness behaviours; detect potential and actual health problems early; determine eligibility for health insurance, military service, and new employment; or make recommendations for admission to a health care facility. When time, personnel, and health care settings constrain nurses' availability, or when clients' conditions or responses warrant the shortest, most relevant examination, nurses conduct a focused physical examination, guided by the symptom/sign analysis. Acutely ill clients, for example, require nursing assessments that are focused, efficient, and concentrated only on the involved body systems or regions.

After mastering physical examination techniques, nurses can integrate physical assessment into their daily routine, focusing their assessment if restricted by time, resources, and client condition. During a bed bath, nurses assess the condition of the integumentary system. They observe ambulatory clients for their gait, balance, and range of motion. When performing oral hygiene on debilitated clients, they observe the structures of the oral cavity. By integrating assessment skills into all encounters with clients, nurses make efficient use of the available

Box 28-4 Focus on Primary Health Care

This chapter focuses on assessing an individual's health. However, assessment can also be used more broadly to consider the health of families, and groups or aggregates, such as 3 year olds in a daycare centre or older adults in an exercise group. Nurses may be involved in assessing the health of communities or even countries. Assessments are guided by an understanding of primary health care (PHC) which is an approach and a philosophy that encompasses health promotion and illness /injury prevention. Also included are the determinants of health (peace, shelter, education, food, income, stable ecosystem, sustainable resources, social justice, and equality (World Health Organization [WHO], 1986), and human rights, social security, social relations, and empowerment of women (WHO, 1997).

Nurses work closely with people and thus are in an ideal position to lead in the acceptance and use of primary health care. DuGas and Knor (1995) state that Mahler, a former director-general of the World Health Organization, "envisioned nurses becoming resources to people rather than assistants to physicians" (p. 63). The Canadian Nurses Association has been actively promoting primary health care since the 1980s and is the only national health association advocating for the implementation of PHC throughout Canada and the world (McIntyre & Tomlinson, 2003). Generally it has been easier for nurses to implement PHC in community settings rather than in acute care where the hospital/medical model is still dominant (Lemire Rodger & Gallagher, 2000).

Nurses need to be able to clearly differentiate primary health care from "primary care" which is about access to medical care (Ogilvie & Reutter, 2003). Nursing students must understand that PHC exists in "real practice" (Paul & Day, 2003). Examples include the Boyle-McCauley Health Centre and, the Northeast Community Health Centre, both in Edmonton (see chapter 2).

time. Physical assessment should become an automatic behaviour whenever nurse and client interact. The same physical assessment skill that nurses use to assess a condition (e.g., palpation of the client's pulse) can be practised as an evaluation of nursing care (e.g., evaluation of client's tolerance to an exercise plan).

Nurses need to make accurate, detailed, objective measurements while performing physical assessments. After mastering the techniques and sequences, the nurse must determine which body systems and regions to assess in the focused examination, and interpret the findings to make decisions about clients' care or referral. Nurses' measurements and observations help determine whether the expected outcomes of care are being met or if client status is stable, improving, or deteriorating.

Physical examination by nurses serves many purposes, which are summarized in Box 28-5.

Box 28-5 Purposes of Physical Examination by Nurses

- Gathering baseline data about clients' health status
- Supplementing, confirming, or refuting data obtained in the health history
- Providing learning opportunities for clients' self-examinations or understanding of the body and body changes
- Identifying potential and actual health problems
- Determining or confirming nursing diagnoses
- Monitoring clients' response to nursing interventions
- Making clinical judgments about clients' changing health status and management of their care
- Determining eligibility for employment, insurance, or admission to a health care facility
- Evaluating the physiological outcomes of care

Infection Control Practices

Standard precautions/routine practices must always be followed during examinations to protect nurses and clients from contact with blood, body fluids, and body substances that can transmit infectious agents (see chapter 29). Examples of transmissible agents include human immunodeficiency virus (HIV), tuberculosis bacilli, hepatitis A–E viruses, *C. difficile,* Epstein-Barr virus, cytomegalovirus, and human T-cell lymphotrophic virus types I and II.

Safety Alert: Hand hygiene is completed before equipment preparation and before and after the examination. The nurse also must wear disposable gloves if the nurse or client has nonintact skin or if there is the possibility of exposure to the client's blood, body fluids, or other body substances.

Cultural Sensitivity and Responsiveness

In Canada's multicultural society, clients bring many cultural differences to their interactions with nurses (Box 28-6). Nurses demonstrate **cultural sensitivity** in respecting and responding to differences (see chapter 9). Nurses need to consider clients' health beliefs, use of alternative therapies, nutritional habits, relationships with family and community, and level of comfort with a nurse's physical closeness and examination.

Nurses must be culturally aware and responsive to avoid stereotyping their clients on the basis of gender or race. With education, experience, and sensitivity, nurses distinguish between the cultural and the physical characteristics of their clients. They learn the common disorders of the ethnic populations in their service area. For example, Black Canadians may experience sickle cell disease and have a higher incidence of hypertension and prostate cancer, Jewish Canadians may present with Tay-Sachs disease, Aboriginal individuals have higher rates of diabetes, Canadians of Middle Eastern background may be at risk for major or minor thalassemia. Nurses also know the biological variations that are observable during physical

Cultural Aspects of Care Box 28-6

Cultural heritage influences the following aspects of health care:

- Interpretation of symptoms
- Decision to consult with family or community members
- Tendency to seek professional health care
- Preference for alternative medicine
- Willingness to assume responsibility for health
- Expectation of health professionals
- Acceptance of health professional by gender
- Response to health professionals' assessments

Box 28-7 Examples of Diseases Acquired by Canadians During Travel

Ascariasis	Japanese encephalitis
Chagas' disease	Malaria
Cholera	Rabies
Cryptosporidiasis	Salmonella
Dengue fever	SARS (sudden acute respiratory syndrome)
Filariasis	Shigellosis
Giardiasis	Schistosomiasis
Hepatitis (A–E)	STIs (sexually transmitted infections)
HIV/AIDS	Tetanus
Hookworm	Yellow fever

assessment; for example, Aboriginal and Asian Canadians generally have limited body hair, dry ear wax, fewer apocrine glands, and unobservable body odour. Blood types of Caucasian clients commonly include RH negative, in contrast to Blacks and Asians who present as RH negative less often and Inuit clients who demonstrate no evidence of RH-negative blood. Recognizing clients' cultural and biological diversity assists nurses to respect clients' uniqueness, consider alternate explanations for their presenting symptoms, make accurate observations about clients' health status, and provide culturally responsive care.

Mobility

In addition to being multicultural, Canadians are a mobile people. Canadians who travel for work, study, family reasons, or pleasure are at risk for environmental or infectious diseases (Box 28-7). Nurses inquire about client travel when completing a health history and consider possible explanations for observations made during the physical examination of symptomatic clients who report recent travel.

Analyzing Signs and Symptoms

Gathering information (data) from clients is an essential skill that improves with increased knowledge and repeated practice. A substantial database provides the foundation for the diagnosis, treatment and intervention, referral, and education of clients. Data are primarily collected from the health history and the physical examination, although other data such as diagnostic tests and laboratory results may be required. The health history is usually taken first, followed by a physical examination. Nurses collect data on clients' signs and symptoms, as this is vital for making a thorough assessment.

A **sign** is an action or physical manifestation of something that can be observed by others. In health care, a sign is a physical finding, expression, or bodily movement that may be observed by the examiner using visual, olfactory, tactile, and auditory senses. Although signs are usually used to indicate disease or impairment, they can also indicate healthy function. Because signs can be seen, measured, felt, heard, or smelled by an examiner, they are considered to be objective data. Objective data come from varied sources and may be collected at any time during the health history and physical examination but are usually collected during the physical examination. The assessment techniques of inspection, palpation, percussion, and auscultation provide the examiner with objective data. Measurements of blood pressure, height, weight, visual acuity, and temperature are examples of objective data. Other objective data include diagnostic test results (e.g., X-rays, electrocardiogram, computed tomography scan, pulmonary function tests, ultrasound) and laboratory findings (e.g., blood work, urine biochemistry, hair and nail analysis, cytology smears). Because objective data are observable, health professionals can validate the findings. For example, if a client reports that he or she has an itchy patch of skin and the examiner sees an area of dryness, the objective data validate the client's subjective report. Signs are observed, but health professionals must depend on clients to describe their symptoms.

Symptoms are sensations or emotions that are perceived or experienced and reported by the person but are not observable by others. They are subjective because they are perceived only by the client and cannot always be verified by the examiner. Subjective data come from clients, family members, or significant others. Subjective data may be collected at any time throughout the health history and physical examination but are usually collected during the health history. Subjective data provide essential information about how the client is feeling. Some essential data can only be collected through client reports. Nausea, numbness, and tingling are examples of data that are not observable by others. These symptoms are important information for examiners. It is essential to collect subjective and objective data to ensure adequate information is available to guide diagnosis, treatment and interventions, referrals, and client education. The examiner must guide the client to describe the symptom or sign as fully and accurately as possible in a process called *analysis of a symptom/sign.*

Analysis of a symptom/sign is a systematic way of collecting more information about a sensation or emotion or physical manifestation that is perceived or experienced by another individual. Accuracy of the information depends on two major factors: reliability of the informant, and interpretation of the information by the examiner. Other important points to remember when analyzing symptoms and signs are as follows:

- Cultural response to situation
- Underlying disease or dysfunction
- Language barriers
- Socio-economic factors
- Ethical/legal issues

When a client reports a symptom/sign, the examiner needs to obtain full information (Table 28-1). The statement "I have a headache" is not sufficient to aid in the diagnosis or treatment of the client. When clients report a concern that affects their "well-being," an analysis of the symptom or sign should lead to comprehensive information about the symptom or sign. The process includes elaborating on several characteristics of the symptom or sign reported by the client. All characteristics contribute to a substantive database and provide important information. Examiners should first ask the client a broad question about the symptom or sign. For example, "Describe your headache." When the client has provided as much information about the symptom or sign as possible, the examiner uses direct questions to elicit essential information about the characteristics.

Physical Examination Modes

Physical examination techniques incorporate the basic examination modes of inspection, palpation, percussion, and auscultation.

Inspection

Inspection is always the first basic examination mode used in the physical examination of the client.

General Inspection. General inspection precedes local inspection and the other three basic examination modes. This avoids examiner distortion or neglect of significant signs.

Examiners use their senses of sight (visual), hearing (auditory), and smell (olfactory) during inspection. From the first moment that a client is encountered until the last, examiners have the opportunity to use these senses. Even when the client is not immediately visible (for example, is behind a screen or a curtain), examiners can still use the senses of hearing and smell (Table 28-2).

General inspection is most productive when examiners assess in a thorough, unhurried manner, know the client characteristics to be scrutinized, and allow time to integrate the information acquired into a global picture of the client. When examiners plan a general inspection, they minimize the risk of discounting, selectively devaluing, or failing to detect significant client signs.

General inspection is likely the examination mode by which nurses detect the majority of physical signs. Nurses selectively focus their attention on numerous client characteristics (Table 28-3).

The secret to general inspection is paying attention to the client using all senses, observing movements, and looking carefully at the body area or activity chosen for scrutiny. The quality of the general inspection depends on the nurse's willingness to take the time to be thorough and pay attention to detail. Experienced nurses acquire the skills to make several observations almost simultaneously and detect early warnings of unexpected findings.

In this chapter, notice that findings are not called *normal* or *abnormal*. Rather, they are called *expected* and *unexpected*. This terminology emphasizes the continuum of findings that can be encountered, the need to be precise in reporting, and the risk that what one health professional describes as "normal" is at a different point on the continuum for the individual who reads the record. Experienced nurses recognize a range of expected findings in physical assessments. They consider age, developmental stage, gender, biological variations, ethnicity, and occupation when interpreting findings as expected or unexpected.

As part of the general inspection, examiners measure clients' vital signs and height and weight.

Vital Signs. **Vital signs** are indicators of clients' circulatory, respiratory, endocrine, and neural functions; changes can indicate alterations in physiological functioning. Vital signs include blood pressure, heart rate and rhythm, respirations, oxygen saturation, and temperature. Because pain affects vital signs, nurses must conduct a complete symptom analysis for any reported pain and observe for the signs of pain (see chapter 38).

Nurses must know when to take vital signs, what range of results to expect, how measurements are to be taken, rationale for techniques, how to record measurements correctly, and when to report findings to the nurse in charge, nurse practitioner, or physician (see chapter 27). Nurses assess vital sign changes in light of other physical examination findings, using clinical judgment to determine the frequency of measurement.

Height, Weight, and Circumference. Height and weight are routinely measured during health screenings, visits to primary care providers, and admissions to health care facilities. Weight measurements are the basis for drug dosage determinations, lifting requirements, or care plans to assist clients with position changes. The health history can suggest possible causes for weight changes (Table 28-4).

Nurses measure weight and height in order to monitor growth and development, trends over time, and relationship to a nutritional assessment and fluid balance. Ambulatory clients may use a standing scale for weight (Figure 28–1) and height (Figure 28–2).

The standing scale must be calibrated at each use, but an electronic scale automatically adjusts to display weight within seconds. Nurses compare observations with standardized tables, taking age-related changes into consideration (Table 28-5). Nurses compare data with a weight classification system devised for adults who are 18 years of age and older, except pregnant and lactating

Table 28-1 Characteristics of Symptoms and Signs

Characteristic	Explanation	Sample Questions
Location	The specific anatomical area that is affected	"Describe where your pain is" (symptom) "Where is your rash?" (sign)
• Localization	Occurs in one specific area of the body	"Is your pain in one spot?" (symptom) "Is the rash only on your left elbow?" (sign)
• Generalization	Occurs over larger area of the body, or over whole body	"Is the rash confined to your chest and back or does it cover other areas as well?" (sign)
• Radiation	Moves to another area or from another area	"Where else do you have pain?" (symptom) "Where else is the rash?" (sign) "Does the tingling move from your back down your legs?" (symptom) "Have you noticed the redness moving along your arm?" (sign)
Quality	The nature or feature of a symptom/sign Refers to colour, consistency (thick, thin, hard, soft), and type (crushing, throbbing, aching, burning, cutting, stabbing) of a symptom or sign	"Describe what the sputum looks like" (sign) "What colour is the rash?" (sign) "Is it itchy?" (symptom) "Describe what your pain feels like" (symptom)
Timing		
• Onset (slow or fast)	When the symptom/sign began and the speed of onset	"When did you first notice the pain?" (symptom) "Did the pain get worse gradually throughout the week?" (symptom)
• Duration	The length of time the symptom/sign occurs	"How long does the pain usually last" (symptom)
• Constancy	Whether the symptom/sign is constant or intermittent	"Is the rash always itchy or only sometimes itchy?" (symptom)
• Time of day/ month/year		"Does the rash appear at every time of year, or mainly in the winter?" (sign)
Intensity/severity	Quantity of a symptom/sign	"On a scale of 0 to 10 with 0 being no pain and 10 being the worst pain, how would you rate your pain?" (symptom) "How many towels did you soak with blood?" (sign) "Compared with a golf ball, how big is the lump?" (sign) "What effect does the stiffness in your back have on your usual activities?" (symptom)
Aggravating factors	Activities or exposures that make the symptom/sign worse	"What makes the pain worse?" (symptom) "What makes the rash worse?" (sign)
Alleviating factors	Activities or exposures that make the symptom/sign better	"What makes the pain better?" (symptom) "What makes the rash better?" (sign)
Associated symptoms/signs	Other symptoms that may be related	"Are you experiencing any other symptoms, like nausea or dizziness?"
Environmental factors	Anything in the client's surroundings that may be related to the symptom/sign	"What is going on in your life, at home, or at work that might be affecting this?" "Are you doing any renovations at home or at work?" "What recent travel have you had?" "Have you made any major changes in your life that might be affecting how you are feeling?" "Is anyone else sick at home?"
Significance to client	The impact of the symptom/sign on the client's lifestyle and well-being	"What effect will this have on your present lifestyle? Will you be able to continue working with a sore back?"
Client perspective	What the client thinks is happening	"What do you think is causing your pain?" (symptom) "What do you think your rash is from?" (sign)

Adapted from "Symptom Analysis," by T. C. Stephen, 1997, in *Adult Health Assessment Series* [CD-ROM], Edmonton, AB: DataStar Education Systems & Services.

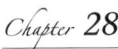

Table 28-2 Assessment of Characteristic Odours During General Inspection

Odour	Site or Source	Potential Causes
Alcohol	Oral cavity	Ingestion of alcohol
	Breath	Diabetes
Ammonia	Urine	Urinary tract infection
Body odour	Skin	Excess perspiration
		Foul-smelling perspiration
	Intertriginous areas	Inadequate hygiene
	Clothing	Vomiting of undigested food
	Wound	Abscess
Feces	Rectal area	Incontinence
		Obstruction
	Clothing	Malabsorption syndrome
Halitosis	Oral cavity	Inadequate dental hygiene
		Dental abscess
		Gum disease
	Stomach	Nervousness or anxiety
Sweet, fruity	Oral cavity	Diabetic acidosis (ketones)
	Breath	Ingestion/inhalation of solvent
Stale urine	Skin	Uremic acidosis
	Clothing	Incontinence
Thick odour (sweet, heavy)	Wound drainage	Bacterial infection
	Vagina	Inadequate hygiene
Mustiness	Cast area	Infection
Fetid and sweet	Mucus secretions	Bacterial infection
	Tracheostomy	

women (Health Canada, 2003; see *www.hc-sc.gc.ca/hpfb-dgpsa/onpp-bppn/cg_bwc_introduction_e.html*). The Canadian system (Tables 28-6A and 28-6B) is based on body weight using the body mass index (BMI) and the amount of abdominal fat measured using waist circumference. The BMI is an index using weight in kilograms and height in centimetres squared (kg/m^2).

Local Inspection. Local inspection *always follows* general inspection. It begins when examiners select an anatomical region or body part and focus their attention on specific client characteristics. Observations made during a local inspection build upon those made during the general inspection. If clinical indicators of abuse are noted (Box 28-8), nurses need to be sensitive to the fact that clients may feel further victimized. Although the procedures are routine for nurses, clients may feel stress and anxiety.

> ***Safety Alert:*** The risk for further abuse is high once the victim has reported the abuse or tries to leave the abusive situation. Provide counselling options for these individuals.

Nurses must be aware of red flags for suspicion of substance abuse. Nurses approach the client in a caring and non-judgmental way, because substance abuse involves both emotional and lifestyle issues. Behaviours that indicate possible substance abuse include those listed in Box 28-9. When substance abuse is considered, the nurse should ask the following **CAGE questions:** Have you ever felt the need to *Cut down* on your drinking or drug use? Have people *Annoyed* you by criticizing your drinking or drug use? Have you ever felt bad or *Guilty* about your drinking or drug use? Have you ever used or had a drink first thing in the morning as an *Eye-opener* to steady your nerves or feel normal? If answers to two or more of the CAGE (a mnemonic for the four questions) questions are positive, the nurse should seriously suspect abuse and consider how to motivate the client to seek treatment (Stuart & Laraia, 2001).

In addition to considering client characteristics to assess during local inspection (Table 28-7), examiners must also consider the lighting and the adequacy of client exposure. Nurses consider client comfort by draping to avoid unnecessary exposure but ensure that the area to be examined is sufficiently exposed for accurate assessment.

Diffuse natural lighting is preferred for local inspection, but artificial lighting that is appropriately directed is usually adequate. Nurses commonly use a penlight for inspection. **Direct lighting** (perpendicular) is used to detect colour of the skin and mucous membranes and to examine the characteristics of skin lesions (type, configuration, distribution, colour). **Oblique (tangential) lighting** is created when nurses shine the penlight at an angle that emphasizes movement, pulsations, and contour in the body region being examined.

Palpation

Palpation is the second basic examination mode used in physical assessment. Involving the sense of touch, it requires knowledge of the sensory properties of the hand, application of light, and deep palpation techniques with the fingers and hands.

Palpation is based on tactile, temperature, kinesthetic, and vibratory sensations and is a technique developed with experience and education. Sensory discrimination depends upon the appropriate use of the examiner's hands. For example, the ball of the hand (see Figure 28–4, *A*) detects vibrations. Anatomical areas of the hand vary in their receptiveness to sensations (Table 28-8). The ulnar edge of the hand (the side with the little finger) has dual sensory properties.

Palpation Techniques. During palpation, examiners vary the pressure, movement, and position of their palpating hand or hands depending on the type of data they want to collect. Bones, tendons, muscles, superficial arteries, salivary ducts, abdominal viscera, and structures accessible through body orifices are all subject to palpation. Using information gained from the history and inspection, examiners select key areas for palpation and determine the amount of pressure to exert. Two types of pressure are used: **light** and **deep**

Table 28-3 Client Characteristics to Be Assessed During General Inspection

Client Characteristic	Focus of Assessment
Gender	Body type, sexual development, type of clothing
Race	Integument, body type
Body type	Shape, muscularity, obesity, thinness
Apparent age	Face, posture, motor activity, gait, type of clothing
Level of consciousness	Eyes, verbal response, motor response (see Glasgow Coma Scale, Table 28-18)
Orientation	Personal identity, place, time
Signs of distress	Anxiety, difficulty breathing, perspiration, pallor, restlessness, dilated pupils, agitation, consciousness Indicators of nociceptive and neuropathic pain (see chapter 38)
Outstanding anatomical malformations	Head, neck, torso, limbs
Appearance of health	Physical, mental, emotional
Posture	Vertical alignment (coronal and median planes)
Affect and mood	Congruence of verbal and non-verbal communication Facial expression, voice, demeanour, emotion
Motor activity and gait	Coordination, balance, arm and head movement, mobility Purposeful movements, tremors
Signs of client abuse	All socio-economic levels Children, women, elderly (see Box 28-8 for clinical indicators)
Signs of substance abuse	All socio-economic levels Men and women Childhood, adolescence, adulthood Alcohol, medications, illegal drugs (see Box 28-9 for clinical indicators)
Clothing	Amount, appropriateness for weather and temperature, fastened correctly, right side out, context
Facial expression at rest and during interaction	Symmetry, congruence with non-verbal communication
Odours	Physical activity, body and oral hygiene, disease (see Table 28-2 for causes)
Personal grooming and hygiene	Cleanliness of hair, skin, nails, clothing Cosmetics
Cognitive functions	Orientation, short- and long-term memory, attention, learning ability
Insight and judgment	Awareness of normality Comparison and evaluation of alternatives for action
Sexual development	Age, gender, type of clothing (see chapter 23)
Speech and language	Clarity, pace, inflection, tone, fluency
Thought processes and content	Logic, coherence, relevance, insight, judgment Patterns (e.g., compulsions, obsessions, phobias, anxieties, delusions)

Table 28-4 Health History for Weight Assessment

Assessment Category	Rationale
Ask about total weight lost or gained; compare with usual weight, note time period for loss (e.g., gradual, sudden, desired, undesired).	Determines severity of problem and may reveal if related to disease process, change in eating pattern, or pregnancy.
If weight loss desired, ask about eating pattern, diet plan followed, usual daily calorie intake, and appetite.	Helps to determine appropriateness of diet plan followed.
If weight loss undesired, ask about anorexia, vomiting, diarrhea, thirst, frequent urination, and change in lifestyle or activity.	Focuses on problems that may cause weight loss (e.g., gastrointestinal problems).
Assess if client has noted changes in social aspects of eating: more meals in restaurants, rushing to eat meals, stress at work, or skipping meals.	Lifestyle changes can contribute to weight changes.
Assess if client takes chemotherapy, diuretics, insulin, psychotropics, steroids, non-prescription diet pills, or laxatives.	Weight gain or loss can be side effect of these medications.

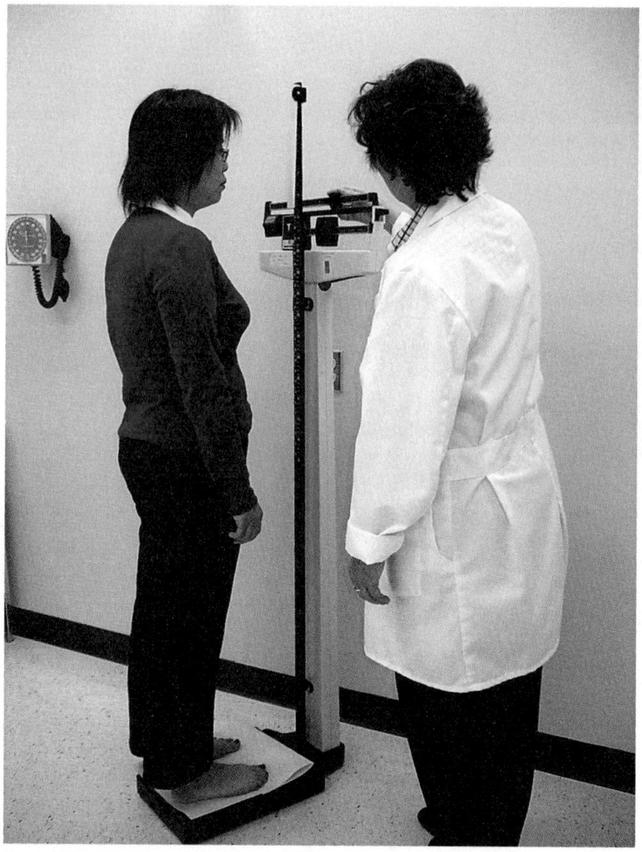

FIGURE **28–1** Weight measurement. (From *Physical Examination Images* [CD-ROM], by D. L. Skillen, R. A. Day, M. C. Anderson, T. C. Stephen, J. A. Gilbert, and L. W. Day, 2004, Edmonton, AB: Faculty of Nursing, University of Alberta.)

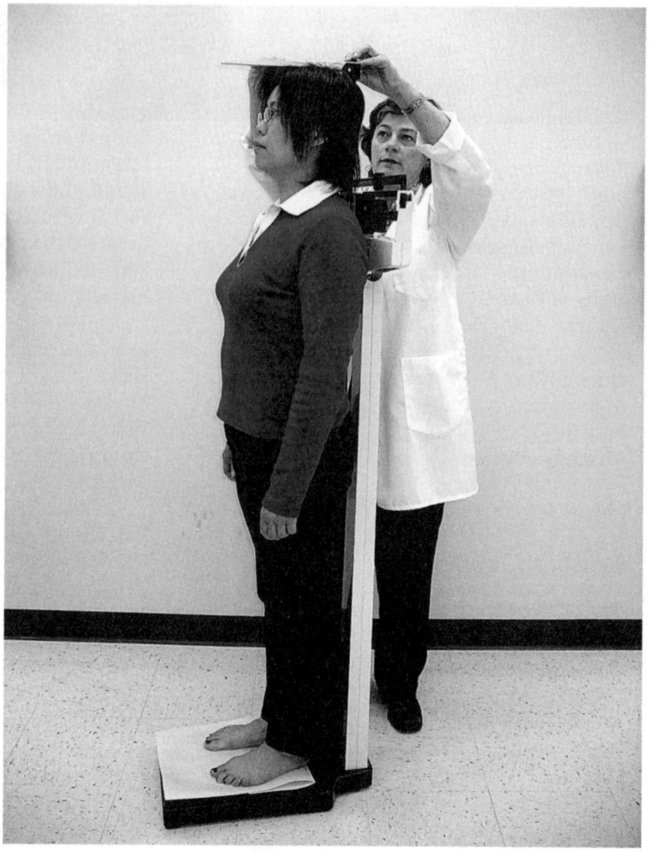

FIGURE **28–2** Height measurement. (From *Physical Examination Images* [CD-ROM], by D. L. Skillen, R. A. Day, M. C. Anderson, T. C. Stephen, J. A. Gilbert, and L. W. Day, 2004, Edmonton, AB: Faculty of Nursing, University of Alberta.)

Table 28-5 Height and Weight Table: Weights for People 25 to 59 Years According to Build*

Men				Women			
HEIGHT cm	Small Frame	Medium Frame	Large Frame	HEIGHT† cm	Small Frame	Medium Frame	Large Frame
157.48	58.06-60.78	59.42-63.95	62.59-68.04	147.32	46.26-50.34	49.44-54.88	53.52-59.42
160.02	58.96-61.68	60.32-64.86	63.50-69.40	149.86	46.26-50.34	50.34-55.79	54.43-60.78
162.56	59.87-62.59	61.23-65-77	64.41-70.76	152.40	46.72-51.25	51.25-57.15	55.33-62.14
165.10	60.78-63.50	62.14-67.13	65.31-72.57	154.94	47.17-52.16	52.16-58.51	56.70-63.50
167.64	61.68-64.41	63.05-68.49	66.22-74.39	157.48	48.08-53.52	53.52-59.87	58.06-64.86
170.18	62.59-65.77	64.41-65.31	67.58-76.20	160.02	48.98-54.88	54.88-61.23	59.42-66.67
172.72	63.50-67.13	65.77-66.22	68.94-78.01	162.56	50.34-56.24	56.24-62.59	60.78-68.49
175.26	64.41-68-49	67.13-67.58	70.30-79.83	165.10	51.71-57.60	57.60-63.95	62.14-70.30
177.80	65.31-69-85	68.49-73.93	71.66-81.64	167.64	53.07-58.96	58.96-65.31	63.50-72.12
180.34	66.22-71-21	69.85-75.29	73.02-83.46	170.18	54.43-60.32	60.32-66.67	64.86-73.93
182.88	67.58-72.57	71.21-77.11	74.39-85.27	172.72	55.79-61.68	61.68-68.04	66.22-75.75
185.42	68.94-74.39	72.57-78.92	76.20-87.09	175.26	57.15-63.05	63.05-69.40	67.58-77-11
187.96	70.30-76.20	74.39-80.74	78.01-89.35	177.80	58.51-64.41	64.41-70.76	68.94-78.47
190.50	71.66-78.01	75.75-82.55	79.83-93.89	180.34	59.87-65.77	65.77-72.12	70.30-79.83
193.04	73.48-79.83	77.56-84.82	82.10-93.89	182.88	62.59-68.49	67.13-73.48	71.66-81.19

Courtesy *Statistical Bulletin,* Metropolitan Life Insurance Company, 2000, New York: Metropolitan.
*Indoor clothing weighing 2.3 kg for men and 1.4 kg for women.
†Shoes with 2.5 cm heels.

Table 28-6A Health Risk Classification According to Body Mass Index (BMI)*

Classification	BMI Category (kg/m²)	Risk of Developing Health Problems
Underweight	<18.5	Increased
Normal weight	18.5–24.9	Least
Overweight	25.0–29.9	Increased
Obese		
Class I	30.0–34.9	High
Class II	35.0–39.9	Very high
Class III	≥40.0	Extremely high

*For use with adults age 18 years and older. Not for use with pregnant and lactating women. Note: For people 65 years and older, the normal weight range may begin slightly above BMI 18.5 and extend into the overweight weight range.
Adapted from *Obesity: Preventing and Managing the Global Epidemic: Report of a WHO Consultation on Obesity* (p. 9), World Health Organization, 2000, Geneva, Switzerland: Author.

Table 28-6B Health Risk Classification According to Waist Circumference (WC)*

WC Cut-off Points		Health Risk (Relative to WC Below Cut-off Point)
Men	≥102 cm	Increased risk of developing health problems**
Women	≥88 cm	

For BMIs in the 18.5 to 34.9 range, use WC as an additional indicator of health risk. For BMIs ≥35, WC measurement does not provide additional information regarding level of risk. *For use among adults age 18 years and older. Not for use with pregnant and lactating women. **Risk for Type 2 diabetes, coronary heart disease, hypertension.
Adapted from *Obesity: Preventing and Managing the Global Epidemic: Report of a WHO Consultation on Obesity* (p. 9), World Health Organization, 2000, Geneva, Switzerland: Author.

(Figure 28–3). Light palpation may be used to detect the characteristics of the skin surface or of structures located immediately adjacent to the surface to a depth of about 1 cm. Deep palpation is used on structures that are deeper than 1 cm but less than 5 cm from the skin surface. Generally, nurses use light palpation throughout a physical examination and deep palpation according to their discretion.

Safety Alert. To avoid injuring clients during deep palpation, nursing students should be supervised.

Nurses begin palpation with warm hands and light pressure to encourage clients' confidence, relaxation, and co-operation. Clients may perceive deep palpation at the beginning as roughness. Therefore, light palpitation always precedes deep palpitation. Nurses perform light palpation using gentle pressure with fingers together and extended. Fingernails should be short to ensure client comfort. By conducting light palpation first, nurses may discover tender areas and prevent unnecessary discomfort or muscular rigidity. Clients who experience tenderness to palpation may voluntarily increase muscular resistance, which inhibits detection of important and useful findings. Nurses always palpate tender areas last.

Nurses conduct deep palpation by using firm, discontinuous pressure; continuous pressure exerted on examiners' finger pads or fingertips can reduce tactile sensitivity. To avoid constant pressure on the nerve endings, which dulls the sensitivity, examiners apply firm hand pressure with fingers together and extended, but alternate between applying and releasing the pressure. They may need to use two hands (bimanual) to achieve the firm pressure required for deep palpation of the abdomen and reaching deeper structures such as the liver or colon. The hand on top exerts the pressure; the hand below stays relaxed to retain sensitivity for receiving tactile sensations. Pressure is always discontinuous during deep palpation, whether one or two hands are used.

Movements of Palpation. The type of data collected by light and deep palpation depends on the position and motion of the palpating hand(s). During light palpation, nurses use gliding, circular (rotary), direct (perpendicular), dipping, and grasping (pincer action; Table 28-9 and Figure 28–4). During light and deep palpation of the abdomen, expected findings may include feces in the colon, bulkiness of the cecum in the right lower quadrant and of the descending colon in the left lower quadrant, and bladder distended with urine, pregnant uterus, or mobile right kidney.

Percussion

Sounds produced when body tissues are tapped (percussed) assist nurses to interpret the status of underlying structures and changes in client condition. When aware of the characteristics of sound and the mechanisms that underlie sound production in the body, nurses apply the principles and acquire the techniques for percussion of body tissues (Figure 28–5).

Characteristics of Sound. **Audible sounds** are perceived in terms of the characteristics of *pitch* (high, low), *intensity* (loud, soft), *duration* (short, long), and *quality* or *nature* (varied). Pitch refers to the *frequency* of sound pressure waves. Frequency is a measure of the number of wave cycles per second (cps) and is usually expressed in Hertz (Hz) in accordance with the international unit for measuring frequency of sound pressure waves.

The intensity (loudness) of sound is measured in decibels (dBs) on the "A" scale, using an instrument that is calibrated to the human hearing curve. Intensity may be measured objectively and independently of frequency (pitch). Loudness is the term used to indicate human perception of the intensity. This is the physiological perception of sound. The intensity is dependent upon the

Text continued on p. 631

Box 28-8 Clinical Indicators of Abuse

Physical Findings	Behavioural Findings
Child Sexual Abuse	
Vaginal or penile discharge Blood on underclothing Pain, itching, or unusual odour in genital area Genital injuries Difficulty in sitting or walking Pain while urinating; recurrent urinary tract infections Foreign bodies in rectum, urethra, or vagina Sexually transmitted infections Pregnancy in young adolescent	Problem with sleeping or eating Fear of certain people or places Play activities recreate the abuse situation Regressed behaviour Sexual acting out Knowledge of explicit sexual matters Preoccupation with other's or own genitals Profound and rapid personality changes Rapidly declining school performance Poor relationship with peers
Domestic Abuse	
Injuries and trauma are inconsistent with reported cause Multiple injuries involving head, face, neck, breasts, abdomen, and genitalia (black eyes, orbital fractures, broken nose, fractured skull, lip lacerations, broken teeth, strangulation marks) X-ray films show old and new fractures in different stages of healing Abrasions, lacerations, bruises/welts Burns Human bites	Attempted suicide Eating or sleeping disorders Anxiety Panic attacks Pattern of substance abuse (follows physical abuse) Low self-esteem Depression Sense of helplessness Guilt Increased forgetfulness Stress-related complaints (headache, anxiety)
Older Adult Abuse	
Injuries and trauma are inconsistent with reported cause (cigarette burn, scratch, bruise, or bite) Hematomas Bruises at various stages of resolution Bruises, chafing, excoriation on wrist and legs (restraints) Burns Fractures inconsistent with cause described Dried blood	Dependent on caregiver Physically and/or cognitively impaired Combative Wandering Verbally belligerent Minimal social support Prolonged interval between injury and medical treatment

Data from "Domestic Violence: How to Screen and Intervene," by M. Gerard, 2000, *RN, 63*(12), pp. 52–56; "Elder Abuse and Neglect," by S. Hoban and K. Kearney, 2000, *American Journal of Nursing, 100*(11), pp. 49–50; "Domestic Violence: How to Ask and How to Listen," by A. Kramer, 2002, *The Nursing Clinics of North America, 37,* pp. 189–210; and *Wong's Essentials of Pediatric Nursing* (6th ed.), by D. L. Wong and M. Hockenberry-Eaton, 2001, St. Louis, MO: Mosby.

Box 28-9 Red Flags for Suspicion of Client Substance Abuse

- Frequently missed appointments
- Frequent requests for written excuses for work
- Chief complaints of insomnia, "bad nerves," or pain that does not fit a particular pattern
- Frequent reports of lost prescriptions (e.g., tranquilizers or pain medications) or requests for frequent refills
- Frequent emergency department visits
- History of changing doctors or bringing in medication bottles prescribed by several different providers
- History of gastrointestinal bleeds, peptic ulcers, pancreatitis, cellulitis, or frequent pulmonary infections
- Frequent sexually transmitted infections (STIs), complicated pregnancies, multiple abortions, or sexual dysfunction
- Complaints of chest pains or palpitations or history of admissions to rule out myocardial infarctions
- History of activities that place the client at risk for human immunodeficiency virus (HIV) infections (multiple sexual partners, multiple rapes)
- Family history of addiction; history of childhood sexual, physical, or emotional abuse; or social and financial or marital problems

Adapted from "Recognition and Diagnosis," by S. Master and J. K. Terpstra, 1992, in *Prescribing Drugs With Abuse Liability* (p. 18), edited by S. H. Schnoll, P. K. Horvatich, and J. K. Terpstra, Richmond, VA: DSAM, MCV-VCU; and *Source Book of Substance Abuse and Addiction,* by L. Friedman et al., 1996, Baltimore: Williams & Wilkins.

Table 28-7 Client Characteristics to Be Assessed During Local Inspection

Alignment	Depressions	Lesion characteristics	Pigmentation	Secretions
Closure	Development	Lustre	Pulsations	Shape
Colour	Elevations	Mass	Range of Motion	Size
Contour	Hair characteristics	Mobility	Reaction to light	Sounds
Coordination	Hygiene	Moisture	Reflections	Spacing
Contraction	Integrity	Movements	Reflexes	Symmetry
Curvatures	Inversion	Parasites	Rhythm	Vascularity

Adapted from *A Primer on Physical Examination Techniques* [WebCT], by D. L. Skillen, 2004a, Edmonton, AB: Faculty of Nursing, University of Alberta.

Table 28-8 Sensory Properties of the Hand for Specific Characteristics

Anatomical Area of Hand	Specific Characteristics to Be Assessed	Rationale
Finger pads	Consistency Contour Moisture Position Texture	Sensory nerve fibres are abundant in the finger pads and facilitate tactile discriminations.
Finger tips	Elasticity Fluid content of tissues Mobility Pulsatility Thickness Tissue turgor Vascularity	Sensory nerve fibres are particularly abundant in the fingertips and facilitate fine tactile discriminations.
Dorsal surface (back of hand)	Temperature	Skin on dorsal surfaces is thinner.
Ball of hand, palmar surface	Vibrations	Metacarpophalangeal joints (ball of hand) on skin surface are sensitive to vibrations.
Ulnar edge (side of hand)	Temperature	Skin on ulnar edge is thinner, facilitating sensitivity to vibrations.
	Vibrations	Contact of fifth finger lengthwise on skin surface.

Adapted from *A Primer on Physical Examination Techniques* [WebCT], by D. L. Skillen, 2004a, Edmonton, AB: Faculty of Nursing, University of Alberta.

A

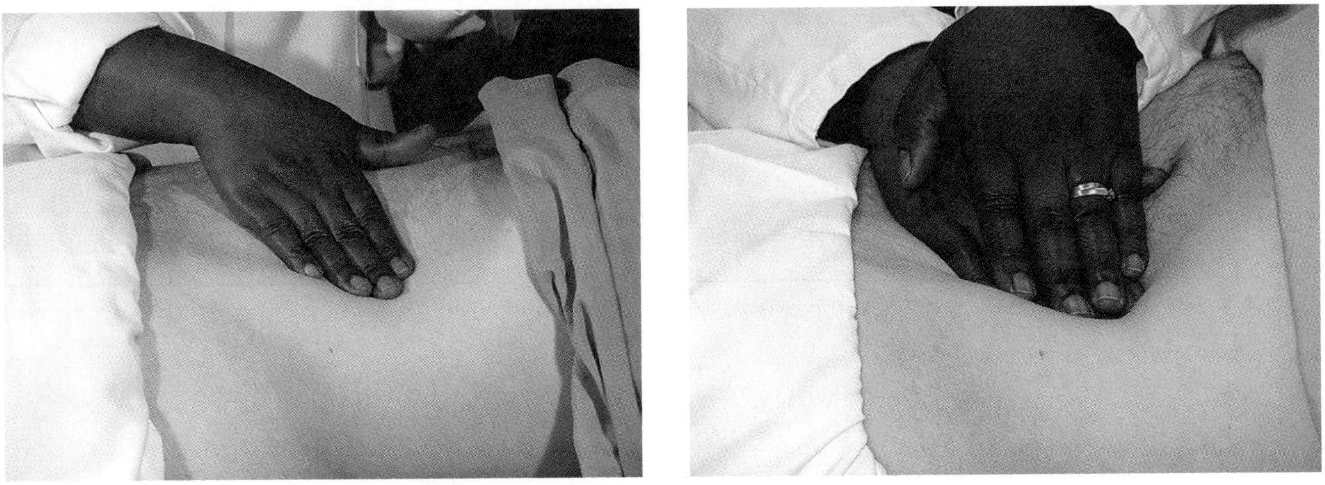

B

FIGURE **28–3** **A,** Light palpation. **B,** Deep palpation. (From *Physical Examination Images* [CD-ROM], by D. L. Skillen, R. A. Day, M. C. Anderson, T. C. Stephen, J. A. Gilbert, and L. W. Day, 2004, Edmonton, AB: Faculty of Nursing, University of Alberta.)

Table 28-9 Movements of the Hand for Palpation of Specific Characteristics

Palpation Movement	Techniques and Rationale	Specific Characteristics to be Assessed
Gliding	Slide finger pads over skin surface in both horizontal and vertical planes.	Moisture Surface contour Tenderness Texture
Circular movements	Roll surface tissue over underlying structures with finger pads to accentuate structural characteristics or characteristics of masses.	Consistency Contour Discreteness of a mass Mobility Shape Size Tenderness
Grasping	Grasp skin surfaces with the finger pads (pincer action) to gather data about structures immediately below the skin surface.	Amplitude Association with respiration (e.g., abdominal mass movement with respiration) Consistency Elasticity Mobility Position Pulsations Shape Size Tenderness Tissue turgor Thickness
Direct perpendicular pressure	Direct pressure of fingertips, pads, ulnar surfaces, or palmar surfaces detects blanching, fluid content, tenderness, guarding, pulsations, resistance, or an association with respiration.	Blood vessels Excursion Fremitus Masses Muscle Pulsations Rate Rhythm Skin lesions Subcutaneous tissue Swelling Tenderness
Dipping	Use finger pads during palpation of the abdomen while visualizing the underlying structures. Failure to imagine underlying structures may lead to the conclusion that an abnormality has been palpated.	Consistency Contour Elasticity Guarding Masses Mobility of underlying structure Resistance Shape Size Status of underlying viscera Tenderness

Adapted from *A Primer on Physical Examination Techniques* [WebCT], by D. L. Skillen, 2004a, Edmonton, AB: Faculty of Nursing, University of Alberta.

A

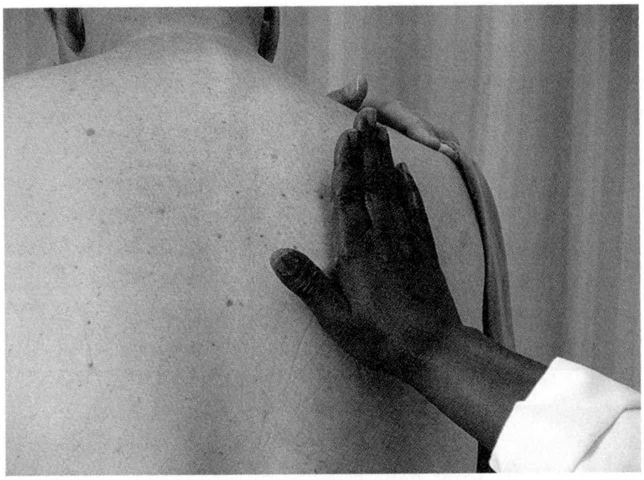

B

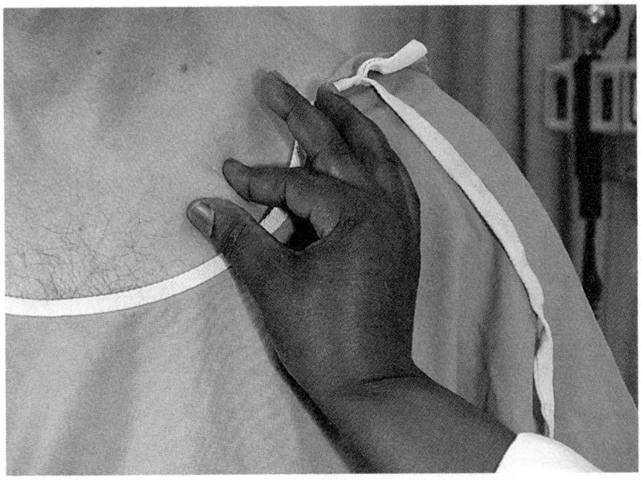

FIGURE 28–4 Movements of palpation. **A,** Ball of hand for vibrations. **B,** Grasping for tissue mobility. (From *Physical Examination Images* [CD-ROM], by D. L. Skillen, R. A. Day, M. C. Anderson, T. C. Stephen, J. A. Gilbert, and L. W. Day, 2004, Edmonton, AB: Faculty of Nursing, University of Alberta.)

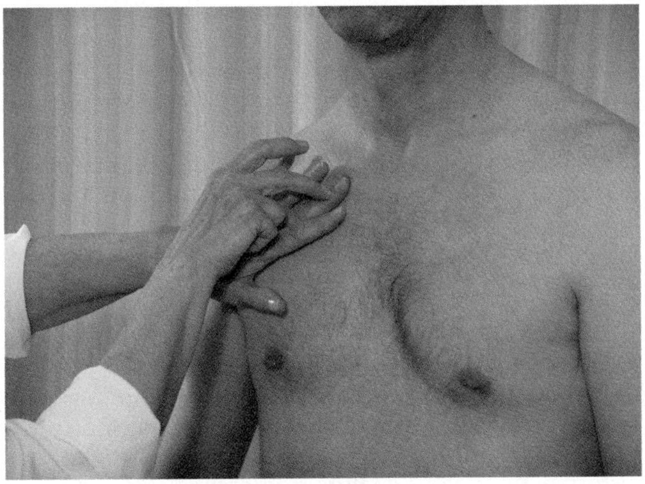

FIGURE 28–5 Indirect percussion. (From *Physical Examination Images* [CD-ROM], by D. L. Skillen, R. A. Day, M. C. Anderson, T. C. Stephen, J. A. Gilbert, and L. W. Day, 2004, Edmonton, AB: Faculty of Nursing, University of Alberta.)

amplitude of the vibrations or sound waves produced by stimulating the source. A freely vibrating source of sound is capable of producing a loud sound for which the intensity varies according to the force applied to set vibrations in motion. For example, a relatively loud sound is produced by striking a drum because of its capacity to vibrate freely. In contrast, when tissues of the human forearm are tapped, the sound is always of low intensity because relatively dense tissues do not vibrate freely. The force used to increase vibration may affect intensity, but not frequency (high, medium, or low pitch) of the vibrating structure. Curiously, two sounds of equal intensity but different frequency will not be perceived as equally loud. The duration of sound is the length of time in seconds, minutes, or hours that a sound is perceived by the ear. Soft tissue (muscle, adipose tissue) may dampen the duration. The quality of sound (its nature, timbre) pertains to its musical nature or its blowing, gurgling, or clicking quality.

During physical examination, examiners use a tuning fork of 1024 or 512 Hz to test hearing, but a tuning fork of 128 or 256 Hz to test vibration. A 1024 Hz tuning fork produces a sound that is higher pitched, more musical, of longer duration, and within the range of human hearing. A 256 Hz tuning fork produces a buzzing noise that is lower pitched, of shorter duration, and possibly outside hearing range.

Sound Transmission in the Body. Audible sound is a travelling pressure wave that moves more quickly through solids and fluids than it does through gases in the body. Sounds detected using percussion and auscultation depend on tissue density and elasticity of body structures. Elasticity permits vibration of body structures, which then creates sound waves that are transmitted to the exterior of the body and perceived as sound by the examiner. Sounds detected during percussion or auscultation are interpreted according to the characteristics of pitch, intensity, quality, and duration. In dense tissue, sounds have a higher pitch, softer intensity, shorter duration, and are less musical in quality. In less dense tissue, sounds have a lower pitch, louder intensity, longer duration, and more musical quality.

Sounds originating in elastic body tissues travel through body structures and tissues to the exterior body surface for detection by the examiner's ear. Gases are poor transmitters of sound, fluids are better, and solids are best. Knowledge of the sound transmission capabilities of various media permits examiners to detect deviations from expected findings in body tissues. For example, breath sounds are altered by lung and other tissue changes. The pitch, intensity, musical quality, and duration of sounds vary as they are transmitted through solids, fluid, and air-filled tissues.

Percussion Notes. Sounds produced in the body as a result of percussion of body surfaces are described as flat,

Table 28-10 **Characteristics of Percussion Notes**

Percussion Note	Pitch	Intensity	Duration	Quality	Tissue Density	Example
Flat	High	Soft	Short	Flat noise	Dense	Thigh muscle scapula
Dull	Medium	Medium	Moderate	Thud-like noise	Dense	Heart, liver, distended urinary bladder
Resonant	Low	Loud	Long	Hollow noise	Less dense	Air-filled lung
Hyperresonant	High	Loud	Longer than resonance	Pronounced hollow noise	Less dense	Hyperinflated lung, child's thin chest
Tympanic	High	Loud	Moderate	Musical, drum-like	Less Dense	Gas in bowel, gastric air bubble, cheek puffed out

dull, resonant, hyperresonant, and tympanic (Table 28-10). Each of the five percussion notes is characterized by pitch, intensity, duration, and quality.

Simulating Sounds. By puffing out their own cheek, learners can simulate tympany. They create a flat percussion note by percussing the scapula of another adult. When percussing their chest just inferior to the clavicle, learners hear resonance on themselves; by percussing their anterior thigh, they hear dullness. They can percuss hyperresonance on the chest of a thin child.

Percussion Techniques. Percussion is used to determine the density of underlying tissues (if air filled, fluid filled, or solid) and to locate and estimate the size of body organs. Knowing how density influences sound, nurses can map the size and location of underlying organs. Variations in percussion notes occur over tissues and organs of varied densities. Percussion also elicits tenderness if present in underlying structures and stimulates reflex action of a partially stretched deep tendon.

Two types of percussion are used: indirect and direct. **Indirect (mediated) percussion** is the most common (Procedure 28-1). With the middle finger of the dominant hand (plexor finger), examiners tap on the middle finger of the non-dominant hand (pleximeter finger) placed on a body surface (see Figure 28–5). This elicits a percussion note. Indirect (mediated) percussion may also involve striking the dorsum of one hand with the ulnar edge of the fist of the other hand, for example, fist percussion of the kidney in the costovertebral angle to detect tenderness.

Direct (non-mediated) percussion is used less commonly. It involves direct percussion with the plexor finger over body surfaces, for example, percussion over the frontal sinuses for tenderness or on the clavicle to detect resonance of apical lung tissue.

Learners need to practise percussion techniques repetitively until achieving a clear percussion note before attempting to distinguish among the five percussion notes (see Table 28-10). To increase the strength or coordination of the plexor finger, some examiners brace the plexor with the thumb of the same hand.

When comparing symmetrical areas, examiners use consistent technique to ensure accuracy of findings and avoid misinterpretations (Box 28-10). The results of percussion vary according to the technique used. To perceive differences among percussion notes most accurately, examiners percuss from areas of lesser density to areas of greater density. It is easier to detect the change from a resonant to a dull note than from dullness to resonance or hyperresonance.

Auscultation

Auscultation is listening to the sounds made by the body. Examiners use stethoscopes to auscultate sounds created by vibration or movement of underlying tissues. The stethoscope was invented by René Laennec in 1816 to exclude external environmental sounds and augment internal body sounds transmitted to the skin surface. Examiners use stethoscopes to auscultate sounds created by vibration or movement of underlying tissues. The binaural stethoscope is the most popular, and has right and left earpieces, single tubing, and a combination bell/diaphragm chestpiece. Differences among stethoscopes include earpiece shape, tubing length, chestpiece characteristics, and adjustability of tension springs. The quality of the stethoscope affects sounds transmitted to the ear. Examiners may interpret incorrectly the sounds distorted by a poor-quality stethoscope; this compromises the quality of their client assessment and care.

Examiners use the chestpieces of the stethoscope to detect the pitch, duration, intensity, and quality of body sounds. Stethoscopes may be equipped with a single chestpiece (a bell or a diaphragm), a paired chestpiece (a bell with a diaphragm), or an adult diaphragm paired with a pediatric diaphragm.

The bell chestpiece has an outer rim, usually bordered by rubber material, and a hollow centre that is not covered by a flat surface. If a chestpiece has a flat surface joining its outer rim, it is a diaphragm. The bell accentuates low-frequency sounds, filtering out high-pitched sounds. The bell is an open system that requires a complete seal with the skin but light pressure. Without a perfect seal, sound leaks occur and environmental noise distorts the sound perceived. If the bell is applied with firm pressure, the skin functions like a diaphragm that accentuates high-pitched sounds.

The diaphragm chestpiece picks up high frequency sounds (think "di-hi") and filters out low-pitched sounds. Clinically more suitable for detecting high-pitched visceral sounds, it does not require a complete seal with the skin surface because it is a closed system. Sound leaks will

Procedure 28-1 Critical Components of Indirect Percussion Techniques

Equipment

- None

Steps	Rationale
1. Trim the fingernail short on the plexor finger.	Perpendicular blows to pleximeter will not draw blood and will cause less soreness.
2. Place pleximeter finger (finger being struck) on the skin surface over the area to be percussed.	Contact with skin surface permits blow to pleximeter to set underlying body structures vibrating to produce a percussion note.
3. Place pleximeter firmly.	Body structures will not vibrate fully if finger not firm.
4. Do not move pleximeter.	Movement reduces and diffuses underlying vibrations.
5. Limit contact of pleximeter to one small area on the skin; preferably only the distal interphalangeal joint (DIP) touches the skin surface.	Limiting the area of contact produces clearer percussion note.
6. Strike a sharp, perpendicular blow to the DIP joint of the stationary pleximeter with the plexor finger (striking finger).	Striking sharply produces a clearer percussion note.
7. Use brisk arc-like wrist action with relaxed wrist.	Produces sharp perpendicular blow.
8. Limit movement to wrist action, avoiding movement at elbow.	Produces sharp perpendicular blow.
9. Limit percussion to one or two sharp blows.	Examiner detects percussion note more accurately.
10. Select the appropriate force of blow to achieve a clear percussion note.	Clarity facilitates interpretation of percussion note.
11. Use the lightest blow possible to achieve a clear percussion note.	Note elicited is restricted to a small body area. Examiners adjust the force of the blow according to body build of clients, using a more forceful blow to percuss over a heavily muscled or obese client, and a less forceful blow if client is emaciated or very thin.

Adapted from *A Primer on Physical Examination Techniques* [WebCT], by D. L. Skillen, 2004a, Edmonton, AB: Faculty of Nursing, University of Alberta.

Box 28-10 Summary of Important Percussion Techniques

- Firm pleximeter finger on the skin surface
- Only the distal interphalangeal (DIP) joint touches the skin
- A sharp, perpendicular blow with the plexor finger and wrist action
- The lightest blow to achieve a clear percussion note
- Consistent technique when comparing symmetrical areas
- Force of the blow adjusted in accordance with client body build
- Percussion from an area of lesser density to an area of greater density

not occur if an incomplete seal is made on the skin surface. For accuracy and hygiene, examiners use their own stethoscope. If they must share a stethoscope, they clean the earpieces with alcohol before use. Earpieces should be large enough to fit snugly in the external opening of the ear for blocking outside noise. An earpiece that is too small may enter further into the auditory canal and obstruct sound transmission. The composition of earpieces (rubber or plastic) also affects the fit and comfort. Examiners should insert earpieces facing forward, medially toward the nose, and pointing somewhat inferiorly so that they fit the natural curvature of adult ear canals. Earpieces need to be comfortable enough to be worn for long periods of time.

To maximize sound conduction, examiners require short flexible tubing that is thick-walled with about a 3 mm diameter for transmitting sounds. A desirable tubing length is about 30 cm, but some authorities accept tubing as long as 50 cm. If too long, tubing does not transmit sound effectively.

An electronic stethoscope amplifies sound and has a different shape. Examiners may adjust it for low-frequency sounds (bell function) or for high-frequency sounds (diaphragm function). Nurses with reduced hearing acuity require a stethoscope with greater sound amplification or must ask colleagues to double-check their findings.

Auscultation Techniques. A learner must be familiar with a stethoscope before using it on a client (Box 28-11).

To maximize the sound volume of the diaphragm chestpiece, nurses should apply it with enough pressure so that it can move in synchrony with body movements from breathing and avoid creation of frictional noise. Nurses may close their eyes to reduce environmental stimuli and improve their focus on a particular sound. They avoid activities such as sliding or moving fingers on the chestpiece, rubbing the tubing, moving the chestpiece on the skin, or breathing on the tubing, which contribute to extraneous noise that obscures detection of significant sounds. The stethoscope is always placed on naked skin because clothing obscures sound. Coarse hair on the skin of a hirsute individual can also create frictional noise. By wetting the hair so that it lies closer to the skin, the examiner reduces the friction. Box 28-12 presents a summary of critical auscultation skills.

Box 28-11 Exercises to Increase Familiarity With the Stethoscope

Ensure that the earpiece follows the contour of the ear canal. Learn what fit is best for you by comparing amplification of sounds with the earpieces in both directions.

Place the earpieces in your ears with the tips of the earpieces turned toward the face. *Lightly* blow into the diaphragm. Again place the earpieces in your ears, this time with the ends turned toward the back of the head. *Lightly* blow into the diaphragm. You will find that clearer sounds are heard with the earpiece turned toward the face. After you have learned the right fit for the loudest amplification, wear the stethoscope the same way each time.

Put on the stethoscope and lightly blow into the diaphragm. If the sound is barely audible, lightly blow into the bell. Sound is carried through only one part of the chestpiece at a time. If the sound is greatly amplified through the diaphragm, the diaphragm is in position for use. If the sound is barely audible through the diaphragm, the bell is in position for use. Rotation of the diaphragm and bell places the chestpiece in the desired position. Leave the diaphragm in position for the next exercise.

Place the diaphragm over the anterior part of your chest. Ask a friend to speak in a normal conversational tone. Environmental noise seriously detracts from hearing the noise created by body organs. When a stethoscope is used, the client and the examiner should remain quiet.

Put the stethoscope on and gently tap the tubing. It is often difficult to avoid stretching or moving the stethoscope's tubing. The examiner should be in a position so that the tubing hangs free. Moving or touching the tubing creates extraneous sounds.

Care of the stethoscope: Earpieces should be removed regularly and cleaned of cerumen (earwax). The bell and diaphragm should be kept free of dust, lint, and body oils. The tubing should be kept away from nurses' body oils. Avoid draping the stethoscope around the neck next to the skin. The entire stethoscope (diaphragm, tubing, etc.) can be wiped clean with alcohol or soapy water. Be sure to dry all parts thoroughly. Follow the manufacturer's recommendations.

During auscultation, more than one sound may be heard. Concentrate on one sound at a time and allow sufficient time to listen carefully. Consider the body area or structure being auscultated and the causes of sounds. For example, the first heart sound "lub" is caused by closure of the mitral valve. Nurses know the types of sounds arising from each body structure and the location where they can be heard best. They are familiar with the areas of the body that are not expected to emit sounds. This knowledge helps them to discriminate between what *should be* heard and what *is* heard.

Location, timing, rate, and rhythm of sound are specific characteristics that are considered during auscultation, depending on the body system being auscultated.

When examining the respiratory system, the location of breath sounds is assessed according to the underlying lobes of the lungs or large airways. The right lower lobe

Box 28-12 Summary of Critical Auscultation Skills

- Insert the earpieces anteriorly, nasally, and inferiorly.
- Place stethoscope on bare skin.
- Avoid frictional noise by applying chestpiece to move in synchrony with client's respiration.
- Use a stethoscope with an earpiece that fits snugly in the opening of the ear.
- Make a complete seal for the bell using light pressure.
- Concentrate on one sound at a time.
- Ensure a short tubing length.
- Dampen hair on hirsute clients.

of the posterior thorax is an example of a peripheral location. The types of sounds include vesicular breath sounds, bronchovesicular breath sounds, and tracheal breath sounds. It is important to establish the timing of breath sounds relative to inspiration and expiration. The rate of sounds is assessed during a defined period of time, usually 1 minute, when assessing all three systems (respiratory, cardiovascular, and gastrointestinal).

When examining the cardiovascular system, the location of cardiac sounds is assessed according to anatomical location on the precordium and the underlying structures of the heart and great vessels. The types of sounds include single first and second heart sounds, split heart sounds, fixed split sounds, murmurs, clicks, and opening snaps. It is important to establish the timing of heart sounds relative to systole and diastole. The rhythm of sounds applies to assessment of the cardiac cycle. In the well adult, the rhythm of the first and second heart sounds is regular and can be heard with the stethoscope. The rate and rhythm can be observed on the electrocardiogram.

Location of gastrointestinal system sounds is assessed according to the abdominal quadrants or regions. The types of sounds include clicks, gurgles, and borborygmi. The rate of sounds in the abdomen should be checked during a 1-minute period. A silent abdomen should be assessed for a longer period of time.

Anatomical Terms

Anatomical Position

To avoid errors in communication among health professionals internationally, nurses use the anatomical position for verbal and written documentation (Box 28-13). The anatomical position has been adopted throughout the world to standardize descriptions of observations, facilitate clear communication, and promote accuracy. Whether clients are standing, sitting, prone, supine, or lying on one side, their examiners *imagine* that they are in the anatomical position when describing findings (Figure 28–6).

The use of the anatomical position by professionals in varied disciplines and national or international jurisdictions transmits information in a mode that promotes client health care. Errors are reduced in collegial discussions or follow-up activities when examiners document findings using standard methods of description. This record is a legal document that directs subsequent activities by health professionals for clients. Clearly communicated findings, using the anatomical position, facilitate accurate comparison of client change over time whether examiners change or remain constant.

Box 28-13 Standardized Anatomical Position

Examiners imagine the client to be in the following position:
- Upright (erect)
- Head, eyes, and toes facing forward (anteriorly)
- Heels and great toes touching
- Arms hanging by the sides with palms facing forward (anteriorly)

Anatomical Planes

Use four major and imaginary *planes* to divide the body and make precise descriptions (see Figure 28-6). Start by imagining the client in the anatomical position. Next, consider the four imaginary planes (Table 28-11):
- Median
- Coronal (Frontal)
- Sagittal
- Horizontal (Transverse)

Anatomical Surfaces

Anatomical planes are reference points for anatomical surfaces that are used to describe body structures in relation to one other. When referring to anatomical surfaces, imagine clients in the anatomical position (Table 28-12): upright, arms hanging at sides, palms of hands facing anteriorly, feet together, great toes touching, and head facing anteriorly.

Nurses use anatomical surfaces to describe their observations and frequently combine terms to indicate location. For example, they might record that a wound dressing was changed on the medial surface of the right forearm. They may also use anatomical surfaces to indicate direction. For example, the diameter from the front of the chest to the back (anteroposterior diameter of the thorax) is less than the lateral diameter. When assessing the shape of the thorax, the two directions are compared in length.

The position of function determines whether a surface is ventral or dorsal when describing the tongue, penis, hand, or foot.

Anatomical Quadrants and Regions

Anatomical Quadrants. Quadrants are created by imaginary intersecting vertical and horizontal lines in the median and horizontal planes (Figure 28–7). The abdomen and breasts are commonly described in terms of their quadrants. The labels for breast quadrants (Figure 28–8) are different from the abdominal quadrants: upper outer quadrant (UOQ), upper inner quadrant (UIQ), lower outer

Table 28-11 Imaginary Anatomical Planes

Name of Plane	Location of Plane	Result of Imaginary Plane
Median	Passes vertically through the body from back to front	Right and left symmetrical halves
Coronal (Frontal)	Beginning at the coronal suture of the skull, the plane passes vertically through the body at right angles to the median plane, posteriorly through the ankles and feet	Anterior and posterior regions
Sagittal	Passes vertically through the body, parallel to the median plane	Sections of right and left symmetrical halves
Midsagittal	Passes vertically through the median plane	Separation of right and left symmetrical halves
Horizontal (Transverse)	Passes through the body at right angles to the sagittal, median, and coronal planes through the umbilicus anteriorly and the intervertebral disc between third lumbar vertebra (L3) and fourth lumbar vertebra (L4) Parallel to the surface on which the individual stands	Superior and inferior regions

Adapted from *A Primer on Physical Examination Techniques* [WebCT], by D. L. Skillen, 2004a, Edmonton, AB: Faculty of Nursing, University of Alberta.

A

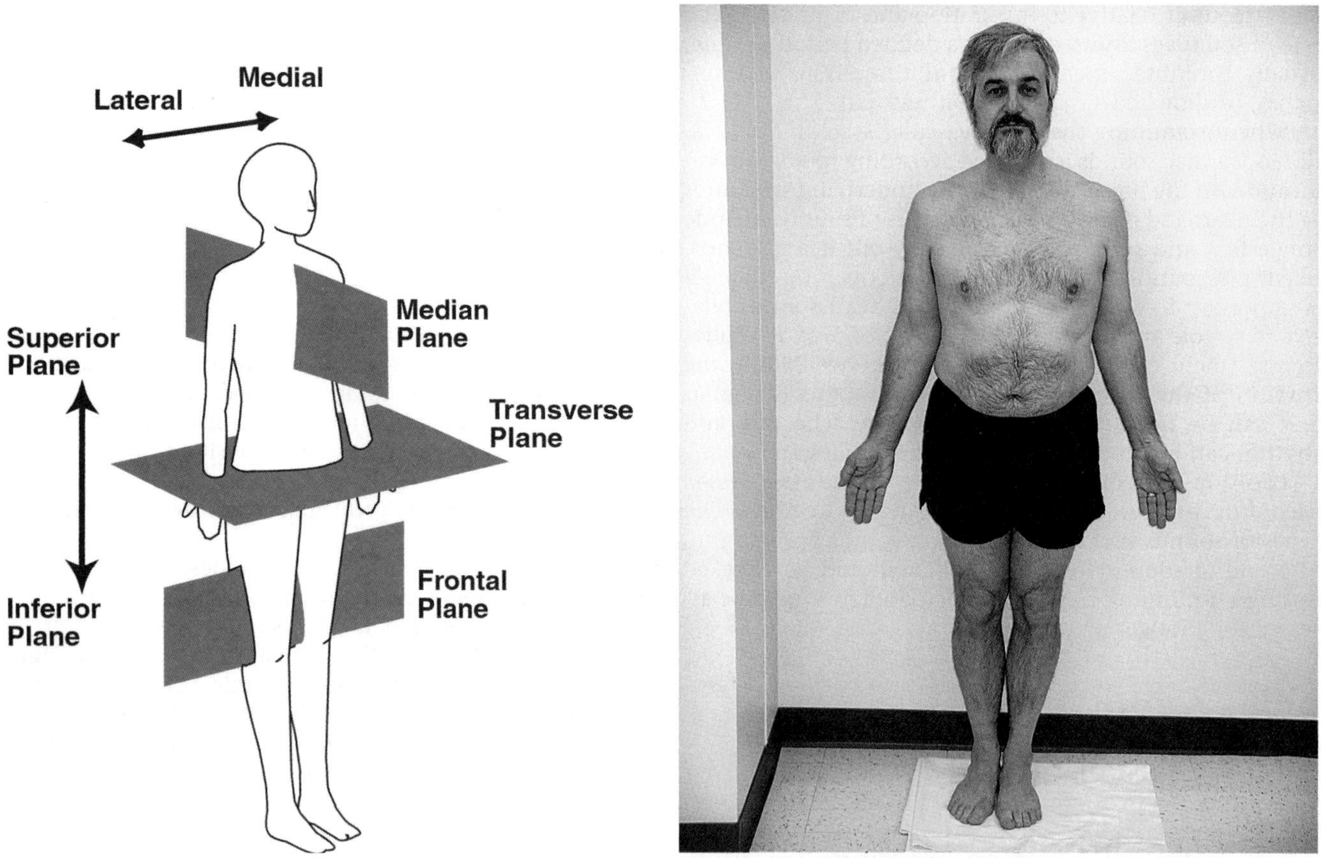

B

FIGURE **28–6** **A,** Anatomical position planes. **B,** Anatomical position. (From *Physical Examination Images* [CD-ROM], by D. L. Skillen, R. A. Day, M. C. Anderson, T. C. Stephen, J. A. Gilbert, and L. W. Day, 2004, Edmonton, AB: Faculty of Nursing, University of Alberta.)

Table 28-12 Anatomical Surfaces

Name of Surface	Location of Surface	Additional Information
Anterior	Front of the body	In neuroanatomy and embryology, the term is ventral
Dorsal (posterior)	Back of the body	It is helpful to think of the dorsal fin of a fish. The term dorsal can be confusing. For example, • the superior surface of the foot or tongue is the dorsal surface or dorsum • the anterior view of the flaccid (non-erect) penis is also referred to as the dorsum
Inferior	Lower parts of the body	Observations are closer to the client's feet than to the head. To illustrate, • the knee is inferior to the hip
Lateral	Surfaces farthest away from the median plane	In the anatomical position, • the little toe is lateral to the great toe
Medial	Surfaces closest to the median plane	In the anatomical position, • the little finger is medial to the thumb • the surfaces of the arms and legs closest to the torso are medial surfaces
Palmar	Anterior surfaces of the hands	Palmar surfaces of the fingers
Plantar	Inferior surfaces of the feet	Includes soles of the toes
Superior	Upper parts of the body	Includes torso above umbilicus and intervertebral disc between L3 and L4, arms, and the head and neck. Structures may be described as superior to another structure. To illustrate, • shoulders are superior to the elbows
Inferior	Lower parts of the body	Includes torso below the umbilicus and the intervertebral disc between L3 and L4, the legs, and feet Structures may be described as inferior to another structure. For example, • the ankle is inferior to the knee

Adapted from *A Primer on Physical Examination Techniques* [WebCT], by D. L. Skillen, 2004a, Edmonton, AB: Faculty of Nursing, University of Alberta.

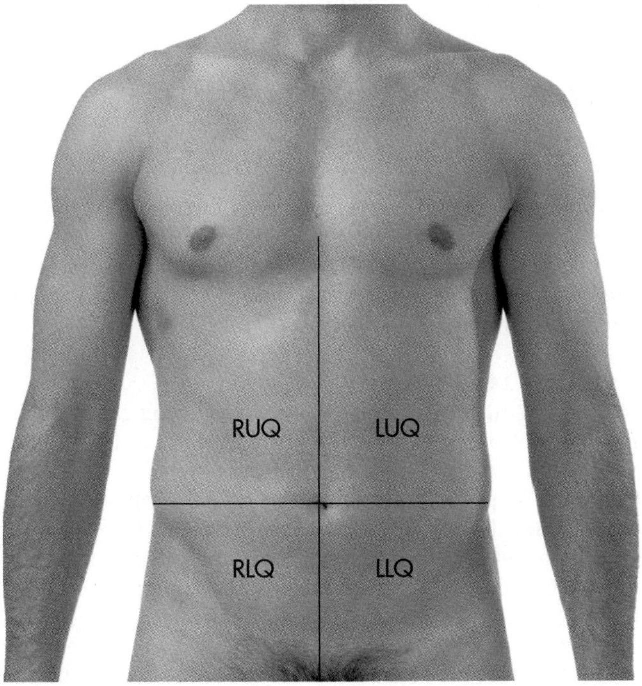

FIGURE **28–7** Four quadrants of the abdomen. (From *Mosby's Guide to Physical Examination,* 5th ed., p. 536, by H. M. Seidel et al., 2003, St. Louis, MO: Mosby.)

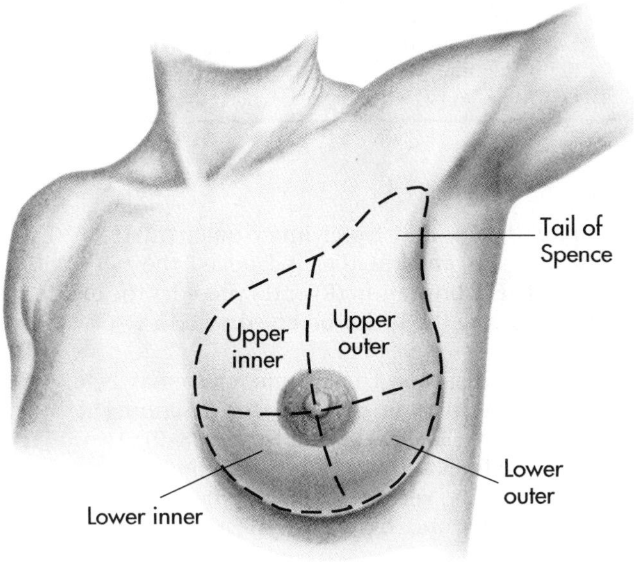

FIGURE **28–8** Breast quadrants. (From *Mosby's Guide to Physical Examination,* 5th ed., p. 497, by H. M. Seidel et al., 2003, St. Louis, MO: Mosby.)

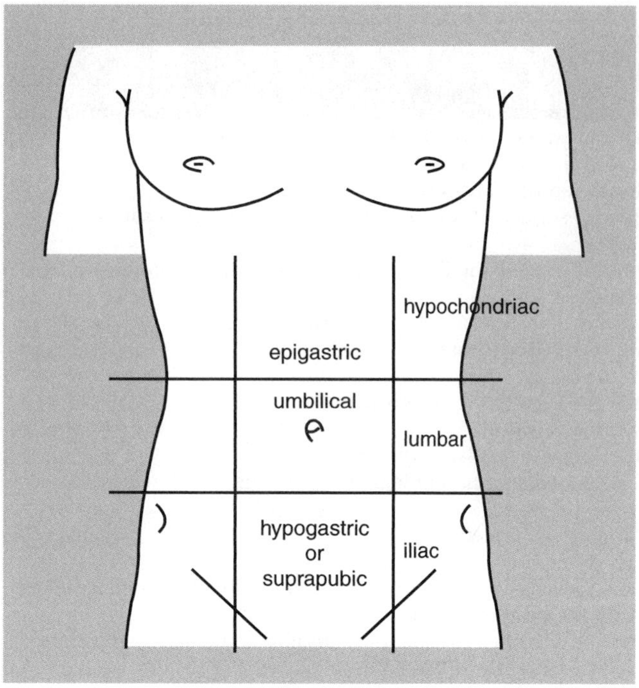

FIGURE **28–9** Nine abdominal regions. (From *Physical Examination Images* [CD-ROM], by D. L. Skillen, R. A. Day, M. C. Anderson, T. C. Stephen, J. A. Gilbert, and L. W. Day, 2004, Edmonton, AB: Faculty of Nursing, University of Alberta.)

Box 28-14 Anatomical Regions of the Abdomen

1. Epigastric
2. Umbilical
3. Suprapubic (or hypogastric)
4. Right hypochondriac
5. Left hypochondriac
6. Right lateral (or right lumbar)
7. Left lateral (or left lumbar)
8. Right inguinal (or right iliac)
9. Left inguinal (or left iliac)

quadrant (LOQ), and lower inner quadrant (LIQ). Each breast also has an area that is labelled the tail (Tail of Spence). The abbreviation (R) or (L) precedes the quadrant label to indicate the breast observed.

Anatomical Regions. The abdomen also may be divided systematically into nine regions for describing findings more precisely (Box 28-14 and Figure 28–9). Two imaginary vertical lines and two imaginary horizontal lines create the 9 regions. Vertical lines are parallel to the median (sagittal) plane; horizontal lines are parallel to the horizontal plane.

Anatomical Terms of Comparison

When using terms of comparison, nurses draw from their knowledge of the anatomical position, planes, surfaces, quadrants, and regions to describe the position of one structure in relation to another structure (Table 28-13). When making comparisons, nurses avoid using the words *on, over, above,* and *under* to describe location. For example, by documenting a mass as lying "under" the umbilicus, it is not clear if it is located inferior, posterior, or deep to the umbilicus. Precision is needed for client safety and management.

Anatomical terms of comparison include the following:

- Proximal and distal
- Ipsilateral and contralateral
- Superficial and deep
- Interior and exterior

Anatomical Terms of Movement

Movements that occur at the articulations of bones and range of motion (ROM) are described in relation to the anatomical planes. The most common planes of reference for movements are the median and coronal (frontal) planes. The median plane creates the imaginary right and left body halves; the coronal plane creates the imaginary anterior and posterior body halves. Guided by the standardized anatomical terms of movement, position, and plane, examiners systematically inspect body structures for the type and ROM. They frequently compare the movements made by symmetrical areas of the body such as the arms, shoulders, hips, and legs, and describe the range of client motion relative to a neutral position, often the midline.

Common terms of movement include flexion and extension, abduction and adduction, dorsiflexion and plantarflexion, medial and lateral rotation, internal and external rotation, eversion and inversion, and supination and pronation (Table 28-14). Less common terms of movement include opposition, protraction, retraction, elevation, depression, and circumduction.

Preparation for the Physical Examination

Preparation of the client, environment, and nurse ensures a smooth examination with few interruptions. An unorganized approach can reduce client confidence in the examiner, create client discomfort or embarrassment, and cause errors or missed observations.

Client Preparation

Nurses attend to the physical and psychological preparation of their clients to ensure a successful assessment.

Physical Preparation of the Client. Client physical comfort is essential for a physical examination. Clients need to be dressed and draped appropriately. In hospital, they may use a simple gown or disposable sheet; in ambulatory settings, they are advised about what clothing to remove and which way to put on a gown (open at the front or at the back). As well, they are given a light drape for cover. They need privacy for undressing and time to do so. Examiners respect a client's dignity and avoid client embarrassment by knocking before entering a room where a client is changing. Physical preparation also ensures that clients have had an opportunity to empty the

Table 28-13 Anatomical Terms of Comparison

Contrasting Terms	Location	Additional Information
Proximal	Nearest to the trunk of the body	A proximal point is nearest to the origin of a structure. When describing a nerve, muscle, or vessel, the term proximal refers to the point nearest to the origin of the structure. When the term proximal is used to describe an area of an arm or leg, it is synonymous with superior (a term of relationship). For example, the upper arm is the proximal region of the arm; the elbow is proximal to the wrist.
Distal	Farthest from the trunk of the body	When describing a nerve, muscle, or vessel, the term distal refers to the point farthest from the origin of the structure. If referring to an area of an arm or leg, inferior is a synonym for distal. For example, the hand is the most distal part of the arm and the wrist is distal to the elbow.
Ipsilateral	The structure is on the same side of the median plane as another observation.	The term ipsilateral is used in neurologic assessments. For example, an immobile right arm is ipsilateral to the right cerebral hemisphere.
Contralateral	The structure is on the opposite side of the median plane from another observation.	The term contralateral is used in neurologic assessments. For example, an immobile left arm is contralateral to the right cerebral hemisphere.
Superficial	Proximity to the surface of the body	For example, the superficial temporal artery passes in front of the ear and is palpable.
Deep	Distance from the surface of the body	For example, the pectoralis major muscle is distant from the skin.
Interior	Location within a structure or in relation to the body core	The term interior has more than one meaning: • Interior can indicate the location of a structure within another structure. • Interior can also indicate location with respect to the body surface. • For example, the cochlea of the ear may be described in both ways.
Exterior	Location outside a structure or in relation to the body surface	The term exterior also has more than one meaning: • Exterior can indicate location of a peripheral structure. • Exterior can also refer to a structure that is nearer to the surface of the body.

Adapted from *A Primer on Physical Examination Techniques* [WebCT], by D. L. Skillen, 2004a, Edmonton, AB: Faculty of Nursing, University of Alberta.

bladder or bowel. This facilitates examination of the abdomen, genitalia, and rectum and provides an opportunity to collect urine or fecal specimens if needed. Nurses explain in advance the proper methods for collecting and labelling specimens.

Nurses ensure that clients are warm by eliminating drafts, providing warm blankets, and controlling room temperature. Seriously ill or older clients are more susceptible to chills. Offering sips of water, tissues, and a pillow can promote clients' comfort. Clients' safety is paramount. The physical examination is conducted so that clients are not at risk of losing their balance, falling, or hurting themselves with equipment.

During the physical examination, nurses ask clients to assume proper positions so that body parts are accessible and clients remain comfortable (Table 28-15). Clients' ability to assume positions will depend on their physical strength, mobility, ease of breathing, age, and degree of wellness. Examiners explain the positions required and assist clients to attain them, adjusting drapes so that only the body area to be examined is exposed and no body parts are uncovered unnecessarily. Some required positions are uncomfortable for clients and may cause embarrassment; therefore, clients are kept in those positions no longer than necessary. Clients may be unable to assume certain positions. For example, a client with rheumatoid arthritis may be unable to get into a lithotomy position but able to lie in the left lateral position for an examination of the genitalia. A client with difficulty breathing may not tolerate lying flat. Nurses choose the position that provides the greatest accessibility and accuracy for assessment. If clients are too weak or physically unable to assume a position, nurses select an alternate. They use extra care so that older clients do not look into a source of light. Specifically, nurses avoid standing in front of a window, which makes it difficult for clients to see their face.

Psychological Preparation of the Client. Nurses convey an open, receptive, and professional approach to clients to instill confidence and encourage their ease at being asked sensitive questions about body functions or being exposed and examined. Nurses provide an explanation in general terms so that clients know what to expect and then explain in more detail as they examine each body system or region. Clients may be anxious about loss of

Table 28-14 Common Terms of Movement

Movement	Description	Additional Information
Flexion	A bending movement that reduces the angle between parts	• Plantar flexion is a bending movement of the foot at the ankle posteriorly toward the floor ("plant" the foot down). • Dorsiflexion is a bending movement anteriorly (upward) of the foot at the ankle. • Lateral flexion of the spine is a movement (sideways) laterally away from the midline position in the coronal plane.
Extension	A movement that increases the angle between parts	• Extension is a movement in the coronal or sagittal planes. • Extension (straightening) of the knee or extension of the spine increases the angle in the sagittal plane.
Abduction	A movement that increases the angle between body parts	• Abduction is a movement away from the median plane. • Arms swing out and away from the body.
Adduction	A movement that decreases the angle between body parts	• Adduction is a movement toward the median plane. • Outstretched leg swings back beside the other leg.
Medial Rotation	Movement around the long axis of a body part toward the median	• The cervical spine rotates medially when the client turns his head to look directly forward or anteriorly.
Lateral rotation	Movement around the long axis of a body part away from the median	• When the client turns her head to look back, she is rotating the cervical spine laterally.
Internal rotation	A combination of movements of a ball-and-socket joint in an anterior direction	• When the client moves his hands to the small of his back, his shoulders rotate internally.
External rotation	A combination of movements of a ball-and-socket joint in a posterior direction	• When the client places her hands behind her head, elbows pointing out to the side, she is externally rotating her shoulders.
Eversion	Movement of the foot when the sole of the foot (plantar surface) is turned away from the median plane	• Soles of feet are everted when turned away from each other.
Inversion	Movement that involves the turning of the plantar surface of the foot (sole) toward the median plane	• Soles of feet are inverted when facing each other.
Supination	Lateral rotation of a structure around the long axis of the radius	• Think of supination as the position of the hand to carry a bowl of soup in the palm. • When the elbow is flexed at a right angle, the radius is in a lateral rotation around its long axis and the palm of the hand is turned upward.
Pronation	Medial rotation around the long axis of the radius	• The pronated palm of the hand faces downward; therefore, a bowl of soup would be dropped because it would be upside down.

Adapted from *A Primer on Physical Examination Techniques* [WebCT], by D. L. Skillen, 2004a, Edmonton, AB: Faculty of Nursing, University of Alberta.

privacy or about the possibility that the examiner will find something unexpected. Clear explanations in advance assist clients to relax and co-operate with the examination. The terminology that nurses use is in accordance with clients' level of understanding; they avoid confusing clients or increasing their fears. They use a calm tone of voice and relaxed facial expressions. When client and nurse are not the same gender, it may be necessary to have a third person of the client's gender in the room, especially when examination of the genitalia or breast is required. The third person acts as a witness to proper conduct and assures the client that the examiner will behave ethically.

Nurses observe clients' emotional responses throughout the examination. Clients may physically demonstrate fear or concern in their facial expressions, in tensing at the examiner's touch, or pulling up on the drape; some may verbalize their embarrassment or discomfort. Not all cultures in Canada will be verbal. Nurses must closely observe Inuit clients, for example, as some may only indicate discomfort with a wrinkled up nose. This also indicates "No" in contrast to "Yes" that is transmitted silently with raised eyebrows.

Examiners must remain calm, clearly explain each step of their assessment, and encourage clients to ask questions. If fears result from client misconceptions, nurses must clarify the purpose and procedure of the examination. They may decide to stop their examination and ask if the client feels anxious or uncomfortable. No client should be forced to continue. Postponement of the examination to a later date may help a client to be more relaxed and co-operative and findings to be more accurate.

Assessment According to Age Groups

Nurses adapt their interview styles and approaches to the chronological and developmental age of clients. Table 28-16 summarizes the focus by age for conducting the physical assessment of children, adolescents, and aging adults. Nurses use primary prevention with children who have competent parenting and no serious health problems. Foster children,

Table 28-15 Positions for Examination

Position	Areas Assessed	Rationale	Limitations
Sitting 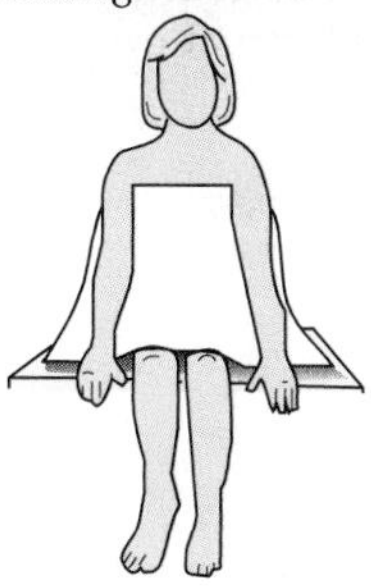	Head and neck, back, posterior thorax and lungs, anterior thorax and lungs, breasts, axillae, heart ,vital signs, and upper extremities	Sitting upright provides full expansion of lungs and provides better visualization of symmetry of upper body parts.	Physically weakened client may be unable to sit. Examiner should use supine position with head of bed elevated instead.
Supine 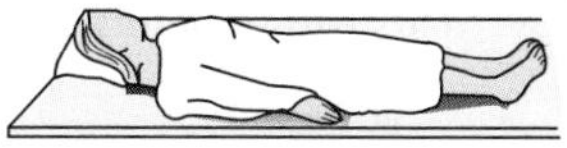	Head and neck, anterior thorax and lungs, breasts, axillae, heart, abdomen, extremities, pulses	This is most normally relaxed position. It provides easy access to pulse sites.	If client becomes short of breath easily, examiner may need to raise head of the bed.
Dorsal recumbent 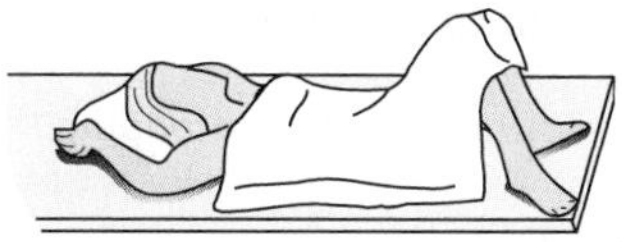	Head and neck, anterior thorax and lungs, breasts, axillae, heart, abdomen	Position is used for abdominal assessment because it promotes relaxation of abdominal muscles.	Clients with painful disorders are more comfortable with knees flexed.
Lithotomy* 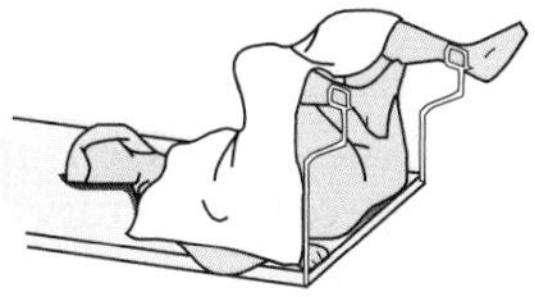	Female genitalia and genital tract	This position provides maximal exposure of genitalia and facilitates insertion of vaginal speculum.	Lithotomy position is embarrassing and uncomfortable; therefore, examiner minimizes time that client spends in it. Client is kept well draped.
Sims' 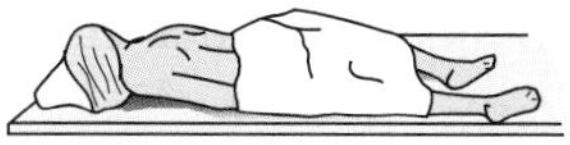	Rectum and vagina	Flexion of hip and knee improves exposure of rectal area.	Joint deformities may hinder client's ability to bend hip and knee.
Prone 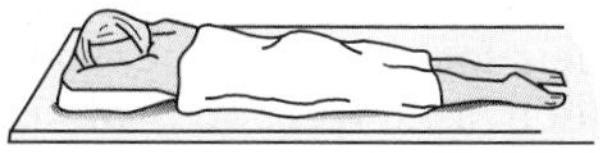	Musculoskeletal system	This position is used only to assess extension of hip joint.	This position is poorly tolerated in clients with respiratory difficulties.
Lateral recumbent 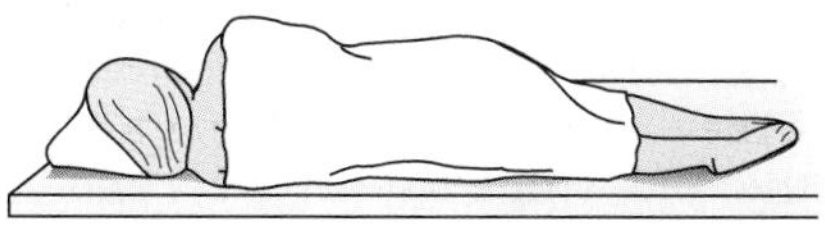	Heart	This position aids in detecting murmurs.	This position is poorly tolerated in clients with respiratory difficulties.
Knee-chest* 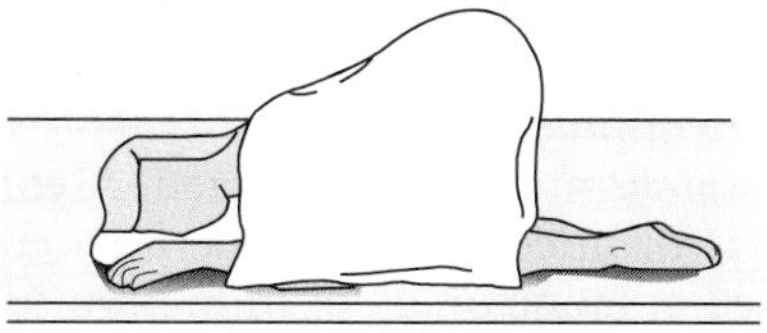	Rectum	This position provides maximal exposure of rectal area.	This position is embarrassing and uncomfortable.

*Clients with arthritis or other joint deformities may be unable to assume this position.

Table 28-16 Assessment of Three Age Groups

Age Group	Focus	Tips for Nurses
Children	Health promotion Illness prevention Growth and development Sensory screening Dental health Behaviour	Gather all or part of the history information from parents or guardians. Provide time for play to become acquainted, meeting children at own level. Perform the examination in a non-threatening area. Offer support to parents and do not pass judgment. Call children by first name; parents by Mr. and Mrs. Use open-ended questions. Observe parent-child interactions.
Adolescents	Confidentiality Counselling for transitions	Establish rapport. Treat as adult and individual. Respect right to privacy and confidentiality. Gather historical information from parent but speak to adolescent alone.
Older adults	Functional assessments • Activities of daily living • Complex instrumental activities Mental status Physical health and safety	Avoid stereotyping older adults. Consider space requirements for examination of clients with mobility aids (e.g., cane, walker). Be patient and allow for pauses. Recognize that clients who see illness as a threat to independence may withhold information. Perform examination near bathroom facilities in case of client urgency to void. Be alert to client fatigue: sighing, grimacing, irritability, head drooping, leaning on object. Avoid shouting; ensure client sees examiner's face.

children who are chronically ill or disabled, and children adopted from countries outside Canada are among those who may require additional examination visits. Adolescents may respond better to nurses who focus on them as individuals rather than on their problems; chatting informally and using more closed questions initially may assist examiners to develop rapport. Adolescents' behaviour is associated with their developmental stage and not necessarily their chronological age. Older adults may require data collection over more than one session because of sensory or physical limitations.

> ***Safety Alert:*** Examiners must remember that aging human bodies do not always respond vigorously to injury or disease and may not display the signs and symptoms expected.

Nurses conduct **screening** (shortened assessments to detect deviations) with clients according to age groups and known risk factors (Table 28-17).

Environment Preparation

The physical environment for client examination may include a northern health centre, examination room in a physician's office, hospital inpatient room, emergency room, or a stretcher in a corridor. It could also be the home of a neighbour, a public health clinic room, bedroom of a home health care client, room of a resident in a continuing care lodge, summer cottage, boat, path, or car. The need for a physical examination cannot always be anticipated. Under the Canadian Nurses Association *Code of Ethics for Registered Nurses* (2002), nurses provide initial assessment and emergency care wherever needed. Regardless of the setting where a physical examination must take place, nurses ensure privacy to the extent possible and respect the dignity of the individual. They use room curtains, dividers, and sheets or blankets held up by assistants to provide some element of visual privacy.

Ideally, the environment is soundproof so that clients feel comfortable discussing their concerns. At minimum, nurses speak in a soft voice if clients are not hearing impaired. They consider the hard-of-hearing client whose privacy is jeopardized by a raised voice and choose their questions and comments carefully. They ensure that clients can see their face as they speak and eliminate sources of noise such as televisions, radios, and telephone conversations by closing a door or turning off the source.

Nurses consider client comfort when noting the temperature of the environment and adapting their examination accordingly. They may decide to drape a client who is sensitive to the cold with a flannel sheet and uncover only small areas at a time.

Adequate lighting is required for proper illumination of body parts or regions. Primary lighting can be either daylight or artificial if the light is direct enough to reveal skin colour without distortion from shadows.

At all times, client safety must be considered. A confused, weak, combative, or unco-operative client should not be left unsupervised or alone on an examination surface above floor level. Wherever an examination is conducted, nurses assist clients to move without risk of falling or injury. To prevent an ergonomic hazard and ensure safe access to clients on a stretcher, bed, or wide surface, nurses position clients closer to them.

Table 28-17 Recommended Preventive Screenings

Disease or Condition	Age Group in Years	Screening Measures
Breast cancer	20 to 39	• Familiarity with how breasts look and feel through regular self-examination • Ability to recognize monthly breast changes • Annual physical exam by physician, nurse practitioner, or other health professional • Awareness of risk factors for breast cancer and early detection guidelines for all age groups
	40 to 49	• Clinical breast exam by a trained health professional at least every 2 years • Regular breast self-examination • Discussion of risk for breast cancer and the risks and benefits of mammography with physician
	50 to 69	• Mammography every 2 years between the ages of 50 and 69 (women) • Clinical breast examination by a trained health professional at least every 2 years • Regular breast self-examination and report of any changes to physician.
	70 and over	• Talking to physician about a screening program • Clinical breast examination by a trained professional at least every 2 years • Regular breast self-examination and report of any changes to physician
Colorectal cancer	50 and over	• Fecal occult blood test (FOBT) at least every 2 years • FOBT blood testing helps identify polyps early before they become cancerous
Ear disorders	All ages	• Periodic hearing checks as needed
	Over age 65	• Regular hearing checks
Eye disorders	40 and under	• Complete eye examination every 3 to 5 years (more if positive history)
	40 to 64	• Complete eye examination every 2 years
	65 and up	• Complete eye examination every year
Heart and vascular disorders	Men 45 to 65, Women 45 to 65	• Regular measurement of total blood cholesterol levels and triglycerides; blood pressure screenings
Obesity	All ages	• Periodic height and weight measurements.
Oral cavity and cancer of pharynx	All ages	• Regular dental examinations every 6 months
Ovarian cancer	18 and over, or on becoming sexually active	• Annual pelvic examination by health care professional
Prostate cancer	50 and over	• Digital rectal examination (DRE): DRE is a physical examination in which a physician or nurse practitioner palpates the prostate by inserting a finger in the rectum. • Prostate-specific antigen (PSA): The PSA test measures the level of a protein, the prostate-specific antigen in the blood. • Men at higher risk because of family history or African ancestry should discuss the need for testing at an earlier age.
Skin cancer	All ages	• Learning what to look for and checking skin regularly, as most skin cancers can be cured if caught early enough • Making sure to check or have checked "hard-to-get-at" places such as the back, back of neck and ears, and backs of legs
Testicular cancer	15 and over	• Testicular self-examination (TSE), performed regularly, informs what is usual for testicles and detects any changes.
Uterine cancer	18 and up, or on becoming sexually active	• Annual pelvic examination by health care professional plus an annual Pap test
Cervical cancer	Women on becoming sexually active; continue even if sexual activities stop	• Pap test and pelvic examination every 1 to 3 years depending on provincial screening guidelines
Endometrial cancer	18 and up, or on becoming sexually active	• Endometrial biopsy at age 35 for high-risk clients. • At menopause, women at average and high risk are informed of high risks and the signs and symptoms to report.

From Canadian Cancer Society (2004) and American Cancer Society (2003).

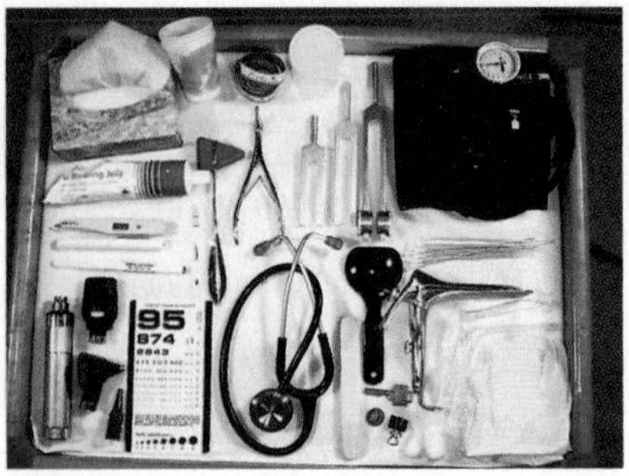

FIGURE **28–10** Equipment and supplies used during a physical examination. (From *Physical Examination Images* [CD-ROM], by D. L. Skillen, R. A. Day, M. C. Anderson, T. C. Stephen, J. A. Gilbert, and L. W. Day, 2004, Edmonton, AB: Faculty of Nursing, University of Alberta.)

After performing hand hygiene, nurses assemble all of the necessary equipment for the examination. Equipment should be clean or sterile, as required, readily available, functioning properly, and arranged in order for easy use. Replacement bulbs and batteries should be available for equipment such as the otoscope or ophthalmoscope. Equipment should be warm as appropriate. For example, nurses run warm water over a vaginal speculum before insertion. They rub the diaphragm of the stethoscope briskly between their hands before applying it directly to skin. They rub their own hands together briskly or run them under warm water before placing otherwise cold hands on the client.

Whether preparing a tray, cart, table, countertop, or portable nurse's bag with equipment for assessment outside a health care facility, nurses consider all possible equipment needs for their particular setting in terms of efficiency or prompt attention in an urgent situation (Figure 28–10). In northern, rural, or remote areas of Canada, they carry additional equipment for initiating client care or preparing for client transport to a health care facility. This equipment includes, at minimum, oxygen, fracture immobilization, cervical collars, backboards, delivery packs, and medications.

Nurse Preparation

For satisfactory physical assessment of clients, nurses require the appropriate knowledge, skills, and attitudes. Regardless of adult client age, a basic physical examination follows a similar approach. Nurses must know how to conduct a complete physical examination to be able to select the techniques and skills according to the needs and circumstances of the client. After mastery of the techniques and skills, the challenge for nurses is to focus the examination when indicated and interpret the findings in light of client age (including developmental stage), gender, biology, and occupation.

Nurses use their judgment and experience to ensure that an examination is relevant but focused according to the circumstances. For example, a client who arrives at a clinic with symptoms of a severe chest cold will not routinely require a neurological assessment. A client who enters the emergency room with an acute illness requires an assessment of the body systems most likely involved. In contrast, when a client is admitted to hospital, a complete physical examination is usually performed. Nurse practitioners may routinely conduct complete examinations upon admission. Clients who approach examiners about specific symptoms, signs, or needs will often require only a focused examination. Nurses dedicated to client health promotion and illness prevention may include specific screening examinations, depending on the client's age or health risk. In evidence-based practice, nurses remain current on the screening measures, procedures, and age groups considered at risk in order to detect client problems as early as possible (see Table 28-17).

The Registered Nurses Association of Ontario is one example of a Canadian professional nursing association that has introduced guidelines for best practice, which are developed from evidence-based nursing research (see *http://www.rnao.org/bestpractices/*).

For safety and comfort, nurses consider the hazards to which they and their clients might be exposed during the physical examination. Occupational and environmental hazards create biological, chemical, ergonomic, physical, and psychosocial risks (Skillen, 1996). Canadian nurses must be aware of their provincial regulations with respect to protection of themselves and their clients, and promotion of health, safety, and wellness. For example, standard precautions/routine practices are required to protect examiners and clients against contact with blood, body fluids, and body substances that can transmit infectious agents. Although individuals with open skin lesions or draining wounds are quickly identified, standard precautions/routine practices should always be used throughout an examination. Depending on the situation, masks and safety glasses may be needed in addition to gloves and gown (see chapter 29). Before initiating a physical examination, nurses perform hand hygiene, introduce themselves, explain what they are going to do, and take steps to promote client comfort.

In the following sections, the criteria, techniques, skills, and sequencing for the entire head-to-toe physical examination are presented. Assessment of mental and emotional status, a component of the examination of the central nervous system (CNS), may be integrated with the health history interview. The brain (brainstem, diencephalon, cerebrum, and cerebellum) and the spinal cord (cervical, thoracic, lumbar, sacral, and coccygeal segments) form the CNS. Mental status cannot be assessed from a physical examination and is inferred from client behaviours and responses to questioning. Because behaviours and responses are evident early in the encounter with the nurse, the mental and emotional status assessment is presented next.

Assessing Mental and Emotional Status

Much can be learned about mental capacity and emotional state by simply interacting with the client, especially during the history. The nurse asks questions throughout the examination, and observes the appropriateness of the client's affective response and ideas. Special

Box 28-15 Mini-Mental State Examination Sample Questions

Orientation to time
"What is the date?"
Registration
"Listen carefully. I am going to say three words. You say them back after I stop.
Ready? Here they are . . .
HOUSE (pause), CAR (pause), LAKE (pause). Now repeat those words back to me."
[Repeat up to 5 times, but score only the first trial.]
Naming
"What is this?" [Point to a pencil or pen.]
Reading
"Please read this and do what it says." [Show examinee the words on the stimulus form.]
CLOSE YOUR EYES

Box 28-16 Clinical Criteria for Delirium

Definition: An acute disturbance of consciousness that is accompanied by a change in cognition. It cannot be accounted for by a pre-existing or evolving dementia. Delirium develops over a short period of time, usually hours to days, and tends to fluctuate during the course of the day. It is usually a direct physiological consequence of a general medical condition.
There is reduced clarity of awareness of the environment.
Ability to focus, sustain, or shift attention is impaired (questions must be repeated).
Person is easily distracted by irrelevant stimuli.
There is an accompanying change in cognition (memory impairment, disorientation, or language disturbance).
Recent memory is most commonly affected.
Disorientation is usually shown, with client disoriented to time or place.
Language disturbance may involve impaired ability to name objects or ability to write; speech may be rambling.
Perceptual disturbances may include misinterpretation, illusions, or hallucinations.

Adapted from *Diagnostic and Statistical Manual of Mental Disorders* (4th ed. Rev.), American Psychiatric Association, 2000, Washington, DC: Author; and *Principles and Practice of Psychiatric Nursing* (7th ed.), by G. Stuart and M. Laraia, 2001, St. Louis, MO: Mosby.

assessment tools are available to screen a client's current **mental status.** Kahn and Goldfarb's mental status questionnaire (MSQ; 1960) is a widely used 10-item instrument (Kahn et al., 1960). Folstein, Folstein, and McHugh (1975) developed the Mini-Mental State Exam (MMSE) to assess orientation and cognitive function in older adults. Box 28-15 presents sample questions from the examination. A maximum score on the MMSE is 30. When a client has a score of 25 or less, the score is suggestive of delirium, dementia, or possible depression, and the client requires further evaluation (Kennedy-Malone, Fletcher, & Plank, 2000).

To ensure an objective assessment, the nurse considers the client's values, beliefs, cultural and educational background, and previous experiences. Such factors influence client response to questions. Alterations in mental or emotional status may reflect a disturbance in cerebral functioning. The cerebral cortex controls and integrates emotional and intellectual functioning. Primary brain disorders, medication, and metabolic changes are examples of factors that may change cerebral function.

A common mental disorder affecting older adults is **delirium,** an acute confusional disorder characterized by changing levels of disorientation, consciousness, and sleep-wake cycle. Delirium is often caused by infection, dehydration, surgical procedure, or adverse medication effects and is amenable to treatment. This acute condition is often misdiagnosed as a form of dementia such as Alzheimer's disease. If the client already has a dementia (organic loss of intellectual function), symptoms of delirium may go untreated if attributed to the dementia. When delirium occurs, nurses may think it is common older adult behaviour. Fortunately, when correctly assessed, the condition can be reversed with treatment of the underlying cause—CNS, metabolic, and cardiopulmonary disorders; systemic illnesses; and sensory deprivation or overload (Stuart & Laraia, 2001). To recognize delirium early, nurses should obtain a full history of the client's behaviour before it develops. Box 28-16 contains criteria for delirium.

Level of Consciousness

The level of consciousness exists along a continuum from full awakening, alertness, and co-operation to unresponsiveness to any form of external stimuli. A fully conscious client responds to questions spontaneously. As consciousness lowers, a client may show irritability, a shortened attention span, or unwillingness to co-operate. To avoid ambiguity in assessment of the level of consciousness, the Glasgow Coma Scale (GCS) measures consciousness by an objective numerical scale in three domains: spontaneity of eye opening, best verbal response, and best motor response (Table 28-18). Caution is needed in using the scale with clients who have sensory losses (e.g., vision or hearing) or motor paralysis. As consciousness deteriorates, clients become disoriented to name, time, and place. Nurses ask short, to-the-point questions regarding information that the client knows (e.g., "Tell me your name," "What's the name of this place?" and "What day is this?"). The client's ability to understand and answer questions has a direct effect on the nurse's ability to perform a complete examination. The client must be aroused to full alertness before a history can be taken.

Table 28-18 Glasgow Coma Scale

Action	Response	Score
Eyes open	Spontaneously	4
	To speech	3
	To pain	2
	None	1
Best verbal response	Oriented	5
	Confused	4
	Inappropriate words	3
	Incomprehensible sounds	2
	None	1
Best motor response	Obeys commands	6
	Localized pain	5
	Flexion withdrawal	4
	Abnormal flexion	3
	Abnormal extension	2
	Flaccid	1
	TOTAL SCORE	15

A client may be unable to follow simple commands, such as "Squeeze my finger" or "Move your toes." As level of consciousness declines, the client may become responsive only to painful stimuli. The nurse tests for response to pain by applying firm pressure with the thumb over the root of the fingernail. The client should withdraw the hand from the painful stimulus, but a client with serious neurological impairment exhibits abnormal posturing in response to pain. A flaccid response indicates the absence of muscle tone in the extremities and severe injury to brain tissue.

The GCS allows the nurse to evaluate a client's neurological status over time. The client who is oriented and able to respond to commands would score a full 15 points. A client unresponsive to pain, who fails to open eyes or move in any way to stimulation, would score 3 points. A client with a score of 8 points or less is in a coma. Nurses record findings and observe for trends.

Behaviour and Appearance

Behaviour, moods, hygiene, grooming, and choice of dress reveal relevant information about mental status. The nurse must be aware of mannerisms and actions during the entire assessment, noting non-verbal and verbal behaviour. Does the client respond appropriately to directions? Does the client's mood vary with no apparent cause? Does the client show concern about appearance? Is the client's hair clean and neatly groomed, and are the nails trimmed and clean? The client is expected to behave in a manner expressing alertness to the examination. Nurses remember that making eye contact and expressing feelings that correspond to the situation are culturally bound.

Choice and fit of clothing may reflect socio-economic background or personal taste rather than deficiency in self-concept or self-care. The nurse avoids being judgmental and focuses assessment on the appropriateness of clothing for the weather. Older adults may neglect their appearance because of a lack of energy, finances, or reduced vision.

Language

An individual's ability to understand spoken or written words and to express the self with writing, words, or gestures is a function of the cerebral cortex. The nurse assesses the client's voice inflection, tone, and manner of speech. The voice should have inflections, be clear and strong, and increase in volume appropriately. Speech should be fluent. Rate of speech, content, and use of words are appropriate to the situation. When communication is clearly ineffective (e.g., omission or addition of letters and words, misuse of words, or hesitations), the nurse assesses for aphasia caused by an injury to the cerebral cortex. Aphasia is the loss of the ability to understand or express speech. Language capabilities can be assessed by the following simple techniques:

- Ask the client to name a familiar object to which the nurse points (naming).
- Ask the client to respond to simple verbal and written commands, such as "Stand up" or "Sit down" (word comprehension).
- Ask the client to read simple sentences out loud (reading comprehension)

Expect the client to correctly name objects, to follow commands, and to read sentences correctly. Allow extra time for older adults to respond, as processing information may be slowed.

Intellectual Function

Intellectual function includes memory (recent, immediate, and past), knowledge, abstract thinking, association, and judgment. Each aspect of intellectual function is tested with a specific technique. However, culture and education influence the ability to respond to test questions. The nurse should not ask questions related to concepts or ideas with which the client is unfamiliar. Before beginning the tests, nurses ask permission of the client.

Memory. The nurse assesses immediate recall and recent and remote memory. Often a problem with memory becomes apparent when taking the health history. To assess immediate recall, the nurse has the client repeat a series of numbers (e.g., *7, 4, 1*) in the order they are presented or in reverse order. The nurse gradually increases the number of digits (e.g., *7, 4, 1, 8, 6*) until the client fails to repeat the digits correctly. Expect digit span to be five to eight digits forward and four to six digits backward.

To test recent memory, the nurse says clearly and slowly the name of three unrelated objects (MMSE, see Box 28-15). After the nurse says all three, the client is asked to repeat each. This is continued until the client is successful. Later in the assessment, the nurse asks the client to repeat the three words again; the client should be able to repeat them. Another test is to ask the client to recall events of the same day (e.g., what was eaten for breakfast). Information may need to be validated with a family member.

To assess past memory, it is best to ask open-ended questions such as the mother's maiden name, a birthday, or a special date in history. A client should have immediate recall of such information. With older adults, a nurse determines if the client has a hearing loss before attributing failure of recall to confusion. The ability to retrieve stored memories should remain intact. Nurses use effective communication techniques throughout the examination to ensure clients' clear understanding of directions.

Knowledge. The nurse can assess knowledge by asking what clients know about their illnesses or the reason for seeking health care. By assessing knowledge, the nurse determines clients' abilities to learn or understand. If an opportunity to teach exists, the nurse can test understanding by asking for feedback during a follow-up visit. Although older adults can learn new tasks, they need more time to do so.

Abstract Thinking. Interpreting abstract ideas or concepts reflects a capacity for abstract thinking. A higher level of intellectual functioning is required for individuals to explain phrases such as "A stitch in time saves nine" or "Don't count your chickens before they're hatched." The nurse notes whether explanations are relevant and concrete. The client with altered mentation will likely interpret the phrase literally or merely rephrase the words. Older adults should be able to complete this task successfully.

Association. Another higher level of intellectual functioning involves identifying similarities or associations between concepts: A dog is to a beagle as a cat is to a Siamese. Alternately, nurses ask what is similar between an apple and a pear, expecting a response such as "They are both fruits." Questions should be appropriate to clients' level of intelligence and cultural background. It is sufficient to use simple concepts. Older adults are expected to successfully complete this task.

Judgment. Judgment requires a comparison and evaluation of facts and ideas to understand their relationships and to form appropriate conclusions. The nurse attempts to measure the ability to make logical decisions. By assessing judgment, the nurse also measures the ability to organize thought processes. The nurse may choose to ask clients why they decided to seek health care or how they plan to adjust to limitations after returning home. A simpler test would involve asking what clients would do if locked out of their homes or becoming ill suddenly when alone at home. Clients are expected to provide an answer that is logical and a realistic solution to the problem. If not, their safety may be an issue. Cognitively intact adults of all ages should be able to perform this task.

Assessing Cranial Nerve Function

Twelve paired cranial nerves are part of the peripheral nervous system that also includes the spinal and peripheral nerves. Cranial nerve function is assessed when the peripheral nervous system is examined or when measures are used to assess the integrity of structures in the head and neck.

Nurses may test a single cranial nerve, assess a related group of cranial nerves, or examine all 12 cranial nerves at one time. For example, a test of the oculomotor nerve measures pupillary response to light. Assessment of the vagus and glossopharyngeal nerves reveals integrity of the gag reflex. The cochlear branch of the eighth cranial nerve is tested during the hearing examination and the function of the ninth and tenth nerves is assessed during examination of the pharynx. Dysfunction in any cranial nerve reflects an alteration at some point along its distribution. Assessment of cranial nerves is easy after nurses are familiar with the nerve functions. Nursing students can use a simple mnemonic (memory aid), "On old Olympus' towering tops, a Finn and German viewed some hops" to remember the order of the 12 pairs of nerves. The first letter of each word in the phrase is the same as the first letter of the names of the cranial nerves (Table 28-19). Eight cranial nerves have either sensory or motor functions; four have both sensory and motor functions. Nurses know the functions of the cranial nerves before they examine the head and neck when each cranial nerve is tested.

Assessing Sensory and Motor Function

Sensory Function

Nurses need to distinguish between the sensory and motor functions of the nervous system before examining the head and neck, torso, or extremities. Sensory pathways of the CNS conduct sensations of pain, temperature, position, vibration, crude touch, and fine touch. Different nerve pathways relay the sensations. Most of the peripheral nerves have sensory and motor fibres. For most clients, screening of sensory function is sufficient unless the client reports symptoms of reduced sensation, motor impairment, or paralysis. Screening is conducted throughout the physical examination.

> ***Safety Alert:*** When a client has impaired sensation, the risk of skin breakdown is greater. If decreased sensation is identified, it is important that nurses do a complete skin and tissue assessment of the area affected by the sensory loss. They teach clients to avoid pressure, thermal, and/or chemical trauma to the affected area.

Usually a client has sensory responses to all stimuli that are tested. Sensations along the surface of the body are felt equally on both sides of the face, trunk, and extremities. A nurse can assess the major sensory nerves by knowing the sensory dermatomes (Figure 28–11). Some areas of the skin are innervated by specific dorsal root cutaneous nerves. For example, if the nurse notes reduced sensation when checking for light touch in an area of the skin such as the lower neck, the nurse can determine that a lesion of the fourth cervical spinal cord segment may exist.

All sensory testing is performed with the eyes closed so that the client is unable to see when or where the nurse uses a stimulus. Stimuli are applied in a random, unpredictable order to maintain the client's attention

Table 28-19 Cranial Nerve Function and Assessment

Number	Name	Type	Function	Method
I	Olfactory	Sensory	Sense of smell	Ask client to identify different non-irritating aromas such as coffee and vanilla.
II	Optic	Sensory	Visual acuity	Use Snellen chart or ask client to read printed material while wearing glasses.
III	Oculomotor	Motor	Extraocular eye movement	Assess directions of gaze.
			Pupil constriction and dilation	Measure pupillary reaction to light reflex and accommodation.
IV	Trochlear	Motor	Upward and downward movement of eyeball	Assess directions of gaze.
V	Trigeminal	Sensory and motor	Sensory nerve to skin of face	Lightly touch cornea with wisp of cotton. Assess corneal reflex. Measure sensation of light pain and touch across skin of face.
			Motor nerve to muscles of jaw	Palpate temples as client clenches teeth.
VI	Abducens	Motor	Lateral movement of eyeballs	Assess directions of gaze.
VII	Facial	Sensory and motor	Facial expression	As client smiles, frowns, puffs out cheeks, and raises and lowers eyebrows, look for asymmetry.
			Taste	Have client identify salty or sweet taste on front of tongue.
VIII	Auditory	Sensory	Hearing	Assess ability to hear spoken word.
IX	Glossopharyngeal	Sensory and motor	Taste	Ask client to identify sour or sweet taste on back of tongue.
			Ability to swallow	Use tongue blade to elicit gag reflex.
X	Vagus	Sensory and motor	Sensation of pharynx	Ask client to say "ah." Observe movement of palate and pharynx.
			Movement of vocal chords	Assess speech for hoarseness.
XI	Spinal accessory	Motor	Movement of head and shoulders	Ask client to shrug shoulders and turn head against passive resistance.
XII	Hypoglossal	Motor	Position of tongue	Ask client to stick out tongue to midline and move it from side to side.

and prevent client detection of a predictable pattern. Nurses ask the client to indicate when and where each stimulus is felt, and what it is. While applying stimuli to the client's face, arms, torso, and legs, they compare results for symmetrical areas. Relevant details for testing sensory function are provided in each section of the physical examination.

Motor Function

Motor pathways of the CNS consist of upper and lower motor neurons and their synapses. Higher motor neurons affect movement through lower motor neurons. Three primary motor pathways mediate muscle tone, posture, muscular activity, reflex activity, balance, coordination, gait, and equilibrium. These pathways are the cerebellar system, corticospinal tract, and basal ganglia system. Assessment of central and peripheral nervous system motor function occurs primarily during examination of the extremities, and to a lesser extent during examination of the head and neck or torso. Relevant details for testing motor function are provided in each section.

Assessing the Integumentary System

The **integument** includes the skin, hair, scalp, nails, sebaceous glands, and sweat glands (apocrine and eccrine). Inspection (including olfaction) and palpation are used to assess the function and integrity of the integumentary system.

Skin

Assessment of the skin reveals a variety of conditions, including changes in circulation, hydration, integrity of tissues, nutrition, and oxygenation. The skin (epidermis, dermis, and subcutaneous tissues) provides the body's external protection, regulates body temperature, synthesizes vitamin D, excretes some metabolic wastes (e.g., sugars, uric acid, urea), absorbs certain chemicals, and acts as a sensory organ for pain, temperature, pressure, and touch.

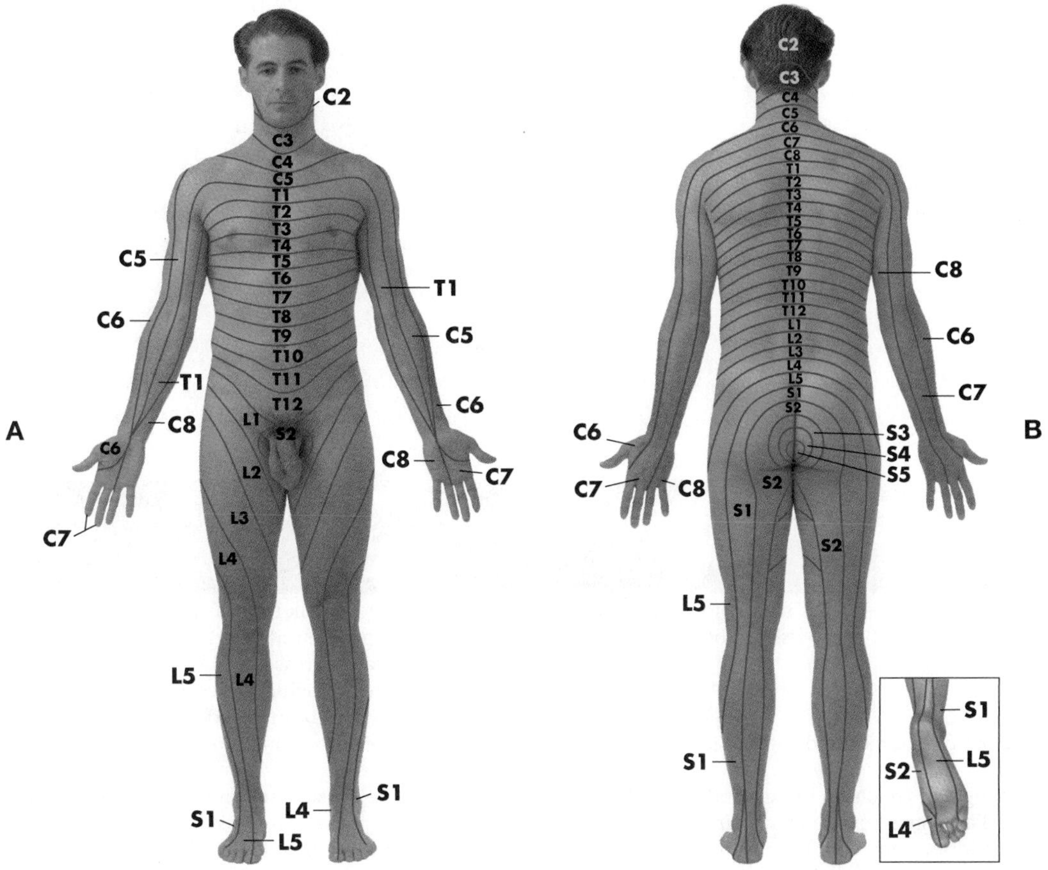

FIGURE **28–11** Dermatomes of the body, the body surface areas innervated by particular spinal nerves; C1 usually has no cutaneous distribution. **A,** Anterior view. **B,** Posterior view. It only appears that there is a distinct separation of surface area controlled by each dermatome; there is almost always overlap between spinal nerves. (From *Mosby's Guide to Physical Examination,* 5th ed., p. 775, by H. M. Seidel et al., 2003, St. Louis, MO: Mosby.)

Safety Alert: The ability of the skin to absorb certain chemicals creates risks for clients who are exposed to chemicals in their work, studies, hobbies, or recreation. Nurses inquire about exposures when conducting a health history. Protective functions of the skin become impaired with compromised mobility, circulation, nutrition, and hydration. Friction and moisture increase the risk of skin breakdown in bedridden clients who are already compromised. Nurses consider the effects when providing nursing care.

Figure 28–12 presents a cross-section of the skin. The thin, avascular epidermis is divided into two layers: the basal cell layer where melanin and keratin are formed, and the outer horny cell layer where dead keratinized cells are shed. The underlying dermis supplies its nutrition. Connective and elastic tissue predominate in the dermis where blood vessels, nerves, lymphatics, hair follicles, sebaceous glands, and sweat glands are located. Except for the skin on the palms and soles, all skin has sebaceous glands. Widely distributed in the skin, the eccrine sweat glands open directly onto skin surfaces to help control body temperature. The apocrine sweat glands mainly open into hair follicles in the axillae and genital area, are stimulated by stress, and produce body odour. The subcutaneous layer is composed of adipose tissue, which contributes to skin mobility.

During the health history (see chapter 12), nurses use open-ended questions to inquire about the skin (e.g., colour, pigmentation, rashes, **lesions,** itching, bruising, dryness, moisture), hair (e.g., loss, dryness, oiliness), nails (e.g., brittleness, colour, shape), changes in known lesions, workplace and lifestyle exposures to chemicals, and previous history of skin disease (including familial predisposition, allergies). Table 28-20 presents the health history for skin assessment.

Nurses have an important role in counselling clients about protecting their skin and avoiding harmful exposures (Box 28-17). See the Slip! Slap! Slop! message that originated in Australia at *www.mydr.com.au/default.asp?article=2570.* Nurses ensure that clients are informed about thorough self-examination of the skin (Box 28-18).

Cutaneous malignancies are the most commonly identified neoplasms (Figure 28–13, *A–C*). Approximately 4,200 new cases of **melanoma,** an aggressive form of skin cancer, may be diagnosed in 2004 (Canadian Cancer

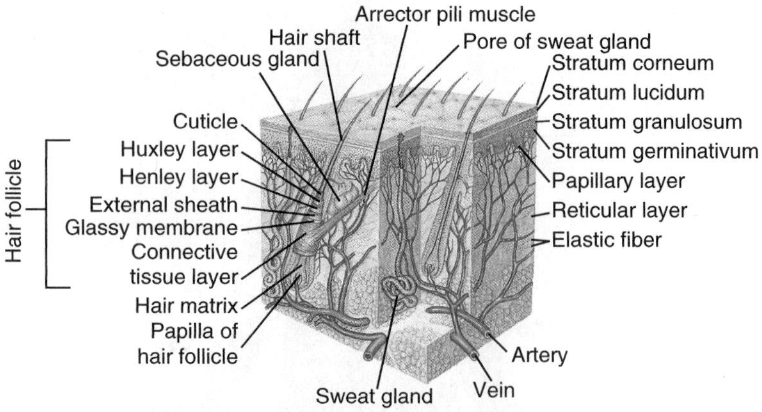

FIGURE **28–12** Cross-section of skin. (From *Mosby's Guide to Physical Examination,* 5th ed., p. 164, Figure 7-1, by H. M. Seidel et al., 2003, St. Louis, MO: Mosby.)

Table 28-20 Health History for Skin Assessment

Assessment Category	Rationale
Question client as to knowledge of risk factors for skin cancer and question client on presence of those risk factors.	Knowledge of risk factors, such as skin tones, sun exposure, exposure to hazardous toxins, and sunburns early in life can increase level of self-care and reduce risk of skin cancer, including reduction of time spent outdoors and in tanning booths.
Inquire about number of and nature of skin lesions, moles, and freckles.	Presence of more than 40 moles increases risk of skin cancer.
Ask client about changes in condition of skin and ask when last skin self-assessment and assessment by an examiner were conducted.	Regular self-assessment and clinical examination of skin ensures proper care of skin.
Inquire about use of lotions and creams on skin surfaces and regular hygiene practices.	Good hygiene practices and use of appropriate lotions can ensure proper skin care
Ask client about presence of allergies.	Skin rashes commonly occur related to allergic response.
Question client on use of hats, sunglasses, protective lotions, and long-sleeved clothing during times of sun exposure.	Protecting skin surfaces is the best prevention of skin cancer.
Inquire about skin exposure to chemical substances in work, study, hobbies, and recreation.	Skin absorption of toxic chemicals contributes to organic or systemic conditions and malignancies.

Society [CCS], 2004a). In addition, 76,000 new cases of the highly curable non-melanoma (basal cell and squamous cell) cancers will be seen (CCS, 2004a). Basal cell carcinomas frequently occur in sun-damaged skin.

In hospital settings, the majority of clients are older, debilitated, or young but seriously ill. Consequently, significant risks for skin lesions result from trauma to the skin during bedside care, exposure to pressure during immobilization, or reaction to treatment medications. Individuals most at risk are chronically ill, neurologically impaired, orthopedic clients, or clients with diminished mental status, poor tissue oxygenation, low cardiac output, or inadequate nutrition. In long-term care facilities, clients may be at risk for similar problems related to their level of mobility and multiple chronic illnesses.

Nurses must routinely assess the skin for early indications of change or development of lesions. **Primary lesions** can quickly deteriorate to become **secondary lesions** that require more extensive nursing care. The development of a pressure ulcer, for example, can lengthen a hospital stay unless it is prevented or discovered early and treated properly (see chapter 43). The condition of the client's skin reveals the need for nursing care. The nurse uses assessment findings to select the hygiene measures required to maintain integrity of the integument (see chapter 34). Adequate nutrition and hydration become goals of therapy if the nurse identifies alterations in the integument (see chapter 39).

Inspection of Skin. Nurses use inspection to observe colour, hygiene (including odours), and lesions. Although nurses observe each part of the body during an examination, it helps when they make a brief but careful visual sweep of the entire body. This informs them of the distribution and extent of any lesions, as well as the overall symmetry of skin colour. Because the nurse inspects all skin surfaces, the client must assume several positions.

Colour. For accurate inspection of skin colour and identification of the type, colour, configuration, and distribution of skin lesions, adequate illumination is required. Diffuse natural lighting or halogen lighting is preferable (Bennett, 1995). For detecting skin changes in dark-skinned clients, sunlight is best (Talbot & Curtis, 1996). Despite individual variations, skin colour is usually uniform over the body, although ambient temperature

Client Teaching Box 28-17

Health Promotion for Skin Assessment

Objectives

- Client will perform a monthly self-examination of the skin.
- Client will identify factors that increase the risk of skin cancer.
- Client will follow hygiene practices that promote maintenance of healthy skin.

Teaching Strategies

- Instruct client how to conduct a monthly self-examination of all skin surfaces, particularly noting moles and lesions.
- Inform client of the recognition of melanoma by following rule set out by the Canadian Dermatology Association (ABCDE): A–asymmetry: one half different from the other half; B–borders: irregular; C–colour: more than one colour (tan, brown, black, white, red, or blue); D–diameter: larger than 6 mm (diameter of a pencil eraser); E–elevation: raised to palpation.
- Encourage client to report any changes in skin lesions to family physician.
- Inform client about health promotion techniques to protect skin: Avoid exposure to sun, particularly between the hours of 10 AM and 3 PM (11 AM to 4 PM in northern Canadian regions), wear sun screen (SPF of 15 or greater), cover all skin surfaces with lightweight clothing, wear a wide-brimmed hat and sunglasses, and avoid use of tanning booths and sun lamps.
- Inform client that medications such as oral contraceptives, antibiotics, immunosuppressive agents, anti-inflammatories and anti-hypertensives can make the skin more sensitive to the sun.
- Instruct client to report any lesion that bleeds or fails to heal to a nurse or physician.
- For treatment of excessively dry skin, inform client to avoid hot water, harsh soaps, and drying agents such as rubbing alcohol. Use a mild soap and pat, rather than rub, the skin after bathing.

Evaluation

- Ask client to demonstrate how skin self-examination is performed at home.
- Have client describe danger signs for melanoma.
- Have client describe health promotion techniques to ensure healthy skin.

Adapted from *A Syllabus for Adult Health Assessment,* edited by D. L. Skillen and R. A. Day (pp. 76–77), 2004, Edmonton, AB: Faculty of Nursing, University of Alberta.

may affect findings. A warm environment may cause superficial vasodilation, resulting in increased redness of the skin. A cool environment may cause sensitive clients to develop **cyanosis** (bluish discolouration) around the lips and nail beds (Talbot & Curtis, 1996). Skin pigmentation ranges in tone from ivory or light pink to ruddy pink in light skin and from light to deep brown or olive in dark skin. Pigmentation from melanin is more pronounced in sun-exposed areas. While inspecting the skin, the nurse is aware that cosmetics or tanning agents may mask colour. Table 28-21 lists colour variations, underlying causes, and the assessment focus.

It is more difficult to note changes such as pallor or cyanosis in clients with dark skin. Usually colour hues are best seen in the palms, soles, lips, tongue, hard palate, earlobes, and nail beds where pigmentation is less. Skin creases and folds are darker than the rest of the body in the dark-skinned client. Nurses observe for loss of the underlying red tones in darker skin and remember that melanin in the lips may be mistaken for cyanosis. In the dark-skinned client, erythema is not easily observed; therefore, the nurse must use palpation after inspection to detect heat and warmth (e.g., presence of skin inflammation; Talbot & Curtis, 1996). Findings should be verified with clinical manifestations.

Odours. Using the sense of smell during inspection, the nurse may note generalized body odour; odour in the **intertriginous** (skin fold) areas such as the axillae, groin, or under breasts; or odour in a particular body area (see Table 28-2).

Box 28-18 Client Instructions for Skin Self-Examination

Always use a good light, positioned to minimize distracting glare.

Be aware of the locations and appearance of moles and birthmarks.

Examine your back and other hard-to-see areas of the body using full-length and hand-held mirrors. Ask a friend or relative to help inspect those areas that are difficult to see, such as the scalp and back.

Begin with your face and scalp and proceed downward, examining your head, neck, shoulders, back, chest, arms, legs, and so on. Concentrate especially on areas where dysplastic nevi (those with unexpected changes) are most common—the shoulders and back—and areas where ordinary moles are rarely found—the scalp, breast, and buttocks. Check the soles of your feet and between the toes.

See rather than feel any early signs of mole change. Compare photographs of your moles (if you have them) with the appearance of those same moles on self-examination. Monitor change in size by measuring. It can be simply done with a small ruler or even by comparing them to the size of your thumb and fingernail.

Consult your physician promptly if any pigmented skin spots look like melanoma, if new moles have appeared, or if any existing moles have changed.

From *Mosby's Guide to Physical Examination* (5th ed., p. 169), by H. M. Seidel et al., 2003, St. Louis, MO: Mosby.

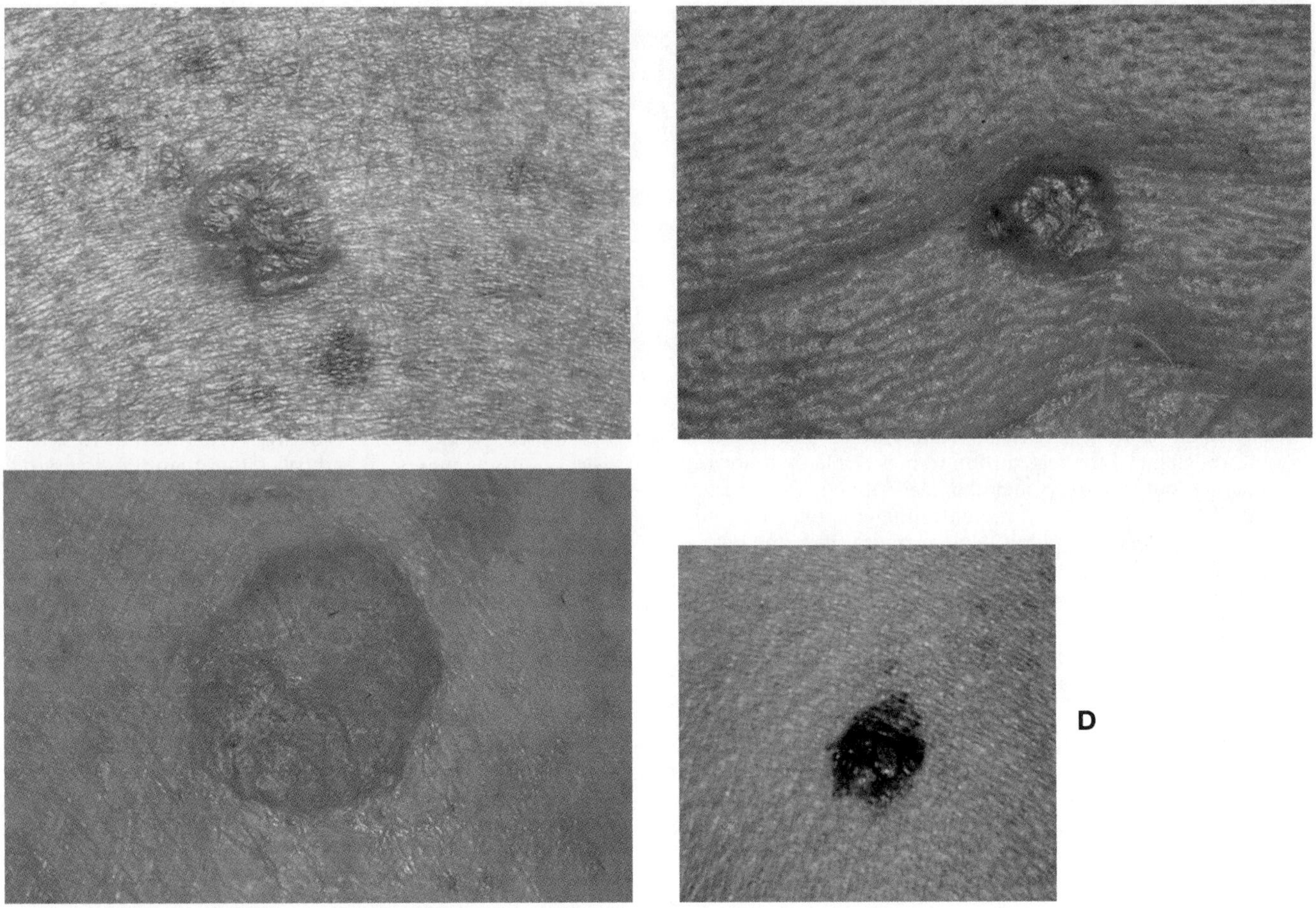

FIGURE **28–13** **A** and **B,** Two common presentations of basal cell carcinoma. **C,** Squamous cell carcinoma. **D,** Malignant melanoma. (From *Mosby's Guide to Physical Examination,* 5th ed., pp. 209–210, by H. M. Seidel et al., 2003, St. Louis, MO: Mosby.)

Table 28-21 Inspection of Skin Colour

Colour	Underlying Cause	Focus of Assessment
Bluish (cyanosis)	Increased amount of deoxygenated hemoglobin, which is associated with hypoxia (e.g., congenital heart disease, advanced lung disease, abnormal hemoglobins)	Lips, oral mucosa, sclera, palpebral conjunctiva, tongue, nails, palms, soles, dorsum of hands and feet
	Cold environment, anxiety	Nails, hands, feet
White (pallor)	Decreased amount of oxyhemoglobin, which is associated with anemia, decreased blood flow (prolonged elevation, immobilization, or edema)	Fingernails, lips, mucous membranes of mouth and palpebral conjunctivae, ear lobes, face, palms, soles
	Fainting, shock, arterial insufficiency or occlusion	Eyes, skin
	Lack of pigmentation from congenital condition (e.g., albinism) or autoimmune condition (e.g., vitiligo) causing loss of pigment	Head, neck, torso, arms, legs
Yellow-orange (**jaundice**)	Increased deposit of bilirubin in tissues associated with liver disease or excessive destruction of red blood cells	Palpebral conjunctivae, lips, hard palate, undersurface of tongue, tympanic membrane, skin
	High levels of carotene in diet	Face, palms, soles
Red (erythema)	Increased visibility of oxyhemoglobin associated with dilation or increased blood flow, fever, direct trauma, pressure, blushing, or alcohol intake	Face, sacrum, shoulders, elbows, hips, buttocks, knees, scrotum, heels, area of trauma
Tan-brown (pigmentation)	Increased melanin in skin (e.g., suntan, tanning sessions indoors)	Areas exposed to sun or tanning agent: face, neck, arms, legs, torso
	(e.g., pregnancy)	Face, areolae, nipples
	(e.g., age-related change)	Dorsum of hands

Box 28-19 Types of Skin Lesions

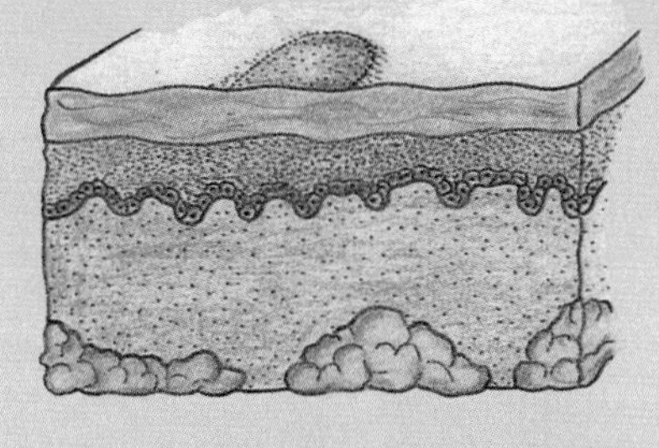

Macule: Flat, non-palpable change in skin colour, smaller than 1 cm (e.g., freckle, petechia)

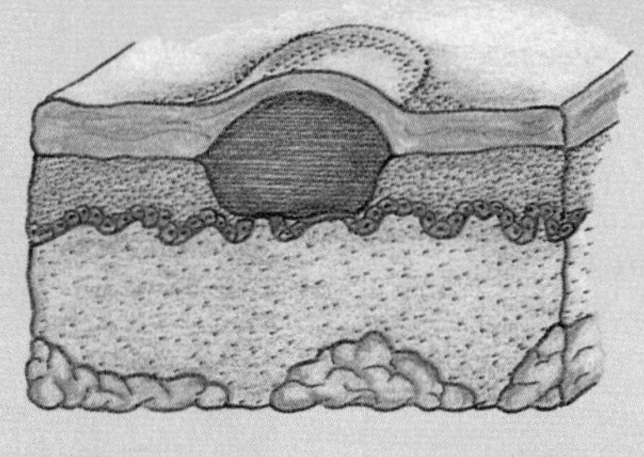

Papule: Palpable, circumscribed, solid elevation in skin, smaller than 0.5 cm (e.g., elevated nevus)

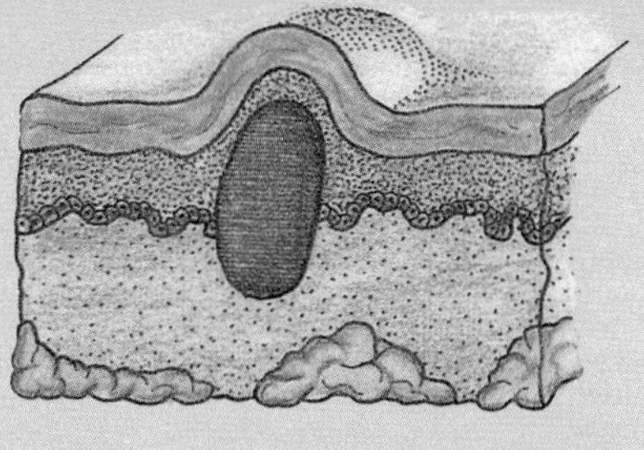

Nodule: Elevated solid mass, deeper and firmer than papule, 0.5–2 cm (e.g., wart)

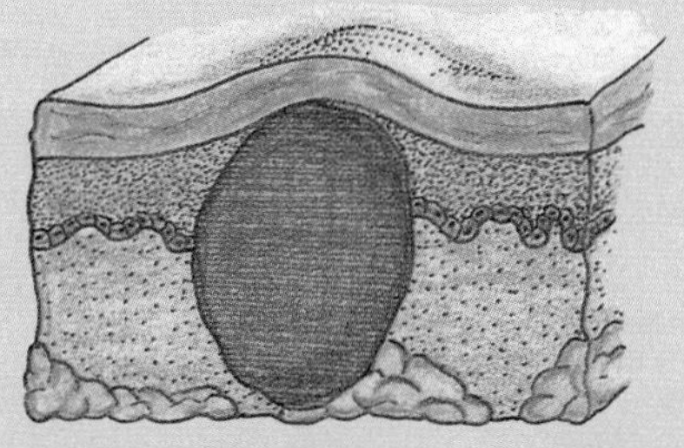

Tumour: Solid mass that may extend deep through subcutaneous tissue, larger than 1–2 cm (e.g., epithelioma)

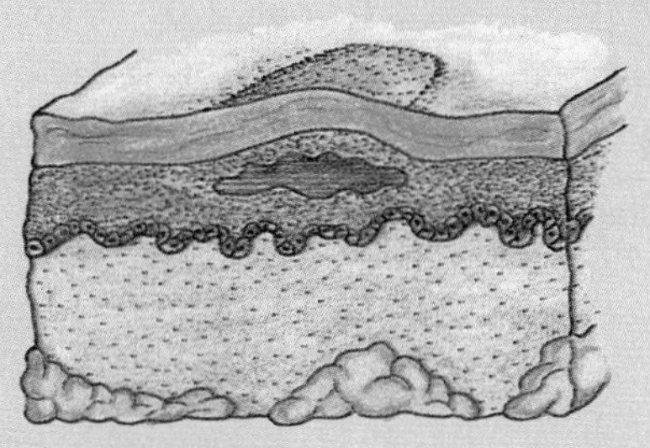

Wheal: Irregularly shaped, elevated area or superficial localized edema; varies in size (e.g., hive, mosquito bite)

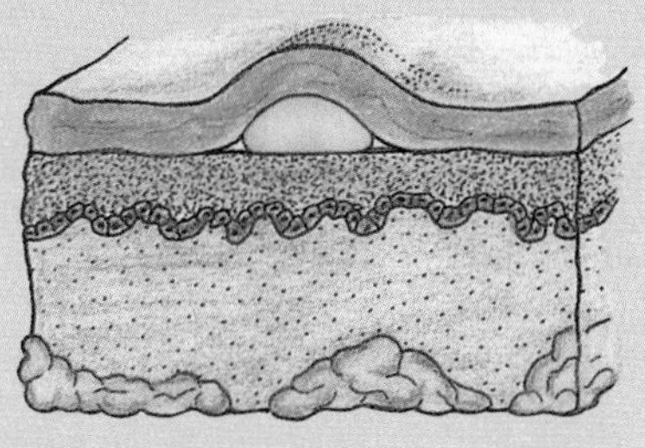

Vesicle: Circumscribed elevation of skin filled with serous fluid, smaller than 0.5 cm (e.g., herpes simplex, chickenpox)

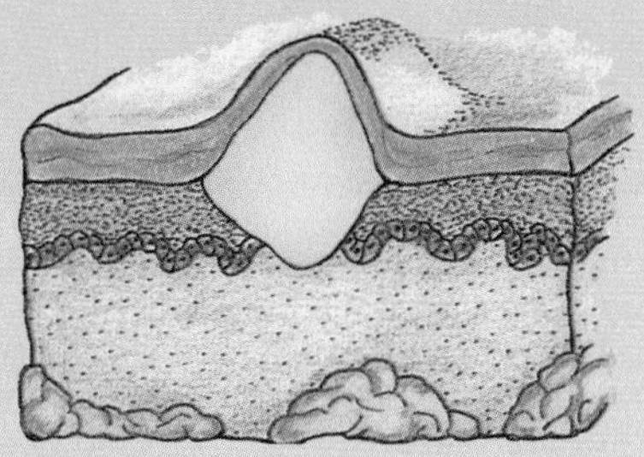

Pustule: Circumscribed elevation of skin similar to vesicle but filled with pus; varies in size (e.g., acne, staphylococcal infection)

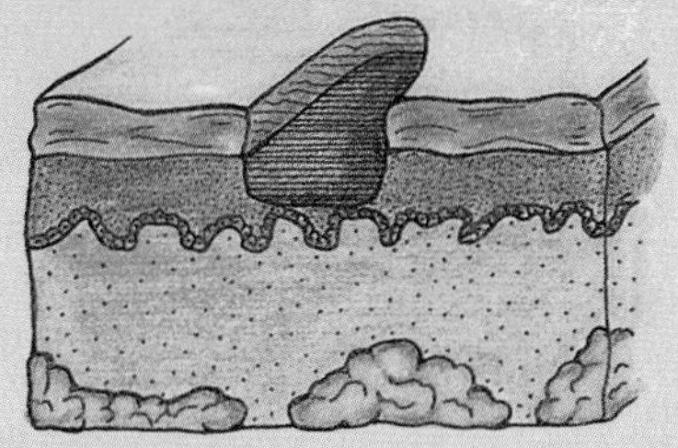

Ulcer: Deep loss of skin surface that may extend to dermis and frequently bleeds and scars; varies in size (e.g., venous stasis ulcer)

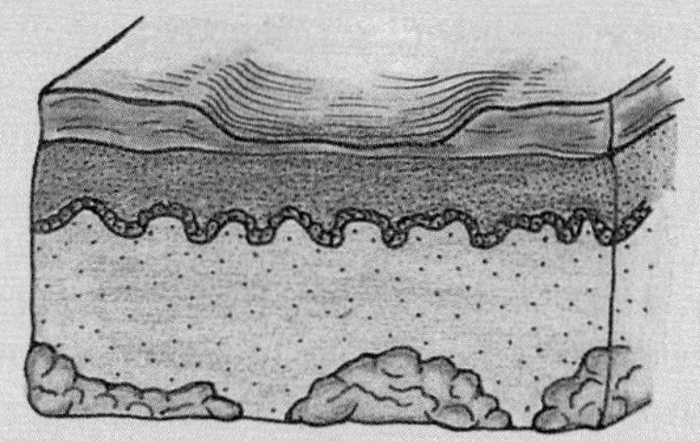

Atrophy: Thinning of skin with loss or normal skin furrow, with skin appearing shiny and translucent; varies in size (e.g., arterial insufficiency)

Lesions. The nurse expects to encounter skin pigmentation in the form of freckles, moles, and birthmarks during inspection, noting their distribution. Nurses may also encounter primary and secondary skin lesions that require further examination during palpation (Box 28-19). For example, **petechiae** are pinpoint-sized red or purple spots on the skin caused by small hemorrhages in the skin layers. They may indicate serious blood-clotting disorders, drug reactions, or liver disease. Any lesion is inspected for colour, location, size, shape, type, grouping (e.g., clustered, linear, circular), and distribution (localized or generalized). Using a small, clear, flexible ruler, nurses measure length, width, and depth dimensions of lesions. Exudate is assessed for amount, colour, odour, and consistency. Tattoos and body piercings are documented.

During skin inspection, nurses may also observe indications of substance abuse in skin colour, perspiration, and lesions (Box 28-20). A pattern of findings that is becoming more common is associated with clients who are chemically dependent or abusers of intravenous drugs. Clients who repeatedly and recently injected drugs intravenously may have edematous, reddened, and warm areas along the arms and legs. Old injection sites appear as hyperpigmented, shiny, or scarred areas.

Palpation of Skin. During palpation of the skin, nurses assess moisture, temperature, texture, thickness, mobility, **turgor,** and lesions. They require disposable gloves for palpation if open, moist, or draining lesions are present or if unexpected findings were found in inspection.

Box 28-20 Physical Findings of the Skin Indicative of Substance Abuse

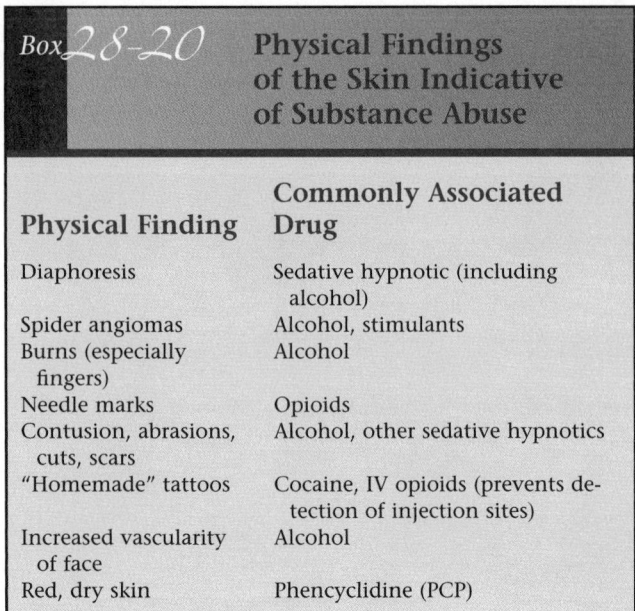

Physical Finding	Commonly Associated Drug
Diaphoresis	Sedative hypnotic (including alcohol)
Spider angiomas	Alcohol, stimulants
Burns (especially fingers)	Alcohol
Needle marks	Opioids
Contusion, abrasions, cuts, scars	Alcohol, other sedative hypnotics
"Homemade" tattoos	Cocaine, IV opioids (prevents detection of injection sites)
Increased vascularity of face	Alcohol
Red, dry skin	Phencyclidine (PCP)

Adapted from "Primary Care Screening for Substance Abuse," by I. Caulker-Burnett, 1994, *The Nurse Practitioner, 19*(6), pp. 42–48; and *Source Book of Substance Abuse and Addiction,* by L. Friedman et al., 1996, Baltimore: Williams & Wilkins.

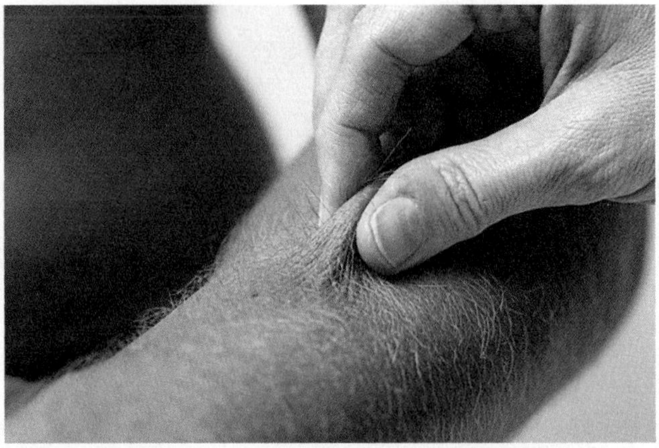

FIGURE **28–14** Assessment for skin turgor on arm. (From *Mosby's guide to physical examination,* 5th ed.; by H. M. Seidel et al., 2003, St. Louis, MO: Mosby.)

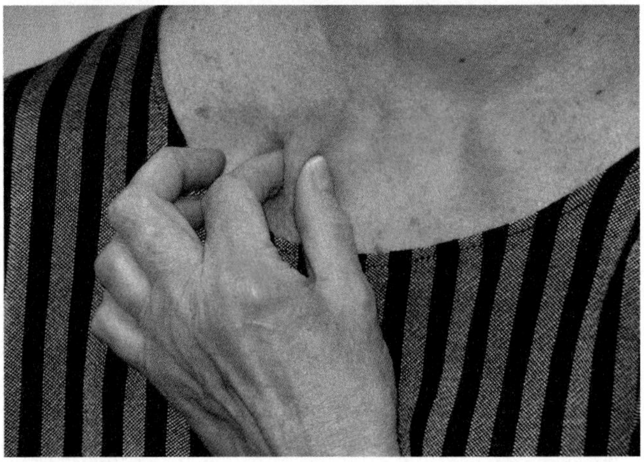

FIGURE **28–15** Assessment for skin turgor in subclavicular area. (From *Physical Examination Images* [CD-ROM], by D. L. Skillen, R. A. Day, M. C. Anderson, T. C. Stephen, J. A. Gilbert, and L. W. Day, 2004, Edmonton, AB: Faculty of Nursing, University of Alberta.)

Nurses use ungloved fingertips to palpate skin surfaces for moisture (wetness and oiliness). The hydration of skin and mucous membranes reveals body fluid imbalances, changes in the environment, and regulation of body temperature. Minimal perspiration or oiliness is expected, except for the intertriginous areas (e.g., axillae, inguinal regions). Increased perspiration may be associated with activity, warm environments, obesity, anxiety, or excitement. Dry skin may result from low humidity, exposure to sun, stress, smoking, excessive perspiration, and dehydration (Hardy, 1996). Excessive dryness can aggravate existing inflammatory conditions such as eczema and dermatitis. Both flaking and scaling are associated with unexpected levels of dryness (Hardy, 1996). Flakes resembling dandruff appear when the skin surface is lightly rubbed. Fish-like scales are easily rubbed off the skin surface.

Skin temperature depends on the amount of blood circulating through the dermis. Increased or decreased skin temperature indicates an increase or decrease in blood flow. If an examination room is cold, the client's skin temperature and colour may be affected. Nurses assess temperature most accurately by palpating the skin with the dorsum (back) of the hand and comparing symmetrical body parts, expecting skin temperature to be warm. Localized erythema or redness of the skin is often accompanied by an increase in skin temperature. A nurse can identify a stage I pressure ulcer early when noting warmth and erythema on an area of the skin (see chapter 43). Nurses always assess skin temperature for clients at risk for impaired circulation, such as after a cast application or vascular surgery.

The character of the skin surface and deeper portions is its texture. The nurse strokes the skin lightly with the fingertips and finger pads to assess for smoothness, thickness, and firmness. Skin texture is expected to be smooth, soft, and uniform, although skin on the palms and soles tends to be thicker. Localized changes may result from trauma, surgical wounds, or lesions. When irregularities in texture such as scars or **induration** (hardening) are found, the nurse asks about recent injury. Deeper palpation may reveal irregularities such as tenderness or localized areas of induration commonly caused by repeated intramuscular or subcutaneous injections. If the client has diabetes or receives vitamin B_{12} or iron injections, indurated areas may be palpated.

The elasticity of skin is assessed when the nurse uses fingertips and pads to grasp a fold of skin in the area under the clavicle or on the back of the forearm and release it (Figures 28-14 and 28-15). The nurse notes the ease with which the skin moves and the speed at which it returns to place. Usually it lifts easily into a fold (mobility) and falls back immediately to its resting position (turgor). If the skin fold remains pinched, the nurse evaluates the client's hydration and takes further action. Clients with reduced skin turgor do not have resilience to the normal wear and tear on the skin and are predisposed to skin breakdown.

Skin circulation affects the appearance of superficial blood vessels. After a client has been lying or sitting in

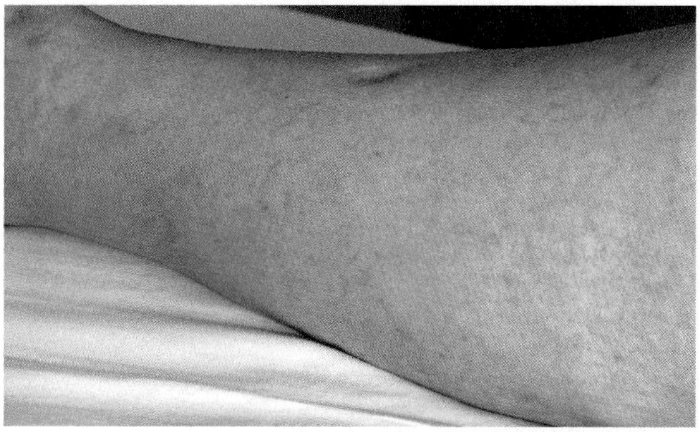

FIGURE **28–16** Pitting edema in leg. (From *Physical Examination Images* [CD-ROM], by D. L. Skillen, R. A. Day, M. C. Anderson, T. C. Stephen, J. A. Gilbert, and L. W. Day, 2004, Edmonton, AB: Faculty of Nursing, University of Alberta.)

one position, localized pressure areas appear as pale, pink, or reddened areas (see chapter 43). Areas are assessed for blanching to pressure.

Areas of the skin become swollen or edematous from fluid buildup in the tissues. Direct trauma and impaired venous return are two common causes of edema. Edematous areas are first inspected for location, colour, and shape. For the client with dependent edema caused by poor venous return, typical sites of edema are the feet, ankles, and sacrum. **Edema** separates the skin surface from the pigmented and vascular layers, masking skin colour. Edematous skin looks stretched and shiny. The nurse palpates areas of edema to determine mobility, consistency, tenderness, and extent. When pressure from the examiner's thumb leaves an indentation in the edematous area, it is called pitting edema (Figure 28–16). To assess the degree of pitting edema, the nurse presses the edematous area firmly with the thumb for 5 seconds and releases. The depth of pitting, recorded in millimetres, determines the degree of edema (see Figure 28–101; Seidel et al., 2003). For example, 1 degree of edema equals a 2-mm depth, 2 degrees equals a 4-mm depth, and so on.

Palpation determines the lesion's mobility, contour (flat, raised, or depressed), and consistency (soft or indurated). Classification of lesions as primary or secondary provides a description including size and elevation (see Box 28-19). Primary lesions occur as initial spontaneous manifestations of a pathological process (e.g., wheal of an insect bite); secondary lesions are alterations in primary lesions (e.g., a pressure ulcer).

Age-Related Changes in Skin. In older adults, skin pigmentation increases unevenly, causing discoloured areas. The skin becomes wrinkled because of decreased collagen, subcutaneous fat, and sweat glands. Very dry skin is common in older adults. Capillaries become more fragile and skin loses elasticity. Age-related skin lesions may appear as skin tags, thickenings (senile keratosis), ruby red papules (cherry angiomas), and atrophic warts.

Documentation. Nurses record their findings from inspection and palpation of the skin (Table 28-22).

Hair and Scalp

Two types of hair are on the body: terminal and vellus. Terminal hair is long, coarse, thick, and easily visible on the scalp, in eyebrows or beards, and in axillae and pubic areas. Clients from Aboriginal and Asian backgrounds have less terminal hair on the body and are assessed using relevant norms. Vellus hair is short, soft, inconspicuous, and lightly pigmented, covering the entire body except for the palms and soles. Nurses examine the type and distribution of body hair during the physical examination. Table 28-23 presents the health history and Box 28-21 presents the client teaching and health promotion during assessment of the hair and scalp.

Inspection of Hair and Scalp. Clients are sensitive about personal appearance. Before separating the hair for inspection, nurses explain the need to examine the scalp and use gloves from the beginning if expecting to encounter lesions or lice. During inspection, nurses examine the colour, distribution, and quantity of body hair. Colour varies widely and may result from rinses or dyes. Distribution and quantity are expected to change with age and vary according to biological variations and genetics. Unexpected changes result from inadequate nutrition, hormonal or endocrine disturbances, or excessive use of chemical agents. For example, hirsutism in women appears as hair growth on the upper lip, chin, cheeks, and coarser vellus hair over the body. In thyroid disorders, hair thinning or loss (alopecia) occurs. Nurses recognize that a change in hair growth can negatively affect body image and emotional well-being of both men and women.

While separating scalp hair, the nurse examines for colour, evidence of dryness, and skin lesions. Moles on the scalp may bleed with combing or brushing. The nurse inquires about recent trauma if lesions are observed. Inspection of scalp hair follicles may reveal lice or other parasites. The three types of lice are head (pediculus humanus capitis), body (pediculus humanus corporis), and crab lice (pediculus pubis). They attach their waxy, yellowish eggs firmly to hair and are difficult to see. If visible, head and body lice have very small greyish-white bodies and crab lice have red legs. Bites or pustular eruptions in the hair follicles and skin irritations behind the ears and in the warm intertriginous area signal their presence. Nurses teach about treating the environment and using a medicated shampoo, in a non-judgmental and calm manner.

Palpation of Hair and Scalp. During palpation, the scalp hair is examined for its thickness, texture, and lubrication. Scalp hair may be coarse, fine, curly, or straight. It is expected to be shiny, smooth, pliant, and evenly or symmetrically distributed. Hair is lubricated by the sebaceous glands. Excessive oiliness is associated with androgen hormone stimulation; unexpected dryness may result from of a thyroid condition or self-care practices.

Age-Related Changes in Hair. With aging, the hair is drier and more brittle, and loses pigment, becoming dull grey, white, or yellow. The number of scalp hairs decreases in a generalized pattern and the hair diameter diminishes. Hairline recession starts as a result of genetics, beginning at the temples and then at the vertex. In women, the pattern

Table 28-22 Examples of Documentation for Skin

Specific Characteristic	Expected Findings	Unexpected Findings
Colour	Uniformly olive	De-pigmented areas on face, arms, upper chest
Odour	Free of odour	Strong odour of perspiration
Lesions	Occasional nevus on extremities and torso	Brown macule 0.8 × 0.4 cm, flexor surface, (R) forearm
Moisture	Minimally moist (R) (L)	Oily skin and hair on head, face, and upper torso
Temperature	Warm bilaterally	Cool hands to elbows; cool feet to knees bilaterally
Texture	Smooth bilaterally	Rough bilaterally
Turgor	Skin mobile, skin fold returns to place quickly	Skin fold tent remains in place after release by examiner, subclavicular area
Vascularity	Occasional red papules noted on torso	Several spider angiomas over nose
Edema	Edema not present bilaterally at ankles	Dark pigmented areas on (R) (L) legs around ankles; 3 mm pitting edema

Adapted from *First Year Student Lab Guide* (p. 19), by J. Chambers et al., 2004, Edmonton, AB: Faculty of Nursing, University of Alberta.

Table 28-23 Health History for Hair and Scalp Assessment

Assessment Category	Rationale
Ask client about usual hygiene routine.	Hygiene practices contribute to health status of hair and scalp.
Question client about alterations in hair or scalp.	Changes in nutrition can affect condition of hair. Chemicals and heat can cause dryness and brittleness. Changes are felt by the client during self-care.
Inquire about current disease conditions, treatments, or medications that may affect integrity of hair and scalp.	Chemotherapy destroys cells that multiply rapidly (e.g., hair cells, tumour cells). Vasodilators may cause excessive hair growth.

Client Teaching

Box 28-21

Health Promotion for Hair and Scalp Assessment

Objective

- Client will learn and perform proper hygiene and assessment techniques for care of scalp and hair.

Teaching Strategies

- Inform client about basic hygiene practices for care of scalp and hair (see chapter 34).
- Inform at-risk client about signs and symptoms of head lice—itchy scalp, presence of nits at base of hair shaft.
- Teach at-risk client the required treatment for head lice—shampoo thoroughly with recommended medicated shampoo, available at drugstores; comb thoroughly with fine-toothed comb and discard comb. Remove any detectable nits with fingernails. Clean all linens and items that have come in head contact with client, using hot water and drying in hot dryer for at least 20 minutes. Soak combs, brushes, and hair accessories in lice-killing products for 10 minutes. Vacuum rugs, furniture, and car. Seal non-washable items in a plastic bag for 14 days.
- Inform client of health-promotion techniques to reduce the transmission of head lice—do not share personal items with others; avoid physical contact with infested individuals and their belongings, especially bed linens and clothing.
- Inform client that partner must be notified if lice were sexually transmitted.

Evaluation

- Have client describe methods of proper hygiene for hair and scalp.
- Have at-risk client describe signs and symptoms of head lice.
- Have client at risk describe the required treatment to reduce transmission of head lice.

Table 28-24 Examples of Documentation for Hair and Scalp

Specific Characteristic	Expected Findings	Unexpected Findings
Colour	Brown	Purple tips, coloured red
Texture	Coarse and curly	Limp
Moisture	Dry	Very dry
Distribution	Evenly distributed over skull	Sparsely distributed postauricular and occipital areas
Quantity	Uniformly thick	Unevenly thin areas over skull
Scalp	Uniformly pinkish white	Whitish scales and yellowish crusts on vertex

Adapted from *First Year Student Lab Guide* (p. 55), by J. Chambers et al., 2004, Edmonton, AB: Faculty of Nursing, University of Alberta.

Table 28-25 Health History for Nail Assessment

Assessment Category	Rationale
Inquire about usual nail care regime.	Frequent manicures or exposure to chemicals may damage nails. Neglected nail care may contribute to infections.
Inquire about recent changes in nails and changes over time.	Systemic conditions may affect colour, growth, or shape; local trauma may affect shape and growth. Stress (physical or psychological) or systemic disease may change nails slowly.
Determine risks for nail problems.	Disease conditions such as diabetes and trauma can affect vascularity of peripheral tissues, including nails. Poor vision, inability to bend over, or lack of coordination may affect nail care practices.

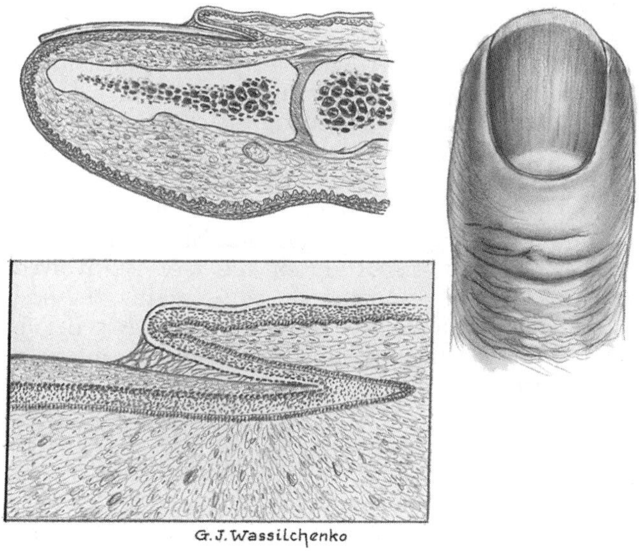

FIGURE **28–17** Anatomic structures of the nail. (From *Mosby's Guide to Physical Examination,* 5th ed., p. 165, Figure 7–2, by H. M. Seidel et al., 2003, St. Louis, MO: Mosby.)

is similar but the hair loss is less severe. As men age, they lose facial hair. In contrast, as women age, they may develop hair on the chin and upper lip. Older adults lose hair on the torso, axillae, pubic area, and legs.

Documentation. Nurses record their findings for inspection and palpation of the hair and scalp (Table 28-24).

Nails

The nail condition reflects a client's general state of health, nutritional status, occupation, and level of self-care. The psychological state may be revealed by evidence of nail biting or picking. Nails usually grow at a constant rate, but direct injury or generalized disease can impair growth. The most visible portion of the nails is the nail plate of keratin that covers the nail bed (Figure 28–17). The vascularity of the underlying epithelial cells in the nail bed and the state of the circulating blood create nail colour. The semilunar, opaque white area at the base of the nail bed is the lunula from which the nail plate develops. Nail folds overlap the lateral and proximal borders of the nail plate. The cuticle protects the nail matrix where new keratin cells develop. Before assessing the nails, the nurse gathers a brief history (Table 28-25).

Inspection of Nails. The nurse inspects the nail bed for colour, cleanliness, and length; the nail plate for contour and surface; the angle between the nail and the nail bed in degrees; and the lateral and proximal nail folds for colour, shape, and integrity. Nails are expected to be smooth, pink, transparent, well rounded, and convex.

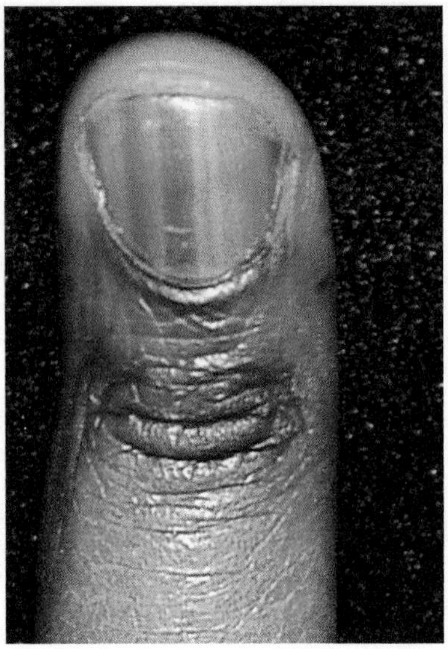

FIGURE **28–18** Pigmented bands in nail of client with dark skin. (From *Mosby's guide to physical examination*, 5th ed.; by H. M. Seidel et al., 2003, St. Louis, MO: Mosby.)

Cuticles are smooth, intact, and clear. In darker-skinned clients (Figure 28–18), longitudinal bands of brown or black pigment may be seen. Bands in nail beds can be caused by nutrient and electrolyte changes. Splinter hemorrhages may indicate trauma or chronic conditions.

The nail bed angle is about 160 degrees, although the angle in clients with chronic oxygenation problems from heart or lung conditions may increase. For example, in clubbing, the distal phalanx is rounded and bulbous when inspected. Looking across the nail, the angle is 180 degrees or greater, and the nail plate is convex. Figure 28–19, *A* and *B* present some of the unexpected findings on inspection.

If nails are ragged, dirty, and poorly kept, the nurse considers the client's reported frequency of nail care, ability to perform care, and type of employment. Work such as farming, mining, or mechanics (e.g., oil and gas industry) may cause dirty nails despite clients' excellent nail care. Jagged, bitten, or broken nail edges or cuticles can predispose to infection and risks because of exposure to substances and infectious agents in the workplace. Inspection of the skin around the nails on the feet or hands may uncover thickenings of the epidermis such as calluses or corns because of friction or pressure. Pressure from shoes, tools, and instruments contributes to the thickening.

Palpation of Nails. The nurse palpates the nail base for firmness, and the nail plate for thickness, texture, smoothness, and capillary return. When an angle of 180 degrees or more has been noted during inspection, the nurse will palpate a base that feels spongy or floating. By pressing firmly, quickly, and gently on the nail plate, the nurse checks **capillary return.** With pressure, the nail bed blanches; on release of pressure, the pink colour returns within 1 or 2 seconds unless circulatory insufficiency delays it. Reduced amounts of oxyhemoglobin will contribute to continual pallor of the nail beds; increased amounts of deoxygenated hemoglobin will create a bluish colour. During inspection and palpation of the nails, the nurse takes advantage of teaching opportunities with the client (Box 28-22).

> ***Safety Alert:*** Clients with impaired circulation are at greater risk for localized infection. Observe the condition of the nails on hands and feet to identify early signs of infection.

Age-Related Changes to Nails. Nails become harder and thicker and nail growth slows. Nails are more brittle, dull, and opaque and develop longitudinal striations. If calcium uptake or intake is insufficient, nails may turn yellow. Cuticles become thinner and narrower.

Documentation. Nurses record their findings from inspection and palpation of the nails (Table 28-26).

Assessing the Head and Neck

Assessment of the head and neck includes the head, eyes, ears, nose, mouth, pharynx, and neck (lymph nodes, carotid arteries, thyroid gland, and trachea). Carotid arteries may also be assessed during examination of the peripheral arteries. Assessment of the head and neck requires inspection and palpation in close sequence and auscultation.

Head

Inspection. The history screens for intracranial injury and local or congenital deformities (Table 28-27).

The nurse begins by inspecting the client's head position and all facial features, expecting the head to be held upright and still. It is common for slight asymmetry of features to exist. When there is facial asymmetry, the nurse notes if all features on one side of the face are affected or if only a portion of the face is involved. Inspection continues with the nurse noting the size, shape, and contour of the skull. The skull is generally round with prominences in the frontal area anteriorly and the occipital area posteriorly.

Palpation. Local skull deformities are typically caused by trauma. The nurse palpates the skull for nodules, masses, and tenderness. Gentle rotation of the fingertips down the midline of the scalp and then along the sides of the head reveals abnormalities. The nurse notes the pulse characteristics of the temporal arteries bilaterally, then assesses movement in the temporomandibular joint (TMJ) space. The TMJ movements are expected to be smooth, although it is not unusual to hear or feel a click or snap. At this time, the motor and sensory branches of cranial nerve V (trigeminal) and the motor function of cranial nerve VII (facial) may also be tested (Procedure 28-2). Cranial nerves are part of the peripheral nervous system and emerge as 12 pairs from the skull. They have motor and sensory functions that are addressed in the section on assessing the extremities.

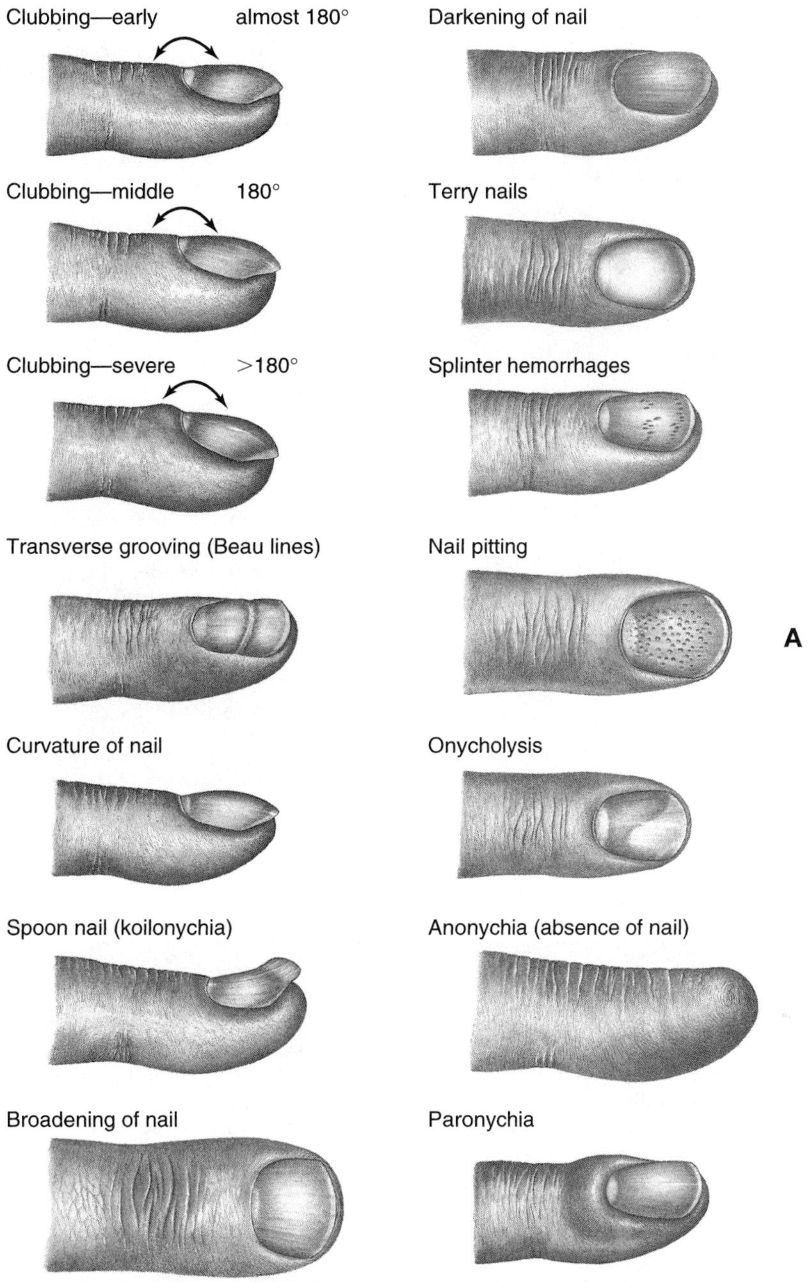

FIGURE **28–19** **A,** Nails: Unexpected findings and appearance. (From *Mosby's Guide to Physical Examination,* 5th ed., p. 188, Figure 7–15, by H. M. Seidel et al., 2003, St. Louis, MO: Mosby.) *Continued*

B

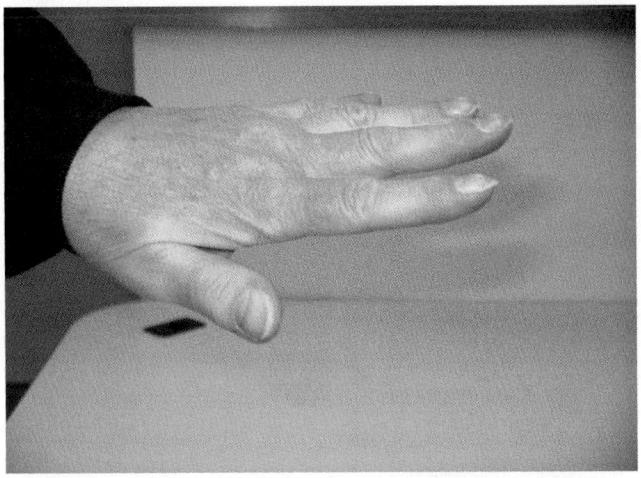

FIGURE **28–19, cont'd** **B,** Clubbing. (From *Physical Examination Images* [CD-ROM], by D. L. Skillen, R. A. Day, M. C. Anderson, T. C. Stephen, J. A. Gilbert, and L. W. Day, 2004. Edmonton, AB: Faculty of Nursing, University of Alberta.)

Client Teaching — Box 28-22

Nail Assessment

Objective

- Client will know proper techniques for care of fingernails and toenails.

Teaching Strategies

- Inform client of need to clean and maintain length of nails.
- If client is diabetic, instruct client to file nails instead of cutting them, wash feet daily in warm water, and inspect all surfaces with good lighting, noting any lesions or cracks in the skin. Instruct to soften dry feet with lotion (not between toes) and caution about using sharp objects around nails and cuticles.
- Encourage regular checkups with a podiatrist or nurse with foot care certificate.
- Instruct to avoid self-selected preparations to treat corns, calluses, and ingrown toenails.

Evaluation

- Have client explain necessary practices to ensure healthy nails.

Table 28-26 Examples of Documentation for Nails

Focus of Assessment	Expected Findings	Unexpected Findings
Nail plate	Smooth and trimmed (R)(L)	Pinpoint pitting thumbs, index fingers (R) (L)
Nail bed	Pink bilaterally	Purplish (R)(L)
	Capillary return <2 seconds	Capillary return >5 seconds
Nail base	Firm bilaterally	Spongy and soft in fingers bilaterally
Nail folds	Smooth, colour of surrounding skin, non-tender (R) (L)	Inflamed and swollen (L) index and middle fingers
Nail angle	160 degrees with nail base (R) (L)	Over 180 degrees with nail base bilaterally, thumbs and index fingers

Adapted from *First Year Student Lab Guide* (p. 19), by J. Chambers et al., 2004, Edmonton, AB: Faculty of Nursing, University of Alberta.

Table 28-27 Health History for Head Assessment

Assessment Category	Rationale
Ask if client has history of headache or trauma to head, documenting results of a symptom analysis.	Characteristics of headache can help to determine causative factors and nature of trauma will guide examination.
Inquire about client's occupational history for use of safety helmets.	Certain occupations can create risks for head injury.
Question client about participation in sporting events and use of protective equipment.	Many sporting activities have the potential for creating head injuries without proper protective equipment.

Procedure 28-2 Assessing the Face

Equipment

- Splintered tongue blade
- Cotton ball

Examination Skill and Focus	Steps	Rationale
Inspection:		
Skin, face, lips	**1.** Inspect skin, face, and lips.	
Palpation:		
Temporal arteries	**1.** Palpate temporal arteries with fingertips or pads.	Fine tactile discrimination is required.
Temporomandibular joint	**2.** Position index fingertips in front of each tragus.	Fingertips will slip into joint space when mouth opens.
	3. Instruct client to open and close jaw with fingertips in position.	
Cranial nerve (CN) V (trigeminal) Motor function	**1.** Instruct client to clench teeth.	Assesses motor function of paired CN V.
	2. Palpate temporal and masseter muscles with fingertips or pads.	
	3. Note strength and symmetry of contraction.	Comparison detects differences.
Sensory function	**1.** Demonstrate how sharp, dull, and light touch feels before beginning tests.	Client must clearly understand what is being tested.
	2. Instruct client to close eyes and indicate when touched.	Ensures that sensation rather than vision is being tested.
	3. Test side to side, varying rhythm, touching ophthalmic, maxillary, and mandibular regions lightly with cotton ball.	Prevents client's anticipation of being touched and tests all three sensory branches of the nerve.
	4. Repeat with splintered tongue blade. Use dull to check client's reliability at least once.	Validates client is sensing pain, not pressure.
	5. Compare sides.	Comparison detects differences.
CN VII (facial) Motor function	**1.** Instruct client to: a. show upper and lower teeth b. puff out cheeks c. smile	Tests functions of paired CN VII.
	2. Observe for symmetry.	Comparison detects differences.
	3. Instruct client to: a. frown b. raise eyebrows c. close eyes tight and resist opening by examiner	
	4. Attempt to open client's closed eyes, exerting pressure on bony orbit, avoiding pressure on eye.	
	5. Observe for symmetry and strength of motion.	

From *A Syllabus for Adult Health Assessment* (pp. 31, 34–35), edited by D. L. Skillen and R. A. Day, 2004, Edmonton, AB: Faculty of Nursing, University of Alberta.

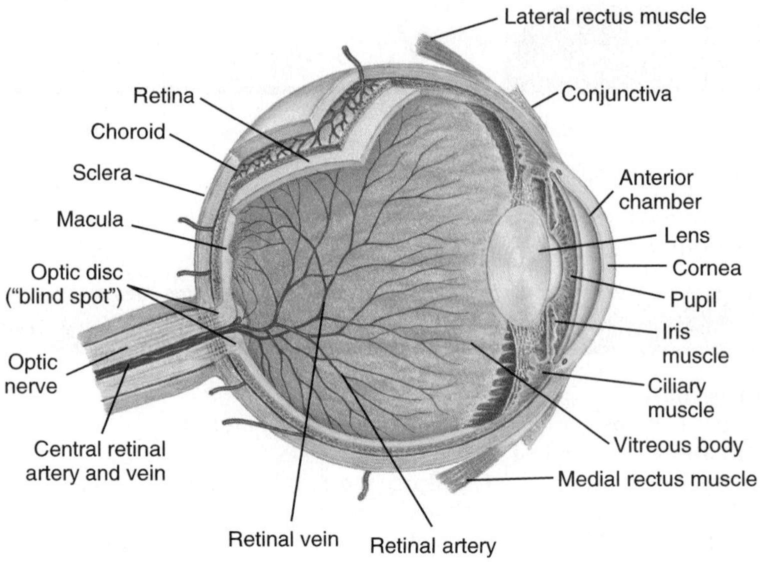

FIGURE **28–20** Anatomy of the human eye. (From *Mosby's Guide to Physical Examination,* 5th ed., p. 279, Figure 10–1, by H. M. Seidel et al., 2003, St. Louis, MO: Mosby.)

Eyes

Assessment of the eyes includes visual acuity, visual fields, extraocular movements, and external and internal eye structures. Figure 28–20 shows a cross-section of the eye. When examiners detect visual alterations, they assess the level of assistance that clients require when ambulating or performing self-care activities. Clients with visual problems may also need special aids for reading instructions such as medication labels. Table 28-28 contains the health history that guides the eye examination. Box 28-23 is an overview of relevant client teaching and health promotion information.

Visual Acuity. Assessment of visual acuity (ability to see small details) tests central vision. Ask clients to read printed material under adequate lighting. Clients who wear glasses for distance should wear them during the examination. Determine which language clients speak and whether they are able to read.

Assessment of distant vision requires the Snellen chart (paper chart or projection screen), which should be well lighted (Figure 28–21). It has standardized numbers at the end of each line of the chart. The numerator is the number 20 (the distance the client stands away from the chart). The denominator is the distance from which the client can read the line of the chart. Vision is expected to be 20/20. The larger the denominator, the poorer the client's visual acuity. A value of 20/40, for example, means that the client standing 20 feet away reads a line that a person with unaffected vision reads from 40 feet away.

Vision is tested without corrective lenses first, but contact lenses are left in place. The client sits or stands 20 feet (6.1 m) away from the chart and tries to read all letters out loud beginning at any line with each eye separately (opposite eye covered with index card or eye cover; Figure 28–22) and then with both eyes open. The client should avoid applying pressure to the covered eye. Note the lowest line that the client can read more than half the letters correctly and record the visual acuity for that line (Bickley & Szilagyi, 2003). Repeat testing with the client wearing corrective lenses. Do the test rapidly enough that the client does not memorize the chart (Seidel et al., 2003) or have the client do part of the test by starting the letters from right to left. Observe for signs of straining (head turning, squinting, frowning) while clients read the chart. Record visual acuity as without correction or with correction (glasses or contact lenses).

If clients cannot see even the largest letters or figures of a Snellen chart, the nurse tests their ability to count upraised fingers or distinguish light. Holding a hand 30 cm (1 foot) from the face, nurses instruct clients to count the upraised fingers. For light perception, nurses shine a penlight into the client's eye and then turn the light off. If clients note when the light is turned on or off, light perception is intact.

If clients are unable to read, the nurse uses an *E* chart or one with pictures of familiar objects. The client says or points to the direction in which each *E* is pointing or names the object. Visual acuity is scored for each eye and for both eyes.

Near vision can be assessed by asking clients to read a hand-held card containing a vision screening chart. They are instructed to hold the card a comfortable distance (about 30 cm) from the eyes and read the smallest line possible.

Inspection of External Eye Structures

Position and Alignment. Nurses stand directly in front of the client at eye level, asking the client to look at their face. They inspect the external structures, position, and alignment (Procedure 28-3). Expected findings include the eyes being parallel to each other without bulging or protrusion. Bulging **(exophthalmos)** is usually caused by hyperthyroidism if both eyes are involved. If one eye protrudes, tumours or inflammation of the orbit can be the cause. Crossed eyes **(strabismus)** result from neuromuscular injury or inherited conditions.

Eyebrows. Eyebrows are inspected for symmetry, size, distribution, hair texture, alignment, and movement. Loss or absence of hair may indicate a hormonal disturbance or be the result of waxing or plucking. The brows should rise and lower symmetrically. Paralysis of the facial nerve prevents movement of eyebrows.

Table 28-28 Health History for Eye Assessment

Assessment Categories	Rationale
Ask if client has history of eye disease, eye trauma, diabetes, hypertension, or eye surgery.	Some disease conditions can cause risk for partial or complete vision loss.
Inquire about family history of eye disorders.	Some eye disorders are hereditary.
Question client about use of protective eyewear for occupational or recreational activities as well as protection while exposed to sun.	Some occupations and recreational events create risk for eye injuries. Sun exposure can damage eyes or surrounding tissues.
Ask client about use of glasses or contact lenses.	Vision should be tested with glasses; contact lens use leads to questions about lens hygiene.
Inquire if client has regular examinations by an eye specialist.	Regular eye examinations reveal preventative care taken by client.
Ask client about use of medications for eye problems.	Certain medications may cause visual disturbances.

Client Teaching Box 28-23

Health Promotion for Eye Assessment

Objectives

- Client will understand need for regular eye examinations and recognize age-related changes.
- Client will be able to recognize warning signs and symptoms of eye disease.
- Client will take appropriate measures to protect eyes while working, during recreational events, and with sun exposure.

Teaching Strategies

- Encourage client to have eyes examined regularly, particularly if experiencing difficulties with sight.
- Inform older adults of the expected age-related changes to eyes and the necessary precautions to take, such as avoiding night driving, increasing lighting in home to reduce risk of falls, and wearing appropriate corrective lenses.
- Describe typical symptoms of eye disease (see Box 28-24).
- Encourage client to wear protective eyewear for hazardous work, recreational events, and whenever eyes are exposed to sun.

Evaluation

- Have client report date of last eye examination.
- Have client describe common symptoms related to eye disease.
- Have client share details about the home environment and driving practices.

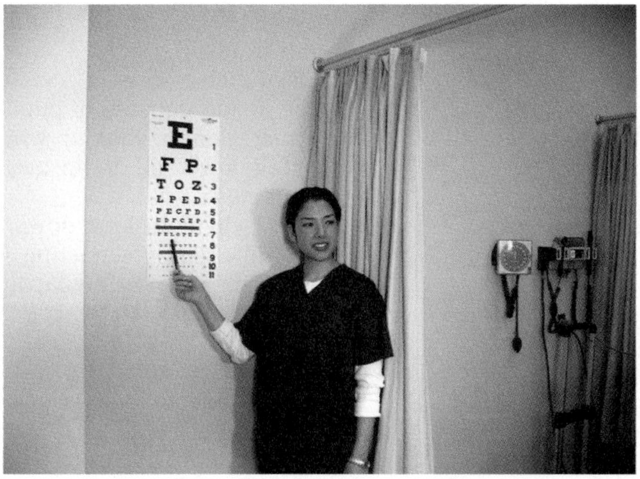

FIGURE 28–21 Snellen chart and nursing student. (From *Physical Examination Images* [CD-ROM], by D. L. Skillen, R. A. Day, M. C. Anderson, T. C. Stephen, J. A. Gilbert, and L. W. Day, 2004, Edmonton, AB: Faculty of Nursing, University of Alberta.)

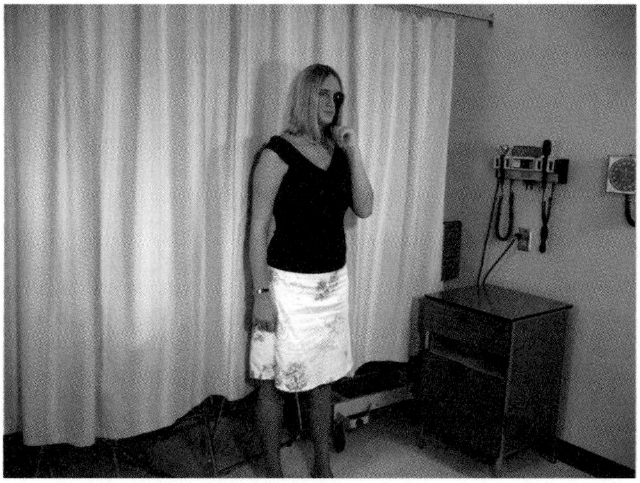
FIGURE 28–22 Client covers eye for Snellen chart. (From *Physical Examination Images* [CD-ROM], by D. L. Skillen, R. A. Day, M. C. Anderson, T. C. Stephen, J. A. Gilbert, and L. W. Day, 2004, Edmonton, AB: Faculty of Nursing, University of Alberta.)

Eyelids. Eyelids are inspected for position, colour, condition of lid surface, and condition of the eyelashes. The client's ability to open, close, and blink eyelids is assessed. When eyes are open in a relaxed position, the lids do not cover the pupil and sclera cannot be seen above the iris. Lids lie close to the eyeball. An unexpected drooping of the lid over the pupil is called **ptosis** (pronounced "toe-sis") and is caused by edema or impairment of the third cranial nerve. Defects in the position of the lid margins may also be observed. Eyelashes are expected to be distributed evenly and curved outward away from the eye. Redness

Procedure 28-3 Inspecting the External Structures of the Eyes

Equipment

- Penlight
- Cotton ball

Examination Skill and Focus	Steps	Rationale
Inspection:		
Eyebrows, lids, lashes	**1.** Inspect eyebrows, lids, lashes.	
Cornea	**1.** Use tangential lighting, with penlight, to inspect cornea.	Tangential lighting shows contour better than direct lighting.
Lens, iris, pupils	**1.** Inspect: • lens from anterior view • iris of each eye • size, shape, equality of pupils	
Sclera, conjunctiva	**1.** Instruct client to look up while gently retracting lower lid to inspect sclera and conjunctiva. **2.** Instruct client to look down and side to side while gently retracting upper lid to view sclera and possibly lacrimal gland.	Ensures adequate exposure of the conjunctivae.
Lacrimal sacs/glands	**1.** Inspect lacrimal sac puncta/gland regions bilaterally.	
Pupillary reaction CN II, III (optic, oculomotor)	Test each eye separately. **1.** Instruct client to look past examiner.	Prevents a false reflex from accommodation.
Pupillary reaction to light; direct, consensual reactions	**2.** Shine a bright light from temporal region on each pupil in turn.	Using tangential lighting prevents a false reflex from accommodation.
	3. Inspect for direct and consensual reactions.	The afferent nerve synapses with both sides of the brain.
Near reaction (accommodation) Dilatation	Test each eye separately. **1.** Instruct client to look into distance with each eye. **2.** Observe pupil for dilatation.	Pupils dilate when looking into the distance.
Constriction	**3.** Instruct client to look at examiner's finger held 10 cm from client's eye. **4.** Observe for pupillary constriction while client focuses on finger. **5.** Repeat for other eye.	Pupils constrict when looking at a near object.
Convergence CN III, IV (oculomotor, trochlear)	**1.** Instruct client to follow finger.	
Convergence	**2.** From directly in front of client, move finger to within 5 to 8 cm from bridge of client's nose.	Convergence occurs within 5-to 8-cm range.
	3. Observe convergence.	Assesses the ability of both eyes to converge.
Corneal reflex CN V, VII (trigeminal, facial)	Test each eye separately. **1.** Ask client if wearing contact lenses. **2.** Instruct client to look up and away from examiner	Contact lenses obstruct the cornea and result in an inaccurate assessment.
	3. Approach from side with fine wisp of cotton **4.** Touch cornea, avoiding eyelashes and sclera	Long-term contact lens wearers may have a decreased corneal reflex.
Bilateral blink	**5.** Observe for bilateral blink.	CN V, VII integrity observed.

From *A Syllabus for Adult Health Assessment* (pp. 29–31), edited by D. L. Skillen and R. A. Day, 2004, Edmonton, AB: Faculty of Nursing, University of Alberta.

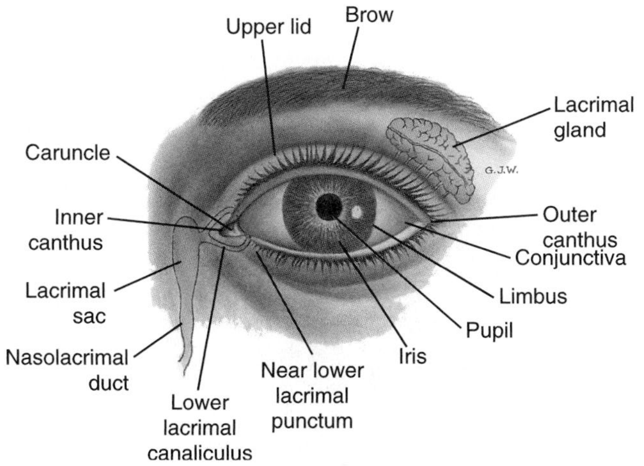

FIGURE **28–23** Important landmarks of the left external eye. (From *Mosby's Guide to Physical Examination,* 5th ed., p. 281, Figure 10-3, by H. M. Seidel et al., 2003, St. Louis, MO: Mosby.)

along the lid margins suggests blepharitis. An erythematous or yellow swelling on an eyelash follicle indicates an acute suppurative inflammation (hordeolum or sty).

Eyelids are expected to be smooth and the colour of the skin. Redness indicates inflammation or infection. Lid edema may be due to allergies or heart or kidney failure, and edema may prevent them from closing. Lesions are inspected for specific characteristics, including discomfort or drainage. Gloves are worn if drainage is present.

The lids close symmetrically. Failure to close exposes corneas to drying, a common condition in unconscious clients or clients with facial nerve paralysis. Usually a person blinks involuntarily and bilaterally up to 20 times a minute, lubricating the cornea. An unexpected finding is absent or infrequent, rapid, or monocular (one-eyed) blinking.

Lacrimal Apparatus. The anterior surface of the eye, made up of the sensitive cornea and conjunctivae, is lubricated by tears secreted from the lacrimal gland (Figure 28–23), which lies in the upper outer wall of each anterior orbit. Tears from the gland flow across the eye surface to the lacrimal duct in the nasal corner (inner canthus) of the eye. The lacrimal gland can be the site of tumours or infections and is inspected for edema and redness. The flow of tears may be blocked if the nasolacrimal duct becomes obstructed. If the client reports excessive tearing, the nurse looks for evidence of edema in the inner canthus.

Palpation. Although the lacrimal gland is not usually felt, the area is palpated gently to detect tenderness. Mild palpation of the duct at the lower eyelid just inside the lower orbital rim (not on the nose) may cause a regurgitation of tears.

Conjunctivae and Sclerae. Bulbar conjunctivae cover the exposed surface of the eyeballs up to the outer edge of the cornea; palpebral conjunctivae are the delicate membranes lining the eyelids. Usually the conjunctivae are transparent, enabling examiners to view the tiny underlying blood vessels that give a light pink colour. Sclerae are seen under the bulbar conjunctivae and are the colour of white porcelain in Caucasians and light yellow in African-Canadians. Sclerae may become pigmented and appear

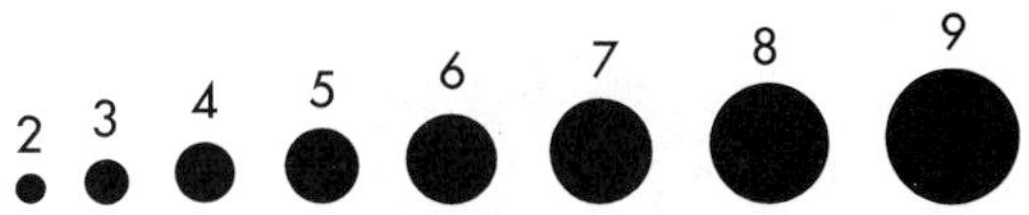

FIGURE **28–24** Chart depicting pupillary size in millimetres.

yellow or green if liver disease is present. Examiners inspect the conjunctivae for colour, texture, edema, and lesions. Localized bright red blood surrounded by clear conjunctiva usually indicates subconjunctival hemorrhage.

To expose the bulbar conjunctivae, the eyelids must be retracted without placing pressure directly on the eyeball. Clients may begin to blink, making the examination difficult. The conjunctivae should be free of erythema, which can indicate an allergic or infectious **conjunctivitis.**

Palpation. Pale conjunctivae result from anemia; a fiery red appearance is from inflammation (conjunctivitis), which is highly contagious. The crusty drainage that collects on eyelid margins can easily spread from one eye to the other. Nurses wear gloves during the examination and perform hand hygiene before and after palpation.

Corneas. The cornea is the transparent and colourless cover of the pupil and iris. From a side view, it looks like the crystal of a wristwatch. As the client looks straight ahead, the cornea is examined for clarity and texture and is expected to be shiny, transparent, and smooth. Any irregularity in the surface may indicate an abrasion or tear that warrants immediate examination by a physician. Iris colour and details are easy to see.

The corneal reflex is assessed using the bilateral blink test. Expected findings include a brisk, bilateral blink when each cornea is touched with a wisp of cotton. Other findings may indicate impairment of the fifth and/or seventh cranial nerves.

Pupils and Irises. The nurse observes the pupils for size, shape, equality, accommodation (near reaction), and reaction to light. Pupils are expected to be black, round, regular, and equal in size (3 to 7 mm in diameter; Figure 28–24). The iris should be clearly visible and intact. A thin white ring along the corneal margin **(arcus senilis)** is not expected in anyone under age 40.

Cloudy pupils indicate cataracts. Dilated pupils can result from glaucoma, trauma, neurological disorders, eye medications (e.g., atropine), or withdrawal from opioids. Constricted pupils may be caused by inflammation of the iris or use of drugs (e.g., pilocarpine, morphine, or cocaine). Pinpoint pupils are a common sign of opioid intoxication. When a beam of light is shone through the pupil on to the retina, the third cranial nerve is stimulated and innervates the muscles of the iris to constrict. Any abnormality along the nerve pathways from the retina to the iris alters pupillary ability to react to light. Changes in intracranial pressure, locally applied ophthalmic medications, lesions along nerve pathways, and direct trauma to the eye may alter pupillary reaction.

Pupillary reflexes are easier to visualize when tested in a dimly lit room (Figure 28–25). A directly illuminated pupil constricts, and the opposite pupil constricts consensually. Observe the speed and equality of responses.

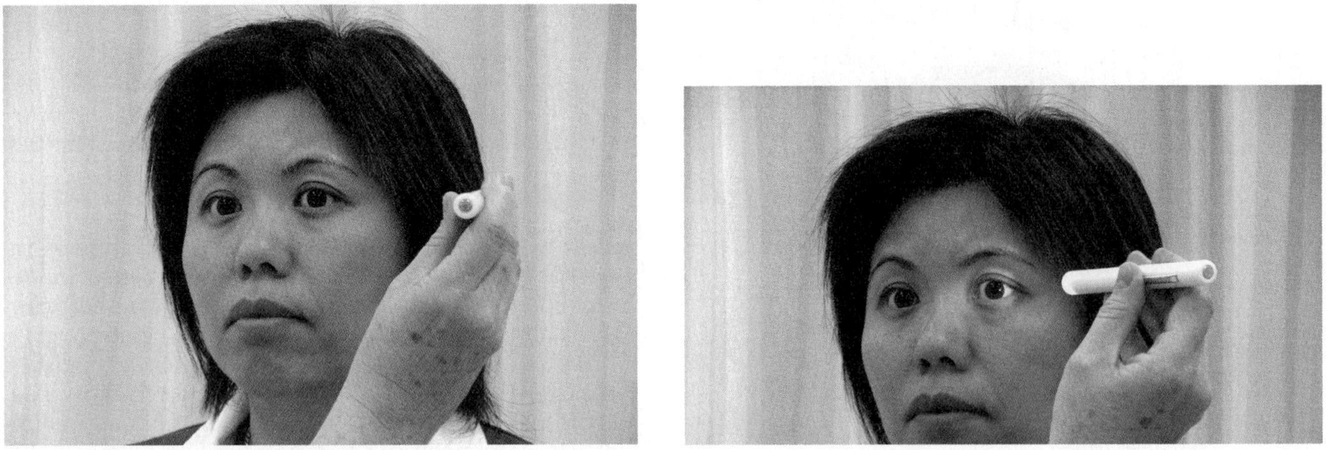

FIGURE **28–25** Direct and consensual pupillary constriction. **A,** First, shine the light behind the client. **B,** Next, shine the light on one pupil for direct and consensual constriction. (From *Physical Examination Images* [CD-ROM], by D. L. Skillen, R. A. Day, M. C. Anderson, T. C. Stephen, J. A. Gilbert, and L. W. Day, 2004, Edmonton, AB: Faculty of Nursing, University of Alberta.)

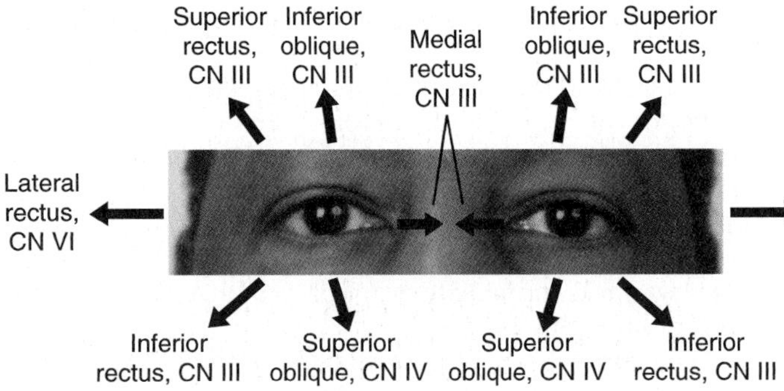

FIGURE **28–26** Cranial nerves and extraocular muscles associated with the six cardinal fields of gaze. (From *Mosby's Guide to Physical Examination,* 5th ed., p. 291, Figure 10–20, by H. M. Seidel et al., 2003, St. Louis, MO: Mosby.)

When testing for accommodation (near reaction), expect the pupils to converge and accommodate by constricting when looking at close objects with equal pupillary responses. To remember this response, nurses should think of "constrict" with up "close" and "dilate" with "distance."

Visual Fields. Assess visual fields to determine clients' peripheral vision (Procedure 28-4). When a client looks straight ahead, expect that all objects in the periphery can be seen. The visual field of each eye includes 180 degrees. Clients with visual field problems may be at risk for injury because they cannot see all of the objects surrounding them.

Extraocular Movements. Six small muscles move the eyes in parallel directions in each of the six directions of gaze (Figure 28–26 and Procedure 28-4). Parallel eye movement, position of the upper eyelid in relation to the iris, and the presence of unexpected movements during conjugate movement are assessed. As eyes move through each direction of gaze, the upper eyelids cover the iris only slightly. By periodically stopping movement of the finger, the nurse assesses **nystagmus,** an involuntary, rhythmical oscillation of the eyes. Local injury to the eye muscles or supporting structures and disorders of the cranial nerves that innervate muscles can be detected. The nurse can also assess the extraocular muscles of the eyes by using the corneal light reflex test (see Procedure 28-4). A weakness or imbalance of the extraocular muscles may cause misalignment. Expect the light to reflect on the cornea in the same spot on both eyes. If muscle impairment is present, the light is reflected from a different spot on each eye. The cover test can replace the corneal light reflection test.

Inspection and Internal Eye Structures

Funduscopic Examination. The internal eye is observed with the ophthalmoscope to inspect the fundus, which includes the retina, choroid, optic nerve disc, macula, fovea centralis, and retinal vessels. The ophthalmoscope has a battery tube light source, two dials or disks, and a keyhole viewer (Figure 28–27). The dial at the top of the battery tube changes the light image. Five lenses are available, but the small white light is used for general examination. To adjust the focus, the examiner rotates the dial at the top of the viewer clockwise.

The nurse should practise holding the ophthalmoscope in each hand, using the index finger to rotate the lens dial (putting the "digit on the widget"). Nurses turn the white light on, rotate the lens dial to *0,* look through the keyhole, and focus on near objects such as the palm of the hand. Reading a newspaper with the ophthalmoscope is useful practice. During an examination, both examiner eyes are open when looking through the keyhole.

The examination is done in a dimly lit room. The nurse and client stand or sit in comfortable positions facing each

Procedure 28-4 Assessing Visual Fields and Extraocular Movements

Equipment

- Penlight

Examination Skill and Focus	Steps	Rationale
Visual fields by confrontation CN II (optic)	**1.** Position self 60 cm away from client with eyes level.	Ensures comfortable distance for focus.
Visual fields	**2.** Instruct client to cover one eye and to look at examiner's eye directly opposite.	Tests each eye separately.
	3. Cover own eye opposite to client's covered eye.	Allows comparison to examiner's field of vision.
	4. Instruct client to indicate when wiggling finger seen.	
	5. Test temporal, inferotemporal, and superotemporal fields of vision by placing wiggling finger somewhat behind client and slowly moving it within client's visual field.	Assesses all fields for each eye.
	6. Test nasal, superior, and inferior fields of vision in turn by maintaining wiggling finger equidistant between client and self. Test eight different positions for each eye.	
	7. Slowly move wiggling finger within visual fields.	
	8. Compare client's visual field against own. X = Temporal X_1 = Inferotemporal X_2 = Superotemporal	

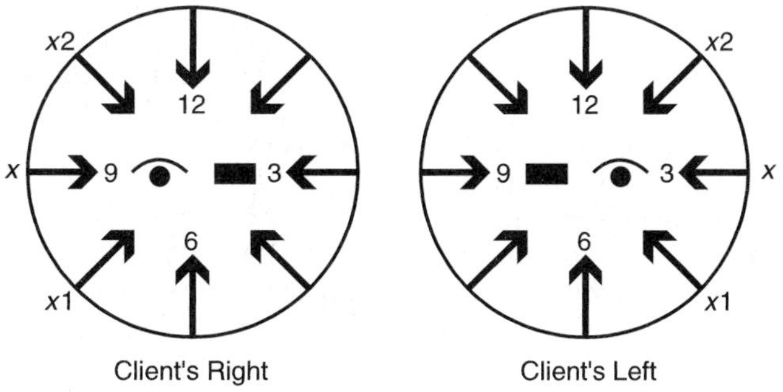

STEP **6**

From *A Syllabus for Adult Health Assessment* (p. 32), edited by D. L. Skillen and R. A. Day, 2004, Edmonton, AB: Faculty of Nursing, University of Alberta.

Continued

Procedure 28-4 Assessing Visual Fields and Extraocular Movements, cont'd

Equipment

- Splintered tongue blade
- Cotton ball

Examination Skill and Focus	Steps	Rationale
Extraocular muscles and movements CN III, IV, VI (oculomotor, trochlear, abducens)	**1.** Inspect extraocular muscle function by performing: a. Cardinal directions test **AND** b. Cover test **OR** c. Corneal reflection test	
a. Cardinal directions (extraocular movements)	**1.** Ask client if wearing contact lenses.	Contacts may be dislodged with lateral and medial directions.
	2. Position self so client can focus.	
	3. Instruct client to follow finger or pen (consider age) without moving head.	Ensures movement of eyes is assessed, not movement of head.
	4. Move finger slowly avoiding straight up and down midline position to client's (R) in line with shoulder, upward to (R) of midline, downward to (R) of midline, to client's (L) in line with shoulder, upward to (L) of midline, downward to (L) of midline.	Assesses all directions.
Parallel tracking, nystagmus, lid lag	**5.** Avoid fixation of extreme lateral points.	Uncomfortable for client
	6. Observe for parallel tracking (conjugate movements), nystagmus, and lid lag.	
b. Cover test	**1.** Keep eyes level with those of client.	
	2. Instruct client to look at examiner.	
	3. Hold opaque cover over one eye for 5 to 10 seconds before removing it quickly, without warning and without touching.	Gives enough time for eye to deviate from original position before cover is removed.
	4. Observe eye that was covered.	Movement of the eye after uncovering indicates it moved while covered.
	5. Repeat with other eye.	
c. Corneal reflections	**1.** Stand at least 0.6 m away from client.	
	2. Shine penlight from midline of examiner directly onto bridge of client's nose; ask client to look directly at light.	Ensures comfortable distance for focus.
	3. Observe site on each cornea from which light is reflected.	Observe symmetry to assess alignment.

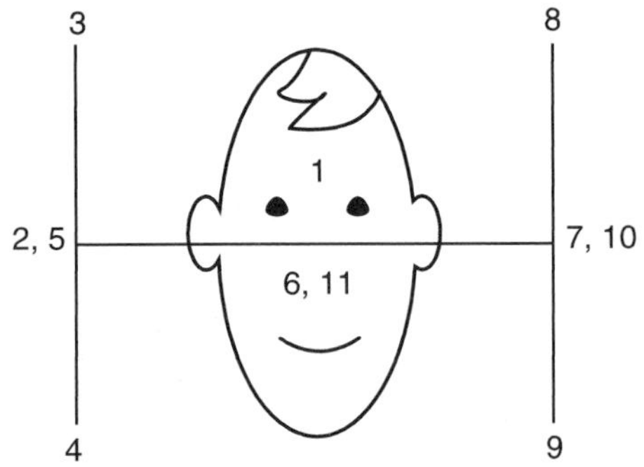

From *A Syllabus for Adult Health Assessment* (p. 32), edited by D. L. Skillen and R. A. Day, 2004, Edmonton, AB: Faculty of Nursing, University of Alberta.

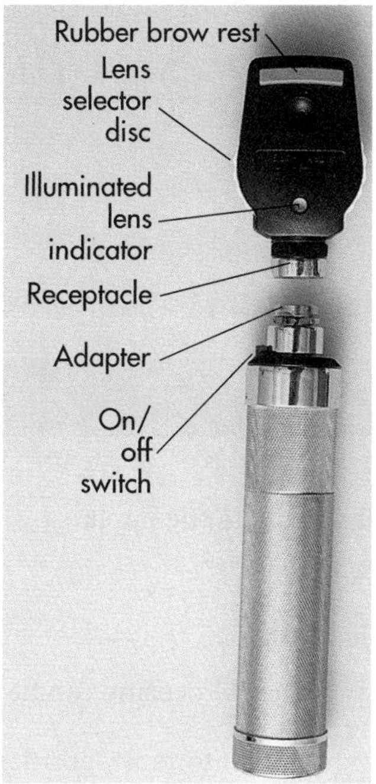

FIGURE **28–27** Ophthalmoscope. (From *Mosby's Guide to Physical Examination,* 5th ed., p. 69, by H. M. Seidel et al., 2003, St. Louis, MO: Mosby.)

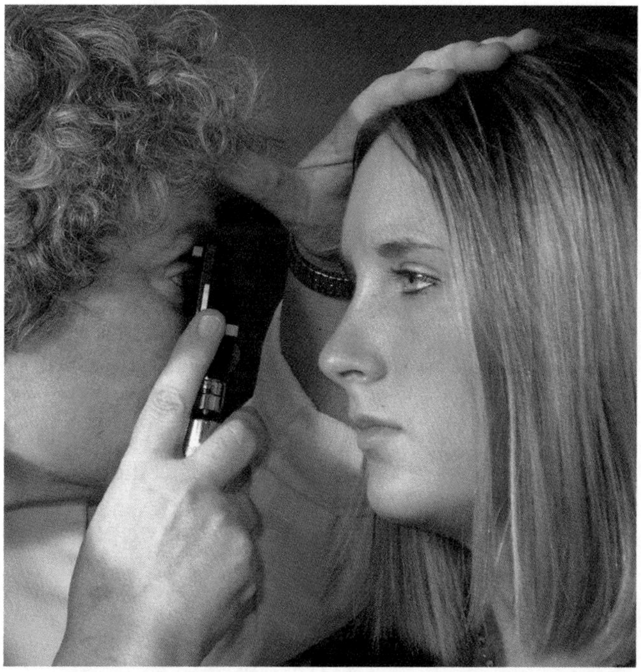

FIGURE **28–28** Ophthalmoscopic examination. (From *Physical Examination Images* [CD-ROM], by D. L. Skillen, R. A. Day, M. C. Anderson, T. C. Stephen, J. A. Gilbert, and L. W. Day, 2004, Edmonton, AB: Faculty of Nursing, University of Alberta.)

other with their eyes at the same height. The client removes eyeglasses, but contact lenses may be left in place, and the examiner may decide to keep eyeglasses on, especially if the correction in diopters is high. The nurse holds the ophthalmoscope against his or her face (Figure 28–28 and Procedure 28-5). A bright orange glow in the pupil, called the red reflex, can usually be seen. The light from the ophthalmoscope causes the pupil to constrict. Moving slowly toward the pupil while keeping the light focused on the red reflex, the nurse begins to see structures of the fundus. Rotating the lens dial brings the internal structures into focus. These structures are inspected for size, colour, and disc clarity; integrity of the vessels; presence of retinal lesions; and appearance of the macula and fovea (Figure 28–29). Expect to see the following structures:

- Clear, yellow optic nerve disc
- Reddish-pink retina (Caucasions) or darkened retina (Black Canadians)
- Light red arterioles and dark red veins
- A 3:2 vein-to-artery ratio in size proportion
- Avascular macula

If any unexpected findings are observed, the client should be referred for further examination. Box 28-24 describes common types of visual problems. The fundus should not be illuminated for extended periods. The bright light of the ophthalmoscope is very irritating and can cause discomfort and tearing.

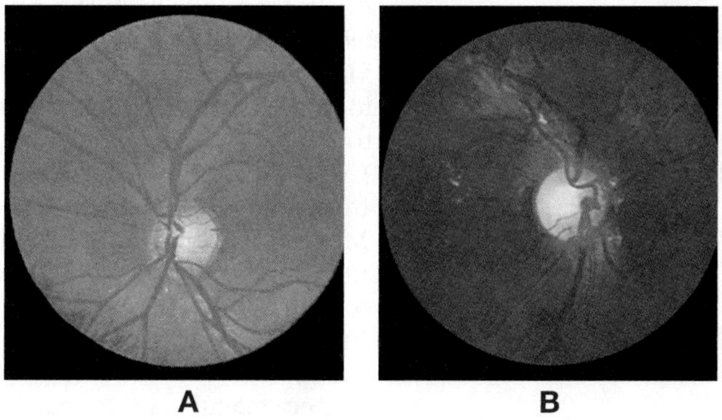

FIGURE **28–29** Fundus of **A,** White client and **B,** Black client. (Courtesy MEDCOM, Cypress, CA.)

Age-Related Changes. Age-related changes occur in the external and internal structures of the eyes as well as in visual acuity. Aging causes loss of the lateral third of the eyebrows, and older adults frequently have lid margins that turn out (ectropion) or in (entropion). An entropion may cause lashes to irritate the conjunctiva and cornea, increasing the risk of infection. The elastic tissues around the eyes atrophy, which results in wrinkles or crow's feet. Orbital fat decreases, which results in the eyes appearing sunken. Other changes include decreased tear production, loss of the lustre in the cornea, and fading of the iris. A thin white ring along the margin of the cornea (arcus senilis) is common with aging. A gradual decline in visual acuity begins after 50 years of age, resulting in the need for visual aids. Changes in the lens reduce peripheral vision and alter accommodation.

Documentation. Nurses record their findings from inspection and palpation of the eyes (Table 28-29).

Procedure 28-5 Assessing the Internal Structures of the Eyes

Equipment

- Ophthalmoscope

Examination Skill and Focus	Steps	Rationale
Fundus	Both eyes	
Inspection by ophthalmoscope	**1.** Instruct client to look slightly up and over examiner's shoulder at specific point on wall.	Helps to dilate the pupil.
	2. Turn lens disc of ophthalmoscope to 0 diopters.	
	3. Maintain index finger on lens disc for refocusing during examination.	Ensures that refocusing can be done easily.
	4. Use (R) hand, (R) eye for client's (R) eye. **5.** Use (L) hand, (L) eye for client's (L) eye.	Avoids uncomfortable positioning of client and examiner.
	6. Shine **small** light beam on pupil from about 40 cm away from client and 15 degrees lateral to midline.	Small light beam reduces amount of pupil constriction. Angle increases likelihood of seeing the optic disc.
	7. Place hand on client's forehead above eye being examined with thumb extended.	Stabilizes the ophthalmoscope and ensures correct distance from eye.
Red reflex	**8.** Observe for red reflex.	
	9. Move in toward client while maintaining focus on pupil and until eyelashes almost touch.	
Disc, cups, arterioles	**10.** Inspect disc, cup, arterioles, veins, crossings, adjusting lens disc if necessary.	Adjusts lens until structures are in focus.
Veins, crossings	**11.** Move head and ophthalmoscope as one unit and follow vessels peripherally in four directions.	Ensures proper visualization of structures.
Macula	**12.** Instruct client to briefly look directly at the light.	Increases the opportunity to see macula and fovea.
	13. Inspect macula and fovea.	

From *A Syllabus for Adult Health Assessment* (p. 33), edited by D. L. Skillen and R. A. Day, 2004, Edmonton, AB: Faculty of Nursing, University of Alberta.

Ears

The ear has three parts: external, middle, and inner ear structures (Figure 28–30). The external ear is inspected and palpated; the middle ear structures are inspected with an otoscope; and the inner ear is assessed by measuring hearing acuity and sound conduction. External ear structures consist of the auricle, tragus, outer ear canal, and tympanic membrane (eardrum). The ear canal is usually curved and approximately 2.54 cm long in an adult. It is lined with skin containing fine hairs, nerve endings, and glands secreting cerumen (earwax). The middle ear is an air-filled cavity that contains three bony ossicles (malleus, incus, and stapes). The eustachian tube connects the middle ear to the nasopharynx and stabilizes pressure between the outer atmosphere and the middle ear. The inner ear contains the cochlea, vestibule, and semicircular canals. The nurse assesses the integrity of ear structures and the condition of hearing.

Health history data (Table 28-30) aid in identifying risks for hearing disorders. An understanding of the mechanisms for sound transmission helps nurses identify the nature of hearing disorders. Sound travels through the ear by air and bone conduction in the following sequence:

1. Sound waves in the air enter the external ear, passing through the outer ear canal;

Box 28-24 Common Eye and Visual Problems

Hyperopia

Hyperopia is farsightedness, a refractive error in which rays of light enter the eye and focus behind the retina. People are able to clearly see distant objects but not close objects.

Strabismus

Strabismus is a congenital problem in which the eyes appear crossed. The muscles controlling movement of the eyes are not coordinated.

Myopia

Myopia is nearsightedness, a refractive error in which rays of light enter the eye and focus in front of the retina. People are able to clearly see close objects but not distant objects.

Cataracts

A cataract is an increased opacity of the lens, which blocks light rays from entering the eye. Cataracts may develop slowly and progressively after the age of 35 years or suddenly after trauma. Cataracts are one of the most common eye disorders. By age 70, most adults have some evidence of visual impairment from cataracts.

Presbyopia

Presbyopia is impaired near vision in middle-aged and older adults and is caused by loss of elasticity of the lens associated with the aging process.

Glaucoma

Glaucoma is intraocular structural damage resulting from elevated intraocular pressure. It is caused by obstruction of the outflow of aqueous humor. Without treatment, the disorder can cause blindness.

Astigmatism

Astigmatism is a condition in which parallel light rays do not focus on a single point on the retina. An uneven curvature of the cornea or lens causes light to be focused on different points.

Macular Degeneration

Macular degeneration is blurred central vision often occurring suddenly, caused by a progressive degeneration of the centre of the retina. It is the most common visual impairment of individuals over age 50 and the most common cause of blindness in older adults. There is no cure.

Retinopathy

Retinopathy is a non-inflammatory eye disorder resulting from changes in retinal blood vessels. It is a leading cause of blindness.

2. Sound waves reach the tympanic membrane, causing it to vibrate;
3. Vibrations are transmitted through the middle ear by the bony ossicular chain to the oval window at the opening of the inner ear;
4. The cochlea receives the sound vibration; and
5. Nerve impulses from the cochlea travel to the auditory (eighth cranial) nerve and cerebral cortex.

Disorders of the ear result from several types of problems, including mechanical dysfunction (blockage by earwax or foreign body), trauma (foreign bodies or noise exposure), neurological disorders (auditory nerve damage), acute illnesses (viral infection), and toxic effects of medications. Box 28-25 contains client teaching and health promotion opportunities.

External Ear Structures

Auricles and Tragus. Begin by inspecting the auricle size, shape, symmetry, landmarks, position, and colour (Figure 28–31 and Procedure 28-6). Expect the auricles to be level with each other. The upper point of attachment is in a straight line with the lateral canthus (corner of the eye). The position of the auricle should also be almost vertical. Ears that are at an unusual angle or low set may indicate a chromosome abnormality (e.g., Down syndrome). Auricle colour should be the same as that of the face, without moles, cysts, deformities, or nodules. Any redness is a sign of inflammation or fever; extreme pallor can indicate frostbite.

Palpate the auricles for texture, tenderness, and skin lesions, expecting smoothness and freedom from lesions. Tenderness is assessed when the tragus and mastoid process are palpated (see Procedure 28-6). If palpation of the external ear produces pain, an external ear infection is likely; if palpation of the auricle and tragus does not influence the pain, the client could have a middle ear infection. Tenderness in the mastoid area can indicate an infection (mastoiditis).

Hearing Acuity. Often nurses can tell if a client has hearing loss from the response to conversation. Three types of hearing loss occur: conductive, sensorineural, and mixed. A conduction loss interrupts sound waves travelling from the outer ear to the cochlea of the inner ear, preventing transmission through the outer and middle ear structures. Swelling of the auditory canal and perforations in the tympanic membrane can cause conduction loss. A sensorineural loss involves the inner ear, auditory nerve, or hearing centre of the brain. Sound is still conducted through the outer and middle ear structures,

Table 28-29 Examples of Documentation for Eye Assessment

Focus of Assessment	Expected Findings	Unexpected Findings
Eyebrows/lids/lashes	Full, lie close to eye, colour consistent with complexion, complete closure over sclera; no scaling, edema, lesions, or lid lag; symmetrical palpebral folds; curl outward, equal hair distribution	Patchy areas of eyebrows; redness noted on lateral half of (R) eyelid; asymmetrical movement of eyelids during blinking.
Cornea/lens	Clear, transparent, shiny	Small opacity (L) cornea
Corneal reflex	Brisk bilateral blinking	Bilateral blinking absent
Iris	Blue, green, brown; circular, equal size, shape, and colour; flat when viewed from side	(R) blue and (L) brown
Conjunctiva/sclera	Pink/white/clear	Yellowish opacity on (L) inferior, medial surface; engorged blood vessels noted in (L) eye
Lacrimal sacs/glands	No swelling or redness	Tenderness noted upon palpation; yellowish discharge from (R) eye; excessive tearing noted
Pupils (Cranial nerves II and III)	Equal and round at 3 mm	Unequal
Pupillary reaction to light	PERRLA (pupils equal, round, reactive to light, and accommodation)	Sluggish, fixed, unequal
Near reaction (accommodation)	Pupils dilate with distant gaze, constrict with near gaze	Pupils remain dilated with near gaze
Convergence	Present to 5 cm	Focus breaks at 10 cm
Confrontation	Full visual fields bilaterally	(L) inferotemporal field absent
Extraocular muscles	Parallel movement in six positions of gaze; no nystagmus or lid lag; gaze maintained in cover test; corneal light reflected symmetrically	(L) eye unable to follow six positions; corneal light reflected asymmetrically
Funduscopy (lens)	Clear, full red reflex bilaterally	Red reflex absent (R)
Funduscopy (vessels)	Arterioles 2/3 size of veins, smooth crossings; arterioles have bright light reflections	Arterioles and veins equal in size; A/V nicking present
Funduscopy (disc)	Round, margins well-defined, yellowish pink colour	Irregular-shaped border in (L) eye

From "Documentation" by T. C. Stephen in *Health Assessment Self-Test Modules* (WebCT Vista), 2004, Edmonton, AB: Faculty of Nursing, University of Alberta.

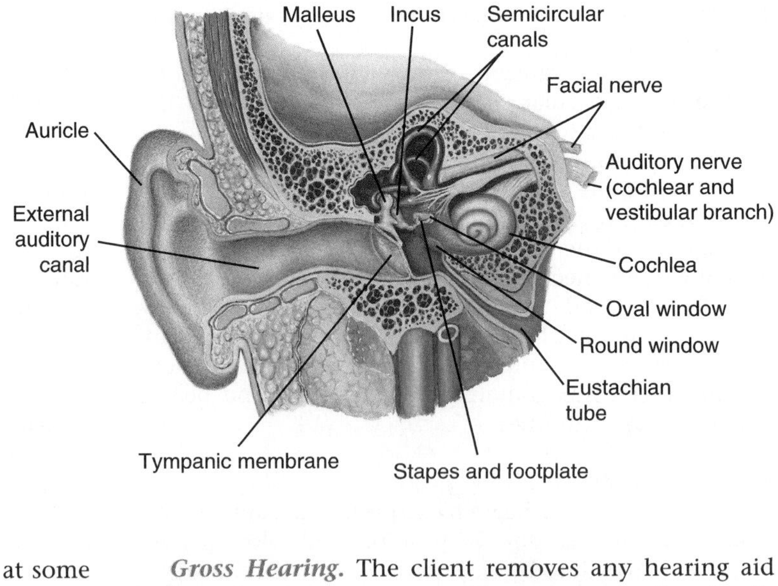

FIGURE **28–30** Anatomy of the ear. (From *Mosby's Guide to Physical Examination,* 5th ed., p. 314, Figure 11–2, by H. M. Seidel et al., 2003, St. Louis, MO: Mosby.)

but transmission of sound becomes interrupted at some point beyond the bony ossicles. A mixed loss involves a combination of conduction and sensorineural loss. Clients who work or live around loud noises are at risk for hearing loss. Adolescents risk premature hearing loss from continued exposure to loud music at home, in the car, or at concert events.

Gross Hearing. The client removes any hearing aid before a hearing assessment. The nurse notes the client's response to questions. If suspecting hearing loss, the nurse checks the client's response to the whispered voice (Procedure 28-7). Clients usually hear numbers clearly when whispered, responding correctly at least 50% of the time (Seidel et al., 2003).

Table 28-30 Health History for Ear Assessment

Assessment Category	Rationale
Document behaviours that suggest hearing loss, such as failure to respond when spoken to, requests to repeat commands, leaning forward to hear or inattentiveness.	Clients with hearing loss may compensate with certain behavioural cues.
Ask if client is experiencing any hearing difficulties or illnesses related to their ears and conduct a symptom analysis.	Different symptoms reveal the cause of ear problems, such as pain from an ear infection.
Inquire about excess accumulation of cerumen in ear canals.	Excessive amounts can interfere with client's ability to hear adequately.
Question client as to risks for hearing impairment, such as head trauma or excessive occupational or recreational noise, and client's use of protective ear equipment.	Prolonged exposure to loud noises can temporarily or permanently alter hearing.
Ask client about medication use, such as large doses of aspirin or other ototoxic drugs.	Some medications have a side effect of ringing in the ears or hearing loss.
Ask if client uses a hearing aid.	Alerts examiner to adjust tone of voice.
Inquire about regularity of hearing tests.	Date of last hearing test will reveal preventative care of ears.

Client Teaching — Box 28-25

Ear Assessment

Objectives

- Client will practise and understand rationale for proper techniques to care for ears.
- Client will follow preventative guidelines for screening of hearing loss.
- Client will understand age-related changes to hearing.

Teaching Strategies

- Inform client of the proper way to clean ears (see chapter 34), avoiding use of cotton-tipped applicators and sharp objects as cleaning instruments.
- Inform client to never insert a pointed object into ear canal.
- Encourage client to have regular hearing tests, particularly over the age of 65 years.
- Inform client that a decrease in hearing acuity is expected with aging (see chapter 44).
- With a client who has reduced hearing ability, avoid shouting, and use direct eye contact.

Evaluation

- Have client explain proper cleaning technique for ears.
- Have client report date of last hearing test.

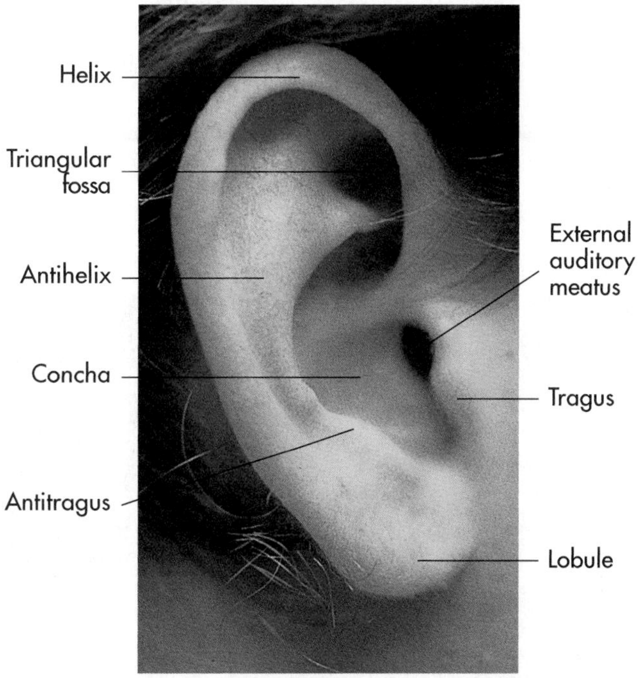

FIGURE 28–31 Anatomical structures of the auricle. (From *Mosby's Guide to Physical Examination,* 5th ed., p. 315, by H. M. Seidel et al., 2003, St. Louis, MO: Mosby.)

Weber Test. To assess hearing acuity, examiners can perform tests using a tuning fork or audiometer. The Weber test assesses for lateralization of sound (see Procedure 28-7 and Figure 28–32). Clients with unimpaired hearing are expected to hear sound equally in both ears with the Weber test. If clients have conduction deafness, the sound is heard best in the impaired ear. If clients have sensorineural hearing loss, the sound is identified only in the unimpaired ear.

Rinné Test. The Rinné test compares air and bone conduction (see Procedure 28-7 and Figure 28–33). Air-conducted sound should be heard twice as long as bone-conducted sound. For clients with conduction deafness, bone-conducted sound can be heard longer. In sensorineural loss, sound is reduced and heard for a short time through air and bone.

Procedure 28-6 Inspecting and Palpating the Ears

Equipment

- None

Examination Skill and Focus	Steps	Rationale
Inspection:	Ears fully exposed	
Auricle, mastoid surface	**1.** Inspect auricle and mastoid bilaterally, adjusting hair where necessary for clear vision.	Ensure that all areas are visible.
Alignment	**1.** Inspect alignment of ears from anterior and lateral views (angle of attachment, horizontal, vertical).	Allows comparison between ears and with alignment of eyes.
Palpation:	**1.** Inquire about tenderness during palpation.	Tenderness may indicate inflammatory or infectious process.
Mastoid surface	**2.** Palpate both mastoid surfaces of temporal bones with pads of fingers.	
Auricle	**3.** Pull up on each auricle.	
Tragus	**4.** Press on each tragus with fingertip.	

From *A Syllabus for Adult Health Assessment* (p. 28), edited by D. L. Skillen and R. A. Day, 2004, Edmonton, AB: Faculty of Nursing, University of Alberta.

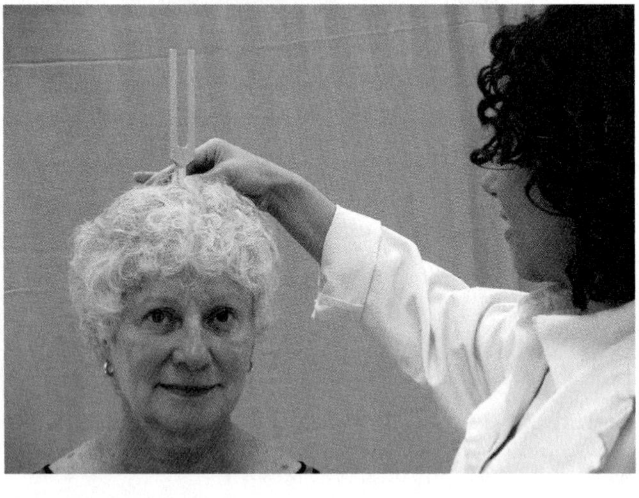

FIGURE **28–32** Weber test by nursing student. (From *Physical Examination Images* [CD-ROM], by D. L. Skillen, R. A. Day, M. C. Anderson, T. C. Stephen, J. A. Gilbert, and L. W. Day, 2004, Edmonton, AB: Faculty of Nursing, University of Alberta.)

Otoscopic Examination

External Ear Canals and Eardrums. The opening of the ear canal is inspected for size and discharge. Discharge may be accompanied by an odour. Yellow or green foul-smelling discharge may indicate infection or a foreign body. The meatus should not be swollen or occluded. A yellow, waxy substance called **cerumen** is commonly present.

Deeper structures of the external and middle ear are observed only with an **otoscope,** which is an ophthalmoscope with a special ear speculum attached to the battery tube (Procedure 28-8). Speculums come in different sizes to conform to the different sizes of ear canals. For best visualization, the largest speculum that fits comfortably into the ear canal is used. Before insertion, the examiner checks for foreign bodies in the opening of the auditory canal. Clients must not move their heads during the examination to avoid damage to the canal and tympanic membrane. The nurse holds the handle of the otoscope in the space between the thumb and index finger, supported on the middle finger. This leaves the ulnar side of the hand to brace against the client's head, stabilizing the otoscope as it is inserted into the canal (Seidel et al., 2003).

Two grips on the otoscope may be used. In one, the nurse holds the battery tube the length of the client's face with the fingers against the face or neck. In the other, the inverted otoscope is lightly braced against the side of the client's head or cheek. This grip, used with children and any adult who might move unexpectedly, prevents accidental movement of the otoscope deeper into the ear canal. The nurse straightens the ear canal in adults by pulling the auricle upward, backward, and slightly out (Figure 28–34). The speculum is inserted slightly down and forward 1.0 to 1.5 cm into the ear canal, avoiding contact

Procedure 28-7 Assessing Hearing Acuity

Equipment

• Tuning fork (512 Hz or 1024 Hz)

Examination Skill and Focus	Steps	Rationale
CN VIII (acoustic) Test hearing Gross hearing Cranial nerve VIII	Each ear separately **1.** Mask hearing in one ear by moving fingertip in client's auditory canal.	Ensures that the ear being tested can hear the examiner without help from the other ear.
	2. Stand 0.3 to 0.6 m from client (ensuring that client cannot lip-read). **3.** Exhale fully and direct whisper toward ear being tested. **4.** Start with three low whispered, two-syllable, equally accented numbers or words. **Only if** client does not identify first numbers or words in low whispers, gradually increase intensity of whispering (while changing numbers or words) to spoken voice.	
Weber test	**1.** Select tuning fork of 512 or 1024 Hz.	Assesses sound within human speech range.
	2. Activate tuning fork using: a. thumb and finger **OR** b. reflex hammer **OR** c. other part of hand	Creates a sound for testing.
	3. Hold base of vibrating tuning fork. **4.** Press end of base of vibrating tuning fork firmly on: a. midline of skull **OR** b. midline of forehead	
	5. Ask client, "Where do you hear the sound?"	Assesses for lateralization of sound.
Rinné test	**1.** Select tuning fork of 512 or 1024 Hz. **2.** Activate tuning fork using: a. thumb and finger **OR** b. reflex hammer **OR** c. other part of hand **3.** Hold base of vibrating tuning fork and place end on mastoid surface level with ear canal. **4.** Request client to indicate when sound is no longer heard.	
	5. Following client response, place vibrating tuning fork about 2.54 cm from auditory meatus of same ear with "U" facing forward (anteriorly).	Assesses bone conduction of sound.
	6. Ask client if sound is heard.	Assesses whether air conduction is longer than bone conduction.

From *A Syllabus for Adult Health Assessment* (pp. 28–29), edited by D. L. Skillen and R. A. Day, 2004, Edmonton, AB: Faculty of Nursing, University of Alberta.

A

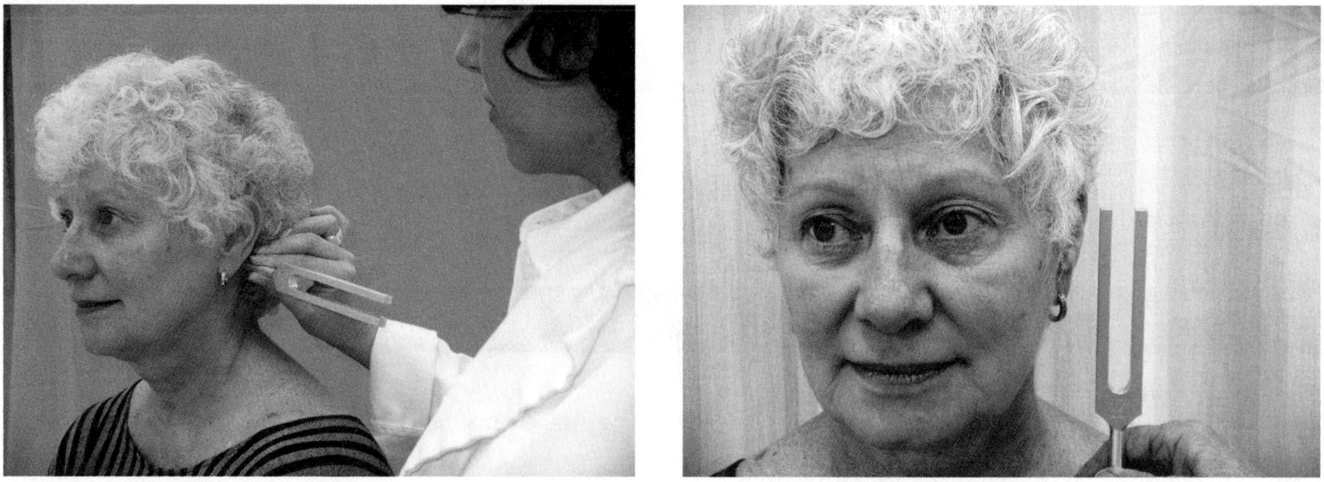

B

FIGURE **28–33** Rinné test. **A,** Bone conduction. **B,** Air conduction. (From *Physical Examination Images* [CD-ROM], by D. L. Skillen, R. A. Day, M. C. Anderson, T. C. Stephen, J. A. Gilbert, and L. W. Day, 2004, Edmonton, AB: Faculty of Nursing, University of Alberta.)

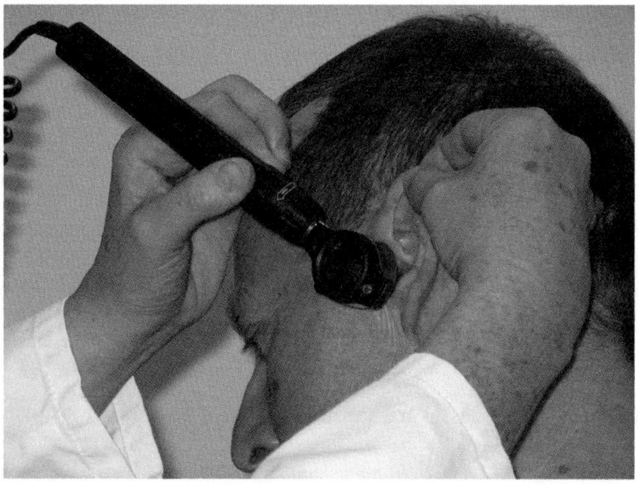

FIGURE **28–34** Otoscopic examination. (From *Physical Examination Images* [CD-ROM], by D. L. Skillen, R. A. Day, M. C. Anderson, T. C. Stephen, J. A. Gilbert, and L. W. Day, 2004, Edmonton, AB: Faculty of Nursing, University of Alberta.)

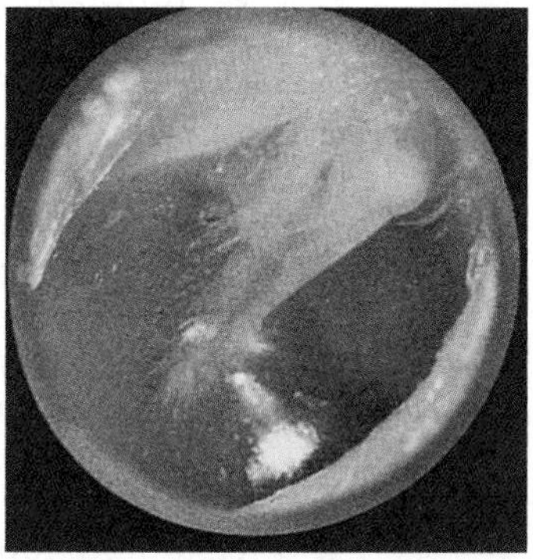

FIGURE **28–35** Healthy right tympanic membrane. (Courtesy Dr. Richard A. Buckingham, Abraham Lincoln School of Medicine, University of Illinois, Chicago, IL.)

with the sensitive lining of the ear canal. The skin of the lining has little subcutaneous fat between it and the underlying bone. The canal usually has limited cerumen and is uniformly pink with tiny hairs in its outer third. The examiner observes for colour, discharge, scaling, lesions, foreign bodies, and cerumen. The cerumen is expected to be dry (light brown to grey and flaky) or moist (dark yellow or brown) and sticky. Dry cerumen occurs in Asian and Aboriginal clients about 85% of the time (Seidel et al., 2003). In other adults, accumulated cerumen is common and can create a mild hearing loss. A reddened canal with discharge is a sign of inflammation or infection.

The light from the otoscope allows visualization of the tympanic membrane (Figure 28–35). Moving the otoscope slowly permits the entire tympanic membrane and its periphery to be seen. Because the tympanic membrane is angled away from the ear canal (toward the examiner), the light reflected from the otoscope appears as a cone. A ring of fibrous cartilage surrounds the oval membrane. The umbo is near the centre of the membrane, and the attachment of the malleus is behind it. A knob-like structure at the top of the tympanic membrane is created by the underlying short process of the malleus. Nurses should check carefully to make sure that there are no tears or breaks in the membrane. The tympanic membrane is translucent, shiny, and pearly grey. It is taut, except for the small triangular pars flaccida near the top. A pink or red bulging membrane indicates inflammation. A white colour reveals pus behind the tympanic membrane.

Age-Related Changes. Aging can affect hearing. Older adults have reduced ability to hear high-frequency sounds

Procedure 28-8 Otoscopy

Equipment
- Otoscope

Examination Skill and Focus	Steps	Rationale
Inspection by otoscopy:	**Otoscopic examination** (each ear, tender ear last)	
	1. Select largest ear speculum that fits in canal.	
	2. Brace hand against head when holding otoscope.	Stabilizes otoscope to prevent injuring client.
	3. Lift auricle upward, backward, and slightly out from head **before inserting** speculum.	Helps straighten ear canal of adult for better visualization.
	4. Instruct client to tilt head slightly toward other shoulder.	
	5. Insert speculum gently and not deeply.	
Auditory canal	**6.** Inspect auditory canal.	
Tympanic membrane, cone of light, umbo, handle of the malleus, short process	**7.** Inspect tympanic membrane, handle of malleus, umbo, cone of light, short process (structures and vascularity).	
	8. Adjust position of speculum in order to visualize drum entirely.	
	9. Remove speculum before releasing auricle.	Prevents possible trauma to ear canal.

From *A Syllabus for Adult Health Assessment* (p. 29), edited by D. L. Skillen and R. A. Day, 2004, Edmonton, AB: Faculty of Nursing, University of Alberta.

and consonants (e.g., *s, z, t,* and *g*). Deterioration of the cochlea and thickening of the tympanic membrane gradually reduces hearing acuity. The tympanic membrane may be whiter and duller than in younger adults. Older adults are especially at risk for hearing loss due to ototoxicity (injury to auditory nerve) that results from high-maintenance doses of antibiotics (e.g., the aminoglycosides). Other changes are the appearance of coarse hairs at the auditory opening and pendulous earlobes with linear creases.

Documentation. Nurses record their findings from inspection and palpation of the ears (Table 28-31).

Nose

The nose consists of bone, cartilage, nares, and septum, all of which can be examined with the client in a sitting position. The nose is expected to be smooth, symmetrical, placed in the centre of the face, and the same skin colour as the face. Air usually passes freely through both nostrils as a person breathes. The nasal septum is highly sensitive to touch and care must be taken to avoid direct contact with it. The health history guides the examination of the nose and paranasal sinuses (Table 28-32).

Data collected during the health history alert the nurse to client learning needs and opportunities for teaching during the physical examination (Box 28-26).

Inspection. The nurse begins by inspecting the nose from two perspectives for size, shape, skin characteristics, midline alignment, and the presence of deformity. To assess **patency** of the nares (open, no obstruction), the nurse inspects the nature of breathing sounds during full respirations. To assess ability to smell (function of cranial nerve I, the olfactory nerve), the nurse uses pungent odours (e.g., coffee, spices, alcohol). Noiseless breathing and odour identification are expected findings.

Palpation. Palpation of the nose follows inspection as the nurse notes any tenderness, masses, or underlying deviations. Nasal structures are usually firm, stable, and non-tender.

Inspection With Nasal Speculum. The nurse uses a nasal speculum to inspect the vestibule, septum, and inferior and middle turbinates and recalls that the septum is very sensitive. While illuminating the anterior nares (vestibule),

Table 28-31 Examples of Documentation for Ear Assessment

Area of Assessment	Expected Findings	Unexpected Findings
Auricle	Pink, smooth, intact, complete bilaterally	2 mm nodule on superior (R) auricle
Mastoid	Smooth, hard, non-tender (R) (L)	Tenderness noted on (L)
Gross hearing test (cranial nerve VIII)	Correctly identified three numbers bilaterally at a distance of 50 cm	Unable to identify numbers whispered in (L) ear after three attempts
Weber test	Heard in (R) and (L) equally	Lateralizes to (R) ear
Rinné test	AC > BC bilaterally; 2:1 ratio	AC = BC bilaterally
Otoscope (canal)	Pink, smooth, clear bilaterally	Obstructed bilaterally
Otoscope (cerumen)	Soft, light amber bilaterally	Small amount of hard, thick, dark, dry, brown (L)
Otoscope (tympanic membrane)	Intact, shiny, pearly grey bilaterally	Reddened black circular area centrally at umbo (R)
Otoscope (landmarks)	Cone of light shiny bilaterally; (R) at 5 o'clock (L) at 7 o'clock; well-defined handle of malleus, umbo, and annulus (R) (L)	Landmarks not visible in (R) or (L)

From *First Year Student Lab Guide* (p. 55), by J. Chambers et al., 2004, Edmonton, AB: Faculty of Nursing, University of Alberta.

Table 28-32 Health History for Nose and Sinus Assessment

Assessment Category	Rationale
Ask client about history of nasal trauma.	Past trauma may create tissue alteration, leading to impaired air entry.
Inquire about history of nosebleeds, postnasal drip, allergies, and nasal discharge.	History is helpful in determining nature of nasal conditions.
Question client about use of nasal sprays, medications, or illicit drugs.	Overuse of over-the-counter nasal sprays can cause damage to nasal mucosa and symptoms to recur (rebound). Cocaine damages septum.
Ask if client snores at night or experiences any breathing difficulties when sleeping.	Snoring or breathing difficulties may be caused by obstruction of the nostrils.

Client Teaching — Box 28-26

Nose and Sinus Assessment

Objectives

- Client will safely use over-the-counter nasal sprays.
- Older adult will take safety precautions with loss of smell (olfaction).

Teaching Strategies

- Caution client against overuse of over-the-counter nasal sprays that can lead to "rebound" effect, causing nasal congestion.
- Instruct older adults to install smoke detectors on each floor of home.
- Instruct older adults to check dated food labels to ensure against spoilage.

Evaluation

- Have client explain proper use of over-the-counter nasal sprays.
- Inspect client's home during visit and look for smoke detectors.
- Ask to check some food items in the refrigerator.

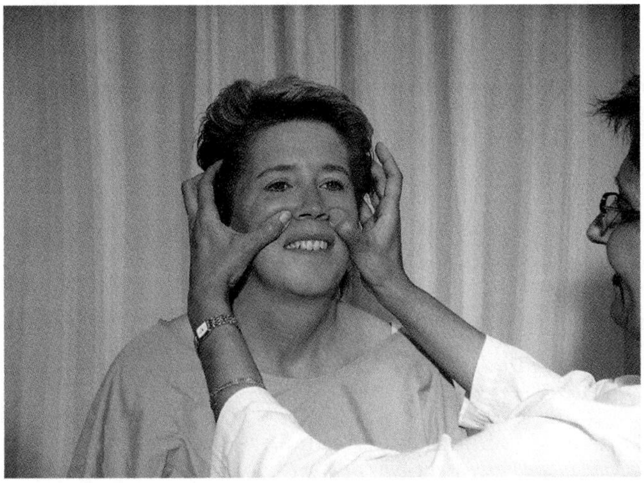

FIGURE **28–36** Palpation of maxillary sinuses. (From *Physical Examination Images* [CD-ROM], by D. L. Skillen, R. A. Day, M. C. Anderson, T. C. Stephen, J. A. Gilbert, and L. W. Day, 2004, Edmonton, AB: Faculty of Nursing, University of Alberta.)

the nurse inspects the mucosa for colour, lesions, discharge, swelling, and evidence of bleeding. The mucosa are expected to be pink and moist with clear mucus and no lesions. When clients have allergies, the mucosa may be pale pink and boggy. The septum is inspected for alignment, perforation, or bleeding. It is expected to be intact and aligned midline. Hair and red mucous membranes line the vestibule. The mucosa and inferior turbinates are inspected for colour, dryness, bleeding, and irritation.

Paranasal Sinuses

Paired sinuses in the frontal and maxillary facial areas are assessed by inspection and palpation (Figure 28–36 and Procedure 28-9). The skin over the sinuses is usually the same colour as the surrounding skin of the face and neither sinus area is expected to be tender to palpation. After inspecting the skin overlying the frontal and maxillary sinuses, the nurse assesses for tenderness most effectively by palpating both areas. Gentle pressure elicits tenderness easily if sinus irritation is present and reveals the severity of sinus irritation. Pressure should not be applied near the eyes.

Mouth and Pharynx

After the health history interview for the mouth and pharynx (Table 28-33), the nurse assesses for overall health of the mouth and pharynx and the status of oral hygiene. The data provide guidance for client teaching and health promotion (Box 28-27). Procedure 28-10 outlines the focus, procedures, and rationale for techniques used to assess the mouth and pharynx.

Inspection of the Mouth

Lips. Nurses inspect the lips for colour, texture, hydration, contour, and lesions, with the client's mouth closed. Lips are expected to be moist, smooth, and symmetrical at rest (Figure 28–37). Clients should remove lipstick prior to the examination.

Buccal Mucosa, Gums, and Teeth. The quality of dental hygiene is easily determined by inspecting the teeth when the position and alignment of teeth are also noted. To examine the posterior surface of the teeth, nurses examine clients with the mouth open and relaxed lips. Nurses may need a tongue depressor to retract lips and cheeks, especially when viewing the molars. Healthy teeth are smooth, white, and shiny. To view the mucosa and gums, the nurse asks the client to first remove any dentures. The nurse views the inner oral mucosa by having the client open and relax the mouth slightly, gently retracting the client's lower lip away from the teeth. This process is repeated with the upper lip. With a penlight, the nurse inspects the mucosa for colour, hydration, texture, and lesions such as ulcers, abrasions, or cysts. Mucous membrane is pinkish-red, smooth, and moist. If lesions are present, the nurse palpates them with a gloved hand for tenderness, size, and consistency. The nurse palpates the cheek with one finger inside the mouth and the thumb on the cheek to check for lesions or thickening. Gums are inspected for colour, edema, retraction, or bleeding. Gums around the back molars are inspected because the area is difficult to reach when cleaning teeth. Healthy gums are pink, smooth, moist, tight around each tooth, and non-tender.

Tongue and Floor of Mouth. Using penlight illumination, the nurse examines the ventral and dorsal surfaces of the tongue for colour, size, position, texture, coating, or lesions. The tongue is medium or dull red in colour, moist, slightly rough on the dorsal surface, and smooth along lateral margins. The ventral surface is highly vascular (Figure 28–38). The floor of the mouth is inspected for nodules, ulcerations, or white patches and palpated for lesions or indurations with a gloved hand. During testing of cranial nerve XII (hypoglossal), the nurse observes for symmetry, purposeful movements, and stillness at rest.

Safety Alert: Clients who chew tobacco or smoke cigarettes, cigars, or pipes have an increased risk of oral cancer. They may have leukoplakia or other lesions anywhere in the oral cavity at an early age.

Palates. The nurse inspects the hard and soft palates for colour, shape, symmetry, texture, and any lesions. The hard palate (roof of the mouth) is dome-shaped, whitish pink, and located superiorly. A benign enlargement (torus palatinus) may be present in the midline of Aboriginal and Asian clients (Overfield, 1995; Figure 28–39). The soft palate is light pink, smooth, and located posteriorly. The uvula (Figure 28–40) is midline, pink, and rises with the soft palate. The soft palate and uvula are innervated by cranial nerve X (vagus) and rise midline as the client says "ah."

Pharynx. The nurse inspects the arch formed by the anterior and posterior pillars, soft palate, and uvula. If present, the tonsils are seen in the cavities between the anterior and posterior pillars and are oval, with a rough surface or crypts. When present, the tonsils are graded on a 4-point scale (1 = visible, 4 = touching each other; Figure 28–41).

Procedure 28-9 Assessing the Nose and Paranasal Sinuses

Equipment

- Penlight
- Nasal speculum

Examination Skill and Focus	Steps	Rationale
Inspection:		
Nose	1. Inspect nose from anterior view and profile.	Abnormalities can best be noted with full inspection.
Frontal and maxillary sinuses	2. Inspect frontal and maxillary sinus regions.	
Palpation:		
Nose	1. Palpate entire length of nose with finger pads.	Abnormalities might only be detectable by palpation.
	2. Inquire of tenderness.	
Frontal, maxillary sinuses	3. Palpate maxillary sinuses simultaneously by pressing upward on maxillae with thumbs and ask about tenderness.	Congested or irritated sinuses create tenderness.
	4. Palpate frontal sinuses by pressing upward, inferior to the supraorbital ridge, from medial border of eyebrow to mid-eyebrow, using thumbs and ask about tenderness	
Test for patency:	1. Occlude each nostril in turn.	Assessment focuses on one nostril.
	2. Instruct client to breathe with mouth closed.	
	3. Listen to complete inspiration for each nostril.	Obstructed breathing may only occur in one phase of respiration.
Test of smell (Cranial nerve): CNI	1. Instruct client to close eyes.	Smell sensation is affected by abnormalities in cranial nerve I.
	2. Occlude one nostril (naris).	
	3. Hold pungent odour for client identification at opposite nostril. Ask client what odour is.	
	4. Change pungent odour and repeat on other side.	
Inspection with nasal speculum:	Both nostrils	
Nose	1. Instruct to tilt head back slightly.	
	2. Insert nasal speculum posteriorly in horizontal plane into vestibule of nares.	
	3. Stabilize speculum with index finger.	Prevents injury with client unexpected movement.
	4. Avoid touching septum.	Contact with nasal septum creates tenderness.
Mucous membrane, septum, inferior and middle turbinates	5. Inspect mucous membrane, septum, and inferior turbinates moving speculum slowly upward.	Middle turbinates become visible.
	6. Inspect middle turbinates and mucous membranes.	
	7. Offer client a tissue if needed.	

From *A Syllabus for Adult Health Assessment* (pp. 33–34), edited by D. L. Skillen and R. A. Day, 2004, Edmonton, AB: Faculty of Nursing, University of Alberta.

Table 28-33 Health History for Mouth and Pharyngeal Assessment

Assessment Category	Rationale
Ask if client wears dentures or other dental appliances and if they are comfortable.	Poorly fitting dental appliances irritate gums and mucosa, causing open sores.
Inquire about tobacco habits (smoking, chewing).	Tobacco use increases the risk of mouth and throat cancers.
Question client about usual dental hygiene practices, including dental checkups, cleaning, use of fluoride toothpaste, and frequency of brushing and flossing.	Good hygiene and regular dental care provide protection from mouth diseases. Examiner can assess need for further education.
Question client about appetite or recent changes in appetite.	Mouth disease can result in client having poor appetite and nutritional intake.

Client Teaching Box 28-27

Health Promotion for Mouth and Pharyngeal Assessment

Objectives

- Client will practise proper oral hygiene and dental care.
- Client will describe warning signs of oral cancers.
- Client will understand and practise self-care related to expected changes with age.

Teaching Strategies

- Discuss proper techniques for oral hygiene, including brushing and flossing teeth (see chapter 34).
- Inform client of warning signs of oral cancer, including a sore that bleeds easily and does not heal, a lump or thickening, and difficulty chewing or swallowing.
- Encourage regular dental examination every 6 months for all adults.
- Instruct older adults who are having difficulty chewing and changes in teeth to eat soft foods or cut food into small pieces.

Evaluation

- Have client illustrate brushing and oral hygiene techniques.
- Have client identify when to have regular dental examinations.
- Have client state the warning signs of oral cancers.

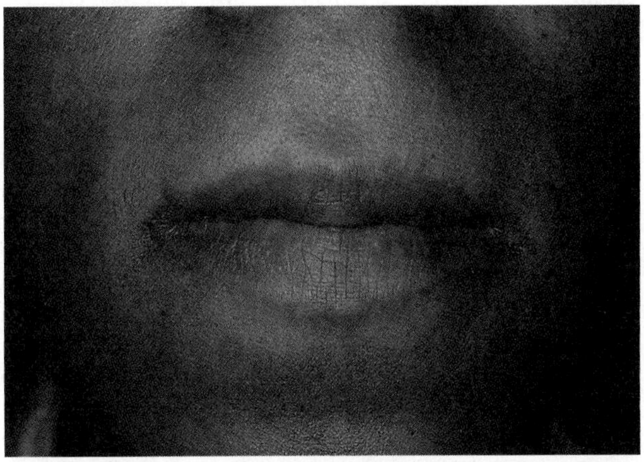

FIGURE 28–37 The lips are normally pink, symmetrical, smooth, and moist.

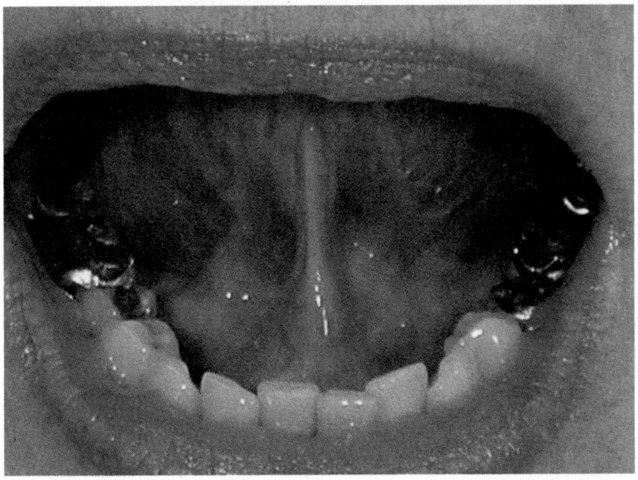

FIGURE 28–38 Inspection of undersurface of tongue. (From *Physical Examination Images* [CD-ROM], by D. L. Skillen, R. A. Day, M. C. Anderson, T. C. Stephen, J. A. Gilbert, and L. W. Day, 2004, Edmonton, AB: Faculty of Nursing, University of Alberta.)

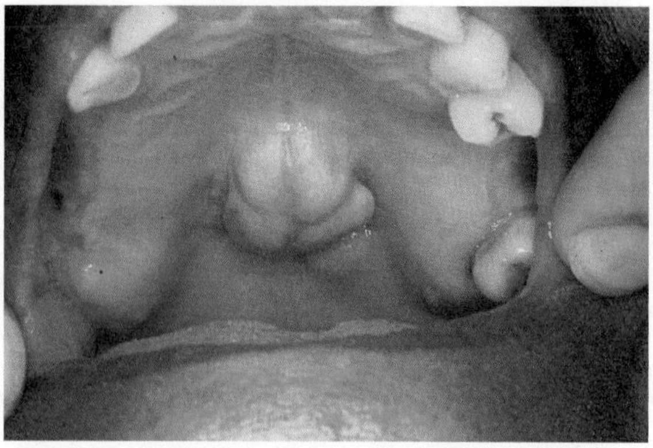

FIGURE **28–39** Torus palatinus (viewed with a mirror). (Courtesy Drs. Abelson and Cameron, Lutherville, MD.)

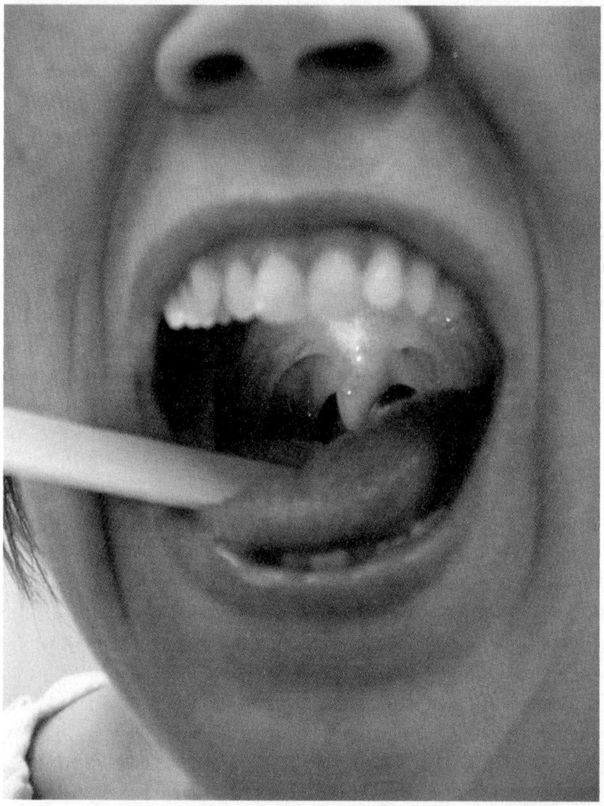

FIGURE **28–40** Uvula. (From *Physical Examination Images* [CD-ROM], by D. L. Skillen, R. A. Day, M. C. Anderson, T. C. Stephen, J. A. Gilbert, and L. W. Day, 2004, Edmonton, AB: Faculty of Nursing, University of Alberta.)

The posterior pharynx lies behind the pillars and tonsils. Pharyngeal tissues are expected to be pink and smooth. The nurse tests the gag reflex on the posterior pharyngeal wall bilaterally to assess the function of cranial nerves IX and X.

Age-Related Changes. In older adults, loose or missing teeth are common due to increased bone resorption. Teeth often feel rough when tooth enamel calcifies. Yellow or darkened teeth are also common because of general wear and tear that exposes the darker, underlying dentin. Oral mucosa become drier when salivation is decreased. Gums often appear pale. Tonsillar tissue is not usually seen in older adults. Bony ridges of the jaw that surround each tooth gradually resorb, especially in the lower jaw.

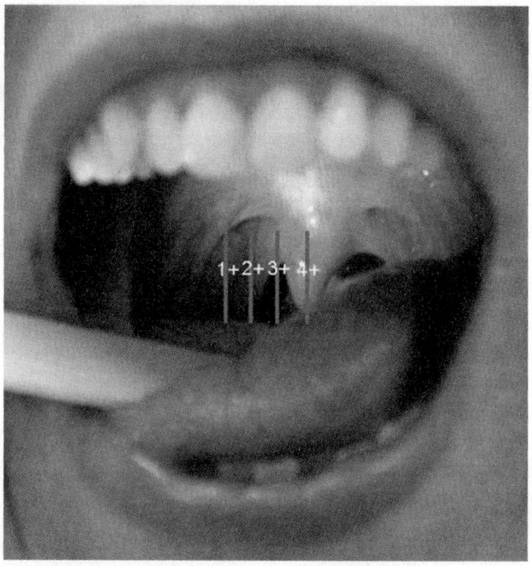

FIGURE **28–41** How to grade tonsil size. (From *Physical Examination Images* [CD-ROM], by D. L. Skillen, R. A. Day, M. C. Anderson, T. C. Stephen, J. A. Gilbert, and L. W. Day, 2004, Edmonton, AB: Faculty of Nursing, University of Alberta.)

Documentation. Nurses record their findings from inspection and palpation of the nose, sinuses, mouth, and pharynx (Table 28-34).

Neck

Muscles, lymph nodes, carotid arteries, jugular veins, thyroid gland, and trachea are located within the neck (Figures 28–42 and 28–43). Each structure can be examined as part of the assessment of the neck or during a systems approach. For example, the examination of the jugular veins and carotid arteries can be part of a cardiovascular assessment or part of a regional assessment of the head and neck.

The two major neck muscles are the sternomastoid and trapezius. The sternomastoid muscles begin at the sternum and the medial aspect of the clavicle, lie diagonally across the neck, and end at the mastoid process behind the ears. The two trapezius muscles begin at the occipital bone and the vertebrae and end at the scapula and the distal end of the clavicle. The sternomastoid and trapezius muscles are useful guideposts for locating and describing neck structures, functions, and findings. The neck is divided into two imaginary triangles by the sternomastoids (Figure 28–44). The anterior triangle lies in front of the sternomastoid muscle and contains the trachea, thyroid gland, carotid artery, and the anterior cervical lymph nodes. The posterior triangle lies between the trapezius muscles (at the back), the sternomastoid muscle (in the front), and the clavicle (at the bottom). The posterior

Procedure 28-10 Assessing the Mouth and Pharynx

Equipment

- Disposable gloves
- Penlight
- Tongue blade

Examination Skill and Focus	Steps	Rationale
Inspection:		
Mouth	**1.** Ask client to remove dentures.	Permits full inspection of area.
	2. Instruct client to sip some water.	
	3. Use penlight and tongue blade to inspect:	
	• buccal mucosa bilaterally	
gums	• upper and lower gums	
teeth	• upper and lower teeth	
tongue	• dorsal and ventral surfaces and sides of tongue	
floor of mouth	• floor of mouth	
uvula, palates	• uvula, soft and hard palates	
tonsils, tonsillar pillars	• tonsils, tonsillar pillars	
posterior pharynx	• posterior pharyngeal wall	
	4. If lesion present, palpate with gloved hand.	Gloves reduce transmission of micro-organisms.
Cranial nerve (CN) IX, X (glossopharyngeal, vagus)	**1.** Depress tongue with tongue blade and instruct client to say "ah."	
	2. Watch uvula and soft palate rise during "ah."	
Motor and sensory Uvula, soft palate, gag reflex	**3.** Touch each side of posterior pharyngeal wall to elicit gag reflex (ability to swallow is tested during examination of the thyroid).	Cranial nerves are in pairs.
CN XII (hypoglossal)	**1.** Observe tongue at rest on floor of mouth.	
Motor function	**2.** Instruct client to protrude tongue and observe.	
Symmetry and strength	**3.** Instruct client to a. wag tongue laterally b. stick tongue into each cheek	
	4. Palpate for strength in each cheek.	

From *A Syllabus for Adult Health Assessment* (pp. 35–36), edited by D. L. Skillen and R. A. Day, 2004, Edmonton, AB: Faculty of Nursing, University of Alberta.

Table 28-34 Examples of Documentation for Assessment of Nose, Sinuses, Mouth, and Pharynx

Focus of Assessment	Expected Findings	Unexpected Findings
Nose	Air entry easy and effortless (R)(L).	Obstructed air entry (L).
	Nose smooth, symmetrical, and located at centre of face.	Nose deviates to left.
	Nasal structures firm, stable, without tenderness.	Tenderness present over nasal structures.
	Nasal mucosa pink, moist, with clear mucus bilaterally.	Nasal mucosa deep red with purulent mucus (R).
	Frontal and maxillary sinuses non-tender. (R) (L)	(R) maxillary sinus tender to palpation.
		Noisy air entry (L); air entry occluded by mucus (R).
	Accurate identification of pungent odours (R) (L).	Unable to correctly identify odours bilaterally.
Lips	Pink, moist, symmetrical, smooth	Dry, cracked, with pustules present on upper lip.
Mouth	Oral mucosa glistening, pink, soft, moist and smooth.	Dry buccal mucosa.
	Gums pink, smooth, moist, with tight margins around each tooth.	Bleeding upper gums, margins receded around majority of teeth.
	Tongue medium or dull red in colour, moist, slightly rough on dorsal surface, smooth along lateral margins and highly vascular on ventral surface.	Excessive dryness and cracking on dorsal surface of tongue.
	Gag reflex present bilaterally.	Absent gag reflex (L).
	Uvula and soft palate rise centrally when client says "ah."	Uvula deviates to (R); soft palate asymmetric rise.
Carotid arteries	No bruit heard over either artery.	(R) bruit present.
Head	Head held upright and still, face symmetrical, intact, round skull, full, smooth and non-tender temporomandibular joint (TMJ) movements.	Head tilts to (L) side; marked asymmetrical facial features; pronounced (L) TMJ clicking or grinding.

Adapted from *First Year Student Lab Guide* (p. 56), by J. Chambers et al., 2004, Edmonton, AB: Faculty of Nursing, University of Alberta.

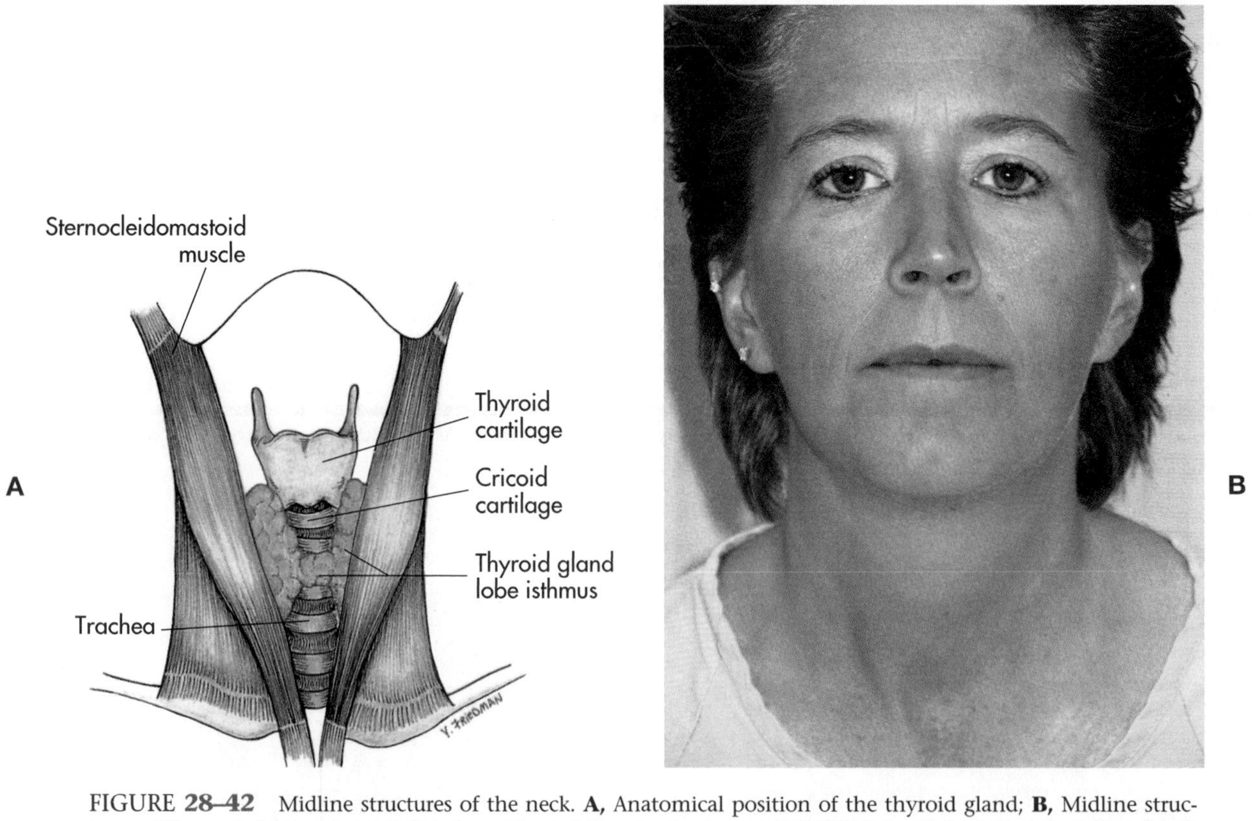

FIGURE 28–42 Midline structures of the neck. **A,** Anatomical position of the thyroid gland; **B,** Midline structures of the neck (external view). (B is from *Physical Examination Images* [CD-ROM], by D. L. Skillen, R. A. Day, M. C. Anderson, T. C. Stephen, J. A. Gilbert, and L. W. Day, 2004, Edmonton, AB: Faculty of Nursing, University of Alberta.)

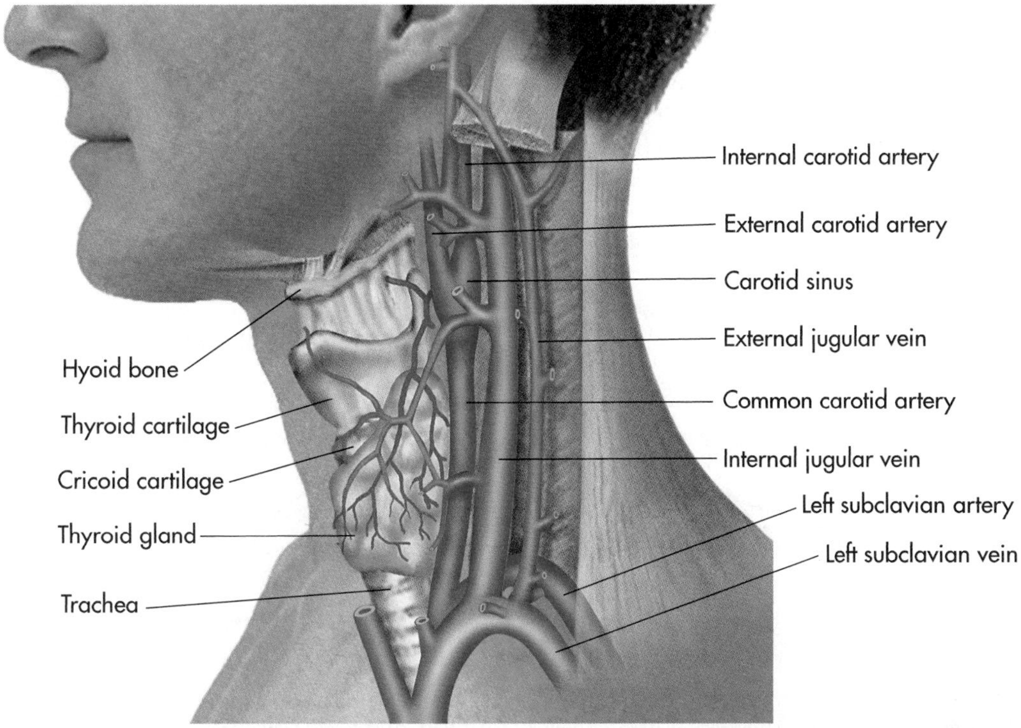

FIGURE **28–43** Arteries and veins of neck. (From *Mosby's Guide to Physical Examination,* 5th ed., p. 253, Figure 9–3b, by H. M. Seidel et al., 2003, St. Louis, MO: Mosby.)

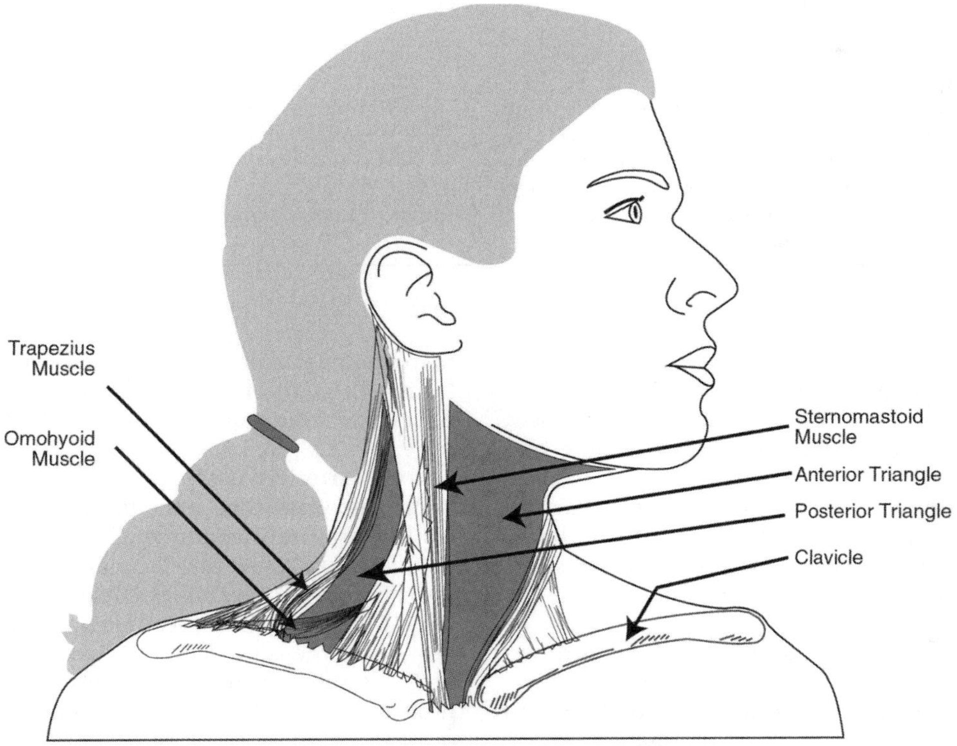

FIGURE **28–44** Neck muscles, anterior triangle, and posterior triangle. (From *Physical Examination Images* [CD-ROM], by D. L. Skillen, R. A. Day, M. C. Anderson, T. C. Stephen, J. A. Gilbert, and L. W. Day, 2004, Edmonton, AB: Faculty of Nursing, University of Alberta.)

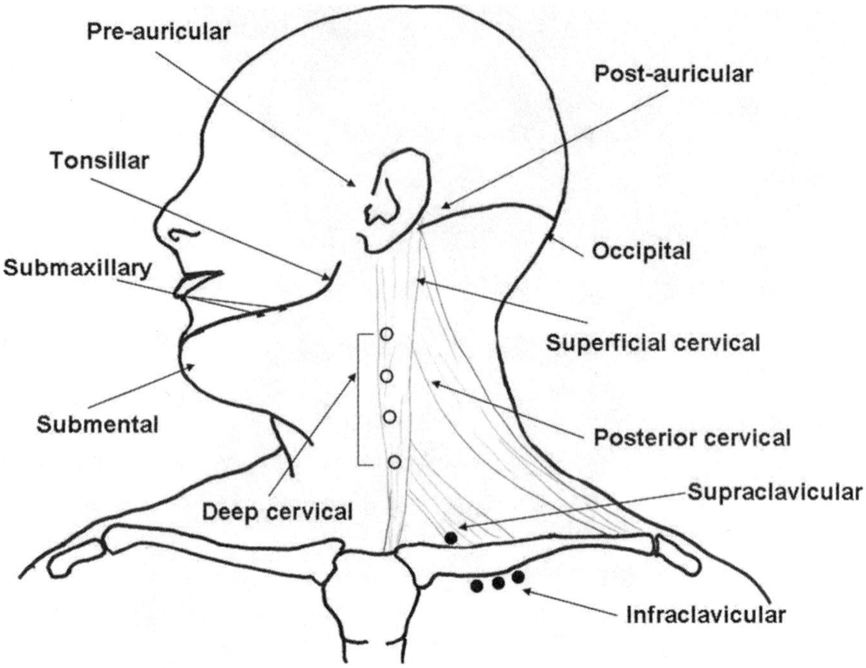

FIGURE **28–45** Lymph nodes of the head and neck. (From *Physical Examination Images* [CD-ROM], by D. L. Skillen, R. A. Day, M. C. Anderson, T. C. Stephen, J. A. Gilbert, and L. W. Day, 2004, Edmonton, AB: Faculty of Nursing, University of Alberta.)

Table 28-35 Health History for Neck Assessment

Assessment Category	Rationale
Ask client about any history of recent cold, infection, or trauma to neck.	Colds and infection can cause lymph node swelling.
Ask client if experiencing any pain or restriction with neck movement.	Muscle strain or trauma to neck may create painful or restricted movement.
Inquire about history of thyroid problems or thyroid treatments.	Disease or medications may influence tissue growth of gland.
Ask client about any current symptoms of thyroid problems, such as a change in temperature preference; swelling in neck; change in texture of hair, skin, nails; and emotional instability.	These symptoms may indicate the presence of thyroid disease.
Inquire about any enlarged lymph nodes and document results of a symptom analysis, as necessary.	Specific signs and symptoms will guide examination.

lymph nodes are located in the posterior triangle. Figure 28–45 presents the lymph nodes of the head and neck.

Table 28-35 contains the health history for the neck examination. Box 28-28 presents client teaching and health promotion during the neck assessment.

The examination of the neck is best performed with the client in a sitting position, with the neck fully exposed. Nurses use mainly inspection and palpation skills, along with auscultation of the carotid arteries.

Inspection. The nurse inspects the neck from two perspectives, noting the client's position. The head may be observed to be directly over the neck, slightly backward (extension) or forward (flexion); this information may be useful in health teaching. The structures of the neck (muscles, arteries, veins, thyroid cartilage, cricoid cartilage, thyroid) are examined for symmetry, alignment, and integrity. The skin of the neck is inspected for lesions and the carotid arteries and jugular veins for pulsations.

Carotid Arteries. When the left ventricle of the heart pumps blood into the aorta, pressure waves are transmitted through the arterial system. These pressure waves are manifested as pulses that are palpable in arteries close to the skin or lying over bones. Nurses assess carotid arteries for information about heart function and pathological changes in the aortic valve.

The carotid arteries supply oxygenated blood to the head and neck (see Figure 28–43) and are protected by the overlying sternomastoid muscle. The carotid sinus is located in the upper third of the neck, level with the superior border of the thyroid cartilage (see Figure 28–42). The sinus

Client Teaching — Box 28-28

Neck Assessment

Objectives

- Client will know signs and symptoms of irregularity in thyroid shape and/or function.
- Client will seek medical attention if a mass is noted in the neck.

Teaching Strategies

- Instruct client about the lymph nodes and how infection can commonly cause node tenderness and enlargement.
- Instruct client about signs and symptoms of thyroid irregularity, including swelling in neck; change in temperature preference; changes in condition of hair, nails, and skin; or change in emotional stability.
- Encourage client to seek further investigation if swelling noted in the neck.

Evaluation

- Have client state the signs and symptoms of thyroid irregularities.

sends impulses along the vagus nerve. Stimulation of the carotid sinus by activities such as palpation, massage, or turning the head quickly can cause a reflex drop in heart rate and blood pressure, causing **syncope** (fainting) or circulatory arrest. This effect can be a particular problem for older adults.

Inspection. To examine the carotid arteries, the nurse has the client sit or lie supine with the head of the bed elevated 30 degrees. With the client's head turned slightly away from the artery being examined, the nurse inspects first for obvious pulsation of each artery (Procedure 28-11).

Palpation. Nurses always palpate the carotid arteries one at a time (Figure 28–46).

Safety Alert: If both arteries are occluded during palpation, the client can lose consciousness as a result of inadequate blood circulation to the brain. It is important to avoid vigorous palpation or massage of the carotids.

For palpation of the carotid pulse, the client turns the head slightly toward the side being examined. This position relaxes the neck muscles for easier palpation. To avoid the carotid sinus, nurses palpate the carotid pulse in the lower third of the neck, level with the cricoid cartilage. The nurse slides the index and middle fingers or the thumb around the medial edge of the sternomastoid muscle. Gentle palpation avoids occlusion of circulation. In the past, the use of the thumb to assess pulses was discouraged. It is now acceptable practice to use the thumb to palpate large arteries such as the carotids (Bickley & Szilagyi, 2003). During palpation of the carotid arteries, the examiner may become aware of feeling vibrations or a thrill. The carotid pulse is a strong pulse, with a thrusting quality. Carotid pulsation does not change with breathing or with a change in position from sitting to supine. Both carotid arteries should be equal in pulse rate, rhythm, and

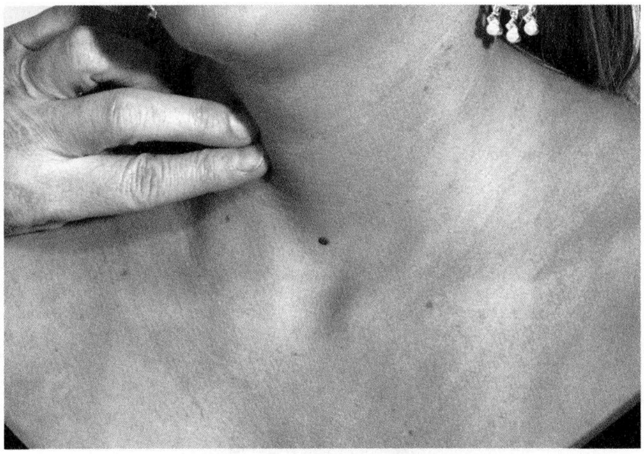
A

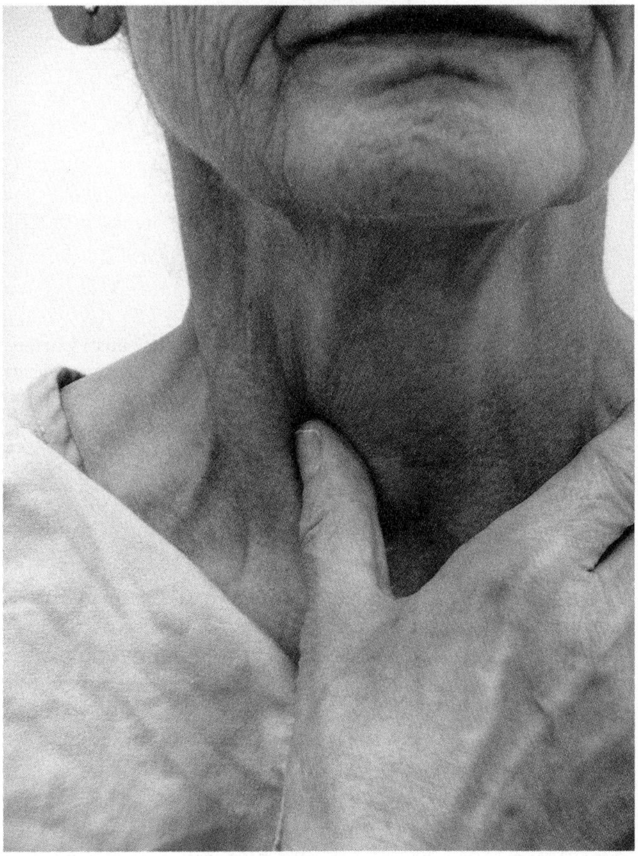
B

FIGURE **28–46** **A,** Palpation of carotid artery with finger pads. **B,** Palpation of carotid artery with thumb. (From *Physical Examination Images* [CD-ROM], by D. L. Skillen, R. A. Day, M. C. Anderson, T. C. Stephen, J. A. Gilbert, and L. W. Day, 2004, Edmonton, AB: Faculty of Nursing, University of Alberta.)

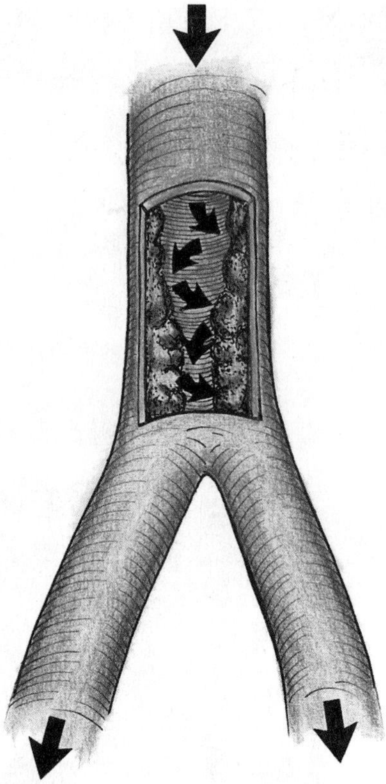

FIGURE **28–47** Occlusion or narrowing of the carotid artery disrupts blood flow. The resultant turbulence creates a sound (bruit) that the nurse can auscultate.

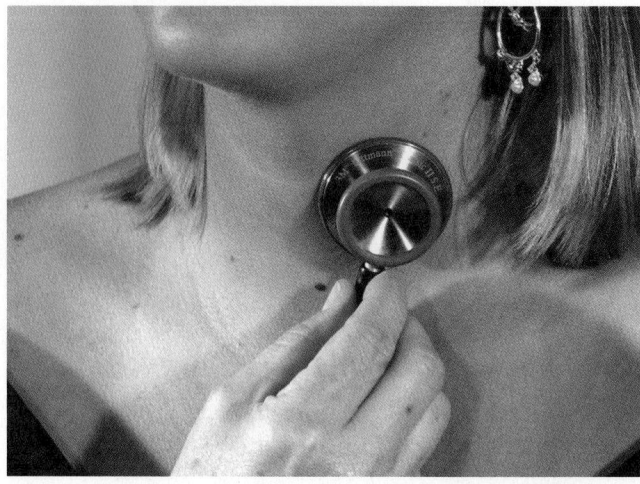

FIGURE **28–48** Auscultation of the carotid artery. (From *Physical Examination Images* [CD-ROM], by D. L. Skillen, R. A. Day, M. C. Anderson, T. C. Stephen, J. A. Gilbert, and L. W. Day, 2004, Edmonton, AB: Faculty of Nursing, University of Alberta.)

strength. Unequal or diminished carotid pulsations can indicate atherosclerosis or aortic arch disease.

Auscultation. The carotid is the most commonly auscultated artery for bruits. Others might include the temporal, femoral, renal, and abdominal arteries. As blood passes through a narrowed section, turbulence is created, causing a blowing or swishing sound. The sound is called a **bruit** (pronounced "brew-ee"; Figure 28–47). Auscultation is especially important for middle-aged and older clients if a thrill is present or for clients suspected of having cerebrovascular disease manifested by carotid artery obstruction. When the lumen of a blood vessel is narrowed, its blood flow is disturbed. During carotid auscultation, the diaphragm of the stethoscope is placed over the artery at the medial end of the clavicle and medial margin of the sternomastoid (Figure 28–48). The nurse asks the client to hold the breath for a moment so that breath sounds do not obscure a bruit. No sound is usually heard during carotid auscultation.

Jugular Veins. The most accessible veins are the internal and external jugular veins in the neck. Both drain bilaterally from the head and neck into the superior vena cava. The external jugular vein lies superficially and can be seen just above the clavicle. The internal jugular vein lies deeper, along the carotid artery (see Figure 28–43), and only its pulsations are visible.

Usually, when a client lies supine, the external jugular vein distends and becomes easily visible. In contrast, the jugular veins usually flatten when the client is sitting. Clients with heart disease, however, may have distended jugular veins when sitting.

The jugular veins are inspected to assess venous pressures, which are influenced by blood volume, capacity of the right atrium to receive blood and send it to the right ventricle, and ability of the right ventricle to contract and force blood into the pulmonary artery. Any factor that creates a greater blood volume within the venous system causes elevated venous pressure. With the client supine at a 30- or 45-degree angle (Figure 28–49), nurses assess venous pressure by locating first the external jugular and then the internal jugular veins (Procedure 28-11). Authorities vary on the required angle. It is best to examine the right internal jugular vein because it follows a more direct anatomical path to the right atrium of the heart (see Figure 28–43). The column of blood inside the internal jugular vein serves as a manometer, reflecting pressure in the right atrium. The higher the column, the greater the venous pressure. Nurses assess venous pressure by measuring the vertical distance between the sternal angle (angle of Louis) and the highest level of the visible point of the internal jugular vein pulsation (Figure 28–50). Bilateral pressures higher than 2.5 cm are considered elevated and are a sign of right-sided heart failure. One-sided pressure elevation can be caused by obstruction.

Range of Motion of the Neck

Inspection. Nurses inspect for symmetry of the neck muscles and range of motion of cervical vertebrae and neck muscles by watching the client perform four moves: flexion, extension, lateral flexion, and rotation (see Procedure 28-11). Flexion, lateral flexion, and rotation are performed to test the function of the sternomastoid muscles; extension and rotation test the trapezius muscles. The neck

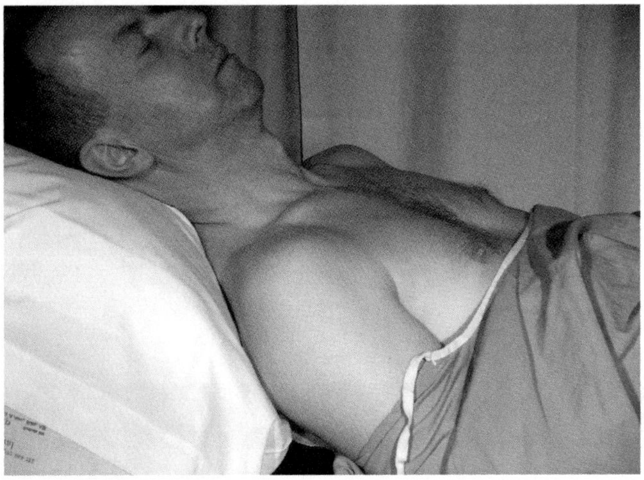

FIGURE **28–49** Position to assess jugular vein distension. (From *Physical Examination Images* [CD-ROM], by D. L. Skillen, R. A. Day, M. C. Anderson, T. C. Stephen, J. A. Gilbert, and L. W. Day, 2004, Edmonton, AB: Faculty of Nursing, University of Alberta.)

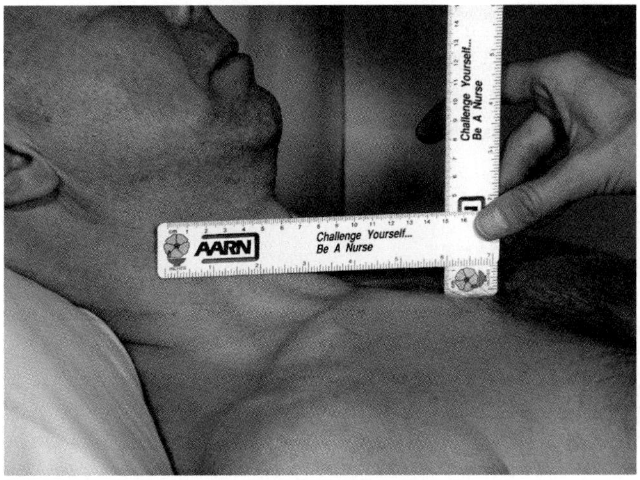

FIGURE **28–50** Measurement of jugular venous pressure. (From *Physical Examination Images* [CD-ROM], by D. L. Skillen, R. A. Day, M. C. Anderson, T. C. Stephen, J. A. Gilbert, and L. W. Day, 2004, Edmonton, AB: Faculty of Nursing, University of Alberta.)

should move freely without discomfort or dizziness. Muscle strength and function are tested during assessment of the musculoskeletal system.

Age-Related Changes. In older adults, the cervical concave curvature of the neck increases and the head and jaw move forward. Range of motion of the neck needs to be done slowly, as older adults are more likely to experience dizziness when turning the head.

Documentation. Nurses record their findings from inspection, palpation, and auscultation of the neck (Table 28-36).

Lymph Nodes. The lymphatic system consists of vessels and lymph nodes and is separate from the cardiovascular system. Lymph, a clear watery liquid, moves from tissue spaces into the lymphatic system. Lymph nodes are clusters of lymphatic tissue that occur at intervals and look like beads on a string. Lymph nodes filter the lymph, trap foreign organisms and damaged cells, and provide a partial barrier to the growth of cancer (malignant) cells within the body. The superficial lymph nodes are the only component of the lymphatic system that is accessible for examination. They are located in the head, neck, axillae, arms, and inguinal regions. Nurses need to be competent in assessing lymph nodes, particularly when caring for clients with severe infections, possible cancer, and those with reduced immunity evidenced by allergies, autoimmune diseases (e.g., lupus erythematosus), or human immunodeficiency virus (HIV) infection.

The head and neck are well supplied with lymph nodes (see Figure 28–45). Although different names exist for these nodes, one commonly used system is provided here. The fact that the names refer to nearby structures aids in learning the location of the nodes. To avoid overlooking any single node or chain of nodes, nurses use a methodical approach of inspection and palpation to systematically examine lymph nodes and evaluate each node or chain for the following:

- Location
- Enlargement
- Size
- Shape (round, regular, irregular)
- Consistency (soft, firm, hard)
- Delineation (are the borders clearly defined or not?)
- Mobility
- Surface characteristics
- Tenderness
- Skin warmth over the nodes

For inspection and palpation, the examiner asks the client to flex the neck slightly forward (Procedure 28-12), which relaxes tissues and muscles. Lymph nodes are not usually visible, but if visible they are examined for swelling, erythema, or red streaks. During palpation, the nurse faces or stands to the side of the client for easy access to all nodes. It is important to press underlying tissue in each area and not simply move the fingers over the skin. However, if too much pressure is applied, small nodes may be missed and palpable nodes obliterated. The nodes can be examined in sets of three. The preauricular (Figure 28–51), postauricular, and occipital nodes are one set. Another set of three is formed by the tonsillar, submaxillary, and submental (Figure 28–51, *B*) lymph nodes. The third set includes the superficial, deep, and posterior cervical nodes. See Procedure 28-12 for the sets of three listed in sequence.

Usually lymph nodes are not easily palpable. However, small, mobile, non-tender nodes are common. Lymph nodes that are large, fixed in position, inflamed, or tender indicate a problem such as local infection, systemic disease, or neoplasm (cancer; Seidel et al., 2003). When enlarged nodes are found, the nurse explores adjacent areas and regions drained by the nodes for signs of infection or malignancy. Noting which nodes are enlarged may help locate the site of an infection. For example, ear infections

Procedure 28-11 Assessing Neck Veins and Arteries and Range of Motion

Equipment

- Stethoscope
- Rulers (2)
- Light source

Examination Skill and Focus	Steps	Rationale
Inspection:	Neck fully exposed. Sitting position or supine at 30-degree angle	Ensures visibility.
Neck, carotid arteries, jugular veins	**1.** Use tangential lighting on neck.	Casting shadows improves visualization of pulsations.
	2. Inspect neck.	Pulsations of the carotid arteries and the level of pulsations of the external and internal jugular veins are visible.
	3. Inspect carotid arteries and jugular veins.	
Palpation: Carotid arteries	**1.** Palpate each carotid artery **separately** (at the level of the cricoid cartilage), using thumb or index and middle fingers.	Avoids decreasing blood flow to the brain.
	2. Assess amplitude, contour, and presence of thrills (humming vibrations).	
	3. Avoid carotid sinus.	Pressure on the carotid sinus (level with top border of thyroid cartilage) can cause syncope.
Auscultation: Carotid arteries	**1.** Instruct client to hold breath while holding own breath.	Holding own breath limits how long client holds breath.
	2. Use diaphragm of stethoscope to auscultate over each carotid artery.	Stethoscopes amplify a bruit.
Inspection: Jugular veins	Neck and upper thorax exposed	Ensures visibility.
	Client in supine position with head on pillow and elevated 45 degrees.	Avoids hyperextension or flexion of neck to prevent kinking or stretching of veins. Uses a standardized position for measuring jugular venous pressure.
	1. Use tangential lighting on neck.	Improves visibility of pulsations.
	2. Locate external jugular first and then the internal jugular veins.	External jugular is easier to find.
	3. Repeat on other side.	
	4. Locate sternal angle (angle of Louis).	
	5. Use (R) internal jugular vein to measure jugular venous pressure.	Vein is directly attached to superior vena cava.
	6. Line up bottom edge of ruler with the top of the highest point of pulsations of the (R) internal jugular vein, holding it horizontal.	
	7. Stand a second ruler on end on the sternal angle (angle of Louis), perpendicular to the first ruler.	
	8. Measure the vertical distance between the sternal angle and the second ruler and the highest level of internal jugular vein pulsation (first ruler).	
	9. Repeat on other side.	

From *A Syllabus for Adult Health Assessment* (pp. 36–37), edited by D. L. Skillen and R. A. Day, 2004, Edmonton, AB: Faculty of Nursing, University of Alberta.

Examination Skill and Focus	Steps	Rationale
Inspection: Range of motion of neck	Client in sitting or standing position **1.** Inspect range of motion of cervical vertebrae by instructing client to: a. touch chin to chest (flexion) b. look up at ceiling (extension) c. touch ear to shoulder bilaterally (lateral flexion) while examiner restricts shoulder movement d. turn head to each side, looking over shoulder (rotation)	Client demonstrates active range of motion (four movements) and any restrictions are noted.

From *A Syllabus for Adult Health Assessment* (pp. 36–37), edited by D. L. Skillen and R. A. Day, 2004, Edmonton, AB: Faculty of Nursing, University of Alberta.

Table 28-36 Examples of Documentation for Assessment of Carotid Arteries, Jugular Veins, and Range of Motion of Neck

Focus of Assessment	Expected Findings	Unexpected Findings
Carotid arteries	Smooth contour, 2+ strength bilaterally, no bruits heard over (R) or (L) arteries	Full and bounding pulses
Jugular veins	At a 45-degree angle, no distension. Jugular venous pressure (JVP) <2 cm bilaterally	Unilateral distension of (L) external jugular vein
Range of motion (ROM) of neck	Full ROM bilaterally without discomfort or dizziness	Restricted (L) lateral flexion and (L) rotation

Adapted from *First Year Student Lab Guide* (p. 56), by J. Chambers et al., 2004, Edmonton, AB: Faculty of Nursing, University of Alberta.

usually drain to the preauricular or deep cervical nodes. After a serious infection, a node may remain permanently enlarged but not be tender. Malignancy is mainly associated with non-tender hard nodes with irregular borders, fixed to the skin and surrounding tissue.

Trachea. The trachea is located in the midline of neck and above the suprasternal notch (see Figure 28–42). Masses in the neck or mediastinum and pulmonary abnormalities can cause the trachea to deviate from the midline to the side (see Procedure 28-12). Nurses assess the position of the trachea using gentle pressure to avoid causing the client to cough (Figure 28–52).

Thyroid Gland. The thyroid gland lies in the middle and front of the neck and is fixed to the trachea. The gland consists of two irregular, cone-shaped lobes that lie behind the sternomastoid muscles. The lobes are connected by a bridge of tissue (thyroid isthmus), which is located over the second and third tracheal rings (see Figure 28–42). Nurses assess the thyroid gland using inspection, palpation, and auscultation (Procedure 28-12).

Inspection. The examiner stands in front of the client to inspect the area of the lower neck overlying the thyroid gland for visible masses, symmetry, and any fullness. Usually a hollow or groove is seen on each side of the neck between the trachea and sternomastoid. At the level of the thyroid isthmus, the examiner observes for fullness and the disappearance of the natural grooves. When the client swallows, examiners look for upward movement of the isthmus and any bulging of the thyroid gland. It is unusual to see the thyroid gland.

Palpation. It helps examiners to begin palpation by identifying the midline structures from the front. For the posterior approach, the examiner has the client sit so that the neck is more accessible. With both hands placed around the neck, two fingers of each hand rest on the sides of the trachea just below the cricoid cartilage. This positioning permits the examiner to assess for enlargement and movement of the thyroid isthmus while the client swallows. The examiner moves the fingers between the sternomastoid and trachea to gently palpate each thyroid lobe separately for enlargement, masses, or nodules (Figure 28–53). Lobes are usually small, smooth, and free of nodules, but in extremely thin individuals they may be palpated more easily. Enlargement is a manifestation of thyroid dysfunction. Masses or nodules may indicate malignancy, but not all nodules are malignant.

A

B

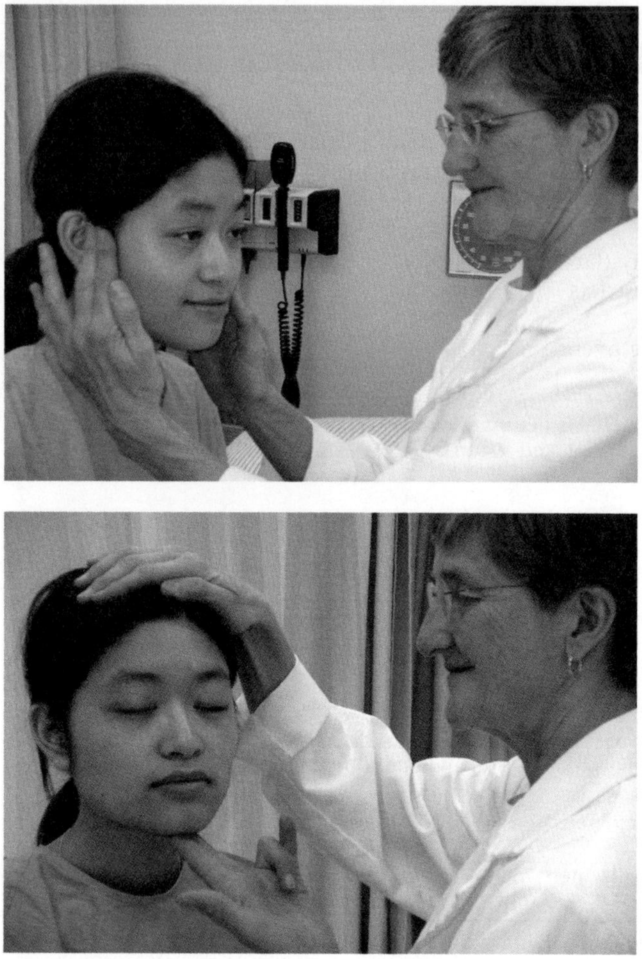

FIGURE **28–51** **A,** Palpation of preauricular lymph nodes. **B,** Palpation of submental lymph nodes. (From *Physical Examination Images* [CD-ROM], by D. L. Skillen, R. A. Day, M. C. Anderson, T. C. Stephen, J. A. Gilbert, and L. W. Day, 2004, Edmonton, AB: Faculty of Nursing, University of Alberta.)

Auscultation. When the gland appears enlarged, the examiner places the bell of the stethoscope over the thyroid. When enlarged, blood flow through the thyroid arteries increases and causes a fine vibration. If auscultated, the vibration is heard as a soft, rushing sound, or bruit.

Cranial Nerves. Nurses assess the motor function of cranial nerves IX (glossopharyngeal) and X (vagus) by watching the client swallow water as part of the thyroid examination or as part of the neurological examination. Nurses assess cranial nerve XI (spinal accessory) by observing the client shrug the shoulders (movement) and testing muscle strength of shoulders and neck.

Age-Related Changes. In older adults, the submandibular (submaxillary) salivary gland may prolapse and be incorrectly identified as a tumour. The fact that the prolapse occurs bilaterally and the glands feel soft helps to rule out a tumour (Jarvis, 2004).

Documentation. Nurses record their findings from inspection and palpation of the lymph nodes, trachea, and thyroid gland (Table 28-37).

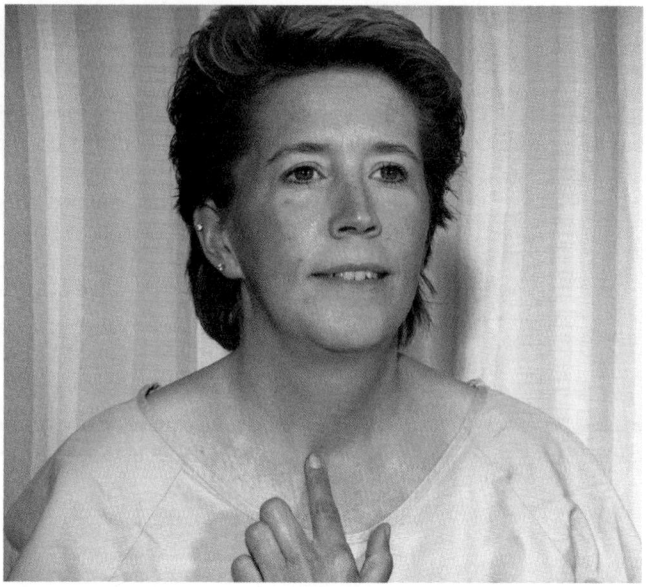

FIGURE **28–52** Examination of tracheal position. (From *Physical Examination Images* [CD-ROM], by D. L. Skillen, R. A. Day, M. C. Anderson, T. C. Stephen, J. A. Gilbert, and L. W. Day, 2004, Edmonton, AB: Faculty of Nursing, University of Alberta.)

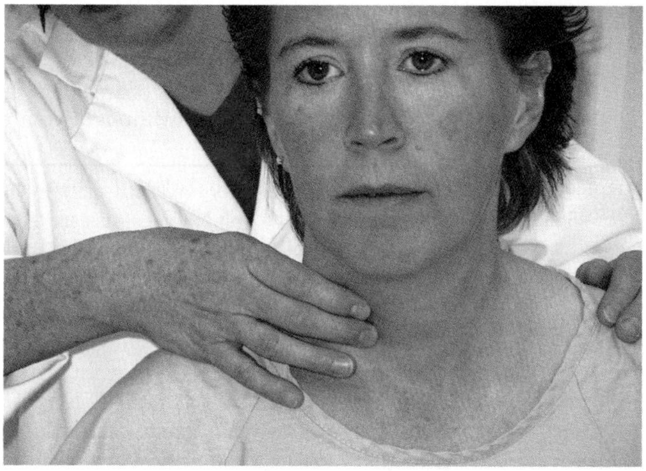

FIGURE **28–53** Palpation of right thyroid lobe. (From *Physical Examination Images* [CD-ROM], by D. L. Skillen, R. A. Day, M. C. Anderson, T. C. Stephen, J. A. Gilbert, and L. W. Day, 2004, Edmonton, AB: Faculty of Nursing, University of Alberta.)

Assessing the Torso

The torso includes the spine, thorax, lungs, heart, breasts, abdomen, female and male genitalia, inguinal regions, anus, rectum, and prostate. Guided by the health history interview, nurses focus their physical examination on the relevant structures of the torso.

Assessing the Spine

The vertebral column has four curvatures: cervical, thoracic, lumbar, and sacral, which ease the impact of active movements and distribute weight from the upper to the lower body. Muscle attachments occur at the transverse processes and the spinous processes, which project

Procedure 28-12 Assessing Lymph Nodes of the Neck, Trachea, and Thyroid Gland

Equipment

- Stethoscope
- Glass of water

Examination Skill and Focus	Steps	Rationale
Inspection: Lymph nodes	**1.** Inspect area of each set of lymph nodes.	Assesses swelling, changes in skin.
Palpation: Lymph nodes	Client sitting and examiner standing in front of client	
	1. Palpate lymph nodes (bilaterally) using finger pads in circular (rotary) motion to move the skin over the underlying structure. May palpate simultaneously: • preauricular • postauricular • occipital • tonsillar • submaxillary • submental (braces top of head with one hand) • superficial cervical • deep cervical • posterior cervical • supraclavicular	Finger pads are useful in assessing characteristics of nodes.
Palpation: Trachea	Client sitting or supine	
	1. Locate trachea above suprasternal notch with index finger and compare spacing from sternomastoid on each side.	Assesses for deviation of the trachea from the midline.
Inspection: Cricoid cartilage and below thyroid	Client sitting, examiner in front	
	1. Instruct client to extend head slightly.	Tightens skin to improve visualization.
	2. Direct tangential lighting from tip of chin toward thyroid region.	Assists in seeing movement and masses.
	3. Inspect region below cricoid cartilage at rest.	Inspects at level of thyroid isthmus.
	4. Ask client to hold water in mouth.	Water helps the client swallow.
	5. Instruct client to extend head slightly again.	Extension makes muscles and skin more taut for visibility.
Inspection: Thyroid gland Movement Cranial nerve (CN) IX, X	**6.** Inspect for isthmus and thyroid gland movement during swallowing.	Isthmus and thyroid gland rise with swallowing. Motor function of cranial nerves IX and X is intact if client can swallow.

From *A Syllabus for Adult Health Assessment* (pp. 36–37), edited by D. L. Skillen and R. A. Day, 2004, Edmonton, AB: Faculty of Nursing, University of Alberta.

Continued

Procedure 28-12 Assessing Lymph Nodes of the Neck, Trachea, and Thyroid Gland—cont'd

Examination Skill and Focus	Steps	Rationale
Palpation: Thyroid	**1.** From the front, palpate down midline to identify each structure.	Ensures examiner is aware of the location of structures before examining the client from behind.
	2. From behind, place index fingers just below cricoid cartilage on neck.	
	3. Instruct client to flex head **slightly** toward the side being examined.	
	4. Instruct client to swallow water while palpating for glandular tissues (isthmus and lobes) first on one side and then the other.	
Auscultation: Thyroid gland	**1.** Place bell of stethoscope lightly over thyroid lobe.	
	2. Ask client to hold breath while holding own breath.	Holding own breath limits how long client holds breath.
	3. Listen for bruit.	Increased blood flow in an enlarged thyroid can be heard better if client holds breath.
	4. Let client breathe and then ask to hold breath again.	
	5. Repeat auscultation on other side.	
Test motor function of CN XI (spinal accessory)	Client in sitting position	
	1. Observe client shrug shoulders.	Assesses active movement.
	2. Instruct client to shrug shoulders which applying resistance with hands on client's shoulders.	Assesses muscle strength.
	3. Instruct client to look straight ahead.	
	4. Place hand on side of face, then instruct client to turn head to the same side against resistance. Observe opposite sternomastoid contraction and force against hand.	Assesses muscle strength.
	5. Repeat on other side.	

From *A Syllabus for Adult Health Assessment* (pp. 36–37), edited by D. L. Skillen and R. A. Day, 2004, Edmonton, AB: Faculty of Nursing, University of Alberta.

posteriorly. The trapezius and latissimus dorsi are large muscles attached to each side of the spine. Coordination of the 24 vertebrae, vertebral discs, muscles, and interconnecting ligaments contributes to healthy back mechanics. After conducting the health history, nurses use inspection and palpation to examine the spine.

Inspection. The nurse conducts inspection with the client standing and draped (Procedure 28-13). The expected standing posture is an upright stance with parallel alignment of shoulders and hips (Figure 28–54).

When viewing the client from the side, the nurse expects to see a slight convex curve in the thoracic region and a concave curve in the lumbar area. Neither a severe **lordosis** (exaggerated concave curvature in the lumbar spine; Figure 28–55, *A*) nor a **kyphosis** (exaggerated convex curvature of the thoracic spine; Figure 28–55, *B*) is desired. An important deviation to detect early in youth is a lateral curvature of the spine called **scoliosis** (Figure 28–55, *C*).

After examining the spinal curvatures, the nurse assesses the alignment of the spine, which is expected to be vertical. Landmarks facilitate assessment of the alignment (shoulders, spinous processes, paravertebral muscles, scapulae, iliac crests, and posterior superior iliac spines) and are expected to be symmetrically aligned horizontally. The gluteal folds may also be examined for horizontal alignment.

Table 28-37 Examples of Documentation for Assessment of Lymph Nodes, Trachea, and Thyroid

Focus of Assessment	Expected Findings	Unexpected Findings
Neck	Symmetrical, smooth, no fullness over thyroid	Fullness over thyroid
Lymph nodes	Bilaterally non-palpable	(L) preauricular node 3 × 3 mm, mobile, non-tender, soft, circumscribed
Tracheal position	Midline, posterior to suprasternal notch	Shifted to the left of midline
Thyroid	Isthmus smooth, lobes non-palpable, lobes and isthmus move upward with swallowing	Lobes palpable bilaterally, bruit present bilaterally
Cranial nerves IX, X	Motor function of both nerves intact	Unable to swallow
Cranial nerve XI	Motor function intact (R)(L) Muscle strength strong (R)(L)	Unable to shrug (L) shoulder

Adapted from *First Year Student Lab Guide* (p. 56), by J. Chambers et al., 2004, Edmonton, AB: Faculty of Nursing, University of Alberta.

A 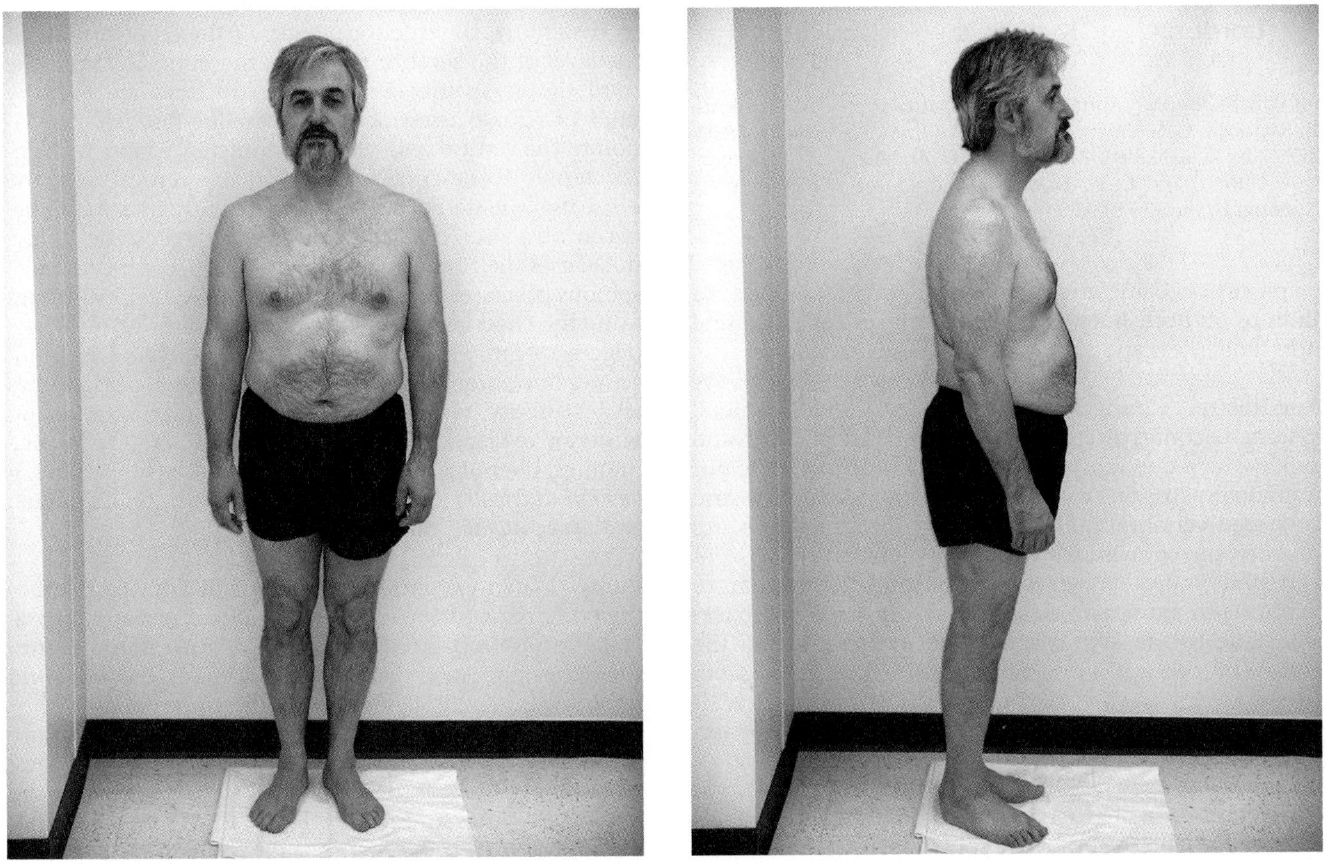 B

FIGURE 28–54 Standing posture. **A,** Anterior view. **B,** Lateral view. (From *Physical Examination Images* [CD-ROM], by D. L. Skillen, R. A. Day, M. C. Anderson, T. C. Stephen, J. A. Gilbert, and L. W. Day, 2004, Edmonton, AB: Faculty of Nursing, University of Alberta.)

Range of Motion. By inspecting range of motion (ROM) of the spine (see Procedure 28-13), the nurse assesses flexibility, ease of movement, symmetry, and curvatures in the client's back. Clients are expected to demonstrate full flexion (hands should almost touch toes) and extension (backward lean from hips), as well as symmetrical lateral bending (hand at side almost reaches knee) and rotation of the spine. Restriction or asymmetry is unexpected.

Palpation. Palpation of the spinous processes and paravertebral muscles begins by tracking two fingers down the spine, expecting vertical alignment of the spinous processes without obvious protrusions of vertebral discs

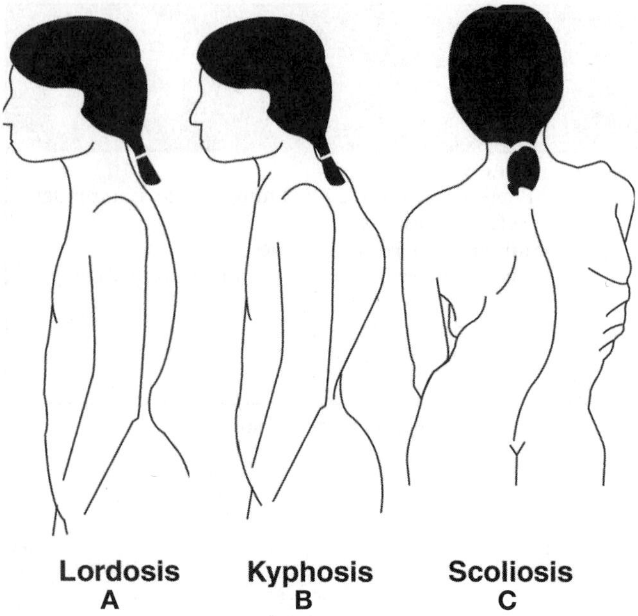

FIGURE **28–55** Abnormalities of the spine. **A,** Lordosis. **B,** Kyphosis. **C,** Scoliosis. (From *Physical Examination Images* [CD-ROM], by D. L. Skillen, R. A. Day, M. C. Anderson, T. C. Stephen, J. A. Gilbert, and L. W. Day, 2004, Edmonton, AB: Faculty of Nursing, University of Alberta.)

or processes. Using circular motions with finger pads or thumbs on both sides of the spine, nurses expect to find non-tenderness and similar muscle bulk bilaterally.

Age-Related Changes. Change in the musculoskeletal system becomes increasingly evident in posture and gait as the older adult reaches 80 years or more. Height is gradually lost due to thinning intervertebral discs and collapsed vertebral bodies from osteoporosis. Knee and hip flexion contributes to loss of height. Collapse of vertebral bodies makes a significant contribution to kyphosis in aging adults. They may tilt the head backward due to the kyphosis or bend forward due to the collapsed cervical vertebral bodies. They may seem stooped with flexion at the knees and hips and with limbs (especially arms) appearing longer in proportion to the trunk.

Documentation. Nurses record their findings from inspection and palpation of the spine (Table 28-38).

Assessing the Thorax and Lungs

Accurate physical assessment of the thorax and lungs requires knowledge of anatomical terms, landmarks, underlying structures, and ventilatory and respiratory functions of the lungs. Nurses assess the thorax and lungs posteriorly, anteriorly, and laterally on both sides. During the thorax and lung assessment, the nurse is alert to alterations in other body systems that may be caused by alterations in the respiratory system. For example, reduced oxygenation of the blood can change the client's mental alertness due to the sensitivity of the brain to lowered oxygen levels. Similarly, alterations in other body systems can cause respiratory alterations.

Thorax. The thorax is a bony structure created by the sternum, clavicle, ribs, thoracic spine, scapulae, and vertebrae (Figures 28–56 and 28–57). The non-palpable costochondral junctions connect ribs with costal cartilage. Anteriorly, the manubrium, body of the sternum, and xiphoid process are midline structures that nurses use to identify underlying structures.

The suprasternal notch on the manubrium forms the superior border of that midline structure and guides identification of the **sternal angle,** a bony prominence or ridge where the manubrium joins the body of the sternum (angle of Louis). The left and right second ribs articulate with this prominence. Anteriorly, the nurse counts the ribs and intercostal spaces (spaces between ribs) starting from the sternal angle and second rib. The number of each intercostal space corresponds to the rib just above it. Laterally, the fourth, fifth, and sixth ribs and posteriorly, the spinous process of the third thoracic vertebra help nurses visualize the lobes of the lungs.

Posteriorly, the inferior margin of the scapula lying at the level of the seventh rib assists the nurse to locate the third thoracic vertebra. Thoracic structures are used by nurses to guide assessment and describe findings in relation to the vertical axis, chest circumference, and anatomical terms. To describe findings on the vertical axis, the nurse uses the sternal angle, numbered ribs, interspaces between ribs, and costal margins anteriorly. Posteriorly, the nurse uses the ribs, interspaces, inferior tip of the scapula, spinous processes, and costal margin. To describe findings using the chest circumference, the nurse uses vertical lines (Figure 28–58). The vertebral line posteriorly and the midsternal line anteriorly are very precise. Other vertical lines are less precise, but very useful: midclavicular, anterior and posterior axillary, midaxillary, and scapular. To describe findings, the nurse uses the anatomical terms *supraclavicular, infraclavicular, interscapular, infrascapular, bases, apices,* and *upper, middle,* and *lower lung fields.*

Lungs. When examining the lungs, the nurse imagines the underlying lungs, trachea, bronchial tree, and pleura. Oblique and horizontal fissures divide the right lung into the right upper lobe (RUL), right middle lobe (RML), and right lower lobe (RLL; Figure 28–59).

In the anterior thorax, the apex of the RUL and left upper lobe (LUL) rises 2 to 4 cm above the medial clavicles. The lower borders of the lungs cross the eighth ribs in the midaxillary lines and the sixth ribs in the midclavicular lines (MCLs). In the posterior thorax, the lower border of the lungs is at approximately the 10th thoracic (T10) spinous process and descends to the T12 spinous process with deep inspiration (Swartz, 2002). The trachea bifurcates anteriorly at the level of the sternal angle into right and left main bronchi and posteriorly at the level of the fourth thoracic (T4) spinous process. The right main bronchus is somewhat straighter than the left.

Lungs are covered by serous membranes, the visceral pleura. The rib cage and the superior surface of the diaphragm are lined by parietal pleura. Between the pleura is a potential space. Pleural fluid permits surfaces to move without friction during respiration.

Respiration depends on an intact brainstem and the muscles of respiration. During inspiration, the diaphragm

Procedure 28-13 Assessing the Spine

Equipment

- None

Examination Skill and Focus	Steps	Rationale
Spine Inspection: Curvatures Vertical alignment	Client standing, loosely draped, feet together. Pants should rest just below sacroiliac joints. **1.** Inspect from side (profile). **2.** Inspect from back, midline.	Adequate exposure ensures spinal curves are visible. Permits assessment of thoracic and lumbar curvatures and vertebral alignment.
	1. Inspect symmetry of shoulders, scapulae, iliac crests, sacroiliac joints, and gluteal folds.	Comparison facilitates identification of horizontal alignment of these structures.
Palpation:	**2.** Palpate structures to confirm symmetry.	
Inspection: Range of motion	**1.** Instruct client to touch toes (flexion). **2.** Place hand on posterior superior iliac spine, fingers pointing toward midline. **3.** Instruct client to bend backward as far as possible (extension). **4.** Place hands on client's hips. **5.** Instruct client to bend sideways as far as possible (lateral bending). **6.** Repeat on other side. **7.** Place hand on client's hip and other hand on opposite shoulder. **8.** Rotate trunk by pulling shoulder, then hip (rotation). **9.** Repeat on other side.	Flexion, extension, lateral bending, and rotation are movements that are possible if the spine and musculature are intact. ***Safety Alert:*** During extension and lateral bending, examiner limits possibility of injury by stabilizing client at hips.
Palpation: Spinous processes	Client standing **1.** Palpate spinous processes from C_1 to L_5. **2.** Use finger pads or thumbs in rotary motion. **3.** Inquire about tenderness. **4.** Assess alignment by running two fingers down spine C_1 to L_5.	Spinous processes are landmarks for the 24 vertebrae that form the vertebral column. Rotary motion detects deviations or tenderness. Both the thumbs and finger pads are sensitive to characteristics to be assessed. Palpation assists identification of vertical alignment.
Paravertebral muscles	**1.** Palpate paravertebral muscles bilaterally from level of C_1 to L_5. **2.** Use finger pads or thumbs. **3.** Inquire about tenderness.	Paravertebral muscles attach to all spinous processes.

From *A Syllabus for Adult Health Assessment* (p. 38), edited by D. L. Skillen and R. A. Day, 2004, Edmonton, AB: Faculty of Nursing, University of Alberta.

Table 28-38 Examples of Documentation for Spine Assessment

Focus of Assessment	Expected Findings	Unexpected Findings
Spinal curvatures	Thoracic curve convex, lumbar curve concave. Spinal vertebrae vertically aligned.	Thoracic convex curvature accentuated (slight kyphosis), lumbar curve concave. Spinal vertebrae curve laterally to right in thoracic area.
Symmetry	Shoulders, scapulae, iliac crests, sacroiliac joints, and gluteal folds horizontally aligned.	(R) shoulder higher than (L) shoulder, (L) scapulae protrudes slightly, iliac crest on (L) higher than on (R), sacroiliac joints and gluteal folds horizontally aligned.
Range of motion (ROM)	Touches toes (R)(L) in flexion, full ROM in extension, lateral bending and rotation. Lateral bending and rotation symmetrical.	Touches knees in forward flexion, (R) lateral bend deeper than on (L), minimal rotation on (R), fuller on (L).
Spinous processes	Non-tender to palpation from C_1 to L_5. No protrusions evident.	Tender area over T10 spinous process.
Paravertebral muscles	Non-tender bilaterally from C_1 to L_5, without spasm; equal muscle bulk.	Tenderness over paravertebral muscles, (L) side at L3

Adapted from "Documentation" by M.C. Anderson in *Health Assessment Self-Test Modules* (WebCT Vista), 2004, Edmonton, AB: Faculty of Nursing, University of Alberta.

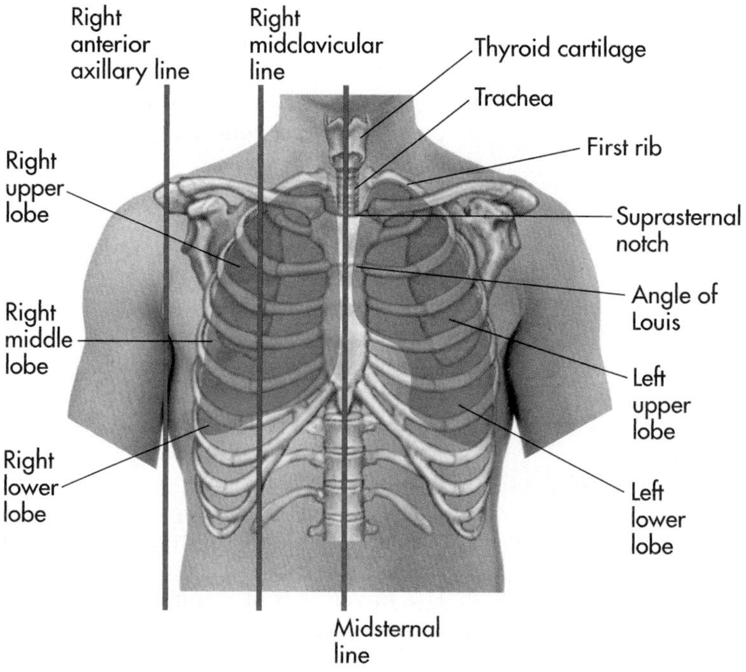

FIGURE **28–56** Anterior thorax. (From *Mosby's Guide to Physical Examination,* 5th ed., p. 369, Figure 12–10A, by H. M. Seidel et al., 2003, St. Louis, MO: Mosby.)

contracts and descends, enlarging the thoracic cavity and compressing the contents of the abdomen. The parasternal and scalene muscles contribute to thoracic expansion; the intercostal muscles elevate the ribs and sternum. The intrathoracic pressure falls, causing air to be drawn through the trachea, bronchi, and bronchioles into the alveoli (air sacs). In the expanded state of the lungs, oxygen diffuses into the blood and carbon dioxide diffuses out of the blood at the alveolar level. During expiration, a primarily passive activity, the diaphragm relaxes, intrathoracic pressure increases, the thoracic cage returns to its former position, and the air in the alveoli and tracheobronchial tree flows in the opposite direction.

The act of breathing is usually quiet, effortless, and automatic. Respiratory rates in healthy adults vary from 12 to 20 respirations per minute. When respiration requires effort due to exercise or disease, breathing is audible and effort is visible. Accessory muscles then facilitate the respiratory effort. In the neck, the sternomastoid and scalene muscles assist with inspiration. In the interspaces between the ribs, muscles retract during inspiration; abdominal muscles contract during expiration.

Before initiating the physical examination, the nurse conducts a health history interview (Table 28-39) and uses the data to focus the respiratory assessment and plan teaching opportunities (Box 28-29).

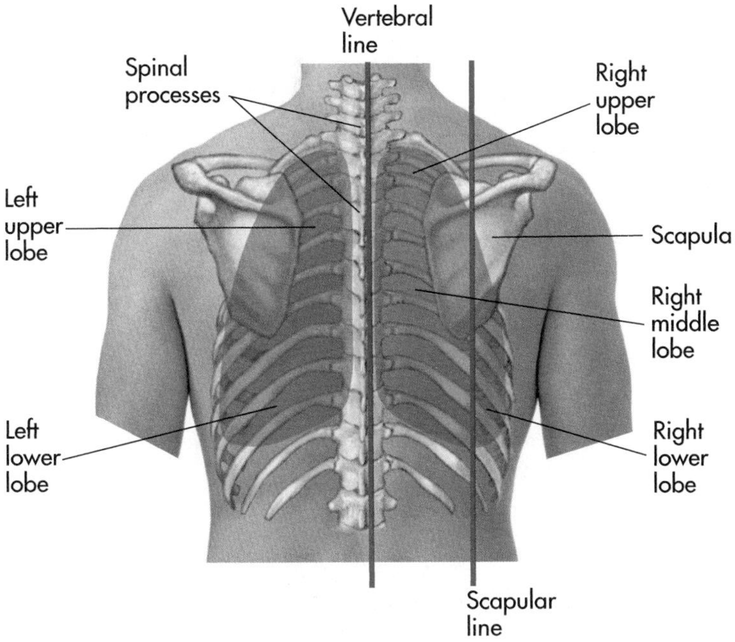

FIGURE 28–57 Posterior thorax. (From *Mosby's Guide to Physical Examination,* 5th ed., p. 369, Figure 12–10C, by H. M. Seidel et al., 2003, St. Louis, MO: Mosby.)

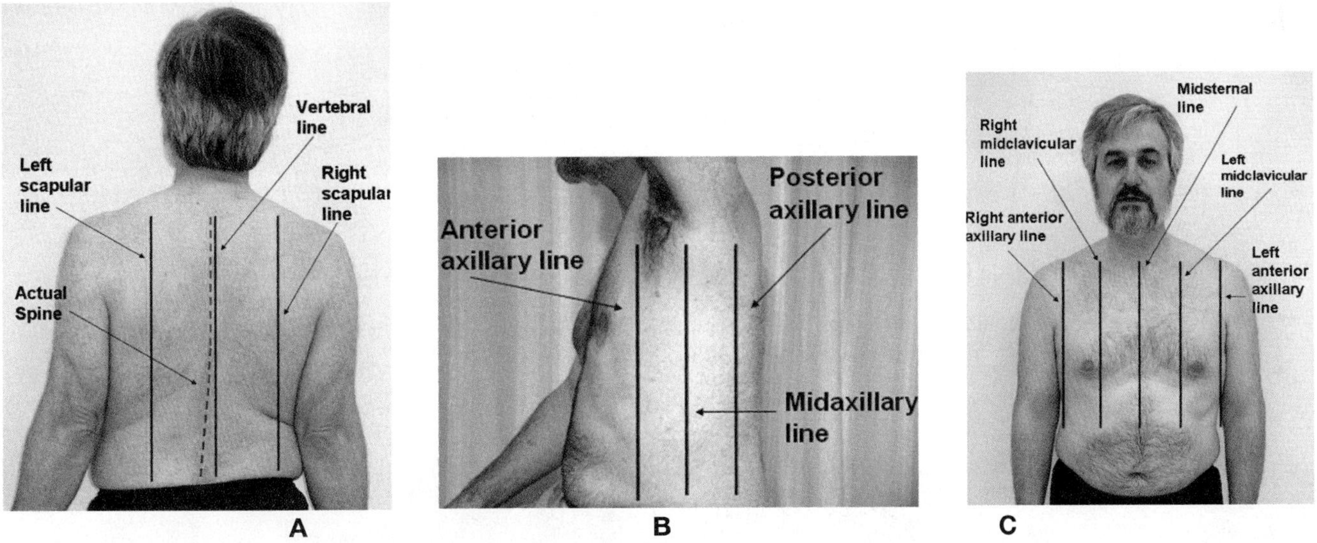

FIGURE 28–58 **A,** Posterior vertical lines. **B,** Lateral vertical lines. **C,** Anterior vertical lines. (From *Physical Examination Images* [CD-ROM], by D. L. Skillen, R. A. Day, M. C. Anderson, T. C. Stephen, J. A. Gilbert, and L. W. Day, 2004, Edmonton, AB: Faculty of Nursing, University of Alberta.)

Posterior Thorax and Lung Fields. Nurses use inspection, palpation, percussion, and auscultation to assess the thorax and the lungs (Procedure 28-14). It is essential that the nurse palpate, percuss, and auscultate on symmetric areas of the thorax to compare sides. The nurse drapes the female client's anterior chest while examining the posterior chest. Bedridden clients may remain supine and be assisted onto their side, but ambulatory clients are best examined in the sitting position during assessment of the posterior thorax.

Inspection. In the midline position, nurses examine the posterior thorax for shape, skin condition, and movement at rest and during respiration. They expect the scapulae to be symmetrical and closely attached to the thoracic wall. Nurses routinely inspect rate, rhythm, depth, and effort of breathing. They always observe for any indication of respiratory difficulty. That includes inspection of client colour (lips, nails), displacement of the trachea from midline, audible sounds of breathing, and client's position to aid breathing. They expect to identify a lateral diameter (Lat) wider than the anteroposterior diameter (AP) and estimate the ratio between them when recording findings. The AP:Lat ratio is from 1:2 to 5:7. Deformities, asymmetry of movement, or use of accessory respiratory muscles are unexpected findings.

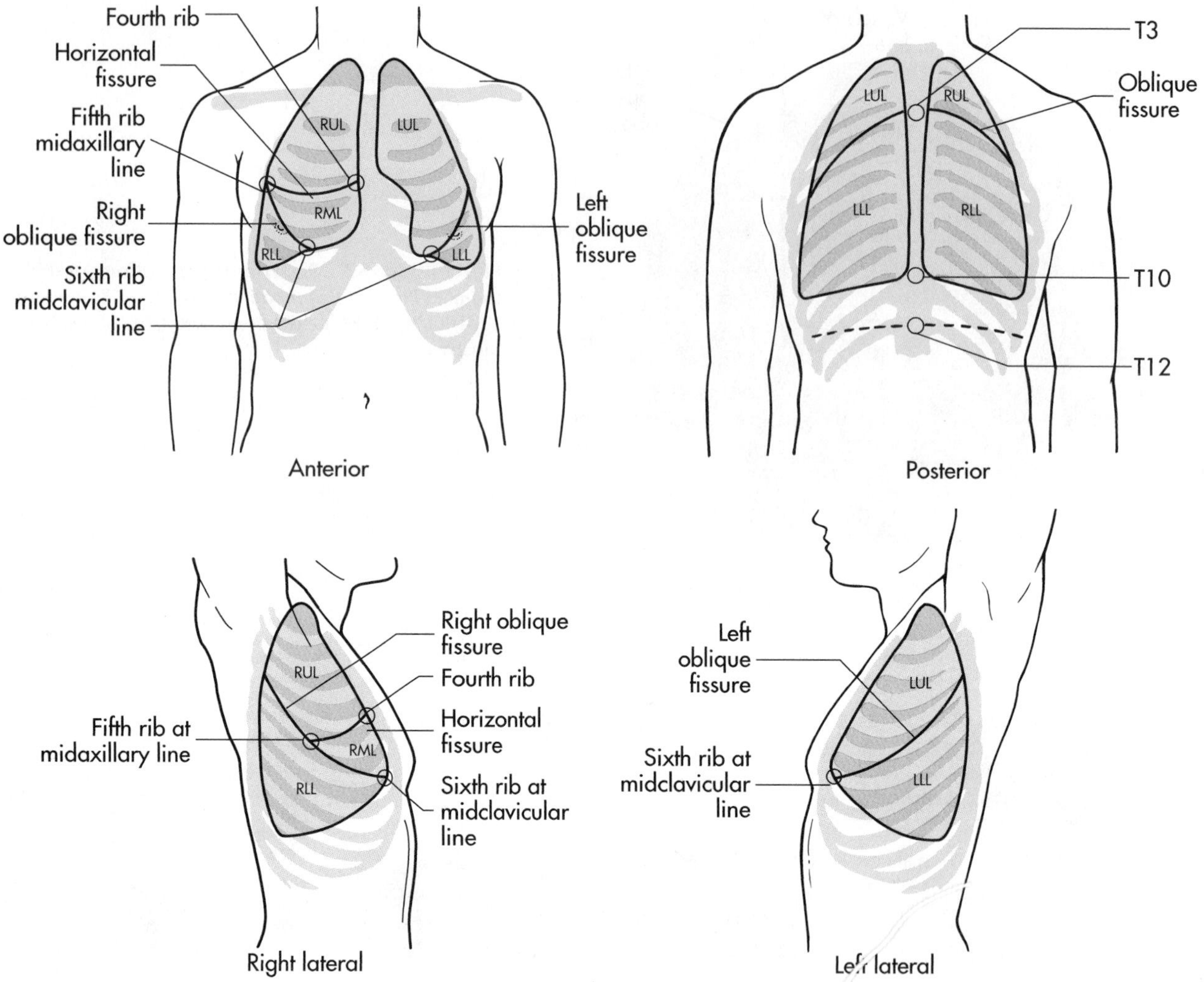

FIGURE 28–59 Visualizing the lungs from the surface. (From *Mosby's Guide to Physical Examination,* 5th ed., p. 361, Box 12-1, by H. M. Seidel et al., 2003, St. Louis, MO: Mosby.)

Table 28-39 Health History for Lung Assessment

Assessment Category	Rationale
Ask client about tobacco use, including duration, amount, frequency of use in pack-years,* age started smoking, type of tobacco, and efforts to quit.	Smoking is a risk factor for lung cancer, other lung diseases, and heart disease.
Inquire about cough, sputum, chest pain, activity tolerance, shortness of breath, recurrent infections.	Symptoms may help nurse localize objective data.
Question client on working environment pollutants (e.g., asbestos, coal dust, second-hand smoke, chemicals).	These exposures increase potential for lung disease.
Inquire about history of substance abuse, HIV infection, low income, residential living, or recent immigration.	These are risk factors for tuberculosis.
Ask client about persistent cough, fatigue, hemoptysis, unexplained weight loss, night sweats, or fever.	These signs and symptoms are associated with tuberculosis and HIV infection.
Ask about any voice hoarseness.	This may indicate a laryngeal disorder or lifestyle issue (use of cocaine/opioids).
Inquire about family history of cancer, tuberculosis, allergies, or chronic obstructive pulmonary disease.	These conditions place client at risk for lung disease.
Ask about allergies to pollutants, dust, or other airborne irritants, and to foods, drugs, or chemical irritants.	Allergic responses can cause signs and symptoms such as dyspnea and wheezes.

*Pack-years = number of years smoked × number of packs per day.

Client Teaching Box 28-29

Health Promotion for Lung Assessment

Objectives

- Client will know risk factors, signs, and symptoms of lung disease.
- Older adults will receive preventative immunization annually against influenza and pneumonia.

Teaching Strategies

- Explain risk factors for lung disease to client, including smoking and exposure to environmental pollution or chemical irritants.
- Share brochures on lung cancer from the Canadian Cancer Society with client.
- Inform about warning signs for lung disease, including a persistent cough, chest pains, sputum streaked with blood, and recurring lung infections (e.g., bronchitis, pneumonia).
- Counsel older adults about benefits of influenza and pneumonia vaccinations for reducing susceptibility to respiratory infection.
- Encourage clients at risk for tuberculosis to have regular skin testing.

Evaluation

- Have client describe risk factors for lung cancer and signs and symptoms of lung disease.
- Review immunization records to ensure current vaccinations against influenza and pneumonia and regular tuberculin skin testing.

Clients who lean forward, supporting their arms against a chair, pillow, their knees, or some other structure, may be doing so because they are having difficulty breathing. This position is common in clients with chronic obstructive pulmonary disease because it aids expiration. Nurses watch for pursed lips during expiration and for clients who may splint or hold the chest wall to minimize localized pain aggravated by respirations. This causes them to bend toward the affected side and impairs ventilatory movement.

Palpation. The nurse explores skin lesions noted during inspection and palpates the chest for tenderness, masses, and skin temperature. The thoracic muscles and skeleton are expected to be non-tender. Nurses assess symmetry of chest expansion by examining respiratory expansion (Figure 28–60). Pain, postural deformity, or fatigue may limit chest expansion. Nurses evaluate symmetry of chest vibrations by assessing **tactile fremitus,** a palpable vibration generated by asking clients to repeat certain sounds during thoracic palpation. If fremitus is faint, it may be necessary to ask clients to speak in a louder or deeper voice. For palpation, either the ball of the hand or ulnar edge will detect the vibrations of sound waves. Nurses may use one hand or both hands simultaneously, unless one is more sensitive to vibrations than the other. They systematically compare thoracic regions as they palpate from apices to bases (Figure 28–61). Palpable vibrations are expected to be present bilaterally and equal, with greater intensity over the apices and interscapular areas and reduced intensity over lung bases. When there are lung lesions, collapsed lung tissues, or accumulations of mucus, vibration intensity decreases.

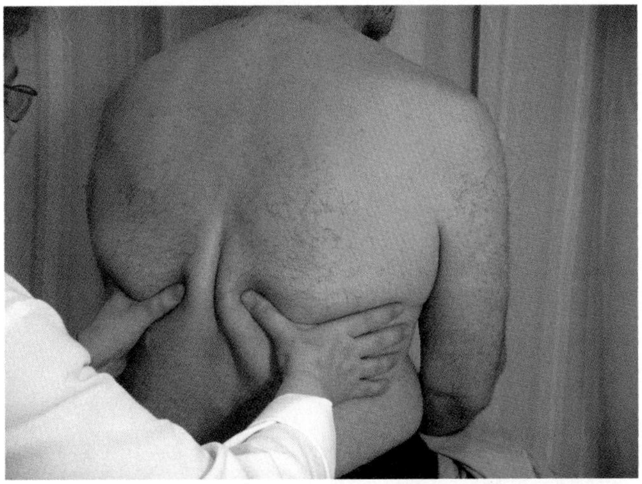

FIGURE **28–60** Respiratory expansion. (From *Physical Examination Images* [CD-ROM], by D. L. Skillen, R. A. Day, M. C. Anderson, T. C. Stephen, J. A. Gilbert, and L. W. Day, 2004, Edmonton, AB: Faculty of Nursing, University of Alberta.)

Percussion. Percussion over the intercostal spaces identifies underlying tissues as air-filled, fluid-filled, or solid. Nurses percuss the posterior thorax in all areas used for palpation and auscultation (see Figure 28–61), comparing sides. As lungs are filled with air, a resonant percussion note is expected for all thoracic regions. Percussion over the scapulae, ribs, or spine will produce a dull percussion note. In adults with hyperinflated lungs, the percussion note may be hyperresonant. When lung tissue is consolidated or contains fluid, the percussion note will be dull. A lung mass causes a flat sound. A dull or flat sound may suggest atelectasis, pleural effusion, pneumothorax, or asthma.

Auscultation. Recognizing sounds created by inspiratory and expiratory airflow (Table 28-40) permits nurses to detect sounds caused by narrowed or obstructed airways. Using the diaphragm chestpiece, nurses listen to an entire inspiration and expiration at each position of the stethoscope. If sounds are faint, as in obese clients, they ask the client to breathe harder. Nurses always systematically move the stethoscope from the right to the left and back (see Figure 28–61, A) to compare the sounds in one region of the chest with sounds in the same region on the other side. Nurses never fully auscultate one side (i.e., from apex to base) before auscultating any of the other side. They always compare symmetric regions to detect unexpected **adventitious sounds,** which may be superimposed over expected sounds. Four types of adventitious sounds are crackles, rhonchi, wheezes, and pleural friction rub. Each sound has specific characteristics (Table 28-41).

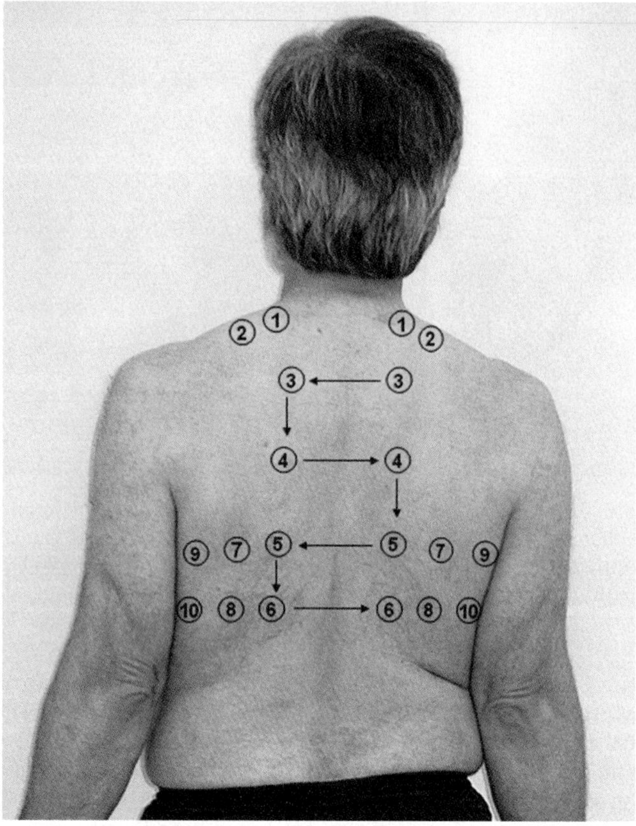

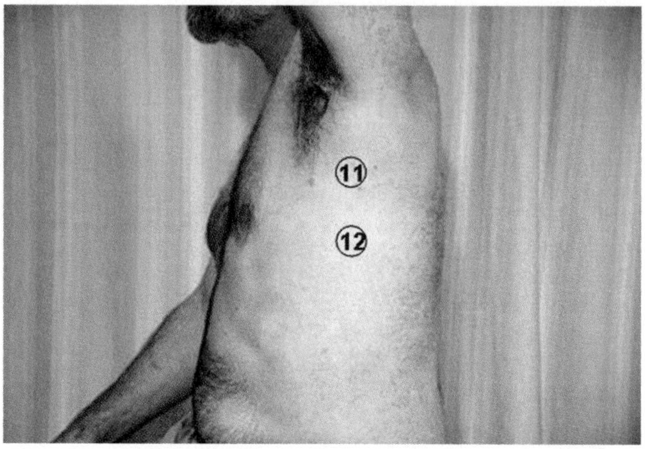

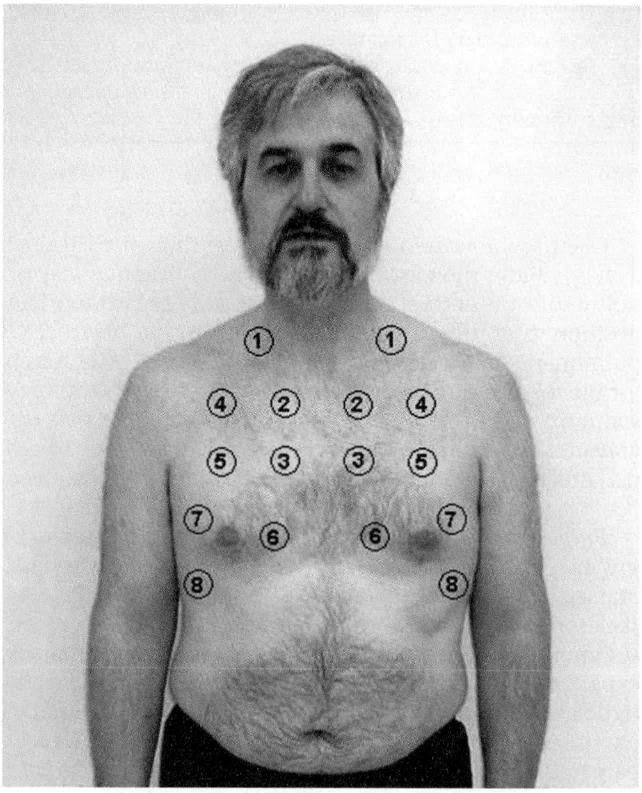

FIGURE **28–61** **A,** Sites on posterior thorax. **B,** Sites on lateral thorax. **C,** Sites on anterior thorax. (From *Physical Examination Images* [CD-ROM], by D. L. Skillen, R. A. Day, M. C. Anderson, T. C. Stephen, J. A. Gilbert, and L. W. Day, 2004, Edmonton, AB: Faculty of Nursing, University of Alberta.)

Table 28-40 Expected Breath Sounds

Description	Location	Origin
Vesicular		
Vesicular sounds are soft, breezy, and low pitched. Inspiratory phase is three times longer than expiratory phase.	Best heard over lung's periphery (except over scapula)	Created by air moving through smaller airways
Bronchovesicular		
Bronchovesicular sounds are blowing sounds that are medium pitched and of medium intensity. Inspiratory phase is equal to expiratory phase.	Best heard posteriorly between scapulae and anteriorly over bronchioles lateral to sternum at first and second intercostal spaces	Created by air moving through large airways
Bronchial		
Bronchial sounds are loud and high pitched with hollow quality. Expiration lasts longer than inspiration (3:2 ratio).	Best heard over trachea	Created by air moving through trachea close to chest wall

Table 28-41 Adventitious Breath Sounds

Sound	Site Auscultated	Cause	Character
Crackles 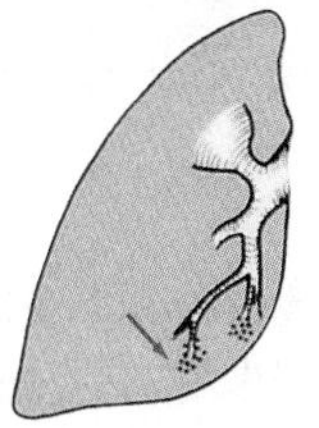	Are most commonly heard in dependent lobes; right and left lung bases	Random, sudden reinflation of groups of alveoli; disruptive passage of air	Fine crackles are high-pitched fine, short, interrupted crackling sounds heard during end of inspiration, usually not cleared with coughing. Medium crackles are lower, more moist sounds heard during middle of inspiration; not cleared with coughing. Coarse crackles are loud, bubbly sounds heard during inspiration; not cleared with coughing.
Rhonchi (sonorous wheeze) 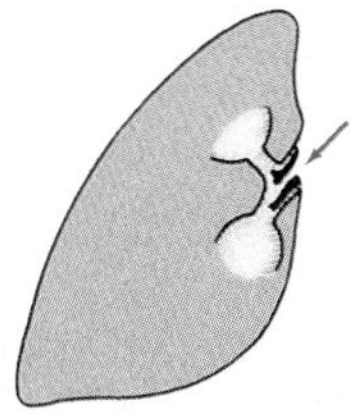	Are primarily heard over trachea and bronchi; if loud enough, can be heard over most lung fields	Muscular spasm, fluid, or mucus in larger airways, causing turbulence	Are loud, low-pitched, rumbling coarse sounds heard most often during inspiration and expiration; may be cleared by coughing.
Wheezes (sibilant wheeze) 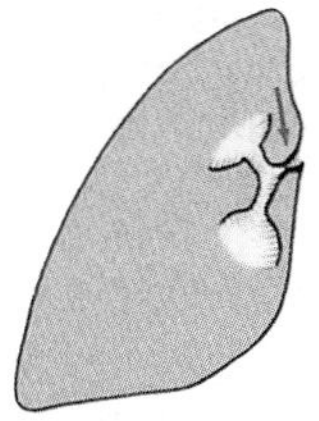	Can be heard over all lung fields	High-velocity airflow through severely narrowed bronchus	Are high-pitched, continuous musical sounds like a squeak heard continuously during inspiration or expiration; usually louder on expiration.
Pleural friction rub 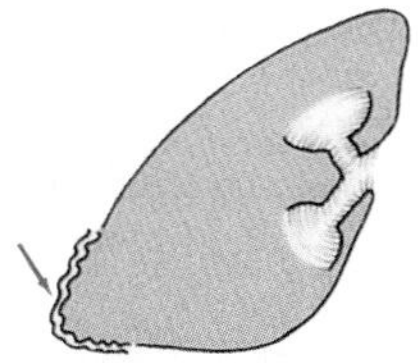	Is heard over anterior lateral lung field (if client is sitting upright)	Inflamed pleura, parietal pleura rubbing against visceral pleura	Has dry, grating quality heard best during inspiration; does not clear with coughing; heard loudest over lower lateral anterior surface.

Data from *Mosby's Guide to Physical Examination* (5th ed., pp. 385–386), by H. M. Seidel et al., 2003, St. Louis, MO: Mosby.

Procedure 28-14 Examination of the Posterior Thorax and Lungs

Equipment

- Stethoscope

Examination Skill and Focus	Steps	Rationale
Thorax Inspection: Anteroposterior/Lateral (AP/lateral) Posterior lung fields	Client sitting disrobed to waist **1.** Inspect from side (profile). **2.** Inspect posterior thorax from midline.	Ensures chest is fully visible. Assesses anteroposterior diameter in relation to lateral diameter.
Palpation: Chest expansion	**1.** Place thumbs at level of and parallel to 10th ribs.	
	2. Wrap hands **loosely** around lateral rib cage.	Loosely wrapped hands permit unrestricted movement of thorax.
	3. Slide hands medially to raise skin folds between thumb and spine.	
	4. Instruct client to inhale deeply and exhale.	As client inhales, a flattened skin fold indicates symmetrical movement of the thorax.
	5. Compare sides.	
Tactile fremitus	**1.** Instruct client to round shoulders with arms folded across chest, hands on shoulders.	As shoulders are rounded, the scapulae separate, increasing access to posterior lung fields.
	2. Palpate and compare symmetrical areas: • Upper (apices and interscapular) • Lower • Lateral (in midaxillary line)	Ensures all posterior lung fields are fully assessed including the lateral lung fields.
	3. Ask client to repeat "99" **OR** words (blue moon) in a deep voice.	A deep voice produces vibrations that carry more effectively to the periphery.
	4. Use ball of hand (palm at base of fingers) **OR** ulnar aspect of hand.	The ulnar surface and ball of the hand are equally sensitive to vibrations.
	5. Use one **OR** two hands to assess fremitus in symmetrical areas (upper, lower, and lateral).	
Percussion: Posterior chest	**1.** Instruct client to continue rounding shoulders.	As shoulders are rounded, the scapulae separate, increasing access to posterior lung fields.
	2. Percuss and compare symmetrical areas at 5-cm intervals over: • upper (apices and interscapular) • lower • **lateral (in midaxillary line)**	Ensures all posterior lung fields are fully assessed.
	3. Press distal phalanx and joint of middle (pleximeter) finger **firmly** over intercostals space (avoiding contact with other fingers).	Any contact on the thorax from fingers other than the pleximeter finger dampens the percussion note.
	4. Aim at distal phalanx or interphalangeal joint.	Avoids percussing over bone (ribs).

From *A Syllabus for Adult Health Assessment* (pp. 39–40), edited by D. L. Skillen and R. A. Day, 2004, Edmonton, AB: Faculty of Nursing, University of Alberta.

Examination Skill and Focus	Steps	Rationale
	5. Strike pleximeter a sharp perpendicular blow with tip of middle (plexor) finger (may support plexor finger with thumb).	Consistent quick sharp blows are most effective in eliciting the desired percussion note. No more than one or two blows per site facilitate identification of the percussion note.
	6. Use wrist action only.	
Auscultation: Posterior lung fields	1. Instruct client to continue rounding shoulders.	Ensures access to posterior lung fields.
	2. Auscultate with diaphragm of stethoscope.	Enhances breath sounds for auscultation.
	3. Instruct client to breathe through open mouth, more deeply than usual, and inform if dizzy.	Dizziness alerts nurse to client hyperventilation and need to rest.
	4. Listen to at least ONE full breath in each area.	Assesses both inspiratory and expiratory breath sounds. Timing in respiratory cycle assists with interpretation of findings.
	5. Listen to and compare symmetrical areas: • upper (apices and interscapular) • lower • lateral (in midaxillary line)	Comparison aids detection of differences. Ensures all posterior lung fields are fully assessed, including lateral lung fields.

From *A Syllabus for Adult Health Assessment* (pp. 39–40), edited by D. L. Skillen and R. A. Day, 2004, Edmonton, AB: Faculty of Nursing, University of Alberta.

Anterior and Lateral Thorax and Lung Fields

Anterior Thorax. The anterior thorax is inspected, palpated, percussed, and auscultated for most of the same features as the posterior thorax. Clients may sit or lie down with head elevated. The supine position facilitates displacement of the female breasts for the examination. In the anterior thorax, the nurse observes for the width of the costal angle between the right and left costal margins, which is usually greater than 90 degrees. The anterior thorax is commonly where respiratory rate, rhythm, and effort are assessed. In men, respirations are often diaphragmatic; in women, they are usually thoracic or costal.

Nurses assess respiratory expansion using the same techniques as for the posterior thorax. When assessing for tactile fremitus, they know that findings will differ because of the heart and female breast tissue. They feel fremitus best next to the sternum at the second intercostal space, at the level of the bronchial bifurcation. They avoid palpating over the heart and breast tissue for tactile fremitus. Instead, they gently retract breast tissue or have the client lift up the breasts for palpation.

Percussion of the anterior thorax follows a systematic pattern. Nurses begin percussion above the clavicles and move from side to side as they approach the lower thorax. Female breasts are displaced as needed. Proceeding downward, nurses detect heart and liver dullness, and the tympanic gastric air bubble.

Auscultation of the anterior thorax follows the same pattern as percussion. Vesicular sounds are heard in the apices, below the clavicles, and over the peripheral lung fields. Bronchovesicular sounds are heard below the clavicles. Bronchial sounds can be heard over the trachea as loud, high pitched, and hollow. Nurses pay special attention to the lower lobes, where mucus commonly collects in adults with illness or disease.

Lateral Thorax. Using the same systematic pattern, nurses inspect, palpate, percuss, and auscultate the lateral lung fields on both sides (see Figure 28–61, *B*). This procedure usually occurs as an extension of the assessment of the posterior thorax when nurses ask the client to lift arms away from the chest. Nurses do not assess respiratory expansion in the lateral thorax, because it is included in the techniques used for the anterior and posterior thorax. In the lateral thorax, percussion notes are expected to be resonant and breath sounds vesicular. The nurse keeps a mental picture of the structures underlying the lateral rib cage and considers the potential source of unexpected findings.

Age-Related Changes. Mobility of the thorax diminishes as costal cartilages become increasingly calcified. Muscles of respiration lose strength. Elastic properties of the lung tissue diminish, affecting extensibility and recoil. Small airways are more likely to close early, reducing the amount of air that can be expelled during expiration and increasing the amount of residual air that remains in the lungs. At the alveolar level, the surface area for oxygen and carbon dioxide exchange is reduced. Ventilation of the lung bases decreases. Skeletal changes increase the anteroposterior diameter and emphasize the thoracic curvature with little effect on function in healthy older adults, but creating more of a barrel-shaped chest.

Documentation. Nurses record their findings from inspection, palpation, percussion, and auscultation of the thorax and lungs (Table 28-42).

Assessing the Heart

Cardiac function is assessed through the anterior thorax. The nurse visualizes the location of the heart chambers and valves and the direction in which the great vessels arise from the heart in relation to the sternum and ribs. In adults, the heart lies posterior to the **precordium** (area of the thorax that lies over the heart), is rotated so that the right ventricle forms most of its anterior surface, and extends almost to the xiphoid process, where it rests on the diaphragm. A small portion of the right atrium extends to the right of the sternum (Figure 28–62). The superior border of the heart, formed mostly by the great vessels, is called the "base" of the heart and is located at about the right and left second interspaces close to the sternum. The left ventricle lies posterior to the right ventricle, its left lateral border extending beyond the right ventricle. The left

Table 28-42 **Examples of Documentation for Posterior Thorax and Lung Assessment**

Focus of Assessment	Expected Findings	Unexpected Findings
Thorax shape	Elliptical; AP:Lat ratio is 1:2	AP:Lat ratio is 1:1
Thorax symmetry	Shoulders, scapulae, iliac crests, and posterior superior iliac spines aligned horizontally; muscle development symmetrical; non-tender bilaterally	(R) shoulder higher than (L); vertebral column deviates to (R) in upper vertebral line; unequal muscle mass (L) > (R)
Skin	Intact; pink; smooth; warm; scattered freckles over shoulders and upper thorax	Brown-black, irregular-shaped papule, 8 mm × 7 mm, with raised borders, over (L) inferior scapula
Respiratory expansion	Symmetrical upward and outward movement on inspiration; equal movement during expiration	Reduced upward and outward movement (R) thorax
Tactile fremitus	Vibrations equally palpable and intense over apices and interscapular areas; less intense (R) (L) lower lung fields	Vibrations faint over entire thorax
Percussion	Resonant throughout (R)(L)	Dullness percussed (R) apex
Breath sounds	Vesicular sounds over lung fields (R)(L); bronchovesicular breath sounds over (R) interscapular area; no adventitious sounds heard	Fine crackles (L)(R) bases; expiratory wheeze throughout posterior chest, (L) > (R)

Adapted from *First Year Student Lab Guide* (p. 68), by J. Chambers et al., 2004, Edmonton, AB: Faculty of Nursing, University of Alberta.

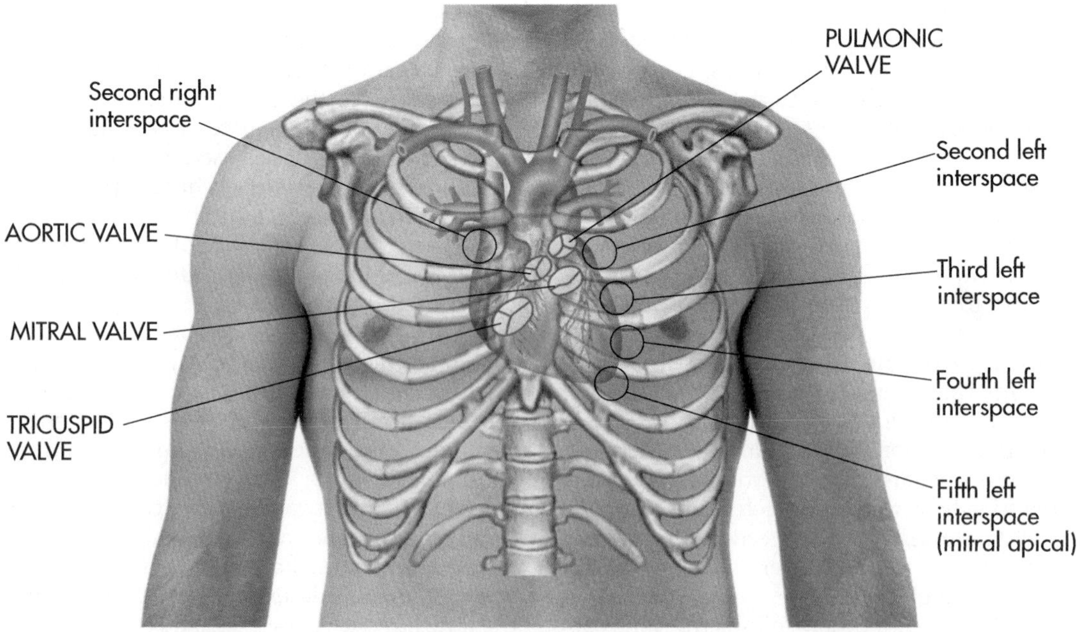

FIGURE 28–62 Position of the heart and great vessels in the thorax. Note the location of the point of maximum impulse (PMI) and areas for auscultation of the heart. (From *Mosby's Guide to Physical Examination,* 5th ed., p. 433, Figure 13–15, by H. M. Seidel et al., 2003, St. Louis, MO: Mosby.)

ventricle forms the left lateral border and the bottom tip or "apex" of the heart. The apex is located just medial to the left MCL at approximately the fifth intercostal space. Contraction of the left ventricle produces the **apical impulse** or **point of maximal impulse (PMI).**

To understand the significance of cardiac assessment findings, nurses must understand the dynamics of the cardiac cycle (Figure 28–63), which has two phases: systole and diastole. Events occurring on the left side of the heart slightly precede those on the right side. At the onset of systole, the ventricles begin to contract, increasing pressure in the ventricles and causing closure of the mitral and tricuspid valves. Further contraction of the ventricles opens the aortic and pulmonic valves when blood is ejected from the left ventricle into the aorta and from the right ventricle into the pulmonary artery. At the beginning of diastole, as pressure in the ventricles drops below that in the aorta and pulmonary arteries, the aortic and pulmonic valves close. As the ventricles relax, pressure drops in the ventricles and the mitral and tricuspid valves open, allowing the ventricles to fill with blood. Late in diastole, the atria contract, pushing an additional amount of blood into the ventricles.

Because the left side of the heart is a high-pressure system, closure of the mitral and aortic valves creates louder auscultatory sounds than those created by closure of the right heart valves (tricuspid and pulmonic). Closure of the mitral and aortic valves is heard with a stethoscope over the entire precordium. Closure of the mitral and tricuspid valves marks the beginning of systole and creates S_1 ("lub"), usually loudest at the apex (mitral area). At the beginning of diastole, the aortic and pulmonic valves

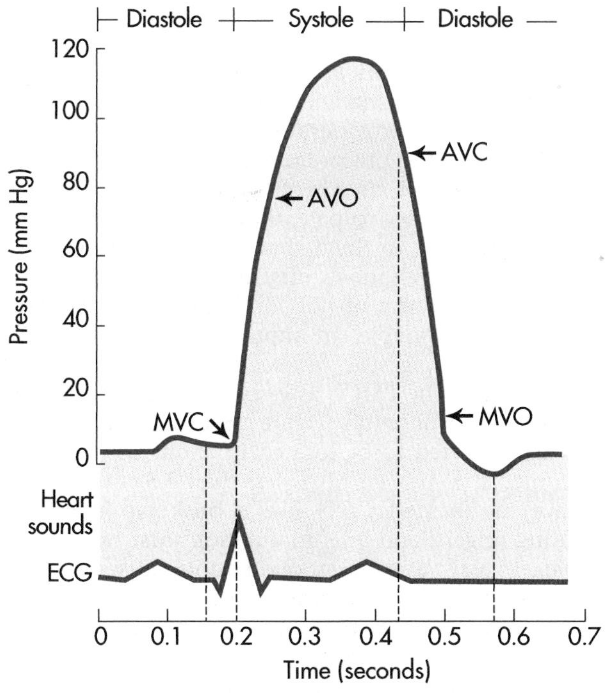

FIGURE 28–63 Cardiac cycle. *MVC,* Mitral valve closes; *AVO,* aortic valve opens; *AVC,* aortic valve closes; *MVO,* mitral valve opens.

close together, creating the second heart sound, S_2 ("dub"). Because sound is carried in the direction of blood flow, S_2 is usually loudest at the base of the heart in the second right interspace (aortic area) and second left interspace (pulmonic area). As systole is usually shorter than diastole, S_1 is followed by S_2 ("lub-dub"), then by a slightly longer interval before S_1 is heard again.

As the ventricular pressures fall below atrial pressures, the mitral and tricuspid valves open, allowing the ventricles to fill. The rapid filling of the left ventricle may create a third heart sound (S_3), more often in children and young adults. After 40 years of age, an S_3 is considered pathological and likely associated with congestive heart failure or regurgitant valves. Near the end of diastole when the atria contract to enhance ventricular filling, a fourth heart sound (S_4) may be heard in some healthy older adults and trained athletes. More commonly, it is due to a pathological condition such as hypertensive heart disease in which the left ventricular wall stiffens, increasing resistance to ventricular filling following atrial contraction. A useful way to think of the timing of S_3 and S_4 heart sounds is diagrammed below (Swartz, 2002).

SLOSH' –	ing	in	a	STIFF'	wall
S_1	S_2	S_3	S_4	S_1	S_2

Events on the left side of the heart usually occur slightly before those on the right side; however, following a deep inspiration, S_2 may split, making closure of the aortic valve (A_2) heard first and then pulmonic valve (P_2) closure audible in the left second and third interspaces close to the sternum. The reason for this physiological splitting of the second heart sound is understood currently as follows. Deep inspiration increases the capacity of the pulmonary vasculature, prolongs right ventricular contraction, and delays closure of the pulmonic valve. The left ventricle contracts comparatively earlier, followed by aortic valve closure (Bickley & Szilagyi, 2003; Seidel et al., 2003).

Nurses are guided by the health history interview (Table 28-43) and seek opportunities for client teaching and health promotion throughout their examination (Box 28-30).

Before assessing the heart, the nurse ensures that the client is relaxed, comfortable, and lying flat with the upper body elevated 30 degrees in a quiet environment with good lighting. To relieve the client's anxiety, the nurse provides the client with ongoing explanations of procedures. The client should not talk during auscultation. The nurse stands at the client's right side and exposes the precordium.

Inspection. Using tangential lighting, examiners inspect the entire precordium for pulsations or lifts. They begin at the base of the heart near the second right and left interspaces and progress downward to the apex or, alternatively, they begin inspection at the apex and progress upward to the base of the heart. They also inspect the epigastric region. An absence of pulsations over the precordium and epigastric region is expected. In thin clients, they may see pulsations at the PMI (left ventricular contraction) or in the epigastric area (aortic pulsations). Pulsation or lifts seen at other locations usually indicate cardiac pathology.

Table 28-43 Health History for Heart Assessment

Assessment Category	Rationale
Ask client about risk factors such as smoking, alcohol or drug use, exercise habits, dietary patterns, and stress levels.	These factors are related to heart disease.
Inquire about medication use for cardiovascular function and if client knows dosage, purpose, and side effects.	Examiner can assess client knowledge and plan teaching as needed.
Ask client about history of chest pain, palpitations, fatigue, cough, dyspnea, leg pains or cramps, edema of extremities, fainting, and orthopnea. Inquire whether these happen at rest and/or during activity and conduct a symptom analysis.	These can be symptoms of heart disease.
Question client about family history of cardiac problems.	Presence of family history of heart disease increases risk of heart disease.
Inquire about the presence of conditions such as diabetes, lung disease, obesity, or hypertension.	These disorders can affect heart function.
Question client about usual habits for ingesting caffeine-containing drinks (coffee, tea, soft drinks) or chocolate.	Caffeine can cause cardiac arrhythmia.

Client Teaching — *Box 28-30*

Health Promotion for Heart Assessment

Objectives

- Client will know risk factors for heart disease and take appropriate actions to eliminate risks from lifestyle.
- Client will know signs and symptoms of heart disease and seek appropriate treatment, as needed.

Teaching Strategies

- Explain risk factors for heart disease, including high dietary intake of saturated fats or cholesterol, lack of regular aerobic exercise, excess weight, stressful lifestyle, hypertension, and family history of heart disease.
- Refer client as necessary for appropriate counselling to reduce risks, including dietary counselling, exercise counselling, and learning of stress-reduction techniques.
- Encourage client to have regular checkups, including measurement of blood pressure and blood cholesterol levels, and to follow the advice of the examiner related to medication, dietary alterations, and further blood or cardiac function testing.

Evaluation

- Have client state the risk factors for heart disease and the signs and symptoms of heart disease.
- Have client describe their lifestyle choices, including dietary and exercise patterns.
- Have client state time of last checkup for blood pressure and cholesterol measurement.

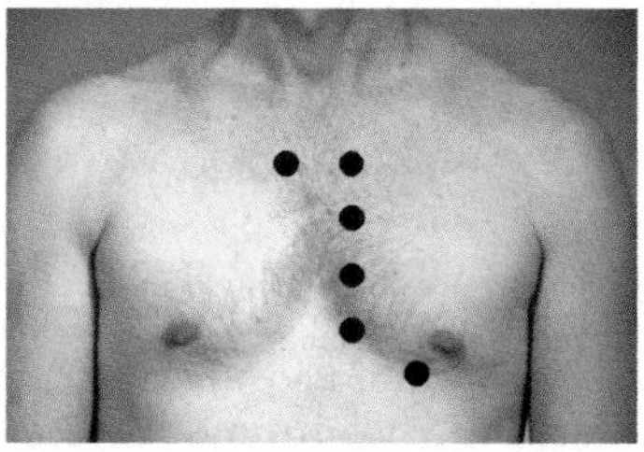

FIGURE **28–64** Landmarks on precordium. (From *Physical Examination Images* [CD-ROM], by D. L. Skillen, R. A. Day, M. C. Anderson, T. C. Stephen, J. A. Gilbert, and L. W. Day, 2004, Edmonton, AB: Faculty of Nursing, University of Alberta.)

Palpation. Six anatomical landmarks on the precordium are important for palpation and auscultation (Figure 28–64). Using their fingertips, nurses first locate the angle of Louis (sternal angle). Then they glide their fingers beside the angle to feel the attached second ribs on each side and just below, the right and left second intercostal spaces. They often mark at least the left second interspace with a water-soluble marker as a reference point.

Procedure 28-15 provides the procedure and techniques for palpation of the precordium and epigastric area. Each time that nurses ask the client to exhale and briefly hold the breath while they palpate, they hold their own breath; this is a reminder to them that clients need to breathe. They palpate for pulsations, lifts, or thrills when the breath is held. The presence of pulsations may indicate cardiac pathology. For example, an impulse against the palpating fingertip in the epigastric area suggests enlargement of the right ventricle. The PMI is assessed for location, diameter, amplitude, and duration (Figure 28–65, *A*). Apical pulsations are expected to be located in about the fifth interspace, medial to the left MCL; less than 2.5 cm (or one interspace) in diameter; feel like a brisk tap against the palpating fingers; and brief in duration (first two thirds of systole). To assist assessment of duration, nurses may identify systole by listening to heart sounds. If the PMI is lateral to the left MCL, larger than 2.5 cm, and palpated during most of systole, nurses suspect an enlarged left ventricle.

If the PMI is not initially palpable, the nurse asks the client to exhale fully and hold before palpating again. If the PMI still cannot be found, the nurse asks the client to roll onto the left side (left lateral recumbent position),

A 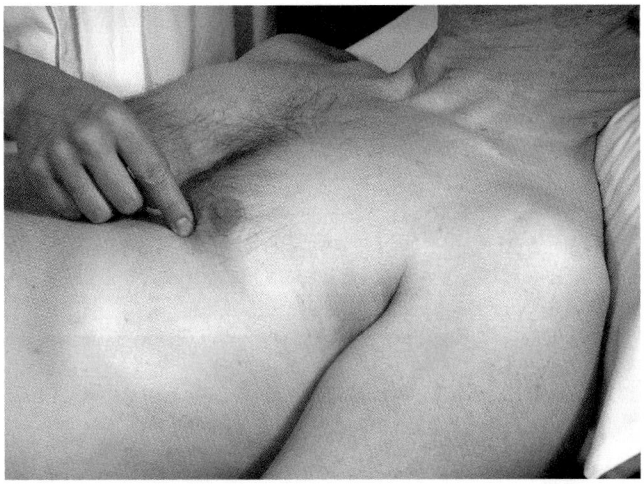 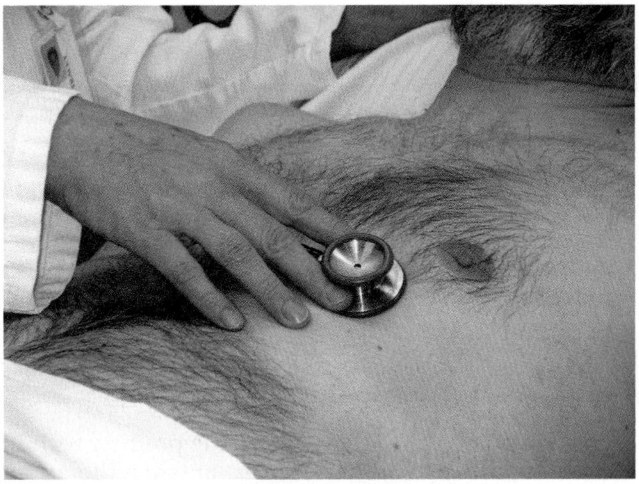 B

FIGURE **28–65** **A,** Palpation of apical impulse. **B,** Auscultation of apex. (From *Physical Examination Images* [CD-ROM], by D. L. Skillen, R. A. Day, M. C. Anderson, T. C. Stephen, J. A. Gilbert, and L. W. Day, 2004, Edmonton, AB: Faculty of Nursing, University of Alberta.)

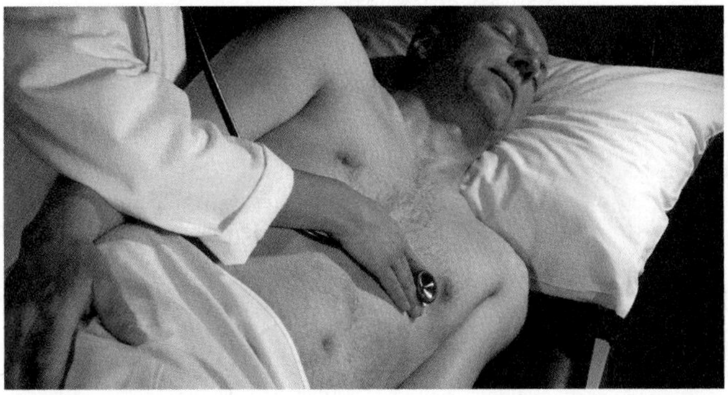

FIGURE **28–66** Left lateral recumbent position. (From *Physical Examination Images* [CD-ROM], by D. L. Skillen, R. A. Day, M. C. Anderson, T. C. Stephen, J. A. Gilbert, and L. W. Day, 2004, Edmonton, AB: Faculty of Nursing, University of Alberta.)

supports the client's back with the left hand flat on the table, and encourages the client to rest back on that arm (Figure 28–66). This manoeuvre brings the heart closer to the chest wall to enhance palpation but may increase the diameter of the PMI. Palpation of the PMI may be difficult if the anterior-posterior diameter is enlarged or if clients are very muscular or overweight.

Auscultation. Auscultation of the heart allows detection of expected heart sounds, extra heart sounds, and murmurs. The nursing student first becomes skilled at hearing and interpreting expected heart sounds using the techniques and procedures in Procedure 28-15. At each location, nurses identify the "lub-dub" sound created primarily by closure of the mitral (S_1) and then the aortic valves (S_2). Each combination of S_1 and S_2 or "lub-dub" counts as one heartbeat.

Systole is the period between the "lub" and "dub" and is usually shorter than diastole. If the heart rate is rapid, systole and diastole may last about the same length, making it difficult to distinguish one from the other. To overcome this problem, nurses palpate the carotid pulse as they auscultate. The carotid pulse occurs during early systole. At the apex, they assess heart rate and rhythm with the diaphragm of the stethoscope (see Figure 28–65, *B*).

When auscultating, the nurse listens carefully to assess the character of the heartbeats. As described earlier, S_1 is expected to be louder at the apex and S_2 louder at the base of the heart. These sounds are relatively high pitched and are heard best with the diaphragm of the stethoscope ("di-hi"). The bell of the stethoscope is better suited to pick up lower pitched sounds such as an S_3 and S_4. Nurses listen for the interval between S_1 and S_2 (systole) and then the time between S_2 and the next S_1 (diastole). They expect regular intervals of time between each beat, and a distinct silent pause during systole and during diastole. Failure of the heart to beat at regular successive intervals is a dysrhythmia.

When the heart rhythm is irregular, the nurse compares apical and radial pulse rates simultaneously to determine if a pulse deficit exists. The apical pulse is auscultated first and then the radial pulse is immediately palpated (one-examiner technique). When two examiners are available, they assess the apical and radial pulses at the same time. A pulse deficit is present when the radial pulse is slower than the apical pulse; a pulse deficit is caused by ineffective contractions fail to send pulse waves to the periphery.

When able to identify S_1 from S_2 and diastole from systole, the nurse listens for sounds that occur during diastole and/or systole. The nurse listens during diastole for an S_3 or S_4 with the bell of the stethoscope placed at the apex. These are extra heart sounds. The nurse also assesses for physiological splitting, listening for the two components of S_2: aortic closure (A_2) followed by pulmonic closure (P_2). A physiological split may or may not be present. Finally, nurses assess for a murmur. Murmurs are sustained swishing or blowing-like sounds heard at the beginning, middle, or end of the systolic or diastolic phase. They are created by turbulent blood flow over a stenosed or incompetent heart valve. The intensity of the murmur varies from barely audible to a sound that can be heard without the aid of a stethoscope. Identification of murmurs is beyond the scope of this chapter.

Procedure 28-15 Assessing the Heart

Equipment

- Penlight
- Stethoscope
- Water-soluble marker

Examination Skill and Focus	Steps	Rationale
Inspection:	Client in supine position with head elevated 30 degrees, anterior thorax and epigastric area exposed, examiner at client's right side	Provides best access to precordium.
Precordium	**1.** Inspect precordium tangentially using penlight.	Enhances the visibility of pulsations.
Palpation:	**1.** Landmark using sternal angle.	Assists in accurate site locations for palpation and auscultation.
	2. Palpate, proceeding from the apex to the base **OR** the base to the apex.	Either direction is acceptable as long as it is consistent.
Apical area	**1.** Use finger pads to palpate 5th interspace medial to (L) MCL.	
	2. Ask client to exhale and hold if unable to locate apical area in 1 above.	Exhalation brings the left ventricle closer to chest wall, enhancing possible palpation.
	3. Analyze impulses in apical area using fingertips, then one finger.	Analyzes the apical impulse for location, size, amplitude, and duration.
Right ventricular area	**1.** Place tips of curved fingers in (L) 3rd, 4th, and 5th interspaces close to sternum.	
	2. Ask client to exhale and hold breath.	Exhalation brings the chest wall closer to the right ventricle and the palpating fingers.
Epigastric area (subxiphoid)	**1.** Press index finger of flattened hand under (L) costal margin and up toward left shoulder.	
	2. Ask client to inhale and hold.	Inhalation brings the right ventricle closer to the palpating finger and also moves the hand away from the aorta.
Left 2nd interspace (pulmonic area)	**1.** Place index finger pad in 2nd (L) interspace.	
	2. Ask client to exhale and hold breath, palpate firmly.	Exhalation brings the chest wall closer to the heart and the pulmonary artery.
Right 2nd interspace (aortic area)	**1.** Place index finger pad in 2nd (R) interspace.	
	2. Ask client to exhale and hold breath, palpate firmly.	Exhalation brings chest wall closer to the heart and the aorta.
Auscultation:	**1.** Use diaphragm and bell to listen to all six areas.	The diaphragm picks up sounds that are higher pitched such as S_1 and S_2. The bell picks up lower-pitched sounds such as S_3 and S_4.
	2. Apply bell lightly to the chest wall.	Applying the bell lightly, just enough pressure to assure a full seal with the skin, prevents stretching the underlying skin and creating a diaphragm.
	3. Auscultate proceeding from apex to base **OR** base to apex.	
	4. Listen for 5 seconds in each area with diaphragm and bell.	Five seconds allows time for careful assessment of the heart sounds.

Examination Skill and Focus	Steps	Rationale
Right 2nd interspace Left 2nd, 3rd, 4th, 5th interspace Apex	**5.** Auscultate: • right 2nd interspace close to sternum • left 2nd interspace close to sternum • left 3rd interspace close to sternum • left 4th interspace close to sternum • left 5th interspace close to sternum • apex	
Apical rate	**6.** Listen for 1 minute at apex for rate, using diaphragm.	

Table 28-44 Examples of Documentation for Heart Assessment

Focus of Assessment	Expected Findings	Unexpected Findings
Inspection	No pulsations evident in (R) or (L) 2nd intercostal space (ICS), along (L) sternal border, or epigastric region. Pulsations evident in 5th ICS, medial to (L) midclavicular line (MCL).	Regular pulsation evident in 2nd (R) ICS and in 5th ICS in MCL; pulsation evident in epigastric region.
Palpation	No palpable pulsations or lifts in aortic or pulmonic areas, along (L) sternal border, or epigastric region. Point of maximal impulse (PMI) palpable in 5th ICS, medial to (L) MCL.	Palpable lift in 2nd (R) ICS. (R) ventricle pulsations palpable in epigastrium. PMI palpable in 5th to 6th ICS lateral to (L) MCL.
Apical impulse	PMI palpable in 5th ICS, medial to (L) MCL as light tap, 2 cm in diameter; spans first half systole.	PMI palpable in 5th to 6th ICS lateral to (L) MCL, 2.5 cm in diameter, feels sluggish/ sustained, spans fully two thirds systole.
Auscultation	S_1 louder than S_2 at apex, S_2 louder than S_1 at 2nd (R) interspace, splitting of S_2 evident in 2nd (L) interspace following deep inspiration, no extra heart sounds or murmurs.	S_2 louder than S_1 at apex, S_2 louder than S_1 at base, S_3 and S_4 evident at apex.
Rate/rhythm	76 bpm, regular rhythm.	88 bpm, regular irregular rhythm.

Adapted from *First Year Student Lab Guide* (p. 63), by J. Chambers et al. (2004), Edmonton AB: Faculty of Nursing, University of Alberta.

Age-Related Changes. It is difficult to differentiate between age-related and disease-related changes in the heart. Cardiovascular function in older adults varies widely. Both age-related and disease-related changes are influenced by lifestyle and environment. Some authorities believe that age-related change in the myocardium includes slight hypertrophy of the left ventricle. It develops gradually over the years in response to increased peripheral vascular resistance and elevated systolic blood pressure from stiffening of the arteries. Over the long term, circulatory efficiency may be impaired. In addition, thickening of the atrioventricular and aortic valves is common. In the aortic valve, thickening is often accompanied by calcification, an age-related change called *aortic sclerosis*. In at least one third of people over the age of 60 years, aortic sclerosis results in a mild aortic systolic murmur heard best with the diaphragm in the right second interspace. If the condition worsens, aortic stenosis, a pathological condition, may develop. Degenerative changes in the sinus node and myocardial pacemaker cells result in more frequent ectopic beats (Miller, 1999).

Documentation. Nurses record their findings from inspection, palpation, and auscultation of the heart (Table 28-44).

Assessing the Breasts

It is important to examine the breasts of both female and male clients. A small amount of glandular tissue, the potential site for the growth of cancer cells, is located in the male breast. In contrast, the majority of the female breast is glandular.

Female Breasts. The breasts are located anterior to the pectoralis major and serratus anterior muscles. They usually extend from the sternum to the midaxillary line, and from the clavicle and second rib to the sixth rib (Figure 28–67). The nipple is situated below the centre of the breast. It is round, usually protrudes, and the surface may be either smooth or wrinkled. The areolae surround the nipples and are usually round or oval and bilaterally nearly equal. Their colour ranges from pink to brown. In light-skinned women, the areola turns brown during pregnancy and remains dark. In dark-skinned women,

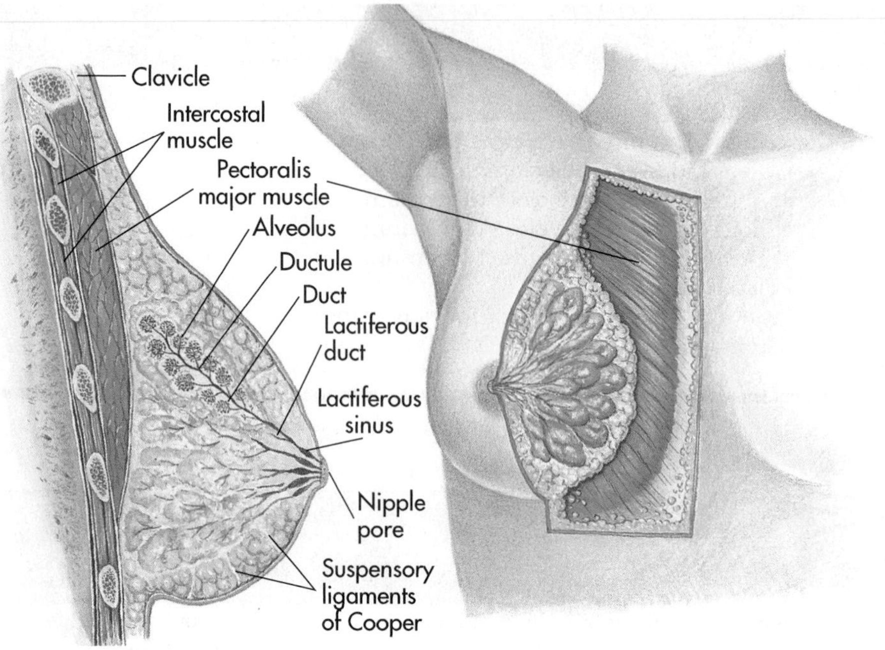

FIGURE **28–67** Anatomy of the breast showing position and major structures. (From *Mosby's Guide to Physical Examination,* 5th ed., p. 497, by H. M. Seidel et al., 2003, St. Louis, MO: Mosby.)

the areola is brown before pregnancy (Seidel et al., 1999). To assist in describing the location of findings, imaginary lines can be drawn through the centre of the nipple to divide the breast into four quadrants and the axillary Tail of Spence (see Figure 28–8).

Breasts consist of glandular tissue, fibrous supportive ligaments, and adipose tissue (fat). The proportion of the three types varies according to age, nutritional status, time in menstrual cycle, pregnancy, and lactation (Jarvis, 2004). Glandular tissue is organized into lobes that end in ducts that open on the nipple surface. The largest portion of glandular tissue is in the upper outer quadrant and tail of each breast. Fibrous suspensory ligaments connect to skin and fascia underlying the breast to support it and maintain its upright position. Fatty tissue is located superficially and to the sides of the breast.

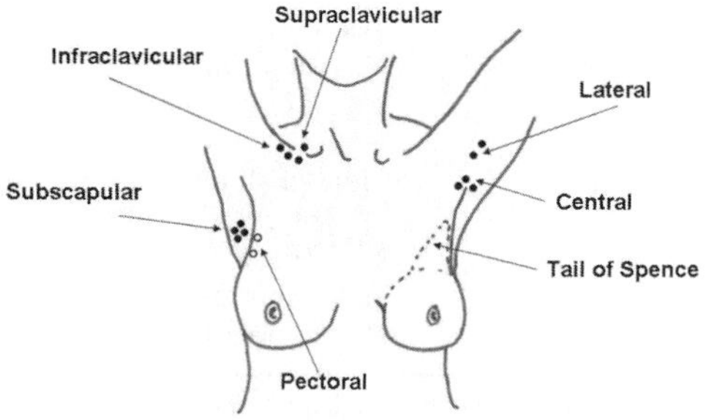

FIGURE **28–68** Lymph nodes of axillae and thorax. (From *Physical Examination Images* [CD-ROM], by D. L. Skillen. R. A. Day, M. C. Anderson, T. C. Stephenn, J. A. Gilbert, and L. W. Day, 2004, Edmonton, AB: Faculty of Nursing, University of Alberta.)

Lymphatics. A large portion of lymph from the breasts drains into axillary lymph nodes. If cancerous lesions **metastasize** (spread), the nodes are commonly involved (Figure 28–68).

The central nodes are located along the chest wall and high up in the axillae. Lymph from the other three sets of axillary nodes (pectoral, subscapular, and lateral) drains into the central nodes. Pectoral nodes are located at the edge of the pectoralis major muscle along the anterior axillary line. Lymph from the anterior chest wall and much of the breast drain into these nodes. Subscapular nodes are found along the lateral border of the scapula, deep in the posterior axillary fold. Lymph from the posterior chest wall and part of the arm drain into these nodes. Lateral nodes are located along the upper part of the humerus of the arm and drain much of the arm. Lymph collected in the central nodes then drains to infraclavicular nodes (below the clavicle) and supraclavicular nodes (above the clavicle). However, some lymph drains directly into the infraclavicular nodes and also deep into the chest. This is why a tumour in one breast may spread to nodes on the opposite side, as well as to those on the same side.

Breast Cancer. Breast cancer was projected to affect an estimated 21,200 women in Canada in 2004 (CCS, 2004a). The disease is second to lung cancer as the leading cause of death in women with cancer. However, current mortality rates for breast cancer are at the lowest point in Canada since 1950 and a decline has also been reported in the United States, the United Kingdom, and Australia. During their lifetimes, 1 in 8.8 women are expected to develop breast cancer, and 1 in 27.4 women are expected to die from it (CCS, 2004a).

Early detection is the key to cure. As most breast lumps are found by the woman herself (often by accident),

Table 28-45 Health History for Breast Assessment

Assessment Category	Rationale
Ask client about presence of risk factors, such as age over 40, personal or family history of breast cancer, onset of menarche before age 12 or menopause after age 50, never pregnant, or having first child after age 30.	These are risk factors for breast cancer.
Inquire about use of oral contraceptives, hormone replacement, steroids, or caffeine.	These medications can affect breast tissue.
Ask if client performs monthly breast self-examination.	This facilitates early detection of breast changes.
Question client on discovery of any lumps, thickening of tissue, pain, discharge or tissue distortion, nipple retraction, or change in breast generally. Conduct a symptom analysis as necessary.	These are potential signs and symptoms of breast disease and conducting a symptom analysis will help determine the nature of the problem.

Box 28-31 Expected Changes in the Breast During a Woman's Lifespan

Puberty (8 to 20 years)*

Breasts mature in five stages. One breast may grow more rapidly than the other. The ages at which changes occur and rate of developmental progression vary.

Stage 1 (Preadolescent)
- This stage involves elevation of the nipple only.

Stage 2
- The breast and nipple elevate as a small mound, and the areolar diameters enlarge.

Stage 3
- There is further enlargement and elevation of the breast and areola, with no separation of contour.

Stage 4
- The areola and nipple project into the secondary mound above the level of the breast (may not occur in all girls).

Stage 5 (Mature Breast)
- Only the nipple projects, and the areola recedes (may vary in some women).

Young Adulthood (20 to 30 years)

- Breasts reach full (non-pregnant) size. Shape is generally symmetrical. Breasts may be unequal in size.

Pregnancy

- Breast size gradually enlarges to two to three times the previous size. Nipples enlarge and may become erect. Areolae darken and diameters increase. Superficial veins become prominent. A yellowish fluid (colostrum) may be expelled from the nipples.

Menopause

- Breasts shrink. Tissue becomes softer, sometimes flabby.

Older Adulthood†

- Breasts become elongated, pendulous, and flaccid as a result of glandular tissue atrophy. The skin of the breasts tends to wrinkle, appearing loose and flabby.
- Nipples become smaller, flatter, and lose erectile ability. Nipples may invert because of shrinkage of fibrotic changes.
- Ligaments supporting the breast tissue weaken, causing the breasts to sag and the nipples to lower.
- Breast tissue may feel stringy and nodular.

*Data from *Whaley and Wong's Nursing Care of Infants and Children* (6th ed.), by D. L. Wong et al., 1999, St. Louis, MO: Mosby.
†Data from *Toward Healthy Aging* (5th ed.), by P. Ebersole and P. Hess, 1998, St. Louis, MO: Mosby.

nurses have a major responsibility to teach health behaviours such as breast self-examination (BSE). Studies suggest that only a minority of women actually perform BSE. Nurses need to be aware of barriers to performing BSE and should regularly incorporate factors that would increase the likelihood of a woman performing BSE into teaching strategies. The Canadian Cancer Society (2004b) recommends the following guidelines for the early detection of breast cancer:
- BSE should be performed monthly by women 20 years of age and older.
- Examination by a health care provider should be performed every 3 years from ages 20 to 39, and at least every 2 years for women between the ages of 40 and 59.
- Women with a family history of breast cancer should have a yearly examination by a health care provider.
- Asymptomatic women should have a baseline screening mammogram by age 40; women aged 50 to 69 should have a mammogram every 2 years.

Examination of the Breasts. The client's history (Table 28-45) should alert the nurse to any signs of breast disease and expected developmental changes. Because of its glandular structure, the breast undergoes changes throughout a woman's life. Knowledge of these changes (Box 28-31) helps nurses complete an accurate assessment and include client teaching and health promotion (Box 28-32).

Client Teaching Box 28-32

Health Promotion for Female Breast Assessment

Objectives

- Client will perform breast self-examination (BSE; see Box 28-33).
- Client will have screening mammography performed at recommended intervals.
- Client will identify risk factors for breast cancer.
- Client will identify signs and symptoms of breast cancer and fibrocystic disease.

Teaching Strategies

- Teach BSE procedure to client and have her practise, allowing time to ask questions (see Box 28-33).
- Explain recommended frequency of mammogram and assessment by health care provider, particularly annual mammogram and clinical examination after the age of 50 years.
- Inform client of risk factors for breast cancer, including being a woman, previous history of breast cancer, age over 50 years, family history of breast cancer (first-degree relative).
- Inform client of signs and symptoms of breast cancer, including unilateral solitary mass, nipple ulceration, inversion or discharge, dimpling, reddened area, edematous, change in size or shape of breast, **peau d'orange** (orange peel) texture to skin, painless lump.
- Inform client of signs and symptoms of fibrocystic disease including one or more (often painful) lumps; lump characteristics change according to menstrual cycle.
- Encourage client to reduce intake of caffeine. This may reduce symptoms of fibrocystic disease.

Evaluation

- Have client demonstrate BSE.
- Have client state date of last mammography and checkup.
- Have client state signs and symptoms of breast cancer compared with fibrocystic disease.

Nurses teach women how to perform a BSE. While assessing the client's breasts, nurses use many of the same techniques that the client will use in the home (Box 28-33). It may be difficult for the client to learn to palpate for lymph nodes. Lying down with the arm abducted makes the area more accessible. The client is instructed to use her left hand for the right axillary and clavicular areas. The nurse can take the client's fingerpads and move them in the proper circular fashion. The client then uses her right hand to palpate for nodes on the left side.

If the female client already performs BSE, the nurse can ask about the method used and when she does the examination in relation to her menstrual cycle. The best time for a BSE is 7 days from the start of the last menstrual period when the breasts of women who are premenopausal are no longer swollen or tender from hormone elevations. If the woman has already completed menopause, she should check her breasts the same time each month. It is important that pregnant women also check their breasts monthly.

Older women may require special attention when reviewing the need for regular BSE. Some may ignore changes in their breasts, assuming they are a part of aging. Others are not aware that cancer of the breast occurs in older women and may avoid having a breast examination or mammogram. In addition, physiological factors can affect the ease with which older women perform BSE. Musculoskeletal limitations, diminished peripheral sensation, reduced eyesight, and changes in joint range of motion can limit inspection and palpation abilities. In these circumstances, nurses teach family members to perform regular breast examinations.

Inspection. The client removes the gown or drape to allow simultaneous visualization of both breasts. If possible, the nurse places a mirror in front of the client so that she can see what to look for when performing a BSE. To recognize abnormalities, the client needs to be familiar with the usual appearance of her breasts. The breasts are inspected for size and symmetry. One breast is commonly larger than the other. However, a difference in size may be caused by inflammation or a mass. Breasts vary in shape from convex to conical or pendulous. Nurses observe the contour or shape of the breasts and note masses, flattening, retraction, or dimpling. Retraction or dimpling may result from tumour invasion of underlying ligaments. The ligaments become fibrotic and pull the overlying skin inward toward the tumour. Edema also changes the contour of the breasts. To bring out retraction or changes in the shape of the breasts, the client is asked to assume different positions (see Box 28-33). Each manoeuvre causes a contraction of the pectoral muscles that will accentuate retraction.

The overlying skin is carefully inspected for colour and venous pattern. Venous patterns are more easily seen in thin clients or pregnant women. The presence of lesions, edema, or inflammation is also noted. The client is asked to lift each breast while the nurse examines lower and lateral aspects for colour and texture changes. The breasts are the colour of neighbouring skin and venous patterns are the same bilaterally. The skin of the axillae is examined for signs of a rash, infection, or increased pigmentation. For women with large breasts, the nurse should be sure to look carefully at the undersurface, a common site for redness and excoriation caused by rubbing of skin surfaces.

The examiner inspects the nipple and areola for size, colour, shape, discharge, and the direction in which the nipples point. They usually point in symmetrical directions, are everted, and have no drainage. Their surface may be either smooth or wrinkled. If the nipples are inverted, the nurse asks if this has been a lifetime history. A recent inversion or inward turning of the nipple may indicate an underlying growth. Ulcerations and rashes on the breasts or nipples are noted. Bleeding or discharge from the nipple is a concern, particularly if it is persistent only on one side. A clear yellow discharge that occurs 2 days after childbirth is expected. It is not recommended that nurses squeeze the nipples to test for discharge. While inspecting the breasts,

Box 28-33 Breast Self-Examination

Breast self-examination (BSE) should be done once a month so that you become familiar with the usual appearance and feel of your breasts. Familiarity makes it easier to notice any changes in the breast from one month to another. Early discovery of a change from what is "normal" is the main idea behind BSE.

If you menstruate, the best time to do BSE is 7 days from the start of your period, when your breasts are least likely to be tender or swollen. If you no longer menstruate, pick a day, such as the first day of the month, to remind yourself that it is time to do BSE.

Here is how to do BSE:

1. Stand or sit before a mirror, arms at sides. Inspect both breasts for anything unusual, such as any discharge from nipples, puckering, dimpling, or scaling of the skin.

The next two steps are designed to emphasize any change in the shape or contour of your breasts. As you do them, you should be able to feel your chest muscles tighten.

2. Watching closely in the mirror, clasp hands behind your head and press hands forward.
3. Next, press hands firmly on hips and bow slightly toward your mirror as you pull your shoulders and elbows forward.
4. Alternatively press hands together in front above or below breast.
5. Inspect breasts as you lean forward.

Some women do the next part of the examination in the shower. Fingers glide over soapy skin, making it easy to appreciate the texture underneath.

6. Raise your left arm. Use three of your fingers of your right hand to explore your left breast firmly, carefully, and thoroughly. Beginning at the outer edge, press the flat part of your fingers in small circles, moving the circles slowly around the breast. Gradually work toward the nipple. Be sure to cover the entire breast. Pay special attention to the area between the breast and the armpit, including the armpit itself. Feel for any unusual lump or mass under the skin. Repeat the exam on your right breast.
7. Step 6 should be repeated lying down. Lie flat on your back, left arm at your side and a pillow or folded towel under your left shoulder. This position flattens the breast and makes it easier to examine. Use the same circular motion described earlier. Repeat on your right breast.

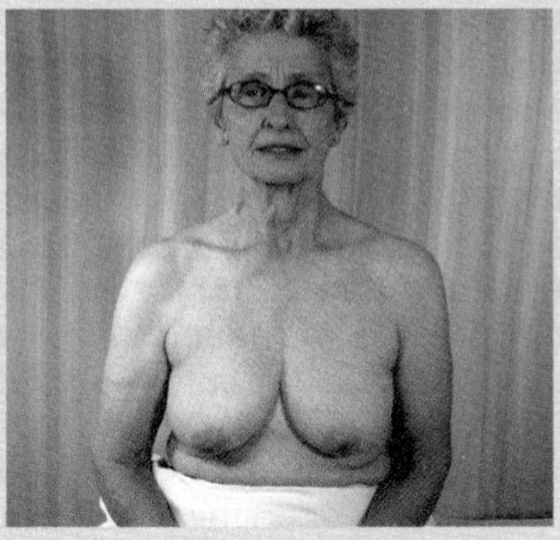

1 Arms at sides

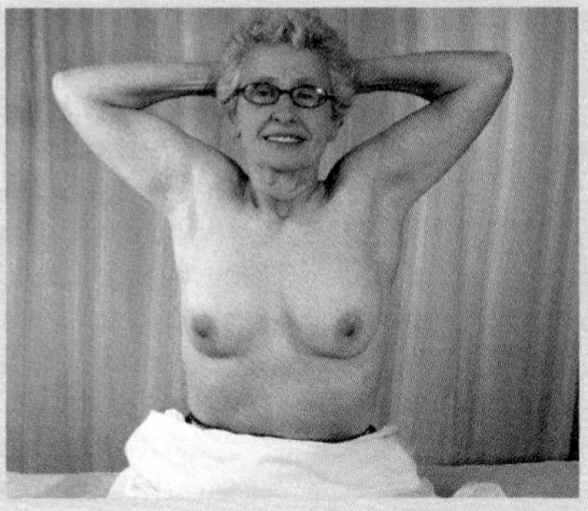

2 Arms above head

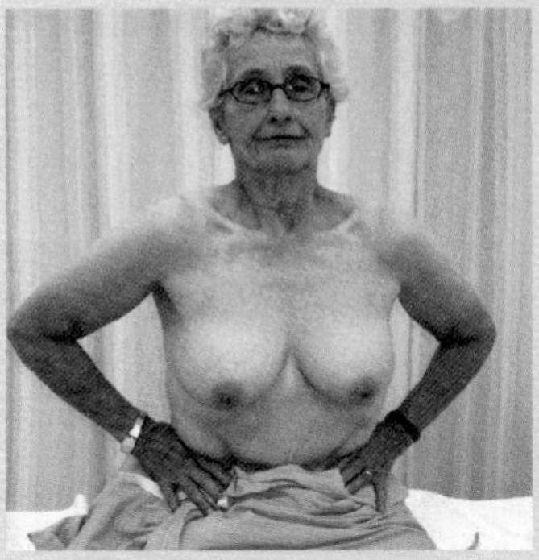

3 Pressing on hips

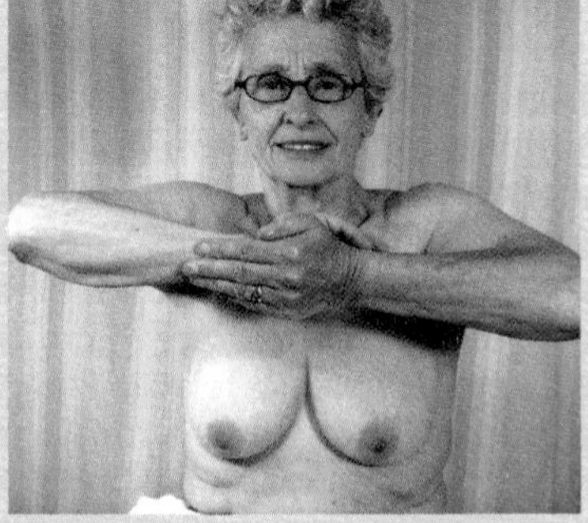

4 Pressing in front below or above breasts

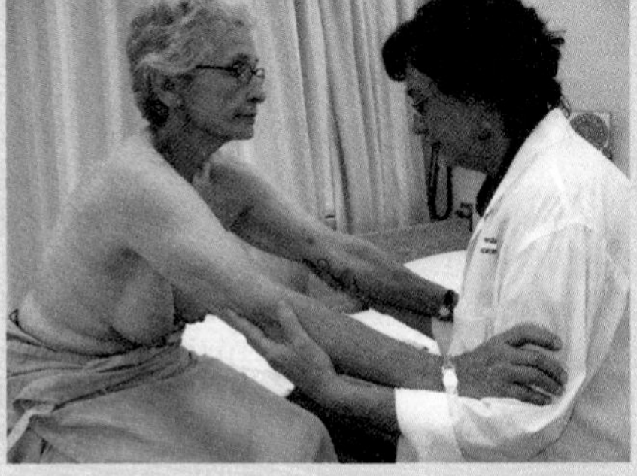

5 Arms forward and leaning forward

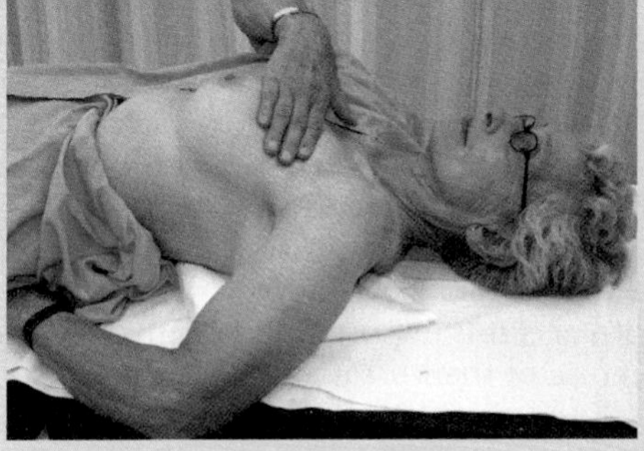

6 Lying position

Photos From *Physical Examination Images* [CD-ROM], by D. L. Skillen, R. A. Day, M. C. Anderson, T. C. Stephen, J. A. Gilbert, and L. W. Day, 2004, Edmonton, AB: Faculty of Nursing, University of Alberta.

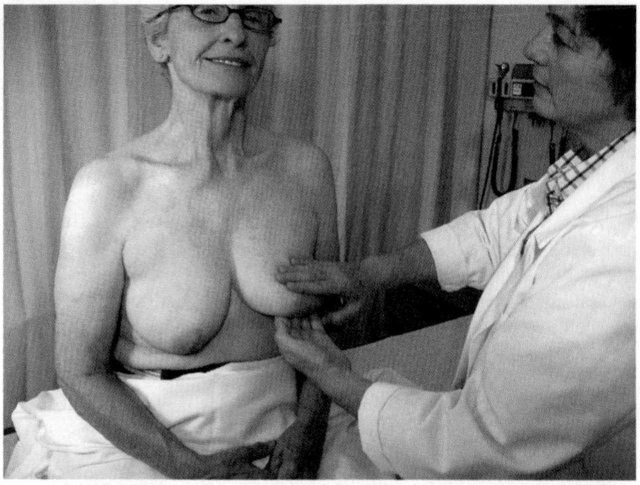

FIGURE **28–69** Bimanual breast palpation. (From *Physical Examination Images* [CD-ROM], by D. L. Skillen, R. A. Day, M. C. Anderson, T. C. Stephen, J. A. Gilbert, and L. W. Day, 2004, Edmonton, AB: Faculty of Nursing, University of Alberta.)

nurses inform the client of observed characteristics and the significance of unusual signs and symptoms. If the breasts are large and pendulous, nurses use a bimanual technique for palpation while the client is still sitting for inspection (Figure 28–69 and Procedure 28-16).

Palpation. Palpation is used to determine the condition of underlying breast tissue and lymph nodes. The lymph nodes are best palpated with the client sitting, although the examination can be performed with the client supine. Easy access is gained to the axillary nodes with the client's arms at her sides and the muscles relaxed. Although lymph nodes are not usually palpable, the central nodes are the most likely to be felt (Figure 28–70, *A*). Each axillary area is carefully assessed to avoid missing enlarged nodes (Figure 28–70, *A–F*). As well, infraclavicular and supraclavicular nodes are assessed. A palpable node feels like a small mass that may be hard, tender, and immobile. The nurse notes the number, size, consistency, and mobility. One or two small, soft, non-tender nodes may be found.

Palpation of the breast is best performed with the client lying supine, with no pillow under the head and with one arm out from the side (alternating with each breast). The supine position allows the breast tissue to flatten evenly against the chest wall (see Box 28-33). If the breasts are large, the examiner may place a small pillow or towel under the shoulder blade to further position breast tissue. As consistency of breast tissue varies widely with age, it is important for clients to be familiar with the texture of their breasts by doing monthly BSE.

If the client presents with a breast mass, the nurse examines the opposite breast first to determine if a mass is present in the symmetrical position in the other breast and to ensure an objective comparison of breast tissue.

The nurse uses the pads of four fingers, making constant small circles, to compress breast tissue gently against the chest wall, noting tissue consistency (Figure 28–71; see Procedure 28-16). The approach recommended by the Canadian Cancer Society is to palpate in horizontal lines back and forth, systematically covering the area from below the clavicle to 3 cm below the breast and from the midsternal line to the midaxillary line (see Procedure 28-16) Other approaches such as palpating along vertical lines (American Cancer Society, 2004b) or circles beginning at the nipple may be used. It is essential to examine the entire breast and tail, directing attention to any areas of tenderness.

During palpation, nurses note the consistency of breast tissue. It usually feels dense, firm, and elastic. With menopause, breast tissue shrinks and becomes softer. Glandular tissue usually feels lobular. The lower edge of each breast may feel firm and hard. This is the inframammary ridge and not a tumour. It may help to move the client's hand so that she can feel common tissue variations. Nurses palpate masses to determine the following:

- Location in relation to quadrants
- Diameter in centimetres
- Shape
- Consistency (soft, firm, or hard)
- Tenderness
- Mobility
- Discreteness (whether boundaries of mass are clear or not).

Cancerous lesions tend to be hard, fixed, irregular in shape and usually, but not always, painless. A common **benign** (non-cancerous) condition of the breast is **fibrocystic breast disease.** This condition is characterized by lumpy, painful breasts and sometimes nipple discharge. Symptoms are more apparent during the menstrual period. When palpated, the cysts (lumps) are soft, well-differentiated, moveable, and in both breasts. Deep cysts may feel hard. Another non-cancerous condition is fibroadenoma, which is the presence of a round, very mobile, firm, and circumscribed mass that occurs mainly in young women.

After the nurse completes the examination, the client should demonstrate self-palpation. Observing client technique emphasizes the importance of a systematic approach. Clients are urged to inform a health care provider if they discover an unusual mass.

Age-Related Changes. See Box 28-31 for a summary of age-related changes to the female breast.

Male Breasts. Examination of the male breast is relatively easy in supine or sitting positions. The nipple and areola are inspected for nodules, edema, and ulceration. An enlarged male breast may result from obesity or glandular enlargement. Fatty tissue feels soft, whereas glandular tissue is firm. Gynecomastia is a temporary, unilateral, enlargement of undeveloped breast tissue, which feels smooth, firm and mobile. It is a usual occurrence in puberty. Breast enlargement in young males may indicate steroid use. Any masses are palpated for the same characteristics as in the female breast. Because breast cancer in men is relatively rare, routine self-examinations are unnecessary.

Documentation. Nurses record their findings from inspection and palpation of the breasts and axillae (Table 28-46).

Procedure 28-16 Assessing Breasts and Axillae

Equipment

- Small pillow or towel
- Gloves (if signs of infection or discharge are present)

Examination Skill and Focus	Steps	Rationale
Inspection: Breast, areola, nipple	Client in **sitting** position disrobed to waist	Both breasts need to be visible.
	1. Inspect breast, areola, and nipple bilaterally from anterior and lateral view: • with arms at side • with arms raised over head • with hands pressed against hips **OR** with hands pressed together, not obstructing view of breasts.	Different positions may allow examiner to see changes in contour of breasts. Contraction of pectoral muscles may make masses or skin changes more visible.
	2. Inspect with client leaning forward, and then with breasts lifted.	Masses may be seen more easily in this position. Skin underneath breasts is checked for rashes.
Palpation: Large breasts	**1.** With the client leaning forward, palpate breast tissue between the examiner's hands.	This position brings the breast tissue away from the chest wall and allows examiner to feel masses that may not be accessible when the client is in the supine position.
Inspection: Axillae	**1.** Inspect skin of axillae with arms raised over head.	Permits examination of total skin surface of axillae.
	2. **Only** if signs of infection, put on gloves for palpation.	Gloves are needed to prevent transmission of organisms.
Palpation: Axillary lymph nodes	**1.** Assist client to dry axillae.	
	2. Support client's (L) hand and wrist with examiner's (L) hand to examine (L) axilla and reverse for (R) axilla.	
	3. Instruct client to relax arm.	Keeps client's arm close to side to reduce tension on axilla.
Central lymph nodes	**4.** Cup fingers together.	
	5. Reach as high as possible into apex of (L) axilla.	
	6. Press fingers against chest wall.	Nodes may be felt as tissue pressed against chest wall.
	7. Bring finger pads down over ribs and feel for central nodes (Figure 28–70, *A*).	
Pectoral lymph nodes	**8.** Slide fingers under anterior axillary fold, palpating chest wall with finger pads for pectoral nodes.	
	9. Grasp anterior axillary folds (pectoral) and palpate with finger pads, using thumbs as anchor (Figure 28–70, *B* and *C*).	
	10. Slide fingers under posterior axillary fold, palpating chest wall with finger pads for subscapular nodes.	
Subscapular lymph nodes	**11.** Turn hands and feel inside posterior axillary folds with finger pads (subscapular) (Figure 28–70, *D* and *E*).	

From *A Syllabus for Adult Health Assessment* (pp. 43–44), edited by D. L. Skillen and R. A. Day, 2004, Edmonton, AB: Faculty of Nursing, University of Alberta.

Continued

Procedure 28-16 Assessing Breasts and Axillae—cont'd

Examination Skill and Focus	Steps	Rationale
Lateral lymph nodes	**12.** Feel along upper humerus with finger pads (lateral) (Figure 28–70, *F*). **13.** Repeat on (R) side.	
Palpation: Infraclavicular lymph nodes	**1.** Palpate bilaterally for infraclavicular nodes below clavicle in 1st interspace with finger pads.	
Palpation: Supraclavicular lymph nodes	**1.** Palpate bilaterally for supraclavicular nodes above clavicle with finger pads.	
Inspection: Breast, areola, nipple	Client supine, with pillow removed from under head. Use small pillow under client's shoulder on side examined **only if breasts are large.** **1.** Inspect breasts bilaterally.	Use pillow with large breasts to shift breast tissue medially.
Palpation: Breast, areola, nipple, and tail of Spence	Ask client to move arm away from chest on side being examined. **1.** Palpate each breast. **2.** Use flat of 2nd, 3rd, and 4th fingers in a rotary motion to compress breast tissue. **3.** Flex, from the wrist, not the fingers.	Allow fingers to stay flat and in contact with the skin.
	4. Apply moderate pressure, keeping constant contact with skin. **5.** Move back and forth across breast in straight lines, making constant small circles. **6.** Slide hand down one finger width for each pass. **7.** Cover full area from below clavicle to 3 cm below breast, from midaxillary line to midsternal line: • glandular tissue • areolar area • nipple • tail of Spence	

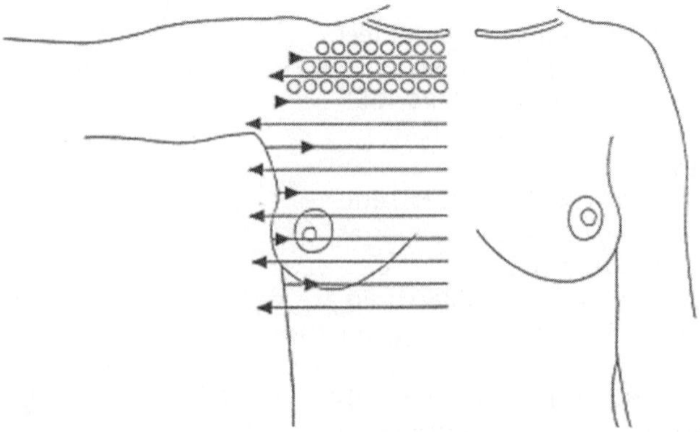

From *A Syllabus for Adult Health Assessment* (pp. 43–44), edited by D. L. Skillen and R. A. Day, 2004, Edmonton, AB: Faculty of Nursing, University of Alberta.
Adapted from *Breast Self-Examination: What You Can Do* [Brochure], Canadian Cancer Society Alberta/NWT Division, 2002, Calgary, AB: Author.

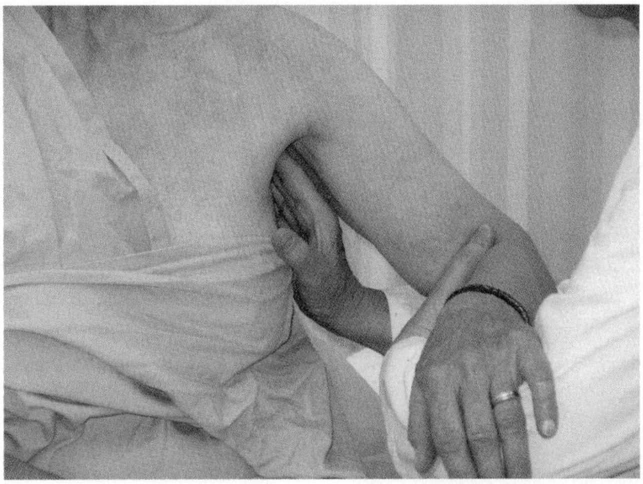

A

B

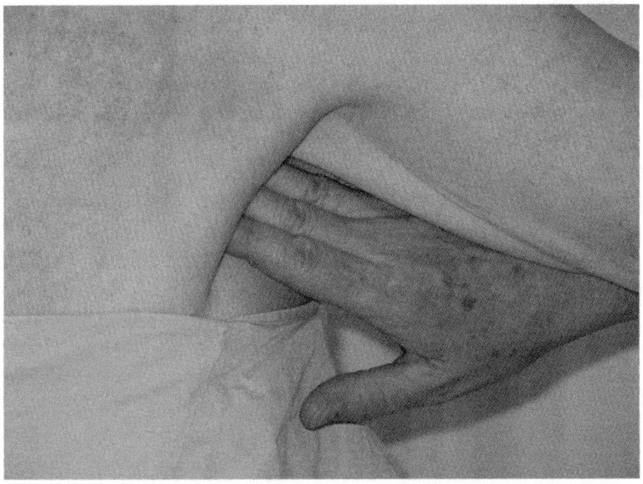

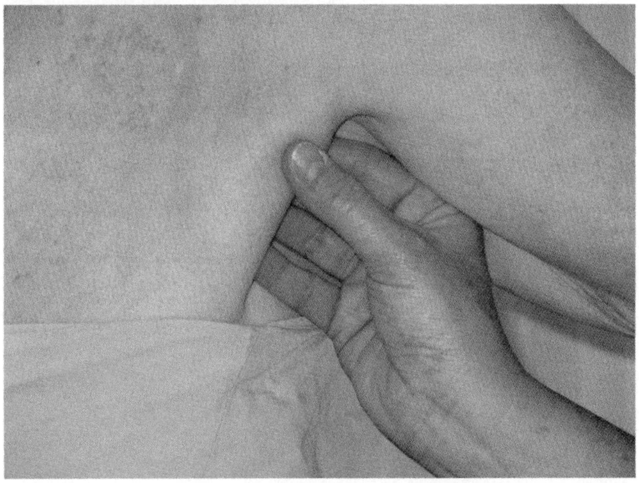

C

D

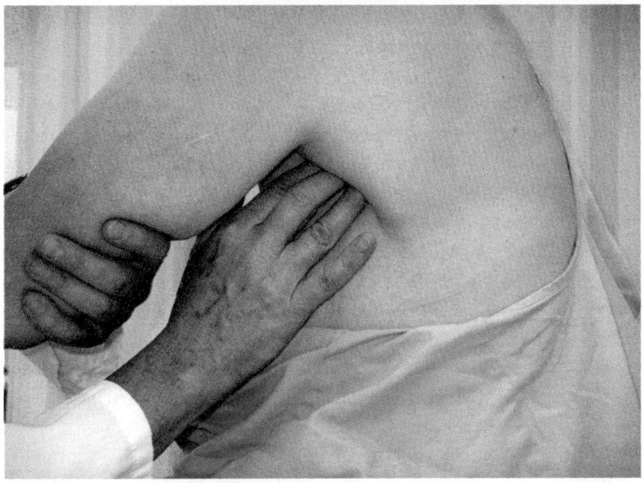

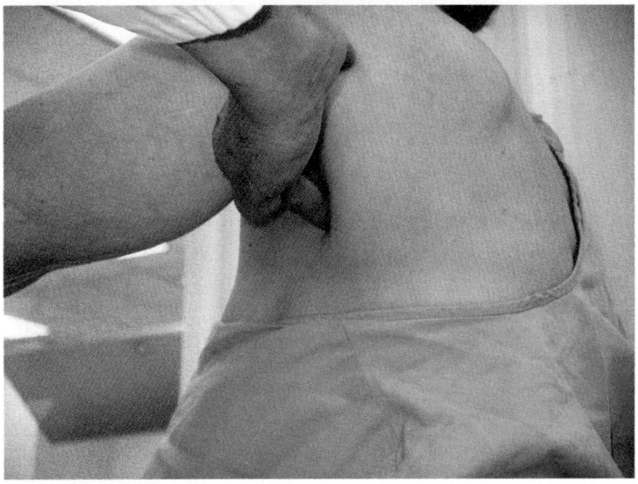

E

F

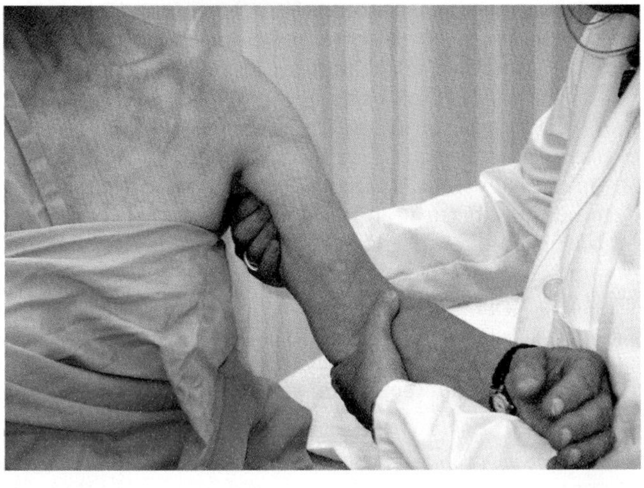

FIGURE **28–70** **A,** Palpation of central lymph nodes. **B** and **C,** Palpation of pectoral lymph nodes. **D** and **E,** Palpation of subscapular lymph nodes. **F,** Palpation of lateral lymph nodes. (From *Physical Examination Images* [CD-ROM], by D. L. Skillen, R. A. Day, M. C. Anderson, T. C. Stephen, J. A. Gilbert, and L. W. Day, 2004, Edmonton, AB: Faculty of Nursing, University of Alberta.)

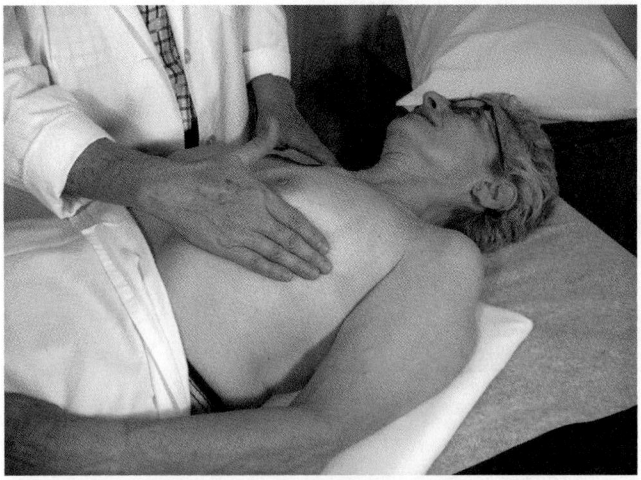

FIGURE **28–71** Palpation technique. (From *Physical Examination Images* [CD-ROM], by D. L. Skillen, R. A. Day, M. C. Anderson, T. C. Stephen, J. A. Gilbert, and L. W. Day, 2004, Edmonton, AB: Faculty of Nursing, University of Alberta.)

Safety Alert: All men, especially men who have a first-degree relative (e.g., mother or sister) with breast cancer are at risk for breast cancer and should palpate their breasts at regular intervals. They may also be scheduled for routine mammograms.

Assessing the Abdomen

The abdominal examination can be complex because of the organs located within and near the abdominal cavity. A thorough health history (Table 28-47) helps the nurse interpret physical signs and plan for teaching and health promotion (Box 28-34). The examination includes an assessment of structures of the lower gastrointestinal (GI) tract in addition to the liver, stomach, spleen, kidneys, and bladder. Abdominal pain is a common symptom that clients report when seeking medical care. An accurate assessment requires that client history data be matched with a careful assessment of the location of physical symptoms.

Landmarks help map out the abdominal region. The xiphoid process (tip of the sternum) marks the upper boundary of the abdominal region; the symphysis pubis delineates the lower boundary. Costal margins are used to landmark for the liver and stomach. Kidney percussion posteriorly requires the landmark of the costovertebral angle (see Thorax).

The abdomen is divided into four imaginary quadrants (Figure 28–72, *A*). Nurses can record assessment findings in relation to each quadrant. For example, nurses may determine that a client is experiencing tenderness over the left lower quadrant (LLQ) with expected bowel sounds present. A system of dividing the abdomen into nine regions (see Figure 28–9) is not used as often, but some terms remain in common use: hypogastric, epigastric, umbilical, and suprapubic (Jarvis, 2004).

It is important to visualize the location of the abdominal organs during examination of the abdomen. For example, the liver is in the right upper quadrant (RUQ) with the lower border of the liver extending just below the costal margin. This knowledge is essential when percussing and palpating for the liver. The stomach and spleen are in the left upper quadrant (LUQ). Posteriorly, the kidneys are located between the T12 and L3 vertebrae and are protected by the lower ribs and heavy back muscles (Figure 28–72).

Clients must be relaxed for abdominal examinations. Tightened abdominal muscles hinder accuracy of palpation and auscultation. To promote relaxation, the nurse asks the client to void before beginning. The nurse also ensures that the room, stethoscope, and his or her hands are warm. Maintaining conversation except during auscultation helps distract clients. The client lies supine or in the dorsal recumbent position with arms at the sides and knees slightly bent; if the client places the arms under the head, the abdominal muscles tighten. The abdomen is exposed from just above the xiphoid process to the symphysis pubis, and the client's upper chest and legs are draped. The nurse asks clients to report pain and tender areas before beginning assessment, then proceeds calmly and slowly and checks regularly for any discomfort. Nurses always examine tender areas last.

The sequence of the abdominal examination differs slightly from other assessments, as auscultation immediately follows inspection. It is important to auscultate before palpation and percussion because palpation and percussion may alter bowel sound frequency.

Inspection. The entire abdomen is inspected for skin characteristics, contour, symmetry, pulsations, and peristalsis (Procedure 28-17). Skin characteristics include colour, scars, venous patterns, lesions, and **striae** (stretch marks). The skin is subject to the same colour variations as the rest of the body. Venous patterns are usually faint, except in thin clients. Striae result from stretching of tissue by obesity or pregnancy. An artificial opening may indicate a drainage site resulting from surgery or an ostomy (see chapters 40 and 41). Scars indicate past trauma or surgery that may have created permanent changes in underlying organ anatomy. Bruising may indicate accidental injury, physical abuse, or a type of bleeding disorder. Nurses ask specifically about the history of any marks. They ask if the client self-administers injections (e.g., heparin or insulin). Unexpected findings include generalized colour changes such as jaundice or cyanosis, or a glistening, taut appearance (ascites).

When examining the umbilicus, the position, shape, and colour, as well as signs of inflammation, discharge, or protruding masses are noted. Usually, the umbilicus is a flat or concave hemisphere positioned in the midline midway between the xiphoid process and the symphysis pubis. The colour is the same as that of the surrounding skin. Underlying masses can cause displacement; an everted (pouched-out) umbilicus usually indicates abdominal distension. **Hernias** (anterior protrusions of abdominal organs through muscle) cause protrusion of the umbilicus. There should be no discharge emitted from the umbilical area.

Nurses inspect for abdominal contour, symmetry, and surface motion, noting masses, bulging, or distension. They expect the abdomen to be flat or rounded (Figure 28–73). The contour should remain smooth and symmetrical at rest

Table 28-46 Examples of Documentation for Breast and Axillary Assessment

Focus of Assessment	Expected Findings	Unexpected Findings
Axillae	Skin smooth, intact, no palpable lymph nodes bilaterally, no tenderness	Faint red rash over both axillae (client states she shaved underarms yesterday)
Nipples	Colour darker than breast, no rashes or discharge bilaterally, everted bilaterally, point in opposite directions	(R) nipple inverted for 3 months
Areola	Symmetrical, round, colour darker than breast	0.5-cm scratch on (L) areola. No bleeding or discharge
Breasts	Breasts are lobular, (R) slightly larger than (L), colour similar to body. Firm and smooth. No masses, lesions, edema, dimpling, retraction or peau d'orange (orange peel) skin noted bilaterally	2-cm mass in lower inner aspect of (R) breast. Round, firm, clear margins, moveable and non-tender

Adapted from *First Year Student Lab Guide* (p. 74), by J. Chambers et al., 2004, Edmonton, AB: Faculty of Nursing, University of Alberta.

Table 28-47 Health History for Abdominal Assessment

Assessment Category	Rationale
Ask client about usual dietary habits, bowel routine, characteristics of stool, and use of laxatives.	Information about usual habits helps to determine if irregularities are present.
Question client about any recent weight changes or intolerance to diet (e.g., nausea, vomiting, cramping, especially in last 24 hours).	Data may indicate alterations in upper GI tract (stomach or gallbladder) or lower colon.
Ask client about medication use, including anti-inflammatory medications or antibiotics.	Some medications irritate gastric mucosal lining, causing pain, nausea, or vomiting.
Inquire about any problems with flatulence, belching, swallowing, heartburn, diarrhea, or constipation.	These signs and symptoms may indicate changes within the gastrointestinal tract.
Ask if female client is pregnant, noting date of last menstrual period.	Pregnancy affects shape and contour of abdomen.
Inquire about family or personal history of hypertension, alcoholism, kidney or heart disease, abdominal trauma, or surgeries.	Data may reveal identifiable alterations during physical examination.
Carefully observe client's movements and positioning, such as lying still with knees drawn up, restlessness, and lying on side during health history; conduct symptom analysis as necessary.	Positions assumed by client may reveal nature and source of pain.
Ask client about knowledge and presence of the following risk factors: health care occupation, hemodialysis client, IV drug user, household or sexual contact with hepatitis B virus (HBV) carrier, international traveller in area of high HBV infection rate, heterosexual person with more than one sexual partner in last 6 months, sexually active homosexual or bisexual male.	Risk factors for exposure to HBV.

Client Teaching

Box 28-34

Abdominal Assessment

Objectives

- Client will maintain healthy bowel elimination pattern.
- Client will identify signs and symptoms of colon cancer and understand recommended screening measures.
- Clients at risk of hepatitis B virus will receive immunization.

Teaching Strategies

- Inform client of the factors that promote bowel elimination, including diet, regular exercise, establishment of regular elimination schedule, and adequate fluid intake (see chapter 41).
- Caution client about dangers of excessive use of laxatives or enemas.
- Inform client of warning signs for colon cancer, including rectal bleeding, black or tarry stools, blood in stool, and a change in bowel habits.
- Encourage client to have stool tested for presence of blood yearly after the age of 50 years and to seek further testing as recommended by examiner.
- If client is a health care worker or has contact with blood or body fluids of hepatitis B-infected people, encourage immunization series and standard precautions/routine practices.

Evaluation

- Have client state signs and symptoms of colon cancer.

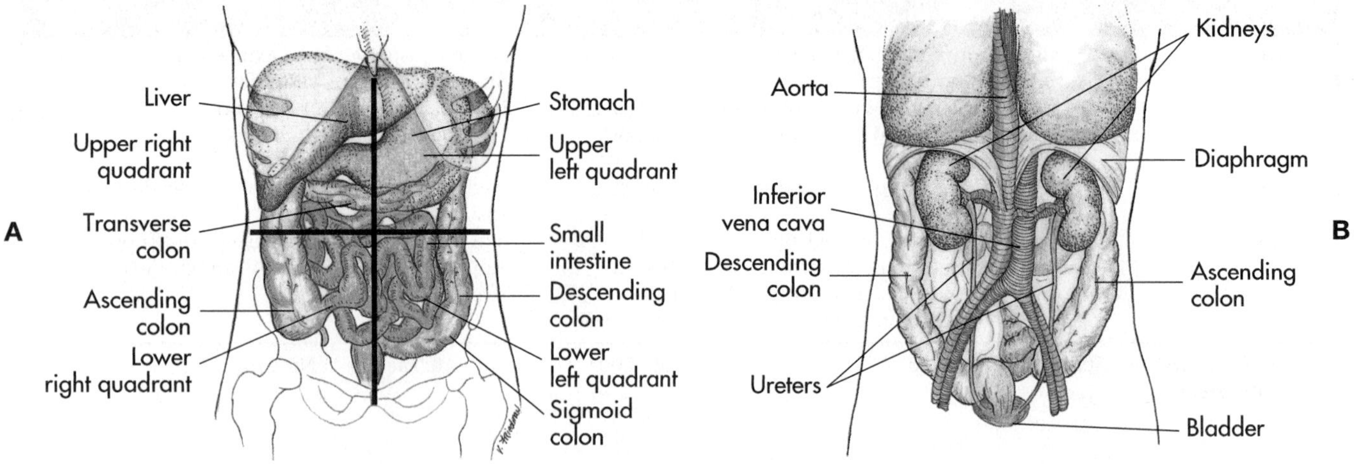

FIGURE **28–72** Abdominal quadrants. **A,** Anterior view of abdomen divided by quadrants. **B,** Posterior view of abdominal section.

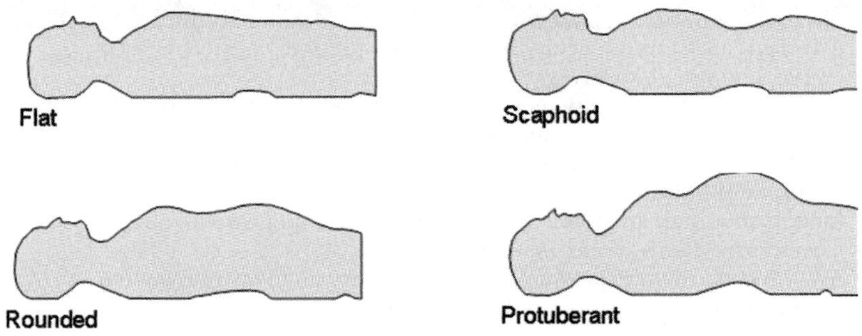

FIGURE **28–73** Contours of the abdomen. (From *Physical Examination Images* [CD-ROM], by D. L. Skillen, R. A. Day, M. C. Anderson, T. C. Stephen, J. A. Gilbert, and L. W. Day, 2004, Edmonton, AB: Faculty of Nursing, University of Alberta.)

and with a deep breath. Masses or asymmetry may indicate an underlying pathological condition.

Intestinal gas, a tumour, or fluid in the abdominal cavity may cause **distension** (swelling). When distension is generalized, the entire abdomen protrudes. The skin often appears taut, as if it were stretched over the abdomen. The nurse asks the client if the abdomen feels unusually tight. The nurse is careful to not confuse distension with obesity. In obesity, the abdomen is large, rolls of adipose tissue are often present along the flanks, and the client does not complain of tightness in the abdomen. If abdominal distension is expected, the nurse measures the abdominal girth by placing a tape measure around the abdomen at the level of the umbilicus. A felt pen is used to indicate where the tape measure was applied. Consecutive measurements show any increase or decrease in distension.

The nurse should remember that men typically breathe abdominally and women breathe more costally. If clients have severe pain, respiratory movement is diminished; to guard against the pain they tighten abdominal muscles. By looking closely across the abdomen from the side, the nurse may detect peristaltic movements and aortic pulsations. It may take several minutes to see a peristaltic wave. In contrast, aortic pulsations occur with each beat of systole and appear in the midline above the umbilicus (epigastric area).

Auscultation. Auscultation always precedes percussion and palpation during the abdominal assessment because manipulation of the abdomen may alter the frequency and intensity of bowel sounds (Procedure 28-18). Auscultation is easier if the client is not talking.

Peristalsis (intestinal motility) is a function of the small and large intestine. Bowel sounds are the audible passage of air and fluid created by peristalsis. Air and fluid move through the intestines, creating soft gurgling or clicking sounds that occur irregularly 5 to 35 times per minute (Seidel et al., 2003). Sounds may last 0.5 seconds to several seconds. It usually takes 5 to 20 seconds to hear a bowel sound. The best time to auscultate is between meals, as bowel sounds tend to be increased right after a meal is consumed or long after a meal is eaten. Sounds are generally described as absent, audible, hyperactive, or hypoactive. Absence of sounds indicates cessation of GI motility that may result from late-stage bowel obstruction, paralytic ileus, or peritonitis. Absent sounds are expected postoperatively following general anaesthesia; nurses should listen for 5 minutes before determining that bowel sounds are absent (Seidel et al., 2003). Loud, growling hyperactive sounds **(borborygmi)** indicate increased motility of the GI tract. Altered motility results from anxiety, diarrhea, bleeding, bowel inflammation, excessive ingestion of laxatives, and reaction to certain foods (see chapter 41).

The presence of bruits can reveal aneurysms or stenosed blood vessels in the abdomen. With the diaphragm, nurses auscultate for aortic, renal, and iliac sounds (Procedure 28-18). No vascular sounds are expected over the aorta (just lateral to midline), renal, or iliac areas (Figure 28–74).

Procedure 28-17 Inspecting the Abdomen

Equipment

- None

Examination Skill and Focus	Steps	Rationale
Inspection: Abdomen	Abdomen fully exposed, bladder empty, draped	Ensures client comfort, abdomen completely visible.
	Client with arms at sides **OR** folded across chest	Relaxes abdominal muscles.
	1. Inspect tangentially from "R" side and from foot of table.	Aids assessment of contour and movements.
	2. Inspect across abdomen.	
	3. Ask client to inhale deeply and hold breath.	Aids assessment of symmetry.
	4. Inspect for symmetry.	

From *A Syllabus for Adult Health Assessment* (p. 45), edited by D. L. Skillen and R. A. Day, 2004, Edmonton, AB: Faculty of Nursing, University of Alberta.

Procedure 28-18 Auscultating the Abdomen

Equipment

- Stethoscope

Examination Skill and Focus	Steps	Rationale
Auscultation: Bowel sounds	**1.** Inquire about abdominal tenderness and ask to indicate area.	Tender areas are assessed last.
	2. Auscultate prior to percussion and palpation.	Percussion and palpation may change bowel sounds.
	3. Place diaphragm gently.	
	4. Listen in all four quadrants.	Ensures no sounds are missed.
Auscultation:	**1.** Press diaphragm **gently** against abdomen.	
Aorta	**2.** Listen slightly "L" of midline in epigastric region (aorta).	Area where aortic, renal, and iliac sounds are heard best if they are present.
Renal arteries	**3.** Listen to "L" and "R" of midline just superior to umbilicus (renal).	
Iliac arteries	**4.** Listen just above inguinal ligament midway between anterior superior iliac spine and symphysis pubis (iliac).	

From *A Syllabus for Adult Health Assessment* (p. 45), edited by D. L. Skillen and R. A. Day, 2004, Edmonton, AB: Faculty of Nursing, University of Alberta.

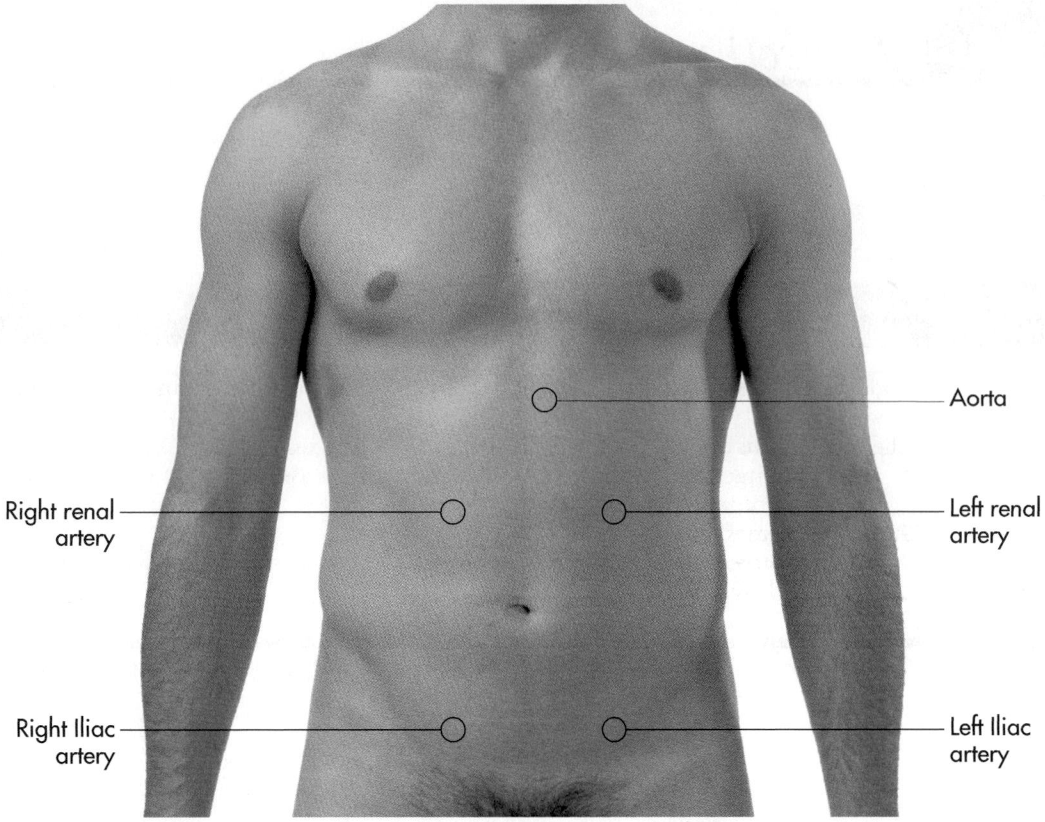

FIGURE **28–74** Sites to auscultate for bruits: renal arteries, iliac arteries, and aorta. (Adapted from *Health Assessment for Nursing Practice,* p. 451, by J. Thompson and S. Wilson, 1996, St. Louis, MO: Mosby.)

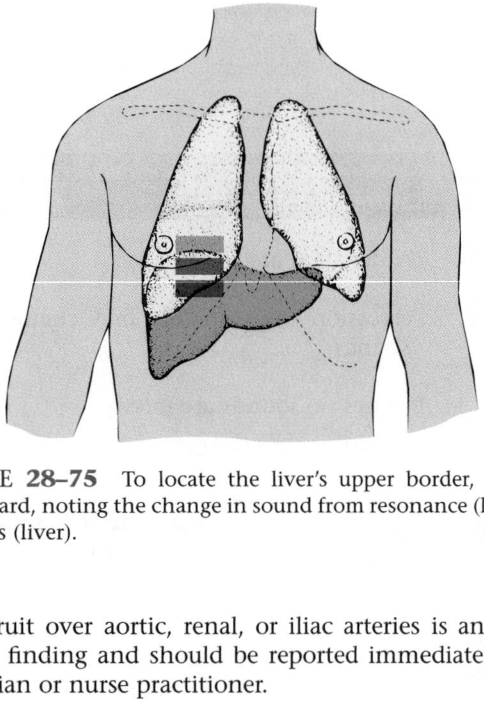

FIGURE **28–75** To locate the liver's upper border, percuss downward, noting the change in sound from resonance (lung) to dullness (liver).

Any bruit over aortic, renal, or iliac arteries is an unexpected finding and should be reported immediately to a physician or nurse practitioner.

Percussion. Percussion of the abdomen maps out underlying organs, bone, and masses and helps reveal the presence of air in the stomach and intestines. The beginning student uses this skill in a limited fashion. Practice is needed to ensure accuracy (Procedure 28-19). Potentially painful areas are always percussed last. Nurses systematically percuss each abdominal quadrant for tympany and dullness (see Table 28-10). Tympany usually predominates because of air in the stomach and intestines. Dullness is heard over organs such as the liver, spleen, pancreas, kidneys, pregnant uterus, and distended bladder, or over a tumour.

Percussion allows the nurse to identify borders of the liver to detect organ enlargement. The percussion note changes from tympanic to dull at the lower border of the liver near the right costal margin. The percussion note changes from resonant to dull at the upper border of the liver (usually found in the fifth, sixth, or seventh intercostal space; Figure 28–75). The liver span (distance) between the upper and lower borders is from 6 to 12 cm in the right MCL. Liver enlargement occurs in diseases such as cirrhosis, cancer, and hepatitis.

With the client sitting or standing, the nurse uses direct or indirect percussion to assess for kidney inflammation (see Procedure 28-19). If the kidneys are inflamed, the client reports tenderness during percussion, sometimes exquisite tenderness. When assessing the spleen (see Procedure 28-19), there should be a tympanic note that remains tympanic when the client takes a deep breath. An unexpected finding is a change to a dull note with a deep breath, which suggests splenic enlargement.

Procedure 28-19 Percussing the Abdomen

Equipment

- Skin marker
- Tape measure

Examination Skill and Focus	Steps	Rationale
Percussion: Abdomen	**1.** Place distal phalanx and joint of middle (pleximeter) finger on abdominal wall (avoiding contact with other fingers).	Ensures best percussion note achieved.
	2. Aim at distal phalanx or interphalangeal joint.	
	3. Strike pleximeter a sharp, light blow with tip of middle (plexor) finger.	
	4. Percuss lightly over entire abdomen.	Percussion notes vary from tympany to dullness.
	5. Inquire about areas of tenderness.	
	6. Observe client's facial reactions during percussion.	Facial expressions may be only client indication of tenderness.
Percussion: Liver	**1.** Percuss in right midclavicular line from lung resonance to liver dullness (upper border); mark level.	
	2. Start at level below umbilicus in right midclavicular line and percuss upward to liver dullness (lower border); mark level.	Identifies upper and lower borders for measurement.
	3. Measure vertical span of liver dullness in centimetres.	
	4. Request client to inhale deeply.	
	5. Percuss upward toward lower border.	Identifies the lowest border of the liver when the diaphragm descends during inhalation, pushing the liver downward.
	6. Identify new level of dullness; mark level.	
Splenic percussion sign	**1.** Percuss lowest interspace in left anterior axillary line.	
	2. Instruct client to take a deep breath, and repeat percussion in lowest interspace of left anterior axillary line.	Note should remain tympanic. If the note changes to dull, splenic enlargement may be present.
	3. Note any change in percussion.	
Percussion: Bladder	Percuss downward in midline from umbilicus to the pelvic brim.	Tympany changes to dull over a distended bladder.
Percussion: Kidney	Client sitting or standing.	
	Inform client of procedure.	
	1. Inquire about kidney tenderness.	If area is tender to palpation, percussion should not be done.
	2. If tender, press in each costovertebral angle in turn with fingertips.	
	3. Inquire about tenderness.	
	4. If not tender, place palm (fingers not touching client) of non-dominate hand over each costovertebral angle in turn.	Palm of hand is positioned over the lower pole of kidney.
	5. Strike dorsum of hand with ulnar surface of fist.	Blunt, indirect percussion is used to elicit kidney tenderness.
	6. Inquire about tenderness.	

From *A Syllabus for Adult Health Assessment* (pp. 38–39, 45–46), edited by D. L. Skillen and R. A. Day, 2004, Edmonton, AB: Faculty of Nursing, University of Alberta.

A 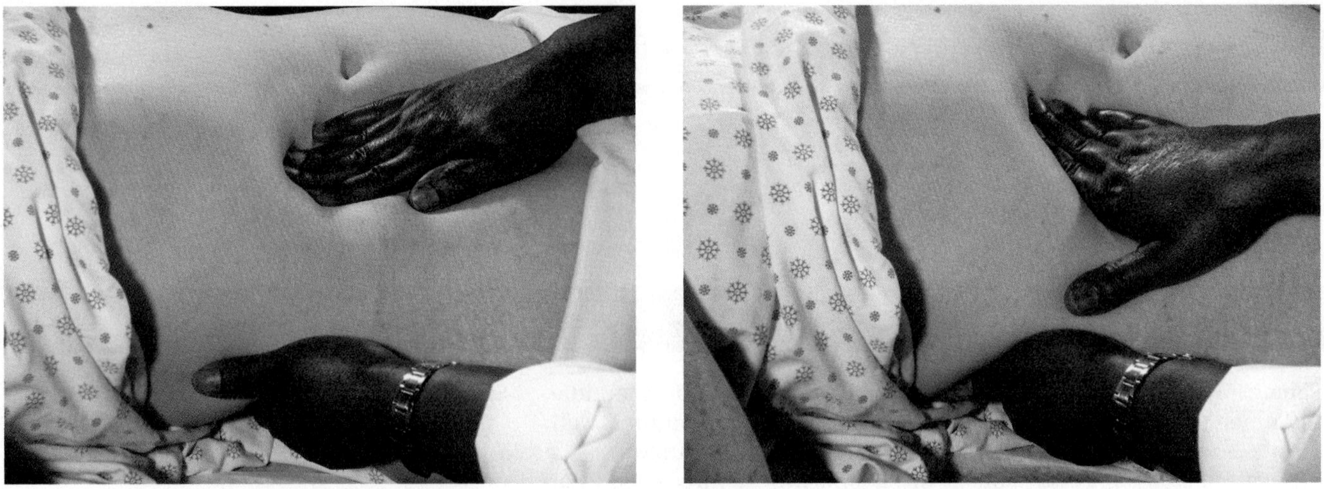 B

FIGURE **28–76** Liver palpation. **A,** Hand is parallel to rectus abdominus muscle. **B,** Hand is oblique to rectus abdominus muscle. (From *Physical Examination Images* [CD-ROM], by D. L. Skillen, R. A. Day, M. C. Anderson, T. C. Stephen, J. A. Gilbert, and L. W. Day, 2004, Edmonton, AB: Faculty of Nursing, University of Alberta.)

Palpation. With palpation, beginning nurses are primarily concerned with detecting areas of abdominal tenderness, unexpected distension, or masses (Procedure 28-20). As nurses become more skilled, they learn to palpate for specific organs such as the liver. Light and deep palpation (see Figure 28–3) are used, but learners must be supervised during deep palpation. Nurses always palpate lightly over each quadrant, using smooth coordinated movements and avoiding quick jabs. They leave painful areas to the last. All quadrants are surveyed systematically. The pads of the fingertips depress approximately 1.3 cm in a gentle dipping motion during light palpation. Systematic palpation of each quadrant assesses for muscular resistance, distension, tenderness, and superficial organs or masses. While palpating, the nurse observes the client's face for signs of discomfort. The abdomen is expected to be smooth, consistently soft, non-tender, and without masses. If the nurse palpates a sensitive area, guarding or muscle tenseness may occur. Although a distended bladder is easy to detect with light palpation, the client is more comfortable if it is detected during percussion. Masses are assessed for size, location, shape, consistency, tenderness, pulsation, and mobility.

Safety Alert: Deep palpation is never used over a surgical incision or over extremely tender organs. It is also unwise to use deep palpation on unexpected masses. Deep pressure may cause tenderness in the healthy client over the cecum, sigmoid colon, aorta, and the midline near the xiphoid process (Seidel et al., 2003).

With experience, nurses can perform deep palpation to delineate abdominal organs and detect less obvious masses. Short fingernails are needed. It is important for the client to be relaxed as the nurse's hands are depressed approximately 2.5 to 7.5 cm into the abdomen. The liver lies in the right upper quadrant under the rib cage. The nurse uses deep palpation to locate the lower edge of the liver. This technique detects liver enlargement (see Procedure 28-20 and Figure 28–76). The liver may not be palpable, but if it is palpable, it is non-tender and has a firm, regular, and sharp edge. Unexpected findings include an irregular edge or a boggy or tender liver.

Lymphatics. Most lymphatics from the lower extremities, the external genitalia, and the abdominal wall drain into the inguinal lymph nodes, but lymphatics from the testes drain into the abdomen where enlarged lymph nodes are not accessible to the examiner. The inguinal area lies between the anterior superior iliac spine and the symphysis pubis. The inguinal ligament runs between them; the inguinal canal lies about parallel to the ligament and is the conduit for the vas deferens through the abdominal muscles. The horizontal and vertical chains of inguinal lymph nodes are assessed for tenderness and inflammation (see Procedure 28-20). Non-tender, mobile, horizontal or vertical nodes less than 1 cm in size may be found. Nodes that are larger than 1 cm, tender, and non-mobile (fixed) require further examination to rule out local, systemic, or malignant disease.

Age-Related Changes. Older adults often have increased adipose tissue distributed on the abdomen and hips. They frequently lack abdominal tone, which makes the organs easier to palpate and pulsations and peristalsis easier to visualize. Salivation decreases because of medications, dehydration, disease processes, or radiation therapy (Miller, 1999), resulting in a dry mouth. An impaired sense of taste is most likely a result of declining health, side effects of medications, and age-related decline in the sense of smell. Difficulty with swallowing may occur with a disease process. The incidence of gallstones increases with age, and older clients frequently report constipation, although age-related change in the large intestine should not affect fecal movement through the large bowel adversely (Miller, 1999). Liver changes structurally, but most liver functions do not change (Jarvis, 2004).

Documentation. Nurses record their findings from inspection, auscultation, percussion, and palpation of the abdomen (Table 28-48).

Procedure 28-20 Palpating the Abdomen

Equipment

- None

Examination Skill and Focus	Steps	Rationale
Palpation	**1.** Use flat of four fingers held together, in a light dipping motion.	
Light abdominal palpation	**2.** Palpate over entire abdomen, more than once in each of four quadrants.	Ensures entire abdomen is palpated.
	3. Inquire about tenderness.	
Deep abdominal palpation	**1.** Palpate deeply **after** light palpation.	If light palpation identifies unexpected findings, deep palpation may be contraindicated.
	2. Palpate over entire abdomen, more than once in each quadrant. Use flat of four fingers of one hand **OR** use two hands, one placed on top of the other and pressure exerted with top hand.	Using two hands allows the top hand to exert the pressure and the bottom hand to feel.
	3. Inquire about tenderness.	
	4. Observe client's facial reactions during palpation.	
Palpation: Liver	**1.** Place (L) hand behind client parallel to and supporting 11th and 12th ribs and soft tissue below.	
	2. Press (L) hand forward while client relaxes.	
	3. Place (R) hand on client's abdomen: • below lower border of liver dullness percussed upon deep inspiration • lateral to rectus muscle with hand held parallel or obliquely to midline of body **OR** parallel to costal margin.	Percussed level of liver may be where palpable.
	4. Palpate deeply with flat of four fingers.	
	5. Instruct client to take a deep breath and try to feel liver edge as it comes down to meet fingertips **OR** lateral edge of index finger.	During inhalation, the diaphragm descends, pushing the liver down toward the hand.
	6. If liver not palpable, • inch hand closer to (R) costal margin and repeat procedure • exert more pressure inward upon expiration and repeat procedure	
Inguinal nodes: horizontal	**1.** Palpate inferior to inguinal ligament from symphysis pubis to anterior superior iliac spine.	Lymph nodes are in chains.
vertical	**2.** Palpate medial to femoral canal from superior ramus to an area 5 cm distally.	Ensures both chains of nodes are palpated.

From *A Syllabus for Adult Health Assessment* (p. 46), edited by D. L. Skillen and R. A. Day, 2004, Edmonton, AB: Faculty of Nursing, University of Alberta.

Table 28-48 Examples of Documentation for Abdominal Assessment

Focus of Assessment	Expected Findings	Unexpected Findings
Skin	Pink, smooth, intact, striae present	10 cm surgical scar RLQ
Umbilicus	Pink, flat, round	Yellowish discharge
Contour and symmetry	Rounded, symmetrical	Concave, 3 cm bulge noted in LUQ
Movement or pulsations	Pulsations visible in aortic region <1 cm diameter	Pulsations visible in epigastric area ~4 cm
Bowel sounds	Bowel sounds present in all four quadrants	Bowel sounds absent in all four quadrants
Vascular sounds	No vascular sounds auscultated in aortic, iliac, or renal areas	Bruits noted in aortic area
Percussion	Dullness in RUQ, tympany in LUQ, LLQ, and RLQ	Dullness noted in LUQ, RUQ, and LLQ
Liver size	Liver span measures 8 cm at midclavicular line	Liver span measures 14 cm at midclavicular line
Kidney tenderness	Client reports no tenderness on direct percussion	Client reports tenderness on (R) side on direct percussion
Splenic percussion note	Percussion note remains tympanic before and after inhalation	Percussion notes change from tympanic to dull on inhalation
Palpation	Soft, non-tender	Tenderness reported in RUQ
Liver	Not palpable	Irregular edge
Inguinal nodes	Not palpable	Tender nodes ~2 cm palpated on (L) horizontal chain

From Documentation" by T. S. Stephen in *Health Assessment Self-Test Modules* (WebCT Vista), 2004, Edmonton, AB: Faculty of Nursing, University of Alberta.

Assessing the Female Genitalia and Reproductive Tract

External Genitalia. The external genitalia are the mons pubis, labia majora, labia minora, clitoris, urethral meatus, and vaginal orifice (Figure 28–77). The mons pubis is a pad of fatty tissue that lies anterior to the symphysis pubis. During adolescence, hair grows along the labia and becomes darker, coarser, and curlier as it spreads over the symphysis pubis. Hair growth eventually forms a triangle over the adult perineum and along the medial thighs. Labia majora are folds of fatty tissue that are located from the mons pubis to the perineum (area between vaginal orifice and anus). The inner surfaces appear dark pink and moist. Labia majora may be gaping or closed. After childbirth, the labia majora are separated and more prominent. The labia minora are smaller folds, which are joined anteriorly at the clitoris, forming a hood or prepuce, and posteriorly by the frenulum. The clitoris is erectile tissue 0.5 cm wide that varies in length from 2 cm or less.

Together, the labial structures form the vestibule, which has several openings. The urethral meatus is anterior to the vaginal orifice, pink, and at times difficult to locate. It may appear as a small slit or pinhole opening 2.5 cm below the clitoris, just above the vaginal canal. In women who have had several vaginal childbirths, the opening to the vaginal canal often extends upward, interfering with the view of the meatus. Small glands (Skene's) surround the urethral meatus. The vaginal orifice (introitus) is a thin vertical slit or a large orifice, with moist tissue. The hymen is just inside the introitus. In virgins, the hymen may restrict the opening of the vagina. Only remnants of the hymen remain after sexual intercourse. Bartholin's glands are located on either side of the vaginal orifice and provide lubrication during sexual intercourse.

Internal Genitalia. The internal genitalia consist of the vagina, cervix, uterus, fallopian tubes, and ovaries (Figure 28–78). The vagina begins at the vaginal orifice and extends back into the pelvis. The vaginal walls are usually pink throughout, moist, and with folds of tissue (rugae) that allow the canal to expand in childbirth. Secretions are thin, clear or cloudy, and odourless. The cervix extends into the end of the vagina. It is glistening pink, smooth, and round, with a diameter of 2.5 to 3 cm in a young woman. An opening (os) in the cervix increases in size after childbirth. The surface of the cervix at the os is lined with layers of vaginal squamous cells that meet a different group of cells, the columnar cells. The columnar cells secrete mucus and line the passageway that leads up into the central cavity of the uterus. Squamous cells have a protective role for the cervix; columnar cells have a role in reproduction (helping sperm to enter the uterus for fertilization). The space around the cervix is called the anterior fornix in front and the posterior fornix in the back. The uterus is pear-shaped and measures "5.5 to 8 cm long by 3.5 to 4 cm wide and 2 to 2.5 cm thick" (Jarvis, 2004, p. 767). The fallopian tubes extend out from the fundus or top of the uterus and curve down toward the ovaries. The ovaries lie on each side of the uterus in line with the anterior superior iliac spine.

Nurses collect a history from female clients about the genitalia and reproductive tract (Table 28-49) and this history guides their client teaching and health promotion (Box 28-35).

An examination of the female genitalia can be embarrassing for many women unless the nurse uses a calm, relaxed approach. For adolescents, the gynecological examination can be one of the most difficult experiences. Cultural background also contributes to apprehension. Nurses need to provide very thorough explanations in advance about the reason for the procedures so that clients

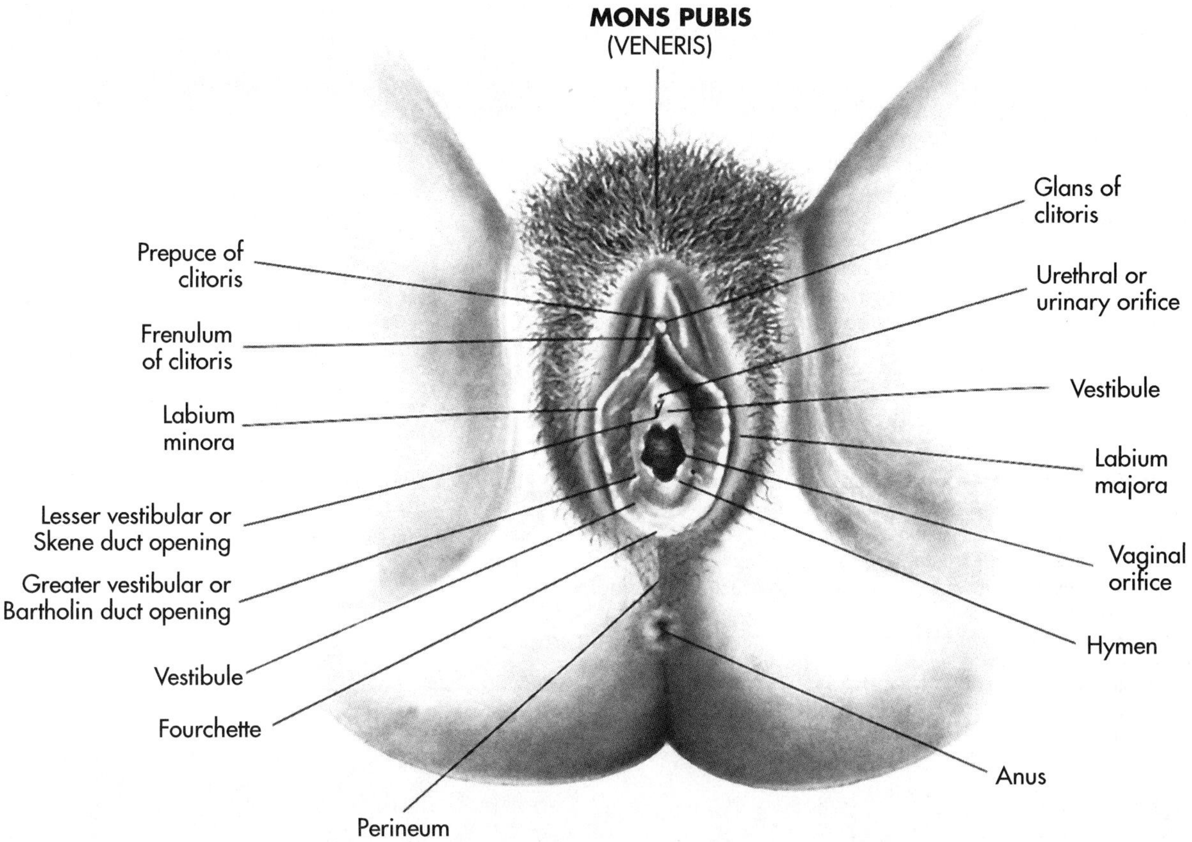

FIGURE 28–77 External female genitalia. (From Lowdermilk, D.L., Perry S.E., & Bobak I.M.(2000) *Maternity and women's health care,* 7th ed., St Louis: Mosby.)

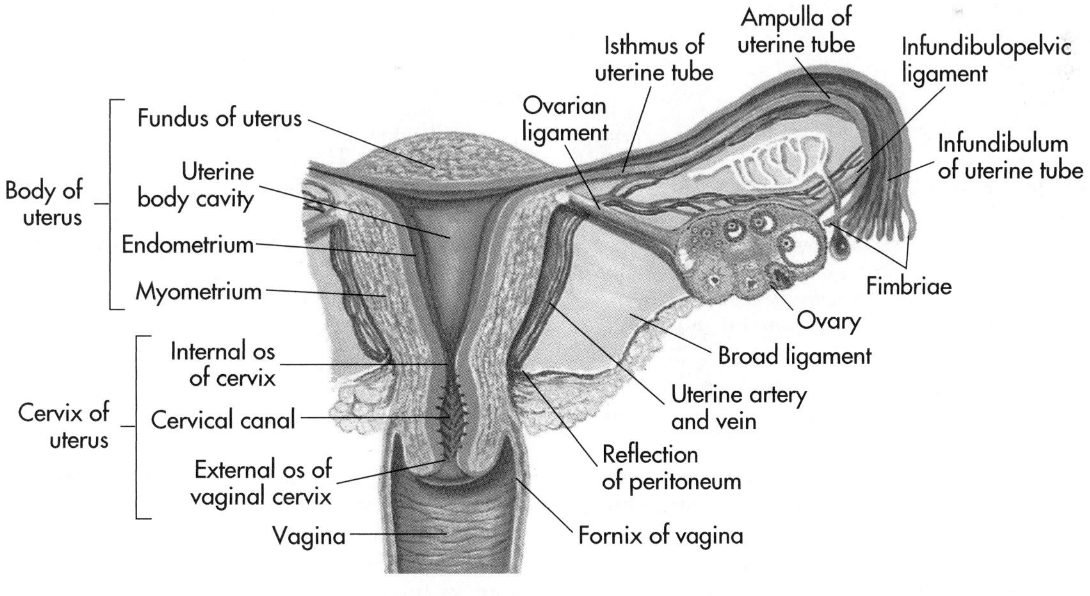

FIGURE 28–78 Internal female genitalia. (From *Mosby's Guide to Physical Examination,* 5th ed., p. 587, Figure 17–4, by H. M. Seidel et al., 2003, St. Louis, MO: Mosby.)

Table 28-49 Health History for Female Genitalia and Reproductive Tract Assessment

Assessment Category	Rationale
Ask client about history of previous illness, surgery or sexually transmitted infections (STIs) involving reproductive organs.	Illness or surgery can influence appearance and position of organs being examined.
Inquire about client's menstrual history, including age of onset, frequency, duration, characteristics of flow, presence of dysmenorrhea (painful menstruation), pelvic pain, premenstrual symptoms.	This information helps to reveal level of reproductive health.
Ask client about obstetrical history, including number of pregnancies, abortions, or miscarriages.	Observed physical findings will vary, depending on woman's history of pregnancy.
Inquire about client's contraceptive and safer sex practices.	Use of certain types of contraceptives may influence reproductive health (e.g., sensitivity reaction to spermicidal jelly). Helps to determine reproductive risks. Sexual history reveals risk for and understanding of STIs.
Ask client about history of genitourinary problems, including burning during urination, frequency, urgency, nocturia, hematuria or incontinence.	Urinary problems may be associated with gynecological disorders.
Ask client if post-menopausal, obese, or infertile; had early menarche (before the age of 12 years); had late menopause (after age 50); has history of hypertension, diabetes, or liver disease; or has family history of endometrial, breast, or colon cancer.	These are risk factors for endometrial cancer.
Ask client about presence of vaginal discharge, painful or swollen tissues, or genital lesions.	These signs and symptoms may indicate STIs.

Client Teaching — Box 28-35

Female Genitalia and Reproductive Tract Assessment

Objectives

- Client will pursue routine gynecological examinations as indicated by age and circumstances and will know self-examination techniques.
- Client will know safer sex practices.
- Client will know and use measures to prevent acquisition and transmission of sexually transmitted infections (STIs).

Teaching Strategies

- Instruct client about purpose and recommended frequency of Pap smears and gynecological examinations (annually after the age of 18 years or when sexually active).
- Inform client about genital self-examination, including use of a mirror to visualize external genitalia, looking for bumps, sores, blisters, or warts (cauliflower-like lesions).
- Inform client of warning signs of STIs, including pain or burning on urination, pain in pelvic area, bleeding between menstruation, itchy rash around vagina, and changes in vaginal discharge.
- Teach client measures to prevent STIs, including use of condoms, restricting sexual partners, and avoiding sex with people who have multiple partners.
- Reinforce the need for proper perineal hygiene and safer sex methods, teaching a variety of contraceptive methods, including the use of condoms.

Evaluation

- Have client state when last gynecological examination occurred.
- Have client state ways to prevent transmission of STIs as well as safer sex practices.
- Have client state warning signs of STIs

are prepared. The position assumed during the examination (lithotomy) is an added source of embarrassment. Comfort is established with correct positioning and draping. Adolescents may choose to have a parent present.

The client may require a complete examination of the female reproductive organs, which includes assessment of the external genitalia and a vaginal examination. Nurses frequently will examine external genitalia during routine hygiene measures or urinary catheter care. They perform parts of the vaginal examination in areas such as obstetrics, family planning clinics, or sexually transmitted infection (STI) clinics. The more complete examinations are performed by experienced nurse practitioners and midwives, but it is important for nurses to understand the procedure because they will often be required to assist physicians or other health care providers.

The examination should be part of each woman's preventive health care, as uterine cancers have a high incidence rate and ovarian cancer causes more deaths than any other cancer of the female reproductive system (CCS, 2004a). Young adults and adolescents should be examined because of the increasing incidence of STIs. The average age of menarche has declined, and the majority of teenagers (male and female) are sexually active by the age of 19 years (Hockenberry et al., 2003). Clients who are at risk for contracting an STI should learn to perform a genital self-examination (Box 28-35) to detect any STI signs or symptoms. Many women do not know they have an STI and some STIs remain undetected for years. As nurses collect the history (see Table 28-49), they also assess the client's level of anxiety and previous experience with a vaginal examination. They can easily combine the rectal and anal examination with the client in the lithotomy or dorsal recumbent position.

Examination of External Genitalia

Preparation of the Client. Before the examination begins, the necessary equipment is prepared and the client empties her bladder so that urine is not accidentally expelled while being examined and a urine specimen can be collected if required. For an external genitalia assessment, the nurse assists the client to assume the lithotomy position in bed or on an examination table. The nurse also assists the client into stirrups if a speculum examination is to be performed (see Table 28-15). The client stabilizes each foot in a stirrup and slides her buttocks down to the edge of the examining table. The nurse places a hand at the edge of the table and instructs the client to move until touching it. To prevent the client from tightening the abdominal muscles, the nurse ensures that the client's arms are either at her sides or folded across her chest.

A woman with joint pain or deformity may be unable to assume a lithotomy position. In this case, the client may assume the side-lying position, where the client lies on her left side with her right thigh and knee drawn up to her chest. Alternatively, the nurse may have the client abduct only one leg or have another nurse assist in separating the thighs. The client is given a square sheet or drape. She holds one corner over her sternum, the adjacent corners fall over each knee, and the fourth corner covers the perineum. When the examination begins, the examiner lifts the drape to expose the perineum. A male examiner always has a female present during the examination. A female examiner may prefer to work alone but should have a female attendant if the client is particularly anxious or requires assistance.

Inspection and Palpation. The perineal area must be well illuminated. The nurse gloves both hands to prevent spread of micro-organisms. The perineum is extremely sensitive and tender and should not be touched suddenly without warning the client. It is best to touch the neighbouring thigh first before advancing to the perineum. Procedure 28-21 presents the procedures and techniques for examination of the external female genitalia.

The nurse inspects the surfaces of the labia majora, which are usually clear of edema, inflammation, lesions, or lacerations. To inspect the remaining external structures, the nurse gently retracts the labia minora outwardly, using a firm hold to avoid repeated retraction of sensitive tissues (Figure 28–79). The nurse looks for atrophy, inflammation, or adhesions. If inflamed, the clitoris is bright red. In young women it is a common site for syphilitic lesions (chancres), which are small open ulcers that drain serous material. Older women may have malignant changes that result in dry, scaly, nodular lesions. The nurse carefully examines the urethral orifice for colour and position and notes any polyps, discharge, or fistulas. With the labia still retracted, the nurse examines

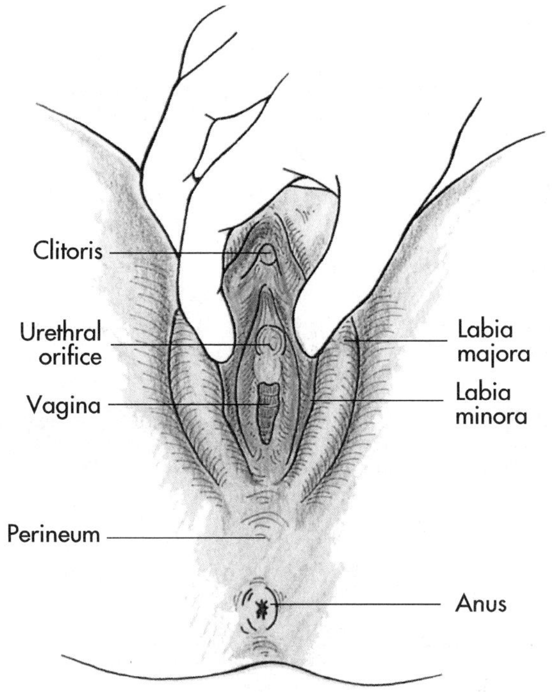

FIGURE **28–79** Female external genitalia.

Skene's and Bartholin's glands for tenderness and discharge (Figure 28–20; Procedure 28-21).

The nurse also assesses the adequacy of the muscle support. If clients lack adequate muscular support, the vaginal walls bulge and block the introitus. With the gloved index and middle fingers in the vaginal orifice, the nurse palpates tension in the muscles by asking the client to constrict or try to close the vaginal orifice. A woman who has undergone vaginal childbirth has less muscle tone than one who has not. The nurse may also inspect the anus at this time, looking for lesions and hemorrhoids (see Procedure 28-24). If performing only the external examination, the nurse discards the gloves and offers the client perineal hygiene.

Examination of Internal Genitalia

Speculum Examination. An examination of the internal genitalia requires much skill and practice. Beginning students will probably only observe the procedure or assist the examiner. A plastic or metal speculum is used. Consisting of two blades and an adjustable thumbscrew, the speculum is inserted into the vagina to assess the internal genitalia for cancerous lesions and other abnormalities. During the assessment, the examiner collects a **Papanicolaou (Pap) smear** to test for cervical and vaginal cancer. To assist an examiner, the nurse ensures that the client is comfortably positioned in the stirrups. The examiner selects the appropriate size of speculum (small, medium, or large) for the client. The smallest is used with a virgin. If a woman is sexually active, a medium-sized speculum is best. For women who have had children vaginally, the examiner uses a medium or large speculum.

Cervix. The examiner explains the procedure and carefully inserts the speculum until fully visualizing the

Procedure 28-21 Assessing the External Female Genitalia

Equipment

- Examination table with stirrups
- Vaginal speculum (correct size)
- Adjustable light source
- Sink
- Clean disposable gloves
- Glass microscopic slides
- Spatula
- Cotton-tipped applicators and/or cytobrush
- Fixative spray
- Culture media

Examination Skill and Focus	Steps	Rationale
Inspection: Pubic hair	Client in lithotomy position, with feet in stirrups, draped with pubis and genitalia exposed, nurse gloved, and light coming over nurse's shoulder.	Position allows for visibility and access to structures. Gloves prevent transmission of microorganisms.
	1. Inspect hair, hair distribution and skin of pubis.	Good light is essential to improve visibility.
Labia majora	**1.** Inspect labia majora.	
	2. Use thumb and index finger of non-dominant hand inside labia minora to gently but firmly retract tissues forward.	Position improves visibility. Repeated re-positioning can damage sensitive tissues.
	3. Inspect labia minora.	
Palpation: Labia minora	**1.** With other hand, palpate labia minora between thumb and index finger on one side.	
	2. Repeat on other side.	
Inspection: Clitoris	**1.** Inspect clitoris.	Location of the meatus is essential for procedures such as inserting a urinary catheter through the meatus to the bladder.
Urethral meatus	**1.** Locate urethral meatus above vaginal canal.	
	2. Inspect meatus.	
Vaginal orifice (introitus)	**1.** With the labia minora still retracted, inspect the introitus.	
	2. With the labia minora still retracted, and using the dominant hand, first dip the index finger into a basin of warm water for lubrication.	Water is the only lubricant if specimens are to be collected.
	3. With the palm facing upward, insert index finger into the vagina as far as the proximal interphalangeal joint (second finger joint).	
Palpation: Skene's glands	**4.** Exert upward pressure by moving fingers outward (milking action) on either side of urethra and directly over the urethra (see Figure 28–80).	Milking the glands causes any discharge to appear.
	5. Inquire about tenderness	
	6. Culture any discharge.	
	7. Remove retracting hand.	
	8. Insert index finger into posterior vaginal opening toward the (L) side and palpate the posterior labia majora between the index finger and the thumb.	

From "Female External and Internal Genital Examination," by R. A. Day, 2004a, in *A Syllabus for Adult Health Assessment* (pp. 92–95), edited by D. L. Skillen and R. A. Day, 2004, Edmonton, AB: Faculty of Nursing, University of Alberta.

Examination Skill and Focus	Steps	Rationale
	9. Repeat on other side.	Prevents contamination.
	10. Culture any discharge.	Bartholin's glands are not usually palpable.
	11. Change gloves.	
Bartholin's glands		
Perineum, vaginal orifice	**1.** Insert first two fingers into vagina and instruct client to squeeze examiner's fingers.	Assesses vaginal tone (important for sexual satisfaction and prevention of urinary incontinence).
	2. Instruct client to strain downward as if voiding. Determine if any structures touch examining fingers.	Bulging of vaginal walls may indicate a prolapse of the bladder (cystocele) or the rectum (rectocele).
	3. Remove fingers from vagina and use first two fingers of both hands to separate the vaginal orifice.	Permits detection of urine and/or bulging of vaginal walls.
	4. Instruct client to bear down.	
	5. Inspect vaginal orifice.	
Inspection: Anus	See Procedure 28-24 "Inspecting the Anus, Rectum, and Prostate" section	

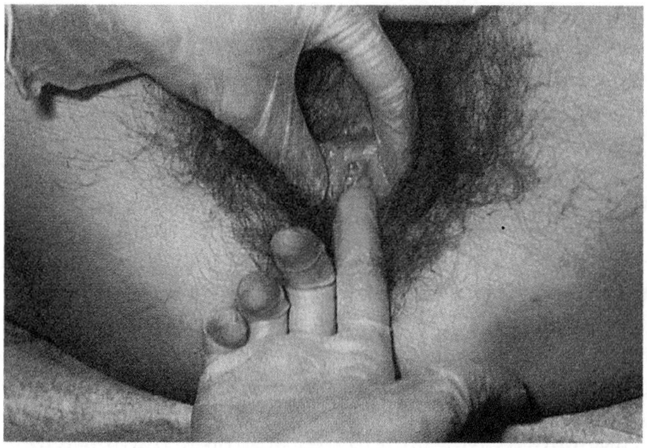

FIGURE **28–80** Milking the urethra and paraurethral Skene's glands.

cervix (Figure 28–81 and Procedure 28-22). If a woman has never been examined, the examiner first inserts two fingers gently into the vagina to explore for abnormalities. The cervix is inspected for colour, appearance of the cervical os, position, size, surface characteristics, and discharge.

Papanicolaou Smear. A Pap smear is a simple, painless screening test for cervical cancer and has no side effects. Smears are taken from the endocervix and ectocervix. The test should be performed annually during the pelvic examination of women who are, or have been, sexually active, and in women who have reached the age of 18 years. After three or more consecutive annual examinations with expected findings, the test may be done less often (e.g., every 1 to 3 years), based on provincial screening guidelines and health care provider discretion. Women at high risk for cervical cancer and those over 40 years should have annual checkups.

Vagina. After specimens are collected, the examiner loosens the speculum thumbscrew but keeps the blades open with the thumb. The examiner then views the vaginal walls while slowly withdrawing the speculum and noting colour, surface characteristics, and secretions. The walls are usually pink, moist, smooth or rugated and free from lesions or discharge. Although secretions are expected to be thin, clear or cloudy, and odourless, women commonly acquire yeast infections that cause a thick, white, patchy, malodorous, curd-like discharge. Following speculum withdrawal, the nurse assists the client to a sitting position, and allows the client to perform hygiene measures and to dress. In a hospital, the client may need assistance with perineal hygiene. The nurse makes sure the gloves, speculum, and other disposable equipment are appropriately discarded in a receptacle.

Age-Related Changes. With aging, pubic hair may diminish and become grey. When a woman reaches menopause (often between 46 and 55 years of age), the labia majora become thinned, and with advancing age, they become atrophied. Sex organs such as the clitoris also atrophy. Cervical diameter is narrower. Vaginal secretions are decreased, sometimes leading to painful sexual intercourse. With the thinning of tissues, urinary infections may increase.

Documentation. Nurses record their findings from inspection and palpation of the female genitalia (Table 28-50).

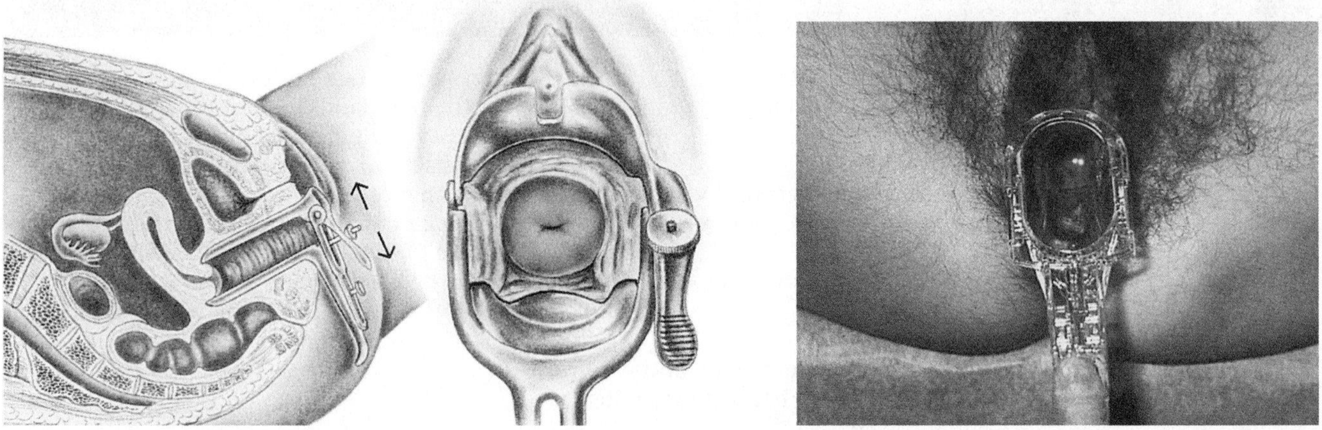

A B C

FIGURE **28–81** **A,** Angle of speculum insertion. **B,** View of cervix. **C,** Vaginal speculum in place with cervix in full view.

Assessing the Male Genitalia

The examination of the external male genitalia includes assessment of the penis, scrotum, external inguinal ring, and inguinal canal. The testis, epididymis, and vas deferens are the internal genital structures that are assessed. Figure 28–82 presents the external and internal male genitalia and the relationship to the rectum, anus, and prostate.

The shaft of the penis contains the urethra and columns of erectile tissue: corpus cavernosum (two) and corpus spongiosum (one). The urethra is located ventrally in the shaft and opens into the urethral meatus, somewhat ventrally on the cone-shaped glans penis. The dorsal vein is usually apparent. At the base of the glans is the corona. In men who are not circumcised, the prepuce (foreskin) covers the glans; secretions of the glans may collect under the prepuce. The scrotum is a wrinkled pouch with two compartments, each containing a testis (testicle). The testes are ovoid, somewhat rubbery, range in length from 3.5 to 5.5 cm, and produce testosterone and spermatozoa. One testis, commonly the left, lies lower in the scrotum. The epididymis is located posteriorly and laterally on the superior margin of each testis and has the shape of a comma. The vas deferens (cord-like structure) transmits the sperm from the testes and epididymis via a circuitous route to the urethra, along with secretions from the seminal vesicles, prostate, and the vas deferens. The vas deferens, blood vessels, nerves, and muscle fibres form the spermatic cord.

Lymphatics from the penis and scrotal sac drain into the inguinal lymph nodes, but lymphatics from the testes drain into the abdomen. The inguinal area lies between the anterior superior iliac spine and the symphysis pubis. The inguinal ligament runs between them; the inguinal canal lies about parallel to the ligament and transmits the vas deferens through the abdominal muscles. The external inguinal ring (medial opening of the canal) lies superior and lateral to the pubic tubercle and is accessible to the examining finger.

The nurse conducts a health history (Table 28-51) to ensure completeness of the subsequent examination. Box 28-36 presents client teaching and health promotion topics that the nurse may address during the male genitalia assessment.

Nurses use a calm, gentle approach to lessen client anxiety about the inspection and palpation of the genitalia and inguinal regions. Clients' modesty must be respected and dignity preserved. Boys and adolescents may worry about their genitals being normal. Adolescents and adult males often fear they will have an erection while being examined. Gentle manipulation of the genitalia reduces the risk of discomfort or erection. By avoiding discussion of the client's sexual activity during the actual examination, the nurse further reduces the risk. Nurses avoid joking and non-verbal expressions that may convey concern or worry. They delay teaching until the examination is completed. It is essential that males understand how to perform the genital self-examination as a routine part of self-care (Box 28-37). Because the incidence of STIs in adolescents and young adults is high, an assessment of the genitalia should be a routine part of any health maintenance examination for this age group.

Penis

Inspection. The nurse applies disposable gloves at the beginning of the examination to indicate routine practice and prevent infection from unexpected discharge or skin lesions (Procedure 28-23). The nurse begins by assessing the sexual maturity of the client, noting the size and shape of the penis and testes, colour and texture of the scrotal skin, and character and distribution of pubic hair. In the adult male, coarse and curly pubic hair extends from the base of the penis over the pubic area, medial thighs, and toward the umbilicus. The penis reaches the bottom of the scrotum, testicles are fully grown, and scrotal skin is darker and rugated.

The nurse inspects the skin covering the genitalia for evidence of rashes, lesions, lice, or excoriations. Inspection for inflammation and swelling of the shaft, corona, prepuce, glans, and urethral meatus of the penis follows (Figure 28–83). The area between the foreskin and

Text continued on p. 739

Procedure 28-22 Assessing the Internal Female Genitalia

(NOTE: This procedure is usually performed by advanced nurse practitioners or nurse-midwives. Beginning students will only observe the procedure or assist the examiner.)

Equipment

- Examination table with stirrups
- Vaginal speculum (correct size)
- Adjustable light source
- Sink
- Clean disposable gloves
- Glass microscopic slides
- Spatula
- Cotton-tipped applicators and/or cytobrush
- Fixative spray
- Culture media

Examination Skill and Focus	Steps	Rationale
Inspection: Cervix	Client continues in lithotomy position, with feet in stirrups, draped with pubis and genitalia exposed, nurse newly gloved, in a sitting position and with light coming over nurse's shoulder.	
	1. Select appropriate size speculum and lubricate with warm water.	Size of speculum depends on factors such as age, history of sexual intercourse, vaginal births.
	2. Hold speculum in dominant hand, with blades closed.	
	3. Insert first two fingers of non-dominant hand into vagina and press downward.	
	4. Insert speculum obliquely.	Avoids pressure on the urethra.
	5. Instruct client to bear down.	Relaxes the perineal muscles and opens the introitus (Jarvis, 2004).
	6. When the speculum has passed the inserted fingers, continue to insert downward toward the table at a 45-degree angle.	Speculum follows the usual slope of the vagina.
	7. Rotate speculum blades to horizontal position.	Avoids catching hair or pinching the labia.
	8. After full insertion, open blades slowly and move to visualize cervix.	
	9. Lock blades in open position.	Hands are now free to collect specimens.
Papanicolaou (Pap) smear	**1.** Inspect cervix and os. If blood is visible, delay taking specimens.	Presence of blood may invalidate tests.
	2. Use a spatula or cotton-tipped applicator rotated 360 degrees against the surface of the cervix (endocervix).	
	3. Remove and gently spread specimen on glass slide.	Gentle action avoids damaging cells.
	4. Spray specimen with cytological fixative immediately and label.	
Other specimens	**5.** Use cotton-tipped applicator or cytobrush to collect a specimen from inside the cervical os (endocervix). (Rotate one or two full turns).	Collects cells from the squamocolumnar junction.
	6. Spread specimen gently on glass slide.	
	7. Spray specimen with cytological fixative immediately and label. If unusual vaginal discharge is present, collect specimens for culture and test specifically for sexually transmitted infections.	

From "Female External and Internal Genital Examination," by R. A. Day, 2004a, in *A Syllabus for Adult Health Assessment* (pp. 92–95), edited by D. L. Skillen and R. A. Day, 2004, Edmonton, AB: Faculty of Nursing, University of Alberta.

Continued

Procedure 28-22 *Assessing the Internal Female Genitalia—cont'd*

Examination Skill and Focus	Steps	Rationale
	8. Inspect walls of vagina while slowly withdrawing speculum.	
	9. After passing the cervix, loosen thumbscrew on speculum but keep blades open with thumb.	
	10. As speculum approaches the vaginal opening, close blades carefully.	Avoids pinching walls of vagina.
	11. Turn blades obliquely and remove speculum.	
Bimanual exam: Vagina	Examiner in standing position.	
	1. Make "the 'obstetric' position with the first two fingers extended, the last two flexed into palm and the thumb abducted" (Jarvis, 2004, p.783).	
	2. Use water-based lubricant on first two fingers of dominant hand.	Lubricant can be used after specimens have been taken.
	3. Insert fingers into vagina and again press downward.	
	4. Allow time for walls of vagina to relax, then insert fingers completely.	
	5. Palpate vaginal walls in all directions.	Assesses for consistency, contour, and mobility.
Cervix	**1.** Palpate cervix.	Use of both hands facilitates assessment for tenderness or masses.
	2. Place fingers on either side of cervix and move it gently from side to side.	
Uterus	Place other hand on abdomen, halfway between the umbilicus and symphysis pubis. Press down firmly to push the pelvic organs closer to the examining fingers.	
	1. Palpate to determine position.	
	2. Palpate walls of uterus with fingers in fornices.	
	3. Move the uterus carefully between abdominal hand and intravaginal hand.	
	4. Attempt to feel the ovaries between the abdominal hand and the intravaginal hand.	
Other manoeuvres	**1.** In the rectovaginal examination, insert one finger into the vagina and one into the rectum and repeat from 1 (obstetric position) above.	This technique provides additional information about the septum between the rectum and the vagina, the rectal wall, and the anal sphincter.
	2. If stool is present when removing gloved finger, test for occult (hidden) blood.	
Completion of examination	**1.** Provide client with tissues to clean areas examined.	
	2. Assist client to move upward on examining table.	
	3. Assist client to sit up.	Reduces risk of client falling.

From "Female External and Internal Genital Examination," by R. A. Day, 2004a, in *A Syllabus for Adult Health Assessment* (pp. 92–95), edited by D. L. Skillen and R. A. Day, 2004, Edmonton, AB: Faculty of Nursing, University of Alberta.

Table 28-50 Examples of Documentation for Female Genitalia Assessment

Focus of Assessment	Expected Findings	Unexpected Findings
Pubic hair	Uniform and thick triangular distribution of coarse, curly hair over pubis, medial thighs; free of parasites	Pubic skin excoriations bilaterally
External genitalia	No swelling, lesions, or discharge noted. No urethral swelling or discharge	Labia minora bright red bilaterally
Vaginal walls	Rugated, free of excoriations, no bulging of walls	White, curd-like discharge on vaginal walls
Cervix	Pink, no lesions, scant clear discharge	Nodule 1 cm × 0.5 cm, anterior surface of cervix, (L) side
Uterus	Midline, firm, mobile, no masses	Enlarged, tender on palpation
Ovaries	Non-palpable bilaterally	Enlarged, painful (R) ovary

Adapted from "Documentation" by R. A. Day in *Health Assessment Self-Test Modules* (WebCT Vista), 2004b, Edmonton, AB: Faculty of Nursing, University of Alberta.

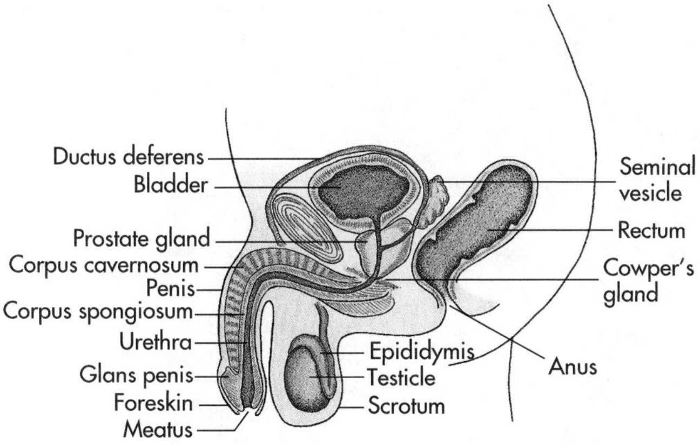

FIGURE **28–82** External and internal male sex organs.

Table 28-51 Health History for Male Genitalia Assessment

Assessment Category	Rationale
Ask client about usual urinary elimination patterns, including frequency of voiding, nocturia, urine characteristics, burning, urgency, hematuria, difficulty starting stream, daily fluid intake.	Urinary problems can be related to genitourinary problems due to anatomical proximity.
Inquire about client's sexual history, safer sex practices, and sexual orientation.	History and practices reveal level of risk for sexually transmitted infections (STIs), including HIV/AIDS.
Ask client about history of surgery or illness involving urinary or reproductive organs, including STIs.	Alterations may underlie reported symptoms or changes.
Inquire about presence of penile swelling, genital lesions, urethral discharge, pain in testicle or scrotum.	These signs and symptoms are associated with STIs.
Inquire about irregular or painless lumps or painless enlargement of testis, a feeling of heaviness in scrotum, or dull ache in abdomen.	These signs and symptoms are associated with testicular cancer.
Inquire about history of undescended testis as child and frequency of self-testicular examination.	Risk for testicular cancer increases in men who had an undescended testis in early childhood. Frequency of examination indicates potential for early detection.
Ask client about any enlargements noted in inguinal area, duration, association with lifting, coughing, or straining.	These signs and symptoms are associated with hernias.
Ask client about current medication use (e.g., antihypertensives, sedatives, diuretics, or tranquilizers), alcohol intake. Also inquire about satisfaction with sexual life, any difficulty achieving erection or ejaculation.	Medications or alcohol may affect sexual performance.

Client Teaching Box 28-36

Health Promotion for Male Genitalia Assessment

Objectives

- Client will describe safer sex methods and methods to prevent transmission of sexually transmitted infections (STIs).
- Client will know how to perform genital self-examination.

Teaching Strategies

- Instruct client how to perform a genital self-examination (see Box 28-37).
- Inform client of measures to prevent STIs, including use of condoms, avoiding sex with a partner who is infected, restricting number of sexual partners, and avoiding sex with people who have multiple partners.

Evaluation

- Have client state safer sex methods to prevent transmission of STIs.
- Have client describe methods for genital self-examination.

Box 28-37 Male Genital Self-Examination

All men aged 15 years and older should perform this examination monthly using the following steps.

Genital Examination

- Perform the examination after a warm bath or shower when the scrotal sac is relaxed.
- Stand naked in front of a mirror and hold the penis in your hand and examine the head. Pull back the foreskin if uncircumcised. Inspect and palpate the entire head of the penis in a clockwise motion, looking carefully for any bumps, sores, or blisters. Look also for any bumpy warts (see illustration). Look at the opening at the end of the penis for discharge. Look along the entire shaft of the penis for the same signs. Be sure to separate pubic hair at the base of the penis and carefully examine the skin underneath.

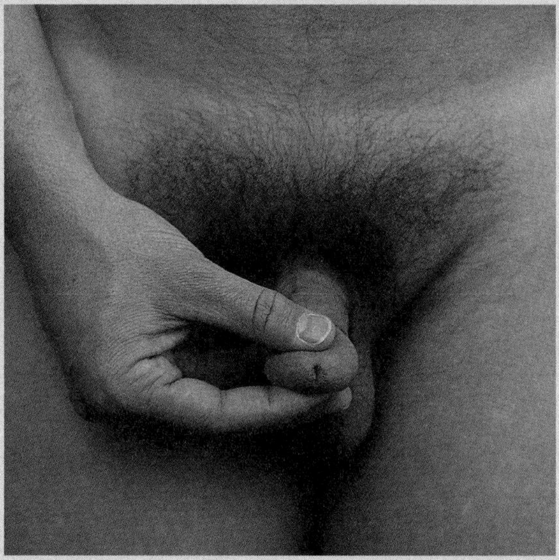

Testicular Self-Examination

- Look for swelling or lumps in the skin of the scrotum while looking in the mirror.
- Using both hands, placing the index and middle fingers under the testicles and the thumb on top (see illustration). Gently roll the testicle, feeling for lumps, thickening, or a change in consistency (hardening).
- Find the epididymis (a cord-like structure on the top and back of the testicle; it is not a lump).
- Feel for small, pea-sized lumps on the front and side of the testicle. The lumps are usually painless and are abnormal. Call your physician if you find a lump.

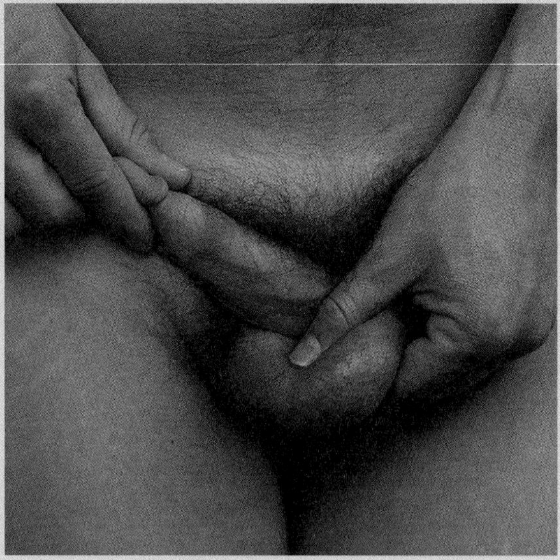

Illustrations from *Mosby's Guide to Physical Examination* (5th ed., p. 659), by H. M. Seidel et al., 2003, St. Louis, MO: Mosby.

A 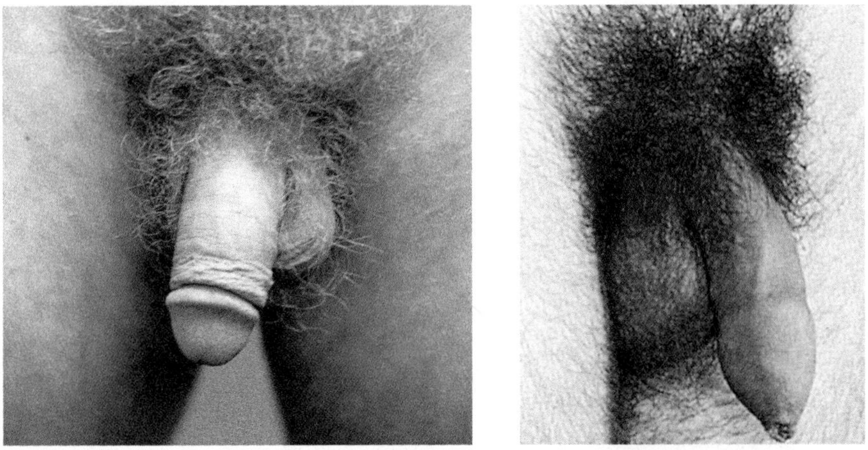 B

FIGURE 28–83 **A,** Circumcised male genitalia. **B,** Uncircumcised male genitalia. (From *Mosby's Guide to Physical Examination* (5th ed., p. 655, Figure 18–5), by H. M. Seidel et al., 2003, St. Louis, MO: Mosby.)

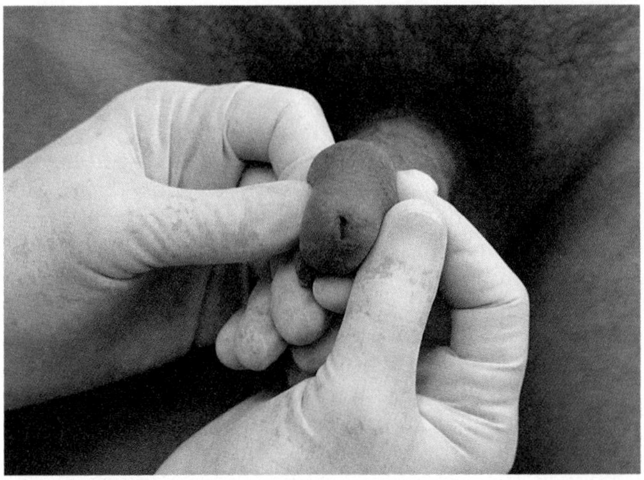

FIGURE 28–84 Examination of the urethral orifice. (From *Mosby's Guide to Physical Examination,* 5th ed., p. 656, Figure 18–8, by H. M. Seidel et al., 2003, St. Louis, MO: Mosby.)

glans is a common site for venereal lesions, and the nurse either retracts the prepuce for inspection or asks the client to do so. The foreskin should retract easily.

Lesions are inspected for size, shape, location, colour, type, and discharge. A small amount of thick, white secretion between the glans and foreskin is expected. If there is evidence of discharge, the nurse takes a culture. The urethral meatus is slit-like and should be positioned on the ventral surface only millimetres from the tip of the glans. In some congenital conditions, the meatus is displaced along the ventral penile shaft. Its opening is expected to be glistening, pink, and without discharge, but the meatus is inspected for lesions, edema, and inflammation (Figure 28–84). When inspection of the penis is completed, the foreskin is returned to its original position. It should never be left retracted because of the risk for impeded arterial circulation.

Palpation. The shaft is palpated between the thumb and first two fingers to detect any localized areas of hardness (induration) and tenderness on dorsal or lateral surfaces. These indicate a risk in older males for fibrotic plaques associated with painful erections.

Scrotum

Inspection. The nurse must be particularly cautious when examining the scrotum because of the sensitivity of structures lying within the scrotal sac. The nurse inspects the scrotum size, shape, and symmetry while observing for lesions or edema. Bedridden clients who are compromised and subject to friction or moisture in the scrotal area may have excoriated skin. The scrotal skin is coarse, rugated, loose, and usually more deeply pigmented than the body skin. Tightening of the skin may reveal edema. The scrotum size generally changes with temperature variations as the dartos muscle contracts in cold and relaxes in warm temperatures. Nurses consider occupational history (e.g., exposure to heat as baker) to assess effects on the scrotum and its contents. They also consider testicular cancer that is a known risk of solid tumour among young men ages 18 to 34 years or more. Early detection is critical. Clients must learn to perform testicular self-examination and to appreciate its importance (see Box 28-37).

Palpation. The nurse gently palpates the testicles and epididymis between the thumb and first two fingers. Scrotal structures are sensitive to gentle compression but are not tender. They feel smooth, rubbery, and free of nodules. The most common signs of testicular cancer are a painless enlargement of one testis and the appearance of a palpable, small, pea-sized, hard lump on the anterior or lateral testicle. Size, shape, consistency, and tenderness of the scrotal organs are noted. The nurse palpates the vas deferens separately, feeling for nodules or swelling. It is expected to be smooth and discrete. The external inguinal ring provides the opening for the spermatic cord to pass into the inguinal canal.

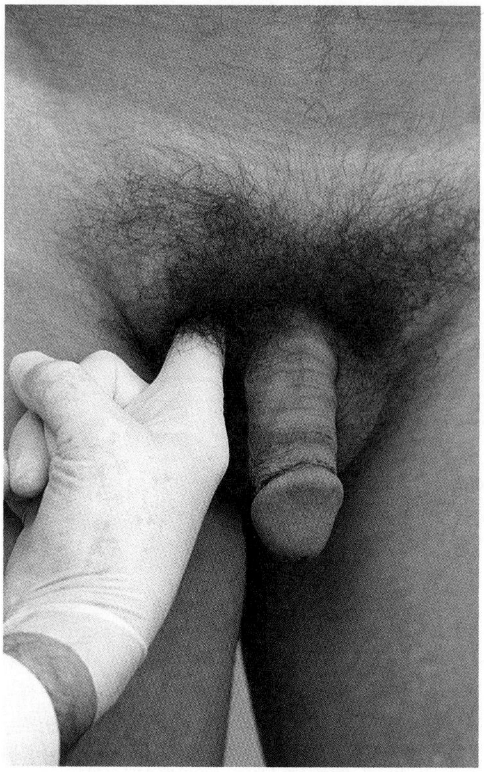

FIGURE **28–85** Checking for inguinal hernia; gloved finger inserted through inguinal canal. (From *Mosby's Guide to Physical Examination,* 5th ed., p. 658, Figure 18–12, by H. M. Seidel et al., 2003, St. Louis, MO: Mosby.)

Inguinal Region

Inspection. During inspection, the nurse asks the standing client to strain or bear down. The manoeuvre helps make an expansile impulse, enlargement, or bulge more obvious. When a portion of intestine or abdominal tissue protrudes through the inguinal or femoral canal, it creates a hernia. Intestinal loops can even enter the scrotum and be auscultated for bowel sounds.

Palpation. The nurse next palpates the external inguinal ring and medial inguinal canal to be sure a hernia is not present (Figure 28–85). The femoral canals are also assessed for a hernia. If a bulge or expansile impulse is observed, the nurse notes its relationship to the pubic tubercle. This will help distinguish an inguinal hernia from a femoral hernia. The nurse completes the examination by palpating for inguinal lymph nodes (see Assessing the Abdomen). A non-tender, mobile, horizontal or vertical node less than 1 cm in size may be found. Nodes that are larger than 1 cm, tender, and non-mobile require further examination.

Age-Related Changes. With aging, pubic hair diminishes and becomes grey. The penis decreases in size. The testicles are less firm to palpation and may also reduce in size during a prolonged illness. Production of spermatozoa and testosterone declines. Muscle tone of the dartos muscles in the scrotum decreases, causing scrotal contents to hang lower and the scrotal sac to be more pendulous. Sexual function continues, but the sexual response is less intense and slower. Erections are slower and less firm; ejaculation occurs more quickly and is less forceful. The refractory state when men physiologically cannot ejaculate is lengthened.

Documentation. Nurses record their findings from inspection and palpation of the male genitalia (Table 28-52).

Assessing the Anus, Rectum, and Prostate

Anus and Rectum. A good time to perform the rectal examination with men and women is after the genital examination. Usually the examination is not performed in young children or adolescents.

The anus is a tightly closed, hairless, moist, visible structure that is the external opening of the anal canal. This is the termination of the GI tract. The anal canal is surrounded by the internal sphincter muscle (under involuntary control) and the external sphincter muscle (under voluntary control). The canal is 3.8 cm long and extends in a line toward the umbilicus before turning into the mucus-lined rectum. The somatic sensory nerves in the anal canal are very sensitive to a poorly directed examining finger or instrument. At the anorectal junction, the rectum dilates and turns posteriorly into the hollow of the coccyx and sacrum. The rectum is about 12 cm long and joins with the sigmoid colon as the distal end of the GI tract. The rectum contains three transverse Valves of Houston; the inferior valve (fold) may be palpable. The upper portion of the rectum is covered by peritoneum, which is only accessible to the examiner's finger on the anterior rectal surface. This permits the examiner to assess for peritoneal inflammation through the rectum (e.g., in suspected appendicitis). In men, the peritoneum reflects on itself to form the rectovesical pouch; in women, the reflection is the rectouterine pouch. The examination can detect colorectal cancer in its early stages. In men, the rectal examination can also detect prostate tumours.

The nurse collects a thorough history (Table 28-53) to detect the client's learning needs and risk for bowel, rectal, or prostate disease. Subsequent client teaching contributes to client self-care (Box 28-38).

Nurses use a calm, slow-paced, gentle approach to explain about the rectal examination. They inform clients that they may feel as if their bowels will move but that it will not happen. This helps clients relax if concerned about discomfort or embarrassment. When examined by male nurses, men may be asked to bend forward with hips flexed and upper body resting across an examination table; in contrast, they will be examined by female nurses in the left lateral side-lying (Sims') position. Women can be examined immediately after examination of the genitalia while they are still in a dorsal recumbent position; otherwise the Sims' position is used. Non-ambulatory clients are examined in the Sims' position.

Anus

Inspection. The nurse begins by inspecting the perianal and sacrococcygeal areas. The skin should be smooth and uninterrupted. Anal tissues are usually moist and hairless

Procedure 28-23 Assessing the Male Genitalia and Inguinal Regions

Equipment

- Disposable gloves
- Glass slide
- Culture media

Examination Skill and Focus	Steps	Rationale
Inspection:	Client standing or supine, pubis and genitalia exposed, nurse gloved.	Visibility is essential. Gloves prevent transmission of microorganisms.
Pubic hair	**1.** Inspect hair and skin of pubis.	
Penis Skin	**1.** Inspect shaft of penis.	
prepuce	**2.** Ask client to retract prepuce (foreskin) if present.	Visibility is essential to assess uncircumcised male.
glans, corona	**3.** Inspect glans and corona.	
urethral meatus	**4.** Inspect location of meatus.	Congenital displacements occur.
	5. Compress glans gently.	Compression exposes meatus for full inspection.
	6. Inspect meatus.	Culture any discharge and obtain glass smear.
	7. Replace prepuce if retracted.	Retracted prepuce creates risk for arterial constriction.
Palpation: Shaft	**1.** Palpate shaft between thumb and first two fingers.	Induration (hardened plaque) is palpable.
	2. Inquire about tenderness.	
Inspection: Scrotum	**1.** Inspect anterior and lateral surfaces.	Visibility is essential for detection of changes.
	2. Lift scrotum gently to inspect posterior surface.	
Palpation	**1.** Use thumb and first two fingers of examining hand.	Manoeuvre captures mobile structures for examination.
	2. Palpate one side in sequence: a. testis b. epididymis c. spermatic cord (and vas deferens)	Sequence permits structures to be located easily.
	3. Repeat on other side.	Comparison permits detection of differences.
Inspection: Inguinal region Pubic tubercle to anterior superior iliac spine (inguinal canal)	Client standing. **1.** Inspect (L) (R) inguinal regions. **2.** Instruct client to strain or bear down.	Position permits hernia visibility and full effects of gravity and increased intra-abdominal pressure with bearing down.
	3. Inspect regions using tangential lighting.	Increases detection of contours, bulges, enlarged nodes.
	4. Compare regions.	Permits detection of differences.
Femoral canal	**1.** Inspect (L) (R) femoral regions.	Expansile impulses and bulges are more readily detected.
	2. Use tangential lighting.	
Palpation:	**3.** Instruct client to cough or strain down (R) (L).	
	4. Use tangential lighting.	
	5. Compare regions.	

From "Male Genitalia Examination," by D. L. Skillen, in *A Syllabus for Adult Health Assessment* (pp. 89–90), edited by D. L. Skillen and R. A. Day, 2004b, Edmonton, AB: Faculty of Nursing, University of Alberta.

Continued

Procedure 28-23 Assessing the Male Genitalia and Inguinal Regions—cont'd

Examination Skill and Focus	Steps	Rationale
Inguinal ring, inguinal canal	Client remains standing.	Position permits oblique direction of finger in inguinal canal and reduces palmar contact with penis.
	1. Stand on (R) side of client.	
	2. Place index finger of (R) hand against scrotal skin on (R) side.	
	3. Place finger low on scrotum.	Starting low on scrotum permits enough mobility through loose scrotal skin to reach inguinal canal.
	4. Move finger toward inguinal ring by invaginating scrotal skin over finger.	
	5. Assess possibility of passage through inguinal ring.	Passage is not to be forced through a narrow opening.
	6. Insert index finger superiorly and obliquely along vas deferens into inguinal canal, following spermatic cord.	Following natural direction of canal reduces discomfort.
	7. When index finger can not move further, instruct client to cough and strain down.	Increased intra-abdominal pressure will emphasize a hernia.
	8. Assess for bulging pressure against finger.	Location of pressure on finger assists with differentiation of direct and indirect hernias.
	9. Observe relationship to pubic tubercle.	Assists with differentiation of inguinal from femoral hernia.
Femoral canal	**10.** Repeat on (L) side with (L) index finger.	Hernias may be bilateral.
	1. Place finger pads on anterior thigh in region of femoral canal.	
	2. Instruct client to cough and strain down.	
	3. Assess for bulge or impulse against fingers.	Finger pads will feel pressure of a hernia.
	4. Observe relationship to pubic tubercle.	
Inguinal lymph nodes	**5.** Repeat on opposite thigh.	Hernias may be bilateral.
	See Procedure 28-20	

From "Male Genitalia Examination," by D. L. Skillen, in *A Syllabus for Adult Health Assessment* (pp. 89–90), edited by D. L. Skillen and R. A. Day, 2004b, Edmonton, AB: Faculty of Nursing, University of Alberta.

compared with perianal skin, and the tissue is coarser and more darkly pigmented. The nurse looks for lesions, rashes, inflammation, excoriation, linear splits (fissures), scars, and protrusions (skin or mucosa). A tuft of hair or dimple midline near the coccyx may indicate a pilonidal cyst. Protrusions from the anus may be hemorrhoids. External hemorrhoids are dilated or thrombosed veins that appear as bluish protrusions; internal hemorrhoids are reddish. The anal lining is expected to be intact.

Rectum

Palpation. Some institutions may not permit nurses to perform digital examinations. Where it is permitted, nursing students should have a qualified examiner present during the first examination. The nurse assesses the tone of the anal sphincter, which is expected to be tight. A weak sphincter may indicate a neurological problem or be associated with anal intercourse. With lubricant and gentle pressure, the nurse assesses the anal canal and lower rectum for smooth, non-tender surfaces. To avoid injury to mucosal tissues, the nurse never forces digital insertion. Beyond the anal canal, the nurse palpates the entire rectal wall for tenderness, irregularities, polyps, masses, or nodules. The wall should feel even and smooth. When the client bears down, high lesions within the rectum descend against the fingertip. Acute rectal pain is an unexpected finding that may be associated with irritation, fissures, inflamed or thrombosed hemorrhoids, or rock-hard constipation. Procedure 28-24 presents the techniques and procedures.

Anterior Rectal Surface. On the anterior surface of the rectum in women, the nurse can assess the posterior region of the cervix, which feels like a small round mass. Nurses should not mistake a retroverted uterus or a tampon in the vagina for a tumour. In men, the nurse will be

Table 28-52 Examples of Documentation for Male Genitalia

Focus of Assessment	Expected Findings	Unexpected Findings
Pubic hair	Uniform and thick distribution of coarse, curly, red hair over pubis, medial thighs, and midway to umbilicus; free of parasites	Pubic skin excoriations bilaterally
Penis	Circumcised (or uncircumcised), free of lesions; reaches bottom of scrotum; meatus slit-like, pink, glistening; corona smooth and pink	Non-tender indurated areas along dorsal surface; tight, non-retractable prepuce; profuse yellow discharge from meatus
Scrotum	Darker skin, rugated, free of excoriations	Generalized pitting edema; scrotal skin tight; excoriations posterior scrotal surface
Testicle	Palpated bilaterally; firm, 4.0 cm long bilaterally	Testicles 2 cm in length bilaterally; painless non-mobile nodule 1 cm × 0.5 cm, anterior surface (L)
Epididymis	Smooth, comma-shaped, non-tender, on postero-lateral testicular surface bilaterally	Firm, enlarged, indurated, tender (L) epididymis
Spermatic cord	Smooth, non-tender (R) (L)	(R) Tender, swollen, retracted
Inguinal canal	No bulge on straining, bilaterally; no pressure on index finger at external inguinal ring (L) (R)	Soft swelling (R) inguinal area, superior to pubic tubercle, increases with increased intra-abdominal pressure and reduces when supine
Femoral canal	No impulse or bulge on cough, bilaterally	Firm, non-reducible, tender swelling (R)
Inguinal lymph nodes	Non-palpable horizontal and vertical nodes bilaterally	One tender, fixed, (L) horizontal node 1.5 cm × 1.0 cm

Adapted from "Documentation" by D. L. Skillen in *Health Assessment Self-Test Modules* (WebCT Vista), 2004c, Edmonton, AB: Faculty of Nursing, University of Alberta.

Table 28-53 Health History for Anal and Rectal Assessment

Assessment Category	Rationale
Question about dietary intake of fat and fibre.	High fat or low fibre intake may be linked to bowel cancer and characteristics of stool.
Ask client about history of rectal bleeding, black or tarry stools, rectal pain, or change in bowel habits.	These are warning signs of colorectal cancer or other gastrointestinal disorders.
Inquire about family or personal history of colorectal cancer, polyps, inflammatory bowel disease, or age over 40.	These are risk factors for colorectal cancer.
Question client about medication use, including laxative or cathartic medications, iron supplements, or codeine.	These medications affect characteristics of stool and bowel habits.
Inquire about any screening for colorectal cancer.	Will help determine client's level of health-promoting behaviours.
Ask male client if weak or interrupted urine flow, inability to urinate, difficulty in starting or stopping flow; ask men and women about polyuria, nocturia, hematuria, dysuria, pain in lower back, pelvis or upper thighs.	These are warning signs of prostate cancer, prostate enlargement, or urinary infection.

able to palpate the prostate through the anterior rectal surface (Figure 28–86). The nurse explains to male and female clients that they may feel the need to pass urine when being palpated, but they will not.

Prostate

Palpation. The prostate gland is palpable anteriorly as a rounded, heart-shaped structure about 2.5 to 4 cm in diameter with less than 1 cm protrusion into the rectum (Figure 28–86). A small median groove separates the gland into two lateral lobes. The surface is smooth, elastic or rubbery, and non-tender. The nurse palpates the size, shape, and consistency (see Procedure 28-24). The gland usually is firm, without bogginess, tenderness, or nodules. Hardness or nodules may indicate the presence of a cancerous lesion. Prostate enlargement is classified by the amount of projection into the rectum: grade I is 1 to 2 cm protrusion; grade II, 2 to 3 cm; grade III, 3 to 4 cm; grade IV, more than 4 cm (Seidel et al., 2003).

Age-Related Changes. Usually, the prostate starts to enlarge in middle life. When straining down, the older adult may have some relaxation of the perianal musculature, with decreased control of the external sphincter muscle.

Documentation. Nurses record their findings from inspection and palpation of the anus, rectum, cervix, and prostate (Table 28-54).

Client Teaching Box 28-38

Health Promotion for Rectal and Anal Assessment

Objectives

- Client will have regular rectal digital examination performed appropriate for age.
- Client will know signs and symptoms of colorectal and prostate cancer.
- Client will increase dietary fibre and reduce fat.

Teaching Strategies

- Discuss the guidelines for early detection of colorectal cancer, including stool examination for presence of blood, following the advice of a physician after baseline examination (Canadian Task Force on Preventive Health Care, 2001).
- Inform client of warning signs of colorectal cancer (see Table 28-53).
- Inquire about client's current dietary habits and provide information about ways to reduce dietary fat and increase dietary fibre.
- Warn client about overuse of laxatives, cathartic medications, codeine, and enemas.
- Discuss the recommended guidelines for early detection of prostate cancer, including digital rectal examination yearly after the age of 50 years and the benefits and risks of a yearly prostate-specific antigen (PSA) blood test for men 50 years and over (Canadian Cancer Society, 2004b).
- Inform client of the warning signs of prostate enlargement and possible cancer, including frequent, difficult, or painful urination; urine that contains blood or pus; pain in the lower back, pelvic area, or upper thighs; and pain during ejaculation

Evaluation

- Have client state date of last digital rectal examination and/or PSA blood test.
- Have client state the warning signs of colorectal and prostate cancer.
- Have client state which foods are high in fibre and low in fat.

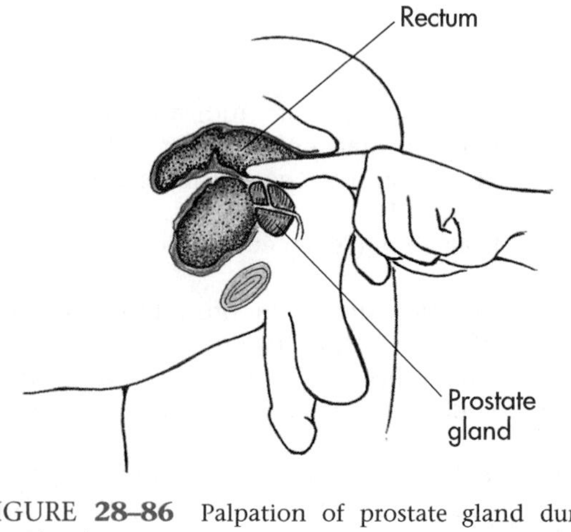

FIGURE **28–86** Palpation of prostate gland during rectal examination.

Assessing the Extremities

To assess integrity of the extremities, nurses integrate physical examination findings from four body systems: integumentary, neurological, musculoskeletal, and peripheral vascular. A comprehensive physical examination of the extremities makes full use of inspection and palpation, as well as limited percussion. In practice, the examination is focused according to the chief complaint or reason for the examination. Inspection and palpation of the integument and pulses of the extremities, including blood pressure, contribute to a comprehensive assessment of the integumentary and vascular systems. Examination of musculoskeletal function includes assessment of joints and surrounding tissues and range of motion. Assessment of the neurological system includes examination of cranial nerves, sensation, coordination, muscle tone, muscle strength, and reflexes. Nurses integrate aspects of the musculoskeletal and neurological examinations when observing client gait, movements in bed, and other activities that require coordination. Nurses usually test function of cranial nerves during examination of the head and neck. Tables 28-55, 28-56, and 28-57 contain the health history assessment for the vascular, musculoskeletal, and neurological systems in upper and lower extremities. See Tables 28-20, 28-23, and 28-25 for the integumentary system health history. Boxes 28-39, 28-40, and 28-41 present the client teaching and health promotion opportunities to be used during assessment of the extremities. See Boxes 28-17, 28-21, and 28-22 for teaching and health promotion activities regarding the integument.

Assessing the Upper Extremities

Inspection

Integument and Muscle Mass. Clients can be seated on the examining table or lying in bed during examination of the upper extremities. Sleeves of the gown must be rolled up to fully expose the arms and part of the shoulders. Nurses begin by inspecting the integument and muscle mass of the hands, arms, and shoulders, critically comparing findings for both sides (Procedure 28-25). Expected findings include symmetrical muscle development without wasting or **fasciculations** (localized twitching of muscle cells innervated by a single motor neuron). Nurses inspect for signs of skin **inflammation** (swelling and redness) and note any lesions including scars, nevi, freckles, and petechiae, or changes in skin colour due to sun or chemical exposure. Depending on clients' work, calluses and thickened epidermis may be expected findings on palmar surfaces as a result of pressure and friction. Nails are assessed for surface integrity and colour (see Figures 28–17, 28–18, and 28–19). Nail beds may be cyanosed (indicating hypoxia) or pale (indicating anemia).

Range of Motion. Arms are inspected for active range of motion (ROM). While performing active ROM, the client voluntarily moves the limb against gravity without assistance (see Procedure 28-25). Examiners can demonstrate the desired ROM or fully instruct the client. They observe ROM at the fingers, wrists (Figure 28–87), elbows,

Procedure 28-24 Assessing the Anus, Rectum, Prostate, and Cervix

Equipment

- Disposable gloves
- Lubricant
- Culture media
- Occult blood test

Examination Skill and Focus	Steps	Rationale
Inspection:	Client forward bending or in Sims' position	Position permits directing index finger toward umbilicus, promotes client comfort, and protects modesty.
Anus	Anal area exposed	Exposure permits inspection.
	Nurse gloved	Gloves prevent transmission of microorganisms.
Palpation	**1.** Spread buttocks apart.	Separation exposes perianal and sacrococcygeal regions.
	2. Inspect perianal and sacrococcygeal regions.	
	3. Lubricate index finger of dominant hand by dropping lubricant onto gloved finger.	Lubrication facilitates insertion of finger.
	4. Place finger pad across anus.	
	5. Instruct client to bear down.	External sphincter relaxes for insertion of finger.
	6. Assess tone of anal sphincter.	Detects neurological problem or lifestyle practice.
Palpation: Rectum	**1.** Flex fingertip and insert gently into anal canal.	Somatic nerve fibres supply anal canal.
(NOTE: Some agencies do not permit nurses to perform digital exams. Check agency policy.)		
	2. Insert finger in direction of umbilicus.	Using natural angle reduces discomfort.
Prostate (male)	**1.** Turn the hand to position finger for assessing all rectal surfaces.	Systematic assessment detects alterations.
	2. Instruct client to bear down.	High lesions in the rectum descend to fingertip.
	3. Reposition hand so that finger palpates anterior rectal surface.	Prostate is only accessible through anterior surface.
	4. Locate median groove (sulcus) of prostate gland.	Identifies lobes for palpating finger.
	5. Sweep index finger across prostate lobe from superior to inferior surface.	Systematic assessment detects alterations.
	6. Repeat on other lobe beginning at superior surface.	Comparisons facilitate identification of differences.
	7. Withdraw finger.	
	8. Examine colour of material on glove.	
	9. Make smear to test for occult blood.	Blood in feces needs to be identified early.
	10. Offer client tissues.	Client can remove lubricant before dressing.
Cervix (female)	**1.** Reposition hand so that finger palpates anterior rectal surface.	Cervix is only accessible through anterior surface.
	2. Locate rounded protrusion of cervix.	Other surfaces are smooth and even.
	3. Sweep index finger across protrusion.	Systematic assessment detects alterations.
	4. Withdraw finger.	
	5. Examine colour of material on glove.	
	6. Make smear to test for occult blood.	Blood in feces needs to be identified early.
	7. Offer client tissues.	Client can remove lubricant before dressing.

Adapted from "Anus, Rectum, and Prostate Examination," by D. L. Skillen, in *A Syllabus for Adult Health Assessment* (p. 96), edited by D. L. Skillen and R. A. Day, 2004, Edmonton, AB: Faculty of Nursing, University of Alberta.

Table 28-54 Examples of Documentation for Anus, Rectum, and Prostate

Focus of Assessment	Expected Findings	Unexpected Findings
Perianal and sacrococcygeal area	Skin smooth and uniform, without lesions	Inflammation surrounding tuft of hair midline superior to coccyx; tender to palpation
Anus	Pigmented, tightly closed, without lesions Anal canal smooth and non-tender	Stellate linear splits in anal circumference; firm shiny blue skin sac at opening of anus; anus loosely closed; tender fissure palpated on posterior midline at anal margin
Rectum	All surfaces smooth and uniform, stool on glove brown	Soft, slightly mobile mass on posterior surface; single firm nodule with rolled edge on posterolateral surface (L)
Prostate	Smooth rubbery non-tender (R) (L) lobes; protrude < 0.5 cm into lumen; median sulcus palpable; lobes about 3.0 cm long	Symmetric, non-tender enlargement, grade I; median sulcus not palpable; boggy tender prostate lobes, asymmetric in size; single hard nodule on superior surface (R) lobe, about 1.0×1.0 cm

Adapted from "Documentation" by D. L. Skillen in *Health Assessment Self-Test Modules* (WebCT Vista), 2004, Edmonton, AB: Faculty of Nursing, University of Alberta.

Table 28-55 Health History for Vascular Assessment of the Extremities

Assessment Category	Rationale
Ask if client experiences legs cramps, numbness or tingling in extremities, cold hands or feet, leg pains, swelling or cyanosis of feet, ankles, or hands. Conduct a symptom analysis as required.	These signs and symptoms indicate vascular disease.
Ask client about use of tight-fitting hosiery or sitting or lying with crossed legs.	These can impair venous return.
Inquire about any history of heart disease, hypertension, diabetes, or varicose veins and any related treatments.	These can affect findings during physical examination.

Table 28-56 Health History for Musculoskeletal Assessment of the Extremities

Assessment Category	Rationale
Inquire about usual activity pattern, including type of exercise usually performed and if alterations in usual habits have occurred; inquire about the effect of the alterations on activities of daily living, including bathing, feeding, dressing, toileting, ambulating, recreational, and sexual activities.	Provides baseline assessment for further investigation related to need for assistance.
Conduct a symptom analysis if pain or disability is reported.	Helps to determine nature of alteration.
Question client about involvement in sports events, including contact or competitive events.	These are risk factors for sports injuries.
Inquire about history of heavy alcohol use, smoking; constant dieting; calcium intake less than 500 mg daily; thin and light body frame; nulliparous status; menopause before age 45; family history of osteoporosis; menopause status; Caucasian, Asian, or northern European ancestry.	These are risk factors for osteoporosis.

Table 28-57 Health History for Neurological Assessment of the Extremities

Assessment Category	Rationale
Ask client about use of medications, including analgesics, antipsychotics, antidepressants, nervous system stimulants, alcohol, sedative-hypnotics, or recreational drugs.	These medications can alter level of consciousness or cause behavioural changes.
Ask about history of seizures or convulsions and conduct symptom analysis as necessary.	Characteristics of seizures help to determine origin.
Inquire about presence of headaches, tremors, dizziness, vertigo, numbness or tingling of body part, visual changes, weakness, pain, changes in speech, or changes in hearing, vision, taste, smell, touch.	These signs and symptoms may indicate a pathological condition.
Ask client or family members about any recent changes in behaviour, including mood changes, irritability, or memory loss, or change in activity level.	May indicate presence of pathology. Client may not notice changes immediately.
Inquire about past history of head or spinal cord injury, hypertension, or psychiatric disorders.	May provide information to guide assessment.
If elderly client displays sudden onset of confusion (delirium; see Box 28-15), review medications, gather information about possible serious infections, metabolic disturbances, heart failure, or severe anemia.	These conditions are potentially reversible.

Client Teaching Box 28-39

Vascular Assessment of the Extremities

Objectives

- Client will know normal blood pressure range for age and compare it with own blood pressure measurement.
- Client will know signs and symptoms of vascular problems.

Teaching Strategies

- Inform client of his or her blood pressure measurement and the normal ranges for adult blood pressure measurements and discuss implications of abnormalities.
- Instruct client about the signs and symptoms of vascular disease (see Table 28-55)
- Encourage clients at risk to avoid wearing tight clothing over extremities, avoid sitting or standing for long periods, to walk frequently, and to elevate feet when sitting.
- Encourage client not to smoke, as smoking causes vasoconstriction.
- Encourage regular monitoring of blood pressure.

Evaluation

- Ask client to identify if blood pressure reading is within normal limits.
- Have client state signs and symptoms of vascular disease and state actions to reduce risk of vascular disease.

and shoulders. In the well adult, a bilaterally symmetrical, full ROM is expected without assistance at each joint. Movements should be comparable to an accepted norm. Any restrictions to full ROM are documented. If the client is unable to perform active ROM, the examiner attempts to move the supported joint through a passive ROM without client assistance. If the examiner achieves passive ROM, the client lacks the muscle strength to move the joint. If the examiner cannot achieve passive ROM, the problem lies within the joint. An examiner *never* forces a joint if there is pain or muscle spasm.

Examiners use a goniometer if a precise measure of the degree of motion at a joint is required. The instrument has two flexible arms with a 180-degree protractor in the centre. The centre of the protractor is positioned over the centre of the joint being measured (Figure 28–88). The goniometer arms extend along the body parts on each side of the protractor. A measurement is taken of the joint angle in a neutral position before moving the joint. The angle is measured after moving the joint through a full ROM to determine the degree of movement and compared with the expected degree of that joint movement.

Palpation. Nurses use the dorsum of the hand to palpate the hands, forearms, and upper arms for temperature, expecting uniform warmth and slight moisture bilaterally (Procedure 28-26). The hands may be cooler than the upper arms if ambient air temperature is cool. In a warm environment or if clients are anxious, the palms, axillae, and skin may be noticeably moist. The skin is expected to be mobile (the nurse pinches up a fold of skin easily). If turgor (elasticity) is intact, the fold will immediately return to the original position when released. In conditions such as dehydration, decreased skin turgor causes skin to remain "tented" when released. Nail plates are firm and uniformly thick. **Capillary refill,** a test of blood circulation

Client Teaching — Box 28-40

Musculoskeletal Assessment of Extremities

Objectives

- Female clients will follow measures to prevent or minimize osteoporosis.
- Client will assume proper body posture when standing, sitting, walking, lying, and lifting.
- Client will perform self-care measures including care appropriate to level of activity.

Teaching Strategies

- Encourage clients to ensure adequate intake of calcium. Recommended daily calcium requirements are as follows: men, premenopausal women, and post-menopausal women on estrogen = 1000 mg; post-menopausal women not on estrogen = 1500 mg; men and women over 65 years old = 1500 mg.
- Encourage clients to engage in proper daily exercise habits. Encourage client to follow a low-impact or higher intensity water exercise program three times weekly to reduce bone demineralization that occurs with age.
- Instruct client in proper postural alignment while standing, walking, sitting, lying, lifting.
- Encourage proper warm-up, stretching, and cool-down activities before and following exercise, proper lifting techniques, and back-strengthening exercises.
- Encourage use of back support device for heavy lifting activities.
- If client is unable to perform self-care activities, inform about assistive devices, such as canes, walkers, elevated chairs, and zippers instead of buttons on clothing.
- Encourage older clients to pace activities to compensate for loss of muscle strength.

Evaluation

- Observe client's posture in a variety of positions.
- Have client state actions to reduce risk of osteoporosis.
- Have client state proper warm-up, stretching, and cool-down activities for exercising.
- Have client or family describe use of assistive devices for self-care in the home.

Client Teaching — Box 28-41

Neurological Assessment of the Extremities

Objectives

- Client and client's family will understand the relationship of client's behavioural and mental changes to physical status.
- Clients with sensory or motor impairment will select safety measures for self-care.
- Older client will routinely inspect skin for injuries.

Teaching Strategies

- Explain to client and family the neurological implications of any behavioural or mental impairment shown by client.
- Encourage older clients to take adequate time to complete tasks, as reaction time slows.
- If client has sensory impairment, advise on measures to ensure safety, such as use of ambulation aids and safety bars in bathrooms and on stairs.
- Teach proper skin assessment technique based on the fact that with increased age, pain sensation may be reduced.

Evaluation

- Have client and/or family members state behaviours that result from neurological impairments.
- Have client explain safety measures to avoid injury from sensory limitations.
- Have client report findings of skin assessment.

to the fingers, is assessed by pressing firmly, quickly, and gently on the nail plate. Pressure on the nail bed causes blanching; when pressure is released, the colour turns pink almost instantly (1 to 2 seconds).

Joints. Examiners palpate the interphalangeal joints (IP), metacarpophalangeal (MCP) joints (Figure 28–89), wrists, elbows, and shoulders, noting size, shape, tenderness, and temperature. Warm, swollen, tender, or boggy joints may indicate inflammation and the presence of fluid in the joint. For assessment of the shoulder joint (see Procedure 28-26), knowledge of the surface landmarks created by the bony structure of the shoulder girdle is essential. The sternoclavicular (SC) joint, acromion, clavicle, and acromioclavicular (AC) joint are useful landmarks. The AC joint can be detected by asking the client to externally rotate the arm. Joints are expected to be non-tender, to move smoothly, and be free of crepitations (grating sensations). The crepitations result from roughened articular cartilage and suggest osteoarthritis. Another useful shoulder landmark is the greater tubercle of the humerus, a bony prominence at the lateral aspect of the humerus (Figure 28–90). Examiners locate the greater tubercle by palpating over the lateral border of the acromion process, which forms the crest of the shoulder. Medial to the greater tubercle is the bicipital groove where the long head of the biceps tendon lies. Asking the client to externally rotate the arm makes the groove and lesser tubercle more accessible. By gently palpating the biceps tendon, it rolls beneath the finger pads during external rotation of the arm; it is non-tender.

Muscle Tone. Muscle tone is the slight muscular tension (contraction) retained in a voluntarily relaxed muscle. Muscle tone is assessed prior to assessing muscle strength because knowledge of the state of muscle tone will guide assessment of muscle strength and interpretation of results (Procedure 28-27). The client relaxes the arm as the examiner moves the supported arm through a modified ROM (Figure 28–91). This may be difficult if the

A

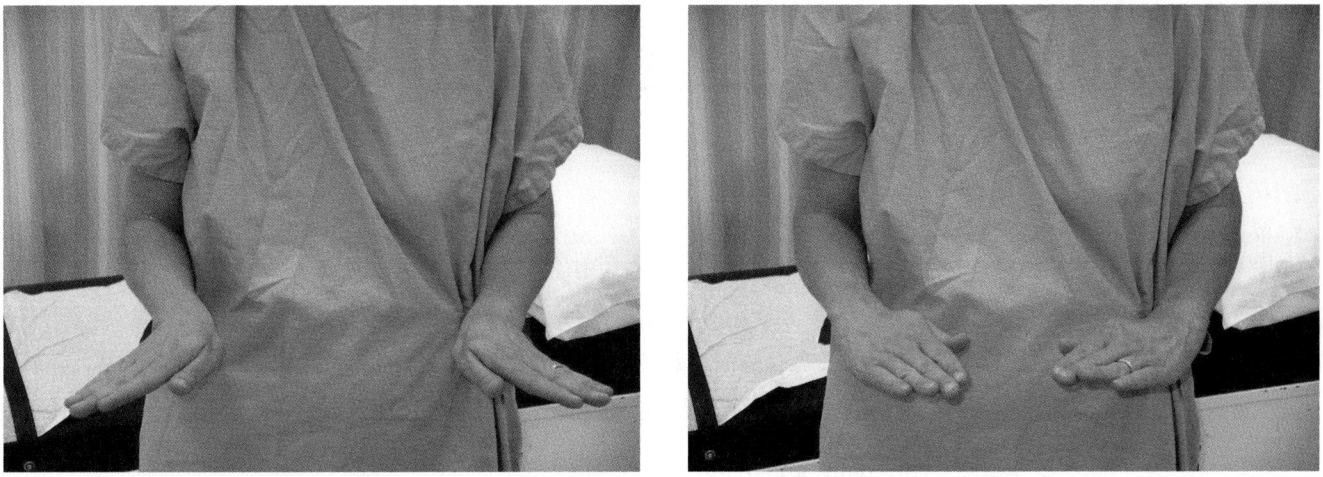

B

FIGURE 28–87 Wrists. **A,** Ulnar deviation. **B,** Radial deviation. (From *Physical Examination Images* [CD-ROM], by D. L. Skillen, R. A. Day, M. C. Anderson, T. C. Stephen, J. A. Gilbert, and L. W. Day, 2004, Edmonton, AB: Faculty of Nursing, University of Alberta.)

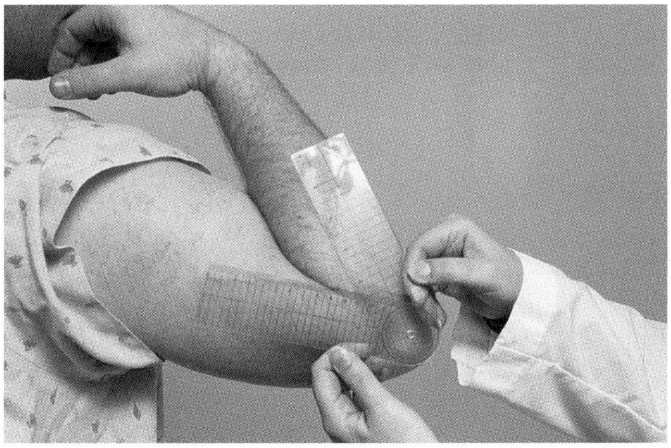

FIGURE 28–88 After the client flexes the arm, the goniometer is used to measure the degree of joint flexion. (From *Mosby's Guide to Physical Examination,* 5th ed., p. 79, by H. M. Seidel et al., 2003, St. Louis, MO: Mosby.)

client has arm pain. A mild, even resistance as the arm is moved smoothly through the entire range is expected. An increase or decrease in muscle tone signals a possible neurological deficit and alterations during strength testing. In a muscle with increased tone (hypertonicity), the passive stretch of a muscle is met with considerable resistance. Continued movement eventually causes the muscle to relax. A muscle with little or no tone (hypotonicity) feels flabby or flaccid. The involved extremity may hang loosely in a position determined by gravity.

Muscle Strength. Strength of muscle groups is assessed from the fingers to the shoulder girdle (see Procedure 28-27). The examiner asks the client to either extend or flex muscles around a joint and then applies an opposing force. For example, when testing the strength of wrist extension, the examiner asks the client to extend the wrist and then resist as the examiner attempts to flex the wrist (Figure 28–92). When possible, examiners simultaneously test muscle strength of the limbs, as this technique provides the best comparison. Clients are expected to demonstrate strength commensurate with the muscle mass present. The examiner would expect a man to exhibit greater strength than a woman because of muscle mass. Clients are expected to sustain the effort against the resistance, with strength and resistance equal bilaterally. Muscle strength can be graded from 0 (no active movement) to 5+ (strong active sustained resistance). See Table 28-58 for a grading scheme. If weakness is identified, the size of the muscle can be compared with its counterpart by measuring the circumference of the muscle body with a tape measure. An atrophied muscle (reduced in size) may feel soft when palpated and contract with less force (muscle weakness).

Peripheral Pulses. The brachial and radial pulses are palpated with finger pads or thumbs, as both are sensitive to arterial pulsations. Access to the arteries improves if clients slightly flex the arm at the elbow and wrist (Figure 28–93). Nurses expect arterial walls to be elastic and easily palpable; they apply firm pressure, but avoid occluding the pulse. When a pulse is difficult to find, they vary the pressure and feel all around the area. A hard, inelastic artery suggests arteriosclerosis. Nurses assess pulses for rate, rhythm, amplitude, and equality (see chapter 27). The amplitude (force at which blood is ejected against the arterial wall) may be graded on a scale of 0 (absent) to 4+ (bounding; Table 28-59). The expected amplitude is 2+. Pulse amplitude should remain consistent between pulsations. Any unexpected variability in amplitude suggests pathology such as atrial fibrillation.

Nurses assess all peripheral pulses for equality and symmetry, and always compare the pulse of one arm with the same pulse on the other arm (Procedure 28-28). Nursing students can practise locating pulses on a friend.

Procedure 28-25 Inspecting the Upper Extremities

Equipment

- Reflex hammer
- Splintered tongue blade/cotton-tip applicator
- Tuning fork (128 Hz)
- Cotton ball

Examination Skill and Focus	Steps	Rationale
Skin, nails, hair, symmetry	**1.** Fully expose the hands and arms of the seated or supine client. **2.** Inspect skin, nails, and symmetry of both arms and hands.	Full visualization of arms is essential for inspection.
Range of motion (ROM)	The examiner inspects the ROM. Each arm is tested, either separately or simultaneously, and compared. Only if the client is unable to perform active ROM does the examiner attempt passive ROM.	
Thumbs	**1.** Instruct client to supinate hands and **2.** Touch base of 5th finger with thumb (flexion) **3.** Move thumb back and forth away from fingers (extension). **4.** Move thumb anteriorly away from palm (abduction). **5.** Move thumb back down (adduction). **6.** Touch tip of thumb to each fingertip (opposition)	Full ROM of the thumbs includes flexion, extension, abduction, adduction, and opposition.
Fingers	**1.** Instruct client to make a fist (flexion), thumb across knuckles. **2.** Straighten fingers (extension). **3.** Spread extended fingers (abduction). **4.** Close extended fingers together (adduction).	Full ROM of the fingers at the distal interphalangeal and proximal interphalangeal joints includes flexion and extension and at the metacarpophalangeal joints, flexion, extension, abduction, and adduction.
Wrists	**1.** Instruct client to flex wrist and **2.** Extend wrist. **3.** Stabilize client's forearm and hand in supination and instruct client to **4.** Move hand medially (ulnar deviation). **5.** Move hand laterally (radial deviation).	Full ROM at the wrist includes flexion, extension, and ulnar and radial deviation.
Elbows	**1.** Instruct client to bend elbows (flexion) and **2.** Straighten elbows (extension). **3.** Instruct client to hold flexed elbows close to sides and turn palms upward (supination), and **4.** Turn palms downward (pronation).	Full ROM at the elbows includes flexion, extension, supination, and pronation. Holding flexed elbows close to sides ensures that only ROM of elbow is tested.

From *A Syllabus for Adult Health Assessment* (pp. 47–48), edited by D. L. Skillen and R. A. Day, 2004, Edmonton, AB: Faculty of Nursing, University of Alberta.

Examination Skill and Focus	Steps	Rationale
Shoulders	**1.** Instruct client to extend arms forward (flexion), and **2.** Extend straightened arms as far back as possible (extension). **3.** Instruct client to bring straightened arms across anterior midline (adduction). **4.** Instruct client to lift arms laterally in an arc starting from sides and ending with both arms extended above head, palms facing (abduction). **5.** Instruct client to place hands behind own neck (external rotation), and **6.** Place hands behind small of back (internal rotation).	Full range of movement at the shoulders includes flexion, extension, adduction, abduction, external rotation, and internal rotation.

From *A Syllabus for Adult Health Assessment* (pp. 47–48), edited by D. L. Skillen and R. A. Day, 2004, Edmonton, AB: Faculty of Nursing, University of Alberta.

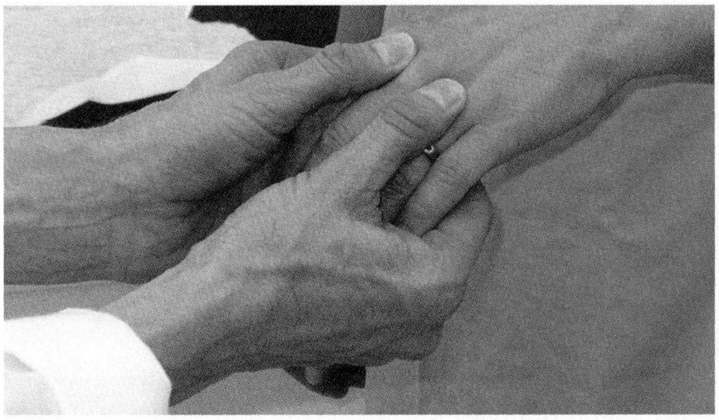

FIGURE **28–89** Palpation of metacarpophalangeal joints. (From *Physical Examination Images* [CD-ROM], by D. L. Skillen, R. A. Day, M. C. Anderson, T. C. Stephen, J. A. Gilbert, and L. W. Day, 2004, Edmonton, AB: Faculty of Nursing, University of Alberta.)

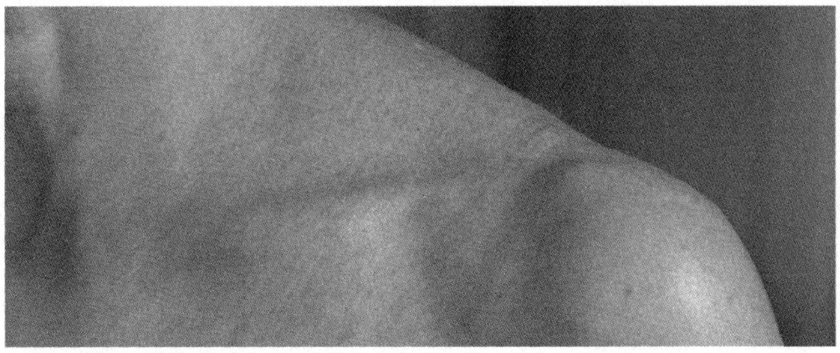

FIGURE **28–90** Landmarks of the shoulder. (From *Physical Examination Images* [CD-ROM], by D. L. Skillen, R. A. Day, M. C. Anderson, T. C. Stephen, J. A. Gilbert, and L. W. Day, 2004, Edmonton, AB: Faculty of Nursing, University of Alberta.)

Procedure 28-26 Palpating Temperature and Joints of the Upper Extremities

Equipment

- None

Examination Skill and Focus	Steps	Rationale
Palpation: Temperature	**1.** Use dorsum of hands or fingers to compare temperature of each hand with forearm and upper arm above it.	Dorsal skin is thin and sensitive to temperature.
	2. Compare sides.	Comparison permits detection of alterations.
Palpation: Joints	Examiner instructs the client to indicate if there is any tenderness during joint palpation. Both limbs are palpated separately and compared.	Single or multiple joints may swell and become inflamed due to trauma or chronic conditions such as arthritis.
Fingers		
Interphalangeal (IP) joints	**1.** Palpate with thumb and index finger of one hand all of the distal and proximal IP joints of fingers and thumb of both hands at the medial and lateral aspects of each joint.	Palpation may elicit tenderness and detect bogginess.
Metacarpophalangeal (MCP) joints	**1.** Palpate with thumbs of both hands the MCP joints of both hands just distal to and on each side of the knuckle.	
Wrists	**1.** Palpate medial and lateral surfaces of each wrist (distal radius and ulna).	
	2. Palpate each wrist with thumbs dorsally and fingers ventrally.	
Elbows	**1.** Support the left slightly flexed arm with the left hand and forearm.	Palpation can also detect the presence of nodules around the elbow.
	2. Palpate a. the olecranon process b. the groove on either side of the olecranon process c. the lateral and medial epicondyles.	
	3. Inquire about tenderness.	
	4. Repeat on the right side.	
Shoulders	**1.** Cup a hand over each of the client's exposed shoulders and	Crepitus in the shoulder may be felt (and sometimes heard) during range of motion (ROM) testing.
	2. Feel for crepitus during adduction, abduction, external and internal rotation.	
	3. Palpate the sternoclavicular (SC) joint.	Joints in the shoulder girdle are subject to injury. Palpation of the SC and AC joints and the biceps tendon may elicit tenderness.
	4. Palpate the acromioclavicular (AC) joint.	
	5. Palpate the biceps groove for long head of biceps tendon.	
	6. Inquire about tenderness during 3, 4, 5 above.	

From *A Syllabus for Adult Health Assessment*, edited by D. L. Skillen and R. A. Day, 2004, Edmonton, AB: Faculty of Nursing, University of Alberta.

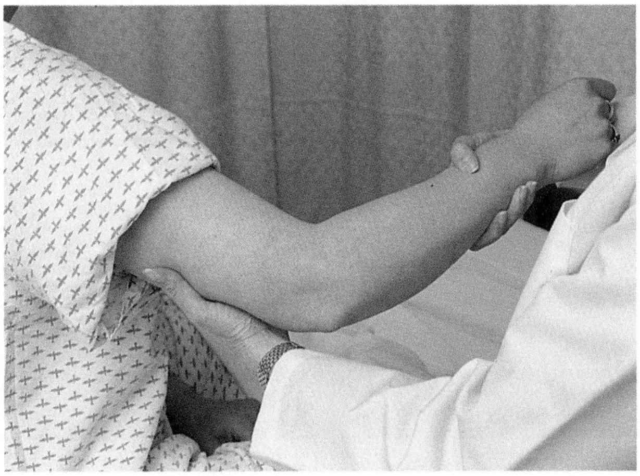

FIGURE **28–91** The nurse assesses muscle tone.

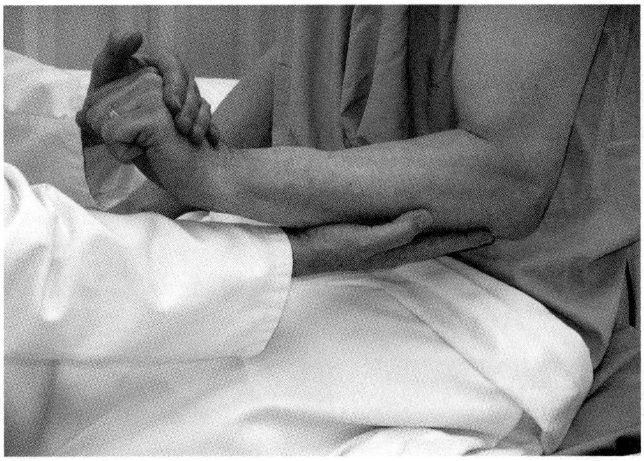

FIGURE **28–92** Wrist extension. (From *Physical Examination Images* [CD-ROM], by D. L. Skillen, R. A. Day, M. C. Anderson, T. C. Stephen, J. A. Gilbert, and L. W. Day, 2004, Edmonton, AB: Faculty of Nursing, University of Alberta.)

Table 28-58 Muscle Strength

Muscle Function Level	Scales		
	Grade	% Normal	Lovett Scale
No evidence of contractility	0	0	0 (zero)
Slight contractility, no movement	1	10	T (trace)
Full range of motion, gravity eliminated*	2	25	P (poor)
Full range of motion with gravity	3	50	F (fair)
Full range of motion against gravity, some resistance	4	75	G (good)
Full range of motion against gravity, full resistance	5	100	N (normal)

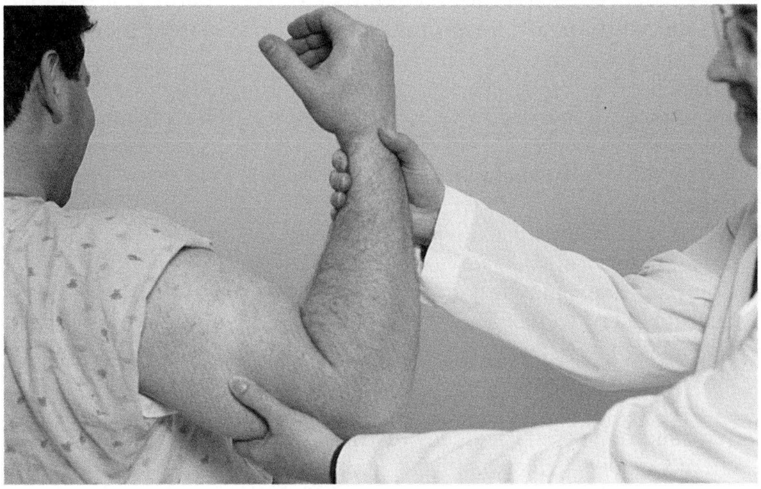

*Passive movement.

From *Health and Physical Assessment* (3rd ed., p. 433), by V. H. Barkauskas, L. C. Baumann, and C. S. Darling-Fisher, 2002, St. Louis, MO: Mosby.

Procedure 28-27 Assessing Muscle Tone and Strength of Upper Extremities

Equipment

- None

Examination Skill and Focus	Steps	Rationale
Palpation: Muscle tone	**1.** Support the relaxed arm at the hand and elbow.	The client must voluntarily relax the arm.
	2. Move each arm (fingers, wrist, elbow, shoulder) through a modified passive range of motion (ROM).	
	3. Attend to the resistance offered.	
	4. Test muscle tone prior to testing muscle strength.	Results of muscle strength testing may be misinterpreted without knowledge of the residual tension (muscle tone).
Muscle strength	**1.** Place two crossed fingers in each hand of client.	The examiner avoids self-injury during testing of grip.
Fingers	**2.** Instruct client to squeeze firmly (grip).	Grip tests integrity of the C_{7-8} and T_1 nerves.
	3. Compare sides; may test simultaneously.	
	4. Try, against resistance, to force client's outspread fingers of each hand together (abduction).	Abduction tests integrity of C_8, T_1, and the ulnar nerve.
	5. Instruct client to touch thumb to little fingertip.	
	6. Resist pull of examiner's thumb against client's thumb (opposition).	Opposition tests integrity of C_8, T_1, and the median nerve.
	7. Compare sides; may test simultaneously.	Comparison detects alterations.
Wrists	**1.** Instruct client to hold flexed elbows close to sides with forearm in pronation.	Holding flexed elbows close to the body isolates movement at the wrist.
	2. Instruct client to make a fist and flex wrists.	
	3. Try to pull client's fist up against resistance (flexion).	Flexion and extension at the wrist tests the integrity of C_{6-8} and the radial nerve.
	4. Instruct client to make a fist and extend wrist.	
	5. Try to pull client's fist down against resistance (extension).	
	6. Compare sides; may test simultaneously.	
Elbows	**1.** Instruct client to flex arm at the elbow.	These manoeuvres test the strength of the biceps (C_{5-6}) and triceps (C_{6-8}) muscles.
	2. Try, against resistance, to extend client's flexed elbows (biceps).	
	3. Instruct client to flex arm at the elbow.	
	4. Try, against resistance, to further flex client's elbows (triceps).	
	5. Compare sides; may test simultaneously.	
Shoulders	**1.** Instruct client to raise both extended arms above the head.	This manoeuvre tests the strength of the shoulder girdle, primarily the abductor muscles (deltoid and supraspinatus, C_{5-6}).
	2. Try, against resistance, to force client's arms to sides.	
	3. Compare sides; may test simultaneously.	

From *A Syllabus for Adult Health Assessment* (pp. 49–50), edited by D. L. Skillen and R. A. Day, 2004, Edmonton, AB: Faculty of Nursing, University of Alberta.

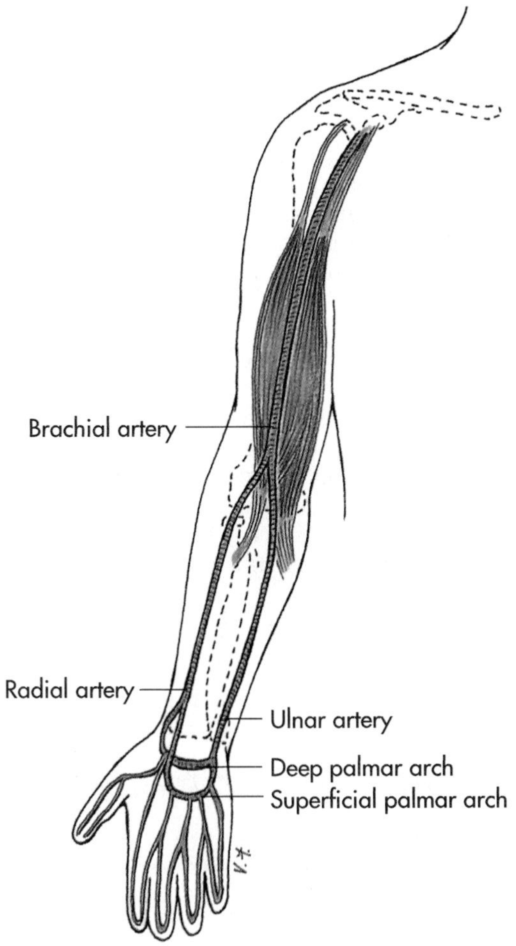

FIGURE **28–93** Anatomical position of brachial, radial, and ulnar arteries.

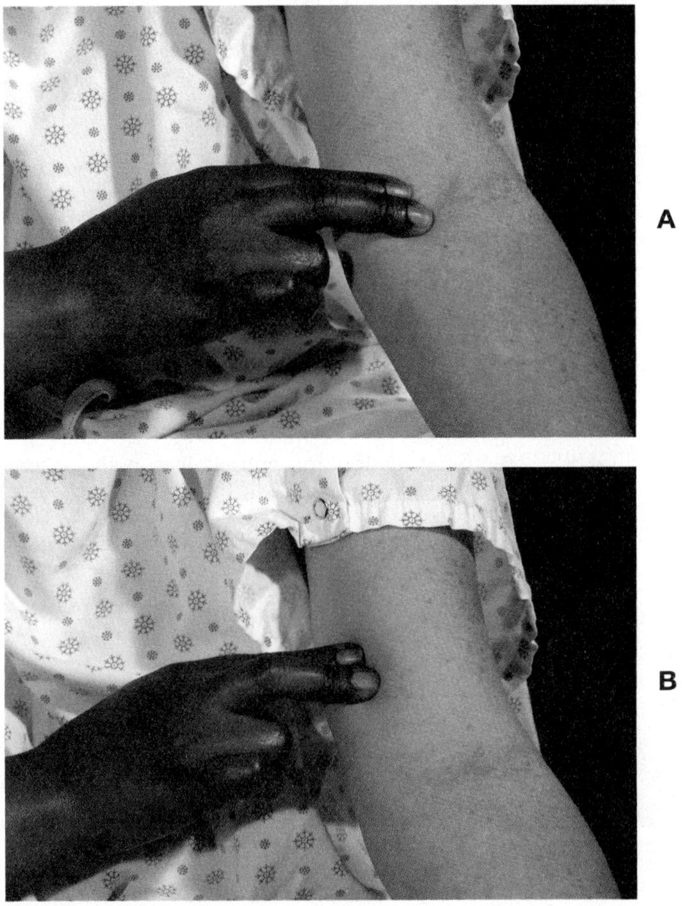

FIGURE **28–94** **A,** Brachial palpation in antecubital fossa. **B,** Brachial palpation between biceps and triceps muscles. (From *Physical Examination Images* [CD-ROM], by D. L. Skillen, R. A. Day, M. C. Anderson, T. C. Stephen, J. A. Gilbert, and L. W. Day, 2004, Edmonton, AB: Faculty of Nursing, University of Alberta.)

An inequality may indicate a local obstruction or abnormally positioned artery. The brachial artery may be palpated in two locations (Figure 28–94). The brachial artery channels blood to the radial and ulnar arteries of the forearm and hand. If brachial circulation becomes blocked, the hands do not receive adequate blood flow. If circulation becomes impaired in the radial or ulnar arteries, the hand still receives adequate perfusion because of an interconnection between radial and ulnar arteries that guards against arterial occlusion (Figure 28–95).

Epitrochlear Nodes. Epitrochlear nodes are located between the biceps and triceps muscles about 3 cm above the medial epicondyle on the inner aspect of the forearm (Figure 28–95). They drain the medial aspect of forearms and hands. A palpable epitrochlear node is not expected in most adults (see Procedure 28-28). If one is palpated, its size, consistency, mobility, and tenderness are documented.

Coordination. Coordinated body movements are smooth, rapid, and accurate. Coordination is achieved through the integrated function of four components of the nervous system. The motor system provides strength; the cerebellar system manages rhythmic movements and upright posture; the vestibular system contributes to balance by integrating eye, head, and body movements; and the sensory system contributes to position sense. Two different rapid alternating tests and one point-to-point test are used to assess coordination of the upper extremities. The examiner may demonstrate each manoeuvre as

Table 28-59 Grading of Peripheral Pulses

Description of Amplitude	Grade
Absent, not palpable	0
Pulse diminished, barely palpable	1+
Easily palpable, brisk, expected	2+
Full pulse, increased	3+
Strong, bounding pulse, cannot be obliterated	4+

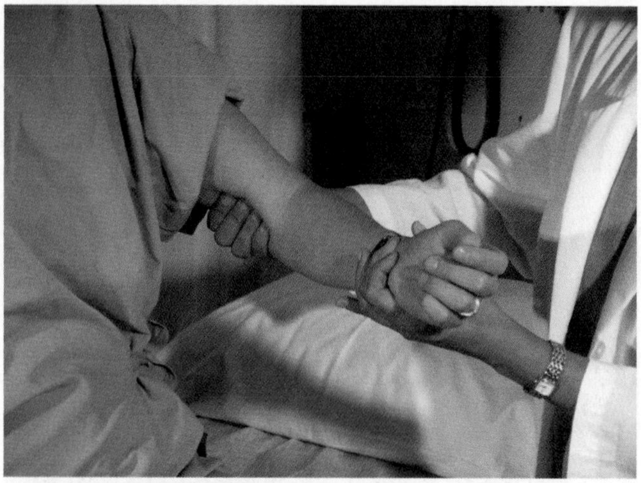

FIGURE **28–95** Palpation for epitrochlear node. (From *Physical Examination Images* [CD-ROM], by D. L. Skillen, R. A. Day, M. C. Anderson, T. C. Stephen, J. A. Gilbert, and L. W. Day, 2004, Edmonton, AB: Faculty of Nursing, University of Alberta.)

well as provide verbal instructions (Procedure 28-29). Examiners expect rapid alternating movements to be smoothly, rhythmically, and rapidly performed with either hand. The dominant hand often has slightly more dexterity than the non-dominant hand. Performance of point-to-point testing is expected to be smooth, accurate, and without tremor. Deviations suggest pathology within the cerebellar and/or motor system. If point-to-point testing is accurate with eyes open, but not with eyes closed, a deviation in position sense is possible.

Sensory System. Assessment of the sensory system tests the integrity of the sensory nerve tracts within the spinal column, medulla, and sensory cortex. The sensations of pain and temperature are both carried in the spinothalamic tracts; if pain sensation is intact, temperature is usually not tested. Position and vibration sensations are carried in the posterior columns. The sensation of touch is carried in both spinal tracts. The fibres for crude touch are carried in the spinothalamic tracts; the fibres for fine touch

Procedure 28-28 *Palpating Pulses and Epitrochlear Nodes in Upper Extremities*

Equipment

- None

Examination Skill and Focus	Steps	Rationale
Palpation: Brachial pulse	**1.** Palpate brachial artery with finger pads or thumbs at the antecubital crease (fossa) **OR** above elbow in groove between biceps and triceps muscles.	The brachial pulse is accessible at either site.
	2. Compare sides.	Comparison detects alterations.
Radial pulse	**1.** Palpate radial artery with finger pads on the lateral flexor surface of wrist.	Slight flexion at the wrist may increase access to the radial artery.
	2. Compare sides.	
Palpation: Epitrochlear nodes	**1.** Support client's right forearm with examiner right hand as client flexes elbow about 90 degrees.	With the client's arm flexed at 90 degrees, access to nodes is increased.
	2. Palpate for epitrochlear node in groove between biceps and triceps muscles with finger pads of the left hand medially and approximately 3 cm above the medial epicondyle.	
	3. Reverse hand position to examine client's left arm.	

From *A Syllabus for Adult Health Assessment* (p. 50), edited by D. L. Skillen and R. A. Day, 2004, Edmonton, AB: Faculty of Nursing, University of Alberta.

are in the posterior columns. Nurses expect clients to perceive sensory stimuli equally on both sides of the body. They assess the major sensory nerves by knowing the sensory dermatome zones (Figure 28–96). The dermatomes are innervated by specific dorsal root cutaneous nerves. For example, a client with reduced pain sensation along the medial aspect of the arm and little finger of the right hand may have a neurological lesion at the eighth cervical spinal cord segment. Clients must close their eyes during all sensory testing so that they are unable to see when or where a stimulus is applied (Procedure 28-30).

Pain and Light Touch. When testing pain and light touch on the upper extremities, the nurse systematically assesses the dermatomes of the shoulder (C_4), upper arm (C_6 and T_1), forearm (C_5 and T_1), and hand (C_{6-8}; see Procedure 28-30). A splintered tongue blade or cotton-tipped applicator is used as the pain stimulus and discarded. The blunt end is occasionally substituted to test validity of the client's response. Areas stimulated with the blunt end must be tested with the sharp end as the blunt end only tests pressure. When testing light touch, a cotton wisp is applied lightly. The rhythm or pace of dermatome testing is varied to ensure clients respond to an actual touch sensation rather than an anticipated touch. The sensations of pain and light touch in both arms are compared by applying the stimulus first on one arm and then on the symmetrical dermatome on the other arm. The examiner expects pain and light touch sensations to be intact bilaterally over dermatomes C_4–C_8 and T_1. If a deviation is identified, the nurse maps out the area of sensory loss (hyposensitivity) or hypersensitivity by testing from

Procedure 28-29 Inspecting Coordination in the Upper Extremities

Equipment

- None

Examination Skill and Focus	Steps	Rationale
Coordination	Test each hand separately.	Testing each hand separately ensures that coordination in one hand is not affected by the other.
Rapid alternating testing	**1.** Instruct client to pat thigh as rapidly as possible, alternating between palm and dorsum of hand. **2.** Compare sides. **3.** Instruct client to touch distal joint of thumb with index fingertip repeatedly as rapidly as possible. **4.** Compare sides.	Two methods of rapid alternating testing are available.
Point-to-point testing	**1.** Instruct client to extend arm.	
	2. Instruct client to alternately touch client's nose, then examiner's finger with fully extended arm. **3.** Alter finger position. **4.** Hold finger in one place	Comparison detects alterations.
	5. Instruct client to raise extended arm over head and lower it to touch finger.	Ensures client, with eyes open, touches examiner's finger.
	6. After several tries, instruct client to close eyes and repeat. **7.** Repeat 5 and 6 with other arm.	Tests position sense.

From *A Syllabus for Adult Health Assessment* (p. 50), edited by D. L. Skillen and R. A. Day, 2004, Edmonton, AB: Faculty of Nursing, University of Alberta.

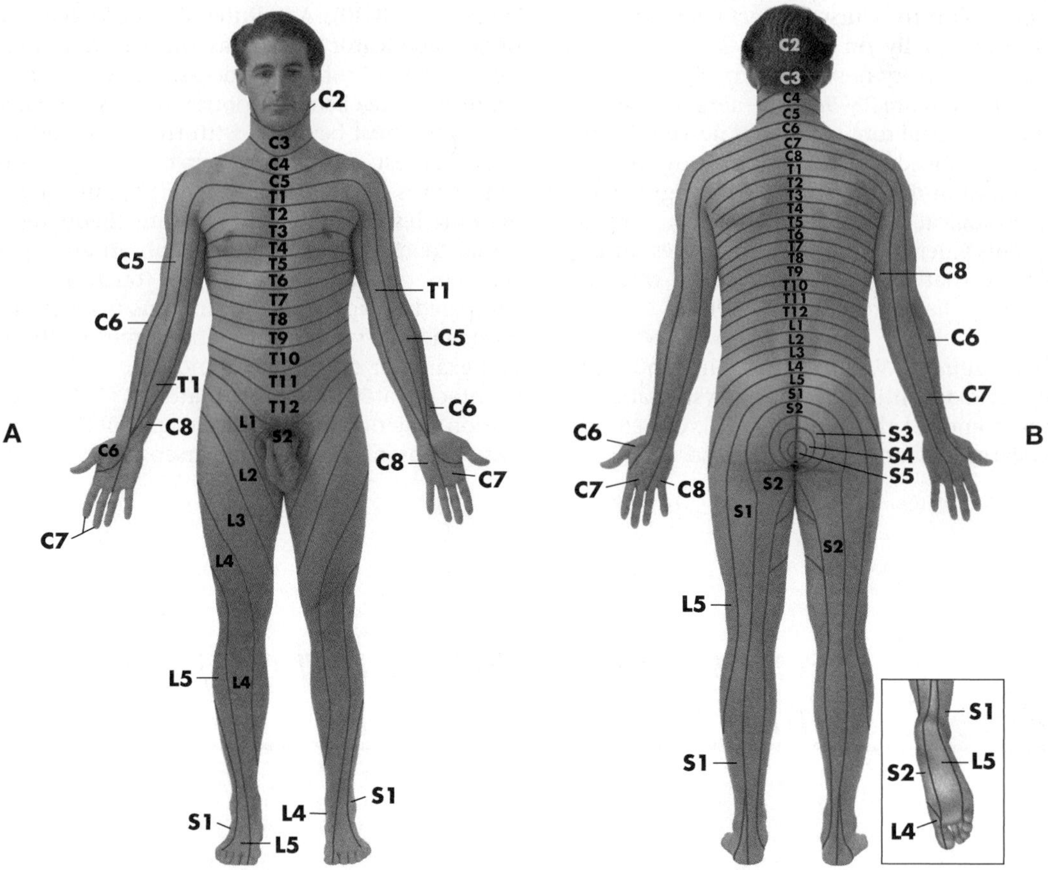

FIGURE **28–96** Dermatomes of the body, the body surface areas innervated by particular spinal nerves; C1 usually has no cutaneous distribution. **A,** Anterior view. **B,** Posterior view. It appears that there is a distinct separation of surface area controlled by each dermatome, but there is almost always overlap between spinal nerves. (From *Mosby's Guide to Physical Examination,* 5th ed., p. 775, by H. M. Seidel et al., 2003, St. Louis, MO: Mosby.)

the area of decreased sensitivity and moving proximally until the client reports a change in sensory perception.

Vibration Sense. Testing vibration sense assesses the integrity of the posterior columns of the sensory system (see Procedure 28-30). Grasping the stem of the 128-Hz tuning fork, the examiner causes it to vibrate by tapping the tines of the fork on the heel of the hand. To validate the client's reporting, the examiner asks the client to state when the vibrations stop, and holds the tines. The examiner expects the client to report a buzz-like sensation at the distal interphalangeal (DIP) joint and to correctly indicate when the vibration has been stopped. If the vibration is not felt, the examiner continues testing by progressing upward through the proximal interphalangeal (PIP) joint, MCP joint, wrist, and elbow until vibrations are felt.

Position Sense. Testing position sense also assesses the integrity of the posterior columns of the sensory system. To test this sensation, the examiner focuses on one digit separated from the other fingers (see Procedure 28-30). This ensures that tactile information from other digits does not influence the client's perception of position sense. The client's eyes must be closed. The nurse always returns the digit to the neutral position before testing again. Clients are expected to identify whether the digit is "up" or "down."

Discriminative Sensation. Discriminative sensation undergoes three tests of fine touch that require a higher level of sensory cortex function because clients must analyze and interpret the stimulus with eyes closed. The sensation of light touch and position sense need to be intact or nearly intact for tests of discriminative sensation to be effective (see Procedure 28-30). Unexpected findings suggest pathology in the sensory cortex and posterior columns. A test for stereognosis occurs when the examiner places a small familiar object such as a key, paper clip, or coin in the client's palm. The client manipulates the object in that palm and is expected to report what it is. A test for graphesthesia is conducted when the examiner uses a blunt object to draw a single number or letter on the client's palm. The examiner must draw a large letter or number so that it correctly faces the client (Figure 28–97). The client is expected to report what was drawn. A test for extinction occurs when the examiner touches both arms in symmetrical places at the same time. The client is expected to report that two places were touched and identify where touched. If the client identifies only one location, extinction is impaired.

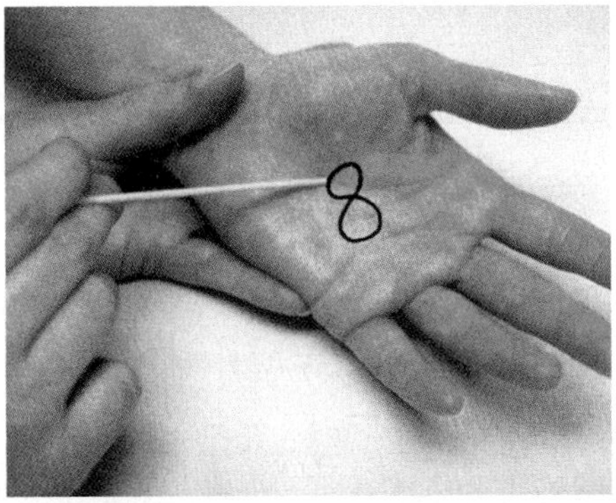

FIGURE **28–97** Graphesthesia. (From *Mosby's Guide to Physical Examination,* 5th ed., p. 795, Figure 21–25c), by H. M. Seidel et al., 2003, St. Louis, MO: Mosby.)

Reflexes. The neurological system has defence mechanisms (reflexes) that facilitate quick reactions to potentially harmful situations and contribute to the maintenance of muscle tone and balance. Reflexes range from monosynaptic to polysynaptic. The monosynaptic reflex arc pathway is shown in Figure 28–98. Each muscle contains a small sensory unit (muscle spindle) that detects changes in the length of muscle fibres. By tapping the tendon of a partially stretched muscle with the reflex hammer, the nurse lengthens the spindle. The spindle sends nerve impulses along afferent nerve pathways to the dorsal horn of the spinal cord segment. Within milliseconds, the impulses reach the spinal cord and synapse with the efferent motor neuron in the spinal cord. A motor nerve sends impulses back to the muscle, causing the monosynaptic reflex response.

Two categories of reflexes are tested: deep tendon, elicited by mildly stretching a muscle and tapping a tendon, and cutaneous reflexes, elicited by stimulating the skin superficially. In the upper extremities, the biceps (Figure 28–99, *A*), triceps (Figure 28–99, *B*), and brachioradialis (supinator) deep tendon reflexes are tested. To achieve the correct technique, the examiner holds the reflex hammer somewhat loosely between the thumb and fingers and swings the head of the hammer in an arc using a rapid wrist (not elbow). Nurses use only as much force as is required to elicit an expected response and they apply the same force bilaterally for comparison purposes. Either the pointed or flat end of the head of a reflex hammer is effective as long as it is directed accurately. The flat end is best used for the brachioradialis reflex, as it will cause less discomfort.

The reflexes in the two arms are compared. If the reflex is symmetrically absent or diminished, an augmentation or reinforcement technique can be used. Just before striking the tendon, the examiner asks the client to clench the teeth or instructs the client to press down firmly on the thigh with the free hand. This technique increases the likelihood of the reflex arc being completed.

The reflex can be affected by the examiner's technique and it is important to practise the technique to ensure consistency (Procedure 28-31). Examiners expect a reflex response at all sites and grade the response on a scale of 0 (no response) to 4+ (hyperactive). Table 28-60 contains the grading scale. An average response is graded as 2+. A hyperactive response, accompanied by clonus (rapidly alternating involuntary contraction and relaxation of skeletal muscle), or an absent response may signal a neuromuscular deviation. Some individuals may exhibit symmetrically diminished or even absent deep tendon reflexes and be without pathology.

Documentation. Nurses record their findings from inspection and palpation of the upper extremities (Table 28-61).

Assessing the Lower Extremities

Examination of the integumentary, peripheral vascular, musculoskeletal, and neurological systems continues in the assessment of the lower extremities. Although many techniques and procedures are identical to the assessment of upper extremities, some components of the lower extremity examination are different. For example, during the **general survey,** nurses observe the client's balance, gait, and posture. They assess these more critically during their examination of the lower extremities and add inspection of heel walking, toe walking, and shallow knee bends by the client. For much of the lower extremities examination, clients are supine on the examining table or bed, but they are assessed for balance, posture, and gait when standing and walking. Their legs are fully exposed with socks or stockings removed, and they are draped to avoid unnecessary exposure of the inguinal regions and genitalia.

Inspection

Integument and Muscles. Nurses inspect the integument and muscle mass of the legs, anteriorly and posteriorly (Procedure 28-32). Expected findings include symmetrical muscle development without wasting or fasciculations. Vellus hair distribution is bilaterally uniform over the toes, lower legs, and thighs. Terminal hair over the lower extremities of males is usually fully evident, whereas females may shave their lower legs and toes. In the lower extremities, nurses may observe depositions of hemosiderin (brown iron-rich pigmentation) around the ankles, which indicate compromised venous return. Thin shiny skin, decreased hair growth, absent hair over the great toes, thickened nails, and edema of lower legs and ankles can indicate vascular disease. Table 28-62 is a comparison of venous and arterial insufficiency. Often toenails are thickened and oddly shaped due to trauma. Fungal infections along the nail fold affect some individuals. Soles of the feet may become callused due to pressure; heels may be callused, dry, rough, and cracked due to harsh, dry conditions. Nurses note any deviations in the surface integrity or colour of the nail plate (see Figure 28–17).

Range of Motion. Nurses inspect the legs for active ROM by beginning at the toes and progressing proximally to the ankle, knee, and hip (see Procedure 28-32). In well adults, a full ROM is expected at the toes, ankles, knees, and hips. Figure 28–100 shows four expected

Procedure 28-30 Assessing Sensation of the Upper Extremities

Equipment

- Tongue blade
- Cotton ball
- 128 Hz tuning fork
- Familiar small objects

Examination Skill and Focus	Steps	Rationale
Inspection and palpation: Sensation	Both arms are tested.	
	The examiner demonstrates how sharp, dull, and light touch feel before beginning tests.	The client is made aware of the expected sensation to be perceived.
Superficial pain	**1.** Instruct client to close eyes and report with each touch whether it is "sharp" or "dull."	The eyes must remain closed throughout testing to ensure vision does not influence perception.
	2. Touch client's arms lightly and alternately in corresponding areas with sharp end of splintered tongue blade (occasionally using blunt end), covering C_4 to C_8 and T_1 dermatomes in upper arms, forearms, and hands.	The blunt end of the tongue blade ("dull") is used to validate the perception of pressure. The area stimulated by the blunt end must be further tested with the sharp end. All dermatomes are tested.
	3. Compare sides.	Comparisons detect asymmetry.
Light touch	**1.** Instruct client to close eyes and report each time touch of the cotton wisp is perceived.	
	2. Touch client's arms lightly, avoiding pressure, alternately in corresponding areas with cotton wisp, testing C_4 to C_8 and T_1 dermatomes in upper arms, forearms, and hands.	The touch must be light, as light touch is being tested, not pressure.
	3. Vary the intervals between touches.	By varying the rhythm of the touches, the examiner is more certain that the client is responding to the touch.
	4. Compare sides.	
Vibration	**1.** Instruct client to close eyes and describe the sensation felt.	
	2. Place vibrating 128 Hz tuning fork firmly over distal interphalangeal (DIP) joint of one finger and proceed proximally to proximal interphalangeal (PIP) and metacarpophalangeal (MCP) joints, etc., until vibrations are felt and reported.	Vibrations from the 128 Hz tuning fork can be felt through bone.
	3. Stop vibration and ask what is felt.	Asking the client to report cessation of the vibrations validates its perception.
	4. Compare sides.	
Position sense	**1.** Demonstrate "up" and "down" position of a finger.	Isolating the test finger ensures that adjacent digits do not influence the sensation felt.
	2. Instruct client to close eyes and identify position of finger.	
	3. Grasp distal phalanx by medial and lateral aspects and move it "up" or "down." Ensure that adjacent digits are not involved.	
	4. Compare sides.	

From *A Syllabus for Adult Health Assessment* (pp. 50–52), edited by D. L. Skillen and R. A. Day, 2004, Edmonton, AB: Faculty of Nursing, University of Alberta.

Examination Skill and Focus	Steps	Rationale
Inspection and palpation: Tactile discrimination	Both sides are tested.	
Stereognosis	**1.** Instruct client to close eyes and identify object placed in palm. **2.** Place a small familiar object in each palm in turn. The object can only be manipulated by the hand being tested. **3.** Compare sides.	Coins, safety pins, and keys are familiar objects. Each hand is tested separately.
Graphesthesia	**1.** Instruct client to close eyes and identify what number is drawn on the skin. **2.** With palm facing client, draw number with a blunt object on palm of hand. **3.** Compare sides.	Ensures that the number is drawn facing the client and in one connected movement.
Extinction	**1.** Instruct client to close eyes and identify where touched. **2.** Touch client in corresponding area of both arms simultaneously. **3.** Ask client where touched.	Corresponding areas of both arms must be touched simultaneously to accurately assess extinction.

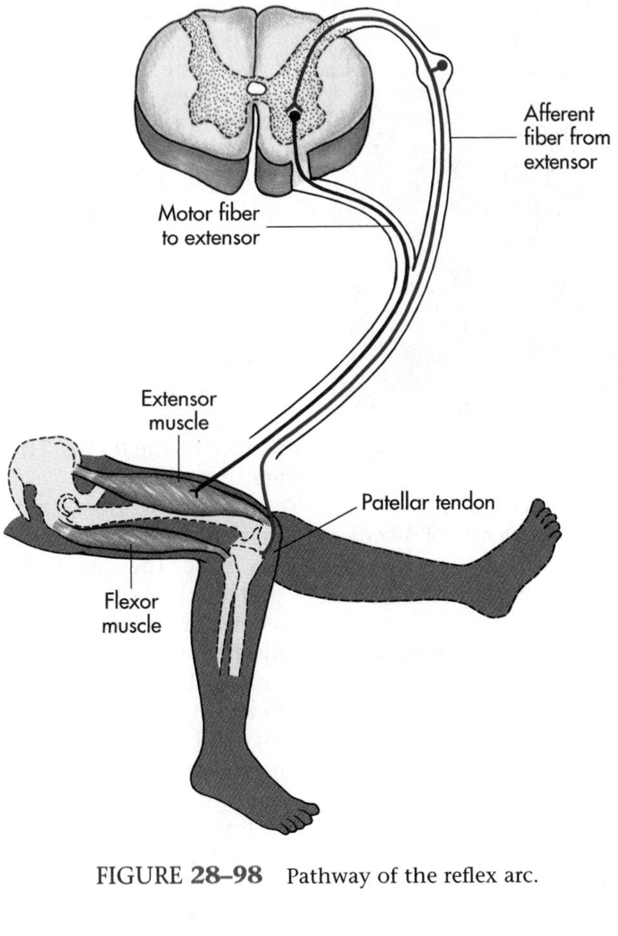

FIGURE **28–98** Pathway of the reflex arc.

A

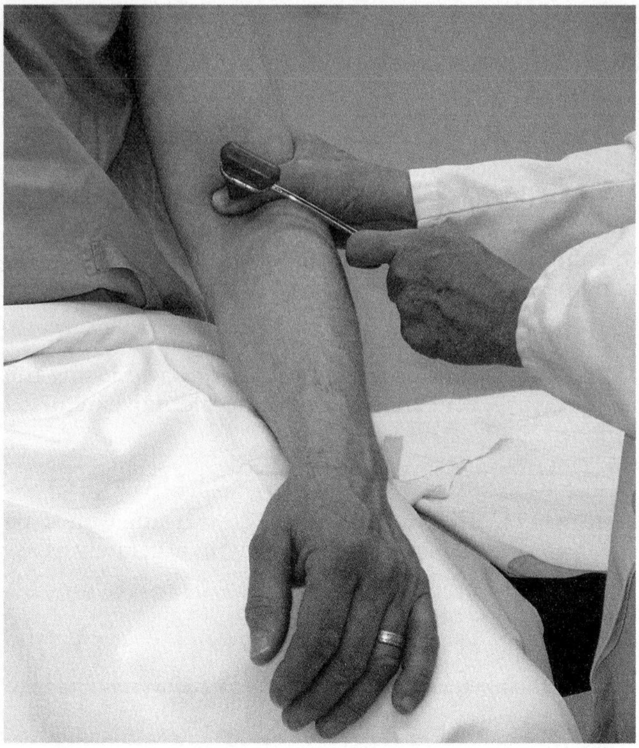

B

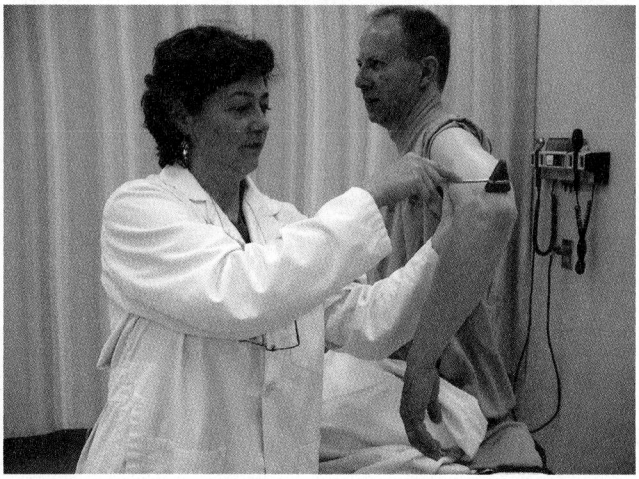

FIGURE **28–99** **A,** Biceps reflex. **B,** Triceps reflex. (From *Physical Examination Images* [CD-ROM], by D. L. Skillen, R. A. Day, M. C. Anderson, T. C. Stephen, J. A. Gilbert, and L. W. Day, 2004, Edmonton, AB: Faculty of Nursing, University of Alberta.)

movements at the hip: abduction, adduction, internal rotation, and external rotation.

Palpation

Temperature. Nurses palpate both legs simultaneously beginning with the dorsum of the feet and moving proximally to the shins and thighs to assess changes in warmth (Procedure 28-33). The skin is expected to be uniformly warm. If ambient air temperature is cool, both feet may feel cooler than shins and thighs. If one leg is cooler than the other, nurses are alert to additional indications

Table 28-60 Grading of Reflexes

Description of Response	Grade
No response (absent)	0
Somewhat diminished with slight muscle contraction	1+
Average, as expected, visible muscle twitch with movement of arm or leg	2+
Brisker than expected, exaggerated but acceptable	3+
Very brisk, with clonus; often associated with spinal cord disorders	4+

of arterial insufficiency such as absent hair on toes and thin, shiny skin over shins (see Table 28-62).

Peripheral Edema. Nurses assess the dorsum of the foot, ankle, and lower leg for the presence of edema (see Procedure 28-33). Although edema is not expected, at the end of the day, especially if an individual must stand during working hours, slight edema (1+) is not unusual. Figure 28–101 is a system for grading the extent of edema. Table 28-63 contains further guidance for grading. Figure 28–102 is an example of pitting edema.

Joints. The examiner palpates each joint separately for temperature, warmth, tenderness, and swelling or bogginess. None is expected. Palpation begins at the DIP joints and progresses proximally to the metatarsophalangeal (MTP) joints, ankles, and knees (see Procedure 28-33). Excessive warmth, redness, tenderness, swelling, and/or bogginess indicate an inflammatory process, often with the production of fluid in and around the joint.

The knee joint is subject to wear and injury, making it a frequent site for degenerative change such as osteoarthritis. The examiner begins by feeling for crepitations. These crackling or grating sounds produced by the rubbing together of roughened bony surfaces indicate a degenerative process. The patella is expected to glide smoothly over the trochlear groove on the distal anterior surface of the femur. The femoral and tibial joint surfaces are smooth.

The tibiofemoral joint of the knee is lined with a synovial capsule. The upper part, the suprapatellar pouch, lies under the quadriceps muscle and patella. It extends posteriorly to the popliteal fossa and laterally to fill the joint space. If inflamed, the synovial capsule produces fluid, causing bulging of the capsule evident on inspection and palpation. By asking the client to flex the knee to about 90 degrees and to keep the foot on the examining table, the examiner obtains access to the tibiofemoral joint space (Figure 28–103). The tibial tuberosity on the anterior surface of the tibia is where the patellar tendon inserts. Slightly superior are the lateral and medial condyles of the tibia. The examiner palpates the joint spaces created by the medial femoral epicondyle and tibial condyle, and the lateral femoral epicondyle and tibial condyle. The specific characteristics to be assessed are

Procedure 28-31 Assessing Deep Tendon Reflexes of the Upper Extremities

Equipment

- Percussion hammer

Examination Skill and Focus	Steps	Rationale
Inspection and percussion: Deep tendon reflexes	Both sides are tested and compared. **Only if** responses are symmetrically diminished or absent does examiner use reinforcement (augmentation).	Failure to ensure that reflexes are symmetrically diminished before reinforcement is used could mask unequal reflexes.
	The examiner strikes the slightly stretched tendon briskly with reflex hammer held loosely and swung freely in an arc.	A consistent force applied by the reflex hammer assists in obtaining accurate results.
Biceps reflex	**1.** Position client with arm supported and relaxed, elbow flexed and palm downward on thigh (seated client) or abdomen (supine client).	A relaxed arm ensures a valid response.
	2. Use hammer to tap own thumb placed over biceps tendon at antecubital fossa (crease).	Pressure of the thumb on the biceps tendon provides a slight stretch. Forearm flexion implies intact reflex arc at C_{5-6}.
	3. Compare flexion of forearm on each side.	
Triceps reflex	**1.** Position client with arm supported and relaxed, elbow flexed **OR** abducted and flexed in a right angle, in "hang-to-dry" position.	Forearm flexion suggests intact reflex arc at C_{6-7}.
	2. Use hammer to tap the triceps tendon 2 to 5 cm above elbow.	
	3. Compare extension of forearm on each side.	
Brachioradialis reflex	**1.** Position client with arm resting on lap (sitting) or abdomen (supine) and palm down.	
	2. Use hammer to tap the brachioradialis tendon 2 to 5 cm above wrist.	The tap of the reflex hammer generates the needed slight stretch of the tendon.
	3. Compare flexion and supination of hand on each side.	Flexion and supination of the hand suggests intact reflex arc at C_{5-6}.

From *A Syllabus for Adult Health Assessment* (pp. 50–52), edited by D. L. Skillen and R. A. Day, 2004, Edmonton, AB: Faculty of Nursing, University of Alberta.

warmth, tenderness, swelling, and presence of fluid (boggy sensation). None are expected. Joint margins are expected to be smooth to palpation, non-tender, and without swelling.

Muscle Tone. Although slightly more difficult to test because the leg is naturally longer and heavier than the arm, muscle tone of the leg is also assessed (Procedure 28-34). The nurse supports the relaxed leg through a full ROM. Pain in any joint of the legs may make the manoeuvre difficult to perform. The nurse expects to feel a mild, even resistance to movement through the entire range. By assessing muscle tone prior to muscle strength, the nurse is able to interpret findings most accurately.

Muscle Strength. Beginning at the feet and moving proximally to the hips, nurses assess the strength of muscle groups in the legs (see Procedure 28-34). The client is expected to demonstrate sustained strength commensurate with the muscle mass present. For example, Figure 28–104, *A* is a demonstration of assessment of knee flexion strength; Figure 28–104, *B* is assessment of knee extension

Text continued on p. 769

Table 28-61 Examples of Documentation for Upper Extremities

Focus of Assessment	Expected Findings	Unexpected Findings
Skin	Pink tones, moist, elastic, scattered nevi bilaterally. No other lesions visible. Fine evenly distributed blond hair over both arms and proximal and distal phalanges. Skin temperature uniformly warm over arms and hands. Turgor and mobility intact.	Deeply tanned skin tones to mid-upper arms. Skin dry, remains "tented" when skin fold released. (R) forearm 2.0 × 2.0 cm irregular purple coloration. Temperature uniformly warm over arms and (R) hand; (L) hand cooler than (R).
Muscles	Muscle mass symmetrical size and contour without atrophy or fasciculations—hands, forearms, upper arm, and shoulder girdle.	Muscle wasting evident between tendons on dorsum of hands, and on thenar surfaces of palms (base of thumbs).
Nails	Short, rounded, manicured without polish. Nail bed firm. No lesions around cuticles.	Nail beds spongy to pressure; angle greater than 180 degrees; free edges of nail ragged and bitten to nail beds.
Range of motion (ROM)	Full ROM—thumbs, fingers, wrists, elbows, and shoulders. No discomfort reported with ROM.	Full ROM fingers, wrists, elbows bilaterally and (R) thumb; opposition at (L) thumb impaired; ROM of shoulders intact bilaterally except for impaired internal and external rotation, producing discomfort, especially external rotation (R) side.
Joints	Distal interphalangeal (DIP), proximal interphalangeal (PIP), and metacarpophalangeal (MCP) joints without tenderness, swelling, or bogginess to palpation bilaterally. Wrists, elbows, and shoulder girdle without tenderness or swelling to palpation bilaterally. All joints same temperature as surrounding skin.	DIP joints, index fingers, enlarged bilaterally but not painful to palpation; remaining DIP, PIP, MCP joints no tenderness, swelling, or bogginess; tenderness (R) acromioclavicular joint, remaining shoulder joints non-tender.
Muscle tone	Slight tension felt to passive movements bilaterally.	(R) arm flaccid to passive movements; lead-pipe rigidity (resistance throughout range in both directions) evident bilaterally.
Muscle strength	Strong, sustained (5+) bilaterally in the fingers, wrists, elbows, and shoulders.	Muscle strength (R) side is 0/5 in all muscle groups; extremity is flaccid; flexion at elbows is 4+ (R), 5+ (L).
Coordination	Performs rapid alternating movements rapidly, smoothly, with even rhythm, dominant (R) side slightly faster than (L). Point-to-point testing smooth and accurate with eyes open and closed bilaterally.	(L) side, alternating movements hesitant and uncoordinated; point-to-point testing inaccurate with eyes open and closed.
Pulses	Radial and brachial pulses 2+ bilaterally. Rhythm regular.	Radial pulse 1+ (R), 2+ (L).
Epitrochlear nodes	Non-palpable bilaterally.	Non-palpable (R); bean-sized, smooth, firm, mobile node (L).
Sensation	Superficial pain and light touch intact bilaterally over dermatomes C_4 to C_8 and T_1; vibration and position senses intact bilaterally at fingers.	Superficial pain decreased C_6 to C_8 (L); intact beginning at wrist; intact (R) side; position sense intact (R), impaired at fingers (L), intact at wrist.
Tactile discrimination	Stereognosis, graphesthesia, and extinction intact bilaterally.	Stereognosis intact (R), impaired (L); extinction impaired- perceived only on (L).
Reflexes	Biceps, triceps, and brachioradialis reflexes 2+ bilaterally.	Biceps reflexes 2+ bilaterally; triceps reflex 1+ (R), 0 on (L); brachioradialis reflexes absent (R)(L).

From "Documentation" by M. C. Anderson in *Health Assessment Self-Test Modules* (WebCT Vista), 2004, Edmonton, AB: Faculty of Nursing, University of Alberta.

Table 28-62 Signs of Venous and Arterial Insufficiency

Assessment Criterion	Venous	Arterial
Colour	Expected or cyanotic	Pale; worsened by elevation of extremity; dusky red when extremity is lowered
Temperature	Expected	Cool (blood flow blocked to extremity)
Pulse	Expected	Decreased or absent
Edema	Often marked	Absent or mild
Skin changes	Brown pigmentation around ankles	Thin, shiny skin; decreased hair growth; thickened nails

A B C D

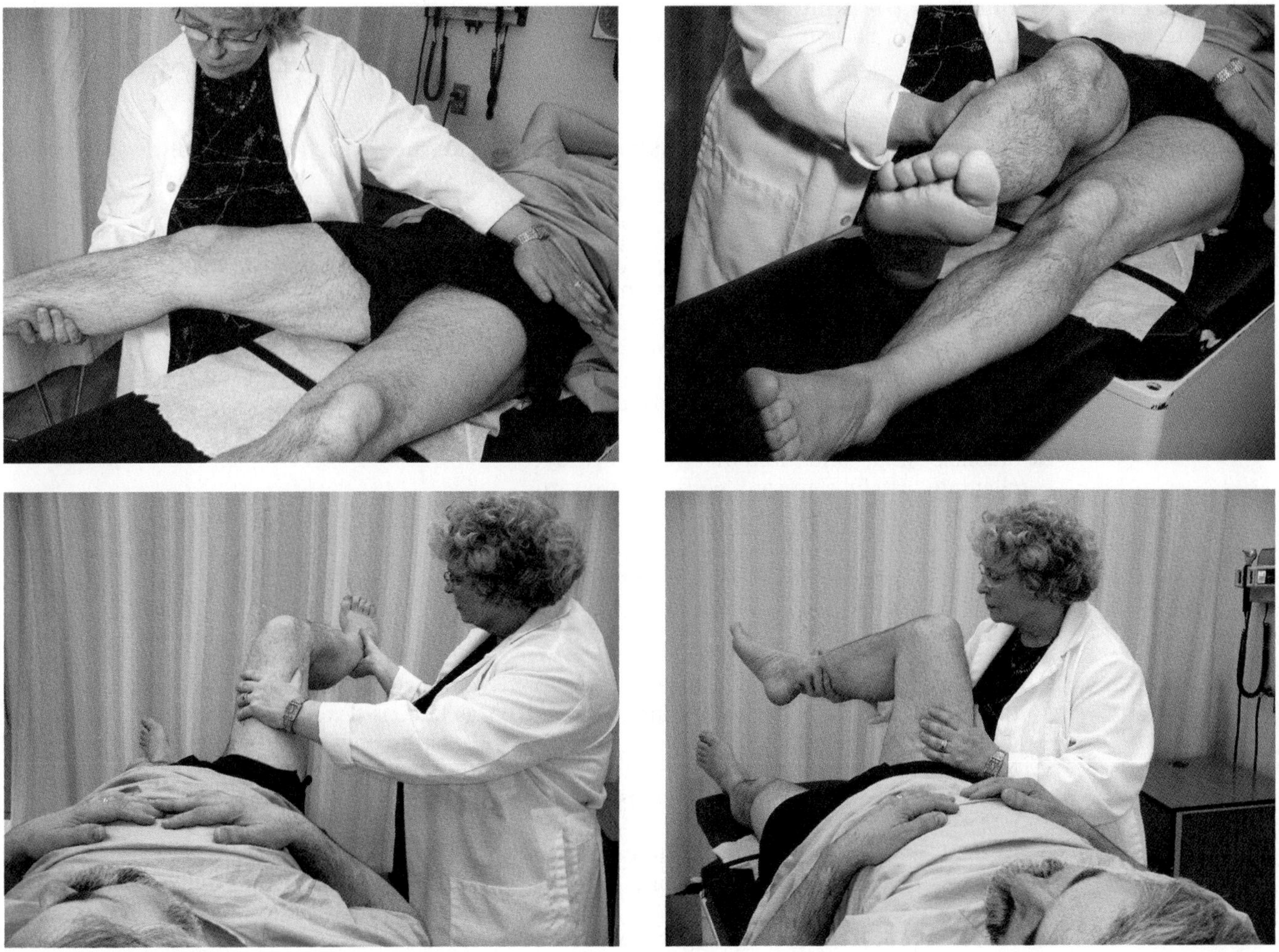

FIGURE **28–100** **A,** Hip abduction. **B,** Hip adduction. **C,** Hip internal rotation. **D,** Hip external rotation. (From *Physical Examination Images* [CD-ROM], by D. L. Skillen, R. A. Day, M. C. Anderson, T. C. Stephen, J. A. Gilbert, and L. W. Day, 2004, Edmonton, AB: Faculty of Nursing, University of Alberta.)

Procedure 28-32 Inspecting the Lower Extremities Including Range of Motion

Equipment

- None

Examination Skill and Focus	Steps	Rationale
Skin, nails, hair, symmetry	**1.** Fully expose legs and feet of supine client. **2.** Inspect skin, nails, muscle mass, and symmetry of both legs and feet. **3.** Inspect knee for expected depressions on either side of patella.	Full visibility of the legs is essential. Symmetry of skin condition and hair distribution provides clues for vascular perfusion.
Range of motion (ROM)	Test each leg either separately or simultaneously and compare. Only if client is unable to perform active ROM does the examiner attempt passive ROM.	Assessment of active ROM is always attempted first to establish client ability. In passive ROM, the examiner attempts to move limb without assistance from the client.
Toes	**1.** Instruct client to bend toes downward (flexion). **2.** Instruct client to straighten toes and point upward (extension).	Flexion and extension are possible at the toes.
Ankles	**1.** Instruct client to bring foot upward toward shin (dorsi-flexion). **2.** Instruct client to bend foot downward away from shin (plantar-flexion). **3.** Stabilize ankle and hold heel and instruct client to tilt foot inward with sole toward midline (inversion). **4.** Stabilize ankle and hold heel and instruct client to tilt foot outward with sole facing laterally (eversion). **5.** Repeat on other foot.	Movement at the ankle includes dorsiflexion, plantar flexion, inversion, and eversion.
Hips and knees	**1.** Place hand under lumbar spine. **2.** Instruct client to bring each knee in turn up toward chest and press firmly onto the abdomen (flexion at hip and knee). **3.** Note when back touches hand. **4.** Observe that opposite thigh remains flat on table. **5.** Instruct client to straighten leg (extension).	ROM at the hip and knee includes flexion and extension. Lumbar spine should flatten as knee is flexed onto abdomen. This stabilizes the pelvis; further flexion originates at the hip.
Hips	**1.** Stabilize pelvis by pressing on one anterior superior iliac crest with left hand. **2.** Grasp opposite ankle with right hand and move leg over other leg (adduction). **3.** Repeat on other side.	ROM at the hip includes flexion, extension, adduction, abduction, and internal and external rotation.
	4. Stabilize pelvis by pressing on one anterior superior iliac crest with left hand. **5.** Grasp opposite leg at ankle and abduct leg until iliac spine moves (abduction). **6.** Repeat on other side. **7.** Flex leg at hip and knee to 90 degrees.	At the end of range for either abduction or adduction, the pelvis begins to move and is felt by the left hand on the anterior superior iliac crest.

From *A Syllabus for Adult Health Assessment* (pp. 52–53), edited by D. L. Skillen and R.A. Day, 2004, Edmonton, AB: Faculty of Nursing, University of Alberta.

Examination Skill and Focus	Steps	Rationale
	8. Support thigh with left hand and ankle with right hand. **9.** Turn lower leg medially (external rotation), then laterally (internal rotation). **10.** Repeat on other side.	

Table 28-63 Description and Grading of Dependent Edema

Description	Depression	Grade
Slight pitting, disappears rapidly	2 mm	1+
Deeper pitting, disappears in 10 to 15 seconds	4 mm	2+
Visibly swollen, dependent extremity, pitting takes more than 60 seconds to disappear	6 mm	3+
Grossly swollen and distorted dependent extremity, pitting may take 3 minutes to disappear	8 mm	4+

Adapted from *Nursing Health Assessment: Clinical Pocket Guide* (p. 170), by P. M. Dillon, 2004, Philadelphia, F. A. Davis.

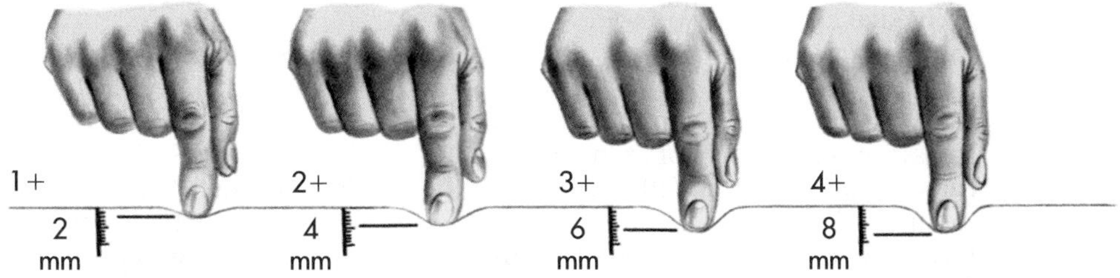

FIGURE **28–101** Assessing for pitting edema. (From *Mosby's Guide to Physical Examination* (5th ed., p. 484), by H. M. Seidel et al., 2003, St. Louis, MO: Mosby.)

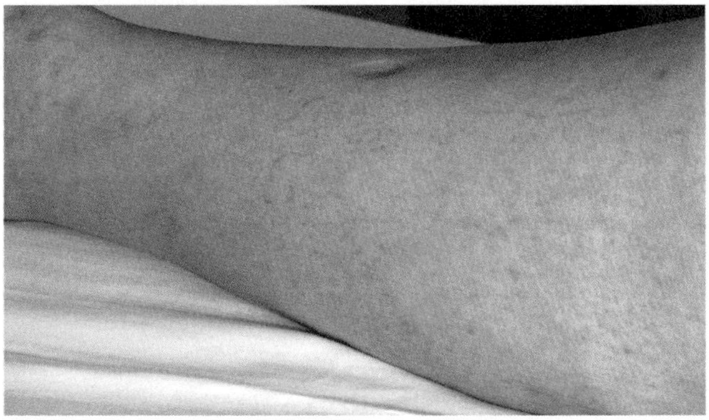

FIGURE **28–102** Pitting edema. (From *Physical Examination Images* [CD-ROM], by D. L. Skillen, R. A. Day, M. C. Anderson, T. C. Stephen, J. A. Gilbert, and L. W. Day, 2004, Edmonton, AB: Faculty of Nursing, University of Alberta.)

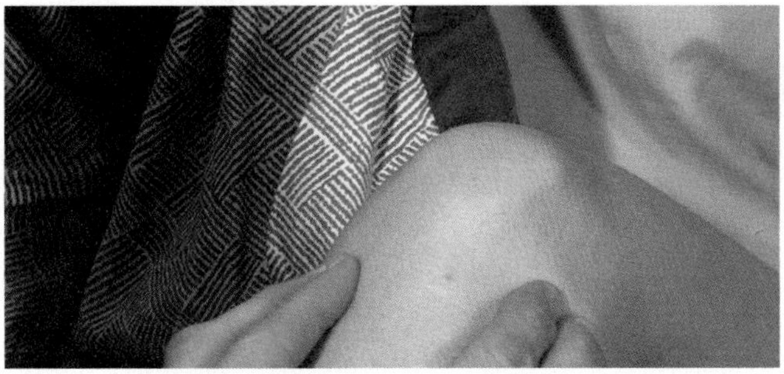

FIGURE **28–103** Palpation of the tibiofemoral joint. (From *Physical Examination Images* [CD-ROM], by D. L. Skillen, R. A. Day, M. C. Anderson, T. C. Stephen, J. A. Gilbert, and L. W. Day, 2004, Edmonton, AB: Faculty of Nursing, University of Alberta.)

Procedure 28-33 Palpating Joints and Skin Surface for Temperature and Edema

Equipment

- none

Examination Skill and Focus	Steps	Rationale
Temperature	**1.** Use dorsum of hands or fingers to compare temperature of each foot with lower leg and thigh above it.	Thin dorsal skin increases sensitivity to temperature.
	2. Compare sides.	
Edema	**1.** Press firmly and gently with thumb for 5 seconds over dorsum of each foot and/or medial malleolus.	Fluid in tissues disperses under pressure, leaving a depression that can be graded.
	2. Assess for extent of depression in the skin.	
	3. Press firmly and gently with thumb for 5 seconds over each shin.	
	4. Assess for extent of depression in the skin.	
Feet		
Interphalangeal (IP) joints	**1.** Palpate with thumb and index finger of one hand all of the distal and proximal interphalangeal (IP) joints of the toes.	Single or multiple joints may swell and become inflamed due to trauma or chronic conditions such as arthritis.
Metatarsophalangeal (MTP) joints	**2.** Compress each forefoot just proximal to MTP joints with thumb and fingers placed on medial and lateral surfaces.	
Heel	**3.** Palpate each heel.	Palpation may elicit tenderness and detect bogginess (spongy feel due to fluid).
Ankles	**1.** Place thumbs dorsally and fingers ventrally.	
Ankle joint	**2.** Palpate anterior aspect of each ankle joint.	
Achilles tendon	**3.** Palpate along each Achilles tendon with thumb and fingers.	Palpation can elicit tenderness and swelling around the Achilles tendon.
Knees	**1.** Instruct client to bend knees (flexion).	Crepitations may be felt and even heard.
Knees	**2.** Cup hands over each knee in turn as client returns leg to resting position (extension).	An inflamed synovial capsule produces fluid, distending the capsule.
Suprapatellar pouch	**3.** Note any crepitations.	
	4. Palpate each side of quadriceps in progressive steps, from 10 cm above superior border of patella to patellar pouch.	
Patella	**5.** Continue palpation along sides of patella.	Distension is evident because hollows on either side of the patella bulge and are boggy to palpation.
Tibiofemoral joint	**6.** Instruct client to slightly flex knee.	
	7. Palpate tibiofemoral joints (inferior, medial, and lateral to patella).	

From *A Syllabus for Adult Health Assessment* (pp. 53–54), edited by D. L. Skillen and R. A. Day, 2004, Edmonton, AB: Faculty of Nursing, University of Alberta.

A B

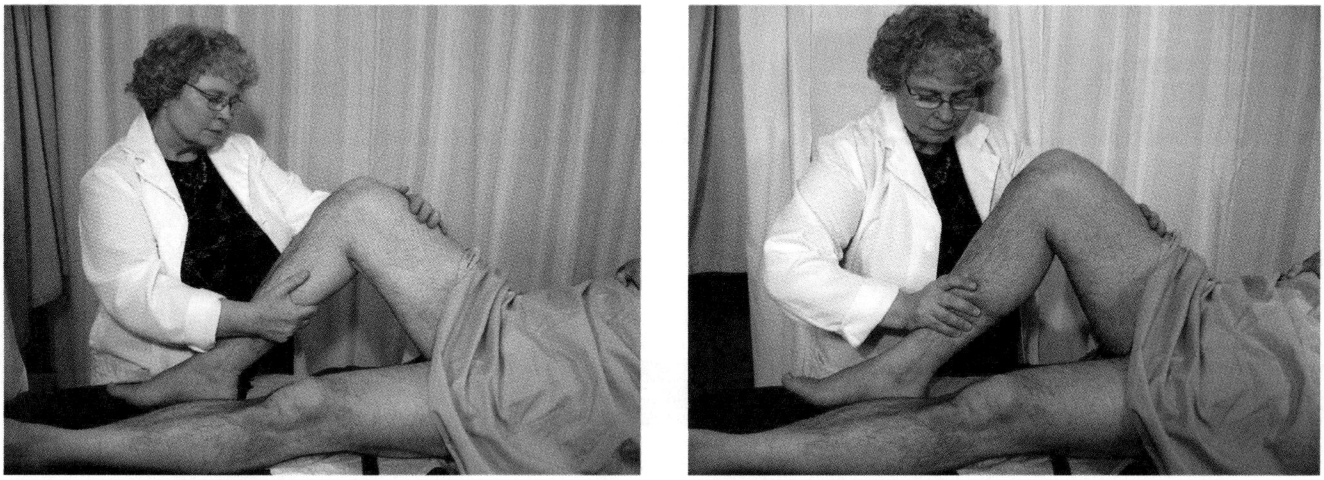

FIGURE **28–104** **A,** Assessment of knee flexion strength. **B,** Assessment of knee extension strength. (From *Physical Examination Images* [CD-ROM], by D. L. Skillen, R. A. Day, M. C. Anderson, T. C. Stephen, J. A. Gilbert, and L. W. Day, 2004, Edmonton, AB: Faculty of Nursing, University of Alberta.)

strength. Nurses expect to observe equal strength and resistance bilaterally. Muscle strength can be graded from 0 to 5+ (see Table 28-58). If weakness is identified, nurses compare the size of the muscle on that leg with the counterpart on the opposite leg (see upper extremities).

Peripheral Pulses. The peripheral pulses in the lower extremities are also assessed for rate, rhythm, amplitude, and equality (Procedure 28-35). An interconnection between the posterior tibial and dorsalis pedis arteries guards against local arterial occlusion (Figure 28–105). In the leg, the popliteal pulse is located behind the knee in the popliteal fossa and may be difficult to palpate (Figure 28–106). Nurses expect this pulse to feel diffuse and difficult to locate in some individuals. The posterior tibial pulses are located behind and below the medial malleoli and are palpated with the finger pads, but may be obscured by edema or fat (Figure 28–107, *A*). The dorsalis pedis pulse is located on the dorsum of the foot lateral to the extensor tendon of the great toe, but may be congenitally absent (Figure 28–107, *B*). These pulses may be palpated simultaneously with the finger pads. The amplitude of the pulses in the legs and feet is expected to attain a grade of 2+ bilaterally, but 1+ is acceptable in the feet. Inequality of symmetrical pulses may indicate local obstruction due to atherosclerosis or an abnormally positioned artery.

Ultrasound Stethoscope. If the nurse cannot palpate a pulse, an ultrasound stethoscope is useful for amplifying the sounds of a pulse wave. Factors that weaken a pulse or make palpation difficult include obesity, reduced stroke volume, diminished blood volume, or arterial obstruction. A thin layer of transmission gel is first applied to the skin at the pulse site or directly onto the transducer tip of the probe. The nurse turns the volume to "on," places the tip of the probe at a 45- to 90-degree angle on the skin, and moves the probe until a pulsating "whooshing sound" is heard, indicating that arterial blood flow is present.

Coordination. When assessing coordination in the lower extremities, one rapid alternating test and one point-to-point test are used. Each leg must be tested separately, as the dexterity in one leg can affect dexterity in the other (Procedure 28-36). Nurses expect rapid alternating movements (rhythmic patting of the foot against the examiner's hand) to be smooth and rhythmical, but not as rapid or dextrous as the same test performed by the hands. In contrast, performance of point-to-point testing is expected to be smooth, accurate, and without tremor. The client should be able to accurately and smoothly run the heel of the foot down the shin and off the great toe of the opposite foot. Deviations suggest pathology within the cerebellar and/or motor system. If point-to-point testing is accurate with eyes open, but not with eyes closed, a deviation in position sense is possible.

Sensory System. Nurses assess the integrity of the sensory system in the lower extremities in a similar sequence and with the same techniques that they use when examining the upper extremities. Despite their supine position, clients must close their eyes during all sensory testing to avoid seeing the stimulus.

Pain and Light Touch. Nurses test for pain and light touch on the lower extremity dermatomes over the anterior aspect of both thighs (L_2 and L_3), the medial and lateral aspects of the lower legs (L_4 and L_5), and the little toes (S_1). Again, a splintered tongue blade or cotton-tipped applicator is used as the pain stimulus, and a cotton wisp is used as the light touch stimulus. Nurses vary the rhythm of testing and occasionally use the blunt end of the blade to touch a dermatome to validate accuracy of client responses. The sensations of pain and light touch are expected to be intact bilaterally from L_2 to S_1.

Vibration Sense. The nurse expects the client to report a buzz-like sensation at the DIP joint on the great toes when the vibrating tuning fork is on the joint. If vibrating

Procedure 28-34 Assessing Muscle Tone and Muscle Strength of the Lower Extremities

Equipment

- None

Examination Skill and Focus	Steps	Rationale
Muscle tone Legs	**1.** Support the leg at the foot and lower thigh. **2.** Move each leg (ankle, knee, hip) through a modified range of motion (ROM). **3.** Assess resistance offered. **4.** Test muscle tone prior to testing muscle strength.	Assessment of tone permits examiner to interpret muscle strength results accurately.
Muscle strength Feet	**1.** May test separately or simultaneously. **2.** Place hands on client's soles of feet. **3.** Ask client to plantar-flex foot against the resistance offered. **4.** Compare sides. **5.** Place hands on dorsum of client's feet. **6.** Ask client to dorsiflex feet against resistance offered. **7.** Compare sides.	Primarily tests strength of plantar flexion (L_{4-5}) and dorsi-flexion (S_1) at the ankle.
Legs	**1.** Instruct client to flex knee. **2.** Place left hand at knee and grasp client's ankle with right hand. **3.** Instruct client to keep foot in contact with table as you attempt to straighten client's leg (flexion at knee). **4.** Compare sides. **5.** Instruct client to flex knee. **6.** Support client's flexed knee with left hand and push against lower shin with right hand as client attempts to straighten leg (extension at knee). **7.** Compare sides.	Flexion tests strength of hamstring muscles (L_{4-5}, S_{1-2}) and extension tests strength of quadriceps muscles (L_{2-4}).
Hip	**1.** Place both hands on client's thigh. **2.** Try to force thigh downward as client raises leg against hand (flexion). **3.** Place hand under client's thigh. **4.** Instruct client to force thigh downward on examiner's hand (extension). **5.** Compares sides. **6.** Place both hands firmly on surface between client's knees, and **7.** Instruct client to bring legs together (adduction). **8.** Place hands firmly on surface at lateral aspect of client's knees, and **9.** Instruct client to spread legs (abduction). **10.** Compare sides.	Flexion tests strength of iliopsoas muscle (L_{2-4}), extension tests strength of the gluteus maximus muscle (S_1), adduction tests strength of the adductors (L_{2-4}), and abduction tests strength of the gluteus medium and minimus muscles (L_{4-5}, S_1) of the hip.

From *A Syllabus for Adult Health Assessment* (pp. 54–55), edited by D. L. Skillen and R. A. Day, 2004, Edmonton, AB: Faculty of Nursing, University of Alberta.

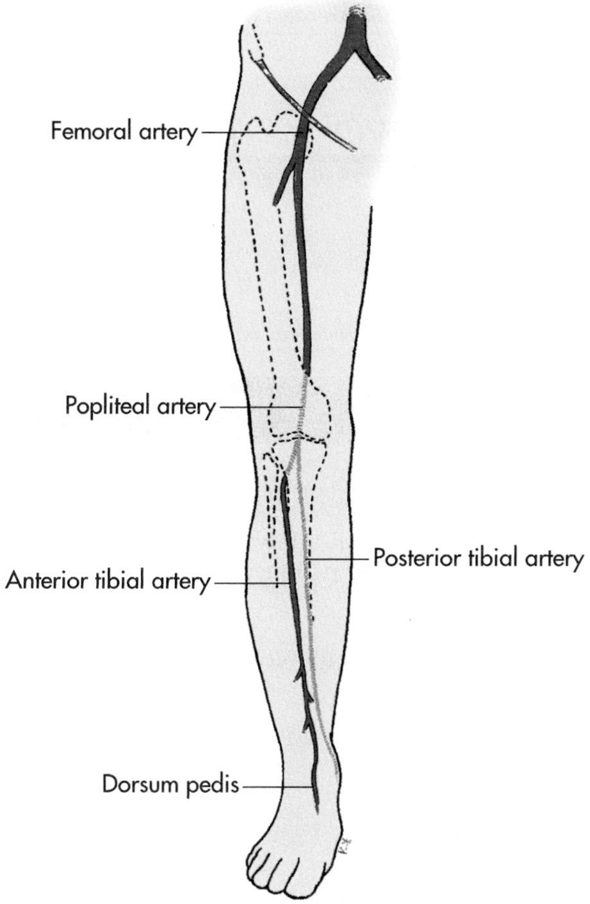

FIGURE **28–105** Anatomical position of femoral, popliteal, dorsalis pedis, and posterior tibial arteries.

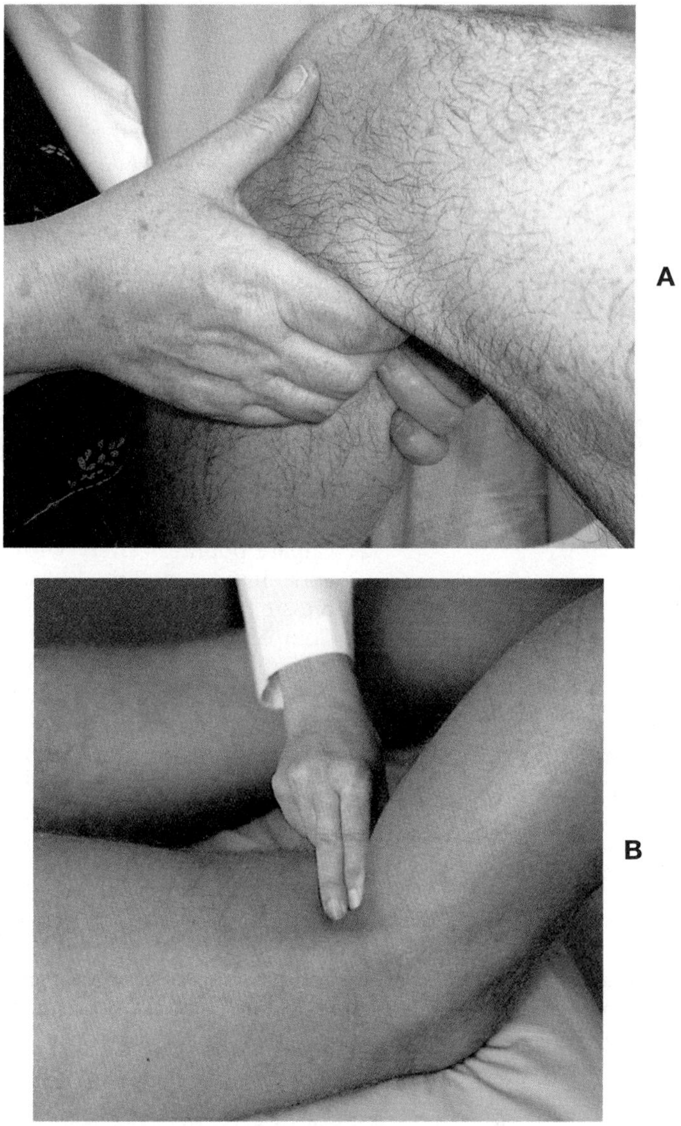

FIGURE **28–106** **A,** Palpation of popliteal artery. **B,** Palpation of popliteal pulse. (A is from *Physical Examination Images* [CD-ROM], by D. L. Skillen, R. A. Day, M. C. Anderson, T. C. Stephen, J. A. Gilbert, and L. W. Day, 2004, Edmonton, AB: Faculty of Nursing, University of Alberta.)

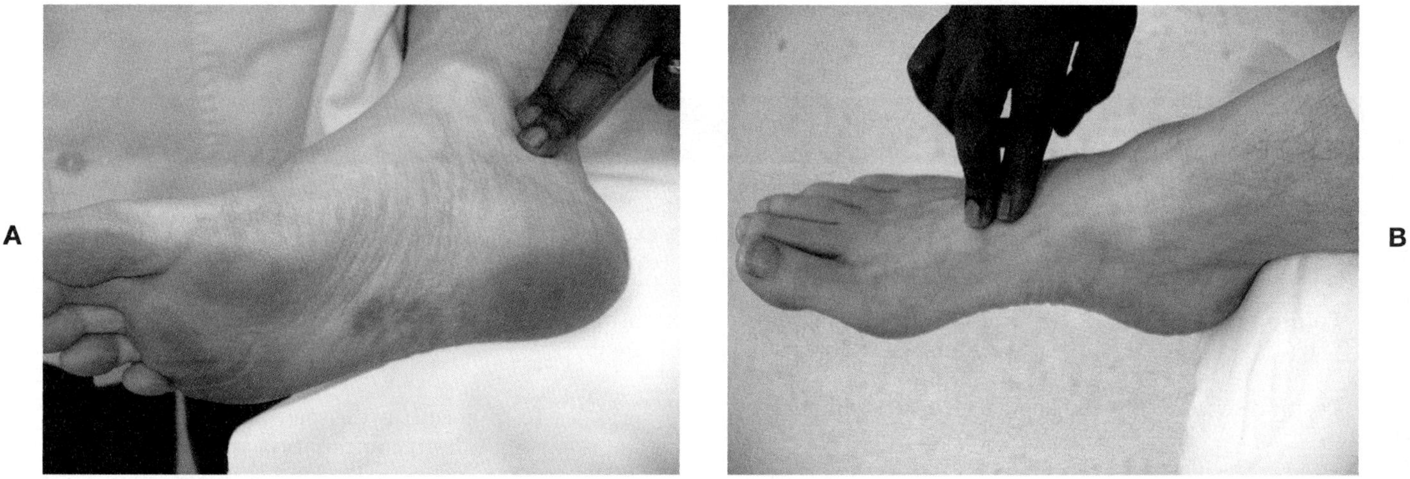

FIGURE **28–107** **A,** Palpation of posterior tibial artery. **B,** Palpation of dorsalis pedis artery. (From *Physical Examination Images* [CD-ROM], by D. L. Skillen, R. A. Day, M. C. Anderson, T. C. Stephen, J. A. Gilbert, and L. W. Day, 2004, Edmonton, AB: Faculty of Nursing, University of Alberta.)

Procedure 28-35 Assessing Pulses in the Lower Extremities

Equipment

• None

Examination Skill and Focus	Steps	Rationale
Popliteal pulses	**1.** Instruct client to flex leg slightly and relax muscles.	
	2. Palpate popliteal artery with fingertips of both hands midline in popliteal fossa, pressing deeply.	The popliteal artery is more deeply situated than other peripheral pulses.
	3. Compare sides.	
	4. If unable to palpate, ask client to lie prone on examining surface with legs flexed at knee and palpate.	The pulse amplitude in both arteries should be equal.
Posterior tibial pulses	**1.** Palpate posterior tibial artery behind and below medial malleolus with finger pads.	
	2. Compare sides. May palpate simultaneously.	
Dorsalis pedis pulses	**1.** Palpate dorsalis pedis artery with finger pads on dorsum of foot just lateral to extensor tendon of great toe.	
	2. Compare sides. May palpate simultaneously.	

From *A Syllabus for Adult Health Assessment* (p. 55), edited by D. L. Skillen and R. A. Day, 2004, Edmonton, AB: Faculty of Nursing, University of Alberta.

Procedure 28-36 Assessing Coordination of the Lower Extremities

Equipment

• None

Examination Skill and Focus	Steps	Rationale
Coordination	Test each leg separately.	
Rapid alternating movements	**1.** Instruct client to pat foot against examiner's hand as rapidly as possible (rhythmic patting).	
Point-to-point test	**2.** Instruct client to place heel on opposite knee and run heel down shin and off great toe.	
Position sense	**3.** Repeat each side with eyes closed.	
	4. Compare sides.	Testing with eyes open and then closed assesses both coordination and position sense.

From *A Syllabus for Adult Health Assessment* (p. 55), edited by D. L. Skillen and R. A. Day, 2004, Edmonton, AB: Faculty of Nursing, University of Alberta.

sensations are not felt, the nurse progressively tests upward over the PIP joints, MCP joints, medial malleolus, patella, and superior anterior iliac spine until the client reports the sensation.

Position Sense. The examiner grasps the distal phalanx of the great toe on its medial and lateral aspects and moves it up or down. With the eyes closed, the client should accurately report whether the toe was moved up or down. If unable to do so, position sense is impaired.

Discriminative Sensations. In the lower extremities, the only test of discriminative sensation is extinction (Procedure 28-37). The examiner touches the client's legs in symmetrical places at the same time. The client should be able to identify that both places on the body were touched and where. If the client can only identify one location, extinction is not intact.

Reflexes. In the lower extremities, the patellar and ankle deep tendon reflexes are tested, and the plantar superficial reflex is assessed (Procedure 28-38 and Figure 28–108). The client is encouraged to relax the leg on which the reflex is being tested. Nurses compare the reflexes of the legs. Only if a reflex is symmetrically absent or diminished will nurses use a reinforcement technique (augmentation) by asking the client to lock fingers together and pull hard without breaking the grasp. They signal the client to perform this manoeuvre just before striking the tendon. A response is expected at all sites and is graded on a scale of 0 (no response) to 4+ (hyperactive; see Table 28-60). Some individuals may consistently exhibit diminished or even absent deep tendon reflexes in the legs. The plantar superficial reflex is stimulated when nurses use a continuous firm stroke on the sole of the foot with a blunt object, such as the end of the handle of the reflex hammer. They expect the toes to flex bilaterally.

Inspection and Palpation. The client is asked to stand for the examiner to complete the examination of the lower extremities (Figure 28–109 and Procedure 28-39). The examiner assesses symmetry of muscle development, evidence of distended saphenous veins (varicose veins), and integrity of the arches and popliteal fossa. Arches of the feet should curve upward. The popliteal fossa is assessed for swelling or bogginess, and there should be none. Muscle development is expected to be symmetrical and without wasting. Although the veins in the legs may become more evident upon standing, they should not appear distended and tortuous, which would suggest the presence of varicose veins.

Coordination. In the standing position, the nurse assesses the client's cerebellar function, position sense, muscle strength, posture, balance, and gait (see Procedure 28-39). The Romberg test performed with eyes open assesses cerebellar function; with eyes closed, it assesses position sense. The nurse tests muscle strength and coordination by asking the client to perform tandem walking, shallow knee bends, hopping in one place, heel walking, and toe walking. The client is expected to perform these tests without difficulty, showing strength and coordinated movement. To assess balance, posture, and gait, the nurse asks the client to walk. Clients are expected to walk unassisted, evenly paced, with the heel striking first followed by a push off with the toe, with arms swinging easily opposite to legs, and the head leading on the turn.

Age-Related Changes for Extremities. Age-related change in the integumentary, peripheral vascular, musculoskeletal, and nervous systems must be considered when assessing the upper and lower extremities of an older adult. With increasing age, the epidermis, dermis, and subcutaneous skin layers thin, and vascularity decreases. The skin, especially over the dorsal surface of the hands, forearms, and lower legs, becomes more transparent, thin, fragile, and loose. Mobility of the skin increases and turgor decreases. The rate of epidermal proliferation slows down and delays wound healing. Skin on the extremities is often dry (xerosis), flaky, and itchy because eccrine sweat glands decrease in number, producing less sweat, and the sebaceous glands produce less sebum. Skin lesions commonly seen in older adults include actinic lentigines, actinic keratosis, seborrheic keratosis, and actinic purpura.

Fingernails and toenails grow more slowly and lose their lustre. Fingernails usually thin and split more easily, whereas toenails thicken as a result of trauma, fungal infection, or vascular insufficiency. Longitudinal ridging is commonly seen in all nails. Changes in the nails reflect the effects of health and environment as well as aging. Growth of hair on the lower legs and feet decreases but is also adversely affected by vascular disease.

Age-related change in the peripheral vascular and lymphatic systems is difficult to differentiate from disease processes. Arteries and veins thicken, becoming less elastic. In the arteries, this is called arteriosclerosis, and it causes increases in peripheral vascular resistance and systolic blood pressure. Because veins become less elastic, they dilate more readily, which increases susceptibility to venous stasis and varicose veins.

Skeletal muscle mass decreases due to deterioration of muscle fibres, resulting in loss of strength and endurance. An exercise program can minimize this decline. Whereas bones and muscles benefit from exercise, joints and articular surfaces are adversely affected by years of accumulated use. Articular surfaces thin and are subject to fraying and cracking. Elastic fibres degenerate and contribute to loss of tensile strength in the ligaments. The result of these changes is loss of joint stability, decreased range of motion, and pain. Osteoarthritis is the deterioration that occurs at the joint surface.

Hands reflect age-related musculoskeletal change quite graphically. Many older adults develop enlarged interphalangeal (IP) joints called Heberden's nodes at the distal joints and Bouchard's nodes at the proximal joints. The hands appear bony because of loss of subcutaneous fat and muscle mass between metacarpals. Muscle mass is also lost in the base of the thumb (thenar eminence) on the palm. Grip strength is maintained.

Pain sensation remains intact, but pressure, vibration, and position sense may be diminished due to a decline in density of cutaneous nerve endings (Miller, 1999). The abil-

Procedure 28-37 Assessing Sensation and Tactile Discrimination of the Lower Extremities

Equipment

- splintered tongue blade
- cotton ball
- 128 Hz tuning fork

Examination Skill and Focus	Steps	Rationale
Tests of sensation	Both sides are tested and compared. Demonstrate how sharp, dull, and light touch feels before beginning tests.	The client is made aware of the expected sensation to be perceived.
Superficial pain	**1.** Instruct client to close eyes and report with each touch whether it is "sharp" or "dull."	The blunt end of tongue blade tests pressure and is used to validate perception of pain stimulated by the sharp end.
	2. Touch client's legs lightly and alternately in corresponding areas with sharp end of splintered tongue blade (occasionally using blunt end), covering L_2 to S_1 dermatomes in thighs, legs, and feet. **3.** Compare sides.	Corresponding areas are stimulated to accurately compare the sensations felt between legs.
Light touch	**1.** Instruct client to close eyes and report each time touch is perceived (avoids pressure). **2.** Touch client's legs lightly in turn in corresponding areas with cotton wisp, covering L_2 to S_1 dermatomes in thighs, legs, and feet. **3.** Compare sides.	Varying the pace ensures the client is responding to the stimulus.
Vibration	**1.** Instruct client to close eyes and describe sensation felt. **2.** Place vibrating 128 Hz tuning fork firmly over distal interphalangeal (DIP) joint of great toe. **3.** Proceed proximally until vibrations felt. **4.** Stop vibrations and ask what is felt. **5.** Compare sides.	Asking the client to report when the felt sensation stops validates that the client felt a sensation.
Position sense	**1.** Demonstrate "up" and "down" position of great toe.	
	2. Instruct client to close eyes and identify position of great toe. **3.** Grasp great toe by medial and lateral aspects and move it "up" or "down," avoiding contact with other toes. **4.** Proceed proximally if necessary. **5.** Compare sides.	Isolating the toe being tested ensures that adjacent digits do not influence the sensation felt.
Test for tactile discrimination		
Extinction	**1.** Instruct client to close eyes and identify where touched. **2.** Touch client in corresponding areas of legs simultaneously. **3.** Ask client where touched.	Corresponding areas of both legs must be touched simultaneously to accurately assess extinction.

From *A Syllabus for Adult Health Assessment* (pp. 55–56), edited by D. L. Skillen and R. A. Day, 2004, Edmonton, AB: Faculty of Nursing, University of Alberta.

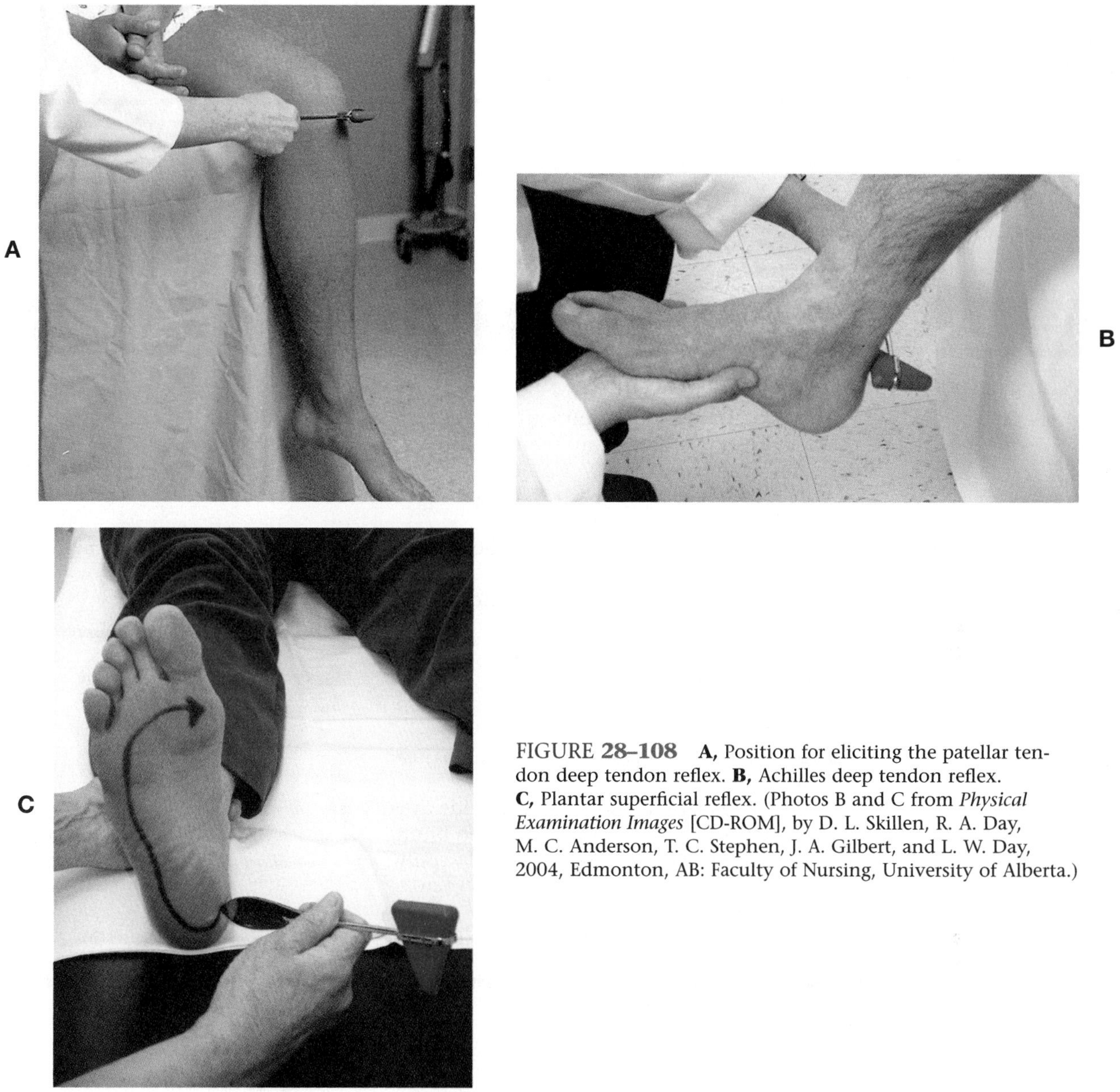

FIGURE **28–108** **A,** Position for eliciting the patellar tendon deep tendon reflex. **B,** Achilles deep tendon reflex. **C,** Plantar superficial reflex. (Photos B and C from *Physical Examination Images* [CD-ROM], by D. L. Skillen, R. A. Day, M. C. Anderson, T. C. Stephen, J. A. Gilbert, and L. W. Day, 2004, Edmonton, AB: Faculty of Nursing, University of Alberta.)

ity to perform tandem walking, walking on heels or toes, and deep knee bends may be diminished, in part due to loss of muscle strength, but also to difficulty in maintaining balance. Swaying may occur during the Romberg test, especially with eyes closed, due to changes in vision and position sense. Gait is usually slower, with a shorter stride, decreased steppage height, and decreased arm swing.

Documentation. Nurses record their findings from inspection and palpation of the lower extremities (Table 28-64).

After the Examination

Nurses' physical assessment findings are integrated into the plan of care and shared with their clients. First, they review all of their findings before clients dress or receive assistance with dressing, in case they need to recheck any information or gather additional data. Next, they ensure that the client assumes a comfortable position. For example, the hospital client may require a clean gown and assistance in returning to bed and with positioning. In the home or clinic, the client needs time to dress and then meet with the nurse for the summary of assessment findings. When nurses discover unexpected findings such as a mass or a highly irregular heart rate, they check with the client's physician or nurse practitioner before revealing those findings. They may have a peer or instructor double-check their findings if they have any doubts. They explain the type of unexpected findings and the need for the physician or nurse practitioner to conduct an additional examination. Definitive medical diagnoses are beyond the responsibility of the nurse.

Many institutions have special forms for recording examination data (see chapter 13). Documentation is

Procedure 28-38 Assessing Deep Tendon and Superficial Reflexes of the Lower Extremities

Equipment

- reflex hammer

Examination Skill and Focus	Steps	Rationale
Deep tendon reflexes	Both sides are tested. **Only if** responses are symmetrically diminished or absent does examiner use reinforcement (augmentation). Strike tendon briskly with hammer held loosely and swung freely in an arc.	Failure to ensure reflexes are symmetrically diminished before reinforcement may mask unequal reflexes. The same force applied by the reflex hammer between limbs ensures accurate comparison.
Patellar reflex	**1.** Position client so that leg is relaxed and knee is flexed. **2.** Use hammer to tap patellar tendon just below patella. **3.** Compare extension on each side.	Assesses integrity of the reflex arc at L_{2-4}.
Ankle reflex	**1.** Position client so that knee is flexed and foot is supported in dorsiflexed position by examiner. **2.** Use hammer to tap Achilles tendon just above the heel. **3.** Compare plantar flexion on each side.	Assesses integrity of the reflex arc primarily at S_1.
Superficial reflex Plantar reflex	**1.** Stroke the lateral aspect of sole with blunt pointed object beginning at heel, laterally along sole, and curving medially across ball of the foot. **2.** Compare toe movement on each side.	Assesses integrity of the reflex arc at L_5 and S_1.

From *A Syllabus for Adult Health Assessment* (p. 56), edited by D. L. Skillen and R. A. Day, 2004, Edmonton, AB: Faculty of Nursing, University of Alberta.

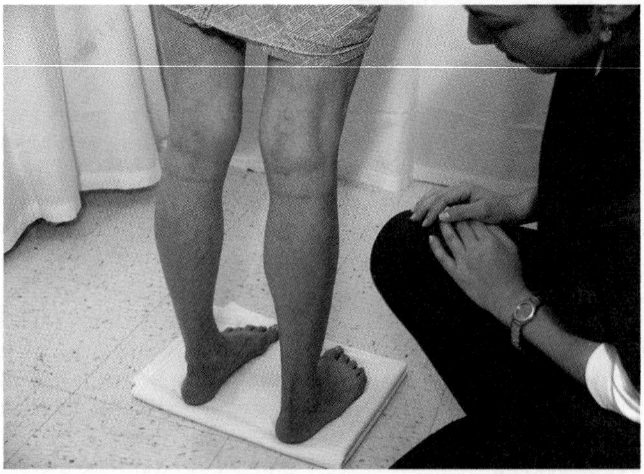

FIGURE **28–109** Inspection when client is standing. (From *Physical Examination Images* [CD-ROM], by D. L. Skillen, R. A. Day, M. C. Anderson, T. C. Stephen, J. A. Gilbert, and L. W. Day, 2004, Edmonton, AB: Faculty of Nursing, University of Alberta.)

Procedure 28-39 Inspecting the Legs and Assessing Coordination in Standing Position

Equipment

- None

Examination Skill and Focus	Steps	Rationale
Legs and feet Symmetry, veins, arches, and popliteal fossae	**1.** Inspect both legs, noting symmetry, veins, arches, and popliteal fossae. **2.** Palpate popliteal fossae.	The effects of gravity are maximized for assessing integrity of venous return, arches of the feet, and popliteal fossae.
Cerebellar tests, position sense	**1.** Instruct client to stand without support, arms at sides and feet together, first with eyes open, then closed for 20 seconds (Romberg test). **2.** Protect client from falling.	Performance of Romberg test, with eyes open, assesses cerebellar function; with eyes closed, tests position sense. ***Safety Alert:*** Because some sway is expected, especially with eyes closed, client must be protected from falling.
	3. Instruct client to walk in straight line by placing heel of foot directly before toes of other foot (tandem walking).	The tandem walk and heel/toe walk test coordination (balance) and motor strength.
Muscle strength Shallow knee bend	**4.** Instruct client to hop in place on one foot, then the other. **5.** Instruct client to stand on one foot and do a shallow knee bend, first on one leg, then the other. **6.** Support elbow if risk of falling.	Hopping and shallow knee bends demonstrate strength and coordination of legs.
Heel walk	**7.** Instruct client to walk on heels.	
Toe walk	**8.** Instruct client to walk on toes.	
Gait, balance, and posture	**1.** Instruct client to walk away and then back toward examiner. **2.** Inspect during walking for posture, gait (stance and swing), balance, arm swing, leg movement, and position of head on turning.	Critical observation of gait assesses integrity of the motor and cerebellar components of the nervous and musculoskeletal systems.

From *A Syllabus for Adult Health Assessment* (p. 57), edited by D. L. Skillen and R. A. Day, 2004, Edmonton, AB: Faculty of Nursing, University of Alberta.

required by law and is part of nursing legislation. All skills performed on a client must be recorded, even if appearing to be minimal, such as taking the blood pressure extra times. The nurse chooses to record findings from the physical assessment either during the examination or at the end. If entries are made periodically during the examination, the nurse reviews them for accuracy and thoroughness. If entry of the findings is delayed, the nurse charts that it is a late entry and records the time that the assessment was actually performed. In clinical situations where the status of a critically ill client is constantly changing, it is extremely important to document the times. Nurses communicate significant findings to appropriate medical and nursing personnel. Initially, they may do this verbally, but they ensure that the findings are also written.

The client often needs a number of ancillary examinations, such as X-ray examinations, laboratory tests, or ultrasonography, after a physical examination. Nurses explain the purpose of these tests and the sensations that the client can expect. The tests provide additional screening information to rule out the presence of abnormalities

Table 28-64 Examples of Documentation for Lower Extremities

Focus of Assessment	Expected Findings	Unexpected Findings
Skin	Brownish hair over proximal and distal phalanges. Skin pink, moist, elastic. Skin temperature uniformly warm over thighs, cooler over shins and feet.	Fine evenly distributed white hair over thighs, no hair over shins or phalanges (denies shaving legs). Thick cracked calluses over heels bilaterally. Brownish pigmentation over medial malleoli. (R) leg cooler than (L).
Muscle development	Muscle mass symmetrical in size and contour without atrophy or fasciculations in the legs. Standing: arches high bilaterally; popliteal fossae without swelling.	Muscle wasting evident in (R) calf; muscle mass less on right than (L) calf. Standing: arches flat bilaterally; mobile 2 × 2 cm swelling in (R) popliteal fossa; small saphenous veins distended and torturous (R)>(L).
Nails	Nails short, firm, uniformly thick, cut straight across. No evidence of lesions around cuticles.	Nails on great toes thick and curved. Nail margin on (R) great toe reddened, no discharge.
Range of motion (ROM)	Full ROM in feet, ankles, knees, and hips. No discomfort reported during ROM.	Flexion at (L) knee less than on right. External rotation at (L) hip decreased compared with (R) hip. External rotation at (L) hip causes slight discomfort.
Joints	Distal interphalangeal (DIP), proximal interphalangeal (PIP), and metacarpophalangeal (MTP) joints without tenderness, swelling, or bogginess to palpation bilaterally. Ankles and knees free of tenderness and swelling to palpation bilaterally. No crepitations at knees.	Crepitations evident in both knees. Swelling and bogginess in (R) knee, both sides of patella.
Muscle tone	Slight tension felt during passive stretch bilaterally.	(L) leg becomes spastic when stretched.
Muscle strength	Muscular strength 5+ bilaterally at ankle, knee, and hip	Muscle strength (L) leg 2+ (with gravity eliminated) at ankles, knee, and hip.
Coordination	Performs rapid alternating movements of feet rapidly, smoothly, with slight uneven rhythm. Point-to-point testing smooth and accurate with eyes open and closed bilaterally.	Alternating movements in (R) foot rapid and smooth; point-to-point testing (R) leg accurate with eyes open and closed. (L) side, alternating movements are hesitant and uncoordinated, point-to-point testing inaccurate with eyes open and closed.
Pulses	Dorsalis pedis and posterior tibial pulses 2+ bilaterally. Popliteal pulses 1+ bilaterally. Rhythm is regular.	Popliteal pulses 1+ bilaterally. Posterior and dorsalis pedis pulses 1+ (R), absent (L).
Sensation	Superficial pain and light touch intact bilaterally over dermatomes L_2 to S_1. Vibration and position senses intact bilaterally at toes.	Superficial pain decreased over L_4 to S_1 from toes to mid-calf bilaterally. Vibration and position sense absent at toes.
Reflexes	Patellar and ankle reflexes 2+ without reinforcement. (R)(L) plantar reflexes: toes plantar flex bilaterally.	Patellar reflex 1+ bilaterally, ankle reflex 1+ (R) absent (L). Plantar reflexes: toes dorsiflex bilaterally.
Posture/gait/balance	Gait coordinated, heel strike with push-off at toe, arm swing opposite to leg, head leads on turn.	Gait hesitant, uses cane in (R) hand, drags toes on (L). (L) hand held close to side.
Cerebellar/muscle strength	Minimal sway during Romberg with eyes open and closed; tandem walking smooth, coordinated; stands on one foot followed by shallow knee bend without assistance bilaterally; coordinated walking on heels and toes.	Romberg-minimal sway with eyes open, sway noticeable with eyes closed; tandem walk unsteady; requires assistance with standing on foot; unable to perform shallow knee bend or hop bilaterally; unable to walk on heels or toes.

From "Documentation" by M. C. Anderson in *Health Assessment Self-Test Modules* (WebCT Vista), 2004, Edmonton, AB: Faculty of Nursing, University of Alberta.

and help in the diagnosis of specific abnormalities found during the examination.

With sensitivity and skill, nurses bring closure to the interview and assessment. They provide extra time to explain the results of the assessment to an older client and/or family member. They offer the client an opportunity to ask questions or mention anything else. The parting comments of a client may be very significant and nurses are alert to what the client says when their time together is coming to a close. Nurses review their findings with the client, summarizing positive health aspects, potential and actual health problems identified, and agreed-upon plans for action.

Key Concepts

- When a client presents with a symptom or sign, the nurse uses symptom/sign analysis to gather data about the symptom or sign.
- Assessment data are used to make nursing diagnoses, select appropriate nursing interventions, and evaluate outcomes of nursing care.
- Physical assessment of different age groups requires the nurse to apply principles of growth and development and understand age-related changes.
- Client teaching is integrated throughout the examination to help clients learn about health promotion and disease prevention.
- Physical examination modes of inspection, palpation, percussion, and auscultation are used to assess the client's baseline functional abilities and to serve as a basis for comparison with subsequent assessments.
- Inspection requires good lighting, full exposure of the body part, and a careful comparison of the part with its counterpart on the opposite side of the body.
- Palpation involves the use of parts of the hand to detect different types of physical characteristics.
- Percussion is the detection of differences in the density of underlying tissues by listening to audible sounds produced while striking the body's surface.
- Auscultation with a stethoscope facilitates assessment of the character of sounds created in various body organs.
- Physical examination is performed only after proper preparation of the client (both physically and psychologically), the environment, and the equipment.
- Throughout the examination, the nurse ensures that the client is warm, comfortable, and informed of each step of the process.
- The nurse uses a systematic approach when conducting a physical assessment and learns to integrate the assessments of different body systems simultaneously.
- During assessments of the skin, breast, and genitalia, the nurse explains the techniques for self-examination.
- The nurse continually assesses the client's cognitive function (mental status and intellectual function) throughout the examination.
- At the end of the examination, the nurse provides for the client's comfort, reviews findings, facilitates closure, and documents the assessment findings.

Key Terms

Adventitious sounds, *p. 702*
Anatomical position, *p. 635*
Apical impulse, *p. 707*
Arcus senilis, *p. 665*
Audible sounds, *p. 627*
Auscultation, *p. 619*
Benign, *p. 716*
Borborygmi, *p. 722*
Bruit, *p. 688*
CAGE questions, *p. 624*
Capillary refill, *p. 747*
Capillary return, *p. 658*
Cerumen, *p. 674*
Conjunctivitis, *p. 665*
Cultural sensitivity, *p. 620*
Cyanosis, *p. 650*
Delirium, *p. 645*
Direct lighting, *p. 624*
Distension, *p. 722*
Edema, *p. 655*
Exophthalmos, *p. 662*
Fasciculations, *p. 744*
Fibrocystic breast disease, *p. 716*
General survey, *p. 759*
Health history, *p. 619*
Hernias, *p. 720*
Induration, *p. 654*
Inflammation, *p. 744*
Inspection, *p. 619*
  General, *p. 622*
  Local, *p. 624*
Integument, *p. 648*
Intertriginous, *p. 651*
Jaundice, *p. 652*
Kyphosis, *p. 694*
Lesions, *p. 650*
  Primary, *p. 650*
  Secondary, *p. 650*
Lordosis, *p. 694*
Melanoma, *p. 650*
Mental status, *p. 645*
Metastasize, *p. 712*
Nystagmus, *p. 666*
Objective data, *p. 619*
Oblique (tangential) lighting, *p. 624*
Otoscope, *p. 674*
Palpation, *p. 619*
  Deep, *p. 627*
  Light, *p. 624*
Papanicolaou (Pap) smear, *p. 731*
Patency, *p. 677*
Peau d'orange skin, *p. 714*
Percussion, *p. 619*
  Direct (non-mediated), *p. 632*
  Indirect (mediated), *p. 632*
Peristalsis, *p. 722*
Petechiae, *p. 651*
Physical assessment, *p. 617*
Point of maximal impulse (PMI), *p. 707*
Precordium, *p. 706*
Ptosis, *p. 662*
Scoliosis, *p. 694*
Screening, *p. 642*
Sign, *p. 641*
Standard precautions/ routine practices, *p. 620*
Sternal angle, *p. 696*
Strabismus, *p. 662*
Striae, *p. 720*
Subjective data, *p. 619*
Symptom/sign analysis, *p. 619*
Symptoms, *p. 621*
Syncope, *p. 687*
Tactile fremitus, *p. 702*
Turgor, *p. 653*
Vital signs, *p. 622*

Critical Thinking Exercises

1. Examine the image of the eyes.

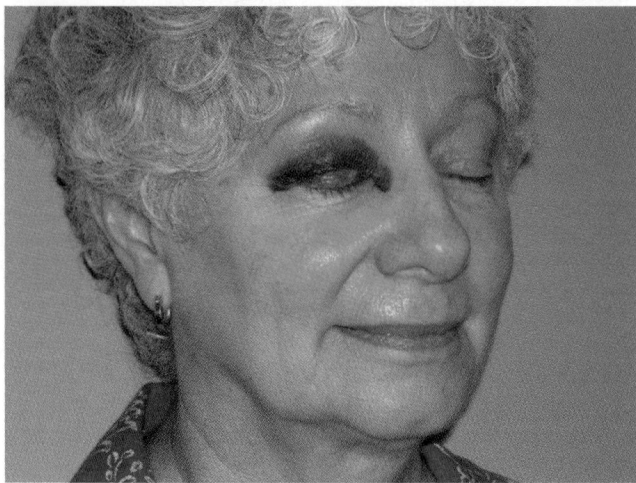

(From *Physical Examination Images* [CD-ROM], by D. L. Skillen, R. A. Day, M. C. Anderson, T. C. Stephen, J. A. Gilbert, and L. W. Day, 2004, Edmonton, AB: Faculty of Nursing, University of Alberta.)

   a. What questions will you ask to complete a symptom and sign analysis?
   b. If you suspect physical abuse, what questions would you ask?
   c. If you suspect a fall related to substance abuse, what questions would you ask?
   d. What techniques will you use to examine the right eye?
   e. What age-related change might influence the sign observed in this client?
   f. What is your documentation for inspection?

2. Examine the image of the right breast.

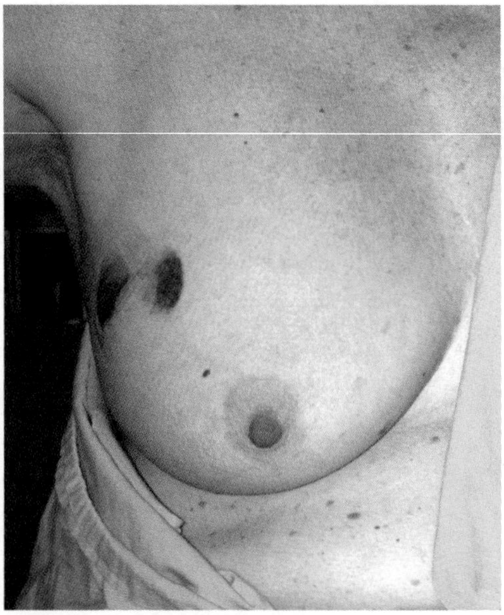

(From *Physical Examination Images* [CD-ROM], by D. L. Skillen, R. A. Day, M. C. Anderson, T. C. Stephen, J. A. Gilbert, and L. W. Day, 2004, Edmonton, AB: Faculty of Nursing, University of Alberta.)

   a. What questions will you ask when taking a health history?
   b. What specific characteristics will you assess in the breast?
   c. What examination mode(s) will you use with this client?
   d. What do you expect to find when you examine the breast?
   e. What is your documentation for inspection?

3. Examine the image of the left leg in a female client.

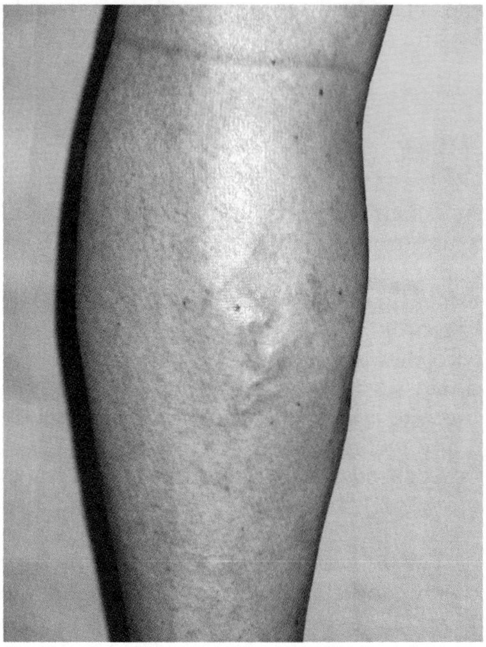

(From *Physical Examination Images* [CD-ROM], by D. L. Skillen, R. A. Day, M. C. Anderson, T. C. Stephen, J. A. Gilbert, and L. W. Day, 2004, Edmonton, AB: Faculty of Nursing, University of Alberta.)

   a. What questions will you ask in your health history?
   b. What anatomical structures are accessible to examination?
   c. What system(s) will you examine?
   d. What teaching and health promotion activities will you integrate in your assessment?
   e. What specific characteristics are you going to assess during your examination?
   f. What aspects of your assessment would change if this were a male client?

Review Questions

1. Your analysis of a symptom includes a focus on all the following characteristics EXCEPT:
   1. quality or nature
   2. intensity or severity
   3. location and radiation
   4. diagnosis or hypothesis
2. Recent memory is measured by asking the client to recall events that occurred:
   1. one week ago
   2. one month ago

3. three minutes ago
4. within the past 24 hours

3. To ensure a thorough inspection of the tympanic membrane, you do all the following EXCEPT:
   1. straighten the ear canal
   2. instruct client to keep head straight in midline position
   3. use the largest ear speculum that the canal will accommodate
   4. move the otoscope slowly to see as much of the tympanic membrane as possible.
4. When palpating the lymph nodes of the neck, you assess for which of the following characteristics?
   1. congruency, induration, size, turgor
   2. enlargement, integrity, shape, moisture
   3. consistency, delineation, mobility, tenderness
   4. configuration, discreteness, temperature, colour
5. If you identify adventitious breath sounds during auscultation of the lungs, you assess all the following characteristics of those unexpected sounds EXCEPT:
   1. location in the lung fields
   2. timing during the respiratory phases
   3. ratio of inspiratory phase to expiratory phase
   4. persistence after several deep inspirations and coughs
6. When palpating the precordium of a client, you expect to detect all the following characteristics of apical pulsations EXCEPT:
   1. solation to one interspace
   2. prominence of pulsation in early systole
   3. brisk tapping against the palpating finger
   4. detection of pulsation 4 cm lateral to the (L) MCL
7. Indirect percussion includes all the following techniques EXCEPT:
   1. use of brisk arc-like and relaxed wrist action
   2. variation of force of percussion to compare sides
   3. application of pleximeter finger firmly to skin surface
   4. use of lightest blow to achieve clear percussion notes
8. Inspection of the spine includes assessment of all the following characteristics EXCEPT:
   1. bilateral lateral bending
   2. curvatures and prominences
   3. attachments of paravertebral muscles
   4. alignment of shoulders and iliac crests
9. When examining the external genitalia of an elderly male, you expect to detect all the following age-related changes EXCEPT:
   1. sparser pubic hair
   2. pendulous scrotal sac
   3. smooth rubbery testicles
   4. small noncircumcised penis
10. When conducting a point-to-point test of the upper extremities, you observe that the client performs the test accurately with eyes open, but inaccurately with eyes closed. This finding suggests a:
    1. vestibular anomaly
    2. position sense deficit
    3. cerebellar dysfunction
    4. discriminatory sensory loss

References

American Cancer Society. (2004a). Cancer facts and figures 2004. Retrieved January 24, 2005, from *http://www.cancer.org/docroot/STT/stt_0.2004.asp?sitearea=STT&level=1*

American Cancer Society. (2004b). Cancer prevention and early detection: Facts and figures 2004. Retrieved January 24, 2005 from *http://www.cancer.org/downloads/STT/CPE2004PWsecured.pdf*

American Psychiatric Association. (2000). *Diagnostic and statistical manual of mental disorders* (4th ed. Rev.). Washington, DC: Author.

Anderson, M. C. (2004). Documentation. In *Health Assessment Self-Test Modules (WebCT Vista).* Edmonton, AB: Faculty of Nursing, University of Alberta.

Barkauskas, V. H., Baumann, L. C., & Darling-Fisher, C. S. (2002). *Health and physical assessment* (3rd ed.). St. Louis, MO: Mosby.

Bennett, M. A. (1995). Report of the task force on the implications for darkly pigmented intact skin in the prediction and prevention of pressure ulcers. *Advances in Wound Care, 8*(6), 34–35.

Bickley, L. S., & Szilagyi, P.G. (2003). *Bates guide to physical examination and history taking* (8th ed.). Philadelphia: Lippincott Williams & Wilkins.

Canadian Cancer Society. (2004a). *Canadian cancer statistics 2004.* Toronto, ON: Author.

Canadian Cancer Society. (2004b). *Screening and early detection.* Retrieved January 23, 2005, from *http://www.cancer.ca/ccs/internet/standard/0,3182,3172_12851_langId-en,00.html*

Canadian Cancer Society/Alberta/NWT Division. (2002). *Breast self-examination: You're worth it* [Brochure]. Calgary, AB: Author.

Canadian Nurses Association. (2002). *Code of ethics for registered nurses.* Ottawa, ON: Author.

Canadian Task Force on Preventive Health Care. (2001). Colorectal cancer screening. Recommendation statement from The Canadian Task Force on Preventive Health Care. *CMAJ, 165,* 206–208.

Caulker-Burnett, I. (1994). Primary care screening for substance abuse. *The Nurse Practitioner, 19*(6), 42–48.

Chambers, J., et al. (2004). *First Year Student Lab Guide.* Edmonton, AB: Faculty of Nursing, University of Alberta.

Day, R. A. (2004a). Female external and internal genital examination. In D. L Skillen & R. A. Day (Eds.), *A syllabus for adult health assessment* (pp. 92–95). Edmonton, AB: Faculty of Nursing, University of Alberta.

Day, R. A. (2004b). Documentation. In *Health Assessment Self-Test Modules (WebCT Vista).* Edmonton, AB: Faculty of Nursing, University of Alberta.

Day, R., & Payne, L. (1987). Computer-managed instruction: An alternative teaching strategy. *Journal of Nursing Education, 26,* 30–36.

Dillon, P. M. (2004). *Nursing health assessment: Clinical pocket guide.* Philadelphia: F. A. Davis.

DuGas, B.W., & Knor, E.R. (1995). *Nursing foundations. A Canadian perspective.* Scarborough, ON: Appleton & Lang Canada.

Ebersole, P., & Hess, P. (1998). *Toward healthy aging* (5th ed.). St. Louis, MO: Mosby.

Folstein, M. F., Folstein, S., & McHugh, P. R. (1975). "Mini-mental state": A practical method for grading the cognitive state of patients for the clinician. *Journal of Psychiatric Research, 12,* 189–198.

Friedman, L., et al. (Eds.). (1996). *Source book of substance abuse and addiction.* Baltimore: Williams & Wilkins.

Gerard, M. (2000). Domestic violence: How to screen and intervene. *RN, 63*(12), 52–56.

Hardy, M. A. (1996). What can you do about your patient's dry skin? *Journal of Gerontological Nursing, 22*(5), 10–18.

Health Canada. (2003). Canadian guidelines for body weight classification in adults. Ottawa, ON: Author.

Hoban, S., & Kearney, K. (2000). Elder abuse and neglect. *American Journal of Nursing, 100*(11), 49–50.

Hockenberry, M. J., et al. (2003). *Wong's nursing care of infants and children* (7th ed.). St. Louis, MO: Mosby.

Jarvis, C. (2004). *Physical examination and health assessment* (4th ed.). St Louis, MO: Elsevier Science.

Kahn, R. L., et al. (1960). Brief objective measures for the determination of mental status of the aged. *The American Journal of Psychiatry, 117,* 326–328.

Kennedy-Malone, L., Fletcher, K. R., & Plank, L. M. (2000). *Management guidelines for gerontological nurse practitioners.* Philadelphia: F. A. Davis.

Kramer, A. (2002). Domestic violence: How to ask and how to listen. *The Nursing Clinics of North America, 37,* 189–210.

Lemire Rodger, G., & Gallagher, S. (2000). The move toward primary health care in Canada: Community health nursing from 1985 to 1995. In M.J. Stewart (Ed.). *Community Nursing: Promoting Canadians' Health* (2nd ed., pp. 33–55). Toronto: W.B. Saunders.

Lowdermilk, D. L., Perry, S. E., & Bobak, I. M. (2000). *Maternity and women's health care* (7th ed.). St. Louis, MO: Mosby.

McIntyre, M., & Thomlinson, E. (2003). *Realities of Canadian nursing. Professional, practice, and power issues.* Philadelphia: Lippincott, Williams & Wilkins.

Master, S., & Terpstra, J. K. (1992). Recognition and diagnosis. In S. H. Schnoll, P. K. Horvatich, & J. K. Terpstra (Eds.), *Prescribing drugs with abuse liability* (p. 18). Richmond, VA: Division of Substance Abuse Medicine, Medical College of Virginia.

Metropolitan Life Insurance Company. (2000). *Statistical bulletin.* New York: Metropolitan.

Miller, C. A. (1999). *Nursing care of older adults. Theory and practice* (3rd ed.). Philadelphia: Lippincott.

Ogilvie, L., & Reutter, L. (2003). Primary health care: Complexities and possibilities from a nursing perspective. In J. C. Ross Kerr & M. Wood (Eds.). *Canadian nursing issues and perspectives* (4th ed., pp. 441–465). Toronto: Mosby.

Overfield, T. (1995). Biologic variation in health and illness: Race, age, and sex differences (2nd ed.). New York: CRC Press.

Paul, P., & Day, R. A. (2003). *Primary health care in nursing programs at the Faculty of Nursing,* University of Alberta, Edmonton, Canada. New York: Strategic Health Development Area, Human Resources Unit PAHO/WHO.

Seidel, H. M., et al. (2003). *Mosby's guide to physical examination* (5th ed.). St. Louis, MO: Mosby.

Skillen, D. L. (1996). Toward a social structural understanding of occupational hazards in public health. *International Journal of Health Services, 26*(1), 111–146.

Skillen, D. L. (2004a). *A primer on physical examination techniques* [WebCT]. Edmonton, AB: Faculty of Nursing, University of Alberta.

Skillen, D. L. (2004b). Male Genital Examination. In D. L. Skillen & R. A. Day (Eds.), *A syllabus for adult health assessment* (pp. 89–90). Edmonton, AB: Faculty of Nursing, University of Alberta.

Skillen, D. L., (2004c). Documentation. In *Health Assessment Self-Test Modules (WebCT Vista).* Edmonton, AB: Faculty of Nursing, University of Alberta.

Skillen, D. L. (2004d). Anus, Rectum, and Prostate Examination. In D. L. Skillen & R. A. Day (Eds.), *A syllabus for adult health assessment* (pp. 89–90). Edmonton, AB: Faculty of Nursing, University of Alberta.

Skillen, D. L., Anderson, M. C., & Knight, C. L. (2001). The created environment for physical assessment by case managers. *Western Journal of Nursing Research, 32*(1), 72–89.

Skillen, D. L., & Day, R. A. (Eds.). (2004). *A syllabus for adult health assessment.* Edmonton, AB: Faculty of Nursing, University of Alberta.

Skillen, D. L., et al. (2004). *Physical examination images* [CD-ROM]. Edmonton, AB: Faculty of Nursing, University of Alberta.

Skillen, D. L., Seglie, J., & Anderson, M. (1998). Beyond bandaids: Are OHNs using physical assessment skills? *AOHNA Newsletter, 19*(1), 5, 10.

Stephen, T. C. (1997). Symptom analysis. In *Adult health assessment series* [CD-ROM]. Edmonton, AB: DataStar Education Systems & Services.

Stephen, T. C. (2004). Documentation. In *Health Assessment Self-Test Modules (WebCT Vista).* Edmonton, AB: Faculty of Nursing, University of Alberta.

Stuart, G., & Laraia, M. (2001). *Principles and practice of psychiatric nursing* (7th ed.). St. Louis, MO: Mosby.

Swartz, M. H. (2002). *Textbook of physical diagnosis: History and examination* (4th ed.). Philadelphia: W. B. Saunders.

Talbot, L., & Curtis, L. (1996). The challenges of assessing skin indicators in people of color. *Home Healthcare Nurse, 14,* 167–171.

Wong, D. L., & Hockenberry-Eaton, M. (2001). *Wong's essentials of pediatric nursing* (6th ed.). St. Louis, MO: Mosby.

Wong, D. L., et al. (1999). *Whaley and Wong's nursing care of infants and children* (6th ed.). St. Louis, MO: Mosby.

World Health Organization. (1978). Primary health care: Report of the international conference on primary health care. Alma -Ata, USSR, Geneva: Author.

World Health Organization (1986). Ottawa Charter for health promotion. Ottawa: Canadian Public Health Association

World Health Organization. (1997). The Jakarta Declaration on health promotion into the 21st century. Retrieved January 24, 2005 from *http://www.who.int/hpr/NPH/docs/jakarta_declaration_en.pdf*

World Health Organization. (2000). Obesity: Preventing and managing the global epidemic: Report of a WHO consultation on obesity. Geneva, Switzerland: Author.

Recommended Web Sites

Canadian Cancer Society:
http://www.cancer.ca/
This site provides access to current cancer statistics and information about screening and early detection.

Public Health Agency of Canada:
http://www.phac-aspc.gc.ca/
This site provides information about chronic diseases, emergency preparedness, health promotion, immunization, infectious diseases, injury prevention, travel health, and surveillance.

29

Infection Control

Leah W. Frederick, MS, RN, CIC
Jennifer Medves, RN, PhD (Canadian author)

Objectives

Mastery of content in this chapter will enable the student to:

- Define the key terms listed.
- Explain the relationship of the chain of infection to transmission of infection.
- Identify the body's normal defences against infection.
- Discuss the events in the inflammatory response.
- Describe the signs and symptoms of localized and systemic infections.
- Identify clients most at risk for infection.
- Explain conditions that promote the transmission of nosocomial infection.
- Explain the difference between medical and surgical asepsis.
- Give an example for preventing infection for each element of the infection chain.
- Perform proper procedures for hand hygiene.
- Explain the rationale and practices for standard precautions/routine practices.
- Explain the rationale and practices for transmission-based (isolation) precautions.
- Explain how infection control measures may differ in the home versus the hospital.
- Properly don a surgical mask, sterile gown, and sterile gloves.

Good health depends in part on a safe environment. Practices or techniques that control or prevent transmission of infection help to protect clients and health care workers from disease. Clients in all health care settings are at risk for acquiring infections because they often have lower resistance to infectious **micro-organisms,** increased exposure to numbers and types of disease-causing micro-organisms, and undergo **invasive** procedures. In acute care or ambulatory care facilities, clients can be exposed to pathogens, some of which may be resistant to most antibiotics. By practising infection prevention and control techniques, the nurse can avoid spreading micro-organisms to clients.

In all settings, clients and their families must be able to recognize sources of infections and be able to institute protective measures. Client teaching should include information concerning infections, modes of transmission, and methods of prevention.

Health care workers can protect themselves from contact with infectious material or exposure to a communicable disease by having knowledge of the infectious process and appropriate barrier protection. Diseases such as hepatitis B and C, acquired immunodeficiency syndrome (AIDS), sudden acute respiratory syndrome (SARS), and tuberculosis (TB) have resulted in a greater emphasis on infection control techniques. There are two foci to infection control: (1) protecting clients from acquiring infections, and (2) protecting health care workers from becoming infected. Many of the techniques used to protect clients also provide effective protection for nurses. Nevertheless, nurses must remain constantly vigilant to prevent the spread of infection while providing care.

Scientific Knowledge Base

Micro-organisms live and grow on inanimate objects and in air, water, food, soil, plants, and animals. They also live and grow in and on people. Most micro-organisms are non-pathogens, meaning they do not cause a person to be ill. However, some micro-organisms are **pathogens,** meaning they are capable of causing disease. An infection is a disease state resulting from the entry and multiplication of a pathogen in the tissues of a host, causing the body to manifest clinical signs and symptoms. If the infection can be transmitted from one person to another, it is a **communicable** (infectious, contagious) disease.

Chain of Infection

The presence of a pathogen does not mean that an infection will begin. Development of an infection occurs in a cycle that depends on the presence of all of the following elements:

- An infectious agent (pathogen)
- A reservoir (source for pathogen growth)
- A portal of exit from the reservoir
- A mode of transmission
- A portal of entry to a host
- A susceptible host

An infection will develop if this chain remains intact (Figure 29–1). Nurses follow infection prevention and control practices to break the chain so that infection will not develop.

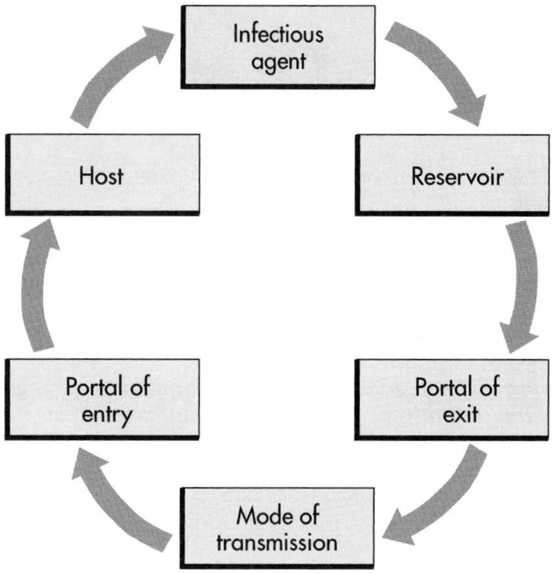

FIGURE **29–1** Chain of infection.

Infectious Agent. Micro-organisms include bacteria, viruses, fungi, and protozoa (Table 29-1). Micro-organisms on the skin are called resident or transient flora. Resident organisms are considered permanent residents of the skin, where they survive and multiply without causing harm. Resident organisms are not easily removed by handwashing with plain soaps unless considerable friction is used. Resident micro-organisms in deep skin layers are usually killed only by performing hand hygiene with products containing antimicrobial ingredients.

Transient micro-organisms attach to the skin when a person has contact with another person or object. For example, when a nurse touches a bedpan or a contaminated dressing, transient bacteria adhere to the nurse's skin. The organisms attach loosely to the skin in dirt and grease or under fingernails. These organisms may be readily transmitted unless removed by handwashing (Larson, 1996).

The potential for micro-organisms to cause disease depends on the following factors:

- Sufficient number of organisms
- **Virulence,** or ability to produce disease
- Ability to enter and survive in the host
- Susceptibility of the host

Resident skin micro-organisms are usually nonpathogenic. However, they can cause serious infection when surgery or other invasive procedures allow them to enter deep tissues or when a client is severely **immunocompromised** (has an impaired immune system).

Reservoir. A reservoir is a place where a pathogen can survive but may or may not multiply. For example, hepatitis A virus survives in shellfish but does not multiply; *Pseudomonas* organisms may survive and multiply in nebulizer reservoirs used in the care of clients with respiratory problems. The most common reservoir is the human body. A variety of micro-organisms live on the skin and within the body cavities, fluids, and discharges. When a pathogen is present on or in the body but does not cause harm, the pathogen is **colonizing** the site. **Carriers** are people or animals who show no symptoms of illness but who have pathogens on or in their bodies that can be transferred to others. For example, a person can be a carrier of hepatitis B virus without having signs or symptoms of infection. Animals, food, water, insects, and inanimate objects can also be reservoirs for infectious organisms. For example, the bacterium *Legionella pneumophila,* which causes Legionnaires' disease, lives in contaminated water and water systems. To thrive, pathogens require a reservoir that provides food, oxygen (or no oxygen, depending on the pathogen), water, appropriate temperature and pH, and minimal light.

Food. Micro-organisms require nourishment. Some, such as *Clostridium perfringens,* the microbe that causes gas gangrene, thrive on organic matter. Others, such as *Escherichia coli,* consume undigested foodstuff in the bowel. Carbon dioxide and inorganic material such as soil provide nourishment for other organisms.

Oxygen. **Aerobic** bacteria require oxygen for survival and for multiplication sufficient to cause disease. Aerobic organisms cause more infections than **anaerobic** organisms (i.e., organisms that can only survive in the absence of

Table 29-1 Common Pathogens and Resulting Major Infections

Organism	Major Reservoir(s)	Major Infections
Bacteria		
C. difficile	Colon	Colitis, diarrhea
Escherichia coli	Colon	Gastroenteritis, urinary tract infection
Staphylococcus aureus	Skin, hair, anterior nares	Wound infection, pneumonia, food poisoning, cellulitis
Streptococcus (beta-hemolytic group A) organisms	Oropharynx, skin, perianal area	"Strep throat," rheumatic fever, scarlet fever, impetigo, wound infection
Streptococcus (beta-hemolytic group B) organisms	Adult genitalia	Urinary tract infection, wound infection, postpartum sepsis, neonatal sepsis
Mycobacterium tuberculosis	Droplet nuclei from lungs	Tuberculosis
Neisseria gonorrhoeae	Genitourinary tract, rectum, mouth	Gonorrhea, pelvic inflammatory disease, infectious arthritis, conjunctivitis
Rickettsia rickettsii	Wood tick	Rocky Mountain spotted fever
Staphylococcus epidermidis	Skin	Wound infection, bacteremia
Viruses		
Hepatitis A virus	Feces	Hepatitis A
Hepatitis B virus	Blood and body fluids	Hepatitis B
Hepatitis C virus	Blood	Hepatitis C
Herpes simplex virus (type I)	Lesions of mouth or skin, saliva, genitalia	Cold sores, aseptic meningitis, genital herpes, herpetic whitlow
HIV	Blood, semen, vaginal secretions, breast milk (also isolated in saliva, tears, and urine, but not proved to be sources of transmission)	AIDS
Fungi		
Aspergillus organisms	Soil, dust, mouth, skin, colon, genital tract	Aspergillosis, pneumonia, sepsis
Candida albicans	Mouth, skin, colon, genital tract	Candidiasis, pneumonia, sepsis
Protozoa		
Plasmodium falciparum	Blood	Malaria

oxygen). Examples of aerobic organisms are *Staphylococcus aureus* and strains of *Streptococcus organisms*.

The gastrointestinal tract is colonized by large numbers of anaerobic bacteria, which can cause infections if the bowel is damaged. Infections deep within the pleural cavity, in a joint, or in a deep sinus tract are typically caused by anaerobes. Bacteria that cause tetanus, gas gangrene, and botulism are anaerobes.

Water. Most organisms require water or moisture for survival. For example, micro-organisms thrive in the moist drainage from a surgical wound. However, some bacteria assume a form called a *spore.* Spores remain viable even when deprived of water; they are resistant to drying. Spore-forming bacteria, such as those that cause anthrax, botulism, and tetanus, can live without water.

Temperature. Micro-organisms can live only in certain temperature ranges. The ideal temperature for most human pathogens is 35° C (Keroack & Rosen-Kotilainen, 1996). However, some can survive temperature extremes that would be fatal to humans. Cold temperatures tend to prevent growth and reproduction of bacteria.

pH. The acidity of an environment determines the viability of micro-organisms. Most micro-organisms prefer an environment within a pH range of 5 to 8. Bacteria in particular thrive in urine with an alkaline pH. Most organisms cannot survive the acid environment of the stomach. Acid-reducing medications (e.g., antacids and H_2 blockers) may cause an overgrowth of gastrointestinal organisms, which can contribute to nosocomial pneumonia in a client receiving these medications (Centers for Disease Control and Prevention [CDC], 2003b).

Minimal Light. Micro-organisms thrive in dark environments such as those under dressings and within body cavities. Ultraviolet light may be effective in killing certain forms of bacteria (e.g., *Mycobacterium tuberculosis*).

Portal of Exit. After micro-organisms find a site in which to grow and multiply, they must find a portal of exit if they are to enter another host and cause disease. A *portal of exit* is the path by which the pathogen leaves the reservoir (Sorrentino, 2004). Exits in the human body include body openings (mouth; nose; rectal, vaginal, and urethral openings; and artificial openings such as ostomies), breaks in the skin (a scrape, cut, or other wound), and breaks in the mucous membranes (the skin in the mouth, eyes, nose, vagina, and rectum). Pathogens are carried through portals of exit by blood, body fluids, excretions, and secretions (e.g., urine, stool, vomitus, saliva, mucus, pus, vaginal discharge,

Table 29-2 Modes of Transmission

Mode of transmission	Examples of Organisms
Contact Transmission	
The transfer of microbes by physical touch. May be by direct contact, indirect contact, or droplet.	
Direct contact	
Physical skin-to-skin contact between an infected or colonized individual and a susceptible host (e.g., touching client)	Hepatitis A virus, *Shigella, Staphylococcus,* Herpes simplex
Indirect contact	
Contact between a susceptible host and a contaminated intermediate object (e.g., touching soiled linen, equipment, dressings; transferring pathogens to a client via hands that are not washed between clients)	Hepatitis B virus, hepatitis C virus, *Staphylococcus,* respiratory syncytial virus (RSV), *Pseudomonas*
Droplet transmission	
Large particles (droplets) from the respiratory system of an infected source are propelled up to 1 m through the air and are deposited onto a susceptible host (e.g., coughing, sneezing, or talking produces droplets)	Influenza virus, rubella virus, SARS virus
Airborne Transmission	
Small airborne particles (droplet nuclei) containing microbes remain suspended in the air for long periods of time; air currents can then transmit these particles long distances (> 1 m), and a susceptible host may then inhale them (e.g., coughing and sneezing produces droplets as well as aeorsolized airborne particles)	*Mycobacterium tuberculosis* (TB), varicella zoster virus (chickenpox), *Aspergillus,* measles virus
Vehicle Transmission	
A single contaminated source (e.g., water, drugs, blood, food, equipment) transmits infection to multiple hosts, possibly resulting in an outbreak	*Pseudomonas* (water, drugs), *Escherichia coli* (food, water), Hepatitis B and C virus (blood), HIV (blood), *Salmonella* (food)
Vectorborne Transmission	
Insects (fleas, mites, ticks, mosquitoes) or pests (mice) transmit microbes to humans	*Vibrio cholerae, Plasmodium falciparum* (malaria), West Nile virus

Adapted from Health Canada. (1999). Routine practices and additional precautions for preventing the transmission of infection in health care. *Canada Communicable Disease Report, 25S4.*

semen, wound drainage, bile, and sputum). For example, pathogens that infect the respiratory tract, such as *M. tuberculosis,* can be released from the body through the mouth and nose when an infected person sneezes, coughs, talks, or even breathes. In clients with artificial airways such as tracheostomy or endotracheal tubes (see chapter 35), organisms easily exit the respiratory tract through these devices. Similarly, when a client has a urinary tract infection, micro-organisms exit during urination or through urinary diversions such as ileal conduits, urostomies, and suprapubic drains (see chapter 40).

Modes of Transmission. There are many modes for transmission of micro-organisms from the reservoir to the host. Certain infectious diseases tend to be transmitted more commonly by specific modes (Table 29-2). However, the same micro-organism may be transmitted by more than one mode. For example, herpes zoster may be spread by the airborne route or by direct contact.

Indirect contact is a major mode of transmission in health care facilities. In particular, the health care worker's hands can easily pick up microbes from one person, place, or thing and then transmit them to other people, places, or things. However, almost any object within the environment (e.g., a stethoscope or thermometer) can become a means of indirectly transmitting pathogens. All health care workers providing direct care (e.g., nurses, physiotherapists, and physicians) or performing diagnostic and support services (e.g., laboratory technicians, respiratory therapists, and dietary workers) must follow practices to minimize the spread of infection. Each group follows procedures for handling equipment and supplies used by a client. For example, respiratory therapists perform hand hygiene before working with each client and dispose of contaminated therapy equipment in a prescribed manner. Certain medical devices and diagnostic procedures provide avenues for the spread of pathogens. Invasive procedures such as cystoscopy (visualization of the bladder) facilitate diagnosis of problems but also increase the risk of transmitting infection. Because so many factors can promote the spread of infection to a client, all health care workers must be conscientious in using infection control practices, such as proper handwashing and ensuring that equipment has been adequately disinfected or sterilized.

Portal of Entry. Organisms can enter the body through the same routes they use for exiting (i.e., body openings and breaks in the skin or mucous membranes). For example, when a needle pierces the skin, organisms enter the body. More organisms enter the body as long as the device is in place. Any obstruction to the flow of urine from a urinary catheter allows organisms to travel up the urethra. Factors that reduce the body's defences enhance the chances of pathogens entering the body.

Susceptible Host. Whether a person acquires an infection depends on susceptibility to an infectious agent. **Susceptibility** depends on the individual degree of resistance to a pathogen. Although everyone is constantly in contact with large numbers of micro-organisms, an infection does not develop until an individual becomes susceptible to the strength and numbers of micro-organisms capable of producing infection. The more virulent an organism, the greater is the likelihood of a person's susceptibility. Organisms with resistance to antibiotics are becoming more common in acute care settings. This is believed to be associated with the frequent and sometimes inappropriate use of antibiotics. A person's resistance to an infectious agent is enhanced by vaccines or by actually contracting the disease.

The Infectious Process

By understanding the chain of infection, the nurse intervenes to prevent infections from developing. When the client acquires an infection, the nurse observes signs and symptoms of infection and takes appropriate actions to prevent its spread. Infections follow a progressive course (Box 29-1). The severity of the client's illness depends on the extent of the infection, the **pathogenicity** of the micro-organisms, and the susceptibility of the host.

If infection is **localized** (e.g., a wound infection), proper care controls the spread and minimizes the illness. The client may experience localized symptoms such as pain and tenderness at the wound site. An infection that affects the entire body instead of just a single organ or part is **systemic** and can be fatal.

The course of an infection influences the level of nursing care provided. The nurse is responsible for properly administering antibiotics and monitoring the response to drug therapy (see chapter 30). Supportive therapy includes providing adequate nutrition and rest to bolster defences against the infectious process. The complexity of care further depends on body systems affected by the infection.

Regardless of whether infection is localized or systemic, the nurse plays a critical role in minimizing its spread. For example, the organism causing a simple wound infection can spread to involve an intravenous (IV) needle insertion site if the nurse uses improper technique during an IV dressing change. Nurses who have breaks in their own skin can also acquire infections from clients if their techniques for controlling infection transmission are inadequate.

Defences Against Infection

The body has normal defences against infection. Normal body flora that reside inside and outside of the body protect a person from several pathogens. Each organ system has defence mechanisms that defend against exposure to infectious micro-organisms. The **inflammatory response** is a protective reaction that neutralizes pathogens and repairs body cells. The immune system is composed of separate cells and molecules that help the body resist disease. Certain responses of the immune system are non-specific, and protect against micro-organisms regardless of prior exposure (such as normal flora, body system defences, and inflammation) whereas others are specific defences against specific pathogens. If any of the body's defences fail, an infection can quickly progress to a serious health problem.

Normal Flora. The body normally contains micro-organisms that reside on the surface and deep layers of skin, in the saliva and oral mucosa, and in the gastrointestinal and genitourinary tracts. A person normally excretes trillions of microbes daily through the intestines. The skin also has a large population of resident flora. **Normal flora** do not usually cause disease when residing in their usual area of the body but instead participate in maintaining health.

Normal flora of the large intestine exist in large numbers without causing injury. Normal flora also secrete

Box 29-1 Course of Infection, by Stage

Incubation Period

- Interval between entrance of pathogen into body and appearance of first symptoms (e.g., chickenpox, 2–3 weeks; common cold, 1–2 days; influenza, 1–3 days; mumps, 15–18 days)

Prodromal Stage

- Interval from onset of non-specific signs and symptoms (malaise, low-grade fever, fatigue) to more specific symptoms (During this time, micro-organisms grow and multiply, and client may be more capable of spreading disease to others.)

Illness Stage

- Interval when client manifests signs and symptoms specific to type of infection (e.g., common cold manifested by sore throat, sinus congestion, rhinitis; mumps manifested by earache, high fever, parotid and salivary gland swelling)

Convalescence

- Interval when acute symptoms of infection disappear and the body tries to replenish its resources and return to a state of homeostasis; length of recovery depends on severity of infection and client's general state of health (recovery may take several days to months.)

antibacterial substances within the intestine's walls. The skin's normal flora exert a protective action by inhibiting multiplication of organisms landing on the skin. The mouth and pharynx are also protected by flora that impair growth of invading microbes. The mass of normal flora maintains a sensitive balance with other micro-organisms to prevent infection. Any factor that disrupts this balance places a person at increased risk for acquiring an infectious disease. For example, recent studies have determined that when a client acquires micro-organisms within the hospital, the person's resident flora changes, which may lead to an infection (Green, 1996; Health Canada, 1999). Also, the use of **broad-spectrum antibiotics** for the treatment of infection can lead to **superinfection.** A superinfection develops when broad-spectrum antibiotics eliminate a wide range of micro-organisms, not just those causing infection. Normal bacterial flora are eliminated, reducing the body's defences and thus allowing disease-producing micro-organisms to multiply.

Body System Defences. A number of the body's organ systems have unique defences against infection (Table 29-3). The skin, respiratory tract, and gastrointestinal tract are easily accessible to micro-organisms. Pathogenic organisms

Table 29-3 Normal Defence Mechanisms Against Infection

Defence Mechanisms	Action	Factors That May Alter Defence
Skin		
Intact multilayered surface (body's first line of defence against infection)	Provides barrier to micro-organisms and antibacterial activity	Cuts, abrasions, wounds, areas of maceration (softening of the skin due to moisture)
Shedding of outer layer of skin cells	Removes organisms that adhere to skin's outer layers	Failure to bathe regularly
Sebum	Contains fatty acid that kills some bacteria	Excessive bathing
Mouth		
Intact multilayered mucosa	Provides mechanical barrier to micro-organisms	Lacerations, trauma, extracted teeth
Saliva	Washes away particles containing micro-organisms, contains microbial inhibitors (e.g., lysozyme)	Poor oral hygiene, dehydration
Eye		
Tearing and blinking	Blinking prevents entry of particles containing pathogens, and tearing helps to wash particles away	Injury
Respiratory Tract		
Cilia lining upper airway, coated by mucus	Trap inhaled microbes and sweep them outward in mucus to be expectorated or swallowed	Smoking, high concentration of oxygen and carbon dioxide, decreased humidity, cold air
Macrophages	Engulf and destroy micro-organisms that reach lung's alveoli	Smoking
Urinary Tract		
Flushing action of urine flow	Washes away micro-organisms on lining of bladder and urethra	Obstruction to normal flow by urinary catheter placement, obstruction from growth or tumour, delayed micturition
Intact multilayered epithelium	Provides barrier to micro-organisms	Introduction of urinary catheter, continual movement of catheter in urethra
Gastrointestinal Tract		
Acidity of gastric secretions	Acids destroy some micro-organisms	Administration of antacids to neutralize acids
Increased peristalsis in small intestine	Prevents retention of bacterial contents	Delayed motility resulting from impaction of fecal contents in large bowel or mechanical obstruction by masses
Vagina		
At puberty, normal flora causing vaginal secretions to achieve low pH	Inhibit growth of many micro-organisms	Use of antibiotics or oral contraceptives, which disrupt normal flora

easily adhere to the skin's surface, are inhaled into the lungs, or are ingested with food. Each organ system has defence mechanisms physiologically suited to its structure and function. For example, the lungs cannot completely control the entrance of micro-organisms; however, the airways are lined with hairlike projections, or cilia, that rhythmically beat to move a blanket of mucus and adherent or trapped organisms up to the pharynx to be removed. Conditions that impair an organ's specialized defences increase susceptibility to infection.

Inflammation. Inflammation is the body's cellular response to injury or infection. Inflammation is a protective vascular reaction that delivers fluid, blood products, and nutrients to interstitial tissues in an area of injury. The process neutralizes and eliminates pathogens or dead **(necrotic)** tissues and establishes a means of repairing body cells and tissues. Signs of localized inflammation may include swelling, redness, heat, pain or tenderness, and loss of function in the affected body part. When inflammation becomes systemic, other signs and symptoms develop, including fever, leukocytosis, malaise, anorexia, nausea, vomiting, and lymph node enlargement.

The inflammatory response may be triggered by physical agents, chemical agents, or micro-organisms. Mechanical trauma, temperature extremes, and radiation are examples of physical agents. Chemical agents include external and internal irritants such as harsh poisons or gastric acid. Micro-organisms may trigger this response, as previously discussed.

After tissues are injured, a series of well-coordinated events occurs. The inflammatory response includes the following:

- Vascular and cellular responses
- Formation of inflammatory **exudates** (fluid and cells that are discharged from cells or blood vessels, e.g., pus or serum)
- Tissue repair

Vascular and Cellular Responses. Acute inflammation is an immediate response to cellular injury. Arterioles supplying the infected or injured area dilate, allowing more blood into the local circulation. The increase in local blood flow causes the characteristic redness of inflammation. The symptom of localized warmth results from a greater volume of blood at the inflammatory site. Local vasodilation delivers blood and white blood cells (WBCs) to injured tissues.

Injury causes tissue necrosis, and as a result, the body releases histamine, bradykinin, prostaglandin, and serotonin. These chemical mediators increase the permeability of small blood vessels. Fluid, protein, and cells enter interstitial spaces. Accumulated fluid appears as localized swelling **(edema).**

Another symptom of inflammation is pain. The swelling of inflamed tissues increases pressure on nerve endings, causing pain. Chemical substances such as histamine stimulate nerve endings. As a result of physiological changes occurring with inflammation, the involved body part usually undergoes a temporary loss of function. For example, a localized infection of the hand causes the fingers to become swollen, painful, and discoloured. Joints may become stiff as a result of swelling, but function of the fingers returns when inflammation subsides.

The cellular response of inflammation involves WBCs arriving at the site. WBCs pass through blood vessels and into the tissues. Through the process of **phagocytosis,** specialized WBCs, called neutrophils and monocytes, ingest and destroy micro-organisms or other small particles. As inflammation becomes systemic, other signs and symptoms develop. **Leukocytosis,** or an increase in the number of circulating WBCs, is the body's response to WBCs leaving blood vessels. A serum WBC count is normally 5,000 to 10,000/mm^3 but may rise to 15,000 to 20,000/mm^3 and higher during inflammation. Fever is caused by phagocytic release of pyrogens from bacterial cells that cause a rise in the hypothalamic set point (see chapter 27). Other systemic signs and symptoms include malaise, anorexia, and lymph node enlargement.

Inflammatory Exudate. Accumulation of fluid, dead tissue cells, and WBCs forms an exudate at the site of inflammation (see chapter 43). Exudate may be **serous** (clear, watery plasma), **sanguineous** (bloody drainage), **serosanguineous** (thin, watery drainage that is blood-tinged), or **purulent** (thick drainage that contains pus). Eventually, the exudate is cleared away through lymphatic drainage. Platelets and plasma proteins such as fibrinogen form a meshlike matrix at the site of inflammation to prevent its spread.

Tissue Repair. When there is injury to tissues, healing involves the inflammation, proliferation, and remodeling stages (see chapter 43). Damaged cells are eventually replaced with healthy new cells. The new cells undergo a gradual maturation until they take on the same structural characteristics and appearance as the previous cells. However, unless a wound is minor, the healed wound usually does not have the tensile strength of the tissue it replaces and scarring may occur.

Nosocomial Infections

Clients in health care settings have an increased risk of acquiring infections. A **nosocomial infection** is an infection acquired after admission to a health care facility. Nosocomial infections are especially common in hospitals (Forster et al., 2004). A hospital is one of the most likely places for acquiring an infection because it harbours a high population of virulent strains of micro-organisms that may be resistant to antibiotics. Also, clients in hospitals are at risk for infections because they have a high acuity of illness and frequently undergo aggressive treatments, many of which compromise immunity (Health Canada, 1999).

Iatrogenic infections are a type of nosocomial infection resulting from a diagnostic or therapeutic procedure. A urinary tract infection that develops after catheter insertion is an example of an iatrogenic nosocomial infection. The incidence of nosocomial infections can be reduced if nurses use critical thinking when practising aseptic techniques. The nurse should always consider the client's risks for infection and anticipate how the approach to care may increase or decrease the chances of infection transmission.

Box 29-2 Sites for and Causes of Nosocomial Infections

Urinary Tract

Inappropriate and unsterile catheterization techniques
Inadequate monitoring of indwelling urinary catheters
Obstruction or blockages in tubing
Improper specimen collection technique
Urine in catheter or drainage tube being allowed to re-enter bladder (reflux)
Improper hand hygiene

Surgical or Traumatic Wounds

Improper skin preparation (shaving and bathing) before surgery
Failure to cleanse skin surface properly
Failure to use aseptic technique during dressing changes
Use of contaminated antiseptic solutions
Improper hand hygiene

Respiratory Tract

Contaminated respiratory therapy equipment
Failure to use aseptic technique while suctioning airway
Improper disposal of secretions
Improper hand hygiene

Bloodstream

Contamination of IV fluids by tubing or needle changes
Insertion of drug additives to IV fluid
Addition of connecting tube or stopcocks to IV system
Improper care of needle insertion site
Contaminated needles or catheters
Failure to change IV access site when inflammation first appears
Improper technique during administration of multiple blood products
Improper care of peritoneal or hemodialysis shunts
Improper hand hygiene

Nosocomial infections may be exogenous or endogenous. An **exogenous infection** arises from micro-organisms external to the individual that do not exist as normal flora; examples are *Salmonella* organisms and *Clostridium tetani*. An **endogenous infection** can occur when part of the client's flora becomes altered and overgrowth results. Examples are infections caused by enterococci, yeasts, and streptococci. When sufficient numbers of micro-organisms normally found in one body cavity or lining are transferred to another body site, an endogenous infection develops. For example, transmission of enterococci, normally found in fecal material, from the hands to the skin is a common cause of wound infections. The number of micro-organisms needed to cause a nosocomial infection depends on the virulence of the organism, the host's susceptibility, and the site affected.

The risk of infection is influenced by the number of health care workers having direct contact with a client, the type and number of invasive procedures, the therapy received, and the length of hospitalization. Major sites for nosocomial infection include surgical or traumatic wounds, urinary and respiratory tracts, and the bloodstream (Box 29-2).

Older adults have increased susceptibility to these infections because of their affinity to chronic disease and the aging process itself (Box 29-3). Extended stays in health care institutions, increased disability, and prolonged recovery times are all potential outcomes of nosocomial infections. Nosocomial infections decrease the client's quality of life and increase costs to the health care system. Therefore, prevention of nosocomial infection is an important part of managed care.

Focus on Older Adults — Box 29-3

- An age-related decline in immune system function, termed *immune senescence,* increases the body's susceptibility to infection and lessens the strength of the overall immune response (Eliopoulos, 2001).
- Chronic disease, prevalent among older adults, allows infectious agents to readily invade; hospitalization and institutionalization because of these chronic diseases also increase older adults' exposure to pathogens (Eliopoulos, 2001).
- Risks associated with the development of nosocomial infections in older clients include poor nutrition, unintentional weight loss, and low serum albumin levels (Lueckenotte, 2000).
- Age-related changes in immunity contribute to the increased risk of acquiring pneumonia and influenza in older adulthood, both of which have significant age-related increases in mortality rates (Miller, 1999).

Data from *Gerontologic Nursing* (5th ed., by C. Eliopoulos, 2001, Philadelphia: Lippincott; *Nursing Care of Older Adults: Theory and Practice* (3rd ed., by Miller, 1999, Philadelphia: Lippincott; and *Gerontologic Nursing* (2nd ed., by Lueckenotte, 2000, St. Louis, MO: Mosby.

The Nursing Process in Infection Control

NP Assessment

The nurse assesses the client's defence mechanisms, susceptibility, and knowledge of infections. A review of disease history with the client and family may reveal an exposure to a communicable disease. A thorough review of the client's clinical condition may detect signs and symptoms of actual infection or risk for infection. An analysis of laboratory findings provides information about a client's defence against infection. By knowing the factors that increase susceptibility or risk for infection, the nurse is better able to plan preventive therapy that includes aseptic techniques. By recognizing early signs and symptoms of infection, the nurse can alert others on the health

Box 29-4 Risk Factors for Infection

Inadequate Primary Defences

Broken skin or mucosa
Traumatized tissue
Decreased ciliary action
Obstructed urine outflow
Altered peristalsis
Change in pH of secretions
Decreased mobility

Inadequate Secondary Defences

Reduced hemoglobin level
Suppression of WBCs (drug or disease related)
Suppressed inflammatory response (drug or disease related)
Low WBC count (leukopenia)

care team to the potential need for therapy and initiate supportive nursing measures.

Status of Defence Mechanisms. A review of physical assessment findings and the client's medical condition reveals the status of normal defence mechanisms against infection. For example, any break in the skin or mucosa is a potential site for infection. Similarly, a chronic smoker is at greater risk for acquiring a respiratory tract infection after general surgery because the cilia of the lung are less likely to propel retained mucus from the lung's airways. Any reduction in the body's primary or secondary defences against infection places a client at risk (Box 29-4).

Client Susceptibility. Many factors influence susceptibility to infection. The nurse gathers information about each factor through the client's and family's history.

Age. Throughout the lifespan, susceptibility to infection changes. An infant has immature defences against infection. Born with only the antibodies provided by the mother, the infant's immune system is incapable of producing the necessary immunoglobulins and WBCs to adequately fight some infections. However, breast-fed infants have greater immunity than bottle-fed infants because they receive the mother's antibodies through the breast milk. As the child grows, the immune system matures, but the child is still susceptible to organisms that cause the common cold, intestinal infections, and, if not vaccinated, infectious diseases such as mumps and measles.

The young or middle-age adult has refined defences against infection. Normal flora, body system defences, inflammation, and the immune response provide protection against invading micro-organisms. Viruses are the most common cause of infectious illness in young or middle-age adults.

Defences against infection may change with aging (Gantz, Tkatch, & Makris, 2000). The immune response, particularly cell-mediated immunity, declines. Older adults also undergo alterations in the structure and function of the skin, urinary tract, and lungs. For example, the skin loses its turgor and the epithelium thins. As a result, the skin is more easily abraded or torn. This increases the potential for invasion by pathogens (Table 29-4).

Nutritional Status. When protein intake is inadequate as a result of poor diet or debilitating disease, the rate of protein breakdown exceeds that of tissue synthesis (see chapter 39). A reduction in the intake of protein and other nutrients such as carbohydrates and fats reduces the body's defences against infection and impairs wound healing (see chapter 43).

Clients with illnesses or problems that increase protein requirements are at further risk. These problems include traumatic injury, extensive burns, and conditions causing fever. Clients who have had surgery also require increased protein.

The nurse assesses clients' dietary intakes and abilities to tolerate solid foods. Clients who have difficulty with swallowing, who experience alterations in digestion, or who are too confused or weak to feed themselves are at risk for inadequate dietary intake. A dietitian may be called to assess the nutritional adequacy of the diet. In preparation for discharge, the nurse evaluates the client's and family's understanding of nutritional needs.

Stress. The body responds to emotional or physical stress by the general adaptation syndrome (see chapter 26). During the alarm stage, the basal metabolic rate increases as the body uses energy stores. Adrenocorticotropic hormone acts to increase serum glucose levels and decrease unnecessary anti-inflammatory responses through the release of cortisone. If stress continues or becomes intense, elevated cortisone levels result in decreased resistance to infection. Continued stress leads to exhaustion, wherein energy stores are depleted and the body has no resistance to invading organisms. The same conditions that increase nutritional requirements, such as surgery or trauma, also increase physiological stress.

Disease Process. Clients with diseases of the immune system are at particular risk for infection. Leukemia, AIDS, lymphoma, and aplastic anemia are conditions that compromise a host by weakening defences against infectious organisms. Clients with leukemia, for example, are unable to produce normal WBCs to effectively ward off infection.

Clients with chronic diseases such as diabetes mellitus and multiple sclerosis are also more susceptible to infection because of general debilitation and nutritional impairment. Diseases that impair body system defences, such as emphysema and bronchitis (which impair ciliary action and thicken mucus), cancer (which alters the immune response), and peripheral vascular disease (which reduces blood flow to injured tissues), increase susceptibility to infection. Clients with burns have a very high susceptibility to infection because of the damage to skin surfaces. The greater the depth and extent of the burns, the higher the risk for infection.

Medical Therapy. Some drugs and medical therapies compromise immunity to infection. The nurse assesses

Table 29-4 Assessing the Risk of Infection in Older Adults

Component	Possible Changes With Age	Possible Outcome
Skin	Thinner dermal and epidermal layers, decreased collagen strength, decreased skin elasticity, decreased sweat	Pressure ulcers
Peripheral nerves	Reduced sensitivity, particularly in clients with history of alcohol abuse, vitamin B_{12} deficiency, and diabetes mellitus	Pressure ulcers, clients unaware of trauma to skin leading to infection
Circulation	Congestive heart failure, calcified mitral and aortic valves	Pneumonia, bacterial endocarditis
Peripheral circulation	Loss of elasticity of veins (prone to distension), less effective venous valves, blood pooling in lower extremities	Venous stasis ulcers
Mouth	Dehydration, reduction in saliva production, functional inability to maintain oral hygiene	Parotid gland infection, periodontal disease, localized abscess, bacteremia (i.e., bacteria in the blood)
Gastrointestinal tract	Loss of ability to secrete stomach acid in 30% of people over age 70	Salmonella diarrhea
Pulmonary system	Increased colonization of oropharynx, impaired mucociliary clearance, decreased macrophage function, decreased cough reflex	Viral and bacterial pneumonia
Urinary tract	Prostatic hypertrophy or hyperplasia, urethral strictures, age-related hormonal changes in vaginal wall, pelvic floor relaxation, ureterocele or cystocele, degeneration of nerves leading to neurogenic bladder, use of tricyclic antidepressants, dehydration	Asymptomatic bacteriuria (i.e., bacteria in the urine), cystitis, pyelonephritis
Nutrition	Malnutrition, vitamin deficiency (vitamin A, vitamin C, pyridoxine, and riboflavin), protein and caloric deficiencies	Impaired immune response to infection
Drug therapy	Corticosteroid and cytotoxic drugs	Impaired immune response to infection
Long-term care residency	Exposure to nosocomial infections, including influenza, *Proteus* and *Providencia* organisms with an indwelling catheter, tuberculosis, and wound infections (incidence of bacteremia after admission is 50%.)	Frequent serious infection, increased risk of pneumonia

Data from "Geriatric Infections," by N. M. Gantz, L. S. Tkatch, and A. T. Makris, in *APIC Text of Infection Control and Epidemiology,* 2000, Washington, DC: Association for Professionals in Infection Control and Epidemiology.

the client's history to determine whether the client takes medications at home that increase infection susceptibility. A review of therapies received within the health care setting further reveals risks. Adrenal corticosteroids, prescribed for several conditions, are anti-inflammatory drugs that cause protein breakdown and impair the inflammatory response against bacteria and other pathogens. Cytotoxic or antineoplastic drugs attack cancer cells but cause side effects of bone marrow depression and normal cell toxicity. With bone marrow depression, the body is unable to produce lymphocytes and sufficient WBCs. When normal cells become altered by antineoplastic agents, cellular defences against infection fail. Cyclosporine and other immunosuppressant drugs, which decrease the body's immune response, are commonly taken by organ transplant recipients. The immunosuppressants prevent organ and tissue rejection, but they also increase susceptibility to infection.

Clients with cancer who are receiving radiotherapy are also at risk for infection. The massive doses of radiation, which destroy cancerous cells, can also depress the bone marrow and destroy normal cells.

Clinical Appearance. The signs and symptoms of infection may be local or systemic. Localized infections are most common in areas of skin or mucous membrane breakdown, such as surgical and traumatic wounds, pressure ulcers, and mouth lesions. Infections also develop locally in cavities beneath the skin; an example is an abscess.

To assess an area for localized infection, the nurse first inspects the area for redness and swelling caused by inflammation. Because there may be drainage from open lesions or wounds, the nurse wears disposable gloves. Infected drainage may be yellow, green, or brown, depending on the pathogen. The nurse asks the client about pain or tenderness around the site. The client may complain of tightness and pain caused by edema. If the infected area is large enough, movement of a body part may be restricted. Gentle palpation of an infected area usually results in some degree of tenderness.

Systemic infections cause more generalized symptoms than local infection. They usually result in fever, fatigue, and malaise. Lymph nodes that drain the area of infection often become enlarged, swollen, and tender during palpation. For example, an abscess in the peritoneal cavity may cause enlargement of lymph nodes in the groin. An infection of the upper respiratory tract may cause cervical lymph node enlargement. If an infection is serious and widespread, all major lymph nodes may enlarge. Systemic infections commonly cause loss of appetite, nausea, and vomiting.

Table 29-5 Laboratory Tests to Screen for Infection

Laboratory Value	Normal (Adult) Values	Indication of Infection
WBC count	4–11 × 10^9/L	Increased in acute infection, decreased in certain viral or overwhelming infections
Erythrocyte sedimentation rate	Up to 15 mm/hour for men and 20 mm/hour for women	Elevated in presence of inflammatory process
Iron level	60–90 g/100 mL	Decreased in chronic infection
Cultures of urine and blood	Normally sterile, without micro-organism growth	Presence of infectious micro-organism growth
Cultures and gram stain of wound, sputum, and throat	No WBCs on gram stain, possible normal flora	Presence of infectious micro-organism growth and WBCs on gram stain
Differential Count (Percentage of Each Type of WBC)		
Neutrophils	55%–70%	Increased in acute suppurative infection, decreased in overwhelming bacterial infection (older adult)
Lymphocytes	20%–40%	Increased in chronic bacterial and viral infection, decreased in sepsis
Monocytes	2%–8%	Increased in protozoal, rickettsial, and tuberculosis infections
Eosinophils	1%–4%	Increased in parasitic infection
Basophils	0.5%–1%	Normal during infection

Systemic infections may develop after treatment for localized infection has failed. The nurse should be alert for changes in the client's level of activity and responsiveness. As systemic infections develop, the client may become lethargic and complain of a loss of energy. An elevation in body temperature may lead to episodes of increased heart and respiratory rates and low blood pressure. Involvement of major body systems may produce specific signs. For example, a pulmonary infection may result in a productive cough with purulent sputum. A urinary tract infection may result in cloudy, foul-smelling urine.

An infection in older adults may not present with typical signs and symptoms. Fever, pain, and swelling are often absent in older adults because they tend to have lower body temperatures, decreased pain sensation, and less immune response to infection. As a result, older adults often have advanced infection before it is identified. Atypical symptoms such as a change in behaviour (e.g., new or increased confusion, incontinence, or agitation) may be the only symptoms of an infectious illness (Gantz et al., 2000). For example, as many as 20% of older adults with pneumonia do not have the typical signs and symptoms of fever, shaking, chills, and rusty productive sputum. The only symptoms may be an increased, unexplained heart rate, confusion, or generalized fatigue.

Laboratory Data. A review of laboratory test results may confirm infection (Table 29-5). Laboratory values, however, are not enough to detect infection. Other clinical signs must be assessed. Factors other than infection may alter test values. For example, trauma and physical stress can cause an elevation in the number of neutrophils. A culture result may show growth of an organism in the absence of overt signs of infection.

Clients With Infection. A client with infection may have a variety of health problems. The nurse assesses ways that the infection affects the client's and family's needs. These needs may be physical, psychological, social, or economical. For example, a client with a chronic disease such as AIDS may experience serious psychological problems as a result of self-imposed isolation or rejection by family and friends. The nurse, using a case-management approach, determines the client's and family's ability to adjust to the disease and the available resources needed for managing health care challenges (Grimes & Grimes, 1994).

NP Nursing Diagnosis

During assessment, the nurse gathers objective findings, such as an open incision or a reduced caloric intake, and subjective data, such as a client's complaint of tenderness over a surgical wound site (Box 29-5). Then the nurse interprets the data carefully, looking for clusters of defining characteristics or risk factors that create a pattern suggesting a specific nursing diagnosis. The following are examples of nursing diagnoses that may apply:

- Disturbed body image
- Risk for infection
- Risk for injury
- Imbalanced nutrition: less than body requirements
- Impaired oral mucous membrane
- Risk for impaired skin integrity
- Social isolation
- Impaired tissue integrity

It may be necessary for the nurse to validate data (e.g., by inspecting the integrity of a wound more carefully). Likewise, additional data such as laboratory findings may be helpful. The selection of appropriate nursing diagnoses depends on analyzing and organizing data correctly.

The diagnosis must have the appropriate etiological factor for the nurse to establish an appropriate and well-thought-out plan. For example, minimizing the *risk for*

Nursing Diagnostic Process — Box 29-5

Assessment Activities	Defining Characteristics	Nursing Diagnosis
Check results of laboratory tests.	WBC count 3.9×10^9/L	Risk for infection related to lowered immunity
Review current medications.	Client receiving azathioprine (Imuran), an immunosuppressant	
Identify potential sites of infection.	IV catheter in right forearm, in place for 3 days Foley catheter draining amber-coloured urine	

infection related to broken skin requires good hygiene measures and wound care. Minimizing the *risk for infection related to malnutrition* requires good nutritional support and fluid balance.

The nurse may diagnose a risk for infection or make diagnoses that result from the effects of infection on health status. The nurse's success in planning appropriate nursing interventions depends on the accuracy of the diagnosis and the ability to meet the client's needs.

Planning

Goals and Outcomes. The client's care plan is based on each nursing diagnosis and related factor (see Care Plan). The nurse develops a plan that sets attainable outcomes so that interventions are purposeful and directed. The nurse caring for the client with the nursing diagnosis of *risk for infection related to broken skin* implements skin and wound care measures to promote healing. The expected outcomes of "reduction in wound size by 1 cm" and "absence of drainage" set targets for measuring the client's improvement. Once outcomes are met, the goal of "skin intact and without drainage" can be reached. Interventions are selected in collaboration with the client, the family, and others on the health care team. The nurse directs the care in the acute care setting and may involve other professionals in assisting with instruction on procedures that need to be followed after discharge. Common goals of care relating to infection may include the following:

- Preventing exposure to infectious organisms
- Controlling or reducing the extent of infection
- Maintaining resistance to infection
- Educating the client and family about infection control techniques

Setting Priorities. The nurse, in collaboration with the client, establishes priorities for the goals of care. For example, a client has an open wound, has cancer, and cannot tolerate solid foods. The priority of administering therapies that promote wound healing exceeds the goal of educating the client to assume self-care therapies at home. When the client's condition improves, the priorities will change, and client education becomes an essential intervention.

Continuity of Care. The development of a care plan includes infection prevention practices. The nurse may initiate appropriate referrals, such as to a dietitian, infection control professional, or home care nurse, to collaborate in the client's care. When care is being administered in the home, the nurse ensures the environment supports good infection control practices. For example, if a client does not have running water, the nurse will bring a waterless antimicrobial solution during visits to ensure adequate hand hygiene. Educating clients and families is also an important aspect of prevention.

Implementation

By recognizing and assessing a client's risk factors and implementing appropriate measures, the nurse can reduce the risk of infection.

Health Promotion. The nurse may prevent an infection from developing or spreading by minimizing the numbers and kinds of organisms transmitted to potential infection sites. Eliminating reservoirs of infection, controlling portals of exit and entry, and avoiding actions that transmit micro-organisms prevent pathogens from finding a new site in which to grow. Proper use of sterile supplies, barrier protection, and proper hand hygiene are examples of methods that nurses use to control the spread of micro-organisms. A final preventive measure is to strengthen a potential host's defences against infection. Nutritional support, rest, maintenance of physiological protective mechanisms, and receiving recommended immunizations protect a client from invasion by pathogens (Box 29-6).

Being vigilant about infection control helps the nurse to apply good medical-surgical aseptic practices at the right time and in the right clinical situation. When a client develops an infection, the nurse continues preventive care so that health care personnel and other clients are not exposed to the infection. Clients with communicable diseases may require isolation precautions that control the environment by forming barriers against transmission of infection (see Isolation Guidelines).

Acute Care Measures. Treatment of an infectious process includes eliminating the infectious organisms and supporting the client's defences. To identify the causative

Nursing Care Plan

Risk for Infection

Assessment

Mrs. Spicer was admitted to the medical nursing unit 3 days ago with a diagnosis of lymphoma. She received her first dose of multi-agent chemotherapy yesterday. Jess Ralston is the student nurse caring for Mrs. Spicer. He begins his shift by conducting a focused assessment.

Assessment Activities	Findings/Defining Characteristics
Review client's chart for laboratory data reflecting immune function.	Data show a reduction in number of WBCs (leukopenia).
Ask client to describe appetite and review food intake for last 24 hours. Weigh client. Measure height.	Client reports she has not had an interest in eating for a couple of weeks. She has lost approximately 2.5 kg. Her current weight is 57 kg, height 170 cm. Her food intake yesterday consisted of a small cup of applesauce, $^{1}/_{2}$ bowl of soup, some crackers, and two glasses of juice. Client states, "I get full easily and lose interest in food."
Palpate client's cervical and clavicular lymph nodes.	Lymph nodes are enlarged and painless.
Review effects of chemotherapy in drug reference.	Multi-agent chemotherapy causes drug-induced pancytopenia.

Nursing Diagnosis: Risk for infection related to immunosuppression and reduced food intake.

Planning

Goal	Expected Outcomes*
	Risk Detection
Client will remain free of infection.	Client will remain afebrile. Client will develop no signs or symptoms of local infection (e.g., remains free of cough, cloudy or foul-smelling urine, or purulent drainage from open wound or normal body opening).
	Knowledge: Infection Control
Client will become knowledgeable of infection risks.	Client will identify routines to follow in the home that reduce transmission of micro-organisms. Client will identify signs and symptoms to report to health care provider indicating infection.

*Outcome classification labels from *Nursing Outcomes Classification (NOC)* (3rd ed.), edited by S. Moorhead, M. Johnson, and M. Maas, 2004, St. Louis, MO: Mosby.

Interventions†	Rationale
Prevention and Early Detection	
Monitor client's body temperature routinely, inspect oral cavity for lesions, inspect urethral and vaginal orifices for drainage or discharge, inspect IV access site for drainage, and observe client for evidence of cough.	Interventions are designed to prevent and ensure early detection of infection in a client at risk (Dochterman & Bulechek, 2004).
Practise hand hygiene routinely before caring for client, between clients, and before any invasive procedures.	Rigorous hand hygiene reduces bacterial counts on the hands (Boyce & Pittet, 2002).
Teach client how to perform hand hygiene correctly.	Client can easily come in contact with infectious agents that can cause infection.
Consult with dietitian in providing a high-calorie, high-protein, low-bacteria diet. Minimize intake of salads, undercooked meat, pepper, paprika, and raw fruits and vegetables. Offer small frequent meals.	Maintaining calorie and protein intake will prevent weight loss. Foods high in bacteria should be avoided because they increase risk for gastrointestinal infection (Ignatavicius & Workman, 2002).
Infection Control	
Instruct client to report the following to physician: temperature greater than 38°C, persistent cough with or without sputum, pus or foul-smelling drainage from body site, presence of abscess, urine that is cloudy or foul smelling, or burning on urination.	Signs and symptoms are indicative of local or systemic infection.

†Intervention classification labels from *Nursing Interventions Classification (NIC)* (4th ed.), edited by J. M. Dochterman and G. M. Bulechek, 2004, St. Louis, MO: Mosby.

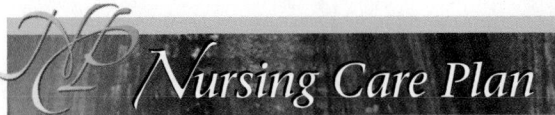

Nursing Care Plan

Risk for Infection—cont'd

Interventions†—cont'd	Rationale
Infection Controls—cont'd Teach client to follow these activities at home: • Avoid crowds and large gatherings of people. • Bathe daily. • Do not share personal hygiene items with family (toothbrush, washcloth, deodorant stick). • Take temperature twice daily. • Do not drink water that has been standing for longer than 15 minutes. • Do not reuse cups or glasses without washing.	These measures are designed to prevent infection in clients with impaired immune function (Ignatavicius & Workman, 2002).

†Intervention classification labels from *Nursing Interventions Classification (NIC)* (4th ed.), edited by J. M. Dochterman and G. M. Bulechek, 2004, St. Louis, MO: Mosby.

Evaluation

Nursing Actions	Client Response/Finding	Achievement of Outcome
Compare client's body temperature and other physical findings with baseline data.	Client remains afebrile and denies having cough or burning on urination. No signs of drainage or discharge from body site.	Client has no active infection at this time.
Ask client to describe signs and symptoms to report to health care provider.	Client able to identify temperature range to report. Client able to describe cough. Unable to identify signs of urinary infection or local discharge.	Client has partial understanding of signs and symptoms to report. Will require additional instruction. Offer information sheet.
Ask client to explain the measures to take at home to reduce exposure to infectious agents.	Client able to discuss need to avoid sharing personal hygiene articles. Asked for a listing of other precautions and requested that husband be included in discussion.	Client has partial understanding of restrictions. Will obtain printed guidelines and include husband in discussion this evening.

Box 29-6

Focus on Primary Health Care

Immunizations

Immunizations are an essential component of disease prevention. The nurse encourages proper immunization of infants, children, those at risk, and older adults. In Canada, most provinces provide free-of-charge immunization to infants against measles, mumps, rubella, diphtheria, tetanus, acellular pertussis, and poliomyelitis. Parents may have to pay to have their infant or child vaccinated for haemophilus influenza type b (Hib), varicella, and hepatitis B.

Older adults and those who are at risk (including health care workers) are offered influenza vaccinations each year. The nurse should remind clients of the importance of having a tetanus-diphtheria booster every 10 years.

In most provinces and territories, public health nurses or community nurses hold free immunization clinics for those at risk when there is an outbreak of a potentially deadly infection such as bacterial meningitis.

From *Canadian Immunization Guide* (6th ed.) Health Canada, 2002, Ottawa, ON: Author.

organism, the nurse may collect specimens of body fluids or drainage from infected body sites for cultures. When the disease process or causative organism has been identified, the physician prescribes the treatment that is most effective for the situation. The nurse properly administers antibiotics and other treatments, watching for adverse reactions and assessing the progress of the infection.

Systemic infections require measures to prevent complications of fever (see chapter 27). Maintaining intake of fluids prevents dehydration resulting from diaphoresis. The client's increased metabolic rate requires an adequate nutritional intake. Rest preserves energy for the healing process.

Localized infections often require measures to remove debris to promote healing. The nurse applies principles of wound care to remove infected drainage from wound sites and support the integrity of healing wounds. Special dressings can be applied to facilitate removal of infectious drainage and promote healing of wound margins. Drainage tubes may be inserted to remove infected drainage from body cavities. The nurse uses medical and surgical aseptic techniques to manage wounds and ensure correct handling of all drainage or body fluids (see chapter 43).

During the course of infection, the nurse supports the client's body defence mechanisms. For example, if a client has infectious diarrhea, the nurse must maintain skin integrity to prevent breakdown and the entrance of micro-organisms. Other routine hygiene measures such as bathing and oral care protect the skin and mucous membranes from invasion and overgrowth of micro-organisms.

Asepsis. The nurse's efforts to minimize the onset and spread of infection are based on the principles of aseptic technique. **Asepsis** is the absence of pathogenic (disease-producing) micro-organisms. Aseptic technique refers to practices that keep a client as free from pathogens as possible. The two types of aseptic technique are medical asepsis and surgical asepsis.

Medical asepsis, or clean technique, includes procedures used to reduce and prevent the spread of micro-organisms. Hand hygiene, using clean gloves (i.e., disposable gloves) to prevent direct contact with blood or body fluids, and cleaning the environment routinely are examples of medical asepsis. Principles of medical asepsis are commonly followed in the home, as in washing hands before preparing food.

After an object becomes unsterile or unclean, it is considered contaminated. In medical asepsis, an area or object is considered contaminated if it contains or is suspected of containing pathogens. For example, a used bedpan, the floor, and a used dressing are contaminated.

The nurse follows certain principles and procedures, including **standard precautions** (also known as **routine practices**) to prevent infection and control its spread (see Isolation Guidelines). During daily routine care, the nurse uses basic medical aseptic techniques to break the infection chain. Because infections are readily transmissible between clients and caregivers, it may become necessary for the nurse to follow **isolation precautions** as appropriate (see Isolation Guidelines).

The nurse is responsible for providing the client with a safe environment. The effectiveness of infection control practices depends on the nurse's conscientiousness and consistency in using effective aseptic technique. It is easy to forget key procedural steps or, when hurried, to take shortcuts that break aseptic procedures. However, the nurse's failure to be meticulous will place the client at risk for an infection that can seriously impair recovery or lead to death.

Control or Elimination of Infectious Agents. Proper cleansing, disinfection, and sterilization of contaminated objects significantly reduce and often eliminate micro-organisms. In health care centres, a sterile processing department disinfects and sterilizes reusable supplies. However, the nurse also may be required to perform these functions. Many principles of cleaning and disinfection also apply to the home.

Cleaning. Cleaning is the physical removal of foreign material (e.g., dust, soil, and organic material such as blood, secretions, excretions, and microorganisms) from objects and surfaces (Health Canada, 1998). Generally, cleaning involves use of water and mechanical action with detergents or enzymatic products. When an object comes in contact with infectious or potentially infectious material, the object is contaminated. Reusable objects must be cleaned thoroughly before reuse and then either disinfected or sterilized according to the manufacturer's recommendations.

When cleaning equipment that is soiled by organic material such as blood, fecal matter, mucus, or pus, the nurse should take appropriate measures to protect self-contamination. These may include wearing a mask and protective eyewear (or a face shield), and waterproof gloves. These barriers provide protection from infectious organisms. A brush and detergent or soap are needed for cleaning. The following steps ensure that an object is clean:

1. Rinse a contaminated object or article with cold running water to remove organic material. Hot water causes the protein in organic material to coagulate and stick to objects, making removal difficult.
2. After rinsing, wash the object with soap and warm water. Soap or detergent reduces the surface tension of water and emulsifies dirt or remaining material. Rinse the object thoroughly to remove the emulsified dirt.
3. Use a brush to remove dirt or material in grooves or seams. Friction dislodges contaminated material for easy removal. Open any hinged items for cleaning.
4. Rinse the object in warm water.
5. Dry the object and prepare it for disinfection or sterilization if indicated by the intended use of the item.
6. The brush, gloves, and sink in which the equipment is cleaned should be considered contaminated and should be cleaned and dried.

Disinfection and Sterilization. **Disinfection** is the elimination of all pathogens except bacterial spores (Health Canada, 1998). Disinfectants are used on inanimate objects; antiseptics are used on living tissue. Disinfection usually involves chemicals, heat, or ultraviolet light. An item must be thoroughly cleaned before it is disinfected. Examples of disinfectants are alcohols, chlorines, glutaraldehydes, and phenols. These chemicals can be caustic and toxic to tissues.

Sterilization is the destruction of all micro-organisms, including spores. Steam under pressure, ethylene oxide gas, hydrogen peroxide plasma, and chemicals are the most common sterilizing agents. Items must be cleaned thoroughly before they can be sterilized.

Whether an item is to be simply cleaned, or cleaned and disinfected or sterilized, depends on the intended use of the item. There are three categories of device classification (Box 29-7). Nurses should be familiar with agency policy and procedures for cleaning, handling, and delivering care items for eventual disinfection and sterilization. Workers especially trained in disinfection and sterilization should perform most of the procedures. Efficacy of the disinfecting or sterilizing method is influenced by the following factors:

- *Concentration of solution and duration of contact.* A weakened concentration or shortened exposure time may lessen effectiveness.
- *Type and number of pathogens.* Certain organisms are killed more easily than others by disruption. The greater the number of pathogens on an object, the longer the required disinfecting time.
- *Surface areas to treat.* All dirty surfaces and areas must be fully exposed to disinfecting and sterilizing agents.
- *Temperature of the environment.* Disinfectants tend to work best at room temperature.
- *Presence of soap.* Soap may cause certain disinfectants to be ineffective. Thorough rinsing of an object is necessary before disinfecting.

Box 29-7 Categories for Sterilization, Disinfection, and Cleaning

Critical Items

Critical items are instruments and devices that enter sterile tissue or the vascular system. They present a high risk of infection if the items are contaminated with micro-organisms, including bacterial spores. Critical items must be thoroughly cleaned and sterilized. Examples of these items include:

- Surgical instruments
- Intravascular catheters
- Urinary catheters
- Needles

Semi-critical Items

Semi-critical items are devices that come in contact with mucous membranes or nonintact skin but do not penetrate them. These items also present risk of infection and must be free of all micro-organisms (except bacterial spores). Semi-critical items must be thoroughly cleaned and disinfected. Examples of these items include:

- Electronic thermometers
- Respiratory therapy equipment
- Endotracheal tubes
- Gastrointestinal endoscopes
- Vaginal and nasal specula

Non-critical Items

Non-critical items are items that either touch only intact skin but not mucous membranes or do not directly touch the client. Non-critical items must be cleaned or cleaned and disinfected. Examples of these items include:

- Bedpans, urinals, commodes
- Blood pressure cuffs
- Linens
- Stethoscopes
- Eating utensils

- *Presence of organic materials.* Disinfectants can become inactivated unless blood, saliva, pus, or body excretions are washed off.

Table 29-6 lists processes for disinfection and sterilization and their characteristics. Selection of the method for disinfecting or sterilizing an item depends on the intended use of the item and the nature of the item (e.g., some delicate instruments requiring sterilization cannot tolerate steam and must be processed using gas or plasma).

Control or Elimination of Reservoirs. To control or eliminate reservoir sites for infection, the nurse eliminates or controls sources of body fluids, drainage, or solutions that might harbour micro-organisms. The nurse also carefully discards articles that become contaminated with infectious material (Box 29-8). All health care institutions must have guidelines for the disposal of infectious waste according to provincial or territorial laws.

Control of Portals of Exit. The nurse follows measures to minimize or prevent infectious organisms from exiting the body. To control organisms exiting via the respiratory tract, the nurse should wear a mask as needed, avoid talking directly into clients' faces, and never talk, sneeze, or cough directly over surgical wounds or sterile dressing fields. The nurse should cover the mouth or nose when sneezing or coughing. The nurse is also responsible for teaching clients to protect others when they sneeze or cough and for providing clients with disposable wipes or tissues to control the spread of micro-organisms.

A nurse who has an upper respiratory tract infection should consider not working and may be required to remain at home. If the nurse continues to work with clients, he or she should wear a mask when working closely with the client and pay special attention to hand hygiene. The same nurse should not be caring for clients who are highly susceptible to infection (e.g., an immunosuppressed client or a neonate).

Another way of controlling the exit of micro-organisms is through the careful handling of blood, body fluids, secretions, or excretions (e.g., urine, feces, vomitus, exudate). Contaminated fluids can easily splash while being discarded or cleaned up. The nurse should always wear disposable gloves when handling blood, body fluids, secretions, or excretions. Masks, gowns, and protective eyewear are worn if there is a possibility of splashing or contact with any fluids. The nurse appropriately disposes of disposable soiled items in impervious plastic bags. Laboratory specimens from all clients are handled as if they were infectious.

Control of Transmission. Effective control of infection requires a nurse to remain aware of the modes of transmission and ways to control them. In the hospital, home, or long-term care facility, a client should have a personal set of care items. Sharing bedpans, urinals, bath basins, and eating utensils can easily lead to transmission of infection. Thermometers, even when individually used, warrant special care. Because the client's own mucus can become a source for micro-organism growth, the electronic thermometer is used with a disposable sheath over the probe; the sheath is discarded after use. Single-use chemical strip thermometers present less risk of infection than other thermometers. Use of electronic thermometers for rectal temperatures has been associated with nosocomial diarrhea (Jernigan, et al., 1998). The organism *Clostridium difficile* is able to survive on inanimate surfaces such as the thermometer probe. In institutions where nosocomial diarrhea occurs, electronic thermometers are not recommended for rectal temperatures.

To prevent transmission of micro-organisms through indirect contact, soiled items and equipment must not touch the nurse's clothing. A common error is to carry dirty linen in the arms against the uniform. Fluid-resistant linen bags should be used, or soiled linen should be carried with hands held out from the body. Laundry hampers should be replaced before they are overflowing.

Hand Hygiene. Hand hygiene is the most important and most basic technique in preventing transmission of infections. **Hand hygiene** includes using an instant alcohol hand antiseptic before and after providing client care, handwashing with soap and water when hands are visibly soiled, and performing a surgical scrub when

Table 29-6 Examples of Disinfection and Sterilization Processes

Characteristics	Examples of Use
Moist Heat	
Steam is moist heat under pressure. When exposed to high pressure, water vapour can attain temperature above boiling point to kill pathogens and spores.	Autoclave is used to sterilize surgical instruments, parenteral solutions, and surgical dressings.
Chemicals	
A number of chemical disinfectants are used in health care, including alcohols, chlorines, formaldehyde, glutaraldehyde, hydrogen peroxide, iodophors, phenolics, and quaternary ammonium compounds. Each product performs in a unique manner and is used for a specific purpose.	Chemicals are used for disinfection of instruments and equipment such as thermometers and endoscopes. Use the appropriate facility-approved disinfectant in a safe manner (e.g., gloves, proper ventilation) for the approved purpose.
Ethylene Oxide Gas	
This gas destroys spores and micro-organisms by altering cells' metabolic processes. Fumes are released within an autoclave-like chamber. Ethylene oxide gas is toxic to humans, and aeration time varies with products.	This gas sterilizes some rubber and plastic items.
Boiling Water	
Boiling is least expensive for use in home. Bacterial spores and some viruses resist boiling. It is not used in hospitals.	The items (e.g., glass baby bottles) should be boiled for at least 15 minutes.

Box 29-8 Infection Control to Reduce Reservoir Sites

Bathing

Use soap and water to remove drainage, dried secretions, or excess perspiration.

Dressing Changes

Change dressings that become wet and/or soiled (see chapter 43).

Contaminated Articles

Place tissues, soiled dressings, or soiled linen in moisture-resistant bags for proper disposal.

Contaminated Needles

Engage safety features of all sharp devices and dispose of in puncture-proof container. Place syringes, uncapped hypodermic needles, and IV needles in puncture-proof containers, which should be located in client rooms or treatment areas so that exposed, contaminated equipment need not be carried a distance (see chapter 30).

Do not recap needles or attempt to break them.

Bedside Unit

Keep table surfaces clean and dry.

Bottled Solutions

Do not leave bottled solutions open for prolonged periods.

Keep solutions tightly capped.

Date bottles when opened and discard according to facility policy.

Surgical Wounds

Keep drainage tubes and collection bags patent to prevent accumulation of serous fluid under the skin surface.

Drainage Bottles and Bags

Empty and dispose of drainage suction bottles according to agency policy.

Empty all drainage systems on each shift unless otherwise ordered by a physician.

Never raise a drainage system (e.g., urinary drainage bag) above the level of the site being drained, unless the drainage system is clamped off.

necessary. The components of good **handwashing** include using an adequate amount of soap, rubbing the hands together to lather the soap and create friction, and rinsing under a stream of water (Health Canada, 1998). The purpose is to remove soil and transient organisms from the hands and to reduce total microbial counts over time.

Contaminated hands are a prime cause of cross-infection. For example, a nurse caring for a client who has excessive pulmonary secretions assists the client in expectorating mucus and disposes of the tissues in a bedside container. The client's roommate asks the nurse to open containers of food on the meal tray. The nurse then leaves the client's room to pour a dose of medication that is due in 5 minutes. If the nurse fails to perform hand hygiene before opening the containers of food or pouring the medication, organisms from the first client's mucus could easily be transmitted to the roommate's food or to the medication container. Decreased nosocomial infection rates have been reported with improved handwashing compliance (Pittet et al., 2000).

The decision regarding when and what type of hand hygiene should occur depends on the following: the intensity of contact with clients or contaminated objects, the degree or amount of contamination that could occur with that contact, the susceptibility of the client or the health care worker to infection, and the procedure or activity to be performed (Larson, 1996). For example, prolonged and direct contact with a client's wound drainage would require thorough hand hygiene.

Washing times of at least 10 seconds are needed to remove most transient micro-organisms from the skin (Larson, 1996; Health Canada, 1998). If the hands are visibly soiled, more time may be needed. Routine handwashing may be performed with plain soap. Plain soap with water can physically remove a certain level of microbes, but antiseptic agents are necessary to kill or inhibit micro-organisms and reduce the level still further (Larson, 1996). Skill 29-1 lists the steps for hand hygiene.

The use of alcohol-based waterless antiseptics is recommended by the CDC (2002) to improve hand hygiene practices, protect health care worker's hands, and reduce transmission of pathogens to clients and personnel in health care settings. Alcohols have excellent germicidal activity and are more effective than either plain soap or antimicrobial soap and water. Emollients are added to alcohol-based antiseptics to prevent drying of the skin. Recent research has found that they may be used more effectively than water because they are quick and available at the bedside (Girou et al., 2002; Parienti et al., 2002).

The CDC (2002) recommends the following:

- Wash hands with plain soap or antimicrobial soap and water when hands are visibly soiled.
- If hands are not visibly soiled, use an alcohol-based waterless antiseptic agent for routinely decontaminating hands in all other clinical situations:
  - Before direct contact with each client (e.g., taking a pulse or blood pressure, lifting a client)
  - After direct contact with each client
  - Before donning sterile gloves
  - After removing gloves (i.e., after removing sterile gloves or clean, non-sterile gloves)
  - After contact with body fluids or excretions, mucous membranes, non-intact skin, or wound dressings, as long as hands are not visibly soiled (if visibly soiled, wash with soap and water)
  - When moving from a contaminated body site to a clean body site during client care
  - After contact with inanimate objects (including medical equipment) in the immediate vicinity of the client

Alternatively, if antiseptic agents are not available, the nurse may wash hands in all clinical situations (CDC, 2002). Also, health care workers are advised to wash hands with soap and water if client exposure to *C. difficile* is suspected or proven. The physical action of washing and rinsing hands under such circumstances is recommended because antiseptic agents have poor activity against spores (Louie & Meddings, 2004).

The nurse instructs clients and visitors about the proper technique and times for hand hygiene. Teaching hand hygiene is particularly important if health care is to continue at home. Clients should wash their hands before eating or handling food; after handling contaminated equipment, linen, or organic material; and after elimination. Visitors are encouraged to wash their hands before eating or handling food, after coming in contact with infected clients, and after handling contaminated equipment or organic material.

Control of Portals of Entry. Many measures that control the exit of micro-organisms likewise control their entrance. Maintaining the integrity of skin and mucous membranes reduces the chances of micro-organisms reaching a host. The client's skin should be kept well lubricated by using lotion as appropriate. Immobilized and debilitated clients are particularly susceptible to skin breakdown. Clients should not be positioned on tubes or objects that might cause breaks in the skin. Dry, wrinkle-free linen also reduces the chances of skin breakdown. Frequent turning and positioning are needed before a client's skin becomes reddened. Frequent oral hygiene prevents drying of mucous membranes. A water-soluble ointment keeps the client's lips well lubricated.

After elimination, a woman should clean the rectum and perineum by wiping from the urinary meatus toward the rectum. Cleansing in a direction from the least to the most contaminated area helps reduce genitourinary infections. Meticulous and frequent perineal care is especially important in women who wear incontinent pads.

Clients, health care workers, and even housekeepers are at risk for acquiring infections from accidental needle sticks. After administering an injection or inserting an IV catheter, the nurse should engage any safety device and carefully dispose of needles in a puncture-resistant box (see chapter 30). A stray needle lying in bed linen or carelessly thrown into a wastebasket is a prime source for exposure to blood-borne pathogens. Hepatitis B and hepatitis C are the infections most commonly transmitted by contaminated needles. A needle stick should be reported immediately. Health care agencies require the victim of a needle stick to complete an injury report and seek appropriate treatment. The Canadian Needle Stick Surveillance Network (CNSSN) has the mandate to monitor health care workers exposed to needle sticks and the subsequent outcomes of these exposures (2003).

Another cause for entrance of micro-organisms into a host is improper handling and management of urinary catheters and drainage sets (see chapter 40). The point of connection between a catheter and drainage tube should remain closed and intact. As long as such systems are closed, their contents are considered sterile. Outflow spigots on drainage bags should also remain closed to prevent entrance of bacteria. Movement of the catheter at the urethra should be minimized by stabilizing the catheter with tape to reduce chances of micro-organisms ascending the urethra into the bladder. Urine-measuring containers should not be shared between clients.

Text continued on p. 806

Research Highlight

Box 29-9

Pathogens and Artificial Fingernails

Research Focus

Some health care workers have artificial or manicured nails. Researchers posed the question as to whether bacteria can reside in higher than normal numbers on artificial nail material.

Research Abstract

In two separate studies, the identity and quantity of microbial flora from health care workers (HCWs) wearing artificial nails was compared with HCWs with normal nails. In both studies, nail surfaces were swabbed and subungual (area under nails) debris was collected to obtain material for culture. In the first study, 12 HCWs who did not normally wear artificial nails wore polished artificial nails on their non-dominant hand for 15 days. Identity and quantity of microflora were compared between the artificial nails and the polished normal nails of the other hand. Potential pathogens were isolated from more samples obtained from artificial nails than normal nails. Colonization of artificial nails increased over time. More organisms were found on the surface of artificial nails than on normal nails.

In the second study, the flora of the nails of 30 HCWs who wore permanent acrylic artificial nails were compared with that of HCWs who had normal nails. HCWs wearing artificial nails were more likely to have a pathogen isolated than the other group.

In this study, artificial nails were more likely to harbour pathogens, especially gram-negative bacilli and yeasts, than were normal nails. The longer artificial nails were worn, the more likely that a pathogen was isolated.

Evidence-Based Practice

- Nurses should not wear artificial nails when performing client care.

Reference

Hedderwick, S. A., et al. (2000). Pathogenic organisms associated with artificial fingernails worn by healthcare workers. *Infection Control and Hospital Epidemiology, 21*(8), 505–509.

Skill 29-1 Hand Hygiene

View Video

Delegation Considerations

- Monitor UCP in proper method of hand hygiene.
- Instruct UCP to report any skin irritation from soaps or antimicrobials.

Equipment

- Easy-to-reach sink with warm running water
- Antimicrobial or regular soap
- Alcohol-based waterless antiseptic
- Paper towels or air dryer
- Clean orangewood stick (optional)

Steps	Rationale
1. Inspect surface of hands for breaks or cuts in skin or cuticles. Report and cover lesions before providing client care.	Open cuts or wounds can harbour high concentrations of micro-organisms. Agency policy may prevent nurses from caring for high-risk clients. If dermatitis occurs, additional interventions may be needed.
2. Inspect hands for heavy soiling.	Requires lengthier handwashing.
3. Inspect nails for length and presence of artificial acrylics or chipped nail polish.	Nails should be short and filed because most microbes on hands come from beneath the fingernails. Nails should be free of artificial applications and chipped or old nail polish (Gruendemann & Mangum, 2001; Health Canada, 1998; CDC, 2002; Box 29-9).
4. Assess client's risk for or extent of infection (e.g., WBC count, extent of open wounds, known medical diagnosis).	Use of alcohol-based waterless antiseptic is encouraged for clients who are immunosuppressed (Health Canada, 1998; CDC, 2002).
5. Push wristwatch and long uniform sleeves above wrists. Avoid wearing rings. If worn, remove during procedure.	Provides complete access to fingers, hands, wrists. Wearing of rings increases number of micro-organisms on hands (Garner, 1996).
6. If hands are visibly dirty or contaminated with protein-containing material, use water and plain soap or antimicrobial soap for handwashing:	
a. Stand in front of sink, keeping hands and uniform away from sink surface. (If hands touch sink during handwashing, repeat procedure.)	Inside of sink is a contaminated area. Reaching over sink increases risk of touching edge, which is contaminated.

Steps	Rationale
b. Turn on water. Turn faucet on or push knee pedals laterally or press pedals with foot to regulate flow and temperature (see illustration).	
c. Avoid splashing water against uniform.	Micro-organisms travel and grow in moisture.
d. Regulate flow of water so that temperature is warm.	Warm water removes less of the protective oils than hot water.
e. Wet hands and wrists thoroughly under running water. Keep hands and forearms lower than elbows during washing.	Hands are the most contaminated parts to be washed. Water flows from least to most contaminated area, rinsing micro-organisms into the sink.
f. Apply a small amount of soap, lathering thoroughly (see illustration). Soap granules and leaflet preparations may be used.	Use of antimicrobial soaps exclusively can be drying to hands and can cause skin irritations. The decision whether to use an antimicrobial soap or alcohol-based hand antiseptic should depend on the procedure to be performed and the client's immune status.
g. Wash hands using plenty of lather and friction for at least 10 to 15 seconds. Interlace fingers, and rub palms and back of hands with circular motion at least five times each. Keep fingertips down to facilitate removal of micro-organisms. Rub knuckles of one hand into the palm of the other; repeat with other hand (see illustration).	Soap cleanses by emulsifying fat and oil and lowering surface tension. Friction and rubbing mechanically loosen and remove dirt and transient bacteria. Interlacing fingers and thumbs and rubbing knuckles ensures that all surfaces are cleansed.
h. Rub thumb on one hand with the palm of the other hand; repeat with other hand (see illustration).	Thumbs are frequently missed areas.
i. Work the fingertips on one hand into the palm of the other. Massage soap into nail spaces; repeat with other hand (see illustration).	Fingertips are frequently missed areas.

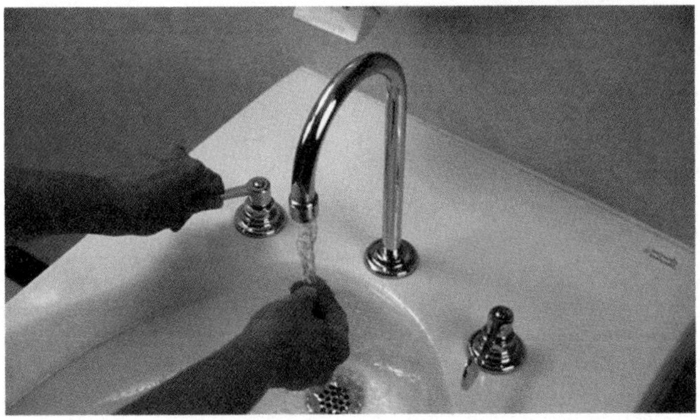

STEP **6b** Turning on water.

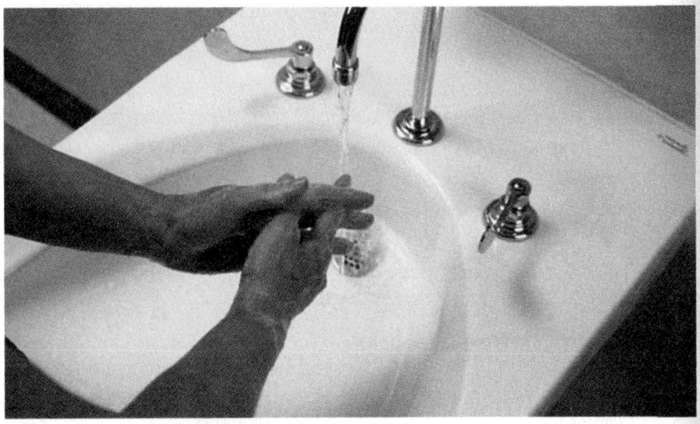

STEP **6f** Lathering hands thoroughly.

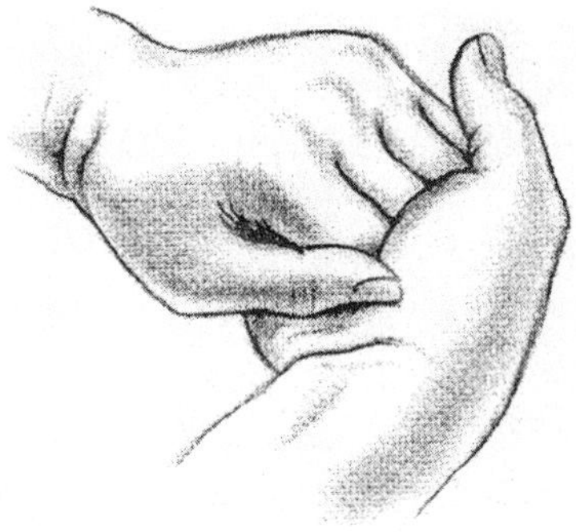

STEP **6g** Rubbing the knuckles of one hand into the palm of the other. (From Susan MacMillan, *Demonstration of a Proper Medical Handwash* (brochure), © May 1996, Infection Prevention Control at St. Michael's Hospital, Toronto, ON.)

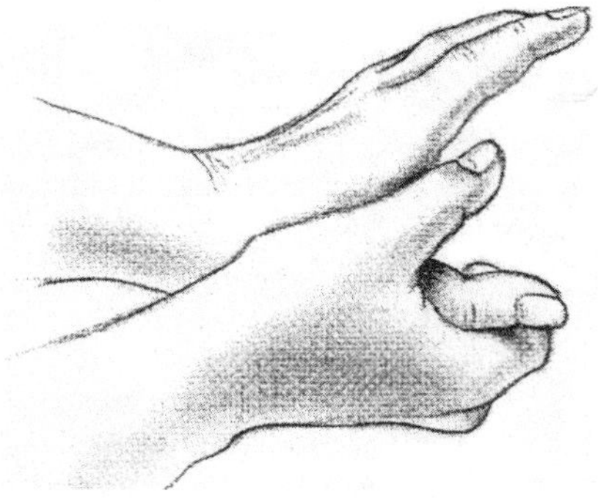

STEP **6h** Rubbing the thumb into the palm of the other hand. (From Susan MacMillan, *Demonstration of a Proper Medical Handwash* (brochure), © May 1996, Infection Prevention Control at St. Michael's Hospital, Toronto, ON.)

Skill 29-1 Hand Hygiene—cont'd

Steps	Rationale
j. Areas under fingernails are often soiled. Clean them with orangewood stick or fingernails of other hand and additional soap.	Areas under nails can be highly contaminated, which will increase the risk of infection.

Critical Decision Point: Do not tear or cut skin under or around nail.

Steps	Rationale
k. Rinse hands and wrists thoroughly, keeping hands down and elbows up (see illustration).	Rinsing mechanically washes away dirt and micro-organisms.
l. *Optional:* Repeat steps a through j and extend period of washing if hands are heavily soiled.	
m. Dry hands thoroughly from fingers to wrists and forearms with paper towel, single-use cloth, or warm air dryer.	Drying from cleanest (fingertips) to least clean (forearms) area avoids contamination. Drying hands prevents chapping and roughened skin.
n. If used, discard paper towel in proper receptacle.	Prevents transfer of micro-organisms.
o. Turn off water with foot or knee pedals. To turn off hand faucet, use clean, dry paper towel; avoid touching handles with hands (see illustration).	Faucets are contaminated. Using paper towels to touch faucet prevents contamination of hands.
p. If hands are dry or chapped, a small amount of lotion or barrier cream can be applied.	Use agency-provided container of lotion because many lotions may interfere with antimicrobial action or disintegrate gloves.

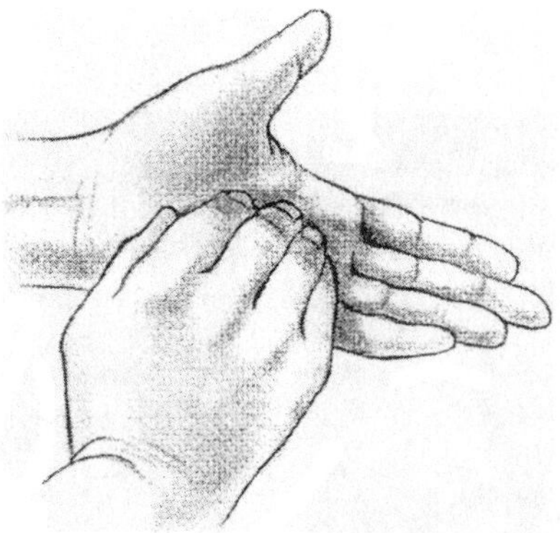

STEP **6i** Working the fingertips into the palm of the other hand. (From Susan MacMillan, *Demonstration of a Proper Medical Handwash* (brochure), © May 1996, Infection Prevention Control at St. Michael's Hospital, Toronto, ON.)

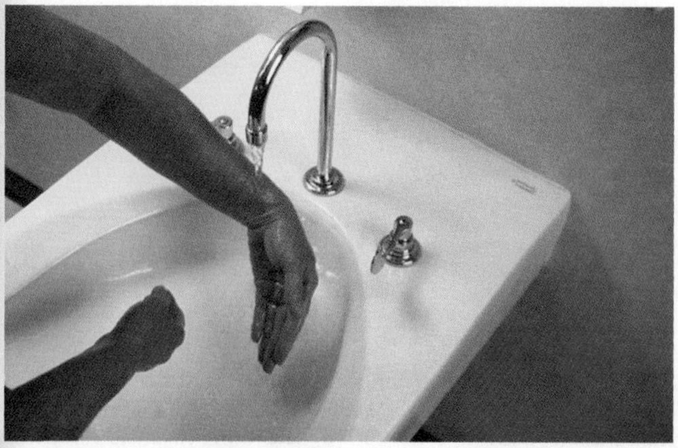

STEP **6k** Rinsing hands.

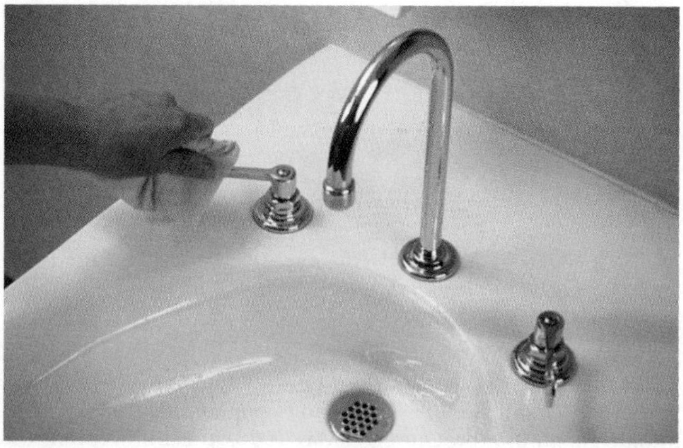

STEP **6o** Turning off faucet.

Steps	Rationale

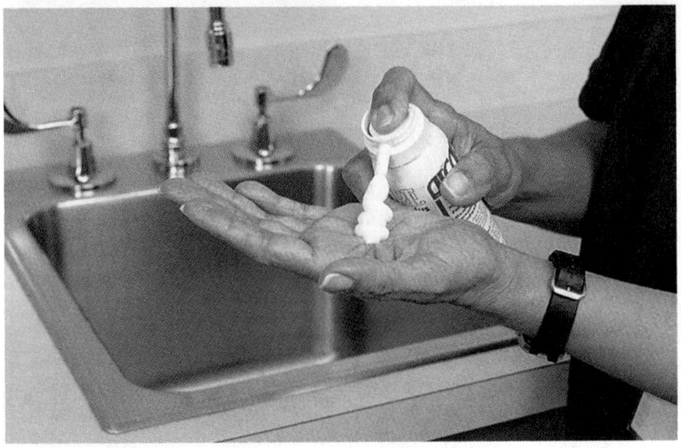

STEP **7a** Apply waterless antiseptic to palm of hand.

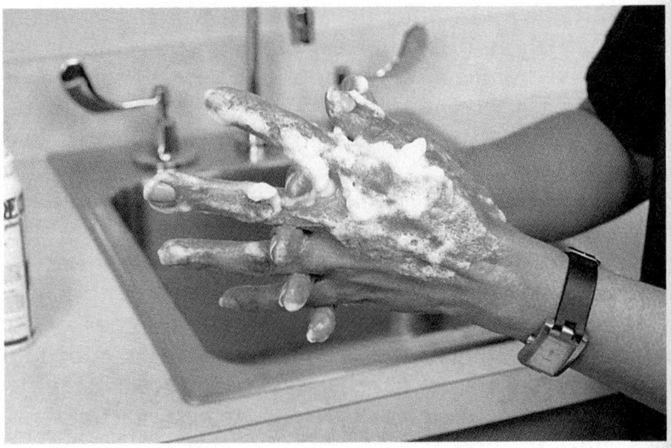

STEP **7b** Rub hands thoroughly.

Steps	Rationale
q. Inspect surfaces of hands for obvious signs of soil or other contaminants.	Determines if handwashing is adequate.
r. Inspect hands for dermatitis or cracked skin.	Indicates complications from excessive handwashing.
7. If hands are not visibly soiled, use an alcohol-based waterless antiseptic for routine decontamination of hands in all clinical situations.	
a. Apply an ample amount of product to palm of one hand (see illustration).	Enough product is needed to thoroughly cover the hands.
b. Rub hands together, covering all surfaces of hands and fingers with antiseptic (see illustration).	
c. Rub hands together for several seconds until alcohol is dry. Allow hands to dry before applying gloves.	Drying ensures full antiseptic effect (Health Canada, 1998).
d. If hands are dry or chapped, a small amount of lotion or barrier cream can be applied.	Use the agency-provided container of lotion because many lotions may interfere with antimicrobial action or disintegrate gloves.

Recording and Reporting

- It is not necessary to record or report this procedure.
- Report any dermatitis to employee health and/or infection control per agency policy.

Home Care Considerations

- Evaluate the hand-washing facilities in the home to determine the possibility of contamination, the proximity of the facilities to the client, and available supplies in the area.
- Evaluate the availability of warm running water and soap when conducting home visits and anticipate the need for alternative hand-washing products such as alcohol-based hand rubs and detergent-containing towels.
- Instruct the client and primary caregiver in proper techniques and situations for handwashing.

The nurse may care for clients with closed drainage systems that collect wound drainage, bile, or other body fluids. In each example, the site from which a drainage tube exits should remain clear of excess moisture or accumulated drainage. All tubing should remain connected throughout use. Drainage receptacles should only be opened when it is necessary to discard or measure the volume of drainage.

At times, the nurse obtains specimens from drainage tubes or IV tubing ports. The nurse disinfects tubes and ports by wiping the surface outward with alcohol or an iodine solution before entering the system. Temporarily placing squares of sterile gauze around the ends of an open drainage tube, such as a urinary catheter, adds further protection against bacteria. However, keeping drainage tubes closed and secure is the best practice.

A final method for reducing the entrance of micro-organisms is the technique for cleansing wounds (see chapter 43). A surgical wound is considered to be sterile. To prevent entrance of micro-organisms into the wound, the nurse should clean outward from a wound site. When applying an antiseptic or cleaning with soap and water, the nurse wipes around the wound edge first and then cleans outward away from the wound. Clean gauze should be used for each revolution around the wound's circumference.

Protection of the Susceptible Host. A client's resistance to infection improves as the nurse protects normal body defences against infection. Nurses intervene to maintain the body's normal reparative processes (Box 29-10). Nurses also protect themselves and others by following their agency's isolation guidelines.

Isolation Guidelines. The risk of transmitting nosocomial infection or infectious disease among clients is high. When a client has a suspected or known infection, health care workers become alerted and follow infection control practices. However, health care workers may not be aware that clients have infections. The majority of organisms causing nosocomial infections are found in the colonized body substances of clients regardless of whether a culture has confirmed infection and a diagnosis has been made (Garner, 1996). Body substances such as feces, saliva, mucus, and wound drainage always contain potentially infectious organisms.

The US Centers for Disease Control and Prevention (CDC) issued isolation guidelines in 1996 that contain a two-tiered approach (Garner, 1996). These CDC guidelines have been adopted by most Canadian health care agencies. Some Canadian agencies have adopted Health Canada's isolation guidelines (1999), which also contain a similar two-tiered approach. The Health Canada guidelines were written to accommodate acute, long-term care, home care, and ambulatory care settings, whereas the CDC guidelines were written specifically for acute care settings. Nevertheless, the CDC guidelines and Health Canada's guidelines are essentially interchangeable.

The first tier of the isolation guidelines contains precautions designed to care for all clients in any setting regardless of their diagnosis or presumed infectiousness. In the CDC's guidelines, this tier is called *standard precautions* (Table 29-7); in Health Canada's guidelines, it is called *routine practices*. Standard precautions/routine practices apply when a health care worker is or potentially may be exposed to (a) blood; (b) all body fluids, secretions, and excretions except sweat; (c) non-intact skin; or (d) mucous membranes. Standard precautions/routine practices include the appropriate use of gowns, gloves, masks, eyewear, and other protective devices or clothing. Barrier protection is indicated for use with all clients because every client has the potential to transmit infection via blood and body fluids, and the risk for infection transmission can be unknown. Standard precautions/routine practices also include rules on appropriate hand washing, cleaning of equipment, and disposal of contaminated linen and sharps.

The second tier of the isolation guidelines is *transmission-based precautions* (in the Health Canada guidelines, the second tier is called *additional precautions*). These precautions are designed to contain pathogens in one area, usually the client's room; therefore, they are often called *isolation precautions*. Only clients infected or colonized with certain highly transmissible or epidemiologically significant pathogens are placed under isolation precautions. These precautions are followed in addition to standard precautions/routine practices. There are three categories of isolation precautions: airborne precautions, droplet precautions, and contact precautions (see Table 29-7). The one used depends on how the pathogen is spread. For example, a client diagnosed with (or suspected of having) active TB would require the use of airborne precautions, using a special mask and ventilated

Box 29-10 Infection Control: Protecting the Susceptible Host

Protecting Normal Defence Mechanisms

Regular bathing removes transient micro-organisms from the skin's surface. Lubrication helps keep the skin hydrated and intact.

Regular oral hygiene removes proteins in the saliva that attract micro-organisms. Flossing removes tartar and plaque that can cause germ infection.

Maintenance of adequate fluid intake promotes normal urine formation and a resultant outflow of urine to flush the bladder and urethral lining of micro-organisms.

For physically dependent or immobilized clients, the nurse encourages routine coughing and deep breathing to keep lower airways clear of mucus.

The nurse encourages proper immunization of children and adult clients (see Box 29-6).

Maintaining Healing Processes

The nurse promotes intake of adequate fluids and a well-balanced diet containing essential proteins, vitamins, carbohydrates, and fats. The nurse also uses measures to increase the client's appetite.

The nurse promotes a client's comfort and sleep so that energy stores are replaced daily.

The nurse assists the client in learning techniques to reduce stress.

Table 29-7 Centers for Disease Control and Prevention (CDC) Isolation Guidelines

Standard Precautions (Tier One)

- Standard precautions apply to blood, all body fluids, secretions, excretions (except sweat), non-intact skin, and mucous membranes.
- Hands are washed between client contacts; after contact with blood, body fluids, secretions, and excretions and after contact with equipment or articles contaminated by them; and immediately after gloves are removed. (Refer to agency policy for use of alcohol-based waterless antiseptics.)
- Gloves are worn when touching blood, body fluids, secretions, excretions, non-intact skin, mucous membranes, or contaminated items. Gloves should be removed and hand hygiene performed between client care. Gloves should also be changed between procedures on the same client and after contact with material that may be highly contaminated.
- Masks, eye protection, or face shields are worn if client care activities may generate splashes or sprays of blood or body fluid.
- Gowns are worn if soiling of clothing is likely from blood or body fluid. Remove used gowns as soon as possible. Perform hand hygiene after removing gown.
- Client care equipment is properly cleaned and reprocessed, and single-use items are discarded.
- Contaminated linen is placed in leak-proof bag and handled so as to prevent skin and mucous membrane exposure.
- All sharp instruments and needles are discarded in a puncture-resistant container. Safety devices must be enabled after use to prevent injury. Never recap a used needle.
- A private room is unnecessary unless the client's hygiene is unacceptable. Check with an infection control professional.

Transmission-Based (Isolation) Precautions (Tier Two)

Category	Description/Disease	Barrier Protection
Airborne precautions	For known or suspected infections caused by microbes transmitted by airborne droplets; examples: measles, chickenpox (varicella), disseminated zoster, TB	Private room (room door kept closed), negative-pressure airflow of at least six exchanges per hour, respiratory protection device (e.g., N95 respirator) must be worn when the client has TB or when the client has varicella, disseminated zoster, or measles and the worker is not immune
Droplet precautions	For known or suspected infections caused by microbes transmitted by droplets produced by coughing, sneezing, or talking; Examples: diphtheria (pharyngeal), rubella, influenza, pertussis, mumps, mycoplasmal pneumonia, meningococcal pneumonia or sepsis	Private room or cohort clients (room door closed unless bed is more than 1 m from the door), mask is worn when within 1 m of the client
Contact precautions	For known or suspected infections caused by direct or indirect contact; Examples: colonization or infection with multidrug-resistant organism; *C. difficile;* major wound infections; gastrointestinal, respiratory, or skin infections	Private room or cohort clients (door can be open); gloves, gowns

Adapted from "Guidelines for Isolation Precautions in Hospitals," by J. S. Garner, 1996, *Infection Control and Hospital Epidemiology, 17*(1), p. 54.

room, in conjunction with standard precautions/routine practices.

Regardless of the category of isolation precaution, the nurse must observe the following basic principles (Box 29-11):

- The nurse should observe thorough hand hygiene before entering and leaving the room of a client in isolation.
- Contaminated supplies and equipment should be disposed of in a manner that prevents spread of microorganisms to other people as indicated by the mode of transmission of the organism.
- Knowledge of a disease process and the mode of infection transmission should be applied when using protective barriers.
- All people who might be exposed during transport of a client outside the isolation room must be protected.

Psychological Implications of Isolation Precautions. When a client requires isolation in a private room, loneliness may develop because normal social relationships become disrupted. This situation can be psychologically harmful, especially for children (Box 29-12).

As a result of the infectious process, clients' body images are altered. They may feel unclean, rejected, lonely, or guilty. Infection prevention and control practices further intensify these beliefs of difference or undesirability. Isolation in a private room limits sensory contact. Unless the nurse acts to minimize feelings of psychological and physical isolation, clients' emotional states can interfere with recovery.

Before isolation measures are instituted, the client and family must understand the nature of the disease or condition, the purposes of isolation, and steps for carrying out specific precautions. If they are able to participate in maintaining infection prevention, the chances of reducing the spread of infection are increased. The client and family should be taught to perform hand hygiene and use barrier protection if appropriate. Each procedure should be demonstrated, and the client and family should be

Box 29-11 Procedural Guidelines

Caring for a Client on Isolation Precautions

Equipment

- Barrier protection determined by type of isolation
- Supplies necessary for procedures performed in room

Delegation considerations. Care of a client in isolation can be delegated to unregulated care providers (UCPs) when necessary procedures are within the UCP's competence.

1. Assess isolation indications (e.g., current laboratory test results or client's history of exposure).
2. Review agency policies and precautions necessary for the specific isolation category and consider care measures to be performed while in client's room.
3. Review nurses' notes or confer with colleagues regarding client's emotional state and adjustment to isolation.
4. Perform hand hygiene and prepare all equipment to be taken into client's room.
5. Prepare for entrance into isolation room:
   a. Apply either surgical mask or respirator around mouth and nose if needed. (Type will depend on type of isolation and facility policy.)
   b. Apply eyewear or goggles snugly around face and eyes (when needed).
   c. Apply gown (when needed), being sure it covers all outer garments. Pull sleeves down to wrist. Tie securely at neck and waist (see illustration).
   d. Apply disposable gloves. (NOTE: Unpowdered, latex-free gloves should be worn if the client or the health care worker has a latex allergy.) If gloves are worn with gown, bring glove cuffs over edge of gown sleeves.
6. Enter client's room. Arrange supplies and equipment. (If equipment will be removed from room for reuse, place on clean paper towel.)
7. Explain purpose of isolation and necessary precautions to client and family. Offer opportunity to ask questions. Assess for evidence of emotional problems that may be caused by being in isolation.
8. Assess vital signs:
   a. If client is infected or colonized with a resistant organism (e.g., VRE [vancomycin-resistant enterococcus], MRSA [methicillin-resistant *S. aureus*]), equipment remains in room. Proceed to assess vital signs. Avoid contact of stethoscope or blood pressure cuff with infectious material.
   b. If stethoscope is to be reused, clean diaphragm or bell with alcohol. Set aside on clean surface.
   c. Individual or disposable thermometers should be used.
9. Administer medications:
   a. Give oral medication in wrapper or cup.
   b. Dispose of wrapper or cup in plastic-lined receptacle.
   c. Administer injection.
   d. Discard syringe and uncapped needle or sheathed needle into special container.
   e. If gloves are not worn and hands contact contaminated article or body fluids, wash hands immediately.

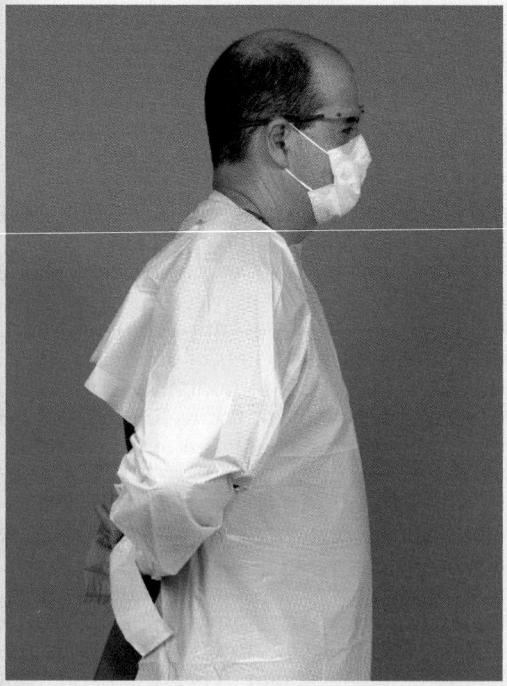

STEP **5c** Tying gown at waist.

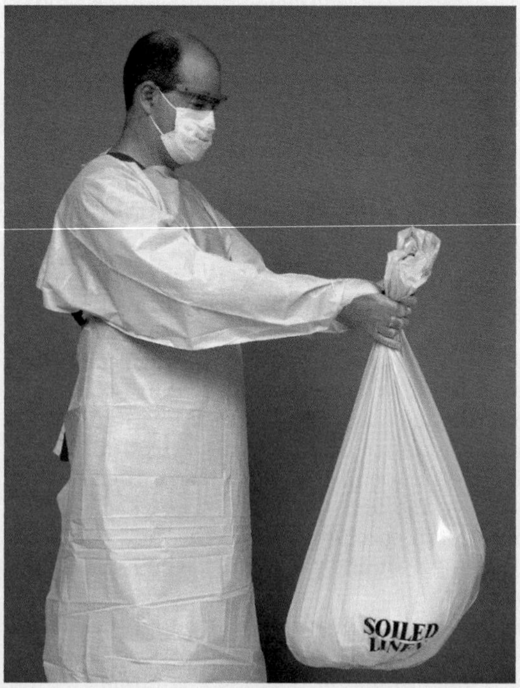

STEP **12b** Tie linen securely.

Box 29-11 Procedural Guidelines

Caring for a Client on Isolation Precautions—cont'd

10. Administer hygiene, encouraging the client to discuss questions or concerns about isolation. Informal teaching can be used at this time:
    a. Prevent gown from becoming wet.
    b. Remove linen from bed; avoid contact with gown. Place in impervious linen bag.
    c. Change gloves and wash hands if they become excessively soiled and further care is necessary.
11. Collect specimens:
    a. Place specimen containers on clean paper towel in client's bathroom.
    b. Follow procedure for collecting specimen of body fluids.
    c. Transfer specimen to container without soiling outside of container. Place container in plastic bag and place label on outside of bag or as per agency policy.
12. Dispose of linen and garbage bags as they become full:
    a. Use sturdy, moisture-resistant single bags to contain soiled articles.
    b. Tie bags securely at top in knot (see illustration).
13. Resupply room as needed.
14. Leave isolation room.
    a. Remove gloves. Remove one glove by grasping cuff and pulling glove inside out over hand. Discard glove. With ungloved hand, tuck finger inside cuff of remaining glove and pull it off, inside out.
    b. Untie *top* mask string and then bottom strings, pull mask away from face and drop into waste receptacle (see illustration). (Do not touch outer surface of mask.)
    c. Untie waist and neck strings of gown. Allow gown to fall from shoulders. Remove hands from sleeves without touching outside of gown (see illustration). Hold gown inside at shoulder seams and fold inside out; discard in laundry bag.
    d. Remove eyewear or goggles.
    e. Perform hand hygiene.
    f. Explain to client when you plan to return to room. Ask whether client requires any personal care items, books, or magazines.
    g. Leave room and close door, if necessary. (Door should be closed if client is on airborne precautions.)
    h. All contaminated supplies and equipment should be disposed of in a manner that prevents spread of micro-organisms to other people (see agency policy).

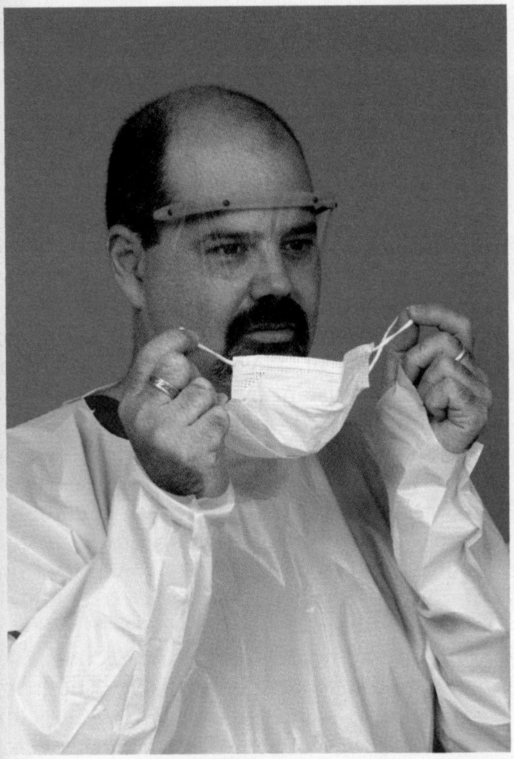

STEP **14b** Remove mask away from face.

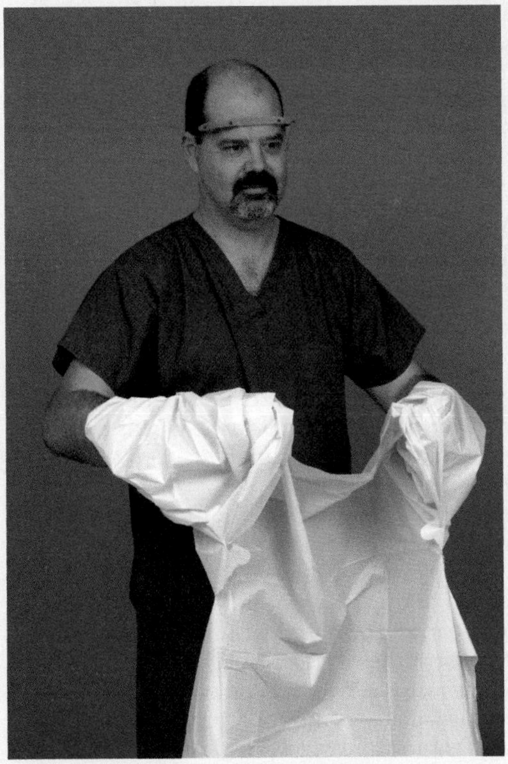

STEP **14c** Remove hands from sleeves without touching outside of gown.

Research Highlight — Box 29-12

Adverse Effects of Isolation

Research Focus

Researchers looked at whether clients who are in isolation in single rooms experience adverse effects as a result of isolation.

Research Abstract

A Canadian and an American hospital were included in a study to examine the likelihood of adverse events. Clients who were cared for in isolation due to MRSA (methicillin-resistant *Staphylococcus aureus*) were compared with those who were not. The research found that (a) isolated clients were more likely to complain about care than were non-isolated controls (8% versus 1%), (b) charting of vital signs were not recorded as ordered as often for isolated clients as for non-isolated clients (51% versus 31%), (c) nurses were less likely to record nursing notes for isolated clients (14% versus 10%), and (d) clients in isolation were eight times more likely to experience falls, pressure ulcers, and fluid or electrolyte disorders.

Evidence-Based Practice

- Nursing staff must be extra vigilant to ensure the standard of care is similar for all clients, including those on isolation precautions.
- Care should be taken to ensure both physical and psychological factors are addressed when planning and carrying out care for isolated clients.
- Recording of observations and completing nursing notes is critical.

Reference

Stelfox, H. T., Bates, D. W., & Redelmeier, D. A. (2003). Safety of patients isolated for infection control. *Journal of the American Medical Association, 290*(14), 1899–1905.

given an opportunity to practise. It is also important to explain how infectious organisms can be transmitted so that the client understands the difference between contaminated and clean objects.

The nurse also takes measures to improve the client's sensory stimulation during isolation. The room environment should be clean and pleasant. Drapes or shades should be opened and excess supplies and equipment removed. The nurse must listen to the client's concerns or interests. If the nurse rushes through care or shows a lack of interest, the client will feel rejected and even more isolated. Mealtime is a particularly good opportunity for conversation. Providing comfort measures such as repositioning, a back massage, or a tepid sponge bath increases physical stimulation. Depending on the client's condition, the nurse should encourage the client to walk and sit up in a chair. Recreational activities such as board games or cards may be an option to keep the client mentally stimulated.

The nurse must explain to the family the client's risk for depression or loneliness. Visiting family members should be taught principles of isolation and encouraged to avoid expressions or actions that convey revulsion, fear, or disgust. The nurse discusses ways to provide meaningful stimulation.

Protective Environment. Private rooms used for isolation may have negative-pressure airflow to prevent infectious particles from flowing out of the room. There are also special rooms with positive-pressure airflow that are used for highly susceptible clients, such as organ transplant recipients. On the door or wall outside the room, the nurse posts a card listing precautions for the isolation category according to agency policy. The card is a handy reference for health care workers and visitors and alerts anyone who might enter the room that special precautions must be followed.

The isolation room or an adjoining anteroom should contain hand hygiene, bathing, and toilet facilities. Soap and antiseptic solutions are made available. Personnel and visitors perform hand hygiene before approaching the client's bedside and again before leaving the room. If toilet facilities are unavailable, there are special procedures for handling portable commodes, bedpans, or urinals. Personal protective equipment should be stored in an anteroom between the room and hallway or in a convenient location close to the point of use.

All client care rooms, including those used for isolation, contain an impervious bag for soiled or contaminated linen, as well as a waste receptacle with plastic liners. Impervious receptacles prevent transmission of micro-organisms by preventing seepage and soiling of the outside surface. A disposable rigid container should be available in the room to discard used needles, syringes, and sharp objects.

The nurse must remain aware of infection prevention and control techniques while working with clients in protected environments. Depending on the micro-organism and the mode of transmission, the nurse must evaluate what articles or equipment may be taken into an isolation room. For example, Health Canada (1997) recommends the dedicated use of articles such as stethoscopes, sphygmomanometers, or rectal thermometers in the isolation room of a client infected or colonized with vancomycin-resistant enterococci (VRE). These devices should not be used on other clients unless they are first adequately cleaned and disinfected. If after bringing any article into the room, the nurse exposes an article to infected material and then touches or removes the article, the risk of transmitting infection to other clients or personnel is increased. Box 29-11 describes the procedures commonly performed in a protective environment.

Personal Protective Equipment. Personal protective equipment (gowns, masks, protective eyewear, and gloves) should be readily available. The primary reason for gowning is to prevent contaminating clothes during contact with the client. Gowns or cover-ups protect health care workers and visitors from coming in contact with infected material, blood, or body fluid. Gowns may also be required for contact precautions, depending on the expected amount of exposure to infectious material. Gowns used for barrier protection are made of a fluid-resistant material and should be changed immediately if damaged or heavily contaminated. Depending on agency policy, isolation gowns can be disposable or reusable.

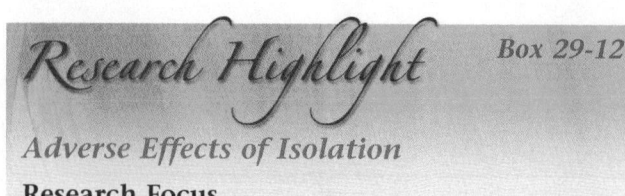

Box 29-13 Procedural Guidelines

Donning a Surgical-Type Mask

1. Find top edge of mask (usually has a thin metal strip along edge). Pliable metal fits snugly against bridge of nose
2. Hold mask by top two strings or loops. Tie two top ties at top of back of head (see illustration), with ties above ears. (*Alternative:* Slip loops over each ear.)

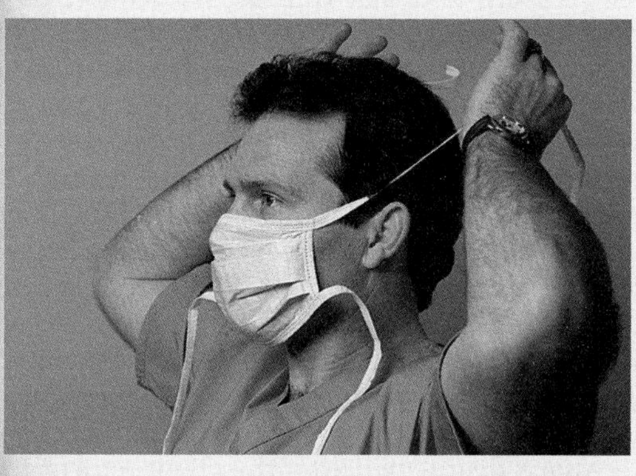

3. Tie two lower ties snugly around neck with mask well under chin (see illustration).

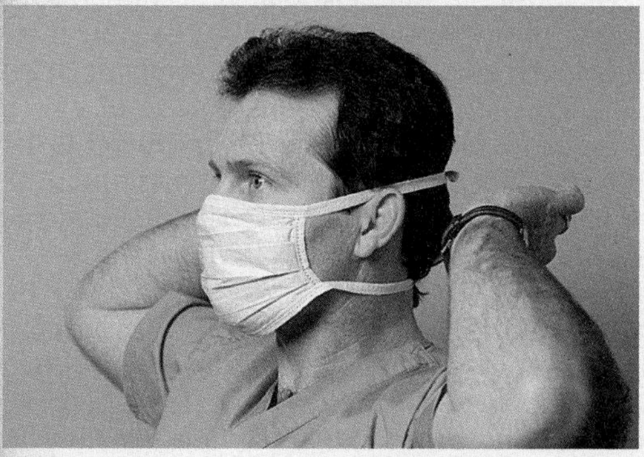

4. Gently pinch upper metal band around bridge of nose.

NOTE: Mask should be changed if wet, moist, or contaminated.

Isolation gowns usually open at the back and have ties or snaps at the neck and waist to keep the gown closed and secure. Gowns should be long enough to cover all outer garments. Long sleeves with tight-fitting cuffs provide added protection. There is no special technique required for applying clean gowns as long as they are fastened securely. However, the nurse must carefully remove gowns to minimize contamination of the hands and uniform and then discard gowns after removal.

Full face protection (with eyes, nose, and mouth covered) should be worn when splashing or spraying of blood or body fluid into the face is possible. Masks should also be worn when working with a client placed on droplet precautions. The mask protects the nurse from inhaling

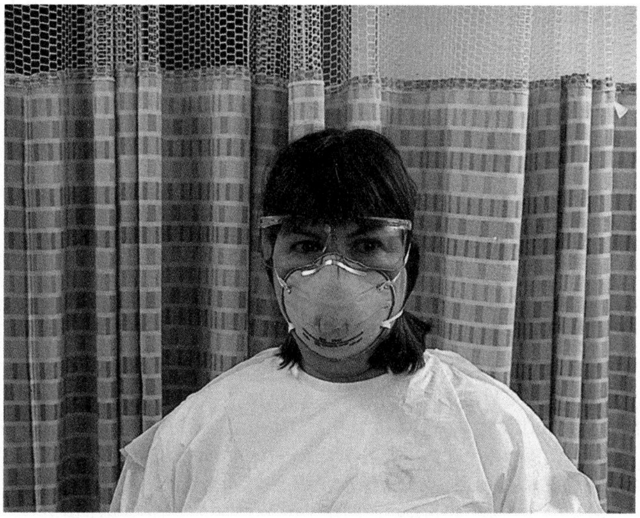

FIGURE **29–2** Nurse wearing fitted TB mask and goggles.

micro-organisms from a client's respiratory tract and prevents transmission of pathogens from the nurse's respiratory tract to the client. The surgical mask protects a wearer from inhaling large-particle aerosols that travel short distances (1 m). At times, a client who is susceptible to infection wears a mask to prevent inhalation of pathogens. Clients on droplet or airborne precautions who are transported outside of their rooms should wear masks to protect other clients and personnel. According to the CDC (Garner, 1996), masks may prevent transmission of infection by direct contact with mucous membranes. A mask discourages the wearer from touching the eyes, nose, or mouth.

A properly applied mask fits snugly over the mouth and nose so that pathogens and body fluids cannot enter or escape through the sides (Box 29-13). If a person wears glasses, the top edge of the mask fits below the glasses so that they will not cloud over as the person exhales. Talking should be kept to a minimum while wearing a mask to reduce respiratory airflow. A mask that has become moist may not provide a barrier to micro-organisms and thus may be ineffective. It should be discarded. A mask should never be reused. Clients and family members should be warned that a mask can cause a sensation of smothering. If family members become uncomfortable, they should leave the room and discard the mask.

Specially fitted respiratory protective devices or masks are required when caring for a client with known or suspected TB or when the client has varicella, disseminated zoster, or measles and the worker is not immune (Figure 29–2). The mask must have a higher filtration rating than the regular surgical mask and be fitted snugly to the wearer's face to prevent leakage around the sides. The nurse should be aware of agency policy regarding the type of respiratory protective device required.

Gloves help to prevent the transmission of pathogens by direct and indirect contact. Clean, non-sterile gloves (also called disposable gloves) should be worn when there is potential for contact with blood, body fluid, secretions, excretions, or contaminated items. Clean gloves should be donned just before touching mucous membranes and non-intact skin. Gloves should be changed between tasks and procedures on the same client after contact with material that may contain a high concentration of micro-organisms. Gloves should be removed promptly after use, before touching non-contaminated items and environmental surfaces, and before going to another client. Hand hygiene should be performed immediately after removing gloves to avoid transfer of micro-organisms to other clients or environments. Because of allergy or sensitivity to latex gloves, facilities provide non-latex gloves for health care staff who are allergic or sensitive to latex. When full protective apparel is needed, the nurse first performs hand hygiene, then applies a mask and eyewear or goggles (as needed), applies a gown, and then puts on gloves. Disposable gloves are easily applied and are designed to fit either hand. The glove's thin rubber can be easily torn. The glove cuffs should be pulled up over the wrists or over the cuffs of the gown. If a break or tear is detected in a glove while providing care, the nurse should change gloves if care is not completed. If the nurse does not plan to have more contact with the client, reapplying gloves is unnecessary.

Family members visiting clients who are on a category of isolation requiring use of gloves must know when and how to apply gloves properly. The nurse demonstrates application of gloves to family members and explains the reason for use of gloves. The nurse emphasizes the importance of hand hygiene following the removal of gloves.

When participating in a procedure that may potentially create droplets or splashing or spraying of blood or other body fluids, a nurse must wear protective eyewear, a mask, or a face shield (Garner, 1996). Examples of such procedures include irrigation of a large abdominal wound or insertion of an arterial catheter in which the nurse assists a physician. Eyewear may be available in the form of plastic glasses or goggles (see Figure 29–2). The eyewear should fit snugly around the face so that fluids cannot enter between the face and the glasses.

Specimen Collection. Many laboratory studies may be required when a client is suspected of having an infectious disease. Body fluids and secretions suspected of containing infectious organisms are collected for culture and sensitivity tests. The specimen is placed in a medium that promotes growth of organisms. A laboratory technologist then identifies the micro-organisms growing in the culture. Additional test results indicate antibiotics to which the organisms are resistant or sensitive. Sensitivity reports determine the antibiotics used in treatment.

The nurse obtains all culture specimens using disposable gloves and sterile equipment. Collecting fresh material from the site of infection, such as wound drainage, ensures that the specimen is not contaminated by neighbouring microbes. All specimen containers should be sealed tightly to prevent spillage and contamination of the outside of the container. Box 29-14 describes techniques for collecting specimens from the client with a suspected infection.

Bagging Waste or Linen. Nurses use special bagging procedures for removing contaminated items from the client's environment. Bagging contaminated items and ensuring the outside of the bag is not contaminated prevents accidental exposure of personnel and prevents contamination of the surrounding environment.

Health Canada (1999) recommends a single bag for discarding items if the bag is impervious and sturdy and if the article can be placed in the bag without contaminating the outside of the bag. Soiled linen should be placed in an impervious laundry bag in the client's room. Health Canada recommends double bagging if it is impossible to prevent contamination of the bag's outer surface. Double bagging is not otherwise recommended. Studies have shown that double bagging is not necessary to control infection (Maki, Alvarado, & Hassemer,1986; Weinstein et al., 1989). Use of one standard-sized linen bag that is not overfilled, that is tied securely, and that is intact is adequate to prevent infection transmission. The same rule applies to garbage bags.

Transporting Clients. Before transferring clients to wheelchairs or stretchers, the nurse gives them clean gowns to serve as robes. Clients infected with organisms transmitted by the airborne route should leave their rooms only for essential purposes, such as diagnostic procedures or surgery. These clients must also wear masks. Personnel transporting these clients should also wear barrier protection as needed.

At times a client being transported may drain body fluids onto a stretcher or wheelchair. When this occurs, the nurse must be sure to have the equipment cleaned and, if necessary, disinfected after the client returns to the room. An extra layer of sheets may be used to cover the stretcher or seat of the wheelchair.

Personnel in diagnostic or procedural areas or the operating room should be notified that the client is on isolation precautions. The nurse explains ways that the client can help prevent transmission of infection during transport. A client on airborne or droplet isolation is provided with a mask and given tissues and a bag to allow proper disposal of secretions. The nurse records the type of isolation on the client's chart.

Role of the Infection Control Professional. Many hospitals employ professionals, most of whom are nurses, who are specially trained in infection prevention and control. These individuals are responsible for advising hospital personnel regarding infection prevention and control and for monitoring infections within the hospital. The Community and Hospital Infection Control Association of Canada (CHICA-Canada) is a voluntary multidisciplinary association of infection control professionals. Its mission is to promote excellence in the practice of infection prevention and control (CHICA-Canada, 2004). Duties of an infection control professional include the following:

- Provide staff education on infection prevention and control.
- Develop and review infection prevention and control policies and procedures.
- Recommend appropriate isolation procedures.
- Screen client records for community-acquired infections that may be reportable to the public health department.
- Consult with employee health departments concerning recommendations to prevent and control the spread of infection among personnel, such as TB testing.
- Gather statistics regarding the **epidemiology** (cause and effect) of nosocomial infections.

Box 29-14 Specimen Collection Techniques*

Wound Specimen

Clean site with sterile water or saline prior to wound specimen collection. Wear gloves and use cotton-tipped swab or syringe to collect as much drainage as possible. Have clean test tube or culture tube on clean paper towel. After swabbing centre of wound site, grasp collection tube by holding it with paper towel. Carefully insert swab without touching outside of tube. After securing tube's top, transfer tube into bag for transport and then perform hand hygiene.

Stool Specimen

Wearing gloves, use clean cup with seal top (need not be sterile) and tongue blade to collect small amount of stool, approximately the size of a walnut. Place cup on clean paper towel in client's bathroom. Using tongue blade, collect needed amount of feces from client's bedpan. Transfer feces to cup without touching cup's outside surface. Dispose of tongue blade, and place seal on cup. Transfer specimen into clean bag for transport. Remove gloves and perform hand hygiene.

Blood Specimen

Wearing gloves, use syringe and culture media bottles to collect up to 10 mL of blood per culture bottle (check agency policy). After prepping, perform venipuncture at two different sites to decrease likelihood of both specimens being contaminated with skin flora. Place blood culture bottles on bedside table or other surface; swab off bottle tops with alcohol. Inject appropriate amount of blood into each bottle. Remove gloves and transfer specimen into clean, labelled bag for transport. Perform hand hygiene.

Urine Specimen

Wearing gloves, use syringe and sterile cup to collect 1 to 5 mL of urine. Place cup or tube on clean towel in client's bathroom. If client has a urinary catheter, use syringe to collect specimen. Have client follow procedure to obtain a clean voided specimen (see chapter 40) if not catheterized. Transfer urine into sterile container by injecting urine from syringe or pouring it from used collection cup. Secure top of container and transfer specimen into clean, labelled bag for transport. Remove gloves and perform hand hygiene.

*Agency policies may differ on type of containers and amount of specimen material required.
From *Diagnostic Testing and Nursing Implications: A Case Study Approach* (5th ed.), by Pagana and T. J. Pagana, 1998, St. Louis, MO: Mosby.

- Notify the public health department of incidences of communicable diseases within the facility.
- Confer with all hospital departments to investigate unusual events or clusters of infection.
- Recommend education for clients and families.
- Identify infection control problems with equipment.
- Monitor antibiotic-resistant organisms in the institution.

An infection control professional can be a valuable resource for assisting nurses in controlling nosocomial infections.

Infection Prevention and Control for Hospital Personnel. Health care workers are continually at risk for exposure to infectious micro-organisms. Each agency ensures there are protocols in place to advise staff and monitor infection protocols. Hospitals offer regularly scheduled staff education programs. Each province and territory has rules and procedures to ensure health care workers are not unnecessarily exposed to pathogens.

Client Education. Often clients must learn to use infection control practices at home (Box 29-15). Preventive technique becomes almost second nature to the nurse who practises it daily. However, the client is less aware of factors that promote the spread of infection or ways to prevent its transmission. The home environment does not always lend itself to infection prevention. Often a nurse must help a client adapt according to the resources available to maintain hygienic techniques. Generally, clients in a home care setting have a decreased risk of infection because of less exposure to resistant organisms such as those found in a hospital and because of fewer invasive procedures.

After clients are at home, nurses determine their compliance with infection control practices. The nurse educates clients about infection and techniques to prevent or control its spread. Family members caring for clients must be involved in the teaching plan. The nurse teaches clients and family members a common-sense approach to controlling and preventing infection. Topics to address in a teaching session include the following:

- Clients' susceptibility to infection
- The chain of infection, with specific reference to means of transmission
- Hygienic practices that minimize organism growth and spread, emphasizing handwashing
- Preventive health care (e.g., diet, immunizations, and exercise)
- Proper methods for handling and storage of food
- Family members who are at risk for acquiring infection

Surgical Asepsis. **Surgical asepsis,** or sterile technique, requires the use of different precautions from those of medical asepsis. Surgical asepsis includes procedures used to eliminate all micro-organisms, including pathogens and spores, from an object or area. In surgical asepsis, an area or object is considered contaminated if touched by any object that is not sterile. The nurse working with a sterile field or with sterile equipment must understand that the slightest break in technique results in contamination. Surgical asepsis should be used in the following situations:

- During procedures that require intentional perforation of the client's skin (e.g., insertion of IV catheters or administration of injections)
- When the skin's integrity is broken as a result of trauma, surgical incision, or burns

Client Teaching — Box 29-15

Infection Control

Objective

- Client will assume self-care using proper infection control techniques.

Teaching Strategies

- Instruct client about cleaning equipment using soap and water and disinfecting with an appropriate disinfectant.
- Demonstrate proper hand hygiene, explaining that it should be done before and after all treatments and when infected body fluids are contacted.
- Instruct client about the signs and symptoms of wound infection.
- For clients who receive tube feedings at home, explain the importance of preparing enough formula for only 8 hours (commercially prepared) or 4 hours (home prepared). Tell client that contaminated enteral feeding can cause infections. Rinse feeding bag and tubing with mild soap and water daily and dry.
- Instruct client to place contaminated dressings and other disposable items containing infectious body fluids in impervious plastic bags and to place needles in a puncture-proof and leak-proof container, such as an empty bleach bottle with the opening taped shut or a coffee can with the lid taped closed. Glass containers should not be used. The local municipality or public health department should be contacted before disposal (Health Canada, 1998).
- Instruct client (or family) to separate noticeably soiled linen from other laundry, wash in water that is as hot as the fabric will tolerate, add 250 mL of bleach to detergent, and set dryer temperature as high as fabric will allow.

Evaluation

- Ask client or family member to describe techniques used to reduce transmission of infection.
- Have client demonstrate select techniques.
- Ask client to explain the risks for infection based on the condition.

- During procedures that involve insertion of catheters or surgical instruments into sterile body cavities

Although surgical asepsis is commonly practised in the operating room, labour and delivery area, and major diagnostic areas, the nurse may also use surgical aseptic techniques at the client's bedside. This includes, for example, inserting IV or urinary catheters, suctioning the tracheobronchial airway, and reapplying sterile dressings. A nurse in an operating room follows a series of steps to maintain sterile technique, including applying a mask, protective eyewear, and a cap; performing a surgical hand scrub; and applying a sterile gown and gloves. In contrast, a nurse performing a dressing change at a client's bedside may only perform hand hygiene and apply sterile gloves. (See Principles of Surgical Asepsis.)

Client Preparation. Because surgical asepsis requires exact techniques, the nurse must have the client's cooperation. Therefore, the nurse must prepare the client before any procedure. Some clients may fear moving or touching objects during a sterile procedure, whereas others may even try to assist. The nurse explains how a procedure is to be performed and what the client can do to avoid contaminating sterile items, including the following:

- Avoid sudden movements of body parts covered by sterile drapes.
- Refrain from touching sterile supplies, drapes, or the nurse's gloves and gown.
- Avoid coughing, sneezing, or talking over a sterile area.

Certain sterile procedures may last an extended time. The nurse assesses the client's needs and anticipates factors that may disrupt a procedure. If a client is in pain, the nurse tries to administer analgesics no more than half an hour before a sterile procedure begins. The nurse gives the client the opportunity to void. Often clients must assume uncomfortable positions during sterile procedures. The nurse helps the client to assume the most comfortable position possible. Finally, the client's condition may result in actions or events that contaminate a sterile field; for example, a client with a respiratory infection transmits organisms by coughing or breathing. The nurse anticipates such a problem and offers the client a mask.

Principles of Surgical Asepsis. When beginning a surgically aseptic procedure, the nurse follows certain principles to ensure maintenance of asepsis. Failure to follow these principles places clients at risk for infection. The following principles are important:

1. *A sterile object remains sterile only when touched by another sterile object.* This principle guides the nurse in placement of sterile objects and how to handle them.
   a. Sterile touching sterile remains sterile; for example, sterile gloves are worn or sterile forceps are used to handle objects on a sterile field.
   b. Sterile touching clean becomes contaminated; for example, if the tip of a syringe or other sterile object touches the surface of a clean disposable glove, the object is contaminated.
   c. Sterile touching contaminated becomes contaminated; for example, when the nurse touches a sterile object with an ungloved hand, the object is contaminated.
   d. Sterile touching questionable is contaminated; for example, when a tear or break in the covering or packaging of a sterile object is found, it is discarded regardless of whether the object itself appears untouched.
2. *Only sterile objects may be placed on a sterile field.* All items are properly sterilized before use. Sterile objects are kept in clean, dry storage areas. The package or container holding a sterile object must be intact and dry. A package that is torn, punctured, wet, or open is considered to be contaminated.
3. *A sterile object or field out of the range of vision or an object held below a person's waist is contaminated.* Nurses never turn their backs on a sterile tray or leave it unattended. Contamination can occur accidentally by a dangling piece of clothing, falling hair, or an unknowing client touching a sterile object. Any object held below waist level is considered contaminated because it cannot be viewed at all times. Sterile objects

should be kept in front with the hands as close together as possible.

4. *A sterile object or field becomes contaminated by prolonged exposure to air.* The nurse avoids activities that may create air currents, such as excessive movements or rearranging linen after a sterile object or field becomes exposed. When sterile packages are being opened, it is important to minimize the number of people walking into the area. Micro-organisms travel by droplet through the air. No one should talk, laugh, sneeze, or cough over a sterile field or when gathering and using sterile equipment. Micro-organisms travelling through the air can fall on sterile items or fields if the nurse reaches over the work area. When opening sterile packages, the nurse holds the item or piece of equipment as close as possible to the sterile field without touching the sterile surface. Keeping movement or rearranging of sterile items to a minimum also reduces contamination by air transmission.
5. *When a sterile surface comes in contact with a wet, contaminated surface, the sterile object or field becomes contaminated by capillary action.* If moisture seeps through a sterile package's protective covering, micro-organisms travel to the sterile object. When stored sterile packages become wet, the nurse discards the objects immediately or sends the equipment for resterilization. When working with a sterile field or tray, the nurse may have to pour sterile solutions. Any spill can be a source of contamination unless the object or field rests on a sterile surface that cannot be penetrated by moisture. Urinary catheterization trays contain sterile supplies that rest in a sterile, plastic container. In this example, sterile solutions spilled within the container will not contaminate the catheter or other objects. In contrast, if a nurse places a piece of sterile gauze in its wrapper on a client's bedside table and the table surface is wet, the gauze is considered contaminated.
6. *Fluid flows in the direction of gravity.* A sterile object becomes contaminated if gravity causes a contaminated liquid to flow over the object's surface. To avoid contamination during a surgical hand scrub, the nurse holds the hands above the elbows. This allows water to flow downward without contaminating the nurse's hands and fingers. The principle of water flow by gravity is also the reason for drying from fingers to elbows with hands held up, after the scrub.
7. *The edges of a sterile field or container are considered to be contaminated.* Frequently a nurse places sterile objects on a sterile towel or drape (Figure 29–3). Because the edge of the drape touches an unsterile surface, such as a table or bed linen, a 2.5-cm border around the drape is considered contaminated. Objects placed on the sterile field must be inside this border. The edges of sterile containers become exposed to air after they are open and are thus contaminated. After a sterile needle is removed from its protective cap or after forceps are removed from a container, the objects must not touch the container's edge. The lip of an opened bottle of solution also becomes contaminated after it is exposed to air. When pouring a sterile liquid, the nurse first pours a small amount of solution to wash away micro-organisms on the bottle lip. This small amount of solution is then discarded, and the nurse pours a second time on the same side to fill a container with the desired amount of solution.

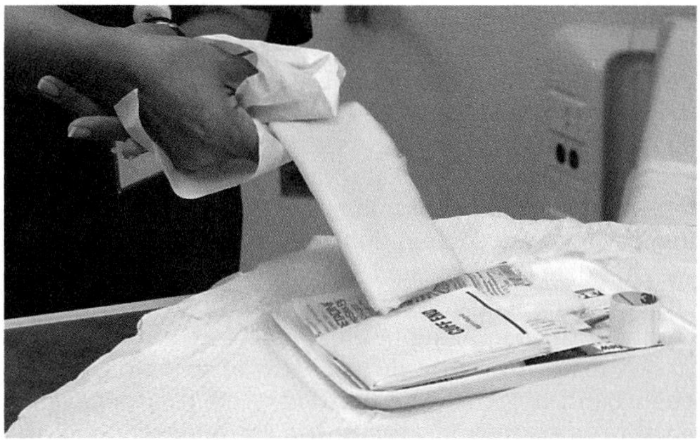

FIGURE **29–3** Placing sterile item on sterile field.

Performing Sterile Procedures. All necessary equipment should be assembled before a procedure. Thus the nurse avoids having to leave a sterile area to obtain equipment. A few extra supplies should be available in case objects accidentally become contaminated. Before the sterile procedure, each step should be explained so that the client can co-operate fully. If an object becomes contaminated during the procedure, the nurse should not hesitate to discard it immediately.

Donning and Removing Caps, Masks, and Eyewear. For sterile procedures on a general nursing division, the nurse may wear a surgical mask and eyewear without a cap. Eyewear is worn as a part of standard precautions/routine practices if there is a risk of fluid or blood splashing into the nurse's eyes. For sterile surgical procedures, the nurse first applies a clean cap that covers all of the hair and then the surgical mask and eyewear. A mask must fit snugly around the face and nose to prevent contamination by droplet nuclei. After a mask is worn for several hours, the area over the mouth and nose often becomes moist. Because moisture promotes the spread of micro-organisms, the mask should be changed if it becomes moist.

Protective glasses or goggles should fit snugly around the forehead and face to fully protect the eyes. Eyewear needs to be worn only for procedures that create the risk of body fluids splashing into the eyes. Before removing a mask, eyewear, and cap, the nurse removes sterile gloves to prevent contamination of the hair, neck, and facial area. After untying the mask, the nurse holds it by the ties and discards it with the cap. Masks should not be worn hanging from the neck after removal. Eyewear is removed and cleaned later for reuse. After removing all protective wear, the nurse performs hand hygiene thoroughly.

Opening Sterile Packages. Sterile items such as syringes, gauze dressings, or catheters are packaged in paper or plastic containers and are impervious to micro-organisms as long as they are dry and intact. Some institutions wrap reusable supplies in a double thickness of paper, linen, or muslin. These packages are permeable to steam and thus allow for steam autoclaving. Sterile items are kept in clean, enclosed storage cabinets and are separated from dirty equipment.

Sterile supplies have chemical tapes indicating that a sterilization process has taken place. The tapes change colour during the sterilization process. Failure of the tapes to change colour means that the item is not sterile. A sterile item should never be used if the integrity of the packaging is compromised. Health care facilities may apply the date processed and a lot number to the item after processing ("event-related expiration"), or they may apply an expiration date ("date-related expiration") to the item. With either system, it is important for the nurse to check the integrity of the packaging of the item before use.

Before opening a sterile item, the nurse performs thorough hand hygiene. The nurse inspects the supplies for package integrity and sterility and assembles the supplies in the work area, such as the bedside table or treatment room, before opening packages. A bedside table or countertop provides a large, clean working area for opening items. The work area should be above waist level. Sterile supplies should not be opened in a confined space where a dirty object might fall on or strike them.

Opening a Sterile Item on a Flat Surface. Sterile packaged items must be opened without contaminating the contents. Commercially packaged items are usually designed so that the nurse only has to tear away or separate the paper or plastic cover. The item is held in one hand while the wrapper is pulled away with the other (Figure 29–4). Care is then taken to keep the inner contents sterile before use. When opening items processed by the facility and packed in paper or linen, the nurse observes the following steps:

1. Place the item flat in the centre of the work surface.
2. Remove the sterilization tape or seal.
3. Grasp the outer surface of the tip of the outermost flap.
4. Open the outer flap away from the body, keeping the arm outstretched and away from the sterile field (Figure 29–5, *A*).
5. Grasp the outside surface of the first side flap.
6. Open the side flap, allowing it to lie flat on the table surface. Keep the arm to the side and not over the sterile surface (Figure 29–5, *B*). Do not allow the flaps to spring back over the sterile contents.
7. Grasp the outside surface of the second side flap and allow it to lie flat on the table surface (Figure 29–5, *C*).
8. Grasp the outside surface of the last and innermost flap.
9. Stand away from the sterile package and pull the flap back, allowing it to fall flat on the surface (Figure 29–5, *D*).
10. Use the inner surface of the package (except for the 2.5-cm border around the edges) as a sterile field to add additional sterile items. The 2.5-cm border can be grasped to manoeuvre the field on the table surface.

If the sterile supplies are not for immediate use, the nurse can close the sterile package. In this case, the nurse should touch only the wrapper's outside surface. To close a package, the order of unwrapping is reversed, and the nurse does not touch the inside contents or reach over the field.

Opening a Sterile Item While Holding It. To open a small, sterile item, the package is held in the non-dominant hand while the top flap is opened and pulled away from the nurse. Using the dominant hand, the nurse carefully opens the sides and top flaps away from the enclosed sterile item in the same order previously mentioned. The nurse opens the item in a hand so that the item can be handed to a person wearing sterile gloves or transferred to a sterile field.

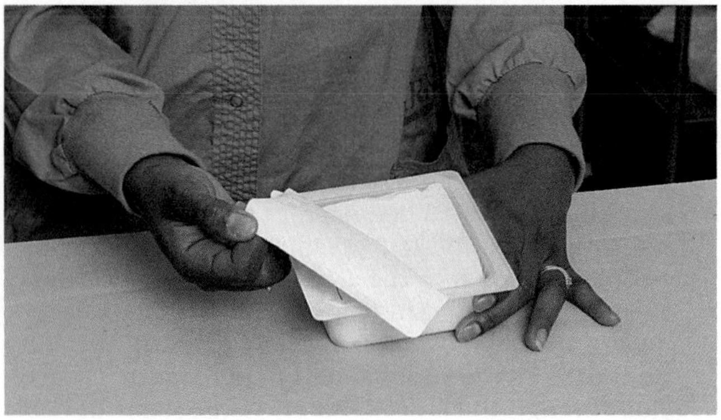

FIGURE **29–4** Nurse opening sterile package on work area above waist level.

Preparing a Sterile Field. When performing sterile procedures, the nurse needs a sterile work area that provides room for handling and placing of sterile items. A **sterile field** is an area free of micro-organisms and prepared to receive sterile items. The field may be prepared by using the inner surface of a sterile wrapper as the work surface or by using a sterile drape or dressing tray. Skill 29-2 describes preparation of a sterile field. After the surface for the field is created, the nurse adds sterile items by placing them directly on the field or by transferring them with a sterile forceps. When transferring sterile items, the nurse must carefully place objects on to the sterile field. An object that comes in contact with the 2.5-cm border must be discarded.

The nurse may choose to wear sterile gloves while preparing items on the field. If this is done, the nurse can touch the entire drape, but sterile items must be handed over by an assistant. The nurse's gloves cannot touch the wrappers of sterile items.

Pouring Sterile Solutions. Often the nurse must pour sterile solutions into sterile containers. A bottle containing a sterile solution is sterile on the inside and contaminated on the outside; the outside neck of the bottle is also contaminated, but the inside of the bottle cap is considered sterile. After a cap or lid is removed, it is held in the hand or placed sterile side (inside) up on a clean surface. This means that the inside of the lid can be seen as it rests on the table surface. A bottle cap or lid should never rest on a sterile surface, even though the inside of the cap is sterile. The outer edge of the cap is unsterile and would contaminate the surface. Likewise, placing a sterile cap down on an unsterile surface increases the chances of the inside of the cap becoming contaminated.

The nurse checks the label of the bottle to ensure it is the correct solution. The bottle should be held with its label in the palm of the hand to prevent the possibility of the solution wetting and fading the label. Before pouring the solution into the container, the nurse pours a small amount (1 to 2 mL) into a disposable cap or plastic-lined waste receptacle. The discarded solution cleans the lip of the bottle. The edge of the bottle is kept away from the edge or inside of the receiving container. The nurse pours the solution slowly to avoid splashing the underlying

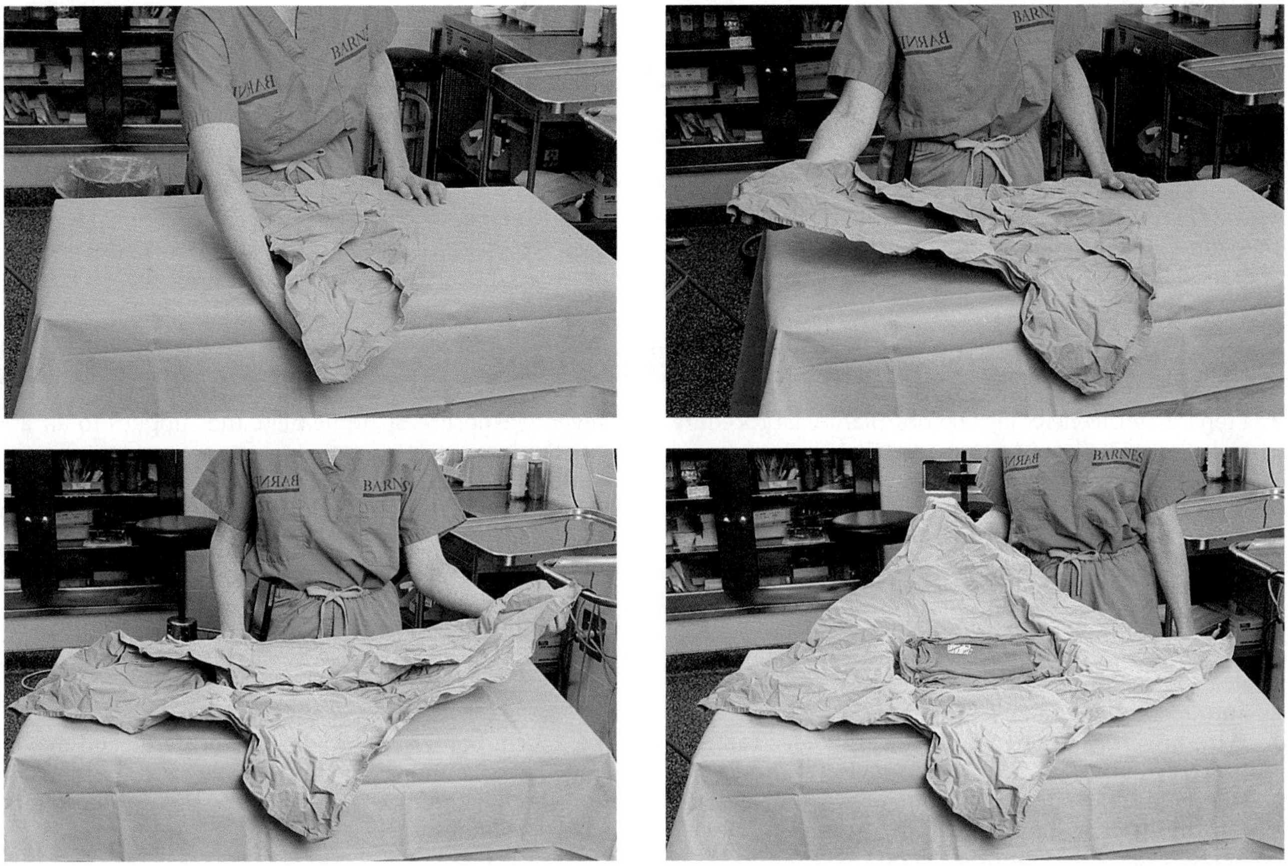

FIGURE **29–5** Opening sterile packaged items on a flat surface. **A,** The nurse opens the top flap away from the body. **B,** The nurse's arm is kept out away from the sterile field while opening a side flap. **C,** The second side flap is opened. **D,** The back flap is opened.

drape or field. The bottle should never be held so high above the container that even slow pouring will cause splashing. The bottle should be held outside the edge of the sterile field.

Surgical Scrub. Clients undergoing operative procedures are at an increased risk for infection. Nurses working in operating rooms perform surgical hand antisepsis to decrease and suppress the growth of skin micro-organisms in case of glove tears (Operating Room Nurses Association of Canada [ORNAC], 2003).

During surgical hand antisepsis, the nurse scrubs from fingertips to elbows with an antiseptic soap before each operation. The optimum duration of the surgical hand scrub is unclear, although research indicates that it may be dependent on the type of antimicrobial product. The usual scrub time for both the initial and the subsequent scrub is 5 minutes (Meeker & Rothrock, 1999). Larson (1996) recommended that at least 2 minutes of friction be used for surgical handwashing. The nurse should follow the agency's policy for length of scrub time. For many years, preoperative handwashing protocols required nurses to scrub with a brush. However, this practice may damage the skin and can result in increased shedding of bacteria from the hands. Scrubbing with a disposable sponge or combination sponge-brush has been shown to reduce bacterial counts on the hands as effectively as scrubbing with a brush. However, several studies suggest that neither a brush nor a sponge is necessary to reduce bacterial counts on the hands, especially when an alcohol-based product is used.

For maximum elimination of bacteria, all jewellery should be removed and the nails should be kept clean and short (ORNAC, 2003). Artificial nails should not be worn, because they may harbour a greater number of bacteria. Similarly, nail polish should be avoided because it conceals soil under the nails and chipped nail polish may increase bacterial load (Health Canada, 1998). Freshly applied polish (not chipped or worn for more than 4 days) may be acceptable, if permitted by facility policy (Gruendemann & Mangum, 2001). Nurses who have active skin infections, open lesions or cuts, or respiratory infections should be excluded from the surgical team. Skill 29-3 describes the steps for surgical hand hygiene.

Applying Sterile Gloves. Sterile gloves are an additional barrier to bacterial transfer. There are two gloving methods: open and closed. Nurses who work on general nursing divisions use open gloving before procedures such as dressing changes or urinary catheter insertions. The closed gloving method, which is performed after nurses apply sterile gowns, is practised in operating rooms and special treatment areas. Skills 29-4 and 29-5 review the steps of each sterile gloving technique. The proper glove size should be selected; the glove should not stretch so tightly that it can easily tear, yet it should be tight enough that objects can be picked up easily.

Text continued on p. 828

Skill 29-2 *Preparation of a Sterile Field*

Delegation Considerations

Delegation of the preparation of a sterile field is inappropriate unless unregulated care providers have received specialized training. Operating room technicians are usually trained for this skill.

Equipment

- Sterile drape
- Assorted sterile supplies

Steps	Rationale
1. Prepare sterile field just before planned procedure. Supplies are to be used immediately.	Prevents exposure of sterile field and supplies to air and contamination.
2. Select clean work surface above waist level.	Sterile object held below waist is contaminated.
3. Assemble necessary equipment.	Preparation of equipment in advance prevents break in technique.
4. Check dates or labels on supplies for sterility of equipment.	Equipment stored beyond expiration date is considered unsterile.
5. Perform hand hygiene thoroughly. *Option:* procedure may be performed with gloves.	Reduces microbial counts on skin.
6. Place pack containing sterile drape on work surface and open as described in Figure 29–5.	Ensures sterility of packaged drape.
7. With fingertips of one hand, pick up folded top edge of sterile drape.	The 2.5-cm border around drape is unsterile and may be touched with fingers or clean gloves.
8. Gently lift drape up from its outer cover and let it unfold by itself without touching any object. Discard outer cover with your other hand.	If sterile object touches any other non-sterile object, it becomes contaminated.
9. With other hand, grasp adjacent corner of drape and hold it straight up and away from your body (see illustration).	Drape can now be properly placed while using two hands. Drape must be held away from unsterile surfaces.
10. Holding drape, first position and lay bottom half over intended work surface (see illustration).	Prevents nurse from reaching over sterile field.
11. Allow top half of drape to be placed over work surface last (see illustration).	Creates flat, sterile work surface.

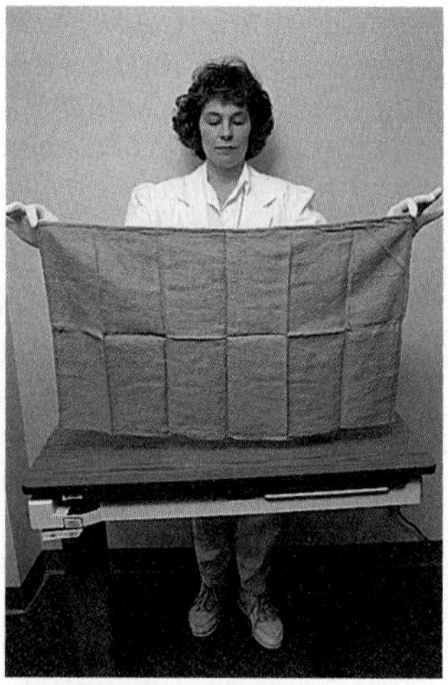

STEP **9** Hold drape straight up and away from body.

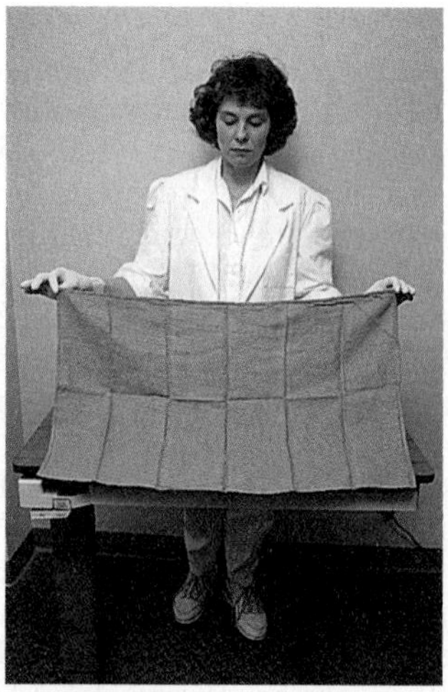

STEP **10** Lay bottom half over work surface.

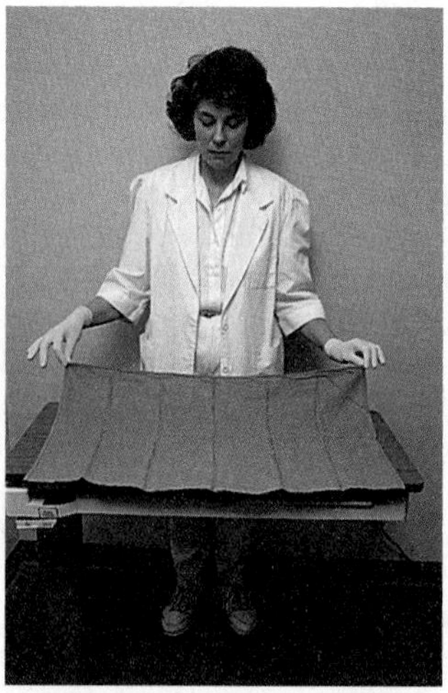

STEP **11** Place top half of drape over work surface.

Steps	Rationale
12. Grasp 2.5-cm border around edge to position as needed.	
Adding Sterile Items	
13. Open sterile item (following package directions) while holding outside wrapper in non-dominant hand.	Frees dominant hand for unwrapping outer wrapper.
14. Carefully peel wrapper onto non-dominant hand.	Item remains sterile.
15. Being sure wrapper does not fall down on sterile field, place item onto field at angle. Do not hold arm over sterile field (see illustration).	Prevents reaching over field and contaminating its surface.
16. Dispose of outer wrapper.	Prevents accidental contamination of sterile field.
17. Perform procedure using sterile technique.	Prevents transmission of infection to client.

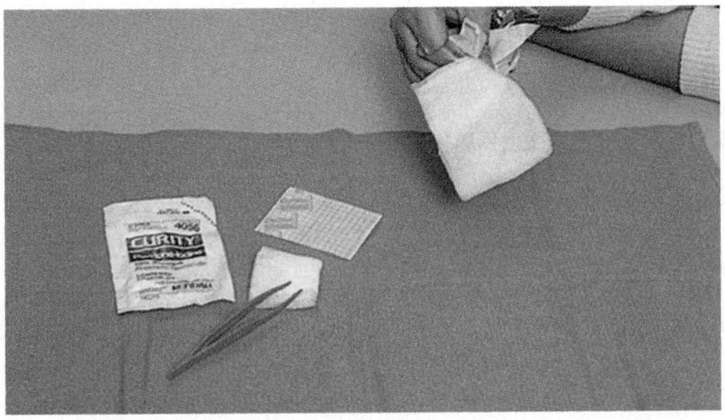

STEP **15** Adding item to sterile field.

Recording and Reporting

- It is not necessary to record or report this procedure.

Skill 29-3 Surgical Hand Hygiene: Preparing for Gowning

Delegation Considerations

The role of the scrub nurse can be delegated to a surgical technologist or licensed practical nurse.

Unregulated care providers can help the registered nurse in the circulating nurse role by opening sterile supplies, setting up sterile fields, and running errands under the direction of the registered nurse.

Equipment

- Deep sink with foot or knee controls for dispensing water and soap (faucets should be high enough for hands and forearms to fit comfortably)
- Antimicrobial detergent or alcohol-based waterless antiseptic, according to agency policy (non-irritating, broad-spectrum, fast-acting, effective in reducing skin micro-organisms, and having a residual effect; Association of periOperative Nurses [AORN], 2004; ORNAC, 2003)
- Surgical scrub sponge with plastic nail pick
- Paper mask and cap or hood
- Sterile towel
- Proper scrub attire
- Protective eyewear (glasses or goggles)

Steps	Rationale
1. Consult agency policy regarding required length of time and antiseptic to use for hand antisepsis.	Guidelines vary regarding ideal time needed and antiseptic to use for surgical scrub.
2. Be sure fingernails are short, clean, and healthy. Artificial nails should be removed. Natural nails should be less than 0.5 cm long.	Long nails and chipped or old polish increase number of bacteria residing on nails. Long fingernails can puncture gloves, causing contamination. Artificial nails are known to harbour gram-negative micro-organisms and fungus (Hedderwick et al., 2000).

Critical Decision Point: Remove nail polish if chipped or worn longer than 4 days because it may harbour micro-organisms (AORN, 2004; ORNAC, 2003).

Steps	Rationale
3. Inspect hands for presence of abrasions, cuts, or open lesions.	These conditions increase likelihood of more micro-organisms residing on skin surfaces.
4. Apply surgical shoe covers, cap or hood, face mask, and protective eyewear.	Mask prevents escape into air of micro-organisms that can contaminate hands. Other protective wear prevents exposure to blood and body fluid splashes during the procedure.
5. Surgical handwashing:	
a. Turn on water using knee or foot controls and adjust to comfortable temperature.	
b. Wet hands and arms under running lukewarm water and lather with detergent to 5 cm above elbows. (Hands need to be above elbows at all times.)	Water runs by gravity from fingertips to elbows. Hands become cleanest part of upper extremity. Keeping hands elevated allows water to flow from least to most contaminated areas. Washing a wide area reduces risk of contaminating overlying gown that the nurse later applies.
c. Rinse hands and arms thoroughly under running water. **Remember to keep hands above elbows.**	Rinsing removes transient bacteria from fingers, hands, and forearms.
d. Under running water, clean under nails of both hands with nail pick. Discard after use (see illustration).	Removes dirt and organic material that harbour large numbers of micro-organisms.
e. Wet clean sponge and apply antimicrobial detergent. Scrub nails of one hand with 15 strokes. Holding sponge perpendicular, scrub palm, each side of thumb and fingers, and posterior side of hand with 10 strokes each. The arm is mentally divided into thirds, and each third is scrubbed 10 times (see illustration). The duration of scrub is determined by the manufacturer's recommendations for the scrub agent used, which is usually 2 to 6 minutes (ORNAC, 2003). Rinse sponge and repeat sequence for other arm. A two-sponge method may be substituted. Check agency policy.	Friction loosens resident bacteria that adhere to skin surfaces. Ensures coverage of all surfaces. Scrubbing is performed from cleanest area (hands) to marginal area (upper arms).

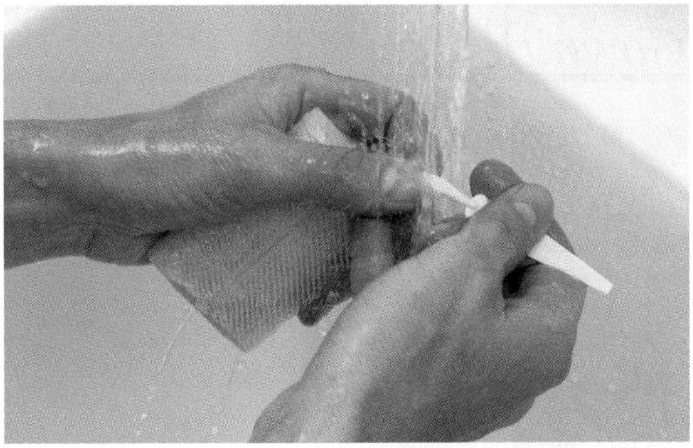

STEP **5d** Cleaning under fingernails.

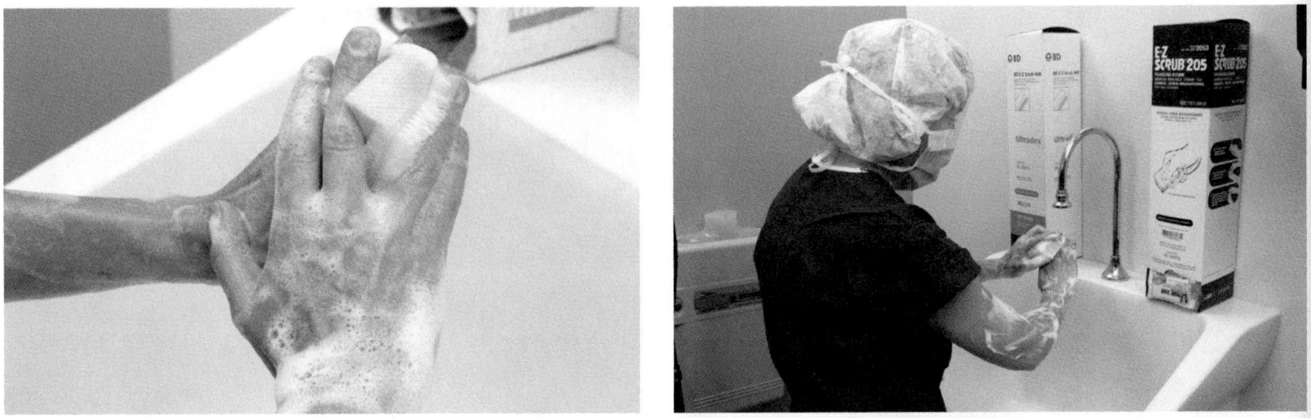

A B

STEP **5e** **A,** Scrubbing side of fingers. **B,** Scrubbing forearms.

Steps	Rationale
f. Discard sponge and rinse hands and arms thoroughly (see illustration). Turn off water with foot or knee control and back into room entrance with hands elevated in front of and away from the body.	After touching skin, sponge is considered contaminated. Rinsing removes resident bacteria. Prevents accidental contamination.
g. Walk up to sterile tray and lean forward slightly to pick up a sterile towel (see illustration). Dry one hand thoroughly, moving from fingers to elbow. Dry in a rotating motion. Dry from cleanest to least clean area (see illustration).	Drying prevents chapping and facilitates donning of gloves. Leaning forward prevents accidental contact of arms with scrub attire.
h. Repeat drying method for other hand by carefully reversing towel or using a new sterile towel.	Prevents accidental contamination.
i. Discard towel.	Prevents accidental contamination.
j. Proceed with sterile gowning (see Skill 29-4).	
6. Alternate method of surgical hand hygiene using alcohol-based antiseptic:	
a. Wash hands with soap and water for 10-15 seconds to remove soil.	Removes dirt and organic material that harbour large numbers of micro-organisms.
b. Under running water, clean under nails of both hands with nail pick. Discard after use and dry hands with a paper towel.	

Skill 29-3 Surgical Hand Hygiene: Preparing for Gowning—cont'd

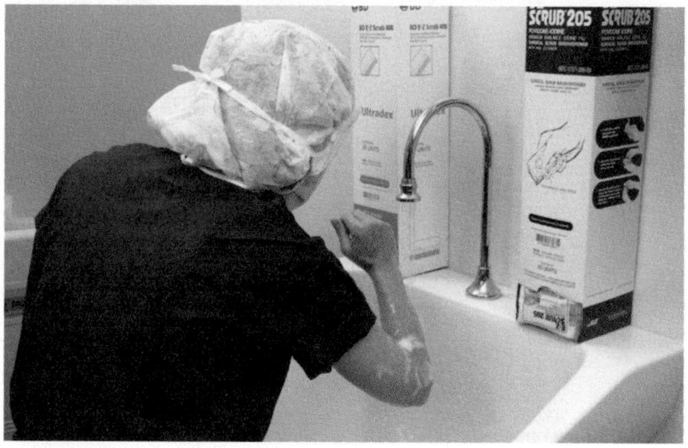

STEP **5f** Rinsing arms.

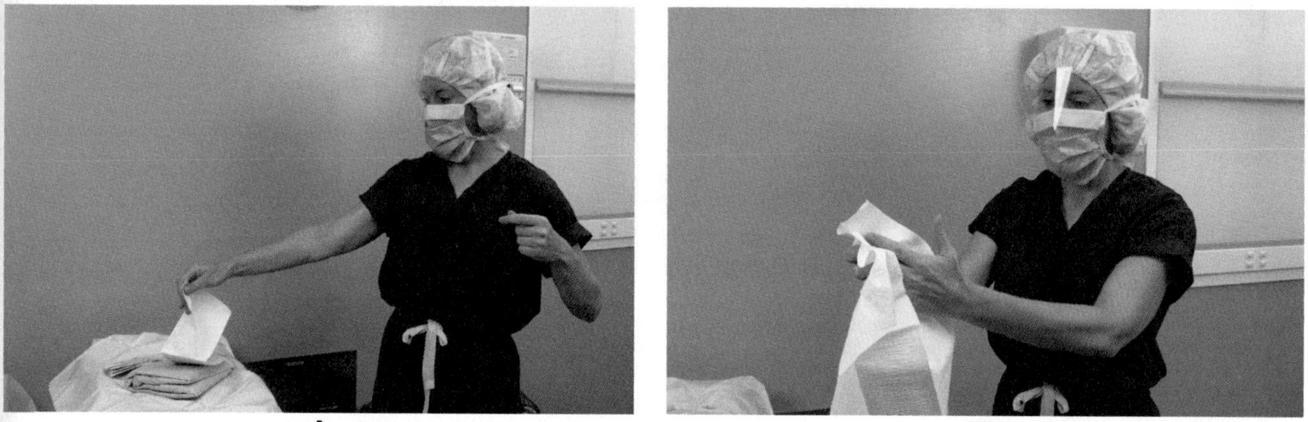

A **B**

STEP **5g** **A,** Grasping sterile towel. **B,** Drying sequence.

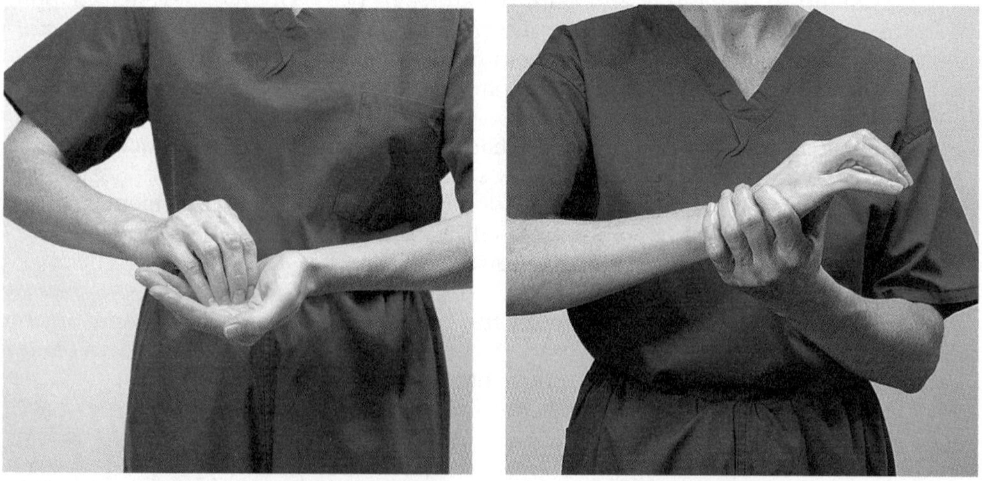

STEP **6c** Application of antimicrobial agent for brushless hand scrub. Nurse using 3M Avagard. (Photo courtesy of 3M Health Care.)

Steps	Rationale
c. Apply enough alcohol-based waterless antiseptic to one palm to cover both hands thoroughly (see illustration). Spread the antiseptic over all surfaces of the hands and fingernails. Follow product instructions for length of time to rub over hand surfaces. Allow to air-dry.	Ensures coverage of all surfaces. Air-drying ensures complete antisepsis is achieved.
d. Repeat the process and allow hands to air-dry before applying sterile gloves.	

Recording and Reporting

- It is not necessary to record or report this procedure.
- Report any dermatitis to employee health or infection control per agency policy.

Skill 29-4 Applying a Sterile Gown and Performing Closed Gloving

Delegation Considerations

The role of the scrub nurse can be delegated to a surgical technician.

Equipment

- Surgical cap
- Surgical mask
- Eyewear
- Foot covers
- Sterile gown (prepared by circulating nurse)

Steps	Rationale
Gowning	
1. Before entering operating room or treatment area, apply cap, face mask, and eyewear. Foot covers are also required in operating room.	Prevents hair and air droplet nuclei from contaminating sterile work areas. Eyewear protects mucous membranes of eye. Foot covers are paper or cloth and fit over work shoes.
2. Perform thorough surgical hand hygiene (see Skill 29-3).	Removes transient and resident bacteria from fingers, hands, and forearms.
3. Ask circulating nurse to assist by opening sterile pack containing sterile gown (folded inside out).	Gown's outer surface remains sterile.
4. Have circulating nurse prepare glove package by peeling outer wrapper open while keeping inner contents sterile. Inner glove package is then placed on sterile field created by sterile outer wrapper.	Keeps gloves sterile and allows nurse who has scrubbed to handle sterile items.
5. Reach down to sterile gown package; lift folded gown directly upward and step back away from table.	Provides wide margin of safety, avoiding contamination of gown.
6. Holding folded gown, locate neckband. With both hands, grasp inside front of gown just below neckband.	Clean hands may touch inside of gown without contaminating outer surface.
7. Allow gown to unfold, keeping inside of gown toward body. Do not touch outside of gown with bare hands.	Outside of gown will be sterile surface.
8. With hands at shoulder level, slip both arms into armholes simultaneously (see illustration). Ask circulating nurse to bring gown over shoulders by reaching inside to arm seams and pulling gown on, leaving sleeves covering hands.	Careful application prevents contamination. Gown covers hands to prepare for closed gloving.

Skill 29-4 Applying a Sterile Gown and Performing Closed Gloving—cont'd

Steps	Rationale
9. Have circulating nurse securely tie back of gown at neck and waist (see illustration). (If gown is a wrap-around style, sterile flap to cover gown is not touched until the nurse has gloved.)	Gown must completely enclose underlying garments.
10. Closed gloving:	
a. With hands covered by gown sleeves, open inner sterile glove package (see illustration).	Hands remain clean. Sterile gown cuff will touch sterile glove surface.
b. With dominant hand inside gown cuff, pick up glove for non-dominant hand by grasping folded cuff.	Sterile gown touches sterile glove.
c. Extend non-dominant forearm with palm up and place palm of glove against palm of non-dominant hand. Glove fingers will point toward elbow.	Positions glove for application over cuffed hand, keeping glove sterile.

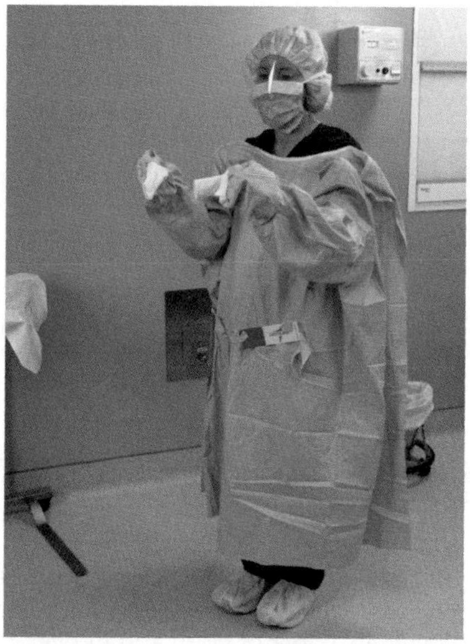

STEP **8** Placing arms in sleeves.

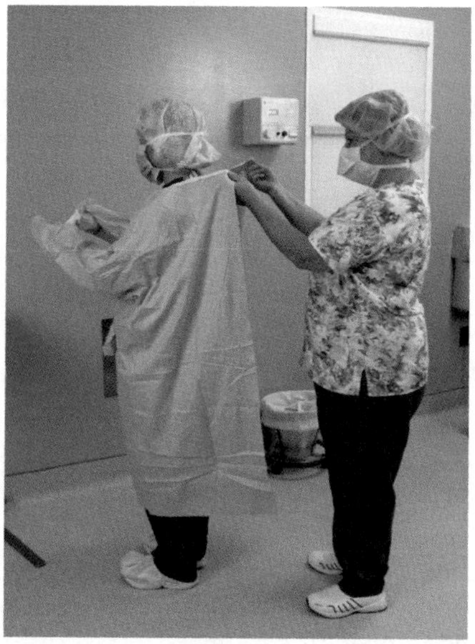

STEP **9** Circulating nurse ties scrub gown.

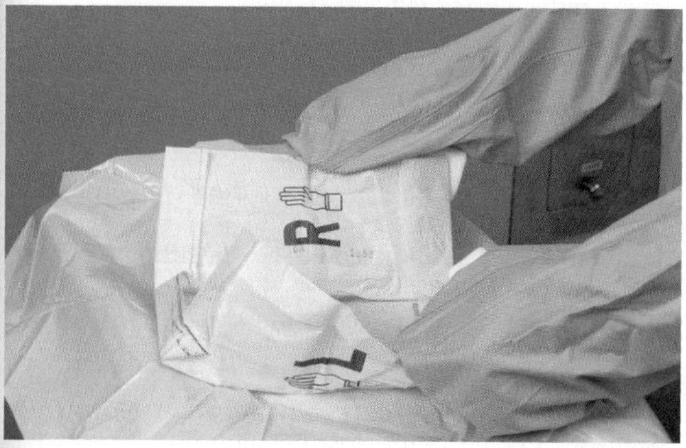

STEP **10a** Scrub nurse opens glove package.

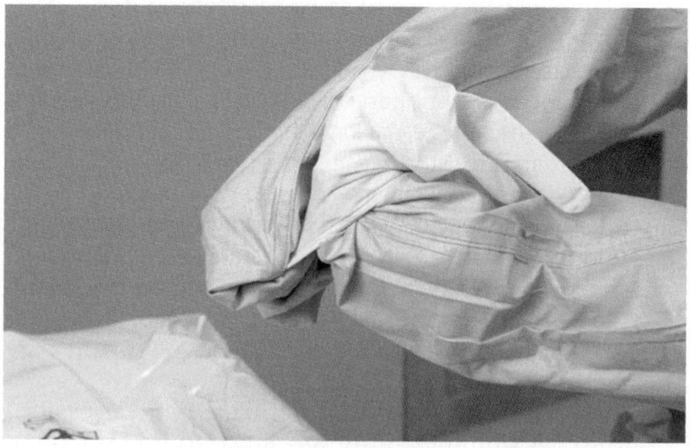

STEP **10d** Glove applied to left hand as right hand remains inside cuff.

Steps	Rationale
d. Grasp back of glove cuff with covered dominant hand and turn glove cuff over end of non-dominant hand and gown cuff (see illustration).	Seal created by glove cuff over gown prevents exit of microorganisms over operative sterile field.
e. Grasp top of glove and underlying gown sleeve with covered dominant hand. Carefully extend fingers into glove, being sure glove's cuff covers gown's cuff.	
f. Glove dominant hand in same manner, reversing hands (see illustration). Use gloved non-dominant hand to pull on glove. Keep hand inside sleeve (see illustration).	Sterile touches sterile.
g. Be sure fingers are fully extended into both gloves.	Ensures that nurse has full dexterity while using gloved hand.
11. For wraparound sterile gowns: Take gloved hand and release fastener or ties in front of gown.	Front of gown is sterile.
12. Hand tie to sterile team member who stands still (see illustration). Allowing margin of safety, turn around to the left, covering back with extended gown flap. Take back tie from team member and secure tie to gown.	Contact with team member could contaminate gown and gloves. Gown must enclose undergarments.

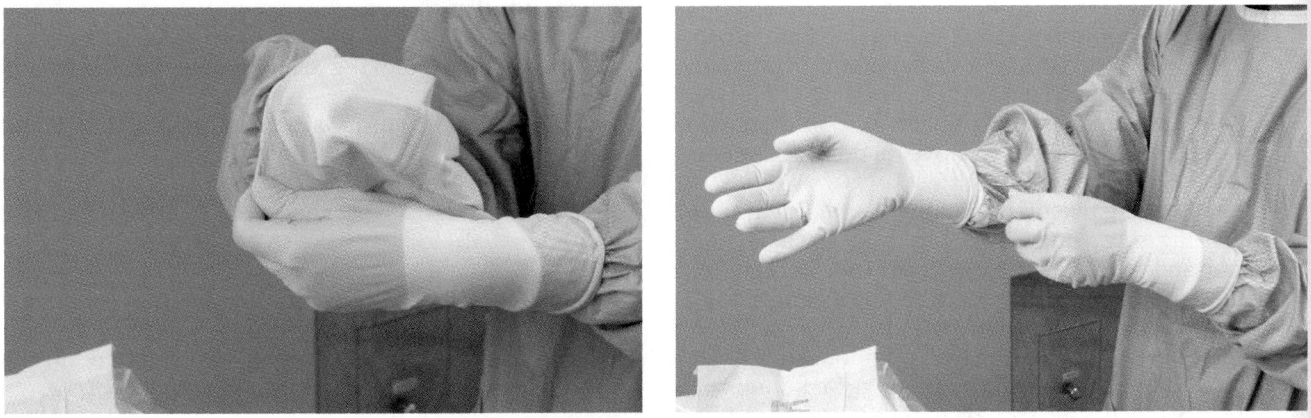

STEP **10f** Second glove applied

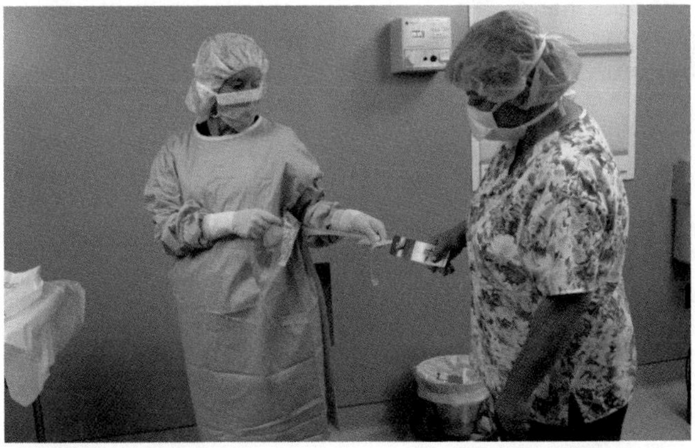

STEP **12** Handing tie to sterile team member.

Recording and Reporting

- It is not necessary to record or report this procedure.

Skill 29-5 Open Gloving

View Video

Delegation Considerations

Delegation of open gloving depends on whether unregulated care providers have received special training and are competent to perform the sterile procedure.

Equipment

- Sterile gloves (proper size)

Steps	Rationale
1. Perform thorough hand hygiene.	Removes bacteria from skin surfaces and reduces transmission of infection.
2. Remove outer glove package wrapper by carefully separating and peeling apart sides.	Prevents inner glove package from accidentally opening and touching contaminated objects.
3. Grasp inner package and lay it on clean, flat surface just above waist level. Open package, keeping gloves on wrapper's inside surface (see illustration).	Sterile object held below waist is contaminated. Inner surface of glove package is sterile.
4. If gloves are not prepowdered, take packet of powder and apply lightly to hands over sink or wastebasket	Powder allows gloves to slip on easily. (Some staff members do not use powder for fear of promoting growth of micro-organisms.)
5. Identify right and left glove. Each glove has cuff approximately 5 cm wide. Glove dominant hand first.	Proper identification of gloves prevents contamination by improper fit. Gloving of dominant hand first improves dexterity.
6. With thumb and first two fingers of non-dominant hand, grasp edge of cuff of glove for dominant hand. Touch only glove's inside surface.	Inner edge of cuff will lie against skin and thus is not sterile.
7. Carefully pull glove over dominant hand, leaving cuff and being sure cuff does not roll up wrist. Be sure thumb and fingers are in proper spaces (see illustration).	If glove's outer surface touches hand or wrist, then it is contaminated.
8. With gloved dominant hand, slip fingers underneath second glove's cuff (see illustration).	Cuff protects gloved fingers. Sterile touching sterile prevents glove contamination.
9. Carefully pull second glove over non-dominant hand. Do not allow fingers and thumb of gloved dominant hand to touch any part of exposed non-dominant hand. Keep thumb of dominant hand abducted back (see illustration).	Contact of gloved hand with exposed hand results in contamination.
10. After second glove is on, interlock hands. The cuffs usually fall down after application. Be sure to touch only sterile sides (see illustration).	Ensures smooth fit over fingers.

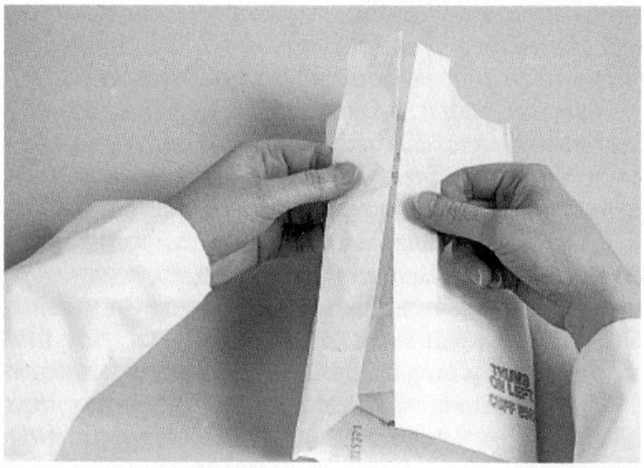

STEP **3** Opening package.

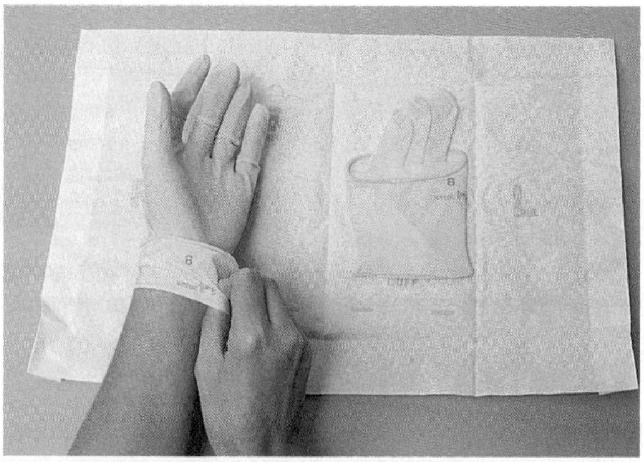

STEP **7** Pulling glove over dominant hand.

Steps	Rationale

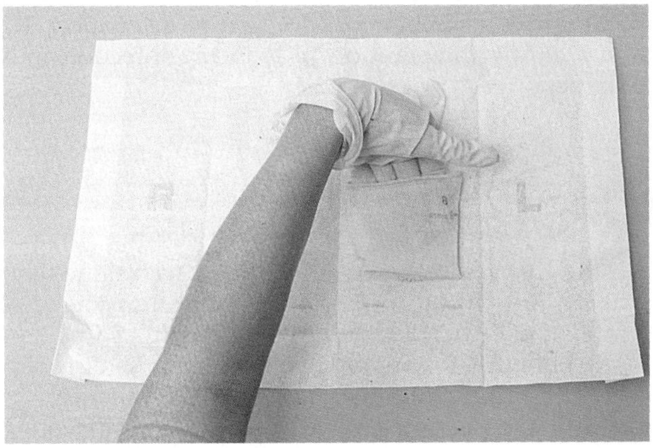

STEP **8** Slipping fingers underneath second glove's cuff.

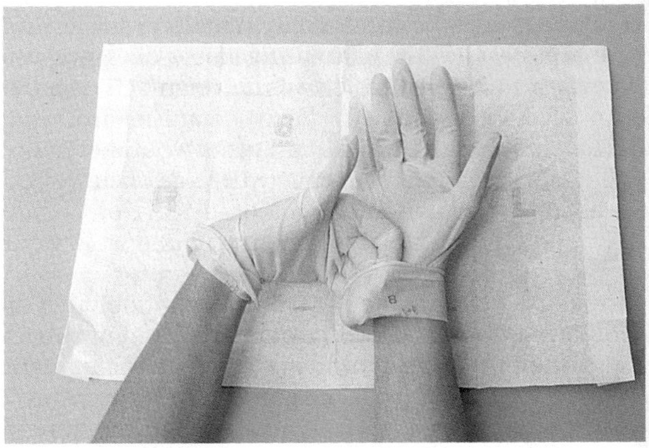

STEP **9** Pulling second glove over non-dominant hand.

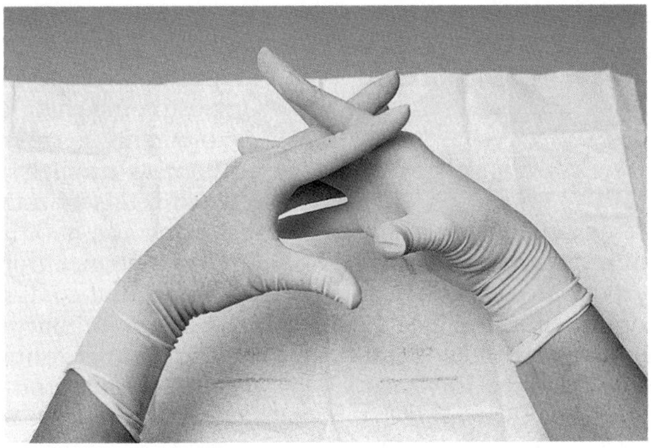

STEP **10** Hands interlocked.

Glove Disposal

Steps	Rationale
11. Grasp outside of one cuff with other gloved hand; avoid touching wrist.	Minimizes contamination of underlying skin.
12. Pull glove off, turning it inside out. Discard in receptacle.	Outside of glove does not touch skin surface.
13. Take fingers of bare hand and tuck inside remaining glove cuff. Peel glove off, inside out. Discard in receptacle.	

Recording and Reporting

- It is not necessary to record or report this procedure.

Donning a Sterile Gown. Nurses must wear sterile gowns when assisting at the sterile field in the operating room, delivery room, and special treatment areas so that sterile objects can be comfortably handled with less risk of contamination. The circulating nurse does not usually wear a sterile gown. The sterile gown acts as a barrier to decrease shedding of micro-organisms from skin surfaces into the air and thus prevents wound contamination. Nurses caring for clients with large open wounds or assisting physicians during major invasive procedures (e.g., inserting an arterial catheter) may also wear sterile gowns.

The nurse does not apply a sterile gown until after applying a mask and surgical cap and performing surgical handwashing. The nurse picks up the gown from a sterile pack, or an assistant hands the gown to the nurse. Only a certain portion of the gown—the area from the anterior waist to, but not including, the collar and the anterior surface of the sleeves—is considered sterile. The back of the gown, the area under the arms, the collar, the area below the waist, and the underside of the sleeves are not sterile because the nurse cannot keep these areas in constant view and ensure their sterility. Skill 29-4 reviews the steps for applying a sterile gown.

NP Evaluation

The success of the nurse who practises infection control techniques is measured by determining whether the goals for reducing or preventing infection are achieved. A comparison of the client's response, such as absence of fever or development of wound drainage, with expected outcomes determines the success of nursing interventions. Similarly, the nurse determines whether interventions should be revised or eliminated. Correctly assessing wounds for healing and conducting a physical assessment of body systems (see chapter 28) are important skills in evaluation. The nurse closely monitors clients, especially those at risk, for signs and symptoms of infection. For example, a client who has undergone a surgical procedure is at risk for infection at the surgical site, as well as at other invasive sites, such as the venipuncture or central line sites. In addition, the client is at risk for a respiratory tract infection as a result of decreased mobility and for a urinary tract infection if an indwelling catheter is present. The nurse closely monitors all invasive and surgical sites for swelling, erythema, or purulent drainage. Breath sounds are monitored for changes, and sputum character is checked for purulence. Laboratory test results are reviewed for leukocytes in the urine, which may indicate a urinary tract infection. The absence of signs or symptoms of infection is the expected outcome of infection prevention and monitoring activities.

The client at risk for infection must understand the measures needed to reduce or prevent micro-organism growth and spread. Providing clients or family members the opportunity to discuss infection control measures or to demonstrate procedures will reveal their ability to comply with therapy. The nurse may determine that clients require new information or that previously instructed information needs reinforcement.

The nurse documents the client's response to therapies for infection control. A clear description of any signs and symptoms of systemic or local infection is necessary to give all nurses a baseline for comparative evaluation. The efficacy of any intervention in reducing infection must also be reported.

Key Concepts

- Hand hygiene is the most important technique to use in preventing and controlling transmission of infection.
- The potential for micro-organisms to cause disease depends on the number of organisms, virulence, ability to enter and survive in a host, and susceptibility of the host.
- Normal body flora help to resist infection by releasing antibacterial substances and inhibiting multiplication of pathogenic micro-organisms.
- The signs of local inflammation and infection are identical.
- An infection can develop as long as the six elements composing the chain of infection are uninterrupted.
- Micro-organisms are transmitted by direct and indirect contact, droplets, airborne particles, and contaminated vehicles and vectors.
- Advancing age, poor nutrition, stress, diseases of the immune system, chronic disease, and treatments or conditions that compromise the immune response increase susceptibility to infection.
- The major sites for nosocomial infections include the urinary and respiratory tracts, bloodstream, and surgical or traumatic wounds.
- The US Centers for Disease Control and Prevention now recommends use of alcohol-based waterless antiseptics as an alternative to handwashing to more effectively reduce transmission of pathogens.
- Invasive procedures, medical therapies, long hospitalization, and contact with health care personnel increase a hospitalized client's risk for acquiring a nosocomial infection.
- Isolation practices may prevent personnel and clients from acquiring infections and may prevent transmission of micro-organisms to other people.
- Standard precautions/routine practices use generic barrier techniques when caring for all clients.
- Transmission-based (isolation) precautions are used for clients with specific, highly transmissible infections.
- Proper cleansing requires mechanical removal of soil from an object or area.
- A client in isolation is subject to sensory deprivation because of the restricted environment.
- An infection control professional monitors the incidence of infection within an institution and provides educational and consultative services to maintain infection prevention.
- Surgical asepsis requires more stringent techniques than medical asepsis and is directed at eliminating all micro-organisms.

- If the skin is broken, or if the nurse performs an invasive procedure into a body cavity normally free of micro-organisms, surgical aseptic practices are followed.

Key Terms

Aerobic, *p. 785*
Anaerobic, *p. 785*
Asepsis, *p. 789*
Broad-spectrum antibiotics, *p. 789*
Carriers, *p. 785*
Colonizing, *p. 785*
Communicable, *p. 785*
Disinfection, *p. 798*
Edema, *p. 790*
Endogenous infection, *p. 791*
Epidemiology, *p. 812*
Exogenous infection, *p. 791*
Exudates, *p. 790*
Hand hygiene, *p. 799*
Handwashing, *p. 800*
Iatrogenic infections, *p. 790*
Immunocompromised, *p. 785*
Inflammatory response, *p. 788*
Invasive, *p. 784*
Isolation precautions, *p. 798*
Leukocytosis, *p. 790*
Localized, *p. 788*
Medical asepsis, *p. 798*
Micro-organisms, *p. 784*
Necrotic, *p. 790*
Normal flora, *p. 788*
Nosocomial infection, *p. 790*
Pathogen, *p. 785*
Pathogenicity, *p. 788*
Phagocytosis, *p. 790*
Purulent, *p. 790*
Routine practices, *p. 798*
Sanguineous, *p. 790*
Serosanguineous, *p. 790*
Serous, *p. 790*
Standard precautions, *p. 798*
Sterile field, *p. 816*
Sterilization, *p. 798*
Superinfection, *p. 789*
Surgical asepsis, *p. 813*
Susceptibility, *p. 788*
Systemic, *p. 788*
Virulence, *p. 785*

Critical Thinking Exercises

1. Mrs. Jaycock had an indwelling urethral catheter for 1 week. The catheter has now been out for 24 hours. She complains of frequency and pain on urination. Mrs. Jaycock suggests reinsertion of the catheter because of the need to get up frequently. What can frequency or pain on urination indicate? Should the catheter be reinserted? Why or why not? Describe at least one appropriate assessment measure and independent nursing action for Mrs. Jaycock.
2. You are caring for Mr. Huang, who has a large, open, and draining abdominal wound. You notice another health care worker changing Mr. Huang's dressing without wearing gloves or using sterile supplies or sterile technique. When you question the health care worker regarding this practice, the person says, "Don't worry, the wound is already infected, and the antibiotics and draining will take care of any contaminants." How would you respond to this comment? What would your next steps be in following up on this incident?
3. Mrs. Niles is 83 years of age and lives alone. She has difficulty walking and relies on a church volunteer group to deliver lunches during the week. Her fixed income limits her ability to buy food. Last week, Mrs. Niles's 79-year-old sister died. The two sisters had been very close. Explain the factors that might increase Mrs. Niles's risk for infection.
4. Mr. Vargas is admitted to the facility with a history of recent weight loss, a cough that has persisted for 2 months, and hemoptysis. His chest X-ray film shows a cavity in one lung, and his physician suspects TB. What type of isolation precautions would you use for Mr. Vargas? What protection would you use to provide care? What education would you provide for the client and his family?

Review Questions

1. If an infection can be transmitted from one person to another, it is a
   1. Communicable disease
   2. Portal of entry to a host
   3. Portal of exit from the reservoir
   4. Susceptible host
2. The mode of transmission for Hepatitis A is
   1. Direct contact
   2. Droplet transmission
   3. Airborne transmission
   4. Vehicle transmission
3. The interval when a client manifests signs and symptoms specific to a type of infection is the
   1. Incubation period
   2. Convalescence
   3. Prodromal stage
   4. Illness stage
4. The most important and basic way to break the chain of infection is by
   1. Wearing gloves
   2. Practising hand hygiene
   3. Placing clients in isolation
   4. Providing private rooms for clients
5. The minimal hand washing time required to remove most transient microorganisms is
   1. 1. 5 seconds
   2. 10 seconds
   3. 60 seconds
   4. 3 minutes
6. A client is on isolation precautions for pulmonary TB. The nurse notes the client seems to be angry, but the nurse knows this is a normal response to isolation. The best intervention is to
   1. Provide a dark, quiet room to calm the client
   2. Explain the isolation procedures and provide meaningful stimulation
   3. Reduce the level of precautions to keep the client from becoming angry
   4. Limit family and other caregiver visits to reduce the risk of spreading the infection
7. A gown should be worn when
   1. The client's hygiene is poor
   2. The client has AIDS or hepatitis
   3. The nurse is assisting with medication administration
   4. Blood or body fluids may get on the nurse's clothing from a task the nurse plans to perform

8. The nurse has dressed a client's wound and now plans to administer a medication to the client. It is important to
   1. Remove gloves and perform hand hygiene before leaving the room
   2. Remove gloves and perform hand hygiene before administering the medication
   3. Leave the gloves on to administer the medication
   4. Leave the medication on the bedside table to avoid having to remove gloves before leaving the client's room

9. To sterilize surgical instruments, parenteral solutions, and surgical dressings
   1. Soap and water are used
   2. Chemicals are used for disinfection
   3. An autoclave is used
   4. Ethylene oxide gas is used

10. When performing a surgical hand hygiene, hands must be kept
   1. Above elbows
   2. Below elbows
   3. At a 45-degree angle
   4. In a comfortable position

References

Association of periOperative Registered Nurses. (2004). Hand antisepsis, surgical. In *Standards, recommended practices, and guidelines*. Denver, CO: Author.

Boyce, J. M., & Pittet, D. (2002). Guideline for hand hygiene in health-care settings. Recommendations of the Healthcare Infection Control Practices Advisory Committee and the HIPAC/SHEA/APIC/IDSA Hand Hygiene Task Force. *American Journal of Infection Control, 30*(8), S1–S46.

Canadian Needle Stick Surveillance Network. (2003). Update — surveillance of health care workers exposed to blood, body fluids and bloodborne pathogens in Canadian Hospital settings: 1 April 2000, to 31 March, 2002. Canada Communicable Disease Report, 29-34. Retrieved May 13, 2004, from *http://www.hc-sc.gc.ca/pphb-dgspsp/publicat/ccdr-rmtc/03vol29/dr2924ea.html*

Centers for Disease Control and Prevention. (2002). Guideline for hand hygiene in health-care settings. Retrieved January 12, 2005, from *http://www.cdc.gov/mmwr/preview/mmwrhtml/rr5116a1.htm*

Centers for Disease Control and Prevention. (2003). Guidelines for preventing health-care-associated pneumonia. Available from *http://www.cdc.gov/ncidod/hip/pneumonia/*

Community and Hospital Infection Control Association–Canada. (2004). Web site. Retrieved January 12, 2005, from *http://www.chica.org*

Dochterman, J. M., & Bulechek, G. M. (Eds.). (2004). *Nursing interventions classification (NIC)* (4th ed.). St. Louis, MO: Mosby.

Eliopoulos, C. (2001). *Gerontologic nursing* (5th ed.). Philadelphia: Lippincott.

Forster, A. J., et al. (2004). Ottawa Hospital Patient Safety Study: Incidence and timing of adverse events in patients admitted to a Canadian teaching hospital. *Canadian Medical Association Journal, 170*(8), 1235–1240.

Gantz, N. M., Tkatch, L. S., & Makris, A. T. (2000). Geriatric infections. In *APIC text of infection control and epidemiology.* Washington, DC: Association for Professionals in Infection Control and Epidemiology.

Garner, J. S. (1996). Guideline for isolation precautions in hospitals. The Hospital Infection Control Practices Advisory Committee. *Infection Control and Hospital Epidemiology, 17*(1), 54–80.

Girou, E., et al. (2002). Efficacy of handrubbing with alcohol based solution versus standard handwashing with antiseptic soap: Randomized clinical trial. *BMJ, 325,* 362–365.

Green, J. N. (1996). The microbiology of colonization, including techniques for assessing measuring colonization. *Infection Control and Hospital Epidemiology, 17,* 114–118.

Grimes, D., & Grimes, R. (1994). *AIDS and HIV infections.* St. Louis, MO: Mosby.

Health Canada. (1997). *Infection control guidelines: Preventing the spread of vancomycin-resistant enterococci (VRE) in Canada.* Canada Communicable Disease Report, 23S8. Retrieved April 27, 2004, from *http://www.phac-aspc.gc.ca/publicat/ccdr-rmtc/97vol23/23s8/vreindxe.html*

Health Canada. (1998). *Infection control guidelines: Handwashing, cleaning, disinfection and sterilization in health care* [Supplement]. Canada Communicable Disease Report, 24S8. Retrieved January 24, 2005, *http://www.hc-sc.gc.ca/pphb-dgspsp/publicat/ccdr-rmtc/98pdf/cdr24s8e.pdf*

Health Canada. (1999). *Infection control guidelines: Routine practices and additional precautions for preventing the transmission of infection in health care.* Canada Communicable Disease Report, 25S4. Retrieved January 24, 2005, from *www.hc-sc.gc.ca/hpb/lcdc/publicat/ccdr-rmtc/99pdf/cdr25s4e.pdf*

Health Canada. (2000). *Canadian immunization guide* (6th ed.; catalogue number H49-8/2002E). Ottawa, ON: Author.

Hedderwick, S. A., et al. (2000). Pathogenic organisms associated with artificial fingernails worn by healthcare workers. *Infection Control and Hospital Epidemiology, 21*(8), 505–509.

Ignatavicius, D., & Workman, M. L. (2002). *Medical-surgical nursing: Critical thinking for collaborative care.* Philadelphia: Saunders.

Jernigan, J. A., et al. (1998). A randomized crossover study of disposable thermometers for prevention of *Clostridium difficile* and other nosocomial infections. *Infection Control and Hospital Epidemiology, 19*(7), 494–499.

Keroack, M. A., & Rosen-Kotilainen, H. (1996). Microbiology/laboratory diagnostics. In *APIC infection control and applied epidemiology: Principles and practice.* St. Louis, MO: Mosby.

Larson, E. (1996). APIC guideline for handwashing and hand antisepsis in health-care settings. In *APIC infection control and applied epidemiology: Principles and practice* St. Louis, MO: Mosby.

Louie, T.J., & Meddings, J. (2004). *Clostridium difficile* infection in hospitals: risk factors and responses. *CMAJ, 171*(1), 45–46.

Lueckenotte, A. G. (2000). *Gerontologic nursing* (2nd ed.). St. Louis, MO: Mosby.

Maki, D. G., Alvarado, C., & Hassemer, C. (1986). Double-bagging of items from isolation rooms is unnecessary as an infection control measure: A comparative study of surface contamination with single- and double-bagging. *Infection Control, 7*(11), 535–537.

Meeker, M. H., & Rothrock, J. C. (1999). *Alexander's care of the patient in surgery* (11th ed.). St. Louis, MO: Mosby.

Miller, C. A. (1999). *Nursing care of older adults: Theory and practice* (3rd ed.). Philadelphia: Lippincott.

Moorhead, S., Johnson, M., & Maas, M. (Eds.). (2004). *Nursing outcomes classification (NOC)* (3rd ed.). St. Louis, MO: Mosby.

Operating Room Nurses Association of Canada. (2003). *Recommended standards, guidelines and position statements for perioperative registered nursing practice* (5th ed.). Ottawa: Author

Parienti, J. J., et al. (2002). Hand-rubbing with an aqueous alcoholic solution vs traditional surgical hand-scrubbing and 30-day surgical site infection rates: A randomized equivalence study. *Journal of the American Medical Association, 288*(6), 722–727.

Pittet, D., et al. (2000). Effectiveness of a hospital wide programme to improve compliance with hand hygiene. Infection Control Programme. *Lancet, 356,* 1307–1312.

Sorrentino, SA. (2004). *Mosby's Canadian textbook for the support worker.* Toronto: Elsevier Canada.

Weinstein, S. A., et al. (1989). Bacterial surface contamination of patient's linen: Isolation precautions versus standard care. *American Journal of Infection Control, 17*(5), 264–267.

Recommended Web Sites

Community and Hospital Infection Control Association of Canada:

http://www.chica.org

Community and Hospital Infection Control Association of Canada (CHICA–Canada) is a national, multidisciplinary, voluntary association of infection control professionals committed to improving infection prevention and control.

Public Health Agency of Canada:

http://www.phac-aspc.gc.ca/new_e.html

This federal government site provides links to documents related to infection control practices, including the *Communicable Disease Report.*

30

Medication Administration

Amy Hall, RN, BSN, MS, PhD
Debbie Fraser Askin, RNC, MN (Canadian author)

Objectives

Mastery of content in this chapter will enable the student to:

- Define the key terms listed.
- Discuss the nurse's role and responsibilities in medication administration.
- Describe the physiological mechanisms of medication action, including absorption, distribution, metabolism, and excretion of medications.
- Differentiate among different types of medication actions.
- Discuss developmental factors that influence pharmacokinetics.
- Discuss factors that influence medication actions.
- Discuss methods of educating a client about prescribed medications.
- Describe the roles of the prescriber, pharmacist, and nurse in medication administration.
- Describe factors to consider when choosing routes of medication administration.
- Correctly calculate a prescribed medication dose.
- Discuss factors to include in assessing a client's needs for and response to medication therapy.
- Explain the six rights of medication administration.
- Correctly prepare and administer subcutaneous, intramuscular, and intradermal injections and intravenous medications; oral and topical skin preparations; eye, ear, and nose drops; vaginal instillations; rectal suppositories; and inhalants.

Clients with acute or chronic health alterations restore or maintain their health using a variety of strategies. A medication is a substance used in the diagnosis, treatment, cure, relief, or prevention of health alterations. In fact, medications have traditionally been the primary modality that clients associate with restoration of health. No matter where clients receive their health care—hospitals, clinics, or home—the nurse plays an essential role in preparing and administering medications, teaching clients about medications, and evaluating clients' responses to medications.

In the primary care setting, the client often self-administers medications. The nurse is responsible for evaluating the effects of the medications on the client's health status, teaching clients about their medications and their side effects, ensuring client compliance with the medication regimen, and evaluating client technique when the client administers medications that are not given by mouth.

In both acute and restorative care settings, nurses spend a great deal of time administering medications to clients. The nurse also ensures that clients are adequately prepared to administer their medications when they are discharged. In the home care setting, clients usually administer their own medications. When clients cannot administer their own medications, family members or support people may be responsible for doing so. The nurse assesses the effect that the medications have in restoring or maintaining health and provides continued education to the client, family, or home care personnel on medication purpose, regimen, and side effects.

Scientific Knowledge Base

Medications administered to clients are used to prevent, diagnose, or treat disease or health conditions. Because medication administration and evaluation are essential to nursing practice, nurses need to have knowledge about the actions and effects of the medications they deliver to clients. This knowledge requires an understanding of the life sciences. Moreover, to safely and accurately administer medications, nurses must have an understanding of pharmacokinetics (the study of drug concentrations), growth and development, human anatomy, nutrition, and mathematics. All of the nurse's previous learning is important and can be applied to medication administration. The nursing process provides the framework for nurses to organize their thoughts and actions and is the foundation for medication administration.

Pharmacological Concepts

Drug Names. A medication may have as many as three different names. A medication's chemical name provides an exact description of the medication's composition and molecular structure. Chemical names are rarely used in clinical practice. An example of a chemical name is N-acetyl-para-aminophenol, which is commonly known as Tylenol. The generic or non-proprietary name is given by the manufacturer who first develops the medication and is protected by law. Acetaminophen is the generic name for Tylenol. The generic name becomes the official name that is listed in official publications such as the *Compendium of Pharmaceuticals and Specialties* (CPS), the *Canadian Formulary* (CF), or the *United States Pharmacopeia* (USP). In addition to the drug name, the Health Protection Branch of the federal government also assigns an eight-digit number to all drug products approved for distribution in Canada. This Drug Identification Number (DIN) is used by various groups and agencies to track drug information across the country.

The trade name, brand name, or proprietary name is the name under which a manufacturer markets a medication. The trade name has the symbol ™ at the upper right of the name, indicating that the manufacturer has trademarked the medication's name (e.g., Tempra™, Motrin™). Manufacturers choose names that are easy to pronounce, spell, and remember so that laypersons will recognize trade names. Many companies may produce the same medication, and similarities in trade names can be confusing. In fact, similarities in drug names are a common cause of medical errors. Hospitals and clinic pharmacies attempt to consistently dispense medications with the same trade names so that nurses can become familiar with them. However, medications are available under a variety of different nomenclatures or names, and nurses must be careful to obtain the exact name and spelling for a particular medication.

Classification. Nurses learn to categorize medications with similar characteristics by their class. Medication classification indicates the effect of the medication on a body system, the symptoms the medication relieves, or the medication's desired effect. For example, clients who have Type 2 diabetes often take medications to lower their blood glucose level. This class of medication is called oral hypoglycemic agents. Usually, each class contains more than one medication that can be prescribed for the type of health problem. For example, there are over 12 different oral hypoglycemic agents. These medications are divided into three classifications of oral agents: first- and second-generation sulfonylureas and a miscellaneous group (McKenry & Salerno, 2003). The physical and chemical composition of medications within a class may differ slightly. A prescriber chooses a particular oral hypoglycemic medication on the basis of client characteristics, cost, efficacy, dosing frequency, or prescriber experience with the medication. One medication may also be part of more than one class. For example, aspirin is an analgesic, an antipyretic, and an anti-inflammatory medication.

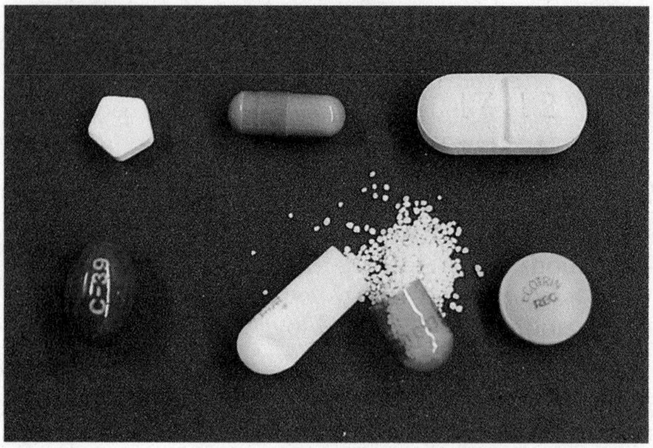

FIGURE **30–1** Forms of oral medications. *Top row:* Uniquely shaped tablet, capsule, scored tablet. *Bottom row:* Gelatin-coated liquid, extended-release capsule, enteric-coated tablet.

Medication Forms. Medications are available in a variety of forms, or preparations (Figure 30–1). The form of the medication determines its route of administration. The composition of a medication is designed to enhance its absorption and metabolism. Many medications are made in several forms such as tablets, capsules, elixirs, and suppositories. When administering a medication, the nurse must be certain to use the proper form (Table 30-1).

Medication Legislation and Standards

Canadian Drug Legislation. Regulation of drug standards began in Canada in 1884 with the *Adulteration Act,* which set the conditions under which adulteration of a drug might occur. The *Food and Drugs Act* of 1920 replaced this act and with amendments in 1950, gave the federal government control of the manufacture and sale of all drugs except narcotics, as well as food, cosmetics, and certain medical devices.

The federal government first attempted to control narcotic substances in 1908 with the *Opium Act.* Cocaine and morphine came under the jurisdiction of this act in 1911. In 1961, the *Narcotic Control Act,* which controls

Table 30-1 Forms of Medication

Form	Description
Caplet	Solid dosage form for oral use; shaped like capsule and coated for ease of swallowing
Capsule	Solid dosage form for oral use; medication in powder, liquid, or oil form and encased by gelatin shell; capsule coloured to aid in product identification
Elixir	Clear fluid containing water and/or alcohol; designed for oral use; usually has sweetener added
Enteric-coated tablet	Tablet for oral use coated with materials that do not dissolve in stomach; coatings dissolve in intestine, where medication is absorbed
Extract	Concentrated medication form made by removing active portion of medication from its other components (e.g., fluid extract is medication made into solution from vegetable source)
Glycerite	Solution of medication combined with glycerine for external use; contains at least 50% glycerine
Intraocular disk	A small, flexible oval consisting of two soft, outer layers and a middle layer containing medication; when moistened by ocular fluid, releases medication for up to 1 week
Liniment	Preparation usually containing alcohol, oil, or soapy emollient that is applied to skin
Lotion	Medication in liquid suspension applied externally to protect skin
Ointment (salve, cream, or unguent)	Semisolid, externally applied preparation, usually containing one or more medications
Paste	Semisolid preparation, thicker and stiffer than ointment; absorbed through skin more slowly than ointment
Pill	Solid dosage form containing one or more medications, shaped into globules, ovoids, or oblong shapes; true pills rarely used because they have been replaced by tablets
Solution	Liquid preparation that may be used orally, parenterally, or externally; can also be instilled into body organ or cavity (e.g., bladder irrigations); contains water with one or more dissolved compounds; must be sterile for parenteral use
Suppository	Solid dosage form mixed with gelatin and shaped in form of pellet for insertion into body cavity (rectum or vagina); melts when it reaches body temperature, releasing medication for absorption
Suspension	Finely divided drug particles dispersed in liquid medium; must be shaken prior to administration; when suspension is left standing, particles settle to bottom of container; commonly oral medication and not given intravenously
Syrup	Medication dissolved in concentrated sugar solution; may contain flavouring to make medication more palatable
Tablet	Powdered dosage form compressed into hard disks or cylinders; in addition to primary medication, contains binders (adhesive to allow powder to stick together), disintegrators (to promote tablet dissolution), lubricants (for ease of manufacturing), and fillers (for convenient tablet size)
Tincture	Alcohol or water-alcohol medication solution
Transdermal disk or patch	Medication contained within semipermeable membrane disk or patch, which allows medications to be absorbed through skin slowly over long period
Troche (lozenge)	Flat, round dosage form containing medication, flavouring, sugar, and mucilage; dissolves in mouth to release medication

the manufacture, distribution, and sale of narcotic drugs, was enacted. This act was repealed in 1996 and replaced by the *Controlled Drugs and Substances Act.* The federal government has also passed legislation that regulates the manufacture and sale of herbs and other natural health products. This legislation addresses the content of these products as well as the packaging, labelling, distribution, and storage.

Drug Standards. Official publications, such as the *British Pharmacopoeia* (BP) and the *Canadian Formulary,* set standards for drug strength, quality, purity, packaging, safety, labelling, and dosage form. Physicians, nurses, and pharmacists depend on these standards to ensure that clients receive pure drugs in safe and effective dosages. Accepted standards must be met in the following areas:

- *Purity:* Manufacturers must meet purity standards for the type and concentration of other substances allowed in drug products.
- *Potency:* The concentration of active drug in the preparation affects strength, or potency.
- *Bioavailability:* The ability of a drug to be released from its dosage form and dissolved, absorbed, and transported by the body to its site of action is its bioavailability.
- *Efficacy:* Detailed laboratory studies can help determine a drug's effectiveness.
- *Safety:* All drugs should be continually evaluated to determine their side effects.

Control. Administration of the *Food and Drugs Act* and the *Controlled Drugs and Substances Act* is carried out by the Health Protection Branch (HPB) of the federal government. Before a new drug can be marketed in Canada, an application for approval must be made to the HPB. After intensive testing to ensure the drug's effectiveness and safety in humans, the HPB reviews the application. A Drug Identification Number and Notification of Compliance are issued by the HPB, allowing the manufacturer to sell the drug in Canada. Stringent controls are applied to this new drug until sufficient information has been accumulated to ensure its safety and efficacy. Only then is the drug released for general use. Monitoring is ongoing with respect to any reported adverse effects, safety concerns, or changes in the indications for a particular drug's use.

Provincial and Local Regulation of Medication. The provincial governments do not directly regulate the manufacture or sale of drugs. However, given that the provincial governments have most of the legislative responsibility for health care, provincial legislation indirectly affects the use and sale of drugs within provincial boundaries. In addition, each province has medical, dental, pharmacy, and nursing practice acts that dictate each professional's role in the ordering, dispensing, and administration of drugs. In particular, some provincial pharmacy acts contain schedules indicating which drugs can be sold without prescription, behind the counter, or by prescription only. The National Association of Pharmacy Regulatory Authorities facilitates the activities of provincial regulatory authorities and promotes the harmonization of the practice of drug sales across the country.

Health care institutions establish policies that conform to federal and provincial regulations. The size of an institution, the types of services it provides, and the types of professional personnel it employs influence policies for drug control, distribution, and administration. Institutional policies are often more restrictive than government controls. An institution is primarily concerned with preventing health problems resulting from drug use. For example, a common institutional policy is the automatic discontinuation of antibiotic therapy after a set number of days. Although a physician may reorder an antibiotic, this policy helps to control unnecessarily prolonged drug therapy, which may lead to sensitivity or toxic reactions.

Medication Regulation and Nursing Practice. Federal and provincial legislation governs nursing practice, including the administration of medications.

Nurses must know the regulations affecting drug administration in their practice areas. When moving from one province to another, nurses may discover significant differences in the laws governing drug administration. For example, laws vary concerning the prescription and administration of drugs. In the past, only physicians prescribed medications. Today, several provinces are revising nursing practice acts to include the prescription of medications by nurses in advanced practice. In most cases, this privilege is limited to nurse practitioners, clinical nurse specialists, and nurse midwives.

Before assuming the responsibility of administering intravenous (IV) medications, the nurse should be aware of the relevant administrative policies of the employing institution. Because IV injection of medications may cause serious adverse effects, nurses who perform this function must be qualified through proper training, education, and experience.

The nurse is responsible for following legal provisions when administering **controlled substances** (drugs that affect the mind or behaviour), which can be dispensed only with a prescription. Violations of the *Narcotic Control Act* are punishable by fines, imprisonment, and loss of nurse licensure or registration. Hospitals and other health care institutions have policies for the proper storage and distribution of controlled substances, including **narcotics** (Box 30-1).

Box 30-1 Guidelines for Safe Narcotic Administration and Control

- Store all narcotics in a locked, secure cabinet or container. (Computerized, locked cabinets are now available.)
- Nurses in charge carry a set of keys (or a special computer entry code) for the narcotics cabinet.
- During an institution's change of shift, the nurse going off duty counts all narcotics with the nurse coming on duty. Both nurses sign the narcotic record to indicate that the count is correct.
- Discrepancies in narcotic counts are reported immediately.
- A special inventory record is used each time a narcotic is dispensed and provides an accurate ongoing count of narcotics used and remaining.
- The record is used to document the client's name, date, time of medication administration, name of medication, dose, and signature of nurse dispensing the medication.
- If only one part of a premeasured dose of a controlled substance is given, a second nurse witnesses disposal of the unused portion and documents such on the record form.

Pharmacokinetics as the Basis of Medication Actions

For medications to be therapeutic, they must be taken into a client's body; absorbed and distributed to cells, tissues, or a specific organ; and alter physiological functions. **Pharmacokinetics** is the study of how medications enter the body, reach their site of action, are metabolized, and exit the body. The nurse uses knowledge of pharmacokinetics when timing medication administration, selecting the route of administration, judging the client's risk for alterations in medication action, and observing the client's response.

Absorption. Absorption refers to passage of medication molecules into the blood from its site of administration. Factors that influence medication absorption are the route of administration, ability of the medication to dissolve, blood flow to the site of administration, body surface area, and lipid solubility of medication.

Route of Administration. Medications can be administered through various routes. Each route has a different rate of absorption. When medications are placed on the skin, absorption is slow due to the physical makeup of the skin. Medications placed on the mucous membranes and respiratory airways are quickly absorbed because these tissues contain many blood vessels. Because orally administered medications must pass through the gastrointestinal (GI) tract to be absorbed, the overall rate of absorption may be slowed. IV **injection** produces the most rapid absorption because this route provides immediate access to the systemic circulation.

Ability of the Medication to Dissolve. The ability of an oral medication to dissolve depends largely on its form or preparation. Solutions and suspensions already in a liquid state are absorbed more readily than tablets or capsules. Acidic medications pass through the gastric mucosa rapidly. Medications that are basic are not absorbed before reaching the small intestine.

Blood Flow to the Site of Administration. When the site of administration contains a rich blood supply, medications are absorbed more rapidly because as blood comes into contact with the site of administration, the medication is absorbed. Therefore, areas that have more blood supply will experience enhanced absorption, facilitating the passage of the medication into the bloodstream.

Body Surface Area. When a medication is in contact with a large surface area, the medication will be absorbed at a faster rate. This explains why the majority of medications are absorbed in the small intestine rather than the stomach.

Lipid Solubility of a Medication. Medications that are highly lipid soluble are absorbed more easily. They readily cross the cell membrane because it is made of a lipid layer. Another factor that may affect absorption of medication is whether or not food is in the stomach. Some oral medications are absorbed more easily when administered between meals because food can change the structure of a medication and impair its absorption. Some medications when administered together may interfere with each other so as to impair the absorption of one or both.

Safe medication administration requires knowledge of factors that may alter or impair absorption of the prescribed medications. This information is based on an understanding of medication pharmacokinetics, the nursing history, the physical examination, and knowledge gained through daily interactions with clients. The nurse uses this knowledge to ensure that all prescribed medications are administered at the correct time. Because medications can interact with food, it may be appropriate for the nurse to administer medications before or after meals, with meals, or on an empty stomach. Some medications interact with each other. If this occurs, the nurse ensures that they are not given at the same time. The nurse consults and collaborates with the client's prescribers to ensure that the client achieves the therapeutic effect of all medications. Before administering any medication, the nurse should consult pharmacology books or drug references, package inserts, or pharmacists to identify medication-medication interactions or medication-nutrient interactions.

Distribution. After a medication is absorbed, it is distributed within the body to tissues and organs and to its specific site of action. The rate and extent of distribution depend on the physical and chemical properties of medications and the physiology of the person taking the medication.

Circulation. Once a medication enters the bloodstream, it is carried throughout the tissues and organs of the body. How fast it reaches the site depends on the vascularity of the various tissues and organs. When conditions exist that limit blood flow or intended sites of actions are poorly perfused, the distribution of a medication is inhibited. For example, clients in congestive heart failure have impaired circulation, which impairs medication delivery to the intended site of action. Therefore, the efficacy of medications in these clients can be delayed or altered.

Membrane Permeability. To be distributed to an organ, a medication must pass through all of the organ's tissues and biologic membranes. Some membranes may serve as barriers to the passage of medications. For example, the blood-brain barrier allows only fat-soluble medications to pass into the brain and cerebral spinal fluid. Therefore, central nervous system infections require treatment with antibiotics injected directly into the subarachnoid space in the spinal cord. Older clients may experience adverse effects (e.g., confusion) as a result of the change in the permeability of the blood-brain barrier, with easier passage of fat-soluble medications. The placental membrane also has a non-selective barrier to medications. Fat-soluble and non-fat-soluble agents may cross the placenta and produce fetal deformities, respiratory depression, and, with narcotic abuse, withdrawal symptoms.

Protein Binding. The degree to which medications bind to serum proteins such as albumin affects medication distribution. Most medications bind to this protein to some extent. When medications bind to albumin, they cannot exert any pharmacological activity. The unbound or "free" medication is the active form of the medication. Older adults have a decrease in albumin in the bloodstream, probably caused by a change in liver function. The same is true for clients with liver disease or malnutrition. Because of the potential for more medication being unbound, the older adult may be at risk for an increase in medication activity or toxicity, or both.

Metabolism. After a medication reaches its site of action, it becomes metabolized into a less active or inactive form that is more easily excreted. **Biotransformation** occurs under the influence of enzymes that **detoxify,** degrade (break down), and remove biologically active chemicals. Most biotransformation occurs within the liver, although the lungs, kidneys, blood, and intestines also metabolize medications. The liver is especially important because its specialized structure oxidizes and transforms many toxic substances. The liver degrades many harmful chemicals before they become distributed to the tissues. If a decrease in liver function occurs, such as with aging or liver disease, a medication may be eliminated more slowly, resulting in an accumulation of the medication. If the organs that metabolize medications are altered, clients are at risk for medication toxicity. For example, a small sedative dose of a barbiturate may cause a client with liver disease to lapse into a hepatic coma.

Excretion. After medications are metabolized, they exit the body through the kidneys, liver, bowel, lungs, and exocrine glands. The chemical makeup of a medication determines the organ of excretion. Gaseous and volatile compounds, such as nitrous oxide and alcohol, exit through the lungs. Deep breathing and coughing (see chapter 35) help the post-operative client to eliminate anaesthetic gases more rapidly. The exocrine glands excrete lipid-soluble medications. When medications exit through sweat glands, the skin may become irritated. The nurse assists the client in good hygiene practices (see chapter 34) to promote cleanliness and skin integrity.

If a medication is excreted through the mammary glands, there is a risk that a nursing infant will ingest the chemicals. Mothers should check on the safety of any medication used while breast-feeding.

The GI tract is another route for medication excretion. Many medications enter the hepatic circulation to be broken down by the liver and excreted into the bile. After chemicals enter the intestines through the biliary tract, the intestines may reabsorb them. Factors that increase peristalsis (e.g., laxatives and enemas) accelerate medication excretion through the feces, whereas factors that slow peristalsis (e.g., inactivity and improper diet) may prolong a medication's effects.

The kidneys are the main organs for medication excretion. Some medications escape extensive metabolism and exit unchanged in the urine. Other medications must undergo biotransformation in the liver before being excreted by the kidney. If renal function declines, a client is at risk for medication toxicity. If the kidney cannot adequately excrete a medication, it may be necessary to reduce the dose. Maintenance of an adequate fluid intake (50 mL/kg/day) promotes proper elimination of medications for the average adult.

Types of Medication Action

Medications vary considerably in the way they act and their types of action. Factors other than characteristics of the medication also influence medication actions. A client may not respond in the same way to each successive dose of a medication. Likewise, the same medication dosage may cause very different responses in different clients. Therefore, it is essential for the nurse to understand all the effects that medications can have when taken by or given to clients.

Therapeutic Effects. The **therapeutic effect** is the expected or predictable physiological response that a medication causes. Each medication has a desired therapeutic effect for which it is prescribed. For example, nitroglycerine is used to reduce the cardiac workload and increase myocardial oxygen supply. A single medication may have many therapeutic effects. For example, aspirin reduces platelet aggregation (clumping) and is an analgesic, antipyretic, and anti-inflammatory. It is important for the nurse to know for which therapeutic effect a medication is prescribed. This will enable the nurse to properly teach the client about the medication's intended effect and to accurately evaluate the medication's desired effect.

Side Effects. **Side effects** are the unintended, secondary effects that a medication predictably will cause. Side effects may be harmless or injurious. If the side effects are serious enough to negate the beneficial effects of a medication's therapeutic action, the prescriber may discontinue the medication. Clients often stop taking medications because of side effects.

Adverse Effects. **Adverse effects** are generally considered to be severe, negative responses to medication. For example, a client may become comatose when a drug is ingested. When adverse responses to medications occur, the prescriber must discontinue the medication. Some adverse effects are unexpected effects that were not discovered during drug testing. When this situation occurs, health care providers should report the adverse effect to the Health Protection Branch of the federal government. This reporting system is voluntary.

Toxic Effects. **Toxic effects** may develop after prolonged intake of a medication or when a medication accumulates in the blood because of impaired metabolism or excretion. Excess amounts of a medication within the body may have lethal effects, depending on the medication's action. For example, toxic levels of morphine, an opioid, may cause severe respiratory depression and death. Antidotes are available to treat specific types of medication toxicity. For example, Narcan is used to reverse the effects of opioid toxicity.

Idiosyncratic Reactions. Medications may cause unpredictable effects such as an **idiosyncratic reaction,** in which a client overreacts to a medication or has a reaction different from normal. For example, a child receiving an antihistamine (Benadryl) may become extremely agitated or excited instead of drowsy. Usually it is impossible to predict if a client might have an idiosyncratic response to a medication.

Allergic Reactions. Allergic reactions are another unpredictable response to a medication; they make up 5% to 10% of all medication reactions. A client can become sensitized immunologically to the initial dose of a medication. With repeated administration, the client develops an allergic response to the medication, its chemical preservatives, or a metabolite. The medication or chemical acts as an antigen, triggering the release of the body's antibodies. A client's **medication allergy** may be mild or severe. Allergic symptoms vary, depending on the individual and the medication. Among the different classes of medications, antibiotics cause a high incidence of allergic reactions. Common, mild allergy symptoms are summarized in Table 30-2. Severe or **anaphylactic reactions** are characterized by circulatory collapse, sudden constriction of bronchiolar muscles, edema of the pharynx and larynx, and severe wheezing and shortness of breath. Antihistamines, epinephrine, and bronchodilators may be used to treat anaphylactic reactions.

The client may also become severely hypotensive, necessitating emergency resuscitation measures. A client with a known history of an allergy to a medication should avoid exposure to that medication in the future. Clients might also wear a MedicAlert bracelet or medal, which has emergency medical information engraved on

Table 30-2 Mild Allergic Reactions

Symptom	Description
Urticaria	Raised, irregularly shaped skin eruptions with varying sizes and shapes; eruptions have reddened margins and pale centre
Rash	Small, raised vesicles that are usually reddened; often distributed over entire body
Pruritus	Itching of skin; accompanies most rashes
Rhinitis	Inflammation of mucous membranes lining nose; causes swelling and clear, watery discharge

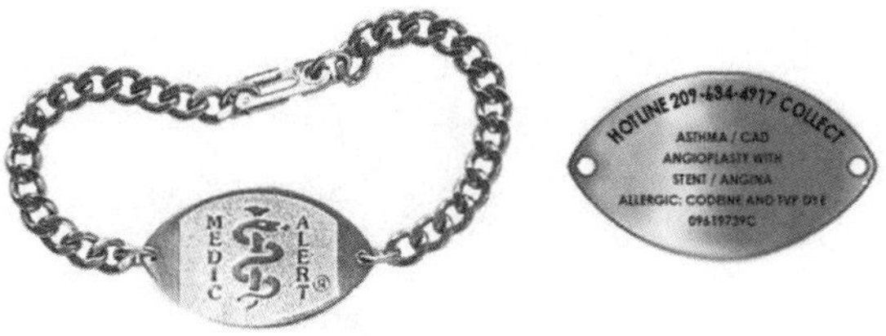

FIGURE **30–2** A MedicAlert bracelet has the person's emergency medical information, including drug allergies, engraved on the back.

the back, including any medication allergies (Figure 30–2). These bracelets alert health care workers to the allergy if the client is unconscious when receiving medical care.

Medication Interactions

When one medication modifies the action of another, a **medication interaction** occurs. Medication interactions are common in individuals taking several medications. A medication may potentiate or diminish the action of other medications and may alter the way in which another medication is absorbed, metabolized, or eliminated from the body. When two medications have a **synergistic effect,** or act synergistically, the effect of the two medications combined is greater than the effect of the medications when given separately. For example, alcohol is a central nervous system depressant that has a synergistic effect on antihistamines, antidepressants, barbiturates, and narcotic analgesics.

A medication interaction is not always undesirable. Often a prescriber combines medications to create an interaction that will have a beneficial effect on the client's condition. For example, a client with hypertension (high blood pressure) that cannot be controlled with one medication typically receives several medications such as diuretics and vasodilators that act together to control the blood pressure.

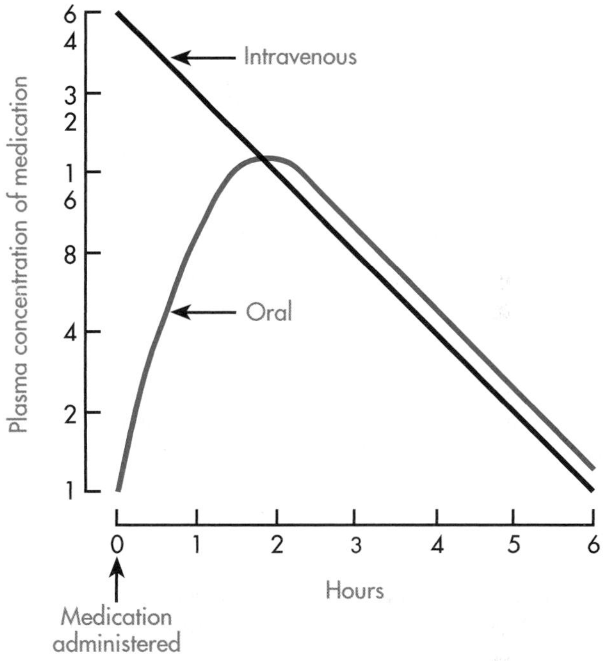

FIGURE **30–3** Curve showing therapeutic blood levels of medication. (From *Pharmacological Basis of Nursing Practice,* 6th ed., by J. F. Clark, S. F. Queener, and V. B. Karb, 1998, St. Louis, MO: Mosby.)

Medication Dose Responses

After a nurse administers a medication, it undergoes absorption, distribution, metabolism, and excretion. Except when administered intravenously, medications take time to enter the bloodstream. The quantity and distribution of a medication in different body compartments change constantly. When a medication is prescribed, the goal is a constant blood level within a safe therapeutic range. Repeated doses are required to achieve a constant therapeutic **concentration** of a medication because a portion of a drug is always being excreted. The highest serum concentration (**peak** concentration) of a medication usually occurs just before the last of it is absorbed (McKenry & Salerno, 2003). After peaking, the serum medication concentration falls progressively. With IV **infusions,** the peak concentration occurs quickly, but the serum level also begins to fall immediately (Figure 30–3). The point at which the lowest amount of drug is detected in the serum is called the trough concentration. Some medications (e.g., vancomycin) are dosed on the basis of peak and trough serum levels. The trough level is generally drawn 30 minutes before the drug is administered, and the peak level is drawn whenever the drug is expected to reach its peak concentration. The time it takes for a drug to reach its peak concentration varies depending on the medication's pharmacokinetics.

All medications have a **serum half-life,** which is the time it takes for excretion processes to lower the serum medication concentration by half. To maintain a therapeutic plateau, the client must receive regular fixed doses. For example, it has been shown that pain medications are most effective when they are given "around the clock" rather than when the client intermittently complains of pain. In this way, an almost constant level of pain medication is maintained. After an initial medication dose, the client receives each successive dose when the previous dose reaches its half-life.

Table 30-3 Common Dosage Administration Schedules

Dosage Schedule	Abbreviation*
Before meals	AC, ac
As desired	ad lib
Twice a day	BID, bid
Hour	h (hr)
At bedtime	
After meals	PC, pc
Whenever there is a need	prn
Every morning, every am	Qam
Every day, daily	
Every hour	Qh
Every 2 hours	q2h
Every 4 hours	q4h
Every 6 hours	q6h
Every 8 hours	q8h
Four times a day	QID, qid
Every other day	
Give immediately	STAT
Three times a day	TID, tid

*Some terms are safer to write out than abbreviate (see Table 30-8). Follow agency policy regarding abbreviations.

The client and nurse must follow regular dosage schedules and adhere to prescribed doses and dosage intervals. Some agencies set schedules for medication administration. However, the nurse can alter this schedule with knowledge about a medication. For example, at some agencies, medications that are to be taken once a day are given at 9:00 A.M. However, if the nurse knows that the medication works best when given before bedtime, the nurse administers the medication before the client goes to sleep. Table 30-3 lists common dosage schedules used in acute care settings.

When teaching clients about dosage schedules, the nurse uses language that is familiar to the client. For example, when teaching a client about medication dosing twice a day (bid), the nurse instructs the client to take a medication in the morning and again in the evening. Knowledge of the time intervals of medication action also helps the nurse to anticipate a medication's effect. With this knowledge, the nurse can instruct the client when to expect a response. Table 30-4 lists common terms associated with medication actions.

Routes of Administration

The route prescribed for administering a medication depends on the medication's properties and desired effect and on the client's physical and mental condition (Table 30-5). A nurse collaborates with the prescriber in determining the best route for a client's medication, as in the following hypothetical situation:

Mr. Huels has progressively worsened physically. His temperature is 39.2°C. He complains of nausea and is unable to tolerate oral fluids. The nurse checks Mr. Huels's order, which reads, "Acetaminophen 1,000 mg orally for temperature above 38.5°C." The nurse believes that because Mr. Huels is nauseated, he will not be able to tolerate an oral dose of acetaminophen. By consulting the physician, the nurse acquires an order for a rectal suppository instead. A rectal suppository enables the nurse to administer the appropriate medication without increasing the client's symptoms of nausea.

Table 30-4 Terms Associated With Medication Actions

Term	Meaning
Onset	Time it takes after a medication is administered for it to produce a response
Peak	Time it takes for a medication to reach its highest effective concentration
Trough	Minimum blood serum concentration of medication reached just before the next scheduled dose
Duration	Time during which the medication is present in concentration great enough to produce a response
Plateau	Blood serum concentration of a medication reached and maintained after repeated fixed doses

Oral Routes. The oral route is the easiest and the most commonly used. Medications are given by mouth and swallowed with fluid. Oral medications have a slower onset of action and a more prolonged effect than parenteral medications. Clients generally prefer the oral route.

Sublingual Administration. Some medications are designed to be readily absorbed after being placed under the tongue to dissolve (Figure 30–4). A medication given by the **sublingual** route should not be swallowed, or the desired effect will not be achieved. Nitroglycerine is commonly given sublingually. The client should not take a drink until the medication is completely dissolved.

Buccal Administration. Administration of a medication by the **buccal** route involves placing the solid medication in the mouth and against the mucous membranes of the cheek until the medication dissolves (Figure 30–5). Clients should be taught to alternate cheeks with each subsequent dose to avoid mucosal irritation. Clients are also warned not to chew or swallow the medication or to take any liquids with it. A buccal medication acts locally on the mucosa or systemically as it is swallowed in a person's saliva.

Parenteral Routes. **Parenteral administration** involves injecting a medication into body tissues. The following are the four major sites of injection:

1. **Intradermal (ID):** Injection into the dermis just under the epidermis
2. **Subcutaneous (Sub-Q):** Injection into tissues just below the dermis of the skin
3. **Intramuscular (IM):** Injection into a muscle
4. **Intravenous (IV):** Injection into a vein

Some medications are administered into body cavities other than the four types listed above. These routes of

Table 30-5 Factors Indicating Choice of Administration Routes

Advantages	Disadvantages or Contraindications
Oral, Buccal, Sublingual Routes	
Routes are convenient and comfortable for client.	These routes are avoided when client has alterations in gastrointestinal function (e.g., nausea, vomiting), reduced motility (after general anaesthesia or bowel inflammation), and surgical resection of portion of gastrointestinal tract.
Routes are economical.	Some medications are destroyed by gastric secretions. Oral administration is contraindicated in clients unable to swallow (e.g., clients with neuromuscular disorders, esophageal strictures, mouth lesions).
Routes are easy to administer.	Oral medications may irritate lining of gastrointestinal tract, discolour teeth, or have unpleasant taste.
Medications may produce local or systemic effects.	Unconscious or confused client is unable or unwilling to swallow or hold medication under tongue.
Routes rarely cause anxiety for client.	Oral medications cannot be given when client has gastric suction and are contraindicated in clients before some tests or surgery.
Subcutaneous (Sub-Q), Intramuscular (IM), Intravenous (IV), Intradermal (ID) Routes	
Routes provide means of administration when oral medications are contraindicated.	There is risk of introducing infection, and some medications are expensive. Clients must experience repeated needle sticks. The Sub-Q, IM, and ID routes are avoided in clients with bleeding tendencies.
More rapid absorption occurs than with topical or oral routes.	There is risk of tissue damage with Sub-Q injections.
IV infusion provides medication delivery when client is critically ill or long-term therapy is required. If peripheral perfusion is poor, IV route is preferred over injections.	IM and IV routes are dangerous because of rapid absorption. These routes cause considerable anxiety in many clients, especially children.
Skin	
Topical	
Topical skin applications primarily provide local effect.	Clients with skin abrasions are at risk for rapid medication absorption and systemic effects.
Route is painless.	
Limited side effects occur.	
Transdermal	
Transdermal applications provide prolonged systemic effects with limited side effects.	Application leaves oily or pasty substance on skin and may soil clothing.
Mucous membranes*	
Therapeutic effects are provided by local application to involved sites.	Mucous membranes are highly sensitive to some medication concentrations.
Aqueous solutions are readily absorbed and capable of causing systemic effects.	Insertion of rectal and vaginal medication often causes embarrassment.
Mucous membranes provide route of administration when oral medications are contraindicated.	Client with ruptured eardrum cannot receive irrigations. Rectal suppositories are contraindicated if client has had rectal surgery or if active rectal bleeding is present.
Inhalation	
Inhalation provides rapid relief for local respiratory problems.	Some local agents can cause serious systemic effects.
Route provides easy access for introduction of general anaesthetic gases.	

*Includes eyes, ears, nose, vagina, rectum, and ostomy.

medication administration include epidural, intrathecal, intraosseous, intraperitoneal, intrapleural, and intraarterial. Depending on agency policy, nurses may or may not be responsible for the administration of medications through these advanced techniques. Additional education or certification may be required to administer medications through some routes. Whether or not the nurse actually administers the medication by these routes, the nurse remains responsible for monitoring the integrity of the system of medication delivery, understanding the therapeutic value of the medication, and evaluating the client's response to the therapy.

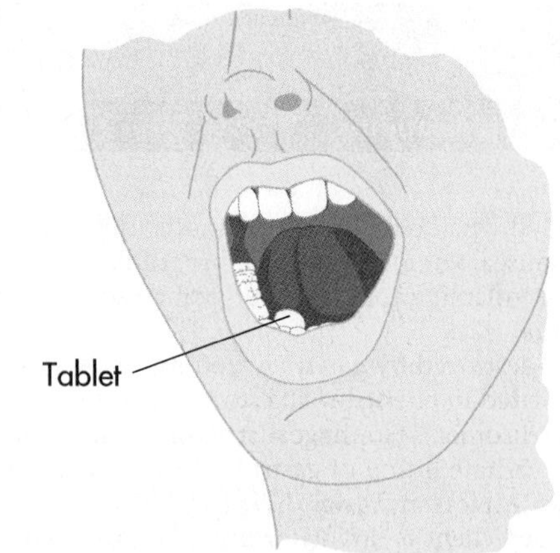

FIGURE **30–4** Sublingual administration of a tablet.

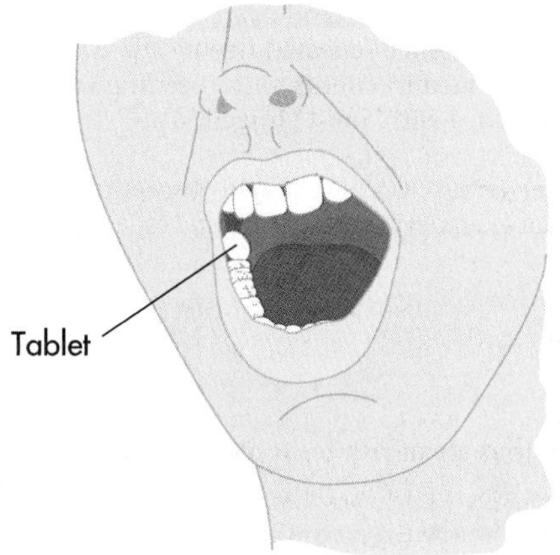

FIGURE **30–5** Buccal administration of a tablet.

Epidural. Medications are administered in the epidural space via a catheter, which has been placed by an anaesthesiologist. This technique of medication administration is most commonly used for the administration of analgesia post-operatively (see chapter 38). Nurses who have received extra education in the epidural route can administer medications in bolus form or by continuous infusion.

Intrathecal. Intrathecal medications are administered through a catheter that has been placed into the subarachnoid space or into one of the ventricles of the brain. Intrathecal administration is often associated with long-term medication administration through catheters that have been surgically implanted. In most institutions, a physician usually injects medications into intrathecal catheters. However, specially educated nurses may also do so.

Intraosseous. This method of medication administration involves the infusion of medication directly into the bone marrow. It is most commonly used in infants and toddlers who have poor access to their intravascular space. This method is most popular when an emergency arises and IV access is impossible. The physician inserts an intraosseous infusion needle into the bone, usually the tibia, for the administration of medication by the nurse.

Intraperitoneal. Medications are administered into the peritoneal cavity, where they are absorbed into the circulation. Chemotherapeutic agents, insulin, and antibiotics may be administered in this fashion. One method of dialysis also uses the peritoneal route for the removal of fluid, electrolytes, and waste products. Nurses often initiate and teach clients how to manage peritoneal dialysis.

Intrapleural. Medications are administered through the chest wall and directly into the pleural space through an injection or through a chest tube that has been inserted by the physician. Chemotherapeutic agents are the most common medications administered via this method. Physicians also instill medications that help resolve persistent pleural effusion. This is called pleurodesis. This technique promotes adhesion between the visceral and parietal pleura. Increasingly, newer indications of this method of medication delivery are being used. One such indication is for the instillation of analgesic agents through specially designed intrapleural catheters (Clarke, 1999).

Intraarterial. This method calls for medications to be administered directly into the arteries. Intraarterial infusions are common in clients who have arterial clots. The nurse will manage a continuous infusion of clot-dissolving agents. The nurse must carefully monitor the integrity of this infusion to prevent inadvertent disconnection of the system and subsequent bleeding.

Other methods of medication administration that are usually limited to physician administration are **intracardiac,** injection of a medication directly into cardiac tissue, and **intraarticular,** injection of a medication into a joint.

Topical Administration. Medications applied to the skin and mucous membranes generally have local effects. The topical medication is applied to the skin by painting or spreading it over an area, applying moist dressings, soaking body parts in a solution, or giving medicated baths. Systemic effects can occur if a client's skin is thin or broken down, if the medication concentration is high, or if contact with the skin is prolonged.

Some medications (e.g., nitroglycerine, scopolamine, estrogens) have systemic effects because they are applied topically by a **transdermal disk** or patch. The disk secures the medicated ointment to the skin. These topical applications may be applied for as little as 24 hours or as long as 7 days.

Medications can be applied to mucous membranes in a variety of ways: (a) by directly applying a liquid or ointment (e.g., eye drops, gargling, swabbing the throat); (b) by inserting a medication into a body cavity (e.g., placing a suppository in the rectum or vagina or inserting medicated packing into the vagina); (c) by instilling fluid into a body cavity (e.g., ear drops, nose drops, or bladder and rectal **instillation** [fluid is retained]); (d) by irrigating a

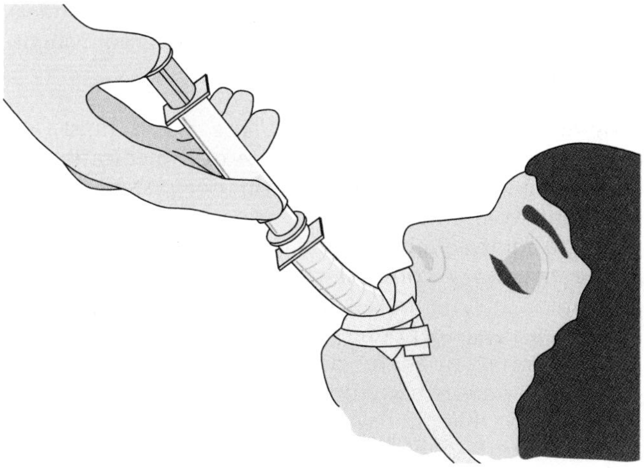

FIGURE **30–6** Medication being instilled through an endotracheal tube.

body cavity (e.g., flushing eye, ear, vagina, bladder, or rectum with medicated fluid [fluid is not retained]); and (e) by spraying (e.g., instillation into nose and throat).

Inhalation Route. The deeper passages of the respiratory tract provide a large surface area for medication absorption. Medications can be administered through the nasal passages, oral passage, or endotracheal or tracheostomy tubes. Endotracheal tubes are inserted into the client's mouth and go to the trachea (Figure 30–6), whereas tracheostomy tubes directly enter the trachea through an incision made in the neck. Medications that are administered by the **inhalation** route are readily absorbed and work rapidly because of the rich vascular alveolar capillary network present in the pulmonary tissue. Inhaled medications may have local or systemic effects.

Intraocular Route. Intraocular medication delivery involves inserting a medication in a form similar to a contact lens directly into the client's eye. The eye medication disk has two soft outer layers that have medication enclosed in them. The disk can remain in the client's eye for up to 1 week. Pilocarpine, a medication used to treat glaucoma, is the most common medication disk.

Systems of Medication Measurement

The proper administration of a medication depends on the nurse's ability to compute medication doses accurately and measure medications correctly. A careless mistake in placing a decimal point or adding a zero to a dose can lead to a fatal error. The nurse is responsible for checking the accuracy of the dose before giving a medication.

The metric, apothecary, and household systems of measurement are used in medication therapy. Most nations, including Canada, use the metric system as their standard of measurement. Prescriptions to be self-administered are often written in household measures for clients. The apothecary system is rarely used.

Metric System. As a decimal system, the **metric system** (Système international d'unités, or SI) is the most logically organized. Metric units can easily be converted and computed through simple multiplication and division. Each basic unit of measurement is organized into units of 10. Multiplying or dividing by 10 forms secondary units. In multiplication, the decimal point moves to the right; in division, the decimal moves to the left. For example:

$$10.0 \text{ mg} \times 10 = 100 \text{ mg}$$
$$10.0 \text{ mg}/10 = 1 \text{ mg}$$

When designating a metric dosage, it is important to *not* write a zero alone after a decimal point (e.g., write 5 mg—not 5.0 mg).

The basic units of measurement in the metric system are the metre (length), the litre (volume), and the gram (weight). For medication calculations, the nurse uses only the volume and weight units. In the metric system, lowercase or capital letters are used to designate basic units:

Gram = g
Litre = L

Lowercase letters are used for abbreviations for other units:

Milligram = mg
Millilitre = mL

A system of Latin prefixes designates subdivision of the basic units: *deci-* (1/10 or 0.1), *centi-* (1/100 or 0.01), and *milli-* (1/1,000 or 0.001). Greek prefixes designate multiples of the basic units: *deka-* (10), *hecto-* (100), and *kilo-* (1,000). When writing medication doses in metric units, prescribers and nurses use fractions or multiples of a unit. Fractions should be converted to decimal form. A zero is always placed in front of the decimal to prevent error.

500 mg or 0.5 g, *not* $^1/_2$ g
10 mL or 0.01 L, *not* $^1/_{100}$ L

Solutions. The nurse uses solutions of various concentrations for injections, **irrigations,** and infusions. A **solution** is a given mass of solid substance dissolved in a known volume of fluid or a given volume of liquid dissolved in a known volume of another fluid. When a solid is dissolved in a fluid, the concentration is in units of mass per units of volume (e.g., g/mL, g/L, mg/mL). A concentration of a solution may also be expressed as a percentage. A 10% solution, for example, is 10 g of solid dissolved in 100 mL of solution. A proportion also expresses concentrations. A 1/1,000 solution represents a solution containing 1 g of solid in 1,000 mL of liquid or 1 mL of liquid mixed with 1,000 mL of another liquid.

Household Measurements. Household units of measure are familiar to most people. The disadvantage of household measures is their inaccuracy. Household utensils such as teaspoons and cups often vary in size. Scales to measure pints or quarts are often not well calibrated. Household measures include drops, teaspoons, tablespoons, cups, pints, and quarts for volume, and ounces

Table 30-6 Equivalents of Measurement

Metric	Apothecary	Household
1 mL	15–16 minims (m)	15 drops (gtt)
4–5 mL	1 fluidram (f2)	1 teaspoon (tsp)
16 mL	4 fluidrams (f2)	1 tablespoon (tbsp)
30 mL	1 fluid ounce (f3)	2 tablespoons (tbsp)
240 mL	8 fluid ounces (f3)	1 cup (c)
480 mL (approximately 500 mL)	1 pint (pt)	1 pint (pt)
960 mL (approximately 1 L)	1 quart (qt)	1 quart (qt)
3840 mL (approximately 5 L)	1 gallon (gal)	1 gallon (gal)

and pounds for weight. Although ounces and pounds are considered household measures, they are also used in the apothecary system.

The advantage of household measurements is their convenience and familiarity. When the accuracy of a medication dose is not critical, it is safe to use household measures. For example, many over-the-counter medications can safely be measured by this method. Table 30-6 gives common equivalents of metric and household units.

Clinical Calculations

To administer medications, the nurse must have an understanding of basic arithmetic to calculate medication doses, mix solutions, and perform a variety of other activities. This skill is essential because medications are not always dispensed in the unit of measure in which they are ordered. This occurs because medication companies package and bottle certain standard equivalents. For example, the prescriber may order 250 mg of a medication that is available only in grams. The nurse is responsible for converting available units of volume and weight to the desired doses. Therefore, the nurse should be aware of approximate equivalents in all major measurement systems.

Conversions Within One System. Converting measurements within one system is relatively easy. In the metric system, the nurse simply divides or multiplies. To change milligrams to grams, the nurse divides by 1,000, moving the decimal three places to the left.

$$1000 \text{ mg} = 1 \text{ g}$$
$$350 \text{ mg} = 0.35 \text{ g}$$

To convert litres to millilitres, the nurse multiplies by 1,000 or moves the decimal three places to the right.

$$1 \text{ L} = 1000 \text{ mL}$$
$$0.25 \text{ L} = 250 \text{ mL}$$

To convert units of measurement within the apothecary or household system, the nurse must consult an equivalence table. For example, when converting fluid ounces to quarts, the nurse must first know that 32 oz is the equivalent of 1 qt. To convert 8 oz to a quart measurement, the nurse divides 8 by 32 to get the equivalent, $^1/_4$ or 0.25 qt.

Conversion Between Systems. The nurse must frequently determine the proper dose of a medication by converting weights or volumes from one system of measurement to another. Often, metric units must be converted to equivalent household measures for use at home. Before making a conversion, the nurse compares the measurement system available with that ordered. For example, the prescriber orders Robitussin 30 mL. To provide proper instruction to the client, the nurse must convert "mL" to common household measurement. To convert millilitres to tablespoons, the nurse must know the equivalent or refer to a table such as Table 30-6. Tables of equivalent measurements are available in all health care institutions. The pharmacist is also a good resource.

Dose Calculations. There are many formulas that can be used to calculate medication doses. The following basic formula can be applied when preparing solid or liquid forms:

$$\frac{\text{Dose ordered}}{\text{Dose on hand}} \times \text{Amount on hand} = \begin{array}{l}\text{Amount}\\\text{to administer}\end{array}$$

The dose ordered is the amount of medication prescribed. The dose on hand is the weight or volume of medication available in units supplied by the pharmacy; it may be expressed on the medication label as the contents of a tablet or capsule or as the amount of medication dissolved per unit volume of liquid. The amount on hand is the basic unit or quantity of the medication that contains the dose on hand. For solid medications, the amount on hand may be one capsule; the amount of liquid on hand may be a millilitre or litre depending on the container. The amount to administer is the actual amount of available medication the nurse will administer. The amount to administer is always expressed in the same unit as the amount on hand.

The following example illustrates how to apply the formula. The prescriber orders the client to receive morphine 2 mg IV. Thus, the dose ordered is 2 mg. The medication is available in a vial containing 10 mg in an amount on hand of 1 mL. The formula is applied as follows:

$$2 \text{ mg}/10 \text{ mg} \times 1 \text{ mL} = \begin{array}{l}\text{Volume in millilitres}\\\text{to administer}\end{array}$$

To simplify the $^2/_{10}$ fraction, divide numerator and denominator by 2:

$$^1/_5 \times 1 \text{ mL} = {}^1/_5 \text{ mL to administer}$$

Syringes are calibrated only in decimals. After converting the fraction $^1/_5$ to 0.2, the nurse accurately prepares the correct dose.

Another example demonstrates how the formula applies with solid dose forms. The physician orders 0.125 mg orally (PO) of digoxin. The medication is available in tablets containing 0.25 mg.

Table 30-7 Ways to Prevent Medication Administration Errors

Precaution	Rationale
Read medication labels carefully.	Many products come in similar containers, colours, and shapes.
Question administration of multiple tablets or vials for single dose.	Most doses are one or two tablets or capsules or one single-dose vial. Incorrect interpretation of order may result in excessively high dose.
Be aware of medications with similar names.	Many medication names sound alike (e.g., digoxin and digitoxin, Keflex and Keflin, Orinase and Ornade).
Check decimal point.	Some medications come in quantities that are multiples of one another (e.g., Coumadin in 2.5- and 25-mg tables, Thorazine in 30- and 300-mg spansules).
Question abrupt and excessive increases in dosages.	Most dosages are increased gradually so that physician can monitor therapeutic effect and response.
When new or unfamiliar medication is ordered, consult resource.	If prescriber is also unfamiliar with drug, there is greater risk of inaccurate dosages being ordered.
Do not administer medication ordered by nickname or unofficial abbreviation.	Many prescribers refer to commonly ordered medications by nicknames or unofficial abbreviations. If nurse or pharmacist is unfamiliar with name, wrong medication may be dispensed and administered.
Do not attempt to decipher illegible writing.	When in doubt, ask prescriber. Unless nurse questions order that is difficult to read, chance of misinterpretation is great.
Know clients with same last names. Also have clients state their full names. Check name bands carefully.	It is common to have two or more clients with same or similar last names. Special labels on Kardex or medication book can warn of potential problem.
Do not confuse equivalents.	When in a hurry, it may be easy to misread equivalents (e.g., milligram instead of millilitre).

FIGURE **30–7** Scored medication tablet. (Courtesy Mosby's GenRx 1999.)

$$0.125\text{ mg}/0.250\text{ mg} \times 1\text{ tablet} = \text{Number of tablets to administer}$$

The fraction $^{0.125}/_{0.250}$ equals $^{1}/_{2}$ or 0.5. Therefore,

$$0.5 \times 1\text{ tablet} = 0.5\text{ or }^{1}/_{2}\text{ tablet to be administered}$$

Many tablets come with scores or indentations across the centre of the tablet (Figure 30–7). A scored tablet is easy to break in half for divided doses. In some institutions, pharmacists are responsible for scoring tablets. The potential for giving an incorrect dose is high when the nurse estimates amounts by breaking unscored tablets. Therefore, the nurse should not cut unscored tablets.

Often, liquid medications come prepared in volumes greater than 1 mL. In applying the formula, the nurse must be careful to use the correct concentration to avoid a medication error. For example, the order is "erythromycin suspension 250 mg PO." The pharmacy delivers 100-mL bottles with the label stating, "5 mL contains 125 mg of erythromycin." Thus, the appropriate concentration to use in this example to obtain the correct dose of medication is 125 mg in 5 mL.

$$250\text{ mg}/125\text{ mg} \times 5\text{ mL} \times \text{Volume to administer}$$

The fraction $^{250}/_{125}$ equals 2. Therefore,

$$2 \times 5\text{ mL} = 10\text{ mL to administer}$$

The nurse should always double-check calculations or confer with another professional if an answer seems unreasonable (Table 30-7).

Pediatric Doses. Calculating children's medication doses requires caution. Children metabolize medications at different rates when compared with adults. For example, premature and newborn infants are especially vulnerable to adverse effects of medications because their livers and kidneys have not matured to full functioning levels. After the newborn period, the liver metabolizes some drugs more quickly, which may require that the child have larger doses or more frequent administration (Hockenberry et al., 2003). Other factors that influence medication dosages in children include the difficulty in evaluating the desired effect and the hydration status of the child. In most cases, the prescriber will calculate the dose for a child before ordering the medication. However, it is the nurse's responsibility to be aware of the safe dosage range for any medication administered to a child. Therefore, nurses should be aware of the formulas used to calculate pediatric doses and recheck all doses before administration. Drug package inserts or medication references often list the normal ranges for pediatric doses.

Various formulas are used to determine appropriate medication dosages for children. These formulas often take the child's age, weight, body surface area, and/or the medication amount into consideration. However, the most accurate method of calculating pediatric doses is based on a child's body surface area (Hockenberry et al., 2003). Body surface area is estimated from the child's height and weight. A standard nomogram (e.g., the West nomogram) can be used to estimate a child's body surface area (Figure 30–8).

The nurse uses the following formula to calculate a pediatric dose. The formula is a ratio of the child's body

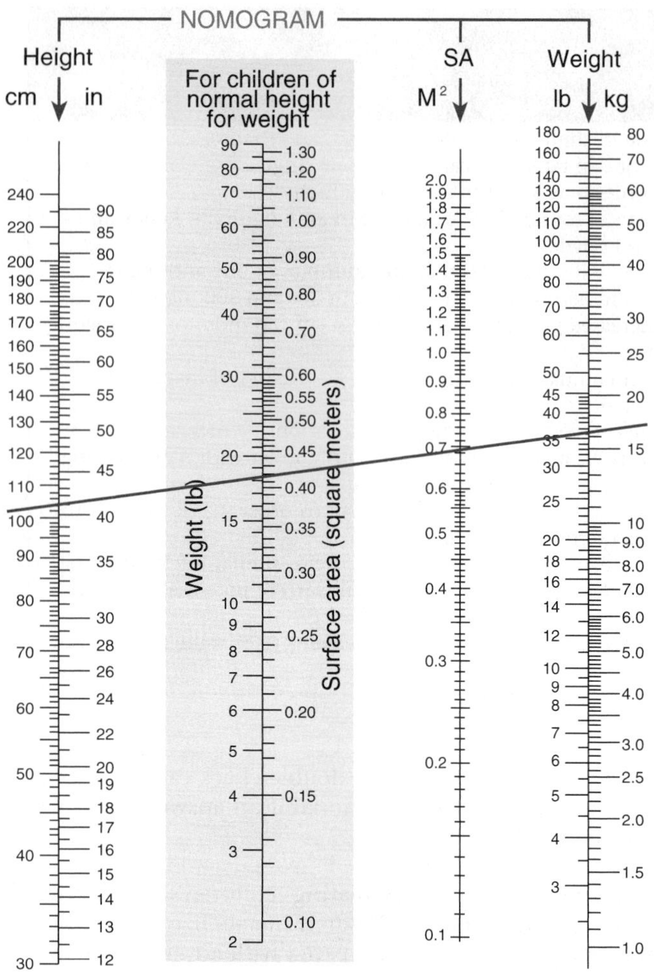

FIGURE **30–8** West nomogram for estimation of surface areas in children. A straight line is drawn between height and weight. The point where the line crosses the surface area column is the estimated body surface area. (From *Nelson Textbook of Pediatrics,* 13th ed., edited by R. E. Behrman and V. C. Vaughan, 1987, Philadelphia: Saunders; modified from data of Boyd E, by West CD.)

surface area compared with the body surface area of an average adult (1.7 square metres, or 1.7 m^2).

$$\text{Child's dose} = \frac{\text{Surface area of child}}{1.7\ m^2} \times \text{Normal adult dose}$$

For example, a prescriber orders ampicillin for a child weighing 12 kg. The normal adult dose for ampicillin is 250 mg. The West nomogram (see Figure 30–8) shows that this child weighing 12 kg has a surface area of 0.54 m^2. Using this information, the nurse calculates the appropriate child's dose:

$$\text{Child's dose} = 0.54m^2/1.7\ m^2 \times 250\ mg$$

The m^2 units are canceled out.

$$\text{Child's dose} = 0.54/1.7 \times 250\ mg$$
$$0.54/1.7 = 0.3$$
$$\text{Child's dose} = 0.3 \times 250\ mg = 75\ mg$$

An alternative method to determine dosages of medications for children involves basing the amount of medication to administer (usually in milligrams) on how much the child weighs (usually in kilograms). For example, a prescriber orders 5 mg/kg to be given to a child weighing 14 kg. Using this information, the nurse calculates the appropriate dosage based on the following calculation:

$$\text{Child's dose} = 5\ mg/kg \times 14\ kg = 70\ mg \text{ to be delivered}$$

Nursing Knowledge Base

The nurse does not have sole responsibility for medication administration. The prescriber (physician, nurse practitioner, or midwife) and pharmacist also help to ensure the right medication gets to the right client. However, the nurse who administers medications is accountable for knowing what medications are prescribed, their therapeutic and non-therapeutic effects, and the medications' associated nursing implications. The nurse is also responsible for knowing why the client needs the medication and determining if the client requires supervision with administration and education about the medication and its effects.

Prescriber's Role

The prescriber writes a medication order on a form in the client's medical record, in an order book, on a legal prescription pad, by a facsimile (fax) machine, or through a computer terminal. There should be a documented diagnosis, condition, or indication for use for each medication ordered.

Where allowed, a prescriber may also order a medication by talking directly to the nurse or by telephone. When medications or medical treatments are ordered this way, it is called a **verbal order.** When the nurse receives a verbal order, he or she immediately enters it into the client's medical record, indicating the time and the name of the prescriber who gave the order. The nurse then signs the record. Most institutions require a prescriber's signature within 24 hours after the order is made.

Institutional policies vary regarding the personnel who can take verbal or telephone orders. Generally, nursing students cannot take these types of medication orders. Nursing students only give newly ordered medications after the order has been written and verified by a registered nurse. Common abbreviations are used when writing orders. However, caution must be exercised in the use of abbreviations because some abbreviations can result in confusion and the potential for medication errors (Table 30-8). It is important for nurses to know their agency's policies on abbreviations.

The abbreviations indicate dosage frequencies or times, routes of administration, and special information for giving the medication (see Table 30-3).

Types of Orders

Four types of medication orders are common in acute care settings: standing, prn, single (one-time), and STAT orders. These medication orders are based on the frequency and/or urgency of medication administration. Some conditions change the status of a client's medication orders.

Table 30-8 Dangerous Abbreviations Used in Medication Administration

Abbreviation	Practice Problem	Preferred Term
U (for unit)	Mistaken as zero, four, or cc.	Write "unit"
IU (for international unit)	Mistaken as IV or 10.	Write "international unit"
Q.D. (once daily), Q.O.D. (every other day)	Mistaken for each other or mistaken for QID (four times daily).	Write "daily" and "every other day"
MS, MSO_4 (morphine sulphate) $MgSO_4$	Mistaken for one another.	Write "morphine sulphate" or "magnesium sulphate"
μg	Mistaken for mg. Resulting in 1000-fold dosing overdose	Write "mcg"
H.S. (bedtime)	Mistaken for either half strength or hour of sleep. q H.S. mistaken for every hour.	Write out "half strength" or "at bedtime"
T.I.W. (for three times a week)	Mistaken for three times a day or twice weekly.	Write "three times weekly"
S.C. or S.Q. (subcutaneous)	Mistaken as SL for sublingual or "5 every."	Write "Sub-Q", "subQ", or "subcutaneously"
D/C (discharge)	Interpreted as discontinue.	Write "discharge"
cc (for cubic centimetre)	Mistaken for U (units) when poorly written.	Write "mL" for millilitres

Adapted from *2004 National Patient Safety Goals—FAQs,* Joint Commission for Accreditation of Healthcare Organizations, 2004. Retrieved December 10, 2003, from *http://www.jcaho.org/accredited+organizations/patient+safety/04+npsg/04_faqs.htm*

For example, surgery automatically cancels all of a client's preoperative medications (see chapter 45). Because the client's condition changes after surgery, the prescriber must write new orders. When a client is transferred to another health care agency or a different service within a hospital or is discharged, the prescriber should review the medications and write new orders as indicated.

A prescription is a medication order for clients to take outside the hospital.

Standing Orders or Routine Medication Orders. A standing order is carried out until the prescriber cancels it by another order or until a prescribed number of days elapse. A standing order may indicate a final date or number of treatments or doses. Many institutions have policies for automatically discontinuing standing orders. The following are examples of standing orders: "tetracycline 500 mg PO q6h" and "Decadron 10 mg daily × 5 days."

prn Orders. The prescriber may order a medication when a client requires it. This is a prn order. The nurse uses objective and subjective assessment and discretion in determining whether or not the client needs the medication. Often, the prescriber sets minimum intervals for the time of administration. This means the medication cannot be given any more often than what is prescribed. An example is "morphine sulphate 2 mg IV q 1-2 h prn for incisional pain." When medications are administered, the nurse documents the assessment made and the time of medication administration. The nurse should make frequent evaluation of the effectiveness of the medication and record findings in the appropriate record.

Single (One-Time) Orders. A prescriber will often order a medication to be given only once at a specified time. This order is common for preoperative medications or medications given before diagnostic examinations, for example, "Versed 25 mg IM on call to OR" and "Valium 10 mg PO at 0900."

STAT Orders. A STAT order signifies that a single dose of a medication is to be given immediately and only once. STAT orders are often written for emergencies when the client's condition changes suddenly. For example, "Give Apresoline 10 mg IV STAT."

Prescriptions. The prescriber writes **prescriptions** for clients who are to take medications outside the hospital. The prescription includes more detailed information than a regular order because the client must understand how to take the medication and when to refill the prescription if necessary. The parts of a prescription are included in Figure 30–9.

Pharmacist's Role

The pharmacist prepares and distributes prescribed medications. Pharmacists work with nurses, physicians, and other health care providers to evaluate the efficacy of clients' medication. The pharmacist is responsible for filling prescriptions accurately and for being sure that prescriptions are valid. The pharmacist in a health care agency rarely has to mix compounds or solutions, except in the case of IV additive solutions. Most medication companies deliver medications in a form ready for use. Dispensing the correct medication, in the proper dosage and amount, with an accurate label is the pharmacist's main task. The pharmacist can also provide information about medication side effects, toxicity, interactions, and incompatibilities.

Distribution Systems

Systems for storing and distributing medications vary. Pharmacists provide the medications, but nurses distribute medications to clients. Institutions providing nursing care have a special area for stocking and dispensing medications. Special medication rooms, portable locked carts,

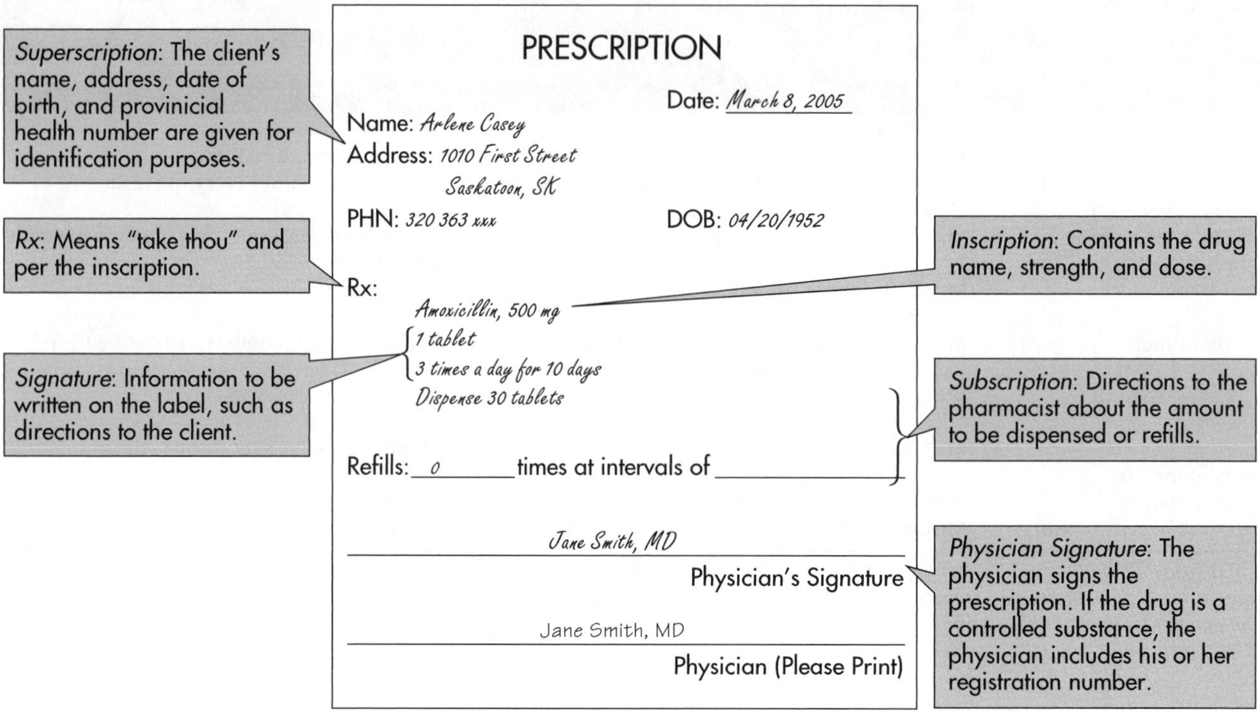

FIGURE **30–9** Sample medication prescription.

computerized medication cabinets, and individual storage units next to clients' rooms are examples of storage areas used. Nurses must make sure that all medications are in locked containers in a room (e.g., medication room) or are under constant surveillance.

Stock Supply. With a stock system, medications are available in quantity in larger, multidose containers. This system is time-consuming and costly because a nurse must dispense each medication separately for each client. This type of system of medication delivery has been associated with a high rate of medication errors and is not commonly used today.

Unit Dose. The unit-dose system uses portable carts containing a drawer with a 24-hour supply of medications for each client. Each drawer is labelled with the name of the client in the designated room. The unit dose is the ordered dose of medication the client receives at one time. Each tablet or capsule is wrapped in a foil or paper container. At a designated time each day, the pharmacist refills the drawers in the cart with a fresh supply. The cart also contains limited amounts of prn and stock medications for special situations. Controlled substances are not kept in the individual client drawer but in a larger locker drawer in the cart. The unit-dose system is designed to reduce the number of medication errors and saves steps in dispensing medications.

Automated Dispensing Systems. Automated medication dispensing systems (AMDSs) are used successfully throughout the country (Figure 30–10). The systems are designed to achieve computerized control of narcotics and unit dose medication dispensing. Each nurse has a security code allowing access to the system. All procedures connected to an AMDS are controlled electronically via a client's profile. The client's name and drug profile must be accessed before the AMDS will dispense a medication. The nurse enters the client's identification number into the computer and selects the desired medication, dosage, and route from a list displayed on the computer screen. The system causes the drawer containing the medication to open, and records it. Nurses may also scan bar codes to identify the client, medication (name, dosage, route), and the nurse administering the medication. This information is then automatically recorded on a computerized database.

Nurse's Role

Because the nurse spends the most time with clients, the nurse is the most appropriate health care worker to administer medications. Medication administration requires knowledge and a set of skills that is unique to the nurse. The nurse assesses the client's ability to self-administer medications, determines whether a client should receive a medication at a given time, administers medications correctly, and monitors the effects of prescribed medications. Client and family education about proper medication administration and monitoring is an integral part of the nurse's role. The nurse uses the nursing process to integrate medication therapy into care.

Critical Thinking

Knowledge

The nurse uses the knowledge learned from many disciplines when administering medications. It is this knowledge that helps the nurse to understand why a particular medication has been prescribed for a client and how this

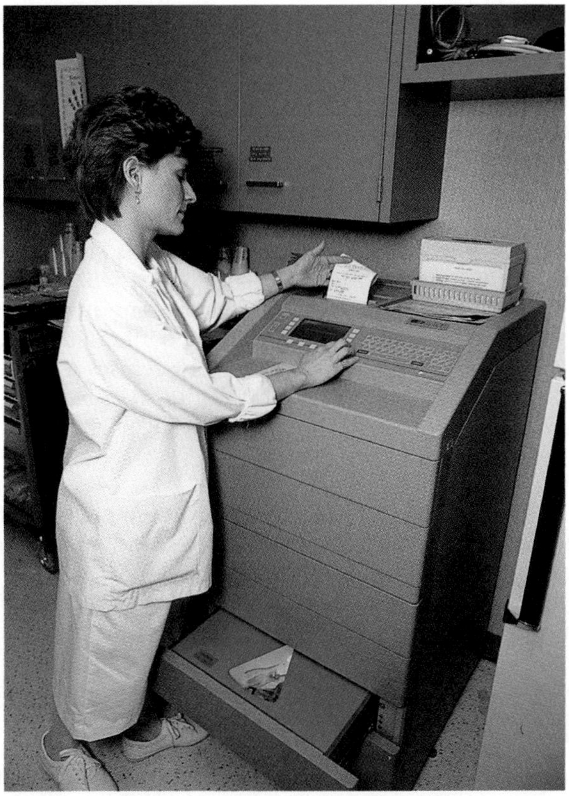

FIGURE **30–10** Nurse using automated medication dispensing system.

Case Study Box 30-2

The physician writes an order for a medication. The nurse receives the order and checks for completeness and appropriateness. The nurse may question the order if the written order is illegible, the dose seems unusually low or high, or the medication seems inappropriate for the client's condition. The order is sent to the pharmacy, where it is read and prepared by either a pharmacist or a pharmacy technician. If the technician prepares the medication, the pharmacist checks the technician's work. The pharmacist also verifies that the medication is the appropriate dosage and that there are no medication interactions or medication allergies. When a medication order seems inappropriate, for example, a medication order written for 2000 mg when the proper dosage calls for 200 mg, the pharmacist may ask the nurse to clarify the order from the prescriber or the pharmacist may call the prescriber directly for order clarification. When the order is appropriate, the medications are sent to the nursing unit.

The nurse receives the medication and checks the administration record against what the pharmacy has sent and the prescriber ordered. Before administration, the nurse performs the six rights of medication administration. The nurse allows the client to be the final check by reviewing the name of the medication, the dosage, and why he or she is receiving the medication.

medication will exert a therapeutic effect. For example, in physiology, the nurse learns that potassium is a major intracellular ion. When clients do not have enough potassium in their body, they may experience signs and symptoms that are associated with hypokalemia, such as muscle fatigue or weakness. Medications may be prescribed to restore the client's potassium level to normal.

Experience

The nursing student often has limited experience with medication administration as it applies to professional practice. The clinical experience provides the student with the opportunity to use the nursing process as it applies to medication administration. As the student nurse gains experiences in medication administration, psychomotor skills ("the how-to") become more refined. However, psychomotor skills represent a small part of medication administration. Client attitudes, knowledge, physical and mental status, and responses can make medication administration a complex experience.

Attitudes

To administer medication safely to clients, the nurse requires certain essential cognitive skills. The nurse accepts full responsibility for all actions that are taken, including the administration of medications. When a nurse administers a medication to the client, the nurse accepts the responsibility that the nursing actions in administering the medication should not harm the client in any way. The nurse does not assume that the medication that is ordered for the client is the correct medication or the correct dose. The nurse could be held accountable for administering an ordered medication that is knowingly inappropriate for the client. Because of this, the nurse should be familiar with the therapeutic effect, usual dosage, laboratory interferences, and side effects of all medications that are administered. The nurse is also responsible for ensuring that clients who will self-administer medications have been properly informed about all aspects of self-administration.

Demonstrating accountability and acting responsibly in professional practice means that the nurse acknowledges when errors in professional practice occur. Most of the errors made by nurses are medication errors. A **medication error** is any event that could cause or lead to a client receiving inappropriate medication therapy or failing to receive appropriate medication therapy. Most medication errors occur when a nurse fails to follow routine procedures such as checking dose calculations, deciphering illegible handwriting, or administering medications with which the nurse is unfamiliar (see Table 30-7). Hospital medication delivery systems should be designed so that there is a system of checks and balances. This system will help to reduce medication errors. Consider the example in Box 30-2, which illustrates the crucial role that nurses play in the prevention of medication errors.

Unfortunately, many medication errors are never identified. When an error occurs, it should be acknowledged immediately and reported to the appropriate hospital personnel (e.g., nurse manager and physician). Measures to counteract the effects of the error may be necessary. The nurse is also responsible for completing an incident report describing the nature of the incident. Incident reports assist administrative personnel in identifying hospital system problems that contribute to medication errors. References to incident reports should *not* be made in a client's permanent record.

Nurses administer a wide variety of medications, and new medications are constantly approved for dispensation. As a result, nurses do not always have knowledge about the medications that they are asked to administer. Critical thinkers admit what they do not know and try to acquire the knowledge needed for safe administration of unfamiliar medications. This may mean consulting expert nurses, a pharmacist, or a medication book.

Institutional policy may place limitations on the nurse's ability to administer medications in certain units of the acute care setting. Nurses may be limited by certain medication routes or dosages. Most institutions have nursing procedure manuals with policies that define the classes of medications that nurses employed by the agency may and may not administer. The types and dosages of medications that nurses may deliver can also vary from unit to unit within the same facility. For example, Dilantin, a powerful medication that is administered to treat seizures, may be administered by mouth or IV push. In large dosages, Dilantin can also affect the rhythm of the heart. Therefore, some institutions place limits on how much Dilantin can be given to a client on a nursing unit that does not have the ability to monitor the client's heart rate and rhythm. Not all prescribers are aware of all of the limitations and may prescribe medications that cannot be given in a particular health care setting. Nurses must recognize these limitations and ensure that the prescriber is informed. Nurses must also ensure that the client receives the medications as prescribed and within the time prescribed in the appropriate environment.

Standards

Standards are those actions that ensure safe nursing practice. To ensure safe medication administration, the nurse should be aware of a nursing standard called the six rights of medication administration. All medication errors can be linked, in some way, to an inconsistency in adhering to the following six rights of medication administration:

1. The right medication
2. The right dose
3. The right client
4. The right route
5. The right time
6. The right documentation

Right Medication. When medications are first ordered, the nurse compares the medication recording form or computer orders with the prescriber's written orders. When administering medications, the nurse compares the label of the medication container with the medication form. The nurse does this three times: (1) before removing the container from the drawer or shelf, (2) as the amount of medication ordered is removed from the container, and (3) before returning the container to storage. With unit-dose prepackaged medications, the nurse checks the label with the medicine form a third time even though there is no permanent container. Unit-dose medications may be checked before opening at the client's bedside.

Nurses administer only the medications that they prepare. If an error occurs, the nurse who administers the medication is responsible. If a client questions the medication, the nurse must not ignore these concerns. An alert client will know whether a medication is different from those received before. In most cases, the client's medication order has been changed; however, the client's questions might reveal an error. The nurse should withhold the medication until the preparation can be rechecked against the prescriber's orders.

Clients who self-administer medications should keep them in their original labelled containers, separate from other medications, to avoid confusion. The nurse never prepares medications from unmarked containers or containers with illegible labels. If a client refuses a medication, the nurse should discard it rather than return it to the original container. Unit-dose packaged medications can be saved if they are unopened.

Right Dose. The unit-dose system is designed to minimize errors. The chance of error increases when a medication must be prepared from a larger volume or strength than needed or when the prescriber orders a system of measurement different from what the pharmacist supplies. When performing medication calculations or conversions, the nurse should have another qualified nurse check the calculated doses.

After calculating doses, the nurse prepares the medication using standard measurement devices. Graduated cups, syringes, and scaled droppers can be used to measure medications accurately. At home, clients should use measuring spoons and cups, rather than household spoons and cups, which vary in volume.

When it is necessary to break a scored tablet, the break should be even. A tablet may be cut in half by using a knife or a cutting device. Tablets that do not break evenly are discarded. The two halves are given in successive doses if the second half was repackaged and labelled.

Often a nurse prepares a tablet by crushing it so that it can be mixed in food. The crushing device should always be cleaned completely before the tablet is crushed. Remnants of previously crushed medications may increase a medication's concentration or result in the client receiving a portion of an unprescribed medication. Crushed medications should be mixed with very small amounts of food or liquid. The client's favourite foods or liquids should not be used because a medication may alter their taste and decrease the client's desire for them.

> ***Safety Alert.*** Not all medications can be crushed. Some medications, such as time-released or extended-release capsules, have special coatings to prevent the medication from being absorbed too quickly. Refer to a medication manual or some other reference before crushing a medication to ensure that the medication can be safely crushed.

Right Client. Medication errors often occur because one client gets a drug intended for another client. An important step in administering medications safely is being sure the medication is given to the right client. It is difficult to remember every client's name and face. To identify a client correctly, the nurse checks the medication administration form against the client's identification

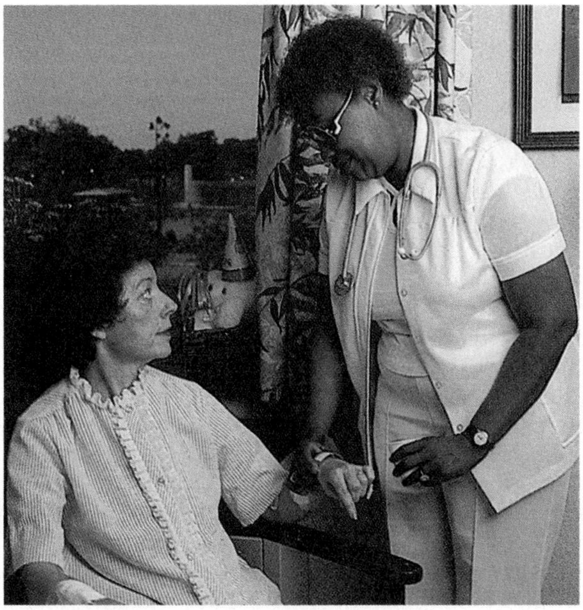

FIGURE **30–11** Before administering any medications, the nurse checks the client's identification bracelet.

bracelet and asks the client to state his or her name to ensure that the client's identification bracelet has the correct information (Figure 30–11).

If an identification bracelet is missing or becomes smudged or illegible, the nurse must acquire a new one for the client. When asking the client's name, the nurse should not merely speak the name and assume that the client's response indicates that he or she is the right person. Instead, the nurse asks the client to state his or her full name. To avoid making the client feel uneasy, the nurse simply states that the question is routine for giving a medication.

Right Route. If a prescriber's order does not designate a route of administration, the nurse consults the prescriber. Likewise, if the specified route is not the recommended route, the nurse should alert the prescriber immediately.

When the nurse administers injections, precautions are necessary to ensure that the medications are given correctly. It is also important to prepare injections only from preparations designed for parenteral use. The injection of a liquid designed for oral use can produce local complications, such as a sterile abscess, or fatal systemic effects. Medication companies label parenteral medications for "injectable use only."

Right Time. The nurse must know why a medication is ordered for certain times of the day and whether the time schedule can be altered. For example, two medications are ordered, one q8h (every eight hours) and the other tid (three times a day). Both medications are to be given three times within a 24-hour period. The prescriber intends the q8h medication to be given around the clock to maintain therapeutic blood levels of the medication. In contrast, the tid medication is given during the waking hours. Each institution has a recommended time schedule for medications ordered at frequent intervals. The nurse may alter these recommended times if necessary or appropriate.

The prescriber often gives specific instructions about when to administer a medication. A preoperative medication to be given on call means that the nurse is to administer the medication when the operating room notifies the nursing unit. A medication ordered pc (after meals) is to be given within half an hour after a meal, when the client has a full stomach. A STAT medication is to be given immediately.

Medications that must act at certain times are given priority. For example, insulin should be given at a precise interval before a meal. Antibiotics should be given on time around the clock to maintain therapeutic blood levels. All routinely ordered medications should be given within 60 minutes of the times ordered (30 minutes before or after the prescribed time).

Some medications require the nurse's clinical judgment in determining the proper time for administration. A prn sleeping medication should be administered when the client is prepared for bed or at a time appropriate for maximum benefit. A nurse also uses judgment when administering prn analgesics. For example, the nurse may need to obtain a STAT order from the prescriber if the client requires a medication before the prn interval has elapsed.

At home, a client may have to take several medications throughout the day. The nurse helps to plan schedules based on preferred medication intervals, the medications' pharmacokinetics, and the client's daily schedule. For clients who have difficulty remembering when to take medications, the nurse can make a chart that lists the times when each medication is to be taken or can prepare a special container to hold each timed dose.

Right Documentation. This right has been added to the traditional five rights of medication administration by several authors to enhance medication safety (Aschenbrenner, Cleveland, & Venable, 2002). Documentation is an important part of safe medication administration. Because medication errors may result from inaccurate documentation, nurses must ensure that the appropriate documentation exists before giving medications. The documentation for the medication should clearly reflect the client's name, the name of the ordered medication, the time the medication was administered, and the medication's dosage, route, and frequency. If any of these pieces of information are missing, the nurse must contact the prescriber to verify the order. After the nurse administers the medication, the medication administration record (MAR) is completed per agency policy to verify that the medication was given as ordered. Accurate documentation serves as a way for health care providers to communicate with each other.

Professional standards influence the activities of medication administration. Provincial nursing associations have developed standards of nursing practice that apply to the practice of medication administration. Other professional nursing standards may also apply.

Maintaining Clients' Rights. Because of the potential risks related to medication administration, a client has the right to the following:

- To be informed of the medication's name, purpose, action, and potential undesired effects
- To refuse a medication regardless of the consequences
- To have qualified nurses or physicians assess a medication history, including allergies
- To be properly advised of the experimental nature of medication therapy and to give written consent for its use
- To receive labelled medications safely without discomfort in accordance with the six rights of medication administration
- To receive appropriate supportive therapy in relation to medication therapy
- To not receive unnecessary medications

The nurse must be aware of these rights and handle all inquiries by clients and families courteously and professionally. A nurse should not become defensive if a client refuses medication therapy. The nurse must have the necessary knowledge and skill to satisfy the responsibilities of safe and effective medication administration.

Nursing Process and Medication Administration

NP Assessment

To determine the need for and potential response to medication therapy, the nurse assesses many factors.

History. Prior to administering medications, the nurse obtains or reviews the client's medical history. The history may provide indications or contraindications for medication therapy. Disease or illness may place clients at risk for adverse medication effects. For example, if a client has a gastric ulcer, compounds containing aspirin will increase the likelihood of bleeding. Long-term health problems such as diabetes or arthritis, which require medications, suggest to the nurse the type of medications a client is taking. A client's surgical history may indicate use of medications. For example, after a thyroidectomy, a client may require hormone replacement.

History of Allergies. If the client has a history of allergies to medication, the nurse informs other members of the health care team. Food allergies should also be carefully documented because many medications have ingredients also found in food sources. One example is shellfish. If clients are allergic to shellfish, the client may be sensitive to any product containing iodine, such as Betadine or dyes used in radiological testing. Another example is dye used in food products (e.g., candy, carbonated beverages). In a hospital, clients wear identification bands listing the medications to which they are allergic. All allergies should be noted on the nurse's admission notes, medication records, and physician's history.

Medication Data. The nurse assesses information about each medication that the client takes, including length of time the medication has been taken, the current dosage, and whether or not the client has experienced adverse effects from the medication. In addition, the nurse reviews medication data, including action, purpose, normal dosages, routes, side effects, and nursing implications for administration and monitoring. Common questions to ask include the following: Is the smallest possible dose ordered? (a question pertinent to older adults), Can a certain medication interact with other medications being used? Are there special instructions for administering the medication? Often, several resources must be consulted to gather needed information. Pharmacology textbooks, nursing journals, the *Compendium of Pharmaceuticals and Specialties* (CPS), medication package inserts, and the pharmacist are valuable resources. Helpful medication resources can also be downloaded to personal hand-held computers. The nurse is responsible for knowing as much as possible about each medication given. Many nursing students prepare or purchase cards containing medication data to use as a quick resource.

Diet History. A diet history reveals normal eating patterns and food preferences. The nurse can then plan the dosage schedule more effectively and advise the client in avoiding foods that may interact with medications.

Client's Perceptual or Coordination Problems. For a client with perceptual or fine motor limitations, self-administration may be difficult. For example, a client with arthritis may have difficulty manipulating a syringe. The nurse must assess the client's ability to prepare doses and take medications correctly. If the client is unable to self-administer medications, the nurse may need to assess whether family or friends will be available to assist.

Client's Current Condition. The ongoing physical or mental status of a client may affect whether a medication is given or how it is administered. The nurse should assess a client carefully before giving any medication. For example, the nurse checks blood pressure before giving an antihypertensive. A client who is nauseated may be unable to swallow a tablet. Assessment findings also serve as a baseline in evaluating the effects of medication therapy.

Client's Attitude Toward Medication Use. The client's attitude about medications may reveal a level of medication dependence or drug avoidance. Clients may not express their feelings about taking a particular medication, particularly if dependence is a problem. The nurse should observe the client's behaviour for evidence of medication dependence or avoidance. The nurse should also be aware that the client's cultural beliefs about Western medicine could interfere with medication compliance (Box 30-3, and see chapter 9).

Client's Knowledge and Understanding of Medication Therapy. The client's knowledge and understanding of medication therapy influence the willingness or ability to follow a medication regimen. Unless a client understands a medication's purpose, the importance of regular dosage schedules and proper administration methods, and the possible side effects, compliance is unlikely. When assessing knowledge of a medication, the nurse asks, What is it for? How is it taken? When is it taken? What side effects

Cultural Aspects of Care — Box 30-3

Health beliefs vary by culture. These beliefs often influence how clients manage and respond to drug therapy. Significant differences in values, beliefs, and attitudes may affect a client's compliance with drug therapy. For example, cultures attach different symbolic meanings to medications and drug therapy. Herbal remedies and alternative therapies are common in various cultures and ethnic groups and may interfere with prescribed medications. In addition, there is often a marked difference in health beliefs between health providers and clients, which further affects a client's compliance with medical therapy. Demographic changes in both age and race are factors that currently affect nursing practice in medication administration. In addition to the psychosocial aspect of medication therapy, pharmacological research has shown that different ethnic and racial groups experience differences in drug response, metabolism, and side effects.

Implications for Practice

- Carefully assess cultural beliefs, attitudes, and values when administering and teaching clients about their medications.
- Conflicts between medications and cultural beliefs need to be resolved to achieve optimal client outcomes.
- When assessing medication history, nurses should investigate if the client practises any alternative therapies or is taking any herbal preparations.
- Consider cultural influences on drug response, metabolism, and side effects if a client is not responding to drug therapy as expected. A change in the client's medication may be warranted.

Data from *Transcultural Concepts in Nursing Care* (4th ed.), by M. M. Andrews and J. S. Boyle, 2003, Philadelphia: Lippincott; and *Mosby's Pharmacology in Nursing Revised and Updated* (21st ed.), by L. M. McKenry and E. Salerno, 2003, St. Louis, MO: Mosby.

have there been? Has the client ever stopped taking doses? Is there anything else the client does not understand and would like to know about the medication? When the client has a history of poor compliance, the nurse should also review resources available for purchase of medications.

Client's Learning Needs. By assessing the client's level of knowledge about a medication and the resources available to take medications regularly, the nurse determines the need for instruction (see chapter 17). It may be necessary for the nurse to explain the action and purpose of the medication, expected side effects, correct administration techniques, and ways to help the client to remember the medication regimen. If a client has been placed on a newly prescribed medication, instruction may need to be more involved.

Nursing Diagnosis

Assessment provides data about the client's condition, ability to self-administer medications, and medication use patterns, which can be used to determine actual or potential problems with medication therapy. Certain data are defining characteristics, which when clustered together reveal nursing diagnoses. For example, *non-compliance related to a medication regimen* may be indicated when a client admits that he or she is not taking prescribed medications correctly, or by evidence that a medication has not reversed symptoms as expected. The following is a list of nursing diagnoses that may be used during the administration of medications:

- Anxiety
- Health maintenance, ineffective
- Health-seeking behaviours
- Deficient knowledge (medications)
- Non-compliance (medications)
- Disturbed visual sensory perception
- Impaired swallowing
- Effective therapeutic regimen management
- Ineffective therapeutic regimen management

Once the diagnosis is selected, the nurse identifies the related factor, which drives the selection of nursing interventions. For example, the related factors of inadequate resources and lack of knowledge require different interventions. If the client's non-compliance is related to inadequate finances, the nurse will collaborate with family members, social workers, or community agencies to help a client receive necessary medications. If the related factor is lack of knowledge, the nurse will implement an extensive teaching plan and follow-up.

Planning

The nurse organizes care activities to ensure the safe administration of medications. Hurrying to give clients medications can lead to errors. It is important for the nurse to minimize distractions or interruptions when preparing and administering medications.

Goals and Outcomes. Setting goals and related outcomes will help the nurse plan to use time wisely during medication administration. For example, the nurse might establish the following goal and related outcomes for a client with newly diagnosed Type 2 diabetes:

Goal: The client will safely administer all ordered medications before discharge.

Outcomes:

- The client will verbalize understanding of desired effects and adverse effects of medications.
- The client will state signs, symptoms, and treatment of hypoglycemia.
- The client will establish a daily routine that will coordinate timing of medication with mealtimes.

Setting Priorities. The nurse prioritizes care when administering medications. The nurse uses information gathered from the client's assessment in determining which medications should be given first and if it is appropriate to administer prn medications. For example, if a client is in pain, it is important that the nurse provide pain medication as soon as possible. If the client is experiencing an elevated blood pressure, the blood pressure medications should be administered before other medications.

The nurse also prioritizes when providing client education about medications. The most important information about the medications should be provided first. For example, if an oral hypoglycemic medication causes hypoglycemia as a side effect, the client must be able to identify and treat the hypoglycemia before taking the medication independently.

Continuity of Care. Whenever possible, the nurse collaborates with the client's family or friends when giving instruction. Family members will often reinforce the importance of medication regimens in the home setting. When clients are hospitalized, it is important for the nurse to not postpone instruction until the day of discharge. In order for the client to understand medications and self-administration guidelines, there must be time for questions and discussion. Early planning is critical.

In the community, the nurse ensures that the client knows where and how to obtain medications. The nurse also ensures that clients know how to read medication labels. Whether a client attempts self-administration or the nurse assumes responsibility for administering medications, the following goals and expected outcomes must be met: (a) the client and family understand medication therapy, (b) the client gains therapeutic effect of the prescribed medications without discomfort or complications, (c) the client has no complications related to the route of administration, and (d) the client safely self-administers medications.

NP Implementation

Health Promotion. The nurse, in promoting or maintaining the client's health, identifies factors that may improve or diminish well-being. Health beliefs, personal motivations, socio-economic factors, and habits (e.g., smoking) can influence the client's compliance with the medication regimen.

Teaching the client and family about the benefit of a medication and the knowledge needed to take it correctly is an essential component of primary health care and can promote adherence to the regimen (Box 30-4). Integrating the client's health beliefs and cultural practices into the treatment plan can assist the nurse in establishing a schedule or routine with the client. The nurse may make referrals to community resources if the client is unable to afford, or get out to obtain, necessary medications. All clients should also learn the basic guidelines for medication safety. These guidelines ensure the proper use and storage of medications in the home (Box 30-5).

Acute Care. Clients are often hospitalized to receive expert nursing observation and documentation of responses to medications. When a nurse receives a medication order, several nursing interventions are essential for safe and effective medication administration.

Receiving Medication Orders. A medication order is required for any medication to be administered by a nurse. Before any other interventions, the nurse ensures that the medication order contains all of the elements in Box 30-6. If the medication order is incomplete, the nurse should inform the prescriber and ensure completeness before carrying out the medication order. Some medication orders can be given verbally or by telephone by the prescriber to the nurse. A verbal order is a medication or treatment order received by the nurse in the presence of the prescriber. Verbal orders are entered into the client's medical record by the registered nurse and transcribed in the same way as if the prescriber wrote the order himself or herself. Telephone orders are medication or treatment orders given to the nurse by the prescriber, generally after the nurse updates the prescriber about a change in the client's condition. The nurse follows institutional policy regarding the receiving, recording, and transcription of verbal and telephone orders. Generally, the prescriber must sign verbal and telephone orders within 24 hours.

Box 30-4

Focus on Primary Health Care

Improving Drug Compliance

When a client is discharged from hospital or sent home from a clinic visit, part of his or her ongoing treatment may include taking regular medications at home. In cases of chronic illness, the success of treatment may depend on the client's compliance with drug therapy. Nurses can play an important role in assisting clients to comply with their medication regimen.

The following suggestions may improve client compliance:

- Ensure that the client and family understand the reason for the medication, how to take the medication properly, and the possible consequences of non-compliance.
- Ensure that the client and family can recognize symptoms of medication side effects or toxicity. Family members or friends should be informed of medication side effects, such as changes in behaviour, because they are often the first people to recognize such effects.
- Teach proper self-administration of medications to clients for all routes. For example, demonstrate how to accurately measure a liquid medication. Offer extra help to clients who depend on daily injections. For example, demonstrate how to prepare and administer an injection correctly using aseptic technique. Family members or friends should also be taught to give injections in case the client becomes ill or physically unable to handle a syringe. Provide specially designed equipment as necessary, such as syringes with enlarged calibrated scales for easier reading or Braille-labelled medication vials for clients with visual alterations.
- Help the client to address any economic issues that might affect compliance.
- Explore with the client factors influencing his or her ability to comply; for some clients, keeping a daily log may be helpful.
- Provide a written schedule that includes the name of the medication and a description or picture of the pill.
- Encourage clients to take their pills in conjunction with something they do every day, such as brushing their teeth or having breakfast.
- Help clients to organize their pills into a box with daily dividers. If compliance is a major concern, home care nurses, public health nurses, or family members can check and refill the box on a weekly basis.
- Work with the client's pharmacist to ensure that the pharmacy calls to remind the client when a refill is due.

Client Teaching Box 30-5

Safe Medication Administration

Objective

- Client will correctly administer subcutaneous insulin.

Teaching Strategies

- Instruct client in how to determine that insulin is not out of date.
- Instruct client to keep medication in its original labelled container.
- Instruct client to keep insulin refrigerated.
- Instruct client in how to rotate insulin injection sites.
- Instruct client in how to determine the amount of insulin from the results of home capillary glucose monitoring.
- Demonstrate to client how to prepare a single insulin preparation.
- Demonstrate to client how to administer subcutaneous insulin injection.
- Instruct client in how to keep a daily log book for insulin injections, including results of home capillary glucose monitoring, type and amount of insulin given, expiration date on insulin vial, time of insulin injection, and injection site used.

Evaluation

- Ask client to describe procedure used at home for determining the correct dose of insulin needed and injection site.
- Observe client preparing insulin dose from results of capillary glucose monitoring.
- Observe client selecting injection site.
- Observe client self-administering insulin injection.
- Review client log book for insulin injections.

Student nurses are prohibited from receiving verbal and telephone orders.

Correct Transcription and Communication of Orders. The nurse or a designated unit secretary writes the prescriber's complete order on the appropriate medication form, the MAR. The transcribed order includes the client's name, room, and bed number and medication name, dose, frequency, and route of administration. Each time a medication dose is prepared, the nurse refers to the medication form. With the unit-dose system, only one transcription is necessary, limiting the opportunity for errors. When transcribing orders, the nurse should be sure that names, dosages, and symbols are legible. The nurse rewrites any smudged or illegible transcriptions.

Some institutions have prescribed order entry. The prescriber is able to enter an order directly into the computer, preventing the need for transcription of orders. Computer interfaces transfer the order to the MAR, the pharmacy record, and automated dispensing system. The computer printout may be used as the MAR, recording which medications are given to the client (Figure 30–12).

Box 30-6 Components of Medication Orders

A medication order is incomplete unless it has the following parts:

- **Client's full name:** The client's full name distinguishes the client from other people with the same last name. In the acute care setting, clients may also be assigned special identification numbers (e.g., medical record number) to help distinguish clients with the same names. This number may be included on the order form.
- **Date that the order is written:** The day, month, year, and time must be included. Designating the time that an order is written helps clarify when certain orders are to stop automatically. If an incident occurs involving a medication error, it is easier to document what happened when this information is available.
- **Medication name:** The prescriber will order a generic or trade name medication. Correct spelling is essential in preventing confusion with medications with similar spelling.
- **Dose:** The amount or strength of the medication is included.
- **Route of administration:** The prescriber uses accepted abbreviations for medication routes. Accuracy is important because some medications are administered by more than one route.
- **Time and frequency of administration:** The nurse needs to know when to initiate medication therapy. Orders for multiple doses establish a routine schedule for medication administration.
- **Signature of prescriber:** The signature makes the order a legal request.

A registered nurse checks all transcribed orders against the original order for accuracy and thoroughness. If an order seems incorrect or inappropriate, the nurse consults the prescriber. The nurse who gives the wrong medication or an incorrect dose is legally responsible for the error.

Accurate Dose Calculation and Measurement. When measuring liquid medications, the nurse uses standard measuring containers. The procedure for medication measurement is systematic to lessen the chance of error. The nurse calculates each dose when preparing the medication, pays close attention to the process of calculation, and avoids interference from other nursing activities.

Correct Administration. For safe administration, the nurse uses aseptic technique and proper procedures when handling and giving medications. For example, certain medications require the nurse to perform assessments (e.g., assessing heart rate before giving antidysrhythmic medications). The nurse must monitor when a client is receiving the first dose of a medication new to the client. The nurse documents the client's response on the appropriate record form according to agency policy.

Recording Medication Administration. After administering a medication, the nurse records it immediately on the appropriate record form (see Figure 30–12). The nurse *never* charts a medication before administering it.

Room: 3700-03

Patient: PDM, Pharmacy
Birth: 11/30/79 Admit: 01/03/05
MRN: 2000403 Acct: 900015
A Doctor: Jim Smith

Age: 20 y Ht: 1 m 57 cm Wt: 56.79 kg

MEDICATION ADMINISTRATION RECORD

Date: 01/18/00 – 01/19/00

ADEs/Nondrug allergies: Latex – Zosyn – Amoxicillin – Insulins – Darvocet – Lugols soln. – Antihi +

Medication	0800	0900	1000	1100	1200	1300	1400	1500	1600	1700	1800	1900	2000	2100	2200	2300	2400	0100	0200	0300	0400	0500	0600	0700
P00014 Bacitracin ointment AKA: Bacitracin ointment Dose: Apply STRGH: 30 gm/tube TID Topical: Right lower leg For external use only Testing			RL 10																					
P00029 Insulin/human regular AKA: Humulin R Dose: 15 units Strgh: 1 ml = 100 units AC Sub-Q	RL 0730																							
P00030 Fexofenadine 60 mg/psuedo 120 mg AKA: Allegra–D Sr Tab Dose: 1 tab STRGH: 60/120/tab BID Oral Auto Sub: 1 Allegra–D Tab bid For Claritin–D 12 hr and 24 hr Per P&T Comm			RL 10																					
P00036 Aspirin AKA: Aspirin 325 mg Tab Dose: 2 tab 650 mg STRGH: 325 mg/tab Q3–4h Oral Testing						RL 1315																		
P00039 Haloperidol tablet AKA: Haldol 0.5 mg tab Dose: 1 mg STRGH: 1 mg/tab QHS Oral																								
P00035 Zolpidem AKA: Ambien 5 mg tab Dose: 5 mg STRGH: 5/tab QHS PRN Oral MR × 1 Testing																								

Circle = Dose not given
Initials = Dose given
Deltoid = R.D., L.D.
Vastus Lateralis = R.V.L., L.V.L.
Lower Abdominal = R.L.A., L.L.A.
Anterior Gluteal = R.A.G., L.A.G.
Posterior Gluteal = R.P.G., L.P.G.

Page: 01 (continued)

Initials and signature Rita Lassater RL	**Initials and signature**	**Initials and signature**
Initials and signature	**Initials and signature**	**Initials and signature**
Initials and signature	**Initials and signature**	**Initials and signature**

FIGURE **30–12** Example of medication administration record (MAR).

Recording immediately after administration prevents errors.

The recording of a medication includes the name of the medication, dose, route, and exact time of administration. Often the medication forms are prepared, and the nurse need record only the time. Agency policies may also require that the nurse record the location of an injection.

If a client refuses a medication or is undergoing tests or procedures that result in a missed dose, the nurse explains in the nurse's notes the reason the medication was not given. Some agencies require the nurse to circle the prescribed administration time on the medication record when a dose is missed.

Restorative Care. Because of the numerous types of restorative care settings, medication administration activities vary. Clients with functional limitations may require the nurse to fully administer all medications. In the home setting, clients usually administer their own medications. Regardless of the type of medication activity, the nurse remains responsible for instructing clients and families in medication action, administration, and side effects. The nurse is also responsible for monitoring compliance with medication and determines the effectiveness of medications that have been prescribed.

Special Considerations for Administering Medications to Specific Age Groups. A client's developmental level is a factor in the way that nurses administer medications. Knowledge of a client's developmental needs helps the nurse to anticipate responses to medication therapy.

Infants and Children. Children vary in age, weight, surface area, and the ability to absorb, metabolize, and excrete medications. Children's medication doses are lower than those of adults; therefore, special caution is needed when preparing medications for them. Medications are usually not prepared and packaged in standardized dose ranges for children. Preparing an ordered dose from an available amount requires careful calculation (see Pediatric Doses).

The child's parents are valuable resources for learning the best way to administer medications to the child. Sometimes it is less traumatic for the child if a parent gives the medication and the nurse supervises.

All children require special psychological preparation before receiving medications. Supportive care is needed if a child is expected to co-operate. The nurse explains the procedure to a child, using short words and simple language appropriate to the child's level of comprehension. Long explanations may increase a child's anxiety, especially for painful procedures such as an injection. The young child who refuses to co-operate or resists consistently despite explanation and encouragement may require physical coercion. If so, it is carried out quickly and carefully (Hockenberry et al., 2003). If it is possible to involve the child, the nurse may have greater success giving a medication (Cromling, 2002). For example, saying "It's time to take your tablet now. Do you want it with water or juice?" allows a child to make a choice. The child should not be given the option of not taking a medication. After a medication is given, the nurse praises the child and may even offer a simple reward such as a star or token. Box 30-7 lists tips for effective medication administration for children.

Box 30-7 Tips for Administering Medications to Children

Oral Medications

- Liquid forms are safer to swallow to avoid aspiration.
- Use droppers for administering liquids to infants; straws may help older children swallow pills.
- Offer juice, a soft drink, or a frozen juice bar after a medication is swallowed.
- Carbonated beverages poured over finely crushed ice reduce nausea.
- When mixing medications with palatable flavourings such as syrup or applesauce, use only a small amount. The child may refuse to take all of a larger mixture. Avoid mixing a medication with foods or liquids that the child is taking well because the child may in turn refuse them.
- A plastic, disposable syringe is the most accurate device for preparing liquid doses, especially those less than 10 mL. (Cups, spoons, and droppers are inaccurate.)
- When administering liquid medications, a spoon, plastic cup, or oral syringe (without needle) is useful.

Injections

- Be careful when selecting IM injection sites because infants and small children have underdeveloped muscles.
- Children can be unpredictable and uncooperative. Someone should be available to restrain a child if needed.
- Always awakens a sleeping child before giving an injection.
- Distracting the child with conversation, a ringing bell, or a toy may reduce pain perception.
- Give the injection quickly and do not argue with the child.
- If time allows, use a eutectic mixture of local anaesthetics (EMLA) cream.

Older Adults. Older adults also require special consideration during medication administration (Box 30-8). In addition to physiological changes of aging (Figure 30–13), behavioural and economic factors influence an older person's use of medications. Ebersole and Hess (1998) described five behavioural patterns of medication use characteristic of the older client: polypharmacy, self-prescribing of medications, use of over-the-counter (OTC) medications, misuse of medications, and noncompliance.

Polypharmacy. **Polypharmacy** means that the client is taking many medications, prescribed or not, in an attempt to treat several disorders simultaneously. Some of the medications taken may have similar effects (Maas et al., 2001). When this occurs, there is a high risk of medication interactions with other medications and with foods that the client may eat. There is also an increased risk of the client having an adverse reaction to the medications.

Self-Prescribing of Medications. A variety of symptoms can be experienced by older adult clients (e.g., pain, constipation, insomnia, and indigestion). All of these symptoms

Focus on Older Adults — Box 30-8

- Simplify the drug therapy plan whenever possible (McKenry & Salerno, 2003).
- Keep instructions clear and simple and provide written material in large print (Maas et al., 2001).
- Assess functional status to determine if client will require assistance in taking medications (McKenry & Salerno, 2003).
- Have client drink a little fluid *before* taking oral medications to ease swallowing, and encourage the client to drink at least 150 to 180 mL of fluid after taking medications (Ebersole & Hess, 1998).
- Older adults may have a greater sensitivity to drugs, especially those that act on the central nervous system. Therefore, carefully monitor clients' responses to medications and anticipate dosage adjustments as needed (McKenry & Salerno, 2003).
- If the client has difficulty swallowing a capsule or tablet:
  - Ask the physician to substitute a liquid medication if possible (Ebersole & Hess, 1998).
  - Have the client sit up straight and tuck the chin to decrease risk of aspiration (McKenry & Salerno, 2003).
- Teach alternatives to medications, such as proper diet instead of vitamins and exercise instead of laxatives (Ebersole & Hess, 1998).
- Review medication history, including over-the-counter medications, on a frequent basis (Maas et al., 2001).

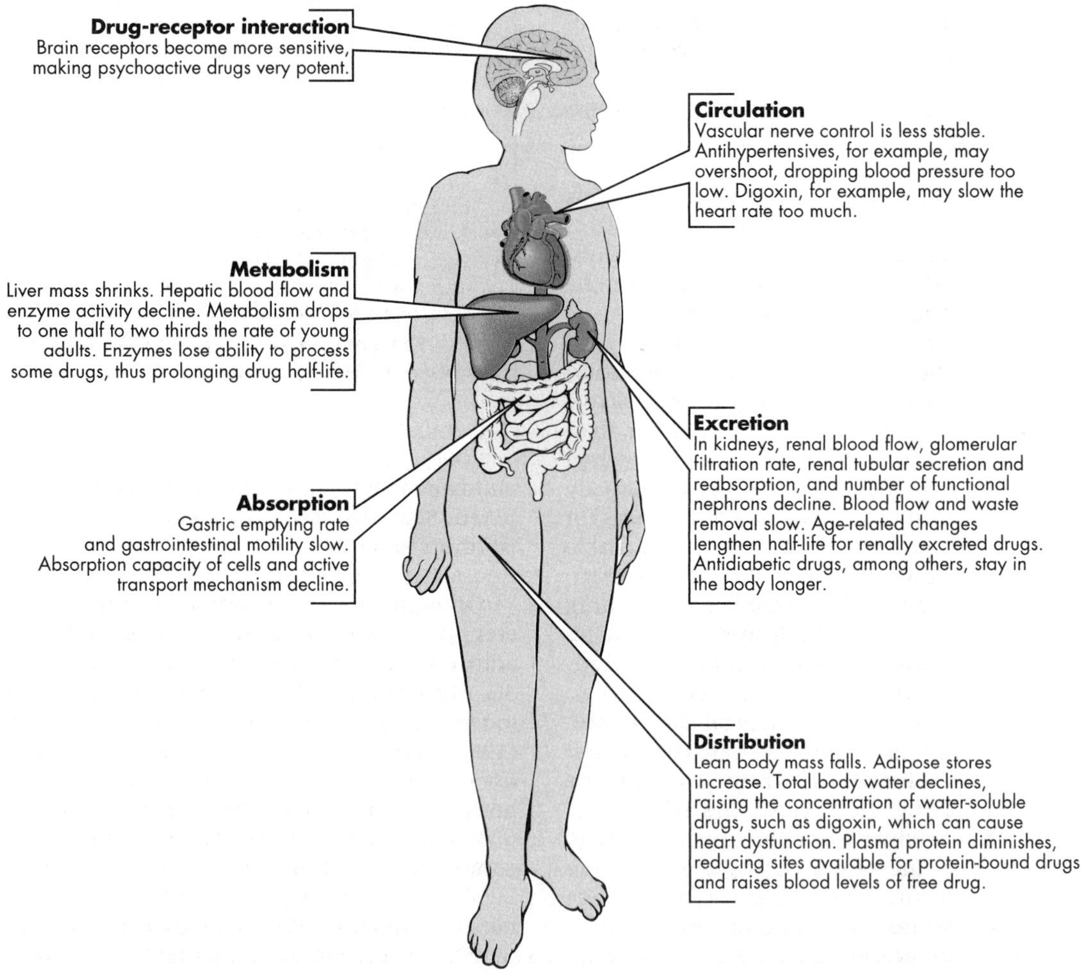

Drug-receptor interaction
Brain receptors become more sensitive, making psychoactive drugs very potent.
Circulation
Vascular nerve control is less stable. Antihypertensives, for example, may overshoot, dropping blood pressure too low. Digoxin, for example, may slow the heart rate too much.
Metabolism
Liver mass shrinks. Hepatic blood flow and enzyme activity decline. Metabolism drops to one half to two thirds the rate of young adults. Enzymes lose ability to process some drugs, thus prolonging drug half-life.
Excretion
In kidneys, renal blood flow, glomerular filtration rate, renal tubular secretion and reabsorption, and number of functional nephrons decline. Blood flow and waste removal slow. Age-related changes lengthen half-life for renally excreted drugs. Antidiabetic drugs, among others, stay in the body longer.
Absorption
Gastric emptying rate and gastrointestinal motility slow. Absorption capacity of cells and active transport mechanism decline.
Distribution
Lean body mass falls. Adipose stores increase. Total body water declines, raising the concentration of water-soluble drugs, such as digoxin, which can cause heart dysfunction. Plasma protein diminishes, reducing sites available for protein-bound drugs and raises blood levels of free drug.

FIGURE **30–13** Aging body and drug use. (From *Medical-Surgical Nursing,* 5th ed., by S. M. Lewis, M. M. Heitkemper, and S. R. Dirksen, 2000, St. Louis, MO: Mosby.)

are amenable to OTC medications. Older adults often attempt to seek relief from the problems by using OTC preparations, folk medicines, and herbs.

Over-the-Counter Medications. It is known that OTC medications are used by 75% of older adults to relieve symptoms. Many of these OTC preparations have ingredients that, when used inappropriately, may cause undesirable side effects or adverse reactions or may be contraindicated in the client's condition.

Misuse of Medications. Forms of misuse by older adults include overuse, underuse, erratic use, and contraindicated use.

Non-compliance. Non-compliance is defined as a deliberate misuse of medication. Many older adults intentionally do not adhere to their medication regimen, either by not taking the medication at all or by altering the dose. Non-compliance generally occurs either because of drug ineffectiveness, uncomfortable side effects, or the prohibitive cost of the medicine (see Box 30-4).

NP Evaluation

The nurse monitors a client's response to medications on an ongoing basis. This requires that the nurse know the therapeutic action and common side effects of each medication. A change in a client's condition can be physiologically related to health status or may result from medications or both. The nurse must be alert for reactions in a client taking several medications. The goal of safe and effective medication administration involves a careful evaluation of technique and the client's response to therapy and ability to assume responsibility for self-care.

To evaluate the effectiveness of nursing interventions when meeting established goals of care, the nurse uses evaluative measures to identify whether client outcomes were met. Many different evaluation measures can be used in the context of medication administration: direct observation of behaviour or response, rating scales and checklists, and oral questioning. The type of measurement used varies with the action being evaluated, the reading skill and knowledge level of the client, and the client's cognitive and psychomotor ability. The most common type of measurement that the nurse uses is a physiological measure. Examples of physiological measure are blood pressure, heart rate, and visual acuity. Client statements can also be used as evaluative measures. Table 30-9 contains examples of goals, expected outcomes, and corresponding evaluative measures.

Medication Administration

Medication administration is an essential part of nursing practice, which requires a sound knowledge base. Nurses must be prepared to administer medications using a variety of routes. The following sections explain the steps involved in administering medications using various routes.

Oral Administration

The easiest and most desirable way to administer medications is by mouth (Skill 30-1). Clients usually are able to ingest or self-administer oral medications with few problems. Most tablets and capsules should be swallowed and administered with approximately 60 to 100 mL of fluid (as allowed). There may, however, be situations that contraindicate the client's receiving medications by mouth.

The primary contraindications to giving oral medications include the presence of gastrointestinal (GI) alterations, the inability of a client to swallow food or fluids, and the use of gastric suction. An important precaution to take when administering any oral preparation is to protect clients from aspiration. Aspiration occurs when food, fluid, or medication intended for GI administration is inadvertently administered into the respiratory tract. The nurse protects the client from aspiration by assessing the client's ability to manage oral medications. Box 30-9 provides techniques the nurse can use to protect the client from aspirating. Properly positioning the client is also essential in preventing aspiration. The nurse positions the client in a seated position when administering oral medications, if not contraindicated by the client's condition. Appropriate personnel (e.g., speech therapist)

Table 30-9 Example Evaluation for Client Goals

Goal	Expected Outcomes	Evaluative Measure With Example
Client and family understand medication therapy.	Client and family describe information about medication, dosage, schedule, purpose, and adverse effects.	Written measurement: Have client write out medication schedule for a 24-hour period. Oral questioning: Ask client to describe purpose, dosage, and adverse effects of each prescribed medication.
	Client and family identify situations that require medical intervention.	Oral questioning: Have family describe what to do when a client has adverse effects from a medication.
	Client and family demonstrate appropriate administration technique.	Direct observation: Have client demonstrate filling of an insulin syringe and self-injection.
Client safely self-administers medications.	Client follows prescribed treatment regimen.	Anecdotal notes: Have family keep log of client's compliance with therapy for 1 week.
	Client performs administration techniques correctly.	Direct observation: For example, observe client instill eye drops.
	Client identifies available resources for obtaining necessary medication.	Oral questioning: Ask family to identify how to contact local pharmacy or community clinic for necessary medications.

Box 30-9 Protecting the Client From Aspiration

- Determine the client's ability to swallow.
- Assess the client's cough.
- Determine the presence of a gag reflex.
- Prepare oral medications in the form that is easiest to swallow.
- Allow the client to self-administer medications if possible.
- If the client has unilateral weakness, place the medication in the stronger side of the mouth.
- Administer pills one at a time, ensuring that each medication is properly swallowed before the next one is introduced.
- Thicken regular liquids or offer fruit nectars if the client cannot tolerate thin liquids.
- Avoid straws because they decrease the control the client has over volume intake, which increases the risk of aspiration.
- Have client hold and drink from cup if possible.
- Time medications to coincide with mealtimes or when the client is well rested and awake if possible.
- Administer medications using another route if risk of aspiration is severe.

Adapted from "Dysphagia: Going Down and Staying Down," by T. J. Galvan, 2001, *American Journal of Nursing, 101*(1), p. 37.

should evaluate clients who have difficulty swallowing before oral medications are given.

For clients with nasogastric feeding tubes, liquid medications are preferred, but some tablets can be crushed and capsules opened to mix in a solution for administration (Box 30-10).

Topical Medication Applications

Topical medications are those that are applied locally, most often to intact skin. They can be in the form of lotions, pastes, or ointments (see Table 30-1). They can also be applied to mucous membranes.

Skin Applications. Because many locally applied medications such as lotions, pastes, and ointments can create systemic and local effects, the nurse should apply these medications using gloves and applicators. Sterile technique is used if the client has an open wound.

Skin encrustation and dead tissues harbour microorganisms and block contact of medications with the tissues to be treated. Simply applying new medications over previously applied medications does little to prevent infection or offer therapeutic benefit. Before applying medications, the nurse cleans the skin thoroughly by washing the area gently with soap and water, soaking an involved site, or locally debriding tissue (see chapter 43).

When applying ointments or pastes, the nurse spreads the medication evenly over the involved surface and covers the area well without applying an overly thick layer. Opaque ointments prevent visualization of underlying skin. Prescribers may order a gauze dressing to be applied over the medication to prevent soiling of clothes and wiping away of the medication. Each type of medication, whether an ointment, lotion, powder, or other type, should be applied in a specific way to ensure proper penetration and absorption. The nurse applies lotions and creams by smearing them lightly onto the skin's surface; rubbing may cause irritation. A liniment is applied by rubbing it gently but firmly into the skin. A powder is dusted lightly to cover the affected area with a thin layer. During any application, the nurse should assess the skin thoroughly. To record administration, the nurse should note the area applied, name of medication, and condition of skin.

Nasal Instillation. Clients with nasal sinus alterations may receive medications by spray, drops, or tampons (Skill 30-2). The most commonly administered form of nasal instillation is decongestant spray or drops, used to relieve symptoms of sinus congestion and colds. Clients must be cautioned to avoid abuse of medications because overuse can lead to a rebound effect in which the nasal congestion worsens. When excess decongestant solution is swallowed, serious systemic effects may also develop, especially in children. Saline drops are safer as a decongestant for children than nasal preparations that contain sympathomimetics (e.g., Afrin or Neo-Synephrine).

It is easier to have the client self-administer sprays because the client can control the spray and inhale as it enters the nasal passages. For clients who use nasal sprays repeatedly, the nurse checks the nares for irritation. The nurse learns the proper way of positioning clients to permit the medication to reach the affected sinus.

Severe nosebleeds are usually treated with packing or nasal tampons treated with epinephrine to reduce blood flow. Usually a physician or advanced practice clinician places nasal tampons.

Eye Instillation. Common medications used by clients are eye drops and ointments, including over-the-counter preparations such as artificial tears and vasoconstrictors (e.g., Visine and Murine). However, many clients receive prescribed **ophthalmic** medications for eye conditions, such as glaucoma, and after cataract extraction. A large percentage of clients receiving eye medications are older adults. Age-related problems, including poor vision, hand tremors, and difficulty grasping or manipulating containers, affect the ease with which the older adult can self-administer eye medications. The nurse instructs clients and family members about the proper techniques for administering eye medications (Skill 30-3). The nurse may determine the client and family's ability to self-administer through a return demonstration of the procedure. Showing clients each step of the procedure for instilling eye drops can improve their compliance. The following principles can be followed when administering eye medications:

- The cornea of the eye is richly supplied with pain fibres and thus very sensitive to anything applied to it. Avoid instilling any form of eye medication directly onto the cornea.
- The risk of transmitting infection from one eye to the other is high. Avoid touching the eyelids or other eye structures with eyedroppers or ointment tubes.
- Use eye medication only for the client's affected eye. Never allow a client to use another client's eye medications.

Text continued on p. 872

Skill 30-1 Administering Oral Medications

View Video

Delegation Considerations

Administering oral medications should not be delegated to unregulated care providers (UCPs). The nurse must instruct the UCP about potential side effects of medications and to report their occurrence to the nurse.

Equipment

- Medication cart or tray
- Disposable medication cups
- Glass of water, juice, or preferred liquid
- Drinking straw
- Pill-crushing device (optional)
- Paper towels
- MAR

Steps	Rationale
1. Assess for any contraindications to client receiving oral medication: Is client suffering from nausea/vomiting? Is client diagnosed as having bowel inflammation or reduced peristalsis? Has client had recent gastrointestinal (GI) surgery? Does client have gastric suction? Check the client's swallow, cough, and gag reflexes.	Alterations in GI function interfere with medication distribution, absorption, and excretion. Clients with GI suction might not receive benefit from the medication because it may be suctioned from the GI tract before it can be absorbed.
2. Assess client's medical history, history of allergies, medication history, and diet history. Client's food and drug allergies should be listed on *each* page of the MAR and should be prominently displayed on the client's medical record. This information may also be on an identification bracelet.	These factors can influence how certain medications act. Information also reflects client's need for medications.
3. Gather physical examination and laboratory data that may influence medication administration.	Physical examination or laboratory data may contraindicate medication administration.

Critical Decision Point: If there are any contraindications to the client receiving oral medications, or if in doubt of the client's ability to swallow oral medications, temporarily withhold medication and inform prescriber.

Steps	Rationale
4. Assess client's knowledge regarding health and medication use.	Determines client's need for medication education. Also assists in identifying client's adherence to medication therapy at home. Assessment may reveal medication use problems such as medication tolerance. This occurs when a client desires more and more medication to achieve the desired effect. Other medication use problems are noncompliance, abuse, addiction, or dependence.
5. Assess client's preferences for fluids.	Offering fluids during medication administration increases client's fluid intake. Fluids ease swallowing and facilitate absorption from the GI tract. Fluid restrictions must be maintained when applicable.
6. Check accuracy and completeness of each MAR with prescriber's written medication order. Check client's name, medication name and dose, route of administration, time for administration, and indication for medication.	The order sheet is the most reliable source and only legal record of medications client is to receive.
7. Prepare medications:	
a. Perform hand hygiene.	Reduces transfer of micro-organisms.
b. If medication cart is used, move it outside client's room.	Organization of equipment saves time and reduces error.
c. Unlock medicine drawer or cart.	Medications are safeguarded when locked in cabinet or cart. Prevents preparation error.
d. Prepare medication for one client at a time. Keep all pages of MAR for one client together.	Reading label and comparing it with transcribed order reduces error.

Skill 30-1 Administering Oral Medications—cont'd

Steps	Rationale
e. Select correct medication from stock supply or unit-dose drawer. Compare label of medication with MAR (see illustration). Check expiration date on all medication labels.	
f. Calculate medication dose as necessary. Double-check calculation.	Double-checking reduces risk of error.
g. To prepare tablets or capsules from a floor stock bottle, pour required number into bottle cap and transfer medication to medication cap. Do not touch medication with fingers. Extra tablets or capsules may be returned to bottle.	Maintains clean technique required of medication administration. Tablets that are prescored can be split to ensure accurate dose is given to client.

Critical Decision Point: Medications that need to be broken to administer half the dose can be broken, using a gloved hand, or cut with a pill-splitting device. Tablets that are to be broken in half must be prescored. Prescored tablets are identified by a manufactured line that transverses the centre of the tablet.

Steps	Rationale
h. To prepare unit-dose tablets or capsules, place packaged tablet or capsule directly into medicine cup. (Do not remove wrapper; see illustration.)	Wrapper maintains cleanliness of medications and identifies medication name and dose.

Critical Decision Point: If preparing narcotics, check narcotic record for previous drug count and compare with supply available and uphold controlled substance laws.

Steps	Rationale
i. All tablets or capsules to be given to client at same time may be placed in one medicine cup except for those requiring preadministration assessments (e.g., pulse rate or blood pressure).	Keeping medications that require preadministration assessments separate from others makes it easier for the nurse to withhold medications as necessary.

Critical Decision Point: Not all medications can be crushed (e.g., capsules, enteric-coated drugs). Consult with pharmacist when in doubt. Choking or aspiration of particles of medication or soft food can also occur.

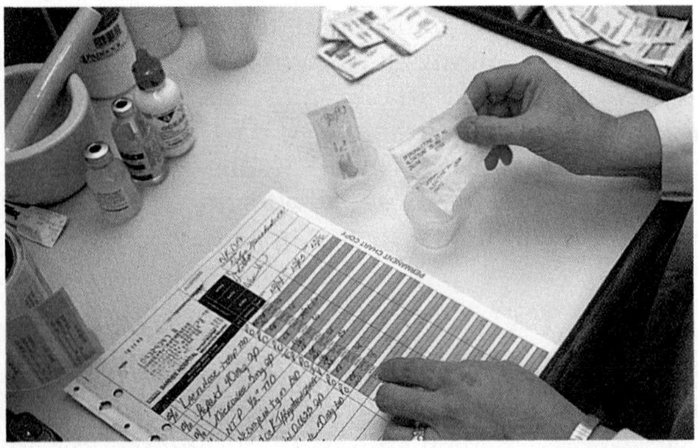

STEP **7e** The nurse verifies each medication with the MAR.

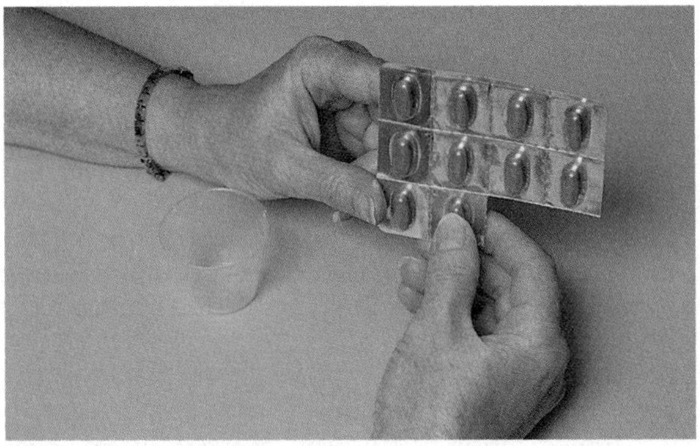

STEP **7h** Place tablet into medicine cup without removing wrapper.

Steps	Rationale

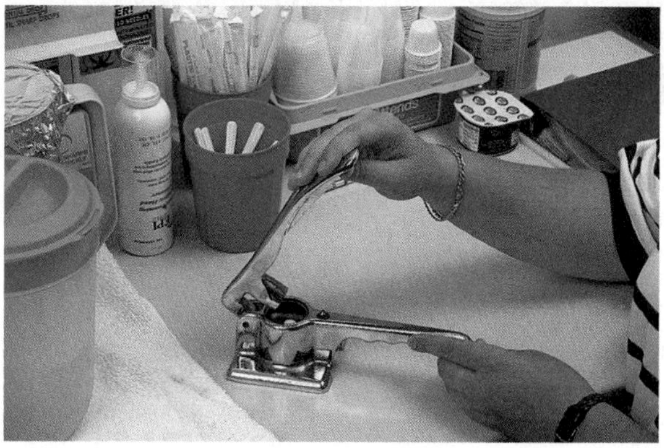

STEP **7j** Pill-crushing device used to crush pills when necessary.

A B

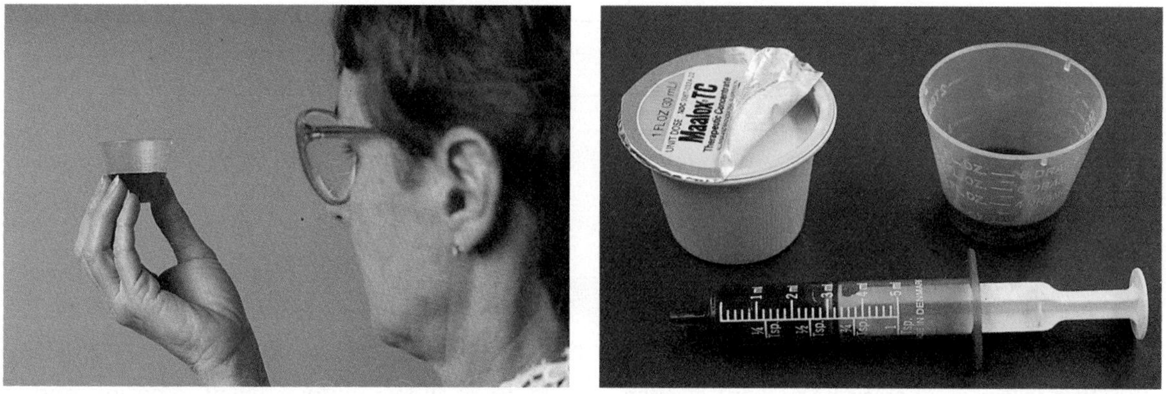

STEP **7k(3)** **A,** Pour the desired volume of liquid so that base of meniscus is level with line on scale. **B,** Use needleless syringe to draw up volumes less than 10 mL.

Steps	Rationale
j. If the client has difficulty swallowing, and liquid medications are not an option, use pill-crushing device such as a mortar and pestle to grind pills (see illustration). If a pill-crushing device is not available, place tablet between two medication cups and grind with a blunt instrument. Mix ground tablet in small amount of soft food (custard or applesauce).	Large tablets can be difficult to swallow. Ground tablet mixed with palatable soft food is usually easier to swallow.
k. To prepare liquids:	
(1) Gently shake container. If medication is in a unit-dose container with correct amount to administer, no further preparation is needed. If medication is in a multidose bottle, remove bottle cap from container and place cap upside down.	Shaking container ensures medication is mixed before administration. Placing cap of bottle upside down prevents contamination of inside of cap.
(2) Hold multidose bottle with label against palm of hand while pouring.	Spilled liquid will not soil or fade label.
(3) Hold medication cup at eye level and fill to desired level on scale (see illustration). Scale should be even with fluid level at its surface or base of meniscus, not edges. Draw up volumes of less than 10 mL in syringe without needle (see illustration).	Ensures accuracy of measurement.
(4) Discard any excess liquid into sink. Wipe lip and neck of bottle with paper towel.	Prevents contamination of bottle's contents and prevents bottle cap from sticking.

Skill 30-1 *Administering Oral Medications—cont'd*

Steps	Rationale
l. Compare MAR with prepared medication and container.	Reading label second time reduces error.
m. Return stock containers or unused unit-dose medications to shelf or drawer and read label again.	Third check of label reduces administration errors.
n. Do not leave medications unattended.	Nurse is responsible for safekeeping of drugs.
8. Administering medications:	
a. Take medications to client at correct time.	Medications are administered within 30 minutes before or after prescribed time to ensure intended therapeutic effect. STAT or single-order medications should be given at time ordered.
b. Identify client by comparing name on MAR with name on client's identification bracelet. Ask client to state name.	Identification bracelets are made at time of client's admission and are most reliable source of identification.

Critical Decision Point: Client identification bracelets that are missing, illegible, or faded must be replaced.

Steps	Rationale
c. Explain purpose of each medication and its action to client. Allow client to ask any questions about drugs.	Client has right to be informed, and client's understanding of purpose of each medication improves compliance with medication therapy.
d. Assist client to sitting position (or side-lying position if sitting is contraindicated).	Sitting position prevents aspiration during swallowing (Galvan, 2001).
e. Administer medications:	
(1) **For tablets:** Client may wish to hold solid medications in hand or cup before placing in mouth.	Client can become familiar with medications by seeing each drug.
(2) Offer water or juice to help client swallow medications. Give cold carbonated water if available and not contraindicated.	Choice of fluid promotes client's comfort and can improve fluid intake. Carbonated water helps passage of tablet through esophagus.
(3) **For sublingual-administered medications:** Have client place medication under tongue and allow it to dissolve completely (see Figure 30–4). Caution client against swallowing tablet.	Medication is absorbed through blood vessels of undersurface of tongue. If swallowed, medication is destroyed by gastric juices or so rapidly detoxified by liver that therapeutic blood levels are not attained.
(4) **For buccal medications:** Have client place medication in mouth against mucous membranes of the cheek until it dissolves (see Figure 30–5). Avoid administering liquids until buccal medication has dissolved.	Buccal medications act locally on mucosa or systemically as they are swallowed in saliva.
(5) **For powdered medications:** Mix with liquids at bedside and give to client to drink.	When prepared in advance, powdered medications may thicken and even harden, making swallowing difficult.
(6) Caution client against chewing or swallowing lozenges.	Medication acts through slow absorption through oral mucosa, not gastric mucosa.
(7) Give effervescent powders and tablets immediately after dissolving.	Effervescence improves unpleasant taste of medication and often relieves GI problems.
f. If client is unable to hold medications, place medication cup to the lips and gently introduce each drug into the mouth, one at a time. Do not rush.	Administering single tablet or capsule eases swallowing and decreases risk of aspiration.
g. If tablet or capsule falls to the floor, discard it and repeat preparation.	Medication is contaminated when it touches floor.
h. Stay until client has completely swallowed each medication. Ask client to open mouth if uncertain whether medication has been swallowed.	Nurse is responsible for ensuring that client receives ordered dosage. If left unattended, client may not take dose or may save medications, causing risk to health.
i. For highly acidic medications (e.g., aspirin), offer client non-fat snack (e.g., crackers) if not contraindicated by client's condition.	Reduces gastric irritation.

Steps	Rationale
j. Assist client in returning to comfortable position.	Maintains client's comfort.
k. Dispose of soiled supplies and perform hand hygiene.	Reduces transmission of micro-organisms.
9. Evaluate client's response to medications at times that correlate with the medication's onset, peak, and duration.	Evaluates medication's therapeutic benefit and can detect onset of side effects or allergic reactions.
10. Ask client or family member to identify medication name and explain purpose, action, dosage schedule, and potential side effects of drug.	Determines level of knowledge gained by client and family.

Unexpected Outcomes and Related Interventions

- Client exhibits adverse effects (side effect, toxic effect, allergic reaction).
  - Symptoms such as urticaria, rash, pruritus, rhinitis, and wheezing may indicate allergic reaction.
  - Always notify prescriber and pharmacy when the client exhibits adverse effects. Withhold further doses.
- Client refuses medication.
  - Explore reasons why client does not want medication.
  - Educate if misunderstandings of medication therapy are apparent.
  - Do not force client to take medication; clients have the right to refuse treatment.
  - If client continues to refuse medication despite educational attempts, record why the drug was withheld on client's chart and notify prescriber.

Recording and Reporting

- Record administration of oral medications on MAR, using nurse's initials or signature.
- Record the reason any drug is withheld and follow agency's policy for proper recording.

Home Care Considerations

- Instruct clients on all aspects of medication administration, including dosage, desired effect, when to take medications, anticipated side effects, and whether to take medication with or without food to ensure safe medication administration at home.

Box 30-10 Procedural Guidelines

Giving Medications Through a Nasogastric Tube, Intestinal Tube, Gastrostomy Tube, or Small-Bore Feeding Tube

- Investigate and use alternative routes of medication administration if possible (e.g., transdermal, rectal).
- Avoid complicated medication regimens that frequently interrupt enteral feedings.
- Avoid giving elixirs or medications with a pH of less than 4.
- Verify that the medication is compatible with the enteral feeding before administration. If the medication is incompatible with the feeding, stop the feeding 1 to 2 hours before medication is given, and restart the feeding 1 to 2 hours after the medication is given. Never add medications directly to the tube feeding.
- Verify tube placement before administering medications (see chapters 39 and 40).
- Administer medications in a liquid form (suspension, elixir, or solution) whenever possible to prevent tube obstruction.
- Before crushing tablets, be sure they can be crushed. Buccal, sublingual, enteric-coated, or sustained released medications cannot be crushed. Read medication labels carefully before crushing a tablet or opening a capsule.
- Dissolve crushed tablets, gelatin capsules, and powders in 15 to 30 mL of warm water. Dissolve and administer each medication separately, flushing between 1 and 30 mL of water between each medication. Irrigate the tube after all medication is given. Unless contraindicated, the total amount of liquid volume administered to the client for each medication may range from 60 to 150 mL of water.
- Do not use pigtail vent for irrigation or instillation of fluid.
- Do not give whole or undissolved medications through the feeding tube.
- Continually evaluate the client's response to medication therapy. If the desired effect is not achieved, a different medication or route of administration may be indicated because of problems with the drug bioavailability when given by the enteral route.

Adapted from "Drug Administration via a Nasogastric Tube," by E. Bryson, 2002, *Nursing Times, 97*(16), p. 51; and "A Guide to Enteral Drug Administration in Palliative Care," by P. J. Gilbar, 1999, *Journal of Pain and Symptom Management, 17*(3), p. 197.

Skill 30-2 Administering Nasal Instillations

Delegation Considerations

Administration of nasal drops and ointments should not be delegated to unregulated care providers (UCPs). The nurse must instruct the UCP about potential side effects of medications and to report their occurrence to the nurse.

Equipment

- Prepared medication with clean dropper or spray container
- Facial tissue
- Small pillow (optional)
- Washcloth (optional)
- Disposable gloves (optional, only if client has extensive nasal drainage)
- MAR
- Penlight (to inspect nares; if ointment is to be applied to a specific lesion inside the nares)

Steps	Rationale
1. For nasal drops, determine which sinus is affected by referring to medical record.	Affects client's position during drug instillation.
2. Assess client's history of hypertension, heart disease, diabetes mellitus, and hyperthyroidism.	These conditions can contraindicate use of decongestants that stimulate central nervous system. Side effects of transient hypertension, tachycardia, palpitations, and headache may occur.
3. Review physician's order, including client's name, medication name, dosage, route, time of administration and indication.	
4. Determine whether client has any known allergies to nasal instillations.	
5. Identify client; compare name on MAR with client's identification bracelet. Ask client to state name.	Ensures that correct client receives medication.
6. Perform hand hygiene. Using a penlight, inspect condition of nose and sinuses. Palpate sinuses for tenderness.	Prevents infection. Provides baseline to monitor effects of medication. Presence of discharge interferes with medication absorption.
7. Assess client's knowledge regarding use of nasal instillations and technique for instillation and willingness to learn self-administration.	May necessitate health teaching regarding use of medications. Motivation influences teaching approach.
8. Explain procedure to client regarding positioning and sensations to expect, such as burning or stinging of mucosa or choking sensation as medication trickles into throat.	Helps client anticipate experience of procedure to reduce anxiety.
9. Arrange supplies and medications at bedside. Apply gloves if client has nasal drainage.	Reduces transmission of micro-organisms, ensures smooth, orderly procedure, and prevents exposure to body fluids (Health Canada, 1999).
10. Instruct client to clear or blow nose gently unless contraindicated (e.g., risk of increased intracranial pressure or nosebleeds).	Removes mucus and secretions that can block distribution of medication.
11. Administer nasal drops:	
a. Assist client to supine position.	Position provides access to nasal passages.
b. Position head properly:	
(1) For access to posterior pharynx, tilt client's head backward.	

Steps	Rationale

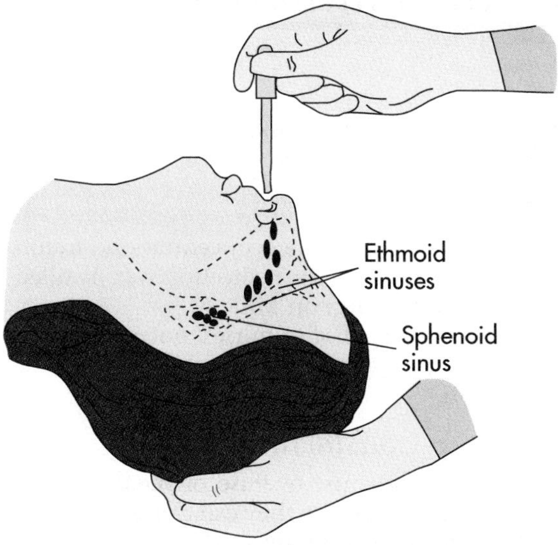

STEP **11b(2)** Position for instilling nose drops into ethmoid or sphenoid sinus.

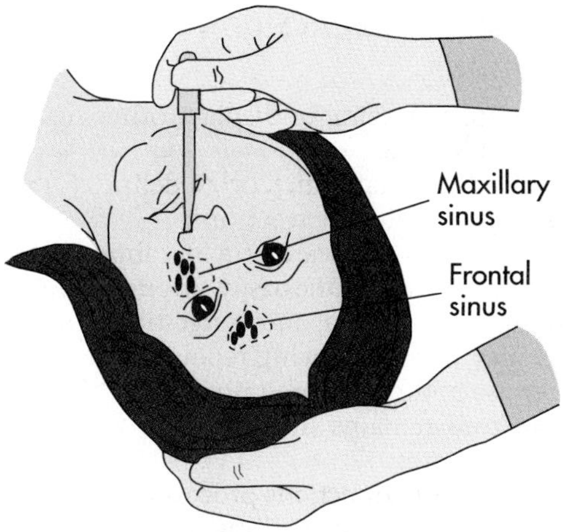

STEP **11b(3)** Position for instilling nose drops into frontal and maxillary sinus.

Steps	Rationale
(2) For access to ethmoid or sphenoid sinus, tilt head back over edge of bed or place small pillow under client's shoulder and tilt head back (see illustration).	
(3) For access to frontal and maxillary sinus, tilt head back over edge of bed or pillow with head turned toward side to be treated (see illustration).	Position allows medication to drain into affected sinus.
c. Support client's head with non-dominant hand.	Prevents straining of neck muscles.
d. Instruct client to breathe through mouth.	Mouth breathing reduces chance of aspirating nasal drops into trachea and lungs.
e. Hold dropper 1 cm above nares and instill prescribed number of drops toward midline of ethmoid bone.	Avoids contamination of dropper. Instilling toward ethmoid bone facilitates distribution of medication over nasal mucosa.
f. Have client remain in supine position 5 minutes.	Prevents premature loss of medication through nares.
g. Offer facial tissue to blot runny nose, but caution client against blowing nose for several minutes.	Allows maximal amount of medication to be absorbed.
12. Assist client to a comfortable position after medication is absorbed.	Restores comfort.
13. Dispose of soiled supplies in proper container and perform hand hygiene.	Maintains neat, orderly environment. Reduces spread of micro-organisms.
14. Observe client for onset of side effects 15 to 30 minutes after administration.	Drugs absorbed through mucosa can cause systemic reaction.
15. Ask if client is able to breathe through nose after decongestant administration. May be necessary to have client occlude one nostril at a time and breathe deeply.	Determines effectiveness of decongestant medication.
16. Reinspect condition of nasal passages between the instillations.	Condition of mucosa reveals response to medication.
17. Ask client to review risks of overuse of decongestants and methods for administration.	Feedback ensures that client can self-administer medications properly.
18. Have client demonstrate self-medication.	Feedback demonstrates learning.

Skill 30-2 Administering Nasal Instillations—cont'd

Unexpected Outcomes and Related Interventions

- Client begins wheezing or displays other signs of allergic reaction to drug.
  - Follow institutional policy or guidelines for appropriate response to allergic reactions.
  - Notify client's health care provider immediately.
- Client is unable to breathe easily through nasal passages. Mucosa appears swollen, and congestion is unrelieved.
  - Client may be experiencing rebound effect. Stop medication use and notify prescriber.
- Nasal mucosa remains inflamed and tender with discharge from nares.
  - Inflammatory or infectious process remains. May need to consider alternative therapy.
- Client complains of sinus headache. Sinuses remain congested.
  - May need to consider alternative therapy.
- Client is unable to explain technique and risks of drug therapy.
  - Further explanation is required.
- Client is unable to self-administer medication.
  - Reinstruction is necessary.

Recording and Reporting

- Record medication name, concentration, number of drops, nostril into which medication was instilled, and time of administration on MAR.
- Record client's response in nurses' notes.
- Report any unusual systemic effects to nurse in charge or physician.

Home Care Considerations

- Caution clients against overuse of nasal spray decongestants at home because they can cause rebound effect, worsening mucosal swelling.
- Nasal applicators should be rinsed after each use.
- Clients should discard over-the-counter nasal sprays or nose drops after one illness because the bottles can become easily contaminated with bacteria after use.
- Each family member should have a different dropper or spray applicator.

Skill 30-3 Administering Ophthalmic Medications

View Video

Delegation Considerations

Administration of eye drops and ointments should not be delegated to unregulated care providers (UCPs). The nurse should instruct the UCP about potential side effects of medications and to report their occurrence to the nurse.

Equipment

- Medication bottle with sterile eyedropper or ointment tube or medicated intraocular disk
- Cotton ball or tissue
- Washbasin filled with warm water and washcloth if eyes have crust or drainage
- Eye patch and tape (optional)
- Clean gloves
- MAR

Steps	Rationale
1. Review prescriber's medication order for number of drops (if a liquid) and eye (right = O.D.; left = O.S.; both = O.U.) to receive medication.	Ensures correct administration of medication.
2. Identify client. Compare name on MAR with client identification bracelet. Ask client to state name.	Ensures that correct client receives medication.
3. Assess condition of external eye structures. (May also be done just before drug instillation.)	Provides baseline to later determine if local response to medications occurs. Also indicates need to clean eye before medication application.
4. Determine whether client has any known allergies to eye medications. Also ask if client has allergy to latex.	Protects client from risk of allergic medication response. If client has latex allergy, use non-latex gloves.
5. Determine whether client has any symptoms of visual alterations.	Certain eye medications act to either lessen or increase these symptoms. Nurse must be able to recognize change in client's condition after drop is administered.

Steps	Rationale
6. Assess client's level of consciousness and ability to follow directions.	If client becomes restless or combative during procedure, a greater risk of accidental eye injury exists.
7. Assess client's knowledge regarding medication therapy and desire to self-administer medication.	Client's level of understanding may indicate need for health teaching. Motivation influences teaching approach.
8. Assess client's ability to manipulate and hold dropper.	Reflects client's ability to learn to self-administer medication.
9. Explain procedure to client.	Relieves anxiety about medication being instilled into eye.
10. Perform hand hygiene and arrange supplies at bedside; apply disposable gloves.	Reduces transmission of micro-organisms, ensures a smooth, orderly procedure, and follows Health Canada (1999) recommendations to prevent accidental exposure to body fluids.
11. Ask client to lie supine or sit back in chair with head slightly hyperextended.	Position provides easy access to eye for medication instillation and minimizes drainage of medication through tear duct.

Critical Decision Point: Do not hyperextend the neck of a client with cervical spine injury.

Steps	Rationale
12. If crusts or drainage are present along eyelid margins or inner canthus, gently wash away. Soak any crusts that are dried and difficult to remove by applying damp washcloth or cotton ball over eye for a few minutes. Always wipe clean from inner to outer canthus.	Crusts or drainage harbours micro-organisms. Soaking allows easy removal and prevents pressure from being applied directly over eye. Cleansing from inner to outer canthus avoids entrance of micro-organism into lacrimal duct.
13. Hold cotton ball or clean tissue in non-dominant hand on client's cheekbone just below lower eyelid.	Cotton or tissue absorbs medication that escapes eye.
14. With tissue or cotton resting below lower lid, gently press downward with thumb or forefinger against bony orbit.	Technique exposes lower conjunctival sac. Retraction against bony orbit prevents pressure and trauma to eyeball and prevents fingers from touching eye.
15. Ask client to look at ceiling and explain steps to client.	Action retracts sensitive cornea up and away from conjunctival sac and reduces stimulation of blink reflex.
A. **Instill eye drops:**	
(1) With dominant hand resting on client's forehead, hold filled medication eyedropper or ophthalmic solution approximately 1 to 2 cm above conjunctival sac (see illustration).	Helps prevent accidental contact of eyedropper with eye structures, thus reducing risk of injury to eye and transfer of infection to dropper (McConnell, 2001). Ophthalmic medications are sterile.
(2) Drop prescribed number of medication drops into conjunctival sac.	Conjunctival sac normally holds 1 or 2 drops. Provides even distribution of medication across eye.
(3) If client blinks or closes eye or if drops land on outer lid margins, repeat procedure.	Therapeutic effect of drug is obtained only when drops enter conjunctival sac.
(4) After instilling drops, ask client to close eye gently.	Helps to distribute medication. Squinting or squeezing of eyelids forces medication from conjunctival sac.
(5) When administering medications that cause systemic effects, apply gentle pressure with your finger and clean tissue on the client's nasolacrimal duct for 30 to 60 seconds.	Prevents overflow of medication into nasal and pharyngeal passages. Prevents absorption into systemic circulation (McConnell, 2001).

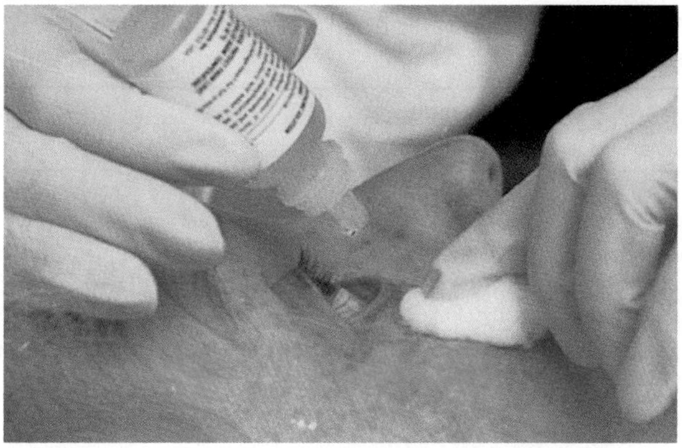

STEP **15A(1)** Hold eyedropper above conjunctival sac.

Skill 30-3 Administering Ophthalmic Medications—cont'd

Steps	Rationale

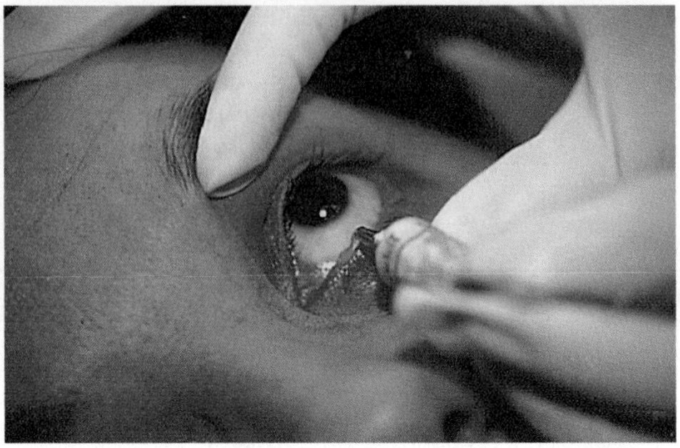

STEP **15B(1)** Apply ointment along lower eyelid.

Steps	Rationale
B. Instill eye ointment:	
(1) Holding ointment applicator above lower lid margin, apply thin stream of ointment evenly along inner edge of lower eyelid on conjunctiva (see illustration) from the inner canthus to outer canthus.	Distributes medication evenly across eye and lid margin.
(2) Have client close eye and rub lid lightly in circular motion with cotton ball, if rubbing is not contraindicated.	Further distributes medication without traumatizing eye.
C. Intraocular disk	
(1) Application:	
a. Open package containing the disk. Gently press fingertip against the disk so that it adheres to finger. Position the convex side of the disk on fingertip (see illustration).	Allows nurse to inspect disk for damage or deformity.
b. With other hand, gently pull the client's lower eyelid away from the eye. Ask client to look up.	Prepares conjunctival sac for receiving medicated disk.
c. Place the disk in the conjunctival sac, so that it floats on the sclera between the iris and lower eyelid (see illustration).	Ensures delivery of medication.
d. Pull the client's lower eyelid out and over the disk (see illustration).	Ensures accurate medication delivery.

Critical Decision Point: You should not be able to see the disk at this time. Repeat step 15C(1)d if you can see the disk.

Steps	Rationale
(2) Removal:	
a. Perform hand hygiene and apply gloves.	Prevents transfer of micro-organisms and follows Health Canada (1999) recommendations for prevention of accidental exposure to body fluids.
b. Explain procedure to client.	Relieves anxiety about manipulation of disk in eye.
c. Gently pull on the client's lower eyelid.	Exposes intraocular disk.
d. Using forefinger and thumb of opposite hand, pinch the disk and lift it out of the client's eye (see illustration).	

Steps	Rationale

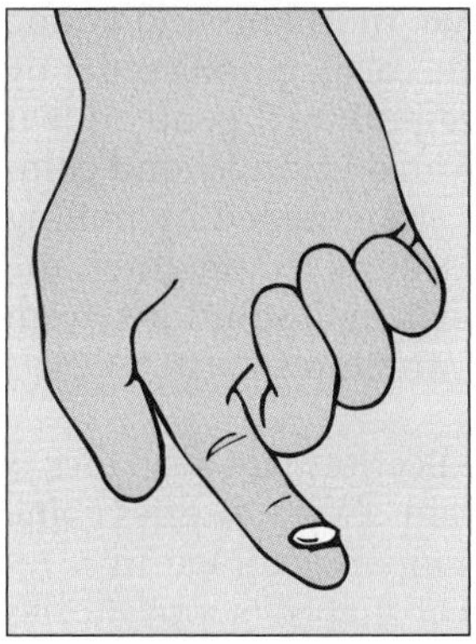

STEP **15C(1)a** Gently position the convex side of the disk against fingertips.

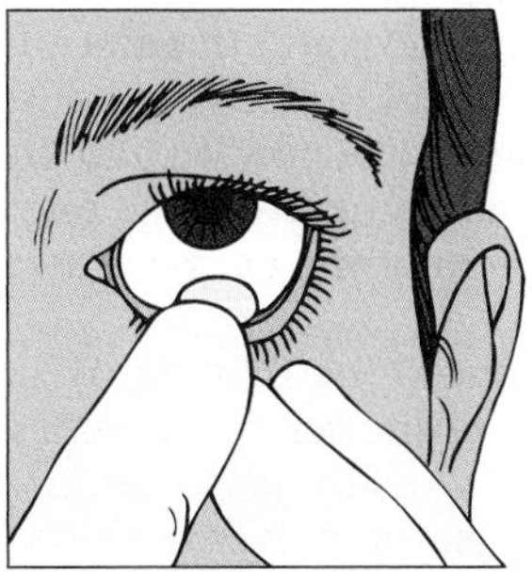

STEP **15C(1)c** Place disk in the conjunctival sac between the iris and lower eyelid.

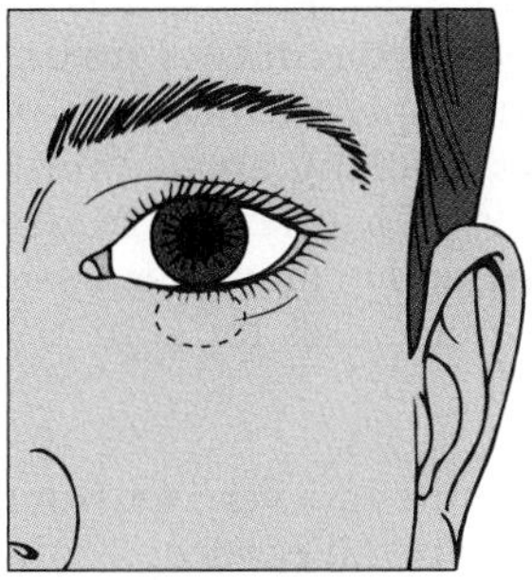

STEP **15C(1)d** Gently pull lower eyelid over the disk.

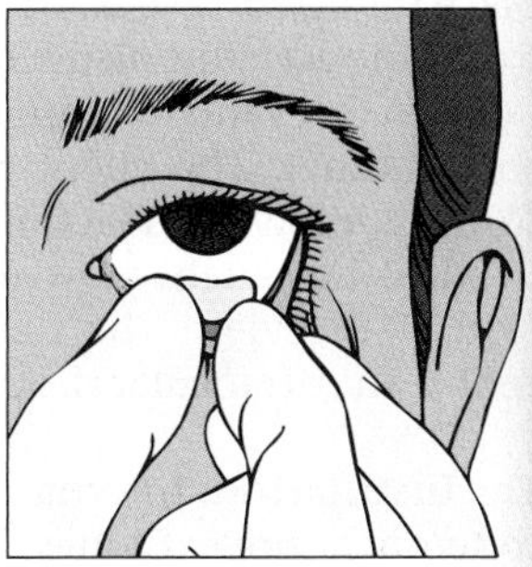

STEP **15C(2)d** Carefully pinch the disk to remove it from client's eye

Steps	Rationale
16. If excess medication is on eyelid, gently wipe it from inner to outer canthus.	Promotes comfort and prevents trauma to eye.
17. If client had eye patch, apply clean one by placing it over affected eye so that entire eye is covered. Tape securely without applying pressure to eye.	Clean eye patch reduces chance of infection.

Critical Decision Point: If client receives more than one eye medication to the same eye at the same time, wait at least 5 minutes before administering the next medication to avoid interaction between medications ("Using Eye Drops," 2000).

Steps	Rationale
18. Remove gloves, dispose of soiled supplies in proper receptacle, and perform hand hygiene.	Maintains neat environment at bedside and reduces transmission of micro-organisms.
19. Note client's response to instillation; ask if any discomfort was felt.	Determines if procedure was performed correctly and safely.
20. Observe response to medication by assessing visual changes and noting any side effects.	Evaluates effects of medication.
21. Ask client to discuss medication's purpose, action, side effects, and technique of administration.	Determines client's level of understanding.
22. Have client demonstrate self-administration of next dose.	Provides feedback regarding competency with skill.

Unexpected Outcomes and Related Interventions

- Client cannot instill drops without supervision.
  - Reinforce teaching and allow client to self-administer drops as much as possible to enhance confidence.
  - If client cannot self-administer drops, teach others, such as family members, to instill drops into the client's eye.
- Client displays signs of allergic reaction (e.g., tearing, reddened sclera) or systemic response (e.g., bradycardia) to medication.
  - Hold medication and speak with prescriber.
  - Follow institutional policy or guidelines for reporting of adverse or allergic reaction to medications.

Recording and Reporting

- Record on MAR: medication, concentration, number of drops, time of administration, and eye (left, right, or both) that received medication.
- Record appearance of eye in nurses' notes.

Home Care Considerations

- Clients with chronic health care problems should consult with their health care provider before using over-the-counter eye medication.
- When using eye drops at home, clients should not share medications with other family members because risk of infection transmission is high.

Intraocular Administration. Some medications are administered intraocularly. Medications delivered this way resemble a contact lens. The nurse places the medication into the conjunctival sac, where it remains in place for up to 1 week. Currently, medications such as pilocarpine are administered this way. Experiments are underway to evaluate administering other medications in this manner. The client requires teaching about monitoring for adverse reactions to the disk. Clients will also need to be taught how to insert and remove the disk. Skill 30-3 reviews the steps the nurse uses for administering an intraocular disk.

Ear Instillation. Internal ear structures are very sensitive to temperature extremes. Failure to instill ear drops or irrigating fluid at room temperature may cause vertigo (severe dizziness) or nausea. Although the structures of the outer ear are not sterile, sterile drops and solutions are used in case the eardrum is ruptured. The entrance of non-sterile solutions into middle ear structures could result in infection. With ear drainage, the nurse should assess to be sure the client does not have a ruptured eardrum. A nurse should never occlude the ear canal with the dropper or irrigating syringe. Forcing medication into an occluded ear canal creates pressure that may injure the eardrum. Box 30-11 reviews guidelines for administering ear drops.

External ear structures of children differ from those of adults. When instilling drops or irrigating solutions, the nurse must straighten the ear canal. In infants and young children, the nurse straightens the cartilaginous canal by grasping the auricle of the ear and pulling it gently down and backward. In adults, the ear canal is longer and composed of underlying bone and is straightened by pulling the auricle upward and outward. Failure to straighten the canal properly may prevent medicinal solutions from reaching the deeper external ear structures.

Vaginal Instillation. Vaginal medications are available as suppositories, foam, jellies, or creams. Suppositories come individually packaged in foil wrappers. Storage in a refrigerator prevents the solid, oval-shaped suppositories from melting. After a suppository is inserted into the vaginal cavity, body temperature causes it to melt and be distributed and absorbed. Foam, jellies, and creams are administered with an applicator inserter (Skill 30-4). A suppository is given with a gloved hand in accordance with standard precautions/routine practices (see chapter 29). Clients often prefer administering their own vaginal medications and should be given privacy. After instillation of the medication, a client may wish to wear a perineal pad to collect drainage. Because vaginal medications are often given to treat infection, discharge may be foul smelling. Aseptic technique should be followed, and

Box 30-11 *Procedural Guidelines*

Administering Ear Medications

Ear Drops

1. Have client assume side-lying position (if not contraindicated by client's condition) with ear to be treated facing up, or client may sit in chair or at the bedside.
2. Perform hand hygiene. Apply gloves if drainage is present.
3. Straighten ear canal by pulling auricle down and back (children) or upward and outward (adult).

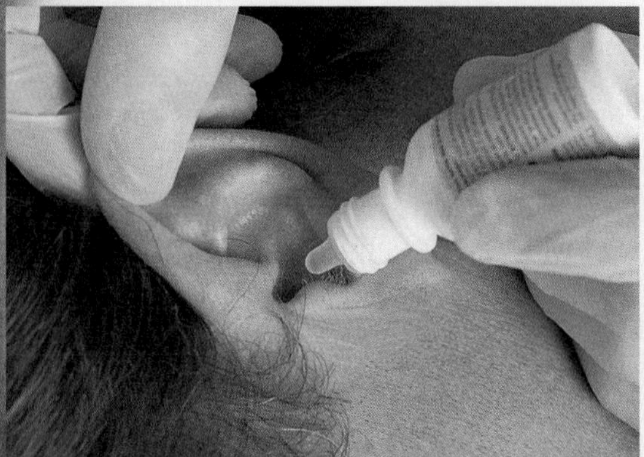

STEP **4** Placing ear drop in ear.

4. Instill prescribed drops holding dropper 1 cm above ear canal (see illustration).
5. Ask client to remain in side-lying position 2 to 3 minutes. Apply gentle massage or pressure to tragus of ear with finger, unless contraindicated due to pain.
6. Sometimes the prescriber orders insertion of portion of cotton ball into outermost part of canal. Do not press cotton into canal. Remove cotton after 15 minutes.

Ear Irrigations

1. Assess the tympanic membrane or review medical record for history of eardrum perforation, which would contraindicate ear irrigation.
2. Assist client in assuming sitting or lying position with head tilted or turned toward affected ear. Place towel under client's head and shoulder and have client hold basin under affected ear.
3. Perform hand hygiene. Apply gloves if drainage is present.
4. Fill irrigating syringe with solution (approximately 50 mL).
5. Gently grasp auricle and straighten ear canal by pulling it down and back (children) or upward and outward (adult).
6. Slowly instill irrigating solution by holding tip of syringe 1 cm above opening of ear canal. Allow fluid to drain out during instillation. Continue until canal is cleansed or all solution is used.

Skill 30-4 Administering Vaginal Medications

Delegation Considerations

Administering medications by the vaginal route should not be delegated to unregulated care providers (UCPs). The nurse should instruct the UCP about the following:

- To report any new or increased vaginal discharge or bleeding
- Potential side effects of medications and to report their occurrence to the nurse

Equipment

- Vaginal creams, foam, jelly, or suppositories, or irrigating solutions with applicator (if required)
- Disposable gloves
- Towels and/or washcloth
- Perineal pad
- Drape or sheet
- Water-soluble lubricating jelly
- MAR

Steps	Rationale
1. Review physician's order, including client's name, medication name, form (cream or suppository), route, dosage, time of administration, and drug indication.	Ensures safe and correct administration of medication.
2. Review client's history of allergies, including latex.	Protects client from risk of allergic medication response.
3. Perform hand hygiene.	Reduces transfer of micro-organisms.

Critical Decision Point: Rectal and vaginal suppositories may be stored near one another in the refrigerator. Vaginal suppositories are larger and more oval.

Steps	Rationale
4. Identify client; compare name on MAR with identification bracelet, and ask client's name.	Ensures that correct client receives medication.
5. Inspect condition of external genitalia and vaginal canal (see chapter 28). (May perform just before insertion.)	Findings provide baseline to monitor effect of medication.
6. Assess client's ability to manipulate applicator or suppository and to position self to insert medication.	Mobility restriction indicates level of assistance required from nurse.
7. Explain procedure to client. Be specific if client plans to self-administer medication.	Promotes understanding. Will enable client to self-administer medication if physically able.
8. Arrange supplies at bedside.	Ensures smooth procedure.
9. Close room curtain or door.	Provides privacy.
10. Assist client to lie in dorsal recumbent position.	Provides easy access to and good exposure of vaginal canal. Also allows suppository to dissolve without escaping through orifice.
11. Keep abdomen and lower extremities draped.	Minimizes client embarrassment.
12. Apply disposable gloves.	Prevents transmission of micro-organisms and follows Health Canada (1999) recommendations to prevent accidental exposure to body fluids.
13. Ensure vaginal orifice is well illuminated by room light or gooseneck lamp. Cleanse area with towel or washcloth if necessary.	Proper insertion requires visualization of external genitalia.
14. Insert suppository with gloved hand:	
a. Remove suppository from foil wrapper and apply liberal amount of sterile water-based lubricating jelly to smooth or rounded end. Lubricate gloved index finger of dominant hand.	Lubrication reduces friction against mucosal surfaces during insertion.
b. With non-dominant gloved hand, gently retract labial folds.	Exposes vaginal orifice.
c. Insert rounded end of suppository along posterior wall of vaginal canal entire length of finger (7.5 to 10 cm) (see illustration).	Proper placement ensures equal distribution of medication along walls of vaginal cavity.
d. Withdraw finger and wipe away remaining lubricant from around orifice and labia.	Maintains comfort.
15. Apply cream or foam:	
a. Fill cream or foam applicator following package directions.	Dose is prescribed by volume in applicator.

Skill 30-4 Administering Vaginal Medications—cont'd

Steps	Rationale

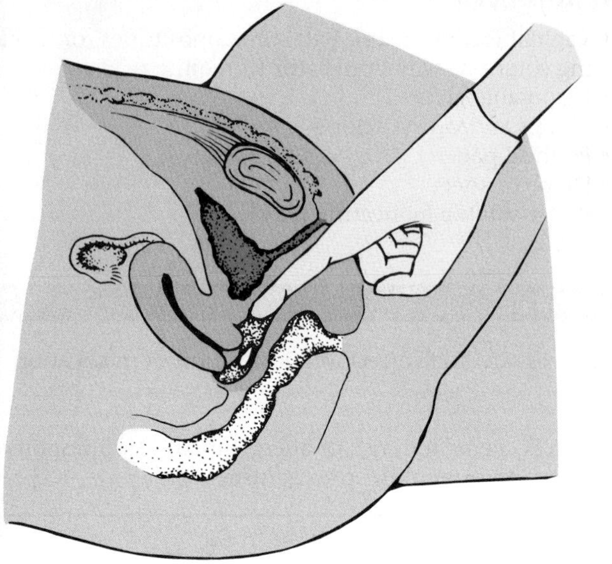

STEP **14c** Insertion of suppository into the vaginal canal.

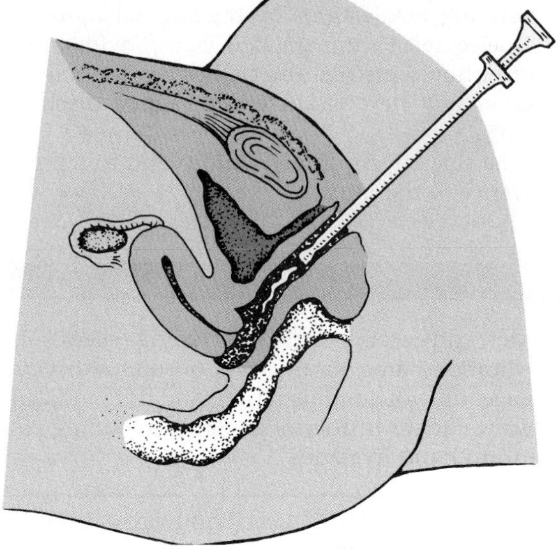

STEP **15c** Instillation of medication in vaginal canal.

Steps	Rationale
b. With non-dominant gloved hand, gently retract labial folds.	Exposes vaginal orifice.
c. With dominant gloved hand, insert applicator approximately 5 to 7.5 cm. Push applicator plunger to deposit medication into vagina (see illustration).	Allows equal distribution of medication along vaginal walls.
d. Withdraw applicator and place on paper towel. Wipe off residual cream from labia or vaginal orifice.	Residual cream on applicator may contain micro-organisms.
16. Dispose of supplies, remove gloves, and perform hand hygiene.	Maintains neat environment and reduces transfer of micro-organisms.
17. Instruct client to remain on back for at least 10 minutes.	Medication will be distributed and absorbed evenly throughout vaginal cavity and not be lost through orifice.
18. If applicator is used, wearing gloves, wash with soap and warm water, rinse, and store for future use.	Vaginal cavity is not sterile. Soap and water assist in removal of bacteria and residual cream. Gloves prevent transfer of micro-organisms.
19. Offer client perineal pad when she resumes ambulation.	Prevents vaginal discharge from spreading to clothing.
20. Inspect appearance of discharge of vaginal canal and condition of external genitalia between applications.	Evaluates whether vaginal medication effectively reduced irritation or inflammation of tissues.

Unexpected Outcomes and Related Interventions

- Client cannot self-administer medication without supervision.
  - Reinforce teaching and allow client to self-administer medication as much as possible to enhance confidence.
  - If client is unable to administer medication, teach significant other medication administration.
- Client displays signs of allergic reaction (e.g., redness, itching) to medication.
  - Hold medication and speak with prescriber.
  - Follow institutional policy or guidelines for reporting of adverse or allergic reaction to medications.

Recording and Reporting

- Record medication name, dose, route, and time of administration on MAR.
- Record character of discharge on nurses' notes.

Home Care Considerations

- Clients should perform regular perineal hygiene when receiving vaginal medications.
- Clients should be instructed to take all of the medication as prescribed, for the prescribed amount of time, to ensure effectiveness of the treatment.
- Women who have a vaginal yeast infection should abstain from sexual intercourse until treatment is completed and the infection is resolved.

the client should be offered frequent opportunities to maintain perineal hygiene (see chapter 34).

Rectal Instillation. Rectal suppositories are thinner and more bullet-shaped than vaginal suppositories. The rounded end prevents anal trauma during insertion. Rectal suppositories contain medications that exert local effects such as promoting defecation or systemic effects such as reducing nausea. Rectal suppositories are usually stored in the refrigerator until administered.

During administration, the nurse must place the suppository past the internal anal sphincter and against the rectal mucosa (Skill 30-5). Otherwise, the suppository may be expelled before it can dissolve and be absorbed into the mucosa. With practice, a nurse learns to recognize the sensation of the sphincter relaxing around the finger. The suppository should not be forced into a mass of fecal material. It may be necessary to clear the rectum with a small cleansing enema before inserting a suppository.

Administering Medications by Inhalation

Medications administered with hand-held inhalers are dispersed through an aerosol spray, mist, or powder that penetrates lung airways. The alveolocapillary network absorbs medications rapidly. **Metered-dose inhalers (MDIs)** and dry powder inhalers (DPIs) are usually designed to produce local effects such as bronchodilatation. However, some medications can create serious systemic side effects.

Clients who receive medications by inhalation frequently suffer chronic respiratory disease such as chronic asthma, emphysema, or bronchitis. Medications given by inhalation provide these clients with control of airway obstruction. Because these clients depend on medications for disease control, they must learn about them and ways to administer them safely (Skill 30-6).

An MDI delivers a measured dose of medication with each push of a canister. Approximately 2 to 5 kg of pressure must be used to activate the aerosol. This is important for the nurse to know because hand strength diminishes with age and from the effects of chronic respiratory disease. The nurse evaluates whether clients have enough hand strength to use the MDI appropriately. A spacer may be used with the MDI. The spacer allows the particles of medication to slow down and break into smaller pieces, which improves the drug's absorption in the client's airway. Spacers are especially helpful when the client has difficulty coordinating the steps involved in self-administering inhaled medications (Togger & Brenner, 2001).

DPIs are becoming more widely available. They hold dry, powdered medication and create an aerosol when the client inhales through a reservoir that contains a dose of the medication. DPIs require less manual dexterity, and because the device is activated with the client's breath, there is no need to coordinate puffs with inhalation, as when using an MDI. They also do not require a spacer. However, the medication inside the DPI may clump if the client is in a humid climate, and some clients cannot inspire fast enough to administer the entire dose of the medication (Togger & Brenner, 2001). Skill 30-6 describes the steps required to administer medication through MDIs and DPIs.

The nurse must teach the client to recognize when the MDI or DPI is empty and needs to be replaced. Floating the MDI to determine how much medication is left is no longer recommended because extra propellant may cause buoyancy even if no medication is remaining. To calculate the number of days a canister will last, the nurse helps the client determine how many doses the canister contains and how many puffs are inhaled daily. Then, the number of doses in the canister is divided by the number of puffs taken daily. Some DPIs have mechanisms that indicate how many doses are left. These mechanisms are not foolproof, but they can help the client predict when the medication needs to be refilled (Togger & Brenner, 2001).

Administering Medications by Irrigations

Medications may be used to irrigate or wash out a body cavity and are delivered through a stream of solution. Irrigations most commonly use sterile water, saline, or antiseptic solutions on the eye, ear, throat, vagina, and urinary tract. If there is a break in the skin or mucosa, the nurse uses aseptic technique. When the cavity to be irrigated is not sterile, as in the case of the ear canal (see Box 30-11) or vagina, clean technique is acceptable. In health care settings, however, sterile solutions are usually used. Irrigations can cleanse an area, instill a medication, or apply hot or cold to injured tissue.

Administering Parenteral Medications

Parenteral administration of medications is the administration of medications by injection. Parenteral administration is an invasive procedure that must be performed using aseptic techniques (Box 30-12). After a needle pierces the skin, there is risk of infection. Each type of injection requires certain skills to ensure that the medication reaches the proper location. The effects of a parenterally administered medication can develop rapidly, depending on the rate of medication absorption. The nurse closely observes the client's response.

Equipment. A variety of syringes and needles are available, each designed to deliver a certain volume of medication to a specific type of tissue. The nurse uses judgment when determining the syringe or needle that will be most effective.

Syringes. Syringes consist of a cylindrical barrel with a tip designed to fit the hub of a hypodermic needle and a close-fitting plunger. Syringes, in general, are classified as being Luer-Lok or non-Luer-Lok. This nomenclature is based on the design of the syringe's tip. Luer-Lok syringes (Figure 30–14, *A*) require special needles, which are twisted onto the tip and lock themselves in place. This design prevents the inadvertent removal of the needle. Non-Luer-Lok syringes (Figure 30–14, *B–D*) require needles that slip onto the tip. In the clinical setting, all syringes now have safety devices to prevent needle-stick injury. The illustrations in this section are used to

Text continued on p. 881

Skill 30-5 Administering Rectal Suppositories

View Video

Delegation Considerations

Administering medications by the rectal route should not be delegated to unregulated care providers (UCPs). The nurse must instruct the UCP about the following:

- Expected fecal discharge or bowel movement and to report occurrence to the nurse
- Potential side effects of medications and to report their occurrence to the nurse

Equipment

- Rectal suppository
- Water-soluble lubricating jelly
- Clean gloves
- Drape or sheet
- Tissue
- MAR

Steps	Rationale
1. Review prescriber's order, including client's name, medication name, form, route, time of administration, and drug indication.	Ensures safe and correct administration of medication.
2. Review medical record for rectal surgery, bleeding, and history of allergies.	Conditions contraindicate use of suppository. Prevents allergic response to medication.
3. Perform hand hygiene.	Reduces transfer of micro-organisms.
4. Apply disposable gloves.	Prevents contact with infected fecal material, following Health Canada (1999) guidelines for body substance isolation.
5. Identify client; check name on MAR with client's identification bracelet and ask client's name.	Ensures that correct client receives medication.
6. Explain procedure. Be specific if client wishes to self-administer medication.	Promotes understanding and co-operation. Will enable client to self-administer medication if physically able.
7. Arrange supplies at bedside.	Ensures smooth procedure.
8. Close room curtain or door.	Maintains privacy and minimizes embarrassment.
9. Assist client in assuming Sims' position. Keep client draped with only anal area exposed.	Exposes anus and helps client relax external anal sphincter. Maintains privacy and facilitates relaxation.
10. Examine condition of anus externally and palpate rectal walls as needed (see chapter 28). Dispose of gloves in proper receptacle if soiled.	Determines presence of active rectal bleeding. Palpation determines whether rectum is filled with feces, which may interfere with suppository placement. Reduces transmission of infection.

Critical Decision Point: Generally, rectal suppository is contraindicated in the presence of active rectal bleeding. Unless suppository is for constipation, medication placed in a rectum filled with feces may be poorly absorbed or prematurely expelled with defecation.

Steps	Rationale
11. Apply disposable gloves (if previous gloves were discarded).	Prevents transmission of micro-organisms and follows Health Canada (1999) guidelines to prevent accidental exposure to body substances.
12. Remove suppository from wrapper and lubricate rounded end (see illustration) with sterile water-soluble lubricating jelly. Lubricate index finger of dominant hand with a water-soluble lubricant.	Lubrication reduces friction as suppository enters rectal canal.

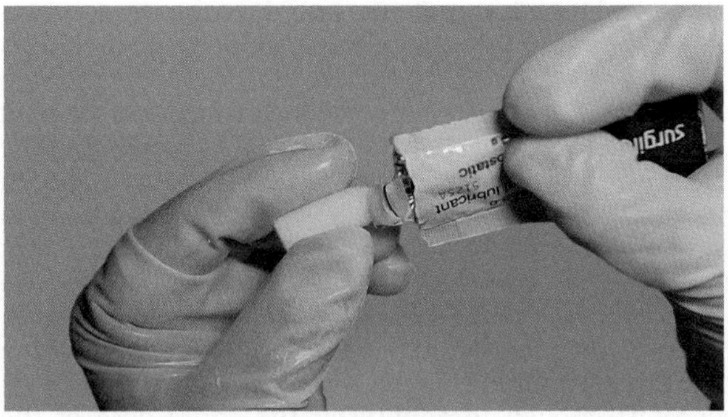

STEP **12** Remove suppository from wrapper.

Steps	Rationale
13. Ask client to take slow deep breaths through mouth and relax anal sphincter.	Forcing suppository through constricted sphincter causes pain.
14. Retract buttocks with non-dominant hand. Insert suppository gently through anus, past internal sphincter and against rectal wall, 10 cm in adults, 5 cm in children and infants. May need to apply gentle pressure to hold buttocks together momentarily.	Suppository must be placed against rectal mucosa for eventual absorption and therapeutic action.
15. Withdraw finger and wipe anal area with tissue.	Provides comfort.
16. Discard gloves in appropriate receptacle.	Reduces transfer of micro-organisms.
17. Ask client to remain flat or on side for 5 minutes.	Prevents expulsion of suppository.
18. If suppository contains laxative or fecal softener, place call light within reach.	Provides client with sense of control over elimination. Allows client to obtain assistance to bedpan or toilet.
19. Perform hand hygiene.	Prevents transfer of micro-organisms.
20. Observe for effects of suppository (e.g., bowel movement, relief of nausea) at times that correlate with the medication's onset, peak, and duration.	Evaluates effectiveness of medication and relief of client's symptoms.

Unexpected Outcomes and Related Interventions

- Suppository falls out shortly after administration.
  - Reinsert suppository, if possible.
- Client refuses medication.
  - Explore reasons why client does not want medication and clarify misunderstandings about medication.
  - Do not force client to take medication.
  - If client refuses to take medication despite educational efforts, record in client's chart why drug was withheld and notify prescriber.

Recording and Reporting

- Record administration of medication on MAR according to institutional policy.
- Report occurrence of rectal bleeding to physician.

Home Care Considerations

- Long-term use of laxatives often results in poor bowel tone and may result in dependency. Clients should be advised not to overuse laxatives, and they should be instructed on use of non-pharmacological measures, such as increasing fibre and fluid intake, to promote healthy bowel elimination.
- Some clients are not able to self-administer rectal medications. In this case, a family member or significant other will need to learn how to give the medication and will need to be available to administer the medication as scheduled.

Skill 30-6 *Using Metered-Dose or Dry Powder Inhalers*

View Video

Delegation Considerations

Administering a metered-dose inhaler (MDI) or dry powder inhaler (DPI) and supervising clients who self-administer them should not be delegated to unregulated care providers (UCPs). The nurse must instruct the UCP about the following:

- The need to report to the nurse any change in client's respiratory status or increased coughing
- Potential side effects of medications and to report their occurrence to the nurse

Equipment

- MDI or DPI
- Spacer (optional with MDI)
- Facial tissues (optional)
- Washbasin or sink with warm water
- Paper towel
- MAR

Steps	Rationale
1. Review prescriber's order, including client's name, medication name, number of inhalations, and drug indication.	Ensures safe and correct administration of medication.
2. Identify client; compare name on MAR with client's identification bracelet, and ask client's name.	Ensures that correct client receives medication.
3. Assess client's ability to hold, manipulate, and depress canister and inhaler.	Any impairment of grasp or coordination interferes with client's ability to use MDI or DPI correctly.
4. Assess client's readiness to learn: client asks questions about medication, disease, or complications; requests education in use of inhaler; is mentally alert; participates in own care.	Affects client's ability to understand explanations and actively participate in teaching process.
5. Assess client's ability to learn: client should not be fatigued, in pain, or in respiratory distress; assess level of understanding of technical vocabulary terms.	Mental or physical limitations affect client's ability to learn and methods nurse uses for instruction.
6. Assess client's knowledge and understanding of disease and purpose and action of prescribed medications.	Knowledge of disease is essential for client to realistically understand use of inhaler.
7. Determine medication schedule and number of inhalations prescribed for each dose.	Influences explanations nurse provides for use of inhaler.
8. If previously instructed in self-administration of inhaled medicine, assess client's technique in using an inhaler.	Nurse's instruction may require only simple reinforcement, depending on client's level of dexterity.
9. Instruct client in comfortable environment by sitting in chair in hospital room or sitting at kitchen table in home.	Client will be more likely to remain receptive to nurse's explanations.
10. Provide adequate time for teaching session.	Prevents interruptions. Instruction should occur when client is receptive.
11. Perform hand hygiene and arrange equipment needed.	Reduces transfer of micro-organisms and saves time.
12. Allow client opportunity to manipulate inhaler, canister, and spacer device. Explain and demonstrate how canister fits into inhaler.	Client must be familiar with how to use equipment.

Critical Decision Point: If client is using an MDI with or without a spacer and the inhaler is new or has not been used for several days, push a "test spray" into the air (MayoClinic.com, 2000).

Steps	Rationale
13. Explain what metered dose is, and warn client about overuse of inhaler, including medication side effects.	Client must not arbitrarily administer excessive inhalations because of risk of serious side effects. If medication is given in recommended doses, side effects are uncommon.
14. Explain steps for administering inhaled dose of medication of MDI (demonstrate steps when possible): a. Insert MDI canister into the holder. b. Remove mouthpiece cover from inhaler.	Use of simple, step-by-step explanations allows client to ask questions at any point during procedure.

Steps	Rationale
c. Shake inhaler vigorously 5 or 6 times.	Ensures fine particles are aerosolized.
d. Have client take a deep breath and exhale.	Empties lungs and prepares the client's airway to receive the medication (Togger & Brenner, 2001).
e. Instruct the client to position the inhaler in one of two ways. (1) Close mouth around MDI with opening toward back of throat (see illustration) (2) Position the device 2 to 4 cm in front of the mouth (see illustration).	Directs aerosol spray toward airway. Positioning the mouthpiece in front of mouth is considered the best way to deliver the medication.
f. With the inhaler properly positioned, have client hold inhaler with thumb at the mouthpiece and the index finger and middle finger at the top. This is called a three-point or lateral hand position.	MDIs work best when clients use a three-point or lateral hand position to activate canisters.
g. Instruct client to tilt head back slightly, inhale slowly and deeply through mouth for 3 to 5 seconds while depressing canister fully.	Medication is distributed to airways during inhalation. Inhalation through mouth rather than nose draws medication more effectively into airways.
h. Hold breath for approximately 10 seconds.	Allows tiny drops of aerosol spray to reach deeper branches of airways.
i. Remove MDI from mouth and exhale through pursed lips.	Keeps small airways open during exhalation.
15. Explain steps to administer MDI using a spacer such as an Aerochamber (demonstrate when possible):	
a. Remove mouthpiece cover from MDI and mouthpiece of spacer. Inspect spacer for foreign objects and ensure valve is intact if spacer has one.	Inhaler fits into end of spacer.
b. Insert MDI into end of spacer.	Spacer traps medication released from the MDI; the client then inhales the drug from the device. These devices break up and slow down the medication particles, enhancing the amount of medication received by client (Togger & Brenner, 2001).
c. Shake inhaler vigorously 5 or 6 times.	Ensures fine particles are aerosolized.
d. Have client exhale completely before closing mouth around mouthpiece of the spacer. Avoid covering small exhalation slots with the lips (see illustration).	Empties lungs and prepares them for the medication (National Heart, Lung and Blood Institute, 1995).

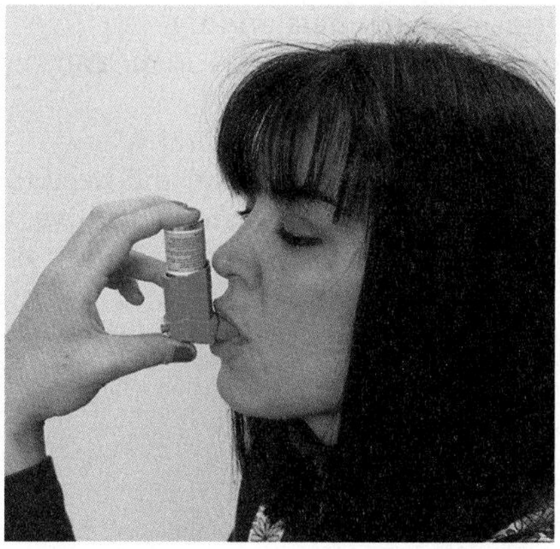

STEP **14e(1)** The client opens lips and places inhaler in mouth with opening toward back of throat.

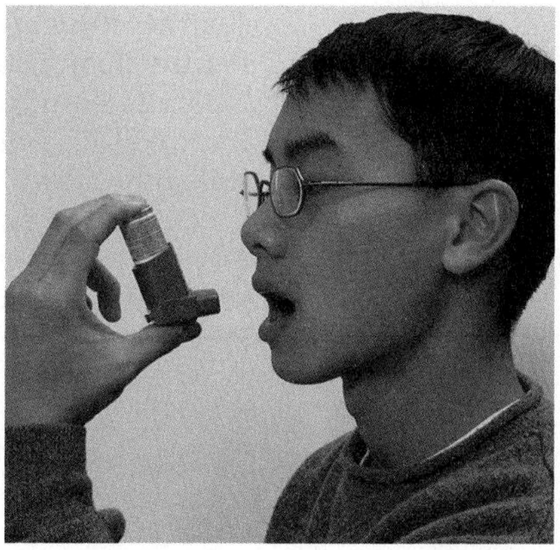

STEP **14e(2)** The client positions the mouthpiece 2 to 4 cm away from the mouth. This is considered the best way to deliver the medication.

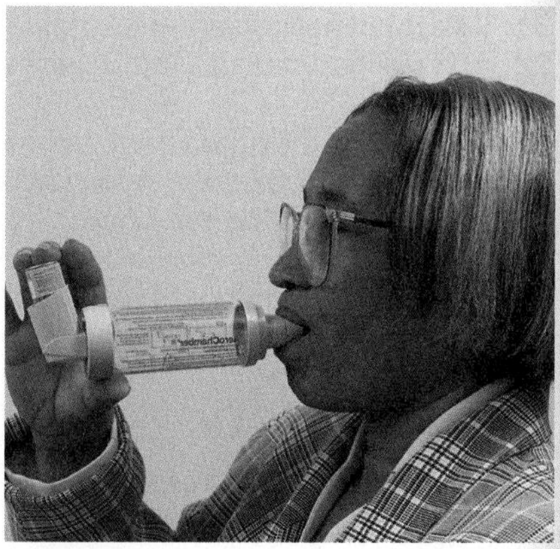

STEP **15d** Have the client place mouthpiece in mouth and close lips, being careful to keep exhalation slots exposed.

Skill 30-6 Using Metered-Dose or Dry Powder Inhalers—cont'd

Steps	Rationale
e. Have client depress medication canister, spraying one puff into spacer.	Emits spray that allows finer particles to be inhaled. Large droplets are retained in spacer.
f. Instruct client to inhale deeply and slowly through the mouth for 3 to 5 seconds.	Maximizes amount of medication that enters the lung.
g. Have client hold breath for 10 seconds.	Ensures full medication distribution.
h. Remove MDI and spacer before exhaling.	Allows client to exhale normally.
16. Explain steps to administer DPI (demonstrate when possible):	
a. Remove cover from mouthpiece. Do not shake the DPI (Epstein et al., 2001).	
b. Hold inhaler upright and turn wheel to the right and then to the left until a click is heard.	Primes inhaler, ensuring medication will be delivered to client (Epstein et al., 2001).
c. Exhale away from inhaler prior to inhalation.	Prevents loss of powder.
d. Position mouthpiece between the lips.	Prevents medication from escaping through mouth.
e. Inhale deeply and forcefully through the mouth.	Creates aerosol (Togger & Brenner, 2001).
f. Hold breath for 5 to 10 seconds.	Ensures full medication distribution.
17. Instruct client to wait at least 20 to 30 seconds between inhalations of the same medication and 2 to 5 minutes between inhalations or as ordered by prescriber.	Medications must be inhaled sequentially. First inhalation opens airways and reduces inflammation. Second or third inhalation penetrates deeper airways.
18. Instruct client against repeating inhalations before next scheduled dose.	Medications are prescribed at intervals during day to provide constant drug levels and minimize side effects. Beta-adrenergic MDIs are used either on an "as needed" basis or regularly every 4 to 6 hours.
19. Explain that client may feel gagging sensation in throat caused by droplets of medication on pharynx or tongue.	Results when inhalant is sprayed and inhaled incorrectly.
20. Instruct client in cleaning inhaler:	
a. Once a day, inhaler and cap should be rinsed in warm running water. Inhaler must be completely dry before using.	Accumulation of spray around mouthpiece can interfere with proper distribution during use.
b. Twice a week, the L-shaped plastic mouthpiece should be washed with mild dishwashing soap and warm water. Rinse and dry well before putting canister back inside mouthpiece (National Heart, Lung and Blood Institute, 1995).	Removes residual medication. Inhalers holding cromolyn or nedocromil should not be placed in water (National Heart, Lung, and Blood Institute, 1995).
21. Ask if client has any questions.	Clarifies misconceptions or misunderstanding.
22. Have client explain and demonstrate steps in use of inhaler.	Return demonstration provides feedback for measuring client's learning.
23. Ask client to explain medication schedule.	Improves likelihood of compliance with therapy.
24. Ask client to describe side effects of medication and criteria for calling prescriber.	Will allow client to recognize signs of overuse and need to seek medical support when medications are ineffective.
25. After medication instillation, assess client's respirations and auscultate lungs.	Determines status of breathing pattern and adequacy of ventilation.

Unexpected Outcomes and Related Interventions

- Client needs a bronchodilator more than every 4 hours.
  - May indicate respiratory problems; reassessment of type of medication and delivery methods needed; notify health care provider if respiratory status does not improve.
- Client experiences cardiac dysrhythmias, especially if receiving beta-adrenergics
  - If client experiences symptoms with the dysrhythmias (e.g., light-headedness, syncope), withhold all further doses of medication and discuss with prescriber.
- Client is not able to self-administer medication properly.
  - Alternative delivery routes or methods of medication administration may need to be explored.
- Client experiences paroxysms of coughing.
  - Aerosolized particles irritate posterior pharynx. Notify prescriber; may need to reassess type of medication or delivery method.

Recording and Reporting

- Document in nurse's notes what skills were taught and client's ability to perform skills.
- Record time when client used MDI or DPI and the amount of puffs.
- Report any undesirable effects from medication.

Home Care Considerations

- Remind clients to carry their prescribed inhalers to use emergently in case of an acute asthma attack.

Box 30-12 Preventing Infection During an Injection

- To prevent contamination of solution, draw medication from ampule quickly. Do not allow it to stand open.
- To prevent needle contamination, avoid letting needle touch contaminated surface (e.g., outer edges of ampule or vial, outer surface of needle cap, nurse's hands, countertop, table surface).
- To prevent syringe contamination, avoid touching length of plunger or inner part of barrel. Keep tip of syringe covered with cap or needle.
- To prepare skin, wash skin soiled with dirt, drainage, or feces with soap and water and then dry. Use friction and a circular motion while cleaning with an antiseptic swab. Swab from centre of site, and move outward in a 5-cm radius.

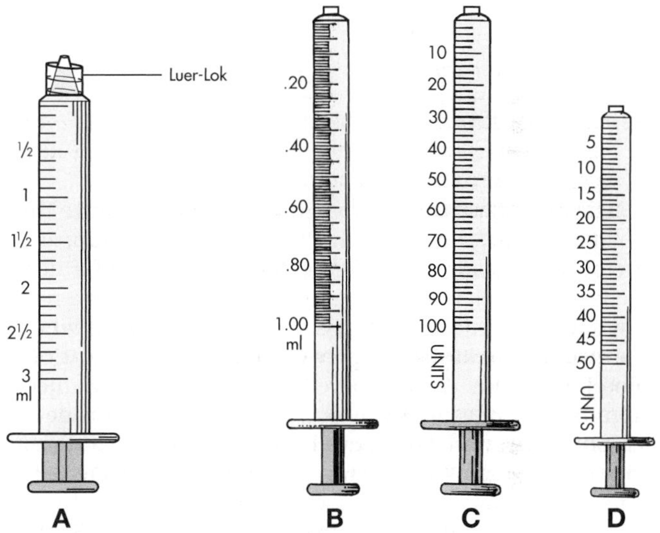

FIGURE **30–14** Types of syringes. **A,** Luer-lok syringe marked in 0.1 (tenths). **B,** Tuberculin syringe marked in 0.01 (hundredths) for doses of less than 1 mL. **C,** Insulin syringe marked in units (100). **D,** Insulin syringe marked in units (50).

demonstrate different syringes, needles, and parts of the syringe.

The nurse fills a syringe by aspiration, pulling the plunger outward while the needle tip remains immersed in the prepared solution. The nurse may handle the outside of the syringe barrel and the handle of the plunger. To maintain sterility, the nurse avoids letting any unsterile object touch the tip or inside of the barrel, the hub, the shaft of the plunger, or the needle (Figure 30–15).

Syringes come in a number of sizes, from 0.5 mL to 60 mL. A 2- to 3-mL syringe is usually adequate for a sub-Q or IM injection. A larger volume creates discomfort. The nurse uses large syringes to administer certain IV medications, add medications to IV solutions, and irrigate wounds or drainage tubes. Syringes may come prepackaged with a needle attached. However, the nurse may change needle sizes. The hypodermic has two scales along the barrel; one is divided into minims and the other into tenths of a millilitre.

Insulin syringes (see Figure 30–14, *C* and *D,* are available in sizes that hold 0.3 mL to 1 mL and are calibrated in units. Each millilitre of solution contains 100 units of insulin. Insulin syringes that hold 0.3 mL are known as low-dose syringes (30 units per 0.3 mL). Most insulin syringes are U-100s (100 units per 1 mL).

The tuberculin syringe (see Figure 30–14, *B*) has a long, thin barrel with a preattached thin needle. The syringe is calibrated in sixteenths of a minim and hundredths of a millilitre and has a capacity of 1 mL. The nurse uses a tuberculin syringe to prepare small amounts of medications. A tuberculin syringe is also useful when preparing small, precise doses for infants or young children.

Needles. Needles come packaged in individual sheaths to allow flexibility in choosing the right needle for a client. Some needles are preattached to standard-sized syringes. Most needles are made of stainless steel and are disposable.

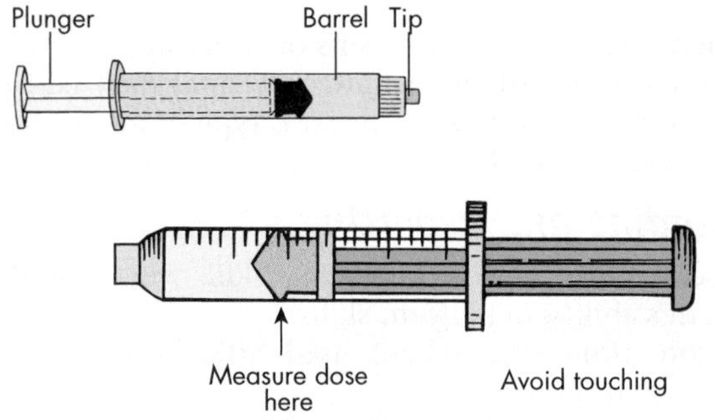

FIGURE **30–15** Parts of a syringe.

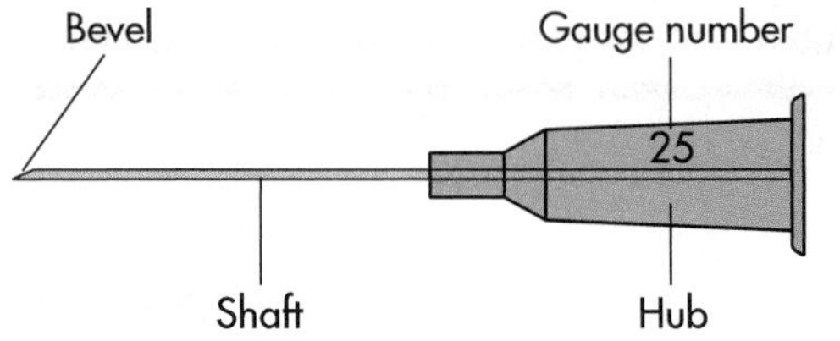

FIGURE **30–16** Parts of the needle.

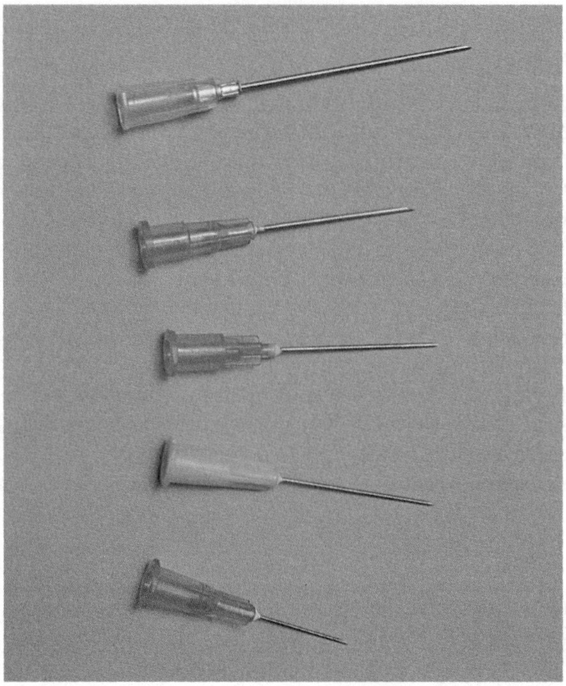

FIGURE **30–17** Needles. *Top to bottom:* 19 gauge, 3.8-cm length; 20 gauge, 2.5-cm length; 21 gauge, 2.5-cm length; 23 gauge, 2.5-cm length; and 25 gauge, 1.6-cm length.

The needle has three parts: the hub, which fits onto the tip of a syringe; the shaft, which connects to the hub; and the bevel, or slanted tip (Figure 30–16). The tip of a needle, or the bevel, is always slanted. The bevel creates a narrow slit when injected into tissue and quickly closes when the needle is removed to prevent leakage of medication, blood, or serum. A short bevelled tip is best for IV injections because it is not easily occluded against the inside of a blood vessel wall. Long bevelled tips are sharper and narrower, minimizing discomfort when entering tissue used for subcutaneous or intramuscular (IM) injections.

Needles vary in length from 0.6 to 7.6 cm (Figure 30–17). The nurse chooses the needle length according to the client's size and weight and the type of tissue into which the medication is to be injected. A child or slender adult generally requires a shorter needle. The nurse uses longer needles (2.5 to 3.8 cm) for IM injections and a shorter needle (1 to 1.6 cm) for subcutaneous injections.

Needle diameter is measured by gauge. As the gauge becomes smaller, the needle diameter becomes larger (see Figure 30–17). The selection of a gauge depends on the viscosity of fluid to be injected or infused. An IM injection usually requires an 18- to 27-gauge needle, depending on the viscosity of the medication (Nicoll & Hesby, 2002). Subcutaneous injections require smaller diameter needles such as a 25-gauge needle. A 26-gauge needle is used for an intradermal injection.

Disposable Injection Units. Disposable, single-dose, prefilled syringes are available for some medications. The nurse must be careful to check the medication and concentration because all prefilled syringes appear very similar. With these syringes, the nurse does not have to prepare medication doses, except perhaps to expel portions of unneeded medications.

The Tubex and Carpuject injection systems include reusable plastic mechanisms that hold prefilled, disposable, sterile cartridge-needle units (Figure 30–18). The nurse slips the cartridge into the syringe, secures it (following package directions), and checks for air bubbles in the syringe. The nurse advances the plunger to expel excess medication as in a regular syringe. A new type of injection system involves screwing a plunger-like device into the end of a prefilled vial containing a needle. After the medication is given, the entire unit is disposed of in a receptacle. This design reduces the risk of needle-stick injuries.

Preparing an Injection From an Ampule. Ampules contain single doses of medication in a liquid. Ampules are available in several sizes, from 1 mL to 10 mL or more (Figure 30–19, *A*). An ampule is made of glass with a constricted neck that must be snapped off to allow access to the medication. A coloured ring around the neck indicates where the ampule is prescored to be broken easily. Aspiration of the medication into a syringe (Skill 30-7) is sometimes completed with a filter needle to prevent small glass fragments from entering the syringe (Koschel, 2001). The filter needle is then replaced with an appropriate-sized needle for administration.

Preparing an Injection From a Vial. A vial is a single-dose or multidose container with a rubber seal at the top (see Figure 30–19, *B*). A metal cap protects the seal until it is ready for use. Vials contain liquid or dry forms of medications. Medications that are unstable in solution are packaged dry. The vial label specifies the solvent or

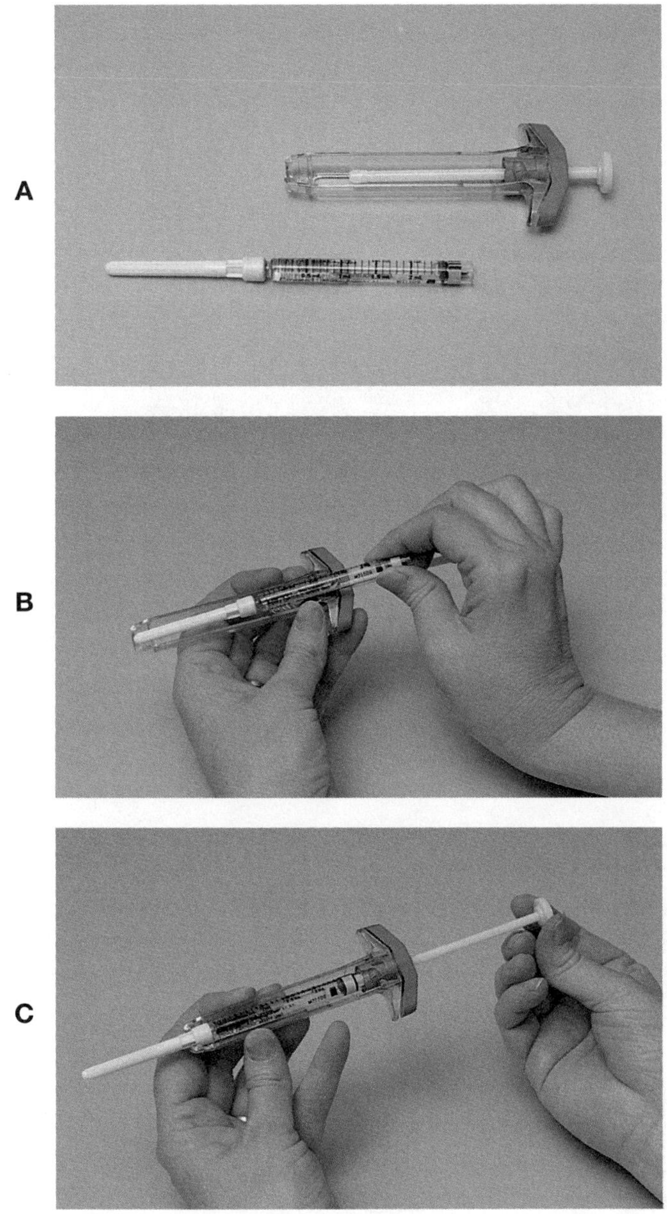

FIGURE **30–18** Disposable injection unit. **A,** Carpuject syringe and prefilled sterile cartridge with needle. **B,** Assembling the Carpuject. **C,** Cartridge locks at needle end; plunger screws into opposite end.

diluent used to dissolve the medication and the amount of diluent needed to prepare a desired medication concentration. Normal saline and sterile distilled water are solutions commonly used to dissolve medications.

Unlike the ampule, the vial is a closed system, and air must be injected into it to permit easy withdrawal of the solution. Failure to inject air when withdrawing creates a vacuum within the vial that makes withdrawal difficult (see Skill 30-7).

To prepare a powdered medication, the nurse draws up the amount of diluent or solvent recommended on the vial's label. The nurse injects the diluent into the vial in the same manner as injecting air into the vial. Most powdered medications dissolve easily, but it may be necessary to withdraw the needle to mix the contents thoroughly. Gently rolling the vial between the hands will dissolve the powdered medication. The needle is reinserted to draw up the dissolved medication. After mixing multidose vials, the nurse makes a label that includes the date and time of mixing and the concentration of medication per millilitre. Multidose vials may require refrigeration after the contents are reconstituted.

Mixing Medications. If two medications are compatible, it is possible to mix them in one injection if the total dose is within accepted limits. Medications are mixed so that a client will not have to receive more than one injection at a time. Most nursing units have charts that list common compatible medications. If there is any uncertainty about medication compatibilities, a pharmacist should be consulted.

Mixing Medications From Two Vials. The nurse applies these principles when mixing medications from two vials:

- Do not contaminate one medication with another.
- Ensure the final dose is accurate.
- Maintain aseptic technique.

Only one syringe is needed to mix medications from two vials (Figure 30–20). The nurse takes a syringe with a needle attached and aspirates the volume of air equivalent to the first medication's dose (vial A). The nurse injects the air into vial A, making sure the needle does not touch the solution. The nurse withdraws the needle, aspirates air equivalent to the second medication's dose (vial B), and then injects the volume of air into vial B. The nurse immediately withdraws the medication from vial B into the syringe. The nurse then inserts the needle back into vial A, being careful not to push the plunger and expel the medication within the syringe into the vial. The nurse withdraws the desired amount of medication from vial A into the syringe. After withdrawing the necessary amount, the nurse withdraws the needle and applies a new needle.

Mixing Medications From One Vial and One Ampule. When mixing medication from both a vial and an ampule, the nurse prepares medication from the vial first and then, using the same syringe and filter needle, withdraws medication from the ampule. The medications are prepared in this order because it is not necessary to add air to withdraw medication from an ampule.

Insulin Preparation. Insulin is the hormone used to treat diabetes. It must be administered by injection because it is a protein and therefore would be broken down and destroyed in the gastrointestinal tract. Most clients with diabetes requiring insulin learn to self-administer injections.

When preparing insulin, a 100-unit insulin syringe is used. If the client is to receive 100-unit insulin, the nurse simply places the ordered number of units in the syringe. However, when 500-unit insulin is ordered, a medication calculation must be performed to correctly prepare the insulin (Box 30-13).

Text continued on p. 889

A

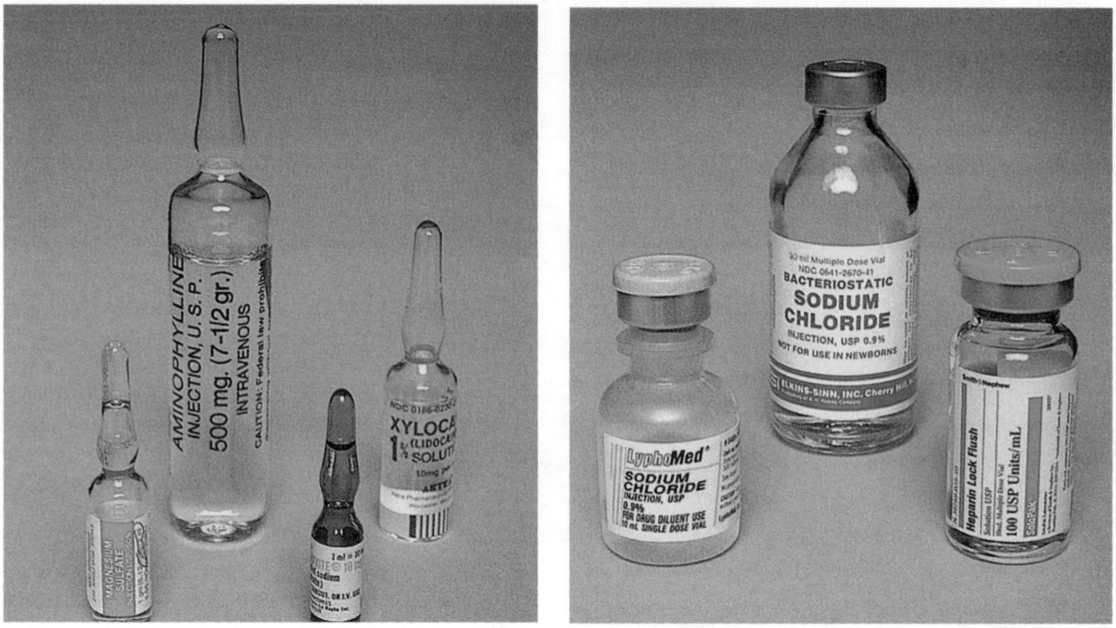

B

FIGURE **30–19** **A,** Medication in ampules. **B,** Medication in vials.

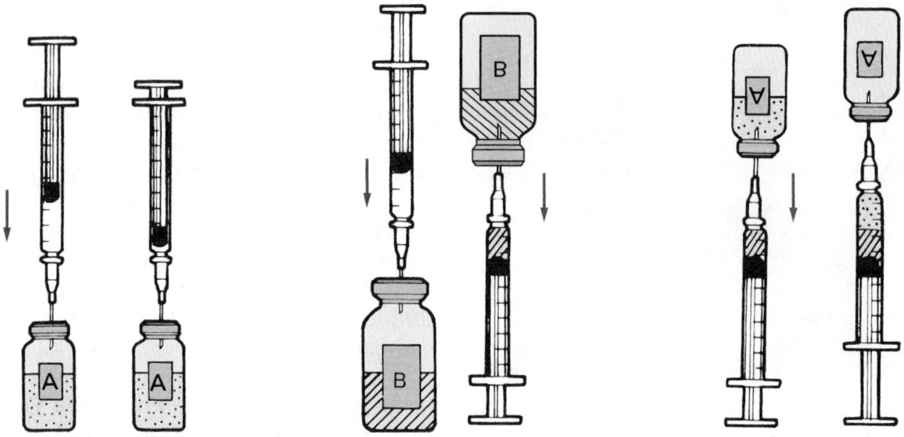

A B C

FIGURE **30–20** Mixing medications from two vials. **A,** Injecting air into vial A. **B,** Injecting air into vial B and withdrawing dose. **C,** Withdrawing medication from vial A; medications are now mixed.

Skill 30-7 *Preparing Injections*

View Video

Delegation Considerations

Preparing injections from ampules and vials should not be delegated to unregulated care providers.

Equipment

- MAR
- **Medication in an ampule**
  - Syringe, needle, and filter needle
  - Small gauze pad or unopened alcohol swab
- **Medication in a vial**
  - Syringe
  - Needles:
    - Blunt tip vial access cannula (if needleless system used)
    - Filter needle (if indicated)
    - Needle for drawing up medication (if needed) and needle for injection
  - Small gauze pad or alcohol swab
  - Diluent (e.g., normal saline or sterile water) (if indicated)

Steps	Rationale
1. Check client's name and medication order, including medication name, dose, route of administration, time of administration, and drug indication.	Ensures correct administration of medication.
2. Review pertinent information related to medication, including action, purpose, side effects, and nursing implications.	Allows nurse to administer medication properly and to monitor client's response.
3. Assess client's body build, muscle size, and weight.	Determines type and size of syringe and needles for injection.
4. Perform hand hygiene and assemble supplies.	Reduces transmission of micro-organisms and saves nurse's time.
5. Check medication order against MAR and check date of expiration for medication vial or ampule.	Ensures correct medication and dose are prepared. Medication potency may increase or decrease when outdated.
6. Prepare medication:	
A. **Ampule preparation**	
(1) Tap top of ampule lightly and quickly with finger until fluid moves from neck of ampule (see illustration).	Dislodges any fluid that collects above neck of ampule. All solution moves into lower chamber.
(2) Place small gauze pad or unopened alcohol swab around neck of ampule (see illustration).	Placing pad around neck of ampule protects nurse's fingers from trauma as glass tip is broken off.
(3) Snap neck of ampule quickly and firmly away from hands (see illustration).	Protects nurse's fingers and face from shattering glass.

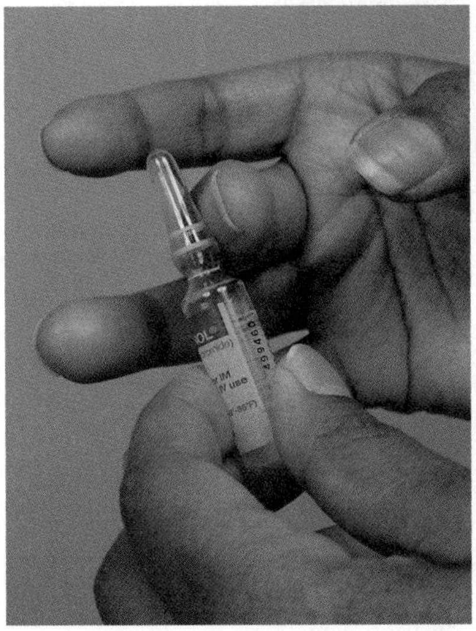

STEP **6A(1)** Tapping ampule moves fluid down neck.

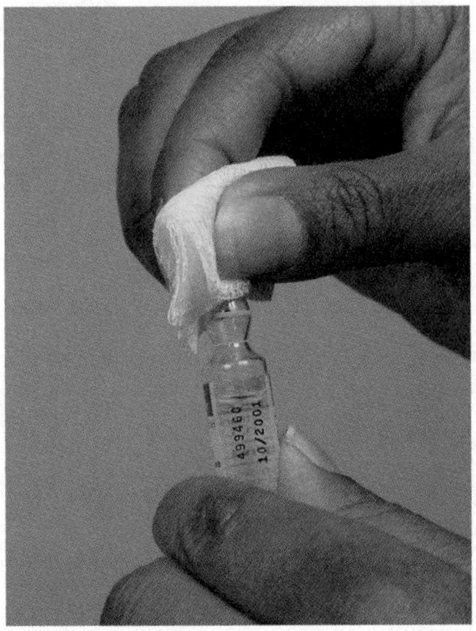

STEP **6A(2)** Gauze pad placed around neck of ampule.

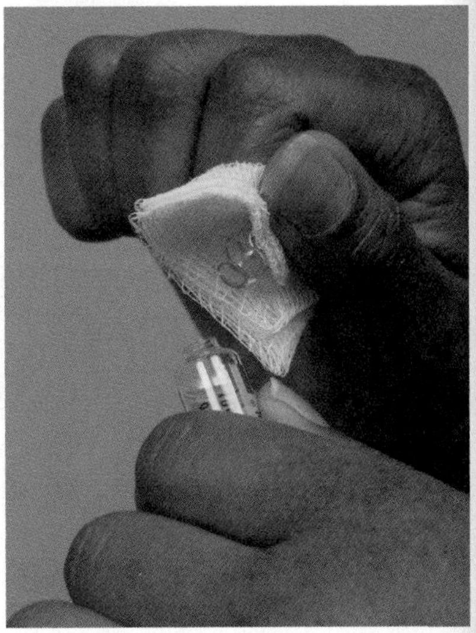

STEP **6A(3)** Snapping neck away from hands.

Skill 30-7 Preparing Injections—cont'd

Steps	Rationale
(4) Draw up medication quickly, using filter needle long enough to reach bottom of ampule.	System is open to airborne contaminants. Needle must be long enough to access medication for preparation. Filter needles are used to filter out any fragments of glass (Nicoll & Hesby, 2002).
(5) Hold ampule upside down, or set it on a flat surface. Insert filter needle into centre of ampule opening. Do not allow needle tip or shaft to touch rim of ampule.	Broken rim of ampule is considered contaminated. When ampule is inverted, solution dribbles out if needle tip or shaft touches rim of ampule.
(6) Aspirate medication into syringe by gently pulling back on plunger (see illustration).	Withdrawal of plunger creates negative pressure within syringe barrel, which pulls fluid into syringe.
(7) Keep needle tip under surface of liquid. Tip ampule to bring all fluid within reach of the needle.	Prevents aspiration of air bubbles.
(8) If air bubbles are aspirated, do not expel air into ampule.	Air pressure may force fluid out of ampule and medication will be lost.
(9) To expel excess air bubbles, remove needle from ampule. Hold syringe with needle pointing up. Tap side of syringe to cause bubbles to rise toward needle. Draw back slightly on plunger, and then push plunger upward to eject air. Do not eject fluid.	Withdrawing plunger too far will remove it from barrel. Holding syringe vertically allows fluid to settle in bottom of barrel. Pulling back on plunger allows fluid within needle to enter barrel so that fluid is not expelled. Air at top of barrel and within needle is then expelled.
(10) If syringe contains excess fluid, use sink for disposal. Hold syringe vertically with needle tip up and slanted slightly toward sink. Slowly eject excess fluid into sink. Recheck fluid level in syringe by holding it vertically.	Medication is safely dispersed into sink. Position of needle allows medication to be expelled without flowing down needle shaft. Rechecking fluid level ensures proper dose.
(11) Cover needle with its safety sheath or cap. Replace filter needle with needle for injection.	Prevents contamination of needle. Filter needles cannot be used for injection.

A 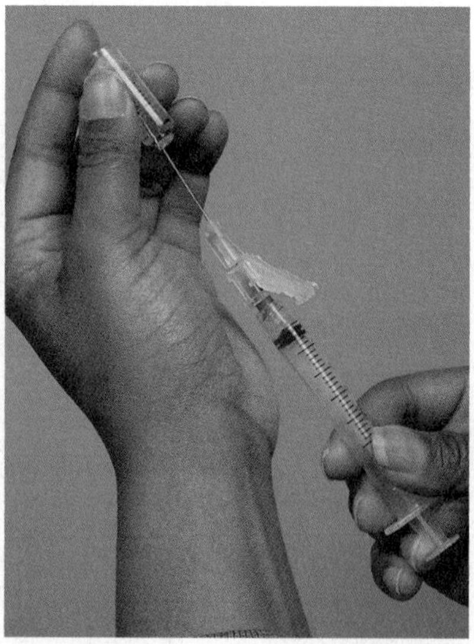 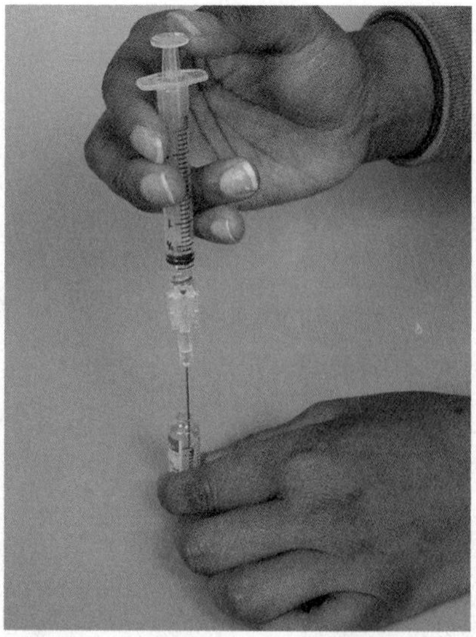 B

STEP **6A(6)** **A,** Medication aspirated with ampule inverted. **B,** Medication aspirated with ampule on flat surface.

Steps	Rationale
B. Vial containing a solution	
(1) Remove cap covering top of unused vial to expose sterile rubber seal. If a multidose vial has been used before, cap is already removed. Firmly and briskly wipe surface of rubber seal with alcohol swab and allow it to dry.	Vial comes packaged with seal that cannot be replaced after cap removal. Not all drug manufacturers guarantee that caps of unused vials are sterile. Therefore seals must be swabbed with alcohol before preparing medication. Allowing alcohol to dry prevents needle from being coated with alcohol and mixing with medication.
(2) Pick up syringe and remove needle cap or cap covering needleless vial access device (see illustration). Pull back on plunger to draw amount of air into syringe equivalent to volume of medication to be aspirated from vial.	Air must first be injected into vial to prevent buildup of negative pressure in vial when aspirating medication.

Critical Decision Point: Some medications and some institutions require that a filter needle be used when preparing medications from a vial. Check agency policy to determine if use of filter needle is indicated (Nicoll & Hesby, 2002).

Steps	Rationale
(3) With vial on flat surface, insert tip of needle with bevelled tip entering first through centre of rubber seal (see illustration). Apply pressure to tip of needle during insertion.	Centre of seal is thinner and easier to penetrate. Injecting bevelled tip first and using firm pressure prevent coring of rubber seal, which could enter vial or needle.
(4) Inject air into the vial's airspace, holding on to plunger. Hold plunger with firm pressure; plunger may be forced backward by air pressure within the vial.	Air must be injected before aspirating fluid. Injecting into vial's airspace prevents formation of bubbles and inaccuracy in dose.
(5) Invert vial while keeping firm hold on syringe and plunger (see illustration). Hold vial between thumb and middle fingers of non-dominant hand. Grasp end of syringe barrel and plunger with thumb and forefinger of dominant hand to counteract pressure in vial.	Inverting vial allows fluid to settle in lower half of container. Position of hands prevents forceful movement of plunger and permits easy manipulation of syringe.
(6) Keep tip of needle below fluid level.	Prevents aspiration of air.
(7) Allow air pressure from the vial to fill syringe gradually with medication. If necessary, pull back slightly on plunger to obtain correct amount of solution.	Positive pressure within vial forces fluid into syringe (unless vial has been used several times).
(8) When desired volume has been obtained, position needle into vial's airspace; tap side of syringe barrel carefully to dislodge any air bubbles. Eject any air remaining at top of syringe into vial.	Forcefully striking barrel while needle is inserted in vial may bend needle. Accumulation of air displaces medication and causes dose errors.

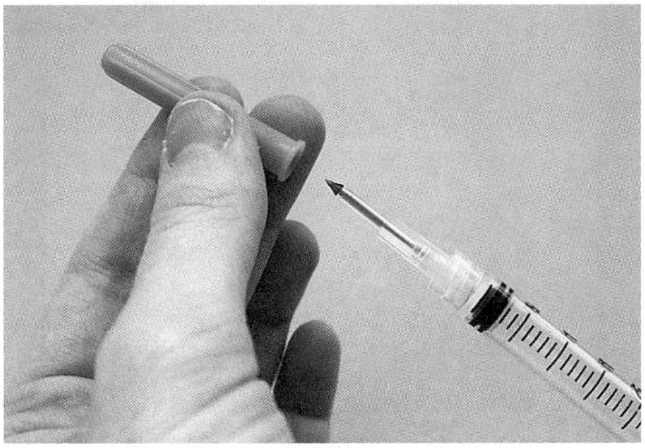

STEP **6B(2)** Syringe with needleless adapter.

Skill 30-7 Preparing Injections—cont'd

Steps	Rationale
(9) Remove needle from vial by pulling back on barrel of syringe.	Accidentally pulling plunger rather than barrel causes plunger to separate from barrel, resulting in loss of medication.
(10) Hold syringe at eye level, at 90-degree angle, to ensure correct volume and absence of air bubbles. Remove any remaining air by tapping barrel to dislodge any air bubbles (see illustration). Draw back slightly on plunger; then push plunger upward to eject air. Do not eject fluid. Recheck volume of medication.	Holding syringe vertically allows fluid to settle in bottom of barrel. Pulling back on plunger allows fluid within needle to enter barrel so that fluid is not expelled. Air at top of barrel and within needle is then expelled.
(11) If medication is to be injected into client's tissue, change needle to appropriate gauge and length according to route of medication.	Inserting needle through a rubber stopper may dull bevelled tip. New needle is sharper. Because no fluid is along shaft, needle will not track medication through tissues.
(12) For multidose vial, make label that includes date of mixing, concentration of medication per millilitre, and nurse's initials.	Ensures that future doses will be prepared correctly. Some medications must be discarded after certain number of days after mixing of vial.
C. Vial containing a powder (reconstituting medications)	
(1) Remove cap covering vial of powdered medication and cap covering vial of proper diluent. Firmly swab both seals with alcohol swab and allow to dry.	Not all drug manufacturers guarantee that caps of unused vials are sterile. Therefore, seals must be swabbed with alcohol before preparing medication. Allowing alcohol to dry prevents needle from being coated with alcohol and mixing with medication.
(2) Draw up diluent into syringe following steps 6B(2) through 6B(10).	Prepares diluent for injection into vial containing powdered medication.
(3) Insert tip of needle through centre of rubber seal of vial of powdered medication. Inject diluent into vial. Remove needle.	Diluent begins to dissolve and reconstitute medication.
(4) Mix medication thoroughly. Roll in palms. Do not shake.	Ensures proper dispersal of medication throughout solution. Shaking produces bubbles.

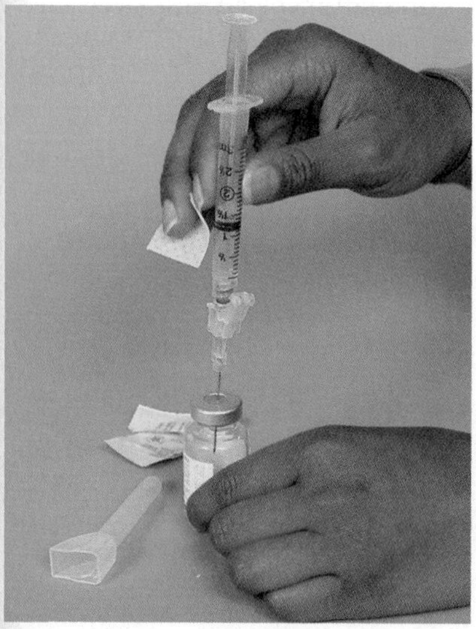

STEP **6B(3)** Insert adapter through centre of vial diaphragm (with vial flat on table).

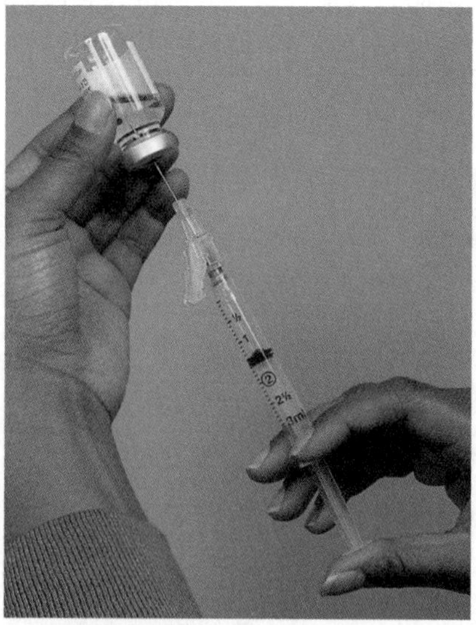

STEP **6B(5)** Withdraw fluid with vial inverted.

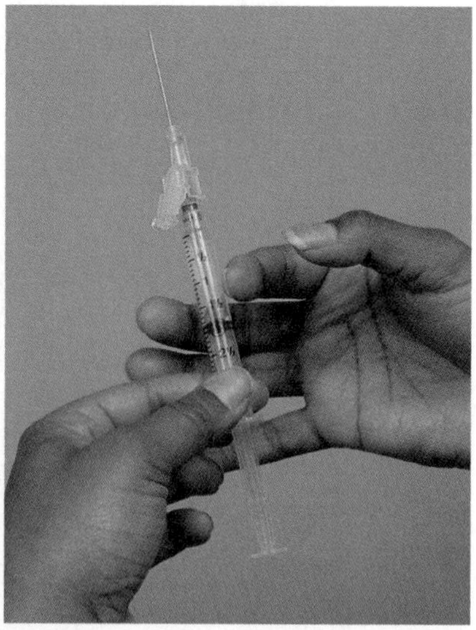

STEP **6B(10)** Hold syringe upright, tap barrel to dislodge air bubbles.

Steps	Rationale
(5) Reconstituted medication in vial is ready to be drawn into new syringe. Read label carefully to determine dose after reconstitution.	Once diluent has been added, concentration of medication (mg/mL) determines dose to be given.
(6) Prepare medication in syringe following steps 6B(2) through 6B(12).	

Critical Decision Point: Some institutions may require prepared parenteral medications to be verified for accuracy by another nurse. Check agency policy.

7. Dispose of soiled supplies. Place broken ampule and/or used vials and used needle in puncture-proof and leak-proof container. Clean work area and perform hand hygiene.	Proper disposal of glass and needle prevents accidental injury to staff. Controls transmission of infection.

Unexpected Outcomes and Related Interventions

- Air bubbles remain in syringe.
  - Expel air from syringe, and add medication to syringe until correct dose is prepared.
- Incorrect dose is prepared.
  - Discard prepared dose and prepare corrected new dose.

Case Study Box 30-13

Mr. Dodds has severe insulin resistance and requires an unusually high regular insulin dosage to control his blood glucose levels. Therefore, the physician has ordered that he begin taking 20 units of U-500 insulin. The nurse goes through the following medication calculation steps to determine how much insulin to prepare in the U-100 syringe:

- U-500 insulin is five times as strong as U-100 insulin.
- Therefore, the amount of U-500 insulin should be divided by 5.
- Dosage of U-500 insulin/5 = amount of insulin to draw into U-100 syringe.
- 20 units of U-500 insulin/5 = 4 units of insulin to draw into U-100 syringe.

Insulin is classified by rate of action, including rapid, short, intermediate, and long acting. Each type has a different onset, peak, and duration of action (Table 30-10). Some insulins come in a stable premixed solution (e.g., 70/30 insulin is 70% NPH and 30% regular). Clients receiving these insulins do not need to mix insulins.

A client with diabetes may require more than one type of insulin. For example, by receiving a short-acting (regular) and an intermediate-acting (NPH) insulin, a client receives more sustained control of blood glucose levels over 24 hours. Only regular insulin can be given intravenously.

Insulin is ordered by specific dose at select times or by a sliding scale. A sliding scale dictates a certain dose based on the client's blood glucose level (Box 30-14). Usually, rapid or short-acting insulins are used for sliding scales. If more than one type of insulin is required to manage the client's diabetes, the nurse can mix two different types of insulin into one syringe if they are compatible (Box 30-15), using the steps demonstrated in Figure 30–20. This minimizes the discomfort to the client associated with multiple injections.

Before withdrawing insulin from a vial, the nurse should rotate the vial at least 1 minute between both hands. This resuspends the modified insulin preparations and helps to warm the medication. The nurse should not shake insulin vials. Shaking causes bubbles to form, which take up space and alter the dose.

Administering Injections

Each injection route differs depending on the type of tissues the medication enters. The characteristics of the tissues influence the rate of medication absorption and thus the onset of medication action. Before injecting a medication, the nurse should know the volume of the medication to administer, the medication's characteristics and viscosity, and the location of anatomical structures underlying injection sites (Skill 30-8).

If a nurse does not administer injections correctly, negative client outcomes result. Failure to select an injection site in relation to anatomical landmarks can result in nerve or bone damage during needle insertion. Inability to maintain stability of the needle and syringe unit could result in pain for the client and possibly tissue damage. If the nurse fails to aspirate the syringe before injecting a medication, the medication may accidentally be injected directly into an artery or vein. Injecting too large a volume

Table 30-10 A Comparison of Insulin Preparations

Type	Onset	Peak	Duration	Colour	Route
Rapid-acting (Insulin lispro, insulin aspart)	15 min	1 hour	2–4 hours	Clear	Sub-Q
Short-acting (Regular)	30 min	2–4 hours	6–8 hours	Clear	IV or Sub-Q
Intermediate-acting (NPH, Lente)	1–2.5 hours	6–12 hours	18 hours	Cloudy	Sub-Q
Long-acting (Ultralente)	4–8 hours	None	24–36 hours	Cloudy	Sub-Q
Long-acting (Insulin glargine)	1 hour	None	24 hours	Clear	Sub-Q*

****Cannot*** be mixed with other insulins.
Adapted from "Insulin Therapy," by S. Strowig, 2001, *RN, 64*(9), p. 38.

Box 30-14 Example of Sliding Scale Insulin Order

Give regular insulin Sub-Q:
2 units for glucose 11.1 to 13.13 mmol/L
4 units for glucose 13.4 to 13.8 mmol/L
6 units for glucose 13.9 to 16.7 mmol/L
For glucose greater than 16.8 mmol/L, call physician

of medication for the site selected causes extreme pain and may result in local tissue damage.

Many clients, particularly children, fear injections. Clients with serious or chronic illness often are given several injections daily. The nurse may be able to minimize the client's discomfort in the following ways:

- Use a sharp-bevelled needle in the smallest suitable length and gauge.
- Position the client as comfortably as possible to reduce muscular tension.
- Select the proper injection site, using anatomical landmarks.
- Divert the client's attention from the injection through conversation.
- Insert the needle quickly and smoothly to minimize tissue pulling.
- Hold the syringe steady while the needle remains in tissues.
- Inject the medication slowly and steadily.

Subcutaneous Injections. Subcutaneous injections involve placing medications into the loose connective tissue under the dermis (see Skill 30-8). Because subcutaneous tissue is not as richly supplied with blood as the muscles, medication absorption is somewhat slower than with intramuscular (IM) injections. However, medications are absorbed completely if the client's circulatory status is normal. Because subcutaneous tissue contains pain receptors, the client may experience some discomfort.

The best subcutaneous injection sites include the outer posterior aspect of the upper arms, the abdomen from below the costal margins to the iliac crests, and the anterior aspects of the thighs (Figure 30–21). The site most frequently recommended for heparin injections is the abdomen (Figure 30–22). Other sites include the scapular areas of the upper back and the upper ventral or dorsal gluteal areas. The injection site chosen should be free of skin lesions, bony prominences, and large underlying muscles or nerves.

Box 30-15 Procedural Guidelines

Mixing Two Kinds of Insulin in One Syringe

- Lente insulins (Semilente, Lente, Ultralente) may be mixed with each other, in any ratio.
- Because Lente insulin binds with regular insulin, mixing of regular and Lente insulin is not recommended except for clients already adequately controlled on such a mixture.
- Insulin glargine (Lantus) *cannot* be mixed with other insulins.
- Insulin should not be mixed with any other medications unless approved by the prescriber.

To prepare insulin from two vials, the nurse or client follows these steps:

1. With an insulin syringe and needle, inject air, equal to the dose of insulin to be withdrawn, into the vial of intermediate- or long-acting (cloudy) insulin. Do not touch the tip of the needle to the solution.
2. Remove the syringe from the vial of cloudy insulin.
3. With the same syringe, inject air, equal to the dose of insulin to be withdrawn, into the vial of rapid- or short-acting insulin (clear vial). Then withdraw the correct dose into the syringe.
4. Remove the syringe from the clear insulin vial after carefully removing air bubbles in the syringe to ensure correct dose.
5. Return to the vial of intermediate- or long-acting (cloudy) insulin, and withdraw the correct dose.
6. Administer mixture of insulins within 5 minutes of preparing it. Rapid- or short-acting insulin can bind with intermediate- or long-acting insulin, thus reducing the action of the faster-acting insulin.

Adapted from "Insulin Therapy," by S. Strowig, 2001, *RN, 64*(9), p. 38.

Text continued on p. 896

Skill 30-8 Administering Injections

View Video

Delegation Considerations

Administering injections should not be delegated to unregulated care providers (UCPs). The nurse should instruct the UCP about the following:

- Potential medication side effects and to report their occurrence to the nurse
- Any impact of medication on client's vital signs or level of consciousness (e.g., sedation)

Equipment

- Proper size syringe and needle:
  - *Sub-Q:* Syringe (1 to 3 mL) and needle (27 to 25 gauge, 1 to 1.6 cm)
  - *IM:* Syringe 2 to 3 mL for adult, 0.5 to 1 mL for infants and small children.
  - Needle, length corresponding to site of injection and age of client according to following guidelines (Nicoll & Hesby, 2002):
    - *Children:* 1.6 to 3.2 cm (based on size of child)
    - *Vastus lateralis (adults):* 2.5 to 3.8 cm
    - *Deltoid (adults):* 2.5 to 3.8 cm
    - *Ventrogluteal (adults):* 3.8 cm
  - *ID:* 1-mL tuberculin syringe with preattached 26- or 27-gauge needle
- Small gauze pad and/or alcohol swab
- Vial or ampule of medication or skin test solution
- Disposable gloves
- MAR

Steps	Rationale
For All Injections	
1. Review prescriber's medication order for client's name, medication name, dose, time, route of administration, and drug indications.	Ensures safe and correct administration of medication.
2. Assess client's history of allergies and know substances client is allergic to and normal allergic reaction.	Certain substances have similar compositions; nurse should not administer any substance to which client is known to be allergic.
3. Check date of expiration for medication.	Drug potency may increase or decrease when outdated.
4. Observe verbal and non-verbal responses toward receiving injection.	Injections can be painful. Clients may have anxiety, which can increase pain.
5. Assess for contraindications.	
A. For subcutaneous injections Assess for factors such as circulatory shock or reduced local tissue perfusion. Assess adequacy of client's adipose tissue.	Reduced tissue perfusion interferes with medication absorption and distribution. Physiological changes of aging or client illness may influence the amount of subcutaneous tissue a client possesses. This influences methods for administering injections.
B. For intramuscular injections Assess for factors such as muscle atrophy, reduced blood flow, or circulatory shock.	Atrophied muscle absorbs medication poorly. Factors interfering with blood flow to muscles impair medication absorption.

Critical Decision Point: Because of documented adverse effects of IM injections, other routes of medication administration are safer. Verify that IM injection is necessary and explore alternative medication routes if possible (Nicoll & Hesby, 2002; Rodger & King, 2000).

Steps	Rationale
6. Aseptically prepare correct medication dose from ampule or vial (see Skill 30-7). Check carefully. Be sure all air is expelled.	Ensures that medication is sterile. Preparation techniques differ for ampule and vial.
7. Identify client; check identification bracelet with MAR and ask client's name.	Ensures correct client receives ordered medication.
8. Explain steps of procedure and tell client injection will cause a slight burning or sting.	Helps minimize client's anxiety.
9. Close room curtain or door.	Provides privacy.
10. Perform hand hygiene; apply disposable gloves.	Reduces transfer of micro-organisms.
11. Keep sheet or gown draped over body parts not requiring exposure.	Respects dignity of client.

Skill 30-8 Administering Injections—cont'd

Steps	Rationale
12. Select appropriate injection site. Inspect skin surface over sites for bruises, inflammation, or edema.	Injection sites should be free of abnormalities that may interfere with medication absorption. Site used repeatedly can become hardened from lipohypertrophy (increased growth in fatty tissue). Do not use an area that is bruised or has signs associated with infection.
a. *Sub-Q:* Palpate sites for masses or tenderness. Avoid these areas. For daily insulin, rotate site daily. Be sure needle is correct size by grasping skinfold at site with thumb and forefinger. Measure fold from top to bottom. Needle should be one-half length.	Sub-Q injections can be inadvertently given in the muscle, especially in the abdomen and thigh sites. Appropriate size of needle ensures that medication will be injected in the subcutaneous tissue.
b. *IM:* Note integrity and size of muscle and palpate for tenderness or hardness. Avoid these areas. If injections are given frequently, rotate sites.	The ventrogluteal site is the preferred site for children older than 7 months and adults unless there are contraindications to this site. In infants younger than 7 months, the vastus lateralis should be used (Nicoll & Hesby, 2002; Rodger & King, 2000).
c. *ID:* Note lesions or discolorations of forearm. Select site three to four fingerwidths below antecubital space and a handwidth above wrist. If forearm cannot be used, inspect the upper back. If necessary, sites for Sub-Q injections may be used (Workman, 1999).	An ID site should be clear so that results of skin test can be seen and interpreted correctly.
13. Assist client to comfortable position:	
a. *Sub-Q:* Have client relax arm, leg, or abdomen, depending on site chosen for injection.	Relaxation of site minimizes discomfort.
b. *IM:* Have client lie flat, on side, or prone, depending on site chosen.	Reduces strain on muscle and minimizes discomfort of injections.
c. *ID:* Have client extend elbow and support it and forearm on flat surface.	Stabilizes injection site for easiest accessibility.
d. Talk with client about subject of interest.	Distraction reduces anxiety.

Critical Decision Point: Ensure that client's position is not contraindicated by medical condition.

14. Relocate site using anatomical landmarks.	Injection into correct anatomical site prevents injury to nerves, bones, and blood vessels.
15. Cleanse site with an antiseptic swab. Apply swab at centre of the site and rotate outward in a circular direction for about 5 cm (see illustration).	Mechanical action of swab removes secretions containing micro-organisms.

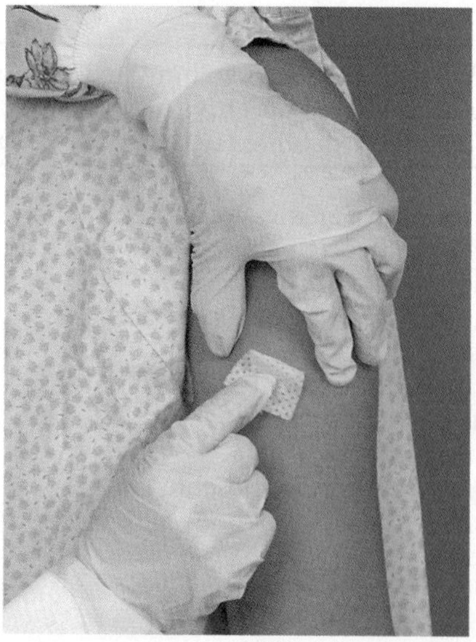

STEP **15** Cleanse site with circular motion.

Steps	Rationale
16. Hold swab or gauze between third and fourth fingers of non-dominant hand.	Gauze or swab remains readily accessible when needle is withdrawn.
17. Remove needle cap or sheath from needle by pulling it straight off.	Preventing needle from touching sides of cap prevents contamination.
18. Hold syringe between thumb and forefinger of dominant hand	
a. *Sub-Q:* Hold as dart, palm down or hold syringe across tops of fingertips (see illustration).	Quick, smooth injection requires proper manipulation of syringe parts.
b. *IM:* Hold as dart, palm down.	
c. *ID:* Hold bevel of needle pointing up.	With bevel up, medication is less likely to be deposited into tissues below dermis.
19. Administer injection:	
A. **Subcutaneous**	
(1) For average-size client, spread skin tightly across injection site or pinch skin with non-dominant hand.	Needle penetrates tight skin easier than loose skin. Pinching skin elevates subcutaneous tissue and may desensitize area.
(2) Inject needle quickly and firmly at 45- to 90-degree angle. Then release skin, if pinched.	Quick, firm insertion minimizes discomfort. (Injecting medication into compressed tissue irritates nerve fibres.)
(3) For obese client, pinch skin at site and inject needle at 90-degree angle below tissue fold.	Obese clients have fatty layer of tissue above subcutaneous layer.

Critical Decision Point: Piercing a blood vessel during a Sub-Q injection is very rare, so aspiration is not necessary when administering Sub-Q injections (McConnell, 2000; Peragallo-Dittko, 1997).

Steps	Rationale
(4) Inject medication slowly (see illustration).	Minimizes discomfort. Injecting heparin over 30 seconds may create less bruising (Chan, 2001).
B. **Intramuscular**	
(1) Position non-dominant hand at proper anatomical landmarks and pull skin down to administer in a Z-track.	Z-track creates zigzag path through tissues that seals needle track to avoid tracking of medication. Z-track should be used for all IM injections (Nicoll & Hesby, 2002).
(2) If client's muscle mass is small, grasp body of muscle between thumb and fingers.	Ensures that medication reaches muscle mass (Hockenberry et al., 2003).

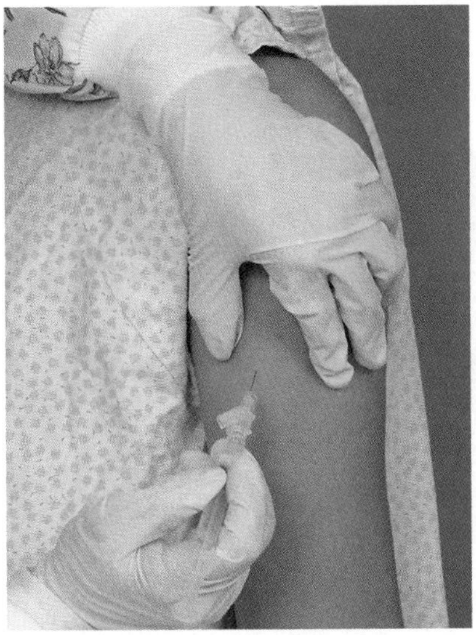

STEP **18a** Hold syringe as if grasping a dart.

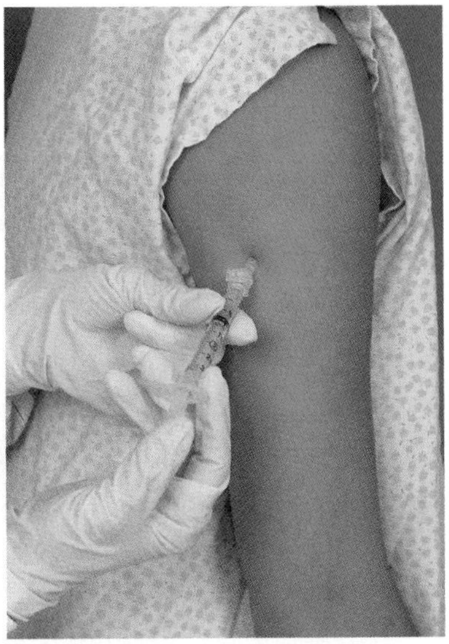

STEP **19A(4)** Inject medication slowly.

Skill 30-8 Administering Injections—cont'd

Steps	Rationale
(3) Insert needle quickly at 90-degree angle into muscle. After needle pierces skin, grasp lower end of syringe barrel with non-dominant hand to stabilize syringe. Continue to hold skin tightly with non-dominant hand. Move dominant hand to end of plunger. Do not move syringe.	Smooth manipulation of syringe reduces discomfort from needle movement. Skin must remain pulled until after drug is injected to ensure Z-track administration.
(4) Pull back on plunger 5 to 10 seconds. If no blood appears, inject medicine slowly, at a rate of 10 sec/mL.	Slow injection rate reduces pain and tissue trauma (Nicoll & Hesby, 2002).

Critical Decision Point: If blood appears in syringe, remove needle and dispose of medication and syringe properly. Prepare another dose of medication for injection.

Steps	Rationale
(5) Wait 10 seconds, and then smoothly and steadily withdraw needle and release skin. Apply gentle pressure with dry gauze if desired.	Allows time for medication to absorb into muscle before removing syringe. Some advocate use of dry gauze to minimize client discomfort (Nicoll & Hesby, 2002).
C. **Intradermal**	
(1) With non-dominant hand, stretch skin over site with forefinger or thumb.	Needle pierces tight skin more easily.
(2) With needle almost against client's skin, insert it slowly with bevel up at a 5- to 15-degree angle until resistance is felt. Then advance needle through epidermis to approximately 3 mm below skin surface. Needle tip can be seen through skin.	Ensures needle tip is in dermis.
(3) Inject medication slowly. Normally, resistance is felt. If not, needle is too deep; remove and begin again.	Slow injection minimizes discomfort at site. Dermal layer is tight and does not expand easily when solution is injected.
(4) While injecting medication, notice that small bleb approximately 6 mm in diameter (resembling mosquito bite) appears on skin's surface (see illustration).	Bleb indicates medication is deposited in dermis.
20. Withdraw needle while applying alcohol swab or gauze gently over site.	Support of tissue around injection site minimizes discomfort during needle withdrawal. Dry gauze may minimize client discomfort associated with alcohol on nonintact skin.

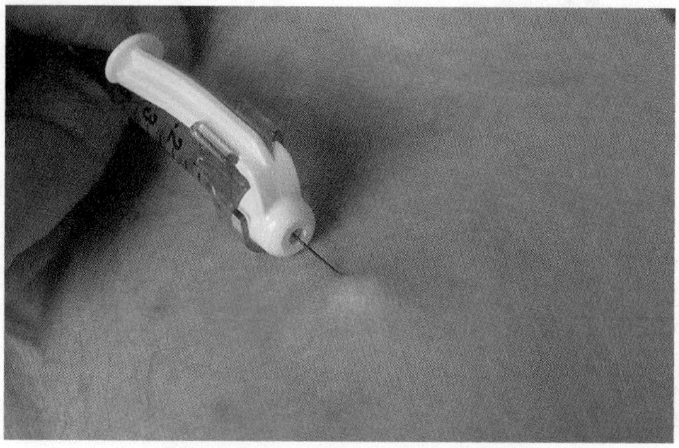

STEP **19C(4)** Injection creates a small bleb.

Steps	Rationale
21. Apply gentle pressure. Do not massage site. Apply bandage if needed.	Massage may cause underlying tissue damage. Massage of ID site may disperse medication into underlying tissue layers and alter test results.
22. Assist client to comfortable position.	Gives client sense of well-being.
23. Discard uncapped needle or needle enclosed in safety shield and attached syringe into puncture and leak-proof receptacle. When nurse is unable to leave client's bedside, a one-handed technique can be used to recap a needle.	Prevents injury to client and health care personnel. Recapping needles increases risk of needle-stick injury (Health Canada, 1997).
24. Remove disposable gloves and perform hand hygiene.	Reduces transmission of micro-organisms.
25. Stay with client 3 to 5 minutes and observe for any allergic reactions.	Severe anaphylactic reaction is characterized by dyspnea, wheezing, and circulatory collapse.
26. Periodically return to client's room to ask if client feels any acute pain, burning, numbness, or tingling at injection site.	Continued discomfort may indicate injury to underlying bones or nerves.
27. Inspect site, noting any bruising or induration.	Bruising or induration indicates complication associated with injection. Document findings and notify health care provider. Provide warm compress to site.
28. Observe client's response to medication at times that correlate with the medication's onset, peak, and duration.	IM medications are rapidly absorbed. Adverse effects of parenteral medications may develop rapidly. Nurse's observations determine efficacy of medication action.
29. Ask client to explain purpose and effects of medication.	Evaluates client's understanding of information taught.
30. *For ID injections,* use skin pencil and draw circle around perimeter of injection site. Read site within 48 to 72 hours of injection.	Pencil mark makes site easy to find. Site must be read at various intervals to determine test results. Refer to manufacturer's directions to determine when to read the test's results.

Unexpected Outcomes and Related Interventions

- Raised, reddened, or hard zone (induration) forms around ID test site.
  - Notify client's health care provider.
  - Document sensitivity to injected allergen or positive test if tuberculin skin testing was completed.
- Hypertrophy of skin develops from repeated Sub-Q injections.
  - Do not use this site for future injections.
  - Instruct client not to use site for 6 months.
- Client develops signs and symptoms of allergy or side effects.
  - Follow institutional policy or guidelines for appropriate response to adverse drug reactions.
  - Notify client's health care provider immediately.
- Client complains of localized pain, numbness, tingling, or burning at injection site.
  - Potential injury to nerve or tissues may have occurred.
  - Assess injection site.
  - Document findings.
  - Notify client's health care provider.

Recording and Reporting

- Chart medication dose, route, site, time, and date given in medication record.
- Report any undesirable effects from medication to nurse in charge or physician.
- Record client's response to medications in nurses' notes.

Home Care Considerations

- Assess the client's readiness to learn before instructing on self-injections. Some clients are hesitant to administer injections to themselves; relieve any anxiety before teaching this skill to a client.
- Some clients prefer to reuse their syringes to save costs. This practice is safe and practical if the needle is not contaminated during the preparation and administration of the injection. Needles should be recapped immediately after use.
- Clients can often purchase or obtain sharps boxes for home use. If this is not feasible, a hard plastic bottle that cannot be seen through (e.g., a fabric softener bottle or detergent bottle) may be used to safely store syringes after use. Disposal of needles used in the home varies among communities. Check with local authorities to verify how to dispose of needles.

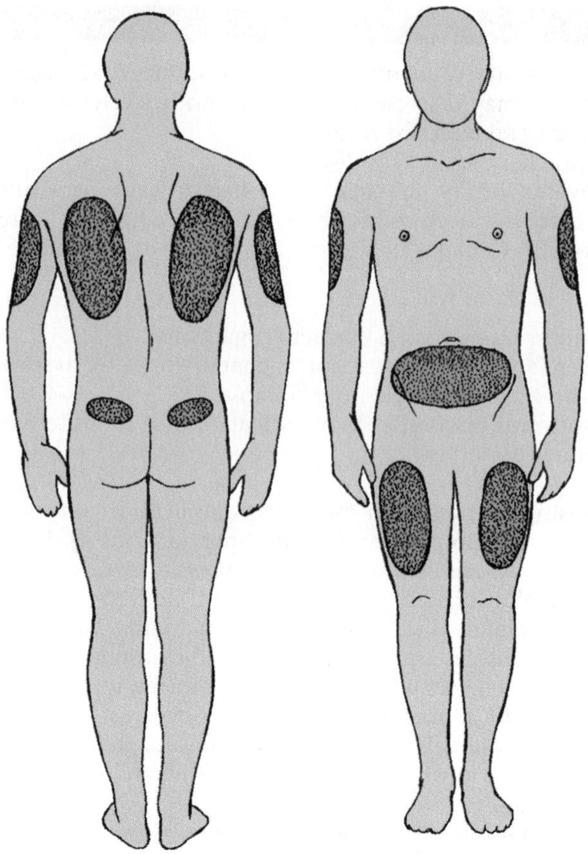

FIGURE 30–21 Sites recommended for subcutaneous injections.

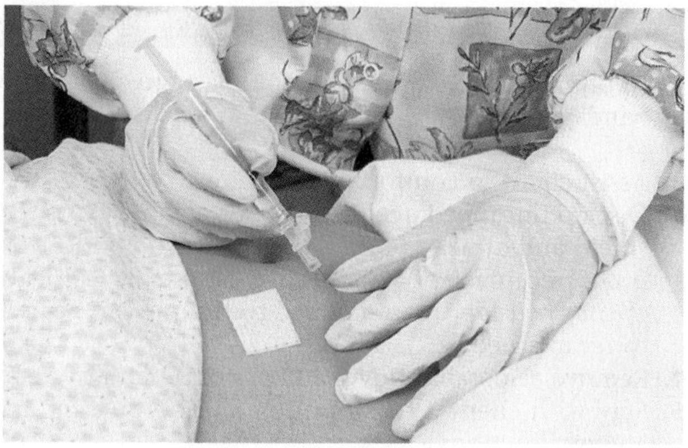

FIGURE 30–22 Giving sub-Q heparin in the abdomen.

Clients with diabetes should practise intrasite rotation of insulin injections. Use of the same part of the body for a sequence of injections provides more consistency in the absorption of the insulin. For example, if the morning insulin is injected into the client's arm, then a subsequent injection should also be given in the arm. The injections are to be given at least 2.5 cm away from the previous site. No injection site should be used again for at least 1 month.

Only small doses (0.5 to 1 mL) of water-soluble medications should be given subcutaneously because the tissue is sensitive to irritating solutions and large volumes of medications. Collection of medications within the tissues can cause sterile abscesses, which appear as hardened, painful lumps under the skin.

A client's body weight indicates the depth of the subcutaneous layer. Therefore, the nurse must choose the needle length and angle of insertion based on weight. Generally, a 25-gauge 1.6-cm needle inserted at a 45-degree angle (Figure 30–23) or a 1.3-cm needle inserted at a 90-degree angle deposits medications into the subcutaneous tissue of a normal-size client. A child may require only a 1.3-cm needle. If the client is obese, the nurse often pinches the tissue and uses a needle long enough to insert through fatty tissue at the base of the skinfold. The preferred needle length is one half the width of the skinfold. With this method, the angle of insertion may be between 45 and 90 degrees. Thin clients may have insufficient tissue for subcutaneous injections. The upper abdomen is the best site for injection with this client.

Insulin syringes generally come with 26- to 29-gauge needles. To ensure that the insulin reaches the subcutaneous tissue, the nurse follows this rule: If 5 cm of tissue can be grasped, the needle should be inserted at a 90-degree angle; if 2.5 cm of tissue can be grasped, the needle should be inserted at a 45-degree angle.

Intramuscular Injections. The IM route provides faster medication absorption than the subcutaneous because of a muscle's greater vascularity. However, IM injections are associated with many risks. Therefore, whenever administering a medication by the IM route, the nurse must first verify that the injection is justified (Nicoll & Hesby, 2002).

The nurse uses a longer and heavier-gauge needle to pass through subcutaneous tissue and penetrate deep muscle tissue (see Skill 30-8). Weight and the amount of adipose tissue can influence needle size selection. For example, an obese client may require a needle 7.5 cm long, and a thin client may only require a 1.3- to 2.5-cm needle.

The angle of insertion for an IM injection is 90 degrees (see Figure 30–23). Muscle is less sensitive to irritating and viscous medications. A normal, well-developed client can tolerate 3 mL of medication into a larger muscle without severe muscle discomfort. A larger volume of medication is unlikely to be absorbed properly. Children, older adults, and thin clients can tolerate only 2 mL of an IM injection. Hockenberry and others (2003) recommended giving no more than 1 mL to small children and older infants.

The nurse assesses the integrity of a muscle before giving an injection. The muscle should be free of tenderness. Repeated injections in the same muscle can cause severe discomfort. With the client relaxed, the nurse can palpate the muscle to rule out any hardened lesions. The nurse can minimize discomfort during an injection by helping the client assume a position that will help reduce muscle strain. Other interventions, such as distraction and applying pressure to the IM site, may be used to decrease pain during an IM injection (Box 30-16).

Sites. When selecting an IM site, the nurse considers the following: Is the area free of infection or necrosis? Are there local areas of bruising or abrasions? What is the

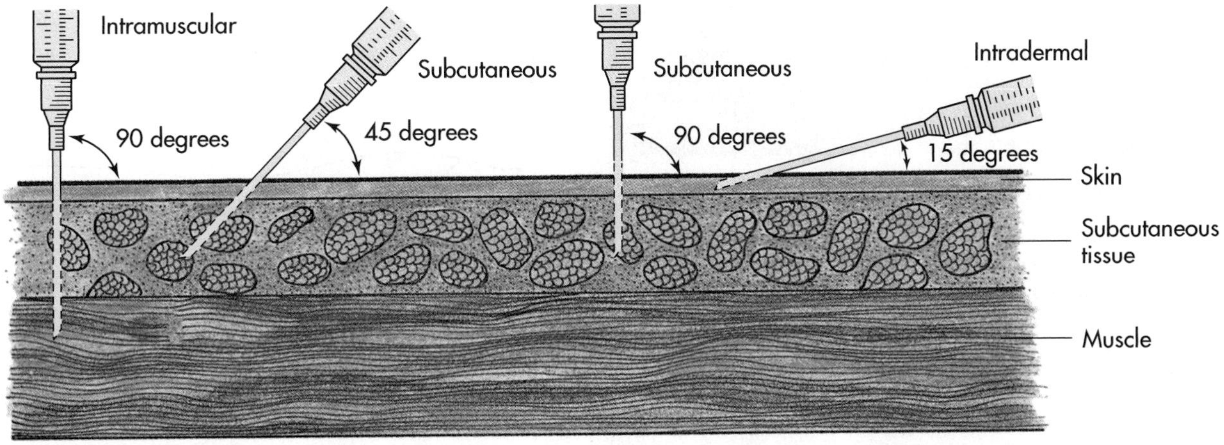

FIGURE **30–23** Comparison of angles of insertion for intramuscular (90 degrees), subcutaneous (45 and 90 degrees), and intradermal (15 degrees) injections.

Research Highlight — *Box 30-16*

Reducing Pain During Intramuscular Injections

Research Focus

Intramuscular injections are often associated with pain. Touch and massage has been used to decrease perceptions of pain. Further research is necessary to determine if the application of pressure at an injection site will decrease the client's perception of pain.

Research Abstract

The purpose of this study was to determine if the application of pressure at an intramuscular injection site would reduce the client's experience of pain. This study used an experimental design with intrasubject comparison. The 74 participants were Chinese students who were participating in an immunization program. Each participant received the hepatitis A vaccine and the hepatitis B vaccine, one in each arm. Pressure was applied to one arm for 10 seconds before the injection and was not applied to the other arm. The arm that received the pressure was determined randomly. After each injection, the participants ranked their pain on a Cantonese 0-to-10 pain scale. A pressure-sensing device measured the amount of pressure exerted. Females in this study reported higher levels of pain for all injections when compared with males. However, male and female participants both reported significantly less pain when they received a pressure of about 200 mm Hg for 10 seconds before the immunization.

Evidence-Based Practice

- Applying pressure at the site of an IM injection may reduce the pain experienced by the client.
- The findings of this study support the gate-control theory of the physiology of pain.
- The gender difference in the report of pain supports that men and women experience and report pain differently.
- Further research is needed to support these results with other client populations, medication types, and injection sites.

Reference

Chung, J., Ng, W. M. Y., & Wong, T. K. S. (2002). An experimental study on the use of manual pressure to reduce pain in intramuscular injections. *Journal of Clinical Nursing, 11*(4), 457–461.

location of underlying bones, nerves, and major blood vessels? What volume of medication is to be administered? Each site has certain advantages and disadvantages. The characteristics of each IM site and indications for use of each site are listed in Box 30-17.

Ventrogluteal. The ventrogluteal muscle involves the gluteus medius, is situated deep and away from major nerves and blood vessels, and is a safe site for all clients because it is a large muscle that is well-developed in adults and young children, including those who do not walk (Nicoll & Hesby, 2002). Research has shown that injuries such as fibrosis, nerve damage, abscess, tissue necrosis, muscle contraction, gangrene, and pain have been associated with all of the common IM sites except the ventrogluteal site. The only published case study of a complication at the ventrogluteal site reported a local reaction to the medication, which is not a complication associated with the site itself (Nicoll & Hesby, 2002).

Safety Alert. Research that has investigated complications associated with IM injection sites indicates that the ventrogluteal site is the preferred site for most injections given to adults and children over 7 months (Hockenberry et al., 2003; Nicoll & Hesby, 2002).

Box 30-17 Characteristics of Intramuscular Sites and Indications for Usage

Vastus Lateralis

- Lacks major nerves and blood vessels
- Rapid drug absorption
- Preferred site for infants (less than 12 months) receiving immunizations
- May also be used in older children and toddlers receiving immunizations

Ventrogluteal

- A deep site, situated away from major nerves and blood vessels
- Less chance of contamination in incontinent clients or infants
- Easily identified by any prominent bony landmark
- Preferred site for medications (e.g., antibiotics) that are larger in volume, more viscous, and irritating for adults, children, and infants

Deltoid

- Easily accessible but muscle not well-developed in most clients
- Used for small amounts of medications
- Not used in infants or children with underdeveloped muscles
- Potential for injury to radial and ulnar nerves or brachial artery
- May be used for immunizations for toddlers, older children, and adults
- Recommended site for hepatitis B vaccine and rabies injections

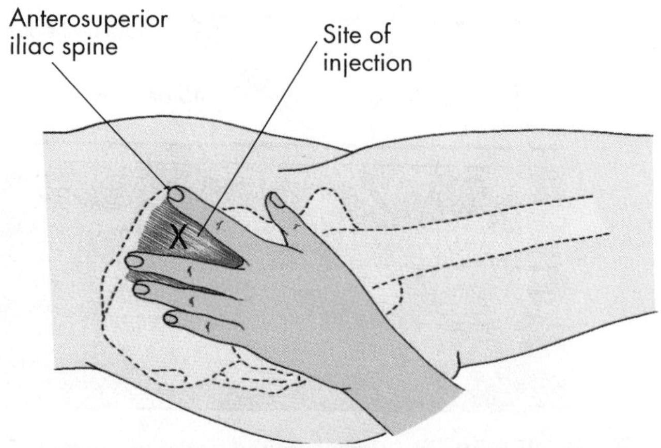

A

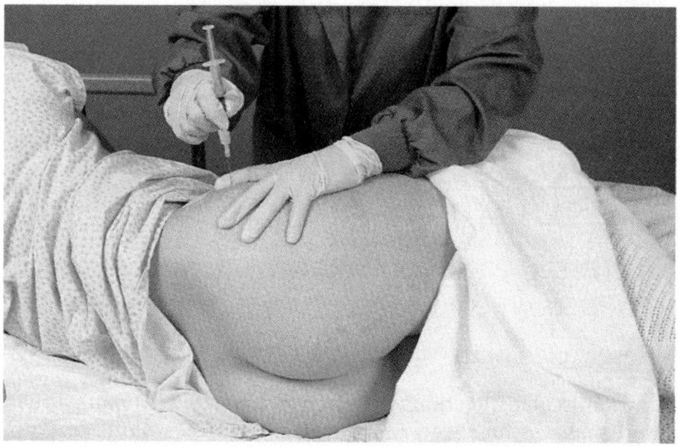

B

FIGURE **30–24** **A,** Landmarks for ventrogluteal site. **B,** Giving IM injection in ventrogluteal muscle.

The nurse locates the ventrogluteal muscle by placing the heel of the hand over the greater trochanter of the client's hip with the wrist perpendicular to the femur. The right hand is used for the left hip, and the left hand is used for the right hip. The nurse points the thumb toward the client's groin and fingers toward the client's head, points the index finger to the anterior superior iliac spine, and extends the middle finger back along the iliac crest toward the buttock. The index finger, the middle finger, and the iliac crest form a V-shaped triangle, and the injection site is the centre of the triangle (Figure 30–24). The client may lie on his or her side or back. Flexing of the knee and hip helps the client relax this muscle.

Vastus Lateralis. The vastus lateralis muscle is another injection site. The muscle is thick and well-developed, is located on the anterior lateral aspect of the thigh, and extends in an adult from a handbreadth above the knee to a handbreadth below the greater trochanter of the femur (Figure 30–25). The middle third of the muscle is the suggested site for injection. The width of the muscle usually extends from the midline of the thigh to the midline of the thigh's outer side. With young children or cachectic clients, it helps to grasp the body of the muscle during injection to be sure that the medication is deposited in muscle tissue. To help relax the muscle, the nurse asks the client to lie flat with the knee slightly flexed or in a sitting position.

Dorsogluteal. The dorsogluteal muscle has been a traditional site for IM injections. However, studies have demonstrated that the exact location of the sciatic nerve varies from one person to another. If a needle hits a sciatic nerve, the client may experience permanent or partial paralysis of the involved leg. Therefore this site should *not* be used (Beyea & Nicoll, 1996; Rodger & King, 2000).

Deltoid. Although the deltoid site is easily accessible, the muscle is not well-developed in many clients. There is a potential for injury when using this site because the axillary, radial, brachial, and ulnar nerves and brachial artery lie within the upper arm along the humerus (Figure 30–26, *A*). The nurse should use this site only for small medication volumes, when giving immunizations, or when other sites are inaccessible because of dressings or casts (Nicoll & Hesby, 2002).

To locate the deltoid muscle, the nurse fully exposes the client's upper arm and shoulder. A tight-fitting sleeve should not be rolled up. The nurse has the client relax the

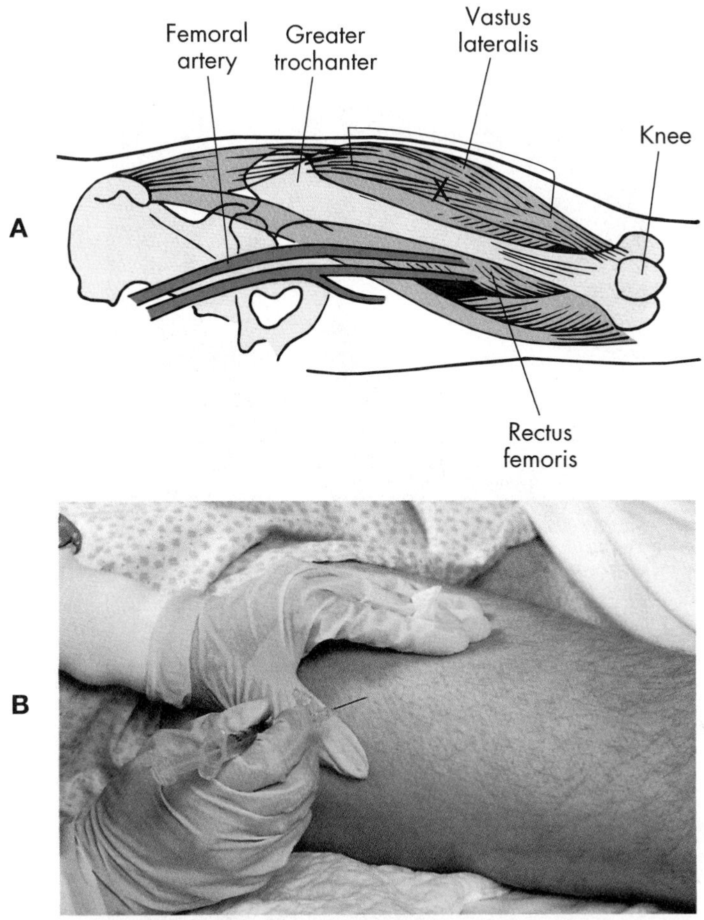

FIGURE **30–25** **A,** Landmarks for vastus lateralis site. **B,** Giving IM injection in vastus lateralis muscle.

arm at the side and flex the elbow. The client may sit, stand, or lie down (Figure 30–26, *B*). The nurse palpates the lower edge of the acromion process, which forms the base of a triangle in line with the midpoint of the lateral aspect of the upper arm. The injection site is in the centre of the triangle, about 3 to 5 cm below the acromion process (Nicoll & Hesby, 2002). The nurse may also locate the site by placing four fingers across the deltoid muscle, with the top finger along the acromion process. The injection site is then three fingerwidths below the acromion process.

Special Techniques in IM Injections

Air-Lock Technique. The use of an air bubble is a topic that draws heated debate among nurses. Historically, nurses believed that the air bubble was required to ensure that the correct dose of medication was prepared in the syringe. Additionally, nurses were told that the air bubble would ensure that the medication would remain in the muscle. However, neither of these two arguments for the use of the air bubble is supported today. Therefore drawing up an air bubble is no longer recommended (Nicoll & Hesby, 2002).

Z-Track Method. It is recommended that when administering IM injections the **Z-track method** be used to minimize local skin irritation by sealing the medication

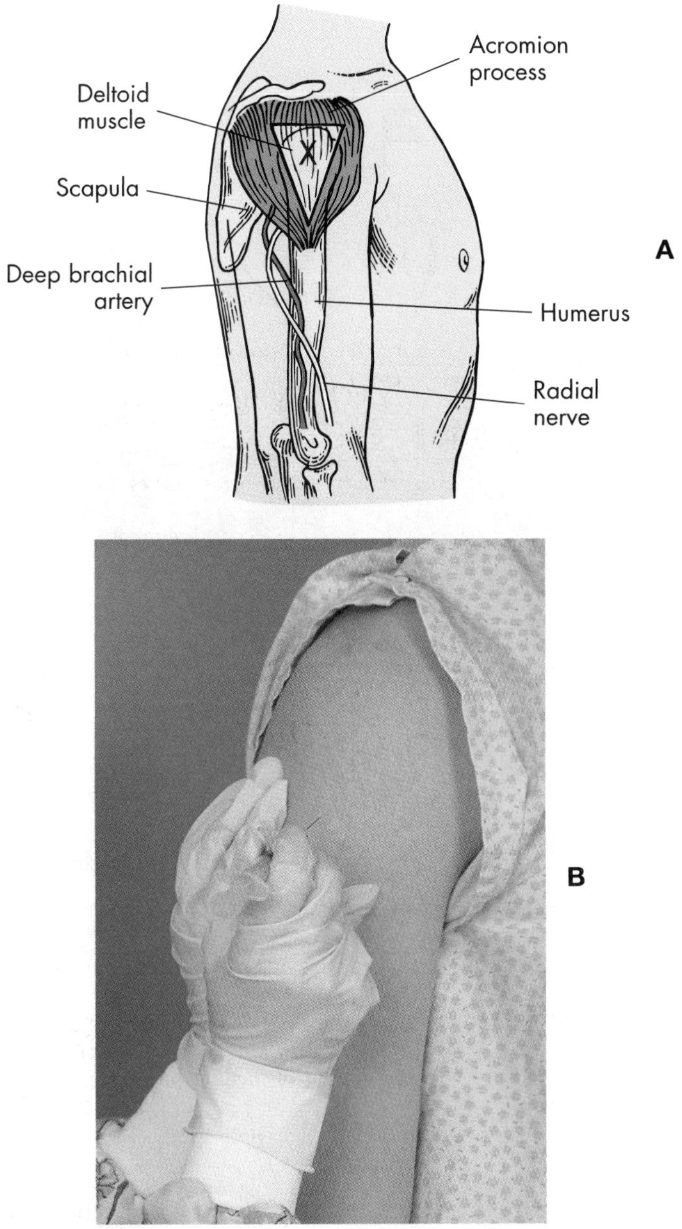

FIGURE **30–26** **A,** Landmarks for deltoid site. **B,** Giving IM injection in deltoid muscle.

in muscle tissue. The nurse selects an IM site, preferably in a large, deep muscle such as the ventrogluteal muscle. A new needle must be applied to the syringe after preparing the medication so that no solution remains on the outside needle shaft. After preparing the site with an antiseptic swab, the nurse pulls the overlying skin and subcutaneous tissues approximately 2.5 to 3.5 cm laterally to the side. Holding the skin taut with the non-dominant hand, the nurse injects the needle deep into the muscle. With practice, the nurse learns to hold the syringe and aspirate with one hand. The nurse injects the medication slowly if there is no blood return on aspiration. The needle remains inserted for 10 seconds to allow the medication to disperse evenly. The nurse then releases the skin after withdrawing the needle. This leaves a zigzag path that seals the

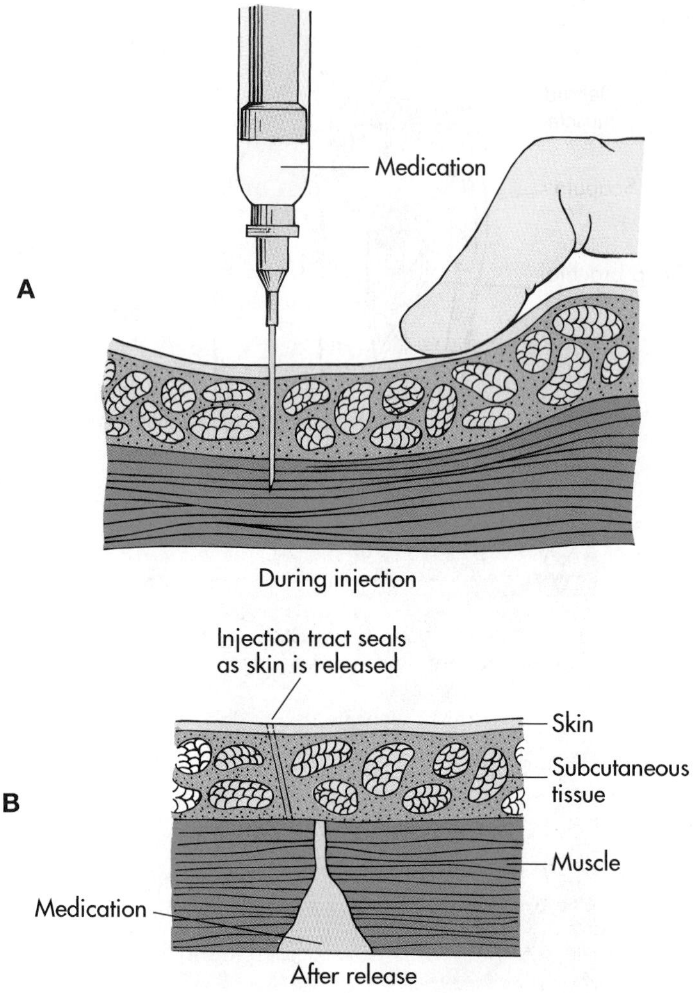

FIGURE **30–27** **A,** Pulling on overlying skin during IM injection moves tissue to prevent later tracking. **B,** The Z-track left after injection prevents the deposit of medication through sensitive tissue.

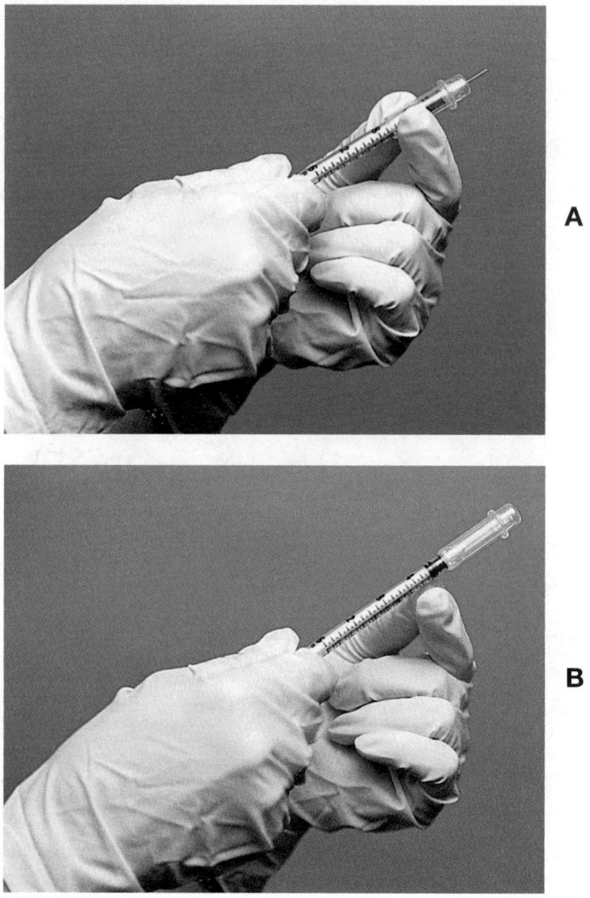

FIGURE **30–28** Needle with plastic guard to prevent needle sticks. **A,** Position of guard before injection. **B,** After injection, the guard locks in place, covering the needle.

needle track where tissue planes slide across each other (Figure 30–27). The medication cannot escape from the muscle tissue. Injections using this technique cause less discomfort and fewer lesions at the injection site (Nicoll & Hesby, 2002).

Intradermal Injections. The nurse typically gives intradermal injections for skin testing (e.g., tuberculin screening and allergy tests). Because these medications are potent, they are injected into the dermis, where blood supply is reduced and medication absorption occurs slowly. A client may have a severe anaphylactic reaction if the medications enter the circulation too rapidly.

Skin testing requires that the nurse be able to see the injection sites clearly for changes in colour and tissue integrity. Intradermal sites should be lightly pigmented, free of lesions, and relatively hairless. The inner forearm and upper back are ideal locations.

The nurse uses a tuberculin or small hypodermic syringe for skin testing. The angle of insertion for an intradermal injection is 5 to 15 degrees (see Figure 30–23), and the bevel of the needle is pointed up. As the nurse injects the medication, a small bleb resembling a mosquito bite should appear on the skin's surface (see Skill 30-8). If a bleb does not appear or if the site bleeds after needle withdrawal, there is a good chance the medication entered subcutaneous tissues. In this case, test results will not be valid.

Safety in Administering Medications by Injection

Needleless Devices. Needlestick injuries occur frequently in all health care settings. Some hospitals report that one third of nursing staff suffer such injuries each year (Canadian Centre for Occupational Health and Safety [CCOHS], 2000). However, because many workers do not report their injuries, the incidence of such injuries is probably even higher. These injuries commonly occur when needles are recapped, IV lines and needles are mishandled, or needles are left at a client's bedside. The risk of exposure of health care workers to blood-borne pathogens has led to the development of "needleless devices" or special needle safety devices.

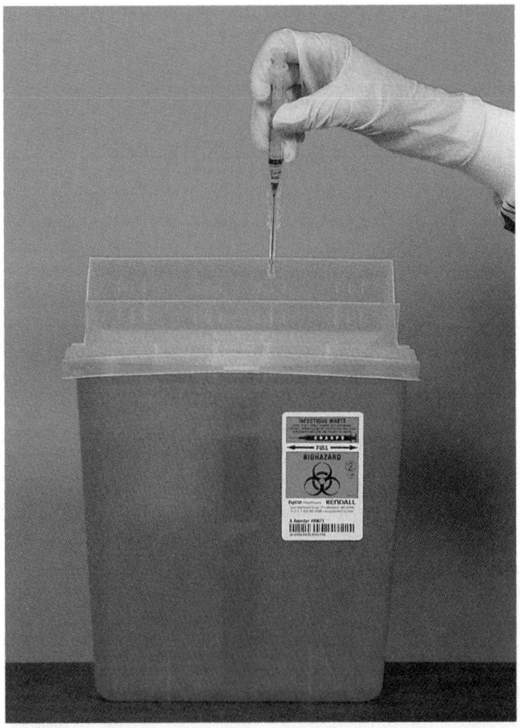

FIGURE **30–29** Sharps disposal using only one hand.

Special syringes are designed with a sheath or guard that covers the needle after it is withdrawn from the skin (Figure 30–28). The needle is immediately covered, eliminating the chance for a needle-stick injury. The syringe and sheath are disposed of together in a receptacle. "Needleless" devices should be used whenever possible to reduce the risk to health care workers of needle sticks and sharps injuries (CCOHS, 2000; Health Canada, 1997, 1999).

Needles and other instruments that are considered "sharps" are always disposed of into clearly marked, appropriate containers (Figure 30–29). Containers should be puncture proof and leak proof. A needle should never be forced into a full needle disposable receptacle. Used needles and syringes are never placed in a wastebasket, in the nurse's pocket, on a client's meal tray, or at the client's bedside. Box 30-18 summarizes recommendations for the prevention of needlestick injuries.

One-Handed Needle Recapping Technique. In administering injections, it may be necessary, for client safety reasons, to recap a contaminated needle. For example, the nurse may be assisting with emergency measures at the bedside and cannot reach a disposable container. If a commercially made recapping device is not available, then the nurse should use the one-handed needle recapping technique that is described in Box 30-19.

IV Administration. The nurse administers medications intravenously by the following methods:

- As mixtures within large volumes of IV fluids
- By injection of a bolus, or small volume, of medication through an existing IV infusion line or intermittent venous access (heparin or saline lock)
- By "piggyback" infusion of a solution containing the prescribed medication and a small volume of IV fluid through an existing IV line

In all three methods, the client has either an existing IV infusion line or an IV access site such as an intermittent infusion (sometime called a heparin or saline lock). In most institutions, policies and procedures list people who may give IV medications and the situations in which they may be given. These policies are based on the medication, capability and availability of staff, and type of monitoring equipment available.

Box 30-18 Recommendations for the Prevention of Needlestick Injuries

- Avoid using needles when effective needless systems or Sharps With Engineered Sharps Injury Protections (SESIP) safety devices are available.
- Never move an exposed needletip toward an unprotected hand.
- Do not recap needles (except for in certain situations, and then use the one-handed technique).
- Plan safe handling and disposal of needles before beginning the procedure.
- Immediately dispose of needles, needleless systems, and SESIP into puncture-proof disposal containers located near the area of use.
- Maintain an exposure control plan (ECP) that includes the following:
  - Assessment and implementation of innovations in procedures and technological developments to reduce risks of exposure to contaminated sharps
  - Employee training addressing risks, hazards, recommended precautions, and the importance of hepatitis B vaccination where appropriate
  - Documentation of consideration and use of appropriate, commercially available, and effective safer devices
  - Selection of devices that do not jeopardize client or employee safety or are determined to be medically inadvisable
  - Documentation of input from employees in ECP as to methods to reduce exposure
  - Annual re-examination of ECP
- Maintain a sharps injury log that protects the privacy of those who have had sharps injuries and includes the following:
  - Type and brand of device involved in the incident
  - Location of the incident (e.g., department or work area)
  - Description of the incident
  - Record of every incident where a needle was found at the bedside or thrown into garbage

Data from *Needlestick Injuries,* CCOHS, 2000, retrieved November 11, 2004, from *http://www.ccohs.ca/oshanswers/diseases/needlestick_injuries.html;* "Occupational Exposure to Bloodborne Pathogens: Needlestick and Other Sharp Injuries—Final Rule" (CFR 29, part 1910), Occupational Safety and Health Administration, 2001, *Federal Register, 66,* p. 5317; and *NIOSH alert: Preventing needlestick injuries in health care settings* (DHHS [NIOSH] Publication No. 2000-108), National Institute for Occupational Safety and Health, 1999, Cincinnati, OH: Author.

Box 30-19 Procedural Guidelines

One-Handed Needle Recapping Technique

Needles should never be recapped. **This procedure should be used only when a sharps disposal box is unavailable and the nurse cannot leave the client's room.** Needlestick injuries place the health care worker at risk for blood-borne pathogens. After using a needle, the health care worker should dispose of it in the nearest designated container.

1. Before giving the injection, place the needle cover on a solid, immovable object such as the rim of a bedside table. The open end of the cap should face the nurse and be within reach of the nurse's dominant, or injection, hand.
2. Give the injection.
3. Place the tip of the needle at the entrance of the cap. *Gently* slide the needle into the needle cover (see illustrations).
4. Once the needle is inside the cover, use the object's resistance to completely cover the needle (see illustration).
5. Dispose of the needle at the first opportunity.
6. Perform hand hygiene.

A

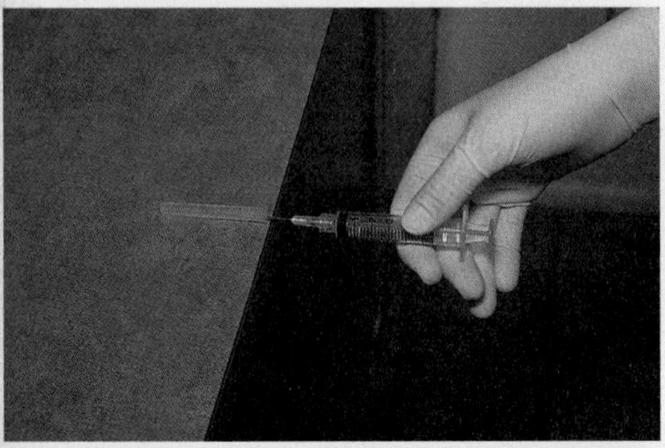

B

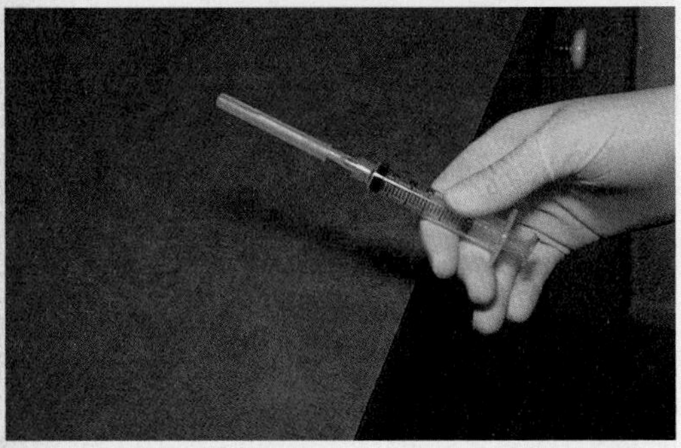

STEP **3** **A,** Place needle tip at entrance of the cap. **B,** Slide needle into the cover.

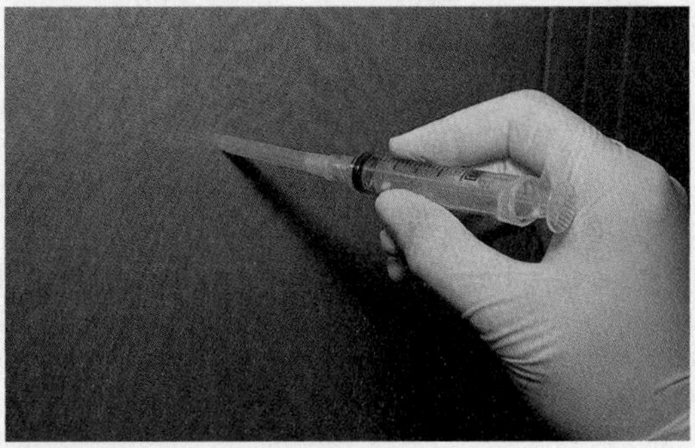

STEP **4** Place needle cover against resistance to secure.

Chapter 36 describes the technique for performing venipuncture and establishing continuous IV fluid infusions. Medication administration is only one reason for supplying IV fluids. IV fluid therapy is used primarily for fluid replacement in clients unable to take oral fluids and as a means of supplying electrolytes and nutrients.

When using any method of IV medication administration, the nurse must observe clients closely for symptoms of adverse reactions. After a medication enters the bloodstream, it begins to act immediately, and there is no way to stop its action. Thus, the nurse takes special care to avoid errors in dose calculation and preparation. The nurse should double-check the six rights of safe medication administration and know the desired action and side effects. If the medication has an antidote, it must be available during administration. When administering potent medications, the nurse assesses vital signs before, during, and after infusion.

Administering medications by the IV route has advantages. Often the nurse uses the IV route in emergencies when a fast-acting medication must be delivered quickly. The IV route is also best when it is necessary to establish constant therapeutic blood levels. Some medications are highly alkaline and irritating to muscle and subcutaneous tissue. These medications cause less discomfort when given intravenously.

> ***Safety Alert.*** Because IV medications are immediately available to the bloodstream once they are administered, the nurse must verify the prescribed rate of administration so that the medication is given over the appropriate amount of time. Clients may experience severe adverse reactions if IV medications are administered too quickly. Verify the rate of administration with a drug reference or a pharmacist before giving any IV medication.

Large-Volume Infusions. Of the three methods of administering IV medications, mixing medications in large volumes of fluids is the safest and easiest. Medications are diluted in large volumes (500 mL or 1,000 mL) of compatible IV fluids such as normal saline or lactated Ringer's solution (Skill 30-9). In most institutions, the pharmacist adds medications to the primary container of IV solution to ensure asepsis. Because the medication is not in a concentrated form, the risk of side effects or fatal reactions is minimal when infused over the prescribed time frame. Vitamins and potassium chloride are two types of medications commonly added to IV fluids. However, there is a danger with continuous infusion: If the IV fluid is infused too rapidly, the client may suffer circulatory fluid overload.

IV Bolus. An IV bolus, or "push," involves introducing a concentrated dose of a medication directly into the systemic circulation (Skill 30-10). An advantage of a bolus is that it requires only a small amount of fluid to deliver the medication; therefore, it is useful to use when the client is on restricted fluid. However, an IV bolus is the most dangerous method for administering medications because there is no time to correct errors. In addition, a bolus may cause direct irritation to the lining of blood vessels. Therefore, some authors have added three additional "rights" to administering IV push medications: the right dilution or flush, the right speed, and the right monitoring (Zurlinden, 2002).

Before administering a bolus, the nurse confirms placement of the IV line. This involves obtaining a blood return through the IV catheter or needle. The inability to obtain a blood return suggests that the needle or catheter is in the client's tissues or resting against the vein wall. A medication should never be given intravenously if the insertion site appears puffy or edematous or the IV fluid cannot flow at the proper rate. Accidental injection of a medication into the tissues around a vein can cause pain, sloughing of tissues, and abscesses, depending on the medication's composition.

The rate of administration of an IV bolus medication is usually determined by the amount of medication that can be given per minute. The nurse should look up each medication to determine the recommended concentration and rate of administration. The purpose for which a medication is prescribed, and any potential adverse effects related to the rate or route of administration, must be considered when a nurse gives a medication IV push.

Volume-Controlled Infusions. Another way of administering IV medications is through small amounts (50 to 100 mL) of compatible IV fluids. The fluid is within a secondary fluid container separate from the primary fluid bag. The container connects directly to the primary IV line or to separate tubing that inserts into the primary line. Three types of containers are volume-control administration sets (e.g., Volutrol or Pediatrol), piggyback and/or tandem set, and mini-infusors. Using volume-controlled infusions has several advantages:

- It reduces risk of rapid-dose infusion by IV push. Medications are diluted and infused over longer time intervals (e.g., 30 to 60 minutes).
- It allows for administration of medications (e.g., antibiotics) that are stable for a limited time in solution.
- It allows for control of IV fluid intake.

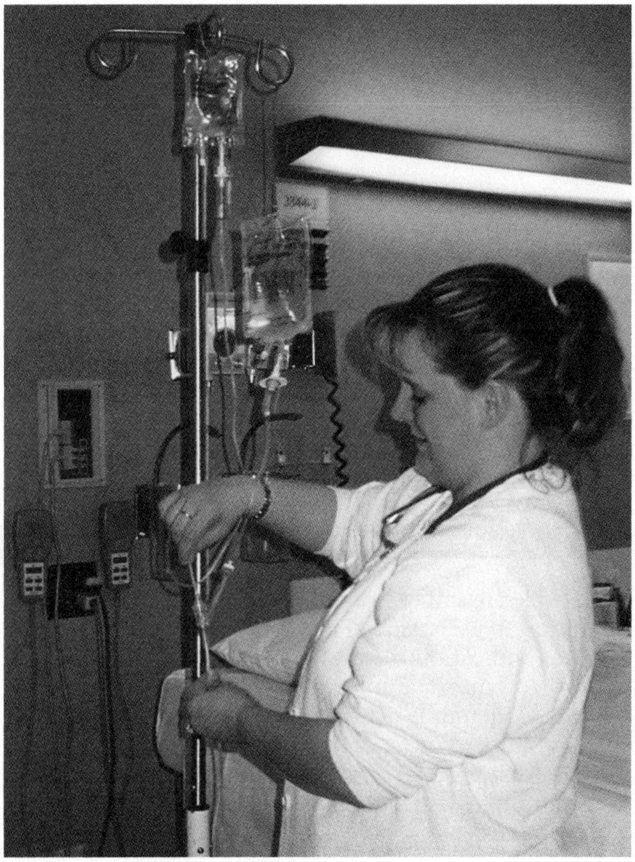

FIGURE **30–30** Piggyback set-up.

Volume-Control Administration. Volume-control administration (Volutrol, Buretrol, Pediatrol) sets are small (50 to 150 mL) containers that attach just below the primary infusion bag or bottle. The set is attached and filled in a manner similar to that used with a regular IV infusion. However, the priming filling of the set is different, depending on the type of filter (floating valve or membrane) within the set. The nurse should follow package directions for priming sets (see chapter 36).

Piggyback. A piggyback is a small (25 to 250 mL) IV bag or bottle connected to short tubing lines that connects to the *upper* Y-port of a primary infusion line or to an intermittent venous access (Figure 30–30). The piggyback tubing is a microdrip or macrodrip system (chapter 36). The set is called a piggyback because the small bag or bottle is set higher than the primary infusion bag or bottle. In the piggyback set-up, the main line does not infuse when the piggybacked medication is infusing. The port of the primary IV line contains a back-check valve that automatically stops flow of the primary infusion once the piggyback infusion flows. After the piggyback solution infuses and the solution within the tubing falls below the level of the primary infusion drip chamber, the back-check valve opens and the primary infusion again flows.

Tandem. A tandem set-up is a small (25 to 100 mL) IV bag or bottle connected to a short tubing line to the *lower* Y-port of a primary infusion line or to an intermittent

Text continued on p. 910

Skill 30-9 Adding Medications to Intravenous Fluid Containers

Delegation Considerations

Adding medications to IV fluid containers should not be delegated to unregulated care providers. (In some institutions, the pharmacist may add medications to primary containers of IV solutions to ensure asepsis.)

Equipment

- Vial or ampule of prescribed medication
- Syringe of appropriate size (5 to 20 mL)
- Sterile needle (2.5 to 3.8 cm, 19 to 21 gauge) with special filters (optional)
- Correct diluent if indicated (e.g., sterile water, normal saline)
- Sterile IV fluid container (bag or bottle, 25 to 1,000 mL in volume)
- Alcohol or antiseptic swab
- Label to attach to IV bag or bottle
- MAR

Steps	Rationale
1. Check prescriber's order to determine type of IV solution to use, name of medication, dosage, route, and drug indication.	Client's overall physical condition dictates type of IV solution used. Ensures safe and accurate medication administration.
2. Collect information necessary to administer drug safely, including action, purpose, side effects, normal dose, time of peak onset, and nursing implications.	Allows nurse to give medication safely and to monitor client's response to therapy.
3. When more than one medication is to be added to IV solution, assess for compatibility of medications.	Medications often are incompatible when mixed together. Chemical reactions that occur result in clouding or crystallization of IV fluids. Check hospital policy for approved medication compatibility list.
4. Assess client's systemic fluid balance, as reflected by skin hydration and turgor, body weight, pulse, and blood pressure.	Danger of continuous IV infusions is that fluids may infuse too rapidly, causing circulatory overload (Hockenberry et al., 2003).
5. Assess client's history of medication allergies.	IV administration of medications causes rapid effects. Allergic response can be immediate.
6. Perform hand hygiene.	Reduces transfer of micro-organisms.
7. Assess IV insertion site for signs of infiltration or phlebitis (see chapter 36).	An intact, properly functioning site ensures medication is given safely.
8. Assemble supplies in medication room.	Ensures procedure will be orderly, with less likelihood of contaminating supplies.
9. Prepare prescribed medication from vial or ampule (see Skill 30-7).	Ensures accurate delivery of medication.
10. Identify client by reading identification bracelet and asking name. Compare with MAR or medication order.	Ensures correct client receives medication.
11. Assess client's understanding of purpose of medication therapy.	May reveal need for education.
12. Add medication to new container (usually done in medication room or at medication cart):	
a. *Solution in a bag:* Locate medication injection port on plastic IV solution bag. Port has small rubber stopper at end. Do not select port for the IV tubing insertion or air vent.	Medication injection port is self-sealing to prevent introduction of micro-organisms after repeated use.
b. *Solution in a bottle:* Locate injection site on IV solution bottle, which is often covered by a metal or plastic cap.	Accidental injection of medication through main tubing port or air vent can alter pressure within bottle and cause fluid leaks through air vent. Cap seals bottle to maintain its sterility.
c. Wipe off port or injection site with alcohol or antiseptic swab (see illustration).	Reduces risk of introducing micro-organisms into bag during needle insertion.
d. Remove needle cap or sheath from syringe and insert needle of syringe or needleless device through centre of injection port or site; inject medication (see illustration).	Injection of needle into sides of port may produce leak and lead to fluid contamination.

Steps	Rationale

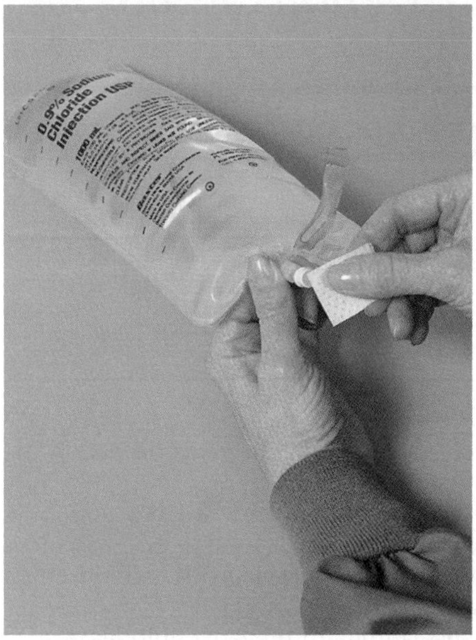

STEP **12c** Cleanse injection port with antiseptic swab.

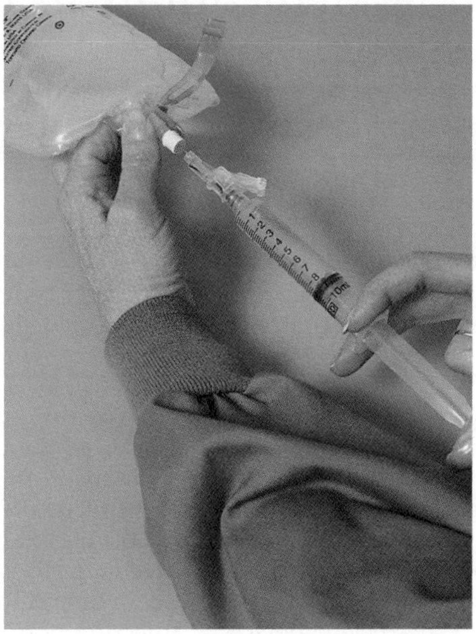

STEP **12d** Inject medication through port.

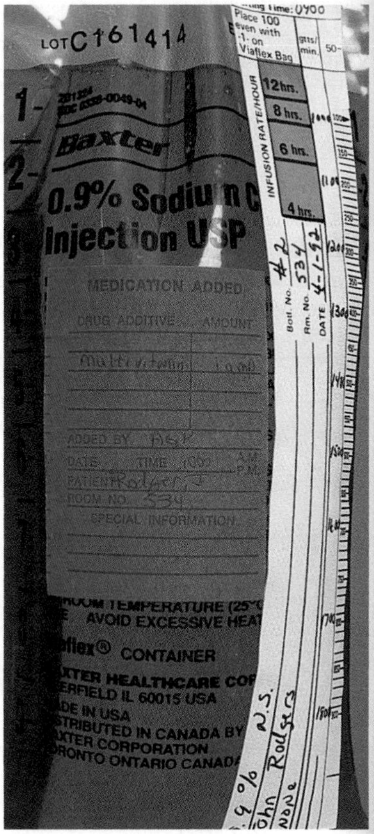

STEP **12g** Affix label to IV bag.

Steps	Rationale
e. Withdraw syringe from bag or bottle.	Open tubing port in bottle provides direct route for microorganisms to enter solution. Bags have self-sealing port.
f. Mix medication and IV solution by holding bag or bottle and turning it gently end to end.	Allows even distribution of medication.
g. Complete medication label with name and dose of medication, date, time, and nurse's initials. Apply it to bottle or bag. *Optional (check agency policy): Apply a flow strip that identifies the time the solution was hung and intervals indicating fluid levels (see illustration).* Spike bag or bottle with IV tubing.	Label can be easily read during infusion of solution. Informs nurses and physicians of contents of bag or bottle.

Critical Decision Point: Do not use felt-tip markers to draw on flow strip. The ink can penetrate the plastic and leak into the IV solution.

Steps	Rationale
13. Bring assembled items to client's bedside.	Ensures correct client receives ordered medication.
14. Prepare client by explaining that medication is to be given through existing IV line or one to be started. Explain that no discomfort should be felt during medication infusion. Encourage client to report symptoms of discomfort.	Most IV medications do not cause discomfort when diluted. However, potassium chloride can be irritating. Pain at insertion site may be early indication of infiltration.
15. Regulate infusion at ordered rate.	Prevents rapid infusion of fluid.

Critical Decision Point: Some medications (e.g., potassium chloride) can cause serious adverse reactions, including fatal cardiac dysrhythmias. These medications should be infused on an IV pump. Check institutional guidelines or policies indicating which IV medications require administration on an IV pump.

Skill 30-9 Adding Medications to Intravenous Fluid Containers—cont'd

Steps	Rationale
16. Add medication to existing container:	
Critical Decision Point: Because there is no way to know exactly how much IV fluid is in an existing hanging IV container, there is no way to determine the exact concentration of the medication in the IV solution. Therefore it is recommended that medications be added to new IV fluid containers whenever possible.	
a. Prepare vented IV bottle or plastic bag:	
(1) Check volume of solution remaining in bottle or bag.	Proper minimal volume (see drug insert) is needed to dilute medication adequately.
(2) Close off IV infusion clamp.	Prevents medication from directly entering circulation as it is injected into bag or bottle.
(3) Wipe off medication port with an alcohol or antiseptic swab.	Mechanically removes micro-organisms that could enter container during needle insertion.
(4) Insert syringe needle or needleless device through injection port and inject medication.	Injection port is self-sealing and prevents fluid leaks.
(5) Withdraw syringe from bag or bottle.	
(6) Lower bag or bottle from IV pole and gently mix. Rehang bag.	Ensures medication is evenly distributed.
b. Complete medication label and apply it to bag or bottle.	Informs nurses and physicians of contents of bag or bottle.
c. Regulate infusion to desired rate. Use IV pump if indicated.	Prevents rapid infusion of fluid.
17. Properly dispose of equipment and supplies. Do not cap needle of syringe. Specially sheathed needles are discarded as a unit with needle covered.	Proper disposal of needle prevents injury to nurse and client. Capping of needles increases risk of needle-stick injuries.
18. Perform hand hygiene.	Reduces transmission of micro-organisms.
19. Observe client for signs or symptoms of medication reaction.	IV medications can cause rapid effects.
20. Observe for signs and symptoms of fluid volume excess.	Rapid uncontrolled infusion can cause circulatory overload.
21. Periodically return to client's room to assess IV insertion site and rate of infusion.	Over time, IV site may become infiltrated or needle malpositioned. Flow rate may change according to client's position or volume left in container.
22. Observe for signs or symptoms of IV infiltration.	Infiltrated medications can injure tissue.

Unexpected Outcomes and Related Interventions

- Client has adverse or allergic reaction to medication.
  - Follow institutional policy or guidelines for appropriate response and reporting of adverse drug reactions.
  - Notify client's health care provider immediately.
- Client develops signs of fluid volume overload (e.g., abnormal breath sounds, shortness of breath, intake greater than output).
  - Circulatory regulation may be compromised.
  - Stop IV infusion.
  - Notify client's health care provider immediately.
- IV site becomes swollen, warm, reddened, and tender to touch (see chapter 36).
  - Indicates phlebitis.
  - Stop IV infusion and discontinue IV.
  - Treat IV site as indicated by institutional policy.
  - Insert new IV site if continuation of IV therapy is indicated.
- IV site becomes cool, pale, and swollen (see chapter 36).
  - Indicates signs of infiltration.
  - Some IV medications are extremely harmful to subcutaneous tissue.
  - Provide IV extravasation care (e.g., inject phentolamine [Regitine] around the IV infiltration site) as indicated by institutional policy, or use a medication reference manual or consult a pharmacist to determine appropriate follow-up care.

Recording and Reporting

- Record solution and medication added to parenteral fluid on appropriate form.
- Report any adverse effects to client's health care provider, and document adverse effects according to institutional policy.

Skill 30-10 Administering Medications by Intravenous Bolus

View Video

Delegation Considerations

Administering medications by IV bolus should not be delegated to unregulated care providers (UCPs). The nurse should instruct the UCP to do the following:

- Report any unexpected drug reactions to the nurse.
- Report discomfort at infusion site as soon as possible.
- Obtain any required vital signs and report these findings to the nurse.

Equipment

- Watch with second hand
- MAR
- Disposable gloves
- Antiseptic swab
- **IV push (existing line)**
  - Medication in vial or ampule
  - Syringe for medication preparation
  - Needleless device or sterile needle (21 to 25 gauge)
- **IV push (IV lock)**
  - Medication in vial or ampule
  - Syringe for medication preparation
  - Vial of appropriate flush solution (saline most common, but heparin may also be used; if heparin is used, most common concentration is 10 to 100 units; check agency policy)
  - Needleless device or sterile needle (21 to 25 gauge)

Steps	Rationale
1. Check the prescriber's order for name of medication to be administered, dosage, route, and drug indication.	Ensures safe and accurate medication administration.

Critical Decision Point: Some IV medications can only be pushed safely when the client is being continuously monitored for dysrhythmias, blood pressure changes, or other adverse effects. Therefore, some medications can only be pushed in specific areas within a health care agency. Confirm institutional guidelines regarding requirements for special monitoring and verify that these requirements are available before giving medication (Zurlinden, 2002).

Steps	Rationale
2. Perform hand hygiene. Assess IV or saline (heparin) lock insertion site for signs of infiltration or phlebitis (see chapter 36).	Confirming the placement of the IV catheter and the integrity of the surrounding tissue ensures that the medication is administered safely.
3. If medication is to be pushed into an IV line, assess the patency of the line by noting infusion rate.	The IV line must be patent, and fluids must infuse easily for medication to reach venous circulation effectively.
4. Prepare ordered medication from vial or ampule (see Skill 30-7).	

Critical Decision Point: Some IV medications require dilution before administration. Verify with agency policy. If a small amount of medication is given (e.g., less than 1 mL), dilute medication in 5 to 10 mL of normal saline or sterile water so that the medication does not collect in the "dead spaces" (e.g., Y-site injection port, IV cap) of the IV delivery system.

Steps	Rationale
5. Perform hand hygiene. Apply gloves.	Reduces transmission of infection. During IV bolus administration, risk of blood exposure is low. However, nurse may manipulate IV dressing or expose site while completing other activities. Gloves reduce exposure (Health Canada, 1999).
6. Check client's identification by looking at identification bracelet and asking name.	Ensures that medication is administered to correct client.
7. Administer medication by IV push (existing line):	
a. Select injection port of IV tubing closest to client. Whenever possible, injection port should accept a needleless syringe. Use IV filter if required by medication reference or agency policy.	Health Canada (1999), the CCOHS (2000), and the CDC (NIOSH, 1999) strongly recommend that all IV injection sites be needleless to prevent needle-stick injuries.
b. Clean off injection port with antiseptic swab. Allow to dry.	Prevents introduction of micro-organisms during needle insertion.

Skill 30-10 Administering Medications by Intravenous Bolus—cont'd

Steps	Rationale
c. Connect syringe to IV line. Insert needleless tip or small-gauge needle of syringe containing prepared drug through centre of injection port.	Prevents damage to port's diaphragm and subsequent leakage.
d. Occlude IV line by pinching tubing just above injection port. Pull back gently on syringe's plunger to aspirate blood return.	Final check that medication is being delivered into the bloodstream.

Critical Decision Point: In some cases, especially with a smaller gauge IV needle, blood return may not be aspirated, even if IV is patent. If IV site does not show signs of infiltration, and IV fluid is infusing without difficulty, proceed with IV push.

Steps	Rationale
e. Release tubing and inject medication within amount of time recommended by institutional policy, pharmacist, or medication reference manual. Use watch to time administration (see illustration). IV line may be pinched while pushing medication and released when not pushing medication (see illustration). Allow IV fluids to infuse when not pushing medication.	Ensures safe medication infusion. Rapid injection of IV medication can prove fatal.

Critical Decision Point: If IV medication is incompatible with IV fluids, stop the IV fluids, clamp the IV line, flush with 10 mL of normal saline or sterile water, give the IV bolus over the appropriate amount of time, flush with another 10 mL of normal saline or sterile water at the same rate as the medication was administered, and then restart the IV fluids at the prescribed rate. If IV that is currently hanging is a medication (e.g., ranitidine), disconnect IV and administer IV push as outlined in step 8 to avoid giving a sudden bolus of the medication in the existing IV line to the client and to avoid creating potential risks associated with IV incompatibilities. Some IV medications and fluids cannot be stopped. Verify institutional policy regarding the temporary stopping of IV fluids or continuous IV medications. If unable to stop IV infusion, start a new IV site (see chapter 36) and administer medication using the IV lock method.

Steps	Rationale
f. After injecting medication, release tubing, withdraw syringe, and recheck fluid infusion rate.	Injection of bolus may alter rate of fluid infusion. Rapid fluid infusion can cause circulatory overload.

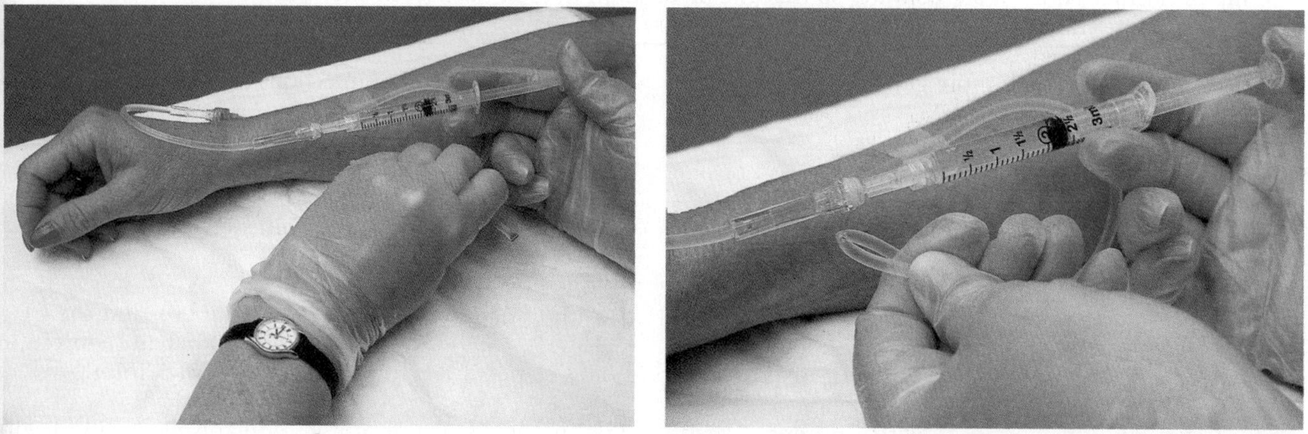

A B

STEP **7e** **A,** Timing IV push medication. **B,** IV line pinched off for medication infusion (optional).

Steps	Rationale
8. Administering medications by IV push (IV lock or a needleless system)	
A. Prepare flush solutions according to agency policy	
(1) Saline flush method (preferred method):	
• Prepare two syringes with 2 to 3 mL of normal saline (0.9%) in syringe.	Normal saline has been found to be effective in keeping IV locks patent and is compatible with a wide range of medications.
(2) Heparin flush method (traditional method):	
• Prepare one syringe with ordered amount of heparin flush solution.	
• Prepare two syringes with 2 to 3 mL of normal saline.	
B. Administer medication:	
(1) Clean lock's injection port with antiseptic swab.	Prevents introduction of micro-organisms during needle insertion.
(2) Insert syringe containing normal saline into injection port of IV lock (see illustration).	
(3) Pull back gently on syringe plunger and look for blood return.	Determines whether IV needle or catheter is positioned in vein.

Critical Decision Point: At times a saline (or heparin) lock will not yield a blood return even though the lock is patent. If IV site does not show signs of infiltration, proceed with IV push.

Steps	Rationale
(4) Flush IV lock with 1 mL saline by pushing slowly on plunger.	Clears IV lock of blood.

Critical Decision Point: Observe closely the area of skin above the IV catheter. Note any puffiness or swelling as the IV lock is flushed, which could indicate infiltration into the vein, requiring removal of the catheter.

Steps	Rationale
(5) Remove saline-filled syringe.	
(6) Clean lock's injection port with antiseptic swab.	Prevents transmission of infection.
(7) Insert syringe containing prepared medication into injection port of IV lock.	
(8) Inject medication within amount of time recommended by institutional policy, pharmacist, or medication reference manual. Use a watch to time administration.	Rapid injection of IV medication can result in death (Zurlinden, 2002).
(9) After administering bolus, withdraw syringe.	
(10) Clean lock's injection port with antiseptic swab.	Prevents transmission of micro-organisms.

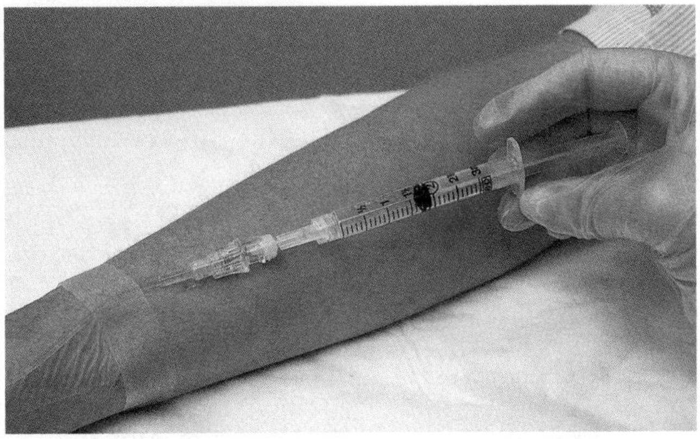

STEP **8B(2)** Syringe inserted into injection port.

Skill 30-10 Administering Medications by Intravenous Bolus—cont'd

Steps	Rationale
(11) Attach syringe with normal saline and inject normal saline flush at the same rate that the medication was delivered.	Irrigation with saline prevents occlusion of IV access device and ensures all medication is delivered. Flushing IV site at same rate as medication ensures that any medication remaining within IV needle is delivered at the correct rate.
(12) *Heparin flush option:* Insert needle of syringe containing heparin through diaphragm.	Maintains patency of needle by inhibiting clot formation.
9. Dispose of uncapped needles and syringes in puncture-proof and leak-proof container.	Reduces accidental needle sticks.
10. Remove and dispose of gloves. Perform hand hygiene.	Reduces the transmission of micro-organisms.
11. Observe client closely for adverse reaction as drug is administered and for several minutes thereafter.	IV medications act rapidly.

Unexpected Outcomes and Related Interventions

- Client develops adverse reaction to medication.
  - Stop delivering medication immediately and follow institutional policy or guidelines for appropriate response and reporting of adverse drug reactions.
  - Notify client's health care provider of adverse effects immediately.
- IV site becomes puffy.
  - Immediately discontinue administration of injection and discontinue site.
  - Follow institutional guidelines on appropriate extravasation care.

Recording and Reporting

- Record medication, dose, time, and route on appropriate form.
- Report any adverse reactions immediately to health care provider because they could be life-threatening. Client's response may indicate need for additional medical therapy.

venous access. The tandem set is placed at the same height as the primary infusion bag or bottle. In the tandem set-up, the tandem and the main line infuse simultaneously. The nurse must monitor the tandem set-up closely. If it is not immediately clamped when the medication is infused, the IV solution from the primary line will back up into the tandem line.

Mini-infusion Pump. The mini-infusion pump is battery operated and allows medications to be given in very small amounts of fluid (5 to 60 mL) within controlled infusion times using standard syringes (Skill 30-11).

Intermittent Venous Access. An intermittent venous access (commonly called a heparin lock or saline lock) is an IV catheter with a small chamber covered by a rubber diaphragm or a specially designed cap (Figure 30–31). Special rubber-seal injection caps accept needle safety devices and can be inserted into most IV catheters (see chapter 36). Advantages to intermittent venous access include the following:

- Cost savings resulting from the omission of continuous IV therapy

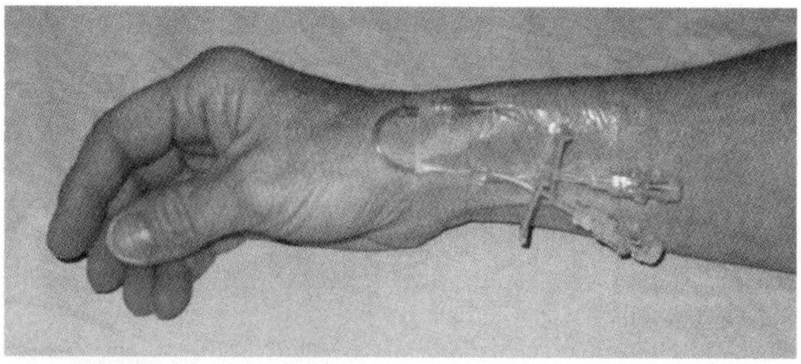

FIGURE **30–31** Intermittent lock covered with a rubber diaphragm.

- Convenience to the nurse by eliminating constant monitoring of flow rates
- Increased mobility, safety, and comfort for the client

Before administering an IV bolus or piggyback medication, the nurse must assess the patency and placement of the IV site. After the medication has been administered through an intermittent venous access, the access must

Text continued on p. 916

Skill 30-11 Administering Intravenous Medications by Piggyback, Intermittent Intravenous Infusion Sets, and Mini-infusion Pumps

View Video

Delegation Considerations

Administering medications by IV fluid by piggyback, intermittent IV infusion sets, and mini-infusion pumps should not be delegated to unregulated care providers (UCPs). The nurse must instruct the UCP to immediately report the following:

- Any unexpected drug reactions
- Discomfort at infusion site

Equipment

- Antiseptic swab
- IV pole
- MAR
- Medication label
- **Piggyback, Tandem, or Mini-infusion Pump**
  - Medication prepared in 5- to 150-mL labelled infusion bag or syringe
  - Short microdrip or macrodrip tubing set for piggyback (may have needleless system attachment)
  - Needleless device or stopcocks if available
  - Needles (21 or 23 gauge, only if stopcocks or other needleless methods are not available)
  - Mini-infusion pump
  - Adhesive tape (optional)
- **Volume-Control Administration Set**
  - Volutrol or Buretrol
  - Infusion tubing (may have needleless system attachment)
  - Syringe (1 to 20 mL)
  - Vial or ampule of ordered medication

Steps	Rationale
1. Check prescriber's order to determine type of IV solution to be used, name of medication, dose, route, time of administration, and drug indication.	Client's overall physical condition dictates type of IV solution used. Ensures safe and accurate medication administration.
2. Collect information necessary to administer medication safely, including action, purpose, side effects, normal dose, time of peak onset, and nursing implications.	Allows nurse to give medication safely and to monitor client's response to therapy.
3. Assess compatibility of drug with existing IV solution.	Drugs that are incompatible with IV solutions may result in clouding or crystallization of solution in IV tubing, which may harm the client.

Critical Decision Point: Never administer IV medications through tubing that is infusing blood, blood products, or parenteral nutrition solutions.

Steps	Rationale
4. Assess patency of client's existing IV infusion line by noting infusion rate of main IV line.	IV line must be patent and fluids must infuse easily for medication to reach venous circulation effectively.

Critical Decision Point: If the client's IV site is saline locked, cleanse the port with alcohol and assess the patency of the IV line by flushing it with 2 to 3 mL of sterile normal saline. Attach appropriate IV tubing to the saline lock, and administer the medication via piggyback, tandem, mini-infusion, or volume-control administration set. When the infusion is completed, disconnect the tubing, cleanse the port with alcohol, and flush the IV line with 2 to 3 mL sterile normal saline. Maintain sterility of IV tubing between intermittent infusions.

Steps	Rationale
5. Perform hand hygiene. Assess IV insertion site for signs of infiltration or phlebitis: redness, pallor, swelling, tenderness on palpation.	Confirmation of placement of IV needle or catheter and integrity of surrounding tissues ensures medication is administered safely.
6. Assess client's history of medication allergies.	Effects of medications can develop rapidly after IV infusion. Nurse should be aware of clients at risk.
7. Assess client's understanding of purpose of medication therapy.	May reveal need for education.
8. Assemble supplies at bedside. Prepare client by informing client that medication will be given through IV equipment.	Medication preparation usually is not required. Nurse may assemble infusion tubing and bag of medication in medication room or client's room. Allows client to understand procedure and minimizes anxiety.
9. Perform hand hygiene.	Reduces transmission of infection.

Skill 30-11 Administering Intravenous Medications by Piggyback, Intermittent Intravenous Infusion Sets, and Mini-infusion Pumps—cont'd

Steps	Rationale
10. Check client's identification by looking at identification bracelet and asking client's name.	Ensures medication is administered to correct client.
11. Explain purpose of medication and side effects to client and explain that medication is to be given through existing IV line. Encourage client to report symptoms of discomfort at site.	Keeps client informed of planned therapies. Clients who can verbalize pain at the IV site can help detect IV infiltrations early, lessening damage to surrounding tissues.
12. Administer infusion:	
A. **Piggyback or tandem infusion**	
(1) Connect infusion tubing to medication bag (see chapter 36). Allow solution to fill tubing by opening regulator flow clamp. Once tubing is full, close clamp and cap end of tubing.	Infusion tubing should be filled with solution and free of air bubbles to prevent air embolus.
(2) Hang piggyback medication bag above level of primary fluid bag. (Hook may be used to lower main bag.) Hang tandem infusion at same level as primary fluid bag.	Height of fluid bag affects rate of flow to client.
(3) Connect tubing of piggyback or tandem infusion to appropriate connector on primary infusion line:	
(a) *Stopcock:* Wipe off stopcock port with alcohol swab and connect tubing. Turn stopcock to open position.	Stopcock eliminates need for needle.
(b) *Needleless system:* Wipe off needleless port, and insert tip of piggyback or tandem infusion tubing (see illustrations).	The CDC strongly recommends needleless connections to prevent accidental needle-stick injuries (NIOSH, 1999). Establishes route for IV medication to enter main IV line.
(c) *Tubing port:* Connect sterile needle to end of piggyback or tandem infusion tubing, remove cap, cleanse injection port on main IV line, and insert needle through centre of port. Secure by taping connection.	Prevents introduction of micro-organisms during needle insertion.

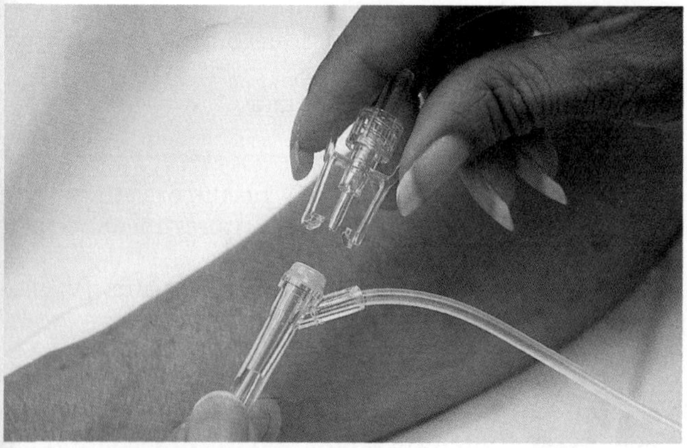
A

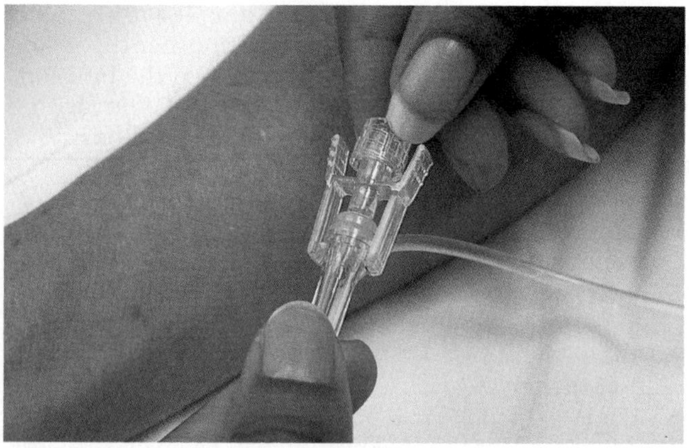
B

STEP **12A(3)(b)** **A,** Needleless lever lock cannula system. **B,** Blunt-ended cannula inserts into port and locks.

Steps	Rationale
(4) Regulate flow rate of medication solution by adjusting regulator clamp. (Infusion times vary. Refer to medication reference or institutional policy for safe flow rate.)	Provides slow, intermittent infusion of medication and maintains therapeutic blood levels.
(5) After medication has infused, check flow regulator on primary infusion. The primary infusion should automatically begin to flow after the piggyback or tandem solution is empty.	Back-check valve on piggyback stops flow of the primary infusion until second medication infuses. The tandem and primary infusions flow together until the tandem set empties. Checking flow rate ensures proper administration of IV fluids.
(6) Regulate main infusion line to desired rate, if necessary.	Infusion of piggyback may interfere with the main line infusion rate.
(7) Leave IV piggyback bag and tubing in place for future medication administration or discard in appropriate containers.	Establishment of secondary line produces route for micro-organisms to enter main line. Repeated changes in tubing increase risk of infection transmission (check agency policy).
B. Volume-control administration set (e.g., Volutrol)	
(1) Assemble supplies in medication room.	Controls risk of contaminating IV solution.
(2) Prepare medication from vial or ampule (see Skill 30-7).	Ensures medication is sterile.
(3) Fill Volutrol with desired amount of fluid (50 to 100 mL) by opening clamp between Volutrol and main IV bag (see illustration).	Small volume of fluid dilutes IV medication and reduces risk of too-rapid infusion.
(4) Close clamp and check to be sure that clamp on air vent of Volutrol chamber is open.	Prevents additional leakage of fluid into Volutrol. Air vent allows fluid in Volutrol to exit at regulated rate.
(5) Clean injection port on top of Volutrol with antiseptic swab.	Prevents introduction of micro-organisms during needle insertion.

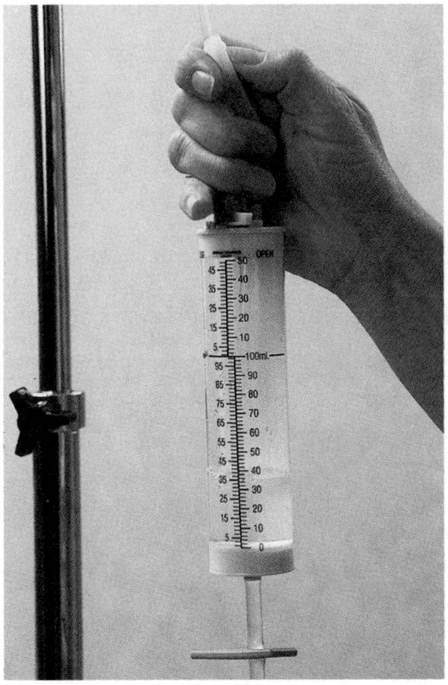

STEP **12B(3)** Filling volume-control administration device.

Skill 30-11 Administering Intravenous Medications by Piggyback, Intermittent Intravenous Infusion Sets, and Mini-infusion Pumps—cont'd

Steps	Rationale

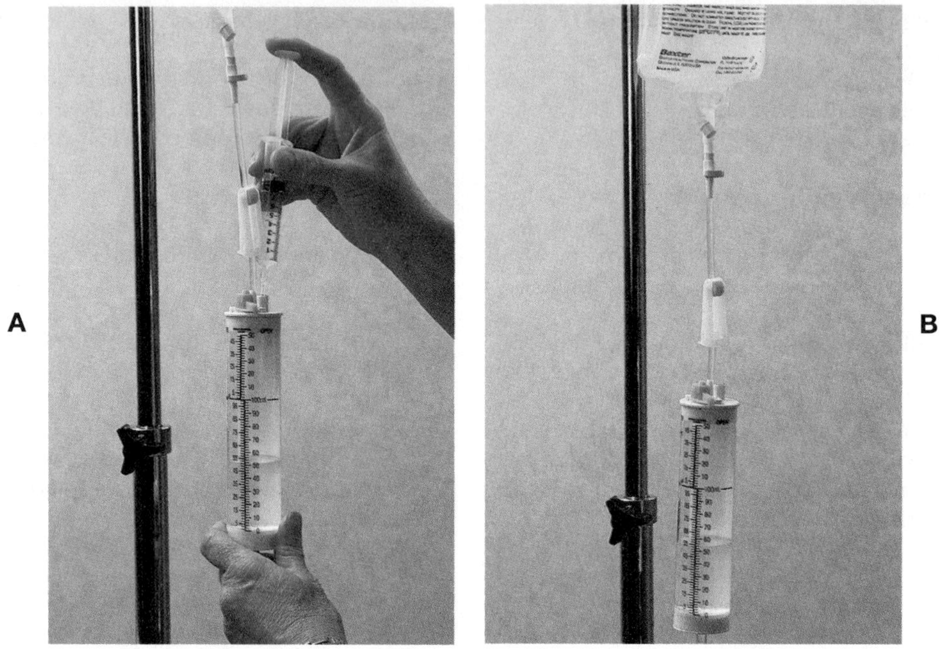

STEP **12B(6)** **A,** Medication injected into device. **B,** Prepared device.

Steps	Rationale
(6) Remove needle cap or sheath and insert syringe needle through port, then inject medication (see illustrations). Gently rotate Volutrol between hands.	Rotating mixes medication with solution in Volutrol to ensure equal distribution.
(7) Regulate IV infusion rate to allow medication to infuse in time recommended by institutional policy, a pharmacist, or a medication reference manual.	For optimal therapeutic effect, medication should infuse in prescribed time interval.
(8) Label Volutrol with name of medication, dosage, total volume including diluent, and time of administration.	Alerts nurses to medication being infused. Prevents other medications from being added to Volutrol.
(9) Dispose of uncapped needle or needle enclosed in safety shield and syringe in proper container.	Prevents accidental needle sticks.
C. Mini-infusion administration	
(1) Connect prefilled syringe to mini-infusion tubing.	Special tubing designed to fit syringe delivers medication to main IV line.
(2) Carefully apply pressure to syringe plunger, allowing tubing to fill with medication.	Ensures that tubing is free of air bubbles to prevent air embolus.
(3) Place syringe into mini-infusor pump (follow product directions). Be sure syringe is secure (see illustration).	

Steps	Rationale

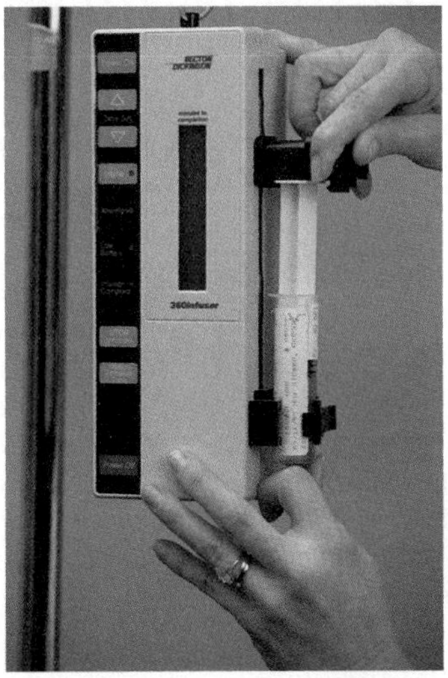

STEP **12C(3)** Securing syringe into mini-infusor.

Steps	Rationale
(4) Connect mini-infusion tubing to main IV line.	
(a) *Stopcock:* Wipe off stopcock port with alcohol swab and connect tubing. Turn stopcock to open position.	Stopcock reduces risk of needle-stick injuries.
(b) *Needleless system:* Wipe off needleless port and insert tip of mini-infusor tubing.	Needleless system reduces risk of needle-stick injuries.
(c) *Tubing port:* Connect sterile needle to mini-infusion tubing, remove cap, cleanse injection port on main IV line, and insert needle through centre of port. Consider placing tape where IV tubing enters port to secure connection.	Cleansing reduces transmission of micro-organisms.
(5) Explain purpose of medication and side effects to client and explain that medication is to be given through existing IV line. Ask client to report symptoms of discomfort at site.	Informs client of planned therapies.
(6) Hang infusion pump with syringe on IV pole alongside main IV bag. Set pump to deliver medication within time recommended by institutional policy, pharmacist, or medication reference manual. Press button on pump to begin infusion. *Optional:* Set alarm.	Pump automatically delivers medication at safe, constant rate based on volume in syringe. (Alarm is used if medication is delivered into heparin/saline lock.)
(7) After medication has infused, check flow regulator on primary infusion. The infusion should automatically begin to flow once the pump stops. Regulate main infusion line to desired rate as needed. (NOTE: If stopcock is used, turn off mini-infusion line.)	Maintains patency of primary IV line.
13. Observe client for signs of adverse reactions.	IV medications act rapidly.
14. During infusion, periodically check infusion rate and condition of IV site.	IV must remain patent for proper medication administration. Development of infiltration necessitates discontinuing infusion.
15. Ask client to explain purpose and side effects of medication.	Evaluates client's understanding of instruction.

Skill 30-11 Administering Intravenous Medications by Piggyback, Intermittent Intravenous Infusion Sets, and Mini-infusion Pumps—cont'd

Unexpected Outcomes and Related Interventions

- Client develops adverse drug reaction.
  - Stop medication infusion immediately.
  - Follow institutional policy or guidelines for appropriate response and reporting of adverse drug reactions.
  - Notify client's health care provider of adverse effects immediately.
- Medication does not infuse over desired period.
  - Determine reason (e.g., improper calculation of flow rate, wrong positioning of IV needle at insertion site, or infiltration).
  - Take corrective action as indicated.
- IV site becomes swollen, warm, reddened, and tender to touch (see chapter 36).
  - Indicates phlebitis.
  - Stop IV infusion.
  - Discontinue IV.
  - Treat IV site as indicated by institutional policy.
  - Insert new IV site if continuation of therapy is indicated.
- IV site becomes cool, pale, and swollen (see chapter 36).
  - Indicates signs of infiltration.
  - Some IV medications are extremely harmful to subcutaneous tissue.
  - Provide IV extravasation care (e.g., injecting phentolamine [Regitine] around IV infiltration site) as indicated by institutional policy or use a medication reference or consult a pharmacist to determine appropriate follow-up care.

Recording and Reporting

- Record medication, dose, route, and time administered on MAR.
- Record volume of fluid in medication bag or Volutrol on intake and output form.
- Report any adverse reactions to nurse in charge or physician.

Home Care Considerations

- Teach client and caregiver to dispose of needles and contaminated equipment in puncture-proof containers (e.g., coffee can)
- Instruct family about community resources to obtain supplies.

be flushed with a solution to keep it patent. Generally, normal saline is an effective flush solution for peripheral catheters. Some institutions require the use of heparin. Nurses must verify and follow the institution's policies regarding the care and maintenance of the IV site.

Administration of IV Therapy in the Home. Sometimes clients may be discharged from an acute care setting and continue to receive IV therapy in the home setting. Medications such as antibiotics, chemotherapy, total parenteral nutrition, pain medications, and blood transfusions may be given in the home. Most clients who have home IV therapy will have a central venous catheter inserted prior to discharge (see chapter 36). In addition, clients who need to receive IV therapy in the home have home care nurses who assist in the management of the IV therapy.

However, clients and their families need to be carefully assessed as to their ability to manage this therapy at home. Instruction on IV care management must be provided while the client is still in the hospital. Clients and families need to be taught how to recognize problems and what to do when these problems occur. It is important for the family to recognize signs of infection and complications and to know that when these signs occur, the home care nurse or physician must be notified. In addition, clients and their families need information regarding maintenance of IV administration equipment, including the infusion pump.

Key Concepts

- Learning medication classifications improves understanding of nursing implications for administering medications with similar characteristics.
- Federal medication legislation regulates the production, distribution, prescription, and administration of medications.
- All controlled substances are handled according to strict procedures.
- The nurse applies understanding of the physiology of medication action when timing administration, selecting routes, initiating actions to promote medication efficacy, and observing responses to medications.
- The older adult's body undergoes structural and functional changes that alter medication actions and influence the manner in which nurses provide medication therapy.

- Children's medication doses are computed based on body surface area or weight.
- Medications given parenterally are absorbed more quickly than medications administered by other routes.
- Each medication order should include the client's name, the order date, the medication name, dosage, route, time of administration, drug indication, and the prescriber's signature.
- A medication history reveals allergies, medications that a client is taking, and the client's compliance with therapy.
- The nursing process should be used when administering medication.
- The six rights of medication administration ensure accurate preparation and administration of medication doses.
- The six rights of medication administration are the right medication, right dose, right client, right route, right time, and right documentation.
- Nurses administer only the medications that they prepare, and prepared medications are never left unattended.
- Medications should be charted immediately after administration.
- A nurse uses clinical judgment in determining the best time to administer prn medications.
- The nurse reports a medication error immediately.
- When preparing medications, the nurse checks the medication container label against the medication administration record (MAR) three times.
- The Z-track method for intramuscular injections protects subcutaneous tissues from irritating parenteral fluids.
- Failure to select injection sites by anatomical landmarks may lead to tissue, bone, or nerve damage.

Key Terms

Absorption, *p. 836*
Adverse effects, *p. 838*
Anaphylactic reactions, *p. 838*
Biotransformation, *p. 837*
Buccal, *p. 840*
Concentration, *p. 839*
Controlled substances, *p. 836*
Detoxify, *p. 837*
Idiosyncratic reaction, *p. 838*
Infusions, *p. 839*
Inhalation, *p. 843*
Injection, *p. 836*
Instillation, *p. 842*
Intraarticular, *p. 842*
Intracardiac, *p. 842*
Intradermal (ID), *p. 840*
Intramuscular (IM), *p. 840*
Intravenous (IV), *p. 840*
Irrigations, *p. 843*
Medication allergy, *p. 838*
Medication error, *p. 849*
Medication interaction, *p. 839*
Metered-dose inhalers (MDIs), *p. 875*
Metric system, *p. 843*
Narcotics, *p. 836*
Ophthalmic, *p. 860*
Parenteral administration, *p. 840*
Peak, *p. 839*
Pharmacokinetics, *p. 836*
Polypharmacy, *p. 857*
Prescriptions, *p. 847*
Serum half-life, *p. 839*
Side effects, *p. 838*
Solution, *p. 843*
Subcutaneous (Sub-Q), *p. 840*
Sublingual, *p. 840*
Synergistic effect, *p. 839*
Therapeutic effect, *p. 838*
Toxic effects, *p. 838*
Transdermal disk, *p. 842*
Verbal order, *p. 846*
Z-track method, *p. 899*

Critical Thinking Exercises

1. Mrs. Nguyen, a 69-year-old woman, has recently experienced a stroke and has right-sided weakness. The neurological clinical nurse specialist wrote orders to start oral medications today. What steps should the nurse take to ensure that it is safe for this client to receive her oral medications? What should the nurse do if the client is unable to swallow?
2. Marissa is a 25-year-old who just delivered a healthy infant. She is to receive RhoGAM 300 mcg IM today. What size needle and which injection site and technique should the nurse use when administering this medication?
3. Jack, a 70-year-old retired farmer, has been experiencing new respiratory difficulties. His physician has ordered for him to start using an albuterol inhaler with a spacer. What steps will the nurse take to ensure that he can self-administer his MDI?
4. The nurse receives an order to give Furosemide (Lasix) 40 mg IV push. The nurse has never given this medication while working on this unit. What steps should the nurse take before administering the Lasix?

Review Questions

1. Which of the following rights has been added to the traditional five rights of medication administration?
   1. Right documentation
   2. Right route
   3. Right medication
   4. Right time
2. The nurse is having difficulty reading a physician's order for a medication. The nurse knows the physician is very busy and does not like to be called. The nurse should
   1. Call a pharmacist to interpret the order
   2. Call the physician to have the order clarified
   3. Consult the unit manager to help interpret the order
   4. Ask the unit secretary to interpret the physician's handwriting
3. A client has a gastrointestinal alteration. Which method of medication administration should NOT be used?
   1. Oral
   2. Topical
   3. Inhalation
   4. Injection
4. Most medication errors occur when the nurse
   1. Fails to follow routine procedures
   2. Is responsible for administering numerous medications
   3. Is caring for too many clients
   4. Is administering unfamiliar medications

5. A client is to receive cephalexin (Keflex) 500 mg PO. The pharmacy has sent 250-mg tablets. The nurse should give
   1. $^1/_2$ tablet
   2. 1 tablet
   3. $1^1/_2$ tablets
   4. 2 tablets
6. A medication injection into the loose connective tissue under the dermis is a(n)
   1. Intramuscular injection
   2. Intravenous injection
   3. Subcutaneous injection
   4. Intradermal injection
7. The nurse is responsible for following legal provisions when administering controlled substances or narcotics. Failure to do so may result in
   1. Fines, imprisonment, and loss of nurse licensure
   2. Loss of employment
   3. Medication errors
   4. Poor health outcomes resulting from narcotic use
8. Pharmacokinetics is the study of how medications
   1. Are derived from plants
   2. Enter the body, reach their site of action, are metabolized, and exit the body
   3. Are used for certain disease processes
   4. Are manufactured and distributed to pharmaceutical companies
9. Official publications such as the following set standards for medication strength, quality, purity, packaging, safety, labelling, and dose form.
   1. *Physicians Reference Guide*
   2. *Nurse's Drug Guide*
   3. *Narcotic Control Act*
   4. The *Canadian Formulary* (CF)
10. Administration of the *Food and Drugs Act* and the *Controlled Drugs and Substances Act* is carried out by the
    1. Health Protection Branch (HPB)
    2. Nurse or physician dispensing and prescribing medications
    3. *Canadian Formulary*
    4. Health care institutions

References

Andrews, M. M., & Boyle, J. S. (2003). *Transcultural concepts in nursing care* (4th ed.). Philadelphia: Lippincott.

Aschenbrenner, D. S., Cleveland, L. W., & Venable, S. J. (2002). *Drug therapy in nursing*. Philadelphia: Lippincott.

Behrman, R. E., & Vaughan, V. C. (Eds.). (1987). *Nelson textbook of pediatrics* (13th ed.). Philadelphia: Saunders.

Beyea, S. C., & Nicoll, L. H. (1996). Back to basics: Administering IM injections the right way. *American Journal of Nursing, 96*(1), 34–35.

Bryson, E. (2002). Drug administration via a nasogastric tube. *Nursing Times, 97*(16), 51.

Canadian Centre for Occupational Health and Safety. (2000). *Needlestick injuries*. Retrieved November 11, 2004, from *http://www.ccohs.ca/oshanswers/diseases/needlestick_injuries.html*

Chan, H. (2001). Effects of injection duration on site-pain intensity and bruising associated with subcutaneous heparin. *Journal of Advanced Nursing, 35*(6), 882–892.

Chung, J., Ng, W. M. Y., & Wong, T. K. S. (2002). An experimental study on the use of manual pressure to reduce pain in intramuscular injections. *Journal of Clinical Nursing, 11*(4), 457–461.

Clark, J. F., Queener, S. F., & Karb, V. B. (1998). *Pharmacological basis of nursing practice* (6th ed.). St. Louis, MO: Mosby.

Clarke, K. (1999). Effective pain relief with intrapleural analgesia. *Nursing Times, 95*(12), 49–50.

Cromling, T. (2002). Giving meds to children needn't be a hassle. *RN, 65*(3), 28hf1.

Ebersole, P., & Hess, P. (1998). *Toward healthy aging: Human needs and nursing response* (5th ed.). St. Louis, MO: Mosby.

Epstein, S., et al. (2001). Patient handling of a dry-powder inhaler in clinical practice. *Chest, 120*(5), 1480–1484.

Galvan, T. J. (2001). Dysphagia: Going down and staying down. *American Journal of Nursing, 101*(1), 37–42.

Gilbar, P. J. (1999). A guide to enteral drug administration in palliative care. *Journal of Pain and Symptom Management, 17*(3), 197–207.

Health Canada. (1997). Preventing the transmission of bloodborne pathogens in health care and public service settings. *Canada Communicable Disease Report, 23S3*, 1–43.

Health Canada. (1999). Routine practices and additional precautions for preventing the transmission of infection in health care [Electronic version]. *Canada Communicable Disease Report, 25S4*, 1–142.

Hockenberry, M. J., et al. (2003). *Wong's nursing care of infants and children* (7th ed.). St. Louis, MO: Mosby.

Joint Commission on Accreditation of Healthcare Organizations. (2004). *2004 National patient safety goals-FAQs*. Retrieved January 14, 2005, from *http://www.jcaho.org/accredited+organizations/patient+safety/04+npsg/04_faqs.htm*

Koschel, M. J. (2001). Filter needles: Question of practice. *American Journal of Nursing, 101*(1), 75.

Lewis, S. M., Heitkemper, M. M., & Dirksen, S. R. (2000). *Medical-surgical nursing* (5th ed.). St. Louis, MO: Mosby.

Maas, M. L., et al. (Eds.). (2001). *Nursing care of older adults: Diagnoses, outcomes, and interventions*. St. Louis, MO: Mosby.

MayoClinic.com. (2000). *Asthma center.* Retrieved January 20, 2005, from *http://www.mayoclinic.com/findinformation/conditioncenters/centers.cfm?objectid=E18882D8-7680-40D3-A3ECE1A2C708A3C3*

McConnell, E. A. (2000). Administering subcutaneous heparin. *Nursing, 30*(6), 17.

McConnell, E. A. (2001). Clinical do's and don'ts: Instilling eyedrops. *Nursing, 31*(9), 17.

McKenry, L. M., & Salerno, E. (2003). *Mosby's pharmacology in nursing revised and updated* (21st ed.). St. Louis, MO: Mosby.

National Heart, Lung, and Blood Institute. (1995, October). *Nurses: Partners in asthma care* (NIH Publication No. 95-3308). Retrieved January 20, 2005, from *http://www.nhlbi.nih.gov/health/prof/lung/asthma/nurs_gde.htm*

National Institute for Occupational Safety and Health. (1999, November). *NIOSH alert: Preventing needle-stick injuries in health care settings* (DHHS [NIOSH] Publication No. 2000-108). Cincinnati, OH: Author.

Nicoll, L. H., & Hesby, A. (2002). Intramuscular injection: An integrative research review and guideline for evidence-based practice. *Applied Nursing Research, 16*(2), 149–162.

Occupational Safety and Health Administration. (2001, January 18). Occupational exposure to bloodborne pathogens: Needlestick and other sharps injuries—Final rule (CFR 29, 1910). *Federal Register, 66*, 5317–5325.

Peragallo-Dittko, V. (1997). Research for practice: Rethinking subcutaneous injection technique. *American Journal of Nursing, 97*(5), 71–72.

Rodger, M. A., & King, L. (2000). Drawing up and administering intramuscular injections: A review of the literature. *Journal of Advanced Nursing, 31*(3), 574–582.
Strowig, S. (2001). Insulin therapy. *RN, 64*(9), 38–44.
Togger, D, & Brenner, P. (2001). Metered dose inhalers. *American Journal of Nursing, 101*(10), 26–32.
Using eye drops. (2000). *RN, 63*(4), Suppl. 23.
Workman, B. (1999). Safe injection techniques. *Nursing Standard, 13*(39), 47–53.
Zurlinden, J. (2002). Double check IV push. *Nursing Spectrum, 15*(25IL), 16.

Recommended Web Sites

Canadian Pharmacists Association:
http://www.pharmacists.ca
The Canadian Pharmacists Association (CPhA) is a national organization of pharmacists. CPhA's Web site provides links to drug information, client information, and resources.

Health Canada: Drug Products:
http://www.hc-sc.gc.ca/english/protection/drugs.html
This site provides access to government reports, resources, and programs about the safety and effectiveness of pharmaceutical drugs and other therapeutic products.

Health Canada Therapeutic Products Directorate:
http://www.hc-sc.gc.ca/hpfb-dgpsa/tpd-dpt/
Health Canada's Therapeutic Products Directorate is the Canadian federal authority that regulates pharmaceutical drugs and medical devices for human use. This site provides access to information on reporting adverse reaction information.

Saskatchewan Drug Information Service:
http://www.usask.ca/pharmacy-nutrition/services/sdis.shtml
Operating from the University of Saskatchewan, the Saskatchewan Drug Information Service (SDIS) aims to provide health care professionals and lay people with access to objective and concise information on drugs and drug therapy.

31

Complementary and Alternative Therapies

Steve Kilkus, RN, MSN
Jean McClennon-Leong, RN, MN, APNP (Canadian author)

Objectives

Mastery of content in this chapter will enable the student to:

- Define the key terms listed.
- Differentiate between complementary and alternative therapies.
- Describe clinical applications of relaxation therapies.
- Discuss the relaxation response and its effect on somatic ailments.
- Identify the principles and effectiveness of imagery, meditation, and breathwork.
- Describe the purpose and principles of biofeedback.
- Describe methods of and psycho-physiological responses to therapeutic touch.
- Explain the scope of chiropractic therapy.
- Discuss the principles and applications of acupuncture.
- Describe safe and unsafe herbal therapies.

Over the past century, the health of North Americans has steadily improved. Scientific and medical changes have provided the knowledge and technology to successfully alter the course of many illnesses. However, despite the success of traditional Western medicine, known as **allopathic medicine,** many conditions such as arthritis, chronic back pain, gastrointestinal problems, allergies, headaches, and insomnia are difficult to treat, and more clients are exploring alternative methods to relieve their symptoms. Up to three quarters of clients visit primary care practitioners for stress, pain, and health conditions for which there are no known causes or cures (Fontaine, 2000). Although allopathic medicine effectively treats numerous physical ailments such as bacterial infections, structural abnormalities, and acute emergencies, it is less effective in preventing disease, decreasing stress-induced illnesses, managing chronic disease, and caring for individuals' emotional and spiritual needs.

Clients increasingly seek unconventional treatments, in part because they perceive that treatments offered by allopathic professionals are not effective. As well, many clients are attracted to holistic approaches to health care (Fontaine, 2000; Pelletier, 2000). Today, the public has greater access to information about personal health through the Internet and journals such as the *Annals of Behavioral Medicine, Alternative Therapies in Health and Medicine, Journal of Alternative and Complementary Medicine,* and *Holistic Nursing.*

Complementary or Alternative Medicine Therapies in Health Care

Unconventional therapies are frequently referred to as complementary or alternative medicine (CAM) therapies. **Complementary therapies** are those therapies used in addition to conventional treatment recommended by the person's health care provider. As the name implies, complementary therapies complement the conventional treatment. Many of the complementary therapies, such as acupuncture, contain diagnostic and therapeutic methods specific to their field, whereas others, such as imagery and breathwork, are

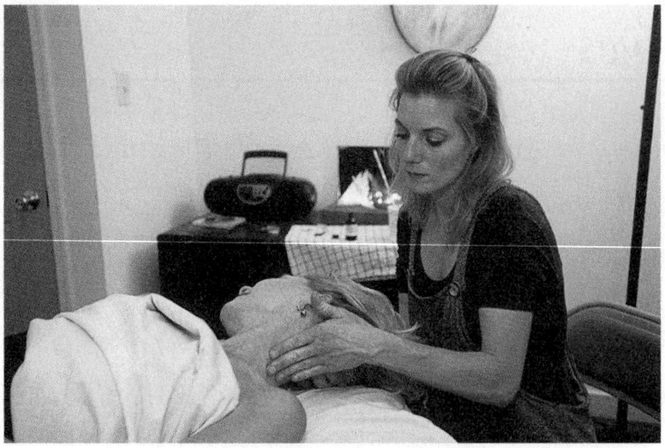

FIGURE **31–1** Massage therapy can effectively relieve tension.

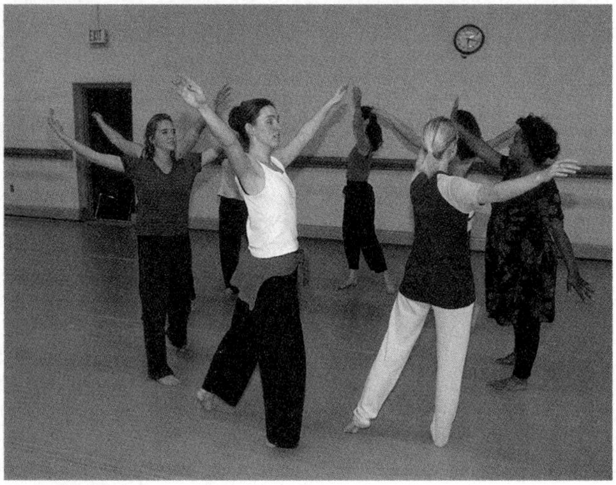

FIGURE **31–2** Young adults participating in dance therapy.

generally easily learned and applied. Complementary therapies also include relaxation; exercise; massage (Figure 31–1); reflexology; prayer; biofeedback; hypnotherapy; shamanism; creative therapies, including art, music, or dance therapy (Figure 31–2); acupuncture and Chinese medicine; Ayurveda medicine; meditation; chiropractic therapy; osteopathy; herbalism; and homeopathy (Fontaine, 2000; Pelletier, 2000).

Alternative therapies, on the other hand, may include the same interventions as complementary therapies but frequently become the primary treatment that replaces allopathic medical care. Both complementary and alternative therapies vary in the degree to which they are compatible with allopathic medicine. For example, chiropractic and Feldenkrais (gentle body-movement therapy) practitioners frequently use diagnostic terminology and methods similar to those used by allopathic practitioners. They base interventions on conventional pathophysiology, anatomy, and kinesiology but at the same time, explore mind-body connections that may cause or contribute to the physiological condition. Some alternative therapies are not supported by scientific data, such as use of shark cartilage and coffee enemas, and must be regarded with caution. Even established therapies have only been tested on small or limited populations. Nurses should make well-informed decisions when considering alternative therapies.

Complementary and alternative therapies are often organized into five categories that researchers find useful (Box 31-1). Some types of complementary and alternative therapies are presented in Table 31-1. This list is not exhaustive.

Public Interest in CAM Therapies

Increasingly, the boundaries between CAM and allopathic medicine are being eroded. The interest in CAM is evident in the increased number of articles about it in respected medical journals and the development of several journals specific to CAM. Some universities are adding courses about CAM therapies to medical and nursing curricula, and colleges are offering certificate courses in a variety of alternative therapies (York University Centre for Health Studies [YUCHS], 1999). **Integrative medical programs** are being developed that give health care consumers access to both allopathic and complementary practitioners. In some institutions, for example, nurses practise massage, Reiki, and therapeutic touch.

There is growing demand for alternative medicines and the services of alternative health care providers in Canada and worldwide (YUCHS, 1999). One survey reported that half of Canadians had used alternative therapies in the previous year (Ramsay, Walker, & Alexander, 1999). Of these, 88% thought the care they received was either somewhat or very helpful. Chiropractic, relaxation, massage, prayer, and herbal medicine were some of the most commonly used therapies. Most respondents (81%) reported using alternative therapies to prevent illness or to maintain wellness. In another study, 40% to 80% of Canadians with HIV/AIDS reported using complementary therapies. The main reasons for use were to enhance immune response, improve nutrition, and prevent infection (Pawluch et al. 1998, as cited in YUCHS, 1999).

Although CAM therapies are less expensive and less invasive than allopathic medicine and their use could save the health care system money, clients (or their private insurance plans) must pay for these therapies. Therefore, many people cannot afford CAM therapies. People who use CAM therapies are typically well-educated professionals.

CAM Therapies and Holistic Nursing

Holistic nursing regards and treats the mind, body, and spirit of the client. Nurses can use holistic interventions such as relaxation therapy, imagery, music therapy, simple touch (especially helpful with older clients; Box 31-2), massage, and prayer (Box 31-3). Such interventions affect the whole person (mind-body-spirit) and are economical, non-invasive, non-pharmacological complements to medical care. Holistic interventions can be used to augment standard treatments, replace ineffective or debilitating interventions, and promote and maintain health (Dossey, Keegan, & Guzzetta, 2000). The Canadian Holistic Nurses Association develops standards for practice for holistic nursing and promotes holistic nursing

Box 31-1 Categories of Complementary and Alternative Medicine (CAM) Therapies

1. Alternative Medical Systems

Alternative medical systems encompass both theories and practices. Often, they have evolved earlier than the conventional Western medical approach. Examples of alternative medical systems that have developed in Western cultures include homeopathic medicine and naturopathic medicine. Systems that have developed in non-Western cultures include traditional Chinese medicine and Ayurveda (a system from India).

2. Mind-Body Interventions

Mind-body medicine uses a variety of techniques designed to enhance the mind's capacity to affect bodily function and symptoms. Some techniques that were considered CAM in the past have become mainstream (e.g., client support groups and cognitive-behavioural therapy). Other mind-body techniques that are still considered CAM include meditation, prayer, mental healing, and art, music, and dance therapies.

3. Biologically Based Therapies

Biologically based therapies in CAM use substances found in nature, such as herbs, foods, and vitamins. Examples include dietary supplements, herbal products, and other so-called natural but as yet scientifically unproven therapies (e.g., shark cartilage to treat cancer). Some uses of dietary supplements have been incorporated into conventional medicine. For example, folic acid is used to prevent certain birth defects, and a regiment of vitamins and zinc can slow the progression of an eye disease called age-related macular degeneration.

4. Manipulative and Body-Based Therapies

Manipulative and body-based methods in CAM are based on manipulation and/or movement of one or more parts of the body. Examples include massage and chiropractic or osteopathic manipulation.

5. Energy Therapies

Energy therapies involve the use of energy fields. There are two types of energy therapies:

- **Biofield therapies** are intended to affect energy fields that purportedly surround and penetrate the human body. The existence of such fields has not been scientifically proven. Biofield therapies involve applying pressure and/or manipulating the body by placing the hands in or through these fields. Examples include Qi gong, Reiki, and therapeutic touch.
- **Bioelectromagnetic-based therapies** involve the unconventional use of electromagnetic fields, such as pulsed, magnetic, or alternating or direct current fields.

From *What Is Complementary and Alternative Medicine?* (NCCAM publication no. D156), National Center for Complementary and Alternative Medicine, 2002, *http://altmed.od.nih.gov/health/whatiscam/#11*

practice, education, research, and administration (Canadian Holistic Nurses Association, 2000).

Growing appreciation for the importance of healing the spirit as well as the body has influenced the development of such hospital programs as music, art, and recreation therapy. At the University of Alberta Hospital in Edmonton, an "Artists in the Wards Program" connects local artists with individual clients at the bedside. This program aims "to support the growth of individuals' creative spirits, which may aid physical, spiritual, emotional and mental healing." The hospital also houses the McMullen Art Gallery (Figure 31–3). As well, many hospitals provide space for spiritual practice. In fact, chaplains are widely regarded as part of the health care team, and many hospitals are now providing space for a variety of spiritual practices. For instance, the University of Alberta Hospital offers both a chapel and a teepee. Built specifically for Aboriginal clients and their families, the teepee is used for prayer, reflection, and healing ceremonies (Figure 31–4). A few hospitals have or are considering the construction of labyrinths on their grounds. Clients use these labyrinths for walking, meditation, and prayer (see Table 31-1).

The following sections present several types of complementary and alternative medicine therapies. The therapies are organized into two types. The first are nursing-accessible therapies. These are therapies that a nurse can begin to learn and apply in client care. The second type includes training-specific therapies, such as chiropractic therapy or acupressure, which a nurse cannot perform without additional training and/or certification.

Nursing-Accessible Therapies

Some CAM therapies and techniques use natural processes such as breathing, concentration, and simple touch to help clients feel better and cope with chronic conditions. Nurses can learn these kinds of techniques with minimum preparation, and many of these procedures can be used with clients as independent nursing practice (Dossey et al., 2000). Adequate assessment and the client's permission are prerequisite for implementation. Some CAM therapies may alter physiological responses such that physician-prescribed therapies, such as drug doses, may need to be changed. CAM therapies should be chosen according to the client's functional status, belief or religious perspectives, access to health care, and insurance coverage.

These therapies are designed to teach individuals ways to change their behaviour to alter physical responses to stress and relieve symptoms such as muscle tension, gastrointestinal discomfort, pain, or sleep disturbances. One of the principles of these therapies is that the individual must be actively involved in the treatment. Clients achieve better responses if they practice the techniques or exercises daily. The client must commit to implementing and maintaining the therapy until a desired outcome is achieved.

Table 31-1 Complementary and Alternative Therapies

Types	Descriptions
Alternative Medical Systems	
Acupuncture	Traditional Chinese method to produce analgesia or alter the body's function system by inserting thin needles along a series of channels, called meridians. Direct needle manipulation of energetic meridians influences internal organs.
Ayurveda	Traditional Hindu system of medicine dating to ancient India. Combination of remedies such as herbs, purgative, and rubbing oils used to treat disease.
Homeopathic medicine	System of medical treatments based on the theory that certain diseases can be cured with small doses of substances that, in a healthy person, would produce symptoms similar to those of disease. Prescribed substances called *remedies* are made from naturally occurring plant, animal, or mineral substances.
Latin American practices	*Curanderismo* medical system, which includes a humoral model for classifying food, activity, drugs, illnesses, and a series of folk illnesses.
Traditional Aboriginal medicine	Goals of healing practices include promoting harmony within a community and in the physical and spiritual worlds through sweating and purging, herbal remedies, and shamanic healing.
Naturopathic medicine	System of therapeutics based on natural foods, light, warmth, massage, fresh air, regular exercise, and avoidance of medications. Recognizes the body's inherent healing abilities. Treatments integrate traditional natural therapies with modern diagnostic sciences. Includes botanical (plant) medicine.
Traditional Chinese (Oriental) medicine	Set of systematic techniques and methods including acupuncture, herbal medicines, massage, acupressure, moxibustion (use of heat from burning herbs), Qigong (balancing energy flow through movement), and oriental massage. Fundamental concepts embedded in Taoism, Confucianism, and Buddhism.
Biologically Based Therapies	
Ayurvedic herbs	Traditional Hindu system of herbs.
Gerson therapy	A low-salt, organic diet of fruit juice, raw vegetables, and nutritional supplements, plus coffee enemas to detoxify the liver. Used primarily in the treatment of cancer. Based on the belief that disease is caused by the accumulation of toxic substances that disrupt the body's immune system. Note: This therapy poses health risks because coffee enemas can cause an electrolyte imbalance.
Macrobiotic diet	Predominantly vegan diet (fish, but no animal products), initially used to manage a variety of cancers. Emphasis is on whole cereal grains, vegetables, and unprocessed foods.
Orthomolecular medicine (megavitamin)	Increased intake of nutrients such as vitamin C and beta-carotene. Used to treat cancer, schizophrenia, and certain chronic diseases such as hypercholesterolemia and coronary artery disease.
European phytomedicines	Products developed under strict quality control in sophisticated pharmaceutical factories, packaged as tablets or capsules. Examples include gingko biloba, milk thistle, and bilberry. Herbs have a wide variety of uses.
Traditional Chinese herbal remedies	Herbs considered backbone of medicine. More than 50,000 medicinal plant species, many of which have been studied extensively.
The "Zone"	Dietary program that requires eating a 30:40:30 ratio of protein, carbohydrates, and fats. Used to balance insulin and other hormones for optimal health.
Manipulative and Body-Based Methods	
Acupressure	Therapeutic technique of applying digital pressure in a specified way on designated body points to relieve pain, produce analgesia, or regulate function.
Chiropractic medicine	Therapy that involves manipulation of the spinal column; may include physiotherapy and diet therapy.
Feldenkrais method	Therapy based on establishing good self-image through awareness and correction of body movements. Technique integrates impact of physics on body's movement patterns with how people move, behave, and interact.
Tai chi	Technique that incorporates breath, movement, and meditation to cleanse, strengthen, and circulate vital energy and blood. Used to stimulate immune system and maintain balance.
Massage therapy	Manipulation of soft tissue through stroking, rubbing, or kneading to increase circulation and improve muscle tone and relaxation.
Simple touch	Touching the client in appropriate, gentle ways to stimulate connection, display acceptance, and give appreciation.

Continued

Table 31-1 Complementary and Alternative Therapies—cont'd

Types	Descriptions
Mind-Body Interventions	
Aromatherapy	Using essential plant oils to promote relaxation or stimulation, thereby enhancing overall well-being.
Art therapy	Use of art to reconcile emotional conflicts, foster self-awareness, and express frequently subconscious concerns.
Biofeedback	Using instruments to provide a person with visual or auditory information about autonomic physiological body functions, such as muscle tension, skin temperature, and brain wave activity.
Breathwork	Using any of a variety of breathing patterns to relax, invigorate, or open emotional channels.
Dance therapy	Using dance to treat social, emotional, cognitive, or physical problems.
Hypnotherapy	Induction of trance states and use of therapeutic suggestion to treat paralysis, headaches, addictions, pain, and phobias.
Imagery	Therapeutic technique used to treat pathological conditions by concentrating on an image or series of images.
Labyrinth meditation	Labyrinths are ancient spiritual symbols found in almost every religious tradition. Walking the labyrinth is regarded as an ancient spiritual act of meditation, a time for reflection and prayer, and a pilgrimage.
Meditation	Self-directed practice to relax the body and calm the mind by focusing on rhythmic breathing.
Music therapy	Use of music to meet physical, psychological, cognitive, and social needs of people with disabilities and illness. Used to improve physical movement, communication, emotional expression, and memory. Also used for pain management.
Prayer therapies	Variety of techniques used in multiple cultures that incorporate caring, compassion, love, and empathy. Prayer can be verbal or silent, a solitary or group activity, and include chanting, visualizations, and rituals.
Psychotherapy	Treatment of mental and emotional disorders by psychological techniques.
Yoga	Use of exercise, postures, regulated breathing, and meditation to attain physical and mental well-being. Focuses on the body's musculature, posture, breathing, and consciousness.
Energy Therapies	
Qigong	Derived from ancient Chinese practice of breathing, movement, and meditation. Believed to promote strength, balance, and optimal function. Involves assuming basic postures; is used for stress-related conditions, fatigue, and musculoskeletal stiffness.
Reiki therapy	Derived from ancient Buddhist practices in which practitioner places hand on or above body and transfers "universal life energy" to the client. This energy provides strength, harmony, and balance to treat health issues.
Therapeutic touch	Directing a practitioner's balanced energies toward those of a client. Involves laying of practitioner's hands on or close to a client's body.

Focus on Older Adults

Box 31-2

- Touch is a primary need, as necessary as food, growth, or shelter. Touch can be thought of as a nutrient transmitted through the skin. "Skin hunger" has been described as a form of malnutrition that has reached epidemic proportions, especially among older adults (Fontaine, 2000).
- Older adults need touch as much as or more than any other age group. However, skin hunger or poverty of touch is often acute among older adults, who often have fewer family members or friends to touch them.
- Simple touch could be an enhanced form of communication when other senses are reduced (Dossey et al., 2000).
- Simple touch helps older adult clients feel more connected to and accepted by those around them and to their environment. Self-esteem and sense of worth are enhanced.
- A nurse who reacts aversely to the skin changes of older people may have difficulty touching an older client. The nurse's reluctance may then communicate a negative message to the older adult (Dossey et al., 2000).

Research Highlight Box 31-3

Use of Prayer

Research Focus

People use prayer to cope with distressing symptoms, anxiety-provoking medical procedures, and the illness experience in general. However, no research has explored the lived experience of using prayer to cope with illness. Some research suggests that prayer is highly valued by those who use it, but there is minimal empirical knowledge about clients' prayer experiences and perspectives that nurses can use to support their clients.

Research Abstract

Because prayer appears to be a significant coping strategy for people with cancer, this study sought to describe the experience of prayer among people with cancer. Thirty people with cancer were interviewed about why, when, and how they prayed, as well as what they prayed for and what they expected the prayers to achieve. Findings detailed how people with cancer used prayer to ease the physical, emotional, and spiritual distress of illness. Researchers observed a range of approaches to prayer and topics for prayer, which were often determined by illness circumstances.

Evidence-Based Practice

- Nurses can promote coping by recognizing and facilitating client's use of prayer.
- Clients are likely to pray at times of symptom distress, emotional distress, and during diagnostic and therapeutic processes. At such times, nurses can help by fostering a condition and environment conducive to prayer.
- Although there are commonalities in prayer experiences, it typically is unique to individuals. Therefore nursing strategies for facilitating prayer must be designed with sensitivity to the uniqueness of each client.
- The nurse can help the client to relax, offer spiritual reading material, place the client with a view of nature, offer a notebook for journaling, or guard the client's room from intruders.

Reference

Taylor, E. J., & Outlaw, F. H. (2002). Use of prayer among persons with cancer. *Holistic Nursing Practice, 16*(3), 46–60.

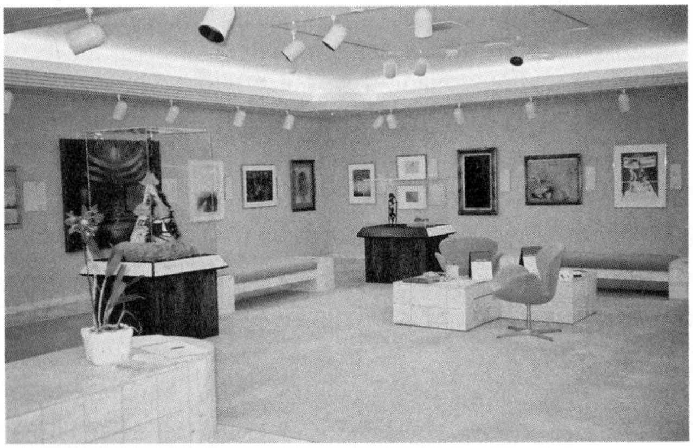

FIGURE **31–3** McMullen Art Gallery, University of Alberta Hospital, is open to visitors, staff, and clients. (Courtesy of the University of Alberta Hospital.)

Relaxation Therapy

People are exposed to stressful situations in everyday life that evoke the **stress response** (see chapter 26). The biochemical functions of major organ systems are modulated by the mind. Thoughts and feelings influence the production of chemicals (i.e., neurotransmitters, neurohormones, and peptides) that circulate in the body and convey messages to various body systems. Physiologically, the stress response causes increased heart, respiratory, and metabolism rates; tightened muscles; and a general sense of foreboding, fear, nervousness, irritability, and negative mood. Other physiological responses include elevated blood pressure, dilated pupils, stronger cardiac contractions, and increased levels of blood glucose, serum cholesterol, circulating free fatty acids, and triglycerides. Although these responses effectively prepare a person for short-term stress, long-term stress can cause structural damage and chronic illness such as angina, tension headaches, cardiac arrhythmias, pain, ulcers, and atrophy of immune system organs (Dossey et al., 2000).

Relaxation is a state of generalized decreased cognitive, physiological, and/or behavioural arousal. The process of relaxation elongates the muscle fibres and reduces the neural impulses sent to the brain, thus decreasing the brain's activity. Relaxation is characterized by decreased heart and respiratory rates, blood pressure, and oxygen consumption and increased alpha brain activity and peripheral skin temperature Relaxation can be achieved with a variety of techniques that incorporate a repetitive mental focus and the adoption of a calm, peaceful attitude (Benson, 1975). Teaching strategies for relaxation are listed in Box 31-4.

Relaxation helps individuals develop the cognitive skills to reduce negative responses to situations. Cognitive skills include focus (the ability to identify, differentiate, and return attention to simple stimuli for an extended period), passivity (the ability to stop unnecessary goal-directed and analytic activity), and receptivity (the ability to tolerate and accept experiences that may be uncertain, unfamiliar, or paradoxical). With relaxation therapy, the client learns to monitor and consciously release tension.

Progressive relaxation involves teaching individuals to effectively rest and reduce physical tension. The client learns to detect subtle localized sensations of muscle tension in one muscle group (e.g., the forearm muscle). In addition, the client learns to differentiate between

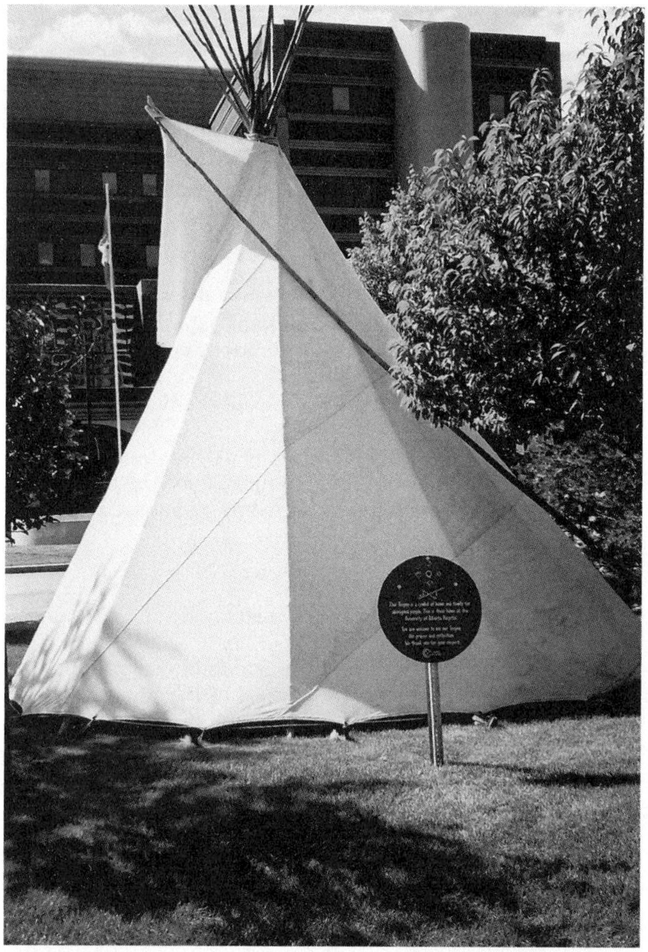

FIGURE 31–4 This teepee outside the University of Alberta Hospital in Edmonton is available for prayer, meditation, and sacred ceremony. (Courtesy of the University of Alberta Hospital.)

high-intensity tension (strong fist clenching) and subtle tension (Dossey et al., 2000). Progressive relaxation is then practised using different muscle groups. One active progressive relaxation technique involves the use of slow, deep abdominal breathing while tightening and relaxing an ordered succession of muscle groups. When guiding a client, the nurse may elect to begin with the muscles in the face, followed by those in the arms, hands, abdomen, legs, and feet.

Passive relaxation involves teaching individuals to relax muscle groups without actively contracting the muscles. One passive relaxation technique incorporates slow, abdominal breathing exercises with imagining warmth and relaxation flowing through specific muscle groups; muscle tension is then released during expiration. Passive relaxation is useful for people who find that active muscle contracting leads to discomfort or exhaustion.

Clinical Applications of Relaxation Therapy. Relaxation techniques lower heart rate and blood pressure, decrease muscle tension, improve well-being, and reduce symptom distress in people experiencing a variety of situations (e.g., complications from medical treatment or grieving the loss of a significant other; Jacobs, 2001). The type of relaxation intervention should be matched to the individual's functional status, the energy expenditure of the relaxation technique, and the motivation of the individual for frequent practice.

Relaxation, alone or in combination with deep breathing, imagery, yoga (Figure 31–5), and music, has been shown to reduce pain (Astin et al., 2002; Good et al., 2001), improve chronic fatigue syndrome (Deale et al., 2001), control hypertension (Yung, French, & Leung, 2001), improve preterm labour outcomes (Janke, 1999), contribute significantly to cancer palliative care (Ernst, 2001), and increase survival following cardiac arrest (Cowan, Pike, & Budzynski, 2001). However, more studies are needed to validate the effects of relaxation therapy. For example, other variables or activities that may also lead to reduced physiological activity and pain level should be controlled in studies to determine if an individual's improved response is due to the relaxation therapy alone. Such variables may include a healthy support network, a positive attitude including humour, and other behavioural therapies such as yoga and tai chi.

Relaxation is a valuable technique because it enables individuals to exert some control over their lives. People may experience a decreased feeling of helplessness and a more positive psychological state overall, which helps them to have a less negative view of their situation.

Limitations of Relaxation Therapy. Some clients using relaxation training have reported fearing loss of control, feeling like they are floating, and experiencing relaxation-induced anxiety related to these feelings. During relaxation training, individuals learn to distinguish between low and high levels of muscle tension. During the first months of training, when learning to focus on sensations and tension, some clients report increased sensitivity in detecting muscle tension. Usually these feelings abate with training. However, nurses should monitor clients for worsening symptoms or the development of new symptoms (Dossey et al., 2000).

An important consideration when choosing which relaxation technique to use is the physiological and psychological status of the client. Clients with advanced disease such as cancer may seek relaxation training to reduce their stress response. However, techniques such as active progressive relaxation training require a moderate expenditure of energy, which can amplify a person's existing fatigue and limit the person's ability to complete individual relaxation sessions and practice. Therefore, active progressive relaxation is not appropriate for clients with advanced disease or with decreased energy reserves. Passive relaxation or imagery is more appropriate for these individuals.

Meditation and Breathing

Meditation is any activity that limits stimulus input by directing attention to a single unchanging or repetitive stimulus (Pelletier, 2000). It is a general term for a range of practices that relax the body and still the mind. The root word, *meditari,* means to consider. In 1975, Dr. Herbert Benson wrote *The Relaxation Response,* which drew the attention of Western health care practitioners to the physical and psychological benefits of relaxation. As Benson noted,

Client Teaching **Box 31-4**

Relaxation

Objective

- The client will demonstrate decreased anxiety, tension, and other manifestations of the stress response as a result of the relaxation intervention.

Teaching Strategies

Meditation and Rhythmic Breathing (Eliciting the Relaxation Response)

1. Provide a quiet environment.
2. Help the client get comfortable while seated or lying on back. Have client remain as still as possible and encourage to move only if necessary to remain comfortable.
3. Instruct the client to close eyes and to hold a receptive attitude—"There is nothing more important for me to do for the next 15 minutes" or "What will be, will be."
4. Instruct client to breathe in and out slowly and deeply using the abdominal muscles, keeping the chest still.
5. At the beginning of every out-breath, have client repeat the number "one" silently in his or her mind. Continue for period of meditation.
6. Explain that when the mind wanders, bring it back to counting the out-breath without judgment.
7. Have client practise for 5, 10, 15, or 20 minutes per session. Practise daily for at least one session.

Progressive Relaxation

1. Follow steps 1, 2, 3, and 4 of meditation and rhythmic breathing.
2. Once the client is breathing slowly and comfortably, instruct client to tighten and relax an ordered succession of muscle groups, tensing them and then relaxing them, while feeling each part relax.
3. Instruct client to tense and then relax the calves, knees, and so on.

Relaxation by Sensory Pacing

1. Follow steps 1, 2, 3, and 4 of meditation and rhythmic breathing.
2. Instruct client to slowly repeat and finish, either in a low voice or to self, each of the following sentences:
   Now I am aware of seeing . . .
   Now I am aware of feeling . . .
   Now I am aware of hearing . . .
   Instruct client to repeat and complete each sentence four times, then three times, then twice, and finally once.

Relaxation by Colour Exchange

1. Follow steps 1, 2, 3, and 4 of meditation and rhythmic breathing.
2. Instruct client to notice any tension, tightness, aches, or pains in the body and to give that sensation the first colour that comes to mind.
3. Instruct client to breathe in pure white light from the universe and send the light to a tense or painful place in the body, letting the white light surround the colour of the discomfort.
4. Instruct client to exhale the colour of the discomfort and let the white light take its place.
5. Instruct client to continue breathing in the white light and exhaling the colour of the discomfort, allowing the white light to fill the entire body and bring about a sense of peace, well-being, and energy.

Modified Autogenic Relaxation

1. Follow steps 1, 2, 3, and 4 of meditation and rhythmic breathing.
2. Instruct client to repeat each of the following phrases to self four times, saying the first part of the phrases while breathing in for 2 to 3 seconds, holding the breath for 2 to 3 seconds, then saying the last part of the phrases while breathing out for 2 to 3 seconds.

Breathing In	Breathing Out
I am	relaxed.
My arms and legs	are heavy and warm.
My heartbeat	is calm and regular.
My breathing	is free and easy.
My abdomen	is loose and warm.
My forehead	is cool.
My mind	is quiet and still.

Relaxing With Music

1. Provide client with a CD player and headset.
2. Ask client to select a favourite CD of slow, quiet music.
3. Instruct client to get into a comfortable position (either sitting or lying down but with arms and legs uncrossed) and to close eyes and listen to the music through the headset.
4. Instruct client to imagine floating or drifting with the music while listening.

Evaluation

- Assess client's vital signs, particularly respiratory pattern.
- Ask client to describe level of tension or uneasiness felt.
- Observe client for presence of behaviours that display anxiety.

the components of meditation are simple: a quiet space, comfortable position, receptive attitude, and focus of attention. He described meditation as a process that anyone can use to calm down, cope with stress, and, for those with spiritual inclinations, feel as one with God or the universe. Meditation is compatible with most religious practices and can be practised alone or in groups. Most meditation techniques involve slow, relaxed, deep, usually abdominal, breathing (see Box 31-4). It evokes a restful state, lowers oxygen consumption, reduces respiratory and heart rates, and reduces anxiety.

Clinical Applications of Meditation. There are many indications for meditation (Box 31-5). There is evidence that meditation improves breathing patterns in clients with asthma, manages stress-related illnesses, lowers

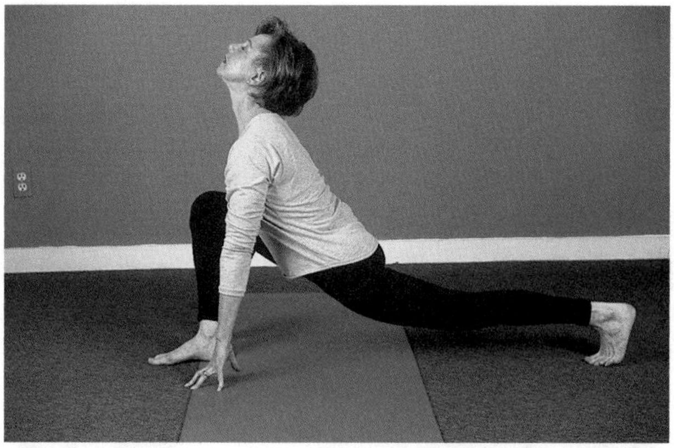

FIGURE **31–5** Yoga focuses on muscles, posture, breathing, and consciousness.

Box 31-5 Indications for Meditation

- Anxiety or tension
- Chronic bereavement
- Chronic fatigue syndrome
- Chronic pain
- Drug abuse (alcohol or tobacco)
- Hypertension
- Irritability
- Low self-esteem; self-blame
- Mild depression
- Psycho-physiological disorders
- Sleep disorders

blood pressure (King, Carr, & D'Cruz, 2002; Lee et al., 2000) and blood glucose levels, decreases episodes of angina pectoris (Cunningham, Brown, & Kaski, 2000), and lowers cholesterol. It is also used to reduce anxiety (Speca et al., 2000), sleep-onset insomnia, stuttering, the symptoms of irritable bowel syndrome (Keefer & Blanchard, 2001, 2002; Shannahoff-Khalsa, 2002), and even the incidence of dental caries by reducing salivary bacteria (Pelletier, 2000). Meditation also increases productivity and sense of self, improves mood, and reduces irritability (Dossey et al., 2000).

When considering meditation, nurses should consider the client's degree of self-discipline, although it actually requires less self-discipline than most other behavioural therapies.

Limitations of Meditation. Although meditation has a number of physiological and psychological benefits, it may be contraindicated in some clients. For example, someone with a strong fear of losing control may perceive meditation as a form of mind control and thus may be resistant to learning the technique. Some clients are sensitive to meditation and require shorter sessions than the typical 15 to 20 minutes.

Meditation can also augment the effects of certain drugs. For example, individuals taking anti-hypertensive, thyroid-regulating, antidepressant, or anti-anxiety medications should be monitored. Prolonged practice of meditation techniques may, in some cases, lead to the reduced need for certain medications, and some doses of medications may need to be adjusted (Pelletier, 2000). Individuals learning meditation, therefore, should be monitored closely for physiological changes with respect to their medications.

Imagery

Imagery or visualization techniques, which are frequently used with relaxation training, help create mental images to stimulate physical changes, improve perceived well-being, and/or enhance self-awareness. Frequently, imagery is used with relaxation training. Imagery can be self-directed or guided by a practitioner (Dossey et al., 2000). For example, the client may be directed to begin slow, abdominal breathing while focusing on the rhythm of breathing. The client is then instructed to visualize ocean waves coming to shore with each inhalation, then receding with each exhalation. Next, the client is instructed to notice the smells, sounds, and temperatures that he or she is experiencing. As the session progresses, the client may be instructed to visualize warmth entering the body during inspiration and tension leaving the body during expiration. Imagery scenarios should be individualized for each client and/or left up to the client to develop.

Imagery can evoke powerful psycho-physiological responses, such as alterations in immune function (Fontaine, 2000). Many imagery techniques involve visual imagery, but they can also include the auditory, proprioceptive, gustatory, and olfactory senses. An example of this involves visualizing a lemon being sliced in half and squeezing the lemon juice under the tongue. This visualization has been observed to produce increased salivation as effectively as the actual event. People typically respond to their environment according to the way they perceive it, as well as by their own visualizations and expectancies. Therefore, individuals can learn to regulate themselves by selecting appropriate visualizations and expectations (Dossey et al., 2000).

Creative visualization is a form of self-directed imagery based on the principle of mind-body connectivity (i.e., every mental image leads to physical or emotional responses; Gawain, 2002). Client teaching strategies for creative visualization are listed in Box 31-6.

Clinical Applications of Imagery. Imagery has been used to visualize cancer cells being destroyed by immune system cells, to control or relieve pain, and to achieve calmness and serenity. It has also been used in the treatment of chronic conditions such as asthma, hypertension, functional urinary disorders, menstrual and premenstrual syndromes, gastrointestinal disorders such as irritable bowel syndrome, and rheumatoid arthritis (Dossey et al., 2000; Fontaine, 2000).

Limitations of Imagery. Imagery has few side effects. However, it is probably one of the least clearly defined interventions and can range from being highly structured to consisting of spontaneous daydreams by the individual (Pelletier, 2000).

Client Teaching Box 31-6

Creative Visualization

Objective

The client will demonstrate skills in creative visualization.

Teaching Strategies

- Set goals that can be accomplished, because confidence and increased self-esteem are achieved through success.
- Create clear images developed in the present tense (e.g., imagine you are floating on a soft, white cloud).
- Frequently visualize the image. Visualization should be done throughout the day, but especially upon awakening or before sleep, when the mind is usually more relaxed.
- While focusing on the image, repeat encouraging statements, such as positive affirmations to alleviate doubts about one's ability to achieve one's goals.

Evaluation

- Observe client for anxiety.
- Ask client if the experience was helpful.
- Ask client if he or she uses positive self-dialogue with visualization (e.g., "I am feeling stronger").
- Note if client reports images of desired health habits, feelings, and desires for healing.
- Note if client reports improved coping with daily stressors.

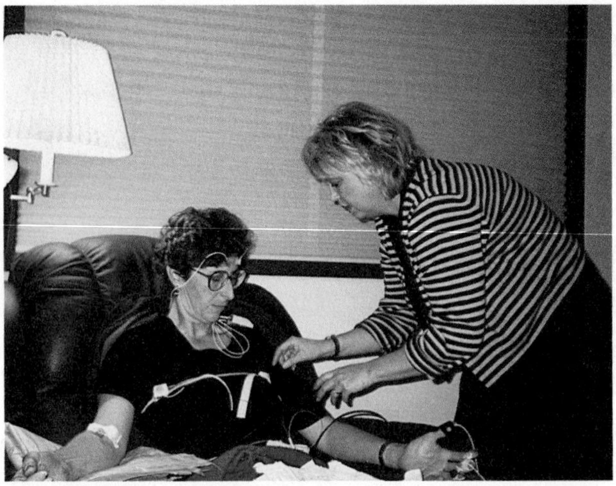

FIGURE **31–6** Biofeedback monitoring. Electrodes are placed on the frontalis and trapezius muscles and the fingers of the left hand. Pneumograph measurements are also made.

Training-Specific Therapies

Training-specific therapies are CAM treatments that may be administered by nurses, but only after the nurse completes a specific course of study and training. A nurse must have a certification, degree, or licence beyond that of registered nurse to administer most of these therapies. Several training-specific therapies are recognized as being very effective and are recommended by Western health care practitioners (e.g., biofeedback and therapeutic touch). But many have not been studied in a systematic way to establish their effectiveness. Many of these unproven techniques are very popular in our society and used by many people from other cultures who live in Canada. Many have positive effects, but some have negative effects, too. Some may have harmful results when used with standard Western medical therapies. Therefore, the nurse should acquire at least a passing knowledge of such treatments and know their possible harmful interactions.

Biofeedback

Biofeedback techniques are frequently used in addition to relaxation interventions to assist individuals in learning how to control specific autonomic nervous system responses. **Biofeedback** is a group of therapeutic procedures that use electronic or electromechanical instruments to measure, process, and provide information about neuromuscular and autonomic nervous system activity (Figure 31–6). This information, or feedback, is provided in physical, physiological, auditory, and/or visual feedback signals. For example, clients may hear a sound if their pulse rate or blood pressure increases out of their therapeutic zone. Practitioners help clients develop awareness of and voluntary control over physiological responses (Pelletier, 2000).

Biofeedback is considered to complement traditional relaxation programs because it can immediately demonstrate to clients their ability to control some physiological responses. It can also help individuals to focus on and monitor specific body parts. By providing immediate feedback in terms of what stress relaxation behaviours work most effectively, it helps the client control physiological functions that are most difficult to control. Eventually, the client will be able to notice positive physiological changes without the need for instrument feedback. Biofeedback demonstrates to the client the relationship between thoughts, feelings, and physiological responses.

Clinical Applications of Biofeedback. Biofeedback has numerous applications. It has successfully treated migraine headaches (Sarafino & Goehring, 2000; Scharff, Marcus, & Masek, 2002), phantom limb pain (Belleggia & Birbaumer, 2001), abdominal pain, temporomandibular pain (Crider & Glaros, 1999), urinary incontinence (Abdelghany et al., 2001), hypertension (Nakao et al., 1999), and some anxiety disorders (Moore, 2000).

One of the most critical components of any behavioural program is adherence to the treatment regimen. Clients who are compliant with appointments, practice times, and goal setting tend to be the most successful.

Limitations of Biofeedback. Although biofeedback has demonstrated effectiveness in a number of client populations, there are several precautions. During relaxation therapy and/or biofeedback sessions, repressed emotions or feelings may be uncovered that clients cannot cope with alone. For this reason, practitioners should be

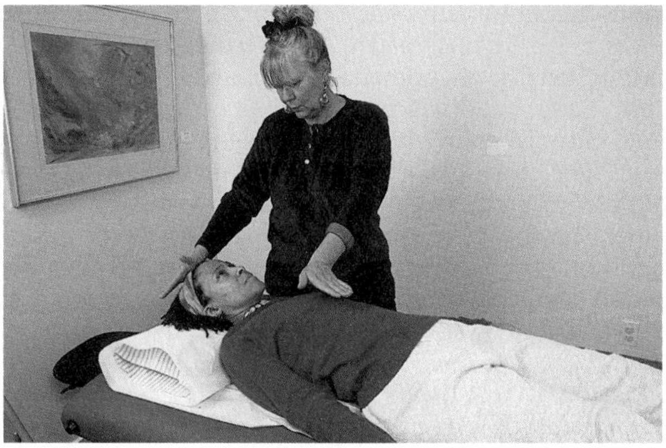

FIGURE 31–7 In therapeutic touch, the practitioner directs the practitioner's own energy to help or heal another.

trained in traditional psychological methods or be able to refer clients to qualified professionals.

Therapeutic Touch

Therapeutic touch (TT) is a training-specific therapy that was developed in the 1970s by a nurse, Dr. Dolores Krieger. Although the philosophical and religious assumptions of TT are different from those of other Eastern healing modalities, they are similar in that both involve trained practitioners who attempt to direct their own balanced energies in an intentional and motivated manner toward those of the client (Krieger, Peper, & Ancoli, 1979).

TT consists of placing the practitioner's hands either on or close to the body of a person (Figure 31–7). The practitioner scans the client's body and diagnoses areas of accumulated tensions. The practitioner then attempts to redirect these energies in order to bring the person back into energy balance (Krieger, 1975; Krieger et al., 1979).

TT consists of five phases: centring, assessment, unruffling, treatment, and evaluation. Centring is the process whereby the practitioner becomes aware and fully present during the entire treatment. The next phase involves the assessment of the client, in which the practitioner moves his or her hands (roughly 5 to 15 cm from the body) in a rhythmic and symmetrical movement from the head to the toes. During this phase, the practitioner notices the quality of **energy flow** and detects accumulations of energy. Physiological indicators of energy imbalance are perceived as congestion, pressure, warmth, coolness, blockage, pulling or drawing, or static or tingling (Krieger, 1975). During the third phase, the practitioner "unruffles" the energy flow or facilitates the symmetrical and rhythmical flow of energy through the body with long downward strokes over the energy field located over the entire body. This rebalancing of energy is achieved either by the practitioner touching the body or by maintaining the hands in a position a few centimetres away from the body. The final phase consists of an evaluation of the client and a reassessment of the energy field. If rebalance is achieved, the practitioner detects a more symmetrical, freely flowing energy field (Krieger et al., 1979).

Clinical Applications of Therapeutic Touch. Early studies found that TT was able to increase hemoglobin levels in several clients (Krieger, 1975; Krieger et al., 1979). Other studies have found it reduced anxiety levels in hospitalized clients with cardiovascular disease, reduced headache pain, and improved mood in bereaved adults (Krieger, 1975; Krieger et al., 1979). Research has also shown that TT can improve outcomes in postpartum women (Kiernan, 2002), reduce pain and shorten hospital stay following abdominal surgery (Smyth, 2001), help treat drug addiction (Hagemaster, 2000), and reduce or eliminate phantom limb pain (Leskowitz, 2000).

Limitations of Therapeutic Touch. Although some studies have demonstrated that TT produces positive outcomes, others have not. TT may be contraindicated in certain client populations. For example, people who are sensitive to human interaction and touch (e.g., those who have been physically abused or have psychiatric disorders) may misinterpret the intent of the treatment and may feel threatened and anxious by the treatment. Other clients who are sensitive to energy repatterning may also need to avoid TT. These include premature infants, newborns, children, pregnant women, older or debilitated people, or those in critical, unstable conditions (Fontaine, 2000).

Chiropractic Therapy

Chiropractic therapy was developed in 1895 and has become the third-largest independently practised health profession in the Western world (Pelletier, 2000). Chiropractors graduate from well-established preparatory programs similar to medical schools. The central tenet of the chiropractic profession is spinal manipulation directed at certain joints by practitioners using their hands or an instrument. Manipulation is defined as the forceful passive movement of a joint beyond its active limit of motion. Chiropractic therapy is considered a holistic therapy that does not typically use drugs or surgery.

The basic principles of chiropractic therapy incorporate the idea that human beings have an innate healing potential, and the goal of this healing profession is to harness this potential. Chiropractic therapy promotes both a natural diet and regular exercise as critical components for the body to function properly (Fontaine, 2000).

Clinical Applications of Chiropractic Therapy. The basic goals of chiropractic therapy focus on restoring the structural and functional imbalances that may result in pain. One of the major structural distortions that chiropractors treat is vertebral subluxation, in which the joint mobility is decreased due to slight changes in the position of the articulating bones. A more severe form of subluxation, called fixation, exists when joint motion is restricted. Chiropractic interventions treat musculoskeletal abnormalities, headaches, dysmenorrhea, blood pressure, vertigo, tinnitus, and visual disorders (Pelletier, 2000).

Limitations of Chiropractic Therapy. Several diseases or joint conditions should not be treated with manipulation. If a malignancy is suspected or determined through diagnostic testing, the client should be referred to a medical physician for further evaluation and treatment. Bone and joint infections also require pharmaceutical or surgical intervention, and the structural integrity of the bone may be compromised if excessive force is used. Contraindications for chiropractic therapy include acute myelopathy, fractures, dislocations, rheumatoid arthritis, and osteoporosis. Severe complications secondary to neck and spine manipulation are rare; however, some research suggests this type of manipulation on infants and children be avoided (Stewart et al., 2002).

Traditional Chinese Medicine

Traditional Chinese medicine (TCM) comprises several healing modalities, including herbs, acupuncture, moxibustion, diet, exercise, and meditation. TCM is several thousand years old and has its roots in Taoism. A major concept in Chinese medicine is the **yin and yang,** which represent opposing, yet complementary, phenomena that exist in a state of dynamic equilibrium. Examples are night/day, hot/cold, and shady/sunny. Yin represents shade, cold, and inhibition, whereas yang represents fire, light, and excitement. Yin also represents the inner part of the body, specifically the viscera, liver, heart, spleen, lung, and kidney, whereas yang represents the outer part, specifically the bowels, stomach, and bladder. When there is an imbalance in these paired opposites, then it is thought that disease occurs (Fontaine, 2000).

Qi (pronounced *chi*) is defined as the body's vital energy. Disease is classified into three major categories: external causes, internal causes, and neither internal nor external causes (Table 31-2). Regardless of the cause, it is thought that yin and yang go out of balance, thus altering the movement of *qi*. The body has several forms of *qi* that directly influence its physiological functions and help maintain homeostasis.

Channels of energy run in regular patterns through the body and over its surface. These channels, called **meridians,** are like rivers flowing through the body. An obstruction of these meridians is like a dam that backs up the flow in one part of the body and restricts it in others, eventually leading to disease. Twelve primary and eight secondary channels have been identified. Located along the channels are **acupoints,** or holes through which *qi* can be influenced by the insertion of needles, a process known as **acupuncture**.

Another important component of Chinese medicine involves five elements: earth, metal, water, wood, and fire. Various health phenomena are organized according to these phases and interact with each other. In Chinese medicine, outward manifestations reflect the internal environment. There are two primary areas that are assessed in Chinese medicine: the tongue and several pulses. The colour, shape, and coating of the tongue reflect the general condition of the internal organs. The pulses provide information about the condition and balance of *qi,* blood, ying and yang, and the internal organs (Fontaine, 2000).

Acupuncture

Acupuncture is a method of stimulating certain points (acupoints) on the body by the insertion of special needles to modify the perception of pain, normalize physiological functions, or treat or prevent disease (Figure 31–8). Acupuncture is used to regulate the flow of *qi*. According to Chinese traditional medicine, acupuncture needles unblock obstructed energy and re-establish the flow of *qi* through the meridians, thereby stimulating and activating the body's self-healing abilities. Effects of needles may be enhanced by application of heat or weak electrical currents to the needles (Fontaine, 2000).

Clinical Applications of Acupuncture. Acupuncture is the primary treatment used by practitioners of Chinese medicine. Many allopathic physicians and health care professionals are also being trained and certified in acupuncture.

Acupuncture is used to treat low back pain, myofascial pain, simple and migraine headaches, sciatica, shoulder pain, tennis elbow, osteoarthritis, whiplash, and musculoskeletal sprains. Other problems that have been successfully treated include sinusitis, gastrointestinal disorders, perimenstrual symptoms, neurological disorders, chronic pulmonary diseases (including asthma), hypertension, smoking and other addictions, and clinical depression (Pelletier, 2000).

Limitations of Acupuncture. Acupuncture is considered a safe therapy when the practitioner has been appropriately trained and uses sterilized needles. Although complications have been noted, they are rare if appropriate steps are taken to ensure the safety of the equipment and

Table 31-2 Three Causes of Disease According to Traditional Chinese Medicine

Cause of Disease	Influences
External causes, or "the six evils"	Wind, cold, fire, damp, summer heat, dryness
Internal causes, or internal damage by seven effects	Joy, anger, anxiety, thought, sorrow, fear, fright
Non-external, non-internal causes	Dietary irregularities, excessive sexual activity, taxation fatigue, trauma, parasites

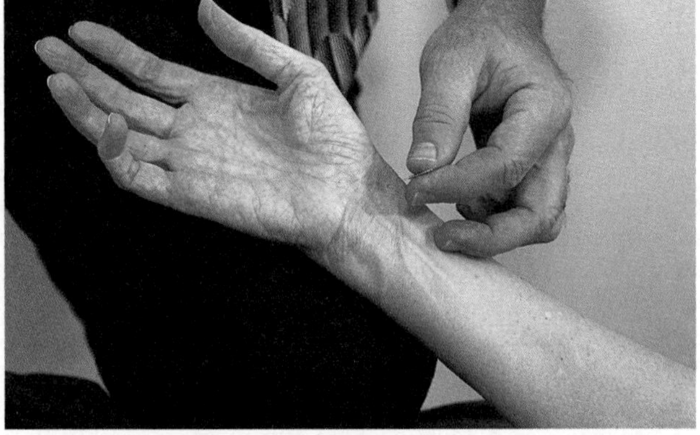

FIGURE **31–8** Acupuncture.

the client. These complications include puncture of an internal organ, bleeding, fainting, seizures, miscarriage, post-treatment drowsiness, and infections from needles being left in place for an extended length of time and from contaminated and broken needles.

Acupuncture should be used with caution in pregnant clients and those who have a history of seizures, are hepatitis carriers, or are infected with HIV. Treatment is contraindicated in people with bleeding disorders, thrombocytopenia, or skin infections. Semi-permanent needles should not be used with people who have valvular heart disease because of the increased risk of infection. Electroacupuncture should be avoided in people who have pacemakers, are pregnant, or have cardiac arrhythmias or epilepsy (Fontaine, 2000).

Herbal Therapies

An estimated 25,000 plant species are used medicinally throughout the world. **Herbal therapy** is the oldest form of medicine; archeological evidence suggests that Neanderthals used herbal remedies 60,000 years ago. Herbal therapy was widespread for thousands of years, but its popularity declined with the development of modern scientific medicine in the early eighteenth century. However, because approximately 80% of the world's population live in developing countries, herbal medicine constitutes a prominent part of health care worldwide. In countries that use predominantly allopathic medicine, growing concern about the complications and limitations of scientific medicine and consumer interest in natural foods have contributed to increased interest in herbal medicine (Fontaine, 2000).

Herbal substances used in Chinese medicine are taken from plants, animals, or minerals, whereas those used in Western herbal medicine are prepared primarily from plant materials. The active ingredients are prepared in tinctures or extracts, elixirs, syrups, capsules, pills, tablets, lozenges, powders, ointments or creams, drops, and suppositories. Many people think, incorrectly, that because herbs are natural plants, they will not cause harm or side effects. As with other medications, some herbal substances contain powerful chemicals and should be examined for interaction and compatibility with other prescribed or unprescribed substances. As well, many herbs are sold with claims that they can "cure" certain ailments, such as pau d'arco for curing cancer, when their efficacy has not been determined through clinical trials. Herbs are generally classified as beneficial, harmful, or neutral, in which case they have no effects on the specific ailment.

The philosophy of herbal therapy is different from that of conventional drug therapy. The goal of herbal therapy is to restore balance within the individual by facilitating the person's self-healing ability. Drug therapy, on the other hand, is aimed at the treatment of specific diseases or symptoms. Herbal therapy is also prescribed on an individual basis with unique herbal concoctions tailored for each person (Kuhn & Winston, 2001). Many herbal medicines are sold as food or food supplements in health food stores and through private companies.

The federal *Food and Drugs Act* states that all drugs have to be proven safe and effective before being sold to the public. In 2004, Health Canada launched a six-year program to regulate all over-the-counter natural health products, including herbal therapies and homeopathic medicines. Natural health products that have been approved for sale under the new regulations have been assigned a Drug Identification Number (DIN; DIN-HM for homeopathic medicines) or Natural Product Number (NPN). These numbers certify that the product has passed a review of their formulation, labelling, and instructions for use. Health Canada advises Canadians only to use health products that carry a DIN, DIN-HM, or NPN on the label.

Clinical Applications of Herbal Therapy. A number of herbs have been determined to be safe and effective for a variety of conditions (Table 31-3). Milk thistle, for example, can effectively treat certain liver and gallbladder conditions and its antioxidant properties are thought to protect the liver and facilitate regeneration of liver cells. St. John's Wort is effective as a mild antidepressant and sedative, along with offering some protection against viruses. Clinical trials investigating the effectiveness of St. John's Wort against AIDS have begun (Kuhn & Winston, 2001; Skidmore-Roth, 2003).

Limitations of Herbal Therapy. Although herbal medicine has been shown to provide beneficial effects for a variety of conditions, a number of problems may exist. Concentrations of active ingredients can vary considerably and contamination with other herbs or chemicals, including pesticides and heavy metals, may also occur. Some herbs have also been found to contain toxic products that can cause cancer. Comfrey, for example, has been used for its wound-healing properties. However, various species of comfrey contain highly carcinogenic pyrrolizidine alkaloids, and it has produced liver cancer in small animals. Other unsafe herbs are listed in Table 31-4.

Not all companies follow strict quality control and manufacturing guidelines, which set standards for acceptable levels of pesticides, residual solvents, bacterial levels, and heavy metals. For this reason, herbal medicine should be purchased only from reputable manufacturers (Box 31-7). In addition, labels on herbal products should contain the scientific name of the botanical, the name and address of the manufacturer, batch or lot number, date of manufacture, and expiration date. If the product has been assessed by Health Canada for safety and effectiveness, it will also have a DIN, DIN-HM, or NPN on its label.

Concurrent use of herbal or other natural products with prescription or over-the-counter medications should be monitored. Herbs may interfere with medications metabolized within a narrow therapeutic range. Pharmacokinetic interactions occur when an herb inhibits or enhances a particular medication's site of action. For example, theophylline in combination with St. John's Wort may elevate serum blood levels of theophylline, leading to negative side effects (Bonakdar, 2003).

Despite the increased use of herbal products, there has not been a parallel increase in reports of toxicity. Nonetheless, herbal products should be avoided or used with extreme caution in pregnant women, nursing mothers, infants or young children, or older adults with liver or cardiovascular disease (Fontaine, 2000).

Table 31-3 Herbs in Common Use and Considered Safe (NOTE: Data Do Not Support the Use of These Herbs in Infants or Children, or During Pregnancy or Lactation.)

Common Name	Effects	Examples of Uses	Warnings	Other
Astragalus (*Huang-qi*)	Stimulates immune system Cardiotonic Antioxidant	Cancer and tonic *qi* (vital energy—in Chinese medicine) Ischemic heart disease Congestive heart failure	People with autoimmune disease or who are immunosuppressed should use with caution	No adverse side effects No studies on long-term use
Bilberry (fruit only)	Vasoprotective Anti-edema Antioxidant Anti-platelet	To improve night vision Diabetic and hypertensive retinopathy Dysmenorrhea Nosebleeds Traditionally used for diarrhea, peripheral vascular disorders, diabetes	Possible interactions with ASA and warfarin due to anti-platelet activity	Most effective form: dried extract in tablet or capsule Long-term use of large doses can be poisonous Monitor for bleeding
Black cohosh	Inhibits estradiol binding to estrogen receptors, thereby exerting a weak estrogenic effect	Menopausal hot flashes Premenstrual syndrome	Contraindicated in women with a history of breast cancer	Safely used in studies lasting up to 6 months Many active constituents, glycosides, tannins, and sugars Is promising in the relief of hot flashes related to menopause
Chamomile (German or Hungarian)	Topically: Anti-inflammatory, aids wound healing Oral: With pectin, anti-diarrheal/anti-spasmodic	Eczema Eye irritation Throat discomfort Hemorrhoids Gastrointestinal spasms Inflammatory conditions Insomnia Menstrual disorders Migraines	Contraindicated if allergies to daisy family May potentiate effect of anticoagulants May cause abortions	
Echinacea	Topically: Anaesthetic and anti-inflammatory Orally: Stimulates immune system	Prevents yeast, *Trichomonas,* vaginal infections Wound healing Prevents/treats upper respiratory infection, colds, urinary tract infection, septicemia, and boils	Contraindicated in conjunction with cancer treatment or in people with autoimmune disease, multiple sclerosis, tuberculosis, diabetes, asthma, leukemia, HIV/AIDS, lupus, or allergies to daisy family Not to be used longer than 8 weeks	Chemical constituents differ a great deal among roots, leaves, flowers, and between species
Evening primrose oil	Anti-inflammatory May lower blood pressure	Atopic dermatitis Premenstrual syndrome Menopausal hot flashes Rheumatoid arthritis Raynaud's disease Source of essential fatty acids	Contraindicated in clients with seizure disorders Large doses may cause loose stools and abdominal pain	Active ingredient is omega-6 essential fatty acid, gamma-linoleic acid Studies have shown positive effect on atopic dermatitis

Adapted from *Herbs: Everyday Reference for Health Professionals,* edited by F. Chandler, 2000, Ottawa, ON: Canadian Pharmacists Association and the Canadian Medical Association; *Professionals Handbook of Complementary and Alternative Medicines,* by C. W. Fetrow and J. R. Avila, 1999, Springhouse, PA: Springhouse; and *Natural Medicines Comprehensive Database* (5th ed), The Pharmacists Letter, 2003, Stockton, CA: Therapeutic Research Faculty Staff.

Table 31-3 Herbs in Common Use and Considered Safe (NOTE: Data Do Not Support the Use of These Herbs in Infants or Children, or During Pregnancy or Lactation.)—cont'd

Common Name	Effects	Examples of Uses	Warnings	Other
Garlic	Lowers blood pressure and blood lipids Stimulates immune system Inhibits platelet aggregation Antibacterial	Hypertension Cold and flu prevention Athlete's foot (topically)	May prolong bleeding time Possibly interacts with anticoagulants	Not recommended for use during pregnancy due to effect on bleeding time
Ginger	Anti-emetic	Motionsickness Nausea and vomiting	Client must use with caution if at risk for hemorrhage	
Ginkgo biloba	Inhibits platelet-activating factor Antimicrobial Anti-tumour Bronchodilator Arterial and vasodilator Decreases capillary fragility Anti-oxidant	Dementia Poor circulation	Ingestion may increase risk of serious bleeding Clients taking drugs affecting hemostasis must use with caution Can cause contact dermatitis	Claims to improve mental alertness and brain function are not supported in clinical trials
Hawthorn	Increases cardiac blood flow Decreases dyspnea and palpitations Lowers of cholesterol	Coronary artery disease Angina	Potentiates digitalis effects Contraindicated if client is using cardiac drugs	
Milk thistle	Antioxidant Protects liver cells Anti-inflammatory Anti-carcinogenic Inhibits hepatic cholesterol synthesis	Chronic hepatitis Cirrhosis Alcohol liver disease	No known contraindications	
Saw palmetto	Androgen receptor blocker; anti-inflammatory	Benign prostatic hyperplasia Urinary problems	May interact with oral contraceptives	
St. John's wort	Antidepressant Antiviral	Mild to moderate depression Anxiety Fatigue Sedative Wound healing (topical) Peptic ulcers Chronic gastritis in depressed alcoholics	Not appropriate for severe depression May interact with medications prescribed for heart conditions and asthma May interact with alcohol and over-the-counter cold and flu medications Avoid foods containing tyramines, such as aged cheese and red wine The client must protect against ultraviolet exposure when using this herb	Has been used for more than 2000 years Studies support use in mild to moderate depression
Valerian	Smooth muscle relaxant Vasodilator in angina Possible antidepressant	Muscle spasms Sleep disorders Restlessness	May cause headaches or gastrointestinal disturbances	Studies support use in insomnia Client must avoid using concurrently with other sedatives

Table 31-4 Unsafe Herbs

Common name	Effects	Comments
Aristolochia (also known as birthwort, snakeroot, snakeweed, sangree root)	Appetite stimulant Promotion of menstruation Aphrodisiac	Contains aristocholic acid, which causes kidney damage and cancer
Borage	Diuretic Anti-diarrheal	Contains toxic pyrrolizidine alkaloids
Calamus	Fever Digestive aid	Contains varying amounts of carcinogenic *cis*-isoasarone Indian type most toxic North American type non-toxic
Chaparral	Anti-cancer	No proven efficacy May induce severe liver toxicity
Coltsfoot	Anti-tussive Demulcent	Contains carcinogenic pyrrolizidine alkaloids
Comfrey	Wound healing	Contains large number of toxic pyrrolizidine alkaloids May induce venoocclusive disease
Ehpedra *(ma huang)*	Central nervous system stimulant Anorectic Bronchodilator Cardiac stimulation	Unsafe for people with hypertension, diabetes, or thyroid disease Avoid consumption with caffeine
Germander	Anorectic	Causes hepatotoxicity because of diterpenoid derivatives
Kava	Used for nervous anxiety, stress Sleep aid	Hepatotoxicity and liver failure in at least 68 documented cases of liver toxicity following use
Life root (ragwort)	Menstrual flow stimulant	Hepatotoxic Contains toxic pyrrolizidine alkaloids
Pokeroot	Anti-rheumatic Anti-cancer	May be fatal in children
Sassafras	Stimulant/tonic Anti-spasmodic Anti-rheumatic	Volatile oil Contains safrole, a liver carcinogen
Yohimbe	Used for impotence, as an aphrodisiac	May cause kidney damage, cancer, hypertension, and cardiac conduction disorders

Adapted from "Group Rates Efficacy of Herbs," by T. Kirn, April 2004, *Family Practice News, 34*(8), p. 26; and *Natural Medicines Comprehensive Database* (5th ed.), The Pharmacists Letter, 2003, Stockton, CA: Therapeutic Research Faculty Staff.

Focus on Primary Health Care — Box 31-7

Educating Clients About Purchasing Herbal Remedies

Many people who buy herbal products are unaware of the lack of regulation. It is difficult to make informed decisions when faced with hundreds of products. When clients choose to use herbal therapies, they should purchase these products only from reputable manufacturers to ensure safety, appropriate use, and response.

Nurses can help clients make informed choices about herbal products by offering these guidelines:

- Avoid hype: Be wary of supplements that offer a "cure" or a "secret formula."
- Examine the label: All products should indicate the
  - scientific name of the botanical
  - quantity, concentration, expiration date, and manufacture's name
  - other key ingredients
  - Natural Product Number (NPN) or Drug Identification Number (DIN), indicating that Health Canada has reviewed its formulation.
- Ensure that the product is supported by published research. Avoid "multi-ingredient" formulations when possible; otherwise, determining potential cross-reactions with other medicines will be very difficult. Also, consumers often pay a lot more for these secondary products that may not necessarily be at established therapeutic levels.
- Look for well-educated service staff that can answer consumers' questions.
- Be cautious about "mega-doses" of anything: Even excess ingestion of certain vitamins can be toxic.
- Be skeptical about cheap herbals. Consumers must pay for the manufacturer's investments in ensuring quality and purity. Very inexpensive herbal products are often of inferior quality.

Nursing Role In Complementary and Alternative Therapies

Nurses are essential participants in the integrative medicine approach. Indeed, many nurses already practise, for instance, the use of simple touch. As essential participants, nurses who provide CAM therapies must have the knowledge and skill necessary to provide care in a safe and ethical way through self-study, certificate courses offered by community colleges, or study with expert practitioners. They should understand provincial legislation about complementary therapies, practise within the scope of these laws, and be able to make appropriate recommendations about CAM therapies to allopathic primary care providers. It is also important for nurses to keep abreast of the current research in the field of CAM therapy to provide accurate information to clients and other health care professionals.

Nurses should advise clients about when to use conventional or CAM therapy. For example, if a client complains of right lower abdominal pain, nausea, and vomiting—signs of a potential appendicitis—the nurse should recommend an allopathic assessment. However, if the client has a chronic gastrointestinal disorder and is diagnosed with irritable bowel syndrome, he or she may benefit from relaxation and herbal therapy. Because nurses work very closely with their clients, they are in a unique position of becoming familiar with clients' religious and cultural viewpoints. Nurses may be able to determine which CAM therapies would be best suited to these beliefs.

Nurses should encourage clients to inform all caregivers, including other health practitioners, about medications and therapies they receive. In particular, complete information about the use of herbal medication should be added to the medical record to prevent potential drug and herb interactions.

Key Concepts

- Complementary therapy is used in conjunction with allopathic medicine, whereas alternative therapy is generally used without conventional care.
- Integrative medical programs use a multidisciplinary (both allopathic and complementary) treatment approach, providing holistic care to clients.
- The stress response is an adaptive response that allows individuals to react to stressful situations.
- A chronic stress response may be maladaptive, leading to chronic muscle tension and mood and immune changes.
- Relaxation is a beneficial state characterized by improved mood, relaxed muscle tension, lowered blood pressure, and decreased pulse and respiratory rates.
- CAM therapies require commitment and regular involvement by the client to be most effective and have prolonged beneficial outcomes.
- CAM therapies should be chosen according to the client's functional status, belief or religious perspectives, access to health care, and insurance coverage.
- Some CAM therapies may alter physiological responses such that routine medication doses may need changing.
- Imagery is usually visual but can also involve the auditory, proprioceptive, gustatory, and olfactory senses.
- Many complementary and alternative therapies lack a scientific basis but are thought to be effective based on observed positive outcomes in a number of clients.
- Not all herbal therapies are safe.

Key Terms

Acupoints, *p. 932*
Acupuncture, *p. 932*
Allopathic medicine, *p. 921*
Alternative therapies, *p. 922*
Biofeedback, *p. 930*
Chiropractic therapy, *p. 931*
Complementary therapies, *p. 921*
Creative visualization, *p. 929*
Energy flow, *p. 931*
Herbal therapy, *p. 933*
Imagery, *p. 929*
Integrative medical programs, *p. 922*
Meditation, *p. 927*
Meridians, *p. 932*
Passive relaxation, *p. 927*
Progressive relaxation, *p. 926*
Qi, *p. 932*
Relaxation, *p. 926*
Stress response, *p. 926*
Therapeutic touch, *p. 931*
Traditional Chinese medicine, *p. 932*
Yin and yang, *p. 932*

Critical Thinking Exercises

Client Profile: Margaret is a 76-year-old Catholic woman diagnosed with a slow-growing renal tumour. Surgery is scheduled in 2 weeks, and Margaret is afraid of both the procedure and the outcome. Is it cancer? Will the surgery result in a disability? After surgery, Margaret becomes depressed.

1. What specific nursing-accessible CAM interventions can the nurse offer Margaret to prepare for the surgery and reduce her anxiety?
2. What CAM therapies may be appropriate to help her deal with her depression?

Review Questions

1. Despite the success of allopathic medicine (traditional Western medicine), many clients with conditions such as the following find relief in complementary therapies:
   1. Heart disease and pancreatitis
   2. Ulcers and hepatitis
   3. Chronic back pain and arthritis
   4. Lupus and diabetes

2. Many of complementary therapies, such as acupuncture, have diagnostic and therapeutic methods specific to their field. Others can be easily learned as used as part of independent nursing practice. Which of the following therapies belongs in the latter category?
   1. Massage therapy
   2. Chinese medicine
   3. Shamanism
   4. Breathwork and imagery
3. It is estimated that half of Canadians have used a CAM therapy within the last year, and of these,
   1. Most used CAM therapy to prevent illness or maintain wellness
   2. Few found these therapies helpful
   3. Most had their CAM therapy financed by Medicare
   4. Most are from lower socio-economic backgrounds
4. Holistic nursing regards and treats the
   1. Mind, body, and spirit
   2. Disease, spirit, and family
   3. Desires and emotions
   4. Muscles, nerves, and spine disorders
5. After an adequate assessment, if the nurse wants to implement a CAM therapy whose permission is required?
   1. The client's
   2. The physician's
   3. The family's
   4. No permission must be given.
6. One of the principles of CAM therapies is that the individual becomes
   1. Actively involved in the treatment
   2. A total believer in what is being taught
   3. Submissive to the practitioner
   4. Less competent in his or her own care
7. St. John's Wort is effectively used as a(n)
   1. Anti-oxidant
   2. Anti-inflammatory
   3. Mild anti-depressant and sedative
   4. Vasodilator
8. Meditation may augment the effects of certain drugs, such as
   1. Anti-hypertensive and thyroid-regulating medications
   2. Insulin and vitamins
   3. Prednisone
   4. Cough syrups and aspirin
9. Biofeedback techniques are frequently used in addition to relaxation interventions to assist individuals to do which of the following?
   1. Eat less food
   2. Learn to control specific autonomic nervous system responses
   3. Control diabetes
   4. Live longer with HIV
10. Therapeutic touch is a training-specific therapy that was developed by a(n)
    1. Physician
    2. Nurse
    3. Physiotherapist
    4. Ancient Scandinavian culture

References

Abdelghany, S., et al. (2001). Biofeedback and electrical stimulation therapy for treating urinary incontinence and voiding dysfunction: One center's experience. *Urologic Nursing, 21*(6), 401–405, 410.

Astin, J., et al. (2002). Psychological interventions for rheumatoid arthritis: A meta-analysis of randomized controlled trials. *Arthritis and Rheumatism, 47*(3), 291–302.

Belleggia, G., & Birbaumer, N. (2001). Treatment of phantom limb pain with combined EMG and thermal biofeedback: A case report. *Applied Psychophysiology and Biofeedback, 26*(2), 141–146.

Benson, H. (1975). *The relaxation response*. New York: Avon.

Bonakdar, R. A. (2003, January). Herb-drug interactions: What physicians need to know. *Patient Care, 37*(1), 58–69.

Canadian Holistic Nurses Association. Web site. Accessed January 25, 2005 from *http://mypage.direct.ca/h/hutchings/chna.html#PH*

Chandler, F. (Ed.). (2000). *Herbs: Everyday reference for health professionals*. Ottawa, ON: Canadian Pharmacists Association and the Canadian Medical Association.

Cowan, M., Pike, K., & Budzynski, H. (2001). Psychosocial nursing therapy following sudden cardiac arrest: Impact on two-year survival. *Nursing Research, 50*(2), 68–76.

Crider, A., & Glaros, A. (1999). A meta-analysis of EMG biofeedback treatment of temporomandibular disorders. *Journal of Orofacial Pain, 13*(1), 29–37.

Cunningham, C., Brown, S., & Kaski, J. (2000). Effects of transcendental meditation on symptoms and electrocardiographic changes in patients with cardiac syndrome X. *The American Journal of Cardiology, 85*(5), 653–655.

Deale, A., et al. (2001). Long-term outcome of cognitive behavior therapy versus relaxation therapy for chronic fatigue syndrome: A five-year follow-up study. *The American Journal of Psychiatry, 158*(12), 2038–2042.

Dossey, B., Keegan, L., & Guzzetta, C. (2000). *Holistic nursing: A handbook for practice* (3rd ed.). Gaithersburg, MD: Aspen.

Ernst, E. (2001). Complementary therapies in palliative cancer care. *Cancer, 91*(11), 2181–2185.

Fetrow, C. W., & Avila, J. R. (1999). *Professionals' handbook of complementary and alternative medicines*. Springhouse, PA: Springhouse.

Fontaine, K. (2000). *Healing practices: Alternative therapies for nursing*. Upper Saddle River, NJ: Prentice Hall.

Gawain, S. (2002). *Creative visualization* (25th anniversary edition). New York: New World Library.

Good, M., et al. (2001). Relaxation and music to reduce postsurgical pain. *Journal of Advanced Nursing, 33*(3), 208–215.

Hagemaster, J. (2000). Use of therapeutic touch in treatment of drug addictions. *Holistic Nursing Practice, 14*(3), 14–20.

Jacobs, G. D. (2001). Clinical applications of the relaxation response and mind-body interventions. *Journal of Alternative and Complementary Medicine, 7*(Suppl. 1), S93–101.

Janke, J. (1999). The effect of relaxation therapy on preterm labor outcomes. *Journal of Obstetric, Gynecologic, and Neonatal Nursing, 28*(3), 255–263.

Keefer, L., & Blanchard, E. (2001). The effects of relaxation response meditation on the symptoms of irritable bowel syndrome. *Behaviour Research and Therapy, 39*(7), 801–811.

Keefer, L., & Blanchard, E. (2002). A one-year follow-up of relaxation response meditation as a treatment for irritable bowel syndrome. *Behaviour Research and Therapy, 40*(5), 541.

Kiernan, J. (2002). The experience of Therapeutic Touch in the lives of five postpartum women. *MCN. The American Journal of Maternal Child Nursing, 27*(1), 47–53.

King, M., Carr, T., & D'Cruz, C. (2002). Transcendental meditation, hypertension and heart disease. *Australian Family Physician, 31*(2), 164–168.

Kirn, T. (2004, April). Group rates efficacy of herbs. *Family Practice News, 34*(8), 26.

Krieger, D. (1975). Therapeutic touch: The imprimatur of nursing. *American Journal of Nursing, 75*, 784–787.

Krieger, D., Peper, E., & Ancoli, S. (1979). Therapeutic touch: Searching for evidence of physiological change. *American Journal of Nursing, 79*, 660–662.

Kuhn, M., & Winston, D. (2001). *Herbal therapy and supplements: A scientific and traditional approach.* New York: Lippincott, Williams & Wilkins.

Lee, M., et al. (2000). Effect of Qi-training on blood pressure, heart rate and respiration rate. *Clinical Physiology, 20*(3), 173–176.

Leskowitz, E. (2000). Phantom limb pain treated with therapeutic touch: A case report. *Archives of Physical Medicine and Rehabilitation, 81*(4), 522–524.

Moore, N. (2000). A review of EEG biofeedback treatment of anxiety disorders, *Clinical Electroencephalography, 31*(1), 1-6.

Nakao, M., et al. (1999). Blood pressure biofeedback treatment, organ damage and sympathetic activity in mild hypertension. *Psychotherapy and Psychosomatics, 68*(6), 341–347.

National Center for Complementary and Alternative Medicine. (2002). *What is complementary and alternative medicine?* (NCCAM publication no. D156). Retrieved January 25, 2005, from *http://altmed.od.nih.gov/health/whatiscam/#11*

Pelletier, K. (2000). *The best alternative medicine: What works? What does not?* New York: Simon & Schuster.

The Pharmacists Letter. (2003). *Natural medicines comprehensive database* (5th ed). Stockton, CA: Therapeutic Research Faculty Staff.

Ramsay, C., Walker, M., & Alexander, J. (1999). *Public policy sources number 21: Alternative medicine in Canda—Use and public attitudes.* Vancouver, BC: The Fraser Institute.

Sarafino, E., & Goehring, P. (2000). Age comparisons in acquiring biofeedback control and success in reducing headache pain. *Annals of Behavioral Medicine, 22*(1), 10–16.

Scharff, L., Marcus, D., & Masek, B. (2002). A controlled study of minimal contact controlled biofeedback treatment in children with migraine. *Journal of Pediatric Psychology, 27*(2), 109–119.

Shannahoff-Khalsa, D. (2002). Complementary healthcare practices: Stress management for gastrointestinal disorders—The use of kundalini yoga meditation techniques. *Gastroenterology Nursing, 25*(3), 126–129.

Skidmore-Roth, L. (2003). *Handbook of herbs and supplements.* St. Louis, MO: Mosby.

Smyth, P. (2001). Therapeutic touch for a patient after a Whipple procedure. *Critical Care Nursing Clinics of North America, 13*(3), 357–363.

Speca, M., et al. (2000). A randomized, wait-list controlled clinical trial: The effect of a mindfulness meditation-based stress reduction program on mood and symptoms of stress in cancer outpatients. *Psychosomomatic Medicine, 62*(5), 613–622.

Stewart, B., et al. (2002, February). *Statement of concern to the Canadian public from Canadian neurologists regarding the debilitating and fatal damage manipulation of the neck may cause to the nervous system.* Retrieved June 27, 2004, from *http://www.chirobase.org/15News/neurol.html*

York University Centre for Health Studies. (1999). *Complementary and alternative health practices and therapies: A Canadian overview.* Toronto, ON: Author.

Yung, P., French, P., & Leung, B. (2001). Relaxation training as complementary therapy for mild hypertension control and the implications of evidence-based medicine. *Complementary Therapies in Nursing and Midwifery, 7*(2), 59–65.

Recommended Web Sites

Canadian College of Naturopathic Medicine:
http://www.ccnm.edu

The Web site of the Canadian College of Naturopathic Medicine (CCNM) has detailed information about Canada's only 4-year, full-time professional college of naturopathic medicine. It also includes job postings and a resource centre with links to CCNM and other free journals.

Canadian Health Network:
http://www.canadian-health-network.ca

Canadian Health Network (CHN) is a national, non-profit, bilingual Web-based health information network offered by Health Canada, national and provincial/territorial non-profit organizations and universities, hospitals, libraries, and community organizations. Information is organized in an index.

Chinese Medicine and Acupuncture Association of Canada:
http://www.cmaac.ca

This organization aims to raise the profile and reputation of Chinese medicine and acupuncture. Its Web site includes the organization's history and a Canada-wide members' index.

Health Care Information Resources:
http://www-hsl.mcmaster.ca/tomflem/top.html

Maintained by Tom Flemming at McMaster University Health Sciences Library, this Web site has an extensive list of links to allopathic and alternative therapy sites about everything from clinical practice guidelines to industry-specific associations. Flemming marks Canadian-run sites with the icon of a Canadian flag.

M. D. Anderson Cancer Center:
http://www.mdanderson.org/departments/cimer

The M. D. Anderson Cancer Center Complementary/Integrative Medicine Education Resources (CIMER) Web site offers information to both health professionals and the public about complementary medicine and how it can be integrated into allopathic medicine.

32

Activity and Exercise

Rita Wunderlich, BSN, MSN(r), PhD
Ann Brokenshire, RN, BScN, MEd (Canadian author)

Objectives

Mastery of content in this chapter will enable the student to:

- Define the key terms listed.
- Describe the role of the musculoskeletal and nervous systems in the regulation of movement.
- Discuss physiological and pathological influences on body alignment and joint mobility.
- Describe how to maintain and use proper body mechanics.
- Describe how exercise and activity benefit physiological and psychological functioning.
- Describe the benefits of implementing an exercise program for the purpose of health promotion.
- Describe the benefits of implementing exercise and activity during the acute, restorative, and continuing care of clients.
- Describe important factors to consider when planning an exercise program for clients across the lifespan and for those with specific chronic illnesses.
- Assess clients for impaired mobility and activity intolerance.
- Formulate nursing diagnoses for clients experiencing problems with impaired mobility and activity intolerance.
- Write a nursing care plan for a client with impaired mobility and activity intolerance.
- Describe the interventions for maintaining activity tolerance and mobility during the acute, restorative, and continuing care of clients.
- Evaluate the nursing care plan for maintaining activity and exercise for clients across the lifespan and with specific chronic illnesses.

Walking, turning, lifting, and carrying are essential when providing nursing care. Such activities require muscle exertion by the nurse. To reduce the risk of injury to the client or nurse, the nurse must know and practise proper **body mechanics.** This includes knowledge of the actions of various muscle groups, understanding of the factors involved in the coordination of body movement, and familiarity with the integrated functioning of the skeletal, muscular, and nervous systems.

In addition, nurses must promote activity and **exercise** because of the beneficial impact on wellness, prevention of illness, and restoration of optimal functioning. A program of regular physical activity and exercise has the potential to enhance all dimensions of wellness (Box 32-1). This chapter provides the student with information about exercise and activity as it relates to health promotion, the acute phase of illness, and the restorative and continuing care of clients. Nursing strategies are included to help plan an individualized exercise and activity program for a variety of clients with specific disease entities and needs.

Box 32-1 The Gift of Exercise

The other day I was looking for a gift to give to a friend. This friend is very important to me and I want her to be around for a long time; I want her to live a long and healthy life. I thought how great it would be if I could give her a gift that would improve the quality of her life.

So I sat down and made a list of what I would look for in this special gift:

It would help her to be stronger, firmer, leaner, more flexible, and energetic.

It would help lower her risk of dying from heart disease, help lower blood pressure and improve lipid profile, control blood glucose level, fight obesity, and help her to age more gracefully.

It would help improve immune function, concentration and task performance, and the quality of sleep.

It would help reduce stress, improve mood, enhance self-esteem, and increase optimism and confidence.

It would help to increase self-awareness and control over choices in her life.

It would be fun but also challenging.

It would allow for socialization but also time alone, depending on her needs.

It would come in all different modes and styles and adapt to various environments and weather conditions.

Finally, it would have a good *Consumer Reports* rating, supported by scientific data from reputable sources.

After completing my list, I realized that the only gift that meets all the criteria is the gift of exercise. Have a happy and healthy life, my friend.

From "Exercise," by J. S. Huddleston, in *Health Promotion Throughout the Lifespan* (5th ed.), edited by C. L. Edelman and C. L. Mandle, 2002, St. Louis, MO: Mosby.

Scientific Knowledge Base

Activity and exercise are important to all individuals' well-being. The nurse is able to provide a more individualized approach to care by knowing the physiology and regulation of body mechanics, exercise, and activity.

Overview of Body Mechanics, Exercise, and Activity

The coordinated efforts of the musculoskeletal and nervous systems to maintain body alignment, balance, and **posture** during lifting, bending, moving, and performing **activities of daily living (ADLs)** provide the foundation for body mechanics. The proper implementation of these activities reduces the risk of injury to the musculoskeletal system and facilitates body movements, allowing physical mobility without muscle strain and excessive use of muscle energy.

Body Alignment. Body alignment refers to the relationship of one body part to another body part along a horizontal or vertical line. Correct alignment reduces the strain on musculoskeletal structures, maintains adequate **muscle tone,** and contributes to balance. The nervous system is responsible for muscle tone and regulates and coordinates the amount of pull exerted by the individual muscles (Thibodeau & Patton, 2002).

Body Balance. Body balance is achieved when a relatively low **centre of gravity** is balanced over a wide, stable base of support and a vertical line falls from the centre of gravity through the base of support. The base of support is the foundation. When the vertical line from the centre of gravity does not fall through the base of support, the body loses balance. Body balance is also enhanced by proper posture, or the body position that most favours function, requires the least muscular work to maintain, and places the least strain on muscles, ligaments, and bones (Thibodeau & Patton, 2002).

The nurse uses balance to maintain proper body alignment and posture by using two simple techniques. First, the base of support is widened by separating the feet to a comfortable distance. Second, balance is increased by bringing the centre of gravity closer to the base of support. This is achieved by bending the knees and flexing the hips until the person is squatting and still maintaining proper back alignment by keeping the trunk erect.

Coordinated Body Movement. Coordinated body movement is a result of weight, centre of gravity, and balance. Weight is the force exerted on a body by gravity. When an object is lifted, the lifter must overcome the object's weight and be aware of its centre of gravity. In symmetrical objects, the centre of gravity is located at the exact centre of the object. The force of weight is always directed downward. An object that is unbalanced has its centre of gravity away from the midline and falls without support. Because people are not geometrically perfect, their centres of gravity are usually at 55% to 57% of standing height and are located in the midline. Like unbalanced objects, clients who fail to maintain a balance with their centre of gravity are unsteady, which places them at risk for falling. Nurses must be able to identify such clients and intervene to prevent the risk of falls.

Friction. Friction is a force that occurs in a direction to oppose movement. As the nurse turns, transfers, or moves a client up in bed, friction must be overcome. A nurse can reduce friction by following some basic principles:

- The greater the surface area of the object to be moved, the greater the friction. If a client is unable to assist in moving up in bed, the client's arms should be placed across the chest. This placement decreases surface area and reduces friction.
- A passive or immobilized client produces greater friction to movement (see chapter 42). Thus, when possible, the nurse should use some of the client's strength and mobility when lifting, transferring, or moving the client up in bed. This can be done by explaining the procedure and telling the client when to move. For instance, friction is decreased if clients can bend their knees as the nurse assists them in moving up in the bed.

- Friction can also be reduced by lifting rather than pushing a client. Lifting has an upward component and decreases the pressure between the client and the bed or the chair. The use of a lift sheet reduces friction because the client is more easily moved along the bed's surface.

Exercise and Activity. Exercise is physical activity for the purpose of conditioning the body, improving health, and maintaining fitness, or it may be used as a therapeutic measure. When a person exercises, physiological changes occur in body systems (Box 32-2). The exercise program chosen and developed for a client depends on the individual's **activity tolerance,** or the kind and amount of exercise or activity that the person is able to perform. Physiological, emotional, and developmental factors influence the client's activity tolerance.

A program of regular physical activity and exercise promotes physical and psychological health. An active lifestyle is important for maintaining and promoting health; it is also an essential treatment modality for chronic illnesses (Flood & Constance, 2002; Konradi & Anglin, 2001). Regular physical activity and exercise enhances functioning of all body systems, including cardiopulmonary functioning (endurance), musculoskeletal fitness (flexibility and bone integrity), weight control and maintenance (body image), and psychological well-being (Burbank et al., 2002; Huddleston, 2002).

The best program of physical activity includes a combination of exercises that produce different physiological and psychological benefits. Isotonic, isometric, and resistive isometric are three categories of exercise classified according to the type of muscle contraction involved. Isotonic exercises cause muscle contraction and change in muscle length **(isotonic contraction).** Examples of isotonic exercises are walking, swimming, dance aerobics, jogging, bicycling, and moving arms and legs with light resistance. The benefits of isotonic exercises are increased circulation and respiratory functioning; increased osteoblastic activity (activity by bone-forming cells), thus combating osteoporosis; and increased muscle tone, mass, and strength.

Isometric exercises involve tightening or tensing of muscles without moving body parts **(isometric contraction).** Examples of isometric exercises are quadriceps set exercises and contraction of the gluteal muscles. This form of exercise is ideal for clients who are unable to tolerate an increase in activity that is expected during isotonic exercises. Immobilized clients in bed can easily accomplish isometric exercises. The benefits are increased muscle mass, tone, and strength, thus decreasing the potential for muscle wasting; increased circulation to the involved body part; and increased osteoblastic activity.

Isometric exercises may also be resistive. Resistive isometric exercises are those in which the individual contracts the muscle while pushing against a stationary object or resisting the movement of an object (Hoeman, 2002). A gradual increase in the amount of resistance and length of time that the muscle contraction is held will increase muscle strength and endurance. Examples of resistive isometric exercises are push-ups, pushing against a footboard to move up in bed, and hip lifting. In hip lifting, the client, who is in a sitting position, pushes with the hands against a surface such as the seat of a chair and raises the hips. Resistive isometric exercises help to promote muscle strength and provide sufficient stress against bone to promote osteoblastic activity.

Box 32-2 Effects of Exercise

Cardiovascular System

Increased cardiac output
Improved myocardial contraction, thereby strengthening cardiac muscle
Decreased resting heart rate
Improved venous return

Pulmonary System

Increased respiratory rate and depth followed by a quicker return to resting state
Improved alveolar ventilation
Decreased work of breathing
Improved diaphragmatic excursion

Metabolic System

Increased basal metabolic rate
Increased use of glucose and fatty acids
Increased triglyceride breakdown
Increased gastric motility
Increased production of body heat

Musculoskeletal System

Improved muscle tone
Increased joint mobility
Improved muscle tolerance to physical exercise
Possible increase in muscle mass
Reduced bone loss

Activity Tolerance

Improved tolerance
Decreased fatigue

Psychosocial Factors

Improved tolerance to stress
Reports of "feeling better"
Reports of decrease in illness (e.g., colds, influenza)

Data from *Understanding Pathophysiology* (2nd ed.), by S. E. Huether and K. L. McCance, 2000, St. Louis, MO: Mosby; and *Rehabilitation Nursing: Process, Application, and Outcomes* (3rd ed.), by S. P. Hoeman, 2002, St. Louis, MO: Mosby.

Regulation of Movement

Coordinated body movement involves the integrated functioning of the skeletal, muscular, and nervous systems. Because these three systems co-operate so closely in the mechanical support of the body, they are often considered as a single functional unit.

Skeletal System. Bones perform five functions in the body: support, protection, movement, mineral storage, and hematopoiesis (blood cell formation). In the discussion of body mechanics, two of these functions—support and movement—are most important (see chapter 42). In support, bones serve as the framework and contribute to the shape, alignment, and positioning of the body parts. In movement, bones, together with their joints, constitute levers for muscle attachment. As muscles contract and shorten, they pull on bones, producing joint movement (Thibodeau & Patton, 2002).

Joints. An articulation, or **joint,** is the connection between bones. Each joint is classified according to its structure and degree of mobility. Depending on the connective structures, joints are classified as fibrous, cartilaginous, or synovial (Huether & McCance, 2000). **Fibrous joints** fit closely together and are fixed, permitting little if any movement, such as the syndesmosis (united by ligaments) between the tibia and fibula. **Cartilaginous joints** have little movement but are elastic, such as the synchondrosis (united by cartilage) that attaches the ribs to the costal cartilage. **Synovial joints,** or true joints, are freely moveable and are the most mobile, numerous, and anatomically complex of the body's joints, such as the hinge type at the elbow.

Ligaments, Tendons, and Cartilage. Ligaments, tendons, and cartilage are structures that support the skeletal system (see chapter 42). **Ligaments** are white, shiny, flexible bands of fibrous tissue that bind joints and connect bones and cartilage. Ligaments are elastic and aid joint flexibility and support. **Tendons** are white, glistening, fibrous bands of tissue that connect muscle to bone. **Cartilage** is non-vascular, supporting connective tissue with the flexibility of a firm, plastic material. The gristle-like nature of cartilage permits it to sustain weight and serve as a shock absorber between articulating bones.

Skeletal Muscle. Walking, talking, running, breathing, and participating in physical activity require the contraction of skeletal muscles. There are over 600 skeletal muscles in the body. In addition to facilitating movement, these muscles determine the form and contour of the body. Most muscles span at least one joint and attach to both articulating bones. When contraction occurs, one bone is fixed while the other moves. The origin is the point of attachment that remains still; the insertion is the point that moves when the muscle contracts (Thibodeau & Patton, 2002).

Muscles Concerned With Movement. The muscles of movement are located near the skeletal region, where movement is caused by a lever system (Thibodeau & Patton, 2002). The lever system makes the work of moving a weight or load easier. It occurs when specific bones, such as the humerus, ulna, and radius, and the associated joints, such as the elbow, act as a lever. Thus, the force applied to one end of the bone to lift a weight at another point tends to rotate the bone in the direction opposite that of the applied force. Muscles that attach to bones of leverage provide the necessary strength to move the object.

Muscles Concerned With Posture. Gravity pulls on parts of the body all the time; the only way the body can be held in position is for muscles to exert pull on bones in the opposite direction. Muscles accomplish this counterforce by maintaining a low level of sustained contraction. Poor posture places more work on muscles to counteract the force of gravity. This leads to fatigue and can eventually interfere with bodily functions and cause deformities.

Muscle Groups. The antagonistic, synergistic, and anti-gravity muscle groups are coordinated by the nervous system and maintain posture and initiate movement. **Antagonistic muscles** bring about movement at the joint. During movement, the active mover muscle contracts while its antagonist relaxes. For example, during flexion of the arm the active mover (the biceps brachii) contracts and its antagonist (the triceps brachii) relaxes. During extension of the arm the active mover, now the triceps brachii, contracts and the new antagonist, the biceps brachii, relaxes.

Synergistic muscles contract to accomplish the same movement. When the arm is flexed, the strength of the contraction of the biceps brachii is increased by contraction of the synergistic muscle, the brachialis. Thus, with synergistic muscle activity, there are now two active movers—the biceps brachii and the brachialis—which contract while the antagonistic muscle, the triceps brachii, relaxes.

Anti-gravity muscles are involved with joint stabilization. These muscles continuously oppose the effect of gravity on the body and permit a person to maintain an upright or sitting posture. In an adult, the anti-gravity muscles are the extensors of the leg, the gluteus maximus, the quadriceps femoris, the soleus muscles, and the muscles of the back.

Skeletal muscles support posture and carry out voluntary movement. The muscles are attached to the skeleton by tendons, which provide strength and permit motion. The movement of the extremities is voluntary and requires coordination from the nervous system.

Nervous System. Movement and posture are regulated by the nervous system. The major voluntary motor area, located in the cerebral cortex, is the precentral gyrus, or motor strip. A majority of motor fibres descend from the motor strip and cross at the level of the medulla. Thus, the motor fibres from the right motor strip initiate voluntary movement for the left side of the body, and the motor fibres from the left motor strip initiate voluntary movement for the right side of the body.

Transmission of the impulse from the nervous system to the musculoskeletal system is an electrochemical event and requires a neurotransmitter. Neurotransmitters are chemicals (e.g., acetylcholine) that transfer the electric impulse from the nerve across the myoneural junction to stimulate the muscle, causing movement.

Movement can be impaired by disorders that alter neurotransmitter production, as in Parkinson's disease; alter transfer from the neurotransmitter to the muscle, as in myasthenia gravis; or alter activation of muscle activity, as in multiple sclerosis (Huether & McCance, 2000).

Proprioception. **Proprioception** is the awareness of the position of the body and its parts (Huether & McCance, 2000). Proprioception is monitored by proprioceptors located on nerve endings in muscles, tendons, and joints. Posture is regulated by the nervous system and requires coordination of proprioception and balance. As a person carries out ADLs, proprioceptors monitor muscle activity and body position. For example, the proprioceptors on the soles of the feet contribute to correct posture while standing or walking. In standing, pressure is continuous on the bottom of the feet. The proprioceptors monitor the pressure, communicating this information through the nervous system to the anti-gravity muscles. The standing person remains upright until deciding to change position. As a person walks, the proprioceptors on the bottom of the feet monitor pressure changes. Thus, when the bottom of the moving foot comes in contact with the walking surface, the individual automatically moves the stationary foot forward. The proprioceptors allow people to walk without having to watch their feet.

Balance. A person must have adequate balance when standing, running, lifting, or performing ADLs. Balance is controlled by the nervous system, specifically by the cerebellum and the inner ear. The major function of the cerebellum is to coordinate all voluntary movement, particularly highly skilled movements, such as those required in skiing.

Within the inner ear are the semicircular canals, three fluid-filled structures that assist in maintaining balance. Fluid within the canals has a certain inertia, and when the head is suddenly rotated in one direction, the fluid remains stationary for a moment, whereas the canal turns with the head. This allows a person to change position suddenly without losing balance.

Principles of Body Mechanics

Using principles of body mechanics during routine activities also prevents injury (Box 32-3). The nurse teaches colleagues and clients' families to lift, transfer, or position clients properly. A nurse who is teaching a client's family to transfer the client from bed to chair can increase and reinforce the family's knowledge by consistently demonstrating proper body mechanics.

Whether the nurse is moving an immobilized client, assisting a client from the bed to the chair, or teaching a client to carry out ADLs efficiently, knowledge of basic principles of body mechanics is crucial. The nurse also incorporates knowledge of physiological and pathological influences on body alignment and mobility.

Pathological Influences on Body Mechanics. Many pathological conditions affect body alignment and mobility. These conditions include congenital abnormalities; disorders of bones, joints, and muscles; central nervous system damage; and musculoskeletal trauma.

Congenital Abnormalities. Congenital abnormalities affect musculoskeletal alignment, balance, and appearance. For example, osteogenesis imperfecta is an inherited disorder characterized by bones that are porous, short, bowed, and deformed; as a result, children with this disorder experience curvature of the spine and shortness of stature (Wong & Hockenberry-Eaton, 2001). Scoliosis is a structural curvature of the spine associated with vertebral rotation. Muscles, ligaments, and other soft tissues become shortened. Balance and mobility are affected in proportion to the severity of abnormal spinal curvatures (Wong & Hockenberry-Eaton, 2001).

Box 32-3 Principles of Body Mechanics

- The wider the base of support, the greater the stability.
- The lower the centre of gravity, the greater the stability.
- The equilibrium of an object is maintained as long as the line of gravity passes through its base of support. Facing the direction of movement prevents abnormal twisting of the spine.
- Dividing balanced activity between arms and legs reduces the risk of back injury.
- Leverage, rolling, turning, or pivoting requires less work than lifting.
- When friction is reduced between the object to be moved and the surface on which it is moved, less force is required to move it.
- Reducing the force of work reduces the risk of injury.
- Maintaining good body mechanics reduces fatigue of the muscle groups.
- Alternating periods of rest and activity helps to reduce fatigue.

Disorders of Bones, Joints, and Muscles. Osteoporosis is a well-known and well-publicized disorder of aging in which the density or mass of bone is reduced. The bone remains biochemically normal but has difficulty maintaining integrity and support. The cause is uncertain, and theories vary from hormonal imbalances to insufficient intake of nutrients, including calcium (Huether & McCance, 2000; Lewis et al., 2000).

Osteomalacia is an uncommon metabolic disease characterized by inadequate and delayed mineralization, resulting in compact and spongy bone (Lewis et al., 2000). Mineral calcification and deposition do not occur. Replaced bone consists of soft material rather than rigid bone.

Joint mobility can be altered by inflammatory and non-inflammatory joint diseases and by articular disruption. Inflammatory joint disease (e.g., arthritis) is characterized by inflammation or destruction of the synovial membrane and articular cartilage and by systemic signs of inflammation. Non-inflammatory diseases have none of these characteristics, and the synovial fluid is normal (Huether & McCance, 2000). Joint degeneration, which can occur with inflammatory and non-inflammatory disease, is marked by changes in articular cartilage combined with overgrowth of bone at the articular ends. Degenerative changes commonly affect weight-bearing joints.

Articular disruption may be as mild as a sprain or as severe as dislocation. Articular disruption involves trauma to the articular capsules, such as a tear in a sprain or a separation in a dislocation. Articular disruption usually results from trauma but can also be congenital, as with developmental dysplasia of the hip (Wong & Hockenberry-Eaton, 2001).

Central Nervous System Damage. Damage to any component of the central nervous system that regulates voluntary movement results in impaired body alignment and mobility. For example, the motor strip in the cerebrum can be damaged by trauma from a head injury. The amount of voluntary motor impairment is directly related to the amount of destruction of the motor strip. A client with a right-sided cerebral hemorrhage and damage to the right motor strip may have left-sided **hemiplegia.** However, a client with a right-sided head injury may only have cerebral edema (but not destruction) of the motor strip. With extensive physiotherapy, voluntary movement gradually returns to the left side.

Musculoskeletal Trauma. Musculoskeletal trauma can result in bruises, contusions, sprains, and fractures. A fracture is a disruption of bone tissue continuity. Fractures most commonly result from direct external trauma. They can also occur because of deformity of the bone, as with pathological fractures of osteoporosis (see chapter 42).

Safety Alert. The first 6 to 12 hours is the most crucial period of time for treating soft tissue injuries (Lewis et al., 2000). Basic treatment of soft tissue injuries is summarized by the acronym *RICES:*

R– Rest: Minimizes the potential for further damage to a joint already unstable from injury.
I – Ice: Reduces pain threshold; should not be applied for longer than 30 minutes at a time.
C – Compression: A wet elastic wrap should be applied to hold ice in place and provide compression.
E – Elevate: The injured part should be held several centimeters above the heart to facilitate venous return and reduce swelling.
S – Support: Usual initial treatment is immobilization either by application of a brace or a cast.

(Smeltzer & Bare, 2003)

Nursing Knowledge Base

This section is concerned with knowledge from areas of nursing practice that enable the nurse to meet the holistic needs of the client. Developmental changes, behavioural aspects, family and social support, cultural and ethnic origin, and environmental issues are important aspects of an individual and must be incorporated into the plan of care whether the client is seeking health promotion, acute care, or restorative and continuing care.

Developmental Changes

Throughout the lifespan, the body's appearance and functioning undergo change. The greatest change and impact on the maturational process is observed at both ends of the developmental spectrum.

Infants Through School-Age Children. The newborn infant's spine is flexed and lacks the anteroposterior curves of the adult. The first spinal curve occurs when the infant extends the neck from the prone position. As growth and stability increase, the thoracic spine straightens and the lumbar spinal curve appears, which allows sitting and standing.

The toddler's posture is awkward because of the slight swayback and protruding abdomen. As the child walks, the legs and feet are usually far apart and the feet are slightly everted. Toward the end of toddlerhood, posture appears less awkward, curves in the cervical and lumbar vertebrae are accentuated, and foot eversion disappears.

By the third year, the body is slimmer, taller, and better balanced. Abdominal protrusion is decreased, the feet are not as far apart, and the arms and legs have increased in length. The child appears more coordinated. The musculoskeletal system continues to grow and develop until adolescence (see chapter 19).

Adolescence. The period of adolescence is usually initiated by a tremendous growth spurt. Growth is frequently uneven. As a result, the adolescent may appear awkward and uncoordinated. Adolescent girls usually grow and develop earlier than boys. In girls, hips widen and fat is deposited in the upper arms, thighs, and buttocks. The adolescent boy's changes in shape are usually a result of long-bone growth and increased muscle mass (see chapter 19).

Young to Middle Adults. An adult who has correct posture and body alignment feels good, looks good, and generally appears self-confident. The healthy adult also has the necessary musculoskeletal development and coordination to carry out ADLs. Normal changes in posture and body alignment in adulthood occur mainly in pregnant women. These changes result from the body's adaptive response to weight gain and the growing fetus (see chapter 20). The centre of gravity shifts toward the anterior. The pregnant woman leans back and is slightly swaybacked. She may complain of back pain.

Older Adults. A progressive loss of bone mass occurs with the older adult. Some of the possible causes of this loss include physical inactivity, hormonal changes, and increased osteoclastic activity (activity by cells responsible for bone tissue absorption). The effect of bone loss is weaker bones, causing vertebrae to be softer and long shaft bones to be less resistant to bending.

In addition, older adults may walk more slowly and appear less coordinated. They may also take smaller steps, keeping their feet closer together, which decreases the base of support. Thus, body balance may become unstable, and they are at greater risk for falls and injuries (see chapter 21).

Safety Alert. Falls and the resulting injuries are among the most debilitating medical problems that prevent the older adult from remaining independent. Regular exercise that promotes strengthening, flexibility, and balance can help prevent falls in the older adult (Burbank et al., 2002; Connelly, 2000; Huddleston, 2002; Resnick, 1999).

Box 32-4 General Strategies for Initiating and Maintaining an Exercise Program

An exercise program is most likely to be initiated and maintained when the individual:
- Perceives a net benefit
- Chooses an enjoyable activity
- Feels competent doing the activity
- Feels safe doing the activity
- Can easily access the activity on a regular basis
- Can fit the activity into the daily schedule
- Feels that the activity does not generate financial or social costs that he or she is unwilling to bear
- Experiences a minimum of negative consequences such as injury, loss of time, negative peer pressure, and problems with self-identity
- Is able to successfully address issues of competing time demands
- Recognizes the need to balance the use of labour-saving devices and sedentary activities with activities that involve a higher level of physical exertion

Data from *Messaging Workbook for the Physical Activity Intervention Policy Framework,* Ontario Ministry of Citizenship, Culture and Recreation and the Ministry of Health, 1995, Toronto, ON: Queen's Printer for Ontario; and "Build Self-Efficacy to Promote Exercise Adherence," by J. Schlicht et al., 1999, *American College of Sport Medicine's Health Fitness Journal, 3*(6), p. 27.

Behavioural Aspects

Clients are more likely to incorporate an exercise program into their daily lives if this is supported and assisted by family and friends, nurses, physicians, and other members of the health care team. The nurse should take into consideration the client's knowledge of exercise and activity, barriers to a program of exercise and physical activity, and current exercise habits. Clients are more open to developing an exercise program if they are at the stage of readiness to change their behaviour (Prochaska, Norcross, & DiClemente, 1994). Information on the benefits of regular exercise may be helpful to the client who is not at the stage of readiness to act. Clients' decisions to change behaviour and include a daily exercise routine in their lives may occur gradually with repeated information that is individualized to their needs and lifestyle (Box 32-4). Once the client has reached the stage of readiness, the nurse must develop in collaboration with the client an exercise program that is customized to fit his or her needs; the nurse then provides continued follow-up support and assistance until the exercise program becomes a daily routine.

Environmental Issues

Work Site. A common barrier for many clients is the lack of time that is needed to engage in a daily exercise program. Work sites have the potential to help their employees overcome the obstacle of time constraints by offering opportunities, reminders, and rewards for those committed to physical fitness (Health Canada, 2001). Reminders such as signs could be used to encourage employees to use the stairs instead of elevators. Rewards such as free parking or discounted parking fees could be given to employees who walk from distant lots (Canadian Fitness and Lifestyle Research Institute, 2002a; Health Canada, 2001).

Schools. It has become increasingly clear that children are becoming less active, resulting in an increase in childhood obesity (Anderson, 2000). Children and adolescents spend a great deal of their time in school; however, in Canada today most children do not receive the recommended five periods of physical activity per week. Physical education has become an optional subject in most secondary schools (Canadian Association for Health, Physical Education, Recreation and Dance [CAHPERD], 1998). Only 18% of teenagers are accumulating enough daily activity to meet the international guidelines for optimal growth and development (Canadian Fitness and Lifestyle Research Institute, 2002b). Schools can provide a foundation for lifetime commitment to exercise and physical fitness by incorporating physical activity into a child's daily routine. The CAHPERD (1998) recommended that all schools provide daily physical activity programs, not limited to competitive sports or physical education classes, that are appropriate for boys and girls of all skill levels and from diverse backgrounds.

Community. The community's support of physical fitness can be instrumental in promoting the health of its members. Examples of community involvement to promote physical fitness are the provision of walking trails and track facilities in community parks and physical fitness classes offered by trained professionals. This may be a difficult task because of cost restraints. However, success in implementing physical fitness programs is dependent on a collaborative effort between public health agencies, parks and recreational associations, provincial and local government agencies, health care agencies, and community members (Box 32-5).

Cultural and Ethnic Influences

Exercise and physical fitness is beneficial to all people. When developing a physical fitness program for culturally diverse populations, the nurse must consider what motivates and what is deemed appropriate and enjoyable. The nurse must also have knowledge of what specific disease entities are associated with different cultural and ethnic origins (Box 32-6).

Family and Social Support

Social support can be used as a motivational tool to encourage and promote exercise and physical fitness. The client can engage a friend or significant other to participate in a "buddy system" whereby they walk together each day at a specified time. This companionship provides for socialization and increases the enjoyment for some clients. Therefore, they may develop a lifelong commitment to physical fitness. Parents can support their children in sports and physical activity by providing encouragement, praise, and transportation and by participating themselves (Health Canada, 2002b, 2002c).

Focus on Primary Health Care — Box 32-5

Exercise Programs to Prevent Gestational Diabetes

Exercise should be an essential primary prevention strategy in populations at high risk for diabetes. In the epidemic of diabetes affecting indigenous peoples worldwide, Aboriginal women of child-bearing age may be regarded as a priority target group for initiatives of this nature. Regular exercise could help to maintain a healthy body weight prior to pregnancy (pre-pregnancy obesity is a major risk factor for gestational diabetes mellitus). This could reduce the risk for later development of non-insulin-dependent diabetes in women and their children.

In a recent study in Saskatoon, Saskatchewan, researchers developed a weekly fitness program with incentives aimed at accommodating the needs of urban Aboriginal prenatal women. During its 2-year course, the program attracted 69 participants of various ages, stages of pregnancy, and education and fitness levels. Water aerobics and walking were the most preferred activities. Snacks and designated social time proved to be important incentives for attendance. While engaged in the program, 91% of participants reported improved fitness levels and 89% reported heightened self-esteem.

Although exercise programs for this target population are challenging to design, they are necessary and feasible.

Adapted from "Description and Evaluation of a Prenatal Exercise Program for Urban Aboriginal Women," by H. Klomp, R. Dyck, and S. Sheppard, 2003, *Canadian Journal of Diabetes, 27*(3), pp. 231–238.

Cultural Aspects of Care — Box 32-6

Epidemiological studies of ethnic groups indicate that physical inactivity is one of the risk factors associated with non-insulin-dependent diabetes mellitus (NIDDM). In Canada, NIDDM is between 3.6 and 5.3 times more prevalent in the Aboriginal population. Physical activity has been identified as having an important role in the prevention and treatment of NIDDM, yet Aboriginal people have a disproportionate number of poor, unemployed, and disadvantaged individuals who lack access to recreation and leisure activities.

Implications for Practice

- Because physical inactivity is a modifiable risk factor for the development of NIDDM, prevention and treatment programs need to focus heavily upon exercise and be tailored to the activity tolerance of the individual client.
- Motivational factors incorporated into the exercise program such as providing a healthy snack or meal for the participants and furnishing each client with a log to monitor weight loss and blood glucose levels will enhance compliance.
- Promotion of physical activity should be supported through recognition that a symbiotic relationship exists between cultural values and traditional leisure pursuits. The strong spiritual connection to the land lends itself to outdoor and/or wilderness recreation in the form of traditional games and activities such as lacrosse and hunting.
- Ensure that members of Aboriginal groups collaborate in the planning and educational program initiatives.
- Development of an exercise/prevention program should attempt to remove potential barriers such as transportation and cost to facilitate commitment to the program.

Data from "Exercise," by J. S. Huddleston, in *Health Promotion Throughout the Lifespan* (5th ed.), edited by C. L. Edelman and C. L. Mandle, 2002, St. Louis, MO: Mosby; "Type 2 Diabetes Mellitus in Canada's First Nations: Status of an Epidemic in Progress," by T. Young et al., 2000, *CMAJ, 163*(5), pp. 561–566; and "Contemporary Issues in Recreation and Leisure for Aboriginal Peoples in Canada," by D. Dawson, G. Karlis, and D. Georgescu, 1998, *Journal of Leisurability, 25*(1), retrieved May 25, 2004, from *http://www.lin.ca/resource/html/Vol25/v25n1a2.htm*

Critical Thinking

Successful critical thinking requires a synthesis of knowledge, experience, information gathered from clients, critical thinking attitudes, and intellectual and professional standards. Clients' conditions are always changing. Clinical judgments require the nurse to anticipate the information necessary, analyze the data, and make decisions regarding client care.

To understand activity tolerance and physical fitness and the impact on the client, the nurse must integrate knowledge from nursing and other disciplines, previous experiences, and information gathered from clients. As the nurse begins the process of problem solving for client care, a variety of concepts must be considered together to provide the best outcome for the client. Knowledge of the musculoskeletal system and health alterations that create problems for the client in the area of activity, exercise, and body mechanics lays the foundation for planning and decision making. Guidelines may also be incorporated, such as those found at the Canadian Diabetes Association (2003) and in *Canada's Physical Activity Guide to Healthy Active Living,* developed by Health Canada (2003a) in conjunction with the Canadian Society for Exercise Physiology (Health Canada, 2002a). Guidelines have also been created for children, youth, and older adults (Health Canada 2002b, 2002c, 2002d). Nurses' experiences and ability to think creatively and critically enhance their approach to each new client situation.

Nursing Process

NP Assessment

After taking a health history, the nurse begins the physical examination with an assessment of body alignment and posture. This can be carried out with the client standing, sitting, lying down, or moving. Through assessment, the nurse will be able to determine normal physiological changes in growth and development; deviations related to poor posture, trauma, muscle damage,

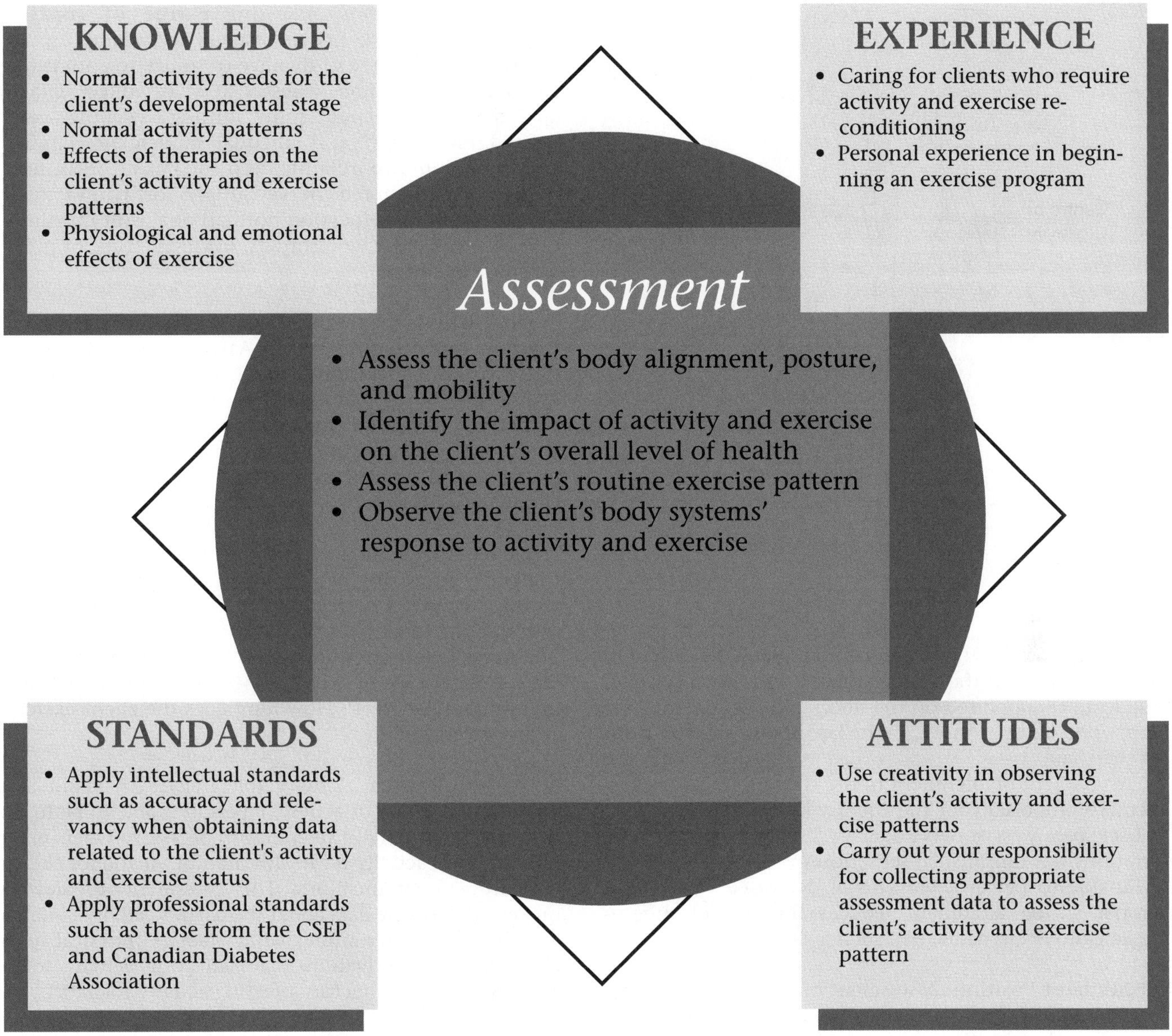
KNOWLEDGE
• Normal activity needs for the client's developmental stage
• Normal activity patterns
• Effects of therapies on the client's activity and exercise patterns
• Physiological and emotional effects of exercise
EXPERIENCE
• Caring for clients who require activity and exercise reconditioning
• Personal experience in beginning an exercise program
Assessment
• Assess the client's body alignment, posture, and mobility
• Identify the impact of activity and exercise on the client's overall level of health
• Assess the client's routine exercise pattern
• Observe the client's body systems' response to activity and exercise
STANDARDS
• Apply intellectual standards such as accuracy and relevancy when obtaining data related to the client's activity and exercise status
• Apply professional standards such as those from the CSEP and Canadian Diabetes Association
ATTITUDES
• Use creativity in observing the client's activity and exercise patterns
• Carry out your responsibility for collecting appropriate assessment data to assess the client's activity and exercise pattern

FIGURE **32–1** Critical thinking model for activity and exercise assessment.

or nerve dysfunction; and any learning needs of clients. In addition, during assessment, the nurse can provide opportunities for clients to observe their posture and obtain important information about other factors that contribute to poor alignment, such as inactivity, fatigue, malnutrition, and psychological problems. The nurse must consider all of the elements that build toward making appropriate nursing diagnoses, including the client strengths (Figure 32–1).

The first step in assessing body alignment is to put the client at ease so that unnatural or rigid positions are not assumed. When assessing body alignment of an immobilized or unconscious client, pillows and positioning supports should be removed from the bed if not contraindicated and the client placed in the supine position.

Standing. Assessment for the standing client includes the following: the head is erect and midline; body parts are symmetrical; the spine should be straight with normal curvatures (cervical concave, thoracic convex, lumbar concave); the abdomen is comfortably tucked; the knees should be in a straight line between the hips and ankles and should be slightly flexed; the feet should be flat on the floor and pointed directly forward and slightly apart to maintain a wide base of support; and the arms should hang comfortably at the sides (Figure 32–2). The client's centre of gravity is in the midline, and the line of gravity is from the middle of the forehead to a midpoint between the feet. Laterally, the line of gravity runs vertically from the middle of the skull to the posterior third of the foot (Wilson & Giddens, 2001).

Sitting. Assessment of the client in the sitting position includes the following: the head is erect and the neck and vertebral column are in straight alignment; the body weight is distributed on the buttocks and thighs; the

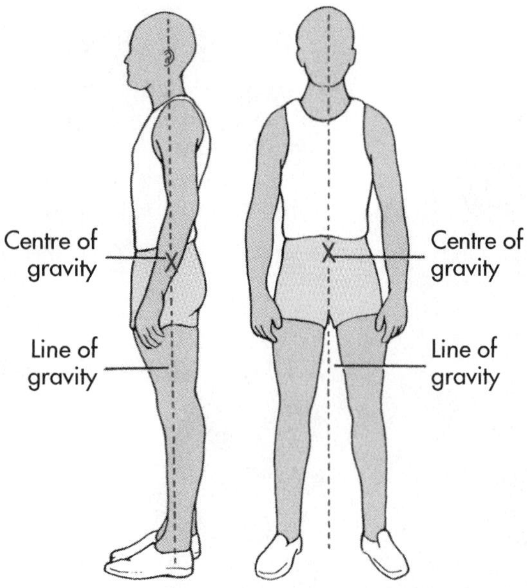

FIGURE **32–2** Correct body alignment when standing.

thighs are parallel and in a horizontal plane (be careful to avoid pressure on the popliteal nerve and blood supply); the feet are supported on the floor; and the forearms are supported on the armrest, in the lap, or on a table in front of the chair.

Assessment of alignment in the sitting position is particularly important for the client with muscle weakness, muscle paralysis, or nerve damage. A client with these alterations has diminished sensation in affected areas and is unable to perceive pressure or decreased circulation. Proper sitting alignment reduces the risk of musculoskeletal system damage in such a client.

Recumbent Position. Assessment of the client in the recumbent position requires that the client be placed in the supine position with all but one pillow and all positioning supports removed from the bed.

Conditions that create a risk of damage to the musculoskeletal system when lying down include impaired mobility (e.g., traction), decreased sensation (e.g., **hemiparesis** from a stroke), impaired circulation (e.g., diabetes), and lack of voluntary muscle control (e.g., spinal cord injuries).

When a client is unable to change position voluntarily, the nurse assesses the position of body parts while the client is lying down. This is best done with the nurse positioned at the foot or head of bed. The vertebrae should be in straight alignment without any observable curves. The extremities should be in alignment and not crossed over one another. The head and neck should be aligned without excessive flexion or extension.

Mobility. Assessment of mobility enables the nurse to determine the client's coordination and balance while walking, the ability to carry out ADLs, and the ability to participate in an exercise program. The assessment of **mobility** has three components: range of motion, gait, and exercise.

Range of Motion. Assessing **range of motion (ROM)** is one of the first assessment techniques used to determine the degree of damage or injury to a joint (see chapter 28). The nurse assesses ROM to collect data to answer questions about joint stiffness, swelling, pain, limited movement, and unequal movement. Limited ROM may indicate inflammation such as arthritis, fluid in the joint, altered nerve supply, or contractures. Increased mobility (beyond normal) of a joint may indicate connective tissue disorders, ligament tears, or possible joint fractures.

Gait. **Gait** is the manner or style of walking, including rhythm, cadence, and speed. Assessing gait allows the nurse to draw conclusions about balance, posture, and the ability to walk without assistance. The nurse should note conformity; a regular, smooth rhythm; symmetry in the length of leg swing; smooth swaying related to the gait phase; and a smooth, symmetrical arm swing (Wilson & Giddens, 2001).

Exercise. Exercise is physical activity for conditioning the body, improving health, maintaining fitness, or providing therapy for correcting a deformity or restoring the overall body to a maximal state of health (see Box 32-2). The nurse determines how much the client regularly exercises. What type of exercise does the client prefer? How many times per week? How long does the client exercise at any given time?

Activity Tolerance. Activity tolerance is the kind and amount of exercise or activity a person is able to perform. Assessment of activity tolerance is necessary when planning physical activity for health promotion and for clients with acute or chronic illness. This assessment provides the nurse with baseline data about the client's activity patterns and assists in determining which factors (physical, psychological, or motivational) are affecting activity tolerance. Box 32-7 lists factors affecting activity tolerance.

Client Expectations. In assessing the client's expectations concerning activity and exercise, the nurse will first need insight into the client's perception of what is normal or acceptable in regard to physical fitness. For example, one of the factors affecting physical activity is freedom from pain. If exercising is painful or tiresome to the client, compliance and commitment to the desired interventions may be lacking. Clients may be content with their present physical activity and fitness and may not perceive a need for improvement. Unless there is a real threat to health maintenance, forcing the client to accept the nurse's perspective is a breach of standards of care.

Nursing Diagnosis

Assessment of the client's activity tolerance, physical fitness, body alignment, and joint mobility provides related clusters of data or defining characteristics that help the nurse identify nursing diagnoses. The nurse must be accurate when identifying diagnoses. For example, a client who reports being tired or weakened could be potentially

Box 32-7 Factors Influencing Activity Tolerance

Physiological Factors

Skeletal abnormalities
Muscular impairments
Endocrine or metabolic illnesses (e.g., diabetes mellitus or thyroid disease)
Hypoxemia
Decreased cardiac function
Decreased endurance
Impaired physical stability
Pain
Sleep pattern disturbance
Prior exercise patterns
Infectious processes and fever

Emotional Factors

Anxiety
Depression
Chemical addictions
Motivation

Developmental Factors

Age
Sex

Pregnancy

Physical growth and development of muscle and skeletal support

Adapted from *Medical-Surgical Nursing: Health and Illness Perspectives* (7th ed.), by W. J. Phipps et al., 2003, St. Louis, MO: Mosby.

Nursing Diagnostic Process — Box 32-8

Assessment Activities	Defining Characteristics	Nursing Diagnosis
Observe client's gait.	Shuffled gait	Impaired physical mobility related to decreased muscle strength and control
Determine muscle mass and strength of upper and lower extremities.	Uncoordinated gait Client reports slower walking speed	
Observe client performing tasks such as feeding, dressing, or recreational activities.	Uncoordinated movements Limited fine motor coordination	
Measure range of joint motion.	Reduced joint motion in lower and/or upper extremities Stiffness in joints	

diagnosed as having activity intolerance or fatigue. Further review of assessed defining characteristics (e.g., abnormal heart rate or dyspnea) can lead to the definitive diagnosis (activity intolerance).

When activity and exercise are problems for a client, nursing diagnoses often focus on the individual's ability to move. The diagnostic label should direct nursing interventions. This requires the correct selection of the related factors. For example, activity intolerance related to excess weight gain and lack of cardiovascular fitness will require very different interventions if the related factor is prolonged bed rest. Box 32-8 provides an example of how the diagnostic process leads to accurate diagnosis selection. The following are examples of nursing diagnoses related to activity and exercise:

- Activity intolerance
- Disturbed body image
- Ineffective coping
- Impaired gas exchange
- Risk for injury
- Impaired physical mobility
- Imbalanced nutrition: more than body requirements
- Acute or chronic pain
- Impaired skin integrity

Planning

During planning, the nurse synthesizes information from multiple resources (Figure 32–3). Critical thinking ensures that the client's care plan integrates all that the nurse knows about the individual, as well as key critical thinking elements. Professional standards are especially important to consider when the nurse develops a care plan. These standards often establish scientifically proven guidelines for selecting effective nursing interventions.

Concept maps assist in the planning of care. Figure 32–4 shows the relationship between a client's medical

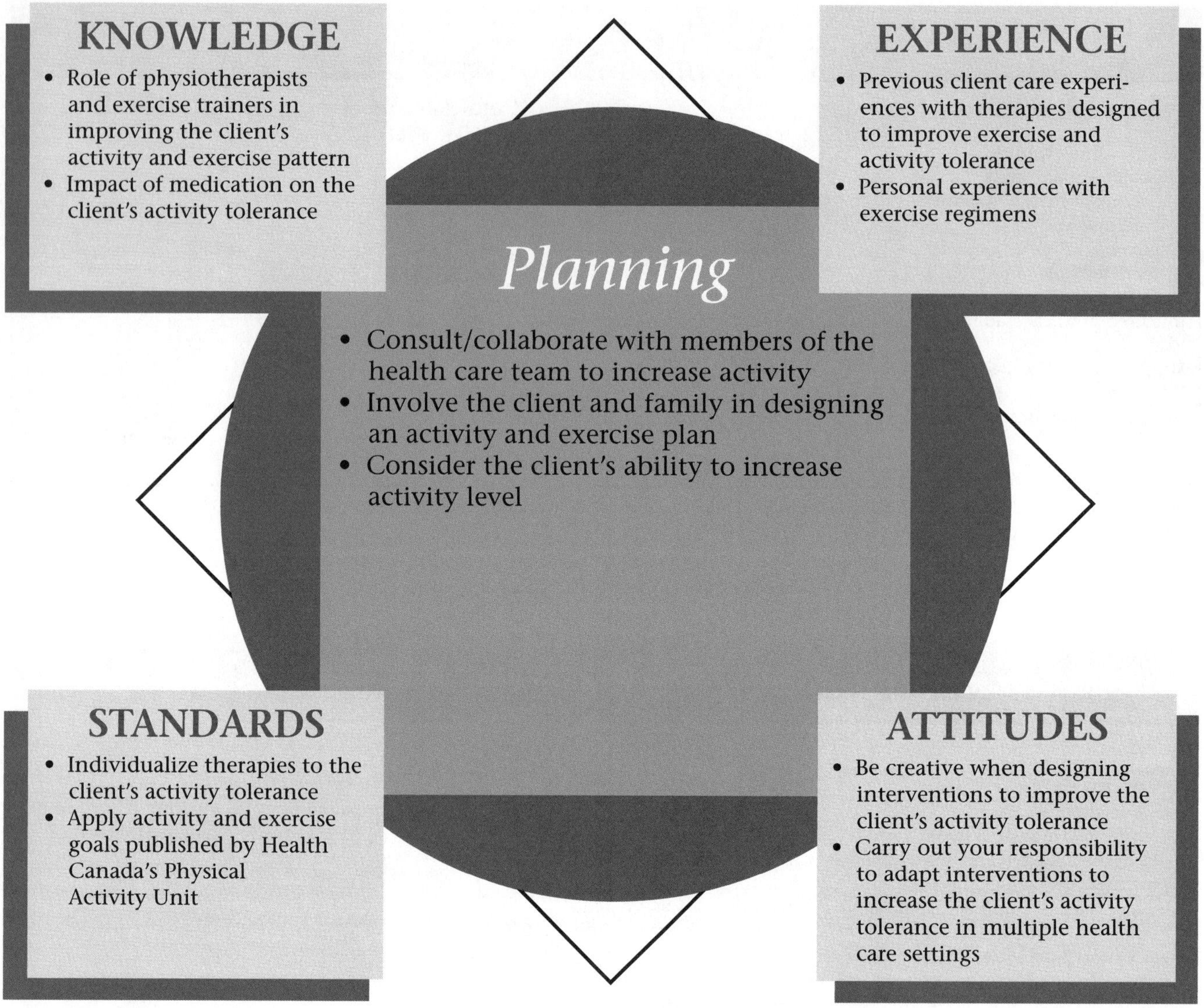

KNOWLEDGE
• Role of physiotherapists and exercise trainers in improving the client's activity and exercise pattern
• Impact of medication on the client's activity tolerance
EXPERIENCE
• Previous client care experiences with therapies designed to improve exercise and activity tolerance
• Personal experience with exercise regimens
Planning
• Consult/collaborate with members of the health care team to increase activity
• Involve the client and family in designing an activity and exercise plan
• Consider the client's ability to increase activity level
STANDARDS
• Individualize therapies to the client's activity tolerance
• Apply activity and exercise goals published by Health Canada's Physical Activity Unit
ATTITUDES
• Be creative when designing interventions to improve the client's activity tolerance
• Carry out your responsibility to adapt interventions to increase the client's activity tolerance in multiple health care settings

FIGURE **32–3** Critical thinking model for activity and exercise planning.

diagnosis of congestive heart failure and the identified nursing diagnosis.

Goals and Outcomes. Once the nursing diagnoses have been defined, the nurse and client set goals and expected outcomes to direct interventions. The plan should include consideration of any risks for injury to the client. It should also take into consideration pre-existing health concerns. It is especially important to have knowledge of the client's home environment when planning therapies to maintain or improve activity, body alignment, and mobility. The client's family should be included in the care plan. For some clients, family members may be the providers of care. The general goal related to exercise and activity is to improve or maintain the client's motor function and independence. The following are examples of outcomes for clients with deficits in activity and exercise (Ackley & Ladwig, 2002):

- Participates in prescribed physical activity while maintaining appropriate heart rate, blood pressure, and breathing rate
- Verbalizes an understanding of the need to gradually increase activity based on tolerance and symptoms
- Expresses understanding of balancing rest and activity

Setting Priorities. Care planning is individualized to the client, taking into consideration the client's most immediate needs. The immediacy of any problem is determined by the effect that the problem has on the client's mental and physical health. There are many tasks associated with the care of clients with activity intolerance, improper body mechanics, and/or impaired mobility, such as turning, transferring, and positioning. It is easy to overlook the complications associated with these health alterations. Therefore, to prevent complications and potential injury, the nurse must be vigilant in monitoring

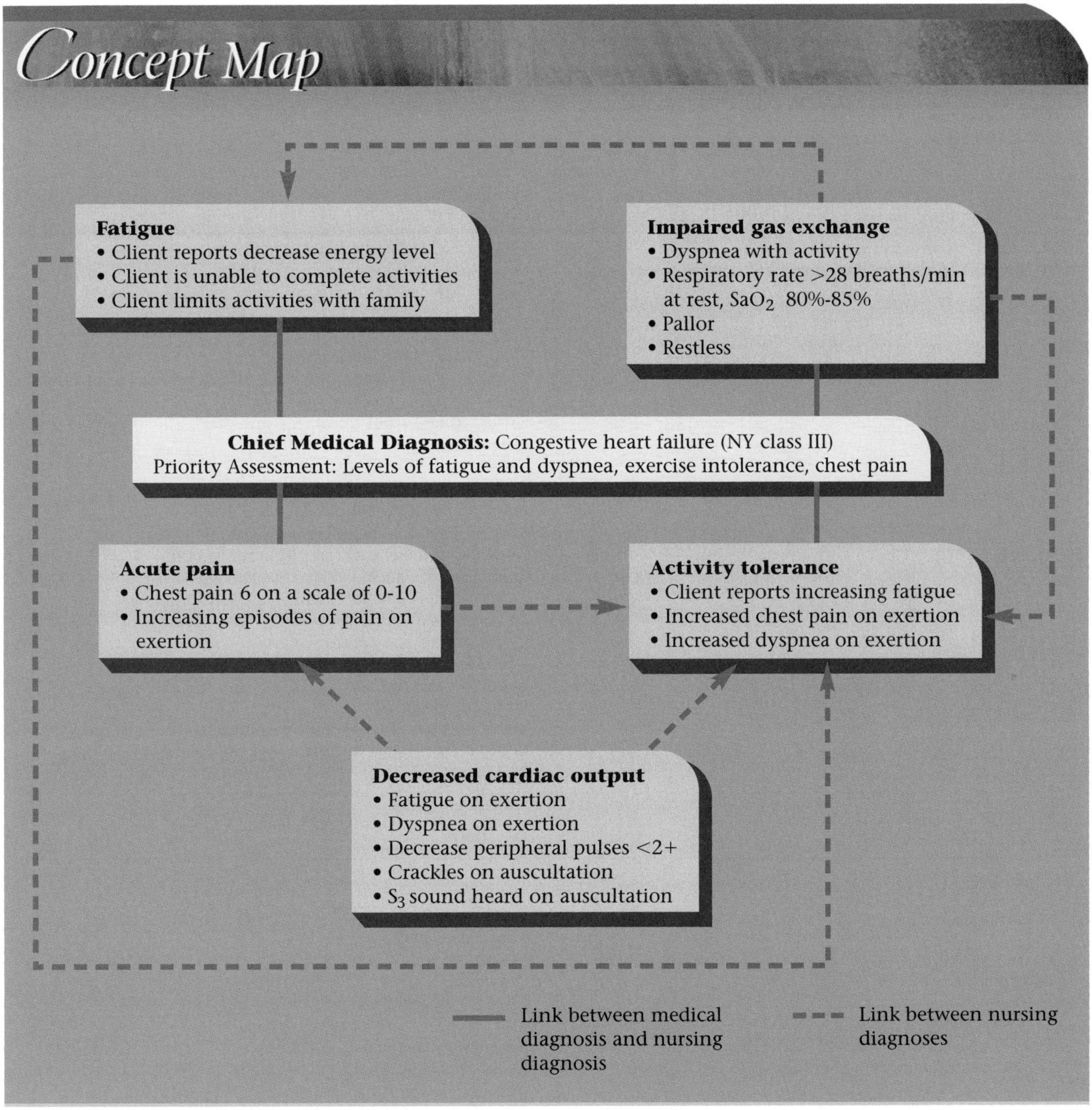
Concept Map
Fatigue
• Client reports decrease energy level
• Client is unable to complete activities
• Client limits activities with family
Impaired gas exchange
• Dyspnea with activity
• Respiratory rate >28 breaths/min at rest, SaO_2 80%-85%
• Pallor
• Restless
Chief Medical Diagnosis: Congestive heart failure (NY class III)
Priority Assessment: Levels of fatigue and dyspnea, exercise intolerance, chest pain
Acute pain
• Chest pain 6 on a scale of 0-10
• Increasing episodes of pain on exertion
Activity tolerance
• Client reports increasing fatigue
• Increased chest pain on exertion
• Increased dyspnea on exertion
Decreased cardiac output
• Fatigue on exertion
• Dyspnea on exertion
• Decrease peripheral pulses <2+
• Crackles on auscultation
• S_3 sound heard on auscultation
Link between medical diagnosis and nursing diagnosis
Link between nursing diagnoses

FIGURE **32–4** Concept map for a client with congestive heart failure and decreased activity.

the client and supervising unregulated care providers in carrying out activities.

Continuity of Care. Planning also involves an understanding of the client's need to maintain motor function and independence. Collaboration with other members of the health care team, for example, physiotherapists and occupational therapists, will be especially important for these clients. Long-term rehabilitation may be necessary, and discharge planning is begun when a client enters the health care system. In addition, the nurse always individualizes a care plan directed at meeting the actual or potential needs of the client (see Care Plan) and ensures that the plan is communicated to home care providers.

NP Implementation

Health Promotion. A sedentary lifestyle contributes to the development of health-related problems. Nurses promote health by encouraging clients to engage in a regular exercise program (Box 32-9). A holistic approach is taken

Nursing Care Plan

Activity Intolerance

Assessment

Mrs. Mary Smith is a 45-year-old homemaker. She has enrolled in a cardiovascular disease prevention (CDP) program prescribed by her physician and conducted by Erich Sieple, a registered nurse. Erich's assessment included a discussion of Mrs. Smith's current health status, as well as a pertinent physical examination.

Assessment Activities	Findings/Defining Characteristics
Ask Mary what prompted her physician to recommend a CDP program.	She responds, "I gained 23 kg over the past year. I become easily fatigued and lack the energy to keep up with even simple household chores. I don't want to leave the house anymore."
Ask Mary about her exercise and eating habits.	She responds, "I want to exercise but with the demands of child care and taking care of my aging parents, I just don't feel like it. I feel pulled in every direction, that increases my stress, then I want to eat, eat, and eat!"
Perform baseline assessment.	Height: 160 cm Weight: 102 kg Blood pressure: 152/90 mm Hg (at rest) Pulse: 96 beats per minute (at rest) Breathing rate: 20 breaths per minute (at rest)
Assess endurance.	Level 2–3 = moderately to substantially compromised. Erich rated Mary's endurance using the nursing outcomes classification (NOC; Moorhead, Johnson, & Maas, 2004): 1 extremely compromised 2 substantially compromised 3 moderately compromised 4 mildly compromised 5 not compromised Blood pressure: 164/96 mm Hg (climbing 10 steps) Pulse: 120 beats per minute (climbing 10 steps) Breathing rate: 36 breaths per minute (climbing 10 steps)

Nursing Diagnosis: Activity intolerance related to excessive weight gain, inactivity, and lack of cardiovascular fitness.

Planning

Goal	Expected Outcomes*
	Health Beliefs
Client will develop a plan of exercise incorporating isotonic and isometric exercises.	Client will state the physiological and psychological effects of exercise. Client will commit to performing physical exercise at home.
	Activity Tolerance
Client's activity tolerance will improve.	Client will perform and record exercise patterns three to four times over the next 2 weeks. Client's level of fatigue associated with exercise will remain the same or decrease.
	Cardiovascular Pump Effectiveness
Client's cardiopulmonary response to exercise will improve.	Client's resting diastolic blood pressure will remain below 80 mm Hg. Client's systolic blood pressure will be below 140 mm Hg. Client's resting heart rate will range between 75 and 85 beats per minute.

*Outcome classification labels from *Nursing Outcomes Classification (NOC)* (3rd ed.), edited by S. Moorhead, M. Johnson, and M. L. Maas, 2004, St. Louis, MO: Mosby.

Continued

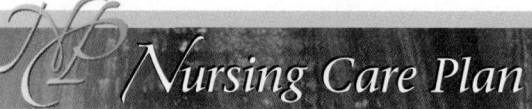

Nursing Care Plan

Activity Intolerance —cont'd

Interventions†	Rationale
Exercise Promotion	
• Instruct the client about the physiological benefits of a regular exercise program.	Physical activity and exercise protect against the development of cardiovascular disease (CVD) and decrease other risk factors associated with CVD, such as obesity, hypertension, and hyperlipidemia (Adams et al., 1999; Konradi & Anglin, 2001; Manson et al., 1999).
• Instruct the client about the psychological benefits of a regular exercise program.	Physical activity and exercise increase self-esteem, feelings of enjoyment, self-confidence, and mood while decreasing physical and psychological stress, anxiety, and depression (School of Physical and Health Education, 2004).
• Develop a progressive plan of exercise with the client, such as 3 to 5 km of brisk walking and quadriceps, biceps, and gluteal muscle isometric exercises three to four times per week.	Cross training (combination of exercise activities) provides variety to combat boredom and increases potential for total body conditioning (Huddleston, 2002).
• Instruct client to use an exercise log and to record the day, time, duration, and responses (pulse, feelings, shortness of breath, daily weight).	Keeping a log may increase adherence to exercise prescription (Kim, McFarland, & McLane, 1997).
• Schedule weekly meetings with the client for follow-up and review of exercise log, progress, and barriers.	Clients are more likely to increase physical activity and remain compliant with an exercise program if they are counselled by a health care professional (Huddleston, 2002).

†Intervention classification labels from *Nursing Interventions Classification (NIC)* (4th ed.), edited by J. M. Dochterman and G. M. Bulecheck, 2004, St. Louis, MO: Mosby.

Evaluation

Nursing Actions	Client Response/Finding	Achievement of Outcome
Review client's exercise log at each visit.	She responds, "I make time to exercise because of this log. I hate missing a day and leaving a blank page, this represents failure. I want to succeed."	Client reports enjoying exercise, as well as observing some personal benefits of exercise.
	Exercise log documents activity four times per week.	The exercise log is facilitating adherence to the exercise prescription.
Record weight, blood pressure, and pulse.	Weight, 95 kg. Resting heart rate remaining between 80 and 85 beats per minute. Blood pressure, 146/86 mm Hg.	Improved cardiovascular effects of exercise: • Heart rate is within normal range. • Blood pressure is lower but not at expected range. Monitor blood pressure as client continues to lose weight.
Ask client if exercise is helping to lower fatigue level.	She responds, "At first, finding time to exercise was hard, but once I started feeling less tired and even less stressed, it was easy to integrate exercise into my daily activities."	Achieved improved activity tolerance with exercise.

to develop and implement a plan to enhance the client's overall physical fitness. The recommendations for physical activity and fitness should be discussed with the client and a program of exercise designed in collaboration with the client (Box 32-10).

Before starting an exercise program, clients should calculate their maximum heart rate by subtracting their current age in years from 220 and should then obtain their target heart rate by taking 60% to 90% of the maximum. No matter what exercise prescription is implemented for the client, a warm-up and cool-down period must be included in the program (Huddleston, 2002). The warm-up period usually lasts about 5 to 10 minutes and may include stretching, calisthenics, and/or the aerobic activity performed at a lower intensity. The warm-up activity prepares the body and decreases the potential for injury. The cool-down period follows the exercise routine and usually lasts about 5 to 10 minutes. The cool-down period allows the body to readjust gradually to baseline functioning and provides an opportunity to combine movement such as stretching with relaxation-enhancing mind-body awareness (Huddleston, 2002).

Many clients find it difficult to incorporate an exercise program into their daily lives because of time constraints.

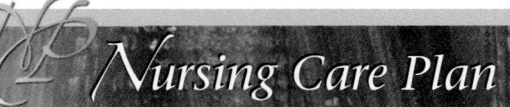

Box 32-9 Procedural Guidelines

Helping Clients to Exercise

Assisting clients in exercising is an important nursing activity. When there are specialized rehabilitation needs, such as with a client who has experienced a stroke or trauma, physiotherapy and/or occupational therapy are consulted and collaborated with to develop an exercise plan. Nurses can teach family members or unregulated care providers to help prepare the client for exercise (e.g., shoes, clothing, hygiene).

1. Assess for any medical limitations (e.g., weight-bearing status, untreated fracture, cardiovascular disease).
2. Teach clients breathing skills to help reduce anxiety and to fully oxygenate tissues and expand lungs.
3. Assess for client's physiological and psychological limitations for learning and implementing an exercise program.
4. Assess for joint limitations and do not force a muscle or a joint during exercise.
5. Encourage each client to move at his or her own pace.
6. Assess for proper posture, body alignment, and good body mechanics during exercise.
7. Monitor vital signs before, during, and after exercise.
8. Assess for pain, shortness of breath, or a change in vital signs. If present, stop exercise.
9. Ensure that the client wears rubber-soled shoes and comfortable clothing.
10. Assess pre-hospitalization mobility status.
11. Document client's progress and provide feedback as the client exercises.

For these clients, it is beneficial to reinforce that many ADLs can be used to accumulate the recommended 30 minutes or more per day of moderate-intensity physical activity.

Other clients may benefit from a prescribed exercise and physical fitness program carefully designed to meet their needs and expectations. An exercise prescription may incorporate a combination of aerobic exercise, stretching and flexibility exercises, and resistance training. Aerobic exercise includes such activities as walking, running, bicycling, aerobic dance, jumping rope, and cross-country skiing. Recommended frequency of aerobic exercise is 3 to 5 times per week or every other day. Cross training is recommended for the client who prefers to exercise every day. For example, the client may run one day and do yoga the next day.

Stretching and flexibility exercises include active ROM that allows for stretching of all muscle groups and joints. This form of exercise is ideal for warm-up and cool-down periods. Benefits include increased flexibility, improved circulation and posture, and an opportunity for relaxation.

Resistance training increases muscle strength and endurance and is associated with improved performance of daily activities and avoidance of injuries and disability (Pate et al., 1995). People lose about 1/4 kg of muscle mass per year from lack of use (Huddleston, 2002). Formal resistance training includes weight training, but the same benefits can be obtained by performing ADLs such as pushing a vacuum cleaner, raking leaves, shovelling snow, and kneading bread. Some clients may use weight training to bulk up their muscles. However, the purpose of weight training from a health perspective is to develop tone and strength and to stimulate and maintain healthy bone (Hass et al., 2000; Huddleston, 2002).

Box 32-10 Recommendations for Exercise

Adults should accumulate 30 minutes or more a day of moderate-intensity (brisk) physical activity on most (or all) days of the week for a weekly total of 3 to 4 hours.

The activity does not have to be continuous; benefits can be realized with short bouts of activity (10 minutes minimum) over the course of the day.

This amount of activity will expend about 150 to 200 calories per day (the equivalent of walking 3 km briskly) or 1,000 to 1,400 calories per week.

All types of activity can be applied to the daily total (e.g., raking leaves, dancing, gardening).

Lower-intensity activities should be done more often, for longer periods of time, or both. More vigorous activities should be done for shorter periods of time or less frequently.

Data from "Moderate-Intensity Exercise: For Our Patients, for Ourselves," by D. B. Konradi and L. T. Anglin, 2001, *Orthopedic Nursing, 20*(1), pp. 47–54; *Handbook to Canada's Physical Activity Guide to Healthy Active Living* [Electronic version], Health Canada, 2002a, Ottawa, ON: Author; and "Exercise," by J. S. Huddleston, in *Health Promotion Throughout the Lifespan,* (5th ed.), edited by C. L. Edelman and C. L. Mandle, 2002, St. Louis, MO: Mosby.

Body Mechanics. The Canadian Centre for Occupational Health and Safety has published numerous guidelines related to ergonomic standards for preventing musculoskeletal injuries in the workplace (2004). More than half of all back pain in health care settings is associated with manual lifting tasks (Workers Health and Safety Centre, 2003). The most common back injury is strain on the lumbar muscle group, which includes the muscles around the lumbar vertebrae. Injury to these areas affects the ability to bend forward, backward, and from side to side. The ability to rotate the hips and lower back is also decreased. To protect the client and the nurse, the

Table 32-1 Body Mechanics for Health Care Workers

Action	Rationale
When planning to move a client, arrange for adequate help. Use mechanical aids if help is unavailable.	Two workers lifting together divide the workload by 50%.
Encourage client to assist as much as possible.	This promotes client's independence and strength while minimizing workload.
Keep back, neck, pelvis, and feet aligned. Avoid twisting.	This reduces risk of injury to lumbar vertebrae and muscle groups. Twisting increases risk of injury.
Flex knees; keep feet wide apart.	A broad base of support increases stability.
Position self close to client (or object being lifted).	The force is minimized. Five kilograms held at waist height close to body is equal to 45 kg held at arms' length.
Use arms and legs (not back).	The leg muscles are stronger, larger muscles capable of greater work without injury.
Slide client toward yourself using a pull sheet.	Sliding requires less effort than lifting. Pull sheet minimizes shearing forces, which can damage client's skin.
Set (tighten) abdominal and gluteal muscles in preparation for move.	Preparing muscles for the load minimizes strain and stabilizes the trunk.
Person on a lift team with the heaviest load coordinates efforts of the lift team involved by counting to three.	Simultaneous lifting minimizes the load for any one lift.

nurse must learn and master proper body mechanics (Table 32-1).

Lifting Techniques. Before lifting, the nurse should assess the weight to be lifted and what assistance, if any, is needed. If help is needed, the nurse should assess if a second person is adequate or if mechanical assistance is needed. Once the amount of needed assistance is determined, these steps are followed:

1. Tighten gluteal, abdominal, pelvic, and leg muscles; this provides balance and protects the back.
2. Bend at the knees; this helps to maintain centre of gravity and lets the strong muscles of the legs do the lifting (Figure 32–5).
3. Keep the weight to be lifted as close to the body as possible; this places the weight in the same plane as the lifter and close to the centre of gravity for balance.
4. Maintain the trunk erect and the knees bent so that multiple muscle groups work together in a synchronized manner (Occupational Health & Safety Agency for Healthcare in British Columbia [OHSAH], 2003).
5. Avoid twisting. Twisting can overload your spine and lead to serious injury.

The best height for lifting vertically is approximately 60 cm off the ground and close to the lifter's centre of gravity (OHSAH, 2003).

To reach an object overhead, do the following:

1. Use a safe, stable step stool or ladder for elevation. Avoid standing on tiptoes with the feet together. This decreases the base of support, elevates the centre of gravity, and decreases balance.
2. Stand as close to the shelf as possible. This decreases the amount of time the nurse must support the weight of the object with the arms.
3. Transfer the weight of the object from the shelf to the arms and over the base of support. This maintains the nurse's base of support and aligns the weight of the object close to the nurse's centre of gravity.

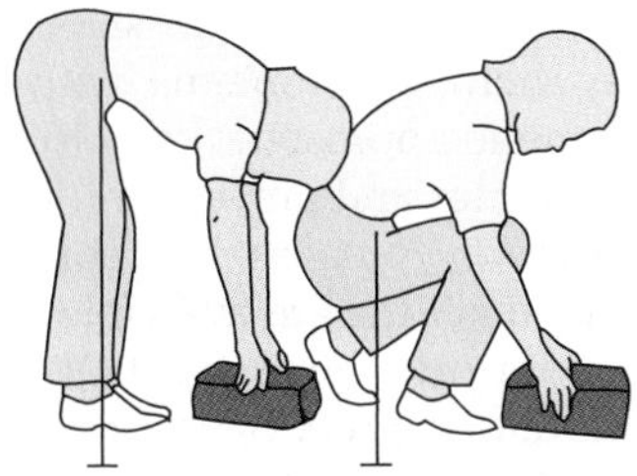

FIGURE **32–5** Incorrect **(A)** and correct **(B)** body position for lifting.

Acute Care. Hospitalized clients can be encouraged to do stretching and isometric exercises, active ROM exercises, and low-intensity walking, depending on their condition. The longer the period of inactivity, or **immobility,** the greater are the physiological changes (see chapter 42). The nurse is responsible for maintaining musculoskeletal function by implementing passive ROM in those clients who are unable to perform physical activity for themselves.

Musculoskeletal System. The musculoskeletal system can be maintained during the acute care of the client by encouraging the use of stretching and isometric-type exercises. Review of the client's chart and collaboration with the physician is undertaken to alert the nurse to any possible contraindications before initiating isometric exercises. An isometric exercise program is designed for the specific needs of a client. For example, an exercise program may be implemented that includes biceps and triceps isometric exercises to prepare the client for crutch walking. The nurse needs to tell the client to stop the activity if pain, fatigue, or discomfort is experienced and needs to reinforce this as necessary.

Generally, the muscle group is tightened (contracted) for 10 seconds and then completely relaxed for several seconds. Repetitions are gradually increased for each muscle group until the isometric exercise can be repeated 8 to 10 times. Clients should be instructed to perform the exercises slowly and increase repetitions as their physical condition improves. Muscle groups (quadriceps and gluteal) used for walking should be exercised isometrically four times per day until the client is ambulatory (Hoeman, 2002).

Joint Mobility. The easiest intervention to maintain or improve joint mobility for clients and one that can be co-ordinated with other activities is the use of ROM exercises (see chapter 42). In active ROM exercises, the client is able to move his or her joints independently. With passive ROM exercises, the nurse moves each joint in clients who are unable to perform these exercises themselves. The use of ROM exercises enables the nurse to systematically assess and improve the client's joint mobility.

Joints that are not moved periodically can develop contractures, a permanent shortening of a muscle followed by the eventual shortening of associated ligaments and tendons. Over time, the joint may become fixed in one position and the client loses normal use of the joint. For the client who does not have voluntary motor control, passive ROM exercises are the exercises of choice.

Older adults often experience a decline in physical activity in association with musculoskeletal changes that may predispose them to problems with mobility. The nurse can recommend approaches to help older adults use proper body mechanics and prevent injury (Box 32-11).

Mechanical devices such as the continuous passive movement (CPM) machine are available to place specific joints through continuous passive ROM. The machine can be set to certain degrees of joint mobility with increasing joint mobility or flexion as the goal. The most common clients who use the CPM machine are those who have undergone some form of total joint replacement surgery (e.g., knee).

Unless contraindicated, the nursing care plan should include exercising each joint through as nearly a full ROM as possible. Passive ROM exercises should be initiated as soon as the client loses the ability to move the extremity or joint. Chapter 42 details ROM exercises for each area and illustrates the motion of each joint.

Focus on Older Adults — Box 32-11

- Encourage the older client to avoid prolonged sitting, to get up and stretch. Frequent stretching diminishes the potential for joint contractures.
- Be sure that the older client maintains proper body alignment when sitting to minimize joint and muscle stress.
- Teach clients how to use stronger joints or larger muscle groups. Efficient distribution of the workload decreases joint stress and pain.
- Provide resources for planned exercise programs, such as Health Canada's *Physical Activity Guide for Older Adults* (2002d). Weight-bearing and resistance exercise slow further bone loss and prevent fractures in the older adult with osteoporosis (Brown, Josse, & The Scientific Advisory Council of the Osteoporosis Society of Canada, 2002; Burbank et al., 2002; Phipps et al., 2003).
- Recommend tai chi, a Chinese traditional conditioning exercise that increases balance and strength. This form of exercise has resulted in reduced fear of falling and increased sense of well-being in older adults (Chewning, Yu, & Johnson, 2000).
- Advise clients that is never too late to begin an exercise program (Burbank et al., 2002; Health Canada, 2002d; Huddleston, 2002). However, remind the client to consult a health care provider before beginning an exercise program, particularly if the client has heart or lung disease and other chronic illnesses.
- Exercise is extremely beneficial to older adults, but adjustments may have to be made to an exercise program for those in advanced age to prevent problems.
- When developing an exercise program for older adults, consider not only current activity level, range of motion, muscle strength and tone, and response to physical activity, but also their interests, capacities, and limitations (Eliopoulos, 2001).
- Older adults who are unable to participate in a formal exercise program can achieve the benefits of improved joint mobility and enhanced circulation by simply stretching and exaggerating movements during the performance of routine daily activities (Eliopoulos, 2001).

Walking. Joint mobility is also increased by walking. Distances walked should be measured in metres instead of charting "ambulated to nurses' station and back." In good walking posture, the head is erect; the cervical, thoracic, and lumbar vertebrae are aligned; the hips and knees have appropriate flexion; and the arms swing freely in alternation with the legs. Illness or trauma can reduce activity tolerance, resulting in the need for assistance with walking or the use of mechanical devices such as crutches, canes, or walkers.

Helping a Client to Walk. Helping a client to walk requires preparation. The nurse assesses the client's activity tolerance, strength, coordination, and balance to determine the type of assistance needed. The nurse should also assess the client's orientation, motivation, and level of co-operation and determine if there are any signs of distress that might preclude attempts at ambulation.

The nurse evaluates the environment for safety before ambulation; this includes the removal of obstacles and ensuring that the floor is clean and dry. The client should also wear supportive, non-skid shoes. Resting points should be established in the event that the client's activity tolerance is less than was estimated or the client becomes dizzy.

The client should be assisted to a position of sitting at the side of the bed and should rest for 1 to 2 minutes before standing. Reduce the risk of orthostatic hypotension (and the risk of falling) by advising the client to keep his or her head up, to take a deep breath or two, and to rotate the ankles a few times while sitting.

Several methods are used for assisting a client with ambulation. The nurse provides support at the waist so that the client's centre of gravity remains midline. This can be achieved when the nurse places both hands at the client's waist or uses a gait belt. A **gait belt** is a belt that is placed around the lower rib cage to provide stability and has handles attached for the nurse to hold while the client ambulates.

If the client has a syncopal episode or begins to fall, the nurse should assume a wide base of support with one

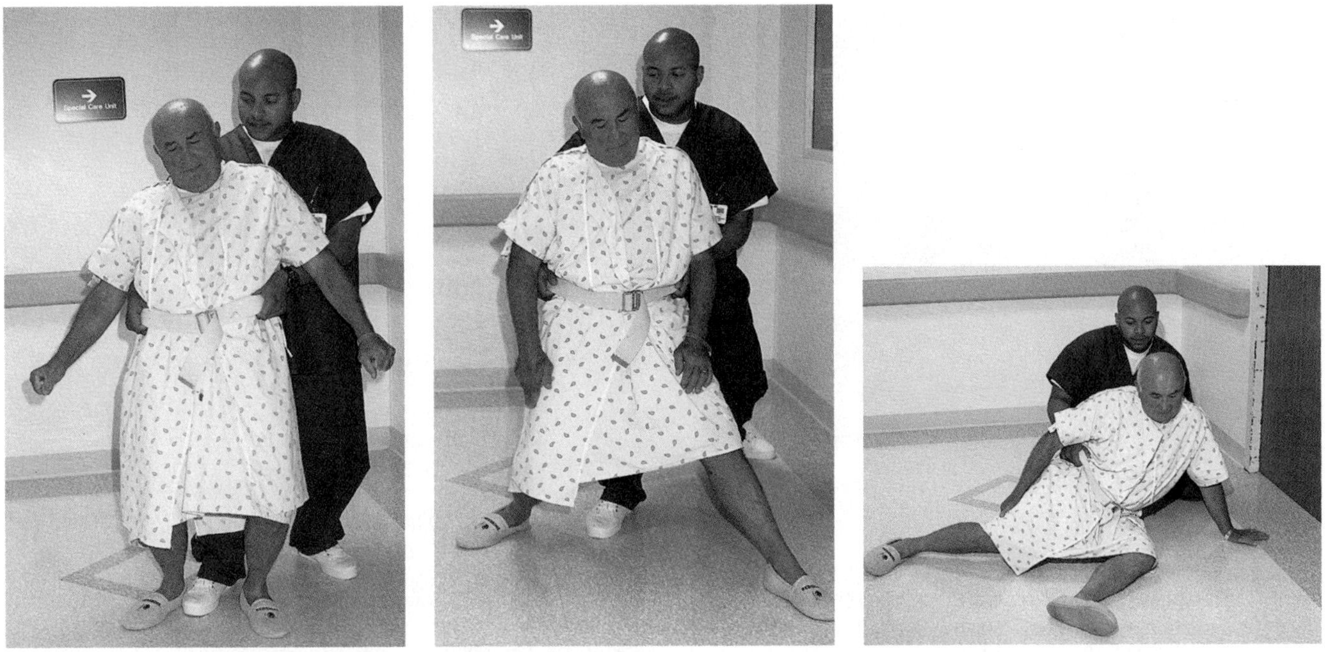

A B C

FIGURE **32–6** **A,** Stand with feet apart to provide a broad base of support. **B,** Extend one leg and let client slide against it to the floor. **C,** Bend knees to lower body as client slides to the floor.

foot in front of the other, thus supporting the client's body weight (Figure 32–6, A). The nurse then extends one leg and lets the client slide against the leg and gently lowers the client to the floor, protecting the client's head (Figure 32–6, *B* and *C*). Although lowering a client to the floor is not difficult, the student should practise this technique with a friend or classmate before attempting it in a clinical setting. When the client next ambulates, the nurse proceeds more slowly, monitoring for complaints of dizziness, as well as the client's blood pressure before, during, and after ambulation.

Restorative and Continuing Care. Restorative and continuing care involves implementing activity and exercise strategies to assist the client in ADLs after acute care is no longer warranted. The nurse, in collaboration with other health care professionals such as physiotherapists, promotes activity and exercise by teaching clients to use an assistive device that is most appropriate for their condition. Assistive devices for walking include walkers, canes, and crutches. Restorative care also includes activities that promote optimal functioning in clients with certain chronic illnesses.

Assistive Devices for Walking

Walkers. Walkers are extremely light, moveable devices that are about waist high and made of metal tubing (Figure 32–7). They have four widely placed, sturdy, rubber-tipped legs. The client holds the handgrips on the upper bars, takes a step, moves the walker forward, and takes another step.

Canes. Canes are lightweight, easily moveable devices that are made of wood or metal. They provide less support than a walker and are less stable. A person's cane length is equal to the distance between the greater trochanter and the floor (Hoeman, 2002). Two common types of canes are the single straight-legged cane and the quad cane. The single straight-legged cane is more common and is used to support and balance a client with decreased leg strength. This cane should be kept on the stronger side of the body.

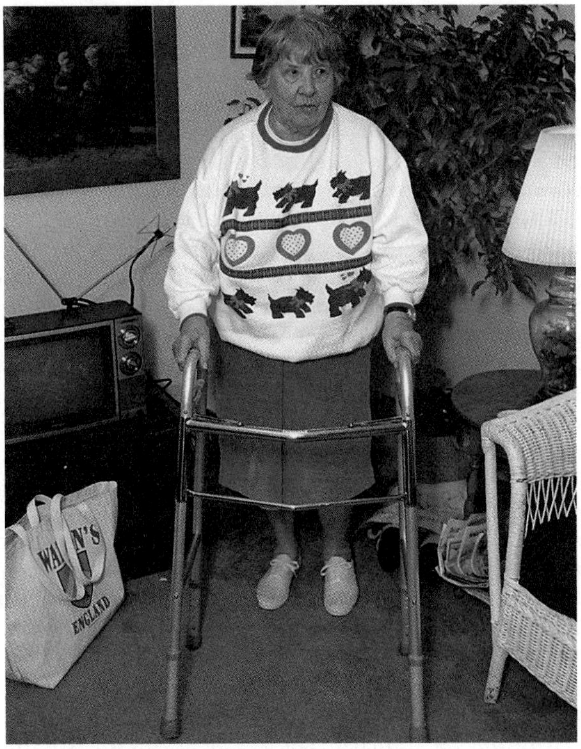

FIGURE **32–7** Client using a walker.

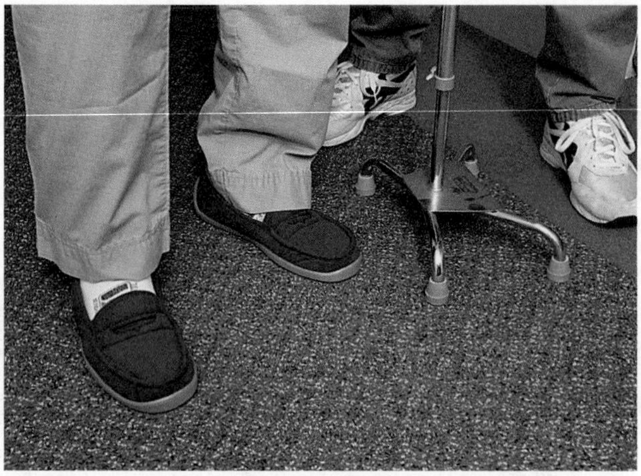

FIGURE **32–8** Bottom of quad cane.

For maximum support when walking, the client places the cane forward 15 to 25 cm, keeping body weight on both legs. The weaker leg is moved forward to the cane so that body weight is divided between the cane and the stronger leg. The stronger leg is then advanced past the cane so that the weaker leg and the body weight are supported by the cane and weaker leg. During walking, the client continually repeats these three steps. The client must be taught that two points of support, such as both feet or one foot and the cane, are present at all times.

The quad cane provides the most support and is used when there is partial or complete leg paralysis or some hemiplegia (Figure 32–8). The same three steps that are used with the straight-legged cane are taught to the client.

Crutches. Crutches are often needed to increase mobility. The nurse begins crutch instruction with guidelines for safe use (Box 32-12). The use of crutches may be temporary, such as after ligament damage to the knee. However, client with paralysis of the lower extremities may need crutches permanently. A crutch is a wooden or metal staff. The two types of crutches are the double adjustable Lofstrand, or forearm, crutch (Figure 32–9) and the axillary wooden or metal crutch. The forearm crutch has a handgrip and a metal band that fits around the client's forearm. The metal band and the handgrip are adjusted to fit the client's height. The axillary crutch has a padded curved surface at the top, which fits under the axilla. A handgrip in the form of a crossbar is held at the level of the palms to support the body. It is important that crutches be measured for the appropriate length and that clients be taught to use their crutches safely, to achieve a stable gait, to ascend and descend stairs, and to rise from a sitting position.

Measuring for Crutches. The axillary crutch is the more common crutch used. Measurements include the client's height, the angle of elbow flexion, and the distance between the crutch pad and the axilla. When crutches are fitted, the length of the crutch should be from three to four fingerwidths from the axilla to a point 15 cm lateral to the client's heel (Hoeman, 2002; Figure 32–10).

The handgrips should be positioned so that the client's body weight is not supported by the axillae. Pressure on the axillae increases risk to underlying nerves, which could result in partial paralysis of the arm. Correct position of the handgrips is determined with the client upright, supporting weight by the handgrips with the elbows slightly flexed at 30 degrees (Hoeman, 2002). Elbow flexion may be verified with a goniometer (Figure 32–11).

When the height and placement of the handgrips have been determined, the nurse should again verify that the distance between the crutch pad and the client's axilla is three to four fingerwidths (Figure 32–12).

Crutch Gait. The **crutch gait** is assumed by alternately bearing weight on one or both legs and on the crutches. The gait selected by the physician is determined by assessing the client's physical and functional abilities and the disease or injury that resulted in the need for crutches. This section summarizes the basic crutch stance and the four standard gaits: four-point alternating gait, three-point alternating gait, two-point gait, and swing-through gait.

The basic crutch stance is the tripod position, formed when the crutches are placed 15 cm in front of and 15 cm to the side of each foot (Figure 32–13). This position improves the client's balance by providing a wider base of support. The body alignment of the client in the tripod position includes an erect head and neck, straight vertebrae,

Client Teaching — Box 32-12

Crutch Safety

Objective

- Client will state and demonstrate safe crutch walking.

Teaching Strategies

- Teach client with axillary crutches about the dangers of pressure on the axillae, which occurs when leaning on the crutches to support body weight.
- Explain why client must use crutches that were measured for him or her.
- Show client how to routinely inspect crutch tips. Rubber tips should be securely attached to the crutches. When tips are worn, they should be replaced. Rubber crutch tips increase surface friction and help prevent slipping.
- Explain that the crutch tips should remain dry. Water decreases surface friction and increases the risk of slipping.
- Show client how to inspect the structure of the crutches.
- Cracks in a wooden crutch decrease its ability to support weight. Bends in aluminum crutches can alter body alignment.
- Provide client with a list of medical supply companies in the community for obtaining repairs, new rubber tips, handgrips, and crutch pads.
- Instruct client to have spare crutches and tips readily available.

Evaluation

- Client states principles of crutch safety.
- Client correctly demonstrates proper use of crutches.

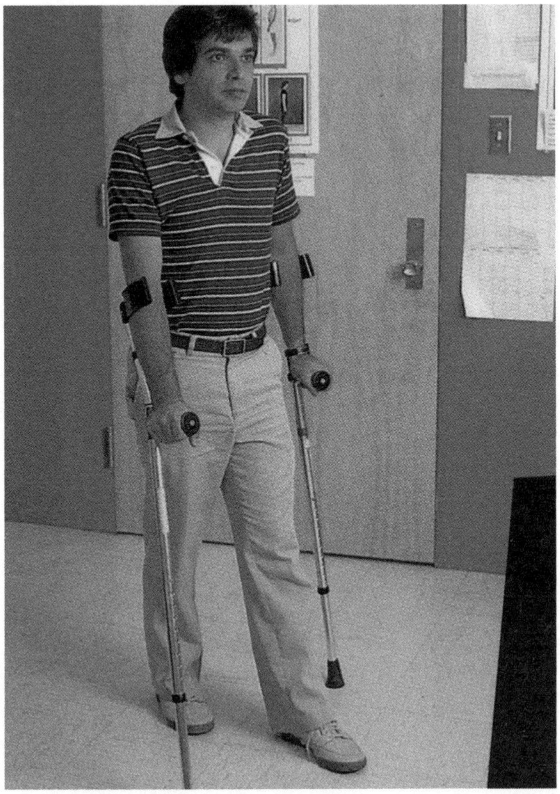

FIGURE **32–9** Double adjustable Lofstrand or forearm crutch.

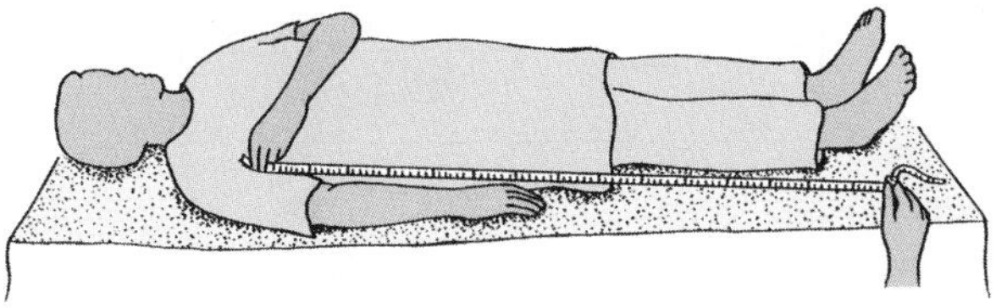

FIGURE **32–10** Measuring crutch length.

and extended hips and knees. The tripod position is assumed before crutch walking.

Four-point alternating, or four-point, gait gives stability to the client but requires weight bearing on both legs. Each leg is moved alternately with each opposing crutch so that three points of support are on the floor at all times (Figure 32–14).

Three-point alternating, or three-point, gait requires the client to bear all of the weight on one foot. In a three-point gait, weight is borne on both crutches and then on the unaffected leg, and the sequence is repeated (Figure 32–15). The affected leg does not touch the ground during the early phase of the three-point gait. Gradually, the client progresses to touchdown and full weight bearing on the affected leg.

The two-point gait requires at least partial weight bearing on each foot (Figure 32–16). The client moves a crutch at the same time as the opposing leg, so that the crutch movements are similar to arm motion during normal walking.

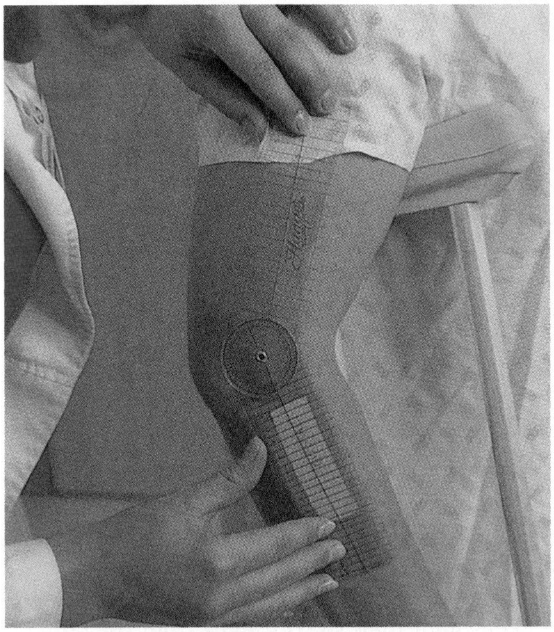

FIGURE **32–11** Using the goniometer to verify correct degree of elbow flexion for crutch use.

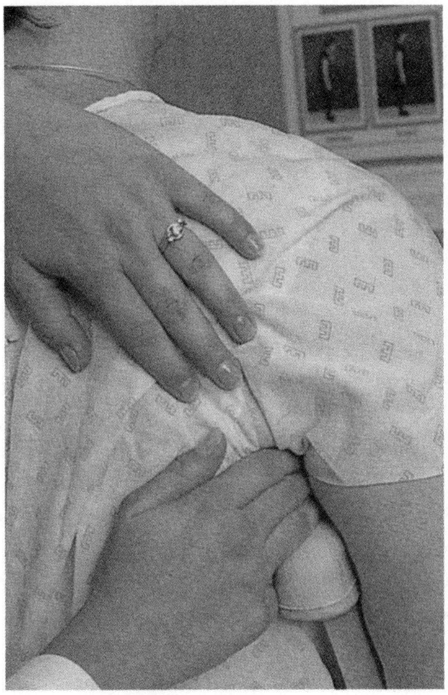

FIGURE **32–12** Verifying correct distance between crutch pads and axilla.

The swing-through, or swing-through gait, is frequently used by clients with paraplegia who wear weight-supporting braces on their legs. With weight placed on the supported legs, the client places the crutches one stride in front and then swings to or through the crutches while they support the client's weight.

Crutch Walking on Stairs. When ascending stairs on crutches, the client usually uses a modified three-point gait (Figure 32–17). The client stands at the bottom of the

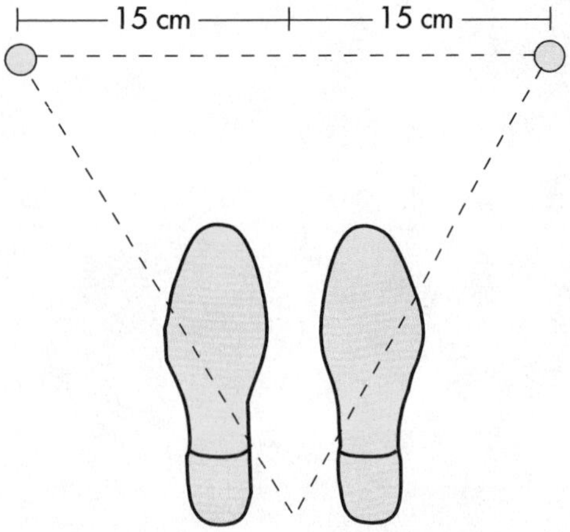

FIGURE **32–13** Tripod position, basic crutch stance.

stairs and transfers body weight to the crutches. The unaffected leg is advanced between the crutches to the stairs. The client then shifts weight from the crutches to the unaffected leg. Finally, the client aligns both crutches on the stairs. This sequence is repeated until the client reaches the top of the stairs.

To descend the stairs (Figure 32–18), a three-phase sequence is also used. The client transfers body weight to the unaffected leg. The crutches are placed on the stairs, and the client begins to transfer body weight to the crutches, moving the affected leg forward. Finally, the unaffected leg is moved to the stairs with the crutches. Again, the client repeats the sequence until reaching the bottom of the stairs.

Because in most cases clients will need to use crutches for some time, they should be adequately taught to use crutches on stairs before discharge. This instruction applies to all crutch-dependent clients, not only those who have stairs in their homes.

Sitting in a Chair With Crutches. As with crutch walking and crutch walking up and down stairs, the procedure for sitting in a chair involves phases and requires the client to transfer weight (Figure 32–19). First, the client gets positioned at the centre front of the chair with the posterior aspect of the legs touching the chair. Then the client holds both crutches in the hand opposite the affected leg. If both legs are affected, as with a client with paraplegia who wears weight-supporting braces, the crutches are held in the hand on the client's stronger side. With both crutches in one hand, the client supports body weight on the unaffected leg and the crutches. While still holding the crutches, the client grasps the arm of the chair with the remaining hand and lowers his or her body into the chair. To stand, the procedure is reversed, and the client, when fully erect, should assume the tripod position before beginning to walk.

Restoration of Activity in Clients With Chronic Illness. Health Canada's Physical Activity Unit (2003b) addressed the role of physical activity in disease prevention and in the treatment of chronic disabling conditions. With this role in mind, the nurse implements a plan of care designed to increase activity and exercise in clients with

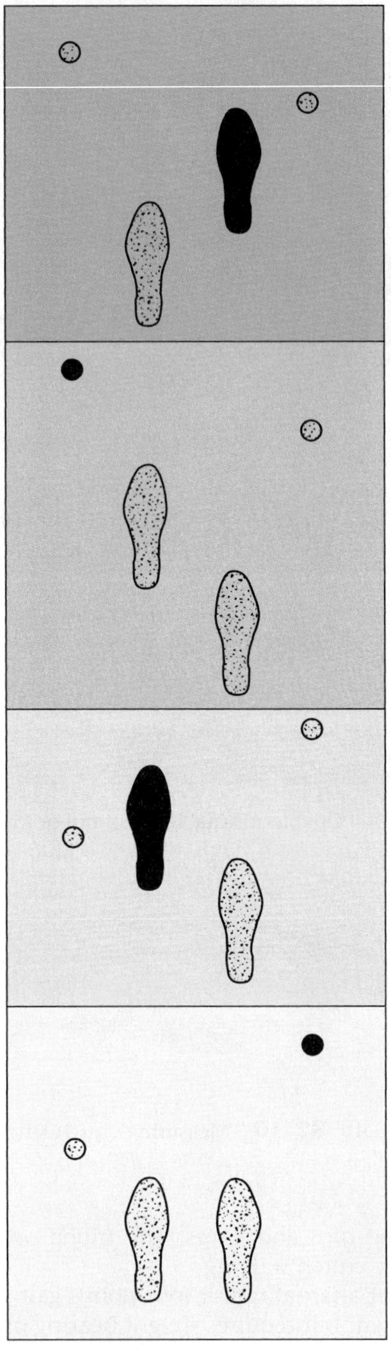

FIGURE **32–14** Four-point alternating gait. Solid feet and crutch tips show foot and crutch tip moved in each of the four phases. (Read from bottom to top.)

specific disease conditions and chronic illnesses such as coronary heart disease (CHD), hypertension, chronic obstructive pulmonary disease (COPD), and diabetes mellitus (Box 32-13).

Coronary Heart Disease (CHD). Activity and exercise have been shown to play a role in secondary prevention or recurrence of CHD. Cardiac rehabilitation is becoming an integral part of comprehensive care of clients who have been diagnosed with CHD. Nurses are involved in

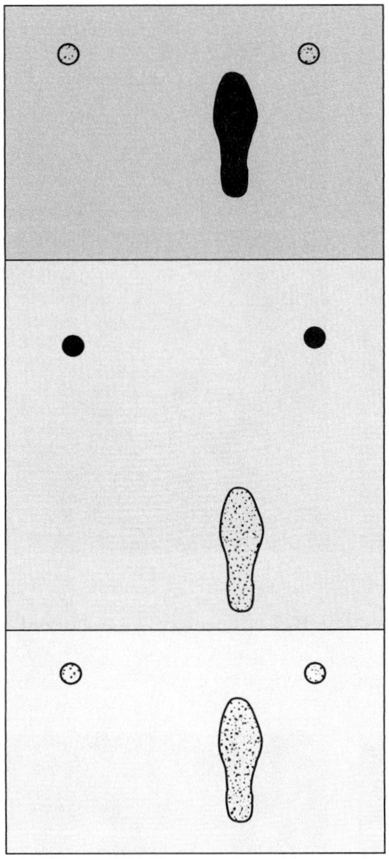

FIGURE **32–15** Three-point gait with weight borne on unaffected leg. Solid foot and crutch tips show weight bearing in each phase. (Read from bottom to top.)

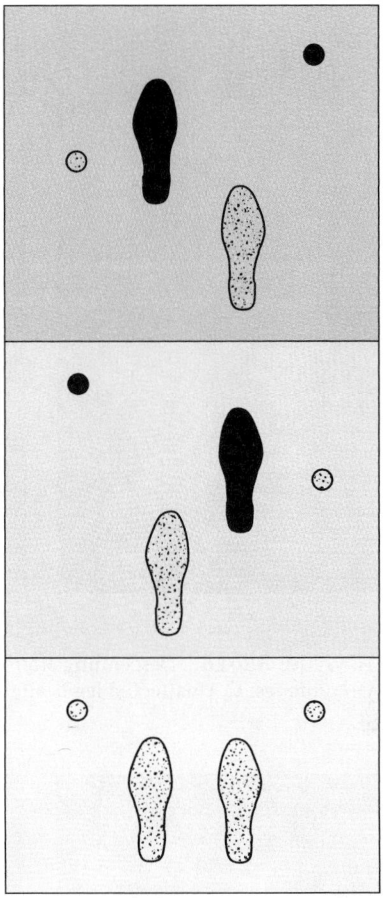

FIGURE **32–16** Two-point gait with weight borne partially on each foot and each crutch advancing with opposing leg. Solid areas indicate leg and crutch tips bearing weight. (Read from bottom to top.)

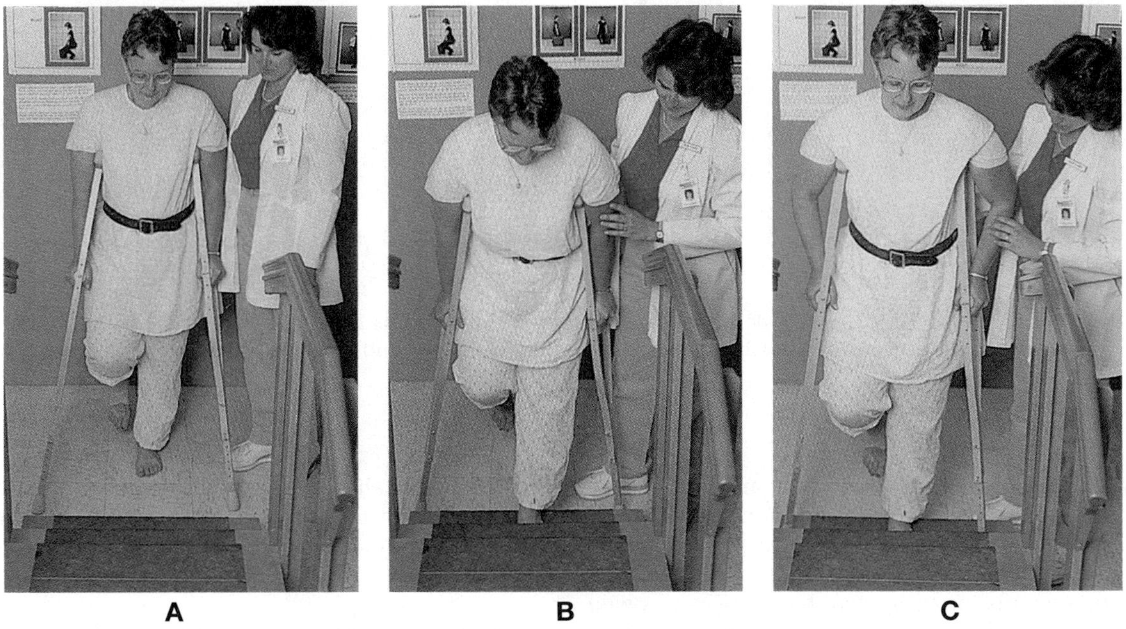

FIGURE **32–17** Ascending stairs. **A,** Weight is placed on crutch. **B,** Weight is transferred from crutches to unaffected leg on stairs. **C,** Crutches are aligned with unaffected leg on stairs.

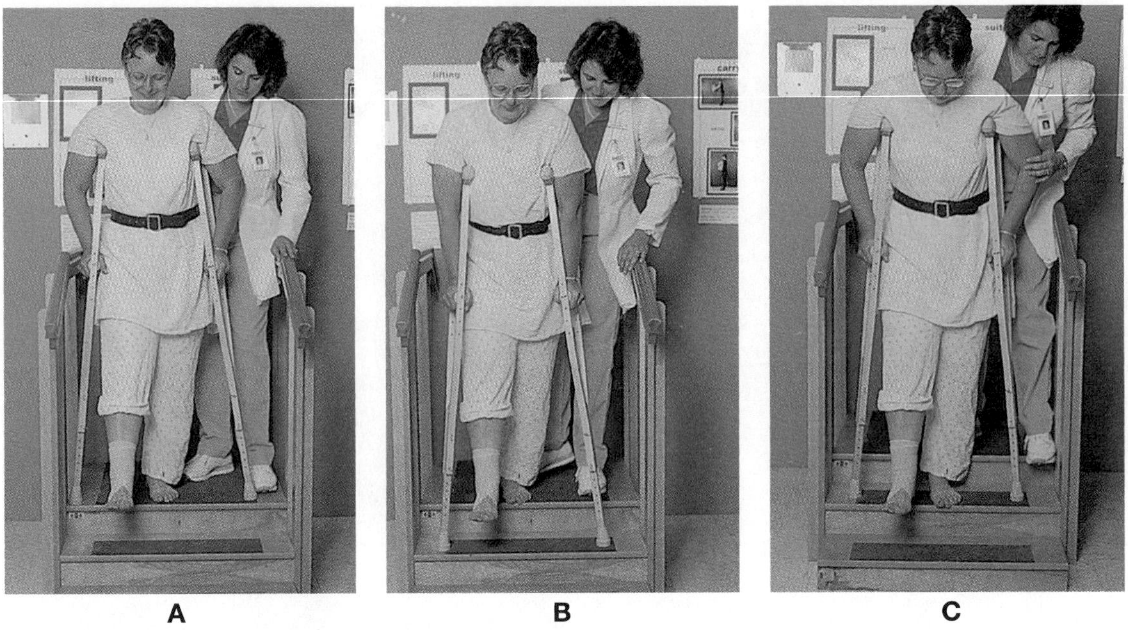

FIGURE 32–18 Descending stairs. **A,** Body weight is on unaffected leg. **B,** Body weight is transferred to crutches. **C,** Unaffected leg is aligned on stairs with crutches.

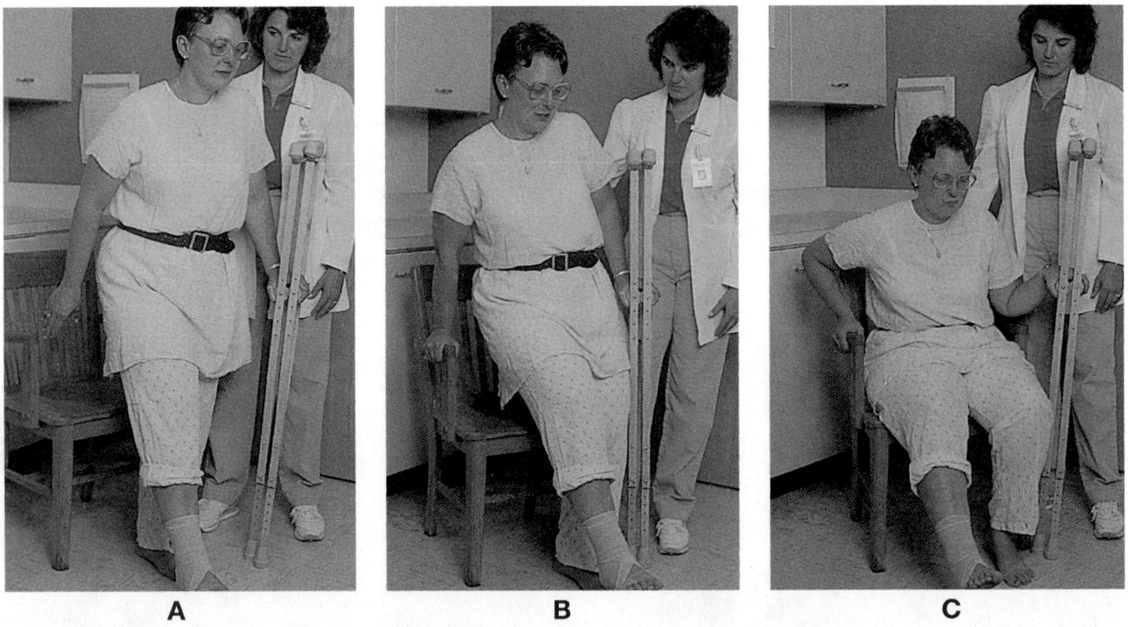

FIGURE 32–19 Sitting in a chair. **A,** Both crutches are held by one hand. Client transfers weight to crutches and unaffected leg. **B,** Client grasps arm of chair with free hand and begins to lower herself into chair. **C,** Client completely lowers herself into chair.

many aspects of cardiac rehabilitation and may assist clients in developing a program of exercise that fits their needs and level of functioning. Increased physical activity appears to benefit individuals with myocardial infarction, angina pectoris, or congestive heart failure, as well as clients who have had a coronary artery bypass graft or percutaneous transluminal coronary angioplasty. Clients with CHD benefit from exercise and activity in terms of reduced mortality and morbidity, improved quality of life, improved left ventricular function, increased functional capacity, and psychological well-being (Konradi & Anglin, 2001; Thompson & Bowman, 1998).

Hypertension. Exercise is instrumental in the reduction of systolic and diastolic blood pressure readings. Low- to moderate-intensity aerobic exercise (brisk walking,

Research Highlight

Box 32-13

Energy Requirements of Tai Chi

Research Focus

Developing alternative exercise strategies for clients with very low functional capacities is a challenge because of the increased risk for complications. Tai chi c'hih, a modified version of tai chi, may be an approach to health promotion in older adults and clients with chronic illness.

Research Abstract

The purpose of this study was to determine the energy cost of tai chi c'hih, which is a form of exercise consisting of a series of slow balanced movements and breathing. The objective of this study was to measure the energy costs and cardiovascular effects to assist in the planning of a safe exercise prescription for clients with very low energy reserves. Twenty-six healthy adults participated in the completion of surveys to estimate functional capacity and exercise participation, in a select series of nine tai chi c'hih movements, and in oxygen consumption testing during the exercise program. The results of the study indicated that the energy requirements for this alternative form of exercise were comparable with low-level exercises for people with low exercise tolerance.

Evidence-Based Practice

- Before initiating exercise, clients should consult their primary care provider.
- Encouraging clients with chronic illness to exercise has the potential to maintain and improve activity tolerance.
- Tai chi c'hih promotes feelings of relaxation and increased energy, thus making it an ideal alternative exercise prescription for clients with chronic illness.

Reference

Fontana, J. A., et al. (2000). The energy costs of a modified form of tai chi exercise. *Nursing Research, 49*(2), 91–96.

bicycling) appears to be the most effective in lowering blood pressure, whereas weight training and high-intensity aerobics seem to have minimal benefits (Huddleston, 2002; Konradi & Anglin, 2001).

Chronic Obstructive Pulmonary Disease (COPD). Pulmonary rehabilitation is a beneficial therapeutic tool to help clients with COPD reach an optimal level of functioning. Some clients are fearful of participating in exercise because of the potential of worsening dyspnea (difficulty breathing). This aversion to physical activity sets up a progressive deconditioning in which minimal physical exertion results in dyspnea. A program of graded exercise for peripheral muscle conditioning improves exercise tolerance (Beers & Berkow, 2005). Many people with COPD enjoy walking, water aerobics, and riding a stationary bike. Specific breathing techniques can reduce the work of breathing and can be applied in times of anxiety or stress when inefficient breathing patterns appear.

Diabetes Mellitus. Along with diet, glucose monitoring, and medication, exercise is an important component in the care of clients with diabetes mellitus. Individuals with Type 1 diabetes are encouraged to exercise because it leads to improved cardiovascular fitness and psychological well-being. The nurse instructs the client with Type 1 diabetes about certain risks and precautions regarding exercise. Instruction should include the need for a pre-exercise physical examination and precautions to monitor blood glucose immediately before and after exercise. The nurse also instructs clients to avoid injecting insulin into muscles that will be active during exercise, to perform low- to moderate-intensity exercises, to carry a concentrated form of carbohydrates (sugar packets, hard candy), and to wear a medical alert bracelet. The client with Type 2 diabetes who decides to participate in a regular program of exercise should include low-intensity warm-up and cool-down exercises, should include aerobic exercise at 50% to 75% of maximal oxygen uptake, and should exercise for 20 to 45 minutes 3 days per week (Canadian Diabetes Association, 2003; Flood & Constance, 2002).

NP Evaluation

Client Care. For activity and exercise, the effectiveness of nursing interventions is measured by the success of meeting the client's expected outcomes and goals of care. The client is the only one who will experience the effectiveness and benefits of activity and exercise (Figure 32–20). To evaluate the effectiveness of nursing interventions to enhance activity and exercise, the nurse can make comparisons with baseline measures that include pulse, blood pressure, strength, endurance, and psychological well-being. Actual outcomes are compared with expected outcomes to determine the client's health status and progression. Continuous evaluation allows the nurse to determine whether new or revised therapies are required and if new nursing diagnoses have developed.

Client Expectations. For the nurse to evaluate the client's perception of nursing care, the nurse must first have assessed the client's expectations concerning activity and exercise. Because what the nurse thinks is acceptable or anticipated may be different from what the client and family members think, it is important for the nurse to ask clients if their expectations of care have been met. Working closely with the client will enable the nurse to redefine those expectations that can be realistically met within the limits of the client's conditions and treatment.

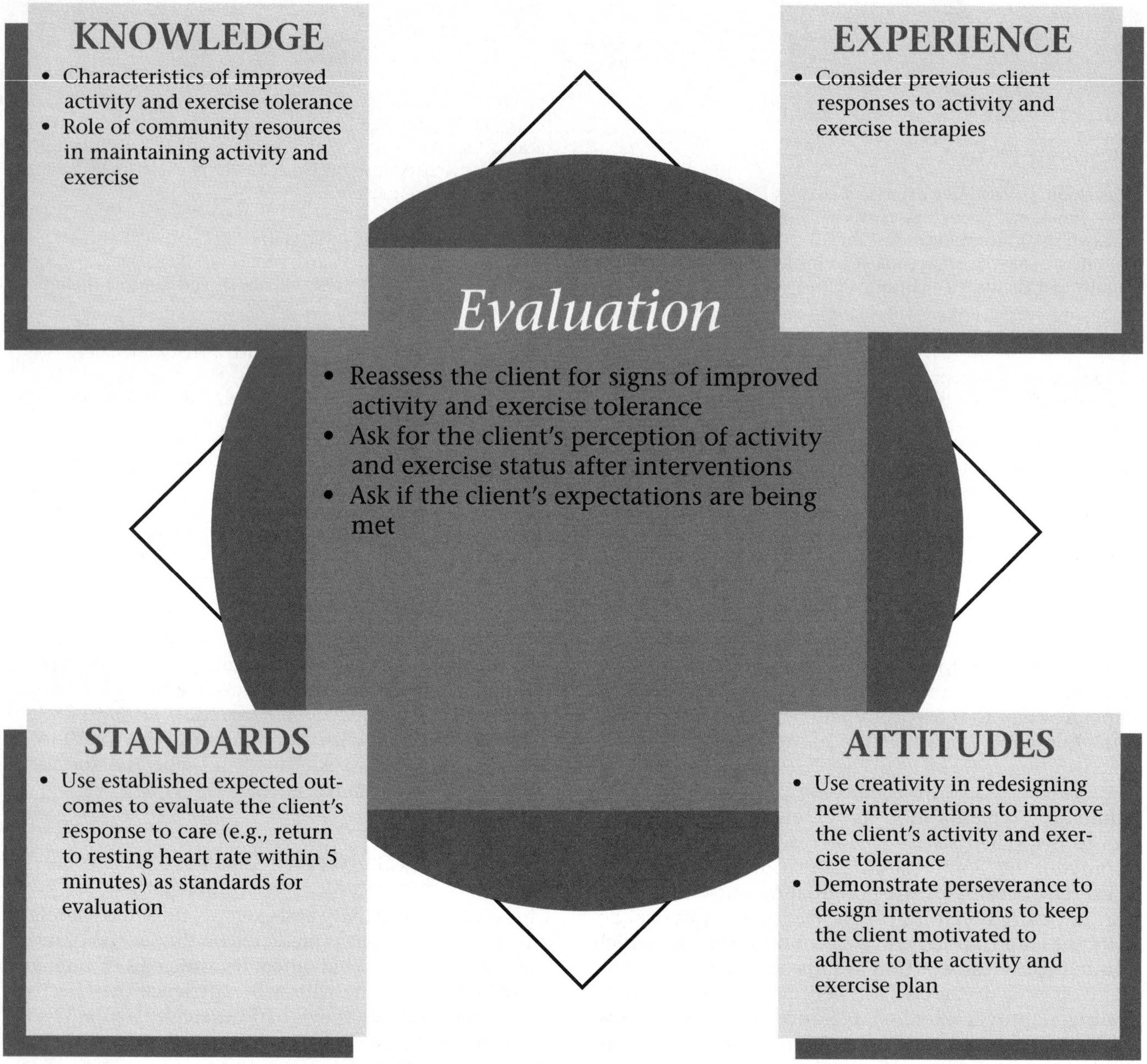
KNOWLEDGE
• Characteristics of improved activity and exercise tolerance
• Role of community resources in maintaining activity and exercise
EXPERIENCE
• Consider previous client responses to activity and exercise therapies
Evaluation
• Reassess the client for signs of improved activity and exercise tolerance
• Ask for the client's perception of activity and exercise status after interventions
• Ask if the client's expectations are being met
STANDARDS
• Use established expected outcomes to evaluate the client's response to care (e.g., return to resting heart rate within 5 minutes) as standards for evaluation
ATTITUDES
• Use creativity in redesigning new interventions to improve the client's activity and exercise tolerance
• Demonstrate perseverance to design interventions to keep the client motivated to adhere to the activity and exercise plan

FIGURE **32–20** Critical thinking model for activity and exercise evaluation.

Key Concepts

- Exercise is physical activity for the purpose of conditioning the body, improving health, and maintaining fitness, or it may be used as a therapeutic measure.
- Activity tolerance is the kind and amount of exercise or work that a person is able to perform. Physiological, emotional, and developmental factors influence the client's activity tolerance.
- The best program of physical activity includes a combination of exercises that produce different physiological and psychological benefits. Isotonic, isometric, and resistive isometric are three categories of exercise classified according to the type of muscle contraction involved.
- Body mechanics are the coordinated efforts of the musculoskeletal and nervous systems as the person moves, lifts, bends, stands, sits, lies down, and completes daily activities.
- Coordinated body movement requires integrated functioning of the skeletal system, skeletal muscles, and nervous system.
- The skeleton provides bony support structure for movement, attachment of ligaments and muscles, protection of vital organs, some regulation of calcium, and production of red blood cells.

- Muscles primarily associated with movement are located near the skeletal region, where movement results from leverage, which is characteristic of movements of the upper extremities.
- Coordination and regulation of muscle groups depend on muscle tone and activity of antagonistic, synergistic, and anti-gravity muscles.
- Balance is assisted through nervous system control in the cerebellum and inner ear function.
- Body balance is achieved when there is a wide base of support, the centre of gravity falls within the base of support, and a vertical line falls from the centre of gravity through the base of support.
- Developmental changes, behavioural aspects, environmental issues, cultural and ethnic origin, and family and social support influence the client's perception and motivation to engage in physical activity and exercise.
- Ability to engage in normal physical activity and exercise depends on intact and functioning nervous and musculoskeletal systems.
- The nurse uses the nursing process to provide care for clients who are experiencing or are at risk for activity intolerance and impaired physical mobility.
- After identifying nursing diagnoses, the nurse plans and implements interventions to increase activity and exercise in collaboration with the client when possible.
- Range-of-motion exercises incorporated into daily activities can include one or all of the body joints.
- Assistive devices to promote walking include walkers, canes, and crutches.

Key Terms

Activities of daily living (ADLs), *p. 942*
Activity tolerance, *p. 943*
Antagonistic muscles, *p. 944*
Anti-gravity muscles, *p. 944*
Body mechanics, *p. 941*
Cartilage, *p. 944*
Cartilaginous joints, *p. 944*
Centre of gravity, *p. 942*
Crutch gait, *p. 960*
Exercise, *p. 941*
Fibrous joints, *p. 944*
Gait, *p. 950*
Gait belt, *p. 958*
Hemiparesis, *p. 950*
Hemiplegia, *p. 946*
Immobility, *p. 957*
Isometric contraction, *p. 943*
Isotonic contraction, *p. 943*
Joint, *p. 944*
Ligaments, *p. 944*
Mobility, *p. 950*
Muscle tone, *p. 942*
Posture, *p. 942*
Proprioception, *p. 945*
Range of motion (ROM), *p. 950*
Synergistic muscles, *p. 944*
Synovial joints, *p. 944*
Tendons, *p. 944*

Critical Thinking Exercises

1. Ms. Moushey is 52 years old. She sustained a fracture of the left femur and must use crutches for 1 week until her follow-up visit at the orthopedic clinic. Her physician has ordered no weight bearing on the left leg. You are conducting the first home visit after her discharge from the hospital. What is the appropriate crutch gait for Ms. Moushey? List several teaching strategies that focus on crutch safety.
2. Mr. Neel has just undergone extensive abdominal surgery. What assessment parameters need to be considered before ambulation of this client? What precautions should you take before ambulating him for the first time?
3. The family of Mrs. Wong made the decision to care for her at home. She is a person with quadriplegia, weighs 72 kg, and requires total care. You are her nurse and responsible for instructing her family on several aspects of her care. Develop a list of basic principles describing body mechanics to protect Mrs. Wong's family members from injury.

Review Questions

1. Nurses must know and practise proper body mechanics in order to
   1. Increase their muscle strength
   2. Restore optimal client functioning
   3. Reduce the risk of injury
   4. Assess the body alignment of clients
2. Proprioception is
   1. Awareness of the position of the body
   2. Needed for anti-gravity
   3. Located within the semicircular canals
   4. The individual's perception of movement at the joint
3. Balance is controlled by the nervous system, specifically by the
   1. Cerebrum and pons
   2. Cerebellum and inner ear
   3. Eye and ear
   4. Cerebral cortex and gyrus
4. A client with a right-sided cerebral hemorrhage may have
   1. Left-sided hemiplegia
   2. Right-sided hemiplegia
   3. Bilateral hemiplegia
   4. Degenerative hemiplegia
5. Older adults are at greater risk for falls and injuries partly because
   1. They may take smaller steps, decreasing their base of support
   2. Their centre of gravity shifts toward the anterior
   3. They tend to walk more quickly, with wide strides
   4. Total bone mass decreases
6. Clients are more open to developing an exercise program if they
   1. Have been diagnosed with a chronic disease such as diabetes
   2. Are ordered by the physician to begin an exercise program
   3. Have been requested to exercise by a family member
   4. Are at the stage of readiness to change their behaviour

7. The result of children being less physically active outside of school has been
   1. An increase in juvenile arthritis
   2. An increase in obesity
   3. Improved school attendance and grades
   4. An increase in school-based fitness activities
8. A principle of good body mechanics includes
   1. Keeping the knees in a locked position
   2. Bending at the knees
   3. Bending at the waist
   4. Holding objects away from the body for improved leverage
9. A client begins to fall during ambulation. To prevent injury to the client the nurse should
   1. Call for assistance
   2. Slide the client down the nurse's body and leg to the floor
   3. Instruct the client to sit in the nearest chair
   4. Allow the client to fall to prevent injury to the nurse
10. The three-point alternating gait when using crutches
    1. Requires at least partial weight bearing on each foot
    2. Is frequently used by clients with paraplegia who wear weight-supporting braces on their legs
    3. Requires weight to be borne on both crutches and then on the unaffected leg
    4. Requires each leg to be moved alternately with each opposing crutch

References

Ackley, B. J., & Ladwig, G. B. (2002). *Nursing diagnosis handbook: A guide to planning care* (5th ed.). St. Louis, MO: Mosby.

Adams, K. J., et al. (1999). Combined high-intensity strength and aerobic training in diverse phase II cardiac rehabilitation patients. *Journal of Cardiopulmonary Rehabilitation, 19,* 209–215.

Anderson, R. (2000). The spread of the childhood obesity epidemic. *Canadian Medical Association Journal, 163*(11), 1461–1462.

Beers, M., & Berkow, R. (Eds.).(1999). Chronic obstructive airway disorders. *The Merck Manual of Diagnosis and Therapy* (17th ed.). Whitehouse Station, NJ: Merck & Co, pp. 568–582.

Brown, J., Josse, R. G., & The Scientific Advisory Council of the Osteoporosis Society of Canada. (2002, November 12). 2002 Clinical practice guidelines for the diagnosis and management of osteoporosis in Canada [Electronic version]. *Canadian Medical Association Journal, 167,* 1–38.

Burbank, P. M., et al. (2002). Exercise and older adults: Changing behaviour with the transtheoretical model. *Orthopedic Nursing, 21*(4), 51–61.

Canadian Association for Health, Physical Education, Recreation and Dance. 1998. *Making the case for physical education in Canada: A presentation kit for leaders.* Retrieved February 1, 2005, from *http://www.cahperd.ca/e/advocacy/index.htm*

Canadian Centre for Occupational Health and Safety. (2004). *OSH answers: Ergonomics/human factors.* Retrieved February 1, 2005, from *http://www.ccohs.ca/oshanswers/ergonomics/*

Canadian Diabetes Association. (2003). *2003 Clinical practice guidelines.* Retrieved May 23, 2004, from *http://www.diabetes.ca/cpg2003/download.aspx*

Canadian Fitness and Lifestyle Research Institute. (2002a). *2002 Capacity study. Increasing physical activity: Building active workplaces.* Retrieved February 1, 2005, from *http://www.cflri.ca/cflri/cflri.html*

Canadian Fitness and Lifestyle Research Institute. (2002b). *2002 Physical activity monitor. Increasing physical activity: Assessing recent trends.* Retrieved February 1, 2005, from *http://www.cflri.ca/cflri/cflri.html*

Connelly, D. M. (2000). Resisted exercise training of institutionalized older adults for improved strength and functional mobility: A review. *Topics in Geriatric Rehabilitation, 15*(3), 6–27.

Dawson, D., Karlis, G., & Georgescu, D. (1998). Contemporary issues in recreation and leisure for aboriginal peoples in Canada. *Journal of Leisurability, 25*(1). Retrieved February 1, 2005, from *http://www.lin.ca/resource/html/Vol25/v25n1a2.htm*

Dochterman, J. M., & Bulecheck, G. M. (Eds.). (2004). *Nursing interventions classification (NIC)* (4th ed.). St. Louis, MO: Mosby.

Eliopoulos, C. (2001). *Gerontologic nursing* (5th ed.). Philadelphia: Lippincott Williams & Wilkins.

Flood, L., & Constance, A. (2002). Diabetes and exercise safety. *American Journal of Nursing, 102*(6), 47–55.

Fontana, J. A. (2000). The energy costs of a modified form of tai chi exercise. *Nurse Researcher, 49*(2), 91.

Hass, C. J., et al. (2000). Single versus multiple sets in long-term recreational weightlifters. *Medicine and Science in Sports and Exercise, 32,* 235–242.

Health Canada. (2001). *The business case for active living at work.* Retrieved February 1, 2005, from *http://www.hc-sc.gc.ca/hppb/fitness/work/main_a_e.html*

Health Canada. (2002a). *Handbook to Canada's physical activity guide to healthy active living* [Electronic version]. Ottawa, ON: Author.

Health Canada. (2002b). *Family guide to physical activity for children* [Electronic version]. Ottawa, ON: Author.

Health Canada. (2002c). *Family guide to physical activity for youth* [Electronic version]. Ottawa, ON: Author.

Health Canada. (2002d). *Physical activity guide for older adults* [Electronic version]. Ottawa, ON: Author.

Health Canada. (2003a). *Canada's physical activity guide to healthy active living.* Retrieved month day, year February 1, 2005, from *http://www.hc-sc.gc.ca/hppb/fitness/downloads.html*

Health Canada. (2003b). Public Health Agency of Canada, Physical Activity Unit Web site. Retrieved February 1, 2005, from *http://www.phac-aspc.gc.ca/pau-uap/fitness/about.html*

Hoeman, S. P. (2002). *Rehabilitation nursing: Process, application, and outcomes* (3rd ed.). St. Louis, MO: Mosby.

Huddleston, J. S. (2002). Exercise. In C. L. Edelman & C. L. Mandle (Eds.), *Health promotion throughout the lifespan* (5th ed., pp. 280–307). St. Louis, MO: Mosby.

Huether, S. E., & McCance, K. L. (2000). *Understanding pathophysiology* (2nd ed.). St. Louis, MO: Mosby.

Kim, M. J., McFarland, G. K., & McLane, A. M. (1997). *Pocket guide to nursing diagnoses* (7th ed.). St. Louis, MO: Mosby.

Klomp, H., Dyck, R., & Sheppard, S. (2003). Description and evaluation of a prenatal exercise program for urban aboriginal women. *Canadian Journal of Diabetes, 27*(3), 231–238.

Konradi, D. B., & Anglin, L. T. (2001). Moderate-intensity exercise: For our patients, for ourselves. *Orthopedic Nursing, 20*(1), 47–54.

Lewis, S. M., et al. (2000). *Medical-surgical nursing assessment and management of clinical problems* (5th ed.). St. Louis, MO: Mosby.

Manson, J. E., et al. (1999). A prospective study of walking as compared with vigorous exercise in the prevention of coronary disease in women. *New England Journal of Medicine, 341,* 650–658.

Moorhead, S., Johnson, M., & Maas, M. L. (Eds.). (2004). *Nursing outcomes classification (NOC)* (3rd ed.). St. Louis, MO: Mosby.

Occupational Health & Safety Agency for Healthcare in British Columbia. (2003). *Reference guidelines for safe patient handling.* Retrieved February 1, 2005, from *http://www.ohsah.bc.ca/index.php?section_id=309&section_copy_id=1155*

Ontario Ministry of Citizenship, Culture and Recreation and the Ministry of Health. (1995). *Messaging workbook for the physical activity intervention policy framework.* Toronto, ON: Queen's Printer for Ontario.

Pate, R, R., et al. (1995). Physical activity and public health: A recommendation from the Centres for Disease Control and Prevention and the American College of Sports Medicine. *Journal of the American Medical Association, 273*(5), 402–407.

Phipps, W. J., et al. (2003). *Medical-surgical nursing: Health and illness perspectives* (7th ed.). St. Louis, MO: Mosby.

Prochaska, J. O., Norcross, J. C., & DiClemente, C. C. (1994). *Changing for good.* New York: William Morrow.

Resnick, B. (1999). Falls in a community of older adults: Putting research into practice. *Clinical Nursing Research, 8*(3), 251–266.

Schlicht, J., Godin J., & Camaione DC (1999). Build self-efficacy to promote exercise adherence. *American College of Sport Medicine's Health and Fitness Journal, 3*(6), 27–31.

School of Physical and Health Education. (2004). Psychological benefits of sport and exercise (class notes). Retrieved February 1, 2005, from *http://www.phe.queensu.ca/courses/phed165/*

Smeltzer, S., & Bare, B. (2003). *Brunner and Suddarth's textbook of medical-surgical nursing* (10th ed.). Philadelphia: Lippincott Williams & Wilkins.

Thibodeau, G. A., & Patton, K. T. (2002). *Anatomy and physiology* (5th ed.). St. Louis, MO: Mosby.

Thompson, D. R., & Bowman, G. S. (1998). Evidence for the effectiveness of cardiac rehabilitation. *Intensive & Critical Care Nursing, 14,* 38–48.

Wilson, S. F., & Giddens, J. F. (2001). *Health assessment for nursing practice* (2nd ed.). St. Louis, MO: Mosby.

Wong, D. L., & Hockenberry-Eaton, M. (2001). *Wong's essentials of pediatric nursing* (6th ed.). St. Louis, MO: Mosby.

Workers Health and Safety Centre. (2003, Summer). Patient lifting: Getting a handle on it. *Resource Lines.* Retrieved February 1, 2005, from *http://www.whsc.on.ca/Publications/hazardbulletins/summer2003/patient_lifting.html*

Young, T., et al. (2000). Type 2 diabetes mellitus in Canada's first nations: Status of an epidemic in progress. *CMAJ, 163*(5), 561–566.

Recommended Web Sites

Active Living Alliance for Canadians With a Disability:
http://www.ala.ca/content/home.asp
This organization is an alliance of individuals, agencies, and national associations who together promote, support, and enable Canadians with disabilities, across all settings and environments, to lead active, healthy lives.

Canadian Centre for Activity and Aging:
http://www.uwo.ca/actage/
The Centre is a research and community resource institution whose mandate is to investigate the interrelationship of physical activity and aging, and to develop strategies, based on research, to promote the independence of older adults.

Canadian Fitness and Lifestyle Research Institute:
http://www.cflri.ca/
The Institute addresses the well-being of Canadians through research and communication of information about physically active lifestyles to the public and private sectors.

Canadian Health Network:
http://www.canadian-health-network.ca
A network of health information providers including Health Canada and national and provincial/territorial non-profit organizations, this Web site was created to provide information on how to stay healthy and prevent disease.

Health Promotion Online:
http://www.hc-sc.gc.ca/hppb
This site within Health Canada has many useful health promotion resources and guides that will aid health professionals and community leaders in encouraging Canadians to take a more active role in their health.

33

Client Safety

Eileen Costantinou, RN, MSN
Daria Romaniuk, RN, BN, MN (Canadian author)

Objectives

Mastery of content in this chapter will enable the student to:

- Define the key terms listed.
- Describe how unmet basic physiological needs of oxygen, nutrition, temperature, and humidity can threaten clients' safety.
- Discuss the specific risks to safety related to developmental age.
- Identify factors to assess when it becomes necessary to physically restrain a client.
- Describe the four categories of risks in a health care agency.
- Describe assessment activities designed to identify clients' physical, psychosocial, and cognitive status as it pertains to their safety status.
- Identify nursing diagnoses associated with risks to safety.
- Develop care plans for clients whose safety is threatened.
- Describe nursing interventions specific to clients' age for reducing risk of falls, fires, poisonings, and electrical hazards.
- Describe methods to evaluate interventions designed to maintain or promote safety.

Safety, often defined as freedom from psychological and physical injury, is a basic human need that must be met. Health care, provided in a safe manner, and a safe community environment are essential for a client's survival and well-being. While incorporating critical thinking skills when using the nursing process, the nurse is responsible for assessing the client and the environment for hazards that threaten safety, as well as for planning and intervening appropriately to maintain a safe environment. By doing this, the nurse is not only a provider of safe care, but is also an active participant in health promotion.

Scientific Knowledge Base

Environmental Safety

A client's **environment** includes all of the many physical and psychosocial factors that influence or affect life and survival of that client. This broad definition of environment crosses the continuum of care for settings in which the nurse and client interact (e.g., the home, community centre, school, clinic, hospital, and long-term care facility). Safety in health care settings reduces the incidence of illness and injury, shortens the length of treatment and/or hospitalization, improves or maintains a client's functional status, and increases the client's sense of well-being. A safe environment affords protection to the staff as well, allowing them to function at an optimal level. A safe environment is an environment in which basic needs are met, physical hazards are reduced, transmission of pathogens is reduced, sanitation is maintained, and pollution is controlled. In addition, a safe environment is one where there is a plan to respond to possible terrorist attack.

Basic Needs. Physiological needs, including the need for sufficient oxygen, nutrition, and optimum temperature and humidity, influence a person's safety.

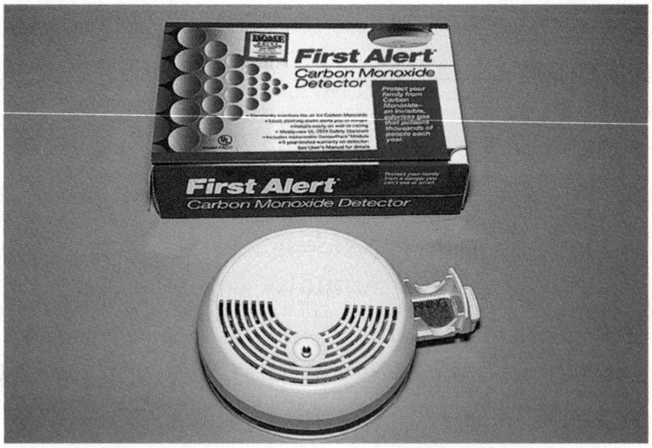

FIGURE **33–1** Carbon monoxide detector.

Oxygen. The nurse must be aware of factors in a client's environment that decrease the amount of available oxygen. A common environmental hazard in the home is an improperly functioning heating system. A furnace that is not properly vented or a car left running inside a closed garage may introduce carbon monoxide into the environment. **Carbon monoxide** is a colourless, odourless, poisonous gas produced by the combustion of carbon or organic fuels. Carbon monoxide binds strongly with hemoglobin, preventing the formation of oxyhemoglobin and thus reducing the supply of oxygen delivered to tissues (see chapter 35). Exposure can cause nausea, headache, drowsiness, confusion, loss of consiousness, and death (Technical Standards and Safety Authority, 2004). Annual inspections of heating systems, chimneys, and appliances should be done in private homes and institutions. Carbon monoxide detectors (Figure 33–1) are available for home or institutional use at a reasonable cost but should not be used as a replacement for proper use and maintenance of fuel-burning appliances.

Nutrition. Meeting nutritional needs adequately and safely requires environmental controls and knowledge. In the home, the client needs a refrigerator with a freezer compartment to keep perishable foods fresh. An adequate, clean water supply is needed for drinking and to wash dishes and fresh produce. Provisions for garbage collection are necessary to maintain sanitary conditions.

Foods that are inadequately prepared or stored, or are subject to unsanitary conditions, increase the client's risk for infections and food poisoning. Bacterial food infections result from eating food contaminated by bacteria such as *Escherichia coli or Salmonella, Shigella,* or *Listeria* organisms. **Food poisoning** is caused by ingestion of bacterial toxins produced in food; staphylococcal and clostridial bacteria are the most common causes. Although most food-borne diseases are bacterial, the hepatitis A virus is spread by fecal contamination of food, water, or milk (Williams, 2000).

For illnesses caused by bacterial contamination, the onset of symptoms may be very rapid or may take a week or longer. The average incubation period for hepatitis A is 28 to 30 days (Health Canada, 2004a). Preventive measures include thorough handwashing before handling food, adequate cooking, and proper storage and refrigeration of perishable foods.

For consumer protection, commercially processed and packaged foods are subject to the provisions of the *Food and Drug Act,* which regulates the manufacture, processing, and distribution of foods, drugs, and cosmetics. The Act protects consumers from the sale of impure or dangerous substances. Ensuring safe food supplies for Canadians is a joint effort among Health Canada, the Canadian Food Inspection Agency, and provincial, territorial, and municipal organizations.

Temperature and Humidity. The comfort zone for environmental temperature varies among individuals, but the usual comfort range is between 18.3° and 23.9° C. Temperature extremes that frequently occur during the winter and summer affect not only comfort and productivity, but also safety.

Exposure to severe cold for prolonged periods may cause frostbite and hypothermia. Frostbite occurs when a surface area of the skin freezes as a result of exposure to extremely cold temperatures. **Hypothermia** occurs when the core body temperature is 35° C or below (see chapter 27). Older adults, the young, clients with cardiovascular conditions, clients who have ingested drugs or alcohol in excess, and the homeless are at high risk for hypothermia.

Exposure to extreme heat can raise the core body temperature, resulting in heatstroke or heat exhaustion. Chronically ill clients, older adults, and infants are at greatest risk for injury from extreme heat. These clients should avoid extremely hot, humid environments.

The relative humidity of the air in the environment may affect the client's health and safety. **Relative humidity** is the amount of water vapour in the air compared with the maximum amount of water vapour that the air could contain at the same temperature. The comfort zone varies from person to person, but most people are comfortable when the humidity is between 60% and 70%. Increasing the environmental humidity can have therapeutic benefits for clients with upper respiratory tract infections because humidity helps to liquefy pulmonary secretions and improve breathing. It is important to follow the manufacturer's directions regarding the cleaning and maintenance of home humidifiers to prevent water contamination.

Physical Hazards. Physical hazards in the environment place clients at risk for accidental injury and death. In Canada, accidental injuries are the leading cause of death for people between the ages of 1 and 44 years (Federal, Provincial, and Territorial Advisory Committee on Population Health, 1999). Accidental injuries are also a major cause of disability. Motor vehicle accidents are the leading cause of accidental injury, followed by falls (Canadian Institute for Health Information [CIHI], 2003). Other causes of injury and death include poisonings, suffocation, drownings, fires, burns, and machinery accidents. Among older adults (aged 65 and over), falls are the most common cause of hospital admissions for trauma (CIHI, 2003). Many physical hazards, especially those contributing to falls, can be minimized through adequate lighting, reduction of obstacles, control of bathroom hazards, and security measures.

Lighting. Adequate lighting reduces physical hazards by illuminating areas in which a person moves and works. Outside the home, there should be adequate lighting on all walkways. Outdoor lighting also helps protect the home and its inhabitants from crime. Well-lighted garages, walkways, and doorways discourage intruders from entering the premises or hiding in shadows.

Inside the house, halls, staircases, and individual rooms should be adequately lit so that residents can safely carry out activities of daily living. Night lights in dark halls, bathrooms, and the rooms of children and older adults help maintain safety by reducing the risk of falls. A night light in a guest room can help orient an overnight guest who needs to get up in the middle of the night. Artificial lighting should be soft and non-glaring because glare is a major problem for older adults (Ebersole & Hess, 2003).

Obstacles. Injuries in the home frequently result from tripping over or coming into contact with common household objects, including doormats, small rugs on the stairs and floor, wet spots on the floor, and clutter on bedside tables, closet shelves, and bookshelves. The risk of falls from obstacles is present for all age groups; however, it is greatest for older adults. Falls are usually a result of a combination of intrinsic risk factors (e.g., illness, drug therapy, or alcohol use) and extrinsic or environmental factors. In some cases, an obstacle or extrinsic factor may be the only cause of a fall. Intrinsic factors may be difficult to modify or eliminate, but extrinsic factors are usually not.

Bathroom Hazards. Accidents such as falls, burns, and poisoning frequently occur in the bathroom. Secure, easily seen grab bars and non-slip, coloured adhesive tape on the bottom of the tub are useful in reducing falls in the bathtub. An elevated toilet seat with armrests and non-slip strips on the floor in front of the toilet are also helpful. Lowering the thermostat setting on the water heater reduces the risk of scalding. In the medicine cabinet, medications should be clearly marked and out of the reach of children. Child-resistant caps should be on all medication containers when there are children living in the home or visiting the home. Medication not in use or out of date should be taken to a pharmacy or municipal waste disposal depot for proper disposal (Health Canada, 2004b).

Fire. Fire is the third leading cause of accidental death in Canada, after falls and motor vehicle accidents (Canada Safety Council, 2004). Most fire deaths occur in the home, and most deaths are due to smoke inhalation. The most common causes of fire are careless smoking and cooking accidents. Smoke detectors (Figure 33–2), along with carbon monoxide detectors, should be placed strategically throughout the home and checked regularly. Multi-purpose fire extinguishers should be installed near the kitchen and any workshop areas.

Lead Poisoning. Individuals may be exposed to lead from various sources. Although Canadian regulations have restricted the lead content of paint since 1976, older homes may still have high lead levels because of old paint. Lead may also be found in contaminated water systems and in household articles such as vinyl blinds and candles. Exposure to lead may occur through oral ingestion, inhalation, or through the skin. Fetuses, infants, and children are more vulnerable to lead poisoning than adults because lead is more easily absorbed into growing bodies. As well, small children are more sensitive to the damaging effects of lead. Exposure to excessive levels of lead can lead to vomiting, headaches, anemia, appetite loss, slowed speech development, and learning and behavioural problems (Health Canada, 2002).

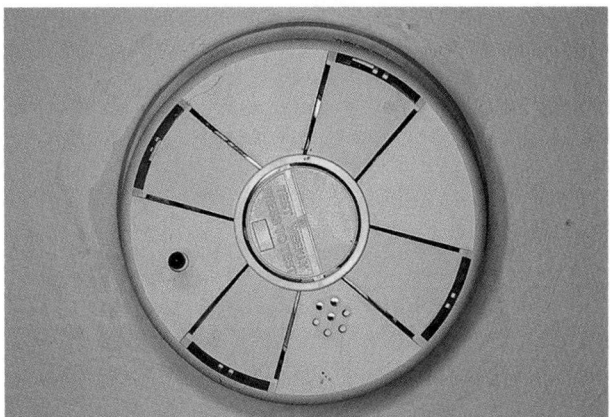

FIGURE **33–2** Smoke and fire detector.

Security. An insecure home places the client at risk for injury or burglary. Inadequate locks on doors and windows make the home susceptible to intruders. Clients need to take precautions to secure their homes. When assessing the home for safety, the nurse guides the client to evaluate doors and windows for the presence and quality of locks. Clients should be encouraged to join block associations and work closely with law enforcement personnel to reduce crime in their neighbourhoods.

Transmission of Pathogens. A **pathogen** is a microorganism capable of producing an illness. One of the most effective methods for limiting the transmission of pathogens is the aseptic practice of hand hygiene (see chapter 29). Clients must be instructed in proper hand-hygiene techniques and encouraged to use them frequently in the home and hospital.

The transmission of disease from person to person can also be reduced, and in some cases prevented, by immunization. **Immunization** is the process by which resistance to an infectious disease is produced or augmented. Active immunity is acquired by injecting a small amount of attenuated (weakened) or dead organisms or modified toxins from the organism (toxoids) into the body. Passive immunity occurs when antibodies produced by other people or animals can be introduced into a person's bloodstream for protection against a pathogen.

The human immunodeficiency virus (HIV)—the pathogen that causes acquired immunodeficiency syndrome (AIDS)—and the hepatitis B virus are transmitted through blood and other body fluids. Drug abusers frequently share syringes and needles, which increases the risk of acquiring these viruses. Safer sex practices (see chapter 23), including the correct use of condoms and engaging in monogamous relationships, reduce the risk for both of these diseases, as well as for other sexually transmitted infections. Nurses use standard precautions (or routine practices) when caring for all clients to prevent the spread of infection and contact with blood and body fluids (see chapter 29).

At the community level, the transmission of disease is also controlled by adequate disposal of human waste through proper construction and repair of sewers and drains. Insect and rodent control (e.g., spraying for mosquitoes) is also necessary to reduce the transmission of disease.

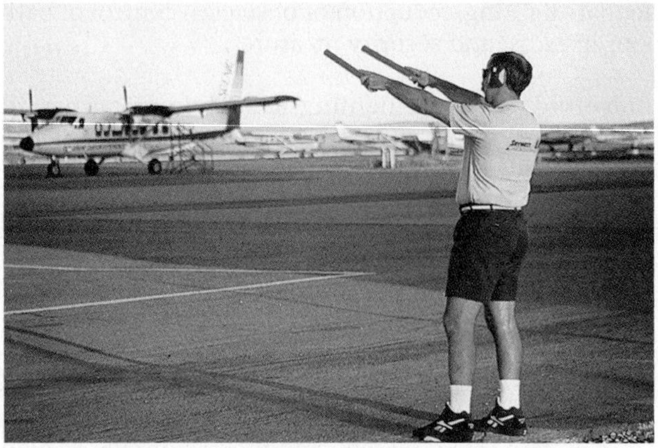

FIGURE **33–3** Protective device to reduce hearing loss.

Pollution. A healthy environment is free of pollution. A **pollutant** is a harmful chemical or waste material discharged into the water, soil, or air. People commonly think of pollution only in terms of air, land, or water pollution, but excessive noise can also be a form of pollution that presents health risks. **Air pollution** is the contamination of the atmosphere with a harmful chemical. Prolonged exposure to air pollution increases the risk of pulmonary disease. In urban areas, industrial waste and vehicle exhaust are common contributors to air pollution. Cigarette smoke is a common cause of air pollution. **Land pollution** of soil can be caused by improper disposal of radioactive and bioactive waste products (e.g., dioxin).

Water pollution is the contamination of lakes, rivers, and streams, usually by industrial pollutants. Water treatment facilities filter harmful contaminants from the water, but these systems may contain flaws. If water becomes contaminated, the public should use bottled or boiled water for drinking and cooking. Flooding frequently causes damage to water treatment stations and also requires the use of bottled or boiled water.

Noise pollution occurs when the noise level in an environment becomes uncomfortable to the inhabitants of the environment. Noise levels are measured in units of sound intensity called decibels. Tolerance for noise varies from individual to individual and is influenced by health status. Irreversible hearing loss may result from constant exposure to high sound intensity. Clients working in environments with high noise levels need to wear protective devices to reduce hearing loss (Figure 33–3). Adolescents should limit their exposure to intense noise such as that encountered at rock concerts.

A health care facility can also be polluted by noise. The sounds of machines, people talking, intercoms, and paging systems can create increased noise levels. Even when the noise level is not high enough to affect hearing acuity, it may produce a syndrome called *sensory overload,* which is a marked increase in the intensity of auditory and visual stimuli. It disrupts processing of information, and the client no longer perceives the environment in a meaningful way (see chapter 44).

Terrorism. A new potential environmental health threat is the possibility of a terrorist attack. The terrorist attacks in the United States on September 11, 2001, raised awareness of this threat for Canadians. If a terrorist health threat were to occur in Canada, Health Canada would work with provincial, territorial, and local health officials to address the situation. St. John and Giroux (2002) emphasized the importance of a strong public health infrastructure in dealing with a terrorist health threat. Health care facilities must have well-rehearsed plans to deal with such an attack (Kollek, 2003). Nurses must be prepared through education and training to be able to respond to an attack by taking the necessary steps to initiate an agency's emergency management plan.

Nursing Knowledge Base

Nurses, in addition to being knowledgeable about the environment, must be familiar with a client's developmental level; mobility, sensory, and cognitive status; and lifestyle choices. Nurses must also be aware of common safety precautions and of the special risks to safety that are found in agency settings.

Risks at Developmental Stages

A client's developmental stage presents specific threats to safety. Clients throughout all developmental stages may be subject to abuse. Child abuse, domestic violence, and abuse of older adults are serious threats to safety. These topics are discussed in chapters 19 and 28.

Infant, Toddler, and Preschooler. Injuries are the leading cause of death in children over the age of 1 year and cause more death and disabilities than do all diseases combined (Wong, 2003). The nature of the injury sustained is closely related to normal growth and development. For example, the incidence of poisoning is highest in late infancy and toddlerhood because of a child's increased level of oral activity and the growing ability to explore the environment. Accidents involving children are mostly preventable, and parents need to be aware of specific dangers at each stage of growth and development. Accident prevention thus requires health education for parents and the removal of dangers whenever possible.

School-Age Child. When a child enters school, the environment expands to include the school, transportation to and from school, school friends, and after-school activities. Parents, teachers, and nurses must instruct the child in safe practices to follow at school or play. Using examples when discussing safe practices is an effective way to teach the school-age child.

Because school-age children are participating in more activities outside their home and neighbourhood environments, they are at greater risk of injury from strangers. A child should be warned repeatedly not to accept candy, food, gifts, or rides from strangers. In addition, a child needs to know what to do if a stranger approaches. Frequently, neighbourhoods have a "block parent" program. In block parent homes, the owner ensures that an adult is home during the times when children are walking to and from school. If a stranger approaches a child, the child can run to that home (identified by a sign), and the adult will protect the child and call the proper authorities. Nurses can work with school systems or neighbourhoods to initiate such a system to protect children.

Sports safety is stressed in school sports, but parents and health professionals can reinforce these safety tips by insisting that children wear protective gear while participating in sports such as skateboarding and snowboarding. For example, schools provide hard batting helmets for baseball games, and parents should also provide this equipment when children are playing baseball in their own backyards.

Bicycle-related injuries, including scooters, are a major cause of death and disability among children. Children 5 to 14 years of age account for one third of bicyclists hospitalized as a result of bicycle injuries (CIHI, 2004a). Bikes should be in good working order and the proper size for the child. The child should be taught the rules of the road and cautioned not to engage in dangerous stunts or activities while bike riding. A properly fitted helmet should be worn. Because most fatalities from bicycle accidents are related to head injuries, most provinces have implemented laws requiring bicycle helmets for children (Figure 33–4).

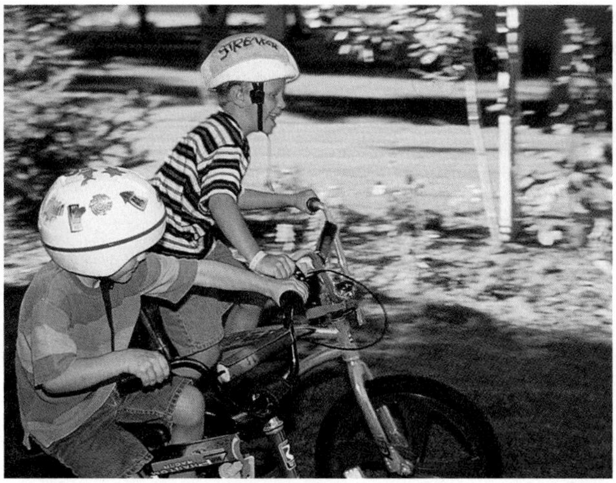

FIGURE 33–4 Proper bicycle safety equipment for school-age child.

Adolescent. As children enter adolescence, they develop greater independence and begin to develop a sense of identity and their own values. In addition, adolescents begin to separate emotionally from their families, and peers generally have a stronger influence. The struggle toward identity may cause the teenager to experience shyness, fear, and anxiety, with resulting dysfunction at home or school. In an attempt to relieve the tensions associated with physical and psychosocial changes, as well as peer pressures, adolescents may begin to act impulsively and engage in risk-taking behaviours such as smoking and using drugs. In addition to the health risks posed by nicotine and other drugs, the ingestion of drugs, including alcohol, increases the incidence of accidents such as drowning and motor vehicle accidents.

When adolescents learn to drive, their environment expands and so does their potential for injury. The risk of motor vehicle accidents is higher among teen drivers than any other age group. Teens are more likely to speed, run red lights, ride with intoxicated drivers, and drive after using alcohol and drugs. The young driver must be taught to comply with rules and regulations regarding use of a car.

Safety Alert. Reinforce to new drivers and parents of new drivers the need to consistently wear safety belts and to never ride in a car with a driver who has been drinking. Assist parents and teen in developing a plan of action to be used if the teen is with a driver who drinks at an outing.

Because adolescence is a time when mature sexual physical characteristics develop, adolescents may begin to have physical relationships with others. They need prompt, accurate instruction about abstinence and/or safer sexual practices and birth control (see chapter 23).

Adult. The threats to an adult's safety are frequently related to lifestyle habits. For example, the client who consumes excessive alcohol is at greater risk for motor vehicle accidents. The long-term smoker has a greater risk of cardiovascular or pulmonary disease. Likewise, the adult experiencing a high level of stress is more likely to have an accident or illness such as headaches, gastrointestinal (GI) disorders, and infections (see chapter 26).

Older Adult. The physiological changes that occur during the aging process increase the client's risk for falls (Box 33-1). In 2001 to 2002, 85% of injury hospitalizations for adults 65 years and older were due to falls (CIHI, 2004a). Older adults are more likely to fall in the bedroom, bathroom, and kitchen. Falls most often occur while transferring from beds, chairs, and toilets; getting into or out of bathtubs; tripping over carpet edges or doorway thresholds; slipping on wet surfaces; and descending stairs (Tideiksaar, 1989). Icy walkways and obstacles in the yard are also common causes of outdoor falls in older adults.

Individual Risk Factors

Other risk factors posing threats to safety include lifestyle, impaired mobility, sensory or communication impairment, and lack of safety awareness.

Box 33-1 Changes Associated With Aging That Increase the Risk of Accidents

Musculoskeletal Changes

Muscle strength and function decrease, joints become less mobile, bones are brittle due to osteoporosis, postural changes (e.g., kyphosis) are common, and range of motion is limited.

Nervous System Changes

All voluntary or automatic reflexes slow to some extent, ability to respond to multiple stimuli decreases, and sensitivity to touch is decreased.

Sensory Changes

Peripheral vision and lens accommodation decrease, lens may develop opacity (cataracts), stimuli threshold for light touch and pain increases, transmission of hot and cold impulses is delayed, and hearing is impaired as high-frequency tones become less perceptible.

Genitourinary Changes

Nocturia and occurrences of incontinence increase.

Adapted from *Toward Healthy Aging* (6th ed.), by P. Ebersole and P. Hess, 2003, St. Louis, MO: Mosby.

Lifestyle. Lifestyle can increase safety risks. People who drive or operate machinery while under the influence of chemical substances (drugs or alcohol), who work at inherently dangerous jobs, or who are risk takers are at greater risk of injury. In addition, people experiencing stress, anxiety, fatigue, or alcohol or drug withdrawal, or those taking prescribed medications may be more accident prone. Because of these factors, clients may be too preoccupied to notice the source of potential accidents, such as cluttered stairs or a stop sign.

Impaired Mobility. Impaired mobility due to muscle weakness, paralysis, or poor coordination or balance is a major factor in client falls. Immobilization predisposes the client to additional physiological and emotional hazards, which in turn can further restrict mobility and independence.

Sensory or Communication Impairment. Clients with visual, hearing, tactile, or communication impairment, such as aphasia or a language barrier, are at greater risk for injury. Such clients may not be able to perceive a potential danger or express their need for assistance (see chapter 44).

Lack of Safety Awareness. Some clients are unaware of safety precautions, such as keeping medicine or poisons away from children or reading the expiration date on food products. A complete nursing assessment, including a home inspection, will help the nurse identify the client's level of knowledge regarding home safety so that deficiencies can be corrected with an individualized nursing care plan.

Risks in the Health Care Agency

Environmental safety pertains to the health care agency as well as to the client's home and community. There are specific risks in health care agencies that must also be addressed.

In a study of Canadian hospitals, Baker et al. (2004) found that 7.5% of clients were affected by medical errors during their hospital stay. The most common errors were related to surgical procedures and drug or fluid administration. In 15.9% of these cases, the errors resulted in the client's death. One study on adverse drug events showed that 78% were due to system failures such as lack of knowledge about a drug, lack of information about a client, failure to follow established procedures, transcription errors, faulty drug identification and checking, faulty dose checking, inadequate monitoring, preparation errors, drug stocking and delivery problems, and lack of standardization (Agency for Healthcare Research and Quality , 2000). Providing safe care is an important concern for Canadian nurses, with individual and system factors influencing that care (Canadian Nurses Association and University of Toronto Faculty of Nursing, 2004). It is essential that nurses and health care facilities build safety into processes of care and take a systems approach when taking on efforts to reduce medical errors.

Various forms of chemicals used in health care settings are a source of environmental risk for both the client and the health care worker. Chemicals such as mercury and those found in some medications, anaesthetic gases, cleaning solutions, and disinfectants can be potentially toxic if ingested or inhaled. The **Workplace Hazardous Materials Information System (WHMIS)** sets the standard for control of hazardous substances in workplaces across Canada (Health Canada, 2003). A hazardous substance is any product or material that could cause physical or medical problems. WHMIS consists of three main elements: worker education programs, cautionary labelling of products, and provision of **Material Safety Data Sheets (MSDSs).** Cautionary labels include information needed to safely handle the hazardous substance, including a description of physical and health hazards, safety and first aid measures, and hazard symbols, which depict the types of hazard that the product presents (Figure 33–5). MSDSs are available to provide detailed information about the substance, any health hazards imposed, precautions for safe handling and use, and steps to take in case the substance is released or spilled. Nurses must understand WHMIS labelling requirements and be aware of the location of MSDSs in the area where they are working.

Specific risks to a client's safety within the health care environment also include falls, client-inherent accidents, procedure-related accidents, and equipment-related accidents. The nurse must assess for these four potential problem areas and, considering the developmental level of the client, take steps to prevent or minimize accidents.

An accident necessitates the filing of an incident report (also called adverse occurrence report), a confidential document that completely describes any client accident occurring on the premises of a health care agency (see

Symbol	Name	Description
	Flammable and Combustible Material	Product may catch fire when exposed to heat, sparks, or flame.
	Oxidizing Material	Product may cause a fire or explosion if exposed to combustible material.
	Compressed Gas	Product is under high pressure. May explode or burst when heated, dropped, or damaged.
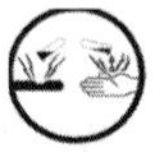	Corrosive Material	Product can cause burns to eyes, skin or respiratory system.
	Dangerously Reactive Material	Product may react with light, heat, extreme temperatures, or vibration causing explosion, fire, or release of poisonous gases.
	Poisonous and Infectious Material: Immediate and Serious Toxic Effects	Product may be fatal or cause serious or permanent damage if exposed to even once.
	Poisonous and Infectious Material: Other Toxic Effects	Product may cause cancer, birth defects, or other permanent damage if exposed to repeatedly.
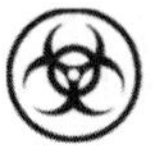	Poisonous and Infectious Material: Biohazardous and Infectious Material	Product may cause disease, serious illness, or death.

FIGURE **33–5** WHMIS hazard symbols. (Adapted from the Canadian Centre for Occupational Health and Safety, retrieved December 8, 2004, from *http://www.ccohs.ca/oshanswers/legisl/ msds_lab.html*).

chapter 8). The report documents the accident, client assessment, and interventions carried out for the client. In addition to completing the incident report, the nurse must objectively document the incident in the client's medical record. Because this is a confidential document, completion of the incident report should not be mentioned in the medical record because this eliminates the health care agency's protective clause.

Falls. Falls account for up to 90% of all reported incidents in hospitals. The risk for falling is significantly higher in older clients. In addition to age, a history of previous falls, gait disturbance, balance and mobility problems, postural hypotension, sensory impairment, urinary and bladder dysfunction, and certain medical diagnostic categories (e.g., cancer and cardiovascular, neurological, and cerebrovascular diseases) increase the risk. One of the more common factors precipitating a fall is a client's attempt to get out of bed to toilet. Drug use and drug interactions are also implicated in falls. Hip fractures are among the most serious fall-related injuries. The older adult with a hip fracture may have a long period of recovery and may not be able to return to the previous level of functioning, even losing his or her ability to live independently (SMARTRISK, 1998). Falls that result in injuries can extend a client's length of stay in the health care environment, placing the client at an even greater risk for other complications.

Client-Inherent Accidents. Client-inherent accidents are accidents (other than falls) in which the client is the primary reason for the accident. Examples of client-inherent accidents are self-inflicted cuts, injuries, and burns; ingestion or injection of foreign substances; self-mutilation or fire setting; and pinching fingers in drawers or doors.

A client-inherent accident may occur as a result of a seizure. A **seizure** is a hyperexcitation and disorderly discharge of neurons in the brain leading to a sudden, violent, involuntary series of muscle contractions that may be paroxysmal and episodic, as in a seizure disorder, or transient and acute, such as following a head injury. A generalized tonic-clonic seizure lasts approximately 2 minutes (no longer than 5 minutes) and is characterized by a cry, loss of consciousness with falling, tonicity (rigidity), clonicity (jerking), and incontinence (Beare & Meyers, 1998). During a fall, or as a result of muscle jerking, musculoskeletal injuries can occur. Before a convulsive episode, a few clients may report an **aura,** which serves as a warning or sense that a seizure is about to occur. An aura may be a bright light, smell, or taste. During the seizure, the client may have shallow breathing, cyanosis, and possibly loss of bladder and bowel control. Following the seizure, there is a postictal phase during which the client may have amnesia or confusion and may fall into a deep sleep.

Continuous seizures that last 15 minutes or a series of seizures over a 20- to 30-minute period in which the client does not regain consciousness between attacks is status epilepticus. This condition is a medical emergency and requires intensive monitoring and treatment. It is important that the nurse observe the client carefully before, during, and after the seizure so that the episode can be documented accurately (Beare & Meyers, 1998).

Procedure-Related Accidents. Procedure-related accidents occur during therapy. They include medication and fluid administration errors, improper application of external devices, and accidents related to improper performance of procedures (e.g., Foley catheter insertion).

The nurse can prevent many procedure-related accidents. For example, strictly following the procedure for administering medications will prevent medication errors (see chapter 30). Proper administration of intravenous (IV) fluids prevents fluid overload or deficit (see chapter 36). The potential for infection is reduced when surgical asepsis is used for sterile dressing changes or any invasive procedure, such as insertion of a Foley catheter. Finally, correct use of body mechanics and transfer techniques reduces the risk of injuries when moving and lifting clients (see chapter 42).

Equipment-Related Accidents. Equipment-related accidents result from the malfunction, disrepair, or misuse of equipment or from an electrical hazard. For example, too-rapid infusion of IV fluids may result from a dysfunctional IV pump. To avoid accidents, the nurse should not operate monitoring or therapy equipment without instruction. A checklist should be used to assess potential electrical hazards to reduce the risk of electrical fires, electrocution, or injury from faulty equipment. In health care settings, clinical engineering staff makes regular safety checks of equipment.

Critical Thinking

Successful critical thinking requires a synthesis of knowledge, experience, information gathered from clients, critical thinking attitudes, and intellectual and professional standards. Clinical judgments require the nurse to anticipate necessary information, analyze the data, and make decisions regarding client care. Critical thinking is an ongoing process. During assessment (Figure 33–6), the nurse must consider all critical thinking elements, as well as information about the specific client, to make appropriate nursing diagnoses.

In the case of safety, the nurse integrates knowledge from nursing and other scientific disciplines, previous experiences in caring for clients who had an injury or were at risk, critical thinking attitudes such as perseverance, and any standards of practice that are applicable. Agency guidelines and professional nursing associations provide standards for nursing activities such as medication administration, fall prevention, and infection control to guide nurses in the provision of safe care. For example, the Registered Nurses Association of Ontario (2005) has a Best Nursing Practice Guideline for preventing falls and fall injuries in the older adult. Nurses refer to all of this information and experience as they conduct a detailed assessment of a specific client. For example, while assessing a client's home environment, the nurse will consider typical locations within the home where dangers commonly exist. If a client has a visual impairment, the nurse will apply previous experiences in caring for clients with visual changes to anticipate how to thoroughly assess the client's needs. Critical thinking directs the nurse to anticipate what needs to be assessed and how to make conclusions about available data.

Safety and the Nursing Process

NP Assessment

To conduct a thorough client assessment, the nurse considers possible threats to the client's safety, including the client's immediate environment, as well as any individual risk factors.

Health History. By conducting a health history, the nurse will gather data about the client's level of wellness to determine if any underlying conditions exist that pose threats to safety. For example, the nurse will give special attention to assessing the client's gait, muscle strength and coordination, balance, and vision. A review of the client's developmental status must be considered as assessment information is analyzed. The nurse will also review if the client has been exposed to any environmental hazards or is taking medications or undergoing procedures that pose risks. For example, use of diuretics increases the frequency of voiding and may result in the client having to use toilet facilities more often. Falls often occur with clients who must get out of bed quickly because of urinary urgency.

Client's Home Environment. When caring for a client in the home, a home hazard assessment is necessary (Box 33-2). The nurse should walk through the home with the client and discuss how the client normally conducts daily activities. Key areas to inspect are the bathroom, kitchen, and areas with stairs. For example, when assessing adequacy of lighting, the nurse inspects areas where the client moves and works, such as outside walkways, steps, interior halls, and doorways. Getting a sense of the client's routines helps the nurse recognize hazards that are not as obvious.

Assessment for risks of food infections or poisoning involves obtaining a detailed dietary assessment for the past week; conducting an examination of GI and central nervous system function; observing for a fever; and analyzing the results of cultures of feces and vomitus. Suspected food and water sources are also studied. The nurse should also assess the client's handwashing practices. It is useful for the nurse to ask clients when they routinely wash their hands. This question can then prompt a helpful discussion about the purpose and importance of handwashing.

Assessment of the environmental comfort of a client's home should include a review of when the client normally has heating and cooling systems serviced. Does the client have a functional furnace or space heater? Does the home have air conditioning or fans? Clients who use space heaters must be informed of the risk for fires.

When clients live in older homes, the nurse should encourage inspections for the presence of lead in paint, dust, or soil. Because lead can also come from the solder of plumbing fixtures in a home, water from each faucet should also be tested. Local health offices can assist a homeowner in locating a trained lead inspector who will

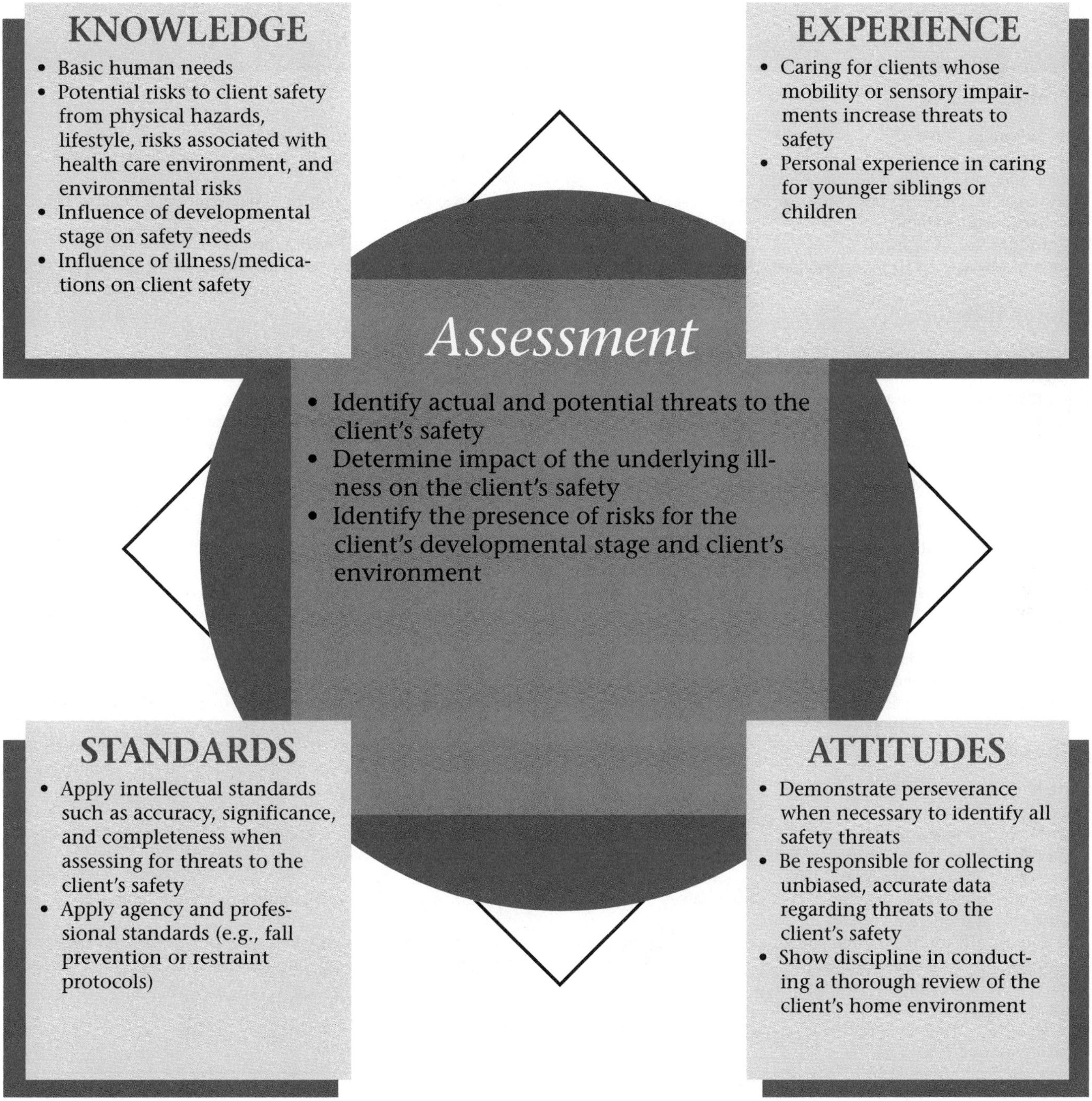
KNOWLEDGE
• Basic human needs
• Potential risks to client safety from physical hazards, lifestyle, risks associated with health care environment, and environmental risks
• Influence of developmental stage on safety needs
• Influence of illness/medications on client safety
EXPERIENCE
• Caring for clients whose mobility or sensory impairments increase threats to safety
• Personal experience in caring for younger siblings or children
Assessment
• Identify actual and potential threats to the client's safety
• Determine impact of the underlying illness on the client's safety
• Identify the presence of risks for the client's developmental stage and client's environment
STANDARDS
• Apply intellectual standards such as accuracy, significance, and completeness when assessing for threats to the client's safety
• Apply agency and professional standards (e.g., fall prevention or restraint protocols)
ATTITUDES
• Demonstrate perseverance when necessary to identify all safety threats
• Be responsible for collecting unbiased, accurate data regarding threats to the client's safety
• Show discipline in conducting a thorough review of the client's home environment

FIGURE **33–6** Critical thinking model for safety assessment.

take samples from various locations and have them analyzed at a laboratory for content of lead.

Health Care Environment. When the client is cared for within a health care facility, the nurse must determine if any hazards exist in the immediate care environment. Does the placement of equipment or furniture pose barriers when the client attempts to ambulate? Does positioning of the client's bed allow the client to reach items on a bedside table or stand? Does the client need assistance with ambulation? Is the client aware of activity restrictions? Has the client been taught to use the call system, and is the call bell within reach? The nurse also collaborates with clinical engineering staff to make sure that equipment has been assessed to ensure proper function and condition.

Risk for Falls. Assessment of a client's fall risk factors is essential in determining specific needs and developing targeted interventions to prevent falls. The nurse begins by asking clients if they have had a history of falls. A fall assessment tool (Table 33-1) can help the nurse assess for

Box 33-2 Home Hazard Assessment

Home Exterior

Are sidewalks uneven?
Are steps in good repair?
Is ice and snow removal adequate?
Do steps and balconies have securely fastened railings?
Is there adequate lighting?
Is outdoor furniture sturdy?
Are window screens in high-rise apartments properly secured?

Home Interior

Do all rooms, stairways, and halls have adequate, non-glare lighting?
Are night lights available?
Are area rugs secured?
Are wooden floors non-slippery?
Are floors where water accumulates covered by non-slip floor mats?
Is furniture placed appropriately to permit mobility? Is furniture sturdy enough to provide support for getting up and down?
Are temperature and humidity within normal range? Are there any steps or thresholds that may pose a hazard? Are step edges clearly marked with coloured tape? Are handrails available and secure?
In homes with young children, are window guards and electrical outlet covers installed?
Can all doors and windows with security gates and locks be opened from the inside without a key?

Kitchen

Are handwashing facilities available?
Is the pilot light on for the gas stove?
Are the stovetop and oven clean?
Are the dials on the stove readable?
Are storage areas within easy reach?
Are fluids such as cleaners and bleach in original containers and stored properly?
In homes with young children, are safety locks on cabinets and corner counter protectors installed?
Is the water temperature within normal range?
Are there clean areas for food storage and preparation? Is refrigeration adequate? Are the refrigerator and freezer temperatures correct?

Bathroom

Are handwashing facilities available?
Are there skid-proof strips or surfaces in the tub or shower? Are bath mats secured?
Does the client need grab bars near the bathtub and toilet? Does the client need an elevated toilet seat?
Is the medicine cabinet well lighted?
Are medications in their original containers?
Are medication containers child resistant if children live in the home or visit?
Have outdated medications been discarded?

Bedroom

Are beds of adequate height to allow getting on and off easily?
Is day and night lighting adequate?
Are floor coverings non-skid?
Does the client have a telephone nearby?
Are emergency numbers visible near the telephone?

Electrical and Fire Hazards

Are smoke and carbon monoxide detectors installed? Are the batteries for all detectors tested every month and changed twice a year?
Have furnaces, chimneys, and stoves been checked for proper ventilation?
Are extension cords in good condition and used appropriately?
Are appliances in good working order?
Are electrical appliances located away from water sources? Is there a multi-purpose fire extinguisher near the cooking area, and does client understand how to use it?
Are combustible items such as oil-based paints, gasoline, and oily rags being stored in a garage and/or basement? Are electrical outlets overloaded?
Are flashlights available?
Is there a first aid kit available to the adult members of the household?
Does everyone in the family know the fire escape plan and have easy access to emergency phone numbers?

Adapted from "Home Safe Home: Practical Tips for Fall-Proofing," by R. Tideiksaar, 1989, *Geriatric Nursing, 11*(6), pp. 280–284; and *Toward Healthy Aging* (6th ed.), by P. Ebersole and P. Hess, 2003, St. Louis, MO: Mosby.

potential risks before accidents and injuries result. The illustrated tool has weighted risk factors. A client's risk of falling increases dramatically as the number of risk factors increases. Initial and daily assessment of fall risk is important in identifying clients who are at risk of falling. In many cases, family members can be important resources in assessing a client's fall risk. Families often are able to report on the client's level of confusion and ability to ambulate.

Risk for Medical Errors. Nurses must also be alert to factors within their own environment that create conditions in which medical errors are more likely to occur. Studies have shown that overwork and fatigue cause a significant decrease in alertness and concentration, leading to errors (Leonard et al., 1998). It is important for nurses to be aware of these factors and to include checks and balances when working under stressful conditions. For example, to reduce the potential for a medical error, it is essential for the nurse to check the client's identification bracelet before beginning any procedure or administering a medication (see chapter 30).

The National Steering Committee on Patient Safety (2002) made recommendations to improve the safety of Canada's health care system. At the core of these recommendations was the need to nurture a culture of safety within the system. The Canadian Patient Safety Institute

Table 33-1 Fall Assessment Tool

Directions: Circle the score for the risk factor that corresponds to the client. The tool should be administered on admission to the facility or agency and again at specified intervals and when warranted by changes in health status. Scores of 15 and higher indicate high risk, and preventive measures should be implemented.

Client Factors	Date Admit	Initial Score	Date	Reassessed Score
History of falls		15		15
Confusion		5		5
Age (over 65)		5		5
Impaired judgment		5		5
Sensory deficit		5		5
Unable to ambulate independently		5		5
Decreased level of cooperation		5		5
Increased anxiety/emotional lability		5		5
Incontinence/urgency		5		5
Cardiovascular/respiratory disease affecting perfusion and oxygenation		5		5
Medications affecting blood pressure or level of consciousness		5		5
Postural hypotension with dizziness		5		5
Environmental Factors				
First week on unit/facility/services, etc.		5		5
Attached equipment (e.g., IV pole, chest tubes, appliances, oxygen, tubing, etc.)		5		5

Adapted from *Try This: Best Practices in Nursing Care to Older Adults,* by B. Farmer, 2000, New York: The Hartford Institute for Geriatric Nursing, New York University.

Nursing Diagnostic Process — Box 33-3

Assessment Activities	Defining Characteristics	Nursing Diagnosis
Observe client's mobility and body alignment.	Uncoordinated gait Poor posture	Risk for injury related to impaired mobility, decreased vision, poorly lighted home, and cluttered environment
Ask client about visual acuity.	Reports difficulty seeing at night Reports tripping over rugs and furniture	
Complete a home hazard appraisal.	Poorly lighted home Rooms filled with small items Excessive amount of furniture for size of room Rugs not secure	

(CPSI) was established in 2003 to provide leadership in the development of such a culture.

Client Expectations. Clients generally expect to be safe in their home and in the health care setting. However, there are times when a client's view of what is safe does not agree with that of the nurse. For this reason, any assessment must include the client's understanding of his or her perception of risk factors. This will be important later as the nurse attempts to make changes in the client's environment. Clients usually do not purposefully put themselves in jeopardy. When clients are uninformed or inexperienced, threats to their safety can occur. Clients must always be consulted on ways to reduce hazards in their environment.

Nursing Diagnosis

After completing an assessment of the client's safety status, the nurse reviews any clusters of data to determine if there are patterns suggesting that safety is threatened. Identification of defining characteristics from the data guide the nurse in identifying appropriate nursing diagnoses. The diagnostic process requires accurate recognition of defining characteristics, as well as the related factors (Box 33-3).

The related factor becomes the basis for selecting nursing therapies. For example, *risk for injury related to impaired mobility* and *risk for injury related to barriers in the home environment* require different nursing interventions. The client with altered mobility may require ambulatory aids and physiotherapy. When the related factor is barriers in the home, the nurse intervenes to recommend changes that will create a safer environment. At times, as in the example in Box 33-3, multiple related factors may apply. Examples of nursing diagnoses that may apply for clients whose safety is threatened include the following:

- Risk for imbalanced body temperature
- Impaired home maintenance
- Risk for injury
- Deficient knowledge
- Risk for poisoning
- Disturbed sensory/perception
- Risk for suffocation
- Disturbed thought processes
- Risk for trauma

Planning

During planning, the nurse critically synthesizes information from multiple sources (Figure 33–7). Critical thinking ensures that the client's plan of care integrates all that the nurse has learned about the client, as well as the key critical thinking elements. For example, the nurse will reflect on knowledge regarding the services that other disciplines (e.g., occupational therapy) can provide in helping clients return to their home environments safely. The nurse will also reflect on any previous experience whereby a client benefited from safety interventions. Such experience helps the nurse adapt approaches with a new client. Applying critical thinking attitudes such as creativity helps the nurse and client collaborate in planning interventions that are relevant and most useful, particularly when changes are made in the home environment.

Goals and Outcomes. Planning and goal setting need to be done in collaboration with the client, family, and other members of the health care team (see Care Plan). The client who is an active participant in reducing threats to safety will be more alert to potential hazards. Goals and outcomes must be measurable and realistic, with consideration of the resources available to the client. The overall goal for a client with a threat to safety is remaining free from injury. The following are examples of expected outcomes that focus on the client's need for safety:

- Modifiable hazards will be reduced in the home environment by 100% within 1 month.
- Client does not suffer a fall or injury.
- Client identifies risks associated with visual impairment.

Setting Priorities. Nursing interventions are prioritized to provide safe and efficient care. For example, the client described in the concept map (Figure 33–8) has several nursing diagnoses. The client's mobility problem is an obvious priority because of its influence on skin integrity and risks for falls. The nurse plans individualized interventions based on the severity of risk factors and the client's developmental stage, level of health, lifestyle, and culture (Box 33-4). Planning also involves an understanding of the client's need to maintain independence within physical and cognitive capabilities. The nurse and client collaborate to establish ways of maintaining the client's active involvement within the home and health care environment. Education of the client and family is also an important intervention to reduce safety risks over the long term.

Continuity of Care. Clients need to learn how to identify and select resources within their community that enhance safety (e.g., block parent homes, local police departments, and neighbours willing to check on a client's well-being). Collaboration with the client and family and other disciplines such as social work and occupational and physiotherapy may become an important part of the nurse's plan of care. For example, a hospitalized client may need to go to a rehabilitation facility to gain strength and endurance before being discharged home. The nurse must be sure that the client and family understand the need for resources and are willing to make changes that will promote their safety.

Implementation

Nursing interventions are directed toward maintaining the client's safety in all settings. Nursing measures for providing a safe environment include health promotion, developmental interventions, general preventive measures, and environmental interventions.

Health Promotion. To promote an individual's health, it is necessary for the individual to be in a safe environment and to practise a lifestyle that minimizes risk of injury. Edelman and Mandle (1998) described passive and active strategies aimed at health promotion. Passive strategies are implemented through public health and government legislative interventions (e.g., sanitation and clean water laws; see chapter 4). Active strategies are those in which the individual is actively involved through changes in lifestyle (e.g., wearing seat belts or installing outdoor lighting) and participation in wellness programs.

The nurse participates by supporting legislation and working in community-based settings. Because environmental and community values have the greatest influence on health promotion, community and home health nurses can assess and recommend safety measures in the home (see Box 33-2), school, neighbourhood, and workplace.

Developmental Interventions

Infant, Toddler, and Preschooler. Infants, toddlers, and preschoolers depend on adults to protect them from injury. Growing children are curious and completely trusting of their environment and do not perceive themselves to be in danger. Nurses are frequently in a position to educate parents or guardians about reducing risks of injuries for young children (see chapter 19). Nurses working in prenatal and postpartum settings can easily incorporate safety into the care plan of the child-bearing family. Community health nurses can assess the home and show parents how to promote safety in their homes (Table 33-2). Nurses can educate parents that children under 5 years of age are also

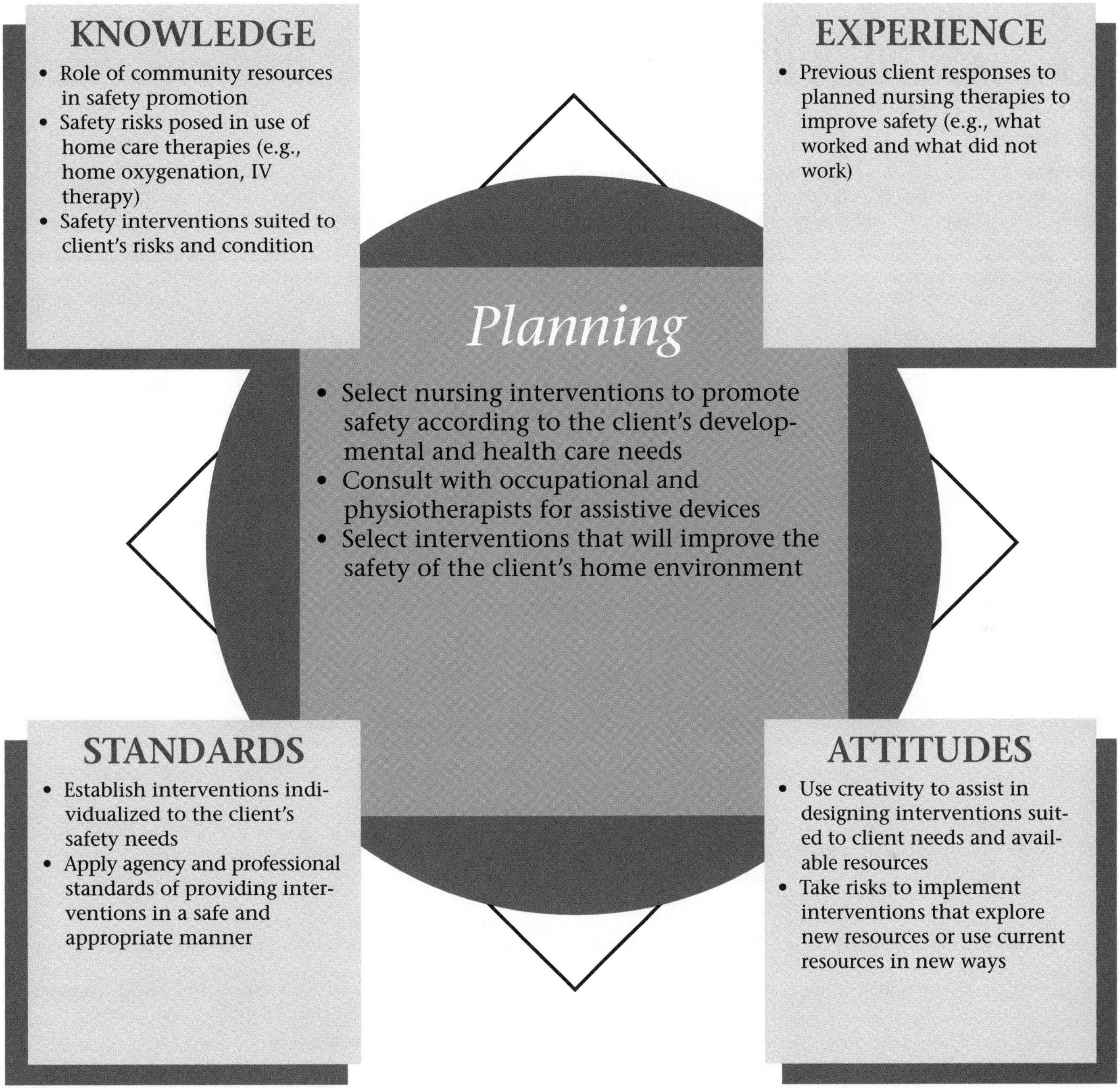
KNOWLEDGE
• Role of community resources in safety promotion
• Safety risks posed in use of home care therapies (e.g., home oxygenation, IV therapy)
• Safety interventions suited to client's risks and condition
EXPERIENCE
• Previous client responses to planned nursing therapies to improve safety (e.g., what worked and what did not work)
Planning
• Select nursing interventions to promote safety according to the client's developmental and health care needs
• Consult with occupational and physiotherapists for assistive devices
• Select interventions that will improve the safety of the client's home environment
STANDARDS
• Establish interventions individualized to the client's safety needs
• Apply agency and professional standards of providing interventions in a safe and appropriate manner
ATTITUDES
• Use creativity to assist in designing interventions suited to client needs and available resources
• Take risks to implement interventions that explore new resources or use current resources in new ways

FIGURE **33–7** Critical thinking model for safety planning.

more susceptible to diseases such as measles, mumps, and chickenpox. Immunizations, given before the age of 2 years and at recommended intervals, can protect a child from life-threatening diseases.

School-Age Child. School-age children increasingly explore their environment (see chapter 19). They have friends outside their immediate neighbourhood, and they become more active in school, church, and community activities. The school-age child needs specific teaching regarding safety in school and at play. See Table 33-2 for nursing interventions to help guide the parent in providing for the safety of the school-age child.

Adolescent. Risks to the safety of adolescents involve many factors outside the home environment, particularly their almost constant involvement with members of their peer group (see chapter 19). Adults serve as role models for adolescents and, through providing examples, setting expectations, and providing education, can help adolescents minimize risks to their safety. This age group has a high incidence of suicide because of feelings of decreased self-worth and hopelessness. The nurse must be aware of the risks posed at this time and be prepared to teach adolescents and their parents measures to prevent accidents and injury (see Table 33-2).

Adult. Risks to young and middle-age adults frequently result from lifestyle factors such as child rearing, high stress levels, inadequate nutrition, use of firearms, excessive alcohol intake, and substance abuse (see chapter 20).

Nursing Care Plan

Risk for Injury

Assessment

Mr. Key, a visiting nurse, is seeing Ms. Cohen, an 85-year-old woman, at her home. The client has been recovering from a mild stroke affecting her left side. Ms. Cohen lives alone but received regular assistance from her daughter and son, who both live within 16 km. Mr Key's assessment included a discussion of Ms. Cohen's health problem and how the stroke has affected her, as well as a pertinent physical examination.

Assessment Activities	Findings/Defining Characteristics
Ask Ms. Cohen how the stroke has affected her mobility.	She responds, "I bump into things, and I'm afraid I'm going to fall."
Conduct a home hazard assessment.	Cabinets in kitchen are in disarray and full of breakable items that could fall out. Throw rugs are on floors; bathroom lighting is poor (40-watt bulb); bathtub lacks safety strips or grab bars; home cluttered with furniture and small objects.
Observe Ms. Cohen's gait and posture.	Ms. Cohen has kyphosis and has a hesitant, uncoordinated gait. She frequently holds walls for support.
Assess Ms. Cohen's muscle strength.	Left arm and leg weaker than right.
Assess visual acuity with corrective lenses.	Ms. Cohen has trouble reading and seeing familiar objects at a distance while wearing current glasses.

Nursing Diagnosis: Risk for injury related to impaired mobility, decreased visual acuity, and physical environmental hazards.

Planning

Goal	Expected Outcomes*
	Risk Control
Home will be free of hazards within 1 month.	Modifiable hazards in kitchen and hallway will be reduced in the home within 1 week. Revisions to bathroom completed in 1 month.
	Knowledge: Personal Safety
Client and family will be knowledgeable of potential hazards for Ms. Cohen's age group within 1 week.	Client and daughter will identify risks and the steps to avoid them in the home at the conclusion of a teaching session next week.
	Safety Behaviour: Fall Prevention
Ms. Cohen will express greater sense of feeling safe from falls in 1 month.	Ms. Cohen will report improved vision with the aid of new eyeglasses.
Client will be free of injury within 2 weeks.	Client will be able to safely ambulate throughout the home and perform personal care activities within 2 weeks.

*Outcome classification labels from *Nursing Outcomes Classification (NIC)* (3rd ed.), edited by S. Moorhead, M. Johnson, and M. L. Maas, 2004, St. Louis, MO: Mosby.

Interventions†	Rationale
Fall Prevention	
• Review findings from home hazard assessment with client and daughter.	Fall risks for homebound older adults include visual disturbances, unsteady gait, and postural changes (Lueckenotte, 2000). Evaluation of home hazards will highlight extrinsic factors that may lead to falls (Tideiksaar, 1989).
• Establish a list of priorities to modify. Have Ms. Cohen's son assist in installing bathroom safety devices.	Modification of environment reduces fall risk.
• Install lighting (75-watt bulbs, non-glare) throughout the home. Have son install blinds over kitchen windows.	With aging, the pupil loses the ability to adjust to light, causing sensitivity to glare. Glare can make it difficult to clearly see a walking path (Lueckenotte, 2000).
• Discuss with client and daughter the normal changes of aging, effects of recent stroke, associated risks for injury, and how to reduce risks.	Education regarding hazards can reduce fear of falling (American Geriatrics Society, British Geriatrics Society, & American Academy of Orthopaedic Surgeons Panel on Falls Prevention, 2001).

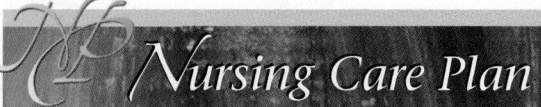

Nursing Care Plan

Risk for Injury—cont'd

Interventions†—cont'd	Rationale
Fall Prevention—cont'd	
• Encourage daughter to schedule vision testing for new prescription within 2 to 4 weeks.	Improved visual acuity reduces incidence of falls (Ebersole & Hess, 2001).
• Refer to a physiotherapist to assess need for assistive devices for kyphosis, left-sided weakness, and gait.	Exercise often improves gait, balance, and flexibility. Modifying gait problems by increasing lower extremity strength reduces fall risk (Schoenfelder, 2000).

†Intervention classification labels from *Nursing Intervention Classifications (NIC)* (4th ed.), edited by J. M. Dochterman and G. M. Bulechek, 2004, St. Louis, MO: Mosby.

Evaluation

Nursing Actions	Client Response/Finding	Achievement of Outcome
Ask client and family to identify risks.	Ms. Cohen and daughter able to identify risks during a walk through the home and expressed a greater sense of safety as a result of changes made.	Client and daughter are more knowledgeable of potential hazards.
Observe environment for elimination of hazards.	Throw rugs have been removed. Lighting has increased to 75 watts except in bathroom and bedroom.	Environmental hazards have been partially reduced.
Reassess Ms. Cohen's visual acuity.	Ms. Cohen has new glasses and says she can read better, and see distant objects more clearly.	Ms. Cohen's vision has improved, enabling her to ambulate more safely.
Observe Ms. Cohen's gait and posture.	Ms. Cohen's gait remains hesitant and uncoordinated; she reports that her daughter has not had time to take her to the physiotherapist.	Outcome of safe ambulation has not been totally achieved; continue to encourage Ms. Cohen and daughter to go to physiotherapy appointment.

In this fast-paced society, there also appears to be more expression of anger, which can quickly precipitate accidents (e.g., "road rage"). Adults need to have the opportunity to discuss the choices they have made in their lifestyle and the types of threats to safety that exist. Given information about threats to their well-being, adults may make necessary modifications in lifestyle practices. Useful resources are stress management centres, employee assistance programs, and health promotion activities, which can be found in many communities and hospitals. In addition, neighbourhood centres, community clinics, and outpatient clinics are equipped to assist adults in modifying lifestyle habits that present risks to health (e.g., smoking, overeating, lack of exercise, and alcoholism).

Older Adult. Nursing interventions for older adults are designed to reduce the risk of falls and other accidents and to compensate for the physiological changes of aging (Box 33-5).

Advancing age and the concurrent physiological changes in vision, hearing, mobility, reflexes, circulation, and the ability to make quick judgments all predispose older adults to falls (see chapter 21). Hospitalization, confusion, multiple medical problems, sedating medications, generalized weakness, postural instability, and an unfamiliar environment are major contributors to falling (Ebersole & Hess, 2001). Certain disease states common to older adults, such as arthritis and cerebrovascular accidents, also increase chances of injury.

Older adults are more likely to have motor vehicle accidents because of three specific physiological changes. First, changes in visual acuity, depth perception, and poor peripheral vision prevent the client from quickly observing situations in which an accident is likely to occur. Second, decreased hearing acuity alters the older adult's ability to hear emergency vehicle sirens or car and truck horns. Third, because of decreased nervous system response, older adults may be unable to react as quickly as they once could to avoid an accident (Ebersole & Hess, 2001). A decline in these skills may account for the most common types of accidents, including right-of-way and turning accidents. The nurse can educate clients regarding safe driving (e.g., driving shorter distances or only in daylight, using side and rear-view mirrors carefully, and looking behind them toward their "blind spot" before changing lanes). If hearing is a problem, the client might try to keep a window rolled down while driving or reduce the volume of the radio or CD or cassette player. Eventually, counselling may be necessary to help clients make the decision of when to stop driving. At that time, the nurse should help locate resources in the community that provide transportation.

Burns and scalds are also more apt to occur with older people because they may forget and leave hot water running or become confused when turning the dials on a stove or other heating appliance. Nursing measures for preventing burns are designed to minimize the risk from

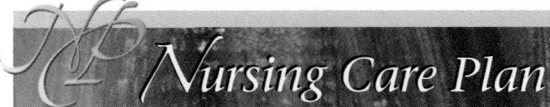

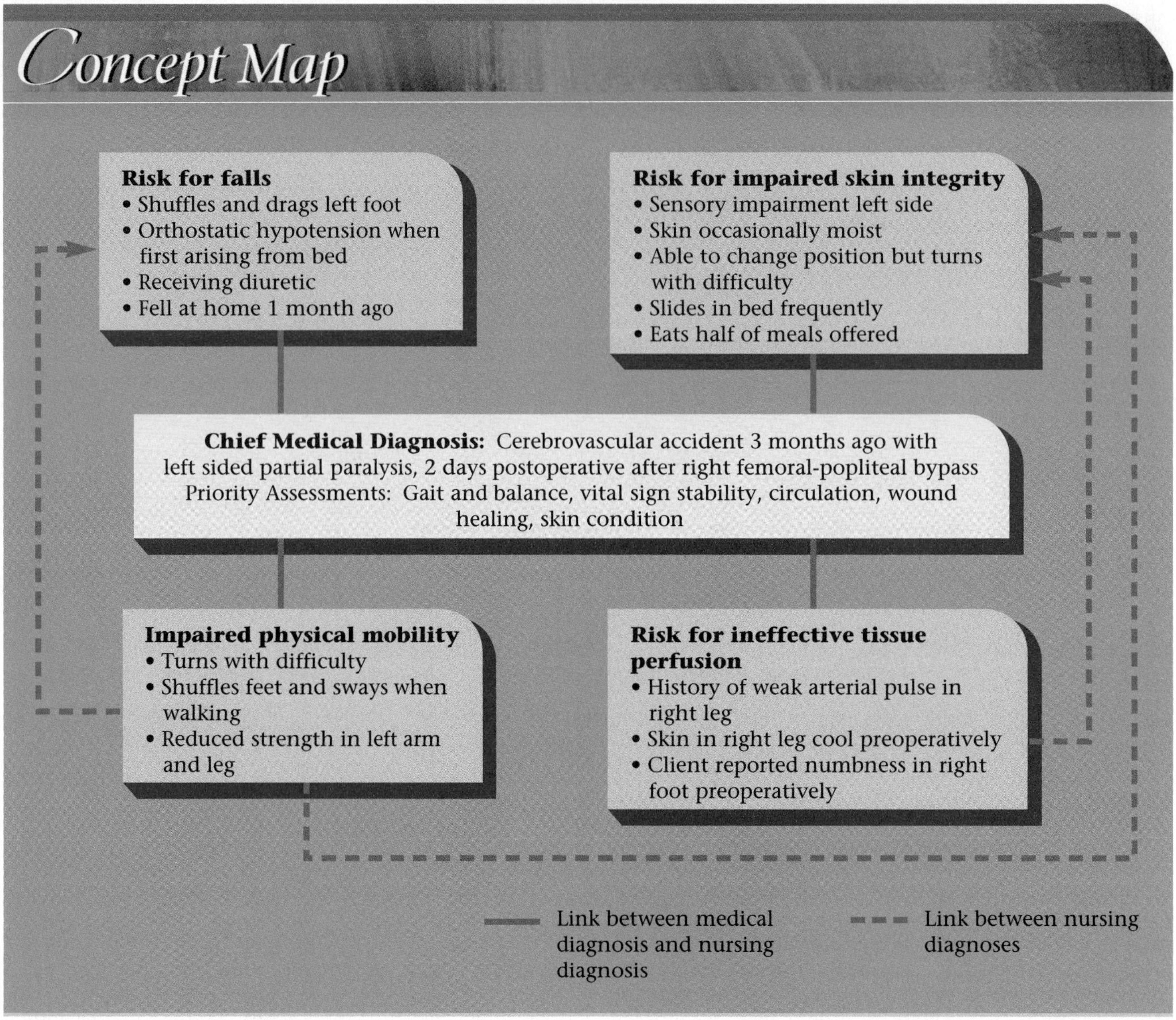
Concept Map
Risk for falls
• Shuffles and drags left foot
• Orthostatic hypotension when first arising from bed
• Receiving diuretic
• Fell at home 1 month ago
Risk for impaired skin integrity
• Sensory impairment left side
• Skin occasionally moist
• Able to change position but turns with difficulty
• Slides in bed frequently
• Eats half of meals offered
Chief Medical Diagnosis: Cerebrovascular accident 3 months ago with left sided partial paralysis, 2 days postoperative after right femoral-popliteal bypass
Priority Assessments: Gait and balance, vital sign stability, circulation, wound healing, skin condition
Impaired physical mobility
• Turns with difficulty
• Shuffles feet and sways when walking
• Reduced strength in left arm and leg
Risk for ineffective tissue perfusion
• History of weak arterial pulse in right leg
• Skin in right leg cool preoperatively
• Client reported numbness in right foot preoperatively
Link between medical diagnosis and nursing diagnosis
Link between nursing diagnoses

FIGURE **33–8** Concept map for a client with a cerebrovascular accident 3 months ago with left-sided paralysis, 2 days post-operative after right femoral-popliteal bypass.

impaired vision. Hot water faucets and dials can be colour-coded to make it easier for the adult to know what has been turned on. Recommending a reduction in temperature of the water heater can also be very beneficial.

Pedestrian accidents can be reduced for older adults and for all other age groups by persuading people to wear reflectors on garments when walking at night; to stand on the sidewalk and not in the street when waiting to cross a street; to always cross at corners and not in the middle of the block (particularly if the street is a major one); to cross with the traffic light and not against it; and to look left, right, and left again before entering the street or crosswalk.

General Preventive Measures. Nurses can contribute to a safer environment by helping the client meet basic needs related to oxygen, nutrition, temperature, and humidity. To ensure that oxygen availability is not threatened, the nurse might recommend that the client be sure to periodically have the furnace inspected for proper functioning. To achieve a comfortable level of humidity in the home, the client might attach a humidifier to the furnace or, in the case of clients who have upper respiratory tract infections, use a room humidifier where the client sleeps. The nurse can teach basic techniques for food handling (e.g., handwashing and checking for spoilage) and preparation (e.g., keeping food refrigerated before serving) so that nutritional needs are met safely. It is also helpful to have family members label the date when leftovers are saved. Older adults may benefit from Meals on Wheels services. These services provide fresh nutritious meals to older adults who have difficulty preparing their own food. Client education for older adults or clients who enjoy outdoor activities should include ways to prevent and

Cultural Aspects of Care

Box 33-4

Cultural phenomena affecting health and safety include personal space, social organizations, communication, and environmental control. While conducting a home assessment for risks to safety, nurses must realize that they have entered the client's territory and that the client's attitude toward his or her residence and belongings must be appreciated. For example, clients from Western Europe and the British Isles may be considered aloof and distant in terms of space. It may be very difficult for them to have an outsider in their home who is suggesting changes with regard to their personal belongings to reduce physical hazards. It is particularly difficult to determine a client's attitude toward his or her home environment when another language is spoken.

Another culturally sensitive issue is the client's sense of environmental control. The nurse must be aware of health beliefs and practices that will affect the outcome of interventions. For example, reliance on family and religious organizations, as opposed to community resources, may affect the client's compliance with nursing interventions and referrals.

Nurses and health care providers need to learn to ask questions sensitively and show respect for different cultural beliefs. Adapting to different cultural beliefs and practices requires flexibility and a respect for others' viewpoints. Respect for the belief systems of others and the effects of those beliefs on the client's well-being are critically important to competent care. Nurses must have the ability and knowledge to communicate and to understand health behaviours influenced by culture.

Implications for Practice

- Resistance to change long-standing habits can interfere with a cultural group's acceptance of injury prevention practices. Include family members who have a strong influence, such as a dominant male or older woman, when providing safety education.
- Evaluate the use of traditional ethnic remedies or foods that contain lead because they can increase a client's risk for lead poisoning.
- Living in rural areas and in manufactured housing places the client at greater risk for fire-related injuries and death.
- Stress the importance of having working smoke detectors and a multi-purpose fire extinguisher.
- Assess the client's smoking and drinking habits. Residential fire deaths can be attributed to the use of cigarettes and alcohol.
- Clients who live in poverty and have low educational levels are at greater risk for injury and disease. Assist the client and family in identifying community resources such as the local health office or clinic.
- Be aware of family patterns and how the client and family interact with each other. Family disruption and weak intergenerational ties can increase a client's risk for injury from violent behaviour.

treat frostbite, hypothermia, heatstroke, and heat exhaustion (see chapter 27).

Adequate lighting and security measures in and around the home, including the use of night lights, exterior lighting, and locks on windows and doors, enable clients to reduce the risk of injury from crime. The local police department and community organizations often have safety classes available for residents to learn how to take precautions to minimize the chance of becoming involved in a crime. For example, some useful tips include always parking the car near a bright light or busy public area, carrying a whistle attached to the car keys, keeping car doors locked while driving, and always paying attention while driving to notice if anyone starts to follow the car.

To prevent the transmission of pathogens, nurses can teach aseptic practices. Medical asepsis, which includes hand hygiene and environmental cleanliness, reduces the transfer of organisms (see chapter 29). Clients and family members need to learn thorough hand hygiene (handwashing or use of hand rub) and when to use it (e.g., before and after caring for a family member, before food preparation, before preparing a medication for a family member, and after contacting any body fluids). When clients require dressing changes or the use of syringes and needles, families should be shown how to properly dispose of contaminated items in the home. Most communities have regulations for the disposal of biohazardous waste.

Acute Care. A number of specific safety measures are applicable to clients in the acute care environment. The nurse takes measures to help clients avoid falls, injuries from use of restraints and side rails, fires, poisoning, and electrical hazards. Special precautions are necessary to prevent injury in clients susceptible to having seizures. Radiation injuries are also a specific safety concern.

Controlling the spread of infection through the consistent use of standard precautions/routine practices maintains the safety of both clients and staff (see chapter 29). The importance of these measures was clearly illustrated during the severe acute respiratory syndrome (SARS) outbreak in Toronto in 2003. Beginning with one individual admitted to an emergency department, the illness spread to several clients and staff before its infectious nature was recognized and precautions instituted. Maintaining the safety of staff caring for SARS-infected clients was a significant challenge during the outbreak (Hynes-Gay et al., 2003).

Falls. Modifications in the home and health care environment can easily reduce the risk of falls (Table 33-3). A heavy or debilitated client in a bed or wheelchair or on a toilet should be properly supported and secured. Side rails may be necessary. Safety bars near toilets, locks on beds and wheelchairs, and call lights are additional safety features found in health care settings (Figures 33-11 and 33-12). Excess furniture and equipment should be removed, and a weakened client should wear rubber-soled

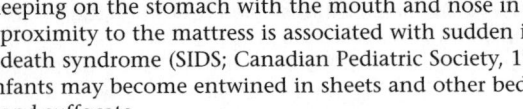

Table 33-2 Interventions to Promote Safety for Children and Adolescents

Intervention	Rationale
Infants and Toddlers	
Have infants sleep on their backs. Teach parents the mnemonic "back to sleep."	Sleeping on the stomach with the mouth and nose in close proximity to the mattress is associated with sudden infant death syndrome (SIDS; Canadian Pediatric Society, 1999).
Do not fill cribs with pillows, large stuffed toys, or comforters. Sheets should fit snugly.	Infants may become entwined in sheets and other bedding and suffocate.
Pacifiers should not be attached to string or ribbon and placed around a child's neck.	Choking may occur.
All instructions for preparing and storing formula must be followed.	Proper formula preparation and storage prevents contamination. A formula may come in a concentrated form, or it may already be diluted and ready to use. Following directions ensures proper concentration of the formula. Undiluted formula can cause fluid and electrolyte disturbances; very diluted formula will not provide sufficient nutrients.
Use large, soft toys without small parts, such as buttons.	Small parts can become dislodged.
Playpens with mesh sides should not be left with a side down; spaces between crib slats should be less than 6 cm apart.	A child's head may become wedged in the lowered mesh side or in between crib slats.
Never leave crib sides down or leave babies unattended on changing tables or in infant seats, swings, strollers, or high chairs.	Infants and toddlers can roll or move and fall from changing tables or out of accessories such as infant seats or swings.
Discontinue using accessories such as infant seats and swings when the child becomes too active.	When physically active or too big, the child can fall out of or tip over these accessories and suffer an injury.
Never leave a child alone in the bathroom.	Accidental drowning may occur.
Baby-proof the home; remove small or sharp objects and toxic or poisonous substances, including plants; install safety locks on floor-level cabinets.	Babies explore their world with their hands and mouth. Choking and poisoning may occur.
Remove plastic bags from the cleaners or grocery store from the home.	Suffocation may occur if plastic covers the nose and mouth.
Electrical outlets should have covers (Figure 33–9).	Crawling babies may insert objects into outlets and experience an electrical shock.
Window guards should be on all windows.	This prevents children from falling out of windows.
Install keyless locks (e.g., deadbolts) on doors above a child's reach, even when they are standing on a chair.	This prevents a toddler from leaving the house and wandering off. Death from exposure, car accidents, and drowning may occur. Keyless locks allow for rapid exit in case of fire.
Children weighing less than 36 kg or under 8 years of age should always be in an age/weight-appropriate car seat that has been installed according to the manufacturer's instructions (Figure 33–10). This includes car seats and booster seats. In cars with a passenger air bag, children under 12 years should be in the back seat. All passengers should have seat belts on.	In case of a sudden stop or crash, an unrestrained child may suffer severe head injuries and death.

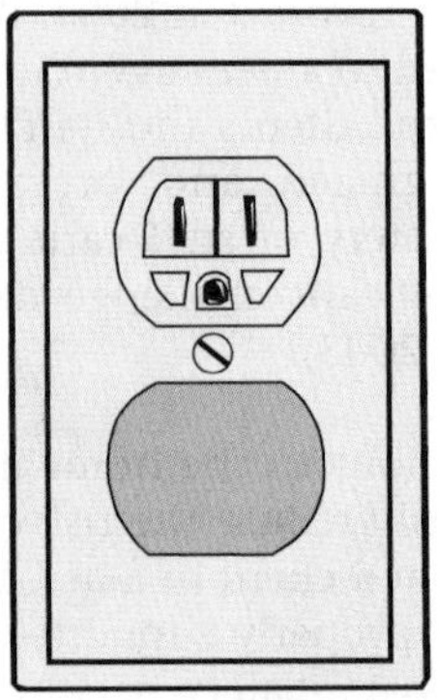

FIGURE **33–9** Safety covers for electrical outlets.

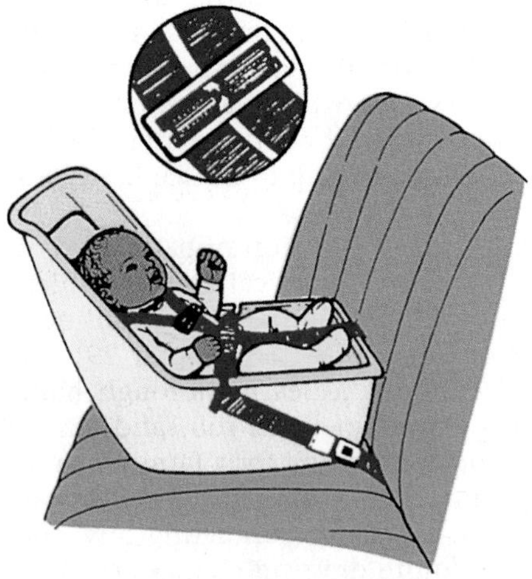

FIGURE **33–10** Infant car seat.

Adapted from *Wong's Nursing Care of Infants and Children* (7th ed.), by D. L. Wong, 2003, St. Louis, MO: Mosby.

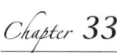

Table 33-2 Interventions to Promote Safety for Children and Adolescents—cont'd

Intervention	Rationale
Infants and Toddlers—*cont'd*	
Caregivers should learn cardiopulmonary resuscitation and the Heimlich manoeuvre.	Caregivers should be prepared to intervene in acute emergencies, such as choking.
Preschoolers	
Teach children to swim at an early age, but always provide supervision near water.	Learning to swim is a useful skill that may someday save a child's life. However, all children need constant supervision near water.
Teach children how to cross streets and walk in parking lots. Instruct them to never run out after a ball or toy.	Pedestrian accidents involving young children are common.
Teach children not to talk to, go with, or accept any item from a stranger.	This reduces the risk of injury and stranger abduction.
Teach children basic physical safety rules, such as proper use of safety scissors, never running with an object in their mouth or hand, and never attempting to use the stove or oven unassisted.	Risk of injury is lowered if children are taught basic safety procedures.
Teach children not to eat items found in the street or grass.	Poisoning may occur.
Remove doors from unused refrigerators and freezers. Instruct children not to play or hide in a car trunk or unused appliances.	If a child cannot freely exit from appliances and car trunks, asphyxiation may occur.
School-Age Children	
Teach children the safe use of equipment for play and work.	The child needs to learn the safe, appropriate use of implements to avoid injury.
Teach children proper bicycle safety, including use of helmet and rules of the road.	This may reduce injuries from falling off a bike or being hit by a car.
Teach children proper techniques for specific sports, as well as the need to wear proper safety gear (e.g., eyewear, mouth guards).	Using proper sports techniques, correct equipment, and protective gear prevents injuries.
Teach children not to operate electrical equipment while unsupervised.	If an electrical mishap were to occur, no one would be available to help.
Children should never have access to firearms or other weapons. All firearms should be kept in locked cabinets.	Children are often fascinated by firearms and weapons and may attempt to play with them.
Teach children safe use of the Internet.	Children are vulnerable to being exploited by predators over the Internet.
Adolescents	
Encourage enrolment in driver's education classes.	Many injuries in this age group are related to motor vehicle accidents.
Provide information about the effects of using alcohol and drugs.	Adolescents are prone to risk-taking behaviours and are subject to peer pressures.
Provide sex education, emphasizing safer sex practices and abstinence.	Many adolescents begin sexual relationships. Pregnancy and sexually transmitted infections may result.
Refer adolescents to community and school-sponsored activities.	The adolescent needs to socialize with peers, yet needs some supervision.
Encourage mentoring relationships between adults and adolescents.	Adolescents are in need of role models after whom they can pattern their behaviour.
Teach them safe use of the Internet.	Avoids overuse and possible exposure to inappropriate Web sites.

shoes or slippers for walking or transferring. When clients use assistive aids such as canes, crutches, or walkers, it is important to routinely check the condition of rubber tips and the integrity of the aid.

The risk of injury in the home may be reduced by removing all obstacles from halls and other heavily travelled areas. Necessary objects such as clocks, glasses, tissues, or medications should remain on bedside tables within reach of the client but out of the reach of children. Care should also be taken to ensure that end tables are secure and have stable, straight legs. Non-essential items should be placed in drawers to eliminate clutter. If small area rugs are used, they should be secured with a non-slip pad or skid-resistant adhesive strips. Carpeting on the stairs should be secured with carpet tacks.

Because falls cannot always be prevented, client-specific modifications may be necessary to reduce the risk of injury related to a fall. Research has shown that the use of an

Focus on Older Adults — Box 33-5

- The older adult experiences alterations in vision and hearing. The nurse should encourage yearly vision and hearing examinations and frequent cleansing of glasses and hearing aids as a means of preventing falls and burns.
- Older adults may have slowed reaction time. Teach clients safety tips for avoiding motor vehicle accidents. Driving may need to be restricted to daylight hours or suspended.
- Range of motion, flexibility, and strength are decreased. The nurse should encourage supervised exercise classes for older adults and teach them to seek assistance with household tasks as needed. Safety features, such as grab bars in the bathroom, may be needed.
- Reflexes are slowed, and the ability to respond to multiple stimuli is reduced. The nurse should provide adequate, meaningful stimuli but prevent sensory overload.
- Nocturia and incontinence are more frequent in older adults. The nurse should institute a regular toileting schedule for the client. A recommended frequency is every 3 hours. Diuretics should be given in the morning. Assistance should be provided, along with adequate lighting, to clients who need to go to the bathroom at night.
- Memory may be impaired. Clients should use medication organizers, which can be purchased at any drugstore at a very reasonable cost. These dispensers can be filled once a week with the proper medications to be taken at a specific time during the day.
- The family plays a significant role in the care of older adults. Often, family members serve as informal caregivers for older adults. Family caregivers frequently provide 10 hours or more of unpaid assistance per week (Vanier Institute of the Family, 2000). Encourage the family to allow the older adult to remain as independent as possible and provide help only for those things that are necessary.
- The high prevalence of chronic conditions in older adults results in the use of a high number of prescription and over-the-counter medications. Coupled with age-related changes in pharmacokinetics, there is a greater risk of serious adverse effects. Medications typically prescribed for older adults include anticholinergics, diuretics, anxiolytic and hypnotic agents, antidepressants, antihypertensives, vasodilators, analgesics, and laxatives, all of which may themselves pose risks or may interact to increase the risk for falls. The nurse should review the client's drug profile to ensure that any of the above noted drugs are used cautiously and assess the client regularly for any adverse effects that may increase fall risk.

external hip protector can considerably reduce the risk of hip fractures among ambulatory older adults (Box 33-6).

Restraints. A physical **restraint** is a mechanical or physical device that is used to immobilize a client or extremity, restricts the freedom of movement or normal access to a person's body, and is not a usual part of treatment plans indicated by the person's condition or symptoms (Zusman, 2001). The optimal goal for all clients is a restraint-free environment; however, clients who are at risk for injury to self or others may need restraints temporarily.

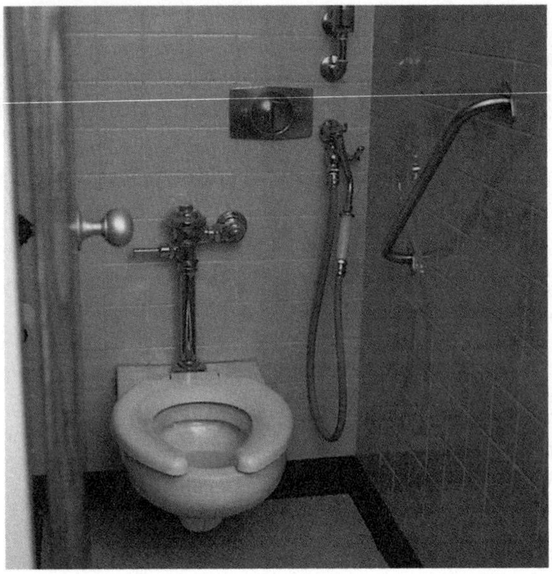

FIGURE **33–11** Safety bars around toilets and showers.

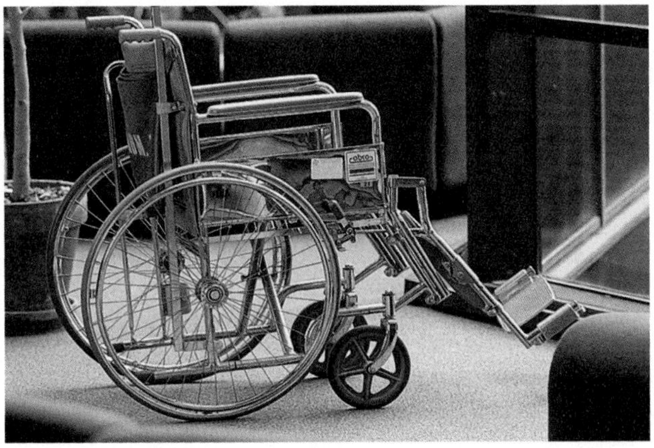

FIGURE **33–12** Safety locks on wheelchairs.

Whenever a client is restrained, there is a natural tendency for the client to try to remove the restraint. When this occurs, client injury is common. Restrained clients can easily become entangled in a restraint device when attempting to get out of the device. In some cases, death has resulted from strangulation or asphyxiation. As a result, long-term care facilities and many health care facilities have banned the use of the jacket (vest) restraint. This text will discuss proper use of the vest restraint because if it becomes necessary for a nurse to apply a vest restraint, it must be done safely. The use of any restraint is also associated with serious complications, including pressure ulcers, constipation, pneumonia, urinary and fecal incontinence, and urinary retention (see chapter 42). Contractures, nerve damage, and circulatory impairment are also potential hazards. In addition, restrained clients can experience humiliation, fear, anger, and a loss of self-esteem.

Table 33-3 Measures to Prevent Falls by Older Adults

Measure	Rationale
Stairs	
Install treads with uniform depth of 22.5 cm and 22.5-cm risers (vertical face of steps).	If stairs are of uniform size, older adults do not have to continually adjust vision.
Install uniform-textured or plain-coloured surfaces on each tread, and mark edge of tread with contrasting colour.	Uniform textures or colour help to decrease vertigo. Marking edge of tread provides obvious visual cue to end of stair.
Ensure proper lighting of each tread. Block sun or light bulb glare with translucent shades or screen, or use lower-wattage or non-glare bulbs.	Older adults' vision is unable to adjust quickly to changes in lighting.
Ensure adequate headroom so that users do not have to duck to negotiate stairs.	Sudden changes in head position may result in dizziness.
Remove protruding objects from staircase walls.	Decreased peripheral vision may prevent client from seeing object.
Maintain outdoor walkways and stairs in good condition and free of holes, cracks, and splinters.	Decreased visual acuity can prevent client from seeing any structural defect.
Handrails	
Install smooth but slip-resistant handrail at least 5 cm from wall.	5-cm distance allows client to grasp handrail firmly for support.
Secure handrail firmly so that user's weight is supported, especially at bottom and top of stairway.	Older adults have greatest risk of falling at top and bottom of stairs, because centre of gravity is being shifted and balance is unstable.
Install grab rails in bathroom near toilet and tub.	This enables client to have support while rising from sitting to standing position.
Floors	
Ensure that clients wear properly fitting shoes or slippers with non-skid surface.	Reduces chances of slipping.
Secure all carpeting, mats, and tile; place non-skid backing under small rugs.	Sudden slip may cause dizziness and inability to regain balance.
Place bath mats or non-skid strips on bathtub or shower stall floors.	Wet surfaces increase the risk of falling.
Secure electrical cords against baseboards.	Prevents tripping.
Maintain proper illumination inside and outside where the client moves and walks.	Reduces the risk of falling due to eye strain.
Health Care Facility	
Orientation	
Place disoriented clients in room near nurses' station.	Provides for more frequent observation by nursing staff.
Maintain close supervision of confused clients.	Confused clients often attempt to wander out of bed or room.
Show the client how to use the call light at the bedside and in bathroom, and place within easy reach.	Location and use of the call light is essential to client safety.
Place bedside tables and over-bed tables close to client.	Prevents client from searching or overreaching for items such as eyeglasses, dentures, hearing aid, or telephone.
Remove clutter from bedside tables, hallways, bathrooms, and grooming areas.	Eliminates potential hazards and promotes client independence.
Leave one side rail up and one down on the side where the oriented and ambulatory client gets out of bed.	Client can use the side rail for support when getting in and out of bed and to position self once in bed.
Transport	
Lock beds and wheelchairs when transferring a client from a bed to a wheelchair or back to bed.	Provides stability and support during transfer.
Place side rails in the up position and secure safety straps around the client when transporting by stretcher.	Prevents the client from rolling off the stretcher.

Research Highlight

Box 33-6

Preventing Hip Fractures From Falls

Research Focus

Hip fractures in older adults are a major cause of disability, functional impairment, and death. Frequency of hip fractures is expected to increase because the number and age of older adults is also increasing. Nurses play a key role in the prevention of falls and injuries related to falls.

Research Abstract

This article describes an investigation into the effect of an anatomically designed external hip protector in the prevention of hip fractures among older adults. The hip protector is shaped to cover the proximal femur and designed to shunt the energy of an impact away from the hip to the soft tissues surrounding the hip. Two protectors are worn with the use of a stretchy undergarment containing a pocket on each side for placement of the protector. In this study, 1,801 ambulatory, but frail, older adults (1,409 women and 392 men) with a mean age of 82 years were randomly assigned (in a 1:2 ratio) either to a group that wore a hip protector or to a control group that did not wear a hip protector; 643 subjects entered the hip protector group, whereas 1,148 subjects entered the control group. All fractures, including pelvic, leg, and arm fractures, were recorded until the end of the first full month (2 years later) after 62 hip fractures had occurred in the control group. The risk of fracture in the two groups was compared. In the hip protector group, the risk of fracture was also analyzed according to whether the protector had been worn at the time of the fall.

A total of 1,404 falls occurred in the hip protector group. Of those falls, 74% (1,034) occurred while subjects wore the hip protector. The results showed that 13 subjects in the hip protector group had a hip fracture, compared with 67 subjects in the control group. In the hip protector group, 4 of those subjects were wearing the hip protector, whereas 9 subjects did not wear their hip protector. In the hip protector group, 2 subjects had pelvic fractures, as compared with 12 subjects in the control group. The risk of other fractures was similar in the two groups. The results of this trial indicate that the risk of hip fracture among ambulatory older adults can be reduced by more than 80% if the protector is worn at the time of a fall.

Evidenced-Based Practice

- Identify clients who are at high risk for hip fractures (previous fall or fracture, impaired balance or mobility, use of a walking aid, cognitive impairment, impaired vision, poor nutrition, disease or medication known to predispose a person to a fall and/or fracture).
- Use hip protectors on those clients who are at high risk for hip fractures.
- Provide frequent reminders to the client and family about the importance of fall prevention strategies and ways to reduce the risk of injury.

Reference

Kannus, P., et al. (2000). Prevention of hip fracture in elderly people with use of a hip protector. *New England Journal of Medicine, 343,* 1506–1513.

Safety Alert. Routine assessment of a client in restraint is critical to prevent injury. The restraint must be moved and the client repositioned at regular intervals, according to agency policy. Restraints are used only after other alternatives have been tried, and the least restrictive method of restraint is used. The use of restraints must be part of the client's medical treatment. Restraints are considered a short-term intervention, and once they have been applied, regular assessments are needed to determine whether or not they should be continued. All assessments and interventions must be clearly documented.

A least-restraint approach is recommended to ensure highest quality care. This approach ensures that all alternative interventions are attempted before moving to the use of restraints (College of Nurses of Ontario, 2004). Restraints do not prevent falls or injury and may actually increase the severity of injury (Registered Nurses Association of Ontario, 2005). It is imperative that nurses try alternative measures instead of restraints (Box 33-7). Using a restraint-use algorithm provides evidenced-based guidelines for determining if a restraint is appropriate and what interventions might be used (Figure 33–13).

The use of restraints involves a psychological adjustment for the client and family. If restraints must be used, the nurse assists family members and clients by explaining the purpose of restraints, the client's expected care while restrained, the precautions to be taken to avoid injury, and the temporary and protective aspects of restraints. Informed consent from family members may also be required before using restraints, as is the case in long-term care settings.

For legal purposes, the nurse must know agency policy and procedures for appropriate use and monitoring of restraints. The use of a restraint must be clinically justified and be a part of the client's prescribed medical treatment and care plan. A physician's order may or may not be required, depending on provincial/territorial legislation and agency policy. Assessment of clients who are restrained must be ongoing. Proper documentation, including the behaviours that necessitated the application of restraints, the procedure used in restraining, the condition of the body part restrained (e.g., circulation to hand), and the evaluation of the client response, is essential. Restraints must be periodically removed, and the nurse must assess the client to determine if the restraints continue to be needed.

Box 33-7 Alternatives to Restraints

- Orient clients and families to surroundings; explain all procedures and treatments to them.
- Encourage family and friends to stay, or use trained sitters for clients who need continuous supervision.
- Assign confused or disoriented clients to rooms near the nurses' station. Observe these clients frequently. Institute reality orientation measures (e.g., frequent reminders of person, time, and place; use of environmental aids such as clocks or calendars [see chapter 44]).
- Provide appropriate visual and auditory stimuli (e.g., family pictures, clock, radio).
- Eliminate bothersome treatments as soon as possible. For example, discontinue tube feedings and begin oral feedings as quickly as allowed by the client's condition.
- Use relaxation techniques (e.g., music suited to client's taste, massage).
- Institute exercise and ambulation schedules as allowed by the client's condition.
- Provide scheduled toileting, especially during peak fall times such as 6 to 8 AM and 4 to 6 PM.
- Consult with physiotherapists and occupational therapists to enhance clients' abilities to carry out activities of daily living.
- Evaluate all medications that clients are receiving to determine if the medication is having the desired therapeutic effect.
- Conduct ongoing assessment and evaluation of clients' care and their ongoing response to care.

Adapted from "The Advanced Practice Nurse and Changing Perspectives on Physical Restraint," by C. A. Quinn, 1996, *Clinical Nurse Specialist, 10*(5), pp. 220–225.

Skill 33-1 includes guidelines for the proper use and application of restraints. Use of restraints must meet the following objectives:

- Reduce the risk of client injury
- Prevent interruption of therapy such as traction, IV infusions, nasogastric tube feeding, or Foley catheterization
- Prevent the confused or combative client from removing life-support equipment
- Reduce the risk of injury to others by the client

In keeping with current trends toward health promotion, improved assessment techniques and modifications of the environment are offered as alternatives to restraints. An **Ambularm** is a device worn on the leg that signals when the leg is in a dependent position, such as over the side rail or on the floor (Figure 33–14). The device is used for clients who climb out of bed unassisted and are in danger of falling. There are also devices that can be placed on the client's mattress or attached to the client's nightgown or chair that sound an alarm when triggered. The devices allow a zone of free movement. When the safe zone is exceeded, an alarm sounds. The alarm can be designed to signal at the central nurses' station so that staff are alerted quickly when a client is up and out of bed. There are also alarms that can be placed on doors to alert staff or family members when a confused or disoriented client, prone to wandering, opens a door.

Another alternative to a restraint is the Vail Enclosed Bed (Figure 33–15). The bed is a soft-sided, self-contained enclosed bed that is much less restrictive than physical restraints. It allows for freedom of movement and thus reduces the side effects caused by physical restraints such as pressure ulcers and loss of dignity. A vinyl top covers the padded upper frame of the bed and the nylon-net canopy surrounds the mattress and completely encloses the client in the bed. Zippers on the four sides of the enclosure provide access to the client. The Vail Enclosed Bed works well for clients who are restless and unpredictable, cognitively impaired, and at risk for injury if they were to fall or get out of bed, such as clients on anticoagulant therapy at risk for intracranial bleed. The bed may also be a safer alternative to side rails.

Side Rails. Side rails may help to increase a client's mobility and/or stability when in bed or when moving from bed to chair. Side rails also help prevent the unconscious client from falling out of bed or from a stretcher (Figure 33–16). However, raised side rails that cannot be opened by the client are considered a restraint (College of Nurses of Ontario, 2004). The use of side rails alone for a disoriented client may cause more confusion and further injury. A confused client who is determined to get out of bed attempts to climb over the side rail or climbs out at the foot of the bed. Either attempt usually results in a fall or injury. Nursing interventions to reduce a client's confusion should first focus on the cause of the confusion. Frequently nurses mistake a client's attempt to explore his or her environment or to self-toilet as confusion. A thorough assessment is essential. Whenever side rails are used, the bed should be maintained in the lowest position possible.

> *Safety Alert.* Side rails have the potential to cause entrapment of the head and body, especially in older adult clients who are confused and restless. Entrapment has resulted in death from asphyxiation and injuries such as fractures and lacerations (Capezuti, 2000). Hazards can be prevented by assessing for excessive gaps and openings between the bed frame and mattress and using side rail netting, protective padding, and/or antiskid mats to prevent the mattress from being pushed to one side.

Fires. A fire is always possible in the home or health care facility. Accidental home fires typically result from smoking in bed, placing cigarettes in trash cans, cooking accidents, or faulty wiring or appliances. Institutional fires typically result from electrical or anaesthetic-related causes. Although smoking is usually not allowed in the

Text continued on p. 1001

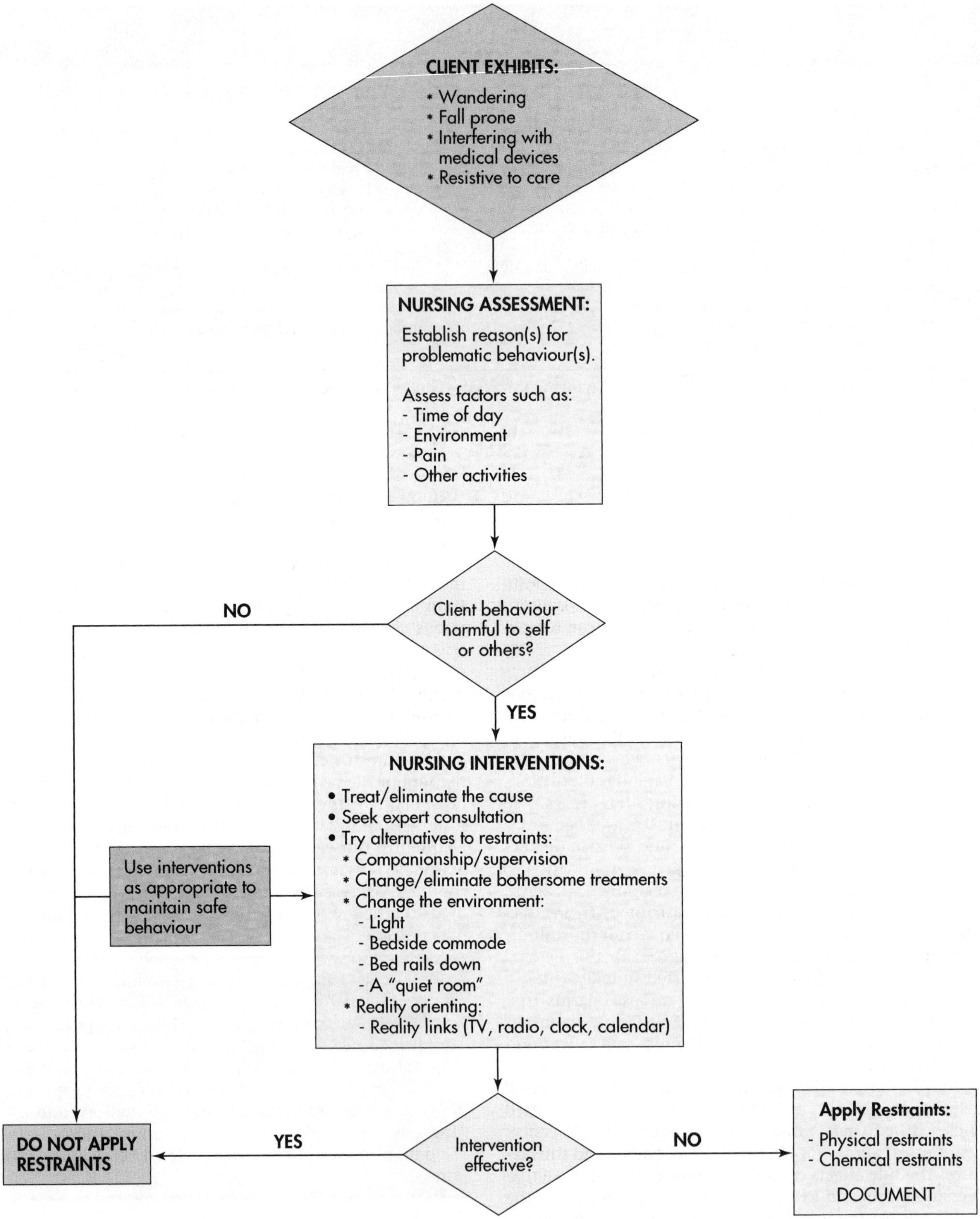

FIGURE **33–13** Restraint-use algorithm. (Developed from "Restraints"—a research-based protocol by L. Ledford, MA, ARNP and J. Mentals, MS, RNCS, GNP. Copyright 1998, University of Iowa Gerontological Nursing Interventions Research Center.)

Skill 33-1 Applying Restraints

View Video

Delegation Considerations

The application of restraints can be delegated to trained unregulated care providers (UCPs). However, the nurse is always responsible for assessment of client's safety needs, selection of appropriate alternative interventions, evaluation of effectiveness of restraint, and ongoing assessment to prevent complications of restraint use.

- Have the UCP inform the nurse of any redness, excoriation, or constriction of circulation under the restraint.
- Have the UCP ask for assistance if the client has any mobility restrictions that might affect how to remove or reapply a restraint.
- Instruct the UCP on when and how to change client's position and provide range of motion, skin care, toileting, and opportunities for socialization.

Equipment

- Proper restraint: jacket, mitten, belt, extremity
- Padding (if needed)

Steps	Rationale
1. Assess whether client needs a restraint. Does the client continually try to interrupt needed therapy? Is the client at risk for injuring self or others?	Restraints are used only when other measures have failed to prevent interruption of therapy such as traction, IV infusions, or nasogastric tube feedings; to prevent a confused or combative client from self-injury by falling out of bed or a wheelchair; to prevent a client from removing a urinary catheter, surgical drain, or life support equipment; and to reduce risk of injury to others by the client.
2. Assess client's behaviour, such as confusion, disorientation, agitation, restlessness, combativeness, or inability to follow directions. Consult with gerontological nurse specialist if available.	If client's behaviour continues despite attempts to eliminate cause of behaviour, use of physical restraint may be necessary.
3. Review agency policies regarding restraints. Consider the purpose, type, location, and duration of restraint. Determine if signed consent for use of restraint is needed.	The least restrictive type of restraint must be ordered. A physician's order may or may not be necessary—check provincial/territorial legislation and agency policy. Because restraints limit the client's ability to move freely, the nurse must make clinical judgments appropriate to the client's condition and agency policy.
4. Review manufacturer's instructions before entering client's room. Determine the most appropriate size restraint.	The nurse should be familiar with all devices used for client care and protection. Incorrect application of a restraining device may result in client injury or death.
5. Perform hand hygiene, and gather equipment.	Reduces transmission of micro-organisms; promotes organization.
6. Introduce self to client and family. Assess their feelings about restraint use. Explain that restraint is temporary and designed to protect client from injury.	Helps minimize client anxiety during application of the device, and helps minimize family concern during maintenance of restraint.
7. Inspect area where restraint is to be placed. Assess condition of skin underlying area where restraint is to be applied.	Restraints may compress and interfere with functioning of devices or tubes. Provides baseline assessment data regarding skin integrity.
8. Approach client in a calm, confident manner. Explain what you plan to do.	Reduces client anxiety and promotes co-operation.
9. Adjust bed to proper height, and lower side rail on side of client contact.	Allows nurse to use proper body mechanics and prevent injury.
10. Provide privacy. Make sure client is comfortable and in proper body alignment. Drape client as needed.	Privacy protects self-esteem. Proper body alignment promotes comfort and prevents contractures and neurovascular injury.
11. Pad skin and bony prominences (if necessary) before applying restraints.	Padding reduces friction and pressure on skin and underlying tissue.

Skill 33-1 Applying Restraints—cont'd

Steps	Rationale
12. Apply appropriate size restraint, making sure it is not over an IV line or other device (e.g., dialysis shunt).	IV lines and other therapeutic devices may become occluded.
A. **Jacket (vest or Posey) restraint:** Front and back of garment should be labelled as such. Apply over clothing or hospital gown (see illustration). Place client's hands through armholes or sleeves, and secure according to manufacturer's directions. Place straps at client's hips.	Restrains client while lying or reclining in bed and while sitting in chair or wheelchair. Proper application prevents suffocation or choking. Clothing or gown prevents friction against skin.

Critical Decision Point: Check agency policy. Some health care facilities no longer use vest restraints because they have been known to cause death due to strangulation.

Steps	Rationale
B. **Belt restraint:** Device that secures client to bed or stretcher. Apply over clothes or gown. Remove wrinkles from front and back of restraint while placing it around client's waist. Bring ties through slots in belt. Avoid placing belt across the chest or too tightly across the abdomen (see illustration).	Restrains centre of gravity and prevents client from rolling off stretcher or sitting up while on stretcher or from falling out of bed. Tight application may interfere with ventilation.

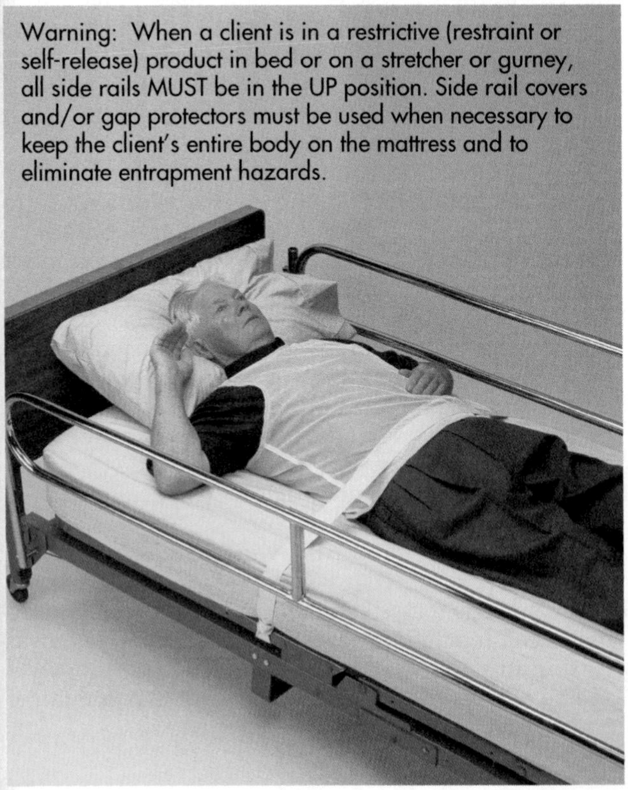
Warning: When a client is in a restrictive (restraint or self-release) product in bed or on a stretcher or gurney, all side rails MUST be in the UP position. Side rail covers and/or gap protectors must be used when necessary to keep the client's entire body on the mattress and to eliminate entrapment hazards.

STEP **12A** Vest restraint securely attached to bed frame. (Courtesy JT Posey Co., Arcadia, CA.)

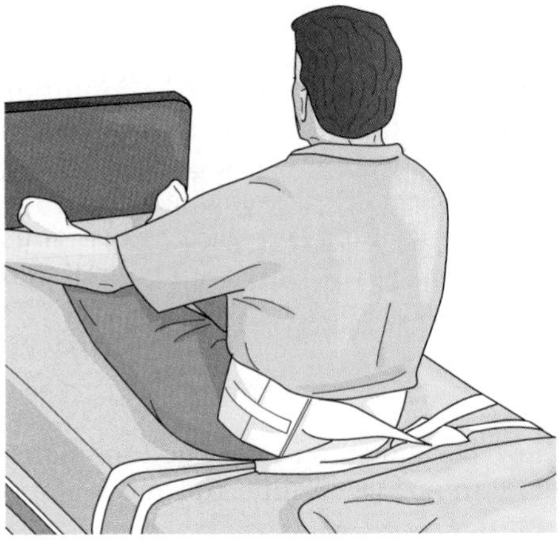

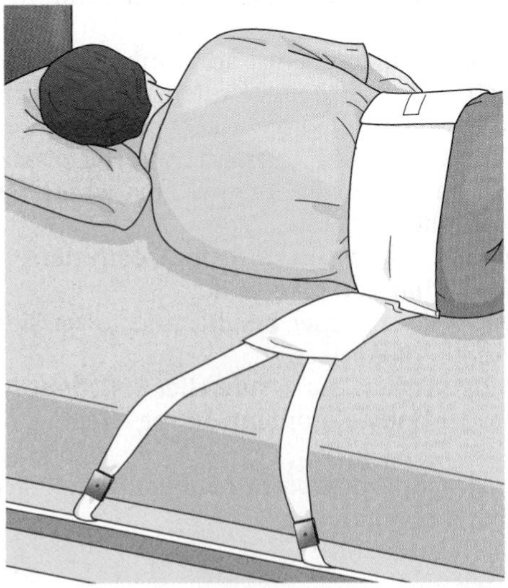

STEP **12B** Belt restraint tied to the bed frame and to an area that does not cause the restraint to tighten when the side rail is raised or lowered. (From *Mosby's Textbook for Nursing Assistants,* 5th ed., p. 4, by S. A. Sorrentino, 2000, St. Louis, MO: Mosby.)

Steps	Rationale
C. **Extremity (ankle or wrist) restraint:** Restraint designed to immobilize one or all extremities. Commercially available limb restraints are composed of sheepskin or foam padding (see illustration). Limb restraint is wrapped around wrist or ankle with soft part toward skin and secured snugly in place by Velcro straps.	Maintains immobilization of extremity to protect client from injury from fall or accidental removal of therapeutic device (e.g., IV tube or Foley catheter). Tight application may interfere with circulation.
D. **Mitten restraint:** Thumbless mitten device to restrain client's hands (see illustration). Place hand in mitten, being sure end is brought all the way up over the wrist.	Prevents clients from dislodging invasive equipment, removing dressings, or scratching, yet allows greater movement than a wrist restraint.
E. **Elbow restraint:** Piece of fabric with slots in which tongue blades are placed so that elbow joint remains rigid (see illustration).	Commonly used with infants and children to prevent elbow flexion (e.g., when an IV line is in place).
F. **Mummy restraint:** Blanket or sheet that is opened on bed or crib with one corner folded toward centre. Child is placed on blanket with shoulders at fold and feet toward opposite corner (see illustration for Step 12F-1). With child's right arm straight down against body, right side of blanket is pulled firmly across right shoulder and chest and secured beneath left side of body (see illustration for Step 12F-2). Left arm is placed straight against body, and left side of blanket is brought across shoulder and chest and locked beneath child's body on right side (see illustration for Step 12F-3). Lower corner is folded and brought over body and tucked or fastened securely with safety pins (see illustration for Step 12F-4).	Maintains short-term restraint of small child or infant for examination or treatment involving head and neck. Effectively controls movement of torso and extremities.

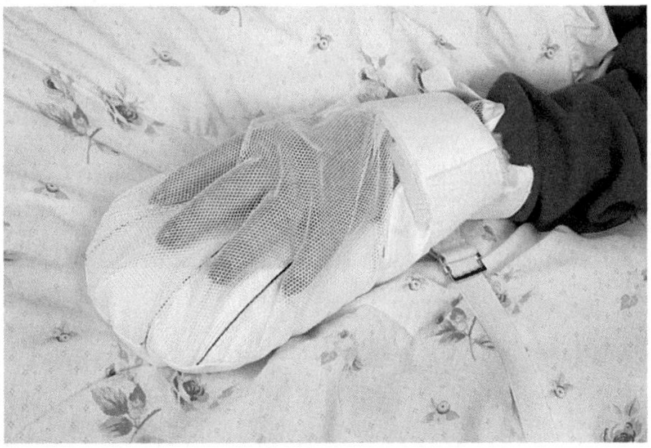

STEP **12D** Mitten restraint.

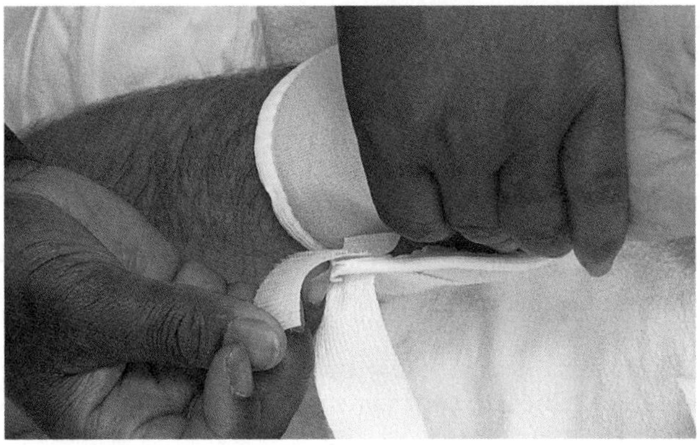

STEP **12C** Extremity restraint being applied to wrist.

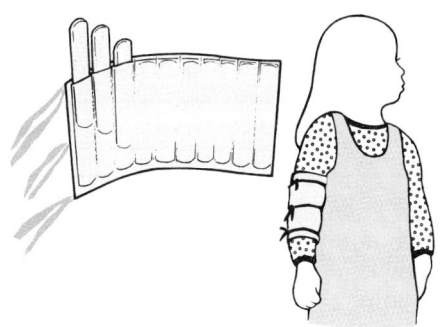

STEP **12E** Elbow restraint.

Skill 33-1 Applying Restraints—cont'd

Steps	Rationale

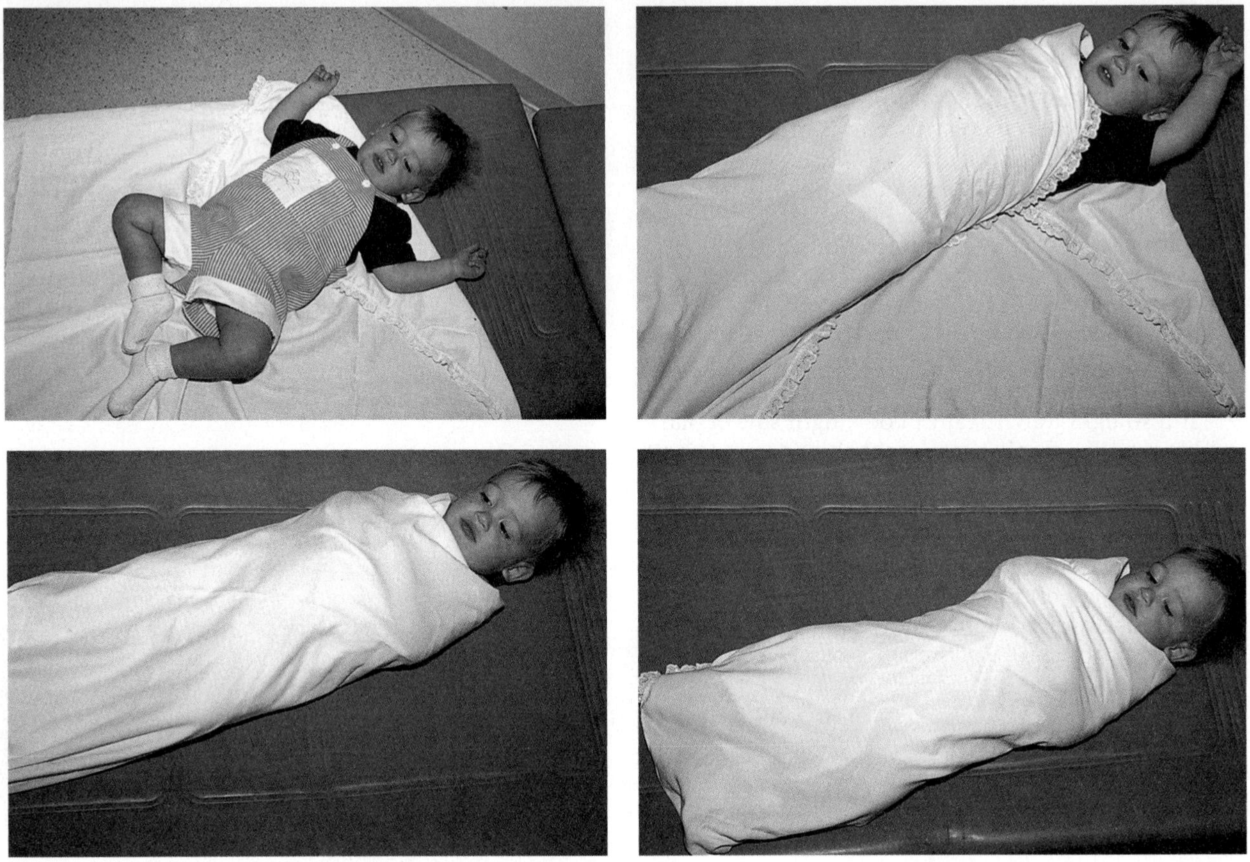

1 2 3 4

STEP **12F** Mummy restraint.

Steps	Rationale
13. Attach restraints to bed frame, which moves when the head of bed is raised or lowered (see illustration).	Client may be injured if restraint is secured to side rail and it is lowered.

Critical Decision Point: Do not attach end of restraint to side rails.

Steps	Rationale
14. When a jacket restraint is used on a client in a wheelchair, it should be secured by placing ties under armrests and securing at the back of chair (see illustration).	Prevents client from sliding restraint ties up the back of the chair.

Critical Decision Point: If ties are not under armrests, clients may be able to slide ties up the back of the chair and free themselves.

Steps	Rationale
15. Secure restraints with a quick-release tie (see illustration). Do not tie in a knot.	Allows for quick release in an emergency.
16. Insert two fingers under the secured restraint (see illustration).	A tight restraint may cause constriction and impede circulation. Checking for constriction prevents neurovascular injury.
17. Proper placement of restraint, skin integrity, pulses, temperature, colour, and sensation of the restrained body part should be assessed at least every hour or according to agency policy.	Frequent assessment prevents complications, such as suffocation, skin breakdown, and impaired circulation.

Steps	Rationale

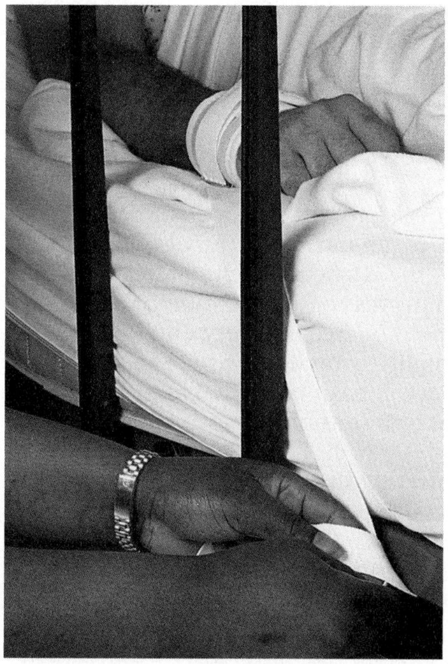

STEP **13** Tie restraint strap to bed frame.

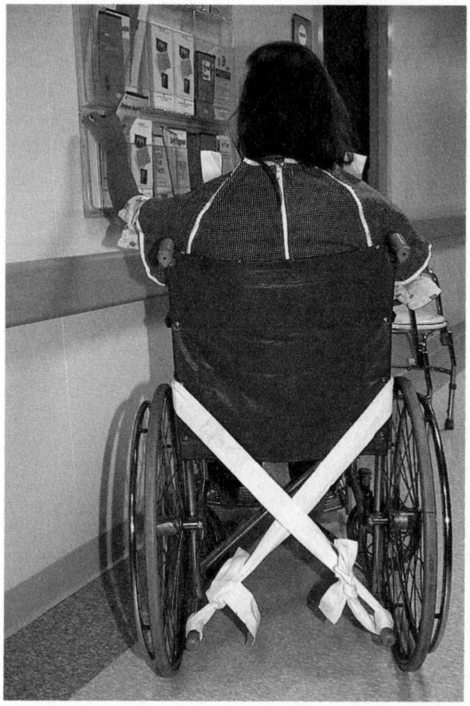

STEP **14** Straps of vest restraint secured at back of chair.

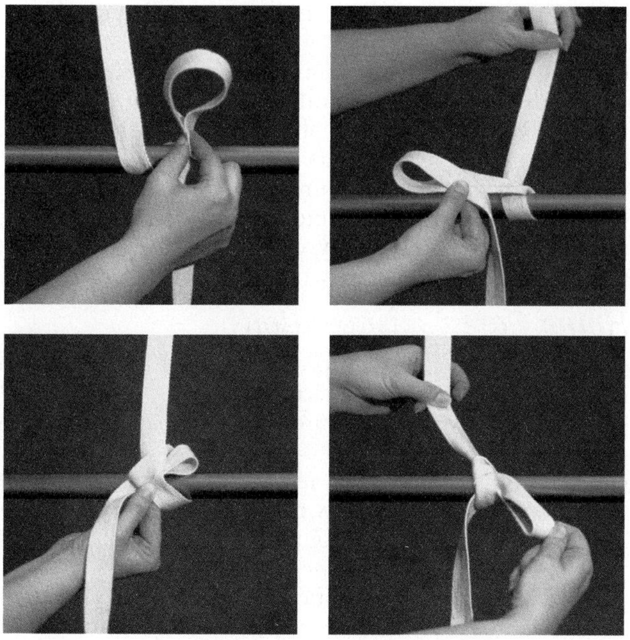

STEP **15** The Posey quick-release tie. (Courtesy JT Posey Co., Arcadia, CA.)

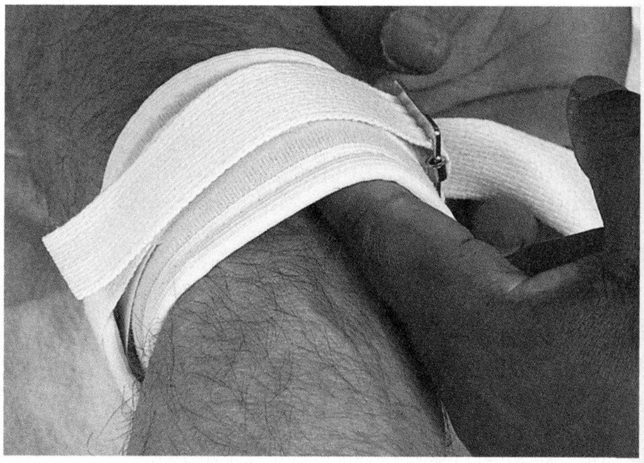

STEP **16** Place two fingers under restraint to check tightness.

Skill 33-1 Applying Restraints—cont'd

18. Restraints should be removed at regular intervals (see agency policy). If client is violent and non-compliant, remove one restraint at a time and/or have staff assistance while removing restraints. Client should not be left unattended at this time.
Provides opportunity to change client's position and perform full range of motion, toileting, and exercise and to provide food or fluids.

19. Secure call light or intercom system within reach.
Allows client, family, or caregiver to obtain assistance quickly.

20. Leave bed or chair with wheels locked. Bed should be in lowest position.
Locked wheels prevent bed or chair from moving if client attempts to get out. If client falls when bed is in lowest position, the chances of injury are reduced.

21. Perform hand hygiene.
Reduces transmission of micro-organisms.

22. Inspect client for any injury, including all hazards of immobility, while restraints are in use.
Client should be free of injury and not exhibit any signs of immobility complications.

23. Observe IV catheters, urinary catheters, and drainage tubes to ensure that they are positioned correctly and that therapy remains uninterrupted.
Reinsertion can be uncomfortable and can increase risk of infection or interrupt therapy.

24. Regularly reassess client's need for continued use of restraint (for medical or surgical reason) with the intent of discontinuing restraint at the earliest possible time (see agency-specific policy).
Use of restraints should be seen as a temporary measure and discontinued as soon as possible (Strumpf et al., 1998).

25. Provide appropriate sensory stimulation and reorient client as needed.
Use of restraints can further increase disorientation.

Unexpected Outcomes and Related Interventions

- Client has signs of impaired skin integrity.
  - Assess skin and provide appropriate therapy.
  - Notify the physician and reassess the need for continued use of the restraint.
  - Ensure correct application of restraint. Pad skin under a restraint and remove restraint more frequently.
- Client has altered neurovascular status to an extremity (cyanosis, pallor, coldness of the skin, or complaints of tingling, pain, or numbness).
  - Remove restraint immediately, stay with the client, and notify the physician.
  - Protect extremity from further injury (e.g., pressure from tubing or encumbrance, positioning).
- Client has increased confusion, disorientation, or agitation.
  - Identify reason for change in behaviour, and attempt to eliminate cause.
  - Attempt a restraint alternative.
- Client escapes from the restraint device and suffers a fall or injury.
  - Attend to client's immediate physical needs, and inform physician.
  - Reassess type of restraint used, correct application, and if alternatives can be used.

Recording and Reporting

- Record behaviours that place client at risk for injury.
- Describe restraint alternatives attempted and client's response.
- Record client's and/or family's understanding of and consent to restraint application.
- Record type and location of restraint and time applied.
- Record time of assessments and releases.
- Document client's behaviour after application of restraint.
- Document specific assessments related to orientation, oxygenation, skin integrity, circulation, and positioning.
- Describe client's response when restraints were removed.

Home Care Considerations

- Plan care with family. If possible, use of an Ambularm may free client from physical restraints.
- Instruct family (or other caregiver) in use of alternatives to restraints (see Box 33-7).
- A physical restraint may require a physician order. It should not be sent home with family unless the device is needed to protect client from injury. If physical restraints are necessary, the family (or other caregiver) must be instructed in proper application, care needed while in restraints, and complications to look for. Also inform caregiver whom to contact if any abnormal findings occur.
- A client who needs to be restrained in bed should have a hospital bed and will require constant supervision in the home.

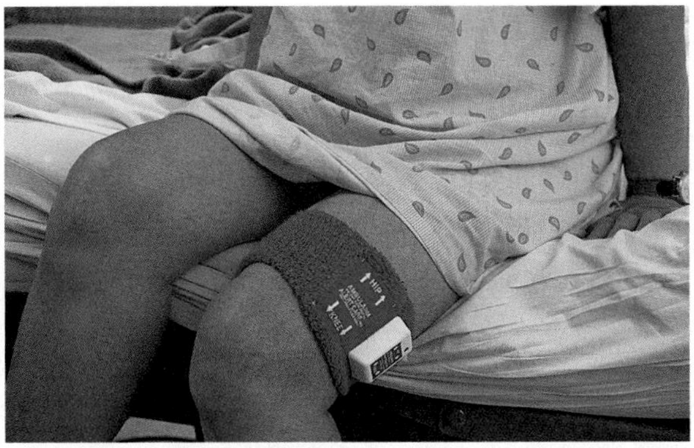

FIGURE **33–14** Client wearing an Ambularm device.

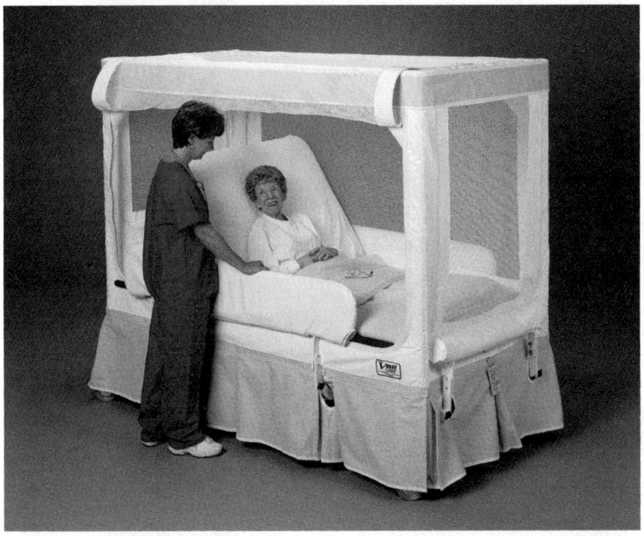

FIGURE **33–15** The Vail Enclosed Bed. (Courtesy Vail Products, Inc., Toledo, OH.)

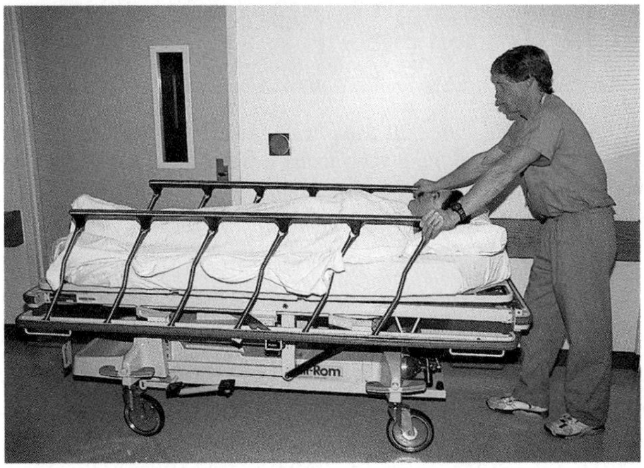

FIGURE **33–16** Side rails in the *up* position on a stretcher.

Box 33-8 Fire Intervention Guidelines for Nurses Working in Health Care Agencies

Keep the phone number for reporting fires visible on the telephone at all times.
Know the agency's mnemonic, fire drill, and evacuation plan.
Know the location of all fire alarms, exits, extinguishers, and oxygen shut-off.
Use the mnemonic RACE to set priorities in case of fire:
- **R** Rescue and remove all clients in immediate danger.
- **A** Activate the alarm. Always do this before attempting to extinguish even a minor fire.
- **C** Confine the fire by closing doors and windows and turning off oxygen and electrical equipment.
- **E** Extinguish the fire using an extinguisher (see Box 33-9).

health care setting, smoking-related fires continue to pose a significant risk as a result of unauthorized smoking in bed.

The interventions described here are directed toward fires occurring in health care agencies, but the same principles apply for fires in the home (Box 33-8). Homes should be equipped with smoke and fire alarms. It is important to have a plan of action in the event of fire, including a route of exit and identification of a location where family members will meet. All clients, even young children, should be familiar with the phrase "stop, drop, and roll," which describes the actions to be followed when a client's clothing and skin are burning.

If a fire occurs in a health care agency, the nurse protects clients from immediate injury, reports the exact location of the fire, and contains the fire and extinguishes it if possible. All personnel are mobilized to evacuate clients. Clients who are close to the fire, regardless of its size, are at risk of injury and should be moved to another area. If a client is receiving oxygen but not life support, the nurse discontinues the oxygen because it is combustible and can fuel an existing fire. If the client is on life support, the nurse may need to maintain the client's respiratory status manually with an Ambu-bag (see chapter 35) until the client is moved away from the fire. Ambulatory clients can be directed to walk by themselves to a safe area and in some cases may be able to assist in moving clients in wheelchairs. Bedridden clients are generally moved from the scene of a fire by a stretcher, their bed, or a wheelchair. If none of these methods is appropriate, clients must be carried from the area. If a client must be carried, the nurse should be careful not to overextend physical limits for lifting because injury to the nurse can result in further injury to the client. If fire department personnel are on the scene, they can help evacuate the clients.

After a fire has been reported and clients are out of danger, nurses and other personnel must take measures to contain or put out the fire, such as closing doors and windows, placing wet towels along the base of doors, turning off oxygen and electrical equipment, and using a fire extinguisher. Fire extinguishers are categorized as

Client Teaching Box 33-9

Correct Use of a Fire Extinguisher in the Home

Objectives

- Client will correctly place the extinguisher in the home.
- Client will describe when it is appropriate to use a home fire extinguisher.
- Client will demonstrate the correct technique when using a fire extinguisher.
- Client will state when fire extinguishers need to be replaced.

Teaching Strategies

- Discuss correct location of the extinguisher. It is recommended that one be placed on each level of the home, near an exit, in clear view, away from stoves and heating appliances, and above the reach of small children. Keep a fire extinguisher in the kitchen, near the furnace, and in the garage. The instructions should be read when the extinguisher is purchased and kept available for periodic review.
- Describe the steps to take before using the extinguisher. Attempt to fight the fire only when all occupants have left the home, the fire department has been called, the fire is confined to a small area, there is an exit route readily available, the extinguisher is the right type for the fire (see discussion in text for a description of the types of extinguishers), and the client knows how to use the extinguisher.
- Instruct the client to memorize the mnemonic PASS: Pull the pin to unlock handle, Aim low at the base of the fire, Squeeze the handle, and Sweep the unit from side to side (see Figure 33–17).

Evaluation

- Client can correctly place an extinguisher in the home.
- Client correctly lists the steps to take before attempting to use an extinguisher.
- Client demonstrates correct use of the extinguisher while reciting the instructions with the mnemonic PASS.

Adapted from *Home Fire Prevention and Preparedness Fact Sheet,* 2002, Itasca, IL: National Safety Council.

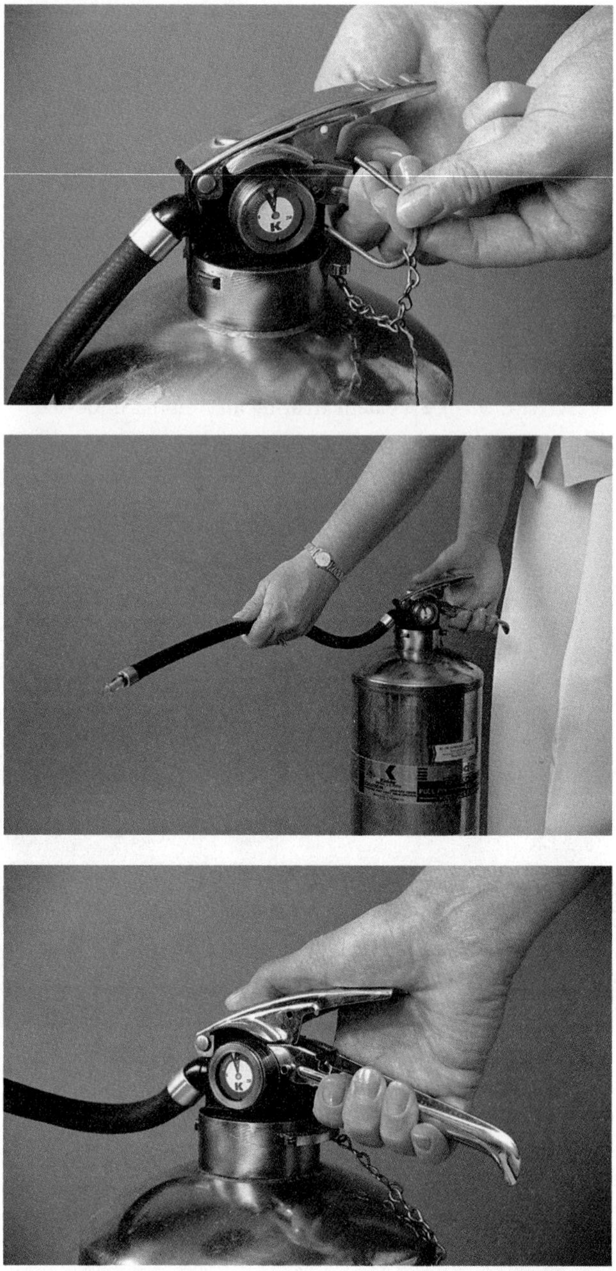

A

B

C

FIGURE **33–17** **A,** Pull the pin. **B,** Aim at the base of the fire. **C,** Squeeze the handle. Sweep from side to side to coat the area evenly. (Adapted from *Mosby's Assisting With Patient Care,* by S. A. Sorrentino, 1999, St. Louis, MO: Mosby.)

type A, used for ordinary combustibles (e.g., wood, cloth, paper, and many plastic items); type B, used for flammable liquids (e.g., gasoline, grease, paint, and anaesthetic gas); and type C, used for electrical equipment. The correct use of an extinguisher is discussed in Box 33-9 and demonstrated in Figure 33–17.

The best intervention is to prevent fires. Nursing measures include complying with the agency's smoking policies and keeping combustible materials away from heat sources. Some agencies have fire doors that are held open by magnets and close automatically when a fire alarm sounds. It is important to keep equipment away from these doors.

Poisoning. A **poison** is any substance that impairs health or destroys life when ingested, inhaled, or otherwise absorbed by the body. Specific antidotes or treatments are available for only some types of poisons. The capacity of body tissue to recover from the poison determines the reversibility of the effect. Poisons can impair the respiratory, circulatory, central nervous, hepatic, GI, and renal systems of the body.

The toddler, preschooler, young school-age child, and older adult must be protected from accidental poisoning. Using child-resistant caps, placing medications and cleaning fluids and powders out of the reach of children, leaving potentially poisonous materials in original containers,

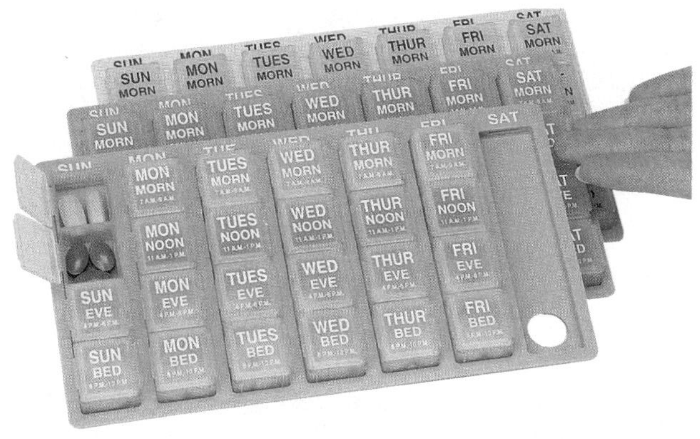

FIGURE **33–18** One-Day-At-A-Time medicine organizer. (Courtesy Apothecary Products, Inc., Burnsville, MN.)

and removing poisonous plants from the home prevent accidental ingestion of poisonous materials. Poisoning can also result from swallowing miniature button or disk batteries commonly found in games, cameras, calculators, and watches. In older adults, diminished eyesight and impaired memory may result in accidental ingestion of poisonous substances or in accidental overdose of prescribed medications. To prevent medication errors on the part of clients in the home, the nurse should recommend the use of medication organizers that are filled once a week by the client and/or family. These organizers have the day and time on each box, so that the client knows when and what to take at any given time (Figure 33–18). This information is particularly useful for clients who may forget whether they have taken their medications.

Guidelines for intervening in accidental poisoning should be adhered to. The poison control centre phone number should be visible on the telephone in homes with young children. In all cases of suspected poisoning, this number should be called immediately (Box 33-10).

Electrical Hazards. Electrical equipment must be maintained in good working order and should be grounded. The third (longer) prong in an electrical plug is the ground. Theoretically, the ground prong carries any stray electrical current back to the ground—hence its name. The other two prongs carry the power to the piece of electrical equipment. Improperly grounded or malfunctioning electrical equipment increases the risk of electrical injury and fire. Educating both the client and the family can reduce the risk for electrical hazards in the home environment (Box 33-11).

If a client receives an electrical shock in a health care setting, the nurse should immediately determine whether the client has a pulse. If the client has no pulse, cardiopulmonary resuscitation should be initiated and emergency personnel should be notified. If the client has a pulse and remains alert and oriented, the nurse should quickly obtain vital signs and assess the skin for signs of thermal injury. The client's physician must be notified. If an electrical shock occurs in the home, the nurse follows the same procedure but has the client go to the emergency department and then notifies the client's physician.

Box 33-10 Procedural Guidelines

Interventions for Accidental Poisoning

1. Assess for airway patency, breathing, and circulation (ABCs) in all clients in whom accidental poisoning is suspected.
2. Remove any visible materials from areas such as the mouth and eyes to terminate exposure.
3. Identify the type and amount of substance ingested, if possible. This may help to determine the antidote.
4. Call your local poison control centre before attempting any interventions.
5. If directed by a physician, give oral fluids to assist vomiting.
6. If directed, save vomitus for laboratory analysis, which may assist with further treatment.
7. Position the victim with the head to the side to prevent aspiration of vomitus, and assist in keeping the airway open.
8. Never induce vomiting in an unconscious person or in a person experiencing convulsions, because aspiration may occur.
9. Never induce vomiting if any of the following substances have been ingested: lye, household cleaners, hair care products, grease or petroleum products, or furniture polish. Vomiting may increase internal burns.
10. If instructed to take the victim to the emergency department, call an ambulance. Emergency equipment may be needed en route.
11. In the case of convulsions, cessation of breathing, or unconsciousness, call 911.
12. Do not administer syrup of ipecac to induce vomiting. It has not been proven effective in preventing poisoning (American Academy of Pediatrics, 2004).

From *Don't Treat Swallowed Poison With Syrup of Ipecac Says AAP* [News release], American Academy of Pediatrics, 2004, retrieved December 4, 2004, from *www.aap.org/advocacy/archives/novpoison.htm*

Seizures. Clients who have experienced some form of neurological injury or metabolic disturbance are at risk for a seizure. A seizure involves a hyperexcitation of neurons in the brain, leading to a sudden, violent, involuntary series of contractions of a group of muscles. The client often loses consciousness. **Seizure precautions** are nursing interventions during and after a seizure and include protecting the client from traumatic injury, positioning for adequate ventilation and drainage of oral secretions, and providing privacy and support following the seizure (Skill 33-2).

During a seizure, a client's jaw muscles can become tense. However, significant injury to the client's oral cavity is rare, even during the most violent seizures. Injury may instead occur from a caregiver forcing an object into the client's mouth and from the teeth biting down on a hard object. Soft objects may break in the mouth during a seizure and be aspirated. Therefore, Epilepsy Canada recommends not inserting objects into the person's mouth during a seizure (2004). The exception is in the case of

Client Teaching — Box 33-11

Prevention of Electrical Hazards

Objective

- Client will recognize electrical hazards in the home and eliminate them.

Teaching Strategies

- Discuss grounding appliances and other equipment.
- Provide examples of common hazards: frayed cords, damaged equipment, and overloaded outlets.
- Discuss guidelines to prevent electrical shocks:
  - Use extension cords only when necessary, and use electrical tape to secure the cord to the floor where it will not be stepped on.
  - Do not run wires under carpeting.
  - Grasp the plug, not the cord, when unplugging items.
  - Keep electrical items away from water.
  - Do not operate unfamiliar equipment.
  - Disconnect items before cleaning.

Evaluation

- Have client list electrical hazards existing in the home.
- Review steps the client will take to eliminate these hazards.
- Check the home after the client has had an opportunity to eliminate hazards.

Skill 33-2 Seizure Precautions

Delegation Considerations

Assessment of a client's need for seizure precautions cannot be delegated. If a seizure occurs, the nurse must constantly assess the client's airway patency, adequacy of breathing, and circulatory status. Clinical judgments must be made quickly. Setting up seizure precautions and protecting clients at risk for seizures may be delegated to unregulated care providers (UCPs).

- Have the UCP protect at-risk clients from falls by assisting with ambulation and transfer.
- Caution the UCP against any attempt to restrain client's extremities during a seizure.

Equipment

- Oral airway
- Padding for side rails and headboard
- Suction machine, oral suction equipment
- Disposable gloves

Steps	Rationale
1. Assess seizure history, noting frequency of seizures, presence of aura, and sequence of events, if known. Assess for medical and surgical conditions that may lead to seizures or exacerbate existing seizure condition. Assess medication history.	This enables the nurse to anticipate onset of seizure activity. Seizure medications must be taken as prescribed and not stopped suddenly, because this may precipitate seizure activity.
2. Inspect client's environment for potential safety hazards if risk for seizure exists: bedside stand or table, IV pole or other medical equipment.	Prevents client from sustaining injury by striking head or body on furniture or equipment.
3. Perform hand hygiene and prepare bed with padded side rails and headboard, bed in low position, and client positioned in side-lying position when possible (see illustration).	Minimizes risks associated with seizure activity.
4. For clients with a history of seizures, an airway (see illustration), suction apparatus, disposable gloves, and pillows should be visible in the hospital setting for immediate use.	This ensures prompt, organized intervention.
5. When a seizure begins, position client safely. If client is standing or sitting, guide client to floor and protect head by cradling in nurse's lap or placing a pillow under head. Clear surrounding area of furniture. If client is in bed, raise side rails, add padding, and put bed in low position.	Protects client from traumatic injury, especially head injury.

Steps	Rationale

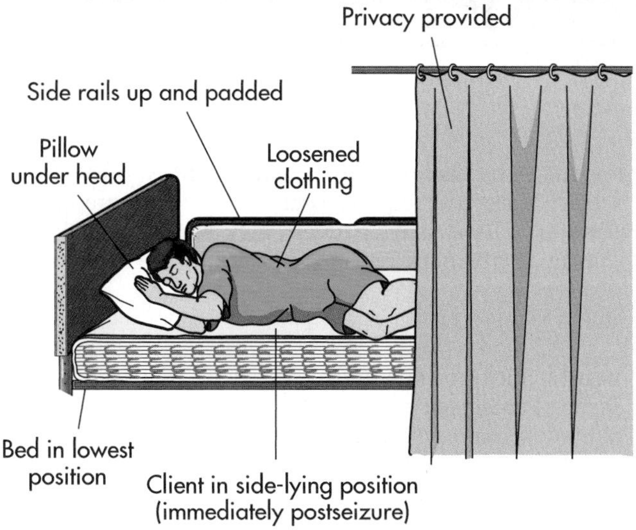

STEP **3** Provide client privacy. Put bed in lowest position with side rails up and padded. Position client in side-lying position, with pillow under head and loosened clothing.

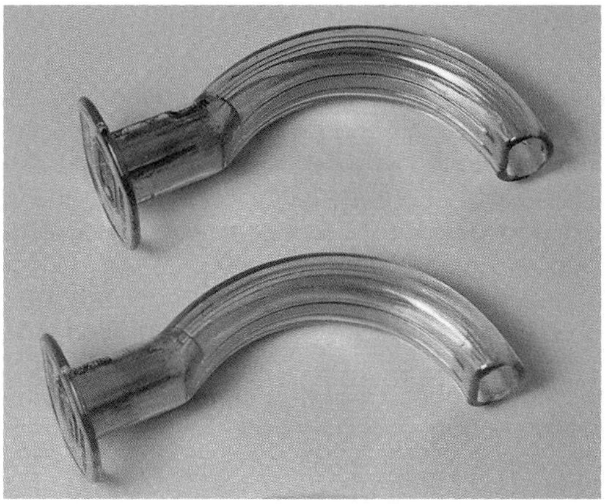

STEP **4** Oral airways.

Steps	Rationale
6. Provide privacy.	Embarrassment is common after a seizure, especially if others witnessed the seizure.
7. If possible, turn client on side, with head flexed slightly forward.	Prevents tongue and dentures from blocking the airway and promotes drainage of secretions, thus reducing risk of aspiration.
8. Do not restrain client. Loosen clothing.	Prevents musculoskeletal injury.
9. Do not put anything into the client's mouth such as fingers, tongue depressor, or medicine.	

Critical Decision Point: Putting something in the client's mouth could result in injury to the jaw, tongue, or teeth and cause stimulation of the gag reflex, causing vomiting, aspiration, and respiratory distress (National Institute of Neurological Disorders and Stroke, 2001).

Steps	Rationale
10. Stay with client, observing the sequence and timing of seizure activity.	Continued observation is necessary to ensure adequate ventilation during and following seizure activity. Accurate, specific observations will assist in documentation, diagnosis, and treatment of the seizure disorder.
11. After the seizure is over, explain what happened and answer client's questions. Foster an atmosphere of acceptance and respect.	Informing clients of the type of seizure activity experienced will assist them in participating knowledgeably in their care.
12. Following seizure, perform hand hygiene and assist client to position of comfort in bed with padded side rails up and bed in low position. Place call light within reach, and provide a quiet, non-stimulating environment.	Provides for continued safety. Clients are often confused and sleepy following a seizure.

Skill 33-2 Seizure Precautions—cont'd

Status Epilepticus

Steps	Rationale
13. For a client experiencing status epilepticus, put on disposable gloves and insert an oral airway (see illustration for Step 4) when the jaw is relaxed between seizure activity. Hold airway with curved side up, insert downward until airway reaches back of throat, then rotate and follow natural curve of the tongue. Do not place fingers near or in client's mouth.	Prevents transmission of infection. Client is in continual seizure state and requires oral airway to ensure airway patency. Client may inadvertently bite nurse's fingers during a seizure if caution is not used.
14. Access oxygen and suction equipment. Prepare for IV insertion.	Intensive monitoring and treatment are required for this medical emergency.
15. Use pillows/pads to protect client from injuring self.	Traumatic injury will be avoided.

Unexpected Outcomes and Related Interventions

- Client suffers traumatic injury.
  - Continue to protect client from further injury.
  - Notify the physician immediately.
  - Ensure environment is free of safety hazards.
- Client verbalizes feelings of embarrassment and humiliation.
  - Offer support, and allow client to verbalize feelings.
  - Encourage client and family to participate in decision making and planning care.

Recording and Reporting

- Record the timing of seizure activity and sequence of events. Record presence of aura (if any), level of consciousness, posture, colour, movements of extremities, incontinence, and patterns of sleep following the seizure.
- Document client's response and expected or unexpected outcomes.
- Report to physician immediately as seizure begins.
- Status epilepticus is an emergency situation requiring immediate medical management.

Home Care Considerations

- Communicate with client and family to identify precipitating factors.
- Teach family to care for the client during a seizure.
- Client's home should be assessed for environmental hazards in light of seizure condition.
- Provide family with guidelines to detect status epilepticus.
- Until a seizure condition is well controlled (usually for at least 1 year), the client should not take a tub bath or engage in activities such as swimming unless a knowledgeable family member is present. Driving may also be restricted during this time.
- Client should wear a medical alert bracelet or tag and have an ID card noting the presence of a seizure disorder and listing the medications taken.
- Referral to a support group or Epilepsy Canada may help to improve client's self-esteem and coping ability.

status epilepticus, a medical emergency whereby a person has continual seizures without interruption. An adequate airway is maintained with an oral airway. Clients experiencing a seizure are never restrained but are placed on seizure precautions.

Radiation. Radiation is a health hazard in the health care setting and the community. Radiation and radioactive materials are used in the diagnosis and treatment of clients. Hospitals have strict guidelines on the care of clients who are receiving radiation and radioactive materials. The nurse must be familiar with established agency protocols. The nurse's exposure to radiation can be reduced by limiting time spent near the source, making the distance from the source as great as possible, and using shielding devices such as lead aprons. Staff working near radiation wear devices that track the accumulative exposure to radiation.

The community may be at risk for radiation exposure because of incorrect disposal and transportation of radioactive waste products. The Canadian Nuclear Safety Commission ensures that disposal of radioactive waste does not pose a danger for the public or the environment. If a radioactive leak occurs, these agencies institute measures to prevent exposure of surrounding neighbourhoods, to clean up radioactive leaks as quickly as possible, and to ensure that injured parties receive prompt medical care.

NP Evaluation

Client Care. The components of critical thinking are applied to the evaluation step of the nursing process (Figure 33–19). The actual care delivered by the health care team is evaluated on the basis of expected outcomes. If the

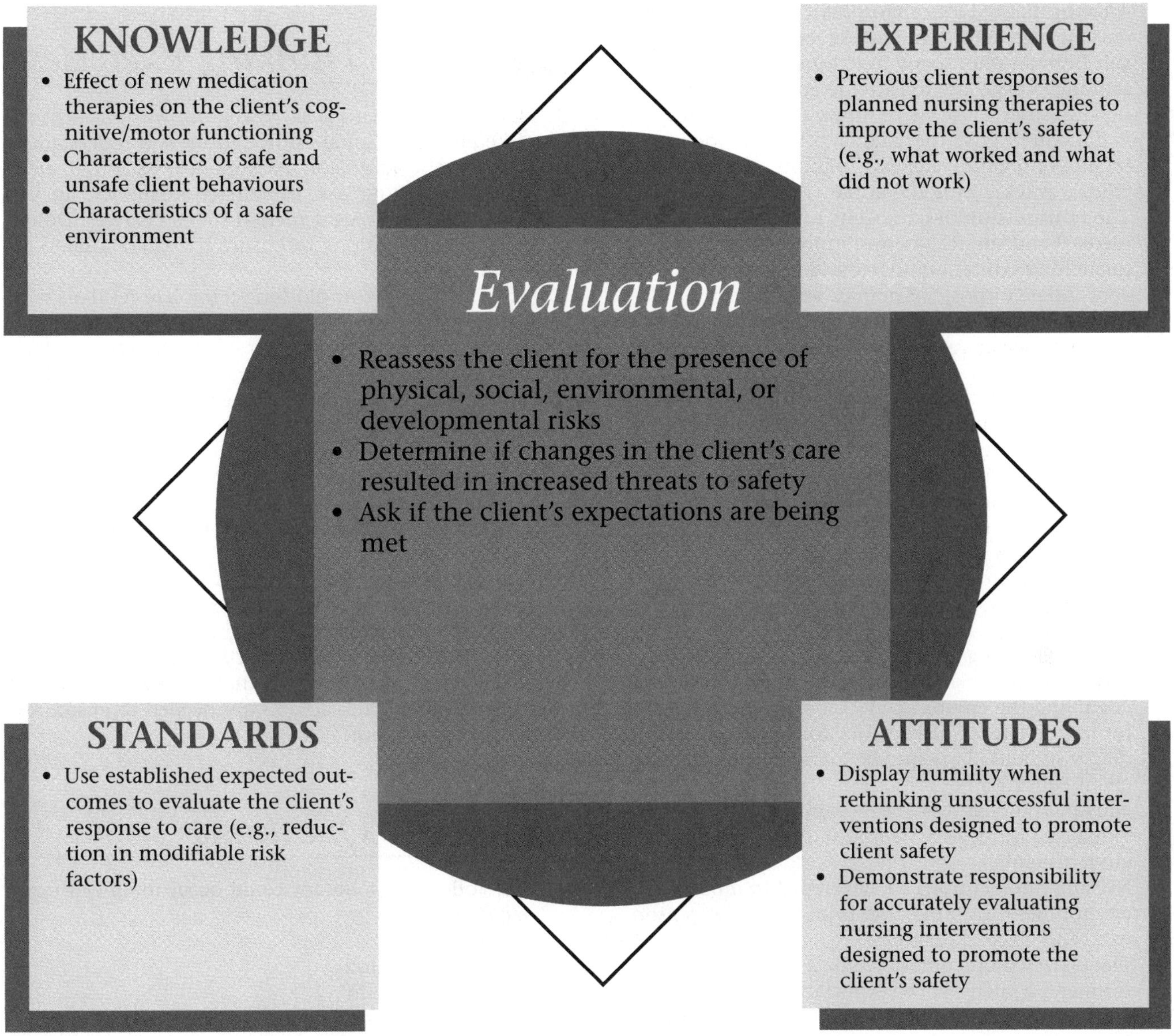
KNOWLEDGE
• Effect of new medication therapies on the client's cognitive/motor functioning
• Characteristics of safe and unsafe client behaviours
• Characteristics of a safe environment
EXPERIENCE
• Previous client responses to planned nursing therapies to improve the client's safety (e.g., what worked and what did not work)
Evaluation
• Reassess the client for the presence of physical, social, environmental, or developmental risks
• Determine if changes in the client's care resulted in increased threats to safety
• Ask if the client's expectations are being met
STANDARDS
• Use established expected outcomes to evaluate the client's response to care (e.g., reduction in modifiable risk factors)
ATTITUDES
• Display humility when rethinking unsuccessful interventions designed to promote client safety
• Demonstrate responsibility for accurately evaluating nursing interventions designed to promote the client's safety

FIGURE **33–19** Critical thinking model for safety evaluation.

client's goals have been met, the nursing interventions can be considered effective and appropriate. If not, the nurse determines whether new risks to the client have developed or whether previous risks remain. The client and family need to participate to find permanent ways to reduce risks to safety. The nurse continually assesses the client's and family's need for additional support services such as home care, physiotherapy, counselling, and further teaching.

Client Expectations. When the nurse has developed a good relationship with a client and the client feels safe and secure in the environment, the client will most likely demonstrate satisfaction. The nurse must determine, however, if client expectations have been met. Is the client satisfied with any changes made to the environment? Does the client believe that his or her safety is ensured? If client expectations have not been met, the nurse must reassess not only the client and the environment, but also the client's expressed desires.

Key Concepts

- A safe environment is essential to promoting, maintaining, and restoring health.
- In the community, a safe environment is one in which basic needs are achievable, physical hazards are reduced, transmission of pathogens is reduced, pollution is controlled, and sanitation is maintained.
- In a health care agency, a safe environment is one that minimizes falls, client-inherent accidents, procedure-inherent accidents, and equipment-related accidents.

- A factor that reduces atmospheric oxygen is the presence of high carbon monoxide levels, which may result from an improperly functioning furnace.
- Prolonged exposure to extreme environmental temperatures can cause client injury or even death.
- Reduction of physical hazards in the environment includes providing adequate lighting, decreasing clutter, and securing the home.
- The transmission of pathogens is reduced through medical and surgical asepsis, immunization, adequate food sanitation, insect and rodent control, and appropriate disposal of human waste.
- Children less than 5 years of age are at greatest risk for home accidents that may result in severe injury and death.
- The school-age child is at risk for injury at home, at school, and while travelling to and from school.
- Adolescents are at risk for injury from automobile accidents, suicide, and substance abuse.
- Threats to an adult's safety are frequently associated with lifestyle habits.
- Risks of injury for older clients are directly related to the physiological changes of the aging process; falls are the greatest cause of accidental injury in older adults.
- By incorporating critical thinking skills in the application of the nursing process, the nurse assesses the client and the environment to determine risk factors for injury; clusters risk factors; formulates a nursing diagnosis; and plans specific interventions, including client education.
- Nursing interventions for promoting safety are individualized for developmental stage, lifestyle, and environment.
- Nursing interventions are developed to modify the environment for protection from falls, fires, poisonings, and electrical hazards.
- The expected outcomes include a safe physical environment, a client whose expectations have been met and who is knowledgeable about safety factors and precautions, and a client free of injury.

Key Terms

Air pollution, *p. 974*
Ambularm, *p. 993*
Aura, *p. 977*
Carbon monoxide, *p. 972*
Environment, *p. 971*
Food poisoning, *p. 972*
Hypothermia, *p. 972*
Immunization, *p. 973*
Land pollution, *p. 974*
Material Safety Data Sheets (MSDS), *p. 976*
Noise pollution, *p. 974*
Pathogen, *p. 973*
Poison, *p. 1002*
Pollutant, *p. 974*
Relative humidity, *p. 972*
Restraint, *p. 990*
Seizure, *p. 977*
Seizure precautions, *p. 1003*
Status epilepticus, *p. 1006*
Water pollution, *p. 974*
Workplace Hazardous Materials Information System (WHMIS), *p. 976*

Critical Thinking Exercises

1. Mrs. Santiago, who is 88 years old, was recently admitted to the hospital. Although she was independent at home, the admission assessment reveals that she is at risk for falling due to urinary frequency, an unsteady gait, and recent mental status changes. Design specific interventions to ensure the client's safety in the hospital.
2. Mrs. Patel, a 76-year-old long-term care resident with Alzheimer's disease, has been refusing food and fluids for the past month. The family has agreed to placement of a nasogatric tube to improve her fluid and nutritional status. Shortly after the first tube feeding was started, Mrs. Patel became more restless, and she has been picking at the tube.
   a. What might be precipitating Mrs. Patel's behaviour of picking at the tube?
   b. What approaches can be used to eliminate interference with the treatment?
   c. If a restraint is necessary to avoid disruption of therapy, what interventions are necessary to ensure the client's safety while in restraints?
3. A family member reports that a lit cigarette dropped on the client's mattress, but they were able to put out the small fire. What actions are needed to ensure the safety of this client?

Review Questions

1. The following pollutant could occur in a health care facility:
   1. Air pollution
   2. Water pollution
   3. Noise pollution
   4. Bioactive waste pollution

2. Accidental injuries are the leading cause of death for which age group?
   1. 1 to 12 months
   2. 1 to 44 years
   3. 45 to 64 years
   4. 65 years and over

3. What are the three leading causes of accidental death in Canada?
   1. Motor vehicle accidents, fire, poisoning
   2. Suffocation, falls, drownings
   3. Falls, motor vehicle accidents, fire
   4. Falls, motor vehicle accidents, machinery accidents

4. Adolescents are at a greater risk for injury from
   1. Poisoning
   2. Motor vehicle accidents, suicide, and substance abuse
   3. Home accidents
   4. Falls

5. The physiological changes caused by aging increase the older client's risk for
   1. Falls
   2. Suicide
   3. Alcoholism
   4. Seizures
6. WHMIS is a system to control hazardous substances in the workplace and involves
   1. Environmental interventions
   2. Worker education programs, cautionary labelling of products, and provision of Material Safety Data Sheets (MSDSs)
   3. Client education programs
   4. Risk assessment
7. Medication and fluid administration errors and improper application of external devices are examples of
   1. Client-inherent accidents
   2. Procedure-related accidents
   3. Equipment-related accidents
   4. Environmental-related accidents
8. Which of the following statements about restraints is NOT true?
   1. Restraints are used only after other alternatives have been tried.
   2. The least restrictive method of restraint is used.
   3. Restraints are considered a long-term intervention.
   4. Use of restraints must be part of the clients' medical treatment.
9. When teaching parents about responding to poisoning in children, the nurse should instruct them to
   1. Give oral fluids
   2. Induce vomiting
   3. Call the local poison control centre
   4. Drive the child to the emergency department
10. Seizure precautions include the following, EXCEPT
   1. Positioning for adequate ventilation and drainage of oral secretions
   2. Protecting the client from traumatic injury
   3. Providing privacy and support following the seizure
   4. Inserting a tongue depressor into the mouth to protect the jaw

References

Agency for Healthcare Research and Quality. (2000). Reducing errors in health care: Translating research into practice. AHRQ publication No. 00-PO58. Retrieved March 14, 2005, from *http://www.ahrq.gov/research/errors.htm*

American Academy of Pediatrics. (2004). *Don't treat swallowed poison with syrup of ipecac says AAP* [News release]. Retrieved December 4, 2004, from *www.aap.org/advocacy/archives/novpoison.htm*

American Geriatrics Society, British Geriatrics Society, & American Academy of Orthopaedic Surgeons Panel on Falls Prevention. (2001). Guideline for the prevention of falls in older persons. *Journal of the American Geriatrics Society, 49*(5), 664–672.

Baker, G. R., et al. (2004). The Canadian adverse events study: The incidence of adverse events among hospital patients in Canada [Electronic version]. *Canadian Medical Association Journal, 170*(11), 1678–1686.

Beare, P., & Meyers, J. (1998). *Adult health nursing* (3rd ed.). St. Louis, MO: Mosby.

Canada Safety Council. (2004). *Home fire safety basics.* Retrieved August 9, 2004, from *http://www.safety-council.org/info/home/homefire.htm*

Canadian Centre for Occupational Health and Safety. *WHMIS labeling requirements.* Retrieved December 8, 2004, from *http://www.ccohs.ca/oshanswers/legisl/msds_lab.html*

Canadian Institute for Health Information. (2003). *National trauma registry report: Major injury in Canada* [Electronic version]. Ottawa, ON: Author.

Canadian Institute for Health Information. (2004a). *National trauma registry report: Injury hospitalizations* [Electronic version]. Ottawa, ON: Author.

Canadian Institute for Health Information. (2004b). *National trauma registry report: Major injury in Canada* [Electronic version]. Ottawa, ON: Author.

Canadian Nurses Association & University of Toronto Faculty of Nursing. (2004). *Nurses and patient safety: A discussion paper* [Electronic version]. Ottawa, ON: Author.

Canadian Pediatric Society. (1999). *Reducing the risk of sudden infant death syndrome in Canada.* Retrieved May 30, 2004, from *http://www.cps.ca/english/statements/IP/cps98-01.htm*

Capezuti, E. (2000). Preventing falls and injuries while reducing siderail use. *Annals of Long-Term Care, 8*(6), 57–63.

College of Nurses of Ontario. (2004). *Practice standard: Restraints* [Electronic version]. Toronto, ON: Author.

Dochterman, J. M., & Bulechek, G. M. (Eds.). (2004). *Nursing interventions classification (NIC)* (4th ed.). St. Louis, MO: Mosby.

Ebersole, P., & Hess, P. (2001). *Geriatric nursing and healthy aging.* St. Louis, MO: Mosby.

Ebersole, P., & Hess, P. (2003). *Toward healthy aging* (6th ed.). St. Louis, MO: Mosby.

Edelman, C. L., & Mandle, C. L. (1998). *Health promotion throughout the lifespan* (4th ed.). St. Louis, MO: Mosby.

Epilepsy Canada. (2004). *First aid for seizure treatment.* Retrieved May 28, 2004, from *http://www.epilepsy.ca/eng/content/firstaid.html*

Farmer, B. (2000). *Try this: Best practices in nursing care to older adults.* New York: The Hartford Institute for Geriatric Nursing, New York University.

Federal, Provincial, and Territorial Advisory Committee on Population Health. (1999, September). *Statistical report on the health of Canadians.* Prepared for the Meeting of Ministers of Health. Charlottetown, PE: Author.

Health Canada. (2002). *Lead information package: Some commonly asked questions about lead and human health.* Retrieved May 26, 2004, from *http://www.hc-sc.gc.ca/hecs-sesc/toxics_management/publications/leadQandA/print.htm*

Health Canada. (2003). Workplace Hazardous Materials Information System Web site. Retrieved May 25, 2004, from *http://www.hc-sc.gc.ca/hecs-sesc/whmis/*

Health Canada. (2004a). *Hepatitis: A fact sheet.* Retrieved May 25, 2004, from *http://www.hc-sc.gc.ca/pphb-dgspsp/hcai-iamss/bbp-pts/hepatitis/hep_a_e.html*

Health Canada. (2004b). *Proper use and disposal of medication.* Retrieved February 24, 2005, from *www.hc-sc.gc.ca/english/pdf/iyh/medication_disposal_e.pdf*

Home fire prevention and preparedness fact sheet. (2002). Itasca, IL: National Safety Council.

Hynes-Gay, P., et al. (2003). Severe acute respiratory syndrome: The Mount Sinai experience. *Canadian Nurse, 99*(5), 17–19.

Kollek, D. (2003). Canadian emergency department preparedness for a nuclear, biological or chemical event. *Canadian Journal of Emergency Medicine, 5*(1). Retrieved May 26, 2004, from *http://www.caep.ca/004.cjem-jcmu/004-00.cjem/vol-5.2003/v51-018.htm#main*

Ledford, L., & Mentals, J. (1998). *"Restraints"—A research-based protocol.* City: University of Iowa Gerontological Nursing Interventions Research Center.

Leonard, C., et al. (1998). The effect of fatigue, sleep deprivation and onerous working hours on the physical wellbeing of pre-registration house officers. *Irish Journal of Medical Science, 167*(1), 22–25.

Lueckenotte, A. G. (2000). *Gerontologic nursing.* St. Louis, MO: Mosby.

Moorhead, S., Johnson, M., & Maas, M. L. (Eds.). (2004). *Nursing outcomes classification (NIC)* (3rd ed.). St. Louis, MO: Mosby.

National Steering Committee on Patient Safety. (2002). *Building a safer system: A national integrated strategy for improving patient safety in Canadian health care* [Electronic version]. Ottawa, ON: Author.

Quinn, C. A. (1996). The advanced practice nurse and changing perspectives on physical restraint. *Clinical Nurse Specialist, 10*(5), 220–225.

Registered Nurses Association of Ontario. (2005). *Nursing best practice guideline: Prevention of falls and fall injuries in the older adult* (Revised; Electronic version). Toronto, ON: Author.

Schoenfelder, D. P. (2000). A fall prevention program for elderly individuals: Exercise in long-term care settings. *Journal of Gerontological Nursing, 26*(3), 43–51.

SMARTRISK. (1998). *The economic burden of unintentional injury in Canada* [Electronic version]. City, ON: Author.

Sorrentino, S. A. (1999). *Mosby's assisting with patient care.* St. Louis, MO: Mosby.

Sorrentino, S. A. (2000). *Mosby's textbook for nursing assistants* (5th ed.). St. Louis, MO: Mosby.

St. John, R., & Giroux, C. (2002). Terrorism and public health: The little known equation. *Canadian Journal of Public Health, 93*(3), 165–166. Retrieved May 26, 2003, from *http://gateway.proquest.com/openurl?url_ver=Z39.88-2004&res_dat=xri:pqd&rft_val_fmt=info:ofi/fmt:kev:mtx:journal&genre=article&rft_dat=xri:pqd:did=000000124842681&svc_dat=xri:pqil:fmt=text&req_dat=xri:pqil:pq_clntid=10120*

Strumpf, N., et al. (1998). *Restraint free care: Individualized approaches for frail elders.* New York: Springer.

Technical Standards and Safety Authority. (2004). *Danger! Carbon monoxide: What you need to know to protect you and your family from the "silent killer."* Retrieved May 25, 2004, from *http://www.tssa.org/about_tssa/carbon_monoxide.asp*

Tideiksaar, R. (1989). Home safe home: Practical tips for fall-proofing. *Geriatric Nursing, 11*(6), 280–284.

Vanier Institute of the Family. (2000). *Profiling Canada's families II.* Nepean, ON: Author.

Williams, S. R. (2000). *Basic nutrition and diet therapy* (11th ed.). St. Louis, MO: Mosby.

Wong, D. L. (2003). *Wong's nursing care of infants and children* (7th ed.). St. Louis, MO: Mosby.

Zusman, J. (2001). *Restraint and seclusion: Understanding the JCAHO standards and federal regulations* (3rd ed.). Marblehead, MA: Opus Communications.

Recommended Web Sites

Canada Safety Council:
http://www.safety-council.org/

The Canada Safety Council is a national, non-government, charitable organization dedicated to providing safety education. Its mission is to reduce preventable deaths and injuries in public and private places throughout Canada.

Canadian Patient Safety Institute:
http://www.hc-sc.gc.ca/english/care/cpsi.html

Part of Health Canada, the Canadian Patient Safety Institute has been a leader in addressing client safety issues in Canadian health care agencies. This Web site provides links to various topics relevant to promoting client safety.

Safe Kids Canada:
http://www.sickkids.ca/safekidscanada.

Part of the national injury prevention program at Toronto's Hospital for Sick Children, Safe Kids Canada offers information on a range of safety topics in order to prevent accidental injuries in children.

SMARTRISK:
http://www.smartrisk.ca/

SMARTRISK is a national non-profit organization dedicated to preventing injuries and saving lives. Founded in 1992, SMARTRISK has become one of the leading injury prevention groups in Canada and enjoys international recognition and support.

Workplace Hazardous Materials Information System:
http://www.hc-sc.gc.ca/hecs-sesc/whmis/

This site is developed and maintained by Health Canada's Workplace Hazardous Materials Information System (WHMIS) Division and includes policies and information related to WHMIS.

34

Hygiene

Anne Griffin Perry, RN, MSN, EdD, FAAN
Susanna Edwards, RN, BScN, MSc, PhD(pc) (Canadian author)

Objectives

Mastery of content in this chapter will enable the student to:

- Define the key terms listed.
- Describe factors that influence personal hygiene practices.
- Discuss the role that critical thinking plays in the provision of hygiene care.
- Conduct a comprehensive assessment of a client's total hygiene needs.
- Discuss conditions that place clients at risk for impaired skin integrity.
- Discuss factors that influence the condition of the nails and feet.
- Explain the importance of foot care for the diabetic client.
- Discuss conditions that place clients at risk for impaired oral mucous membranes.
- List common hair and scalp problems and their related interventions.
- Describe how hygiene care for the older client may differ from that for the younger client.
- Discuss the different approaches used in maintaining a client's comfort during hygiene care.
- Successfully perform hygiene procedures for the care of the skin, perineum, feet and nails, mouth, eyes, ears, and nose.

Personal hygiene affects an individual's comfort, safety, and well-being. Well people are capable of meeting their own hygiene needs. People who are ill or have disabilities may require various levels of assistance. A variety of personal, social, and cultural factors influence hygiene practices. In agency or home care settings, the nurse determines a client's ability to perform self-care and provides hygiene care according to the client's needs and preferences. In the home setting, the nurse also assists in helping the client and family adapt hygiene techniques and approaches.

Because hygiene care requires close contact with the client, the nurse uses communication skills (see chapter 14) to promote a caring therapeutic relationship and to use the time with the client for teaching and counselling. The nurse can integrate other nursing activities during hygiene care, including client assessment and interventions such as range-of-motion exercises, application of dressings, or inspection and care of intravenous (IV) sites. During hygiene care, the nurse tries to preserve as much of the client's independence as possible, ensure privacy, convey respect, and foster the client's physical comfort.

Scientific Knowledge Base

Proper hygiene care requires an understanding of the anatomy and physiology of the integument, oral cavity, and the eyes, ears, and nose. The skin and mucosa cells exchange oxygen, nutrients, and fluids with underlying blood vessels. The cells require adequate nutrition, hydration, and circulation to resist injury and disease. Good hygiene techniques promote the normal structure and function of body tissues.

In addition, the nurse must apply knowledge of pathophysiology to provide good preventive hygiene care. The nurse learns to recognize disease states that create changes in the integument, oral cavity, and sensory organs. For example, diabetes mellitus results in chronic vascular changes that impair healing of the skin and mucosa. In the early stages of acquired immunodeficiency syndrome (AIDS), fungal infections of the oral cavity are common. As a result of a stroke, paralysis of the trigeminal nerve eliminates the blink reflex, causing risk of corneal drying. In the presence of conditions such as these, the nurse adapts hygiene practices to anticipate client needs and minimize any harmful effects. By integrating knowledge of anatomy, physiology, and pathophysiology during hygiene care, nurses can recognize abnormalities and initiate appropriate actions to prevent further injury.

The Skin

The skin is an active organ with the functions of protection, secretion, excretion, temperature regulation, and sensation (Table 34-1). The skin has three primary layers: epidermis, dermis, and subcutaneous. The **epidermis** (outer layer) is composed of several thin layers of cells undergoing different stages of maturation. It shields underlying tissue against water loss and injury and prevents entry of disease-producing micro-organisms. The innermost layer of the epidermis generates new cells to replace the dead cells that are continuously shed from the skin's outer surface. Bacteria commonly reside on the outer epidermis. These resident bacteria are normal flora (see chapter 29) that do not cause disease but instead inhibit the multiplication of disease-causing micro-organisms.

The **dermis** is a thicker skin layer containing bundles of collagen and elastic fibres to support the epidermis. Nerve fibres, blood vessels, sweat glands, sebaceous glands, and hair follicles course through the dermal layers. Sebaceous glands secrete sebum, an oily, odorous fluid, into the hair follicles.

The subcutaneous tissue layer contains blood vessels, nerves, lymph, and loose connective tissue filled with fat cells. The fatty tissue is a heat insulator for the body. Subcutaneous tissue also supports upper skin layers to withstand stresses and pressure without injury. Very little subcutaneous tissue underlies the oral mucosa.

The skin often reflects a change in physical condition by alterations in colour, thickness, texture, turgor, temperature, and hydration (Box 34-1; see chapter 28). As long as the skin remains intact and healthy, its physiological function remains optimal.

Table 34-1 Function of the Skin and Implications for Care

Function/Description	Implications for Care
Protection	
The epidermis is a relatively impermeable layer that prevents entrance of micro-organisms. Although micro-organisms reside on skin surface and in hair follicles, relative dryness of skin's surface inhibits bacterial growth. Sebum removes bacteria from hair follicles. Acidic pH of skin further retards bacterial growth.	Weakening of epidermis occurs by scraping or stripping its surface (e.g., use of dry razors, tape removal, or improper turning or positioning techniques). Excessive dryness causes cracks and breaks in skin and mucosa that allow bacteria to enter. Emollients soften skin and prevent moisture loss, and hydration of mucosa prevents dryness. Constant exposure of skin to moisture can cause maceration (softening), which interrupts dermal integrity and promotes ulcer formation and bacterial growth. Bed linen and clothing should be kept dry. Misuse of soap, detergents, cosmetics, deodorant, and depilatories can cause chemical irritation. Alkaline soaps neutralize the protective acid condition of skin. Cleansing of skin removes excess oil, sweat, dead skin cells, and dirt that can promote bacterial growth. Bath water should not be excessively hot or cold.
Sensation	
Skin contains sensory organs for touch, pain, heat, cold, and pressure.	Friction should be minimized to avoid loss of stratum corneum, which can result in development of pressure ulcers. Smoothing linen removes sources of mechanical irritation. The nurse can prevent accidental injury of the client's skin by removing jewellery before giving care.
Temperature Regulation	
Body temperature is controlled by radiation, evaporation, conduction, and convection.	Factors that interfere with heat loss can alter temperature control. Wet bed linen or gowns interfere with convection and conduction. Excess blankets or bed coverings can interfere with heat loss through radiation and conduction. Coverings can promote heat conservation.
Excretion and Secretion	
Sweat promotes heat loss by evaporation. Sebum lubricates skin and hair.	Perspiration and oil can harbour micro-organisms. Bathing removes excess body secretions, although if excessive, it can cause drying of skin.

Cultural Aspects of Care Box 34-1

Identifying changes in skin colour and determining if these changes are normal reactive hyperemia or abnormal reactive hyperemia is important in evaluating clients' risks for pressure ulcers (see chapter 43). When the client's natural skin contains more melanin, it is more difficult to determine abnormal reactive hyperemia and cyanosis. There are normal hyperpigmentation areas, such a Mongolian spots, which may be on the sacrum of African, Aboriginal, and Asian clients. These areas should not be confused with skin colour changes such as abnormal reactive hyperemia or cyanosis.

Implications for Practice

- For dark-skinned clients, assess baseline skin tone by asking the client or family to point out an area of baseline skin colour for that person.
- Frequently assess for changes in baseline skin tone and skin temperature over pressure areas.
- Use natural light sources when possible because fluorescent light sources cast a bluish hue on darkly pigmented skin tones.
- Examine body sites with least melanin for underlying skin colour identification.

Data from "Detection of Cyanosis in the Person With Dark Skin," by F. C. Gaskin, 1986, *Journal of National Black Nurses' Association, 1,* pp. 52–60; "Report of the Task Force on the Implications for Darkly Pigmented Intact Skin in the Prediction and Prevention of Pressure Ulcers," by M. A. Bennet, 1995, *Advances in Wound Care, 8*(6), pp. 34–35; and "Draft Definition of Stage I Pressure Ulcers: Inclusion of Persons With Darkly Pigmented Skin," by C. T. Henderson, et al., 1997, *Advances in Wound Care, 10*(5), pp. 16–19.

The Feet, Hands, and Nails

The feet, hands, and nails often require special attention to prevent infection. Any injury or deformity to the foot, including growths or injuries to the overlying skin, can be painful and thus interfere with a client's normal ability to walk and bear weight. The hand, in contrast to the foot, is constructed largely for manipulation rather than support.

Dexterity exists in the hand because of the wide range of movement between the thumb and fingers. Any condition that interferes with movement of the hand (e.g., superficial or deep pain or joint inflammation) can impair a client's self-help abilities.

The nails are epithelial tissues that grow from the root of the nail bed, located in the skin at the nail groove, hidden by the fold of skin called the **cuticle.** The visible part of the nail is the nail body. It has a crescent-shaped white area known as the **lunula.** Under the nail lies a layer of epithelium called the nail bed (Figure 34–1). A healthy nail for light-skinned individuals is transparent, smooth, and convex, with a pink nail bed and translucent white tip. Disease can cause changes in the shape, thickness, and curvature of the nail (see chapter 28).

The Oral Cavity

The oral cavity is lined with mucous membranes continuous with the skin. The oral or buccal cavity consists of the lips surrounding the opening of the mouth, the cheeks running along the side walls of the cavity, the tongue and its muscles, and the hard and soft palate. The oral mucosa is normally light pink and moist. The floor of the mouth and the undersurface of the tongue are richly supplied with blood vessels. Any type of ulceration or trauma can result in significant bleeding. There are three pairs of salivary glands that secrete about 1 liter of saliva a day. The **buccal glands** found in the mucosa lining the cheeks and mouth maintain the hygiene and comfort of oral tissues. Salivary secretion in the mouth can be impaired through the effects of medications, exposure to radiation, and mouth breathing.

The teeth are the organs of chewing, or **mastication.** They are designed to cut, tear, and grind ingested food so that it can be mixed with saliva and swallowed. A normal tooth consists of the crown, neck, and root (Figure 34–2). The periodontal membrane lies just below the gum margins, surrounds a tooth, and holds it firmly in place. Healthy teeth appear white, smooth, shiny, and properly aligned.

Difficulty in chewing can develop when surrounding gum tissues become inflamed or infected or when teeth are lost or become loosened. Regular oral hygiene is necessary to maintain the integrity of tooth surfaces and to prevent **gingivitis,** or gum inflammation.

The Hair

Hair growth, distribution, and pattern can indicate a person's general health status. Hormonal changes, emotional and physical stress, aging, infection, and certain illnesses can affect hair characteristics. The hair shaft itself is inert and cannot be directly affected by physiological factors. However, changes in its colour or condition are caused by hormonal and nutrient deficiencies of the hair follicle (Figure 34–3).

The Eyes, Ears, and Nose

When nurses provide hygiene care, the eyes, ears, and nose require careful attention. Chapter 28 describes the structure and function of these organs. Cleansing of the sensitive sensory tissues should be done in a way that prevents injury and discomfort for the client, such as using care not to get soap in the client's eyes. In addition, the time that a nurse spends with a client during hygiene provides an excellent opportunity to ask if there have been any changes in vision, hearing, or sense of smell.

Nursing Knowledge Base

A client's personal preferences for hygiene are influenced by a number of factors. No two individuals perform hygiene in the same manner, and it is important that the nurse individualize the client's care from knowledge about the client's unique hygiene practices and preferences.

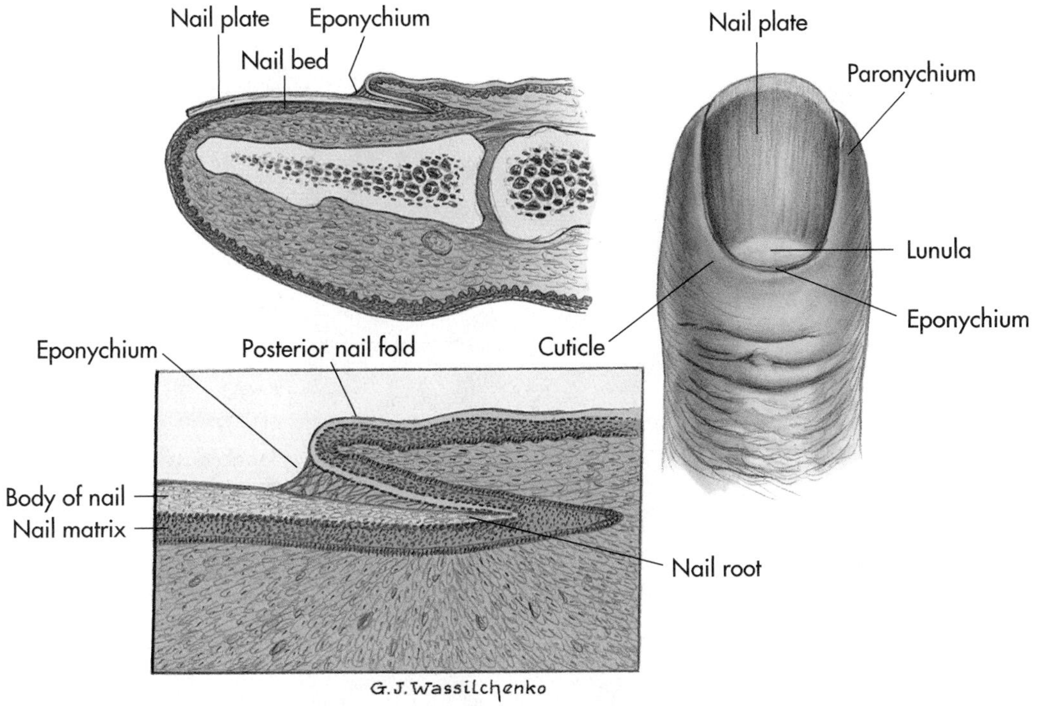

FIGURE 34–1 Anatomic structure of a normal nail. (From *Mosby's Clinical Nursing,* 4th ed., edited by J. M. Thompson et al., 1997, St. Louis, MO: Mosby.)

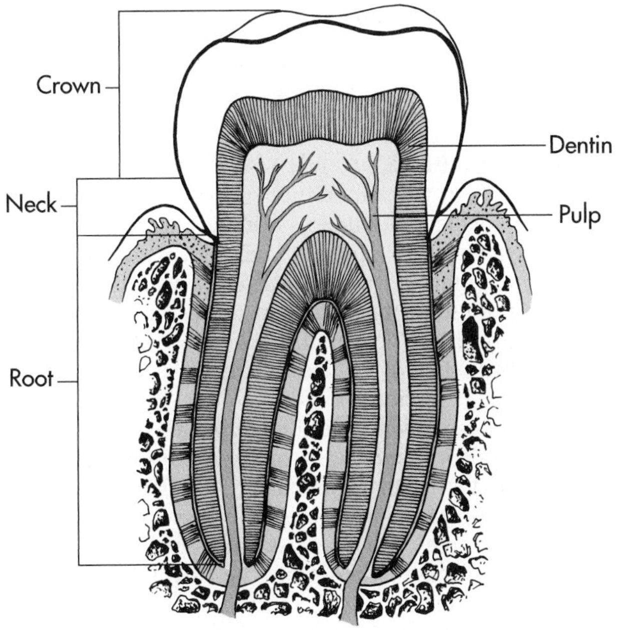

FIGURE 34–2 A normal tooth.

Hygiene care is never routine; the care requires intimate contact with the client and communication skills to promote the therapeutic relationship. In addition, during this care, the nurse can learn about the client's health promotion practices and needs, emotional needs, and health care education needs.

Social Practices

Social groups influence hygiene preferences and practices, including the type of hygiene products used and the nature and frequency of personal care. During childhood, hygiene is influenced by family customs. This may include, for example, the frequency of bathing, the time of day bathing is performed, and the type of oral hygiene practised. As children enter their adolescent years, personal hygiene may be influenced by peer group behaviour and they may become more interested in their personal appearance. For example, girls may begin to wear makeup and boys may begin shaving. During the adult years, involvement with friends and work groups shape the expectations people have about their personal appearance. Older adults' hygiene practices may change because of living conditions and available resources.

Personal Preferences

Each client has individual preferences about when to bathe, shave, and perform hair care. Clients select different products according to personal preferences, needs, and financial resources. These preferences should assist the nurse in delivering individualized care for the client. In addition, the nurse should also assist the client in developing new hygiene practices when indicated by an illness or condition.

Body Image

A client's general appearance may reflect the importance that hygiene holds for that person. Body image is a person's subjective concept of his or her physical appearance (see chapter 22). These images can change frequently.

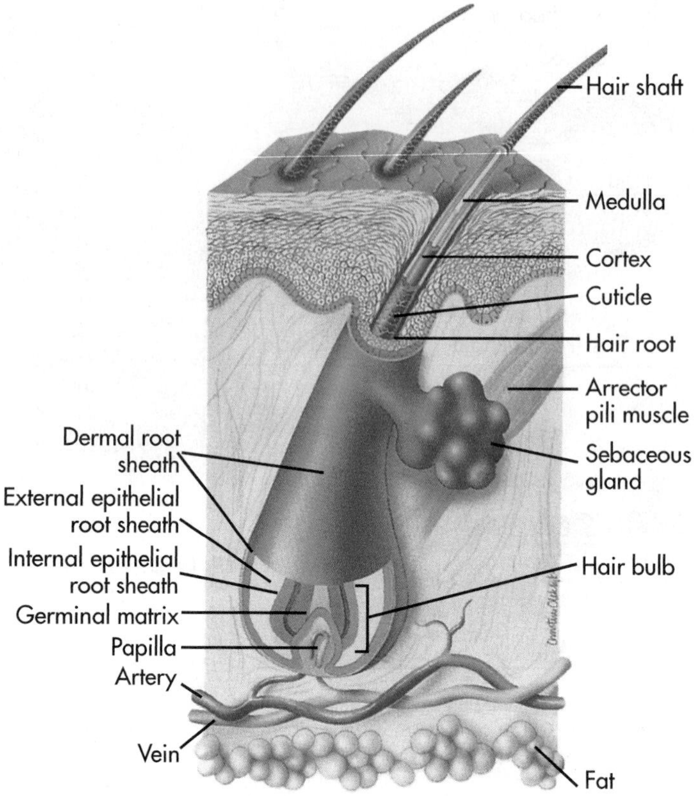

FIGURE **34–3** Hair follicle and relationship of a follicle and related structures to the epidermal and dermal layers of the skin. (From *Anatomy and Physiology* (4th ed.), by G. A. Thibodeau and K. T. Patton, 1999, St. Louis, MO: Mosby.)

When clients undergo surgery, illness, or a change in physical or mental health status, body image can alter dramatically. For this reason, the nurse will take extra effort to promote the client's hygienic comfort and appearance.

Body image affects the way in which hygiene is maintained. If a client is neatly groomed, the nurse considers the details of grooming when planning care and consults the client before making decisions about how hygiene care is to be provided. Clients who appear unkempt or uninterested in hygiene may require an assessment of their hygiene practices or additional education about the importance of hygiene.

Socio-economic Status

A person's economic resources influence the type and extent of hygiene practices used. The nurse should be sensitive in considering that the client's economic status may influence his or her ability to regularly maintain hygiene. When clients have the added problem of a lack of socio-economic resources, it becomes difficult to participate and take a responsible role in health promotion activities such as basic hygiene.

When basic care items are not affordable, the nurse looks for alternatives. It is also important to assess if use of these products is an acceptable practice among the client's social or cultural group. For example, not all clients may choose to use deodorant or cosmetics.

Health Beliefs and Motivation

Knowledge about the importance of hygiene and its implications for well-being influences hygiene practices. However, knowledge alone is not enough. The client also must be motivated to maintain self-care. Health motivation is a generalized state of intent that results in behaviours to maintain or improve health (Champion, 1984). Motivation is part of an individual's health beliefs or attitudes that influence health-related behaviours.

Studies have shown that clients' health beliefs predict the likelihood of assuming health promotion behaviour (Champion, 1984). In regard to a client's hygiene practices, it is important for the nurse to know if a client, for example, perceives being at risk for dental disease, perceives dental disease to be serious, perceives brushing and flossing to be effective in reducing risk, and perceives any negative implications from following recommended hygiene practices. When clients recognize that there is a risk and reasonable action can be taken with no negative consequence, they are more receptive to counselling and teaching efforts.

Cultural Variables

A client's cultural beliefs and personal values influence hygiene care. People from diverse cultural backgrounds follow different self-care practices (see chapter 9). The nurse must not convey feelings of disapproval when caring for clients whose hygienic practices are different from the nurse's. In some cultures, it is customary to bathe once a week, whereas in North America it is common to bathe or shower daily.

Physical Condition

Clients with certain types of physical limitations or disabilities often lack the physical energy and dexterity to perform hygiene care. A client in traction or a cast or who has an intravenous line or other device connected to the body will need assistance with hygiene. Illnesses that cause pain may limit the dexterity and range of motion needed to perform certain measures.

Clients under the effects of sedation will not have the mental clarity or coordination to perform self-care. Chronic illnesses, such as cardiac disease, cancer, neurological disorders, and certain psychiatric conditions, may exhaust or incapacitate a client. A weakened grasp resulting from arthritis, stroke, or muscular disorders can prevent a client from using a toothbrush, washcloth, or comb.

Critical Thinking

Successful critical thinking requires synthesis of knowledge, experience, information gathered from clients, critical thinking attitudes, and intellectual and professional standards. Clinical judgments require the nurse to anticipate the information necessary to analyze data and make decisions regarding client care. A client's condition is always changing, requiring ongoing critical thinking. During assessment, the nurse must consider all contributing factors needed to make a nursing diagnosis (Figure 34–4).

Because hygiene care is so important for a client to feel comfortable, refreshed, and renewed, the nurse avoids making hygiene care a simple routine. Instead, the nurse integrates knowledge from nursing and other disciplines, previous experiences, and information gathered from clients. In addition, attitudes such as curiosity and humility are required to design a plan of care that will meet the client's hygiene needs. The nurse uses agency and professional nursing standards and guidelines, such as those from the Canadian Diabetes Association (2003), when planning care to meet the client's hygiene needs.

Nursing Process

NP Assessment

Nursing assessment is an ongoing process. The nurse may not assess all body regions before administering hygiene; however, the nurse does routinely assess the client's condition whenever client care is given. For example, during oral care, the condition of the teeth and mucosa can be inspected. When a client has had a repeated problem (e.g., dry skin or inflamed oral mucosa), then it is important to conduct an assessment before care is administered because variations in technique may be necessary. Hygiene care is an opportunity for the nurse to make assessment findings for a variety of health care problems and thus helps set health care priorities.

Physical Examination. While assisting a client with personal hygiene, the nurse carefully assesses the integument, oral cavity structures, and the eyes, ears, and nose (see chapter 28). Using the skills of inspection and palpation, the nurse looks for alterations in the integrity and function of tissues. The assessment also reveals the type and extent of hygiene care required. Special attention is given to the characteristics most influenced by hygiene measures. Is the skin intact, especially over bony prominences? Is the skin dry from too much bathing? Are there calluses on the feet that may benefit from soaking? Is there a coating of the tongue that requires frequent brushing and hydration? Over time, the nurse's assessment provides the baseline for determining whether hygienic measures maintain or improve the client's condition.

Skin. While inspecting the skin, the nurse thoroughly examines its colour, texture, thickness, turgor, temperature, and hydration. The skin should be smooth, warm, supple, and have good turgor. The nurse pays special attention to the presence and condition of any lesions (see chapter 28). In addition, it is important to assess for dryness indicated by flaking, redness, scaling, and cracking. There are tools available to assess the degrees of dryness to have a baseline in determining if bathing is beneficial (Handy, 1996). Certain common skin problems affect how hygiene is administered (Table 34-2). Special care is also given to assess less obvious or difficult-to-reach skin surfaces, such as under the female client's breasts, under the male client's scrotum, or around the female's perineal tissues. The nurse who observes skin problems should explain proper skin care with the client and use the time to instruct on specific hygiene techniques.

Certain conditions place clients at risk for impaired skin integrity (Box 34-2). Nurses must be particularly alert when assessing clients with reduced sensation, vascular insufficiency, and immobility. Nurses must be sure to assess both extremities and assist in turning a client so that a skin surface can be fully viewed. The development of pressure ulcers is a common complication that can extend hospital stays and threaten the well-being of the long-term care client. When caring for clients with darkly pigmented skin, nurses should be aware of assessment techniques and skin characteristics unique to highly pigmented skin (Box 34-3).

Feet and Nails. Assessment of the feet involves a thorough examination of all skin surfaces, including areas between the toes and over the soles of the feet. The heels, soles, and sides of the feet are prone to irritation from poorly fitting shoes. In addition, the nurse inspects the shape and size of toes and shape of the foot. The toes are normally straight and flat. The feet should be in straight alignment with the ankle and tibia. Inspection of the feet for lesions includes noting areas of dryness, inflammation, or cracking.

The nurse assesses the client's gait. Painful foot disorders or decreased sensation can cause limping or an unnatural

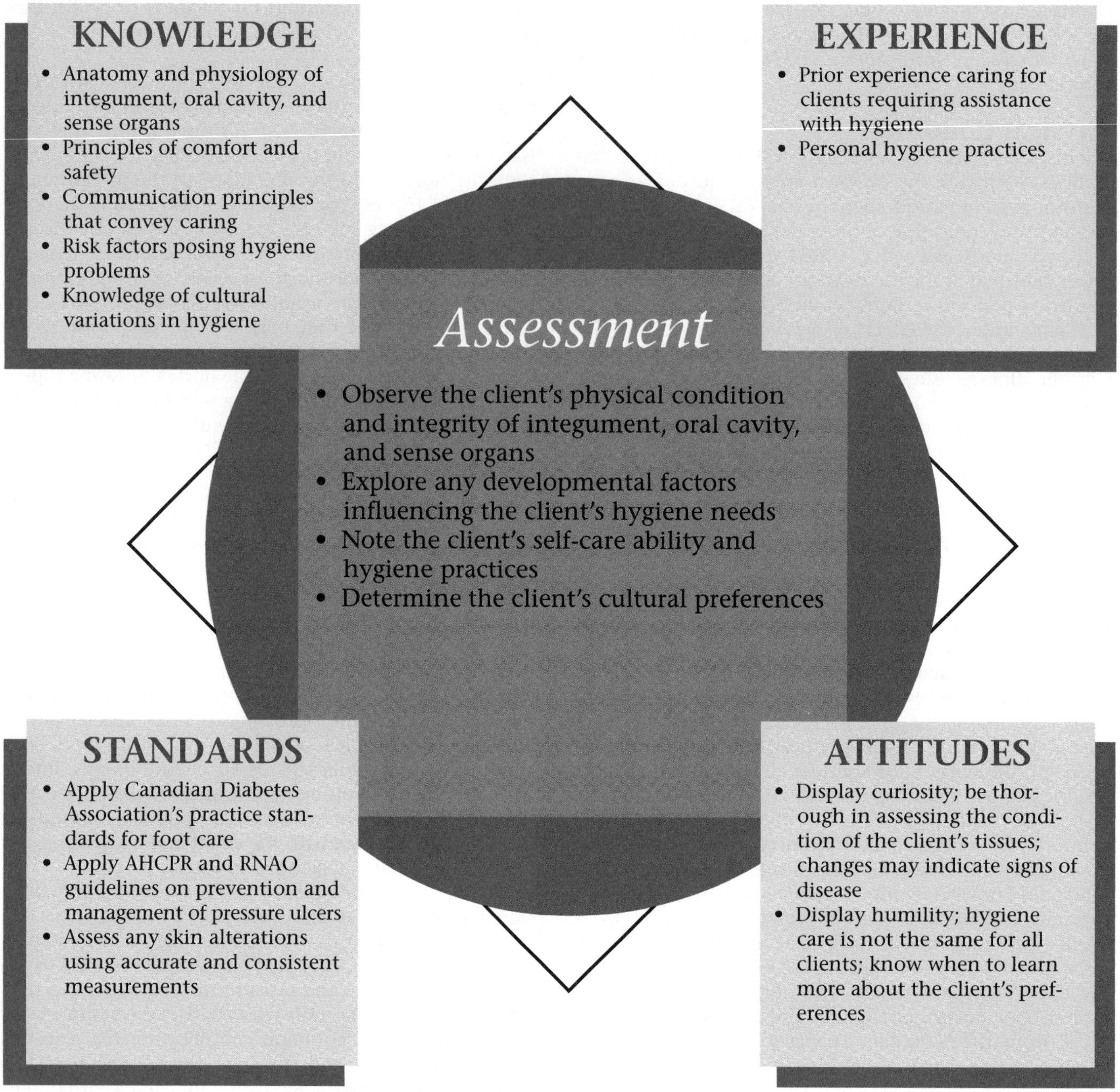
KNOWLEDGE
• Anatomy and physiology of integument, oral cavity, and sense organs
• Principles of comfort and safety
• Communication principles that convey caring
• Risk factors posing hygiene problems
• Knowledge of cultural variations in hygiene
EXPERIENCE
• Prior experience caring for clients requiring assistance with hygiene
• Personal hygiene practices
Assessment
• Observe the client's physical condition and integrity of integument, oral cavity, and sense organs
• Explore any developmental factors influencing the client's hygiene needs
• Note the client's self-care ability and hygiene practices
• Determine the client's cultural preferences
STANDARDS
• Apply Canadian Diabetes Association's practice standards for foot care
• Apply AHCPR and RNAO guidelines on prevention and management of pressure ulcers
• Assess any skin alterations using accurate and consistent measurements
ATTITUDES
• Display curiosity; be thorough in assessing the condition of the client's tissues; changes may indicate signs of disease
• Display humility; hygiene care is not the same for all clients; know when to learn more about the client's preferences

FIGURE **34-4** Critical thinking model for hygiene assessment.

gait. The nurse asks whether the client has foot discomfort and determines factors that aggravate the pain. Foot problems may result from bone or muscular alterations or wearing poor fitting footwear rather than skin disorders.

Clients with peripheral vascular disease, such as diabetes mellitus and other diseases that affect peripheral circulation and sensation, should be assessed for the adequacy of circulation to the feet (see chapter 28). Inspection and daily foot care can prevent the development of foot ulcers and subsequent complications that may lead to amputation (Canadian Diabetes Association, 2003; Neil, 2002). Palpation of the dorsalis pedis and posterior tibial pulses indicates whether adequate blood flow is reaching peripheral tissues. Edema and changes in skin colour, texture, and temperature can indicate whether the client requires special hygiene care. People with diabetes mellitus should also be checked for **neuropathy,** degeneration of the peripheral nerves characterized by a loss of sensation. The nurse assesses the client's sensation to light touch, pinprick, and temperature.

The nurse inspects the condition of the fingernails and toenails, looking for lesions, dryness, inflammation, or cracking (Table 34-3). The nail is surrounded by a cuticle, which slowly grows over the nail and must be regularly pushed back. The skin around the nail beds and cuticles should be smooth and without inflammation. The nurse

Table 34-2 Common Skin Problems

Characteristics	Implications	Interventions
Dry Skin		
Flaky, rough texture on exposed areas such as hands, arms, legs, or face	Skin may become infected if epidermal layer is allowed to crack.	Have client bathe less frequently and rinse body of all soap because residue left on skin can cause irritation and breakdown. Add moisture to air through use of humidifier. Increase fluid intake when skin is dry. Use a non-allergenic moisturizing cream to aid healing because cream can form a protective barrier and assist with maintaining fluid within the skin. Use creams to clean skin that is dry or allergic to soaps and detergents.
Acne		
Inflammatory, papulopustular skin eruption, usually involving bacterial breakdown of sebum; appears on face, neck, shoulders, and back	Infected material within pustule can spread if area is squeezed or picked. Permanent scarring can result.	Wash hair and skin thoroughly each day with soap to remove oil. Use cosmetics sparingly because oily cosmetics or creams accumulate in pores and tend to make condition worse. Use prescribed topical or oral antibiotics for severe forms of acne.
Skin Rashes		
Skin eruption that may result from overexposure to sun or moisture or from allergic reaction (may be flat or raised, localized or systemic, pruritic or nonpruritic)	If skin is continually scratched, inflammation and infection may occur. Rashes can also cause discomfort.	Wash area thoroughly and apply antiseptic spray or lotion to prevent further itching and aid in healing process. Apply warm or cold soaks to relieve inflammation, if indicated.
Contact Dermatitis		
Inflammation of skin characterized by abrupt onset with erythema, pruritus, pain, and appearance of scaly oozing lesions (seen on face, neck, hands, forearms, and genitalia)	Dermatitis is often difficult to eliminate because the person is usually in continual contact with substance causing skin reaction. Substance may be hard to identify.	Avoid causative agents (e.g., cleansers and soaps).
Abrasion		
Scraping or rubbing away of epidermis that may result in localized bleeding and later weeping of serous fluid	Infection occurs easily because of loss of protective skin layer.	Be careful not to scratch client with jewellery or fingernails. Wash abrasions with mild soap and water; dry thoroughly and gently. Observe for retained moisture in dressings or bandages because excess moisture can increase the risk of infection.

should ask women whether they frequently polish their nails and use polish remover because chemicals in these products can cause excessive nail dryness. Disease can change the shape and curvature of the nails. Inflammatory lesions and fungus of the nail bed can cause thickened, horny nails, which can separate from the nail bed.

Oral Cavity. The nurse inspects all areas carefully for colour, hydration, texture, and lesions (see chapter 28). Clients who do not follow regular oral hygiene practices may have receding gum tissue, inflamed gums, a coated tongue, discoloured teeth (particularly along gum margins), dental caries, missing teeth, and **halitosis** (bad breath). Localized pain and infection are common symptoms of gum disease and certain tooth disorders.

Clients in acute care settings require complete oral assessment. Identification of risks for infection and other conditions identify the type and frequency of oral care. Proper oral care has been shown to reduce pneumonia in long-term care residents because it reduces the bacterial count in oral secretions, which may be aspirated and cause a bacterial infection (Research update, 2002). It is especially important to examine the oral cavity of clients receiving radiation or chemotherapy. Both treatments can reduce the amount of saliva, resulting in drying and inflammation of the oral mucosal tissues. The

Box 34-2 Risk Factors for Skin Impairment

Immobilization

When restricted from moving freely, dependent body parts are exposed to pressure, reducing circulation to affected body parts. The nurse should know which clients require assistance to turn and change positions.

Reduced Sensation

Clients with paralysis, circulatory insufficiency, or local nerve damage are unable to sense an injury to the skin. During a bath, assess the status of sensory nerve function by checking for pain, tactile sensation, and temperature sensation.

Nutrition and Hydration Alterations

Clients with limited caloric and protein intake can develop thinner, less elastic skin, with loss of subcutaneous tissue. This can result in impaired or delayed wound healing.

Secretions and Excretions on the Skin

Moisture on the skin's surface serves as a medium for bacterial growth and can cause irritation, soften epidermal cells, and lead to skin maceration. Presence of perspiration, urine, watery fecal material, and wound drainage on the skin can result in breakdown and infection.

Vascular Insufficiency

Inadequate arterial supply to tissues and impaired venous return decrease circulation to the extremities. Inadequate blood flow can cause ischemia and breakdown. Risk of infection also exists because delivery of nutrients, oxygen, and white blood cells to injured tissues is inadequate.

External Devices

An external device applied to or around the skin exerts pressure or friction on the skin. The nurse assesses all surfaces exposed to casts, cloth restraints, bandages and dressings, tubing, or orthopedic braces.

Box 34-3 Skin Assessment for the Client With Darkly Pigmented, Intact Skin

- Assess localized skin colour changes.
  - Colour darker than surrounding skin, purplish, bluish, eggplant
  - Taut
  - Shiny
  - Induration
- Assess for edema (non-pitting, swelling).
- Importance of lighting for skin assessment:
  - Use natural or halogen light.
  - Avoid fluorescent lamps, which can give the skin a bluish tone.
- Assess skin temperature.
  - Initially may feel warmer than surrounding skin.
  - Subsequently may feel cooler than surrounding skin.
  - Use the back of your hand and fingers and, if the client's condition permits, do not use gloves when doing this assessment.

Data from "Report of the Task Force on the Implications for Darkly Pigmented Intact Skin in the Prediction and Prevention of Pressure Ulcers," by M. A. Bennet, 1995, *Advances in Wound Care, 8*(6), pp. 34–35.

nurse's assessment serves as a basis for preventive care for clients as they undergo treatment.

Hair. Before performing hair care, the nurse assesses the condition of the hair and scalp. Healthy hair is clean, shiny, and untangled, and the scalp is clear of lesions. The hair of dark-skinned clients is usually thicker, drier, and curlier than that of lighter skinned clients. Table 34-4 summarizes hair and scalp problems that the nurse may identify. In community and home care settings, it is particularly important to inspect the hair for lice so that appropriate treatment can be provided. If pediculosis capitis (head lice) is suspected, the nurse guards against self-infestations by handwashing and use of gloves or tongue blades to inspect the client's hair. The loss of hair **(alopecia)** can result from the effects of chemotherapy medications, hormonal changes, or improper hair care practices. Clients at risk for scalp problems are those who have experienced head trauma and those who practise poor hygiene.

Eyes, Ears, and Nose. The nurse's examination assesses the condition and function of the eyes, ears, and nose (see chapter 28). Normally the eyes are free of infection and irritation. The sclerae are visible anteriorly as the white portion of the eye. The conjunctivae (the lining of the eyelids) are clear, pink, and without inflammation. The eyelid margins are in close approximation with the eyeball, and the lashes are turned outward. The lid margins are without inflammation, drainage, or lesions. The eyebrows should be symmetrical.

The nurse also determines if the client wears contact lenses. This is especially significant for clients who enter hospitals or other agencies unresponsive or in a confused state. To determine if a contact lens is present, the nurse should stand to the side of the client's eye and observe the cornea for the presence of a soft or rigid lens. The sclera should be observed to detect whether a contact lens has shifted off of the client's cornea. An undetected lens can cause severe corneal injury when left in place too long.

Assessment of the external ear structures is done using an otoscope to inspect the auricle, external ear canal, and

Table 34-3 Common Foot and Nail Problems

Characteristics	Implications	Interventions
Callus		
Thickened portion of epidermis consists of mass of horny, keratotic cells. Callus is usually flat, painless, and found on the undersurface of the foot or on the palm of the hand. Problems are caused by local friction or pressure.	Condition may cause discomfort when wearing tight shoes.	Nurse advises client to wear gloves when using tools or objects that may create friction on palmar surfaces. Soft-sole shoes with insoles are recommended. Nurse soaks callus in warm water and Epsom salts to soften cell layers. Applications of creams or lotions can reduce re-formation. Encourage client to see a podiatrist.
Corns		
Keratosis is caused by friction and pressure from ill-fitting or loose shoes. It is seen mainly on or between toes or over a bony prominence. A corn is usually cone shaped, round, and raised. Soft corns are macerated.	The conical shape compresses the underlying dermis, making it thin and tender. Pain is aggravated when tight shoes are worn. Tissue can become attached to bone if allowed to grow. Client may suffer alteration in gait resulting from pain.	Surgical removal may be necessary, depending on severity of pain and size of the corn. The nurse avoids use of oval corn pads, which can increase the pressure on toes and reduce circulation. Warm water soaks can soften corns before gentle rubbing with a callus file or pumice stone (consult with physician). Wider and softer shoes are suggested.
Plantar Warts		
A fungating lesion appears on the sole of foot and is caused by the papilloma virus.	Warts may be contagious. They are painful and make walking difficult.	Treatment ordered by physician may include applications of salicylic acid, electrodesiccation (burning with electrical spark), or freezing with solid carbon dioxide.
Athlete's Foot (Tinea Pedis)		
Athlete's foot is fungal infection of the foot; scaliness and cracking of skin occurs between toes and on soles of feet. Small blisters containing fluid may appear. The problem can be induced by wearing constricting footwear.	Athlete's foot can spread to other body parts, especially hands. It is contagious and frequently recurs.	Feet should be well ventilated. Drying feet well after bathing and applying powder helps to prevent infection. Wearing clean socks or stockings reduces the incidence. The physician may treat the condition with antifungal topical applications.
Ingrown Nails		
Toenail or fingernail grows inward into soft tissue around nail. Ingrown nail often results from improper nail trimming.	Ingrown nails can cause localized pain when pressure is applied.	Treatment is frequent hot soaks in antiseptic solution and removal of the portion of nail that has grown into skin. Instruct the client regarding proper nail-trimming techniques and provide a referral to a podiatrist.
Ram's Horn Nails		
Ram's horn nails are unusually long curved nails.	Attempts by the nurse to cut nails may result in damage to nail bed with risk of infection.	The nurse refers the client to podiatrist.
Paronychia		
Inflammation of tissue surrounding nail occurs after hangnail or other injury. It occurs in people who frequently have their hands in water and is common in clients with diabetes.	The area can become infected.	Treatment is hot compresses or soaks and local application of antibiotic ointments. Paronychia can be prevented by careful manicuring.
Foot Odours		
Foot odours are the result of excess perspiration promoting micro-organism growth.	Condition may cause discomfort because of excess perspiration.	Frequent washing, use of foot deodorants and powders, and wearing clean footwear prevents or reduces problem.

Table 34-4 Hair and Scalp Problems

Characteristics	Implications	Interventions
Dandruff		
Scaling of scalp is accompanied by itching. In severe cases, dandruff is found on eyebrows.	Dandruff causes person embarrassment. If dandruff enters eyes, conjunctivitis may develop.	Shampoo regularly with medicated shampoo. In severe cases, obtain physician's advice.
Ticks		
Small, grey-brown parasites burrow into skin and suck blood.	Ticks transmit several diseases to people. Most common are Rocky Mountain spotted fever, Tularemia, and Lyme disease.	Do not pull ticks from skin because sucking apparatus remains and may become infected. Suffocate tick by placing a drop of oil or ether on tick or covering it with petrolatum for ease of removal.
Pediculosis (Lice)		
A tiny, greyish-white ecoparasite insect that can infest mammals, including humans.		
Pediculosis Capitis (Head Lice)		
Head lice require a source of human blood to survive. Transmission is by direct contact (i.e., head to head). The parasite is found on scalp attached to hair strands. Eggs look like oval particles, similar to dandruff. Bites or pustules may be observed behind ears and at hairline. Itching at the hairline is the most common symptom.	Contacts of the clients (e.g., family members and classmates) should be examined and treated. Although no current evidence exists of transmission by shared articles, families may wish to wash bedding and combs in hot water. Dry cleaning or storing items in plastic bags for 10 days is also effective (Infectious Diseases and Immunization Committee, Canadian Pediatric Society, 2003).	Check entire scalp. Use a medicated shampoo for eliminating lice. Follow product directions carefully; repeat of application is required 7 to 10 days after the first to ensure that surviving eggs are killed. Seek physician advice if treatment is ineffective; a new medication may be required for effective chemical eradication. Some products can cause neurotoxicity and should not be used with children under 6 years of age. **Caution is advised against use of products containing Lindane.** This product has been withdrawn for use in some countries. Manual removal of lice with a fine-toothed comb can assist with removal of nits (the empty eggshell).
Pediculosis Corporis (Body Lice)		
Body lice differ from head lice in that body lice parasites tend to cling to clothing and may not be easily seen. They suck blood and lay eggs on clothing and furniture	Client itches constantly. Scratches seen on skin may become infected. Hemorrhagic spots may appear on skin where lice are sucking blood.	Bathe or shower thoroughly. After skin is dried, apply recommended pediculicide lotion. After 8 to 12 hours, take another bath or shower. Bag infested clothing or linen until laundered in hot water. Vacuum rooms thoroughly and throw away bag after completion.
Pediculosis Pubis (Crab Lice)		
Crab lice parasites are found in pubic hair. Crab lice are greyish white with red legs.	Lice may spread through bed linen, clothing, or furniture or between people via sexual contact.	Cleanse as for body lice. Treatment of sexual partners is recommended, but contact tracing and reporting to public health authorities is not required (Health Canada, 1998).
Hair Loss (Alopecia)		
Alopecia occurs in people of all races. Balding patches are seen in periphery of hairline. Hair becomes brittle and broken. Condition is caused by genetics and use of hair curlers, hot comb, hair picks, tight braiding.	Patches of uneven hair growth and loss alter client's appearance.	Stop hair-care practices that damage hair.

tympanic membrane. While performing hygiene measures, the nurse is most concerned with noting the presence of accumulated **cerumen** or drainage in the ear canal, local inflammation, tenderness on palpation, or the client's report of pain (see chapter 28).

The nurse inspects the nares for signs of inflammation, discharge, lesions, edema, and deformity (see chapter 28). The nasal mucosa is normally pink and clear and has little or no discharge. A clear, watery discharge may be the result of allergies. If clients have any form of tubing exiting the nose (e.g., nasogastric), the nurse should look at the nares surfaces that come in contact with the tubing for tissue sloughing, localized tenderness, inflammation, and bleeding.

Developmental Changes. The normal process of aging influences the condition of body tissues and structures and thus the manner in which hygiene measures are performed. Chapter 44 addresses the changes in hearing, vision, and olfaction across the lifespan as a result of growth and development.

Skin. The neonate's skin is relatively immature at birth. The epidermis and dermis are loosely bound together, and the skin is very thin. Friction against the skin layers can cause bruising. The nurse must handle the neonate carefully during bathing. Any break in the skin can easily lead to infection.

A toddler's skin layers are more tightly bound together. Thus, the child has a greater resistance to infection and skin irritation. However, because of the child's active play and the absence of established hygiene habits, greater attention is needed from parents and caregivers to provide thorough hygiene and to begin teaching good hygiene habits.

During adolescence, the growth and maturation of the integument increases. In girls, estrogen secretion causes the skin to become soft, smooth, and thicker, with increased vascularity. In boys, male hormones produce an increased thickness of the skin with some darkening in colour. Sebaceous glands become more active, predisposing adolescents to **acne. Eccrine** and **apocrine** sweat glands become fully functional during puberty. Adolescents usually begin to use antiperspirants. More frequent bathing and shampooing also become necessary to reduce body odours and eliminate oily hair. Sweating is usually more pronounced in boys.

The condition of the adult's skin depends on hygiene practices and exposure to environmental irritants. Normally the skin is elastic, well hydrated, firm, and smooth. When an adult practises frequent bathing or is exposed to an environment with low humidity, the skin can become very dry and flaky.

With aging, the skin loses its resiliency and moisture, and sebaceous and sweat glands become less active. The epithelium thins and elastic collagen fibres shrink, making the skin fragile and subject to bruising and breaking. These changes warrant caution when turning and repositioning older adults (Lueckenotte, 2000).

Typically, an older adult's skin becomes drier and wrinkled. Because the skin may become excessively dry, older adults should avoid bathing daily and using very hot water or harsh soaps.

Feet and Nails. While standing, the foot provides body support and absorbs shock. With aging, the feet begin to show signs of wear and tear. This may occur earlier if a person has failed to wear comfortable, supportive footwear. The cushioning layer of fat on the soles of the feet becomes thin.

Chronic foot problems are a common result of poor foot care, improper fit of footwear, aging, and systemic disease. Older adults often have dry feet because of a decrease in sebaceous gland secretion, dehydration of epidermal cells, and poor condition of footwear. Fissures that result in itching frequently develop (Bryant & Beinlich, 1999). One of the most common problems for older adults is foot pain (Lueckenotte, 2000). Painful feet can be the result of congenital deformities, weak structure, injuries, and diseases such as diabetes, rheumatoid arthritis, or osteoarthritis. After 55 years of age, arthritis is a common cause of changes in the feet. Additional common foot problems include hammer and claw toes (flexion contractures), bunions, corns, calluses, loss of sensation, and pathological nail conditions (Boyer, 2001).

Fungal infections occur under toenails, causing dark yellow streaks or total discolouration. The nails can also become opaque, scaly, and hypertrophied. If foot or nail problems stay unresolved, the client can easily become disabled. The nurse applies knowledge of typical changes in the feet and nails when anticipating the type of hygiene that a client will require.

Oral Cavity. Infants begin teething at approximately 6 to 8 months of age (Wong, 1999). The first permanent (secondary) teeth erupt at about 6 years of age. From adolescence, when all of the permanent teeth are in place, through middle adulthood, the teeth and gums will remain healthy if the person avoids fermentable carbohydrates and sticky sweets. Regular dental care and hygiene practices such as brushing and flossing help to prevent **caries** and periodontal disease.

As a person grows older, there are numerous factors that can result in poor oral care. These include age-related changes of the mouth, chronic disease such as diabetes, physical disabilities involving hand grasp or strength affecting the ability to perform oral care, lack of attention to oral care, and prescribed medications that have oral side effects. Aging teeth become brittle, drier, and darker in colour. Teeth become uneven, jagged, and fractured. Gums lose vascularity and tissue elasticity, which can cause dentures to fit poorly. Often older adults are **edentulous** and wear complete or partial dentures. It is important for the nurse to determine if older clients wear dentures and the condition of underlying supportive gum tissue.

Eyes, Ears, and Nose. Although the structure of the eyes do not have marked developmental changes, altered visual acuity can occur at several points during the aging process; for example, when children start school or when clients reach middle age, there may be changes in visual acuity. As clients age, they are also at risk for changes in visual clarity (e.g., caused by glaucoma) and visual field losses (e.g., caused by macular degeneration or glaucoma).

Structures of the ears do not change as the client ages; however, changes in hearing acuity or balance may occur with aging. In the young child, changes in hearing acuity may result from foreign objects being placed in the ear; this may be a temporary change and is resolved once the object is removed. Changes may also result from repeated ear infections or exposure to loud noise, such as when the child listens to loud music on headphones.

Older adults may have changes in the structure and function of the small bones in the inner ear that affect changes in hearing acuity. Aging may result in increased cerumen production, which can also impede hearing acuity. In addition, there may be age-related changes in the movement of fluid through the semicircular canals, and the client may experience positional dizziness or balance problems.

Although changes in the sense of smell can occur at any time, it seems to be more common in older adults. It is important to remember that changes in the sense of smell may also affect taste and the client's appetite.

New and acute changes in the structure and function of the eyes, ears, and nose must be fully assessed and evaluated. Timely evaluation of these changes may identify other illnesses or verify that they are age related.

Use of Sensory Aids. When clients wear eyeglasses, contact lenses, artificial eyes, or hearing aids, the nurse assesses their knowledge and asks them to describe the methods that are used for routine care (Box 34-4). The nurse compares information gathered from the client with what the nurse knows is the proper care technique. Any differences in client practice with standard practice may indicate a need for client education.

Box 34-4 Assessing a Client's Use of Sensory Aids

Eyeglasses

Purpose for wearing glasses (e.g., reading, distance, or both)
Methods used to clean glasses
Presence of symptoms (e.g., blurred vision, photophobia, headaches, irritation)

Contact Lenses

Type of lens worn
Frequency and duration of time lenses are worn (including sleep time)
Presence of symptoms (e.g., burning, excess tearing, redness, irritation, swelling, sensitivity to light)
Techniques used by the client to cleanse, store, insert, and remove lenses
Use of eye drops or ointments
Use of emergency identification bracelet or card that warns others to remove client's lenses in case of emergency

Artificial Eye

Method used to insert and remove eye
Method for cleansing eye
Presence of symptoms (e.g., drainage, inflammation, pain involving the orbit)

Hearing Aid

Type of aid worn
Methods used to cleanse aid
Client's ability to change battery and adjust hearing aid volume

Self-Care Ability. Clients with physical or cognitive impairments need assistance with all or some aspects of personal hygiene. Assessment of the client's physical and cognitive status determines specifically what aspects of hygiene care can be performed independently, those that require some assistance, and those that require total assistance.

The nurse's assessment must include measurement of a client's muscle strength, flexibility and dexterity, balance, coordination, and activity tolerance needed to perform activities such as bathing, brushing teeth, and bending over to inspect the feet. The degree of assistance needed by a client during hygiene care may also depend on vision, the ability to sit without support, hand grasp strength, the range of motion in the client's extremities, or the presence of equipment, such as an IV line, dressings, or traction. Painful conditions of the upper extremities pose special problems. The nurse can assess self-care ability by asking clients to perform activities such as brushing teeth or combing the hair. The nurse observes the client carefully and notes whether the client can perform the task thoroughly and correctly (Figure 34–5).

When clients have self-care limitations, part of the nurse's assessment is to determine if family or friends are available to assist. Assisting with hygiene measures can at times be unpleasant. The nurse's assessment should include how the family assists, how often this assistance is provided, and what their feelings are about being caregivers. In addition, the nurse also assesses the home environment and its influence on the client's hygiene practices. Are there barriers in the home that may affect the client's self-care abilities? Water faucets that are too tight to easily adjust, bathtubs with high sides, and a bathroom too small to fit a wheelchair in front of a sink are a few examples.

Hygiene Practices. Assessment of hygiene practices reveals the client's grooming preferences. For example, a client may choose to groom the hair in a certain style or choose to trim nails in a certain way. When a client has a physical disability, special precautions may be needed to perform grooming without injury. Asking the client to assist or teach how to perform preferred grooming practices gives the client a greater sense of independence and helps the nurse avoid causing the client discomfort or injury.

Cultural Factors. A client's cultural background is an influential factor when determining hygiene needs. Culture plays a role not only in hygiene practices and preferences, but also in sensitivity to personal space (see chapter 9). For example, some clients may view tasks associated with

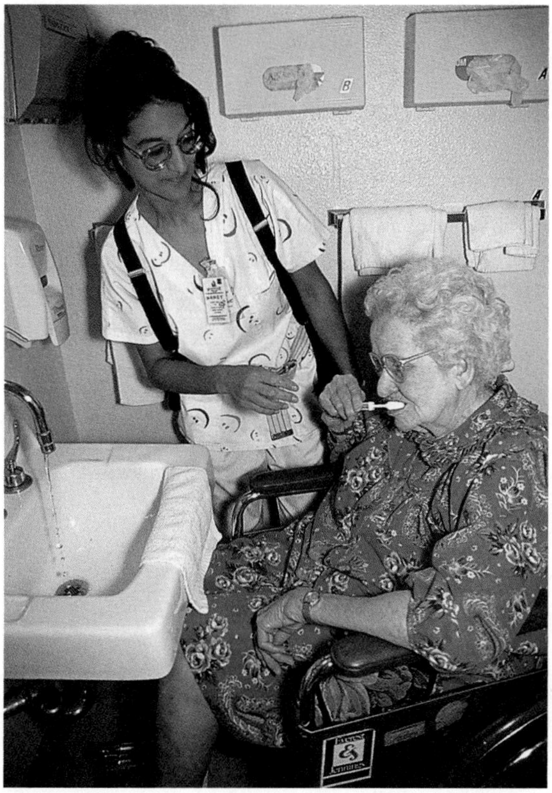

FIGURE **34–5** The nurse observes client brushing teeth. Observation allows the nurse to determine how much assistance the client may need.

closeness and touch as being offensive or impolite. The nurse should ask clients what would make them feel most comfortable during a bath. Instead of a full bath from the nurse, perhaps the client would prefer only a partial bath, with a family member completing the bathing of more private body parts. The client may also defer part of the hygiene care. If, in the nurse's judgment, hygiene is critical to prevent developing or worsening problems, such as skin breakdown, the nurse must take the time to understand the client's concerns and negotiate a mutually satisfactory solution to the problem.

Clients at Risk for Hygiene Problems. Some clients present risks that require more attentive and rigorous hygiene care (Table 34-5). These risks may result from side effects of medications, a lack of knowledge, an inability to perform hygiene, or a physical condition that potentially injures the skin or other structures. An immobilized client who has a fever, for example, will require more frequent bathing to minimize perspiration on the skin and more frequent turning and positioning to reduce the chance of skin breakdown.

The nurse anticipates whether a client is predisposed to such risks and follows through with a complete assessment. For example, if a client is receiving chemotherapy, there is the risk of the medication destroying normal flora in the mouth, allowing for the overgrowth of opportunistic bacteria. Therefore, the oral examination should be more thorough and detailed, with the nurse examining all surfaces of the tongue and mucosa. If a client is diaphoretic, the nurse gives special attention to body areas, such as a woman's breasts and perineal area, where moisture may collect and irritate skin surfaces. The nurse anticipates problems created by these risks and provides appropriate preventive care. The nurse's assessment will include a review of the client's medical and surgical history, medications, and specific risk factors.

Special Considerations in Hygiene Assessment. Depending on the type of hygiene a nurse plans to provide, there are focused assessments that are important to conduct. Before giving foot care, the nurse assesses the type of footwear worn by a client. Children or young adults who frequently fail to wear socks may have excess perspiration that promotes fungal growth. Tight or poorly fitting shoes, socks, garters, or knee-high nylon stockings may cause skin irritation and interfere with circulation to the feet. The nurse also assesses whether clients wear clean footwear daily because repeated use of soiled footwear can lead to infection. If the client has diabetes mellitus or other peripheral vascular disease, it is extremely important that correct footwear be worn. Extra wide and extra deep shoes will accommodate bunions or hammer toes. Cushioned inner soles help redistribute pressure on the metatarsal head. Rocker-bottom shoes help with ambulation (Strauss, Hart, & Winant, 1998).

It is also important to assess a client's eating patterns before oral care. Identifying problems may help the nurse to locate abnormalities. The nurse asks a client if problems are noted with chewing, denture fit, or swallowing. A client may have changed the type of food in the diet as a result of chewing difficulties. The presence of an ulcer or irritation may impair chewing and cause a client to avoid eating. This is common in an older adult with poorly fitting dentures.

Client Expectations. As is the case in any nursing assessment, it is important to know what a client expects from nursing care. For hygiene care, the client may simply expect to have hygiene preferences and practices applied in the health care setting. The nurse can assess the client's expectations by asking questions such as, "To make you most comfortable and feel at home, how can I best perform your bath and personal care?" or "How can we help you care for your teeth, nails, and hair, now that you are at home?"

Understanding a client's expectations and applying them in practice is important in establishing a caring relationship. Truly individualizing hygiene care shows the nurse's respect for the client's needs. As the nurse learns what the client expects, this information can be incorporated into goal development (see Planning).

ND Nursing Diagnosis

The nurse's assessment will reveal the condition of the skin, oral cavity, and other tissues, as well as the client's need for and ability to meet personal hygiene needs. The nurse reviews all data gathered, considers previous clients cared for, reviews knowledge pertaining to pre-existing

Table 34-5 **Risk Factors for Hygiene Problems**

Risks	Hygiene Implications
Oral Problems	
Clients who are unable to use upper extremities because of paralysis, weakness, or restriction (e.g., cast or dressing)	Client lacks upper extremity strength or dexterity needed to brush teeth (Lewis et al., 2000).
Dehydration, inability to take fluids or food by mouth (NPO)	Causes excess drying and fragility of mucosa; increases accumulation of secretions on tongue and gums.
Presence of nasogastric or oxygen tubes; mouth breathers	Causes drying of mucosa.
Chemotherapeutic drugs	Drugs kill rapidly multiplying cells, including normal cells lining oral cavity. Ulcers and inflammation can develop.
Over-the-counter lozenges, cough drops, antacids, and chewable vitamins	Medications may contain large amounts of sugar. Repeated use increases sugar or acid content in mouth.
Radiation therapy to head and neck	Reduces salivary flow and lowers pH of saliva; can lead to stomatitis and tooth decay (Lewis et al., 2000).
Oral surgery, trauma to mouth, placement of oral airway	Cause trauma to oral cavity with swelling, ulcerations, inflammation, and bleeding.
Immunosuppression; alters blood clotting	Predisposes to inflammation and bleeding gums.
Diabetes mellitus	Prone to dryness of mouth, gingivitis, periodontal disease, and loss of teeth.
Skin Problems	
Immobilization	Dependent body parts are exposed to pressure from underlying surfaces. The inability to turn or change position increases risk for pressure ulcers.
Reduced sensation due to stroke, spinal cord injury, diabetes, local nerve damage	Client does not receive normal transmission of nerve impulses when excessive heat or cold, pressure, friction, or chemical irritants are applied to skin.
Limited protein or caloric intake and reduced hydration (e.g., caused by fever, burns, gastrointestinal alterations, poorly fitting dentures)	Limited caloric and protein intake predispose to impaired tissue synthesis. Skin becomes thinner, less elastic, and smoother with a loss of subcutaneous tissue. Poor wound healing may result. Reduced hydration impairs skin turgor.
Excessive secretions or excretions on the skin from perspiration, urine, watery fecal material, and wound drainage	Moisture is a medium for bacterial growth and can cause local skin irritation, softening of epidermal cells, and skin maceration.
Presence of external devices (e.g., casts, restraint, bandage, dressing)	Device can exert pressure or friction against skin's surface.
Vascular insufficiency	Arterial blood supply to tissues is inadequate, or venous return is impaired, causing decreased circulation to extremities. Tissue ischemia and breakdown may occur. Risk for infection is high.
Foot Problems	
Client unable to bend over or has reduced visual acuity	Client is unable to fully visualize entire surface of each foot, impairing ability to adequately assess condition of skin and nails.
Eye Care Problems	
Reduced dexterity and hand coordination	Physical limitations create inability to safely insert or remove contact lenses.

conditions, and then looks for clusters of data suggesting a problem trend. For example, an older adult with degenerative arthritis presents to the home care nurse with pain in the joints, weakness, mobility limitations in the dominant hand, and a generally unkempt appearance. Closer review of assessment data reveals defining characteristics of an inability to wash body parts and difficulty turning and regulating a water faucet. The nursing diagnosis of *bathing/hygiene self-care deficit* is supported and becomes part of the nurse's plan of care. The nurse's accurate selection of nursing diagnoses requires critical thinking to identify actual or potential health problems. Assessment activities must be thorough in revealing all appropriate defining characteristics so that an accurate diagnosis can be made (Box 34-5).

The focus of nursing interventions depends on whether a client has an actual alteration (e.g., impaired tissue integrity) or is at risk for a problem (e.g., risk for impaired oral mucous membrane). The client with an actual alteration will require extensive hygiene care, which is often more thorough than routine care. For example, if the client has skin breakdown, the nurse must initiate care more frequently to keep intact skin surfaces clean and dry and to eliminate factors such as moisture or drainage that can worsen the condition of the skin. The nurse would also provide care to promote healing of injured skin surfaces (see chapter 43). If the client is at risk for a problem, the nurse will institute preventive measures. In the case of risk for impaired oral mucous

Nursing Diagnostic Process — Box 34-5

Assessment Activities	Defining Characteristics	Nursing Diagnosis
Observe client's attempt to bathe self either in bed or at bathroom sink. (NOTE: Be sure positioning does not restrict potential movement.)	Unable to wash body or body parts	Self-care deficit, bathing/hygiene related to upper extremity weakness and generalized fatigue
Assess client's upper extremity strength, range of motion, and coordination.	Restricted upper extremity range of motion and strength Coordination adequate	
Ask client about level of fatigue after bathing.	Complains of fatigue and needs to rest after bathing	
Obtain vital signs after bathing.	Pulse elevated from 90 to 110 beats per minute, blood pressure stable, respirations elevated from 16 to 22 breaths per minute	

membranes, the nurse will keep the mucosa well hydrated, minimize foods irritating to tissues, and provide cleansing that soothes and reduces tissue inflammation.

The identification of related factors guides the nurse in the selection of nursing interventions. Diagnoses of *impaired oral mucous membrane related to malnutrition* and *impaired oral mucous membrane related to chemical trauma* require very different interventions. When malnutrition is a causal factor, the nurse will confer with a dietitian for appropriate dietary supplements and incorporate client education into the plan. When mucosa are injured as a result of chemical trauma from chemotherapy, techniques for cleansing and hydrating inflamed tissues and eliminating sources of irritation will be the focus of nursing care. Although there are many possible nursing diagnoses associated with hygiene problems, the following are a few of the more common diagnoses:

- Impaired dentition
- Fatigue
- Ineffective health maintenance
- Risk for infection
- Deficient knowledge about hygiene practices
- Impaired physical mobility
- Impaired oral mucous membrane
- Self-care deficit, bathing/hygiene, dressing/grooming, toileting
- Chronic low self-esteem
- Risk for impaired skin integrity
- Ineffective tissue perfusion

Planning

During planning, the nurse synthesizes information from multiple resources (Figure 34–6). Critical thinking ensures that the client's plan of care integrates all that the nurse knows about the individual client and key critical thinking elements.

There are situations when clients have multiple nursing diagnoses. The concept map (Figure 34–7) shows graphically how numerous nursing diagnoses can be interrelated.

Previous experience with other clients can be very useful in knowing how to adapt hygiene techniques for special needs. Professional nursing standards and evidence-based clinical guidelines are especially important to consider when the nurse develops a care plan. For example, the Canadian Diabetes Association's clinical practice recommendations offer valuable foot care guidelines for diabetic clients.

Goals and Outcomes. The nurse and client work together to identify goals and expected outcomes and to develop an individualized care plan based on the client's nursing diagnoses (see Care Plan). Goals are established with the client's self-care abilities and resources in mind and focus on maintaining or improving the condition of the skin and mucosa, oral mucosa, or dental hygiene, for example. Outcomes should be measurable and achievable within client limitations. The nurse works further with the client to then select hygiene measures that are appropriate and realistic.

When providing for client hygiene, nurses care for a variety of clients with different self-care abilities and needs. For example, for a client who has one-sided paralysis following a cerebral vascular accident, the nurse and client might develop the following goal: "Client's musculoskeletal system remains free of breakdown or contractures." A series of realistic individualized expected outcomes would then be established to assist the client in meeting this goal. These outcomes may include the following:

- Client's skin is clean, dry, and intact without signs of inflammation.
- Client's skin remains elastic and well hydrated.
- Client's range of joint motion remains within normal limits on both affected and unaffected side.
- Client tolerated bathing without excessive fatigue.

Setting Priorities. The client's condition influences the plan for delivering hygiene. A seriously ill client usually needs a daily bath because body secretions accumulate. An older client at home may require a visit from a home care aide to assist with a tub bath. Clients who are normally

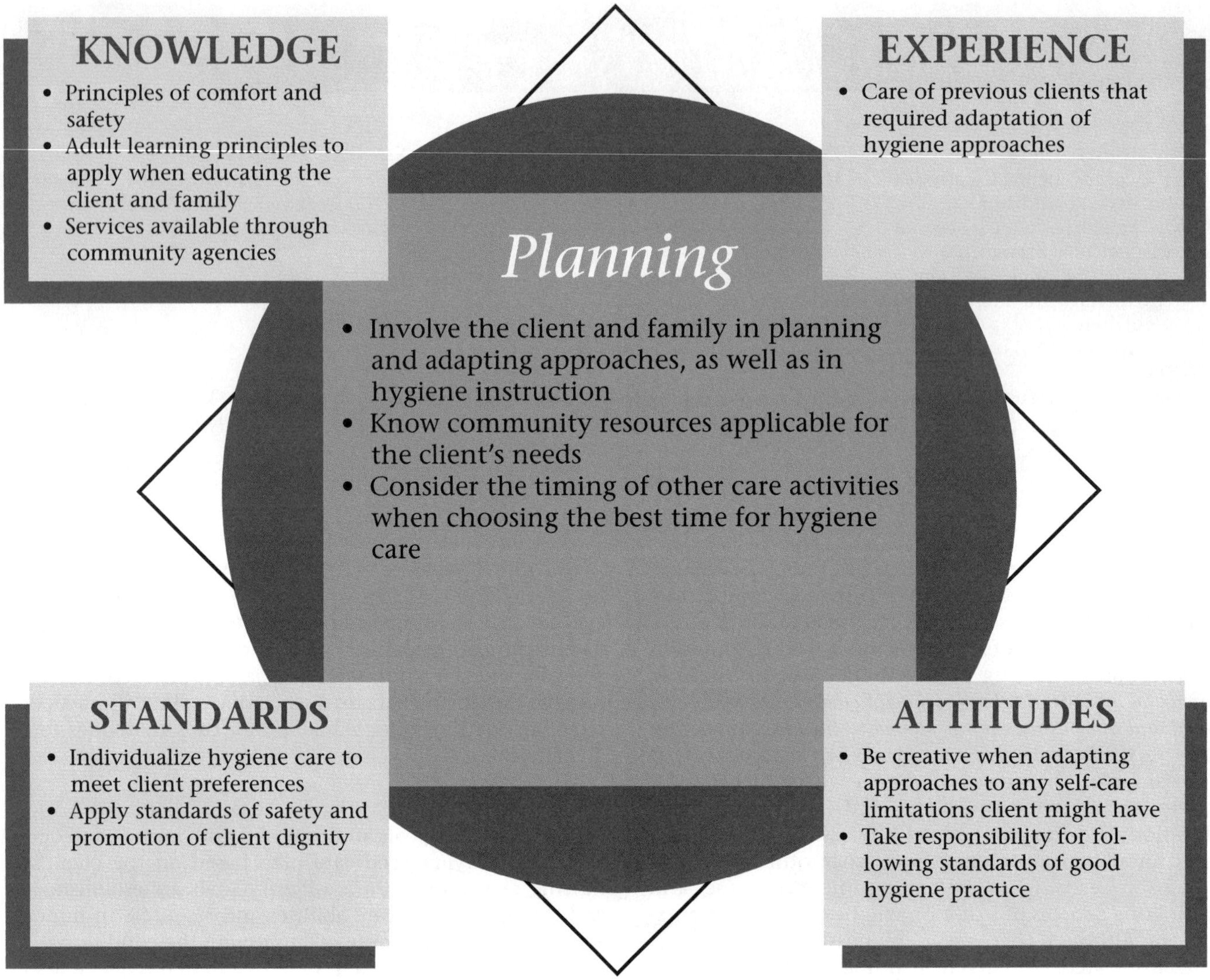
KNOWLEDGE
• Principles of comfort and safety
• Adult learning principles to apply when educating the client and family
• Services available through community agencies
EXPERIENCE
• Care of previous clients that required adaptation of hygiene approaches
Planning
• Involve the client and family in planning and adapting approaches, as well as in hygiene instruction
• Know community resources applicable for the client's needs
• Consider the timing of other care activities when choosing the best time for hygiene care
STANDARDS
• Individualize hygiene care to meet client preferences
• Apply standards of safety and promotion of client dignity
ATTITUDES
• Be creative when adapting approaches to any self-care limitations client might have
• Take responsibility for following standards of good hygiene practice

FIGURE **34–6** Critical thinking model for hygiene planning.

inactive during the day and have skin that tends to be dry may need to bathe only twice a week. The nurse must plan for necessary assistance for clients who are weakened or possess poor coordination. For example, a partially paralyzed client who has had difficulty getting out of a tub should have a tub chair, handrails, or extra personnel available for help.

Timing is also important in planning hygiene. Being interrupted in the middle of a bath to have X-rays taken can frustrate and embarrass a client. Following extensive diagnostic tests (e.g., a stress test), it may be best to delay hygiene and allow a client to rest.

Continuity of Care. It is important to plan for care throughout the hospital stay, discharge to a rehabilitation facility, and home. When a client needs assistance as a result of a self-care limitation, the family becomes a valuable resource to the nurse. Family members can usually assist with hygiene measures but may need guidance in adapting techniques to fit client limitations. The nurse must be aware of equipment and procedures used in the agency so that the client and family are knowledgeable about the care, have the skill needed to provide the care, and have access to necessary equipment. In addition, various community resources may be needed. For example, the nurse involved in the care of a homeless client may need to be aware of the location of clothing distribution centres for basic hygiene supplies or a shelter where bathing facilities are available. Frequently, the nurse will consult with social workers or staff in local area churches and schools to be sure clients have the resources they need to maintain hygiene.

NP Implementation

Providing hygiene is a very basic part of a client's care. The nurse learns to use caring practices that help to alleviate the client's anxiety and promote comfort and relaxation while performing each hygiene measure. For example,

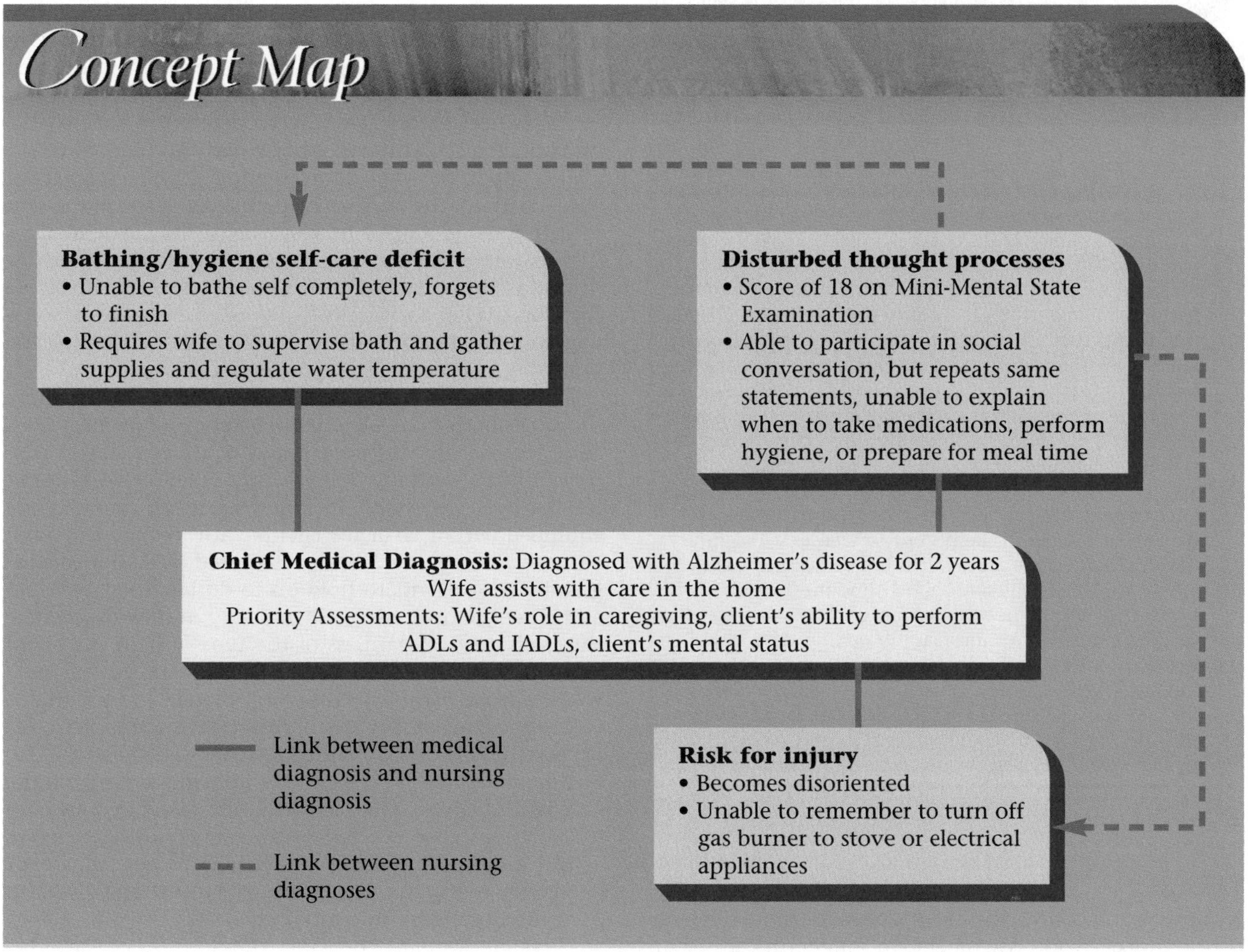
Concept Map
Bathing/hygiene self-care deficit
• Unable to bathe self completely, forgets to finish
• Requires wife to supervise bath and gather supplies and regulate water temperature
Disturbed thought processes
• Score of 18 on Mini-Mental State Examination
• Able to participate in social conversation, but repeats same statements, unable to explain when to take medications, perform hygiene, or prepare for meal time
Chief Medical Diagnosis: Diagnosed with Alzheimer's disease for 2 years
Wife assists with care in the home
Priority Assessments: Wife's role in caregiving, client's ability to perform ADLs and IADLs, client's mental status
Link between medical diagnosis and nursing diagnosis
Link between nursing diagnoses
Risk for injury
• Becomes disoriented
• Unable to remember to turn off gas burner to stove or electrical appliances

FIGURE **34–7** Concept map for client with Alzheimer's disease and hygiene needs.

while giving a client a bath and changing a gown, the nurse uses a gentle approach in turning and repositioning. Using a soft, gentle voice while conversing with the client helps to relieve any fears or concerns. For clients with symptoms such as pain or nausea, administering symptom relief therapies before hygiene helps to prepare the client for the procedure.

Another important part of implementation is helping clients to administer their own hygiene. This includes educating clients on proper hygiene techniques and connecting clients with the community resources necessary to enable them to perform hygiene care. The same clients at risk for hygiene problems are those in greatest need of understanding their risks, knowing the implications, and then having the information they need to make choices about when and how hygiene is performed.

Health Promotion. In primary health care settings, nurses educate and counsel clients and families on proper hygiene techniques. A new mother will need assistance in learning how to bathe her newborn infant. An older adult will need to become informed on the importance of regular ear care to avoid any hearing deficits resulting from accumulated cerumen. When assisting clients, the nurse maintains the standards for hygiene illustrated in this chapter and incorporates adaptations as needed to the client's lifestyle, living arrangements, and preferences. Guidelines to help the nurse in educating clients about hygiene are included in Box 34-6.

Acute and Restorative Care. Nursing knowledge and skills needed for performing hygiene care are consistent across all health care settings where acute care and restorative care are provided. In addition, some of the skills in this section are applicable in areas of health promotion.

In health care settings where clients receive direct nursing care, nurses provide a variety of scheduled hygiene measures (Box 34-7). Times may change because of factors affecting the nurse's organization or scheduling of care such as client preferences, planned diagnostic and

Box 34-6 Educating Clients about Hygiene Care

- Make instructions relevant. After assessing a client's knowledge, motivation, and health beliefs, provide information that relates to the client's situation and will be most useful in resolving the client's problem. For example, when offering foot care instruction to a client with diabetes mellitus, explain how the circulation to the feet can be impaired and how that poses a risk for poor healing and infection should the skin become cut or broken.
- Adapt instruction of techniques to the client's personal bathing facilities. Not all clients will have the ideal situation that exists in a health care setting (e.g., easily accessible shower or a bedside table to place over a bed). Use the facilities or equipment that the client has so that personal care items are easy to reach, the client's safety is ensured, and the client feels comfortable when performing hygiene. For example, a young mother may have more room and feel that bathing an infant will be safer if she uses her kitchen sink and counter rather than her bathroom sink.
- Be sure to teach the client steps to take to avoid injury. Almost any hygiene procedure can pose risks (e.g., cutting a nail too close to the skin, failing to adjust the water temperature of the bath, or using tap water for contact lens care). Any instruction must clearly outline safety risks.
- Reinforce infection-control practices. Damage to the skin, mucosa, eyes, or other tissues creates an immediate risk for infection. Be sure the client understands the relationship between healthy and intact skin and tissues, hand hygiene practices, and the prevention of infection.

treatment procedures, the client's need for more hygiene, or the nurse's work assignment. In long-term care facilities, the schedule for hygiene may be less frequent.

Bathing and Skin Care. Bathing and skin care are a part of total hygiene. The extent of a client's bath and the methods used for bathing depend on the client's physical abilities, health problems, and the degree of hygiene required. If a client is physically dependent or cognitively impaired, the nurse increases skin assessment and provides skin care directed toward reducing the risk for skin breakdown. When bathing cognitively impaired clients, the nurse must consider their special needs and challenges (Box 34-8). These clients can easily become afraid, use physical and verbal aggressive behaviours to avoid bathing, and may also display self-injurious behaviours (Hall & Buckwalter, 2001).

A **complete bed bath** is for clients who are totally dependent and require total hygiene care (Skill 34-1). It is an activity that can be exhausting for a client, even if the nurse provides all of the care. Turning during a complete bed bath and receiving back care have been shown to increase oxygen consumption in healthy adults (Verderber & Gallagher, 1994). The nurse must anticipate and assess whether clients are physically able to tolerate a complete bath. Measuring heart rate before, during, and after the bath provides a measure of the client's physical tolerance. A **partial bed bath** involves bathing only body parts that would cause discomfort or odour if not bathed. This includes perineal care. Aging or dependent clients in need of only partial hygiene or self-sufficient bedridden clients unable to reach all body parts receive partial bed baths. Nurses assess carefully to determine that clients can sufficiently bathe other body parts on their own.

It is important when administering either a complete or partial bath for the nurse to assess the condition of the skin to determine if soap is necessary or if the client requires daily bathing. Clients with excessively dry skin are predisposed to skin impairment. The nurse may decide to skip a bath for a day or bathe only badly soiled areas. Use of soaps that contain emollients is another option. Lubricating the skin with lotion can also help reduce dryness.

The tub bath or shower can be used to give a more thorough bath than a bed bath. Safety is of primary concern because the surface of a tub or shower stall is slippery. In some settings, a physician's order for a shower or tub bath is necessary. In some agencies, showers are equipped with a chair for clients with weakness or poor balance. Both tubs and showers should be equipped with grab bars for clients to hold on to during entry and exit and when manoeuvring. Clients vary in how much help they will need. Regardless of the type of bath the client receives, the nurse should use the following guidelines:

- *Provide privacy.* Close the door, or pull room curtains around the bathing area. While bathing the client, expose only the areas being bathed.
- *Maintain safety.* Keep side rails up while away from the client's bedside. (This is critical for dependent and unconscious clients.) NOTE: When side rails are used as a restraint, a physician's order may be needed. Check agency policy. Place the call light in the client's reach if leaving the room temporarily.
- *Maintain warmth.* The room should be kept warm because the client is partially uncovered and may easily be chilled. Wet skin causes an excess loss of heat through convection. Control drafts, and keep windows closed. Keep client covered, only exposing the body part being washed during the bath.
- *Promote independence.* Encourage the client to participate in as much of the bathing activities as possible. Offer assistance when needed.
- *Anticipate needs.* Bring a new set of clothing and hygiene products to the bedside or bathroom.

Bag Baths. An innovative approach to the traditional bed bath was developed because of nurses' concern for clients who are predisposed to dry skin and the risk for infection. When washbasins are not cleaned and dried completely after use, there is the risk of contamination by gram-negative organisms. Successive uses of the basin may cause the client's skin to harbour more gram-negative organisms. The "bag bath" is a specially prepared package containing 10 washcloths that are pre-moistened in a mixture of water and a non-rinsable cleanser. A bag is warmed in a microwave before use, and then the nurse uses a different cloth for each part of the client's body. In this technique, the skin is allowed to air-dry because

Nursing Care Plan

Ineffective Tissue Perfusion, Improper Foot Care/Hygiene

Assessment

Mrs. Wyatt is a 77-year-old who has had diabetes mellitus for 20 years. She was recently hospitalized for an acute exacerbation of the disease. The nurse, Jeannette, makes the initial home visit for Mrs. Wyatt. Jeannette's assessment reveals that Mrs. Wyatt has an unbalanced gait and appears to limp. Mrs. Wyatt continues to be very independent in making decisions about her care. She tells Jeannette, "It is important for me to be able to care for myself."

Assessment Activities	Findings/Defining Characteristics
Ask Mrs. Wyatt about the comfort of her shoes.	Mrs. Wyatt complains that in the winter her shoes feel tight with socks so she eliminates wearing any type of sock.
Observe Mrs. Wyatt's feet.	Mrs. Wyatt has bilateral heel blisters. Her toenails are long, tissue surrounding nail is peeling, and the nails are dirty. There is tissue inflammation between left great and second toes.
Palpate lower extremities.	Popliteal pulses are within normal limits. Dorsalis pedis pulses are weak. Feet are pale and cool to touch. Capillary refill time of great toe is increased in left foot at >2 seconds.
Ask Mrs. Wyatt about routine foot and nail care.	She cannot describe any specific foot care practice.

Nursing Diagnosis: Ineffective peripheral tissue perfusion related to improper diabetic foot care and nail hygiene practices.

Planning

Goal	Expected Outcomes*
Skin integrity in both feet will improve within 1 month.	**Skin Integrity** Blisters will heal within 2 weeks. Tissue inflammation on left toes will resolve within 10 days.
Client will have improved peripheral circulation to both feet.	**Tissue Perfusion: Peripheral** Within 3 months, feet will be warm to touch, capillary refill brisk.
Client will be able to complete diabetic foot care regimen within 1 month.	**Deficient Knowledge: Treatment Regimen** Client is able to accurately inspect tissue integrity of feet and toenails within 1 month. Client describes correct preventive diabetic foot care practices. Client has improved diabetic foot care and nail hygiene within 2 weeks.

*Outcome classification labels from *Nursing Outcomes Classification (NOC)* (3rd ed.), edited by S. Moorhead, M. Johnson, and M. Maas, 2004, St. Louis, MO: Mosby.

Interventions†	Rationale
Skin Surveillance	
Review with client how to assess feet for breaks in skin, friction from shoes, and how to avoid foot injury.	Injury to diabetic foot from improper nail care, friction from poorly fitting shoes, and minor injuries to the foot increase the client's risk for infection, impaired mobility, and amputation (Strauss, Hart, & Winant, 1998).
Instruct client to observe feet for reddened areas, abrasions, blisters, and swollen areas immediately after removing shoes.	Improperly fitting shoes produce friction, redness, and swelling. Observation for these conditions immediately after removing shoes promotes timely identification of early foot problems (Bryant & Beinlich, 1999).

†Intervention classification labels from *Nursing Interventions Classification (NIC)* (4th ed.), edited by J. M. Dochterman and G. M. Bulechek, 2004, St. Louis, MO: Mosby.

Continued

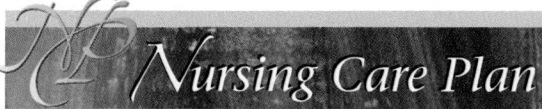

Nursing Care Plan

Ineffective Tissue Perfusion, Improper Foot Care/Hygiene—cont'd

Interventions†—cont'd	Rationale
Skin Care	
Show client how to clean and apply moisturizers and other skin care products to feet daily.	Proper foot care practices include daily cleaning and moisturizing of the feet (Boyer, 2001).
Demonstrate to client how to apply moleskin over blistered areas.	Moleskin preparations are useful in avoiding pressure and friction. Avoiding pressure and friction then allows the area to heal.
Explain that client should see a podiatrist every 4 to 6 weeks for toenail care.	Regular nail care, callus removal, and inspection of feet by a professional reduces the risk for peripheral tissue injury and subsequent immobility and morbidity (Green, Aliabadi, & Green, 2002).
Refer client to orthotic footwear specialist.	Orthotic footwear specialist can evaluate client's walk patterns and create footwear individualized to client's walk, weight, and other individual needs. Specialized footwear can reduce the risk of impaired skin integrity of the feet.

†Intervention classification labels from *Nursing Interventions Classification (NIC)* (4th ed.), edited by J. M. Dochterman and G. M. Bulechek, 2004, St. Louis, MO: Mosby.

Evaluation

Nursing Actions	Client Response/Finding	Achievement of Outcome
Observe client's feet	Blisters are healed.	Resolution of foot blisters has been achieved.
	Inflammation between toes on left foot has resolved.	Resolution of tissue inflammation has occurred, and no new foot injury is observed.
	Toenails are clean and properly trimmed, and no cracks around nail tissue are observed.	Mrs. Wyatt has improved diabetic foot and nail hygiene.
Palpate lower extremities.	Pulses are equal bilaterally; capillary refill is still sluggish.	Tissue perfusion to feet has not improved.
Ask client about frequency of foot inspection.	Mrs. Wyatt states she observes her feet daily after removing her shoes and immediately before bed.	Mrs. Wyatt inspects feet daily; because no new foot injuries are observed, Mrs. Wyatt appears to have achieved this outcome.
Observe client's foot care practice.	Mrs. Wyatt correctly washed and moisturized feet but was not wearing socks with her shoes. She states that she does not consistently wear socks.	Mrs. Wyatt is able to perform diabetic foot hygiene practice but is not consistent in preventive practice.
Ask client about podiatrist appointment.	Mrs. Wyatt has been to the podiatrist twice and will be returning every 6 weeks for toenail trimming and care.	Mrs. Wyatt has improved diabetic foot and nail hygiene practice.

towel drying removes the emollient that is left behind after the water/cleanser solution evaporates. Staff members who have used the bag bath report shorter bathing times and client and nurse satisfaction (Skewes, 1994).

Perineal Care. **Perineal care** is usually part of the complete bed bath (Skill 34-2). Clients most in need of perineal care are those at greatest risk for acquiring an infection (e.g., clients who have in-dwelling urinary catheters, clients who are recovering from rectal or genital surgery or childbirth, or uncircumcised males). In addition, women who are having a menstrual period will require good perineal care. A client able to perform self-care should be encouraged to do so. Nurses can become embarrassed when providing perineal care, particularly for clients of the opposite sex. Similarly, the client may feel embarrassed, but this should not cause the nurse to overlook the client's hygiene needs. A professional, dignified, and sensitive approach can reduce embarrassment and put the client at ease.

If a client performs self-care, various problems such as vaginal and urethral discharge, skin irritation, and unpleasant odours may go unnoticed. The nurse must be alert for complaints of burning during urination or localized soreness, excoriation, or pain in the perineum. The nurse also inspects the client's bed linen for signs of discharge. Clients most at risk for skin breakdown in the perineal area are those with urinary or fecal incontinence,

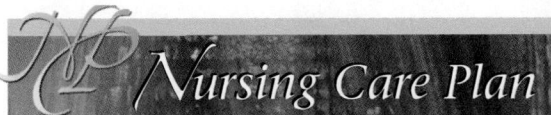

Box 34-7 Hygiene Care Schedule in Acute and Long-Term Care Settings

Early Morning Care

Nursing personnel on the night shift may provide basic hygiene to clients getting ready for breakfast, scheduled tests, or early morning surgery. Early morning care, or AM care, includes offering a bedpan or urinal if the client is not ambulatory, washing the client's hands and face, and assisting with oral care.

Routine Morning Care

In care performed after breakfast, the nurse assists by offering a bedpan or urinal to clients confined to bed; providing a bath or shower; providing perineal care; providing oral, foot, nail, and hair care; giving a back rub; changing the client's gown or pyjamas; changing the bed linens; and straightening the client's bedside unit and room. This is often referred to as "complete AM care."

Afternoon Care

Hospitalized clients often undergo many exhausting diagnostic tests or procedures in the morning. In rehabilitation centres, clients may participate in physiotherapy during the morning. Afternoon hygiene care includes washing the hands and face, assisting with oral care, offering a bedpan or urinal, and straightening bed linen.

Evening, or Hour-Before-Sleep, Care

Before bedtime, the nurse offers personal hygiene care that helps a client relax to promote sleep. Evening care, or PM care, may include changing soiled bed linens, gowns, or pyjamas; assisting the client in washing the face and hands; providing oral hygiene; giving a back massage; and offering the bedpan or urinal to non-ambulatory clients. Some clients may enjoy a beverage such as juice.

rectal and perineal surgical dressings, or in-dwelling urinary catheters, as well as those who are morbidly obese.

Back Rub. A back rub or back massage usually follows the client's bath. It promotes relaxation, relieves muscular tension, and stimulates skin circulation. Labyak and Metzger (1997) evaluated the efficacy of massage and its effects on the physiological measures of relaxation. Their analysis showed that the long, slow, gliding strokes **(effleurage)** of a massage are associated with a reduction in heart rate and respiratory rate. Males seem to achieve greater reductions in systolic and diastolic blood pressure during a back rub than females. Because effleurage causes an immediate rise in blood pressure and heart rate in clients who have had coronary artery bypass surgery, the researchers do not recommend the therapy for those clients within the first 48 hours of their surgery. Clients generally report that they are more comfortable following a back rub and find the experience pleasant, regardless of the length of the massage. A back rub of 3 minutes' duration can actually enhance client comfort and relaxation and thus be very therapeutic (Labyak & Metzger, 1997).

When providing a back rub, the nurse can enhance relaxation by reducing any noise and ensuring that the client is comfortable. Because some individuals may dislike physical contact, it is important to ask whether a client would like a back rub or if the client prefers gentle instead of heavy massage. The nurse should consult the medical record for any contraindications to a massage (e.g., fractured ribs, burns of the skin, and heart surgery).

Foot and Nail Care. Foot and nail care should be incorporated into a person's regular hygiene routine. Routine care involves soaking to soften cuticles and layers of horny cells, thorough cleansing, drying, and proper nail trimming. The exception involves clients with diabetes mellitus who do not soak their nails because of the risk of infection. When the nurse administers care, the client may remain in bed or sit in a chair (Skill 34-3). In some

Text continued on p. 1048

Evidence-Based Practice Guideline — Box 34-8

Bathing Clients With Dementia

Provide individualized and flexible client-centred care

- Obtain bathing history: what works, what doesn't work.
- Identify preferences from the client, other caregivers, or family.
- Determine method that is least distressing to the client (e.g., soaking feet in the bathtub).
- Prepare bath environment in advance.
- Minimize the time the client is unclothed.
- Use distraction and negotiation instead of demands (e.g., give the client a washcloth to keep hands occupied).
- Minimize noise in bathing area.
- Be sure bathing environment is warm.
- Assess if the client requires glasses or a hearing aid, which can assist with communication (remove aids as required during bathing after communicating your intent to the client).
- Set priorities as to which body parts need bathing and which can be "skipped" (e.g., separate hair washing from bathing).
- Use as few staff as possible.
- If client fears water, coloured water or a bubble bath may help.
- Reward client after bathing; praise and rewards should be realistic.

Adapted from "Understanding Alzheimer Disease: The Link Between Brain and Behaviour," Alzheimer Society of Canada, Module 4 in *The Alzheimer Journey* [Video and workbook series], 2003, retrieved May 30, 2004, from *http://www.alzheimer.ca/english/disease/whatisit-video.htm;* and "Research-Based Protocol: Bathing Persons With Dementia," by G. R. Hall and K. C. Buckwalter, in *Series on Evidence-Based Practice for Older Adults,* edited by M.G. Titler (Series Ed.), 2001, Iowa City, IA: The University of Iowa College of Nursing Gerontological Nursing Interventions Research Center, Research Dissemination Core.

Skill 34-1 Bathing a Client

Delegation Considerations

Skills of bathing may be delegated to unregulated care providers (UCPs).

- Instruct the UCP on the importance of not massaging reddened skin areas.
- Clarify the early signs of impaired skin integrity for select clients and their situation.
- Have the UCP report changes in the client's skin to the nurse.

Equipment

- Two washcloths
- Two bath towels
- Bath blanket
- Soap and soap dish
- Toiletry items (deodorant, powder, lotion, cologne)
- Clean hospital gown or client's own pyjamas or gown
- Linen bag
- Disposable gloves (when risk for contacting body fluids)

Steps	Rationale
1. Assess client's tolerance for activity, discomfort level, cognitive ability, and musculoskeletal function.	Determines client's ability to perform self-care and level of assistance required from nurse. Also determines type of bath to administer (e.g., tub bath or partial bed bath).

Critical Decision Point: Clients whose level of independence and mobility change frequently may require more or less assistance during bathing.

Steps	Rationale
2. Assess client's bathing preferences: frequency and time of day preferred for bathing, type of hygiene products, and other factors related to client preferences.	Client participates in plan of care. Promotes client's comfort and provides opportunity to include cultural or personal hygiene preferences in hygiene care.
3. Ask if client has noticed any problems or unusual marks on skin.	Provides information to direct physical assessment of skin during bathing.
4. Review orders for specific precautions concerning client's movement or positioning.	Prevents accidental injury to client during bathing activities. Determines level of assistance required by client.
5. Explain procedure, and ask client for suggestions on how to prepare supplies. If partial bath, ask how much of bath client wishes to complete.	Promotes client's co-operation and participation.
6. Adjust room temperature and ventilation, close room doors and windows, and draw room divider curtain.	Warm room that is free of drafts prevents rapid loss of body heat during bathing. Privacy ensures client's mental and physical comfort.
7. Perform hand hygiene. Prepare equipment and supplies.	Reduces transmission of micro-organisms and avoids interrupting procedure or leaving client unattended to retrieve missing equipment.
8. Offer client bedpan or urinal. Provide towel and washcloth.	Client will feel more comfortable after voiding. Prevents interruption of bath.
9. Perform hand hygiene. If client's skin is soiled with drainage or body secretions, apply disposable gloves. Ensure client is not allergic to latex.	Reduces transmission of micro-organisms.
10. Bathe client.	
A. **Complete or partial bed bath**	
(1) Place hospital bed at appropriate level. If raised, lower side rail closest to you, and assist client in assuming comfortable position, maintaining body alignment. Bring client toward side closest to you.	Raising the height of the bed to appropriate position for the nurse facilitates proper body mechanics. Aids nurse's access to client. Maintains client's comfort throughout procedure. Nurse does not have to reach across bed, thus minimizing strain on back muscles.
(2) Loosen top covers at foot of bed. Place bath blanket over top sheet. Fold and remove top sheet from under blanket. If possible, have client hold bath blanket while withdrawing sheet. *Optional:* Use top sheet when bath blanket is not available.	Removal of top linens prevents them from becoming soiled or moist during bath. Blanket provides warmth and privacy.
(3) If top sheet is to be reused, fold it for replacement later. If not, dispose in linen bag, taking care not to allow linen to contact uniform.	Proper disposal prevents transmission of micro-organisms.

Steps	Rationale
(4) Remove client's gown or pyjamas. If an extremity is injured or has reduced mobility, begin removal from *unaffected* side. If client has intravenous (IV) tube, remove gown from arm *without* IV first; then lower IV container or remove from pump and slide gown covering affected arm over tubing and container. Rehang IV container and check flow rate (see illustrations) or reset pump rate. Do not disconnect tubing.	Provides full exposure of body parts during bathing. Undressing unaffected side first allows easier manipulation of gown over body part with reduced range of motion (ROM).

Critical Decision Point: If available, be sure that clients with an IV or upper extremity injury have a gown with snap or tie sleeves, which ensures there is easy access to upper extremities during hygiene.

Critical Decision Point: When an IV pump is used, it may be appropriate to manually adjust the IV flow rate to a keep vein open (KVO) flow and remove the IV tubing from the pump (check agency policy). When the bath is complete, the nurse resets the pump to the prescribed IV flow rate (see chapter 36).

(5) Pull side rail up. Fill washbasin two-thirds full with warm water. Have client place fingers in water to test temperature tolerance.	Raising side rail maintains client's safety as nurse leaves bedside. Warm water promotes comfort, relaxes muscles, and prevents unnecessary chilling. Testing temperature prevents accidental burns.

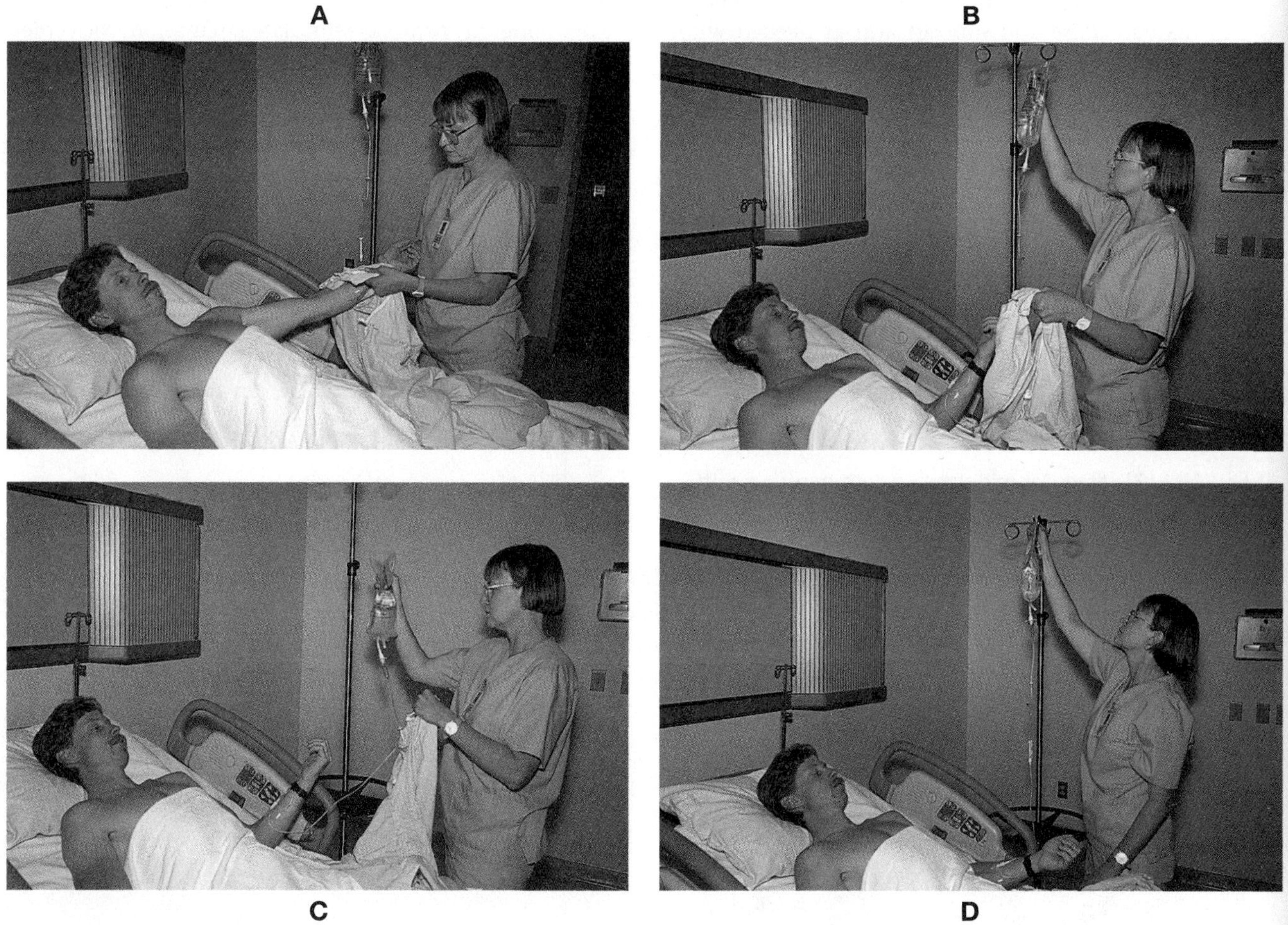

STEP **10A(4)** **A,** Remove client's gown. **B,** Remove IV from pole. **C,** Slide IV tubing through arm of client's gown. **D,** Rehang IV bag.

Skill 34-1 Bathing a Client—cont'd

Steps	Rationale
(6) Remove pillow if allowed, and raise head of bed 30 to 45 degrees. Place bath towel under client's head. Place second bath towel over client's chest.	Removal of pillow makes it easier to wash client's ears and neck. Placement of towels prevents soiling of bed linen and bath blanket.
(7) Immerse washcloth in water and wring thoroughly. If desired, fold washcloth around fingers of nurse's hand to form mitt (see illustration).	Mitt retains water and heat better than loosely held washcloth; keeps cold edges from brushing against client and prevents splashing.
(8) Wash client's eyes with plain warm water. Inquire if client is wearing contact lenses. Use different section of mitt for each eye. Move mitt from inner to outer canthus (see illustration). Soak any crusts on eyelid for 2 to 3 minutes with damp cloth before attempting removal. Dry eye thoroughly but gently.	Soap irritates eyes. Use of separate sections of mitt reduces infection transmission. Bathing eye from inner to outer canthus prevents secretions from entering nasolacrimal duct. Pressure can cause internal injury.
(9) Ask if client prefers to use soap on face. Wash, rinse, and thoroughly dry the forehead, cheeks, nose, neck, and ears. (Men may wish to shave at this point or after bath.)	Soap tends to dry face, which is exposed to air more than other body parts.
(10) Remove bath blanket from client's arm that is closest to nurse. Place bath towel lengthwise under arm.	Prevents soiling of bed.
(11) Bathe arm with soap and water using long, firm strokes from distal to proximal areas (fingers to axilla). Raise and support arm as needed while thoroughly washing axilla (see illustration).	Soap lowers surface tension and facilitates removal of debris and bacteria when friction is applied during washing. Long, firm strokes stimulate circulation. Movement of arm exposes axilla and exercises joint's normal ROM.
(12) Rinse and dry arm and axilla thoroughly. If client uses deodorant or talcum powder, apply it.	Alkaline residue from soap discourages growth of normal skin bacteria (Barnes, 1987). Excess moisture causes skin maceration or softening. Deodorant controls body odour.

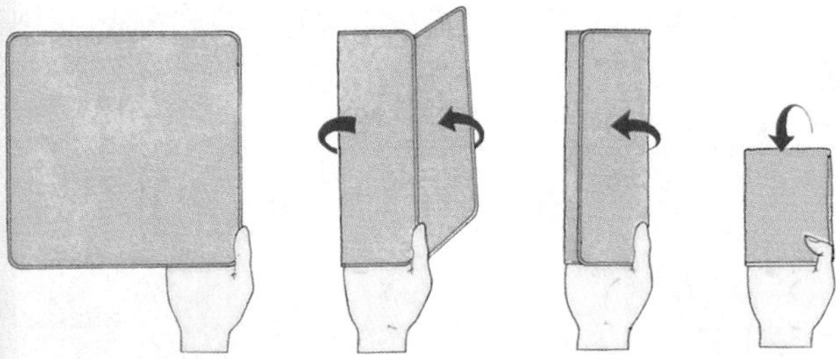

STEP **10A(7)** Steps for folding washcloth to form a mitt.

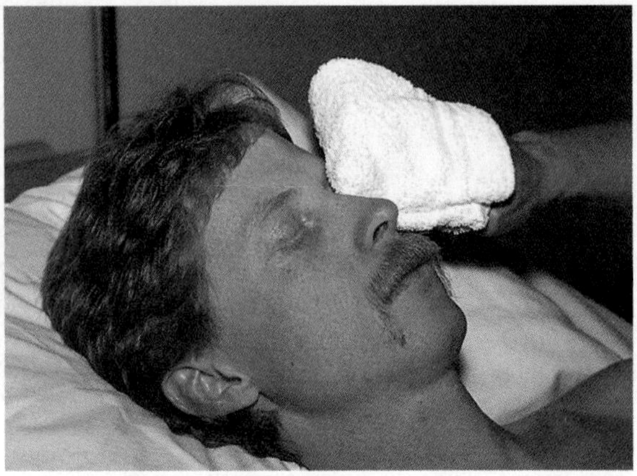

STEP **10A(8)** Wash eye from inner to outer canthus.

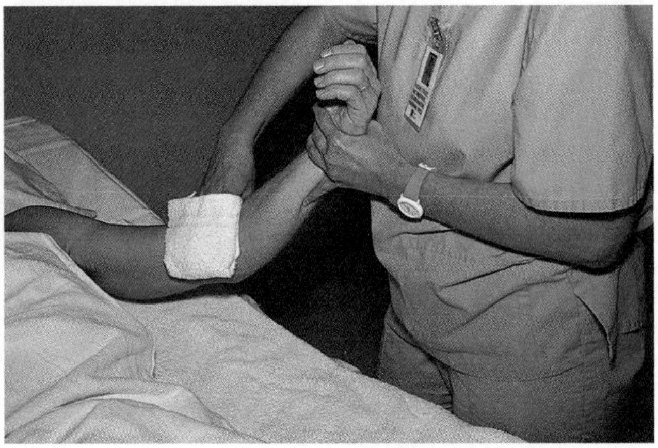

STEP **10A(11)** Washing from fingers to axilla.

Steps	Rationale
(13) Fold bath towel in half, and lay it on bed beside client. Place basin on towel. Immerse client's hand in water. Allow hand to soak for 3 to 5 minutes before washing hand and fingernails (see Skill 34-3). Remove basin and dry hand well.	Soaking softens cuticles and calluses of hand, loosens debris beneath nails, and enhances feeling of cleanliness. Thorough drying removes moisture from between fingers. NOTE: Do not soak if client is diabetic or if client is cognitively impaired and unable to understand procedure.
(14) Raise side rail, and move to other side of bed. Lower side rail, and repeat Steps 10 through 13 for other arm.	
(15) Check temperature of bath water, and change water if necessary.	Warm water maintains client's comfort.

Critical Decision Point: If a client is at risk for falls, be sure two side rails are up before obtaining fresh water or other supplies. Remember, side rails cannot be used as a restraint unless ordered.

Steps	Rationale
(16) Cover client's chest with bath towel, and fold bath blanket down to umbilicus. With one hand, lift edge of towel away from chest. With washcloth or mitted hand, bathe chest using long, firm strokes. Take special care to wash skinfolds under female client's breasts. It may be necessary to lift breast upward while bathing underneath it. Keep client's chest covered between wash and rinse periods. Dry well.	Draping prevents unnecessary exposure of body parts. Towel maintains warmth and privacy. Secretions and dirt collect easily in areas of tight skinfolds. Skinfolds are susceptible to excoriation if breasts are pendulous.
(17) Place bath towel lengthwise over chest and abdomen. (Two towels may be needed.) Fold blanket down to just above pubic region.	Prevents chilling and exposure of body parts.
(18) With one hand, lift bath towel. With mitted hand, bathe abdomen, giving special attention to bathing umbilicus and abdominal folds. Stroke from side to side. Keep abdomen covered between washing and rinsing. Dry well.	Moisture and sediment that collect in skinfolds predispose skin to maceration and irritation.
(19) Apply clean gown or pyjama top. If one extremity is injured or immobilized, always dress affected side first. This step may be omitted until completion of bath; gown should not become soiled during remainder of bath.	Maintains client's warmth and comfort. Dressing affected side first allows easier manipulation of gown over body part with reduced ROM.
(20) Cover chest and abdomen with top of bath blanket. Expose near leg by folding blanket toward midline. Be sure other leg and perineum are draped.	Prevents unnecessary exposure.
(21) Bend client's leg at knee by positioning nurse's arm under leg. While grasping client's heel, elevate leg from mattress slightly, and slide bath towel lengthwise under leg. Ask client to hold foot still. Place bath basin on towel on bed, and secure its position next to foot to be washed.	Towel prevents soiling of bed linen. Support of joint and extremity during lifting prevents strain on musculoskeletal structures. Sudden movement by client could spill bath water. (Omit this step if client is unable to hold leg in basin.)
(22) With one hand supporting lower leg, raise it and slide basin under lifted foot. Make sure foot is firmly placed on bottom of basin. Allow foot to soak while washing leg. If client is unable to hold leg, do not immerse; simply wash with washcloth (see illustration).	Proper positioning of foot prevents pressure being applied from edge of basin against calf. Soaking softens calluses and rough skin.
(23) Unless contraindicated, use long, firm strokes in washing from ankle to knee and from knee to thigh. Dry well.	Promotes venous return.

Critical Decision Point: Clients with history of deep vein thromboses or hypercoagulation disorders should not have their lower extremities washed with long firm strokes.

Skill 34-1 Bathing a Client—cont'd

Steps	Rationale

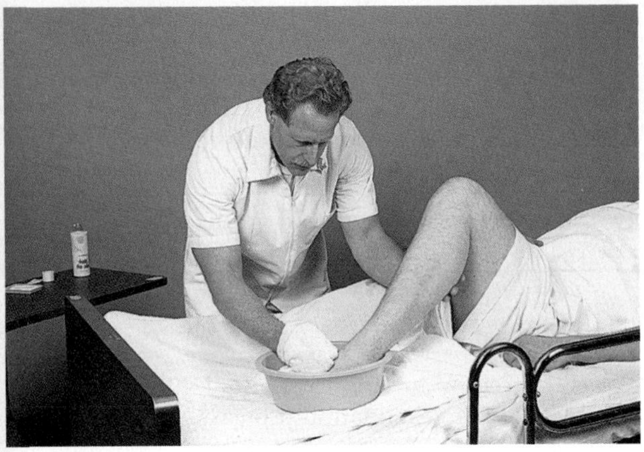

STEP **10A(22)** Supporting client's leg and foot in water basin.

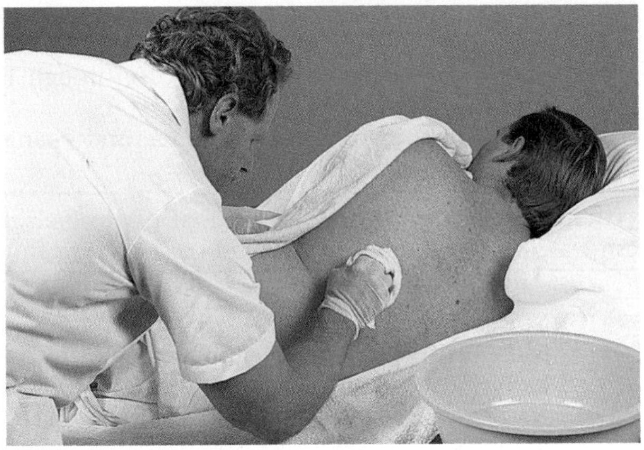

STEP **10A(28)** Washing client's back.

Steps	Rationale
(24) Cleanse foot, making sure to bathe between toes. Clean and clip nails as per physician orders (see Skill 34-3). Dry well. If skin is dry, apply lotion.	Secretions and moisture may be present between toes. Lotion helps retain moisture and soften skin.

Critical Decision Point: Do not massage any reddened area on client's skin because massaging causes breaks in the skin's surface capillaries and increased risk of skin breakdown (Agency for Health Care Policy Research, 1992).

Steps	Rationale
(25) Raise side rail, and move to other side of the bed. Lower side rail, and repeat steps 20 through 24 for other leg and foot.	
(26) Cover client with bath blanket, raise side rail for client's safety, and change bath water.	Decreased bath water temperature can cause chilling. Clean water reduces micro-organism transmission.
(27) Lower side rail. Assist client in assuming prone or side-lying position (as applicable). Place towel lengthwise along client's side.	Exposes back and buttocks for bathing.
(28) Keep client draped by sliding bath blanket over shoulders and thighs. Wash, rinse, and dry back from neck to buttocks using long, firm strokes (see illustration). Pay special attention to folds of buttocks and anus. Give a back rub (see chapter 38). Change bath water.	Maintains warmth and prevents unnecessary exposure. Skinfolds near buttocks and anus may contain fecal secretions that harbour micro-organisms. Changing water prevents transfer of micro-organisms from anal area to genitalia.
(29) Apply disposable gloves if not done previously.	Prevents contact with micro-organisms in body secretions.
(30) Assist client in assuming side-lying or supine position. Cover chest and upper extremities with towel and lower extremities with bath blanket. Expose only genitalia. (If client can wash, covering entire body with bath blanket may be preferable.) Provide perineal care (see Skill 34-2). Pay special attention to skinfolds.	Maintains client's privacy. Clients capable of performing partial bath usually prefer to wash their own genitalia.
(31) Dispose of gloves in receptacle.	Prevents transmission of infection.
(32) Apply additional body lotion or oil as desired. Observe skin, paying particular attention to areas that were previously soiled, reddened, or showed early signs of breakdown.	Moisturizing lotion prevents dry, chapped skin. Techniques used during bathing should leave skin clean and clear.
(33) Assist client in dressing. Comb client's hair. Women may want to apply makeup.	Promotes client's body image.

Steps	Rationale
(34) Make client's bed (see Skill 34-6).	Provides clean environment.
(35) Remove soiled linen, and place in linen bag. Clean and replace bathing equipment. Replace call light and personal possessions. Leave room as clean and comfortable as possible.	Prevents transmission of infection. Clean environment promotes client's comfort. Keeping call light and articles of care within reach promotes client's safety.
(36) Perform hand hygiene.	Reduces transmission of micro-organisms.
B. **Tub or whirlpool bath or shower; verify with agency policy if a physician's order is needed.**	
(1) Consider client's condition, and review orders for precautions concerning client's movement or positioning.	Prevents accidental injury to client during bathing.
(2) Check tub or shower for cleanliness. Use cleaning techniques outlined in agency policy. Place rubber mat on tub or shower bottom. Place disposable bath mat or towel on floor in front of tub or shower.	Cleaning prevents transmission of micro-organisms. Mats prevent slipping and falling.
(3) Collect all hygienic aids, toiletry items, and linens requested by client. Place within easy reach of tub or shower.	Placing items close at hand prevents possible falls when client reaches for equipment.
(4) Assist client to bathroom if necessary. Have client wear robe and slippers to bathroom.	Assistance prevents accidental falls. Wearing robe and slippers prevents chilling.
(5) Demonstrate how to use call signal for assistance.	Bathrooms are equipped with signalling devices in case client feels faint or weak or needs immediate assistance. Clients prefer privacy during bath if safety is not jeopardized.
(6) Place "occupied" sign on bathroom door.	Maintains client's privacy.
(7) Provide shower seat or tub chair if needed (see illustration). Fill bathtub halfway with warm water. If sensation is normal, ask client to test water, and adjust temperature if water is too warm. Explain which faucet controls hot water. If client is taking shower, turn shower on, and adjust water temperature before client enters shower stall.	Adjusting water temperature prevents accidental burns. Older adults and clients with neurological alterations (e.g., spinal cord injury) are at high risk for burns as a result of reduced sensation. Use of assistive devices facilitates bathing and minimizes physical exertion.
(8) Instruct client to use safety bars when getting in and out of tub or shower. Caution client against use of bath oil in tub water.	Prevents slipping and falling. Oil causes tub surfaces to become slippery.
(9) Instruct client not to remain in tub longer than 20 minutes. Check on client every 5 minutes. Observe ROM during bath.	Prolonged exposure to warm water may cause vasodilation and pooling of blood, leading to light-headedness or dizziness. Measures joint mobility.
(10) Return to bathroom when client signals, and knock before entering.	Provides privacy.

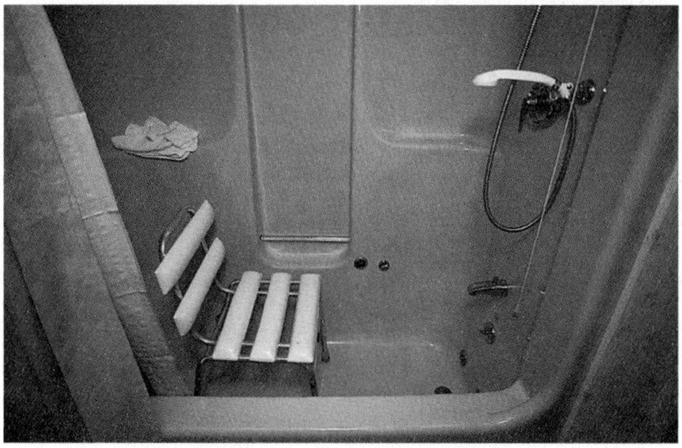

STEP **10B(7)** Shower seat for client safety.

Skill 34-1 Bathing a Client—cont'd

Steps	Rationale
(11) For client who is unsteady, drain tub of water before client attempts to get out of it. Place bath towel over client's shoulders. Assist client in getting out of tub as needed, and assist with drying. If client is weak or unstable, have UCPs assist.	Prevents accidental falls. Client may become chilled as water drains.

Critical Decision Point: Weak or unstable clients need extra assistance in getting out of a tub. Planning for additional personnel is essential before attempting to assist the client from tub.

Steps	Rationale
(12) Observe skin, paying particular attention to areas that were previously soiled, reddened, or showed early signs of breakdown.	Techniques used during bathing should leave skin clean and clear.
(13) Assist client as needed in donning clean gown or pyjamas, slippers, and robe. (In home setting, client may don regular clothing.)	Maintains warmth to prevent chilling.
(14) Assist client to room and comfortable position in bed or chair.	Maintains relaxation gained from bathing.
(15) Clean tub or shower according to agency policy. Whirlpool baths may require special cleansing. Remove soiled linen and place in linen bag. Discard disposable equipment in proper receptacle. Place "unoccupied" sign on bathroom door. Return supplies to storage area.	Prevents transmission of infection through soiled linen and moisture.
(16) Perform hand hygiene.	Reduces transfer of micro-organisms.
11. Ask client to rate level of comfort.	Evaluates success of bath in promoting client's comfort.

Unexpected Outcomes and Related Interventions

- Areas of excessive dryness, rashes, irritation, or signs of a pressure ulcer appear on skin.
  - Review agency skin care policy regarding special cleansing and moisturizing products.
  - Limit frequency of complete baths.
  - Complete pressure ulcer assessment (see chapter 43).
  - Obtain special bed surface if client is at risk for skin breakdown.
- Client becomes excessively fatigued and unable to cooperate or participate in bathing.
  - Reschedule bathing to a time when client is more rested.
  - Clients with cardiopulmonary conditions and breathing difficulties require pillow or elevated head of bed during bathing.
  - Notify physician about changes in client's fatigue level.
  - Schedule rest periods.
- Client seems unusually restless or complains of discomfort.
  - Consider analgesia before bathing.
  - Schedule rest periods before bathing.

Recording and Reporting

- Record condition of skin and any significant findings (e.g., reddened areas, bruises, nevi, or joint or muscle pain).
- Report evidence of alterations in skin integrity, break in suture line, or increased wound secretions to nurse in charge or physician.
- Record procedure, amount of assistance, and client participation.

Home Care Considerations

- Assess client's tub and shower area for the need for safety devices (e.g., grab bars).
- Assess client for the need for assistive bathing devices (e.g., shower chair, hand-held shower).

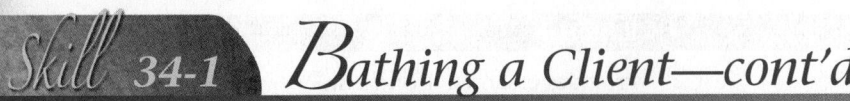

Skill 34-2 Perineal Care

View Video

Delegation Considerations

Skills of perineal care can be delegated to unregulated care providers (UCPs).

- Inform the UCP when the client has physical restrictions that will affect proper way to position for procedure.
- Provide information about proper positioning of in-dwelling catheter during perineal care.
- Instruct the UCP to inform nurse if any perineal drainage, excoriation, or rash is observed.

Equipment

- Washbasin
- Soap dish with soap
- Two or three washcloths
- Bath towel
- Bath blanket
- Waterproof pad or bedpan
- Toilet tissue or diaper wipes
- Disposable gloves

Additional supplies are needed when pericare is given other than during a bath:

- Cotton balls or swabs
- A solution bottle or container filled with warm water or prescribed rinsing solution
- Waterproof bag

Steps	Rationale
1. Identify clients at risk for developing infection of genitalia, urinary tract, or reproductive tract (e.g., uncircumcised male, clients with an in-dwelling catheter or fecal incontinence).	Secretions that accumulate on surface of skin surrounding female and male genitalia act as reservoir for infection. Tissues traumatized by surgery or by presence of foreign object provide route for introduction of infectious organisms.
2. Assess client's cognitive and musculoskeletal function.	Determines client's ability to perform self-care and determines level of assistance required from nurse.
3. Apply disposable gloves and assess genitalia for signs of inflammation, skin breakdown, or infection (see chapter 28). Discard gloves. Perform hand hygiene.	Reduces infection. Determines extent of perineal care required by client.

Critical Decision Point: Assessment of genitalia may be deferred until perineal care is administered.

Steps	Rationale
4. Assess client's knowledge of importance of perineal hygiene.	Clients at risk for infection in perineal area may be unaware of importance of cleanliness. Reflects client's need for education.
5. Explain procedure and its purpose to client.	Helps minimize anxiety during procedure that is often embarrassing to nurse and client.
6. Perfrom hand hygiene. Prepare necessary equipment and supplies.	Reduces transmission of micro-organisms and promotes organization.
7. Pull curtain around client's bed, or close room door. Assemble supplies at bedside.	Maintains client's privacy and ensures orderly procedure.
8. Raise bed to comfortable working position. If raised, lower side rail, and assist client in assuming side-lying position, placing towel lengthwise along client's side and keeping client covered with bath blanket or top sheet.	Facilitates good body mechanics. Provides easy access to genitalia.
9. Apply disposable gloves.	Prevents transmission of micro-organisms.
10. If fecal material is present, enclose in a fold of underpad or toilet tissue, and remove with disposable wipes or tissue. Cleanse buttocks and anus, washing front to back (see illustration). Cleanse, rinse, and dry area thoroughly. If needed, place an absorbent pad under client's buttocks. Remove and discard underpad and replace with clean one.	Cleansing reduces transmission of micro-organisms from anus to urethra or genitalia.
11. Change gloves when they are soiled. Perform hand hygiene.	

Skill 34-2 *Perineal Care—cont'd*

Steps	Rationale

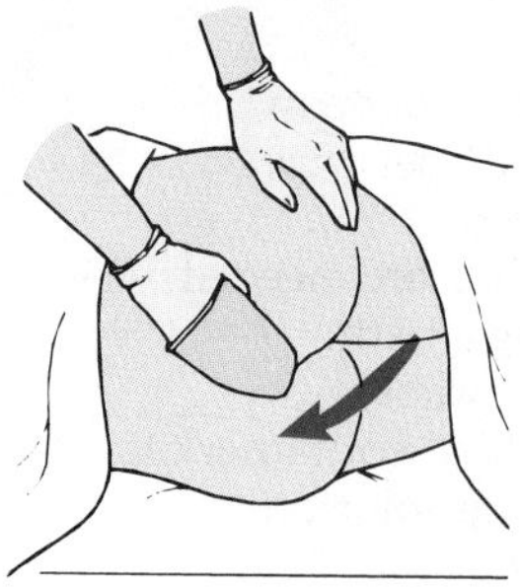

STEP **10** Cleanse buttocks from front to back.

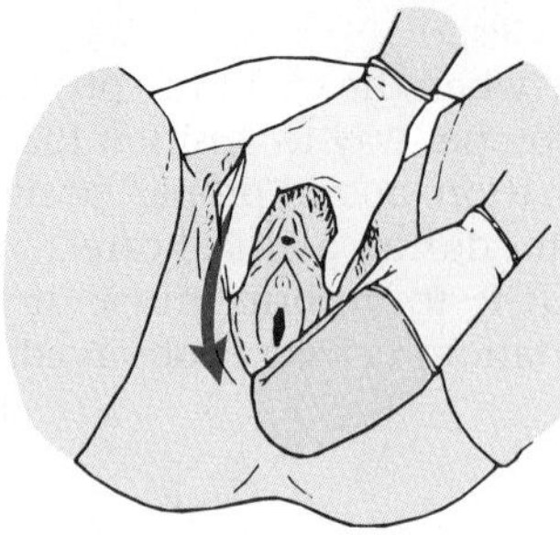

STEP **15A(5)** Cleanse from perineum to rectum (front to back).

Steps	Rationale
12. Fold top bed linen down toward foot of bed, and raise client's gown above genital area. Prepare bed linen to protect client's privacy.	Exposes perineal area for easy accessibility.
a. "Diamond" drape client by placing bath blanket with one corner between client's legs, one corner pointing toward each side of bed, and one corner over client's chest. Tuck side corners around client's legs and under hips.	Prevents unnecessary exposure of body parts and maintains client's warmth and comfort during procedure.
13. Raise side rail. Fill washbasin with warm water.	Prevents client from falling. Proper water temperature prevents burns to perineum.
14. Place washbasin and toilet tissue on overbed table. Place washcloths in basin.	Equipment placed within nurse's reach prevents accidental spills.
15. Provide perineal care.	
A. **Female perineal care**	
(1) Assist client to dorsal recumbent position.	Provides easy access to genitalia.
(2) Lower side rail, and help client flex knees and spread legs. Note restrictions or limitations in client's positioning.	Provides full exposure of female genitalia. Minimize degree of abduction in female if position causes pain because of arthritis or reduced joint mobility.
(3) Fold lower corner of bath blanket up between client's legs onto abdomen. Wash and dry client's upper thighs.	Minimizes transmission of micro-organisms. Keeping client draped until procedure begins minimizes anxiety. Buildup of perineal secretions can soil surrounding skin surfaces.
(4) Wash labia majora. Use non-dominant hand to gently retract labia from thigh; with dominant hand, wash carefully in skinfolds. Wipe in direction from perineum to rectum (front to back). Repeat on opposite side using separate section of washcloth. Rinse and dry area thoroughly.	Skinfolds may contain body secretions that harbour micro-organisms. Wiping from perineum to rectum (front to back) reduces chance of transmitting fecal organisms to urinary meatus.
(5) Separate labia with non-dominant hand to expose urethral meatus and vaginal orifice. With dominant hand, wash downward from pubic area toward rectum in one smooth stroke (see illustration). Use separate section of cloth for each stroke. Cleanse thoroughly around labia minora, clitoris, and vaginal orifice.	Cleansing method reduces transfer of micro-organisms to urinary meatus. (For menstruating women or clients with in-dwelling urinary catheters, cleanse with cotton balls.)
(6) If client uses bedpan, pour warm water over perineal area. Dry perineal area thoroughly, using front-to-back method.	Rinsing removes soap and micro-organisms more effectively than wiping. Retained moisture harbours micro-organisms.
(7) Fold lower corner of bath blanket back between client's legs and over perineum. Ask client to lower legs and assume comfortable position.	

Steps	Rationale

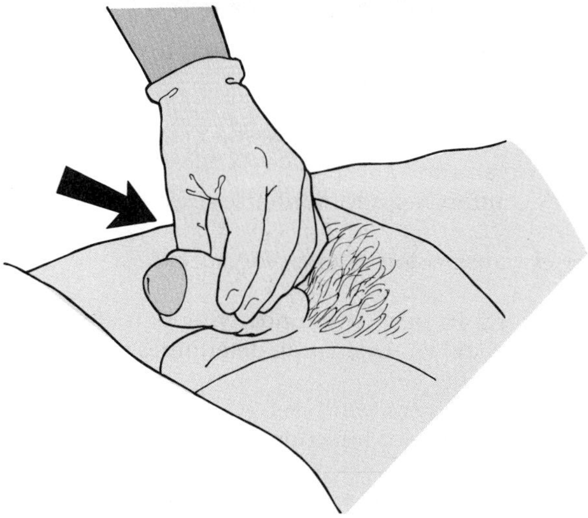

STEP **15B(3)** Retract foreskin.

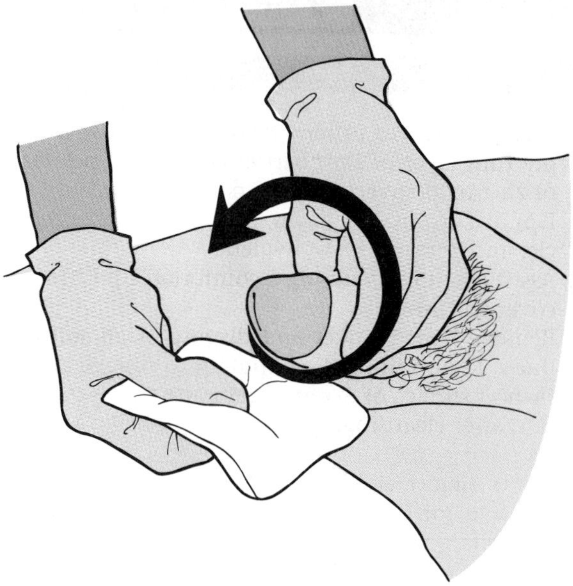

STEP **15B(4)** Use circular motion to cleanse tip of penis.

Steps	Rationale
B. Male perineal care	
(1) Lower side rails, and assist client to supine position. Note restriction in mobility.	Provides full exposure of male genitalia.
(2) Fold lower corner of bath blanket up between client's legs and onto abdomen. Wash and dry client's upper thighs.	Minimizes transmission of micro-organisms. Keeping client draped until procedure begins minimizes anxiety. Buildup of perineal secretions can soil surrounding skin surfaces.
(3) Gently raise penis, and place bath towel underneath. Gently grasp shaft of penis. If client is uncircumcised, retract foreskin (see illustration). If client has an erection, defer procedure until later.	Towel prevents moisture from collecting in inguinal area. Gentle but firm handling reduces chance of client having an erection. Secretions capable of harbouring micro-organisms collect underneath foreskin. Cleansing the penis can lead to an erection, which can embarrass both client and nurse. It is important to assess if the procedure can be continued or deferred until a later time.
(4) Wash tip of penis at urethral meatus first. Using circular motion, cleanse from meatus outward (see illustration). Discard washcloth, and repeat with clean cloth until penis is clean. Rinse and dry gently.	Direction of cleansing moves from area of least contamination to area of most contamination, preventing micro-organisms from entering urethra
(5) Return foreskin to its natural position	Tightening of foreskin around shaft of penis can cause local edema and discomfort.

Critical Decision Point: After administering male perineal care, make sure the foreskin is in its natural position. This is extremely important in those clients with decreased sensation in their lower extremities.

Steps	Rationale
(6) Wash shaft of penis with gentle but firm downward strokes. Pay special attention to underlying surface of penis. Rinse and dry penis thoroughly. Instruct client to spread legs apart slightly.	Underlying surface of penis may have greater accumulation of secretions. Abduction of legs provides easier access to scrotal tissues.
(7) Gently cleanse scrotum. Lift it carefully, and wash underlying skinfolds. Rinse and dry.	Pressure on scrotal tissues can be painful to client. Secretions collect between skinfolds.
(8) Fold bath blanket back over client's perineum, and assist client in turning to side-lying position.	Draping promotes comfort and minimizes client's anxiety. Side-lying position provides access to anal area.

Skill 34-2 Perineal Care—cont'd

Steps	Rationale
16. If client has had urinary or bowel incontinence, apply thin layer of skin barrier containing petrolatum or zinc oxide over anal and perineal skin.	Protects skin from excess moisture and toxins from urine or stool (Maklebust, 1991).
17. Remove disposable gloves, dispose in proper receptacle, and perform hand hygiene.	Moisture and body secretions on gloves can harbour micro-organisms.
18. Assist client in assuming a comfortable position, and cover with sheet.	Client's comfort helps to minimize stress of procedure.
19. Remove bath blanket and dispose of all soiled bed linen. Return unused equipment to storage area.	Reduces transmission of micro-organisms.
20. Inspect surface of external genitalia and surrounding skin after cleansing.	Thick secretions may cover underlying skin lesions or areas of breakdown. Evaluation determines need for additional hygiene.
21. Ask if client feels sense of cleanliness.	Evaluates client's comfort level.
22. Observe for abnormal drainage or discharge from genitalia.	Evaluates presence of infection.

Unexpected Outcomes and Related Interventions

- Skin and genitalia may be inflamed, with localized tenderness, swelling, and presence of foul-smelling discharge.
  - Bathe area frequently to keep clean and dry.
  - Obtain order for sitz bath.
  - Apply protective barrier.
  - Notify physician and apply prescribed antibacterial or antifungal ointment/cream.
- Client expresses discomfort.
  - Increase frequency of perineal care.
  - Assess perineum for signs of irritation or discharge.
- Client unable to perform perineal care correctly.
  - Review perineal care.
  - Position client and have client observe cleansing procedure.

Recording and Reporting

- Record procedure and presence of any abnormal findings (e.g., character and amount of discharge or condition of genitalia).
- Record appearance of suture line, if present.
- Report any break in suture line or presence of abnormalities to nurse in charge or physician.

Home Care Considerations

- Instruct caregivers to daily assess client's perineal area for signs of infection and skin breakdown.

Skill 34-3 Performing Nail and Foot Care

Delegation Considerations

The skill of nail and foot care of the non-diabetic client can be delegated to unregulated care providers (UCPs). If the client is diabetic, this skill should not be delegated.
- Instruct the UCP that if client's nails need clipping, this must be performed by the nurse.
- Instruct the UCP on any special considerations for client positioning.

Equipment

- Washbasin
- Emesis basin
- Washcloth
- Bath or face towel
- Nail clippers
- Orange stick
- Emery board or nail file
- Body lotion
- Disposable bath mat
- Paper towels
- Disposable gloves

Steps	Rationale
1. Inspect all surfaces of fingers, toes, feet, and nails. Pay particular attention to areas of dryness, inflammation, or cracking. Also inspect areas between toes, heels, and soles of feet.	Integrity of feet and nails determines frequency and level of hygiene required. Heels, soles, and sides of feet are prone to irritation from ill-fitting shoes.

Critical Decision Point: Client with peripheral vascular diseases or diabetes mellitus, older adults, and clients whose immune system is suppressed may require nail care from a specialist to reduce the risk of infection.

Steps	Rationale
2. Assess colour and temperature of toes, feet, and fingers. Assess capillary refill of nails. Palpate radial and ulnar pulse of each hand and dorsalis pedis pulse of foot; note character of pulses (see chapter 28).	Assesses adequacy of blood flow to extremities. Circulatory alterations may change integrity of nails and increase client's chance of localized infection when break in skin integrity occurs (Bryant & Beinlich, 1999).
3. Observe client's walking gait. Have client walk down hall or walk straight line (if able).	Structural as well as painful disorders of feet can cause limping or unnatural gait. These disorders may be the result of impaired circulation, improper fitting shoes, or structural foot abnormalities (e.g., bunions; Bryant & Beinlich, 1999).
4. Ask female clients about whether they use nail polish and polish remover frequently.	Chemicals in these products can cause excessive dryness.
5. Assess type of footwear worn by clients: Are socks worn? Are shoes tight or ill fitting? Are garters or knee-high nylons worn? Is footwear clean?	Types of shoes and footwear may predispose client to foot and nail problems (e.g., infection, areas of friction, ulcerations). These conditions decrease mobility and increase the risk for amputation in the diabetic client (Pinzur, Slovenkai, & Trepman, 1999).
6. Identify client's risk for foot or nail problems:	Certain conditions increase likelihood of foot or nail problems.
a. Older adult	Poor vision, lack of coordination, or inability to bend over contributes to difficulty in performing foot and nail care. Normal physiological changes of aging also result in nail and foot problems (Lueckenotte, 2000).
b. Diabetes mellitus	Vascular changes associated with diabetes mellitus reduce blood flow to peripheral tissues. Breaks in skin integrity places a diabetic client at high risk for skin infection. Meticulous foot assessment reduces the diabetic client's risk of debilitating foot problems (Canadian Diabetes Association, 2003).

Skill 34-3 *Performing Nail and Foot Care—cont'd*

Steps	Rationale
c. Heart failure, renal disease	Both conditions can increase tissue edema, particularly in dependent areas (e.g., feet). Edema reduces blood flow to neighbouring tissues.
d. Cerebrovascular accident (stroke)	Presence of residual foot or leg weakness or paralysis results in altered walking patterns. Altered gait pattern causes increased friction and pressure on feet.
7. Assess type of home remedies client uses for existing foot problems:	Certain preparations or applications may cause more injury to soft tissue than the initial foot problem (Neil, 2002).
a. Over-the-counter liquid preparations to remove corns	Liquid preparations can cause burns and ulcerations.
b. Cutting of corns or calluses with razor blade or scissors	Cutting of corns or calluses may result in infection caused by a break in skin integrity. The diabetic client or any client with decreased peripheral circulation has an increased risk for infection secondary to a break in skin integrity (Canadian Diabetes Association, 2003; Green et al., 2002).
c. Use of oval corn pads	Oval pads may exert pressure on toes, thereby decreasing circulation to surrounding tissues.
d. Application of adhesive tape	Skin of older adult is thin and delicate and prone to tearing when adhesive tape is removed.
8. Assess client's ability to care for nails or feet: visual alterations, fatigue, musculoskeletal weakness.	Determines client's ability to perform self-care and degree of assistance required from nurse (Neil, 2002).
9. Assess client's knowledge of foot and nail care practices.	Determines client's need for health teaching.
10. Explain procedure to client, including fact that proper soaking requires several minutes.	Client must be willing to place fingers and feet in basins for 10 to 20 minutes. Client may become anxious or fatigued.

Critical Decision Point: Clients with diabetes do not soak hands and feet. Soaking increases their risk of infection due to maceration of the skin.

Steps	Rationale
11. Obtain physician's order for cutting nails if agency policy requires it.	Client's skin may be accidentally cut. Certain clients are more at risk for infection, depending on their medical condition.
12. Perform hand hygiene. Arrange equipment on overbed table.	Reduces transmission of micro-organisms. Easy access to equipment prevents delays.
13. Pull curtain around bed or close room door (if desired).	Maintaining client's privacy reduces anxiety.
14. Assist ambulatory client to sit in bedside chair. Help bed-bound client to supine position with head of bed elevated. Place disposable bath mat on floor under client's feet or place towel on mattress.	Sitting in chair facilitates immersing feet in basin. Bath mat protects feet from exposure to soil or debris.
15. Fill washbasin with warm water. Test water temperature.	Warm water softens nails and thickened epidermal cells, reduces inflammation of skin, and promotes local circulation. Proper water temperature prevents burns.
16. Place basin on bath mat or towel and help client place feet in basin. Place call light within client's reach.	Clients with muscular weakness or tremors may have difficulty positioning feet. Client's safety is maintained.
17. Adjust overbed table to low position, and place it over client's lap. (Client may sit in chair or lie in bed.)	Easy access prevents accidental spills.
18. Fill emesis basin with warm water, and place basin on paper towels on overbed table.	Warm water softens nails and thickened epidermal cells.
19. Instruct client to place fingers in emesis basin and place arms in comfortable position.	Prolonged positioning can cause discomfort unless normal anatomical alignment is maintained.
20. Allow client's feet and fingernails to soak for 10 to 20 minutes. Re-warm water after 10 minutes.	Softening of corns, calluses, and cuticles ensures easy removal of dead cells and easy manipulation of cuticle.
21. Clean gently under fingernails with orange stick or wooden end of cotton-tipped swab while fingers are immersed (see illustration). Remove emesis basin, and dry fingers thoroughly.	Orange stick removes debris under nails that harbours micro-organisms. Thorough drying impedes fungal growth and prevents maceration of tissues.

Steps	Rationale

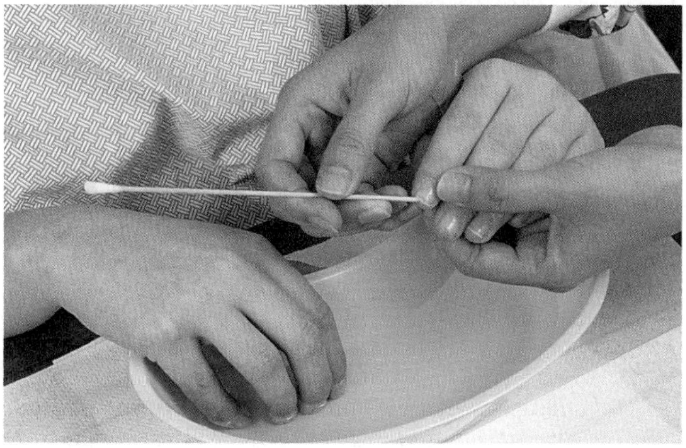

STEP **21** Clean fingernails with end of cotton-tipped swab or an orange stick.

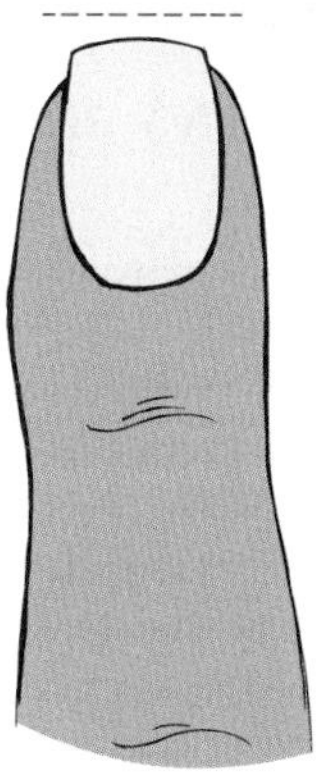

STEP **22** Using nail clippers, trim nails straight across.

Steps	Rationale
22. Using nail clippers, clip fingernails straight across and even with tops of fingers (see illustration). Shape nails with emery board or file. If client has circulatory problems, do not cut nail; file the nail only.	Cutting straight across prevents splitting of nail margins and formation of sharp nail spikes that can irritate lateral nail margins. Filing prevents cutting nail too close to nail bed
23. Push cuticle back gently with orange stick.	Reduces incidence of inflamed cuticles.
24. Move overbed table away from client.	Provides easier access to feet.
25. Put on disposable gloves, and scrub callused areas of feet with washcloth.	Gloves prevent transmission of fungal infection. Friction removes dead skin layers.
26. Clean gently under nails with orange stick. Remove feet from basin, and dry thoroughly.	Removal of debris and excess moisture reduces chances of infection.
27. Clean and trim toenails using procedures in steps 22 and 23. Do not file corners of toenails.	Shaping corners of toenails may damage tissues.
28. Apply lotion to feet and hands, and assist client back to bed and into comfortable position	Lotion lubricates dry skin by helping to retain moisture.
29. Remove disposable gloves and place in receptacle. Clean and return equipment and supplies to proper place. Dispose of soiled linen in hamper. Perform hand hygiene.	Reduces transmission of infection.
30. Inspect nails and surrounding skin surfaces after soaking and nail trimming.	Evaluates condition of skin and nails. Allows nurse to note any remaining rough nail edges.
31. Ask client to explain or demonstrate nail care.	Evaluates client's level of learning techniques.
32. Observe client's walk after toenail care.	Evaluates level of comfort and mobility achieved.
33. Record procedure and observations (e.g., breaks in skin, inflammation, ulcerations).	Documents procedure, client's response, and presence of abnormalities requiring additional therapy.
34. Report any breaks in skin or ulcerations to nurse in charge or physician.	These abnormalities can seriously increase client's risk of infection and must be carefully observed.

Skill 34-3 Performing Nail and Foot Care—cont'd

Unexpected Outcomes and Related Interventions

- Cuticles and surrounding tissues are inflamed and tender to touch.
  - Repeated soakings may be needed to relieve inflammation and loosen layers of cells from calluses or corns.
  - Client with diabetes or peripheral vascular disease may require referral to a podiatrist.
  - Evaluate need for antifungal cream.
- Localized areas of tenderness occur on feet with calluses or corns at point of friction.
  - Change in footwear may be needed.
  - Refer to a podiatrist.
- Ulcer appears between toes or other pressure areas in foot.
  - Notify physician.
  - Refer to a podiatrist.
  - Increase frequency of foot assessment and hygiene.

Recording and Reporting

- Record procedure and observations (e.g., breaks in skin, inflammation, ulcerations).
- Report any breaks in skin or ulcerations to nurse in charge or physician. These breaks are serious in clients with diabetes, peripheral vascular disease, and illnesses that impair circulation. Special foot care treatments may be needed.

Home Care Considerations

- If the client has diabetes or decreased peripheral circulation, alternative therapies or foot soaking should only be done after consulting with a physician.
- Alternative therapies: moleskin applied to areas of feet that are under friction is less likely to cause pressure than corn pads; spot adhesive bandages can guard against friction, but they do not have padding to protect against pressure.
- If client is ambulatory, instruct to soak feet in bathtub.
- When client's mobility is limited, a large basin or pan can be used.

settings or with specific clients, such as a person with diabetes mellitus, a physician's order is needed to trim a client's toenails. Before implementing this procedure, check agency policy to determine if a physician's order is needed.

The nurse takes time during the procedure to teach the client and family proper techniques for cleaning and nail trimming. Measures to prevent infection and promote good circulation should be stressed. Clients learn to protect the feet from injury, keep the feet clean and dry, and wear footwear that fits properly. The nurse instructs clients on the proper way to inspect all surfaces of the feet and hands for lesions, dryness, or signs of infection. It is important for clients to know the appearance of any abnormalities and the importance of reporting these conditions to their caregiver (Boyer, 2001).

A client with diabetes mellitus or peripheral vascular disease is at risk for foot and nail problems as a result of poor peripheral blood supply to the feet. In addition, sensation in the feet can be reduced. These clients are especially at risk for the development of chronic foot ulcers. These lesions typically heal very slowly and once present are difficult to treat. Over time, circulation can become compromised enough to cause ischemia and sloughing of tissue. Although ongoing foot care can help prevent toe amputation, studies show that many clients have not learned proper care (Bryant & Beinlich, 1999; Canadian Diabetes Association, 2003; Box 34-9).

The client must be given information to understand how circulation directly affects the health and integrity of tissues. The nurse advises clients to use the following guidelines in a routine foot and nail care program (Canadian Diabetes Association, 2003; Pinzur et al., 1999):

- Inspect the feet daily, including the tops and soles of the feet, the heels, and the areas between the toes. Use a mirror to help inspect the feet thoroughly or ask a family member to check daily.
- All clients with diabetes mellitus should receive a thorough foot examination at least once a year. People with one or more high-risk foot conditions should be evaluated more frequently and referred to a specialist as necessary (Canadian Diabetes Association, 2003).
- Wash the feet daily using lukewarm water; ***do not soak.*** Clients with reduced sensation may want to use a bath thermometer at home to test water temperature. Thoroughly pat the feet dry, and dry well between toes.
- Do not cut corns or calluses or use commercial removers. Consult a physician or podiatrist.
- If the feet perspire excessively, apply a non-allergenic foot powder.
- If dryness is noted along the feet or between the toes, rub a non-allergenic lotion gently into the skin, wiping off any excess.
- File the toenails straight across and square; do not use scissors or clippers. Consult a podiatrist as needed.
- Do not use over-the-counter preparations to treat athlete's foot or ingrown toenails. Consult a physician or podiatrist.
- Elastic stockings, knee-high hose, constricting garters, and crossing the legs while sitting can cause impaired circulation to the lower extremities.

Box 34-9

Research Highlight

Foot Care Practices of Rural Adults

Research Focus

Foot injuries are debilitating and painful; however, to the diabetic population, foot injuries, even minor injuries, can result in long-term disability or even death. When clients are taught proper foot care practices and they implement them, the risk for developing foot ulcers and the subsequent complications are greatly reduced.

Research Abstract

The purpose of this study was to determine knowledge about foot care practices in a sample of adults who had either Type 1 or Type 2 diabetes mellitus. These adults all lived in an impoverished rural area that had little access to health care, and going barefoot and wading in local streams were normal activities. Thirty-seven of the adults were ulcer free, whereas the remaining adults had a foot ulcer present. Factors surveyed included foot inspection, foot cleaning, nail care, and use of proper footwear. The scores of both groups were low, and it appeared to the investigators that the foot care practices for both groups were the same. These two groups of clients were inconsistent in preventive foot care practices, but the lowest scores ranged in foot inspection and wearing proper footwear. The investigators concluded that ongoing assessment and use of preventive practices was necessary to reduce the risk of foot ulcers in this risk population. In addition, the assessment of these practices at the point of client contact either in the home or clinic environment was essential in increasing the client's adherence to foot care practice protocols.

Evidence-Based Practice

- Use of an assessment designed to evaluate foot care practices helps to increase the client's awareness of potential disease-related complications.
- Each point of client contact is an effective method to reinforce foot care practices.
- When possible, conducting an assessment of foot care practices in the client's home environment can assist the nurse in determining true foot care practices and in correcting any client misconceptions at that time.

Reference

Neil, J. A. (2002). Assessing foot care knowledge in a rural population with diabetes. *Ostomy/Wound Management, 48*(1), 50–56.

- Wear clean socks or stockings daily. Change socks twice a day if feet perspire heavily. Socks should be dry and free of holes or repairs that might cause pressure on the tissue.
- Do not walk barefoot.
- Wear properly fitted shoes with porous uppers if possible. The soles of shoes should be flexible and non-slipping. Shoes should be sturdy, closed in, and not restrictive to the feet. Clients with increased plantar pressure (e.g., erythema or callus) should use footwear that cushions and redistributes pressure. Clients with bony deformity (e.g., bunion or Charcot's joint) may need extra wide or extra deep shoes with cushioned insoles.
- Do not wear new shoes for an extended time. Wear them for short periods over several days to break them in.
- Exercise regularly to improve circulation to the lower extremities. Walk slowly and elevate, rotate, flex, and extend the feet at the ankles. Dangle the feet over the side of the bed for one minute, then extend both legs and hold them parallel to the bed while lying supine for one minute, and, finally, rest one minute.
- Do not apply hot water bottles or heating pads to the feet; use extra coverings instead.
- Minor cuts should be washed immediately and dried thoroughly. Use only mild antiseptics (e.g., Neosporin ointment). Avoid iodine or Mercurochrome. Contact a physician to treat cuts or lacerations.

Any client who requires regular, thorough foot care should have a caregiver or family member able to provide care during times when the client is incapacitated. Clients with visual difficulties, physical constraints preventing movement, or cognitive problems that impair their ability to assess the condition of the feet will need caregiver or family assistance (American Diabetes Association, 1999; Canadian Diabetes Association, 2003).

Oral Hygiene. Oral hygiene helps to maintain the healthy state of the mouth, teeth, gums, and lips (Ring, 2002). Brushing cleans the teeth of food particles, plaque, and bacteria. It also massages the gums and relieves discomfort resulting from unpleasant odours and tastes. Flossing further helps remove plaque and tartar from between teeth to reduce gum inflammation and infection. Complete oral hygiene enhances well-being and comfort and stimulates the appetite. Clients also benefit from a proper diet, which excludes foods promoting plaque formation and tooth decay and promotes healthy periodontal structures (Hornick, 2002). Plaque-forming foods include carbonated beverages, breads, and starches. In addition, oral hygiene immediately following a meal further reduces plaque. The nurse assists clients in maintaining good oral hygiene by teaching the importance of correct techniques and a routine daily schedule.

Clients of all ages should be advised to have a dental checkup at least every six months. Education about common gum and tooth disorders and methods of prevention can motivate clients to follow good oral hygiene practices. The nurse also assists in performing hygiene for weakened or disabled clients. When clients have variations in oral mucosal integrity, the nurse adapts hygiene techniques to ensure thorough and effective care (Box 34-10).

Focus on Older Adults **Box 34-10**

- Many older adults are edentulous (without teeth), and the teeth that are present are often diseased or decayed (Lueckenotte, 2000).
- The periodontal membrane weakens, making it more prone to infection; periodontal disease can predispose the older adult to systemic infection.
- The presence of chronic illnesses (e.g., diabetes mellitus, renal insufficiency, and cardiovascular diseases) increases the older adult's risk for periodontal disease (Bush & Donley, 2002).
- Dentures or partial plates may not fit properly, causing pain and discomfort, which can in turn affect digestive processes, enjoyment of food, and nutritional status.
- Weaker jaw muscles and shrinkage of the bony structure of the mouth may increase the work of chewing and lead to increased fatigue when eating (Lueckenotte, 2000).
- Dry mouth can be caused by an age-related decline in saliva secretion, as well as by medications that are frequently used by older adults (e.g., antihypertensives, diuretics, anti-inflammatories, and antidepressants; Eliopoulos, 2001).
- Poor nutritional status in some older adults can increase the risk for and severity of dental problems (e.g., caries, periodontal disease, receding gums, and tooth degeneration; Hornick, 2002).
- Financial limitations and the belief that dentures eliminate the need for routine dental care are reasons why some older adults do not seek dental care (Eliopoulos, 2001).

Data from *Gerontologic Nursing* (5th ed.), by C. Eliopoulos, 2001, Philadelphia: Lippincott Williams & Wilkins.

Brushing and Flossing. Thorough tooth brushing at least four times a day (after meals and at bedtime) is basic to an effective oral hygiene program. A toothbrush should have a straight handle and brush small enough to reach all areas of the mouth. An even, rounded brushing surface with soft, multi-tufted, nylon bristles is best. Rounded soft bristles stimulate the gums without causing abrasion and bleeding. Older adult clients with reduced dexterity and grip may require an enlarged handle with an easier grip or an electric toothbrush (Felder et al., 1994). One simple way to devise an enlarged brush handle is to pierce a soft rubber ball and push the brush handle through or glue a short piece of plastic tubing around the handle. Clients should know to obtain a new toothbrush every 3 months or following a cold or strep throat to minimize growth of micro-organisms on the brush surfaces.

All tooth surfaces should be brushed thoroughly with fluoride toothpaste. Commercially made foam rubber toothbrushes are useful for clients with sensitive gums. However, swabbing fails to cleanse teeth adequately because plaque accumulates around the base of the teeth. Foam rubber swabs should be used in moderation. Electric toothbrushes can be used, but the nurse working in an agency setting should check for electrical hazards. Lemon-glycerine sponges should not be used because they dry mucous membranes and erode teeth enamel. Moi-Stir is a salivary supplement that improves moisture and texture of the tongue and mucosa (Poland et al., 1987).

When teaching clients about mouth care, the nurse should recommend they do not share toothbrushes with family members or drink directly from a bottle of mouthwash. Cross contamination occurs easily. The use of disclosure tablets or drops to stain the plaque that collects at the gum line can be useful for showing clients how effectively they brush. Many clients can perform their own oral care and should be encouraged to do so. The nurse observes the client to be sure proper techniques are used.

Clients will experience conditions that threaten the integrity of oral mucosa. For example, mucosal changes associated with aging, use of chemotherapeutic drugs, or dehydration requires the nurse to adapt oral hygiene approaches. More frequent mouth care and use of anti-infective agents are examples of ways the nurse will revise approaches to meet client needs. Unconscious clients and those with artificial airways (e.g., endotracheal or tracheal tubes) need more frequent and specialized oral hygiene. These clients have an increased risk of aspiration and subsequently aspiration pneumonia, and they also have more problems with dry and inflamed oral mucosa.

The amount of assistance needed by the client when brushing the teeth may vary. When assisting with or providing oral hygiene, the nurse determines the amount of assistance needed and individual oral hygiene preferences (Skill 34-4).

Flossing. Dental flossing removes plaque and tartar between teeth. Flossing involves inserting waxed or unwaxed dental floss between all tooth surfaces, one at a time. The seesaw motion used to pull floss between teeth removes plaque and tartar from tooth enamel. To prevent bleeding, clients who are receiving chemotherapy or radiation or who are on anticoagulant therapy should use unwaxed floss and avoid vigorous flossing near the gumline. If toothpaste is applied to the teeth before flossing, fluoride can come in direct contact with tooth surfaces, aiding in cavity prevention. Flossing once a day is sufficient. Because it is important to clean all teeth surfaces thoroughly, the nurse should not rush to complete flossing. Placing a mirror in front of the client will help the nurse to demonstrate the proper method for holding the floss and cleaning between the teeth. Flossing a client's teeth is not realistic, nor appropriate in all care settings. However, flossing may be done more frequently in rehabilitation and long-term care settings.

Clients With Special Needs. Some clients require special oral hygiene methods because of their level of dependence on the nurse or the presence of oral mucosa problems. Unconscious clients are susceptible to drying of mucous-thickened salivary secretions because they are unable to eat or drink, frequently breathe through the mouth, and often receive oxygen therapy. The unconscious client also cannot swallow salivary secretions that accumulate in the mouth. These secretions often contain gram-negative bacteria that can cause pneumonia if aspirated into the lungs. While providing hygiene to an unconscious client, the nurse must protect the client from choking and aspiration. The safest technique for reducing the risk of aspiration and subsequent pneumonia is to have two nurses provide the care. The nurse may delegate unregulated care providers to participate. One nurse does

Skill 34-4 Providing Oral Hygiene

View Video

Delegation Considerations

Skills of brushing teeth can be delegated to unregulated care providers (UCPs).

- Instruct the UCP on how to adapt the procedure for a client who is at risk of aspiration. These clients include those with an impaired level of consciousness or impaired swallowing, and those who are confused.
- Instruct the UCP to immediately report to the nurse excessive client coughing or choking during or after oral hygiene.
- Instruct the UCP to report any bleeding of oral mucosa or gums, lesions, or client report of pain to the nurse.

Equipment

- Soft-bristled toothbrush
- Non-abrasive fluoride toothpaste or dentifrice
- Dental floss
- Water glass with cool water
- Normal saline or an essential oil antiseptic mouthwash (optional; follow client's preference)
- Emesis basin
- Tongue blade
- Face towel
- Paper towels
- Disposable gloves

Steps	Rationale
1. Perform hand hygiene and apply disposable gloves.	Reduces transmission of micro-organisms.
2. Inspect integrity of lips, teeth, buccal mucosa, gums, palate, and tongue (see chapter 28).	Determines status of client's oral cavity and extent of need for oral hygiene.
3. Identify presence of common oral problems:	Helps determine type of hygiene client requires and information client requires for self-care.
a. Dental caries—chalky white discolouration of tooth or presence of brown or black discolouration	
b. Gingivitis—inflammation of gums	
c. Periodontitis—receding gum lines, inflammation, gaps between teeth	Receding gums occur with aging, and as a result older clients require meticulous oral hygiene (Walton, Miller, & Tordecilla, 2002).
d. Halitosis—bad breath	
e. Cheilosis—cracking of lips	
f. Stomatitis—inflammation of the mouth	Clients receiving immunosuppressive chemotherapy (e.g., cancer chemotherapy, anti-rejection medication post-organ transplant) and clients with suppressed immune function are at risk for stomatitis (Fulton, Middleton, & McPhail, 2002).
4. Remove gloves and perform hand hygiene.	Prevents spread of micro-organisms.
5. Assess risk for oral hygiene problems (see Table 34-5).	Certain conditions increase likelihood of impaired oral cavity integrity and need for preventive care.
6. Assess client's risk for aspiration: impaired swallowing, reduced gag reflex.	Accumulation of secretions and dentifrice can increase client's risk for aspiration because of reduced ability to control oral secretions.
7. Determine client's oral hygiene practices:	Allows nurse to identify errors in technique, deficiencies in preventive oral hygiene, and client's level of knowledge regarding dental care.
a. Frequency of toothbrushing and flossing	
b. Type of toothpaste or dentifrice used	
c. Last dental visit	
d. Frequency of dental visits	
e. Type of mouthwash or moistening preparation	Lemon-glycerine preparations can be detrimental. Glycerine is an astringent that dries and shrinks mucous membranes and gums. Lemon exhausts salivary reflex and can erode tooth enamel (Poland et al., 1987). Mouthwash provides pleasant aftertaste but can dry mucosa after extended use if it has an alcohol base.
8. Assess client's ability to grasp and manipulate toothbrush. (For older adult, try 30-second toothbrush assessment.)	Toothbrush test useful in assessing dexterity and strength. Determines level of assistance required.
9. Prepare equipment at bedside.	

Skill 34-4 *Providing Oral Hygiene—cont'd*

Steps	Rationale
10. Explain procedure to client and discuss preferences regarding use of hygiene aids.	Some clients feel uncomfortable about having the nurse care for their basic needs. Client involvement with procedure minimizes anxiety.
11. Place paper towels on overbed table, and arrange other equipment within easy reach.	
12. Raise bed to comfortable working position. Raise head of bed (if allowed) and lower side rail. Move client, or help client move closer. Side-lying position can be used.	Raising bed and positioning client prevent nurse from straining muscles. Semi-Fowler's position helps prevent client from choking or aspirating.
13. Place towel over client's chest.	
14. Apply gloves.	Prevents contact with micro-organisms or blood in saliva.
15. Apply toothpaste to brush, holding brush over emesis basin. Pour small amount of water over toothpaste.	Moisture aids in distribution of toothpaste over tooth surfaces.
16. Client may assist by brushing. Hold toothbrush bristles at 45-degree angle to gum line (see illustration). Be sure tips of bristles rest against and penetrate under gum line. Brush inner and outer surfaces of upper and lower teeth by brushing from gum to crown of each tooth. Clean biting surfaces of teeth by holding top of bristles parallel with teeth and brushing gently back and forth (see illustration). Brush sides of teeth by moving bristles back and forth (see illustration).	Angle allows brush to reach all tooth surfaces and to clean under gum line where plaque and tartar accumulate. Back-and-forth motion dislodges food particles caught between teeth and along chewing surfaces.
17. Have client hold brush at 45-degree angle and lightly brush over surface and sides of tongue (see illustration). Avoid initiating gag reflex.	Micro-organisms collect and grow on tongue's surface and contribute to bad breath. Gagging may cause aspiration of toothpaste.
18. Allow client to rinse mouth thoroughly by taking several sips of water, swishing water across all tooth surfaces, and spitting into emesis basin.	Irrigation removes food particles.
19. Allow client to gargle to rinse mouth with mouthwash as desired.	An essential oil antiseptic mouthwash can be effective in reducing plaque and gingivitis (Bauroth et al., 2003).
20. Assist in wiping client's mouth.	Promotes sense of comfort.
21. Allow client to floss.	Reduces tartar on tooth surfaces.
22. Allow client to rinse mouth thoroughly with cool water and spit into emesis basin. Assist in wiping client's mouth.	Irrigation removes plaque and tartar from oral cavity.

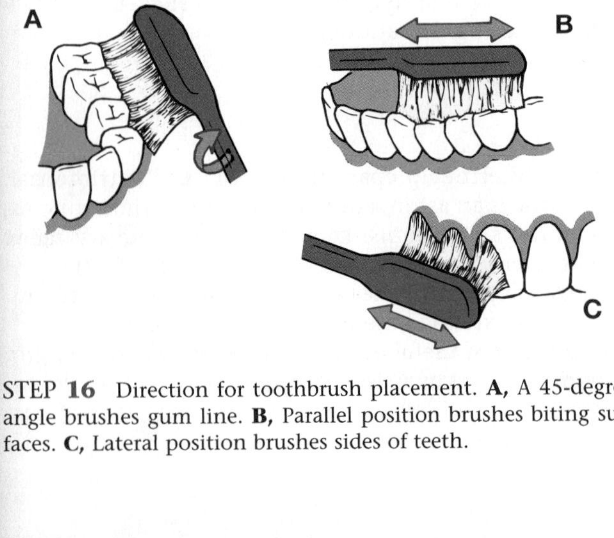

STEP **16** Direction for toothbrush placement. **A,** A 45-degree angle brushes gum line. **B,** Parallel position brushes biting surfaces. **C,** Lateral position brushes sides of teeth.

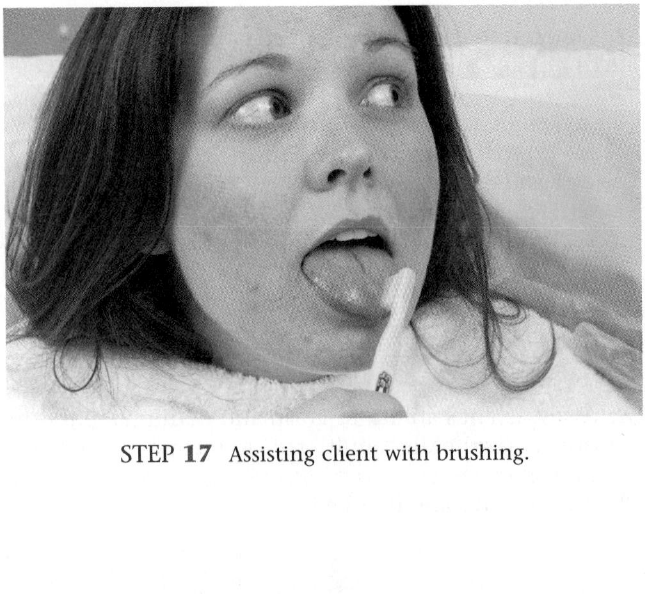
STEP **17** Assisting client with brushing.

Steps	Rationale
23. Assist client to comfortable position, remove emesis basin and bedside table, raise side rail, and lower bed to original position.	Provides for client comfort and safety.
24. Wipe off overbed table, discard soiled linen and paper towels in appropriate containers, remove soiled gloves, and return equipment to proper place.	Proper disposal of soiled equipment prevents spread of infection.
25. Perform hand hygiene.	Reduces transmission of micro-organisms.
26. Ask client if any area of oral cavity feels uncomfortable or irritated.	Pain indicates more chronic problem.
27. Apply gloves and inspect condition of oral cavity.	Determines effectiveness of hygiene and rinsing.
28. Ask client to describe proper hygiene techniques.	Evaluates client's learning.
29. Observe client brushing.	Evaluates client's ability to use correct technique.

Unexpected Outcomes and Related Interventions

- Oral mucosa is dry and inflamed.
  - Increase frequency of oral hygiene.
  - Increase client's hydration.
  - Apply protectant to client's lips.
- Gum margins are retracted from teeth, with localized areas of inflammation. Bleeding occurs around gum margins.
  - Determine if client has underlying bleeding tendency (e.g., anticoagulant therapy).
  - Report findings to physician.
  - Use soft-bristled toothbrush.
  - Increase frequency of oral hygiene.
- Teeth show signs of dental caries.
  - Refer client to dentist.
  - Teach client oral hygiene.

Recording and Reporting

- Record procedure on flow sheet. Note condition of oral cavity in nurses' notes.
- Report bleeding or presence of lesions to nurse in charge or physician.

Home Care Considerations

- Teach client and caregiver to assess oral cavity daily to determine any effects of medications on the oral cavity (e.g., reddened, inflamed gums).

the actual cleaning, and the other removes secretions with suction equipment. While cleansing the oral cavity, the nurse should never use fingers to hold the client's mouth open. A human bite is highly contaminated. It may be necessary to perform mouth care at least every 2 hours. The nurse explains the steps of mouth care and the sensations the client will feel. The nurse also tells the client when the procedure is completed (Skill 34-5).

Clients who receive chemotherapy, radiation, or nasogastric tube intubation or clients who have an infection of the mouth can suffer from **stomatitis.** Inflammation of the oral mucosa can cause oral burning, pain, and change in food tolerance. Gentle brushing and flossing are important in preventing bleeding of the gums. Clients should be advised to avoid alcohol and commercial mouthwash and to stop smoking. Normal saline rinses (approximately 30 mL) upon awaking in the morning, after each meal, and at bedtime can effectively clean the oral cavity. The rinses can be increased to every 2 hours if necessary. The physician may order a mild oral analgesic for pain control.

Clients with diabetes mellitus frequently have periodontal disease. Visits to the dentist are needed every 3 to 4 months. All tissues should be handled gently with a minimum of trauma. Clients should learn to follow rigid cleansing schedules, at least four times a day.

Denture Care. Clients should be encouraged to clean their dentures on a regular basis to avoid gingival infection and irritation. When clients become disabled, the nurse or family caregiver can assume responsibility for denture care (Box 34-11). Dentures are the client's personal property and need to be handled with care because they can be easily broken. Dentures must be removed at night to give the gums a rest and prevent bacterial buildup. Dentures should be kept covered in water when they are not worn to prevent warping, and they should always be stored in an enclosed, labelled cup with the cup placed in the client's bedside stand. Discourage clients from removing their dentures and placing them on a napkin or tissue because they could be easily thrown away.

Hair and Scalp Care. A person's appearance and feeling of well-being often depend on the way the hair looks and feels. Illness or disability may prevent a client from maintaining daily hair care. An immobilized client's hair soon

Skill 34-5 Performing Mouth Care for an Unconscious or Debilitated Client

View Video

Delegation Considerations

The skill of brushing teeth of an unconscious or debilitated client can be delegated to unregulated care providers (UCPs). The nurse must first assess the client for the gag reflex and inform the UCP about the proper way to position clients for mouth care.

- The UCP must be able to safely use oral suctioning for clearing oral secretions (see chapter 35).
- Instruct the UCP to report to the nurse any bleeding of mucosa or gums, painful reaction by the client, or excessive coughing or choking.

Equipment

- Anti-infective solution (e.g., commercial diluted hydrogen peroxide solution) that loosens crusts
- Small soft-bristled toothbrush
- Sponge toothette or tongue blade wrapped in single layer of gauze
- Padded tongue blade
- Face towel
- Paper towels
- Emesis basin
- Water glass with cool water
- Water-soluble lip lubricant
- Small-bulb syringe (optional)
- Suction machine equipment (optional)
- Disposable gloves (three pairs)

Steps	Rationale
1. Perform hand hygiene. Apply disposable gloves.	Reduces transmission of micro-organisms. Gloves prevent contact with micro-organisms in blood or saliva.
2. Assess client's risk for oral hygiene problems (see Table 34-5).	Impaired levels of consciousness increase the likelihood of alterations in integrity of oral cavity structures and may require more frequent care. Proper oral care is shown to reduce the risk of pneumonia (Research update, 2002).
3. Test for presence of gag reflex by placing tongue blade on back half of client's tongue.	Reveals whether client is at risk for aspiration.

Critical Decision Point: Clients with impaired gag reflex require oral care as well. The nurse determines the type of suction apparatus needed at the bedside to protect the client's airway against aspiration.

Steps	Rationale
4. Inspect condition of oral cavity (see chapter 28).	Determines condition of oral cavity and need for hygiene.
5. Remove gloves. Perform hand hygiene.	Prevents spread of infection.
6. Explain procedure to client.	Allows debilitated client to anticipate procedure without anxiety. Unconscious client may retain ability to hear.
7. Apply disposable gloves.	Reduces transfer of micro-organisms.
8. Place paper towels on overbed table and arrange equipment. If needed, turn on suction machine, and connect tubing to suction catheter.	Prevents soiling of tabletop. Equipment prepared in advance ensures smooth, safe procedure.
9. Pull curtain around bed, or close room door.	Provides privacy.
10. Raise bed to the appropriate height for nurse; lower head of bed and then lower side rail.	Use of good body mechanics with bed in elevated position reduces the risk of injury to the nurse.
11. Position client on side (Sims' position) with head turned well toward dependent side. Move client close to side of bed. Then raise side rail.	Turning the client's head to the side allows secretions to drain from mouth instead of collecting in back of pharynx. Prevents aspiration. Moving the client close to the side of the bed facilitates proper body mechanics as the nurse performs this skill.
12. Place towel under client's head and emesis basin under chin.	Prevents soiling of bed linen.
13. Carefully separate upper and lower teeth with padded tongue blade by inserting blade, quickly but gently, between back molars. Insert when client is relaxed, if possible. Do not use force (see illustration).	Prevents client from biting down on nurse's fingers and provides access to oral cavity.

Steps	Rationale

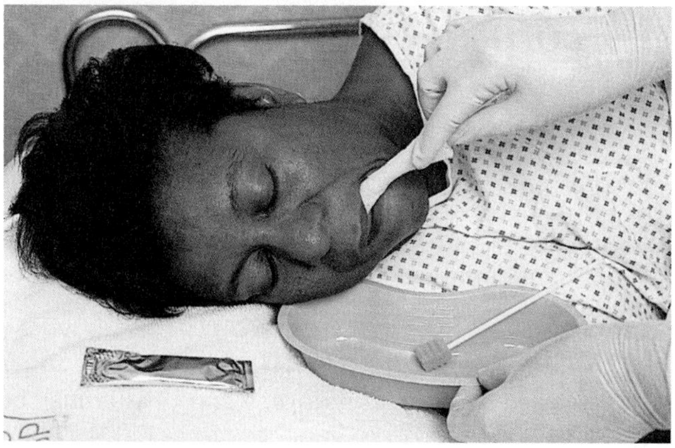

STEP **13** Separate upper and lower teeth with padded tongue blade.

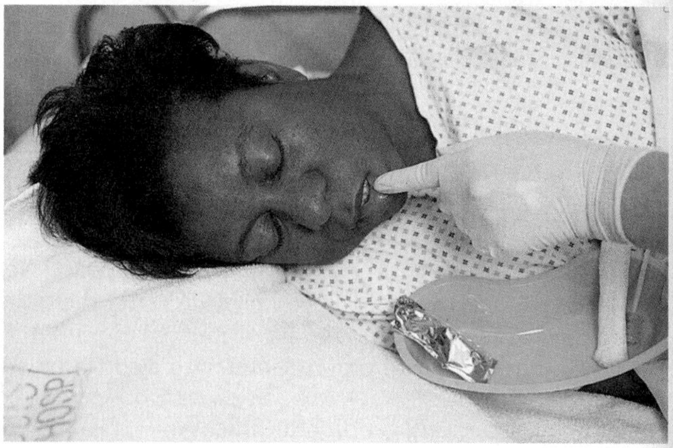

STEP **16** Application of water-soluble moisturizer to lips.

Critical Decision Point: Never use fingers to separate client's teeth.

Steps	Rationale
14. Clean mouth using brush or sponge toothettes moistened with commercial hydrogen peroxide solution if client condition can tolerate; otherwise moisten with water. Clean chewing and inner tooth surfaces first. Clean outer tooth surfaces. Swab roof of mouth, gums, and inside cheeks. Gently swab or brush tongue but avoid stimulating gag reflex (if present). Moisten clean swab or toothette with water to rinse. (Bulb syringe may also be used to rinse.) Repeat rinse several times.	Brushing action removes food particles between teeth and along chewing surfaces. Swabbing helps remove secretions and crusts from mucosa and moistens mucosa. Repeated rinsing removes peroxide that can be irritating to mucosa.
15. Suction secretions as they accumulate, if necessary.	Suction removes secretions and fluid that can collect in posterior pharynx.
16. Apply thin layer of water-soluble jelly to lips (see illustration).	Lubricates lips to prevent drying and cracking.
17. Inform client that procedure is completed.	Provides meaningful stimulation to unconscious or less responsive client.
18. Reposition client comfortably, raise side rail as appropriate or as ordered, and return bed to original position.	Maintains client's comfort and safety. Raising all four side rails may be considered a restraint, and a physician's order is needed.
19. Clean equipment and return to its proper place. Place soiled linen in proper receptacle.	Proper disposal of soiled equipment prevents spread of infection.
20. Remove and discard gloves. Perform hand hygiene.	Reduces transmission of micro-organisms.
21. Apply clean gloves, and inspect oral cavity.	Determines efficacy of cleansing. Once thick secretions are removed, underlying inflammation or lesions may be revealed.
22. Ask debilitated client if mouth feels clean.	Evaluates level of comfort.
23. Assess client's respirations on an ongoing basis.	Ensures early recognition of aspiration.

Skill 34-5 Performing Mouth Care for an Unconscious or Debilitated Client—cont'd

Unexpected Outcomes and Related Interventions

- Secretions or crusts remain on oral mucosa, tongue, or gums.
  - Increase frequency of oral hygiene.
  - A pediatric-size toothbrush may provide better hygiene.
- Localized inflammation of gums or mucosa is present.
  - Increase frequency of oral hygiene with a soft-bristled toothbrush.
  - Apply moisturizing gel on oral mucosa.
  - Chemotherapy and radiation can cause stomatitis. Antiseptic mouthwashes provide relief, promote oral hygiene, and improve healing (Fulton et al., 2002).
- Client aspirated secretions.
  - Suction oral airway.
  - Perform tracheal bronchial suctioning.
  - Notify physician.

Recording and Reporting

- Record procedure, including pertinent observations (e.g., presence of bleeding gums, dry mucosa, ulcerations, crusts on tongue).
- Report any unusual findings to nurse in charge or physician.

Home Care Considerations

- Irrigate cavity with bulb syringe; a gravy baster may be substituted.
- Mouth care should be given at least twice a day. Caregivers can get non-prescription oral care solutions (e.g., carbamide peroxide solutions) at most pharmacies.
- Have caregivers demonstrate positioning of client to prevent aspiration.

becomes tangled. Dressings may leave sticky blood or antiseptic solutions on the hair. In the clinic and home care setting, nurses will encounter clients who have head lice. Proper hair care is important to the client's body image. Brushing, combing, and shampooing are basic hygiene measures for all clients.

Brushing and Combing. Frequent brushing helps to keep hair clean and distributes oil evenly along hair shafts. Combing prevents hair from tangling. The client should be encouraged to maintain routine hair care. However, clients with limited mobility or weakness and those who are confused require help. Clients in a hospital or long-term care facility appreciate the opportunity to have their hair brushed and combed before being seen by others.

When caring for clients from different cultures, it is important to learn as much as possible from them or their family about preferred hair care practices. Cultural preferences will affect how hair is combed and styled.

Long hair can easily become matted after a client is confined to bed, even for a short period. When lacerations or incisions involve the scalp, blood and topical medications can also cause tangling. Frequent brushing and combing keeps long hair neatly groomed. Braiding can help to avoid repeated tangles; however, braids should be unbraided periodically and hair combed to ensure good hygiene. Braids made too tightly can lead to bald patches. The nurse obtains permission from the client before braiding his or her hair.

To brush hair, the nurse parts the hair into two sections and separates each into two more sections. It is easier to brush smaller sections of hair. Brushing from the scalp toward the hair ends minimizes pulling. Moistening the hair with water or alcohol frees tangles for easier combing. Never cut a client's hair without written consent.

Clients who develop head lice require special considerations in the way combing is performed. The lice are small, about the size of a sesame seed. Bright light or natural sunlight is necessary for the lice to be seen. Thorough combing is recommended and may remove nits (empty eggshells) if infestation is extensive. Follow these steps:

- Apply disposable gown and gloves.
- Use a grooming comb or hairbrush to remove tangles.
- Divide the client's hair in sections and fasten off hair that is not being combed.
- Comb out from the scalp to the end of the hair (special fine-toothed combs are available in drugstores).
- Dip the comb in a cup of water or use a paper towel to remove nits between each passing.
- After combing, look through the hair carefully for attached live lice.
- Live lice may be caught with tweezers or comb.
- Move to next section of hair after combing thoroughly.
- Instruct family to clean the comb with an old toothbrush and dental floss and boil the comb (if possible). The ideal would be to discard the comb after each use, but some client's financial situations may prevent the purchase of multiple combs.
- Instruct family to comb and screen for lice daily.
- Instruct family to contain client's clothes and wash in hot water.
- Instruct caregivers on how to prevent transmission of lice:
  - Do not share bed linens.
  - Avoid placing bare hand on client's head.
  - Immediately wash hands after providing hair care.
  - Contain all hair care products.

Box 34-11 Procedural Guidelines

Care of Dentures

Equipment: Soft-bristled toothbrush or denture toothbrush, denture cleaning agent or toothpaste, denture adhesive (optional), glass of water, emesis basin or sink, washcloth, disposable gloves, denture cup (if dentures are to be stored after cleaning).

Delegation Considerations: The skill of denture care can be delegated to unregulated care providers (UCPs). The nurse instructs the UCP to do the following:

- Inform the nurse if cracks are found in the dentures.
- Inform the nurse if the client complains of oral discomfort.

1. Ask client if dentures fit and if there is any gum or mucous membrane tenderness or irritation.
2. Ask client about preferences for denture care and products used. If client is unable to care for own dentures, the nurse must provide this care. Clean dentures for client during routine mouth care.
3. Fill emesis basin with tepid water, or if using sink, place washcloth in bottom of sink and fill sink with 2.5 cm of water.
4. Remove dentures: If client is unable to do this independently, perform hand hygiene and apply gloves, grasp upper plate at front with thumb and index finger wrapped in gauze, and pull downward. Gently lift lower denture from jaw, and rotate one side downward to remove from client's mouth. Place dentures in emesis basin or sink.
5. Apply cleaning agent to brush and brush surfaces of dentures (see illustration). Hold dentures close to water. Hold brush horizontally, and use back-and-forth motion to cleanse biting surfaces. Use short strokes from top of denture to biting surfaces to clean outer and inner teeth surfaces. Hold brush vertically, and use short strokes to clean inner tooth surfaces. Hold brush horizontally, and use back-and-forth motion to clean undersurface of dentures.

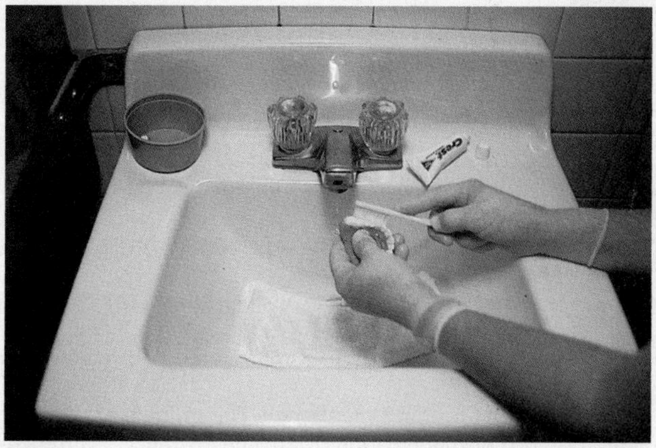

STEP **5** Brushing dentures.

6. Rinse thoroughly in tepid water.
7. Some clients use an adhesive to seal dentures in place. Apply a thin layer to undersurface before inserting.
8. If client needs assistance with insertion of dentures, moisten upper denture and press firmly to seal it in place. Then insert moistened lower denture. Ask if dentures feel comfortable.
9. Some clients prefer to have their dentures stored to give the gums a rest and to reduce risk of infection. Keeping dentures moist will prevent warping and facilitate easier insertion. Store in a secure place to prevent loss.
10. Remove and discard gloves and perform hand hygiene.

If a pediculicidal shampoo is ordered, instruct the client and caregiver on proper use of shampoo. These shampoos may have neurological side effects. The very young and very old have increased susceptibility to the toxic effects of seizure, dizziness, headache, paresthesia, and death. This type of medication should never be used on clients infected with Human Immunodeficiency Virus (HIV), those with neurological conditions, the neonate, or clients who weigh less than 50 kg (Zurlinden, 2003). As with any medication preparation, it is important to review and understand pertinent information. Most side effects associated with pediculicidal shampoos occur from applying too much medicated shampoo, leaving the shampoo in place too long, or repeated shampooing too soon. Many clients have been over-treated because they incorrectly believed that continued itching meant that lice survived the initial treatment. They did not know that itching was a common side effect of the shampoo (Zurlinden, 2003).

Shampooing. Frequency of shampooing depends on a person's daily routines and the condition of the hair. The nurse should remind clients in hospitals or long-term care facilities that staying in bed, excess perspiration, or treatments that leave blood or solutions in the hair may require more frequent shampooing. For clients at home, the nurse is challenged to find ways that the client can shampoo the hair without causing injury.

If the client is able to take a shower or bath, the hair can usually be shampooed without difficulty. A shower or tub chair may be used for the ambulatory, weight-bearing client who becomes tired or faint. Hand-held shower nozzles allow clients to easily wash the hair in the tub or shower. Clients allowed to sit in a chair may choose to be shampooed in front of a sink or over a washbasin. However, bending is limited or contraindicated in certain conditions (e.g., eye surgery or neck injury). In these situations, the nurse needs to teach the client the degree of bending allowed.

If a client is unable to sit but can be moved, the nurse may transfer the client to a stretcher for transportation to a sink or shower equipped with a hand-held nozzle. Long-term care facilities are commonly equipped with

Box 34-12 Procedural Guidelines

Shampooing Hair of Bed-Bound Client

Equipment: Bath towels, washcloths, shampoo and hair conditioner (optional), water pitcher, plastic shampoo trough, washbasin, bath blanket, waterproof pad, clean comb and brush, hair dryer *(optional),* disposable gloves *(optional)*

Delegation Considerations: The skill of shampooing hair can be delegated to unregulated care providers (UCPs).

- Instruct the UCP about any precautions needed in positioning the client.
- Instruct the UCP to inform the nurse if the client reports neck pain.
- Instruct the UCP to inform the nurse of any new skin lesions.

1. Before washing client's hair, determine that there are no contraindications to this procedure. Certain medical conditions, such as head and neck injuries, spinal cord injuries, and arthritis, could place the client at risk for injury during shampooing because of positioning and manipulation of client's head and neck.
2. Apply gloves if needed. Inspect the hair and scalp before initiating the procedure. This determines the presence of any conditions that may require the use of special shampoos or treatments (e.g., for dandruff or the removal of dried blood).
3. Place waterproof pad under client's shoulders, neck, and head (see illustration). Position client supine, with head and shoulders at top edge of bed. Place plastic trough under client's head and washbasin at end of trough. Be sure trough spout extends beyond edge of mattress.
4. Place rolled towel under client's neck and bath towel over client's shoulders.
5. Brush and comb client's hair.
6. Obtain warm water.
7. Offer client the option of holding face towel or washcloth over eyes.
8. Slowly pour water from water pitcher over hair until it is completely wet (see illustration). If hair contains matted blood, don gloves, apply peroxide to dissolve clots, and then rinse hair with saline. Apply small amount of shampoo.
9. Work up lather with both hands. Start at hairline, and work toward back of neck. Lift head slightly with one hand to wash back of head. Shampoo sides of head. Massage scalp by applying pressure with fingertips.
10. Rinse hair with water. Make sure water drains into basin. Repeat rinsing until hair is free of soap.
11. Apply conditioner or cream rinse if requested, and rinse hair thoroughly.
12. Wrap client's head in bath towel. Dry client's face with cloth used to protect eyes. Dry off any moisture along neck or shoulders.
13. Dry client's hair and scalp. Use second towel if first becomes saturated.
14. Comb hair to remove tangles, and dry with dryer if desired.
15. Apply oil preparation or conditioning product to hair, if desired by client.
16. Assist client to comfortable position, and complete styling of hair.

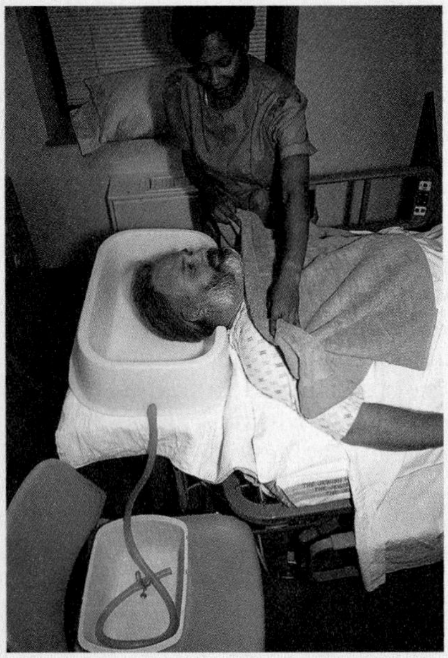

STEP **3** Pad under shoulders, neck, and head.

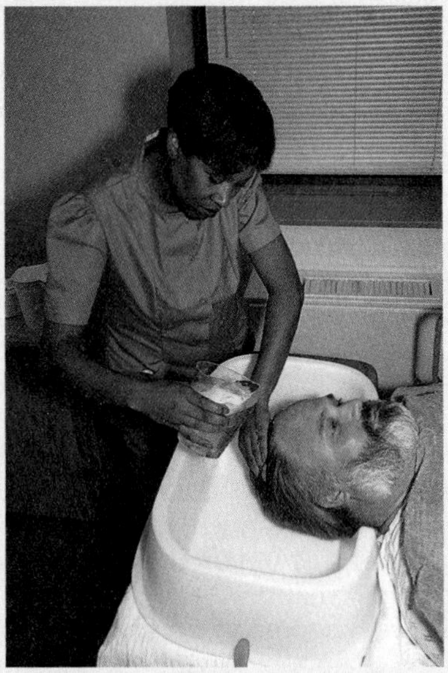

STEP **8** Pouring water over hair.

this option. Caution is again needed when the client's head and neck are positioned, particularly in clients with any form of head or neck injury.

If the client is unable to sit in a chair or be transferred to a stretcher, shampooing must be done with the client in bed (Box 34-12). A special shampoo trough can be positioned under the client's head to catch water and suds. After shampooing, clients like having their hair styled and dried. Most health care centres have portable hair dryers. Dry shampoos that reduce the need to wet the client's hair are also available but are not highly effective. These dry shampoo preparations vary, and the application procedures, listed on the container, should be followed exactly. In most agencies, a physician's order is necessary to shampoo the dependent client.

Shaving. Shaving facial hair can be done after the bath or shampoo. Women may prefer to shave their legs or axillae while bathing. When assisting a client, the nurse should take care to avoid cutting the client with a razor blade. Clients prone to bleeding (e.g., those receiving anticoagulants or high doses of aspirin or those with low platelet counts) must use an electric razor. Before using an electric razor, the nurse should check for frayed cords or other electrical hazards. Razor blades and electric razors should be used on only one client because of infection-control considerations.

When a razor blade is used for shaving, the skin must be softened to prevent pulling, scraping, or cuts. Placing a warm washcloth over the male client's face for a few seconds, followed by application of shaving cream or a lathering of mild soap, softens the skin. If the client is unable to shave, the nurse may perform the shave. To avoid causing discomfort or razor cuts, the nurse gently pulls the skin taut and uses short, firm razor strokes in the direction that the hair grows (Figure 34–8). Short downward strokes work best to remove hair over the upper lip. A client usually can explain to the nurse the best way to move the razor across the skin. In the case of dark-skinned clients, facial hair tends to be curly and can become ingrown unless shaved close to the skin.

Moustache and Beard Care. Clients with moustaches or beards require daily grooming. Keeping these areas clean is important because food particles and mucus can easily collect in the hair. If the client is unable to carry out self-care, the nurse should do so at the client's request. Beards can be gently combed out. A shaggy or unkempt moustache or beard can be trimmed. For cultural or religious reasons, shaving off a moustache or beard cannot be performed without the client's consent.

Hair and Scalp Health. To best promote and restore hair and scalp health, clients should be instructed to keep hair clean, combed, and brushed regularly. Clients may also need to know how to check for and remove parasites, such as lice (see Table 34-4). The nurse should tell clients that they need to notify their primary caregiver of changes in the texture and distribution of hair, which may indicate a serious systemic problem.

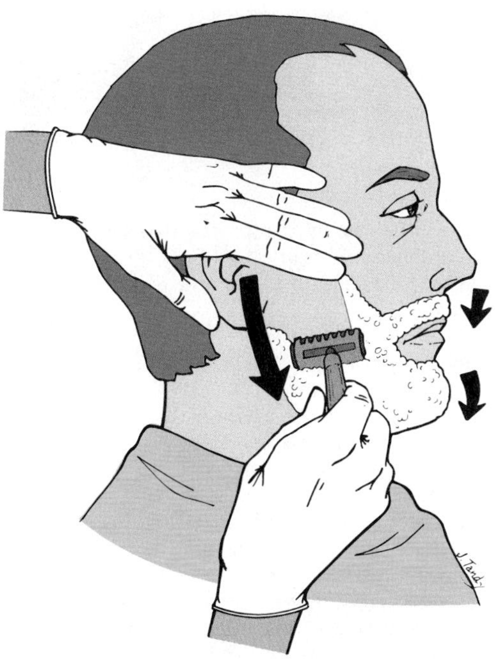

FIGURE **34–8** Shave in the direction of hair growth. Use longer strokes on the larger areas of the face. Use short strokes around the chin and lips. (From *Assisting With Patient Care,* by S. A. Sorrentino, 1999, St. Louis, MO: Mosby.)

Care of the Eyes, Ears, and Nose. Special attention is given to cleansing the eyes, ears, and nose during a routine bath and when drainage or discharge accumulate. This aspect of hygiene not only makes the client more comfortable, but also improves sensory reception (see chapter 44). Care focuses on preventing infection and maintaining normal sensory function. In addition, care of the eyes, ears, and nose requires approaches that consider the client's special needs.

Basic Eye Care. Cleansing the eyes simply involves washing with a clean washcloth moistened in water. Soap may cause burning and irritation (see Skill 34-1). Direct pressure should never be applied over the eyeball because it may cause serious injury.

Unconscious clients often require more frequent eye care. When cleansing the client's eyes, obtain a clean washcloth and cleanse from inner canthus to outer canthus. Use a different section of the washcloth for each eye.

Secretions may collect along the lid margins and inner canthus when the blink reflex is absent or when the eye does not totally close. It may be necessary to place an eye patch over the involved eye to prevent corneal drying and irritation. Lubricating eye drops may be given according to the physician's orders.

Eyeglasses. Glasses are made of hardened glass or plastic that is impact resistant to prevent shattering. Nevertheless, because of the cost, the nurse should be careful when cleaning glasses and should protect them from breakage or other damage when they are not worn. Glasses should be put in a case in a drawer of the

Client Teaching

Box 34-13

Contact Lens Care

Objectives

- Client will be able to identify warning signs of corneal irritation and eye infection.
- Client will be able to clean and care for contact lenses correctly.

Teaching Strategies

- Encourage client to see a vision care specialist (**ophthalmologist** or **optometrist**) regularly: every 3 to 5 years before the age of 40 years, every 2 years after age 40, and yearly after age 65.
- Plastic lenses scratch easily. Special cleaning solutions and drying tissues are recommended.
- Never use fingernail on lens to remove dirt or debris that does not loosen during washing.
- Follow recommendations of lens manufacturer or eye care practitioner when cleaning and disinfecting lenses.
- Encourage client to remember the mnemonic RSVP: *R*edness, *S*ensitivity, *V*ision problems, and *P*ain. If one of these problems occurs, remove contact lenses immediately. If problems continue, contact vision care specialist (Lewis et al., 2000).
- Lenses become very slippery once cleaning solution is applied.
- If lens is dropped on a hard surface, moisten finger with cleaning or wetting solution and gently touch lens to pick it up. Then clean, rinse, and disinfect lens.
- Lens should be kept moist or wet when not worn.
- Use fresh solution daily when storing and disinfecting lenses.
- Do not wipe lens with tissue or towel.
- Thoroughly wash and rinse lens storage case on a daily basis. Clean periodically with soap or liquid detergent; rinse thoroughly with warm water and air-dry.
- To avoid mix-up, always start with the same lens when removing or inserting lenses.
- Disposable or planned replacement lenses should be thrown away after prescribed wearing period.

Evaluation

- Have client identify warning signs of corneal irritation and eye infection.
- Ask client to describe methods of contact lens care that can lead to infection.
- Ask client to describe techniques to use in cleaning and storing contact lenses.

bedside table when not in use and labelled with the client's name.

Cool water is sufficient for cleaning glass lenses. A soft cloth is best for drying to prevent scratching the lens. Paper towels can scratch a lens. Plastic lenses in particular are scratched easily, and special cleansing solutions and drying tissues are available. Use whatever the client's eye care specialist recommends.

Contact Lenses. A contact lens is a small, round, transparent, and sometimes coloured disk that fits directly over the cornea of the eye. Contact lenses are designed specifically to correct refractive errors of the eye or abnormalities in the cornea's shape. They are relatively easy to apply and remove.

Contact lenses are available as daily wear, extended wear, and disposable. In terms of a client's hygiene care, it is important to know that all lenses must be removed periodically to prevent ocular infection and corneal ulcers or abrasions. Common infectious agents are *Pseudomonas aeruginosa* and staphylococci. Client education must include a discussion of proper lens care techniques (Box 34-13).

Daily-wear lenses should be removed overnight for cleaning and disinfection and should not be worn for more than 10 to 14 hours daily (Cohen & Krachmer, 1992). It is recommended that all extended-wear lenses be worn no longer than six consecutive nights without cleaning and disinfecting (Johnson & Johnson Vision Products, 1994).

Disposable lenses are available for daily wear and extended wear. Extended wear disposable lenses are usually replaced every 1 to 2 weeks. Pain, tearing, discomfort, and redness of the conjunctivae may be symptoms of lens over-wear. Persistence of symptoms even after lens removal is abnormal, however, and may indicate serious ocular damage.

As contact lenses are worn, they accumulate secretions and foreign matter. This material deteriorates and then irritates the eye, causing distorted vision and risk for infection. Once removed, contact lenses should be cleaned and thoroughly disinfected. Clients should be cautioned to never use saliva, homemade saline, or tap water when cleaning lenses as these solutions may contain microorganisms that can cause serious infection.

Artificial Eyes. Clients with artificial eyes have had an **enucleation** of an entire eyeball as a result of tumour growth, severe infection, or eye trauma. Some artificial eyes are permanently implanted. Others can be removed for routine cleaning. Clients with artificial eyes usually prefer to care for their own eyes. The nurse should respect the client's wishes and help by assembling needed equipment.

Clients may at times require assistance in prosthesis removal and cleansing. To remove an artificial eye, the nurse retracts the lower eyelid and exerts slight pressure just below the eye (Figure 34–9). This action causes the artificial eye to rise from the socket because the suction holding the eye in place has been broken. The nurse may also use a small, rubber bulb syringe or medicine dropper bulb to create a suction effect. The suction created by placing the bulb tip directly over the eye and squeezing lifts the eye from the socket.

The artificial eye is usually made of glass or plastic. Warm normal saline cleanses the prosthesis effectively. The nurse also cleanses the edges of the eye socket and

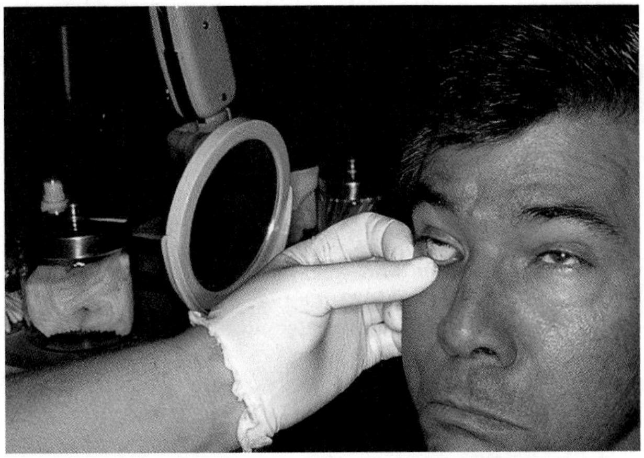

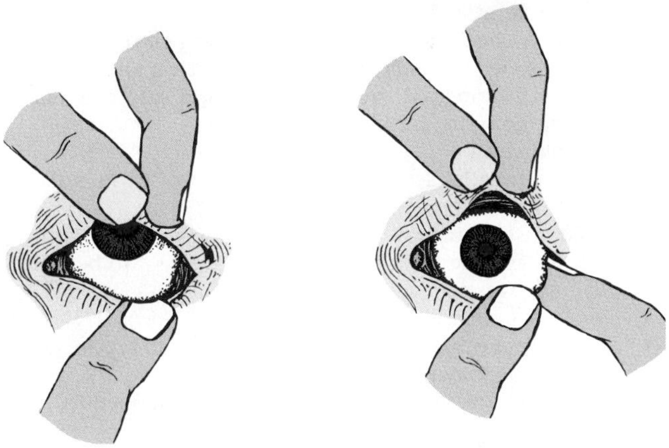

FIGURE **34–9** Removal of prosthetic eye.

surrounding tissues with soft gauze moistened in saline or clean tap water. Signs of infection should be reported immediately because bacteria can spread to the neighbouring eye, underlying sinuses, or even underlying brain tissue. To reinsert the eye, the nurse retracts the upper and lower lids and gently slips the eye into the socket, fitting it neatly under the upper eyelid. An artificial eye may be stored in a labelled container filled with tap water or saline.

Ear Care. Routine ear care involves cleansing the ear with the end of a moistened washcloth, rotated gently into the ear canal. When cerumen is visible, gentle, downward retraction at the entrance of the ear canal may cause the wax to loosen and slip out. The nurse warns clients never to use sharp objects such as bobby pins or paper clips to remove earwax. The use of such objects can traumatize the ear canal and rupture the tympanic membrane. Use of cotton-tipped applicators should also be avoided because they can cause earwax to become impacted within the canal.

Children and older adults commonly have impacted cerumen. Excessive or impacted cerumen can usually be removed only by irrigation, which usually requires a physician's order. If a client has a history of a perforated eardrum or if perforation is discovered during assessment, the procedure is contraindicated. Before irrigation, first instill three drops of glycerine at bedtime to soften the wax and three drops of hydrogen peroxide twice a day to loosen the wax. Then the instillation of approximately 250 mL of warm water (37°C) into the ear canal mechanically washes away loosened wax. Cold or hot water causes nausea or vomiting.

The client may sit or lie on his or her side with the affected ear up. The nurse places a small curved basin under the affected ear to catch the irrigating solution. A bulb-irrigating syringe can be used to irrigate the ear canal. The tip of the syringe should not occlude the canal to avoid exerting pressure against the tympanic membrane. Gentle irrigation directed at the top of the canal loosens the cerumen from the sides of the canal. After the canal is clear, the nurse wipes off any moisture from the ear and inspects the canal for remaining cerumen.

Hearing Aid Care. Hearing aids are instruments made up of miniature parts working together as a system to amplify sound in a controlled manner. The aid receives normal low-intensity sound inputs and delivers them to the client's ear as louder outputs. The new class of hearing aids can reduce background noise interference. Computer chips placed in the aids allow for fine adjustments to the specific client's hearing needs. Hearing aids are used by both hard-of-hearing (slight or moderate hearing loss) and deaf people (severe or prolonged hearing loss).

There are three popular types of hearing aids. An in-the-canal (ITC) aid is the newest, smallest, and least visible hearing aid and fits entirely in the ear canal. It has cosmetic appeal, is easy to manipulate and place in the ear, does not interfere with wearing eyeglasses or using the telephone, and can be worn during most physical exercise. However, it requires adequate ear diameter and depth for proper fit. It does not accommodate progressive hearing loss, and it requires manual dexterity to operate, insert, remove, and change batteries. Also, cerumen tends to plug this model more than the others.

An in-the-ear (ITE, or intra-aural) aid (Figure 34–10, *A*) fits into the external auditory canal and allows for better fine tuning. It is more powerful and stronger and therefore is useful for a wider range of hearing loss than the ITC aid. It is easy to position and adjust and does not interfere with eyeglass wearing. It is, however, more noticeable than the ITC aid and is not recommended for people with moisture or skin problems in the ear canal.

A behind-the-ear (BTE, or post-aural) aid (Figure 34–10, *B*) hooks around and behind the ear and is connected by a short, clear, hollow plastic tube to an ear mould inserted into the external auditory canal. It allows for fine tuning. It is the largest of the three aids and is useful for clients with rapidly progressive hearing loss or manual dexterity difficulties or those who find partial ear occlusion intolerable. Disadvantages are that it is more visible, may interfere with wearing eyeglasses and using a phone, and is more difficult to keep in place during physical exercise. Box 34-14 reviews client education guidelines for the care and use of a hearing aid.

Nasal Care. The client can usually remove secretions from the nose by gently blowing into a soft tissue. The nurse cautions the client against harsh blowing that creates

A

B

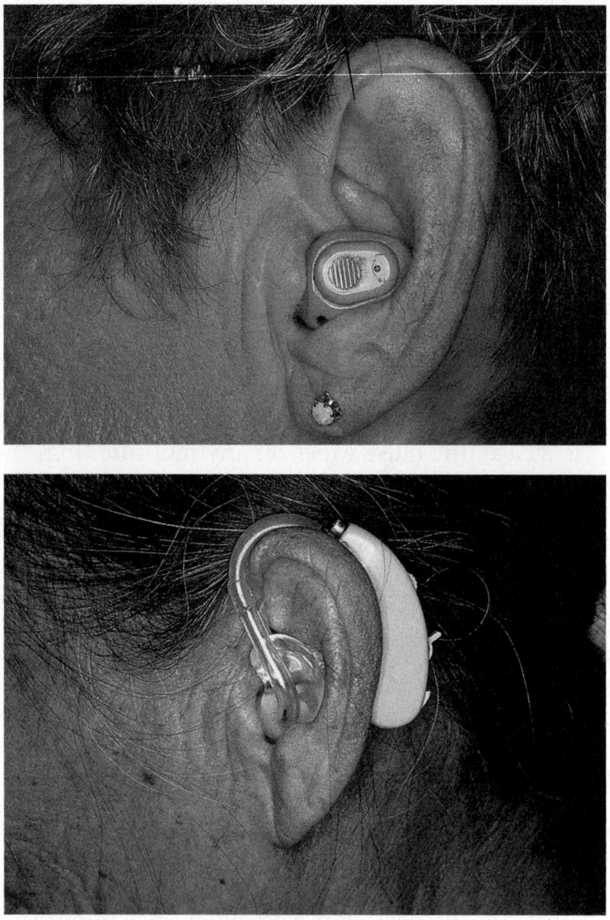

FIGURE **34–10** Two common types of hearing aids. **A,** In the ear. **B,** Behind the ear.

pressure capable of injuring the eardrum, nasal mucosa, and even sensitive eye structures. Bleeding from the nares is a sign of harsh blowing.

If the client is unable to remove nasal secretions, the nurse assists by using a wet washcloth or a cotton-tipped applicator moistened in water or saline. The applicator should never be inserted beyond the length of the cotton tip. Excessive nasal secretions can also be removed by gentle suctioning.

When clients have nasogastric, feeding, or endotracheal tubes inserted through the nose, the nurse should change the tape anchoring the tube at least once a day. When tape becomes moist from nasal secretions, the skin and mucosa can easily become macerated. Friction from a tube can cause tissue sloughing. After carefully removing the tape, the nurse maintains hold of the tubing and thoroughly cleanses and dries the nasal surface (see chapter 39).

Client's Room Environment. Attempting to make a client's room as comfortable as the home is one of the nurse's priorities. The client's room should be comfortable, safe, and large enough to allow the client and visitors to move about freely. The nurse can control room temperature, ventilation, noise, and odours to create a more comfortable environment. Keeping the room neat and orderly also contributes to the client's sense of well-being.

Box 34-14 Care and Use of Hearing Aids

- Initially wear a hearing aid 15 to 20 minutes; then gradually increase time until 10 to 12 hours.
- Once inserted, turn the aid slowly to one-third to one-half volume.
- A whistling sound indicates incorrect ear mould insertion, improper fit of aid, and buildup of earwax or fluid.
- Adjust volume to a comfortable level for talking at a distance of 1 metre.
- Do not wear aid under heat lamps, a hair dryer; or in very wet, cold weather.
- Batteries last 1 week with daily wearing of 10 to 12 hours.
- Remove or disconnect battery when not in use.
- Replace ear moulds every 2 or 3 years.
- Routinely check battery compartment: Is it clean? Are batteries inserted properly? Is compartment shut all the way?
- Dials on hearing aid should be clean and easy to rotate, creating no static during adjusting.
- Keep aid clean.
- Aids are usually cleaned with a soft cloth; see manufacturer's instructions.
- Avoid use of hairspray and perfume while wearing hearing aids; the residue from the spray can cause aid to become oily and greasy.
- Do not submerse in water.
- Routinely check cord or tubing (depending on type of aid) for cracking, fraying, and poor connections.
- Routine follow-up with audiologist is recommended to evaluate effectiveness of current aid.
- Newer computerized hearing aids can have frequencies easily adjusted.

Data from *Toward Healthy Aging* (5th ed.), by P. Ebersole and P. Hess, 2000, St. Louis, MO: Mosby; *Gerontologic Nursing* (2nd ed.), by A. G. Lueckenotte, 2000, St. Louis, MO: Mosby; and *Hearing Aids* (Publication No. 99-4340), National Institute on Deafness and Other Communication Disorders, 2001, retrieved December 12, 2004 from *http://www.nidcd.nih.gov/health/hearing/ hearingaid.asp*

Maintaining Comfort. The nature of what constitutes a comfortable environment depends on the client's age, severity of illness, and level of normal daily activity. Depending on the client's age and physical condition, the room temperature should be maintained between 20° C and 23° C. Infants, older adults, and the acutely ill may need a warmer room. However, certain ill clients benefit from cooler room temperatures to lower the body's metabolic demands.

A good ventilation system keeps stale air and odours from lingering in the room. The nurse must protect the acutely ill, infants, and older adults from drafts by ensuring that they are adequately dressed and covered with a lightweight blanket.

Good ventilation also reduces lingering odours caused by draining wounds, vomitus, bowel movements, and unemptied urinals. Room deodorizers can help remove many unpleasant odours but should be used with discretion in consideration of the client's possible embarrassment. Nurses should always empty and rinse bedpans or urinals promptly. Thorough hygiene measures are the best way to control body or breath odours. Before using room deodorizers, the nurse should determine that the client is not allergic to or sensitive to the deodorizer itself.

Ill clients seem to be more sensitive to common hospital noises (e.g., intravenous pump alarms, suction apparatus, or stretchers exiting an elevator). Until the client is familiar with hospital noises, the nurse should try to control the noise level. This can also help the client sleep (see chapter 37). The nurse also explains the source of any unfamiliar noise to the client and family members.

Proper lighting is necessary for everyone's safety and comfort. A brightly lit room is usually stimulating, and a darkened room is best for rest and sleep. Room lighting can be adjusted by closing or opening drapes, regulating overbed and floor lights, and closing or opening room doors. When entering a client's room at night, refrain from abruptly turning on an overhead light unless necessary.

Room Equipment. Although there may be variation across health care settings, a typical hospital room contains the following basic pieces of furniture: overbed table, bedside stand, chairs, lamp, and bed (Figure 34–11). Long-term care and rehabilitation facilities may have similar equipment. The overbed table rolls on wheels and can be adjusted to various heights over the bed or a chair. The table provides ideal working space for the nurse performing procedures. It also provides a surface on which to place meal trays, toiletry items, and objects frequently used by the client. The bedpan and urinal should not be placed on the overbed table. The bedside stand is used to store the client's personal possessions and hygiene equipment. The telephone, water pitcher, and drinking cup are commonly found on top of the bedside stand.

Most hospital rooms contain an armless straight-backed chair or an upholstered lounge chair with arms. Straight-backed chairs are convenient when temporarily transferring the client from the bed, such as during bed making. Lounge chairs tend to be more comfortable when a client is willing and able to sit for an extended period.

Each room usually has an overbed light and a floor or table lamp. Moveable lights that extend over the bed from the wall should be positioned for easy reach but moved aside when not in use. Additional portable lighting is used to provide extra light during bedside procedures.

Other equipment usually found in a client's room includes a call light, a television set, a wall-mounted blood pressure gauge, oxygen and vacuum wall outlets, and personal care items. Special equipment designed for comfort or positioning clients includes footboards and foot boots, special mattresses, and bed boards (see chapters 42 and 43). Check agency policy and manufacturer's directions before applying comfort and positioning equipment.

Beds. Seriously ill clients may remain in bed for a long time. Because a bed is the piece of equipment used most by a hospitalized client, it should be designed for comfort, safety, and adaptability for changing positions.

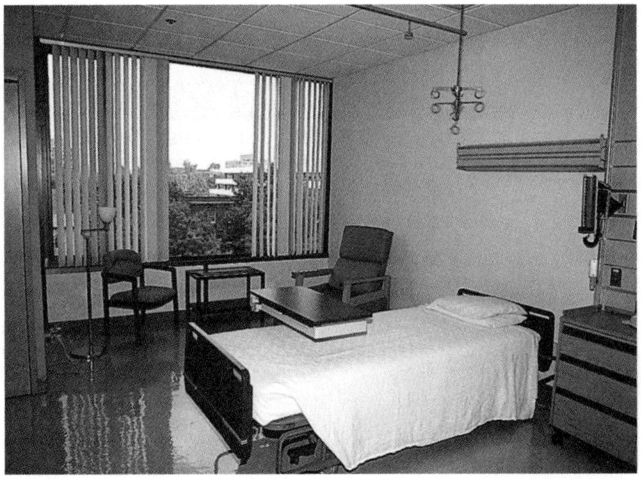

FIGURE **34–11** Typical hospital room.

The typical hospital bed has a firm mattress on a metal frame that can be raised and lowered horizontally. Many hospitals are converting the standard hospital bed to one in which the mattress surface can be electronically adjusted for client comfort. Different bed positions are used to promote client comfort, minimize symptoms, promote lung expansion, and improve access during certain procedures (Table 34-6).

The position of a bed is usually changed by electrical controls incorporated into the client's call light and in a panel on the side or foot of the bed (Figure 34–12). It is important for the nurse to become familiar with use of the bed controls. Ease in raising and lowering a bed and in changing position of the head and foot eliminates undue musculoskeletal strain on the nurse. Nurses should instruct clients on the proper use of controls and caution them against raising the bed to a position that might cause harm.

Beds contain safety features such as locks on the wheels or casters. Wheels should be locked when the bed is stationary to prevent accidental movement. Side rails protect clients from accidental falls. The headboard can be removed from most beds. This is important when the medical team must have easy access to the head, such as during cardiopulmonary resuscitation.

Bed Making. A client's bed should be kept clean and comfortable. This requires frequent inspections to be sure linen is clean, dry, and free of wrinkles. When clients are diaphoretic, have draining wounds, or are incontinent, the nurse should check frequently for soiled linen.

The nurse usually makes a bed in the morning after the client's bath or while the client is bathing in a shower, sitting in a chair eating, or out of the room for procedures or tests. Throughout the day, the nurse straightens linen that becomes loose or wrinkled. The bed linen should also be checked for food particles after meals and for wetness or soiling. Linen that becomes soiled or wet should be changed.

When changing bed linen, the nurse follows principles of medical asepsis by keeping soiled linen away from the uniform (Figure 34–13). Soiled linen is placed in special

Table 34-6 Common Bed Positions

Position	Description	Uses
Fowler's 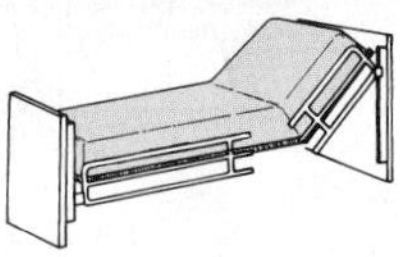	Head of bed raised to angle of 45 degrees or more; semi-sitting position; foot of bed may also be raised at knee	Is preferred while client eats Is used during nasogastric tube insertion and nasotracheal suction Promotes lung expansion
Semi-Fowler's 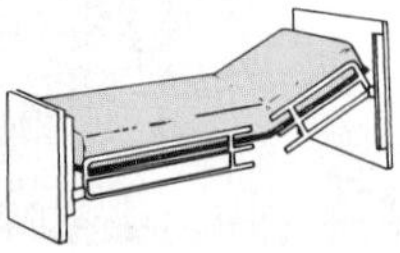	Head of bed raised approximately 30 degrees; inclination less than Fowler's position; foot of bed may also be raised at knee	Promotes lung expansion Used when clients receive gastric feedings to reduce regurgitation and risk of aspiration
Trendelenburg's 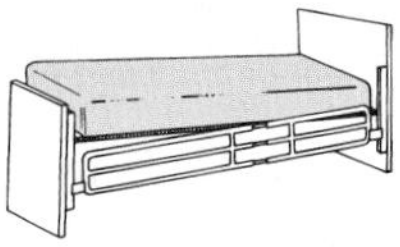	Entire bed fame tilted with head of bed down	Is used for postural drainage Facilitates venous return in clients with poor peripheral perfusion
Reverse Trendelenburg's 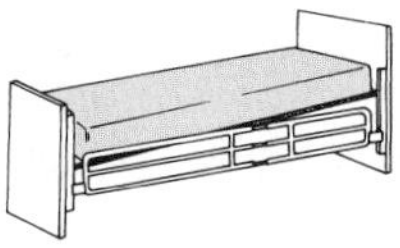	Entire bed frame tilted with foot of bed down	Is used infrequently Promotes gastric emptying Prevents esophageal reflux
Flat 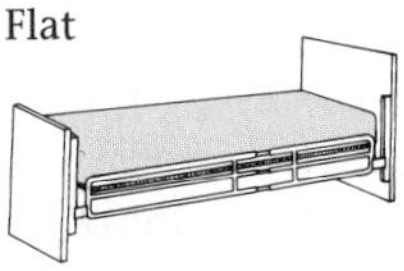	Entire bed frame horizontally parallel with floor	Is used for clients with vertebral injuries and in cervical traction Is used for clients who are hypotensive Is generally preferred by clients for sleeping

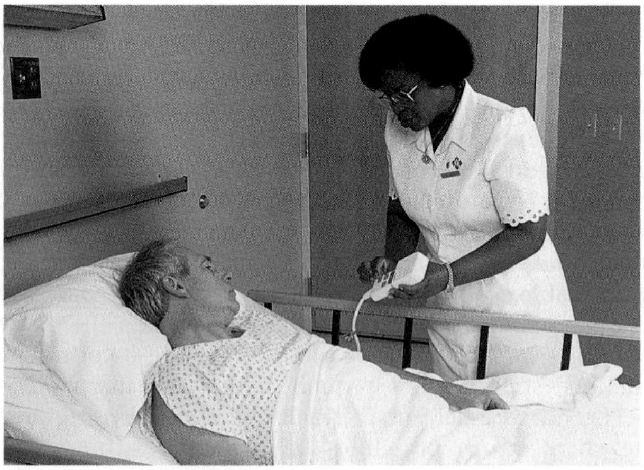

FIGURE **34–12** Nurse instructing client in use of call light and bed controls.

linen bags before discarding in a hamper. To avoid air currents, which can spread micro-organisms, the nurse never shakes the linen. To avoid transmitting infection, the nurse should not place soiled linen on the floor. If clean linen touches the floor, it is immediately discarded.

During bed making, the nurse uses proper body mechanics (see chapter 32). The bed should always be raised to the appropriate height before changing linen so that the nurse does not have to bend or stretch over the mattress. The nurse also moves back and forth to opposite sides of the bed while applying new linen. Body mechanics is also important when turning or repositioning the client in bed.

When clients are confined to bed, the nurse organizes bed-making activities to conserve time and energy (Skill 34-6). The client's privacy, comfort, and safety are all important when making a bed. Using side rails to aid positioning and turning, keeping call lights within the client's reach, and maintaining the proper bed position help promote comfort and safety. After making a bed, the nurse always returns it to the lowest horizontal position to prevent accidental falls should the client get in and out of the bed alone.

When possible, the nurse should make the bed while it is unoccupied (Box 34-15). The nurse uses judgment in regard to when is the best time to have the client sit up in a chair while the bed is made. When making an unoccupied bed, the nurse follows the same basic principles as for occupied bed making.

An unoccupied bed can be open or closed. In an open bed, the top covers are folded back so that a client can

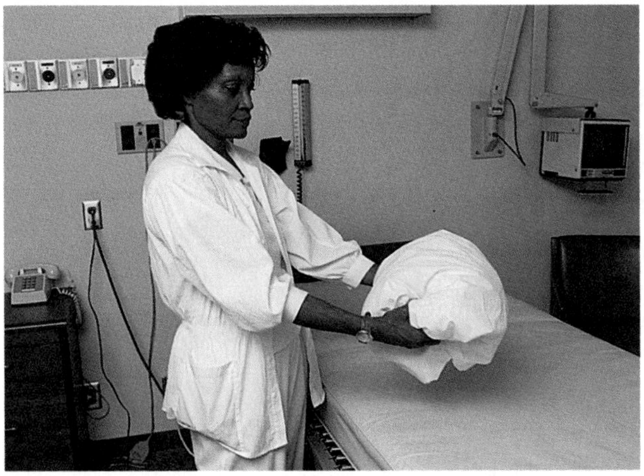

FIGURE 34–13 Holding linen away from the uniform prevents contact with micro-organisms.

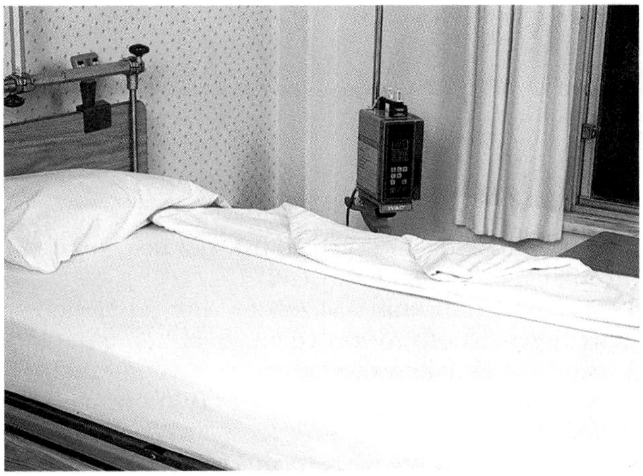

FIGURE 34–14 Surgical or recovery bed.

easily get into bed. In a closed bed, the top sheet, blanket, and bedspread are drawn up to the head of the mattress and under the pillows. A closed bed is prepared in a hospital room before a new client is admitted to that room. A surgical, recovery, or post-operative bed is a modified version of the open bed. The top bed linen is arranged for easy transfer of the client from a stretcher to the bed. The top sheets and spread are not tucked or mitred at the corners. Instead, the top sheets are folded to one side or folded to the bottom third of the bed (Figure 34–14). This makes it easier to transfer the client into the bed.

Linens. In any health care agency, it is important to have an adequate supply of linen to care appropriately for clients. Many agencies have what are called "nurse servers," either within or just outside a client's room, where a daily supply of linen is stored. Because of the importance of cost control in health care, it is important to not bring excess linen into a client's room. Linen brought into a client's room, if unused, must be discarded for laundering. This can increase an agency's costs. Excess linen lying around a client's room creates clutter and obstacles for client care activities.

Before bed making, it is important to collect necessary bed linens and the client's personal items. In this way, the nurse will have all equipment accessible to prepare the bed and room. Linens are pressed and folded to prevent the spread of micro-organisms and to make bed making easier. When fitted sheets are not available, flat sheets usually are pressed with a centre crease to be placed down the centre of the bed. The linens unfold easily to the sides, with creases often fitting over the mattress edge. A complete linen change is not always necessary. The nurse may reuse the mattress pad, sheet, blanket, and bedspread for the same client if they are not wet or soiled.

Disposal of linen must be done to minimize the spread of infection (see chapter 29). Agency policies provide guidelines for the proper way to bag and dispose of soiled linen. After a client is discharged, all bed linen is sent to the laundry, the mattress and bed are cleansed by housekeeping staff, and new bed linen is applied.

Evaluation

Client Care. Evaluation of hygiene measures occurs both during and after each particular skill. For example, as the nurse bathes a client, close inspection of the skin reveals if drainage or other soiling is effectively removed from the skin's surface. Once the bath is completed, the nurse will ask if the client's comfort and relaxation have improved. When evaluating for the effectiveness of hygiene measures, the nurse observes for changes in the client's behaviour. Does the client assume a more relaxed position? Is the client free of body odour? Is the client able to fall asleep? Does the client's facial expression convey a sense of comfort?

Frequently it takes time for hygiene care to result in an improvement in the client's condition. The presence of oral lesions, a scalp infestation, or skin excoriation will often require repeated measures and a combination of nursing interventions. The nurse will evaluate for improvement in the client's condition over time and determine if existing therapies are effective.

Throughout evaluation, the nurse considers the goals of care and evaluates whether expected outcomes are achieved. A critical thinking approach ensures that the nurse considers all factors when evaluating the client's care (Figure 34–16). The nurse's knowledge base and experience provide important perspectives when the nurse analyzes observations made about a client. For example, once the nurse has seen how dehydration of the oral mucosa clears with repeated hygiene, it will help in recognizing when another client's progress is slow. The standards for evaluation are the expected outcomes established in the planning stage of the client's care. If outcomes are not met, the care plan may need to be revised. The nurse continues to apply critical thinking attitudes when considering all evaluation findings.

Client Expectations. The final portion of the evaluation considers whether or not the client's expectations were met through hygiene care. The nurse might ask, Do you feel

Text continued on p. 1074

Skill 34-6 Making an Occupied Bed

View Video

Delegation Considerations

The skill of making an occupied bed can be delegated to unregulated care providers (UCPs).

- Before delegating this skill, review any precautions or activity restrictions for the client.
- Be sure the UCP knows what to do if wound drainage, dressing material, drainage tubes, or IV tubing becomes dislodged or is found in the linens.
- Instruct the UCP in what to do if client becomes fatigued.

Equipment *(Figure 34–15)*

- Linen bag(s)
- Mattress pad (needs to be changed only when soiled)
- Bottom sheet (flat or fitted)
- Drawsheet
- Top sheet
- Blanket
- Bedspread
- Waterproof pads and/or bath blankets (optional)
- Pillowcases
- Bedside chair or table
- Disposable gloves (optional)
- Towel
- Disinfectant

Steps	Rationale
1. Assess potential for client incontinence or for excess drainage on bed linen.	Determines need for protective waterproof pads or extra bath blankets on bed.
2. Check chart for orders or specific precautions concerning movement and positioning.	Ensures client safety and use of proper body mechanics.
3. Explain procedure to the client, noting that the client will be asked to turn on side and roll over linen.	Minimizes anxiety and promotes co-operation.
4. Perform hand hygiene, and apply gloves (gloves are worn only if linen is soiled or there is risk for contact with body secretions).	Reduces transmission of micro-organisms.
5. Assemble equipment, and arrange on bedside chair or table. Remove unnecessary equipment such as a dietary tray or items used for hygiene.	Assembling all equipment provides for smooth procedure and assists in increasing client's comfort. Placing linen on clean surface minimizes spread of infection.
6. Draw room curtain around bed or close door.	Maintains client's privacy.
7. Adjust bed height to comfortable working position. Lower any raised side rail on one side of bed. Remove call light.	Minimizes strain on back. It is easier to remove and apply linen evenly to bed in flat position. Provides easy access to bed and linen.
8. Loosen top linen at foot of bed.	Makes linen easier to remove.

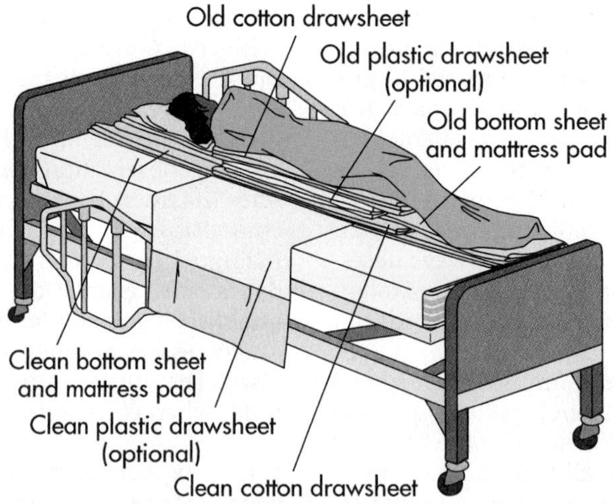

FIGURE **34–15** Equipment for making occupied bed.

Steps	Rationale
9. Remove bedspread and blanket separately. If spread and blanket are soiled, place them in linen bag. Keep soiled linen away from uniform.	Reduces transmission of micro-organisms.
10. If blanket and spread are to be reused, fold them by bringing the top and bottom edges together. Fold farthest side over onto nearer bottom edge. Bring top and bottom edges together again. Place folded linen over back of chair.	Folding method facilitates replacement and minimizes wrinkles.
11. Cover client with bath blanket in the following manner: Unfold bath blanket over top sheet. Ask client to hold top edge of bath blanket. If client is unable to help, tuck top of bath blanket under shoulder. Grasp top sheet under bath blanket at client's shoulders and bring sheet down to foot of bed. Remove sheet and discard in linen bag.	Bath blanket provides warmth and keeps body parts covered during linen removal.
12. With assistance from another nurse, slide mattress toward head of bed.	If mattress slides toward foot of bed when head of bed is raised, it is difficult to tuck in linen. In addition, it is uncomfortable for the client because the client's feet may be pressed against or hang over the foot of the bed.
13. Position client on the far side of the bed, turned onto side and facing away from you. Be sure side rail in front of client is up. Adjust pillow under client's head.	Turning client onto side provides space for placement of clean linen. Side rail ensures client's safety from forward falls from the bed surface and helps client in moving.
14. Loosen bottom linens, moving from head to foot. With seam side down (facing the mattress), fanfold bottom sheet and drawsheet toward client—first drawsheet, then bottom sheet. Tuck edges of linen just under buttocks, back, and shoulders. Do not fanfold mattress pad if it is to be reused (see illustration).	Prepares for removal of all bottom linen simultaneously. Provides maximum workspace for placing clean linen. Later, when client turns to other side, soiled linen can be removed easily.
15. Wipe off any moisture on exposed mattress with towel and appropriate disinfectant.	Reduces transmission of micro-organisms.
16. Apply clean linen to exposed half of bed:	
a. Place clean mattress pad on bed by folding it lengthwise with centre crease in middle of bed. Fanfold top layer over mattress. (If pad is reused, simply smooth out any wrinkles.)	Applying linen over bed in successive layers minimizes energy and time used in bed making.
b. Unfold bottom sheet lengthwise so that centre crease is situated lengthwise along centre of bed. Fanfold sheet's top layer toward centre of bed alongside the client. Smooth bottom layer of sheet over mattress, and bring edge over closest side of mattress. Pull fitted sheet smoothly over mattress ends. Allow edge of flat unfitted sheet to hang about 25 cm over mattress edge. Lower hem of bottom flat sheet should lie seam down and even with bottom edge of mattress (see illustration).	Proper positioning of linen on one side ensures that adequate linen will be available to cover opposite side of bed. Keeping seam edges down eliminates irritation to client's skin.

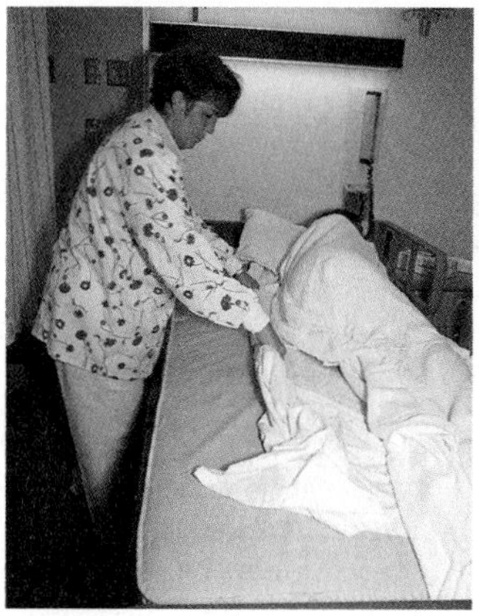

STEP **14** Old linen tucked under client.

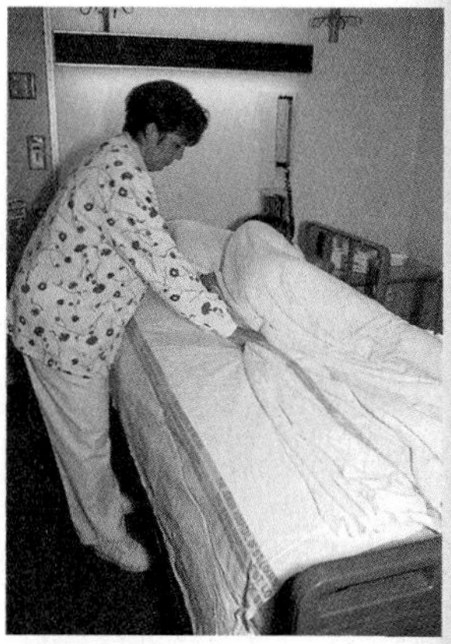

STEP **16b** Clean linen applied to bed.

Skill 34-6 Making an Occupied Bed—cont'd

Steps	Rationale
17. Mitre bottom flat sheet at head of bed:	
a. Face head of bed diagonally. Place hand away from head of bed under top corner of mattress, near mattress edge, and lift.	Ensures secure flat sheet will not loosen easily.
b. With other hand, tuck top edge of bottom sheet smoothly under mattress so that side edges of sheet above and below mattress would meet if brought together.	
c. Face side of bed and pick up top edge of sheet at approximately 45 cm from top of mattress (see illustration).	
d. Lift sheet, and lay it on top of mattress to form a neat triangular fold, with lower base of triangle even with mattress side edge (see illustration).	
e. Tuck lower edge of sheet, which is hanging free below the mattress, under mattress. Tuck with palms down, without pulling triangular fold (see illustration).	
f. Hold portion of sheet covering side of mattress in place with one hand. With the other hand, pick up top of triangular linen fold and bring it down over side of mattress (see illustrations). Tuck this portion under mattress (see illustration).	Mitred corner cannot be loosened easily even if client moves frequently in bed.
18. Tuck remaining portion of sheet under mattress, moving toward foot of bed. Keep linen smooth.	Folds of linen are source of irritation.

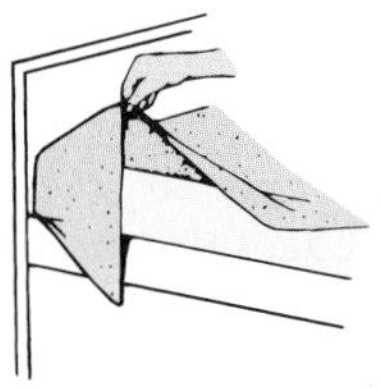

STEP **17c** Top edge of sheet picked up.

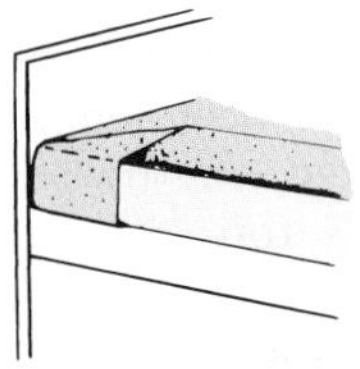

STEP **17e** Lower edge of sheet tucked under mattress.

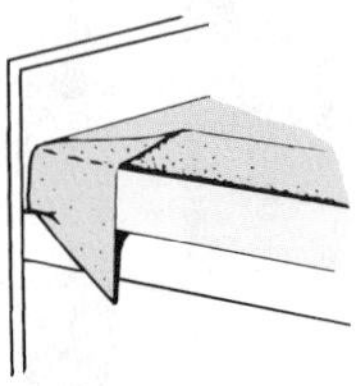

STEP **17d** Sheet on top of mattress in a triangular fold.

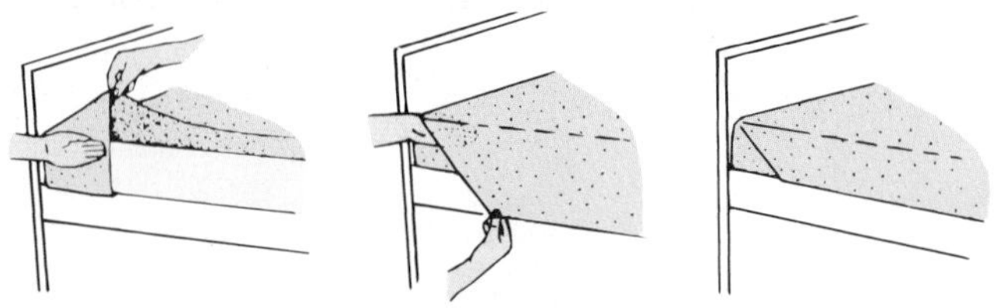

A **B** **C**

STEP **17f** **A** and **B,** Triangular fold placed over side of mattress. **C,** Linen tucked under mattress.

Steps	Rationale

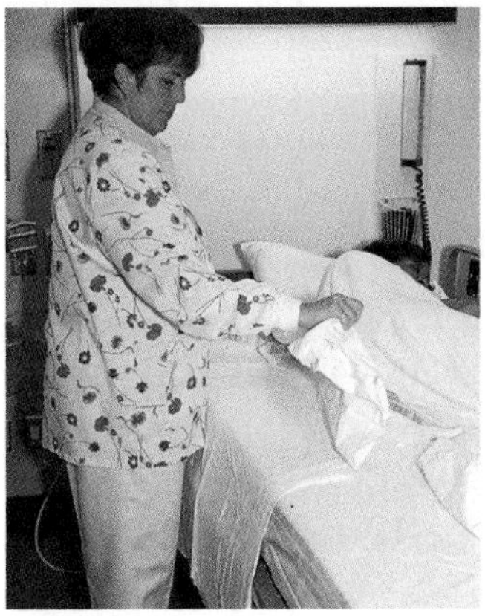

STEP **19** Optional draw sheet.

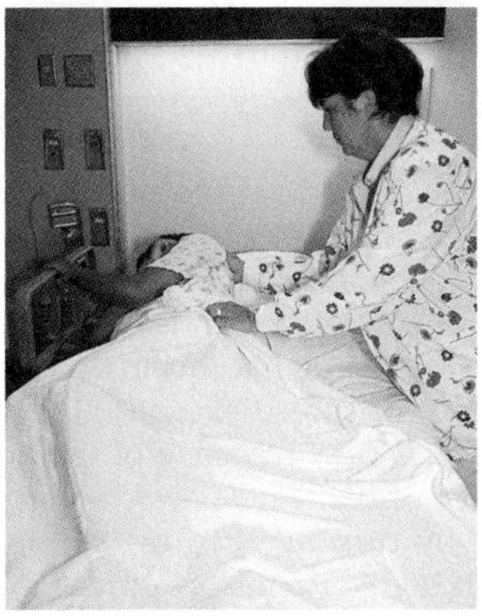

STEP **22** Assisting client to roll over folds of linen.

19. *(Optional)* Open drawsheet so that it unfolds in half. Lay centrefold along middle of bed lengthwise, and position sheet so that it will be under the client's buttocks and torso (see illustration). Fanfold top layer toward client, with edge along client's back. Smooth bottom layer out over mattress, and tuck excess edge under mattress (keep palms down).
Drawsheet is used to lift and reposition client. Placement under client's torso distributes most of client's body weight over sheet.

20. Place waterproof pad over drawsheet, with centrefold against client's side. Fanfold top layer toward client.
Protects bed linen from being soiled.

21. Have client roll slowly toward you, over the layers of linen. Raise side rail on working side, and go to other side of bed.
Positions client for removal and placement of linens. Maintains client's safety and body alignment during turning.

22. Lower side rail. Assist client in positioning on other side, over folds of linen. Loosen edges of soiled linen from under mattress (see illustration).
Exposes opposite side of bed for removal of soiled linen and placement of clean linen. Makes linen easier to remove.

23. Remove soiled linen by folding it into a bundle or square, with soiled side turned in. Discard in linen bag. If necessary, wipe mattress with antiseptic solution, and dry mattress surface before applying new linen.
Reduces transmission of micro-organisms.

24. Pull clean, fanfolded linen smoothly over edge of mattress from head to foot of bed.
Smooth linen will not irritate client's skin.

25. Assist client in rolling back into supine position. Reposition pillow.
Maintains client's comfort.

26. Pull fitted sheet smoothly over mattress ends. Mitre top corner of bottom sheet (see step 17). When tucking corner, be sure that sheet is smooth and free of wrinkles.
Wrinkles and folds can cause irritation to skin.

27. Facing side of bed, grasp remaining edge of bottom flat sheet. Lean back; keeping back straight, pull while tucking excess linen under mattress. Proceed from head to foot of bed. (Avoid lifting mattress during tucking to ensure fit.)
Proper use of body mechanics while tucking linen prevents injury.

28. Smooth fanfolded drawsheet out over bottom sheet. Grasp edge of sheet with palms down, lean back, and tuck sheet under mattress. Tuck from middle to top and then to bottom.
Tucking first at top or bottom may pull sheet sideways, causing poor fit.

29. Place top sheet over client with centrefold lengthwise down middle of bed. Open sheet from head to foot, and unfold over client.
Sheet should be equally distributed over bed by correctly positioning centrefold.

30. Ask client to hold clean top sheet, or tuck sheet around client's shoulders. Remove bath blanket and discard in linen bag.
Sheet prevents exposure of body parts. Having client hold sheet encourages client participation in care.

Skill 34-6 *Making an Occupied Bed—cont'd*

Steps	Rationale
31. Place blanket on bed, unfolding it so that crease runs lengthwise along middle of bed. Unfold blanket to cover client. Top edge should be parallel with edge of top sheet and 15 to 20 cm from top sheet's edge.	Blanket should be placed to cover client completely and provide adequate warmth.
32. Place spread over bed according to step 31. Be sure that top edge of spread extends about 2.5 cm above blanket's edge. Tuck top edge of spread over and under top edge of blanket.	Gives bed neat appearance and provides extra warmth.
33. Make cuff by turning edge of top sheet down over top edge of blanket and spread.	Protect client's face from rubbing against blanket or spread.
34. Standing on one side at foot of bed, lift mattress corner slightly with one hand and tuck linens under mattress. Top sheet and blanket are tucked under together. Be sure that linens are loose enough to allow movement of client's feet. Making a horizontal toe pleat is an option (see illustration).	Makes neat-appearing bed. Pressure ulcers can develop on client's toes and heels from feet rubbing against tight-fitting bed sheets.
35. Make modified mitred corner with top sheet, blanket, and spread (see illustration in Box 34-15):	Ensures top covers will not loosen easily.
a. Pick up side edge of top sheet, blanket, and spread approximately 45 cm from foot of mattress. Lift linen to form triangular fold, and lay it on bed.	
b. Tuck lower edge of sheet, which is hanging free below mattress, under mattress. Do not pull triangular fold.	
c. Pick up triangular fold, and bring it down over mattress while holding linen in place along side of mattress. Do not tuck tip of triangle.	Secures top linen but keeps even edge of blanket and top sheet draped over mattress.
36. Raise side rail. Make other side of bed; spread sheet, blanket, and bedspread out evenly. Fold top edge of spread over blanket and make cuff with top sheet (see step 33); make modified mitred corner at foot of bed (see step 35).	Side rail protects client from accidental falls.
37. Change pillowcase:	
a. Have client raise head. While supporting neck with one hand, remove pillow. Allow client to lower head.	Support of neck muscles prevents injury during flexion and extension of neck.
b. Remove soiled case by grasping pillow at open end with one hand and pulling case back over pillow with the other hand. Discard case in linen bag.	Pillows slide out easily, thus minimizing contact with soiled linen.

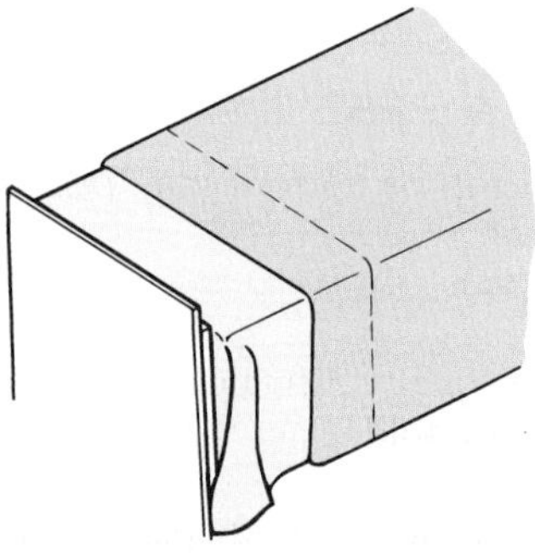

STEP **34** Optional toe pleat.

Steps	Rationale
c. Grasp clean pillowcase at centre of closed end. Gather case, turning it inside out over the hand holding it. With the same hand, pick up middle of one end of the pillow. Pull pillowcase down over pillow with the other hand.	Eases sliding of pillowcase over pillow.
d. Be sure pillow corners fit evenly into corners of pillowcase. Place pillow under client's head.	Poorly fitting case constricts fluffing and expansion of pillow and interferes with client comfort.
38. Place call light within client's reach, and return bed to comfortable position.	Ensures client safety and comfort.
39. Open room curtains, and rearrange furniture. Place personal items within easy reach on overbed table or bedside stand. Return bed to a comfortable height.	Promotes sense of well-being.
40. Discard dirty linen in hamper or chute and perform hand hygiene.	Prevents transmission of micro-organisms.
41. Ask if client feels comfortable.	Ensures bed linens are clean and smooth.
42. Inspect skin for areas of irritation.	Folds in linen can cause pressure on skin.
43. Observe client for signs of fatigue, dyspnea, pain, or discomfort.	Provides data about client's level of activity tolerance and ability to participate in other procedures.

Unexpected Outcomes and Related Interventions

- Client feels discomfort from linen fold.
  - Tighten sheets.
  - Change client's position frequently.
- Client's skin shows signs of breakdown.
  - Institute skin care measures to reduce risk of pressure ulcer (see chapter 43).
  - Change client's position frequently.

Recording and Reporting

- Making an occupied bed need not be recorded.

Box 34-15 Procedural Guidelines

Making an Unoccupied Bed

Equipment: Linen bag, mattress pad (change only when soiled), bottom sheet (flat or fitted), drawsheet (optional), top sheet, blanket, bedspread, waterproof pads (optional), pillowcases, bedside chair or table, disposable gloves (if linen is soiled), washcloth, antiseptic cleanser.

Delegation Considerations: The skill of making an unoccupied bed can be delegated to unregulated care providers.

1. Determine if client has been incontinent or if excess drainage is on linen. Gloves will be necessary.
2. Assess activity orders or restrictions in mobility to plan whether client can get out of bed for procedure. Assist to bedside chair or recliner.
3. Raise bed to comfortable working position. Lower side rails on both sides of bed.
4. Remove soiled linen and place in linen bag. Avoid shaking or fanning linen.
5. Reposition mattress and wipe off any moisture using a washcloth moistened in antiseptic solution. Dry thoroughly.
6. Apply all bottom linen on one side of bed before moving to opposite side.
7. Be sure fitted sheet is placed smoothly over mattress. To apply a flat unfitted sheet, allow about 25 cm to hang over mattress edge. Lower hem of sheet should lie seam down, even with bottom edge of mattress. Pull remaining top portion of sheet over top edge of mattress.
8. While standing at head of bed, mitre top corner of bottom sheet (see Skill 34-6, step 17).
9. Tuck remaining portion of unfitted sheet under mattress.
10. *Optional:* Apply drawsheet, laying centre fold along middle of bed lengthwise. Smooth drawsheet over mattress and tuck excess edge under mattress, keeping palms down.
11. Move to opposite side of bed and spread bottom sheet smoothly over edge of mattress from head to foot of bed.
12. Apply fitted sheet smoothly over each mattress corner. For an unfitted sheet, mitre top corner of bottom sheet (see Step 8) making sure corner is taut.
13. Grasp remaining edge of unfitted bottom sheet and tuck tightly under mattress while moving from head to foot of bed. Smooth folded drawsheet over bottom sheet and tuck under mattress, first at middle, then at top, and then at bottom.
14. If needed, apply waterproof pad over bottom sheet or drawsheet.
15. Place top sheet over bed with vertical centre fold lengthwise down middle of bed. Open sheet out from head to foot, being sure top edge of sheet is even with top edge of mattress.
16. Make horizontal toe pleat: Stand at foot of bed and fanfold in sheet 5 to 10 cm across bed. Pull sheet up from bottom to make fold approximately 15 cm from bottom edge of mattress (see Skill 34-6, step 34).
17. Tuck in remaining portion of sheet under foot of mattress. Place blanket over bed with top edge parallel to top edge of sheet and 15 to 20 cm down from edge of sheet. (*Optional:* Apply additional spread over bed.)
18. Make cuff by turning edge of top sheet down over top edge of blanket and spread.
19. Standing on one side at foot of bed, lift mattress corner slightly with one hand, and with other hand tuck top sheet, blanket, and spread under mattress. Be sure toe pleats are not pulled out.
20. Make modified mitred corner with top sheet, blanket, and spread. After triangular fold is made, do not tuck tip of triangle (see illustration).
21. Go to other side of bed. Spread sheet, blanket, and spread out evenly. Make cuff with top sheet and blanket. Make modified corner at foot of bed.
22. Apply clean pillowcase.
23. Place call light within client's reach on bed rail or pillow and return bed to height allowing for client transfer. Assist client to bed.
24. Arrange client's room. Remove and discard supplies. Perform hand hygiene.

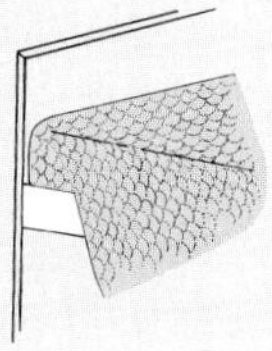

STEP **20** Modified mitred corner.

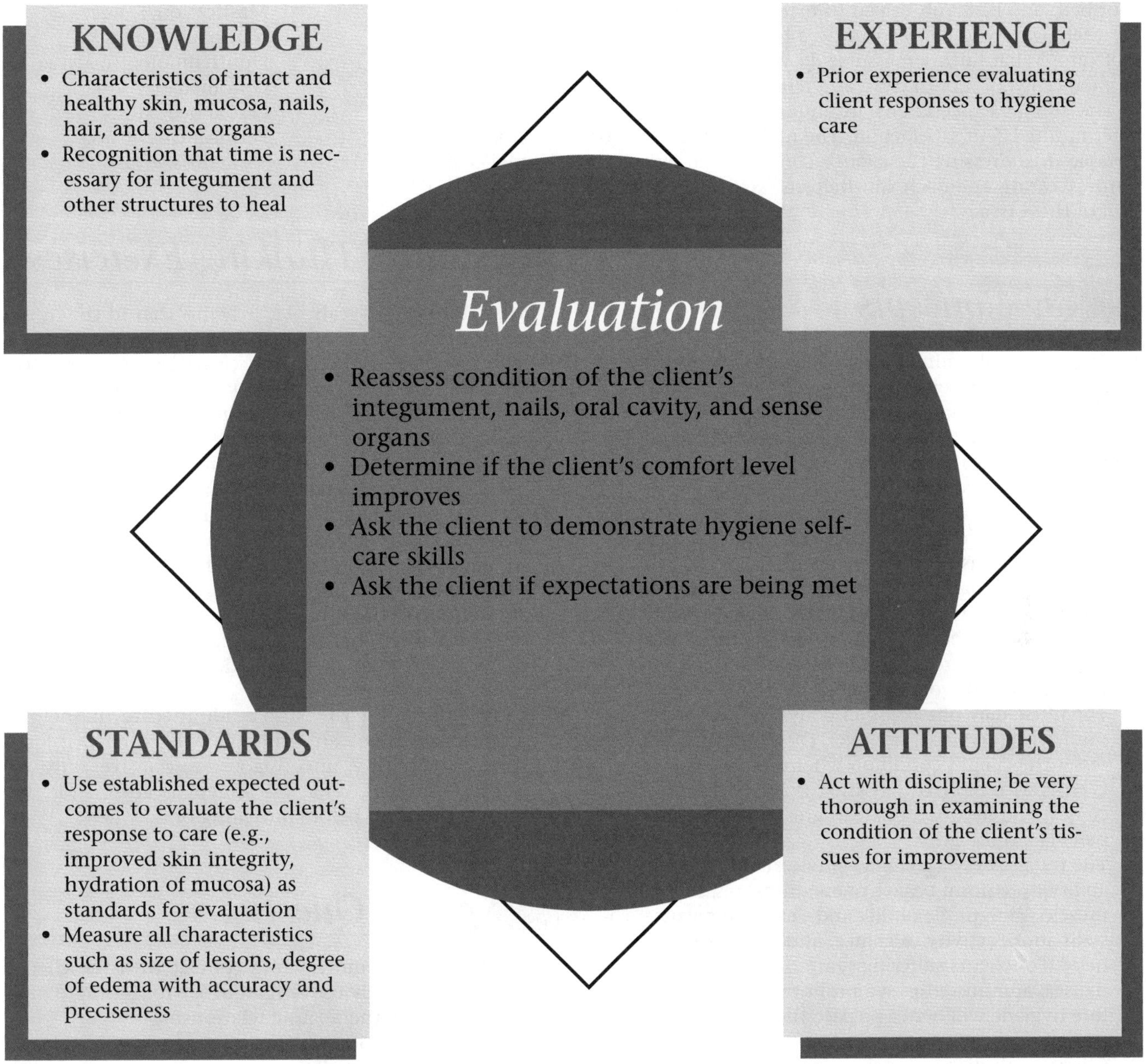
KNOWLEDGE
• Characteristics of intact and healthy skin, mucosa, nails, hair, and sense organs
• Recognition that time is necessary for integument and other structures to heal
EXPERIENCE
• Prior experience evaluating client responses to hygiene care
Evaluation
• Reassess condition of the client's integument, nails, oral cavity, and sense organs
• Determine if the client's comfort level improves
• Ask the client to demonstrate hygiene self-care skills
• Ask the client if expectations are being met
STANDARDS
• Use established expected outcomes to evaluate the client's response to care (e.g., improved skin integrity, hydration of mucosa) as standards for evaluation
• Measure all characteristics such as size of lesions, degree of edema with accuracy and preciseness
ATTITUDES
• Act with discipline; be very thorough in examining the condition of the client's tissues for improvement

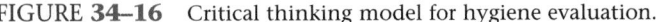

FIGURE **34–16** Critical thinking model for hygiene evaluation.

your bath and back rub helped to make you comfortable? Are there ways you feel we can do a better job with your foot care? What further measures do you think are necessary to keep your mouth clean and refreshed?

The client's expectations are important guidelines in determining client satisfaction. The nurse must feel comfortable in addressing the client's concerns and expectations. A caring approach can help in facilitating discussion of these issues.

Key Concepts

- The nurse determines a client's ability to perform self-care and provides hygiene care according to the client's needs and preferences.
- During hygiene, the nurse integrates other activities such as physical assessment, wound care, and range-of-motion exercises.
- While providing daily hygiene needs, the nurse uses teaching and communication skills in developing a caring relationship with the client.
- Various personal, socio-cultural, economic, and developmental factors influence clients' hygiene practices.
- Clients' health beliefs predict the likelihood of assuming health promotion behaviour, such as the maintenance of good hygiene.
- The nurse may not assess all body regions before administering hygiene; however, the nurse routinely assesses the client's condition whenever care is given.
- Clients with reduced sensation, vascular insufficiency, and immobility are at greater risk for impaired skin integrity.
- The nurse assesses a client's physical and cognitive ability to perform basic hygiene measures, including muscle strength, flexibility and dexterity, balance, coordination, activity tolerance, and ability to comprehend. For clients suffering symptoms such as pain or nausea, administering symptom relief therapies before hygiene will better prepare the client for any procedure.
- Clients with diabetes mellitus require special nail and foot care.
- When administering oral care to unconscious clients, the nurse takes measures to prevent aspiration.
- The client's room should be comfortable, safe, and large enough to allow the client and visitors to move about freely.
- Evaluation of hygiene care is based on the client's sense of comfort, relaxation, well-being, and understanding of hygiene techniques.

Key Terms

Acne, *p. 1023*
Alopecia, *p. 1020*
Apocrine, *p. 1023*
Buccal glands, *p. 1014*
Caries, *p. 1023*
Cerumen, *p. 1023*
Complete bed bath, *p. 1030*
Cuticle, *p. 1014*
Dermis, *p. 1013*
Eccrine, *p. 1023*
Edentulous, *p. 1023*
Effleurage, *p. 1033*
Enucleation, *p. 1060*
Epidermis, *p. 1013*
Gingivitis, *p. 1014*
Halitosis, *p. 1019*
Lunula, *p. 1014*
Mastication, *p. 1014*
Neuropathy, *p. 1018*
Ophthalmologist, *p. 1060*
Optometrist, *p. 1060*
Partial bed bath, *p. 1030*
Perineal care, *p. 1032*
Stomatitis, *p. 1053*

Critical Thinking Exercises

1. Mrs. Truman, 62-years-old, is being seen in the internal medicine clinic for management of her diabetes mellitus. During the nurse's conversation with Mrs. Truman, the client says, "You know, last week I found a sore on my left foot; I didn't even know it was there." What type of assessment should the nurse conduct for Mrs. Truman, and what recommendations are needed for Mrs. Truman's foot care regimen?
2. Mr. Paes suffered abdominal trauma in a motorcycle accident. Abdominal surgery resulted in an ileostomy, which is leaking liquid fecal material on his skin. In addition, he has a post-operative infection, is diaphoretic and has a high fever, and has a nasogastric tube in place. What factors must you consider when providing hygiene care? Include rationales for assessments and interventions.
3. Tony Vitale is an 18-year-old admitted to the neurosurgical intensive care unit following a head injury. Tony is currently unconscious, responsive only to painful stimulus. What assessment is critical for the nurse to perform before providing oral hygiene?

Review Questions

1. Hygiene care requires close contact with the client; the nurse initially uses which of the following to promote a caring therapeutic relationship?
   1. Communication skills
   2. Therapeutic touch
   3. Assessment skills
   4. Fundamental skills
2. A client's personal preferences for hygiene are influenced by a number of factors. The nurse must recognize that
   1. Hygiene care is a routine procedure
   2. The nurse is in charge of the care
   3. No two individuals perform hygiene care in the same manner
   4. Hygiene has no influence on client outcomes
3. Head lice are transmitted by
   1. Poor hygiene
   2. Poor housekeeping
   3. Infested classrooms
   4. Direct contact (head to head)
4. Clients most in need of perineal care are those at greatest risk of
   1. Acquiring an infection
   2. Death

3. Needing to be institutionalized
4. Falling

5. In addition to bathing, the following intervention may best promote client comfort
   1. Back rub
   2. Books on tape
   3. Snacks
   4. Postural drainage
6. Clients will experience conditions that threaten the integrity of oral mucosa; therefore
   1. Less oral hygiene is needed
   2. More frequent mouth care is needed
   3. No mouth care should be performed
   4. No anti-infective agents should be used
7. Unconscious clients and clients with artificial airways require specialized oral hygiene because of their increased risk of
   1. Dental caries
   2. Mouth odour
   3. Aspiration
   4. Mouth ulcerations
8. Depending on the client's age and physical condition, the room temperature should be maintained between
   1. 17° and 19°C
   2. 20° and 23°C
   3. 24° and 26°C
   4. 26° and 28°C
9. To trim the toenails of a client with circulatory difficulties, the nurse
   1. Cuts the nail in a curve
   2. Files the nail straight across
   3. Calls a foot specialist
   4. Cuts the nails to the cuticles
10. An open bed is prepared
    1. With the top sheet, blanket, and bedspread drawn up and under the pillows
    2. In a hospital room before a new client is admitted
    3. While the bed is occupied
    4. With the top covers folded back

References

Agency for Health Care Policy and Research. (1992). *Pressure ulcers in adults: Prediction and prevention* (Publication No. 92-0047, 92-0050). Rockville, MD: U.S. Department of Health and Human Services, Public Health Service.

Alzheimer Society of Canada. (2002). Understanding Alzheimer disease: The link between brain and behaviour. Module 4 in *The Alzheimer journey* [Video and workbook series]. Retrieved May 30, 2004, from *http://www.alzheimer.ca/english/disease/whatisit-video.htm*

American Diabetes Association. (1999). Position statement on preventive foot care in people with diabetes: Clinical practice recommendations 1999. *Diabetes Care,* 22(Suppl. 1).

Barnes, S. H. (1987). Patient and family education for the patient with a pressure necrosis. *The Nursing Clinics of North America, 22,* 463–474.

Bauroth, K., et al. (2003). The efficacy of an essential oil antiseptic mouthwash vs. dental flossing in controlling interproximal gingivitis: A comparative study. *Journal of the American Dental Association, 134*(3), 359–365.

Bennett, M. A. (1995). Report of the Task Force on the Implications for Darkly Pigmented Intact Skin in the Prediction and Prevention of Pressure Ulcers. *Advances in Wound Care, 8*(6), 34–35.

Boyer, L. (2001). News from NNGF: Home care nurse's thoughts on dry skin and foot care in the older person. *World Council of Enterostomal Therapists Journal, 21*(1), 9.

Bryant, J. L., & Beinlich, N. R. (1999). Foot care: Focus on the elderly. *Orthopedic Nursing, 18*(6), 53–60.

Bush, B. C., & Donley, T. G. (2002). A model for dental hygiene education concerning the relationship between periodontal health and systemic health. *Education for Health, 15*(1), 19–26.

Canadian Diabetes Association. (2003). *2003 Clinical practice guidelines for the prevention and management of diabetes in Canada.* Retrieved May 26, 2004, from *http://www.diabetes.ca/cpg2003/chapters.aspx*

Champion, V. L. (1984). Instrument development for health belief model constructs. *Advances in Nursing Science, 6*(3), 73–85.

Cohen, E., & Krachmer, J. (1992). Red eyes and contact lenses. *Patient Care, 26*(9), 143–146.

Dochterman, J. M., & Bulecheck, G. M. (Eds.). (2004). *Nursing interventions classification (NIC)* (4th ed.). St. Louis, MO: Mosby.

Ebersole, P., & Hess, P. (2000). *Toward healthy aging* (5th ed.). St. Louis, MO: Mosby.

Eliopoulos, C. (2001). *Gerontologic nursing* (5th ed.). Philadelphia: Lippincott Williams & Wilkins.

Felder, R., et al. (1994). Dexterity testing as a prediction of oral care ability. *Journal of the American Geriatrics Society, 42*(10), 1081–1086.

Fulton, J. S., Middleton, G. J., & McPhail, J. T. (2002). Management of oral complications. *Seminars in Oncology Nursing, 18,* 28–35.

Gaskin, F. C. (1986). Detection of cyanosis in the person with dark skin. *Journal of National Black Nurses' Association, 1,* 52–60.

Green, M. F., Aliabadi, Z., & Green, B. T. (2002). Diabetic foot: Evaluation and management. *The Southern Medical Journal, 95*(1), 95–101.

Hall, G. R., & Buckwalter, K. C. (2001). Research-based protocol: Bathing persons with dementia. In M. G. Titler (Series Ed.), *Series on evidence-based practice for older adults.* Iowa City, IA: The University of Iowa Gerontological Nursing Interventions Research Center, Research Dissemination Core.

Handy, M. (1996). A pilot study of the diagnosis and treatment of impaired skin integrity: Dry skin in older persons. *Nursing Diagnosis, 1*(2), 57–63.

Health Canada. (1998). *Canadian STD guidelines: 1998 edition* (Catalogue No. H49-119/1998E). Retrieved February 10, 2005, from *www.phac-aspc.gc.ca/publicat/std-mts98/pdf/std98_e.pdf*

Henderson, C. T., et al. (1997). Draft definition of stage I pressure ulcers: Inclusion of persons with darkly pigmented skin. *Advances in Wound Care, 10*(5), 16–19.

Hornick, B. (2002). Diet and nutrition implications for oral health. *Journal of Dental Hygiene, 76*(1), 67–78.

Infectious Diseases and Immunization Committee, Canadian Pediatric Society. (2003). Head lice infestations: A clinical update. Accessed February 10, 2005, from *http://www.cps.ca/english/publications/InfectiousDiseases.htm*

Johnson & Johnson Vision Products. (1994). *Your guide to healthy contact lens wear.* New Brunswick, NJ: Johnson & Johnson.

Labyak, S. E., & Metzger, B. L. (1997). The effects of effleurage backrub on the physiological components of relaxation: A meta-analysis. *Nursing Research, 46,* 59–62.

Lewis, S. L., et al. (2000). *Medical surgical nursing: Assessment and management of clinical problems* (5th ed.). St. Louis, MO: Mosby.

Lueckenotte, A. G. (2000). *Gerontologic nursing* (2nd ed.). St. Louis, MO: Mosby.

Maklebust, J. (1991). Pressure ulcer update. *RN, 41*(12), 56–63.

Moorhead, S., Johnson, M., & Maas, M. (Eds.). (2004). *Nursing outcomes classification (NOC)* (3rd ed.). St. Louis, MO: Mosby.

National Institute on Deafness and Other Communication Disorders. (2001). *Hearing aids* (Publication No. 99-4340). Retrieved December 12, 2004, from *http://www.nidcd.nih.gov/health/hearing/hearingaid.asp*

Neil, J. A. (2002). Assessing foot care knowledge in a rural population with diabetes. *Ostomy/Wound Management, 48*(1), 50–56.

Pinzur, M. S., Slovenkai, M. P., & Trepman, E. (1999). Guidelines for diabetic foot care. The Diabetes Committee of the American Orthopaedic Foot and Ankle Society. *Foot & Ankle International, 20,* 695–702.

Poland, J. M., et al. (1987). Comparing Moi-Stir to lemon-glycerin swabs. *American Journal of Nursing, 87,* 422, 424.

Research update: Oral care prevents pneumonia in nursing homes. (2002). *Australian Nursing Journal, 9*(11), 18.

Ring, T. (2002). Trends in dental hygiene education. *Access, 16*(7), 16.

Skewes, S. M. (1994). No more bed baths! *RN, 57,* 34–35.

Sorrentino, S. A. (1999). *Assisting with patient care.* St. Louis, MO: Mosby.

Strauss, M. B., Hart, J. D., & Winant, D. M. (1998). Preventive foot care: A user-friendly system for patients and physicians. *Postgraduate Medicine, 103*(5), 233–236.

Thibodeau, G. A., & Patton, K. T. (1999). *Anatomy and physiology* (4th ed.). St. Louis, MO: Mosby.

Thompson, J. M., et al. (Eds.). (1997). *Mosby's clinical nursing* (4th ed.). St. Louis. MO: Mosby.

Verderber, A., & Gallagher, K. J. (1994). Effects of bathing, passive range-of-motion exercises, and turning on oxygen consumption in healthy men and women. *American Journal of Critical Care, 3,* 374–381.

Walton, J. C., Miller, J., & Tordecilla, L. (2002). Elder oral assessment and care. *ORL-Head and Neck Nursing, 20*(2), 12–19.

Wong, D. L. (1999). *Wong and Whaley's clinical manual of pediatric nursing* (5th ed.). St. Louis, MO: Mosby.

Zurlinden, J. (2003). Drug news: New warnings for Lindane Shampoo and Lotion. *Nursing Spectrum—Midwestern Edition, 40*(6), 10.

Recommended Web Sites

Canadian Dental Association:
http://www.cda-adc.ca

The Canadian Dental Association Web site offers information on maintaining optimal oral health, including oral hygiene for older adults.

Canadian Health Network:
http://www.canadian-health-network.ca

The Canadian Health Network is a national, non-profit, Web-based information service. Its goal is to help Canadians stay healthy and prevent disease. It offers links to a variety of hygiene-related topics.

35

Cardiopulmonary Functioning and Oxygenation

Pamela Becker Weilitz, RN, MSN(R), BC, ANP, M-SCNS
Zoraida DeCastro Beekhoo, RN, MA (Canadian author)

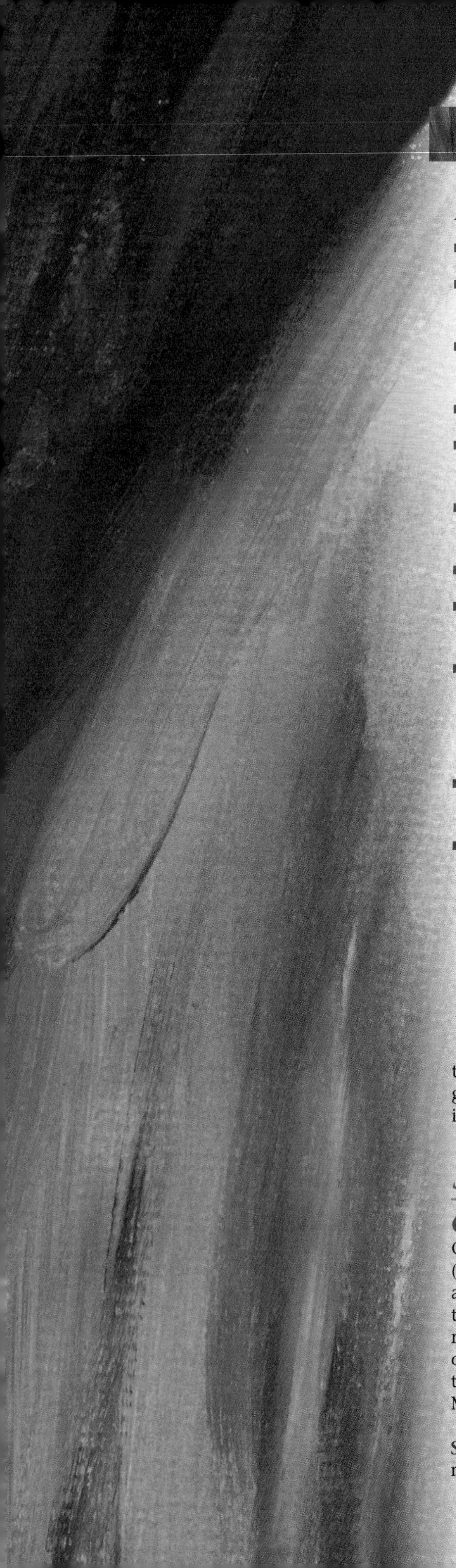

Objectives

Mastery of content in this chapter will enable the student to:

- Define the key terms listed.
- Describe the structure and function of the cardiopulmonary system.
- Identify the physiological processes of cardiac output, myocardial blood flow, and coronary artery circulation.
- Diagram the electrical conduction system of the heart.
- Describe the relationship of cardiac output, preload, afterload, contractility, and heart rate.
- Identify the physiological processes involved in ventilation, perfusion, and exchange of respiratory gases.
- Describe the neural and chemical regulation of respiration.
- Describe the impact of a client's level of health, age, lifestyle, and environment on tissue oxygenation.
- Identify and describe clinical outcomes as a result of disturbances in conduction, altered cardiac output, impaired valvular function, myocardial ischemia, and impaired tissue perfusion.
- Identify and describe clinical outcomes of hyperventilation, hypoventilation, and hypoxemia.
- Identify nursing care interventions in the primary care, acute care, and restorative and continuing care settings that promote oxygenation.

Oxygen is required to sustain life. The cardiac and respiratory systems function to supply the body's oxygen demands. Blood is oxygenated through the mechanisms of ventilation, perfusion, and transport of respiratory gases. Neural and chemical regulators control the rate and depth of respiration in response to changing tissue oxygen demands.

Scientific Knowledge Base

Cardiovascular Physiology

Cardiopulmonary physiology involves delivery of (a) deoxygenated blood (blood high in carbon dioxide and low in oxygen) to the right side of the heart and to the pulmonary circulation and (b) oxygenated blood from the lungs to the left side of the heart and the tissues. The cardiac system delivers oxygen, nutrients, and other substances to the tissues and removes the waste products of cellular metabolism through the cardiac pump, the circulatory vascular system, and the integration of other systems (e.g., respiratory, digestive, and renal; McCance & Huether, 2001).

Structure and Function. The right ventricle pumps blood through the pulmonary circulation. The left ventricle pumps blood to the systemic circulation

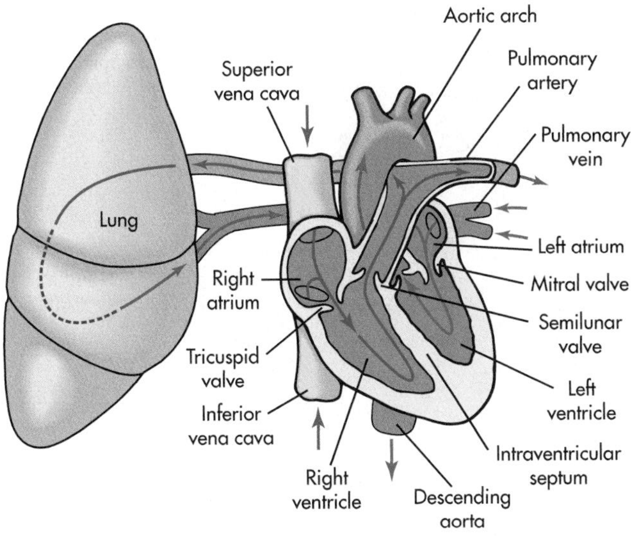

FIGURE **35–1** Schematic representation of blood flow through the heart. Arrows indicate direction of flow. (From *Medical-Surgical Nursing: Assessment and Management of Clinical Problems,* 5th ed., by S. M. Lewis et al., 2000, St. Louis, MO: Mosby.)

Box 35-1 Coronary Arteries

Right Coronary Artery

Right Atrium, Anterior Right Ventricle

Supplies

- Posterior aspect of septum (90% of population)
- Posterior papillary muscle
- Sinus and atrioventricular nodes (80% to 90% of population)
- Inferior aspect of left ventricle

Left Coronary Arteries

Left Anterior Descending Artery

Supplies

- Anterior left ventricular wall
- Anterior interventricular septum (septal branches supply conduction system, bundle of His, and bundle branches)
- Anterior papillary muscle
- Left ventricular apex
- Right ventricle

Circumflex Artery

Supplies

- Left atrium
- Posterior surfaces of left ventricle
- Posterior aspects of septum

(Figure 35–1). The circulatory system exchanges respiratory gases, nutrients, and waste products between the blood and the tissues.

Myocardial Pump. The pumping action of the heart is essential to maintaining oxygen delivery. Coronary artery disease and cardiomyopathic (enlarged heart) conditions result in a diminished stroke volume (i.e., the volume of blood ejected from the ventricles) and decreased pump effectiveness. Hemorrhage and dehydration decrease pump effectiveness by decreasing the amount of blood ejected from the ventricles, thereby reducing circulating blood volume. The four chambers of the heart fill with blood during diastole and empty during systole.

The myocardial (cardiac muscle) fibres have contractile properties that enable them to stretch during filling. In a healthy heart, this stretch is proportionally related to the strength of contraction. As the myocardium stretches, the strength of the subsequent contraction increases; this is known as the Frank-Starling (Starling's) law of the heart. In the diseased heart, Starling's law does not apply because the stretch of the myocardium is beyond the heart's physiological limits. The subsequent contractile response results in insufficient ventricular ejection (volume), and blood begins to "back up" in the pulmonary (left heart failure) or systemic circulation (right heart failure).

Myocardial Blood Flow. To maintain adequate blood flow to the pulmonary and systemic circulation, myocardial blood flow must supply sufficient oxygen and nutrients to the myocardium itself. Blood flow through the heart is unidirectional. There are four heart valves that ensure this forward blood flow (see Figure 35–1). During ventricular diastole, the atrioventricular (mitral and tricuspid) valves open and blood flows from the higher pressure atria into the relaxed ventricles. This represents S_1, or the first heart sound. After ventricular filling, the systolic phase begins.

During the systolic phase, semilunar (aortic and pulmonic) valves open and blood flows from the ventricles into the aorta and pulmonary artery. Closure of aortic and pulmonic valves represents S_2, or the second heart sound. Clients with valvular disease may have backflow or regurgitation of blood through the incompetent valve, causing a murmur that is heard on auscultation (see chapter 28).

Coronary Artery Circulation. Blood in the atria and ventricles does not supply oxygen and nutrients to the myocardium itself. The coronary circulation is the branch of the systemic circulation that supplies the myocardium with oxygen and nutrients and removes waste. The coronary arteries fill during ventricular diastole (McCance & Huether, 2001). The right and left coronary arteries arise from the aorta just above and behind the aortic valve through openings called the coronary ostia (coronary openings). The left coronary artery, the most abundant blood supply, feeds the left ventricular myocardium, which is more muscular and does most of the heart's work (Box 35-1).

Systemic Circulation. The arteries and veins of the systemic circulation deliver nutrients and oxygen to and remove waste from the tissues. Oxygenated blood flows from the left ventricle by way of the aorta and into large systemic arteries. These arteries branch into smaller arteries, into arterioles, and finally into the smallest vessels, the capillaries. At the capillary level, the exchange of respiratory gases, nutrients, and wastes occurs, and the tissues are oxygenated. The waste products exit the capillary network by way of the venules that join to form veins. These veins form larger veins, which carry deoxygenated blood to the right side of the heart, where it is returned to pulmonary circulation.

Blood Flow Regulation. The amount of blood ejected from the left ventricle each minute is the **cardiac output.** The normal cardiac output is 4 to 6 L/minute in the healthy 68-kg adult at rest. The circulating volume of blood changes according to the oxygen and metabolic needs of the body. For example, during exercise, pregnancy, and fever, the cardiac output increases, but during sleep it decreases. Cardiac output is represented by the following formula:

$$\text{Cardiac output (CO)} = \text{Stroke volume (SV)} \times \text{Heart rate (HR)}$$

Cardiac output in the older adult may be affected by increased arterial wall tension and moderate myocardial hypertrophy due to an increased systolic blood pressure.

Cardiac index (CI) is the adequacy of the cardiac output for an individual. It takes into account the body surface area (BSA) of the client. The CI is determined by dividing the cardiac output by the BSA. The normal range is 2.5 to 4 L/minute/m^3. Both cardiac output and the CI are measured with invasive pulmonary artery catheters.

Stroke volume is the amount of blood ejected from the left ventricle with each contraction. It can be affected by the amount of blood in the left ventricle at the end of diastole (preload), the resistance to left ventricular ejection (afterload), and myocardial contractility.

Preload is essentially the end-diastolic volume. The ventricles stretch when filling with blood. The more stretch on the ventricular muscle, the greater the contraction and the greater the stroke volume (Starling's law). In clinical situations, the preload and subsequent stroke volume can be manipulated by changing the amount of circulating blood volume. For example, in the client with hemorrhagic shock, fluid therapy and replacement of blood increases volume, thus increasing the preload and cardiac output. If volume is not replaced, preload decreases, the cardiac output decreases, and ultimately the venous return to the right atrium decreases, further decreasing preload and cardiac output.

Afterload is the resistance to left ventricular ejection: the work that the heart must overcome to fully eject blood from the left ventricle. The diastolic aortic pressure is a good clinical measure of afterload. In a client with an acute hypertensive crisis, the afterload is increased, increasing the cardiac workload. Afterload in this situation can be manipulated by decreasing systemic blood pressure.

The measurement and monitoring of these cardiopulmonary hemodynamics is usually performed in critical care units. Some step-down or special care units may also have the capability to measure and monitor hemodynamics.

Myocardial contractility also affects stroke volume and cardiac output. Poor contraction decreases the amount of blood ejected by the ventricles during each

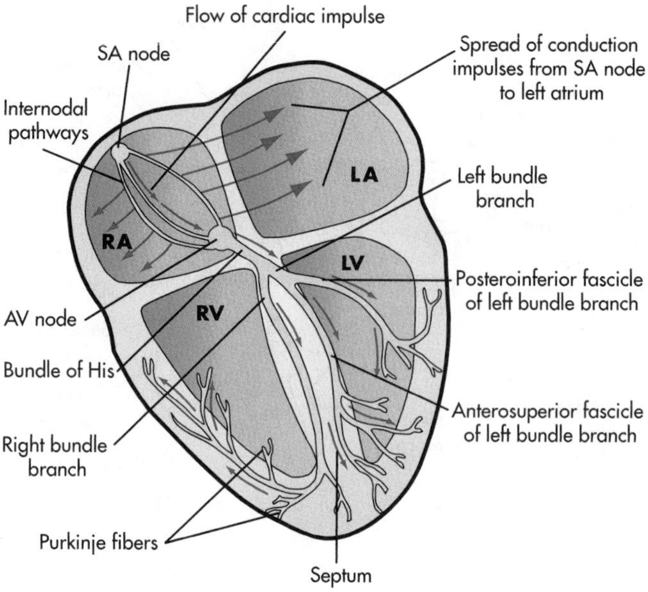

FIGURE **35–2** Conduction system of the heart. *LA,* Left atrium; *LV,* left ventricle; *RA,* right atrium; *RV,* right ventricle; *SA,* sinoatrial; *AV,* atrioventricular. (From *Medical-Surgical Nursing: Assessment and Management of Clinical Problems,* 5th ed., by S. M. Lewis et al., 2000, St. Louis, MO: Mosby.)

contraction. Drugs that can increase the force of myocardial contraction include digitalis preparations, epinephrine, and sympathomimetic drugs (drugs that mimic the effects of the sympathetic nervous system). Injury to the myocardial muscle, such as an acute myocardial infarction (AMI) can cause a decrease in myocardial contractility. The myocardium of the older adult is more rigid and slower in recovering its contractility (Lueckenotte, 2000).

Heart rate affects blood flow because of the interaction between rate and diastolic filling time. With a sustained heart rate greater than 160 beats per minute, diastolic filling time decreases, decreasing stroke volume and cardiac output. The heart rate of the older adult is slow to increase under stress. The stroke volume may increase to increase the cardiac output and blood pressure (Lueckenotte, 2000).

Conduction System. The rhythmic relaxation and contraction of the atria and ventricles depend on continuous, organized transmission of electrical impulses. These impulses are generated and transmitted by way of the cardiac conduction system (Figure 35–2).

The heart's conduction system generates the necessary action potentials that conduct the impulses required to initiate the electrical chain of events resulting in the heartbeat. The autonomic nervous system influences the rate of impulse generation, the speed of transmission through the conductive pathway, and the strength of atrial and ventricular contractions. Sympathetic nerve fibres, which increase the rate of impulse generation and the speed of impulse transmission, innervate all parts of the atria and ventricles. The parasympathetic fibres originating from the vagus nerve decrease the rate and also innervate all parts of the atria and ventricles, as well as

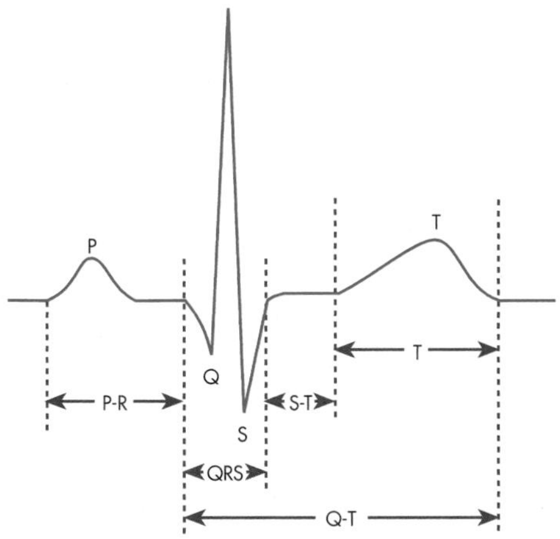

FIGURE **35–3** Normal ECG waveform.

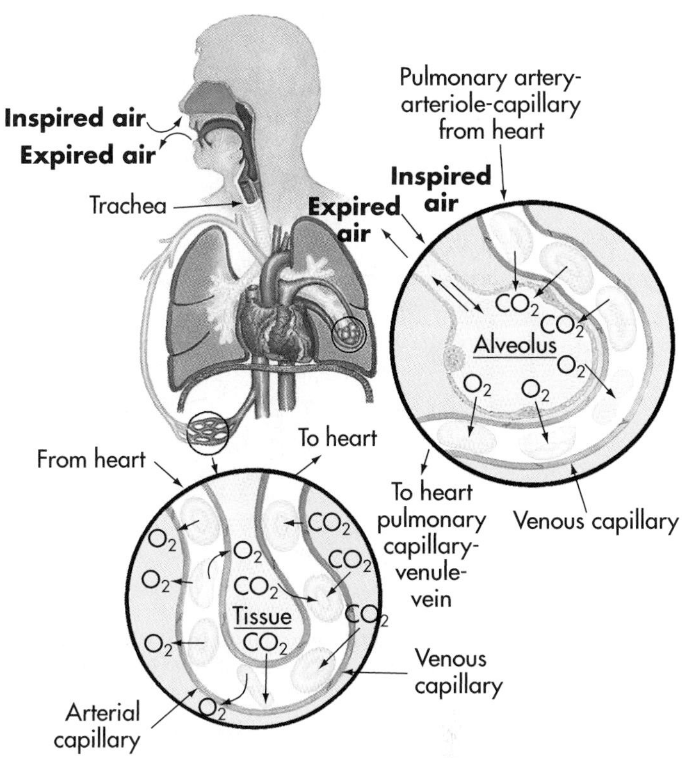

FIGURE **35–4** Structures of the pulmonary system. The circle denotes the alveoli. (From *Mosby's Clinical Nursing,* 3rd ed., edited by J. Thompson et al., 1993, St. Louis, MO: Mosby-Year Book.)

the sinoatrial (SA) and atrioventricular (AV) nodes (McCance & Huether, 2001).

The conduction system originates with the SA node, the "pacemaker" of the heart. The SA node is in the right atrium next to the entrance of the superior vena cava (McCance & Huether, 2001). Impulses are initiated at the SA node at an intrinsic rate of 60 to 100 beats per minute. The resting adult rate is approximately 75 beats per minute.

The electrical impulses are then transmitted through the atria along intraatrial pathways to the AV node. The AV node mediates impulses between the atria and the ventricles. The intrinsic rate of the normal AV node is 40 to 60 beats per minute. The AV node assists atrial emptying by delaying the impulse before transmitting it through the bundle of His and the ventricular Purkinje network. The intrinsic rate of the bundle of His and the ventricular Purkinje network is 20 to 40 beats per minute.

An **electrocardiogram (ECG)** reflects the electrical activity of the conduction system. An ECG monitors the regularity and path of the electrical impulse through the conduction system; however, it does not reflect muscular work of the heart. The normal sequence on the ECG is called **normal sinus rhythm** (**NSR;** Figure 35–3).

NSR implies that the impulse originates at the SA node and follows the normal sequence through the conduction system. The P wave represents the electrical conduction through both atria. Atrial contraction follows the P wave. The PR interval represents the impulse travel time through the AV node, through the bundle of His, and to the Purkinje fibres. The normal length for the PR interval is 0.12 to 0.20 seconds. An increase in the time (i.e., >0.20 seconds) indicates that there is a block in the impulse transmission through the AV node; a decrease (i.e., <0.12 seconds) indicates the initiation of the electrical impulse from a source other than the SA node.

The QRS complex indicates that the electrical impulse has travelled through the ventricles. Normal QRS duration is 0.06 to 0.12 seconds. An increase in QRS duration indicates a delay in conduction time through the ventricles. Ventricular contraction usually follows the QRS complex.

The QT interval represents the time needed for ventricular depolarization and repolarization. The normal QT interval is 0.12 to 0.42 seconds. Changes in electrolyte values, such as hypocalcemia, or therapy with drugs such as disopyramide, amiodarone, and theophylline (Theo-Dur) can increase the QT interval. Shortening of the QT interval occurs with digitalis therapy, hyperkalemia, and hypercalcemia.

Respiratory Physiology

Most cells in the body obtain their energy from chemical reactions involving oxygen and the elimination of carbon dioxide. The exchange of respiratory gases occurs between environmental air and the blood (Figure 35–4). There are three steps in the process of oxygenation: ventilation, perfusion, and diffusion (McCance & Huether, 2001).

Structure and Function. Conditions or diseases that change the structure and function of the lung can alter respiration. The respiratory muscles, pleural space, lungs, and alveoli (Figure 35–5) are essential for ventilation, perfusion, and exchange of respiratory gases. Gases are moved into and out of the lungs through pressure changes. Intrapleural pressure is negative or less than atmospheric pressure, which is 760 mm Hg at sea level. For air to flow into the lungs, intrapleural pressure must become more negative, setting up a pressure gradient between the atmosphere and the alveoli. The diaphragm and external intercostal muscles contract to create a negative pleural pressure and increase the size of the thorax for inspiration. Relaxation of the diaphragm and contraction of the internal intercostal muscles allows air from the lung to escape.

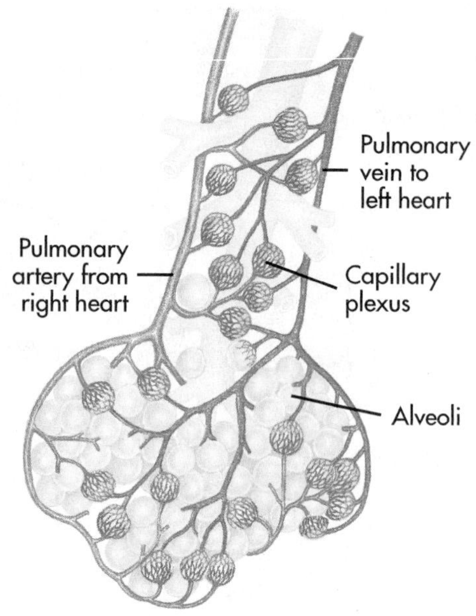

FIGURE **35–5** Alveoli at the terminal end of the lower airway. (From *Mosby's Clinical Nursing,* 3rd ed., edited by J. Thompson et al., 1993, St. Louis, MO: Mosby-Year Book.)

The coordination of the respiratory muscles is essential for effective respiration and gas exchange. The lung transfers oxygen from the atmosphere into the alveoli, where the oxygen is exchanged for carbon dioxide. The alveoli transfer oxygen and carbon dioxide to and from the blood through the alveolar membrane.

Ventilation is the process of moving gases into and out of the lungs. Ventilation requires coordination of the muscular and elastic properties of the lung and thorax, as well as intact innervation. The major inspiratory muscle of respiration is the diaphragm. It is innervated by the phrenic nerve, which exits the spinal cord at the fourth cervical vertebra. Perfusion relates to the ability of the cardiovascular system to pump oxygenated blood to the tissues and return deoxygenated blood to the lungs. Last, diffusion is responsible for moving the molecules from one area to another. For the exchange of respiratory gases to occur, the organs, nerves, and muscles of respiration must be intact and the central nervous system able to regulate the respiratory cycle.

Work of Breathing. Breathing is the effort required for expanding and contracting the lungs. In the healthy individual, breathing is quiet and accomplished with minimal effort. The amount of energy expended on breathing depends on the rate and depth of breathing, the ease in which the lungs can be expanded (compliance), and airway resistance (Jevon & Ewens, 2001).

Inspiration is an active process, stimulated by chemical receptors in the aorta. **Expiration** is a passive process that depends on the elastic recoil properties of the lungs, requiring little or no muscle work. Elastic recoil is produced by elastic fibres in lung tissue and by surface tension in the fluid film lining the alveoli. Surfactant is a chemical produced in the lungs that maintains the surface tension of the alveoli and keeps them from collapsing. Clients with advanced chronic obstructive pulmonary disease (COPD) lose the elastic recoil of the lungs and thorax. As a result, the client's work of breathing is increased. In addition, clients with certain pulmonary diseases can have decreased surfactant production and in turn may develop atelectasis.

Accessory muscles of respiration can increase lung volume during inspiration. Clients with COPD, especially emphysema, frequently use these muscles to increase lung volume. Prolonged use of the accessory muscles of respiration does not promote effective ventilation and causes fatigue. During assessment, the nurse may observe elevation of the client's clavicles during inspiration.

Compliance is the ability of the lungs to distend or to expand in response to increased intraalveolar pressure. Compliance is decreased in diseases such as pulmonary edema, interstitial and pleural fibrosis, and congenital or traumatic structural abnormalities such as kyphosis or fractured ribs.

Airway resistance is the pressure difference between the mouth and the alveoli in relation to the rate of flow of inspired gas. Airway resistance can be increased by an airway obstruction, small airway disease (such as asthma), and tracheal edema. When resistance is increased, the amount of air travelling through the anatomical airways is decreased.

Decreased lung compliance, increased airway resistance, active expiration, or the use of accessory muscles increases the work of breathing, resulting in increased energy expenditure. To meet this expenditure, the body increases its metabolic rate, and the need for oxygen, as well as for the elimination of carbon dioxide, increases. This sequence is a vicious cycle for a client with impaired ventilation, causing further deterioration of respiratory status and the ability to oxygenate adequately.

Lung Volumes and Capacities. Spirometry is used to measure the volume of air entering or leaving the lungs. Variations in lung volumes may be associated with health states such as pregnancy, exercise, obesity, or obstructive and restrictive conditions of the lungs. The amount of surfactant, degree of compliance, and strength of respiratory muscles can affect pressures and volumes within the lungs.

Pulmonary Circulation. The primary function of the pulmonary circulation is to move blood to and from the alveolocapillary membrane for gas exchange to occur. The pulmonary circulation is a reservoir for blood so that the lung can increase its blood volume without large increases in pulmonary artery or venous pressures. The pulmonary circulation also acts as a filter, removing small thrombi before they can reach vital organs.

The pulmonary circulation begins at the pulmonary artery, which receives poorly oxygenated mixed venous blood from the right ventricle. Blood flow through this system depends on the pumping ability of the right ventricle, which has an output of approximately 4 to 6 L/minute. The flow continues from the pulmonary artery through the pulmonary arterioles to the pulmonary capillaries, where blood comes in contact with the alveolocapillary membrane and the exchange of respiratory gases occurs. The oxygen-rich blood then circulates through the pulmonary venules and pulmonary veins, returning to the left atrium.

Pressure and resistance within the pulmonary circulatory system is lower than that within the systemic circulatory system. The walls of the pulmonary vessels are thinner and contain less smooth muscle. The lung accepts the total cardiac output from the right ventricle and, except in cases of alveolar hypoxia or cor pulmonale, does not direct blood flow from one region to another.

Respiratory Gas Exchange. Respiratory gases are exchanged in the alveoli and the capillaries of the body tissues. Oxygen is transferred from the lungs to the blood, and carbon dioxide is transferred from the blood to the alveoli to be exhaled as a waste product. At the tissue level, oxygen is transferred from the blood to tissues, and carbon dioxide is transferred from tissues to the blood to return to the alveoli and be exhaled. This transfer is dependent on the process of diffusion.

Diffusion is the movement of molecules from an area of higher concentration to an area of lower concentration. Diffusion of respiratory gases occurs at the alveolocapillary membrane, and the rate of diffusion can be affected by the thickness of the membrane. Increased thickness of the membrane impedes diffusion because gases take longer to transfer across. Clients with pulmonary edema, pulmonary infiltrates, or a pulmonary effusion have an increased thickness of the alveolocapillary membrane, resulting in slowed diffusion, slowed exchange of respiratory gases, and impaired delivery of oxygen to tissues. The surface area of the membrane can be altered as a result of chronic disease (e.g., emphysema), acute disease (e.g., pneumothorax), or surgical process (e.g., lobectomy). The alveolocapillary membrane can be destroyed or may thicken, changing the rate of diffusion. When fewer alveoli are functioning, the surface area is decreased.

Oxygen Transport. The oxygen transport system consists of the lungs and cardiovascular system. Delivery depends on the amount of oxygen entering the lungs (ventilation), blood flow to the lungs and tissues (perfusion), rate of diffusion, and oxygen-carrying capacity. The capacity of the blood to carry oxygen is influenced by the amount of dissolved oxygen in the plasma, amount of hemoglobin, and tendency of hemoglobin to bind with oxygen. Only a relatively small amount of required oxygen, less than 1%, is dissolved in the plasma. Most oxygen is transported by hemoglobin, which serves as a carrier for oxygen and carbon dioxide. The hemoglobin molecule combines with oxygen to form oxyhemoglobin. The formation of oxyhemoglobin is easily reversible, allowing hemoglobin and oxygen to dissociate, which frees oxygen to enter tissues.

Carbon Dioxide Transport. Carbon dioxide diffuses into red blood cells and is rapidly hydrated into carbonic acid (H_2CO_3) because of the presence of carbonic anhydrase. The carbonic acid then dissociates into hydrogen (H^{+-}) and bicarbonate (HCO_3^-) ions. The hydrogen ion is buffered by hemoglobin, and the HCO_3^- diffuses into the plasma (see chapter 36). In addition, some of the carbon dioxide in red blood cells reacts with amino acid groups, forming carbamino compounds. This reaction can occur rapidly without the presence of an enzyme. Reduced hemoglobin (deoxyhemoglobin) can combine with carbon dioxide more easily than oxyhemoglobin, and therefore venous blood transports the majority of carbon dioxide.

> **Box 35-2 Physiological Processes of Oxygenation**
>
> **Neural Regulation**
>
> Maintains rhythm and depth of respiration and balance between inspiration and expiration.
>
> **Cerebral Cortex**
> Voluntary control of respiration delivers impulses to the respiratory motor neurons by way of the spinal cord; accommodates speaking, eating, and swimming.
>
> **Medulla Oblongata**
> Automatic control of respiration occurs continuously.
>
> **Chemical Regulation**
>
> Maintains appropriate rate and depth of respirations depending on changes in the blood's carbon dioxide (CO_2), oxygen (O_2), and hydrogen ion (H^+) concentration.
>
> **Chemoreceptors**
> Located in the medulla, aortic body, and carotid body. Changes in chemical content of O_2, CO_2, and H^+ stimulate chemoreceptors, which in turn stimulate neural regulators to adjust the rate and depth of ventilation to maintain normal arterial blood gas levels. Chemical regulation can occur during physical exercise and in some illnesses. It is a short-term adaptive mechanism.

Regulation of Respiration. Regulation of respiration is necessary to ensure sufficient oxygen intake and carbon dioxide elimination to meet the body's demands (e.g., during exercise, infection, or pregnancy). Neural and chemical regulators control the process of respiration. Neural regulation includes the central nervous system control of respiratory rate, depth, and rhythm. Chemical regulation involves the influence of chemicals such as carbon dioxide and hydrogen ions on the rate and depth of respiration (Box 35-2).

Factors Affecting Oxygenation

Adequacy of circulation, ventilation, perfusion, and transport of respiratory gases to the tissues is influenced by four types of factors: (1) physiological, (2) developmental, (3) lifestyle, and (4) environmental. Developmental, lifestyle, and environmental factors will be presented in a later section.

Physiological Factors. Any condition that affects cardiopulmonary functioning directly affects the body's ability to meet oxygen demands. The general classifications of cardiac disorders include disturbances in conduction, impaired valvular function, myocardial hypoxia,

Table 35-1 Physiological Processes Affecting Oxygenation

Process	Effect on Oxygenation
Anemia	Decreases oxygen-carrying capacity of blood
Toxic inhalant	Decreases oxygen-carrying capacity of blood
Airway obstruction	Limits delivery of inspired oxygen to alveoli
High altitude	Atmospheric oxygen concentration is lower and inspiratory oxygen concentration decreases
Fever	Increases metabolic rate and tissue oxygen demand
Decreased chest wall motion (e.g., from musculoskeletal impairments)	Prevents lowering of diaphragm and reduces anteroposterior diameter of thorax on inspiration, reducing volume of air inspired

cardiomyopathic conditions, and peripheral tissue hypoxia. Respiratory disorders include hyperventilation, hypoventilation, and hypoxia.

Other physiological processes affecting a client's oxygenation include alterations that affect the oxygen-carrying capacity of blood, such as anemia, increases in the body's metabolic demands (e.g., pregnancy, fever, infection), and alterations that affect chest wall movement or the central nervous system (Table 35-1).

Decreased Oxygen-Carrying Capacity. Hemoglobin carries 99% of the oxygen to tissues (Lewis et al., 2000). Anemia and inhalation of toxic substances decreases the oxygen-carrying capacity of blood by reducing the amount of available hemoglobin to transport oxygen. **Anemia,** a lower than normal hemoglobin level, is a result of decreased hemoglobin production, increased red blood cell destruction, and/or blood loss. Clients will have complaints of fatigue, decreased activity tolerance, and increased breathlessness, as well as pallor (especially seen in the conjunctiva of the eye) and an increased heart rate.

Carbon monoxide is the most common toxic inhalant that decreases the oxygen-carrying capacity of blood. The affinity for hemoglobin to bind with carbon monoxide is greater than 200 times its affinity to bind with oxygen, creating a functional anemia. Because of the bond's strength, carbon monoxide is not easily dissociated from hemoglobin, making the hemoglobin unavailable for oxygen transport.

Decreased Inspired Oxygen Concentration. When the concentration of inspired oxygen declines, the oxygen-carrying capacity of the blood is decreased. Decreases in the fraction of inspired oxygen concentration (FIO_2) can be caused by an upper or lower airway obstruction limiting delivery of inspired oxygen to alveoli; decreased environmental oxygen, such as at high altitudes; or decreased inspiration as a result of an incorrect oxygen concentration setting on respiratory therapy equipment.

Hypovolemia. **Hypovolemia** is caused by conditions such as shock and severe dehydration resulting from extracellular fluid loss and reduced circulating blood volume. With a significant fluid loss, the body tries to adapt by increasing the heart rate and peripheral vasoconstriction to increase the volume of blood returned to the heart and, in turn, increase the cardiac output.

Increased Metabolic Rate. Increased metabolic activity causes increased oxygen demand. When body systems are unable to meet this increased demand, the level of oxygenation declines. An increased metabolic rate is a normal physiological response to pregnancy, wound healing, and exercise because the body is building tissue. Most people can meet the increased oxygen demand and do not display signs of oxygen deprivation. Fever increases the tissues' need for oxygen, and as a result, carbon dioxide production also increases. If the febrile state persists, the metabolic rate remains high and the body begins to break down protein stores, resulting in muscle wasting and decreased muscle mass. Respiratory muscles such as the diaphragm and intercostal muscles are also wasted. The body attempts to adapt to the increased carbon dioxide levels by increasing the rate and depth of respiration. The client's work of breathing increases, and the client will eventually display signs and symptoms of hypoxemia. Those clients with pulmonary diseases are at greater risk for hypoxemia and hypercapnia. Assessment findings include an increased rate and depth of respiration, use of the accessory muscles of respiration, pursed-lip breathing, and decreased activity tolerance.

Conditions Affecting Chest Wall Movement. Any condition that reduces chest wall movement can result in decreased ventilation. If the diaphragm cannot fully descend with breathing, the volume of inspired air decreases and less oxygen is delivered to the alveoli and subsequently to tissues.

Pregnancy. As the fetus grows during pregnancy, the greater size of the uterus pushes abdominal contents upward against the diaphragm. In the last trimester of pregnancy, the inspiratory capacity declines, resulting in dyspnea on exertion and increased fatigue.

Obesity. Morbidly obese clients have reduced lung volumes from the heavy lower thorax and abdomen, particularly when in the recumbent and supine positions. Morbidly obese clients have a reduction in compliance as a result of encroachment of the abdomen into the chest, increased work of breathing, and decreased lung volumes, and they may have fatigue and carbon dioxide retention. In some clients, an obesity-hypoventilation syndrome develops in which oxygenation is decreased and carbon dioxide is retained, resulting in daytime sleepiness. Morbidly obese clients may also develop obstructive sleep apnea, characterized by excessive daytime somnolence and loud snoring and apneic periods during sleep. The obese client is also susceptible to pneumonia after an upper respiratory tract infection because the lungs cannot fully expand and pulmonary secretions are not mobilized in the lower lobes.

Musculoskeletal Abnormalities. Musculoskeletal impairments in the thoracic region reduce oxygenation. Such impairments may result from abnormal structural configurations, trauma, muscular diseases, and diseases of the central nervous system. Abnormal structural configurations impairing oxygenation include those that affect the rib cage, such as pectus excavatum, and those that affect the vertebral column, such as kyphosis, lordorsis, or scoliosis.

Trauma. The person with multiple rib fractures can develop a flail chest, a condition in which fractures cause instability in part of the chest wall. The unstable chest wall allows the lung underlying the injured area to contract on inspiration and bulge on expiration, resulting in hypoxia. Chest wall or upper abdominal incisions may also decrease chest wall movement as the client uses shallow respirations to minimize chest wall movement to avoid pain. Excessive or high doses of narcotic analgesics may depress the respiratory centre, further decreasing respiratory rate and chest wall expansion.

Neuromuscular Diseases. Diseases such as muscular dystrophy affect oxygenation of tissues by decreasing the client's ability to expand and contract the chest wall. Ventilation is impaired, and atelectasis, hypercapnia, and hypoxemia can occur. Myasthenia gravis, Guillain-Barré syndrome, and poliomyelitis affect respiratory functioning and result in hypoventilation. Myasthenia gravis interferes with normal transmission of impulses from nerves to muscles, involving the whole body, including muscles of respiration. Guillain-Barré syndrome and poliomyelitis cause inflammation and paralysis of muscle groups. Guillain-Barré syndrome usually results in an ascending pattern of paralysis. Respiratory muscles become paralyzed as paralysis ascends to the thoracic region. Poliomyelitis may lead to general or local paralysis. Both may reverse, but poliomyelitis usually results in more residual paralysis.

Central Nervous System Alterations. Diseases or trauma involving the medulla oblongata and spinal cord may result in impaired respiration. When the medulla oblongata is affected, neural regulation of respiration is damaged and abnormal breathing patterns may develop. If the phrenic nerve is damaged, the diaphragm may not descend, thus reducing inspiratory lung volumes and causing hypoxemia. Cervical trauma at C3 to C5 can result in paralysis of the phrenic nerve. Spinal cord trauma below the fifth cervical vertebra usually leaves the phrenic nerve intact but damages nerves that innervate the intercostal muscles, preventing anteroposterior chest expansion.

Influences of Chronic Disease. Oxygenation can be decreased as a direct consequence of chronic disease. It can also be decreased as a secondary effect, as with anemia. The physiological response to chronic hypoxemia is the development of a secondary polycythemia. This adaptive response is the body's attempt to increase the amount of circulating hemoglobin to increase the available oxygen-binding sites.

Alterations in Cardiac Functioning

Illnesses and conditions that affect cardiac rhythm, strength of contraction, blood flow through the chambers, myocardial blood flow, and peripheral circulation cause alterations in cardiac functioning. Older adults experience alterations in cardiac function due to calcification of the conduction pathways, thicker and stiffer heart valves from lipid accumulation and fibrosis, and a decrease in the number of pacemaker cells in the SA node (Lueckenotte, 2000).

Disturbances in Conduction. Some disturbances in conduction are a result of electrical impulses that do not originate from the SA node. These rhythm disturbances are called **dysrhythmias,** meaning a deviation from the normal sinus heart rhythm (Table 35-2). Dysrhythmias may occur as a primary conduction disturbance; as a response to ischemia, valvular abnormality, anxiety, or drug toxicity; as a result of caffeine, alcohol, or tobacco use; or as a complication of acid-base or electrolyte imbalance (see chapter 36).

Dysrhythmias are classified by cardiac response and site of impulse origin. Cardiac response can be tachycardiac (greater than 100 beats per minute), bradycardiac (less than 60 beats per minute), a premature (early) beat, or a blocked (delayed or absent) beat. Tachydysrhythmias and bradydysrhythmias can lower cardiac output and blood pressure. Tachydysrhythmias reduce cardiac output by decreasing diastolic filling time. Bradydysrhythmias lower cardiac output because of the decreased heart rate.

Atrial fibrillation is a common type of dysrhythmia in older adults. The electrical impulse in the atria is chaotic and originates from multiple sites. The rhythm is irregular because of the multiple pacemaker sites and the unpredictable conduction to the ventricles. The QRS complex is normal; however, it occurs at irregular intervals. Atrial fibrillation is often described as an irregularly irregular rhythm.

Abnormal impulses originating above the ventricles are referred to as supraventricular dysrhythmias. The abnormality on the waveform is the configuration and placement of the P wave. Ventricular conduction usually remains normal, and a normal QRS complex is observed.

Ventricular dysrhythmias represent an ectopic site of impulse formation within the ventricles. It is ectopic in that the impulse originates in the ventricle, not the SA node. The configuration of the QRS complex is usually widened and bizarre. P waves may or may not be present; often they are buried in the QRS complex. **Ventricular tachycardia** and **ventricular fibrillation** are life-threatening rhythms that require immediate intervention. Ventricular tachycardia is considered a life-threatening dysrhythmia because of the decreased cardiac output and the potential to deteriorate into ventricular fibrillation (Lewis et al., 2000).

Table 35-2 Common Basic Cardiac Dysrhythmias

Rhythm Characteristics and Etiology	Clinical Significance and Management
Sinus Tachycardia	
Regular rhythm, rate 100 to 180 beats/minute (higher in infants), normal P wave, normal QRS complex. Rate increase may be normal response to exercise, emotion, or stressors such as pain, fever, pump failure, hyperthyroidism, and certain drugs (e.g., caffeine, nitrates, epinephrine, nicotine).	Client with damaged heart may not be able to sustain increased myocardial oxygen consumption by increased heart rate. Correct underlying factors; discontinue drugs producing the side effect.
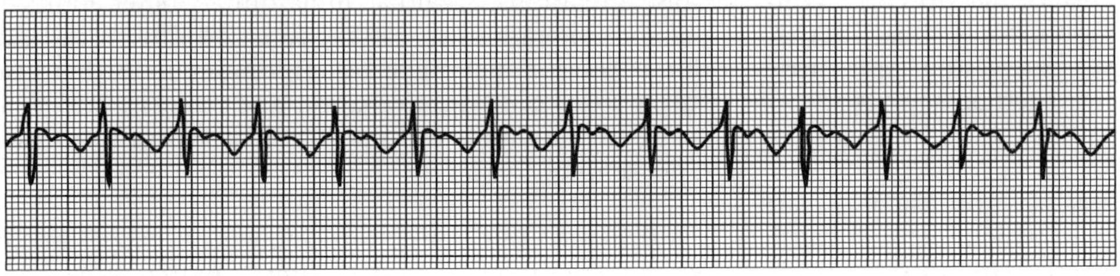	
Sinus Bradycardia	
Regular rhythm, rate less than 60 beats/minute, normal P wave, normal PR interval, normal QRS complex. Rate decrease may be normal response to sleep or in well-conditioned athlete; abnormal drops in rate may be caused by diminished blood flow to SA node, vagal stimulation, hypothyroidism, increased intracranial pressure, or pharmacological agents (e.g., digoxin, propranolol, quinidine, procainamide).	No clinical significance unless associated with signs and symptoms of reduced cardiac output such as dizziness or syncope or presence of chest pain. Bradycardia with hypotension and decreased cardiac output is treated with atropine; a pacemaker may be required.
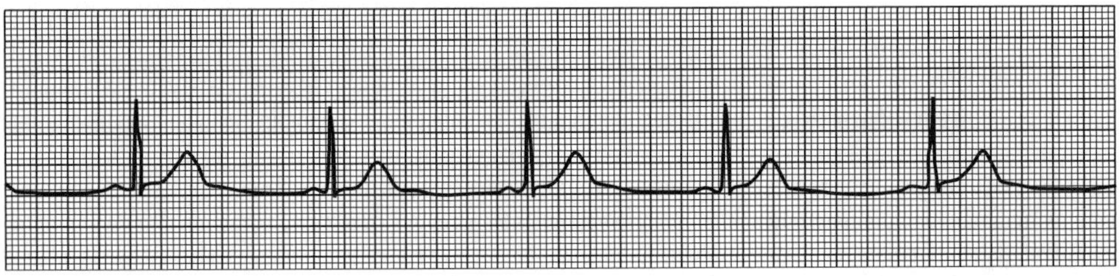	
Sinus Dysrhythmia	
Sinus rhythm with cyclic variation; slows during inspiration and increases with expiration; rate of 60 to 100 beats/minute; normal P wave; normal PR interval; normal QRS complex. Caused by vagal impulses; occurs commonly in children, young adults, and older adults; usually disappears as heart rate increases.	No clinical significance unless dizziness occurs with decreased rate. No management indicated unless heart rate decreases and symptoms occur.
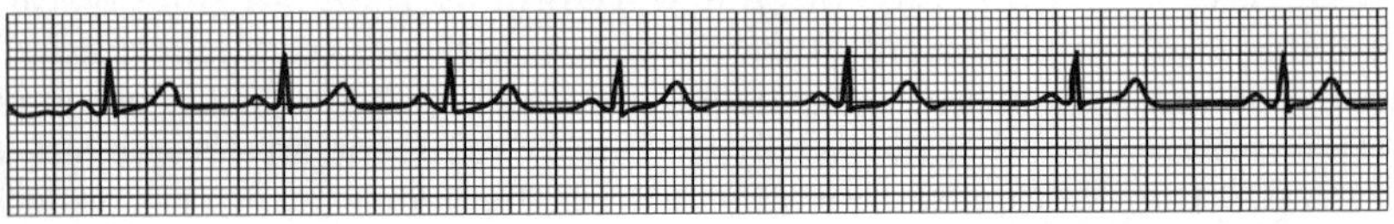	

Table 35-2 Common Basic Cardiac Dysrhythmias—cont'd

Rhythm Characteristics and Etiology	Clinical Significance and Management
Atrial Fibrillation (A-fib)	
Chaotic, irregular atrial activity resulting in an irregular ventricular response. No identifiable P waves. Irregular ventricular response resulting in an irregular cardiac rate and rhythm. The rate is determined by the conduction of the multiple atrial impulses across the AV node. Caused by aging, calcification of the SA node, or changes in myocardial blood supply.	There is a loss of the atrial kick (portion of the cardiac output squeezed in the ventricles with a coordinated atrial contraction), pooling of blood in the atria, and development of microemboli. The client may complain of fatigue, a fluttering in the chest, or shortness of breath if the ventricular response is rapid. Commonly occurring dysrhythmia in the aging and older adult.

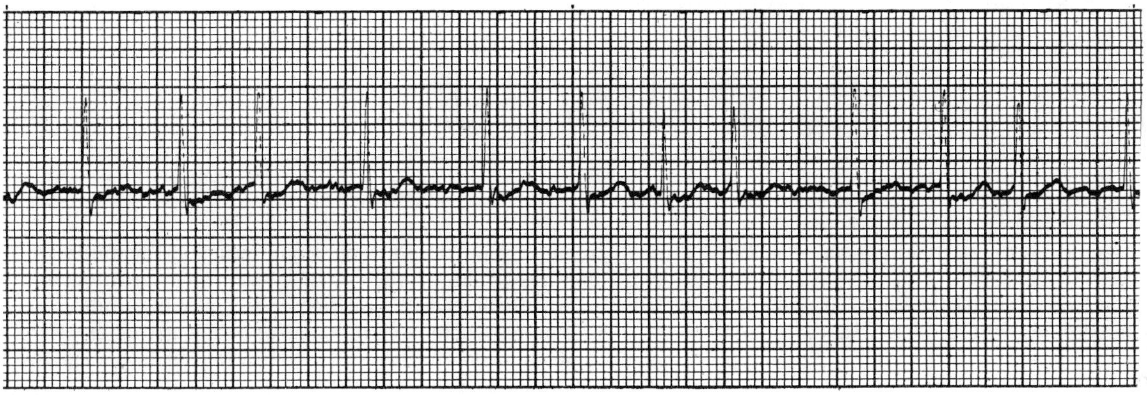

Rhythm Characteristics and Etiology	Clinical Significance and Management
Paroxysmal Supraventricular Tachycardia (PSVT)	
Sudden, rapid onset of tachycardia with stimulus originating above AV node; regular rhythm; rate 150 to 250 beats/minute; P wave uniform, possibly buried in preceding T wave; PR interval variable, often difficult to measure; normal QRS complex. May begin and end spontaneously or be precipitated by excitement, fatigue, caffeine, smoking, or alcohol use.	Usually no significant impairment; client complains of palpitations and shortness of breath; if persistent or occurring in client with pre-existing organic heart disease, may cause decrease in cardiac output and/or blood pressure, resulting in pump failure or shock. Treatment includes Valsalva manoeuvre or vagal stimulation by carotid sinus massage, adenosine, diltiazem, digitalis, or beta-adrenergic blockers.

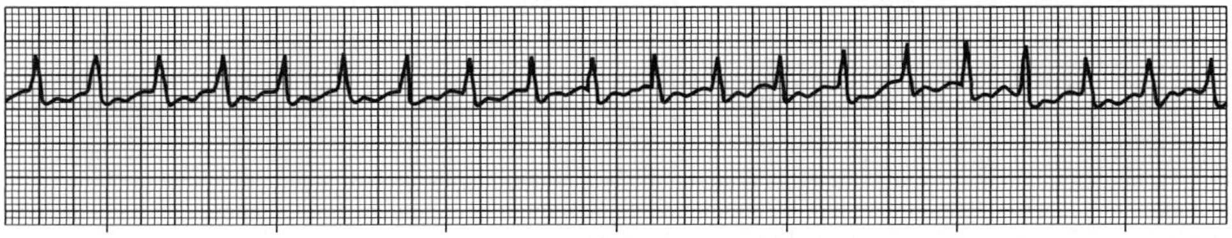

Rhythm Characteristics and Etiology	Clinical Significance and Management
Premature Ventricular Contractions (PVCs)	
Irregular rhythm with ectopic beats followed by full compensatory pause; rate normal or increased rate P wave absent in ectopic beat; PR interval absent; QRS complex widened and distorted; T wave in opposition to R wave. Caused by changes in the normal pacemaker of the heart such as decrease in blood flow, ischemia, or embolus.	PVCs occurring more than 6/minute, in pairs, or with multiple configurations indicates increased ventricular irritability. Treat underlying cause such as myocardial infarction, hypoxia, hypocalcemia, or acidosis.

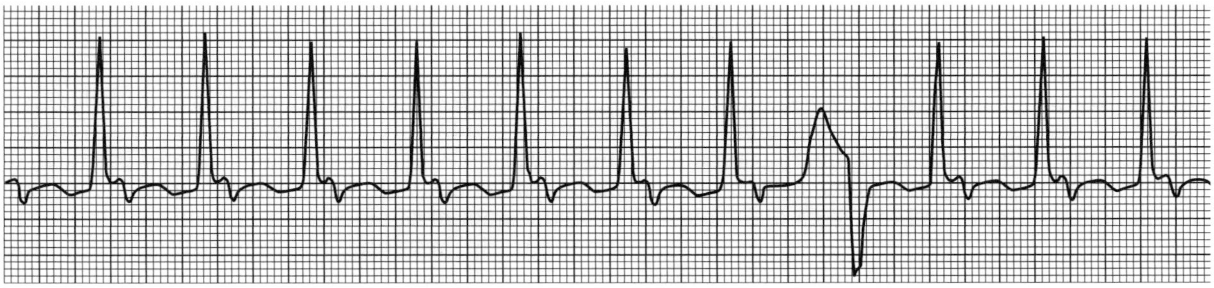

Continued

Table 35-2 Common Basic Cardiac Dysrhythmias—cont'd

Rhythm Characteristics and Etiology	Clinical Significance and Management
Ventricular Tachycardia	
Rhythm slightly irregular, rate 100 to 200 beats/minute, P wave absent, PR interval absent, QRS complex wide and bizarre, >0.12 seconds. Caused by changes in the normal pacemaker of the heart such as decrease in blood flow, ischemia, or embolus.	Results in a decreased cardiac output due to decreased ventricular filling time; may lead to severe hypotension and loss of pulse and consciousness. If refractory to defibrillation, amiodarone 300 mg IV followed by an additional 150 mg IV in 3 to 5 minutes (American Heart Association [AHA], 2000).
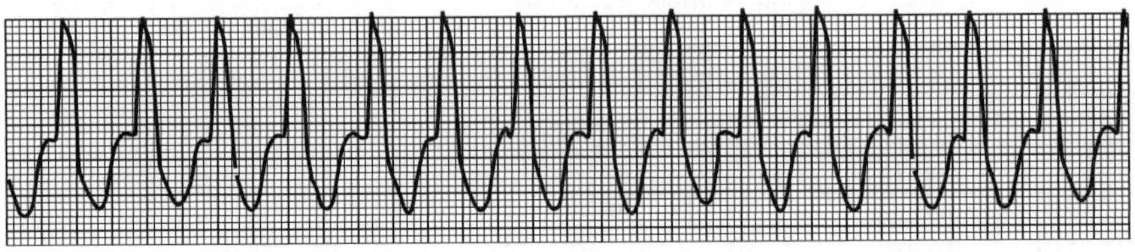	
Ventricular Fibrillation	
Uncoordinated electrical activity. No identifiable P, QRS, or T wave. Causes include sudden cardiac death, electrical shock, acute myocardial infarction, drowning, or trauma.	Acute loss of pulse and respiration. Immediate defibrillation after assessment of ABCs of CPR. Availability of automated external defibrillator is recommended in public and/or private places where large numbers of people gather or where there are people who are at high risk for heart attack (AHA, 2003; Box 35-3).
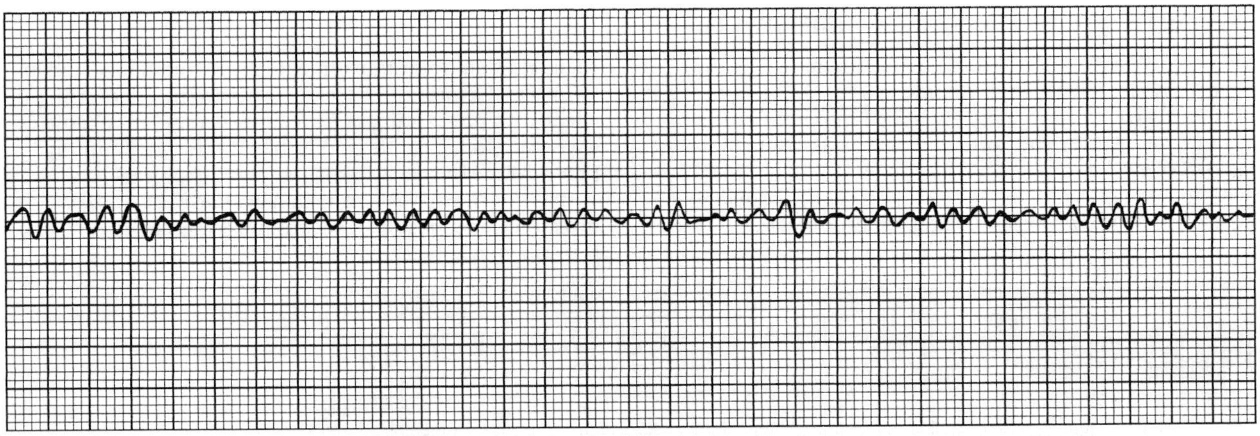	

Adapted from *Cardiovascular disorders,* by M. M. Canobbio, 1990. St. Louis, MO: Mosby.
PSVT management: Vagal stimulation such as carotid sinus massage or Valsalva maneuver to decrease ventricular response with medication to block AV conduction; adenosine 6 mg IV over 1-3 seconds; adenosine 12 mg IV over 1-3 seconds; assess complex width; narrow-check blood pressure, normal verapamil 2.5-5 mg IV; if blood pressure low or unstable, proceed to synchronized cardioversion; wide complex, lidocaine 1-1.5 mg/kg IV push, procainamide 20-30 mg/min; synchronized cardioversion if resistant to drug therapy (ECC, 1992).
Sinus bradycardia management: Correct underlying causes. If symptomatic (e.g., hypotension, chest pain, decreased level of consciousness, shortness of breath), administer atropine 0.04 mg/kg IV; transcutaneous pacing if available; dopamine 5-20 mcg/kg/min; epinephrine 2-10 mcg/min; temporary transvenous pacemaker if resistant to drug therapy (ECC, 1992).

Altered Cardiac Output. Failure of the myocardium to eject sufficient volume to the systemic and pulmonary circulations can result in heart failure. Primary coronary artery disease, cardiomyopathic conditions, valvular disorders, and pulmonary disease lead to myocardial pump failure.

Left-Sided Heart Failure. Left-sided heart failure is an abnormal condition characterized by impaired functioning of the left ventricle as a result of elevated pressures and pulmonary congestion. If left ventricular failure is significant, the amount of blood ejected from the left ventricle drops greatly, resulting in decreased cardiac output.

Box 35-3 Automated External Defibrillator (AED)

- A device used to administer an electrical shock through the chest wall to the heart.
- Built-in computers assess the victim's heart rhythm and determine if defibrillation is needed.
- The AED delivers a shock to the victim.
- Can be used by non-medical personnel.
- Used to strengthen the chain of survival. Every minute of a sudden cardiac arrest with defibrillation decreases the survival rate by 7% to 10% (American Heart Association, 2003).

Assessment findings may include decreased activity tolerance, breathlessness, dizziness, and confusion as a result of tissue hypoxia from the diminished cardiac output. As the left ventricle continues to fail, blood begins to pool in the pulmonary circulation, causing pulmonary congestion. Clinical findings include crackles on auscultation, hypoxia, shortness of breath on exertion and often at rest, cough, and paroxysmal nocturnal dyspnea.

Right-Sided Heart Failure. Right-sided heart failure results from impaired functioning of the right ventricle characterized by venous congestion in the systemic circulation. Right-sided heart failure more commonly results from pulmonary disease or as a result of long-term left-sided failure. The primary pathological factor in right-sided failure is elevated pulmonary vascular resistance (PVR). As the PVR continues to rise, the right ventricle must generate more work, and the oxygen demand of the heart increases. As the failure continues, the amount of blood ejected from the right ventricle declines, and blood begins to "back up" in the systemic circulation. Clinically, the client has weight gain, distended neck veins, hepatomegaly and splenomegaly, and dependent peripheral edema.

Impaired Valvular Function. Valvular heart disease is an acquired or congenital disorder of a cardiac valve characterized by stenosis and obstructed blood flow or valvular degeneration and regurgitation of blood. When stenosis occurs in the semilunar valves (aortic and pulmonic valves), the adjacent ventricles must work harder to move the ventricular volume beyond the stenotic valve. Over time, the stenosis can cause the ventricle to hypertrophy (enlarge), and if the condition is untreated, left- or right-sided heart failure can occur. If stenosis occurs in the atrioventricular valves (mitral and tricuspid valves), the atrial pressure rises, causing the atria to hypertrophy. When regurgitation occurs, there is a backflow of blood into an adjacent chamber. For example, in mitral regurgitation, the mitral leaflets do not close completely. When the ventricles contract, blood escapes back into the atria, causing a murmur, or "whooshing" sound (see chapter 28).

Myocardial Ischemia. **Myocardial ischemia** results when the supply of blood to the myocardium from the coronary arteries is insufficient to meet the oxygen demands of the organ. Common manifestations of this ischemia include angina pectoris, myocardial infarction, and acute coronary syndrome.

Angina Pectoris. **Angina pectoris** is usually a transient imbalance between myocardial oxygen supply and demand. The condition results in chest pain that is aching, sharp, tingling, or burning, or that feels like pressure. The chest pain may be left sided or substernal and may radiate to the left or both arms, and to the jaw, neck, and back. In some clients, anginal pain may not radiate. The pain can last from 1 to 15 minutes. Clients report that pain is often precipitated by activities that increase myocardial oxygen demand (e.g., exercise, anxiety, or stress). The pain is usually relieved with rest and coronary vasodilators, the most common being a nitroglycerine preparation.

Myocardial Infarction. **Myocardial infarction (MI)** results from sudden decreases in coronary blood flow or an increase in myocardial oxygen demand without adequate coronary perfusion. Infarction occurs because of ischemia (which is reversible) and necrosis (which is not reversible) of myocardial tissue.

Chest pain associated with MI in men is usually described as crushing, squeezing, or stabbing. The pain may be retrosternal and left precordial, and it may radiate down the left arm to the neck, jaws, teeth, epigastric area, and back. The pain occurs at rest or exertion, lasts more than 30 minutes, and is unrelieved by rest, position change, or sublingual nitroglycerine administration.

Current research indicates that there is a significant difference between men and women in relation to coronary artery disease. It is known that women and men do not present the same type of symptoms (Anderson & Kessenich, 2001). The most common initial symptom in women is angina. Women may also present with complaints of epigastric pain and radiation through to the back and into the jaw. Women tend to have fewer Q waves and ST segment changes with chest pain when compared with men. The initial signs and symptoms in women may include a sensation of choking, shortness of breath, variant angina, and vasospasm (Denke, 2001).

Acute Coronary Syndrome. Acute coronary syndrome (ACS) includes unstable angina, non-ST segment elevation MI, and ST-segment elevation MI. There is an imbalance in the oxygen supply and demand to the myocardium. Causes include non-occlusive thrombus on pre-existing plaque, coronary vasospasm, arterial narrowing from atherosclerosis, inflammation or infection, and secondary unstable angina from anemia, fever, or hypoxemia (Granger & Miller, 2001). Symptoms may not be constant and may present atypically. Clients with classic AMI symptoms are more easily identified. Intermediate risk factors for ACS include male gender, age greater than 70 years with diabetes mellitus, extracardiac vascular disease, fixed Q waves, and previous abnormal ST segment and T-wave changes (Granger & Miller, 2001).

Alterations in Respiratory Functioning

Illnesses and conditions that affect ventilation or oxygen transport cause alterations in respiratory functioning. The three primary alterations are hyperventilation, hypoventilation, and hypoxia.

The goal of ventilation is to produce a normal arterial carbon dioxide tension ($PaCO_2$) between 35 and 45 mm Hg and maintain a normal arterial oxygen tension (PaO_2) between 80 and 100 mm Hg. Hyperventilation and hypoventilation refer to alveolar ventilation and not to the client's respiratory rate. Arterial oxygen levels can be monitored using a non-invasive oxygen saturation monitor. The normal range is 95% to 100%. Hypoxia refers to a decrease in the amount of arterial oxygen.

Hyperventilation. **Hyperventilation** is a state of ventilation in excess of that required to eliminate the normal venous carbon dioxide produced by cellular metabolism. Anxiety, infections, drugs, or an acid-base imbalance can induce hyperventilation, as well as hypoxia associated with pulmonary embolus or shock. Acute anxiety can lead to hyperventilation and may cause loss of consciousness from excess carbon dioxide exhalation. Fever can cause hyperventilation. As a client's body temperature increases, there is an increase in the metabolic rate, thereby increasing carbon dioxide production. The clinical response is an increased rate and depth of respiration.

Hyperventilation may also be chemically induced. Salicylate (aspirin) poisoning causes excessive stimulation of the respiratory centre as the body's attempt to compensate for excess carbon dioxide. Amphetamines also increase ventilation by raising carbon dioxide production. Hyperventilation can also occur as the body tries to compensate for metabolic acidosis by producing a respiratory alkalosis. For example, the diabetic client who has gone into diabetic ketoacidosis is producing large amounts of metabolic acids. The respiratory system tries to correct the acid-base balance by over-breathing. Ventilation increases to reduce the amount of carbon dioxide available to form carbonic acid (see chapter 36). Hemoglobin does not release oxygen to tissues as readily, and tissue hypoxia results. As symptoms worsen, the client may become more agitated, which further increases the respiratory rate and can result in respiratory alkalosis.

Hypoventilation. **Hypoventilation** occurs when alveolar ventilation is inadequate to meet the body's oxygen demand or to eliminate sufficient carbon dioxide. As alveolar ventilation decreases, $PaCO_2$ is elevated. Severe atelectasis can produce hypoventilation. **Atelectasis** is a collapse of the alveoli that prevents normal respiratory exchange of oxygen and carbon dioxide. As alveoli collapse, less of the lung can be ventilated and hypoventilation occurs.

In clients with COPD, the inappropriate administration of excessive oxygen can result in hypoventilation. These clients have adapted to a high carbon dioxide level, and their carbon dioxide-sensitive chemoreceptors are essentially not functioning. Their stimulus to breathe is a decreased PaO_2. If excessive oxygen is administered, the oxygen requirement is satisfied and the stimulus to breathe is negated. High concentrations of oxygen (e.g., greater than 24% to 28% [1 to 3 L/minute]) prevent the PaO_2 from falling and obliterate the stimulus to breathe, resulting in hypoventilation. The excessive retention of carbon dioxide may lead to respiratory arrest.

Signs and symptoms of hypoventilation include mental status changes, dysrhythmias, and potential cardiac arrest. Treatment requires improving tissue oxygenation, restoring ventilatory function, treating the underlying cause of the hypoventilation, and achieving acid-base balance. If untreated, the client's status can rapidly decline, leading to convulsions, unconsciousness, and death.

Hypoxia. **Hypoxia** is inadequate tissue oxygenation at the cellular level. This can result from a deficiency in oxygen delivery or oxygen utilization at the cellular level. Hypoxia can be caused by (a) a decreased hemoglobin level and lowered oxygen-carrying capacity of the blood; (b) a diminished concentration of inspired oxygen, which may occur at high altitudes; (c) the inability of the tissues to extract oxygen from the blood, as with cyanide poisoning; (d) decreased diffusion of oxygen from the alveoli to the blood, as in pneumonia; (e) poor tissue perfusion with oxygenated blood, as with shock; and (f) impaired ventilation, as with multiple rib fractures or chest trauma.

The clinical signs and symptoms of hypoxia include apprehension, restlessness, inability to concentrate, declining level of consciousness, dizziness, and behavioural changes. The client with hypoxia is unable to lie down and appears fatigued and agitated. Vital sign changes include an increased pulse rate and increased rate and depth of respiration. The client with a narcotic overdose, such as a heroin overdose, may display signs of hypoventilation. During early stages of hypoxia, the blood pressure is elevated unless the condition is caused by shock. As the hypoxia worsens, the respiratory rate may decline as a result of respiratory muscle fatigue.

Cyanosis, blue discolouration of the skin and mucous membranes caused by the presence of desaturated hemoglobin in capillaries, is a late sign of hypoxia. The presence or absence of cyanosis is not a reliable measure of oxygenation status. Central cyanosis, observed in the tongue, soft palate, and conjunctiva of the eye, where blood flow is high, indicates hypoxemia. Peripheral cyanosis, seen in the extremities, nail beds, and earlobes, is often a result of vasoconstriction and stagnant blood flow. Hypoxia is a life-threatening condition. Untreated, it can produce cardiac dysrhythmias that result in death. Hypoxia is managed by administration of oxygen and treatment of the underlying cause, such as airway obstruction.

Nursing Knowledge Base

Developmental Factors

The developmental stage of the client and the normal aging process can affect tissue oxygenation.

Infants and Toddlers. Infants and toddlers are at risk for upper respiratory tract infections as a result of frequent exposure to other children and exposure to second-hand smoke. In addition, during the teething process, some infants develop nasal congestion, which encourages bacterial

Box 35-4

Focus on Older Adults

- The tuberculin skin test is an unreliable indicator of tuberculosis in older clients. They frequently display false-positive or false-negative skin test reactions.
  - Older clients are at an increased risk for reactivation of dormant organisms that have been present for decades as a result of age-related changes in the immune system.
  - The standard 5-TU Mantoux test is given and repeated or repeated with the 250-TU strength to create a booster effect.
  - If the older client has a positive reaction, a complete history is necessary to determine any risk factors.
- Older adults often have atypical signs and symptoms of coronary artery disease (Lueckenotte, 2000).
- The incidence of atrial fibrillation increases with age and is the leading contributing factor for stroke in the older adult (Lueckenotte, 2000).
- Mental status changes are often the first signs of respiratory problems and may include forgetfulness and irritability.
- Older adults may not complain of dyspnea until it affects the activities of daily living that are important to them.
- Changes in the older adult's cough mechanism may lead to retention of pulmonary secretions, airway plugging, and atelectasis if cough suppressants are not used with caution.

Box35-5

Focus on Primary Health Care

Positive Lifestyle Practices for Cardiopulmonary Health Promotion

As part of a primary health care focus, the nurse teaches young to older adults about the following lifestyle practices that promote cardiopulmonary health:

- Maintain ideal body weight.
- Eat a low-fat, low-salt, calorie-appropriate diet.
- Engage in regular aerobic exercise of 1 hour daily.
- Use a filter mask when exposed to occupational hazards.
- Use stress-reduction techniques.
- Reduce exposure to secondary infections.
- Be smoke free.
- Avoid second-hand smoke and other pollutants.
- Have annual visits with health care provider.
  - Monitor blood pressure.
  - Monitor cholesterol and triglyceride levels.
  - Get an annual influenza vaccine if at risk for the development of influenza.
  - Get a pneumococcal vaccine if appropriate.

growth and increases the potential for respiratory tract infection. Upper respiratory tract infections are usually not dangerous, and infants or toddlers recover with little difficulty.

School-Age Children and Adolescents. School-age children and adolescents are exposed to respiratory infections and respiratory risk factors such as second-hand smoke and cigarette smoking. A healthy child usually does not have adverse pulmonary effects from respiratory infections. A person who starts smoking in adolescence and continues to smoke into middle age, however, has an increased risk for cardiopulmonary disease and lung cancer.

Young and Middle-Age Adults. Young and middle-age adults are exposed to multiple cardiopulmonary risk factors: an unhealthy diet, lack of exercise, stress, over-the-counter and prescription drugs not used as intended, illegal drugs, and smoking. Reducing these modifiable factors may decrease the client's risk for cardiac or pulmonary diseases. This is also the time when lifelong habits and lifestyles are established. It is important to help these clients make good choices and informed decisions about the rest of their lives and their health care practices.

Older Adults. The cardiac and respiratory systems undergo changes throughout the aging process (Box 35-4). The changes are associated with calcification of the heart valves, SA node, and costal cartilages. The arterial system develops atherosclerotic plaques. Osteoporosis leads to changes in the size and shape of the thorax.

The trachea and large bronchi become enlarged from calcification of the airways. The alveoli enlarge, decreasing the surface area available for gas exchange. The number of functional cilia is reduced, causing a decrease in the effectiveness of the cough mechanism, putting the older adult at increased risk for respiratory infections (Lueckenotte, 2000). Ventilation and transfer of respiratory gases decline with age because the lungs are unable to expand fully, leading to lower oxygenation levels.

Lifestyle Risk Factors

Lifestyle modifications that influence cardiopulmonary functioning are frequently difficult because a client is being asked to change a habit or behaviour that may be enjoyed, such as cigarette smoking or eating certain foods; however, these changes can be achieved with encouragement, support, and time (Box 35-5). Risk factor modification is important, including smoking cessation, weight reduction, a low-cholesterol and low-sodium diet, management of hypertension, and moderate exercise. Although it may be difficult to get older adults to change long-term behaviour, developing healthy behaviours can slow or halt the progression of their cardiopulmonary disease (Lueckenotte, 2000).

Poor Nutrition. Nutrition affects cardiopulmonary function in several ways. Severe obesity decreases lung expansion, and the increased body weight increases oxygen demands to meet metabolic needs. The malnourished client may experience respiratory muscle wasting, resulting in decreased muscle strength and respiratory excursion. Cough efficiency is reduced secondary to respiratory muscle weakness, putting the client at risk for retention of pulmonary secretions. Diets high in fat increase cholesterol and atherogenesis in the coronary arteries.

Clients who are morbidly obese and/or malnourished are at risk for anemia. Diets high in carbohydrates may play a role in increasing the carbon dioxide load for clients with carbon dioxide retention. As carbohydrates are metabolized, an increased load of carbon dioxide is created and excreted via the lungs.

Dietary restriction of sodium has been shown to be beneficial in reducing antihypertensive medication requirements and may cause left ventricular hypertrophy to regress (Joint National Committee [JNC], 2003). Diets high in potassium may prevent hypertension and help improve control in clients with hypertension. A 2000-calorie diet high in fibre, potassium, calcium, and magnesium, with an emphasis on fruits, vegetables, and low-fat dairy foods and low in saturated and total fat is recommended to help prevent and reduce the effects of hypertension (JNC, 2003).

Inadequate Exercise. Exercise increases the body's metabolic activity and oxygen demand. The rate and depth of respiration increase, enabling the person to inhale more oxygen and exhale excess carbon dioxide. A physical exercise program has many benefits (see chapter 32). People who exercise for 1 hour daily have a lower pulse rate and blood pressure, decreased cholesterol level, increased blood flow, and greater oxygen extraction by working muscles. Fully conditioned people can increase oxygen consumption by 10% to 20% because of increased cardiac output and increased efficiency of the myocardial muscle (JNC, 2003).

Smoking. Cigarette smoking is associated with a number of diseases, including heart disease, chronic obstructive lung disease, and lung cancer. Cigarette smoking can worsen peripheral vascular and coronary artery diseases (JNC, 2003). Inhaled nicotine causes vasoconstriction of peripheral and coronary blood vessels, increasing blood pressure and decreasing blood flow to peripheral vessels. Women who take birth control pills and smoke cigarettes are at increased risk for cardiovascular problems such as thrombophlebitis and pulmonary emboli.

Cigarette smoking is the major cause of lung cancer, accounting for 85% of all new cases of lung cancer in Canada. Exposure to second-hand smoke also increases the non-smoker's risk of lung cancer and cardiovascular disease by 20% (Health Canada, 2002). Lung cancer is the leading cause of death for both men and women. It is estimated that 1 in 11 men and 1 in 18 women will develop lung cancer in their lifetime (National Cancer Institute of Canada, 2004). The 5-year survival rate for all clients with lung cancer is only 15%, regardless of the diagnosis (Canadian Cancer Society, 2004). If lung cancer is detected when the disease is still localized, the survival rate is 49%. However, lung cancer is often diagnosed only when it has reached an advanced stage.

Substance Abuse. Excessive use of alcohol and other drugs can impair tissue oxygenation in two ways. First, the person who chronically abuses substances often has a poor nutritional intake. With the resultant decrease in intake of iron-rich foods, hemoglobin production declines. Second, excessive use of alcohol and certain other drugs can depress the respiratory centre, reducing the rate and depth of respiration and the amount of inhaled oxygen. Substance abuse by either smoking or inhaling, such as crack cocaine or inhaling fumes from paint or glue cans, causes direct injury to lung tissue that can lead to permanent lung damage and impaired oxygenation.

Stress. A continuous state of stress or severe anxiety increases the body's metabolic rate and the oxygen demand. The body responds to anxiety and other stresses with an increased rate and depth of respiration. Most people can adapt, but some, particularly those with chronic illnesses or acute life-threatening illnesses such as a myocardial infarction, cannot tolerate the oxygen demands associated with anxiety (see chapter 26).

Environmental Factors

The environment can also influence oxygenation. The incidence of pulmonary disease is higher in smoggy, urban areas than in rural areas. In addition, the client's workplace may increase the risk for pulmonary disease. Occupational pollutants include asbestos, talcum powder, dust, and airborne fibres. Asbestosis is an occupational lung disease that develops after exposure to asbestos. The lung in asbestosis is characterized by diffuse interstitial fibrosis, creating a restrictive lung disease. It can also cause pleural mesotheliomas and pleural plaques. Clients at risk for developing asbestosis include those working with textiles, fireproofing, or milling, or in the production of paints, plastics, or some prefabricated construction. Clients exposed to asbestos who also smoke are at increased risk of developing lung cancer.

Critical Thinking

Successful critical thinking requires a synthesis of knowledge, experience, information gathered from clients, critical thinking attitudes, and intellectual and professional standards. Clinical judgments require the nurse to anticipate the information necessary, analyze the data, and make decisions regarding the client's care. During assessment, the nurse must consider all elements that build toward making an appropriate nursing diagnosis (Figure 35–6).

To understand the oxygen demands of a client and the ability of the client's body to meet those demands, the nurse integrates knowledge from nursing and other disciplines, previous experiences, and information gathered from clients. The use of professional standards, such as those developed by the Heart and Stroke Foundation of Canada, the Canadian Lung Association, the Canadian Thoracic Society, and the Canadian Infectious Diseases Society, provide valuable guidelines for care and management of clients with altered oxygenation.

Nursing Process

NP Assessment

The nursing assessment of a client's cardiopulmonary functioning includes an in-depth history of the client's normal and present cardiopulmonary function, past impairments in circulatory or respiratory functioning, and measures that the client uses to optimize oxygenation. The history should

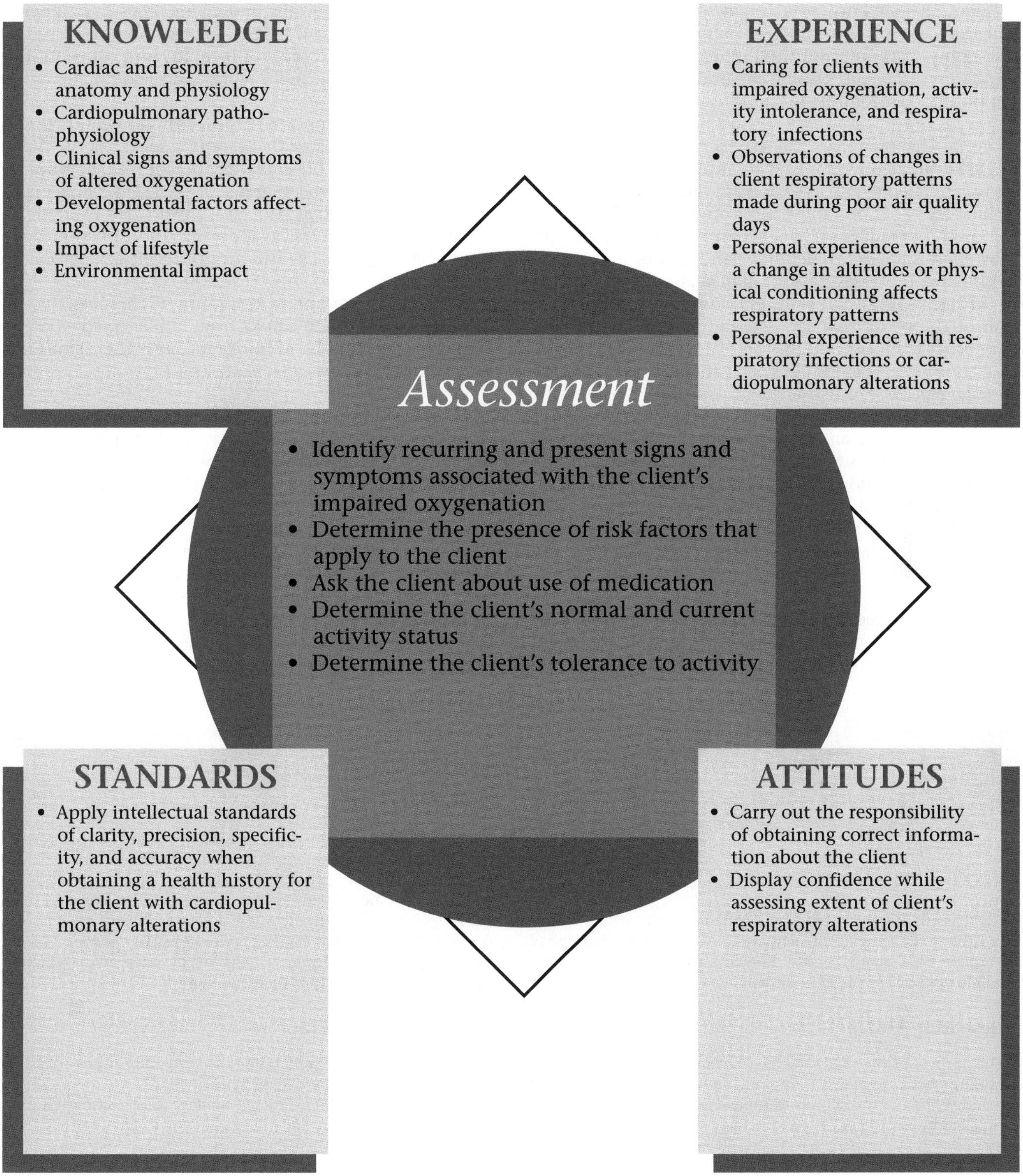
KNOWLEDGE
• Cardiac and respiratory anatomy and physiology
• Cardiopulmonary pathophysiology
• Clinical signs and symptoms of altered oxygenation
• Developmental factors affecting oxygenation
• Impact of lifestyle
• Environmental impact
EXPERIENCE
• Caring for clients with impaired oxygenation, activity intolerance, and respiratory infections
• Observations of changes in client respiratory patterns made during poor air quality days
• Personal experience with how a change in altitudes or physical conditioning affects respiratory patterns
• Personal experience with respiratory infections or cardiopulmonary alterations
Assessment
• Identify recurring and present signs and symptoms associated with the client's impaired oxygenation
• Determine the presence of risk factors that apply to the client
• Ask the client about use of medication
• Determine the client's normal and current activity status
• Determine the client's tolerance to activity
STANDARDS
• Apply intellectual standards of clarity, precision, specificity, and accuracy when obtaining a health history for the client with cardiopulmonary alterations
ATTITUDES
• Carry out the responsibility of obtaining correct information about the client
• Display confidence while assessing extent of client's respiratory alterations

FIGURE **35–6** Critical thinking model for oxygenation assessment.

include a review of drug, food, and other allergies, such as pet dander, mould, and environmental triggers.

Physical examination of the client's cardiopulmonary status reveals the extent of existing signs and symptoms. A review of laboratory and diagnostic test results provides valuable data on respiratory and ventilatory parameters.

Health History. The health history should focus on the client's ability to meet oxygen needs. The health history for cardiac function includes pain and characteristics of pain, dyspnea, fatigue, peripheral circulation, cardiac risk factors, and the presence of past or concurrent cardiac conditions. The health history for respiratory function includes the presence of a cough, shortness of breath, wheezing, pain, environmental exposures, frequency of respiratory tract infections, pulmonary risk factors, past respiratory problems, current medication use, and smoking history or second-hand smoke exposure.

Pain. The presence of chest pain needs to be thoroughly evaluated with regard to location, duration, radiation, and frequency. Cardiac pain does not occur with respiratory variations and is most often on the left side of the chest and radiates to the left arm in men. Chest pain in women is much less definitive and may be a sensation of choking, breathlessness, or pain that radiates through to the back. Pericardial pain resulting from an inflammation of the pericardial sac is usually non-radiating and may occur with inspiration.

Pleuritic chest pain is peripheral and may radiate to the scapular regions. It is worsened by inspiratory manoeuvres, such as coughing, yawning, and sighing. Pleuritic pain is often caused from an inflammation or infection in the pleural space and is described as knifelike, lasting from a minute to hours and always in association with inspiration.

Musculoskeletal pain may be present following exercise, rib trauma, and prolonged coughing episodes. This pain is also aggravated by inspiratory movements and may easily be confused with pleuritic chest pain.

Fatigue. Fatigue is a subjective sensation in which the client reports a loss of endurance. Fatigue in the client with cardiopulmonary alterations is often an early sign of a worsening of the chronic underlying process. To provide an objective measure of fatigue, the client may be asked to rate the fatigue on a scale of 0 to 10, with 10 being the worst level of fatigue and 0 representing no fatigue.

Smoking. It is important to determine clients' direct and secondary exposure to cigarette smoke. Ask the client about any history of smoking; include the number of years smoked and the number of packages smoked per day. This is recorded as pack-year history. For example, if a client smoked two packs a day for 20 years, the client would have a 40 pack-year history (packages per day × years smoked).

It is also important to determine if the client is exposed to second-hand smoke from family or co-workers. Exposure to second-hand smoke increases the client's risk for chronic lung or cardiac diseases.

Dyspnea. **Dyspnea** is a clinical sign of hypoxia and manifests as breathlessness. It is the subjective sensation of difficult or uncomfortable breathing (Box 35-6). Dyspnea is shortness of breath associated with exercise or excitement, but in some clients dyspnea may be present without any relation to activity or exercise. Dyspnea is associated with many conditions, such as pulmonary diseases, cardiovascular diseases, neuromuscular conditions, and anemia. In addition, dyspnea may occur in the pregnant woman in the final months of pregnancy. Environmental factors, such as pollution, cold air, and smoking, may also cause or worsen dyspnea.

Research Highlight — *Box 35-6*

The Efficacy of Exercise Training in Clients With Dyspnea

Research Focus

Clients with dyspnea often have a difficult time controlling their breathing. Assisting clients with dyspnea self-management may improve their quality of life. Knowing what interventions are helpful will be beneficial in developing a plan of care.

Research Abstract

The purpose of this study was to determine (a) whether exercise training adds benefit to dyspnea self-management and (b) whether there is a response to supervised exercise training sessions in dyspnea, exercise performance, and health-related quality of life. Subjects with COPD, aged 58 to 74 years, with a forced expiratory volume at 1 second (FEV_1) ranging from 30.8% to 58.8% of predicted, were randomized into three groups. All three groups participated in a dyspnea self-management program, which included individualized education about dyspnea management strategies, a home-walking prescription, and daily logs. One group received no additional exercise supervision, another group had exposure to exercise (30 minutes every other week for 8 weeks), and the third group had supervised exercise training (30 minutes, 3 times per week for 8 weeks). Outcomes were measured at baseline and at every 2-month interval as part of a 1-year longitudinal randomized clinical trial using the Chronic Respiratory Questionnaire (CRQ), Shortness of Breath Questionnaire, and Baseline/Transitional Dyspnea Index. Outcomes measured included dyspnea during laboratory exercise and with activities of daily living, exercise performance and endurance testing, a 6-minute walk, and a quality of life survey (SF-36). The group that had supervised exercise training had a significantly greater improvement in dyspnea management than the group that had no exercise training.

Evidence-Based Practice

- Supervised exercise (rehabilitation) programs improve dyspnea management for clients with COPD.
- Simply providing dyspnea self-management techniques information does not have a significant impact on clients' ability to manage their dyspnea.
- A prescription for exercise is not an effective tool in helping clients with COPD learn to manage their dyspnea.
- Individualized programs for dyspnea self-management lead to better management of the client's dyspnea and improvement in quality of life.

Reference

Stulbarg, M. S., et al. (2002). Exercise training improves outcomes of a dyspnea self-management program. *Journal of Cardiopulmonary Rehabilitation, 22*(2), 109–121.

Dyspnea can be associated with clinical signs such as exaggerated respiratory effort, use of the accessory muscles of respiration, nasal flaring, and marked increases in the rate and depth of respirations (Jevon & Ewens, 2001). The use of a visual analog scale (VAS) can help clients to make an objective assessment of their dyspnea. The VAS is a 100-mm vertical line with end points of 0 and 10. Zero is equated with no dyspnea and 10 is equated with the worst breathlessness the client has experienced. Studies have validated the use of the VAS to evaluate a client's dyspnea in the clinical setting. The nurse can evaluate the effectiveness of nursing interventions by monitoring the client's assessment of their dyspnea.

If the client has a history of dyspnea, the nurse determines the circumstances under which it occurred, such as with exertion, stress, or respiratory tract infection. The nurse also determines whether the client's perception of dyspnea affects the ability to lie flat. **Orthopnea** is an abnormal condition in which the person must use multiple pillows when lying down or must sit with the arms elevated and leaning forward to breathe. The number of pillows required for sleeping, such as two- or three-pillow orthopnea, usually quantifies the presence of orthopnea.

Cough. Cough is a sudden, audible expulsion of air from the lungs. The person breathes in, the glottis is partially closed, and the accessory muscles of expiration contract to expel the air forcibly. Coughing is a protective reflex to clear the trachea, bronchi, and lungs of irritants and secretions. The carina, the point of bifurcation of the right and left mainstem bronchus, is the most sensitive area for cough production. A cough is difficult to evaluate, and almost everyone has periods of coughing. Clients with a chronic cough tend to deny, underestimate, or minimize their coughing, often because they are so accustomed to it that they are unaware of how frequently it occurs.

Coughing is classified according to the time when the client most frequently coughs. Clients with chronic sinusitis may cough only in the early morning or immediately after rising from sleep. This clears the airway of mucus resulting from sinus drainage. Clients with chronic bronchitis generally produce sputum all day, although greater amounts are produced after rising from a semi-recumbent or flat position. This is a result of the dependent accumulation of sputum in the airways and is associated with reduced mobility (see chapter 42). Once the nurse determines that the client has a cough, it must be identified as productive or non-productive and its frequency must be assessed. A productive cough results in sputum production, material coughed up from the lungs that may be swallowed or expectorated. Sputum contains mucus, cellular debris, and micro-organisms, and it may contain pus or blood. The nurse must collect data about the type and quantity of sputum. The client is instructed to try to produce some sputum, being careful not to simply clear the throat to produce a sample of saliva. The nurse then inspects it for colour, consistency, odour, and amount (Box 35-7).

If **hemoptysis** (bloody sputum) is reported, the nurse determines if it is associated with coughing and bleeding from the upper respiratory tract, from sinus drainage, or from the gastrointestinal tract **(hematemesis).** In addition, the hemoptysis should be described according to amount, colour, and duration and whether it is mixed with sputum. When the client reports bloody or blood-tinged sputum, diagnostic tests, such as examination of sputum specimens, chest X-ray examinations, **bronchoscopy,** and other X-ray studies, should be performed.

Wheezing. **Wheezing** is characterized by a high-pitched musical sound caused by high-velocity movement of air through a narrowed airway. Wheezing may be associated with asthma, acute bronchitis, or pneumonia. Wheezing can occur on inspiration, expiration, or both. The nurse should determine any precipitating factors, such as respiratory infection, allergens, exercise, or stress.

Environmental or Geographical Exposures. Environmental exposure to many inhaled substances is closely linked with respiratory disease. The nurse should investigate exposures in the client's home and workplace. The most common environmental exposures in the home are cigarette smoke, carbon monoxide, and radon. The nurse should determine whether a client who is a non-smoker is passively exposed to smoke.

Carbon monoxide poisoning can result from a blocked furnace flue or fireplace. The client may have vague complaints of general malaise, flu-like symptoms, and excessive sleepiness. Clients are particularly at risk in the late fall when they turn the heat on or begin to use the fireplace again. Radon gas, a radioactive substance that can damage lung tissue and cause lung cancer, enters homes through the ground. When homes are under-ventilated, this gas is not able to escape into the atmosphere and becomes trapped in the home.

An employment history is obtained to assess exposure to substances such as asbestos, coal, cotton fibres, fumes, or chemical inhalants. This is particularly important with middle-age and older adults, who may have worked in

Box 35-7 Sputum Characteristics

Colour

- Clear
- White
- Yellow
- Green
- Brown
- Red
- Streaked with blood

Changes in Colour

- Same colour throughout the day
- Clearing with coughing
- Progressively darker

Odour

- None
- Foul

Quantity

- Same as usual
- Increased
- Decreased

Consistency

- Frothy
- Watery
- Tenacious, thick

Presence of Blood

- Occasional
- Early morning
- Bright or dark red
- Blood tinged

places without regulations to protect workers from carcinogens such as asbestos.

Exposure to pathogens may occur during travel. Schistosomiasis can be acquired in Asia, Africa, the Caribbean, and South America. This is infection of a human with a species of fluke found in fresh water that has been contaminated by human feces. Coccidioidomycosis is a fungal disease caused by inhalation of *Coccidioides immitis,* a wind-borne spore carried on dust particles.

Respiratory Infections. A health history should contain information about the client's frequency and duration of respiratory tract infections. Although everyone occasionally experiences a cold, for some people it can result in bronchitis or pneumonia. On average, clients will have four colds per year. The nurse should determine if the client has had a pneumococcal or flu vaccine in the past and should also ask about any known exposure to tuberculosis (TB) and the results of the tuberculin skin test.

The client's risk for human immunodeficiency virus (HIV) infection is determined. Clients with a history of intravenous (IV) drug use and multiple unprotected sexual partners are at risk of developing HIV infection. Clients may not display any symptoms of HIV infection until they present with *Pneumocystis carinii* (PCP) or *Mycoplasma* pneumonia. Presentation with PCP or *Mycoplasma* pneumonia indicates a significant depression of the client's immune system and progression to acquired immunodeficiency syndrome (AIDS).

Allergies. When obtaining a respiratory system history, the nurse inquires about airborne allergens. The client's allergic response may be watery eyes, sneezing, runny nose, or respiratory symptoms, such as cough or wheezing. The nurse also asks the client specific questions about the type of allergens, response to these allergens, and successful and unsuccessful relief measures. In addition, the impact environmental air quality and second-hand smoke exposure has on the client's allergy and symptoms is determined.

Safe nursing practice also includes obtaining information about food, drug, or insect sting allergies. These data are usually obtained on initial history and physical. However, the nurse should always double-check this information with the client, especially when obtaining information about respiratory allergens.

Health Risks. The nurse must also investigate familial risk factors, such as a family history of lung cancer or cardiovascular disease. Documentation should include which blood relatives have had the disease and their present level of health or age at time of death. Other family risk factors include the presence of infectious diseases, particularly TB. The nurse should determine who in the client's household has been infected and the status of treatment.

Medications. The health history should also list medications the client is using. These include prescribed, over-the-counter, folk medicine, herbal medicines, alternative therapies, and illicit drugs and substances. Such medications may have adverse effects by themselves or because of interactions with other drugs. A person using a prescribed bronchodilator drug, for example, may decide that using an over-the-counter inhalant as well will be beneficial. Many of these contain ephedrine or *ma huang,* a natural chemical that acts like epinephrine. This product may react with the prescribed medication by potentiating or decreasing the effect of the prescribed medication. Clients taking warfarin (Coumadin) for blood thinning will prolong the prothrombin time/international normalized ratio (INR) results if they are taking gingko biloba, garlic, or ginseng with the anticoagulant. The drug interaction could precipitate a life-threatening bleed.

Safety Alert: During history taking, have clients include all over-the-counter and herbal supplements they are taking to ensure that there are no medication interactions.

When clients are prescribed drugs for which toxic levels can be monitored by blood analyses, the nurse needs to review these laboratory values. Common drugs that can be monitored include theophylline (theophylline levels), digitalis preparations (digitalis levels), anticoagulants such as warfarin (Coumadin; INR level), and phenobarbital (phenobarbital levels). Toxic effects of these medications can impair cardiopulmonary functioning.

It is important to determine whether a client uses illicit drugs. Illicit drugs, particularly parenterally administered narcotics, which are often diluted with talcum powder, can cause pulmonary disorders resulting from the irritant effect of the powder on lung tissues.

As with all medication, the nurse assesses the client's knowledge and ability to apply the six rights of medication administration (see chapter 30). Of particular importance is the nurse's assessment of the client's understanding of potential side effects of the medications. Clients should be able to recognize adverse reactions and be aware of the dangers in combining prescribed medications with over-the-counter drugs.

Physical Examination. The physical examination performed to assess the client's level of tissue oxygenation includes evaluation of the cardiopulmonary system (see chapter 28). Special consideration should be given when assessing the older client because changes in the cardiopulmonary system occur with the aging process (Table 35-3). These changes may result in changes in the client's activity tolerance, level of fatigue, or transient changes in vital signs and may not be associated with a specific cardiopulmonary disease.

Inspection. Using inspection techniques, the nurse performs a head-to-toe observation of the client for skin and mucous membrane colour, general appearance, level of consciousness, adequacy of systemic circulation, breathing patterns, and chest wall movement (Table 35-4). Any abnormalities should be investigated during palpation, percussion, and auscultation.

Inspection includes observations of the nails for clubbing. Clubbed nails, obliteration of the normal angle between the base of the nail and the skin, are seen in clients with prolonged oxygen deficiency, endocarditis, and congenital heart defects.

Table 35-3 Assessment Findings in the Aging Cardiopulmonary System

Function	Pathophysiological Change	Key Clinical Findings
Heart		
Muscle contraction	Thickening of the ventricular wall, increased collagen and decreased elastin in the heart muscle	Decreased cardiac output Diminished cardiac reserve
Blood flow	Heart valves become thicker and stiffer, more often in the mitral and aortic valves	Systolic ejection murmur
Conduction system	The SA node becomes fibrotic from calcification; the number of pacemaker cells in the SA node decreases	Increased PR, QRS, and Q-T intervals, decreased amplitude of the QRS complex
Arterial vessel compliance	Vessels become calcified, loss of arterial distensibility, decreased elastin in the vessel walls, more tortuous vessels	Hypertension, with an increase in systolic blood pressure Fluctuation in blood pressure
Lungs		
Breathing mechanics	Decreased chest wall compliance, loss of elastic recoil	Prolonged exhalation phase
	Decreased respiratory muscle mass/strength	Decreased vital capacity (volume of air exhaled after a maximal inhalation; normal range is 4500–4800 mL)
Oxygenation	Increased ventilation/perfusion mismatch Decreased alveolar surface area Decreased carbon dioxide diffusion capacity	Decreased PaO_2 Decreased cardiac output Slightly increased $PaCO_2$
Breathing control/ breathing pattern	Decreased responsiveness of central and peripheral chemoreceptors to hypoxemia and hypercapnia	Increased respiratory rate Decreased tidal volume (volume of air inhaled or exhaled per breath; normally 5–10 mL/kg)
Lung defence mechanisms	Decreased number of cilia Decreased IgA production and humoral and cellular immunity	Decreased airway clearance Diminished cough reflex
Sleep and breathing	Decreased respiratory drive Decreased tone of upper airway muscles	Increased risk of aspiration and infection Increased risk of arterial oxygen desaturation Snoring, obstructive sleep apnea

Observe the chest wall movement for retraction, sinking in of soft tissues of the chest between the intercostal spaces. Also observe for paradoxical breathing, asynchronous breathing, and the client's breathing pattern (Table 35-5). In paradoxical breathing, the chest wall contracts during inspiration and expands during exhalation. Infants can experience sternal and substernal chest wall retractions with only a slight inspiratory effort because of the pliability of the chest wall. Note the anteroposterior diameter of the chest wall. Conditions such as emphysema, advancing age, and COPD can cause the chest to assume a rounded shape.

Palpation. Palpation of the chest provides assessment data in several areas. It documents the type and amount of thoracic excursion, elicits any areas of tenderness, and can identify tactile fremitus, thrills, heaves, and the cardiac point of maximal impulse (PMI). Palpation also allows the nurse to feel for abnormal masses or lumps in the axilla and breast tissue. Palpation of the extremities provides data about the peripheral circulation, the presence and quality of peripheral pulses, skin temperature, colour, and capillary refill (see chapter 28).

Palpation should also include the feet and legs to assess the presence or absence of peripheral edema. Clients with alterations in their cardiac function, such as those with congestive heart failure or hypertension, often have pedal or lower extremity edema. Edema is graded from 1+ to 4+, depending on the depth of visible indentation after firm application of a finger (see chapter 28).

Palpation of the pulses in the neck and extremities is performed to assess arterial blood flow (see chapter 28). A scale of 0 (absent pulse) to 3+ (full, bounding pulse) is used to describe what is palpated. The normal pulse is graded at 2+, and a weak, thready pulse is graded as 1+.

Percussion. Percussion allows the nurse to detect the presence of abnormal fluid or air in the lungs. It is also used to determine diaphragmatic excursion (see chapter 28).

Auscultation. Auscultation enables the nurse to identify normal and abnormal heart and lung sounds (see chapter 28). Auscultation of the cardiovascular system should include assessment for normal S_1 and S_2 sounds, the presence of abnormal S_3 and S_4 sounds (gallops), and murmurs or rubs. Auscultation is also used to identify a bruit over the carotid arteries, abdominal aorta, and femoral arteries.

Auscultation of lung sounds involves listening for movement of air throughout all lung fields: anterior, posterior, and lateral. Adventitious breath sounds occur with

Table 35-4 Inspection of Cardiopulmonary Status

Abnormality	Cause
Eyes	
Xanthelasma (yellow lipid lesions on eyelids)	Hyperlipidemia
Corneal arcus (whitish opaque ring around junction of cornea and sclera)	Hyperlipidemia in young to middle adults, normal finding in older adults with arcus senilis
Pale conjunctivae	Anemia
Cyanotic conjunctivae	Hypoxemia
Petechiae on conjunctivae	Fat embolus or bacterial endocarditis
Mouth and Lips	
Cyanotic mucous membranes	Decreased oxygenation (hypoxia)
Pursed-lip breathing	Associated with chronic lung disease
Neck Veins	
Distension	Associated with right-sided heart failure
Nose	
Flaring nares	Air hunger, dyspnea
Chest	
Retractions	Increased work of breathing, dyspnea
Asymmetry	Chest wall injury
Skin	
Peripheral cyanosis	Vasoconstriction and diminished blood flow
Central cyanosis	Hypoxemia
Decreased skin turgor	Dehydration (normal finding in older adults as a result of decreased skin elasticity)
Dependent edema	Associated with right- and left-sided heart failure
Periorbital edema	Associated with kidney disease
Fingertips and Nail Beds	
Cyanosis	Decreased cardiac output or hypoxia
Splinter hemorrhages	Bacterial endocarditis
Clubbing	Chronic hypoxemia

From *Health Assessment Pocket Guide Series,* by P. A. Potter and P. B. Weilitz, 2003, St. Louis, MO: Mosby.

collapse of a lung segment, fluid in a lung segment, or narrowing or obstruction of an airway. Auscultation also evaluates the client's response to interventions for improving the respiratory status.

Diagnostic Tests. There are a variety of diagnostic tests to monitor cardiopulmonary functioning. Some of these tests can be obtained through screening, simple blood specimens, X-ray films, or other non-invasive means. One such screening mechanism is TB skin testing (Box 35-8). This is a simple test that is usually required annually for health care workers to monitor possible TB exposure. In contrast, invasive diagnostic tests, such as a thoracentesis, can be quite painful, depending on the client's tolerance for pain.

Tables 35-6 and 35-7 and Box 35-9 summarize diagnostic testing used in the assessment and evaluation of the client with cardiopulmonary alterations. The primary role of the nurse with diagnostic tests is to prepare the client. The nurse explains the procedure to the client and tells the client what to expect, thereby reducing anxiety. The client must understand the importance of following instructions, such as holding the breath as requested and not coughing during the procedure. After any procedure, the nurse monitors the client for signs of changes in cardiopulmonary functioning, sudden shortness of breath, pain, oxygen desaturation, and anxiety. The nurse also promotes the client's comfort and encourages the client to rest after the test because many clients find these tests to be tiring.

Client Expectations. The nurse asks clients what they expect from the encounter and what their priority is for management of their health. Identifying expectations involves clients in the decision-making process and allows them to participate in their care and to know what will happen to them. For example, planning a smoking cessation or weight-reduction program for a client who is not ready for the change will be frustrating for both the client and the nurse. Short-term realistic goals are established that build to

Table 35-5 Assessment of Breathing Pattern

Pattern and Rate (Breaths per Minute)	Clinical Significance
Eupnea (12-20) 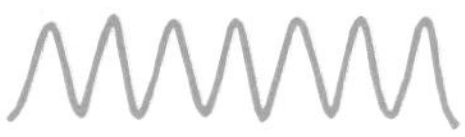	Normal rate in the adult
Tachypnea (>35) 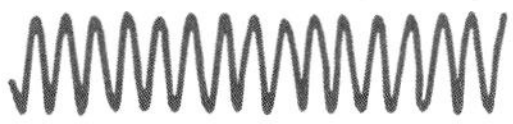	Can result from anxiety or response to pain or fever, respiratory failure, shortness of breath, or a respiratory infection. May lead to respiratory alkalosis, paresthesia, tetany, and confusion
Bradypnea (<10) 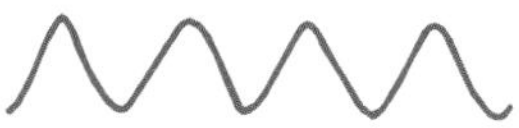	Results from sleep, respiratory depression, drug overdose, or central nervous system lesion
Apnea (absence of respiration >15 seconds) 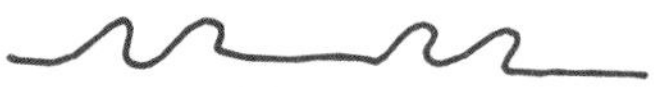	May be intermittent, such as in sleep apnea, or prolonged, as in a respiratory arrest
Kussmaul's respirations (usually >35, may be slow or normal) 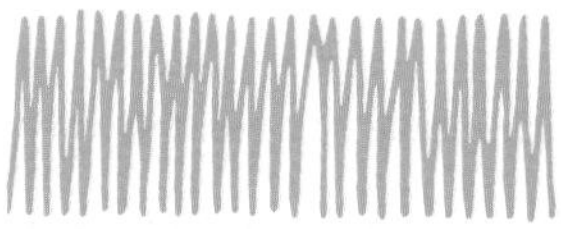	Tachypnea pattern associated with metabolic imbalance such as diabetic ketoacidosis, metabolic acidosis, or renal failure

Box 35-8 Tuberculosis Skin Testing

- Skin testing is used to determine past exposure to *Mycobacterium tuberculosis*.
- The antigen is injected intradermally (see chapter 30). Afterward, the injection site may be circled, and the client is instructed not to wash it off.
- Tuberculin skin tests are read at 72 hours.
- *Positive results:* A palpable, elevated, hardened, reddened area around the injection site, caused by edema and inflammation from the antigen-antibody reaction. The site is measured in millimetres. A positive test result is when the site is ≥10 mm. (In HIV+ clients only, a positive test is when the site is ≥5 mm.)
- Reddened flat areas are ***not*** positive reactions and are not measured.
- TB testing in older adults is less reliable (see Box 35-4).

a larger goal. For example, reducing the fat in the client's diet may start out with replacing food such as whole milk with 2% milk and gradually introducing skim milk. A sudden change from whole to skim milk will most likely fail, because the change is too much. A plan for adding exercise to the client's lifestyle may start with a commitment to exercise once a week for 20 minutes, or the client may commit to a weight-reduction plan of 2 kg per month.

It is important to remember that the goals and expectations of the nurse may not always coincide with those of the client. By addressing the client's concerns and expectations, the nurse will establish a relationship that can address other health care goals and expected outcomes. Knowing the mindset of the clients and respecting their wishes will go a long way in helping clients to make significant lifestyle changes to benefit their health.

NP Nursing Diagnosis

Clients with an altered level of oxygenation can have nursing diagnoses that are primarily from a cardiovascular or pulmonary origin. Each nursing diagnosis is based on specific defining characteristics and the related etiology (Box 35-10). The nurse uses the information gathered in the nursing assessment to identify and cluster the defining characteristics. The clustered defining characteristics support the nursing diagnosis.

Nursing diagnoses appropriate for the client with alterations in oxygenation include, but are not limited to, the following:

- Activity intolerance
- Risk for activity intolerance
- Ineffective airway clearance
- Anxiety
- Ineffective breathing pattern
- Decreased cardiac output

Table 35-6 Cardiopulmonary Diagnostic Blood Studies

Test and Normal Values	Interpretation
Complete Blood Count (CBC)	
Normal values for a CBC vary with age and gender.	A CBC determines the number and type of red and white blood cells per cubic millimetre of blood.
Cardiac Enzymes	
MB-CK 10 to 13 units/L; a serial MB-CK with 50% increase between two samples 4 hours apart, or a single MB-CK elevation twofold is diagnostic for an acute myocardial infarction.	Cardiac enzymes are used to diagnose acute myocardial infarcts.
Plasma Cardiac Troponin I	
$<$0.3 mg/mL	Value elevates within 4 to 6 hours of a cardiac event and remains elevated for 10 to 14 days.
Plasma Cardiac Troponin T	
$<$0.2 mg/mL	
Serum Electrolytes	
Potassium (K^+) 3.5 to 5 mmol/L	Clients on diuretic therapy are at risk for hypokalemia (low potassium). Clients receiving angiotensin-converting enzyme inhibitors are at risk for hyperkalemia (elevated potassium).
Cholesterol	
Fasting cholesterol $\leq$200 mg/100 mL	Contributing factors include sedentary lifestyle with intake of saturated fatty acids, familial hypercholesterolemia.
Low-density lipoprotein (LDL) cholesterol (bad cholesterol) $\leq$130 mg/100 mL	High LDL cholesterol (hypercholesterolemia) is caused by excessive intake of saturated fatty acids, dietary cholesterol intake, and obesity. Familial hypercholesterolemia and hyperlipidemia are also contributing factors, as well as hypothyroidism, nephrotic syndrome, and diabetes mellitus.
High-density lipoprotein (HDL) cholesterol (good cholesterol) $>$40 mg/100 mL	Low HDL cholesterol is caused by factors such as cigarette smoking, obesity, lack of regular exercise, beta-adrenergic blocking agents, genetic disorders of HDL metabolism, hypertriglyceridemia, and Type 2 diabetes.
Triglycerides $\leq$130 mg/100 mL	Obesity, excessive alcohol intake, diabetes mellitus, beta-adrenergic blocking agents, and genetic predisposition cause hypertriglyceridemia.

Table 35-7 Cardiac Function Diagnostic Tests

Test	Significance
12-Lead electrocardiogram (ECG)	Graphic recording of the electrical activity of the heart used to detect abnormal electrical activity and the electrical position of the heart. The ECG includes 12 leads: I, II, III, AVR, AVL, AVF, V_{1-6}. Provides a 360-degree view of the heart.
Holter monitor	Portable ECG worn by the client. The test produces a continuous ECG tracing over a period of time. Clients keep a diary of activity, noting when they experience rapid heartbeats or dizziness. Evaluation of the ECG recording along with the diary provides information about the heart's electrical activity during activities of daily living.
ECG exercise stress test	ECG is monitored while the client walks on a treadmill at a specified speed and duration of time. Used to evaluate the cardiac response to physical stress. The test is not a valuable tool for evaluation of cardiac response in women because of an increased false-positive finding.
Thallium stress test	An ECG stress test with the addition of talliuym-201-injected IV. Determines coronary blood flow changes with increased activity.
Electrophysiological study	Invasive measure of intracardiac electrical pathways. Provides more specific information about difficult-to-treat dysrhythmias. Assesses adequacy of antidysrhythmic medication.
Echocardiography	Non-invasive measure of heart structure and heart wall motion. Graphically demonstrates overall cardiac performance.
Scintigraphy	Radionuclide angiography. Used to evaluate cardiac structure, myocardial perfusion, and contractility.
Cardiac catheterization and angiography	Used to visualize cardiac chambers, valves, the great vessels, and coronary arteries. Pressures and volumes within the four chambers of the heart can also be measured.

Box 35-9 Common Respiratory Tests and Methods

Oxygenation Tests

- *Pulse Oximetry.* A **pulse oximeter** is a device used to measure pulse rate and oxygen concentration in arterial blood. A sensor is attached to the client's finger, toe, nose, earlobe, or forehead. Accuracy is directly related to the perfusion of the probe area, a systolic blood pressure >90 mm Hg, and the hemoglobin level. Decreased levels correlate well with arterial oxygen levels and are used to trend oxygenation over time. Normal SaO_2 values are 98% to 100%. An SaO_2 below 70% is life-threatening.
- *Arterial Blood Gas.* A radial or femoral artery is punctured to obtain arterial blood. Tests measure the oxygen concentration in the blood, the hydrogen ion concentration (pH), partial pressure of carbon dioxide, and the partial pressure of oxygen. Normal values are as follows:
  - pH 7.35–7.45
  - $PaCO_2$ 35–45 mm Hg
  - PaO_2 80–100 mm Hg
  - SaO_2 95–100%

Pulmonary Function Tests

Pulmonary function tests measure lung volume (the amount of air moving into and out of the lungs) and capacity (how much air the lungs can hold). Respiratory therapists usually conduct these tests. The client takes as deep a breath as possible and forcefully exhales into a mouthpiece attached to a machine. Pulmonary readings are recorded and compared with previous readings and with average normal values, which vary depending on the client's age, gender, weight, height, and race. These tests are used to diagnose and monitor pulmonary disease and conditions (e.g., asthma, emphysema). They are also used to evaluate post-operative lung conditions.

Imaging

- *Chest X-Ray Examination.* Usually posteroanterior and lateral films are taken to adequately visualize all of the lung fields. A radiograph of the thorax is used to observe the lung fields for fluid, infiltrates (e.g., pneumonia), masses (e.g., lung cancer), fractures, pneumothorax, and other abnormal processes.
- *Computed Tomography (CT) Scan.* A CT scan allows visualization of fine detail of the lungs and other structures in the thorax. It is often used as part of the assessment of clients with pneumonia, lung masses, and suspected pulmonary emboli.
- *Ventilation/Perfusion (Nuclear Medicine) Lung Scan.* This scan is used to detect pulmonary emboli. The results from two separate scans are compared: the perfusion scan uses an injected radioactive tracer to measure pulmonary blood flow, and the ventilation scan shows the pulmonary distribution of a different inhaled tracer. Mismatches (areas of ventilation without corresponding perfusion or blood flow) indicate pulmonary emboli.

Methods of Obtaining Respiratory Specimens for Analysis

Specimens are cultured to detect for the presence of blood, microbes, and abnormal cells. A variety of methods are used to obtain respiratory specimens.

- *Sputum Tests:* Sputum is mucus from the respiratory system that is expectorated through the mouth. Sputum specimens are obtained when the client coughs up sputum from the bronchi and trachea; specimens are easier to obtain in the morning when the secretions are coughed up upon awakening. Sputum tests include (a) *Sputum culture and sensitivity (C and S).* Sputum C and S is used to identify a specific microorganism growing in the sputum and to identify drug resistance and sensitivities. (b) *Sputum for acid-fast bacillus (AFB).* This test is used to screen for the presence of AFB for detection of TB by early morning specimens on three consecutive days. (c) *Sputum for cytology.* Cytology is used to identify abnormal lung cancer and differentiates the type of cancer cells (small cell, oat cell, large cell).
- *Tracheal Aspiration via Endotracheal Tube in Intubated Clients.* Secretions are collected by passing a flexible suction catheter through the endotracheal tube.
- *Bronchoscopy.* A narrow, flexible, fibre-optic scope is passed into the trachea and bronchi to enable visual examination of the tracheobronchial tree. Performed to obtain fluid, sputum, or biopsy samples; also performed to remove mucous plugs or foreign bodies.
- *Thoracentesis.* A needle is passed through the chest wall to aspirate fluid for diagnostic or therapeutic purposes. The procedure is performed using aseptic technique and local anaesthetic. The client usually sits upright with the anterior thorax supported by pillows or an overbed table.
- *Nasopharyngeal Aspirate or Swab.* This swab is used to detect respiratory viruses. Aspirates are the best specimens from young children, whereas swabs can be used for obtaining samples from older children and adults.

- Impaired comfort
- Impaired verbal communication
- Ineffective individual coping
- Fatigue
- Fear
- Risk for imbalanced fluid volume
- Impaired gas exchange
- Ineffective health maintenance
- Risk for infection
- Deficient (specify) knowledge
- Risk for impaired skin integrity
- Disturbed sleep pattern
- Ineffective tissue perfusion
- Impaired spontaneous ventilation

NP Planning

During planning, the nurse again synthesizes information from multiple sources (Figure 35–7). Critical thinking ensures that the client's plan of care integrates all that the nurse knows about the individual, as well as key critical thinking elements. Professional standards are especially important to consider when the nurse develops a care

Nursing Diagnostic Process — Box 35-10

Assessment Activities	Defining Characteristics	Nursing Diagnosis
Ask client or family about client's mood, attentiveness, memory, and activity level.	Confusion Decreased activity Fatigue Irritability Restlessness Sleepiness	Impaired gas exchange related to decreased lung expansion
Observe client's respirations.	Dyspnea Impaired gas exchange related to collapsed alveoli Nasal flaring Tachypnea Use of accessory muscles	
Inspect skin and mucous membranes.	Diaphoresis Pallor Moist skin Abnormal lung sounds may be present	
Auscultate chest.	Decreased respiratory excursion Distant lung sounds	

plan. These standards often establish scientifically proven guidelines for selecting effective nursing interventions.

Goals and Outcomes. The nurse develops an individualized care plan for each nursing diagnosis (see Care Plan). The nurse and client set realistic expectations for care. Goals are to be individualized and realistic with measurable outcomes.

Clients with impaired oxygenation require a nursing care plan directed toward meeting the actual or potential oxygenation needs of the client. Individual outcomes are derived from client-centred needs. For example, the goal of maintaining a patent airway can be evaluated by specific outcomes for the client. These might include the following expected outcomes:

- Client's lungs are clear to auscultation.
- Client achieves maintenance and promotion of bilateral lung expansion.
- Client coughs productively.
- Tissue oxygenation (SaO_2) is maintained or improved.

Often a client with cardiopulmonary disease has multiple nursing diagnoses (Figure 35–8). In this case, the nurse identifies when goals or outcomes apply to more than one diagnosis. The presence of multiple diagnoses also makes priority setting a critical activity.

Setting Priorities. The client's level of health, age, lifestyle, and environmental risks affect the level of tissue oxygenation. Clients with severe impairments in oxygenation frequently require nursing interventions in multiple areas. The nurse must consider what is the most important goal to reach in the limited amount of time the client is seen in the hospital or primary care setting. For example, in an acute care setting, maintaining a patent airway has a higher priority than improving the client's exercise tolerance. The need for a patent airway is an immediate need. In a second example, when caring for a client who has an abdominal incision, pain control may have a greater priority than coughing and deep breathing. Again, in this situation, controlling the client's pain ultimately will facilitate coughing and deep breathing.

However, in a community-based or primary setting, the priority may focus on smoking cessation, exercise, and/or diet modifications. Both the client and nurse need to be focused on the same goal and expected outcomes to be successful. In addition to being individualized, each goal should be realistic and attainable for the client.

Continuity of Care. The time a nurse gets to spend with the client in any setting is limited. Therefore, the nurse must rely on collaboration with family members, colleagues, and other specialists to accomplish the goals and outcomes that have been determined. Some clients may need to improve their exercise and activity tolerance; for some clients their continuity of care may involve enrolling in a community-based cardiopulmonary rehabilitation program. Another client may have the same health care need but is unable to leave the home, and home physiotherapy is needed.

Collaboration with physiotherapists, nutritionists, and community-based nurses may be valuable for a client with congestive heart failure or chronic lung conditions and is an essential component of primary health care. These professionals work with the client and the community to optimize resources to assist the client in attaining the highest level of wellness. In addition, professionals can help to identify community resources and support systems for both the client and family in preventing and managing symptoms related to cardiopulmonary diseases.

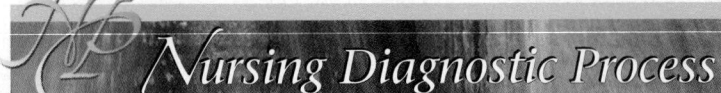

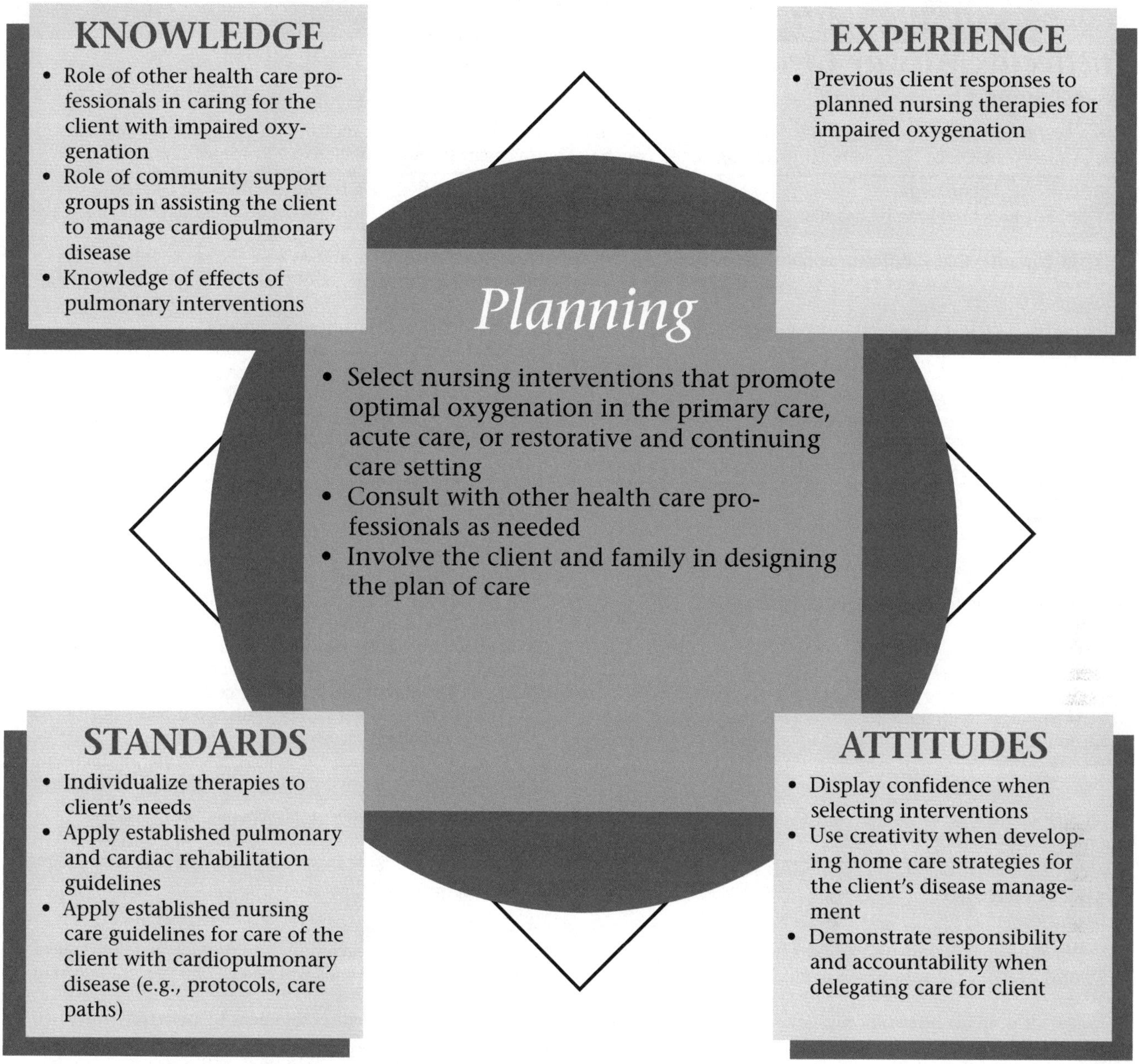
KNOWLEDGE
• Role of other health care professionals in caring for the client with impaired oxygenation
• Role of community support groups in assisting the client to manage cardiopulmonary disease
• Knowledge of effects of pulmonary interventions
EXPERIENCE
• Previous client responses to planned nursing therapies for impaired oxygenation
Planning
• Select nursing interventions that promote optimal oxygenation in the primary care, acute care, or restorative and continuing care setting
• Consult with other health care professionals as needed
• Involve the client and family in designing the plan of care
STANDARDS
• Individualize therapies to client's needs
• Apply established pulmonary and cardiac rehabilitation guidelines
• Apply established nursing care guidelines for care of the client with cardiopulmonary disease (e.g., protocols, care paths)
ATTITUDES
• Display confidence when selecting interventions
• Use creativity when developing home care strategies for the client's disease management
• Demonstrate responsibility and accountability when delegating care for client

FIGURE **35–7** Critical thinking model for oxygenation planning.

Implementation

Nursing interventions for promoting and maintaining adequate oxygenation include independent nursing actions such as health promotion and disease prevention behaviours, positioning, and coughing techniques. Interdependent or dependent interventions include oxygen therapy, lung inflation techniques, hydration, medication administration, and chest physiotherapy (CPT).

Health Promotion. Maintaining the client's optimal level of health is important in reducing the number and severity of respiratory symptoms. Prevention of respiratory infections is foremost in maintaining optimal health. Providing cardiopulmonary-related health information (Box 35-11) is an important nursing responsibility and part of a primary health care model.

Vaccinations. Annual influenza vaccines are recommended for older clients and clients with chronic illnesses. This includes clients older than 65 years of age; clients of any age with chronic disease of the heart, lung, or kidneys; clients with diabetes; and clients with immunosuppression or severe forms of anemia. The vaccine is also recommended for people in close or frequent contact with anyone in the high-risk groups. The vaccine has been shown to be 70% to 90% effective in healthy young adults (Zimmerman & Ball, 2001). The vaccine is most

Nursing Care Plan

Ineffective Airway Clearance/Retained Secretions

Assessment

Mr. Edwards, an older adult with a history of COPD, comes to the primary care office with complaints of continued coughing. He continues to smoke 2 to 3 cigarettes a day, an improvement from his previous 10 to 15 per day.

Assessment Activities	Findings/Defining Characteristics
Ask Mr. Edwards how long he has had this cough.	He replies, "I have a morning cough every day, but this cough is different. It started about a week ago."
Ask Mr. Edwards what is different about this cough.	He replies, "My ribs are getting sore. I can't cough up anything, my mouth is dry, and I have become more fatigued over the past week."
Observe Mr. Edwards's skin and mucous membranes.	His skin and mucous membranes are dry.
Auscultate lung fields.	Abnormal lung sounds in the upper lobes. The lower lobes are clear.
Ask Mr. Edwards how many glasses of water he drinks daily.	Over last week has drunk two to three glasses a day.
Ask Mr. Edwards to produce a sputum sample.	He is unable to produce a sputum sample for evaluation.

Nursing Diagnosis: Ineffective airway clearance related to retained secretions and reduced fluid intake.

Planning

Goal	Expected Outcomes*
	Respiratory Status: Airway Patency
Client will be able to effectively clear secretions.	Lung sounds will be normal in 48 hours. Sputum will be thin, white, and watery. Respiratory rate will be within 20 to 24 breaths per minute in 48 hours. Client will be able to clear airway by coughing.
Client will increase oral hydration to 1000 mL of water every 24 hours.	Oral mucous membranes will be pink and moist. Client will verbalize that his mouth is not dry. Client will notice an increase in ease of sputum production. Client will report that his sputum is thin, white, and watery.

*Outcome classification labels from *Nursing outcomes classification (NOC)* (3rd ed.), edited by S. Moorhead, M. Johnson, and M. Maas, 2004, St. Louis, MO: Mosby.

Interventions† / Rationale

Interventions†	Rationale
Airway Management	
Increase fluids to 1000 mL in 24 hours if not contraindicated by cardiovascular disease (Lewis et al., 2000).	Fluids help to liquefy secretions and promote ease of removal (Snow et al., 2001). Fluids will relieve oral mucosa and skin dryness.
Have client deep breathe and cough every 2 hours four to five times (Lewis et al., 2000).	Retained secretions predisposes client to atelectasis and pneumonia (Day et al., 2002).
Teach client effective cough techniques.	Coughing techniques will help to clear the airway effectively and decrease fatigue from ineffective coughing (Snow et al., 2001).
Consider chest physiotherapy (CPT) if there is evidence of infiltrates on chest X-ray film.	Standards for CPT include sputum production greater than 30 mL/day or infiltrates on chest X-ray film.

†Intervention classification labels from *Nursing interventions classification (NIC)* (4th ed.), edited by J. M. Dochterman and G. M. Bulechek, 2004, St. Louis, MO: Mosby.

Evaluation

Nursing Actions	Client Response/Finding	Achievement of Outcome
Ask Mr. Edwards if he can deep breathe and cough.	Mr. Edwards reports, "It is easier to cough up my secretions now."	Client is able to clear airway by coughing.
Assess the chest for adventitious lung sounds.	Mr. Edwards reports that he has not heard any wheezing or rattling in his chest.	Lungs clear to auscultation in all fields.
Assess respiratory rate.	No use of accessory muscles of respiration. Normal breathing pattern and respiratory rate.	Respiratory rate is between 20 and 24 breaths per minute.
Assess client's level of hydration.	Mucous membranes are moist. Mr. Edwards reports "My mouth isn't so dry anymore."	Oral mucous membranes are pink and moist.
Observe appearance of sputum.	Sputum is thin, white, and watery.	Sputum is thin, white, and watery.

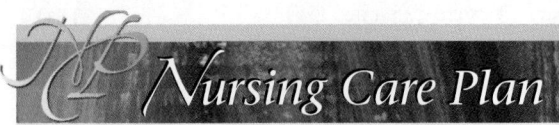

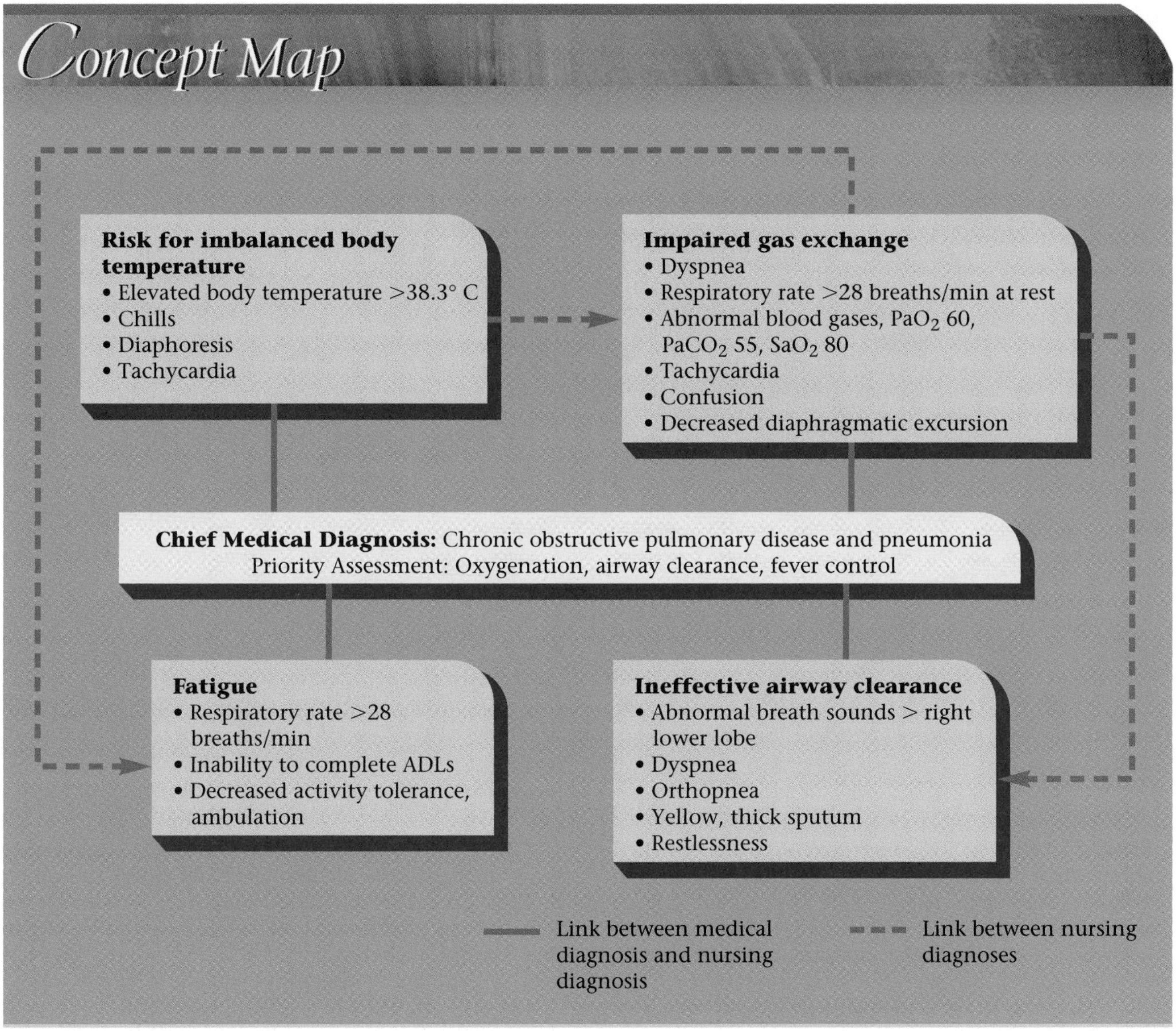

FIGURE **35–8** Concept map for a client with chronic obstructive pulmonary disease and pneumonia.

effective in reducing the severity of illness and the risk of serious complications and death. Studies have shown a 70% reduction in the number of older adults requiring hospitalization for pneumonia and an 85% reduction in mortality for those not in long-term care facilities (Centers for Disease Control and Prevention [CDC], 2002).

Influenza occurs from November until April. The incidence is usually very low until December and peaks between January and March. Vaccines should be given between September and mid-November. It takes about 1 to 2 weeks after vaccination for antibody development and protection that lasts for approximately 6 months in most adults (CDC, 2002).

The value of vaccination of immunocompromised clients is not completely understood. HIV-positive clients may receive the flu vaccine; however, they may require a second vaccine to gain protection. People who should not be vaccinated include those with a known hypersensitivity to eggs or other components of the vaccine and adults with an acute febrile illness. The vaccines are formulated annually based on worldwide surveillance data.

Pneumococcal vaccine is recommended for clients at increased risk of developing pneumonia, those with chronic illnesses or immunosuppression (such as HIV/AIDS), those living in special environments such as long-term care facilities, and clients over the age of 65 years. HIV-positive clients can also receive the pneumococcal vaccination. Revaccination has been recommended for clients at 65 years of age (CDC, 2002).

Both the influenza vaccine and pneumococcal vaccine can be administered to pregnant women after the first trimester. However, in all cases, it is important to consult the client's obstetrician before administering either vaccine.

Client Teaching — Box 35-11

Cardiovascular Disease

Objectives

- Client will be able to verbalize risk factors associated with cardiovascular disease.
- Client will be able to demonstrate health promotion behaviours.

Teaching Strategies

- Teach risk factors that cannot be changed and those that can, such as smoking, alcohol intake, high blood pressure, and blood cholesterol levels.
- Educate the client about other risk factors for cardiovascular disease, such as diabetes, obesity, physical inactivity, stress, and oral contraceptives.
- Educate the client about the importance of regular blood pressure monitoring and adherence to a medication regimen.
- Educate client about the importance of blood cholesterol monitoring and maintaining a fasting total cholesterol and triglyceride level less than 200 mg/100 mL.
- Educate the client about low-fat, low-salt, and calorie-appropriate diets. Provide sample menus.
- Discuss strategies for stress reduction, such as realistic goal setting, relaxation techniques, exercise, proper diet, and rest.
- Educate client about the benefits of exercising for 1 hour daily to help reduce weight and lower blood pressure.
- Set realistic goals with the client for follow-up for blood pressure monitoring.
- Determine the cultural, religious, or economic issues that may interfere with client's ability to complete the plan of care.
- Determine age-related issues that may prevent client from achieving the goals.

Evaluation

- Have client verbalize his or her risk factors for cardiovascular disease.
- Ask client to verbalize what he or she will do to reduce stress.
- Client can list his or her medications, use, and dosage and reports that he or she has been taking the medication as prescribed.
- Obtain client's weight and blood pressure and measure for presence of pedal edema.
- Monitor the serum cholesterol (total, high- and low-density lipids) and triglyceride levels.
- Client returns for follow-up as scheduled.

Adapted from *Mosby's Handbook of Patient Teaching,* by M. M. Canobbio, 2000, St. Louis, MO: Mosby.

Healthy Lifestyle Behaviour. Identification and elimination of risk factors for cardiopulmonary disease is an important part of primary health care. Clients are encouraged to eat a healthy, low-fat, high-fibre diet; monitor their cholesterol, triglyceride, high-density lipoprotein (HDL), and low-density lipoprotein (LDL) levels; reduce stress; exercise; and maintain a body weight in proportion to their height.

Elimination of cigarettes and other tobacco, reduction of pollutants, monitoring of air quality, and adequate hydration are additional healthy behaviours. Clients should be encouraged to examine their habits and make changes to achieve their goals.

Exercise is a key factor in promoting and maintaining a healthy heart and lungs. Clients should be encouraged to exercise three to four times a week for 20 to 30 minutes. Aerobic exercise is necessary to improve lung function, strengthen muscles, and achieve the desired outcome. Walking is one of the most efficient ways to achieve a good aerobic workout. Many shopping malls have programs that allow people to enter the mall before the shops open and use the enclosed area for walking. Some even have measured the distances to help people plan their activity and measure their progress. Clients should be taught how to take their pulse and pace themselves. It is better to walk 15 minutes every day than to walk to exhaustion to achieve a goal. Clients should plan a time interval and walk for the designated time. Gradually they will notice that the distance increases as their endurance and fitness improve.

Clients with cardiopulmonary alterations need to minimize their risk for infection, especially during the winter months. Clients are taught to avoid large, crowded places; to keep their mouth and nose covered; and to be sure to dress warmly, including a scarf, hat, and gloves. This is especially important during the peak of the influenza season.

Clients with known cardiac disease and those with multiple risk factors should be cautioned to avoid exertion in cold weather. Shovelling snow is especially risky and has been known to precipitate a cardiac event in many clients. Other activities such as hanging holiday lights and decorations in the extreme cold can precipitate chest pain and bronchospasm. Clients are advised to avoid alcohol, because it blunts the respiratory drive when used in excess and may contribute to exposure to the cold by making the client feel warm when the client is really not protected.

Clients should also be taught to plan for the hot summer months. Activities should be limited to early in the day or late in the evening, when temperatures are lower. Care should be taken to maintain adequate hydration and sodium intake, especially in those clients who are taking diuretics. Caffeinated and alcoholic beverages should be limited or avoided completely, because they act as diuretics and can contribute to dehydration.

Environmental Pollutants. Avoiding exposure to second-hand smoke is essential to maintaining optimal cardiopulmonary function. Most businesses and restaurants now ban smoking or have separate areas designated as smoking areas. If clients are exposed to second-hand smoke in their home environments, counselling and support may be necessary to assist the smoker in successful smoking cessation or alterations in behaviour patterns, such as smoking outside.

Exposure to chemicals and pollutants in the work environment must also be considered. Clients such as farmers, painters, carpenters, and others benefit from the use of particulate filter masks to reduce inhalation of particles.

Acute Care. Clients with acute pulmonary illnesses require nursing interventions directed toward halting the pathological process (e.g., respiratory tract infection), shortening the duration and severity of the illness (e.g., hospitalization with pneumonia), and preventing complications from the illness or treatments (e.g., nosocomial infection resulting from invasive procedures).

Dyspnea Management. Dyspnea is difficult to quantify and to treat. Treatment modalities need to be individualized for each client, and more than one therapy is usually implemented. The underlying process that causes or worsens dyspnea must be treated and stabilized initially, and then four additional therapies—pharmacological measures, oxygen therapy, physical techniques, and psychosocial techniques—are implemented. Pharmacological agents may include bronchodilators, steroids, mucolytics, and low-dose antianxiety medications. Oxygen therapy can reduce dyspnea associated with exercise. Physical techniques, such as cardiopulmonary reconditioning through exercise, breathing techniques, and cough control, can help to reduce dyspnea. Relaxation techniques, biofeedback, and meditation are physiological measures that can lessen the sensation of dyspnea.

Airway Maintenance. The airway is patent when the trachea, bronchi, and large airways are free from obstructions. Airway maintenance requires adequate hydration to prevent thick, tenacious secretions. Proper coughing techniques remove secretions and keep the airway open. A variety of interventions, such as suctioning, CPT, and nebulizer therapy, assist the client in managing alterations in airway clearance.

Mobilization of Pulmonary Secretions. The ability of a client to mobilize pulmonary secretions may make the difference between a short-term illness and a long recovery involving complications. Nursing interventions that promote mobilization of pulmonary secretions assist the client in achieving and maintaining a clear airway and help promote lung expansion and gas exchange.

Humidification. **Humidification** is the process of adding water to gas. Temperature is the most important factor affecting the amount of water vapour a gas can hold. The percentage of water in the gas in relation to its capacity for water is the relative humidity. Air or oxygen with a high relative humidity keeps the airways moist and helps loosen and mobilize pulmonary secretions. Humidification is necessary for clients receiving oxygen therapy at greater than 4 L/minute. Bubbling oxygen through water can add humidity to the oxygen delivered to the upper airways, as with a nasal cannula or face mask.

Nebulization. **Nebulization** is a process of adding moisture or medications to inspired air by mixing particles of varying sizes with the air. A nebulizer uses the aerosol principle to suspend a maximum number of water drops or particles of the desired size in inspired air. The moisture added to the respiratory system through nebulization improves clearance of pulmonary secretions. Nebulization is often used for administration of bronchodilators and mucolytic agents.

When the thin layer of fluid that supports the mucous layer over the cilia is allowed to dry, the cilia are damaged and cannot adequately clear the airway. Humidification through nebulization enhances mucociliary clearance, the body's natural mechanism for removing mucus and cellular debris from the respiratory tract.

The major types of nebulizers are the jet-aerosol nebulizer and the ultrasonic nebulizer. A jet-aerosol nebulizer uses gas under pressure, and the ultrasonic nebulizer uses high-frequency vibrations to break up the water or medication into fine drops or particles. When inspired with air or administered oxygen, the drops of particles are then deposited throughout the tracheobronchial tree.

Chest Physiotherapy. **Chest physiotherapy (CPT)** is a group of therapies used in combination to mobilize pulmonary secretions. These therapies include postural drainage, chest percussion, and vibration. CPT should be followed by productive coughing and suctioning of the client who has a decreased ability to cough. CPT is recommended for clients who produce greater than 30 mL of sputum per day or have evidence of atelectasis by chest X-ray examination. This procedure can be safely used with infants and young children; however, conditions and diseases unique to children may at times contraindicate this procedure. CPT is used for a select group of clients. Box 35-12 describes the guidelines to determine if CPT is indicated for the client.

Chest percussion involves striking the chest wall over the area being drained. The hand is positioned so that the fingers and thumb touch and the hands are cupped (Figure 35–9). Percussion on the surface of the chest wall sends waves of varying amplitude and frequency through the chest, changing the consistency and location of the sputum. Chest percussion is performed by striking the chest wall alternately with cupped hands (Figure 35–10). Percussion is performed over a single layer of clothing, not over buttons, snaps, or zippers. The single layer of clothing prevents slapping the client's skin. Thicker or multiple layers of material dampen the vibrations.

Percussion is contraindicated in clients with bleeding disorders, osteoporosis, or fractured ribs. Caution should be taken to percuss the lung fields and not the scapular regions, or trauma may occur to the skin and underlying musculoskeletal structures.

Vibration is a fine, shaking pressure applied to the chest wall only during exhalation. This technique is thought to increase the velocity and turbulence of exhaled air, facilitating secretion removal. Vibration increases the exhalation of trapped air and may shake mucus loose and induce a cough.

Postural drainage is the use of positioning techniques that draw secretions from specific segments of the lungs and bronchi into the trachea. Coughing or suctioning normally removes secretions from the trachea. The procedure for postural drainage can include most lung segments (Table 35-8). Because clients may not require

Box 35-12 Guidelines for Chest Physiotherapy

Nursing care and selection of chest physiotherapy (CPT) skills are based on specific assessment findings. The following guidelines help the nurse in physical assessment and subsequent decision making:

- Know the client's normal range of vital signs. Conditions such as atelectasis and pneumonia requiring CPT can affect vital signs. The degree of change is related to the level of hypoxia, overall cardiopulmonary status, and tolerance to activity.
- Know the client's medications. Certain medications, particularly diuretics and antihypertensives, cause fluid and hemodynamic changes. These changes may decrease the client's tolerance to the positional changes of postural drainage. Steroid medications increase the client's risk of pathological rib fractures and often contraindicate rib shaking.
- Know the client's medical history. Certain conditions such as increased intracranial pressure, spinal cord injuries, and abdominal aneurysm resection contraindicate the positional changes of postural drainage. Thoracic trauma or surgery may also contraindicate percussion, vibration, and rib shaking.
- Know the client's level of cognitive function. Participation in controlled coughing techniques requires the client to follow instructions. Congenital or acquired cognitive limitations may alter the client's ability to learn and participate in these techniques.
- Be aware of the client's exercise tolerance. CPT manoeuvres are fatiguing. When the client is not used to physical activity, initial tolerance to the manoeuvres may be decreased. However, with gradual increases in activity and planned CPT, client tolerance for the procedure improves.

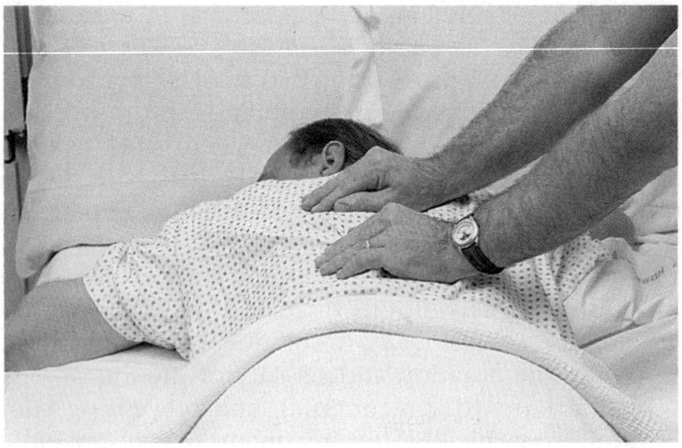

FIGURE **35–9** Hand position for chest wall percussion during chest physiotherapy.

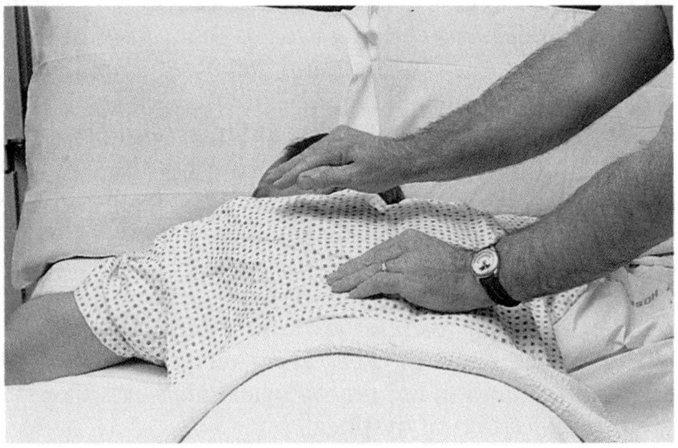

FIGURE **35–10** Chest wall percussion, alternating hand clapping against the client's chest wall.

postural drainage of all lung segments, the procedure is based on clinical assessment findings. For example, clients with left lower lobe atelectasis may require postural drainage of only the affected region, whereas a child with cystic fibrosis may require postural drainage of all lung segments.

Suctioning Techniques. When a client is unable to clear respiratory tract secretions with coughing, the nurse must use suctioning to clear the airways. The suctioning techniques include oropharyngeal and nasopharyngeal suctioning, orotracheal and nasotracheal suctioning, and suctioning an artificial airway.

These techniques are based on common principles. Because the oropharynx and trachea are considered sterile, sterile technique is used for suctioning. The mouth is considered clean, and therefore the suctioning of oral secretions should be performed after suctioning of the oropharynx and trachea. Each type of suctioning requires the use of a rounded-tipped catheter with a number of side holes at the distal end of the catheter. Frequency of suctioning is determined by client assessment and need. If secretions are identified by inspection or auscultation techniques, suctioning is required. Sputum is not produced continuously or every 1 or 2 hours but occurs as a response to a pathological condition. Therefore, there is no rationale for routine suctioning of all clients every 1 to 2 hours. In addition, suctioning reduces the amount of the available dead space in the oropharynx and trachea, often resulting in significant desaturation. The nurse must be careful to monitor the client to ensure adequate oxygenation. Too-frequent suctioning can put the client at risk for development of hypoxemia, hypotension, arrhythmias, and possible trauma to the mucosa of the lungs (Day et al., 2002).

Oropharyngeal and Nasopharyngeal Suctioning. The oropharynx extends behind the mouth from the soft palate above the level of the hyoid bone and contains the tonsils. The nasopharynx is located behind the nose and extends to the level of the soft palate. Oropharyngeal or nasopharyngeal suctioning is used when the client is able to cough effectively but is unable to clear secretions by expectorating or swallowing. The suction procedure is used after the client has coughed (Skill 35-1). As the amount of pulmonary secretions is reduced and the client is less fatigued, the client may be able to expectorate or swallow the mucus and suctioning is no longer required.

Orotracheal and Nasotracheal Suctioning. Orotracheal or nasotracheal suctioning is necessary when the client with pulmonary secretions is unable to manage secretions by

Text continued on p. 1118

Table 35-8 Positions for Postural Drainage

Lung Segment	Position of Client
Adult	
Bilateral 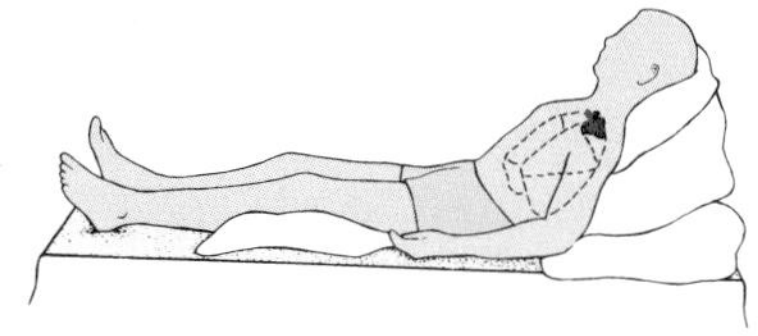	High-Fowler's position
Apical segments Right upper lobe—anterior segment 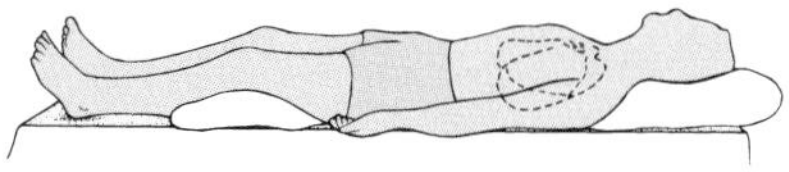	Supine with head of bed elevated 15 to 30 degrees
Left upper lobe—anterior segment 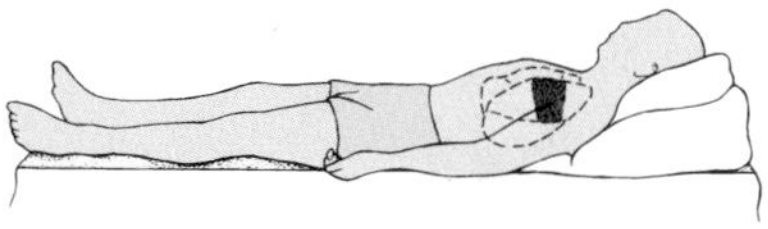	Supine with head elevated
Right upper lobe—posterior segment 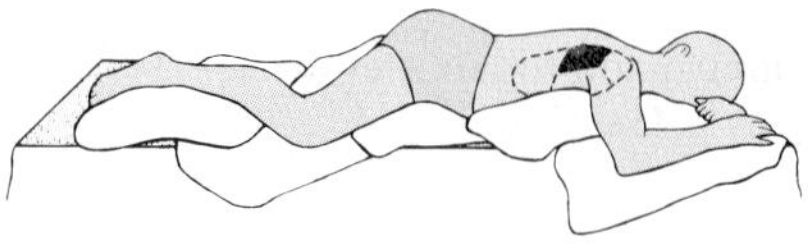	Side lying with right side of chest elevated on pillows
Left upper lobe—posterior segment 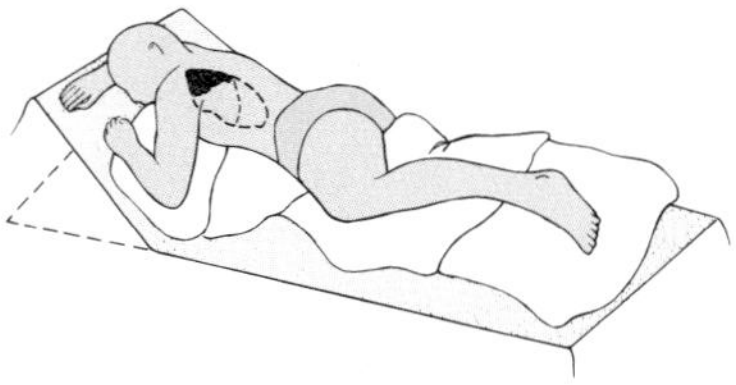	Side lying with left side of chest elevated on pillows
Right middle lobe—anterior segment 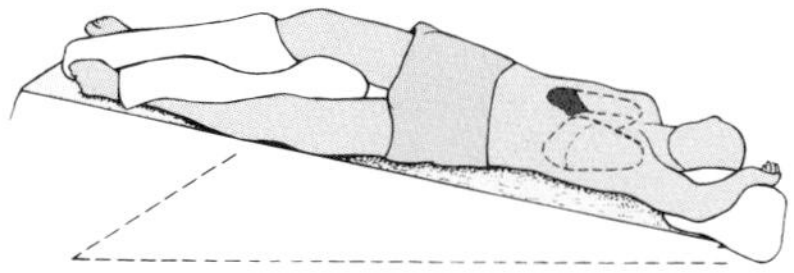	Three-fourths supine position with dependent lung in Trendelenburg's position
Right middle lobe—posterior segment 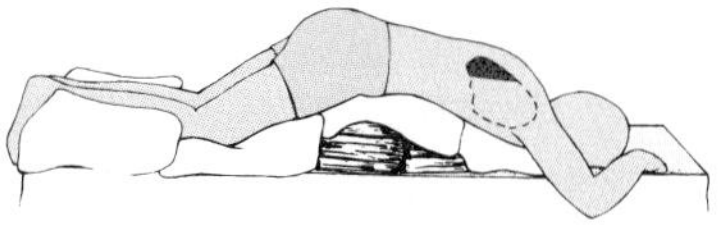	Prone with thorax and abdomen elevated
Both lower lobes—anterior segments 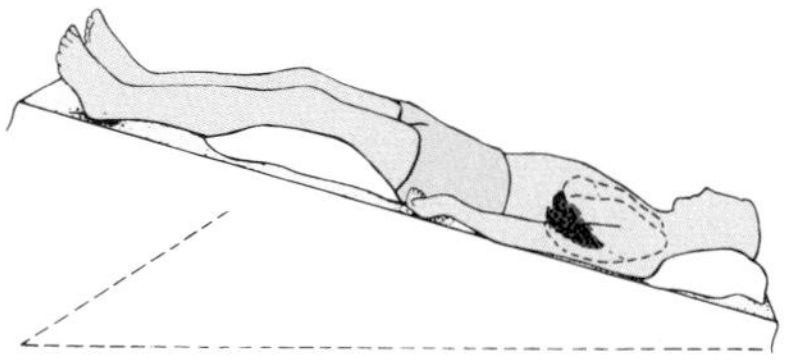	Supine in Trendelenburg's position

Continued

Table 35-8 Positions for Postural Drainage—cont'd

Lung Segment	Position of Client
Adult—cont'd	
Left lower lobe—lateral segment 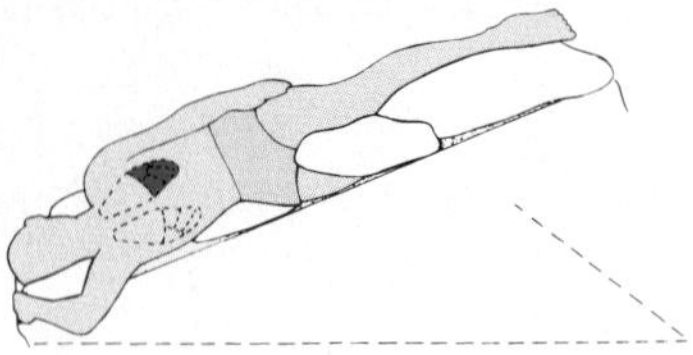	Left lateral in Trendelenburg's position
Right lower lobe—lateral segment 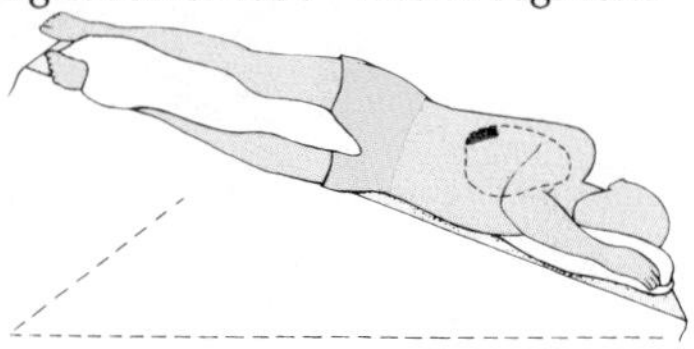	Right side-lying in Trendelenburg's position
Right lower lobe—posterior segment 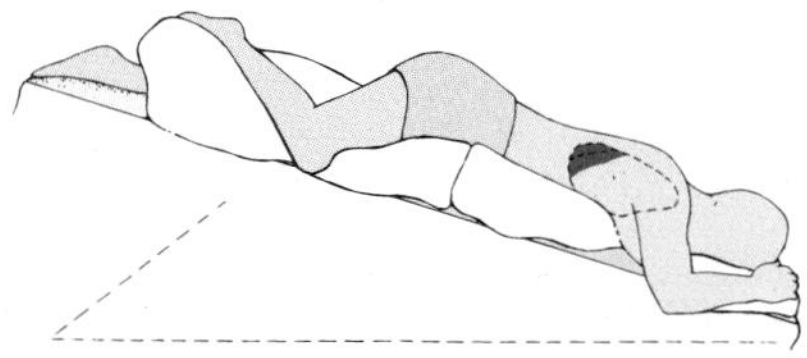	Prone in Trendelenburg's position with abdomen and thorax elevated
Both lower lobes—posterior segments 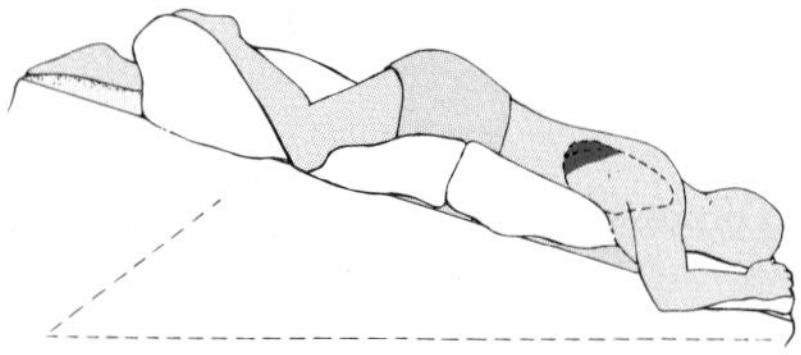	Prone in Trendelenburg's position with abdomen and thorax elevated
Child	
Bilateral—apical segments 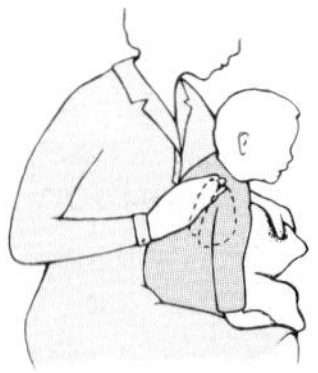	Sitting on nurse's lap, leaning slightly forward, flexed over pillow
Bilateral—middle anterior segments 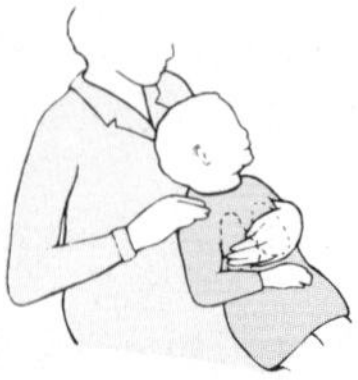	Sitting on nurse's lap, leaning against nurse
Bilateral lobes— anterior segments 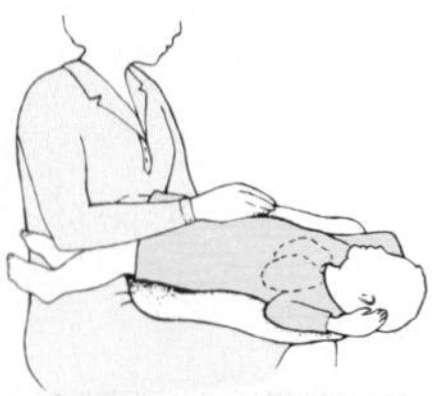	Lying supine on nurse's lap, back supported with pillow

Skill 35-1 Suctioning

View Video

Delegation Considerations

This skill may be delegated to unregulated care providers (UCPs) in special situations. When the nurse assesses that the client is stable, the skill of performing suctioning of an established tracheostomy can be delegated to a UCP when the client has a permanent tracheostomy tube or is receiving home mechanical ventilation. Before delegating this skill, the nurse must do the following:

- Discuss with care provider any unique modifications of the skill, such as the need to reapply any supplemental oxygen equipment following the procedure.
- Instruct the UCP to report any change in client's respiratory status, secretion colour or volume, or unresolved coughing or gagging.
- Instruct the UCP to report any change in client's colour, vital signs, or complaints of pain.

Equipment

- Appropriate-size suction catheter (smallest diameter that will remove secretions effectively) or Yankauer catheter (oral suction)
- Nasal or oral airway (if indicated)
- Two sterile gloves or one sterile and one clean disposable glove, or one disposable (refer to technique)
- Clean towel or paper drape
- Portable or wall suction
- Mask or face shield
- Connecting tube (1.8 metres)

Equipment that will be needed if not using closed-suction catheter:

- Small Y adapter (if catheter does not have a suction-control port)
- Water-soluble lubricant
- Sterile basin
- Sterile normal saline solution or water (about 100 mL)

Steps	Rationale
1. Assess signs and symptoms of upper and lower airway obstruction requiring nasotracheal or orotracheal suctioning, including respiratory rate or adventitious sounds, nasal secretions, drooling, gastric secretions, or vomitus in mouth.	Physical signs and symptoms result from pooling of secretions in upper and lower airways.
2. Assess signs and symptoms associated with hypoxia and hypercapnia: apprehension, anxiety, decreased ability to concentrate, lethargy, decreased level of consciousness (especially acute), increased fatigue, dizziness, behavioural changes (especially irritability), increased pulse rate or rate of breathing, decreased depth of breathing, elevated blood pressure, cardiac dysrhythmias, pallor, cyanosis, and dyspnea.	Physical signs and symptoms resulting from decreased oxygen to tissues indicate need for suctioning.
3. Determine factors that normally influence upper or lower airway functioning:	
a. Fluid status	Fluid overload may increase amount of secretions. Dehydration promotes thicker secretions.
b. Lack of humidity	The environment influences secretion formation and gas exchange, necessitating airway suctioning when client cannot clear secretions effectively.
c. Infection	Clients with respiratory infections are prone to increased secretions that are thicker and sometimes more difficult to expectorate.
d. Anatomy	Abnormal anatomy can impair normal drainage of secretions. For example, nasal swelling, a deviated septum, or facial fractures may impair nasal drainage. Tumours in or around the lower airway may impair secretion removal by occluding or externally compressing the lumen of the airway.
4. Assess client's understanding of procedure.	Reveals need for client instruction and also encourages co-operation.
5. Obtain physician's order if indicated by agency policy.	Some institutions require a physician's order for tracheal suctioning.

Skill 35-1 Suctioning—cont'd

Steps	Rationale
6. Explain to client how procedure will help clear airway and relieve breathing problems and that temporary coughing, sneezing, gagging, or shortness of breath is normal. Encourage client to cough out secretions. Practise coughing, if able. Splint surgical incisions, if necessary.	Encourages co-operation and minimizes risks, anxiety, and pain.
7. Explain importance of and encourage coughing during procedure.	Facilitates secretion removal and may reduce frequency and duration of future suctioning.
8. Help client to assume position comfortable for nurse and client (usually semi-Fowler's or sitting upright with head hyperextended, unless contraindicated).	Reduces stimulation of gag reflex, promotes client comfort and secretion drainage, and prevents aspiration. Position lessens strain on nurse's back. Hyperextension facilitates insertion of catheter into trachea.
9. Place pulse oximeter on client's finger. Take reading and leave pulse oximeter in place.	Provides baseline oxygen level to determine client's response to suctioning.
10. Place towel across client's chest.	Reduces transmission of micro-organisms by protecting gown from secretions.
11. Perform hand hygiene.	Reduces transmission of micro-organisms.
12. Preparation for all types of suctioning:	
a. Open suction kit or catheter with use of aseptic technique. If sterile drape is available, place it across client's chest or on the overbed table. Do not allow the suction catheter to touch any nonsterile surfaces.	Prepares catheter and prevents transmission of micro-organisms. Provides sterile surface on which to lay suction catheter between passes, if needed.
b. Unwrap or open sterile basin and place on bedside table. Fill basin or cup with approximately 100 mL of sterile normal saline solution or water (see illustration)	Unwrap or open sterile cup/basin. Place on bedside table.
c. Connect one end of connecting tubing to suction machine. Place other end in convenient location near client. Check that equipment is functioning properly by suctioning a small amount of water from basin.	
d. Turn on suction device. Set regulator to appropriate negative pressure: wall suction, 80 to 120 mm Hg; portable suction, 7 to 15 mm Hg for adults.	Elevated pressure settings increase risk of trauma to mucosa and can induce greater hypoxia.

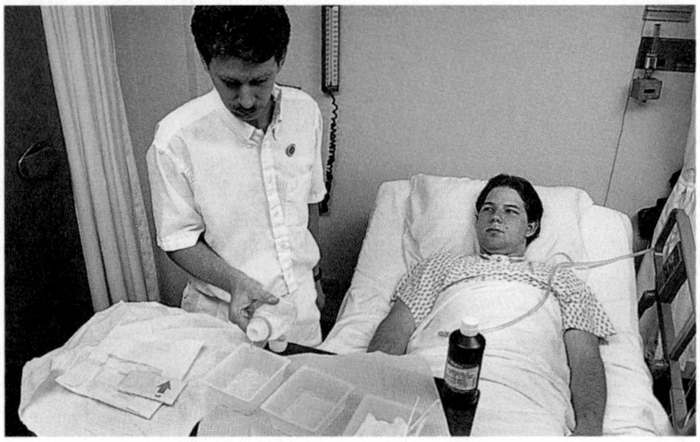

STEP **12b** Pouring sterile saline into basin.

Steps	Rationale
13. Suction airway.	
A. **Oropharyngeal suctioning**	
(1) Apply clean disposable glove to dominant hand.	Suction of oral cavity does not require sterile glove use.
(2) Consider applying mask or face shield.	Suction may cause splashing of body fluids.
(3) Attach suction catheter to connecting tubing. Remove oxygen mask if present.	
(4) Insert catheter into client's mouth. With suction applied, move catheter around mouth, including pharynx and gum line, until secretions are cleared.	If catheter does not have a suction control to apply intermittent suction, take care not to allow suction tip to invaginate oral mucosal surfaces with continuous suction (St. John, 1999).
(5) Encourage client to cough, and repeat suctioning if needed. Replace oxygen mask if used.	Coughing moves secretions from lower to upper airways into mouth.
(6) Suction water from basin through catheter until catheter is cleared of secretions.	Clearing secretions before they dry reduces probability of transmission of micro-organisms and enhances delivery of preset suction pressures.
(7) Place catheter in a clean, dry area for reuse with suction turned off or within client's reach, with suction on, if client is capable of suctioning self.	Facilitates prompt removal of airway secretions when suctioning is needed in the future.
B. **Nasopharyngeal and nasotracheal suctioning**	
(1) If indicated, increase supplemental oxygen therapy to 100% or as ordered by physician. Encourage client's deep breathing.	Preoxygenation and deep breathing assist in reducing suction-induced hypoxemia (Day et al., 2002). Preoxygenation should be used with caution in oxygen-sensitive clients, such as those with chronic heart and lung conditions and those with pneumonia.

Critical Decision Point: Following the suction procedure, the client's oxygen must be readjusted as ordered by physician after procedure to avoid increased risk of oxygen toxicity and absorption atelectasis from prolonged administration of high concentrations of oxygen and increased carbon dioxide retention in clients with chronic obstructive lung diseases (Day et al., 2002).

Steps	Rationale
(2) Open lubricant. Squeeze small amount onto open sterile catheter package without touching package.	Prepares lubricant while maintaining sterility. Water-soluble lubricant is used to avoid lipoid aspiration pneumonia. Excessive lubricant can occlude catheter.
(3) Apply sterile glove to each hand, or apply non-sterile glove to non-dominant hand and sterile glove to dominant hand.	Reduces transmission of micro-organisms and allows nurse to maintain sterility of suction catheter.

Critical Decision Point: A clean technique is used in selected settings, such as the home or long-term care facility, and with clients with an established tracheostomy who do not have an airway infection.

Steps	Rationale
(4) Pick up suction catheter with dominant hand without touching non-sterile surfaces. Pick up connecting tubing with non-dominant hand. Secure catheter to tubing (see illustration).	Maintains catheter sterility. Connects catheter to suction.
(5) Check that the equipment is functioning properly by suctioning small amount of normal saline solution from basin.	Ensures equipment function; lubricates catheter and tubing.
(6) Lightly coat distal 6 to 8 cm of catheter with water-soluble lubricant.	Lubricates catheter for easier insertion.
(7) Remove oxygen delivery device, if applicable, with non-dominant hand. **Without applying suction** and using dominant thumb and forefinger, gently insert catheter into naris during inhalation.	Application of suction pressure while introducing catheter into nasopharyngeal tissues increases risk of damage to mucosa. When advanced into trachea, suction could damage mucosa and increase risk of hypoxia. Proper placement ensures removal of pharyngeal secretions.

Skill 35-1 Suctioning—cont'd

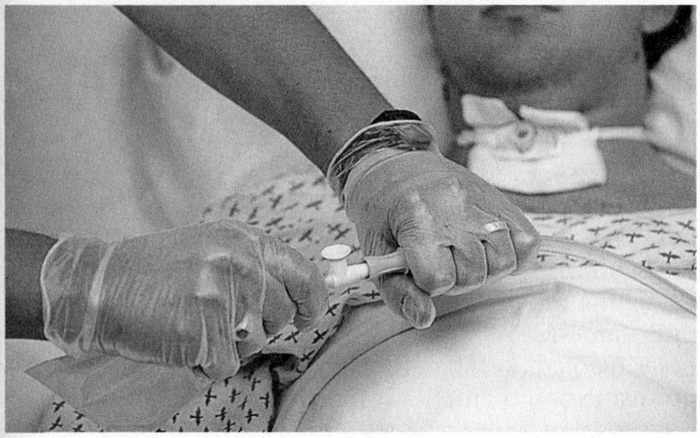

STEP **13B(4)** Attaching catheter to suction.

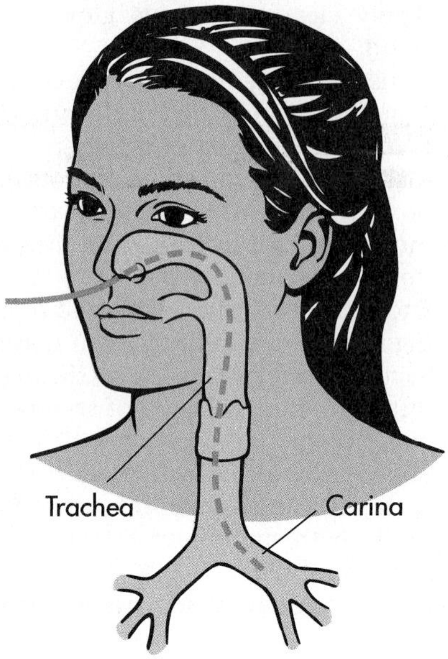

STEP **13B(9)** Distance of insertion of nasotracheal catheter.

(8) *Nasopharyngeal:* Follow natural course of naris; slightly slant catheter downward and advance to back of pharynx. In adults, insert catheter about 16 cm; in older children, 8 to 12 cm; in infants and young children, 4 to 8 cm. Rule of thumb is to insert catheter distance from tip of nose (or mouth) to base of earlobe.

Intermittent suction safely removes pharyngeal secretions.

a. Apply intermittent suction for up to 10 to 15 seconds by placing and releasing nondominant thumb over catheter vent. Slowly withdraw catheter while rotating it back and forth between thumb and forefinger.

(9) *Nasotracheal:* Follow natural course of naris and advance catheter slightly slanted and downward to just above entrance into trachea. Allow client to take a breath. Quickly insert catheter about 16 to 20 cm (in adult) into trachea (see illustration). Client will begin to cough. NOTE: In older children, advance 14 to 20 cm; in young children and infants, 8 to 14 cm.

Ensures catheter will be inserted into trachea with minimum stress to client.

Critical Decision Point: Insert catheter during client inhalation, especially if inserting catheter into trachea because epiglottis is open. **Do not insert during swallowing** or catheter will most likely enter esophagus. **Never** apply suction during insertion. Client should cough. If client gags or becomes nauseated, catheter is most likely in esophagus and must be removed.

Steps	Rationale
a. *Positioning option for nasotracheal suctioning:* In some instances, turning client's head to right helps nurse suction left mainstem bronchus; turning head to left helps nurse suction right mainstem bronchus. If resistance is felt after insertion of catheter for maximum recommended distance, catheter has probably hit carina. Pull catheter back 1 cm before applying suction.	

Critical Decision Point: Use nasal approach and perform tracheal suctioning before pharyngeal suctioning whenever possible. The mouth and pharynx contain more bacteria than the trachea does. If copious oral secretions are present before beginning the procedure, suction mouth with oral suction device.

b. Apply intermittent suction for up to 10 to 15 seconds by placing and releasing non-dominant thumb over vent of catheter and slowly withdrawing catheter while rotating it back and forth between dominant thumb and forefinger. Encourage client to cough. Replace oxygen device, if applicable.	Intermittent suction and rotation of catheter prevent injury to mucosa. If catheter "grabs" mucosa, remove thumb to release suction. Suctioning longer than 10 seconds can cause cardiopulmonary compromise, usually from hypoxemia or vagal overload.

Critical Decision Point: If ordered to monitor client's vital signs and oxygen saturation during procedure, note if there is a 20-beats-per-minute change (either increase or decrease) or if pulse oximetry falls below 90% or 5% from baseline (Akgul & Akyolcu, 2002).

(10) Rinse catheter and connecting tubing with normal saline or water until cleared.	Removes secretions from catheter. Secretions that remain in suction catheter or connecting tubing decrease suctioning efficiency.
(11) Assess for need to repeat suctioning procedure. Allow adequate time between suction passes for ventilation and oxygenation. Ask client to deep breathe and to cough.	Observe for alterations in cardiopulmonary status. Suctioning can induce hypoxemia, dysrhythmias, laryngospasm, and bronchospasm. Deep breathing reventilates and reoxygenates alveoli. Repeated passes clear the airway of excessive secretions but can also remove oxygen and may induce laryngospasm.
C. **Artificial airway suctioning**	
(1) Apply face shield.	Reduces transmission of micro-organisms.
(2) Prepare proper suction catheter.	Suction catheter's outer diameter should not exceed one half of internal diameter of the endotracheal tube (ET) or tracheostomy tube (St. John, 1999).
(3) Apply one sterile glove to each hand, or apply non-sterile glove to non-dominant hand and sterile glove to dominant hand.	Reduces transmission of micro-organisms and allows nurse to maintain sterility of suction catheter.
(4) Pick up suction catheter with dominant hand without touching non-sterile surfaces. Pick up connecting tubing with non-dominant hand. Secure catheter to tubing.	Maintains catheter sterility. Establishes suction.
(5) Check that equipment is functioning properly by suctioning small amount of saline from basin.	Ensures equipment function; lubricates catheter and tubing.
(6) Hyperinflate and/or hyperoxygenate client before suctioning, using manual resuscitation Ambu-bag connected to oxygen source on mechanical ventilator. Some mechanical ventilators have a button that when pushed delivers 100% oxygen for a few minutes and then resets to the previous value.	Hyperinflation decreases the risk for atelectasis caused by negative pressure of suctioning (St. John, 1999). Preoxygenation converts large proportion of resident lung gas to 100% oxygen to offset amount used in metabolic consumption while ventilator or oxygenation is interrupted, as well as to offset volume lost during suction procedure (Day et al., 2002; Wood, 1998).

Skill 35-1 Suctioning—cont'd

Steps	Rationale

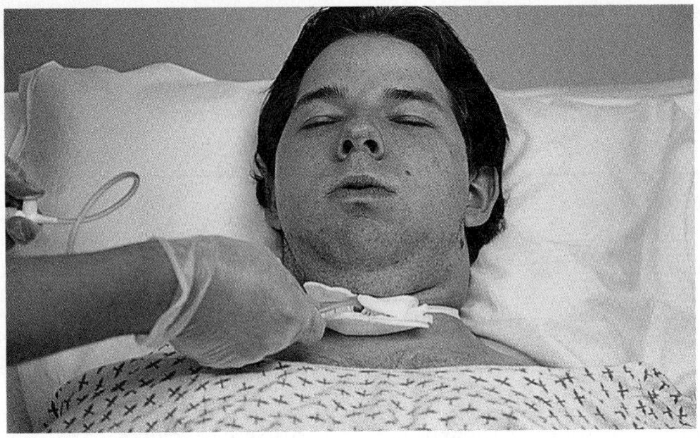

STEP **13C(9)** Suctioning tracheostomy.

Steps	Rationale
(7) If client is receiving mechanical ventilation, open swivel adapter or if necessary remove oxygen or humidity delivery device with non-dominant hand.	Exposes artificial airway.
(8) Without applying suction, gently but quickly insert catheter using dominant thumb and forefinger into artificial airway (best to time catheter insertion with inspiration) until resistance is met or client coughs; then pull back 1 cm.	Application of suction pressure while introducing catheter into trachea increases risk of damage to tracheal mucosa, as well as increased hypoxia related to removal of entrained oxygen present in airways. Pulling back stimulates cough and removes catheter from mucosal wall so that catheter is not resting against tracheal mucosa during suctioning.

Critical Decision Point: If unable to insert catheter past the end of the ET tube, the catheter is probably caught in the Murphy eye (i.e., side hole at the distal end of the ET tube that allows for collateral airflow in the event of main stem intubation). If this happens, rotate the catheter to reposition it away from the Murphy eye, or withdraw it slightly and reinsert with the next inhalation. Usually the catheter meets resistance at the carina. One indication that the catheter is at the carina is acute onset of coughing because the carina contains many cough receptors. The catheter should be pulled back.

Steps	Rationale
(9) Apply intermittent suction by placing and releasing non-dominant thumb over vent of catheter; slowly withdraw catheter while rotating it back and forth between dominant thumb and forefinger (see illustration). Encourage client to cough. Watch for respiratory distress.	Intermittent suction and rotation of catheter prevent injury to tracheal mucosal lining. If catheter "grabs" mucosa, remove thumb to release suction.

Critical Decision Point: If client develops respiratory distress during the suction procedure, immediately withdraw catheter and supply additional oxygen and breaths as needed. Oxygen can be administered directly through the catheter in an emergency. Disconnect suction and attach oxygen at prescribed flow rate through the catheter.

Steps	Rationale
(10) If client is receiving mechanical ventilation, close swivel adapter or replace oxygen delivery device.	Re-establishes the artificial airway.
(11) Encourage client to deep breathe, if able. Some clients respond well to several manual breaths from the mechanical ventilator or Ambu-bag.	Reoxygenates and re-expands alveoli. Suctioning can cause hypoxemia and atelectasis.

Steps	Rationale
(12) Rinse catheter and connecting tubing with normal saline until clear. Use continuous suction.	Removes catheter secretions. Secretions left in tubing decrease suction and provide environment for micro-organism growth. Secretions left in connecting tube decrease suctioning efficiency.
(13) Assess client's cardiopulmonary status for secretion clearance and complications. Repeat steps 13C(6) through (12) once or twice more to clear secretions. Allow adequate time (at least 1 full minute) between suction passes for ventilation and reoxygenation.	Suctioning can induce dysrhythmias, hypoxia, and bronchospasm and impair cerebral circulation or adversely affect hemodynamics (Akgul & Akyolcu, 2002; Kerr et al., 1999). Repeated passes with suction catheter clear airway of excessive secretions and promote improved oxygenation (Wood, 1998).
Perform oropharyngeal and nasopharyngeal suctioning (steps 13A, 13B). After oropharyngeal and nasopharyngeal suctioning is performed, catheter is contaminated; do not reinsert into ET or tracheostomy tube.	Upper airway is considered clean and lower airway is considered sterile. Therefore the same catheter can be used to suction from sterile to clean areas, but not from clean to sterile areas.
14. Complete procedure:	
a. Disconnect catheter from connecting tubing. Roll catheter around fingers of dominant hand. Pull glove off inside out so that catheter remains in glove. Pull off other glove over first glove in same way to contain contaminants. Discard into appropriate receptacle. Turn off suction device.	Reduces transmission of micro-organisms. Clean equipment should not be touched with contaminated gloves.
b. Remove towel and place in laundry or remove drape and discard in appropriate receptacle.	
c. Reposition client as indicated by condition. Nurse may need to reapply clean gloves for client's personal care (e.g., oral hygiene).	Proper positioning based on client's condition promotes comfort, encourages secretion drainage, and reduces risk of aspiration.
d. If indicated, readjust oxygen to original level because client's blood oxygen level should have been returned to baseline.	
e. Discard remainder of normal saline into appropriate receptacle. If basin is disposable, discard into appropriate receptacle. If basin is reusable, rinse and place in soiled utility room.	Solution is contaminated.
f. Remove and discard face shield, and perform hand hygiene.	Reduces transmission of micro-organisms.
g. Place unopened suction kit on suction machine table or at head of bed according to institution preference.	Provides for immediate access of suction catheter and equipment in the event of an emergency or for the next suctioning procedure.
15. Compare client's vital signs and O_2 saturation before and after suctioning.	Identifies physiological effects of suction procedure to restore airway patency.
16. Ask client if breathing is easier and if congestion is decreased.	Provides subjective confirmation that airway obstruction is relieved with suctioning procedure.
17. Observe airway secretions.	Provides data to document presence or absence of respiratory tract infection.

Skill 35-1 Suctioning—cont'd

Steps	Rationale

Unexpected Outcomes and Related Interventions

- Worsening respiratory status
  - Limit length of suctioning.
  - Determine need for more frequent suctioning, possibly of shorter duration.
  - Notify physician.
- Return of bloody secretions
  - Determine amount of suction pressure used. May need to be decreased.
  - Evaluate suctioning frequency.
  - Provide more frequent oral hygiene.
- Unable to pass suction catheter through first naris attempted
  - Try other naris or oral route.
  - Insert nasal airway, especially if suctioning through client naris frequently.
  - Guide catheter along naris floor to avoid turbinates.
  - If obstruction is mucus, apply suction to relieve obstruction, but do not apply suction to mucosa. If obstruction is thought to be a blood clot, consult physician.
  - Increase lubrication of catheter.
- Paroxysms of coughing
  - Administer supplemental oxygen.
  - Allow client to rest between passes of suction catheter.
  - Consult physician regarding need for inhaled bronchodilators or topical anaesthetics.
- No secretions obtained
  - Evaluate client's fluid status.
  - Assess for signs of infection.
  - Determine need for chest physiotherapy.
  - Assess adequacy of humidification on oxygen delivery device.

Recording and Reporting

- Record the amount, consistency, colour, and odour of secretions and client's response to procedure; document client's pre-suctioning and post-suctioning cardiopulmonary status.

Home Care Considerations

- It is necessary to adhere to best practices for infection control while weighing cost-effectiveness in the presence of a chronic situation. If the client has an established tracheostomy or requires long-term nasotracheal suctioning and infection is not present, clean suction technique is appropriate.
- Instruct client and family how to practise infection-control measures when emptying the secretion jar.

coughing and does not have an artificial airway present (see Skill 35-1). A catheter is passed through the mouth or nose into the trachea. The nose is the preferred route because stimulation of the gag reflex is minimal. The procedure is similar to nasopharyngeal suctioning, but the catheter tip is moved farther into the client's trachea. The entire procedure from catheter passage to its removal should be done quickly, lasting no longer than 15 seconds. Unless in respiratory distress, the client should be allowed to rest between passes of the catheter. If the client is using supplemental oxygen, the oxygen cannula or mask should be replaced during rest periods.

Tracheal Suctioning. Tracheal suctioning is accomplished through an artificial airway such as an endotracheal tube or tracheostomy tube (see Skill 35-1). The suction catheter should be no greater than one half the size of the internal diameter of the artificial airway. Secretion removal should be as atraumatic as possible. To avoid trauma to the mucosa of the lung, the nurse should never apply suction pressure while inserting the catheter, and suction pressure should be maintained between 120 and 180 mm Hg. Suction is applied intermittently as the catheter is withdrawn. Rotating the catheter will enhance removal of secretions that have adhered to the sides of the ET. The nurse should wear a mask and goggles and may need to wear a barrier gown to prevent splashes with body fluids.

The two current methods of suctioning are the open and closed methods. Open suctioning involves a sterile catheter that is opened at the time of suctioning. The nurse wears sterile gloves to perform the suction procedure. Closed suctioning involves a multiple-use suction catheter that is encased in a plastic sheath (Figure 35–11). Closed suctioning is most often used on clients who require mechanical ventilation to support their respiratory efforts, because it permits continuous delivery of oxygen while suction is performed, thus reducing the risk of oxygen desaturation. Although sterile gloves are not used in this procedure, nonsterile (i.e., disposable) gloves are recommended to prevent contact with splashes from body fluids.

Artificial Airways. An artificial airway is indicated for clients with decreased level of consciousness or airway obstruction and to aid in removal of tracheobronchial secretions.

Oral Airway. The oral airway, the simplest type of artificial airway, prevents obstruction of the trachea by displacement of the tongue into the oropharynx (Figure 35–12). The oral airway extends from the teeth to the

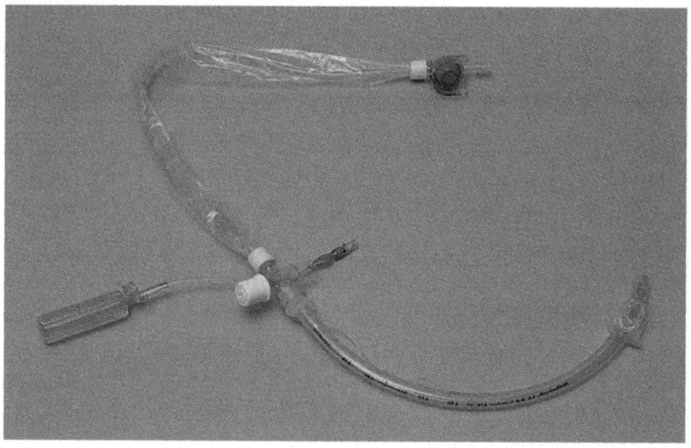

FIGURE **35–11** Ballard tracheal care, closed suction.

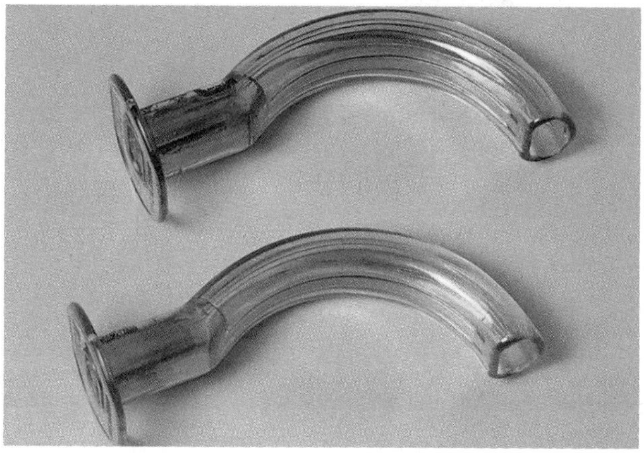

FIGURE **35–12** Artificial oral airways.

oropharynx, maintaining the tongue in the normal position. The correct-size airway must be used. Proper oral airway size is determined by measuring the distance from the corner of the mouth to the angle of the jaw just below the ear. The length is equal to the distance from the flange of the airway to the tip. If the airway is too small, the tongue is not held in the anterior portion of the mouth; if the airway is too large, it may force the tongue toward the epiglottis and obstruct the airway.

The nurse inserts the airway by turning the curve of the airway toward the cheek and placing it over the tongue. When the airway is in the oropharynx, the nurse turns it so that the opening points downward. When correctly placed, the airway moves the tongue forward away from the oropharynx, and the flange, the flat portion of the airway, rests against the client's teeth. Incorrect insertion merely forces the tongue back into the oropharynx.

Endotracheal and Tracheal Airway. The presence of an artificial airway places the client at high risk for infection and airway injury. Sterile technique is used in caring for and maintaining an artificial airway to prevent nosocomial infections. Artificial airways need be cared for and maintained in the correct position to prevent airway damage (Skill 35-2).

Endotracheal tubes (ETs) are used as short-term artificial airways to administer mechanical ventilation, relieve upper airway obstruction, protect against aspiration, or clear secretions. ET tubes are generally removed within 14 days; however, they may be used for a longer period of time if the client is showing progress toward weaning from mechanical ventilation and extubation.

If the client requires long-term assistance from an artificial airway, a tracheostomy is considered. A surgical incision is made into the trachea, and a short artificial airway (a tracheostomy tube) is inserted.

Maintenance and Promotion of Lung Expansion. Nursing interventions to maintain or promote lung expansion include non-invasive and invasive techniques. Non-invasive techniques include positioning and incentive spirometry. Invasive procedures include management of a chest tube.

Positioning. In the healthy, completely mobile person, adequate ventilation and oxygenation are maintained by frequent position changes during daily activities. However, when a person's illness or injury restricts mobility, there is an increased risk for respiratory impairment. Frequent changes of position are simple and cost-effective methods for reducing the risks of stasis of pulmonary secretions and decreased chest wall expansion.

The most effective position for clients with cardiopulmonary diseases is the 45-degree semi-Fowler's position, using gravity to assist in lung expansion and reduce pressure from the abdomen on the diaphragm. When the client uses this position, the nurse needs to ensure that the client does not slide down in bed, which could reduce lung expansion. A client with unilateral lung disease (e.g., pneumothorax, atelectasis, pneumonia, thoracotomy, multiple trauma affecting one lung) should be positioned with the unaffected lung down ("good lung down"). This promotes better perfusion of the healthy lung, improving oxygenation. In the presence of pulmonary abscess or hemorrhage, the client should be placed with the affected lung down to prevent drainage toward the unaffected (healthy) lung.

Incentive Spirometry. **Incentive spirometry** is a method of encouraging voluntary deep breathing by providing visual feedback to clients about inspiratory volume. Incentive spirometry is used to promote deep breathing and to prevent or treat atelectasis in the post-operative client. Studies have shown no respiratory benefit to post-operative incentive spirometry when compared with deep breathing and early ambulation (Fujimoto et al., 2002; Stulbarg et al., 2002).

Flow-oriented incentive spirometers consist of one or more plastic chambers containing freely moving coloured balls. The client inhales slowly and with an even flow to elevate the balls and to keep them floating as long as possible to ensure a maximally sustained inhalation.

Volume-oriented incentive spirometry devices have a bellows that is raised to a predetermined volume by an inhaled breath (Figure 35–13). An achievement light or counter is used to provide feedback. Some devices are constructed so that the light will not turn on unless the bellows is held at a minimum desired volume for a specified period to enhance lung expansion.

Incentive spirometry encourages clients to breathe to their normal inspiratory capacities. A post-operative

Text continued on p. 1127

Skill 35-2 Care of an Artificial Airway

Delegation Considerations

This skill should not be routinely delegated to unregulated care providers (UCPs). It is the responsibility of the nurse to perform endotracheal care. In some settings, clients who have well-established tracheostomy tubes may have the care delegated to UCPs. It is the responsibility of the nurse to assess and ensure that proper artificial airway care is provided. In addition, UCPs may perform other aspects of the client's care. The nurse should instruct the UCP about the following:

- To report any changes in client's respiratory status, level of consciousness, confusion, pain
- Emergency procedures in case the tracheostomy tube inadvertently becomes dislodged when ties are changed
- Expected drainage from tracheostomy

Equipment

- Endotracheal (ET) tube care
  - Towel
  - ET and oropharyngeal suction equipment
  - 2.5 to 3 cm adhesive or waterproof tape (not paper tape) or commercial ET holder (follow manufacturer's instructions for securing)
  - Two pairs of disposable (non-sterile) gloves
  - Adhesive remover swab or acetone on a cotton ball
  - Mouth care supplies (e.g., toothbrush, toothpaste, mouth swabs)
  - Face cleanser (e.g., wet washcloth, towel, soap, shaving supplies)
  - Clean 2 × 2 gauze
  - Tincture of benzoin or liquid adhesive
  - Face shield (if indicated)
- Tracheostomy care
  - Towel
  - Tracheostomy suction supplies
  - Sterile tracheostomy care kit, if available, or three sterile 4 × 4 gauze pads
  - Sterile cotton-tipped applicators
  - Sterile tracheostomy dressing
  - Sterile basin
  - Small sterile brush (or disposable cannula)
  - Tracheostomy ties (e.g., twill tape, manufactured tracheostomy ties, Velcro tracheostomy ties)
  - Hydrogen peroxide
  - Normal saline (NS)
  - Scissors
  - Two sterile gloves
  - Face shield, if indicated

Steps	Rationale
1. Perform pulmonary assessment:	
a. Auscultate lung sounds.	Provides baseline information.
b. Assess condition and potency of airway and surrounding tissues.	Indicates if additional skin care to irritated areas is needed. Identifies potential pressure areas.
c. Note type and size of tube, movement of tube, cuff size.	Movement of tube predisposes client to tracheal trauma or tube dislodgement and may indicate the need for another size airway. Cuff size indicates the amount of air needed to properly inflate cuff. An underinflated cuff increases client's risk for aspiration.
2. Explain procedure to client and family.	Reinforces information given to client and family and provides opportunity to ask additional questions.
3. Position client. Clients usually prefer to be lying down. A client with a long-term well-established tracheostomy may be seated.	Provides access to site and facilitates completion of the procedure.
4. Place towel across client's chest.	Reduces transmission of micro-organisms and protects linens and bedclothes.
5. Perform hand hygiene.	Reduces transmission of micro-organisms.
6. Perform airway care.	
A. **Endotracheal tube care**	
(1) Observe for signs and symptoms of need to perform care of the artificial airway: a. Soiled or loose tape b. Pressure sores on nares, lip, or corner of mouth c. Unstable tube d. Excessive secretions	A client with an artificial airway is at increased risk due to inability to control or difficulty controlling secretions and due to pressure points of the artificial airway.

Steps	Rationale
(2) Identify factors that increase risk of complications from ET tubes: a. Type and size of tube b. Movement of tube up and down trachea c. Cuff size d. Duration of placement	Tube moving up and down trachea disposes client to tracheal trauma or dislodgement. Cuff underinflation may allow aspiration, whereas overinflation may cause ischemia or necrosis of tracheal tissue. Longer duration increases risk of lower airway complications such as pneumonia.
(3) Suction ET tube (see Skill 35-1):	Removes secretions. Diminishes client's need to cough during procedure.

Critical Decision Point: An oral airway should be immediately accessible in the event that the client bites down and obstructs the ET tube.

Steps	Rationale
a. Instruct client not to bite or move ET tube with tongue or pull on tubing; removal of tape can be uncomfortable.	Prepares client for procedure and what to expect.
b. Leave Yankauer suction catheter connected to suction source.	Prepares for oropharyngeal suctioning.
(4) Prepare tape. Cut piece of tape long enough to go completely around client's head from naris to naris plus 15 cm: a. Adult, about 30 to 60 cm b. Lay adhesive side up on bedside table. c. Cut and lay 8 to 16 cm of tape, adhesive side down, in centre of long strip to prevent tape from sticking to hair.	Adhesive tape must be placed around head from cheek to cheek below ears. Avoid over ears, as this may result in a pressure sore.
(5) Have an assistant apply a pair of gloves and hold ET tube firmly so that tube does not move.	Reduces transmission of micro-organisms. Maintains proper tube position and prevents accidental extubation.
a. Carefully remove tape from ET tube and client's face. If tape is difficult to remove, moisten with water or adhesive tape remover. Discard tape in appropriate receptacle if nearby. If not, place soiled tape on bedside table or on distant end of towel.	Provides nurse with access to skin under tape for assessment and hygiene. Reduces transmission of micro-organisms.
b. Use adhesive remover swab to remove excess adhesive left on face after tape removal.	Promotes hygiene. Retained adhesive can cause damage to skin and prevent adhesion of new tape.
c. Remove oral airway or bite block if present.	Provides access and complete observation of client's oral cavity.
d. Clean mouth, gums, and teeth opposite ET tube with mouthwash solution and 4×4 gauze, sponge-tipped applicators, or saline swabs. Brush teeth as indicated. If necessary, administer oropharyngeal suctioning with Yankauer catheter.	Provides oral hygiene and allows for observation of any pressure ulcers.
e. Note "cm" ET tube marking at lips or gums. With help of assistant, move ET tube to opposite side or centre of mouth. Do not change tube depth.	Prevents pressure sore formation at sides of client's mouth. Ensures correct position of tube and allows for quick visual of displaced tube.
f. Repeat oral cleaning as in step d on opposite side of mouth.	Removes secretions from mouth and oropharynx.
g. Clean face and neck with soapy washcloth; rinse and dry. Shave male client as necessary.	Moisture and beard growth prevent adhesive tape adherence.
h. Use tincture of benzoin swab or pour small amount of tincture of benzoin on clean 2×2 gauze and dot on upper lip (oral ET tube) or across nose (nasal ET tube) and cheeks to ear. Allow tincture to dry completely.	Protects and makes skin more receptive to tape.

Skill 35-2 Care of an Artificial Airway—cont'd

Steps	Rationale
i. Slip tape under client's head and neck, adhesive side up. Take care not to twist tape or catch hair. Do not allow tape to stick to itself. It helps to stick tape gently to tongue blade, which serves as a guide as tape is passed behind the client's head. Centre tape so that double-faced tape extends around back of neck from ear to ear.	Positions tape to secure ET tube in proper position.
j. On one side of face, secure tape from ear to naris (nasal ET tube) or edge of mouth (oral ET tube). Tear remaining tape in half lengthwise, forming two pieces that are 1- to 2-cm wide. Secure bottom half of tape across upper lip (oral ET tube) or across top of nose (nasal ET tube; see illustration, *A*). Wrap top half of tape around tube (see illustration, *B*).	Secures tape to face. Using top tape to wrap prevents downward drag on ET tube.
k. Gently pull other side of tape firmly to pick up slack and secure to remaining side of face (see illustration). Assistant can release hold when tube is secure. Nurse may want assistant to help reinsert oral airway.	Secures tape to face and tube. ET tube should be at same depth at the lips. Check earlier assessment for verification of tube depth in centimetres.
l. Clean oral airway in warm soapy water and rinse well. Hydrogen peroxide can aid in removal of crusted secretions. Shake excess water from oral airway.	Promotes hygiene. Reduces transmission of micro-organisms.
m. For unconscious client, reinsert oral airway without pushing tongue into oropharynx.	Prevents client from biting ET tube and allows access for oropharyngeal suctioning. An oral airway in a conscious, co-operative client may cause excessive gagging and pressure ulcers to the mouth and tongue.

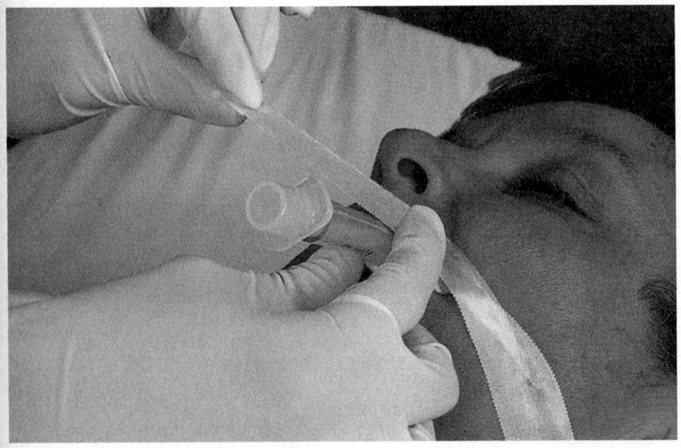

A

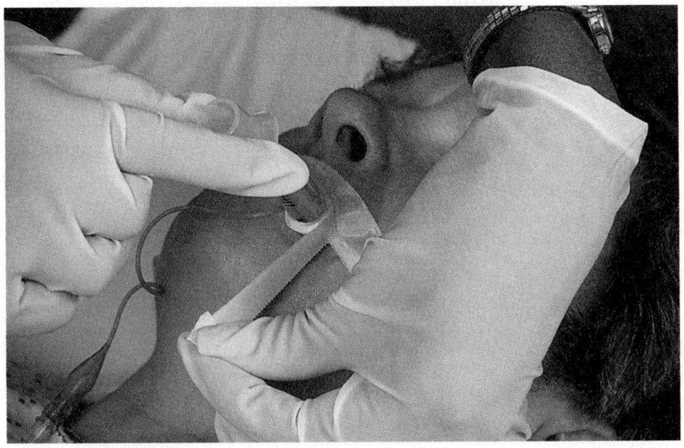

B

STEP **6A(5)j** **A,** Securing bottom half of tape across client's upper lip. **B,** Securing top half of tape around tube.

Steps	Rationale

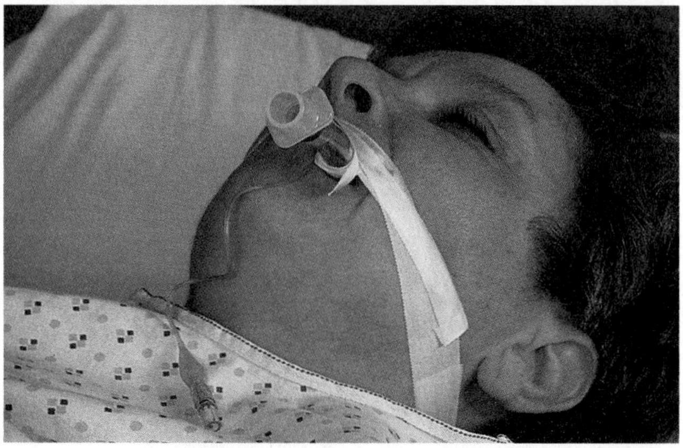

STEP **6A(5)k** Tape securing ET tube.

Steps	Rationale
B. Tracheostomy care	
(1) Observe for signs and symptoms of need to perform tracheostomy care: a. Soiled/loose ties or dressing b. Non-stable tube c. Excessive secretions	A client with a tracheostomy tube is at increased risk due to loss of natural airway protection of the upper airway.
(2) Suction tracheostomy (see Skill 35-1). Before removing gloves, remove soiled tracheostomy dressing and discard in glove with coiled catheter.	Removes secretions so as not to occlude outer cannula while inner cannula is removed. Reduces need for client to cough. Prevents aspiration of retained secretions. Disposal method contains micro-organisms.
(3) Prepare equipment:	
a. Open two packages of cotton-tipped swabs and pour NS on one package and hydrogen peroxide on the other. b. Open sterile tracheostomy package. c. Unwrap sterile basin and pour about 2 cm of hydrogen peroxide into it. d. Open small sterile brush package and place aseptically into sterile basin. e. If using large roll of twill tape, cut appropriate length of tape and lay aside in dry area. Do not recap hydrogen peroxide and NS.	Preparation and organization of equipment allows the nurse to complete tracheostomy care procedure efficiently and then reconnect client to oxygen source in a timely manner.
(4) Apply gloves. Keep dominant hand sterile throughout procedure.	Reduces transmission of micro-organisms.
(5) Remove oxygen source. Apply oxygen source loosely over tracheostomy if client desaturates during procedure.	Helps reduce amount of desaturation.

Critical Decision Point: It is important to stabilize the tracheostomy tube at all times during tracheostomy care to prevent injury and unnecessary discomfort.

Steps	Rationale
(6) If a ***non-disposable inner cannula*** is used:	
a. While touching only the outer aspect of the tube, remove the inner cannula with non-dominant hand. Drop inner cannula into hydrogen peroxide basin.	Removes inner cannula for cleaning. Hydrogen peroxide loosens secretions from inner cannula.
b. Place tracheostomy collar or T tube and ventilator oxygen source over or near outer cannula. (NOTE: T tube and ventilator oxygen devices cannot be attached to all outer cannulas when inner cannula is removed.)	Maintains supply of oxygen to client.

Skill 35-2 Care of an Artificial Airway—cont'd

Steps	Rationale

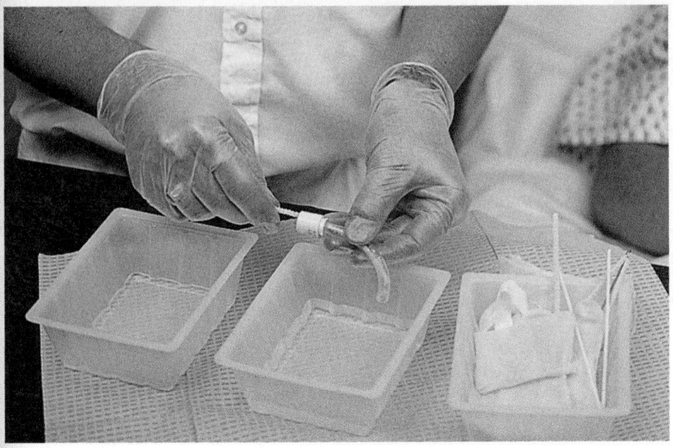

STEP **6B(6)c** Cleaning the tracheostomy inner cannula.

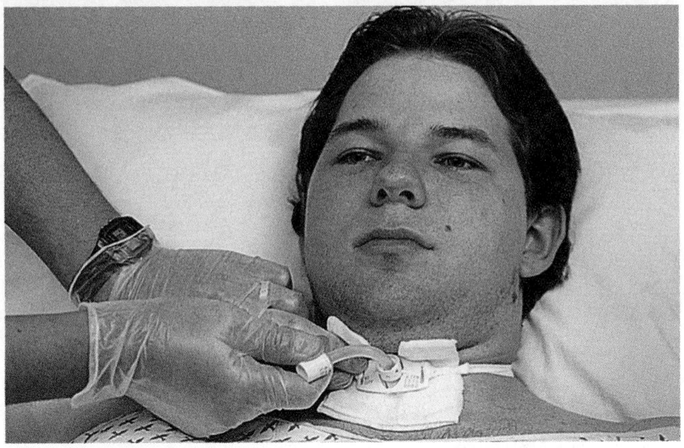

STEP **6B(6)e** Reinserting the inner cannula.

Steps	Rationale
c. To prevent oxygen desaturation in affected clients, quickly pick up inner cannula and use small brush to remove secretions inside and outside cannula (see illustration).	Tracheostomy brush provides mechanical force to remove thick or dried secretions.
d. Hold inner cannula over basin and rinse with NS, using non-dominant hand to pour.	Removes secretions and hydrogen peroxide from inner cannula.
e. Replace inner cannula and secure "locking" mechanism (see illustration). Reapply ventilator or oxygen sources.	
(7) If a ***disposable inner cannula*** is used:	
a. Remove cannula from manufacturer's packaging.	
b. While touching only the outer aspect of the tube, withdraw inner cannula and replace with new cannula. Lock into position.	
c. Dispose of contaminated cannula in appropriate receptacle and apply oxygen source.	Prevents unnecessary oxygen desaturation.
(8) Using hydrogen peroxide-prepared cotton-tipped swabs and 4 × 4 gauze, clean exposed outer cannula surfaces and stoma under faceplate, extending 5 to 10 cm in all directions from stoma (see illustration). Clean in circular motion from stoma site outward, using dominant hand to handle sterile supplies.	Aseptically removes secretions from stoma site.
(9) Using NS-prepared cotton-tipped swabs and 4 × 4 gauze, rinse hydrogen peroxide from tracheostomy tube and skin surfaces.	Rinses hydrogen peroxide from surfaces, preventing possible irritation.
(10) Using dry 4 × 4 gauze, pat lightly at skin and exposed outer cannula surfaces.	Dry surfaces prohibit formation of moist environment from growth of micro-organisms and skin excoriation.

Steps	Rationale

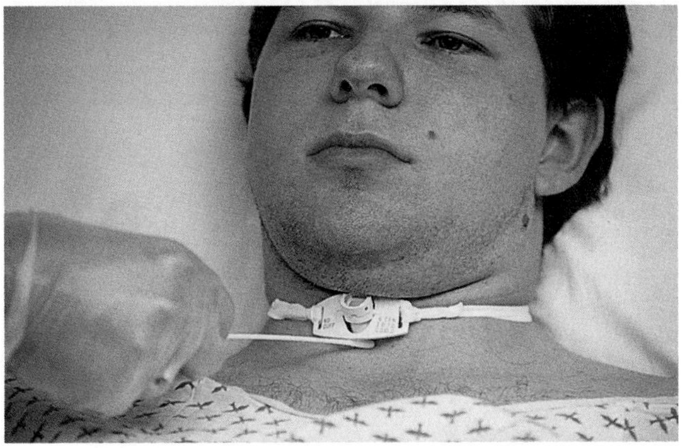

STEP **6B(8)** Cleansing around stoma.

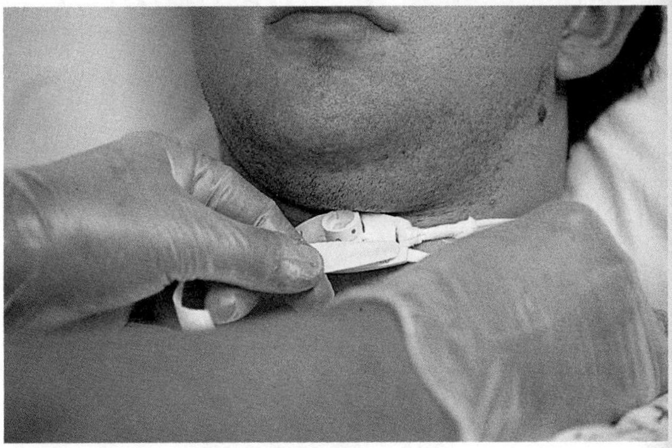

STEP **6B(11)b** Replacing tracheostomy ties when an assistant is not available. Do not remove old tracheostomy ties until new ones are secure.

Steps	Rationale
(11) Instruct assistant, if available, to hold tracheostomy tube securely in place while ties are cut.	Promotes hygiene, reduces transmission of micro-organisms, and secures tracheostomy tube.

Critical Decision Point: Assistant must not release hold on tracheostomy tube until new ties are firmly tied to reduce risk of accidental extubation. If no assistant is present, do not cut old ties until new ties are in place and securely tied. (Follow manufacturer's guidelines for Velcro ties.)

Steps	Rationale
a. Cut length of twill tape long enough to go around client's neck two times, about 60 to 75 cm for an adult. Cut ends on a diagonal.	Cutting ends of tie on a diagonal aids in inserting tie through eyelet.

Critical Decision Point: Secure tracheostomy ties with one-finger slack. For accidental extubation, call for assistance and manually ventilate client with Ambu-bag, if necessary. Tracheostomy obturator should be kept at bedside with a fresh tracheostomy to facilitate reinsertion of the outer cannula, if dislodged. An additional tracheostomy tube of the same size and shape should be kept on hand for emergency replacement. If another tracheostomy tube is not available, insert a size 6 ET tube to keep airway open until physician arrives.

Steps	Rationale
b. Insert one end of tie through faceplate eyelet and pull ends even (see illustration).	
c. Slide both ends of tie behind head and around neck to other eyelet, and insert one tie through second eyelet.	
d. Pull snugly.	Secures tracheostomy tube in place.
e. Tie ends securely in double square knot, allowing space for only one finger in tie.	One-finger slack prevents ties from being too tight when tracheostomy dressing is in place.
f. Insert fresh tracheostomy dressing under clean ties and faceplate (see illustration).	Absorbs drainage. Dressing prevents pressure on clavicle heads.
g. Position client comfortably and assess respiratory status.	Promotes comfort. Some clients may require post-tracheostomy care suctioning.
7. Replace any oxygen delivery devices.	Maintains oxygen therapy.
8. Remove and discard gloves. Perform hand hygiene.	Reduces transmission of infection.
9. Compare respiratory assessments before and after procedure.	Identifies any changes in presence and quality of breath sounds after procedure.
10. Observe depth and position of tubes.	Verifies that position of tube is correct.

Skill 35-2 Care of an Artificial Airway—cont'd

Steps	Rationale

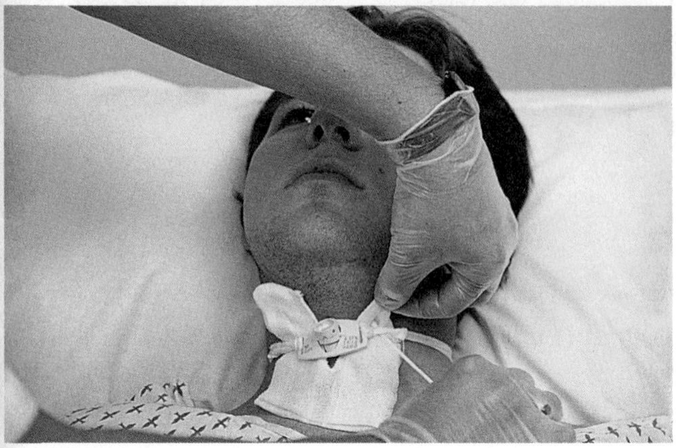

STEP **6B(11)f** Applying tracheostomy dressing.

Steps	Rationale
11. Assess security of tape or commercial ET or tracheostomy tube holder by tugging at tube.	Artificial airway should not move. Client may cough.
12. Assess skin around mouth and oral mucosa (ET tube) and tracheostomy stoma for drainage, pressure, and signs of irritation.	Skin breakdown and/or irritation should not be present.

Unexpected Outcomes and Related Interventions

- Accidental extubation occurs.
  - Call for assistance.
  - Maintain patent airway: Replace old tracheostomy tube with new tube.
  - Observe vital signs and signs of respiratory distress.
- Breath sounds are not equal bilaterally with an ET tube in place.
  - Evaluate ET tube for proper depth. If incorrect, arrange for ET tube to be repositioned as allowed by institution.
  - Obtain order for chest X-ray study to verify placement if applicable.
- Hard, reddened areas with or without excessive or foul-smelling secretions are observed.
  - Indicates infection. Notify physician.
  - Increase frequency of tube care.
  - Remove inner cannula, if applicable, for cleaning and suctioning.
- Tube is not secure, and artificial airway moves in or out or is coughed out by client.
  - Assess client's respiratory status and observe for the presence of mucus plugs.
  - Adjust or apply new ties.
- Breakdown, pressure areas, or stomatitis (tracheostomy tube) are observed.
  - Increase frequency of tube care.
  - Make sure skin areas are clean and dry.

Recording and Reporting

- Record respiratory assessments before and after care.
- Record ET tube care: depth of ET tube, frequency and extent of care, client tolerance, and any complications related to presence of the tube.
- Record tracheostomy care: type and size of tracheostomy tube, frequency and extent of care, client tolerance, and any complications related to presence of the tube.

Home Care Considerations (Tracheostomy Only)

- Instruct caregivers on how to obtain supplies.
- Instruct caregivers on signs and symptoms of respiratory distress, tube dysfunction, and respiratory and stoma infections.

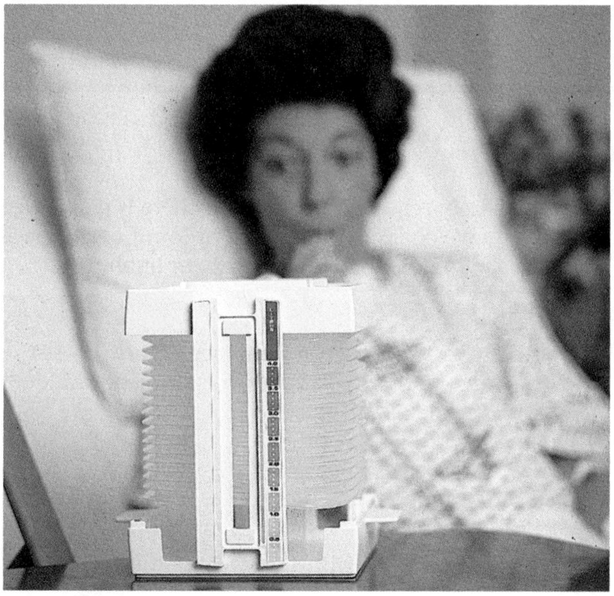

FIGURE **35–13** Volume-oriented spirometer.

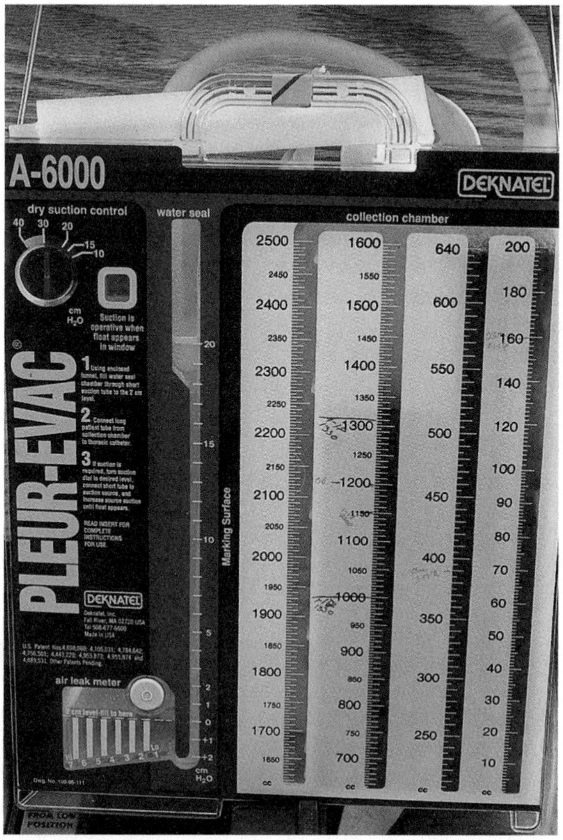

FIGURE **35–14** Disposable, commercial chest drainage system.

inspiratory capacity one half to three fourths of the preoperative volume is acceptable because of postoperative pain. Administration of pain medications before incentive spirometry will help the client achieve deep breathing by reducing pain and splinting (see chapter 45).

Chest Tubes. Chest tubes are inserted to remove air and fluids from the pleural space, to prevent air or fluid from re-entering the pleural space, and to re-establish normal intrapleural and intrapulmonic pressures. A **chest tube** is a catheter inserted through the thorax to remove fluid or air. There are a variety of chest tubes on the market. In addition to the usual disposable waterless system, the traditional reusable glass three-bottle systems may still be used. The newest system available is the mobile chest drain. Regardless of the system used, the principles of client management are the same (Carroll, 2002). Chest tubes are commonly used after chest surgery and chest trauma and for pneumothorax or hemothorax to promote lung re-expansion (Skill 35-3).

A **pneumothorax** is a collection of air in the pleural space. The loss of negative intrapleural pressure causes the lung to collapse. There are a variety of mechanisms for a pneumothorax. It may occur spontaneously or as a result of chest trauma, such as a stabbing or the chest striking the steering wheel in a motor vehicle accident. A pneumothorax may also result from the rupture of an emphysematous bleb on the surface of the lung (a large bulla resulting from the destruction caused by emphysema) or from an invasive procedure, such as insertion of a subclavian IV line.

A client with a pneumothorax usually feels pain as atmospheric air irritates the parietal pleura. The pain may be sharp and pleuritic. Dyspnea is common and worsens as the size of the pneumothorax increases.

A **hemothorax** is an accumulation of blood and fluid in the pleural cavity between the parietal and visceral pleurae, usually as a result of trauma. It produces a counter-pressure and prevents the lung from full expansion. A hemothorax can also be caused by rupture of small blood vessels from inflammatory processes, such as pneumonia or TB. In addition to pain and dyspnea, signs and symptoms of shock can develop if blood loss is severe.

A disposable system, such as a Thora-Sene III or Pleur-Evac chest drainage system (DeKnatel), is a one-piece moulded plastic unit that provides for a single- or multiple-chamber closed drainage system (Figure 35–14). The disposable units appear to be the system of choice because they are cost-effective and some facilitate autotransfusion, a common practice in open-heart surgeries. Knowledge of the basics of chest tube management and troubleshooting manoeuvres reduces the client's risk of complications.

The simplest closed drainage system is the use of a single chamber. The chamber serves as a collector and a water seal. During normal respiration, the fluid will ascend with inspiration and descend with expiration. A single chamber is used for smaller amounts of drainage, such as an empyema—a collection of infected fluid or pus in the pleural space.

The use of two chambers permits the liquid to flow into the collection chamber as air flows into the water-sealed chamber. Fluctuations in the water-seal tube are still anticipated. Use of two chambers allows for more accurate measurement of chest drainage and is used when larger amounts of drainage are expected.

Skill 35-3 Care of Clients With Chest Tubes

Delegation Considerations

This skill should not be delegated to unregulated care providers (UCPs). However, a UCP may assist with other aspects of the client's care and should be informed of the following:

- Proper positioning of the client with chest tubes to facilitate chest tube drainage and optimal function of the system
- How to ambulate and transfer client with chest drainage
- Appropriate set-up of drainage equipment for the type of system to be used
- To report to the nurse of any changes in vital signs, chest pain, sudden shortness of breath, or excessive bubbling in water-seal chamber
- To immediately report to the nurse if there is disconnection of system, change in type and amount of drainage, sudden bleeding, or sudden cessation of bubbling.

Equipment

- Disposable chest drainage system (see Figure 35–14)
- Suction source and set-up (wall canister or portable)
- Disposable (non-sterile) gloves
- 5-cm tape
- Sterile gauze sponges
- Two shodded hemostats

Steps	Rationale
1. Perform hand hygiene and assess client.	Signs and symptoms should reflect improvement in respiratory distress and chest pain after insertion of chest tube.
a. Pulmonary status: Assess for respiratory distress, chest pain, breath sounds over affected lung area, and stable vital signs (see chapter 27). Signs and symptoms of increased respiratory distress and/or chest pain include decreased breath sounds over the affected and non-affected lungs, marked cyanosis, asymmetrical chest movements, presence of subcutaneous emphysema around tube insertion site or neck, hypotension, and tachycardia (Carroll, 2002).	Notify physician immediately.
b. Vital signs	Changes in pulse and blood pressure may indicate infection, respiratory distress, pain.
c. Pain: If possible, ask client to rate level of pain on a scale of 0 to 10.	Chest tubes can be painful and interfere with client's mobility, coughing and deep breathing, and rehabilitation.
2. Observe:	
a. Chest tube dressing and site surrounding tube insertion.	Ensures that dressing is intact and occlusive seal remains without air or fluid leaks and that area surrounding insertion site is free of drainage or skin irritation (Carroll, 2002).
b. Tubing for kinks, dependent loops, or clots.	Maintains a patent, freely draining system, preventing fluid accumulation in chest cavity. The presence of kinks, dependent loops, or clotted drainage increases the client's risk for infection, atelectasis, and tension pneumothorax (Allibone, 2003).
c. Chest drainage system, which should be upright and below level of tube insertion.	Facilitates drainage; system must be in this position to function properly.
3. Provide two shodded hemostats or approved clamps for each chest tube, attached to top of client's bed with adhesive tape. Chest tubes are only clamped under specific circumstances per physician order or nursing policy and procedure: a. To assess air leak b. To quickly empty or change disposable systems; performed by a nurse who has received education in the procedure c. If there is an accidental disconnection of drainage tubing from the drainage collection device or damage to the device	Shodded hemostats have a covering to prevent hemostat from penetrating chest tube once changed. The use of these shodded hemostats or other clamp prevents air from re-entering the pleural space (Allibone, 2003).

Steps	Rationale
d. To assess if client is ready to have chest tube removed (which is done by physician's order); monitor the client for recurrent pneumothorax	
4. Position client.	Permits optimal drainage of fluid and/or air.
a. Semi-Fowler's position to evacuate air (pneumothorax)	Air rises to highest point in chest. Pneumothorax tubes are usually placed on anterior aspect at midclavicular line, second or third intercostal space.
b. High-Fowler's position to drain fluid (hemothorax, effusion)	Permits optimal drainage of fluid. Posterior tubes are placed on midaxillary line, eighth or ninth intercostal space.
5. Maintain tube connection between chest and drainage tubes intact and taped.	Secures chest tube to drainage system and reduces risk of air leak causing breaks in airtight system.
a. Water-sealed vent must be without occlusion.	Permits displaced air to pass into atmosphere.
b. Suction-control chamber vent must be without occlusion when suction is used.	Provides safety factor of releasing excess negative pressure into atmosphere. Too little suction prevents lung re-expansion and increases client risk for infection, atelectasis, and tension pneumothorax. Too much suction damages the lung tissue and perpetuates existing air leaks (Allibone, 2003).
6. Avoid excess tubing; the tubing should be laid horizontally across the client bed or chair before dropping vertically into the drainage bottle. If the client is in a chair and the tubing is coiled, the tubing should be lifted every 15 minutes to promote drainage.	The length of tubing should be tailored to each client to avoid excessive coiling or loop formation. Coiled, looped, or clotted tubing impedes chest tube drainage (Allibone, 2003).
7. Adjust tubing to hang in straight line from top of mattress to drainage chamber. If chest tube is draining fluid, indicate time (e.g., 0900) that drainage was begun on drainage bottle's adhesive tape or on write-on surface of disposable commercial system.	Provides a baseline for continuous assessment of type and quality of drainage.
8. Strip or milk chest tube only if indicated (this means compressing the tube to encourage clots to pass through the tube).	Stripping may cause complications because it creates excessive negative intrapleural pressure (over –100 cm H_2O pressure). Milking causes less of a pressure change.
a. Stripping—compression along length of the tubing beginning at client and continuing until drainage unit is reached	
b. Milking—compressing and releasing the tube sequentially	

Critical Decision Point: Check agency policy before stripping or milking chest tubes. This practice is being discontinued at most institutions because it is believed that stripping the tube greatly increases intrapleural pressure, which could damage the pleural tissue and cause or worsen an existing pneumothorax. However, even though the literature is contradictory, stripping or milking may be done in selected clients (e.g., fresh post-operative thoracic surgery, chest trauma) because the presence of clotted drainage causes decreased re-expansion and increases risk of tension pneumothorax (Allibone, 2003), and the benefits or stripping or milking outweigh the risks.

Steps	Rationale
9. Perform hand hygiene.	Reduces transmission of infection.
10. Evaluate:	
a. Chest tube dressing.	Appearance of drainage may be due to tube occlusion, causing drainage to exit around tube.

Critical Decision Point: Check the dressing carefully because it must remain occlusive. It can come loose from the skin, although this may not be readily apparent.

Steps	Rationale
b. Tubing: should be free of kinks and dependent loops.	Straight and coiled drainage tube positions are optimal for pleural drainage. However, when a dependent loop is unavoidable, periodic lifting and drainage of the tube will promote pleural drainage.

Skill 35-3 Care of Clients With Chest Tubes—cont'd

Steps	Rationale
c. Chest drainage system: should be upright and below level of tube insertion. Note presence of clots or debris in tubing.	System must be in the upright position to function and facilitate proper drainage.
d. Water seal for fluctuations with client's inspiration and expiration.	
(1) Waterless system: diagnostic indicator for fluctuations with client's inspirations and expirations	In the non-mechanically ventilated client, fluid should rise in the water seal or diagnostic indicator with inspiration and fall with expiration. The opposite occurs in the client who is mechanically ventilated. This indicates the system is properly functioning.
(2) Water-seal system: bubbling in the water-seal chamber	When system is initially connected to client, bubbles are expected from the chamber. These are from air that was present in the system and in client's intrapleural space. After a short time, the bubbling stops. Fluid will continue to fluctuate in the water seal on inspiration and expiration until the lung is re-expanded or the system becomes occluded.
e. Waterless system: Bubbling is diagnostic indicator.	Indicates proper functioning of the system.
f. Type and amount of fluid drainage: Nurse should note colour and amount of drainage, client's vital signs, and skin colour. The normal amount of drainage is as follows:	
(1) *In the adult:* less than 50 to 200 mL/hour immediately after surgery in a mediastinal chest tube; approximately 500 mL in first 24 hours.	Dark-red drainage is expected only in the post-operative period, turning serous with time.
(2) Between 100 and 300 mL of fluid may drain in pleural chest tube in an adult during first 3 hours after insertion. This rate will decrease after 2 hours; 500 to 1000 mL can be expected in first 24 hours. Drainage is grossly bloody during first several hours after surgery and then changes to serous. Remember that a sudden gush of drainage may be retained blood and not active bleeding. This increase in drainage can result from client position changes.	Re-expansion of lungs forces drainage into the tube. Coughing can also cause large gushes of drainage or air. Excessive amounts and/or continued presence of frank, bloody drainage during first several hours after surgery should be reported to the physician, along with client's vital signs and respiratory status.

Critical Decision Point: If drainage suddenly increases or if there is more than 100 mL/hour of blood drainage (except for the first 3 hours post-operative), the nurse should inform the physician (Allibone, 2003).

Steps	Rationale
g. Water-sealed system: bubbling in the suction-control chamber (when suction is being used)	Suction-control chamber has constant, gentle bubbling. Tubing to suction source should be free of obstruction, and suction source should be turned on to appropriate setting.
h. Waterless system: The suction control (float ball) indicates the amount of suction that the client's intrapleural space is receiving.	The suction float ball dictates the amount of suction in the system. The float ball allows no more suction than dictated by its setting. If the suction source is set too low, the suction float ball cannot reach the prescribed setting. In this case, the suction must be increased for the float ball to reach the prescribed setting.
i. Lungs: auscultate and observe for symmetry.	Breath sounds should be equal. Decreased breath sounds on the affected side may indicate that air or fluid has re-accumulated in the pleural space. Percuss the area. A hollow sound indicates retained air; a dull/flat sound may indicate the presence of fluid (Carroll, 2002).
j. Pain: ask client to evaluate pain on a level of 0 to 10.	May indicate the need for medication for pain.

Steps	Rationale

Unexpected Outcomes and Related Interventions

- Continuous bubbling is seen in water-sealed chamber, indicating that leak is between client and water seal.
  - Tighten loose connections between client and water seal.
  - Cross-clamp chest tube close to client's chest. If bubbling stops, air leak is inside client's thorax or at chest tube insertion site. Unclamp tube, and notify physician immediately. Reinforce chest dressing. Leaving chest tube clamped causes a tension pneumothorax and mediastinal shift.
  - Gradually move clamps down drainage tubing away from client and toward drainage chamber, moving one clamp at a time. When bubbling stops, leak is in section of tubing or connection distal to the clamp. Replace tubing or secure connection and release clamp.
- Leak is in drainage system.
  - Change drainage system.
- Tension pneumothorax is present.
  - Determine that chest tubes are not clamped, kinked, or occluded. Obstructed chest tubes trap air in intrapleural space when air leak originates within client.
  - Notify physician immediately.
  - Prepare immediately for another chest tube insertion; obtain a flutter (Heimlich) valve or large-gauge needle for short-term emergency release of air in intrapleural space; have emergency equipment (e.g., oxygen, code cart) near client.
- Dependent loops of drainage tubing have trapped fluid.
  - Drain tubing contents into drainage bottle. Coil excess tubing onto mattress, and secure in place or place in a straight line down the length of the bed.

Recording and Reporting

- Record in nurse's notes patency of chest; presence, type, and amount of drainage; presence of fluctuations; client's vital signs; chest dressing status, amount of suction and/or water seal; and level of comfort.

Home Care Considerations

- Client with chronic conditions (e.g., uncomplicated pneumothorax, effusions, empyema) that require a chest tube may be discharged home with smaller mobile chest drains. These systems do not have a suction-control chamber and use a mechanical one-way valve instead of a water-seal chamber (Carroll, 2002).
- Instruct client how to ambulate and remain active with a home chest tube drainage system.
- Provide client with information as to when to contact health care professionals regarding changes in drainage system (e.g., chest pain, breathlessness, change in drainage).

When a volume of air or fluid needs to be evacuated with controlled suction, all three chambers are used. The suction control is marked with centimetre readings to adjust the amount of suction. Usually 15 to 20 cm of water is used for adults. This means that the chamber is filled with sterile water to the 15- or 20-cm water level. Children require less pressure.

Special Considerations. Clamping a chest tube at any time is inadvisable. The nurse should instead handle the chest drainage unit carefully and maintain the drainage device below the client's chest. If the tubing disconnects from the drainage unit, the nurse should instruct the client to exhale as much as possible and to cough. This manoeuvre rids the pleural space of as much air as possible. The nurse needs to cleanse the tips of the tubing and reconnect them quickly. If the drainage unit is broken, the end of the chest tube can be quickly submerged in a container of sterile water to re-establish the seal. Clamping the chest tube may result in a tension pneumothorax. Air pressure builds in the pleural space, collapsing the lung and creating a life-threatening event.

Removal of chest tubes requires client preparation. Clients report various sensations during chest tube removal. The most frequent sensations include burning, pain, and a pulling sensation.

Maintenance and Promotion of Oxygenation. Promotion of lung expansion, mobilization of secretions, and maintenance of a patent airway assists the client in meeting oxygenation needs. Some clients, however, also require oxygen therapy to keep a healthy level of tissue oxygenation.

Oxygen Therapy. Oxygen therapy is cheap, widely available, and used in a variety of settings to relieve or prevent tissue hypoxia (Thomson et al., 2002). The goal of oxygen therapy is to prevent or relieve hypoxia. Any client with impaired tissue oxygenation can benefit from controlled oxygen administration. Oxygen is not a substitute for other treatment, however, and should be used only when indicated. Oxygen should be treated as a drug. It has dangerous side effects, such as atelectasis or oxygen toxicity (Thomson et al., 2002). As with any drug, the dosage or concentration of oxygen should be continuously monitored. The nurse should routinely check the physician's orders to verify that the client is receiving the prescribed oxygen concentration. The six rights of medication administration also pertain to oxygen administration (see chapter 30).

Safety Precautions. Oxygen is a highly combustible gas. Although it will not spontaneously burn or cause an explosion, it can easily cause a fire to ignite in a client's room if it contacts a spark from an open flame or electrical equipment. With increasing use of home oxygen therapy, clients and health care professionals must be aware of the dangers of combustion.

> ***Safety Alert.*** Oxygen in high concentrations has a great combustion potential and readily fuels fire.

The nurse should promote safety by using the following measures:

- "No smoking" signs should be placed on the client's room door and over the bed. The client, visitors, roommates, and all personnel should be informed that smoking is not permitted in areas where oxygen is in use.
- Determine that all electrical equipment in the room is functioning correctly and is properly grounded (see chapter 33). An electrical spark in the presence of oxygen can result in a serious fire.
- Locate the closest fire extinguisher.
- Know the fire procedures and the route for evacuation of the area.
- Check the oxygen level of portable tanks before transporting a client to ensure that there is enough oxygen in the tank.

Supply of Oxygen. Oxygen is supplied to the client's bedside either by oxygen tanks or through a permanent wall-piped system. Oxygen tanks are transported on wide-based carriers that allow the tank to be placed upright at the bedside. Regulators are used to control the amount of oxygen delivered. One common type is an upright flowmeter with a flow adjustment valve at the top. A second type is a cylinder indicator with a flow adjustment handle. In the home setting, oxygen therapy is also supplied in a variety of methods, including refillable cylinders (Cuvelier et al., 2002).

In the hospital or home, oxygen tanks are delivered with the regulator in place. In the hospital, the respiratory care department usually connects the regulator to the oxygen source. Home care vendors are usually responsible for connecting the oxygen tank to the regulator for home use.

Methods of Oxygen Delivery. Oxygen can be delivered to the client by nasal cannula, tracheal catheter, or mask.

Nasal Cannula. A **nasal cannula** is a simple, comfortable device used for oxygen delivery (Skill 35-4). The two cannulas, about 1.5 cm long, protrude from the centre of a disposable tube and are inserted into the nares (Figure 35–15). Oxygen is delivered via the cannulas with a flow rate of up to 6 L/minute. Flow rates greater than 4 L/minute are not often used because of the drying effect on the mucosa and the relatively little increase in delivered oxygen concentration. The nurse must know what flow rate produces a given percentage of inspired oxygen concentration (FiO_2; Table 35-9). The nurse must also be alert for skin breakdown over the ears and in the nares from too tight an application of the nasal cannula.

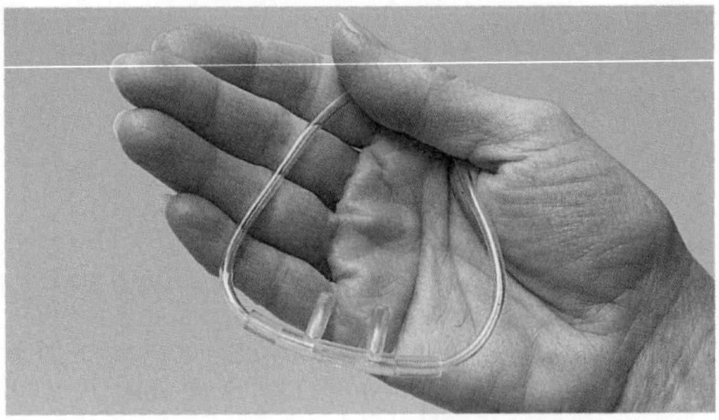

FIGURE **35–15** Nasal cannula.

Table 35-9 Approximate FiO_2 With Different Oxygen Delivery Devices

Oxygen Delivery Device	Required Liter Flow (L/minute)	Approximate Percent Oxygen
Nasal cannula	1–2	24–28
	3–4	32–36
	5–6	40–44
Simple face mask	5–6	40
	6–7	50
	7–8	60
Venturi mask	2	24
	3	28
	4	30
	6	35
	8	40
	10	50
	14	55

Transtracheal Oxygen. Transtracheal oxygen (TTO) is a method of oxygen delivery for clients with chronic lung diseases in which a small, IV-size catheter is inserted directly into the trachea through a surgical tract in the lower neck. Oxygen is delivered directly into the trachea. The advantages of TTO are (a) no oxygen is lost to the atmosphere; (b) clients achieve adequate oxygenation at lower flow rates; (c) oxygen delivery is more efficient and less expensive, (d) there are fewer side effects, such as drying of the nasal mucosa; and (e) clients are more likely to use oxygen because of increased mobility, comfort, and cosmetic improvement.

Once the tracheal stoma is healed, the client is taught to remove and irrigate the catheter with normal saline at least three times a day to maintain a patent catheter. The final oxygen flow rate, usually less than 4 L/minute, is delivered through an 8 Fr catheter through the mature tract.

Oxygen Masks. An oxygen mask is a device used to administer oxygen, humidity, or heated humidity. It is shaped to fit snugly over the mouth and nose and is secured in place with a strap. There are two primary types of oxygen masks: those delivering low concentrations of oxygen and those delivering high concentrations.

The simple face mask (Figure 35–16) is used for short-term oxygen therapy. It fits loosely and delivers oxygen

Skill 35-4 Applying a Nasal Cannula or Oxygen Mask

Delegation Considerations

This skill cannot be delegated to unregulated care providers (UCPs). The nurse is responsible for assessing the client and providing safe and accurate oxygen therapy including adjustment of oxygen flow rate and evaluation of client response. The nurse should instruct the UCP about the following:

- Correct placement and adjustment of delivery device
- The type of equipment and the oxygen flow rate
- Unexpected outcomes associated with the oxygen delivery device (e.g., increased rate of breathing, decreased level of consciousness, increased confusion, pain) and the need to inform the nurse if any occur

Equipment

- Nasal cannula or oxygen mask
- Oxygen tubing
- Humidifier, if indicated
- Sterile water for humidification, if indicated
- Oxygen source
- Oxygen flowmeter
- Appropriate room signs

Steps	Rationale
1. Inspect client for signs and symptoms associated with hypoxia and presence of airway secretions.	Left untreated, hypoxia can produce cardiac dysrhythmias and death. Presence of airway secretions decreases effectiveness of oxygen delivery.

Critical Decision Point: Clients with sudden changes in their vital signs, level of consciousness, or behaviour may be experiencing profound hypoxia. Clients who demonstrate subtle changes over time may have worsening of a chronic or existing condition or a new medical condition (Jevon & Ewens, 2001).

Steps	Rationale
2. Explain to client and family what procedure entails and purpose of oxygen therapy.	Decreases client's anxiety, which reduces oxygen consumption and increases client co-operation.
3. Perform hand hygiene.	Reduces transmission of infection.
4. Attach nasal cannula to oxygen tubing and attach to humidified oxygen source adjusted to prescribed flow rate (see illustration).	Prevents drying of nasal and oral mucous membranes and airway secretions.

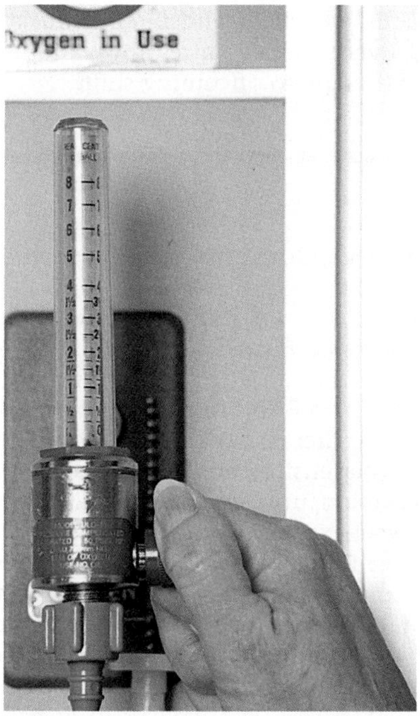

STEP **4** Adjusting flowmeter to prescribed oxygen flow rate.

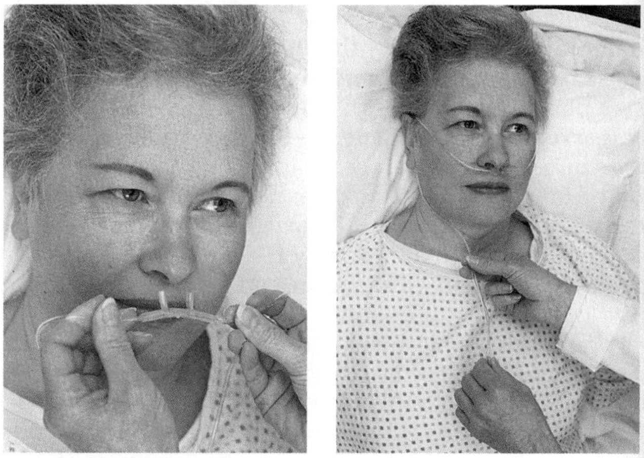

STEP **5** Applying nasal cannula and adjusting fit to client comfort.

Skill 35-4 Applying a Nasal Cannula or Oxygen Mask—cont'd

Steps	Rationale
5. Place tips of cannula into client's nares, and adjust elastic headband or plastic slide until cannula fits snugly and comfortably (see illustration).	Directs flow of oxygen into client's upper respiratory tract. Client is more likely to keep cannula in place if it fits comfortably.
6. Maintain sufficient slack on oxygen tubing and secure to client's clothes.	Allows client to turn head without dislodging cannula and reduces pressure on tips of nares.
7. Check cannula every 8 hours. Keep humidification jar filled at all times.	Ensures patency of cannula and oxygen flow. Prevents inhalation of dehumidified oxygen.
8. Observe client's nares and superior surface of both ears for skin breakdown.	Oxygen therapy can cause drying of nasal mucosa. Pressure on ears from cannula tubing or elastic can cause skin irritation.
9. Perform hand hygiene.	Reduces transmission of micro-organisms.
10. Check oxygen flow rate and physician's orders every 8 hours.	Ensures delivery of prescribed oxygen flow rate and patency of cannula.
11. Inspect client for relief of symptoms associated with hypoxia.	Indicates that hypoxia is corrected or reduced.

Unexpected Outcomes and Related Interventions

- Worsening respiratory status
  - Check that oxygen delivery device is patent, not kinked, and attached to the oxygen flowmeter.
  - Check oxygen level set on flowmeter; determine if delivered amount is consistent with physician order.
  - If not using wall oxygen, determine if the oxygen source contains enough oxygen to deliver the prescribed oxygen amount.
  - Notify physician.
- Dry nasal and upper airway mucosa
  - If oxygen flow rate is greater than 4 L/minute, determine the need for humidification.
  - Assess the client's fluid status and increase fluids if appropriate.
  - Provide frequent oral care.
  - Obtain physician order for use of sterile nasal saline intermittently.
- Skin breakdown over the ears
  - Adjust tightness of elastic strap to looser level.
  - Use good hygiene and skin care around the ears.
  - Place soft, woven 4 × 4 gauze pads between elastic and ears.
  - Reposition elastic strap frequently.

Recording and Reporting

- Record oxygen delivery device and litre flow in medical record; document client and family education; report oxygen delivery device, litre flow, and response to changes in therapy to oncoming shift.

concentrations from 30% to 60%. The mask is contraindicated for clients with carbon dioxide retention because retention can be worsened.

A plastic face mask with a reservoir bag (Figure 35–17) and a Venturi mask (Figure 35–18) are capable of delivering higher concentrations of oxygen. When used as a non-rebreather, the plastic face mask with a reservoir bag can deliver from 80% to 90% oxygen (70% when used as a rebreather), with a flow rate of 10 L/minute. This oxygen mask maintains a high-concentration oxygen supply in the reservoir bag.

The nurse should frequently inspect the bag to make sure it is inflated. If it is deflated, the client may be breathing large amounts of exhaled carbon dioxide.

The Venturi mask can be used to deliver oxygen concentrations of 24% to 55% with oxygen flow rates of 2 to 14 L/minute, depending on which flow-control meter is selected (see Table 35-9).

Home Oxygen Therapy. Indications for home oxygen therapy include a PaO_2 of 55 mm Hg or less or an SaO_2 of 88% or less on room air at rest, on exertion, or with exercise. Clients with a PaO_2 from 56 to 59 mm Hg may also receive oxygen if there is also evidence of cor pulmonale, pulmonary hypertension, erythrocytosis, central nervous system dysfunction, impaired mental status, or increasing hypoxemia with exertion.

Home oxygen therapy has beneficial effect with clients with chronic cardiopulmonary diseases (Snow et al., 2001). This therapy improves clients' exercise tolerance and fatigue levels and in some situations assists in the management of dyspnea (Fujimoto et al., 2002). When home oxygen is required, it is usually delivered by nasal cannula.

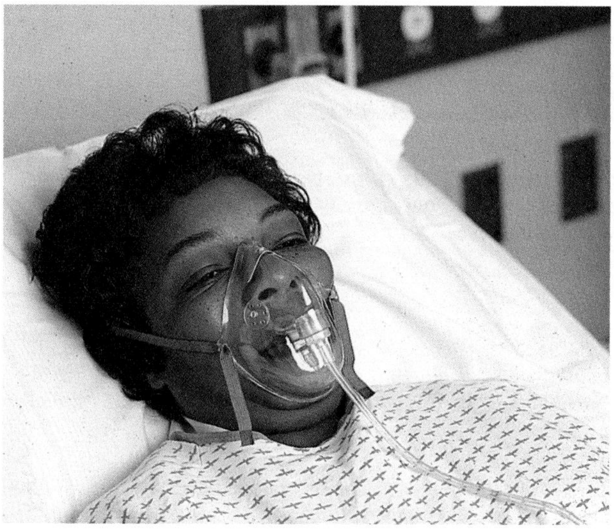

FIGURE **35–16** Simple face mask.

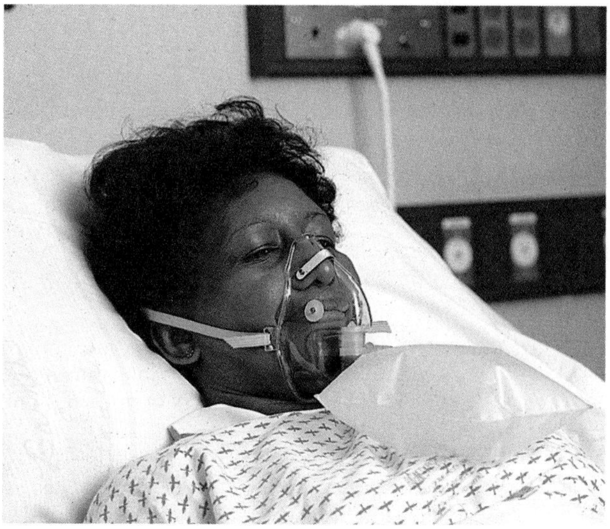

FIGURE **35–17** Plastic face mask with reservoir bag.

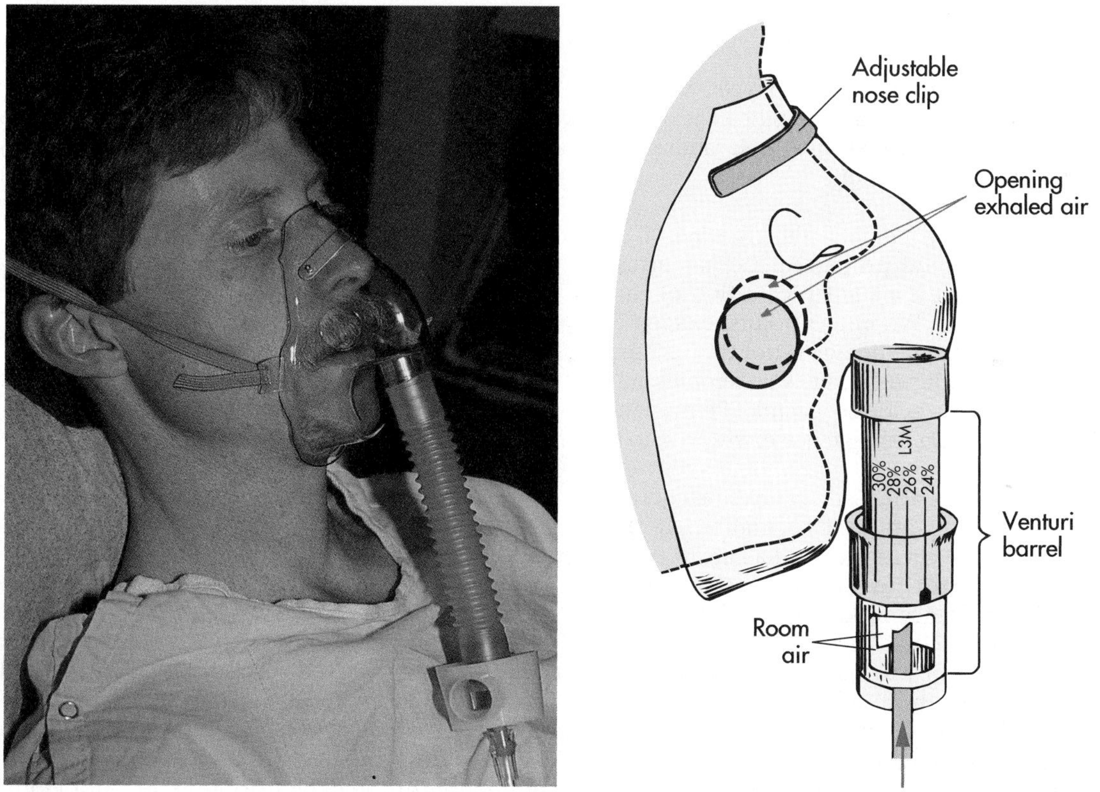

FIGURE **35–18** Venturi mask.

When a client has a permanent tracheostomy, however, a T tube or tracheostomy collar is necessary. Three types of oxygen are used: compressed oxygen, liquid oxygen, and oxygen concentrators. The advantages and disadvantages (Table 35-10) of each type are assessed, along with the client's needs and community resources, before placing a certain delivery system in the home. In the home, the major consideration is the oxygen delivery source.

Clients requiring home oxygen need extensive teaching to be able to continue oxygen therapy at home efficiently and safely (Skill 35-5). This includes oxygen safety, regulation of the amount of oxygen, and how to use the prescribed home oxygen delivery system. The nurse coordinates the efforts of the client and family, home care nurse, home respiratory therapist, and home oxygen equipment vendor. The social worker usually assists with

Table 35-10 Home Oxygen Systems

Primary Use	Advantages	Disadvantages
Compressed Gas Cylinders		
Intermittent therapy Used for exercise or sleep only	100% oxygen, relatively inexpensive, no loss of gas during storage, relatively portable, delivery of up to 15 L/minute	Bulky, possibly unsightly, frequent refilling necessary with continuous use
Liquid Oxygen Systems (Figure 35-19)		
High-litre flows Used with active clients	100% oxygen, conveniently portable, portable units refilled at home, delivery of up to 6 L/minute	Usually weekly delivery necessary for refill, evaporates if not used, potential for frostbite at connections and if liquid is spilled
Oxygen Concentrators		
Moderate-litre flows Homebound clients with limited mobility inside or outside home	Fixed monthly cost, minimal interruption of household by supplier, no refills of "main tank," most units with delivery of up to 4 or 5 L/minute	Oxygen concentration decreases as litre flow increases (usually 85% to 90%), power supply needed, electric bill increase, second system needed for portability, usually E tank gas cylinders

arranging for the home care nurse and oxygen vendor. The nurse must assist the client and family in learning about home oxygen and must ensure their ability to maintain the oxygen delivery system.

Restoration of Cardiopulmonary Functioning. If a client's hypoxia is severe and prolonged, cardiac arrest may result. A cardiac arrest is a sudden cessation of cardiac output and circulation. When this occurs, oxygen is not delivered to tissues, carbon dioxide is not transported from tissues, tissue metabolism becomes anaerobic, and metabolic and respiratory acidosis occurs. Permanent heart, brain, and other tissue damage occur within 4 to 6 minutes.

Cardiopulmonary Resuscitation. Cardiac arrest is characterized by an absence of pulse and respiration. If the nurse determines that the client has cardiac arrest, **cardiopulmonary resuscitation (CPR)** must be initiated. CPR is a basic emergency procedure of artificial respiration and manual external cardiac massage. Most nursing students are required to have successfully completed a CPR course before their clinical experiences.

The "ABCs" of CPR are to establish an ***A***irway, initiate ***B***reathing, and maintain ***C***irculation. When an airway cannot be established, the nurse must reassess proper head position and assess for airway obstruction. There is no clinical benefit to cardiac compressions if an airway cannot be established. The purpose of CPR is to circulate oxygenated blood to the brain to prevent permanent tissue damage (AHA, 2003).

Restorative and Continuing Care. Restorative and continuing care may emphasize cardiopulmonary reconditioning as a structured rehabilitation program. **Cardiopulmonary rehabilitation** is actively helping the client to achieve and maintain an optimal level of health through controlled physical exercise, nutrition counselling, relaxation and stress management techniques, prescribed medications and oxygen, and compliance. As physical reconditioning occurs, the client's complaints of dyspnea, chest pain, fatigue, and activity intolerance should decrease. The client's anxiety, depression, or somatic concerns also often decrease. The client and the rehabilitation team define goals of rehabilitation.

Hydration. Maintenance of adequate systemic hydration keeps mucociliary clearance normal. In clients with adequate hydration, pulmonary secretions are thin, white, watery, and easily removable with minimal coughing. Excessive coughing to clear thick, tenacious secretions is fatiguing and energy depleting. The best way to maintain thin secretions is to provide a fluid intake of 1500 to 2000 mL/day unless contraindicated by cardiac status. The colour, consistency, and ease of secretion expectoration can determine adequacy of hydration.

Coughing Techniques. Coughing is effective for maintaining a patent airway. Coughing permits the client to remove secretions from both the upper and lower airways. The normal series of events in the cough mechanism are deep inhalation, closure of the glottis, active contraction of the expiratory muscles, and glottis opening. Deep inhalation increases the lung volume and airway diameter, allowing the air to pass through partially obstructing mucous plugs or other foreign matter. Contraction of the expiratory muscles against the closed glottis causes a high intrathoracic pressure to develop. When the glottis opens, a large flow of air is expelled at a high speed, providing momentum for mucus to move to the upper airways, where it can be expectorated or swallowed.

The effectiveness of coughing is evaluated by sputum expectoration, the client's report of swallowed sputum, or clearing of adventitious sounds by auscultation. Clients

Skill 35-5 Using Home Liquid Oxygen Equipment

Delegation Considerations

This skill should not be delegated to unregulated care providers (UCPs). However, once the client is stable on home oxygen therapy, UCPs may perform certain aspects of care. The nurse is responsible for assessing the client, checking the device set-up, and providing safe and accurate oxygen therapy. The nurse should instruct the UCP about the following:

- Unique needs of the client (e.g., amount of assistance in applying home nasal cannula or mask) and any assistance needed in filling liquid canisters
- The type of equipment that the client should have in the home and the oxygen flow rate
- Unexpected outcomes associated with the oxygen delivery device (e.g., increased rate of breathing, decreased level of consciousness, increased confusion, pain), and the need to inform the nurse if any occur

Equipment

- Nasal cannula equipment (see Skill 35-4)
- Primary and portable liquid oxygen source for ambulation (see Figure 35–19)

Steps	Rationale
1. Assess:	
a. Client for need for home oxygen therapy.	Candidates for home oxygen have a $PaO_2 \leq 55$ mm Hg or oxygen saturation of 88% on room air, or a PaO_2 of 55 to 59 mm Hg or oxygen saturation of 86% to 89% with evidence of right heart failure, cor pulmonale, or polycythemia.
b. Client or family's ability to use oxygen equipment properly, or for appropriate use of oxygen equipment in home setting.	Physical or cognitive impairments may require instructing family members or significant others on how to operate home oxygen equipment.
c. Client's and family's ability to observe for signs and symptoms of hypoxia: apprehension, anxiety, decreased ability to concentrate, decreased level of consciousness, increased fatigue, dizziness, behavioural changes, increased pulse, increased respiratory rate, pallor, or cyanosis of the mucous membranes.	Hypoxia can occur at home despite use of oxygen therapy. It can be caused by worsening of client's physical condition or another underlying condition, such as a change in the respiratory status.
2. Explain procedure to client and family.	Reinforces information given to client and family; allows opportunity to ask questions.
3. Perform hand hygiene.	Reduces transmission of infection.
4. Demonstrate steps for preparation and completion of oxygen therapy.	Teaches psychomotor skill and enables client to ask questions.

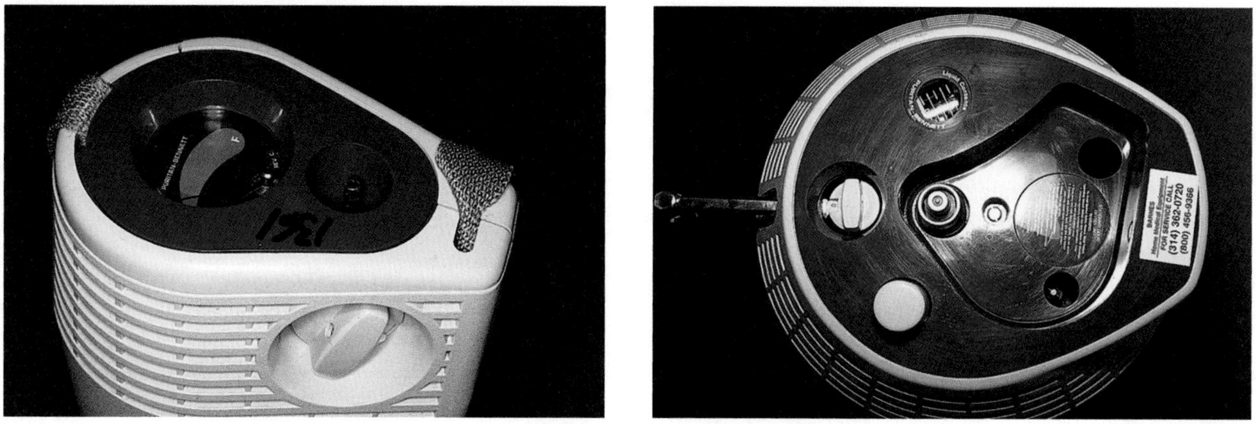

STEP **5b** Oxygen level is verified by the gauges on top of the canisters.

Skill 35-5 Using Home Liquid Oxygen Equipment—cont'd

Steps	Rationale

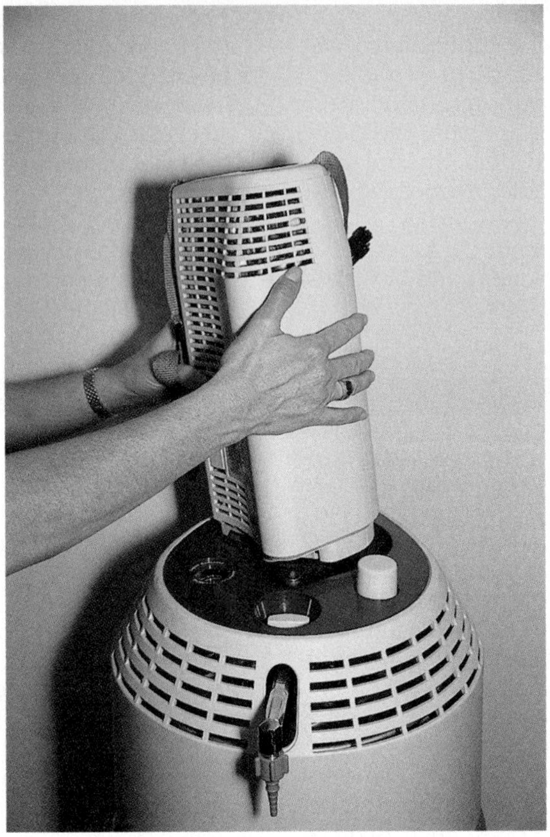

STEP **5c** Refilling portable oxygen delivery system.

Steps	Rationale
5. Prepare primary and portable oxygen: a. Place primary oxygen source in clutter-free environment.	Primary oxygen source replaces compressed oxygen cylinders.

Critical Decision Point: Check oxygen levels in the primary and portable sources to ensure that there is an adequate supply, especially when the nurse is leaving the home.

Steps	Rationale
b. Check oxygen levels of both sources by reading gauge on top (see illustrations).	Ensures adequate amount of oxygen available for use and timely refills of primary source.
c. Refill portable source by placing on top of primary source and pressing down firmly. Check oxygen gauge to determine fullness of portable source (see illustration).	Provides secure connection and prevents leakage of oxygen into room. If not seated securely, the cold liquid oxygen will leak out, creating a snow-like precipitate.
d. Select prescribed rate.	Ensures delivery of prescribed amount of oxygen.
e. Connect nasal cannula and oxygen tubing to oxygen source.	Connects oxygen source to delivery method.
f. Perform hand hygiene.	
6. Have client and family perform each step with guidance from the nurse.	Allows nurse to correct for errors in technique and discuss their implications.

Unexpected Outcomes and Related Interventions

- Client reports no oxygen flow.
  - Check tank pressure gauge. If level of oxygen is low, refill tank if portable, or provide alternate source of oxygen, such as concentrator or H cylinder.
  - Notify home oxygen supplier of need for refill.
  - Reassure client and family.
- Unable to fill portable liquid oxygen from main source.
  - Check to see that portable tank is connected correctly.
  - Determine if valve is frozen.
  - Contact home oxygen supplier for service visit.
  - Provide alternate oxygen source if necessary.

Recording and Reporting

- Record the client's and family's ability to safely use the home oxygen equipment; report the type of home oxygen equipment to be used, the client's and family's understanding of how to use the equipment, knowledge of safety guidelines and unexpected outcomes, and ability to return demonstrate proper use of the oxygen delivery device.

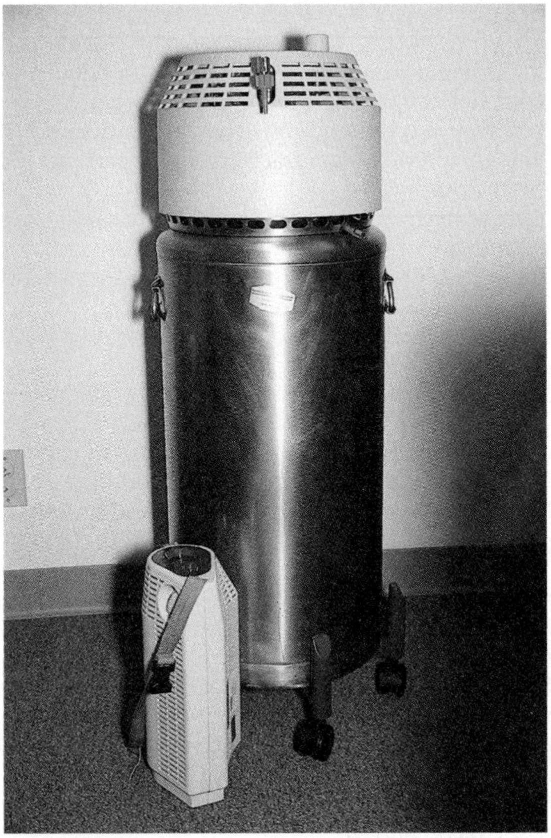

FIGURE **35–19** Primary and portable liquid oxygen source for ambulation.

with chronic pulmonary diseases, upper respiratory tract infections, and lower respiratory tract infections should be encouraged to deep breathe and cough at least every 2 hours while awake. Clients with a large amount of sputum should be encouraged to cough every hour while awake and every 2 to 3 hours while asleep until the acute phase of mucus production has ended. Coughing techniques include deep breathing and coughing for the post-operative client, cascade, huff, and quad coughing.

With the *cascade cough,* the client takes a slow, deep breath and holds it for 2 seconds while contracting expiratory muscles. Then the client opens the mouth and performs a series of coughs throughout exhalation, thereby coughing at progressively lowered lung volumes. This technique promotes airway clearance and a patent airway in clients with large volumes of sputum.

The *huff cough* stimulates a natural cough reflex and is generally effective only for clearing central airways. While exhaling, the client opens the glottis by saying the word *huff.* With practice, the client inhales more air and may be able to progress to the cascade cough.

The *quad cough* technique is used for clients without abdominal muscle control, such as those with spinal cord injuries. While the client breathes out with a maximal expiratory effort, the client or nurse pushes inward and upward on the abdominal muscles toward the diaphragm, causing the cough.

Respiratory Muscle Training. Respiratory muscle training improves muscle strength and endurance, resulting in improved activity tolerance. Respiratory muscle training may prevent respiratory failure in clients with COPD.

One method for respiratory muscle training is the incentive spirometer resistive breathing device (ISRBD). Resistive breathing is achieved by placing a resistive breathing device into a volume-dependent incentive spirometer. Muscle training is achieved when the client uses the ISRBD on a scheduled routine (e.g., twice a day for 15 minutes or four times a day for 15 minutes).

Breathing Exercises. Breathing exercises include techniques to improve ventilation and oxygenation. The three basic techniques are deep breathing and coughing exercises, pursed-lip breathing, and diaphragmatic breathing. Deep breathing and coughing exercises are routine interventions for post-operative clients (see chapter 45).

Pursed-Lip Breathing. **Pursed-lip breathing** involves deep inspiration and prolonged expiration through pursed lips to prevent alveolar collapse. While sitting up, the client is instructed to take a deep breath and to exhale slowly through pursed lips, as if blowing through a straw. The nurse can also have the client blow through a straw into a glass of water to learn the technique. Clients need to gain control of the exhalation phase so that it is longer than inhalation. The client is usually able to perfect this technique by counting the inhalation time and gradually increasing the count during exhalation. In studies using pulse oximetry as a feedback tool, clients have been able to demonstrate an increase in their arterial oxygen saturation during pursed-lip breathing.

Diaphragmatic Breathing. **Diaphragmatic breathing** is more difficult and requires the client to relax intercostal and accessory respiratory muscles while taking deep inspirations. The client concentrates on expanding the diaphragm during controlled inspiration and is taught to place one hand flat below the breastbone above the waist and the other hand 2 to 3 cm below the first hand. The client is asked to inhale while the lower hand moves outward during inspiration. The client observes for inward movement as the diaphragm ascends. These exercises are initially taught with the client in the supine position and then practised while the client sits and stands. The exercise is often used with the pursed-lip breathing technique.

Diaphragmatic breathing is also useful for clients with pulmonary disease, for post-operative clients, and for women in labour to promote relaxation and provide pain control. The exercise improves efficiency of breathing by decreasing air trapping and reducing the work of breathing.

NP Evaluation

Nursing interventions and therapies are evaluated by comparing the client's progress with the goals and expected outcomes of the nursing care plan. The nurse evaluates the actual care given to the client by the health care team on the basis of the expected outcomes (Figure 35–20).

Client Care. The client is the only one who can evaluate his or her degree of breathlessness. The client should be asked to rate his or her breathlessness on a scale of 1 to 10, with 1 being no shortness of breath and 10 being severe shortness of breath. Evaluation of arterial blood gas levels, pulmonary function tests, vital signs, ECG tracings, and physical assessment data provide the nurse with objective measurement of the success of therapies and treatments. Outcomes are compared with expected outcomes to determine the client's health status. Continuous evaluation allows the nurse to determine whether new or revised therapies are required and if new nursing diagnoses have developed and require a new plan of care.

When nursing measures directed to improve oxygenation are unsuccessful, the nurse must immediately modify the nursing care plan. The nurse should not hesitate to notify the physician about a client's deteriorating oxygenation status. Prompt notification can avoid an emergency situation or even the need for CPR.

Client Expectations. It is important for the nurse to ask clients if their expectations of care have been met. For example, the nurse can ask the client, "Do you feel like you will be able to use the breathing techniques we have practised at home?" If the client does not think this will work at home, then the client's expectations for care management have not been met.

The nurse should ask the client whether all questions and needs have been met. If not, the nurse needs to spend more time understanding what the client wants and needs to meet his or her expectations. Working closely with the client will enable the nurse to redefine those client expectations that can be realistically met within the limitations of the client's condition and treatment.

Key Concepts

- The primary function of the heart is to deliver deoxygenated blood to the lungs for oxygenation and to deliver oxygen and nutrients to the tissues.
- Preload, afterload, contractility, and heart rate alter cardiac output.
- Cardiac dysrhythmias are classified by cardiac activity and site of impulse origin.
- The primary function of the lungs is to transfer oxygen from the atmosphere into the alveoli and to transfer carbon dioxide out of the body as a waste product.
- Ventilation is the process of providing adequate oxygenation from the alveoli to the blood.
- Compliance, or the ability of the lungs to expand and contract, depends on the function of musculoskeletal and neurological systems and on other physiological factors.
- The process of inspiration (active process) and expiration (passive process) is caused by changes in intrapleural and intraalveolar pressures and lung volumes.
- Respiration is controlled by the central nervous system and by chemicals within the blood.
- Decreased hemoglobin levels alter the client's ability to transport oxygen.
- Impaired chest wall movement reduces the level of tissue oxygenation.
- Hyperventilation is a respiratory rate greater than that required to maintain normal levels of carbon dioxide.
- Hypoventilation causes carbon dioxide retention.
- Hypoxia occurs if the amount of oxygen delivered to tissues is too low.
- The health history and assessment includes information about the client's cough, dyspnea, fatigue, wheezing, chest pain, environmental exposures, respiratory infection, cardiopulmonary risk factors, and use of medications.

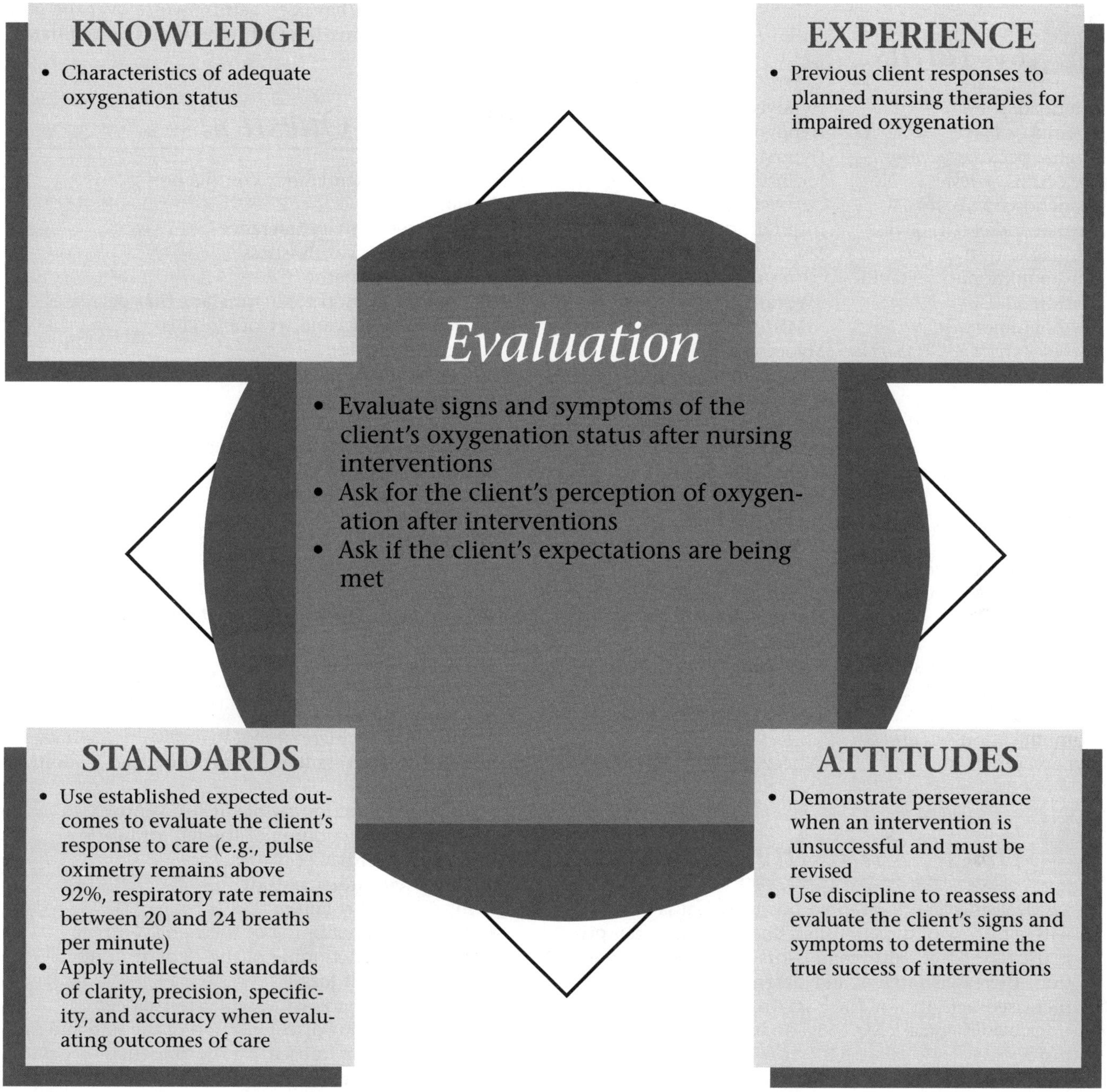
KNOWLEDGE
• Characteristics of adequate oxygenation status
EXPERIENCE
• Previous client responses to planned nursing therapies for impaired oxygenation
Evaluation
• Evaluate signs and symptoms of the client's oxygenation status after nursing interventions
• Ask for the client's perception of oxygenation after interventions
• Ask if the client's expectations are being met
STANDARDS
• Use established expected outcomes to evaluate the client's response to care (e.g., pulse oximetry remains above 92%, respiratory rate remains between 20 and 24 breaths per minute)
• Apply intellectual standards of clarity, precision, specificity, and accuracy when evaluating outcomes of care
ATTITUDES
• Demonstrate perseverance when an intervention is unsuccessful and must be revised
• Use discipline to reassess and evaluate the client's signs and symptoms to determine the true success of interventions

FIGURE **35–20** Critical thinking model for oxygenation evaluation.

- Diagnostic and laboratory tests may be needed to complete the database for a client with decreased oxygenation.
- Breathing exercises improve ventilation, oxygenation, and sensations of dyspnea.
- Nebulization delivers small drops of water or particles of medication to the airways.
- Chest physiotherapy includes postural drainage, percussion, and vibration to mobilize pulmonary secretions.
- Coughing and suctioning techniques are used to maintain a patent airway.
- Oxygen therapy is used to improve levels of tissue oxygenation and is delivered by a nasal cannula, tracheal catheter, or oxygen mask.

Key Terms

Afterload, *p. 1080*
Anemia, *p. 1084*
Angina pectoris, *p. 1089*
Atelectasis, *p. 1090*
Bronchoscopy, *p. 1095*
Cardiac index (CI), *p. 1080*
Cardiac output, *p. 1080*
Cardiopulmonary rehabilitation, *p. 1136*
Cardiopulmonary resuscitation (CPR), *p. 1136*
Chest physiotherapy (CPT), *p. 1107*
Chest tube, *p. 1127*
Cyanosis, *p. 1090*
Diaphragmatic breathing, *p. 1140*
Diffusion, *p. 1083*
Dyspnea, *p. 1094*
Dysrhythmias, *p. 1085*
Electrocardiogram (ECG), *p. 1081*
Expiration, *p. 1082*
Hematemesis, *p. 1095*
Hemoptysis, *p. 1095*
Hemothorax, *p. 1127*
Humidification, *p. 1107*
Hyperventilation, *p. 1090*
Hypoventilation, *p. 1090*
Hypovolemia, *p. 1084*
Hypoxia, *p. 1090*
Incentive spirometry, *p. 1119*
Inspiration, *p. 1082*
Myocardial contractility, *p. 1080*
Myocardial infarction (MI), *p. 1089*
Myocardial ischemia, *p. 1089*
Nasal cannula, *p. 1132*
Nebulization, *p. 1107*
Normal sinus rhythm (NSR), *p. 1081*
Orthopnea, *p. 1095*
Pneumothorax, *p. 1127*
Postural drainage, *p. 1107*
Preload, *p. 1080*
Pulse oximeter, *p. 1101*
Pursed-lip breathing, *p. 1139*
Stroke volume, *p. 1080*
Ventilation, *p. 1082*
Ventricular fibrillation, *p. 1085*
Ventricular tachycardia, *p. 1085*
Wheezing, *p. 1095*

Critical Thinking Exercises

1. Ms. Delgado is a 56-year-old postmenopausal woman with a history of hypertension. She presents to her primary care office with complaints of nausea, indigestion, increased fatigue, and shortness of breath with increased activity for the past 16 hours. What questions would you ask Ms. Delgado in the nursing health history?
2. Mr. Kwan has recently immigrated to Canada. He comes to the clinic because he has been increasingly fatigued, has a persistent cough, has been losing weight, and awakens at night with sweats. What questions would be important to ask when completing the nursing health history?
3. Mrs. Leblanc, age 45 years, has been admitted to the hospital with community-acquired pneumonia. She has a productive cough, fever, chills, crackles and wheezes on auscultation of her chest, and a heart rate of 104 beats per minute. What nursing diagnosis would you consider for this client? What nursing interventions would be appropriate for her? What health promotion interventions need to be initiated before discharge from the hospital?
4. Mr. Chen Lee, age 72 years, has been having chest pain, shortness of breath, and pain down his left arm for about 2 hours. He comes to the emergency department because the pain has been getting worse over the past hour. What nursing interventions would you initiate?

Review Questions

1. Clients with anemia may complain of
   1. Fatigue
   2. Increased activity tolerance
   3. Decreased breathlessness
   4. Increased appetite
2. The most common toxic inhalant that decreases the oxygen-carrying capacity of blood is
   1. Carbon dioxide
   2. Carbon monoxide
   3. Nitrogen
   4. Mustard gas
3. Conditions such as shock and severe dehydration resulting from extracellular fluid loss and reduced circulating blood volume cause
   1. Hypovolemia
   2. Hypervolemia
   3. Uncontrolled bleeding
   4. Hypoxia
4. Fever increases the tissues' need for oxygen, and as a result
   1. Carbon dioxide decreases
   2. Cyanosis occurs
   3. Carbon dioxide increases
   4. Muscle mass increases
5. Left-sided heart failure is an abnormal condition characterized by
   1. Impaired functioning of the left ventricle
   2. Impaired functioning of the left atrium
   3. Lowered cardiac pressures
   4. Increased cardiac output
6. Right-sided heart failure results from
   1. Impaired functioning of the right ventricle
   2. Impaired functioning of the right atrium
   3. Severe weight loss
   4. Lowered pulmonary vascular resistance
7. Cyanosis, the blue discolouration of the skin and mucous membranes caused by the presence of desaturated hemoglobin in capillaries, is a(an)
   1. Early sign of hypoxia
   2. Late sign of hypoxia
   3. Reliable measure of oxygenation status
   4. Non–life-threatening event
8. A person who starts smoking in adolescence and continues to smoke into middle age
   1. Has an increased risk for cardiopulmonary disease and lung cancer
   2. Has an increased risk for obesity and diabetes
   3. Has an increased risk for stress-related illnesses
   4. Has an increased risk for alcoholism
9. A simple and cost-effective method for reducing the risks of stasis of pulmonary secretions and decreased chest wall expansion is
   1. Oxygen humidification
   2. Chest physiotherapy
   3. Frequent changes of position
   4. Anti-infectives

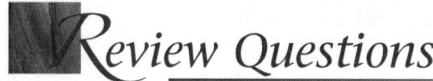

10. The most effective position for clients with cardiopulmonary diseases is the
    1. Supine position
    2. Prone position
    3. High Fowler's
    4. 45-degree semi-Fowler's

References

Akgul, S., & Akyolcu, N. (2002). Effects of normal saline on endotracheal suctioning. *Journal of Clinical Nursing, 11*(6), 826–830.

Allibone, L. (2003). Nursing management of chest drains. *Nursing Standard, 17*(22), 45–54.

American Heart Association (in collaboration with the International Liaison Committee on Resuscitation). (2000). Guidelines 2000 for cardiopulmonary resuscitation and emergency cardiovascular care. VI. Advanced cardiovascular life support. *Circulation, 102*(Suppl. 8), I86–89.

American Heart Association. (2003). *CPR and AEDs.* Retrieved December 18, 2004, from *www.AHA.org*

Anderson, J., & Kessenich, C. R. (2001). Women and coronary heart disease. *The Nurse Practitioner, 26*(8), 12, 18, 21–23.

Canadian Cancer Society. (2004). *Smoking and health.* Retrieved February 8, 2005, from *http://www.cancer.ca/ccs/internet/standard/0,3182,3172_367563_374693_langId-en,00.html*

Canobbio, M. M. (1990). *Cardiovascular disorders.* St. Louis, MO: Mosby.

Canobbio, M. M. (2000). *Mosby's handbook of patient teaching.* St. Louis, MO: Mosby.

Carroll, P. (2002). A guide to mobile chest drains. *RN, 65*(5), 56–60.

Centres for Disease Control and Prevention. (2002). Notice to readers: Recommended adult immunization schedule—United States, 2002–2003. *MMWR Morbity and Mortality Weekly Report, 51*(40), 904–908.

Cuvelier, A., et al. (2002). Refillable oxygen cylinders may be an alternative for ambulatory oxygen therapy in COPD. *Chest, 122*(2), 451–456.

Day, T., et al. (2002). Tracheal suctioning: An exploration of nurses' knowledge and competence in acute and high dependency ward areas. *Journal of Advanced Nursing, 39*(1), 35–45.

Denke, M. A. (2001). Primary prevention of heart disease in women. *Current Artherosclerosis Reports, 3*(2), 136–138.

Dochterman, J. M., & Bulechek, G. M. (Eds.). (2004). *Nursing interventions classification (NIC)* (4th ed.). St. Louis, MO: Mosby.

Fujimoto, K., et al. (2002). Benefits of oxygen on exercise performance and pulmonary hemodynamics in patients with COPD with mild hypoxemia. *Chest, 122*(2), 457–463.

Granger, B. B., & Miller, C. M. (2001). Acute coronary syndrome: Putting the new guidelines to work. *Nursing, 31*(11), 36–42.

Health Canada. (2002). *Go smokefree!* Retrieved Feburary 8, 2005, from *http://www.hc-sc.gc.ca/hecs-sesc/tobacco/index.html*

Jevon, P., & Ewens, B. (2001). Assessment of a breathless patient. *Nursing Standard, 15*(16), 48–53.

Joint National Committee on Prevention, Detection, Evaluation and Treatment of High Blood Pressure. (2003). The seventh report of the Joint National Committee on Prevention, Detection, Evaluation and Treatment of High Blood Pressure (JNC VII). Bethesda, MD: US Department of Health and Human Services, National Heart, Lung, and Blood Institute. Retrieved December 18, 2004, from *www.nhlbi.nih.gov/guidelines/hypertension/express.pdf*

Kerr, M. E., et al. (1999). Effect of endotracheal suctioning on cerebral oxygen in traumatic brain injured patients. *Critical Care Medicine, 27*(2), 2776–2781.

Lewis, S. M., et al. (2000). *Medical-surgical nursing: Assessment and management of clinical problems* (5th ed.). St. Louis, MO: Mosby.

Lueckenotte, A. G. (2000). *Gerontologic nursing* (2nd ed.). St. Louis, MO: Mosby.

McCance, K. L., & Huether, S. E. (2001). *Pathophysiology: The biologic basis for disease in adults and children* (4th ed.). St. Louis, MO: Mosby.

Moorhead, S., Johnson, M., & Maas, M. (Eds.). (2004). *Nursing outcomes classification (NOC)* (3rd ed.). St. Louis, MO: Mosby.

National Cancer Institute of Canada. (2004). *Canadian cancer statistics 2004.* Toronto, ON: Author. Retrieved February 8, 2005, from *http://www.cancer.ca/ccs/internet/standard/0,3182,3172_14279__langId-en,00.html*

Potter, P. A., & Weilitz, P. B. (2003). *Health assessment pocket guide series* (5th ed.). St. Louis, MO: Mosby.

Snow, V., et al. (2001). The evidence base for management of acute exacerbations of COPD: Clinical practice guideline, part 1. *Chest, 119*(4), 1185–1189.

St. John, R. E. (1999). Airway management. *Critical Care Nurse, 19*(4), 79–83.

Stulbarg, M. S., et al. (2002). Exercise training improves outcomes of a dyspnea self-management program. *Journal of Cardiopulmonary Rehabilitation, 22*(2), 109–121.

Thomson, A., et al. (2002). Oxygen therapy in acute medical care: The potential dangers of hyperoxia need to be recognised. *British Medical Journal, 324*(7351), 1406–1407.

Thompson, J., et al. (Eds.). (1993). *Mosby's clinical nursing* (3rd ed.). St. Louis, MO: Mosby-Year Book.

Wood, C. J. (1998). Endotracheal suctioning: A literature review. *Intensive & Critical Care Nursing, 14*(930), 124–136.

Zimmerman, R. K., & Ball, J. A. (2001). Adult vaccination. *Primary Care, 28*(4), 763–790.

Recommended Web Sites

Canadian Lung Association:
http://www.lung.ca/

The Canadian Lung Association is the umbrella group for the 10 provincial lung associations. Its goal is to promote research, education, and healthy living in order to combat lung disease.

Health Canada-Cardiovascular Disease Division:
http://www.hc-sc.gc.ca/english/diseases/heart.html

This Health Canada Web site provides links, information, and resources on the topic of cardiovascular health.

Heart and Stroke Foundation of Canada:
http://www.heartandstroke.ca

The Heart and Stroke Foundation is a national voluntary, nonprofit organization whose mission is to improve the health of Canadians by preventing heart disease and stroke through research, health promotion, and advocacy.

36

Fluid, Electrolyte, and Acid-Base Balances

Jeannette Adams, PhD, MSN, APRN, CRNI
Anita Molzahn, RN, BScN, MN, PhD (Canadian author)

Objectives

Mastery of content in this chapter will enable the student to:

- Define the key terms listed.
- Describe the distribution, composition, movement, and regulation of body fluids.
- Describe the regulation and movement of major electrolytes.
- Describe the processes involved in acid-base balance.
- Describe common disturbances in fluid, electrolyte, and acid-base balances.
- Identify the variables affecting normal fluid, electrolyte, and acid-base balances.
- Discuss the clinical assessment for a client for fluid, electrolyte, and acid-base balances.
- Describe laboratory studies associated with fluid, electrolyte, and acid-base imbalances.
- List and discuss nursing interventions for clients with fluid, electrolyte, and acid-base imbalances.
- Discuss purpose and procedure for initiation and maintenance of intravenous therapy.
- Calculate intravenous flow rate.

Fluid, electrolyte, and acid-base balances within the body are necessary to maintain health and function in all body systems. These balances are maintained by the intake and output of water and electrolytes and regulation by the renal and pulmonary systems. Imbalances may result from many factors, including illnesses, altered fluid intake, or prolonged episodes of vomiting or diarrhea. Acid-base balance is necessary for many physiological processes, and imbalances can alter respiration, metabolism, and the function of the central nervous system. Knowledge and understanding of the mechanisms that contribute to fluid, electrolyte, and acid-base imbalances are essential (Phipps et al., 2003).

Scientific Knowledge Base

Water is the largest single component of the body; 60% of the average adult's weight is fluid. A healthy, mobile, well-oriented adult can usually maintain normal fluid, electrolyte, and acid-base balances because of the body's adaptive physiological mechanisms.

Distribution of Body Fluids

Body fluids are distributed in two distinct compartments, one containing **intracellular fluids** and the other **extracellular fluids** (Table 36-1). Intracellular fluid (ICF) comprises all fluid within body cells. In adults, approximately 40% of body weight is ICF (Phipps et al., 2003).

Extracellular fluid (ECF) is all the fluid outside a cell, which is divided into three smaller compartments: **interstitial fluid, intravascular fluid,** and **transcellular fluids.** Interstitial fluid, which contains lymph, is the fluid between the cells and outside the blood vessels, whereas intravascular fluid is blood plasma. Transcellular fluid consists of cerebrospinal, pleural, peritoneal, and synovial fluids (McCance & Huether, 2002). ECF makes up about 20% of the total body weight.

Composition of Body Fluids

Water that moves through compartments of the body contains minerals or salts, technically known as **electrolytes** (Christensen & Kockrow, 2003). An electrolyte is an element or compound that, when melted or dissolved in aqueous solution, separates into **ions** and is able to carry an electrical current. Positively charged electrolytes are **cations** (e.g., sodium [Na^+], potassium [K^+], calcium [Ca^{2+}]). Negatively charged electrolytes are **anions** (e.g., chloride [Cl^-], bicarbonate [HCO_3^-], sulphate [SO_4^-]).

Electrolytes are vital to many body functions. The value **millimoles per litre (mmol/L)** represents the amount of the specific electrolyte **(solute)** dissolved in a litre of plasma **(solution).** The solution in which a solute is dissolved is called a **solvent** (Speakman & Weldy, 2002).

Minerals (e.g., iron, zinc), which are ingested as compounds, are constituents of all body tissues and fluids and are important in maintaining physiological processes. Minerals also act as catalysts in nerve response, muscle contraction, and metabolism of nutrients. They also regulate electrolyte balance and hormone production and strengthen skeletal structures.

Movement of Body Fluids

Fluids and electrolytes constantly shift between compartments to facilitate body processes such as tissue oxygenation, acid-base balance, and urine formation. Because cell membranes separating the body fluid compartments are selectively permeable, water can pass through them easily. However, most ions and molecules pass through them more slowly. Fluids and solutes move across these membranes by four processes: osmosis, diffusion, filtration, and active transport.

Osmosis. Osmosis is the movement of a pure solvent, such as water, through a semi-permeable membrane from an area of lesser solute concentration to an area of greater solute concentration in an attempt to equalize concentrations on both sides of the membrane (Figure 36–1). The rate of osmosis depends on the concentration of the solutes in the solution, temperature of the solution, electrical charges of the solutes, and differences between the osmotic pressures exerted by the solutions. The concentration of a solution is measured in **osmols,** which reflect the amount of a substance in solution in the form of molecules, ions, or both. Boiling a hot dog is an example of osmosis. The concentration of molecules inside the hot dog is greater than in water. The water passes through the hot dog skin, a semi-permeable membrane, in an attempt to equalize the number of molecules on both sides of the membrane. The skin ruptures when the hot dog cannot hold any more water (Christensen & Kockrow, 2003).

Osmotic pressure is the drawing power for water and depends on the number of molecules in solution. A solution with a high solute concentration has a high osmotic pressure and draws water into itself. If the concentration of the solute is greater on one side of the semi-permeable membrane, the rate of osmosis is faster, and solvent rapidly transfers across the membrane. This continues until equilibrium is reached. The osmotic pressure of a solution is called its osmolarity, which is expressed in osmols, or milliosmols per kilogram (mOsm/kg) of the solution. The normal serum osmolarity is 280 to 295 mOsm/kg. **Osmolarity** is the measure used to evaluate serum and urine in clinical practice. Changes in extracellular osmolarity may result in changes in both ECF and ICF volume.

Solutions are classified as **hypertonic, isotonic,** or **hypotonic.** A solution with the same osmolarity as blood plasma is called isotonic. A hypertonic solution (a solution of higher osmotic pressure), such as 3% sodium chloride, pulls fluid from cells, causing them to shrink; an isotonic solution (a solution of same osmotic pressure), such as 0.9% sodium chloride, expands the body's fluid volume without causing a fluid shift from one compartment to another; and a hypotonic solution (a solution of lower osmotic pressure), such as 0.45% sodium chloride, moves fluid into the cells, causing them to enlarge. Each of these actions occurs through osmosis.

Plasma proteins affect the blood's osmotic pressure, especially the protein albumin (which is naturally produced

Table 36-1 **Electrolyte Distribution in Body Fluid**

Electrolytes	Extracellular (mmol/L)
Sodium (Na^+)	135–145
Potassium (K^+)	3.5–5.0
Calcium (Ca^{2+})	4.5–5.5
Bicarbonate (HCO_3^-)	22–26 (arterial) 24–30 (venous)
Chloride (Cl^-)	95–105
Magnesium (Mg^{2+})	0.6–1.0
Phosphate (PO_4^{3-})	1.0–1.5

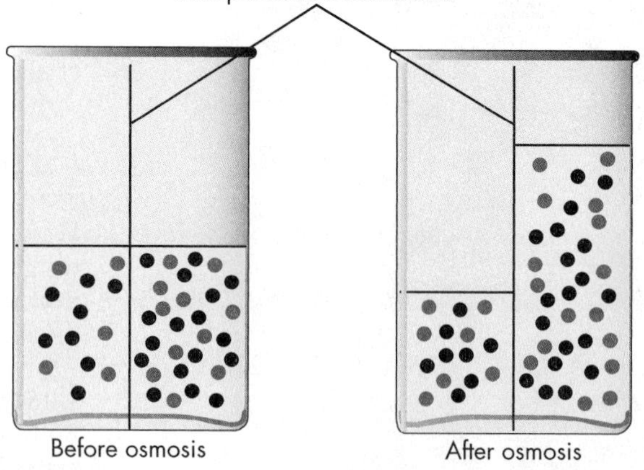

FIGURE **36–1** Osmosis through a semi-permeable membrane. (From *Medical-Surgical Nursing: Assessment and Management of Clinical Problems,* 4th ed., by S. M. Lewis, I. C. Collier, and M. Heitkemper, 2002, St. Louis, MO: Mosby.)

by the body). Albumin exerts **colloid osmotic pressure** or **oncotic pressure,** which tends to keep fluid in the intravascular compartment by pulling water from the interstitial space back into the capillaries (Speakman & Weldy, 2002).

Diffusion. **Diffusion** is the movement of a solute (gas or substance) in a solution across a semi-permeable membrane from an area of higher concentration to an area of lower concentration (Figure 36–2). The result is an even distribution of the solute in a solution. For example, when you pour a small amount of cream into a cup of black coffee, the cream left unmixed will diffuse through the whole cup of coffee (Speakman & Weldy, 2002). A physiological example is the movement of oxygen and carbon dioxide between the alveoli and blood vessels in the lungs. The difference between the two concentrations is known as a **concentration gradient.**

Filtration. **Filtration** is the process by which water and diffusible substances move together in response to fluid pressure, moving from an area of higher pressure to one of lower pressure. This process is active in capillary beds, where **hydrostatic pressure** differences determine the movement of water (Figure 36–3). When there is increased hydrostatic pressure on the venous side of the capillary bed, as occurs in congestive heart failure, the normal movement of water from the interstitial space into the intravascular space by filtration is reversed, resulting in an accumulation of excess fluid in the interstitial space, known as **edema.**

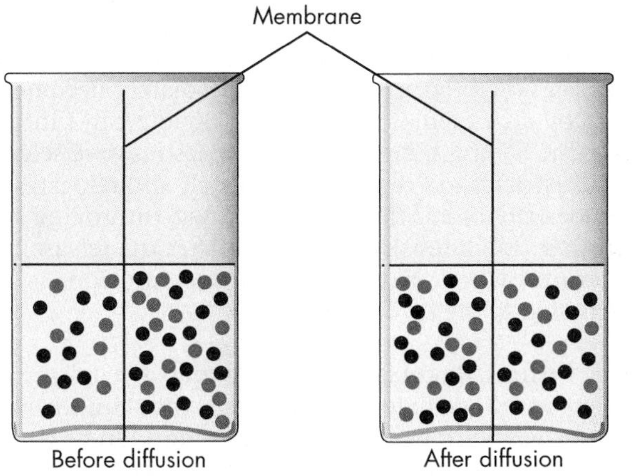

FIGURE 36–2 Diffusion across a semi-permeable membrane. (From *Medical-Surgical Nursing: Assessment and Management of Clinical Problems,* 4th ed., by S. M. Lewis, I. C. Collier, and M. Heitkemper, 2002, St. Louis, MO: Mosby.)

Active Transport. **Active transport** requires metabolic activity and expenditure of energy to move materials across cell membranes, allowing cells to admit larger molecules than they would otherwise be able to admit or to move molecules from areas of lesser concentration to areas of greater concentration "uphill" (Figure 36–4). Examples of active transport are the sodium and potassium pump. Sodium is pumped out of the cell and potassium is pumped in against the concentration gradient. This process enables a higher concentration of potassium in the ICF and a higher concentration of sodium in the ECF.

Active transport is enhanced by carrier molecules within a cell, which bind to incoming molecules. For example, glucose is able to enter cells after it binds with the transport vehicle insulin. Active transport is the mechanism by which cells absorb glucose and other substances to carry out metabolic activities.

Regulation of Body Fluids

Body fluids are regulated by fluid intake, hormonal controls, and fluid output. This physiological balance is termed **homeostasis** (Heitz & Horne, 2001). In health, the body is able to respond to disturbances in fluids and electrolytes to prevent and repair damage.

Fluid Intake. Fluid intake is regulated primarily through the thirst mechanism. The thirst-control centre is located within the brain's hypothalamus. Thirst is one of the major factors that determines fluid intake (Speakman & Weldy, 2002). The **osmoreceptors** continually monitor the serum osmotic pressure, and when osmolality increases, the hypothalamus is stimulated. Eating potato chips is an example; the salt on the chips increases the osmotic pressure of the body fluids and stimulates the thirst mechanism (Phipps et al., 2003). Increased plasma osmolality can occur with any condition that interferes with the oral ingestion of fluids or it can occur with the intake of hypertonic fluids. The hypothalamus will also be

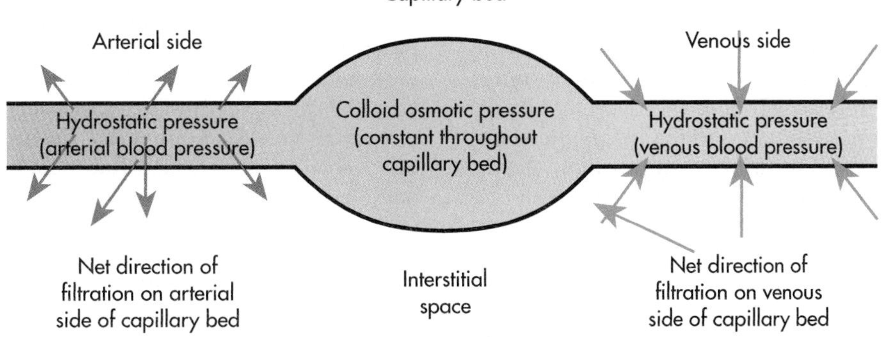

FIGURE 36–3 An example of filtration and hydrostatic pressure.

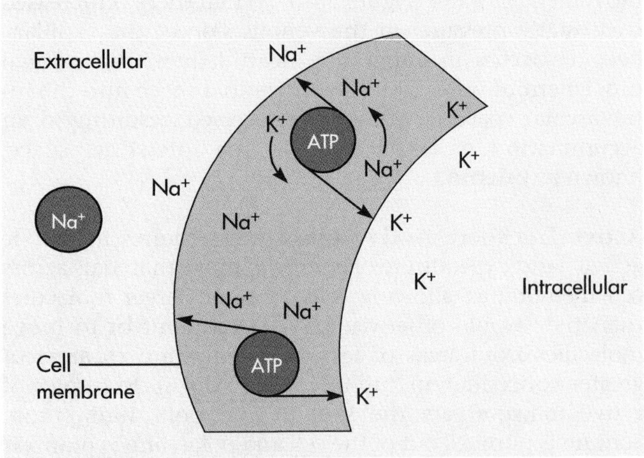

FIGURE 36–4 The sodium-potassium pump. As sodium diffuses into the cell and potassium out of the cell, active transport delivers sodium back to the extracellular compartment and potassium back to the intracellular compartment. (From *Medical-Surgical Nursing: Assessment and Management of Clinical Problems,* 4th ed., by S. M. Lewis, I. C. Collier, and M. Heitkemper, 2002, St. Louis, MO: Mosby.)

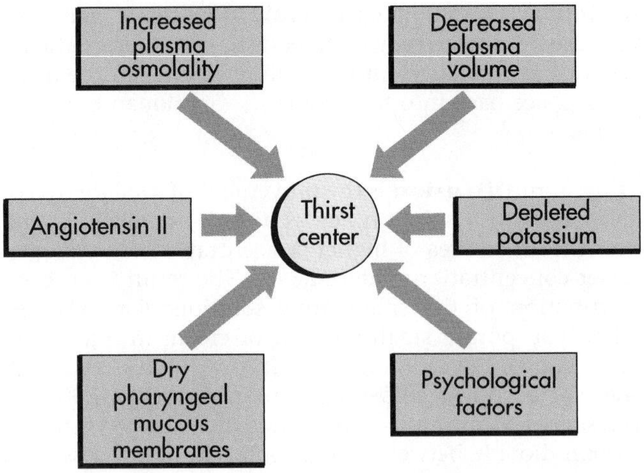

FIGURE 36–5 Stimuli affecting the thirst mechanism.

stimulated when excess fluid is lost and **hypovolemia** occurs, as in excessive vomiting and hemorrhage. In addition, the stimulation of the renin-angiotensin-aldosterone mechanism, potassium depletion, psychological factors, and oropharyngeal dryness initiate the sensation of thirst (Figure 36–5).

The average adult's fluid intake is about 2200 to 2700 mL per day; oral intake accounts for 1100 to 1400 mL, solid foods about 800 to 1000 mL, and oxidative metabolism 300 mL daily (Heitz & Horne, 2001). Water oxidation (oxidative metabolism) is the by-product of cellular metabolism of ingested solid foods. Fluid intake requires an alert state. Infants, clients with neurological or psychological problems, and some older adults who are unable to perceive or respond to the thirst mechanism are at risk for **dehydration.**

Hormonal Regulation. Hormones regulate fluid intake through various mechanisms. **Antidiuretic hormone (ADH)** is stored in the posterior pituitary gland and is released in response to changes in blood osmolarity. The osmoreceptors in the hypothalamus are stimulated to release the hormone ADH when there is an increase in the osmolarity. The ADH works directly on the renal tubules and collecting ducts to make them more permeable to water. This in turn causes water to return to the systemic circulation, which dilutes the blood and decreases its osmolarity. As the body attempts to compensate, the client will experience a decrease in urinary output temporarily. When the blood has been sufficiently diluted, the osmoreceptors stop the release of ADH and urinary output is restored.

Aldosterone is released by the adrenal cortex in response to increased plasma potassium levels or as a part of the renin-angiotensin-aldosterone mechanism to counteract hypovolemia. It acts on the distal portion of the renal tubule to increase the reabsorption (saving) of sodium and the secretion and excretion of potassium and hydrogen. Because sodium retention leads to water retention, the release of aldosterone acts as a volume regulator (Heitz & Horne, 2001).

Renin, a proteolytic enzyme secreted by the kidneys, responds to decreased renal perfusion secondary to a decrease in extracellular volume. Renin acts to produce **angiotensin** I, which causes some vasoconstriction. However, angiotensin I almost immediately becomes reduced by an enzyme that converts angiotensin I into angiotensin II. Angiotensin II then causes massive selective vasoconstriction of many blood vessels and relocates and increases the blood flow to the kidney, improving renal perfusion. Angiotensin II also stimulates the release of aldosterone when the sodium concentration is low (Speakman & Weldy, 2002).

Fluid Output Regulation. Fluid output occurs through four organs of water loss: the kidneys, the skin, the lungs, and the gastrointestinal (GI) tract. The kidneys are the major regulatory organs of fluid balance. They receive approximately 180 L of plasma to filter each day and produce 1200 to 1500 mL of urine (Table 36-2).

Water loss from the skin is regulated by the sympathetic nervous system, which activates sweat glands. Water loss from the skin can be a sensible or insensible loss. An average of 500 to 600 mL of sensible and insensible fluid is lost via the skin each day (Heitz & Horne, 2001). **Insensible water loss** is continuous and is not perceived by the person but can increase significantly with fever or burns (Heitz & Horne, 2001). **Sensible water loss** occurs through excess perspiration and can be perceived by the client or by the nurse through inspection. The amount of sensible perspiration is directly related to the stimulation of the sweat glands.

The lungs expire about 400 mL of water daily. This insensible water loss may increase in response to changes in respiratory rate and depth. In addition, devices for giving oxygen can increase insensible water loss from the lungs.

The GI tract plays a vital role in fluid regulation. Approximately 3 to 6 L of isotonic fluid is moved into the

Table 36-2 Adult Average Daily Fluid Gains and Losses

Fluid Gains	(mL)	Fluid Losses	(mL)
Oral fluids	1100–1400	Kidneys	1200–1500
Solid foods	800–1000	Skin	500–600
Metabolism	300	Lungs	400
		Gastrointestinal	100–200
TOTAL GAINS	2200–2700	TOTAL LOSSES	2200–2700

GI tract and then returns again to the ECF. Under normal conditions, the average adult loses only 100 to 200 mL of the 3 to 6 L each day through feces. However, in the presence of a disease process, for example, diarrhea, the GI tract may become a site of a large amount of fluid loss. This loss may have a significant impact on maintaining normal fluid regulation.

Regulation of Electrolytes

Cations. Major cations within the body fluids include sodium (Na^+), potassium (K^+), calcium (Ca^{2+}), and magnesium (Mg^{2+}). Cations interchange when one cation leaves the cell and is replaced by another. This occurs because cells tend to maintain electrical neutrality.

Sodium Regulation. Sodium is the most abundant cation (90%) in ECF. Sodium ions are the major contributors to maintaining water balance through their effect on serum osmolality, nerve impulse transmission, regulation of acid-base balance, and participation in cellular chemical reactions (McCance & Huether, 2002). Sodium is regulated by dietary intake and aldosterone secretion. The normal extracellular sodium concentration is 135 to 145 mmol/L.

Potassium Regulation. Potassium is the major electrolyte and principal cation in the intracellular compartment (Phipps et al., 2003). It regulates many metabolic activities and is necessary for glycogen deposits in the liver and skeletal muscle, transmission and conduction of nerve impulses, normal cardiac conduction, and skeletal and smooth muscle contraction (McCance & Huether, 2002). A relatively small amount (approximately 2%) of potassium is located within the ECF (Heitz & Horne, 2001). The normal range for serum potassium concentrations is 3.5 to 5 mmol/L. Potassium is regulated by dietary intake and renal excretion. The body conserves potassium poorly, so any condition that increases urine output decreases the serum potassium concentration.

Calcium Regulation. Calcium is stored in bone, plasma, and body cells. Ninety-nine percent of calcium is located in bone, and only 1% is located in ECF. Approximately 50% of calcium in the plasma is bound to protein, primarily albumin, and 40% is free ionized calcium. The remaining small percentage is combined with non-protein anions such as phosphate, citrate, and carbonate (Heitz & Horne, 2001). Normal serum ionized calcium is 1.0 to 1.4 mmol/L. Normal total calcium is 2.1 to 2.6 mmol/L. Calcium is necessary for bone and teeth formation, blood clotting, hormone secretion, cell membrane integrity, cardiac conduction, transmission of nerve impulses, and muscle contraction.

Magnesium Regulation. Magnesium is essential for enzyme activities, neurochemical activities, and cardiac and skeletal muscle excitability. Plasma concentrations of magnesium range from 0.6 to 1.0 mmol/L. Serum magnesium is regulated by dietary intake, renal mechanisms, and actions of the parathyroid hormone (PTH). About 50% to 60% of body magnesium is contained within the bone, and only 1% is contained within the ECF compartment; the rest is located inside the cell (Phipps et al., 2003).

Anions. The three major anions of body fluids are chloride (Cl^-), bicarbonate (HCO_3^-), and phosphate (PO_4^{3-}) ions.

Chloride Regulation. Chloride is the major anion in ECF. The transport of chloride follows sodium. Normal concentrations of chloride range from 95 to 105 mmol/L. Serum chloride is regulated by dietary intake and the kidneys. A person with normal renal function who has a high chloride intake will excrete a higher amount of urine chloride.

Bicarbonate Regulation. Bicarbonate is the major chemical base buffer within the body. The bicarbonate ion is found in ECF and ICF. The bicarbonate ion is an essential component of the carbonic acid-bicarbonate buffering system essential to acid-base balance. The kidneys regulate bicarbonate. Normal arterial bicarbonate levels range between 22 and 26 mmol/L; venous bicarbonate is measured as carbon dioxide content, and the normal value is 24 to 30 mmol/L.

Phosphorus-Phosphate Regulation. Nearly all the phosphorus in the body exists in the form of phosphate (PO_4^{-3}), and the terms phosphorus and phosphate often are used interchangeably (Heitz & Horne, 2001). Phosphate is a buffer anion found primarily in ICF, with a small amount found in ECF. It assists in acid-base regulation. Phosphate and calcium help to develop and maintain bones and teeth. Calcium and phosphate are inversely proportional; if one rises, the other falls. Phosphate also promotes normal neuromuscular action and participates in carbohydrate metabolism. Phosphate is normally absorbed through the GI tract and is regulated by dietary intake, renal excretion, intestinal absorption, and PTH. The normal serum level is 1.0 to 1.5 mmol/L.

Regulation of Acid-Base Balance

For optimal functioning of the cells, metabolic processes maintain a steady balance between acids and bases. Arterial pH is inversely proportional to the hydrogen ion (H^+) concentration (i.e., the greater the concentration, the more acidic the solution and the lower the pH; the lower the concentration, the more alkaline the solution and the higher the pH). The pH is also a reflection of the balance between carbon dioxide (CO_2), which is regulated by the lungs, and bicarbonate (HCO_3^-), a base regulated by the kidneys (Heitz & Horne, 2001). Acid-base balance exists when the net rate at which the body produces acids or bases equals the rate at which acids or bases are excreted. This balance results in a stable concentration of hydrogen ions in body fluids that is expressed as the pH value. Normal hydrogen ion level is necessary to maintain cell membrane integrity and the speed of cellular enzymatic actions. The pH is a scale for measuring the acidity or alkalinity of a fluid. A pH value of 7 is neutral, below 7 is acid, and above 7 is alkaline. Normal values in arterial blood range from 7.35 to 7.45. The three general types of acid-base regulators in the body are chemical, biological, and physiological buffering systems. A **buffer** is a substance or a group of substances that can absorb or release H^+ to correct an acid-base imbalance.

Chemical Regulation. The largest chemical buffer in ECF is the carbonic acid and bicarbonate buffer system (Figure 36–6). This system can be expressed as the following:

$$CO_2 + H_2O \leftrightarrow H_2CO_3 \leftrightarrow H^+ + HCO_3^-$$

Carbon dioxide + Water ↔ Carbonic acid
↔ Hydrogen ion + Bicarbonate

The carbonic acid-bicarbonate buffer system is the first buffering system to react to change in the pH of ECF, and it reacts within seconds. The previous equation demonstrates how hydrogen ions (H^+) and carbon dioxide (CO_2) concentrations are directly related to each other. Whenever carbon dioxide increases, there is an increase in hydrogen ions produced, and whenever hydrogen ions are produced, there is more carbon dioxide produced (Ignatavicius & Workman, 2002). The lungs control the excretion of carbon dioxide, and the kidneys control the excretion of hydrogen and bicarbonate ions.

Biological Regulation. Biological buffering occurs when hydrogen ions are absorbed or released by cells. Biological buffering occurs after chemical buffering and takes 2 to 4 hours. The hydrogen ion has a positive charge and must be exchanged with another positively charged ion, frequently potassium (K^+). In conditions with excess acid, a hydrogen ion enters the cell and a potassium ion leaves the cell and enters the ECF, thus causing an elevated serum potassium.

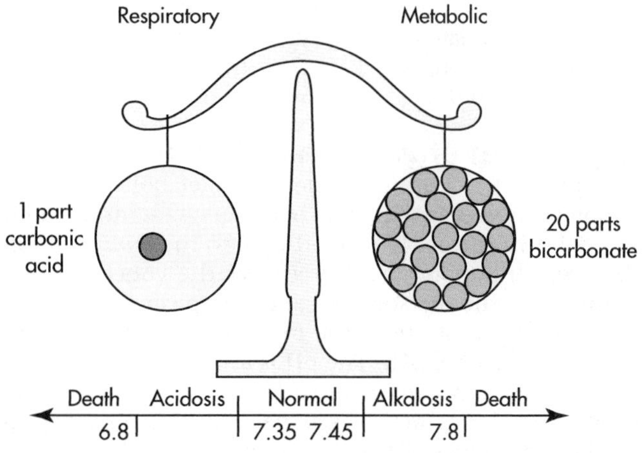

FIGURE **36–6** Carbonic acid-bicarbonate ratio and pH.

An example is the release of fatty acids that occurs with diabetic ketoacidosis and starvation. A second biological buffer is the hemoglobin-oxyhemoglobin system. Carbon dioxide diffuses into the red blood cells (RBCs) and forms carbonic acid. The carbonic acid dissociates into hydrogen and bicarbonate ions. The hydrogen ions attach to hemoglobin, and the bicarbonate ion becomes available for buffering by exchanging with extracellular chloride (Metheney, 2000).

Another biological buffer is the chloride shift within RBCs. When blood is oxygenated in the lungs, bicarbonate diffuses into the cells and chloride travels from the hemoglobin to the plasma to maintain electrical neutrality. The reverse occurs when carbon dioxide moves into the red cells in tissue capillary beds. This process is referred to as the chloride shift and is a reciprocal exchange between these anions (Groer, 2000).

Physiological Regulation. The two physiological buffers in the body are the lungs and the kidneys. The lungs adapt rapidly to an acid-base imbalance; they act to return the pH to normal before the action of the biological buffers. Ordinarily, increased levels of hydrogen ions and carbon dioxide provide the stimulus for respiration. When the concentration of hydrogen ions is altered, the lungs react to correct the imbalance by altering the rate and depth of respiration. For example, when metabolic acidosis is present, respirations are increased, resulting in a greater amount of carbon dioxide being exhaled, which results in a decrease in the acidic level; when metabolic alkalosis is present, the lungs retain carbon dioxide by decreasing the respirations, thereby increasing the acidic level (Phipps et al., 2003).

The kidneys take from a few hours to several days to regulate acid-base imbalance. They reabsorb bicarbonate in cases of acid excess and excrete it in cases of acid deficit. In addition, the kidneys use a phosphate ion (PO_4^{3-}) to excrete hydrogen ions by forming phosphoric acid (H_3PO_4); sulphuric acid (H_2SO_4) may also be excreted. Finally, the kidneys use the ammonia mechanism to regulate acid-base balance. In this mechanism, certain amino acids are chemically changed within the renal tubules into ammonia, which in the presence of hydrogen ions forms ammonium and is excreted in the urine, hence releasing hydrogen ions from the body (Phipps et al., 2003).

Disturbances in Electrolyte, Fluid, and Acid-Base Balances

Disturbances in electrolyte, fluid, or acid-base balances seldom occur alone and can disrupt normal body processes. When there is a loss of body fluids because of burns, illness, or trauma, the client is also at risk for electrolyte imbalances (Table 36-3). In addition, some untreated electrolyte imbalances (e.g., potassium loss) result in acid-base disturbances.

Electrolyte Imbalances

Sodium Imbalances. Hyponatremia is a lower-than-normal concentration of sodium in the blood (serum), which can occur with a net sodium loss or net water excess (see Table 36-3). It occurs frequently in seriously ill clients.

Clinical indicators and treatment depend on the cause of hyponatremia and whether it is associated with a normal, decreased, or increased ECF volume (Heitz & Horne, 2001). The usual situation is a loss of sodium without a loss of fluid, and results in a decrease in the osmolality of ECF. The body initially adapts by reducing water excretion and thus sodium excretion occurs in order to maintain serum osmolality at near normal levels. As the sodium loss continues, the body continues to preserve the blood and interstitial (tissue) volume. As a result, the sodium in ECF becomes diluted.

Hypernatremia is a greater-than-normal concentration of sodium in ECF that can be caused by excess water loss or overall sodium excess (see Table 36-3). When the cause of hypernatremia is an increased aldosterone secretion, sodium is retained and potassium is excreted. When hypernatremia occurs, the body attempts to conserve as much water as possible through renal reabsorption.

Potassium Imbalances. Hypokalemia is one of the most common electrolyte imbalances, in which an inadequate amount of potassium circulates in ECF (see Table 36-3). When severe, hypokalemia can affect cardiac conduction and function. Because the normal amount of serum potassium is so small, there is little tolerance for fluctuations. The most common cause of hypokalemia is the use of potassium-wasting diuretics such as thiazide and loop diuretics.

Hyperkalemia is a greater-than-normal amount of potassium in the blood. Severe hyperkalemia produces marked cardiac conduction abnormalities (see Table 36-3).

The primary cause of hyperkalemia is renal failure, because any decrease in renal function diminishes the amount of potassium the kidney can excrete. Elevations in potassium may also be seen in crushing injuries where cells are broken and potassium is released from with the cells.

Calcium Imbalances. Hypocalcemia represents a drop in serum and/or ionized calcium. It can result from several illnesses, some of which directly affect the thyroid and parathyroid glands (see Table 36-3). Other causes include prolonged bed rest and renal insufficiency (in which the kidneys' inability to excrete phosphorus causes the phosphorus level to rise and the calcium level to decline). Signs and symptoms can be related to a diminished function of the neuromuscular, cardiac, and renal systems.

Hypercalcemia is an increase in the total serum concentration of calcium and/or ionized calcium. Hypercalcemia is frequently a symptom of an underlying disease resulting in excess bone reabsorption with release of calcium.

Table 36-3 Electrolyte Imbalances

Causes	Signs and Symptoms
Hyponatremia	
Kidney disease resulting in salt wasting Adrenal insufficiency GI losses Increased sweating Use of diuretics, especially when combined with low-sodium diet Psychogenic polydipsia Syndrome of inappropriate ADH (SIADH)	*Physical examination:* apprehension, personality change, postural hypotension, postural dizziness, abdominal cramping, nausea and vomiting, diarrhea, tachycardia, convulsions and coma, and fingerprints remaining on sternum after palpation *Laboratory findings:* serum sodium level **below** 135 mmol/L, serum osmolality 280 mOsm/kg, and urine specific gravity **below** 1.010 (if not caused by SIADH)
Hypernatremia	
Ingestion of large amounts of concentrated salt solutions Iatrogenic administration of hypertonic saline solution parenterally Excess aldosterone secretion Diabetes insipidus Increased sensible and insensible water loss Water deprivation	*Physical examination:* thirst, dry and flushed skin, dry and sticky tongue and mucous membranes, fever, agitation, convulsions, restlessness, and irritability *Laboratory findings:* serum sodium levels **above** 145 mmol/L, serum osmolality 295 mOsm/kg, and urine specific gravity 1.030 (if not caused by diabetes insipidus)
Hypokalemia	
Use of potassium-wasting diuretics Diarrhea, vomiting, or other GI losses Alkalosis Excess aldosterone secretion Polyuria Extreme sweating Excessive use of potassium-free intravenous (IV) solutions Treatment of diabetic ketoacidosis with insulin	*Physical examination:* weakness and fatigue, decreased muscle tone, intestinal distension, decreased bowel sounds, ventricular dysrhythmias, paresthesias and weak, irregular pulse *Laboratory findings:* serum potassium level **below** 3.5 mmol/L and electrocardiogram (ECG) abnormalities (e.g., ventricular dysrhythmias)*

*Data from *Mosby's Pocket Guide Series: Fluid, Electrolyte, and Acid-Base Balance* (4th ed.), by U. E. Heitz and M. M. Horne, 2001, St. Louis, MO: Mosby.

Continued

Table 36-3 Electrolyte Imbalances—cont'd

Causes	Signs and Symptoms
Hyperkalemia	
Renal failure Fluid volume deficit Massive cellular damage such as from burns and trauma Iatrogenic administration of large amounts of potassium intravenously Adrenal insufficiency Acidosis, especially diabetic ketoacidosis Rapid infusion of stored blood Use of potassium-sparing diuretics	*Physical examination:* anxiety, dysrhythmias, paresthesia, weakness, abdominal cramps, and diarrhea *Laboratory findings:* serum potassium level **above** 5.0 mmol/L and ECG abnormalities (bradycardia, heart block, dysrhythmias); eventually QRS pattern widens and cardiac arrest occurs*
Hypocalcemia	
Rapid administration of blood transfusions containing citrate Hypoalbuminemia Hypoparathyroidism Vitamin D deficiency Pancreatitis Alkalosis	*Physical examination:* numbness and tingling of fingers and circumoral region, hyperactive reflexes, positive Trousseau's sign (carpopedal spasm with hypoxia), positive Chvostek's sign (contraction of facial muscles when facial nerve is tapped), tetany, muscle cramps, and pathological fractures (chronic hypocalcemia) *Laboratory findings:* serum calcium level **below** 2.1 mmol/L and ECG abnormalities
Hypercalcemia	
Hyperparathyroidism Osteometastasis Paget's disease Osteoporosis Prolonged immobilization Acidosis	*Physical examination:* anorexia, nausea and vomiting, weakness, lethargy, low back pain (from kidney stones), decreased level of consciousness, personality changes, and cardiac arrest *Laboratory findings:* serum calcium level **above** 2.8 mmol/L; X-ray examination showing generalized osteoporosis, widespread bone cavitation, radiopaque urinary stones; elevated blood urea nitrogen (BUN) level above 8.9 mmol/L and elevated creatinine level above 106 mmol/L caused by fluid volume deficit (FVD) or renal damage caused by urolithiasis; ECG abnormalities
Hypomagnesemia	
Inadequate intake: malnutrition and alcoholism Inadequate absorption: diarrhea, vomiting, nasogastric drainage, fistulas; diseases of small intestine Excessive loss resulting from thiazide diuretics Aldosterone excess Polyuria	*Physical examination:* muscular tremors, hyperactive deep tendon reflexes, confusion and disorientation, dysrhythmias, and positive Chvostek's sign and Trousseau's sign *Laboratory findings:* serum magnesium level **below** 0.6 mmol/L
Hypermagnesemia	
Renal failure Excess oral or parenteral intake of magnesium	*Physical examination:* physical findings that are more frequent in acute elevations in magnesium levels: hypoactive deep tendon reflexes, decreased depth and rate of respirations, hypotension, and flushing *Laboratory findings:* serum magnesium level **above** 1.0 mmol/L

*Data from *Mosby's Pocket Guide Series: Fluid, Electrolyte, and Acid-Base Balance* (4th ed.), by U. E. Heitz and M. M. Horne, 2001, St. Louis, MO: Mosby.

Magnesium Imbalances. Disturbances in magnesium levels are summarized in Table 36-3. Symptoms are the result of changes in neuromuscular excitability. Hypomagnesemia, a drop in serum magnesium, occurs with malnutrition and with malabsorption disorders, and signs and symptoms are directly related to the neuromuscular system. Hypermagnesemia is an increase in serum magnesium levels. It depresses skeletal muscles and nerve function. The depression of acetylcholine leads to a sedative effect, which can lead to bradycardia, electrocardiogram changes, cardiac arrhythmias, and decreased respiratory rate and depth (Phipps et al., 2003).

Chloride Imbalances. Hypochloremia occurs when the serum chloride level falls below normal. Vomiting or prolonged and excessive nasogastric or fistula drainage can result in hypochloremia because of the loss of hydrochloric acid. The use of loop and thiazide diuretics also results in increased chloride loss as sodium is excreted. When serum chloride levels fall, metabolic alkalosis results as the body adapts by increasing reabsorption of the bicarbonate ion to maintain electrical neutrality.

Hyperchloremia occurs when the serum chloride level rises above normal, which usually occurs when the serum bicarbonate value falls or sodium level rises. Hypochloremia and hyperchloremia rarely occur as single disease processes but are commonly associated with acid-base imbalance. There is no single set of symptoms associated with these two alterations.

Fluid Disturbances. The basic types of fluid imbalances are isotonic and osmolar. Isotonic deficit and excess exist when water and electrolytes are gained or lost in equal proportions. In contrast, osmolar imbalances are losses or excesses of only water so that the concentration (osmolality) of the serum is affected. Table 36-4 lists the causes and symptoms of common disturbances.

Acid-Base Balance. **Arterial blood gas (ABG)** analysis is the best way to evaluate acid-base balance. Measurement of ABGs involves analysis of six components. Deviation from a normal value will indicate that the client is experiencing an acid-base imbalance. These six components are pH, $PaCO_2$, PaO_2, oxygen saturation, base excess, and HCO_3^-.

pH. pH measures hydrogen ion (H^+) concentration in the body fluids. Even a slight change can be potentially life threatening. An increase in concentration of H^+ makes a solution more acidic; a decrease makes the solution more alkaline. Normal pH value is 7.35 to 7.45 (acidic is 7.35, and alkalotic is 7.45).

$PaCO_2$. $PaCO_2$ is the partial pressure of carbon dioxide in arterial blood and is a reflection of the depth of pulmonary ventilation. The normal range is 35 to 45 mm Hg. When the $PaCO_2$ is less than 35 mm Hg, it is an indication that hyperventilation has occurred. As rate and depth of respiration increase, more carbon dioxide is exhaled and the carbon dioxide concentration decreases. When the $PaCO_2$ is more than 45 mm Hg, hypoventilation has occurred. As rate and depth of respiration decrease, less carbon dioxide is exhaled and more is retained, increasing the concentration of carbon dioxide.

PaO_2. PaO_2 is the partial pressure of oxygen in arterial blood. It has no primary role in acid-base regulation if it is within normal limits. A PaO_2 less than 60 mm Hg can lead to anaerobic metabolism, resulting in lactic acid production and metabolic acidosis. There is a normal decline in PaO_2 in older adults. Hypoxemia also may cause hyperventilation, resulting in respiratory alkalosis (Heitz & Horne, 2001). The normal range is 80 to 100 mm Hg.

Oxygen Saturation. Saturation is the point at which hemoglobin is saturated by oxygen (O_2). When a client is hypoxic and uses up readily available oxygen, the reserve oxygen (oxygen attached to hemoglobin) is drawn from to provide oxygen to the tissues (Ignatavicius & Workman, 2002). Oxygen can be affected by changes in temperature, pH, and $PaCO_2$. When the PaO_2 falls below 60 mm Hg, there is a large drop in saturation (Heitz & Horne, 2001). The normal range is 95% to 99%.

Base Excess. Base excess is the amount of blood buffer (hemoglobin and bicarbonate) that exists. A high value indicates alkalosis and can result from the ingestion of large amounts of sodium bicarbonate solutions (some antacids), citrate excess with rapid blood transfusions, or intravenous infusion of sodium bicarbonate to correct ketoacidosis. A low value indicates acidosis and is usually the result of the elimination of too many bicarbonate ions. An example is diarrhea, where the increased intestinal motility that accompanies diarrhea forces the bicarbonate-containing fluid to be lost instead of being absorbed (Ignatavicius & Workman, 2002). The normal range is ± 2.

Bicarbonate. Serum bicarbonate (HCO_3^-) is the major renal component of acid-base balance and is excreted and reproduced by the kidneys to maintain a normal acid-base environment. It is the principal buffer of the extracellular fluids of the body, and once bicarbonate is in the ECF, it is maintained at a concentration of 20 times that of the fluid concentration of carbonic acid (Ignatavicius & Workman, 2002). The normal range is 22 to 26 mmol/L. Less than 22 mmol/L usually indicates metabolic acidosis; more than 26 mmol/L indicates metabolic alkalosis.

Types of Acid-Base Imbalances. The four primary types of acid-base imbalance are respiratory acidosis, respiratory alkalosis, metabolic acidosis, and metabolic alkalosis (Table 36-5).

Respiratory Acidosis. **Respiratory acidosis** is marked by an increased arterial carbon dioxide concentration ($PaCO_2$), excess carbonic acid (H_2CO_3), and an increased hydrogen ion concentration (decreased pH). With respiratory acidosis, the cerebrospinal fluid and brain cells become acidic, causing neurological changes. Hypoxemia occurs because of respiratory depression, resulting in further neurological impairment. Electrolyte changes such as hyperkalemia and hypercalcemia may accompany the acidosis.

Respiratory Alkalosis. **Respiratory alkalosis** is marked by decreased $PaCO_2$ and increased pH. Like respiratory acidosis, respiratory alkalosis can begin outside the respiratory system (e.g., anxiety with hyperventilation) or within the respiratory system (e.g., initial phase of an asthma attack).

Metabolic Acidosis. **Metabolic acidosis** results because of the high acid content of the blood, which also causes a loss of sodium bicarbonate, the alkaline half of the carbonate buffer system (Speakman & Weldy, 2002). An

Table 36-4 Fluid Disturbances

Causes	Signs and Symptoms
Isotonic Imbalances	
Fluid Volume Deficit (FVD)—Water and Electrolytes Lost in Equal or Isotonic Proportions	
Losses from the GI system, such as from diarrhea, vomiting, or drainage from fistulas or tubes Loss of plasma or whole blood, such as with burns or hemorrhage Excessive perspiration Fever Decreased oral intake of fluids Use of diuretics	*Physical examination:* postural hypotension, tachycardia, dry mucous membranes, poor skin turgor, thirst, confusion, rapid weight loss, slow vein filling, lethargy, oliguria, weak pulse *Laboratory findings:* urine specific gravity greater than 1.030, increased hematocrit level, and increased BUN level (hemoconcentration)
Fluid Volume Excess (FVE)—Water and Sodium Retained in Osotonic Proportions	
Congestive heart failure Renal failure Cirrhosis of the liver Increased serum aldosterone and steroid levels Excessive sodium intake or administration	*Physical examination:* rapid weight gain, edema (especially in dependent areas), hypertension, polyuria (if renal mechanisms are normal), neck vein distension, increased venous pressure, crackles in lungs *Laboratory findings:* decreased hematocrit level and decreased BUN level **below** 1.2 mmol/L (hemodilution)
Osmolar Imbalances	
Hyperosmolar Imbalance—Dehydration	
Diabetes insipidus Interruption of neurologically driven thirst drive Diabetic ketoacidosis Osmotic diuresis Administration of hypertonic parenteral fluids or tube feeding formulas	*Physical examination:* dry and sticky mucous membranes, flushed and dry skin, thirst, elevated body temperature, irritability, convulsions, coma *Laboratory findings:* increased serum sodium level **above** 145 mmol/L and increased serum osmolality **above** 295 mOsm/kg
Hypoosmolar Imbalance—Water Excess	
SIADH Excess water intake	*Physical examination:* decreased level of consciousness, convulsions, coma *Laboratory findings:* decreased serum sodium level **below** 135 mmol/L and decreased serum osmolality **below** 280 mOsm/kg

analysis of serum electrolytes to detect an anion gap may be helpful in attempting to identify the cause of the metabolic acidosis. An **anion gap** reflects unmeasurable anions present in plasma and is calculated by subtracting the sum of chloride and bicarbonate from the amount of plasma sodium concentration (Table 36-6; Heitz & Horne, 2001).

Metabolic Alkalosis. **Metabolic alkalosis** is marked by the heavy loss of acid from the body or by increased levels of bicarbonate. The most common causes are vomiting and gastric suction. Other causes include the overcorrection of metabolic acidosis, potassium deficiency, hyperaldosteronism, and the use of thiazide therapy that causes an increase of renal excreted acid (Phipps et al., 2003).

Nursing Knowledge Base

Fluid and electrolyte imbalances may affect anyone. Infants, severely ill adults, disoriented or immobile clients, and older adults are frequently at greater risk because they cannot respond independently to early symptoms. Over time, the body can no longer maintain fluid and electrolyte or acid-base balance adequately, and the client's health becomes compromised. Prolonged or severe compromises may lead to irreversible chronic health problems (Box 36-1).

Critical Thinking

Successful critical thinking requires a synthesis of knowledge, experience, information gathered from clients, and intellectual and professional standards. The nurse must use clinical judgments to anticipate the information necessary, analyze the data, and make decisions regarding client care. The nurse must adapt critical thinking to the changing needs of the client. During assessment (Figure 36–7), the nurse must consider all elements that build toward making appropriate nursing diagnoses.

To understand how fluid, electrolyte, and acid-base imbalances affect the client, the nurse must integrate knowledge of physiology, pathophysiology, and pharmacology with previous experiences and information gathered from the client. Critical thinking attitudes such as discipline and integrity are also necessary to identify diagnoses and

Table 36-5 Acid-Base Imbalances

Causes	Signs and Symptoms
Respiratory Acidosis	
Hypoventilation Resulting from Primary Respiratory Problems	
Atelectasis (obstruction of small airways often caused by retained mucus) Pneumonia Cystic fibrosis Respiratory failure Airway obstruction Chest wall injury	*Physical examination:* confusion, dizziness, lethargy, headache, ventricular dysrhythmias, warm and flushed skin, muscular twitching, convulsions, and coma *Laboratory findings:* arterial blood gas alterations: pH **below** 7.35, partial pressure of carbon dioxide in arterial blood ($PaCO_2$) **above** 45 mm Hg, arterial partial pressure of oxygen (PaO_2) **less than** 80 mm Hg, and bicarbonate level normal (if uncompensated) or **above** 26 mmol/L (if compensated)
Hypoventilation Resulting from Factors Outside of the Respiratory System	
Drug overdose with a respiratory depressant Paralysis of respiratory muscles caused by various neurological alterations Head injury Obesity	
Respiratory Alkalosis	
Hyperventilation Resulting from Primary Respiratory Problems	
Asthma Pneumonia Inappropriate mechanical ventilator settings	*Physical examination:* dizziness, confusion, dysrhythmias, tachypnea, numbness and tingling of extremities, convulsions, and coma *Laboratory findings:* arterial blood gas alterations: pH **above** 7.45, $PaCO_2$ 35 mm Hg, PaO_2 normal, and bicarbonate level normal (if short lived or uncompensated) or **below** 22 mmol/L (if compensated)
Hyperventilation Resulting from Factors Outside of the Respiratory System	
Anxiety Hypermetabolic states (fever, exercise) Disorders of the central nervous system (head injuries, infections) Salicylate overdose	
Metabolic Acidosis	
High Anion Gap	
Starvation Diabetic ketoacidosis Renal failure Lactic acidosis from heavy exercise Use of drugs (methanol, ethanol, formic acid, paraldehyde, aspirin)	*Physical examination:* headache, lethargy, confusion, dysrhythmias, tachypnea with deep respirations, abdominal cramps, and flushed skin *Laboratory findings:* arterial blood gas alterations: pH **below** 7.35, $PaCO_2$ normal (if uncompensated) or **below** 35 mm Hg (if compensated), PaO_2 normal or increased (with rapid, deep respirations), bicarbonate level **below** 22 mmol/L, and oxygen saturation normal
Normal Anion Gap	
Renal tubular acidosis Diarrhea	
Metabolic Alkalosis	
Excessive vomiting Prolonged gastric suctioning Hypokalemia or hypercalcemia Excess aldosterone Use of drugs (steroids, sodium bicarbonate, diuretics)	*Physical examination:* dizziness; dysrhythmias; numbness and tingling of fingers, toes, and circumoral region; muscle cramps; tetany *Laboratory findings:* arterial blood gas alterations: pH **above** 7.45, $PaCO_2$ normal (if uncompensated) or **above** 45 mm Hg (if compensated), PaO_2 normal, and bicarbonate level above 26 mmol/L

Table 36-6 Anion Gap

Anion Gap Type	Values	Causes
Normal anion gap	12 (±2) mmol/L	Diarrhea, renal tubular acidosis, or pancreatic fistula causing a direct loss of HCO_3^-; addition of chloride-containing acids
Increased anion gap	>14 mmol/L	Lactic acidosis, uremia, diabetic ketoacidosis (DKA), or salicylate and methanol toxicity, resulting in accumulation of nonvolatile acids with decrease in HCO_3^-

From *Mosby's Pocket Guide Series: Fluid, Electrolyte, and Acid-Base Balance* (4th ed.), by U. E. Heitz and M. M. Horne, 2001, St. Louis, MO: Mosby.

Box 36-1 Risk Factors for Fluid, Electrolyte, and Acid-Base Imbalances

Age

Very young
Very old

Chronic Diseases

Cancer
Cardiovascular disease, such as congestive heart failure
Endocrine disease, such as Cushing's disease and diabetes mellitus
Malnutrition
Chronic obstructive pulmonary disease
Renal disease, such as progressive renal failure
HIV/AIDS
Changes in level of consciousness

Trauma

Crush injuries
Head injuries
Burns

Therapies

Diuretics
Steroids
Intravenous (IV) therapy
Total parenteral nutrition (TPN)

Gastrointestinal Losses

Gastroenteritis
Nasogastric suctioning
Fistulas

plan interventions. Professional standards provide valuable guidelines for comprehensive assessment.

Nursing Process

Assessment

The nurse understands the importance of fluid, electrolyte, and acid-base balances to homeostasis dynamics. By gathering assessment data through a history and physical examination and using critical thinking skills, the nurse will identify clients at risk and then identify all appropriate nursing diagnoses.

Health History. The nursing assessment begins with a nursing health history, which is designed to reveal any risk factors or pre-existing conditions that may cause or contribute to a disturbance of fluid, electrolyte, and acid-base balances. The nurse will explore with the client any factors that may cause a disturbance and integrate the information with knowledge of fluid volume regulation, electrolyte concentration, and acid-base regulation.

Age. The nurse first considers the client's age. An infant's proportion of total body water (70% to 80% total body weight) is greater that that of children or adults. Infants are not protected from fluid loss because they ingest and excrete a relatively greater daily water volume than do adults (Heitz & Horne, 2001). Therefore, they are at a greater risk for **fluid volume deficit (FVD)** and hyperosmolar imbalance because body water loss is proportionately greater per kilogram of weight.

Children ages 2 through 12 years have less stable regulatory responses to imbalance, and in childhood illnesses they tend to operate within a more narrow range with less tolerance for large changes. Children frequently respond to illnesses with fevers of higher temperatures and longer duration than those of adults. At any age, fever in childhood can increase the rate of insensible water loss.

Adolescents have increased metabolic processes and increased water production because of the major rapid changes that occur in the anatomical and physiological process. Changes in fluid balance are greater in adolescent girls because of hormonal changes associated with the menstrual cycle.

Older adults experience a number of age-related changes that can affect fluid, electrolyte, and acid-base balances. They have a decreased thirst sensation, which may affect their oral intake of fluids. The kidneys have a decrease in glomerular filtration rate and in the number of filtering nephrons (Lueckenotte, 2000). These changes can mean that in the presence of sodium depletion or overload, the older adult may be unable to maintain homeostasis and the imbalance is instead worsened. In addition, older adults are at risk for decreased excretion of medications, which can lead to imbalances causing metabolic or respiratory acidosis, FVD, and hyperosmolar imbalance, hyponatremia, and hypernatremia (Heitz & Horne, 2001). The changes in lung function that accompany aging can lead to respiratory acidosis and the inability to compensate for metabolic acidosis. Therefore, the older adult who has any condition that involves renal function, fluid and electrolyte balance, or plasma volume and osmolality is more likely to experience more serious consequences (Phipps et al., 2003).

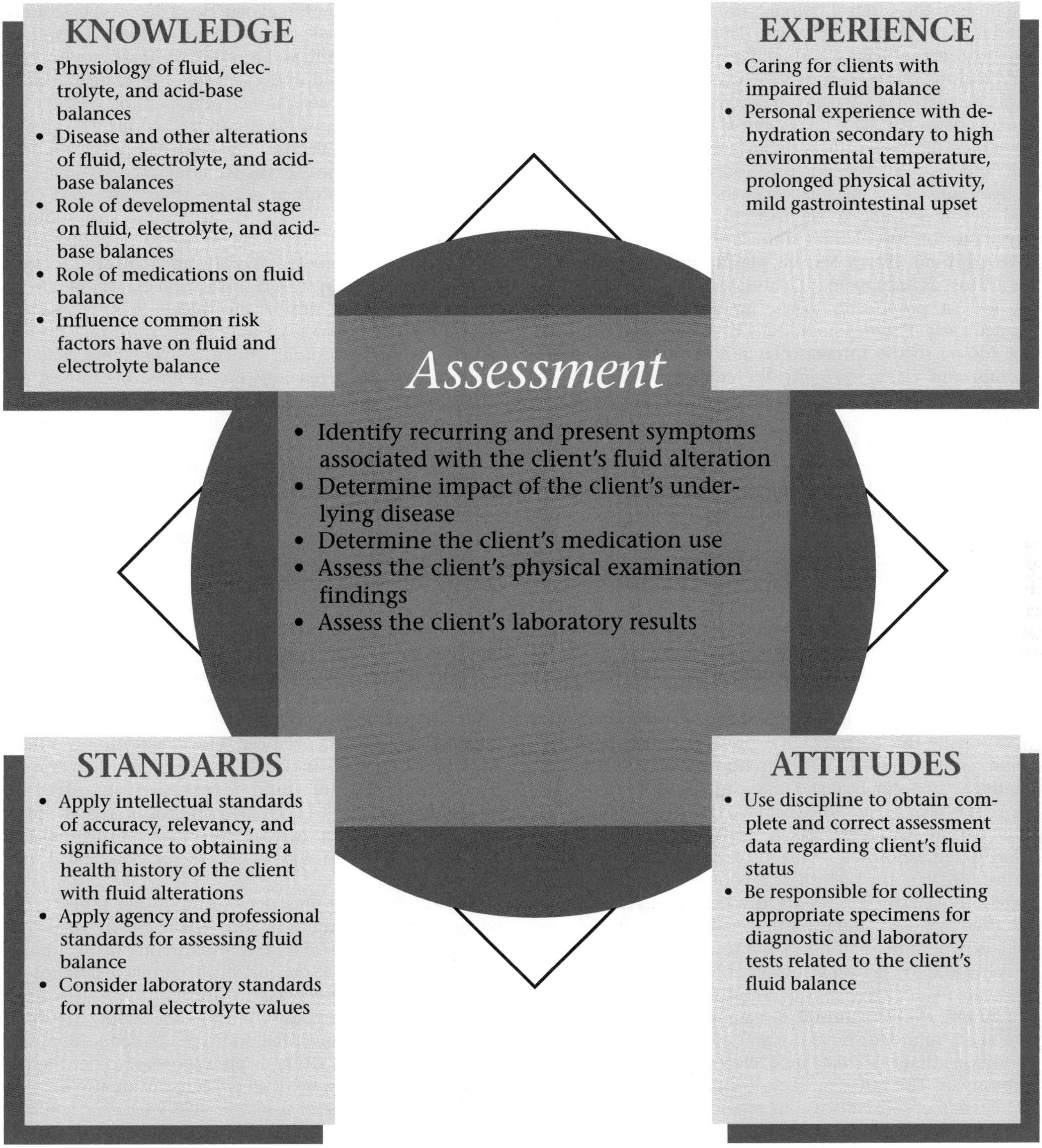
KNOWLEDGE
• Physiology of fluid, electrolyte, and acid-base balances
• Disease and other alterations of fluid, electrolyte, and acid-base balances
• Role of developmental stage on fluid, electrolyte, and acid-base balances
• Role of medications on fluid balance
• Influence common risk factors have on fluid and electrolyte balance
EXPERIENCE
• Caring for clients with impaired fluid balance
• Personal experience with dehydration secondary to high environmental temperature, prolonged physical activity, mild gastrointestinal upset
Assessment
• Identify recurring and present symptoms associated with the client's fluid alteration
• Determine impact of the client's underlying disease
• Determine the client's medication use
• Assess the client's physical examination findings
• Assess the client's laboratory results
STANDARDS
• Apply intellectual standards of accuracy, relevancy, and significance to obtaining a health history of the client with fluid alterations
• Apply agency and professional standards for assessing fluid balance
• Consider laboratory standards for normal electrolyte values
ATTITUDES
• Use discipline to obtain complete and correct assessment data regarding client's fluid status
• Be responsible for collecting appropriate specimens for diagnostic and laboratory tests related to the client's fluid balance

FIGURE **36–7** Critical thinking model for fluid, electrolyte, and acid-base balances assessment.

Prior Medical History

Acute Illness. Recent surgery, head and chest trauma, shock, and second- or third-degree burns are conditions that place clients at high risk for fluid, electrolyte, and acid-base alterations. In addition, the client continues to be at risk during the acute phase until the underlying process is resolved. For example, the stress response of surgery may cause fluid-balance changes in the second to fifth post-operative day, when aldosterone, glucocorticoids, and ADH are increasingly secreted, causing sodium and chloride retention, potassium excretion, and decreased urinary output.

Surgery. The more extensive the surgery and fluid loss during the surgical procedure, the greater the body's response to the surgical trauma. After surgery, clients can exhibit many acid-base changes. The client who is reluctant to breathe deeply and cough may develop respiratory acidosis due to retained $PaCO_2$. The client with nasogastric suction may develop metabolic alkalosis due to the loss of gastric acid, fluids, and electrolytes.

Burns. The greater the body surface burned, the greater the fluid loss. The burned client loses body fluids by one of five routes. First, plasma leaves the intravascular space and becomes trapped edema. This is also called the plasma-to-interstitial fluid shift. It is accompanied by a loss of serum proteins. Second, plasma and interstitial fluids are lost as burn exudate. Third, water vapour and heat are lost in proportion to the amount of skin that is burned away. Fourth, blood leaks from damaged capillaries, adding to the intravascular fluid volume loss. Last, sodium and water shift into the cells, further compromising extracellular fluid volume (Phipps et al., 2003).

Respiratory Disorders. Many alterations in respiratory function predispose the client to respiratory acidosis. For example, the changes involved in pneumonia, sedative overdose, and exacerbated chronic airflow limitation interfere with the elimination of carbon dioxide as the client retains carbon dioxide during hypoventilation. As the carbon dioxide continues to build up in the bloodstream, the body's compensatory mechanisms can no longer adapt and the pH decreases. Likewise, hyperventilation that occurs with such conditions as fever or anxiety causes the client to experience respiratory alkalosis by blowing off too much carbon dioxide with the increased respiratory rate.

Head Injury. Head injury can result in cerebral edema. Occasionally this edema creates pressure on the pituitary gland, and as a result, ADH secretion is changed. Two alterations can occur. Diabetes insipidus occurs when too little ADH is secreted and the client excretes large volumes of diluted urine with a low specific gravity. The second alteration is the syndrome of inappropriate antidiuretic hormone (SIADH), in which there is continued inappropriate secretion of ADH. This results in water intoxication characterized by fluid volume expansion and hyponatremia, as well as hypotonicity of fluids as a result of high urine osmolality and low serum osmolality (Phipps et al., 2003).

Chronic Illness. Chronic disease (e.g., cancer, congestive heart failure, or renal disease) comprises a variety of conditions that can create fluid, electrolyte, and acid-base imbalances. The nurse must review the normal course of the client's chronic disease in order to understand how fluid, electrolyte, and acid-base status may be affected.

Cancer. The types of fluid and electrolyte imbalances that are observed in a client with cancer depend on the type and progression of the cancer. All electrolyte imbalances can occur in the client with cancer and are caused by anatomical distortion and functional impairment from tumour growth and tumour-caused metabolic and endocrine abnormality. In addition, clients with cancer are at risk for fluid and electrolyte imbalances related to the side effects (e.g., diarrhea and anorexia) of their chemotherapeutic and radiological treatments.

Cardiovascular Disease. In the client with cardiovascular disease, a diminished cardiac output reduces kidney perfusion, causing the client to experience a decrease in urinary output. The client will retain sodium and water, resulting in circulatory overload, and run the risk of developing pulmonary edema. Fluid and electrolyte imbalances associated with heart disease can be controlled for a time with medications and fluid and sodium restrictions. The goal of fluid reduction is to decrease the workload of the left ventricle by reducing the excess circulating fluid volume.

Renal Disorders. Kidney disease alters fluid and electrolyte balance by the abnormal retention of sodium, chloride, potassium, and water in the extracellular compartment. The plasma levels of metabolic waste products such as blood urea nitrogen (BUN) and creatinine are elevated because the kidneys are unable to filter and excrete the waste products of cellular metabolism. This elevation is toxic to cellular processes. Metabolic acidosis results when hydrogen ions are retained because of decreased renal function. Because of the renal disorder, the usual renal compensatory mechanisms such as bicarbonate reabsorption are not available; therefore, the body's ability to restore normal acid-base balance is limited.

The severity of fluid and electrolyte imbalance is proportional to the degree of renal failure. Occasionally, acute renal failure–induced shock or a decrease in ECF may be reversible. Although chronic renal failure is progressive, the client may be treated successfully with dietary control of protein and salt intake, diuretic medications, and fluid restrictions. In later stages, treatment with dialysis and/or transplantation may be required.

Gastrointestinal Disturbances. Gastroenteritis and nasogastric suctioning result in a loss of fluid, potassium, and chloride ions. Hydrogen ions are also lost, causing a disturbance in acid-base balance. Timely education of infant and child caregivers is necessary to prevent dehydration when the infant or child is experiencing diarrhea. Gastrointestinal fistulas can also result in a loss of potassium, resulting in an increased risk for hypokalemia. The loss of potassium increases the risk for acid-base disturbances as well.

Regardless of the presence of any disease process, the nurse must determine how long the client has had that disease and the type of treatment currently being administered. In addition to chronic health problems, the nurse determines if the client has a history of new-onset acute illnesses such as diarrhea, vomiting, colostomy, nasogastric suctioning, or intestinal drainage. Any condition that results in the loss of GI fluids predisposes the client to dehydration and a variety of electrolyte disturbances.

Human Immunodeficiency Virus (HIV)/Acquired Immunodeficiency Syndrome (AIDS). The types of fluid and electrolyte imbalances that are observed in a client with HIV/AIDS depend on the stage of the disease and manifestations of the illness, complications (e.g., nephropathy, malignancy, and opportunistic infections), and side effects of antiretroviral therapy. Electrolyte and acid/base imbalances can occur as a result of anorexia, nausea, vomiting, diarrhea, and malignancies. Treatment should focus on improving food and fluid intake, providing comfort measures, and addressing the cause of the imbalance.

Environmental Factors. The nurse should also include certain environmental factors in the health history. Clients who have participated in vigorous exercise or who have become exposed to temperature extremes may have clinical signs of fluid and electrolyte alterations. Exposure to environmental temperatures exceeding 28° to 30° C results in excessive sweating with weight loss. A body weight loss over 7% decreases the ability of the cooling mechanism to conserve water. Loss of fluid from sweating varies and can reach a maximal rate of 2 L/hour (Ignatavicius & Workman, 2002). Inadequate fluid replacement can lead to fluid volume disturbances.

Diet. A client's current dietary history is an important component of nursing assessment. Dietary intake of fluids, salt, potassium, calcium, magnesium, and necessary carbohydrates, fats, and protein helps maintain normal fluid, electrolyte, and acid-base status. Recent changes in appetite or the ability to chew and swallow can affect nutritional status and fluid hydration. When nutritional intake is inadequate, the body tries to preserve its protein stores by breaking down glycogen and fat stores. When excess free fatty acids are released, metabolic acidosis can occur because the liver converts free fatty acids to ketone, a strong acid. However, after those resources are depleted, the body begins to destroy protein stores. Hypoalbuminemia occurs when serum protein levels drop below normal. In hypoalbuminemia, the serum colloid osmotic pressure is decreased, and fluid shifts from the circulating blood volume and enters the interstitial fluid space in the peritoneal cavity. In addition, because rapid water loss can lead to osmolar fluid imbalance, dieting can lead to acidosis.

Lifestyle. Lifestyle factors should also be included in the client's health history. Pre-existing medical risks, such as a history of smoking or alcohol consumption, can further impair the client's ability to adapt to fluid, electrolyte, and acid-base alterations. For example, the consistent use of alcohol and tobacco can ultimately cause respiratory depression, which can result in respiratory acidosis and alteration in maintaining adequate fluid and electrolyte balance.

Medication. A final category to include in the nurse's assessment is a history of medication use (Box 36-2). If the assessment reveals a medication that is likely to cause an electrolyte or acid-base disorder, the nurse will also closely examine laboratory values. In addition, the nurse will assess the client's knowledge of side effects and adherence to medication schedules and the client's knowledge of the potential side effects of over-the-counter medications on fluid, electrolyte, and acid-base balances (Phipps et al., 2003).

Physical Assessment. A thorough examination is necessary because fluid and electrolyte imbalances or acid-base disturbances can affect all body systems. While examining each system, the nurse carefully considers the signs and symptoms to expect as a result of any imbalance. For example, an examination of the oral cavity will likely reveal signs of dehydration if the nurse suspects the client is experiencing a fluid loss. Table 36-7 summarizes possible physical findings for clients with fluid, electrolyte, and acid-base imbalances.

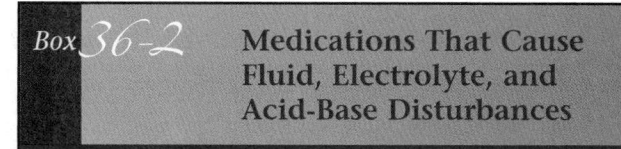

Box 36-2 Medications That Cause Fluid, Electrolyte, and Acid-Base Disturbances

Diuretics—metabolic alkalosis, hyperkalemia, and hypokalemia
Steroids—metabolic alkalosis
Potassium supplements—GI disturbances, including intestinal and gastric ulcers and diarrhea
Respiratory centre depressants such as opioid analgesics—decreased rate and depth of respirations, resulting in respiratory acidosis
Antibiotics—nephrotoxicity (e.g., vancomycin, methicillin, aminoglycosides); hyperkalemia and/or hypernatremia (e.g., azlocillin, carbenicillin, piperacillin, ticarcillin, Unasyn)*
Calcium carbonate (Tums)—mild metabolic alkalosis with nausea and vomiting*
Magnesium hydroxide (Milk of Magnesia)—hypokalemia*

*Data from *Mosby's Pharmacology in Nursing* (21st ed.), by L. M. McKenry and E. Salerno, 2003, St. Louis, MO: Mosby.

Measuring Fluid Intake and Output. Measuring and recording all liquid intake and output (I&O) during a 24-hour period is an important part of the client's assessment database for fluid and electrolyte balance. Recognition of trends in the I&O is important (e.g., a gradually decreasing urine output can indicate that the body is trying to adapt to an FVD or hyperosmolar fluid imbalance). Accurate I&O measurements can identify both clients at risk for and clients who are experiencing fluid, electrolyte, and acid-base disturbances.

For clients in health care settings, I&O measurement is a nursing intervention routinely used for clients following a procedure, clients who are febrile, clients with restricted fluids, or clients who receive diuretic or intravenous (IV) therapy. The nurse also measures I&O for clients with chronic cardiopulmonary or renal illnesses and clients whose health status has deteriorated or has become unstable.

Intake includes all liquids taken by mouth, (e.g., gelatin, ice cream, soup, juice, and water), through nasogastric or jejunostomy feeding tubes (see chapter 39), IV fluids (including both large-volume and intermittent IVs), and blood or its components. Occasionally, clients receive a specific amount of a liquid medication every 1 to 2 hours. A client receiving tube feedings may receive numerous liquid medications, and water may be used to flush the tube for the medications. Over a 24-hour period, these liquids can amount to significant intake and should always be recorded on the I&O record. Output includes urine, diarrhea, vomitus, gastric suction, and drainage from post-surgical wounds or other tubes (see chapter 45).

Ambulatory clients are instructed to save their urine in a calibrated insert, which attaches to the rim of the toilet bowl (Figure 36–8). When a client has an in-dwelling Foley catheter, drainage tube, or suction, output is recorded when the client's condition requires (e.g., at the end of each nursing shift or every hour). Co-operation

Table 36-7 Physical and Behavioural Nursing Assessment for Fluid, Electrolyte, and Acid-Base Imbalances

Assessment	Imbalance
Weight Changes	
2%–5% loss	Mild FVD*
5%–10% loss	Moderate FVD*
10%–15% loss	Severe FVD*
15%–20% loss	Death*
2% gain	Mild fluid volume excess (FVE)
5% gain	Moderate FVE
8% gain	Severe FVE
Head	
History:	
Headache	FVD,* metabolic or respiratory acidosis, metabolic alkalosis
Dizziness	FVD,* respiratory acidosis or alkalosis, hyponatremia
Observation:	
Irritability	Metabolic or respiratory alkalosis, hyperosmolar imbalance, hypernatremia, hypokalemia
Lethargy	FVD,* metabolic acidosis or alkalosis, respiratory acidosis, hypercalcemia
Confusion, disorientation	FVD,* hypomagnesemia, metabolic acidosis, hypokalemia
Eyes	
Inspection:	
Sunken, dry conjunctivae, decreased or absent tearing	FVD
Periorbital edema, papilledema	FVE
History:	
Blurred vision	FVE
Throat and mouth	
Inspection:	
Sticky, dry mucous membranes, dry cracked lips, decreased salivation	FVD, hypernatremia
Longitudinal tongue furrows	
Cardiovascular System	
Inspection:	
Flat neck veins	FVD
Distended neck veins	FVE
Slow venous filling	FVD*
Palpation:	
Edema (dependent body parts: back, sacrum, legs)	FVE*
Dysrhythmias (also noted as ECG changes)	Metabolic acidosis, respiratory alkalosis and acidosis, potassium imbalance, hypomagnesemia
Increased pulse rate	Metabolic alkalosis, respiratory acidosis, hyponatremia, FVD, hypomagnesemia
Decreased pulse rate	Metabolic alkalosis, hypokalemia
Weak pulse	FVD, hypokalemia
Decreased capillary filling	FVD
Bounding pulse	FVE
Auscultation:	
Blood pressure low or without orthostatic changes	FVD, hyponatremia, hyperkalemia, hypermagnesemia
Third heart sound	FVE
Hypertension	FVE

Table 36-7 Physical and Behavioural Nursing Assessment for Fluid, Electrolyte, and Acid-Base Imbalances—cont'd

Assessment	Imbalance
Respiratory System	
Inspection:	
Increased rate	FVE, respiratory alkalosis, metabolic acidosis
Dyspnea	FVE
Auscultation:	
Crackles	FVE
Gastrointestinal System	
History:	
Anorexia	Metabolic acidosis
Abdominal cramps	Metabolic acidosis
Inspection:	
Sunken abdomen	FVD
Distended abdomen	Third-space syndrome
Vomiting	FVD, hypercalcemia, hyponatremia, hypochloremia, metabolic alkalosis
Diarrhea	Hyponatremia, metabolic acidosis
Auscultation:	
Hyperperistalsis with diarrhea, or hypoperistalsis	FVD, hypokalemia
Renal System	
Inspection:	
Oliguria or anuria	FVD, FVE
Diuresis (if kidneys are normal)	FVE
Increased urine specific gravity	FVD
Neuromuscular System	
Inspection:	
Numbness, tingling	Metabolic alkalosis, hypocalcemia, potassium imbalances
Muscle cramps, tetany	Hypocalcemia, metabolic or respiratory alkalosis
Coma	Hyperosmolar or hypoosmolar imbalances, hyponatremia
Tremors	Respiratory acidosis, hypomagnesemia
Palpation:	
Hypotonicity	Hypokalemia, hypercalcemia*
Hypertonicity	Hypocalcemia, hypomagnesemia, metabolic alkalosis
Percussion:	
Decreased or absent deep tendon reflexes	Hypercalcemia, hypermagnesemia
Increased or hyperactive deep tendon reflexes	Hypocalcemia, hypomagnesemia
Skin	
Body temperature:	
Increased	Hypernatremia, hyperosmolar imbalance, metabolic acidosis
Decreased	FVD
Inspection:	
Dry, flushed	FVD, hypernatremia, metabolic acidosis
Palpation:	
Inelastic skin turgor, cold, clammy skin	FVD

*Data from *Mosby's Pocket Guide Series: Fluid, Electrolyte, and Acid-Base Balance* (4th ed.), by U. E. Heitz and M. M. Horne, 2001, St. Louis, MO: Mosby.

from the client and family is essential with I&O measurements. It is important for the client to have good vision and motor skills to ensure accuracy. The nurse teaches the client and family the purpose of the measurements and either to notify the nurse to empty any container with voided fluid or how to measure and empty the container themselves.

In the hospital, forms for recording I&O are attached to the bedside chart or room door (Figure 36–9). The 24-hour total is calculated as directed by agency policy. The nurse who still retains responsibility may delegate I&O recording to unregulated care providers with competent skills in measurement and calculation, not estimation, and timeliness.

A

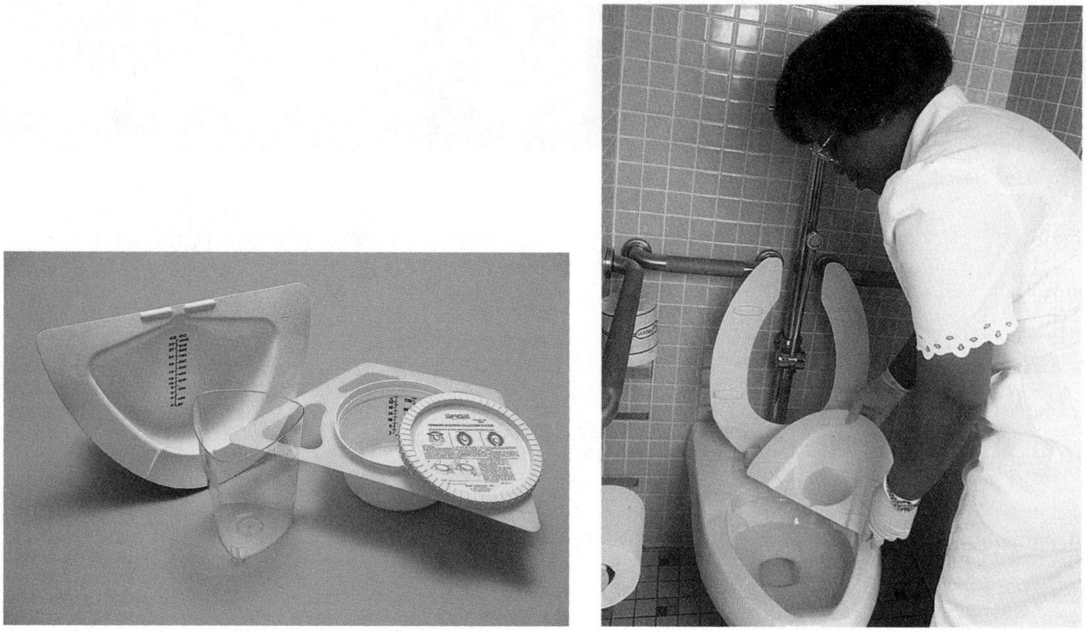

B

FIGURE 36–8 **A,** Graduated measuring containers. Clockwise from far left: "hat" receptacle, specipan, and graduated measuring container. **B,** Emptying collected urine.

Recording I&O is essential for obtaining an accurate database. Daily intake should equal output plus 500 mL (to cover for insensible fluid losses). This information helps maintain an ongoing evaluation of the client's hydration status to prevent severe imbalances.

Laboratory Studies. The nurse reviews laboratory tests to obtain further objective data about fluid, electrolyte, and acid-base balances. These tests include serum and urinary electrolyte levels, hematocrit, blood creatinine level, BUN levels, urine specific gravity, and ABG readings (Box 36-3). Serum electrolyte levels are measured to determine the hydration status, the electrolyte concentration of the blood plasma, and acid-base balance. The frequency with which these electrolyte levels are measured depends on the severity of the client's illness. Serum electrolyte tests are routinely performed on any client entering a hospital to screen for alterations and to serve as a baseline for future comparisons.

Client Expectations. Often a fluid, electrolyte, or acid-base disturbance is so serious or acute that the client's condition prevents a review of his or her expectations. However, if a client is alert enough to discuss care with the nurse, a review of expectations may reveal short-term needs (e.g., provision of comfort from nausea) or long-term needs (e.g., understanding how to prevent alterations from occurring in the future). The client must be able to understand the implications of fluid, electrolyte, or acid-base changes to be able to express expectations of care. The client's trust in the nurse is strengthened through the nurse's competent response to sudden changes in the client's condition.

Nursing Diagnosis

When caring for clients with suspected fluid, electrolyte, and acid-base imbalances, it is particularly important that the nurse be skilled in using critical thinking to formulate nursing diagnoses. The assessment data that establish the risk for or the actual presence of a nursing diagnosis in these areas may be subtle, and patterns and trends emerge only when the nurse consciously assesses for them. The nurse must keep in mind that many body systems may be involved. Clustering of defining characteristics will lead the nurse to selection of the appropriate diagnoses. For example, the nursing diagnosis *deficient fluid volume* is developed in Box 36-4.

An important part of formulating nursing diagnoses is identifying the relevant causative or related factor. The nursing interventions that are chosen must treat or modify the related factor for the diagnosis to be resolved. *Deficient fluid volume related to loss of gastrointestinal fluids via vomiting* will require therapies different than those needed for *deficient fluid volume related to elevated body temperature.*

Possible nursing diagnoses for clients with fluid, electrolyte, and acid-base alterations may include the following:

- Risk for imbalanced body temperature
- Ineffective breathing pattern
- Decreased cardiac output
- Deficient fluid volume
- Risk for deficient fluid volume
- Excess fluid volume
- Impaired gas exchange
- Deficient knowledge regarding disease management

Intake and Output Summary

Client Label	P.O. Intake	Tube Feedings	Hyperalimentation	I.V. Primary	I.V.P.B.	Blood/Blood Products	Other:	Urine	Emesis	G.I. Suction	Drainage	Other: Chest tube
Date: 6-10-XX												
2200–0600	120				50			325			50	75
0600–1400	800							700			75	50
1400–2200	650				50			500			30	50
24Hr. Subtotal	1570				100			1525			155	175
Total Intake/Output	1570/100							1525/330				
Date:												
2200–0600												
0600–1400												
1400–2200												
24Hr. Subtotal												
Total Intake/Output												
Date:												
2200–0600												
0600–1400												
1400–2200												
24Hr. Subtotal												
Total Intake/Output												
Date:												
2200–0600												
0600–1400												
1400–2200												
24Hr. Subtotal												
Total Intake/Output												
Date:												
2200–0600												
0600–1400												
1400–2200												
24Hr. Subtotal												
Total Intake/ Output												
Date:												
2200–0600												
0600–1400												
1400–2200												
24Hr. Subtotals												
Total Intake/Output												
Date:												
2200–0600												
0600–1400												
1400–2200												
24Hr. Subtotals												
Total Intake/Output												

FIGURE 36–9 Twenty-four-hour intake and output record. (Courtesy St. Mary's Health Center, St. Louis, MO.)

Box 36-3 Laboratory Data for Fluid, Electrolyte, and Acid-Base Imbalances

Fluid and Electrolytes

Altered concentrations of sodium, potassium, magnesium, calcium, phosphates, chloride, and bicarbonate (venous CO_2 contentions)
Increase in hematocrit, BUN, sodium, and osmolality in serum (related to loss of ECF fluid or gain of solutes)
Decrease in hematocrit, BUN, sodium, and osmolality in serum (related to gain of ECF fluid or loss of solutes)
Concentrated urine demonstrated by urine specific gravity >1.030
Dilute urine demonstrated by a specific gravity <1.012

Metabolic Alkalosis

pH >7.45
$PaCO_2$ normal or >45 mm Hg if lungs are compensating PaO_2 normal
O_2 saturation (SaO_2) normal
HCO_3^- >26 mmol/L
K^+ <3.5 mmol/L

Metabolic Acidosis

pH <7.35
$PaCO_2$ normal or <35 mm Hg if lungs are compensating

Metabolic Acidosis, cont'd

PaO_2 normal
SaO_2 normal
HCO_3^- <22 mmol/L
K^+ >5.3 mmol/L
K^+ <3.5 mmol/L

Respiratory Alkalosis

pH >7.45
$PaCO_2$ <35 mm Hg
PaO_2 normal
SaO_2 normal
HCO_3^- normal
K^+ <3.5 mmol/L

Respiratory Acidosis

pH <7.35
$PaCO_2$ >45 mm Hg
PaO_2 normal or <80 mm Hg, depending on cause of acidosis
SaO_2 normal or <95%, depending on cause of acidosis
HCO_3^- normal if early respiratory acidosis or >26 mmol/L if kidneys are compensating
K^+ >5.3 mmol/L

Nursing Diagnostic Process Box 36-4

Assessment Activities	Defining Characteristics	Nursing Diagnosis
Assess blood pressure and pulse.	Client is hypotensive with increased heart rate.	Deficient fluid volume related to loss of gastrointestinal fluids via vomiting
Obtain daily weight measurements.	Client experiences sudden weight loss.	
Observe volume of urine output related to intake and specific gravity.	Decreased volume of output in comparison to intake; increased urine specific gravity is present.	
Palpate skin turgor.	Inelastic skin turgor noted.	
Ask if client is thirsty or weak.	Client verbalizes thirst and weakness.	
Inspect mucous membranes for degree of moisture.	Dry mucous membranes are noted.	
Observe for abnormal losses of fluids.	Client is vomiting.	
Assess client's tolerance to changing from lying to sitting position.	Client complains of dizziness when changing position.	

- Impaired mobility
- Impaired oral mucous membrane
- Impaired skin integrity
- Risk for impaired skin integrity
- Ineffective therapeutic regimen management
- Impaired tissue integrity
- Ineffective tissue perfusion

Planning

During the planning process, the nurse uses critical thinking to synthesize information from multiple resources (Figure 36–10) and to ensure that the client's care plan integrates both the nurse's scientific and nursing

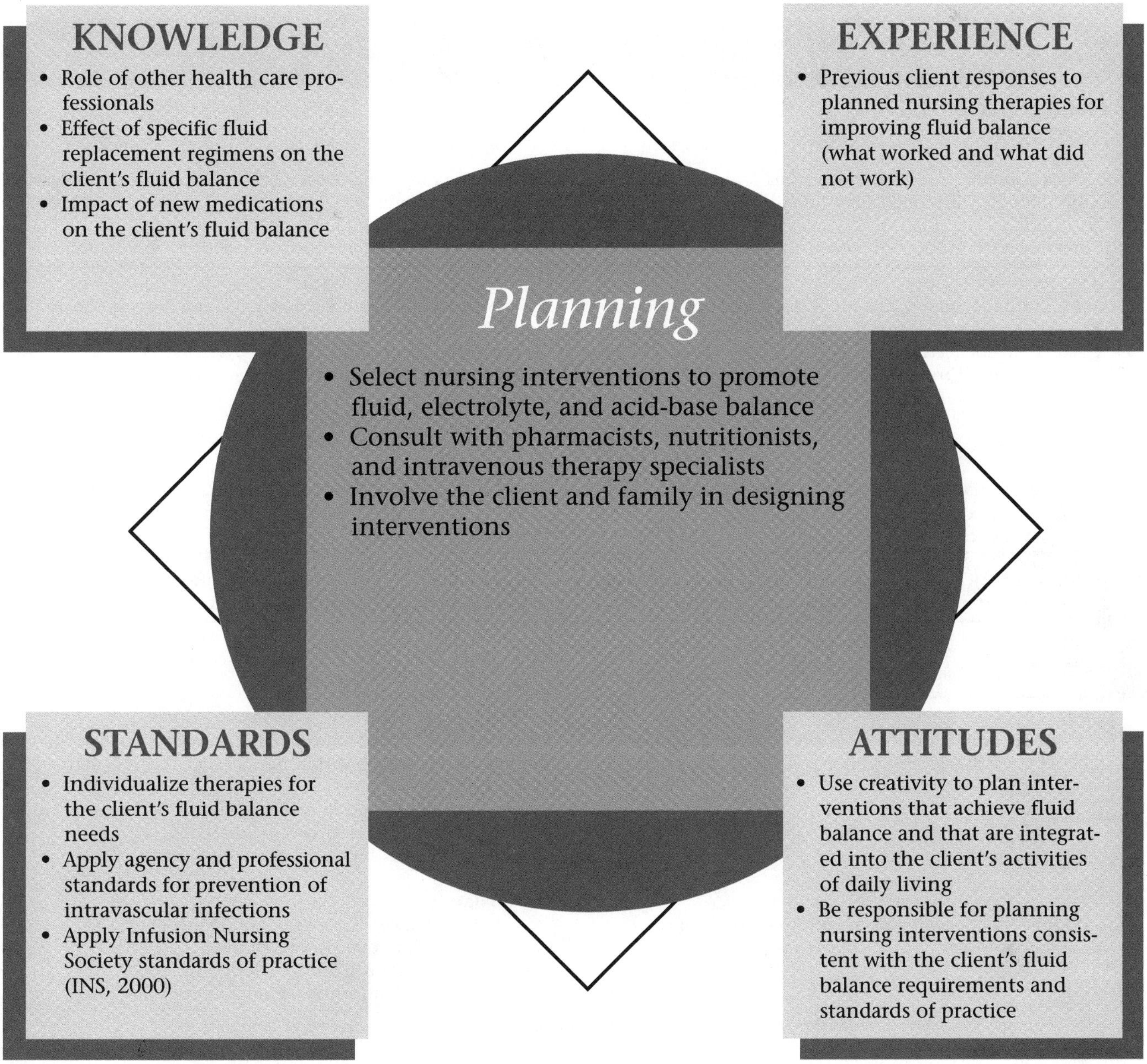
KNOWLEDGE
• Role of other health care professionals
• Effect of specific fluid replacement regimens on the client's fluid balance
• Impact of new medications on the client's fluid balance
EXPERIENCE
• Previous client responses to planned nursing therapies for improving fluid balance (what worked and what did not work)
Planning
• Select nursing interventions to promote fluid, electrolyte, and acid-base balance
• Consult with pharmacists, nutritionists, and intravenous therapy specialists
• Involve the client and family in designing interventions
STANDARDS
• Individualize therapies for the client's fluid balance needs
• Apply agency and professional standards for prevention of intravascular infections
• Apply Infusion Nursing Society standards of practice (INS, 2000)
ATTITUDES
• Use creativity to plan interventions that achieve fluid balance and that are integrated into the client's activities of daily living
• Be responsible for planning nursing interventions consistent with the client's fluid balance requirements and standards of practice

FIGURE **36–10** Critical thinking model for fluid, electrolyte, and acid-base balances planning.

knowledge, as well as all of the knowledge that the nurse has gathered about the individual client.

Goals and Outcomes. The nurse develops an individual care plan for each of the nursing diagnoses (see Care Plan). The nurse and client set expectations for care that are individualized and realistic with measurable outcomes. Goals are designed to achieve and maintain homeostasis. For example, the following related outcomes might be established for the goal "The client will restore hydration status at discharge":

- The client will be free of complications associated with the IV device throughout the duration of IV therapy.
- The client will demonstrate fluid balance by moist, mucous membranes; balanced I&O measurements; and stable daily weights (within 0.5 kg) within 48 hours.
- The client will have serum electrolytes within the normal range within 48 hours.

Setting Priorities. The client's clinical condition will determine which of the diagnoses takes the greatest priority. Many nursing diagnoses in the area of fluid, electrolyte, and acid-base balances are of highest priority, because the consequences for the client can be serious or even life-threatening. For example, in the concept map for the client with gastroenteritis and dehydration (Figure 36–11),

Nursing Care Plan

Fluid and Electrolyte Alterations

Assessment

Mrs. Hilda Bottomley is a 72-year-old woman seen by her physician this morning with complaints of flu-like symptoms and difficulty breathing. She admits that she has not felt like eating and drinking much lately. After an outpatient chest X-ray examination, Mrs. Bottomley has been admitted for respiratory toileting and IV antibiotic and fluid therapy. The physician orders oxygen at 4 L/minute with humidification, respiratory treatments, fluids by mouth and IV, pulse oximetry, and activity with assistance.

Assessment Activities	Findings/Defining Characteristics
Ask Mrs. Bottomley to describe when her respiratory discomfort began and what accompanying signs and symptoms she may have experienced.	She states that she became congested about 2 weeks ago and now she is coughing up mucus, has chills, feels weak, is not interested in eating, and aches all over.
Observe her pulmonary secretions.	Mrs. Bottomley coughed up thick and yellowish-greenish sputum.
Assess Mrs. Bottomley's vital signs.	Mrs. Bottomley's temperature is 36.7° C, her respiratory rate is 28 breaths per minute, and rhonchi breath sounds are present. Other vital signs are within normal limits.
Evaluate her arterial blood gas values and review her chest X-ray report.	Mrs. Bottomley's arterial blood gas results indicate a mild respiratory acidosis, and the chest X-ray film revealed a left lower lobe pneumonia.

Nursing Diagnosis: Ineffective airway clearance related to increased mucus in response to airway infection and manifested by mild respiratory acidosis; risk for deficient fluid volume related to reduced fluid intake.

Planning

Goal	Expected Outcomes*
	Electrolyte and Acid/Base Balance
Client's airway will be free from secretions with normal arterial blood gas (ABG) levels by discharge.	ABG levels will be within normal limits in 24 hours. Respiratory rate will be within normal limits with activity in 24 hours. Temperature will be within normal limits in 24 hours. Breath sounds will be clear on auscultation. Mucus will become thin and clear in 48 hours.
	Fluid Balance
Client's fluid volume will remain within normal limits throughout hospital stay.	Urine output will equal intake of approximately 1,500 mL. Daily weight will not vary more than 0.5 kg. Mucous membranes will remain moist. Vital signs will remain within normal limits.

*Outcome classification labels from *Nursing Outcomes Classification (NOC)* (3rd ed.), edited by S. Moorhead, M. Johnson, and M. L. Maas, 2004, St. Louis, MO: Mosby.

Interventions†	Rationale
Airway Maintenance	
• Schedule coughing and deep breathing exercises every 2 hours while awake.	Cough control exercises and deep breathing promote pulmonary secretion clearance (Woods, 2002).
• Administer chest physiotherapy every 4 hours while awake to affected regions of the lung	Chest physiotherapy, breathing exercises, cough techniques, along with ambulating the client, are effective in promoting airway clearance (Woods, 2002).
• Ambulate client once every 8 hours and encourage client to get out of bed into chair often.	Mobility promotes air exchange and position change prevents settling of secretions in lung tissue.
Fluid Management	
• Provide client with an additional 500 mL of non-caffeinated oral fluids every 8 hours.	Increased fluid intake helps to liquefy pulmonary secretions and in turn facilitate productive coughing (Woods, 2002).

†Intervention classification labels from *Nursing Interventions Classification (NIC)* (4th ed.), edited by J. M. Dochterman and G. M. Bulecheck, 2004, St. Louis, MO: Mosby.

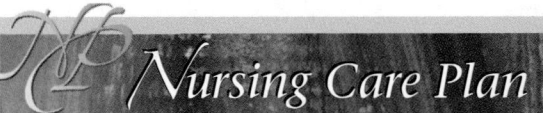

Nursing Care Plan

Fluid and Electrolyte Alterations—cont'd

Evaluation

Nursing Actions	Client Response/Finding	Achievement of Outcome
Monitor ABG levels, vital signs, intake and output (I&O), daily weight and O_2 saturation levels. Assess mucous membranes.	She is able to walk down the hall without respiratory discomfort. Mrs. Bottomley states she is drinking more fluids. She no longer experiences chills and a fever.	Mrs. Bottomley's ABG levels have returned to normal values. Vital signs and O_2 saturation are within normal range. Her I&O measurements are negative for fluid loss or excess. Daily weight remained stable. Mucous membranes are moist.
Auscultate breath sounds.	Mrs. Bottomley denies any discomfort with breathing in or out.	Mrs. Bottomley's breath sounds are clear bilaterally on inspiration and expiration.
Evaluate effectiveness of coughing and deep-breathing exercises.	Mrs. Bottomley demonstrated three deep breaths followed by coughing and said she no longer coughs up sputum.	Mrs. Bottomley is free of sputum production.
Identify methods to provide for adequate rest.	Mrs. Bottomley says she takes naps between her morning and afternoon treatments.	Mrs. Bottomley schedules her activities throughout the day and rests in bed before her respiratory therapy.

nausea and diarrhea have caused a deficient fluid volume. Unless the nurse intervenes to resolve the client's nausea and diarrhea, the fluid imbalance will likely worsen.

Consultation with the client's physician may assist in setting realistic time frames for the goals of care, particularly when the client's physiological status is unstable. During planning, the nurse collaborates as much as possible with the client and family and other members of the health care team, such as IV therapy and pharmacy. The family can be particularly helpful in identifying subtle changes in a client's behaviour associated with imbalances (e.g., anxiety, confusion, or irritability).

Continuity of Care. For clients with acute disturbances, discharge planning must begin early. In the hospital, the nurse ensures that care can continue in the home or long-term care setting with few disruptions. For example, when a client is discharged on IV therapy, the nurse must determine the knowledge and skills of the person who is to assume care-giving responsibilities and make a referral to home IV therapy as soon as possible. The nurse also collaborates closely with other members of the health care team, such as the physician, dietitian, and pharmacist. The dietitian can recommend therapeutic diets to increase or reduce intake of certain electrolytes (See chapter 39). The pharmacist can help identify medications likely to cause electrolyte or acid-base disturbances and describe possible side effects of the client's prescribed drugs. The physician directs the treatment of any fluid, electrolyte, or acid-base alteration.

Implementation

Health Promotion. Health promotion activities in the area of fluid, electrolyte, and acid-base imbalances focus primarily on client teaching (Box 36-5). Clients and caregivers need to recognize risk factors for these imbalances and implement appropriate preventive measures. For example, parents of infants need to understand that GI losses can quickly lead to serious imbalances; therefore, when an infant has vomiting or diarrhea, the parent must recognize the risk and promptly seek health care to restore normal balance. Even the healthy adult is at risk for developing imbalances when subjected to high temperatures. Nurses need to advise clients to increase water intake, maintain adequate ventilation, and refrain from excessive activity during heat waves.

Sometimes it is difficult to separate the effects of age-related changes from changes associated with disease processes. For example, any older adult who has a chronic condition involving renal or respiratory function is more likely to suffer serious consequences when an acute disease process occurs (Phipps et al., 2003).

All clients with a chronic health alteration are at risk for developing changes in their fluid, electrolyte, and acid-base balances. They need to understand their own risk factors and the measures to be taken to avoid imbalances. For example, clients with renal failure must avoid excess intake of fluid, sodium, potassium, and phosphorus. Through diet education, these clients learn the types of foods to avoid and the suitable volume of fluid they are permitted daily (see chapter 39). Clients with chronic health conditions need to be made aware of early signs and symptoms of fluid, electrolyte, and acid-base imbalances. A client with heart disease should be instructed to obtain an accurate body weight each day at the approximate same time and to inform the physician of significant changes of weight from one day to another. Increase in weight, shortness of breath, orthopnea, and dependent edema are all associated with fluid retention.

Acute Care. Although fluid, electrolyte, and/or acid-base imbalance can occur in all settings, changes in the acute care delivery system place more demands on the nurse.

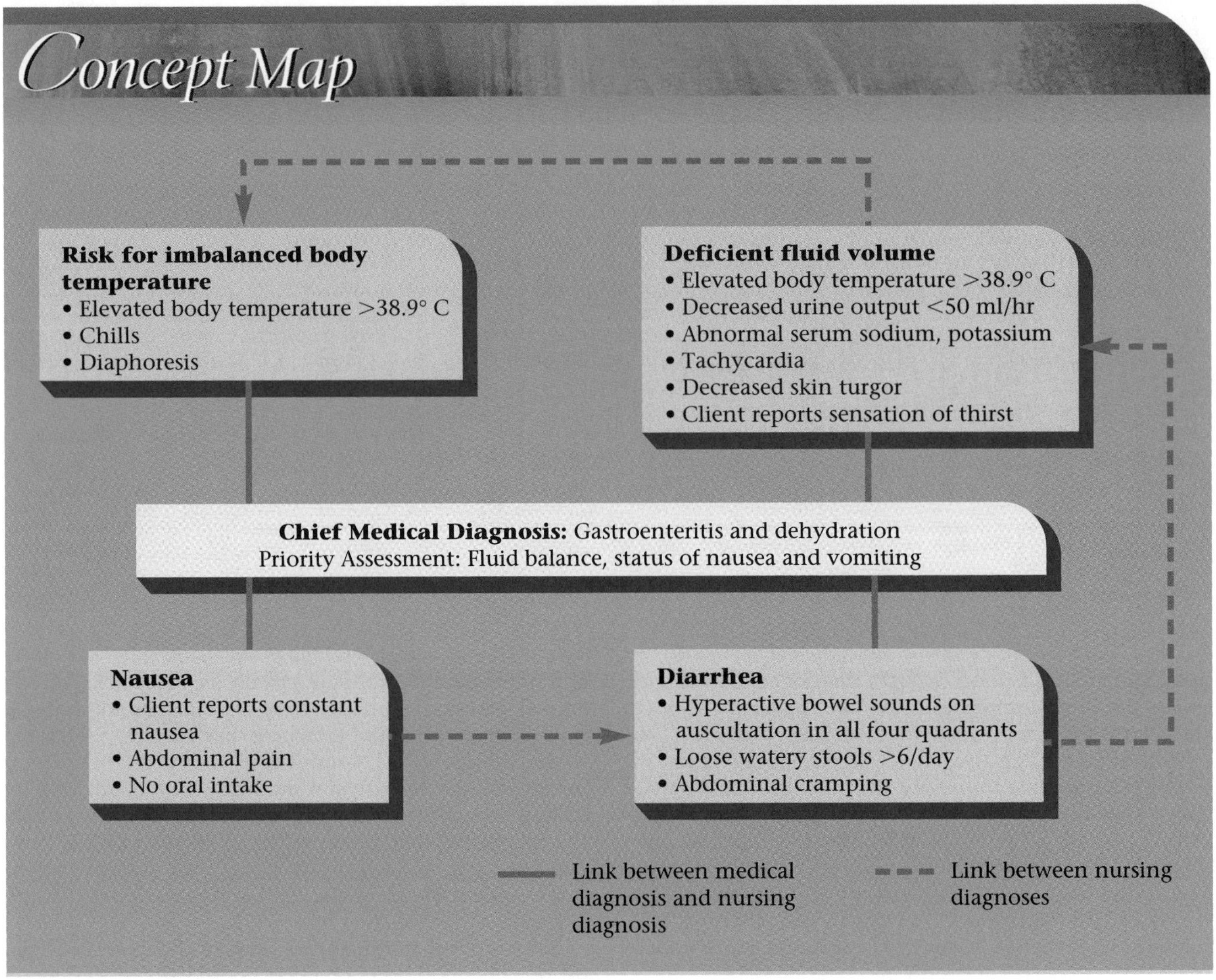

FIGURE **36–11** Concept map for a client with gastroenteritis and dehydration.

Today the nurse must manage the client's complex medical care in a shorter span of time while performing difficult technological skills.

Daily Weights and Intake and Output Measurement. When implementing specific measures to increase or decrease fluid, two nursing interventions are necessary: daily weight and I&O measurements. Clients with fluid and electrolyte alterations may need to be weighed daily. Daily weights are the single most important indicator of fluid status (Heitz & Horne, 2001). Weight should be determined at the same time each day with the same scale after the client voids. The scale should be calibrated each day or routinely. The client should wear the same clothes or clothes that weigh the same; if a bed scale is used, the same number of sheets should be used on the scale with each weighing.

I&O records provide additional information about fluid balance (see Measuring Fluid Intake and Output). I&O measurements, when examined for trends, can indicate whether excess fluid volume is excreted in the form of urine or whether excretion of fluids through the kidneys has diminished. The I&O is not as accurate as daily weights in assessing daily fluid balance unless it has been measured strictly and precisely (Box 36-6).

Enteral Replacement of Fluids. Oral replacement of fluids and electrolytes is appropriate as long as the client is not so physiologically compromised that oral fluids cannot be replaced rapidly. Oral replacement of fluids is contraindicated when the client is vomiting, has a mechanical obstruction of the GI tract, is at risk for aspiration, or has impaired swallowing. Clients unable to tolerate solid foods may still be able to ingest fluids. The nurse should use strategies to encourage fluid intake such as frequently offering small sips of fluid, popsicles, and ice chips.

When replacing fluids by mouth in a client with a fluid deficit, it is wise to choose fluids with adequate calories and electrolyte content (e.g., fruit juices, gelatin, and replacements such as Pedialyte and Gastrolyte). However, liquids containing lactose, caffeine, or low-sodium content may not be appropriate when the client has diarrhea.

A feeding tube may be appropriate when the client's GI tract is healthy but the client cannot ingest fluids (e.g., after oral surgery or with impaired swallowing). Fluids

Client Teaching

Box 36-5

Preventing and Managing Chronic Kidney Disease

Chronic kidney disease is a major burden for individuals and the health care system. The accumulation of waste products and the fluid, electrolyte, and acid base imbalances associated with this disease have many negative results. Primary health care for clients with chronic kidney disease can alleviate some of the morbidity, early mortality, as well as psychosocial and financial challenges for clients and their families.

Cardiovascular disease is a major cause of death of people with chronic kidney disease. Clients should be taught that the progression of kidney disease can be slowed and cardiovascular risk reduced through the following:

- Control of blood pressure
- Control of blood sugar of diabetics
- Control of lipids, antiplatelet therapy
- Renin-angiotensin system antagonism
- Management of anemia
- Control of calcium/phosphate levels (Barrett, 2003; Levin et al., 2001).

In a randomized controlled trial currently in progress, the outcomes associated with primary health care offered by nurses and supervised by physicians using a chronic disease care model are being evaluated (Parfrey et al., 2002). It is hypothesized that client education and empowerment and collaborative nurse-client partnerships will enhance self-management of this disease. It is also hypothesized that nursing interactions and interventions will slow progression of disease, minimize morbidity and mortality, and enhance quality of life for participants. Clinical outcomes will be monitored over a 5-year period, beginning in 2004, to compare the benefits of the nurse-run clinic with the control group receiving standard medical care.

Research Highlight

Box 36-6

Measuring Intake and Output

Research Focus

Continuous fluid intake and output (I&O) measurement is a traditional practice for nurses to monitor the client's cardiovascular and renal function. Validation of this standard of care as an effective determination of fluid balance is questioned.

Research Abstract

The purpose of this study was to determine whether I&O measurements and daily weights revealed redundant information and, if so, which of the two practices was least efficient and could be deleted. A chart audit of clients in three nursing units was conducted to evaluate the efficiency and effectiveness of assessing the client's fluid balance using both a 24-hour I&O and daily weight measurements. Clients were selected who had a physician's order for both I&O and daily weights, the client was treated under this order for at least 48 hours, and the record was complete. The nursing team examined 48-hour records of daily weight and I&O for 73 clients meeting the criteria and correlated the two records. Analyses illustrated the unreliability of weight and fluid balance measurements for determining day-to-day changes in true weight variation. Daily weights alone provide more reliable fluid balance than cumulative I&O measurements. A reduction in personnel resources and costs are realized with elimination of labour-intensive interventions.

Evidenced-Based Practice

- Multiple sources of inaccuracy contribute to unreliable fluid measurements such as inadvertent omission recording, inaccurate measurement, insensible fluid loss, and required multiple recording.
- Sources of error with daily client weights are limited to accuracy of scale and user competency.
- Nursing time and resource expenditure are conserved with only daily weight measurements for evaluating fluid balance.
- Limit the use of combined I&O and daily weights to circumstances where reliability can be ensured.
- Cumulative I&O is best applied for short-term fluid monitoring and for clients in whom acute changes in fluid balance are critical.

Reference

Wise, L., et al. (2000). Evaluating the reliability and utility of cumulative intake and output. *Journal of Nursing Care Quality, 14*(3), 37–42.

can also be replaced through a gastrostomy or jejunostomy feeding tube, or they can be administered via a small-bore nasoenteral feeding tube.

Restriction of Fluids. Clients who retain fluids and have **fluid volume excess (FVE)** require restricted fluid intake. Fluid restriction is often difficult for clients, particularly if they take drugs that dry the oral mucous membranes or if they breathe through the mouth and experience thirst. The nurse should explain the reason that fluids are restricted. In addition, the client needs to know the amount of fluid permitted orally and should understand that ice chips, gelatin, and ice cream are considered fluid. The client should help to decide the amount of fluid with each meal, between meals, before bed, and with medications. Frequently clients on fluid restriction can swallow a number of pills with as little as 30 mL of liquid.

In general, when restricting fluids, allow half of the allotted total oral fluids between 7 AM and 3 PM, the period when clients usually are more active, receive two meals, and take most of their oral medications. Clients on fluid restriction require mouth care frequently to moisten mucous membranes, decrease the chance of mucosal drying and cracking, and maintain comfort (see chapter 34).

Parenteral Replacement of Fluids and Electrolytes. Fluid and electrolytes may be replaced through infusion directly into the blood rather than via the digestive system. Parenteral fluids can also be administered subcutaneously through **hypodermoclysis.** This procedure is particularly useful in older adults in long-term care settings because it is safer, less invasive, less expensive, and better tolerated than IV fluid administration. It can minimize the need for transfers to hospital for rehydration (Dasgupta, Binns, & Rochon, 2000; Slesak et al., 2003). Parenteral replacement includes total parenteral nutrition (TPN), IV fluid and electrolyte therapy **(crystalloids),** and blood and blood component **(colloids)** administration.

Because of the risk for transmission of infectious diseases (e.g., HIV, hepatitis B), standard precautions (or routine practices) must be practised when administering parenteral fluids (see chapter 29).

Vascular Access Devices. **Vascular access devices (VADs)** are catheters, cannulas, or infusion ports designed for repeated access to the vascular system. Peripherally placed catheters are designed for short-term use (e.g., fluid restoration post-operative and short-term antibiotic administration). Devices such as central line catheters, peripherally inserted catheters, and implanted parts are more effective than peripherally placed catheters for administering medications and solutions that are irritating to veins and for the delivery of long-term IV therapy. Increased use of central venous catheters and implanted infusion ports (Figure 36–12) requires nurses to be educated in the care of these devices.

Total Parenteral Nutrition. **Total parenteral nutrition** is a nutritionally adequate hypertonic solution consisting of glucose and other nutrients and electrolytes given through an in-dwelling or central IV catheter that may be inserted peripherally or percutaneously, implanted, or tunnelled. Chapter 39 reviews principles and guidelines for TPN administration, which is used as an intervention in severe cases of malnutrition.

Intravenous Therapy (Crystalloids). The goal of IV fluid administration is to correct or prevent fluid and electrolyte disturbances. It allows direct access to the vascular system, permitting the infusion of continuous fluids over a period of time. Intravenous fluid therapy must be continuously regulated because of continual changes in the client's fluid and electrolyte balance.

When IV fluid administration is required, the nurse must know the correct ordered solution, the equipment needed, the procedures required to initiate an infusion, how to regulate the infusion rate and maintain the system, how to identify and correct problems, and how to discontinue the infusion if necessary.

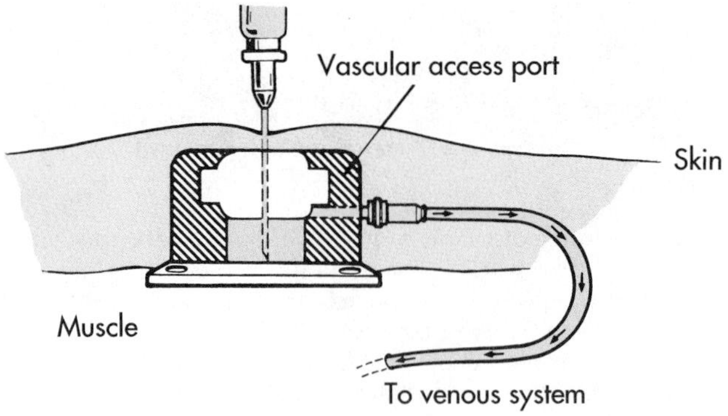

FIGURE **36–12** Example of an implantable vascular access device.

Administration of Intravenous Therapy

Types of Solutions. Many prepared IV solutions are available for use (Table 36-8). Intravenous solutions fall into the following categories: isotonic, hypotonic, and hypertonic. Isotonic solutions are those that have the same effective osmolality as body fluids. Hypotonic solutions are those that have an effective osmolality that is less than body fluids. Hypertonic solutions are those that have an effective osmolality that is greater than body fluids (Heitz & Horne, 2001).

In general, isotonic fluids are used most commonly for extracellular volume replacement (e.g., FVD after prolonged vomiting). The decision to use a hypotonic or hypertonic solution is based on the specific fluid and electrolyte imbalance. For example, the client with a hypertonic fluid imbalance will generally receive a hypotonic IV to dilute the ECF and rehydrate the cells. All IV fluids should be given carefully, especially hypertonic solutions, because these pull fluid into the vascular space by osmosis, resulting in an increased vascular volume that can lead to pulmonary edema, particularly in clients with heart or renal failure. Certain additives, most commonly vitamins and potassium chloride (KCl), are frequently added to IV solutions.

> *Safety Alert. Under no circumstances should potassium chloride (KCl) be given IV push. A direct IV infusion of KCl may be fatal.* If an IV is to have additives added, a physician's order must be obtained that includes the required additives, for example, Bottle 1: 1000 mL $D_5{}^1/_2$ NS with 20 mmol/L KCl at 125 mL/hour.

Clients with normal renal function who are receiving nothing by mouth should have potassium added to IV solutions. The body cannot conserve potassium, and even when the serum level falls, the kidneys continue to excrete potassium. If there is no potassium intake orally or parenterally, hypokalemia can develop quickly. Conversely, the nurse should verify that the client has adequate urine output before administering an IV solution containing potassium, because hyperkalemia can quickly develop.

Table 36-8 Intravenous Solutions

Solution	Concentration	Other Names
Dextrose in Water Solutions		
Dextrose 5% in water*	Isotonic	D_5W
Dextrose 10% in water	Hypertonic	$D_{10}W$
Saline Solutions		
0.45% sodium chloride (half normal saline)	Hypotonic	½ NS 0.45% NS
0.9% sodium chloride† (normal saline)	Isotonic	NS 0.9% NS 0.9% NaCl
3%–5% sodium chloride	Hypertonic	3%–5% NS 3%–5% NaCl
Dextrose in Saline Solutions		
Dextrose 5% in 0.9% sodium chloride	Hypertonic	$D_5$0.9% NaCl $D_5$0.9% NS D_5NS
Dextrose 5% in 0.45% NaCl sodium chloride	Hypertonic	$D_5$0.45% NaCl $D_5$0.45% NS D_5½ NS
Multiple Electrolyte Solutions		
Lactated Ringer's‡	Isotonic	LR
Dextrose 5% in lactated Ringer's	Hypertonic	D_5LR

*Dextrose is quickly metabolized, leaving free water to be distributed evenly in all fluid compartments (Heitz & Horne, 2001).
†Although it is isotonic because the total concentration of electrolytes equals plasma concentration, it contains 154 mmol/L of both sodium and chloride, which is a higher concentration of these electrolytes than is found in the plasma, which can cause FVE (Metheny, 2000).
‡Contains sodium, potassium, calcium, chloride, and lactate.

Equipment. Correct selection and preparation of IV equipment is necessary for safe and quick placement of an IV line. Because fluids are instilled into the bloodstream, sterile technique is necessary; the nurse must therefore have all equipment organized and at the bedside. The nurse who must leave the bedside to obtain another piece of equipment will need to start the procedure over again. Intravenous equipment includes needles or catheters, tourniquet, gloves, dressings, solution containers, various types of tubing, and IV pumps or volume control devices. Injectable medications such as antibiotics may be added to a small IV solution bag and "piggybacked" into the primary line or as a primary intermittent infusion to be administered over a 30- to 60-minute period (see chapter 30). The type and amount of solution depend on the medication added and the client's physiological status. Different types of tubing are used to administer medications or IV fluids. A solution given rapidly needs to be infused with macrodrip tubing, which delivers large drops (standard drop size is 10 or 15 gtt/mL depending on the manufacturer) so that the prescribed rate can be maintained. In contrast, microdrip tubing provides a standard drop size of 60 gtt/mL. Microdrip tubing is used to allow precise regulation of IV fluids even at slow rates. In addition, clients may require IV extension tubing to increase mobility, to decrease manipulation and potential contamination at the insertion site, or to facilitate changes in position.

Safety Alert. Intravenous pumps or volume control devices ensure a prescribed rate. They are vital with children, clients with renal or cardiac failure, and critically ill clients. They are also used for medications that require precise rates. However, many agencies use these devices routinely in most clients.

Initiating the Intravenous Line. After the equipment is collected at the bedside, the nurse prepares to place the IV line by assessing the client for a venipuncture site (Skill 36-1). Common IV puncture sites include the hand and the arm (Figure 36–13). The use of the foot for an IV site is common with children but is avoided in the adult because of the danger of thrombophlebitis (Infusion Nurses Society [INS], 2000). There are variations in IV procedures among agencies, and there may be slight variations in practice from what is presented in this chapter. Nurses should always follow agency procedures.

The nurse assessing the client for potential venipuncture sites for IV infusion should consider conditions and contraindications that exclude certain sites. Because children and older adults have fragile veins, the nurse should

Text continued on p. 1183

Skill 36-1 Initiating a Peripheral Intravenous Infusion

View Video

Delegation Considerations

The skill of initiating intravenous (IV) therapy should not be delegated to unregulated care providers (UCPs). In many provinces, monitoring IV therapy is included within the scope of practice for licensed/registered practical nurses (LPNs/RPNs). However, the delegating nurse is ultimately responsible for assessment and monitoring of the IV. Other aspects of the client's care may be delegated to UCPs. The nurse should instruct the UCP about the following:

- To inform the nurse if the client complains of burning, bleeding, swelling, or coolness at the catheter insertion site
- The prescribed flow rate and to report if rate has slowed or increased
- To inform the nurse if the IV dressing becomes wet
- To inform the nurse if the volume of fluid in the IV bag is low

Equipment

- Correct IV solution (with time tape attached)
- Proper catheter for venipuncture (gauge will vary with client's body size and reason for IV fluid administration). In an adult, a 22-gauge catheter is appropriate for fluid maintenance (Ellenberger, 1999)
- IV start kit (if available): may contain a sterile drape to place under the client's arm, tourniquet, cleansing and antiseptic preparations, dressings, and a small roll of sterile tape
- Local anaesthetic (optional)

For IV fluid infusion

- Administration set (choice depends on type of solution and rate of administration; infants and children, clients with cardiac and renal disease, and certain medications require microdrip tubing, which provides 60 gtt/mL)
- 0.22-μm filter (if required by agency policy or if particulate matter is likely; size appropriate to type of solution)
- Extension tubing (used when a longer IV line is necessary or to avoid manipulation of the catheter insertion site with frequent tubing changes)
- Antiseptic swabs or sticks (chlorhexidine, povidone-iodine, alcohol; see Box 36-8)
- Disposable gloves
- Tourniquet (determine type of tourniquet based on client assessment, e.g., blood pressure cuff [older adult], rubber band [infants]. Tourniquets can be a source of contamination; use a single-use product.)
- Arm board and protective cover, if needed (used to maintain wrist or elbow joint position when over-the-needle catheter [ONC] is placed close to or over a joint; will help prevent infiltration of IV and mechanical phlebitis).
- Non-allergenic tape and sterile tape (for use under the dressing)
- Waterproof pad (to place under client's hand or arm)
- IV pole, rolling or ceiling mounted
- Special client gown with snaps at shoulder seams (makes removal with IV tubing easier), if available
- Needle disposal container (also called sharps container)
- IV site protection device (optional)

For heparin or normal saline lock

- Injection cap (also called IV plug, adapter, hep-lok)
- IV loop or short piece of extension tubing, if necessary
- 1 to 3 mL of sterile normal saline or heparin flush solution (10 to 100 units/mL as ordered or per agency protocol)
- Syringes and 25-gauge needles

Gauge dressing only

- 2 × 2 (5 cm × 5 cm) or 4 × 4 (10 cm × 10 cm) sterile gauze sponge

Transparent dressing only

- Transparent dressing

Steps	Rationale
1. Review physician's order for type and amount of IV fluid, rate of fluid administration, and purpose of infusion. In addition, nurse follows six rights for administration of medications (see chapter 30).	An order requesting the initiation of a peripheral IV access and administration of an IV solution must be made by a physician before the implementation of this procedure. Assists in decision making for selection of appropriate access device.
2. Observe for signs and symptoms indicating fluid or electrolyte imbalances that may be affected by IV fluid administration:	Provides baseline data for later evaluation of change in fluid and electrolyte status.
a. Peripheral edema	Indicates expanded interstitial fluid volume, evident in dependent body parts (e.g., feet and ankles). Excess IV fluids will worsen this condition.
b. Greater than 20% change in body weight	Daily weights assist in documenting fluid retention or loss. Change in body weight of 1 kg corresponds to 1 L of fluid retention or loss.
c. Dry skin and mucous membranes	Frequently associated with fluid volume deficit.
d. Distended neck veins	Frequently associated with fluid volume excess or cardiovascular alterations.

Steps	Rationale
e. Blood pressure changes	Elevations in blood pressure (BP) may indicate volume excess, and decreased pressure may indicate fluid volume deficit. These changes can be more sudden and pronounced in those clients with underlying cardiopulmonary disease.
f. Irregular pulse rhythm; tachycardia	Rate and rhythm change can occur with changes in intravascular volume, as well as changes in potassium, calcium, and/or magnesium.
g. Auscultation of abnormal lung sounds	With fluid volume excess, the cardiovascular system is unable to compensate for this excess and fluid builds up in the lungs, creating abnormal lung sounds.
h. Decreased skin turgor	With decreased fluid volume, the skin when pinched remains in that state for several seconds. This is called "tenting."

Critical Decision Point: Changes in skin turgor are a less reliable indicator for older adult clients because of the natural loss in skin elasticity caused by the normal aging process (Lueckenotte, 2000).

i. Thirst	Symptomatic of fluid volume deficit. Very young, confused, and severely debilitated clients may not be able to indicate their thirst.
j. Anorexia, nausea, and vomiting	May be present with fluid volume excess or deficit. These symptoms may also be present with the client's underlying disease.
k. Decreased urine output	During dehydration, the kidneys attempt to restore fluid balance by reducing urine production.
l. Behavioural changes	May occur with fluid volume deficit and acid-base imbalance. In addition, behavioural changes may be due to fever, the underlying condition, or pre-existing disease.
3. Assess client's previous or perceived experience with IV therapy and arm placement preference.	Determines level of emotional support and instruction necessary. If hypersensitive to venipunctures, a local anaesthetic may be indicated. Anaesthetic cream needs to be applied for 60 minutes. Transdermal anaesthetic may be administered before venipuncture.
4. Determine if client is to undergo any planned surgeries or is to receive blood infusion later.	Allows nurse to place an adequate-size catheter (i.e., 18 or 16 gauge for surgery) and avoids placement in an area that will interfere with medical procedures.
5. Assess laboratory data and client's history of allergies.	May reveal information that affects insertion of devices, such as fluid volume deficit, anemia, or allergy to iodine, adhesive, or latex.
6. Assess for the following risk factors: child or older adult, presence of heart failure or renal failure, or low platelet count.	People at extremes in age develop fluid imbalances more rapidly because they have proportionately larger ECF volume, people with heart failure may require fluid restriction and cannot adapt to sudden increases in vascular volume, and people with renal failure cannot eliminate excess ECF. A low platelet count predisposes clients to bleeding at IV site.
7. Prepare client and family by explaining the procedure, its purpose, and what is expected of the client.	Decreases anxiety and promotes co-operation.
8. Perform hand hygiene.	Reduces transmission of micro-organisms.
9. Assist client to comfortable sitting or supine position.	Enables client to extend arm.
10. Organize equipment on clean clutter-free bedside stand or overbed table.	Reduces risk of contamination and accidents.
11. Change client's gown to the more easily removed gown with snaps at the shoulder, if available.	Use of a special IV gown facilitates safe removal of the gown.
12. Open sterile packages using sterile aseptic technique.	Maintains sterility of equipment and reduces spread of micro-organisms.

Skill 36-1 Initiating a Peripheral Intravenous Infusion—cont'd

Steps	Rationale
13. Check IV solution, using six rights of drug administration (see chapter 30). Make sure prescribed additives, such as potassium and vitamins, have been added. Check solution for colour, clarity, and expiration date. Check bag for leaks, which is best if done before reaching the bedside.	IV solutions are medications and should be carefully checked to reduce risk of error. Solutions that are discoloured, contain particles, or are expired are not to be used. (Some solutions may have slight discolouration [e.g., be pink-tinged] and still be suitable for use.) Leaky bags present an opportunity for infection and must not be used.
14. Open infusion set, maintaining sterility of both ends of tubing. Many sets allow for priming of tubing without removal of end cap.	Prevents bacteria from entering infusion equipment and bloodstream.
15. Place roller clamp about 2 to 5 cm below drip chamber and move roller clamp to "off" position (see illustrations).	Close proximity of roller clamp to drip chamber allows more accurate regulation of flow rate. Moving clamp to "off" prevents accidental spillage of fluid.
16. Remove protective sheath over IV tubing port on plastic IV solution bag (see illustration). For bottled IV solution, remove metal cap and metal and rubber disks beneath cap. Use caution to avoid touching exposed opening.	Provides access for insertion of infusion tubing into solution.
17. Insert infusion set into fluid bag or bottle by removing protector cap from tubing insertion spike (keeping spike sterile), and inserting spike into opening of IV bag (see illustration). Cleanse rubber stopper on glass-bottled solution with antiseptic, and insert spike into black rubber stopper of IV bottle. Hang solution container on IV pole at a minimum height of 90 cm above planned insertion site.	Prevents contamination of solution from contaminated insertion spike. Container heights of approximately 1 m are usually sufficient to overcome venous pressure and other resistance from tubing and catheter.
18. Compress drip chamber and release, allowing it to fill one-third to one-half full (see illustration). Open clamp and prime infusion tubing by filling with IV solution.	Creates vacuum effects; fluid enters drip chamber to prevent air from entering tubing.

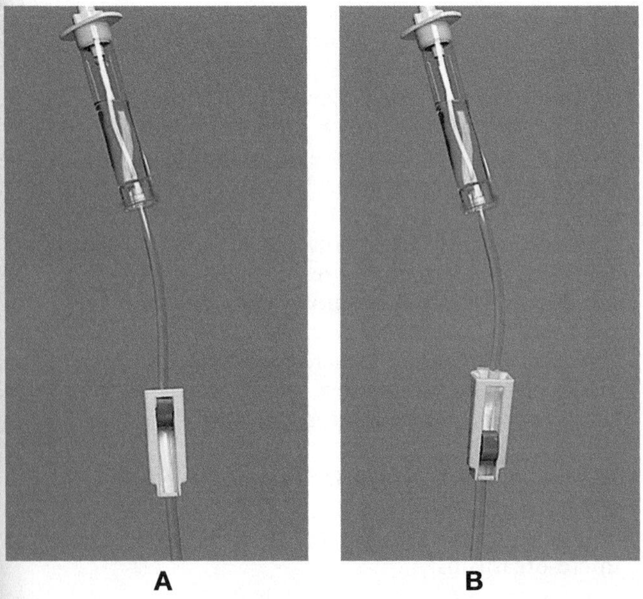

STEP **15** **A,** Roller clamp in open position. **B,** Roller clamp in closed position.

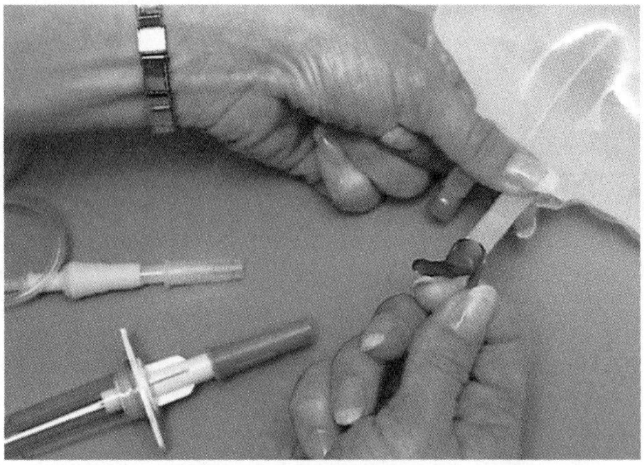

STEP **16** Removing protective sheath from IV bag port.

Steps	Rationale

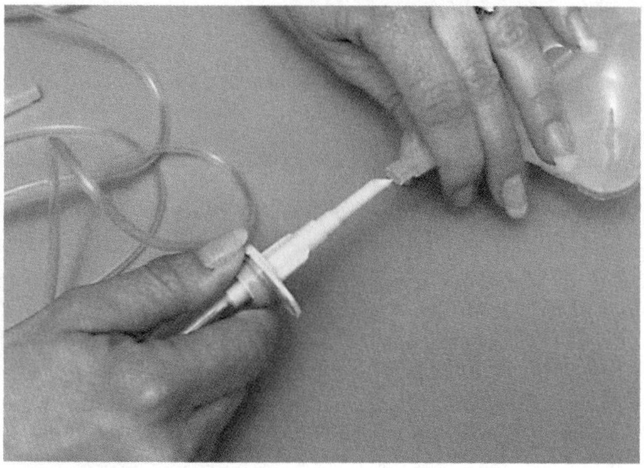

STEP **17** Inserting spike into IV bag.

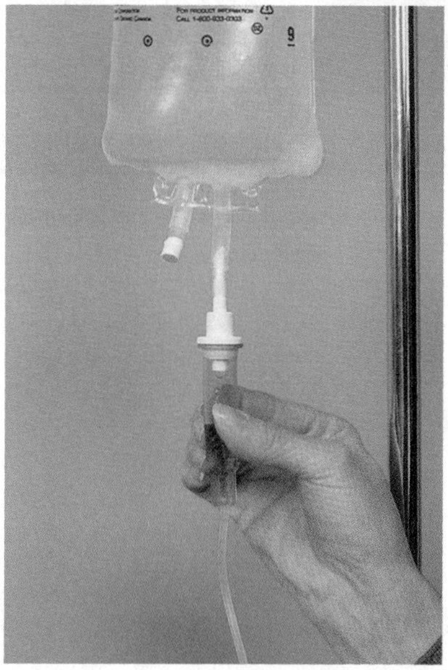

STEP **18** Squeezing drip chamber to fill with fluid.

Steps	Rationale
19. Remove tubing protector cap (some tubing can be primed without removal) and slowly release roller clamp to allow fluid to travel from drip chamber through tubing to needle adapter. Return roller clamp to "off" position after tubing is primed (filled with IV fluid).	Slow fill of tubing decreases turbulence and chance of bubble formation. Removes air from tubing and permits tubing to fill with solution. Closing the clamp prevents accidental loss of fluid.
20. Be certain tubing is clear of air and air bubbles. To remove small air bubbles, firmly tap IV tubing where air bubbles are located. Check entire length of tubing to ensure that all air bubbles are removed (see illustration).	Large air bubbles can act as emboli. Air bubbles may contribute to anxiety related to IV therapy.

Critical Decision Point: Extra extension tubing may be added to IV tubing to allow for more length, which will enable the client to move more freely while still keeping the IV line stable. But remember, adding extensions increases risk for infection.

Steps	Rationale
21. Replace tubing cap protector on end of tubing.	Maintains system sterility.
22. *Optional:* Prepare heparin or normal saline lock for infusion. If a loop or short extension tubing is needed, use sterile technique to connect the IV plug to the loop or short extension tubing. Inject 1 to 3 mL normal saline through the plug and through the loop or short extension tubing.	Removes air to prevent introduction into the vein. Do the same with the saline plug.
23. Apply disposable gloves. Eye protection and mask may be worn (see agency policy) if splash or spray of blood is possible. NOTE: Gloves can be left off to locate vein but must be applied before preparing site.	Reduces transmission of micro-organisms. Decreases exposure to HIV, hepatitis, and other blood-borne organisms (INS, 2000).
24. Identify accessible vein for IV placement. Apply tourniquet 10 to 15 cm above the proposed insertion site (see illustration). Position tourniquet so that ends are away from proposed venipuncture site. Check for presence of radial pulse. OPTION: Apply blood pressure cuff instead of tourniquet. Inflate to a level just below client's normal diastolic pressure. Maintain inflation at that pressure until venipuncture is completed.	Tourniquet should be tight enough to impede venous return but *not* occlude arterial flow.

Skill 36-1 *Initiating a Peripheral Intravenous Infusion—cont'd*

Steps	Rationale

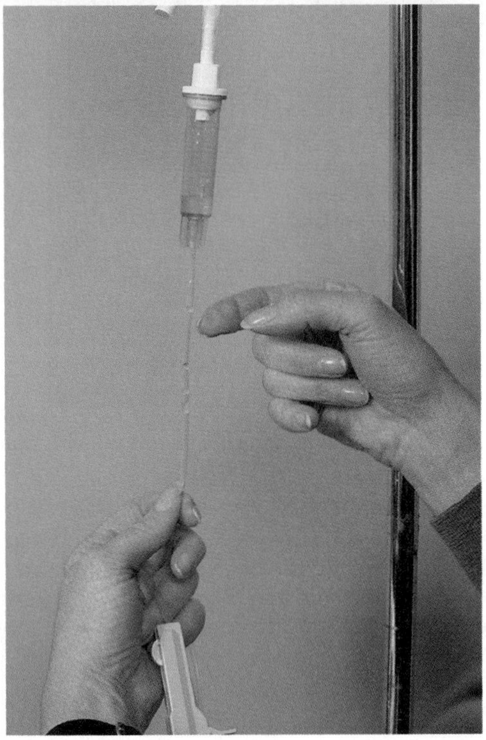

STEP **20** Removing air bubbles from tubing.

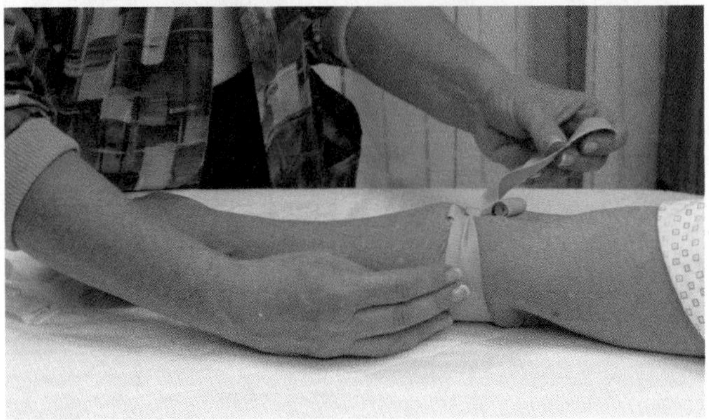

STEP **24** Apply tourniquet.

Steps	Rationale
25. Select the vein. Common IV sites for the adult include cephalic, basilic, and median cubital veins (see Figure 36–13).	
a. Use the most distal site in the non-dominant arm, if possible.	Venipuncture should be performed distal to proximal, which increases the availability of other sites for future IV therapy.
b. Avoid areas that are painful to palpation.	May indicate inflamed vein.
c. Select a vein large enough for catheter placement.	Prevents interruption of venous flow while allowing adequate blood flow around the catheter.
d. Choose a site that will not interfere with client's activities of daily living (ADLs) or planned procedures.	
e. Use the fingertips to palpate the vein by pressing downward and noting the resilient, soft, bouncy feeling as the pressure is released (see illustration).	Fingertips are more sensitive and are better to assess vein condition.
f. Promote venous distension by instructing the client to open and close the fist several times, lowering the client's arm in a dependent position, applying warmth to the arm for several minutes, and/or rubbing or stroking the client's arm from distal to proximal below proposed site.	These activities increase blood flow to the area of insertion. When these techniques are properly used, they foster venous dilation and access to the vein.

Critical Decision Point: Avoid vigorous rubbing and multiple tapping of client's veins. These techniques may cause injury to the vein, such as a hematoma, or cause venous constriction.

Steps	Rationale

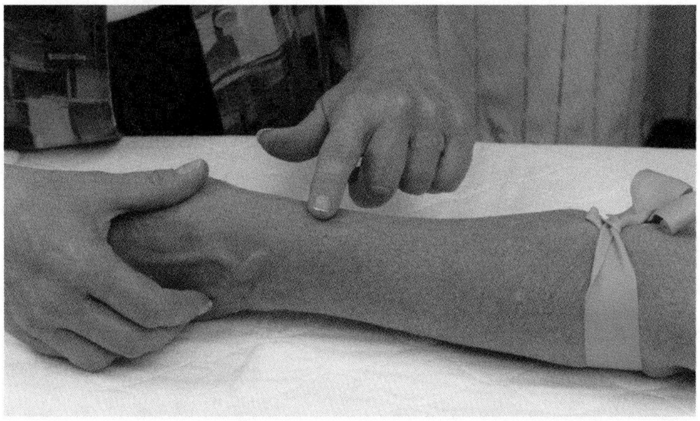

STEP **25e** Palpate vein for resilience.

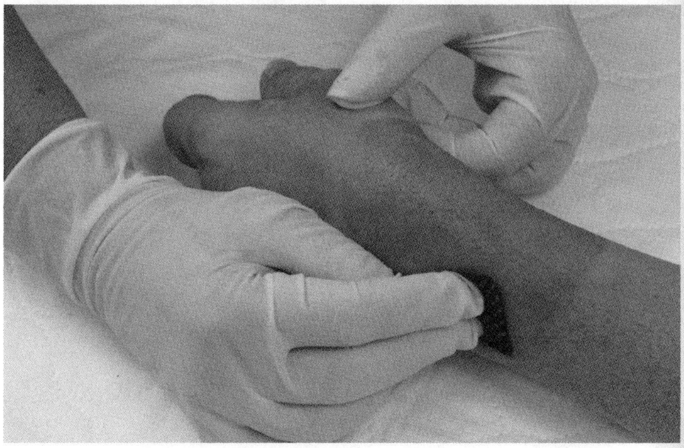

STEP **27** Cleanse site chosen for insertion.

g. Avoid sites distal to previous venipuncture site, sclerosed or hardened cordlike veins, infiltrated site or phlebotic vessels, bruised areas, and areas of venous valves or bifurcation. Avoid veins in antecubital fossa and ventral surface of the wrist.

Such sites increase the risk of infiltration of newly placed IV line and excessive vessel damage.

Veins in the antecubital fossa are used for blood draws and placement in this area limits mobility. Inner wrist contains numerous tendons that could be damaged.

h. Avoid fragile dorsal veins in older adults and vessels in an extremity with compromised circulation (e.g., in cases of mastectomy, dialysis graft, or paralysis).

Venous alterations can increase risk of complications (e.g., infiltration and decreased catheter dwell time).

26. Release tourniquet temporarily and carefully. Clip arm hair with scissors (if necessary). Do not shave area.

Hair impedes venipuncture and adherence of dressing. Shaving can cause microabrasions and predispose client to infection.

27. (If area of insertion appears to need cleansing, use soap and water first.) Cleanse insertion site using firm, circular motion (centre to outward) in concentric circles 5 to 7.5 cm from insertion site. Use antiseptic prep as a single agent or in combination, according to agency policy (see Box 36-8). Avoid touching the cleansed site. Allow the site to dry for at least 2 minutes (see illustration). If skin is touched after cleansing, repeat cleansing procedure.

Chlorhexidine is the antiseptic cleansing agent of choice (Centers for Disease Control and Prevention, 2002). Povidone-iodine is a topical anti-infective that reduces skin surface bacteria; 70% alcohol is another antiseptic cleansing agent. Povidone-iodine must dry to be effective in reducing microbial counts (Millam & Hadaway, 2000). Air-drying prevents chemical reactions between agents and allows time for maximum microbicidal activity of agents (INS, 2000). Touching the cleansed area would introduce organisms from nurse's hand to the site.

28. Reapply tourniquet or BP cuff.

Critical Decision Point: Do not use povidone-iodine if the client is allergic to iodine; use an alternate cleansing agent.

29. Perform venipuncture. Anchor vein by placing thumb over vein beneath insertion site and by stretching the skin against the direction of insertion 5 to 7.5 cm distal to the site (see illustration). Warn client of a sharp stick. Puncture skin and vein, holding catheter at 10- to 30-degree angle with the bevel pointed upward.

The vascular access device (VAD) selected should be the smallest gauge and shortest length that will accommodate the therapy (INS, 2000).

Places needle parallel to vein. When vein is punctured, risk of puncturing posterior vein wall is reduced.

Superficial veins require a smaller angle; deeper veins require a greater angle.

A. **Butterfly needle:** Hold needle at 10- to 30-degree angle with bevel up slightly distal to actual site of venipuncture.

B. **Needleless ONC safety device:** Insert ONC (see illustration) with bevel up at 10- to 30-degree angle slightly distal to actual site of venipuncture in the direction of the vein.

Skill 36-1 Initiating a Peripheral Intravenous Infusion—cont'd

Steps	Rationale

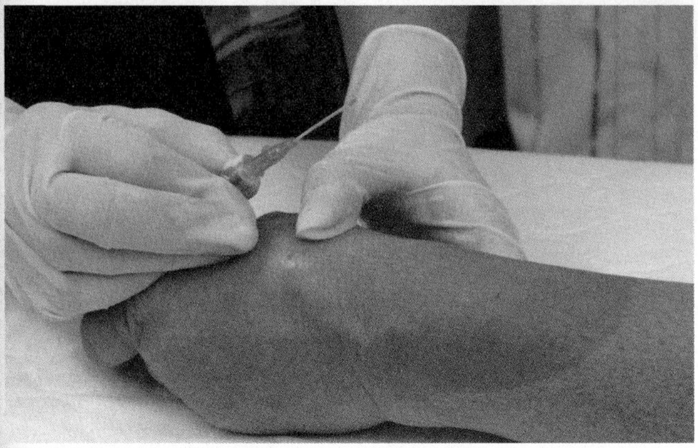

STEP **29** Stabilize vein below insertion site with skin taut.

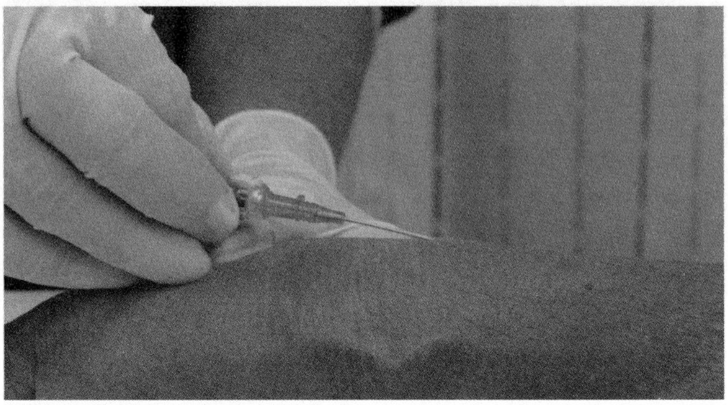

STEP **29B** Puncture skin with catheter at 10- to 30-degree angle. Catheter enters vein.

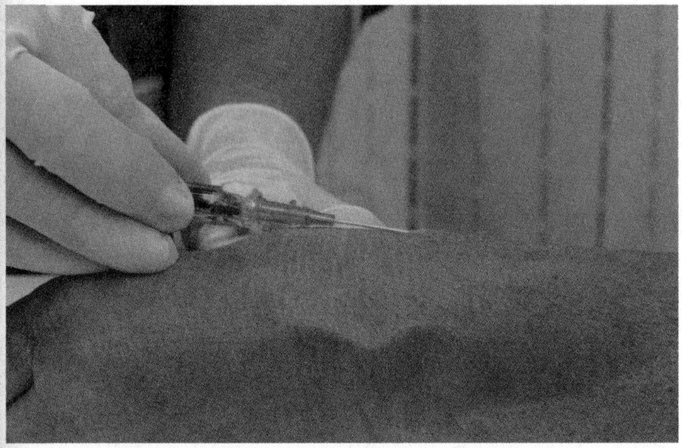

A

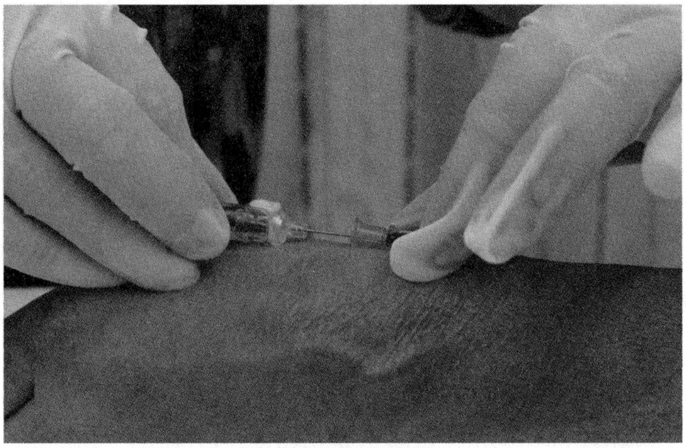

B

STEP **30** **A,** Blood return in flashback chamber, catheter lowered flush with skin. **B,** Advance catheter into vein; use safety device push-tab.

Critical Decision Point: No more than two attempts at inserting an IV should be made by a single nurse (INS, 2000).

Steps	Rationale
30. Look for blood return through tubing of butterfly needle or flashback chamber of ONC, indicating that needle has entered vein (see illustration). Lower catheter/needle until almost flush with skin. Advance butterfly needle until hub rests at venipuncture site. Advance ONC catheter 0.5 cm into vein and then loosen stylet. Advance catheter off the stylet into vein until hub rests at venipuncture site (see illustration). Do not reinsert the stylet once it is loosened. (Advance the safety device by using push-off tab to thread the catheter.)	Increased venous pressure from tourniquet increases backflow of blood into catheter or tubing. Lowering the angle and advancing the cannula slightly allows for full penetration of vein wall, placement of catheter within vein's inner lumen, and easy advancement of catheter off stylet. Threading catheter up to hub reduces the risk of introduction of infectious organisms along the catheter length. Reinsertion of the stylet can cause catheter damage and potential catheter embolization.

Steps	Rationale

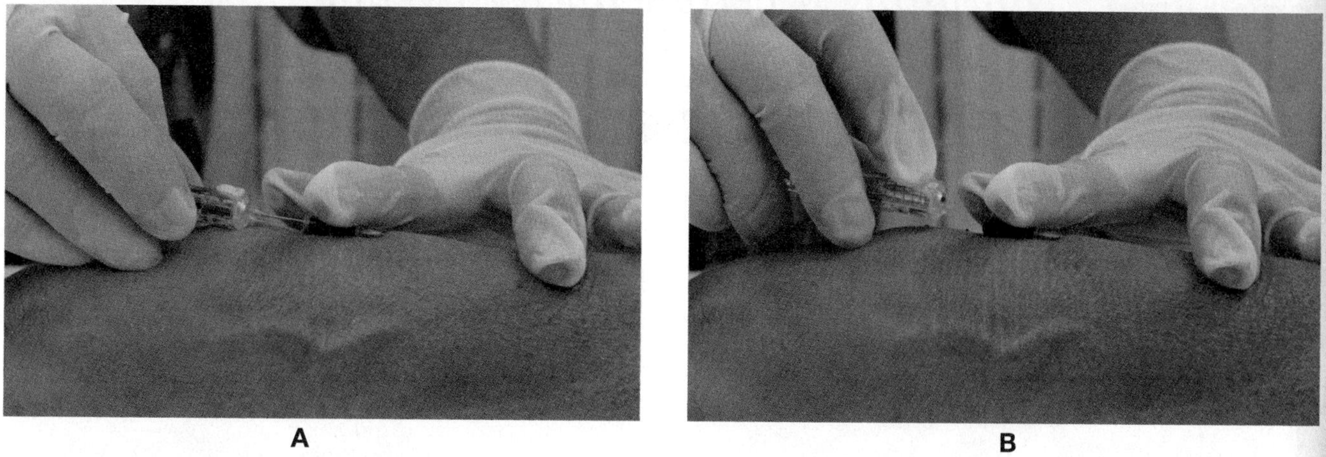

STEP **31** **A,** Apply pressure above insertion site with index finger of non-dominant hand. **B,** Retract the stylet by pushing safety tab.

Steps	Rationale
31. Stabilize the catheter. Apply gentle, but firm, pressure with the index finger of non-dominant hand 3 cm above insertion site (see illustration, *A*). Release tourniquet or BP cuff with dominant hand and retract stylet from ONC (see illustration, *B*). Do not recap the stylet. For a safety device, slide the catheter off the stylet while gliding the protective guard over the stylet. A click indicates the device is locked over the stylet.	Permits venous flow, reduces backflow of blood, and prevents accidental withdrawal or dislodgement.
32. Quickly connect adapter of primed fluid administration set (see illustration) or heparin lock to hub of ONC or butterfly tubing. Be sure connection is secure. Do not touch point of entry of adapter.	Prompt connection of infusion set maintains patency of vein. Maintains sterility.
33. Release roller clamp slowly to begin infusion at a rate to maintain patency of IV line.	Permits venous flow and prevents clotting of vein and obstruction of flow of IV solution.
a. *Intermittent infusion:* Continue to stabilize catheter with non-dominant hand and attach injection cap of adapter. Insert pre-filled flush solution into injection cap. Flush slowly (see illustration). Maintain thumb pressure on syringe during withdrawal or close clamp on extension tubing of injection cap while still flushing last 0.2 to 0.4 mL of flush solution.	Positive pressure in the catheter prevents reflux of blood into the catheter lumen (Phillips, 2001).

Critical Decision Point: Be sure to calculate rate so as not to infuse IV solution too rapidly or too slowly.

Steps	Rationale
34. Tape or secure catheter.	
A. If applying transparent dressing, secure catheter with non-dominant hand while preparing to apply dressing.	
B. If applying a gauze dressing	
(1) Tape the IV catheter. Place narrow piece (1-cm wide) of sterile tape under hub of catheter with adhesive side up (see illustration, *A*) and criss-cross tape over hub to form a chevron (see illustration, *B*).	Securing the catheter and tubing prevents movement and tension on the device, reducing mechanical irritation and possible phlebitis or infection. Tape placed underneath the dressing should be sterile; non-sterile tape is a potential source of pathogenic bacteria.

Skill 36-1 Initiating a Peripheral Intravenous Infusion—cont'd

Steps	Rationale

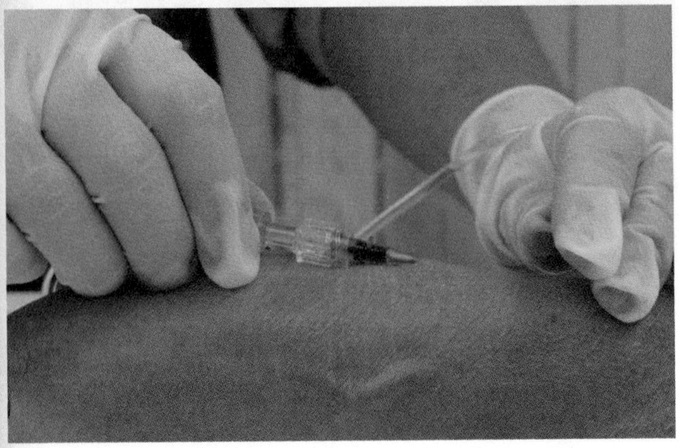

STEP **32** Connect end of IV tubing to catheter tubing. Secure connector.

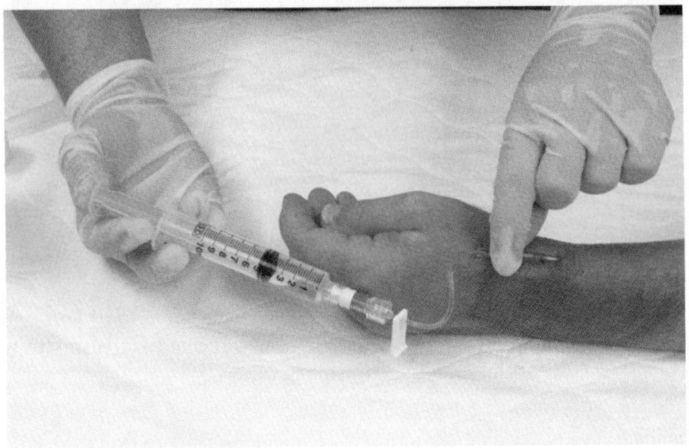

STEP **33a** Flush injection cap slowly.

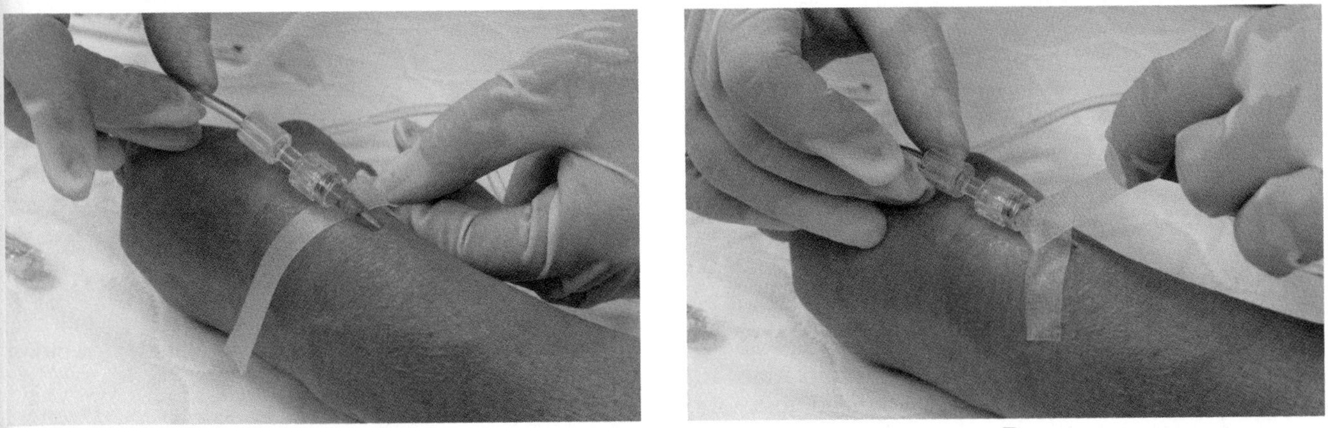

A **B**

STEP **34B(1)** **A,** Place tape under catheter hub. **B,** Criss-cross ends of tape over hub.

Steps	Rationale
(2) Place tape only on the catheter, *never* over the insertion site. Secure the site to allow easy visual inspection and early recognition of infiltration and phlebitis. Avoid applying tape around the extremity.	Taping around extremity could result in a "tourniquet effect" and impede venous return.
35. Apply sterile dressing over site.	
A. Transparent dressing	
(1) Carefully remove adherent backing. Apply one edge of dressing and then gently smooth remaining dressing over site, leaving end of catheter hub uncovered (see illustration). Refer to manufacturer's directions.	Transparent dressings are occlusive to moisture and micro-organisms. Transparent dressings allow continuous inspection of the IV site, are more comfortable, and permit clients to bathe and shower without saturating the dressing (Phillips, 2001).
(2) Take a 2.5-cm piece of tape, and place it from end of hub of the catheter to insertion site, over transparent dressing (see illustration).	

Steps	Rationale

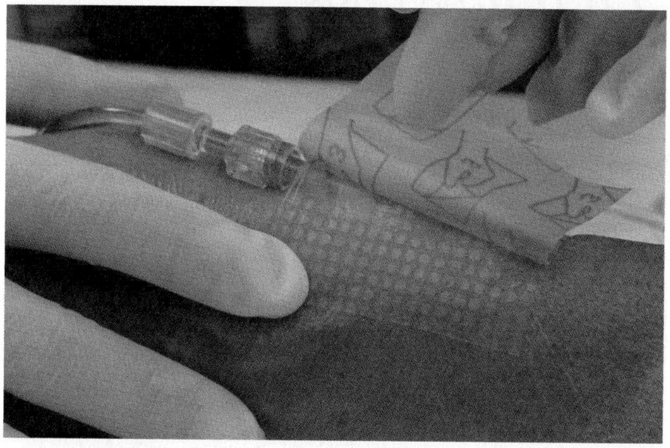

STEP **35A(1)** Apply transparent dressing.

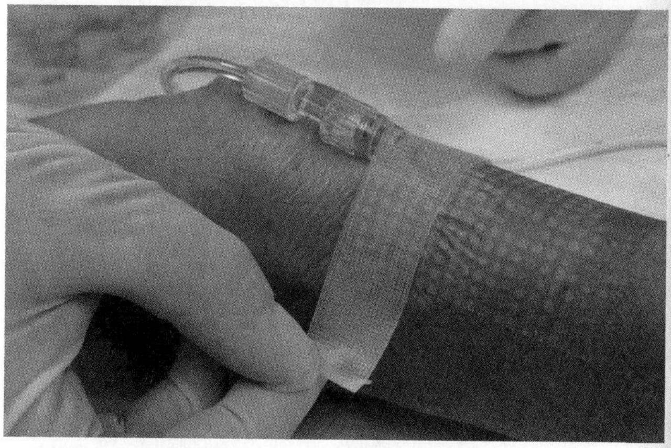

STEP **35A(2)** Place tape over transparent dressing.

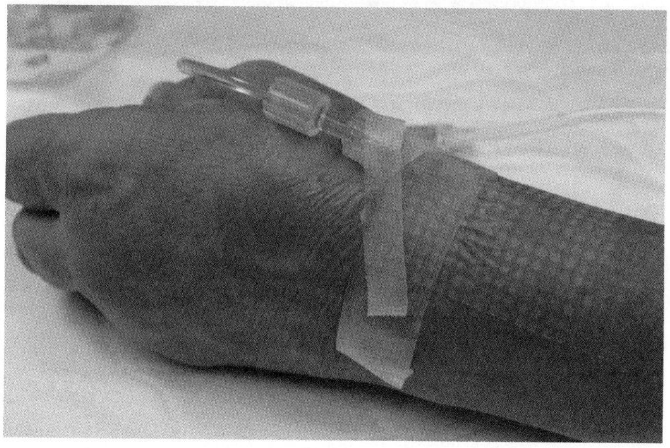

STEP **35A(3)** Apply chevron over tape.

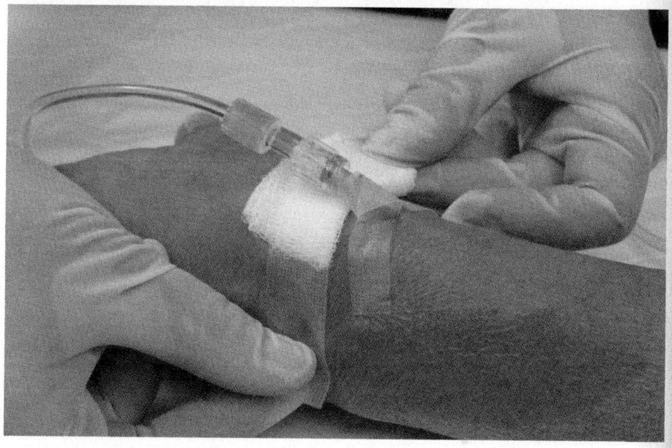

STEP **35B(1)** Fold 2 × 2 gauze in half, cover with 2.5-cm tape, and place under catheter hub.

(3) Then apply chevron and place only over tape, not the transparent dressing (see illustration).

B. Sterile gauze dressing

(1) Fold a 2 × 2 gauze in half and cover with a 2.5-cm-wide piece of sterile tape extending about 2.5 cm from each side. Place it under the tubing/catheter hub junction (see illustration).

Tape on top of tape makes it easier to access hub/tubing junction. Securing loop of tubing reduces risk of dislodging catheter from accidental pull.

Gauze is less expensive than transparent dressing and may also be useful if there is bleeding or excessive moisture at the site.

(2) Place a 2 × 2 gauze pad over venipuncture site and catheter hub. Secure all edges with tape. Do not cover connection between IV tubing and catheter hub (see illustration).

(3) Curl a loop of tubing alongside the arm and place a second piece of tape directly over the padded 2 × 2, securing tubing in two places.

Skill 36-1 Initiating a Peripheral Intravenous Infusion—cont'd

Steps	Rationale
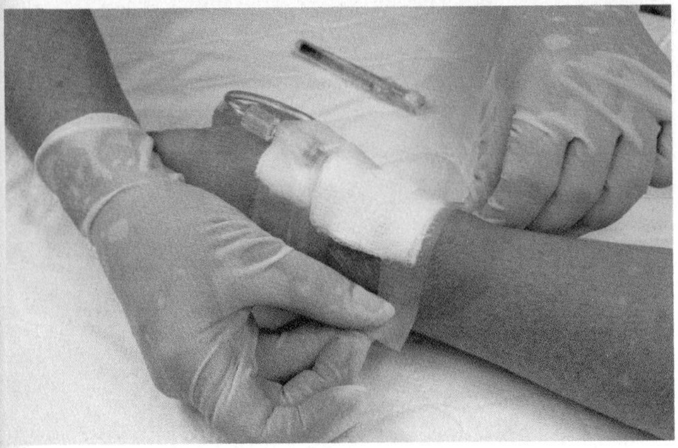 STEP **35B(2)** Apply 2x2 gauze.	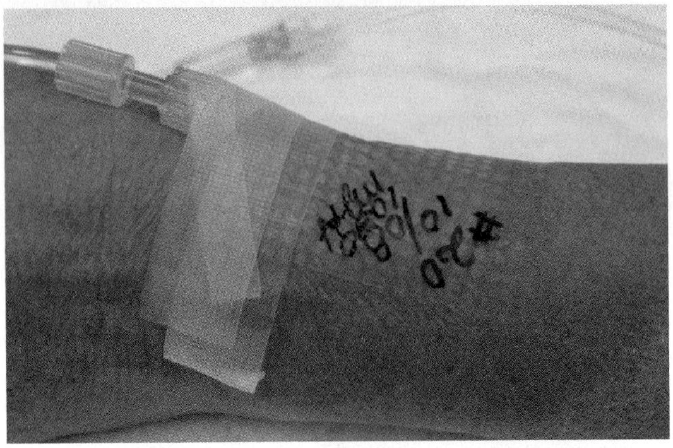 STEP **37** Dressing labelled with date and time.
36. For *IV fluid administration,* adjust flow rate to correct drops per minute (see Skill 36-2) or connect to electronic infusion device (EID).	Maintains correct rate of flow for IV solution. Flow can fluctuate; therefore, it must be checked at intervals.
A. Heparin lock. Flush with 1 to 3 mL of heparin flush solution (10 to 100 units/mL) at prescribed frequency or agency policy.	Maintains patency of IV catheter.
B. Saline lock. Flush with 1 to 3 mL of sterile normal saline at prescribed frequency or agency policy.	Maintains patency of IV catheter.
37. Label dressing with date, time, gauge size and length of catheter, and nurse's initials (see illustration).	Allows for easy recognition of type of device and time interval for site rotation. INS standard for site rotation of peripheral IV access device is every 72 hours (INS, 2000).
38. Dispose of used needles in appropriate sharps container. Discard supplies. Remove gloves and perform hand hygiene.	Reduces transmission of micro-organisms and protects staff from injury.
39. Observe client every hour to determine if fluid is infusing correctly:	
a. Check if correct amount of solution is infused as prescribed by looking at time tape.	Correct administration of fluid volume prevents fluid imbalance.
b. Count flow rate or check rate on infusion pump.	Accurate monitoring of rate furthers ensures correct volume administration.
c. Check patency of IV catheter or needle.	
d. Observe client for signs of discomfort.	
e. Inspect insertion site for absence of phlebitis (Table 36-9), infiltration (Table 36-10), or inflammation.	Provides continuous evaluation of type and amount of fluid delivered to client. Hourly inspection prevents accidental fluid overload or inadequate infusion rate and identifies early incidence of vein inflammation or tissue damage.
40. Observe client every hour to determine response to therapy (i.e., measure vital signs, conduct post-procedure assessments).	IV fluids and additives are given to maintain or restore fluid and electrolyte balance. They can also cause unexpected effects, which can be serious.

Unexpected Outcomes and Related Interventions

- Fluid volume deficit (FVD) as manifested by decreased urine output, dry mucous membranes, hypotension, tachycardia.
  - Notify physician; may require readjustment of infusion rate.
- Fluid volume excess (FVE) as manifested by crackles in the lungs, shortness of breath, edema.
  - Reduce IV flow rate if symptoms appear, and notify physician.
- Electrolyte imbalances as manifested by abnormal serum electrolyte levels, changes in mental status, and alterations in neuromuscular function, changes in vital signs, and other manifestations.
  - Notify physician. Additives in IV or type of IV fluid may be adjusted.
- Infiltration as indicated by swelling and possible pitting edema, pallor, coolness, pain at insertion site, and possible decrease in flow rate.
  - Stop infusion and discontinue IV. Elevate affected extremity. Restart new IV if continued therapy is necessary.
- Phlebitis is indicated by pain, increased skin temperature, erythema along path of vein.
  - Stop infusion and discontinue IV. Restart new IV if continued therapy is necessary.
  - Place moist warm compress over area of phlebitis.
- Bleeding occurs at venipuncture site.
  - Bleeding from vein is usually slow, continuous seepage. Common in clients who have received heparin or have a bleeding disorder or if the IV site is over bend in arm/hand.
  - If bleeding occurs around venipuncture site and catheter is within vein, gauze dressing may be applied over site. Eventually, IV may need to be discontinued.
  - Blood on the dressing can result when the administration set becomes disconnected from the catheter's hub. When blood appears on the dressing, verify that the system is intact and change the dressing.

Recording and Reporting

- Record in nurses' notes number of attempts for insertion, type of fluid, insertion site by vessel, flow rate, size and type of catheter or needle, and when infusion was begun. A special parenteral therapy flow sheet may be used.
- Record client's response to IV fluid, amount infused, and integrity and patency of system every 4 hours or according to agency policy.
- Report the following to oncoming nursing staff: type of fluid, flow rate, status of venipuncture site, amount of fluid remaining in present solution, expected time to hang next IV bag or bottle, and any side effects.

Home Care Considerations

- Teach caregiver to apply pressure with sterile gauze if catheter falls out and, if client is on anticoagulant therapy, to tape several pieces of sterile gauze in place for at least 20 minutes with pressure or until bleeding stops.
- Teach client and caregiver to perform tub bath without getting IV tubing wet and to unplug pump first if one is used. For showering, the client must protect the IV site and dressing from getting wet by covering completely with plastic.
- Teach client and family to monitor I&O using measuring devices.
- Teach client and family to dispose of open and sheathed needles into sharps container. All sharps containers must be stored in safe area away from children.

---

avoid sites easily moved or bumped, such as the dorsal surface of the hand (Box 36-7). Venipuncture is contraindicated in a site that has signs of infection, infiltration, or thrombosis. An infected site is red, tender, swollen, and possibly warm to the touch. Exudate may be present. An infected site is not used because of the danger of introducing bacteria from the skin surface into the bloodstream. Avoid using an extremity with a vascular (dialysis) graft/fistula or on the side of a mastectomy. Place IVs at the most distal point when possible. Using a distal site first allows for the use of proximal sites later if the client needs a venipuncture site change The nurse prepares the skin for IV insertion (Box 36-8).

A **venipuncture** is a technique in which a vein is punctured through the skin by a sharp rigid stylet (e.g., butterfly needle or metal needle), a partially covered plastic catheter (over-the-needle catheter [ONC]), or a needle attached to a syringe. Catheters placed into a central vein such as the subclavian vein and superior vena cava are used to deliver large volumes of fluids and TPN or to administer irritating medications. Peripherally inserted central catheters may be placed by nurses; however, central line catheters require insertion by physicians. Nurses are responsible for maintaining both of them. When veins are fragile or collapse, venipuncture may become extremely difficult, but it may be a life-saving measure as well. For these difficult cases, venipuncture should be performed by an experienced practitioner. The general purposes of venipuncture are to collect a blood specimen, instill a medication, start an IV infusion, or inject a radiopaque or radioactive tracer for special examinations. Skill 36-1 describes venipuncture for IV fluid infusion.

Regulating the Infusion Flow Rate. After the IV infusion is secured and the line is patent, the nurse must regulate the rate of infusion according to the prescriber's orders (Skill 36-2). An infusion rate that is too slow can lead to further cardiovascular and circulatory collapse in a critically ill client who has FVD or hyperosmolar imbalance or who is in shock. An IV that is running too slowly can

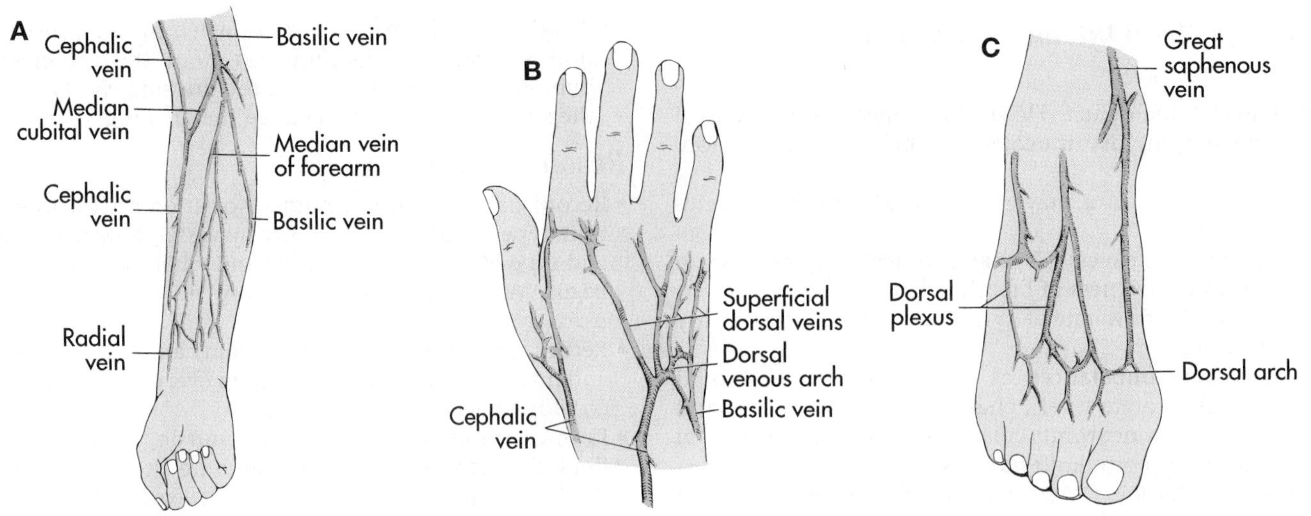

FIGURE **36–13** Common IV sites. **A,** Inner arm. **B,** Dorsal surface of hand. **C,** Dorsal surface of foot (used only for children).

Table 36-9 Phlebitis Scale

Grade	Clinical Criteria
0	No clinical symptoms
1	Erythema at access site with or without pain
2	Pain at access site with erythema and/or edema
3	Pain at access site with erythema and/or edema Streak formation Palpable venous cord
4	Pain at access site with erythema and/or edema Streak formation Palpable venous cord >2.5 cm long Purulent drainage

From "Infusion Nursing Standards of Practice," Infusion Nurses Society, 2000, *Journal of Intravenous Nursing, 23*(6S), p. S56.

Table 36-10 Infiltration Scale

Grade	Clinical Criteria
0	No symptoms Skin blanched Edema, 2.5 cm in any direction Cool to touch With or without pain
1	Skin blanched Edema 2.5 to 15 cm in any direction Cool to touch With or without pain
3	Skin blanched, translucent Gross edema >15 cm in any direction Cool to touch Mild-moderate pain Possible numbness
4	Skin blanched, translucent Skin tight, leaking Skin discoloured, bruised, swollen Gross edema >15 cm in any direction Deep pitting tissue edema Circulatory impairment Moderate to severe pain Infiltration of any amount of blood product, irritant, or vesicant

From "Infusion Nursing Standards of Practice," Infusion Nurses Society, 2000, *Journal of Intravenous Nursing, 23*(6S), p. S57.

also become clotted off more easily. An infusion rate that is too rapid can result in FVE. The nurse calculates the infusion rate to prevent too-slow or too-rapid administration of the IV fluids. Numerous methods are used to ensure an accurate hourly infusion rate for IV therapy. Fluids that run by gravity are adjusted through use of a flow control/regulator clamp. Fluids infused by an electronic infusion device or rate controller are regulated by a mechanical mechanism set at the prescribed rate. Regardless of the device in use, the client requires close monitoring to verify the correct infusion of the IV solution and to detect the occurrence of any complication.

Electronic **infusion pumps** are necessary when administering low hourly volumes (e.g., less than 20 mL/hour) and for clients who are at risk for volume overload such as neonatal, pediatric, and geriatric clients. In addition, when infusing high volumes of IV fluids (more than 150 mL/hour) to clients with impaired renal clearance, older adults, or children, or when infusing drugs or IV fluids that require specific hourly volumes, electronic infusion devices permit accurate infusion. Electronic infusion pumps deliver the infusion via positive pressure. A rate controller used on gravity infusions regulates the infusion but, unlike the electronic pump, is affected by many mechanical and client factors. Recent advances in infusion technology have resulted in a variety of devices available for use to ensure accurate delivery.

Focus on Older Adults

Box 36-7

- Use the smallest gauge catheter or needle possible (e.g., 24 to 26 gauge). This is less traumatizing to the vein and allows better blood flow to provide increased hemodilution of the IV fluids or medications.
- Consider the client's need for independence, mobility, and limitations when selecting the site for the IV catheter.
- Impaired skin integrity leads to susceptibility of tearing, difficulty detecting complications, and venous sclerosis.
- Avoid veins that are easily bumped because there is less subcutaneous support tissue.
- If the client has fragile skin and veins, use minimal or no tourniquet pressure.
- After tourniquet is applied, venous pressure rises rapidly, the vein is overstretched, and puncture with even a thin needle can rupture the wall of vein (Chukhraev & Grekov, 2000).
- Place tourniquet, if used, over the client's sleeve to decrease shearing of fragile skin.
- With loss of supportive tissue, veins tend to lie more superficially; lower insertion angle for venipuncture to 5 to 15 degrees (INS, 2000).
- If the client has lost subcutaneous tissue, the veins lose stability and will roll away from the needle. To stabilize the vein, apply traction to the skin below the projected insertion site.
- Secure the device well with minimal tape or specialized products for protection.
- Nutritional deficiencies promote fluid to migrate into tissues surrounding vessels, making IV access more difficult.
- Multiple medication usage (e.g., anticoagulants, antibiotics, and steroids) increases the likelihood of fragile, transparent skin that bruises and bleeds easily.
- Dehydration related to a lower percentage of body weight as water, diminished thirst mechanism, and social factors of bladder control contribute to difficult IV access (Toth, 2002).

Research Highlight

Box 36-8

IV Skin Preparation

Research Focus

There is frequently debate about the best antiseptics and practices for skin preparation prior to insertion of an IV. This study examines the effectiveness of three methods of skin antisepsis.

Research Summary

The purpose of this study was to compare the efficacy of 0.5% chlorhexidine gluconate in a 70% isopropyl alcohol swab; 70% isopropyl alcohol followed by 10% povidone-iodine; and 10% povidone-iodine followed by 70% isopropyl alcohol. A prospective randomized clinical trial was conducted and data were collected on 244 participants. Clients having their skin prepared with 0.5% chlorhexidine gluconate in isopropyl alcohol had an infection rate of 1.2%; those having their skin prepared with alcohol followed by povidone iodine had an infection rate of 12.5%; and those with povidone iodine followed by alcohol had an infection rate of 9.88%.

Evidence-Based Practice

- Of the three skin preparations, 0.5% chlorhexidine gluconate in 70% isopropyl alcohol is most effective in preventing infections associated with IV therapy.
- Data are not available to support the practice of removing povidone iodine with alcohol.
- Questions remain regarding allowing one product to dry before application of the second product.

Reference

LeBlanc, A., & Cobbett, S. (2000). Traditional practice versus evidence-based practice for IV skin preparation. *Canadian Journal of Infection Control, 15*(1), 9–14.

Many devices have operating and programming capabilities that allow for single- and multiple-solution infusions at different rates. A variety of detectors and alarms respond to air in IV lines, completion of infusion, high and low pressure, low battery power, occlusion, and the inability to deliver at a preset rate.

Safety Alert. An anti-free flow safeguard (preventing bolus infusion in the event of machine malfunction) is an important element of an electronic infusion device and is required. Manufacturer's recommendations for specific device features should always be checked.

Patency of the IV needle or catheter means that there are no clots at the tip of the needle or catheter and that the catheter or needle tip is not against the vein wall. A blocked catheter or needle can affect the rate of infusion of the IV fluids. IV flow rates can also be affected by the patency of the IV needle or catheter, infiltration, a knot or kink in the tubing, the height of the solution, a restrictive IV dressing, and the position of the client's extremity. One way that the nurse may assess patency is by lowering the IV bag below the level of the IV insertion site and observing for a blood return; however, this method does not confirm patency. If no blood return occurs and fluid does not flow easily from the drip chamber

Text continued on p. 1191

Skill 36-2 Regulating Intravenous Flow Rate

Delegation Considerations

In many provinces, regulating and monitoring IV therapy is included within the scope of practice for licensed/registered practical nurses (LPNs/RPNs). The skill of regulating IV therapy should not be delegated to unregulated care providers (UCPs). The nurse should instruct the UCP about the following:

- To inform nurse if client complains of burning, bleeding, swelling, coolness at the catheter insertion site
- The prescribed flow rate and to report if rate has slowed or increased
- To notify nurse if the alarm on an electronic infusion device (EID) sounds
- To inform the nurse if the volume of fluid in the IV bag is low

Equipment

- Watch with second hand
- Paper and pencil or calculator
- IV electronic infusion controller/pump (optional)
- Volume control device (optional)
- Time indicator tape

Steps	Rationale
1. Check client's medical record for correct solution, additives, and time of infusion. Usual order includes solution for 24 hours, usually divided into 2 or 3 L. Occasionally, IV order contains only 1 L to keep vein open (KVO). Order also indicates time over which each litre is to infuse.	Six rights of drug administration ensure correct fluids are given to correct client.
2. Perform hand hygiene. Observe for patency of IV line and needle or catheter	For fluid to infuse at proper rate, IV line and needle must be free of kinks, knots, and clots.
a. Open drip regulator and observe for rapid flow of fluid from solution into drip chamber, then close drip regulator to prescribed rate.	Rapid flow of fluid into drip chamber indicates patency of IV line. Closing drip chamber to prescribed rate prevents fluid overload.
3. Check client's knowledge of how positioning of the IV site affects flow rate.	Fosters client participation in maintaining most effective position of arm with IV equipment.
4. Verify with client how venipuncture site feels (e.g., determine if there is pain or burning).	Pain or burning may be early indication of phlebitis. Includes client in decision making.
5. Have paper and pencil or calculator to calculate flow rate or use calculator.	The beginning student is unfamiliar with IV fluid rates and should use mathematical calculations to obtain correct rate.
6. Know calibration (drop factor) in drops per millilitre (gtt/mL) of infusion set: **A. Microdrip:** 60 gtt/mL **B. Macrodrip:** 15 gtt/mL or 10 gtt/mL depending upon manufacturer (will state on package)	Microdrip tubing, also called pediatric tubing, universally delivers 60 gtt/mL and is used when small or very precise volumes are to be infused. However, there are different commercial parenteral administration sets for macrodrip tubing. Macrodrip tubing should be used when large quantities or fast rates are necessary.

Critical Decision Point: Know which company's infusion set that your agency uses.

7. Calculate flow rate (hourly volume) of prescribed infusion. Flow rate mL/hour = total infusion (volume in mL)/hours of infusion (time to be infused) Example: $\frac{1000\text{ mL}}{8\text{ hour}} = \frac{125\text{ mL}}{1\text{ hour}}$	Once hourly rate has been determined, these formulas give correct flow rate.
8. Read physician's orders and follow six rights for correct solution and proper additives.	IV fluids are medications; following six rights decreases chance of medication error.

Steps	Rationale
9. IV fluids are usually ordered for 24-hour period, indicating how long each litre of fluid should run; for example, IV order for client is: Bottle 1: 1000 mL D_5W with 20 mmol KCl to run 8 hr Bottle 2: 1000 mL D_5W with 20 mmol KCl to run 8 hr Bottle 3: 1000 mL D_5W with 20 mmol KCl to run 8 hr Total 24-hour IV intake: 3000 mL	Determines volume of fluid that should infuse hourly.
10. Place adhesive or fluid indicator tape on IV bottle or bag next to volume markings (see illustration).	Time taping IV bag gives nurse visual cue as to whether fluids are being administered over correct period of time. Time tapes may be required for all IV infusions, including those on therapies infused via electronic infusion devices. Check agency policy.

Critical Decision Point: Do not use felt-tip pens or permanent markers on IV bags, because ink could contaminate the solution (Millam & Hadaway, 2000).

Steps	Rationale
11. After hourly flow rate has been determined, calculate minute rate based on drop factor of infusion set. Microdrip infusion set has a drop factor of 60 gtt/mL. Regular drip or macrodrip infusion set used in this example has drop factor of 15 gtt/mL.	Allows nurse to calculate minute flow rate based on this formula: Total volume × Drop factor/infusion time in minutes When using microdrip, mL/hour always equals gtt/minute.

Use the following formula:

$$\frac{\text{gtt factor}}{60} \times \frac{\text{flow rate}}{1} = \text{Drop rate}$$

Calculate minute flow rates for 120 mL/hour via 15 gtt/mL drop factor:

$$15/60 \times \frac{120}{1} = 30 \text{ gtt/minute}$$

via 60 gtt/mL (microdrip) drop factor:

$$60/60 \times \frac{120}{1} = 120 \text{ gtt/mL.}$$

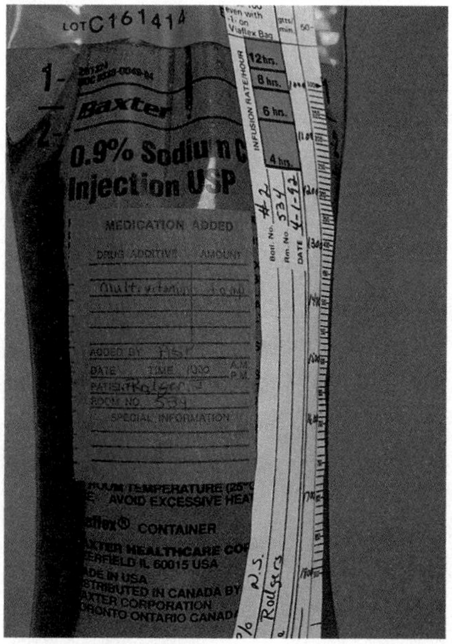

STEP **10** IV fluid bag with time tape.

Skill 36-2 Regulating Intravenous Flow Rate—cont'd

Steps	Rationale
12. Establish flow rate by counting drops in drip chamber for 1 minute by watch, then adjust roller clamp to increase or decrease rate of infusion (see illustration).	Determines if fluids are administered too slowly or too fast.
13. Follow this procedure for infusion controller or pump:	
a. Place electronic eye on half-filled drip chamber below origin of drop and above fluid level in chamber, or consult manufacturer's directions for set-up of the infusion (see illustration). If a controller is used, ensure that IV bag is 1 m above the IV site.	The electronic eye counts the number of drops flowing from administration set to ensure that proper rate infuses. IV controller works by gravity.
b. IV infusion tubing is placed within ridges of control box in direction of flow (i.e., portion of tubing nearest IV bag at top and portion of tubing nearest client at bottom) or consult manufacturer's directions for use of pump (see illustration). Some devices require securing tubing through "air in line" alarm system. Close control chamber door. Turn on pump. Required drops per minute or volume per hour and volume to be infused are selected. Open rate control clamp and press start button.	Infusion pumps move fluid by compressing and milking IV tubing, thus propelling fluid through tubing. Rate control clamp should be open completely while infusion controller or pump is in use.

Critical Decision Point: Special infusion tubing is required for some pumps (check manufacturer's directions).

Steps	Rationale
c. Monitor infusion rates and IV site for complications according to agency policy.	Infusion controllers or pumps are not infallible and do not replace frequent, accurate nursing assessments. Infusion pumps may continue to infuse IV fluids after an infiltration has begun. All EIDs must have free-flow protector device.
d. Assess patency and integrity of system when alarm sounds.	Alarm indicates that electronic eye has not noted precise number of drops from drip chamber, or there is an empty solution bag or bottle, or flow obstruction (e.g., kink in tubing, closed drip regulator, infiltrated or clotted needle, and/or air in the tubing).

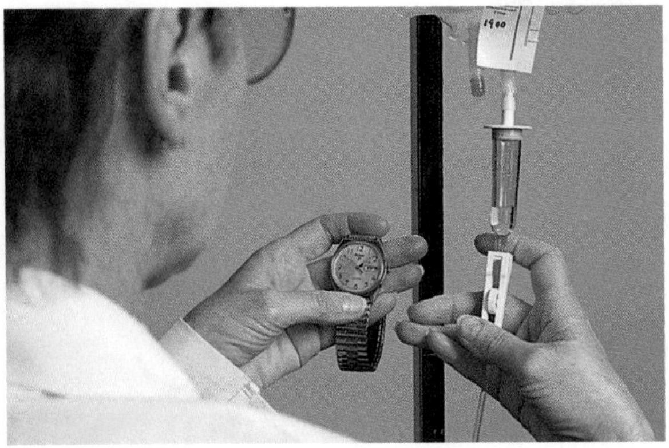

STEP **12** Counting IV drip rate.

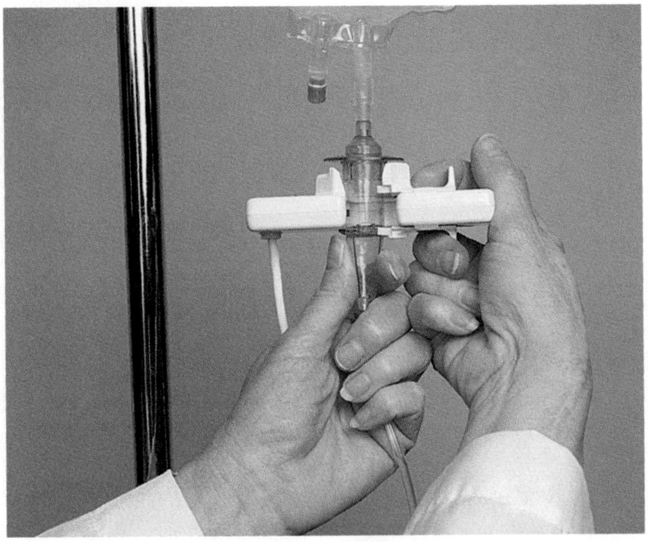

STEP **13a** Place electronic eye above fluid level in drip chamber.

Steps	Rationale

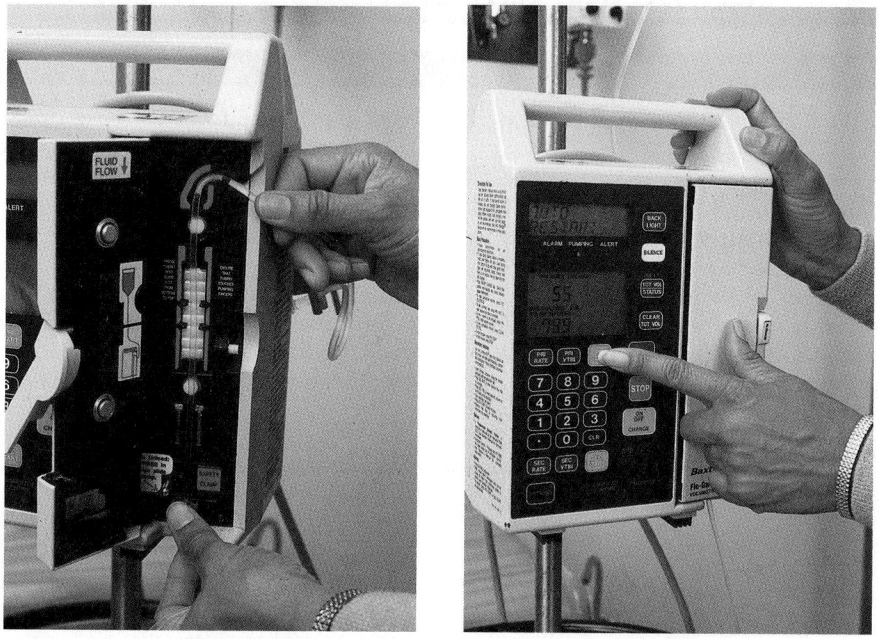

A B

STEP **13b** **A,** Place infusing tubing within ridges of pump. **B,** Press start button to begin infusion.

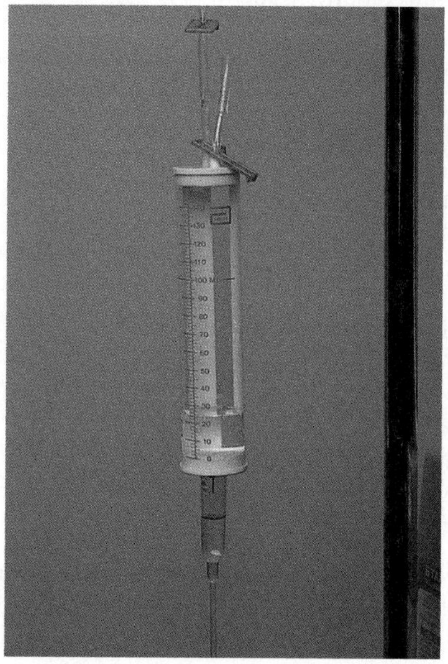

STEP **14a** Volume control device.

Steps	Rationale
14. Follow this procedure for volume control device: a. Place volume control device (see illustration) between IV bag and insertion spike of infusion set using sterile technique.	Reduces risk of sudden increase in fluid volume.

Skill 36-2 Regulating Intravenous Flow Rate—cont'd

Steps	Rationale
b. Place 2 hours' fluid allotment into chamber device.	Prevents IV line from running dry if nurse does not return in exactly 60 minutes. In addition, if there is accidental increase in flow rate, client receives at most only a 2-hour allotment of fluid.
c. Assess system at least hourly; add fluid to volume control device. Regulate flow rate.	Maintains patency of system.
15. Observe client for signs of overhydration or dehydration to determine response to therapy and restoration of fluid and electrolyte balance.	Signs and symptoms of dehydration or over-hydration warrant changing rate of fluid infused.
16. Evaluate infusion site for signs of infiltration, inflammation, clot in catheter, or kink or knot in infusion tubing.	Prevents decrease or cessation of flow rate.

Unexpected Outcomes and Related Interventions

- Sudden infusion of large volume of solution occurs with client having symptoms of dyspnea, crackles in the lung, and increased urine output, indicating fluid overload.
  - Slow infusion to KVO rate, and notify physician immediately. New IV orders will be required. Client may require diuretics.
- IV fluid bag runs empty with subsequent loss of IV line patency.
  - IV will be restarted.
- The IV infusion is slower than ordered.
  - Check client for positional change that might affect rate, height of IV bag, kinking of tubing.
  - An infiltration may be developing at IV site. Check condition of site.
  - If volume infused is deficient, consult physician for new order to provide necessary fluid volume.

Recording and Reporting

- Record name of solution, rate of infusion, drops/minute, and mL/hour in nurses' notes or flow sheet every 4 hours or according to agency policy.
- Immediately record in nurses' notes or flow sheet any new IV fluid rates.
- Document use of any EID or controlling device and number on that device.
- At change of shift or when leaving on break, report rate of infusion to nurse in charge or next nurse assigned to care for client.

Home Care Considerations

- Ensure that client is able and willing to operate the EID (if applicable) and administer IV therapy or that there is a reliable caregiver or nursing support personnel at home to provide this IV therapy care.
- Teach client and primary caregiver to time drops per minute using watch with second hand.
- Ensure that electric outlets are functioning properly, are grounded, and infusion device has back-up power, if required by type of infusate.

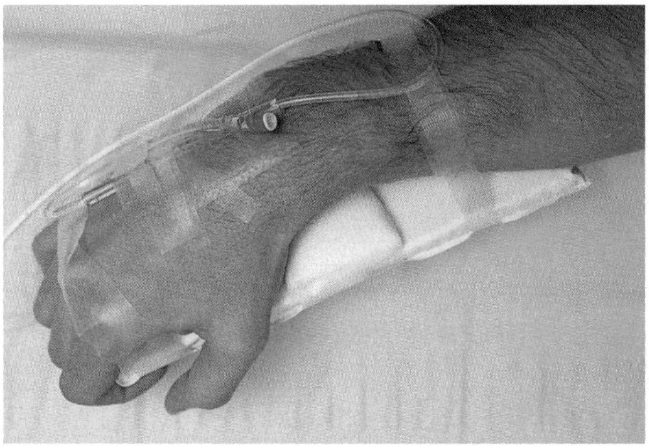

FIGURE **36–14** IV arm board and cover.

when the roller clamp is opened, the nurse should assess potential causes: a too-tight IV dressing may be impeding the flow, a clot may be occluding the cannula of the IV catheter, or the catheter tip may be occluded against the wall of the vein. The tubing and area around the insertion site should be inspected for anything that could obstruct the flow of IV fluids. A knot or kink in the tubing can decrease the flow rate. Occasionally the tubing is kinked under a dressing, which requires the nurse to remove the dressing to locate the problem. The flow rate frequently resumes after the tubing is straightened. The client may also occlude the tubing by lying or sitting on it. The height of the IV bag can also affect flow rates. Raising the bag usually increases the rate because of increased hydrostatic pressure.

The position of the extremity, particularly at the wrist or elbow, can decrease flow rates. Occasionally the use of an arm board helps to keep the joint extended (Figure 36–14). The arm board also provides some protection to the IV site and tubing. Sometimes it is more comfortable for the client to have an infusion started in a new location rather than relying upon a site that causes problems. However, before discontinuing the infusion hampered by an extremity position, the nurse should start the infusion in another site to verify that the client has other accessible veins.

Children, older adults, clients with severe head trauma, and clients susceptible to volume overload must be protected from sudden increases in infusion volumes. The nurse needs to understand that when certain IV controller devices are opened, the IV fluid will infuse rapidly. If this is not controlled, an excessive amount of solution can infuse. Sudden increases can occur accidentally. For example, a restless client may loosen the roller clamp with a sudden movement and increase the flow rate, or the flow rate may be accidentally increased if the client ambulates. A sudden increase in IV infusion rate causes a rapid increase in vascular volume, which can make the client critically ill or even cause death. Volume control devices, such as a Volutrol burette, can prevent sudden excessive increases in the volume of IV solution infused.

Maintaining the System. After the IV line is in place and the flow rate is regulated, the nurse must maintain the system. The nurse keeps in mind agency policy regarding the maintenance of IV lines. Line maintenance is achieved by (a) keeping the system sterile; (b) changing solutions, tubing, and site dressings; and (c) assisting the client with self-care activities so as to not disrupt the system.

The nurse plays an important role in maintaining the integrity of an IV to prevent infection from developing. Figure 36–15 demonstrates the potential sites for contamination of an IV device. The client's microflora and contamination by insertion are initially controlled for in the procedure for IV insertion. However, the other factors are controlled through conscientious use of infection-control principles. This begins with thorough hand hygiene before and after the nurse handles any component of the IV system.

The integrity of the IV system must always be maintained. The nurse never disconnects tubing because it becomes tangled or because it might be more convenient in positioning or moving a client or applying a gown. If a client needs more room to manoeuvre, extension tubing can be added to an IV line. However, the use of extension tubing should be kept to a minimum, as each connection of tubing provides opportunity for contamination. Stopcocks for connecting more than one solution to a single IV site are sources of contamination and should be avoided (Centers for Disease Control and Prevention [CDC], 2002). Whenever an IV line is disconnected from a stopcock, the port should be plugged with a sterile cap. A port should never remain exposed to air because of risk of contamination. A new administration set should be exchanged with the subsequent fluid change. Intravenous tubing also contains injection ports through which adapters can be inserted for medication injections. An injection port must be cleaned thoroughly according to agency policy before accessing the system (INS, 2000).

Clients receiving IV therapy over several days will require changing of solutions. It is important for the nurse to organize tasks so that this can be done in plenty of time before the solution empties and possibly becomes clotted. The CDC (2002) has no recommendation for the hang time of IV fluids. Skill 36-3 reviews steps for changing IV solutions.

Intravenous tubing administration sets can remain sterile for 72 hours (CDC, 2002). The CDC (2002) recommends changing tubing no more frequently than every 72 hours. The INS (2000) recommends 72-hour intervals for continuous tubing changes, adding that 48-hour tubing changes should be considered if the rate of catheter-related infection and phlebitis in an agency exceeds 5%. The exception is tubing containing blood, TPN, blood products, and lipid emulsions, which are more likely to promote bacterial growth. Agency policy may require more frequent tubing changes (e.g., every 24 hours). Whenever possible, schedule tubing changes when it is time to hang a new container to promote aseptic technique. To prevent entry of bacteria into the bloodstream, the nurse must maintain sterility during tubing and solution changes.

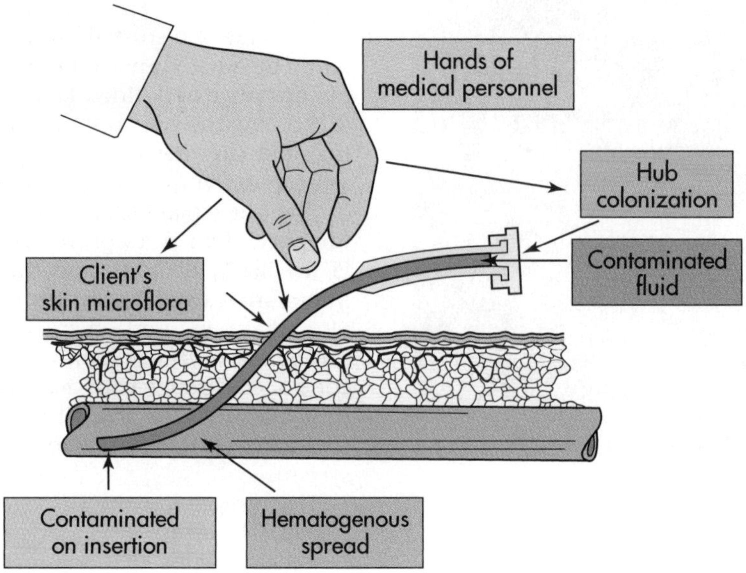

FIGURE **36–15** Potential sites for contamination of an IV device.

The dressings over IV sites are applied to reduce the entrance of bacteria into the insertion site. The two forms of dressings are transparent and gauze. Transparent dressings reliably secure the IV device, allow continuous visual inspection of the IV site, become less easily soiled or moistened, and require less frequent changes than standard gauze (CDC, 2002). Either form of dressing must be changed when the IV device is removed or replaced or when the dressing becomes damp, loosened, or soiled (INS, 2000). Agency policy may require IV dressings to be routinely changed within a certain time frame (e.g., 48 to 72 hours; Skill 36-4).

To prevent the accidental disruption of an IV system, the nurse may need to assist the client with hygiene, comfort measures, meals, and ambulation. Because a client with an infusion in the arm has difficulty meeting hygiene needs, the nurse should help with bathing and changing gowns. It helps to use a gown specifically made with snaps along the top sleeve seam to facilitate changing the gown without disturbing the venipuncture site. Regular gowns are changed as follows:

1. Remove the sleeve of the gown from the arm without the IV, maintaining the client's privacy.
2. Remove the sleeve of the gown from the arm with the IV.
3. Remove the IV solution container from its stand and pass it and the tubing through the sleeve. (If this involves removing the tubing from an IV electronic infusion device, use the roller clamp to slow the infusion to prevent the accidental infusion of a large volume of solution or medication).
4. Place the IV solution container and tubing through the sleeve of the clean gown and hang it on its stand. (If the IV is connected to an electronic infusion device, reassemble and open the roller clamp. Turn the pump on.)
5. Place the arm with the IV through the gown sleeve.
6. Place the arm without the IV through the gown sleeve. (Breaking the integrity of an IV line to change a gown leads to contamination.)

There are now protective devices designed to prevent accidental dislodgement of an IV catheter (Figure 36–16). The device fits comfortably around a client's hand or arm and provides a plastic shield to cover the IV device.

The client with an arm or a hand infusion is able to walk, unless contraindicated. A portable IV pole (a standard IV pole with wheels) is needed. The nurse helps the client get out of bed and places the pole next to the involved arm. The client is instructed to hold on to the pole with the involved hand and to push it while walking. The nurse should assess the equipment to make sure that the IV bag is at the proper height, that there is no tension on the tubing, and that the flow rate is correct. The nurse should instruct the client to report any blood in the tubing, a stoppage in the flow, or increased discomfort. Intravenous medications, especially antibiotics and potassium, can cause discomfort and burning sensations at the IV site. Although discomfort may be relieved by repositioning the extremity, the source of discomfort must always be carefully evaluated and may necessitate starting a new IV line in a larger vein.

Complications of Intravenous Therapy. An **infiltration** occurs when IV fluids enter the surrounding space around the venipuncture site. This is manifested as swelling (from increased tissue fluid) and pallor and coolness (caused by decreased circulation) around the venipuncture site. Fluid may be flowing through the IV line at a decreased rate or may have stopped flowing. Pain may also be present and usually results from edema and increases proportionately as the infiltration continues.

When infiltration occurs, the infusion must be discontinued and, if IV therapy is still necessary, a new cannula is inserted into a vein in another extremity. To reduce discomfort, the nurse raises the extremity, which promotes

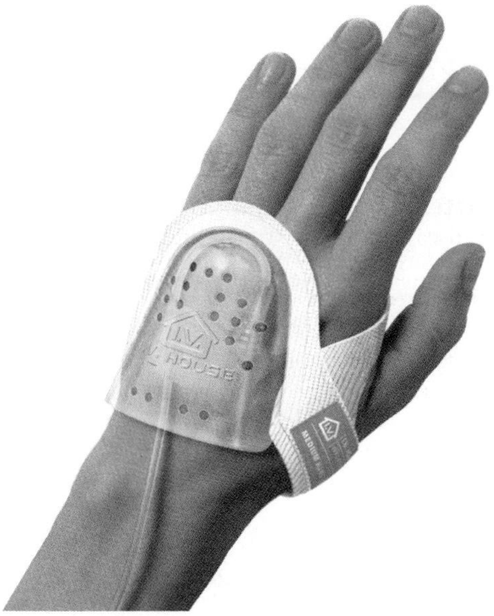

FIGURE **36–16** IV House protective device. (Courtesy IV House, St. Louis, MO.)

venous drainage. To help decrease the edema, the nurse wraps the extremity in a warm, moist towel for 20 minutes while keeping it elevated on a pillow. This promotes venous return, increases circulation, and reduces pain and edema.

Phlebitis is inflammation of the vein. Selected risk factors for phlebitis include the type of catheter material, chemical irritation of additives and drugs given intravenously (e.g., antibiotics), and the anatomical position of the catheter. Signs and symptoms may include pain, edema, **erythema,** increased skin temperature over the vein, and, in some instances, redness travelling along the path of the vein (INS, 2000). Dehydration may also be a contributing factor because of the increase in blood viscosity.

When phlebitis develops, the IV line must be discontinued and a new line inserted in another vein. Warm, moist heat on the site of phlebitis can offer some relief to the client (see chapter 43). Phlebitis can be dangerous, because blood clots (thrombophlebitis) can occur and in some cases may result in emboli. This may result in permanent damage to veins as well as resulting in extended agency care. Phlebitis may be prevented by the routine removal and rotation of IV sites. The CDC recommends replacing peripheral venous catheters and rotating sites at least every 72 to 96 hours (CDC, 2002).

Fluid volume excess occurs when the client has received a too-rapid administration of IV solutions. The assessment findings include shortness of breath, crackles in the lungs, and tachycardia. The nurse should slow the rate of infusion, notify the physician, raise the head of the bed, and monitor vital signs.

Bleeding can occur around the venipuncture site during the infusion or through the catheter needle or tubing if these become inadvertently disconnected. Bleeding is common in clients who have received heparin or who have a bleeding disorder (e.g., leukemia or thrombocytopenia). If bleeding occurs around the venipuncture site and the catheter is within the vein, a pressure dressing may be applied over the site to control the bleeding. Bleeding from a vein is usually a slow, continuous seepage and is not serious.

Discontinuing Intravenous Infusions. Discontinuing an infusion is necessary after the prescribed amount of fluid has been infused, when an infiltration occurs, if phlebitis is present, or if the infusion catheter or needle develops a clot at its tip. The nurse discontinuing an infusion first applies disposable gloves and then removes the tape and dressing in the same manner as for the daily infusion dressing changes. The nurse then moves the roller clamp to the "off"/closed position to prevent continued flow of IV fluid. The site may be cleansed with antiseptic solution(s) before removal. Each solution must be allowed to dry completely. The nurse should check agency policy. The nurse places a sterile 2×2 (5 cm $\times$ 5 cm) gauze pad over the venipuncture site and, using the other hand, with a slow, steady movement, withdraws the cannula by pulling straight back away from the puncture site (Figure 36–17). The catheter should be inspected for intactness and integrity. If necessary, alcohol or soap and water can be used to remove dried blood or other drainage from around the site. The nurse elevates the extremity and applies pressure to the site for 1 to 2 minutes to control bleeding and prevent hematoma formation. Clients who have received heparin require longer pressure because of the action of heparin on blood-clotting mechanisms. If needed, the nurse applies a bandage over a sterile cotton ball or applies a larger sterile dressing over the venipuncture site. The nurse records the amount of fluid infused and the time of the discontinuation as well as the appearance of the insertion site.

Blood Replacement (Colloids). Blood replacement or transfusion is the IV administration of whole blood or a component such as plasma, packed red blood cells (RBCs), or platelets. The objectives for blood transfusions include (a) to increase circulating blood volume after surgery, trauma, or hemorrhage; (b) to increase the number of RBCs and to maintain hemoglobin levels in clients with severe anemia; and (c) to provide selected cellular components as replacement therapy (e.g., clotting factors, platelets, albumin).

Blood Groups and Types. The most important grouping for transfusion purposes is the ABO system, which includes A, B, O, and AB blood types. The determination of blood groups is based on the presence or absence of A and B red cell antigens. Individuals with A antigens, B antigens, or no antigens belong to groups A, B, and O, respectively. The person with A and B antigens has AB blood. Individuals with type A blood naturally produce anti-B antibodies in their plasma. Similarly, type B individuals naturally produce anti-A antibodies. A type O individual has neither type A nor type B antigen and thus is considered a universal blood donor. A type AB individual produces neither antibody, which is why a type AB individual can be a universal recipient and receive any type of blood. If blood that is mismatched with the client's blood is transfused, a **transfusion reaction** occurs. The transfusion reaction is an antigen-antibody reaction and can

Text continued on p. 1201

Skill 36-3 *Maintenance of IV System*

Delegation Considerations

In many provinces, this skill is included within the scope of practice for licensed/registered practical nurses (LPNs/RPNs). The skill of changing IV solutions and tubing should not be delegated to unregulated care providers (UCPs). UCPs may be delegated the task of collecting supplies, assisting with comfort measures, and distracting the client during the procedure.

Equipment

IV infusion
- Bottle/bag of IV solution as ordered by physician
- Time tape
- Infusion tubing and tubing label
- Filter (size appropriate to solution) and extension tubing (if necessary)

Intermittent saline/heparin lock
- Injection cap, loop, or short extension tubing (if necessary)

Normal saline flush
- Syringe filled with normal saline or heparin flush solution (check agency policy)
- 2 sterile 2 × 2 (5 cm × 5 cm) gauze pads
- Tape
- Disposable gloves

Discontinuation of IV
- Disposable gloves
- Alcohol swabs
- Sterile 2 × 2 (5 cm × 5 cm) gauze
- Tape

Steps	Rationale
Changing IV Solution	
1. Check physician's orders.	Ensures that correct solution will be used. IV therapy requires the six rights of medication administration.
2. If order is written for keep vein open (KVO) or to keep open (TKO), contact physician for clarification of the rate of the infusion. Note date and time when solution was last changed.	Orders for KVO do not provide complete information and can result in fluid overload or deficit and electrolyte imbalance. A KVO order should contain a specific infusion rate (INS, 2000). Refer to agency policy. IV tubing and solution should be changed at the same time.
3. Determine the compatibility of all IV fluids and additives by consulting appropriate literature or the pharmacy.	Incompatibilities may lead to precipitate formation and can cause physical, chemical, and therapeutic client changes. Precipitation may occlude patency of catheter.
4. Determine client's understanding of need for continued IV therapy.	Reveals need for client instruction.
5. Assess patency of current IV access site.	If patency is occluded, a new IV access site may be needed. Notify physician.
6. Have next solution prepared and accessible at least 1 hour before needed. Check that solution is correct and properly labelled. Check solution expiration date and for presence of precipitate and discolouration.	Adequate planning reduces risk of clot formation in vein caused by empty IV bag. Checking prevents medication error.
7. Prepare to change solution when less than 50 mL of fluid remains in bottle or bag or when a new type of solution is ordered.	Prevents air from entering tubing and vein from clotting from lack of flow.
8. Prepare client and family by explaining the procedure, its purpose, and what is expected of client.	Decreases anxiety and promotes co-operation.
9. Be sure drip chamber is at least half full.	Provides fluid to vein while bag is changed.
10. Perform hand hygiene.	Reduces transmission of micro-organisms.
11. Prepare new solution for changing. If using plastic bag, remove protective cover from IV tubing port. If using glass bottle, remove metal cap and metal and rubber disks.	Permits quick, smooth, and organized change from old to new solution.
12. Move roller clamp to stop flow rate.	Prevents solution remaining in drip chamber from emptying while changing solutions.
13. Remove old IV fluid container from IV pole.	Brings work to nurse's eye level.
14. Quickly remove spike from old solution bag or bottle and, without touching tip, insert spike into new bag or bottle.	Reduces risk of solution in drip chamber running dry and maintains sterility.

Critical Decision Point: If spike is contaminated, a new IV tubing set is required.

Steps	Rationale
15. Hang new bag or bottle of solution on IV pole.	Gravity assists with delivery of fluid into drip chamber.
16. Check for air in tubing. If bubbles form, they can be removed by closing the roller clamp, stretching the tubing downward, and tapping the tubing with the finger (the bubbles rise in the fluid to the drip chamber, see illustration). For larger amounts of air, swab injection port below the air with alcohol and allow to dry. Connect a syringe to this port and aspirate the air into the syringe. Reduce air in tubing by priming slowly instead of allowing a wide-open flow.	Reduces risk of air embolus. Use of an air-eliminating filter also reduces this risk.
17. Make sure drip chamber is one-third to one-half full. If the drip chamber is too full, pinch off tubing below the drip chamber, invert the container, squeeze the drip chamber (see illustration), hang up the bottle, and release the tubing.	Reduces risk of air entering tubing.
18. Regulate flow to prescribed rate.	Maintains measures to restore fluid balance and deliver IV fluid as ordered.
19. Mark time on label tape and place on bag. Do not use felt-tip pens or permanent markers on IV bags.	Ink from markers may leach through polyvinyl chloride containers.
20. Observe client for signs of overhydration or dehydration to determine response to IV fluid therapy.	Provides ongoing evaluation of client's fluid and electrolyte status.
21. Observe IV system for patency and development of complications (e.g., infiltration or phlebitis).	Provides ongoing evaluation of IV system.
Changing IV Tubing	
22. Determine when new infusion set is needed:	
a. Agency policy will indicate frequency of routine change for IV administration sets and heparin/saline flush tubing.	The CDC (2002) and INS (2000) recommend changing tubing for primary infusions no more frequently than 72-hour intervals or whenever tubing has been compromised.
b. Puncture of infusion tubing requires immediate change.	Punctured tubing results in fluid leakage and bacterial contamination.

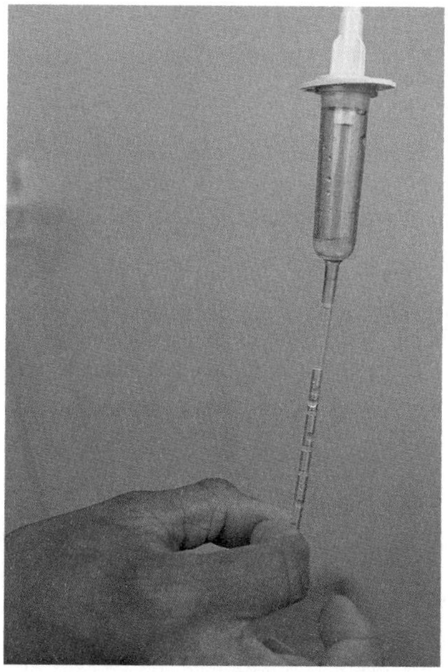

STEP **16** Tap tubing to cause air bubbles to rise up to drip chamber.

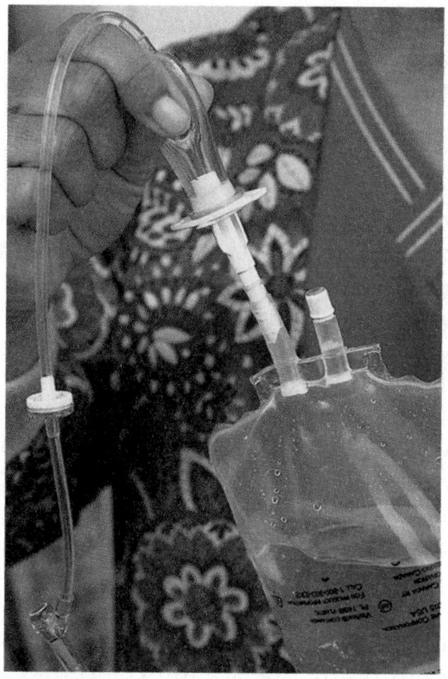

STEP **17** Squeeze drip chamber to remove a portion of fluid. Be sure to leave chamber one-third to one-half full.

Skill 36-3 Maintenance of IV System—cont'd

Steps	Rationale
c. Contamination of tubing requires immediate change.	Contamination of tubing allows entry of bacteria into client's bloodstream.
d. Occlusions in existing tubing can occur after infusion of packed red cells, whole blood, albumin, or other blood components.	Whole blood or blood component product can occlude or partially occlude tubing, because viscous solutions adhere to walls of tubing and decrease the size of the lumen.
23. Prepare client and family by explaining the procedure, its purpose, and what is expected of client.	Decreases anxiety, promotes co-operation, and prevents sudden movement of extremity, which could dislodge IV needle or catheter.
24. Perform hand hygiene.	Reduces transmission of micro-organisms.
25. Open new infusion set, keeping protective coverings over infusion spike and distal adapter. Secure all junctions with Luer-loks, clasping devices, or threaded devices.	Provides nurse with ready access to new infusion set and maintains sterility of infusion set.
26. Apply non-sterile, disposable gloves.	Reduces risk of exposure to HIV, hepatitis, and other blood-borne pathogens.
27. If needle or catheter hub is not visible, remove IV dressing while maintaining stability of catheter. If transparent dressing has to be removed, place small piece of sterile tape across hub temporarily to anchor catheter during disconnection. Do not remove tape securing needle or catheter to skin with gauze dressing.	Needle hub must be accessible to provide smooth transition when removing old and inserting new tubing.
28. For IV continuous infusion:	
a. Move roller clamp on new IV tubing to "off" position.	Prevents spillage of solution after bag or bottle is spiked.
b. Slow rate of infusion by regulating drip rate on old tubing. Be sure rate is at KVO rate.	Prevents complete infusion of solution that remains in tubing, which can increase risk of occlusion of IV catheter or needle.
c. Compress and fill drip chamber of old tubing.	Provides surplus of fluid in drip chamber so there is enough fluid to maintain IV patency while changing tubing.
d. Remove IV container from pole, invert container and remove old tubing from container. Carefully hold container while hanging or taping drip chamber on IV pole 1 m above IV site.	Fluid in drip chamber will run slowly to keep catheter patent.
e. Place insertion spike of new tubing into old solution bag opening and hang solution bag on IV pole.	Permits flow of fluid from solution into new infusion tubing.
f. Compress and release drip chamber on new tubing; fill drip chamber one-third to one-half full.	Allows drip chamber to fill and promotes rapid, smooth flow of solution through new tubing.
g. Slowly open roller clamp, remove protective cap from needle adapter (if necessary), and flush new tubing with solution. Replace cap.	Removes air from tubing and replaces it with fluid.
h. Turn roller clamp on old tubing to "off" position.	Prevents spillage of fluid as tubing is removed from needle hub.
29. For saline/heparin lock:	
a. If a loop or short extension tubing is needed because of an awkward IV site placement, use sterile technique to connect the new injection cap to the loop or tubing.	
b. Swab injection cap with alcohol, povidone-iodine, or chlorhexidine. Insert syringe with 1 to 3 mL saline or heparin flush solution and inject through the injection cap into the loop or short extension tubing (see illustration).	Removes air to prevent introduction into the vein.

Steps	Rationale

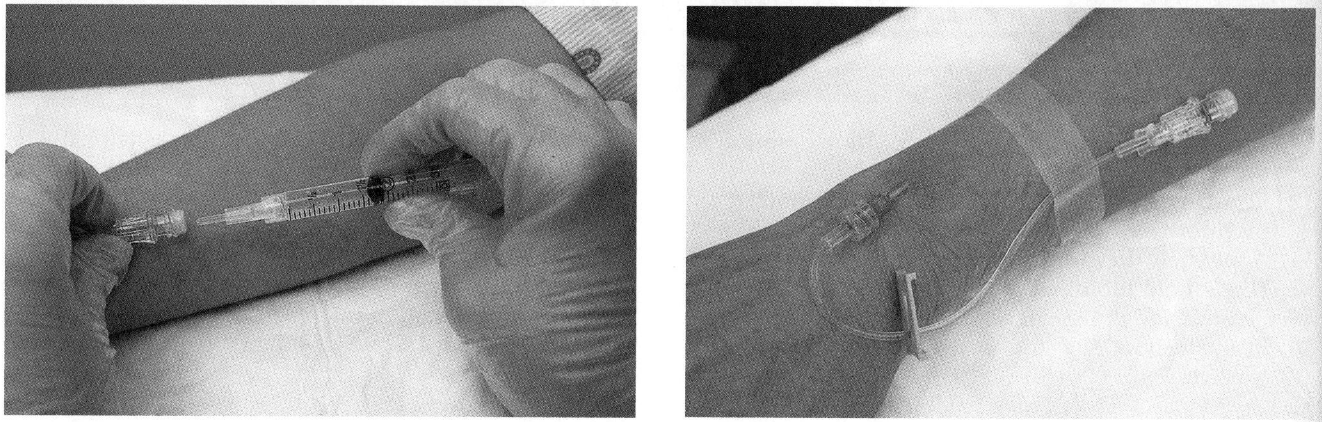

A B

STEP **29b** **A,** Inject saline into injection cap. **B,** Connect to saline lock extension tube.

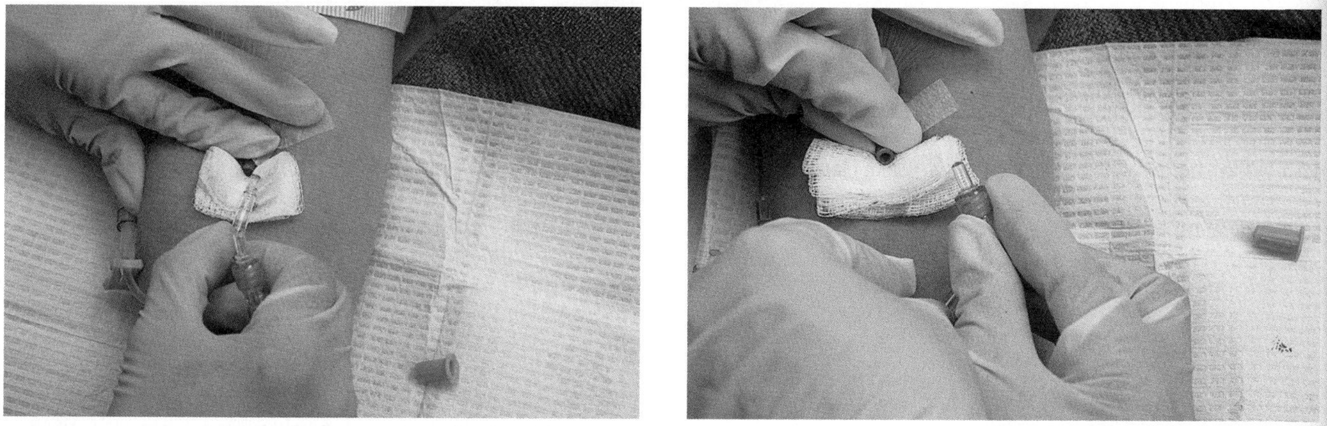

A B

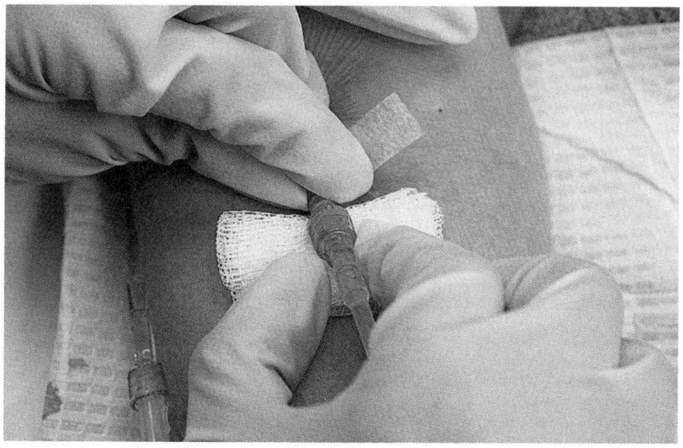

C

STEP **30** **A,** Maintain stability of catheter hub while removing old tubing. **B,** Connect new infusion tubing. **C,** Be sure connection at hub is secure.

Steps	Rationale
30. Stabilize hub of catheter and apply pressure over vein just above catheter tip at least 3 cm above insertion site. Gently disconnect old tubing from catheter hub (see illustration). Maintain stability of hub and quickly insert adapter of new tubing or saline/heparin lock into hub (see illustrations).	Prevents accidental displacement of catheter or needle. Prevents clot formation in catheter or needle and backflow of blood.

Skill 36-3 Maintenance of IV System—cont'd

Steps	Rationale
31. Open roller clamp on new tubing. Allow solution to run rapidly for 30 to 60 seconds.	Permits IV solution to enter catheter to prevent catheter occlusion.
32. Regulate IV drip according to physician's orders and monitor rate hourly.	Maintains infusion flow at prescribed rate.
33. Apply new dressing, if needed.	Reduces risk of bacterial infection from skin.
34. Discard old tubing in proper container.	Reduces accidental transmission of micro-organisms.
35. Remove and dispose of gloves. Perform hand hygiene.	Reduces transmission of micro-organisms.
36. Evaluate flow rate and observe connection site for leakage.	Maintains prescribed rate of flow of IV fluid and determines if fit is secure.
Discontinuing Peripheral IV Access	
37. Check physician's order for discontinuation of IV.	Order is required for discontinuation of fluids/medication.
38. Explain procedure to client. Explain that affected extremity must be held still and how long procedure will take.	Minimizes client's anxiety and discomfort.
39. Perform hand hygiene and apply disposable gloves.	Reduces transmission of micro-organisms.
40. Turn IV tubing roller clamp to "off" position. Remove tape securing tubing.	
41. Remove IV site dressing and tape while stabilizing catheter.	Movement of catheter will cause discomfort.
42. With dry gauze or alcohol swab held over site, apply light pressure and withdraw the catheter, using a slow steady movement, keeping the hub parallel to the skin.	Changing the angle of the catheter inside the vein could cause additional vein irritation, increasing the risk of post-infusion phlebitis.
43. Apply pressure to the site for 2 to 3 minutes, using the dry, sterile gauze pad. Secure with tape.	Dry pad causes less irritation to the puncture site. Subcutaneous hematoma is common complication. When needle is removed, vein wall contracts to stop bleeding. Contraction is enhanced by pressure to site for at least 2 to 3 minutes (Chukhraev & Grekov, 2000).
44. Inspect the catheter for intactness, noting tip integrity and length.	Tips of catheter can break off, causing an embolus, an emergency situation. Notify physician if tip is broken.
45. Discard used supplies.	
46. Remove and discard gloves, and perform hand hygiene.	
47. Instruct client to report any redness, pain, drainage, or swelling that may occur after catheter removal.	Post-infusion phlebitis may occur within 48 to 96 hours after catheter removal.

Unexpected Outcomes and Related Interventions

- Flow rate is incorrect; client receives too little or too much fluid.
  - Readjust infusion rate to ordered rate; evaluate client for adverse effects; notify physician.
- Flow of IV fluid is decreased or absent.
  - Assess IV infusion system for patency.
  - Recalibrate drip rate on new tubing.
  - Assess IV site for infiltration.

Recording and Reporting

- Record changing of tubing and solution on client's record. A special parenteral therapy flow sheet may be used.
- Place a piece of tape or preprinted label with the date and time of tubing change and attach to tubing below the level of drip chamber.

Home Care Considerations

- Emphasize to client and family the importance of changing solutions when IV tubing still contains fluid.

Skill 36-4 Changing a Peripheral Intravenous Dressing

View Video

Delegation Considerations

In many provinces, skill of changing a peripheral IV dressing is included within the scope of practice for licensed/registered practical nurses. This skill should not be delegated to unregulated care providers (UCPs). UCPs may be delegated the task of collecting supplies, assisting with comfort measures, and distracting the client during the procedure.

Equipment

- Antiseptic swab stick (chlorhexidine, povidone-iodine, and/or 70% alcohol, as recommended by the agency)
- Alcohol swab stick
- Adhesive remover (if needed)
- Strips of non-allergenic sterile tape for use underneath the dressing
- Disposable gloves
- Arm board or housing device (if needed)
- For gauze dressing
  - Sterile 2 × 2 (5 cm × 5 cm) gauze pad OR
  - Sterile 4 × 4 (10 cm × 10 cm) gauze pad
- For transparent dressing
  - Sterile transparent dressing

Steps	Rationale
1. Determine when dressing was last changed. Many institutions require the nurse to write date and time on dressing and date the device was first placed.	Provides information regarding length of time present dressing has been in place. In addition, the nurse is able to plan for dressing change. The CDC recommends that, whenever possible, peripheral IV dressings should be scheduled when IV system is changed.
2. Perform hand hygiene. Observe present dressing for moisture and intactness.	Moisture is a medium for bacterial growth and renders dressing contaminated.
3. Observe IV system for proper functioning or complications: kinks in infusion tubing or IV catheter. Palpate the catheter site through the intact dressing for inflammation or subjective complaints of pain or burning.	Unexplained decrease in flow rate requires the nurse to investigate placement and patency of the IV catheter. Pain can be associated with both phlebitis and infiltration.
4. Inspect exposed catheter site for swelling or blanching.	Indicates fluid infusing into surrounding tissues. Will require removal of IV catheter.
5. Assess client's understanding of need for continued IV infusion.	Determines need for client instruction.
6. Explain procedure and purpose to client and family. Explain that affected extremity must be held still and how long procedure will take.	Decreases anxiety, promotes co-operation, and gives client time frame around which personal activities can be planned.
7. Apply disposable gloves	Reduces transmission of micro-organisms.
8. Remove tape, gauze, and/or transparent dressing from old dressing one layer at a time, leaving tape (if present) that secures IV catheter in place. Be cautious if catheter tubing becomes tangled between two layers of dressing. When removing transparent dressing, hold catheter hub and tubing with non-dominant hand.	Prevents accidental displacement of catheter or needle.
9. Observe insertion site for signs and/or symptoms of infection (redness, swelling, and exudate). If present, remove catheter and insert a new IV in another site.	
10. If infiltration, phlebitis, or clot occurs or if ordered by physician, stop infusion and discontinue IV. Restart new IV if continued therapy is necessary. Place moist warm compress over area of phlebitis (see Tables 36-9, 36-10).	
11. If IV is infusing properly, gently remove any tape securing catheter. Stabilize needle or catheter with one hand. Use adhesive remover to cleanse skin and remove adhesive residue, if needed.	Exposes venipuncture site. Stabilization prevents accidental displacement of catheter or needle. Adhesive residue decreases ability of new dressing to adhere tightly to skin.
12. Stabilize catheter at all times with one finger over catheter until tape or dressing is replaced.	Prevents decannulation from vein.

Skill 36-4 Changing a Peripheral Intravenous Dressing—cont'd

Steps	Rationale

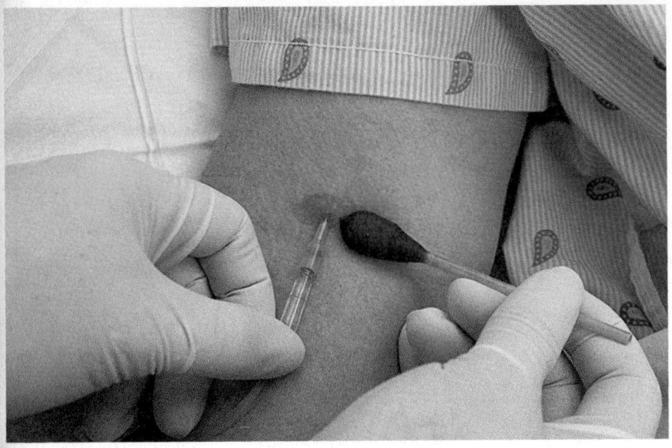

STEP 13 Cleanse peripheral insertion site.

Steps	Rationale
13. Using circular motion, cleanse peripheral IV insertion site with antiseptic swab starting at insertion site and working outward, creating concentric circles (see illustration). Allow swab solution to air-dry completely.	Circular motion prevents cross-contamination from skin bacteria near venipuncture site. Antiseptics may include chlorhexidine, povidone-iodine, and alcohol. CDC recommends 2% chlorhexidine-based solution. Povidone-iodine is a topical anti-infective that reduces skin surface bacteria; the solution must be dry to be effective in reducing microbial counts (CDC, 2002). If antiseptic agents are used in combination, allow each to dry separately.

Critical Decision Point: Do not tape over connection of access tubing or port to IV catheter.

Steps	Rationale
14. Apply new transparent or gauze dressing (See Skill 36-1).	Ensures protection of IV site and reduces chance of infection.
15. Remove and discard gloves.	
16. Anchor IV tubing with additional pieces of tape. When using transparent polyurethane dressing, minimize the tape placed over dressing.	Prevents accidental displacement of IV needle or catheter or separation of IV tubing from needle adapter.
17. Place insertion date (if known), date and time of dressing change, size and gauge of catheter, and initials of nurse directly on dressing. Apply arm board and/or commercial housing device if site is affected by joint motion.	Documents dressing change.
18. Discard used equipment and perform hand hygiene.	Reduces transmission of micro-organisms.
19. Observe functioning and patency of IV system in response to changing dressing.	Validates that IV is patent and functioning correctly.
20. Monitor client's body temperature.	Elevated temperature indicates an infection that may be associated with bacterial contamination of the venipuncture site.

Unexpected Outcomes and Related Interventions

- IV catheter is infiltrated, as evidenced by decreased flow rate or edema, pallor, or decreased temperature around insertion site.
  - Stop infusion and discontinue IV. Restart new IV in other extremity if continued therapy is necessary.
  - Elevate affected extremity.
- Phlebitis is present, as evidenced by erythema and tenderness along vein pathway.
  - Stop infusion and discontinue IV. Restart new IV in other extremity if continued therapy is necessary.
  - Apply warm moist compress to area of phlebitis.
- IV catheter or needle is accidentally removed.
  - Restart IV if continued therapy is needed.
- Client has an elevated temperature.
  - Notify physician. IV may be removed and restarted. Client will be evaluated for source of infection.
- Insertion site is red and/or edematous and/or painful and/or has presence of exudates, indicating infection at venipuncture site.
  - Discontinue IV. Antibiotic therapy may begin.
  - Apply warm moist compress to area of inflammation.

Recording and Reporting

- Record appearance of IV site, type of dressing, and status of IV fluid infusion.
- A special parenteral fluid flow sheet may be used for recording.

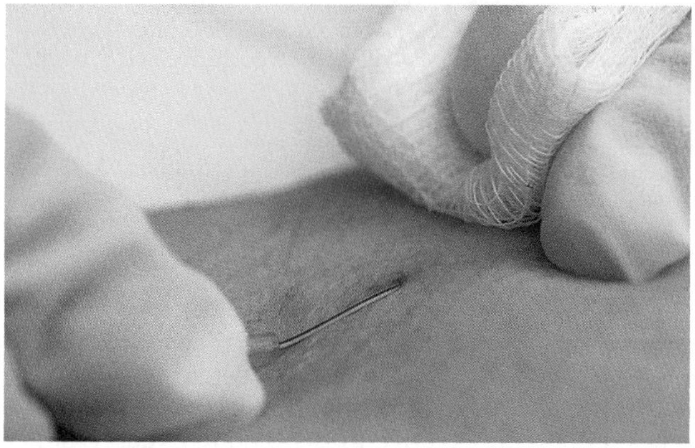

FIGURE **36–17** IV catheter is removed slowly, keeping catheter parallel to vein.

range from a mild response to severe anaphylactic shock, which can be life-threatening.

Another consideration when matching for blood transfusions is the Rh factor, which is an antigenic substance in the erythrocytes of most people. A person with the factor is Rh positive, and a person without it is Rh negative.

Autologous Transfusion. **Autologous transfusion** or autotransfusion is the collection of a client's own blood. The blood for an autologous transfusion can be obtained by preoperative donation up to 5 weeks before the planned surgery (e.g., heart, orthopedic, plastic, or gynecological). Clients can donate 1 to 5 units of their own blood depending on the type of surgery and the ability of the client to maintain an acceptable hematocrit. The blood will be tested for HIV and hepatitis B virus (HBV). Another way to collect blood for an autologous transfusion is during perioperative blood salvage (e.g., during vascular and orthopedic surgery, organ transplant surgery, and traumatic injuries). The blood that has been salvaged is then reinfused during the surgery. Blood can also be salvaged post-operatively from mediastinal and chest-tube drainage and after joint and spinal surgery. Autologous transfusions decrease the risk of complications such as mismatched blood and exposure to bloodborne infectious agents.

Blood Transfusions. Transfusing blood or blood components is a nursing procedure. The nurse is responsible for assessment before, during, and after the transfusion and for regulation of the transfusion. Assessment is critical because of the risk of allergic reactions.

If the client has an IV line in place, the nurse assesses the venipuncture site for signs of infection or infiltration. The nurse also determines the gauge of the IV catheter. A large catheter such as an 18 gauge or 19 gauge is preferred because blood is thicker and stickier than IV fluids, although smaller gauge sizes will accommodate transfusions. The nurse determines whether the IV catheter is patent and functioning properly. The tubing for blood administration has an in-line filter (Figure 36–18). The tubing should be filled with 0.9% normal saline to prevent **hemolysis,** or breakdown of RBCs.

Pre-transfusion assessment also includes obtaining information from the client. The nurse asks whether the client knows the reason for the blood transfusion and whether the client has ever had a previous transfusion or transfusion reaction. A client who has had a transfusion reaction is usually at no greater risk for a reaction with a subsequent transfusion. However, the client may be anxious about the transfusion, requiring nursing intervention. Before giving a transfusion, the nurse explains the procedure and instructs the client to report any side effects (e.g., chills, dizziness, or fever) once the transfusion begins. The nurse also checks to be sure the client has signed an informed consent. Clients with certain cultural backgrounds may abstain from blood transfusions (Box 36-9).

Because of the danger of transfusion reactions, it is very important to use specific precautions in administering blood or blood products. The nurse must obtain the client's baseline vital signs before the transfusion begins. This allows the nurse to determine when changes in vital signs occur, which can indicate that a transfusion reaction is developing. A thorough procedure, which checks identity of the blood products, the client, and the compatibility of the

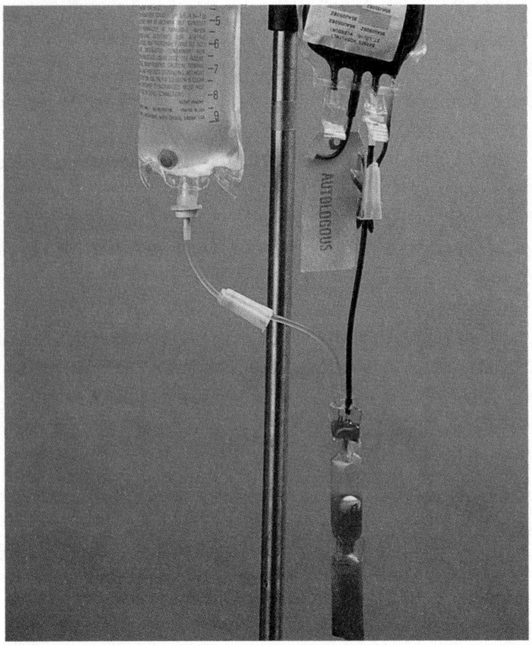

FIGURE **36–18** Tubing for blood administration has an in-line filter.

Cultural Aspects of Care — Box 36-9

When a client's natural skin contains more melanin, it becomes more difficult to determine colour changes. Early assessment for IV complications such as phlebitis and infiltration may not be easily detected.

Clients within certain cultural backgrounds have fear related to the donor process for blood.

Clients with certain religious or personal beliefs may abstain from receiving blood transfusions and/or medications.

Implications for Practice

- Use light palpation to assess for tenderness associated with phlebitis.
- Use light palpation to assess for edema and coolness associated with infiltration.
- Assess clients individually to determine their acceptance or abstinence toward therapeutic regimens.
- Appreciate clients' choice related to their therapy.
- Although some clients will abstain from receiving whole blood or packed red blood cells, there are other blood products or alternatives that they will accept.

Adapted from "Transfusion Alternatives," by C. Rudnicke, 2003, *Journal of Infusion Nursing, 26*(3), pp. 29–33.

blood and the client, is used to ensure that the right client receives the correct type of blood or blood product. The nurse, although not involved in the blood labelling process, is responsible for determining that the blood delivered to the client corresponds to the client's blood type listed in the medical record. Two registered nurses or one registered nurse and a licensed practical nurse (see agency policy) must together check the label on the blood product against the client's identification number, blood group, and complete name. If even a minor discrepancy exists, the blood should not be given and the blood bank should be notified immediately.

Initiation of a transfusion begins slowly to allow for the early detection of a transfusion reaction. The nurse maintains the infusion rate, monitors for side effects, assesses vital signs, and promptly records all findings. The nurse usually stays with the client during the first 15 minutes, the time when a reaction is most likely to occur. The nurse will continue to monitor the client and obtain vital signs periodically during the transfusion as directed by agency policy. If a transfusion reaction is anticipated or suspected, the nurse will obtain vital signs more frequently (Table 36-11).

The rate of transfusion is usually specified in the physician's orders. Ideally a unit of whole blood or packed RBCs is transfused in 2 hours. This time can be lengthened to 4 hours if the client is at risk for FVE. Beyond 4 hours, there is a risk of the blood becoming contaminated.

When clients have a severe blood loss such as with hemorrhage, they may receive rapid transfusions through a central venous catheter. A blood-warming device is often necessary, because the tip of the central venous catheter lies in the superior vena cava, above the right atrium. Rapid administration of cold blood can result in cardiac dysrhythmia (Otto, 2001).

Transfusion Reactions. A transfusion reaction is a systemic response by the body to incompatible blood. Causes include red cell incompatibility or allergic sensitivity to the components of the transfused blood or to the potassium or citrate preservative in the blood. Several types of acute reactions can result from blood transfusions (see Table 36-11).

A second category of reactions includes diseases transmitted by infected blood donors who are asymptomatic. Diseases transmitted through transfusions are malaria, hepatitis, and AIDS. Because all units of blood collected must undergo serological testing and screening for HIV and HBV, the risk of acquiring blood-borne infections from blood transfusions is reduced.

Circulatory overload is a risk when a client receives large volumes of whole blood or packed RBC transfusions for massive hemorrhagic shock or when a client with normal blood volume receives blood. Clients particularly at risk for circulatory overload are older adults and those with cardiopulmonary diseases.

Blood transfusion reactions are life-threatening, but prompt nursing intervention can maintain the client's physiological stability.

> *Safety Alert.* If a blood reaction is suspected, the nurse stops the transfusion immediately.

- The nurse keeps the IV line open by "piggybacking" 0.9% normal saline directly into the IV line and running the saline.
- The nurse should not turn off the blood and simply turn on the 0.9% normal saline that is connected to the Y-tubing infusion set. This would cause blood

Table 36-11 Acute Transfusion Reactions

Reaction	Cause	Clinical Manifestations	Management	Prevention
Acute hemolytic	Infusion of ABO-incompatible whole blood, RBCs, or components containing 10 mL or more of RBCs Antibodies in the recipient's plasma attach to antigens on transfused RBCs, causing RBC destruction	Chills, fever, low back pain, flushing, tachycardia, tachypnea, hypotension, vascular collapse, hemoglobinuria, hemoglobinemia, bleeding, acute renal failure, shock, cardiac arrest, death	Stop transfusion. Treat shock, if present. Draw blood samples for serological testing slowly to avoid hemolysis from the procedure. Send urine specimen to the laboratory. Maintain BP with IV colloid solutions. Give diuretics as prescribed to maintain urine flow. Insert in-dwelling catheter or measure voided amounts to monitor hourly urine output. Dialysis may be required if renal failure occurs. Do not transfuse additional RBC-containing components until transfusion service has provided newly cross-matched units.	Meticulously verify and document client identification from sample collection to component infusion.
Febrile, nonhemolytic (most common)	Sensitization to donor white blood cells, platelets, or plasma proteins	Sudden chills and fever (rise in temperature of greater than 1° C), headache, flushing, anxiety, muscle pain	Give antipyretics as prescribed—avoid aspirin in thrombocytopenic clients. **Safety Alert. Do not restart transfusion.**	Consider leukocyte-poor blood products (filtered, washed, or frozen).
Mild allergic	Sensitivity to foreign plasma proteins	Flushing, itching, urticaria (hives)	Give antihistamine as directed. If symptoms are mild and transient, transfusion may be restarted slowly. **Safety Alert. Do not restart transfusion if fever or pulmonary symptoms develop.**	Treat prophylactically with antihistamines.
Anaphylactic	Infusion of IgA proteins to IgA-deficient recipient who has developed IgA antibody	Anxiety, urticaria, wheezing, progressing to cyanosis, shock, possible cardiac arrest	Initiate CPR, if indicated. Have epinephrine ready for injection (0.4 mL of a 1:1000 solution subcutaneously or 0.1 mL of 1:1000 solution diluted to 10 mL with saline for IV use). **Safety Alert. Do not restart transfusion.**	Transfuse extensively washed RBC products, from which all plasma has been removed. Alternately, use blood from IgA-deficient donor.
Circulatory overload	Fluid administered faster than the circulation can accommodate	Cough, dyspnea, pulmonary congestion (rales), headache, hypertension, tachycardia, distended neck veins	Place client upright with feet in dependent position. Administer prescribed diuretics, oxygen, morphine. Phlebotomy may be indicated.	Adjust transfusion volume and flow rate based on client size and clinical status. Have transfusion service divide unit into smaller aliquots for better spacing of fluid input.
Sepsis	Transfusion of contaminated blood components	Rapid onset of chills, high fever, vomiting, diarrhea, and marked hypotension and shock	Obtain culture of client's blood and send bag with remaining blood to transfusion service for further study. Treat septicemia as directed—antibiotics, IV fluids, vasopressors, steroids.	Collect, process, store, and transfuse blood products according to blood banking standards and infuse within 4 hours of starting time.

ABO, Blood group consisting of groups A, AB, B, and O; *RBCs,* red blood cells; *BP,* blood pressure; *IV,* intravenous; *IgA,* immunoglobulin A; *CPR,* cardiopulmonary resuscitation.

Data from "Transfusion Reaction," by J. Young, 2000, *Nursing, 30*(12); and *AABB Technical Manual* (13th ed.), edited by V. Vengelen-Tyler, 1999, Bethesda, MD: American Association of Blood Banks.

remaining in the Y-tubing to infuse into the client. Even a small amount of mismatched blood can cause a major reaction.

- The nurse has the physician notified immediately.
- The nurse remains with the client, observing signs and symptoms and monitoring vital signs as often as every 5 minutes.
- The nurse prepares to administer emergency drugs such as antihistamines, vasopressors, fluids, and steroids as per physician order or protocol.
- The nurse prepares to perform cardiopulmonary resuscitation.
- The nurse obtains a urine specimen and sends it to the laboratory to determine presence of hemoglobin as a result of RBC hemolysis.
- The blood container, tubing, attached labels, and transfusion record are saved and returned to the laboratory.

Interventions for Acid-Base Imbalances. Nursing interventions to promote acid-base balance support prescribed medical therapies and are aimed at reversing the acid-base imbalance. Such imbalances can be life-threatening and require rapid correction. The nurse must maintain a functional IV line and frequently check the physician's orders for new medications or fluids. Prescribed drugs, such as insulin or sodium bicarbonate, and fluid and electrolyte replacement should be given promptly. Chapter 35 reviews appropriate therapies for clients with respiratory acidosis.

The nurse also monitors clients closely for changes in acid-base balance. Clients with acid-base disturbances usually require repeated ABG analysis. This procedure provides arterial blood samples for analysis of hydrogen ion concentration.

Arterial Blood Gases. Determination of ABG levels requires the removal of a sample of blood from an artery to assess the client's acid-base status and the adequacy of ventilation and oxygenation. Arterial blood is drawn from a peripheral artery (usually the radial) or from an arterial line inserted by a physician. In some agencies, nurses are responsible for radial artery punctures. Beginning nursing students do not draw arterial samples but frequently assist in the sampling process and care for the client after the procedure. After the specimen is obtained, care is taken to prevent air from entering the syringe because this will affect the blood gas analysis. The syringe is submerged in crushed ice and transported immediately to the laboratory to reduce metabolism of cells. The nurse applies pressure to the puncture site for at least 5 minutes to reduce the risk of hematoma formation. The nurse might also reassess the radial pulse after pressure has been removed.

Restorative Care. After experiencing acute alterations in fluid, electrolyte, or acid-base balance, clients often require ongoing maintenance to prevent a recurrence of health alterations. Older adults and the chronically ill require special considerations to prevent complications from developing (see Box 36-7).

Home Intravenous Therapy. Intravenous therapy is often continued in the home setting for clients who are discharged from the hospital and have not completed their prescribed treatment or who require long-term therapy. Preferably, a family member at home can be available if the client suddenly cannot manage the IV or if a problem develops. A home care nurse will work closely with the client and family to ensure that a sterile IV system is maintained and that complications are avoided or recognized promptly. Box 36-10 summarizes client education guidelines for home IV therapy.

Nutritional Support. Most clients who have had electrolyte disorders or metabolic acid-base disturbances require ongoing nutritional support. Depending on the type of disorder, fluid or food intake may be encouraged or restricted (see chapter 39).

Medication Safety. Numerous drugs contain components or create potential side effects that can alter fluid and electrolyte balance. Clients with chronic disease who are receiving multiple medications and those with renal or liver disorders are at significant risk for alterations to develop. Once clients return to a restorative care setting, whether in the home or long-term care, drug safety becomes important. Clients and families must be educated about their drugs' side effects. The nurse should review all medications with clients and encourage them to consult with their pharmacist and physician, especially if they try a new over-the-counter medication or alternative therapy.

NP Evaluation

Client Care. The evaluation of a client's clinical status is especially important if an acute fluid and electrolyte or acid-base disturbance exists. The client's condition can change very quickly, and the nurse must be able to recognize the signs and symptoms of impending problems by being aware of health alterations, the effects of medications and fluids, and the client's presenting clinical status (Figure 36–19).

The nurse will perform evaluative measures and determine if changes have occurred from the last client assessment. For example, the physical signs and symptoms of the assessed condition begin to disappear or lessen in intensity.

For clients with less acute alterations, evaluation likely occurs over a longer period of time. In this situation, the nurse's evaluation may be focused more on behavioural changes (e.g., the client's ability to follow dietary restrictions and medication schedules). The family's ability to anticipate alterations and prevent problems from recurring is also an important element of evaluation.

The client's level of progress determines whether the nurse needs to continue or revise the care plan. If goals are not met, the nurse may need to consult with a physician and discuss additional methods such as increasing the frequency of an intervention (e.g., provide more fluids to a dehydrated client), introducing a new therapy (e.g., initiate insertion of an IV), or discontinuing a particular therapy. Once outcomes have been met, the nurse can resolve the nursing diagnosis and focus on other priorities.

Client Teaching

Box 36-10

Home Intravenous Therapy

Objective

- The client and caregiver will demonstrate understanding and competence with IV therapy for safe delivery in the home setting.

Teaching Strategies

- Explain to client and caregiver the importance of IV therapy in maintaining hydration and access for the delivery of medications.
- Emphasize the risks involved when the IV system is not kept sterile.
- Be sure the client and/or caregiver is able to manipulate the required equipment.
- Instruct client or caregiver in how to change IV solutions, tubing, and dressing when they become soiled or dislodged. (NOTE: The home care nurse may be able to visit frequently enough to perform scheduled tubing and dressing changes.)
- Instruct client and caregiver about signs and symptoms of infiltration, phlebitis, and infection and to notify the home care nurse immediately.
- Instruct client and caregiver to notify the home care nurse if the infusion slows or stops or if blood is seen in the tubing.
- Teach client with caregiver's assistance how to ambulate, perform hygiene, and participate in other activities of daily living without dislodging or disconnecting catheter and tubing.

Evaluation

- Ask client and caregiver why it is necessary to maintain hydration and IV access for the delivery of medications.
- Ask client and caregiver what to do if IV stops.
- Ask the client and caregiver to describe signs and symptoms of complications and the action they should take.
- Observe the client or caregiver changing the IV container, tubing, and dressing.
- Observe the client ambulate and participate in activities of daily living to see how he or she protects and manipulates the IV catheter and apparatus.

Client Expectations. The nurse routinely reviews with the client his or her success in meeting expectations of care. "Tell me if I have helped you feel more comfortable" is a question that the nurse might raise if the client's expectations revolve around comfort and symptom management. If the client's concerns involve having a better understanding of a chronic problem, the nurse's evaluation might focus on the client's satisfaction with educational offerings. Often the client's level of satisfaction with care also depends on the nurse's success in involving family and friends. If the client has concerns about returning home or to a different care setting, it will be important to evaluate if the client feels prepared for the transition from acute care.

Key Concepts

- Body fluids are distributed in ECF and ICF compartments.
- Body fluids are composed of electrolytes, minerals, cells, and water.
- Body fluids are regulated through fluid intake, output, and hormonal regulation.
- Volume disturbances include isotonic and osmolar deficits and excesses.
- Electrolytes are regulated by dietary intake and hormonal controls.
- Acid-base imbalances are buffered by chemical, biological, and physiological buffering, especially the lungs and kidneys.
- Chronic and serious illnesses increase the risk of fluid, electrolyte, and acid-base imbalances.
- Clients who are very young or very old are at greater risk for fluid, electrolyte, and acid-base imbalances.
- Assessment for fluid, electrolyte, and acid-base alterations includes the nursing health history, physical and behavioural assessment, measurements of I&O, daily weights, and specific laboratory data.
- Osmolar imbalances and FVD can be corrected by enteral or parenteral administration of fluid.
- Common complications of IV therapy include infiltration, phlebitis, infection, FVE, and bleeding at the infusion site.
- Blood transfusions are given to replace fluid volume loss from hemorrhage, treat anemia, or replace coagulation factors.
- Blood transfusions can be donor, autologous, or obtained through perioperative salvage.
- Administration of blood or blood products requires the nurse to follow a specific procedure to identify transfusion reactions quickly.
- In addition to transfusion reactions, the risks of transfusion also include hyperkalemia, hypocalcemia, FVE, and infection.
- Treatment for electrolyte disturbances include dietary and pharmacological interventions.
- The body's chemical buffering system responds first to acid-base abnormalities.
- The goals of therapy for acid-base imbalances are to treat the underlying illness and to restore the arterial pH to normal.

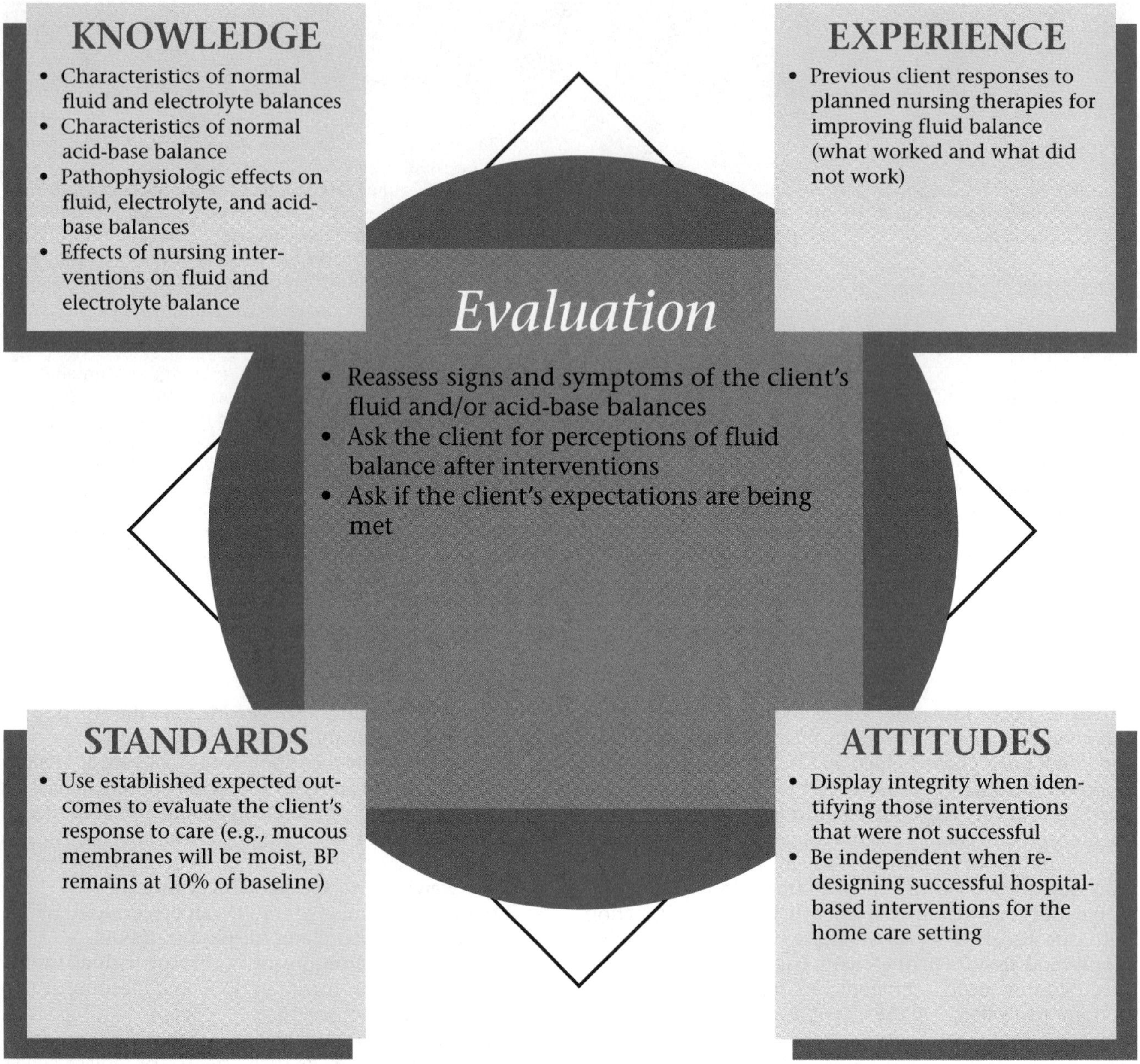
KNOWLEDGE
• Characteristics of normal fluid and electrolyte balances
• Characteristics of normal acid-base balance
• Pathophysiologic effects on fluid, electrolyte, and acid-base balances
• Effects of nursing interventions on fluid and electrolyte balance
EXPERIENCE
• Previous client responses to planned nursing therapies for improving fluid balance (what worked and what did not work)
Evaluation
• Reassess signs and symptoms of the client's fluid and/or acid-base balances
• Ask the client for perceptions of fluid balance after interventions
• Ask if the client's expectations are being met
STANDARDS
• Use established expected outcomes to evaluate the client's response to care (e.g., mucous membranes will be moist, BP remains at 10% of baseline)
ATTITUDES
• Display integrity when identifying those interventions that were not successful
• Be independent when redesigning successful hospital-based interventions for the home care setting

FIGURE **36–19** Critical thinking model for fluid, electrolyte, and acid-base balances evaluation.

Key Terms

Active transport, *p. 1147*
Aldosterone, *p. 1148*
Angiotensin, *p. 1148*
Anion gap, *p. 1154*
Anions, *p. 1146*
Antidiuretic hormone (ADH), *p. 1148*
Arterial blood gas (ABG), *p. 1153*
Autologous transfusion, *p. 1201*
Buffer, *p. 1150*
Cations, *p. 1146*
Colloid osmotic pressure, *p. 1147*
Colloids, *p. 1170*
Concentration gradient, *p. 1147*
Crystalloids, *p. 1170*
Dehydration, *p. 1148*
Diffusion, *p. 1147*
Edema, *p. 1147*
Electrolytes, *p. 1146*
Erythema, *p. 1193*
Extracellular fluids, *p. 1145*
Filtration, *p. 1147*
Fluid volume deficit (FVD), *p. 1156*
Fluid volume excess (FVE), *p. 1169*
Hemolysis, *p. 1201*
Homeostasis, *p. 1147*
Hydrostatic pressure, *p. 1147*
Hypertonic, *p. 1146*
Hypodermoclysis, *p. 1170*
Hypotonic, *p. 1146*
Hypovolemia, *p. 1148*
Infiltration, *p. 1192*
Infusion pumps, *p. 1185*
Insensible water loss, *p. 1148*
Interstitial fluid, *p. 1145*
Intracellular fluids, *p. 1145*
Intravascular fluid, *p. 1145*
Ions, *p. 1146*
Isotonic, *p. 1146*
Metabolic acidosis, *p. 1153*
Metabolic alkalosis, *p. 1154*
Millimoles per litre (mmol/L), *p. 1146*
Oncotic pressure, *p. 1147*
Osmolarity, *p. 1146*
Osmols, *p. 1146*
Osmoreceptors, *p. 1147*
Osmosis, *p. 1146*
Osmotic pressure, *p. 1146*
Phlebitis, *p. 1193*
Renin, *p. 1148*
Respiratory acidosis, *p. 1153*
Respiratory alkalosis, *p. 1153*
Sensible water loss, *p. 1148*
Solute, *p. 1146*
Solution, *p. 1146*
Solvent, *p. 1146*
Total parenteral nutrition, *p. 1170*
Transcellular fluid, *p. 1145*
Transfusion reaction, *p. 1193*
Vascular access devices (VADs), *p. 1170*
Venipuncture, *p. 1183*

Critical Thinking Exercises

1. Mrs. Emanuele is an 81-year-old woman admitted to the hospital with a 3-day history of vomiting and diarrhea. She has had only ice chips since the first episode of vomiting and is now complaining of malaise, cramping muscles, and a temperature of 39° C. Which laboratory findings would you expect to be abnormal on the basis of her complaints? What interventions would you expect the physician to order?
2. Caroline has just received a new client on her unit who is to receive 1 unit of RBCs within the next hour. What nursing actions are necessary before administering blood? What are the signs and symptoms of a transfusion reaction? Can Caroline delegate the administration of blood to a licensed practical nurse or an unregulated care provider?
3. Carlos is caring for Mr. Rossi, a 52-year-old man who has been seen in the emergency department following a motor vehicle accident. Mr. Rossi is complaining of difficulty breathing and has a respiratory rate of 40 breaths per minute. He is transferred to the intensive care unit, intubated, and placed on a ventilator. A nursing student asks Carlos to interpret Mr. Rossi's last ABG results: pH, 7.30; PaO_2, 70; $PaCO_2$, 50; HCO_3^-, 24. What interpretation will Carlos give to the student nurse? What is the relationship between the ABG results and Mr. Rossi being intubated and ventilated?
4. Janelle is the nurse caring for Mrs Kwan, a 59-year-old woman who has just had a total knee replacement. The physician has ordered Ancef 1 g in 50 mL to run over 30 minutes IV piggyback tid. Mrs. Kwan has a continuous infusion of Ringer's lactate at 75 mL/hour in the left forearm. What type of tubing will Janelle use to administer the IV piggyback medication? Calculate the drops per minute of the piggyback using both microtubing (60 drops/mL) and macrotubing (15 drops/mL).
5. A 24-year-old tennis professional was admitted to the clinic with a temperature of 41° C. He has a history of playing in a 5-hour tennis match in 38° C heat. His coach brought him to the clinic because he was weak and lethargic. What assessment findings would the nurse expect to find? What interventions would be necessary? Describe a teaching plan for this client upon discharge.

Review Questions

1. One of the most common electrolyte imbalances is
   1. Hypokalemia
   2. Hyperkalemia
   3. Hyponatremia
   4. Hypocalcemia
2. The client most at risk for fluid volume deficits (FVDs) is a(n)
   1. Older adult
   2. Young to middle adult
   3. Child
   4. Infant
3. One reason that older adults experience fluid and electrolyte imbalance and acid-base imbalances is that they
   1. Eat poor-quality food
   2. Have a decreased thirst sensation
   3. Have more stress response
   4. Have an overly active thirst response
4. Output recorded on an intake and output (I&O) record includes
   1. Urine, vomitus, diarrhea, and drainage from wounds
   2. Diarrhea, gastric suction, and drainage from wounds
   3. Medications, juices, and water
   4. Urine, diarrhea, vomitus, gastric suction, and drainage from wounds or tubes
5. Health promotion activities in the area of fluid and electrolyte imbalances focus primarily on
   1. Client teaching
   2. Dietary intake
   3. Medication regimen
   4. Physician involvement in care

6. Total parenteral nutrition (TPN) is delivered by which of the following methods?
   1. Mouth and rectum
   2. Mouth and intravenous
   3. In-dwelling or central IV catheter
   4. Nasogastric tube
7. The nurse is aware that the following medication is never given directly intravenously:
   1. Potassium chloride (KCl)
   2. Lasix
   3. Dextrose
   4. Calcium gluconate
8. Many factors are initially controlled for in the IV insertion procedure. This nurse understands this begins with
   1. Hand hygiene
   2. Checking sterility of supplies
   3. Assuring the six rights of medication administration
   4. Carefully checking the order for the IV therapy
9. Indications of IV fluid infiltration include
   1. Phlebitis and coolness
   2. Edema and erythema
   3. Pallor and coolness
   4. Pain and erythema
10. The Centers for Disease Control (CDC) recommends that replacing peripheral venous catheters and rotating sites should occur at least every
    1. 72 to 96 hours
    2. 48 to 72 hours
    3. 24 to 48 hours
    4. 48 hours

References

Barrett, B. J. (2003). Applying multiple interventions in chronic kidney disease. *Seminars in Dialysis, 16,* 157–164.

Centers for Disease Control and Prevention. (2002). Guidelines for the prevention of intravascular catheter-related infections. *MMWR Morbidity and Mortality Weekly Report, 51*(RR-10), 1–29.

Christensen, B., & Kockrow, E. (2003). *Foundations of nursing* (4th ed.). St. Louis, MO: Mosby.

Chukhraev, A. M., & Grekov, I. G. (2000). Local complications of nursing interventions on peripheral veins. *Journal of Infusion Nursing, 23*(3), 167–169.

Dasgupta, M., Binns, M. A., & Rochon, P. A. (2000). Subcutaneous fluid infusion in a long-term care setting. *Journal of the American Geriatrics Society, 48,* 795–799.

Dochterman, J. M., & Bulechek, G. M. (Eds.). (2004). *Nursing interventions classification (NIC)* (4th ed.). St. Louis, MO: Mosby.

Ellenberger, A. (1999). An expert answers questions about starting an i.v. line. *Nursing, 99*(3), 56–59.

Groer, M. W. (2000). *Advanced pathophysiology: Application to clinical practice.* St. Louis, MO: Mosby.

Heitz, U. E., & Horne, M. M. (2001). *Mosby's pocket guide series: Fluid, electrolyte, and acid-base balance* (4th ed.). St. Louis, MO: Mosby.

Ignatavicius, D., & Workman, M. J. (2002). *Medical-surgical nursing* (4th ed.). Philadelphia: W. B. Saunders.

Infusion Nurses Society. (2000). Infusion nursing standards of practice. *Journal of Intravenous Nursing, 23*(6S), S1.

Levin, A., et al. (2001). Cardiovascular disease in patients with chronic kidney disease: Getting to the heart of the matter. *American Journal of Kidney Diseases, 38*(6), 1398–1401.

Lewis, S. M., Collier, I. C., & Heitkemper, M. (2002). *Medical-surgical nursing: Assessment and management of clinical problems* (4th ed.). St. Louis, MO: Mosby.

Lueckenotte, A. (2000). *Gerontologic nursing* (2nd ed.). St. Louis, MO: Mosby.

McCance, K. L., & Huether, S. E. (2002). *Pathophysiology: The biologic basis for disease in adults and children* (4th ed.). St. Louis, MO: Mosby.

McKenry, L. M., & Salerno, E. (Eds.). (2003). *Mosby's pharmacology in nursing* (21st ed.). St. Louis, MO: Mosby.

Metheney, N. M. (2000). *Fluid and electrolyte balance: Nursing considerations* (4th ed.). Philadelphia: J. B. Lippincott.

Millam, D. A., & Hadaway, L. C. (2000). On the road to successful IV starts. *Nursing, 30*(4), 34–48.

Moorhead, S., Johnson, M., & Maas, M. (Eds.). (2004). *Nursing outcomes classification (NOC)* (3rd ed.). St. Louis, MO: Mosby.

Otto, S. E. (2001). *Pocket guide to intravenous therapy* (4th ed.). St. Louis, MO: Mosby.

Phillips, D. (2001). *Manual of IV therapeutics* (3rd ed.). Philadelphia: F. A. Davis.

Phipps, W. J., et al. (Eds.). (2003). *Medical-surgical nursing: Health and illness perspectives* (7th ed.). St. Louis, MO: Mosby.

Rudnicke, C. (2003). Transfusion alternatives. *Journal of Infusion Nursing, 26*(3), 29–33.

Slesak, G., et al. (2003). Comparison of subcutaneous and intravenous rehydration in geriatric patients: A randomized trial. *Journal of the American Geriatrics Society, 51*(2), 155–160.

Speakman, E. S., & Weldy, N. J. (2002). *Body fluids and electrolytes: A programmed presentation* (8th ed.). St. Louis, MO: Mosby.

Toth, L. (2002). Monitoring infusion therapy in patients residing in long-term care facilities. *Journal of Vascular Access Devices, 7*(1), 34–38.

Vengelen-Tyler, V. (Ed.). (1999). *AABB technical manual* (13th ed.). Bethesda, MD: American Association of Blood Banks.

Woods, A. W. (2002). Pneumonia. *Nursing, 32*(11), 56–57.

Young, J. (2000). Transfusion reaction. *Nursing, 30*(12), 33.

Recommended Web Sites

Canadian Intravenous Nurses Association:
http://www.cina.ca

This site summarizes the resources available from the Canadian Intravenous Nurses Association. Current newsletters are available and certification procedures are described.

Fluid and Electrolyte Calculator:
http://www.drbradleybeer.com/fec/about.asp

The Fluid & Electrolyte Calculator (FEC) was developed to serve as a tool for health care providers. It is designed to calculate maintenance fluid requirements and replacement of fluids after dehydration. The calculator is designed to run on any device that is running the Palm OS. At this time, the FEC is freely available.

MedCalc: Acid-Base Calculator:
http://www.medcalc.com/acidbase.html

The program provides a calculator for acid-base status and anion gap. Other options also include calculators for creatinine clearance, fractional excretion of sodium, free water deficit, and hypo/hypernatremia.

Nurse CEUs: Acid Base Balance:
http://www.nursingceu.com/NCEU/courses/acidbase2/

This is a continuing education program about acid-base balance for nurses. It provides a good overview, but because this is an American site, the units of measurement will be different than those used in Canada.

37

Sleep

Patricia A. Stockert, RN, BSN, MS, PhD
Kathryn A. Smith Higuchi, RN, BScN, Med, PhD (Canadian author)

Objectives

Mastery of content in this chapter will enable the student to:

- Define the key terms listed.
- Compare the characteristics of rest and sleep.
- Explain the effect that the 24-hour sleep-wake cycle has on biological function.
- Discuss mechanisms that regulate sleep.
- Describe the stages of a normal sleep cycle.
- Explain the functions of sleep and rest.
- Compare the sleep requirements of different age groups.
- Identify factors that normally promote and disrupt sleep.
- Discuss characteristics of common sleep disorders.
- Conduct a sleep history for a client.
- Identify nursing diagnoses appropriate for clients with sleep alterations.
- Identify nursing interventions designed to promote normal sleep cycles for clients of all ages.
- Describe ways to evaluate sleep therapies.

Adequate rest and sleep are as important to health as good nutrition and sufficient exercise. Physical and emotional health depends on the ability to fulfill these basic human needs. Without sufficient rest and sleep, the ability to concentrate and make judgments decreases and irritability increases. Sleep is also associated with healing and restoration (McCance & Huether, 2002). The best quality sleep promotes good health and recovery from illness.

Nurses identify and treat sleep pattern disturbances. To do this, nurses must understand the nature of sleep, factors influencing it, and clients' sleep habits. Some clients have pre-existing sleep disturbances; others develop sleep problems due to illness, anxiety, or hospitalization. Ill people require more sleep and rest than usual. However, illness can disrupt rest and sleep, as can health care routines and the environment of a health care facility. Lack of rest can prevent recovery. Clients need an individualized approach based on their habits, sleep pattern, and sleep problems. Nursing interventions can resolve short- and long-term sleep disturbances.

Scientific Knowledge Base

Physiology of Sleep

Sleep is a cyclical physiological process that alternates with longer periods of wakefulness. The sleep-wake cycle influences and regulates physiological function and behavioural responses.

Circadian Rhythms. Cyclical rhythms are part of everyday life. The most familiar rhythm is the 24-hour, day-night cycle known as the diurnal or **circadian rhythm** (derived from Latin: *circa,* "about," and *dies,* "day"). A woman's menstrual cycle is an infradian rhythm, one that occurs in a cycle longer than 24 hours. Biological cycles lasting less than 24 hours are called ultradian rhythms. Circadian rhythms influence the pattern of major biological and behavioural functions. The fluctuation and predictability of body temperature, heart rate, blood pressure, hormone secretion, sensory acuity, and mood depend on the maintenance of the 24-hour circadian cycle.

Circadian rhythms, including daily sleep-wake cycles, are affected by light and temperature and external factors such as social activities and work routines. All people have **biological clocks** that synchronize their sleep cycles. Some people go to bed early; others stay up late; still others sleep during the day. Different people function best at different times of the day.

Most health care facilities do not adapt care to a client's sleep-wake cycle preferences. Routines may interrupt sleep or keep clients awake. Changes to the sleep-wake cycle can result in poor quality sleep. Reversals in the sleep-wake cycle such as falling asleep during the day can indicate serious illness. Anxiety, restlessness, irritability, and impaired judgment are symptoms of disturbances in the sleep cycle.

The biological rhythm of sleep frequently becomes synchronized with other body functions. Changes in body temperature, for example, correlate with sleep patterns. Normally, body temperature peaks in the afternoon, decreases gradually, and then drops sharply after a person falls asleep. When the sleep-wake cycle is disrupted, other physiological functions may change as well. For example, a person may have decreased appetite (National Sleep Foundation, 2001). A disruption to the usual sleep-wake cycle can adversely influence overall health.

Sleep Regulation. Sleep involves a sequence of physiological states maintained by highly integrated central nervous system (CNS) activity that is associated with changes in the peripheral nervous, endocrine, cardiovascular, respiratory, and muscular systems (McCance & Huether, 2002). Each sequence can be identified by specific physiological responses and patterns of brain activity. Instruments such as the electroencephalogram (EEG), which measures electrical activity in the cerebral cortex, the electromyogram (EMG), which measures muscle tone, and the electrooculogram (EOG), which measures eye movements, provide information about some structural physiological aspects of sleep.

Current theory indicates that sleep is an active inhibitory process. Therefore, the control and regulation of sleep may depend on the interrelationship between two cerebral mechanisms that intermittently activate and suppress the brain's higher centres to control sleep and wakefulness (Jones, 2000). One mechanism causes wakefulness; the other causes sleep.

The ascending reticular activating system (RAS), located in the upper brain stem, is believed to contain special cells that maintain alertness and wakefulness. The RAS receives visual, auditory, pain, and tactile sensory stimuli. Activity from the cerebral cortex, which governs thought, memory, reasoning and voluntary movement (Jarvis, 2004) also stimulates the RAS. Wakefulness results

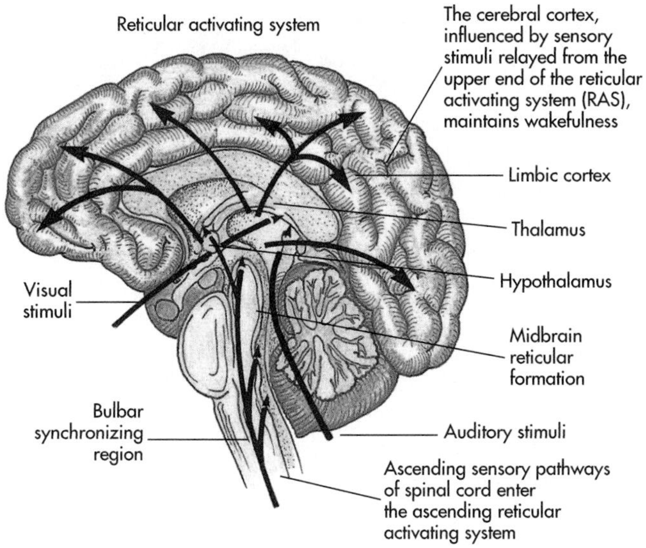

FIGURE **37–1** RAS and BSR control sensory input, intermittently activating and suppressing the brain's higher centres to control sleep and wakefulness.

from neurons in the RAS that release catecholamines such as norepinephrine (Chokroverty, 2000).

Sleep may be produced by the release of serotonin from specialized cells in the raphe sleep system of the pons and medulla. This area of the brain is also called the bulbar synchronizing region (BSR). Whether a person remains awake or falls asleep depends on a balance of impulses received from higher centres, peripheral sensory receptors, and the limbic system (Figure 37–1).

When trying to fall asleep, people close their eyes and assume relaxed positions. Stimuli to the RAS decline. If the room is dark and quiet, activation of the RAS further declines and at some point, the BSR takes over, causing sleep.

Stages of Sleep. EEG, EMG, and EOG signals show that different brain wave, muscle, and eye activity are associated with different stages of sleep (Carskadon & Dement, 2000). Normal sleep involves two phases: **non-rapid eye movement (NREM) sleep** and **rapid eye movement (REM) sleep** (Box 37-1). During NREM, a sleeper progresses through four stages during a typical 90-minute sleep cycle. The quality of sleep from stage 1 through stage 4 becomes increasingly deep. Lighter sleep is characteristic of stages 1 and 2, when a person is more easily aroused. Stages 3 and 4 involve a deeper sleep, called slow-wave sleep, from which a person is more difficult to arouse. REM sleep is the phase at the end of each sleep cycle. Different factors promote or interfere with various stages of the sleep cycle.

Sleep Cycle. The normal adult sleep pattern begins with pre-sleep, with a gradual feeling of sleepiness. This period normally lasts 10 to 30 minutes, but if a person has difficulty falling asleep, it may last an hour or more.

Once asleep, the person usually passes through four to six complete sleep cycles per night, each consisting of

Box 37-1 Stages of the Sleep Cycle

Stage 1: NREM

Includes lightest level of sleep.
Stage lasts a few minutes.
Decreased physiological activity begins with gradual fall in vital signs and metabolism.
Person is easily aroused by sensory stimuli such as noise.
Awakened, person feels as though daydreaming has occurred.

Stage 2: NREM

Period of sound sleep.
Relaxation progresses.
Arousal remains relatively easy.
Stage lasts 10 to 20 minutes.
Body functions continue to slow down.

Stage 3: NREM

Involves initial stages of deep sleep.
Sleeper is difficult to arouse and rarely moves.
Muscles are completely relaxed.
Vital signs decline but remain regular.
Stage lasts 15 to 30 minutes.

Stage 4: NREM

Deepest stage of sleep.
Very difficult to arouse sleeper.
If sleep loss has occurred, sleeper will spend considerable portion of night in this stage.
Vital signs are significantly lower than during waking hours.
Stage lasts approximately 15 to 30 minutes.
Sleepwalking and enuresis may occur.

REM Sleep

Vivid, full-colour dreaming may occur.
Less vivid dreaming may occur in other stages.
Stage usually begins about 90 minutes after sleep has begun.
Typified by autonomic response of rapidly moving eyes, fluctuating heart and respiratory rates, and increased or fluctuating blood pressure.
Loss of skeletal muscle tone occurs.
Gastric secretions increase.
Very difficult to arouse sleeper.
Duration of REM sleep increases with each cycle and averages 20 minutes.

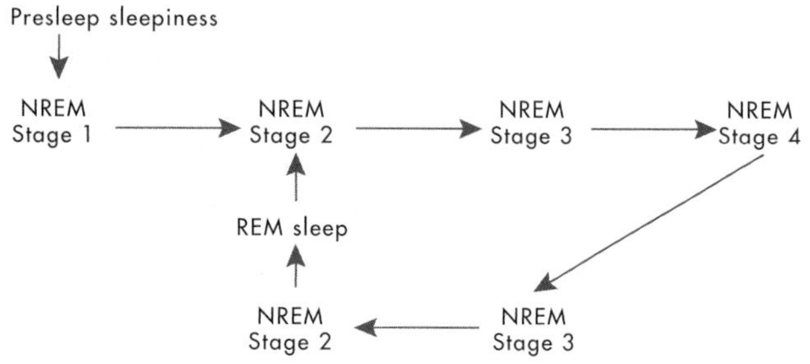

FIGURE **37–2** The stages of the adult sleep cycle.

four stages of NREM sleep and a period of REM sleep (McCance & Huether, 2002). The cyclical pattern usually progresses from stage 1 through stage 4 of NREM, followed by a reversal from stage 4 to 3 to 2, ending with a period of REM sleep (Figure 37–2). REM is usually reached about 90 minutes into the sleep cycle.

With each successive cycle, stages 3 and 4 shorten, and the period of REM lengthens. REM sleep may last up to 60 minutes during the last sleep cycle. Not everyone progresses consistently through the stages of sleep. For example, a sleeper may fluctuate for short intervals between NREM stages 2, 3, and 4 before entering REM stage. The time spent in each stage varies over the lifespan. Newborns and children have more deep sleep. With aging, sleep becomes fragmented and more time is spent in lighter stages (National Sleep Foundation, 2003). Shifts from stage to stage tend to accompany body movements. Shifts to light sleep or wakefulness tend to occur suddenly, whereas shifts to deep sleep tend to be gradual (Carskadon & Dement, 2000; Jones, 2000). The number of sleep cycles depends on the total time that is spent sleeping. In a 1998 survey, Statistics Canada reported that adult women spend an average of 8.2 hours per day in nighttime sleep, whereas adult male counterparts spend an average of 8 hours in night sleep (2005a, 2005b).

Functions of Sleep

The purpose of sleep is unclear, but it is believed to contribute to physiological and psychological restoration (McCance & Huether, 2002). NREM sleep contributes to body tissue restoration (Chokroverty, 2000). During NREM sleep, biological functions slow. A healthy adult's normal heart rate throughout the day averages 70 to 80 beats per minute or less if the person is extremely physically fit. During sleep, the heart rate falls to 60 beats per minute or less, meaning that the heart beats 10 to 20 fewer times in each minute during sleep or 60 to 120 fewer times in each hour. Clearly, restful sleep may be beneficial in preserving cardiac function. Other biological functions that decrease during sleep are respirations, blood pressure, and muscle tone (McCance & Huether, 2002).

Sleep appears to be needed to routinely restore biological processes. During deep slow-wave (NREM stage 4) sleep, the body releases human growth hormone for the repair and renewal of epithelial and specialized cells such as brain cells (Jones, 2000; McCance & Huether, 2002). Protein synthesis and cell division for renewal of tissues such as the skin, bone marrow, gastric mucosa, or brain occur during rest and sleep. NREM sleep may be especially important in children, who experience more stage 4 sleep.

Another theory about the purpose of sleep is that the body conserves energy during sleep. The skeletal muscles relax progressively, and the absence of muscular contraction preserves chemical energy for cellular processes. Lowering of the basal metabolic rate further conserves the body's energy supply (Chokroverty, 2000).

REM sleep is needed for brain tissue restoration and appears to be important for cognitive restoration (Chokroverty, 2000). REM sleep is associated with changes in cerebral blood flow, increased cortical activity, increased oxygen consumption, and epinephrine release. This association may assist with memory storage and learning. During sleep, the brain filters stored information about the day's activities.

The benefits of sleep often go unnoticed until a problem develops from sleep deprivation. Loss of REM sleep can lead to feelings of confusion and suspicion. Various body functions (e.g., mood, motor skills, and memory) can change with prolonged sleep loss (National Sleep Foundation, 2002b). Changes in the natural and cellular immune function also occur with moderate to severe sleep deprivation (Bonnet, 2000). Industrial accidents, such as the Chernobyl nuclear accident, have been attributed to human error associated with sleep deprivation. Traffic, home, and work-related accidents caused by falling asleep also have far-reaching economic and personal effects.

Dreams. Although dreams occur during both NREM and REM sleep, the dreams of REM sleep are more vivid and elaborate and are believed to be functionally important to learning, memory processing, and adaptation to stress (Pagel, 2000). REM dreams may progress in content throughout the night from dreams about current events to emotional dreams of childhood or the past. Personality can influence the quality of dreams. For example, a creative person may have elaborate dreams, and a depressed person may dream of helplessness.

Most people dream about immediate concerns such as marriage or work worries. Sometimes a person is unaware of fears represented in dreams. Objects in dreams hold symbolic significance. For example, an apple may represent a forbidden object, and water may have a sexual meaning. The ability to describe a dream and interpret its significance may help resolve concerns or fears. Clinical psychologists may analyze a client's dreams as part of psychotherapy.

One theory suggests that dreams erase fantasies or nonsensical memories. Because most dreams are forgotten, many people have little dream recall and do not believe they dream at all. To remember a dream, a person must consciously think about it on awakening. People who recall dreams vividly usually awake just after a period of REM sleep.

Physical Illness

Any illness that causes pain, discomfort, anxiety, or depression can result in sleep problems. The person may have to sleep in an unaccustomed or awkward position, or may have trouble falling or staying asleep.

Respiratory disease often interferes with sleep. Chronic lung disease causes shortness of breath; to sleep, clients need their heads raised. Asthma, bronchitis, and allergic rhinitis alter breathing rhythm and disturb sleep. Even the congestion caused by a common cold can impair breathing and the ability to relax.

A connection between heart disease, sleep, and sleep disorders exists. Sleep-related breathing disorders have been linked to high blood pressure and risk of heart diseases and stroke (American Academy of Sleep Medicine, 2002). Hypertension often causes early morning awakening and fatigue. Hypothyroidism decreases stage 4 sleep, whereas people with hyperthyroidism need more time to fall asleep. Also, there is an increased risk of sudden cardiac death in the first hours after wakening.

Nocturia, urination during the night, disrupts sleep and the sleep cycle. This condition is most common in older people with reduced bladder tone or people with cardiac disease, diabetes, urethritis, or prostatic disease.

Older adults often experience restless legs syndrome (RLS), which occurs before sleep onset. People with RLS experience recurrent, rhythmical movements of the feet and legs and an itching sensation deep in the muscles. Relief comes only from moving the legs, which prevents relaxation and sleep. Depending on how severely sleep is disrupted, RLS may be benign. Primary RLS is a central nervous disorder. Secondary RLS is associated with lower levels of iron, pregnancy, and uremia (National Heart, Lung, and Blood Institute, 2000). In contrast, people who have severe leg cramps during the night may have a problem with arterial circulation.

Peptic ulcer disease can cause wakefulness at night. Although research showing a relationship between gastric acid secretion and stages of sleep are conflicting, it has been found that those with duodenal ulcers fail to suppress acid secretion in the first 2 hours of sleep (Orr, 2000).

Sleep Disorders

Sleep disorders are conditions that, if untreated, generally cause disturbed nighttime sleep, resulting in insomnia, abnormal movements or sensation during sleep or when awake at night, or excessive daytime sleepiness (Aldrich & Naylor, 2000). Many adults fall asleep during the day **(hypersomnolence)** as a result of inadequacies in either the quantity or quality of their nighttime sleep (National Sleep Foundation, 2002b).

Sleep disorders are classified into four categories (American Sleep Disorders Association, as cited in Thorpy, 2000; Box 37-2). The **dyssomnias** are primary disorders that originate in different body systems and are subdivided into three major groups: intrinsic, extrinsic, and circadian rhythm disorders. The intrinsic sleep disorders include disorders of initiating and maintaining sleep (e.g., various forms of insomnia) and disorders of excessive sleepiness (e.g., narcolepsy and obstructive sleep apnea). Extrinsic sleep disorders develop from external factors, which, if removed, resolve the disorder. The circadian rhythm sleep disorders arise from a misalignment between the timing of sleep and what is desired by the individual or is a societal norm. Hospitalization, especially in intensive care units, places clients at risk for extrinsic and circadian sleep disorders (Redeker, 2000).

The **parasomnias** are undesirable behaviours that occur mainly during sleep, such as arousal disorders, partial

Box 37-2 Classification of Sleep Disorders

Dyssomnias

Intrinsic Sleep Disorders
Psychophysiological insomnia
Narcolepsy
Periodic limb movement disorder
Sleep apnea syndromes

Extrinsic Sleep Disorders
Inadequate sleep hygiene
Insufficient sleep syndrome
Hypnotic-dependent sleep disorders
Alcohol-dependent sleep disorders

Circadian Rhythm Sleep Disorders
Time-zone change (jet lag) syndrome
Shift-work sleep disorder
Delayed sleep phase syndrome

Parasomnias

Arousal Disorders
Sleepwalking
Sleep terrors

Sleep-Wake Transition Disorders
Sleeptalking
Sleep starts
Nocturnal leg cramps

Parasomnias Usually Associated With REM Sleep
Nightmares
REM sleep behaviour disorder
Sleep paralysis

Parasomnias—cont'd

Other Parasomnias
Sleep bruxism (teeth grinding)
Sleep enuresis (bed wetting)
Sudden infant death syndrome

Sleep Disorders Associated With Medical-Psychiatric Disorders

Associated With Psychiatric Disorders
Mood disorders
Anxiety disorders
Psychoses
Alcoholism

Associated With Neurological Disorders
Dementia
Parkinsonism
Central degenerative disorders

Associated With Other Medical Disorders
Nocturnal cardiac ischemia
Chronic obstructive pulmonary disease
Peptic ulcer disease

Proposed Sleep Disorders

Menstruation-associated sleep disorders
Sleep choking syndrome
Pregnancy-associated sleep disorders

Adapted from American Sleep Disorders, as cited in "Classification of Sleep Disorders," by M. Thorpy, in *Principles and practice of sleep medicine,* (3rd. ed., pp. 547–557), edited by M. H. Kryger, T. Roth, and W. C. Dement, 2000, Philadelphia: W. B. Saunders.

arousals, or disorders during transitions in the sleep cycle or from sleep to wakefulness.

Many medical and psychiatric disorders are also associated with sleep and wake disturbances. These disturbances are divided into those associated with psychiatric, neurological, or other medical specialty disorders. The proposed sleep disorders are newly described disturbances; research does not yet substantiate their existence.

Sleep laboratory studies such as a nighttime **polysomnogram,** the Multiple Sleep Latency Test (MSLT), and actigraphy are often used to diagnose a sleep disorder (Mahowald, 2000). A polysomnogram uses EEG, EMG, and EOG to monitor stages of sleep and wakefulness during nighttime sleep. The MSLT provides objective information about sleepiness and selected aspects of sleep structure by measuring eye movements, muscle-tone changes, and brain electrical activity during at least four napping opportunities spread throughout the day. Sleep-onset REM episodes are also noted because this abnormality is associated with several sleep disorders. The MSLT takes 8 to 10 hours to complete. The actigraph is worn on the wrist and measures sleep-wake patterns over time (Attarian, 2000). Actigraphy data provides information on sleep time, sleep efficiency, number and duration of awakenings, and levels of activity and rest (Redeker, 2000).

Insomnia. The most common sleep-related complaint, **insomnia** is chronic difficulty falling asleep, frequent awakenings from sleep, and/or a short sleep or nonrestorative sleep (Attarian, 2000; Zorick & Walsh, 2000). Chronic insomnia may result in sleepiness, fatigue, anxiety, and depression. The person complains of not being able to sleep. Frequently, however, the person sleeps more than is realized. Insomnia may signal an underlying physical or psychological disorder. Insomnia occurs more frequently in women (Kravitz et al., 2003).

Transient insomnia may result from situational stresses such as family or work problems, jet lag, illness, or loss. Insomnia may recur, but between episodes, the person sleeps well. Insomnia is often associated with poor **sleep hygiene,** which are habits and practices the client uses that are associated with sleep. Temporary insomnia can lead to chronic sleep deficiency, perhaps due to anxiety about obtaining enough sleep. The fear of not being able to sleep can cause wakefulness.

Because there are many causes of insomnia, management involves several approaches (Attarian, 2000). Underlying emotional or medical problems must be treated. Other treatment is often symptomatic, including improved sleep hygiene measures, biofeedback, cognitive techniques, and relaxation techniques. When insomnia develops secondary to inappropriate health behaviours, treatment is directed at changing these behaviours. For example, in drug-dependence insomnia the client is unable to fall asleep because of excessive use of hypnotic medications. This client usually benefits from a gradual withdrawal of the hypnotics.

Sleep Apnea. **Sleep apnea** is characterized by lack of airflow through the nose and mouth for periods of 10 seconds or longer during sleep. There are three types: central, obstructive, and mixed apnea, which has both a central and an obstructive component.

The most common form is obstructive sleep apnea (OSA), which occurs when muscles or structures of the oral cavity or throat relax during sleep. The upper airway becomes partially or completely blocked, diminishing (hypopnea) or stopping (apnea) nasal airflow for up to 30 seconds (Bassiri & Guilleminault, 2000; Dobbin & Strollo, 2002). The person still attempts to breathe; chest and abdominal movement continue, often resulting in loud snoring and snorting. When breathing is diminished, each successive diaphragmatic movement becomes stronger until the obstruction is relieved. Structural abnormalities such as a deviated septum, nasal polyps, certain jaw configurations, or enlarged tonsils predispose a person to obstructive apnea. The effort to breathe during sleep results in arousals from deep sleep often to the stage 2 cycle. In severe cases, hundreds of hypopnea/apnea episodes can occur every hour, resulting in severe interference with deep sleep.

Excessive daytime sleepiness (EDS) is the most common complaint of people with OSA. People with severe OSA may report experiencing a disruption in their daily activities because of sleepiness (National Sleep Foundation, 2002a). Feelings of sleepiness are usually most intense upon awakening from or right before going to sleep, and about 12 hours after the mid-sleep period. EDS often results in impaired waking function, poor work or school performance, accidents, and behavioural or emotional problems.

OSA occurs in middle-aged men, particularly those who are obese (Elliott, 2001). It also occurs in postmenopausal women as well as younger women and children (Mahowald, 2000). Obstructive apnea causes a serious decline in arterial oxygen saturation level, raising the risk of cardiac dysrhythmias, right heart failure, pulmonary hypertension, angina attacks, stroke, and hypertension. Sleep apnea contributes to high blood pressure and increases the risk of heart attack and stroke (National Sleep Foundation, 2002a).

Surgery and anaesthesia disrupt normal sleep patterns. Post-operative clients may reach deep levels of REM sleep, which causes muscle relaxation that can lead to OSA (Cullen, 2001). Clients with OSA who are given opioid analgesics after surgery have an increased risk of developing airway obstruction because normal arousal mechanisms that occur with obstruction are suppressed (Cullen, 2001).

Central sleep apnea (CSA) involves dysfunction in the brain's respiratory control centre. The impulse to breathe temporarily fails, and nasal airflow and chest wall movement cease. The oxygen saturation of the blood falls. The condition occurs in people who breathe normally during the day and in those with brain stem injury, muscular dystrophy, and encephalitis. Less than 10% of sleep apnea is predominantly central in origin. People with CSA tend to awaken during sleep and therefore complain of insomnia and EDS. Mild and intermittent snoring is also present.

Clients with sleep apnea are often significantly sleep deprived. As well as EDS, sleep attacks, fatigue, morning headaches, and decreased sex drive are common (White, 2000). Treatment includes therapy for underlying cardiac or respiratory complications and emotional problems that arise as a result of sleep apnea symptoms. Sleep hygiene and a weight-loss program may help. An effective therapy is use of a nasal continuous positive airway pressure (CPAP) device at night, which requires a mask be worn over the nose. Room air is delivered through the mask at a high pressure. The air pressure prevents airway collapse. The CPAP device is portable and effective particularly for obstructive apnea. In cases of severe sleep apnea, the tonsils, uvula, or portions of the soft palate may be surgically removed. Success with surgical procedures is variable.

Narcolepsy. **Narcolepsy** is a dysfunction of mechanisms that regulate the sleep and wake states. EDS is the most common complaint associated with this disorder. During the day, the person may suddenly feel an overwhelming wave of sleepiness and fall asleep; REM sleep can occur within 15 minutes of falling asleep. **Cataplexy,** or sudden muscle weakness during intense emotions such as anger, sadness, or laughter, may occur at any time during the day. If the cataplectic attack is severe, the person may lose voluntary muscle control and fall. People with narcolepsy may have vivid dreams as they fall asleep that are difficult to distinguish from reality (called hypnagogic hallucinations). Sleep paralysis, or the feeling of being unable to move or talk just before waking or falling asleep, is another symptom (Cohen, Nehring, & Cloninger, 1996). Some studies show a genetic link for narcolepsy (Mahowald, 2000).

Falling asleep uncontrollably can be troubling. A sleep attack can be mistaken for laziness, boredom, or drunkenness. Typically, symptoms begin in adolescence. Narcoleptics are treated with stimulants that may only partially increase wakefulness and reduce sleep attacks, as well as antidepressant medications that suppress cataplexy and the other REM-related symptoms. Taking daytime naps of 20 minutes or less and eliminating behaviours that increase drowsiness (e.g., consuming alcohol or heavy meals) help reduce sleepiness. A new drug for treating narcolepsy is a wakefulness-promoting agent, modafinil, which has little potential for abuse (Zoidis,

Box 37-3 Sleep Deprivation Symptoms

Physiological Symptoms

Ptosis, blurred vision
Fine motor clumsiness
Decreased reflexes
Slowed response time
Decreased reasoning and judgment
Decreased auditory and visual alertness
Cardiac arrhythmias

Psychological Symptoms

Confusion and disorientation
Increased sensitivity to pain
Irritable, withdrawn, apathetic
Excessive sleepiness
Agitation
Hyperactivity
Decreased motivation

2001). Other helpful treatment methods are exercising regularly, eating high-protein light meals, breathing deeply, chewing gum, and taking vitamins (Cohen et al., 1996).

Sleep Deprivation. **Sleep deprivation** is a problem many clients experience as a result of the dyssomnia. Sleep deprivation involves decreases in the quantity and quality of sleep and inconsistency in the timing of sleep. With interrupted or fragmented sleep, changes occur in the sequencing of the sleep cycles, resulting in cumulative sleep deprivation. Causes may include illness with symptoms of fever, difficulty breathing, or pain; emotional stress; medications; environmental disturbances such as frequent nursing care; and variability in the timing of sleep due to shift work. Nurses are prone to sleep deprivation due to long working hours and rotating shifts (Thurston, Tanguay, & Fraser, 2000a, 2000b).

Responses to sleep deprivation vary. Clients may experience a variety of physiological and psychological symptoms (Box 37-3), the severity of which is often related to the duration of sleep deprivation. The most effective treatment for sleep deprivation is elimination of factors that disrupt the sleep pattern. Nurses play an important role in identifying treatable sleep deprivation problems.

Parasomnias. The parasomnias are more common in children than in adults. Sudden infant death syndrome (SIDS) is hypothesized to be related to apnea, hypoxia, and cardiac arrhythmias caused by abnormalities in the autonomic nervous system that are manifested during sleep (Gillis, 2000). The Canadian Paediatric Society (1999) recommends that apparently healthy infants be placed in the supine position during sleep because of an association between the prone position and the occurrence of SIDS.

Parasomnias that occur among older children include somnambulism (sleepwalking), night terrors, nightmares, nocturnal enuresis (bed wetting), body rocking, and tooth grinding (bruxism; D'Cruz & Vaughn, 2001). When adults have these problems, a more serious disorder may be indicated. Specific treatments vary. However, safety and support are paramount. Because sleepwalkers are unaware of their surroundings and are slow to react; they are at risk for falls. They should be gently awakened and led back to bed.

Nursing Knowledge Base

Sleep and Rest

When people are at **rest** they usually feel relaxed, free from anxiety, and physically calm. Rest does not imply inactivity, although it is often thought of as settling in a comfortable chair or lying in bed. When at rest, people are in a state of mental, physical, and spiritual activity that leaves them feeling refreshed, rejuvenated, and ready to resume the activities of the day (Mornhinweg & Voignier, 1996). People have their own habits for obtaining rest. They may rest by reading, doing relaxation exercises, listening to music, taking a walk, or sitting quietly (Mornhinweg & Voignier, 1996).

Nurses frequently care for clients on bed rest in a variety of health care settings. Clients confined to bed may not necessarily feel rested. They still may have emotional worries that prevent complete relaxation. For example, concern over physical limitations or a fear of being unable to return to their usual lifestyle may prevent relaxation.

Normal Sleep Requirements and Patterns

Sleep requirements vary. One person may feel rested after 4 hours of sleep, whereas another requires 10 hours. However, generally people in the same age group have a range of requirements and similar patterns.

Neonates. The neonate up to the age of 3 months averages about 16 hours of sleep a day. The sleep cycle is generally 40 to 50 minutes with wakening occurring after one to two sleep cycles (Renaud, 1996). For the first week, the neonate sleeps almost constantly. Approximately 50% of this sleep is REM sleep, which stimulates the higher brain centres. This is thought to be essential for development.

Infants. Infants usually develop a nighttime pattern of sleep by 3 months of age. The infant may take several naps during the day but usually sleeps an average of 8 to 10 hours at night for a total daily sleep of 15 hours. About 30% of sleep time is spent in the REM cycle. Awakening commonly occurs early in the morning, although it is not unusual for an infant to awaken during the night. If awakening during the night becomes routine, the problem may be with diet because hunger frequently awakens the child. Active (REM) sleep of infants makes up a larger proportion of sleep compared with that of older children.

Toddlers. By the age of 2 years, children usually sleep through the night and take daily naps. Total sleep averages 12 hours a day. After 3 years of age, children often give up daytime naps (Hockenberry et al., 2003). The percentage of REM sleep continues to fall. The toddler may be unwilling to go to bed at night, which may be due to a need for autonomy or a fear of separation from parents.

Preschoolers. Preschoolers sleep an average of 12 hours a night (about 20% is REM). By the age of 5 years, they rarely nap. Some preschoolers have difficulty relaxing after long days. Some have bedtime fears, nightmares, or wake during the night. Partial wakening followed by a normal return to sleep may occur (Hockenberry et al., 2003). While awake, the child may cry, walk around, speak unintelligibly, sleepwalk, or wet the bed. Parents are most successful in getting a preschooler to bed by establishing a consistent ritual that includes some quiet time activity before bedtime.

School-Age Children. Sleep needed during the school years is individualized because of varying activity and health levels. Six-year-olds average 11 to 12 hours of sleep nightly, whereas 11-year-olds sleep 9 to 10 hours (Hockenberry et al., 2003). The 6- or 7-year-old can usually be persuaded to go to bed by encouraging quiet activities. Older children often resist sleep because of lack of awareness of fatigue or a need to be independent. Parents are usually successful in getting the older child to bed by using a firm, consistent approach.

Adolescents. Typically, teenagers sleep $7^1/_2$ hours per night. At a time when sleep needs increase, school, job, and social demands cut down on sleep time (Dahl & Carskadon, 1995). Usually parents are no longer involved in setting a specific bedtime. Because lifestyle demands shorten sleeping time, teens often experience EDS. Poor grades, accidents, behaviour and mood problems, and increased alcohol use can be the result of EDS due to insufficient sleep (Mitler, Dement, & Dinges, 2000).

Young Adults. Young adults average 6 to $8^1/_2$ hours of sleep per night. About 20% of sleep time is spent in REM sleep, which remains consistent throughout life. Job and family stress and social activities interrupt sleep patterns, which may lead to insomnia and the use of sleeping pills. Long-term use of such medications can disrupt sleep patterns and worsen insomnia. Pregnancy increases the need for sleep and rest. Insomnia commonly occurs in the third trimester of pregnancy (Mindell & Jacobson, 2000).

Middle Adults. During middle adulthood, nighttime sleep declines. The amount of stage 4 sleep falls, a decline that continues with aging. Sleep disorders are often first diagnosed in middle life even when symptoms have been present for years. Insomnia is common, probably because of stress. Sleep disturbances are caused by anxiety, depression, or physical ailments. Insomnia is a common symptom of menopause (Kravitz et al., 2003). Adults may use herbal supplements or sleeping medications.

Older Adults. Complaints of sleeping difficulties increase with age. More than 80% of adults 65 years or older report problems with sleep (Schneider, 2002). Episodes of REM sleep tend to shorten. There is a progressive decrease in stages 3 and 4 NREM sleep; some older adults have almost no stage 4 sleep (deep sleep). An older adult awakens more often during the night and may take more time to fall asleep.

Variability in the sleep behaviours of older adults is common. Complaints about difficulties with night-time sleep frequently occur among older adults, often resulting from chronic illness. For example, an older adult with arthritis may have difficulty sleeping because of painful joints. The tendency to nap seems to increase progressively with age, perhaps because of frequent night awakenings. Sleep pattern changes may be due to changes in the CNS that affect sleep regulation. Sensory impairment, which is common with aging, may reduce sensitivity to time cues that maintain circadian rhythms.

Factors Affecting Sleep

Physiological, psychological, and environmental factors can alter the quality and quantity of sleep. Often multiple factors cause a sleep problem.

Drugs and Substances. Sleepiness, insomnia, and fatigue often occur as an effect of commonly prescribed medications (Box 37-4) that alter sleep and impair daytime alertness (McKenry & Salerno, 2003; Schweitzer, 2000). Sleeping medications may create more problems than benefits. Older adults often take several drugs to treat chronic illness, the combined effects of which can disrupt sleep. One substance that may promote sleep is L-tryptophan, a natural protein found in foods such as milk, cheese, and meats.

Lifestyle. Daily routine affects sleep. Shift work plays havoc with sleep schedules. An individual working a rotating shift schedule often has difficulty adjusting to alterations in the sleep schedule. People who work rotating shifts are more likely to report having trouble falling asleep and staying asleep than those who work only daytime shifts, and they also report that their sleep is less refreshing (Thruston et al., 2000a, 2000b). The body's internal clock might be set at 11 PM, but the work schedule forces sleep at 9 AM. The person may sleep only 3 or 4 hours because the body perceives that it is time to be awake and active. Sleepiness during work time can be hazardous. After several weeks of working at night, the biological clock usually adjusts. Other routine changes that disrupt sleep patterns include unaccustomed heavy work and late-night social activities.

Usual Sleep Patterns. In North America, sleep has decreased in the last century (National Sleep Foundation, 2003), leading to sleep deprivation and daytime sleepiness. Many cope with temporary sleep loss, but chronic lack of sleep is more serious and hinders functioning. Sleepiness is most difficult to overcome during sedentary tasks. For example, single-vehicle accidents that occur because a driver falls asleep occur most often between 2 AM and 6 AM (National Sleep Foundation, 2003).

Emotional Stress. Worry over personal problems or situations can disrupt sleep. **Emotional stress** causes tension and often leads to frustration when sleep does not

Box 37-4 Drugs and Their Effect on Sleep

Hypnotics

Interfere with reaching deeper sleep stages
Provide only temporary (1 week) increase in quantity of sleep
Eventually cause "hangover" during day; excess drowsiness, confusion, decreased energy
May worsen sleep apnea in older adults

Diuretics

Nighttime awakenings caused by nocturia

Antidepressants and Stimulants

Suppress REM sleep
Decrease total sleep time

Alcohol

Speeds onset of sleep
Reduces REM sleep
Awakens person during night and causes difficulty returning to sleep

Caffeine

Prevents person from falling asleep
May cause person to awaken during night
Interferes with REM sleep

Beta-Adrenergic Blockers

Cause nightmares
Cause insomnia
Cause awakening from sleep

Benzodiazepines

Alter REM sleep
Increase sleep time
Increase daytime sleepiness

Narcotics

Suppress REM sleep
Cause increased daytime drowsiness

Anticonvulsants

Decrease REM sleep time
May cause daytime drowsiness

come. The person may try too hard to fall asleep, awaken frequently, or oversleep. Continued stress may cause poor sleep habits.

Older clients often feel emotional stress from losses such as retirement, impairment, or the death of a spouse. Older adults and others with depression often experience delays in falling asleep, earlier appearance of REM sleep, frequent awakening, increased total bed time, feelings of sleeping poorly, and early awakening (Beck-Little & Weinrich, 1998).

Environment. The environment influences the ability to fall and remain asleep. Good ventilation is essential. Temperature level affects sleep, as does light. Some clients prefer darkness, whereas others prefer a soft light. The size, firmness, and position of the bed and mattress can affect sleep. If a person usually sleeps with another individual, sleeping alone can cause wakefulness. A restless or snoring roommate or bed partner can also disrupt sleep.

The level of noise that awakens a sleeper depends on the stage of sleep (Webster & Thompson, 1986). Low noises can usually arouse a person from stage 1 sleep, whereas louder noises are necessary to awaken people in stage 3 or 4 sleep. Some people need silence to fall asleep, whereas others prefer background noise such as soft music or television.

In hospitals and other in-patient facilities, noise creates a problem for clients. Noise in hospitals is usually new or strange and so clients are prone to awaken. The problem is greatest during the first night of hospitalization, when clients wake often and have decreased REM sleep and sleep time. Hospitals are noisy, particularly intensive care units (ICUs; Box 37-5). Close proximity of clients, noise from confused or ill clients, the ringing of alarm systems and telephones, as well as disturbances caused by emergencies, make the environment unpleasant. Clients in ICUs for extended time may show the "ICU syndrome" of sleep deprivation (Dines-Kalinowski, 2002). Repeated environmental stimuli (activity, noise, and light) coupled with poor physical status lead to sleep deprivation (Olson et al., 2001).

Exercise and Fatigue. Moderate fatigue can lead to restful sleep, especially if the fatigue results from enjoyable work or activity. Exercising 2 hours or more before bedtime allows the body to cool down and maintains a state of fatigue that promotes relaxation. However, fatigue from exhausting or stressful work can make falling asleep difficult.

Food and Caloric Intake. Good eating habits are important for sleep. Hunger can prevent sleep. Heavy or spicy meals can cause indigestion that interferes with sleep. Caffeine and alcohol consumed in the evening can cause insomnia. Food allergies may cause insomnia. In infants, a milk allergy may cause nighttime waking and crying or colic. Other foods that can result in an insomnia-producing allergy for both children and adults include corn, wheat,

Research Highlight

Box 37-5

Promoting Sleep in an ICU Setting

Research Focus

Noise combined with other environmental factors in intensive care units disrupts normal sleep-wake patterns in clients. This leads to sleep deprivation that is associated with poor client outcomes. Nursing interventions to promote sleep in these clients need to be tested. Little research focusing on the effect of specific nursing interventions is available.

Research Abstract

The purpose of this study was to examine the effect that a "quiet time" protocol to reduce noise and light stimulation had on sleep in clients in a neuroscience critical care unit. The protocol reduced noise and environmental stimuli by limiting visitors, turning down lights, closing blinds, and turning off television. The study also evaluated whether a "quiet time" in the ICU unit was feasible. One hundred twenty-one clients in the treatment group received the "quiet time" protocol. One hundred eighteen clients in the control group received the usual care conditions. Data collection included 1446 observations on the clients in the control group and 1529 observations on the clients in the treatment group. Trained RN observers collected data on clients' sleeping behaviour 8 times each day. Measurement of light and noise were taken at the same time. The results showed that significantly more clients were observed to be asleep during the period in which the "quiet time" protocol was implemented. Light and sound levels were also significantly reduced during the protocol implementation. Implementing the "quiet time" protocol did present a challenge to the nursing staff in the ICU setting because it was difficult for the nurses to organize care to provide the uninterrupted 2-hour rest period and it was difficult to control noise from ventilators, monitor alarms, and other equipment.

Evidence-Based Practice

- Implementing a "quiet time" protocol on ICU units is a low-cost nursing intervention.
- Reduction of environmental stimuli can help promote needed rest and sleep in clients in an ICU.
- Use of "quiet time" protocols can improve sleep in acutely ill clients.

Reference

Olson, D. M., et al. (2001). Quiet time: A nursing intervention to promote sleep in neurocritical care units. *American Journal of Critical Care, 10*(2), 74–78.

nuts, chocolate, eggs, seafood, red and yellow food dyes, and yeast (Hauri & Linde, 1990). Restoration of normal sleep may take up to 2 weeks after the food has been eliminated from the diet.

Weight loss or gain influences sleep patterns. Weight gain can cause longer sleep with fewer interruptions. Weight loss can cause short and fragmented sleep. Certain sleep disorders may be the result of overly restrictive diets.

Critical Thinking

Critical thinking requires synthesizing knowledge, including information from clients, experience, critical thinking attitudes, and professional standards. Clinical judgments require anticipating information needs, analyzing data, and making client care decisions. Nurses adapt their thinking to the changing needs of the client. During assessment (Figure 37–3), the nurse considers all elements involved in making nursing diagnoses.

The nurse integrates nursing knowledge about sleep and disciplines such as pharmacology and psychology. Experience, perseverance, confidence, and discipline are needed to complete a comprehensive assessment and to develop a care plan that manages the sleep problem. Nursing knowledge, attitudes, and skills required to work effectively with clients who have sleep problems are identified in the *List of Competencies* developed by the Canadian Nurses Association (CNA, 2003) and standards of practice developed by each provincial and territorial nursing organization.

Nursing Process

NP Assessment

During the nursing health history, the nurse assesses the client's sleep patterns by gathering information about factors that usually influence sleep. Sleep and restfulness are subjective experiences. Only the client can report if sleep is sufficient and restful.

Sleep Assessment. Most people can accurately estimate their sleep patterns, particularly if changes have occurred. Assessment is aimed at understanding the characteristics of a sleep problem and the client's sleep habits.

Assessing Usual Sleep Patterns. Normal sleep is hard to define because of variability in what individuals perceive as adequate. Clients should describe their usual sleep pattern so that the nurse can determine if recent changes indicate a problem. Knowing a client's usual, preferred sleep pattern also allows a nurse to match sleeping conditions in a health care setting with those in the home. These questions help determine the client's sleep pattern:

- What time do you usually get into bed each night?
- What time do you usually fall asleep? Do you do anything special to help you fall asleep?
- How many times do you awaken at night? Why?
- What time do you typically wake up in the morning?
- What time do you get out of bed for good once you have awakened?
- What is the average number of hours you sleep each night?

The nurse compares these data with the predominant pattern for clients of the same age. From this comparison, the nurse assesses for patterns such as insomnia.

Clients with sleep problems may show patterns very different from usual or the change may be minor. Ill

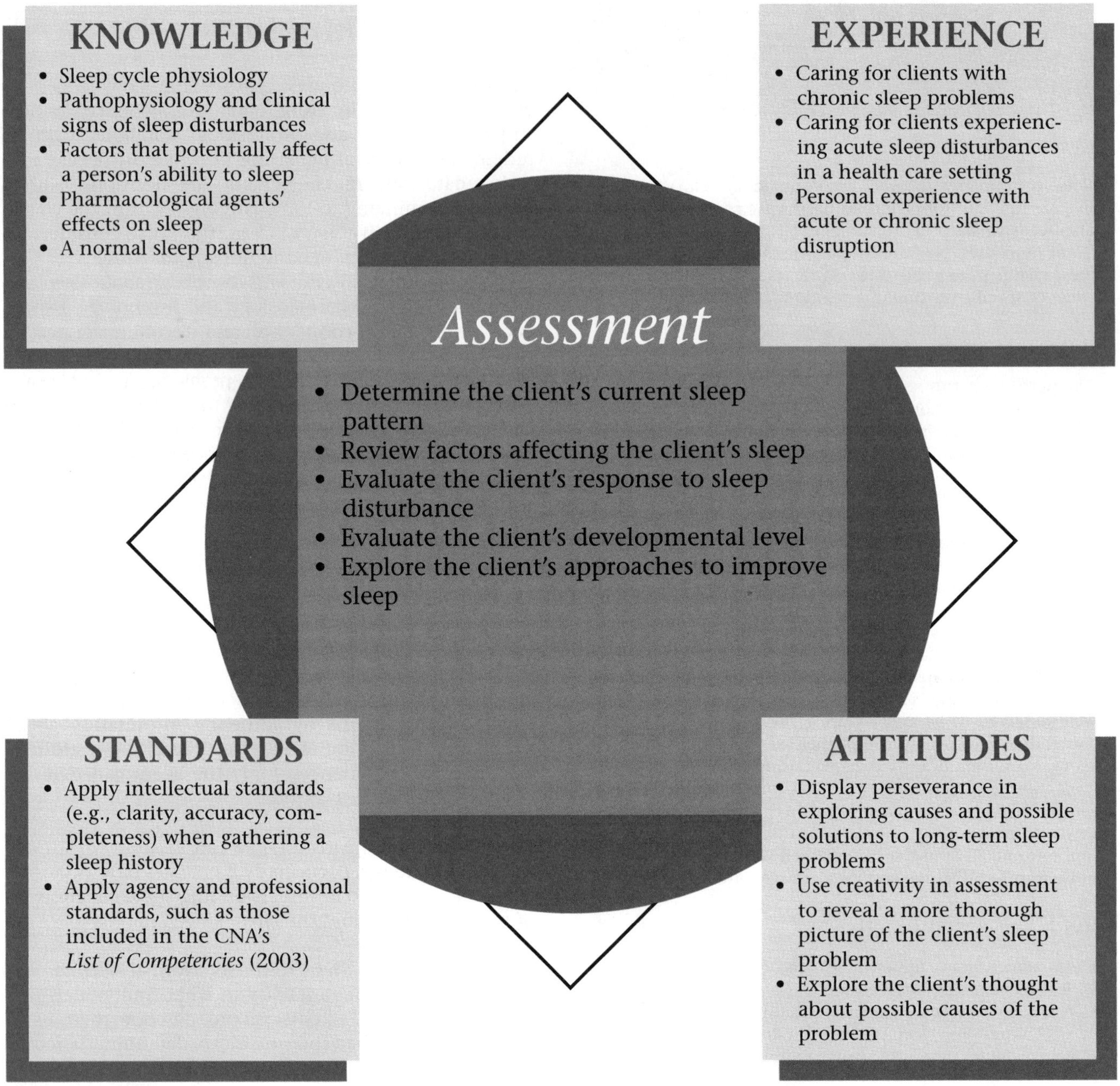
KNOWLEDGE
• Sleep cycle physiology
• Pathophysiology and clinical signs of sleep disturbances
• Factors that potentially affect a person's ability to sleep
• Pharmacological agents' effects on sleep
• A normal sleep pattern
EXPERIENCE
• Caring for clients with chronic sleep problems
• Caring for clients experiencing acute sleep disturbances in a health care setting
• Personal experience with acute or chronic sleep disruption
Assessment
• Determine the client's current sleep pattern
• Review factors affecting the client's sleep
• Evaluate the client's response to sleep disturbance
• Evaluate the client's developmental level
• Explore the client's approaches to improve sleep
STANDARDS
• Apply intellectual standards (e.g., clarity, accuracy, completeness) when gathering a sleep history
• Apply agency and professional standards, such as those included in the CNA's *List of Competencies* (2003)
ATTITUDES
• Display perseverance in exploring causes and possible solutions to long-term sleep problems
• Use creativity in assessment to reveal a more thorough picture of the client's sleep problem
• Explore the client's thought about possible causes of the problem

FIGURE **37–3** Critical thinking model for sleep assessment.

clients in hospital usually need or want more sleep. However, some may require less sleep because they are less active. Ill clients may believe that they should be increasing their amount of sleep, which, in itself, can make sleeping difficult.

Sources for Sleep Assessment. Usually clients can describe sleep problems and report changes from their usual sleep and waking patterns. The client may know the cause of sleep problems, such as a noise or anxiety.

Bed partners can also report on a client's sleep patterns. For example, partners of clients with sleep apnea may complain that snoring keeps them awake. The nurse should ask the bed partner if the client's breathing pauses during sleep and how frequently apneic attacks occur. Some people feel anxious when their partner's breathing seems to stop.

When caring for children, the nurse asks parents about sleep patterns. Hunger, warmth, and separation anxiety may prevent an infant from falling asleep or result in frequent nighttime awakenings. Older children can usually explain their sleep problem. They may relate worries that keep them awake. If children have bad dreams, parents can identify the problem but may not be able to interpret the dreams. Parents can also describe the typical behaviour patterns that foster or impair sleep. For example, stimulation from active play may impair sleep. With chronic sleep problems, parents can relate the duration of the problem, its progression, and children's responses. Parents of infants can describe influences on their infant's sleep, such as eating patterns and the environment. They may be asked to keep a 24-hour log of their infant's waking and sleeping behaviour.

Tools for Sleep Assessment. Subjective reports of sleep are reliable and valid measures (Libman et al., 2000). Several subjective sleep assessment tools are easy and quick to administer.

An effective, brief method for assessing sleep quality is a visual analog scale (Closs, 1988). The nurse draws a horizontal 100-mm line. Opposing statements such as "best night's sleep" and "worst night's sleep" are at opposite ends of the line. Clients place a mark on the line at the point corresponding to their perceptions of the previous night's sleep. The distances of the mark along the line can be measured in millimetres and offer a numerical value for sleep satisfaction. The scale can be repeatedly administered to show change over time. It is a useful assessment tool for individuals, but it is not useful for comparing clients. The Richards-Campbell Sleep Questionnaire, a five-item visual analog scale, measures sleep in critically ill clients (Richards, O'Sullivan, & Phillips, 2000).

Another brief subjective method to assess sleep is a 0 to 10 sleep rating scale similar to the concept of the 0 to 10 pain scale (Richards, 1996). Clients separately rate their sleep on the scale by indicating their sleep quantity with a number between 0 and 10, and then their quality of sleep with 0 being the worst and 10 the best. Other tools are available, such as the St. Mary's Hospital Sleep Questionnaire, the Baekeland-Hoy Sleep Log, the Pittsburgh Sleep Quality Index, the Epworth Sleepiness Scale, and the Verran- Snyder-Halpern Sleep Scale (Elliott, 2001; Leigh et al., 1988; Richardson, 1997; Smyth, 1999).

Sleep History. For clients who report adequate sleep, the sleep history can be brief. Determining the usual bedtime, bedtime rituals, and preferred sleeping environment is sufficient. When a sleep problem is suspected, the history must be detailed. The quality and characteristics of sleep should be explored. The client should describe the sleep problem, including changes in sleep pattern and sleep symptoms experienced during waking hours, use of sleeping and other medications, dietary intake pattern and substances that influence sleep, and recent life events that have affected mental and emotional states.

Description of Sleeping Problems. Open-ended questions help a client to describe a problem. A general description of the problem followed by more focused questions usually reveals specific characteristics that can be used in planning therapies.

To begin, the nurse needs to understand the nature of the sleep problem, its signs and symptoms, its onset and duration, its severity, any predisposing factors or causes, and the overall effect on the client. Assessment questions might include the following:

- *Nature of the problem:* Tell me what type of problem you have with your sleep. Tell me why you think your sleep is inadequate. Describe for me a recent typical night's sleep. How is this sleep different from what you are used to?
- *Signs and symptoms:* Do you have difficulty falling asleep, staying asleep, or waking up? Have you been told that you snore loudly? Do you have headaches when awakening? Does your child awaken from nightmares?
- *Onset and duration:* When did you notice the problem? How long has this problem lasted?
- *Severity:* How long does it take you to fall asleep? How often during the week do you have trouble falling asleep? Tell me how many hours of sleep a night you got this week; compare that to what is usual for you. What do you do when you awaken during the night or too early in the morning?
- *Predisposing factors:* Tell me what you do just before going to bed. Have you recently had any changes at work or at home? How is your mood, and have you noticed any changes recently? What medications or recreational drugs do you take on a regular basis? Are you taking any new prescription or over-the-counter medications? How long have you been taking medications? Do you eat spicy or greasy foods or drink alcohol or caffeinated beverages that could be interfering with your sleep? Do you have a physical illness that might be interfering with your sleep? Does anyone in your family have a history of sleep problems?
- *Effect on client:* How has the loss of sleep affected you? (Ask the client's spouse or friend: Have you noticed any changes in behaviour since the sleep problem started?) Do you feel excessively sleepy, irritable, or have trouble concentrating during waking hours? Do you have trouble staying awake or have you fallen asleep at inappropriate times, for example, while driving, sitting quietly in a meeting, or watching TV?

Proper questioning helps to determine the type of sleep disturbance and the nature of the problem. Box 37-6 gives sample questions if specific sleep disorders are suspected.

As an adjunct to the sleep history, a client and bed partner may be asked to keep a sleep-wake log for 1 to 4 weeks (Attarian, 2000; Beck-Little & Weinrich, 1998). This provides information on day-to-day variations in sleep-wake patterns over extended periods. Entries in the log often include 24-hour information about various waking and sleeping health behaviours such as physical activities, mealtimes, type and amount of intake (alcohol and caffeine), time and length of daytime naps, evening and bedtime routines, the time the client tries to fall asleep, nighttime awakenings, and the time of morning awakening. A partner can help record the estimated times the client falls asleep or awakens. For the sleep-wake log to be helpful, the client must be motivated to make the log. Usually it is not used with acutely ill clients in hospital for a short stay.

Physical and Psychological Illness. The nurse determines whether the client has pre-existing health problems that might disturb sleep (e.g., depression or chronic pain). The nurse also assesses the client's medication history, including the use of over-the-counter and prescribed drugs. The nurse may also assess daily caffeine intake.

Box 37-6 Questions to Ask to Assess for Sleep Disorders

Insomnia

How easily do you fall asleep?
Do you fall asleep and have difficulty staying asleep? How many times do you awaken?
Do you awaken early from sleep?
What time do you awaken for good? What causes you to awaken early?
What do you do to prepare for sleep? To improve your sleep?
What do you think about as you try to fall asleep?
How often do you have trouble sleeping?

Sleep Apnea

Do you snore loudly?
Has anyone ever told you that you often stop breathing for short periods during sleep? (Spouse or bed partner/roommate may report this).
Do you experience headaches after awakening?
Do you have difficulty staying awake during the day?
Does anyone else in your family snore loudly or stop breathing during sleep?

Narcolepsy

Are you tired during the day?
Do you fall asleep at inopportune times? (Friends or relatives may report this.)
Do you have episodes of losing muscle control or falling to the floor?
Have you ever had the feeling of being unable to move or talk just before falling asleep?
Do you have vivid lifelike dreams when going to sleep or waking up?

Recent surgery usually results in sleep disturbance. The client may awaken often during the first night after surgery and receive little deep or REM sleep. Depending on the surgery, the normal sleep cycle may take several days to return.

Current Life Events. Lifestyle may offer a clue to the sleep problem. The nurse should ask questions about work, social activities, recent travel, and mealtime schedules.

Emotional and Mental Status. The nurse should be aware of stress in the client's life. Clients with psychiatric disorders may need mild sedation for adequate rest. The nurse assesses the effectiveness of the medication and its effect on daytime function.

Bedtime Routines. The nurse asks what the client does to prepare for sleep. For example, the client may drink a glass of milk or watch television. The nurse assesses habits that are beneficial compared with those that have been found to disturb sleep. Not all clients are alike. Watching television may promote sleep for one person, whereas another individual may be stimulated to stay awake while watching TV. Sometimes pointing out that a particular habit may be interfering with sleep can help clients to find ways to change or eliminate habits that may be disrupting sleep.

Bedroom Environment. The nurse asks the client to describe preferred bedroom conditions. Changes in the home or facility may be needed to promote sleep. The nurse should ask how the environment can be adapted to accommodate preferences (Andrews & Boyle, 2003).

Behaviours of Sleep Deprivation. Sleep problems can affect behaviour. The nurse observes for irritability, disorientation, yawning, and slurred speech. If sleep deprivation has been prolonged, psychotic behaviour such as delusions and paranoia may develop.

Client Expectations. A poor night's sleep often starts a cycle of anticipatory anxiety, with fear of disturbed sleep as the client tries harder and harder to sleep (Attarian, 2000). The nurse should always ask clients what they expect regarding sleep. This includes asking clients what interventions they currently use and how successful the interventions are. The nurse also asks clients what other interventions to promote sleep they prefer and how they might be implemented. When clients ask the nurse for assistance because of sleep disturbances, they typically expect the nurse to assist them in improving their quantity and quality of sleep.

NP Nursing Diagnosis

The nurse looks for data clusters in the assessment that indicate defining characteristics of a sleep pattern disturbance. If a disturbance is identified, the nurse specifies the condition before designing interventions. Box 37-7 demonstrates how to identify and cluster defining characteristics to make a nursing diagnosis. The assessment should identify related factors or probable causes of the sleep disturbance, such as a noise, caffeine, or stress. These causes become the focus of interventions. For example, if a client has insomnia because of worry about marriage problems, interventions may involve counselling.

Sleep problems may create other problems. For example, snoring or anxiety about breathing problems may lead to marital problems. A nursing diagnosis of *compromised family coping* indicates that the nurse will help the couple understand sleep apnea and obtain medical treatment. Nursing diagnoses for clients with sleep problems may include the following:

- Anxiety
- Ineffective breathing pattern
- Acute confusion
- Compromised family coping
- Ineffective coping
- Fatigue
- Ineffective protection
- Disturbed sensory perception
- Sleep deprivation
- Disturbed sleep pattern

Nursing Diagnostic Process — Box 37-7

Assessment Activities	Defining Characteristics	Nursing Diagnosis
Ask client to explain nature of sleep problem.	Client reports difficulty falling asleep, taking up to an hour. Reports awakening two to three times nightly, with difficulty returning to sleep. Client admits to not feeling well rested.	Disturbed sleep pattern
Observe client's behaviour and ask bed partner if behaviour changes have been noted.	Spouse says client is sometimes lethargic and irritable.	
Determine if client has had recent lifestyle changes.	Spouse reports client recently lost job, and is worried about finding new job.	

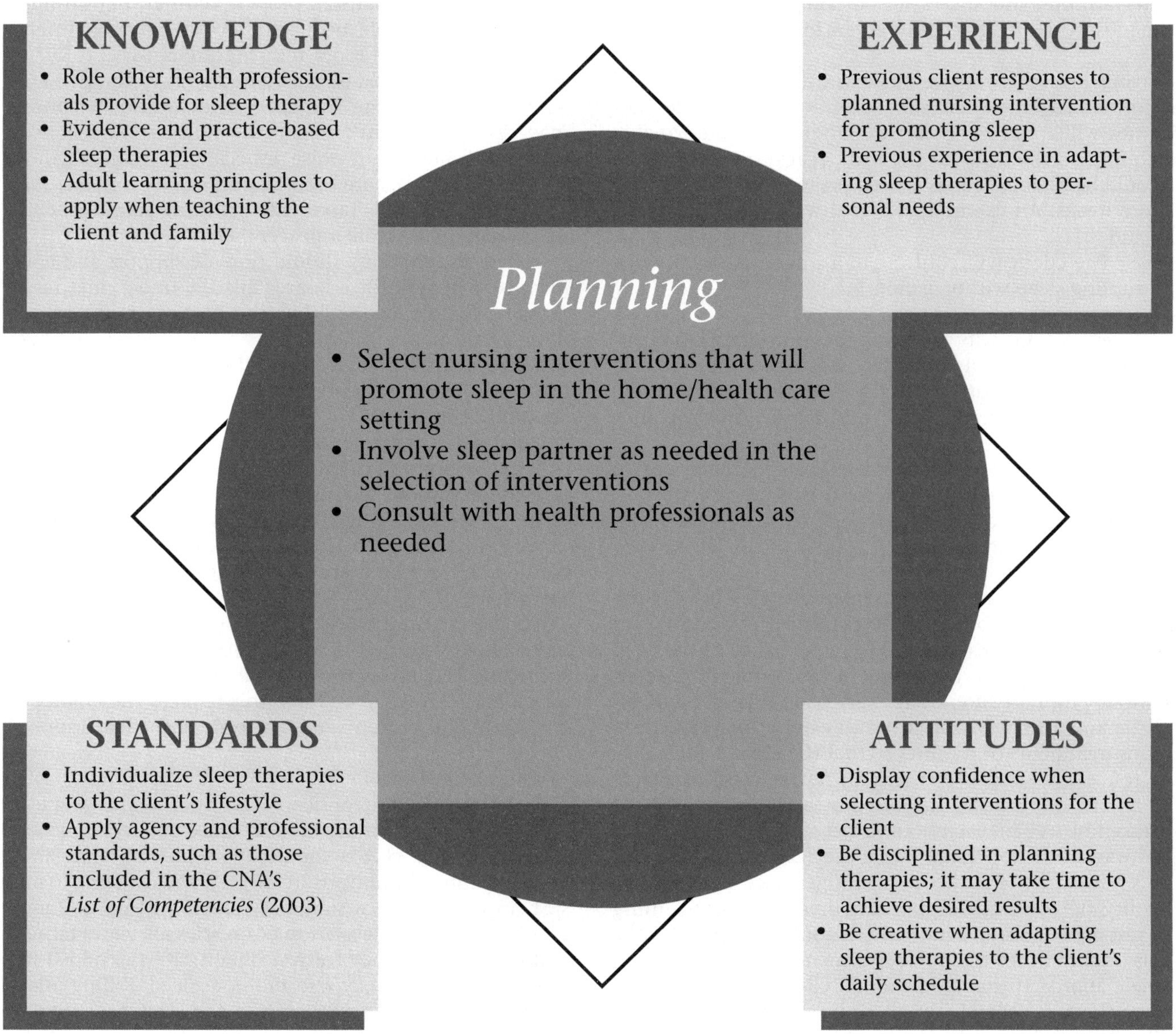
KNOWLEDGE
• Role other health professionals provide for sleep therapy
• Evidence and practice-based sleep therapies
• Adult learning principles to apply when teaching the client and family
EXPERIENCE
• Previous client responses to planned nursing intervention for promoting sleep
• Previous experience in adapting sleep therapies to personal needs
Planning
• Select nursing interventions that will promote sleep in the home/health care setting
• Involve sleep partner as needed in the selection of interventions
• Consult with health professionals as needed
STANDARDS
• Individualize sleep therapies to the client's lifestyle
• Apply agency and professional standards, such as those included in the CNA's List of Competencies (2003)
ATTITUDES
• Display confidence when selecting interventions for the client
• Be disciplined in planning therapies; it may take time to achieve desired results
• Be creative when adapting sleep therapies to the client's daily schedule

FIGURE **37–4** Critical thinking model for sleep planning.

Planning

Goals and Outcomes. During planning, the nurse again synthesizes information to develop an individualized care plan (Figure 37–4; see Care Plan). Professional standards are important to consider when developing a care plan because they often contain scientific guidelines for effective interventions. The care plan should include strategies that work with the client's sleep routines, environment, and lifestyle.

A concept map helps the nurse develop holistic client-centred care. The nurse creates the map after identifying nursing diagnoses. In Figure 37–5, the nursing diagnoses are linked to the client's medical diagnosis of depression following the death of the spouse. The concept map shows the relationships between the nursing diagnoses *dysfunctional grieving, disturbed sleep pattern,* and *impaired social interaction.* This approach helps the nurse to recognize relationships between planned interventions. Interventions and successful outcomes for one nursing diagnosis can affect other interventions.

Setting Priorities. If the nurse and client set goals and priorities together, realistic goals and measurable outcomes will more likely be set. Often the family makes helpful contributions to the plan. A realistic time frame should be established, as a sleep promotion plan may require weeks. An example of a goal with client outcomes includes:

Goal: The client will control environmental sources disrupting sleep within 1 month.

Outcomes:

- Client will identify factors in the immediate home environment that disrupt sleep in 2 weeks.
- Client will report having a discussion with family members about environmental barriers to sleep in 2 weeks.
- Client will report changes made in the bedroom to promote sleep within 4 weeks.
- Client will report having fewer than two awakenings per night within 4 weeks.

Continuity of Care. The nurse partners closely with the client, family, and other members of the health care team to ensure that any therapies, such as a change in the sleep schedule, changes to the bedroom environment, or referral to appropriate interdisciplinary team members, are realistic and achievable. In a health care setting, the nurse plans treatments or routines so that the client will be able to rest. For example, in the ICU, nurses check available electronic monitors to track trends in vital signs without awakening a client each hour. Other staff members should be aware of the care plan so that they can cluster activities at certain times to reduce awakenings. In a long-term care facility, the focus of the plan may involve better planning of rest periods around the activities of the other residents. It is important for the nurse to remember that there is no single approach that works for all clients. The success of sleep therapy depends on an approach that best fits the client's lifestyle and the nature of the disorder.

Implementation

Implementations in a facility are often different from those in a home. Nurses are on hand in a facility, whereas a home-care client may not have nursing care at night. The client's age also influences the therapies that are chosen. Box 37-8 provides principles for promoting sleep in older clients.

Health Promotion. In community health settings, the nurse helps clients develop behaviours conducive to rest and relaxation. This may include suggesting changes in the environment or lifestyle. Clients may need to learn techniques that promote sleep and conditions that interfere with sleep (Zarcone, 2000; Box 37-9). Parents need to know how to promote good sleep habits in their children.

Environmental Controls. All clients require a comfortable room temperature, proper ventilation, minimal noise, a comfortable bed, and proper lighting. Infants sleep best when the room temperature is 18° C to 21° C. at night. Cribs should be positioned away from open windows or drafts. In the home, the television or telephone may disrupt a client's sleep. The nurse should consult with the family about noise, especially if sleep schedules differ. Some clients are used to sleeping with noise, such as the hum of a fan. Tapes with soothing sounds such as waves may help create a peaceful environment.

A bed and mattress should provide support and comfortable firmness. Bed boards placed under mattresses provide support. Extra pillows can help a person position more comfortably. Infants' beds must be safe: to reduce suffocation risk, pillows and stuffed toys should not be put in cribs and loose-fitting plastic mattress covers should not be used.

For any client prone to confusion or falls, safety is critical. In the home, a night light might help the person locate the bathroom. Beds set lower to the floor lessen the chance of falls. Clutter and throw rugs should be removed from the path from the bed to the bathroom. A bedside bell can be useful if a client needs to call family members.

People vary in their need for light at night. Infants and older adults sleep best in softly lit rooms. Light should not shine directly on their eyes. Small table lamps prevent total darkness. For older adults, this reduces the chance of confusion and prevents falls en route to the bathroom.

Promoting Bedtime Routines. Bedtime routines relax clients in preparation for sleep. It is important for people to go to bed when they are tired. Because an alert mind can cause insomnia, clients should avoid mental stimulation before bedtime. Reading, watching TV, and listening to music help a person relax. Slow, deep breathing for 1 or 2 minutes induces calm. Relaxation of muscles alleviates tension and prepares the body for rest (Elliott, 2001). Guided imagery and praying may also promote sleep. Falling asleep and waking up at a consistent time strengthens the rhythm of the sleep-wake cycle.

Nursing Care Plan

Disturbed Sleep Pattern

Assessment

Julie Arnold, a 42-year-old lawyer, is the first client of the day at the neighbourhood clinic where you work. When asked how she is doing, she tells you she is having difficulty sleeping. Julie is married and has two school-age children. Julie's assessment includes a thorough sleep history and a discussion of how the sleep problem is affecting her life. A physical examination is also completed.

Assessment Activities	Findings/Defining Characteristics
Ask Julie to explain the nature of her sleep problem.	Julie says she wakes up once or twice a night. She states, "I feel tired when I wake up, and I have trouble concentrating at work in the afternoon." She also reports that she has less patience with her children at home.
Ask Julie if there have been any recent changes in her life.	Julie says she is feeling pressured at work to complete an important case. She also reports that because of her heavy workload, she has stopped her daily walk.
Ask Julie to describe her bedtime routine.	Julie says she is going to bed between 12 AM and 1 AM, 2 hours later than her usual bedtime. It takes an hour to fall asleep. She used to get 7 to 8 hours of sleep a night and now it is more like 5 to 6 hours. She drinks two to three cups of coffee after dinner while she is working and drinks a glass of wine before bedtime to help her relax because she has been having trouble falling asleep.
Assess Julie for signs of sleep problems.	Julie has dark circles under her eyes; she shifts her position and yawns frequently.

Nursing Diagnosis: Disturbed sleep pattern related to psychological stress from job pressures.

Planning

Goal	Expected Outcomes*
	Sleep
Client will achieve an improved sense of adequate sleep within 2 weeks.	Client will report feeling rested within 2 weeks. Client will verbalize adherence to a regular bedtime routine within 1 week. Client will fall asleep within 30 minutes of going to bed within 2 weeks.
Client will achieve a more normal sleep pattern within 2 weeks.	Client will report sleeping 7 hours nightly within 2 weeks.

*Outcome classification labels from *Nursing Outcomes Classification (NOC)* (3rd ed.), edited by S. Moorhead, M. Johnson, and M. L. Maas, 2004, St. Louis, MO: Mosby.

Interventions†	Rationale
Sleep Enhancement	
Encourage client to establish a bedtime routine and a regular sleep pattern.	Maintaining a consistent schedule helps induce sleep (Schneider, 2002).
Instruct client to limit caffeine, nicotine, and alcohol before bedtime.	Caffeine and nicotine are stimulants and cause difficulty in falling asleep. Alcohol lightens and fragments sleep (Kwentus, 2000).
Assist client in identifying ways to eliminate stressful concerns about work before bedtime, for example, taking time before actual sleep time to read a light novel rather than reviewing briefs related to a stressful case at work.	Excess worry and intense activities before bedtime may stimulate client and prevent sleep (Elliott, 2001).
Adjust environment, have client control noise, temperature, and light in the bedroom.	This develops an environmental conducive to sleep (Kwentus, 2000).

†Intervention classification labels from *Nursing Interventions Classification (NIC)* (4th ed.), edited by J. M. Dochterman and G. M. Bulecheck, 2004, St. Louis, MO: Mosby.

Continued

Nursing Care Plan

Disturbed Sleep Pattern—cont'd

Interventions†	Rationale
Exercise Promotion	
Encourage client to reinstitute walking routinely during the day, but not 2 to 3 hours before bedtime.	Exercise can increase activity levels and the need for sleep. Exercise just before bedtime is a stimulant that prevents sleep (Elliott, 2001).
Simple Relaxation Therapy	
Instruct client on how to perform muscle relaxation before bedtime.	Relaxation therapy can help reduce anxiety, which interferes with sleep (Elliott, 2001).

†Intervention classification labels from *Nursing Interventions Classification (NIC)* (4th ed.), edited by J. M. Dochterman and G. M. Bulecheck, 2004, St. Louis, MO: Mosby.

Evaluation

Nursing Actions	Client Response/Finding	Achievement of Outcome
Ask Julie if she is able to fall asleep and stay asleep.	Julie responds, "It usually takes me 15 to 20 minutes to fall asleep, and I woke up once for only two nights last week."	Julies reports she falls asleep within 30 minutes and wakes up less frequently during the night.
Ask Julie to describe her waking behaviours at work and home during the day.	Julie responds that she has completed her case at work and feels less pressure. She has restarted her walking routine. She reports that she is better able to cope with her children and that she is able to concentrate at work.	Julie reports feeling more rested.
Observe Julie's waking non-verbal expressions and behaviour.	Julie sits in the chair without shifting position. She does not yawn. The circles under her eyes are almost gone.	Julies says she is sleeping an average of 7 hours a night.

Newborns and infants sleep through so much of the day that a routine is hardly necessary. However, quieting activities, such as singing or talking softly, and gentle rocking, help infants fall asleep.

A bedtime routine (e.g., same hour for bedtime, snack or quiet activity) used consistently helps young children avoid delaying sleep. Toddlers and preschoolers may be too excited and full of energy to go to bed. Reading stories, allowing children to sit in a parent's lap while listening to music, or listening to a prayer are routines that can be associated with preparing for bed. Quiet activities such as colouring and reading work well with school-age children.

At home a client should not try to finish office work or resolve family problems before bedtime. The bedroom should not be used as a place to work and should always be associated with sleep. Working toward a consistent time for sleep and wakening helps most clients gain a healthy sleep pattern and strengthens the rhythm of the sleep-wake cycle.

Promoting Comfort. People fall asleep if they are relaxed and comfortable. Minor irritants can keep them awake. Clients should void before bed so that they are not kept awake by a full bladder and should wear loose-fitting nightwear. Soft cotton nightclothes keep infants and children comfortable. Infants should be covered with a light, warm blanket. Older adults often require extra blankets or covers.

Establishing Periods of Rest and Sleep. In the home, nurses frequently care for clients with chronic, debilitating disease. The care plan might call for long afternoon rests. The nurse helps adjust medication schedules, instructs clients to regularly void before rest periods, and suggests unplugging the telephone so that rest periods are uninterrupted. Increasing daytime activity (for those who are able) lessens problems with falling asleep.

Stress Reduction. Clients should not try not to force sleep. Otherwise, insomnia may develop, and soon bedtime is associated with the inability to relax. A client who cannot fall asleep can be encouraged to get up and pursue a relaxing activity, such as reading, rather than staying in bed and thinking about sleep.

Preschoolers often have bedtime fears, awaken at night, or have nightmares. After nightmares, the parent should talk immediately to the child about fears to provide a cooling-down period. One approach is to comfort children and leave them in their own beds so that their fears are not used as excuses to delay bedtime. Keeping a light on in the room may also help.

Bedtime Snacks. Some people enjoy bedtime snacks, whereas others cannot sleep after eating. Dairy products such as warm milk or cocoa, which contain L-tryptophan, may help promote sleep. A full meal before bedtime may interfere with the ability to fall asleep.

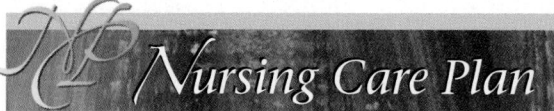

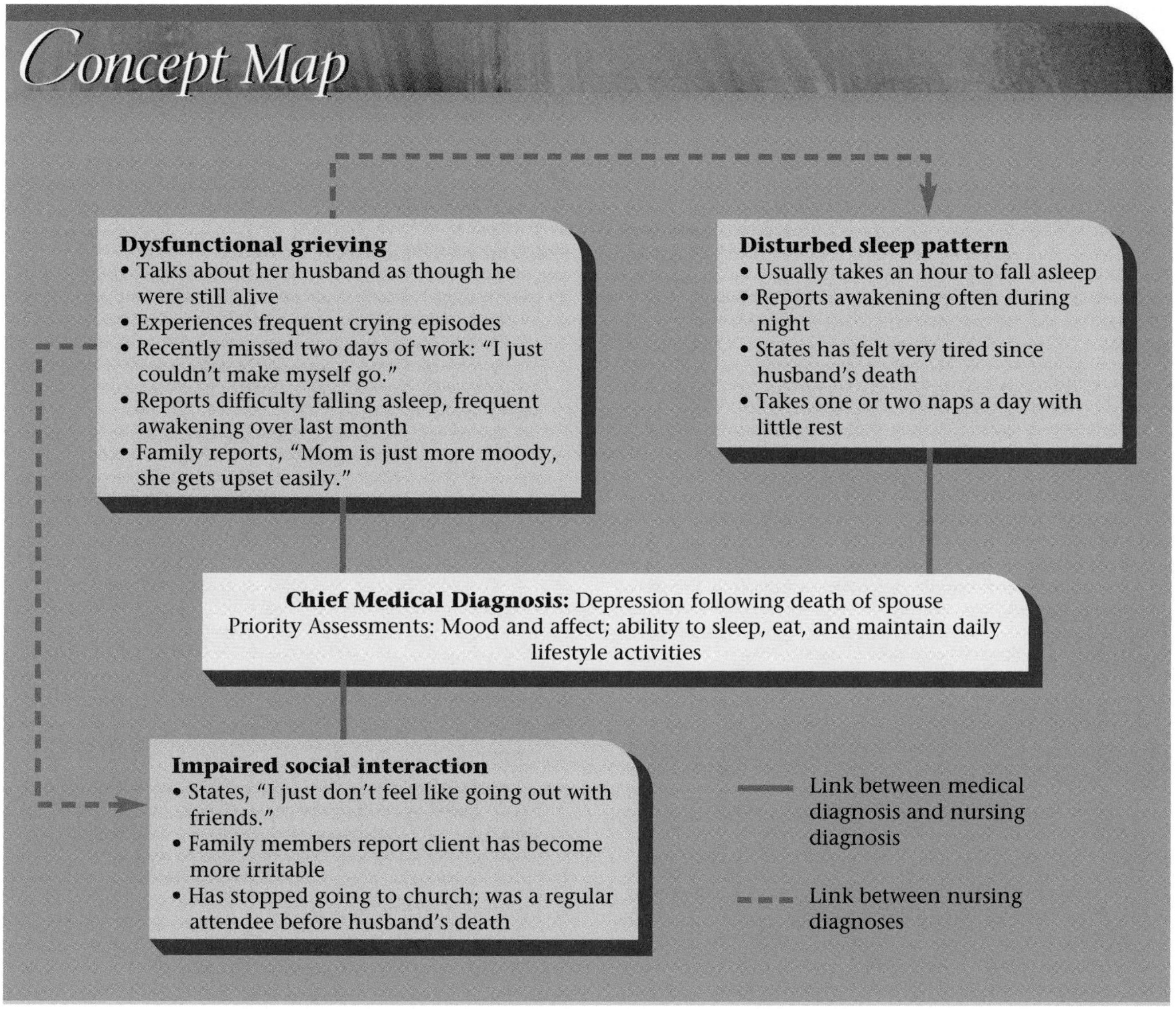

Concept Map
Dysfunctional grieving
• Talks about her husband as though he were still alive
• Experiences frequent crying episodes
• Recently missed two days of work: "I just couldn't make myself go."
• Reports difficulty falling asleep, frequent awakening over last month
• Family reports, "Mom is just more moody, she gets upset easily."
Disturbed sleep pattern
• Usually takes an hour to fall asleep
• Reports awakening often during night
• States has felt very tired since husband's death
• Takes one or two naps a day with little rest
Chief Medical Diagnosis: Depression following death of spouse
Priority Assessments: Mood and affect; ability to sleep, eat, and maintain daily lifestyle activities
Impaired social interaction
• States, "I just don't feel like going out with friends."
• Family members report client has become more irritable
• Has stopped going to church; was a regular attendee before husband's death
Link between medical diagnosis and nursing diagnosis
Link between nursing diagnoses

FIGURE **37–5** Concept map for client with depression following death of spouse.

Nurses should encourage clients to try to refrain from drinking or ingesting caffeine before bedtime. Coffee, tea, cola, and chocolate act as stimulants, causing a person to stay awake or awaken throughout the night. Alcohol can interrupt sleep cycles and reduce the amount of deep sleep. Coffee, tea, colas, and alcohol act as diuretics and may cause a person to awaken in the night to void (Miller, 2004).

Many infants need to be fed in the night. They require special measures to minimize nighttime awakenings for feeding. Hockenberry et al. (2003) recommend offering the last feeding as late as possible. Infants should not be given bottles in bed.

Pharmacological Approaches. Melatonin is a neurohormone produced in the brain that helps control circadian rhythms and promote sleep (Cheng & Umland, 2000). It is a popular nutritional supplement to aid sleep. The recommended dosage is 0.3 to 1 mg taken 2 hours before bedtime. Older adults who have decreased levels of melatonin may find melatonin beneficial as a sleep aid (Elliott, 2001). Several other herbal products assist in sleep. Valerian is effective in mild insomnia. It effects release of neurotransmitters and produces very mild sedation (Cheng & Umland, 2000; Elliott, 2001). Kava helps promote sleep in those whose sleep problems are related to anxiety. Chamomile, passionflower, lemon balm, and lavender are other herbal products with mild sedative effects (Elliott, 2001). Clients should be cautioned about the dosage and use of herbal compounds because active ingredients can vary from product to product. Herbal compounds may create interactions with prescribed medication, and concurrent use should be avoided (Merritt et al., 2000; see chapter 31).

The use of non-prescription sleeping medications is not advisable. Clients should learn the risks of such drugs.

Box 37-8

Focus on Older Adults

Strategies for Promoting Sleep

Sleep-Wake Pattern

- Maintain a regular bedtime and wake-up schedule (Kwentus, 2000).
- Eliminate naps unless they are a routine part of the schedule.
- If naps are used, limit to 20 minutes or less twice a day.
- Go to bed when sleepy.
- Use warm bath and relaxation techniques to promote sleep (Schneider, 2002).
- If unable to sleep in 15 to 30 minutes, get out of bed.

Environment

- Sleep where you sleep best.
- Keep noise to minimum; use soft music to mask noise if necessary.
- Use night light and keep path to bathroom free of obstacles.
- Set room temperature to preference; use socks to promote warmth.

Medications

- Use sedatives and hypnotics as last resort and then only short term if absolutely necessary (Lueckenotte, 2000).
- Adjust medications being taken for other conditions and assess for drug interactions that may cause insomnia or excessive daytime sleepiness (EDS).

Diet

- Limit alcohol, caffeine, and nicotine in late afternoon and evening (Lueckenotte, 2000).
- Consume carbohydrates or milk as a light snack before bedtime (Ebersole & Hess, 2001).
- Decrease fluids 2 to 4 hours before sleep (Lueckenotte, 2000).

Physiological/Illness Factors

- Elevate head of bed and provide extra pillows as preferred.
- Use analgesics 30 minutes before bed to ease aches and pains (Ebersole & Hess, 2001).
- Use therapeutics to control symptoms of chronic conditions as prescribed (Beck-Little & Weinrich, 1998).

Box 37-9

Client Teaching

Sleep Hygiene Habits

Objective

- Client will follow proper sleep hygiene habits at home.

Teaching Strategies

- Advise daily exercise and avoid vigorous exercise within 2 hours of bedtime.
- Caution against sleeping long hours during weekends or holidays to prevent disturbance of normal sleep-wake cycle.
- Advise against using the bedroom for any non-sleep activity, besides sex.
- Advise to try avoiding worrying when going to bed and to use relaxation exercises.
- Advise getting up and doing quiet activity until sleepy enough to go back to bed if client does not fall asleep within 30 minutes of going to bed.
- Recommend limiting caffeine to A.M., and limiting alcohol (more than 1 to 2 drinks a day can interrupt sleep cycle).
- Recommend keeping room dark, well ventilated, quiet, and at a comfortable temperature.
- Instruct that use of earplugs and eyeshades may be helpful.
- Advise avoiding heavy meals for 3 hours before bedtime; a light snack may help.

Evaluation

- Have client complete sleep-wake log for 1 week, and compare it with previous sleep-wake log.
- Ask client to periodically complete visual analog or sleep rating scale for perceptions of quality of sleep.

Over the long term, these drugs can lead to further sleep disruption even when they initially seemed to be effective. Older adults should be cautioned about using over-the-counter antihistamines because of their long duration of action that can cause confusion, constipation, urinary retention, and increased risk of falls (Cheng & Umland, 2000). The nurse can help clients use behavioural and proper sleep hygiene measures to establish sleep patterns that do not require the use of drugs (see Box 37-9).

Acute Care. Nursing interventions in acute care settings focus on controlling environmental factors, relieving physiological or psychological disruptions to sleep, and providing for uninterrupted rest and sleep.

Environmental Controls. In a hospital the nurse can control the environment in several ways, such as closing the curtains between clients in semiprivate rooms, closing bedroom doors, and adjusting bedroom lighting (Miller, 2004). Lights on a hospital nursing unit can be dimmed at night. It is also noteworthy that scheduled bright light exposure may be used to correct disturbances in circadian rhythms in older adults, so alterations in lighting around the clock may affect the quality of night time sleep (Miller, 2004). One of the biggest problems for clients in the hospital is noise. Important ways to reduce noise are to conduct conversations and reports in a private area away from client rooms and to keep necessary conversations to a minimum, especially at night. Additional ways to control noise in the hospital can be found in Box 37-10.

Promoting Comfort. Hospital beds are harder and of a different height, length, and width than regular beds. A clean, dry bed and in a comfortable position helps clients relax. Some clients require special comfort measures such as application of dry or moist heat, use of supportive

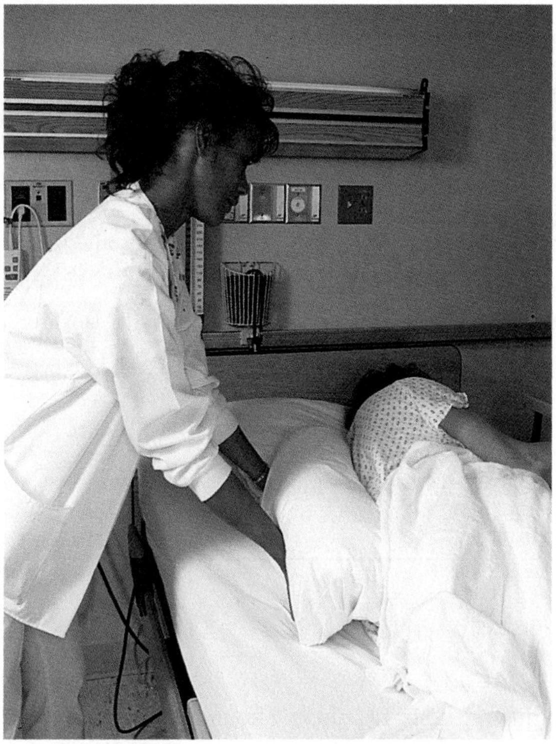

FIGURE **37–6** Positioning client for sleep.

Box 37-10 Control of Noise in the Hospital

- Close doors to client's room when possible.
- Keep doors to work areas on unit closed when in use.
- Reduce volume of nearby telephone and paging equipment.
- Wear rubber-soled shoes. Avoid clogs.
- Turn off bedside oxygen and other equipment that is not in use.
- Turn down alarms and beeps on bedside monitoring equipment.
- Turn off room TV and radio unless client prefers soft music.
- Avoid abrupt loud noise such as flushing a toilet or moving a bed.
- Keep necessary conversations at low levels, particularly at night.
- Conduct conversations and reports in a private area away from client rooms.

dressings or splints, and proper positioning before sleeping (Figure 37–6).

Establishing Periods of Rest and Sleep. In hospitals and other facilities, it is difficult to provide clients with the time needed to rest and sleep. However, the nurse plans care to avoid awakening clients for non-essential tasks. The nurse can schedule assessments, treatments, procedures, and routines for times when clients are awake. For example, a nurse should not wake a stable client to check vital signs. Allowing clients to determine the timing and methods of basic care can promote rest. Routine hygiene measures should not be given during the night for convenience. Blood should be drawn and medications given when the client is awake, unless a drug's therapeutic blood level must be maintained.

When the client's condition demands more frequent monitoring, the nurse can plan activities to allow extended rest periods. This means planning activities so that instead of a nurse or other personnel returning to the room every few minutes, the client may have up to an hour or more to rest quietly. For example, if a client needs frequent dressing changes, is receiving intravenous therapy, and has drainage tubes from several sites, a single visit can be used to change the dressing, regulate the intravenous system, and empty the drainage tubes. The nurse can become the client's advocate for promoting sleep. This may mean becoming a gatekeeper by rescheduling visits by family, asking consultants to reschedule visits, or questioning the frequency of certain procedures.

Stress Reduction. Clients who must have diagnostic testing may have difficulty sleeping because of anxiety. Giving clients control over their health care minimizes uncertainty and anxiety. Providing information about the purpose of procedures and routines and answering questions may give clients the peace of mind to rest or fall asleep. A nurse on the night shift should sit and talk with clients unable to sleep. This helps the nurse determine what is keeping clients awake. Back rubs can be used to help clients relax. If a sedative is indicated, the nurse confers with the physician to be sure that the lowest dosage is used initially. Discontinuing a sedative as soon as possible prevents a dependence that can seriously disrupt the normal sleep cycle. Older adults' metabolism of drugs is slowed, making them more vulnerable to the side effects of sedatives, hypnotics, anti-anxiety drugs, or analgesics.

Restorative or Continuing Care. Nursing interventions used in acute care setting can also be used in the restorative or continuing care environment. Helping a client achieve restful sleep in this environment may take time.

Promoting Comfort. These measures are similar to acute care comfort measures. A warm bath or shower before bed can be relaxing. Clients restricted to bed should be offered the opportunity to void and wash their face and hands. Brushing teeth or cleaning dentures also helps to prepare the client for sleep. Position the client to support dependent body parts and protect pressure points. The nurse can offer a massage to aid in muscle relaxation just before the client goes to sleep (see Chapter 38).

Controlling Physiological Disturbances. For clients with physical illness, the nurse can help control symptoms that disrupt sleep. For example, a client with respiratory abnormalities should sleep with two pillows or in a semi-sitting position to ease breathing. The client may benefit from taking prescribed bronchodilators before sleep to prevent airway obstruction. A client with a hiatal hernia also needs special care. After meals, the client may experience a burning sensation as a result of gastric reflux.

Table 37-1 Pharmacology of Anti-insomnia Agents

Generic Name	Trade Name	Onset of Action (in Minutes)	Oral Dosage* (mg)	Indications
Alprazolam	Apo-Alpraz Novo-Alprazol Xanax	15–60	0.25–0.5 (3 times/day)	Anxiety
Diazepam	Valium	15–45	5–10 at bedtime	Sleep disorder
Flurazepam	Dalmane Apo-Flurazepam	15–45	15–30 at bedtime	Sleep disorder
Lorazepam	Ativan Apo-Lorazepam	15–60	1–4 per day, given in divided dosages	Anxiety, sleep disorder
Oxazepam	Apo-Oxazepam Serax	45–90	10–30 (3–4 times/day)	Anxiety
Temazepam	Apo-Temazepam Restoril	25–27	15–30 at bedtime	Sleep disorder
Triazolam	Apo-Triazo Halcion	15–30	0.125–0.25, give 1–1$^1/_2$ hours before bedtime	Sleep disorder
Zolpidem	Ambien	15–45	5–10 at bedtime	Sleep disorder

*Dosage may be reduced in older adult clients.

To prevent sleep disturbances, the client should eat a small meal several hours before bedtime and sleep in a semi-sitting position. Clients with pain, nausea, or other recurrent symptoms should receive any symptom-relieving medication so that the drug takes effect at bedtime. The nurse should remove or change skin irritants such as moist dressings or drainage tubes.

Pharmacological Approaches. Central nervous system stimulants such as amphetamines, caffeine, nicotine, terbutaline, theophylline, and pemoline should be used sparingly and under medical management (McKenry & Salerno, 2003). Withdrawal from CNS depressants such as alcohol, barbiturates, tricyclic antidepressants (amitriptyline, imipramine, and doxepin), and triazolam can cause insomnia and must be managed.

Medications that are used to induce sleep are called **hypnotics. Sedatives** are medications that produce a calming or soothing effect (McKenry & Salerno, 2003). Hypnotics and sedatives as sleep medications can help if used correctly. Clients taking sleep medications should know about their proper use, as well as risks and side effects. Long-term use of anti-anxiety, sedative, or hypnotic agents can disrupt sleep and lead to more serious problems. One group of drugs considered to be relatively safe is the benzodiazepines (Table 37-1). The benzodiazepines cause relaxation, anti-anxiety, and hypnotic effects by facilitating the action of neurons in the CNS that suppress responsiveness to stimulation, thereby decreasing levels of arousal (Mendelson, 2000). These medications do not cause general CNS depression as sedatives or hypnotics do.

The benzodiazepines are used cautiously with children under 12 years of age and are contraindicated in infants less than 6 months. Pregnant clients should avoid benzodiazepines because their use is associated with risk of congenital anomalies. Nursing mothers should not receive the drugs because they are excreted in breast milk. Short-acting benzodiazepines such as oxazepam or lorazepam are usually recommended. Initial doses should be small, and increments are added gradually, based on client response, for a limited period of time. Nurses should warn clients not to take more than the prescribed dose, especially if the medication seems to become less effective after initial use. If older clients who were recently continent, ambulatory, and alert become incontinent, confused, and/or demonstrate impaired mobility, the use of benzodiazepines should be considered as a possible cause.

Regular use of any sleep medication can lead to tolerance and withdrawal. Rebound insomnia can occur after stopping the medication. Immediately administering a sleeping medication when a client complains of being unable to sleep may be doing the client more harm than good. Alternative approaches to promote sleep must be considered. Routine monitoring of client response to sleeping medications is important.

NP Evaluation

Client Care. The client is the only person who knows if sleep problems are improved and which interventions or therapies are successful (Figure 37-7). The nurse makes comparisons with baseline sleep assessment data to evaluate if sleep has improved.

The nurse determines whether expected outcomes have been met. Evaluative measures may be used shortly after a therapy has been tried (e.g., observing whether a client falls asleep after reducing noise). Other evaluative measures may be used after a client awakens from sleep (e.g., asking a client to describe the number of awakenings during the previous night). The client and bed partner can usually provide accurate evaluative information. Over longer periods, the nurse may use assessment tools such as the visual analog scale or sleep rating scale to determine whether sleep has progressively improved or changed.

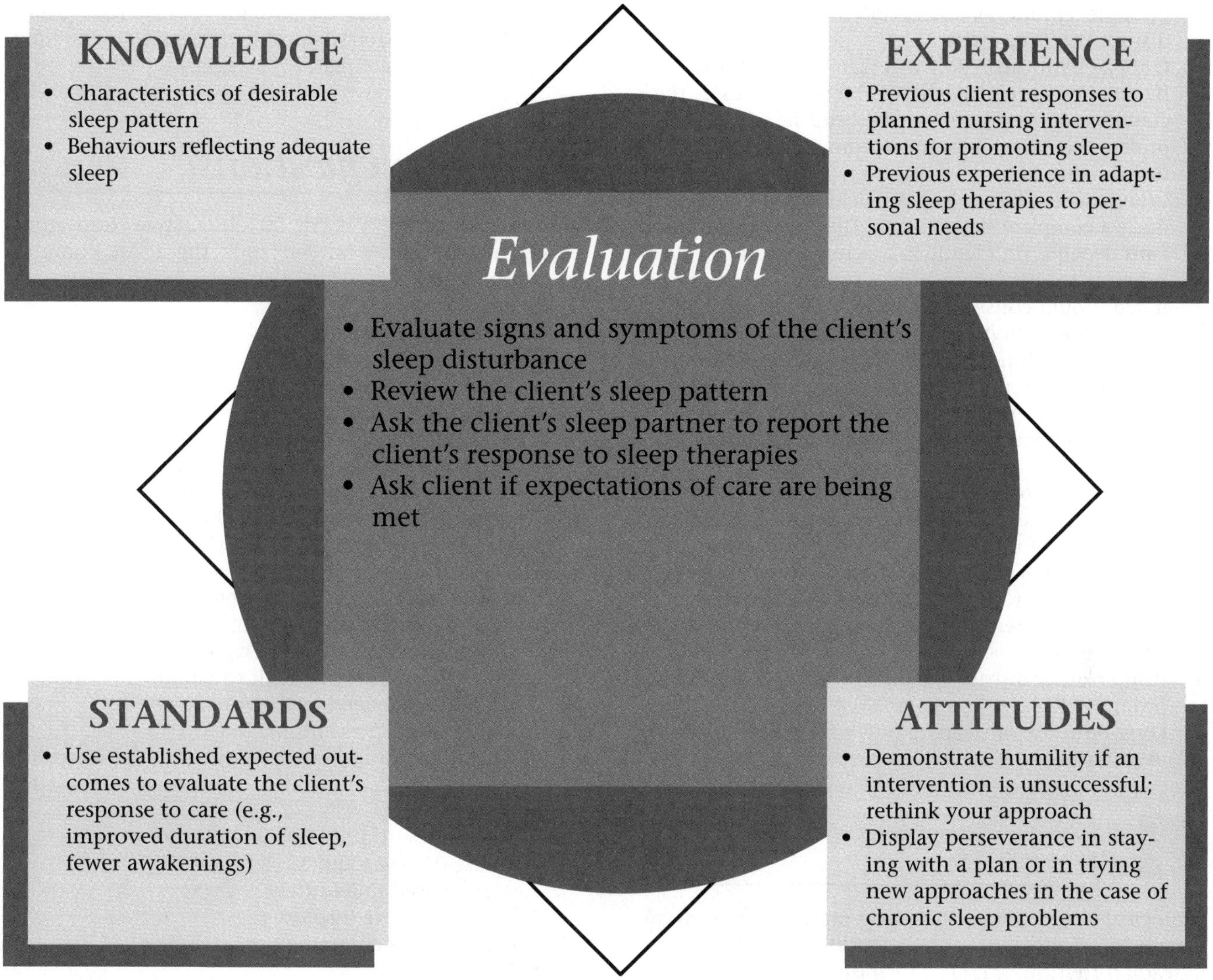
KNOWLEDGE
• Characteristics of desirable sleep pattern
• Behaviours reflecting adequate sleep
EXPERIENCE
• Previous client responses to planned nursing interventions for promoting sleep
• Previous experience in adapting sleep therapies to personal needs
Evaluation
• Evaluate signs and symptoms of the client's sleep disturbance
• Review the client's sleep pattern
• Ask the client's sleep partner to report the client's response to sleep therapies
• Ask client if expectations of care are being met
STANDARDS
• Use established expected outcomes to evaluate the client's response to care (e.g., improved duration of sleep, fewer awakenings)
ATTITUDES
• Demonstrate humility if an intervention is unsuccessful; rethink your approach
• Display perseverance in staying with a plan or in trying new approaches in the case of chronic sleep problems

FIGURE **37–7** Critical thinking model for sleep evaluation.

The nurse also assesses the understanding that clients or family members gain after receiving instruction on sleep habits. Compliance with these practices may best be measured during a home visit, when the environment can be observed. When expected outcomes are not met, the nurse revises the nursing measures or expected outcomes based on the client's needs or preferences.

Client Expectations. Subtle behaviours may indicate the client's satisfaction level with sleep therapy. Signs of sleep problems, such as yawning and restlessness, may be absent. The nurse must ask if the client's sleep needs have been met. A question might be, "Are you feeling more rested?" If the client's expectations have not been met, the nurse needs to spend more time understanding the client's needs and preferences. Working closely with the client and family will help redefine expectations that can be met within the limits of the client's condition and treatment. The nurse has effectively promoted rest and sleep if the client's goals and expectations are met.

Key Concepts

- Sleep is believed to provide physiological and psychological restoration.
- The 24-hour sleep-wake cycle is a circadian rhythm that influences physiological function.
- Sleep control and regulation depends on a balance between regulators within the central nervous system.
- During a typical night's sleep, a person passes through four to six complete sleep cycles. Each sleep cycle contains three NREM stages of sleep and a period of REM sleep.
- Neonates, infants, children, and adolescents require more sleep than do adults.
- The most common sleep disorder is insomnia, which is characterized by the inability to fall asleep, remain asleep during the night, or go back to sleep after awakening earlier than is desired.

- Lifestyle, emotional stress, caffeine, and alcohol can disrupt the sleep pattern.
- Only a client can report whether sleep is restful.
- If a client's sleep is adequate, the nurse assesses the client's usual bedtime, normal bedtime ritual, the preferred environment for sleeping, and usual preferred rising time.
- When a client has a sleep problem, the nurse conducts a complete sleep history. Diagnosing sleep problems depends on identifying factors that impair sleep.
- When planning interventions to promote sleep, the nurse should consider the usual characteristics of the client's home environment and normal lifestyle.
- A regular bedtime routine of relaxing activities prepares a person physically and mentally for sleep.
- An environment with a darkened room, reduced noise, comfortable bed, and good ventilation promotes sleep.
- One of the most important nursing interventions for promoting sleep in hospitalized clients is establishing periods of uninterrupted sleep and rest.
- Noise is one of the most common causes of sleep disturbances in hospitalized clients. The nurse should implement noise-reducing interventions to promote sleep.
- Pain or other disease symptom control is essential to promote sleep.
- Long-term use of sleeping pills may lead to difficulty in initiating and maintaining sleep.

Key Terms

Biological clocks, *p. 1211*
Cataplexy, *p. 1215*
Circadian rhythm, *p. 1210*
Dyssomnias, *p. 1213*
Emotional stress, *p. 1217*
Excessive daytime sleepiness (EDS), *p. 1215*
Hypersomnolence, *p. 1213*
Hypnotics, *p. 1230*
Insomnia, *p. 1214*
Narcolepsy, *p. 1215*
Nocturia, *p. 1213*
Non-rapid eye movement (NREM) sleep, *p. 1211*
Parasomnias, *p. 1213*
Polysomnogram, *p. 1214*
Rapid eye movement (REM) sleep, *p. 1211*
Rest, *p. 1216*
Sedatives, *p. 1230*
Sleep, *p. 1210*
Sleep apnea, *p. 1215*
Sleep deprivation, *p. 1216*
Sleep hygiene, *p. 1214*

Critical Thinking Exercises

1. Mr. Mehta, age 45 years, comes to the doctor for a checkup. He tells you he is not getting enough sleep and that his wife says he snores loudly. What assessment data should you gather from Mr. Mehta?
2. You are doing a presentation to a preschool parents group on sleep and rest. What information should you provide to promote sleep in preschool and school-age children?
3. Mrs. Li, age 85 years, recently moved into a long-term care facility. She reports problems sleeping since moving. Develop a care plan for Mrs. Li.

Review Questions

1. When assessing a client for obstructive sleep apnea (OSA), the nurse understands the most common symptom is
   1. Headache
   2. Early wakening
   3. Impaired reasoning
   4. Excessive daytime sleepiness
2. One priority nursing intervention to promote sleep for a hospitalized client is to
   1. Turn television on low to late-night programming
   2. Avoid awakening the client for non-essential tasks
   3. Give prescribed sleeping medications at dinner
   4. Have the client follow hospital routines
3. The use of non-prescription sleeping medications is not advisable because these medications can
   1. Lead to further sleep disruption even when they initially seemed to be effective
   2. Be expensive and difficult to obtain
   3. Cause severe depression and anxiety
   4. Cause headaches and nausea
4. If a client is using herbal compounds for sleep, the nurse should caution the client that these compounds can
   1. Interfere with prescribed medications
   2. Cause diarrhea and anxiety
   3. Not be used indefinitely
   4. Produce severe insomnia
5. The most vivid dreaming occurs during
   1. REM sleep
   2. Stage 1 NREM sleep
   3. Stage 4 NREM sleep
   4. Transition period from NREM to REM sleep
6. A client taking a beta-adrenergic blocker for hypertension can experience interference with sleep patterns such as
   1. Nocturia
   2. Increased daytime sleepiness
   3. Increased awakening from sleep
   4. Increased difficulty falling asleep
7. The care plan for improving sleep in an older person may include
   1. A nap during the day to make up for lost sleep
   2. Exercise in the evening to increase fatigue
   3. Allowing the client to sleep as late as possible
   4. Decreasing fluids 2 to 4 hours before sleep
8. Healthy infants should be placed in a supine position during sleep to decrease the risk of
   1. Falls
   2. Vomiting
   3. Cradle cap
   4. Sudden infant death syndrome (SIDS)

9. Narcolepsy can be best explained as
   1. A sudden muscle weakness during exercise
   2. Stopping breathing for short intervals during sleep
   3. Frequent awakenings during the night
   4. An overwhelming wave of sleepiness and falling asleep
10. A nursing measure to promote sleep in school-age children is to
    1. Make sure the room is dark and quiet
    2. Encourage evening exercise
    3. Encourage television viewing
    4. Encourage quiet activities prior to bedtime

References

Aldrich, M. S., & Naylor, M. W. (2000). Approach to the patient with disordered sleep. In M. H. Kryger, T. Roth, & W. C. Dement (Eds.), *Principles and practice of sleep medicine* (3rd ed., pp. 521–525). Philadelphia: W. B. Saunders.

American Academy of Sleep Medicine. (2002). *Sleep and heart disease*. Westchester, IL: Author.

Andrews, M. M., & Boyle, J. S. (2003). *Transcultural concepts in nursing care* (4th ed.). Philadelphia: Lippincott.

Attarian, H. P. (2000). Helping patients who say they cannot sleep: Practical ways to evaluate and treat insomnia. *Postgraduate Medicine, 107*(3), 127–130, 133–137, 140–142.

Bassiri, A. G., & Guilleminault, C. (2000). Clinical features and evaluation of obstructive apnea-hypopnea syndrome. In M. H. Kryger, T. Roth, & W. C. Dement (Eds.), *Principles and practice of sleep medicine* (3rd ed., pp. 869–878). Philadelphia: W. B. Saunders.

Beck-Little, R., & Weinrich, S. P. (1998). Assessment and management of sleep disorders in the elderly. *Journal of Gerontological Nursing, 24*(4), 21–29.

Bonnet, M. (2000). Sleep deprivation. In M. H. Kryger, T. Roth, & W. C. Dement (Eds.), *Principles and practice of sleep medicine* (3rd ed., pp. 53–71). Philadelphia: W. B. Saunders.

Canadian Nurses Association. (2003). *List of competencies for the 2005–2009 Canadian Registered Nurse examination*. Ottawa, ON: Author.

Carskadon, M. A., & Dement, W. C. (2000). Normal human sleep: An overview. In M. H. Kryger, T. Roth, & W. C. Dement (Eds.), *Principles and practice of sleep medicine* (3rd ed., pp. 15–25). Philadelphia: W. B. Saunders.

Chokroverty, S. S. (2000). *Clinical companion to sleep disorders in medicine* (2nd ed.). Boston: Butterworth Heinemann.

Cheng, C., & Umland, E. (2000). New and old drugs to treat insomnia. *Patient Care, 34*(11), 34–43.

Closs, S. J. (1988). Assessment of sleep in hospital patients: A review of methods. *Journal of Advanced Nursing, 13,* 501–510.

Cohen, F. L., Nehring, W. M., & Cloninger, L. (1996). Symptom description and management in narcolepsy. *Holistic Nursing Practice, 10*(4), 44–53.

Cullen, D. F. (2001). Obstructive sleep apnea and postoperative analgesia—A potentially dangerous combination. *Journal of Clinical Anesthesia, 13*(2), 83–85.

Dahl, R. E., & Carskadon, M. A. (1995). Sleep and its disorders in adolescence. In E. Ferber & M. Kryger (Eds.), *Principles and practice of sleep medicine in the child* (pp. 19–27). Philadelphia: W. B. Saunders.

D'Cruz, O. F., & Vaughn, B. V. (2001). Parasomnias: An update. *Seminars in Pediatric Neurology, 8*(4), 251–257.

Dines-Kalinowski, C. M. (2002). Nature's nurse: Promoting sleep in the ICU. *Dimensions of Critical Care Nursing, 21*(1), 32–34.

Dobbin, K. R., & Strollo, P. J. (2002). Obstructive sleep apnea: Recognition and management considerations for the aged patient. *AACN Clinical Issues, 13*(1), 103–113.

Dochterman, J. M., & Bulechek, G. M. (Eds.). (2004). *Nursing interventions classification (NIC)* (4th ed.). St. Louis, MO: Mosby.

Ebersole, P., and Hess. P. (2001). *Geriatric nursing and healthy aging*. Toronto, ON: Mosby.

Elliott, A. C. (2001). Primary care assessment and management of sleep disorders. *Journal of the American Academy of Nurse Practitioners, 13,* 409–417.

Gillis, A. M. (2000). Cardiac arrhythmias. In M. H. Kryger, T. Roth, & W. C. Dement (Eds.), *Principles and practice of sleep medicine* (3rd ed., pp. 1014–1029). Philadelphia: W. B. Saunders.

Hauri, P., & Linde, S. (1990). *No more sleepless nights*. New York: Wiley.

Hockenberry, M. J., et al. (2003). *Wong's nursing care of infants and children* (7th ed.). New York: Mosby.

Jarvis, C. (2004). *Physical examination and health assessment* (4th ed.). Toronto, ON: W. B. Saunders.

Jones, B. (2000). Basic mechanisms of sleep-wake states. In M. H. Kryger, T. Roth, & W. C. Dement (Eds.), *Principles and practice of sleep medicine* (3rd ed., pp. 134–154). Philadelphia: W. B. Saunders.

Kravitz, H. M., et al. (2003). Sleep difficulties in women at midlife: A community survey of sleep and the menopausal transition. *Menopause: The Journal of the North American Menopause Society, 10*(1), 19–28.

Kwentus, J. A. (2000). Sleep problems. *Clinical Geriatrics, 8*(8), 64–68, 71–72.

Leigh, T. J., et al. (1988). Factor analysis of the St. Mary's Hospital Sleep Questionnaire. *Sleep, 11*(5), 448–453.

Libman, E., et al. (2000). Sleep questionnaire versus sleep diary: Which measure is better? *International Journal of Rehabilitation and Health, 5*(3), 205–209.

Lueckenotte, A. G. (2000). *Gerontologic Nursing* (2nd ed.). St. Louis, MO: Mosby.

Mahowald, M. W. (2000). What is causing excessive daytime sleepiness? Evaluation to distinguish sleep deprivation from sleep disorders. *Postgraduate Medicine, 107*(3), 108–110, 115–118, 123.

McCance, K. L., & Huether, S. E. (2002). *Pathophysiology: The biologic basis for disease in adults and children* (4th ed.). St. Louis, MO: Mosby.

McKenry, L. M., & Salerno, E. (2003). *Mosby's pharmacology in nursing* (21st ed.). St. Louis, MO: Mosby.

Mendelson, W. B. (2000). Hypnotics: Basic mechanisms and pharmacology. In M. H. Kryger, T. Roth, & W. C. Dement (Eds.), *Principles and practice of sleep medicine* (3rd ed., pp. 407–413). Philadelphia: W. B. Saunders.

Merritt, S. L., et al. (2000). Herbal remedies: Efficacy in controlling sleepiness and promoting sleep. *Nurse Practitioner Forum, 11*(2), 87–100.

Miller, C. A. (2004). *Nursing for wellness in older adults: Theory and practice* (4th ed.). Philadelphia: Lippincott, Williams and Wilkins.

Mindell, J. A., & Jacobson, B. J. (2000). Sleep disturbances during pregnancy. *Journal of Obstetrical, Gynecologic and Neonatal Nursing, 29*(6), 590–597.

Mitler, H., Dement, W. C., & Dinges, D. F. (2000). Sleep medicine, public policy and public health. In M. H. Kryger, T. Roth, & W. C. Dement (Eds.), *Principles and practice of sleep medicine* (3rd ed., pp. 580–588). Philadelphia: W. B. Saunders.

Moorhead, S., Johnson, M., & Maas, M. (Eds.). (2004). *Nursing outcomes classification (NOC)* (3rd ed.). St. Louis, MO: Mosby.

Mornhinweg, G. C., & Voignier R. R. (1996). Rest. *Holistic Nursing Practice, 10*(4), 54–60.

National Heart, Lung, and Blood Institute Working Group on Restless Legs Syndrome. (2000). Restless leg syndrome: Detection and management in primary care. *American Family Physician, 62*(1), 108–114.

National Sleep Foundation. (2001). *Sleep strategies for shiftworkers.* Retrieved May 28, 2004 from *http://www.sleepfoundation.org/publications/shiftworker.cfm*

National Sleep Foundation. (2002a). *Sleep apnea.* Retrieved May 28, 2004 from *http://www.sleepfoundation.org/publications/sleepap.cfm*

National Sleep Foundation. (2002b). *When You Can't Sleep: ABCs of ZZZs.* Retrieved May 28, 2004 from *http://www.sleepfoundation.org/publications/ZZZs.cfm*

National Sleep Foundation. (2003). *Let sleep work for you.* Retrieved May 28, 2004 from *http://www.sleepfoundation.org/publications/letsleepwork.cfm*

Olson, D. M., et al. (2001). Quiet time: A nursing intervention to promote sleep in neurocritical care units. *American Journal of Critical Care, 10*(2), 74–78.

Orr, W. C. (2000). Gastrointestinal physiology. In M. H. Kryger, T. Roth, & W. C. Dement (Eds.), *Principles and practice of sleep medicine* (3rd ed., pp. 279–288). Philadelphia: W. B. Saunders.

Pagel, J. F. (2000). Nightmares and disorders of dreaming. *American Family Physician, 61*(7), 2037–2042, 2044.

Redeker, N. (2000). Sleep in acute care settings: An integrative review. *Image—The Journal of Nursing Scholarship, 32*(1), 31–38.

Renaud, M. T. (1996). Neonatal sleep patterns: Implications for nursing. *Holistic Nursing Practice, 10*(4), 27–32.

Richards, K. C. (1996). Sleep promotion. *Critical Care Nursing Clinics of North America, 8*(1), 39–52.

Richards, K. C., O'Sullivan, P. S., & Phillips, R. L. (2000). Measurement of sleep in critically ill patients. *Journal of Nursing Measurement, 8*(2), 131–144.

Richardson, S. J. (1997). A comparison of tools for assessment of sleep pattern disturbance in critically ill adults. *Dimensions of Critical Care Nursing 16*(5), 226–239.

Schneider, D. L. (2002). Insomnia: Safe and effective therapy for sleep problems in the older patient. *Geriatrics, 57*(5), 24–26, 29, 32.

Schweitzer, P. K. (2000). Drugs that disturb sleep and wakefulness. In M. H. Kryger, T. Roth, & W. C. Dement (Eds.), *Principles and practice of sleep medicine* (3rd ed., pp. 441–461). Philadelphia: W. B. Saunders.

Smyth, C. (1999). Try this: The Pittsburgh Sleep Quality Index (PSQI). *Clinical Nurse Specialist, 14*(3), 139–140.

Statistics Canada (2005a). Average time spent on activities, by sex (female). Retrieved February 10, 2005, from *http://www.statcan/english/Pgdb/famil36c.htm*

Statistics Canada (2005b). Average time spent on activities, by sex (male). Retrieved February 10, 2005, from *http://www.statcan/english/Pgdb/famil36b.htm*

Thorpy, M. (2000). Classification of sleep disorders. In M. H. Kryger, T. Roth, & W. C. Dement (Eds.). *Principles and practice of sleep medicine,* (3rd. ed., pp. 547–557). Philadelphia: W. B. Saunders.

Thurston, N. E., Tanguay, S. M., & Fraser, K. L. (2000a). Sleep and shiftwork I. *Canadian Nurse, 96*(9), 35–36.

Thurston, N. E., Tanguay, S. M., & Fraser, K. L. (2000b). Sleep and shiftwork II. *Canadian Nurse, 96*(10), 31–32.

Webster, R. A., & Thompson, D. R. (1986). Sleep in the hospital. *Journal of Advanced Nursing, 11,* 447–457.

White, D. P. (2000). Central sleep apnea. In M. H. Kryger, T. Roth, & W. C. Dement (Eds.), *Principles and practice of sleep medicine* (3rd ed., pp. 827–839). Philadelphia: W. B. Saunders.

Zarcone, V. P. (2000). Sleep hygiene. In M. H. Kryger, T. Roth, & W. C. Dement (Eds.), *Principles and practice of sleep medicine* (3rd ed., pp. 657–661). Philadelphia: W. B. Saunders.

Zoidis, J. D. (2001). Narcolepsy: Recognition is key to proper management. *RT: The Journal for Respiratory Care Practitioners, 14*(2), 33–34, 36, 74.

Zorick, F., & Walsh, J. (2000). Evaluation and management of insomnia: An overview. In M. H. Kryger, T. Roth, & W. C. Dement (Eds.), *Principles and practice of sleep medicine* (3rd ed., pp. 615–623). Philadelphia: W. B. Saunders.

Recommended Web Sites

Canadian Lung Association:
http://www.lung.ca
This Web site includes educational information on sleep apnea.

Canadian Pediatric Society:
http://www.cps.ca
This site includes educational information about reducing the risk of sudden infant death syndrome (SIDS).

Canadian Sleep Society:
http://www.css.to/sleep/index.htm
This organization is for health care professionals and researchers who are interested in sleep-related conditions. The site also includes information for the public on sleep-related topics and links to other sleep-related organizations and services.

Public Health Agency of Canada: Division of Aging and Seniors:
http://www.phac-aspc.gc.ca/seniors-aines/index_pages/publications_e. htm
This government Web site includes publications that are of interest to older adults and health professionals who work them. Several sleep-related publications are listed under the category: Medication Use.

National Sleep Foundation (U.S.):
http://www.sleepfoundation.org
This organization is for health care professionals and lay people interested in sleep-related topics. The site includes sleep-related educational material as well as research reports.

38

Pain and Comfort

Joan Domigan Wentz, BSN, MSN
Fay F. Warnock, RN, PhD (Canadian author)

Objectives

Mastery of content in this chapter will enable the student to:

- Define the key terms listed.
- Discuss common misconceptions about pain.
- Describe the physiology of pain.
- Identify components of the pain experience.
- Explain how the physiology of pain relates to selecting interventions for pain relief.
- Describe the components of pain assessment.
- Perform an assessment of a client experiencing pain.
- Explain how cultural factors influence the pain experience.
- Describe the appropriate nursing diagnoses, outcomes, and interventions for a client with pain.
- Describe guidelines for selecting and individualizing pain interventions.
- Explain the various pharmacological approaches to treating pain.
- Describe applications for use of non-pharmacological pain interventions.
- Discuss nursing implications for administering analgesics.
- Identify barriers to effective pain management.
- Evaluate a client's response to pain interventions.

Pain is the most common reason for people to seek health care. Despite being a commonly occurring medical symptom, pain is one of the least understood. A person in pain feels distress or suffering and seeks relief. The nurse uses a variety of interventions to bring relief or to restore comfort. However, the nurse cannot see or feel the client's pain. Pain is subjective; no two people experience pain in the same way, and no two painful events create identical responses or feelings in a person. The International Association for the Study of Pain (IASP, 1979) defined pain as "an unpleasant, subjective sensory and emotional experience associated with actual or potential tissue damage, or described in terms of such damage." Thus, physical pain can cause psychological pain and vice versa. However, the IASP definition of pain may be limiting because it does not apply to people who cannot provide verbal self-reports of their pain (Anand & Craig, 1996). These people include infants, small children, the cognitively impaired, and comatose individuals. Thus, when assessing pain or making pain care decisions on behalf of these individuals, the nurse must consider other sources of information, including the individual's behavioural and physiological responses to pain.

Comfort is central to nursing. As Donahue (1989) summarized, "Through comfort and comfort measures . . . nurses provide strength, hope, solace, support, encouragement, and assistance." A variety of nursing theorists refer to comfort as a basic client need for which nursing care is delivered. Comfort is as subjective as pain. Each person has physiological, social, spiritual, psychological, and cultural characteristics that influence how comfort is interpreted and experienced. Pain and pain management options are viewed within the context of comfort.

Pain is a universally shared but private experience that affects health and well-being. Nurses are responsible for understanding the pain experience of all their clients. The nurse, client, family, and health care team must collaborate to find the most effective approach to pain control. According to McCaffery (1979), "Pain is whatever the experiencing person says it is, existing whenever he says it does." For clients who cannot verbally communicate their pain, the nurse must serve as advocate so that they receive optimal pain assessment and treatment.

One should not assume that suffering is a natural part of being in hospital and being ill. The relief from pain is considered a basic human right and is incorporated into the Canadian Pain Society's *Patient Pain Manifesto* (2001). Nurses are ethically responsible for managing pain and relieving suffering. They are also legally and ethically obligated to advocate for change in the care plan when pain relief is inadequate (Registered Nurses Association of Ontario [RNAO], 2002). Effective pain management not only reduces physical discomfort, but also improves quality of life and promotes earlier mobilization and return to work, resulting in fewer hospital/clinic visits, shortened hospital stays, and reduced health care costs.

Scientific Knowledge Base

Pain is part of the human experience. Traditionally, pain has been viewed simply as a symptom of an illness or condition. However, pain itself is now considered to be a separate disease.

Nature of Pain

Pain is much more than a physical sensation caused by a specific stimulus. The experience of pain is personal, complex, and multi-dimensional; it involves physical, emotional, and cognitive components (Melzack & Wall, 1965). The stimulus for pain can be physical and/or mental in nature. Pain is exhausting and saps a person's energy. It can interfere with personal relationships and influence the meaning of life (Davis, Hiemenz, & White, 2002).

Physiology of Pain

There are four processes of nociceptive (normal) pain: transduction, transmission, perception, and modulation (McCaffery & Pasero, 1999). A client in pain cannot discriminate among the processes. However, understanding each process helps the nurse recognize factors that can cause pain, symptoms that accompany pain, and the rationale and actions of select therapies.

Pain is usually caused by thermal, chemical, or mechanical stimuli. The energy of these stimuli is converted to electrical energy. This energy conversion is known as **transduction.** Transduction begins in the periphery when a pain-producing stimulus sends an impulse across a peripheral pain nerve fibre **(nociceptor),** initiating an action potential. Once transduction is complete, transmission of the pain impulse begins.

All cellular damage caused by thermal, mechanical, or chemical stimuli results in the release of excitatory neurotransmitters such as prostaglandins, bradykinin, potassium, histamine, and substance P (Box 38-1). These pain-sensitizing substances surround the pain fibres in the extracellular fluid, creating the spread of the pain message and causing an inflammatory response (Paice, 1994). The pain fibre enters the spinal cord and travels one of several routes until ending within the grey matter of the spinal cord. Within the dorsal horn, substance P is released, causing a synaptic transmission from the afferent (sensory) peripheral nerve to spinothalamic tract nerves (Wall & Melzack, 1999; Figure 38–1).

Nerve impulses resulting from the painful stimulus travel along afferent (sensory) peripheral nerve fibres. Two types of peripheral nerve fibres conduct painful stimuli: the fast, myelinated A-delta fibres and the very small, slow, unmyelinated C fibres. The A fibres send sharp, localized, and distinct sensations that localize the source of the pain and detect its intensity. The C fibres relay impulses that are poorly localized, burning, and persistent (Wall & Melzack, 1999). For example, after stepping on a

Box 38-1 Neurophysiology of Pain: Neuroregulators

Neurotransmitters (Excitatory)

Substance P
- Found in the pain neurons of the dorsal horn (excitatory peptide)
- Needed to transmit pain impulses from the periphery to higher brain centre
- Causes vasodilation and edema

Serotonin
- Released from the brain stem and dorsal horn to inhibit pain transmission

Prostaglandins
- Generated from the breakdown of phospholipids in cell membranes
- Believed to increase sensitivity to pain

Neuromodulators (Inhibitory)

Endorphins and Dynorphins
- Are the body's natural supply of morphine-like substances
- Activated by stress and pain
- Located within the brain, spinal cord, and gastrointestinal tract
- Cause analgesia when they attach to opiate receptors in the brain
- Present in higher levels in people who have less pain than others with a similar injury

Bradykinin
- Released from plasma that leaks from surrounding blood vessels at the site of tissue injury
- Binds to receptors on peripheral nerves, increasing pain stimuli
- Binds to cells that cause the chain reaction producing prostaglandins

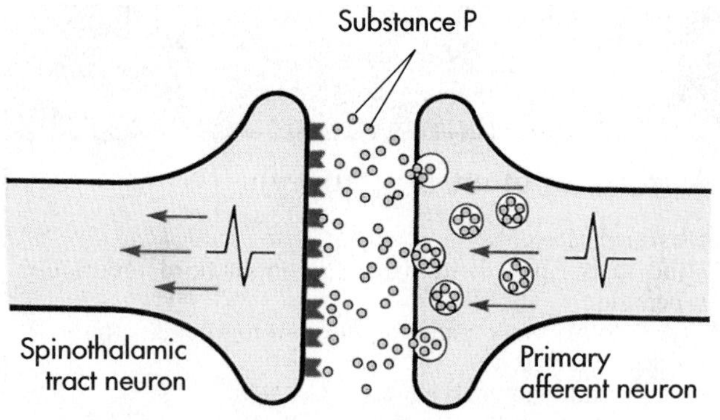

FIGURE **38–1** Substance P and other neurotransmitters are released from primary afferent fibres that terminate in the dorsal horn of the spinal cord. (From "Unraveling the Mystery of Pain," by J. A. Paice, 1991, *Oncology Nursing Forum, 18*(5), p. 843.)

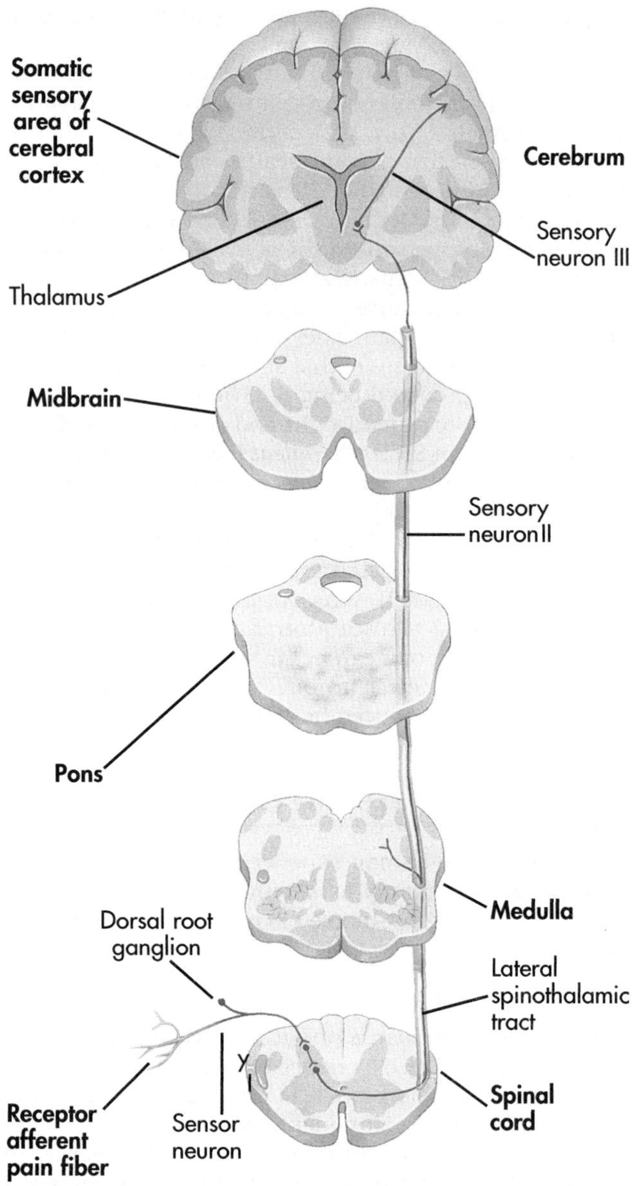

FIGURE **38–2** Spinothalamic pathway that conducts pain stimuli to the brain.

nail, a person initially feels a sharp, localized pain, which is a result of A-fibre transmission. Within a few seconds, the pain becomes more diffuse and widespread, until the whole foot aches because of C-fibre innervation.

Transmission of the pain stimulus continues along the afferent nerve fibres until they end in the dorsal horn of the spinal cord. Pain stimuli continue to travel through nerve fibres in the spinothalamic tracts that cross to the opposite side of the spinal cord. Pain impulses then travel up the spinal cord. Figure 38–2 shows the normal pain reception pathway. After the pain impulse ascends the spinal cord, information is transmitted quickly by the thalamus to higher centres in the brain. These centres include the reticular formation, limbic system, somatosensory cortex, and association cortex.

Once a pain stimulus reaches the cerebral cortex, the brain interprets the quality of the pain and processes information from past experience, knowledge, and cultural associations in the perception of the pain (McCaffery & Pasero, 1999). **Perception** is the point at which a person is aware of pain. The somatosensory cortex identifies the location and intensity of pain, and the association cortex determines how we feel about the pain. There are cells within the limbic system that are believed to control emotion, particularly anxiety. Thus the limbic system may play an active role in processing the emotional reaction to pain and memory of the pain experience. However, the human ability to experience and remember pain does not depend on cognitive ability (explicit memory). The experience of pain is remembered by even the youngest of infants, including those born prematurely (Anand & Scalzo, 2000). Pain studies using animal models (Fitzgerald, 1995) have shown that significant exposure to pain can permanently alter a developing organism's pain mechanism. This suggests physiological and implicit forms of pain memory take place in the first days of life.

As a person becomes aware of pain, a complex reaction unfolds. Psychological and cognitive factors interact with neurophysiological factors in the perception of pain. Perception gives awareness and meaning to pain so that a person can then react. The reaction to pain is the physiological and behavioural responses that occur after pain is perceived.

Once the brain perceives the pain, there is a release of inhibitory neurotransmitters (see Box 38-1) such as endogenous opioids (endorphins and enkephalins), serotonin, norepinephrine, and gamma aminobutyric acid, which work to hinder the transmission of pain and help produce an analgesic effect (Carlton & Coggeshall, 1998). This inhibition of the pain impulse is the fourth phase of the nociceptive process known as **modulation.**

A protective reflex response may also occur with pain reception (Figure 38–3). A-delta fibres send sensory impulses to the spinal cord, where they synapse with spinal motor neurons. The motor impulses travel via a reflex arc along efferent (motor) nerve fibres back to a peripheral muscle near the site of stimulation, thus bypassing the brain. Contraction of the muscle leads to a protective withdrawal from the source of pain. For example, when a person touches a hot iron, a burning sensation is felt, but the

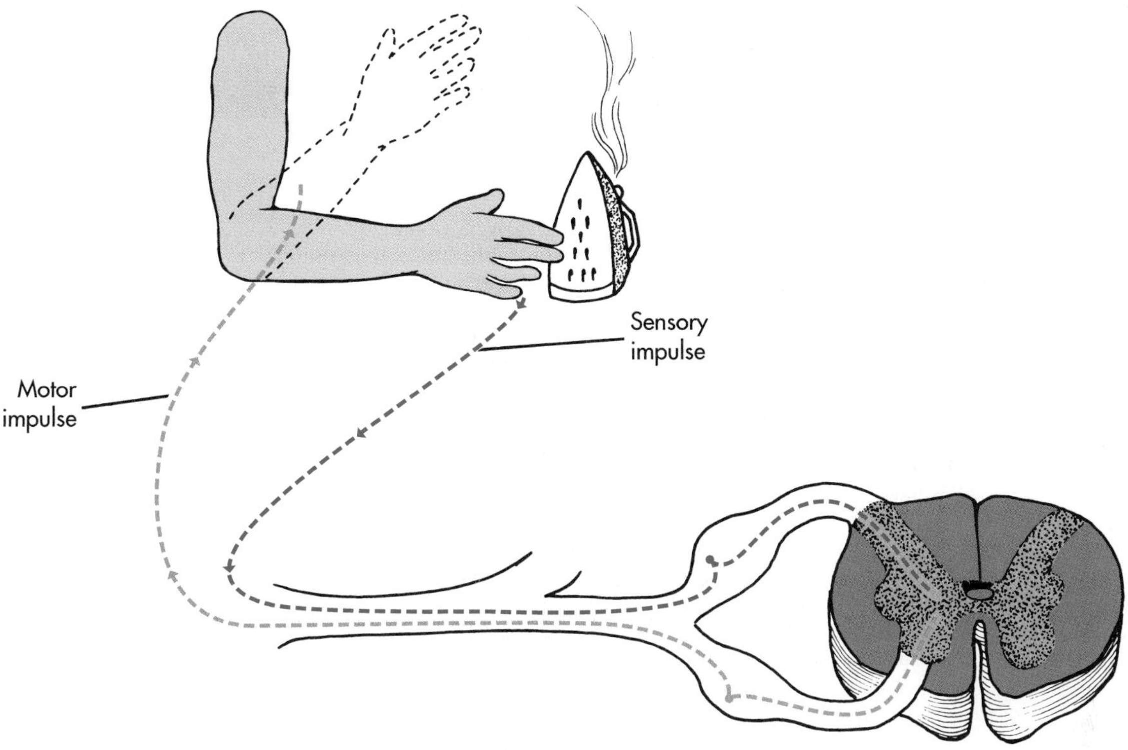

FIGURE **38–3** Protective reflex to pain stimulus.

hand also reflexively withdraws from the iron's surface. When superficial fibres in the skin are stimulated, a person moves away from the pain source. If internal tissues such as muscle or mucous membranes become stimulated, tightening and guarding of muscles occur. This reflex is usually absent below the injury in clients with spinal cord injuries. However, clients with spinal cord injuries can still experience pain (Siddall, Yezierski, & Loeser, 2000).

Gate-Control Theory of Pain. Researchers know that there is no specific pain centre in the nervous system. Melzack and Wall's gate-control theory (1965) was the first to suggest that in addition to the physical sensation, pain has emotional and cognitive dimensions. Melzack and Wall further suggested that pain impulses can be regulated or even blocked by gating mechanisms located along the central nervous system. The theory suggests that pain impulses pass through when a gate is open and that impulses are blocked when a gate is closed. Closing the gate is the basis for pain-relief interventions. Gating mechanisms can be found in substantia gelatinosa cells within the dorsal horn of the spinal cord, thalamus, and limbic system. By understanding what can influence these gates (physiology, emotional and cognitive processes), nurses can gain a useful conceptual framework for pain management. For example, stress, exercise, and other factors increase the release of endorphins, raising an individual's **pain threshold** (the point at which a person feels pain). Because the amount of circulating substances varies with every individual, the response to pain will be different. Recently *N*-methyl-D-aspartate receptors have been implicated in the pain experience (Helmy & Bali, 2001).

Physiological Responses. As pain impulses ascend the spinal cord toward the brain stem and thalamus, the autonomic nervous system becomes stimulated as part of the stress response. Superficial pain and pain of low to moderate intensity elicit the fight-or-flight reaction of the general adaptation syndrome (see chapter 26). Stimulation of the sympathetic branch of the autonomic nervous system results in physiological responses (Table 38-1). If the pain is continuous, severe, or deep, typically involving the visceral organs (e.g., with a myocardial infarction or colic from gallbladder or renal stones), the parasympathetic nervous system goes into action. Sustained physiological responses to pain could cause serious harm to an individual. Except in cases of severe traumatic pain, which may send a person into shock, most people reach a level of adaptation in which physical signs return to normal. Thus clients in pain will *not* always have changes in their vital signs. Therefore, while physiological responses are highly important, they should not be used as sole measures to infer pain.

Behavioural Responses. Once pain is experienced, a cycle of events begins that if left untreated or unrelieved can significantly alter the quality of a person's life. Pain can have a dominating nature, interfering with the ability to relate and to care for oneself. This component of pain reaction helps to explain why the management of pain can be such a challenge.

Pain threatens physical and psychological well-being. Clients may choose not to report pain if they believe their pain would inconvenience others or signal loss of self-control. Some clients will endure severe pain without

Table 38-1 Physiological Reactions to Pain

Response	Cause or Effect
Sympathetic Stimulation*	
Dilation of bronchial tubes and increased respiratory rate	Provides increased oxygen intake
Increased heart rate	Provides increased oxygen transport
Peripheral vasoconstriction (pallor, elevation in blood pressure)	Elevates blood pressure with shift of blood supply from periphery and viscera to skeletal muscles and brain
Increased blood glucose level	Provides additional energy
Diaphoresis	Controls body temperature during stress
Increased muscle tension	Prepares muscles for action
Dilation of pupils	Affords better vision
Decreased gastrointestinal motility	Frees energy for more immediate activity
Parasympathetic Stimulation†	
Pallor	Causes blood supply to shift away from periphery
Muscle tension	Results from fatigue
Decreased heart rate and blood pressure	Results from vagal stimulation
Rapid, irregular breathing	Causes body defences to fail under prolonged stress of pain
Weakness or exhaustion	Results from expenditure of physical energy

*Pain of low to moderate intensity and superficial pain.
†Severe or deep pain.

assistance. Often a nurse must encourage such a client to accept pain-relieving measures so that activity or nutritional intake is not seriously curtailed. The nurse must also educate the individual about the benefits of receiving and accepting analgesics to prevent pain before it occurs. Further, the individual's ability to tolerate pain significantly influences the nurse's perceptions of the degree of the discomfort. Clients deemed to have a low **pain tolerance** (level of pain a person is willing to put up with) may be perceived as whiners. The nurse must, therefore, avoid judging another's pain, and instead teach clients the importance of self-reporting. The nurse should also consider both the immediate context in which a person experiences pain and the person's past experience of pain. Pain assessment and pain care decision making is thus based on a variety of objective measures and observations (e.g., client self-reporting, family feedback, the client's behaviour and physiology, and internal and external environmental factors).

Typical body movements and facial expressions that indicate pain include clenching the teeth, holding the painful part, bent posture, and grimaces. A client may cry or moan, be restless, or make frequent requests. The nurse soon learns to recognize behaviour patterns that reflect pain. This recognition is especially important in clients who cannot report their pain. Lack of pain expression does not necessarily mean that a person has no pain. It is known that children who have pain will sometimes quietly play or watch television (P. A. McGrath, 1990); premature and full-term infants sometimes do not cry, and they exhibit few motor movements following excessive and repeated exposure to pain (Johnston et al., 1999; Warnock & Sandrin, 2004).

Types of Pain

Pain may be categorized by duration or pathology. Acute and chronic pain are categorized by duration.

Acute Pain. **Acute pain** is protective, has an identifiable cause, is of short duration (usually less than 6 months), and has limited tissue damage and emotional response. Acute pain eventually resolves with or without treatment after a damaged area heals. Because acute pain has a predictable ending (healing) and an identifiable cause, health care professionals are usually willing to treat acute pain aggressively. Unrelieved acute pain can progress to chronic pain.

Significant exposure to acute pain may have long-term psychosocial and physiological consequences if it is experienced at critical times of infant development (Anand & Scalzo, 2000). Untreated or poorly treated intra-operative and post-operative pain and stress increase infant mortality and morbidity (Anand, Sippell, & Aynsley-Green, 1987).

Unresolved acute pain in older adults can seriously threaten recovery, resulting in prolonged hospitalization, increased risks of complications from immobility (see chapter 42), and delayed rehabilitation. There cannot be physical or psychological progress as long as acute pain persists, because all energy is focused on pain relief. The nurse's efforts at teaching self-care will often be ineffective until the pain is successfully managed. Complete pain elimination may not be achievable, but reducing pain to an acceptable level is realistic. Primary nursing goals should be to prevent pain and to provide pain relief that allows clients to participate in their recovery.

Chronic Pain. An important difference between chronic and acute pain is that chronic pain is not considered protective and thus serves no purpose. **Chronic pain** is generally defined as pain that has been present for at least 6 months, persists beyond the normal time of healing, may not have an identifiable cause, serves no biological benefit, and leads to great personal suffering (Health and Welfare Canada, 1990; Jovey et al., 2003). Chronic pain can be experienced at any point in life, including early infancy and childhood (P. J. McGrath & Finley, 1999). Chronic pain may be non-cancerous or cancerous. Examples of chronic non-cancer pain include arthritis, low back pain, myofascial pain, headache, and peripheral neuropathy (McCaffery & Pasero, 1999). Chronic non-cancer pains are usually not life-threatening.

The possible unknown cause of non-cancer pain, combined with the unrelenting pain and uncertainty of its duration, frustrates the client, frequently leading to depression and perhaps suicide. For example, an injured area may have healed long ago, yet the pain is ongoing and may not respond to treatment. Chronic non-cancer pain is a major cause of psychological and physical disability, leading to problems such as job loss, the inability to perform simple daily activities, sexual dysfunction, and social isolation from family and friends.

The person with chronic non-cancer pain often does not show overt symptoms and does not adapt to the pain; rather, the person suffers more with time because of physical and mental exhaustion. Chronic non-cancer pain creates the insecurity of never knowing how one will feel from day to day. Symptoms of chronic non-cancer pain include fatigue, insomnia, anorexia, weight loss, apathy, hopelessness, and anger. Caring for the client with chronic non-cancer pain can be challenging. The nurse should emphasize that the pain can successfully be managed, although not necessarily cured, via a comprehensive approach.

Health care professionals are usually reluctant to treat chronic non-cancer pain with opioids, although in 1998, the Canadian Pain Society approved a consensus statement and developed guidelines to support the use of opioid analgesics for the management of chronic non-cancer pain (Jovey et. al, 2003). Often clients with chronic non-cancer pain who "doctor shop" are labelled "drug seekers," when they were actually seeking pain relief. This behaviour is known as **pseudoaddiction.** To break the cycle of poor pain management, the nurse discourages the client from having multiple health care providers for treating pain and refers the client to pain experts. The nurse should emphasize that the pain can be successfully managed, although not necessarily cured, using a comprehensive approach, including non-pharmacological as well as pharmacological strategies.

Cancer Pain. Not all clients with cancer experience pain. But for those who do, the Agency for Healthcare Research and Quality (AHRQ), formerly the Agency for Health Care Policy and Research (AHCPR), reports that up to 90% can have their pain managed (Jacox et al., 1994). Pain in a client with cancer may be acute, chronic, or both. The pain may also be nociceptive and/or neuropathic. Cancer pain may be due to tumour progression and its related pathological process, invasive procedures, toxicities of treatment, infection, and physical limitations. It can be sensed at the actual site of the tumour or distant to the site, which is called referred pain. A new report of pain by a client with existing pain needs to be investigated. Although the need for treatment of cancer pain has become more visible, the issue of undertreatment continues. In a study conducted in a hospice setting, of those clients with pain, only 42% stated they had pain-relief scores of 5 or more on a scale of 1 to 10 (1 being no relief and 10 being complete relief; McMillan, 1996). The importance of establishing an organized and systematic approach to pain assessment and treatment, therefore, cannot be overemphasized; nurses have the potential to play pivotal roles in this endeavour.

Pain by Inferred Pathology Process. Identifying the cause of pain is the first step in successfully treating pain. Nociceptive or normal pain is subdivided into somatic (musculoskeletal) and visceral (internal organ) pain. Neuropathic pain arises from abnormal or damaged pain nerves (Table 38-2). Each of these pathological processes has distinct pain characteristics that are discussed under pain assessment.

Idiopathic Pain. Because not all pain has an identifiable cause, a third category is necessary: idiopathic pain. **Idiopathic pain** is chronic pain in the absence of an identifiable physical or psychological cause or pain perceived as excessive for the extent of organic pathological condition. An example of idiopathic pain is complex regional pain syndrome (CRPS), previously known as reflex sympathetic dystrophy (RSD) and causalgia. The cause is unknown. It is hoped that future technology will identify the cause or causes, thus leading to a more effective treatment.

Nursing Knowledge Base

In *Notes on Nursing: What It Is and What It Is Not,* Florence Nightingale (1859/1969) stated that "pain . . . perpetuates and intensifies itself." Thus nurses have a long history of dealing with the effect of pain on clients. Traditionally, pain was considered a symptom of a disease or condition. If the condition were successfully treated, the pain would cease. Pain is now considered a comorbid medical condition needing treatment. Knowing that pain affects every aspect of a client's life, pain management is one of the most researched concepts in nursing. Through the contributions of nurse researchers and other members of the multidisciplinary pain research team, nursing knowledge of the nature, assessment, and treatment of pain will continue to grow. In this section, factors that influence pain are explored.

Knowledge, Attitudes, and Beliefs

Unless clients have objective signs of pain, a nurse may not believe they are in discomfort. These attitudes about pain are remnants of the traditional medical model of illness, and they are usually based on the personal views, attitudes, and beliefs of health care workers. The traditional medical model suggests that physical problems result from physical causes. Thus pain is viewed as a physical response to organic dysfunction. When no obvious source of pain can be found (e.g., the client with chronic low back pain or neuropathies), nurses and physicians may stereotype pain sufferers as complainers or difficult clients.

McCaffery, Ferrell, and Pasero (2000) studied nurses' attitudes to pain management and found that the nurse's personal opinion about the client's report of pain affected the pain assessment and titration of opioid doses. In a study by Zalon (1993), the greater the client's pain intensity, the worse the nurse's estimation of the pain. Tesler et

Table 38-2 Classification of Pain by Inferred Pathology

Nociceptive Pain	Neuropathic Pain
Normal processing of stimuli that damages normal tissues or has the potential to do so if prolonged; usually responsive to non-opioids and/or opioids. A. Somatic pain: Arises from bone, joint, muscle, skin, or connective tissue. It is usually aching or throbbing in quality and is well localized. B. Visceral pain: Arises from visceral organs, such as the gastrointestinal tract and pancreas. This may be subdivided: 1. Tumour involvement of the organ capsule that causes aching and fairly well localized pain. 2. Obstruction of hollow viscus, which causes intermittent cramping and poorly localized pain.	Abnormal processing of sensory input by the peripheral or central nervous system; treatment usually includes adjuvant analgesics. A. Centrally generated pain 1. Deafferentation pain: Injury to either the peripheral or central nervous system. *Examples:* Phantom pain may reflect injury to the peripheral nervous system; burning pain below the level of a spinal cord lesion reflects injury to the central nervous system. 2. Sympathetically maintained pain: Associated with dysregulation of the autonomic nervous system. *Examples:* Pain associated with reflex sympathetic dystrophy/causalgia (complex regional pain syndrome, type I, type II). B. Peripherally generated pain 1. Painful polyneuropathies: Pain is felt along the distribution of many peripheral nerves. *Examples:* Diabetic neuropathy, alcohol-nutritional neuropathy, and those associated with Guillain-Barré syndrome. 2. Painful mononeuropathies: Usually associated with a known peripheral nerve injury; pain is felt at least partly along the distribution of the damaged nerve. *Examples:* Nerve root compression, nerve entrapment, trigeminal neuralgia.

Adapted from *Pain: Clinical Manual* (2nd ed.), by M. McCaffery and C. Pasero, 1999, St. Louis, MO: Mosby. Data from "Methodological Challenges for Clinical Trials of Cancer Pain Treatments," by M. B. Max and R. K. Portenoy, in *Current and Emerging Issues in Cancer Pain: Research and Practice,* edited by C. R. Chapman and K. M. Foley, 1993, New York: Raven Press; and "Neuropathic Pain," by R. K. Portenoy, in *Pain Management: Theory and Practice,* edited by R. K. Portenoy and R. M. Kanner, 1996, Philadelphia: F. A. Davis. Also see "Pain: An Overview," by J. D. Loeser and P. Melzack, 1999, *The Lancet, 353,* pp. 1607–1609.

Box 38-2 Common Biases and Misconceptions About Pain

The following statements are *false:*
- Drug abusers and alcoholics overreact to discomforts.
- Clients with minor illnesses have less pain than do those with severe physical alteration.
- Administering analgesics regularly will lead to drug addiction.
- The amount of tissue damage in an injury can accurately indicate pain intensity.
- Health care personnel are the best authorities on the nature of a client's pain.
- Psychogenic pain is not real.
- Chronic pain is psychological.
- Clients should expect to have pain in a hospital.
- Clients who cannot speak do not feel pain.

al. (1994) also found that nurses underrated post-operative pain in children when those ratings were compared with the self-reported ratings of the children themselves. Although inaccurate pain assessment in infants and children may be rooted in the nurse's personal biases or lack of knowledge (Porter et al., 1997), variation in pain ratings may also be due to the type of pain scale that the nurse uses to assess pain (Chambers et al., 2002). For example, nurses who use pain scales that incorporate a "happy face" rate pain lower than do nurses who use a visual analog scale (VAS). It is therefore important for nurses to be aware of their personal biases and preferences when assessing and managing clients' pain.

Making assumptions about clients in pain may seriously limit a nurse's ability to offer pain relief. Too often, nurses allow misconceptions about pain (Box 38-2) to affect their willingness to intervene. Some even avoid acknowledging a client's pain because of their own fear and denial. Nurses are entitled to their personal beliefs; however, they must accept the client's report of pain and act according to professional guidelines, standards, position statements, policies and procedures, and evidence-based research findings.

To help a client gain pain relief, the nurse must view the experience from the client's perspective. Pain is tiring, affects relationships, and hampers self-care. Acknowledging prejudices and misconceptions helps the nurse address the client's problem. The nurse who is an active, knowledgeable observer of a client in pain will make a more inclusive assessment of the pain experience and its meaning for the individual. The client makes the diagnosis that

Table 38-3 Pain in Infants

Misconception	Correction
Infants are incapable of feeling pain.	Infants have the anatomical and functional requirements for pain processing by mid to late gestation.
Infants are less sensitive to pain than are older children and adults.	Preterm and term neonates may have a greater sensitivity to pain than older infants and children. This is due to their small skin surface area, high density of cutaneous nerve fibres, and their developing but still immature ability to inhibit transmission of sensory nerve impulses.
Infants are incapable of expressing pain.	Although infants cannot verbalize pain, they respond with behavioural cues and physiological indicators that can be observed by others.
Infants must learn about pain from previous painful experiences.	Pain requires no prior experience; it need not be learned from earlier painful experience (Anand & Craig, 1996). Pain is present with the first insult.
Pain cannot be accurately assessed in infants.	Behavioural cues (i.e., facial expressions, cry, body movements) and physiological indicators of pain can be reliably and validly assessed either alone or in combination. The most valid approach is facial expression (Craig, 1998). However, pain assessment should be based on the use of tools that incorporate composite pain measure (Stevens, 1998b). Inclusive approaches to infant pain assessment includes not only taking into consideration the behavioural and physiological responses of the infant, but also assessing the pain context and how the baby is interacting or failing to interact with the immediate environments (Warnock, 2003).
Because infants cannot demonstrate cognitive awareness, they are insensible and lack memory for pain.	Early exposure to noxious stimuli may have an effect on the infant's future responses to painful events (Grunau et al., 1994; Taddio et al., 1997).
Analgesics and anaesthetics cannot be safely given to infants and neonates because of their immature capacity to metabolize and eliminate drugs and their sensitivity to opioid-induced respiratory depression.	Infants older than 1 month of age metabolize drugs in the same manner as older infants and children. Careful selection of the agent, dosage, administration route, and time; frequent monitoring for desired and undesired effects; and drug titration and weaning can minimize the adverse effects of opioids and non-opioids for pain management in neonates (Stevens, 1998a).

Adapted from *Pain: Clinical Manual* (2nd ed.), by M. McCaffery and C. Pasero, 1999, St. Louis, MO: Mosby.

pain is present, and the nurse works to apply techniques and skills that ultimately give relief.

Factors Influencing Pain

Pain is complex, involving physiological, social, spiritual, psychological, and cultural influences. Each individual's pain experience is different. The nurse considers all factors that affect the client in pain.

Physiological Factors

Age. Age is an important variable that influences pain, particularly in infants and older adults. Developmental differences among these age groups influence how children and older adults react to pain. Young children have difficulty understanding pain and the procedures nurses administer that may cause pain. Young children may have difficulty describing and expressing pain. Cognitively, toddlers and preschoolers are unable to recall explanations about pain or associate pain with experiences that can occur in various situations. With these developmental considerations in mind, the nurse must adapt approaches for assessing a child's pain (including what to ask and the behaviours to observe for) and how to prepare a child for a painful procedure (Table 38-3). One technique is to ask the child the terms he or she most often use to define pain and pain treatment, and to then use those terms when communicating about pain with the child.

Pain is not an inevitable part of aging. However, older adults with pain are at increased risk for developing serious impairments in their functional status. Mobility, activities of daily living (ADLs), social activities outside the home, and activity tolerance can all be reduced. Pain in an older adult requires aggressive assessment, diagnosis, and management (Box 38-3).

The ability of older clients to interpret pain can be complicated by the presence of multiple diseases with vague symptoms that affect similar parts of the body. When there is more than one source of pain, a nurse must make detailed assessments (Herr, 2002a, 2002b). The manifestations of different diseases can cause an atypical presentation of painful conditions. In addition, different diseases can cause similar symptoms. For example, chest pain does not always indicate a heart attack; it may be a symptom of arthritis of the spine or of an abdominal disorder. Not all older adults experience cognitive impairment. However, when older adults are confused, recalling pain experiences and explaining details is difficult. Misconceptions about pain management in the very young and in older adults need to be addressed before nurses can adequately intervene in a client's pain (Miaskowski, 2000; Miaskowski & Levine, 2000; Table 38-4).

Fatigue. Fatigue heightens pain perception, intensifies pain, and decreases coping abilities. This is a common problem for clients with long-term illness or with fatigue as a result of treatment. If fatigue occurs along with sleeplessness, the perception of pain may be even greater. Pain is often experienced less after a restful sleep than at the end of a long day.

Focus on Older Adults — Box 38-3

- With aging, muscle mass decreases, body fat increases, and percentage body water decreases. This results in an increased concentration of water-soluble drugs such as morphine. Also, the volume of distribution for fat-soluble drugs such as fentanyl increases (Popp & Portenoy, 1996).
- Older adults frequently eat poorly, resulting in low serum albumin levels. Many drugs are highly protein bound. In the presence of low serum albumin, more free drug (active form) is available, thus increasing the risk for side and/or toxic effects (Lehn, 2001).
- Decline of liver and renal function is a natural occurrence with aging. This results in reduced metabolism and excretion of drugs. Hence, older adults often experience a greater peak effect and longer duration of analgesics (Kelly, 2003).
- Age-related changes in the skin such as thinning and loss of elasticity could affect the absorption rate of topical analgesics.

Table 38-4 Pain in Older Adults

Misconception	Correction
Pain is a natural outcome of growing old.	Older adults are at greater risk (as much as twofold) than younger adults for many painful conditions; however, pain is not an inevitable result of aging.
Pain perception, or sensitivity, decreases with age.	This assumption is unsafe. Although there is evidence that emotional suffering specifically related to pain may be less in older than in younger clients, no scientific evidence exists that pain perception decreases with age or that age dulls sensitivity to pain.
If the older client does not report pain, he or she does not have pain.	Older clients commonly underreport pain. Reasons include expecting to have pain with increasing age; not wanting to alarm loved ones; being fearful of losing independence; not wanting to distract, anger, or bother caregivers; and believing that caregivers know the older client has pain and are doing all that can be done to relieve it. The absence of a report of pain does not mean the absence of pain.
If an older client appears to be occupied, asleep, or otherwise distracted from pain, he or she does not have pain.	Older clients often believe it is unacceptable to show pain and have learned to use a variety of ways to cope with it instead (e.g., many clients use distraction successfully for short periods of time). Sleeping may be a coping strategy or it may indicate exhaustion, not pain relief. Assumptions about the presence or absence of pain cannot be made solely on the basis of a client's behaviour.
The potential side effects of opioids make them too dangerous to use to relieve pain in older adults.	Opioids may be used safely in older adults. Although the opioid-naive older adult may be more sensitive to opioids, this does not justify withholding the use of them in the management of pain in this population. The key to use of opioids in the older adult is to "start low and go slow." Potentially dangerous opioid-induced side effects can be prevented with slow titration; regular, frequent monitoring and assessment of the client's response; and adjustment of dose and interval between doses when side effects are detected. If necessary, clinically significant respiratory depression can be reversed by an opioid antagonist drug.
Clients with Alzheimer's disease and other cognitive impairments do not feel pain, and their reports of pain are most likely invalid.	No evidence exists that cognitively impaired older adults experience less pain or that their reports of pain are less valid than those of individuals with intact cognitive function. It is probable that clients with dementia or other deficits of cognition suffer significant unrelieved pain and discomfort. Assessment of pain in these clients is challenging but possible. The best approach is to accept the client's report of pain and treat the pain as it would be treated in an individual with intact cognitive function.
Older clients report more pain as they age.	Even though older clients experience a higher incidence of painful conditions than younger clients (e.g., arthritis, osteoporosis, peripheral vascular disease, and cancer), studies have shown that older adults underreport pain. Many older clients grew up valuing the ability to "grin and bear it," and, unfortunately, have been heavily influenced by the "Just Say No" to drugs campaign.

Adapted from *Pain: Clinical Manual* (2nd ed.), by M. McCaffery and C. Pasero, 1999, St. Louis, MO: Mosby. Data from "Care of the Aged: Perspectives on Pain and Discomfort," by R. N. Butler and B. Gastel, in *The Handbook of Pain Assessment,* edited by D. C. Turk and R. Melzack, 1992, New York: Guilford Press; "Are There Special Needs for Pain Assessment in the Elderly?" by S. W. Harkins and D. D. Price, 1993, *American Pain Society Bulletin, 3,* pp. 4–6; "Geriatric Pain," by S. W. Harkins et al., in *Textbook of Pain,* edited by P. D. Wall and R. Melzack, 1999, London: Churchill Livingstone; and "The Management of Persistent Pain in Older Persons," American Geriatrics Society, 2002, *Journal of the American Geriatrics Society, 50*(Suppl. 6), pp. 205–224.

Genes. Recent research on animal models suggests that genetic information passed on by parents might increase or decrease sensitivity to pain. What was historically described as pain threshold or pain tolerance may, in fact, be determined by genetic makeup. In addition, exposure to pain at a young age may increase sensitivity to pain (Ruda et al., 2000).

Neurological Function. A client's neurological function can influence the pain experience. Any factor that interrupts or influences normal pain reception or perception affects the client's awareness and response to pain. For example, clients who have a spinal cord injury, peripheral neuropathy (as in the case of diabetes mellitus), or a neurological disease (e.g., multiple sclerosis) experience altered pain sensation. Certain pharmacological agents influence pain perception and response. **Analgesics** (medications that relieve pain), sedatives, and **anaesthetics** (medications that cause temporary loss of sensation) depress functions of the central nervous system. Because clients at risk for pain insensitivity could suffer injury, they require preventive nursing care. Thus, the nurse must conduct a neurological assessment (see chapter 28).

Social Factors

Attention. The degree to which a client focuses attention on pain can influence pain perception. Increased attention has been associated with increased pain, whereas distraction has been associated with a diminished pain response (Carroll & Seers, 1998). Nurses apply this concept in pain-relief interventions such as relaxation and massage. By focusing a client's attention on other stimuli, the nurse places pain on the periphery of awareness.

Previous Experience. A previous painful experience does not mean that a person will accept pain more easily. If a person has had frequent episodes of pain without relief or has had bouts of severe pain, anxiety or fear may recur. If a person has had repeated experiences with the same type of pain but the pain has been successfully relieved, it becomes easier to interpret the pain sensation. As a result, the client is better prepared to take actions to relieve the pain.

When people have not experienced pain, their perception can impair coping. For example, severe incisional pain is common after abdominal surgery. Unless they know this, clients may view their incisional pain as a serious complication. The resulting fear may cause them to tense up and breathe shallowly. The nurse should prepare the client by explaining the type of pain to expect and methods to reduce it.

Family and Social Support. People in pain often depend on family or friends for support, assistance, or protection. A loved one can help minimize loneliness and fear. An absence of support can make the pain experience more stressful. The presence of parents is especially important for children with pain. The role modelling influence of parents also has a powerful impact on shaping children's attitudes and responses to pain (P. A. McGrath, 1990).

Spiritual Factors. Spiritual questions may include, "Why has this happened to me?" "Why am I suffering?" "Why has God done this to me?" "Is this suffering teaching me something?" People may worry about losing their independence and becoming a burden to family (Otis-Green et al., 2002). Nurses must show clients that their pain and suffering matters. Requesting a clergy consult for a client with chronic pain is a recommended strategy.

Psychological Factors

Anxiety. The relationship between pain and anxiety is complex. Anxiety often heightens the perception of pain, and pain may cause anxiety. Wall and Melzack (1999) reported that painful stimuli activate the portion of the limbic system believed to control emotion, particularly anxiety. The limbic system may process the emotional reaction to pain, aggravating or relieving it.

Critically ill clients, who feel they have lost control of their situation and care, are often anxious. When anxiety goes unnoticed, pain management problems may result. Pharmacological and non-pharmacological approaches to anxiety management are appropriate. However, anxiolytic medications should not be a substitute for analgesia. The potential for these drugs to reduce or prevent post-operative pain is being explored. Some studies show that administering anxiolytic and anti-inflammatory drugs *before* surgery results in lower self-reported pain scores and expedited recovery (Richmond, Bromley, & Woolf, 1993).

Coping Style. Coping style influences the ability to deal with pain. People with internal loci of control perceive themselves as being able to control their environment and the outcome of events (Gil, 1990). People with external loci of control perceive other factors in their environments, such as nurses, as being responsible for the outcome of events. The perception of self-control is key to pain management. For example, clients in acute pain who self-administer small doses of intravenous (IV) pain medication achieve pain control more quickly than do those who receive intermittent doses of pain medication from nurses.

Meaning of Pain. The meaning of pain affects the experience of pain and how one adapts to it. A person will perceive pain differently if it suggests a threat, loss, punishment, or challenge. For example, a woman in labour perceives pain differently than a woman with a history of cancer who is experiencing a new pain and is fearing recurrence.

Cultural Factors. Cultural beliefs affect how people deal with pain. People learn what is expected and accepted by their culture, including the meaning of pain and how to react to pain (Lasch, 2000; Steefel, 2002). Nurses often assume that others share their attitudes. Thus, they try to presume how clients will respond to pain. However, by understanding that pain has different meanings for different cultures, they can design culturally sensitive care.

Some cultures are demonstrative about pain; others are introverted. The nurse should know how much a client has assimilated into Canadian society. For example, if several generations of an Asian client's family have lived

Cultural Aspects of Care — Box 38-4

Culture models our responses, behaviours, and attitudes about pain. Culturally acquired patterns of pain responses may influence the neurophysiological processing of pain information as well as psychological, behavioural, and verbal response to pain. A client's meaning of pain may influence how much pain can be tolerated. Response to pain may be limited by language used to describe or report pain. The degree of pain expression does not necessarily correlate with pain intensity. Preferences for pain coping strategies are usually determined by culture; thus non-traditional interventions to manage pain need to be explored with the client. How people view and respond to pain influence the interventions the nurse chooses.

Implications for Practice

- Be aware of perceived causal factors of pain (fate, lifestyle, punishment, witchcraft).
- Emotional responses to pain (overt, stoic) vary between and within cultures.
- Words used to express pain vary among cultures (hurt, ache, discomfort).
- Personal and social meaning of pain and past pain experiences affect pain perception.
- Definitions of pain change the perception of pain intensity.
- Feelings about pain direct treatment.
- Health care provider beliefs and expectations regarding pain expression sway pain management strategies.
- Therapeutic goals of pain management are influenced by cultural beliefs.

Data from "Culture, Pain, and Culturally Sensitive Pain Care," by K. Lasch, 2000, *Pain Management Nursing, 1*(3 Suppl. 1), pp. S16–22; "Treat Pain in Any Culture," by L. Steefel, 2002, *Nursing Spectrum, 6*(5), p. 8; "Pain Response in Chinese and Non-Chinese Canadian Infants: Is There a Difference?" by C. Rosmus et al., 2000, *Social Science & Medicine, 51*(2), pp. 175–184; "Provisional Educational Needs of Health Care Providers in Palliative Care in Three Nursing Homes in Ontario," by C. Patterson et al., 1997, *Journal of Palliative Care, 13*(3), pp. 13–17; and "Multimeasure Pain Assessment in an Ethnically Diverse Group of Patients With Cancer," by L. Ramer et al., 1999, *Journal of Transcultural Nursing, 10*(2), pp. 94–101.

in Canada, the influence of the Asian culture may be limited. In contrast, a recent immigrant from another culture may have different beliefs from the larger Canadian population. Nurses must explore the impact of cultural differences and include cultural beliefs in the care plan (Box 38-4).

Critical Thinking

Critical thinking requires synthesizing knowledge, experience, information from clients, critical thinking attitudes, and professional standards. Clinical judgments require anticipating information needs, analyzing the data, and making decisions about client care. Nurses adapt their thinking to the changing needs of the client. During assessment, the nurse considers all elements involved in making nursing diagnoses.

The nurse must know pain physiology and factors that influence pain. Experience with clients who have pain sharpens skills. Successful pain management may not mean eliminating pain, but rather attaining mutually agreed upon pain relief goals that allow clients to control their pain.

Nursing Process and Pain

Pain management extends beyond pain relief, encompassing the client's quality of life and ability to work productively, to enjoy recreation, and to function normally in the family and society (Jacox et al., 1994). Pain management should be approached systematically. Nurses should begin by establishing a trusting relationship with the client and family.

NP Assessment

Nurses must monitor pain consistently along with temperature, pulse, respirations, and blood pressure. In some facilities, pain is considered the fifth vital sign. Central to assessment is placing the person suffering from pain at the centre and taking into consideration the trajectory or course of their pain (ability to recover from pain) and the context of pain.

Establishing a nursing diagnosis, deciding on appropriate interventions, and evaluating the client's response (outcomes) to the interventions are contingent on a timely and accurate pain assessment (Figure 38–4). A variety of pain assessment tools are available (RNAO, 2002). However, the goal in using these tools is not to identify how much pain the client can tolerate; rather it is to gauge the effects of pain treatment in order to optimize client function.

AHRQ has established guidelines for assessing clients with acute and cancer pain. The focus is on planning pain management interventions before pain is experienced. Because it involves collaboration, the AHRQ pain treatment flow chart (Figure 38–5) is a useful conceptual approach to acute pain control. However, clients must understand that reporting of pain is necessary if the health care team is to manage the pain effectively.

The nurse must find out the client's discomfort level and its affect on functional ability. The nurse might ask, "What is an acceptable level of pain for you?" The client might answer that a level 2 pain (on a scale of 0 to 10, with 0 being no pain and 10 being the worst pain imaginable) is acceptable. The nurse focuses on decreasing the pain to at least that level. If pain is acute or severe, the client probably cannot describe the experience in detail. During an episode of acute pain, the nurse assesses and responds to the location, severity, and quality of the pain. A more thorough pain assessment can occur when the client is more comfortable (Kim, 2002).

Assessment of chronic pain may best focus on affective, cognitive, and behavioural dimensions of the pain

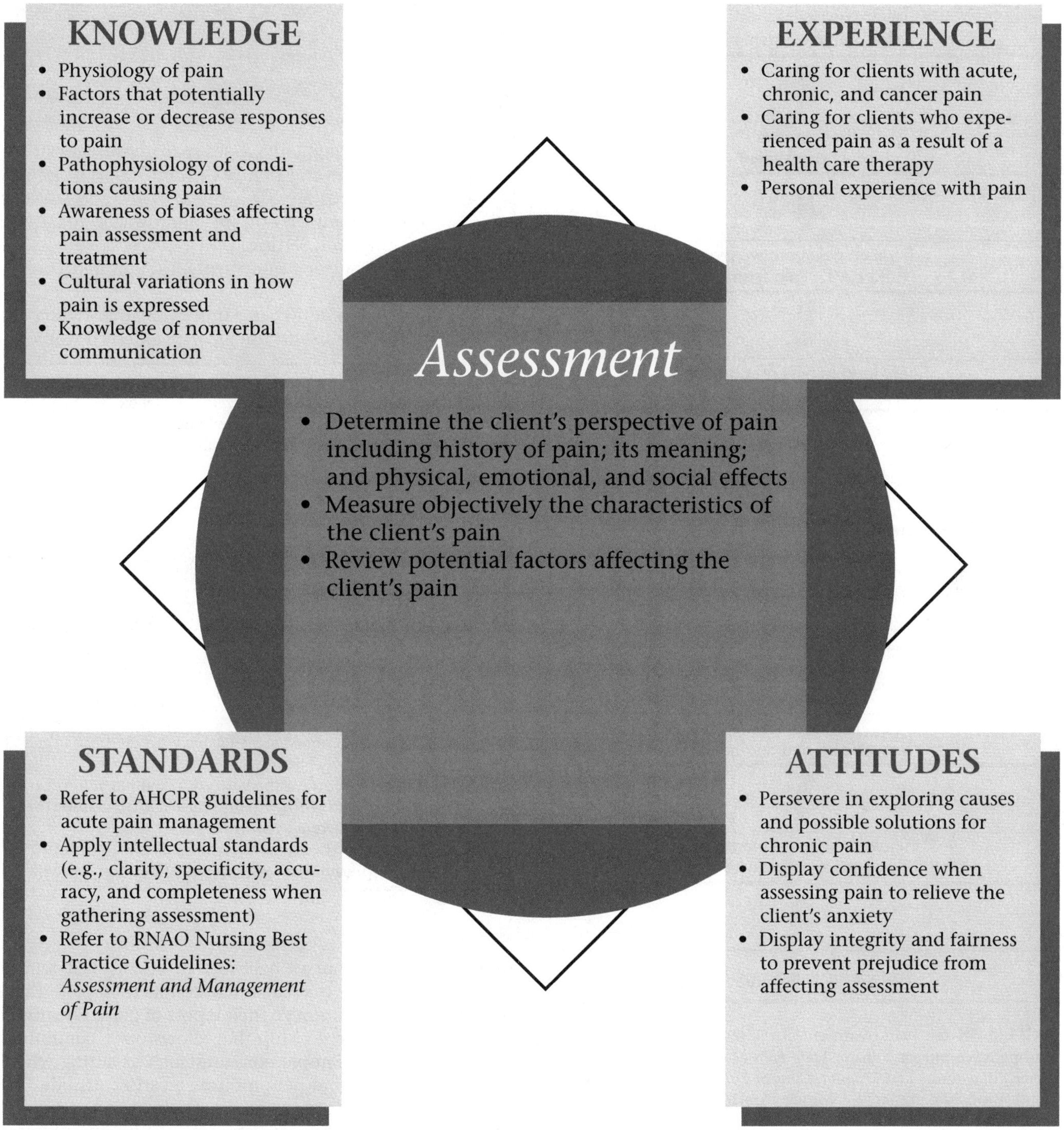
KNOWLEDGE
• Physiology of pain
• Factors that potentially increase or decrease responses to pain
• Pathophysiology of conditions causing pain
• Awareness of biases affecting pain assessment and treatment
• Cultural variations in how pain is expressed
• Knowledge of nonverbal communication
EXPERIENCE
• Caring for clients with acute, chronic, and cancer pain
• Caring for clients who experienced pain as a result of a health care therapy
• Personal experience with pain
Assessment
• Determine the client's perspective of pain including history of pain; its meaning; and physical, emotional, and social effects
• Measure objectively the characteristics of the client's pain
• Review potential factors affecting the client's pain
STANDARDS
• Refer to AHCPR guidelines for acute pain management
• Apply intellectual standards (e.g., clarity, specificity, accuracy, and completeness when gathering assessment)
• Refer to RNAO Nursing Best Practice Guidelines: Assessment and Management of Pain
ATTITUDES
• Persevere in exploring causes and possible solutions for chronic pain
• Display confidence when assessing pain to relieve the client's anxiety
• Display integrity and fairness to prevent prejudice from affecting assessment

FIGURE **38–4** Critical thinking model for pain and comfort assessment.

experience and on its history and context (Lawler, 1997). Assessment of chronic non-cancer pain should focus on function, because complete pain relief may not be possible. In the home setting, family members may assess the pain. The ABCs of pain management is an effective way to manage pain (Box 38-5).

The nurse should be aware of possible errors in pain assessment (Box 38-6). Using the right tools and methods can help the nurse avoid errors and choose the best pain interventions. Failure of clinicians to assess a client's pain, accept the findings, and treat the report of pain is a common cause of unrelieved pain and suffering (McCaffery & Pasero, 1999).

Expression of Pain. A self-report of pain is the single most reliable indicator of the existence and intensity of pain and any related discomfort (AHCPR, 1992; Jovey et al., 2003). Many clients fail to report or discuss discomfort; at the

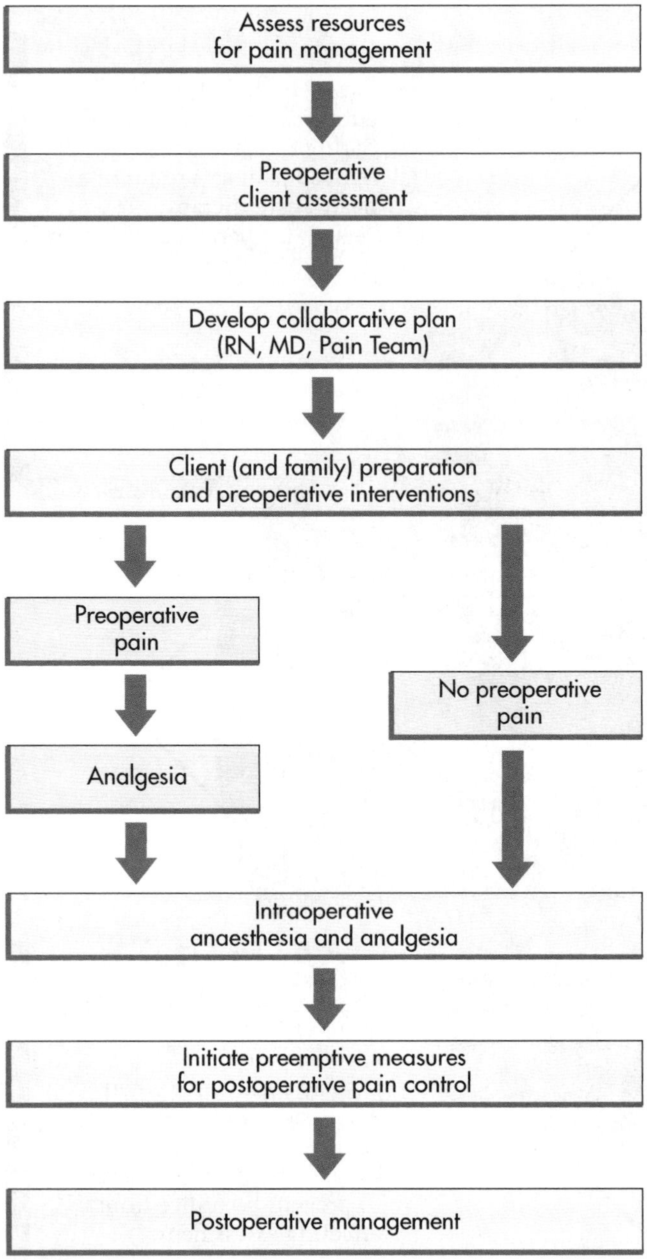

FIGURE **38–5** Pain treatment flow chart: preoperative and intra-operative phases. (From *Acute Pain Management: Operative or Medical Procedures and Trauma. Clinical Practice Guideline,* AHCPR Publication No. 92-0032, Agency for Health Care Policy and Research, Acute Pain Management Guideline Panel, 1992, Rockville, MD: Agency for Health Care Policy and Research, Public Health Service, U.S. Department of Health and Human Services; and *Management of Cancer Pain. Clinical Practice Guideline No. 9,* AHCPR Publication No. 94-0592, by A. Jacox et al., 1994, Rockville, MD: Agency for Health Care Policy and Research, Public Health Service, U.S. Department of Health and Human Services.)

Box 38-5 Routine Clinical Approach to Pain Assessment and Management: *ABCDE*

A *Ask* about pain regularly. *A*ssess pain systematically.
B *Believe* the client and family in their report of pain and what relieves it.
C *Choose* pain control options appropriate for the client, family, and setting.
D *Deliver* interventions in a timely, logical, and coordinated fashion.
E *Empower* clients and their families. *E*nable them to control their course to the greatest extent possible.

From *Management of Cancer Pain. Clinical Practice Guideline No. 9* (AHCPR Publication No. 94-0592), by A. Jacox et al., 1994, Rockville, MD: Agency for Health Care Policy and Research, Public Health Service, U.S. Department of Health and Human Services.

Box 38-6 Possible Sources for Error in Pain Assessment

- Bias, which causes nurses to consistently overestimate or underestimate their clients' pain
- Unclear assessment questions, which lead to unreliable assessment data
- Use of pain assessment tools that have no established reliability or validity
- Expecting self-reports of pain from individuals who cannot rate their pain using a pain scale or who cannot provide a complete verbal account of their pain
- Not considering the pain context and the trajectory or change in an individual's expression of pain over time

same time, many nurses believe that clients will report pain. If clients sense that the nurse doubts their pain, they will share little or minimize their report of pain. The nurse must establish a relationship that allows open communication about pain. Simple measures such as sitting when talking to clients about pain indicate a caring attitude.

Clients unable to communicate effectively often require special attention during assessment. Children, persons who are developmentally delayed, clients who are psychotic, the critically ill, clients with dementia, and clients who do not speak the same language as the nurse all require different approaches. Increasingly, Canadian research is focusing on the development of pain assessment instruments and approaches for use with pre- and nonverbal individuals. For example, a national collaboration is contributing to the development of pain assessment tools for use with cognitively impaired children (Oberlander et al., 1999) and older adults with limited ability to communicate (Fuch-Lacelle & Hadjistavropoulos, in press).

Cognitively impaired clients might require simple assessment approaches involving close observation of

Research Highlight — Box 38-7

Non-verbal Pain Indicators in Cognitively Impaired Older Adults

Research Focus

Assessing pain in a nonverbal client is difficult. Nurses encounter many clients who are unable to express their pain, although this does not mean they do not feel pain. Therefore there remain questions as to how to accurately assess pain in the noncommunicative client.

Research Abstract

The study's purpose was to pilot test the Checklist of Nonverbal Pain Indicators (CNPI) as a measure of pain behaviours in cognitively impaired older adults. Non-verbal behaviours studied were vocalizations, grimaces, bracing, rubbing, and restlessness. The instrument was tested on cognitively intact and impaired older adults with hip fractures. Cognitively intact older adults showed fewer non-verbal indications of pain both at rest and with movement than did the impaired clients. Facial grimaces were the most common observed pain behaviour in both impaired and unimpaired clients at rest. CNPI indicators were observed more frequently with movement. Over half of the sample (56%) showed no non-verbal indications of pain at rest. The CNPI proved to be a reliable and simple tool to assess pain in post-operative cognitively impaired older adults. The tool was more accurate in assessing pain during client movement.

Evidence-Based Practice

- Non-verbal clients require focused, around-the-clock pain assessment.
- Impaired clients may forget about painful areas when resting, thus requesting pain medication less frequently.
- Observing for pain behaviours in cognitively impaired older adults with activity is essential.
- Assessing pain at rest in cognitively impaired older adults may give misleading cues to staff about pain.
- Use of a research-based pain assessment tool for nonverbal older adults should improve accuracy of pain intensity assessment.
- Accurate pain assessment can result in better pain relief in clients unable to verbalize their pain.

Reference

Feldt, K. (2000). The checklist of nonverbal pain indicators (CNPI). *Pain Management Nursing, 1*(1), 13–21.

behaviour changes, especially with movement. Feldt (2000) has designed a tool that focuses on behaviours for use with cognitively impaired older adults (Box 38-7).

A critically ill client who may have a clouded sensorium or the presence of nasogastric tubes or artificial airways may require the nurse to ask specific directive questions that the client can answer with a nod of the head or by writing out a response. If the client speaks a different language, a family member or interpreter may be necessary to describe the client's feelings and sensations. Assessment tools such as the visual analog scale (VAS) have been translated into several languages to aid the nurse when an interpreter or family is not present (McCaffery and Pasero, 1999).

Characteristics of Pain. The nurse assesses common pain characteristics to understand the type and pattern of pain and choose interventions. Use of instruments to quantify the extent and degree of pain depends on a client being sufficiently cognitively alert to be able to understand the nurse's instructions.

Onset and Duration. Questions determine the onset, duration, and sequence of pain. When did the pain begin? How long has it lasted? Does it occur at the same time each day? How often does it recur? Does the client have frequent breakthrough pain or prolonged pain recovery?

Certain types of headaches are characterized by the time of day when they occur. Sudden and severe pain is easier to assess than gradual, mild discomfort. By understanding the time cycle of pain, the nurse knows to intervene before the pain occurs or worsens. Preventing recurrent pain is key.

Location. To assess location, the nurse asks the client to describe or point to all areas of discomfort. The nurse should not assume that pain will always occur in the same location.

When describing pain location, the nurse uses anatomical landmarks and descriptive terminology. The statement "The pain is localized in the upper right abdominal quadrant" is more specific than "The client states the pain is in the abdomen." Pain, classified by location, may be superficial or cutaneous, deep or visceral, referred, or radiating (Table 38-5).

Intensity. A person's pain intensity is subjective. Knowing the severity or intensity of a client's pain is extremely useful. Clients should be asked to describe pain as mild, moderate, or severe. Because the meaning of these terms differ for the nurse and client, this information may be difficult to verify over time.

Descriptive scales are a more objective means of measuring pain intensity (Figure 38–6). When scales are used to rate pain, a 10-cm baseline is recommended (AHCPR, 1992). A verbal descriptor scale (VDS) consists of a line with three- to five-word descriptors equally spaced along the line. The descriptors are ranked from "no pain" to "unbearable pain." The nurse shows the client the scale and asks the client to choose the current intensity of pain. The nurse also asks what rating to give the average pain and the worst pain over the past 24 hours. With a VDS, the client chooses a category for describing pain. A numerical rating scale (NRS) may be used instead of word descriptors. In this case, clients rate pain on a scale of 0 to 10. It is generally assumed that a pain score of 0 to 3 indicates mild pain, 4 to 6 moderate pain, and 7 to 10 severe pain. The scales work best when assessing pain intensity before and after therapeutic interventions.

The visual analog scale (VAS) does not have labelled subdivisions. It consists of a straight line, representing a

Table 38-5 Classification of Pain by Location

Location	Characteristics	Examples of Causes
Superficial or Cutaneous		
Pain resulting from stimulation of skin	Pain is of short duration and is localized. It usually is a sharp sensation.	Needle stick; small cut or laceration
Deep or Visceral		
Pain resulting from stimulation of internal organs	Pain is diffuse and may radiate in several directions. Duration varies but it usually lasts longer than superficial pain. Pain may be sharp, dull, or unique to organ involved.	Crushing sensation (e.g., angina pectoris); burning sensation (e.g., gastric ulcer)
Referred		
Common phenomenon in visceral pain because many organs themselves have no pain receptors; entrance of sensory neurons from affected organ into same spinal cord segment as neurons from areas where pain is felt; perception of pain is in unaffected areas	Pain is felt in part of body separate from source of pain and may assume any characteristic.	Myocardial infarction, which may cause referred pain to jaw, left arm, and left shoulder; kidney stones, which may refer pain to groin
Radiating		
Sensation of pain extending from initial site of injury to another body part	Pain feels as though it travels down or along body part. It may be intermittent or constant.	Low back pain from ruptured intravertebral disk accompanied by pain radiating down leg from sciatic nerve irritation

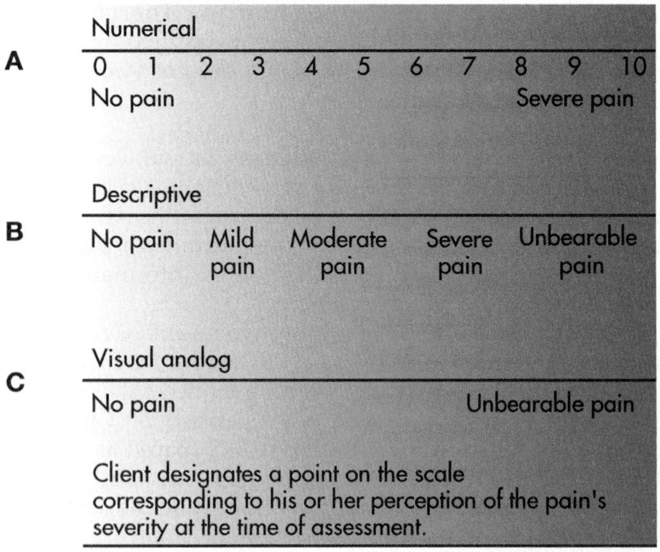

FIGURE **38–6** Sample pain scales. **A,** Numerical rating scale. **B,** Verbal descriptive scale. **C,** Visual analog scale.

continuum of intensity, and has verbal descriptors at each end. This scale gives the client total freedom in identifying the severity of pain. Although the VAS is less biased, it may not be as practical for daily use as an NRS (McCaffery & Pasero, 1999).

Assessing pain intensity in children requires special techniques. Children's verbal statements are most important (Hockenberry et al., 2003). Because young children may not know what the word *pain* means, the nurse may need to use words such as *owie, boo-boo,* or *hurt.* Some unique tools measure pain intensity in children. Beyer, Denyes, and Villarruel (1992) have developed the "Oucher," which consists of two separate scales: a 0 to 100 scale on the left for older children and a six-picture photographic scale on the right for younger children (Figure 38–7). Photographs of the face of a child (in increasing levels of discomfort) cue children into understanding what pain is and its severity. A child simply points to the selection. Ethnic versions of the tool are available. Wong and Baker (1988) developed the FACES scale to assess pain in children (Figure 38–8). The scale consists of six cartoon faces ranging from a smiling face ("no hurt") to increasingly less happy faces, to a final sad, tearful face ("hurts worst"). Children as young as 3 years of age can use the scale. Whatever tool is chosen, the nurse must teach children to use the tool and demonstrate their understanding and ability to use it (Fowler-Kerry & Lander, 1987). Several tools assess pain in neonates, infants, and non-verbal toddlers, such as the Premature Infant Pain Profile (PIPP) and the Neonatal Infant Pain (NIP) Scale (Stevens, 1998b).

A pain scale should be easy to use and should not be time consuming for the client to complete. If clients can read and understand the scale, their pain description should be accurate. Descriptive scales are used both to assess pain severity and evaluate changes in a client's

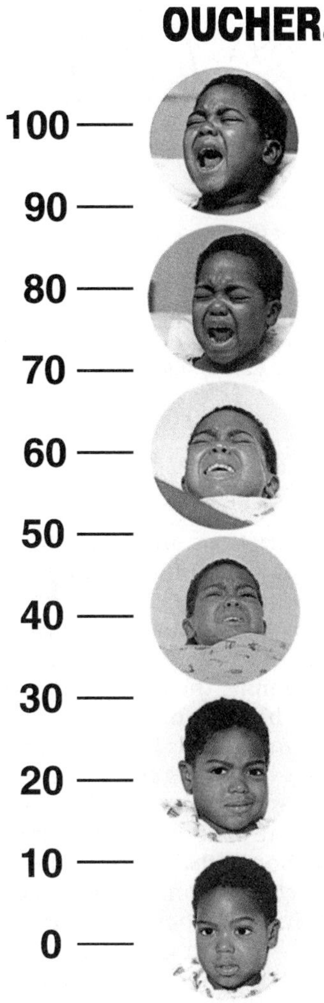

FIGURE **38–7** The Oucher pain scale. (Copyright Denyes Villarrael, 1990).

condition. The nurse can use the scales after an intervention or when symptoms become aggravated to evaluate if the pain has decreased or increased. The nurse must select and consistently use the same scale on the same client. A pain scale cannot be used to compare the pain of one client to that of another client. A rating of 7 or more on a 0 to 10 scale requires immediate attention. However, a numerical value has limited meaning; effective pain assessment requires various approaches, not just a pain assessment tool.

Quality. Another subjective characteristic of pain is its quality. Because there is no common or specific pain vocabulary, the words that describe pain vary. Clients may use *hurt* and *ache,* but reserve the word *pain* for severe discomfort. The nurse should use words other than *pain* to obtain an accurate report. For example, the nurse might say, "Tell me what your discomfort feels like." The client may describe the pain as crushing, throbbing, sharp, or dull. Although a list of descriptive terms is available, the client's own words are usually most accurate.

People describe certain types of pain fairly consistently. They often describe pain associated with a myocardial infarction as crushing or viselike, and the pain of a surgical incision as dull, aching, and throbbing, indicating nociceptive pain. Neuropathic pain is usually described as burning, shooting, or electric-like (Portenoy, 1996). When the client's descriptions fit the pattern forming in the nurse's mind, a clearer analysis can be made. This will lead to better pain management because nociceptive and neuropathic pain are treated differently.

Pain Pattern. Various factors affect the pain pattern. It helps to assess events or conditions that precipitate or aggravate pain. The nurse asks the client to describe activities that cause pain, such as physical movement, and to demonstrate actions that cause pain, such as turning a certain way. In the example of a ruptured intravertebral disk, the low back pain and radiation down the leg is usually aggravated by bending or lifting. Swallowing and talking typically aggravate the pain of pharyngitis. Asking the client if the pain is worse at certain times of day or if it is intermittent, constant, or a combination helps the nurse to plan effective interventions.

Relief Measures. The nurse should find out what relief measures a client uses, such as changing position, ritualistic behaviour (pacing, rocking, rubbing), or applying heat or cold to the painful site. The client's methods often work best. Clients gain comfort from knowing that the nurse is willing to try their relief measures. They also gain a sense of control over the pain instead of feeling as if the pain is controlling them (Haythornthwaite et al., 1998). The nurse should also identify practitioners whose services the client has used (e.g., orthopedist, acupuncturist, chiropractor).

Contributing Symptoms. Some symptoms (depression, anxiety, fatigue, sedation, anorexia, sleep disruption, spiritual distress, guilt) may cause the pain to worsen. The nurse evaluates the effect of such symptoms on the client's pain perception. Treating these symptoms can help manage pain.

Effects of Pain. Pain is stressful. It can alter lifestyle, affect emotional health, impair well-being, and cause suffering.

When a client has acute pain, the nurse should assess vital signs, conduct a focused physical examination, and observe for non-verbal responses to pain. At the initial onset of acute pain, the heart and respiratory rate and blood pressure increase. However, the body adapts quickly to acute pain and the vital signs return to within normal range quickly. The nurse should not confuse signs and symptoms of pain with other pathological changes. Changes in vital signs are more often indicative of problems other than pain. For example, a highly anxious client also has elevated heart and respiratory rates. The nurse performs a physical and neurological assessment on the basis of the client's pain history. The painful area should be examined to see if palpation or manipulation of the site increases pain (Jacox et al., 1994). During a general overview, the nurse looks for clues indicating

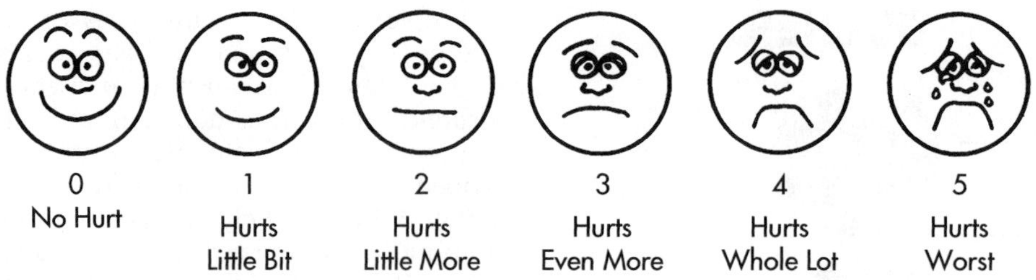

Brief word instructions: Point to each face using the words to describe the pain intensity. Ask the child to choose face that best describes own pain and record the appropriate number.

FIGURE **38–8** Wong-Baker FACES pain rating scale. (From *Wong's Nursing Care of Infants and Children*, 7th ed., by M. J. Hockenberry et al., 2003, St. Louis, MO: Mosby.)

Box 38-8 Behavioural Indicators of Pain

Vocalizations

- Moaning
- Crying
- Gasping
- Grunting

Facial Expressions

- Grimace
- Clenched teeth
- Wrinkled forehead
- Tightly closed or widely opened eyes
- Lip biting

Body Movement

- Restlessness
- Immobilization
- Muscle tension
- Increased hand and finger movements
- Pacing activities
- Rhythmic or rubbing motions
- Protective movement of body parts

Social Interaction

- Avoidance of conversation
- Focus only on activities for pain relief
- Avoidance of social contacts
- Reduced attention span
- Despondent—failure to interact purposefully and meaningfully with immediate environment

pain (e.g., posturing or guarding a painful area). If pain is unrelieved, the nurse looks for signs of physical exhaustion.

Behavioural Effects. When a client has pain, the nurse assesses verbalization, vocal response, facial and body movements, and social interaction. A verbal report of pain is vital to assessment. The nurse must listen and understand. Many clients cannot verbalize discomfort (e.g., infants, clients who are unconscious, disoriented, confused, or aphasic, and clients who speak a foreign language). In these cases, the nurse must be alert for behaviours that indicate pain (Box 38-8).

Groaning, grunting, and crying are vocalizations used to express pain. Some vocalizations may be involuntary and may occur without warning with acute pain. For some clients, vocalizations are culturally acceptable ways to communicate and do not necessarily indicate a higher severity of pain or reduced pain tolerance.

Subtle facial expressions or body movements often reveal more about the character of pain than do precise questions. For example, the client may grimace or begin to toss and turn. The amount of restlessness or protective movement may increase as the assessment progresses. Some non-verbal expressions characterize sources of pain. A person with chest pain often grabs or holds the chest. A person with severe abdominal pain often assumes a fetal position. The non-verbal expression of pain may support or contradict other information about pain. If a woman reports that her labour pains are occurring more frequently and begins to massage her abdomen more frequently, her report is confirmed. If a client complains of severe abdominal pain but grasps the chest, a more detailed assessment may be necessary.

Pre-mature and full-term infants in pain often display characteristic facial actions as described in the Neonatal Facial Coding System (NFCS; Grunau & Craig, 1987). Facial actions of infants in pain include brow lowering, eyes squeezing shut, chin quivering, mouth stretching vertically or horizontally, and lip pursing. Infants in pain may also show a complete lack of response, including no crying or movement (Johnston et al., 1999). The lack of pain response may also occur in older children and adults.

Pain causes the person to attend to the discomfort and fight it or give in to the discomfort and withdraw socially. The extent to which a client interacts with the environment can provide a clue about the intensity or nature of the pain. A person who withdraws completely may be in intense pain.

Influence on Activities of Daily Living. Clients who have daily pain may not be able to carry out routine activities. Inactivity leads to physical deconditioning. The primary goal should be to improve client function.

The nurse asks if pain hinders sleep. Clients may have problems falling asleep. Pain may awaken clients and keep them awake (see chapter 37). Sleeping pills or other medications may be needed to induce sleep.

Depending on the location of the pain, the client may have difficulty performing activities of daily living,

Nursing Diagnostic Process — Box 38-9

Assessment Activities	Defining Characteristics	Nursing Diagnosis
Have client describe pain intensity.	Pain is constant; 5 out of 10	Chronic pain related to chronic physical disability
Assess onset and location of pain.	Present for 7 months in lower lumbar area	
Observe client behaviours.	Grimaces and grunts with movement, rubs flanks frequently; reduced movement	
Assess effect of pain on activities of daily living (ADLs).	Appetite poor; gets little sleep; difficulty dressing	
Review medical history.	Previous trauma; previous exposure to opioids	

including normal hygiene and dressing/grooming activities. For example, clients with severe arthritis may experience pain when grasping eating utensils or lowering themselves to a toilet seat. The nurse assesses the client's need for assistance with self-care activities and collaborates with members of the health care team (e.g., physiotherapy). The nurse also considers the need for family members or friends to assist the client with basic hygiene.

The nurse should assess if pain has affected sexual activity. Conditions such as arthritis and chronic back pain make it difficult to assume positions for intercourse. Prolonged use of opioids for cancer pain affects sexual function and libido (Jacox et al., 1994). The nurse should learn whether a client is physically unable to participate or if pain has reduced the desire for sexual intercourse.

Pain also affects the ability to work. The more physical activity required in a job, the greater the risk of discomfort when the pain is associated with musculoskeletal and certain visceral alterations. Pain may increase if the job is stressful. The nurse assesses clients' ability to work and can often help clients select ways of minimizing or controlling the pain so that they can remain productive.

It is also important to include an assessment of the effect of pain on social activities. The nurse should ask if and how the pain has disrupted the client's regular social activities and if the client wishes to participate.

Client Expectations. Clients who seek health care assistance with pain as a major symptom may have experienced the pain for many hours or days. Hospitalized clients may expect and even accept some pain. Asking clients to describe an acceptable comfort level is a first step in encouraging them to take control of pain. Assessing previous pain experiences and effective home interventions provides a foundation on which the nurse can build. Clients expect that nurses will believe their reports of pain and be prompt in meeting their pain needs.

Nursing Diagnosis

An accurate nursing diagnosis results from thorough data collection and analysis (Box 38-9). A nurse must not diagnose pain simply because it is presumed that a client will have discomfort. Assessment will or will not indicate pain as a (potential) problem. An accurate diagnosis is made only after a complete assessment has been performed. In the diagnosis of pain, the nurse considers the client's withdrawal from communication, grimacing, moaning, and verbalizations of discomfort. A diagnosis of anxiety may be made by observing a client's facial tension and appearance, poor eye contact, restlessness, and verbalizations of feeling scared. The two diagnoses have similar defining characteristics. The nurse sorts out patterns of data to identify pain as the correct diagnosis.

The nursing diagnosis focuses on the nature of the pain so that the nurse can identify the best interventions for relieving pain and minimizing its effect on function. Accurate identification of related factors ensures that appropriate nursing interventions will be chosen. For example, *Acute pain related to physical trauma* versus *acute pain related to natural childbirth processes* require very different nursing interventions.

If pain affects general health and lifestyle, nursing diagnoses other than *acute* or *chronic pain* may be made. For example, a client may have arthritic hand and shoulder pain and, as a result, cannot fasten clothing. The nursing diagnoses would be *self-care deficit: dressing/grooming* and *chronic pain*. The nurse would involve health care team members (e.g., occupational therapist) to provide assistive devices for performing self-care. Examples of other diagnoses that may be applicable to clients at risk for pain include the following:

- Anxiety
- Ineffective coping
- Fatigue
- Fear
- Hopelessness
- Impaired physical mobility
- Imbalanced nutrition: less than body requirements
- Acute pain
- Chronic pain
- Powerlessness
- Ineffective role performance
- Self-care deficit
- Chronic low self-esteem
- Situational low self-esteem
- Risk for situational low self-esteem

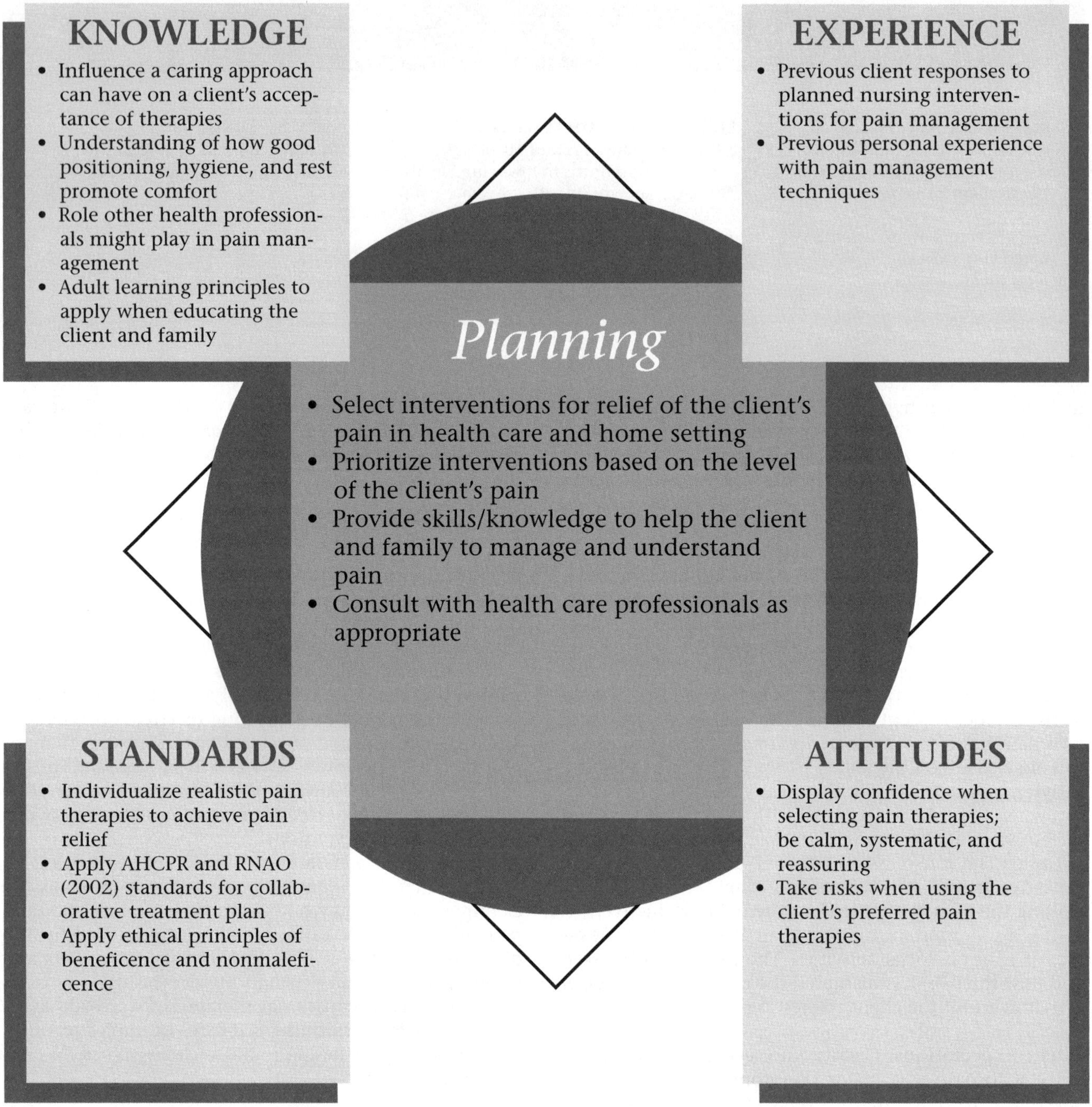
KNOWLEDGE
• Influence a caring approach can have on a client's acceptance of therapies
• Understanding of how good positioning, hygiene, and rest promote comfort
• Role other health professionals might play in pain management
• Adult learning principles to apply when educating the client and family
EXPERIENCE
• Previous client responses to planned nursing interventions for pain management
• Previous personal experience with pain management techniques
Planning
• Select interventions for relief of the client's pain in health care and home setting
• Prioritize interventions based on the level of the client's pain
• Provide skills/knowledge to help the client and family to manage and understand pain
• Consult with health care professionals as appropriate
STANDARDS
• Individualize realistic pain therapies to achieve pain relief
• Apply AHCPR and RNAO (2002) standards for collaborative treatment plan
• Apply ethical principles of beneficence and nonmaleficence
ATTITUDES
• Display confidence when selecting pain therapies; be calm, systematic, and reassuring
• Take risks when using the client's preferred pain therapies

FIGURE **38–9** Critical thinking model for comfort planning.

- Sexual dysfunction
- Disturbed sleep pattern
- Impaired social interaction
- Spiritual distress

Planning

The care plan integrates key client information, critical thinking elements (Figure 38–9) and professional standards, which provide scientifically proven guidelines for selecting nursing interventions (see Care Plan). Professional standards of care regarding pain management are available as agency policies or through professional organizations such as the RNAO and the Canadian Pain Society and its affiliated special interest groups.

A concept map helps with care planning. Clients in pain frequently have interrelated problems. As one problem worsens, others also change. The concept map shows how nursing diagnoses link to one another and to medical diagnoses. For example, when planning care for the client with arthritis, the nurse notes the relationships between *acute*

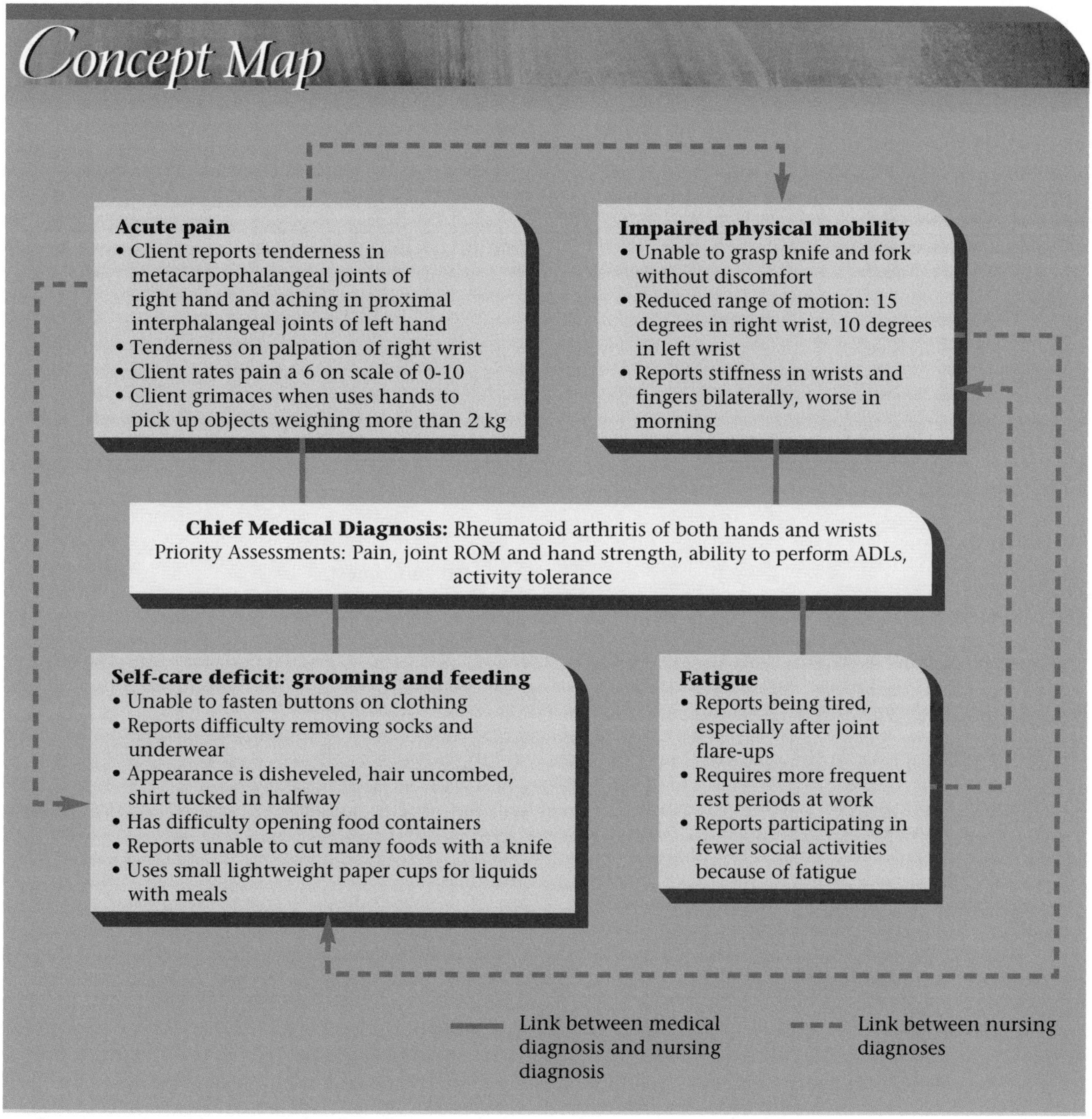
Concept Map
Acute pain
• Client reports tenderness in metacarpophalangeal joints of right hand and aching in proximal interphalangeal joints of left hand
• Tenderness on palpation of right wrist
• Client rates pain a 6 on scale of 0-10
• Client grimaces when uses hands to pick up objects weighing more than 2 kg
Impaired physical mobility
• Unable to grasp knife and fork without discomfort
• Reduced range of motion: 15 degrees in right wrist, 10 degrees in left wrist
• Reports stiffness in wrists and fingers bilaterally, worse in morning
Chief Medical Diagnosis: Rheumatoid arthritis of both hands and wrists
Priority Assessments: Pain, joint ROM and hand strength, ability to perform ADLs, activity tolerance
Self-care deficit: grooming and feeding
• Unable to fasten buttons on clothing
• Reports difficulty removing socks and underwear
• Appearance is disheveled, hair uncombed, shirt tucked in halfway
• Has difficulty opening food containers
• Reports unable to cut many foods with a knife
• Uses small lightweight paper cups for liquids with meals
Fatigue
• Reports being tired, especially after joint flare-ups
• Requires more frequent rest periods at work
• Reports participating in fewer social activities because of fatigue
Link between medical diagnosis and nursing diagnosis
Link between nursing diagnoses

FIGURE **38–10** Concept map for client with pain related to rheumatoid arthritis.

pain, impaired physical mobility, self-care, and *fatigue* (Figure 38–10). Understanding these relationships helps the nurse to develop a holistic and client-centred care plan.

Goals and Outcomes. Goals of pain management permit the client to function to the best possible extent. The nurse and client first identify what the pain has prevented the client from doing. Then a mutually acceptable level of pain that will allow return of function is determined. An indication of success is determined through attainment of goals and outcomes. For example, if the goal is "the client will achieve a satisfactory level of pain relief within 24 hours," the following are possible outcomes:

- Reporting that pain is a 3 or less on a scale of 0 to 10, or does not interfere with ADLs
- Identifying factors that intensify pain and modifying behaviour accordingly
- Using pain relief measures safely

Setting Priorities. Together the nurse and client discuss realistic expectations for the care plan. Interventions

Nursing Care Plan

Acute Pain

Assessment

Mrs. Mays was diagnosed with a cancerous tumour in her left lung 8 months ago. After treatment, she was taking oral analgesics on a prn basis. She is now hospitalized with uncontrollable chest pain and possible pneumonia. Her husband is with her. A PCA of morphine 0.5 mg demand dose with a 10-minute lockout is begun.

Assessment Activities	Findings/Defining Characteristics
Ask Mrs. Mays what she did at home to control her pain.	Her pain escalated from a 3 to a 10, so she doubled her medication and went to bed, but this did not help.
Ask Mrs. Mays what her pain intensity is now.	On a scale of 0 to 10, she reports a 9.
Ask Mrs. Mays what her pain has prevented her from doing.	She responds that she is unable to complete her own hygiene activities or sleep well.
Observe Mrs. Mays's non-verbal behaviour.	She is restless, unfocused, and is very still during the history taking.
Ask Mrs. Mays her pain intensity goal (out of 10).	She says that a pain intensity of 5 out of 10 would help her function better right now. A goal of 3 would be preferred.

Nursing Diagnosis: Acute pain related to a biological injuring agent (tumour).

Planning

Goal	Expected Outcomes*
	Pain Control
Client will obtain an acceptable level of comfort before discharge.	Client will report pain at stated goal or below.
Husband will assist in restoring Mrs. Mays to a pain-free state.	Husband will provide slow-stroke massage to Mrs. Mays before bedtime.
	Pain: Disruptive Effects
Client will actively participate in ADLs.	Mrs. Mays will report sleeping for 5 to 6 hours without interruption from pain. She will complete her own hygiene with minimal assistance. She will walk the hallway with her husband every 4 hours for 15 minutes.
	Medication Response
Mrs. Mays will not experience unmanageable opioid side effects.	Mrs. Mays will report having a normal bowel movement every other day.

*Outcome classification labels from *Nursing Outcomes Classification (NOC)* (3rd ed.), edited by S. Moorhead, M. Johnson, and M. L. Maas, 2004, St. Louis, MO: Mosby.

Interventions†	Rationale
Pain Management	
Begin PCA at ordered dose. Explain to client and spouse how to use the PCA. Emphasize the importance of only the client pushing the button, not the husband.	Client is experiencing an acute episode of her cancer pain. Discouraging the husband from pushing the button will minimize potential toxic effects of the opioid because client must be awake to perceive the pain and push the button (Reiff & Nizolek, 2001).
Monitor IV PCA morphine use. Explain to client and spouse the action of the medication, potential side effects, and the importance of reporting if the pain is not relieved.	Pain is easier to prevent than to treat. Side effects are usually transient, except for constipation. Calculating 24-hour dose of opioid helps determine appropriate oral dose (McCaffery & Pasero, 1999).
Have client select non-pharmacological interventions that have relieved pain in the past (e.g., distraction, music, simple relaxation therapy).	Personal control allows a client to shape immediate circumstances through own actions. (Salerno & Willens, 1996). Non-pharmacological interventions augment pharmacological strategies but should not be used in place of analgesics (McCaffery & Pasero, 1999).
Teach spouse how to perform slow-stroke back massage.	Slow-stroke back massage is easy to do, takes a brief time, and has been shown to induce relaxation (Meek, 1993).

†Intervention classification labels from *Nursing Interventions Classification (NIC)* (4th ed.), edited by J. M. Dochterman and G. M. Bulecheck, 2004, St. Louis, MO: Mosby.

Continued

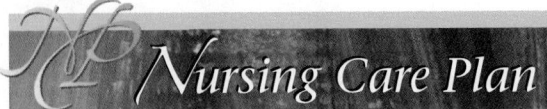

Nursing Care Plan

Acute Pain—cont'd

Evaluation

Nursing Actions	Client Response/Finding	Achievement of Outcome
Ask Mrs. Mays if she attained her pain relief goal most of the time.	She responds, "My pain usually runs around a 3, which is my goal, except when I start walking."	Mrs. Mays reports an acceptable level of comfort, which is a change from the level that indicated unacceptable pain. Instruct her to push her button before ambulating.
Observe Mrs. Mays performing ADLs, walking, and ability to sleep.	She is dressed for breakfast, walking the hallway every 4 hours with her husband. The night nurse's notes indicate Mrs. Mays slept through the night.	Ability to perform ADLs and sleep has improved. Continue to monitor.
Ask Mr. Mays if he was able to give his wife a back rub.	He reported that she did not want a back rub but preferred to have her feet rubbed, which he was happy to do. "She said it made her feel more relaxed."	Non-pharmacological intervention successful, but needs changing from back rub to foot rub in the nursing care plan.
Ask Mrs. Mays when was the last time she had a bowel movement and its consistency.	She has not had a bowel movement in 3 days (since starting the morphine PCA).	Assess her abdomen for bowel sounds and distension. Consult with physician about starting a stimulant laxative once intestinal obstruction is ruled out (McCaffery & Pasero, 1999).

must be appropriate for the nature and type of pain. An intervention that works for one client will not work for all. Priorities are based on pain level (provided via self-report and observation) and its effect on the client's condition over time and within the context of the immediate environment.

Immediate relief should be provided for severe pain. Analgesics can provide rapid relief and lessen the chance of pain worsening. After a client gains some relief, the nurse plans other interventions such as relaxation or the application of cold to enhance the effect of analgesics. Plans should take into account expected occurrences of pain.

Continuity of Care. A comprehensive plan includes a variety of resources for pain control, including nurse specialists, pharmacologists, physiotherapists, occupational therapists, and clergy. An oncology nurse specialist knows the pharmacological and non-pharmacological interventions that work best for chronic non-cancer and cancer pain. Pharmacologists are knowledgeable about pharmacological treatments of pain. Physiotherapists can plan exercises that strengthen muscle groups and lessen pain in affected areas. Occupational therapists can devise splints to support painful body parts. Clergy members can help clients resolve spiritual pain. The family should be involved in the care plan because they may need to administer care in the home after discharge. If the pain management plan is not successful, the nurse should talk with the physician about changing the plan. Pain expert consultation might be necessary.

Implementation

The nature of the pain and how much it affects well-being determine the choice of interventions. Pain therapy requires an individualized approach, perhaps more so than any other client problem. The nurse, client, and oftentimes the family must be partners in using pain-control measures. Nurses administer and monitor interventions ordered by physicians for pain relief and independently use pain-relief measures that complement those prescribed by a physician. Client remedies are often most successful, especially when the client has already had experience with pain. Generally, the least invasive or safest therapy should be tried first. If in doubt about a nursing therapy, the nurse should consult with a physician.

Health Promotion. Clients are better prepared to handle almost any situation when they understand it, including the experience of pain. However, clients with moderate to severe pain may not be able to participate in the decision-making process until the pain is controlled to an acceptable level. Once this is accomplished, teaching may begin.

Teaching clients about pain reduces anxiety and helps them achieve a sense of control. For example, clients in hospital for the first time may know that they must have tests but do not understand them. As a result, they may be anxious. Fears are greater if friends have had unpleasant experiences in similar circumstances. Fear increases the perception of painful stimuli.

When a client is anticipating pain, the nurse needs to explain procedures and associated discomfort. A confident explanation of the procedure helps a client place trust in a nurse. When clients are informed about an upcoming painful experience, they often perceive the actual experience as less unpleasant.

Non-Pharmacological Pain-Relief Interventions. A number of non-pharmacological interventions lessen pain and can be used in combination with pharmacological measures (Titler & Rakel, 2001). Non-pharmacological interventions include cognitive-behavioural and physical approaches. The goals of cognitive-behavioural interventions are to change pain perceptions, alter pain behaviour, and provide a greater sense of control. Relaxation and guided imagery are examples. Physical agents have the goal of providing comfort, correcting physical dysfunction, altering physiological responses, and reducing fears associated with pain-related immobility. The AHCPR guidelines for acute pain management (1992) cited non-pharmacological interventions as being appropriate for clients who meet the following criteria:

- Find such interventions appealing
- Express anxiety or fear
- May benefit from avoiding or reducing drug therapy
- Are likely to experience and need to cope with a prolonged interval of post-operative pain
- Have incomplete pain relief after use of pharmacological interventions

Relaxation and Guided Imagery. These techniques can alter affective-motivationaland cognitive pain perception. **Relaxation** is mental and physical freedom from tension or stress. Relaxation techniques provide clients with self-control, reversing the physical and emotional stress of pain. Relaxation techniques can be used at any phase of health or illness. Clients who successfully use relaxation techniques experience physiological and behavioural changes such as decreased pulse, blood pressure, and respirations; heightened global awareness; decreased oxygen consumption; a sense of peace; and decreased muscle tension and metabolic rate. Relaxation techniques include meditation, yoga, Zen, guided imagery, and progressive relaxation exercises (see chapter 31).

For effective relaxation, the client must participate and co-operate. Relaxation is not taught to clients in severe pain because their concentration is usually impaired. The nurse explains the technique and describes common sensations that the client may experience (e.g., a decrease in temperature or numbness of a body part). The client should use these sensations as feedback. The nurse is a coach, guiding the client slowly through steps of the exercise. The environment should be quiet and free of stimuli. The client may sit in a comfortable chair or lie in bed (Box 38-10). A light sheet or blanket may help the client feel more comfortable. Guided imagery and relaxation exercises may be done together or separately.

Progressive relaxation of the entire body takes about 15 minutes. The client pays attention to the body, noting areas of tension. Tense areas are replaced with warmth and relaxation. Some clients relax better with their eyes closed. Soft background music can help.

Progressive relaxation exercise involves controlled breathing exercises and a series of contractions and relaxation of muscle groups. The client begins by breathing slowly and diaphragmatically, allowing the abdomen to rise slowly and the chest to expand fully. When the client establishes a regular breathing pattern, the nurse coaches the client to locate any area of muscular tension, to think about how it feels, to tense muscles fully, and then to relax them completely. This creates the sensation of removing all discomfort and stress. Gradually the client can relax the muscles without first tensing them. When full relaxation is achieved, pain perception is lowered and anxiety about pain becomes minimal. Chapter 31 offers several relaxation exercise approaches.

If a client becomes agitated or uncomfortable, the nurse stops the exercise. If the client has difficulty relaxing any part of the body, the nurse slows the progression of the exercise and concentrates on the tensed body part. The client must know that the exercise can be stopped at any time. With practice, the client can soon perform relaxation exercises independently.

In **guided imagery,** the client creates an image in the mind, concentrates on that image, and gradually becomes less aware of pain. The nurse coaches the client in forming the image and concentrating on the sensory experience. Initially, the nurse asks the client to think of a pleasant scene or experience that promotes the use of all the senses. The client describes the image, which the nurse records for use during later exercises. The nurse uses information given by the client and does not change the client's image. The following is an example of part of a guided imagery exercise:

> Imagine you are lying on a cool bed of grass with the sounds of rushing water from a nearby stream. It's a balmy day. You turn to see a patch of blue wildflowers in bloom and can smell their fragrance.

The nurse sits close enough to be heard but is not intrusive and speaks in a calm, soft voice. While relaxing, the client focuses on the image, and it becomes unnecessary for the nurse to speak continuously. If the client shows signs of agitation, restlessness, or discomfort, the nurse stops the exercise and tries again when the client is more at ease.

Box 38-10 Body Positions for Relaxation

Sitting

Sit with entire back resting against back of chair.
Place feet flat on floor.
Keep legs separated.
Hang arms at the side or rest on chair arms.
Keep head aligned with spine.

Lying

Keep legs separated with toes pointed slightly outward.
Rest arms at sides without touching sides of body.
Keep head aligned with spine.
Use thin, small pillow under head.

Distraction. The reticular activating system inhibits painful stimuli if a person receives sufficient or excessive sensory input. People who are bored or in isolation tend to focus on their pain and thus perceive it more acutely. Pleasurable stimuli cause the release of endorphins that help a person ignore or become unaware of pain. Distraction directs attention to something else, thus reducing pain awareness and increasing tolerance. However, if distraction works, health care workers or family may question the existence or severity of the pain. Distraction may work best for short, intense pain lasting a few minutes, such as during an invasive procedure or while waiting for an analgesic to work. The nurse assesses activities that the client enjoys, which might include singing, praying, describing photos or pictures aloud, listening to music, and playing games. Most distractions can be used in a hospital, home, or long-term care facility.

Music. Music can decrease physiological pain, stress, and anxiety by diverting attention away from pain and creating a relaxation response. Nurses can use music creatively in many clinical situations. Clients generally prefer to perform (play an instrument or sing) or listen to music. All forms of music are used in music therapy. Clients should select the music they prefer. Popular music does not usually produce deep relaxation because it is short with a steady beat and words. Music produces an altered state of consciousness through sound, silence, space, and time. It must be listened to for at least 15 minutes to be therapeutic. Earphones can help concentration. In an acute care setting, listening to music can significantly reduce a client's post-operative pain. The nurse creates a relaxing setting so that music can be listened to uninterrupted. If pain becomes acute, the nurse suggests increasing the music's volume until the pain subsides.

Clients with Alzheimer's disease or related disorders have been found to benefit significantly from music. They often experience agitation, which worsens with pain. Research shows that music may be used to communicate with these clients even if they cannot understand speech and have problems interpreting environmental stimuli (Gerdner, 2001; Box 38-11.)

Evidence-Based Practice Guideline — Box 38-11

Individualized Music

- Determine if client is able to hear a normal speaking voice at a distance of about 0.5 m. Impaired hearing may distort sound, which may be source of irritation.
- Assess client's personal music preference.
  - Ask client how important music has been in his or her life.
  - Ask if client plays a musical instrument.
  - Ask if client enjoys singing and dancing.
  - Ask client to identify favourite types of music (e.g., country and western, folk, blues, jazz, rock and roll, ethnic).
  - Ask client which of the following is their favourite form of music: vocal, instrumental, or both.
  - Ask client to identify songs that make him or her happy.
  - Have client identify specific artists or performers he or she enjoys listening to.
  - Have client list albums, tapes, CDs he or she has at home.
- If client is unable to provide information because of cognitive impairment, interview a family member who is knowledgeable about the client's music preference.
- Play the music selections:
  - Use an audio cassette player or CD player that functions properly.
  - Plan each music intervention session to last about 30 minutes, in a location where client is comfortable or spends most of time.
  - Set volume at an appropriate level.
  - Headphones may be an option; however, they can be uncomfortable or confusing to people with dementia.

Adapted from Evidence-Based Protocol: "Individualized Music:" by L. Gerdner, in *Series on Evidence-Based Practice for Older Adults,* edited by M. G. Titler (Series), 2001, Iowa City, IA: The University of Iowa College of Nursing Gerontological Nursing Interventions Research Center, Research Dissemination Core. (For more information, see *http://www.nursing.uiowa.edu/centers/gnirc/rtdcore.htm*)

Biofeedback. **Biofeedback** is a behavioural therapy that involves giving individuals information about physiological responses (e.g., blood pressure or tension) and ways to exercise voluntary control over those responses (McGrady et al., 1994). It is used to produce deep relaxation and is especially effective for muscle tension and migraine headaches. In the treatment of headaches, electrodes are attached externally over each temple. The electrodes measure skin tension in microvolts. A polygraph machine visibly records the tension level for the client to see. The client learns to achieve optimal relaxation using feedback from the polygraph while lowering the actual level of tension experienced. The therapy takes several weeks to learn. Chapter 31 describes the benefits and limitations of biofeedback.

Cutaneous Stimulation. **Cutaneous stimulation** is the stimulation of the skin to relieve pain. A massage, warm bath, ice bag, and transcutaneous electrical nerve stimulation (TENS) are simple ways to reduce pain perception. How cutaneous stimulation works is unclear. One suggestion is that it causes release of endorphins, thus blocking the transmission of painful stimuli. The gate-control theory suggests that cutaneous stimulation activates larger, faster-transmitting A-beta sensory nerve fibres. This decreases pain transmission through small-diameter A-delta and C fibres. Synaptic gates close to the transmission of pain impulses. In a review by O'Mathuna (2000), touch and massage influenced autonomic nervous system activity. When a person perceives touch to be relaxing, the relaxation response is elicited.

An advantage to cutaneous stimulation is that the measures can be used in the home, giving clients and families some control over pain symptoms and treatment. The proper use of cutaneous stimulation can reduce pain perception and help to reduce muscle tension that might otherwise increase pain. When using cutaneous stimulation methods, the nurse eliminates sources of environmental noise, helps the client to assume a comfortable position, and explains the purpose of the therapy. Cutaneous stimulation should not be used directly on sensitive skin areas (e.g., burns, bruises, skin rashes, inflammation, and underlying bone fractures).

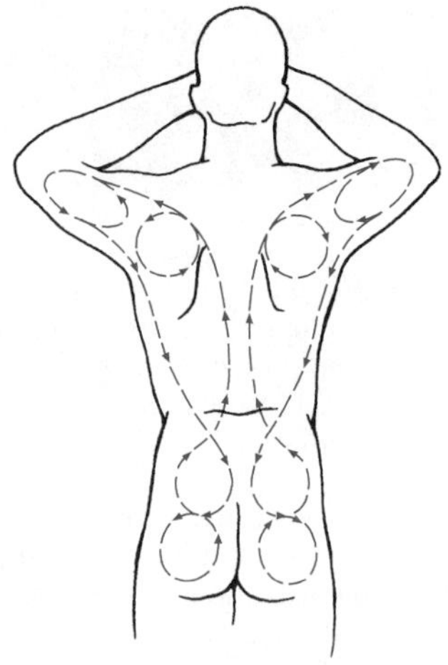

FIGURE **38–11** Back massage pattern.

Massages have been used by nurses for many years as a safe and effective way to produce physical and mental relaxation, reduce pain, and enhance the effectiveness of pain medications (Figure 38–11). Massaging the back and shoulders or the hands and feet for 3 to 5 minutes can help relax muscles and promote sleep and comfort (Grealish, Lomasney, & Whiteman, 2000). Massages communicate caring and can easily be taught to family members or other health care workers (Box 38-12).

Cold and heat applications (see chapter 43) relieve pain and promote healing. The choice of heat or cold varies with clients' conditions. Moist heat can help relieve pain from a tension headache, and cold applications can reduce acute pain from inflamed joints. When using a heat or cold application, the nurse instructs the client to avoid injury to the skin by checking the temperature and avoiding direct application of the cold or hot surface to the skin. Especially at risk are clients with spinal cord or other neurological injury, older adults, and confused clients.

Ice massage and application of cold packs are particularly effective for pain relief. Ice massage involves the use of a large ice cube or a small paper cup filled with water and frozen (water rises out of the cup as it freezes to create a smooth surface of ice for massage). The massage is simple. A nurse or the client can apply the ice with firm pressure to the skin, followed by a slow, steady, circular massage over the area. Cold may be applied near the pain site, on the opposite side of the body corresponding to the pain site, or on a site located between the brain and the pain site. It takes 5 to 10 minutes to apply cold. Each client responds differently to the site of application that is most effective. Application near the actual site of pain tends to work best. A client feels cold, burning, and aching sensations as well as numbness. When numbness occurs, the ice should be removed. Cold is particularly effective for tooth or mouth pain when ice is placed on the web of the hand between the thumb and index finger. This point on the hand is an **acupressure** point that apparently influences nerve pathways to the face and head. Cold applications are also effective before invasive needle punctures.

Heat application might work better for some clients. Heating pads or hot water bottles may be used, but clients should be taught not to lie on the heating element to avoid burns. Commercial pillows that can be warmed in the microwave and that contour to the body can also be used.

Another form of cutaneous stimulation, sometimes called counterstimulation, is **transcutaneous electrical nerve stimulation (TENS),** involving stimulation of the skin with a mild electrical current passed through external electrodes (Sluka, 2001). The therapy requires a physician's order. The TENS unit consists of a battery-powered transmitter, lead wires, and electrodes. The electrodes are placed directly over or near the site of pain. Hair or skin preparations should be removed before attaching the electrodes. When a client feels pain, the transmitter is turned on and a buzzing or tingling sensation is created. The client may adjust the intensity and quality of skin stimulation. The tingling sensation can be applied until pain relief occurs. TENS is effective for post-surgical pain control and reduction of pain caused by post-operative procedures.

Herbals. Although herbals have not been sufficiently studied to recommend for pain relief, many clients self-medicate using herbals. Herbals could have an interaction with prescribed analgesics; thus, the nurse asks the client to report all substances taken to relieve pain (see chapter 31).

Reducing Pain Perception. A simple way to promote comfort is by removing or preventing painful stimuli (Box 38-13). This is especially important for clients who are immobilized or unable to sense discomfort. Pain can also be prevented by anticipating painful events. Before performing procedures, the nurse considers the client's condition, aspects of the procedure that may be uncomfortable, and techniques to avoid causing pain. For example, in a client with severe arthritic knee pain, the nurse knows that extreme flexion of the knee causes pain. Before walking the client to the bathroom, the nurse makes sure that an elevated toilet seat is available. The client can then be seated and can rise with minimal discomfort. It takes only simple consideration of the client's comfort and a little extra time to avoid pain-producing situations.

Acute Care

Acute Pain Management. Some clients have acute pain from invasive procedures (e.g., surgery or endoscopy) or trauma. The AHCPR (1992) has a pain treatment flow chart (Figure 38–12) for the aggressive treatment of post-operative pain and pain from medical procedures and trauma. The systematic approach ensures a quick response to client discomfort. The key to success in pain relief is ongoing evaluation of interventions: Is relief obtained? Are there any unacceptable side effects from the medications? It is the responsibility of the health care team to collaborate to find the combination of therapy that works best for a client.

Pharmacological Pain-Relief Interventions. There are several pharmacological agents that provide pain relief and require a physician's order. The nurse's judgment in their use and management helps ensure the best pain relief possible. Nurses must understand the drugs available for pain relief and their pharmacological effects.

Analgesics. Analgesics are the most common method of pain relief. Although analgesics can effectively relieve pain, nurses and physicians still tend to undertreat clients because of incorrect drug information, concerns

Box 38-12 Procedural Guidelines

Massage

Equipment: Moisturizing lotion, bath towel or blanket

Delegation considerations: The nurse is responsible for assessing any possible contraindication or client response to massage. The skill of administering a massage may be delegated to an unregulated care provider (UCP), providing the client is stable. Before delegation the nurse must:

- Instruct the UCP as to which body parts to massage.
- Instruct the UCP on the importance of not massaging reddened skin areas.
- Clarify the early signs of impaired skin integrity for select clients and their situation and instruct the UCP to report changes in the client's skin to the nurse.

1. Assist client to assume comfortable position.
2. Dim room lights and/or turn on soft music according to client preference.
3. Perform hand hygiene. Warm lotion in hands or place container in warm water.
4. Adjust or remove client's bed clothing.
5. Place small amount of lotion in hands.

Critical Decision Point

Clients who have had neck or spinal trauma and/or surgery should not have back or neck massage without order by their physician.

6. Massage each body part at least 10 minutes.
   a. *Back:* Begin a sacral area massage with a circular motion (see Figure 38–11) while moving upward from buttocks to shoulders. Use a firm smooth stroke over the scapula. Continue in one smooth stroke to upper arms and laterally along sides of back down to iliac crests. Use long, gliding strokes along muscles of spine. Knead any muscles that feel tense or tight. Knead skin by gently grasping tissue between thumb and fingers. Knead upward along one side of the spine from buttocks to shoulders around nape of neck. Knead or stroke downward toward sacrum. Repeat along other side of the back.
   b. *Neck:* Support the neck at the hairline with one hand and massage up with a gliding stroke. Knead muscles on one side. Switch hands to support neck and knead other side. Stretch the neck slightly, with one hand at the top and the other at the bottom.
   c. *Arms:* Use a gliding stroke to massage from the client's wrist or forearm. With thumb and forefinger of both hands, knead muscles from forearm to shoulder. Continue kneading biceps, deltoid, and triceps muscles. Finish with gliding strokes from the wrists to the shoulder.
   d. *Hands:* Slowly open the client's palm; glide fingers over the palmar surface. Use thumbs to apply friction to the palm and move thumbs in a circular motion; stretch the palm outward. Massage each finger using a corkscrew-like motion from base of finger to the tip. Gently knead each muscle in the client's fingers. Glide hands smoothly from fingertips to wrists. Repeat for other hand.
   e. *Feet:* Gently massage the top and bottom of each foot. Using gliding motion, massage from heel to toe. Gently massage the dorsal surface of the foot and each toe. Repeat for other foot.

Critical Decision Point

Do not massage client's legs or calf muscle.

7. Wipe excess lotion off client's back, neck, or extremity. If necessary, retie gown or assist with pyjamas and assist client to comfortable position.
8. Ask client about level of comfort. Note any areas of muscle pain or tension.

about addiction, anxiety over errors in using opioid analgesics, and administration of less medication than was ordered.

There are three types of analgesics: (1) non-steroidal anti-inflammatory drugs (NSAIDs) and non-opioids, (2) **opioids** (traditionally called narcotics), and (3) adjuvants. NSAIDs generally provide relief for mild to moderate acute intermittent pain, such as headache pain. Treatment of mild to moderate post-operative pain should begin with an NSAID unless contraindicated (AHCPR, 1992). Although the exact mechanism of action is unknown, NSAIDs are believed to act by inhibiting the synthesis of prostaglandins (Halverson, 1999), thus inhibiting the cellular responses during inflammation. Most NSAIDs act on peripheral nerve receptors to reduce transmission and reception of pain stimuli. Unlike opioids, NSAIDs do not depress the central nervous system, nor do they interfere with bowel or bladder function (AHCPR, 1992). Chronic NSAID use in the older client, though, is associated with more frequent adverse effects (gastrointestinal bleeding and renal insufficiency) and

Box 38-13 Controlling Painful Stimuli in the Client's Environment

Tighten and smooth wrinkled bed linen.
Loosen constricting bandages (unless specifically applied as a pressure dressing).
Change wet dressings and linens.
Position client in anatomical alignment.
Check temperature of hot or cold applications, including bath water.
Lift client in bed—do not pull.
Position client correctly on bedpan.
Avoid exposing skin or mucous membranes to irritants (e.g., urine, stool, wound drainage).
Prevent urinary retention by keeping Foley catheters patent and free flowing.
Prevent constipation with fluids, diet, and exercise.
Reduce lighting and ambient sound.

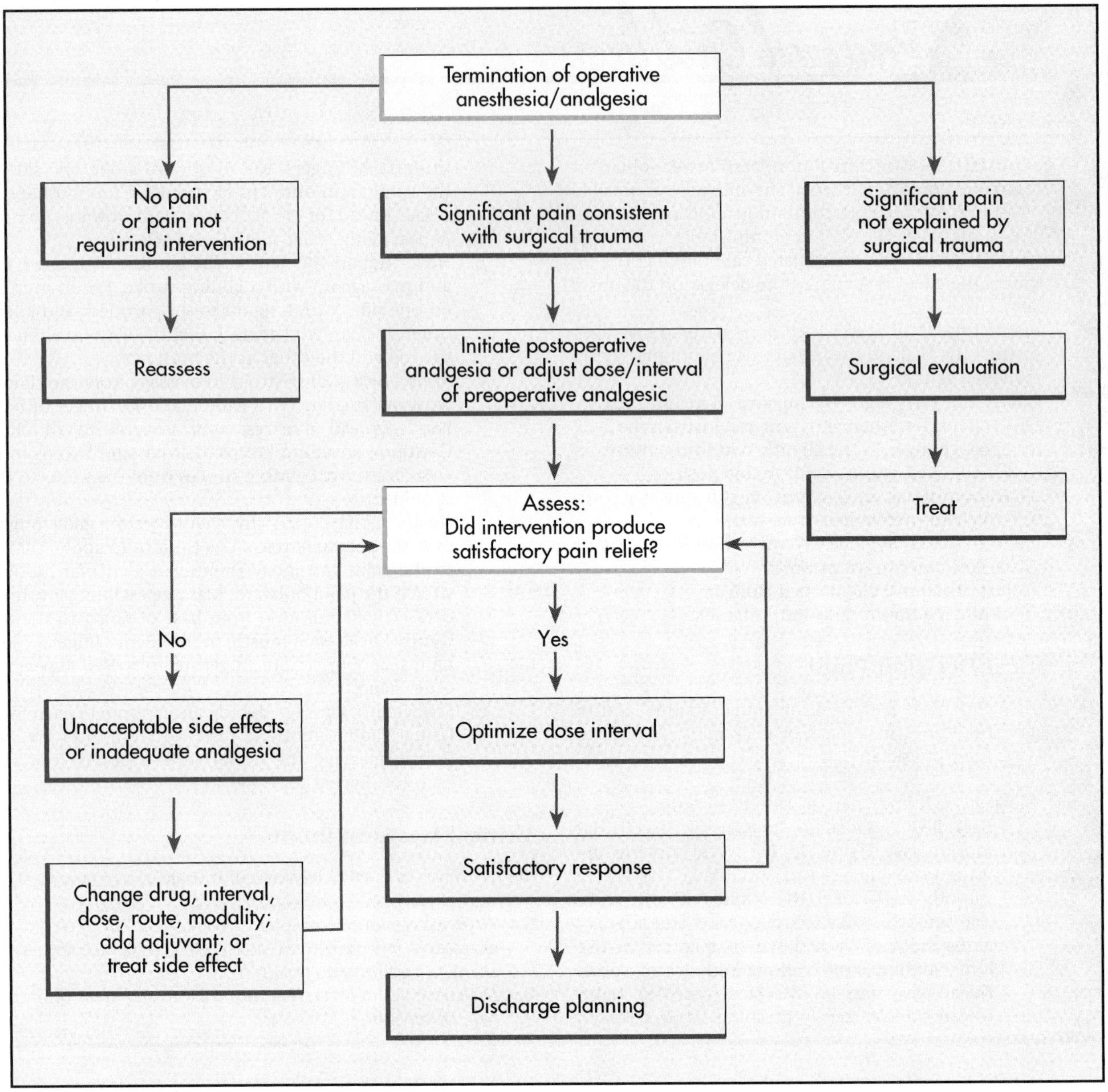

FIGURE **38–12** Pain treatment flow chart: post-operative phase. (From *Acute Pain Management: Operative or Medical Procedures and Trauma. Clinical Practice Guideline,* AHCPR Publication No. 92-0032, Agency for Health Care Policy and Research, Acute Pain Management Guideline Panel, 1992, Rockville, MD: Agency for Health Care Policy and Research, Public Health Service, U.S. Department of Health and Human Services.)

should be avoided. Mild to moderate musculoskeletal pain in older adults is effectively managed with the non-opioid acetaminophen (American Geriatrics Society [AGS], 2002).

Opioid or opioid-like analgesics are generally prescribed for moderate to severe acute pain, such as post-operative pain. They may also be ordered for chronic non-cancer and cancer pain. They act on the central nervous system to produce a combination of depressing and stimulating effects. These analgesics, when given orally or by injection, act on higher centres of the brain and spinal cord by binding with opiate receptors to modify perception of pain. A risk of opioid and opioid-like analgesics is depression of vital nervous system functions. Opiates depress the respiratory centre within the brain stem. However, this is rare (Wheeler et al., 2002). Respiratory depression is only clinically significant if there is a decrease in the rate *and* depth of respirations from the client's baseline assessment (McCaffery & Pasero, 1999). Clients who are breathing deeply rarely have clinical respiratory depression. It is important to note that sedation *always* occurs before respiratory depression. Thus, the nurse should closely monitor opioid-naive clients who are receiving opioids for sedation (Pasero & McCaffery, 2002).

Box 38-14 Nursing Principles for Administering Analgesics

Know the Client's Previous Response to Analgesics

Determine whether the client has allergies.
Know whether client is at risk for using opioids (e.g., history of obstructive sleep apnea).
Identify previous doses and routes of analgesic administration to avoid undertreatment.
Determine whether relief was obtained.
Ask whether a non-opioid was as effective as an opioid.

Select Proper Medications When More Than One Is Ordered

Use non-opioid analgesics or opioid combination drugs for mild to moderate pain.
Know that non-opioids can be given with opioids.
In older adults, avoid combinations of opioids.
Remember that morphine and hydromorphone are the opioids of choice for long-term management of severe pain.
Know that intravenous medications act more quickly and can relieve severe, acute pain within 1 hour and that oral medication may take as long as 2 hours to relieve pain.
Understand that intramuscular analgesics should be avoided, especially in older adults.
Use an opioid with a non-opioid analgesic for severe pain because such combinations treat pain peripherally and centrally.
For chronic pain, give sustained-release oral formulations around the clock.

Know the Accurate Dosage

Recall that 4 g is considered the maximum 24-hour dose for acetaminophen and acetylsalicylic acid (ASA); 3200 mg is the maximum for ibuprofen.
Adjust doses, as appropriate, for children and older clients.
Bear in mind that large doses of opioids are acceptable in opioid-tolerant clients, but not opioid-naive clients.
Recognize that when titrating opioids, it is important to titrate to effect or to uncontrollable side effects.

Assess the Right Time and Interval for Administration

Administer analgesics in anticipation of pain, when pain occurs, and before it increases in severity, as appropriate. The goal is to prevent breakthrough episodes of pain.
An around-the-clock (ATC) administration schedule is usually best because this will prevent occurrences of breakthrough pain, thus helping keep pain under control.
Give analgesics before pain-producing procedures or activities.
Know the average duration of action for a drug and the time of administration so that the peak effect occurs when the pain is most intense.
Use extended-release opioid formulations to treat chronic pain.

Adapted from *Pain: Clinical Manual* (2nd ed.), by M. McCaffery and C. Pasero, 1999, St. Louis, MO: Mosby and *The significance of breakthrough pain in cancer,* by S.M. Colleau, 1999, *Cancer Pain Release, 12.* Retrieved February, 14, 2005, from *http://www.whocancerpain.wisc.edu/eng/12_4/significance.html*

Clients can experience side effects such as nausea, vomiting, constipation, and altered mental processes. Except for constipation, these side effects usually stop once the client has been receiving the opioid around-the-clock (ATC) for 4 to 7 days. One way to maximize pain relief while minimizing drug toxicity is to administer the medication on a regular ATC basis rather than on an as-needed (prn) basis. The Canadian Pain Society (Jovey et al., 2002), the APS (1999), and the AHCPR (1992) have stated that if pain is anticipated for the majority of the day, ATC administration should be considered. This is to prevent breakthrough pain, which is hard to control once it appears.

Opioids are effective in older adults. Although there is controversy about the use of opioids for chronic non-cancer pain in all age groups, the AGS (2002) stated that opioids are probably not used enough with older people. The AGS suggests a "start low" (dose) and "go slow" (upward dose titration) philosophy. In addition, several professional organizations have developed position statements advocating the use of opioids for non-cancer pain after careful client assessment.

The proper use of analgesics requires careful assessment and critical thinking in the application of pharmacological principles and logic (Box 38-14). A person's response to an analgesic is highly individualized. An NSAID may be as or more effective than an opioid for some clients if the pain is due to inflammation. An orally administered analgesic usually has a longer duration of action than an injectable form. Nurses must stay familiar with comparative doses of different analgesics. In addition, nurses must know the route of administration most effective for a client so that controlled, sustained pain relief is achieved.

The nurse should always know the comparative potencies of analgesics in oral and injectable form. If nurses on succeeding shifts choose different routes for the same doses, the client will not receive the same level of analgesia and pain control will be poor. Nurses must provide controlled, sustained pain relief. Equianalgesic charts are available on most nursing units or by contacting pharmacy staff. The charts convert parenteral forms to oral forms and give equivalent doses of different opioids (e.g., morphine to hydromorphone).

Adjuvants are drugs with analgesic properties that were not originally developed to relieve pain. Tricyclic antidepressants and anticonvulsants are used to successfully treat neuropathic pain (Collins et al., 2000). Corticosteroids are used to relieve pain associated with inflammation and bone metastasis. Other adjuvants are bisphosphonates and calcitonin given for bone pain (Jacox et al., 1994). Additional adjuvants are also available.

Although sedatives, antianxiety agents, and muscle relaxants may be ordered with opioids to enhance pain control or relieve other symptoms associated with pain, they have no analgesic effect. However, they can cause drowsiness and impairment of coordination, judgment, and mental alertness and contribute to respiratory depression. It is important for the nurse to avoid attributing these side effects to the opioid. A thorough reassessment must be conducted.

Patient-Controlled Analgesia. Clients benefit from having control over pain therapy. When clients depend on nurses for prn analgesia, an erratic cycle of alternating pain and analgesia often occurs. The client feels pain and asks for medication, but the nurse must first assess the client and then prepare the medication. Within an hour, analgesia finally occurs, but pain relief may last only 30 minutes. Then, gradually, the client again feels discomfort, and the cycle begins again. The client is constantly going in and out of analgesic therapeutic range.

A drug delivery system called **patient-controlled analgesia (PCA)** is a safe method for post-operative and cancer pain management that most clients prefer. It is a drug delivery system that allows clients to self-administer opioids (morphine, hydromorphone, fentanyl) with minimal risk of overdose. The goal is to maintain a constant plasma level of analgesic so that the problems of prn dosing are avoided. Systemic PCA usually involves IV drug administration, but it can also be given subcutaneously. PCAs are portable infusion pumps (usually computerized), containing a chamber for a syringe (Figure 38–13) or bag that delivers a small, preset dose of medication. To receive a demand dose, the client pushes a button attached to the PCA device. The system is designed to deliver no more than a specified number of doses either every hour or every 4 hours (depending on the pump) to avoid overdoses. A typical PCA prescription relies on a series of "loading" doses (e.g., 3 to 5 mg of morphine) repeated every 5 minutes until initial post-operative pain diminishes. On-demand doses typically add 1 mg morphine every 6 minutes, with a total hourly limit of 6 mg (AHCPR, 1992; APS, 1999). Most pumps have locked safety systems that prevent tampering by clients or their family members and are generally safe to be managed in the home. For clients with cancer pain, a low-dose continuous infusion (basal rate) of 0.5 to 1 mg/hour may be programmed to deliver a steady dose of continuous medication.

> ***Safety Alert.*** PCA basal doses are *not* recommended for opioid-naive clients following surgery because of the possibility for respiratory depression.

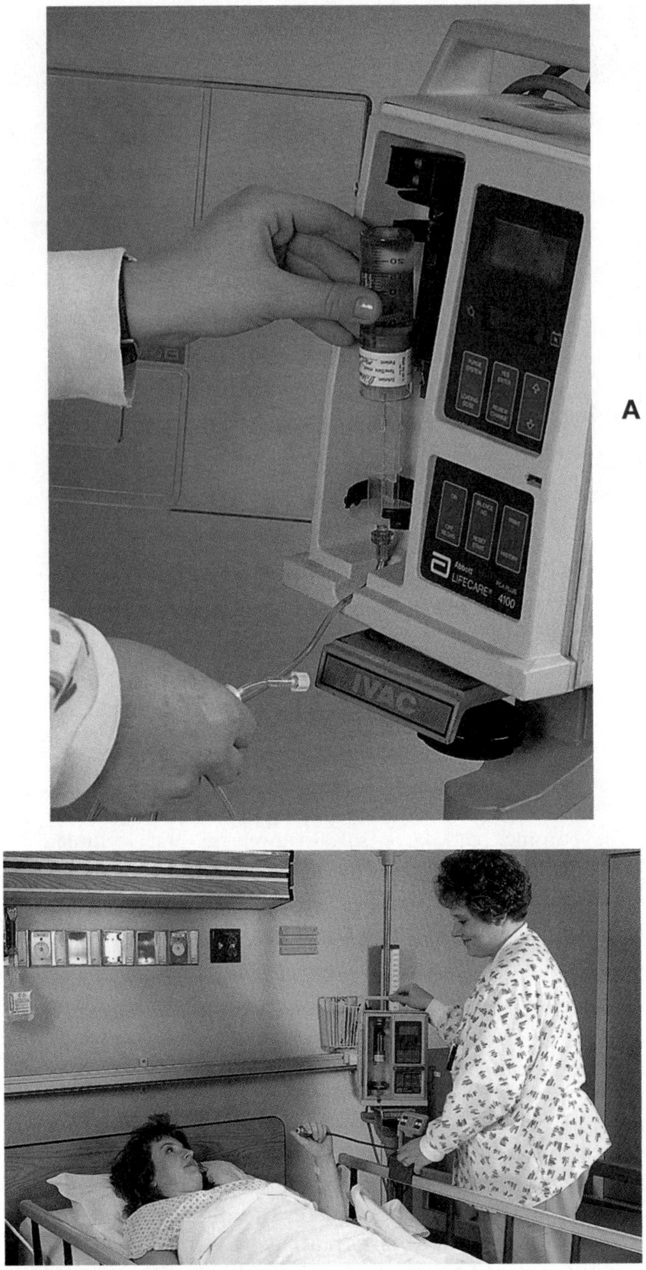

A

B

FIGURE **38–13** **A,** PCA pump with syringe chamber. **B,** Client learns to use PCA pump.

There are many benefits of PCA use. The client gains control over pain, and pain relief does not depend on nurse availability. Clients can also access medication when they need it. This can decrease anxiety and lead to decreased medication use. Small doses of medications are delivered at short intervals, stabilizing serum drug concentrations for sustained pain relief. Client preparation and teaching is critical to the safe and effective use of PCA devices (Box 38-15). Clients must be able to understand the use of the equipment and be physically able to locate and press the button to deliver the dose. Family members must be instructed not to "hit the button" for the client, as this could cause toxic effects (Reiff & Nizolek, 2001). Nurse-controlled analgesia may be implemented in lieu of client-controlled analgesia, with physician approval, after assessing the client.

Nurses must check the IV line and PCA device regularly to ensure proper functioning. Even though clients control administration of analgesics, the nurse must routinely check that the PCA device operates correctly. In opioid-naive clients, do not increase demand or basal dose *and* shorten the interval time simultaneously because this will increase the risk for oversedation and respiratory depression. The nurse also documents drug dosages and tracks any waste of medications according to agency policy (Pasero, 2003).

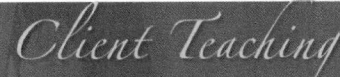

Client Teaching Box 38-15

Preparation for Patient-Controlled Analgesia (PCA)

Objectives

- Client will be able to explain purpose of PCA in managing pain.
- Client will use the PCA device correctly.
- Client achieves pain control.

Teaching Strategies

- Teach the use of PCA before any procedure so that clients can understand how to use it after awakening from anaesthesia or sedation. Reinforce as needed.
- Instruct client on the purpose of PCA, emphasizing that the client controls medication delivery.
- Explain that the pump prevents the risk of overdose.
- Tell family members or friends that they should not operate the PCA device for the client.
- Have the client demonstrate use of the PCA delivery button.

Evaluation

- Ask client to tell you the purpose of the PCA device.
- Observe the client administering a dose.
- Evaluate the severity of the client's pain 15 to 20 minutes after use of the PCA device.

Local Analgesic Infusion Pump. Following orthopedic surgery, to avoid systemic effects of oral analgesics, an application of a local anaesthetic may be appropriate. A catheter from the wound placed during surgery is connected to a pump containing a local anaesthetic (Marcaine). The pump may be set as a demand or continuous mode. The device is usually left in place for 48 hours. The client is taught how to discontinue the pump at home and to bring the catheter to the next physician visit. Oral analgesics may still be needed by the client, but the total dose is often reduced (Pasero, 2000). Safe use of the pump in surgeries other than orthopedic has not yet been established.

Topical Analgesics and Anaesthetics. A topical anaesthetic often used on children is EMLA (eutectic mixture of local anaesthetics). This anaesthetic disk or cream (thickly applied) is placed on the skin 15 minutes before local anaesthetic infiltration or minor procedures (e.g., IV start). EMLA should not be placed around eyes, the tympanic membrane, or over large skin surfaces. The Lidoderm patch is a topical analgesic effective for cutaneous neuropathic pain. Three patches are placed on and around the pain site using a 12-hour on, 12-hour off schedule to avoid lidocaine toxicity.

Local and Regional Anaesthetics and Analgesics. **Local anaesthesia** is the infiltration of a local anaesthetic medication to induce loss of sensation to a localized body part. Physicians use local anaesthesia during brief surgical procedures such as removal of a skin lesion or suturing a wound. Local anaesthetics can be applied topically on skin and mucous membranes or injected subcutaneously or intradermally to anaesthetize a body part. The drugs produce temporary loss of sensation by inhibiting nerve conduction. Local anaesthetics can also block motor and autonomic functions depending on the amount used and the location and depth of an injection. Smaller sensory nerve fibres are more sensitive to local anaesthetics than are large motor fibres. As a result, the client loses sensation before losing motor function, and conversely, motor activity returns before sensation.

Local anaesthetics can cause side effects, depending on their absorption into the circulation. Itching or burning of the skin or a localized rash is common after topical applications. Application to vascular mucous membranes increases the chance of systemic effects, such as a change in heart rate. Injection of anaesthetics increases the risk of systemic side effects, depending on the amount of drug used and the area injected. Each medication produces a different level of anaesthesia as a result of the amount of anaesthetic used and location of the spinal nerve affected.

Regional anaesthesia is the injection of a local anaesthetic to block a group of sensory nerve fibres. Tissues are anaesthetized layer by layer, as the surgeon or anaesthesiologist introduces the agent into deeper structures of the body. Kinds of regional anaesthesia include epidural anaesthesia, pudendal blocks, and spinal anaesthesia.

Whereas an epidural anaesthesia induces temporary loss of sensation, an **epidural analgesia** permits control or reduction of severe pain, without the more serious sedative effects of parenteral or oral narcotics. Epidural analgesia is commonly used for the treatment of acute post-operative pain, labour and delivery pain, and chronic pain, especially that associated with cancer (Cox, 2001). However, intraspinal morphine can produce the same side effects of nausea, mental clouding, and sedation, because it is absorbed via the cerebrospinal fluid into the circulation of the epidural vascular plexus. Epidural analgesia can be short or long term, depending on the client's condition and life expectancy. Short-term therapy is used for pain after intrathoracic, abdominal, and orthopedic surgery. Long-term therapy is used for intractable pain in the lower part of the body, particularly when it is bilateral (Du Pen & Williams, 1992).

Epidural analgesia is administered into the spinal **epidural space** (Figure 38–14). The physician inserts a blunt-tip needle into the level of the vertebral interspace nearest to the area requiring analgesia. When the needle reaches the space, solutions may be freely injected and small catheters may be passed into it. Once a catheter is advanced into the epidural space and the needle is removed, the remainder of the catheter is secured with a dressing and taped along the back of the client (Figure 38–15). If the catheter is only temporary, it is connected to tubing positioned along the spine and over the client's shoulder. The end of the catheter can then be placed on the client's chest for the nurse's access. Epidural analgesia may be anaesthesiology or nurse controlled, depending on agency policy. Clients may also be given control of the demand dose, known as patient-controlled epidural analgesia (PCEA).

Nursing Implications. The nurse provides emotional support to clients receiving local or regional anaesthesia

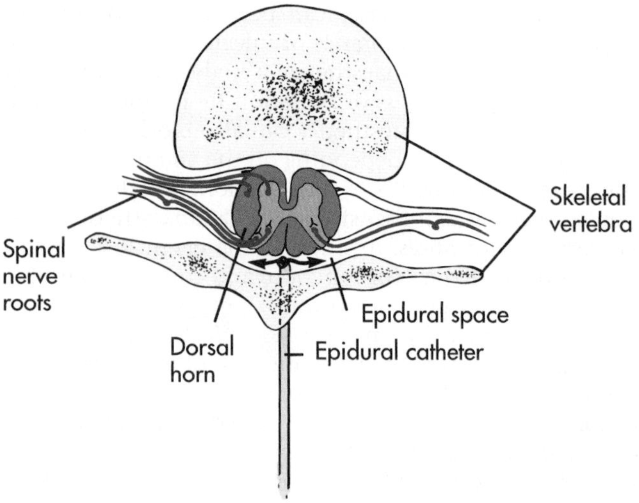

FIGURE **38–14** Anatomical drawing of epidural space.

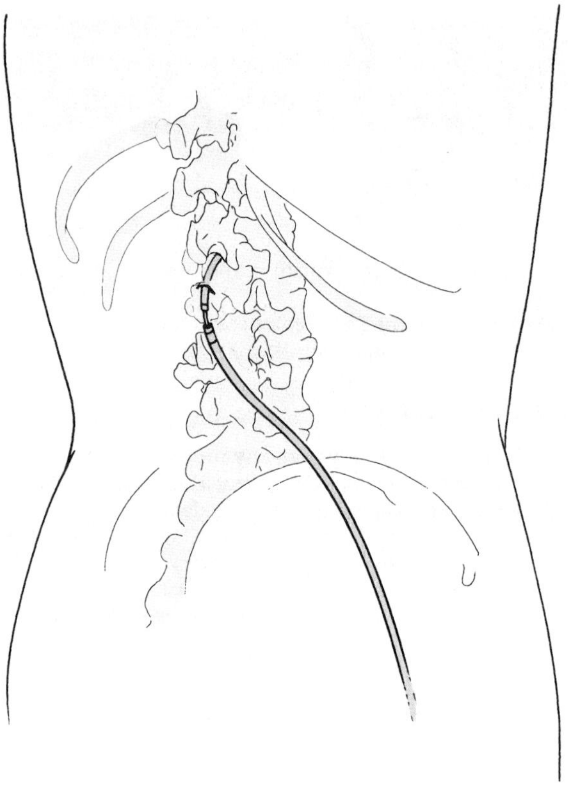

FIGURE **38–15** Epidural catheter taped in place.

by explaining insertion or application sites and warning clients that they will temporarily lose sensory function. In the case of regional anaesthesia, the nurse must explain when motor and autonomic function are expected to be temporarily lost. It is common for clients to fear paralysis because epidural and spinal injections come close to the spinal cord. Autonomic function (bowel and bladder control) may also be temporarily lost. To reassure the client, the nurse explains the sensations to be experienced. Injection can be painful unless the physician first numbs the injection site. The nurse prepares clients for such discomfort. Before a client receives an anaesthetic, the nurse checks for allergies. To monitor systemic effects, the nurse assesses blood pressure and pulse. Spinal anaesthesia may also cause respiratory changes.

After administration of a local anaesthetic, the nurse protects the client from injury until full sensory and motor function return. Until a local anaesthetic is absorbed and metabolized, the client must be careful in using an anaesthetized body part. Clients can easily injure themselves without knowing it. For example, after an injection into a joint, the nurse warns the client to avoid using the joint until function returns. For clients with topical anaesthesia, the nurse avoids applying heat or cold to numb areas. After spinal anaesthesia, the client stays in bed until sensory and motor function return. The nurse helps the client during the first attempt to get out of bed.

For epidural infusions, the catheter is connected to an epidural infusion pump, a port, or reservoir or is capped off for bolus injections. The catheter should be clearly labelled "epidural catheter" to reduce the risk of accidental epidural injection of drugs intended for IV use. Continuous infusions must be administered through electronic infusion devices for proper control. Because of the catheter location, strict surgical asepsis is needed to prevent a serious and potentially fatal infection. Physicians are notified immediately of any signs or symptoms of infection or pain at the insertion site. Thorough nursing care is needed during hygiene procedures to keep the catheter system clean and dry.

The nursing implications for managing epidural analgesia are numerous (Table 38-6). Supplemental doses of opioids or sedative/hypnotics are avoided because of possible additive central nervous system adverse effects. Monitoring of medications' effects differs, depending on whether infusions are intermittent or continuous. Complications of epidural opioid use include nausea and vomiting, urinary retention, constipation, respiratory depression, and **pruritus** (Cox, 2001). When clients are receiving epidural analgesia, monitoring occurs as often as every 15 minutes, including assessment of respiratory rate, respiratory effort, and skin colour. Once stabilized, monitoring can move to every hour (refer to agency policy).

The client must receive thorough education about epidural analgesia in terms of the action of the medication and its advantages and disadvantages. Clients should know about the potential for side effects and should be instructed to notify a health care provider if they develop. If the client requires long-term epidural use, a permanent catheter may be tunnelled through the skin and exit at the client's side. A client on long-term therapy can be taught to safely administer infusions in the home with minimal ongoing intervention by the nurse.

Surgical Interventions for Pain Relief. When a client's pain persists despite medical treatment, surgical interventions may give relief. Neurosurgical treatment is appropriate for clients in whom more conservative treatment is neither tolerated nor effective (Jacox et al., 1994).

Table 38-6 Nursing Care for Clients With Epidural Infusions

Goal	Actions
Prevent catheter displacement.	Secure catheter (if not connected to implanted reservoir) carefully to outside skin.
Maintain catheter function.	Check external dressing around catheter site for dampness or discharge. (Leak of cerebrospinal fluid may develop.) Use transparent dressing to secure catheter and to aid inspection. Inspect catheter for breaks.
Prevent infection.	Use strict aseptic technique when caring for catheter (see chapter 29). Do not routinely change dressing over site. Change infusion tubing every 24 hours.
Monitor for respiratory depression.	Monitor vital signs, especially respirations, per agency policy. Pulse oximetry and apnea monitoring may be used.
Prevent undesirable complications.	Assess for pruritus (itching) and nausea and vomiting. Administer antiemetics as ordered.
Maintain urinary and bowel function.	Monitor intake and output. Assess for bladder and bowel distension. Assess for discomfort, frequency, and urgency.

The risks include new pain symptoms from nerve damage or nerve division, recurrence of pain, and post-operative neurological impairment. Surgery involves resection of either peripheral nerve roots or pain pathways in the spinothalamic tract. For example, a **dorsal rhizotomy** involves surgically cutting the dorsal (posterior) nerve roots as they enter the spinal cord. It is effective for relieving localized acute pain in the area supplied by the nerve root and deep visceral pain. The client loses sensation of pain but retains full motor function. A **chordotomy** is more extensive and involves resection of the spinothalamic tract. The procedure is used to treat unrelieved pain. The risks of the procedure are great because permanent paralysis may result from edema of the spinal cord or accidental resection of motor nerves. After the procedure, the client has a permanent loss of pain and temperature sensation in the affected areas.

When nurses care for these clients, they need to be aware of the area of resection to assess for paresthesia, change in temperature sensation, and loss of motor function. When performed correctly, these procedures can relieve persistent pain without causing serious neurological deficits. Additional invasive pain-relieving procedures available for intractable pain include spinal cord stimulators and vertebroplasty.

Procedure Pain Management. The Thunder Project II (Puntillo et al., 2001) identified several procedures in critical care clients that cause pain:

- Turning
- Wound drain removal
- Tracheal suctioning
- Femoral catheter removal
- Placement of central line
- Changing of non-burn wound dressings

Premedicating clients before painful procedures allows clients to co-operate more fully and reduces the experience of pain. This is also true for clients with abdominal pain who present in the emergency department. APS (1999) recommended medicating the client in pain before conducting an extensive physical examination or diagnostic procedures.

Chronic Non-Cancer and Cancer Pain Management. Cancer pain can be chronic or acute. The AHCPR released clinical practice guidelines for the management of cancer pain (Jacox et al., 1994). The guidelines are designed to treat cancer pain in a more comprehensive and aggressive manner. Similarly, they provide clients and families more options for pain relief. Figure 38–16 is a flow chart depicting cancer pain management from assessment to various treatment options. The best choice of treatment often changes as the client's condition and the characteristics of pain change. Non-pharmacological interventions and pharmacological interventions can be used together.

Various medications and routes of administration can provide relief for clients with cancer pain. Relatively new oral analgesics have fewer side effects. Long-acting or controlled-release medications have successfully managed both cancer and non-cancer pain. These controlled-released medications (e.g., MS Contin, Roxanol SR, and OxyContin) can provide pain relief for 6 to 12 hours. Although most non-cancer and cancer pain can be managed by using oral medications, other routes are sometimes required. Epidural analgesia and intrathecal infusions (administration of opioids via catheters placed within the brain's ventricles) have been highly effective with select clients.

Estimates of addiction in clients with chronic pain range from 1% to 24% (Passik, Kirsh, & Portenoy, 2002). It has been demonstrated that clients with persistent pain requiring prolonged opioid administration can develop an opioid tolerance. As a result, clients require higher doses of opioids to attain pain relief. The higher opioid dose is not lethal because clients also develop a tolerance to respiratory depression.

Clients with chronic pain should be given required analgesics on a regular basis. Prescribing analgesics on a prn basis for chronic pain is ineffective and causes more

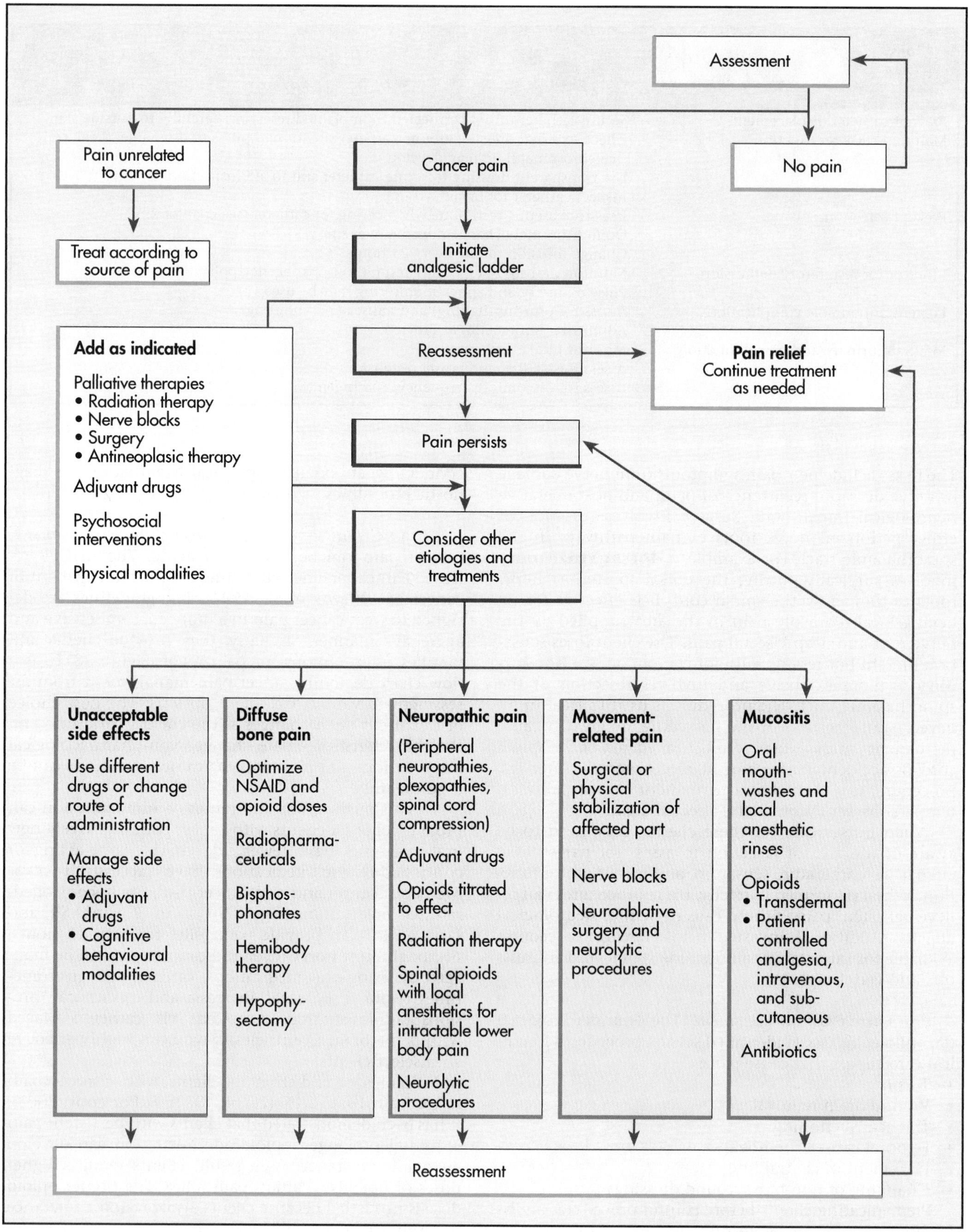

FIGURE **38–16** Flow chart: continuing pain management in clients with cancer. (From *Management of Cancer Pain. Clinical Practice Guideline No. 9,* AHCPR Publication No. 94-0592, by A. Jacox et al., 1994, Rockville, MD: Agency for Health Care Policy and Research, Public Health Service, U.S. Department of Health and Human Services.)

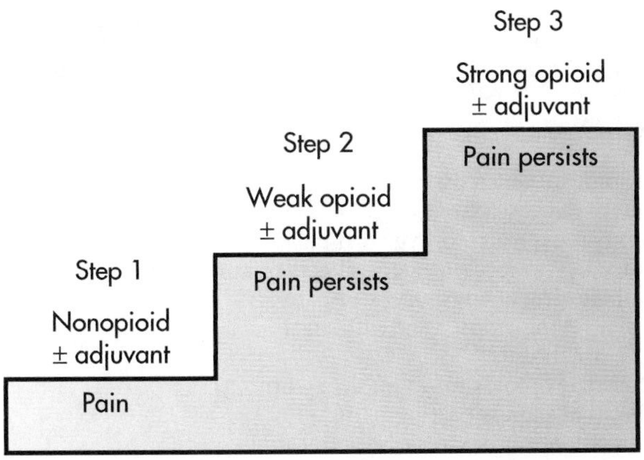

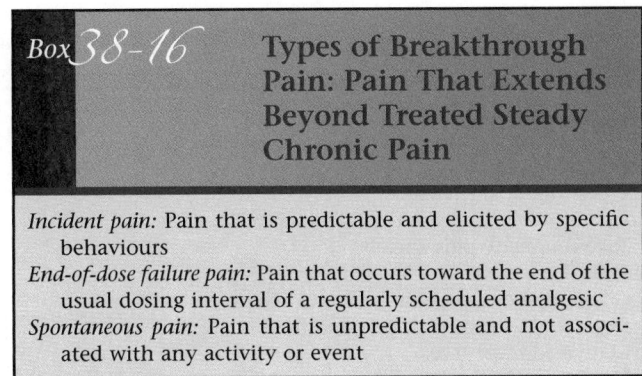

FIGURE **38–17** WHO analgesic ladder is a three-step approach to using drugs in cancer pain management. ± *adjuvant,* With or without adjuvant medications. (From *Cancer Pain Relief and Palliative Care: Report of a WHO Expert Committee,* WHO Tech Rep Series No. 804, World Health Organization, 1990, Geneva, Switzerland: Author.)

suffering. The client with chronic pain must take an analgesic regularly, even when the pain subsides. Regular administration maintains therapeutic drug blood levels for ongoing pain control.

Principles used in administering analgesics to treat chronic non-cancer and cancer pain are different from those used to treat acute pain. The World Health Organization (1990) recommended a three-step approach to managing cancer pain (Figure 38–17). Therapy begins with using NSAIDs and/or adjuvants and progresses to strong opioids if pain persists. However, when a client with cancer first experiences pain, it is best to begin with a higher dosage than will be needed for continued pain relief. The physician can slowly decrease the dosage to the amount needed, thus providing the client with immediate pain relief. Side effects of analgesia, such as nausea and constipation, can be aggressively treated, so that analgesia can be continued. Clients can become tolerant to the side effects of nausea but not to the constipating effects of analgesics. Stimulant laxatives, not simple stool softeners, should be routinely administered both to prevent and to treat constipation.

Transdermal drug systems administer fentanyl at predetermined doses for up to 48 to 72 hours. Fentanyl is about 100 times more potent than morphine.

> ***Safety Alert.*** Fentanyl should *only* be used in clients who are opioid tolerant.

The transdermal route is useful when clients are unable to take drugs orally. Clients find these systems easy to use, and they allow for continuous opioid administration without needles or pumps. Self-adhesive patches release the medication slowly over time, achieving effective analgesia. Caution is needed in administering transdermal patches to adult clients who weigh less than 45 kg (too little subcutaneous tissue for absorption) or who are hyperthermic. Hyperthermia causes more rapid drug absorption. The patch should never be cut; it must be disposed of according to agency policy.

A transmucosal fentanyl "unit" has been developed to treat **breakthrough pain** (Box 38-16) in opioid-tolerant clients. It is placed in the client's mouth and swabbed over the inside of the cheeks and lower gums. The unit needs to be left intact and not chewed, but allowed to dissolve and be absorbed for 15 minutes. No more than two units should be used per breakthrough pain episode. If pain is not relieved, the physician should be notified. Research on breakthrough pain is still developing and nurses need to stay current on best evidence to support treatment approaches. The CIHR has recently funded Canadian researchers to advance pharmacological approaches to treat breakthrough and others kinds of pain experienced by those receiving palliative and end-of-life care. (See Colleau [1999] for a more in-depth discussion on cancer-related breakthrough pain.)

Box 38-16 Types of Breakthrough Pain: Pain That Extends Beyond Treated Steady Chronic Pain

Incident pain: Pain that is predictable and elicited by specific behaviours
End-of-dose failure pain: Pain that occurs toward the end of the usual dosing interval of a regularly scheduled analgesic
Spontaneous pain: Pain that is unpredictable and not associated with any activity or event

Analgesics may be given rectally when clients have nausea and vomiting or are fasting before or after surgery (Jacox et al., 1994). This route is contraindicated if clients have diarrhea or if cancerous lesions involve the anus or rectum. Morphine, hydromorphone, and oxymorphone are available in suppositories.

Another way to treat severe cancer pain in the home or acute care setting is with continuous infusions or a basal rate on a PCA device. This provides improved, uniform pain control with fewer peaks and valleys in plasma concentration, more effective drug action, and lower drug dosages overall. Candidates for continuous infusions include clients with severe pain for whom oral and injectable medications provide minimal relief, clients with severe nausea and vomiting, and clients unable to swallow oral medications. The intramuscular route should not be used for controlling cancer pain because the injection itself is painful and there is inconsistent, erratic absorption of the drug.

When a client is first given continuous-drip morphine sulphate, it is essential that the IV access be patent and that the IV site be without complications (see chapter 36). A central line catheter such as a Groshong or Hickman catheter, an implanted venous access port, or a peripherally inserted central catheter is usually best suited for long-term IV infusion. When IV access is poor, the subcutaneous route with a concentrated dose is possible. When infusions begin, the client continues to be monitored.

Box 38-17 Barriers to Effective Pain Management

Client Barriers

Fear of addiction
Worry about side effects
Fear of tolerance (won't be there when I need it)
Take too many pills already
Fear of injections
Concern about not being a "good" client
Don't want to worry family and friends
May need more tests
Need to suffer to be cured
Pain is for past indiscretions
Inadequate education
Reluctance to discuss pain
Pain is inevitable
Pain is part of aging
Fear of disease progression
Physicians and nurses are doing all that they can
Just forget to take analgesics
Weak in character
Fear of distracting physicians from treating illness
Physicians have more important or ill clients to see
Suffering in silence is noble and expected

Health Care Provider Barriers

Inadequate pain assessment
Concern with addiction
Opiophobia, fear of opioids
Fear of legal repercussions
No visible cause of pain
Clients must learn to live with pain
Reluctance to deal with side effects of analgesics
Not believing client's report of pain
Fear of giving a dose that will kill the client
Time constraints
Belief that opioids may "mask" symptoms
Belief that pain is part of aging
Overestimation of rates of respiratory depression

Health Care System Barriers

Concern with creating "addicts"
Ability to fill prescriptions
Nurse practitioners and physician assistants not used efficiently
Extensive documentation requirements
Poor pain policies and procedures regarding pain management
Lack of money
Inadequate access to pain clinics
Poor understanding of economic impact of unrelieved pain

Clients placed on continuous analgesic infusions are not usually opioid naive, and thus respiratory depression is rare.

In the home, clients may use ambulatory infusion pumps. These are small devices, often no larger than a deck of cards, that contain a 1- to 30-day supply of medication. The pumps are lightweight and allow free movement. The pump is battery powered and worn in a pouch attached to a belt or harness. The bag of medication and IV fluid fits inside the pump.

Although the pumps are programmed by health care professionals, clients or families must be highly motivated to care for the pump properly. The client must show the capacity to learn the procedures and to assume responsibility for proper pump operation (Bernstein et al., 1993). The client must also be physically capable of adjusting the pump (e.g., change batteries). The client and family learn to manage the pump, to observe for side effects, and to maintain function of the central venous catheter. Because the client is initially managed with opioids in the hospital, the risk of side effects is not as great unless the client or family member increases the dosage. A home care nurse makes routine visits to ensure that the client manages the pump correctly. The nurse routinely changes the IV fluid bag and tubing to maintain sterility of the system.

Barriers to Effective Pain Management. Barriers to pain management can be complex, involving the client, health care provider, and health care system (Box 38-17). A deep-seated and often inappropriate concern shared by health care providers and clients is the fear of addiction when long-term opioid use is prescribed to manage pain. There is a difference between **physical dependence, addiction,** and **drug tolerance** (Box 38-18). The nurse needs to clarify the differences for clients and other health care providers. Experiencing a physical dependency does not imply addiction, and drug tolerance in and of itself does not constitute addiction. That is not to say that addiction does not occur or that true addicts should not be treated for pain. The nurse monitors for addiction while managing pain for all clients, including addicts (Newshan, 2000).

Placebos are "sugar pills" with no active ingredient, but they can produce positive or negative responses in 30% to 50% of people who take them (Thompson, 2000). The use of placebos to treat pain is discouraged by many professional organizations. Administering placebos is considered unethical and deceitful (Tucker, 2001), jeopardizing the trust between clients and health care providers. If a placebo is ordered, the nurse must question the order and ask, "Why?" Many health care agencies have policies that limit placebo use to research only.

Restorative and Continuing Care

Pain Clinics, Palliative Care, and Hospices. In recent years, health professionals have recognized pain as a significant health problem (The SUPPORT Principal Investigators, 1995), and as a result, programs have been

Box 38-18 Definitions Related to the Use of Opioids in Pain Treatment

Physical Dependence

A state of adaptation that is manifested by a drug class-specific withdrawal syndrome that can be produced by abrupt cessation, rapid dose reduction, decreasing blood level of the drug, and/or administration of an antagonist.

Drug Tolerance

A state of adaptation in which exposure to a drug induces changes that result in a diminution of one or more of the drug's effects over time.

Addiction

A primary, chronic, neurobiologic disease, with genetic, psychosocial, and environmental factors influencing its development and manifestations. It is characterized by behaviours that include one or more of the following: impaired control over drug use, compulsive use, continued use despite harm, and craving.

Pseudoaddiction

Client behaviours (drug seeking) that may occur when pain is undertreated.

Pseudotolerance

Need to increase opioid dose for reasons other than opioid tolerance: progression of disease, onset of new disorder, increased physical activity, lack of adherence, change in opioid formulation, drug-drug interaction, drug-food interaction (Wall & Melzack, 1999).

Approved by the Boards of Directors of the American Academy of Pain Medicine, The American Pain Society, and the American Society of Addiction Medicine, February 2001.

Also refer to *The Use of Opioids in the Management of Opioid Dependence, Health Canada (http://dsp-psd.communication.gc.ca/Collection/H42-2-57-1992E.pdf);* and *Alberta Palliative Care Resource (http://www.albertapalliative.net/APN/PCHB/F_OpioidAnalgesics. html).*

designed for pain management. Pain clinics may offer several options. A comprehensive pain centre can treat clients on an inpatient or outpatient basis, conduct research into new treatments, and train professionals. Health professionals from various disciplines, such as nursing, medicine, physiotherapy, pastoral care, and dietetics, work with clients to find effective pain-relief measures.

Many hospitals have palliative care teams to assist clients and families to manage their diseases (Ferrell & Coyle, 2001). Learning to live life fully with an incurable condition is the goal of palliative care (see chapter 25). Clients and their family members must be given ongoing assistance in managing their pain at home (Schumacher et al., 2002).

In Canada, palliative and end-of-life care are emerging fields. The CIHR is supporting research and program development in palliative and end-of-life care—including those programs associated with hospice care. Hospices are programs for care of clients at the end of life. The term *hospice* comes from the Latin word *hospes,* which means "a place to rest." Often, hospice programs are affiliated with hospitals. The programs help terminally ill clients continue to live at home in comfort and privacy with the help of a hospice health care team. Pain control is a priority for hospices. Clients receive the proper dosage and form of analgesics that provide pain relief. Under the guidance of hospice nurses, families learn to monitor clients' symptoms and be primary caregivers. A hospice client may be hospitalized in the event of an acute care crisis or family problem.

Hospice programs help nurses overcome their fears of contributing to a client's death when administering large doses of opioids. Recent research suggests that dying clients suffer less and live longer with opioid administration at the end of life (Thorns & Sykes, 2000). It is the disease that is killing the client, not the treatment of pain.

NP Evaluation

Client Care. The evaluation of pain is one of many nursing responsibilities that require critical thinking (Figure 38–18). The client's behavioural responses to pain-relief interventions are not always obvious. The nurse must be an intent observer and know what responses to anticipate on the basis of the type of pain, the intervention, the timing of the interventions, the physiological nature of the injury or disease, and the client's previous responses. The nurse evaluates psychological as well as physiological responses to pain.

If a client continues to have discomfort after an intervention, a different approach may be needed. For example, if an analgesic provides only partial relief, the nurse may add relaxation exercises or guided-imagery exercises. The nurse may also consult with the physician about increasing the dosage, decreasing the interval between doses, or trying different analgesics.

The nurse evaluates the client's perceptions of the effectiveness of interventions. The client may help decide the best times to attempt a treatment. The nurse also evaluates tolerance to therapy and the overall relief obtained. For example, if a nurse administers an analgesic, side effects from the medication and the client's reported pain relief must be assessed. Similarly, after turning a client, the nurse should return to determine whether the client is tolerating the new position and whether pain has subsided. If an intervention aggravates discomfort, the nurse stops it immediately and seeks an alternative. Time and patience are necessary to maximize the effectiveness of pain management. The nurse evaluates the entire pain experience to determine interventions that are most effective and times that they should be administered.

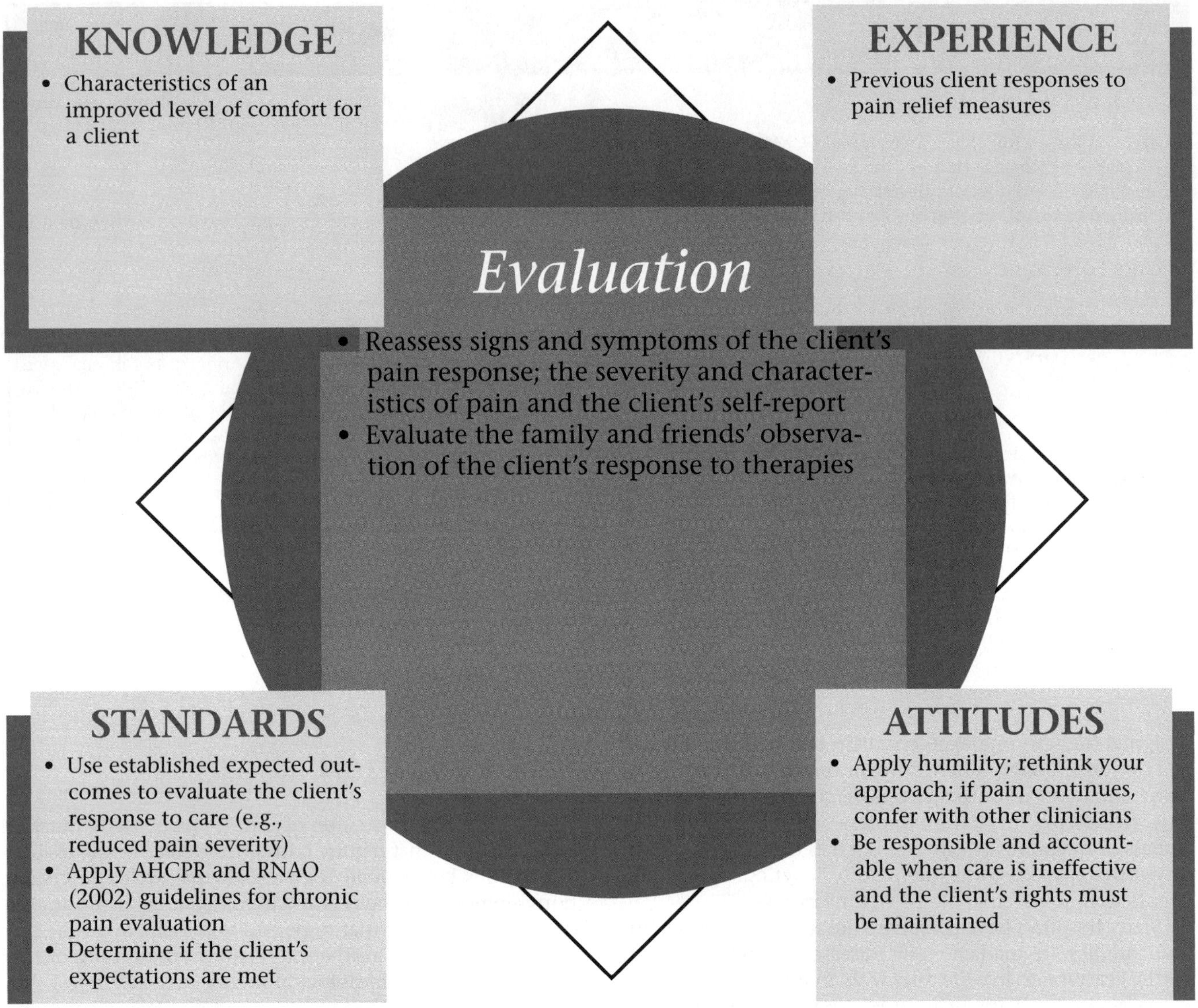
KNOWLEDGE
• Characteristics of an improved level of comfort for a client
EXPERIENCE
• Previous client responses to pain relief measures
Evaluation
• Reassess signs and symptoms of the client's pain response; the severity and characteristics of pain and the client's self-report
• Evaluate the family and friends' observation of the client's response to therapies
STANDARDS
• Use established expected outcomes to evaluate the client's response to care (e.g., reduced pain severity)
• Apply AHCPR and RNAO (2002) guidelines for chronic pain evaluation
• Determine if the client's expectations are met
ATTITUDES
• Apply humility; rethink your approach; if pain continues, confer with other clinicians
• Be responsible and accountable when care is ineffective and the client's rights must be maintained

FIGURE **38–18** Critical thinking model for pain relief evaluation.

Box 38-19 Nurse-Physician Pain Communication

1. Identify physician by name.
2. Give your name.
3. State the general nature of the call.
4. Identify the client by name and diagnosis.
5. State the pain management goal: rating and activities.
6. Summarize the current pain rating and effect of pain on activities.
7. List the current analgesic doses and relevant side effects.
8. Identify non-pharmacological strategies used.
9. Suggest a solution (on the basis of a clinical practice guideline, if possible).

Adapted from *Pain: Clinical Manual* (2nd ed.), by M. McCaffery and C. Pasero, 1999, St. Louis, MO: Mosby.

Client Expectations. The client is the best judge of whether an intervention works. The nurse must continually assess whether the nature of the pain changes and whether individual interventions are effective. The family can be a valuable resource, particularly if the client has cancer and may not be able to express discomfort during the latter stages of terminal illness. The nurse has successfully treated pain when the client's expectations of pain relief are met. The nurse uses evaluative criteria to determine the outcome of pain-relief interventions.

Pain assessment and responses to intervention should be accurately and thoroughly documented so that they can be communicated to others caring for the client. Communication occurs from nurse to nurse, shift to shift, and nurse to other health care providers. The nurse caring for the client is responsible for reporting what has been effective for managing pain. The client is not responsible for communicating this information. Various tools such as a pain flow sheet help centralize information about pain management. Clients expect nurses to be sensitive to their pain and to be diligent in managing that pain. Communicating effectively with physicians (Box 38-19) help nurses to achieve optimal pain relief for clients.

Key Concepts

- Pain is a purely subjective physical and psychosocial experience.
- A nurse's misconceptions about pain often result in doubt about the degree of the client's suffering and in unwillingness to provide relief.
- Knowledge of the nociceptive pain processes of the pain experience—transmission, transduction, perception, and modulation—provides the nurse with guidelines for determining pain-relief measures.
- An interaction of psychological and cognitive factors affects pain perception.
- A person's cultural background influences the meaning of pain and how it is expressed.
- It is common for older clients not to report pain.
- Clients who have chronic pain are unlikely to show behavioural changes.
- The difference between acute and chronic pain involves the concept of harm. Acute pain is protective, thus preventing harm; chronic pain is no longer protective.
- The nurse does not collect an in-depth pain history when the client is experiencing severe discomfort.
- Pain can cause physical signs and symptoms similar to the signs and symptoms of other diseases.
- Clients waiting to undergo invasive tests may gain some pain relief by anticipatory guidance.
- The nurse individualizes pain interventions by collaborating closely with the client, using assessment findings, and trying a variety of interventions.
- Eliminating sources of painful stimuli is a basic nursing measure for promoting comfort.
- Using a regular schedule for analgesic administration is more effective than an as-needed schedule in controlling pain.
- A patient-controlled analgesic device gives clients pain control with low risk of overdose.
- While caring for a client who receives local anaesthesia, the nurse protects the client from injury.
- Nursing implications for administering epidural analgesia include preventing infection and monitoring closely for respiratory depression.
- The goal of pain management is to anticipate and prevent pain rather than treat it.
- Evaluation of the client's pain interventions requires consideration of the changing character of pain, the client's response to interventions, and the client's perceptions of a therapy's effectiveness.

Key Terms

Acupressure, *p. 1260*
Acute pain, *p. 1240*
Addiction, *p. 1270*
Adjuvants, *p. 1263*
Anaesthetic, *p. 1245*
Analgesics, *p. 1245*
Biofeedback, *p. 1259*
Breakthrough pain, *p. 1269*
Chordotomy, *p. 1267*
Chronic pain, *p. 1280*
Cutaneous stimulation, *p. 1259*
Dorsal rhizotomy, *p. 1267*
Drug tolerance, *p. 1270*
Epidural analgesia, *p. 1265*
Epidural space, *p. 1265*
Guided imagery, *p. 1258*
Idiopathic pain, *p. 1240*
Local anaesthesia, *p. 1265*
Modulation, *p. 1238*
Nociceptor, *p. 1237*
Opioids, *p. 1261*
Pain, *p. 1236*
Pain threshold, *p. 1239*
Pain tolerance, *p. 1240*
Patient-controlled analgesia (PCA), *p. 1264*
Perception, *p. 1238*
Physical dependence, *p. 1270*
Placebos, *p. 1270*
Pruritus, *p. 1266*
Pseudoaddiction, *p. 1241*
Regional anaesthesia, *p. 1265*
Relaxation, *p. 1258*
Transcutaneous electrical nerve stimulation (TENS), *p. 1260*
Transduction, *p. 1237*

Critical Thinking Exercises

1. Mr. Gorsky, aged 32 years, is a construction worker who sustained an injury to the lumbar region of his back during a fall 8 months ago. He is 180 cm tall and weighs 127 kg. He continues to report pain intensity as a 5 (on a scale of 0 to 10), increasing with activity; he has limited flexibility and is unable to return to work. He has recently been admitted for treatment at a comprehensive pain clinic. What interventions might the health care team use?
2. Alexis, aged 3 years, is admitted to the pediatric unit for a third-degree burn to her right lower extremity. What tools might be useful when assessing this child's pain?
3. You are caring for an unconscious client who was involved in an automobile accident and sustained multiple injuries. The client has several lacerations, wounds, and surgical incisions, as well as multiple lines and tubes. What measures might you take to promote the client's comfort?
4. Madeleine Tremblay, a 55-year-old woman with metastatic breast cancer to the bone, has been receiving IV morphine sulphate (MSO_4) for a week for severe back and leg pain. Her frequently increased infusion of MSO_4 is not reducing her pain to an acceptable level, and she is becoming increasingly sedated. What other pharmacological interventions might be considered?
5. Ms. Wilkins, aged 65 years, returns from surgery following a small bowel resection. The physician orders a 25-mcg fentanyl patch applied to help manage the post-operative pain. Ms. Wilkins received one dose of morphine 4 mg IV push in the recovery room 1 hour ago, which relieved her pain. What actions would be appropriate for you to take at this time?

Review Questions

1. Pain is viewed as a(n)
   1. Separate disease
   2. Symptom of an illness
   3. Symptom of a condition
   4. Objective finding
2. This type of pain lasts longer than anticipated and a minimum of 6 months, may not have an identifiable cause, and leads to great personal suffering:
   1. Cancer pain
   2. Chronic pain
   3. Acute pain
   4. Idiopathic pain
3. One of the reasons that many nurses avoid acknowledging a client's pain is
   1. Inadequate pain management skills
   2. Insufficient time to respond to the client
   3. Fear that the intervention may cause addiction
   4. Inability to manage their client load
4. Cognitively, this age group is unable to recall explanations about pain or associate pain with experiences that can occur in various situations:
   1. Preschoolers
   2. Adolescents
   3. Young adults
   4. Older adults
5. An 82-year-old man with Alzheimer's disease is restless and moaning. The client's daughter states that the client did not sleep well most of the night. The nurse's first response would be to
   1. Recommend giving the client sleeping medication
   2. Obtain a psychiatric evaluation
   3. Administer pain medication as ordered
   4. Assess and document physical and behavioural data
6. The client requested medication for her abdominal incision pain, which she rates as 5 (scale of 0 to 10, with 10 the worst pain). One hour after administration of her pain medication, she was able to walk in the hall for 10 minutes and rated her pain as a 7. This indicated that the dosage of pain medication was
   1. Adequate
   2. Excessive
   3. Insufficient
   4. Unnecessary
7. When a client is anticipating a painful procedure, the nurse
   1. Teaches about the procedure, avoiding focusing on the associated discomfort
   2. Teaches about the procedure and its associated discomfort
   3. Orders an analgesic
   4. Tells the client that the discomfort will be minimal
8. Relaxation and guided imagery are examples of
   1. Cognitive-behavioural interventions
   2. Physical interventions
   3. Pharmacological interventions
   4. Adjuvants
9. The Canadian Pain Society recommends that if pain is anticipated for the majority of the day, health care professionals should consider administering opioids
   1. On an as-needed (prn) basis
   2. With complementary therapies
   3. On a around-the-clock (ATC) basis
   4. When the pain tolerance level is exceeded
10. One of the reasons that patient-controlled analgesia (PCA) pumps are frequently used for post-operative and cancer pain management is to
    1. Enable family members to control the drug doses
    2. Enable improved nursing control over drug doses
    3. Enable sustained pain relief, with the client in control
    4. Increase medication use

References

Agency for Health Care Policy and Research, Acute Pain Management Guideline Panel. (1992). *Acute pain management: Operative or medical procedures and trauma. Clinical Practice Guideline* (AHCPR Publication No. 92-0032). Rockville, MD: Agency for Health Care Policy and Research, Public Health Service, U.S. Department of Health and Human Services.

American Geriatrics Society. (2002). The management of persistent pain in older persons. *Journal of the American Geriatrics Society, 50*(Suppl. 6), 205–224.

American Pain Society. (1999). *Principles of analgesic use in the treatment of acute and cancer pain* (4th ed.). Glenview, IL: Author.

Anand, K. J. S., & Craig, K. (1996). New perspectives on the definition of pain. *Pain, 67,* 3–6.

Anand, K. J. S., & Scalzo, F. M. (2000). Can adverse neonatal experiences alter brain development and subsequent behavior? *Biology of the Neonate, 77*(2), 69–82.

Anand, K. J. S., Sippell, W. G., & Aynsley-Green, A. (1987). Randomized trial of fentanyl anesthesia in preterm babies undergoing surgery: Effects on the stress response. *Lancet, 1,* 243–248.

Bernstein, L. H., et al. (1993). Portable medicine pumps in primary care. *Patient Care, 27, 91-3, 97-8, 103-4.*

Beyer, J. E., Denyes, M. J., & Villarruel, A. M. (1992). The creation, validation, and continuing development of the Oucher: A measure of pain intensity in children. *Journal of Pediatric Nursing, 7*(5), 335–346.

Butler, R. N., & Gastel, B. (1992). Care of the aged: Perspectives on pain and discomfort. In D. C. Turk & R. Melzack (Eds.), *The handbook of pain assessment.* New York: Guilford Press.

Canadian Pain Society. (2001). *Patient Pain Manifesto.* Retrieved February 19, 2005 from *http://www.canadianpainsociety.ca/contang/4nouvelles-manifeste.htm*

Carlton, S. M., & Coggeshall, R. E. (1998). Noceptive integration: Does it have a peripheral component? *Pain Forum, 7,* 71–78.

Carroll, D., & Seers, K. (1998). Relaxation for the relief of chronic pain: A systematic review. *Journal of Advanced Nursing, 27*(3), 476–487.

Chambers, C. T., von Baeyer, C.L., Montgomery, C., Court, C. & Hardial, J. (2002). Self-Report Measures For Pediatric Pain Assessment: Impact of Scale Format on Nurses' Ratings of Clinically Significant Pain. Poster presented at the Canadian Pain Society Annual Conference, Toronto, ON, 2003.

Collins, S., et al. (2000). Antidepressants and anticonvulsants for diabetic neuropathy and postherpetic neuralgia: A quantitative systematic review. *Journal of Pain and Symptom Management, 206,* 449–458.

Colleau, S. M. (1999). The significance of breakthrough pain in cancer. *Cancer Pain Release, 12.* Retrieved February, 14, 2005 , from *http://www.whocancerpain.wisc.edu/eng/12_4/significance.html*

Cox, F. (2001). Clinical care of patients with epidural infusions. *Professional Nurse, 16*(10), 1429–1432.

Craig, K. D. (1998). The facial display of pain in infants and children. In G. A. Finley & P. J. McGrath (Eds.), *Progress in pain research and management: Vol. 10. Measurement of pain in infants and children* (pp. 103–122). Seattle: IASP Press.

Davis, G., Hiemenz, M. L., & White, T. L. (2002). Barriers to managing chronic pain of older adults with arthritis. *Journal of Nursing Scholarship, 34*(2), 121–126.

Dochterman, J. M., & Bulechek, G. M. (Eds.). (2004). *Nursing interventions classification (NIC)* (4th ed.). St. Louis, MO: Mosby.

Donahue, P. (1989). *Nursing: The finest art.* St. Louis, MO: Mosby.

Du Pen, S. L., & Williams, A. R. (1992). Management of patients receiving combined epidural morphine and bupivacaine for the treatment of cancer pain. *Journal of Pain and Symptom Management, 7*(2), 125–127.

Ferrell, B., & Coyle, N. (2001). *Textbook of palliative nursing.* London: Oxford Press.

Fitzgerald, M. (1995). Pain in infancy: Some unanswered questions. *Pain Reviews, 2*(2), 77–91. 1995.

Fowler-Kerry, S., & Lander, J. R. (1987). Management of injection pain in children. *Pain, 30,* 169–175.

Fuch-Lacelle, S., & Hadjistavropoulos, T. (in press). Development and preliminary validation of the Pain Assessment Checklist for Seniors with Limited Ability to Communicate (PACSLAC). *Pain Management Nursing.*

Gerdner, L. (2001). Evidence-based protocol: Individualized music. In M. G. Titler (Series Ed.), *Series on Evidence-Based Practice for Older Adults.* Iowa City, IA: The University of Iowa College of Nursing Gerontological Nursing Interventions Research Center, Research Dissemination Core.

Gil, K. (1990). Psychologic aspects of acute pain. *Anesthesiology Reports, 2*(2), 246.

Grealish, L., Lomasney, A., & Whiteman, B. (2000). Foot massage: A nursing intervention to modify the distressing symptoms of pain and nausea in patients hospitalized with cancer. *Cancer Nursing, 23*(3), 237–243.

Grunau, R. V., & Craig, K. (1987). Pain expression in neonates: Facial action and cry. *Pain, 28,* 395–410.

Grunau, R. V. E., et al. (1994). Early pain experience, child and family factors, as precursors of somatization: A prospective study of extremely premature and full-term children. *Pain, 56,* 353–359.

Halverson, P. (1999). Nonsteroidal anti-inflammatory drugs: Benefits, risks, and COX-2 selectivity. *Orthopedic Nursing, 18*(6), 21–26.

Harkins, S. W., et al. (1999). Geriatric pain. In P. D. Wall & R. Melzack (Eds.), *Textbook of pain* London: Churchill Livingstone.

Harkins, S. W., & Price, D. D. (1993). Are there special needs for pain assessment in the elderly? *American Pain Society Bulletin, 3,* 4–6.

Haythornthwaite, J., et al. (1998). Pain coping strategies predict perceived control over pain. *Pain, 77*(1), 33–39.

Health and Welfare Canada. (1990). *Guidelines for establishing standards for chronic-pain programs.* Ottawa: Author.

Helmy, S., & Bali, A. (2001). The effect of preemptive use of the NMDA receptor antagonist dextromethorphan on postoperative analgesic requirements. *Anesthesia and Analgesia, 92,* 739–744.

Herr, K. (2002a). Chronic pain: Challenges and assessment strategies. *Journal of Gerontological Nursing, 28*(1), 20–27.

Herr, K. (2002b). Chronic pain in the older patient: Management strategies. *Journal of Gerontological Nursing, 28*(2), 28–34.

Hockenberry, M. J., et al. (2003). *Wong's nursing care of infants and children* (7th ed.). St. Louis, MO: Mosby.

International Association for the Study of Pain, Subcommittee on Taxonomy. (1979). Pain terms: A list with definitions and notes on usage. *Pain, 6,* 249.

Jacox, A., et al. (1994). *Management of cancer pain. Clinical practice guideline no. 9* (AHCPR Publication No. 94-0592). Rockville, MD: Agency for Health Care Policy and Research, Public Health Service, U.S. Department of Health and Human Services.

Johnston, C. C., et al. (1999). Factors explaining lack of response to heel stick in preterm newborns. *Journal of Obstetric, Gynecologic, and Neonatal Nursing, 28,* 587–594.

Jovey, R.D., et al. (2003). *Use of opioid analgesics for the treatment of chronic noncancer pain–A consenus statement and guidelines from the Canadian Pain Society.* Pain Research & Management 8(Suppl A): 3A-14A.

Kelly, A. (2003). *Geriatric pain assessment: Self-directed learning module.* Pensacola, FL: American Society of Pain Management Nurses (ASPMN).

Kim, M. K. (2002). A randomized clinical trial of analgesia in children with acute abdominal pain. *Academic Emergency Medicine, 9*(4), 281–287.

Lasch, K. (2000). Culture, pain, and culturally sensitive pain care. *Pain Management Nursing, 1*(3 Suppl. 1), S16–22.

Lawler, K. (1997). Pain assessment. *Professional Nurse Study Supplement, 13*(Suppl. 1), S5–8.

Lehn, R. (2001). *Pharmacology for nursing care* (4th ed.). Philadelphia: W. B. Saunders.

Loeser, J. D., & Melzack, R. (1999). Pain: An overview. *The Lancet, 353,* 1607–1609.

Max, M. B., & Portenoy, R. K. (1993). Methodological challenges for clinical trials of cancer pain treatments. In C. R. Chapman & K. M. Foley (Eds.), *Current and emerging issues in cancer pain: Research and practice.* New York: Raven Press.

McCaffery, M. (1979). *Nursing management of the patient with pain* (2nd ed.). Philadelphia: Lippincott.

McCaffery, M., Ferrell, B. R., & Pasero, C. (2000). Nurses' personal opinion about patients' pain and their effect of recorded assessments and titration of opioid doses. *Pain Management Nursing, 1*(3), 79–87.

McCaffery, M., & Pasero, C. (1999). *Pain: Clinical manual* (2nd ed.). St. Louis, MO: Mosby.

McGrady, A., et al. (1994). Effect of biofeedback-assisted relaxation on migraine headache and changes in cerebral blood flow velocity in the middle cerebral artery. *Headache, 34*(7), 424–428.

McGrath, P. A. (1990). *Pain in children: Nature, assessment, and treatment.* New York: Guilford Press.

McGrath, P. J., & Finley, G. A. (Eds.). (1999). Chronic and recurrent pain in children and adolescents. Seattle, WA: IASP Press.

McMillan, S. C. (1996). Pain and pain relief experienced by hospice patients with cancer. *Cancer Nursing, 19,* 298–307.

Meek, S. S. (1993). Effects of slow-stroke back massage on relaxation in hospice clients. *Image—The Journal of Nursing Scholarship, 25*(1), 17–21.

Melzack, R., & Wall, P. D. (1965). Pain mechanisms: A new theory. *Science, 150,* 971–979.

Miaskowski, C. (2000). The impact of age on a patient's perception of pain and ways it can be managed. *Pain Management Nursing, 1*(3), 2–7.

Miaskowski, C., & Levine, D. (2000). Does opioid analgesia show a gender preference for females? *Pain Forum, 8,* 34–44.

Moorhead, S., Johnson, M., & Maas, S. (Eds.). (2004). *Nursing outcomes classification (NOC)* (3rd ed.). St. Louis, MO: Mosby.

Newshan, G. (2000). Pain management in the addicted patient: Practical considerations. *Nursing Outlook, 48*(2), 81–85.

Nightingale, F. (1969). *Notes on nursing: What it is and what it is not.* New York: Dover (Original work published 1859).

Oberlander, T. F., O'Donnell, M.E., & Montgomery, C.J. (1999). Pain in children with significant neurological impairment. *Journal of Developmental & Behavioral Pediatrics. 20*(4), 235-243.

O'Mathuna, D. (2000). Evidence-based practice and reviews of therapeutic touch. *Journal of Nursing Scholarship, 32*(3), 279–285.

Otis-Green, S., et al. (2002). An integrated psychosocial model for cancer pain management. *Cancer Practice, 10*(Suppl. 1), 58–65.

Paice, J. A. (1991). Unraveling the mystery of pain. *Oncology Nursing Forum, 18*(5), 843–849.

Paice, J. A. (1994). *The physiology and pharmacologic management of pain: Physiology of pain: Unraveling the mystery.* Baltimore: Williams & Wilkins.

Pasero, C. (2000). Continuous local anesthetics. *American Journal of Nursing, 100*(8), 22–23.

Pasero, C. (2003). *Intravenous patient-controlled analgesia for acute pain management: Self-directed learning module.* Pensacola, FL: American Society of Pain Management Nurses (ASPMN).

Pasero, C., & McCaffery, M. (2002). Monitoring sedation. *American Journal of Nursing, 102*(2), 67–69.

Passik, S.D., Kirsh, K,L & Portenoy, R,K. (1999). Understanding aberrant drug-taking behavior: addiction redefined for palliative care and pain management settings. *Principles and Practice of Supportive Oncology Updates 2*:1–12.

Patterson, C., et al. (1997). Provisional educational needs of health care providers in palliative care in three nursing homes in Ontario. *Journal of Palliative Care, 13*(3), 13–17.

Popp, B., & Portenoy, R. (1996). Management of chronic pain in the elderly: Pharmacology of opioids and other analgesics. In B. A. Ferrell & B. R. Ferrell (Eds.), *Pain in the elderly.* Seattle, WA: IASP Press.

Portenoy, R. K. (1996). Neuropathic pain. In R. K. Portenoy & R. M. Kanner (Eds.), *Pain management: Theory and practice.* Philadelphia: F. A. Davis.

Porter, F. L., et al. (1997). Pain and pain management in newborn infants: A survey of physicians and nurses. *Pediatrics, 100*(4), 626–632.

Puntillo, K., et al. (2001). Patients' perceptions and responses to procedural pain: Results from Thunder Project II. *American Journal of Critical Care, 10*(4), 238–251.

Ramer, L., et al. (1999). Multimeasure pain assessment in an ethnically diverse group of patients with cancer. *Journal of Transcultural Nursing, 10*(2), 94–101.

Registered Nurses Association of Ontario (2002). *Assessment and Management of Pain.* Accessed February 25, 2005, from *http://www.rnao.org/bestpractices/completed_guidelines/BPG_Guide_C2_pain.asp*

Reiff, P., & Nizolek, M. (2001). Troubleshooting tips for PCA. *RN, 64*(4), 33–37.

Richmond, C. E., Bromley, L. M., & Woolf, C. J. (1993). Preoperative morphine pre-empts postoperative pain. *Lancet, 342*(8863), 73–75.

Rosmus, C., et al. (2000). Pain response in Chinese and non-Chinese Canadian infants: Is there a difference? *Social Science & Medicine, 51*(2), 175–184.

Ruda, R., et al. (2000). Altered nociceptive neuronal circuits after neonatal peripheral inflammation. *Science, 289*(5479), 628–631.

Salerno, E., & Willens, J. S. (1996). *Pain management handbook: An interdisciplinary approach.* St. Louis, MO: Mosby.

Schumacher, K., et al. (2002). Putting cancer pain management regimens into practice at home. *Journal of Pain and Symptom Management, 23*(5), 369–382.

Siddall, P., Yezierski, R., & Loeser, J. (2000). Pain following spinal cord injury: Clinical features, prevalence, and taxonomy. *IASP Newsletter.* Retrieved February 14, 2005, from *http://www.iasp-pain.org/TC00-3.html*

Sluka, K. (2001). The basic science mechanisms of TENS and clinical applications. *APS Bulletin, 11*(2).

Steefel, L. (2002). Treat pain in any culture. *Nursing Spectrum, 6*(5).

Stevens, B. (1998a). Composite measures of pain. In G. A. Finley & P. J. McGrath (Eds.), *Progress in pain research and management: Vol. 10. Measurement of pain in infants and children* (pp. 161–178). Seattle: IASP Press.

Stevens, B., & Koren, G. (1998b). Evidence-based pain management for infants. *Current Opinion in Pediatrics, 10*(2), 203–207.

The SUPPORT Principal Investigators. (1995). A controlled trial to improve care for seriously ill hospitalized patients: The study to understand prognoses and preferences for outcomes and risks of treatments (SUPPORT). *Journal of the American Medical Association, 274*(20), 1591–1598.

Taddio, A., Katz, J. Ilersich, A, L, & Koren, G. (1997). Effect of neonatal circumcision on pain response during subsequent routine vaccination. *Lancet, 349,* 599–603.

Tesler, M. D., et al. (1994). Postoperative analgesics for children and adolescents: Prescription and administration. *Journal of Pain and Symptom Management, 9,* 85–95.

Thompson, W. (2000). Placebos: A review of the placebo response. *The American Journal of Gastroenterology, 95*(7), 1637–1643.

Thorns, A., & Sykes, N. (2000). Opioid use in last week of life and implications for end-of-life decision-making. *Lancet, 356*(9927), 398–399.

Titler, M., & Rakel, B. (2001). Nonpharmacological treatment of pain. *Critical Care Nursing Clinics of North America, 13*(2), 221–232.

Tucker, K. (2001). Deceptive placebo administration. *American Journal of Nursing, 101*(8), 55–56.

Wall, P., & Melzack, R. (1999). *Textbook of pain* (4th ed.). London: Churchill Livingstone.

Warnock, F. F. (2003). An ethogram on neonatal distress related pain behavior (newborn male circumcision). *Infant Behavior and Development, 26*(3), 398–420.

Warnock, F., & Sandrin, D. (2004). Comprehensive description of newborn distress behavior in response to acute pain (newborn male circumcision). *Pain, 107*(3), 242–255.

Wheeler, M., et al. (2002). Adverse events associated with postoperative opioid analgesia: A systemic review. *The Journal of Pain, 3*(3), 159–180.

Wong, D. L., & Baker, C. M. (1988). Pain in children: Comparison of assessment scales. *The Oklahoma Nurse, 33*(1), 8.

World Health Organization. (1990). *Cancer pain relief and palliative care: Report of a WHO expert committee* (WHO Tech Rep Series No. 804). Geneva, Switzerland: Author.

Zalon, M. L. (1993). Nurses' assessment of post operative patients' pain. *Pain, 54*(3), 329–334.

Recommended Web Sites

Canadian Pain Society

http://www.canadianpainsociety.ca/index.html

The Canadian Pain Society is an association whose members include physicians, nurses, and other clinicians involved with management of pain. Its aim is to foster and encourage research on pain and to improve the management of clients with acute and chronic pain.

University of Toronto Pain Research Group:
http://www.utoronto.ca/pain/
The University of Toronto Centre for the Study of Pain is a partnership involving the faculties of dentistry, medicine, nursing, and pharmacy. The mission of the Centre is to lead, both nationally and internationally, in pain research, education, and clinical activity.

Pediatric Pain—Science Helping Children:
http://www.pediatric-pain.ca/
The Pediatric Pain Research Lab is located in the IWK Health Centre and the Psychology Department of Dalhousie University in Halifax, Nova Scotia.

International Association for the Study of Pain (IASP):
http://www.iasp-pain.org/
The IASP is the largest multidisciplinary international association in the field of pain. One of the purposes of this site is to call attention to the importance of pain as a field for multidisciplinary scientific enquiry and to promote pain prevention/relief as a priority for health care delivery.

Alberta Palliative Care Resource:
http://www.albertapalliative.net/APN/PCHB/PCHBIdx.html
This site is intended as an educational resource to aid primary care practitioners to care for their palliative clients. It includes sections on management of cancer pain, adjuvant analgesics, and opioid analgesics.

39

Nutrition

Anne Griffin Perry, RN, MSN, EdD, FAAN
Donna Best, RN, BN, MN, ACNP (Canadian author)

Objectives

Mastery of content in this chapter will enable the student to:

- Define the key terms listed.
- Explain why each major nutrient is necessary for good nutrition.
- Explain the importance of a balance between energy intake and energy requirements.
- List the end products of carbohydrate, protein, and fat metabolism.
- Explain the significance of saturated, unsaturated, and polyunsaturated fats.
- Describe *Canada's Food Guide to Healthy Eating,* and discuss its value in planning meals for good nutrition.
- Explain dietary reference intakes.
- List the intakes suggested by *Nutrition Recommendations for Canadians* and *Canada's Guidelines for Healthy Eating.*
- Explain the variance in nutritional requirements throughout growth and development.
- Discuss the major methods of nutritional assessment.
- Identify three major nutritional problems, and describe clients at risk.
- State the goals of enteral and parenteral nutrition.
- Describe the procedure for initiating and maintaining tube feedings.
- Describe the methods to avoid complications of tube feedings.
- Describe the methods to avoid complications of parenteral nutrition.
- Discuss medical nutrition therapy in relation to three medical conditions.
- Discuss diet counselling and client teaching in relation to client expectations.

Food provides sustenance and also holds symbolic meaning. The giving or taking of food is part of ceremonies, social gatherings, holiday traditions, religious events, the celebration of birth, and the mourning of death. The difficulty of the decision to withhold food in a terminal illness, even in the form of intravenous (IV) nutrients, is a testament to the symbolic power of food and feeding.

Florence Nightingale understood the importance of nutrition, stressing the nurse's role in the science and art of feeding during the mid-1800s (Dossey, 1999). Since then, the nurse's role in nutrition and diet therapy has changed. Medical nutrition therapy (MNT) is now recognized as a disease-specific treatment modality when clients are at risk for malnutrition (American Academy of Family Physicians, 1997). In some illnesses, such as Type 2 diabetes mellitus or mild hypertension, diet therapy may be the major treatment for disease control (Campbell et al., 1999; Canadian Diabetes Association, 2003b). Other conditions, such as inflammatory bowel disease, may require specialized nutrition support such as enteral nutrition (EN) or parenteral nutrition (PN).

Scientific Knowledge Base

Nutrients: The Biochemical Units of Nutrition

The body requires fuel to provide energy for cellular metabolism and repair, organ function, growth, and body movement. An individual's energy requirements are influenced by several factors. The energy requirement of a person at rest is called the **basal metabolic rate (BMR).** This is the energy needed to maintain life-sustaining activities (breathing, circulation, heart rate, and temperature) for a specific period of time. The **resting energy expenditure (REE)** is a measurement that accounts for BMR plus energy to digest meals and perform mild activity. REE is a baseline of energy requirement that accounts for approximately 60% to 75% of our daily needs. Factors such as age, body mass, gender, fever, starvation, menstruation, illness, injury, infection, activity level, or thyroid function may affect energy requirements. Factors that affect metabolism include illness, pregnancy, lactation, and activity level.

In general, when energy requirements are completely met by kilocalorie (kcal) intake in food, weight does not change. When the kilocalories ingested exceed energy demands, a person gains weight. If the kilocalories ingested fail to meet energy requirements, a person loses weight.

Nutrients are the elements necessary for body processes and function. Energy needs are met from three categories of nutrients: carbohydrates, proteins, and fats. Other nutrients include water, vitamins, and minerals. Water is a vital body component that acts as a solvent for metabolic processes. Vitamins and minerals do not provide energy but are essential to metabolic processes, including acid–base balance.

Foods are sometimes described according to their **nutrient density,** the proportion of essential nutrients to the number of kilocalories. High-nutrient-density foods, such as fruits and vegetables, provide a large number of nutrients in relationship to kilocalories. Low-nutrient-density foods, such as alcohol or sugar, are high in kilocalories but are nutrient poor.

Carbohydrates.

Carbohydrates are the main source of energy in the diet. Each gram of carbohydrate produces 4 kcal and serves as the main source of fuel (glucose) for the brain, skeletal muscles during exercise, erythrocyte and leukocyte production, and cell function of the renal medulla. Carbohydrates are obtained primarily from plant foods, except for lactose (milk sugar), and are classified according to their carbohydrate units, or **saccharides.**

Monosaccharides such as glucose (dextrose) or fructose cannot be broken down into a more basic carbohydrate unit. Disaccharides such as sucrose, lactose, and maltose are composed of two monosaccharides and water. Both monosaccharides and disaccharides are classified as **simple carbohydrates** and are found primarily in sugars. Polysaccharides such as glycogen are composed of many carbohydrate units and are classified as **complex carbohydrates.** They are insoluble in water and are digested to varying degrees. Starches are polysaccharides.

Some polysaccharides cannot be digested because humans do not have enzymes capable of breaking them down. This dietary fibre is important in disease prevention, as it decreases total and low-density lipoprotein (LDL) cholesterol (Williams, 2001).

Proteins.

Proteins are essential for synthesis (building) of body tissue in growth, maintenance, and repair. Collagen, hormones, enzymes, immune cells, DNA, and RNA are all composed of protein. In addition, blood clotting, fluid regulation, and acid–base balance require proteins. Nutrients and many pharmacological substances are transported in the blood by proteins.

The simplest form of protein is the amino acid. **Essential amino acids** are those that the body cannot synthesize but must have provided in the diet. Others can be synthesized and are classified as **non-essential amino acids. Amino acids** can be linked together to form larger protein molecules. Albumin and insulin are simple proteins because they contain only amino acids or their derivatives. The combination of a simple protein with a non-protein substance produces a complex protein, such as lipoprotein, formed by a combination of a lipid and a simple protein.

Incomplete proteins lack one or more of the nine essential amino acids and include cereals, legumes (beans, peas), and vegetables. **Complementary proteins** are pairs of incomplete proteins that when combined supply the total amount of protein provided by complete protein sources. A complete protein contains all nine essential amino acids in sufficient quantity to support growth and maintain nitrogen balance—its most important function in the body. Complete proteins are also referred to as high-quality proteins.

Protein is the only major nutrient that contains nitrogen (it is 16% nitrogen) and is the only source of nitrogen for the body. Thus nitrogen can be used to determine protein balance in the body.

Nitrogen balance is achieved when the intake and output of nitrogen are equal. When the intake of nitrogen exceeds the output, the body is in positive nitrogen balance, which is required for growth, normal pregnancy, maintenance of lean muscle mass and vital organs, and wound healing. The nitrogen retained by the body is used for building, repair, and replacement of body tissues. Negative nitrogen balance occurs when the body loses more nitrogen than the body gains, for example, with infection, sepsis, burns, fever, starvation, head injury, and trauma. The increased nitrogen loss is the result of body-tissue destruction or loss of nitrogen-containing body fluids. Nutrition during this period must provide nutrients to put clients into positive balance for healing.

Protein can be used to provide energy (4 kcal/g), but because of protein's essential role in growth, maintenance, and repair, adequate kilocalories should be provided in the

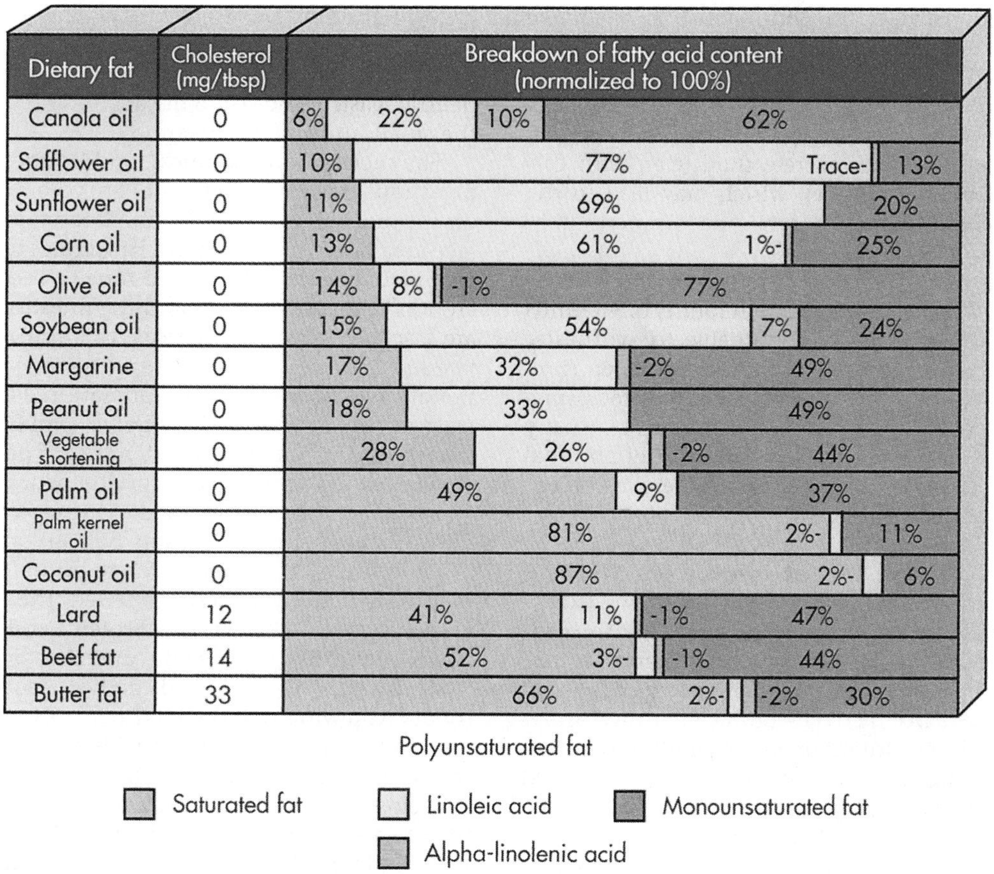
Dietary fat
Cholesterol (mg/tbsp)
Breakdown of fatty acid content (normalized to 100%)
Canola oil 0 6% 22% 10% 62%
Safflower oil 0 10% 77% Trace- 13%
Sunflower oil 0 11% 69% 20%
Corn oil 0 13% 61% 1%- 25%
Olive oil 0 14% 8% -1% 77%
Soybean oil 0 15% 54% 7% 24%
Margarine 0 17% 32% -2% 49%
Peanut oil 0 18% 33% 49%
Vegetable shortening 0 28% 26% -2% 44%
Palm oil 0 49% 9% 37%
Palm kernel oil 0 81% 2%- 11%
Coconut oil 0 87% 2%- 6%
Lard 12 41% 11% -1% 47%
Beef fat 14 52% 3%- -1% 44%
Butter fat 33 66% 2%- -2% 30%
Polyunsaturated fat
Saturated fat
Linoleic acid
Monounsaturated fat
Alpha-linolenic acid

FIGURE 39–1 Comparison of dietary intake of cholesterol, saturated fat, and unsaturated fat. (From *Perspectives in Nutrition,* 3rd ed., by G. M. Wardlaw and P. M. Insesll, 1996, New York: McGraw-Hill.)

diet from non-protein sources. Protein is spared as an energy source when there is sufficient carbohydrate in the diet to meet the energy needs of the body.

Fats. Fats **(lipids)** are the most calorically dense nutrient, providing 9 kcal/g. Fats are composed of triglycerides and fatty acids. **Triglycerides** circulate in the blood and are made up of three fatty acids attached to a glycerol. **Fatty acids** are composed of chains of carbon and hydrogen atoms with an acid group on one end of the chain and a methyl group at the other. Fatty acids can be **saturated,** in which each carbon in the chain has two attached hydrogen atoms, or **unsaturated,** in which an unequal number of hydrogen atoms are attached and the carbon atoms attach to each other with a double bond. **Monounsaturated fatty acids** have one double bond, whereas **polyunsaturated fatty acids** have two or more double carbon bonds.

Most animal fats have high proportions of saturated fatty acids, whereas vegetable fats have higher amounts of unsaturated and polyunsaturated fatty acids (Figure 39–1). The various types of fatty acids have significance for health and the incidence of disease, and are referred to in dietary guidelines from the Heart and Stroke Foundation, The Canadian Cancer Society, and the Canadian Diabetes Association. More recently, trans fatty acids have received attention for their role in the development of coronary artery disease. **Trans fatty acids** are formed by the partial hydrogenation of vegetable oils and are mostly found in prepared foods, snack foods, and margarines. It is recommended that Canadians decrease the proportion of saturated and trans fatty acids to less than 7% of total calories (Genest et al., 2003).

Cholesterol is often discussed in connection with fats, although it is a sterol, not a triglyceride (Williams, 2001). It occurs naturally in animal foods but is also synthesized by the liver. Cholesterol deposits in blood vessel walls cause atherosclerosis, which is the underlying cause of coronary artery disease.

Water. Water is a critical component of the body because cell function depends on a fluid environment. Water composes 60% to 70% of total body weight. The percentage of total body water is greater for lean people than obese people because muscle contains more water than any other tissue except blood. Infants have the greatest percentage of total body water, and older people have the least. When deprived of water, a person cannot survive for more than a few days.

Fluid needs are met by ingesting liquids and solid foods high in water content, such as fresh fruits and vegetables. Water is also produced during digestion when food is oxidized. In a healthy individual, fluid intake from all sources equals fluid output through elimination, respiration, and sweating (see chapters 36 and 40). An ill person can have an increased need for fluid (e.g., with fever or gastrointestinal [GI] losses). An ill person can also have a decreased ability to excrete fluid (e.g., with cardiopulmonary or renal disease), which may lead to the need to restrict fluid intake.

Vitamins. **Vitamins** are organic substances that are essential to normal metabolism. Small amounts of vitamins are present in foods. The body is unable to synthesize most vitamins in the required amounts and depends on dietary intake. Vitamins are affected by food processing, storage, and preparation. Vitamin content is usually highest in fresh foods that are used quickly after minimal exposure to heat, air, or water. Vitamins are classified as fat soluble and water soluble.

Fat-Soluble Vitamins. The **fat-soluble vitamins** (A, D, E, and K) can be stored in the body. With the exception of vitamin D, these vitamins are provided through dietary intake. Vitamin D is provided by dietary intake and can be synthesized in the body with exposure to sunlight. **Hypervitaminosis** of fat-soluble vitamins can result from megadoses (intentional or unintentional) of supplemental vitamins, excessive amounts in fortified food, and large intake of fish oils.

Certain vitamins are currently of considerable interest in their role as antioxidants that neutralize substances called free radicals, which are thought to produce oxidative damage to body cells and tissues. It is believed that oxidative damage increases a person's risk for various cancers. These vitamins include beta-carotene and vitamins A, C, and E (Williams, 2001).

Water-Soluble Vitamins. The **water-soluble vitamins** are vitamins C and B complex (which consists of eight vitamins: thiamine, riboflavin, niacin, vitamin B_6, folate, vitamin B_{12}, pantothenic acid, and biotin). Water-soluble vitamins cannot be stored in the body and must be provided in the daily food intake. Although water-soluble vitamins are not stored, toxicity may still occur with vitamin megadoses.

Minerals. **Minerals** are inorganic elements essential to the body as catalysts in biochemical reactions. Minerals are classified as **macrominerals** when the daily requirement is 100 mg or more and microminerals or **trace elements** when less than 100 mg is needed daily.

Anatomy and Physiology of the Digestive System

Digestion. Digestion of food consists of mechanical breakdown that results from chewing, churning, and mixing with fluid, as well as chemical reactions by which food is reduced to its simplest form. Each part of the GI system has an important digestive or absorptive function (Figure 39–2). Enzymes are an essential component of the chemistry of digestion. **Enzymes** are protein-like substances that act as catalysts to speed up chemical reactions.

Most enzymes have one specific function and function best at a specific pH. The secretions of the GI tract have vastly different pH levels. For example, saliva is relatively neutral, gastric juice is highly acidic, and the secretions of the small intestine are alkaline.

The mechanical, chemical, and hormonal activities of digestion are interdependent. Enzyme activity depends on the mechanical breakdown of food to increase the surface area for chemical action. Hormones regulate the flow of digestive secretions needed for enzyme supply. The secretion of digestive juices and the motility of the GI tract are also regulated by physical, chemical, and hormonal factors, because they are bound to psychological, emotional, and nervous system alterations. Gastrointestinal tract action is increased by nerve stimulation from the parasympathetic nervous system (e.g., the vagus nerve).

Digestion begins in the mouth, where chewing mechanically breaks down food. The food is mixed with saliva, which contains ptyalin (salivary amylase), an enzyme that acts on cooked starch to begin its conversion to maltose. The longer food is chewed, the more starch digestion occurs in the mouth. Proteins and fats are broken down physically but remain unchanged chemically because enzymes in the mouth do not react with these nutrients. Chewing reduces food particles to a size suitable for swallowing, and saliva provides lubrication to further ease swallowing of the food. The epiglottis is a flap of skin that closes over the trachea during swallowing to prevent **aspiration.** Swallowed food enters the esophagus and is moved along by wave-like muscular contractions **(peristalsis)** to the base of the esophagus, above the cardiac sphincter. Pressure from a bolus of food at the cardiac sphincter causes it to relax, allowing the food to enter the fundus, or uppermost portion, of the stomach. Difficulty swallowing is referred to as **dysphagia.**

In the stomach, pepsinogen is secreted by chief cells and then converted by hydrochloric acid (HCl) to pepsin, a protein-splitting enzyme. The stomach's pyloric glands secrete gastrin, a hormone that triggers parietal cells to secrete HCl and intrinsic factor (IF). IF is necessary for absorption of vitamin B_{12} in the ileum. Gastric lipase and amylase are produced to begin fat and starch digestion, respectively. The lining of the stomach is protected from autodigestion by a thick layer of mucus. Alcohol and aspirin are two substances directly absorbed through the lining of the stomach. The stomach acts as a reservoir where food remains for approximately 3 hours, with a range of 1 to 7 hours.

Food leaves the antrum, or distal stomach, via the pyloric sphincter and enters the duodenum. Food has now become an acidic, liquefied mass called **chyme.** Chyme flows into the duodenum and is quickly mixed with bile, intestinal juices, and pancreatic secretions. Secretin and cholecystokinin (CCK) are hormones secreted by the mucosa of the small intestine. Secretin activates release of bicarbonate from the pancreas, raising the pH of chyme. CCK inhibits further gastrin secretion and initiates release of additional digestive enzymes from the pancreas and gallbladder.

Bile is manufactured in the liver and stored in the gallbladder. Bile acts as a detergent, as it emulsifies fat to permit enzyme action while suspending fatty acids in

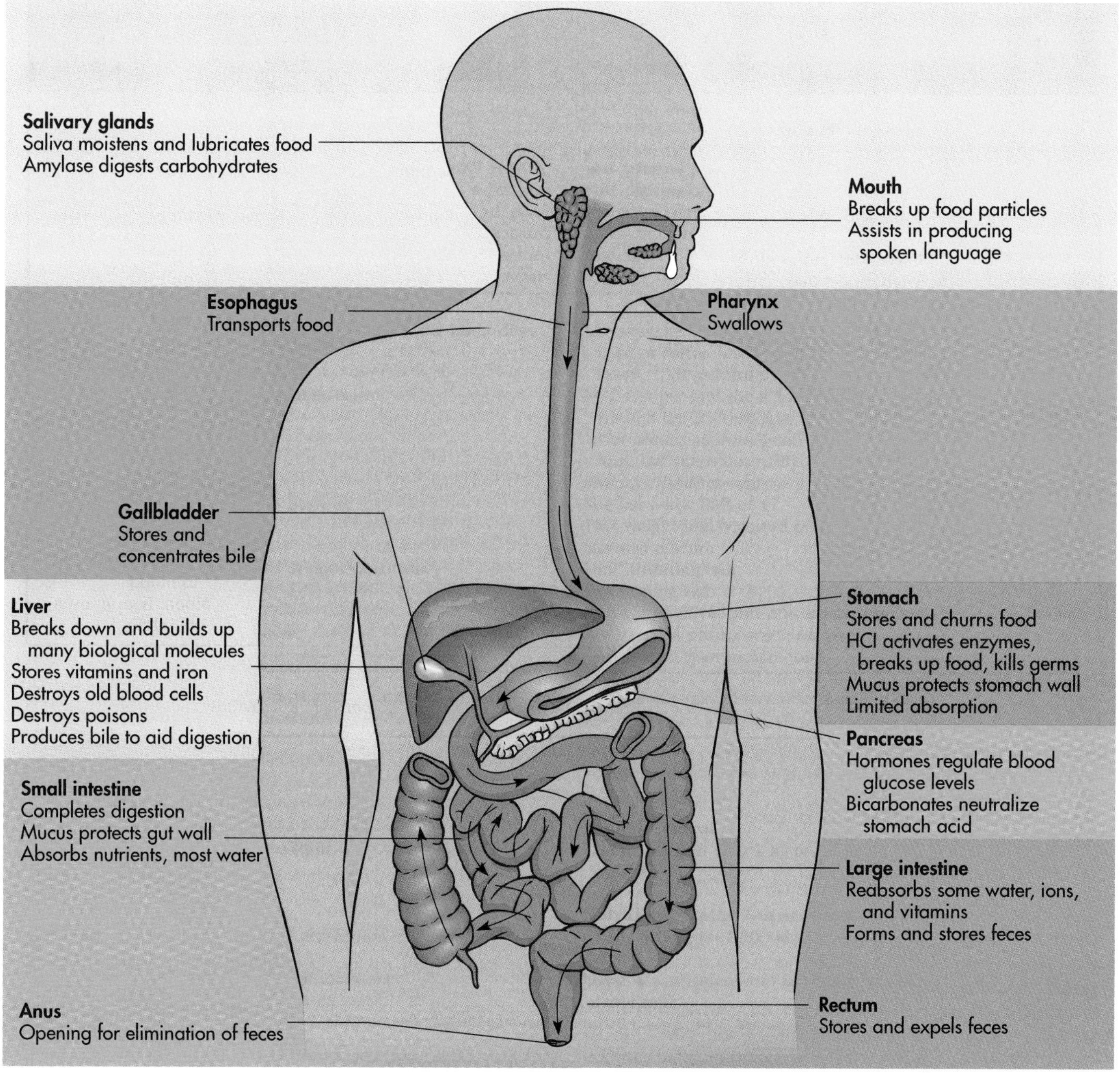

FIGURE **39–2** Summary of digestive system anatomy and organ function. (From Rolin Graphics.)

solution. Pancreatic secretions contain six enzymes: amylase to digest starch; lipase to break down emulsified fats; and trypsin, elastase, chymotrypsin, and carboxypeptidase to break down proteins.

Peristalsis continues in the small intestine, mixing the secretions with the chyme. The mixture becomes increasingly alkaline, inhibiting the action of the gastric enzymes and promoting the action of the duodenal secretions. Epithelial cells in the small intestinal villi secrete enzymes to facilitate digestion. These enzymes include sucrase, lactase, maltase, lipase, and peptidase. The major portion of digestion occurs in the small intestine, producing glucose, fructose, and galactose from carbohydrates; amino acids and dipeptides from proteins; and fatty acids, glycerides, and glycerol from lipids. Approximately 5 hours are required to pass food through the small intestine via peristalsis.

Absorption. The small intestine is the primary absorption site for nutrients. It is lined with finger-like projections called villi, which increase the surface area available for absorption. Nutrients are absorbed by means of passive diffusion, osmosis, active transport, and pinocytosis (Table 39-1).

Table 39-1 **Intestinal Absorption of Major Nutrients**

Nutrient	Form	Absorption Method	Control Agent/Cofactor	Route
Carbohydrate*	Monosaccharides (glucose and galactose)	Competitive	—	Blood
		Selective	—	Blood
		Active transport (via sodium pump)	Sodium	Blood
Fat†	Fatty acids	Fatty acid-bile complex (micelles)	Bile	Lymph
	Glycerides (mono, di)		—	Lymph
	Triglycerides (few; neutral fat)	Pinocytosis	—	Lymph
Protein	Amino acids	Selective	—	Blood
	Dipeptides (some)	Carrier transport systems	Pyridoxine (pyridoxal phosphate)	Blood
	Whole protein (rare)	Pinocytosis	—	Blood
Minerals	Sodium	Active transport via sodium pump	—	Blood
	Calcium	Active transport	Vitamin D	Blood
	Iron	Active transport	Ferritin mechanism (as transferritin)	Blood
Vitamins‡	B_{12}	Carrier transport	Intrinsic factor	Blood
	A	Bile complex	Bile	Blood
	K	Bile complex	Bile	From large intestine to blood
Water§	H_2O	Osmosis	—	Blood, lymph, interstitial fluid

*Carbohydrates, protein, minerals, and water-soluble vitamins are absorbed by villus capillaries within the small intestine, processed within the liver, and released via portal vein circulatory means.
†Fatty acids are absorbed into the lymphatic circulatory system via lacteal ducts at the centre of each microvillus found within the small intestine.
‡Exceptions to vitamin absorption are listed (i.e., B_{12} A, and K). Vitamins A and K are fat soluble and are transported via bile to the blood. Vitamin B_{12} is water soluble but requires specialized transport factor for absorption.
§Water is reabsorbed in the large intestine through capillaries to the blood and flows to the lymphatic system by absorption via large intestinal lymphatic ducts; it serves as a source of interstitial fluid through osmosis.
Adapted from Williams, S.R. (2001). *Basic Nutrition and Diet Therapy* (11th ed.), St. Louis, MO: Mosby.

The main source of water absorption is via the intestine. Approximately 7 L of GI secretions and 1.2 L of oral intake, totalling 8.2 L of fluid, must be managed daily within the GI tract. The small and large intestines reabsorb 8.1 L a day. The remaining 0.1 L is eliminated in feces. In addition to water, electrolytes and minerals are absorbed, and bacteria in the colon synthesize vitamin K and some B complex vitamins. Finally, feces are formed in the colon for elimination.

Metabolism and Storage of Nutrients. **Metabolism** refers to all of the biochemical reactions within the cells of the body. Metabolic processes can be anabolic (building) or catabolic (breaking down). **Anabolism** is the production of more complex biochemical substances by synthesis of nutrients. Anabolism occurs when lean muscle is added through diet and exercise. Amino acids are anabolized into tissues, hormones, and enzymes. **Catabolism** is the breakdown of biochemical substances into simpler substances. Starvation is an example of catabolism, when wasting of body tissues occurs. Normal metabolism and anabolism are physiologically possible when the body is in positive nitrogen balance, whereas catabolism occurs during physiologic states of negative nitrogen balance.

Nutrients absorbed in the intestines, including water, are transported through the circulatory system to body tissues. Through the chemical changes of metabolism, nutrients are converted into a number of substances required by the body. Carbohydrates, protein, and fat undergo metabolism to produce chemical energy and to maintain a balance between anabolism and catabolism. To carry out the body's work, the chemical energy produced by metabolism is converted to other types of energy. Muscle contraction involves mechanical energy, nervous system function involves electrical energy, and the mechanisms of heat production involve thermal energy. All of these forms of energy originate in metabolism. Some of the nutrients required by the body are stored in body tissues. The body's major form of reserve energy is fat, stored as adipose tissue.

Amino acids can be converted to fat and stored or catabolized into energy via gluconeogenesis. All body cells except red blood cells and neurons can oxidize fatty acids into **ketones** for energy in the absence of dietary carbohydrates (glucose). Glycogen, synthesized from glucose, provides energy during brief periods of fasting. Glycogen is stored in small reserves in liver and muscle tissue. For example, blood glucose levels are maintained by this mechanism as we sleep. Nutrient metabolism consists of three main processes:

1. Catabolism of glycogen into glucose, carbon dioxide, and water **(glycogenolysis)**
2. Anabolism of glucose into glycogen for storage **(glycogenesis)**
3. Catabolism of amino acids and glycerol into glucose for energy **(gluconeogenesis)**

Elimination. Chyme is moved by peristaltic action through the ileocecal valve into the large intestine, where it becomes feces. As feces move toward the rectum, water is absorbed in the mucosa. The longer the material stays in the large intestine, the more water is absorbed, causing the feces to become firmer. Exercise and fibre stimulate peristalsis, and water maintains the consistency of stool. Feces contain cellulose and similar indigestible substances, sloughed epithelial cells from the GI tract, digestive secretions, water, and microbes.

Dietary Guidelines

Dietary Reference Intakes. In 1997, the Food and Nutrition Board of the American National Institute of Medicine/National Academy of Sciences, in partnership with Health Canada, initiated **dietary reference intakes (DRIs).** The Food and Nutrition Board (1997) of the National Academy of Sciences published the DRIs in response to the increased public use of nutritional supplements. The DRIs broaden the base of information on nutrients, vitamins and minerals. These DRIs present evidenced-based criteria for minimum to maximum amounts of vitamins and nutrients to avoid deficiencies or toxicities. Because this evidence is continually evolving, clinicians should consult with current resources, such as Web pages and evidenced-based literature, when determining a client's specific nutrition needs or supplementation. The final DRI report is expected in 2005 (Health Canada, 2005).

This new format presents a range of acceptable intakes rather than absolute values. As research has expanded the scientific body of nutrition knowledge, absolute values are no longer sufficient. Studies addressing the reduction of risk of chronic diseases such as cardiovascular disease, cancer, and osteoporosis have launched a need for expanded nutrient information.

Food Guidelines. Health Canada has developed *Canada's Food Guide to Healthy Eating* (Health and Welfare Canada, 1992), which was designed to guide daily nutritional selections (Figure 39–3). These basic plans provide for diets ranging from 1600 to 1800 kcal/day. Additional foods to round out meals and meet energy requirements can be selected from enriched cereals, complex carbohydrates, and additional grains. Health Canada has supplemented the general guidelines in *Canada's Food Guide to Healthy Eating* with *Canada's Guidelines for Healthy Eating* (Table 39-2) and *Nutrition Recommendations for Canadians* (Table 39-3). See Table 39-4 for a summary of recommended intakes according to *Canada's Food Guide to Healthy Eating.* The nutrition recommendations for Canadians are under review and will be revised to ensure that they continue to be scientifically sound and that they continue to address those characteristics of the diet most relevant to the

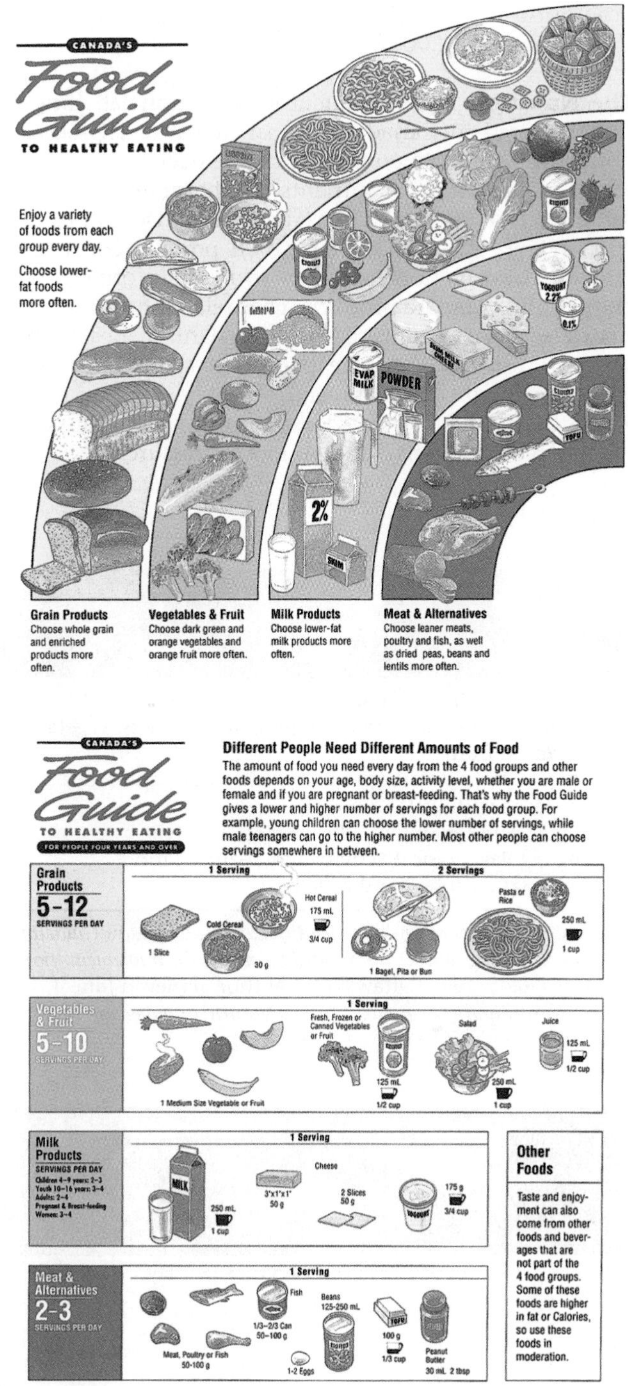

FIGURE **39–3** *Canada's Food Guide to Healthy Eating.* (From *Canada's Food Guide to Healthy Eating,* Catalogue no. H39-252/1992, Health and Welfare Canada, 1992, 1997, Ottawa, ON: Author.)

promotion of health and reduction of chronic disease (Health Canada, 2005).

The Nutrition Label. Mandatory nutrition labelling is now required in Canada on most prepackaged food. A nutrition facts table consisting of the declaration of energy (calories) and 13 nutrients will become mandatory for most prepackaged foods beginning December 12, 2005 (Figure 39–4). This table will provide consumers with the information necessary to make informed food choices and compare products. Diet-related health claims have also been established from recognized health and scientific information. The permitted claims are about the following diet/health relationships:

- A healthy diet low in sodium and high in potassium may reduce the risk of high blood pressure.
- A healthy diet adequate in calcium and vitamin D may reduce the risk of osteoporosis.
- A healthy diet low in saturated fat and trans fat may reduce the risk of heart disease.
- A healthy diet rich in vegetables and fruit may reduce the risk of some types of cancer.

Table 39-2 Canada's Guidelines for Healthy Eating

- Enjoy a VARIETY of foods.
- Emphasize cereals, breads, other grain products, vegetables, and fruits.
- Choose low-fat dairy products, lean meats, and foods prepared with little or no fat.
- Achieve and maintain a healthy body weight by enjoying regular physical activity and healthy eating.
- Limit salt, alcohol, and caffeine.

Adapted from *Action Towards Healthy Eating—Canada's Guidelines for Healthy Eating and Recommended Strategies for Implementation*, Health Canada, 1990, Ottawa: ON: Author; retrieved June 4, 2004, from *http://www.hc-sc.gc.ca/hppb/nutrition/pube/eat/eat03.htm*

Table 39-3 Nutritional Recommendations for Canadians

- The Canadian diet should provide energy consistent with the maintenance of body weight within the recommended range.
- The Canadian diet should include essential nutrients in amounts specified in the Recommended Nutrient Intakes.
- The Canadian diet should include no more than 30% of energy as fat (33 g/1000 kcal or 39 g/5000 kJ) and no more than 10% as saturated fat (11 g/1000 kcal or 13 g/5000 kJ).
- The Canadian diet should provide 55% of energy as carbohydrates (138 g/1000 kcal or 165 g/5000 kJ) from a variety of sources.
- The sodium content of the Canadian diet should be reduced.
- The Canadian diet should include no more than 5% of total energy as alcohol, or two drinks daily, whichever is less.
- The Canadian diet should contain no more caffeine than the equivalent of four cups of regular coffee per day.
- Community water supplies containing less than 1 mg/L should be fluoridated to that level.

Adapted from *Action towards healthy eating: Canada's Guidelines for Healthy Eating and Recommended Strategies for Implementation*, Health Canada, 1990, Ottawa: ON: Author; retrieved June 4, 2004, from *http://www.hc-sc.gc.ca/hppb/nutrition/pube/eat/eat03.htm*

Table 39-4 Summary of Recommended Intakes and Nutritional Values According to *Canada's Food Guide to Healthy Eating*

Grain Products	Vegetables and Fruits	Milk Products	Meat and Alternatives
5–12 servings per day	5–10 servings per day	2–4 servings per day: 4–9 years, 2–3 servings; 10–16 years, 3–4 servings; adults, 2–4 servings; pregnant/lactating, 3–4 servings	2–3 servings per day
Protein		Protein	Protein
		Fat	Fat
Carbohydrate	Carbohydrate		
Fibre	Fibre		
Thiamine	Thiamine		Thiamine
Riboflavin		Riboflavin	Riboflavin
Niacin			Niacin
Folate	Folate		Folate
		Vitamin B_{12}	Vitamin B_{12}
	Vitamin C		
	Vitamin A	Vitamin A	
		Vitamin D	
		Calcium	
Iron	Iron		Iron
Zinc		Zinc	Zinc
Magnesium	Magnesium	Magnesium	Magnesium

Adapted from *Canada's Food Guide to Healthy Eating* (Catalogue no. H39-253/1992E), Health and Welfare Canada, 1992, Ottawa, ON: Author.

The Canadian government defines words used in nutritional claims that describe a product to allow consumers to associate claims with particular standards. Highlights of the new regulations regarding nutrient content claims include the following:

- *Free* claims indicate that the number of calories or the amount of a nutrient is nutritionally insignificant in a specified amount of food.
- Claims for *saturated fatty acids* now include a restriction on levels of both saturated and trans fatty acids.
- The claim *(naming the percent) fat-free* is allowed only if accompanied by the statement *low fat* or *low in fat.*
- The nutrient content claim *light* is allowed only on foods that meet the criteria for either *reduced in fat* or *reduced in calories.*
- A statement that explains what makes the food light must accompany the use of *light;* this is also true if *light* refers to a sensory characteristic such as light in colour.
- The only nutrient content claims that are permitted for foods for children under 2 years of age are *source of protein, excellent source of protein, more protein, no added salt,* and *no added sugar.*

Nutrition for Health: An Agenda for Action. In 1992, the World Health Organization (WHO) endorsed a World Declaration on Nutrition. In 1996, Canada responded to this endorsement and devised *Nutrition for Health: An Agenda for Action.* This document is the combined work of multi-sectoral groups in Canada focused on stimulating and accelerating action by all sectors toward achieving healthier people. The strategic directions recommended by the *Agenda for Action* have arisen from an analysis of Canada's current situation and select high-priority, health-enhancing activities that build on the strength of previous activities. The challenge remains to motivate consumers to put the dietary recommendations into practice. The most current Health Canada information on patterns of consumption indicates a move by most Canadians toward meeting the nutritional recommendations. Health professionals can play a key role in promoting healthy dietary practices.

Nursing Knowledge Base

Nutrition During Human Growth and Development

Infants Through School-Age Children. Infancy is marked by rapid growth with high protein, vitamin, mineral, and energy requirements. The average birth weight of a Canadian baby is currently 3389 g. The infant usually doubles birth weight at 4 to 5 months and triples it at 1 year. An energy intake of approximately 108 kcal/kg of body weight is needed in the first half of infancy and 98 kcal/kg in the second half (U.S. Department of Agriculture [USDA] and U.S. Department of Health and Human Services, 2000). Commercial formulas and human breast milk both provide approximately 20 kcal/30 mL. A full-term newborn is able to digest and absorb simple carbohydrates, proteins, and a moderate amount of emulsified fat. Infants need about 100 to 150 mL/kg/day of fluid because a large portion of total body weight is water.

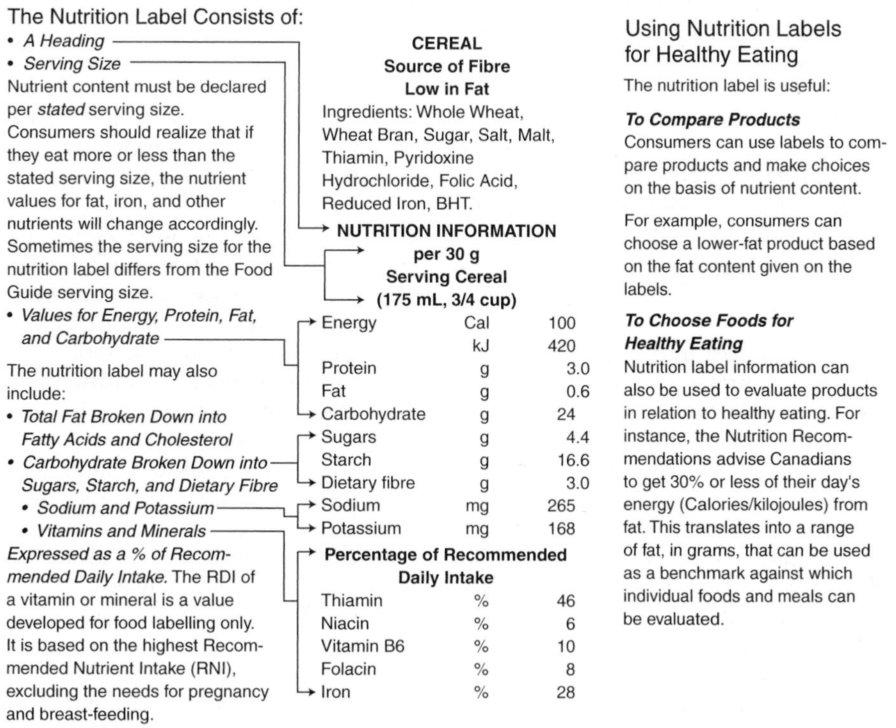
The Nutrition Label Consists of:
• A Heading
• Serving Size
Nutrient content must be declared per stated serving size. Consumers should realize that if they eat more or less than the stated serving size, the nutrient values for fat, iron, and other nutrients will change accordingly. Sometimes the serving size for the nutrition label differs from the Food Guide serving size.
• Values for Energy, Protein, Fat, and Carbohydrate
The nutrition label may also include:
• Total Fat Broken Down into Fatty Acids and Cholesterol
• Carbohydrate Broken Down into Sugars, Starch, and Dietary Fibre
• Sodium and Potassium
• Vitamins and Minerals
Expressed as a % of Recommended Daily Intake. The RDI of a vitamin or mineral is a value developed for food labelling only. It is based on the highest Recommended Nutrient Intake (RNI), excluding the needs for pregnancy and breast-feeding.
CEREAL
Source of Fibre
Low in Fat
Ingredients: Whole Wheat, Wheat Bran, Sugar, Salt, Malt, Thiamin, Pyridoxine Hydrochloride, Folic Acid, Reduced Iron, BHT.
NUTRITION INFORMATION
per 30 g
Serving Cereal
(175 mL, 3/4 cup)
Energy Cal 100
kJ 420
Protein g 3.0
Fat g 0.6
Carbohydrate g 24
Sugars g 4.4
Starch g 16.6
Dietary fibre g 3.0
Sodium mg 265
Potassium mg 168
Percentage of Recommended Daily Intake
Thiamin % 46
Niacin % 6
Vitamin B6 % 10
Folacin % 8
Iron % 28
Using Nutrition Labels for Healthy Eating
The nutrition label is useful:
To Compare Products
Consumers can use labels to compare products and make choices on the basis of nutrient content.
For example, consumers can choose a lower-fat product based on the fat content given on the labels.
To Choose Foods for Healthy Eating
Nutrition label information can also be used to evaluate products in relation to healthy eating. For instance, the Nutrition Recommendations advise Canadians to get 30% or less of their day's energy (Calories/kilojoules) from fat. This translates into a range of fat, in grams, that can be used as a benchmark against which individual foods and meals can be evaluated.

FIGURE **39-4** Sample food label. (From *Food Guide Facts: Background for Educators and Communicators,* Catalogue no. H39-253/10-1992E, Health Canada, 1992, Ottawa, ON: Author.)

Breast-Feeding. The Canadian Paediatric Society Nutrition Committee, Dieticians of Canada, and Health Canada (Joint Working Group, 1998; reaffirmed March 2004) recommend breast-feeding as the optimal method of infant feeding. There are multiple benefits of breast-feeding to both infant and mother. For example, breast-feeding confers immunological protection and reduces allergy risks in the infant, is economical and convenient (breast milk is always fresh and at the correct temperature), and provides an excellent opportunity for mother and infant to interact (Grodner, Anderson, & DeYoung, 2000). Breast-fed infants need supplemental vitamin D. Other vitamin or mineral supplementation is not recommended for the first 6 months (Joint Working Group, 1998).

Multidisciplinary promotion of breast-feeding has resulted in a current 73% initiation rate in Canada (Health Canada, 2002a). Many hospitals and communities have nurse lactation consultants who work individually with mothers for successful breast-feeding in the hospital and at home. The need for health practitioners to promote, protect, and support breast-feeding as the healthiest choice for both infant and mother is well recognized (WHO/UNICEF, 1990).

Formula. Commercially prepared infant formulas, cow's milk-based and iron-fortified, are the most acceptable alternative to breast milk. Infant formulas are designed to contain the approximate nutrient composition of human milk. Protein in the formula is typically supplied as whey, soy, cow's milk base, casein hydrolysate, or elemental amino acids. Specialty formulas are indicated for infants with detected or suspected pathology. The composition, processing, packaging, and labelling of all infant formulas are regulated under Canadian food and drug laws. The addition of nucleotides to infant formula is a new area of research, intended to parallel human milk more closely and boost immune function (Pickering et al., 1998).

Regular cow's milk should not be used for infant formula before 9 to 12 months of age. It may cause gastrointestinal bleeding and is too concentrated for the infant's kidneys to manage. Honey is a potential source of botulism toxin and should not be used in the infant's diet. The toxin can be fatal in children under 1 year of age (Williams & Schlenker, 2003).

Introduction to Solid Food. Breast milk or formula provides sufficient nutrition for the first 4 to 6 months of life. The development of fine motor skills of the hand and fingers parallels the infant's interest in food and self-feeding. Iron-fortified cereals are typically the first semi-solid food to be introduced.

The addition of foods to an infant's diet should be governed by the infant's nutrient needs, physical readiness to handle different forms of foods, and the need to detect and control allergic reactions. New foods should be introduced one at a time, early in the day, approximately 4 to 7 days apart to identify allergies. It is best to introduce new foods before milk or other foods to avoid satiety (Wong, 1997).

The growth rate slows during toddler years (ages 1 to 3 years). The toddler needs fewer kilocalories but an increased amount of protein in relation to body weight; consequently, appetite may decrease at about 18 months of age. Toddlers exhibit strong food preferences and become picky eaters. Small, frequent meals consisting of breakfast, lunch, and dinner, with three interspersed, high-nutrient-density snacks, may improve nutritional intake (Wong, 1997). Calcium and phosphorus are important for healthy bone growth.

Toddlers who consume more than 720 mL of milk daily in lieu of other foods may develop milk anemia, as milk is a poor source of iron. Whole milk should be used until the toddler reaches 2 years of age to help ensure adequate intake of fatty acids necessary for brain and neurological development. Certain foods such as hot dogs, candy, gum, cough drops, raisins, sunflower seeds, fish with bones, peanut butter, marshmallows, nuts, grapes, raw vegetables, and popcorn have been implicated in choking deaths and should be avoided or prepared in a safe manner (Joint Working Group, 1998). Preschoolers' (3 to 5 years) dietary requirements are similar to those of toddlers. They consume slightly more than toddlers, and nutrient density is more important than quantity.

School-age children, 6 to 12 years old, grow at a slower and steadier rate, with a gradual decline in energy requirements per unit of body weight. The school-age child gains 3 to 5 kg in weight and 6 cm in height per year until puberty. Despite better appetites and more varied food intake, school-age children's diets should be carefully assessed for adequate protein and vitamins A and C. School-age children frequently fail to eat a proper breakfast and have an unsupervised intake at school. High fat, sugar, and salt can result from a liberal intake of snack foods. Inappropriate nutrition may play an important role in childhood obesity. The prevalence of childhood obesity in Canada has tripled from 1981 to 1996 (Tremblay & Willms, 2000, 2001). In a 1998 Canadian survey of the eating habits of Grade 6 students, approximately 27% said they did not eat at least one serving of fruit each day, while 55% said they did not have at least one serving of vegetables each day. About 15% of these students ate French fries or potato chips daily and 24% ate candy or chocolate bars daily (Health Canada, 2002b).

Adolescents. During adolescence, physiological age is a better guide to nutritional needs than chronological age. Energy needs increase to meet greater metabolic demands of growth. Daily requirement of protein also increases. Calcium is essential for the rapid bone growth of adolescence, and girls need a continuous source of iron to replace menstrual losses. Boys also need adequate iron for muscle development. Iodine supports increased thyroid activity, and use of iodized table salt assures availability. B complex vitamins are needed to support heightened metabolic activity.

The adolescent's diet is influenced by many factors other than nutritional needs, including concern about body image and appearance, desire for independence, and fad diets. Nutritional and energy deficiencies may occur in adolescent girls (Best, Small, & Brennan, 1994) as a result of dieting and use of oral contraceptives. The adolescent boy's diet may be inadequate in total kilocalories, protein, iron, folic acid, B vitamins, and iodine. Snacks provide approximately 25% of the teenager's total dietary intake. The consumption of fast foods has been associated with excess weight gain, which may be related to the higher energy and fat content of most of these foods. Fast-food restaurants also offer increasingly larger portions, which encourages the ingestion of greater amounts (U.S. Department of Health and Human Services, Centers for Disease Control and Prevention, 2001).

Obese children are at an increased risk for hypertriglyceridemia, hypercholesterolemia, hyperinsulinemia, Type 2 diabetes mellitus, hypertension, respiratory disorders, orthopedic problems, and psychological problems during their youth. Because juvenile obesity frequently continues into adulthood, it could lead to higher rates of morbidity and mortality from cardiovascular disease, diabetes, arthritis-related disability, and some cancers. Thus, preventing and treating obesity in childhood and adolescence is a critical public health issue and an important determinant of health. Increasing physical activity is often more important than curbing intake for countering obesity.

The onset of eating disorders such as **anorexia nervosa** or **bulimia nervosa** often occurs during adolescence. Recognition of eating disorders is essential for early intervention (Table 39-5).

Parents often have more influence on the adolescent diet than they believe. Effective strategies include limiting the amount of unhealthy food choices kept at home and enhancing the appearance and taste of healthy foods. Making healthy food choices more convenient and available and working to change social norms of what foods are "cool" are also ways to promote optimal nutritional health in adolescents (Neumark-Sztainer et al., 1999).

Pregnancy occurring within 4 years of menarche may place mother and fetus at risk because of anatomical and physiological immaturity. Malnutrition at the time of conception increases risk to the adolescent and her fetus. Most teenage girls do not want to gain weight. Counselling related to nutritional needs of pregnancy may be difficult, and suggestions are better tolerated than rigid directions. The diet of pregnant adolescents is often deficient in calcium, iron, and vitamins A and C. Prenatal vitamin and mineral supplements are recommended.

Table 39-5 Potential Assessment for Eating Disorders

Anorexia Nervosa

A. Refusal to maintain body weight over a minimal normal weight for age and height, e.g., weight loss leading to maintenance of body weight less than 85% of ideal body weight (IBW); or failure to make expected weight gain during period of growth, leading to body weight less than 85% of that expected.
B. Intense fear of gaining weight or becoming fat, although underweight.
C. Disturbance in the way in which one's body weight, size, or shape is experienced; e.g., the person claims to "feel fat" even when obviously underweight.
D. In females, absence of at least 3 consecutive menstrual cycles when otherwise expected to occur (primary or secondary amenorrhea). (A woman is considered to have amenorrhea if her periods occur only following hormone administration.)

Bulimia Nervosa

A. Recurrent episodes of binge eating (rapid consumption of a large amount of food in a discrete period of time).
B. A feeling of lack of control over eating behaviour during the eating binges.
C. The person regularly engages in either self-induced vomiting, use of laxatives or diuretics, strict dieting or fasting, or vigorous exercise in order to prevent weight gain.
D. A minimum average of 2 binge eating episodes a week for at least 3 months.

Reprinted with permission from American Psychiatric Association: *Diagnostic and statistical manual of mental disorders,* ed 4 revised, Washington, DC, Copyright 1994, American Psychiatric Association.

Young and Middle Adults. The demands for most nutrients are reduced as the growth period ends. Adults need nutrients for energy, maintenance, and repair, although energy needs usually decline over the years. Obesity may become a problem as a result of decreased physical exercise, frequent dining out, and the increased ability to afford more luxury foods. Adult women who use oral contraceptives may need extra vitamins. Iron and calcium intake continues to be important.

Maintaining good oral health is important throughout adulthood. Poor oral hygiene and periodontal disease are potential risk factors for systemic diseases such as bacteremia, endocarditis, cardiopulmonary disease, diabetes mellitus, and adverse outcomes in pregnancy (Hornick, 2002).

Pregnancy. Poor nutrition during pregnancy can cause low birth weight in infants and decreased chances of survival. Generally, the fetus's needs are met at the expense of the mother. However, if nutrient sources are not available, both suffer. The nutritional status of the mother at the time of conception is important. Significant aspects of fetal growth and development often occur before pregnancy is even suspected.

The energy requirements of pregnancy are related to the mother's body weight and activity. Rigid recommendations about weight gain should be avoided. The quality of nutrition during pregnancy is more important than weight gain per se or kilocalories consumed per day. Food intake in the first trimester should include balanced portions of essential nutrients with emphasis on quality. *Canada's Food Guide to Healthy Eating* recommends pregnant women get the additional nutrients needed for growth by increasing their daily servings of milk and milk products, breads and cereals, and fruits and vegetables (Health and Welfare Canada, 1992). Supplementation is usually recommended along with dietary modification to increase intake of folate, calcium, vitamin D, iron, and essential fatty acids (Health Canada, 2002a).

Calcium intake is especially critical in the third trimester, when fetal bones are mineralized. Iron may be supplemented to provide for increased maternal blood volume, for fetal blood storage, and for blood loss during delivery. Iodine needs increase 15% to 17% because of increased activity of the thyroid gland. Folic acid intake is particularly important for DNA synthesis and the growth of red blood cells. Inadequate intake may lead to fetal neural tube defects, anencephaly, or maternal megaloblastic anemia (Daly et al., 1997; Food and Nutrition Board, 1992). Prenatal care usually includes vitamin and mineral supplementation to ensure daily intakes; however, pregnant women should not take additional supplements beyond prescribed amounts. For example, vitamin A is essential to maternal and fetal health but is teratogenic when consumed in excess (Kessler, 1995).

Pregnant women should drink at least eight glasses of water daily. They should avoid artificial sweeteners, alcohol, excessive caffeine, and all drugs not specifically ordered. Adequate fluid and fibre intake and moderate exercise help prevent constipation, which is commonly associated with pregnancy.

Lactation. Lactating women need 500 kcal/day above the usual allowance because the production of milk increases energy requirements. *Canada's Food Guide to Healthy Eating* suggests lactating women ingest the same nutrient levels as recommended during pregnancy. The need for calcium remains the same as during pregnancy. There is an increased need for vitamins A and C. Daily intake of water-soluble vitamins (B and C) is needed to ensure adequate levels in breast milk. Fluid intake should be adequate but need not be excessive. Caffeine, alcohol, and drugs are excreted in breast milk and should be avoided. Tobacco use can decrease milk production (Joint Working Group, 1998).

Older Adults. Adults 65 years and older have a decreased need for energy because metabolic rate slows with age. However, vitamin and mineral requirements remain unchanged from middle adulthood.

Many factors influence the nutritional status of older adults (Box 39-1). Income is significant because living on a fixed income may reduce the amount of money available to buy food. A large number of older clients benefit from home-delivered or congregate meal services. Health is another important influence. The older adult may be on a therapeutic diet; have difficulty eating because of physical symptoms, lack of teeth, or dentures; or be at risk for drug–nutrient interactions. Thirst sensation may diminish, leading to inadequate fluid intake or dehydration (see chapter 36). Meats may be avoided because of cost or because they are difficult to chew. Cream soups and meat-based vegetable soups are nutrient-dense sources of protein. Cheese, eggs, and peanut butter are also useful high-protein alternatives. Milk continues to be an important food for older adults, who need adequate calcium to protect against osteoporosis (a decrease of bone-mass density). Although research has shown that older men lag behind women in developing osteoporosis by approximately a decade, screening and treatment are necessary for older men as well as older women (Atkinson & Ward, 2001; Ybarra, Ade, & Romeo, 1996). The diet of older adults should contain choices from all food groups and may require a vitamin and mineral supplement.

Focus on Older Adults **Box 39-1**

Factors Affecting Nutritional Status

- Age-related gastrointestinal changes that affect digestion of food and maintenance of nutrition include changes in the teeth and gums, reduced saliva production, atrophy of oral mucosal epithelial cells, increased taste threshold, decreased thirst sensation, reduced gag reflex, and decreased esophageal and colonic peristalsis.
- Presence of co-morbidities increases risk of poor nutrition (Millen et al., 2001).
- Malnutrition in older adults has multiple causes, such as income, educational level, physical functional level to meet activities of daily living, loss, dependency, loneliness, and transportation (Chen, Schilling, & Lyder, 2001).
- Nutrition knowledge may be poor: Older adults may not read food labels or understand nutrient value of foods.
- Medications may have adverse effects such as causing anorexia, xerostomia, early satiety, and impaired smell and taste perception.
- Intake of calcium, vitamin D, and phosphorus may be deficient, increasing risk for osteoporosis. Vitamin B_{12} may not be synthesized because of lack of intrinsic factor in terminal ileum, decreased lean muscle mass, and lower basic energy expenditure (Chen et al., 2001; Lueckenotte, 2000).
- Cognitive impairments related to delirium, dementia, and depression may be present.

Safety Alert. Home-bound older adults with chronic illness have additional nutritional risks. Frequently, this group lives alone with little or no social resources to assist in obtaining or preparing nutritionally sound meals. Increased nutritional screening during regular medical visits may result in more timely recognition of potential nutritional deficiencies and subsequent treatment of these deficiencies (Millen et al., 2001; Todorovic, 2001).

Alternative Food Patterns

Many people follow special patterns of food intake based on religion (Table 39-6), cultural background (Box 39-2) ethics, health beliefs, personal preference, or concern for the efficient use of land to produce food. Such special diets are not necessarily more or less nutritious than diets based on *Canada's Food Guide to Healthy Eating* or other nutritional guidelines because good nutrition depends on a balanced intake of all required nutrients.

Vegetarian Diet. Vegetarianism is the consumption of a diet consisting predominantly of plant foods. Vegetarians may be ovolactovegetarians (avoid meat, fish, and poultry but eat eggs and milk), lactovegetarians (drink milk but avoid eggs), or vegans (consume only plant foods). Vegan, Zen macrobiotic (eat primarily brown rice, other grains, and herb teas), and fruitarian (eat only fruit, nuts, honey, and olive oil) diets can be nutrient poor

Table 39-6 Religious Dietary Restrictions

Islam	Christianity	Hinduism	Judaism	Church of Jesus Christ of Latter-Day Saints (Mormons)	Seventh-Day Adventists Church
Pork Alcohol Caffeine Ramadan fasting sunrise to sunset for month Ritualized methods of animal slaughter required for meat ingestion	Minimal or no alcohol Holy day observances may restrict meat	All meats	Pork Predatory fowl Shellfish (eat only fish with scales) Rare meats Blood (blood sausage, etc.) Mixing of milk or dairy products with meat dishes Must adhere to kosher food preparation methods 24 hours of fasting on Yom Kippur, a day of atonement No leavened bread eaten during Passover (8 days) No cooking on the Sabbath (Saturday)	Alcohol Tobacco Caffeine	Pork Shellfish Alcohol Vegetarian diet encouraged

Cultural Aspects of Care

Box 39-2

Nutrition

The theory of hot and cold foods predominates in many cultures. The origin appears to be from Hippocratic beliefs concerning health and the four humors. Arabs were keepers of this knowledge during the Dark Ages and later influenced the Spanish to adopt this belief system in the later Middle Ages. The foundation of the theory is keeping harmony with nature by balancing "cold," "hot," "wet," and "dry." Some cultures believe hot is warmth, strength, and reassurance, whereas cold is menacing and weak. Classification has nothing to do with spiciness but is a symbolic representation of temperature.

Implications for Practice

- When hot and cold foods are used by clients as part of their cultural health practices, dietary modifications may be needed. For example, a client may wish to increase consumption of hot foods (e.g., rice, grain cereals, alcohol, beef, lamb, chili peppers, chocolate, cheese, temperate zone fruits, eggs, peas, goat's milk, corn husks, oils, onions, pork, radishes, and tamales) or cold foods (e.g., beans, citrus fruits, tropical fruits, dairy products, most vegetables, honey, raisins, chicken, fish, and goat).
- Foods can be rendered hot or cold through preparation methods. Blending of hot and cold food creates a balance.
- Some conditions are considered to be cold and require hot foods, including menstruation, cancer, pneumonia, earache, colds, paralysis, headache, and rheumatism. Others are considered to be hot and require cold foods, including pregnancy, fever, infections, diarrhea, rashes, ulcers, liver problems, constipation, kidney problems, and sore throats.

Adapted from *Transcultural Nursing: Assessment and Intervention* (3rd ed.), by J. N. Giger and R. E. Davidhizar, 1999, St. Louis, MO: Mosby.

and can result in malnutrition. Knowledge related to complementary use of complete and incomplete proteins is necessary. Children who follow a vegetarian diet are especially at risk for protein and vitamin deficiencies, such as vitamin B_{12}.

Critical Thinking

Critical thinking requires drawing together knowledge, experience, information from clients, and intellectual and professional standards. Clinical judgments involve anticipating the required information, analyzing the data, and making decisions regarding client care. Critical thinking is a dynamic process. During assessment (Figure 39–5), the nurse must consider all elements that build toward making appropriate nursing diagnoses.

In the case of nutrition, the nurse must integrate knowledge from nursing and other disciplines, previous experiences, information gathered from clients and families regarding food preferences, and dietary history. Professional standards, such as the DRIs, *Canada's Food Guide to Healthy Eating, Canada's Guidelines for Healthy Eating,* and *Nutrition Recommendations for Canadians,* provide guidelines for assessing and maintaining clients' nutritional status. Other professional standards from the Heart and Stroke

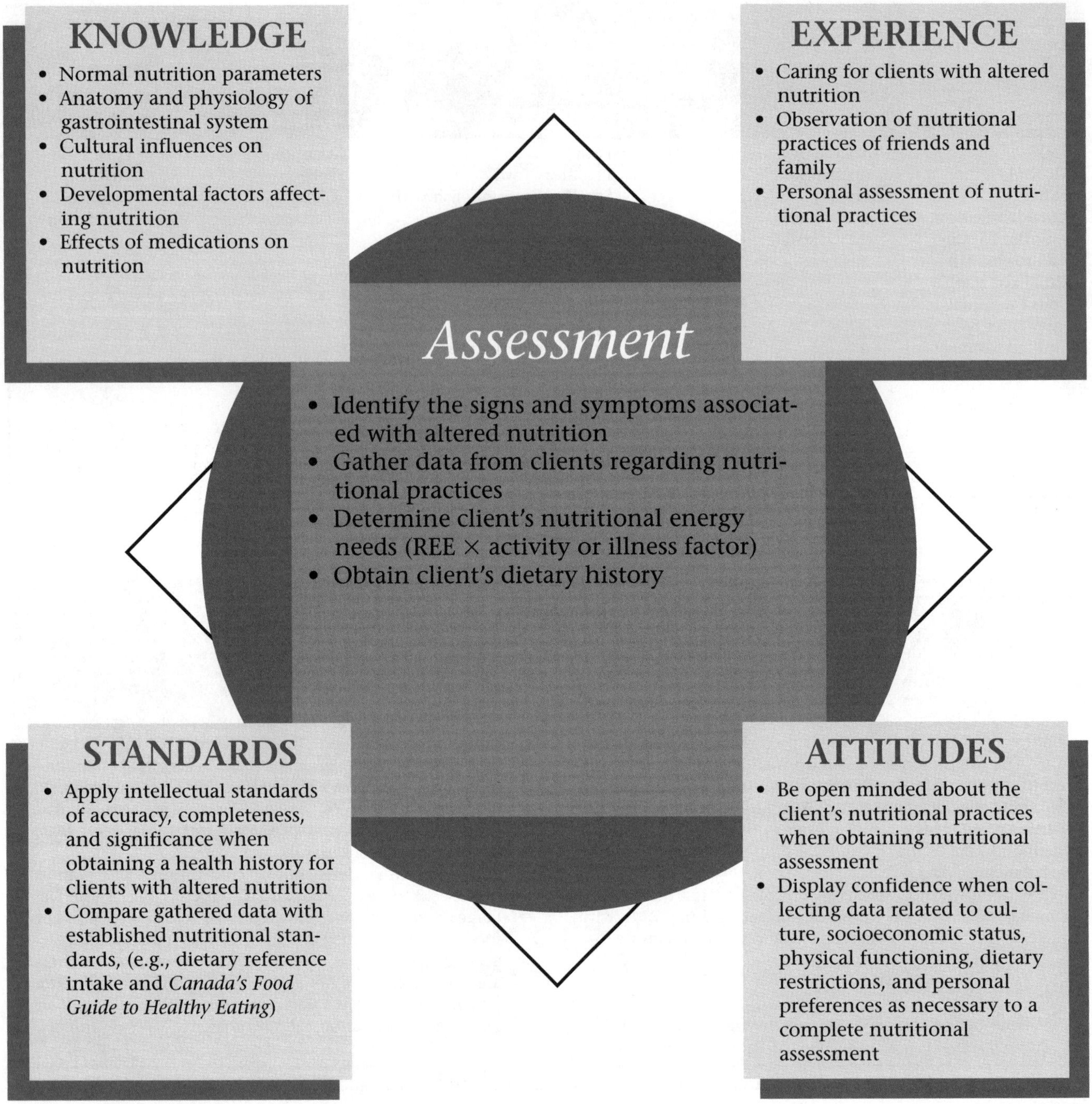
KNOWLEDGE
• Normal nutrition parameters
• Anatomy and physiology of gastrointestinal system
• Cultural influences on nutrition
• Developmental factors affecting nutrition
• Effects of medications on nutrition
EXPERIENCE
• Caring for clients with altered nutrition
• Observation of nutritional practices of friends and family
• Personal assessment of nutritional practices
Assessment
• Identify the signs and symptoms associated with altered nutrition
• Gather data from clients regarding nutritional practices
• Determine client's nutritional energy needs (REE × activity or illness factor)
• Obtain client's dietary history
STANDARDS
• Apply intellectual standards of accuracy, completeness, and significance when obtaining a health history for clients with altered nutrition
• Compare gathered data with established nutritional standards, (e.g., dietary reference intake and Canada's Food Guide to Healthy Eating)
ATTITUDES
• Be open minded about the client's nutritional practices when obtaining nutritional assessment
• Display confidence when collecting data related to culture, socioeconomic status, physical functioning, dietary restrictions, and personal preferences as necessary to a complete nutritional assessment

FIGURE **39–5** Critical thinking model for nutrition assessment.

Foundation of Canada, the Canadian Cancer Society, Canadian Society for Clinical Nutrition, and the Canadian Dietetic Association are available. These standards are research based and are regularly updated.

Nursing Process and Nutrition

Nurses are in an excellent position to recognize signs of poor nutrition and to take steps to initiate change. Close contact with clients and their families enables nurses to make observations about physical status, food intake, weight changes, and response to therapy.

NP Assessment

Early recognition of malnourished or at-risk clients has a strong positive influence on both short- and long-term health outcomes (American Society for Parenteral and Enteral Nutrition [ASPEN], 2001; Evans-Stoner, 1997). Studies have identified 40% to 55% of adult hospitalized

The Warning Signs of poor nutritional health are often overlooked. Use this checklist to find out if you or someone you know is at nutritional risk.

Read the statements below. Circle the number in the yes column for those that apply. For each yes answer, score the number in the box. Total the nutritional score.

DETERMINE YOUR NUTRITIONAL HEALTH

	YES
I have an illness or condition that made me change the kind and/or amount of food I eat.	2
I eat fewer than 2 meals per day.	3
I eat few fruits or vegetables, or milk products.	2
I have 3 or more drinks of beer, liquor or wine almost every day.	2
I have tooth or mouth problems that make it hard for me to eat.	2
I don't always have enough money to buy the food I need.	4
I eat alone most of the time.	1
I take 3 or more different prescribed or over-the-counter drugs a day.	1
Without wanting to, I have lost or gained 10 pounds in the last 6 months.	2
I am not always physically able to shop, cook and/or feed myself.	2
TOTAL	

Total Your Nutritional Score. If it's –

0–2 **Good!** Recheck your nutritional score in 6 months.

3–5 **You are at moderate nutritional risk.** See what can be done to improve your eating habits and lifestyle. Your office on aging, senior nutrition program, senior citizens center or health department can help. Recheck your nutritional score in 3 months.

6 or more **You are at high nutritional risk.** Bring this checklist the next time you see your doctor, dietitian or other qualified health or social service professional. Talk with them about any problems you may have. Ask for help to improve your nutritional health.

These materials developed and distributed by the Nutritional Screening Initiative, a project of:

AMERICAN ACADEMY OF FAMILY PHYSICIANS

THE AMERICAN DIETETIC ASSOCIATION

NATIONAL COUNCIL ON THE AGING

Remember that warning signs suggest risk, but do not represent diagnosis of any condition.

FIGURE **39–6** Nutrition screening tool for older adults. (From the Nutrition Screening Initiative, a project of the American Academy of Family Physicians, the American Dietetic Association, and the National Council of the Aging, Inc. and funded in part by a grant from Ross Products Division, Abbott Laboratories, Inc.).

clients as being either malnourished or at risk for malnutrition and have also found a relationship between malnutrition and adverse outcomes, including mortality (Gallagher-Allred et al., 1996). Nutrition assessment forms are useful in identifying clients in need or at risk. Registered Nurses Association of Ontario (2002), Hennessy and Orr (1996), Kovacevich et al. (1997), and Costello and Todd-Magel (1997) are sources of assessment forms.

Body mass index (BMI) is another nutritional assessment tool. It measures weight corrected for height and serves as an alternative to traditional height–weight relationships. Calculation of BMI is achieved by dividing the client's weight in kilograms by height in metres squared: Weight (kg)/Height^2 (m^2). The BMI is available on Health Canada's Web site at *http://www.hcsc.gc.ca/hppb/nutrition/bmi/index.html.* Although BMI is a valid measurement of weight in relation to health, it is not recommended for use as the sole measurement of body composition or level of fitness (RNAO, 2002).

An **ideal body weight (IBW)** provides an estimate of what a person should weigh. This can be calculated using the BMI as a reference guide. A BMI measuring between 25 and 30 indicates overweight, and greater than 30 defines obesity (Health Canada, 2003). If height cannot be measured with the client standing, position the client lying flat in bed as straight as possible, arms folded on the client's chest, and measure the client lengthwise.

The Nutritional Screening Initiative (1998) is a multidisciplinary U.S. effort begun in 1991 to identify warning signs of malnutrition in older adults. A three-tiered approach was designed for the nutritional assessment of older adults. Ten key risk factors are shown in the checklist to determine nutritional health (Figure 39–6) that serves as the first tier. Second-tier screening aims at prevention, and the third tier involves diagnosis and intervention (Nutritional Screening Initiative, 1998; USDA, 2000).

Assessment of nutritional status is essential because of the need for nutrients, energy, and fluids. Nutrition assessment centres on five major areas: anthropometry, laboratory tests, dietary and health history, clinical observation, and client expectations.

Anthropometry. **Anthropometry** is a measurement system of the size and makeup of the body. Height and weight should be obtained for each client admission to any health care setting. If possible, the client should be weighed at the same time each day, on the same scale, and with the same clothing or linen. Rapid weight gain usually reflects fluid shifts. Five hundred millilitres of fluid equals 0.45 kg. For example, for a client with renal failure or congestive heart failure, a weight increase of 0.9 kg is significant, as it may indicate that the client has retained a litre of fluid. Recent weight changes should be documented.

Anthropometric measurements that aid in identifying nutritional problems include the ratio of height-to-wrist circumference, mid-upper arm circumference (MAC); triceps skin fold (TSF), and mid-upper arm muscle circumference (MAMC). Significant variation may result unless the examiner is skilled and has proper equipment. Values for MAC, TSF, and MAMC are compared with standards and calculated as a percentage of the standard. Changes in values for an individual over time are of greater significance than isolated measurements (Williams, 2001).

Laboratory and Biochemical Tests. No single laboratory or biochemical test is diagnostic for malnutrition. Factors that may alter test results include fluid balance, liver function, kidney function, and the presence of disease. Common laboratory tests used to study nutritional status include measures of plasma proteins such as albumin, transferrin, prealbumin, retinol binding protein, total iron-binding capacity, and hemoglobin. After feeding, the response time for changes in these proteins ranges from hours to weeks. The metabolic half-life of albumin is 21 days, transferrin 8 days, prealbumin 2 days, and retinol binding protein 12 hours. This range demonstrates why albumin level, for example, is not an accurate short-term indicator of serum protein status (Pagana & Pagana, 2005). Furthermore, serum albumin levels are affected by the following factors: hydration; hemorrhage; renal or hepatic disease; high-output drainage of wounds, drains, burns, or the gut; steroid administration; exogenous albumin infusions; age; and trauma, burns, stress, or surgery. In summary, albumin level is a better indicator for chronic illnesses, whereas prealbumin level is preferred for acute conditions.

Nitrogen balance is important to establish serum protein status (see the discussion of protein in this chapter). Nitrogen intake is calculated by dividing 6.25 into the total grams of protein ingested in a day (24 hours). The output of nitrogen is established through laboratory analysis of a 24-hour urinary urea nitrogen. For clients with diarrhea or fistula drainage, a further addition of 2 to 4 g of nitrogen output is estimated. Nitrogen balance is found by subtracting the nitrogen output from the nitrogen intake. A positive (more nitrogen taken in than put out) 2- to 3-g nitrogen balance is ideal for anabolism. In contrast, negative (more nitrogen put out than taken in) nitrogen balance is present when catabolic states exist, seen in either starvation or physiologic stress.

Dietary History and Health History. In addition to the general nursing health history, the nurse obtains a diet history to assess the client's needs (Table 39-7). The dietary history focuses on the client's habitual intake of foods and liquids, as well as information about preferences, allergies, and other relevant areas, such as the client's ability to ob-

Table 39-7 Obtaining a Dietary History

Components of a Dietary History	Areas to Assess and/or Questions to Ask
Diet	
Number of meals per day	How many meals do you eat? Are these scheduled meals or snacks?
Food preferences	What type of food do you like?
Food preparation practices	Who prepares the food?
Food purchasing practices	Who purchases the food?
Unpleasant symptoms	
Indigestion, heartburn, gas	What foods cause indigestion, gas, or heartburn? Does this occur each time you have the food?
Relief practices	What relieves the symptoms?
Allergies	Are you allergic to any foods? Get specific listing of foods and allergic response (e.g., hives, itching, anaphylaxis). Determine what is done to treat allergies (e.g., EpiPen, oral antihistamines).
Taste	Have you noticed any changes in taste? Did these changes occur with medications or following an illness?
Chewing and swallowing	Do you wear dentures? Are the dentures comfortable? Assess the condition of the client's teeth. Do you experience mouth pain or sores (e.g., cold sore, canker sores)? Do you have difficulty swallowing? Do you cough or gag when you swallow?
Appetite	Have you had a change in appetite? Have you noticed a change in weight? Was this change an anticipated change (e.g., client was on a weight-reduction diet)?
Elimination patterns	Frequency of bowel movements. Diarrhea associated with meals or specific foods. Constipation.
Use of medications	What medications do you take? Do you take any over-the-counter medications that your doctor does not prescribe? Do you take any nutritional or herbal supplements?

tain food. The nurse gathers information about the client's illness or activity level to determine energy needs and compares that information with food intake. Nursing assessment of nutrition includes health status; age; cultural background (see Box 39-2); religious food patterns (see Table 39-6); socio-economic status; personal food preference; psychological factors; use of alcohol or illegal drugs; use of vitamin, mineral, or herbal supplements or prescription or over-the-counter drugs; and the client's general nutrition knowledge (Evans-Stoner, 1997).

Outpatient clients may keep a 3- to 7-day food diary, which allows the nurse to calculate nutritional intake and to compare it with DRIs to see if dietary habits are adequate. Food-frequency questionnaires may be used to establish patterns over time.

Clinical Observation. Clinical observation is key to a nutritional assessment. The nurse observes the client for signs of nutritional alterations. Because improper nutrition affects all body systems, clues to malnutrition can be observed during physical assessment (see chapter 28). When the general physical assessment of body systems is complete, the nurse can recheck pertinent areas to evaluate the client's nutritional status. The clinical signs of nutritional status (Table 39-8) provide guidelines for observation during physical assessment.

The nurse must also assess for aspiration risk. Those at risk have decreased levels of alertness, decreased gag and/or cough reflexes, difficulty managing saliva, or a wet gurgly voice. The nurse should assess swallowing before giving food or medications. To check swallow adequacy, the nurse places fingers at the throat at the level of the client's larynx, and asks the person to swallow. The nurse should be able to palpate the movement of the larynx. Clients at risk of aspiration need specialized assistance with feeding.

Client Expectations. Clients rely on health care professionals to identify problems of which they may not be aware. Most nutritional problems develop insidiously over weeks and months, not overnight (American Diabetes Association [ADA], 2002). Lindseth (1997) studied graduate

Table 39-8 Clinical Signs of Nutritional Status

Body Area	Signs of Good Nutrition	Signs of Poor Nutrition
General appearance	Alert; responsive	Listless, apathetic, cachectic appearance
Weight	Weight normal for height, age, body build	Obese or underweight appearance (special concern for underweight)
Posture	Erect posture; straight arms and legs	Sagging shoulders; sunken chest; humped back
Muscles	Well-developed, firm muscles; good tone; some fat under skin	Flaccid appearance, poor tone, underdeveloped tone; tenderness; edema; wasted appearance; inability to walk properly
Nervous system control	Good attention span; lack of irritability or restlessness; normal reflexes; psychological stability	Inattention; irritability; confusion; burning and tingling of hands and feet (paresthesia); loss of position and vibratory sense; weakness and tenderness of muscles (may result in inability to walk); decrease or loss of ankle and knee reflexes; absent vibratory sense
Gastrointestinal function	Good appetite and digestion; normal regular elimination; no palpable organs or masses	Anorexia; indigestion; constipation or diarrhea; liver or spleen enlargement
Cardiovascular function	Normal heart rate and rhythm; lack of murmurs; normal blood pressure for age	Rapid heart rate (above 100 beats/minute), enlarged heart; abnormal rhythm; elevated blood pressure
General vitality	Endurance; energy; good sleep habits; vigorous appearance	Easily fatigued; lack of energy; falling asleep easily; tired and apathetic appearance
Hair	Shiny, lustrous appearance; firmness; strands not easily plucked; healthy scalp	Stringy, dull, brittle, dry, thin, and sparse, depigmented appearance; strands that can be easily plucked
Skin (general)	Smooth and slightly moist skin with good colour	Rough, dry, scaly, pale, pigmented, irritated appearance; bruises; petechiae; subcutaneous fat loss
Face and neck	Uniform colour; smooth, pink, healthy appearance; lack of swelling	Greasy, discoloured, scaly, swollen appearance; dark skin over cheeks and under eyes; lumpiness or flakiness of skin around nose and mouth
Lips	Smoothness; good colour; moist (not chapped or swollen) appearance	Dry, scaly, swollen appearance; redness and swelling (cheilosis); angular lesions at corners of mouth; fissures or scars (stomatitis)
Mouth, oral membranes	Reddish pink mucous membranes in oral cavity	Swollen, boggy oral mucous membranes
Gums	Good pink colour; healthy and red appearance; lack of swelling or bleeding	Spongy gums that bleed easily; marginal redness, inflammation; receding gums
Tongue	Good pink or deep reddish colour; lack of swelling; smoothness, presence of surface papillae; lack of lesions	Swelling, scarlet, and raw appearance; magenta colour, beefiness (glossitis); hyperemic and hypertrophic papillae; atrophic papillae

From *Basic Nutrition and Diet Therapy* (11th ed., p. 7), by S. R. Williams, 2001, St. Louis, MO: Mosby.

Continued

Table 39-8 Clinical Signs of Nutritional Status—cont'd

Body Area	Signs of Good Nutrition	Signs of Poor Nutrition
Teeth	Lack of cavities and pain; bright, straight appearance; lack of crowding; well-shaped jaw; clean appearance with no discoloration	Unfilled caries; absent teeth; worn surfaces; mottling (fluorosis); malpositioned appearance
Eyes	Bright, clear, shiny appearance; lack of sores at corner of membranes; eyelids moist and healthy pink colour; prominent blood vessels or lack of mound of tissue or sclera; lack of fatigue circles beneath eyes	Pale eye membranes (pale conjunctivae); redness of membrane (conjunctival infection); dryness; signs of infection; Bitot's spots, redness and fissuring of eyelid corners (angular palpebritis); dryness of eye membrane (conjunctival xerosis); dull appearance of cornea (corneal xerosis); soft cornea (keratomalacia)
Neck (glands)	Lack of enlargement	Thyroid enlargement
Nails	Firm, pink appearance	Spoon shape (koilonychia); brittleness; ridges
Legs, feet	Lack of tenderness, weakness, or swelling; good colour	Edema; tender calf; tingling; weakness
Skeleton	Lack of malformation	Bowlegs; knock-knees; chest deformity at diaphragm; prominent scapulae and ribs

From *Basic Nutrition and Diet Therapy* (11th ed., p. 7), by S. R. Williams, 2001, St. Louis, MO: Mosby.

Nursing Diagnostic Process — Box 39-3

Assessment Activities	Defining Characteristics	Nursing Diagnosis
Body mass index (BMI)	BMI = 37.7	Imbalanced nutrition: more than body requirements
Obtain height and weight	52-year-old man Height: 180 cm Weight: 122 kg	
Obtain 24-hour food history	Lack of satiety High fat and carbohydrate intake, three to four beers/day	
Fluid	Fluid intake is cola, beer, and juice, all high caloric	
Physical assessment	Short of breath on walking Large abdomen Blood pressure: 125/85 mm Hg Pulse: 102 beats per minute Respirations: 32 breaths per minute	
Laboratory values	Cholesterol and triglycerides elevated. All others within normal limits.	
Medication	None	
Social	Wife and family eat out or have large family dinners two times a week.	

nurses and found scores of 50% to 60% on nutritional knowledge. The poorest scores were for topics related to nutrient requirements for specific populations, body weight versus energy intake, and food sources of specific nutrients. In a similar study, Weigley (1995) found several specific nutrition tasks that were least likely to be performed by nurses. These tasks included development of nutrition plans, reference to diet manuals and research literature, use of nutritional materials in teaching, and use of resources to learn about clients' cultural food habits. A firm knowledge base is important to meet client expectations and needs.

Nursing Diagnosis

Assessment enables the nurse to determine any actual or potential nutrition problems (Box 39-3). Knowledge of normal nutritional parameters, anatomy and physiology of the GI system, and cultural, developmental, pharmacological, and dietary guidelines is necessary for complete assessment. A problem may occur when overall intake is significantly decreased or increased, or when one or more nutrients are not ingested, completely digested, or completely

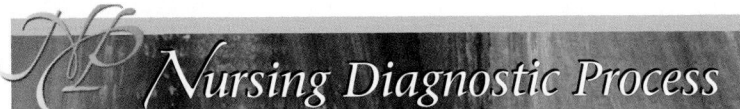

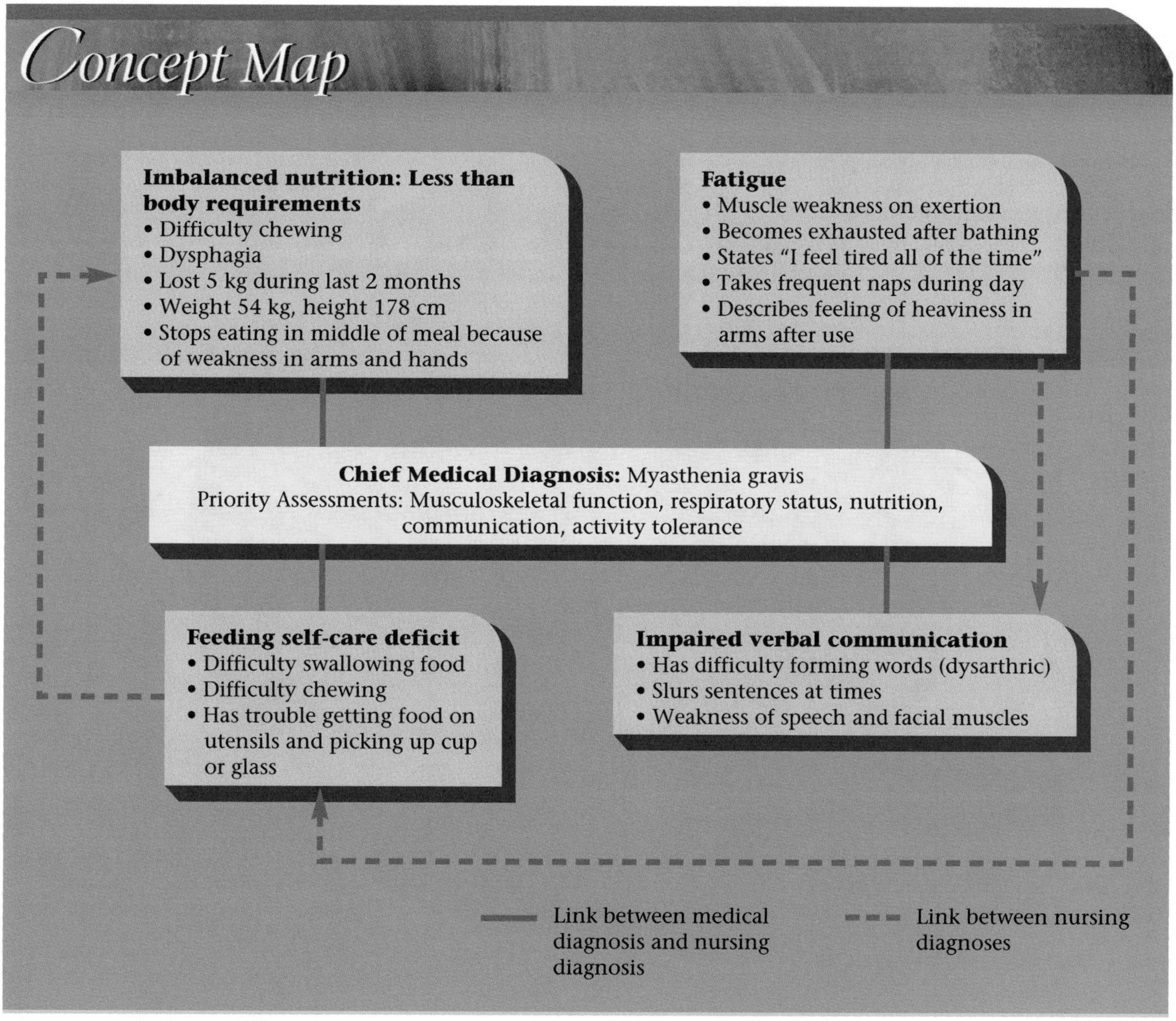

FIGURE **39–7** Concept map for client with myasthenia gravis.

absorbed. Specific diagnoses are related to the actual nutritional problem (e.g., inadequate intake), but may also involve problems that place the client at risk for nutritional deficiencies, such as oral trauma, severe burns, or infections. Some clients have multiple related problems. The concept map in Figure 39–7 shows the relationship of nursing diagnoses in a client with myasthenia gravis.

The nursing diagnostic statement is based on defining characteristics present in the assessment database. The suspected health problem related to the nursing diagnosis is stated. The following are examples of nursing diagnoses of clients with nutritional problems:

- Risk for aspiration in enteral nutrition therapy
- Constipation
- Diarrhea
- Deficient fluid volumes
- Excess fluid volume
- Health maintenance, ineffective
- Health-seeking behaviours (nutrition)
- Risk for infection
- Deficient knowledge (nutrition)
- Ineffective management of therapeutic regimen, individuals
- Imbalanced nutrition: less than body requirements
- Imbalanced nutrition: more than body requirements
- Risk for imbalanced nutrition: more than body requirements
- Feeding self-care deficit

NP Planning

Planning to maintain optimal nutritional status requires a higher level of care than simply correcting problems. Synthesis of client information from multiple sources is necessary to devise an individualized approach to care that is relevant to the client's needs (Figure 39–8). All

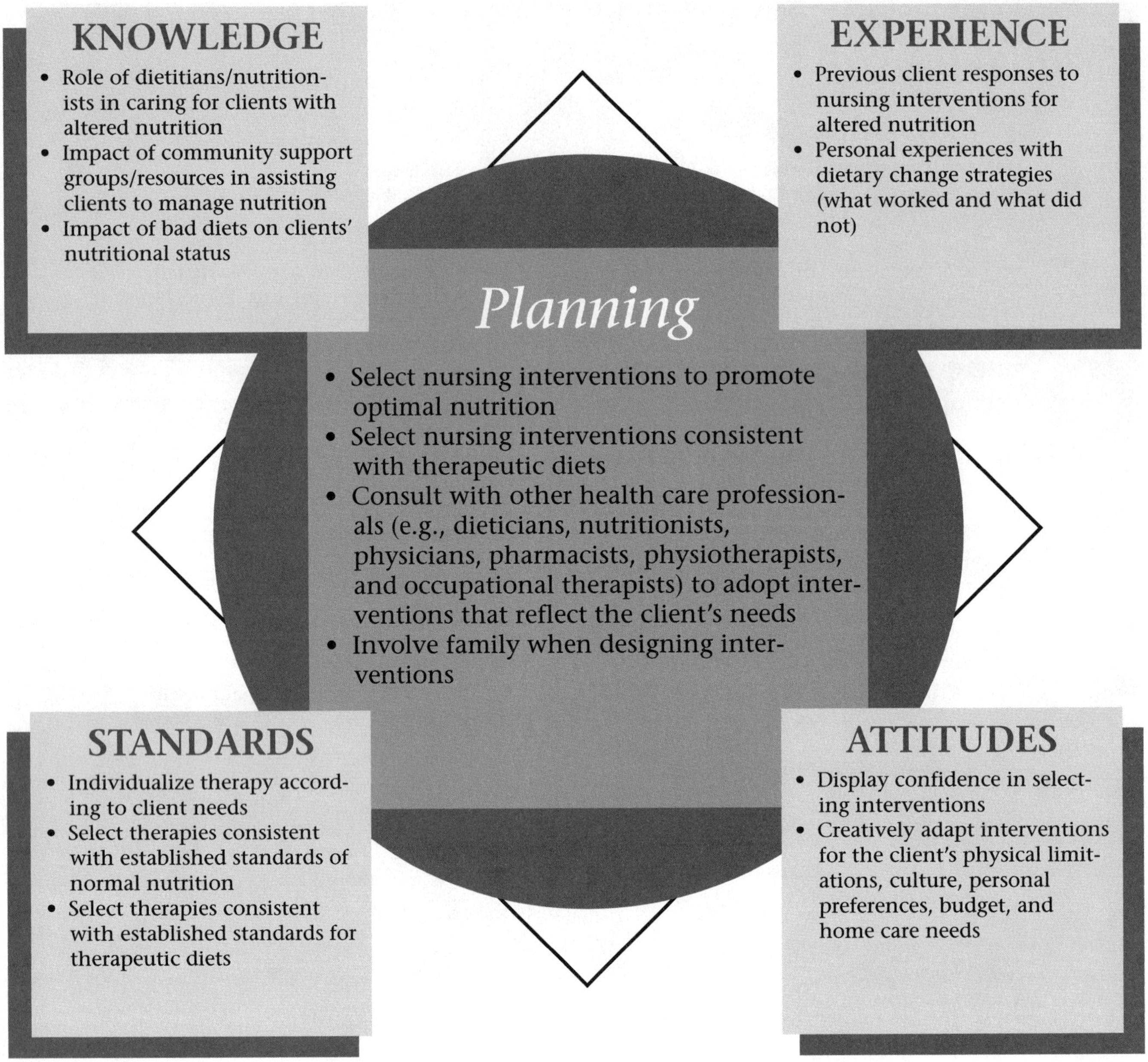
KNOWLEDGE
• Role of dietitians/nutritionists in caring for clients with altered nutrition
• Impact of community support groups/resources in assisting clients to manage nutrition
• Impact of bad diets on clients' nutritional status
EXPERIENCE
• Previous client responses to nursing interventions for altered nutrition
• Personal experiences with dietary change strategies (what worked and what did not)
Planning
• Select nursing interventions to promote optimal nutrition
• Select nursing interventions consistent with therapeutic diets
• Consult with other health care professionals (e.g., dieticians, nutritionists, physicians, pharmacists, physiotherapists, and occupational therapists) to adopt interventions that reflect the client's needs
• Involve family when designing interventions
STANDARDS
• Individualize therapy according to client needs
• Select therapies consistent with established standards of normal nutrition
• Select therapies consistent with established standards for therapeutic diets
ATTITUDES
• Display confidence in selecting interventions
• Creatively adapt interventions for the client's physical limitations, culture, personal preferences, budget, and home care needs

FIGURE **39–8** Critical thinking model for nutrition planning.

data sources are considered in developing a care plan that prevents or minimizes nutritional problems (see Care Plan). Referring to professional standards for nutrition is crucial during this step because published standards are based on scientific findings.

Goals and Outcomes. Goals and outcomes and priorities of care reflect the client's physiological, therapeutic, and individualized needs. Nutritional education and counselling are important for clients on regular diets to prevent disease and promote health. Clients on therapeutic diets must understand the implications of the diet and how the diet assists in controlling their illness. For example, clients with congestive heart failure who follow a low-sodium diet in conjunction with medication therapy and a prescribed exercise program show improvement in their functional activities (Hunt et al., 2001).

Individualized planning is crucial. For example, obese clients usually respond better to regular obtainable goals of moderate weight loss than to one large overwhelming goal (Foster et al., 1997). Mutually planned goals negotiated between the client, dietitian, and nurse help ensure success. An overall goal for an obese client might be "to achieve appropriate BMI height-weight range or be within 10% of ideal body weight (IBW)." The following smaller goals or outcomes can help the person achieve the goal:

- Daily nutritional intake meets the minimal DRIs
- Daily nutritional fat intake is less than 30%

Nursing Care Plan

Imbalanced Nutrition: Less Than Body Requirements

Assessment

Belinda Wong, a nurse practitioner in a Community Health Centre, is seeing 68-year-old Mrs. Cooper, who has a history of congestive heart failure. Recently, Mrs. Cooper noticed a weight loss (15%). She has been taking an antidepressant (Sertraline) for 3 months for an initial episode of depression related to the loss of her husband 6 months ago. Mrs. Cooper was referred for counselling 3 months ago for help with grief and depression. When Belinda inquired about her financial situation, Mrs. Cooper responded that it was tight living on an income from the Canada Pension Plan, but she was able to manage.

Assessment Activities	Findings/Defining Characteristics
Ask Mrs. Cooper about her food intake during the last 2 days.	She says she drinks one juice in the morning and two or three cups of coffee. She may have a sandwich in the late afternoon. "I'm just not interested in food. It has no taste."
Ask Mrs. Cooper about social interaction.	Mrs. Cooper says she is lonely and does not get out much, although her psychologist recommended more socializing. Her friends at church call to ask her to come back to meetings, but she is not ready. She says she tires easily.
Weigh Mrs. Cooper and assess posture.	She has a low BMI of 17. This weight loss occurred over 6 months, down 11 kg. Stooped posture
Observe Mrs. Cooper for signs of poor nutrition.	Dull, thinning hair Dry, scaling skin Pale conjunctivae and mucous membranes
Palpate muscles and extremities.	2 + bilateral pitting ankle edema Generalized poor muscle tone

Nursing Diagnosis: Imbalanced nutrition: less than body requirements related to a decreased ability to ingest food as a result of depression.

Planning

Goals	Expected Outcomes*
	Weight Control
Client will progressively gain weight.	Client will gain ½ to 1 kg per month until goal of 59 kg is reached.
	Nutritional Status: Nutrient Intake
Client will consume adequate nourishment each day.	Client will ingest 1,900 kcal/day, including 50 g of protein per day.
Client will exhibit no signs of malnutrition.	Physical assessment and laboratory values will be within normal limits.

*Outcome classification labels from *Nursing Outcomes Classification (NOC)* (3rd ed.), edited by S. Moorhead, M. Johnson, and M. L. Maas, 2004, St. Louis, MO: Mosby.

Interventions†	Rationale
Nutritional Monitoring	
Monitor client monthly for weight gain, anemia, serum albumin level, and total lymphocyte count (TLC).	Weight gain should be slow and progressive. Serum albumin of 40 g/L and TLC of 1,500/mm^3 are within normal limits (Grodner et al., 2000).
Perform physical assessment of hair, eyes, mouth, skin, and muscle tone.	Provides progressive monitoring for improved nutritional status

†Intervention classification labels from *Nursing Interventions Classification (NIC)* (4th ed.), edited by J. M. Dochterman and G. M. Bulecheck, 2004, St. Louis, MO: Mosby.

Continued

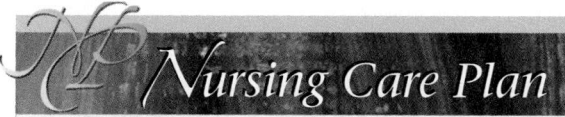

Nursing Care Plan

Imbalanced Nutrition: Less Than Body Requirements—cont'd

Interventions†—cont'd	Rationale
Nutritional Management	
Encourage client to eat small meals and to increase dietary intake and to help offset anorexia secondary to sertraline.	Sertraline is a selective serotonin reuptake inhibitor (SSRI) medication; diminished taste and anorexia is a common effect of SSRIs. Frequent small meals help to reduce anorexia-associated weight loss.
Encourage fluid intake.	Older adults need eight 250-mL glasses per day of fluid from beverage and food sources. Concentrating intake in morning and early afternoon prevents nocturia (Lueckenotte, 2000).
Encourage fibre intake.	Adequate fluid, fibre, and exercise help prevent constipation.
Consult with client about referral for congregate meals (lunch at Senior's Centre) five times per week.	Congregate meal participation encourages good nutrition and promotes socialization with peers (Millen et al., 2001).

†Intervention classification labels from *Nursing Interventions Classification (NIC)* (4th ed.), edited by J. M. Dochterman and G. M. Bulecheck, 2004, St. Louis, MO: Mosby.

Evaluation

Nursing Actions	Client Response/Finding	Achievement of Outcome
Ask Mrs. Cooper to review her diet for the last 2 to 3 days.	Client responds that she ate her main meal at the Senior's Centre, has fruit and grain fibre for breakfast, and in the evening either has soup or a sandwich with fruit.	Mrs. Cooper is selecting more nutritionally rich foods, consistent with current guidelines.
Observe client's appearance.	Skin is less pale, hair appears to be in better condition and styled. Ankle edema is present, but less than 1+.	Mrs. Cooper has improved physical parameters of nutrition; still needs follow-up.
Weigh client.	Weight gain of 2 kg in 4 weeks.	Weight gain is steady; client is still below ideal body weight.
Ask client about appetite and energy level.	Mrs. Cooper responds that on days she eats at the Senior's Centre her appetite seems better and she "wants to do more things." She notes that weekends are very lonely.	Weekday support for nutritional status appears effective, needs to increase client's activity status and nutritional intake during weekends.

- Sugared beverages removed from diet
- Client refrains from eating between meals and after dinner
- Client loses 0.5 to 1 kg per week

The setting of goals and outcomes requires multidisciplinary input. Nurses need to know each discipline's role in providing nutrition support. Nurses frequently collaborate with dietitians to ensure nutrition plans are appropriate and to learn how to obtain accurate data, for example, how to conduct calorie counts. A good care plan requires accurate exchange of information between disciplines.

Setting Priorities. Identifying clients at risk for nutritional problems leads to timely interventions that prevent or minimize nutritional problems. Improving nutritional intake is usually a priority. During acute illness or surgery, food intake is often altered in the perioperative period. The priority of care may be to provide optimal preoperative nutrition support in clients with malnutrition. The priority for the resumption of food intake post-operatively depends on the return of bowel function, the extent of the surgical procedure, and the presence of complications (see chapter 45).

Sometimes other priorities take precedence. For example, clients who have had throat surgery must be out of pain and comfortable before nutritional priorities can be addressed.

The client and family need to collaborate with the nurse in setting care priorities. Food purchase and preparation may involve the family and the care plan may not succeed without their commitment to, involvement in, and understanding of the nutritional priorities.

Continuity of Care. In any health care setting, continuity of care is essential, including continuity of nutritional interventions. Hospital discharge planning should extend nutritional interventions to the home or long-term care facility. Interventions such as enteral tube feedings often supplement a client's oral nutrition in the home or extended setting. These feedings can be administered into the stomach or intestines via a tube inserted through the nose or a percutaneous access (see Skill 39-2 and Skill 39-3). In extended settings, the dietitian monitors the client's nutritional status and intake and makes recommendations for changes. Dietitians select enteral

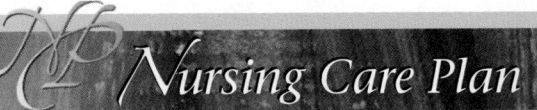

Focus on Primary Health Care — Box 39-4

Case Study

In Saskatoon, an innovative program is aiming to eradicate child hunger and malnutrition. The Child Hunger and Education Program (CHEP) takes a primary health care approach to disease prevention and health promotion in the community. The goal of CHEP is to work with communities to achieve solutions to child hunger and improve access to good food for all. CHEP's philosophy is that food is a basic right and inadequate nutrition adversely affects a child's development, learning ability, health, and participation in the community. Targeting children at risk, CHEP supports community groups in the operation of programs for children at schools and community centres. CHEP's partners include the provincial government, Public Health Services, the Community Clinic, the University of Saskatchewan Kinesiology and Nutrition faculties, Aboriginal organizations, and school boards. Kinesiologists, dietitians, public health nurses, teachers, parents, and volunteers work together on various aspects of the program, which include the following:

- *Meal programs*—Breakfast, lunch, snack, and supper programs are offered at targeted schools. The goal is to provide one third of a child's daily nutrition needs at each meal.
- *Collective cooking programs*—Groups of people pool resources and come together to plan and prepare low-cost nutritious meals for their families. Leadership training workshops enable participants to lead other collective kitchen groups and champion healthy lifestyles in the community.
- *Nutritious food choices programs*—These are programs to bring good nutrition into the whole school community. Classroom and school activities, staff events, fundraising projects and meal programs all focus on good nutrition and creating healthy food environments.
- *The Good Food Box*—This food distribution system provides fresh, nutritious foods at affordable prices. Families, as part of neighbourhood-based groups, each with a volunteer coordinator, pay for and order food boxes ahead of time. The CHEP program worker purchases foods in bulk from local producers and wholesalers. Volunteers and staff pack the boxes and deliver them to the neighbourhood depots.
- *Health promotion program*—This program seeks to prevent Type 2 diabetes among Aboriginal families by improving access to good food and encouraging active living. Groups of adults and youth meet for discussions about health and related issues, to cook meals, to order Good Food Boxes, and to take part in physical activities.

Groups and individuals including producers, Social Services, and community food action organizations meet at workshops and events to work at improving the food system for the Saskatoon region. CHEP also hosts educational and community-building workshops. The CHEP program works to ensure food security for all residents by researching and advocating for policy that will support access to an equitable, healthy, sustainable food system.

From *Child Hunger and Education Program* (n.d.). Accessed December 22, 2004, from *http://www.chep.org*

formulas and dietary modifications required for specific disease states.

When parenteral nutrition (PN), a solution consisting of glucose, amino acids, lipids, minerals, electrolytes, trace elements, and vitamins, is needed, it is given through an in-dwelling peripheral or central venous catheter. The pharmacist is expert in drug-nutrient interactions and mixture of total parenteral nutrition (TPN).

When clients require care in a long-term care or home setting, occupational therapists help them to choose assistive devices, such as large-handled utensils and cups with a space for the nose. They also help rearrange food preparation areas to maximize the client's function. Speech therapists recommend appropriate diet textures and feeding strategies and assist clients with swallowing exercises and techniques to reduce aspiration risk.

NP Implementation

Health Promotion. Nurses are in a key position to educate clients about good nutritional habits. Incorporating knowledge of nutrition into lifestyle prevents the development of many diseases (Box 39-4). Early identification of potential or actual problems is the best way to avoid more serious problems. Outpatient and community-based settings are key locations for nursing assessment of nutritional practices and status. Clients with nutritional problems such as obesity may require help with menu planning and compliance strategies. The nurse frequently educates families about nutrition, tells them about community resources, and provides contact information for a dietitian or nurse so that families can follow up with questions.

A meal plan is built around the family's budget and preferences, with foods chosen based on the dietary prescription and food groups. For those on limited budgets, substitutes can be used. For example, bean or cheese dishes can often replace meat. Food preparation is modified for substances that need to be used sparingly. Baking rather than frying reduces fat intake, and lemon juice or spices add flavour to low-sodium diets.

Menu planning a week in advance helps clients comply with a specific diet, eat nutritiously, and stay within budget. A nurse or dietitian may check menus for content. Often, a simple tip can help, such as avoiding grocery shopping when hungry because it can lead to spontaneous purchases of foods not included in meal plans.

> ***Safety Alert.*** Food safety is also an important public health issue. Food-borne illnesses can occur from poor hygiene practices and improper food storage or preparation. Nurses should educate clients about reducing the risks of food-borne illnesses (Table 39-9; Box 39-5).

Table 39-9 Food Safety

Food-Borne Disease	Organism	Food Source	Symptoms*
Botulism	*Clostridium botulinum*	Improperly home-canned foods, smoked and salted fish, ham, sausage, shellfish	Symptoms are varied from mild discomfort to death in 24 hours, initially nausea, dizziness, progressing to motor (respiratory) paralysis
Escherichia coli	*Escherichia coli* 0157:H7	Undercooked meat (ground beef)	Severe cramps, nausea, vomiting, diarrhea (may be bloody), renal failure. Appears 1–8 days after eating, lasts 1–7 days
Listeriosis	*Listeria* *L. monocytogenes*	Soft cheese, meat (hot dogs, pâté, lunch meats), unpasteurized milk, poultry, seafood	Severe diarrhea, fever, headache, pneumonia, meningitis, endocarditis, appears 3–21 days after infection
Perfringens enteritis	*Clostridium* *C. perfringens*	Cooked meats, meat dishes held at room or warm temperature	Mild diarrhea, vomiting. Appears 8–24 hours after eating, lasts 1–2 days
Salmonellosis	*Salmonella* *S. typhi* *S. paratyphi*	Milk, custards, egg dishes, salad dressings, sandwich fillings, polluted shellfish	Mild to severe diarrhea, cramps, vomiting. Appears 12–24 hours after ingestion, lasts 1–7 days
Shigellosis	*Shigella* *S. dysenteriae*	Milk, milk products, seafood, salads	Mild diarrhea to fatal dysentery. Appears 7–36 hours after ingestion, lasts 3–14 days
Staphylococcus	*Staphylococcus* *S. aureus*	Custards, cream fillings, processed meats, ham, cheese, ice cream, potato salad, sauces, casseroles	Severe abdominal cramps, pain, vomiting, diarrhea, perspiration, headache, fever, prostration. Appears 1–6 hours after ingestion, lasts 1–2 days

*Symptoms are generally most severe for youngest and oldest age groups.
From Basic *Nutrition and Diet Therapy* (11th ed.), by S. R. Williams, 2001, St. Louis, MO: Mosby.

Client Teaching — Box 39-5

Food Safety

Objectives

- Client will be able to verbalize measures to prevent food-borne illness.
- Client will understand the primary types of illness and how they are transmitted.
- Client will not experience food-borne illness.

Teaching Strategies

- Food safety has become an important public health issue in recent years. Populations particularly at risk are older and younger people and immunosuppressed individuals.
- Instruct clients on the following:
  - Wash hands with warm, soapy water before touching or eating food.
  - Cook meat, poultry, fish, and eggs until they are well done.
  - Wash fresh fruits and vegetables thoroughly.
  - Do not eat raw meats or drink unpasteurized milk.
  - Do not buy or consume food that has passed the expiration date.
  - Keep foods properly refrigerated at 7°C and frozen at −13°C.
  - Wash dishes and cutting boards with hot, soapy water.
  - Do not save leftovers for more than 2 days in refrigerator.
  - Wash dishcloths, towels, and sponges regularly, or use paper towels.
  - Clean the inside of refrigerator and microwave regularly to prevent microbial growth.

Evaluation

- Ask client to verbalize measures to prevent food-borne illnesses.
- Observe the client at home for safe practices, if making home visit.

Adapted from "Minimizing HIV/AIDS Malnutrition," by J. K. Keithley and B. Swanson, 1998 *MedSurg Nursing, 7*(5), pp. 256–267.

Acute Care. Many factors influence nutritional intake in acute care settings. Ill or debilitated clients often have loss of appetite **(anorexia).** The ketosis that accompanies starvation can further suppress appetite, as can the pain that results from surgical procedures and trauma. In addition, deficiencies in certain vitamins and minerals can cause anorexia. Nurses can help clients to understand the factors that cause anorexia and use creative approaches to stimulate appetite.

During hospitalizations, diagnostic testing disrupts many mealtimes or requires nothing by mouth (NPO) status before tests. Clients who are NPO and receive only

Table 39-10 Nutrition and the Immune System

Immune/Physiological Component	Malnutrition Effect	Vital Nutrient
Granulocytes and macrocytes	Longer time for phagocytosis kill time and lymphocyte activation	Protein, vitamins A, C, B_{12} B_6 folic acid, thiamine, riboflavin, niacin, zinc, iron
Mucus	Flat microvilli in GI tract, decreased antibody secretion	Vitamins B_{12} B_6 C, biotin
Skin	Integrity compromised, density reduced, wound healing slowed	Protein, vitamins A, B_{12} C, niacin, copper, zinc
T lymphocytes	Depressed T-cell distribution	Protein, arginine, iron, zinc, omega-3 fatty acids, vitamins A, B_{12} B_6 folic acid, thiamine, riboflavin, niacin, pantothenic acid

Total Lymphocyte Count (TLC)

TLC = % lymphocytes × white blood cell count ÷ 100*

*Results <2000 cells/mm³ suggest impaired immunocompetence; results <1500 cells/ mm³ are associated with greater morbidity and mortality.

Adapted from *Foundations and Clinical Applications of Nutrition: A Nursing Approach* (2nd ed.), by M. Grodner, S. Anderson, and S. DeYoung, 2000, St. Louis, MO: Mosby.

standard IV fluids for more than 7 days are at nutritional risk. Clients worried about families, finances, employment, or illnesses are often not able to eat an adequate diet. Mealtimes are often interrupted, or the client is too fatigued or uncomfortable to eat. Both physiological stress and emotional stress influence dietary need and intake. Medications may interfere with taste, cause nausea, interfere with absorption, or affect metabolism.

The nurse must continuously assess the client's nutritional status and plan interventions that promote normal intake, digestion, and metabolism of nutrients.

Advancing Diets. Acute and chronic conditions affect the immune system which, in turn, can affect nutritional status. Clients who have conditions such as human immunodeficiency virus (HIV) infections or cancers or who are undergoing treatments such as chemotherapy may have a decreased immune function. They may require nutritional supplements or diets that are higher in selected nutrients. Table 39-10 gives an overview of the immune system, the malnutrition impact, and what nutrients are beneficial. Clients who are ill, who have had surgery, or who have been NPO have specialized dietary needs. They may have a gradual progression of dietary intake or need therapeutic diets to manage their illness (Box 39-6). For inpatients, a physician will order a therapeutic diet and the dietetic services department will prepare it.

Promoting Appetite. Providing an environment that promotes a client's appetite includes eliminating odours, providing oral hygiene as needed to remove unpleasant tastes, and maintaining client comfort. In addition, certain medications can affect dietary intake and nutrient use. For example, insulin, glucocorticoids, and thyroid hormones affect metabolism. Other medications, such as antifungal agents, can affect taste. Some of the psychotropic medications affect appetite, cause nausea, and may alter taste. Sometimes the nurse and dietician can help the client select foods to reduce the altered taste sensations or nausea. In other situations, medication may need to be changed. Physicians may order pharmacological agents to stimulate appetite (e.g., cyproheptadine [Periactin], megestrol [Megace]) or manage symptoms that interfere with nutrition.

Assisting Clients With Feeding. When helping clients to eat, the nurse must protect their safety, independence, and dignity. People need all of their senses to fully enjoy the taste, smell, and look of a meal. Glasses, hearing aids, and dentures should be functioning and in place. The nurse should assess the client's risk of aspiration. Risk factors for aspiration are decreased alertness, decreased gag and/or cough reflexes, and difficulty managing saliva (see Assessment).

Clients with dysphagia need help with feeding. Dysphagia can result in malnutrition and dehydration. It can also cause aspiration of food particles into the lungs, leading to pneumonia. It is common following stroke and involves up to 50% of stroke clients (Odderson et al., 1995), and up to 20% of dysphagic clients die of aspiration pneumonia within a year of their stroke (Heart and Stroke Foundation of Canada, 2005). Therefore, nurses must understand dysphagia assessment and management (Platt, 2002). Usually a speech language pathologist evaluates clients at risk for dysphagia and provides therapy to improve swallowing. Interventions also include postural changes, feeding strategies, and dietary changes (Logemann, 1999). The client may be ordered a diet of thickened fluids because these are safer to swallow than thin liquids. The client should sit upright at a 75 to 90-degree angle and may be supported by pillows, foam wedges, or rolled towels. A client should not be fed while lying back or with an arched or hyperextended neck because these positions create an open airway. Small bites of food should be placed and chewed on the stronger side of the mouth. Turning the head to the affected side may ease swallowing. Nurses should give clients with dysphagia enough time to chew and should assess swallowing during feeding. They should observe for two completed swallows between mouthfuls. The client's Adam's apple

Box 39-6 Diet Progression and Therapeutic Diets

Clear Liquid

Broth, bouillon, coffee, tea, carbonated beverages, clear fruit juices, gelatin, Popsicles

Thickened Liquid

Fruits thickened with rice flakes or thickening agents are used when thin fluids cannot be safely swallowed and may be aspirated.

Full Liquid

As above with addition of smooth-textured dairy products, custards, refined cooked cereals, vegetable juice, pureed vegetables, all fruit juices

Pureed

All of above with addition of scrambled eggs, pureed meats, vegetables, fruits, mashed potatoes and gravy

Mechanical Soft

All of above with addition of ground or finely diced meats, flaked fish, cottage cheese, cheese, rice, potatoes, pancakes, light breads, cooked vegetables, cooked or canned fruits, bananas, soups, peanut butter

Soft/Low Residue

Addition of low-fibre, easily digested foods, such as pastas, casseroles, moist tender meats, canned cooked fruits and vegetables, desserts, cakes, and cookies without nuts or coconut

High Fibre

Addition of fresh uncooked fruits, steamed vegetables, bran, oatmeal, and dried fruits

Low Sodium

4-g (no added salt), 2-g, 1-g, or 500-mg sodium diets. These diets vary from no added salt to severe sodium restriction (500-mg sodium diet) that requires selective food purchases.

Low Cholesterol

<200 mg/day cholesterol, in keeping with the National Cholesterol Education Program (NCEP) recommendations (2002).

Diabetic

In general, people with diabetes should follow a healthy diet recommended for the general population in *Canada's Guidelines for Healthy Eating* (Canadian Diabetes Society, 2003). This includes consuming a variety of foods from the four food groups (grain products, vegetables and fruits, milk products, meat and alternatives), attaining and maintaining a healthy body weight, decreasing total fat intake to <30% of calories, and ensuring an adequate intake of carbohydrate, protein, essential fatty acids, vitamins, and minerals.

Regular

No restrictions, unless specified

should move up and down. After each meal, the client should rinse the mouth and perform oral hygiene.

Clients with visual deficits also need special assistance. Those with low vision may be able to feed themselves if adequate care and information is given. If the client wears glasses or contact lenses, they should be clean and in place. The location of the food on the plate should be identified as if it were a clock (e.g., meat at 9 o'clock and vegetable at 3 o'clock). The client should be told where the beverage is located in relation to the plate. The nurse should be aware of visual field cuts (right or left) caused by stroke or other vision difficulties and the client's inability to see food or utensils in the location of the blind spot. Food should be positioned within the client's visual field. Other care providers should set the meal tray and plate in the same manner. Clients with impaired vision or decreased motor skill may retain more independence by using large-handled adaptive utensils. These are easier to grip and manipulate.

When a client needs to be fed, a metal teaspoon is usually the best utensil, as it provides an appropriate size serving. The nurse should provide opportunities for clients to direct the order and speed at which they wish to eat. At meals where food intake is less than usual because of illness, fatigue, or other factors, high calorie, nutrient-dense items should be provided first. Small frequent meals, five to six per day, may be required for those who eat slowly. The nurse should heed special requests, such as a request for the food to be warmed up. Small measures help many clients retain a sense of independence.

Clothing and bedding should be protected with napkins, towels, or aprons; these items should not be called "bibs." Because mealtime is usually a social activity, nurses and other care providers should talk to clients during meals. They can use this opportunity to educate clients about therapeutic diets, medications, or adaptive devices.

Enteral Tube Feeding. **Enteral nutrition (EN)** refers to nutrients given via the GI tract. When the client cannot ingest food but is still able to digest and absorb nutrients, enteral tube feeding is indicated. Feeding tubes can be inserted through the nose into the stomach or intestines (nasogastric or nasointestinal tubes), surgically through a stoma into the stomach or jejunum (gastrostomy or jejunostomy tubes), or endoscopically (percutaneous endoscopic gastrostomy or jejunostomy [PEG or PEJ] tubes). Nasoenteral tubes (i.e., nasogastric and nasointestinal tubes) can be inserted by a nurse. All other tubes must be inserted by a physician. If EN therapy is to be administered for less than 4 weeks, nasoenteral tubes may be used. Surgical or endoscopically placed tubes are preferred for long-term feeding (more than 4 weeks) to reduce the discomfort of a nasal tube and to provide a more secure, reliable access (Bowers, 1996). Clients with gastroparesis (decreased or absent innervation to the stomach that results in delayed gastric emptying) or esophageal reflux, at risk for aspiration, or with a history of aspiration pneumonia require placement of tubes beyond the stomach into the intestine (Edwards & Metheny, 2000; Metheny, 2002).

Box 39-7 lists indications for EN. The nurse or the family can give enteral tube feedings in the home setting. The nurse inserts the nasoenteral tube (Skill 39-1), and verification of tube placement by X-ray examination must occur before the client receives the first enteral feeding.

Initiating Enteral Tube Feedings. Enteral formulas are usually one of four types. Polymeric formulas (1.0 to 2.0 kcal/mL) include milk-based blenderized foods prepared by hospital dietary staff or in the client home. The polymeric classification also includes commercially prepared whole nutrient formulas. For this type of formula to be effective, the client's gastrointestinal tract must be able to absorb whole nutrients. Modular formulas (3.8 to 4.0 kcal/mL) are single-macronutrient (e.g., protein, glucose, polymers, or lipids) preparations and are not nutritionally complete. This type of formula is added to other foods for meeting the client's individual nutritional needs. Elemental formulas (1.0 to 3.0 kcal/mL) contain predigested nutrients that are easier for a partially dysfunctional gastrointestinal tract to absorb. Finally, specialty formulas (1.0 to 2.0 kcal/mL) are designed to meet specific nutritional needs in certain illnesses (e.g., liver failure, pulmonary disease, or HIV infection).

Tube feedings are typically started at full strength at slow rates (Box 39-8). The hourly rate is increased every 12 to 24 hours if no signs of intolerance appear (nausea, cramping, vomiting, diarrhea). Studies have demonstrated a beneficial effect of enteral feedings compared with parenteral nutrition. Feeding by the enteral route may reduce sepsis, blunt the hypermetabolic response to trauma, and maintain intestinal structure and function (ASPEN, 2002; Guenter, Ericson, & Jones, 1997). Enteral nutrition has been used successfully within 24 to 48 hours after surgery or trauma to provide fluids, electrolytes, and nutritional support. Gastric ileus may prevent nasogastric feedings, whereas nasointestinal or jejunostomy tubes allow successful postpyloric feeding, where formula is placed directly into the small intestine or jejunum or beyond the pyloric sphincter of the stomach (ASPEN, 2002).

Skill 39-2 describes the procedure for administering feedings via nasoenteral tubes, and Skill 39-3 describes administering feedings via gastrostomy or jejunostomy tubes.

Preventing Complications. A serious complication associated with enteral feeding is aspiration of enteral formula into the tracheobronchial tree. Aspiration of enteral formula into the lungs irritates the bronchial mucosa, resulting in decreased blood supply to affected pulmonary tissue (Metheny, 2002). This leads to necrotizing infection, pneumonia, and potential abscess formation. The high glucose content serves as a bacterial medium for growth, promoting infection. Adult respiratory distress syndrome is also an outcome frequently associated with pulmonary aspiration. Common conditions that increase the risk of aspiration include coughing, nasotracheal suctioning, an artificial airway, decreased level of consciousness, and lying flat during and after feeding.

Nursing research has investigated the problems associated with nasoenteral tube placement, type of feeding instilled, rate of feeding, and complications associated with tube feeding. Small-bore feeding tubes create less discomfort for the client and are currently most often used (Figure 39–9). For the adult, most of these tubes are 8 to 12 Fr and 91 to 109 cm long. A stylet is often used during insertion of a small-bore tube to stiffen it. The stylet is removed when the correct position of the feeding tube is confirmed.

Feeding tube placement used to be checked by injecting air through the tube while auscultating the stomach for a gurgling or bubbling sound or asking the client to speak (Metheny et al., 1998b). These methods have a high degree of inaccuracy. Rombeau and Rolandelli (1997) reported that clients were able to speak despite placement of feeding tubes in the lung. Auscultation has

Text continnued on p. 1310

Box 39-7 Indications for Enteral Nutrition

Cancer

Head and neck
Upper GI
Critical illness/trauma

Neurological and Muscular Disorders

Brain neoplasm
Cerebrovascular accident
Dementia
Myopathy
Parkinson's disease

Gastrointestinal Disorder

Enterocutaneous fistula
Inflammatory bowel disease
Mild pancreatitis

Respiratory Failure With Prolonged Intubation

Inadequate oral intake
Continuous feedings
Supine positioning
Cerebral vascular accident
Local trauma
Anorexia nervosa
Difficulty chewing, swallowing
Severe depression

Skill 39-1 Inserting a Small-Bore Nasoenteric Tube for Enteral Feeding

View Video

Delegation Considerations

This skill requires problem solving and knowledge application unique to a professional nurse. For this reason, this skill should not be delegated to unregulated care providers.

Equipment

- Nasogastric or nasointestinal tube (8 to 12 Fr) with guide wire or stylet
- Stethoscope
- 60-mL or larger Luer-Lok or catheter-tip syringe
- Hypoallergenic tape and tincture of benzoin or tube fixation device
- pH indicator strip (scale 0.0 to 14.0)
- Glass of water and straw
- Emesis basin
- Safety pin
- Rubber band
- Towel
- Facial tissues
- Disposable gloves
- Suction equipment in case of aspiration
- Penlight to check placement of nasopharynx
- Tongue blade

Steps	Rationale
1. Assess client for the need for enteral tube feeding: NPO or insufficient intake for more than 5 days, functional GI tract, unable to ingest sufficient nutrients.	Identifying clients who need tube feedings before they become nutritionally depleted may help to prevent complications related to malnutrition.
2. Perform hand hygiene. Assess patency of nares. Have client close each nostril alternately and breathe. Examine each naris for patency and skin breakdown.	Evaluates nares for patency. Nares may be obstructed or irritated, or septal defect may be present.
3. Assess the gag reflex. Place tongue blade in client's mouth, touching uvula to induce a gag response.	Identifies ability to swallow and determines if there is a risk for aspiration.

Critical Decision Point: Clients with impaired level of consciousness may also have impaired gag reflex, and their risk of aspiration is increased during this type of procedure and subsequent tube feedings.

Steps	Rationale
4. Review client's medical history for nasal problems (e.g., nosebleeds, oral facial surgery, anticoagulation therapy, history of aspiration).	Nasoenteral tubes are contraindicated in clients with recent nasal surgery, facial traumas, or nosebleeds, and in those who are receiving anticoagulation. Tubes are also contraindicated in clients with surgical procedures requiring a transphenoid approach used to remove pituitary tumours because there is a risk for improper tube placement (Metheny, 2002).
5. Review physician's order for type of tube and enteral feeding schedule.	Procedure and tube feedings require a physician's order.
6. Auscultate abdomen for bowel sounds.	Absence of bowel sounds may indicate decreased or absent peristalsis and increased risk for aspiration and/or abdominal distension.
7. Perform hand hygiene.	Reduces transfer of micro-organisms.
8. Explain procedure to client and how to communicate during intubation by raising index finger to indicate gagging or discomfort.	Reduces anxiety and helps client to assist in insertion.
9. Stand on same side of bed as naris for insertion, and assist client to high-Fowler's position unless contraindicated. Place pillow behind head and shoulders.	Allows easier manipulation of tube. Fowler's position reduces risk of aspiration and promotes effective swallowing.
10. Place bath towel over client's chest. Keep facial tissues within reach.	Prevents soiling of gown. Insertion of tube may produce tearing.
11. Determine length of tube to be inserted and mark with tape:	Length approximates distance from nose to stomach in 98% of clients. For duodenal or jejunal placement, an additional 20 to 30 cm is required.
a. Traditional method: Measure distance from tip of nose to earlobe to xiphoid process of sternum (see illustration).	

Steps	Rationale

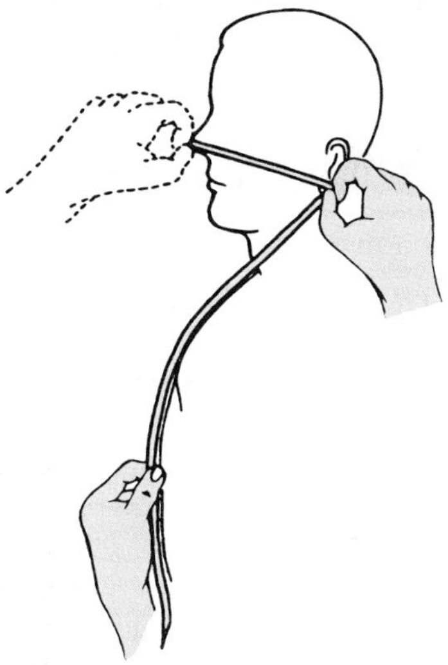

STEP **11a** Length of tube to be inserted is equal to distance from tip of nose to earlobe to xiphoid process.

Steps	Rationale
12. Prepare nasogastric or nasointestinal tube for intubation:	
a. Plastic tubes should not be iced.	Tubes will become stiff and inflexible, causing trauma to mucous membranes.
b. Inject 10 mL of water from 30-mL or larger Luer-Lok or catheter-tip syringe into the tube.	Aids in guide wire or stylet insertion.
c. Make certain that guide wire is securely positioned against weighted tip and that both Luer-Lok connections are snugly fitted together.	Promotes smooth passage of tube into GI tract. Improperly positioned stylet can induce serious trauma.
13. Cut tape 10 cm long or prepare tube fixation device.	To be used to anchor tubing following insertion.
14. Put on gloves.	Reduces transmission of micro-organisms.
15. Dip tube with surface lubricant into glass of water.	Activates lubricant to facilitate passage of tube into naris to GI tract.
16. Insert tube through nostril to back of throat (posterior nasopharynx). Aim back and down toward ear.	Natural contour facilitates passage of tube into GI tract and reduces gagging by client.
17. Have client flex head toward chest after tube has passed through nasopharynx.	Closes off glottis and reduces risk of tube entering trachea.

Critical Decision Point: Encourage client to swallow by giving small sips of water or ice chips when possible. Advance tube as client swallows. Rotate tube 180 degrees while inserting.

Steps	Rationale
18. Emphasize the need to mouth breathe and swallow during the procedure.	Helps facilitate passage of tube and alleviates client's fears during the procedure.
19. When tip of tube reaches the carina (about 25 cm in an adult), stop, hold end of tube near ear and listen for air exchange from the distal portion of the tube.	If air is heard, the tube could be in the respiratory tract; remove tube and start over. This step should never be used for tube verification (Metheny & Titler, 2001).
20. Advance tube each time client swallows until desired length has been passed.	Reduces discomfort and trauma to client.

Critical Decision Point: Do not force tube. If resistance is met or client starts to cough, choke, or become cyanotic, stop advancing the tube and pull tube back.

Steps	Rationale
21. Check for position of tube in back of throat with penlight and tongue blade.	Tube may be coiled, kinked, or entering trachea.
22. Perform measures to verify placement of tube (see Box 39-9).	

Skill 39-1 Inserting a Small-Bore Nasoenteric Tube for Enteral Feeding—cont'd

Steps	Rationale
Critical Decision Point: Auscultation is no longer considered a reliable method for verification of tube placement because a tube inadvertently placed in the lungs, pharynx, or esophagus can transmit a sound similar to that of air entering the stomach (Metheny et al., 1990b; Metheny & Titler, 2001).	
23. After gastric aspirates are obtained, anchor tube to nose and avoid pressure on nares. Mark exit site with indelible ink. Select one of the following options:	A properly secured tube allows the client more mobility and prevents trauma to nasal mucosa.
A. **Apply tape**	
(1) Apply tincture of benzoin or other skin adhesive on tip of client's nose and tube and allow it to become "tacky."	Helps tape adhere better. Protects skin.
(2) Remove gloves and split one end of tape lengthwise 5 cm.	
(3) Place the intact end of tape over bridge of client's nose. Wrap each of the 5-cm strips around tube as it exits nose (see illustration).	Securing tape to nares prevents tissue necrosis.
B. **Apply tube fixation device using shaped adhesive patch**	Secures tube and reduces friction on nares.
(1) Apply wide end of patch to bridge of nose (see illustration).	
(2) Slip connector around tube as it exits nose (see illustration).	
24. Fasten end of nasogastric tube to client's gown by looping rubber band around tube in slipknot. Pin rubber band to gown (see illustration).	Reduces traction on the naris if tube moves.
25. For intestinal placement, position client on right side when possible until radiological confirmation of correct placement has been verified. Remove gloves, perform hand hygiene, and assist client to a comfortable position.	Promotes passage of the tube into the small intestine (duodenum or jejunum).

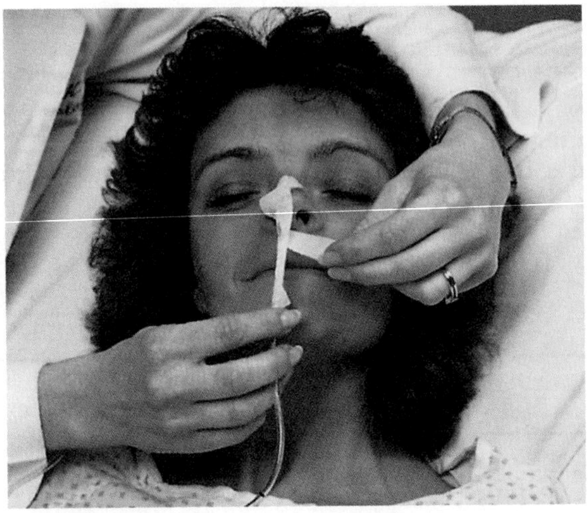

STEP **23A(3)** Wrapping tape to anchor nasoenteral tube.

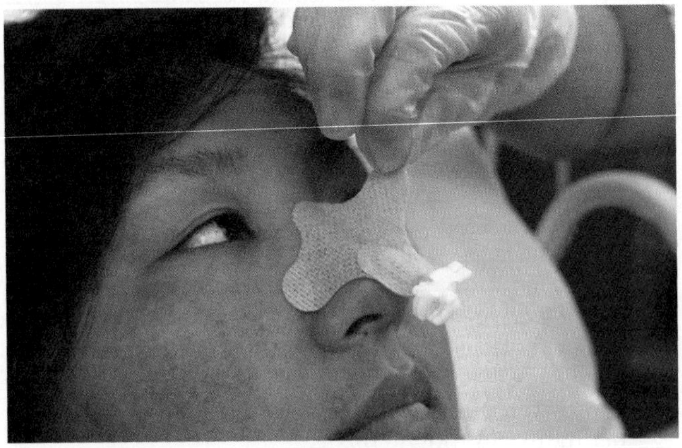

STEP **23B(1)** Applying patch to bridge of nose.

Steps	Rationale

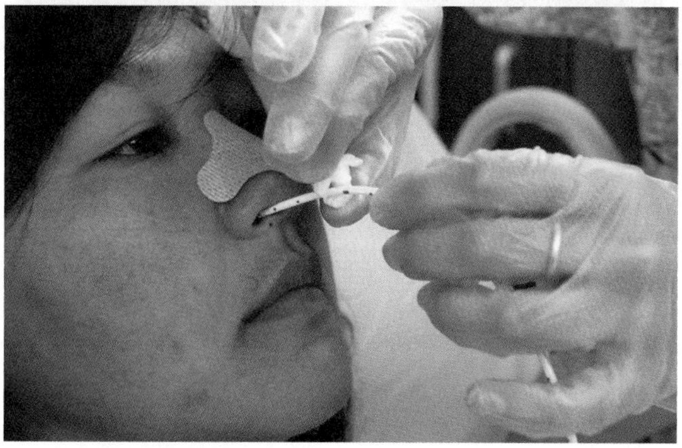

STEP **23B(2)** Slip connector around feeding tube.

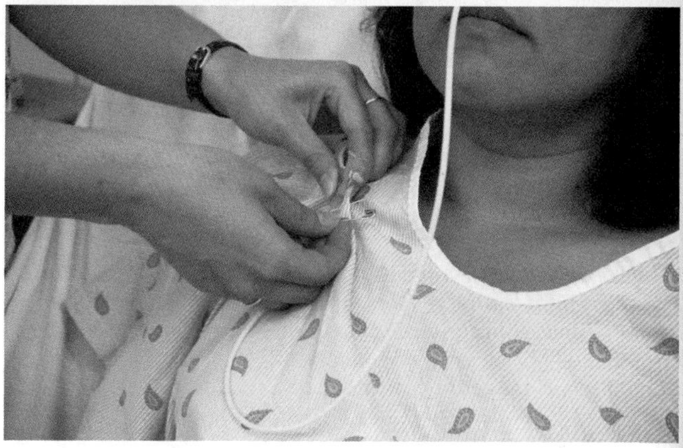

STEP **24** Fastening feeding tube to client's gown.

Critical Decision Point: Leave guide wire or stylet in place until correct position is ensured by X-ray film. Never attempt to reinsert partially or fully removed guide wire or stylet while feeding tube is in place.

Steps	Rationale
26. Obtain X-ray film of abdomen.	Placement of tube is verified by X-ray examination (Metheny, 1988; Metheny & Titler, 2001).
27. Apply clean gloves, and administer oral hygiene (see chapter 34). Cleanse tubing at nostril.	Promotes client comfort and integrity of oral mucous membranes.
28. Remove gloves, dispose of equipment, and perform hand hygiene.	Reduces transmission of micro-organisms.
29. Inspect naris and oropharynx for any irritation after insertion.	In insertion is difficult, irritation of naris or oropharynx may have occurred.
30. Ask if client feels comfortable.	Evaluates clients' level of comfort.
31. Observe client for any difficulty breathing, coughing, or gagging.	Malposition of the tube may cause these symptoms.
32. Auscultate lung sounds.	Abnormal lung sounds can be an early sign of aspiration.

Unexpected Outcomes and Related Interventions

- Aspiration of stomach contents into the respiratory tract (immediate response), evidenced by coughing, dyspnea, cyanosis, auscultation of crackles or wheezes
  - Position client on side.
  - Suction nasotracheally and oral tracheally.
  - Consult physician immediately to order chest X-ray examination.
- Aspiration of stomach contents into respiratory tract (delayed response), evidenced by dyspnea, fever, auscultation of crackles or wheezes
  - Consult physician to obtain order for chest X-ray film.
  - Prepare for possible initiation of antibiotics.
- Displacement of feeding tube to another site (e.g., from duodenum to stomach, mark at exit site if tube is moved); may occur when client coughs or vomits
  - Aspirate GI contents and measure pH (Metheny & Titler, 2001).
  - Remove displaced tube and insert and verify placement of new tube.
  - If there is a question of aspiration, obtain chest X-ray film.
- Clogging of feeding tube
  - Aspirate gastric contents to assess patency of tube.
  - Irrigate tube.
- Irritation of naris and nasal mucosa.
  - Provide hygiene and remove and replace tube.
  - Consider removing tube and inserting into other naris (physician order required).

Recording and Reporting

- Record and report type and size of tube placed, location of distal tip of tube, client's tolerance of procedure, pH value, and confirmation of tube position by X-ray examination.

Box 39-8 Advancing the Rate of Tube Feeding

Intermittent

1. Start formula at full strength for isotonic formulas (300 to 400 mOsm) or at ordered concentration.
2. Infuse bolus of formula over at least 20 to 30 minutes via syringe or feeding container.
3. Begin feedings with no more than 150 to 250 mL at one time. Increase by 50 mL per feeding per day to achieve needed volume and calories in six to eight feedings. (NOTE: Concentrated formulas at full strength may be infused at slower rate until tolerance is achieved.)

Continuous

1. Start formula at full strength for isotonic formulas (300 to 400 mOsm) or at ordered concentration. Usually hypertonic formulas are also started at full strength but at a slower rate.
2. Begin infusion rate at designated rate.
3. Advance rate slowly (e.g., 10 to 20 mL/hour per day) to target rate if tolerated (tolerance indicated by absence of nausea and diarrhea, and low gastric residuals).

repeatedly been shown to be ineffective in detecting tubes accidentally placed in the lung; further, it is not effective in distinguishing between gastric and intestinal placement for stationary feeding tubes (Metheny et al., 1997, 1999). Thus, the nurse must suspect tube displacement in clients at risk and use meticulous assessment skills. Metheny, Aud, and Ignatavicius (1998) reported several cases in which nasoenteral feeding tube displacement in the lung went undetected by auscultation.

At present, the most reliable method for verification of placement of small bore feeding tubes is X-ray examination (Box 39-9). Measuring the pH of secretions withdrawn from the feeding tube may also help to differentiate the location of the tube (Box 39-10). For accurate pH measurements, 30 mL of air is injected into the tube before measurement. Flushing the tube with air clears out formula or medications. Only 5 to 10 mL of gastric fluid is needed for pH testing. A client who takes acid inhibitor medications will usually have an acidic pH value ranging from 4.0 (after 4 hours of fasting) to 6.0 (with continuous EN infusion). In contrast, intestinal aspirate has a pH of 7.8 to 8.0. More precise indicators are needed to help differentiate the source of tube feeding aspirate (Metheny, Smith, & Stewart, 2000).

Adding blue food colouring to enteral formula to assist with the detection of formula aspirated into the lung, presumably by staining the tracheobronchial secretions, is now questioned and should not be used. The U. S. Food and Drug Administration (2003) issued a public health advisory reporting an association between use of Blue No. 1 food colouring and client deaths. Research has determined that the absence of blue-stained tracheobronchial secretions does not rule out pulmonary aspiration (Davis et al., 1995; Metheny, Aud, & Wunderlich, 1999).

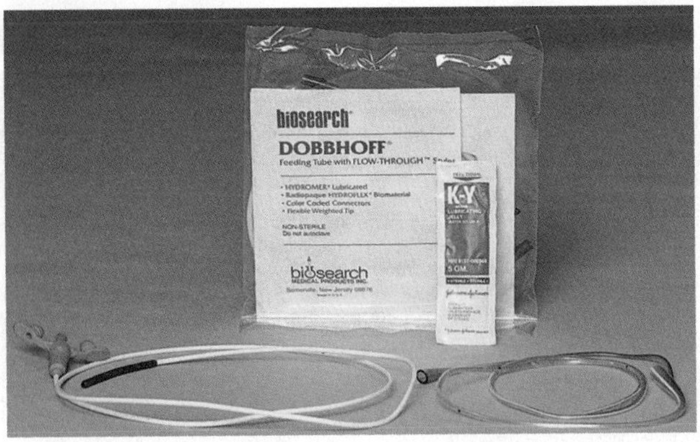

FIGURE **39–9** Enteral tubes, small bore.

Major complications of enteral nutrition are outlined in Table 39-11. Of special note, severely malnourished clients are at risk for electrolyte disturbances from refeeding syndrome because cations such as potassium, magnesium, and phosphate move intracellularly during EN or parenteral nutrition therapy.

Parenteral Nutrition. **Parenteral nutrition (PN)** is a form of specialized nutrition support in which nutrients are provided intravenously. Safe administration of this form of nutrition depends on appropriate assessment of nutrition needs, meticulous management of the central venous catheter (CVC), and careful monitoring to prevent or treat metabolic complications. PN is administered in a variety of settings, including the client's home. Regardless of the setting, the nurse adheres to the same principles of asepsis and infusion management to ensure safe nutrition support.

Clients who are unable to digest or absorb enteral nutrition benefit from PN. Clients in highly stressed physiological states such as sepsis, head injury, or burns are also candidates for PN therapy. Box 39-11 lists other indications for PN. Clinical and laboratory monitoring by a multidisciplinary team is required throughout PN therapy. The need for continued PN is consistently re-evaluated, with the goal of moving toward using the GI tract (ASPEN, 2002). Disuse of the GI tract has been associated with villus atrophy and generalized cell shrinkage. Translocation of bacteria from the local gut to systemic regions has been noted in relation to GI cell shrinkage, resulting in gram-negative septicemia (Panigrahi et al., 1997).

Lipid emulsions provide supplemental kilocalories and prevent essential fatty acid deficiencies. These emulsions can be administered through a separate peripheral line, through the central line by Y-connector tubing (see chapter 36), or as an admixture to the PN solution. The addition of lipid emulsion to the PN solution is called a 3-in-1 admixture and is given over a 24-hour period. The admixture should not be used if oil droplets are observed or if an oil or creamy layer is observed on the surface of the admixture. This observation indicates that the emulsion has broken into large lipid droplets that can cause fat emboli if administered. Lipid emulsions are white and opaque; thus, care should be taken to avoid confusing enteral formula with parenteral lipids.

Text continued on p. 1317

Skill 39-2 Administering Enteral Feedings via Nasoenteric Tubes

View Video

Delegation Considerations

Administration of enteral tube feeding via nasoenteral tube is a procedure that can be delegated to unregulated care providers (UCPs) after the nurse verifies tube placement. The nurse is also responsible for client assessment.

- Ensure that the client is sitting upright in a chair or in bed, and instruct UCP to infuse the feeding slowly.
- Instruct the UCP to report any difficulty infusing the feeding or any discomfort voiced by the client.

Equipment

- Disposable feeding bag and tubing or ready-to-hang system
- 30-mL or larger Luer-Lok or catheter-tip syringe
- Stethoscope
- pH indicator strip (scale 0.0 to 14.0)
- Infusion pump (required for intestinal feedings): use pump designed for tube feedings
- Prescribed enteral feedings
- Disposable gloves
- Equipment to obtain blood glucose by finger stick

Steps	Rationale
1. Assess client's need for enteral tube feedings: impaired swallowing, decreased level of consciousness, head or neck surgery, facial trauma, surgeries of upper alimentary canal	Identify clients who need tube feedings before they become nutritionally depleted.
2. Evaluate client's nutritional status (see Table 39-8). Obtain baseline weight and laboratory values. Assess client for fluid volume excess or deficit, electrolyte abnormalities, and metabolic abnormalities, such as hyperglycemia.	Enteral feedings are to restore or maintain a client's nutritional status. Provides objective data to measure effectiveness of feedings.
3. Verify physician's order for formula, rate, route, and frequency. Laboratory data and bedside assessments, such as finger-stick blood glucose measurement, are also ordered by the physician.	Tube feedings, laboratory tests, and bedside tests must be ordered by physician.
4. Explain procedure to client.	Well-informed client is more co-operative and at ease.
5. Perform hand hygiene.	Reduces transmission of micro-organisms.
6. Auscultate for bowel sounds before feeding.	Absent bowel sounds may indicate decreased ability of GI tract to digest or absorb nutrients.
7. Prepare feeding container to administer formula:	
a. Check expiration date on formula and integrity of container.	Tube feedings administered within the designated shelf life from a container without cracks or breaks reduces the client's risk of obtaining tube-feeding-borne GI infections. In addition, a container without cracks or breaks prevents leakage of tube feeding.
b. Have tube feeding at room temperature.	Cold formula may cause gastric cramping and discomfort because the liquid is not warmed by the mouth and esophagus.
c. Connect tubing to container as needed or prepare ready-to-hang container.	Tubing must be free of contamination to prevent bacterial growth.
d. Shake formula container well, and fill container with formula (see illustration). Open stopcock on tubing and fill with formula to remove air. Hang on intravenous (IV) pole.	Filling the tubing with formula prevents excess air from entering GI tract.
8. For intermittent feeding, have syringe ready and be sure formula is at room temperature.	Cold formula may cause gastric cramping.
9. Place client in high-Fowler's position, or elevate head of bed 30 degrees.	Elevated head helps prevent aspiration.
10. Verify tube placement (see Box 39-9): Consider the results from pH testing together with the aspirate's appearance.	On occasion, colour alone may differentiate gastric from intestinal placement. Because most intestinal aspirates are stained by bile to a distinct yellow colour and most gastric aspirates are not, the difference can often distinguish sites (Metheny et al., 1999). The pH aspirate offers valuable data as well in tracking advancement of a feeding tube (Metheny & Titler, 2001).

Skill 39-2 Administering Enteral Feedings via Nasoenteric Tubes—cont'd

Steps	Rationale

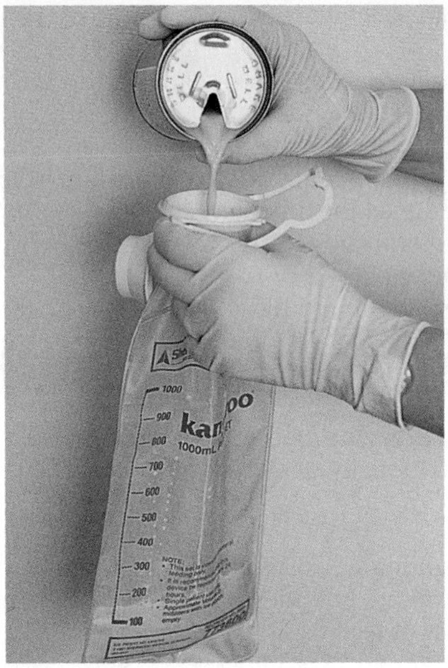

STEP **7d** Pour formula into feeding container.

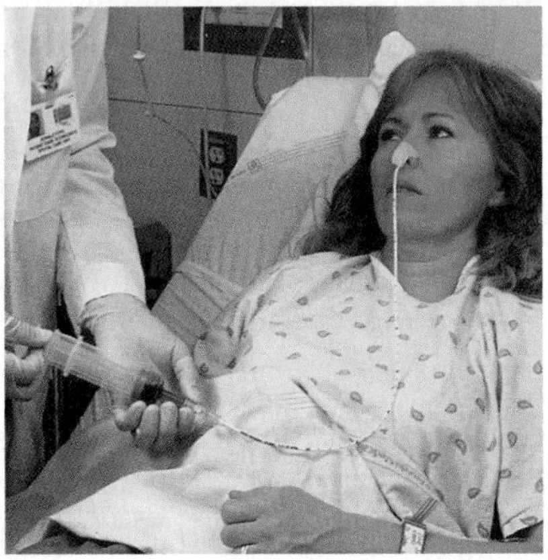

STEP **11b** Check for gastric residual (small-bore tube).

Critical Decision Point: Auscultation is no longer considered a reliable method for verification of placement of tube because a tube inadvertently placed in lungs, pharynx, or esophagus can transmit sound similar to that of air entering stomach (Metheny et al., 1990a, 1990b).

Steps	Rationale
11. Check for gastric residual. a. Draw up 30 mL of air with syringe. Connect to end of feeding tube. Flush tube with air. b. Pull back evenly to aspirate gastric contents (see illustration). c. Return aspirated contents to stomach unless the volume exceeds 100 mL (check agency policy).	Residual volume indicates if gastric emptying is delayed. Delayed gastric emptying may be reflected if 100 mL or more remain in the client's stomach (McClave et al., 1999). Return of aspirate prevents fluid and electrolyte imbalance.
12. Flush tubing with 30 mL of water.	Ensures tube is clear and patent.
13. Initiate feeding: A. **Syringe or intermittent feeding** (1) Pinch proximal end of the feeding tube.	Prevents air from entering client's stomach.
(2) Remove plunger from syringe and attach barrel of syringe to end of tube.	
(3) Fill syringe with measured amount of formula (see illustration). Release tube and hold syringe high enough to allow it to empty gradually by gravity, refill; repeat until prescribed amount has been delivered to the client. (4) If feeding bag is used, hang feeding bag on an IV pole (see illustration). Fill bag with prescribed amount of formula, and allow bag to empty gradually over at least 30 minutes.	Gradual emptying of tube feeding by gravity from syringe or feeding bag reduces risk of abdominal discomfort, vomiting, or diarrhea induced by bolus or too-rapid infusion of tube feedings.

Steps	Rationale

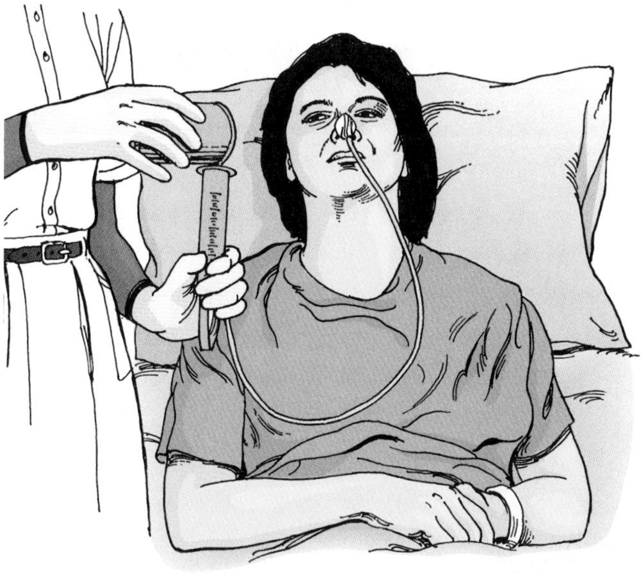

STEP **13A(3)** Fill syringe with formula.

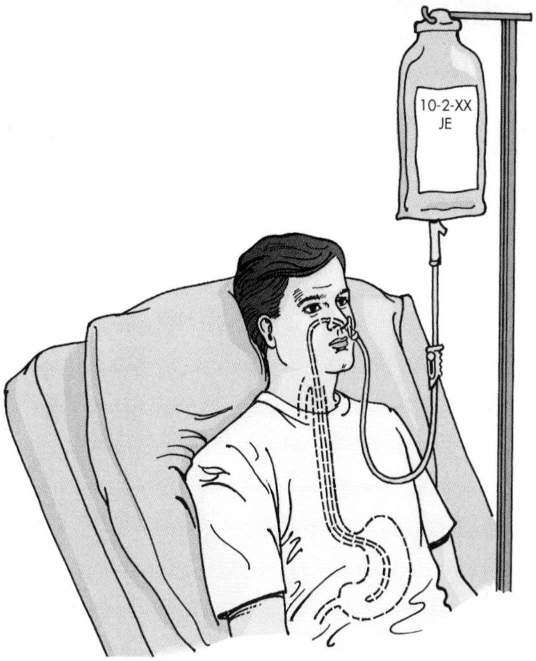

STEP **13A(4)** Administer feeding.

B. Continuous-drip method
(1) Hang feeding bag and tubing on IV pole.
(2) Connect distal end of tubing to the proximal end of the feeding tube.
(3) Connect tubing through infusion pump and set rate (see illustration).

Continuous feeding method is designed to deliver prescribed hourly rate of feeding. This method reduces risk of abdominal discomfort. Clients who receive continuous drip feedings should have residuals checked every 4 hours and tube placement verified.

14. Advance tube feeding gradually (see Box 39-8).

Tube feedings should be advanced gradually to prevent diarrhea and gastric intolerance to formula.

Critical Decision Point: Tube feedings should be infused by feeding pumps and not by intravenous (IV) pump.

15. Following intermittent infusion or at end of continuous infusion, flush nasoenteral tubing with 30 mL of water. Repeat every 4 to 6 hours. Remove gloves and/or perform hand hygiene.

Maintains patency of feeding tube and provides client with a source of water to help maintain fluid and electrolyte balance.

Critical Decision Point: It may be necessary to consult with a dietitian to recommend a total free water requirement per day. This avoids the potential of fluid overload.

16. When tube feedings are not being administered, cap or clamp the proximal end of the feeding tube.

Prevents air from entering stomach between feedings.

17. Rinse bag and tubing with warm water whenever feedings are interrupted.

Rinsing bag and tubing with warm water clears old tube feedings and reduces bacterial growth.

18. Change bag and tubing every 24 hours.

Reduces client's exposure to bacterial growth occurring in bag and tubing.

19. Measure amount of aspirate (residual) every 8 to 12 hours.

Evaluates tolerance of tube feeding.

20. Monitor finger-stick blood glucose every 6 hours until maximum administration rate is reached and maintained for 24 hours.

Alerts nurse to client's tolerance of glucose.

21. Monitor intake and output every 8 hours and do 24-hour totals.

Intake and output are indications of fluid balance or fluid volume excess or deficit.

Skill 39-2 Administering Enteral Feedings via Nasoenteric Tubes—cont'd

Steps	Rationale

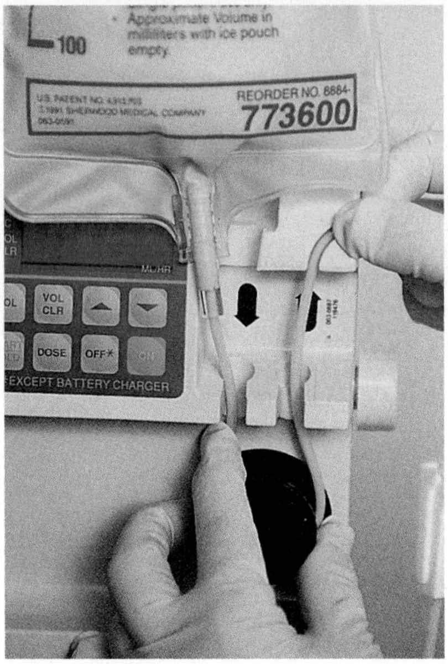

STEP **13B(3)** Connect tubing through infusion pump.

Steps	Rationale
22. Weigh client daily until maximum administration rate is reached and maintained for 24 hours; then weigh client three times per week.	Weight gain is an indicator of improved nutritional status; however, sudden gain of more than 1 kg in 24 hours usually indicates fluid retention.
23. Observe return of normal laboratory values.	Improving laboratory values (e.g., albumin, transferring, and prealbumin) indicate an improved nutritional status.

Unexpected Outcomes and Related Interventions (in addition to those in Skill 39-1)

- Gastric residual exceeds 100 mL (see agency policy).
  - Hold feeding.
  - Notify physician.
  - Maintain client in semi-Fowler's or at least have head of bed elevated 30 degrees.
  - Recheck residual in 1 hour.
- Client develops diarrhea three times or more in 24 hours.
  - Notify physician.
  - Confer with dietitian.
  - Institute skin-care measures.
  - Consider change in antibiotics only for clients receiving antibiotics.
- Client develops nausea and vomiting.
  - Notify physician.
  - Check patency of tube.
  - Aspirate for residual.
  - Auscultate for bowel sounds.

Recording and Reporting

- Record amount and type of feeding and client's response to tube feeding, patency of tube, and any side effects.
- Report client's tolerance and adverse effects.

Home Care Considerations

- Teach client or primary caregiver how to determine correct placement of feeding tube.
- Inform client or primary caregiver of signs associated with pulmonary aspiration, delayed gastric emptying.
- Reinforce signs and symptoms associated with feeding tube complications and when to call physician.

Skill 39-3 Administering Enteral Feedings via Gastrostomy or Jejunostomy Tube

Delegation Considerations

Administration of enteral tube feeding via a gastrostomy or jejunostomy tube is a procedure that can be delegated to an unregulated care provider (UCP) after the nurse verifies tube placement. UCPs should never test the position of the tube or give the first dose of a tube feeding.

- Ensure that the client is sitting upright in a chair or in bed and instruct the UCP to infuse the feeding slowly.
- Instruct the UCP to report any difficulty infusing the feeding or any discomfort voiced by the client.

Equipment

- Disposable feeding container or ready-to-hang bag.
- 30-mL or larger Luer-Lok or catheter-tip syringe
- Formula
- Infusion pump: Use pump designed for tube feedings
- pH indicator strips (scale 0.0 to 14.0)
- Stethoscope
- Disposable gloves
- Equipment to obtain blood glucose by finger stick

Steps	Rationale
1. Assess client's need for enteral tube feedings (see Skill 39-1 and Skill 39-2): impaired swallowing, decreased level of consciousness, surgeries of upper alimentary tract, need for long-term enteral nutrition.	Identifies clients who need tube feedings before they become nutritionally depleted. Enteral feeding preserves the function and mass of the gut, promotes wound healing, diminishes hypermetabolism in burn injuries, and may decrease infection in critically ill clients (Zaloga, 1994).
2. Auscultate for bowel sounds before feeding. Consult physician if bowel sounds are absent.	Absence of bowel sounds may indicate decreased or absent peristalsis and increased risk of aspiration or abdominal distension.
3. Obtain baseline weight and laboratory values.	Enteral feedings are to restore or maintain nutritional status. Provides objective data to measure effectiveness of feedings.
4. Verify physician's order for formula, rate, route, and frequency.	Tube feedings must be ordered by physician.
5. Perform hand hygiene.	Reduces transmission of micro-organisms.
6. Assess gastrostomy/jejunostomy site for breakdown, irritation, or drainage.	Infection, pressure from tube, or drainage of gastric secretions can cause skin breakdown.
7. Explain procedure to client.	Well-informed client is more co-operative and feels more at ease.
8. Prepare feeding container to administer formula:	
a. Have tube feeding at room temperature.	Cold formula may cause gastric cramping and discomfort because the liquid is not warmed by mouth and esophagus.
b. Connect tubing to container as needed, or prepare ready-to-hang bag.	Tubing must be free of contamination to prevent bacterial growth.
c. Shake formula well. Fill container and tubing with formula.	Placement of formula through tubing prevents excess air from entering gastrointestinal tract.
9. For intermittent feeding, have syringe ready and be sure formula is at room temperature.	Cold formula may cause gastric cramping.
10. Elevate head of bed 30 to 45 degrees.	Elevating client's head helps prevent chance of aspiration.
11. Apply gloves and verify tube placement.	
A. **Gastrostomy tube:** Attach syringe and aspirate gastric secretions; observe their appearance and check pH. Return aspirated contents to stomach unless the volume exceeds 100 mL. If the volume is greater than 100 mL on several consecutive occasions, hold feeding and notify physician (McClave et al., 1999).	Fluid from gastric tube of client who has fasted for at least 4 hours usually has a pH of 1 to 4, especially when client is not receiving a gastric-acid inhibitor. Continuous administration of tube feedings may elevate pH (Metheny & Titler, 2001). Gastric residual determines if gastric emptying is delayed. Delayed gastric emptying may be indicated by 100 mL or more remaining in client's stomach from previous feeding (McClave et al., 1999).

Skill 39-3 Administering Enteral Feedings via Gastrostomy or Jejunostomy Tube—cont'd

Steps	Rationale
B. Jejunostomy tube: Aspirate intestinal secretions, observe their appearance, and check pH.	Presence of intestinal fluid indicates that the end of the tube is in the small intestine (i.e., the duodenum or jejunum). Generally the intestinal residual is very small (10 mL or less). If fluid tests acidic on pH test, looks like gastric fluid, or the residual volume is large (more than 10 mL), displacement of the tube into the stomach may have occurred.
12. Flush with 30 mL of water.	
13. Initiate feedings:	Usually gastrostomy and jejunostomy feedings are given continuously to ensure proper absorption. However, initial feedings may be given by bolus to assess client's tolerance to formula. See Box 39-8 for guidelines to advance enteral feedings.
A. Syringe feedings	
(1) Pinch proximal end of gastrostomy/jejunostomy tube.	Prevents excessive air from entering the client's stomach or leaking of gastric contents.
(2) Remove plunger and attach barrel of syringe to end of tube, then fill syringe with formula.	
(3) Release tube and elevate syringe. Allow syringe to empty gradually by gravity. Refill until prescribed amount has been delivered to client.	Gradual administration of tube feedings by gravity reduces the risk of diarrhea induced by bolus tube feedings.
B. Continuous drip method	Continuous-feeding method is designed to deliver a prescribed hourly rate of feeding. This method reduces the risk of diarrhea. Clients who receive continuous-drip feedings should have residuals checked every 8 to 12 hours.
(1) Verify that volume in container is sufficient for length of feeding (4 to 8 hours, check manufacturer's recommendations).	
(2) Hang container on IV pole, and clear tubing of air.	Allows for gravity flow of formula. Prevents accumulation of air in the client's stomach.
(3) Thread tubing into pump according to manufacturer's directions.	
(4) Connect tubing to end of gastrostomy/jejunostomy tube.	
(5) Begin infusion at prescribed rate.	
14. Administer water via feeding tube as ordered with or between feedings.	Provides clients with source of water to help maintain fluid and electrolyte balance.
15. Flush tube with 30 mL of water every 4 to 6 hours and before and after administering medications via feeding tube.	Maintains patency of tube and provides client with some free water. Small jejunal tubes are prone to clogging and are difficult to replace (Simon & Fink, 1999).
16. When tube feedings are not being administered, cap or clamp the proximal end of the gastrostomy/jejunostomy tube.	Prevents excess air from entering the gastrointestinal tract between feedings and prevents leakage of gastric contents.
17. Rinse container and tubing with warm water after all intermittent feedings.	Clears feeding from tubing and reduces bacterial growth in container and tubing.
18. Assess skin around tube exit site. The skin around the tube should be cleansed daily with warm water and mild soap. Tubing exit site is left open to air. If a dressing is needed because of drainage, assess drainage and change dressing as needed.	Report any drainage, redness, swelling, or displacement of the tube to the physician. Leakage of gastric drainage may cause skin irritation. Skin around feeding tube should be cleansed daily with warm water and mild soap. When needed, a small precut gauze dressing may be applied to exit site.
19. Dispose of supplies, and perform hand hygiene.	Prevents transmission of micro-organisms.
20. Evaluate client's tolerance to tube feeding. Measure the amount of aspirate (residual) every 8 to 12 hours.	Evaluates tolerance of tube feeding.

Steps	Rationale
21. Monitor finger-stick blood glucose every 6 hours until maximum administration rate is reached and maintained for 24 hours.	Alerts nurse to client's tolerance of glucose.
22. Monitor intake and output every 24 hours.	Intake and output are indications of fluid balance or fluid volume excess.
23. Weigh client daily until maximum administration rate is reached and maintained for 24 hours; then weigh client three times per week.	Weight gain is an indicator of improved nutritional status; however, a sudden gain of more than 1 kg in 24 hr usually indicates fluid retention.
24. Observe return of normal laboratory values.	Improving laboratory values (albumin, transferring, prealbumin) indicate an improved nutritional status.
25. Inspect stoma site for signs of impaired skin integrity.	Enteral tubes can cause pressure and excoriation at the stoma site. In addition, gastric secretions also cause irritation to client's skin.

Unexpected Outcomes and Related Interventions

- Client aspirates formula when gastric emptying is delayed or formula is administered too rapidly and produces vomiting.
  - Position client in side-lying position.
  - Suction airway.
  - Notify physician.
  - Obtain chest X-ray film.
- Skin around gastrostomy/jejunostomy site breaks down.
  - Institute skin-care practices.
  - Use pressure relief measures around tube.
  - Provide appropriate wound care (see chapter 43).

Recording and Reporting

- Record amount and type of feeding and client's response to tube feeding, patency of tube, and any side effects.
- Report to oncoming nursing staff type of feeding, status of feeding tube, client's tolerance, and adverse effects.

Home Care Considerations

- Teach client or primary caregiver how to determine correct placement of feeding tube.
- Inform client or primary caregiver of signs associated with pulmonary aspiration, delayed gastric emptying.
- Reinforce signs and symptoms associated with feeding tube complications and when to call physician.

Initiating PN. Clients with short-term nutritional needs often receive intravenous solutions of less than 10% dextrose via a peripheral vein in combination with amino acids and lipids. Peripheral solutions are not as calorically dense and therefore are less irritating to the peripheral veins and are usually temporary. PN with greater than 10% dextrose requires a CVC that is placed into a high-flow central vein (such as the superior vena cava) by a physician using sterile technique (see chapter 36). Nurses who have special training insert peripherally inserted central catheters (PICCs) that are started in a vein of the forearm and threaded into the subclavian or superior vena cava vein.

After catheter placement, the catheter is flushed with saline or heparin until the position is radiographically confirmed. The physician sutures the catheter in place and covers the site with a sterile dressing. A PICC is usually stabilized with sterile strips of tape and a sterile dressing. A chest X-ray examination identifies any complications.

Before beginning any parenteral infusion, the nurse verifies the physician's order and inspects the solution for particulate matter or a break in the lipid emulsion. An infusion pump is always used. An initial rate of 40 to 60 mL/hour is recommended. The rate is gradually increased until the client's complete nutrition needs are supplied. Clients who receive PN at home frequently administer the entire daily solution over 12 hours at night. This allows the client to disconnect from the infusion each morning, flush the central line, and have independent mobility during day.

Preventing Complications. Complications of PN include mechanical complications from insertion of the CVC, infection, and metabolic alterations (Table 39-12). Pneumothorax occurs when a puncture insult to the pulmonary system results in accumulation of air in the pleural cavity with subsequent impaired breathing. Pneumothorax is usually accompanied by symptoms of sudden sharp chest pain, dyspnea, and coughing. In relation to PN, pneumothorax most often occurs during CVC placement.

Air embolus can occur during insertion of the catheter or when changing the tubing or cap. Having the client perform a Valsalva manoeuvre (holds his or her breath and "bears down") while assuming a left lateral decubitus position can prevent air embolus. The increased venous pressure created by the manoeuvre prevents air from entering the bloodstream during catheter insertion.

The infusion tubing should be changed every 24 hours with lipids and every 48 hours when lipids are not infused to avoid infection. During CVC dressing changes,

Research Highlight

Box 39-9

Accuracy in Determining Placement of Feeding Tubes

Research Focus

Two possible adverse outcomes of enteral nutrition are (a) accidental placement of a nasoenteral feeding tube into the lung and (b) pulmonary aspiration of gastric contents.

Research Abstract

No one knows the precise incidence of accidental tube misplacements into the lung, but estimates of close to 5% have been cited; clients at highest risk are those with a decreased level of consciousness (LOC), confusion, unco-operativeness, agitation, presence of an endotracheal tube, recent extubation, and poor gag reflex. A feeding tube accidentally inserted into the lung may end in the tracheobronchial tree or perforate into the pleural space. In either event, efforts are made to detect the misplacement before the introduction of tube feedings because inadvertent infusion of formula into the lung promotes tissue consolidation, pneumonia, and respiratory failure. The most accurate method for checking feeding tube placement is X-ray examination; the most effective non-radiological methods include aspirating fluid from the feeding tube and measuring its pH and describing its appearance. Although observing for respiratory distress is helpful in alert clients (especially when firm large-diameter tubes are used), it is of little benefit in those who have a decreased LOC and when small-bore tubes are used. Risk factors for pulmonary aspiration in tube-fed clients include feeding into the stomach when gastric atony is present (resulting in high gastric residual volumes), poor gag reflexes, mechanical ventilation, and flat positioning in bed. Bedside methods used to detect pulmonary aspiration are not well defined.

Evidence-Based Practice

- X-ray verification of feeding tube placement is the most reliable method available to confirm correct feeding tube location and is required in most acute care facilities when small-bore tubes are initially inserted.
- When the X-ray method is not feasible, the next best method involves testing the feeding tube aspirate's pH and observing its appearance. A properly obtained pH of 0 to 4 is a good indication of gastric placement; a pH of 6 or higher could indicate placement in the lung, intestine, or even the stomach when gastric pH is usually high. Intestinal fluid is usually bile-stained (dark golden yellow); in contrast, gastric fluid is usually grassy green, off-white to tan, or clear and colourless.
- The auscultatory method should not be used to determine tube location.
- If the dye method is used to detect aspiration of enteral feedings, the dye should be sterile to reduce the risk of pulmonary infection in the event of aspiration.

References

Metheny, N., Aud, M., & Ignatavicius, D. (1998, Summer). Detection of improperly placed feeding tubes. *Journal of Healthcare Risk Management, 18*(3), 37.

Metheny, N.A., Aud, M.A., & Wunderlich, R.J. (1999). A survey of bedside methods used to detect pulmonary aspiration of enteral formula in intubated tube-fed patients. *American Journal of Critical Care, 8*(3), 160–167.

Metheny, N., & Titler, M. (2001). Assessing placement of feeding tubes. *American Journal of Nursing, 101*(5), 36–45.

sterile mask and gloves are always used, and insertion sites should be assessed for signs and symptoms of infection (see chapter 36).

The PN solution contains most of the major electrolytes, vitamins, and minerals. Supplemental vitamin K must be given as ordered throughout therapy. Vitamin K can be synthesized by microflora found in the jejunum and ileum with normal use of the GI tract; however, because PN circumvents GI use, exogenous vitamin K must be administered.

Electrolyte and mineral imbalances may occur. Administration of concentrated glucose is accompanied by increases in endogenous insulin production, which causes cations (potassium, magnesium, and phosphorus) to move intracellularly. In malnourished or cachectic clients, the resulting low serum (extracellular) levels of electrolytes and edema may cause cardiac dysrhythmias, congestive heart failure, respiratory distress, convulsions, coma, or death. This has been called refeeding syndrome.

Too-rapid administration of hypertonic dextrose can result in an osmotic diuresis and dehydration (see chapter 36). If an infusion falls behind schedule, the nurse should not increase the rate in an attempt to catch up. Sudden discontinuation of the solution can cause hypoglycemia. Usually, 5% to 10% dextrose is infused when PN solution is suddenly discontinued. Diabetic clients are more at risk. The goal is to move clients from PN to EN or oral feeding, or both. Once clients are meeting one third to one half of their kilocalorie needs per day, PN is usually decreased to half the original volume. EN feedings should then be increased to meet needs. When 75% of daily energy needs are consistently met with tube feeding, PN may be discontinued. Clients who make the transition from PN to oral feedings typically have early satiety and decreased appetite. PN should be gradually decreased in response to increased oral intake. If oral intake is inadequate, small frequent meals may prove helpful. Calorie and protein counts are recommended when clients begin taking soft foods. When 75% of needs are being met by reliable dietary intake, PN therapy may be discontinued.

Restorative and Continuing Care. Clients discharged from a hospital with diet prescriptions often need dietary

Box 39-10 Procedural Guidelines

Obtaining GI Aspirate for pH Measurement, Large- and Small-Bore Feeding Tubes: Intermittent and Continuous Feeding

Equipment: Cone tipped or asepto syringe, pH test paper (scale of 1 to 11), paper towel, small medication cup, disposable gloves.

Delegation Considerations: The skill of measuring pH in GI aspirate should not be delegated to unregulated care providers.

1. Perform hand hygiene. Perform measures to verify placement of tube:
   a. For intermittently fed clients, test placement immediately before feeding (usually a period of at least 4 hours will have elapsed since previous feeding). More frequent checking has been associated with increased clogging of small-bore tubes. To avoid clogging, flush tube with 30 mL of water after aspirating for the residual volume (Edwards & Metheny, 2000).
   b. For continuously tube-fed clients, check agency policy. If the client is tolerating the feedings without incident and other indicators of correct location are present (the mark on the tube at the exit site has remained in its original position and the most recent X-ray films confirm tube's correct position), it is reasonable to continue feedings. **If risk of tube displacement is high and the tube has moved, consider the need for an X-ray film to verify placement** (Metheny & Titler, 2001). Plan pH testing at times when feeding may be withheld (e.g., during diagnostic testing, chest physical therapy, or to avoid medication interaction).
   c. Wait at least 1 hour after medication administration by tube or mouth.
2. Apply disposable gloves.
3. Draw up 30 mL of air into syringe, then attach to end of feeding tube. Flush tube with 30 mL of air before attempting to aspirate fluid. It will likely be more difficult to aspirate fluid from the small intestine than from the stomach. Repositioning the client from side to side may be helpful. More than one bolus of air through the tube may be needed in some cases. A burst of air aids in aspirating fluid more easily (Metheny et al., 1993b).
4. Draw back on syringe and obtain 5 to 10 mL of gastric aspirate. Observe appearance of aspirate (see illustration Step 4A).

   Gently mix aspirate in syringe. Then expel a few drops into a clean medicine cup. Dip the pH strip into the fluid or apply a few drops of the fluid to the strip (see illustration Step 4B). Compare the colour of the strip with the colour on the chart provided by the manufacturer (Metheny et al., 1998b).
   a. Gastric fluid usually has a pH range of 1 to 4 (Metheny et al., 1998a).
   b. Intestinal fluid usually has a pH greater than 6.
   c. Client with continuous tube feeding may have a pH of 5 or higher.
   d. pH of pleural fluid from tracheobronchial tree is generally greater than 6.
5. Remove gloves and discard supplies. Perform hand hygiene.

Critical Decision Point

If after repeated attempts, it is not possible to aspirate fluid from a tube that was originally established by X-ray examination to be in desired position, and (a) there are no risk factors for tube dislocation, (b) the tube has remained in original taped position, and (c) the client is not experiencing difficulty, assume the tube is correctly placed (Metheny et al., 1993a).

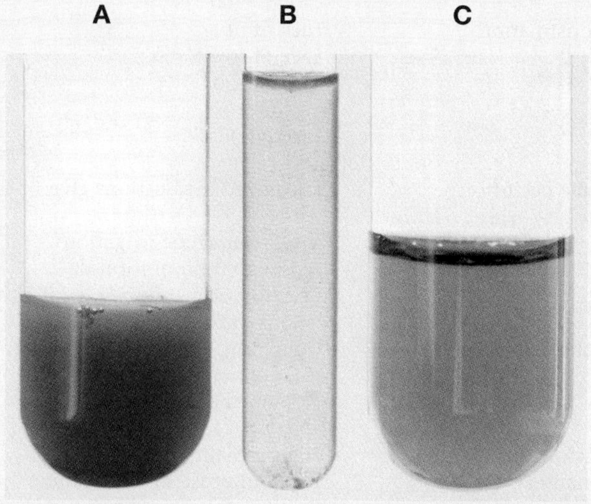

STEP **4A** Gastrointestinal contents. **A,** Stomach. **B,** Stomach. **C,** Intestinal. (Courtesy Dr. Normal Metheny, Professor, St. Louis University School of Nursing.)

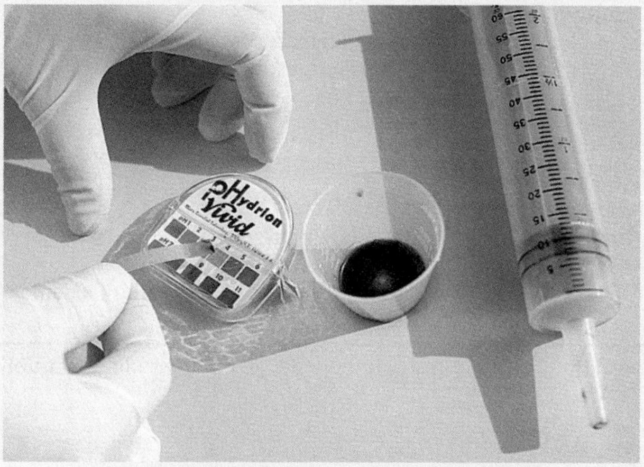

STEP **4B** Comparing pH strip with colour chart.

Table 39-11 Enteral Tube Feeding Complications

Problem	Possible Cause	Intervention
Pulmonary aspiration	Regurgitation of formula	Verify tube placement.
	Feeding tube displaced	Reposition tube and verity tube placement.
	Client in supine position	Elevate head of bed 30 to 45 degrees during feedings and for 2 hours afterward.
	Deficient gag reflex	Reassess for return of normal gag reflex; until then place client on aspiration precautions and place client in supine position.
	Gastroesophageal reflux disease	Verify tube placement.
	Delayed gastric emptying	Lower rate of delivery to increase tolerance.
Diarrhea	Hyperosmolar formula or medications	Deliver formula continuously, lower rate, dilute, or change to isotonic EN.
	Allergy to elixir ingredients (sorbitol)	Liquid medications are often sweetened with sorbitol, consider as possible cause.
	Antibiotic therapy	Antibiotics may destroy normal intestinal flora; physician may change medication; treat symptoms with anti-diarrhea agents.
	Bacterial contamination	Do not hang formula longer than 4–8 hours in bag, wash bag out well when refilling, change tube feeding bags q24h, and use aseptic practices. Check expiration dates.
	Malabsorption	Check for pancreatic insufficiency; use low-fat, lactose-free formula and continuous feedings.
Constipation	Lack of fibre	Select a formula containing fibre.
	Lack of free water	Add water as needed as flushes.*
	Medications	Evaluate side effects; suggest stool softener or bulk-forming laxative.
	Inactivity	Monitor client's ability to ambulate; collaborate with physician for activity order or physiotherapy.
Tube occlusion	Pulverized medications given per tube	Irrigate with 30 mL water before and after each medication per tube.*
	Insufficient tube irrigation	Dilute crushed medications if not liquid.
	Sedimentation of formula	Shake cans well before administering (read label).
	Reaction of incompatible medications or formula	Read pharmacological information on compatibility of drugs and formula.
Tube displacement	Coughing, vomiting	Replace tube and confirm placement before restarting tube feeding.
	Not taped securely	With placement verification, check that tape is secure (nasoenteral).
Abdominal cramping, nausea/vomiting	High osmality of formula	Suggest an isotonic formula, or dilute current formula.
	Rapid increase in rate/volume	Lower rate of delivery to increase tolerance.
	Delayed gastric emptying	
	Lactose intolerance	Suggest use of lactose-free formula.
	Intestinal obstruction	Stop feeding with GI obstruction.
	High-fat formula used	Use greater proportion of carbohydrate.
	Cold formula used	Warm formula to room temperature.
Delayed gastric emptying	Diabetic gastroparesis	Consult with physician regarding medication for increasing gastric motility.
	Prematurity	Check for residual (see agency policy).
	Serious illnesses	
	Inactivity	Consult physician regarding advancing tube to intestinal placement.
		Monitor medications and pathological conditions that may affect GI motility.
Serum electrolyte imbalance	Excess GI losses	Monitor serum electrolyte levels daily.
	Dehydration	Provide free water as per dietitian recommendation.
	Cirrhosis	Know of links with specific pathological condition.
	Congestive heart failure, edema	
	Diabetes mellitus	

*Check first for fluid-restricted conditions that would affect volume of water given.

Table 39-11 Enteral Tube Feeding Complications—cont'd

Problem	Possible Cause	Intervention*
Increased respiratory quotient	Overfeeding of carbohydrates	Balance kilocalorie needs provided from fat, protein, and carbohydrate with greater proportion of fat in formula (to decrease CO^2 production).
Fluid overload	Refeeding syndrome in malnutrition	Restrict fluids if necessary and use either a specialized formula or a diluted enteral formula at first. Monitor levels of serum proteins and electrolytes.
	Excess free water or diluted (hypotonic) formula	Use a more concentrated formula with fluid volume excess without risk of refeeding syndrome.
Hyperosmolar dehydration	Hypertonic formula with insufficient free water	Slow rate of delivery, dilute, or change to isotonic formula.

*Check first for fluid-restricted conditions that would affect volume of water given.

Box 39-11 Indications for Parenteral Nutrition

Non-functional GI Tract

Massive small bowel resection/GI surgery
Paralytic ileus
Intestinal obstruction
Trauma to abdomen, head, or neck
Severe malabsorption
Intolerance to enteral feeding (established by trial)
Chemotherapy, radiation therapy, bone marrow transplantation

Extended Bowel Rest

Enterocutaneous fistula
Inflammatory bowel disease exacerbation
Severe diarrhea
Moderate to severe pancreatitis

Preoperative TPN

Preoperative bowel rest
Treatment for co-morbid severe malnutrition in clients with non-functional GI tracts
Severely catabolic clients when GI tract non-usable for >4 to 5 days

education to plan meals that meet specific therapeutic requirements. Restorative care includes both immediate postsurgical care and routine medical care and therefore includes hospitalized and home care clients. **Medical nutrition therapy (MNT)** is the use of specific nutritional therapies to treat an illness, injury, or condition. MNT may be necessary to assist the body's ability to metabolize certain nutrients, correct nutritional deficiencies related to the disease, and eliminate foods that may exacerbate disease symptoms. The following sections address MNT for some common disease states.

Gastrointestinal Diseases. Peptic ulcers are controlled with regular meals and medications such as cimetidine. Cimetidine is one of a class of drugs that are histamine receptor antagonists that block secretion of hydrochloric acid. *Helicobacter pylori* was first identified by Marshall and Warren in 1984 and is a bacterium that causes peptic ulcers. The presence of bacteria is confirmed by laboratory tests and treated with antibiotics. Stress and overproduction of gastric HCl also contribute to peptic ulcer disease.

Clients are encouraged to avoid foods that increase stomach acidity, such as caffeine, decaffeinated coffee, frequent milk intake, citric acid juices, and certain seasonings (hot chili peppers, chili powder, black pepper). Smoking, alcohol, and ASA are also discouraged.

Inflammatory bowel disease includes Crohn's disease and idiopathic ulcerative colitis. Treatment of acute inflammatory bowel disease may include elemental diets (formula with the nutrients in their simplest form ready for absorption) or PN when symptoms such as diarrhea and weight loss are prevalent. In the chronic stage of the disease, a regular, highly nourishing diet is appropriate. Vitamin and iron supplements may be required to correct or prevent anemia. Irritable bowel syndrome is managed by increasing fibre, reducing fat, avoiding large meals, and avoiding lactose- or sorbitol-containing foods for susceptible individuals.

The treatment of **malabsorption** syndromes, such as celiac disease, includes a gluten-free diet. Gluten is present in wheat, rye, barley, and oats. Short-bowel syndrome results from extensive resection of bowel after which clients have malabsorption from lack of intestinal surface area. These clients may require lifetime feeding with either elemental enteral formulas or PN.

Diverticulitis is nutritionally treated with a moderate- or low-residue diet until the infection subsides. Afterward, a high-fibre diet is generally prescribed for chronic diverticulosis.

Diabetes Mellitus. Type I diabetes mellitus requires both insulin and dietary restrictions for optimal control, beginning with diagnosis (Canadian Diabetes Association, 2003b). In contrast, Type II diabetes mellitus may initially be controlled solely by exercise and diet therapy. If these measures prove ineffective, it is common to add oral medications. Insulin injections may follow if Type II diabetes worsens or fails to respond to these initial interventions.

Table 39-12 Complications of Parenteral Nutrition (PN)

Problem	Signs/Symptoms	Intervention
Air embolism	Tachypnea, apnea, wheezing, hypotension, cyanosis	Turn client to left lateral decubitus position, instruct client to perform Valsalva manoeuvre, and lower head of bed. Cap open end of catheter or tape perforation in catheter wall. Administer oxygen; notify physician. Maintain integrity of closed system to prevent air emboli, and have client perform Valsalva manoeuvre when changing cap.
Catheter occlusion	No flow or sluggish flow through the catheter	Temporarily stop infusion and flush with saline or heparin. If effort to flush is unsuccessful, attempt to aspirate clot; if still unsuccessful, follow protocol for use of thrombolytic agent (e.g., urokinase).
Catheter sepsis	Fever, chills, glucose intolerance, positive blood culture	To prevent, change catheter site dressing if it becomes wet or contaminated, use aseptic technique when changing dressing of handling IV tubing, catheter caps, or PN containers. Do not hang a single container of PN for more than 24 hours, or lipids more than 12 hours; use an in-line 0.22-μm filter to remove bacteria.*
Electrolyte imbalance	Monitor Na, Ca, K, Cl, PO_4, Mg, and CO_2 levels	See chapter 36 for signs of deficiency/toxicity. Check total parenteral nutrition (TPN) for supplemental electrolyte levels. Notify physician of imbalances.
Hypercapnia	Increased oxygen consumption, increased CO_2, respiratory quotient >1.0, minute ventilation	Ventilator-dependent clients are at risk; to prevent monitor parameters; provide 30% to 60% of energy requirements as fat per physician's order.
Hypoglycemia	Diaphoresis, shakiness, confusion, loss of consciousness	To prevent, do not abruptly discontinue TPN but taper rate down to within 10% of infusion rate 1 to 2 hours before stopping. If hyperglycemia is suspected, test blood glucose, administer IV bolus of dextrose per physician order if necessary.
Hyperglycemia	Thirst, headache, lethargy, increased urination	Monitor blood glucose level daily until stable, then as ordered or prn. TPN is initiated slowly and tapered up to maximal infusion rate. Additional insulin may be required during therapy if problem persists (or if client has diabetes mellitus).
Hyperglycemic hyperosmolar non-ketonic dehydration/coma	Hyperglycemia (>500 mg%/dL), glycosuria, serum osmolarity >350 mOsm/L, confusion, azotemia, headache, severe signs of dehydration (see chapter 36), hypernatremia, metabolic acidosis, convulsions, coma	To prevent, monitor blood glucose, BUN, serum osmolarity, glucose in urine, and fluid losses; administer insulin as ordered; replace fluids as needed; maintain consistent infusion rate; and provide 30% of daily energy needs as fat. Clients at risk are hypermetabolic, receiving steroids, older adults, diabetic, have impaired renal or pancreatic function, or are septic.
Pneumothorax	Severe dyspnea, cyanosis, X-ray confirmation	Complication that occurs upon catheter insertion, may evolve slowly afterward. Monitor for first 24 hours for pulmonary distress.
Thrombosis of central vein	Unilateral edema of neck, shoulder and arm; pain	Repeated or traumatic catheter insertions place clients at risk; notify physician.

*With 3-in-1-admixture TPN, filtration is not possible because of large lipid molecules.

In both cases, the diet is individualized according to the client's age, build, weight, and activity level. Current guidelines for nutritional management of diabetes are being revised to reflect the changes in the nutrition recommendations for Canadians (Canadian Diabetes Association, 2003a). *Healthy Eating Is in Store for You* is a project that will help consumers make healthy food choices through better use of the nutrition information on the label of packaged foods. The Canadian Diabetes Association and Dietitians of Canada have joined forces to bring this program to the general public *(http://www.healthyeatingisinstore.ca/)*. Nurses also need to be aware of the signs and symptoms of and interventions for hypoglycemia and hyperglycemia.

Cardiovascular Diseases. Dietary therapy following an acute myocardial infarction includes initial reduction in kilocalories, soft-textured foods, and amounts of fat, sodium, and cholesterol that conform to the American Heart Association recommendations. Magnesium, folic acid, and vitamin B_6 appear to be important for primary prevention of coronary heart disease. Increases in folic aid are associated with a decrease in homocysteine, which is associated with greater risk of coronary artery disease (Rimm et al., 1998).

The National Cholesterol Education Program (2002) recommends the following dietary parameters for cholesterol management:

- Saturated fat: <7% of total calories
- Polyunsaturated fat: up to 10% of total calories
- Monounsaturated fat: up to 20% of total calories
- Total fat: 25% to 35% of total calories
- Carbohydrate: 50% to 60% of total calories

- Fibre: 20 to 30 g/day
- Protein: approximately 15% of total calories
- Cholesterol: <200 mg/day
- Total calories (energy): balance energy intake and expenditure to maintain desirable body weight and to prevent weight gain

Nutritional therapy for hypertension includes kilocalorie reduction to promote weight loss as appropriate, decreased sodium intake, and potassium-rich foods if potassium-wasting diuretics are part of the treatment.

Cancer and Cancer Treatment. Malignant cells compete with normal cells for nutrients, increasing metabolic needs. Most cancer treatments cause nutritional problems. Clients with cancer typically complain of anorexia and taste distortions. Malnutrition in cancer is associated with increased morbidity and mortality. Newer and more effective antiemetic drugs and enhanced nutritional status may improve the client's quality of life.

Radiation therapy is intended to destroy rapidly dividing malignant cells; however, other normal rapidly dividing cells, such as the epithelial lining of the GI tract, are often affected. Radiation therapy can cause anorexia, stomatitis, severe diarrhea, strictures of the intestine, and pain. Radiation treatment of the head and neck region can cause taste and smell disturbances, decreased salivation, and dysphagia. Nutrition management of the client with cancer focuses on maximizing intake of nutrients and fluids. The nurse should use creative approaches to manage alterations in taste and smell such as rinsing the mouth before a meal.

Human Immunodeficiency Virus. HIV-infected clients typically experience body wasting and severe weight loss. The wasting can be related to anorexia, stomatitis, oral thrush infection, nausea, or recurrent vomiting, all resulting in inadequate intake. Factors associated with weight loss and malnutrition are severe diarrhea, GI malabsorption, and altered metabolism of nutrients. Systemic infection results in hypermetabolism from cytokine elevation. Often the medications taken to treat HIV infection cause side effects that alter nutritional status.

Restorative care of acquired immunodeficiency syndrome (AIDS) malnutrition focuses upon maximizing kilocalories and nutrients. Each cause of nutritional depletion should be diagnosed and addressed in the care plan. Individually tailored nutritional support should progress in stages from oral, to enteral, and lastly to parenteral. Good hand hygiene and food safety are essential, including minimization of exposure to *Cryptosporidium* in drinking water, lakes, or swimming pools. Low-fat diets and small, frequent, nutrient-dense meals may be better tolerated (Keithley & Swanson, 1998).

NP Evaluation

Care plans should reflect achievable goals and outcomes. Nurses need to evaluate outcomes of nursing actions and be alert for signs that goals are being met. Adequate time should be allowed to test each nursing approach to a problem. Multidisciplinary collaboration is essential in provision of nutrition support.

Client Care. Effectiveness of nutritional interventions is best measured by meeting the client's expected outcomes and goals of care (Figure 39–10). Nutrition therapy does not always produce rapid results. Ongoing comparisons may be made with baseline measures of weight, serum albumin or prealbumin, and protein and kilocalorie intake. EN therapy is frequently interrupted. Medications may produce unwanted side effects. If gradual weight gain is not observed, or if weight loss continues, the prescription may need to be increased. Changes in condition may also indicate a need to change the nutritional care plan. Multidisciplinary members of the health care team should be consulted, and the client should be an active participant whenever possible. The client's ability to incorporate dietary changes into his or her lifestyle with the least amount of stress or disruption will ensure that outcome measures are met.

Client Expectations. Clients expect competent and accurate care. If outcomes of nutritional therapies are unsuccessful, clients expect nurses to alter the care plan. Expectations held by nurses may differ from those held by clients. For example, Young, Minnick, and Marcantonio (1996) found discrepancies between nursing staff, nursing managers, and clients regarding health care values. Nurses should be aware of these different values. By working closely with clients, the nurse can get to know their expectations and try to meet these expectations within the limits of their conditions and treatments.

Key Concepts

- A balanced diet with carbohydrates, fats, proteins, vitamins, and minerals provides the essential nutrients to carry out the body's normal physiological functioning throughout the lifespan.
- Through digestion, food is broken down into its simplest form for absorption. Digestion and absorption occur mainly in the small intestine.
- Dietary reference intakes (DRIs) provide a range of values that address the needs of groups (estimated average requirement) and individuals (adequate intakes, recommended dietary allowances, and tolerable upper intake level).
- Guidelines for dietary change advocate reduced fat, saturated fat, sodium, refined sugar, and cholesterol and increased intake of complex carbohydrates and fibre.
- Because improper nutrition can affect all body systems, nutritional assessment includes a review of total physical assessment.
- Multidisciplinary collaboration is essential to optimal nutrition.
- Tube feedings can be used for clients who are unable to ingest food but are able to digest and absorb food.

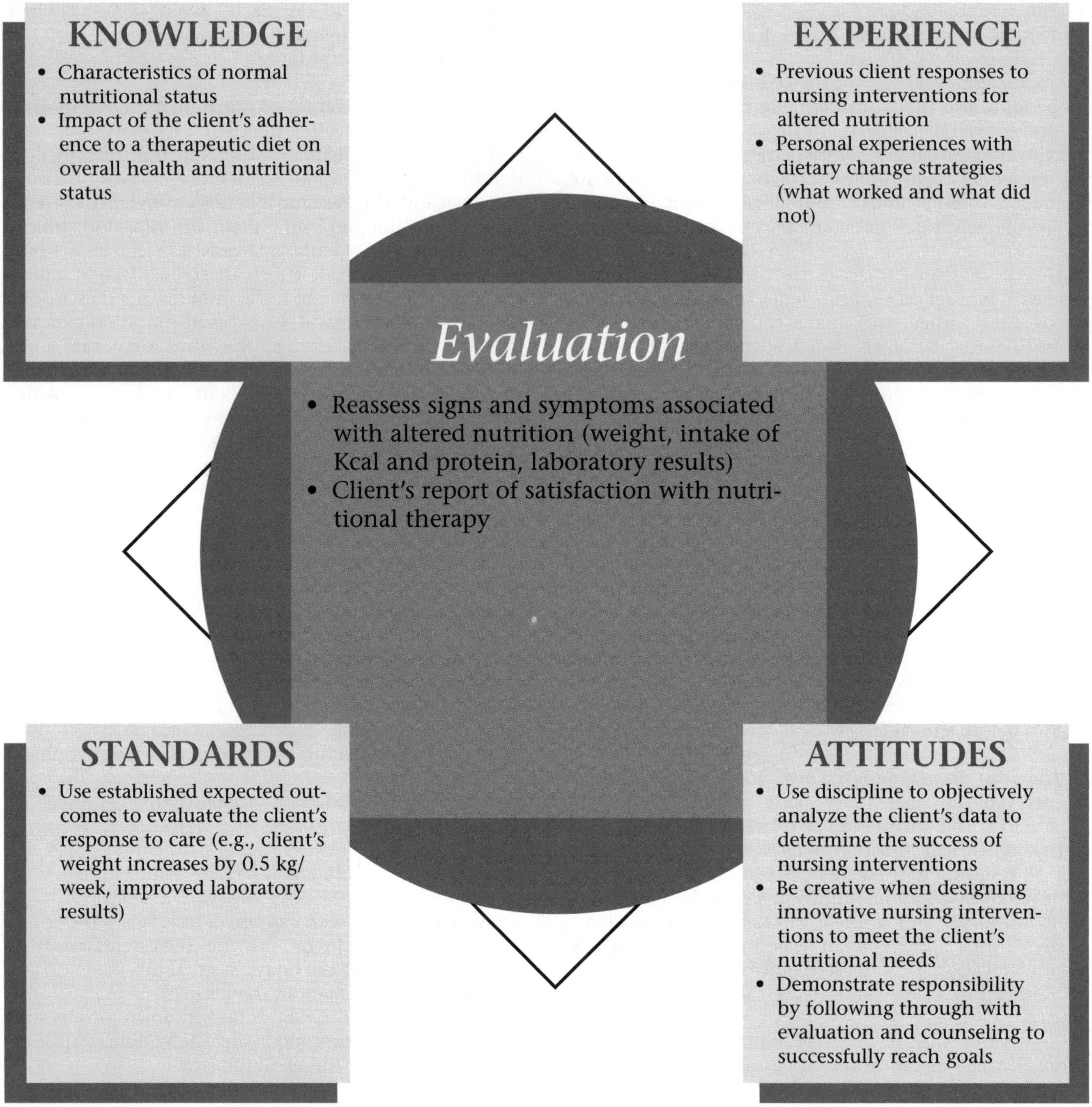
KNOWLEDGE
• Characteristics of normal nutritional status
• Impact of the client's adherence to a therapeutic diet on overall health and nutritional status
EXPERIENCE
• Previous client responses to nursing interventions for altered nutrition
• Personal experiences with dietary change strategies (what worked and what did not)
Evaluation
• Reassess signs and symptoms associated with altered nutrition (weight, intake of Kcal and protein, laboratory results)
• Client's report of satisfaction with nutritional therapy
STANDARDS
• Use established expected outcomes to evaluate the client's response to care (e.g., client's weight increases by 0.5 kg/week, improved laboratory results)
ATTITUDES
• Use discipline to objectively analyze the client's data to determine the success of nursing interventions
• Be creative when designing innovative nursing interventions to meet the client's nutritional needs
• Demonstrate responsibility by following through with evaluation and counseling to successfully reach goals

FIGURE **39–10** Critical thinking model for nutrition evaluation.

- Enteral nutrition may protect intestinal structure and function and enhance immunity.
- Total parenteral nutrition supplies essential nutrients in appropriate amounts to support life through the introduction of a concentrated nutrient solution into the superior vena cava near the right atrium of the heart.
- Medical nutrition therapy is a recognized treatment modality for both acute and chronic disease states.
- Special diets alter the composition, texture, digestibility, and residue of foods to suit the client's particular needs.

Key Terms

Amino acids, *p. 1280*
Anabolism, *p. 1284*
Anorexia, *p. 1302*
Anorexia nervosa, *p. 1289*
Anthropometry, *p. 1293*
Aspiration, *p. 1282*
Basal metabolic rate (BMR), *p. 1280*
Body mass index (BMI), *p. 1293*
Bulimia nervosa, *p. 1289*
Carbohydrates, *p. 1280*
Catabolism, *p. 1284*
Cholesterol, *p. 1281*
Chyme, *p. 1282*
Complementary proteins, *p. 1280*
Complex carbohydrates, *p. 1280*
Dietary reference intakes (DRIs), *p. 1285*
Dysphagia, *p. 1282*
Enteral nutrition (EN), *p. 1304*
Enzymes, *p. 1282*
Essential amino acids, *p. 1280*
Fat-soluble vitamins, *p. 1282*
Fatty acids, *p. 1281*
Gluconeogenesis, *p. 1285*
Glycogenesis, *p. 1285*
Glycogenolysis, *p. 1285*
Hypervitaminosis, *p. 1282*
Ideal body weight (IBW), *p. 1293*
Ketones, *p. 1285*
Lipid emulsions, *p. 1310*
Lipids, *p. 1281*
Macrominerals, *p. 1282*
Malabsorption, *p. 1321*
Medical nutrition therapy (MNT), *p. 1321*
Metabolism, *p. 1284*
Minerals, *p. 1282*
Monounsaturated fatty acids, *p. 1281*
Nitrogen balance, *p. 1280*
Non-essential amino acids, *p. 1280*
Nutrient density, *p. 1280*
Nutrients, *p. 1280*
Parenteral nutrition (PN), *p. 1310*
Peristalsis, *p. 1282*
Polyunsaturated fatty acids, *p. 1281*
Resting energy expenditure (REE), *p. 1280*
Saccharides, *p. 1280*
Saturated (fatty acids), *p. 1281*
Simple carbohydrates, *p. 1280*
Trace elements, *p. 1282*
Trans fatty acids, *p. 1281*
Triglycerides, *p. 1281*
Unsaturated (fatty acids), *p. 1281*
Vegetarianism, *p. 1290*
Vitamins, *p. 1282*
Water-soluble vitamins, *p. 1282*

Critical Thinking Exercises

1. Jean, 35 years old, has just had surgery for a bowel obstruction. Her medical history includes Crohn's disease. Three months ago, Jean's weight was 55.8 kg. Admission weight was 52.2 kg; 3 days after surgery, she now weighs 49.0 kg. Her height is 165 cm. Reported laboratory values are white blood cell count, 8.3; % lymphocytes 13; albumin, 2.3 g/dL. What is Jean's BMI? What is her percent weight loss? What is her total lymphocyte count? Jean remains NPO with nasogastric suction; what intervention(s) would you discuss with her physician?
2. Borys Shihura, 86 years old, was admitted for a viral infection. He lost 3 kg in the week before admission. He has lost an additional 2 kg during the week of hospitalization. His appetite is poor; he has frequent nausea and vomiting. His abdomen is soft, non-tender, and cancer free, and bowel sounds are present. Enteral feedings will be initiated.
   a. What type of tube should be selected?
   b. How will the tube placement be verified?
   c. Describe the type of feeding and initiation of feedings.
   d. What complications should be assessed?
3. Roberta is being treated for breast cancer with chemotherapy as adjunct to a lumpectomy. She has maintained a positive attitude but is concerned about the side effects of the medication. Roberta has bleeding gums, stomatitis, nausea, and diarrhea. As a result, she has no desire to eat. She is 85% of her usual body weight. How could you assist Roberta in improving her nutritional status?

Review Questions

1. The nutrient that provides the body's most preferred energy source is
   1. Fat
   2. Protein
   3. Vitamin
   4. Carbohydrate
2. The nutrient that is needed for tissue repair is
   1. Fat
   2. Protein
   3. Vitamin
   4. Carbohydrate
3. Positive nitrogen balance would occur in
   1. Infection
   2. Starvation
   3. Burn injury
   4. Pregnancy
4. Water composes 60% to 70% of
   1. Total body weight
   2. Digested food
   3. Carbohydrates
   4. Water-soluble vitamins
5. When feeding tubes are first positioned, verification is done by
   1. Auscultation
   2. X-ray confirmation
   3. pH testing of gastric contents
   4. Confirmation of distal mark on feeding tube
6. Parenteral nutrition is used when the client is
   1. NPO
   2. Experiencing a highly stressed physiological state
   3. Recovering from abdominal surgery
   4. Experiencing a condition resulting in gastrointestinal dysfunction
7. The bacteria that causes peptic ulcers is
   1. *Micrococcus*
   2. *Helicobacter pylori*
   3. *Staphylococcus*
   4. *Corynebacteria*

8. Inflammatory bowel disease include(s)
   1. Crohn's disease and idiopathic ulcerative colitis
   2. Celiac disease
   3. Peptic ulcers
   4. Diverticulitis
9. Nutritional therapy for hypertension includes
   1. A moderate or low-residue diet
   2. Reduction in kilocalories, soft-textured foods, and amounts of fat, sodium, and cholesterol
   3. Kilocalorie reduction to promote weight loss as appropriate, decreased sodium intake, and potassium-rich foods if potassium-wasting diuretics are part of the treatment
   4. A high-fibre diet
10. Homebound older adults have an increased risk of
   1. Diverticulitis
   2. Poor nutrition
   3. Food intolerances
   4. Peptic ulcers

References

American Academy of Family Physicians. (1997, November 7). *A position paper on disease state management.* Retrieved June 6, 2004, from *http://www.aafp.org/fpr/may96/paper.html*

American Diabetes Association. (2002). Evidence-based nutrition principles and recommendations for the treatment and prevention of diabetes and related complications. *Diabetes Care, 25*(Suppl. 1), S50–S60. Retrieved June 4, 2004, from *http://care.diabetesjournals.org/*

American Psychiatric Association. (1994). *Diagnostic and statistical manual of mental disorders* (4th revised ed.). Washington, DC: Author.

American Society for Parenteral and Enteral Nutrition. (2001). Standards of practice for nutrition support nurses. *Nutrition in Clinical Practice, 16*(1), 56–62.

American Society for Parenteral and Enteral Nutrition. (2002). Guidelines for the use of parenteral and enteral nutrition in adult and pediatric patients. *Journal of Parenteral and Enteral Nutrition, 26*(1), 1SA–138SA.

Atkinson, S. A., & Ward, W. E. (2001). Clinical nutrition: 2. The role of nutrition in the prevention and treatment of adult osteoporosis. *Canadian Medical Association Journal, 165*(11), 1511–1514.

Best, D. G., Small, S. P., & Brennan, A. L. (1994). You are what you eat. *Canadian Nurse, 90*(8), 17.

Bowers, S. (1996). Tubes: A nurse's guide to enteral feeding devices. *MedSurg Nursing, 5*(5), 313–324.

Campbell, N. R., et al. (1999). Lifestyle modifications to prevent and control hypertension. *Canadian Medical Association Journal, 160*(Suppl. 9), S1–6.

Canadian Diabetes Association. (2003a). *Clinical practice guidelines.* Retrieved June 4, 2004, from *http://www.diabetes.ca/cpg2003*

Canadian Diabetes Association. (2003b). *Evidence-based best practices for the nutritional management of diabetes: nutritional management of diabetes mellitus in the new millennium: A position statement of the Canadian Diabetes Association.* Retrieved June 6, 2004, from *http://www.diabetes.ca/Files/nutritional_guide_eng.pdf*

Canadian Hypertension Education Program. (2004). *The 2004 Canadian recommendations for the management of hypertension.* Retrieved February 22, 2005, from *http://www.hypertension.ca/recommendations_2005/execsummary2005.pdf*

Chen, C. C., Schilling, L. S., & Lyder, C. H. (2001). A concept analysis of malnutrition in the elderly. *Journal of Advanced Nursing, 36*(1), 131–142.

Child hunger and education program. (n.d.). Retrieved December 22, 2004, from *http://www.chep.org*

Costello, M. C., & Todd-Magel, C. (1997). Bridging the gap: Hospital to home nutrition support. *MedSurg Nursing, 6*(6), 328–337.

Daly, S., et al. (1997). Minimum effective dose of folic acid for food fortification to prevent neural tube defects. *Lancet, 350,* 1666–1669.

Davis, A. E., et al. (1995). Preventing feeding-associated aspiration. *MedSurg Nursing, 4*(2), 111–119.

Dochterman, J. M., & Bulechek, G. M. (Eds.). (2004). *Nursing interventions classification (NIC)* (4th ed.). St. Louis, MO: Mosby.

Dossey, B. (1999). *Florence Nightingale: Mystic, visionary, and healer.* Philadelphia: Springhouse.

Edwards, S., & Metheny, N. (2000). Measurement of gastric residual volume: State of the science. *Medsurg Nursing, 9*(3), 125–128.

Evans-Stoner, N. (1997). Nutritional assessment: A practical approach. *The Nursing Clinics of North America, 32*(4), 637–650.

Food and Nutrition Board. (1992). *Nutrition during pregnancy and lactation: An implementation guide.* Washington, DC: National Academy Press.

Food and Nutrition Board. (1997). *Dietary reference intakes for calcium, phosphorus, magnesium, vitamin D, and fluoride.* Washington, DC: National Academy Press.

Food and Nutrition Board. (1998). *Dietary reference intakes: Thiamin, riboflavin, niacin, vitamin B_6 folate, vitamin B_{12} pantothenic acid, biotin, and choline.* Washington, DC: National Academy Press.

Foster, G. D., et al. (1997). What is a reasonable weight loss? Patient expectations of obesity treatment. *Journal of Consulting and Clinical Psychology, 65*(1), 79–85.

Gallagher-Allred, C. R., et al. (1996). Malnutrition and clinical outcomes: The case for medical nutrition therapy. *Journal of the American Dietetic Association, 96*(4), 361–366.

Galvan, T. J. (2001). Dysphagia: Going down and staying down. *American Journal of Nursing, 101*(1), 37–42.

Genest, J., et al. (2003). Recommendations for the management of dyslipidemia and the prevention of cardiovascular disease: Summary of the 2003 update. *Canadian Medical Association Journal, 169*(9), 921–924.

Giger, J. N., & Davidhizar, R. E. (1999). *Transcultural nursing: Assessment and intervention* (3rd ed.). St. Louis, MO: Mosby.

Grodner, M., Anderson, S., & DeYoung, S. (2000). *Foundations and clinical applications of nutrition: A nursing approach* (2nd ed.). St. Louis, MO: Mosby.

Guenter, P., Ericson, M., & Jones, S. (1997). Enteral nutrition therapy. *The Nursing Clinics of North America, 32*(4), 651–668.

Health Canada. (1990). *Actions towards healthy eating—Canada's guidelines for healthy eating and recommended strategies for implementation.* Ottawa, ON: Author. Retrieved June 4, 2004, from *http://www.hc-sc.gc.ca/hppb/nutrition/pube/eat/eat03.htm*

Health Canada. (1992). *Food guide facts: Background for educators and communicators* (Catalogue no. H39-253/10-1992E). Ottawa, ON: Author.

Health Canada. (1998). *Dietary intakes: Questions and answers.* Ottawa, ON: Food Directorate, Health Protection Branch, Health Canada.

Health Canada. (2002a). *Nutrition for a healthy pregnancy: National guidelines for the childbearing years.* Retrieved June 4, 2004, from *http://www.hc-sc.gc.ca/hpfb-dgpsa/onpp-bppn/national_guidelines_06_e.html*

Health Canada. (2003a). *Canadian guidelines for body weight classifications in adults.* Ottawa, ON: Author.

Health Canada. (2002b). *Trends in the health of Canadian youth.* Retrieved June 4, 2004, from *http://www.phac-aspc.gc.ca/dca-dea/7-18yrs-ans/index_e.html*

Health Canada. (2004). *Nutrition Labelling. Nutrition Facts—To Help You Make Informed Food Choices.* Retrieved February 27, 2005 from *http://www.hc-sc.gc.ca/hpfb-dgpsa/onpp-bppn/labelling-etiquetage/cr_tearsheet_e.html*

Health Canada. (2005). *Revision of Canada's Food Guide to Healthy Eating.* Retrieved February 25, 2005, from *http://www.hc-sc.gc.ca/hpfb-dgpsa/onpp-bppn/revision_food_guide_e.html*

Health and Welfare Canada. (1992/1997). *Canada's food guide to healthy eating* (Catalogue no. H39-252/1992). Ottawa, ON: Author.

Heart and Stroke Foundation of Canada (Prepared in collaboration with Centre for Chronic Disease Prevention and Control, Health Canada, & Canadian Cardiovascular Society). (2003). *The growing burden of heart disease and stroke in Canada 2003.* Ottawa, ON: Author. Retrieved June 6, 2004, from *http://www.cvdinfobase.ca/cvdbook/En/Index.htm*

Heart and Stroke Foundation of Canada. (2005). *Swallowing and Feeding Challenges.* Retrieved March 23, 2005, from *http://ww1.heartandstroke.ca/Page.asp?PageID=33&ArticleID=474&Src=stroke&From=SubCategory*

Hennessy, K. A., & Orr, M. E. (1996). *Nutrition support core curriculum* (3rd ed.). Silver Spring, MD: American Society of Parenteral and Enteral Nutrition.

Hornick, B. (2002). Diet and nutrition implications for oral health. *Journal of Dental Hygiene, 76*(1), 67–78.

Hunt, S., et al. (2001). ACC/AHA guidelines for the evaluation and treatment of chronic heart failure in the adult: Executive summary—ACC/AHA practice guidelines. *Circulation, 104,* 2996–3007.

Joint Working Group: Canadian Paediatric Society, Dieticians of Canada, Health Canada. (1998). *Nutrition for healthy term infants.* Ottawa, ON: Minister of Public Works and Government Services Canada.

Keithley, J., & Swanson, B. (1998). Minimizing HIV/AIDS malnutrition. *MedSurg Nursing, 7*(5), 256–267.

Kessler, D. A. (1995). The evolution of national nutrition policy. *Annual Review of Nutrition, 15,* xiii–xxvi.

Kovacevich, D. S., et al. (1997). Nutrition risk classification: A reproducible and valid tool for nurses. *Nutrition in Clinical Practice, 12*(1), 20–25.

Lindseth, G. (1997). Factors affecting graduating nurses' nutritional knowledge: Implications for continuing education. *Journal of Continuing Education in Nursing, 28,* 245–251.

Logemann, J. A., et al. (1989). The benefit of head rotation on pharyngoesophageal dysphagia. *Archives of Physical Medicine and Rehabilitation, 70,* 767–771.

Logemann, J. A. (1999). Behavior management of oropharyngeal dysphagia. *International Journal of Phoniatrics, Speech therapy and Communication Pathology, 51*(4–5), 199–212.

Lueckenotte, A. G. (2000). *Gerontologic nursing* (2nd ed.). St. Louis, MO: Mosby.

McClave, S. A., et al. (1999). Enteral tube feeding in the intensive care unit: Factors impeding adequate delivery. *Critical Care Medicine, 27*(7), 1252–1256.

Metheny, N. (1988). Measures to test placement of nasogastric and nasointestinal feeding tubes: A review. *Nursing Research, 37,* 324–329.

Metheny, N. A. (2002). Inadvertent intracranial nasogastric tube placement. *American Journal of Nursing, 102*(8), 25–27.

Metheny, N., Aud, M., & Ignatavicius, D. (1998, Summer). Detection of improperly placed feeding tubes. *Journal of Health Risk Management, 18*(3), 37.

Metheny, N. A., Aud, M. A., & Wunderlich, R. J. (1999). A survey of bedside methods used to detect pulmonary aspiration of enteral formula in intubated tube-fed patients. *American Journal of Critical Care, 8*(3), 160–167.

Metheny, N., et al. (1990a). Detection of inadvertent respiratory placement of small-bore feeding tubes: A report of 10 cases. *Heart & Lung, 19*(6), 631–638.

Metheny, N., et al. (1990b). Effectiveness of the auscultatory method in predicting feeding tube location. *Nursing Research, 39*(5), 262–267.

Metheny, N., et al. (1993a). Effectiveness of pH measurements in predicting feeding tube placement: An update. *Nursing Research, 42*(6), 324–331.

Metheny, N., et al. (1993b). How to aspirate fluid from small bore feeding tubes. *American Journal of Nursing, 93*(5), 86.

Metheny, N. M., et al. (1997). pH and concentrations of pepsin and trypsin in feeding tube aspirates as predictors of tube placement. *Journal of Parenteral and Enteral Nutrition, 21*(5), 279–285.

Metheny, N., et al. (1998a). pH, color, and feeding tubes. *RN, 61*(1), 25–27.

Metheny, N., et al. (1998b). Testing feeding tube placement: Auscultation vs. pH method. *American Journal of Nursing, 98,* 37–42.

Metheny, N. A., et al. (1999). pH and concentrations of bilirubin in feeding tube aspirates as predictors of tube placement. *Nursing Research, 48*(4), 189–197.

Metheny, N., Smith, L., & Stewart, B. J. (2000). Development of a reliable and valid bedside test for bilirubin and its utilizatin for improving prediction of feeding tube location. *Nursing Research, 49*(6), 302–309.

Metheny, N., & Titler, M. (2001). Assessing placement of feeding tubes. *American Journal of Nursing, 101*(5), 36–45.

Millen, B. E., et al. (2001). Nutritional risk in an urban homebound older population: The nutrition and healthy aging project. *The Journal of Nutrition, Health & Aging, 5*(4), 269–277.

Moorhead, S., Johnson, M., & Maas, M. (Eds.). (2004). *Nursing outcomes classification (NOC)* (3rd ed.). St. Louis, MO: Mosby.

National Cholesterol Education Program. (2002). *Third report of the expert panel on detection, evaluation, and treatment of high blood cholesterol in adults (adult treatment panel III): Final report.* Accessed February 27, 2005, from *http://www.nhlbi.nih.gov/guidelines/cholesterol/atp3_rpt.htm*

Neumark-Sztainer, D., et al. (1999). Factors influencing food choices of adolescents: Findings from focus-group discussions with adolescents. *Journal of the American Dietetic Association, 99*(8), 929–937.

Nutrition Screening Initiative. (1998). *Nutrition Management for Adults.* Washington, DC: Author.

Odderson, I. R., Keaton, J. C., McKenna B. S. (1995). Swallow management in patients on an acute stroke pathway: quality is cost effective. *Archives of Physical Medical Rehabilitation.* 76: 1130–1133.

Pagana, K. D., & Pagana, T. J. (2005). *Mosby's diagnostic and laboratory test reference* (7th ed.). St. Louis, MO: Mosby.

Panigrahi, P., et al. (1997). Role of glutamine in bacterial transcytosis and epithelial cell injury. *Journal of Parenteral and Enteral Nutrition, 21,* 75–80.

Pickering, L. K., et al. (1998). Modulation of the immune system by human milk and infant formula containing nucleotides. *Pediatrics, 101,* 242–249.

Platt, J. (2002). The pivotal role of nursing in dysphagia management. *Perspectives, Journal of the Gerontological Nursing Association (26)*1, 3–6.

Registered Nurses Association of Ontario. (2002). *Assessment and management of stage I to IV pressure ulcers: Appendix F.* Retrieved February 26, 2005, from *http://www.rnao.org/bestpractices/completed_guidelines/BPG_Guide_C2_pressure_ulcer.asp*

Rimm, E. B., et al. (1998). Folate and vitamin B_6 from diet and supplements in relation to risk of coronary heart disease among women. *Journal of the American Medical Assocation, 279*(5), 359–364.

Rombeau, J. L., & Rolandelli, R. H. (Eds.). (1997). *Enteral feeding and tube feeding.* Philadelphia: W. B. Saunders.

Simon, T., & Fink, A. S. (1999). Current management of endoscopic feeding tube dysfunction. *Surgical Endoscopy, 13,* 403–405.

Small, S. P., Best, D. G., & Hustins K. A. (1994). Energy and nutrient intakes of independently-living elderly women. *The Canadian Journal of Nursing Research, 26*(1) 71–81.

Todorovic, V. (2001). Detecting and managing nutrition of older people in the community. *British Journal of Community Nursing, 6*(2), 54–60.

Tremblay, M. S., & Willms, J. D. (2000). Secular trends in the body mass index of Canadian children. *Canadian Medical Association Journal, 163*(11), 1429–1433.

Tremblay, M. S., & Willms, J. D. (2001). Obesity in Canadian Children. *Canadian Medical Association Journal, 164*(7), 1564–1565.

U.S. Department of Agriculture and U.S. Department of Health and Human Services. (2000). *Nutrition and your health: Dietary guidelines for Americans* (5th ed., USDA/DHHS Home and Garden Bulletin No. 232). Washington, DC: U.S. Government Printing Office. Retrieved July 15, 2004, from *http://www.usda.gov/cnpp/DietGd.pdf*

U.S. Department of Health and Human Services, Centers for Disease Control and Prevention. (2001). *The importance of physical activity and good nutrition.* Atlanta, GA: Author.

U.S. Food and Drug Administration. (2003). *FDA public health advisory: Reports of blue discoloration and death in patients receiving enteral feedings tinted with the dye FD&C Blue No. 1* (pp. 1–3). Washington, DC: Author.

Wardlaw, G. M., & Insesll, P. M. (1996). *Perspectives in nutrition* (3rd ed.). New York: McGraw-Hill.

Weigley, E. S. (1995). Nutrition-related activities of entry level nurses. *Nurse Educator, 20,* 3–4.

WHO/UNICEF. (1990, August 1). *Innocenti Declaration: On the protection, promotion and support of breastfeeding.* Presented at Policymakers' Meeting on Breastfeeding, Breastfeeding in the 1990s: A Global Initiative, Florence, Italy.

Williams, S. R. (2001). *Basic Nutrition and diet therapy* (11th ed.). St. Louis, MO: Mosby.

Williams, S. R., & Schlenker, E. D. (2003). *Essentials of Nutrition and Diet Therapy* (8th ed.). St. Louis, MO: Mosby.

Wong, D. L. (1997). *Whaley & Wong's essentials of pediatric nursing* (5th ed.). St. Louis, MO: Mosby.

Working Group on Hypercholesterolemia and Other Dyslipidemias. (2003). Recommendations for the management of dyslipidemia and the prevention of cardiovascular disease: 2003 update. *Canadian Medical Association Journal, 169*(9), 921–924.

Ybarra, J., Ade, R., & Romeo, J. H. (1996). Osteoporosis in men: A review. *The Nursing Clinics of North America, 31*(4), 805–813.

Young, W. B., Minnick, A. F., & Marcantonio, R. (1996). How wide is the gap in defining quality care? Comparison of patient and nurse perceptions of important aspects of patient care. *Journal of Nursing Administrators, 26*(2), 15–20.

Zaloga, G. (1994). Frontiers in critical care nutrition. *New Horizons, 2*(2), 121–130.

Recommended Web Sites

Health Canada Food and Nutrition:
http://www.hc-sc.gc.ca/english/lifestyles/food_nutr.html

Health Canada's Web site provides information for the public on food, nutrition, food safety issues, allergy alerts, food policy and legislation, and other nutrition issues.

Office of Nutrition Policy and Promotion (ONPP):
http://www.hc-sc.gc.ca/hpfb-dgpsa/onpp-bppn/index_e.html

The ONPP promotes the nutritional health and well-being of Canadians. This Web site (part of Health Canada's Web site) contains current information on nutrition and Canadian nutrition policy.

Ontario Public Health Association (OPHA):
http://www.opha.on.ca/resources/multilingual/foodguide.html

Ontario Public Health Association has a nutrition resource centre that presents seven different cultural adaptations of Canada's Food Guide to Health Eating. The adaptations are available for use with the Chinese, Portuguese, Vietnamese, Tamil, Urdu, Punjabi, and Spanish speaking communities.

Dieticians of Canada:
http:///www.dieticians.ca/

Dieticians of Canada is an association of food and nutrition professionals committed to the health and well-being of Canadians. This Web site contains numerous nutritional resources and links to other resources and research abstracts.

National Heart, Lung, and Blood Institute: The DASH Eating Plan:
http://www.nhlbi.nih.gov/health/public/heart/hbp/dash/

The Dietary Approaches to Stop Hypertension (DASH) is an eating plan low in total fat, saturated fat, and cholesterol, and rich in fruits, vegetables, and low fat dairy products. The DASH eating plan is developed for clients with hypertension and is based on clinical studies that showed how elevated blood pressure levels can be reduced with particular eating habits.

40

Urinary Elimination

Judith Ann Kilpatrick, RN, DNSc
Jill Milne, RN, MN, PhD (Canadian author)
Katherine N. Moore, RN, PhD (Canadian author)

Objectives

Mastery of content in this chapter will enable the student to:

- Define the key terms listed.
- Describe the process of urination.
- Identify factors that commonly influence urinary elimination.
- Compare common alterations in urinary elimination.
- Identify two modalities of renal replacement therapy.
- Obtain a nursing health history for a client with urinary elimination problems.
- Identify nursing diagnoses appropriate for clients with alterations in urinary elimination.
- Obtain urine specimens.
- Describe characteristics of normal and abnormal urine.
- Describe the nursing implications of common diagnostic tests of the urinary system.
- Discuss nursing measures to promote normal micturition and reduce episodes of incontinence.
- Insert a urinary catheter.
- Discuss nursing measures to reduce urinary tract infection.
- Irrigate a urinary catheter.

Normal elimination of urinary wastes is a basic function most people take for granted. When the urinary system fails to function properly, virtually all organ systems will be eventually affected. Clients with alterations in urinary elimination may also suffer emotionally from body image changes. The nurse must be understanding and sensitive to all clients' needs. Understanding the reasons for urinary elimination problems and finding acceptable solutions are essential nursing functions.

Scientific Knowledge Base

Urinary elimination depends on the function of the kidneys, ureters, bladder, and urethra. Kidneys remove wastes from the blood to form urine. Ureters transport urine from the kidneys to the bladder. The bladder holds urine until the urge to urinate develops. Urine leaves the body through the urethra. All organs of the urinary system must be intact and functional for successful removal of urinary wastes (Figure 40–1).

Upper Urinary Tract

Kidneys. The kidneys lie on either side of the vertebral column behind the peritoneum and against deep muscles of the back. The kidneys extend from the 12th thoracic to the 3rd lumbar vertebrae. Normally, the left kidney is higher than the right because of the anatomical position of the liver.

Waste products of metabolism that collect in the blood are filtered in the kidneys. Blood reaches each kidney by a renal (kidney) artery that branches

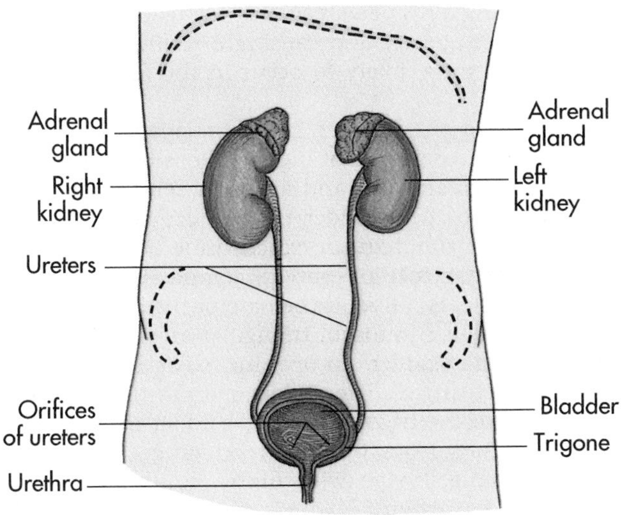

FIGURE 40–1 Organs of the urinary system.

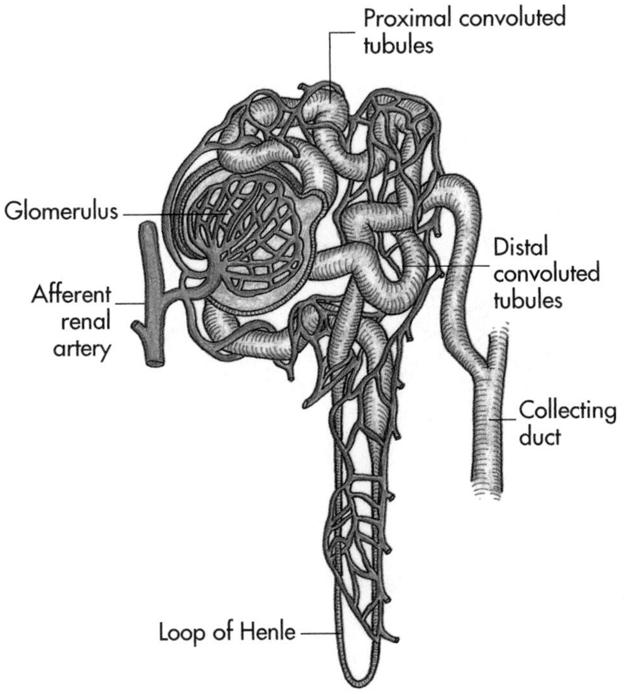

FIGURE 40–2 Renal nephron.

from the abdominal aorta. Approximately 20% to 25% of the cardiac output circulates each minute through the kidneys. The nephron, the functional unit of the kidney, forms the urine. The **nephron** is composed of the glomerulus, Bowman's capsule, proximal convoluted tubule, loop of Henle, distal tubule, and collecting duct (Figure 40–2).

A cluster of blood vessels forms the capillary network of the glomerulus, which is the initial site of filtration of the blood and the beginning of urine formation. The glomerular capillaries permit filtration of water, glucose, amino acids, urea, creatinine, and major electrolytes into Bowman's capsule. Large proteins and blood cells do not normally filter through the glomerulus. The presence of large proteins in the urine **(proteinuria)** is a sign of glomerular injury. The glomerulus filters approximately 125 mL of filtrate per minute.

Not all of the glomerular filtrate is excreted as urine. About 99% of the filtrate is reabsorbed into the plasma, with the remaining 1% excreted as urine (McCance & Huether, 2002). The kidneys play a key role in fluid and electrolyte balance (see chapter 36). Although output does depend on intake, the normal adult urine output is 1500 to 1600 mL/day. An output of less than 30 mL/hour may indicate renal alterations. The kidneys also produce several substances vital to production of red blood cells (RBCs), blood pressure regulation, and bone mineralization.

The kidneys are responsible for maintaining a normal RBC volume by producing erythropoietin. **Erythropoietin** functions within the bone marrow to stimulate RBC production and maturation and prolongs the life of mature RBCs (McCance & Huether, 2002). Clients with chronic alterations in kidney function cannot produce sufficient quantities of this hormone and are therefore prone to anemia.

Renin is another hormone produced by the kidneys. Its major role is the regulation of blood flow in times of renal ischemia (decreased blood supply). Renin is released from juxtaglomerular cells (Figure 40–3). The kidneys also produce prostaglandin E2 and prostacyclin, which are important in maintaining renal blood flow through vasodilation.

Renin functions as an enzyme to convert angiotensinogen (a substance synthesized by the liver) into angiotensin I. Angiotensin I is converted to angiotensin II in the lungs. Angiotensin II causes vasoconstriction and stimulates aldosterone release from the adrenal cortex. Aldosterone causes retention of water, which increases blood volume. Both of these mechanisms increase arterial blood pressure and renal blood flow (McCance & Huether, 2002).

The kidneys also play a role in calcium and phosphate regulation by producing a substance that converts vitamin D into its active form. Clients with chronic alterations in kidney function do not make sufficient amounts of the active vitamin D. They are prone to develop renal bone disease resulting from the demineralization of bone caused by impaired calcium absorption.

Ureters. Urine enters the **renal pelvis** from the collecting ducts and travels to the bladder through ureters. The ureters are tubular structures that enter the urinary bladder in the pelvic cavity at the ureterovesical junction (the juncture of the ureters with the bladder). Urine draining from the ureters to the bladder is usually sterile.

Three layers of tissue form the wall of the ureter. The inner layer is a mucous membrane continuous with the lining of the renal pelvis and urinary bladder. The middle layer consists of smooth muscle fibres that transport urine by peristaltic waves. An outer layer of fibrous connective tissue supports the ureters.

Peristaltic waves cause the urine to enter the bladder in spurts rather than steadily. The ureters enter obliquely through the posterior bladder wall. This arrangement

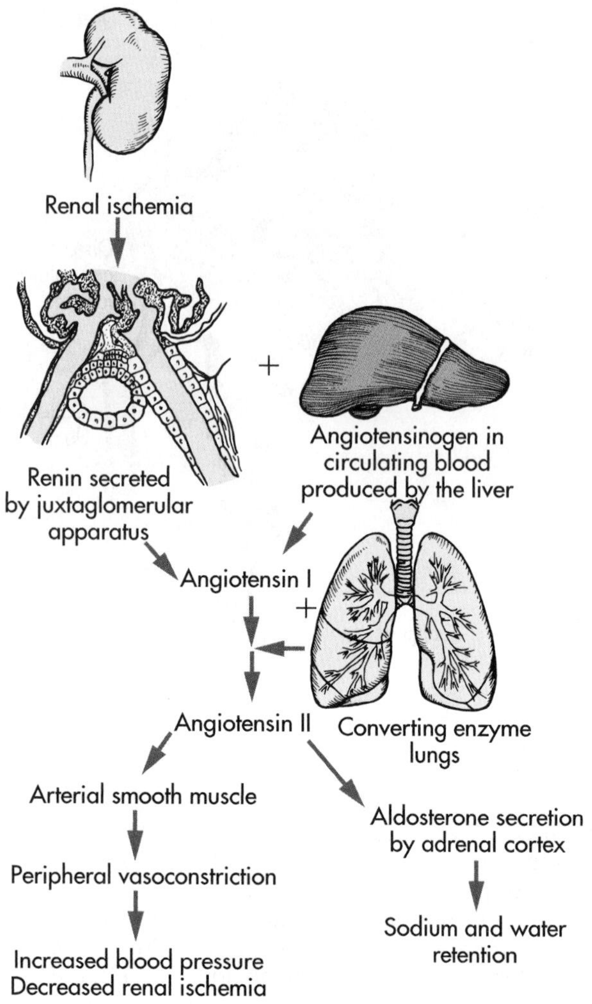

FIGURE **40–3** Physiological effects of renin-angiotensin mechanism.

normally prevents the reflux of urine from the bladder into the ureters during the act of **micturition** (urination) by the compression of the ureter at the ureterovesical junction. An obstruction within a ureter, such as a kidney stone **(renal calculus),** results in strong peristaltic waves that attempt to move the obstruction into the bladder. These strong peristaltic waves result in pain often referred to as renal colic.

Lower Urinary Tract

Bladder. The urinary bladder is a hollow, distensible muscular organ that stores and excretes urine. When empty, the bladder lies behind the symphysis pubis in the pelvic cavity. It rests against the anterior wall of the rectum in men and against the anterior walls of the cervix and vagina in women (Figure 40–4).

The bladder expands as it becomes filled with urine. Pressure within the bladder is usually low, even when partly full, a factor that protects the urinary tract against infection. When the bladder is full, it expands and extends above the symphysis pubis. A greatly distended bladder may reach the umbilicus. In a pregnant woman, the developing fetus pushes against the bladder, reducing the bladder's capacity and causing a feeling of fullness. This effect is more likely to occur in the first and third trimester.

The wall of the bladder has four layers: a mucosal layer, a submucosal layer of highly extensible connective tissue, a muscular layer, and an outer serous layer. The main muscle of the bladder is the **detrusor muscle.** Contraction of the detrusor expels urine from the body. The **bladder neck** or outlet, composed of distinct smooth muscle, is found at the base of the bladder.

The trigone is a smooth, triangular area at the posterior base of the bladder. An opening exists at each of the trigone's three angles. The ureters enter at the two superior corners of the trigone and the bladder neck and the urethra extends from the lower opening. The trigone does not change shape with filling, resulting in pear-shaped bladders when full.

Urethra. Urine travels from the bladder through the urethra (a fibromuscular tube) and passes outside of the body through the **urethral meatus.** Normally, the turbulent flow of urine through the urethra washes it free of bacteria. Mucous membrane lines the urethra, and urethral glands secrete mucus into the urethral canal. Thick layers of smooth muscle surround the urethra. In addition, the urethra descends through a layer of skeletal muscles called the pelvic floor muscles (PFMs). When these muscles are contracted, it is possible to prevent urine flow through the urethra (McCance & Huether, 2002).

In women, the urethra is approximately 4 cm long. The short length of the urethra predisposes women and girls to infection. Bacteria can easily enter the urethra from the perineal area. In men, the urethra, which is both a urinary canal and a passageway for cells and secretions from reproductive organs, is about 20 cm long. The male urethra has three sections: the prostatic urethra, the membranous urethra, and the penile urethra. The prostatic urethra pierces the anterior portion of the **prostate gland** (see Figure 40–4, *A*) and transports urine as well as sperm, seminal fluid, and prostatic secretions.

Urethral Closure. The ability of the urethra to maintain adequate closure pressure between voids is critical to continence. This is accomplished through a combination of factors. Smooth muscle fibres, under involuntary control, extend the length of the urethra from the bladder neck to provide ongoing tonic support and enhance urethral resistance during bladder filling and storage. A circular collar of smooth muscle commonly known as the internal sphincter surrounds the proximal urethra in men; however, its role in maintaining continence is not well understood. No such anatomical smooth muscle sphincter exists in the female urethra (DeLancey et al., 2002). Striated urethral muscle plays a predominant role in urethral closure. The urethral sphincter or **rhabdosphincter,** which has been commonly known as the external sphincter, encircles two thirds of the distal urethra in women and extends from the apex of the prostate to the membranous urethra in men (Creed & Van der Werf, 2001). The urethral sphincter is primarily under voluntary control, which enables contraction in response to sudden

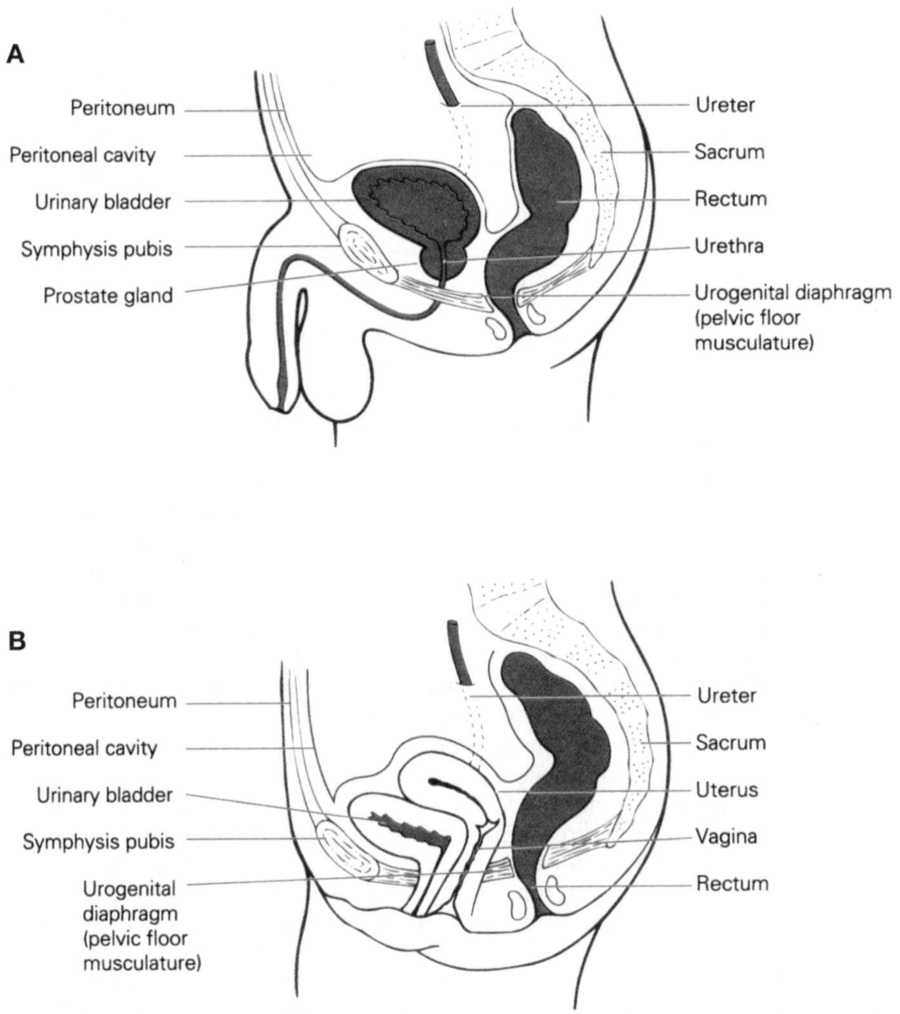

FIGURE **40–4** Anatomical location of bladder and pelvic organs: **A,** In men. **B,** In women. (From "Normal and Abnormal Bladder Function," by K. Getliffe and M. Dolman, in *Promoting Continence,* pp. 22–67, edited by K. Getliffe and M. Dolman, 1997, London: Bailliere Tindall.)

increases in intra-abdominal or detrusor pressure. The striated muscle of the pelvic floor surrounds the urethra and provides additional closure pressure when contracted.

Urethral closure also depends on the relative health and vascularity of mucosal tissue. As the bladder fills, epithelial folds that are pliable and soft are able to fill existing gaps in the urethral lumen. Adequate mucosal secretions reduce surface tension to enable closure, supported by a rich vascular network that nourishes and cushions the epithelial tissue against muscular forces. Because estrogen plays a critical role in the tone and vascularity of urethral tissue, the closure mechanism can be compromised by menopause.

Act of Urination

The act of urination relies on the coordinated effort of the bladder and the urethral closure mechanism. Bladder musculature relaxes to fill and store urine and contracts to expel urine when appropriate. In contrast, the urethra and pelvic floor musculature contract to prevent leakage during filling and storage and relax to allow voiding.

The bladder normally holds as much as 600 mL of urine. However, the desire to urinate can be sensed when the bladder contains a smaller amount of urine (150 to 200 mL in an adult and 50 to 100 mL in a child). As the volume increases, the bladder wall stretches, sending sensory impulses to the micturition centre in the sacral spinal cord. The impulses travel from the micturition centre to the pontine centre. If a person is ready to void, the pontine centre relays the impulses back to the sacral micturition centre to initiate detrusor contraction, sphincter relaxation, and bladder emptying. If a person chooses not to void, the impulses are relayed to the cerebral cortex for voluntary inhibition of a detrusor contraction. If the urge to void has been ignored repeatedly, the bladder capacity may be reached and the resulting pressure on the sphincter may make continued voluntary control impossible.

The extensive and complex role that the central nervous system plays in maintaining function of the lower urinary tract suggests that any disruption to the pathway can impact the ability to maintain continence. For example, damage to the spinal cord above the sacral region causes loss of voluntary control of urination, but the micturition reflex pathway may remain intact, allowing urination to occur reflexively. This condition is called a **reflex bladder.** If bladder emptying is hindered by chronic obstruction such as prostate enlargement, over time, the micturition reflex becomes non-functional and severe urinary retention occurs.

Factors Influencing Urination

Many factors influence the volume and quality of urine and the client's ability to urinate. Some pathophysiological conditions may be acute and reversible (urinary tract infection), whereas others may be chronic and irreversible (slow, progressive development of renal dysfunction). Problems related to the act of urination may be the result of cognitive, functional, or physical means resulting in incontinence, retention, or infection.

Disease Conditions. Disease processes that affect urine elimination may affect renal function (changes in urine volume or quality), the act of urine elimination, or both. Those conditions that affect urine volume and quality are generally categorized as prerenal, renal, or postrenal in origin.

Prerenal alterations decrease circulating blood flow to and through the kidneys with resulting decreased blood flow to renal tissue. In other words, the alterations occur before the urinary system. The decrease in renal blood flow leads to **oliguria** (diminished capacity to form urine) or, less commonly, **anuria** (inability to produce urine). Oliguria may occur when fluid loss through other means is increased (perspiration, diarrhea, or vomiting), or with kidney disease. Selected causes include dehydration, hemorrhage, and congestive heart failure.

Renal alterations result from factors that cause injury directly to the glomeruli or renal tubule, interfering with their normal filtering, reabsorptive, and secretory functions. Selected causes include transfusion reactions, diseases of the glomeruli, and systemic diseases such as diabetes mellitus.

Postrenal alterations result from obstruction to the flow of urine in the urinary collecting system anywhere between the renal pelvis and urethral meatus. Urine is formed by the urinary system but cannot be eliminated by normal means. Urinary obstruction can be caused by calculi (stones), blood clots, or tumours. Calculi are more common in men and should be suspected in clients with asymptomatic hematuria and repeated urinary tract infections (UTIs) that do not respond to antibiotic treatment. Obstructive symptoms in the lower urinary tract, such as hesitancy, intermittent stream, and straining to void, are frequently associated with enlargement of the prostate gland caused by benign prostatic hyperplasia or prostate cancer.

Several diseases or conditions that cause neurological, cognitive, or physical impairment can affect the ability to micturate. Conditions that impact the central or peripheral nervous systems can affect the bladder's ability to store and eliminate urine. Any lesion of peripheral nerves leading to the bladder causes loss of bladder tone, reduced sensation of bladder fullness, and difficulty in controlling urination. For example, Parkinson's disease, stroke, diabetes mellitus, and multiple sclerosis cause neuropathic conditions that alter bladder function. Older men may suffer from benign prostatic hypertrophy, which makes them prone to urinary retention and incontinence.

Clients with cognitive impairments, such as Alzheimer's disease, may lose the ability to sense a full bladder or be unable to recall the procedure for voiding. Diseases or conditions that slow or hinder physical activity also interfere with the ability to void. Rheumatoid arthritis and degenerative joint disease are examples of conditions that make it difficult to reach and use toilet facilities. A client with rheumatoid arthritis often cannot sit on or rise from a toilet without an elevated seat.

Diseases and conditions that cause irreversible damage to the glomeruli or tubules cause permanent alterations in renal function. The resulting decline in kidney function is called end-stage renal disease (ESRD), and the client manifests numerous metabolic disturbances that require treatment for survival. The associated symptoms occur as a result of the **uremic syndrome,** characterized by an increase in nitrogenous wastes in the blood, altered regulatory functions (causing marked fluid and electrolyte abnormalities), nausea, vomiting, headache, coma, and convulsions. The problem may be managed conservatively with medications and a regimen of dietary and fluid restrictions. However, as the uremic symptoms worsen, more aggressive treatment is indicated. These treatments are known as **renal replacement therapies.**

Box 40-1 Indications for Dialysis

Renal failure that can no longer be controlled by conservative management (i.e., dietary modifications and administration of medications to correct electrolyte abnormalities)
Worsening of uremic syndrome associated with ESRD (i.e., nausea, vomiting, neurological changes, pericarditis)
Severe electrolyte and/or fluid abnormalities that cannot be controlled by simpler measures (i.e., hyperkalemia, pulmonary edema)

Renal Replacement Therapies. Dialysis (Box 40-1) and organ transplantation are two methods of renal replacement. Dialysis may take one of two forms, peritoneal or hemodialysis. Both dialysis modalities can be applied for a short or long time but require specialized equipment and nurses with specific training.

Peritoneal dialysis is an indirect method of cleansing the blood of waste products using osmosis and diffusion. The peritoneum functions as a semi-permeable membrane. Excess fluid and waste products are readily removed from the bloodstream when a sterile electrolyte solution (dialysate) is instilled into the peritoneal cavity by gravity via a surgically placed catheter. The dialysate is left in the cavity for a prescribed time interval and then is drained out by gravity, taking accumulated wastes and excess fluid and electrolytes with it.

Hemodialysis involves using a machine equipped with a semi-permeable filtering membrane (artificial kidney) that removes accumulated waste products and excess fluids from the blood. In the dialysis machine, dialysate fluid is pumped through one side of the filter membrane (artificial kidney) while the client's blood passes through the other side. The processes of diffusion, osmosis, and ultra-filtration cleanse the client's blood, which is returned through a specially placed vascular access device (Gore-Tex graft, arteriovenous fistula, or hemodialysis catheter).

Organ transplantation is the replacement of a client's diseased kidneys with a healthy one from a living or cadaver donor of compatible blood and tissue type. The new organ is surgically implanted into the abdomen. Special medications (immunosuppressives) are administered for life to prevent the body from rejecting the transplanted organ. Unlike dialysis, successful organ transplantation offers the client the potential for restoration of normal kidney function.

Fluid Balance. Fluid balance directly affects the quantity of urine produced. The kidneys maintain a sensitive balance between retention and excretion of fluids (see chapter 36). If fluids and the concentration of electrolytes and solutes are in equilibrium, an increase in fluid intake causes an increase in urine production. Ingested fluids increase the body's circulating plasma and thus increase the volume of urine excreted. In a healthy person, the intake of water in food and fluids balances the output of water in urine, feces, and insensible losses in perspiration and respiration. An excessive output of urine is known as **polyuria,** a common symptom of diabetes mellitus.

Ingestion of certain fluids directly affects urine production and excretion. Coffee, tea, cocoa, and cola drinks that contain caffeine promote increased urine formation **(diuresis).** Alcohol inhibits the release of antidiuretic hormone (ADH), resulting in increased water loss in urine. Evidence suggests that caffeine is irritating to bladder mucosa and can precipitate urinary urgency or incontinence (Tomlinson et al., 1999).

Nocturia, excessive urination at night, can be a sign of high intake of fluids in the evening. Clients with peripheral edema (e.g., caused by circulatory problems associated with venous insufficiency) may also experience nocturia because lying down for sleep facilitates reabsorption of pooled fluid and leads to increased urinary output overnight. In such cases, elevating the feet during evening hours reduces edema and enables return of pooled fluid prior to bedtime.

Febrile conditions also affect urine production. The client who becomes diaphoretic (sweats profusely) loses a large amount of fluid through insensible water loss, which decreases urine production. However, the increased body metabolism associated with fever increases accumulation of body wastes. Although urine volume may be reduced, it is highly concentrated.

Medications. Medications may interfere with the production of urine and affect the act of urination. Diuretics prevent reabsorption of water and certain electrolytes to increase urine output. Urinary retention may be caused by use of anticholinergics (e.g., tranquilizers or antidepressants), antihistamines (e.g., Sudafed), or antihypertensives (e.g., Aldomet). The nurse must be aware of the prescribed and over-the counter medications a client is taking and how they may impact bladder function. Clients with alterations in kidney function require dosage alterations in medications excreted by the kidneys.

Pelvic Floor Muscle Tone. The pelvic floor muscle (PFM) is under voluntary as well as involuntary control. The PFM spans the opening in the bony pelvis and combines with connective tissue to provide structural support for the pelvic organs. A well-toned PFM maintains the bladder neck in position to ensure that an increase in intra-abdominal pressure, as occurs with coughing, is transmitted not only to the bladder but also to the bladder neck to maintain closure. Contraction of the PFM results in urethral compression as the urethra is pulled forward toward the symphysis pubis (Delancey et al., 2002). A weak PFM contributes to urethral hypermobility, a major cause of stress urinary incontinence, because it impairs the ability to voluntarily inhibit micturition. Poor control of micturition can result from muscle wasting caused by prolonged immobility, frequent straining in association with urinary or fecal elimination, stretching of muscles during childbirth, menopausal muscle atrophy, or traumatic damage to muscles.

Diagnostic Examination. Examination of the urinary system can influence micturition. Procedures such as an intravenous pyelogram may require that the client limit fluids before the test. A restriction in fluid intake commonly lowers urine output. A laxative used to cleanse the bowel may also limit fluid available for urine production. Diagnostic examinations (i.e., cystoscopy) that involve direct visualization of urinary structures may cause localized edema of the urethral passageway and spasm of the striated muscle. The client often has urinary retention after such a procedure and may pass red or pink urine because of trauma to the urethral or bladder mucosa.

Surgical Procedures. The stress of surgery initially triggers the general adaptation syndrome (see chapter 26). The surgical client is often in an altered state of fluid balance before surgery due to the disease process or preoperative fasting, which aggravates the reduction in urine output. The stress response releases an increased amount of ADH, which increases water reabsorption. Stress also elevates the level of aldosterone, causing retention of sodium and water. Both of these substances reduce urine output in an effort to maintain circulatory volume. The decreased blood pressure following surgery releases renin and thus increases angiotensin II to increase vascular tone. This effect aids in counteracting the effects of ADH and aldosterone.

Anaesthetics and narcotic analgesics may alter the glomerular filtration rate (generally 125 mL/minute), reducing urine output. These pharmacological agents also impair sensory and motor impulses travelling between the bladder, spinal cord, and brain. Clients recovering from anaesthesia and deep analgesia are often unable to sense bladder fullness and are unable to initiate or inhibit micturition. Spinal and epidural anaesthetics, in particular, may cause urinary retention because the person cannot feel the need to void and the bladder muscle and sphincter may not respond (Lewis, Heitkemper, & Dirksen, 2000).

Surgery of lower abdominal and pelvic structures can impair urination because of local trauma to surrounding tissues. The edema and inflammation may obstruct the flow of urine from the kidneys to the bladder or from the bladder or urethra, interfere with relaxation of pelvic and sphincter muscles, or cause discomfort during voiding. After returning from surgery involving the ureters, bladder, and urethra, clients routinely have catheters.

The surgical formation of a **urinary diversion** temporarily or permanently bypasses the bladder and urethra as the exit routes for urine. Permanent urinary diversions may be needed in the client with cancer of the bladder. The client with a urinary diversion has a **stoma** (artificial opening) on the abdomen to drain urine.

Psychological Factors. Anxiety and emotional stress may cause a sense of urgency and increased frequency of urination. Anxiety may prevent a person from being able to urinate completely; as a result, the urge to void may return shortly after voiding. Emotional tension makes it difficult to relax the abdominal and perineal muscles. If the sphincter is not completely relaxed, voiding may also be incomplete.

Attempting to void in a public restroom may also result in a temporary inability to void. Privacy and adequate time to urinate are important to most people, and some may need distractions to relax (e.g., reading). The possibility that incomplete voiding may result from physiological abnormalities, however, must always be considered.

Common Alterations in Urinary Elimination

Most clients with urinary problems have disturbances in the act of micturition that involve a failure to store urine, a failure to empty urine, or both. These disturbances result from infection, impaired bladder function, obstruction to urine outflow, or inability to voluntarily control micturition. Some clients may have permanent or temporary changes in the normal pathway of urinary excretion. The client with a urinary diversion has special challenges because urine drains to the outside through a stoma.

Urinary Tract Infections. Urinary tract infections (UTIs) are responsible for more than 500 000 visits to Canadian doctors every year (Kidney Foundation of Canada, 2004). If left untreated, UTIs can spread to the kidneys, causing kidney infection **(pyelonephritis)** and possibly long-term kidney damage.

Etiology. Although several different micro-organisms may cause UTIs, *Escherichia coli* is the most frequent causative pathogen, accounting for 80% of uncomplicated infections. Between 10% and 20% of UTIs are caused by *Staphylococcus saprophyticus* and approximately 5% by *Klebsiella, Proteus,* and *Enterobacter.*

Bacteria in the urine **(bacteriuria)** may lead to the spread of organisms into the kidneys and bloodstream, leading to **urosepsis** (O'Donnell & Hofmann, 2002). Bacteria usually enter the urinary tract by ascending the urethra. Bacteria inhabit the distal urethra, external genitalia, and vagina in women. Organisms enter the urethral meatus easily and travel up the inner mucosal lining to the bladder. Women are more susceptible to infection because of the short urethra and the proximity of the anus to the urethral meatus.

Infection depends on the virulence of the bacteria and the presence of host defence mechanisms. In a healthy person with good bladder function, organisms are flushed out during voiding. As well, normal urine has a low pH, which inhibits bacterial growth. Although the short length of the female urethra makes women more susceptible to UTIs, organisms such as *Lactobacillus* that occur naturally in the periurethral area inhibit colonization of pathogenic bacteria. In addition, mucous-secreting glands found in the distal two thirds of the female urethra impede bacterial ascension (Shupp-Byrne et al., 2001). In males, the length of the urethra and an antibacterial substance in prostatic secretions reduce susceptibility.

Alterations in any of these defence mechanisms can contribute to a UTI. For example, if the client cannot empty the bladder when voiding or if there is any interference with the free flow of urine, **residual urine** (urine left in the bladder after voiding) becomes more alkaline and is an ideal site for micro-organism growth. Therefore, a kinked, obstructed, or clamped catheter or any condition resulting in urinary retention increases the risk of bladder infection. Risk factors for urinary infection in women include sexual activity, pregnancy, diaphragm or spermicide use, and uterine prolapse. UTIs are less common in men and risk factors include the introduction of instruments into the urinary tract (instrumentation) and congenital abnormalities (Goldman, 2001). Older adults, clients using antibiotics, and clients with progressive underlying disease or decreased immunity are also at increased risk. Clients with diabetes mellitus are especially susceptible to UTIs because the increased sugar in the urine is a good medium for bacterial growth.

One of the most common causes of urinary tract infection, however, is instrumentation. For example, the introduction of a catheter through the urethra provides a direct route for micro-organisms. With an in-dwelling catheter, bacteria ascend along the outside of the catheter on the urethral wall or travel up the catheter's lumen, and bacteriuria is generally inevitable within 2 days. One hundred per cent colonization can be expected after 30 days. Local irritation to the urethra or bladder also predisposes tissues to bacterial invasion.

Signs and Symptoms. Clients with lower UTIs may have pain or burning during urination **(dysuria)** as urine flows over inflamed tissues. Fever, chills, nausea, vomiting, and malaise may develop as the infection worsens. Inflammation of the bladder **(cystitis)** causes a frequent and urgent sensation of the need to void, and may cause **incontinence.** Irritation to bladder and urethral mucosa results in blood-tinged urine **(hematuria).** The urine appears concentrated and cloudy because of the presence of white blood cells (WBCs) or bacteria. If infection spreads to the upper urinary tract (i.e., to the kidneys, causing pyelonephritis), rapid onset of flank or lower back pain, tenderness, fever, and chills can occur.

Lower UTIs can also be asymptomatic, particularly in pregnant women, children, and older adults. In one study, 43% of long-term care residents were found to have asymptomatic infections (Raz et al., 2001).

Urinary Incontinence. **Urinary incontinence** is the involuntary loss of urine that is sufficient to be a problem (Abrams et al., 2002). It is a prevalent condition experienced by one and a half million Canadians of all ages (Angus Reid Group, 1997). Research estimates suggest that 10% to 40% of community-dwelling women (Hannestad et al., 2000; Moller, Lose, & Jorgensen, 2000) and 3% to 10% of community-dwelling men (Bartolotti et al., 2000; Schluman, Claesm, & Mattijs, 1997) are affected. Psychosocial impact ranges from minor lifestyle changes to self-imposed social isolation.

Urinary incontinence may present as any of the following types (Registered Nurses Association of Ontario, 2005):

- *Transient incontinence*—urine loss resulting from causes outside of or affecting the urinary system that resolves when the underlying causes are treated. Causes include **d**ementia or acute confusion, **i**nfection (symptomatic UTI), **a**trophic urethritis or vaginitis in women, **ph**armaceuticals (medications), **e**ndocrine disorders, **re**stricted mobility, and **s**tool impaction (DIAPERS).
- *Urge incontinence*—the loss of urine associated with or immediately preceded by a sudden urgent need to void. The need to void is so sudden that the person cannot get to a toilet in time. Urge incontinence often also presents with **urinary frequency** (need to void more than every 2 hours) and nocturia. Causes include nervous system disorders and outflow obstruction (particularly in men with an enlarged prostate), but urge incontinence may also be idiopathic (of unknown origin).
- *Stress incontinence*—urine loss resulting from increased intra-abdominal pressure (e.g., coughing, sneezing, laughing, lifting). It usually involves a small volume of urine loss (less than 50 mL); it usually occurs in women or in men following radical prostatectomy. Pregnancy and delivery, weak pelvic floor muscles, heavy lifting, and obesity are sometimes contributing factors.
- *Mixed incontinence*—urine loss having features of both stress and urge.
- *Functional incontinence*—the loss of urine that occurs from altered cognitive and/or physical function or environmental factors. The person has bladder control but is unable to reach the toilet. The causes may include confusion, difficulty removing clothing, or immobility. Older clients with restricted mobility are at high risk of this type of incontinence. For example, low-set chairs and beds raised well above the floor may prevent a client from reaching a toilet.
- *Overflow incontinence*—the loss of small and large amounts of urine associated with overdistension of the bladder. The person may feel as if the bladder is never completely empty. Overflow incontinence may be associated with bladder outlet obstruction, fecal impaction, diabetes, spinal cord injury, prostate enlargement, or severe uterine prolapse.
- *Reflex incontinence*—involuntary loss of urine occurring at somewhat predictable intervals. The person is unaware that the bladder is filling and does not feel the urge to void, but the bladder contracts spontaneously. Reflex incontinence may be caused by spinal cord dysfunction (either inhibition of cerebral awareness or impairment of the reflex arc).
- *Total incontinence*—continuous and unpredictable loss of urine. It is caused by damage to the nerves controlling the bladder and may be a result of spinal deformities such as spina bifida or scoliosis, spinal cord injury, or advanced disease such as multiple sclerosis or Alzheimer's disease. Repeated pelvic surgery may also cause total incontinence if it causes scarring of the urethra.

Safety Alert Continued episodes of incontinence create the potential for skin breakdown. The immobilized client who has frequent incontinence is especially at risk for pressure ulcers (see chapter 43). Timely and meticulous skin care is essential.

Overactive Bladder Syndrome. ***Overactive bladder syndrome*** is the term applied to involuntary bladder contractions that are generally associated with symptoms of urgency, frequency, and nocturia (DeLancey et al., 2002). Individuals with overactive bladder may also experience urge incontinence; however, approximately 60% do not (Canadian Continence Foundation, 2001). Similar to urge incontinence, overactive bladder syndrome can be idiopathic but is commonly attributed to changes associated with nervous system disorders and outflow obstruction and may be aggravated by caffeinated beverages.

Urinary Retention. **Urinary retention** is the marked accumulation of urine in the bladder as a result of the inability of the bladder to empty. Normally, urine production slowly fills the bladder and prevents activation of stretch receptors until the bladder distends to a certain level of stretch. The micturition reflex occurs, and the bladder empties. With urinary retention, the bladder becomes unable to respond to the micturition reflex and thus unable to empty. Urine continues to collect in the bladder, stretching its walls and causing feelings of pressure, discomfort, tenderness over the symphysis pubis, restlessness, and diaphoresis. As retention progresses, overflow incontinence may occur. Pressure in the bladder builds to a point at which the urethral sphincter is unable to hold back urine and a small volume escapes (25 to 60 mL). The client may void small amounts of urine two or three times an hour with little relief of discomfort.

Retention results from an underactive or acontractile detrusor muscle, urethral obstruction (more common in men and usually related to prostatic enlargement or urethral stricture), surgical or childbirth trauma, alterations in motor and sensory innervation of the bladder, medication side effects (e.g., anticholinergics), or fecal impaction.

The nurse should be aware of the volume and frequency of voiding to assess this condition in the client. Key signs of urinary retention are absence of urine output over several hours, bladder distension, restlessness, diaphoresis, and moderate to extreme abdominal discomfort. The client under the influence of anaesthetics or

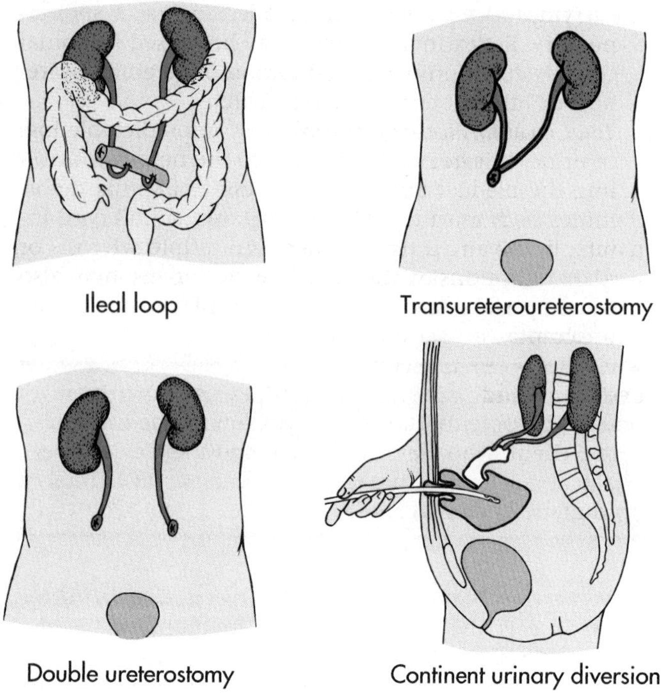

FIGURE **40–5** Types of urinary diversions.

analgesics may feel only pressure, but the alert client has severe pain as the bladder distends beyond its normal capacity. In severe urinary retention, the bladder may hold as much as 2000 to 3000 mL of urine. Intermittent catheterization may be required to empty the bladder and reduce the risk of overflow incontinence and UTI.

Urinary Diversions. A urinary stoma to divert the flow of urine from the kidneys directly to the abdominal surface is created for several reasons, including cancer of the bladder, trauma, radiation injury to the bladder, fistulas, and chronic cystitis. A urinary diversion may be temporary or permanent. The client with an incontinent urinary diversion must wear an ostomy appliance continuously because there is no sphincter control for regulation of urine flow. Local irritation and skin breakdown occur when urine comes in contact with the skin for long periods. Figure 40–5 illustrates several approaches to urinary diversion.

The ileal loop or conduit involves separating a loop of intestinal ileum with its blood supply intact. The ureters are implanted into the isolated segment of ileum. The remaining ileum is reconnected to the rest of the digestive tract. The ileal segment can then be used as a conduit for continuous urine drainage or fashioned into a continent reservoir (McCance & Huether, 2002). The continent pouch is constructed to provide urinary storage in a leak-proof pouch. The portion of the ileum connected to the abdominal wall acts as a continent nipple, requiring intermittent catheterization for emptying. The disadvantage of either an ileal conduit or reservoir is that if urine outflow becomes obstructed, irreversible damage to the kidneys can occur secondary to chronic infections or hydronephrosis.

A **ureterostomy** involves bringing the end of one or both ureters to the abdominal surface. To avoid the need for two collecting devices, a transureteroureterostomy connects the ureters and brings one out through the abdominal wall. In some cases, a tube may need to be placed directly into the renal pelvis to provide urinary drainage. This procedure is called a **nephrostomy.**

It is essential that stoma appliances fit correctly, that the client (or caregiver) is capable of changing the appliance easily, and that skin around the stoma remains protected and intact. Unprotected skin that is in contact with urine will quickly become macerated and break down, causing pain, infection, increased hospital stays, and potential breakdown of the stoma. All clients must be referred to an enterostomal nurse for preoperative stoma siting and assessment and should be followed closely for several months post-operatively. The client should also be referred to the United Ostomy Association of Canada for invaluable sources of advice and networking.

A urinary diversion poses threats to a client's body image, and adjustment takes time. Although a normal lifestyle is possible with a stoma, adjustment can be difficult. The nurse must understand that each person will cope differently.

Nursing Knowledge Base

Urinary elimination is a basic human function that is usually a private process. Nurses are often the first to be aware that a client has elimination problems and must be alert to cues, prepared to discuss relevant assessment and treatment options, and able to provide counselling and support. This requires a sound base of scientific knowledge related to anatomy and physiology, as well as an understanding of concepts such as infection control and hygiene, normal growth and development, and psychosocial considerations.

Infection Control and Hygiene

The urinary tract is usually considered sterile. The nurse must use infection-control principles to help prevent the development and spread of UTIs, as well as to treat existing infections (see chapter 29). Hospital-acquired UTIs are often related to poor hand hygiene, improper catheter care, or faulty catheterization technique (Kunin, 2001). Knowledge of both medical and surgical asepsis must be applied meticulously when providing care involving the urinary tract and external genitalia. Any invasive procedure of the urinary tract such as catheterization requires sterile technique. Procedures such as perineal care or examination of the genitalia require medical asepsis.

Growth and Development

Growth and development factors determine the client's ability to control the act of urination during the lifespan. Infants and young children cannot effectively concentrate urine. Their urine appears light yellow and clear.

Relative to their small body size, infants and children excrete large volumes of urine. For example, a 6-month-old infant who weighs 6 to 8 kg excretes 400 to 500 mL of urine daily. As the neurological system matures, a toddler of 2 to 3 years is able to associate the sensations of bladder filling and urination. A child must be able to recognize the feeling of bladder fullness, hold urine for 1 to 2 hours, and communicate the sense of urgency to an adult. Many toddlers may then be able to control the urethral sphincter, and toilet training can begin. The young child needs parents' understanding, patience, and consistency. A child may not gain full control of micturition until age 4 or 5 years. Daytime control of micturition is easier to accomplish than nighttime control and occurs earlier in the child's development, usually by 2 years of age. Occasional daytime accidents or nocturnal enuresis (bedwetting) may continue until the age of 5 years.

The adult normally voids 1500 to 1600 mL of urine daily, or approximately 300 to 500 mL every 4 hours. During pregnancy, urinary frequency is common and susceptibility to UTIs is increased. In the female, child-bearing and hormonal changes of menopause may contribute to urinary difficulties. In the male, prostate enlargement can begin in the 40s and continue throughout life, resulting in urinary frequency and possibly retention.

Changes in kidney and bladder function also occur with aging. The kidney's ability to concentrate urine or reabsorb water and sodium declines. Alterations in kidney function include a reduction in glomerular filtration rate, from 125 mL per minute for younger adults to 60 mL to 70 mL per minute in adults approximately 80 years of age. The older adult often experiences nocturia due mainly to age-related changes in vasopressin secretion (Miller, 2000). The bladder loses muscle tone and capacity to hold urine, resulting in increased urinary frequency. Because the bladder cannot contract as effectively, an older person often retains urine in the bladder after voiding (residual urine). Older men commonly experience incomplete bladder emptying associated with prostatic enlargement. These changes increase the risk for bacterial growth and development of UTIs.

Physiologic changes occur in continent as well as incontinent older adults. Incontinence should never be accepted as a normal consequence of aging; it should always be investigated. The nurse plays a key role in this investigation and serves as an important advocate on the older client's behalf.

Psychosocial and Cultural Considerations

The nurse must consider that urinary elimination problems may result in alterations of sexuality and self-concept (which includes body image, self-esteem, roles, and identity). The embarrassment associated with elimination problems may delay the person in seeking help. Individuals with incontinence often blame themselves for their condition and go to great lengths, including self-imposed social isolation, to keep others from finding out. Nurses must initiate discussion concerning urinary elimination as a routine part of care. It is important to consider how bothersome symptoms are for each client before planning care. For example, although men tend to feel greater distress than women do about incontinence (Gray, 2003), both men and women who do not find their symptoms problematic are less likely to adhere to therapies. The nurse must always consider the client's expectations and goals to ensure that care is client focused and that interventions are realistic.

Socio-cultural factors may influence the client's expectation of the degree of privacy and location for attending to urinary needs. The nurse's approach to a client's elimination needs must consider cultural, social, and gender habits. If a client prefers privacy, the nurse tries to prevent interruptions as the client voids. A client with less need for privacy should be treated with understanding and acceptance. Ensure that the client is comfortable when he or she is trying to void. Men generally urinate best in a standing position, whereas women generally sit on a toilet. In some cultures, people prefer to squat over a receptacle rather than sit on one. Culture dictates when and where it is appropriate to urinate. In some cultures, only a female should assist a woman with urinary needs.

Critical Thinking

Critical thinking during assessment of urinary elimination requires the integration of evidence-based knowledge from nursing and other disciplines, experiential knowledge, and understanding of the client's perceptions of the alterations in elimination and their impact. Critical thinking also involves an understanding of relevant cultural, environmental, and personal factors, including the unique goals of every client. Empathy, teaching, and ongoing support are needed to assist the client in meeting these goals and maintaining improvement.

Professional standards provide valuable directions for treatment and management of elimination problems. When planning and implementing care for the client with alterations in urinary elimination, the nurse uses standards developed by professional organizations such as the Canadian Nurses Association, Canadian Continence Foundation, the United Ostomy Association of Canada, and the Urology Nurses of Canada. The nurse should also follow clinical care guidelines for management of urinary incontinence as developed by a multidisciplinary team of health care professionals (Canadian Continence Foundation, 2001).

Nursing Process and Alterations in Urinary Function

NP Assessment

To identify a urinary elimination problem and gather data for a care plan, the nurse obtains information by collecting a health history, performing a focused physical assessment, assessing the client's urine, and reviewing information from diagnostic tests and examinations. The nurse uses critical thinking to synthesize this information as assessment proceeds (Figure 40–6). Adequate assessment should result in the formulation of nursing diagnoses appropriate for alterations in urinary elimination.

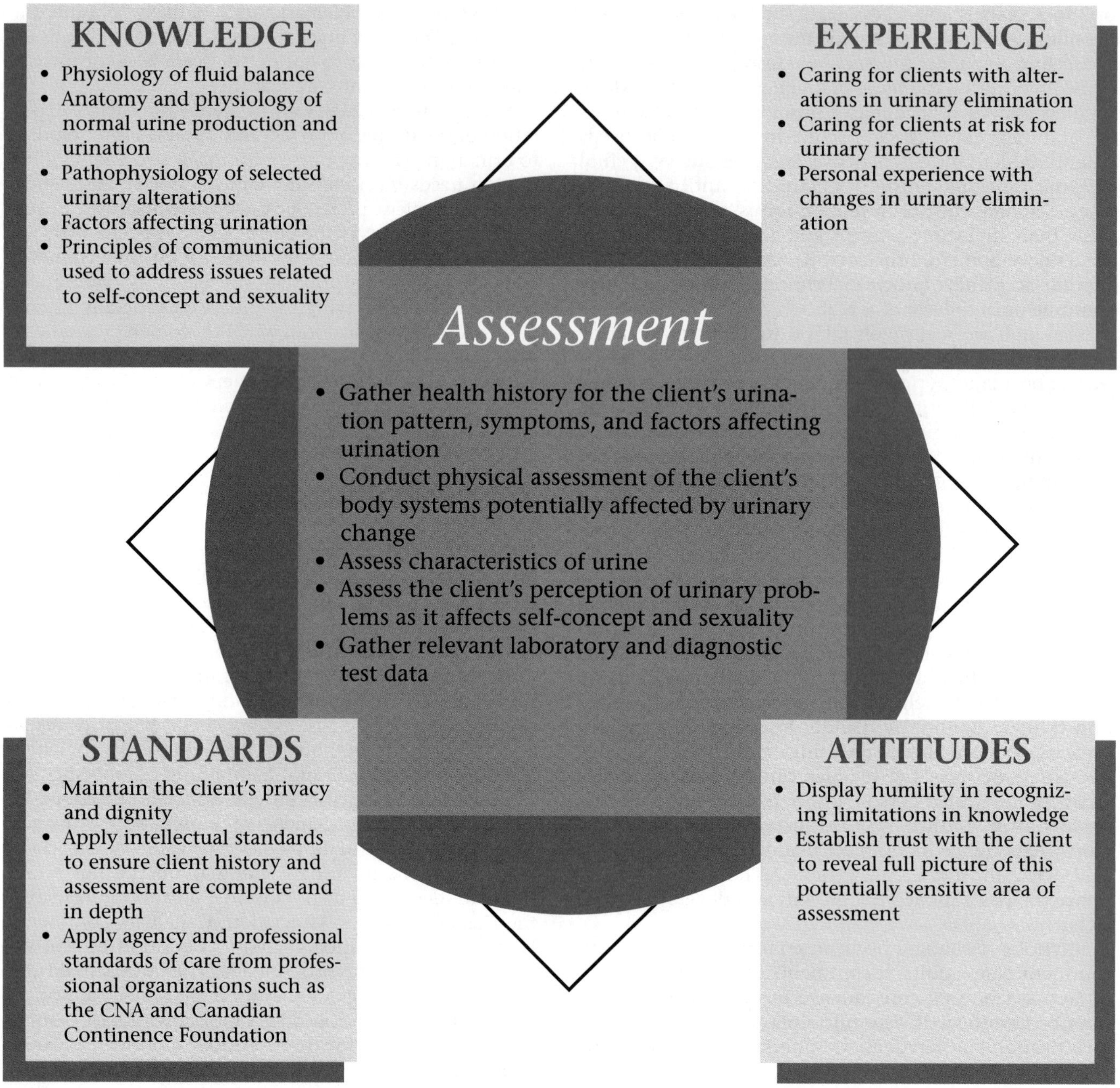
KNOWLEDGE
• Physiology of fluid balance
• Anatomy and physiology of normal urine production and urination
• Pathophysiology of selected urinary alterations
• Factors affecting urination
• Principles of communication used to address issues related to self-concept and sexuality
EXPERIENCE
• Caring for clients with alterations in urinary elimination
• Caring for clients at risk for urinary infection
• Personal experience with changes in urinary elimination
Assessment
• Gather health history for the client's urination pattern, symptoms, and factors affecting urination
• Conduct physical assessment of the client's body systems potentially affected by urinary change
• Assess characteristics of urine
• Assess the client's perception of urinary problems as it affects self-concept and sexuality
• Gather relevant laboratory and diagnostic test data
STANDARDS
• Maintain the client's privacy and dignity
• Apply intellectual standards to ensure client history and assessment are complete and in depth
• Apply agency and professional standards of care from professional organizations such as the CNA and Canadian Continence Foundation
ATTITUDES
• Display humility in recognizing limitations in knowledge
• Establish trust with the client to reveal full picture of this potentially sensitive area of assessment

FIGURE **40–6** Critical thinking model for urinary elimination assessment.

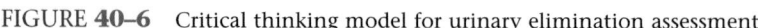

The nurse should be alert to individual needs related to normal changes of aging that predispose older adults to certain elimination problems (Box 40-2).

Health History. The nursing health history includes a review of the client's elimination patterns and symptoms of urinary alterations and an assessment of factors that may affect the ability to urinate normally.

Pattern of Urination. The nurse asks the client about daily voiding patterns, including frequency and times of day, normal volume at each voiding, and any recent changes. Frequency varies among individuals and varies with intake and other types of fluid losses. The common times for urination are on awakening, after meals, and before bedtime. Most people void an average of five or more times a day. The client who voids frequently during the night may have renal disease or prostate enlargement. Information about the pattern of urination establishes a baseline for comparison.

Assessing voiding patterns is an important part of screening for alterations in elimination. A **urinary diary** provides a baseline assessment of urination patterns and is a useful diagnostic tool for urinary incontinence (Figure 40–7). A diary is kept by the client or caregiver for 24 to 72 hours and includes times of urination, the

Focus on Older Adults

Box 40-2

- High-quality nursing care is essential in the care of the older adult. When older adults become dependent on others for personal care, maintenance of their urinary health falls into the domain of nursing practice (Dowd, Kolbaca, & Steiner, 2000).
- Dilute urine discourages bacterial growth; therefore, older adults should be encouraged to increase their fluid intake to at least six to eight glasses a day, unless medically contraindicated (Gray & Krissovich, 2003).
- Fluids that promote an acidic urine (e.g., cranberry juice) should be made available as part of the client's fluid intake because an acidic urine also inhibits bacterial growth and may prevent UTIs (Gray, 2002).
- Restricting fluid intake does not decrease urinary incontinence severity or frequency. However, restriction of fluids 2 hours before sleep, combined with nocturnal toileting, may diminish the severity of incontinence (Gray & Krissovich, 2003).
- In-dwelling catheters should not be used routinely in older adults unless other options have been tried. If a catheter is necessary, it should be used for no longer than 3 days. The risk of infection increases dramatically for catheterized clients (Kunin, 2001).
- Treating asymptomatic bacteriuria in older adults is not generally recommended.
- The nurse should note that incontinence is not a normal part of aging, and efforts should be made to assess incontinence and provide interventions to promote return to continence.

Instructions:

- ❒ Mark the time in the appropriate column each time you void in a toilet or accidentally leak urine. Note how much urine was leaked (a small, moderate, or large amount).
- ❒ In the COMMENTS column, indicate any factors associated with the leakage or the voiding (e.g., "coughing caused leakage," or "don't feel empty after voiding").
- ❒ In the FLUIDS column, describe the type (coffee, tea, juice) and amount (250 mL).
- ❒ In the last column, record the time that you changed a pad. Complete the diary for a full 24 hours.

NAME: ______________________

DAY/DATE: ______________________

TIME	VOIDED IN TOILET	ACCIDENTAL LEAKAGE	COMMENTS	FLUIDS (TYPE, AMOUNT)		PAD CHANGE

FIGURE **40–7** Sample urinary diary. (Adapted from *Urinary Diary,* Women's Continence Center, University of California, 2001, San Francisco; retrieved February 22, 2005, from *http://www.ucsf.edu/wcc/print_diary.html*)

amount urinated, times of leakage, the amount lost, and type and amount of fluid ingested. Recording factors that precipitated urination or leakage such as a strong urge or cough is particularly helpful. The number of pad changes is also useful information that may be noted. The diary can be adjusted to whatever format the client finds most practical (Payne et al., 2002).

Symptoms of Urinary Alterations. Certain symptoms specific to urinary alterations may occur in more than one type of disorder. During assessment, the nurse asks the client about any symptoms related to urination and their onset and duration (Table 40-1). The nurse also assesses whether the client is aware of conditions or factors that precipitate or aggravate symptoms. Likewise, it is important that the nurse determine what the client does when any of these symptoms occur.

Factors Affecting Urination. The nurse summarizes factors associated with the client's medical history, surgical history, and current environment that may affect urination. Medical history includes disease conditions that can affect elimination, such as multiple sclerosis, spinal cord injury, stroke, and diabetes. Another factor to consider is the bowel elimination pattern. Constipation often interferes with normal urine elimination. Medication history, including the name, amount, and frequency of each prescription and over-the-counter medication, should also be noted as part of the history.

Relevant surgical history (e.g., urological and gynecological interventions and pelvic radiation) should be considered because surgery may cause scarring and disruption of neurological pathways. The presence or history of an in-dwelling catheter should be noted because of the potential for infection, catheter blockage, or skin care

Table 40-1 Common Symptoms of Urinary Alterations

Symptoms	Description	Common Causes or Associated Factors
Incontinence	Involuntary loss of urine	Multiple factors: urethral hypermobility, loss of pelvic floor muscle tone, estrogen depletion, fecal impaction, neurological impairment, pelvic organ prolapse
Urgency	Feeling of need to void immediately	Full bladder, bladder irritation or inflammation from infection, tumour, calculi, atrophic vaginitis, caffeine, incompetent urethral sphincter, incomplete emptying, psychological stress
Dysuria	Painful or difficult urination	Bladder inflammation, urethral trauma, urinary tract infection, inflammation of urethra and/or sphincter
Frequency	Voiding at frequent intervals (<2 hours)	Increased fluid intake, bladder infection/inflammation, increased pressure on bladder (pregnancy, psychological stress), incomplete emptying
Hesitancy	Difficulty initiating urination	Hypotonic bladder, anxiety, urethral stricture, obstruction associated with prostate enlargement
Polyuria	Voiding large amounts of urine	Excess fluid intake, diabetes mellitus or insipidus, use of diuretics, post-obstructive diuresis
Oliguria	Diminished urinary output relative to intake (usually 400 mL/24 hours)	Dehydration, renal failure, increased ADH secretion, congestive heart failure
Nocturia	Frequent or excessive urination at night	Excessive fluid intake before bed (especially coffee or alcohol), renal disease, aging process, cardiovascular insufficiency, prostate enlargement, sleep apnea
Dribbling	Leakage of urine despite voluntary control of urination	Stress incontinence, overflow from urinary retention, post-void pooling of urine in the urethra (men)
Hematuria	Blood in the urine	Neoplasms of the kidney or bladder, glomerular disease, infection of kidney or bladder, trauma to urinary structures, calculi, bleeding disorders, UTI
Retention	Accumulation of urine in the bladder, with inability of bladder to empty fully	Urethral obstruction, bladder inflammation, decreased sensory activity, neurogenic bladder, prostate enlargement, post-anaesthesia effects, side effects of medications (e.g., anticholinergics, antidepressants)
Residual urine	Volume of urine remaining after voiding (>100 mL)	Neurogenic bladder, prostate enlargement, trauma, inflammation of urethra, inflammation or irritation of bladder mucosa from infection

problems (Getliffe, 2003). Environmental barriers in the home or health care setting are also evaluated. The client's mobility and ability to dress/undress and toilet independently are assessed. Such aids as elevated toilet seats, grab bars, or a portable commode may be needed.

One of the most important parts of the assessment is the impact of alterations in elimination on the client's lifestyle and quality of life. The impact of urinary incontinence, in particular, can be substantial and it is important to discuss changes the client has made to cope with the condition. It is also important to note whether the client has previously seen a health care professional for help or advice.

Physical Assessment. A physical examination (see chapter 28) provides the nurse with data to determine the presence and severity of urinary elimination problems. The primary structures reviewed include the skin and mucosal membranes, kidneys, bladder, and perineum.

Skin and Mucosal Membranes. The nurse assesses the condition of the skin and mucosal membranes. Problems with urinary elimination are often associated with fluid and electrolyte disturbances. By assessing skin turgor and the oral mucosa, the nurse assesses the client's hydration status. Urinary incontinence increases the risk of skin breakdown (see chapter 43).

Kidneys. Flank pain usually develops if the kidneys become infected or inflamed. The nurse assesses for flank tenderness early in the disease by percussing the costovertebral angle (the angle formed by the spine and the twelfth rib). Auscultation is also performed to detect the presence of a renal artery bruit (sound resulting from turbulent blood flow through a narrowed artery).

Nurses with advanced examination skills learn to palpate the kidneys during abdominal examination. The kidneys' position, shape, and size can reveal renal swelling.

Bladder. In adults, the bladder rests below the symphysis pubis and is difficult to palpate. When distended, the bladder rises above the symphysis pubis at the midline of the abdomen and may extend to just below the umbilicus. On inspection, the nurse may note a swelling or convex curvature of the lower abdomen. The nurse lightly palpates the lower abdomen. The partially filled bladder normally feels smooth and rounded. As the nurse applies light pressure to the bladder, the client may feel the urge to urinate, tenderness, or even pain. Percussion of a full bladder yields a dull percussion note.

The Female Perineum. When examining the female client, the nurse requests that she assume a dorsal recumbent position to provide full exposure of the genitalia. The perineum is inspected for skin integrity and the presence of a rash associated with incontinence and the use of containment pads. The rash may be monilial (maculopapular, red rash), or an ammonia contact perineal dermatitis (papular with macerated skin).

The vaginal vault in females is assessed for signs of vaginitis, a common result of estrogen depletion following menopause (Rutchik & Resnick, 1998). Signs include dry, thin, pale, friable mucosa, and tenderness/sensitivity to touch. Women with vaginal infections are susceptible to UTIs because the vaginal discharge may easily travel to the urethral meatus. The nurse inspects the vaginal orifice carefully for signs of inflammation and describes any drainage.

The nurse assesses the urethral meatus to note the presence of discharge, inflammation, and lesions. Normally the meatus is pink and appears as a small slit-like opening below the clitoris and above the vaginal orifice. It may recede well into the vaginal vault with aging, making catheterization difficult. There is normally no discharge from the meatus. If present, specimens of urethral discharge should be obtained before the client voids.

Pelvic floor muscle strength can be digitally assessed in women by inserting a gloved finger gently into the vagina. The client is asked to squeeze around the finger and hold the contraction (generally 3 to 5 seconds; see chapter 28). Digital assessment is also useful in helping the client to correctly identify the pelvic floor muscles.

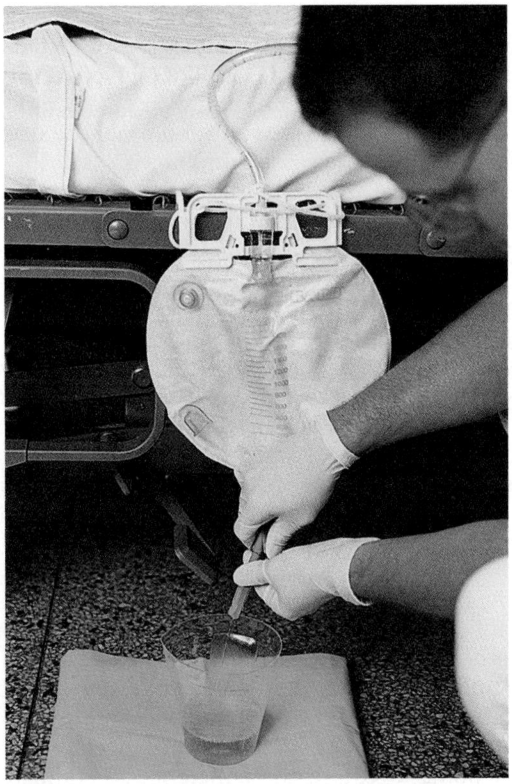

FIGURE **40–8** Urine drainage bag.

The Male Perineum. The male urethral meatus is normally a small opening at the tip of the penis. The nurse inspects the meatus for discharge, inflammation, and lesions. If the foreskin is retracted in uncircumcised men to see the meatus, it must be replaced to avoid constriction of the glans. Disposable gloves should be worn when retracting the foreskin. Pelvic floor muscle strength in men can be digitally assessed by inserting a gloved finger gently into the rectum and, as with women, asking the client to squeeze around the finger (see chapter 28).

Assessment of Urine. Assessment of urine involves measuring the client's fluid intake and urine output and observing characteristics of the urine.

Intake and Output. The nurse assesses the client's average daily fluid intake. If an accurate measurement of fluid intake is needed from the client who is at home, the nurse may ask the client to show a commonly used glass or cup on which the intake estimate is based. In a health care setting, the nurse measures a client's fluid intake either when the physician orders intake and output (I&O) measurements or when nursing judgment warrants a more precise measurement (see chapter 36). A change in urine volume is a significant indicator of fluid alterations or kidney disease. While caring for the client, the nurse assesses volume by measuring urinary output with each voiding (with plastic receptacles, bedpans, or urinals). Special receptacles (urimeters) attach between in-dwelling catheters and drainage bags and are a convenient means of accurately measuring urine volume. A urimeter holds 100 to 200 mL of urine. After measuring urine from a urimeter, the nurse can drain the cylinder into the urinary drainage bag or into a receptacle for disposal. Urimeters are indicated when precise hourly measurements of urine are needed.

When urine from a drainage bag is measured, the urine should be drained into a plastic graduated receptacle for more precise measurement of output (Figure 40–8). Each client should have a graduated receptacle for his or her exclusive use to prevent potential cross-contamination.

The nurse reports any extreme increase or decrease in volume. An hourly output of less than 30 mL for more than 2 hours is cause for concern. Similarly, consistently high volumes of urine (polyuria), over 2000 to 2500 mL daily, should be reported to a physician.

Characteristics of Urine. The nurse inspects the client's urine for colour, clarity, and odour.

Colour. Normal urine ranges from a pale, straw colour to amber, depending on its concentration. Urine is usually more concentrated in the morning or with fluid volume deficits. As the person drinks more fluids, urine becomes less concentrated.

Bleeding from the kidneys or ureters causes urine to become dark red; bleeding from the bladder or urethra causes urine to become bright red. Various medications and foods also change urine colour and will cause a false-positive urinalysis. For example, phenazopyridine, a urinary analgesic, colours the urine bright orange. Eating beets, rhubarb, or blackberries may cause red urine. Special dyes used in intravenous diagnostic studies also discolour urine. Dark amber urine may be the result of high concentrations of bilirubin caused by liver dysfunction or vitamin B. The nurse documents and reports any abnormal colour or sediment, especially if the cause is unknown.

Clarity. Normal urine appears transparent at voiding. Urine that stands several minutes in a container becomes cloudy. Freshly voided urine in clients with renal disease may appear cloudy or foamy because of high protein concentrations. Urine also appears thick and cloudy as a result of bacteria.

Odour. Urine has a characteristic odour. The more concentrated the urine, the stronger the odour. Stagnant urine has an ammonia odour, which is common in clients who are repeatedly incontinent. A sweet or fruity odour occurs from acetone or acetoacetic acid (by-products of incomplete fat metabolism) seen with diabetes mellitus or starvation.

Urine Testing. The nurse often collects urine specimens for laboratory testing. The type of test determines the method of collection. All specimens are labelled with the client's name, date, and time of collection. Specimens should be transported to the laboratory in a timely fashion to ensure accuracy of test results. Agency infection control policies require the adherence to standard precautions/routine practices by all personnel during specimen handling (see chapter 29).

Specimen Collection. The nurse collects random, clean-voided or midstream, sterile, and timed specimens (Table 40-2).

Urine Collection in Children. Specimen collection from infants and children is often difficult. Adolescents and school-age children are usually able to co-operate, although they may be embarrassed. Preschool children and toddlers have difficulty voiding on request. Offering a young child fluids 30 minutes before requesting a specimen may help. The nurse must use terms for urination that the child can understand. A young child may be reluctant to void in unfamiliar receptacles. A potty-chair or specimen hat placed under the toilet seat is usually effective. The nurse must use special collection devices for infants and toddlers who are not toilet trained. Clear plastic, single-use bags with self-adhering material can be attached over the child's urethral meatus. Specimens should not be obtained by squeezing urine from the diaper material because the results may be inaccurate.

Common Urine Tests

Urinalysis. The laboratory performs a **urinalysis** on a specimen obtained by any of the previously described methods. Table 40-3 lists normal values for a urinalysis. The specimen should be examined as soon as possible, preferably within 2 hours. It should be the first voided specimen in the morning to ensure a uniform concentration of constituents. For a quick screening, the nurse can perform certain portions of the urinalysis with special reagent strips. The nurse dips the strips into the urine and then observes for a colour change in the time interval designated on the package (Figure 40–10).

Specific Gravity. The **specific gravity** is the weight or degree of concentration of a substance compared with an equal amount of water. A urine specimen is poured into a special dry, clean cylinder. The weighted urinometer is suspended in the cylinder of urine. The concentration of dissolved substances in the urine aids in determination of a client's fluid balance. This measurement is always done as part of a complete urinalysis. The nurse in a critical care unit may be responsible for doing periodic measurement of specific gravity of urine as part of complete assessment for specific clients.

If questions regarding the accuracy of specific gravity measurements arise, a urine osmolality test should be obtained. Although both tests measure urine concentration, the osmolality test is more accurate because it measures the total number of particles in a solution (see chapter 36).

Urine Culture. A urine culture requires a sterile or clean-voided sample of urine. It takes approximately 24 to 48 hours before the laboratory can report findings of bacterial growth. While awaiting results, a broad-spectrum antibiotic may be ordered as soon as a culture has been obtained. The test for sensitivity determines which specific antibiotics are effective. The results of a urine culture may indicate a change in choice of medication.

Diagnostic Examinations. The urinary system is amenable to accurate diagnostic study by several radiographic techniques. The two approaches for visualization of urinary structures, direct and indirect techniques, can be quite simple or very complex, requiring extensive nursing intervention. These procedures are further subdivided into invasive or non-invasive categories (Table 40-4).

Many of the nursing responsibilities related to diagnostic examinations of the urinary tract are common to many of the studies. The common responsibilities before the study include the following:

- Witnessing a signed consent (if agency policy)
- Assessing client for history of shellfish (iodine) allergy, which predicts allergy to the dye used in specific studies (intravenous pyelogram [IVP] and renal arteriogram)
- Administering bowel cleansing medications (check agency policy)
- Ensuring client receives appropriate pretest diet (clear liquids) or nothing by mouth (NPO), as needed

Common post-procedure interventions may include the following:

- Assessing intake and output
- Observing characteristics of urine (colour, clarity, presence of blood)

Client Expectations. Clients are dependent on their caregivers to recognize and promptly meet their needs. Nurses need to use a skilled and caring approach, to be creative in using a variety of assessment techniques, and to serve as a client advocate. A caring nurse will meet the client's needs in a way that is acceptable and individualized for the client and family situation. Clients with alterations in urinary elimination expect that the nurse will be respectful of privacy needs and sensitive to the impact of urinary impairments on sexuality and self-concept. The nurse should always include the client in the plan of

Table 40-2 Urine Testing

Collection Type/Use of Specimen	Nursing Considerations
Random (routine urinalysis)	Can be collected during normal voiding, from an in-dwelling catheter or urinary diversion collection bag. Collected in a clean specimen cup.
Clean-voided or midstream (culture and sensitivity)	See Skill 40-1. Collected in a sterile specimen cup.
Sterile specimen (culture and sensitivity)	If the client has an in-dwelling catheter, a sterile specimen can be collected using aseptic technique through the special port (Figure 40–9) found on the side of the catheter. If the catheter has been in situ for more than 3 days, it should be changed before the specimen is collected to avoid contamination by organisms in the catheter lumen. The nurse clamps the tubing below the port, allowing fresh, uncontaminated urine to collect in the tube. After the nurse wipes the port with an antimicrobial swab, a sterile syringe needle is inserted and at least 3 to 5 mL of urine is withdrawn. Using sterile aseptic technique, the nurse transfers the urine to a sterile container (see chapter 29).
Timed urine specimens (for measuring levels of adrenal cortical steroids or hormones, creatinine clearance, or protein quantity tests)	Time required may be 2-, 12-, or 24-hour collections. The timed period begins after the client urinates and ends with a final voiding at the end of the time period. The client voids into a clean receptacle, and the urine is transferred to the special collection container, which may contain special preservatives. Each specimen must be free of feces and toilet tissue. Missed specimens make the whole collection inaccurate. Check with agency policy and the laboratory for specific instructions.

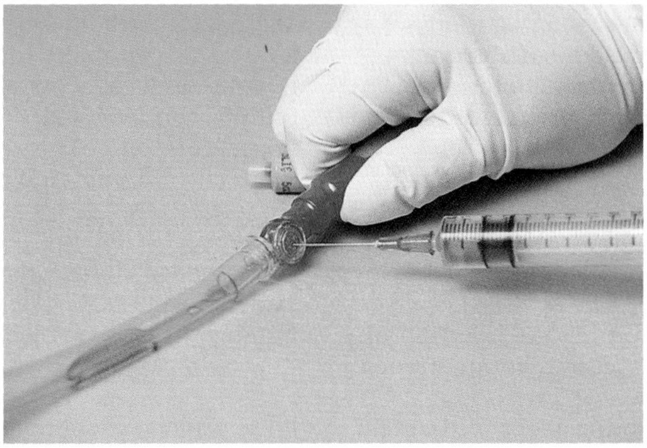

FIGURE **40–9** Urine specimen collection: aspiration from a collection port in drainage tubing on an in-dwelling catheter.

care and develop goals that are mutually acceptable. Cultural practices and personal preferences must also be considered.

Nursing Diagnosis

A thorough assessment of the client's urinary elimination function reveals patterns of data that allow the nurse to make relevant and accurate nursing diagnoses. The diagnosis may focus on a specific alteration or an associated problem such as *impaired skin integrity related to urinary incontinence.* Identification of defining characteristics leads the nurse to select an appropriate diagnosis. Specifying related factors for each diagnosis allows selection of individualized nursing interventions (see chapter 12). One sample of diagnostic reasoning is found in Box 40-3. Nursing diagnoses common to clients with urine elimination alterations include the following:

- Disturbed body image
- Pain (acute, chronic)
- Self-care deficit, toileting
- Impaired skin integrity
- Impaired urinary elimination
- Urinary incontinence (transient, urge, stress, mixed, functional, overflow, reflex, total)
- Urinary retention

Common symptoms that contribute to a nursing diagnosis of impaired urinary elimination, such as frequency, urgency, and nocturia, have been described in Table 40-1.

Text continued on p. 1352

Skill 40-1 Collecting Midstream (Clean-Voided) Urine Specimen

Delegation Considerations

Collecting midstream (clean-voided) urine specimen may be delegated to unregulated care providers (UCPs). If appropriate, an alert client who is physically able may be instructed to collect the specimen. It is the nurse's responsibility to ensure that this specimen is obtained correctly and in a timely manner. Be aware of agency policy regarding specimen collection.

Instruct the UCP to inform the nurse of the following:

- When the specimen was obtained
- If client is unable to initiate a stream or has pain or burning on urination
- If the collected specimen is dark, bloody, or cloudy; is odorous; or contains mucus

Equipment

- Soap or cleansing solution, washcloth, towel, and hand washing basin
- Commercial kit for clean-voided specimen or individual supplies as listed
  - Sterile cotton balls or sterile 2 × 2 or 4 × 4 (5 × 5 cm or 10 × 10 cm) gauze pads
  - Antiseptic solution (e.g., providone-iodine); check for client allergy, if allergic provide an alternative
  - Sterile water
- Sterile specimen collection cup or jar
- Sterile and non-sterile (disposable) gloves
- Bedpan, bedside commode, or specimen hat
- Completed specimen label

Steps	Rationale
1. Assess voiding status of client:	
a. When client last voided	May indicate readiness to void.
b. Level of awareness or developmental stage	Reveals client's ability to co-operate during procedure.
c. Mobility, balance, and physical limitations	Determines level of assistance in acquiring specimen.
2. Assess client's understanding of purpose of test and method of collection.	Information allows clarification and promotes client co-operation.
3. Explain procedure to client:	Helps client understand the procedure.
a. Reason midstream specimen is needed	
b. Ways client and family can assist	
c. Ways to obtain specimen free of feces	Feces change characteristics of urine and may cause abnormal values.
4. Provide fluids to drink ½ hour before collection unless contraindicated (i.e., fluid restriction) if client does not feel urge to void.	Improves likelihood of client being able to void.
5. Provide privacy for client by closing door or bed curtain.	Privacy allows client to relax and produce specimen more quickly.
6. Give client or family members soap, washcloth, and towel to cleanse perineal area.	Client may prefer to wash own perineal area.
7. Perform hand hygiene and apply non-sterile gloves and assist non-ambulatory clients with perineal care. Assist female client onto bedpan.	Prevents transmission of micro-organisms to nurse, provides easy access to perineal area to collect specimen.
8. Change gloves if necessary.	Reduces transfer of infection.
9. Using surgical asepsis, open sterile kit (see illustration) or prepare sterile supplies. Apply sterile gloves after opening sterile specimen cup, placing cap with sterile inside surface up; do not touch inside of container or cap (see chapter 29).	Sterile technique is essential to maintain sterility of equipment and specimen. Sterile gloves prevent the transmission of micro-organisms to the specimen from the nurse or from the client to the nurse. Contaminated specimen is most frequent reason for inaccurate reporting of urine cultures and sensitivities.
10. Pour antiseptic solution over cotton balls or gauze pads unless kit contains prepared gauze pads in antiseptic solution.	Cotton balls or gauze pads will be used to further cleanse the perineum.
11. Assist or allow client to independently cleanse perineum and collect specimen:	
A. Female	
(1) Spread labia with thumb and forefinger of non-dominant hand.	Provides access to urethral meatus.
(2) Cleanse area with cotton ball or gauze, moving from front (above urethral orifice) to back (toward anus; see illustration).	Cleanse from area of least contamination to area of greatest contamination to decrease bacterial levels.

Steps	Rationale
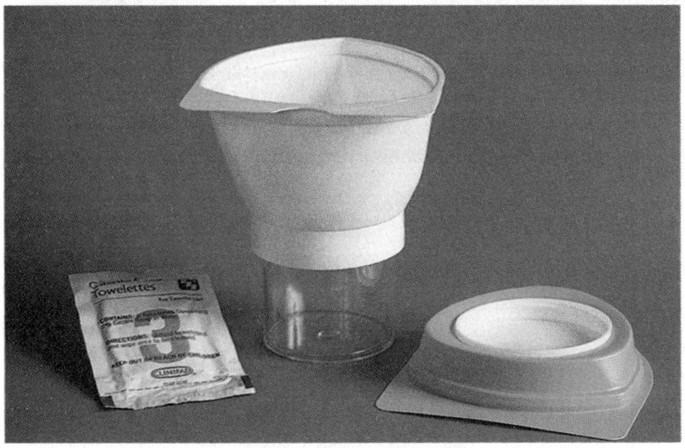 STEP **9** Commercial midstream urine collection kit.	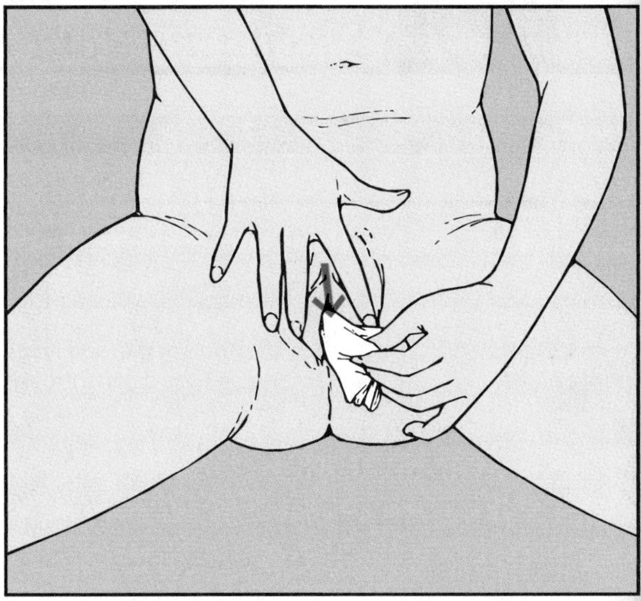 STEP **11A(2)** Cleansing technique (female).
(3) If agency policy indicates, rinse area with sterile water, and dry with dry cotton ball or gauze.	Prevents contamination of specimen with antiseptic solution.
(4) While continuing to hold labia apart, client should initiate stream and after stream is achieved, pass container into stream and collect 30 to 60 mL (see illustration).	Initial stream flushes out micro-organisms that accumulate at urethral meatus and prevents transfer into specimen.
B. Male	
(1) Hold penis with one hand, and using circular motion and antiseptic swab, cleanse end of penis, moving from centre to outside (see illustration). In uncircumcised men, the foreskin should be retracted before cleansing.	Cleanse from area of least contamination to area of greatest contamination to decrease bacterial levels.
(2) If agency procedure indicates, rinse area with sterile water, and dry with cotton or gauze.	Prevents contamination of specimen with antiseptic solution.
(3) After client has initiated urine stream, pass specimen collection container into stream, and collect 30 to 60 mL (see illustration).	Initial stream flushes out micro-organisms that accumulate at urethral meatus and prevents transfer into specimen.
12. Remove specimen container before flow of urine stops and before releasing labia or penis. Client finishes voiding in bedpan or toilet. If foreskin was retracted for specimen collection, it must be replaced over the glans.	Prevents contamination of specimen with skin flora. If foreskin not replaced, swelling and constriction may occur, causing pain and possible obstruction to urine flow.
13. Replace cap securely on specimen container (touch outside only).	Retains sterility of inside of container and prevents spillage of urine.
14. Cleanse any urine from exterior surface of container, and place in a plastic specimen bag.	Prevents transfer of micro-organisms to others.
15. Remove bedpan (if applicable), assist client to comfortable position, and provide handwashing basin if needed.	Promotes relaxing environment.
16. Label specimen, and attach laboratory requisition.	Prevents inaccurate identification that could lead to errors in diagnosis or treatment.

Skill 40-1 Collecting Midstream (Clean-Voided) Urine Specimen—cont'd

Steps	Rationale

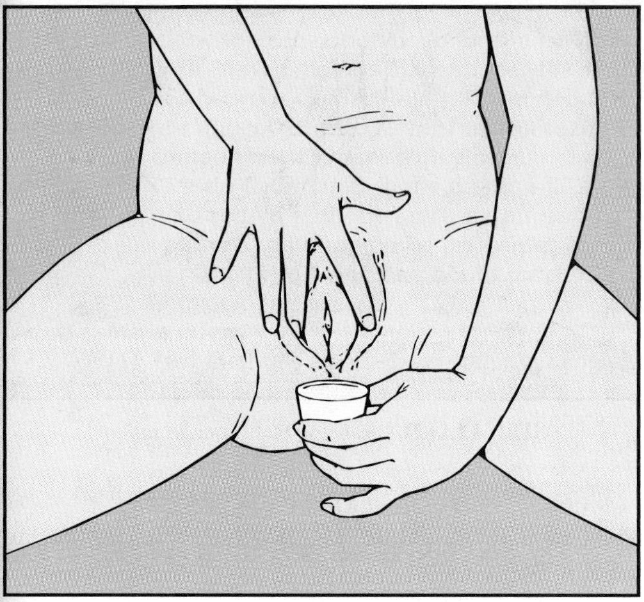

STEP **11A(4)** Specimen collection (female).

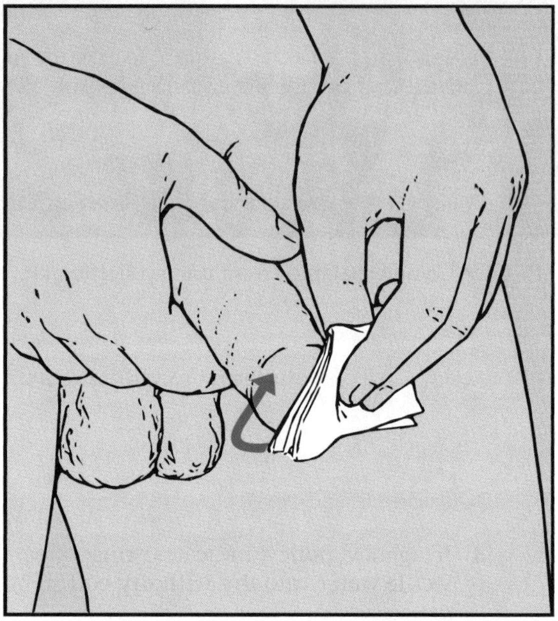

STEP **11B(1)** Cleansing technique (male).

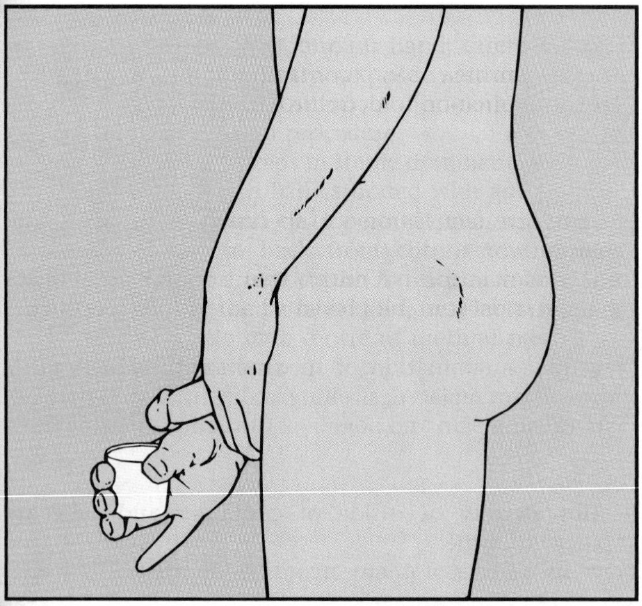

STEP **11B(3)** Specimen collection (male).

Critical Decision Point: If client is menstruating, indicate information on laboratory requisition.

Steps	Rationale
17. Remove gloves, dispose in proper receptacle, and perform hand hygiene.	Reduces transmission of infection.
18. Transport specimen to laboratory within 15 minutes or refrigerate immediately.	Bacteria grow quickly in urine, and specimen should be analyzed immediately to obtain correct results.

Unexpected Outcomes and Related Interventions

- Urine specimen is contaminated with feces or toilet paper.
  - Repeat instruction to client or assist client in obtaining specimen.
  - Obtain a new specimen.
  - Consider using a straight catheterization to obtain specimen.
- Specimen is accidentally discarded.
  - Repeat specimen collection.

Recording and Reporting

- Record date and time urine specimen was obtained in nurses' notes.
- Notify physician of any significant abnormalities.

Home Care Considerations

- If client is to collect specimen as outpatient, proper instruction for collection needs to be given.
- Appropriate equipment will need to be given to client and family.
- Information on storing specimen until time for delivery to doctor's office or hospital laboratory needs to be given.

Table 40-3 Routine Urinalysis

Measurement and Normal Value	Interpretation
pH (4.6–8.0) average 6.0	pH indicates acid-base balance. Urine that stands for several hours becomes alkaline. An acid pH helps protect against bacterial growth.
Protein (none or up to 8 mg/100 mL)	Protein is not normally present in urine. It is seen in renal disease because damage to glomeruli or tubules allows protein to enter urine.
Glucose (none)	Diabetic clients have glucose in urine as a result of inability of tubules to reabsorb high glucose concentrations (180 mg/100 mL). Ingestion of high concentrations of glucose may cause some glucose to appear in urine of healthy people.
Ketones (none)	Clients whose diabetes mellitus is poorly controlled experience breakdown of fatty acids. End products of fat metabolism are ketones. Clients with dehydration, starvation, or excessive aspirin usage also may have **ketonuria.**
Blood (up to 2 RBCs)	Damage to glomeruli or tubules may allow RBCs to enter the urine. Trauma, disease, or surgery of the lower urinary tract also may cause blood to be present. In women, blood in a routine urine specimen may be contaminated with menstrual fluid.
Specific gravity (1.010–1.025)	Specific gravity measures concentration of particles in urine. High specific gravity reflects concentrated urine, and low specific gravity reflects diluted urine. Dehydration, reduced renal blood flow, and increased ADH secretion elevate specific gravity. Overhydration, early renal disease, and inadequate ADH secretion reduce specific gravity.
Microscopic Examination	
WBCs (0–4 per low-power field)	Greater numbers may indicate urinary tract infection.
Bacteria (none)	Bacteria indicate urinary tract infection. (Client may or may not have symptoms.)
Casts (none)	Casts are cylindrical bodies whose shapes take on likeness of objects within the renal tubule. Types include hyaline, WBCs, RBCs, granular cells, and epithelial cells. Their presence is always an abnormal finding and indicates renal alterations.

Adapted from *Mosby's Manual of Diagnostic and Laboratory Tests* (2nd ed.), by K. D. Pagana and T. J. Pagana, 2002, St. Louis, MO: Mosby.

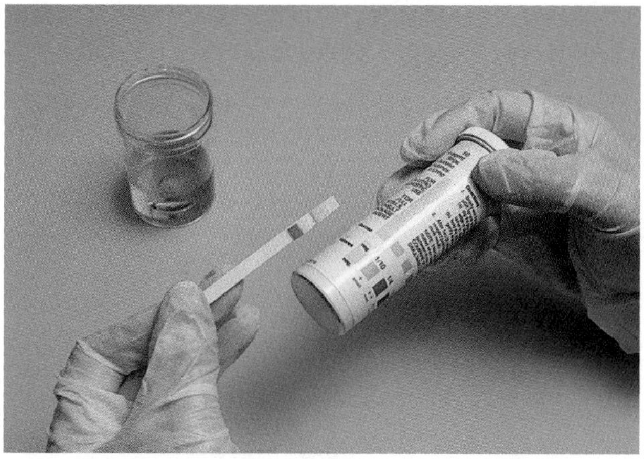

FIGURE **40–10** Checking results of a chemical reagent strip dipped in urine.

Table 40-4 Diagnostic Examinations

Name of Procedure	Purpose and Method of Procedure	Special Nursing Considerations
Non-invasive Procedures		
Abdominal roentgenogram (plain film; kidney, ureter, bladder [KUB], or flat plate)	To determine the size, shape, symmetry, and location of the kidneys; diagnose urinary calculi; preliminary X-ray for intravenous pyelogram (IVP).	No special preparation or precautions; bowel preparation is required if preliminary film prior to IVP.
Computerized axial tomography (CT) scan (Figure 40–11)	A computerized X-ray procedure used to obtain detailed images of structures within a selected plane of the body. The computer reconstructs cross-sectional image and thus allows the physician to view pathologic conditions such as tumours, obstructions.	Bowel cleansing as per agency or physician preference. Assess client for shellfish (iodine) allergy if a CT with contrast is ordered. Prepare client for the procedure (e.g., client will be placed into a large machine, need to lie still, feelings of claustrophobia in some clients).
Intravenous pyelogram (IVP)	To view the collecting ducts and renal pelvis and outline the ureters, bladder, and urethra using dye that is excreted through the urine. A special intravenous injection that converts to a dye in urine is injected intravenously. The client's ability to empty the bladder is assessed through a post-voiding X-ray	Bowel cleansing will be completed as per agency or physician preference. Only clear liquids are permitted until after test completed. Assess client for shellfish and iodine allergy before test. After test, fluid intake is encouraged to dilute and flush dye from client. Observe for late symptoms of allergic reactions (rash, throat tightness, difficulty breathing, etc.).
Retrograde pyelogram	Series of X-rays that provide detailed anatomic views of the ureter, ureteropelvic junction, renal pelvis, and calyces. A ureteral catheter is placed in the lower ureteral segment, and contrast material is injected or infused into the upper urinary tract.	Same as for IVP.
Retrograde urethrogram (RUG)	To obtain oblique X-rays of the male urethra by instilling a small volume of iodine-bound contrast material into the urethra from a retrograde direction.	Assess for iodine allergy before test.
Renal (kidney) scan	To determine renal blood flow, anatomical structure of the kidneys, and excretory function using a radioisotope.	Usually no bowel cleansing needed, but check agency policy. After test, only precaution is rinsing bedpan or urinal after use and flushing the urine, as urine will contain a minute amount of radioisotope. Rinse fluid carefully using a double flush.
Ultrasound		
renal	To identify gross renal structures and structural abnormalities in the kidney using high-frequency, inaudible sound waves.	No bowel cleansing needed.
bladder	To identify structural abnormalities of bladder or lower urinary tract. Also used to estimate the volume of urine in the bladder either pre-void or post-void.	Client may be asked to drink fluids before the test to cause bladder distension for better results. No special care necessary after either study.

Continued

Table 40-4 Diagnostic Examinations—cont'd

Name of Procedure	Purpose and Method of Procedure	Special Nursing Considerations
Invasive Procedures		
Endoscopy	Use of an endoscope will allow for direct visualization, specimen collection, and/or treatment of the interior of the kidney (nephroscopy), ureter (ureteroscopy), bladder (cystosopy), and urethra (cystourethroscopy). Although this procedure may be accomplished using local anaesthesia, it is more commonly performed using general anaesthesia or conscious sedation to avoid unnecessary anxiety and trauma for the client.	Signed consent is obtained. If ordered, a bowel cleansing will be completed. Follow agency policy for preoperative preparation and checklist (see chapter 45). After client's return, assess the vital signs, the characteristics of urine, monitor intake and output (I&O), encourage fluids, and observe for fever, dysuria, and pain in suprapubic region.
Arteriogram (angiography)	Used primarily to visualize the renal arteries and/or their branches to detect narrowing or occlusion. A catheter is placed in one of the femoral arteries and introduced up to the level of the renal arteries. Radiopaque contrast is injected through the catheter while X-ray images are taken in rapid succession.	Signed consent is required. Assess for shellfish (iodine) allergy. Follow agency preprocedure checklist. After the procedure, the nurse must monitor vital signs frequently until stable; bed rest is maintained for prescribed time interval; fluids are encouraged to flush the contrast from the system. The nurse will also monitor the affected extremity for neuro-circulatory function (pulse, skin temperature, sensation, and movement), as well as observe catheter site for bleeding, swelling, increased tenderness, or hematoma formation. Physician must be notified immediately of any post-procedure abnormality.
Urodynamic testing (cystometrogram)	Determines bladder and sphincter function in the case of urinary obstruction or urinary incontinence. A catheter is inserted, the urine drained, and sterile water or contrast liquid is used to fill the bladder. Pressure readings are taken and compared with the client's reported sensations.	The nurse explains the need for the client to report all sensations during the test. After the test, the nurse assesses the client for sensations of sweating, pain, nausea, bladder fullness, or a strong urge to void.

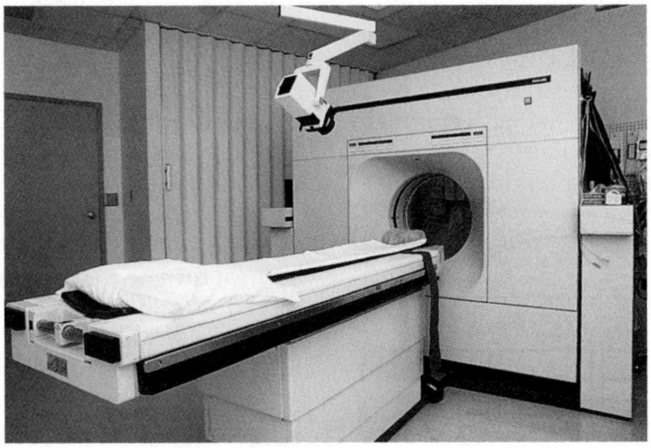

FIGURE **40–11** CT equipment. (From *Renal Disorders,* by D. J. Brundage, 1992, St. Louis, MO: Mosby.)

Nursing Diagnostic Process — Box 40-3

Assessment Activities	Defining Characteristics	Nursing Diagnosis
Have client describe situations that accompany urine leakage.	Client states that she "loses a little urine" whenever she sneezes, coughs, or laughs. Client states she has been having problems for the past year.	Stress urinary incontinence related to decreased pelvic muscle tone and urethral sphincter trauma
Observe client behaviour.	Client is wearing a menstrual minipad continuously. Client is reluctant to interact with others and tries not to cough or laugh.	
Review medical history.	Client is post-menopausal after three vaginal births.	

Each of these symptoms is associated with multiple underlying disorders. The nurse assimilates what has been learned from personal history taking, physical assessment, and diagnostic tests to determine a nursing diagnosis and appropriate plan of care.

Planning

During planning, the nurse integrates the knowledge from assessment and the knowledge related to resources and available therapies to develop an individualized plan of care (see Care Plan). The client's needs should be matched with clinical and professional standards recommended in the literature (Figure 40–12). Building a relationship of trust with the client is important because the implementation of care involves interaction of a very personal nature.

Goals and Outcomes. The plan of care for alterations in elimination must include realistic and individualized goals along with relevant outcomes. The nurse and the client must collaborate in setting goals and outcomes. A general goal might be normal urinary elimination, but the individual goal may differ depending on the problem. The goals may be short term or long term. For example, urinary retention following surgery may require the short-term goal "Client will have normal voiding with complete bladder emptying within 24 hours." Relevant expected outcomes for this goal may include the following:

- Client will void within 8 hours.
- Urinary output of 300 mL or greater will occur with each voiding.
- Client's bladder will not be distended to palpation.
- Client will not continually feel an urge to void.

Conversely, the client with stress incontinence may have a long-term goal that is dependent on weeks of pelvic floor muscle exercise (PFME; also known as Kegel exercises) to achieve urinary control: "Client will achieve full urinary continence within 8 weeks after start of exercise program (Kegel)." Goals must be reasonably achievable for the client situation and be relevant to the client's situation.

Setting Priorities. Urinary elimination is a personal and intimate activity. The nurse must establish a relationship with the client that promotes open discussion. A supportive and collaborative environment allows the client's priorities to become apparent and fosters mutual understanding of realistic goals.

When a client has multiple nursing diagnoses (Figure 40–13), the nurse must recognize the primary health problem and its influence on other problems. In the example of the client with chronic confusion, the resultant incontinence creates several risks. Focusing on the management of incontinence will often help to resolve more than one nursing diagnosis. Although physical care needs may appear to have higher priority, the psychological needs related to self-esteem or sexuality may be of higher priority for the client. Attention to the client's perceived needs may be the most satisfactory and successful approach to accomplishing all of the goals. Reinforcement and praise of good health habits improves compliance with the care plan.

Continuity of Care. The care plan incorporates health promotion activities and therapeutic interventions for clients. Preventive interventions may be required for clients at risk for urinary problems. It is important to consider the client's home environment and normal elimination routines when planning therapies. Consultation with other health care professionals and the client's family is often necessary. For example, the physiotherapist can design an exercise plan to increase strength and endurance so that the client will be able to ambulate to the bathroom. The need for home care services should be explored and appropriate referrals made. The family may need to alter the home environment to make it easier and safer for the client to use the bathroom.

Implementation

Implementation is the action phase of the nursing process. The nurse will carry out the independent and collaborative behaviours needed to assist the client in

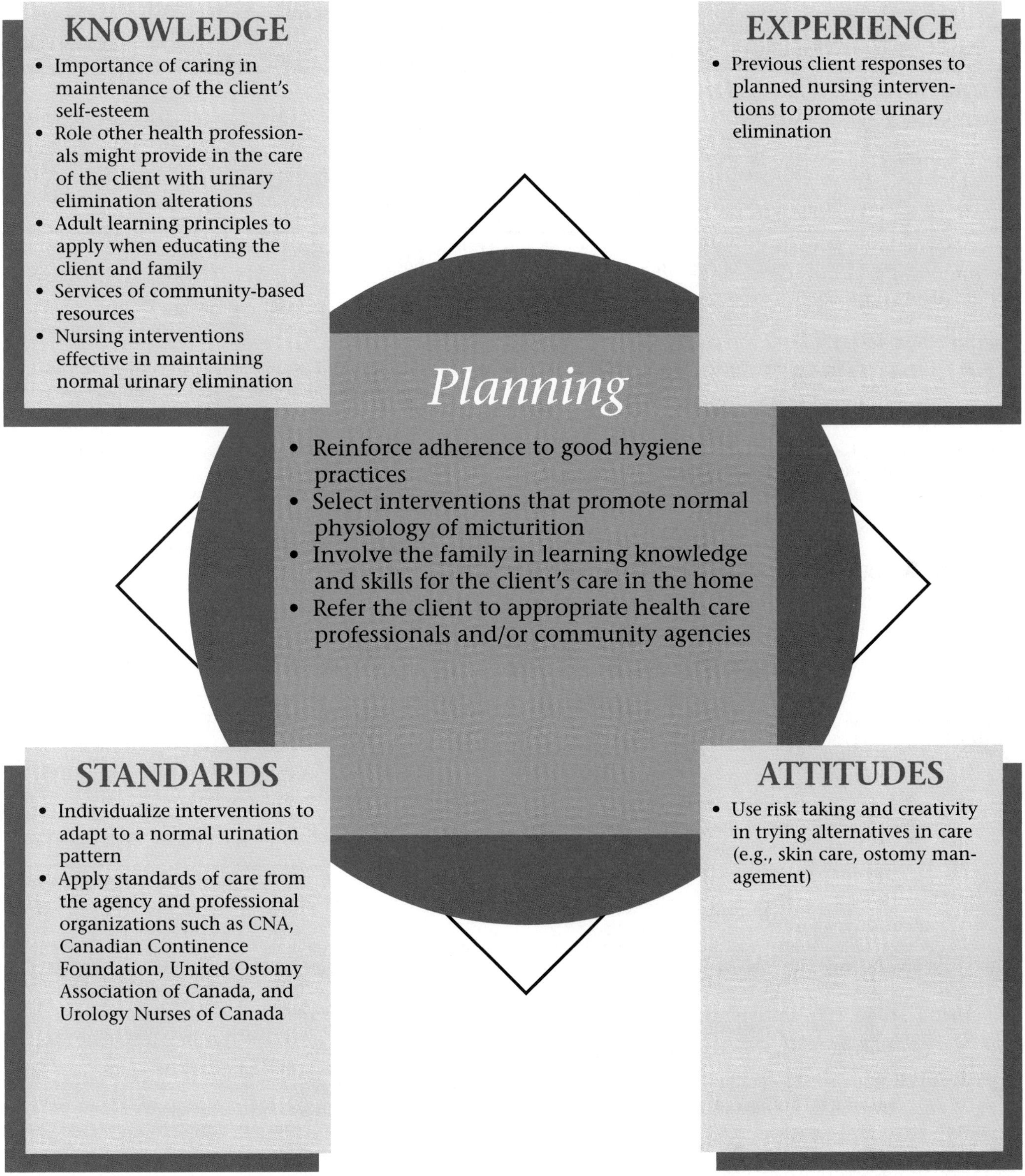
KNOWLEDGE
• Importance of caring in maintenance of the client's self-esteem
• Role other health professionals might provide in the care of the client with urinary elimination alterations
• Adult learning principles to apply when educating the client and family
• Services of community-based resources
• Nursing interventions effective in maintaining normal urinary elimination
EXPERIENCE
• Previous client responses to planned nursing interventions to promote urinary elimination
Planning
• Reinforce adherence to good hygiene practices
• Select interventions that promote normal physiology of micturition
• Involve the family in learning knowledge and skills for the client's care in the home
• Refer the client to appropriate health care professionals and/or community agencies
STANDARDS
• Individualize interventions to adapt to a normal urination pattern
• Apply standards of care from the agency and professional organizations such as CNA, Canadian Continence Foundation, United Ostomy Association of Canada, and Urology Nurses of Canada
ATTITUDES
• Use risk taking and creativity in trying alternatives in care (e.g., skin care, ostomy management)

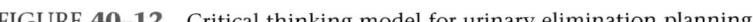

FIGURE **40–12** Critical thinking model for urinary elimination planning.

Nursing Care Plan

Functional Urinary Incontinence

Assessment

Kay, the home care nurse, is seeing Mrs. Grayson, a 75-year-old widow, at her home. Mrs. Grayson has arthritis and was referred by her physician because of urinary incontinence. She lives alone, but her daughter lives less than a 10-minute drive away. Kay's assessment included a discussion of Mrs. Grayson's current health problems with emphasis on the more recent urinary concerns.

Assessment Activities	Findings/Defining Characteristics
Ask Mrs. Grayson about the effects of her arthritis on her mobility.	She responds, "It is hard for me to get up once I'm down. Even when I'm up, I have such pain I have trouble walking."
Observe Mrs. Grayson's gait and ability to get up and down.	You observe that she has difficulty standing to an upright position. She limps on the right side. Mrs. Grayson grimaces as she walks.
Ask Mrs. Grayson about any other effects that her difficulty in walking have had.	Mrs. Grayson begins to cry and states, "You can see the plastic cover on my chair. I'm so embarrassed, sometimes I can't get out of the chair fast enough and I lose my water. I've been wearing those diapers lately."
Ask Mrs. Grayson to complete a 1- to 3-day urinary diary, with several measured voids. Establish diary format she understands and can work with.	Mrs. Grayson completes a 24-hour diary but finds it difficult to maintain for longer. Diary suggests a normal capacity bladder (two voids of 450 mL) and ability to hold urine for 4-hour intervals. Episodes of incontinence occur on way to bathroom.

Nursing Diagnosis: Functional incontinence related to impaired mobility.

Planning

Goal	Expected Outcomes*
	Urinary Continence
Client will have reduced episodes of incontinence within 1 week.	Client will report less frequent episodes of incontinence following initiation of a pattern of timed voiding.
	Independent Toileting
Client will ambulate with less discomfort within 1 week.	Client will demonstrate ability to walk comfortably with a steady gait to bathroom within 1 week.

*Outcome classification labels from *Nursing Outcomes Classification (NOC)* (3rd ed.), edited by S. Moorhead, M. Johnson, and M. L. Maas, 2004, St. Louis, MO: Mosby.

Interventions†	Rationale
Urinary Incontinence Care	
Establish interval for toileting to anticipate need for voiding based on urinary diary data. Interval may vary from 1½ to 4 hours.	Timed voiding (habit training) will empty the bladder before the usual stimuli (bladder stretch) and avoid association with inability to get to bathroom facilities in time (Lyons & Specht, 2001; Wyman, 2003).
Work with client to establish a reasonable, manageable voiding program using environmental cues to minimize or eliminate incontinence episodes.	Uncontrolled incontinence can lead to institutionalization of older adults who prefer to remain in their own homes and contributes to increased illness (urinary tract infections, skin breakdown; Gray, 2003).
Consult with physician to prescribe an alternative antiarthritic.	Reduction in joint pain will increase mobility.

†Intervention classification labels from *Nursing Interventions Classification (NIC)* (4th ed.), edited by J. M. Dochterman and G. M. Bulecheck, 2004, St. Louis, MO: Mosby.

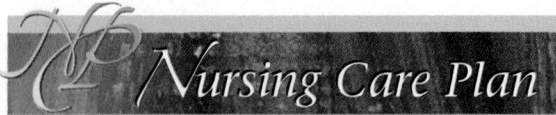

Nursing Care Plan

Functional Urinary Incontinence—cont'd

Evaluation

Nursing Actions	Client Response/Finding	Achievement of Outcome
Ask Mrs. Grayson about degree of continence since starting timed voiding.	She responds, "I'm dry most of the time now."	Mrs. Grayson reports partial success with bladder control. She is satisfied that with time her success will be complete.
Observe Mrs. Grayson's gait and ability to get up and down.	Mrs. Grayson is taking a new arthritis medication. You observe improved ambulation and ease of getting up and down.	Mrs. Grayson reports improved ambulation and increased comfort.

Concept Map

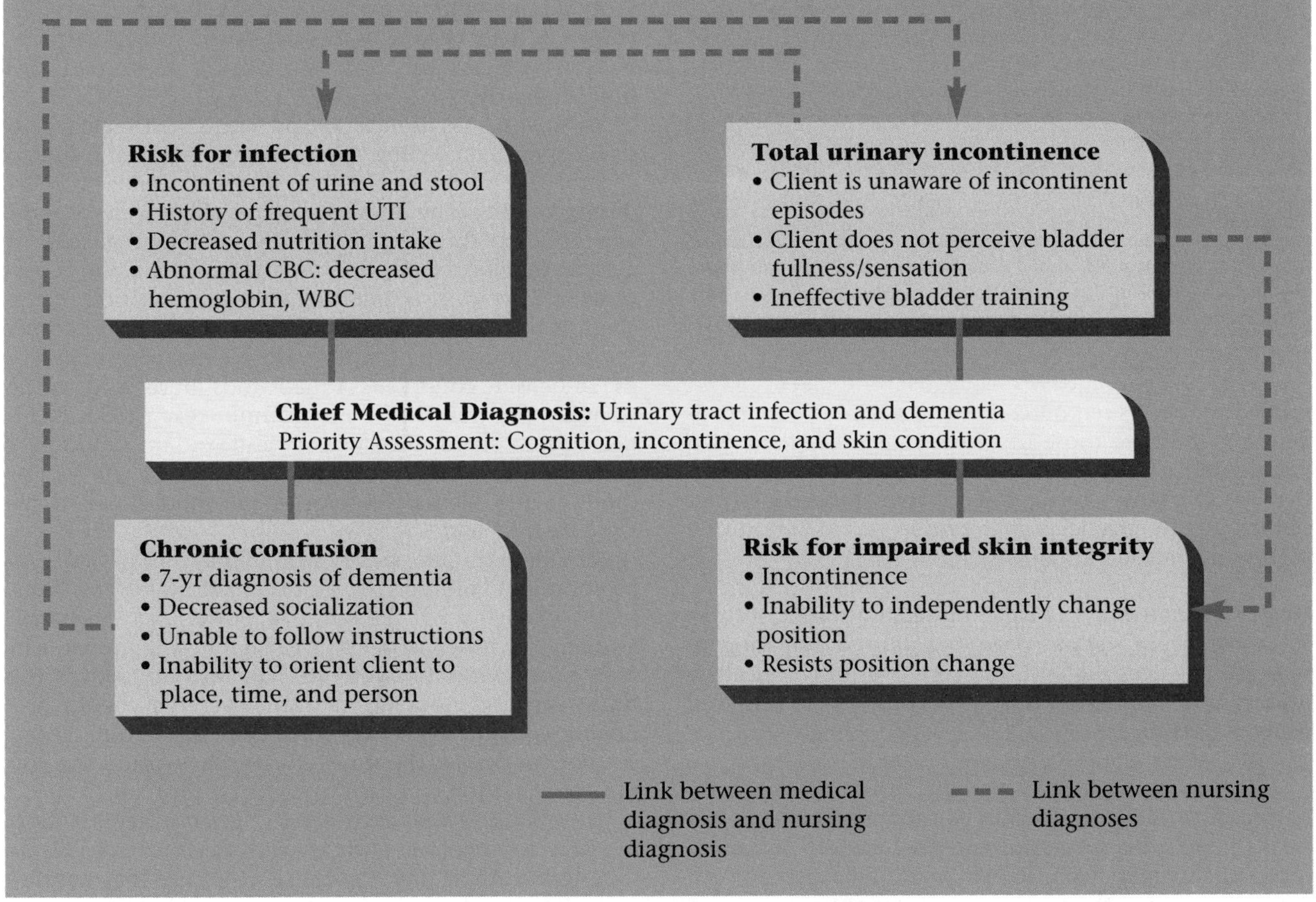
Risk for infection
• Incontinent of urine and stool
• History of frequent UTI
• Decreased nutrition intake
• Abnormal CBC: decreased hemoglobin, WBC
Total urinary incontinence
• Client is unaware of incontinent episodes
• Client does not perceive bladder fullness/sensation
• Ineffective bladder training
Chief Medical Diagnosis: Urinary tract infection and dementia
Priority Assessment: Cognition, incontinence, and skin condition
Chronic confusion
• 7-yr diagnosis of dementia
• Decreased socialization
• Unable to follow instructions
• Inability to orient client to place, time, and person
Risk for impaired skin integrity
• Incontinence
• Inability to independently change position
• Resists position change
Link between medical diagnosis and nursing diagnosis
Link between nursing diagnoses

FIGURE **40–13** Concept map for client with urinary tract infection and dementia.

Box 40-4

Focus on Primary Health Care

Urinary Incontinence

People with urinary incontinence often attempt to manage the condition on their own and do not seek professional help because they are embarrassed, they believe incontinence is a normal part of aging, or they are not aware of the treatment options. Screening for incontinence at the primary health care level should be a fundamental aspect of care provided by all nurses to overcome such barriers. Such routine screening demonstrates that it is acceptable to discuss elimination problems and provides a forum for teaching about bladder health. Health promotion topics that should be taught include the following:

- Basic education about lower urinary tract function.
- Education about promoting good bladder and bowel habits.
- Education about risk factors including smoking, caffeine, weight gain, and fluid restriction.
- Education about preventing UTIs.

When a client is experiencing urinary incontinence, the nurse at the primary health care level provides information about common causes, goals and expectations of treatment, and absorbent products available. The nurse communicates with other health care professionals (particularly the client's family physician) and is aware of how to access additional care at the secondary or tertiary care levels. The nurse is also able to perform a focused assessment that includes relevant medical and surgical history, physical examination, urinalysis, and a 24- to 72-hour bladder diary. The nurse then initiates behavioural interventions that are relevant to the nursing diagnosis.

Adapted from *Promoting a Collaborative Consumer-Focused Approach to Continence Care in Canada,* Canadian Continence Foundation, 2001; retrieved June 16, 2004, from *http://www.continence-fdn.ca*

achieving the desired outcomes and goals. The independent activities are those in which nurses use their own judgment. An example of this is teaching self-care activities to the client. Collaborative activities are those prescribed by the physician and carried out by the nurse, such as medication administration.

Health Promotion. The focus of health promotion is to assist the client in understanding and participating in self-care practices that will preserve and protect healthy urinary system function (Box 40-4). This can be achieved using several means.

Client Education. Success of therapies aimed at eliminating or minimizing urinary elimination problems depends in part on successful client education. Although many clients may need to learn about all aspects of urinary elimination, the nurse first focuses the teaching on the client's specific elimination problems. For example, clients who practise poor hygiene benefit most from learning about normal sterility of the urinary tract and ways to prevent infection. Clients also learn the significance of symptoms of urinary alterations so that early preventive health care can be initiated.

Nurses can easily incorporate teaching when giving nursing care. For example, when attempting to increase the client's fluid intake, a good time to discuss the benefits is while giving fluids with medications or meals. Teaching about perineal hygiene may be appropriate while giving a bath or performing catheter care.

Promoting Regular Micturition. Maintaining regular patterns of urinary elimination can help prevent many urination problems. Clients with urinary incontinence commonly void frequently throughout the day to avoid accidental urine loss. However, frequent voiding (at hourly intervals) may contribute to small-capacity bladders. Conversely, clients who hold their urine for long periods (more than 8 hours) may develop a hypotonic bladder with incomplete emptying. The nurse should reinforce the importance of voiding regularly (approximately every 3 to 4 hours) to help maintain a normal bladder capacity (400 to 500 mL). Because constipated stool in the rectum may compress the urethra and impede emptying, the nurse should emphasize the importance of regular bowel movements and encourage measures to enhance regularity, including diets rich in fibre (see chapter 41).

Many nursing measures have been designed to promote normal voiding in clients at risk for urination difficulties and in clients with established urination problems. The nurse can initiate many of these measures independently.

Stimulating Micturition Reflex. The client's ability to void depends on feeling the urge to urinate, being able to control the urethral sphincter, and being able to relax during voiding. The nurse can help a client learn to relax and stimulate the reflex to void by enabling the client to assume the normal position for voiding. A woman is better able to void in a squatting or sitting position. If the client is unable to use toilet facilities, the nurse positions the client in a sitting position on a bedpan (see chapter 41) or bedside commode. A man voids more easily in the standing position. If the man cannot reach toilet facilities, he may stand at the bedside and void into a urinal (a metal or plastic receptacle for urine; Figure 40–14). At times, it may be necessary for one or more nurses to assist a man in standing.

Providing certain sensory stimuli may also promote relaxation and voiding. The sound of running water helps many clients void though the power of suggestion. Stroking the inner aspect of the thigh may stimulate sensory nerves and promote the micturition reflex. The nurse can also pour warm water over the client's perineum to create the sensation to urinate. If urine output is to be measured, the nurse must first measure the volume of water to be poured over the perineal area.

Maintaining Elimination Habits. Many clients follow routines to promote normal voiding. In a hospital or long-term care facility, the nurse's routines may conflict with those of clients. Integrating clients' habits into the care plan fosters normal voiding and will assist in preventing problems related to urination.

Maintaining Adequate Fluid Intake. Clients with urinary incontinence often reduce fluid intake because they believe this will help keep them dry. In reality, maintaining an adequate fluid intake of 1500 to 2000 mL promotes

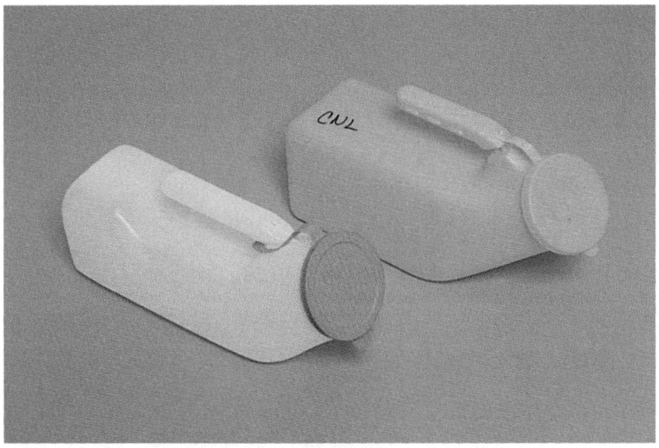

FIGURE **40–14** Types of male urinals.

continence because concentrated urine can irritate the bladder mucosa. Fluid intake should not include caffeinated beverages, which have a diuretic effect. Remind the client that many vegetables and fruits have a high fluid content and can contribute to daily fluid intake. At home, it may help to set a schedule for drinking fluids (e.g., with meals or medications). Fluids should be avoided 2 hours before bedtime to minimize nocturia.

Avoiding Food and Fluids That Can Irritate the Bladder Mucosa. The nurse teaches the client to avoid foods and fluids that may cause symptoms of urgency and frequency, including the following:

- Tobacco
- Alcohol
- Substances containing caffeine, such as coffee, tea, and chocolate
- Carbonated beverages
- Aspartame (artificial sweetener)
- Citrus fruits/juices
- Tomatoes or tomato-based products
- Greasy or spicy foods

Promoting Complete Bladder Emptying. Under normal circumstances, a small amount of urine (<50 mL) remains in the bladder after voiding (residual urine) because urinary sphincters close. Thus, people normally remain continent and dry. People with abnormal residual urine (>50 mL) are able to remain dry when their urethral closure pressure is sufficient to prevent leakage. However, urinary incontinence may occur when too much residual urine is in the bladder or when the sphincters are too weak. As well as contributing to incontinence, residual urine can provide a medium for bacterial growth.

Clients should be encouraged to take their time while voiding and be encouraged to try again when they feel they have not emptied their bladders. Those with consistently elevated post-void residual volumes may require intermittent catheterization.

Preventing Infection. One of the most important considerations for a client with urinary alterations is the need to prevent infection of the urinary system. Good perineal hygiene that includes cleaning the urethral meatus after each voiding or bowel movement is essential. Clients with limited dexterity due to such conditions as arthritis or stroke can benefit from the use of a squirt bottle with warm water to rinse the perineum after defecation.

Maintaining an adequate daily intake of fluids (1500 to 2000 mL) dilutes urine and promotes regular micturition. In contrast, very concentrated or excessively dilute urine can impair host defence mechanisms (Gray & Krissovich, 2003). Urine is normally acidic and tends to inhibit growth of micro-organisms. Meats, eggs, whole-grain breads, cranberries, and prunes increase urine acidity. Cranberry juice has been shown to lower urine pH and decrease bacterial adherence to the bladder wall (Gray, 2002).

Acute Care. Many measures can be used in the acute care setting to decrease the incidence of urinary alterations. Box 40-5 lists some of the many types of interventions for urinary incontinence.

Maintaining Elimination Habits. Clients usually require time to void. Requesting a urine specimen on demand does not contribute to relaxation and normal voiding habits. Clients should be given at least 30 minutes to provide a specimen. Clients normally void upon awakening or before meals; therefore, the nurse should offer the opportunity to use toilet facilities then. Also important is the need to promptly respond to clients' urges to urinate. Delay in assisting clients to the bathroom may interfere with normal micturition and contribute to incontinence. This is particularly the case with clients with overactive bladder.

Safety Alert. Many falls in the older adult are related to the urge to urinate. Anticipate the need and provide for scheduled bathroom visits. Make sure the pathway is clear of any barriers between the bed and the facilities.

Privacy is essential for normal voiding. If the client cannot reach the bathroom, the nurse makes sure that the bedside curtain is closed. The debilitated client at home may prefer using a bedside commode screened by a partition or room divider. Young children are often unable to void in the presence of people other than their parents.

When possible, the nurse should encourage the continued use of special measures that the client uses to void. The client may be able to relax and void more easily while reading or listening to music. Having a cup or glass of fluids may also promote urination.

Medications. Drug therapy, either alone or in combination with other therapies, can help problems of incontinence and retention. The major categories of medication are presented in Table 40-5.

Safety Alert. Alpha blockers may cause postural hypotension and increase the client's risk of fall or injury. Instruct clients taking these medications to plan their nighttime toileting and to get out of bed slowly.

Catheterization. **Catheterization** of the bladder involves introducing a narrow tube through the urethra

Box 40-5 Urinary Incontinence Treatment Options

Transient Incontinence

- Address underlying cause of incontinence (e.g., treat for infection or manage for constipation, as necessary)

Urge Incontinence

- Anticholinergic medications
- Bladder training
- Scheduled toileting
- Biofeedback
- Lifestyle modifications (e.g., selected dietary and fluid modifications)

Stress Incontinence

- Pelvic floor muscle exercises (Kegel)
- Surgery
- Artificial sphincter
- Biofeedback
- Lifestyle modifications (e.g., weight loss, smoking cessation)
- Medications (i.e., estrogen replacement)

Mixed Incontinence

- Interventions as for stress incontinence and urge incontinence

Functional Incontinence

- Habit retraining
- Environmental alterations
- Scheduled toileting
- Condom catheter (men)
- Protective undergarments

Overflow Incontinence

- Intermittent catheterization
- Surgery (i.e., for treatment of obstruction)
- In-dwelling or condom catheter

Reflex Incontinence

- Anticholinergic medications
- Surgery
- Intermittent catheterization
- In-dwelling or condom catheter
- Estrogen replacement

Total Incontinence

- Artificial sphincter
- Surgery (e.g., sling procedure)
- Urinary diversion

Table 40-5 Medications Used to Treat Urinary Incontinence and Retention

Classification	Action	Generic Name	Side Effects	Contraindications/Alerts
Anticholinergics/ antimuscarinics	Inhibit effect of acetylcholine on smooth muscle: antispasmodic	Oxybutynin Oxybutynin XL Tolterodine Tolterodine LA Propantheline bromide	Constipation Dry mouth Blurred vision Confusion and decreased cognition in older adults Retention	Narrow angle glaucoma GI obstruction Ulcerative colitis Myasthenia gravis Retention elevated residual (can be used in conjunction with intermittent catheterization)
Alpha adrenergic blockers	Block alpha-receptors to relax bladder neck/ proximal urethra and reduce symptoms of obstructive voiding	Terazosin Doxazosin Tamsulosin	Postural hypotension Syncope fainting especially first dose	Clients on antihypertensives will require dosage titration
Alpha adrenergic agents	Stimulate alpha receptors at bladder neck/ proximal urethra to increase tone and reduce stress incontinence	Pseudo-Phedrine	Hypertension Insomnia Tremor Agitation	Monoamine oxidase inhibitors Hypertension Narrow angle glaucoma Older clients
Low-dose, topical hormone replacement therapy	Reduces irritation/ atrophic vaginitis Can reduce symptoms of overactive bladder and stress incontinence	Premarin vaginal cream Estradiol ring Vagifem tab	Sore breasts Spotting (rare with very low dose)	History of endometrial, ovarian, breast cancer

Adapted from *Pharmacological Aspects of Nursing Care* (6th ed.), by B. Reiss, M. Evans, and B. Broyles, 2002, Clifton Park, NY: Delmar Learning.

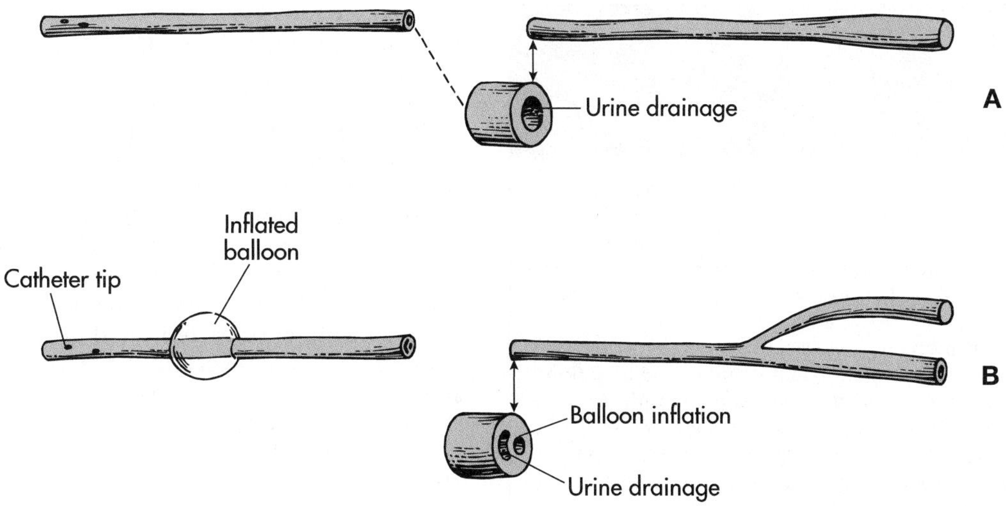

FIGURE **40–15** Types of urinary catheters. **A,** Straight catheter. **B,** In-dwelling (Foley) catheter.

Box 40-6 Indications for Catheterization

Short-Term In-dwelling Catheterization

- Obstruction to urine outflow (e.g., prostate enlargement)
- Surgical repair of bladder, urethra, and surrounding structures
- Prevention of urethral obstruction from blood clots
- Measurement of urinary output in critically ill clients
- Continuous or intermittent bladder irrigations

Long-Term In-dwelling Catheterization

- Severe urinary retention with recurrent episodes of UTI
- Skin rashes, ulcers, or wounds irritated by contact with urine
- Terminal illness when bed linen changes or toileting are painful for client

Intermittent Catheterization

- Relief of discomfort of bladder distension, provision of decompression
- Obtaining sterile urine specimen
- Assessment of residual urine after urination
- Management of urethral strictures
- Long-term management of clients with spinal cord injuries, neuromuscular degeneration, or incompetent bladders

and into the bladder to allow a continuous flow of urine into a drainage receptacle. There are numerous indications for urethral catheterization in acute, community, and long-term care settings (Box 40-6). In acute care, catheterization is particularly useful for careful monitoring of output in hemodynamically unstable clients. Because bladder catheterization carries the risk of UTI, blockage, and trauma to the urethra, it is preferable to rely on other measures for either specimen collection or management of incontinence (Getliffe, 2003).

Types of Catheterization. Catheters may be intermittent or in-dwelling (retention). With the intermittent technique, a straight single-use catheter (Figure 40–15, *A*) is introduced for 5 to 10 minutes, just long enough to drain the bladder. The straight catheter has a single lumen with a small opening about 1.3 cm from the tip. Urine drains from the tip, through the lumen, and to a receptacle. Intermittent catheterization is performed by the client or the nurse and is common in clients who have incomplete bladder emptying due to neurogenic conditions (e.g., spinal cord injury). In hospital, intermittent catheterization is sterile to reduce the risk of nosocomial infections. In the community, clients use clean intermittent catheterization technique and reuse their catheters many times. Catheters are washed with soap and water and left to air-dry until the next use. There is no evidence that UTIs are increased in people who use clean rather than sterile technique (Schlager, Clark, & Anderson, 2001).

The Coudé catheter is a type of catheter that has a curved tip and is used for male clients who have enlarged prostates that partly obstruct the urethra. It is less traumatic during insertion because it is stiffer and easier to control than the straight-tip catheter.

An in-dwelling or Foley catheter (Figure 40–15, *B*) is retained for longer periods in the bladder by means of a small balloon that anchors the catheter against the bladder neck. The catheter remains in place until the client is able to void completely and voluntarily or as long as accurate measurements are needed. In-dwelling catheters are either two lumen (most common; one lumen drains urine and the other lumen carries sterile water to inflate or deflate the balloon) or three lumen (the third lumen allows for irrigation). They can be used on a short-term or long-term basis.

Catheters also come in many different materials (latex, silicone, Teflon) and diameters. Guidelines on how to

Box 40-7 Guidelines for Appropriate Catheter Selection

- The catheter size should be determined by the size of the client's urethral canal. When the French system is used, the larger the gauge number, the larger the catheter size. Generally, children require an 8 to 10 Fr, and adults require a 14 to 16 Fr (Lewis et al., 2000). The smallest effective catheter size is preferred to prevent trauma.
- After urologic procedures (prostatectomy), a 20 to 24 Fr 3 lumen catheter is used to allow clot drainage and irrigation.
- The expected time required for the catheterization will determine the catheter material selection (Teflon- or silicone-coated latex, 100% silicone, hydrophilic-coated latex).
- Plastic catheters are suitable only for intermittent use because of their inflexibility.
- Latex and rubber catheters are recommended for use up to 3 weeks. Be aware of allergies to either of these materials.
- Pure silicon or Teflon catheters are best suited for long-term use (2 to 3 months) because they cause less encrustation at the urethral meatus.
- Silicone catheters have larger interior lumens than other catheters of the same size and may allow more efficient urine drainage.
- Hydrophilic-coated catheters may be more comfortable and less likely to inflame urethral tissue than non-hydrophilic catheters; encrustation may develop more slowly (Cox, 1990).
- For clients who develop encrustations and blockage frequently, the use of an inexpensive catheter changed every 7 to 10 days (depending on their pattern of blockage) may be more economical.
- For short-term use, silver-hydrogel catheters and catheters with anti-infective surfaces are effective in delaying the onset of bacteriuria.
- Balloon size is also important to consider when selecting an indwelling catheter. Balloon sizes range from 3 mL (pediatric) to large post-operative volumes (30 mL). In adults, the 5-mL size allows for optimal drainage, whereas the 30-mL size is used after prostatectomies to provide hemostasis of the prostatic bed (Lewis et al., 2000).
- Only sterile water should be used to inflate the balloon because saline may crystallize, resulting in incomplete deflation of the balloon at the time of removal.
- Leakage of urine around the catheter may be due to bladder spasms secondary to constipation or fecal impaction, a large catheter balloon (30 mL), large catheter (>18 Fr), urinary tract infection, kinking of the catheter, or trauma at the bladder neck from traction on the balloon. A change in lumen size, use of anticholinergic medication, or referral to urologist may be warranted.

make appropriate decisions regarding catheter selection are provided in Box 40-7.

Catheter Insertion. Urethral catheterization of any type requires a physician's order. The nurse must use strict aseptic technique (see chapter 29). Organizing equipment before the procedure prevents interruptions. The steps for inserting in-dwelling and single-use straight catheters are basically the same. The difference lies in the procedure taken to inflate the in-dwelling catheter balloon and secure the catheter. Skill 40-2 lists the steps for inserting in-dwelling and single-use straight catheters in both men and women.

Closed Drainage Systems. After inserting an in-dwelling catheter, the nurse maintains a closed urinary drainage system to minimize the risk of infection. Urinary drainage bags are plastic and can hold about 1000 to 1500 mL of urine. The drainage bag should never be raised above the level of the client's bladder. The bag should hang on the bed frame or wheelchair without touching the floor. Urine in the bag and tubing can become a medium for bacteria, and infection is likely to develop if urine flows back into the bladder. Therefore, do not hang the bag on the bed rail because it can be accidentally raised above the level of the bladder. When the client ambulates, the drainage bag must be held below the client's waist.

If the catheter must be disconnected from the drainage tubing, both tips should be cleansed with an alcohol swab before being reconnected to minimize the transfer of organisms into the tubing.

Most drainage bags contain an anti-reflux valve to prevent urine in the bag from re-entering the drainage tubing and contaminating the client's bladder. A spigot at the base of the bag is used to empty the bag. The spigot should always be clamped, except during emptying, and tucked into the protective pouch on the side of the bag (see agency policy). To keep the drainage system patent, the nurse checks for kinks or bends in the tubing, avoids positioning the client on the drainage tubing, and observes for clots or sediment that may occlude the collecting tubing.

Routine Catheter Care. Clients with in-dwelling catheters have a number of special care needs. Nursing measures are directed at maintaining client comfort, preventing infection, and maintaining unobstructed flow of urine.

Perineal Hygiene. Buildup of secretions or **encrustation** at the catheter insertion site is a source of irritation and potential infection. Nurses provide perineal hygiene (see chapter 34) at least twice daily, after a bowel movement, or as needed for a client with an in-dwelling catheter. Soap and water or skin cleansers are effective in reducing the number or organisms around the urethra and help to maintain skin health and client comfort. The nurse must not accidentally advance the catheter up into the bladder during cleansing or risk introducing bacteria.

Catheter Care. In addition to routine perineal hygiene, many institutions recommend that clients with catheters receive special care three times a day and after defecation or bowel incontinence to help minimize discomfort and infection (Skill 40-3).

Fluid Intake. All clients with catheters should have a daily intake of 2000 to 2500 mL if permitted. This can be met through oral intake or intravenous infusion. A high fluid intake produces a large volume of urine that flushes the bladder and keeps catheter tubing free of sediment.

Preventing Infection. The most important strategy in preventing the onset of infection is performing hand hygiene between clients. Maintaining a closed urinary drainage system is also important (Maki & Tambyah, 2001). A break in the system can lead to introduction of micro-organisms. Sites at risk are the site of catheter insertion, the

Text continued on p. 1371

Skill 40-2 Inserting a Straight or In-dwelling Catheter

View Video

Delegation Considerations

Catheterization is not usually delegated to unregulated care providers (UCPs). However, in some settings, agency policy may permit this skill to be delegated to UCPs who have been properly instructed.

- UCPs routinely assist with positioning the client and maintaining client privacy and comfort, empty urine from the collection bag, and provide perineal care.
- Instruct the UCP to report client discomfort or fever to the nurse.
- Instruct the UCP to report abnormal colour, odour, and amount of urine in drainage bag to the nurse.

Equipment

Catheterization kit containing the following sterile items:

- Gloves (extra pair optional)
- Drapes, one fenestrated
- Lubricant
- Antiseptic cleansing solution
- Cotton balls
- Forceps
- Prefilled syringe with sterile water to inflate the balloon of in-dwelling catheter
- Catheter of correct size and type for procedure (i.e., intermittent or in-dwelling)
- Sterile drainage tubing with collection bag and multipurpose tube holder or tape, safety pin, and elastic band for securing tubing to bed if client is bed bound (for in-dwelling catheter)
- Receptacle or basin (usually bottom of catheterization tray)
- Specimen container
- Blanket

Steps	Rationale
1. Review client's medical record, including physician's order and nurses' notes.	Determines purpose of inserting catheter: preparation for surgery, urinary irrigations, collection of sterile specimens, measurement of residual urine, and size and style of catheter. Assess for previous catheterization, including catheter size, response of client, and time of last catheterization.
2. Close curtain or door.	Offers privacy, reduces embarrassment, and aids in relaxation during procedure.
3. Assess status of client:	
a. Ask client when last voided, or check I&O flow sheet, or palpate bladder.	Determines time of last voiding or potential for bladder fullness.
b. Level of awareness or developmental stage.	Reveals the client's ability to co-operate and level of explanation needed.
c. Mobility and physical limitations of client.	Affect the way that the nurse positions client.
d. Client's gender and age.	Determines catheter size: 8 to 10 Fr is generally used for children, 14 to 16 Fr is indicated for adults, 12 Fr may be considered for young girls.
e. Distended bladder.	Causes pain. Can indicate need to insert catheter if client is unable to void independently.
f. Perform hand hygiene. Inspect perineum for erythema, drainage, and odour.	Reduces infection. Determines condition of the perineum.
g. Any pathological condition that may impair passage of catheter (e.g., enlarged prostate in men).	Obstruction prevents passage of catheter through urethra into the bladder. May require use of coude catheter.
h. Allergies	Procedure risks exposure to antiseptic, tape, latex, and lubricant. Betadine allergies are common; if the client is unaware of allergy, ask if allergic to shellfish.
4. Assess client's knowledge of the purpose for catheterization.	Reveals need for client instruction.
5. Explain procedure to client.	Promotes co-operation.
6. Arrange for extra nursing personnel to assist as necessary.	Client may be unable to assume positioning for procedure.
7. Perform hand hygiene.	Reduces transmission of micro-organisms.
8. Raise bed to appropriate working height.	Promotes use of proper body mechanics.
9. Facing client, stand on left side of bed if right-handed (on right side of bed if left-handed). Clear the bedside table and arrange equipment.	Successful catheter insertion requires nurse to assume comfortable position with all equipment easily accessible.
10. Raise side rail on opposite side of bed, and put side rail down on working side.	Promotes client safety.

Skill 40-2 Inserting a Straight or In-dwelling Catheter—cont'd

Steps	Rationale
11. Place waterproof pad under client.	Prevents soiling of bed linen.
12. Position client	
A. Female client	
(1) Assist to dorsal recumbent position (supine with knees flexed). Ask client to relax thighs so that the hips can be externally rotated.	Provides good visualization of perineal structures. Legs may be supported with pillows to reduce muscle tension and promote comfort.
(2) Position female client in side-lying (Sims') position with upper leg flexed at hip if unable to assume dorsal recumbent position. If this position is used, nurse must take extra precautions to cover rectal area with drape to reduce chance of cross-contamination.	This alternate position is used if client cannot abduct leg at hip joint (e.g., if client has arthritic joints). Support client with pillows if necessary to maintain position.
B. Male client	
(1) Assist to supine position with thighs slightly abducted.	Comfortable position for client that aids in visualization.
13. Drape client.	Avoids unnecessary exposure of body parts and maintains client's comfort.
A. Female client (see illustration)	
(1) Drape with bath blanket. Place blanket diamond fashion over client, with one corner at client's midsection, side corners over each thigh and abdomen, and last corner over perineum.	
B. Male client (see illustration)	
(1) Drape upper trunk with bath blanket, and cover lower extremities with bed sheets, exposing only genitalia.	

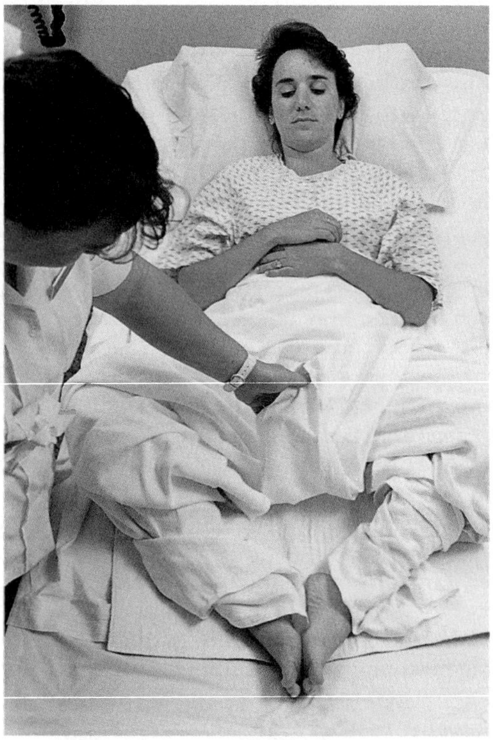

STEP **13A** Draping technique (female).

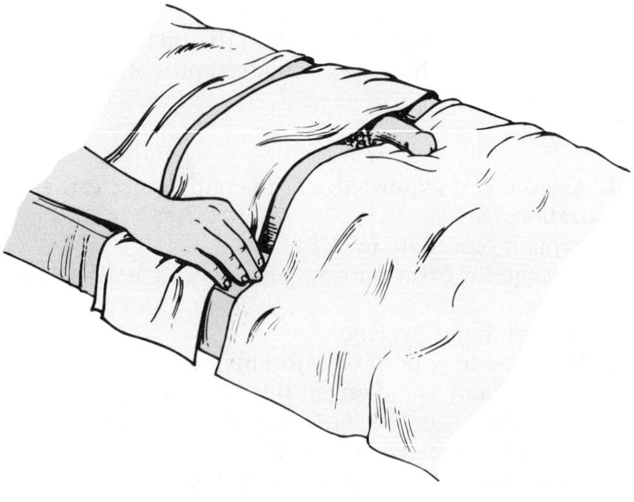

STEP **13B** Draping technique (male).

Steps	Rationale
14. Wearing disposable gloves, wash perineal area with soap and water as needed; dry thoroughly. Remove and discard gloves; perform hand hygiene.	Reduces micro-organisms near urethral meatus and allows further opportunity to visualize perineum and landmarks.
15. Position lamp to illuminate perineal area. (When using flashlight, have an assistant hold it.)	Permits accurate identification and good visualization of urethral meatus.
16. Open package containing drainage system; place drainage bag over edge of bottom bed frame, and bring drainage tube up between side rails and mattress.	Prepare system for eventual connection with catheter.

Critical Decision Point: This step is necessary only when an in-dwelling catheter is to be inserted and drainage system is not part of the catheterization kit.

Steps	Rationale
17. Open catheterization kit according to directions, keeping bottom of container sterile.	Prevents transmission of micro-organisms from table or work area to sterile supplies. The materials in the kit are arranged in sequence of use.
18. Place plastic bag that contained kit within reach of work area to use as a waterproof bag to dispose of used supplies.	
19. Apply sterile gloves (see chapter 29).	Allows nurse to handle sterile supplies without contamination.

Critical Decision Point: If underpad is first item in kit, place pad plastic side down under client, touching only the edges so as to maintain sterility. Then apply sterile gloves.

Steps	Rationale
20. Organize supplies on sterile field. Open inner sterile package containing catheter. Pour sterile antiseptic solution into correct compartment containing sterile cotton balls. Open packet containing lubricant. Remove specimen container (lid should be placed loosely on top) and prefilled syringe from collection compartment of tray, and set them aside on sterile field.	Maintains principles of surgical asepsis and organizes work area.
21. Before inserting in-dwelling catheter, test balloon by injecting fluid from prefilled syringe into balloon port (see illustration).	Checks integrity of balloon. Do not use the catheter if the balloon does not inflate or leaks.
22. Lubricate 2.5 to 5 cm of catheter for women and 12.5 to 17.7 cm for men.	

Critical Decision Point: Some catheters will have a plastic sheath over the catheter that must be removed before lubrication. In some cases, the physician may order local anaesthetic lubricant.

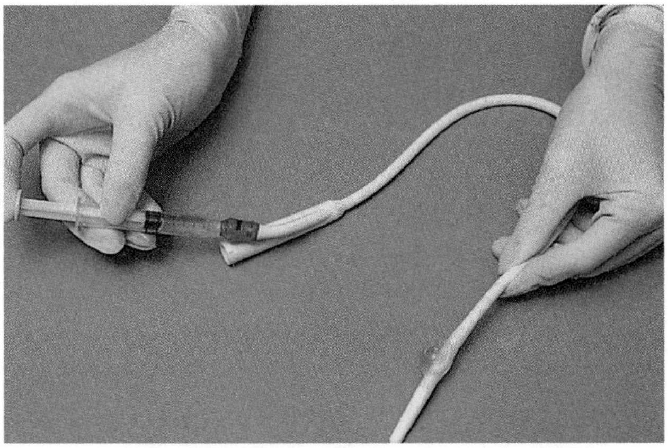

STEP **21** Checking balloon (in-dwelling catheter).

Skill 40-2 Inserting a Straight or In-dwelling Catheter—cont'd

Steps	Rationale
23. Apply sterile drape:	
A. Female client	
(1) Allow top edge of drape to form a cuff over both gloved hands. Place drape down on bed between client's thighs. Slip cuffed edge just under buttocks, taking care not to touch contaminated surface with gloves.	Outer surface of drape covering hands remains sterile. Sterile drape against sterile gloves is sterile.
(2) Pick up fenestrated sterile drape, and allow it to unfold without touching an unsterile object. Apply drape over perineum, exposing labia, and being sure not to touch contaminated surface.	Maintains sterility of work surface.
B. Male client	
(1) Two methods are used for draping, depending on preference. *First method:* Apply drape over thighs and under penis without completely opening fenestrated drape. *Second method:* Apply drape over thighs just below penis. Pick up fenestrated sterile drape, allow it to unfold, and drape it over penis with fenestrated slit resting over penis.	Maintains sterility of work surface.
24. Place sterile tray and contents on sterile drape. Open specimen container.	Provides easy access to supplies during catheter insertion. Maintains aseptic technique during procedure.
25. Cleanse urethral meatus:	
A. Female client	
(1) With non-dominant hand, carefully retract labia to fully expose urethral meatus. Maintain position of non-dominant hand throughout procedure.	Full visualization of urethral meatus is provided. Full retraction prevents contamination of urethral meatus during cleansing.
(2) Using forceps in sterile dominant hand, pick up cotton ball saturated with antiseptic solution and clean perineal area, wiping from front to back from clitoris toward anus. Using a new cotton ball for each area, wipe along the far labial fold, near labial fold, and directly over centre of urethral meatus (see illustration).	Cleansing reduces number of micro-organisms at urethral meatus. Use of a single cotton ball for each wipe prevents transfer of micro-organisms. Cleansing proceeds from area of least contamination to that of most contamination. Dominant hand remains sterile.

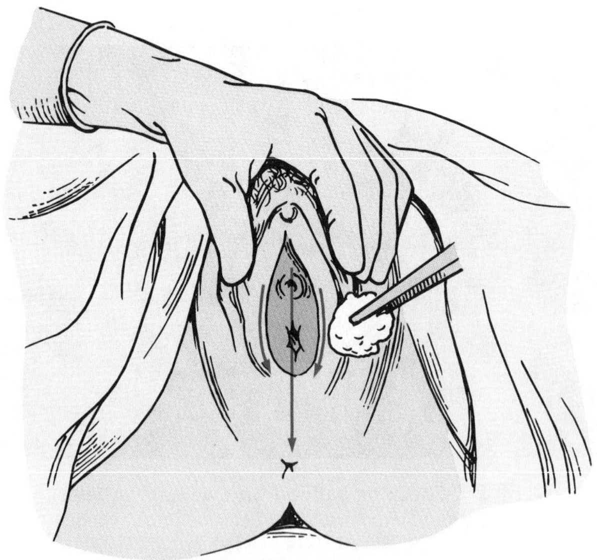

STEP **25A(2)** Cleansing technique (female).

Steps	Rationale

Critical Decision Point: Closure of labia during cleansing requires that the cleansing procedure be repeated because the area has become contaminated.

Steps	Rationale
B. Male client	
(1) If client is not circumcised, retract foreskin with non-dominant hand. Grasp penis at shaft just below glans. Retract urethral meatus between thumb and forefinger. Maintain non-dominant hand in this position throughout procedure.	Accidental release of foreskin or dropping of penis during cleansing requires process to be repeated because area has become contaminated.
(2) With dominant hand, pick up cotton ball with forceps and clean penis. Move in a circular motion from urethral meatus down to base of glans. Repeat cleansing three more times, using a clean cotton ball each time (see illustration).	Reduces number of micro-organisms at urethral meatus and moves from area of least to most contamination. Dominant hand remains sterile.

Critical Decision Point: If foreskin does not remain retracted during insertion, then the cleansing process must be repeated because the area has become contaminated.

Steps	Rationale
26. Pick up catheter with gloved dominant hand 7.5 to 10 cm from catheter tip. Hold end of catheter loosely coiled in palm of dominant hand. (Optional: May grasp catheter with forceps.)	
27. Insert catheter:	
A. Female client	
(1) Ask client to bear down gently as if to void, and slowly insert catheter through urethral meatus (see illustration).	Relaxation of urethral sphincter and pelvic floor muscle aids in insertion of catheter.
(2) Advance catheter a total of 5 to 7.5 cm in adult or until urine flows out of catheter's end. When urine appears, advance catheter another 2.5 to 5 cm. **Do not force against resistance.**	Female urethra is short. Appearance of urine indicates that catheter tip is in bladder or lower urethra. Advancement of catheter ensures bladder placement.
(3) Release labia, and hold catheter securely with non-dominant hand. Slowly inflate balloon if in-dwelling catheter is used (see illustrations; see step 30).	Bladder or sphincter contraction may cause accidental expulsion of catheter.

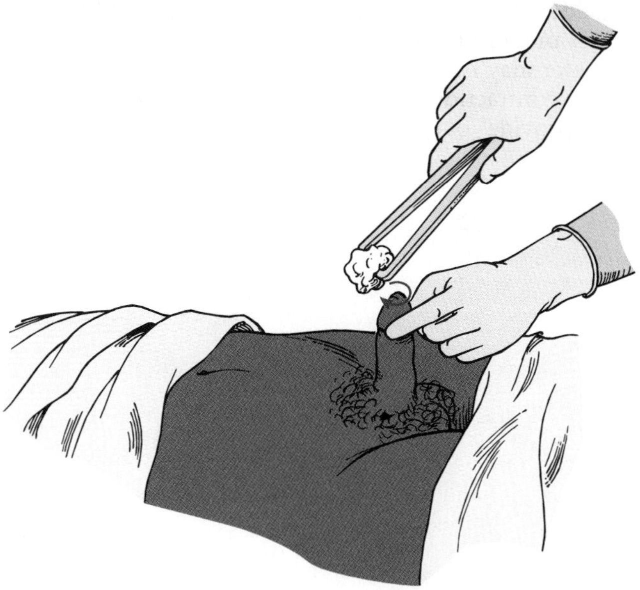

STEP **25B(2)** Cleansing technique (male).

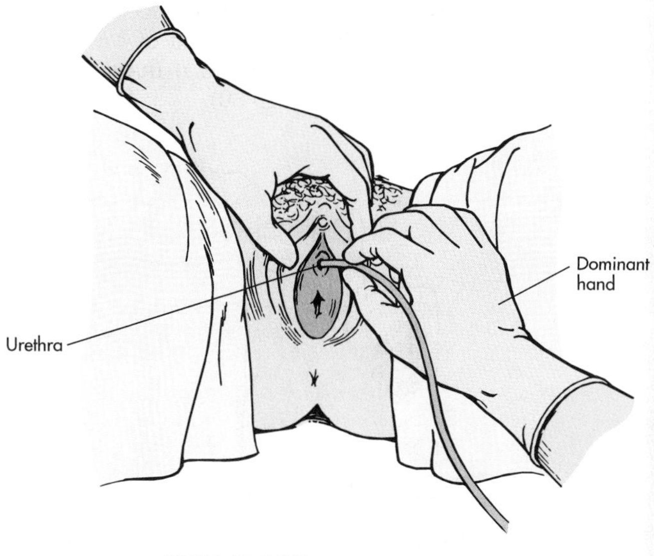

STEP **27A(1)** Inserting the catheter.

Skill 40-2 Inserting a Straight or In-dwelling Catheter—cont'd

Steps	Rationale

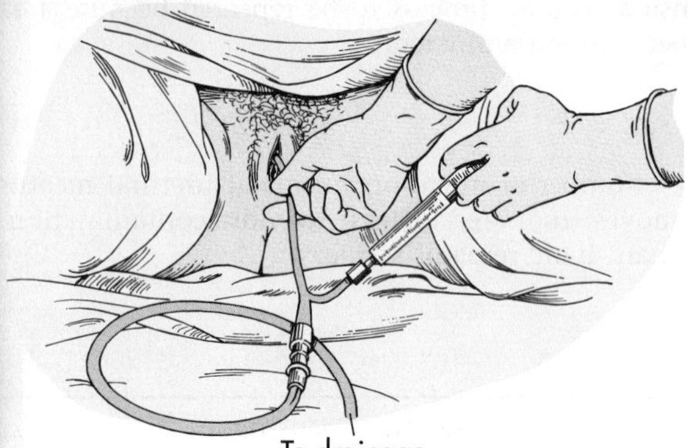

STEP **27A(3)** Inflating the balloon (in-dwelling catheter).

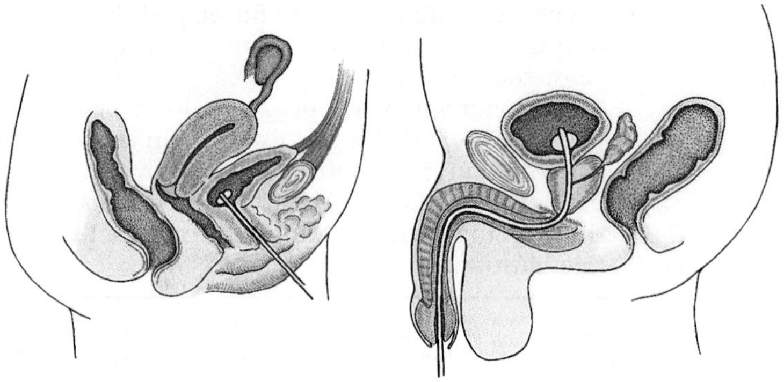

STEP **27A(3)** Placement of inflated balloon in bladder.

Critical Decision Point: If no urine appears, check if catheter is in vagina. If misplaced, leave catheter in vagina as landmark indicating where not to insert, and insert another.

B. Male client

Steps	Rationale
(1) Lift penis to position perpendicular to client's body and apply light traction (see illustration).	Straightens urethral canal to ease catheter insertion.
(2) Ask client to bear down as if to void, and slowly insert catheter through urethral meatus.	Relaxation of urethral sphincter and pelvic floor muscle aids in insertion of catheter.
(3) Advance catheter 17 to 22.5 cm in adult or until urine flows out catheter's end. If resistance is felt, withdraw catheter; do not force it through urethra. When urine appears, advance catheter another 2.5 to 5 cm. **Do not use force against resistance.**	The adult male urethra is long. It is normal to meet resistance at the prostate. When resistance is met, nurse should hold catheter firmly without forcing it. After a few seconds, the muscle relaxes, and the catheter is advanced. Appearance of urine indicates catheter tip is in bladder or urethra. Further advancement of catheter ensures proper placement.
(4) Lower penis and hold catheter securely in non-dominant hand. Place end of catheter in urine tray. Inflate balloon if in-dwelling catheter is used (see step 30).	Catheter may be accidentally expelled by bladder or urethral contraction. Collection of urine prevents soiling and provides output measurement.

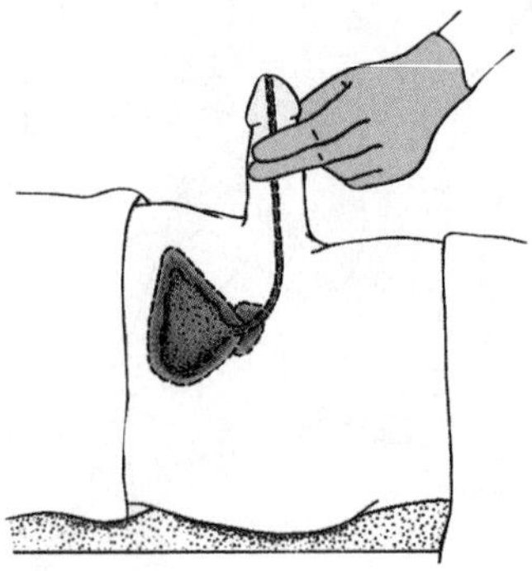

STEP **27B(1)** Position penis perpendicular to body for catheter insertion.

Steps	Rationale
(5) Reduce (or reposition) the foreskin.	Paraphimosis (retraction and constriction of the foreskin behind the glans penis) secondary to catheterization may occur if foreskin is not reduced.
28. Collect urine specimen as needed. Fill specimen cup or jar to desired level (20 to 30 mL) by holding end of catheter in dominant hand over cup.	Allows sterile specimen to be obtained for culture analysis.
29. Allow bladder to empty fully (about 800 to 1000 mL) unless institution policy restricts maximal volume of urine to drain with each catheterization. Check institution policy before beginning catheterization.	As always, the nurse should monitor the client's condition, and if the vital signs change or bleeding occurs, temporarily stop the flow of urine and continue when the client's condition warrants. Retained urine may serve as a reservoir for growth of micro-organisms.

Critical Decision Point: If a straight, single-use catheter was inserted, withdraw it slowly, but smoothly until it is removed.

Steps	Rationale
30. Inflate balloon fully per manufacturer's recommendation and then release catheter with non-dominant hand and pull gently.	Inflation of balloon anchors catheter tip in place above the bladder outlet to prevent removal of the catheter. Note size of balloon on catheter. Most commonly, a 5-mL balloon is used, but a 30-mL balloon may be ordered in some cases. A prefilled syringe may be included with the kit. Use only the amount included. Do not overinflate the balloon.

Critical Decision Point: If resistance to inflation is noted or client complains of pain, the balloon may not be entirely in the bladder. Stop inflation, aspirate the fluid injected into the balloon and advance the catheter a little more before attempting to inflate the balloon again.

Steps	Rationale
31. Attach end of in-dwelling catheter to collecting tube of drainage system. Drainage bag must be below level of bladder; attach bag to bed frame, do not place bag on side rails of bed (see illustration).	
32. Anchor catheter:	
A. Female client	
(1) Secure catheter tubing to inner thigh or abdomen with strip of non-allergenic tape (or multi-purpose tube holders with a Velcro strap). Allow for slack so that movement of thigh does not create tension on catheter (see illustration).	Anchoring catheter to inner thigh reduces pressure on urethra, thus reducing possibility of tissue injury.

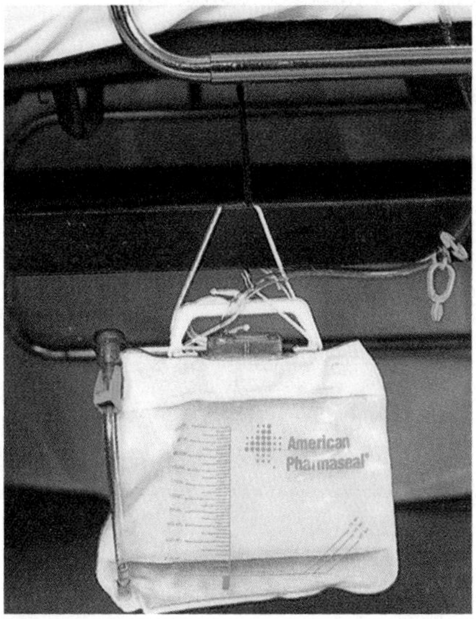

STEP **31** Attach drainage to lower bed frame.

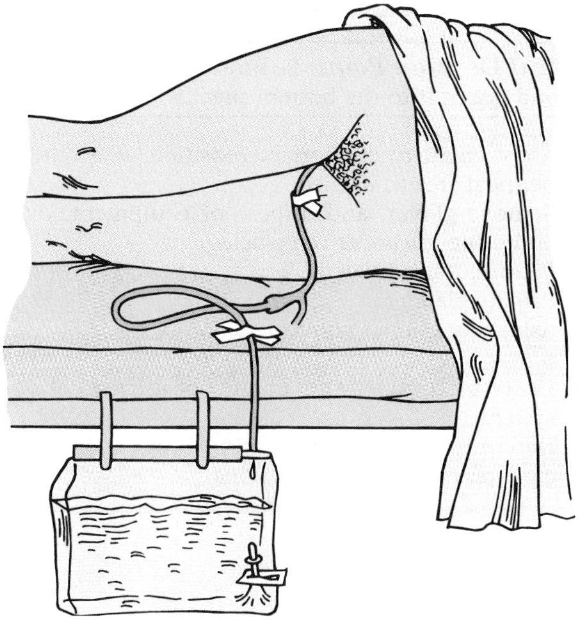

STEP **32A(1)** Tape catheter to inner thigh (female) and coil extra tubing on bed and attach to sheet.

Skill 40-2 *Inserting a Straight or In-dwelling Catheter—cont'd*

Steps	Rationale

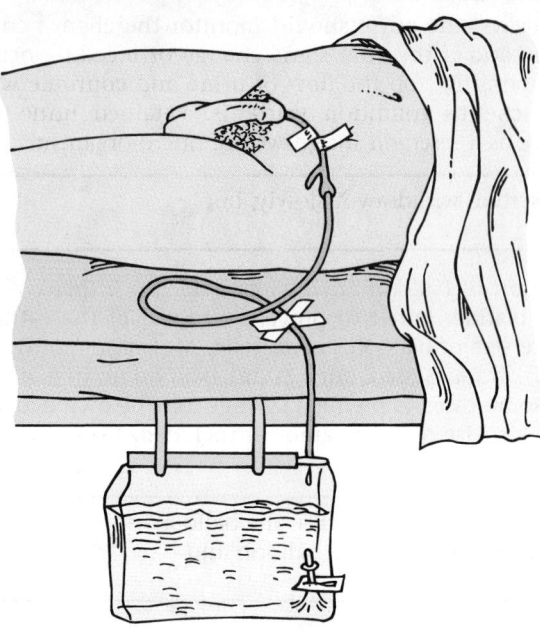

STEP **32B(1)** Tape catheter to lower abdomen (male) and coil extra tubing on bed and attach to sheet.

Steps	Rationale
B. Male client	
(1) Secure catheter tubing to top of thigh or lower abdomen (with penis directed toward chest). Allow slack in catheter so that movement does not create tension on catheter (see illustration).	Anchoring catheter to lower abdomen reduces pressure on urethra at junction of penis and scrotum, thus reducing possibility of tissue injury.

Critical Decision Point: Be sure that there are no obstructions in tubing. Coil excess tubing on bed and fasten it to the bottom sheet with clip from kit or use rubber band and safety pin.

Steps	Rationale
33. Assist client to comfortable position. Wash and dry perineal area as needed.	Maintains comfort and security.
34. Remove gloves, and dispose of equipment, drapes, and urine in proper receptacles.	Reduces transmission of micro-organisms.
35. Perform hand hygiene.	Reduces transmission of micro-organisms.
36. Palpate bladder.	Determines if distension is relieved.
37. Ask about client's comfort.	Determines if client's sensation of discomfort or fullness has been relieved.
38. Observe character and amount of urine in drainage system.	Determines if urine is flowing adequately.
39. Determine that there is no urine leaking from catheter or tubing connections.	Prevents injury to client's skin.

Unexpected Outcomes and Related Interventions

- Urethral or perineal irritation is present.
  - Observe for catheter leaking; replace if necessary.
  - Assess that in-dwelling catheter is anchored properly.
  - Perform perineal hygiene and catheter care more frequently.
- Client has fever and/or odour is present, or client experiences small frequent voidings, burning, or bleeding on voiding.
  - Obtain clean voided urine specimen.
  - Notify physician.
- Client experiences urinary retention and is unable to void after catheter is removed.
  - Provide adequate fluid intake and ensure client privacy.
  - If client unable to void 6 to 8 hours following catheter removal, notify physician.

Recording and Reporting

- Report and record type and size of catheter inserted, amount of fluid used to inflate the balloon, characteristics of urine, amount of urine, reasons for catheterization, specimen collection if appropriate, and client's response to procedure and teaching concepts.
- Initiate I&O record.
- If catheter is definitely in bladder and no urine is produced within an hour, absence of urine should be immediately reported to physician.

Home Care Considerations

- Clients who are at home may use a leg bag during the day and switch to a large-volume bag at night so that sleep can be uninterrupted.
- Clients may catheterize themselves at home using a clean technique.

Skill 40-3 In-dwelling Catheter Care

View Video

Delegation Considerations

Perineal care is often part of routine hygiene care that is delegated to unregulated care providers (UCPs). Proper assessment and care of the perineal area will need professional clinical judgment. If the client has had trauma or surgical procedures that involve the perineal area, this care should not be delegated.

- Instruct the UCP to report client discomfort, perineal pain, perineal discharge, and/or odour to the nurse.

Equipment

- Catheter care kit or individual supplies
  - Disposable gloves
  - Cotton balls or large swabs
  - Clean washcloth and towel
  - Warm water and soap
  - Antibiotic ointment (if agency policy)
- Bath blanket
- Waterproof absorbent pad

Steps	Rationale
1. Assess for episode of bowel incontinence or client discomfort or provide care as per agency routine as part of hygiene measures (see chapter 34).	Accumulation of secretions or feces causes irritation to perineal tissues and acts as a source of bacterial growth.
2. Explain procedure to client. Offer opportunity to perform self-care to able client.	Reduces anxiety and promotes co-operation. Embarrassment may motivate client to perform own hygiene.
3. Close door or bedside curtain.	Maintains client privacy.
4. Perform hand hygiene.	Reduces transmission of infection.
5. Position client:	
A. Female	
(1) Dorsal recumbent position	Ensures easy access to perineal tissues.
B. Male	
(1) Supine or Fowler's position	
6. Place waterproof pad under client.	Protects bed linens from soiling.
7. Drape bath blanket on client so that only perineal area is exposed.	Prevents unnecessary exposure of body parts.
8. Apply gloves.	
9. Remove anchor device to free catheter tubing.	

Skill 40-3 In-dwelling Catheter Care—cont'd

Steps	Rationale
10. With non-dominant hand:	
A. Female	
(1) Gently retract labia to fully expose urethral meatus and catheter insertion site, maintaining position of hand throughout procedure.	Provides full visualization of urethral meatus. Full retraction prevents contamination of meatus during cleansing.
B. Male	
(1) Retract foreskin if not circumcised, and hold penis at shaft just below glans, maintaining position throughout procedure.	Accidental closure of labia or dropping of penis during cleansing requires procedure to be repeated.
11. Assess urethral meatus and surrounding tissue for inflammation, swelling, and discharge. Note amount, colour, odour, and consistency of discharge. Ask client if any burning or discomfort is felt.	Determines presence of local infection and status of hygiene.
12. Cleanse perineal tissue:	
A. Female	
(1) Use clean cloth, soap, and water. Cleanse around urethral meatus and catheter. Cleaning from pubis toward anus, clean labia minora. Use a clean side of cloth for each wipe. Finally, clean around anus. Dry each area well.	Reduces the number of micro-organisms at urethral meatus. Use of clean cloth prevents transfer of micro-organisms.
B. Male	
(1) While spreading urethral meatus, cleanse around catheter first, and then wipe in circular motion around meatus and glans.	Cleansing moves from area of least to most contamination.
13. Reassess urethral meatus for discharge.	Determines if cleansing is complete.
14. With towel, soap, and water, wipe in a circular motion along length of catheter for 10 cm.	Reduces presence of secretions or drainage on exterior of catheter surface.
15. Apply an antibiotic ointment at urethral meatus and along 2.5 cm of catheter if ordered by physician or part of agency policy.	Further reduces growth of micro-organisms at insertion site.
16. In male client, reduce (or reposition) the foreskin.	
17. Place client in a safe, comfortable position.	Promotes comfort.
18. Dispose of contaminated supplies, remove gloves, and perform hand hygiene.	Prevents spread of infection.

Unexpected Outcomes and Related Interventions

- Urethral discharge
  - Increase frequency of in-dwelling catheter care.
  - Apply topical antibiotic ointment per agency policy.
  - Notify physician.
- Accidental catheter dislodgement
  - Notify physician.
  - Assess for urethral trauma.
  - Monitor urine output.

Recording and Reporting

- Report and record presence and characteristics of drainage, condition of perineal tissue, and any discomfort reported by client.
- If infection is suspected, report findings to physician.

Home Care Considerations

- If client is discharged with in-dwelling catheter, the client and family should be taught catheter care and signs and symptoms to report to nurse or physician.

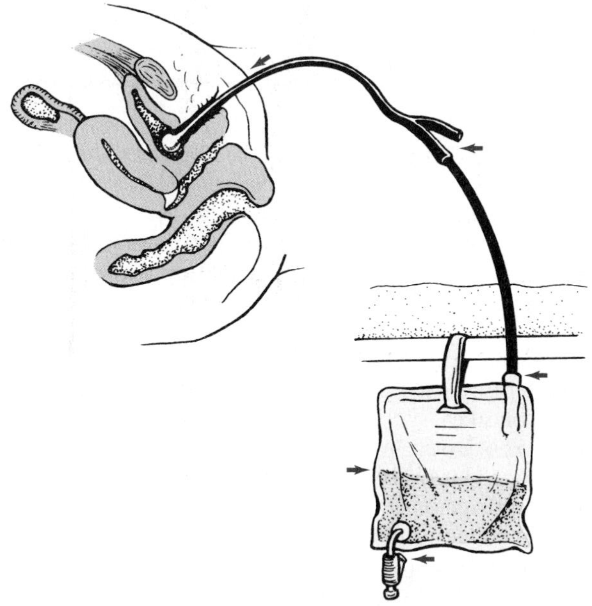

FIGURE **40–16** Potential sites for introduction of infectious organisms into a urinary drainage system.

drainage bag, the spigot, the tube junction, and the junction of the tube and the bag (Figure 40–16).

In addition, the nurse monitors the patency of the system to prevent pooling of urine within the tubing. Bacteria can travel up drainage tubing to grow in pools of urine. If this urine flows back into the client's bladder, an infection will likely develop (Kunin, 2001). The nurse observes the client for symptoms of UTI and documents any changes in condition. Suggestions for ways to prevent infections in catheterized clients are provided in Box 40-8.

Catheter Irrigations and Instillations. To maintain patency of in-dwelling urinary catheters, the nurse may sometimes need to irrigate or flush a catheter. Blood, pus, or sediment can collect within tubing and result in bladder distension and the buildup of stagnant urine. Instillation of a sterile solution ordered by the physician clears the tubing of accumulated material. For clients with bladder infections, a physician may order antiseptic or antibiotic bladder irrigations to wash out the bladder or treat local infection. In both irrigations, sterile aseptic technique is followed.

Before performing catheter irrigation, the nurse assesses the catheter for blockage. If the amount of urine in the drainage bag is less than the client's intake or less than the output during the previous shift, blockage can be expected. If urine does not drain freely, the nurse may milk the tubing. Milking is done by gently squeezing then releasing the drainage tube, starting from the client and working to the drainage bag so that a clot or sediment will not be forced back into the catheter.

Maintenance of a closed system is recommended during intermittent irrigations or instillations. This technique is effective for irrigating a partially blocked catheter or for bladder instillations. A single intermittent irrigation is safer and less likely to introduce infections into the urinary tract than repeated irrigations. There are two additional methods for catheter irrigation. One is a closed bladder irrigation system (Skill 40-4). This system provides for frequent intermittent irrigations or continuous irrigation without disruption of the sterile catheter system through use of a three-way catheter. This method is used most often in clients who have had genitourinary surgery and are at risk for blood clots and mucus fragments occluding the catheter. The other system involves opening the closed drainage system to instill bladder irrigations (see Skill 40-4). This technique poses greater risk for causing infection. However, it may be needed when catheters become blocked and it is undesirable to change the catheter (e.g., after recent bladder or prostate surgery).

Removal of In-dwelling Catheter. When removing an in-dwelling catheter, the nurse promotes normal bladder function and prevents trauma to the urethra.

To remove a catheter, the nurse requires a clean, disposable towel; a discard receptacle; a sterile syringe that is the same size as the volume of solution within the catheter's inflated balloon; and disposable gloves. The end of the catheter contains a label that denotes the volume of solution (5 to 30 mL) within the balloon.

The nurse positions the client in the same position as during catheterization. Some institutions recommend collecting a sterile urine specimen at this time or sending the catheter tip for culture and sensitivity tests. After removing the tape, the nurse places the towel between a female client's thighs or over a male client's thighs. The nurse inserts the syringe into the injection port. Most ports are self-sealing and require that only the tip of the

Text continued on p. 1375

Box 40-8 Preventing Infection in Catheterized Clients

- Follow good hand-hygiene techniques (see chapter 29).
- Do not allow the spigot on the drainage system to touch a contaminated surface.
- Only use sterile technique to collect specimens from a closed drainage system.
- If the drainage tube becomes disconnected, wipe the end of the tubing and catheter with an antimicrobial solution before reconnecting.
- Ensure that each client has a separate receptacle for measuring urine to prevent cross-contamination.
- Prevent pooling of urine in the tubing and reflux of urine into the bladder.
- If it is necessary to raise the bag during transfer of the client to a bed or stretcher, clamp the tubing for the transfer.
- Provide for drainage of urine from the tubing to the bag by positioning the tubing.
- Avoid prolonged kinking or clamping of the tubing.
- Empty the drainage bag at least every 8 hours and record output. If large outputs are noted, empty more frequently.
- Encourage fluid intake (if not contraindicated).
- Remove the catheter as soon as clinically warranted (Kunin, 2001).
- Tape or secure the catheter appropriately for the client (see Skill 40-2).
- Perform routine perineal hygiene per agency policy and after defecation or bowel incontinence (see Skill 40-3).

Skill 40-4 *Closed and Open Catheter Irrigation*

Delegation Considerations

Although closed catheter irrigation carries less risk of infection, neither closed nor open catheter irrigation are usually delegated to unregulated care providers (UCPs). Catheter irrigation is usually done in clients with complications such as urinary tract infections or post-surgically after prostatectomy.

- UCPs may assist with other aspects of client care, such as positioning and measuring intake and output.
- Instruct the UCP to report complaints of pain, discomfort, or fever to the nurse.
- Instruct the UCP to report the presence of clots in the output or a change in output to the nurse.

Equipment

- **Closed intermittent method**
  - Sterile irrigation solution at room temperature
  - Sterile graduated container
  - Sterile 30- to 50-mL syringe
  - Sterile 19- to 22-gauge 2.5-cm needle
  - Antiseptic swab
  - Clamp for catheter or tubing
  - Bath blanket
- **Closed continuous method**
  - Sterile irrigation solution at room temperature
  - Irrigation tubing and clamp (with or without Y connector)
  - IV pole
  - Y connector (optional)
  - Antiseptic swab
  - Bath blanket
- **Open method**
  - Sterile irrigation set with tray
  - Bulb syringe or 60-mL piston-type syringe
  - Sterile collection basin
  - Waterproof drape
  - Sterile solution container
  - Antiseptic swabs
  - Sterile gloves
  - Sterile correct irrigation solution at room temperature
  - Tape or elastic band to resecure catheter
  - Bath blanket

Steps	Rationale
1. Assess physician's order for type of irrigation and irrigation solution to use.	Ensures proper selection of equipment.
2. Assess colour of urine and presence of mucus or sediment.	Determines if client is bleeding, has infection, or is sloughing tissue.
3. Determine type of catheter in place:	
a. Triple lumen (one lumen to inflate balloon, one to instill irrigation solution, one to allow outflow of urine).	Indicates method for irrigation.
b. Double lumen (one lumen to inflate balloon, one to allow outflow of urine).	
4. Determine patency of drainage tubing.	Ensures that drainage tubing is not kinked, clamped incorrectly, or looped.
5. Assess amount of urine in drainage bag (may want to empty drainage bag before irrigation).	If not empty, will need to subtract urine volume from amount drained to determine if all irrigant returned.
6. Explain procedure and purpose to client.	Helps client relax and co-operate during procedure.
7. Perform hand hygiene and apply disposable gloves for closed methods.	Prevents transmission of micro-organisms.
8. Provide privacy by pulling bed curtains closed. Fold back covers so that catheter is exposed. Cover client's upper torso with bath blanket.	Promotes client comfort.
9. Assess lower abdomen for bladder distension.	Detects whether catheter is malfunctioning or blocking urinary drainage.
10. Position client in dorsal recumbent or supine position.	Promotes client comfort and provides easy access to catheter. Promotes flow of irrigating solution into bladder.
11. Closed intermittent irrigation:	
a. Prepare prescribed sterile solution in sterile graduated cup.	Ensures that irrigating fluid remains sterile.
b. Draw sterile solution into syringe using aseptic technique.	

Steps	Rationale

Critical Decision Point: Avoid cold solution as irrigant because it may result in bladder spasm and discomfort.

Steps	Rationale
c. Clamp in-dwelling catheter just below soft injection port.	Occlusion of catheter provides resistance against which irrigant can be forcefully instilled into catheter.
d. Cleanse injection port with antiseptic swab (same port used for specimen collection).	Reduces transmission of infection.
e. Insert needle of syringe through port at 30-degree angle toward bladder.	Ensures that needle tip enters lumen of catheter and flow is directed into bladder.
f. Slowly inject fluid into catheter and bladder.	Slow, continuous pressure dislodges clots and sediment without traumatizing bladder wall.

Critical Decision Point: If catheter does not irrigate easily, the tip may be incorrectly placed in the urethra and not in the bladder. Use slow pressure when injecting fluid. Too much pressure may traumatize the urethal or bladder wall.

Steps	Rationale
g. Withdraw syringe, remove clamp, and allow solution to drain into drainage bag. If ordered by physician, keep clamped to allow solution to remain in bladder for short time (20 to 30 minutes).	Allows drainage by gravity.

Critical Decision Point: If solution is to remain in bladder, do not forget to unclamp tubing at the end of the instillation period.

Steps	Rationale
12. Closed continuous irrigation (see illustration):	
a. Using aseptic technique, insert tip of sterile irrigation tubing into bag of sterile irrigating solution.	Prevents entrance of micro-organisms.
b. Close clamp on tubing and hang bag of solution on IV pole.	

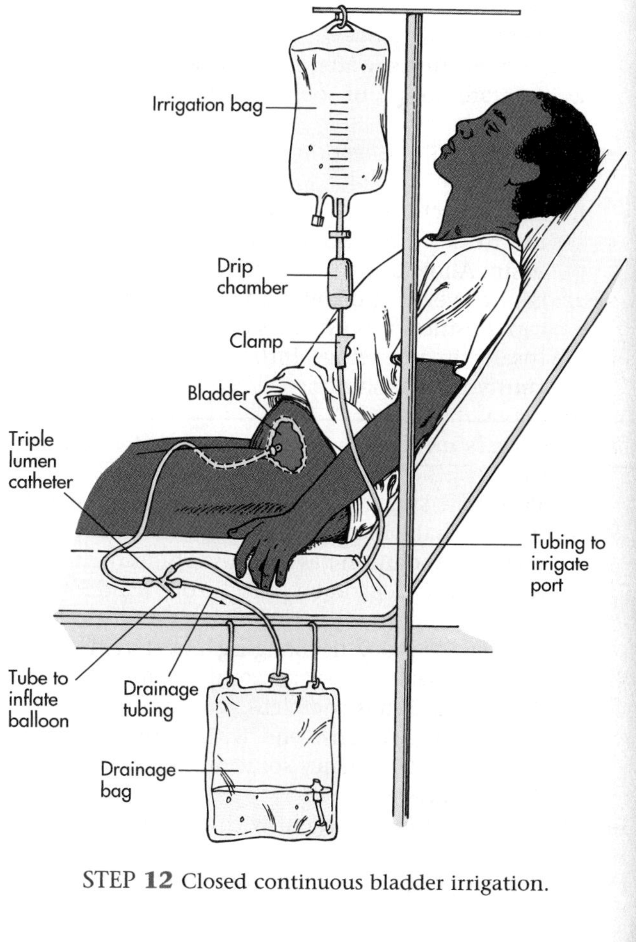

STEP **12** Closed continuous bladder irrigation.

Skill 40-4 Closed and Open Catheter Irrigation—cont'd

Steps	Rationale
c. Open clamp and allow solution to flow through tubing, keeping end of tubing sterile. Close clamp.	Removes air from tubing.
d. Wipe off irrigation port of triple lumen catheter, or attach sterile Y connector to double lumen catheter and then attach to irrigation tubing.	Third lumen or Y connector provides means for irrigation solution to enter bladder. System must remain sterile.
e. Be sure that drainage bag and tubing are securely connected to drainage port of triple lumen catheter or other arm of Y connector.	Ensures that urine and irrigation solution will drain from bladder.
f. For intermittent flow, clamp tubing on drainage system, open clamp on irrigation tubing, and allow prescribed amount of fluid to enter bladder (100 mL is normal for adults). Close irrigation clamp, and then open drainage tubing clamp. (Optional: Leave clamp closed for 20 to 30 minutes if ordered. See previous Critical Decision Point.)	Fluid instills through catheter into bladder, flushing system. Fluid drains out after irrigation is completed.
g. For continuous drainage, calculate drip rate and adjust clamp on irrigation tubing accordingly. Be sure that clamp on drainage tubing is open, and check volume of drainage in drainage bag. Make sure drainage tubing is patent, and avoid kinks.	Ensures continuous, even irrigation of catheter system. Prevents accumulation of solution in bladder, which may cause bladder distension and possible injury.
13. Open irrigation (when double lumen catheter is in place):	
a. Open sterile irrigation tray, establish sterile field, pour required volume of sterile solution into sterile container, and replace cap on large container of solution.	Adheres to principles of surgical asepsis (see chapter 29).
b. Apply sterile gloves.	Reduces transmission of infection.
c. Position sterile waterproof drape under catheter.	Prevents soiling of bed linens.
d. Aspirate 30 mL of solution into sterile irrigating syringe.	Prepares irrigant for instillation into catheter.
e. Move sterile collection close to client's thighs.	Prevents soiling of bed linen and prohibits reaching over sterile field.
f. Disconnect catheter from drainage tubing, allowing urine from catheter to flow into collection basin. Allow urine in tubing to flow into drainage bag. Cover end of tubing with sterile protective cap. Position tubing in a safe place.	Maintains sterility of inner aspect of catheter and drainage tubing and reduces potential of introducing pathogens into bladder.
g. Insert tip of syringe into catheter lumen, and gently instill solution.	Gentle instillation reduces incidence of bladder spasm but clears catheter of obstruction.

Critical Decision Point: If resistance is noted, do not force the irrigation.

Steps	Rationale
h. Withdraw syringe, lower catheter, and allow solution to drain into basin. Repeat instillation until prescribed solution has been used or until drainage is clear (will depend on purpose of irrigation).	Allows drainage to flow by gravity. Provides for adequate flushing of catheter.
i. If solution does not return, have client turn onto side facing you. If changing position does not help, reinsert syringe and gently aspirate solution.	Change of position may move catheter tip in bladder, increasing likelihood that fluid instilled will flow out.
j. After irrigation is complete, remove protector cap from tubing, cleanse end with alcohol swab (or recommended agency solution), and re-establish drainage system.	Reduces entrance of micro-organisms into system.
14. Re-anchor catheter to client with tape or elastic tube holder.	Prevents trauma to urethral tissue.
15. Assist client to comfortable position.	Promotes relaxation and rest.

Steps	Rationale
16. Lower bed to lowest position. Put side rails up if appropriate.	Promotes client safety.
17. Dispose of contaminated supplies, remove gloves, and perform hand hygiene.	Prevents spread of infection.
18. Calculate fluid used to irrigate bladder and catheter and subtract from total output.	Determines accurate urinary output.
19. Assess characteristics of output: viscosity, colour, and presence of matter (e.g., sediment, clots, blood).	Evaluates results of irrigation.

Unexpected Outcomes and Related Interventions

- Irrigating solution does not return or is not flowing at a prescribed rate, which may indicate possible occlusion of catheter.
  - Examine tubing for kinks, clots, or urine sediment.
  - Notify physician if irrigant is retained, client complains of pain, or bladder is distended.
- Cloudy or foul urine, fever
  - Monitor fever.
  - Notify physician.
  - Obtain sterile urine specimen if ordered by physician.
- Increase in bladder spasms; may indicate occlusion of catheter with foreign object (e.g., blood clot)
  - Notify physician.
  - May be instructed to perform intermittent irrigations until clots clear.

Recording and Reporting

- Record type and amount of irrigation solution used, amount returned as drainage, and the character of drainage.
- Record and report any findings such as complaints of bladder spasms, inability to instill fluid into bladder, and/or presence of blood clots.

Home Care Considerations

- If client is discharged with in-dwelling catheter and requires bladder irrigations, either the client or the family must be properly instructed.
- In the home, it is most likely that open irrigation will be required. Because this method carries the highest risk of contamination, the nurse must assess the level of understanding of surgical asepsis by the client and family.

syringe be inserted. The nurse slowly withdraws all of the solution to deflate the balloon totally. If a portion of the solution remains, the partially inflated balloon will traumatize the urethral canal as the catheter is removed. After deflation, the nurse explains that the client may feel a burning sensation as the catheter is withdrawn. The nurse then pulls the catheter out smoothly and slowly.

It is normal for the client to experience some dysuria, especially if the catheter has been in place several days or weeks. Until the bladder regains full tone, the client may also experience urinary frequency or retention.

The nurse assesses the client's urinary function by noting the first voiding after catheter removal and documenting the time and amount of voiding for the next 24 hours. If amounts are small, frequent assessment of bladder distension is necessary. If 8 hours have elapsed without voiding or the client experiences discomfort, it may become necessary to reinsert the catheter.

Alternatives to Urethral Catheterization. There are two alternatives for urinary drainage to avoid the risks associated with catheters inserted through the urethra: suprapubic and condom catheters.

Suprapubic Catheterization. **Suprapubic catheterization** involves surgical placement of a catheter through the abdominal wall above the symphysis pubis and into the urinary bladder. The physician performs the procedure under local or general anaesthesia. The catheter is anchored in place with sutures, a commercially prepared body seal, or both. Urine drains into a urinary drainage bag. Maintenance of the tubing and drainage bag is the same as for an in-dwelling catheter. The suprapubic catheter is relatively painless and reduces the incidence of infection commonly seen with in-dwelling catheters. Women who have undergone a vaginal hysterectomy may also benefit temporarily from the insertion of a suprapubic catheter after surgery.

Sediment, clots, encrustations, or the abdominal wall itself can block the suprapubic catheter. Adequate fluid intake will help to minimize risk of blockage by sediment or infection from stagnation. The suprapubic catheter must remain patent at all times. Nurses must monitor the client's I&O carefully, monitor the appearance of urine, and observe for signs of infection (e.g., fever and chills). The nurse also administers skin care around the insertion site

Condom Catheters. The second alternative to catheterization is the condom catheter (external urinary catheter; Box 40-9), which may be suitable for incontinent or comatose men who still have complete and spontaneous bladder emptying. The condom is a soft, pliable, rubber sheath that slips over the penis. It may be worn at night only or continuously, depending on the client's needs. One method to secure the condom catheter involves

Box 40-9 Procedural Guidelines

Condom Catheter

Equipment: Condom catheter (may come with self-adhesive or elastic adhesive), collection bag, basin with warm water, towel and washcloth, disposable gloves, scissors.

Delegation Considerations: The skill of applying a condom catheter can be delegated to unregulated care providers (UCPs). The registered nurse (RN) is responsible for assessing the condition of the penis over time. The RN informs the UCP to notify the RN of signs of skin irritation or swelling of tissues.

1. Check physician's order.
2. Perform hand hygiene.
3. Assess urinary elimination patterns, client's ability to voluntarily urinate, and continence.
4. Assess mental status of client so that appropriate teaching related to condom catheter care can be implemented.
5. Assess condition of penis and scrotum.
6. Assess client's knowledge of the purpose of the condom catheter.
7. Explain procedure to client.
8. Raise bed to working height and raise far upper side rail.
9. Using sheet, drape client so that only genitals are exposed.
10. Prepare condom catheter and drainage system (see manufacturer's directions).
11. Apply gloves and provide perineal care.
    a. If needed, clip hair at base of penile shaft.
12. Apply skin preparation to penile shaft and allow to dry.
13. Holding penis in non-dominant hand, apply condom by rolling smoothly onto penis. NOTE: Leave a 2.5- to 5-cm space between tip of penis and end of catheter (see illustration).
14. Secure condom catheter:
    a. If using elastic adhesive, wrap the strip of adhesive over the condom catheter to secure it in place by using a spiral technique (see illustration). NOTE: Adhesive tape must never be used.
    b. For self-adhesive catheter, follow manufacturer's directions.
15. Attach catheter to drainage bag and attach drainage bag to lower bed frame.
16. Make client comfortable.
17. Observe urinary drainage, drainage tube patency, condition of penis, and tape placement.

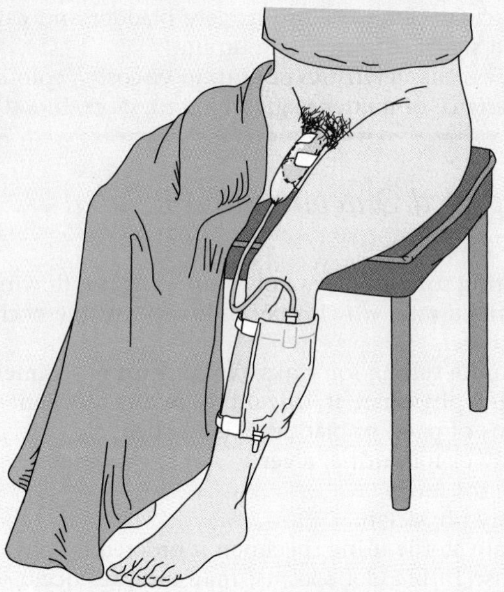

STEP **13** Distance between end of penis and tip of catheter.

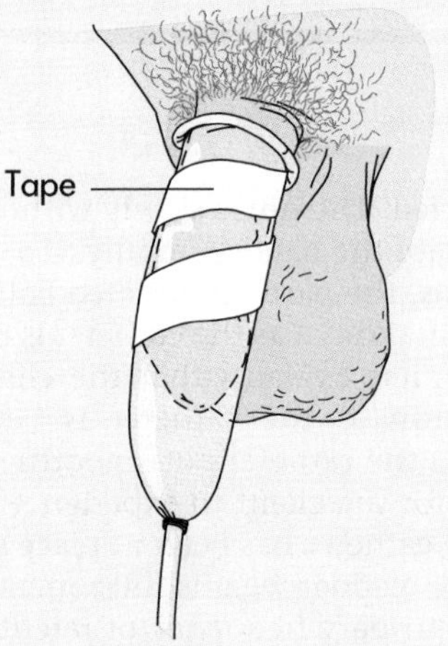

STEP **14A** Elastic tape is applied in spiral fashion to secure the condom catheter to the penis.

using a strip of elastic tape or rubber that encircles the top of the condom to secure it in place. An alternative securing method is to use a self-adhesive condom sheath. Care must be taken to ensure that whatever type or size of condom is used, blood supply to the penis is not impaired. Standard adhesive tape should never be used to secure a condom catheter because it does not expand with change in penis size and is painful to remove.

The end of the condom is attached to plastic drainage tubing that can be attached to the side of the bed or strapped to the client's leg. The condom catheter itself poses little risk of infection. Infections usually result from buildup of secretions around the urethra, trauma to the urethral meatus, or buildup of pressure in the outflow tubing. External catheters must be applied and changed according the manufacturers' directions to prevent abrasion, dermatitis, ischemia, necrosis, edema, and maceration of the penis. Frequent skin assessment is vital.

If the condom catheter is made of opaque material, the nurse should remove it daily to check for skin irritation.

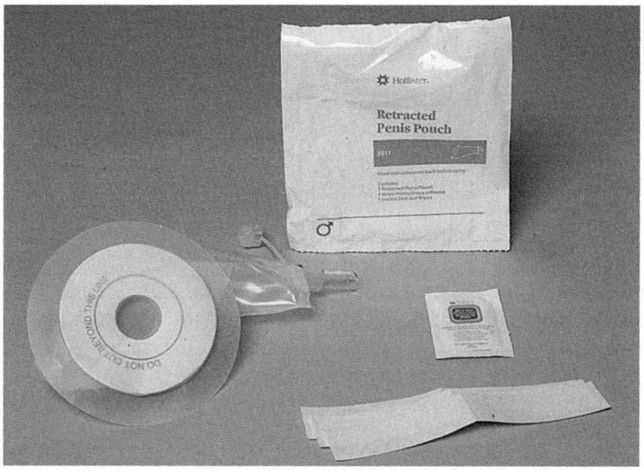

FIGURE **40–17** Retracted penis pouch external urinary device.

Some new condom catheters are transparent, and the skin may be observed through them more easily. With each catheter change, the nurse thoroughly cleans the urethral meatus and penis. The drainage tubing must be checked often for patency.

For a man with a retracted penis, maintaining a conventional external catheter may prove difficult. Special devices are available to help alleviate this problem (Figure 40–17). Manufacturer's guidelines for product application should be consulted.

There are no collection devices for women as effective as the condom catheter is for men; usually the only incontinent devices used are pads and protective clothing. To maintain the client's dignity, pads and protective clothing should not be referred to as adult diapers, and they should be changed frequently to control odour. These devices should be only used temporarily to minimize or prevent episodes of incontinence while treatment is ongoing. Clients should be monitored frequently and good skin care given to prevent irritation caused by urine.

Maintenance of Skin Integrity. Urine is irritating to skin and in continuous contact with the skin becomes alkaline, causing dermatitis and skin breakdown. Continuous exposure of the perineal area or skin around an ostomy leads to gradual maceration and excoriation (see chapter 43). Washing with pH balanced soap and warm water is the best way to remove urine. Body lotion keeps skin moisturized and petroleum-based ointments provide a barrier to the urine. Clients who soil their clothing should receive partial baths and dry clothing and linen immediately after voiding. If the skin becomes irritated or inflamed, the physician may prescribe a cream or spray containing steroids to reduce inflammation. If fungal growth develops, the antifungal drug nystatin, available in cream or powder, is effective.

Promotion of Comfort. Clients with urinary alterations become uncomfortable as a result of the symptoms of urinary problems. Frequent or unpredictable voiding, dysuria, and painful distension are sources of discomfort.

If the client has local discomfort, a warm sitz bath may soothe inflamed tissues near the urethral meatus by improving blood supply. The client is often relaxed after a sitz bath, and voiding occurs easily. Pain of distension cannot be relieved unless the client is able to empty the bladder. Interventions that stimulate micturition or intermittent catheterization may be the only sources of pain relief.

Restorative Care. The following measures may help the incontinent client gain control over urination and are part of restorative and rehabilitative care:

- Learning exercises to strengthen the pelvic floor
- Initiating a voiding schedule
- Using methods to initiate voiding (e.g., running water and stroking the inner thigh)
- Using methods to relax to aid complete bladder emptying (e.g., reading and deep breathing)
- Never ignoring the urge to void (if problem involves infrequent voidings that result in retention)
- Minimizing tea, coffee, other caffeine drinks, and alcohol
- Taking prescribed diuretic medication or fluids that increase diuresis (such as tea or coffee) early in the morning
- Progressively lengthening or shortening periods between voiding as appropriate for control of specific cause of incontinence
- Offering protective undergarments to contain urine and reduce the client's embarrassment (not diapers)
- Following a weight-control program if obesity is a problem
- Providing positive reinforcement when continence is maintained

Numerous therapies can help restore normal urinary voiding function, including surgical, pharmacological, and behavioural options. Behavioural therapies should be the first line of treatment because they are generally noninvasive and have few side effects. Behavioural therapies include lifestyle modification, pelvic floor muscle exercise, bladder training, habit retraining, and prompted voiding (RNAO, 2005). Because all of these therapies require change in daily lifestyle and ongoing adherence to maintain improvement, it is important that the nurse provides support and follow-up to enhance motivation. Cognitive strategies such as educational/motivational audio tapes can also be helpful for the client who is coping with incontinence at home (Box 40-10). If behavioural therapies do not eliminate the urinary alteration, then self-catheterization may restore a measure of control to the client.

Lifestyle Modification. Several lifestyle factors have been associated with urinary incontinence. Smoking has been associated with increased risk of moderate to severe incontinence, likely due to the chronic cough experienced by smokers (Dallosso et al., 2003; Hannestad et al., 2000). Increased weight, particularly in obese and moderately obese individuals, is believed to increase intra-pelvic pressure, and, in one study, women who lost an average of 15 kg experienced a 51% reduction in incontinent episodes (Subak et al., 2002). Caffeine has been indicated

Research Highlight — Box 40-10

Cognitive Measures for Bladder Control

Research Focus

Alterations in urine elimination often include urinary leakage and/or frequency that cause discomfort for clients. Skin breakdown is a common condition resulting from consistent exposure of the skin to urine. Falls may occur secondary to clients' need to use toilet facilities. Because these urinary problems are often manageable by cognitive strategies, research has been done to determine the best methods to use.

Research Abstract

The purpose of this study was to determine if the introduction of an audio tape with reinforcing cognitive strategies would be successful in enhancing the comfort and quality of life for clients with urinary incontinence and/or frequency. Dowd et al. (2000) investigated the use of cognitive strategies with two groups of adults with a history of incontinence and/or frequency. Thirty-one women and nine men entered into the study and were randomly assigned to the treatment group or the control group. Both groups received education about bladder health and recorded incontinence and/or frequency episodes in the urinary diary, but only the treatment group listened to an audio tape that contained relaxation, music, and cognitive strategies. The verbal side of the tape contained instructions for relaxation followed by cognitive strategy statements. These statements focused on concepts of self and on specific aspects of bladder management. Statements such as "I am not alone; many other men and women have loss of urine and are okay" were designed to enhance social comfort. The statements "being physically fit is important" and "I often tighten and relax the muscles that control my urine flow" were designed to enhance physical comfort. Other statements reinforced concepts such as the effect of fluids on output and how to manage the urge to void. Music was on the second side of the tape. Comfort was measured at four intervals during the study using the Urinary Incontinence and Frequency Comfort Questionnaire. The results demonstrated that self-report of increased comfort and decreased urinary episodes were significant, with the treatment group having better results. In addition, after the control group was given the audio-tape treatment, their levels of comfort and episodes of incontinence and/or frequency approximated the levels of the original treatment group.

Evidence-Based Practice

- Incontinence and/or frequency are experienced by adults of all ages, educational levels, economic status, and health status.
- Many adults wrongly believe that urinary incontinence and/or frequency are an expected part of the aging process.
- Clients who take an active part in their management of bladder control have improved self-esteem and fewer physical complications such as skin breakdown.
- Nurses can support the use of this inexpensive non-pharmacological intervention to enhance comfort in community-based and selected institutionalized older adults.

Reference

Dowd, T., Kolcaba, K., Steiner, R. (2000). Using cognitive strategies to enhance bladder control and comfort. *Holistic Nursing Practice, 14*(2), 91–103.

as a risk factor for individuals with overactive bladder, and may irritate the bladder mucosa and cause involuntary detrusor contractions in some clients (Arya, Myers, & Jackson, 2000; Bryant, Dowell, & Fairbrother, 2002). The nurse can play an important role in educating, counselling, and supporting the client to enable lifestyle modification that reduces risk factors for incontinence.

Pelvic Floor Muscle Exercise. **Pelvic floor muscle exercises (PFMEs),** also known as **Kegel exercises,** improve the strength of PFMs and consist of repetitive contractions of muscle groups (Thompson & Smith, 2002). These exercises have demonstrated effectiveness in treating stress incontinence, overactive bladders, and mixed cause of urinary incontinence (Sampselle, 2003). A client begins these exercises during voiding to learn the technique. They are then practised at non-voiding times. Improvement is usually gradual. Clients should be alert and motivated to perform the exercises. The client must continue to use these exercises to maintain effectiveness (Box 40-11). These exercises are non-invasive and carry a low risk of adverse effects. Clients should be aware that it may take 16 to 20 weeks to notice appreciable change, and that improvement in incontinence will depend on both proper and longer-term performance of the exercises.

Bladder Training. The goal of bladder training is to gradually increase the interval between voids and to decrease voiding frequency during waking and sleeping hours (Sampselle, 2003). The overall purpose is to increase bladder capacity and restore a normal pattern of voiding. For bladder training to be successful, clients must be alert, motivated, and physically able to follow a training program. The program includes education, scheduled voiding, and positive reinforcement.

The first step is establishing a baseline. The client and/or caregiver complete a urinary diary to assess maximum voiding intervals. It is not uncommon for the client with frequency or overactive bladder to void small amounts hourly or more often. An initial training schedule for such a client might involve a voiding schedule of every 75 minutes while awake, increasing every 1 to 3 weeks by 15-minute increments toward a 3-hour schedule. The rate of incremental changes will depend on the individual's progress and ability to adhere to a rigid schedule. Urge-suppression techniques, such as counting backward from 100 when the urge to void is felt, are helpful. The

Client Teaching — Box 40-11

Pelvic Floor Muscle Exercises (Kegels)

Objectives

Client will achieve continence or experience fewer episodes of incontinence through increased pelvic floor muscle tone and strength.

Teaching Strategies

- Explain the method to identify proper muscle contraction: female client sits on toilet with knees far apart and tightens muscles to stop the flow of urine; male client tries to stop the flow of urine midstream.
- After muscle is identified, instruct client to sit or stand without tensing muscles of legs, buttocks, back, or abdomen. Remind the client to breathe during the exercise.
- Instruct client to gradually contract the pelvic floor muscle and hold for 3 to 10 seconds, and then to gradually relax the muscle for an equal time period. The client should repeat this exercise at least two or three times, and work up to 10 repetitions as the exercise becomes easier. The client should do this about two to three times a day, or as often as possible.
- Explain that within first week of exercises, the client should assess if proper muscle contraction is occurring by placing two fingers in the vagina (or for men, one finger in the rectum) while contracting the pelvic floor muscle. The client should feel tightening in the vagina or anus during the contraction.
- Teach client and caregiver to keep a 1- to 3-day urinary diary to identify changes in patterns of urinary elimination.

Evaluation

- Ask client if he or she has identified pelvic floor muscle via finger insertion.
- During vaginal or rectal (male) bimanual examination, ask client to do exercises and assess muscle tone.
- Monitor client's urinary diary.
- Ask client and caregiver about degree of satisfaction related to control achieved in urinary elimination.

nurse must be aware that the client who has experienced an episode of incontinence in public will be particularly hesitant to deter voiding for even brief periods.

Habit Retraining and Prompted Voiding. **Habit retraining** and **prompted voiding** are useful strategies for clients with cognitive and/or physical impairment who rely on caregiver assistance. Habit retraining involves assessment of a client's normal pattern of voiding to establish a toileting schedule that pre-empts incontinence (Ostaszkiewicz, Johnston, & Roe, 2004). Such individualized toileting schedules have demonstrated effectiveness, but are labour-intensive. The nurse helps the client to the bathroom before incontinent episodes occur. Fluids and medications are timed to prevent interference with the toileting schedule. When combined with positive reinforcement, this approach is also called prompted voiding (Box 40-12).

Self-Catheterization. Some clients with chronic disorders such as spinal cord injury learn to perform self-catheterization. The client must be able to physically manipulate equipment and assume a position for successful catheterization. The nurse teaches the client the structure of the urinary tract, clean versus sterile technique, the importance of adequate fluid intake, and the frequency of self-catheterization. Generally, the goal is to have clients perform self-catheterization every 6 to 8 hours, but the schedule should be individualized.

Evidence-Based Practice Guideline — Box 40-12

Prompted Voiding for People With Urinary Incontinence

- Approach person at scheduled prompted voiding times.
  - Wait 5 seconds for client to initiate request to toilet.
- Ask person if he or she is wet or dry.
  - Physically assess person to determine continence status.
  - Provide feedback. Praise if client is dry, no comment if client is wet.
- Prompt individual to toilet.
  - Offer assistance with toileting.
- Provide feedback.
- Inform individual of next scheduled prompted voiding session.
- Encourage individual to self-initiate requests to toilet.
- Record result of prompted voiding session.

Adapted from "Evidence-Based Protocol: Prompted Voiding for Persons With Urinary Incontinence," by S. S. Lyons and J. K. P. Specht, in *Series on Evidence-Based Practice for Older Adults,* edited by M. G. Titler (Series Ed.), 2001, Iowa City, IA: The University of Iowa College of Nursing Gerontological Nursing Interventions Research Center, Research Dissemination Core.

Evaluation

Client Care. The client is the best source of evaluation of outcomes and responses to nursing care (Figure 40–18). However, the nurse will also evaluate the effectiveness of nursing interventions through comparisons with baseline data. The nurse evaluates for change in the client's voiding pattern, presence of urinary tract alteration, and physical condition. Outcomes are compared with expected outcomes to determine the client's health status. Continuous evaluation allows the nurse to determine whether new or revised therapies are required or if any new nursing diagnoses have developed.

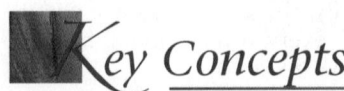

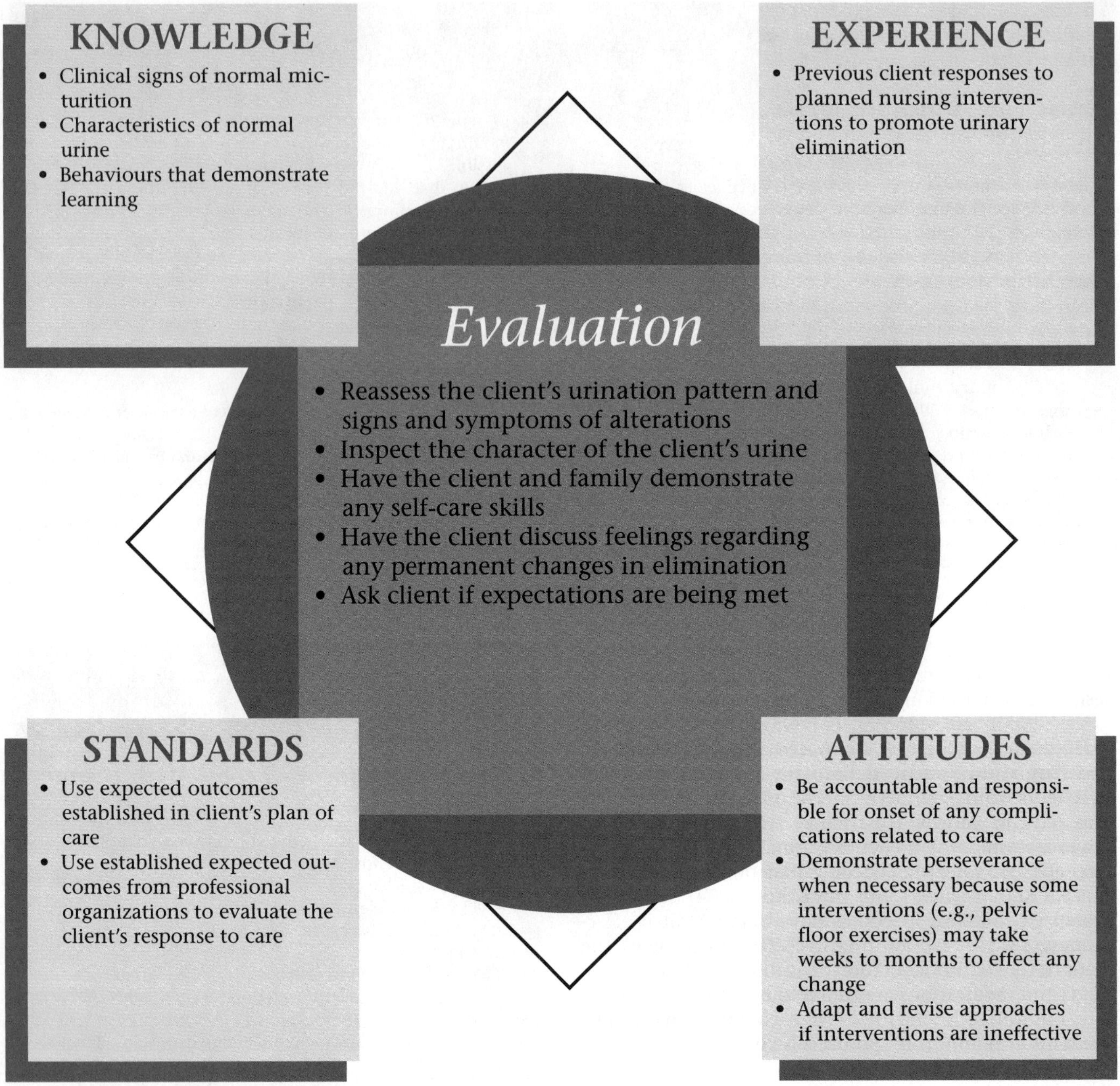
KNOWLEDGE
• Clinical signs of normal micturition
• Characteristics of normal urine
• Behaviours that demonstrate learning
EXPERIENCE
• Previous client responses to planned nursing interventions to promote urinary elimination
Evaluation
• Reassess the client's urination pattern and signs and symptoms of alterations
• Inspect the character of the client's urine
• Have the client and family demonstrate any self-care skills
• Have the client discuss feelings regarding any permanent changes in elimination
• Ask client if expectations are being met
STANDARDS
• Use expected outcomes established in client's plan of care
• Use established expected outcomes from professional organizations to evaluate the client's response to care
ATTITUDES
• Be accountable and responsible for onset of any complications related to care
• Demonstrate perseverance when necessary because some interventions (e.g., pelvic floor exercises) may take weeks to months to effect any change
• Adapt and revise approaches if interventions are ineffective

FIGURE **40–18** Critical thinking model for urinary elimination evaluation.

Client Expectations. If the nurse has developed a trust relationship with a client, indications of the client's degree of satisfaction with his or her care are evident. The client may smile or nod in appreciation. However, the nurse needs to confirm whether the client's expectations have been met to full satisfaction. The nurse may need to ask specifically about the client's degree of urinary control and comfort. If just asked, "How are you feeling today?" the client may reply with a non-committal "OK." However, the nurse needs specific information about how well an intervention has met the need in order to continue or revise the care plan. The nurse can also assist the client in redefining unrealistic client goals when impairment in function is not likely to be altered as completely as the client might like.

Key Concepts

- The act of micturition or voiding is influenced by voluntary control from higher brain centres and involuntary control from the spinal cord.
- Symptoms common to urinary disturbances include urgency, dysuria, polyuria, oliguria, and difficulty in starting the urinary stream.

- When collected properly, a clean-voided urine specimen does not contain bacteria from the urethral meatus.
- Methods of promoting the micturition reflex assist clients in sensing the urge to urinate and controlling urethral sphincter relaxation.
- An increased fluid intake results in increased diluted urine formation that reduces the risk of urinary tract infections.
- An in-dwelling urinary catheter remains in the bladder for an extended period, making the risk of infection greater than with intermittent catheterization.
- Catheter irrigation becomes necessary when the catheter becomes occluded with sediment or blood clots.
- A catheter drainage system should be a closed system positioned to allow free drainage of urine by gravity.
- Incontinence is classified as transient, urge, stress, mixed, functional, overflow, reflex, or total. Each type has specific nursing interventions.
- Specific guidelines for catheter selection should be followed so that the catheter does not cause harm.

Key Terms

Anuria, *p. 1334*
Bacteriuria, *p. 1336*
Bladder neck, *p. 1332*
Catheterization, *p. 1357*
Cystitis, *p. 1336*
Detrusor muscle, *p. 1332*
Diuresis, *p. 1335*
Dysuria, *p. 1336*
Encrustation, *p. 1360*
Erythropoietin, *p. 1331*
Habit retraining, *p. 1379*
Hematuria, *p. 1336*
Incontinence, *p. 1336*
Kegel exercises, *p. 1378*
Ketonuria, *p. 1349*
Micturition, *p. 1332*
Nephron, *p. 1331*
Nephrostomy, *p. 1338*
Nocturia, *p. 1335*
Oliguria, *p. 1334*
Overactive bladder syndrome, *p. 1337*
Pelvic floor muscle exercises (PFMEs), *p. 1378*
Polyuria, *p. 1335*
Prompted voiding, *p. 1379*
Prostate gland, *p. 1332*
Proteinuria, *p. 1331*
Pyelonephritis, *p. 1336*
Reflex bladder, *p. 1334*
Renal calculus, *p. 1332*
Renal pelvis, *p. 1331*
Renal replacement therapies, *p. 1334*
Residual urine, *p. 1336*
Rhabdosphincter, *p. 1332*
Specific gravity, *p. 1344*
Stoma, *p. 1336*
Suprapubic catheterization, *p. 1375*
Uremic syndrome, *p. 1334*
Ureterostomy, *p. 1338*
Urethral meatus, *p. 1332*
Urinalysis, *p. 1344*
Urinary diary, *p. 1340*
Urinary diversion, *p. 1336*
Urinary frequency, *p. 1339*
Urinary incontinence (UI), *p. 1337*
Urinary retention, *p. 1337*
Urosepsis, *p. 1336*

Critical Thinking Exercises

1. Mrs. Rodriquez is a 77-year-old woman who has had problems with urgency for the past 2 years. The episodes are becoming increasingly frequent. She has been attempting to deal with the problem by using an absorbent pad in her underwear but she feels as though everyone knows her problem. The embarrassment of having an odour often keeps her at home. She has given up attending daily mass at church.
   a. How can the nurse help her regain control of her urinary elimination?
   b. What are the actual nursing diagnoses that apply to Mrs. Rodriquez?
   c. For one diagnosis, give one goal/outcome and two nursing interventions.
2. Mrs. Brownell is a 37-year-old woman who has been admitted with back pain radiating down into her groin. She has also noticed blood in her urine for a week, but she was hoping it would go away. She is to undergo an IVP in 4 hours.
   a. What is the purpose of the IVP?
   b. What nursing care is needed before she goes to the X-ray department?
   c. Give at least two nursing responsibilities for care of the client who has undergone an IVP.
3. Mrs. Fenton is a 70-year-old woman with physical limitations related to rheumatoid arthritis. Her daughter, with whom she lives, has brought her to her family practitioner's office. You are the family nurse practitioner in the practice. As you assess Mrs. Fenton, you ask her how she is coping. Mrs. Fenton begins to answer but then starts to cry. "I know when I have to go to the bathroom, but I often don't make it in time." The daughter asks you for suggestions on how to manage, as she noticed that her mother's perineal skin is reddened and sore. What assessments need to be completed before planning interventions for Mrs. Fenton's care?

Review Questions

1. The normal adult urine output is
   1. 1000 mL/day
   2. 1500 to 1600 mL/day
   3. 3000 to 3200 mL/day
   4. 4000 mL/day
2. Renal alterations result from factors that cause injury directly to the glomeruli or renal tubule, interfering with their normal filtering, reabsorptive, and secretory functions. Selected causes include
   1. Transfusion reactions
   2. Dehydration
   3. Hemorrhage
   4. Congestive heart failure

3. Postrenal alterations result from obstruction to the flow of urine in the urinary collecting system caused by
   1. Dehydration
   2. Calculi
   3. Hemorrhage
   4. Diabetes mellitus
4. Which of the following is NOT a risk factor for UTI ?
   1. Catheterization
   2. Antibiotic use
   3. Acidic urine
   4. Spermicide use
5. Hospital-acquired UTIs are often related to poor hand hygiene and
   1. Urinary drainage bags
   2. Poor perineal hygiene
   3. Poor catheterization technique
   4. Poor urinary output
6. The urine appears concentrated and cloudy because of the presence of white blood cells or
   1. Bacteria
   2. Urinary drainage bags
   3. Blood clots
   4. Poor perineal hygiene
7. Prompted voiding is most appropriate for
   1. Clients with cognitive disorders
   2. Clients with small-capacity bladders
   3. Clients with urinary obstruction
   4. Male clients following prostatectomy
8. A client with stress incontinence
   1. Is incontinent following a strong urge to void
   2. Is unaware of the need to void
   3. Loses small amounts of urine with increased intra-abdominal pressure (e.g., coughing)
   4. Exhibits a small-capacity bladder
9. Maintaining an in-dwelling catheter drainage bag lower than the bladder prevents
   1. Urine flowing back into the bladder, likely causing an infection
   2. Urinary retention
   3. Reflex incontinence
   4. Urinary incontinence
10. When applying a condom catheter, it is important to secure the catheter in the penile shaft in such a manner that the catheter is
    1. Tight and draining well
    2. Dependent and draining well
    3. Secured with adhesive tape applied in a circular pattern
    4. Snug and secure, but does not cause constriction to blood flow

References

Abrams, P., et al. (2002). The standardization of terminology of lower urinary tract function: Report from the standardization sub-committee of the International Continence Society. *Neurourology and Urodynamics, 21,* 167–178.

Angus Reid Group. (1997). *Urinary incontinence in the Canadian adult population.* Survey commissioned by the Canadian Continence Foundation. Montreal, Canada.

Arya, L., Myers, D., & Jackson, N. (2000). Dietary caffeine intake and the risk for detrusor instability: A case control study. *Obstetrics and Gynecology, 96,* 85–89.

Bartolotti, A., et al. (2000). Prevalence and risk factors for urinary incontinence in Italy. *European Urology, 37,* 30–35.

Brundage, D. J. (1992). *Renal disorders.* St. Louis, MO: Mosby.

Bryant, C., Dowell, C., & Fairbrother, G. (2002). Caffeine reduction education to improve urinary symptoms. *British Journal of Nursing, 11,* 560–565.

Canadian Continence Foundation. (2001). *Promoting a collaborative consumer-focused approach to continence care in Canada.* Retrieved June 16, 2004, from *http://www.continence-fdn.ca*

Cox, A. J. (1990). Comparison of catheter surface morphologies. *British Journal of Urology, 65*(1), 55–60.

Creed, K., & Van der Werf, B. (2001). The innervation and properties of the urethral striated muscle. *Scandinavian Journal of Urology and Nephrology Supplementum, 207,* 8–11.

Dallosso, H., et al. (2003). The association of diet and other lifestyle factors with overactive bladder and stress incontinence: A longitudinal study in women. *BJU International, 92,* 69–77.

DeLancey, J., et al. (2002). Gross anatomy and cell biology of the lower urinary tract. In P. Abrams et al. (Eds.), *Incontinence* (pp. 19–84). Plymouth, UK: Health Publication Ltd.

Dochterman, J. M., & Bulechek, G. M. (Eds.). (2004). *Nursing interventions classification (NIC)* (4th ed.). St. Louis, MO: Mosby.

Dowd, T., Kolcaba, K., & Steiner, R. (2000). Using cognitive strategies to enhance bladder control and comfort. *Holistic Nursing Practice, 14*(2), 91–103.

Getliffe, K. (2003). Managing recurrent urinary catheter blockage: Problems, promises, and practicalities. *Journal of Wound, Ostomy, and Continence Nursing, 30*(3), 146–151.

Getliffe, K., & Dolman, M. (1997). Normal and abnormal bladder function. In K. Getliffe & M. Dolman (Eds.), *Promoting continence* (pp. 22–67). London: Bailliere Tindall.

Goldman, H. B. (2001). Evaluation and management of recurrent urinary-tract infections. In E. Kursh & J. Ulchaker (Eds.), *Office urology: The clinician's guide* (pp. 105–111). Totawa, NJ: Humana Press.

Gray, M. (2002). Are cranberry juice or cranberry products effective in the prevention or management of urinary tract infection? *Journal of Wound, Ostomy, and Continence Nursing, 29*(3), 122–126.

Gray, M. (2003). Gender, race, and culture in research on UI. *American Journal of Nursing, 103*(Suppl. 3), 20–25.

Gray, M., & Krissovich, M. (2003). Does fluid intake influence the risk for urinary incontinence, urinary tract infection, and bladder cancer? *Journal of Wound, Ostomy, and Continence Nursing, 30*(3), 126–131.

Hannestad, Y., et al. (2000). A community-based epidemiological survey of female urinary incontinence: The Norwegian EPINCONT study. *Journal of Clinical Epidemiology, 53,* 1150–1157.

Kidney Foundation of Canada, Northern Alberta and the Territories Branch. (2004). *Urinary tract infections (UTIs).* Retrieved November 23, 2004, from *http://www.kidney.ab.ca/kidneys/utis.html*

Kunin, C. M. (2001). Nosocomial urinary tract infections and the in-dwelling catheter. *Chest, 120*(1), 10–12.

Lewis, S., Heitkemper, M.,& Dirksen, S. (2000). *Medical-surgical nursing,* ed 5, St. Louis: Mosby.

Lyons, S. S., & Specht, J. K. P. (2001). Evidence-based protocol: Prompted voiding for persons with urinary incontinence. In M. G. Titler (Series Ed.), *Series on evidence-based practice for older adults.* Iowa City, IA: The University of Iowa College of Nursing Gerontological Nursing Interventions Research Center, Research Dissemination Core.

Maki, D. G., & Tambyah, P. A. (2001). Engineering out the risk of infection with urinary catheters [Electronic version]. *Emerging Infectious Disease, 7*(2), 1–6.

McCance, K. L., & Huether, S. E. (2002). *Pathophysiology: The biological basis for disease in adults and children* (4th ed.). St. Louis, MO: Mosby.

Miller, M. (2000). Nocturnal polyuria in older people: Pathophysiology and clinical implications. *Journal of the American Geriatrics Society, 48,* 1321–1329.

Moller, L., Lose, G., & Jorgensen, T. (2000). The prevalence and bothersomeness of lower urinary tract symptoms in women 40–60 years of age. *ACTA Obstetrics and Gynecology in Scandinavia, 79,* 298–305.

Moorhead, S., Johnson, M., & Maas, M. (Eds.). (2004). *Nursing outcomes classification (NOC)* (3rd ed.). St. Louis, MO: Mosby.

O'Donnell, J. A., & Hofmann, M. T. (2002). Urinary tract infections: How to manage nursing home patients with or without chronic catheterization. *Geriatrics, 57*(5), 45, 49–52, 55–56.

Ostaszkiewicz, J., Johnston, L., & Roe, B. (2004). Timed voiding for the management of urinary incontinence in adults. *Cochrane Database of Systematic Reviews, 2.*

Pagana, K. D., & Pagana, T. J. (2002). *Mosby's manual of diagnostic and laboratory tests* (2nd ed.). St. Louis, MO: Mosby.

Payne, C., et al. (2002). Research methodology in urinary incontinence. In P. Abrams et al. (Eds.), *Incontinence* (pp. 1045–1078). Plymouth, UK: Health Publication Ltd.

Raz, R., et al. (2001). Asymptomatic bacteriuria in institutionalized elders in Israel. *Journal of the American Medical Directors Association, 2,* 275–278.

Registered Nurses Association of Ontario. (2005). *Promoting continence using prompted voiding.* (Revised). Retrieved April 7, 2005, from *http://www.rnao.org/bestpractices/completed_guidelines/BPG_Guide_C1_Promote_Continence.asp*

Reiss, B., Evans, M., & Broyles, B. (2002). *Pharmacological aspects of nursing care* (6th ed.). Clifton Park, NY: Delmar Learning.

Rutchik, S., & Resnick, N. (1998). The epidemiology of incontinence in the elderly. *British Journal of Nursing, 82*(Suppl.), 1–4.

Sampselle, C. M. (2003). Behavioral interventions in young and middle-age women. *American Journal of Nursing, 103*(Suppl. 3), 9–19.

Schlager, T. A., Clark, M., & Anderson, S. (2001). Effect of a single-use sterile catheter for each void on the frequency of bacteriuria in children with neurogenic bladder on intermittent catheterization for bladder emptying. *Pediatrics, 108*(4), E71.

Schluman, C., Claesm, H., & Mattijs, J. (1997). Urinary incontinence in Belgium: A population-based epidemiological survey. *European Urology, 32,* 315–320.

Shupp-Byrne, D. E., et al. (2001). Interaction of bladder glycoprotein GP51 with uropathogenic bacteria. *Journal of Urology, 165,* 1342–1346.

Subak, L., et al. (2002). Does weight loss improve incontinence in moderately obese women? *International Urogynecology Journal, 13, 40–43.*

Thompson, D. L., & Smith, D. A. (2002). Continence nursing: A whole person approach. *Holistic Nursing Practice, 16*(2), 14–31.

Tomlinson, B., et al. (1999). Dietary caffeine, fluid intake, and urinary incontinence in older rural women. *International Urogynecology Journal of Pelvic Floor Dysfunction, 10,* 22–28.

Women's Continence Center, University of California. (2001). *Urinary Diary.* San Francisco. Retrieved February 22, 2005, from *http://www.ucsf.edu/wcc/print_diary.html*

Wyman, J. (2003). Treatment of urinary incontinence in men and older women. *American Journal of Nursing, 3*(Suppl.), 26–35.

Recommended Web Sites

Canadian Association for Enterostomal Therapy:
http://www.caet.ca

The Canadian Association for Enterostomal Therapy (CAET) is a professional organization representing Enterostomal Therapy Nurses, who provide services for clients with abdominal stomas (opening), fistulae, draining wound, or selected skin, gastrointestinal, and genitourinary disorders. The CAET promotes education, standards, and research for enterostomal practice.

The Canadian Continence Foundation:
http://www.continence-fdn.ca

The Canadian Continence Foundation is a national, non-profit organization serving the education needs of people experiencing incontinence. The foundation implements and promotes professional education and research to advance incontinent treatment and management.

United Ostomy Association of Canada Inc.:
http://www.ostomycanada.ca

The United Ostomy Association of Canada Inc. is a voluntary organization dedicated to assisting people with bowel or bladder diversions by providing support and information.

Urology Nurses of Canada:
http://www.unc.org

Urology Nurses of Canada (UNC) is the professional organization for urologic nurses in Canada. This Web site offers links to urological-related information, including the UNC professional standards.

41

Bowel Elimination

Anne Griffin Perry, RN, MSN, EdD, FAAN
Jo-Ann E.T. Fox-Threlkeld, RN, BN, MSc, PhD (Canadian author)

Objectives

Mastery of content in this chapter will enable the student to:

- Define the key terms listed.
- Discuss the role of gastrointestinal organs in digestion and elimination.
- Describe the integrated processes of oral pharyngeal swallowing and breathing.
- Describe the functions of the large intestine.
- Explain the physiological aspects of normal defecation.
- Discuss psychological and physiological factors that influence the elimination process.
- Describe common physiological alterations in elimination.
- Assess a client's elimination pattern.
- List nursing diagnoses related to alterations in elimination.
- Describe nursing implications for common diagnostic examinations of the gastrointestinal tract.
- List nursing measures that promote normal elimination.
- List nursing measures included in bowel training.
- Discuss nursing measures required for clients with a bowel diversion.
- Use critical thinking in the provision of care to clients with alterations in bowel elimination.

Food entering the gastrointestinal tract is dissolved by intraluminal water and broken down by mechanical and chemical digestion. Nutrients and water are absorbed from the lumen and the remaining contents are propelled along by contractions of the smooth muscle layers. The material that reaches the colon is further dehydrated and expelled from the anus as stool.

Regular elimination of bowel waste products is essential for normal body functioning. Alterations in elimination are often early indications of problems within either the gastrointestinal or another body system. Because bowel function depends on the balance of several factors, elimination patterns and habits vary among individuals.

To manage the elimination problems of clients, the nurse must understand normal elimination and factors that promote, impede, or cause alterations in elimination. Supportive nursing care respects the client's privacy and emotional needs. Measures designed to promote normal elimination should also minimize discomfort for the client.

Scientific Knowledge Base

The gastrointestinal (GI) tract is a series of hollow, multi-layered, muscular organs lined with mucous membranes. The GI tract begins at the mouth and continues through to the anus. The mucosal and muscle layers are innervated by the intrinsic enteric nervous system with its sensory, interneuronal, and motor fibres. The mucosa contains neurons; mucous, endocrine, and immune cells;

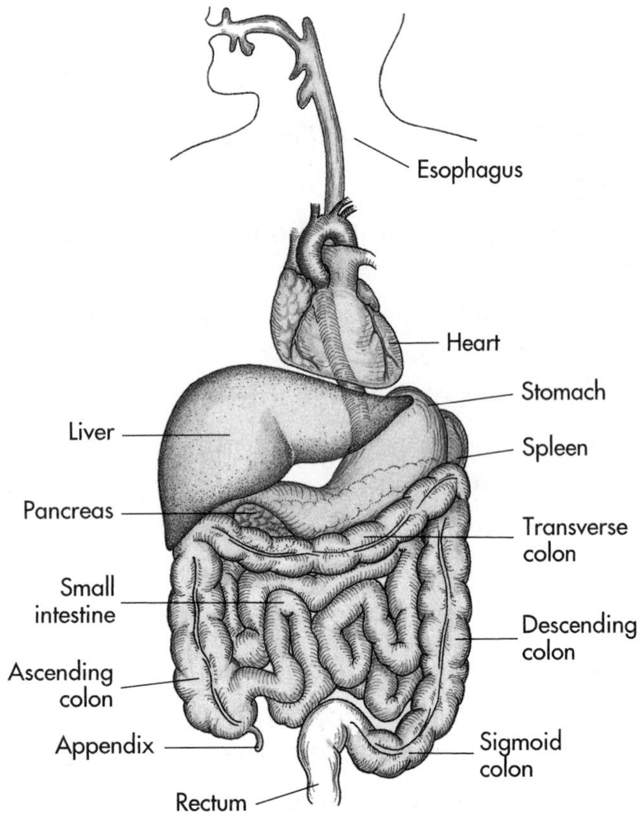

FIGURE **41–1** Organs of the gastrointestinal tract (with the heart as a reference point).

and the crypt ion-secreting cells that mature into the absorptive enterocytes of the villus tip. The central nervous system receives input from the gastrointestinal tract via sensory fibres, which travel in the vagus and sympathetic nerves. Extrinsic sympathetic and parasympathetic motor nerves end on the enteric nervous system and act to modulate the activity of the intrinsic enteric nervous system. The gastrointestinal tract also has a specialized immune system, which prevents bacteria and viruses from the non-sterile lumen from entering the blood stream.

The purposes of the GI tract are to ingest (take in) food, break down the ingested food into absorbable forms (digestion), absorb fluid and nutrients, prepare food for absorption and use by the body's cells, and provide for temporary storage of feces (Figure 41–1). The volume of fluids absorbed by the GI tract is high. Oral fluid intake is about 1.2 L/day; another 7 L enters from the blood from the secretion of digestive enzymes by the mucosa, liver gallbladder, and pancreas and by osmosis as numbers of molecules in the lumen increase by digestion. Absorption from the small and large intestine amounts to 8.1 L/day, leaving 100 mL to be excreted in the feces. Therefore, maintaining fluid and electrolyte balance is a key function of the GI system.

Mouth

The mouth mechanically and chemically breaks down nutrients into usable size and form. The teeth **masticate** food, breaking it down into a soft, moist ball (a **bolus**) suitable for swallowing. Saliva, produced by the salivary glands in the mouth, dilutes and softens the food in the mouth for easier swallowing and commences digestion of carbohydrates with the enzyme ptyalin. (Saliva also contains growth factors, antibacterial agents, and antibodies that are necessary for the maintenance of gum and teeth integrity.) In addition, mucus from the salivary glands lubricates the passage of the bolus through the pharynx and down the esophagus during swallowing.

Swallowing begins with the lips closing and tongue curling with its tip and then the back being pressed to the roof of the mouth (put the tip of your tongue behind your lower teeth and open your mouth and then try to swallow; Figure 41–2). This tips the bolus into the pharynx. The pharyngeal cavity is common to both the gastrointestinal tract and the respiratory tract. The swallowed bolus must cross the nasopharynx and the soft palate approximate with the pharynx to prevent material from entering the back of the nose. To prevent aspiration, the vocal chords in the glottis approximate, the epiglottis moves downward to seal off the trachea, and breathing is inhibited in the central nervous system. The bolus enters the esophagus through the relaxed upper esophageal sphincter. This complex process is under striated muscle control and requires an intact nervous system. Anaesthesia, strokes, and high blood alcohol levels inhibit this close regulation and can lead to aspiration of food or vomited gastric contents into the trachea and lungs.

Esophagus

The esophagus provides a conduit through the chest cavity, which it shares with the lungs, heart, and the large blood vessels. The esophagus enters the abdominal cavity through the diaphragm at the lower esophageal sphincter, which maintains a barrier against the acid proteolytic contents of the stomach. With aging, the esophageal sphincter frequently herniates into the chest cavity, producing a hiatus hernia and regurgitation of gastric contents into the esophagus.

The bolus travels down the relaxed esophagus mainly by gravity to the lower esophageal sphincter, which is opened by the initiation of swallowing in the pharynx and upper esophageal sphincter. A wave of **peristaltic contractions** propels the bolus into the stomach. Peristaltic contractions relax over the bolus and contract behind the bolus, thus moving contents through the length of the GI tract. If the bolus moves slowly or is stuck, a local reflex will relax the area ahead of the bolus and produce a powerful contraction behind the bolus. In the esophagus, this is known as *secondary peristalsis*. Tertiary contractions of the esophagus are frequently simultaneous and produced by irritation of the mucosa by gastric contents. These contractions can be extremely painful and mimic cardiac chest pain.

Stomach

The stomach performs several tasks: storage of swallowed food and liquid, mixing of food with liquid and gastric digestive juices, and the controlled emptying of its contents through the pyloric sphincter into the small intestine. The stomach produces and secretes hydrochloric acid (HCl), mucus, the enzyme pepsin, and intrinsic factor.

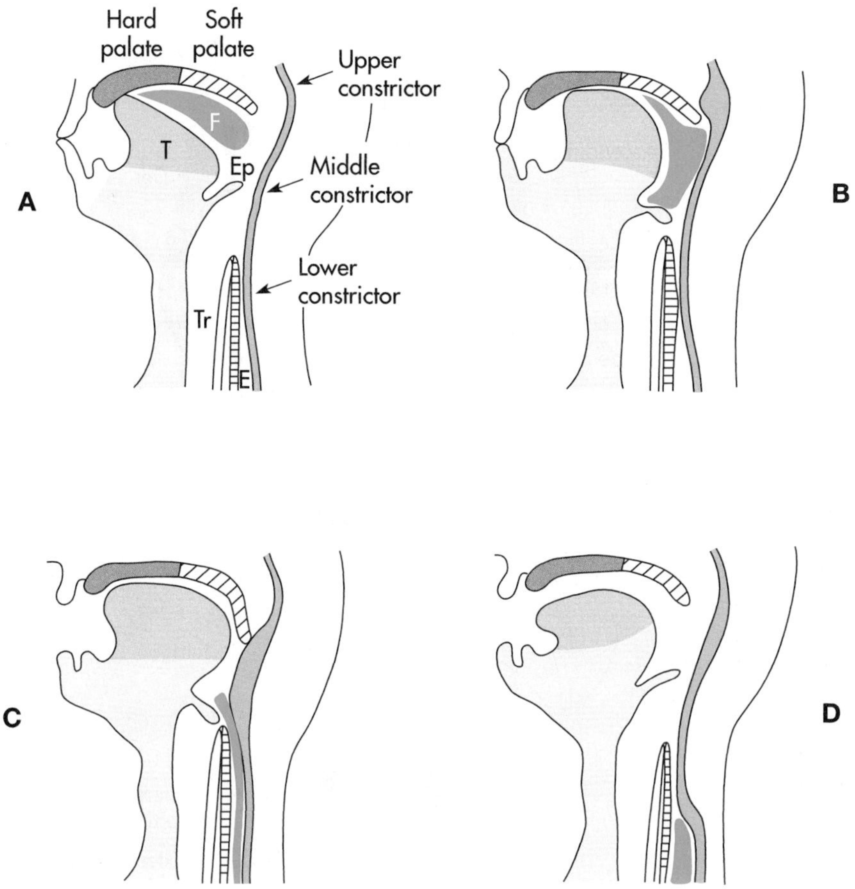

FIGURE **41–2** Oral and pharyngeal events during swallowing. **A,** The bolus (F) is propelled into the pharynx by placement of the tongue (T) on the roof of the hard palate. **B,** Further propulsion is caused by movement of the more distal regions of the tongue against the palate. Contraction of the upper constrictors of the pharynx and the soft palate separate the oropharynx from the nasopharynx. **C,** Contraction of the pharynx and relaxation of the cricopharyngeal muscle propels the bolus through the upper esophageal sphincter. Upward movement of the glottis and downward movement of the epiglottis (EP) seal off the trachea (Tr), and respiratory drive is inhibited in the CNS. **D,** The bolus is now in the esophagus (E) and is propelled into the stomach by a peristaltic contraction. (From *Gastrointestinal Physiology,* 6th ed., Figure 3–1, p. 28, by L. R. Johnson, 2001, St. Louis, MO: Mosby.)

Pepsin and HCl facilitate the digestion of protein and are antibacterial. Mucus protects the stomach mucosa from acidity and enzyme activity. The intrinsic factor is essential in the absorption of vitamin B_{12}.

The rate of emptying of the stomach depends on the content of the dissolved and partially digested bolus **(chyme).** Water diffuses from both the stomach and small intestine and is emptied rapidly. Carbohydrates are emptied only slightly more slowly, particularly if they are not strongly acid. Proteins empty even more slowly and in smaller amounts as determined by the acidity of the chyme. Fats are emptied the slowest of all. The controlled emptying allows the pancreatic secretions and bile to neutralize the chyme and secrete enzymes for luminal digestion.

Small Intestine

Propulsion of contents along the small intestine occurs by segmentation, which facilitates both digestion and absorption (Figure 41–3). Chyme mixes with secretions from the gallbladder (bile) and pancreatic enzymes (amylases, proteolytic enzymes, and lipases) and is exposed to the absorbing surfaces of the mucosa. Reabsorption in the small intestine is so efficient that by the time the chyme reaches the end of the small intestine, it is paste-like in consistency.

The small intestine is divided into three sections: the duodenum, the jejunum, and the ileum. The duodenum is approximately 0.6 m long and continues to process the

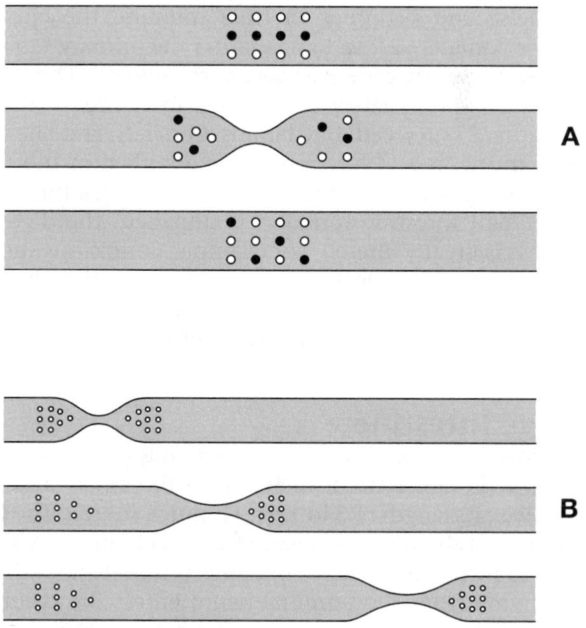

FIGURE **41–3** The influence of contractions on the contents within a region of the intestine. **A,** A contraction that is neither preceded by nor followed by other contractions serves to mix and locally circulate the intestinal contents. **B,** Contractions that have an orad to aborad sequence (left to right) serve to propel contents in an aborad direction. (From *Gastrointestinal Physiology,* 6th ed., Figure 5–3, p. 50, by L. R. Johnson, 2001, St. Louis, MO: Mosby.)

chyme from the stomach. The chyme entering the duodenum is acidic and contains partially digested protein, carbohydrates, and unemulsified fats. The presence of these substances stimulates the release of the hormones secretin and cholecystokinin from the duodenal mucosa. Secretin stimulates the pancreas to secrete bicarbonate to neutralize the acid. Cholecystokinin stimulates the pancreas to secrete the following enzymes: (1) amylases to convert carbohydrates to disaccharides, (2) proteases to further hydrolyze proteins into smaller peptides, and (3) lipases to hydrolyze triglycerides into fatty acids and monoglycerides. The presence of fats in the duodenum further stimulates cholecystokinin release, which causes the gallbladder to contract, which in turn releases bile to emulsify the fats. Any blockage of the release of these enzymes prevents the digestion of fats and proteins, resulting in large, fatty, and foul-smelling stools. This is the case in cystic fibrosis, in which the metabolic error in chloride pumping produces a thick mucus that prevents emptying of the pancreatic and biliary ducts into the duodenum. Undigested fats and proteins reaching the colon are responsible for the changes in fecal appearance.

The mature enterocytes at the tip of the villi, with their digestive enzymes and absorptive capacity, are replaced every 48 to 64 hours. Thus, these cells are very susceptible to damage from radiation and antimetabolic chemotherapy, inflammation, and allergic responses. For example, some individuals may have sensitivity to gluten that damages the villus tip with every exposure to gluten. This damage results in malabsorption of nutrients caused by the lack of mature absorbing enterocytes at the tip of the villus. The treatment is to remove gluten-containing food from the diet.

The second section of the small intestine, the jejunum, is approximately 2.7 m long and has the primary function of absorption of carbohydrates and proteins. The ileum, which is approximately 3.7 m long, specializes in the absorption of water, certain vitamins, iron, fats, and bile salts. Most nutrients and electrolytes are absorbed in the small intestine, specifically by the duodenum and jejunum.

If small intestine function is impaired, the digestive process is greatly altered. For example, conditions such as inflammation, surgical resection, or obstruction can disrupt contractile activity, reduce the area of absorption, or block the passage of chyme. Electrolyte and nutrient deficiencies then develop.

Large Intestine

The lower GI tract is called the large intestine (colon) because it is larger in diameter than the small intestine. However, its length (1.5 to 1.8 m) is much shorter. The large intestine is the primary organ of bowel elimination and is divided into the cecum, colon, and rectum (Figure 41–4).

Chyme from the terminal ileum enters the cecum of the large intestine by waves of peristalsis through the ileocecal sphincter, a circular muscle layer that regulates ileal emptying and prevents regurgitation of fecal contents. After a meal, the gastroilieal reflex causes the terminal ileum to contract regularly, and the sphincter opens with each contraction, thereby pushing the ileal contents into the colon.

The colon is divided into the ascending, transverse, descending, and sigmoid colons. The colon's muscular tissue allows it to accommodate and eliminate large quantities of waste and gas **(flatus).** The colon has three functions: absorption, secretion, and elimination. A volume of water and significant amounts of sodium and chloride are absorbed by the colon daily (Doughty, 2000b).

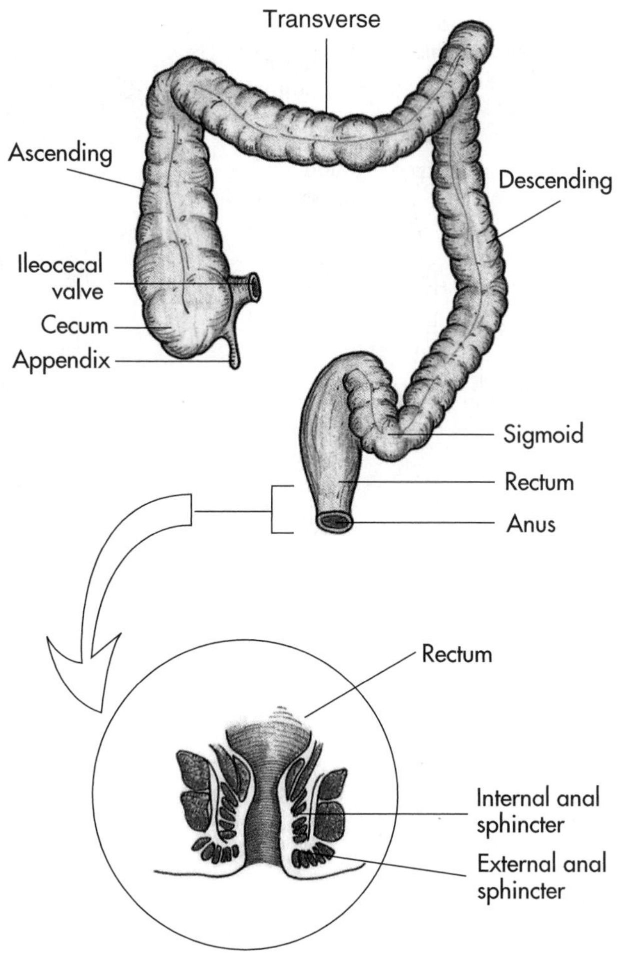

FIGURE **41–4** Divisions of the large intestine.

There are two types of muscle contractions in the colon: slow mixing contractions (similar to segmentation, but slower) and mass **peristalsis** (or mass movement). Slow mixing contractions move contents through the colon and expose the chyme to the mucosa, where active absorption of sodium and chloride causes water absorption and dries the chyme to feces. Intestinal content is the main stimulus for the slow mixing contractions. Mass peristalsis movements then push the feces toward the rectum. The ingestion of food is the main stimulus for mass peristalsis. This is known as the **gastrocolic reflex.** In adults, these mass movements occur only three or four times a day.

When the slow mixing contractions are increased and the mass peristalsis diminished, water continues to be absorbed and the feces are dried out, resulting in constipation. Conversely, when the mixing movements are decreased and the mass peristalsis is increased, there is less time for water to be absorbed and the stool will be watery (diarrhea).

The secretory function of the colon aids in electrolyte balance. Bicarbonate is secreted in exchange for chloride.

About 4 to 9 mmol of potassium is also excreted daily. Serious alterations in colon function (e.g., diarrhea) can cause severe electrolyte disturbances.

The rectum is the final portion of the large intestine. Normally the rectum is empty of waste products **(feces)** until just before defecation. The rectum contains vertical and transverse folds of tissue that may help to temporarily hold fecal contents during **defecation.** Each fold contains an artery and vein that can become distended from pressure during straining. This distension can result in hemorrhoid formation.

Anus

Feces and flatus are expelled from the rectum through the anal canal and anus. Contraction and relaxation of the internal anal sphincter is under autonomic control (unconscious control), and the external anal sphincter is under somatic neural control (conscious control). The anal canal is richly supplied with sensory and motor nerve fibres to help control continence.

Defecation

The physiological factors critical to bowel function and defecation include normal GI tract function, sensory awareness of rectal distension and rectal contents, voluntary sphincter control, and adequate rectal capacity and compliance (Doughty, 2000a). Normal defecation is painless, resulting in passage of soft, formed stool.

Defecation begins with movement in the left colon, moving stool toward the anus. When stool reaches the rectum, the distension causes relaxation of the internal sphincter, and an awareness of the need to defecate. At the time of defecation, the external sphincter relaxes and abdominal muscles contract, increasing intrarectal pressure and forcing the stool out (Doughty, 2000a). Pressure can be exerted to expel feces through a voluntary contraction of the abdominal muscles and diaphragm while maintaining forced expiration against a closed airway. This is termed the **Valsalva manoeuvre.** This will assist in stool passage but has a pronounced effect on the return of blood up the inferior vena cava. (Take your pulse while holding your breath and bearing down. Your pulse will grow weak and thready and speed up because the diaphragm has occluded the return of the blood through the inferior vena cava. When you breathe out, the pulse will feel very full and bounding as the blood return surges up the vena cava). Clients with cardiovascular disease, glaucoma, increased intracranial pressure, or a new surgical wound can be placed at further risk (e.g., cardiac irregularities and elevated blood pressure) with this manoeuvre and should be cautioned to avoid straining to pass stool.

Nursing Knowledge Base

Factors Affecting Bowel Elimination

Many factors influence the process of bowel elimination. Knowledge of these factors enables the nurse to anticipate measures required to maintain a normal elimination pattern.

Age. Developmental changes that affect elimination occur throughout life. An infant has a small stomach capacity and less secretion of digestive enzymes. Some foods such as complex starches are tolerated poorly. Food passes quickly through an infant's intestinal tract because of rapid peristalsis. The infant is unable to control defecation because of a lack of neuromuscular development. This development usually does not take place until 2 to 3 years of age.

Systemic changes in the function of digestion and absorption of nutrients result from changes in older clients' cardiovascular and neurological systems, rather than their GI system. For example, arteriosclerosis may cause decreased splanchnic and mesenteric blood flow, thus decreasing absorption from the small intestine (Lueckenotte, 2000). In addition, there is a decrease in peristalsis and esophageal emptying slows. Older adults often experience changes in the GI system that impairs digestion and elimination (Table 41-1).

Older adults also lose muscle tone in the perineal floor and anal sphincter. Although the integrity of the external sphincter may remain intact, older adults may have difficulty controlling bowel evacuation and are at risk for incontinence. In addition, there is a slowing of nerve impulses to the anal region and some individuals become less aware of the need to defecate and as a result develop irregular bowel movements and are at risk for constipation.

Diet. The food that a person eats influences elimination. Regular daily food intake helps maintain a regular pattern of peristalsis in the colon. **Fibre,** the indigestible residue in the diet, provides the bulk of fecal material. Bulk-forming foods, such as grains, fruits, and vegetables, absorb fluids and increase stool mass. The bowel walls are stretched, creating peristalsis and initiating the defecation reflex. By stimulating peristalsis, bulk foods pass quickly through the intestines, keeping the stool soft. Ingestion of a high-fibre diet or fibre supplementation improves the likelihood of a normal elimination pattern if other factors are normal. Fibre intake can help resolve constipation, and further research has documented the use of supplemental dietary fibre to reduce bowel incontinence (Bliss et al., 2001). However, fibre retains fluid in the GI tract. Therefore, adequate fluid intake is essential. Inadequate fluid intake could lead to serious constipation or impaction.

Gas-producing foods such as onions, cauliflower, and beans stimulate peristalsis. The gas formed distends intestinal walls and increases colon motility. Some spicy foods can increase peristalsis but can also cause indigestion and watery stools.

Milk and milk products are difficult or impossible for many people to digest. **Lactose intolerance** is the inability to digest lactose, the predominant sugar in milk. It is caused by a shortage of the enzyme lactase, which is normally produced by the cells that line the small intestine and is needed to digest lactose. Lactase frequently disappears in adulthood, and as a result, lactose cannot be absorbed and acts as an osmotic laxative, resulting in diarrhea, gaseous distension, and cramping (Mishkin, 1997). It is estimated that up to 75% of the world's population is lactose intolerant. Lactose intolerance is very common among Asian, South American, Black, and Aboriginal adults. The person must learn how much lactose his or her body can tolerate. For example, some people can drink one glass of milk without effect, but not

Table 41-1 Normal Age-Related Changes in the Gastrointestinal Tract

Portion of GI Tract	Functional or Physiological Change	Causes
Mouth	Decreased chewing and decreased salivation, including oral dryness	Degeneration of cells, medications.
Esophagus	Reduced motility, especially in lower third	Degeneration of neural cells.
Stomach	Decrease in:	
	Acid secretions	Degeneration of gastric mucosa. Alkaline gastric medium contributes to malabsorption of iron. Although digestive enzymes are decreased, enough remain available for digestion.
	Motor activity	Delayed gastric emptying, causing fewer hunger contractions.
	Mucosal thickness	Loss of parietal cells also leads to loss of intrinsic factor, which is needed for vitamin B_{12} absorption.
Small intestine	Decreased nutrient absorption	Fewer absorbing cells.
Large intestine	Increase in pouches on the weakened intestinal wall	Weakened musculature. Absorption not significantly affected.
	Constipation	Decreased peristalsis.
	Missed defecation signal	Duller nerve sensations.
	Increasing risk for fecal incontinence	
Liver	Size decreased	Reduced storage capacity and ability to synthesize protein and metabolize medications.

Data from *Gerontologic Nursing* (2nd ed.), by A. G. Lueckenotte, 2000, St. Louis, MO: Mosby.

two. However, young children with lactose intolerance should not eat any foods with lactose. Lactase enzymes are available without a prescription and may help the person who is lactose intolerant.

Fluid Intake. An inadequate fluid intake or disturbances resulting in fluid loss (such as vomiting) affect the character of feces. Fluid liquefies intestinal contents, easing its passage through the colon. Reduced fluid intake slows passage of food through the intestine and can result in hardening of stool contents. Unless there is a medical contraindication, an adult should drink six to eight glasses (1400 to 2000 mL) of non-caffeinated fluid daily. An increase in intake fruit juices softens stool and increases peristalsis. However, too much fruit juice, especially in children, can lead to diarrhea. In very young children, too much fruit juice can also delay toilet training of the bowels.

Older adults are at risk of insufficient intake of fluids and are thus predisposed to constipation (Semla, Beizer, & Highbee, 1997). Sometimes older adults reduce fluid intake in an attempt to reduce micturition (see chapter 40). In addition, an increased ingestion of milk or milk products may slow peristalsis in some people and cause constipation (Anti et al., 1998).

Physical Activity. Physical activity promotes peristalsis, whereas immobilization depresses peristalsis. Early ambulation as illness begins to resolve or as soon as possible after surgery is encouraged to promote maintenance of peristalsis and normal elimination. Maintaining tone of skeletal muscles used during defecation is important. Weakened abdominal and pelvic floor muscles impair the ability to increase intra-abdominal pressure and to control the external sphincter. Muscle tone may be weakened or lost as a result of long-term illness or neurological disease that impairs nerve transmission. As a result of these changes in the abdominal and pelvic floor muscles, there is an increased risk for constipation.

Psychological Factors. The function of almost all body systems can be impaired by prolonged emotional stress (see chapter 26). If an individual becomes anxious, afraid, or angry, the stress response is initiated, which allows the body to restore defences. The digestive process is accelerated, and peristalsis increases. Side effects of increased peristalsis are diarrhea and gaseous distension. If a person becomes depressed, the autonomic nervous system slows impulses and peristalsis can decrease, resulting in constipation. Stress exacerbates a number of diseases of the GI tract, including ulcerative **colitis,** gastric and duodenal ulcers, and **Crohn's disease.**

Personal Habits. Personal elimination habits influence bowel function. Most people benefit from being able to use their own toilet facilities at a time that is most effective and convenient for them. A busy work schedule may prevent the person from going to the bathroom in response to the urge to defecate, thus disrupting regular habits and possibly causing constipation. A person should establish a regular time for elimination. The gastrocolic reflex, initiated by eating food, is frequently stimulated to cause defecation after meals.

Chronically ill and hospitalized clients may not be able to maintain privacy during defecation. In a hospital or long-term care setting, bathroom facilities are often shared with a roommate whose hygienic habits might be quite different. In addition, a chronic illness may limit a client's balance, activity tolerance, or physical activity; therefore, the client may require the use of a bedpan or bedside commode. The sights, sounds, and odours associated with sharing toilet facilities or using bedpans are often embarrassing. Embarrassment prompts clients to ignore the urge

Table 41-2 Medications and the Gastrointestinal System

Medications	Action
Dicyclomine HCl (Bentyl)	Suppresses peristalsis and can decrease gastric emptying.
Narcotic analgesics	Increase mixing segmentation contractions and slow propulsive contractions, often resulting in constipation (McKenry & Salerno, 2001).
Anticholinergic drugs, such as atropine or glycopyrrolate (Robinul)	Inhibit gastric acid secretion and depress GI motility (McKenry & Salerno, 2001). Although useful in treating hyperactive bowel disorders, anticholinergics can cause constipation.
Antibiotics	May produce diarrhea by disrupting the normal bacterial flora in the GI tract. If the diarrhea and associated abdominal cramping become severe, the client might need to change medications (Bartlett, 2002). The client may also benefit by concurrently taking a probiotic acidophilus supplement.
Non-steroidal anti-inflammatory drugs (Motrin and ibuprofen)	Prostaglandin inhibitors that promote gastrointestinal irritation that can range from dyspepsia to life-threatening hemorrhage (Cooke, 1996).
Aspirin	A prostaglandin inhibitor, it can interfere with the formation and production of protective mucus and can predispose clients to gastritis.
Histamine$_2$ (H_2) antagonists	Suppress the secretion of hydrochloric acid and may interfere with the digestion of some foods.
Iron	Can cause discoloration of the stool (black) and lead to constipation (McKenry & Salerno, 2001).

to defecate, which can begin a vicious cycle of constipation and discomfort.

Position During Defecation. Squatting is the normal position during defecation. Toilets are designed to facilitate this posture, allowing the person to lean forward, exert intra-abdominal pressure, and contract the thigh muscles. For the client immobilized in bed, defecation is often difficult. In a supine position, it is impossible to contract the muscles used during defecation. If the client's condition permits, raise the head of the bed; this assists the client to a more normal sitting position on a bedpan, enhancing the ability to defecate.

Pain. Normally the act of defecation is painless. However, a number of conditions, including hemorrhoids, rectal surgery, rectal fistulas, and abdominal surgery, can result in discomfort. In these instances, the client often suppresses the urge to defecate to avoid pain, and constipation may develop.

Pregnancy and Labour. As pregnancy advances, the size of the fetus increases and pressure is exerted on the rectum. A temporary obstruction created by the fetus impairs passage of feces. Slowing of peristalsis during the third trimester often leads to constipation. A pregnant woman's frequent straining during defecation or delivery can result in formation of permanent hemorrhoids. Damage to the perineum extending to the anal sphincters during labour also alters sphincter integrity.

Surgery and Anaesthesia. General anaesthetic agents used during surgery cause temporary cessation of peristalsis (see chapter 45). Inhaled anaesthetic agents block parasympathetic impulses to the enteric nervous system, and the stress of surgery stimulates the sympathetic nervous system. The anaesthetic's action slows or stops integrated contractions. The client who receives local or regional anaesthesia is less at risk for elimination alterations because bowel activity may be affected minimally or not at all.

Any surgery that involves direct manipulation of the bowel temporarily stops peristalsis. This condition, called **paralytic ileus,** usually lasts about 24 to 48 hours. If the client remains inactive or is unable to eat after surgery, return of normal bowel function may be further delayed.

Medications. Medication may have certain expected actions on the bowel; for example, there are medications to promote defecation or control diarrhea. In addition, medications prescribed for acute and chronic conditions may have secondary effects on the client's bowel elimination patterns (Table 41-2). **Laxatives** and **cathartics** soften the stool and promote peristalsis. Although similar to cathartics, laxatives are milder in action. When used correctly, laxatives and cathartics safely maintain normal elimination patterns. However, chronic use of cathartics causes the large intestine to lose muscle tone and become less responsive to stimulation by laxatives. Laxative overuse can also cause serious diarrhea that can lead to dehydration and electrolyte depletion. Mineral oil, a common laxative, decreases fat-soluble vitamin absorption. Laxatives can influence the efficacy of other medications by altering the transit time (i.e., the time the medication remains in the GI tract and is available for absorption).

Diagnostic Tests. Diagnostic examinations involving visualization of GI structures often require that portions of the bowel be empty of contents. The client usually receives a prescribed bowel preparation before the test. Usually, the client is asked to drink a large volume (4 L) of a solution containing a non-absorbable inert molecule such as polyethylene glycol. Other medications, cathartics, and/or enemas may be used. In addition, the client is not allowed to eat or drink after midnight of the day preceding examinations such as a colonoscopy, **endoscopy,** or other testing that requires visualization of the lower GI tract. Following the diagnostic procedure, there may be changes in elimination, such as increased gas or loose stools, until the client resumes a normal eating pattern.

Common Bowel Elimination Problems

The nurse might care for clients who have or are at risk for elimination problems because of emotional stress (anxiety or depression), physiological changes in the GI tract such as surgical alteration of intestinal structures, inflammatory diseases, prescribed therapy, or disorders impairing defecation.

Constipation. **Constipation** is a symptom, not a disease (Box 41-1). The signs of constipation vary among clients, but it usually includes infrequent bowel movements (fewer than three per week), difficult evacuation of feces, inability to defecate at will, and hard feces (Dosh, 2002). Abdominal pain and distension and a sensation of fullness and pressure in the rectum are common. Straining during defecation is an associated sign. When intestinal motility slows, the fecal mass becomes exposed over time to the intestinal walls and most of the fecal water content is absorbed. Little water is left to soften and lubricate the stool. Passage of a dry, hard stool may cause rectal pain.

Constipation can be a significant hazard to health. Straining during defecation may cause problems to the client with recent abdominal, gynecological, or rectal surgery. The effort to pass a stool can cause sutures to separate, reopening the wound. In addition, clients with histories of cardiovascular disease, diseases causing elevated intraocular pressure (glaucoma), and increased intracranial pressure should prevent constipation and avoid using the Valsalva manoeuvre. Exhaling through the mouth during straining avoids a Valsalva manoeuvre. Clients may have constipation from certain medications that they are taking. Some medications that cause constipation include aspirin, antihistamines, diuretics, tranquilizers, hypnotics, antacids with aluminum or calcium, opiates, and drugs used to control Parkinson's disease.

Impaction. Fecal **impaction** results from unrelieved constipation. It is a collection of hardened feces, wedged in the rectum, that cannot be expelled. In cases of severe impaction, the mass can extend up into the sigmoid colon. Clients who are debilitated, confused, or unconscious are most at risk for impaction. They are too weak or unaware of the need to defecate, or they may be dehydrated so that the stool becomes too hard and dry to pass. High intake of fibre or cellulose without fluids also increases the risk of impaction.

An obvious sign of impaction is the inability to pass a stool for several days, despite the repeated urge to defecate. When a continuous oozing of diarrhea stool develops, impaction should be suspected. The liquid portion of feces located higher in the colon seeps around the impacted mass. Loss of appetite (anorexia), nausea and/or vomiting, abdominal distension and cramping, and rectal pain may accompany the condition. The nurse who suspects an impaction can gently perform a digital examination of the rectum and palpate for the impacted mass.

Box 41-1 Common Causes of Constipation

- Irregular bowel habits and ignoring the urge to defecate.
- Chronic illnesses (e.g., Parkinson's disease, multiple sclerosis, rheumatoid arthritis, chronic bowel diseases, depression, eating disorders; Annells & Koch, 2002; Richmond, 2003).
- Low-fibre diet high in animal fats (e.g., meats, dairy products, eggs) and refined sugars (rich desserts). Also, low fluid intake slows peristalsis (Bliss et al., 2001).
- Situational stress (e.g., illness of a family member, death of a loved one, divorce; Dosh, 2002).
- Lengthy bed rest or lack of regular exercise.
- Heavy laxative use causes loss of normal defecation reflex. In addition, the lower colon is completely emptied, requiring time to refill with bulk (Annels & Koch, 2002).
- Older adults experience slowed peristalsis, loss of abdominal muscle elasticity, and reduced intestinal mucous secretion. Older adults often eat low-fibre foods.
- Neurological conditions that block nerve impulse to the colon (e.g., spinal cord injury, tumour).
- Organic illnesses such as hypothyroidism, hypocalcemia, or hypokalemia (Richmond, 2003).

Diarrhea. **Diarrhea** is an increase in the number of stools (several bowel movements per day) and the passage of liquid, unformed feces. It is associated with disorders affecting digestion, absorption, and secretion in the GI tract. Intestinal contents pass through the small and large intestine too quickly to allow the usual absorption of fluid and nutrients. Irritation within the colon can result in an increased mucus secretion. As a result, feces become watery and the client may be unable to control the urge to defecate.

Excess loss of colonic fluid can result in serious fluid and electrolyte or acid-base imbalances. Infants and older adults are particularly susceptible to associated complications (see chapter 36). Because repeated passage of diarrhea stools also exposes the skin of the perineum and buttocks to irritating intestinal contents, meticulous skin care and containment of fecal drainage is needed to prevent skin breakdown (see chapter 34).

Many conditions cause diarrhea. Antibiotic use via any route of administration may cause diarrhea because these medications alter the normal flora in the gastrointestinal tract (Bartlett, 2002). To counteract this effect of antibiotics, the client may be advised to eat active-culture yogurt or take a lactobacillus supplement to reintroduce the normal flora of the colon. Clients receiving enteral nutrition are also at risk for diarrhea, which may be due to the GI response to the nutritional components, frequency, or volume of the enteral feeding. Food allergies and intolerances increase peristalsis and cause diarrhea. Diseases, surgeries, laxatives, chemotherapy, radiotherapy, or diagnostic testing of the lower gastrointestinal tract can also cause diarrhea. The aims of treatment are to remove precipitating conditions and to slow peristalsis.

In addition, communicable food-borne pathogens can cause diarrhea. The risk of food-borne illnesses can be greatly reduced by simple handwashing following the use of the bathroom and before and after preparing foods, and by cleaning and properly storing fresh produce and meats. When diarrhea is the result of a food-borne virus, the goal is usually to rid the system of the pathogen, rather than to slow peristalsis.

Incontinence. **Fecal incontinence** is the inability to control passage of feces and gas from the anus. Incontinence can harm a client's body image (see chapter 22). In many situations, the client is mentally alert but physically unable to avoid defecation. The embarrassment of soiling clothes can lead to self-imposed social isolation. Physical conditions that impair anal sphincter function or control can cause incontinence. Incontinence can occur in a variety of settings. Conditions that create frequent, loose, large-volume, watery stools also predispose to incontinence (Box 41-2).

Flatulence. In most healthy individuals, 100 to 200 mL of gas is present in the GI tract. Gas in the upper GI tract may increase from swallowing of air. Gas production in the colon occurs from bacteria digesting cellulose in the colon.

As gas accumulates in the lumen of the intestines, the bowel wall stretches and distends **(flatulence).** It is a common cause of abdominal fullness, pain, and cramping. Normally, intestinal gas escapes through the mouth (belching) or the anus (passing of flatus). For someone eating a normal diet, 50 to 500 mL of gas is passed 10 to 15 times a day. However, if there is a reduction in intestinal motility resulting from opiates, general anaesthetics, abdominal surgery, or immobilization, flatulence can become severe enough to cause abdominal distension and severe sharp pain.

Hemorrhoids. **Hemorrhoids** are dilated, engorged veins in the lining of the rectum. They are either external or internal. External hemorrhoids are clearly visible as protrusions of skin. If the underlying vein is hardened, there can be a purplish discoloration (thrombosis). This causes increased pain, and the hemorrhoid may need to be excised. Internal hemorrhoids have an outer mucous membrane. Increased venous pressure from straining at defecation, pregnancy, heart failure, and chronic liver disease can cause hemorrhoids.

Bowel Diversions

Certain diseases cause conditions that prevent normal passage of feces through the rectum. The treatment for these disorders may result in the need for a temporary or permanent artificial opening **(stoma)** in the abdominal wall. Surgical openings may be created in the ileum **(ileostomy)** or colon **(colostomy)** with the ends of the intestine brought through the abdominal wall to create the stoma.

Research Highlight — Box 41-2

Factors Associated With Fecal Incontinence

Research Focus

Identifying causes for fecal incontinence of clients in acute care settings is difficult. Nurses care for many clients who are incontinent. This condition is embarrassing for the client. However, it also increases the client's risk of complications secondary to incontinence, such as impaired skin integrity or prolonged hospital stays.

Research Abstract

The purpose of this study was to determine the presence of fecal incontinence in hospitalized clients who were acutely ill and to determine if there was a relationship between fecal incontinence and stool consistency, and between two well-known nosocomial or iatrogenic causes of diarrhea: *Clostridium difficile* and enteral tube feedings. Data from 152 clients were collected on fecal incontinence, stool frequency and consistency, presence of tube feedings and medications, severity of illness, and nutritional information. Rectal swabs and stool specimens were obtained weekly and cultured for nosocomial infections.

Evidence-Based Practice

- The presence of diarrhea was more frequently associated with incontinence.
- Clients who were incontinent of loose, watery diarrhea had little or no warning prior to the incontinence episode.
- Diarrhea is present without a positive stool culture.
- Controlling the diarrhea is beneficial because the more formed a stool becomes, the less frequent the incontinence.
- When clients have organism-related diarrheas, as with *C. difficile,* treatments should be avoided that slow intestinal transit.

Reference

Bliss, D. Z., et al. (2000). Fecal incontinence in hospitalized patients who are acutely ill. *Nursing Research,* 49(2), 101–108.

The standard bowel diversion creates a stoma, or the client has reconstructive surgery that uses the native sphincter for bowel continence. The reconstructive surgery includes a continent stoma procedure, which is rarely done anymore, or the ileoanal pouch anastomosis, which is described later (Colwell et al., 2001).

Ostomies. The location of the ostomy determines the consistency of stool. An ileostomy bypasses the entire large intestine. As a result, stools are frequent and liquid. The same is true for a colostomy of the ascending colon. A colostomy of the transverse colon generally results in a more solid, formed stool. The sigmoid colostomy emits near-normal stool. The location of a colostomy is determined by the client's medical problem and general condition. There are three types of colostomy construction:

loop colostomy, end colostomy, and double-barrel colostomy.

Loop Colostomy. A loop colostomy is usually performed in a medical emergency when closure of the colostomy is anticipated. These are usually temporary large stomas constructed in the transverse colon (Figure 41–5, *A–D*). The surgeon pulls a loop of bowel onto the abdomen (Figure 41–5, *E*). An external supporting device such as a plastic rod, bridge (Figure 41–5, *C* and *D*), or rubber catheter is temporarily placed under the bowel loop to keep it from slipping back (Figure 41–5, *A*). The surgeon then opens the bowel and sutures it to the skin of the abdomen (Figure 41–5, *F*). A communicating wall remains between the proximal and distal bowel. The loop ostomy has two openings through the one stoma (Figure 41–5, *D* and *G*). The proximal end drains stool, whereas the distal portion drains mucus. Within 7 to 10 days, the external supporting device is removed.

End Colostomy. The end colostomy consists of one stoma formed from one end of the bowel with the distal portion of the GI tract either removed or sewn closed (called Hartmann's pouch) and left in the abdominal cavity. For many clients, end colostomies are a result of surgical treatment of colorectal cancer. In such cases, the rectum might also be removed. Clients with diverticulitis who are treated surgically often have a temporary end colostomy with a Hartmann's pouch (Figure 41–6).

Double-Barrel Colostomy. In a double-barrel colostomy (unlike in the loop colostomy), the bowel is surgically severed (Figure 41–7, *A*) and the two ends are brought out onto the abdomen (Figure 41–7, *B*). The double-barrel colostomy consists of two distinct stomas: the proximal functioning stoma and the distal non-functioning stoma.

Alternative Procedures

Ileoanal Pouch Anastomosis. The ileoanal pouch anastomosis is a new surgical procedure that may be used in clients who need to have a colectomy for treatment of ulcerative colitis or familial **polyps.** In this procedure, the colon is removed, a pouch (or reservoir) is created from the end of the small intestine, and the pouch is attached to the client's anus (Figure 41–8). This pouch provides for the collection of waste material, which is similar to the rectum. The client is continent of stool, as stool is evacuated via the anus. When the ileal pouch is created, the client has a temporary ileostomy to allow the anastomosis to heal.

Kock Continent Ileostomy. The Kock continent ileostomy is created using the client's small intestine to create a pouch (Figure 41–9). This procedure is occasionally used in the treatment of ulcerative colitis. The pouch has a continent stoma, a nipple-type valve that is drained with an external catheter, which is placed intermittently in the stoma. The client empties the pouch several times a day. The stoma is covered with a protective dressing or stoma cap (Colwell et al., 2001).

Psychological Considerations. A stoma can cause serious body image changes, particularly if it is permanent. A classic study reported by Walsh et al. (1995) measured the perception of body image in clients who had a stoma. Clients who had a long-standing history of chronic bowel disease such as Crohn's disease or ulcerative colitis had improved quality of life but a lower body image. Conversely, clients who needed an ostomy because of cancer had a higher body image but a reduced quality of life. Clients often perceive a stoma as invasive and disfiguring. However, a well-placed stoma should not interfere with the client's activities and can be concealed with clothing (Banks & Razor, 2003). However, even though clothing may conceal the ostomy, the client feels different. Many clients have difficulty maintaining or initiating normal sexual relations. An important factor in the client's reactions is the character of fecal secretions and the ability to control them. Foul odours, spillage, or leakage of liquid stools and inability to regulate bowel movements impair the client's self-esteem.

Critical Thinking

Successful critical thinking requires a synthesis of knowledge, experience, information gathered from clients, critical thinking attitudes, and intellectual and professional standards. Clinical judgments require the nurse to anticipate the information necessary, analyze the data, and make decisions regarding client care. During assessment (Figure 41–10), the nurse must consider all elements that build toward making appropriate diagnoses.

In the case of bowel elimination, the nurse must integrate the knowledge from nursing and other disciplines to better understand the client's response to bowel elimination interruptions. Often clients respond to disruptions in bowel elimination with fright and embarrassment. Sensitivity on the part of the nurse is essential. For clients with significant interruptions such as a bowel diversion, including information from an enterostomal specialist is an important part of the care plan.

Nursing Process and Bowel Elimination

NP Assessment

Assessment for bowel elimination patterns and abnormalities includes a nursing health history, a physical assessment of the abdomen, inspection of fecal characteristics, and a review of relevant test results. In addition, the nurse needs to determine the client's medical history, pattern and types of fluid and food intake, chewing ability, medications, and recent illnesses and/or stressors.

Health History. The nursing health history provides a review of the client's usual bowel pattern and habits. What a client describes as normal or abnormal may be different from factors and conditions that tend to promote normal elimination. Identifying normal and abnormal patterns, habits, and the client's perception of normal and abnormal in regard to bowel elimination allows the nurse to

Text continued on p. 1398

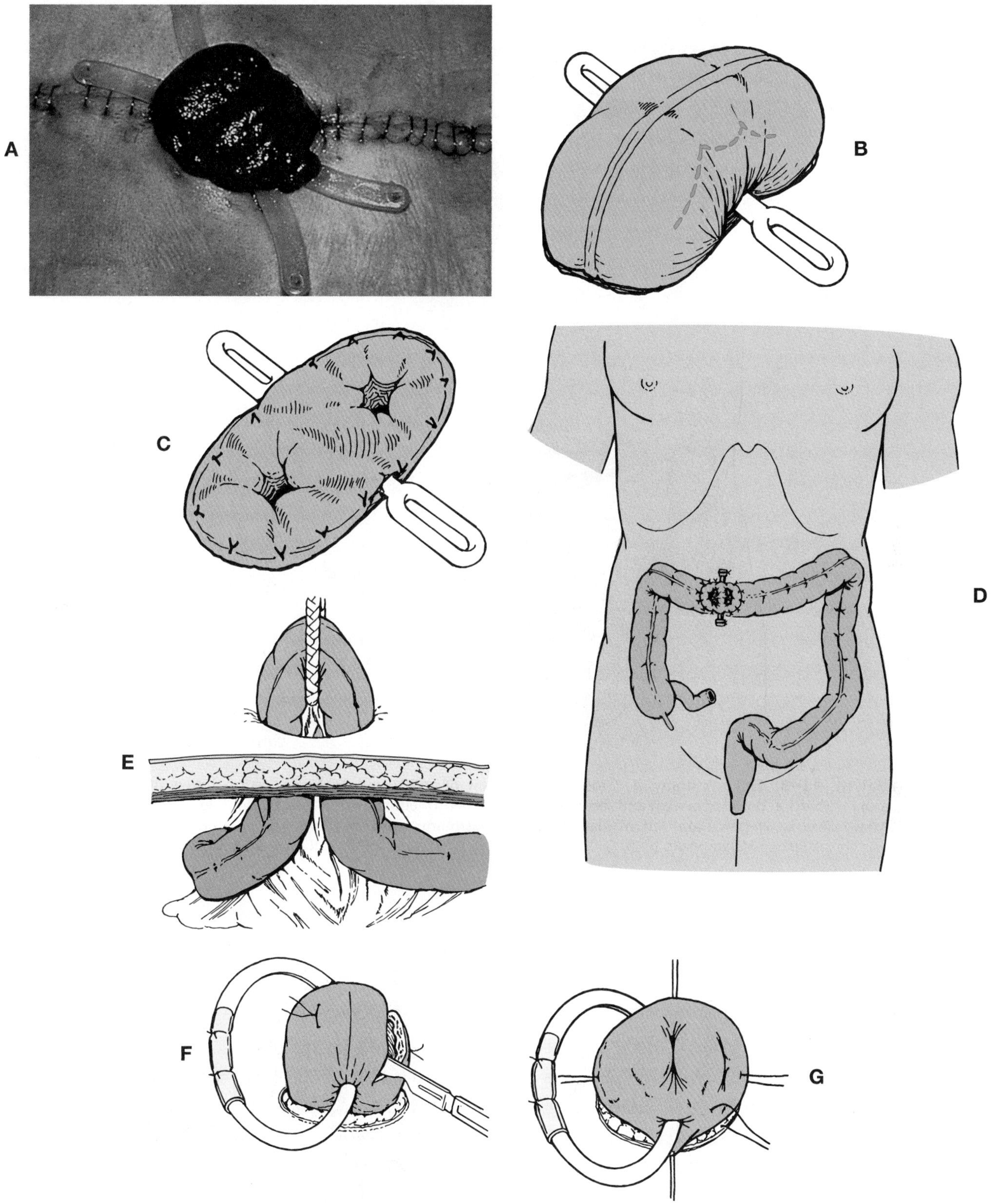

FIGURE **41–5** **A,** Transverse loop colostomy supported with a flexible red rubber catheter. **A, B,** Abdominal view of loop colostomy in transverse colon. **C,** Loop colostomy construction is much the same as construction of loop ileostomy. Stoma is created with longitudinal incision through sacculations in colon. **D,** Loop colostomy matured. **E,** Loop ostomy construction, loop of bowel exteriorized. **F,** Support device placed to maintain position of bowel on abdominal surface. Distal bowel of ileum is incised, mesentery. Stitch placed to designate proximal bowel. **G,** Loop ileostomy matured with protruding functional limb. (**A,** Courtesy Hollister, Inc., Libertyville, IL; **B** to **G,** From *Ostomies and Continent Diversions: Nursing Management,* by B. G. Hampton and R. A. Bryant, 1992, St. Louis, MO: Mosby.)

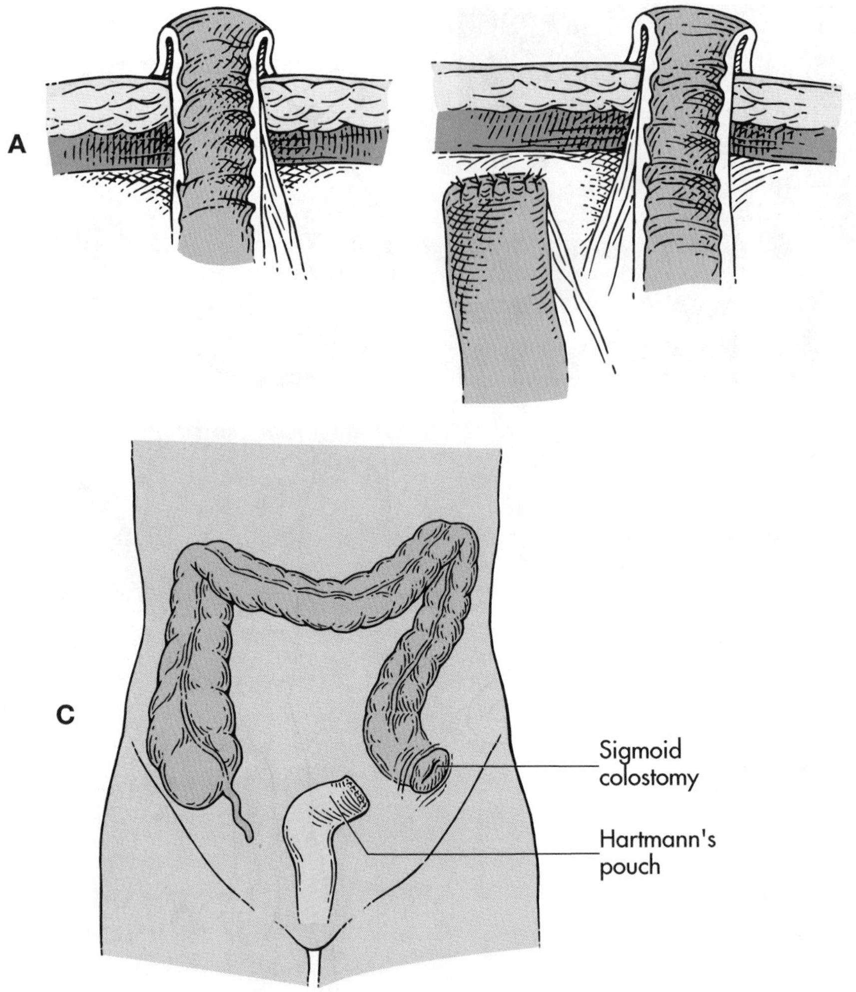

FIGURE **41–6** End colostomy. **A,** Cross-sectional view of end stoma. **B,** Cross-sectional view of end stoma with distal bowel oversewn and secured to anterior peritoneum at stoma site. **C,** Sigmoid colostomy. Distal bowel is oversewn and left in place to create Hartmann's pouch. (From *Ostomies and Continent Diversions: Nursing Management,* by B. G. Hampton and R. A. Bryant, 1992, St. Louis, MO: Mosby.)

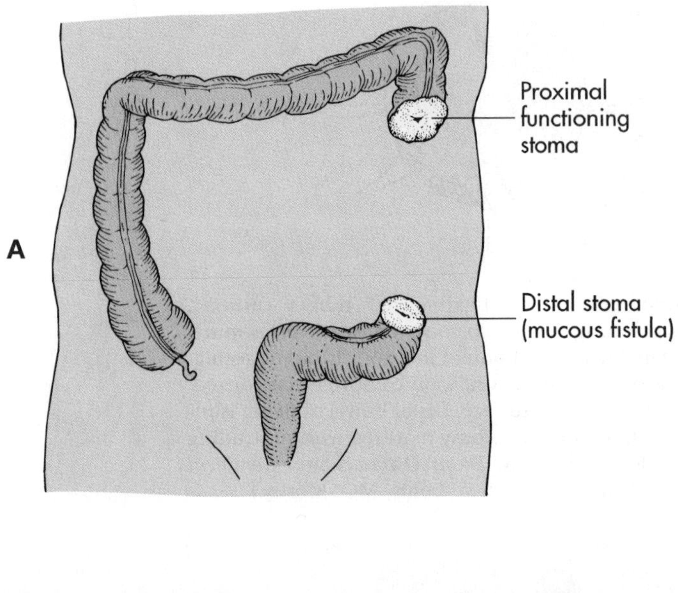

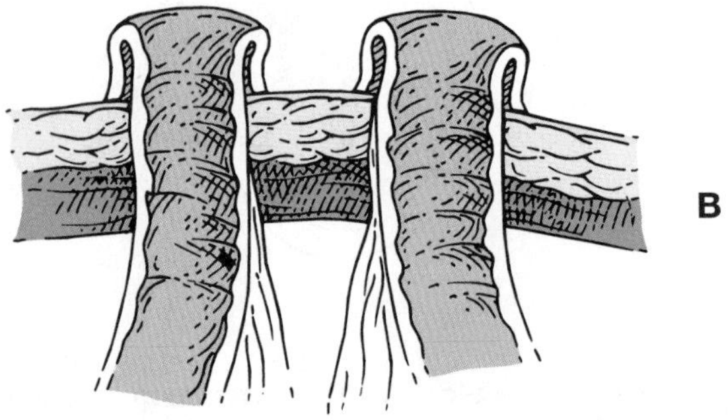

FIGURE **41–7** Double-barrel colostomy. **A,** Double-barrel colostomy in the descending colon. **B,** Cross-sectional view of double-barrel stoma. (From *Ostomies and Continent Diversions: Nursing Management,* by B. G. Hampton and R. A. Bryant, 1992, St. Louis, MO: Mosby.)

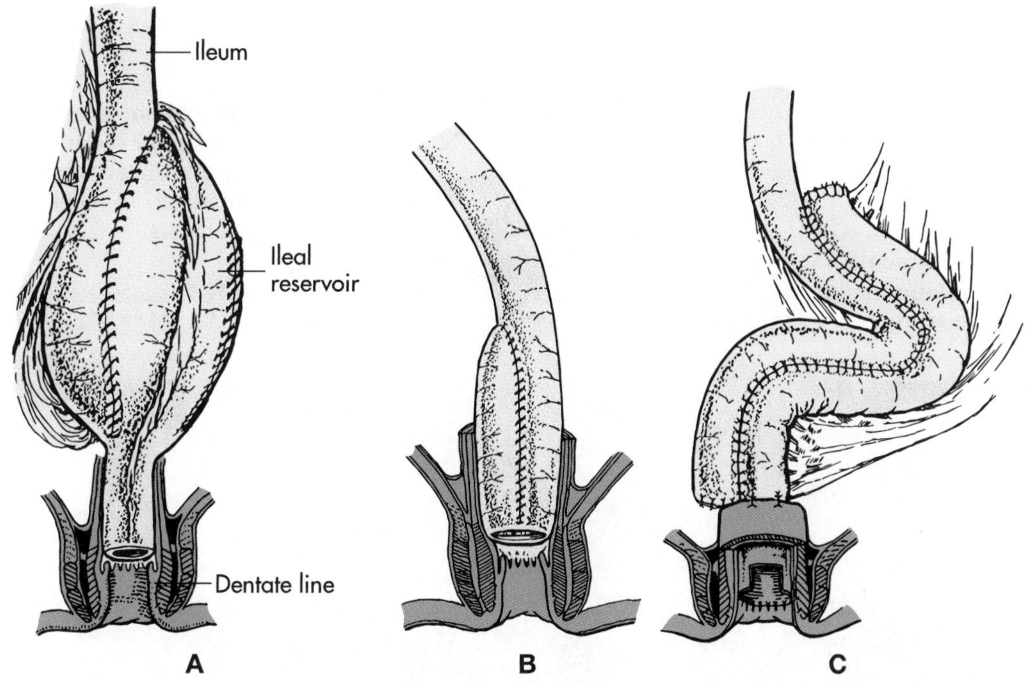

FIGURE **41–8** Ileaoanal reservoirs (IARs). **A,** S-shaped configuration for IAR. Three 10-cm limbs of ileum are used, antimesenteric surface of each limb opened, and adjacent bowel walls anastomosed. **B,** J-shaped configuration for IAR. Distal ileum is aligned in J shape; antimesenteric surface of J shape is opened, and adjacent bowel walls anastomosed. Side-to-end anastomosis of bowel to dentate line is evident. **C,** Lateral or side-by-side ileoanal pouch configuration. (From *Ostomies and Continent Diversions: Nursing Management,* by B. G. Hampton and R. A. Bryant, 1992, St. Louis, MO: Mosby.)

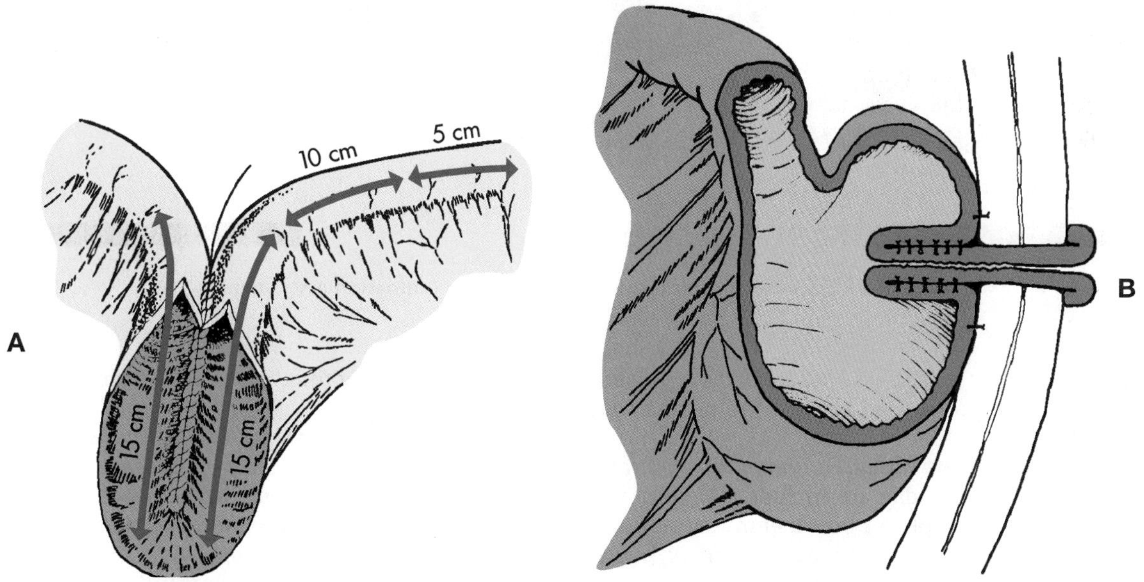

FIGURE **41–9** Construction of Kock continent ileostomy—Kock pouch. **A,** Two 15-cm limbs are used to create pouch, and one 15-cm limb is used to fashion a nipple valve and stoma. **B,** Distal limb is intussuscepted into reservoir to create one-way valve and accomplish continence. Sutures or staples, or both, are placed to stabilize and maintain intussuscepted nipple. Anterior surface of reservoir is anchored to anterior peritoneal wall. (From *Ostomies and Continent Diversions: Nursing Management,* by B. G. Hampton and R. A. Bryant, 1992, St. Louis, MO: Mosby.)

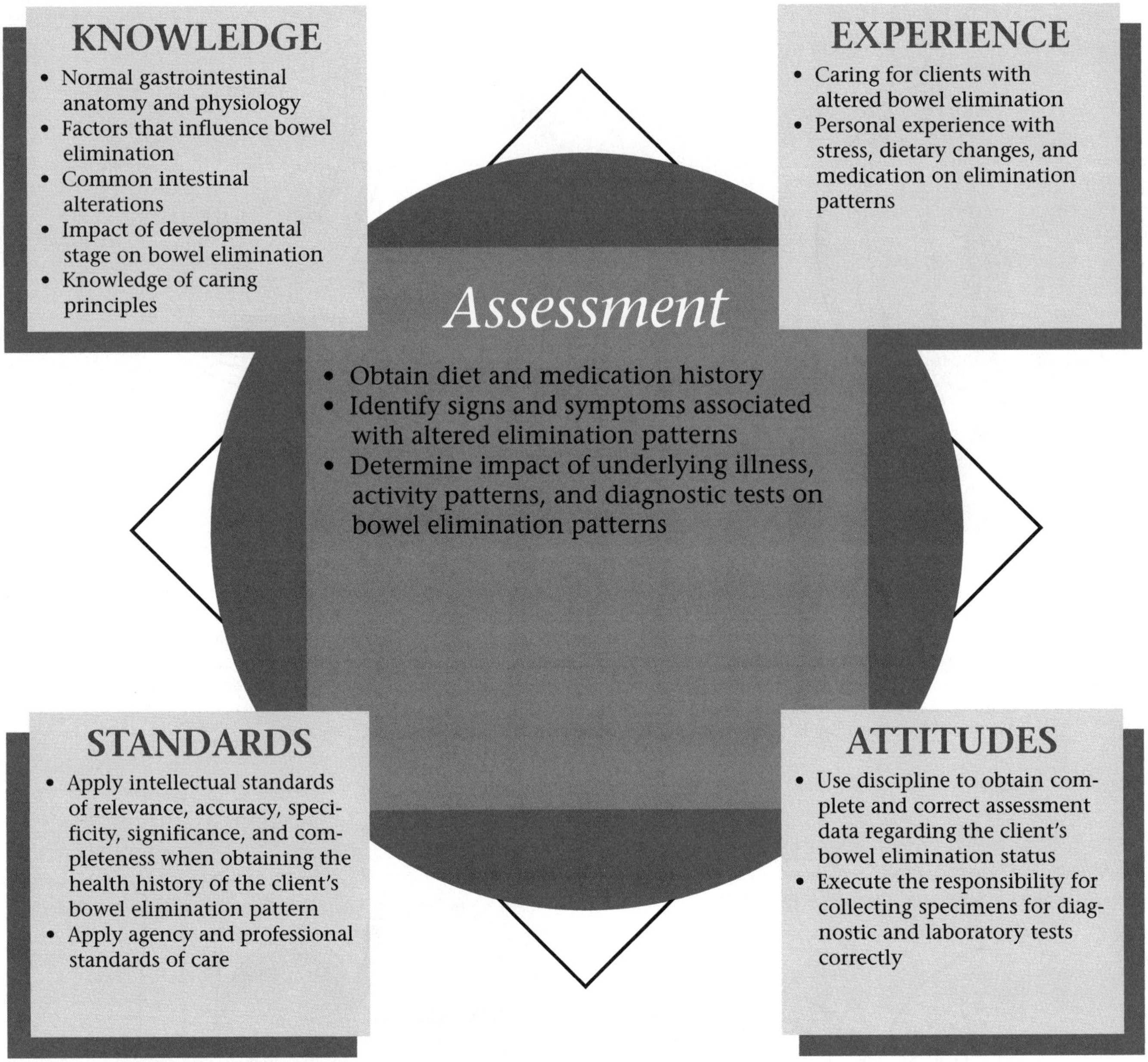
KNOWLEDGE
• Normal gastrointestinal anatomy and physiology
• Factors that influence bowel elimination
• Common intestinal alterations
• Impact of developmental stage on bowel elimination
• Knowledge of caring principles
EXPERIENCE
• Caring for clients with altered bowel elimination
• Personal experience with stress, dietary changes, and medication on elimination patterns
Assessment
• Obtain diet and medication history
• Identify signs and symptoms associated with altered elimination patterns
• Determine impact of underlying illness, activity patterns, and diagnostic tests on bowel elimination patterns
STANDARDS
• Apply intellectual standards of relevance, accuracy, specificity, significance, and completeness when obtaining the health history of the client's bowel elimination pattern
• Apply agency and professional standards of care
ATTITUDES
• Use discipline to obtain complete and correct assessment data regarding the client's bowel elimination status
• Execute the responsibility for collecting specimens for diagnostic and laboratory tests correctly

FIGURE **41–10** Critical thinking model for elimination assessment.

determine the client's problems. Much of the nursing health history can be organized around the factors that affect elimination:

- *Determination of the usual elimination pattern:* Frequency and time of day are included. Having the client or caregiver complete a bowel elimination diary for a week may enable accurate assessment of bowel elimination pattern.
- *Client's description of usual stool characteristics.* Determines whether the stool is normally watery or formed, soft or hard, the typical colour, whether the stool floats or sinks, and the presence of blood. Ask the client to describe the usual shape of the stool and the number of stools per day.
- *Identification of routines followed to promote normal elimination:* Examples are drinking hot liquids, eating specific foods, or taking time to defecate during a certain part of the day.
- *Assessment of the use of artificial aids at home:* Assess whether the client uses enemas, laxatives, or bulk-forming food additives before having a bowel movement. Ask how often client uses them.
- *Assessment of cognitive capacity:* The nurse must assess the client's ability to understand the questions posed to him or her. This is particularly true of older clients and those with memory or other cognitive impairment. It may be necessary for the nurse to carry out a brief mental exam to establish mental status. This is particularly important when the client lives alone and there is no one to corroborate his or her statements.
- *Presence and status of bowel diversions:* If the client has an ostomy, assess frequency of fecal drainage, character of

feces, appearance and condition of the stoma (colour, swelling, and irritation), type of fecal collection device used, and methods used to maintain the ostomy's function.

- *Changes in appetite:* Also include changes in eating patterns and a change in weight (amount of loss or gain). If a change of weight is present, ask if the weight change was planned, such as weight loss with a diet.
- *Diet history:* Determine the client's dietary preferences for a day or a week. Assess the intake of fruits, vegetables, cereals, and breads and also if meals are regular or irregular. In the case of the frail, older client living alone, determine whether assistance is required to provide food (i.e., money, food preparation, or transportation to grocery stores with a full selection of fresh fruits and vegetables).
- *Description of daily fluid intake:* This includes the type and amount of fluid. The client might have to estimate the amount using common household measurements.
- *History of surgery or illnesses affecting the GI tract:* This information can often help explain symptoms, the potential for maintaining or restoring normal bowel elimination pattern, and whether there is a family history of gastrointestinal cancer.
- *Medication history:* Ask for a list of the medications that the client takes. This must include prescribed and over-the-counter medications (such as laxatives, antacids, iron supplements, and analgesics) that might alter defecation or fecal characteristics. In many cases, the community nurse should ask to see the medications.
- *Emotional state:* The client's emotions can significantly alter frequency of defecation. During assessment, observation of the client's emotions, tone of voice, and mannerisms can reveal significant behaviours that indicate stress.
- *History of exercise:* Ask the client to describe the type and amount of daily exercise.
- *History of pain or discomfort:* Ask the client whether there is a history of abdominal or anal pain. The type, frequency, and location of pain may help identify the source of the problem.
- *Social history:* Clients have many different living arrangements. Where clients live may affect their toileting habits. If the client is sharing living quarters, how many bathrooms are there? Do clients have their own bathroom, or do they need to share and thus adjust the time they use the bathroom to accommodate others? If clients live alone, are they capable of ambulating to the toilet safely? If the client is not independent in bowel management, who assists the client and how?
- *Mobility and dexterity:* The client's mobility and dexterity need to be evaluated to determine if the client needs assistive devices or personal assistance.

Physical Assessment. The nurse conducts a physical assessment (see chapter 28) of body systems and functions likely to be influenced by the presence of elimination problems.

Mouth. The nurse inspects the client's teeth, tongue, and gums. Poor dentition or poorly fitting dentures influence the ability to chew (see chapter 39). Sores in the mouth can make eating not only difficult, but also painful. If the mouth is dry, this may indicate dehydration.

Abdomen. The nurse inspects all four abdominal quadrants for contour, shape, symmetry, and skin colour. Inspection also includes noting masses, peristaltic waves, scars, venous patterns, stomas, and lesions. Normally, peristaltic waves are not visible. However, observable peristalsis can be a sign of intestinal obstruction.

Abdominal distension appears as an overall outward protuberance of the abdomen. Intestinal gas, large tumours, or fluid in the peritoneal cavity may cause distension. A distended abdomen feels tight, like a drum, and the skin appears taut, as if stretched.

Percussion detects lesions, fluid, or gas within the abdomen. Familiarity with the five percussion notes (see chapter 28) also permits identification of underlying abdominal structures. Gas or flatulence creates a tympanic note. Masses, tumours, and fluid are dull to percussion.

The nurse auscultates the abdomen with the stethoscope to assess bowel sounds in each quadrant (see chapter 28). Normal bowel sounds occur every 5 to 15 seconds and last a second to several seconds. While auscultating, the nurse notes the character and frequency of bowel sounds. An increase in pitch or a tinkling sound may be heard with abdominal distension. Absent (no auscultated bowel sounds) or hypoactive sounds (fewer than five sounds per minute) occur with paralytic ileus, such as after abdominal surgery. High-pitched and hyperactive bowel sounds (35 or more sounds per minute) occur with small intestine obstruction and inflammatory disorders.

The nurse gently palpates the abdomen for masses or areas of tenderness (see chapter 28). It is important for the client to relax. Tensing abdominal muscles interferes with palpating underlying organs or masses.

Rectum. The nurse inspects the area around the anus for lesions, discolorations, inflammation, and hemorrhoids. Abnormalities should be carefully recorded (see chapter 28).

Laboratory Tests. Laboratory and diagnostic examinations yield useful information concerning elimination problems (Table 41-3). Laboratory analysis of fecal contents can detect pathological conditions such as tumours, bleeding, and infection.

Fecal Specimens. The nurse is directly responsible for ensuring that specimens are accurately obtained, properly labelled in appropriate containers, and transported to the laboratory on time. Institutions provide special containers for fecal specimens. Some tests require specimens to be placed in chemical preservatives.

Medical aseptic technique should be used during collection of stool specimens (see chapter 29). Because about 25% of the solid portion of a stool is bacteria from the colon, the nurse should wear disposable gloves when handling specimens.

Hand hygiene is necessary for anyone who might come in contact with the specimen. Often the client can obtain the specimen if properly instructed. The nurse explains that feces cannot be mixed with urine or water. For

Table 41-3 Laboratory and Diagnostic Tests for Bowel Function

Measurement and Normal Values	Interpretation
Laboratory tests	
• Total bilirubin: 0.1–1.0 mg/dL	• Increased in hepatobiliary diseases, obstructions in bile duct, certain anemias, and following transfusion reactions
• Alkaline phosphatase: 30–85 ImU/mL	• Elevated in obstructive hepatobiliary diseases, hepatobiliary carcinomas, bone tumours, healing fractures
• Amylase: 56–190 IU/L	• Elevated in abnormalities of the pancreas, such as inflammation, tumours, cholecystitis, necrotic bowel, and diabetic ketoacidosis
• Carcinoembryonic antigen: (CEA): <5 ng/mL	• Elevated in the presence of cancer or inflammation of the GI tract or hepatobiliary organs
Direct visualization	
• Endoscopy	• Routine examination (e.g., colonoscopy) for people after 50 years of age. Normally the GI tract should be free of polyps, tumours, inflammation, ulcers, hernias, obstruction, and ulcerations. If a lesion such as a polyp is identified, the physician removes the growth or a portion of the growth and sends it to pathology for analysis. If bleeding is present, the physician may attempt to coagulate the source. In some cases, the identification of an abnormality may indicate the need for follow-up surgery for the client.
Indirect visualization	
• X-ray with contrast medium	• The X-ray may identify the presence of abnormalities in the GI tract. A series of X-rays may be completed to allow for indirect visualization of the entire tract. The presence of tumours, ulcerations, inflammation, or other abnormalities may indicate the need for further diagnostic testing and medical or surgical intervention.

From *Mosby's Diagnostic and Laboratory Test Reference* (5th ed.), by K. D. Pagana and T. J. Pagana, 2001, St. Louis, MO: Mosby.

this reason, the client must defecate into a clean, dry bedpan or special container placed under the toilet seat.

Tests performed by the laboratory for occult (microscopic) blood in the stool and stool cultures require only a small sample. The nurse collects about 2.5 cm of formed stool or 15 to 30 mL of liquid diarrhea stool. Tests for measuring the output of fecal fat require a 3- to 5-day collection of stool. All fecal material must be saved throughout the test period.

After obtaining a specimen, the nurse labels and tightly seals the container and completes laboratory requisition forms. The nurse then records specimen collections in the client's medical record. It is important to avoid delays in sending specimens to the laboratory. Some tests such as measurement for ova and parasites require the stool to be warm. When stool specimens are allowed to stand at room temperature, bacteriological changes that alter test results can occur.

A common laboratory test that can be done at home or at the client's bedside is the **fecal occult blood testing (FOBT),** or guaiac test, which measures microscopic amounts of blood in feces (Box 41-3). It is useful as a diagnostic screening test for colon cancer (Box 41-4). One positive result does not confirm GI bleedings. The test should be repeated at least three times while the client refrains from ingesting foods and medications that can cause false-positive results. For example, red meat, poultry, fish, some raw vegetables, vitamin C, and aspirin or non-steroidal anti-inflammatory medications can cause false-positive results (Ransohoff & Lang, 1997). Clients who are receiving anticoagulants or who have a bleeding disorder or a GI disorder known to cause bleeding (e.g., intestinal tumours, bowel inflammation, or ulcerations) should be regularly screened for fecal occult blood.

Fecal Characteristics. Inspection of fecal characteristics (Table 41-4) reveals information about the nature of elimination alterations. Several factors can influence each characteristic. A key to assessment is knowing whether there have been any recent changes. The client can best provide this information during the nursing health history.

Diagnostic Examinations. A variety of radiological and diagnostic tests may be ordered for the client experiencing altered bowel elimination (Box 41-5). Visualization of GI structures may be by direct or indirect approach. Each test has a prescribed preparation routine to empty the area under study so that visualization is facilitated. Many facilities use conscious sedation during these procedures. Midazolam (Versed) is often the sedative drug of choice, with possible augmentation with Demerol or morphine. It is essential for the nurse to understand the safety precautions involved concerning the use of this form of anaesthesia. In many institutions, special training is required. A crash cart must be present at the bedside, and the client must be monitored continuously with pulse oximetry and frequent vital signs, usually every 15 minutes during and immediately following the procedure (check agency policy).

Client Expectations. Clients expect the nurse to be able to answer all of their questions regarding diagnostic tests and the preparation for those tests. Clients will be concerned

Box 41-3 Procedural Guidelines

Measuring Fecal Occult Blood

Equipment: Hemoccult test paper, Hemoccult developer, and wooden applicator (see illustration).

Delegation Considerations: This skill can be delegated to unregulated care providers. The nurse assesses significance of findings.

1. Explain the purpose of the test and ways client can assist. Client can collect own specimen if possible.
2. Perform hand hygiene.
3. Apply clean disposable gloves.
4. Use tip of wooden applicator (see illustration of equipment) to obtain a small portion of a stool specimen. Be sure that specimen is free of toilet paper.
5. Perform Hemoccult slide test.
   a. Open flap of slide and, using the wooden applicator, thinly smear stool in the first box of the guaiac paper. Apply a second fecal specimen from a different portion of the stool to the slide's second box (see illustration).
   b. Close slide cover and turn the packet over to the reverse side (see illustration). Open cardboard flap and apply two drops of developing solution on each box of guaiac paper. A blue colour indicates a positive guaiac, or presence of fecal occult blood.
   c. Assess colour of the guaiac paper after 30 to 60 seconds.
   d. Dispose of test slide in proper receptacle.
6. Wrap wooden applicator in paper towel, remove gloves, and discard in proper receptacle.
7. Perform hand hygiene.
8. Record results of test, noting any unusual fecal characteristics.

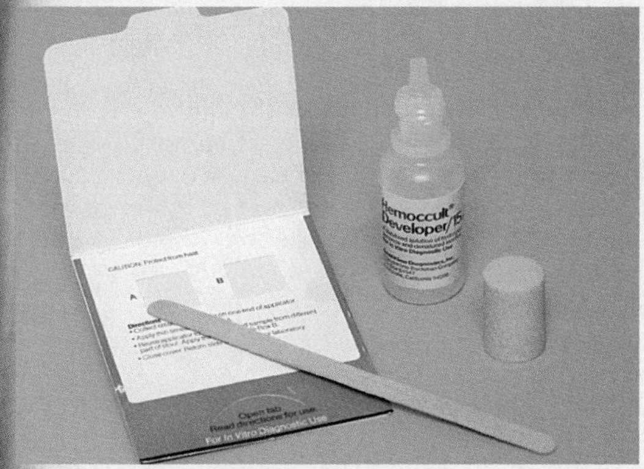

Equipment for performing fecal occult blood testing.

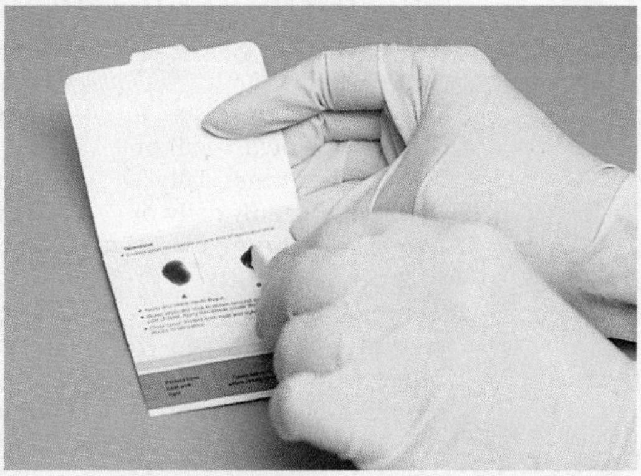

STEP **5a** Application of fecal specimen on guaiac paper.

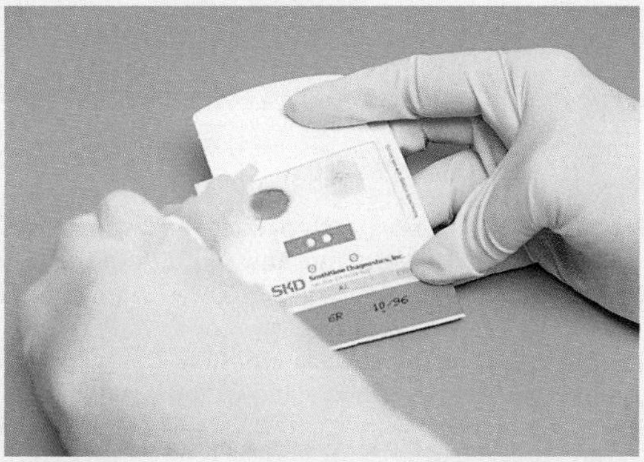

STEP **5b** Application of Hemoccult developing solution on the guaiac paper on the reverse side of the test kit.

Box 41-4 Screening for Colon Cancer

Risk Factors

- Age: over 50 years of age
- Family history: colon polyps or colorectal cancer
- History of inflammatory bowel disease (colitis, Crohn's disease)
- Personal history of polyps
- Diet: high intake of animal fats and low fibre intake
- Obesity and inactivity
- Heavy alcohol consumption or smoking

Warning Signs

- Change in bowel habits for no apparent reason
- Blood in or on the stool
- Sensation of incomplete bowel evacuation

Screening Tests

- Digital rectal examination every year after age 40
- Fecal occult blood test (FOBT) at least every 2 years after age 50
- A positive FOBT should be followed up with a colonoscopy, sigmoidoscopy, and double-contrast barium enema

From Canadian Cancer Society, 2005.

Table 41-4 Fecal Characteristics

Characteristic	Normal	Abnormal	Abnormal Cause
Colour	Infant: yellow; adult: brown	White or clay	Absence of bile
		Black or tarry (melena)	Iron ingestion or upper GI bleeding
		Red	Lower GI bleeding, hemorrhoids
		Pale with fat	Malabsorption of fat
		Translucent mucus	Spastic constipation, colitis, excessive straining
		Bloody mucus	Blood in feces, inflammation, infection
Odour	Pungent; affected by food type	Noxious change	Blood in feces or infection
Consistency	Soft, formed	Liquid	Diarrhea, reduced absorption
		Hard	Constipation
Frequency	*Varies:* Infant four to six times daily (breast-fed) or one to three times daily (bottle-fed); adult daily or two to three times a week	Infant more than six times daily or less than once every 1-2 days; adult more than three times a day or less than once a week	Hypomotility or hypermotility
Amount	150 g per day (adult)		
Shape	Resembles diameter of rectum	Narrow, pencil shaped	Obstruction, rapid peristalsis
Constituents	Undigested food, dead bacteria, fat, bile pigment, cells lining intestinal mucosa, water	Blood, pus, foreign bodies, mucus, worms	Internal bleeding, infection, swallowed objects, irritation, inflammation
		Excess fat	Malabsorption syndrome, enteritis, pancreatic disease, surgical resection of intestine

Box 41-5 Radiologic and Diagnostic Tests

Plain Film of Abdomen/Kidneys, Ureter, Bladder

A simple X-ray film of the abdomen requiring no preparation.

Upper GI/Barium Swallow

An X-ray examination using an opaque contrast medium (barium) to examine the structure and motility of the upper GI tract, including pharynx, esophagus, and stomach.
Client must be allowed nothing by mouth (NPO) after midnight the night before the examination.
Client must remove all jewellery and other metallic objects.
After the test, client must increase fluids to facilitate passage of barium.

Upper Endoscopy

An endoscopic examination of the upper GI tract allowing more direct visualization through a lighted fibre-optic tube that contains a lens, forceps, and brushes for biopsy.
Preparation is similar to that of the upper GI.
Light sedation is required.

Barium Enema

An X-ray examination using an opaque contrast medium to examine the lower GI tract.
Preparation includes NPO after midnight, a bowel preparation such as magnesium citrate, and, in some instances, enemas to empty out any remaining stool particles.

Ultrasound

A technique that uses high-frequency sound waves to echo off body organs, creating a picture.
Preparation depends on the organ to be visualized and may include NPO or no preparation.

Colonoscopy

An endoscopic examination of the entire colon with a long, flexible tube (colonoscope) inserted into the rectum.
Preparation is similar to that of barium enema: clear liquids the day before and then some form of bowel cleanser, such as GoLYTELY. Enemas until clear may also be ordered. Light sedation is required.

Flexible Sigmoidoscopy

An examination of the interior of the sigmoid colon through the use of a flexible or rigid lighted tube.
Preparation is similar to that of a barium enema or colonoscopy.
Light sedation is required.

Computerized Tomography Scan

An X-ray examination of the body from many angles using a scanner analyzed by a computer.
Preparation may be NPO, or nothing may be required.
The client must be informed of the need to lie very still. If claustrophobia is a problem, light sedation may be used.

Magnetic Resonance Imaging

A non-invasive examination that uses magnetic and radio waves to produce a picture of the inside of the body.
Preparation is NPO 4 to 6 hours before examination.
No metallic objects are allowed in the room, including metal objects on clothes.

Enteroclysis

Introduction of contrast material to the jejunum, allowing the entire small intestine to be studied.
Preparation is 24 hours of clear liquid diet and colon cleansing, such as a GoLYTELY or enemas until clear.

about discomfort and exposure. Fear of loss of control over bowel elimination is especially worrisome. Clients will need reassurance that their needs will be met and that the nurse will be supportive. Constipation is more of a problem as people age. Some older clients who may fail to recognize their elimination needs will need the nurse to monitor elimination patterns so that negative consequences will not occur. It is important for the nurse to remember that the client brings to any situation an individual perception of what is "right" for them. In the area of bowel elimination, clients will expect a knowledgeable nurse who can teach them methods of promoting and maintaining a normal bowel elimination pattern.

Nursing Diagnosis

The nurse's assessment of the client's bowel function reveals data that may indicate an actual or potential elimination problem or a problem resulting from elimination alterations. The concept map (Figure 41–11) shows how the nursing diagnosis of constipation may be related to other diagnoses. In this example, a client with cancer has developed constipation as a result of activity intolerance and imbalanced nutrition. Both of those conditions were a result of the client's pain. Examples of diagnoses that may apply to clients with elimination problems include the following:

- Bowel incontinence
- Constipation
- Constipation, risk for
- Constipation, perceived
- Diarrhea

Associated problems, such as body-image changes or skin breakdown, require interventions unrelated to bowel function impairment. However, in some instances, the nurse must direct as much attention to the associated problem as to the elimination problem.

The nurse's ability to identify the correct nursing diagnosis depends not only on the thoroughness of assessment, but also on recognition of defining characteristics and factors

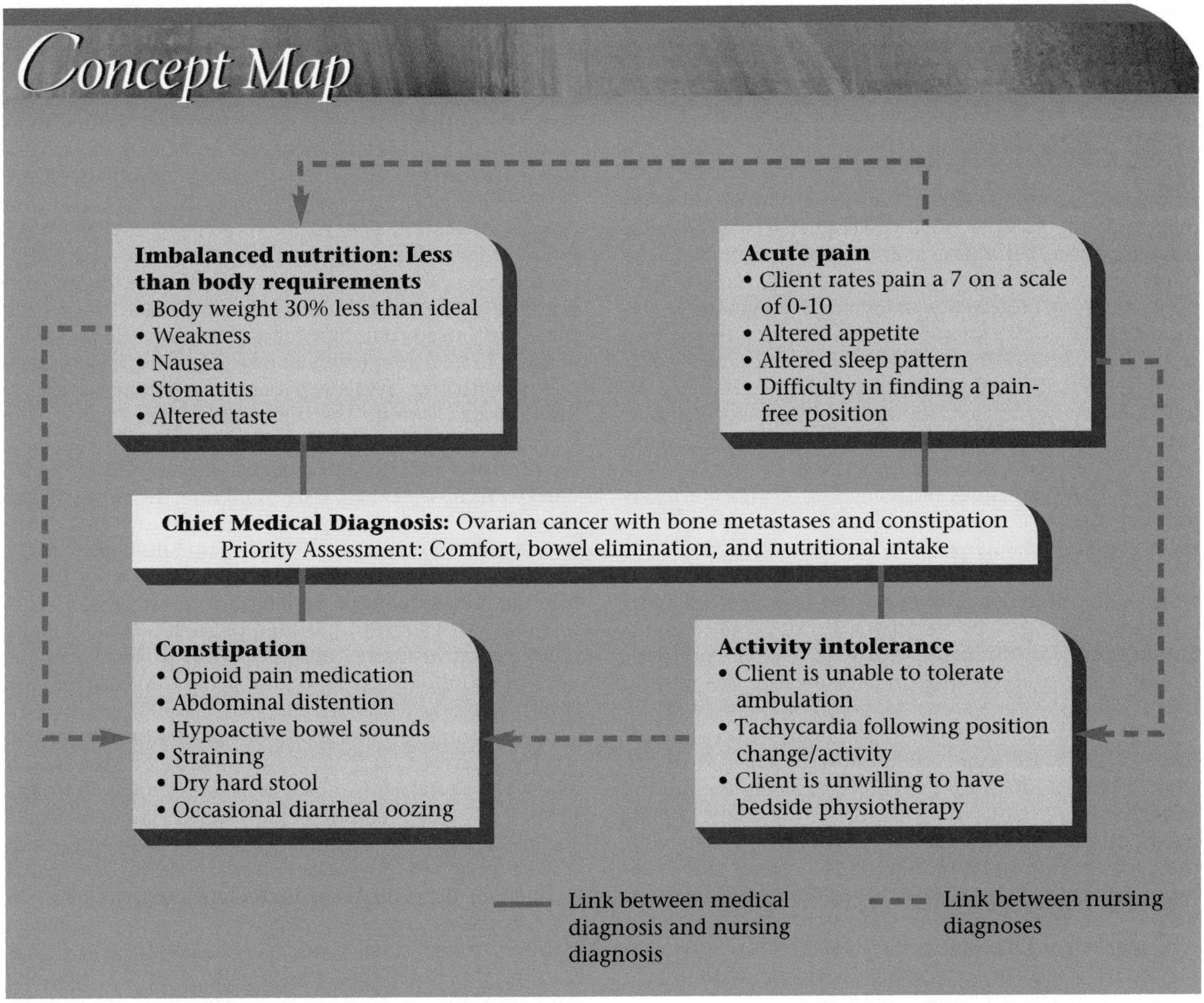

FIGURE **41–11** Concept map for client with ovarian cancer with bone metastases and constipation.

Nursing Diagnostic Process — Box 41-6

Assessment Activities	Defining Characteristics	Nursing Diagnosis
Auscultate bowel sounds.	Bowel sounds are hyperactive and audible without a stethoscope.	Diarrhea related to alteration in gastrointestinal functioning
Assess frequency of stools.	Client reports having more than three loose bowel movements a day, accompanied by muscle cramps.	
Assess hydration status.	Loss of skin turgor and dry mucous membranes.	
Have client describe pain, cramping, or any associated factors.	Pain is colicky in nature and spasmodic.	
Evaluate perianal area for redness and irritation.	Breakdown of perianal tissues.	

that can impair elimination (Box 41-6). The nurse determines the client's risk and institutes measures to ensure maintenance of normal bowel function.

Planning

During the planning of care, the nurse synthesizes information from multiple resources (Figure 41–12). Critical thinking ensures that the plan of care integrates all the nurse knows about the client and the clinical problem. The nurse relies on professional standards. The guidelines on incontinence (see chapter 40) can assist the nurse in protecting the client's skin, promoting continence, and reducing the embarrassment associated with incontinence. In addition, the Agency for Health Care Policy and Research (AHCPR), the Registered Nurses Association of Ontario (RNAO), and the Canadian Association of Wound Care (CAWC) have guidelines on reduction of pressure ulcers that also assist in developing care for clients with bowel incontinence (see chapter 43).

Goals and Outcomes. The nurse and the client establish goals and outcomes by incorporating the client's elimination habits or routines as much as possible and reinforcing those routines that promote health. Pre-existing health concerns are also considered. For example, if the client is at risk for the worsening of heart failure, an outcome of increased fluid intake must be tailored to the client's cardiac function and ability to safely handle the increased fluid. In another example, if the client's bowel habits caused the elimination problem, the nurse helps the client learn new bowel habits. The overall goal of returning the client to a normal bowel elimination pattern may include the following outcomes:

- Client sets regular defecation habits.
- Client is able to list proper fluid and food intake needed to achieve bowel elimination.
- Client implements a regular exercise program.
- Client reports daily passage of soft, formed brown stool.
- Client does not report any discomfort associated with defecation.

Setting Priorities. Defecation patterns vary among individuals. For this reason, the nurse and client must work together closely to plan effective interventions (see Care Plan). What may be a realistic time frame to establish a normal defecation pattern for one client might be very different for another. In the client with a new ostomy resulting from newly diagnosed cancer, the priority of coping with cancer and its treatment may need to precede the client's need to independently manage the bowel diversion. In addition, when a bowel diversion is necessary, coping with the changes in body image may become a high priority for both the client and family.

Continuity of Care. When clients are disabled or debilitated by illness, it is necessary to include the family in the plan of care. Often family members have the same elimination habits as the client. Thus, client and family teaching is an important part of the care plan. Other health team members such as dietitians and enterostomal therapist (ET) nurses can be valuable resources. When clients require surgical intervention, a critical pathway may be used to coordinate the activities of the multidisciplinary health care team.

The client with alterations in bowel elimination will require intervention from many members of the health care team. Certain tasks, such as assisting clients onto the bedpan or bedside commode, are appropriate to delegate to unregulated care providers (UCPs). It will be important for the nurse to remind the UCP to report any abnormal findings or difficulties encountered during the elimination process. Many of the diagnostic tests for evaluation of the gastrointestinal system will be performed by non-nursing personnel. The nurse must maintain ongoing communication with these caregivers to ensure that the client's needs, wants, and concerns are addressed.

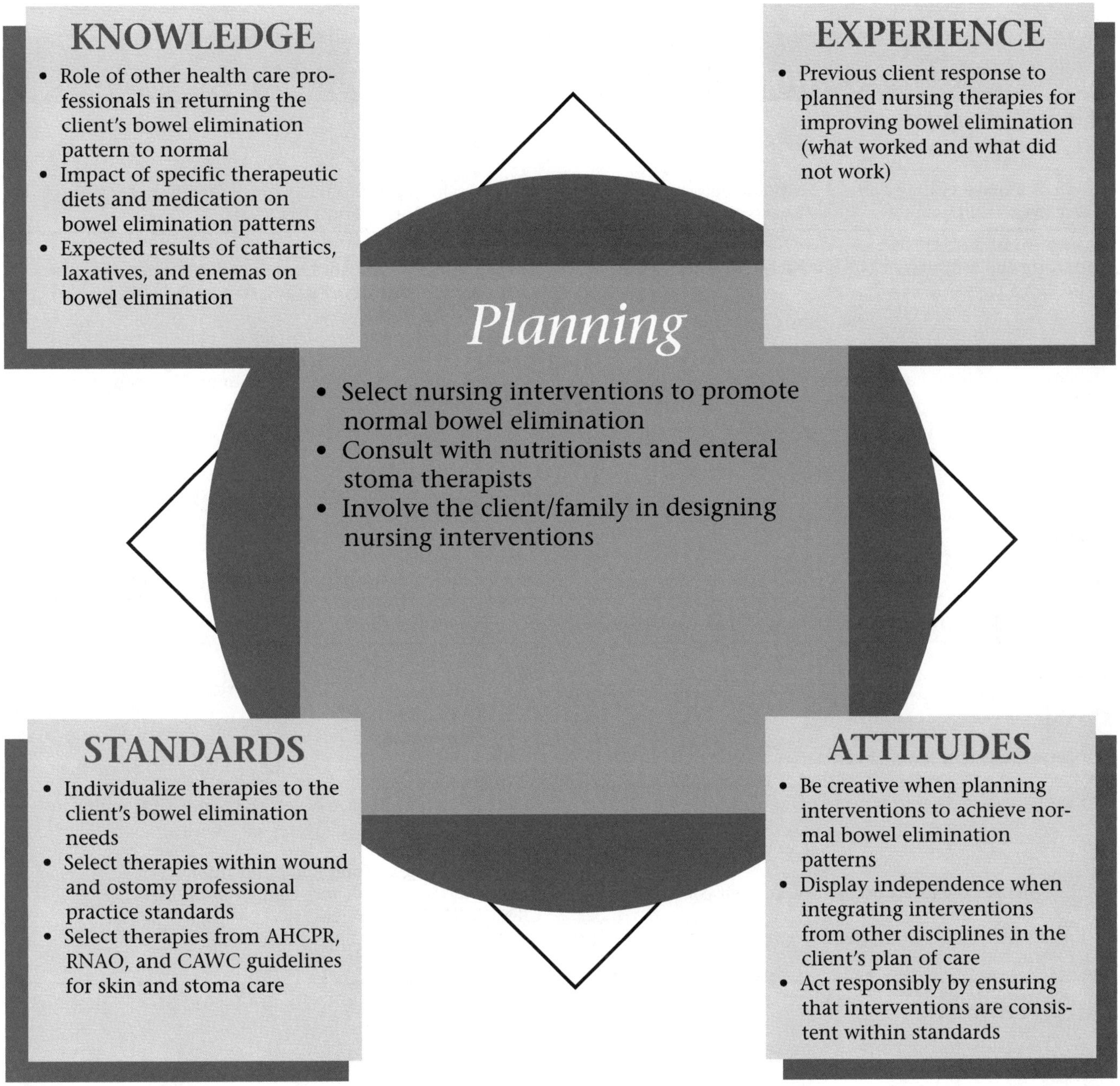
KNOWLEDGE
• Role of other health care professionals in returning the client's bowel elimination pattern to normal
• Impact of specific therapeutic diets and medication on bowel elimination patterns
• Expected results of cathartics, laxatives, and enemas on bowel elimination
EXPERIENCE
• Previous client response to planned nursing therapies for improving bowel elimination (what worked and what did not work)
Planning
• Select nursing interventions to promote normal bowel elimination
• Consult with nutritionists and enteral stoma therapists
• Involve the client/family in designing nursing interventions
STANDARDS
• Individualize therapies to the client's bowel elimination needs
• Select therapies within wound and ostomy professional practice standards
• Select therapies from AHCPR, RNAO, and CAWC guidelines for skin and stoma care
ATTITUDES
• Be creative when planning interventions to achieve normal bowel elimination patterns
• Display independence when integrating interventions from other disciplines in the client's plan of care
• Act responsibly by ensuring that interventions are consistent within standards

FIGURE **41–12** Critical thinking model for elimination planning.

NP Implementation

Success of the nurse's interventions depends on improving the client's and family members' understanding of bowel elimination. In the home, hospital, or long-term care facility, clients capable of learning can be taught effective bowel habits.

The nurse should teach the client and family about proper diet, adequate fluid intake, and factors that stimulate or slow peristalsis, such as emotional stress. This often can best be done during the client's mealtime. The client should also learn the importance of establishing regular bowel routines and regular exercise and taking appropriate measures when elimination problems develop.

Health Promotion. One of the most important habits a nurse can teach regarding bowel habits is to take time for defecation. To establish regular bowel habits, a client must know when the urge to defecate normally occurs. The nurse advises the client to begin establishing a routine during a time when defecation is most likely to occur, usually an hour after a meal. Many evidenced-based interventions are available to reduce the risk of constipation (Box 41-7). If a client is restricted to bed or requires

Nursing Care Plan

Constipation

Assessment

Javier is a nurse visiting Larry at his home on a cattle ranch. Larry lives 40 km from town. He is 22 years old and had surgery 6 days ago for repair of a badly broken right leg. Larry also tells Javier that he "Just doesn't feel good."

Assessment Activities	Findings/Defining Characteristics
Ask Larry about his recent bowel elimination patterns over the last 5 days.	Larry says that he has not had a bowel movement since he left the hospital 4 days ago and that he feels like his abdomen is tight and sore.
Review client's medication.	Client has been prescribed Lortabs for pain. Larry says he is taking one tablet every 6 hours, up to three a day.
Review dietary intake over last day.	Larry has eaten eggs, bacon, and toast and had soup for lunch. For supper Larry had chicken, rice, and corn. He drinks about 6 cups of coffee each day, no water, but will drink a cola.
Ask about any nausea or vomiting.	Client has not felt nauseated.
Auscultate client's abdomen.	Decreased bowel sounds auscultated throughout all four abdominal quadrants.
Palpate abdomen.	While Javier is palpating Larry's abdomen, Larry tells Javier, "It really hurts." On palpation, left lower quadrant is tender and firm.

Nursing Diagnosis: Constipation related to opiate-containing pain medication and decreased fibre intake.

Planning

Goals	Expected Outcomes*
	Bowel Elimination
Client will establish normal defecation.	Client will drink at least 1500 mL of fluid over the next 8 hours.
Client will voice relief from constipation.	Client will report passage of soft stool without straining in next 24 hours.
	Nutritional Status: Food and Fluid Intake
Client will identify measures that will prevent constipation.	Client will increase the fibre content of his diet. Client will increase exercise.

*Outcome classification labels from *Nursing Outcomes Classification (NOC)* (3rd ed.), edited by S. Moorhead, M. Johnson, and M. L. Maas, 2004, St. Louis, MO: Mosby.

Interventions†	Rationale
Constipation/Impaction Management	
Encourage fluid intake of appropriate fluids, fruit juice, water.	Adequate fluid intake is necessary to prevent hard, dry stool.
Encourage activity within the limits of client's mobility regimen.	Even minimal activity (such as leg lifts) increases peristalsis.
Add bran flakes or bran to the diet.	The number of bowel movements is increased with bran (Bliss et al., 2001).
Provide laxative or stool softeners as ordered.	Medications can soften the stool and prevent straining (McKenry & Salerno, 2001).
Provide privacy.	Clients should feel relaxed when moving bowels.

†Intervention classification labels from *Nursing Interventions Classification (NIC)* (4th ed.), edited by J. M. Dochterman and G. M. Bulecheck, 2004, St. Louis, MO: Mosby.

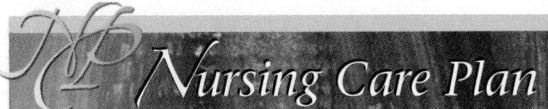

Nursing Care Plan

Constipation—cont'd

Evaluation

Nursing Actions	Client Response/Finding	Achievement of Outcome
Ask client to identify foods high in fibre.	Client able to state appropriate foods. Review of 24-hour diet diary shows client is selecting high-fibre, low-fat foods.	Larry is making excellent progress in introducing high-fibre and low-fat foods into his diet.
Ask client to plan menus to increase fibre.	Review of 24-hour diet diary showed meals planned with high-fibre content. Client reviewed shopping list with bran, oat, and fruit products.	Larry is knowledgeable about fibre content and purchases food that is high in fibre.
Ask client about increased activity.	Client states that he has not changed his activity pattern.	Client has not increased activity pattern and needs to continue to work on this activity.
Observe client's subsequent stool for characteristics such as consistency and colour.	Stools are now every 24 to 48 hours. Larry does not "feel regular." Abdomen is soft and non-distended. Stools are formed and hard, and client reports straining.	Client has not achieved passage of regular, formed stool.

Evidence-Based Practice Guideline Box 41-7

Management of Constipation

- Fluid intake of at least 1.5 L/day is recommended. Preferred fluid is water because it is sodium and calorie free. Client may benefit from one to two glasses of fruit juice as well.
- Coffee, tea, and alcohol should be avoided because of their diuretic properties.
- A high-fibre diet (25 to 30 g/day) reduces constipation; fibre that passes though the colon acts as a sponge. As a result, bulkier and softer stools develop. In addition, the waste moves through the body more easily and results in more regular bowel movements. **A high-fibre diet is not recommended for individuals who are immobile or who do not consume at least 1.5 L of fluid per day.**
- The most beneficial means to prevent constipation is a combination of insoluble and soluble fibre (e.g., bran, fruits, and vegetables).
- Physical activity in combination with adequate fluid intake and a high-fibre diet is beneficial in the management of constipation. For those who are fully mobile, walking once or twice a day for 15 to 20 minutes is sufficient.
- For individuals who are unable to walk, chair or bed exercises such as pelvic tilt, low trunk rotation, and single leg lifts are recommended.
- Laxatives should be used with caution, and a stepwise progression of laxatives is recommended: first bulk-forming laxatives, followed by stool softeners, osmotics, stimulants, suppositories, and enemas as a last resort.

Adapted from "Evidenced-Based Protocol: Management of Constipation," by M. Hinrichs and J. Huseboe, in *Series on Evidence-Based Practice for Older Adults*, edited by M. G. Titler (Series Ed.), 2001, Iowa City, IA: The University of Iowa College of Nursing Gerontological Nursing Interventions Research Center, Research Dissemination Core.

assistance in ambulating, the nurse should offer a bedpan or help the client reach the bathroom in a timely manner.

Many clients have established routines for defecation. In a hospital or long-term care facility, the nurse should make certain that treatment routines do not interfere with the client's routine. It is important to provide privacy. When clients forced to use a bedpan share rooms with other people, the nurse should pull the curtain around the area so that clients can relax, knowing that interruptions will not occur. The call light should always be placed within the clients' reach. Bathroom doors should be closed, although the nurse may stand close by in case the client needs assistance.

Promotion of Normal Defecation. A number of interventions can stimulate the defecation reflex, affect the character of feces, or increase peristalsis to help clients evacuate bowel contents normally and without discomfort.

Sitting Position. The nurse might need to assist clients who have difficulty sitting because of muscular weakness and mobility problems. Regular toilets are too low for clients unable to lower themselves to a sitting position because of joint- or muscle-wasting diseases. Elevated toilet seats for the home are available. With such a seat, less effort is needed to sit or stand. In many provinces, these seats can be acquired through the service agencies for minimal or no cost. The community nurse must assess the client capabilities in the home and the requirement for any additional equipment to facilitate daily living.

Positioning on Bedpan. Clients restricted to bed must use bedpans for defecation. Women use bedpans to pass both urine and feces, whereas men use bedpans only for defecation. Sitting on a bedpan can be extremely uncomfortable. The nurse should help position clients comfortably. Two types of bedpans are available (Figure 41–13). The regular bedpan, made of metal or hard plastic, has a

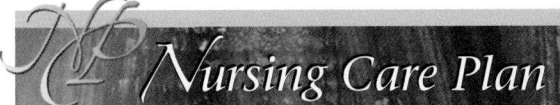

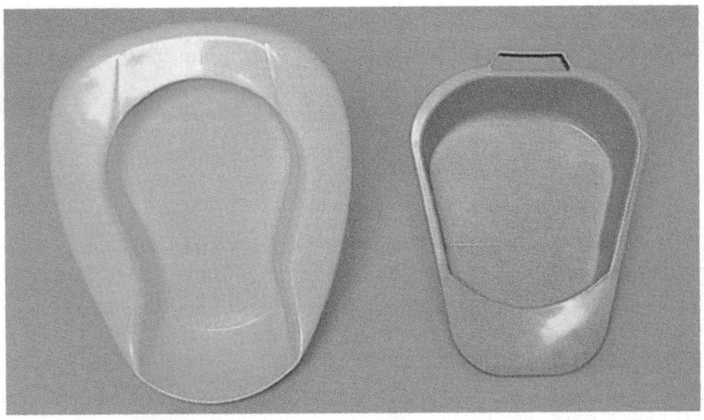

FIGURE **41–13** Types of bedpans. From *left,* regular bedpan and fracture bedpan.

curved smooth upper end and a sharp-edged lower end and is about 5 cm deep. A fracture pan, designed for clients with body or leg casts, has a shallow upper end about 1.3 cm deep. The upper end of the pan fits under the buttocks toward the sacrum, with the lower end just under the upper thighs. The pan should be high enough so that feces enter the pan. A metal bedpan should be warmed with water first, then dried.

When positioning a client, it is important to prevent muscle strain and discomfort. A nurse should never try to lift a client onto a bedpan. A client should never be placed on a bedpan and then left with the bed flat unless activity restrictions demand it. If the bed is flat, the hips remain hyperextended.

Figure 41–14 shows proper and improper positions on bedpans. The best method is to be sure that the client is positioned high in bed. The nurse raises the client's head about 30 degrees to prevent hyperextension of the back and to provide support to the upper torso. The client then raises the hips by bending the knees and lifting the hips upward. The nurse places a hand, palm up, under the client's sacrum, resting the elbow on the mattress and using it as a lever to help in lifting, while slipping the pan under the client. Clients who have had abdominal surgery are hesitant to exert strain on suture lines and may have difficulty positioning on a pan. Gloves should always be worn by the nurse when handling a bedpan.

If the client is immobile or it is unsafe to allow the client to exert such effort, the client can roll onto the bedpan by using the following steps:

1. Lower the head of the bed flat and assist the client to roll onto one side, backside toward you.
2. Apply a little powder to back and buttocks to prevent skin from sticking to the pan.
3. Place the bedpan firmly against the buttocks, down into the mattress with the open rim toward the client's feet (Figure 41–15).
4. Keeping one hand against the bedpan, place the other around the client's far hip. Ask the client to roll back onto the pan, flat in bed. Do not shove the pan under the client.
5. With the client positioned comfortably, raise the head of the bed 30 degrees.

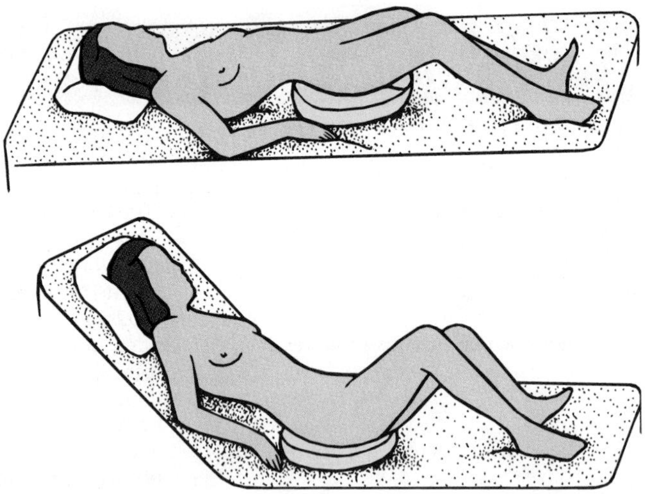

FIGURE **41–14** Positions on a bedpan. *Top,* Improper positioning of client. *Bottom,* Proper position reduces client's back strain.

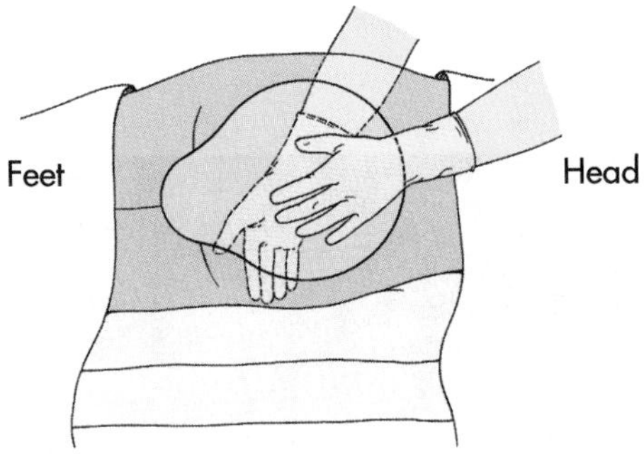

FIGURE **41–15** Positioning an immobilized client on a bedpan.

6. Place a rolled towel or small pillow under the lumbar curve of the client's back for added comfort.
7. Raise the knee gatch or ask the client to bend the knees to assume a squatting position. Do not raise the knee gatch if contraindicated.

Privacy. The nurse should maintain the client's privacy during bowel elimination. This is especially important for a client using a bedpan. The call light and a supply of toilet paper should be within easy reach. When the client finishes, the nurse responds to the call signal immediately and removes the pan. The client might require assistance with wiping. To remove the pan, the nurse asks the client to roll off to the side or to raise the hips. The nurse holds the pan steady to avoid spilling. The nurse should avoid pulling or shoving the pan from under the client's hips because this can pull the client's skin and cause tissue injury such as shearing (see chapter 43). After the pan is removed, the nurse, while wearing gloves, cleans the anal and perineal areas.

After assessing the stool, the nurse should immediately empty the bedpan's contents into the toilet or in a special receptacle in the utility room. A spray faucet attached to most toilets allows the nurse to rinse the bedpan thoroughly. The client uses the same bedpan each time. The nurse should chart the characteristics of the feces.

The nurse should offer the bedpan often. Clients may accidentally soil bedclothes if forced to wait. Many clients try to avoid using a bedpan because it is embarrassing and uncomfortable. They may try to get to the bathroom even though their conditions prohibit ambulation. The nurse must warn clients about the risk of falls or accidents.

Acute Care. The GI system may be affected by any acute illness. Changes in the client's fluid status, mobility patterns, nutrition, and sleep cycle can affect regular bowel habits. Surgical interventions on the GI tract affect bowel elimination. However, surgery on other systems, such as the musculoskeletal and cardiovascular systems, may also affect the client's bowel elimination patterns. The nurse must remain sensitive to the client's elimination needs and intervene to assist the client to maintain as normal bowel elimination habits as possible.

Medications. Medications may be used to initiate and facilitate bowel elimination. Cathartics, laxatives, and occasionally an enema are used to control constipation, whereas antidiarrheal preparations assist the client in resolving diarrhea. All of these medications are available over the counter; stronger preparations are available through prescriptions. Clients must be cautioned not to use these over-the-counter medications on a prolonged basis without consulting their health care provider.

> *Safety Alert.* Excessive use of laxatives, enemas, and/or bulk-forming agents increases the client's risk for diarrhea and abnormal bowel elimination. Excessive use of these agents destroys the client's normal defecation reflex. In addition, the client may develop altered absorption of nutrients, fluid and electrolyte imbalances, and generalized weakness. In the chronically ill or older adult clients, this may result in an increased risk for falls and other injuries.

Cathartics and Laxatives. Often a client is unable to defecate normally because of pain, constipation, or impaction. Cathartics and laxatives have the short-term action of emptying the bowel. They are also used in bowel evacuation for clients undergoing GI tests and abdominal surgery. Although the terms *cathartic* and *laxative* are often used interchangeably, cathartics have a stronger effect on the intestines. Five types of laxatives and cathartics are available (Table 41-5).

Cathartics and laxatives are available in oral, tablet, and powder suppository dosage forms (see chapter 30). Although the oral route is most commonly used, cathartics that are prepared as suppositories are more effective because of their stimulant effect on the rectal mucosa. Cathartic suppositories such as bisacodyl (Dulcolax) can act within 30 minutes. Older adults often get a strong sudden urge to defecate with Dulcolax.

Electrolyte Balance and Antidiarrheal Agents. For clients with diarrhea, frequent passage of liquid stools becomes a problem. When the person has secretory diarrhea, cells at the base of the villi secrete massive amounts of fluid into the lumen of the small intestine. However, the tip of the villi can still absorb sugars and fluids. Therefore, diarrhea can quickly lead to serious electrolyte imbalances, particularly in infants and children (see chapter 36). Therefore, the first course of action is to immediately replace fluids by mouth. It is wise to choose fluids with adequate electrolyte content (e.g., Pedialyte and Gastrolyte). In developing countries without safe water supply or during epidemics of infectious diarrhea (e.g., cholera), millions of lives have been saved by using a cheap, safe, and simple method of replacing water and salts lost through diarrhea. This method is known as oral rehydration therapy (ORT), and involves mixing a very low-cost package of salts (sodium, potassium chloride, citrate/bicarbonate, and glucose) with boiled water.

Many clients will use over-the-counter agents, such as Imodium, to relieve common diarrhea. However, the most effective antidiarrheal agents are prescriptive opiates such as codeine phosphate, opium tincture (Paregoric), and diphenoxylate (Lomotil). Antidiarrheal opiate agents decrease intestinal muscle tone to slow passage of feces. Opiates inhibit peristaltic waves that move feces forward, but they also increase segmental contractions that mix intestinal contents and expose the contents to the mucosal absorbing surface. The further effect of opiates on increasing the absorption of sodium and water also dries out the feces. As a result, more water is absorbed by the colonic mucosa. Antidiarrheal agents should be used with caution because opiates are habit forming.

Enemas. An **enema** is the instillation of a solution into the rectum and sigmoid colon. The primary reason for an enema is to promote defecation by stimulating peristalsis. The volume of fluid instilled breaks up the fecal mass, stretches the rectal wall, and initiates the defecation reflex. Enemas are also given as a vehicle for medications that exert a local effect on rectal mucosa.

The most common use for an enema is temporary relief of constipation. Other indications include removing impacted feces; emptying the bowel before diagnostic tests, surgery, or childbirth; and beginning a program of bowel training.

Cleansing Enemas. Cleansing enemas promote the complete evacuation of feces from the colon. They act by stimulating peristalsis through the infusion of a large volume of solution or through local irritation of the colon's mucosa. Cleansing enemas include tap water, normal saline, low-volume hypertonic saline, and soapsuds solution. Each solution exerts a different osmotic effect, influencing the movement of fluids between the colon and interstitial spaces beyond the intestinal wall. Infants and children should receive only normal saline because they are at risk for fluid imbalance.

A physician may order a high or low cleansing enema. The terms *high* and *low* refer to the height from which, and hence the pressure with which, the fluid is delivered. High enemas are given to cleanse the entire colon. After the enema is infused, the client is asked to turn from the left lateral to the dorsal recumbent to the right lateral position.

Table 41-5 Common Types of Laxatives and Cathartics

Agent/Brand Name	Action	Indications	Risks
Bulk Forming			
Methylcellulose (Cologel, Hydrolose)	High-fibre content absorbs water and increases solid intestinal bulk.	Agents are least irritating, most natural, and safest cathartics. Agents are drugs of choice for chronic constipation (e.g., pregnancy, low-residue diet).	Agents can cause obstruction if not mixed with at least 240 mL of water or juice and swallowed quickly.
Psyllium (Metamucil, Naturacil)	Agents stretch intestinal wall to stimulate peristalsis.	Agents may also be used to relieve mild, watery diarrhea.	Caution is used with bulk-forming laxatives that also contain stimulants. Agents are not used in clients for whom large fluid intake is contraindicated.
Emollient or Wetting			
Docusate sodium (Colace, Disonate) Docusate calcium (Surfak) Docusate potassium (Dialose)	Stool softeners are detergents that lower surface tension of feces, allowing water and fat to penetrate. They may increase secretion of water by intestines.	Agents are used for short-term therapy to relieve straining on defecation (e.g., hemorrhoids, perianal surgery, pregnancy, recovery from myocardial infarction).	Agents are of little value for treatment of chronic constipation.
Saline			
Magnesium citrate or citrate of magnesia (Citroma) Magnesium hydroxide (Milk of Magnesia)	Agents contain salt preparation not absorbed by intestines. Osmotic effect increases pressure in bowel to act as stimulant for peristalsis.	Agents are used only for acute emptying of bowel (e.g., endoscopic examination, suspected poisoning, acute constipation).	Agents are not used in long-term management of constipation. Agents are not used in clients with kidney dysfunction (toxic buildup of magnesium).
Sodium phosphate (Fleet Phospho-Soda, Fleet Enema)	Agents may also lubricate feces.		Phosphate salts are not used for clients on fluid restriction.
Stimulant Cathartics			
Bisacodyl (Dulcolax)	Agents irritate intestinal mucosa to increase motility.	Agents may be used to prepare bowel for diagnostic procedures.	Agents may cause severe cramping.
Castor oil (Neoloid, Purge) Casanthranol (Dialose Plus, Peri-Colace) Danthron (Modane Bulk)	Agents decrease absorption in small bowel and colon.		Agents are not for long-term use. Chronic use may cause fluid and electrolyte imbalances. Agents are avoided during pregnancy and lactation.
Phenolphthalein (Doxidan, Correctol, Ex-Lax)	Phenolphthalein and danthron may cause pink or red urine.		
Lubricants			
Mineral oil (Haley's M-O, Petrogalar Plain)	Agents coat fecal contents, allowing easier passage of stool. Agents reduce water absorption in colon.	Agents are used to prevent straining on defecation (e.g., hemorrhoids, perianal surgery).	Agents decrease absorption of fat-soluble vitamins (A, D, E, and K). Agents can cause dangerous form of pneumonia if aspirated into lungs. Mineral oil when taken with emollients can increase risk for fat emboli.

The position change ensures that fluid reaches the large intestine. A low enema cleanses only the rectum and sigmoid colon.

Tap Water. Tap water is hypotonic and exerts a lower osmotic pressure than fluid in interstitial spaces. After infusion into the colon, tap water escapes from the bowel lumen into interstitial spaces. The net movement of water is low. The infused volume stimulates defecation before large amounts of water leave the bowel. Tap water enemas should not be repeated because water toxicity or circulatory overload can develop if large amounts of water are absorbed.

Normal Saline. Physiologically, normal saline is the safest solution to use because it exerts the same osmotic pressure as fluids in interstitial spaces surrounding the bowel. The volume of infused saline stimulates peristalsis. Giving saline enemas does not create the danger of excess fluid absorption.

Hypertonic Solutions. Hypertonic solutions infused into the bowel exert osmotic pressure that pulls fluids out of interstitial spaces. The colon fills with fluid, and the resultant distension promotes defecation. Clients unable to tolerate large volumes of fluid benefit most from this type of enema, which is, by design, low volume. Contraindications for this type of enema are clients who are dehydrated and young infants. A hypertonic solution of 120 to 180 mL is usually effective. The commercially prepared Fleet Enema is the most commonly used.

Soapsuds. Soapsuds may be added to tap water or saline to create the effect of intestinal irritation to stimulate peristalsis. Only pure castile soap is safe and it comes in a liquid form included in most soapsuds enema kits. Harsh soaps or detergents can cause serious bowel inflammation.

Oil-Retention Enemas. Oil-retention enemas lubricate the rectum and colon. The feces absorb the oil and become softer and easier to pass. To enhance action of the oil, the client retains the enema for several hours if possible.

Other Types of Enemas. Carminative enemas provide relief from gaseous distension. They improve the ability to pass flatus. An example of a carminative enema is MGW solution, which contains 30 mL of magnesium, 60 mL of glycerine, and 90 mL of water.

Medicated enemas contain drugs. An example is sodium polystyrene sulphonate (Kayexalate), used to treat clients with dangerously high serum potassium levels. This drug contains a resin that exchanges sodium ions for potassium ions in the large intestine. Another medicated enema is neomycin solution, an antibiotic used to reduce bacteria in the colon before bowel surgery.

Enema Administration. The nurse administers enemas in commercially packaged, disposable units or with reusable equipment prepared before use. Sterile technique is unnecessary because the colon normally contains bacteria. However, the nurse wears gloves to prevent the transmission of fecal micro-organisms.

The nurse should explain the procedure, including the position to assume, precautions to take to avoid discomfort, and the length of time necessary to retain the solution before defecation. If the client is to receive the enema at home, the nurse explains the procedure to a family member.

Often the physician orders "enemas till clear." This means that the enema is repeated until the client passes fluid that is clear and contains no fecal material. It may be necessary to give as many as three enemas, but the nurse should caution the client against using more than three. Excess enema use seriously depletes fluids and electrolytes. If the enema fails to return a clear solution after three times (check agency policy) or if the client seems to not be tolerating the rigours of repeated enemas, the physician should be notified.

Giving an enema to a client who is unable to contract the external sphincter can pose difficulties. The nurse gives the enema with the client positioned on the bedpan. Giving the enema with the client sitting on the toilet is unsafe because the curved rectal tubing can abrade the rectal wall. Skill 41-1 outlines the steps for an enema administration.

Digital Removal of Stool. For clients with an impaction, the fecal mass may be too large to be passed voluntarily. If enemas fail, the nurse must break up the fecal mass with the fingers and remove it in sections. The procedure can be very uncomfortable for the client. Excess rectal manipulation may cause irritation to the mucosa, bleeding, and stimulation of the vagus nerve, which results in a reflex slowing of the heart rate. Because of the procedure's potential complications, a physician's order is necessary for the nurse to remove a fecal impaction (Box 41-8).

Inserting and Maintaining a Nasogastric Tube. A client's condition or situation may warrant special interventions to decompress the GI tract. Such conditions include surgery, infections of the GI tract, trauma to the GI tract, and conditions in which peristalsis is absent.

A nasogastric (NG) tube is a pliable tube that is inserted through the client's nasopharynx into the stomach. The tube has a hollow lumen that allows removal of gastric secretions and introduction of solutions into the stomach. Nasogastric intubation has several purposes (Table 41-6).

The Levin and Salem sump tubes are the most common for stomach decompression. The Levin tube is a single-lumen tube with holes near the tip. It may be connected to a drainage bag or to an intermittent suction device to drain stomach secretions.

The Salem sump tube is preferable for stomach decompression. The tube has two lumina: one for removal of gastric contents (Figure 41–16) and one to provide an air vent. A blue "pigtail" is the air vent that connects with the second lumen. When the sump tube's main lumen is connected to suction, the air vent permits free, continuous drainage of secretions. The air vent should never be clamped off, connected to suction, or used for irrigation.

Nasogastric tube insertion (Skill 41-2) does not require sterile technique. The nurse simply uses clean technique. The procedure is uncomfortable. The client experiences a burning sensation as the tube passes through the sensitive nasal mucosa. When the tube reaches the back of the pharynx, the client may begin to gag. The nurse must help the client relax to make tube insertion easier. Some institutions

Text continued on p. 1416

Skill 41-1 Administering a Cleansing Enema

View Video

Delegation Considerations

The skill of administering an enema can be delegated to unregulated care providers (UCPs). It is the nurse's responsibility to assess the client for specific considerations such as need for alternative positioning, comfort, and stable vital signs prior to procedure. In addition, it is the nurse's responsibility to determine the client's response to the enema.

- Inform and assist the UCP in proper way to position clients who have mobility restrictions, such as those clients with arthritis or severe fatigue.
- Instruct the UPC how to position clients who also have therapeutic equipment present, such as drains, intravenous catheters, or traction.
- Instruct the UCP in the specific signs and symptoms of clients not tolerating the procedure and when the procedure must be stopped. For example, these signs and symptoms may include abdominal pain more than a pressure sensation, abdominal cramping, abdominal distension, or rectal bleeding.

Equipment

- Disposable gloves
- Water-soluble lubricant
- Waterproof, absorbent pads
- Bath blanket
- Toilet tissue
- Bedpan, bedside commode, or access to toilet
- Washbasin, washcloths, towel, and soap
- Intravenous (IV) pole
- Enema bag administration
  - Enema container
  - Tubing and clamp (if not already attached to container)
  - Appropriate size rectal tube:
    - *Adult:* 22 to 30 Fr
    - *Child:* 12 to 18 Fr
  - Correct volume of warmed solution:
    - *Adult:* 750 to 1000 mL
    - *Child:*
      150 to 250 mL, infant
      250 to 350 mL, toddler
      300 to 500 mL, school-age child
      500 to 750 mL, adolescent
  - Prepackaged enema
- Prepackaged enema container with rectal tip

Steps	Rationale
1. Assess status of client: last bowel movement, normal bowel patterns, hemorrhoids, mobility, external sphincter control, and abdominal pain.	Determines factors indicating need for enema and influencing the type of enema used.
2. Assess for presence of increased intracranial pressure, glaucoma, or recent rectal or prostate surgery.	Conditions contraindicate use of enemas.
3. Check client's medical record to clarify the rationale for the enema.	Determines purpose of enema administration: preparation for special procedure or relief of constipation.
4. Review physician's order for enema.	Order by physician is required. Determines number and type of enemas to be given.
5. Determine client's level of understanding of purpose of enema.	Allows nurse to plan for appropriate teaching measures.
6. Perform hand hygiene. Collect appropriate equipment.	Reduces transmission of micro-organisms.
7. Correctly identify client and explain procedure.	Information promotes client co-operation and reduces anxiety.
8. Assemble enema bag with appropriate solution and rectal tube.	
9. Perform hand hygiene and apply gloves.	Reduces transmission of micro-organisms.
10. Provide privacy by closing curtains around bed or closing door.	Reduces embarrassment for client.
11. Raise bed to appropriate working height for nurse; raise side rail on client's left.	Promotes good body mechanics and client safety.
12. Assist client into left side-lying (Sims') position with right knee flexed. Children may instead be placed in dorsal recumbent position.	Allows enema solution to flow downward by gravity along natural curve of sigmoid colon and rectum, thus improving retention of solution.

Critical Decision Point: If client is suspected of having poor sphincter control, position on bedpan. Client will have difficulty retaining enema solution.

Steps	Rationale
13. Place waterproof pad under hips and buttocks.	Prevents soiling of linen.
14. Cover client with bath blanket, exposing only rectal area, clearly visualizing anus.	Provides warmth, reduces exposure of body parts, and allows client to feel more relaxed and comfortable.
15. Place bedpan or commode in easily accessible position. If client will be expelling contents in toilet, ensure that toilet is free. (If client will be getting up to bathroom to expel enema, place client's slippers and bathrobe in easily accessible position.)	Used in case client is unable to retain enema solution.
16. Administer enema:	
A. **Enema bag**	
(1) Add warmed solution to enema bag: warm tap water as it flows from faucet, place saline container in basin of hot water before adding saline to enema bag, check temperature of solution with bath thermometer or by pouring small amount of solution over inner wrist.	Hot water can burn intestinal mucosa. Cold water can cause abdominal cramping and is difficult to retain.
(2) Raise container, release clamp, and allow solution to flow long enough to fill tubing.	Removes air from tubing.
(3) Reclamp tubing.	Prevents further loss of solution.
(4) Lubricate 6 to 8 cm of tip of rectal tube with lubricating jelly.	Allows smooth insertion of rectal tube without risk of irritation or trauma to mucosa.
(5) Gently separate buttocks and locate anus. Instruct client to relax by breathing out slowly through mouth.	Breathing out promotes relaxation of external anal sphincter.
(6) Insert tip of rectal tube slowly by pointing tip in direction of client's umbilicus (see illustration). Length of insertion varies: *Adult:* 7.5 to 10 cm *Child:* 5 to 7.5 cm *Infant:* 2.5 to 3.75 cm	Careful insertion prevents trauma to rectal mucosa from accidental lodging of tube against rectal wall. Insertion beyond proper limit can cause bowel perforation.

Critical Decision Point: If tube does not pass easily, do not force. Consider allowing a small amount of fluid to infuse and then try reinserting tube slowly.

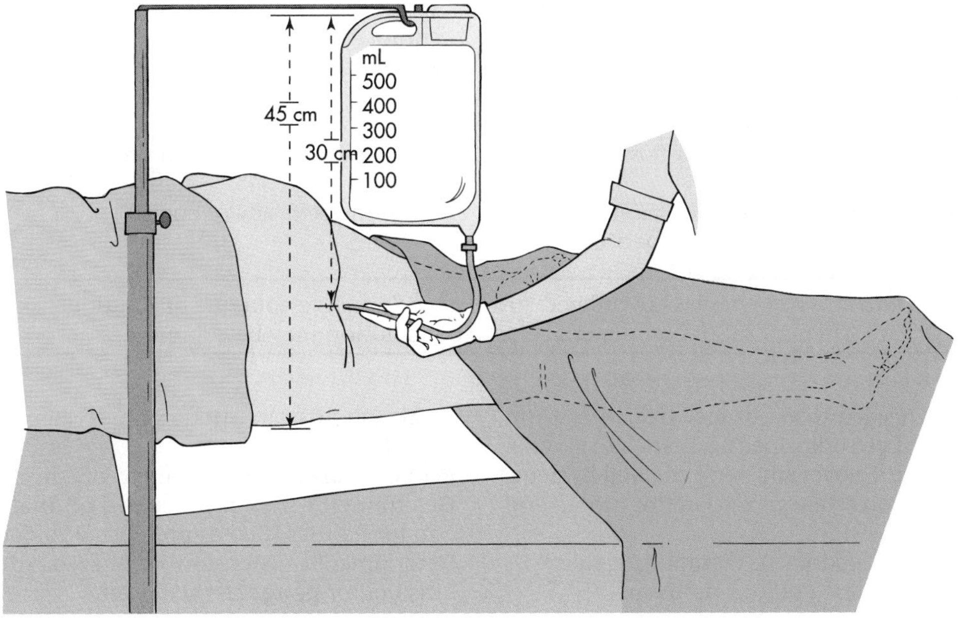

STEP **16A(6)** Insertion of a rectal tube into rectum.

Skill 41-1 Administering a Cleansing Enema—cont'd

Steps	Rationale
(7) Hold tubing in rectum constantly until end of fluid instillation.	Bowel contraction can cause expulsion of rectal tube.
(8) Open regulating clamp and allow solution to enter slowly with container at client's hip level.	Rapid instillation can stimulate evacuation of rectal tube.
(9) Raise height of enema container slowly to appropriate level above anus: 30 to 45 cm for high enema, 30 cm for regular enema, 7.5 cm for low enema (see illustration for step 16A[6]). Instillation time varies with the volume of solution administered.	Allows for continuous, slow instillation of solution. Raising container too high causes rapid instillation and possible painful distension of colon. High pressure can cause rupture of bowel in infant.
(10) Lower container or clamp tubing if client complains of cramping or if fluid escapes around rectal tube.	Temporary cessation of instillation prevents cramping, which may prevent client from retaining all fluid, altering effectiveness of enema.
(11) Clamp tubing after all solution is instilled.	Prevents entrance of air into rectum.
B. **Prepackaged disposable container**	
(1) Remove plastic cap from rectal tip. Tip is already lubricated, but more jelly can be applied as needed.	Lubrication provides for smooth insertion of rectal tube without causing rectal irritation or trauma.
(2) Gently separate buttocks and locate rectum. Instruct client to relax by breathing out slowly through mouth.	Breathing out promotes relaxation of external rectal sphincter.
(3) Insert tip of bottle gently into rectum. *Adult:* 7.5 to 10 cm *Child:* 5 to 7.5 cm *Infant:* 2.5 to 3.75 cm	Gentle insertion prevents trauma to rectal mucosa.
(4) Squeeze bottle until all of solution has entered rectum and colon. Instruct client to retain solution until the urge to defecate occurs, usually 2 to 5 minutes.	Hypertonic solutions require only small volumes to stimulate defecation.
17. Place layers of toilet tissue around tube at anus and gently withdraw rectal tube.	Provides client's comfort and cleanliness.
18. Explain to client that feeling of distension is normal. Ask client to retain solution as long as possible while lying quietly in bed. (For infant or young child, gently hold buttocks together for a few minutes.)	Solution distends bowel. Length of retention varies with type of enema and client's ability to contract rectal sphincter. Longer retention promotes more effective stimulation of peristalsis and defecation.
19. Discard enema container and tubing in proper receptacle or rinse out thoroughly with warm soap and water if container is to be reused.	Reduces transmission and growth of micro-organisms.
20. Assist client to bathroom or help to position client on bedpan.	Normal squatting position promotes defecation.
21. Observe character of feces and solution (caution client against flushing toilet before inspection).	Determines efficacy of enema.

Critical Decision Point: When enemas are ordered "until clear," observe contents of solution passed. Return is "clear" when no solid fecal material exists, but solution may be coloured.

Steps	Rationale
22. Assist client as needed to wash anal area with warm soap and water (if providing perineal care, use gloves).	Fecal contents can irritate skin. Hygiene promotes client's comfort.
23. Remove and discard gloves and perform hand hygiene.	Reduces transmission of micro-organisms.
24. Inspect colour, consistency, amount of stool, and fluid passed.	Determines if stool is evacuated or fluid is retained. Note abnormalities such as presence of blood or mucus.
25. Assess condition of abdomen; cramping, rigidity, or distension can indicate a serious problem.	Determines if distension is relieved. Excess volume can distend or perforate the bowel.

Unexpected Outcomes and Related Interventions

- Abdomen becomes rigid and distended
  - Stop enema if fluid is still being instilled.
  - Notify physician and obtain vital signs.
- Abdominal pain or cramping develops
  - Slow rate of instillation.
- Bleeding occurs
  - Stop enema administration.
  - Notify physician and obtain vital signs.

Recording and Reporting

- Record type and volume of enema given and characteristics of results.
- Report to physician if the client failed to defecate.

Home Care Considerations

- For clients who require enemas for bowel preparation at home, instruct family not to exceed recommended fluid volume levels or number of enemas. Encourage family about the need for slow administration of warmed fluid.
- Instruct family about the negative side effects of tap water enemas.

Box 41-8 Procedural Guidelines

Digital Removal of Stool

Equipment: Disposable gloves, lubricant, towel, washcloth, soap and water, and bedpan.

Delegation considerations: This procedure should not be delegated to unregulated care providers.

1. Explain the procedure to the client.
2. Perform hand hygiene. Take baseline vital signs prior to the procedure. Help the client lie on the left side with knees flexed and back toward you.
3. Drape the trunk and lower extremities with a bath blanket and place a waterproof pad under the buttocks. Keep a bedpan next to the client.
4. Apply disposable gloves and lubricate the index finger of your dominant hand with lubricating jelly.
5. Gently insert the gloved index finger into the rectum and advance the finger slowly along the rectal wall toward the umbilicus.
6. Gently loosen the fecal mass by massaging around it. Work the finger into the hardened mass.
7. Work the feces downward toward the end of the rectum. Remove small pieces at a time and discard into bedpan.
8. Reassess the client's vital signs and look for signs of fatigue. Stop the procedure if the heart rate drops significantly or the rhythm changes.
9. Continue to remove feces and allow the client to rest at intervals.
10. After completion, wash and dry the buttocks and anal area.
11. Remove bedpan and dispose of feces. Remove gloves by turning them inside out, then discard.
12. Assist client to toilet or clean bedpan if urge to defecate develops.
13. Perform hand hygiene. Record results of removal of impaction by describing fecal characteristics.
14. Follow procedure with enemas or cathartics as ordered by physician.
15. Reassess client's vital signs and level of comfort.

Table 41-6 Purposes of Nasogastric Intubation

Purpose	Description	Type of Tube
Decompression	Removal of secretions and gaseous substances from gastrointestinal tract; prevention or relief of abdominal distension	Salem sump, Levin, Miller-Abbott
Feeding (gavage; see chapter 39)	Instillation of liquid nutritional supplements or feedings into stomach for clients unable to swallow fluid	Duo, Dobhoff, Levin
Compression	Internal application of pressure by means of inflated balloon to prevent internal esophageal or gastrointestinal hemorrhage	Sengstaken-Blakemore
Lavage	Irrigation of stomach in cases of active bleeding, poisoning, or gastric dilation	Levin, Ewald, Salem sump

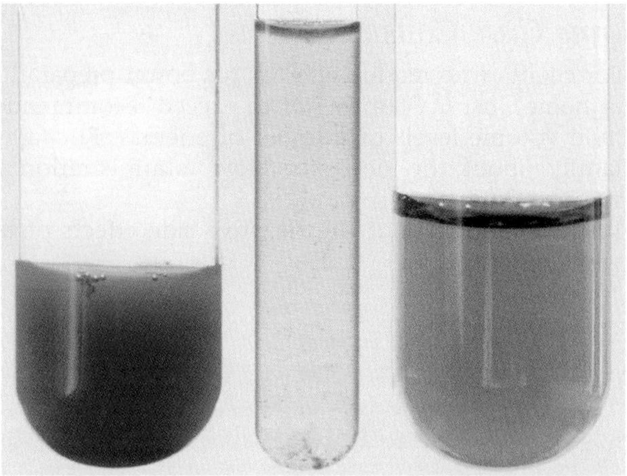

FIGURE **41–16** Gastric contents. **A,** Stomach. **B,** Stomach. **C,** Intestinal. (Courtesy Dr. Norma Metheny, St. Louis University, School of Nursing, St. Louis, MO.)

allow Xylocaine Jelly to be used when inserting the tube, as it increases client comfort during the procedure.

One of the greatest problems in caring for a client with an NG tube is maintaining comfort. The tube is a constant irritation to nasal mucosa. The nurse must assess the condition of the nares and mucosa for inflammation and **excoriation.** The tape used to anchor the tube often becomes soiled. The nurse changes it every day to lessen irritation. Frequent lubrication of the nares also minimizes excoriation. With one nares occluded, the client may breathe through the mouth. Frequent mouth care (at least every 2 hours) helps minimize dehydration. A glass of cool water for rinsing is useful, but the client who is allowed nothing by mouth (NPO) should not swallow the water. The client will frequently complain of a sore throat. An ice bag applied externally to the throat may help. Gargling with topical Xylocaine Jelly or lozenges may be used if ordered by the physician.

After the tube is inserted, the nurse must maintain its patency. If the tip of the tubing rests against the stomach wall or if the tube becomes blocked with thick secretions, regular irrigation is necessary. Flushing the tube with normal saline by way of a catheter-tipped syringe clears blockage within the tube (see Skill 41-2). If an NG tube continues to drain improperly after irrigation, the nurse must reposition it by advancing or withdrawing it slightly. Any change in tube position requires the nurse to verify the placement of the tube in the client's GI tract (see Skill 41-2).

The NG tube can cause distension. The presence of the tube causes many clients to swallow large volumes of air. Channels of gastric secretions also form along the walls of the stomach and bypass the suction holes. Turning the client regularly helps to collapse the channels and promote emptying of stomach contents.

Continuing and Restorative Care. As the client recovers and is able to return home or to a long-term care facility, regular elimination patterns must begin. When clients have a colostomy they must learn to care for the ostomy. Other clients may require bowel training. It is important to remember that ostomy care and bowel training may be initiated or take place in the acute care settings as well. However, because these are long-term care needs, these activities are usually completed in the restorative care settings.

Care of Ostomies. Clients with temporary or permanent bowel diversions have unique elimination needs. People with an ostomy wear a pouch or appliance to collect **effluent** (the stool discharged from an ostomy) from the stomas (Hyland, 2002). These clients must use meticulous skin care to prevent liquid stool from irritating the skin around the stoma (Box 41-9).

Irrigating a Colostomy. Although this practice is not as common as it once was, some clients may be instructed to irrigate their left-sided colostomies in order to regulate colon emptying. Other clients do not want to spend the additional 60 to 90 minutes in the bathroom every day, and they empty their pouch only as necessary (Hyland, 2002).

Specific equipment for irrigating a colostomy should be used. An enema set should never be used to irrigate a colostomy. A special cone-tipped irrigator (Figure 41–17) is used. This device prevents bowel penetration and prevents backflow of the irrigating solution. Clients usually sit on the toilet and place an irrigating sleeve over the stoma. The end of this sleeve extends into the bowl of the toilet. The physician orders the amount and type of solution. For adults, the amount ranges from 500 to 700 mL of tap water. The solution is instilled slowly through the lubricated cone tip. Irrigation should take 5 to 10 minutes. The client then removes the cone tip and waits 30 to 45 minutes for the solution and feces to drain out of the irrigation sleeve. Once the drainage stops, the client applies a stoma cap or a pouch. If a client chooses to irrigate the colostomy, the time of irrigation is individualized to the client's lifestyle.

Pouching Ostomies. Ostomies require a pouch to collect fecal material. An effective pouching system protects the skin, contains fecal material, remains odour free, and is comfortable and inconspicuous. A person wearing a pouch should feel secure in participating in any activity.

Many pouching systems are available. To ensure that a pouch fits well and meets the client's needs, the nurse considers the location of the ostomy; type and size of the stoma; type and amount of ostomy drainage; size and contour of the abdomen; condition of the skin around the stoma; physical activities of the client; client's personal preference, age, and dexterity; and cost of equipment. An **enterostomal therapist (ET)** is a nurse trained to care for wound and ostomy management. The staff nurse collaborates with the ET to be sure the correct pouching system is used. For example, referral to an ET nurse would be appropriate to plan the care of a client who has a high-output ostomy that requires a pouch modification.

A pouching system consists of a pouch and skin barrier. Some pouching systems, such as Squibb-Convatec, Hollister, Coloplast, and Smith & Nephew, are attached to the client's skin from the product's adhesive surface, whereas other pouching systems, such as VIP, are nonadhesive systems. Pouches come in one- and two-piece systems that are disposable or reusable. Some pouches

Text continued on p. 1423

Skill 41-2 Inserting and Maintaining a Nasogastric Tube

View Video

Delegation Considerations

The skill of inserting and maintaining the nasogastric (NG) tube should not be delegated to unregulated care providers (UCPs). The nurse is responsible for the proper function and drainage of the nasogastric tube, all relevant assessments, and determining the client's level of comfort. The nurse may instruct the UCP to do the following:

- Measure and record the drainage
- Provide oral and nasal hygiene
- Perform selected comfort measures

Equipment

- No. 14 or no. 16 Fr NG tube (smaller-lumen catheters are not used for decompression in adults because they must be able to remove thick secretions)
- Water-soluble lubricating jelly
- pH test strips (measure gastric aspirate acidity)
- Tongue blade
- Flashlight
- Emesis basin
- Asepto bulb or catheter-tipped syringe
- 2.5-cm wide hypoallergenic tape (7.5- to 10-cm long) or commercial fixation device
- Safety pin and rubber band
- Clamp, drainage bag, or suction machine or pressure gauge if wall suction is to be used
- Towel
- Glass of water with straw
- Facial tissues
- Normal saline
- Tincture of benzoin (optional)
- Suction equipment
- Disposable gloves

Steps	Rationale
1. Perform hand hygiene. Inspect condition of client's nasal and oral cavity.	Baseline condition of nasal and oral cavity determines need for special nursing measures for oral hygiene after tube placement.
2. Ask if client has had history of nasal surgery and note if deviated nasal septum is present.	Nurse should insert tube into uninvolved nasal passage. Procedure may be contraindicated if surgery is recent.
3. Palpate client's abdomen for distension, pain, and rigidity. Auscultate for bowel sounds.	Baseline determination of level of abdominal distension later serves as comparison once tube is inserted.
4. Assess client's level of consciousness and ability to follow instructions.	Determines client's ability to assist in procedure.

Critical Decision Point: If client is confused, disoriented, or unable to follow commands, obtain assistance from another staff member to insert the tube.

Steps	Rationale
5. Check medical record for surgeon's order, type of NG tube to be placed, and whether tube is to be attached to suction or drainage bag.	Procedure requires physician's order. Adequate decompression depends on NG suction.
6. Perform hand hygiene. Prepare equipment at the bedside. Cut a piece of tape about 10 cm long and split one end in half to form a V, or have NG tube fixator device available.	Reduces transmission of infection. Ensures well-organized procedure. Tape or fixator device will be used to hold the tube in place after insertions.
7. Identify client and explain procedure.	Identification prevents error of placing tube in wrong client. Explanation gains client's co-operation and lessens possibility that client will remove tube.
8. Apply disposable gloves.	Reduces transmission of micro-organisms.
9. Position client in high-Fowler's position with pillows behind head and shoulders. Raise bed to a horizontal level comfortable for the nurse.	Promotes client's ability to swallow during procedure. Good body mechanics prevent injury to nurse and client.
10. Place bath towel over client's chest; give facial tissues to client. Place emesis basin within reach.	Prevents soiling of client's gown. Tube insertion through nasal passages may cause tearing and coughing with increased salivation.
11. Pull curtain around the bed or close room door.	Provides privacy.
12. Stand on client's right side if right-handed, left side if left-handed.	Allows easiest manipulation of tubing.
13. Instruct client to relax and breathe normally while occluding one naris. Then repeat this action for other naris. Select nostril with greater airflow.	Tube passes more easily through naris that is more patent.

Skill 41-2 Inserting and Maintaining a Nasogastric Tube—cont'd

Steps	Rationale
14. Measure distance to insert tube: a. Measure distance from tip of nose to earlobe to xiphoid process (see illustration). b. First mark 50-cm point on tube, then do traditional measurement. Tube insertion should be to midway point between 50 cm and traditional mark.	Approximates distance from naris to stomach. Tube should extend from naris to stomach; distance varies with each client.
15. Mark length of tube to be inserted with small piece of tape placed so that it can easily be removed.	Marks amount of tube to be inserted from nares to stomach.
16. Curve 10 to 15 cm of end of tube tightly around index finger, then release.	Curving tube tip aids insertion and decreases stiffness of tube.
17. Lubricate 7.5 to 10 cm of end of tube with water-soluble lubricating jelly.	Minimizes friction against nasal mucosa and aids insertion of tube.
18. Alert client that procedure is to begin.	Decreases client anxiety and increases client co-operation.
19. Initially instruct client to extend neck back against pillow; insert tube gently and slowly through nares with curved end pointing downward (see illustration).	Facilitates initial passage of tube through naris and maintains clear airway for open naris.
20. Insert tube slowly through naris with curved end pointing downward. Continue to insert tube along floor of nasal passage aiming down toward client's ear. If resistance is met, apply gentle downward pressure to advance tube (do not force past resistance).	Minimizes discomfort of tube rubbing against upper nasal turbinates. Resistance is caused by posterior nasopharynx. Downward pressure helps tube curl around corner of nasopharynx.
21. If resistance is met, try to rotate the tube to see if it advances. If still resistant, withdraw tube, allow client to rest, relubricate tube, and insert into other naris.	Forcing against resistance can cause trauma to mucosa. Helps relieve client's anxiety.

Critical Decision Point: If unable to insert tube in either naris, stop procedure and notify physician.

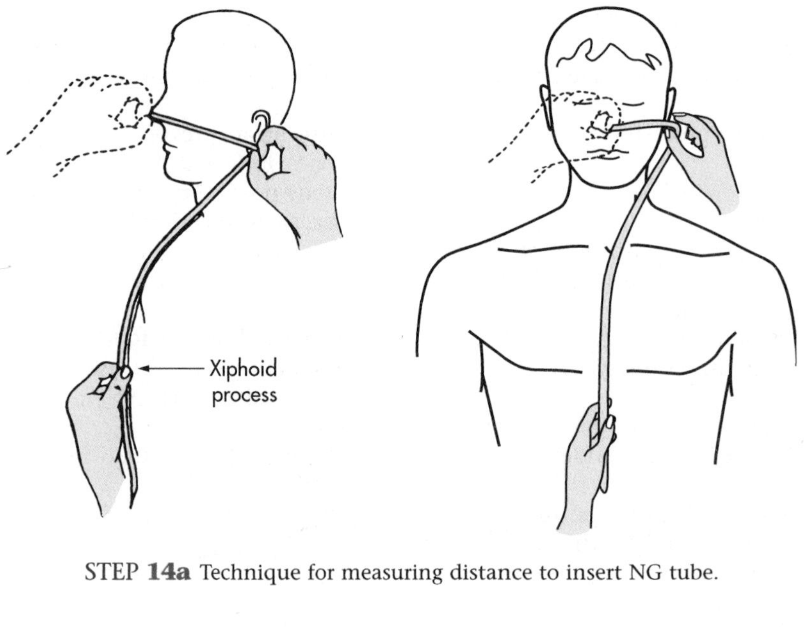

STEP **14a** Technique for measuring distance to insert NG tube.

Steps	Rationale
22. Continue insertion of tube until just past nasopharynx by gently rotating tube toward opposite naris.	Helps prevent coiling of tube in oropharynx.
a. Stop tube advancement, allow client to relax, and provide tissues.	Relieves client's anxiety; tearing is natural response to mucosal irritation, and excessive salivation may occur because of oral stimulation.
b. Explain to client that next step requires that client swallow. Give client glass of water unless contraindicated.	Slipping of water aids passage of NG tube into esophagus.
23. With tube just above oropharynx, instruct client to flex head forward, take a small sip of water, and swallow. Advance tube 2.5 to 5 cm with each swallow of water. If client is not allowed fluids, instruct to dry swallow or suck air through straw.	Flexed position closes off upper airway to trachea and opens esophagus. Swallowing closes epiglottis over trachea and helps move the tube into the esophagus. Swallowing water reduces gagging or choking. Water can be removed later from stomach by suction.
24. If client begins to cough, gag, or choke, withdraw tube slightly (do not remove the tube) and stop tube advancement. Instruct client to breathe easily and take sips of water.	Tube may be displaced into larynx and produce coughing. Swallowing water closes epiglottis over trachea and helps move the tube into the esophagus. Risk for aspiration increases if vomiting occurs.

Critical Decision Point: If vomiting occurs, assist client in clearing airway; oral suctioning may be needed. Do not proceed until airway is cleared.

Steps	Rationale
25. If client continues to gag and cough or complains that tube feels as though it is coiling in the back of throat, check back of oropharynx using tongue blade. If tube has coiled, withdraw it until the tip is back in the oropharynx. Then reinsert with client swallowing.	Tube may coil around itself in the back of the throat and stimulate the gag reflex.
26. Continue to advance tube with swallowing until tape or mark is reached. Temporarily anchor tube to client's cheek with a piece of tape until tube placement is checked.	Tip of tube must be well within stomach for adequate decompression. Tube should be anchored before placement if verified.
27. Verify tube placement. Check agency policy for preferred methods for checking NG tube placement.	
a. Ask client to talk.	Inability to speak can indicate that tube is through client's vocal cords into the lungs.
b. Inspect posterior pharynx for presence of coiled tube.	Tube is pliable and can coil up in back of pharynx instead of advancing into esophagus.
c. Aspirate gently back on syringe to obtain gastric contents, observing colour.	Gastric contents are usually cloudy and green, but may be off-white, tan, bloody, or brown in colour. Aspiration of contents provides means to measure fluid pH and thus determine tube tip placement in gastrointestinal tract (see Figure 41–16). Other common aspirate colours include the following: Duodenal placement (yellow or bile stained), esophagus (may or may not have saliva-appearing aspirate).

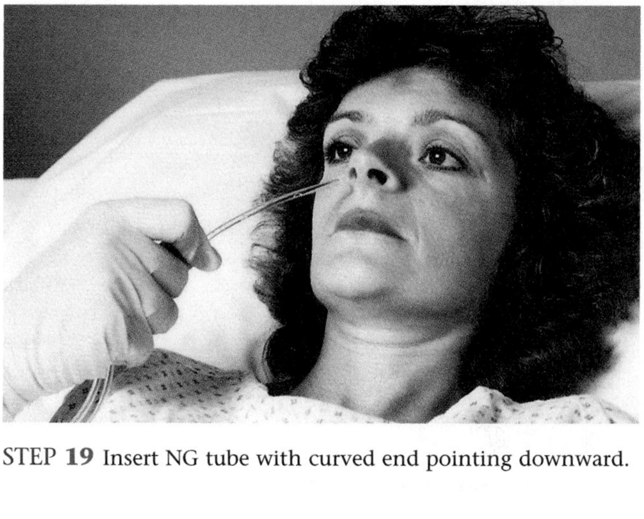

STEP **19** Insert NG tube with curved end pointing downward.

Skill 41-2 Inserting and Maintaining a Nasogastric Tube—cont'd

Steps	Rationale
d. Measure pH of aspirate with colour-coded pH paper with range of whole numbers 1 to 11 (see illustration).	Gastric aspirates have decidedly acidic pH values, preferably 4 or less, compared with intestinal aspirates, which are usually greater than 4, or respiratory secretions, which are usually greater than 5.5 (Metheny & Titler, 2001).
e. Have ordered X-ray examination performed of chest/abdomen.	Placement of tube can be reliably verified by X-ray exam.

Critical Decision Point: Be sure to use gastric (Gastroccult) pH test and not Hemoccult test.

Steps	Rationale
f. If tube is not in stomach, advance another 2.5 to 5 cm and repeat steps 27b, c, and d to check tube position.	Tube must be in stomach to provide decompression.
28. Anchoring tube:	
a. After tube is properly inserted and positioned, either clamp end or connect it to drainage bag or suction machine.	Drainage bag is used for gravity drainage. Intermittent suction, low suction, is most effective for decompression. Client going to the operating room often has tube clamped.
b. Tape tube to nose; avoid putting pressure on nares.	Prevents tissue necrosis. Tape anchors tube securely.
(1) Before taping tube to nose, apply small amount of tincture of benzoin to lower end of nose and allow to dry (optional). Be sure that top end of tape over nose is secure.	Benzoin prevents loosening of tape if client perspires.
(2) Carefully wrap two split ends of tape around tube (see illustration).	
(3) Alternative: Apply tube fixation device using shaped adhesive patch (see illustration).	

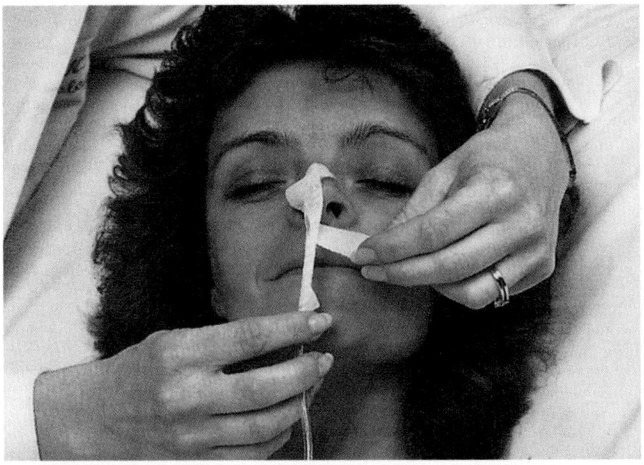

STEP **28b(2)** Tape is crossed over and around NG tube.

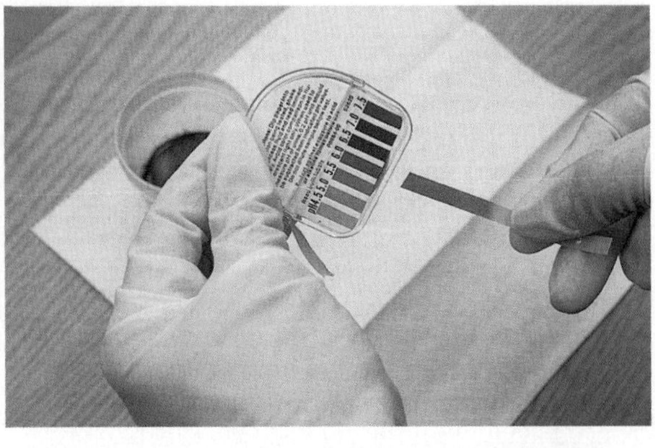

STEP **27d** Checking pH of gastric aspirate.

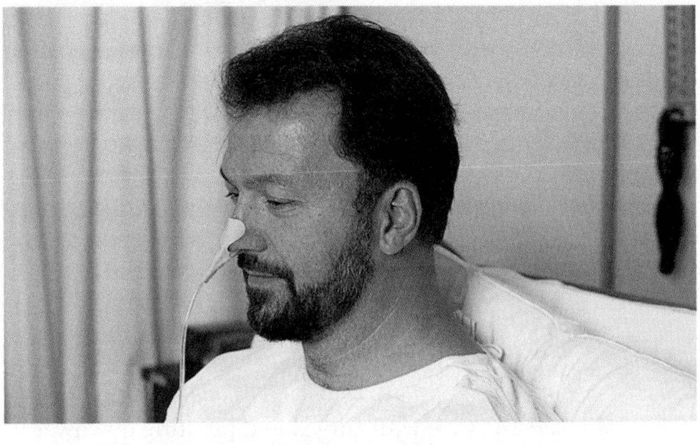

STEP **28b(3)** Client with tube fixation device.

Steps	Rationale
c. Fasten end of NG tube to client's gown by looping rubber band around tube in slip-knot. Pin rubber band to gown (provides slack for movement).	Reduces pressure on the nares if tube moves.
d. Unless physician orders otherwise, head of bed should be elevated 30 degrees.	Helps prevent esophageal reflux and minimizes irritation of tube against posterior pharynx.
e. Explain to client that sensation of tube should decrease somewhat with time.	Adaptation to continued sensory stimulus.
f. Remove gloves and wash hands.	Reduces transmission of micro-organisms.
29. Once placement is confirmed:	
a. Place a mark, either a red mark or tape, on the tube to indicate where the tube exits the nose.	The mark or tube length is to be used as a guide to indicate whether displacement may have occurred.
b. Measurement of the tube length from nares to connector is an alternate method.	
c. Document the tube length in the client record.	
30. Tube irrigation:	
a. Wash hands and apply gloves.	Reduces transmission of micro-organisms.
b. Check for tube placement in stomach (see Step 27). Reconnect NG tube to connecting tube.	Prevents accidental entrance of irrigating solution into lungs.
c. Draw up 30 mL of normal saline into Asepto or catheter-tipped syringe.	Use of saline minimizes loss of electrolytes from stomach fluids.
d. Clamp NG tube. Disconnect from connection tubing and lay end of connection tubing on towel.	Reduces soiling of client's gown and bed linen.
e. Insert tip of irrigating syringe into end of NG tube. Remove clamp. Hold syringe with tip pointed at floor and inject saline slowly and evenly. Do not force solution.	Position of syringe prevents introduction of air into vent tubing, which could cause gastric distension. Solution introduced under pressure can cause gastric trauma.

Critical Decision Point: Do not introduce saline through blue-coloured "pigtail" air vent of Salem sump tube.

Steps	Rationale
f. If resistance occurs, check for kinks in tubing. Turn client onto left side. Repeated resistance should be reported to the physician.	Tip of tube may lie against stomach lining. Repositioning on left side may dislodge tube away from the stomach lining. Buildup of secretions will cause distension.
g. After instilling saline, immediately aspirate or pull back slowly on syringe to withdraw fluid. If amount aspirated is greater than amount instilled, record the difference as output. If amount aspirated is less than amount instilled, record the difference as intake.	Irrigation clears tubing; stomach should remain empty. Fluid remaining in stomach is measured as intake.
h. Reconnect NG tube to drainage or suction (if solution does not return, repeat irrigation.)	Re-establishes drainage collection; may repeat irrigation or repositioning of tube until NG tube drains properly.
i. Remove gloves and perform hand hygiene.	Reduces transmission of micro-organisms.
31. Observe amount and character of contents draining from NG tube. Ask if client feels nauseated.	Determines if tube is decompressing stomach of contents.
32. Palpate client's abdomen periodically, noting any distension, pain, and rigidity and auscultate for the presence of bowel sounds. Turn off suction while auscultating.	Determines success of abdominal decompression and the return of peristalsis. The sound of the suction apparatus may be transmitted to abdomen and be misinterpreted as bowel sounds.
33. Inspect condition of nares and nose.	Evaluates onset of skin and tissue irritation.
34. Observe position of tubing.	Determines if tension is being applied to nasal structures.
35. Ask if client feels sore throat or irritation in pharynx.	Evaluates level of client's discomfort.
36. Discontinuation of NG tube:	
a. Verify order to discontinue NG tube.	Physician's order required for procedure.
b. Explain procedure to client and reassure that removal is less distressing than insertion.	Minimizes anxiety and increases co-operation. Tube passes out smoothly.
c. Perform hand hygiene and apply disposable gloves.	Reduces transmission of micro-organisms.

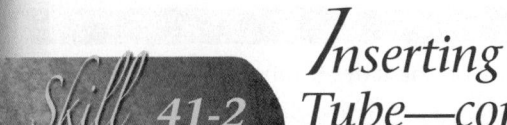

Skill 41-2 *Inserting and Maintaining a Nasogastric Tube—cont'd*

Steps	Rationale
d. Turn off suction and disconnect NG tube from drainage bag or suction. Remove tape from bridge of nose and unpin tube from gown.	Have tube free of connections before removal.
e. Stand on client's right side if right-handed, left side if left-handed.	Allows easiest manipulation of tube.
f. Hand the client facial tissue; place clean towel across chest. Instruct client to take and hold a deep breath.	Client may wish to blow nose after tube is removed. Towel may keep gown from getting soiled. Airway will be temporarily obstructed during tube removal.
g. Clamp or kink tubing securely and then pull tube out steadily and smoothly into towel held in other hand while client holds breath.	Clamping prevents tube contents from draining into oropharynx. Reduces trauma to mucosa and minimizes client's discomfort. Towel covers tube, which can be an unpleasant sight. Holding breath helps to prevent aspiration.
h. Measure amount of drainage and note character of content. Dispose of tube and drainage equipment into proper container.	Provides accurate measure of fluid output. Reduces transfer of micro-organisms.
i. Clean nares and provide mouth care.	Promotes comfort.
j. Position client comfortably and explain procedure for drinking fluids, if not contraindicated.	Depends on physician's order. Sometimes clients are allowed nothing by mouth (NPO) for up to 24 hours. When fluids are allowed, the order usually begins with a small amount of ice chips each hour and increases as client is able to tolerate more.
37. Clean equipment and return to proper place. Place soiled linen in utility room or proper receptacle.	Proper disposal of equipment prevents spread of micro-organisms and ensures proper exchange procedures.
38. Remove gloves and perform hand hygiene.	Reduces transmission of micro-organisms.
39. Inspect condition of nares and nose.	Evaluates onset of skin and tissue irritation.
40. Ask if client feels sore throat or irritation in pharynx.	Evaluates level of client's discomfort.

Unexpected Outcomes and Related Interventions

- Client's abdomen becomes distended and/or painful.
  - Assess patency of tube and irrigate as needed.
- Client complains of sore throat from dry, irritated mucous membranes.
  - Increase frequency of oral hygiene.
  - Ask physician if client may suck on ice chips, throat lozenges.
- Clients develops irritation of skin around nares.
  - Provide skin care to nares.
  - Retape so that tube does not press against nares.
  - Consider switching tube to other nares.
- Client develops signs of pulmonary aspiration: fever, shortness of breath, pulmonary congestion.
  - Perform respiratory assessment.
  - Notify physician.
  - Obtain chest X-ray examination as ordered.

Recording and Reporting

- Record in nurses' notes time and type of NG tube inserted, client's tolerance of procedure, confirmation of placement, character of gastric contents, pH value, whether tube is clamped or connected to drainage device, and amount of suction applied.
- Record in nurses' notes and/or flow sheet amount and character of contents draining from NG tube every shift, unless ordered more frequently by physician.

Client Teaching — Box 41-9

Stomal Care (Incontinent Ostomy)

Objective

- Client will demonstrate the correct procedure for stomal care.

Teaching Strategies

- Teach the client that the drainage from the stoma is very irritating to the skin and contact of the skin with the drainage should be avoided. However, when contact does occur, the client should cleanse the area as soon as possible.
- Show client how to inspect the appearance of the skin and surrounding stoma. The stoma should be moist, shiny, and pink (Hyland, 2002). Bleeding should be minimal. The skin around the stoma, called the peristomal area, should be normal skin tone.
- Skin surrounding the stoma should be cleansed with mild soap and water or even plain water (Hyland, 2002). The client must also dry the area thoroughly.
- Instruct client to avoid the use of creams, ointments, baby wipes, or other moist towelettes on peristomal skin, as these agents can prevent the pouch from adhering securely on the client's skin (Hyland, 2002).
- Instruct client to report excess bleeding or prolonged oozing to the nurse or physician.
- Demonstrate to client how to select and apply a skin barrier and pouch; also instruct client regarding length of wear.
- Demonstrate to client how to empty and change the pouching system.
- Instruct client on how to reduce odour and what commercial agents to use.
- Assist client in determining what ostomy supplies should be carried at all times. Provide client and family with a list of resources to obtain supplies in the community.
- Instruct client that if a yeast infection occurs, the client should thoroughly cleanse the area, pat dry, and apply a prescribed topical agent to the affected region, such as triamcinolone acetonide (Kenalog) spray or nystatin (Mycostatin).

Evaluation

- Client will correctly state skin care procedures.
- Client will correctly perform stoma skin care procedure.

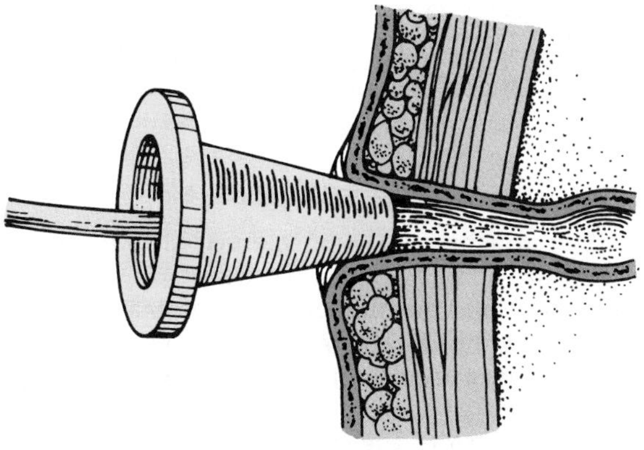

FIGURE **41–17** Ostomy irrigation cone inserted into stoma.

have the opening precut by the manufacturer; others require the stoma opening to be custom cut to the client's specific stoma size.

Skin barriers include wafers, pastes, powders, and liquid film that are applied to the skin around the stoma. Some wafer skin barriers are permanently attached to the ostomy pouch. These are called one-piece pouch systems. In a two-piece system, the pouch can be detached from the skin barrier for emptying or changing. This allows the skin barrier to remain around the client's stoma for several days, thus minimizing the chance of skin damage from too-frequent removal of the skin barrier from the peristomal skin. When using a two-piece pouching system, it is important to remember that the skin barrier and pouch must be the same corresponding size and from the same manufacturer. The pouch from one manufacturer will not fit correctly on the skin barrier from another manufacturer. The nurse must be sure to use an ostomy pouch made for collecting fecal matter (colostomy or ileostomy) and not one for collecting urine.

It is important to measure the stoma size carefully when selecting and cutting out the opening on the wafer skin barrier. A good skin barrier protects the skin, prevents irritation from repeated removal of the pouch, and is comfortable for the client to wear. Skill 41-3 describes steps for applying one type of pouch system.

Nutritional Considerations for Clients With Ostomies. Nutritional therapy is important for clients with ostomies. During the first weeks after surgery, many physicians recommend low-fibre diets, particularly for ileostomy clients, because the small bowel requires time to adapt to the diversion. Low-fibre foods include bread, noodles, rice, cream cheese, eggs (not fried), strained fruit juices, lean meats, fish, and poultry. As ostomies heal, clients can eat almost any food. High-fibre foods such as fresh fruits and vegetables help ensure a more solid stool needed to achieve success at irrigation. Blockage must be avoided. The stoma's surgical construction can affect the likelihood of blockage.

Clients with an ileostomy should eat slowly and chew food completely. Drinking 10 to 12 glasses of water daily also prevents blockage. High-fibre foods that may cause problems include stringy meats, mushrooms, popcorn, fruits such as cherries, and some seafood such as shrimp and crab. Ostomy clients may benefit from avoiding foods that cause gas and odour, including broccoli, cauliflower, dried beans, and Brussels sprouts.

Bowel Training. The client with incontinence is unable to maintain bowel control. A **bowel training** program can help some clients achieve normal defecation, especially those who still have some neuromuscular control.

The training program involves setting up a daily routine. By attempting to defecate at the same time each day and using measures that promote defecation, the client gains control of bowel reflexes. The program requires time, patience, and consistency. The physician determines the client's physical readiness and ability to

Text continued on p. 1429

Skill 41-3 Pouching an Ostomy

Delegation Considerations

The skill of pouching an ostomy, especially a newly established ostomy, should not be delegated to unregulated care providers (UCPs). Pouching of an established ostomy can be delegated to a UCP. The nurse must do the following:

- Assist caregiver in selecting appropriate pouch and skin barrier
- Inform caregiver of the signs of stomal and peristomal skin changes that should be reported to a nurse
- Have caregiver monitor and report characteristics and volume of ostomy output and report changes in volume and/or consistency to the nurse for further assessment

Equipment (Figure 41–18)

- Clear drainable colostomy/ileostomy pouch in correct size for two-piece system or custom cut-to-fit one-piece type with attached skin barrier
- Pouch closure device, such as clamp
- Disposable gloves
- Deodorant specific for an ostomy collection bag
- Gauze pads and washcloths
- Towel or disposable waterproof barrier
- Basin with warm tap water
- Scissors/pen
- Adhesive remover (optional)

Steps	Rationale
1. Perform hand hygiene and auscultate for bowel sounds.	Documents presence of peristalsis.
2. Apply gloves. Observe skin barrier and pouch for leakage and length of time in place. Depending on type of pouching system used (such as with an opaque pouch), the nurse may have to remove the pouch to fully observe the stoma. Clear pouches permit the viewing of the stoma without their removal.	May indicate need for different type of pouch or sealant.

Critical Decision Point: Intact skin barriers with no evidence of leakage do not need to be changed daily and can remain in place for 3 to 5 days.

3. Observe stoma for colour, swelling, trauma, and healing; stoma should be moist and reddish-pink. Assess type of stoma. Stomas can be flush with the skin or be a bud-like protrusion on the abdomen (see illustration for a normal bud stoma).	Stoma characteristics should be one of the factors to consider when selecting an appropriate pouching system.

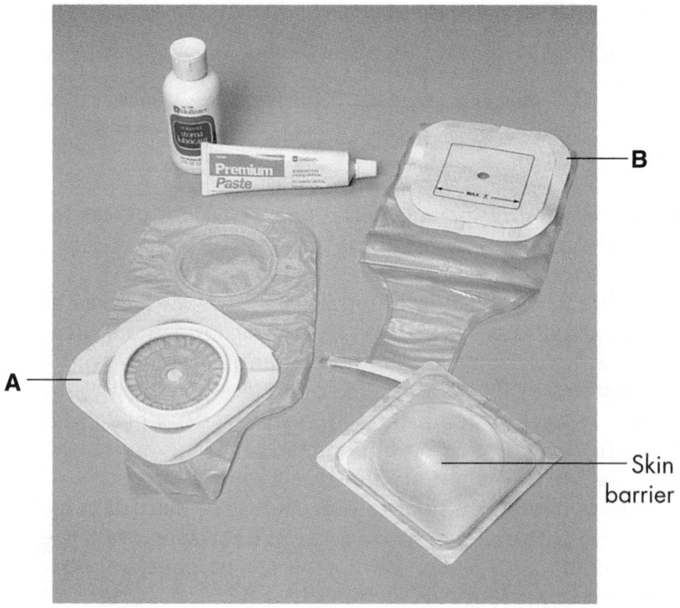

FIGURE **41–18** Ostomy pouches and skin barriers. **A,** Two-piece detachable system. (NOTE: Skin barrier would need to be custom cut according to stoma size). The pouch opening is already precut by the manufacturer to fit the size of the flange on the skin barrier. **B,** One-piece pouch with skin barrier attached. (Permission to use this copyrighted photo has been granted by the owner, Hollister Incorporated.)

Steps	Rationale
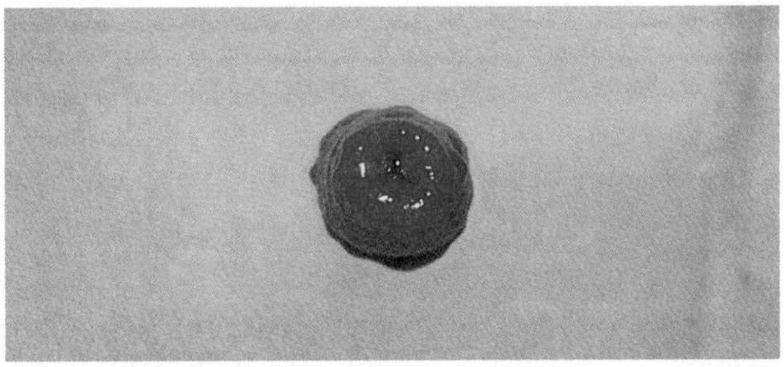 STEP 3 Bud stoma. (Permission to use this copyrighted photo has been granted by the owner, Hollister Incorporated.)	
4. Measure the stoma with each pouching change. Follow pouch manufacturer's directions and measuring guide as to which pouch to use based on client's stoma size. The opening around the appliance should be no more than 2 mm larger than the stoma (Hyland, 2002).	Determines correct size equipment, preventing trauma to stoma. Too large of an opening can permit fecal drainage to ooze from under the appliance, causing skin irritation. Too small of an opening can cause the appliance to cut into the stoma (Hyland, 2002).
5. Observe abdominal incision (if present).	Relationship of abdominal incision to stoma determines proper placement of pouch.
6. Observe effluent from stoma and keep a record of intake and output. Ask client about skin tenderness. Remove gloves and perform hand hygiene.	Effluent from stoma is caustic, and if it comes in contact with the sensitive peristomal skin, the risk of skin breakdown increases (Hyland, 2002).
7. Assess abdomen for best type of pouching system to use. Consider the following: a. Contour and peristomal plane b. Presence of scars, incisions c. Location and type of stoma	Determines pouching system selection and need for other equipment. For a stoma to have an adequate seal with an ostomy appliance, the stoma must be placed within the abdominal rectus muscle, away from abdominal creases and folds, away from the bony understructures, and surrounded by at least 5 cm of smooth surface on all sides (Banks & Razor, 2003).
8. Assess the client's self-care ability to determine the best type of pouching system to use.	Clients who have difficulty using their hands or who have limited vision may find a one-piece system or a precut pouch and skin barrier more desirable to use; others prefer being able to keep the skin barrier in place for several days, changing just the pouch, and therefore prefer the two-piece system.
9. After skin barrier and pouch removal, assess skin around stoma, noting scars, folds, skin breakdown, and peristomal suture line, if present. Keep pouch loosely attached to stoma to collect any drainage while the system is being changed.	Determines need for barrier paste to increase adherence of pouch to skin or to fill in irregularities.

Critical Decision Point: If the skin around the stoma is discoloured, weeping, itchy, or sore, the client should be referred to an ostomy specialist (Hyland, 2002).

Steps	Rationale
10. Determine client's emotional response and knowledge and understanding of an ostomy and its care.	Assists in determining extent to which client is able to participate in care and need for teaching and information clarification.
11. Explain procedure to client; encourage client's interaction and questions.	Lessens anxiety and promotes client's participation.
12. Perform hand hygiene. Assemble equipment and close room curtains or door.	Reduces infection transmission. Optimizes use of time; conserves client's and nurse's energy. Provides privacy.
13. Position client either standing or supine and drape. If seated, position either on or in front of the toilet.	When client is supine, fewer wrinkles allow for ease of application of pouching system; maintains client's dignity.
14. Perform hand hygiene and apply disposable gloves.	Reduces transmission of micro-organisms.
15. Place towel or disposable waterproof barrier under the client.	Protects bed linen.

Skill 41-3 Pouching an Ostomy—cont'd

Steps	Rationale
16. Completely remove used pouch and skin barrier gently by pushing the skin away from the barrier. An adhesive remover may be used to facilitate removal of the skin barrier.	Reduces trauma; jerking irritates the skin and can cause tears.
17. Cleanse peristomal skin gently with warm tap water using gauze pads or clean washcloth; do not scrub the skin; dry completely by patting the skin with gauze or towel.	Avoid use of soap because it leaves a residue on the skin that interferes with pouch adhesion to the skin. Skin must be as dry as skin barrier; pouch does not adhere to wet skin. If blood appears on the gauze pad, do not be alarmed; the stoma, if rubbed, may ooze some blood from the cleaning process. The stoma's surface is a highly vascular mucous membrane. Bleeding into the pouch is abnormal.
18. Measure the stoma for correct size of pouching system needed, using the manufacturer's measuring guide (see illustration).	Ensures accuracy in determining correct pouch size needed. Stoma shrinks and does not reach usual size for 6 to 8 weeks.
19. Select appropriate pouch for client based on client assessment. With a custom cut-to-fit pouch, use an ostomy guide to cut opening on the pouch 2 mm larger than stoma before removing backing (Hyland, 2002). Prepare pouch by removing backing from barrier and adhesive (see illustration). With ileostomy, apply thin circle of barrier paste around opening in pouch; allow to dry.	The paste facilitates seal and protects skin. Size of pouch opening keeps drainage off skin and lessens risk of damage to stoma during peristalsis or activity. Pouch and skin barrier are changed whenever leaking. Can also be changed before or after tub bath or shower. Stool is alkaline and this irritates the skin; fecal bacteria can colonize on the skin and increase risk of infection. Change when client is comfortable; before a meal is better, because this avoids increased peristalsis and chance of evacuation during the pouch change.

Critical Decision Point: If client has a large volume of liquid stool from an ileostomy, consider using a "high-output" pouch that will contain the volume of effluent and reduce the frequency of pouch emptying.

20. Apply the skin barrier and pouch. If creases next to stoma occur, use barrier paste to fill in; let dry 1 to 2 minutes.

Critical Decision Point: If client has surgical incision near stoma, the skin barrier may have to be trimmed for fit.

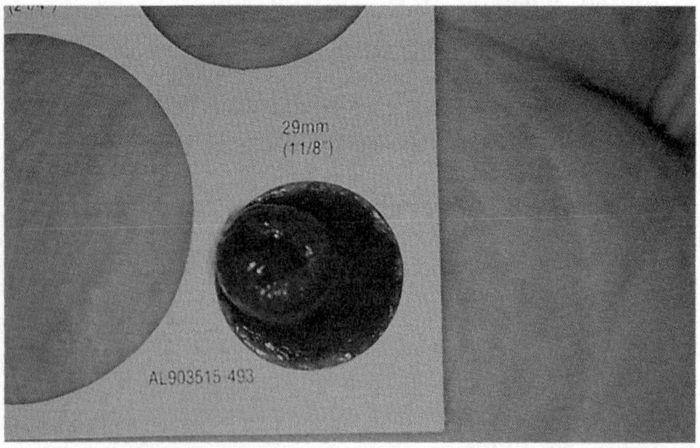

STEP **18** Measuring a stoma.

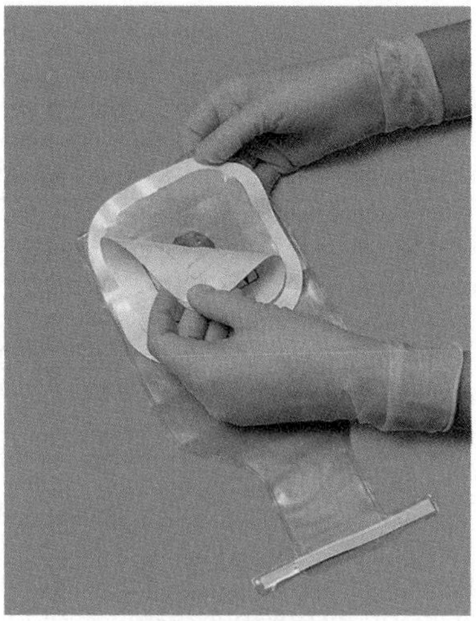

STEP **19** Preparing an ostomy pouch.

Steps	Rationale
A. **For one-piece pouching system**	
(1) Use skin sealant wipes on skin directly under adhesive skin barrier or pouch; allow to dry. Press the adhesive backing of the pouch and/or skin barrier smoothly against the skin, starting from the bottom and working up and around the sides.	
(2) Hold pouch by barrier, centre over stoma, and press down gently on barrier; bottom of pouch should point toward client's knees (see illustration).	
(3) Maintain gentle finger pressure around the barrier for 1 to 2 minutes.	
B. **For two-piece pouching system**	
(1) Apply flange (barrier with adhesive) as in steps above for one-piece system (see illustration). Then snap on pouch and maintain finger pressure.	Creates wrinkle-free, secure seal; decreases irritation from the adhesive on skin.
C. **For both pouching systems, gently tug on the pouch in a downward direction.**	Determines if the pouch is securely attached.
21. Apply non-allergic paper tape around the pectin skin barrier in a "picture frame" method. Half of the tape should be on the skin barrier and half on the client's skin. Some clients may prefer a belt attached to the pouch for extra security rather than tape.	"Picture framing" the pectin skin barrier adds to the security of keeping the pouch system attached securely.

Critical Decision Point: If the client chooses to wear a belt, be sure it is not too tight by placing two fingers between belt and client's skin.

Steps	Rationale
22. Although many ostomy pouches are odour proof, some nurses and clients like to put a small amount of ostomy deodorant into the pouch. Do not use "home remedies," such as aspirin, to control ostomy odour.	Aspirin or other substances can harm the stoma.
23. Fold bottom of drainable open-ended pouches up once and close using a closure device such as a clamp (or follow manufacturer's instructions for closure).	Maintains secure seal to prevent leaking.
24. Properly dispose of old pouch and soiled equipment. Consider spraying deodorant in room if needed.	Lessens odours in room.
25. Remove gloves and perform hand hygiene.	Reduces transmission of micro-organisms.
26. Change one- or two-piece pouch every 3 to 7 days unless leaking; pouch can remain in place for tub bath or shower; after bath, pat adhesive dry.	Avoids unnecessary trauma to skin from too frequent changes. Drying ensures adhesion of pouch.

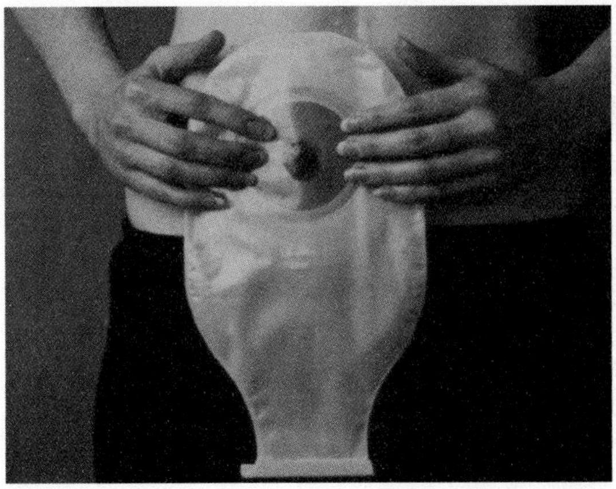

STEP **20A(2)** Applying a one-piece pouch. (Courtesy ConvaTec, Princeton, NJ.)

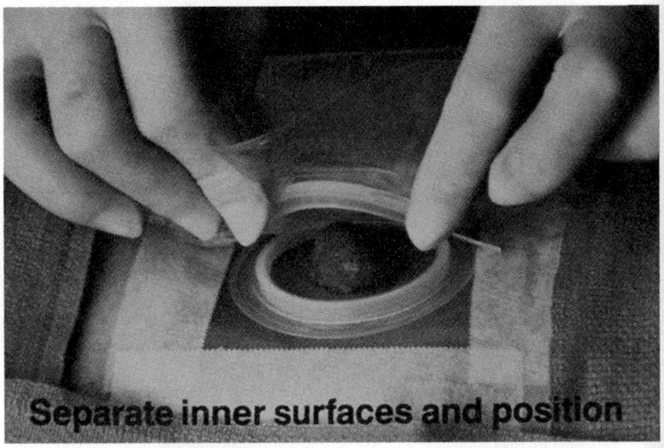

STEP **20B(1)** Application of barrier-paste flange. (Courtesy ConvaTec, Princeton, NJ.)

Skill 41-3 Pouching an Ostomy—cont'd

Steps	Rationale
27. Ask if client feels discomfort around stoma.	Determines presence of skin irritation.
28. Note appearance of stoma around skin and existing incision (if present) while pouch is removed and skin is cleansed. Reinspect condition of skin barrier and adhesive.	Determines condition of tissues and progress of healing. Determines presence of leaks.
29. Auscultate bowel sounds and observe characteristics of stool.	Determines return of peristalsis and bowel elimination.
30. Observe client's non-verbal behaviours as pouch is applied. Ask if client has any questions about pouching.	May indicate emotional response to stoma and readiness for teaching. Determines level of understanding of procedure.

Unexpected Outcomes and Related Interventions

- Client experiences damage to peristomal skin.
  - Assess for and report to physician for treatment:
    - Mechanical damage (Figure 41–19, *A*) due to inappropriate skin care, incorrect tape removal
    - Chemical damage due to effluent coming into contact with peristoma skin or skin reaction to adhesive
    - Damage due to a fungus (candidiasis; Figure 41–19, *B*), usually caused by excessive skin moisture
- Stoma becomes necrotic as manifested by purple or black colour, dry instead of moist, failure to bleed, or tissue sloughing.
  - Assess circulation to stoma.
  - Observe for excessive edema or tension on bowel suture line (if present).
  - Immediately report this finding to the physician.

Recording and Reporting

- Chart type of pouch and skin barrier applied.
- Record amount and appearance of stool, texture, condition of peristomal skin, and sutures.
- Report any of the following to the charge nurse and/or physician:
  - Abnormal appearance of stoma, suture line, peristomal skin, character of output, absence of bowel sounds.
  - No flatus in 24 to 36 hours and no stool by third day.
- Document abdominal distension and excessive tenderness, nature of bowel sounds.
- Record client's level of participation and need for teaching.

Home Care Considerations

- Evaluate the client's home toileting facilities. This includes presence of adequate toileting facilities, flushable toilet, and number and location of toilets.
- Caution the client that most ostomy pouches and barriers cannot be flushed down the toilet; they clog the system. Dispose of used ostomy pouch according to agency policy and local sanitation regulations.

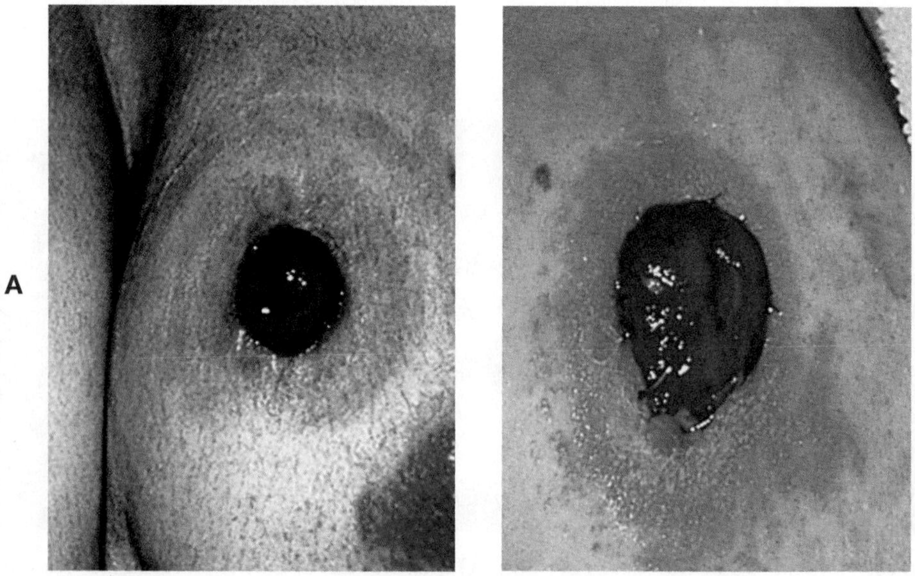

FIGURE **41–19**
A, Mechanical injury.
B, Candidiasis. (Permission to use this copyrighted photo has been granted by the owner, Hollister Incorporated.)

Focus on Older Adults — Box 41-10

- The energy needs of people over 51 years of age are considered to be less because of loss of metabolic tissue with age. Protein needs do not decrease with aging.
- Maintaining a well-balanced diet that is high in fibre will assist in maintaining normal bowel elimination patterns (Bliss et al., 2001).
- Constipation is a common complaint in older clients. Contributing factors are impaired general health, use of medication, and decreased mobility and physical activity.
- If constipation is ignored, significant complications can arise. Instructing clients to establish a specific time for bowel elimination may assist in preventing constipation (Dosh, 2002).
- Clients need to feel at ease during elimination. Lack of privacy may lead the client to ignore the urge to defecate.
- Older adults are known for their concern with their elimination habits.
- Warm liquids and certain juices (prune) stimulate bowel motility.

benefit from bowel training. A successful program includes the following:

- Assessing the normal elimination pattern and recording times when the client is incontinent
- Incorporating principles of gerontologic nursing when providing bowel training programs for the older adult client (Box 41-10)
- Choosing a time in the client's pattern to initiate defecation-control measures
- Giving stool softeners orally every day or a cathartic suppository at least half an hour before the selected defecation time (lower colon must be free of stool so that suppository contacts intestinal mucosa)
- Offering a hot drink (hot tea), or fruit juice (prune juice), or whatever fluids normally stimulate peristalsis for the client before the defecation time
- Assisting the client to the toilet at the designated time
- Avoiding medications, such as analgesics, that may increase constipation
- Providing privacy and setting a time limit for defecation (15 to 20 minutes)
- Instructing the client to lean forward at the hips while sitting on the toilet, to apply manual pressure with the hands over the abdomen, and to bear down but not strain to stimulate colon emptying
- Not criticizing or conveying frustration if the client is unable to defecate
- Providing regular meals with adequate fluids and fibre (Bliss et al., 2001)
- Maintaining normal exercise within the client's physical ability

Clients with cognitive impairment present a special challenge when managing fecal incontinence. A team approach is required (Box 41-11).

Maintenance of Proper Fluid and Food Intake. In choosing a diet for promoting normal elimination, the

Focus on Primary Health Care — Box 41-11

A Team Approach to Managing Fecal Continence in the Cognitively Impaired Client

- Before establishing an appropriate bowel control program for the cognitively impaired client, the physician or nurse must assess the musculoskeletal system for the level of activity that the individual can attain, the rectum and anus for such problems as hemorrhoids or rectal prolapse, and the cognitive status so that the interventions can be matched to cognitive ability.
- Information concerning bowel habits may be provided by the family. If this is not possible, the nurse and unregulated care providers assess the client's frequency and consistency of bowel movements and level of independence in toileting, including the amount of assistance required.
- The dietitian or nutritional staff should assess the client's diet.
- Adequate hydration, six to eight glasses of fluid daily, is an important part of normal bowel routine and is particularly difficult to achieve with cognitively impaired individuals. The team must address creative methods of delivering adequate nutrition and hydration.
- Caregivers should be made aware that sometimes individuals become impacted from use of Metamucil with insufficient fluids. Gentle laxatives for a few days, rather than those that irritate the bowel may be effective. However, a natural dietary cathartic (a mixture of applesauce, pureed prunes, and bran) or simply adding more high-fibre foods to the diet may be preferable to a pharmacological intervention.
- As with all individuals, appropriate exercise and fluid intake should be included in the care plan. A physiotherapist or occupational therapist may be involved in the exercise plan.
- Environmental cues such as having the toilet visible and gentle questioning may facilitate independent function, but these cues may also be stressful and cause belligerence.
- The individual with cognitive impairment may not respond appropriately to the urge to defecate. Caregivers should be aware that the urge to defecate is strongest the first hour after breakfast and offer opportunities for toileting at that time.
- Assisted toileting procedures include stabilizing the client on the toilet or commode by placing a chair next to the toilet for stabilization. A glass of warm water may be given as a drink, a warm pack placed on the abdomen, or the abdomen gently massaged to facilitate bowel emptying.
- For a client who is continually incontinent, appropriate, dignified continence products can be provided.
- Severely cognitively impaired clients may smear the incontinent feces. Emptying the rectum regularly diminishes the problem. However, it may be necessary to give fleet enemas, increase the bulk of the stool with Metamucil, or stimulate the local peristalsis with glycerine suppositories to facilitate rectal emptying.

nurse should consider the frequency of defecation, characteristics of feces, and types of foods that impair or promote defecation. The client with frequent constipation or impaction requires an increased intake of high-fibre foods and more fluids. However, the client should realize that diet therapy provides only long-term relief of elimination problems and may not give immediate relief from problems such as constipation. The community nurse should ascertain whether the client has sufficient income to buy the foods recommended and a method of obtaining these foods. Community services such as Meals on Wheels can be arranged.

When diarrhea is a problem, the nurse can recommend foods with a low fibre content and discourage foods that typically cause gastric upset or abdominal cramping. Diarrhea caused by illness can be debilitating. If the client cannot tolerate foods or liquids orally, intravenous therapy (with potassium supplements) is necessary. The client returns to a normal diet slowly, often beginning with fluids. Excessively hot or cold fluids stimulate peristalsis, causing abdominal cramps and further diarrhea. As the tolerance to liquids improves, solid foods are ordered. It may be necessary to withhold milk products until the enterocyte population has matured following a severe diarrheal episode. Milk products might perpetuate the diarrhea.

Promotion of Regular Exercise. A daily exercise program helps prevent elimination problems. Walking, riding a stationary bicycle, or swimming stimulates peristalsis. Clients who are sedentary at work are most in need of regular exercise. For clients with mobility problems such as arthritis, a passive exercise program may be helpful.

For a client temporarily immobilized, the nurse should attempt ambulation as soon as possible. If the condition permits, the nurse assists a post-operative client in walking to a chair on the evening of the day of surgery. The client should walk farther each day.

Some clients have difficulty passing stool because of weak abdominal and pelvic floor muscles. Exercises help bedridden clients using a bedpan. The client can practise the exercises as follows:

- Lie supine; tighten the abdominal muscles as though pushing them to the floor. Hold them tight to the count of three; relax. Repeat 5 to 10 times as tolerated.
- Flex and contract the thigh muscles by raising one knee slowly toward the chest. Repeat for each leg at least five times and increase frequency as tolerated.

Hemorrhoids. Many clients have discomfort from alterations in elimination. Pain results when hemorrhoid tissues are directly irritated. The primary goal for the client with hemorrhoids is to have soft-formed, painless bowel movements. Proper diet, fluids, and regular exercise improve the likelihood of stools being soft. If the client becomes constipated, passage of hard stools may cause bleeding and irritation. Local heat provides temporary relief to swollen hemorrhoids. A sitz bath is the most effective means of heat application (see chapter 43).

Maintenance of Skin Integrity. The client with diarrhea or fecal incontinence is at risk for skin breakdown when fecal contents remain on the skin. The same problem exists for the client with an ostomy that drains liquid stool. Liquid stool is usually acidic and contains digestive enzymes. Irritation from repeated wiping with toilet tissue aggravates skin breakdown. Bathing the skin after soiling helps but may result in more breakdown unless the skin is thoroughly dried.

When caring for a debilitated, incontinent client who is unable to ask for assistance, the nurse should check often for defecation. The anal areas can be protected with petrolatum, zinc oxide, or another ointment that holds moisture in the skin, preventing drying and cracking. Yeast infections of the skin can develop easily. Several powdered antifungal agents are effective against yeast. Baby powder or cornstarch should not be used because they have no medical properties and they frequently cake on the skin and become difficult to remove.

NP Evaluation

Client Care. The effectiveness of care depends on success in meeting the goals and expected outcomes of care. Optimally, the client will be able to have regular, pain-free defecation of soft, formed stools. The client is the only one who is able to determine if the bowel elimination problems have been relieved and which therapies were the most effective (Figure 41–20). The client will also be able to demonstrate information gained regarding establishment of a normal elimination pattern. The client will be able to demonstrate any skills learned such as ostomy protocols and skin protection. The client will be able to accomplish normal defecation by manipulating components of daily living such as diet, fluid intake, and exercise. The client will have minimal reliance on artificial means of defecation such as enemas and laxative use.

Client Expectations. If the nurse has been successful in establishing a therapeutic relationship with the client, the client will feel more comfortable in discussing the intimate details often associated with bowel elimination. The client will not be as fearful of embarrassment as the nurse assists the client with elimination needs. The client will relate a feeling of comfort and freedom from pain as elimination needs are met within the limits of the client's condition and treatment.

Key Concepts

- Mechanical breakdown of food elements, gastrointestinal motility, and selective absorption and secretion of substances by the large intestine influence the character of feces.
- Food high in fibre content and an increased fluid intake keep feces soft.

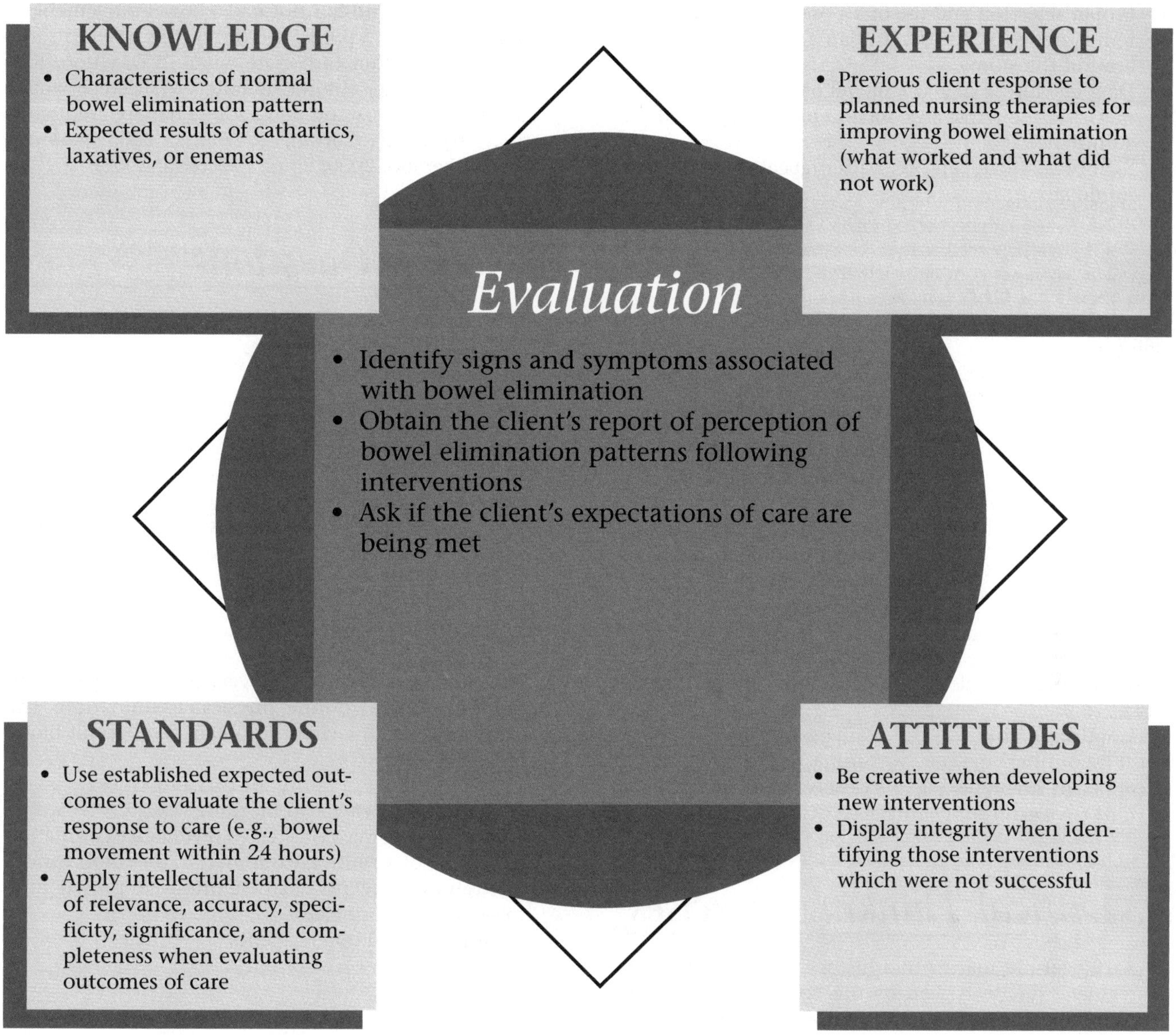
KNOWLEDGE
• Characteristics of normal bowel elimination pattern
• Expected results of cathartics, laxatives, or enemas
EXPERIENCE
• Previous client response to planned nursing therapies for improving bowel elimination (what worked and what did not work)
Evaluation
• Identify signs and symptoms associated with bowel elimination
• Obtain the client's report of perception of bowel elimination patterns following interventions
• Ask if the client's expectations of care are being met
STANDARDS
• Use established expected outcomes to evaluate the client's response to care (e.g., bowel movement within 24 hours)
• Apply intellectual standards of relevance, accuracy, specificity, significance, and completeness when evaluating outcomes of care
ATTITUDES
• Be creative when developing new interventions
• Display integrity when identifying those interventions which were not successful

FIGURE **41–20** Critical thinking model for elimination evaluation.

- Ongoing use of cathartics, laxatives, and enemas affects and delays normal defecation reflexes.
- Vagal stimulation, which slows the heart rate, may occur during straining while defecating, enemas, and digital removal of impacted stool.
- The greatest danger from diarrhea is development of fluid and electrolyte imbalance.
- The location of an ostomy influences consistency of the stool.
- Assessment of elimination patterns should focus on bowel habits, factors that normally influence defecation, recent changes in elimination, and a physical examination.
- Indirect and direct visualization of the lower gastrointestinal tract requires cleansing of the bowel before the procedure.
- The nurse should consider frequency of defecation, fecal characteristics, and effect of foods on gastrointestinal function when selecting a diet promoting normal elimination.
- Proper positioning on a bedpan allows the client to assume a position similar to squatting without experiencing muscle strain.
- Nasogastric intubation decompresses the gastric contents by removing secretions and gaseous products from the gastrointestinal tract.
- The purposes of gastric decompression are to keep the gastrointestinal tract free of secretions, reduce nausea and gas, and decrease the risk of vomiting and aspiration.

- Proper selection and use of an ostomy pouching system is necessary to prevent damage to the skin around the stoma.
- Dangers during digital removal of stool include traumatizing the rectal mucosa and promoting vagal stimulation.
- Skin breakdown can occur after repeated exposure to liquid stool.

Key Terms

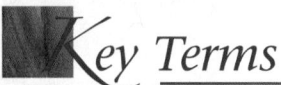

Bolus, *p. 1386*
Bowel training, *p. 1423*
Cathartics, *p. 1391*
Chyme, *p. 1387*
Colitis, *p. 1390*
Colostomy, *p. 1393*
Constipation, *p. 1392*
Crohn's disease, *p. 1390*
Defecation, *p. 1389*
Diarrhea, *p. 1392*
Effluent, *p. 1416*
Endoscopy, *p. 1392*
Enema, *p. 1409*
Enterostomal therapist (ET), *p. 1416*
Excoriation, *p. 1416*
Fecal incontinence, *p. 1393*
Fecal occult blood testing (FOBT), *p. 1400*
Feces, *p. 1389*
Fibre, *p. 1389*
Flatulence, *p. 1393*
Flatus, *p. 1388*
Gastrocolic reflex, *p. 1388*
Hemorrhoids, *p. 1393*
Ileostomy, *p. 1393*
Impaction, *p. 1392*
Lactose intolerance, *p. 1389*
Laxatives, *p. 1391*
Masticate, *p. 1386*
Paralytic ileus, *p. 1391*
Peristalsis, *p. 1388*
Peristaltic contractions, *p. 1386*
Polyps, *p. 1394*
Stoma, *p. 1393*
Valsalva manoeuvre, *p. 1389*

Critical Thinking Exercises

1. A 19-year-old man with a history of good health and regular exercise is seen by the college health service nurse practitioner. He complains of increasing diarrhea and abdominal cramping; he has no weight loss. He states that on rare occasions he had noticed blood on the toilet paper he has used. What additional pieces of assessment data does the nurse need?
2. A long-term care facility has invited you to come and do a presentation concerning prevention of bowel incontinence in their residents. What points of information would you want to include in your presentation?
3. A 22-year-old man is to undergo surgery for Crohn's disease. He will have a new pouching ileostomy. He and his mother need teaching about what this means for his future elimination needs. What would you tell them?
4. Mrs. Edna Pidpahora, 82 years old and a resident in a long-term care facility, has just been assessed for acute confusion in the Emergency Department and has now been admitted to your ward. In her documentation, you see that she has become more confused and forgetful since she has moved into long-term care 4 months ago. She spends most of her time in bed or sitting in a chair in her room. She is occasionally incontinent of urine and has not had a bowel movement in 5 days. She is taking the following medications: Synthroid, calcium carbonate, vitamin D, chlorothiazide, risperidone, chloral hydrate. What steps would you take to understand and address her apparent constipation? (Neil, Curran, & Wattis, 2003; Robson, Kiely, & Lembo, 2000; Spina & Scordo, 2002).

Review Questions

1. Most nutrients and electrolytes are absorbed in the
   1. Colon
   2. Stomach
   3. Esophagus
   4. Small intestine
2. During the nursing assessment, the client reveals that he has diarrhea and cramping every time he has ice cream. He attributes this to the cold nature of the food. However, these symptoms might be associated with
   1. Food allergy
   2. Irritable bowel
   3. Lactose intolerance
   4. Increased peristalsis
3. The nurse is assessing a 55-year-old client who is in the clinic for a routine physical examination. The nurse instructs the client to obtain fecal occult blood testing (FOBT)
   1. When there is a family history of polyps
   2. If client reports rectal bleeding
   3. If a palpable mass is detected on digital examination
   4. As part of a routine examination for colon cancer
4. The following agents decrease intestinal muscle tone to slow passage of feces:
   1. Antidiarrheal opiate agents
   2. Hypertonics
   3. Cathartics
   4. Laxatives
5. Diarrhea that occurs with a fecal impaction is the result of
   1. A clear liquid diet
   2. Irritation of the intestinal mucosa
   3. Seepage of stool around the impaction
   4. Inability of the client to form a stool
6. A cleaning enema is ordered for a 55-year-old client before intestinal surgery. The maximum amount given is
   1. 150 to 200 mL
   2. 200 to 400 mL
   3. 400 to 750 mL
   4. 750 to 1000 mL
7. During the enema, the client begins to complain of pain. The nurse notes blood in the return fluid and rectal bleeding. The nurse's actions are to
   1. Stop the instillation
   2. Slow down the rate of instillation
   3. Stop the instillation, notify the physician, and obtain vital signs
   4. Tell the client to breathe slowly and relax

8. One of the greatest problems in caring for a client with an NG tube is
   1. Dehydration
   2. Maintaining comfort
   3. Constipation
   4. Nutritional therapy
9. The stool discharged from an ostomy is called
   1. Effluent
   2. Cathartics
   3. Colonic fluid
   4. Mucosa
10. A nurse trained to care for ostomy clients is a(n)
    1. Enterostomal therapist
    2. Nurse practitioner
    3. Ostomy practitioner
    4. GI therapist

References

Annells, M., & Koch, T. (2002). Older people seeking solutions to constipation: The laxative mire. *Journal of Clinical Nursing, 11*(5), 603–612.

Anti, M., et al. (1998). Water supplementation enhances the effect of high-fiber diet on stool frequency and laxative consumption in adult patients with functional constipation. *Hepatogastroenterology, 45*(21), 727–732.

Banks, N., & Razor, B. (2003). Preoperative stoma site assessment and marking: Trained RNs can improve ostomy outcomes. *American Journal of Nursing, 103*(3), 64A–64D.

Bartlett, J. G. (2002). Antibiotic-associated diarrhea. *The New England Journal of Medicine, 346*(5), 334–339.

Bliss, D. Z., et al. (2000). Fecal incontinence in hospitalized patients who are acutely ill. *Nursing Research, 49*(2), 101–108.

Bliss, D. Z., et al. (2001). Supplementation with dietary fiber improves fecal incontinence. *Nursing Research, 50*(4), 203–213.

Canadian Cancer Society. (2002). What is Colorectal cancer? Retrieved March 21, 2003, from *http://www.cancer.ca/ccs/internet/standard/0,2939,3172_1075_273118_langId-en,00.html*

Colwell, J., et al. (2001). The state of the standard diversion. *Journal of Wound, Ostomy, and Continence Nursing, 28*, 6–17.

Cooke, C. E. (1996). Disease management: Prevention of NSAID-induced gastropathy. *Drug Benefit Trends, 8*(3), 14–15, 19–22.

Dochterman, J. M., & Bulechek, G. M. (Eds.) (2004). *Nursing interventions classification (NIC)* (4th ed.). St. Louis, MO: Mosby.

Dosh, S. A. (2002). Evaluation and treatment of constipation. *Journal of Family Practice, 51*(6), 555–559.

Doughty, D. (2000a). A physiologic approach to bowel training. *Journal of Wound, Ostomy, and Continence Nursing, 23*(1), 46–56.

Doughty, D. (2000b). *Urinary and fecal incontinence nursing* (2nd ed.). St. Louis, MO: Mosby.

Hampton, B. G., & Bryant, R. A. (1992). *Ostomies and continent diversions: Nursing management.* St. Louis, MO: Mosby.

Hinrichs, M., & Huseboe, J. (2001). *Evidenced-based protocol: Management of constipation.* In M. G. Titler (Series Ed.), *Series on evidence-based practice for older adults.* Iowa City, IA: The University of Iowa, Gerontological Nursing Interventions Research Center, Research Dissemination Core.

Hyland, J. (2002). Basics of ostomies. *Gastroenterology Nursing, 25*(6), 241–244.

Johnson, L. R. (2001). *Gastrointestinal physiology* (6th ed.). St Louis, MO: Mosby.

Lueckenotte, A. G. (2000). *Gerontologic nursing* (2nd ed.). St. Louis, MO: Mosby.

McKenry, L. M., & Salerno, E. (2001). *Pharmacology in nursing* (21st ed.). St. Louis, MO: Mosby.

Mishkin, S. (1997). Dairy sensitivity, lactose malabsorption, and elimination diets in inflammatory bowel disease. *American Journal of Clinical Nutrition, 65*(2), 564–567.

Moorhead, S., Johnson, M., and Maas, M. (Eds.). (2004). *Nursing Outcomes Classification (NOC)* (3rd ed.). St. Louis, MO: Mosby.

Neil, W., Curran, S., & Wattis, J. (2003). Antipsychotic prescribing in older people. *Age and Aging, 32*(5), 475–483.

Pagana, K. D., & Pagana, T. J. (2001). *Mosby's diagnostic and laboratory test reference* (5th ed.). St. Louis, MO: Mosby.

Ransohoff, D. F., & Lang, C. A. (1997). Screening for colorectal cancer with the fecal occult blood test: A background paper. *Annals of Internal Medicine, 126*, 811–822.

Richmond, J. (2003). Prevention of constipation through risk management. *Nursing Standard, 17*(16), 39–46.

Robson, K. M., Kiely, D. K., & Lembo, T. (2000). Development of constipation in nursing home residents. *Diseases of the Colon and Rectum, 43*(7), 940–943.

Selma, T. P., Beizer, J. L., & Highbee, M. D. (1997). *Geriatric dosage handbook.* Hudson, OH: Lexi-Comp.

Spina, E., & Scordo, M. G. (2002). Clinically significant drug interactions with antidepressants in the elderly. *Drugs and Aging, 19*(4), 299–320.

Walsh, B. A., et al. (1995, May). *Psychometric evaluation of body image and quality of life following ostomy surgery.* Oral abstract presented at the Wound, Ostomy, Continence Nurses (WOCN) Society 27th Annual Conference, Denver, CO.

Recommended Web Sites

Canadian Digestive Health Foundation:
http://www.cdhf.ca/
The Canadian Digestive Health Foundation (CDHF) supports research and education in the management and cure of digestive diseases and disorders.

Colorectal Cancer Association of Canada:
http://www.ccac-accc.ca/
Colorectal cancer is the second most common cause of cancer deaths in Canada. The Colorectal Cancer Association of Canada is a non-profit organization that supports people with colorectal cancer, their families, and caregivers.

Registered Nurses Association of Ontario, Prevention of Constipation in the Older Adult Population:
http://www.rnao.org/bestpractices/completed_guidelines/BPG_Guide_C1_Prevent_Constipation.asp
This document is a Registered Nurses of Ontario (RNAO) Best Practice Guideline and offers a professional nursing standard for reducing the frequency and severity of constipation among older adults. It is relevant to all areas of clinical practice including acute care, community care, and long-term care.

Rehydration Project:
http://rehydrate.org/index.html
The Rehydration Project is a private, non-profit, international development group concerned with oral rehydration therapy (ORT). This Web site provides information on diarrhea in developing countries and how ORT can help. It provides a wealth of information, including facts, resources, and links to current research.

42

Mobility and Immobility

Ruth Ludwick, BSN, MSN, PhD, RNC
Nancy C. Panthofer, RN, MSN
Jan Park Dorsay, RN, MN, ACPN(D) (Canadian author)

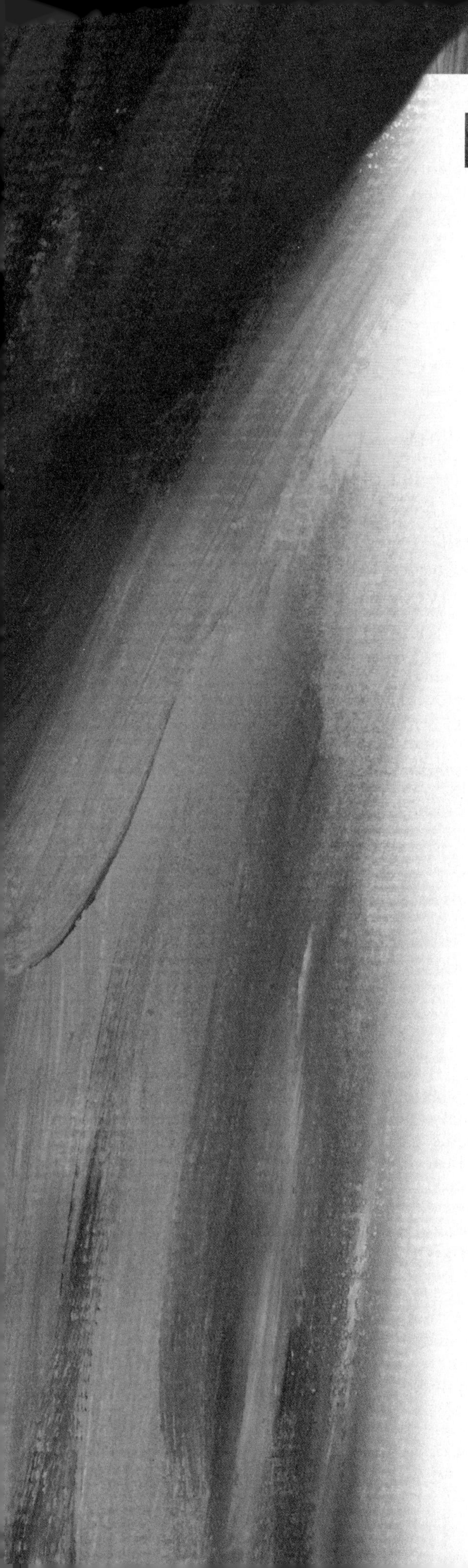

Objectives

Mastery of content in this chapter will enable the student to:

- Define the key terms listed.
- Describe the functions of the musculoskeletal (skeleton, skeletal muscles) and nervous systems in the regulation of movement.
- Discuss physiological and pathological influences on body alignment and joint mobility.
- Identify changes in physiological and psychosocial function associated with immobility.
- Assess for correct and impaired body alignment and mobility.
- State correct nursing diagnoses for impaired body alignment and mobility.
- Develop nursing care plans for clients with impaired body alignment and mobility.
- Describe essential techniques when assisting with active/passive range-of-motion (ROM) exercises, assisting a client to move up in bed, repositioning a client, assisting a client to a sitting position, and transferring a client from a bed to a chair or from a bed to a stretcher.
- Evaluate the nursing care plan for maintaining body alignment and mobility.

Mobility refers to the ability to move easily and independently. To maintain optimal physical mobility, the musculoskeletal and nervous systems of the body must be intact and functioning. Illnesses, surgery, injuries, pain, and aging can temporarily or permanently impair mobility. Nurses need to know the many hazards created by immobility and how to prevent them. They also need to know how to care for clients who are immobile. This care includes positioning the immobile client so that optimal body alignment is attained and helping to move and transfer clients who cannot do so independently. Clinical nursing practice related to mobility requires knowledge of body mechanics and the basic structure and function of bones and muscles.

Scientific Knowledge Base

Physiology and Principles of Body Mechanics

Body mechanics are the coordinated efforts of the musculoskeletal and nervous systems to maintain balance, posture, and body alignment during lifting, bending, moving, and performing activities of daily living (ADLs; see chapter 32). Use of proper body mechanics reduces risk of injury to the musculoskeletal system, facilitates mobility, and allows for efficient use of energy.

Use of proper body mechanics is important to the safety and well-being of the nurse and client. The nurse uses a variety of muscle groups for each nursing activity, such as walking during nursing rounds, administering medications, lifting and transferring clients, and moving objects. The physical forces of weight and friction can influence body movement. Correctly used, these forces increase the nurse's efficiency. Incorrect use can impair the nurse's ability to lift, transfer, and position clients and can cause serious injury. Knowledg of the basic structures and functions of the neuromuscular and skeletal systems and knowledge of physiological and pathological influences on mobility and body alignment are important to a full understanding of body mechanics (see Box 32-3).

Alignment and Balance. The terms ***body alignment*** and ***posture*** are analogous and refer to the positioning of the joints, tendons, ligaments, and muscles while standing, sitting, and lying. Body alignment means that the individual's centre of gravity is stable and body strain is minimized. Correct body alignment reduces strain on musculoskeletal structures and risk for injury, aids in maintaining adequate muscle tone, and contributes to balance. Without balance control, the centre of gravity is displaced, thus creating a risk for falls and subsequent injuries. Balance is enhanced with a wide base of support and correct body posture and when the body's centre of gravity is kept low and within the base of support.

Balance is required for maintaining a static position such as sitting, for performing ADLs, and for moving freely. The ability to balance can be compromised by disease, injury, pain, physical development (e.g., age), life changes (e.g., pregnancy), medications (e.g., in which dizziness is a side effect), and prolonged immobility, which may cause **deconditioning** (loss of muscle strength). Nurses must be alert to impaired balance because it is a major threat to physical safety. Impaired balance can also lead to a client's fear of falls and self-imposed restrictions on activity.

Safety Alert. Impaired balance is a risk factor for falls among older adults. Approximately 5% of falls result in fractures, and 20% require some medical attention. Nursing interventions should be aimed at a thorough client safety assessment and implementing fall prevention strategies (Van Haastregt et al., 2000).

Gravity and Friction. Weight is the force exerted on a body by gravity. To lift safely, the lifter must overcome the weight of the object to be lifted and know its centre of gravity. In a person, the centre of gravity is usually at 55% to 57% of standing height and is located in the midline. People who are unsteady can fall as their centres of gravity become unbalanced because of the gravitational pull of their weight.

Friction is a force that occurs in a direction to oppose movement. As the nurse turns, transfers, or moves a client up in bed, friction must be overcome. The larger the surface area of the object to be moved, the greater is the friction. A larger object produces greater resistance to movement. To decrease surface area and reduce friction when a client is unable to assist in moving up in bed, the nurse should place the client's arms across the chest. This decreases surface area and reduces friction.

Whenever possible, the nurse should use some of the client's strength when lifting, transferring, or moving clients. This can be done by explaining the procedure and telling the client when and what body parts to move. The result should be a synchronized movement in which the client can participate and friction is decreased. Involving the client may have the added bonus of increasing participation in self-care, thus promoting a sense of accomplishment.

Lifting a client, rather than pushing or pulling, can also reduce friction. Lifting has an upward component and decreases the pressure between the client and the bed or chair. Placing the client on a sheet or blanket (drawsheet, pull sheet, or lift sheet) and then pulling this sheet to move the client reduces friction because the client is raised off of the surface and is more easily moved along the bed's surface.

Regulation of Movement

Coordinated body movement involves integrated functioning of the skeletal system, skeletal muscle, and nervous system. Because these three systems co-operate so closely in mechanical support of the body, they are discussed as a single functional unit.

Skeletal System. The skeleton provides attachments for muscles and ligaments and the leverage necessary for movement. It is the body's supporting framework and consists of four types of bones: long, short, flat, and irregular. **Long bones** contribute to height (e.g., the femur, fibula, and tibia in the leg) and length (e.g., the phalanges of the fingers and toes). **Short bones** occur in clusters and, when combined with ligaments and cartilage, permit movement of the extremities. Two examples of short bones are the carpal bones in the foot and the patella in the knee. **Flat bones** provide structural contour, such as bones in the skull and the ribs in the thorax. **Irregular bones** make up the vertebral column and some bones of the skull, such as the mandible.

Bones are further characterized by firmness, rigidity, and elasticity. Firmness results from inorganic salts, such as calcium and phosphate, which are laid down in the bone matrix. Firmness is related to the bone's rigidity, which is necessary to keep long bones straight and enables bones to withstand weight bearing. In addition, bones have a degree of elasticity and skeletal flexibility that changes with age. For example, the newborn has a large amount of cartilage and is highly flexible but is unable to support weight. The toddler's bones are more pliable than those of an older person and are better able to withstand falls. Older adults, especially women, are more susceptible to bone loss (resorption) and osteoporosis.

The skeletal system has several functions. Bones protect vital organs (e.g., the skull around the brain; the ribs around the heart and lungs). Bones also aid in calcium regulation, store calcium, and release it into the circulation as needed. Clients with decreased calcium regulation and metabolism are at risk for developing osteoporosis and **pathological fractures** (fractures caused by weakened bone tissue). In addition, the internal structure of bones contains bone marrow, participates in red blood cell (RBC) production, and acts as a reservoir for blood. Clients with altered bone marrow function or diminished RBC production are usually weakened and fatigue easily, which decreases their mobility and places them at risk of falling.

Joints, ligaments, tendons, and cartilage permit strength and flexibility of the skeleton. Strength enables the skeletal system to support the body.

Joints. **Joints** are the connections between bones. Each joint is classified according to its structure and degree of mobility. There are four classifications of joints: synarthrotic, cartilaginous, fibrous, and synovial. A person's flexibility is demonstrated through **range of motion (ROM),** which is the range of normal movement for a joint.

The **synarthrotic joint** refers to bones jointed by bones. No movement is associated with this type of joint, and the bony tissue that forms between the bones provides strength and stability. The classic example of this type of joint is the sacrum, in which vertebrae are joined (Figure 42–1, *A*).

The **cartilaginous joint,** or synchondrodial joint, has little movement but is elastic and uses cartilage to unite body surfaces. Cartilaginous joints are found when bones are exposed to constant pressure, such as the costosternal joints between the sternum and ribs (Figure 42–1, *B*).

The **fibrous joint,** or syndesmodial joint, is a joint in which two bony surfaces are united by a ligament or membrane. The fibres of ligaments are flexible and stretch, permitting a limited amount of movement. For example, the paired bones of the lower leg (tibia and fibula) are fibrous joints (McCance & Huether, 2002; Figure 42–1, *C*).

The **synovial joint,** or true joint, is a freely moveable joint in which contiguous bony surfaces are covered by articular cartilage and connected by ligaments lined with a synovial membrane. Joining of the humeral radius and ulna by cartilage and ligaments forms a pivotal joint (Figure 42–1, *D*). Other types of synovial joints are the ball-and-socket joints, such as the hip joint, and the hinge joints (e.g., the interphalangeal joints of the fingers).

Ligaments. **Ligaments** are white, shiny, flexible bands of fibrous tissue binding joints together and connecting bones and cartilages. Ligaments are elastic and aid joint flexibility and support (Figure 42–2). In addition, some ligaments have a protective function. For example, ligaments between the vertebral bodies and the ligamentum flavum prevent damage to the spinal cord during movement of the back.

Tendons. **Tendons** are white, fibrous bands of tissue that connect muscle to bone. Tendons are strong, flexible, and inelastic, and they occur in various lengths and thicknesses. The Achilles tendon (tendo calcaneus) is the thickest and strongest tendon in the body. It begins near the middle of the posterior of the leg and attaches the gastrocnemius and soleus muscles in the calf to the calcaneal bone in the back of the foot (Figure 42–3).

Cartilage. **Cartilage** is non-vascular, supporting connective tissue located chiefly in the joints and thorax, trachea, larynx, nose, and ear. The fetus has a large amount of temporary cartilage, which is replaced by bone developed during infancy. Permanent cartilage is **unossified** (not hardened) except in advanced age and diseases such as osteoarthritis.

Skeletal Muscle. Movement of bones and joints involves active processes that must be carefully integrated to achieve coordination. Skeletal muscles, because of their ability to contract and relax, are the working elements of movement. Contractile elements of the skeletal muscle are enhanced by anatomical structure and attachment to the skeleton. Adequate skeletal muscle is necessary for strength and flexibility.

Muscles are made of fibres that contract when stimulated by an electrochemical impulse that travels from the nerve to the muscle across the neuromuscular junction. The electrochemical impulse causes the filaments (predominantly protein molecules of myosin and actin) within the fibre to slide past each other, with the filaments changing length.

Muscle contractions can be categorized by functional purpose: moving, resisting, or stabilizing body parts. In **concentric tension,** increased muscle contraction causes muscle shortening with movement resulting, such as when a client uses an overhead trapeze to pull up in bed. **Eccentric tension** helps control the speed and direction of movement. In the example of the overhead trapeze, the client should slowly lower to the bed. The lowering is controlled when the antagonistic muscles lengthen. Concentric and eccentric muscle actions are necessary for active movement and are therefore referred to as dynamic or **isotonic contraction. Isometric contraction** (static contraction) causes an increase in muscle tension or muscle work but no shortening or active movement of the muscle (e.g., instructing the client in tightening and relaxing a muscle group, as in quadriceps set exercises or pelvic floor muscle exercises). Voluntary movement is a combination of isotonic and isometric contractions. For example, when the nurse lifts a client up in bed, the client's weight causes increased tension in the muscles of the nurse's arms until the tension (isometric) is equal to the weight to be lifted and the weight of the lower arm. When this equilibrium is reached, continued stimulation to the muscles results in muscle shortening (isotonic) and bending of the elbow (active movement), and the client is lifted off the bed.

Although isometric contractions do not result in muscle shortening, energy expenditure is increased. This type of muscle work is comparable to having a car in neutral with the driver continually depressing the accelerator and racing the engine. The driver is not going anywhere but expends a large amount of energy. The nurse must recognize the energy expenditure (increased respiratory rate and increased work on the heart) associated with isometric exercises because they may be contraindicated in certain illnesses or conditions (e.g., myocardial infarction or chronic obstructive pulmonary disease).

Muscle Movement and Posture. Muscles that attach to bones of leverage provide necessary strength to move an object. **Leverage** is an inducing or compelling force and occurs when specific bones, such as the humerus, ulna, and radius, and the associated joint, such as the elbow, act together as a lever. Force is applied to one end of the bone to lift a weight as another point rotates the bone in the opposite direction.

Muscles associated primarily with maintaining posture are short and featherlike in appearance because they converge obliquely at a common tendon. Muscles of the

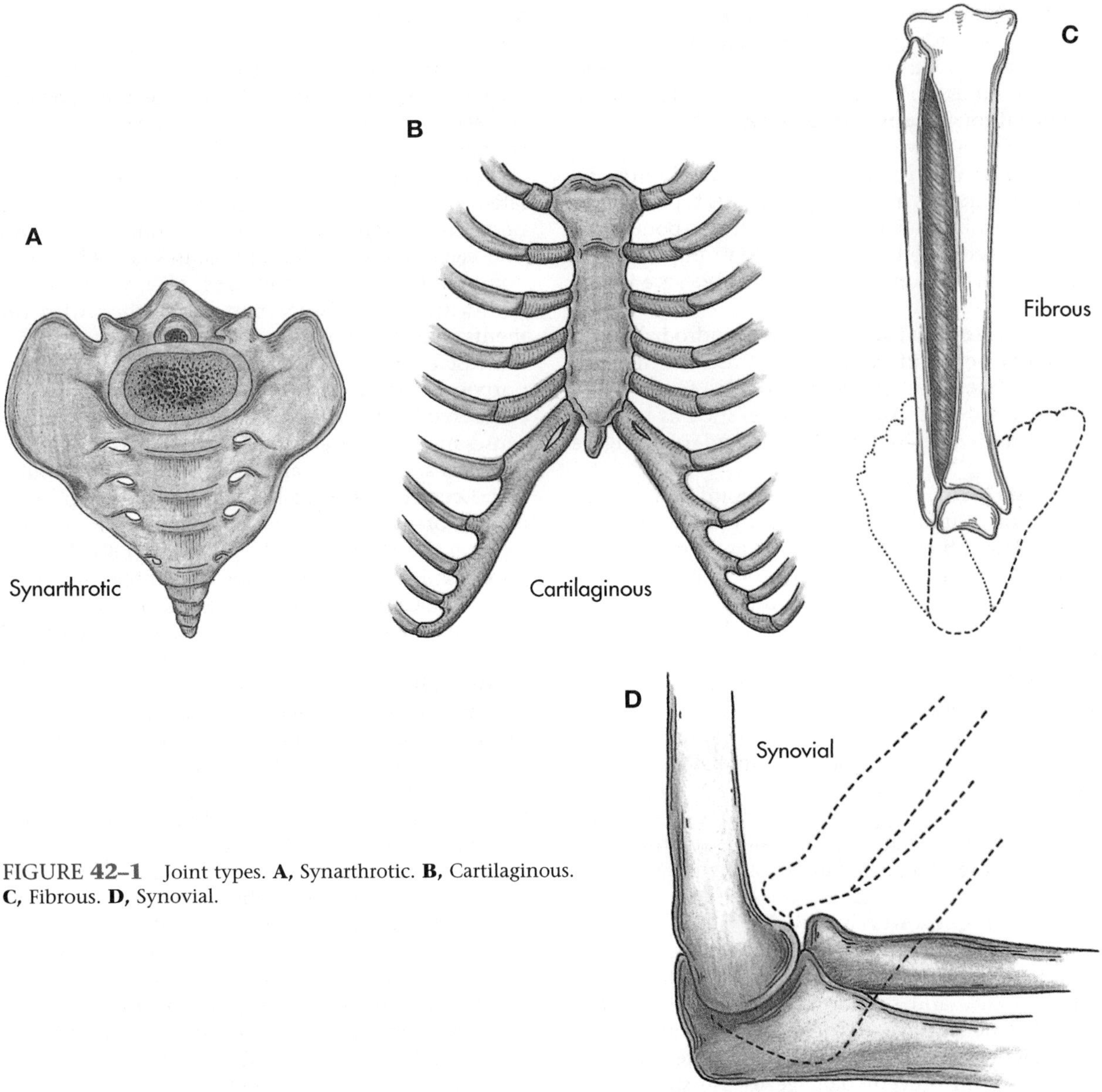

FIGURE **42–1** Joint types. **A,** Synarthrotic. **B,** Cartilaginous. **C,** Fibrous. **D,** Synovial.

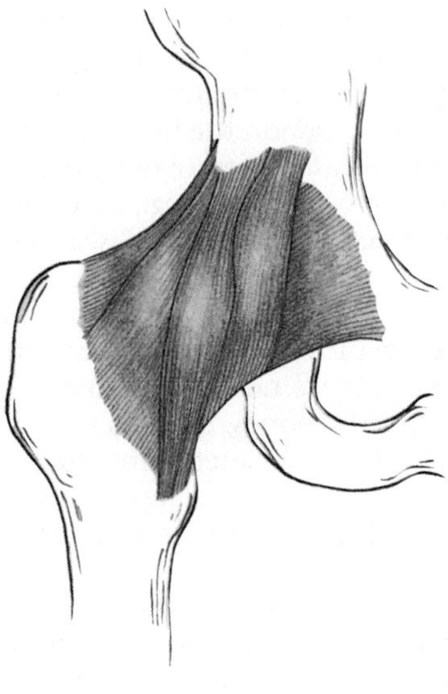

FIGURE **42–2** Ligaments of the hip joint.

lower extremities, trunk, neck, and back affect posture. These muscle groups work together to stabilize and support body weight standing or sitting, and they allow an individual to maintain a sitting or standing posture.

Muscle Regulation of Posture and Movement. Posture and movement can be reflections of personality, discomfort, and mood, as well as musculoskeletal function. For example, a person with a dramatic personality gestures with the hands, a person who is fatigued or depressed may slouch, and a person with abdominal pain may curl into the fetal position.

Posture and movement also depend on the skeleton and the shape and development of skeletal muscles. Coordination and regulation of different muscle groups depend on muscle tone and activity of antagonistic, synergistic, and anti-gravity muscles.

Muscle tone, or tonus, is the normal state of balanced muscle tension. Tension is achieved by alternate contraction and relaxation, without active movement, of neighbouring fibres of a specific muscle group. Good muscle

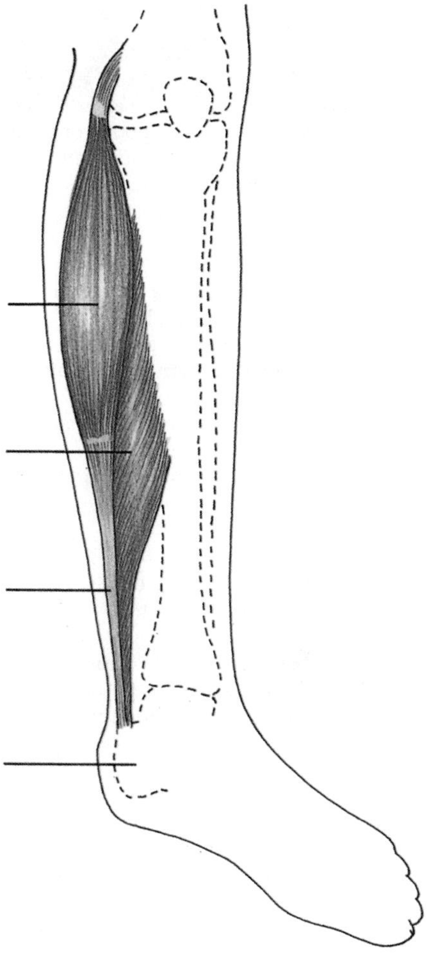

FIGURE **42–3** Tendons and muscles of the lower leg.

tone helps maintain functional positions such as sitting or standing without excess muscle fatigue. Muscle tone is maintained through continual use of muscles. ADLs require muscle action and help maintain muscle tone. Immobility or prolonged bed rest decreases muscle tone.

The antagonistic, synergistic, and anti-gravity muscle groups are coordinated by the nervous system and work together to maintain posture and initiate movement (see chapter 32).

Nervous System. Movement and posture are regulated by the nervous system. The precentral gyrus, or motor strip, is the major voluntary motor area and is located in the cerebral cortex. A majority of motor fibres descend from the motor strip and cross at the level of the medulla. Thus, the motor fibres from the right motor strip initiate voluntary movement for the left side of the body, and motor fibres from the left motor strip initiate voluntary movement for the right side of the body.

During voluntary movement, impulses descend from the motor strip to the spinal cord. An impulse exits the spinal cord through efferent motor nerves and travels through the nerves. Through a complex process, **neurotransmitters,** or chemicals such as acetylcholine, transfer electric impulses from the nerve across the neuromuscular junction to the muscle. The neurotransmitter reaches a muscle and stimulates it, causing movement. Movement can be impaired by disorders that alter neurotransmitter production, alter transfer from the nerve to the muscle, or alter activation of muscle activity. Parkinsonism is an example of such a disorder.

Pathological Influences on Mobility

Many pathological conditions affect mobility. Although a complete description of each is beyond the scope of this chapter, an overview of four pathological influences are presented here: postural abnormalities, impaired muscle development, damage to the central nervous system, and direct trauma to the musculoskeletal system.

Postural Abnormalities. Congenital or acquired postural abnormalities affect the efficiency of the musculoskeletal system, as well as body alignment, balance, and appearance. During assessment, the nurse observes body alignment and ROM (see chapter 32). Postural abnormalities can cause pain, impair alignment or mobility, or both. Knowledge about the characteristics, causes, and treatment of common postural abnormalities (Table 42-1) is necessary for lifting, transfering, and positioning. Some postural abnormalities may limit ROM. Nurses intervene to maintain maximum ROM in unaffected joints and then may design interventions to strengthen affected muscles and joints, improve the client's posture, and adequately use affected and unaffected muscle groups. Referral to and/or collaboration with a physiotherapist may enhance the nurse's interventions for a client with a postural abnormality.

Impaired Muscle Development. Injury and disease can lead to numerous alterations in musculoskeletal function. The muscular dystrophies, for example, are a group of familial disorders that cause degeneration of skeletal muscle fibres. The most prevalent of the muscle diseases in childhood, the muscular dystrophies are characterized by progressive, symmetrical weakness and wasting of skeletal muscle groups, with increasing disability and deformity (McCance & Huether, 2002).

Damage to the Central Nervous System. Damage to any component of the central nervous system that regulates voluntary movement results in impaired body alignment and mobility. The motor strip in the cerebral cortex can be damaged by trauma from a head injury, ischemia from a stroke or brain attack (cerebrovascular accident), tumour, or bacterial infection such as meningitis. Motor impairment is directly related to the amount of destruction of the motor strip. For example, a person with a right-sided cerebral hemorrhage with complete necrosis will likely have destruction of the right motor strip and left-sided hemiplegia. Trauma to the spinal cord also impairs mobility. Common trauma includes transection of the spinal cord in which motor fibres are cut. A complete transection will likely result in a bilateral loss of voluntary motor control below the level of the trauma.

Direct Trauma to the Musculoskeletal System. Direct trauma to the musculoskeletal system can result in bruises, contusions, sprains, and fractures. A fracture is a disruption of bone tissue continuity. Fractures most commonly result

Table 42-1 Postural Abnormalities

Abnormality	Description	Cause	Possible Treatments*
Torticollis	Inclining of head to affected side, in which sternocleidomastoid muscle is contracted	Congenital or acquired condition	Surgery, heat, support, or immobilization, depending on cause and severity, gentle range of motion
Lordosis	Exaggeration of anterior convex curve of lumbar spine	Congenital condition Temporary condition (e.g., pregnancy)	Spine-stretching exercises (based on cause)
Kyphosis	Increased convexity in curvature of thoracic spine	Congenital condition Rickets, osteoporosis Tuberculosis of spine	Spine-stretching exercises, sleeping without pillows, using bed board, bracing, spinal fusion (based on cause and severity)
Kypholordosis	Combination of kyphosis and lordosis	Congenital condition	Similar to methods used in kyphosis or lordosis (based on cause) Immobilization and surgery (based on cause and severity)
Scoliosis	Lateral "S" curvature of spine, unequal heights of hips and shoulders	Congenital condition Poliomyelitis Spastic paralysis Unequal leg length	Immobilization and surgery (based on cause and severity)
Kyphoscoliosis	Abnormal anteroposterior and lateral curvature of spine	Congenital condition Poliomyelitis Cor pulmonale	Immobilization and surgery (based on cause and severity)
Congenital hip dysplasia	Hip instability with limited abduction of hips and, occasionally, adduction contractures (head of femur does not articulate with acetabulum because of abnormal shallowness of acetabulum)	Congenital condition (more common with breech deliveries)	Maintenance of continuous abduction of thigh so that head of femur presses into centre of acetabulum Abduction splints, casting, surgery
Knock-knee (genu valgum)	Legs curved inward so that knees come together as person walks	Congenital condition Rickets	Knee braces, surgery if not corrected by growth
Bowlegs (genu varum)	One or both legs bent outward at knee, which is normal until 2 to 3 years of age	Congenital condition Rickets	Slowing rate of curving if not corrected by growth With rickets, increase of vitamin D, calcium, and phosphorus intake to normal ranges
Clubfoot	95%: medial deviation and plantar flexion of foot (equinovarus) 5%: lateral deviation and dorsiflexion (calcaneovalgus)	Congenital condition	Casts, splints such as Denis-Browne splint, and surgery (based on degree and rigidity of deformity)
Footdrop	Inability to dorsiflex and invert foot because of peroneal nerve damage	Congenital condition Trauma Improper position of immobilized client	None (cannot be corrected) Prevention through physiotherapy Bracing with ankle-foot orthotic
Pigeon-toes	Internal rotation of forefoot or entire foot, common in infants	Congenital condition Habit	Growth, wearing reversed shoes

*Severity of condition and cause will dictate treatment, which must be individualized.
Data from *Pathophysiology: The Biologic Basis for Disease in Adults and Children* (4th ed.), by K. L. McCance and S. E. Huether, 2002, St. Louis, MO: Mosby.

from direct external trauma but can also occur as a consequence of some deformity of the bone (e.g., pathological fractures of osteoporosis, Paget's disease, metastatic cancer, or osteogenesis imperfecta). Young children are usually able to form new bone more easily than adults and, as a result, have few complications after a fracture. Treatment often includes positioning the fractured bone in proper alignment and immobilizing it to promote healing and restore function. Even this temporary immobilization can result in some **muscle atrophy,** loss of tone, and joint stiffness. After the fracture has healed, physiotherapy may be required to regain functional losses.

Nursing Knowledge Base

Mobility-Immobility

Fully understanding mobility requires more than an overview of body mechanics and the regulation of movement by the musculoskeletal and nervous systems. The nurse must also know how mobility and immobility affect the systems of the body and the psychosocial and developmental aspects of clients.

Mobility refers to a person's ability to move about freely, and **immobility** refers to the inability to move about freely. Mobility and immobility are best understood as the end points of a continuum, with many degrees of partial immobility between. Some clients move back and forth on this continuum, but for other clients, immobility is absolute and continues indefinitely. The terms *bed rest* and *impaired physical mobility* are frequently used when discussing clients on the mobility-immobility continuum.

Bed rest is an intervention that restricts clients to bed for therapeutic reasons. Nurses and physicians most often prescribe this intervention. Clients with a wide variety of conditions are placed on bed rest. The general objectives of bed rest are as follows:

- Reduce physical activity and the oxygen needs of the body
- Reduce pain, including post-operative pain, and the need for large doses of analgesics
- Allow ill or debilitated clients to rest
- Allow exhausted clients the opportunity for uninterrupted rest

The duration of bed rest depends on the illness or injury and the client's prior state of health.

Impaired physical mobility is defined by the North American Nursing Diagnosis Association as a state in which the individual experiences or is at risk of experiencing limitation of physical movement (Ackley & Ladwig, 2002). Alterations in the level of physical mobility can result from prescribed restriction of movement in the form of bed rest, physical restriction of movement because of external devices (e.g., a cast or skeletal traction), voluntary restriction of movement, or impairment of motor or skeletal function.

The effects of muscular deconditioning associated with lack of physical activity may be apparent in a matter of days. The normal individual on bed rest loses muscle strength from baseline levels at a rate of 3% a day. Bed rest also is associated with cardiovascular, skeletal, and other organ changes. The term *disuse atrophy* has been used to describe the pathological reduction in normal size of muscle fibres after prolonged inactivity from bed rest, trauma, casting, or local nerve damage (McCance & Huether, 2002).

In a classic study, Deitrick and others (1948) found that even young healthy men put on bed rest had physiological problems. Periods of immobility or prolonged bed rest can cause major physiological, psychological, and social effects. These effects can be gradual or immediate and vary from client to client. The greater the extent and the longer the duration of immobility, the more pronounced the consequences. The client with complete mobility restrictions is continually at risk for hazardous system-wide effects.

Systemic Effects of Immobility. All body systems work more efficiently with some form of movement. Exercise has been shown to have positive outcomes for all major systems of the body. Therefore, when there is an alteration in mobility, each body system is at risk for impairment. The severity of the impairment depends on the client's overall health, degree and length of immobility, and age. For example, older adults with chronic illnesses develop pronounced effects of immobility more quickly than do younger clients with the same immobility problem.

Metabolic Changes. Endocrine metabolism, calcium resorption, and functioning of the gastrointestinal system are altered by changes in mobility.

The endocrine system, made up of hormone-secreting glands, helps to maintain and regulate vital functions such as response to stress and injury, growth and development, reproduction, ionic homeostasis, and energy metabolism. When injury or stress occurs, the endocrine system triggers a series of responses aimed at maintaining blood pressure and preserving life. The endocrine system is important in maintaining homeostasis. Tissues and cells live in an internal environment that the endocrine system helps regulate through maintenance of sodium, potassium, water, and acid-base balance. The endocrine system also helps regulate energy metabolism. The basal metabolic rate (BMR) is increased by thyroid hormone, and energy is made available to cells through the integrated action of gastrointestinal and pancreatic hormones (McCance & Huether, 2002).

Immobility disrupts normal metabolic functioning by decreasing the metabolic rate; altering the metabolism of carbohydrates, fats, and proteins; causing fluid, electrolyte, and calcium imbalances; and causing gastrointestinal disturbances such as decreased appetite and slowing of peristalsis. However, in the presence of an infectious process, immobilized clients may have an increased BMR as a result of fever or wound healing. Fever and repair of wounds increase cellular oxygen requirements (McCance & Huether, 2002).

A deficiency in calories and protein is characteristic of clients with a decreased appetite secondary to immobility. Proteins are constantly being synthesized and broken down into amino acids in the body to be re-formed into other proteins. Amino acids that are not used are excreted. The body can synthesize certain non-essential amino acids but depends on ingested proteins to supply the eight essential amino acids. When more nitrogen (the end product of amino acid breakdown) is excreted than is ingested in proteins, the body is said to have a **negative nitrogen balance** (Figure 42–4). Weight loss, decreased muscle mass, and weakness result from tissue catabolism (tissue breakdown). Protein loss leads to muscle loss.

Another metabolic change is calcium resorption (loss) from bones. As a result, urinary excretion of calcium increases because immobility causes the release of calcium into the circulation. Normally, the kidneys can excrete the excess calcium. However, if the kidneys are unable to respond appropriately, hypercalcemia results (Maher, Salmond, & Pellino, 2002).

Decreased mobility also leads to decreased gastrointestinal motility, which in turn can cause a variety of impairments to gastrointestinal functioning. Difficulty in passing stools (constipation) is a common symptom, although diarrhea may result from a fecal impaction (accumulation of hardened feces). The nurse must be aware that this finding is not normal diarrhea, but rather liquid stool passing around the area of impaction (see chapter 41). Left untreated, fecal impaction can result in a mechanical bowel obstruction that may partially or completely occlude the intestinal lumen, blocking normal propulsion of liquid and gas. The resulting fluid in the intestine produces distension and increases intraluminal

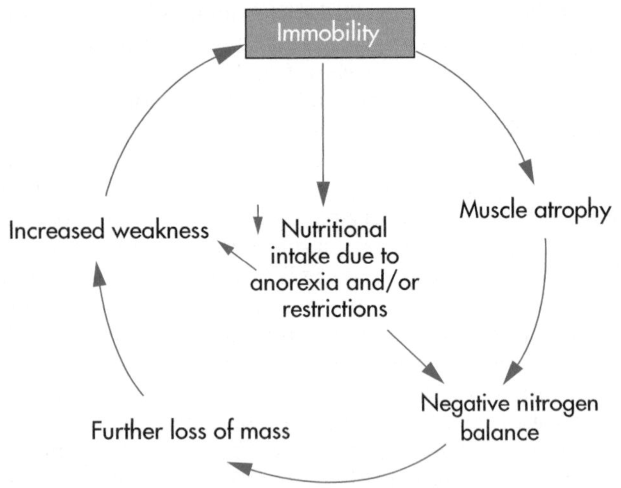

FIGURE **42–4** Factors contributing to negative nitrogen balance associated with immobility. (From *Basic Pathophysiology: A Holistic Approach,* 3rd ed., by M. W. Gröer and M. E. Shekleton, 1989, St. Louis, MO: Mosby.)

pressure. Over time, intestinal function becomes depressed, dehydration occurs, absorption ceases, and fluid and electrolyte disturbances worsen.

Respiratory Changes. Regular aerobic exercise is known to enhance respiratory functioning. Lack of movement and exercise places clients at higher risk for respiratory complications. Post-operative and immobile clients are at high risk for developing pulmonary complications. The most common respiratory complications are **atelectasis** (collapse of alveoli) and **hypostatic pneumonia** (inflammation of the lung from stasis or pooling of secretions). Both decrease oxygenation, prolong recovery, and add to the client's discomfort (Black, Hawks, & Keene, 2001). In atelectasis, secretions block a bronchiole or a bronchus, and the distal lung tissue (alveoli) collapse as the existing air is absorbed, producing hypoventilation. The site of the blockage determines the extent of atelectasis. A lung lobe or even a whole lung may collapse. At some point in the development of these complications, there is a proportional decline in the client's ability to cough productively. Ultimately, the distribution of mucus in the bronchi increases, particularly when the client is in the supine, prone, or lateral position (Figure 42–5). Mucus accumulates in the dependent regions of the airways. Because mucus is an excellent medium for bacterial growth, hypostatic pneumonia may result.

Cardiovascular Changes. The cardiovascular system is also affected by immobilization. The three major changes are orthostatic hypotension, increased cardiac workload, and thrombus formation.

Orthostatic hypotension is a drop of 20 mm Hg or more in systolic blood pressure and of 10 mm Hg in diastolic blood pressure when the client rises from a lying or sitting position to a standing position (Lance et al., 2000). In the immobilized client, decreased circulating fluid volume, pooling of blood in the lower extremities, and decreased autonomic response occur. These factors result in decreased venous return, followed by a decrease in cardiac output, which is reflected by a decline in blood pressure (McCance & Huether, 2002).

As the workload of the heart increases, its oxygen consumption does, too. The heart therefore works harder and less efficiently during periods of prolonged rest. As immobilization increases, cardiac output falls, further decreasing cardiac efficiency and increasing workload.

Clients are also at risk for thrombus formation. A **thrombus** is an accumulation of platelets, fibrin, clotting factors, and the cellular elements of the blood attached to the interior wall of a vein or artery, sometimes occluding the lumen of the vessel (Figure 42–6). There are three factors that contribute to venous thrombus formation: (a) loss of integrity of the vessel wall (e.g., injury), (b) abnormalities of blood flow (e.g., slow blood flow in calf veins associated with bed rest), and (c) alterations in blood constituents (e.g., a change in clotting factors or increased platelet activity). These three factors are sometimes referred to as Virchow's triad (McCance & Huether, 2002).

Musculoskeletal Changes. The effects of immobility on the musculoskeletal system can include temporary or permanent impairment. Restricted mobility may result in loss of endurance, strength, and muscle mass as well as decreased stability and balance. Other effects of restricted mobility affecting the skeletal system are impaired calcium metabolism and impaired joint mobility.

Muscle Effects. Because of protein breakdown, the client loses lean body mass, which is composed partially of muscle. The reduced muscle mass is unable to sustain activity without increased fatigue. If immobility continues and the muscles are not exercised, there is further decrease in muscle mass. Muscle weakness always occurs with immobility. Prolonged immobility often leads to muscle atrophy (or loss of muscle tissue). Therefore, atrophy is widely observed in response to illness, decreased ADLs, and immobilization. Loss of endurance, decreased muscle mass and strength, and joint instability (see Skeletal Effects) put clients at risk for falls.

Skeletal Effects. Immobilization causes two skeletal changes: impaired calcium metabolism and joint abnormalities. Because immobilization results in bone resorption, the bone tissue is less dense, or is atrophied, and **disuse osteoporosis** results. When disuse osteoporosis occurs, the client is at risk for pathological fractures. Immobilization and non-weight-bearing activities increase the rate of bone resorption. Bone resorption also causes calcium to be released in the blood, and hypercalcemia results.

Osteoporosis is a major health concern in Canada. Most affected are women; 25% of women and 12.5% of men have osteoporosis (Brown & Josse, 2002). A 50-year-old woman has a lifetime risk of 40% of an osteoporosis-related fracture. Fifty percent of women who fracture their hip do not return to their previous functional level (Brown & Josse, 2002). Although primary osteoporosis is different in origin from the osteoporosis that results from immobility, it is imperative for nurses to recognize that immobilized clients may be at high risk for accelerated

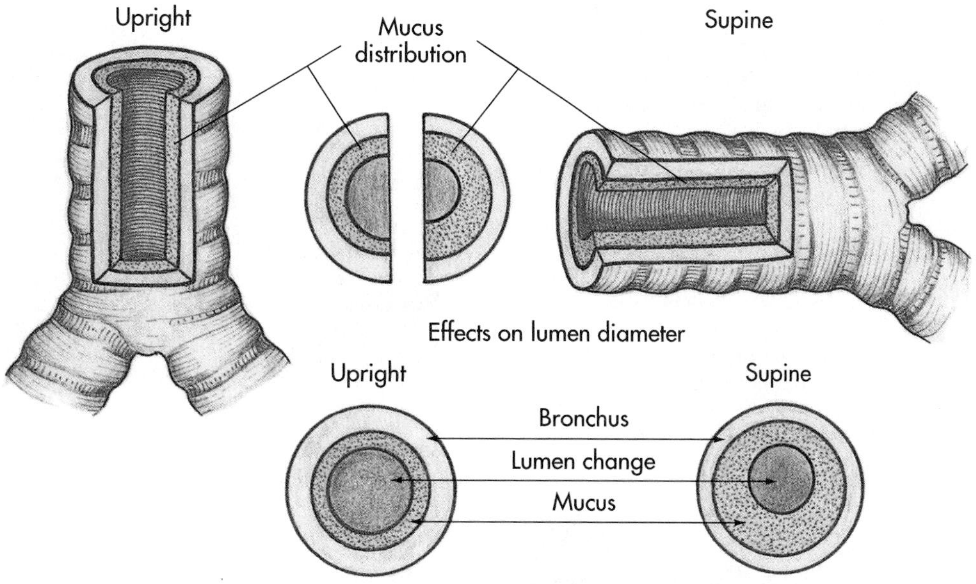

FIGURE **42–5** Effect of recumbency and gravity on distribution of respiratory tract and diameter of bronchiolar lumen. (From *Basic Pathophysiology: A Holistic Approach,* 3rd ed., by M. W. Gröer and M. E. Shekleton, 1989, St. Louis, MO: Mosby.)

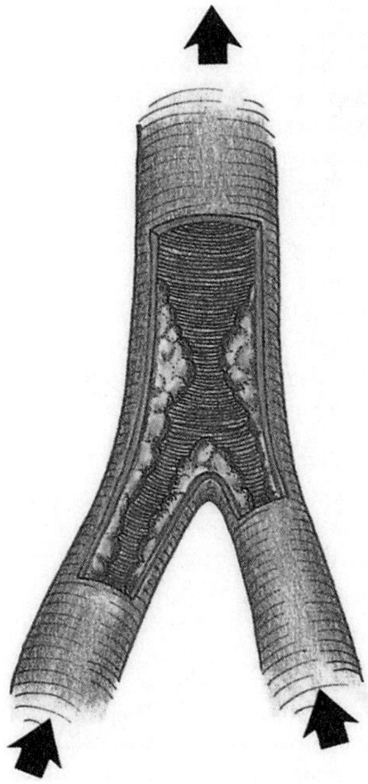

FIGURE **42–6** Thrombus formation in a vessel.

bone loss if they have primary osteoporosis. Important interventions for preventing disability in clients with primary osteoporosis who become immobilized include early client evaluation and consultation and referral with physicians, dietitians, and physiotherapists. For the client with osteoporosis, the goal is to maintain independence with ADLs. Assistive ambulatory devices, adaptive clothing, and safety bars may assist the client with maintaining independence. Client teaching should focus on limiting the severity of the disease through diet and activity (Box 42-1).

Immobility can lead to joint contractures. A **joint contracture** is an abnormal and possibly permanent condition characterized by fixation of the joint. It is caused by disuse, atrophy, and shortening of the muscle fibres. When a contracture occurs, the joint cannot obtain full ROM. Contractures may leave a joint(s) in a nonfunctional position (Figure 42–7). Resnick (2000) found that upper and lower extremity contractures significantly reduce functional performance in older adults.

One common and debilitating contracture is footdrop (Figure 42–8). When **footdrop** occurs, the foot is permanently fixed in plantar flexion. Ambulation is difficult with the foot in this position because the client cannot dorsiflex the foot. The client with footdrop is therefore unable to lift the toes off the ground. Clients who have suffered a cerebral vascular accident with resulting left- or right-sided paralysis (hemiplegia) are susceptible to footdrop.

Urinary Elimination Changes. The client's urinary elimination is altered by immobility. In the upright position, urine flows out of the renal pelvis and into the ureters and bladder because of gravitational forces. When the client is recumbent or flat, the kidneys and the ureters move toward a more level plane. Urine formed by the kidney must enter the bladder unaided by gravity. Because the peristaltic contractions of the ureters are insufficient to overcome gravity, the renal pelvis may fill before urine enters the ureters. This condition is called **urinary stasis** and increases the risk of urinary tract infection and renal calculi (see chapter 40). Renal calculi are calcium stones that lodge in the renal pelvis and pass through the ureters. Immobilized clients are at risk for calculi because of altered calcium metabolism and the resulting hypercalcemia.

Client Teaching — Box 42-1

Clients With Osteoporosis

Objective

- Client will verbalize strategies to prevent or limit the severity of osteoporosis.

Teaching Strategies

- Instruct client and/or caregiver on common risk factors and how to modify lifestyle (e.g., eliminating smoking, caffeine, alcohol).
- Teach client and/or caregiver the current recommended dietary allowances for calcium and vitamin D and review foods high in calcium and vitamin D.
- Instruct clients and/or caregiver on appropriate types of weight-bearing exercises as recommended by physician or physiotherpist to prevent injury or fractures.
- Teach client and/or caregiver about safety, fall prevention, and strategies to create a safe home environment.
- Instruct client and/or caregiver self-administration of appropriate medication as ordered by physician.
- Promote positive self-image in client by providing realistic yet optimistic and positive feedback about changes in appearance and mobility.

Evaluation

- Client and/or caregiver verbalize strategies to modify lifestyle such as stopping smoking, reducing caffeine or alcohol intake, or increasing dietary calcium.
- Client and/or caregiver verbalize foods high in calcium and vitamin D.
- Client and/or caregiver verbalize appropriate weight-bearing exercises.
- Client and/or caregiver verbalize safety strategies to prevent falls.
- Client and/or caregiver verbalize appropriate knowledge about medications.
- Client and/or caregiver express positive but realistic feedback regarding effects of disease.

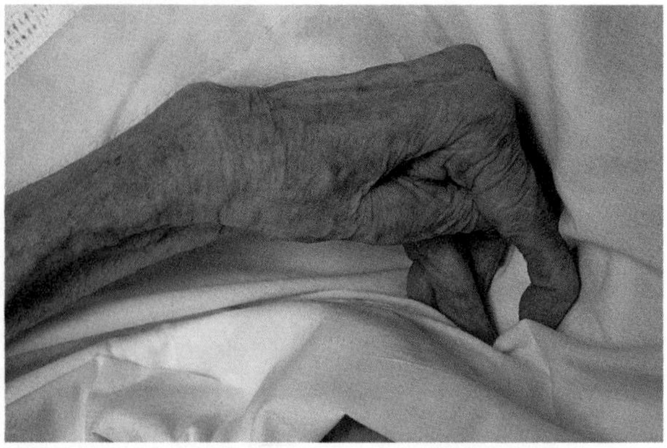

FIGURE **42–7** A contracture of the joints in the fingers. (From *Mosby's Canadian Textbook for the Support Worker,* by S. A. Sorrentino, 2004, Toronto, ON: Elsevier Canada.)

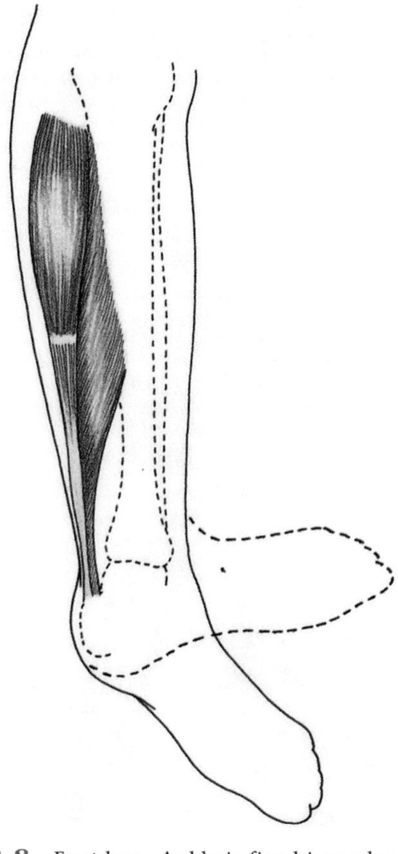

FIGURE **42–8** Footdrop. Ankle is fixed in a plantar flexion. Normally, the ankle is able to flex *(dotted line),* which eases walking.

As the period of immobility continues, fluid intake can diminish, and this increases the risk for dehydration. As a result of decreased fluid intake, urinary output may decline around the fifth or sixth day after immobilization and the urine is often highly concentrated. This concentrated urine increases the risk for calculi formation and infection. Immobility can contribute to decreased access to bathing equipment and inability to perform adequate perineal hygiene, which may also increase the risk of urinary tract contamination by *Escherichia coli* bacteria. Another cause of urinary tract infections in immobilized clients is the use of an indwelling urinary catheter.

Integumentary Changes. The direct effect of pressure on the skin by immobility is compounded by the changes in metabolism that accompany immobility. Any break in the skin's integrity is difficult to heal in the immobilized client. Preventing a pressure ulcer is much less expensive than treating one (Bergquist, 2001). Thus, immobility is a major risk for pressure ulcers and preventive nursing interventions are imperative.

A **pressure ulcer** is an impairment of the skin as a result of prolonged ischemia (decreased blood supply to an area) in tissues (see chapter 43). The ulcer is characterized initially by inflammation and usually forms over a bony prominence. Ischemia develops when the pressure on the skin is greater than the pressure inside the small peripheral blood vessels supplying blood to the skin.

Tissue metabolism depends on the body's receipt of oxygen and nutrients from the blood supply and the elimination of metabolic wastes. Pressure affects cellular metabolism by decreasing or obliterating tissue circulation. When a client lies in bed or sits in a chair, the weight of the body is on bony prominences. The longer the pressure is applied, the longer the period of ischemia and therefore the greater the risk of skin breakdown.

> ***Safety Alert.*** Immobilized clients should be turned every 2 hours at a minimum to prevent skin breakdown. Defloor (2000) reported that the preferred position is a 30-degree lateral position if the client is going to remain in a position for more than 2 hours.

Psychosocial Effects. Immobilization may lead to emotional and behavioural responses, sensory alterations, and changes in coping. These changes are individualized to each client. In addition, immobilized clients may also have social and family difficulties.

Common emotional changes are depression, behavioural changes, sleep-wake disturbances, and impaired coping. The immobilized client can become depressed because of changes in role, self-concept, and other factors. Depression is an affective disorder characterized by exaggerated feelings of sadness, melancholy, dejection, worthlessness, emptiness, and hopelessness out of proportion to reality. Depression can result from worrying about present and future levels of health, finances, and family needs. Because immobilization removes the client from a daily routine, he or she has more time to worry about disability. Worrying can quickly increase the client's depression, causing withdrawal. Assessing behavioural changes throughout restricted mobility helps the nurse to identify changes in self-concept, recognize early signs of depression, and develop nursing interventions.

Behavioural changes resulting from immobilization vary widely, depending on the client. Common behavioural changes include hostility, belligerence, giddiness, fear, and anxiety. Early in the nursing process, the nurse should interview the client's family about normal behavioural patterns to gain baseline data. If unexpected behaviours are observed later, the nurse can intervene to reduce the effects of immobilization on the client's behavioural patterns.

Sleep-wake alterations in the immobile client may occur from nursing care or changes in habit or environment. Disruption of normal sleeping patterns can further cause behavioural changes. Nursing interventions should be used to ensure that the client receives sufficient sleep (see chapter 37). The client who is on bed rest and is able to change position during sleep does not require continuous physical nursing care. Unless other treatment activities are required during the night, the care plan for the physiologically stable client on bed rest should provide for uninterrupted sleep.

Long-term immobility or bed rest can affect usual coping patterns. Such a client may withdraw and become passive. The passive client allows nurses to provide care but is not interested in increasing independence or involvement in care. Early in the care of an immobilized client, the nurse should assess the client's normal coping mechanisms in order to design a nursing care plan that will accommodate the client's coping abilities or help the client develop new ones.

Developmental Changes. Developmental changes tend to be associated with immobility in the very young and in older adults. The immobilized young or middle-age adult who has been healthy may experience few, if any, developmental changes. However, there are exceptions, and clients must be fully assessed for developmental implications. One exception might be a mother who has complications at childbirth and as a result cannot interact with the newborn as expected.

Infants, Toddlers, and Preschoolers. The newborn infant's spine is flexed and lacks the anteroposterior curves of the adult (see chapter 19). As the baby grows, musculoskeletal development permits support of weight for standing and walking. Posture is awkward because the head and upper trunk are carried forward. Because body weight is not evenly distributed along a line of gravity, posture is off balance, and falls occur often. When the infant, toddler, or preschooler is immobilized, it is usually because of trauma or the need to correct a congenital skeletal abnormality. Prolonged immobilization can delay the child's gross motor skills, intellectual development, or musculoskeletal development. Nurses caring for immobilized children should plan activities that provide physical and psychosocial stimuli.

Adolescents. The adolescence stage is usually initiated by a tremendous growth spurt (see chapter 19). Growth is frequently uneven. Prolonged immobilization may alter adolescent growth patterns. In addition, the adolescent may lag behind peers in gaining independence. When immobilization occurs, social isolation must be a concern for this age group.

Adults. An adult who has correct posture and body alignment feels good, looks good, and generally appears self-confident. The healthy adult also has the necessary musculoskeletal development and coordination to carry out ADLs (see chapter 20). When periods of prolonged immobility occur, all physiological systems are at risk. In addition, the role of the adult may change with regard to the family or social structure. The adult may lose identity associated with a job.

Older Adults. Aging is normally associated with a progressive loss of total bone mass, muscle strength, and aerobic capacity. Some of the possible causes of this loss include decreased physical activity, hormonal changes, and actual bone resorption. The effect of bone loss is weaker bones. Older adults may walk more slowly, take smaller steps, and appear less coordinated. Thus, balance is impaired, and they are at greater risk for falls and injuries (see chapter 21). The outcomes of a fall include not only possible injury, but also hospitalization, loss of independence, and psychological effects.

Box 42-2 Hazards of Immobility in Hospitalized Older Adults

For many older adults, admission to the hospital often results in functional decline. Older adults can quickly regress to a dependent state, and rapid intervention of an interdisciplinary health team is required to maintain functional capacity.

Usual aging is associated with decreased muscle strength and aerobic capacity. Placing clients on bed rest without sufficient ambulation leads to loss of mobility and functional decline. Immobility causes weakness, fatigue, and an increased risk for falls. It results in shallow breathing, which may lead to pneumonia, and inadequate turning or repositioning results in skin breakdown and pressure ulcers.

Catheter use and improper pericare lead to urinary tract infections. Older adults are prone to nosocomial infections (infections obtained in the health care environment) because of compromised immune systems. Infections, as well as medications, treatments, and translocation, often cause confusion in older adults.

Hospitalization affects the nutritional status in the older adult. Limited access to fluids causes dehydration. Conversely, fluid overload occurs from improper administration of IV fluids. Treatments and medications cause fluid and electrolyte imbalances, contributing to confusion in the geriatric client.

Finally, multiple interruptions and noise in the environment impair sleep, causing fatigue, depression, and confusion. Any of these factors may thrust vulnerable older adults into a state of irreversible functional decline.

Adapted from *Geriatric Nursing and Healthy Aging,* by P. Ebersole and P. Hess, 2001, St. Louis, MO: Mosby.

Older adults may experience functional status changes secondary to hospitalization and altered mobility status (Box 42-2). Immobilization of older adults may increase their physical dependence on others and accelerate functional losses. Immobilization of some older adults results from a degenerative disease, neurological trauma, or chronic illness. For some older adults, immobilization occurs gradually and progressively, whereas for others—especially those who have had a stroke—immobilization is sudden. When providing nursing care for an older adult, the nurse should develop a care plan that encourages the client to perform as many self-care activities as possible, thereby maintaining the highest level of mobility. Nurses may inadvertently contribute to a client's immobility by providing unnecessary help with activities such as bathing and transferring.

Critical Thinking

Critical thinking requires the nurse to combine knowledge, experiences, client data, critical thinking attitudes, and intellectual and professional standards. Each of these sources must be weighed for its validity and applicability to the client who is facing impaired mobility. The immobile client has multiple needs, and by integrating these sources, the nurse can best judge appropriate nursing diagnoses and subsequent care.

To understand the impact of immobility on the client and family, the nurse must integrate knowledge from nursing and other disciplines, previous experiences, and information gathered from clients. In addition, the use of critical thinking attitudes such as creativity is needed. Standards, such as those developed by provincial nursing associations (e.g., Registered Nurses Association of Ontario [RNAO] *Best Practice Guidelines*), provide valuable guides for managing complications associated with immobility (Figure 42–9). In addition, many agencies may have standards of practice related to lifting and transferring clients and to prevention of falls and pressure sores.

Nursing Process for Impaired Body Alignment and Mobility

By applying the nursing process and using a critical thinking approach, the nurse can develop individualized care plans for clients with mobility impairments or risk for immobility. A care plan is designed to improve the client's functional status, promote self-care, maintain psychological well-being, and reduce the hazards of immobility.

Assessment

Nursing assessment is presented in two sections: mobility and immobility. Both areas are usually assessed during the complete physical examination.

Mobility. Assessment of client mobility focuses on ROM, gait, exercise and activity tolerance, and body alignment. When unsure of the client's abilities, the nurse should begin assessment of mobility with the client in the most supportive position and move to higher levels of mobility according to the client's tolerance. Generally, the nurse starts assessing movement while the client is lying, then proceeds to assessing sitting positions in bed, transfers to chair, and finally gait. This helps to protect the client's safety.

Range of Motion. ROM is the maximum amount of movement available at a joint in one of the four planes of the body: medial, sagittal, frontal, or transverse (see Figure 28-6 and Table 28-11). The medial plane is a line through the axis of the body, separating the body into equal halves, a left side and a right side. The sagittal plane is any plane parallel to the medial. The frontal plane passes through the body from side to side and divides the body into front and back. The transverse plane is a horizontal line that divides the body into upper and lower portions.

Joint mobility is limited by ligaments, muscles, and the nature of the joint. Joint movements are described using the followng terms:

- *Flexion and extension*—flexion is decreasing the angle between two adjoining bones (bending of the joint); extension is increasing the angle between two adjoining

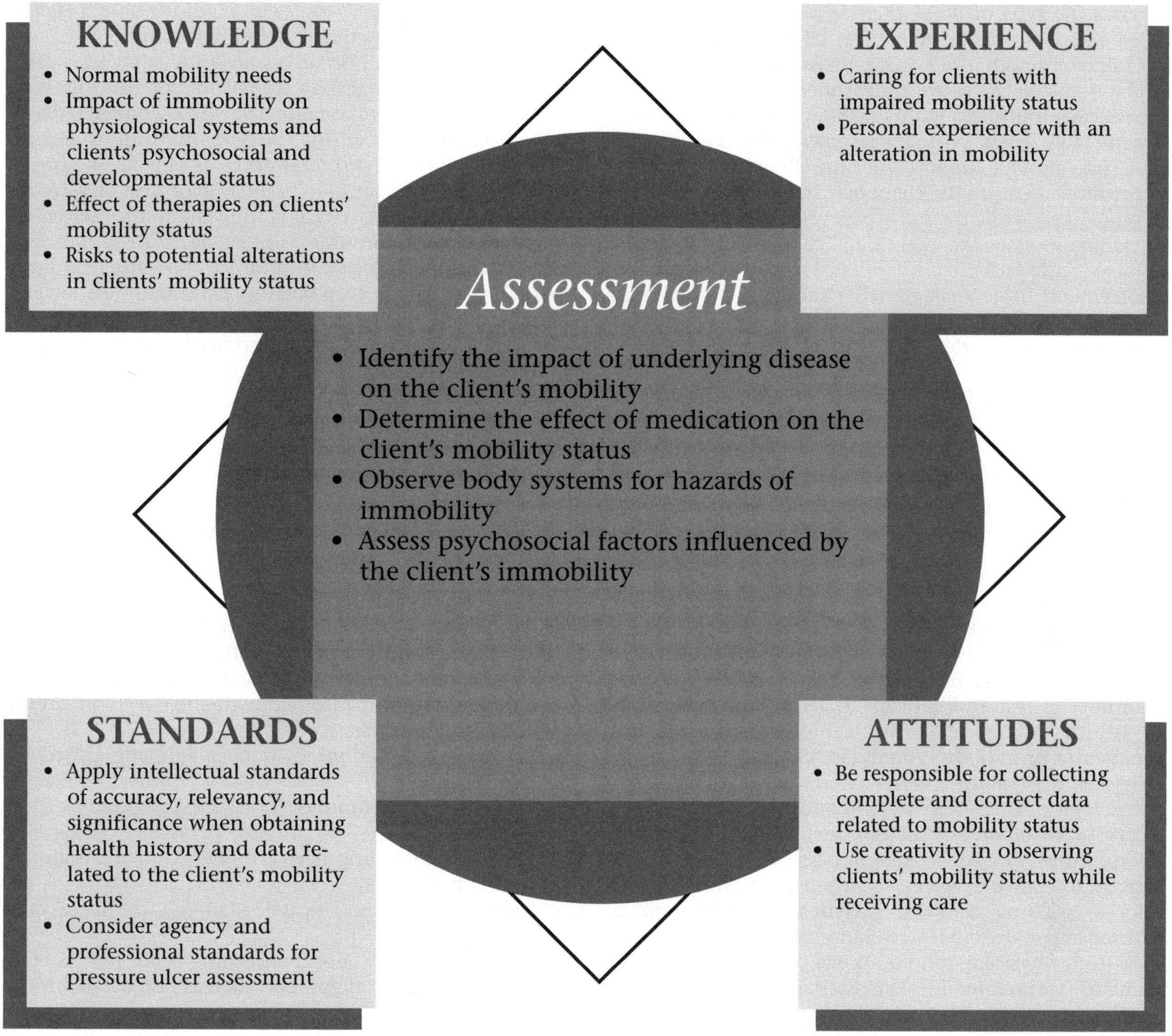
KNOWLEDGE
• Normal mobility needs
• Impact of immobility on physiological systems and clients' psychosocial and developmental status
• Effect of therapies on clients' mobility status
• Risks to potential alterations in clients' mobility status
EXPERIENCE
• Caring for clients with impaired mobility status
• Personal experience with an alteration in mobility
Assessment
• Identify the impact of underlying disease on the client's mobility
• Determine the effect of medication on the client's mobility status
• Observe body systems for hazards of immobility
• Assess psychosocial factors influenced by the client's immobility
STANDARDS
• Apply intellectual standards of accuracy, relevancy, and significance when obtaining health history and data related to the client's mobility status
• Consider agency and professional standards for pressure ulcer assessment
ATTITUDES
• Be responsible for collecting complete and correct data related to mobility status
• Use creativity in observing clients' mobility status while receiving care

FIGURE **42–9** Critical thinking model for immobility assessment.

bones (extending the joint). Examples include the fingers, elbows, and knees.

- *Hyperextension*—movement of a body part beyond its normal resting extended position
- *Dorsiflexion and plantar flexion*—dorsiflexion is the flexion of toes and foot upward; plantar flexion is bending of toes and foot downward
- *Abduction and adduction*—abduction is movement of extremity away from the midline of the body; adduction is movement of extremity toward midline of body (e.g., arms, fingers, and legs)
- *Eversion and inversion*—eversion is turning of body part away from midline; inversion is turning of body part toward midline (e.g., feet)
- *Pronation and supination*—pronation is movement of body part so that front or ventral surface faces downward; supination is movement of body part so that front or ventral surface faces upward (e.g., hands, forearm)
- *Internal and external rotation*—internal rotation is rotation of the joint inward; external otation is rotation of the joint outward (e.g., hip)
- *Circumduction*—the circular movement of a limb in a cone-shaped manner (e.g., shoulder)

When assessing ROM, the nurse asks questions about and physically examines the client for stiffness, swelling, pain, limited movement, and unequal movement. Chapter 28 describes specific techniques for measuring the degrees of motion in a joint. Assessment of ROM is important as a baseline measurement to compare and evaluate whether loss in joint mobility has occurred. Clients whose mobility is restricted require ROM exercises to reduce the hazards of immobility. Thus, the nurse assesses the type of ROM exercise a client can perform. ROM exercises may be active (the client is able to move all joints through their ROM unassisted), passive (the client is unable to move independently, and the nurse moves each joint through its ROM), or somewhere in between (Table 42-2). With a weak client, for example, the nurse may provide support while the client performs most of the movement, or the client may be able to move some joints actively while the nurse passively moves others. The nurse first assesses the client's ability to engage in active ROM exercises and the need for assistance, teaching, or reinforcement. In general, exercises should be as active as health and mobility allow. Contractures may develop in joints not moved periodically through their full ROM.

Gait. The term ***gait*** is used to describe a particular manner or style of walking. The gait cycle begins with the heel strike of one leg and continues to the heel strike of the other leg. Assessing a client's gait allows the nurse to draw conclusions about balance, posture, safety, and ability to walk without assistance. The mechanics of human gait involve coordination of the skeletal, neurological, and muscular systems of the human body.

Exercise and Activity Tolerance. **Exercise** is physical activity for conditioning the body, improving health, and maintaining fitness. It can be used as therapy to correct a deformity or restore the overall body to a maximal state of health. When a person exercises, physiological changes occur in body systems (see chapter 32).

Assessment of the client's energy level includes the physiological effects of exercise and activity tolerance. **Activity tolerance** is the type and amount of exercise or work that a person is able to perform. Assessment of activity tolerance is necessary when planning activities such as walking or ROM exercises or ADLs such as bathing clients. Activity tolerance assessment includes data from physiological, emotional, and developmental domains (see chapter 32). This assessment is applicable in all clinical settings and is quickly completed by the nurse.

As activity is begun, clients should be monitored for symptoms such as dyspnea, fatigue, chest pain, or change in vital signs from baseline. Some clients may be unable to sustain activity because the energy needed to complete the activity creates fatigue and generalized weakness. Even simple tasks such as eating or moving in bed may need to be monitored. When decreased activity tolerance is noted, the nurse should assess the time needed by the client to recover. A decreasing recovery time may indicate improved activity tolerance.

People who are depressed, worried, or anxious are frequently unable to tolerate exercise. Depressed clients are usually not motivated to participate. Clients who are worried or anxious tire easily because they expend a great deal of energy in worry and anxiety. Thus, they may experience physical and emotional exhaustion.

Developmental changes also affect activity tolerance. As the infant enters the toddler stage, the activity level increases and the need for sleep declines. The child entering preschool or primary grades expends mental energy in learning and may require more rest after school or before strenuous play. The adolescent going through puberty may require more rest because much of the body's energy is expended for growth and hormone changes.

Changes may still occur through the adult years, but many of these changes are related to work and lifestyle choices. Pregnancy may cause decrease a woman's energy tolerance, especially during the first and third trimesters. Hormonal changes and fetal development use body energy, and the woman may be unable or unmotivated to carry out physical activities. During the last trimester, fetal development consumes a great deal of the mother's energy, and the size and location of the fetus may limit the ability to take a deep breath, resulting in less oxygen being available for physical activities.

As the person grows older, activity tolerance changes. Muscle mass is reduced, posture changes, and the composition of bones is altered. There are often changes in the cardiopulmonary system, such as decreased maximum heart rate and decreased lung compliance that affect the intensity of exercise. The older adult may still exercise but will do so at a reduced intensity. The more inactive a client becomes, the more pronounced these activity changes are.

Body Alignment. Assessment of body alignment can be carried out with the client standing, sitting, or lying down. This assessment has the following objectives:

- Determining normal physiological changes in body alignment resulting from growth and development for each individual client
- Identifying deviations in body alignment caused by poor posture
- Providing opportunities for clients to observe their posture
- Identifying learning needs of clients for maintaining correct body alignment
- Identifying trauma, muscle damage, or nerve dysfunction
- Obtaining information concerning other factors contributing to poor alignment, such as fatigue, malnutrition, and psychological problems

The first step in assessing body alignment is to put clients at ease so that unnatural or rigid positions are not assumed. When the body alignment of an immobilized or unconscious client is assessed, pillows and positioning supports should be removed from the bed and the client placed in the supine position.

Standing. When the client is standing, the nurse checks for the following signs of good body alignment:

- The head is erect and midline.
- When observed posteriorly, the shoulders and hips are straight and parallel.
- When observed posteriorly, the vertebral column is straight.
- When the client is observed laterally, the head is erect and the spinal curves are aligned in a reversed S pattern. The cervical vertebrae are anteriorly convex, the thoracic vertebrae are posteriorly convex, and the lumbar vertebrae are anteriorly convex.
- When observed laterally, the abdomen is comfortably tucked in and the knees and ankles are slightly flexed. The person appears comfortable and does not seem conscious of the flexion of knees or ankles.

Text continued on p. 1453

Table 42-2 Range-of-Motion Exercises

Body Part	Type of Joint	Type of Movement	Range (Degrees)	Primary Muscles
Neck, cervical spine	Pivotal 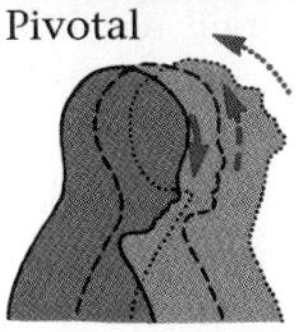	*Flexion:* Bring chin to rest on chest	45	Sternocleidomastoid
		Extension: Return head to erect position	45	Trapezius
		Hyperextension: Bend head back as far as possible	10	Trapezius
	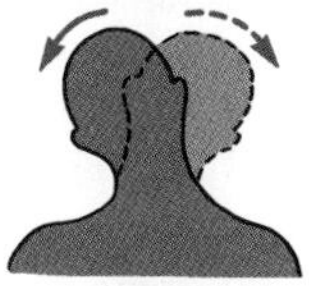	*Lateral flexion:* Tilt head as far as possible toward each shoulder	40–45	Sternocleidomastoid
	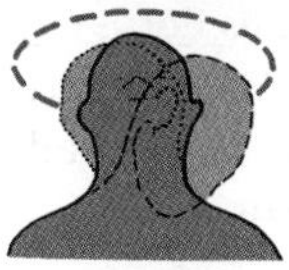	*Rotation:* Turn head as far as possible in circular movement	180	Sternocleidomastoid, trapezius
Shoulder	Ball and socket 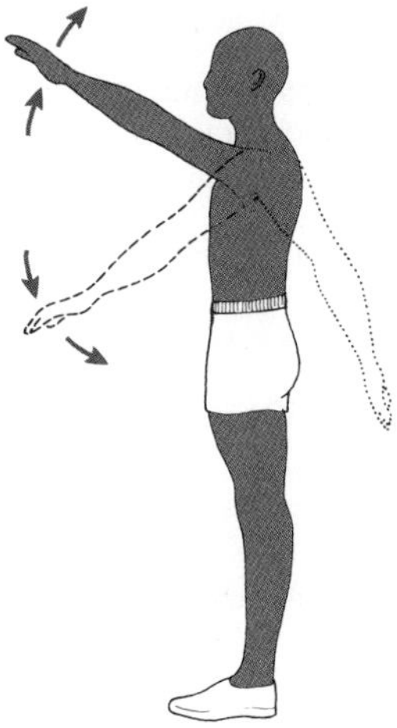	*Flexion:* Raise arm from side position forward to position above head	180 45–60	Coracobrachialis, biceps brachii, deltoid, pectoralis major
		Extension: Return arm to position at side of body	180	Latissimus dorsi, teres major, triceps brachii
		Hyperextension: Move arm behind body, keeping elbow straight	45–60	Latissimus dorsi, teres major, deltoid
	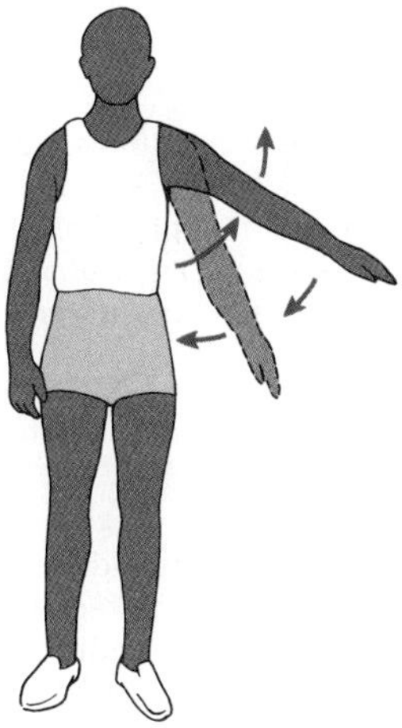	*Abduction:* Raise arm to side to position above head with palm away from head	180	Deltoid, supraspinatus
		Adduction: Lower arm sideways and across body as far as possible	320	Pectoralis major

Continued

Table 42-2 Range-of-Motion Exercises—cont'd

Body Part	Type of Joint	Type of Movement	Range (Degrees)	Primary Muscles
Shoulder,—cont'd	Ball and socket—cont'd 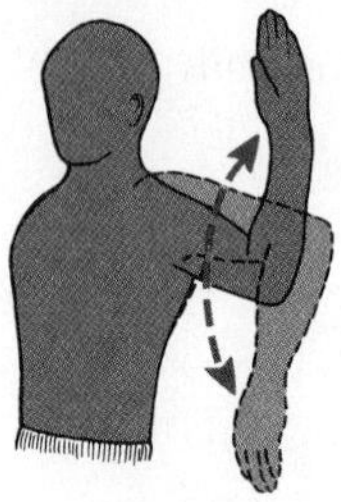	*Internal rotation:* With elbow flexed, rotate shoulder by moving arm until thumb is turned inward and toward back	90	Pectoralis major, latissimus dorsi, teres major, subscapularis
		External rotation: With elbow flexed, move arm until thumb is upward and lateral to head	90	Infraspinatus, teres major, deltoid
	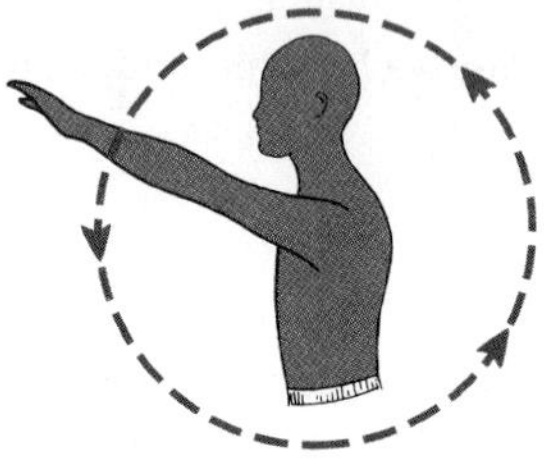	*Circumduction:* Move arm in full circle (Circumduction is combination of all movements of ball-and-socket joint.)	360	Deltoid, coracobrachialis, latissimus dorsi, teres major
Elbow	Hinge 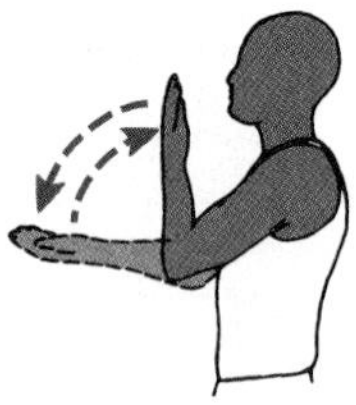	*Flexion:* Bend elbow so that lower arm moves toward its shoulder joint and hand is level with shoulder	150	Biceps brachii, brachialis, brachioradialis
		Extension: Straighten elbow by lowering hand	150	Triceps brachii
Forearm	Pivotal 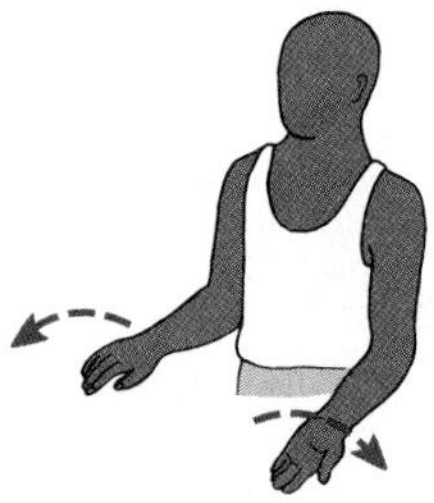	*Supination:* Turn lower arm and hand so that palm is up	70–90	Supinator, biceps brachii
		Pronation: Turn lower arm so that palm is down	70–90	Pronator teres, pronator quadratus
Wrist	Condyloid 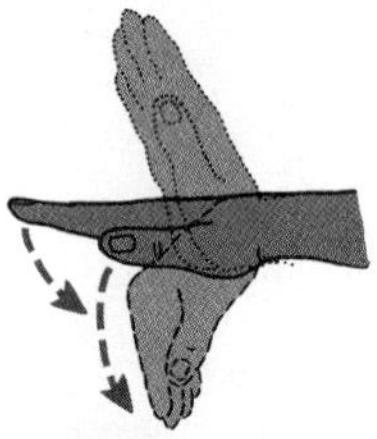	*Flexion:* Move palm toward inner aspect of forearm	80–90	Flexor carpi ulnaris, flexor carpi radialis
		Extension: Move fingers and hand posterior to midline	80–90	Extensor carpi radialis brevis, extensor carpi radialis longus, extensor carpi ulnaris
	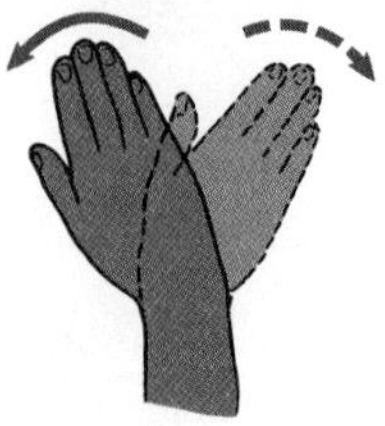	*Hyperextension:* Bring dorsal surface of hand back as far as possible	80–90	Extensor carpi radialis brevis, extensor carpi radialis longus, extensor carpi ulnaris
		Abduction (radial deviation): Bend wrist laterally toward fifth finger	Up to 30	Flexor carpi radialis, extensor carpi radialis brevis, extensor carpi radialis longus
		Adduction (ulnar deviation): Bend wrist medially toward thumb	30–50	Flexor carpi ulnaris, extensor carpi ulnaris

Table 42-2 Range-of-Motion Exercises—cont'd

Body Part	Type of Joint	Type of Movement	Range (Degrees)	Primary Muscles
Fingers	Condyloid hinge 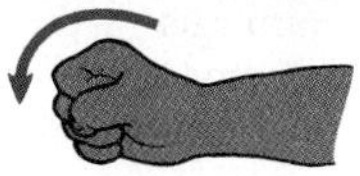	*Flexion:* Make fist	90	Lumbricales, interosseus volaris, interosseus dorsalis
		Extension: Straighten fingers	90	Extensor digiti quinti proprius, extensor digitorum communis, extensor indicis proprius
	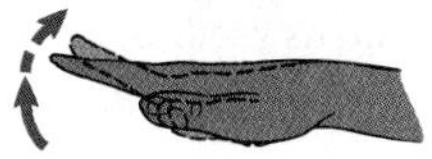	*Hyperextension:* Bend fingers back as far as possible	30–60	
	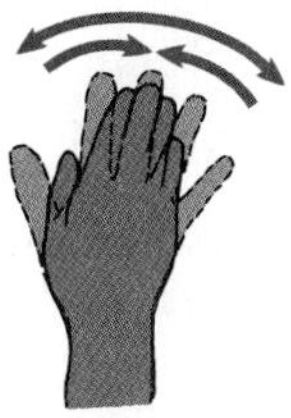	*Abduction:* Spread fingers apart	30	Interosseus dorsalis
		Adduction: Bring fingers together	30	Interosseus volaris
Thumb	Saddle 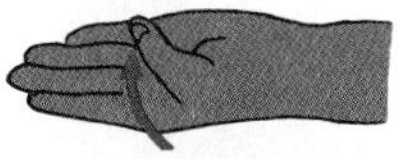	*Flexion:* Move thumb across palmar surface of hand	90	Flexor pollicis brevis
		Extension: Move thumb straight away from hand	90	Extensor pollicis longus, extensor pollicis brevis
	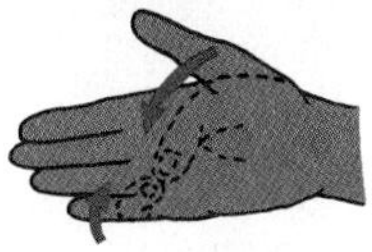	*Abduction:* Extend thumb laterally (usually done when placing fingers in abduction and adduction)	30	Abductor pollicis brevis
		Adduction: Move thumb back toward hand	30	Adductor pollicis obliquus, adductor pollicis transversus
		Opposition: Touch thumb to each finger of same hand		Opponeus pollicis, opponeus digiti minimi
Hip	Ball and socket 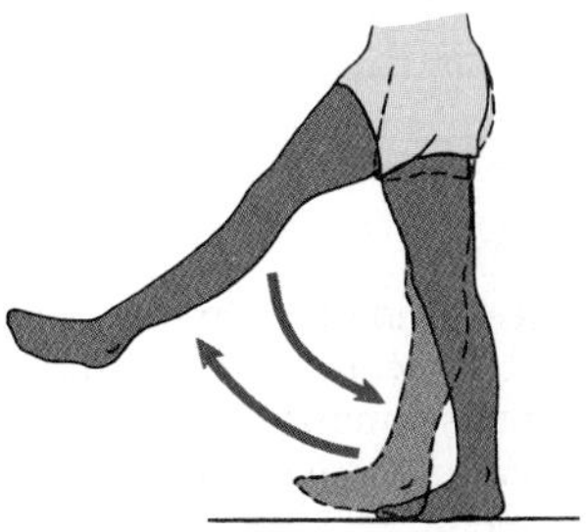	*Flexion:* Move leg forward and up	90–120	Psoas major, iliacus, sartorius
		Extension: Move back beside other leg	90–120	Gluteus maximus, semitendinosus, semimembranosus
	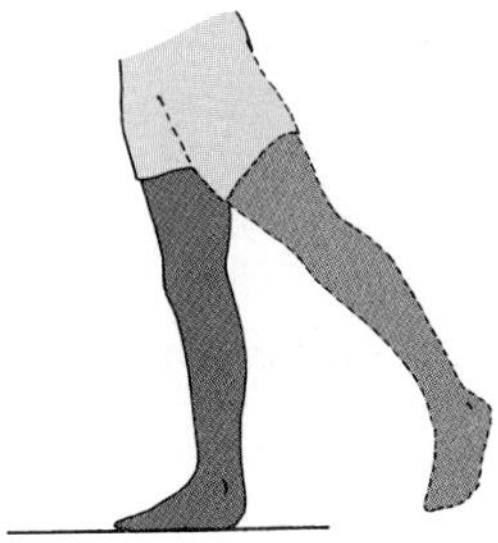	*Hyperextension:* Move leg behind body	30–50	Gluteus maximus, semitendinosus, semimembranosus

Continued

Table 42-2 Range-of-Motion Exercises—cont'd

Body Part	Type of Joint	Type of Movement	Range (Degrees)	Primary Muscles
Knee	Hinge	*Abduction:* Move leg laterally away from body	30–50	Gluteus medius, gluteus minimus
		Adduction: Move leg back toward medial position and beyond if possible	30–50	Adductor longus, adductor brevis, adductor magnus
	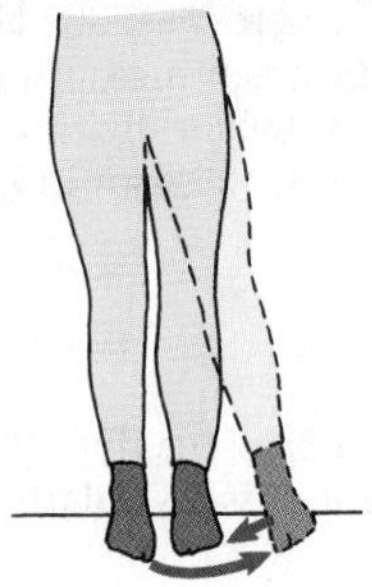	*Internal rotation:* Turn foot and leg toward other leg	90	Gluteus medius, gluteus minimus, tensor fasciae latae
	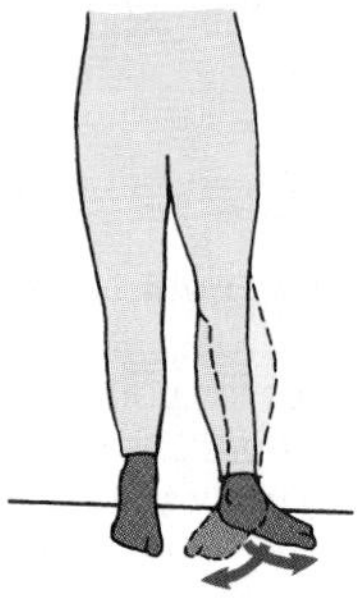	*External rotation:* Turn foot and leg away from other leg	90	Obturatorius internus, obturatorius externus
	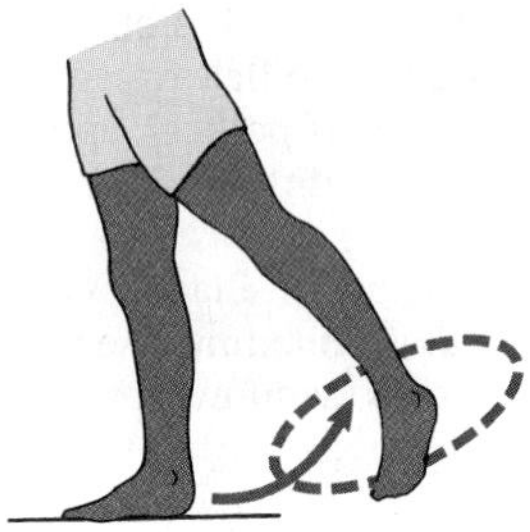	*Circumduction:* Move leg in circle		Psoas major, gluteus maximus, gluteus medius, adductor magnus
Knee	Hinge 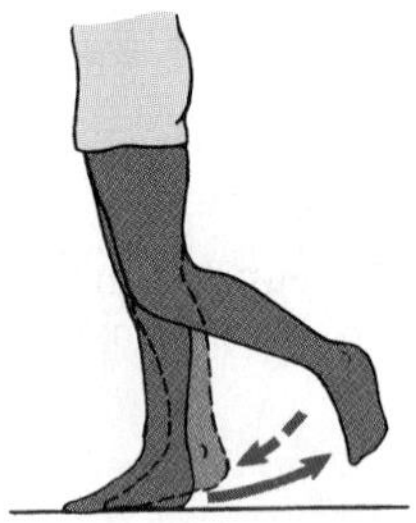	*Flexion:* Bring heel back toward back of thigh	120–130	Biceps femoris, semitendinosus, semimembranosus, sartorius
		Extension: Return leg to floor	120–130	Rectus femoris, vastus lateralis, vastus medialis, vastus intermedius
Ankle	Hinge 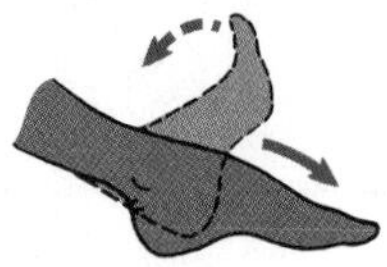	*Dorsal flexion:* Move foot so that toes are pointed upward	20–30	Tibialis anterior
		Plantar flexion: Move foot so that toes are pointed downward	45–50	Gastrocnemius, soleus

Table 42-2 Range-of-Motion Exercises—cont'd

Body Part	Type of Joint	Type of Movement	Range (Degrees)	Primary Muscles
Foot	Gliding 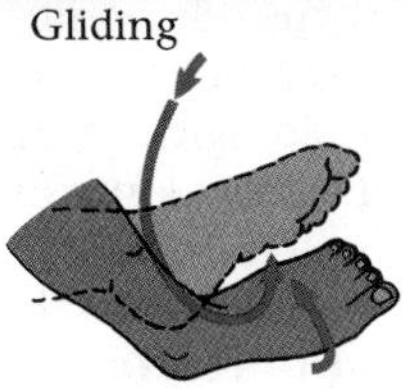	*Inversion:* Turn sole of foot medially	10 or less	Tibialis anterior, tibialis posterior
		Eversion: Turn sole of foot laterally	10 or less	Peroneus longus, peroneus brevis
Toes	Condyloid 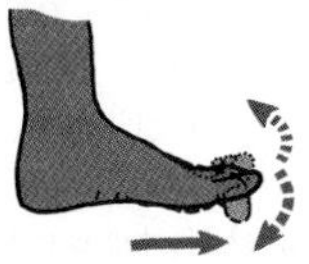	*Flexion:* Curl toes downward	30–60	Flexor digitorum, lumbricalis pedis, flexor hallucis brevis
		Extension: Straighten toes	30–60	Extensor digitorum longus, extensor digitorum brevis, extensor hallucis longus
	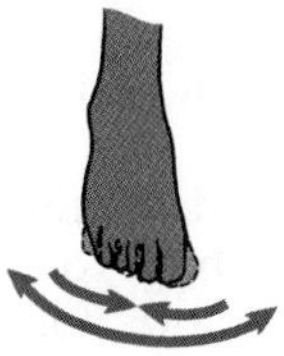	*Abduction:* Spread toes apart	15 or less	Abductor hallucis, interosseus dorsalis
		Adduction: Bring toes together	15 or less	Adductor hallucis, interosseus plantaris

- The arms hang comfortably at the sides.
- The feet are placed slightly apart to achieve a base of support, and the toes are pointed forward.
- When the client is viewed anteriorly, the centre of gravity is in the midline, and the line of gravity is from the middle of the forehead to a midpoint between the feet. Laterally, the line of gravity runs vertically from the middle of the skull to the posterior third of the foot (Figure 42–10).

Sitting. The nurse assesses body alignment when the client is sitting in a chair or wheelchair by observing for the following (Figure 42–11):

- The head is erect, and the neck and vertebral column are in straight alignment.
- The body weight is evenly distributed on the buttocks and thighs.
- The thighs are parallel and in a horizontal plane.
- Both feet are supported on the floor or on wheelchair footrests. With short clients, a footstool is used and the ankles are comfortably flexed.
- A 2.5- to 5-cm space is maintained between the edge of the seat and the popliteal space on the posterior surface of the knee. This space ensures that there is no pressure on the popliteal artery or nerve to decrease circulation or impair nerve function.
- The client's forearms are supported on the armrest, in the lap, or on a table in front of the chair.

It is particularly important to assess alignment when sitting if the client has muscle weakness, muscle paralysis, or nerve damage. Because of these alterations, the client has diminished sensation in the affected area and is unable to perceive pressure or decreased circulation. Proper alignment while sitting reduces the risk of musculoskeletal system damage in such a client. The client with severe respiratory disease may assume a posture of leaning on the table in front of the chair in an attempt to breathe more easily.

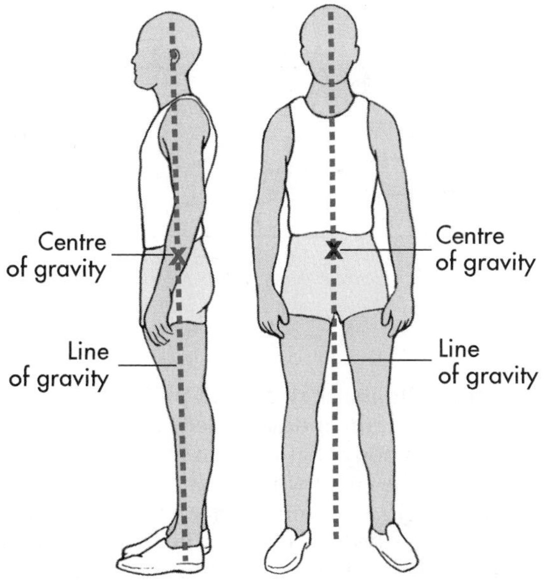

FIGURE **42–10** Correct body alignment when standing.

Lying. People who are conscious have voluntary muscle control and normal perception of pressure. As a result, they usually assume a position of comfort when lying down. Because their ROM, sensation, and circulation are

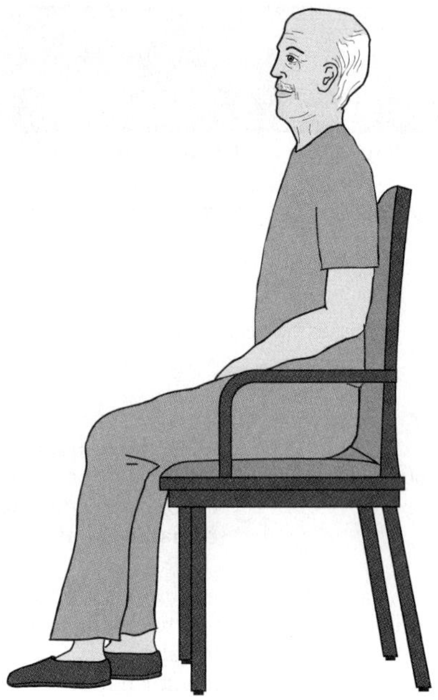

FIGURE **42–11** Correct body alignment when sitting. The client's feet are flat on the floor, the calves do not touch the chair, and the back is straight and against the back of the chair. (From *Mosby's Canadian Textbook for the Support Worker,* by S. A. Sorrentino, 2004, Toronto, ON: Elsevier Canada.)

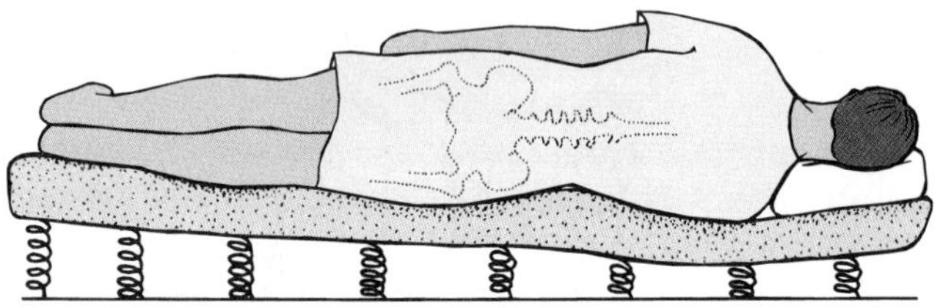

FIGURE **42–12** Correct body alignment when lying down.

within normal limits, they change positions when they perceive muscle strain and decreased circulation.

Assessment of body alignment in the lateral position is best done with the client who is restricted to bed and not able to move well. All positioning supports should be removed from the bed except for the pillow under the head, and the body should be supported by an adequate mattress (Figure 42–12). This position allows for full view of the spine and back and will help provide other baseline body alignment data, such as whether the client can remain positioned without aid. The vertebrae should be aligned, and the position should not cause discomfort. Conditions that create a risk of damage to the musculoskeletal system when lying down include clients with impaired mobility, such as those in traction or with arthritis; clients with decreased sensation, such as those with hemiparesis (one-sided weakness) following stroke or brain attack; clients with impaired circulation, such as those with diabetes; and clients with lack of voluntary muscle control, such as those with spinal cord injuries.

Immobility

Physiological Assessment. The nurse assesses the immobilized client for hazards of immobility by performing a head-to-toe physical assessment (see chapter 28). The nursing assessment should focus on certain physiological areas, as well as on the client's psychosocial and developmental dimensions. The physiological hazards of immobility that may be identified during a nursing assessment are summarized below and in Table 42-3.

Metabolic System. When assessing metabolic functioning, the nurse uses **anthropometric measurements** (measures of height, weight, and skinfold thickness) to evaluate muscle atrophy (see chapter 28). In addition, the nurse may analyze intake and output records for fluid balance. Does fluid intake equal output? Intake and output measurements assist the nurse in determining whether a fluid imbalance exists (see chapter 36). Dehydration and edema can increase the rate of skin breakdown in an immobilized client. Monitoring laboratory data such as electrolytes, serum protein (albumin and total protein) levels, and blood urea nitrogen help the nurse determine metabolic functioning.

Assessing wound healing and monitoring food intake and elimination patterns will help to determine altered gastrointestinal functioning and potential metabolic problems. If an immobilized client has a wound, the rate of healing indicates how well nutrients are being delivered to tissues. Normal progression of healing indicates that metabolic needs of injured tissues are being met. Anorexia occurs commonly in immobilized clients. The client's food intake should be assessed before the meal tray is removed to determine the amount eaten. Nutritional imbalances can be avoided if the nurse assesses the client's dietary patterns and food preferences early in immobilization (see chapter 39).

Respiratory System. A respiratory assessment should be performed at least every 2 hours for clients with restricted activity. The nurse inspects chest wall movements during the full inspiratory-expiratory cycle. If a client has an atelectatic area, chest movement may be asymmetrical. In addition, the nurse auscultates the entire lung region to identify diminished breath sounds, crackles, or wheezes. Auscultation should focus on the dependent lung fields because pulmonary secretions tend to collect in these lower regions. A complete respiratory assessment identifies the presence of secretions and can be used to determine nursing interventions necessary for optimal respiratory function.

Cardiovascular System. Cardiovascular assessment of the immobilized client includes blood pressure monitoring, evaluation of apical and peripheral pulses, and observation for signs of venous stasis (e.g., edema and poor wound healing). All clients should have their vital signs monitored during the first few attempts at sitting or standing.

When getting the client from a supine position into a chair, the nurse moves the client gradually. When performing this procedure, the nurse assesses and documents orthostatic changes. The nurse first obtains baseline blood pressure and pulse measurements with the client in the supine position. The nurse then assists the client to a position sitting at the side of the bed. The client should

Table 42-3 **Physiological Hazards of Immobility**

System	Assessment Techniques	Abnormal Findings
Metabolic	Inspection	Slowed wound healing, abnormal laboratory data
	Inspection	Muscle atrophy
	Anthropometric measurements (mid-upper arm circumference, triceps skinfold measurement)	Decreased amount of subcutaneous fat
	Palpation	Generalized edema
Respiratory	Inspection	Asymmetrical chest wall movement, dyspnea, increased respiratory rate
	Auscultation	Crackles, wheezes, decreased air entry
Cardiovascular	Auscultation	Orthostatic hypotension
	Auscultation, palpation	Increased heart rate, third heart sound, weak peripheral pulses, peripheral edema
Musculoskeletal	Inspection, palpation	Decreased range of motion, erythema, increased diameter in calf or thigh
	Palpation	Joint contracture
	Inspection	Activity intolerance, muscle atrophy, joint contracture
Elimination	Inspection	Decreased urine output, cloudy or concentrated urine, decreased frequency of bowel movements
	Palpation	Distended bladder and abdomen
	Auscultation	Decreased bowel sounds
Skin	Inspection, palpation	Break in skin integrity

remain sitting for 2 minutes before the nurse takes the blood pressure and pulse. The nurse remains with the client in a sitting position and continually monitors the client for dizziness or light-headedness. If there is no dizziness or drop in blood pressure (≥20 mm Hg systolic or 10 mm Hg diastolic), the nurse assists the client to a standing position and retakes the blood pressure and pulse immediately upon the client standing and again after 2 minutes of standing. The client should be monitored closely for dizziness throughout this procedure. The longer the period of immobility, the greater is the risk of hypotension when the client stands (Lance et al., 2000).

The nurse also assesses the apical and peripheral pulses. Recumbency increases cardiac workload and pulse rate. In some clients, particularly older adults, the heart may not tolerate the increased workload, and a form of cardiac failure may develop. A third heart sound, heard at the apex with the bell of the stethoscope, can be an early indication of congestive heart failure. Monitoring peripheral pulses allows the nurse to evaluate the heart's ability to pump blood. The absence of a peripheral pulse in the lower extremities, particularly one that was previously present, should be documented and reported to the physician.

Edema may develop in clients who have had injury or whose heart is unable to handle the increased workload of bed rest. Because edema moves to dependent body regions, assessment of the immobilized client should include the sacrum, legs, and feet. If the heart is unable to tolerate the increased workload, peripheral body regions, such as the hands, feet, nose, and earlobes, will be colder than central body regions.

Finally, the nurse assesses the venous system because deep vein thrombosis (DVT) is a hazard of restricted mobility. A dislodged venous thrombus, called an **embolus,** may travel through the circulatory system to the lungs and impair circulation and oxygenation. Venous emboli that travel to the lungs may be life-threatening. More than 90% of all pulmonary emboli begin in the legs or pelvis (Byrne, 2001).

To assess for a DVT, the nurse removes the client's elastic stockings and/or sequential compression devices (SCDs) every 8 hours and observes the calves for redness, warmth, and tenderness. Homans' sign, or calf pain on dorsiflexion of the foot, indicates a probable thrombus, but this sign is not always present (Maher et al., 2002). However, checking Homans' sign may be contraindicated in a suspected DVT, as some investigators think that vigorous dorsiflexion may dislodge the thrombus. In addition, calf circumference should be measured daily. To do this, the nurse marks a point on each calf 10 cm from the midpatella. The circumference is measured each day using the mark for placement of the tape measure. Unilateral increases in calf diameter can be an early indication of thrombosis. Because DVTs can also occur in the thigh, thigh measurements should be taken daily if the client is prone to thrombosis. In many clients, DVTs can be prevented by active exercise and compression devices in conjunction with prescribed anticoagulant treatment.

Musculoskeletal System. Major musculoskeletal abnormalities that may be identified during nursing assessment include decreased muscle tone and strength, loss of muscle mass, and contractures. The anthropometric measurements described previously may indicate losses in muscle tone and muscle mass. Muscle atrophy is a common complication that arises from bed rest (Takata & Yasui, 2001).

Assessment of ROM is important as a baseline against which later measurements can be compared to evaluate whether a loss in joint mobility has occurred. ROM can be measured with a goniometer (see Figure 32-11).

Disuse osteoporosis (generalized bone loss resulting from the lack of mechanical stress on bones) cannot be identified by physical assessment. However, clients on prolonged bed rest, post-menopausal women, clients taking steroids, and people with increased serum and urine calcium levels have a greater risk for bone demineralization. The risk of disuse osteoporosis should be considered when planning nursing interventions. Not only may falls result in injury, but also falls may occur because of pathological fractures secondary to osteoporosis. Clients who are at risk for osteoporosis should have their diet assessed for calcium intake. Some clients have lactose intolerance and need dietary teaching about alternative sources of calcium (Maher et al., 2002).

Elimination System. The client's elimination status should be evaluated on each shift, and total intake and output should be evaluated every 24 hours and compared over time. The nurse should determine that the client is receiving the correct amount and type of fluids orally or parenterally (see chapter 40). Inadequate intake and output or fluid and electrolyte imbalances can increase the risk for renal system impairment, ranging from recurrent infections to kidney failure. Dehydration can also increase the risk for skin breakdown, thrombus formation, respiratory infections, and constipation.

Assessment of elimination status should also include the adequacy of dietary choices, bowel sounds, and the frequency and consistency of bowel movements (see chapter 41). Accurate assessment enables the nurse to intervene before constipation and fecal impaction occur.

Integumentary System. The nurse must continually assess the client's skin for breakdown and colour changes such as pallor or redness. The skin should be observed when the client is turned, during hygiene measures, and when elimination needs are provided for. At a minimum, assessment should occur every 2 hours (see chapter 43).

Psychosocial Assessment. Many alterations in physiological, socio-cultural, and developmental functioning are related to immobility. Often, these problems are interrelated. Nursing care must focus on all dimensions, not just on physical problems (Box 42-3).

Abrupt changes in personality may have a physiological cause, such as surgery, a medication reaction, a pulmonary embolus, or an acute infection. For example, compromised older clients have confusion as their primary symptom when experiencing a pulmonary emboli or an acute urinary tract infection. Identifying confusion is an important component of the nurse's assessment. Acute confusion in older adults is not normal and should be thoroughly examined (Ludwick, 1999).

Common reactions to immobilization include boredom, feelings of isolation, depression, and anger. The nurse should observe for changes in a client's emotional status. Examples of change that may indicate psychosocial concerns are a co-operative client who becomes less co-operative or an independent client who asks for more help than is necessary. The nurse should try to determine the reasons for such alterations. Identifying how the client usually copes with loss is vital (see chapters 25 and 26). A change in mobility status, whether permanent or not, may cause a grief reaction. Families are a key resource for information about behaviour changes.

Unexplained changes in the sleep-wake cycle must be identified and corrected. Most can be prevented or minimized, such as those occurring because of nursing activities, a noisy environment, or discomfort. They may also occur because of medications such as analgesics, sleeping pills, or cardiovascular drugs (see chapter 37).

Because psychosocial changes usually occur gradually, the nurse should observe the client's behaviour on a daily basis. If behavioural changes occur, the nurse should determine the causes and evaluate the changes as short or long term. Identifying the cause helps the nurse design appropriate nursing interventions. For example, a fear of falling often limits the bariatric (obese) client's mobility; fear may be related to past experiences of falling and not being able to get up (Dumas, 2001). Interventions include encouraging the client to lean forward prior to standing rather than standing straight up, and teaching the client how to get up and down from the floor, with assistance if needed (Dumas, 2001).

Developmental Assessment. Assessment of the immobilized client should include developmental considerations to ensure that the client's needs are identified. The nurse determines whether the young child can meet developmental tasks and is progressing normally. The child's development may regress or be slowed because of immobilization. By identifying a child's overall developmental needs, the nurse can design nursing therapies to maintain normal development. The nurse may also need to assure the parents that developmental delays are usually temporary.

Immobilization of a family member changes the family's functioning. The family's response to this change may lead to problems, stress, and anxieties. Children seeing parents who are immobile may have difficulty understanding what is occurring and may have difficulty coping.

Immobility can have a significant effect on the older adult's levels of health, independence, and functional status. Nursing assessment enables the nurse to determine the older client's ability to meet needs independently and to adapt to developmental changes such as declining physical functioning and altered family and peer relationships. A decline in developmental functioning needs prompt investigation to determine why the change occurred and what can be done to return the client to an optimal level of functioning as soon as possible. Activities that reduce immobility and promote participation in ADLs are vital to prevent functional decline (Ludwick, Dieckman, & Snelson, 1999). Assessment also includes considering the client's home and community to identify factors that are risks to the client's mobility and safety (see chapter 33).

Client Expectations. Clients may have unrealistic expectations of themselves or their caregivers. They may agree with the staff and understand their limitations, or they may set their expectations of themselves too high or too low. Some clients may expect to be waited on, and other clients may want to do as much as possible. The nurse

Research Highlight

Box 42-3

The Meaning of Mobility

Research Focus

It is widely known that decreased mobility contributes to physical and psychological impairment. Little is known, however, about the significance of mobility to residents and nurses in long-term care facilities. The purpose of this study was to determine nurses' and residents' perceptions of mobility in order to develop strategies that would support mobility in the institutionalized adult.

Research Abstract

In this exploratory, qualitative study, focus groups with residents and nursing staff were conducted in three long-term care facilities. Twenty residents and 15 nurses participated in the study. Both groups identified mobility as key to quality of life. Older adults equated mobility with freedom, choice, and independence. Nurses valued mobility and associated it with freedom and autonomy. Both nurses and residents viewed having to wait for assistance as a barrier to mobility. Nurses identified further obstacles such as heavy workload and lack of time. Residents focused on physical barriers such as steep ramps, crowded elevators, and negative attitudes of staff.

Evidence-Based Practice

- Mobility is central to clients' quality of life and well-being.
- Nurses play a key role in assessing and assisting clients with their mobility needs.
- Nurses focus on minimizing obstacles to mobility.
- Nurses coordinate with other health care professionals to meet client's mobility needs.
- Nurses use creative strategies to encourage mobility in older adults.

Reference

Bourret, E., et al. (2002). The meaning of mobility for residents and staff in long-term care facilities. *Journal of Advanced Nursing, 37*(4), 338–345.

should ask clients to explain what they know about their mobility status, what questions they and their families have, and how the immobility is affecting their goals.

Nursing Diagnosis

An immobilized or partially immobilized client may have one or more nursing diagnoses. The two diagnoses most directly related to mobility problems are *impaired physical mobility* and *risk for disuse syndrome*. The diagnosis of *impaired physical mobility* is used for the client who has some limitation but is not completely immobile. The diagnosis of *risk for disuse syndrome* should be considered for the client who is immobile and at risk for multi-system pathophysiology because of inactivity. The list of potential diagnoses is extensive because immobility affects multiple body systems:

- Activity intolerance
- Ineffective airway clearance
- Ineffective breathing pattern
- Ineffective individual coping
- Risk for disuse syndrome
- Risk for fluid volume deficit
- Impaired gas exchange
- Risk for infection
- Risk for injury
- Impaired physical mobility
- Impaired skin integrity
- Risk for impaired skin integrity
- Disturbed sleep pattern
- Social isolation
- Ineffective (peripheral) tissue perfusion
- Impaired urinary elimination

Assessment reveals clusters of data that indicate whether a client is at risk or if an actual problem exists. The clusters of data include defining characteristics that support the diagnostic label and probable cause of the diagnosis. Locating the probable cause of the diagnosis (based on assessment data) is important in planning client-centred goals and subsequent nursing interventions.

Impaired physical mobility related to bed rest would require different interventions than *impaired physical mobility related to pain in the left shoulder.* Thus, the nurse must identify and cluster defining characteristics that support the nursing diagnosis selected (Box 42-4). The diagnosis related to bed rest would require interventions aimed at keeping the client as mobile as possible and encouraging the client to do self-care and ROM exercises in bed. The diagnosis related to pain would require the nurse to assist the client with comfort measures so that the client would then be more willing and able to move. In both situations, the nurse would explain the importance of activity to healthy body functioning.

Often the physiological dimension is the major focus of nursing care for clients with impaired mobility, and the psychosocial and developmental dimensions are neglected. However, all dimensions are important to health. For example, during immobilization, social interaction and stimuli are decreased. Ultimately, the client may become isolated, withdrawn, and bored. Such clients may frequently use the call bell to request minor physical attention when their real need is greater socialization. Nursing diagnoses for health needs in developmental areas reflect changes from the client's normal activities. Immobility can lead to a developmental crisis if the client is unable to resolve problems and continue to mature.

Nursing Diagnostic Process Box 42-4

Assessment Activities	Defining Characteristics	Nursing Diagnosis
Measure range of motion (ROM) during exercises of extremities.	Client has limited ROM with left shoulder. Client has impaired coordination while attempting to perform ROM with left shoulder.	Impaired physical mobility related to left shoulder pain
Observe client use left shoulder in activities of daily living.	Client is reluctant to attempt movement with left shoulder.	
Ask client about perception of pain.	Client complains of sharp pain in shoulder.	
Ask client about endurance and activity tolerance.	Client reports decreased muscle strength in left shoulder.	

Immobility may also lead to complications such as pulmonary emboli or pneumonia. If these conditions develop, the nurse will collaborate with the physician or nurse practitioner for prescribed therapy to intervene.

Planning

During planning, the nurse synthesizes information from resources such as knowledge of the role of respiratory therapy and physiotherapy, professional standards such as RNAO guidelines for prevention of falls and pressure ulcers (2002a, 2002b), attitudes such as creativity and perseverance, and past experiences with immobilized clients (Figure 42–13).

Goals and Outcomes. The nurse develops an individualized care plan for each nursing diagnosis (see Care Plan). The nurse and client set realistic expectations for care. Goals are individualized, realistic, and measurable. They focus on preventing problems or risks to body alignment and mobility. These goals are client centred and should be mutually set with client and family.

The goals and expected outcomes are developed to assist the client in achieving his or her highest level of mobility. In addition, these goals may be written to reduce the hazards of immobility. For example, a client who has left-sided paralysis following a stroke may have two long-term goals. The first, directed toward improved mobility, may be "Client uses walker to ambulate around the home and grocery store." A parallel goal, directed toward the hazards of immobility, may be "Client's skin remains free of pressure." Both of these goals are essential to restoring maximal mobility for this client. Because there is impaired sensation, both the client and caregivers must be aware of the client's need to have the skin free of pressure. Expected outcomes for the second goal could include the following:

- Client's skin colour and temperature return to normal baseline within 20 minutes of position change
- Client's skin remains dry and intact

Setting Priorities. Care planning must take into consideration priority setting so that immediate needs are attended to first. This is particularly important when clients have multiple diagnoses (Figure 42–14). The nurse plans therapies according to severity of risks to the client, and the plan is individualized according to the client's developmental stage, level of health, and lifestyle. The immediacy of any problem is determined by the effect the problem has on the client's mental and physical health.

Potential complications should not be overlooked. Many times actual problems such as pressure ulcers and disuse osteoporosis get addressed only after they develop. Therefore, the nurse must be vigilant in monitoring the client, reinforcing prevention techniques to both client and other caregivers, and supervising unregulated care providers (UCPs) in carrying out activities aimed at preventing complications of impaired mobility.

Continuity of Care. The interventions planned for the client may be done directly by the nurse or delegated to UCPs. UCPs can reinforce leg exercises, use of the incentive spirometer, and coughing and deep breathing (see chapter 35). They may turn and position clients, apply elastic stockings, and assess leg circumferences and height and weight.

Because many of the skills associated with care of the immobile client can be delegated, the nurse must be vigilant in performing routine assessments to identify any developing complications early. The nurse also informs the UCP when clients are at risk for immobility hazards so that complications can be prevented. For example, although turning and positioning of a comatose client may be delegated, the nurse must ensure that it is done correctly and that the position is changed frequently to reduce the risk of poor alignment and future injury to the skin and musculoskeletal system. The frequency of turning is based on client assessment for risk of pressure ulcer development (see chapter 43).

The nurse may need the help of another health team member such as a physiotherapist or occupational therapist when considering mobility needs. For example, physiotherapists are a resource for planning ROM or strengthening exercises, and occupational therapists are a resource for planning ADLs that clients need to modify or relearn. Discharge planning is begun when a

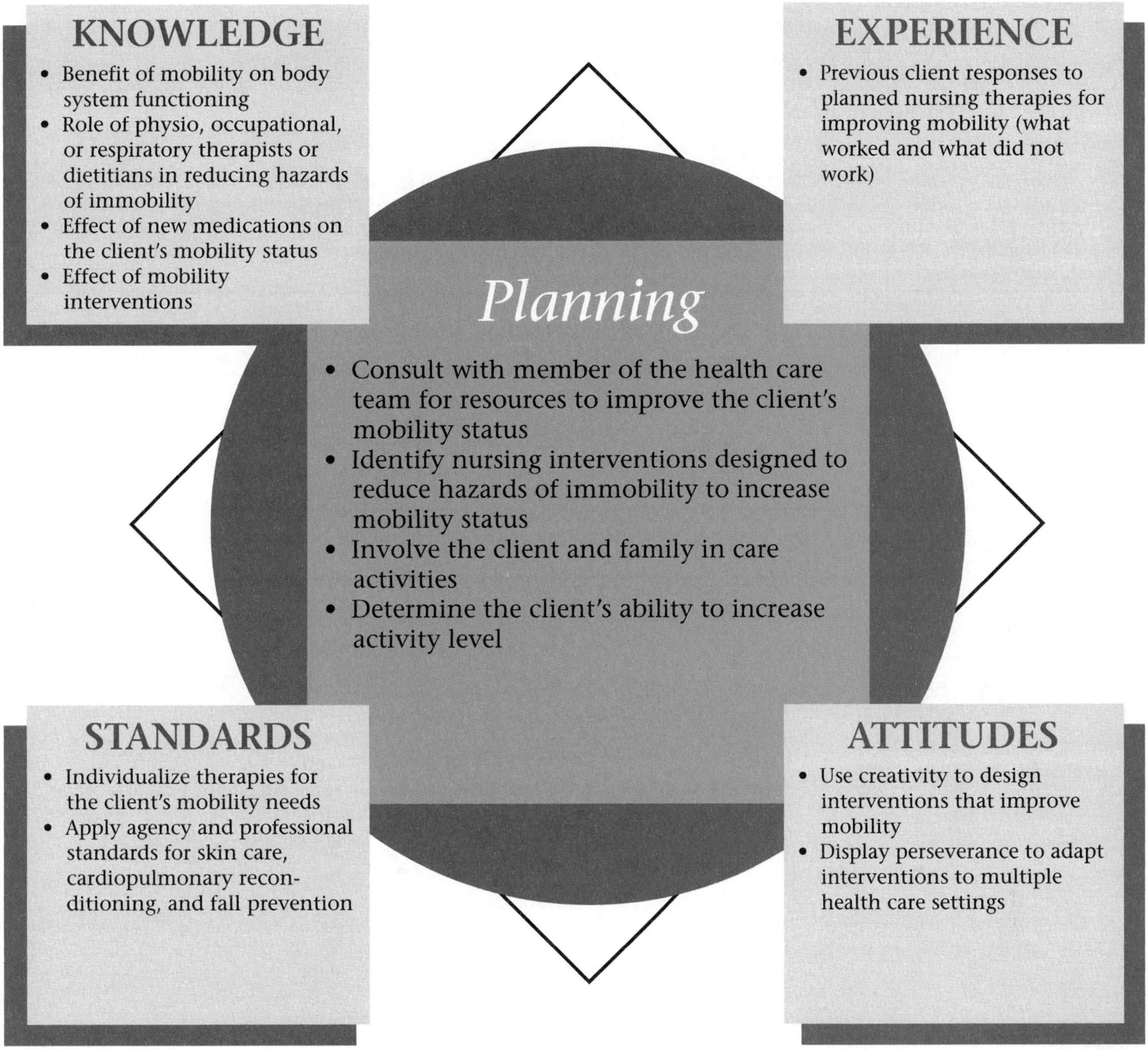
KNOWLEDGE
• Benefit of mobility on body system functioning
• Role of physio, occupational, or respiratory therapists or dietitians in reducing hazards of immobility
• Effect of new medications on the client's mobility status
• Effect of mobility interventions
EXPERIENCE
• Previous client responses to planned nursing therapies for improving mobility (what worked and what did not work)
Planning
• Consult with member of the health care team for resources to improve the client's mobility status
• Identify nursing interventions designed to reduce hazards of immobility to increase mobility status
• Involve the client and family in care activities
• Determine the client's ability to increase activity level
STANDARDS
• Individualize therapies for the client's mobility needs
• Apply agency and professional standards for skin care, cardiopulmonary recon-ditioning, and fall prevention
ATTITUDES
• Use creativity to design interventions that improve mobility
• Display perseverance to adapt interventions to multiple health care settings

FIGURE **42–13** Critical thinking model for immobility planning.

client enters the health care system. In anticipation of the client's discharge from an institution, a referral may be made to help the client remain mobile or regain mobility at home. Therefore, consideration must be given to the client's home environment when planning therapies to maintain or improve body alignment and mobility.

Implementation

Health Promotion. Health promotion activities are an essential part of primary health care and include a variety of interventions that can be divided into education, prevention, and early detection. Promoting exercise should be a key health promotion strategy (Box 42-5). Another issue that is important for preventing injury of clients and nurses is knowledge of proper lifting techniques.

Lifting. Back problems are the most prevalent type of occupational injury across Canada. In 1998, over 25% of occupational injuries were to the back (Association of Workers' Compensation Boards of Canada, 1999). Back injuries are often the direct result of improper lifting and bending. The most common back injury is strain on the lumbar muscle group, which includes the muscles around the lumbar vertebrae. Injury to these areas affects the ability to bend forward, backward, and from side to side and limits the ability to rotate the hips and lower back.

Nurses and UCPs are especially at risk for injury to lumbar muscles when lifting, transferring, or positioning

Nursing Care Plan

Impaired Physical Mobility

Assessment

Ms. Barbara Adams, an 84-year-old client, has been admitted for rehabilitation after a total hip replacement for osteoarthritis. The wound is clean, dry, and intact. Staples will be removed in 2 days. She is not able to transfer from chair to bed. She states that she is "afraid of falling" and frequently refuses to get out of bed. She rates her pain as a 2 on a scale of 0 to 10. She has a history of smoking. She states that she needs pain medication to help her sleep during the night but does not need any during the day. She is to start physiotherapy tomorrow.

Assessment Activities	Findings/Defining Characteristics
Assess Ms. Adams' pain level.	She rates her pain as a 2 on a scale of 0 to 10. She states that she needs pain medication at night to help her sleep, but does not need any during the day.
Assess Ms. Adams' ability to transfer.	She is not able to transfer with help from chair to bed.
Ask Ms. Adams how her surgery has affected her mobility.	She responds that she is "afraid of falling," and she frequently refuses to get out of bed.
Assess Ms. Adams' wound status.	Wound is clean, dry, and intact.

Nursing Diagnosis: Impaired physical mobility related to musculoskeletal impairment from surgery and a fear of falling.

Planning

Goal	Expected Outcomes*
	Tissue Integrity: Skin
Ms. Adams will be free from skin breakdown by discharge.	Client's skin will remain intact. Client's skin will be free of erythema.
	Tissue Perfusion: Peripheral
Ms. Adams will exhibit no evidence of deep vein thrombosis (DVT) by discharge.	Client's calf diameters will remain within 1 cm of baseline through discharge. Client's lower extremity pulses will remain equal. Client will have no complaints of calf pain.
	Mobility Level
Ms. Adams will be able to transfer with assistance within 2 days.	Client will transfer with assistance three times per day within 2 days. Client will state fear of falling during transfer is less within 2 days.

*Outcome classification labels from *Nursing Outcomes Classification (NOC)* (3rd ed.), edited by S. Moorhead, M. Johnson, and M. L. Maas, 2004, St. Louis, MO: Mosby.

Interventions†	Rationale
Circulatory Care	
Administer low-dose heparin as ordered.	Administration of low-dose heparin has been shown to reduce risk for vein thrombosis (Nunnelee, 1997).
Apply intermittent compression stockings as ordered and remove each shift for hygiene.	Application increases venous tone, improving venous return, and reducing venous stasis (Byrne, 2001).
Reinforce antiembolic exercises while awake.	Exercises promote venous return.
Assist client out of bed slowly.	Moving slowly will decrease the likelihood of orthostatic hypotension. Moving the client slowly will also avoid the perception by the client of being rushed, which may cause the client to become fearful.

†Intervention classification labels from *Nursing Interventions Classification (NIC)* (4th ed.), edited by J. M. Dochterman and G. M. Bulecheck, 2004, St. Louis, MO: Mosby.

Nursing Care Plan

Impaired Physical Mobility—cont'd

Interventions†—cont'd	Rationale
Skin Surveillance	
Instruct client to shift position every 1 to $1^1/_2$ hours while awake.	Position changes should occur every 1 to $1^1/_2$ hours or more frequently if needed. Reduces the risk of pressure ulcer development.
When recumbent, place client in 30-degree lateral position.	The 30-degree lateral position reduces pressure from the sacral area and reduces the risk of skin breakdown (RNAO, 2002a).
Keep client's heels off of bed by placing a pad under the lower legs.	Using a thin pad under the lower legs raises the heels just enough so that a paper can slide between the heels and the bed, thereby reducing the pressure on the heels so that tissue blood flow is maintained (Agency for Healthcare Research and Quality, 2003).
Positioning	
Explain positioning procedure to client.	Reduces anxiety.
Refer to physiotherapy for transfer training.	Helps to strengthen muscles used in transfer.
Encourage client to assist in transfer and positioning.	

†Intervention classification labels from *Nursing Interventions Classification (NIC)* (4th ed.), edited by J. M. Dochterman and G. M. Bulecheck, 2004, St. Louis, MO: Mosby.

Evaluation

Nursing Actions	Client Response/Finding	Achievement of Outcome
Ask Ms. Adams if her mobility has improved post-operatively. Observe client transfer from bed to chair.	Client is able to transfer from the chair to the bed with assistance.	Client has achieved goal of transferring with assistance.
Observe Ms. Adams's skin integrity each shift.	Client's wound remains clean, dry, and intact. No breakdown noted on extremities.	Client has achieved outcome that skin will remain intact.
Perform circulatory assessment of extremities every shift.	Client's calf diameters remain within 1 cm of baseline. No evidence of swelling, pain, redness, or warmth.	There is no evidence of a DVT.
Ask Ms. Adams to rate her fear of falling on a scale of 0 to 10.	Client rates fear of falling a 7 on a scale of 0 to 10. Client is getting out of bed every shift.	Outcome of decrease in fear of falling has not been totally achieved. Continue to encourage client.

immobilized clients. Many health care agencies have a "no-lift" policy, whereby manual lifting of the whole or a large part of the weight of the client by a health care worker is prohibited except for in exceptional or life-threatening situations. Therefore, the nurse should not attempt to lift a client without assistance unless the client is a young child or a light-weight adult who is able to help while being moved. Alternatives to manual lifting may include the use of mechanical lifts, drawsheets, slide boards, and other handling aids (Ontario Hospital Association, 2002). Two or more people may be needed to turn or position a client.

Nurses need to be aware of good lifting techniques to protect themselves, those they supervise, and the clients being cared for. Before lifting, the nurse should assess the weight to be lifted and what assistance is needed. If help is needed, the nurse should determine if a second person or mechanical assistance is needed.

Once the amount of assistance is determined, these steps are followed:

1. Keep the weight to be lifted as close to the body as possible; this action places the object in the same plane as the lifter and close to the centre of gravity for balance.
2. Bend at the knees; this helps to maintain the centre of gravity and uses the stronger leg muscles to do the lifting (Figure 42–15). Avoid twisting. Twisting can overload the spine and lead to serious injury.
3. Tighten abdominal muscles and tuck the pelvis; this provides balance and helps protect the back.
4. Maintain the trunk erect and knees bent so that multiple groups work together in a coordinated manner (see chapter 32).

Nurse injuries are not only related to lifting. Many nursing activities involve bending and twisting and so may cause injury. Examples of such activities include

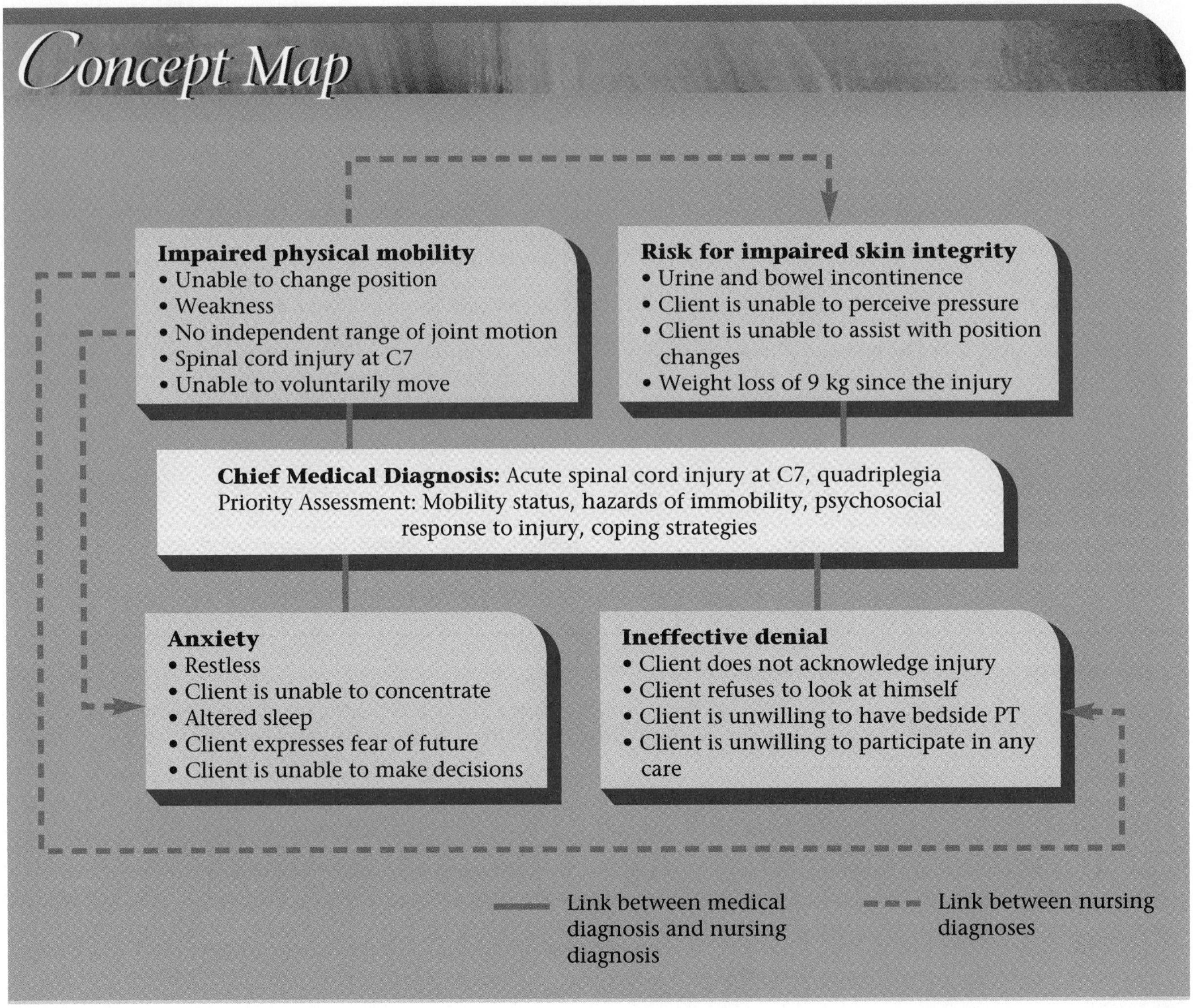
Concept Map
Impaired physical mobility
• Unable to change position
• Weakness
• No independent range of joint motion
• Spinal cord injury at C7
• Unable to voluntarily move
Risk for impaired skin integrity
• Urine and bowel incontinence
• Client is unable to perceive pressure
• Client is unable to assist with position changes
• Weight loss of 9 kg since the injury
Chief Medical Diagnosis: Acute spinal cord injury at C7, quadriplegia
Priority Assessment: Mobility status, hazards of immobility, psychosocial response to injury, coping strategies
Anxiety
• Restless
• Client is unable to concentrate
• Altered sleep
• Client expresses fear of future
• Client is unable to make decisions
Ineffective denial
• Client does not acknowledge injury
• Client refuses to look at himself
• Client is unwilling to have bedside PT
• Client is unwilling to participate in any care
Link between medical diagnosis and nursing diagnosis
Link between nursing diagnoses

FIGURE **42–14** Concept map for client with acute spinal cord injury at C7 and quadriplegia.

bathing, feeding, and dressing and undressing clients (Nelson, Fragala, and Menzel, 2003).

Acute Care. In the acute care setting, the nurse must implement interventions to reduce the hazards of immobility. The nurse also must know proper positioning and transferring techniques to safely move clients.

Immobility Hazards. Clients in acute care settings may demonstrate some problems associated with prolonged immobility, such as impaired respiratory status, orthostatic hypotension, and impaired skin integrity. For these clients, nursing interventions are designed to reduce the impact of immobility on body systems and prepare the client for the restorative phase of care.

Metabolic System. The immobilized client requires a high-protein, high-calorie diet with vitamin B and C supplements. Protein is needed to repair injured tissue and rebuild depleted protein stores. A high-calorie intake provides sufficient fuel to meet metabolic needs and to replace subcutaneous tissue. Supplementation with vitamins C and B complex is needed for skin integrity and wound healing.

If the client is unable to eat, nutrition must be provided parenterally or enterally. Enteral feedings include delivery through a nasogastric, nasointestinal gastrostomy, or jejunostomy tube of high-protein, high-calorie solutions with complete requirements of vitamins, minerals, and electrolytes (see chapter 39). Total parenteral nutrition refers to delivery of nutritional supplements through a central or peripheral intravenous catheter.

Respiratory System. Nursing interventions for the respiratory system are aimed at promoting expansion of the chest and lungs, preventing stasis of pulmonary secretions, maintaining a patent airway, and promoting adequate exchange of respiratory gases.

Promoting Expansion of the Chest and Lungs. Changing the position of the client at least every 2 hours allows the

Focus on Primary Health Care — Box 42-5

Promoting Exercise

Exercise is known to increase mobility and strength, maintain functional performance, reduce the risk of many health problems (e.g., cardiovascular disease, diabetes, and osteoporosis), and enhance perceived quality of life. In the case of older adults, routine completion of activities of daily living prevents contractures and improves independence (Resnick, 2000).

Functional decline from disuse is a major concern as aging occurs. Nurses can contribute to promoting health for many types of clients by encouraging or starting managed exercise programs. All people can enjoy and benefit from exercise. Even hospitalized clients can be encouraged to do stretching, range-of-motion exercises, and light walking within the limits of their condition. However, older adults and people with mobility problems face barriers to physical activity (Cooper et al., 2001). Nurses can do the following to help these clients participate in exercise:

- Educate clients about the importance of exercise in preserving health.
- Encourage clients to pace activities and increase speed and intensity gradually to avoid pain.
- Administer prescribed anti-inflammatory medications 1 to 2 hours before starting exercise program.
- Encourage clients to balance rest and activity and get plenty of sleep.
- Advise clients to avoid caffeine and alcohol before bed.
- Teach clients to use canes or walkers to assist with walking as needed.
- Encourage clients to choose smooth and even walking surfaces.
- Advise clients not to force joints past the point of resistance or pain.
- Teach clients to check legs and feet daily for redness, swelling, blisters, or broken skin.
- Teach clients to wear properly fitting shoes.
- Encourage clients to walk with a companion or group so that exercise is socially rewarding.
- The nurse should also consider cultural influences on choice of physical activity (Box 42-6).

Cultural Aspects of Care — Box 42-6

Cultural influences have an important role on exercise and physical activity. Exercise is often described relative to white middle-class values. Immigrants may be more sedentary and less likely to engage in recommended exercise activities such as joining a fitness club or golfing because they lack financial and social supports or would not feel comfortable in these environments (Im & Choe, 2004). Certain cultures discourage involvement in organized recreational physical activities such as basketball, running, and aerobics (Johnson, 2000). In some cultures, ethnic dancing is a more acceptable activity than organized sports (Jain & Brown, 2001). Other cultures emphasize exercise in terms of activities of daily living such as walking, gardening, and prayer/meditation. As an example, people from Bangladesh view prayer as a structured form of exercise. Muslims value participation in community activities and may consider walking to the mosque as part of their weekly exercise regime (Johnson, 2000).

Implications for Practice

- Nurses must evaluate patterns of daily living and culturally prescribed activities before suggesting specific forms of exercise to clients (Andrews & Boyle, 1999).
- Nurses must help clients plan physical activities that are culturally acceptable (Melillo et al., 2001).
- Exercise programs must be flexible and accommodate family and community responsibilities of the culture (Banks-Wallace, 2000).
- Nurses must encourage culturally specific interventions to facilitate commitment to exercise (Banks-Wallace, 2000).

Data from *Transcultural Concepts in Nursing Care* (3rd ed.), by M. Andrews and J. Boyle, 1999, Philadelphia: Lippincott; "Staggering Under the Weight of Responsibility: The Impact of Culture on Physical Activity Among African American Women," by J. Banks-Wallace, 2000, *The Journal of Multicultural Nursing Health, 6*(3), pp. 24–30; "Cultural Dance: An Opportunity to Encourage Physical Activity and Health in Communities," by S. Jain and D. R. Brown, 2001, *American Journal of Health Education, 32*(4), pp. 216–222; "Perceptions of Barriers to Healthy Physical Activity Among Asian Communities," by M. Johnson, 2000, *Sport Education and Society, 5*(1), pp. 51–70; and "Perceptions of Older Latino Adults Regarding Physical Fitness, Physical Activity, and Exercise," by K. Melillo et al., 2001, *Journal of Gerontological Nursing, 27*(9), pp. 38–46.

dependent lung regions to re-expand. Re-expansion maintains the elastic recoil property of the lungs and clears the dependent lung regions of pulmonary secretions.

The nurse encourages the client to deep breathe and cough every 1 to 2 hours. Alert clients can be taught to deep breathe or yawn every hour or to use an incentive spirometer (see chapter 35). The nurse instructs the client to take in three deep breaths and cough with the third exhalation. This technique produces a more forceful, productive cough without excessive fatigue. These respiratory interventions will aid alveolar expansion and prevent atelectasis. Coughing reduces the stasis of pulmonary secretions. For unconscious clients with an artificial airway, the nurse can expand the chest and lungs by using an Ambu-bag.

If abdominal binders are required, they should be removed every 2 hours to allow the client to breathe deeply.

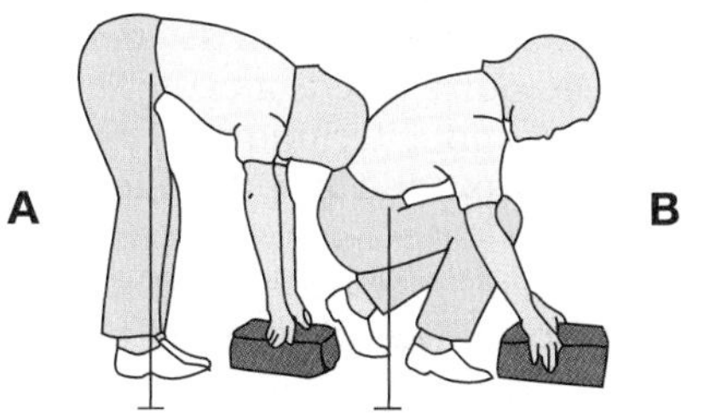

FIGURE **42–15** Body position for lifting. **A,** Incorrect. **B,** Correct.

Binders must be assessed for correct positioning and adjusted as necessary to prevent interference with respirations. Often clients will wear the binder only when ambulating. Specific physician instructions for the use of binders will vary.

Preventing Stasis of Pulmonary Secretions. Stagnant secretions accumulating in the bronchi and lungs may lead to growth of bacteria and subsequent development of pneumonia. Changing the client's position every 2 hours can reduce stagnation of secretions. This change rotates the dependent lung, mobilizing secretions.

The immobile client should take in a minimum of 2000 mL of fluid a day, if not contraindicated, to help keep mucociliary clearance normal. In clients free from infection and with adequate hydration, pulmonary secretions will appear thin, watery, and clear. The client can easily remove the secretions with coughing. Without adequate hydration, the secretions are thick and difficult to remove. Encouraging fluids also benefits in helping with bowel and urine elimination and aids in maintaining circulation and skin integrity.

Chest physiotherapy (**CPT;** percussion and positioning) is an effective method for preventing pulmonary secretion stasis. CPT techniques help the client to drain secretions from specific segments of the bronchi and lungs into the trachea so that the client can cough and expel the secretions. Respiratory assessment findings identify areas of the lungs requiring CPT (see chapter 35).

Maintaining a Patent Airway. Immobilized clients and those on bed rest are generally weakened. If weakness progresses, the cough reflex gradually becomes inefficient. The stasis of secretions in the lungs may be life-threatening for an immobilized client because hypostatic pneumonia can easily develop. Dislodging and mobilizing the stagnant secretions reduce the risk of pneumonia. Assessment findings that indicate this condition include productive cough with greenish yellow sputum; fever; pain on breathing; and crackles, wheezes, and dyspnea. The nurse should actively work with the client to deep breathe and cough every 1 to 2 hours as described earlier in Promoting Expansion of the Chest and Lungs.

In the immobilized client, an obstructed airway is usually a result of a mucous plug. The nurse can implement several therapies (e.g., CPT) to reduce the risk of mucous plugs and to maintain a patent airway. Nasotracheal or orotracheal suction techniques may be used to remove secretions in the upper airways of a client who is unable to cough productively. This procedure must be performed aseptically. The nurse can also suction secretions when clients have artificial airways such as an endotracheal or tracheal tube. The nurse inserts a catheter into the artificial airway using sterile technique. This removes pulmonary secretions from the upper and lower airways (see chapter 35).

Cardiovascular System. The effects of bed rest or immobilization on the cardiovascular system include orthostatic hypotension, increased cardiac workload, and thrombus formation. Nursing therapies are designed to minimize or prevent these alterations.

Reducing Orthostatic Hypotension. After bed rest, clients usually have increased pulse rate and decreased pulse pressure and blood pressure. A large decrease in blood pressure when arising to a sitting or standing position (orthostatic hypotension) can result in light-headedness and fainting (Black et al., 2001). When getting an immobile client up for the first time, the nurse should be assisted by at least one other person. This is a precautionary step in case the client faints. The client will still be expected to do as much of the transfer as the condition allows.

Interventions should be directed toward reducing or eliminating the effects of orthostatic hypotension. The nurse attempts to get the client moving as soon as the physical condition allows, even if this only involves sitting at the side of the bed (dangling) or moving to a chair. Changing position slowly and gradually helps to prevent orthostatic hypotension. Before the client gets up from the bed, the nurse slowly raises the head of the bed so that the client is sitting up for about 10 minutes prior to standing. The nurse then helps the client to sit on the side of the bed for a few minutes before the client stands up. This activity maintains muscle tone and increases venous return. The nurse then helps the client to stand. It is important to ask the client if he or she feels weak, dizzy, or sees spots before the eyes. If any of these symptoms occur, the nurse helps the client sit down again.

Reducing Cardiac Workload. Cardiac workload is increased by immobility. A primary intervention is to discourage clients from holding their breath while bearing down (the Valsalva manoeuvre), as may occur when the client is moving up in bed or straining to defecate. The Valsalva manoeuvre increases intrathoracic pressure, thus decreasing venous return and cardiac output. When the strain is released, venous return and cardiac output immediately increase and systolic blood pressure and pulse pressure rise. These pressure changes produce a reflex bradycardia and a possible decrease in blood pressure that may cause sudden cardiac death in clients with heart disease. The nurse reminds the client to breathe out while moving or being lifted up in bed.

Preventing Thrombus Formation. The most cost-effective way to address the deep vein thrombosis problem is through prevention (prophylaxis). It begins with identifying clients at risk and continues throughout the time clients are immobile or otherwise at risk. This is clearly a collaborative role between nurses and physicians. The nurse can easily identify risk factors during an admission nursing assessment. Many interventions reduce the risk of thrombus formation in the immobilized client. Leg exercises, encouraging fluids, position changes, and teaching should begin when the client becomes immobile. Preoperative clients should be given this information before surgery (see chapter 45). Other interventions such as intermittent pneumatic compression (IPC) and sequential compression devices (SCDs) require a physician's order. Maintenance and administration of prophylaxis is a nursing role, and nurses can determine when the client is fully mobile post-operatively, decreasing the continued risk for DVT.

Medications also require a physician's order. Heparin and low-molecular-weight heparin (LMWH) are the most widely used drugs in the prophylaxis of DVT. Standard heparin is considered the gold standard for treatment be-

Box 42-7 Procedural Guidelines

Application of Sequential Compression Stockings (SCSs)

Equipment: Tape measure, sequential stockings, stockinette, hygiene supplies

Delegation Considerations: The skill of applying SCSs can be delegated to unregulated care providers (UCPs). The nurse is responsible for assessing circulation in the extremities. The nurse instructs the UCP to do the following:

- Notify nurse if client complains of pain in leg.
- Notify nurse if discolouration develops in extremities.

1. Assess client for need for sequential compression stockings.
2. Obtain baseline assessment data about the status of circulation, pulse, and skin integrity on client's lower extremities before initiating sequential compression stockings.
3. Measure client for proper-size stocking by measuring around the largest part of the client's thigh. Review manufacturer's directions regarding measuring for proper fit.
4. Perform hand hygiene. Provide hygiene to lower extremities if needed.
5. Place a protective stockinette over the client's leg.
6. Wrap the stocking around the leg, starting at the ankle, with the opening over the patella (see illustration).
   a. Attach the stockings to the insufflator and verify that the intermittent pressure is between 35 and 45 mm Hg.
7. Record date and time of stocking application and stocking length and size in nurses' notes.
8. Record condition of skin and circulatory assessment.
9. Monitor skin integrity and circulation to client's lower extremities as ordered or according to manufacturer's guidelines.

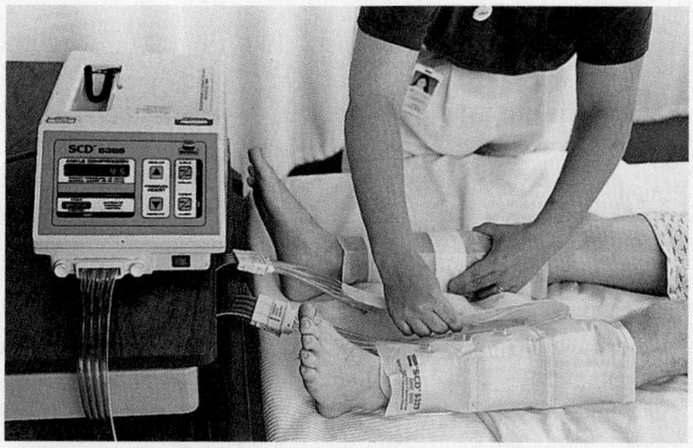

STEP **6** Application of sequential compression stocking.

cause it has been well studied and validated. Common dosage for heparin therapy is 5000 units given subcutaneously 2 hours before surgery and repeated every 8 to 12 hours until the client is fully mobile or discharged. Heparin is an anticoagulant, and it suppresses clot formation. Because of the action of this medication, the nurse must continually assess the client for signs of bleeding, such as increased bruising, guaiac-positive stools, and bleeding gums. Common dosage of Lovenox (LMWH) to prevent DVT is 30 to 40 mg subcutaneously 2 hours before surgery and continued throughout the post-operative period. Although the majority of clients receiving LMWH do not experience side effects, the risk is present (Nunnelee, 1997).

SCD/IPCs consist of sleeves or stockings made of fabric or plastic that are wrapped around the leg and secured with Velcro (Box 42-7). The sleeves are then connected to a pump that alternately inflates and deflates the stocking around the leg. A typical cycle is inflation for 10 to 15 seconds and deflation for 45 to 60 seconds. Inflation pressures average 40 mm Hg. Use of SCD/IPCs on the legs decreases venous stasis by increasing venous return through the deep veins of the legs. For optimal results, use of SCD/IPCs is begun as soon as possible and maintained until the client becomes fully ambulatory. Graded compression stockings can help prevent DVT, but clients must receive the right size, and the SCD/IPCs must be used correctly.

Elastic stockings (sometimes called thromboembolic device hose; TED) also aid in maintaining external pressure on the muscles of the lower extremities and thus may promote venous return (Box 42-8). When considering applying TED stockings, the nurse first assesses the client's suitability for wearing them. The stockings should not be applied if there is any local condition affecting the leg (e.g., any skin lesion, gangrenous condition, or recent vein ligation), because application may compromise circulation. The stockings must be applied properly, and they must be removed and reapplied at least twice a day. The nurse should assess circulation at the toes to ensure that the hose are not too tight. In addition, the stockings should always be clean and dry; it may be useful for the client to have two pairs.

Positioning techniques aid in reducing compression of the leg veins. Proper positioning used with other therapies (e.g., heparin or elastic stockings) aid in reducing the client's risk of thrombus formation. When positioning clients, the nurse uses caution to prevent pressure on the posterior knee and deep veins in the lower extremities. Client teaching should include avoiding crossing the legs, not sitting for prolonged periods of time, not wearing clothing that constricts the legs or waist, not putting pillows under the knees, and avoiding massaging the legs.

ROM exercises are designed to reduce the risk of contractures but may also aid in preventing thrombi. Activity causes contraction of the skeletal muscles, which in turn

Box 42-8 Procedural Guidelines

Application of Thromboembolic Device (TED) Hose

Equipment: Tape measure, TED hose, hygiene supplies

Delegation Considerations: The skill of applying TED hose can be performed by unregulated care providers (UCPs). The nurse is responsible for assessing circulation to the lower extremities. The nurse instructs the UCP to report if the client develops leg pain or discolouration.

1. Assess the need for elastic stockings and condition of the client's skin.
2. Observe for conditions that might contraindicate use of stockings.
3. Perform hand hygiene. Provide hygiene to lower extremities if needed.
4. Use tape measure to measure client's legs to determine proper stocking size (measure according to manufacturer's directions). Elastic stockings come in two lengths: knee length and thigh length.
5. Apply stockings:
   a. Turn elastic stocking inside out up to the heel. Place one hand into sock, holding heel. Pull top of sock with the other hand inside out over foot of sock.
   b. Place client's toes into foot of elastic stocking, making sure that sock is smooth (see illustration).
   c. Slide remaining portion of sock over client's foot, being sure that the toes are covered. Make sure the foot fits into the toe and heel position of the sock (see illustration).
   d. Slide top of sock up over client's calf until sock is completely extended. Be sure sock is smooth and no ridges or wrinkles are present, particularly behind the knee (see illustration).
6. Instruct client not to roll socks partially down.
7. Record date and time of stocking application and stocking length and size in nurses' notes.
8. Record condition of skin and circulatory assessment.

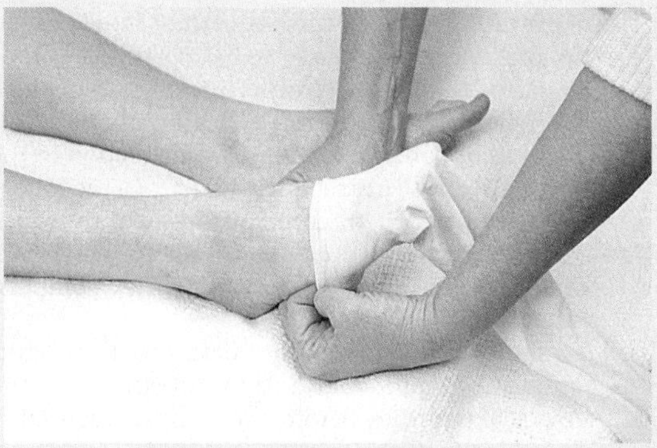

STEP **5b**

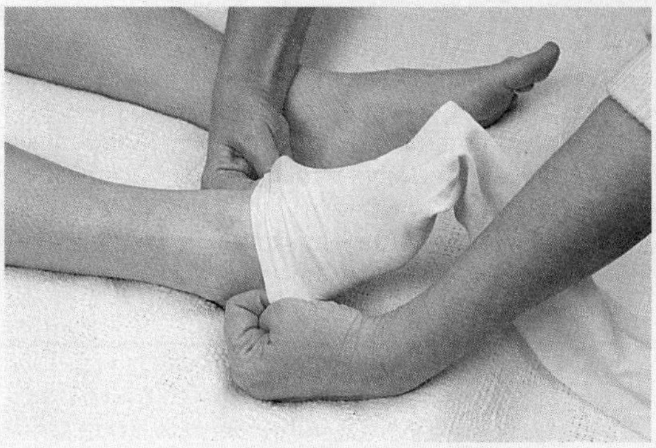

STEP **5c**

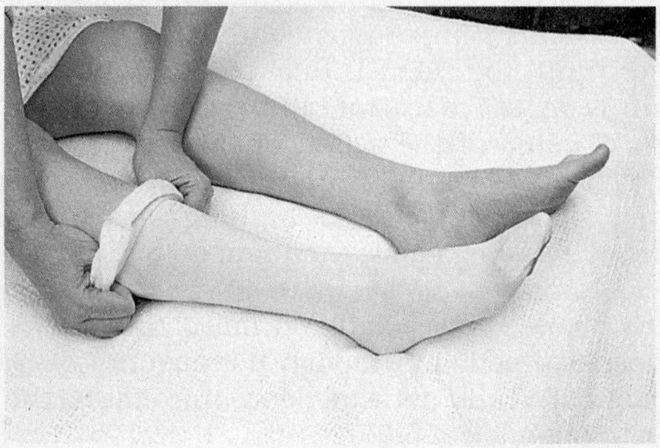

STEP **5d**

exerts pressure on the veins to promote venous return, thereby reducing venous stasis. Specific exercises that help prevent thrombophlebitis are ankle pumps, foot circles, and knee flexion. Ankle pumps, sometimes called calf pumps, include alternating plantar flexion and dorsiflexion. Foot circles require the client to rotate the ankle. Making the letters of the alphabet with their feet every 1 to 2 hours is a good exercise for clients. Knee flexion involves alternately extending and flexing the knee. These exercises are sometimes referred to as antiembolic exercises and should be done hourly while awake.

When DVT is suspected, the nurse should report it immediately. The leg should be elevated with no pressure on the thrombus. The family, client, and all health care personnel should be instructed to not massage the area because of the danger of dislodging the thrombus.

Musculoskeletal System. The immobilized client must receive some exercise to prevent or minimize muscle atrophy

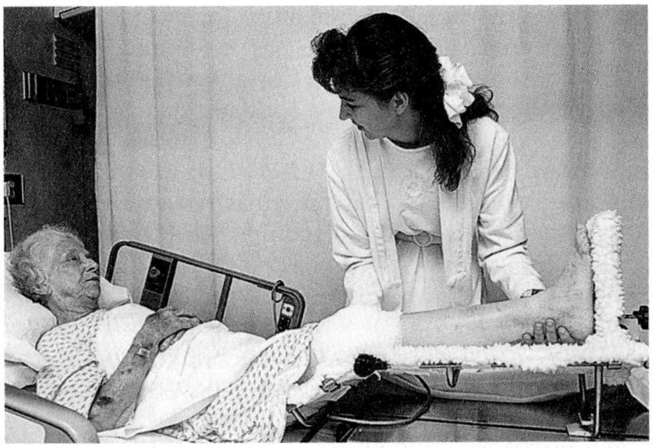

FIGURE **42–16** Continuous passive motion machine.

Focus on Older Adults — Box 42-9

The nurse should base an older client's exercise program on individual assessment data (underlying conditions, medications, present activity level). Before onset of exercise program, consult physician for exercise restrictions. The nurse should modify the exercise program based on the individual's responses. The nurse should also instruct the client to do the following:

- Use correct body mechanics, wear appropriate clothing and footwear, and maintain sufficient hydration.
- Perform a gradual, extended exercise warm-up (e.g., 15 minutes) to maximize flexibility and decrease muscle injury.
- Begin at low level (40% to 50% of predicted maximal heart rate), and follow gentle exercise progression.
- Avoid sudden twisting movements, rapid movements, and rapid transitions from one movement to the next.
- Avoid exercises that tax vision and balance.
- Avoid sustained isometric contractions of greater than 10 seconds.
- Avoid exercise during acute viral infections.
- Stop exercising if cardiac dysrhythmias, angina, or excessive breathlessness occurs.
- Perform cool-down until heart rate returns to resting level to decrease postural hypotension and cardiac dysrhythmias.

Adapted from *Geriatric Nursing and Healthy Aging,* by P. Ebersole and P. Hess, 2001, St. Louis, MO: Mosby.

and joint contractures. If the client is unable to move part or all of the body, the nurse must perform passive ROM exercises for all immobilized joints while bathing the client and at least two or three more times a day (see Restorative Care). If one extremity is paralyzed, the client can be taught to put each joint independently through its ROM. Clients on bed rest should have active ROM exercises incorporated into their daily schedules. Nurses can teach clients to integrate exercises during ADLs. Some orthopedic conditions require frequent passive ROM exercises to restore the injured joint's function after surgery. Clients with such conditions may use automatic equipment (continuous passive motion [CPM]) for passive ROM exercises (Figure 42–16). The CPM machine moves an extremity to a prescribed angle for a prescribed period. This is beneficial when the client must gradually increase the degree and duration of flexion and extension. Studies over the last several years have yielded varying evidence about the effectiveness of CPM in clients with total knee replacements. Short-term benefits were noted in some studies, but long-term improvement in range of motion was questionable (Maher et al., 2002).

Active ROM exercises maintain function of the musculoskeletal system. The nurse should also plan interventions for the gradual return of mobility for clients who will be able to resume normal activity. The best nursing intervention is establishing an individualized progressive exercise program. A progressive exercise program gradually increases the client's physical activity to reverse the deconditioning associated with immobility. Progressive exercise programs are used for clients with musculoskeletal, neurological, cardiopulmonary, renal, and other chronic diseases.

When working with older adults, the nurse must keep in mind gerontological principles that enhance the effectiveness of exercise programs and limit injuries (Box 42-9).

Teaching, referral, and interdisciplinary collaboration are important for clients with limited mobility. Depending on the setting and resources available, the nurse may want to refer the client for physiotherapy. The therapist would set up the specific exercise program, and the nurse would reinforce it.

Elimination System. The nursing interventions for maintaining optimal urinary functioning are directed at keeping the client well hydrated and preventing urinary stasis, calculi, and infections without causing bladder distension.

Adequate hydration (i.e., 2000 to 3000 mL of fluids per day) helps prevent renal calculi and urinary tract infections. The well-hydrated client should void large amounts of dilute urine that is approximately equal to fluid intake. If the client is incontinent, the nurse should modify the care plan to include toileting aids and a hygiene schedule so that the increased urinary output does not cause skin breakdown.

To prevent bladder distension, the nurse assesses the frequency and amount of urinary output. A client who continually dribbles urine and whose bladder is distended may have reflex incontinence. If the immobilized client does not have voluntary control of bladder elimination, bladder training may be necessary. If the client experiences bladder distension, the nurse may be required to insert a straight catheter or an in-dwelling Foley catheter (see chapter 40).

The nurse must also record the frequency and consistency of bowel movements. A diet rich in fluids, fruits, vegetables, and fibre can facilitate normal peristalsis. If a client is unable to maintain regular bowel patterns, stool softeners, cathartics, or enemas may be needed (see chapter 41).

Integumentary System. The major risk to the skin from restricted mobility is the formation of pressure ulcers. Early identification of high-risk clients and their risk factors aids the nurse in preventing pressure ulcers (see chapter 43). Interventions aimed at prevention are positioning, skin care, and the use of therapeutic devices to relieve pressure. The immobilized client's position should be changed according to the client's activity level, perceptual ability, treatment protocols, and daily routines. Although turning every 1 to 2 hours is recommended for preventing ulcers, it may also be necessary to use devices for relieving pressure. The time that a client sits uninterrupted in a chair should be limited to 1 hour or less, but this time interval is individualized. The client should be repositioned frequently because uninterrupted pressure will cause skin breakdown. The nurse should teach clients who are able to do so to shift their weight every 15 minutes. Chair-bound clients should have a device for the chair that reduces pressure; however, donut-shaped devices should not be used (RNAO, 2002b).

Psychosocial Changes. Assessment can identify effects of prolonged immobilization on the client's psychosocial dimension. People who have a tendency toward depression or mood swings are at greater risk for developing psychosocial changes during bed rest or immobilization.

The nurse should anticipate changes in the client's psychosocial status. The nurse can provide routine and informal socialization. Nursing activities can be planned so that the client can talk and interact with staff. If possible, the client should be placed in a room with others who are mobile and interactive. If a private room is required, staff members should be asked to visit throughout the shift to provide meaningful interaction.

The nurse also provides stimuli to maintain a client's orientation. Maintaining a calendar and clock; providing a newspaper, books, radio, or television; and encouraging visits from significant others may reduce the risk of social isolation. Spending time in the room talking and listening to the client also reduces isolation.

Nursing care should encourage immobilized clients to perform as many ADLs as independently as possible. Clients should continue to perform personal grooming if they did so before their mobility was restricted. This type of activity preserves the client's dignity and gives the client a sense of accomplishment.

In institutional health care settings, nursing care given between 2200 hours and 0700 hours should be scheduled to minimize interruptions of sleep. For example, the nurse may administer medications and assess vital signs at the time when the client is turned or receives special skin care.

The nurse should also observe the client's ability to cope with restricted mobility. If the nursing care plan is not improving coping patterns, a clinical nurse specialist, counsellor, social worker, spiritual adviser, or other consultant may be needed. Their recommendations should be incorporated into the care plan.

Developmental Changes in Children. Ideally, immobilized clients continue normal development. Nursing interventions can help. Nursing care should provide mental and physical stimulation, particularly for a young child. Play activities can be incorporated into the care plan. Completing puzzles, for example, helps a child to develop fine motor skills, and reading helps the child to develop cognitively. Parents can be encouraged to stay with a child who is hospitalized. An immobilized child should be placed with children of the same age who are not immobilized, unless a contagious disease is present. The nurse must recognize significant changes from normal behavioural patterns. If these changes continue, the nurse should consult with a clinical nurse, counsellor, or other health care professional whose specialty is children.

Positioning Devices and Techniques. Clients with impaired nervous, skeletal, or muscular system functioning and general weakness often require help from the nurse to attain proper body alignment while in bed or sitting.

Several positioning devices are available for maintaining good body alignment for clients:

- *Pillows*—provide support, elevate body parts, and can splint incisional areas, reducing post-operative pain during activity or coughing and deep breathing. Before using a pillow, the nurse should determine whether it is the proper size. A thick pillow under the client's head increases cervical flexion. A thin pillow under body prominences may be inadequate to protect skin and tissue from damage caused by pressure. When additional pillows are unavailable, or if they are an improper size, the nurse can use folded sheets, blankets, or towels as positioning aids.
- *Wedge (or abductor) pillow*—a triangular-shaped pillow made of heavy foam used to maintain the legs in abduction following total hip replacement surgery.
- *Bed board*—plywood board placed under the entire surface of the mattress. A bed board is useful for increasing back support and alignment, especially with a soft mattress.
- *Footboard*—a flat, plastic or wood panel placed perpendicular to the mattress, parallel to and touching the plantar surfaces of the client's feet. The footboard prevents footdrop by maintaining the feet in dorsiflexion. The nurse determines that it is correctly placed, with the client's feet placed firmly against the board (Figure 42–17).
- *Footboot*—maintains feet in dorsiflexion. Footboots are made of rigid plastic or heavy foam (Figure 42–18). They keep the foot flexed at the proper angle and the weight of the bedsheets off the toes. The nurse should remove the footboots two or three times a day to assess skin integrity and joint mobility.
- *Trochanter roll*—prevents external rotation of the hips when the client is in a supine position. A **trochanter roll** is formed by folding a cotton bath blanket lengthwise to a width that will extend from the greater trochanter of the femur to the lower border of the popliteal space (Figure 42–19). The blanket is placed under the buttocks and then rolled counter-clockwise until the thigh is in neutral position or in inward rotation. When correct alignment of the hip is achieved, the patella faces directly upward.
- *Sandbags*—sand-filled plastic tubes or bags that can be shaped to body contours. Sandbags can be used in place of or in addition to trochanter rolls. They immobilize an extremity or maintain body alignment.
- *Hand rolls*—maintain the thumb in slight adduction and in opposition to the fingers. A hand roll maintains the hand, thumb, and fingers in a functional position, thus preventing contractures (Figure 42–20). The nurse evaluates the hand roll to make sure that the hand is indeed in a functional position. Hand

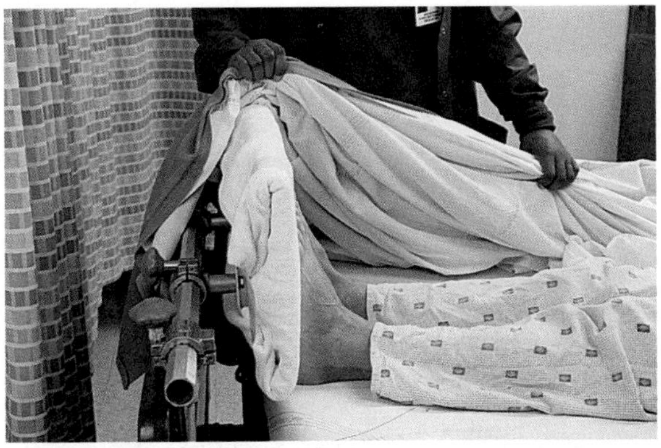

FIGURE **42–17** Footboard. Feet are flush with the board to keep them in normal alignment. (From *Mosby's Canadian Textbook for the Support Worker,* by S. A. Sorrentino, 2004, Toronto, ON: Elsevier Canada.)

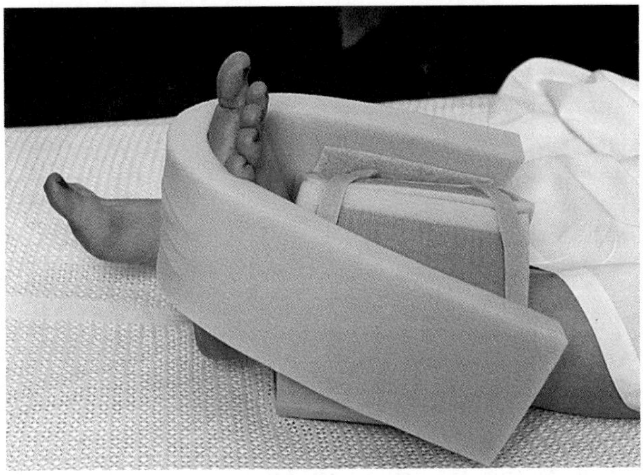

FIGURE **42–18** Foot boot.

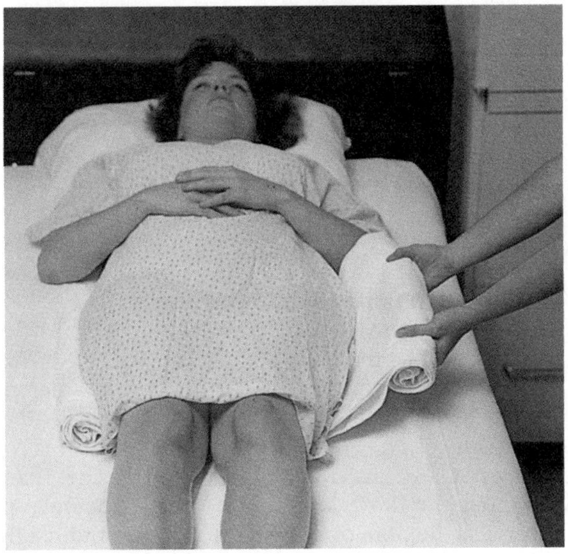

FIGURE **42–19** Trochanter roll.

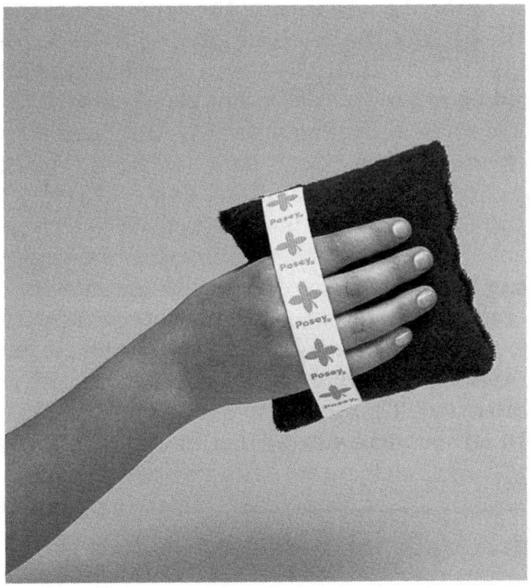

FIGURE **42–20** Hand roll. (Courtesy J.T. Posey, Arcadia, CA.)

rolls are most often used for clients whose arms are paralyzed or who are unconscious. Rolled washcloths should not be used as hand rolls, because they do not keep the thumb well abducted, especially in clients who have a spastic paralysis.

- *Hand-wrist splints*—individually moulded for the client to maintain proper alignment of the thumb (slight adduction) and the wrist (slight dorsiflexion). These splints should be used only by the client for whom the splint was made (Figure 42–21).
- *Trapeze bar*—a triangular device that descends from a securely fastened overhead bar attached to the bed frame. A **trapeze bar** allows the client to use the upper extremities to raise the trunk off the bed, to assist in transfer from bed to wheelchair, or to perform upper arm exercises (Figure 42–22). It is a useful device for helping to increase independence, maintain upper body strength, and decrease the shearing action from sliding across or up and down in bed.

Although procedures for each position has specific guidelines, there are some universal steps that the nurse should follow for clients who require positioning assistance (Skill 42-1). Following the guidelines reduces the risk of injury to the musculoskeletal system. When joints are unsupported, their alignment is impaired. Joints must be positioned in a slightly flexed position or their mobility is decreased. During positioning, the nurse also assesses bony prominences (pressure points; see Figure 43-3). When actual or potential pressure areas exist, nursing interventions involve removal of the pressure, thus decreasing the risk for development of pressure ulcers and further trauma to the musculoskeletal system. In clients at risk for pressure ulcers, the 30-degree lateral position should be used (see Figure 43-18).

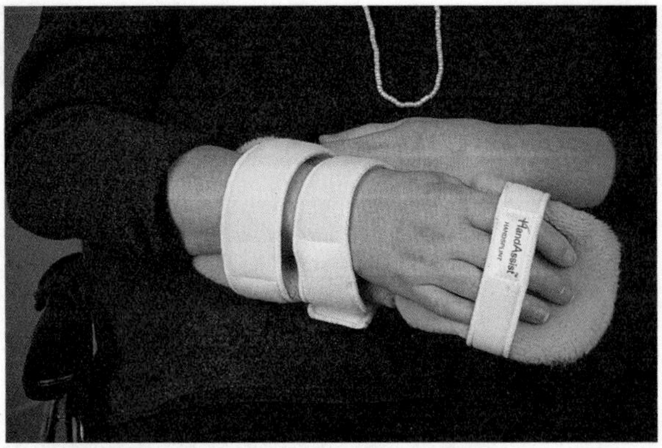

FIGURE **42–21** Hand-wrist splint. (From *Mosby's Canadian Textbook for the Support Worker,* by S. A. Sorrentino, 2004, Toronto, ON: Elsevier Canada.)

Supported Fowler's Position. In the supported Fowler's position, the head of the bed is elevated 45 to 60 degrees and the client's knees are slightly elevated without pressure; the client is sitting up in bed. Do not elevate the head of the bed more than 60 degrees because this would increase shearing force on the client's back and heels. The angle of head and knee elevation and the length of time that the client should remain in the supported Fowler's position vary depending on the client's illness and overall condition. Supports must permit flexion of the hips and knees and proper alignment of the normal curves in the cervical, thoracic, and lumbar vertebrae. The following are common trouble areas for the client in the supported Fowler's position (see Skill 42-1 for preventive measures):

- Excessive cervical flexion because the pillow at the head is too thick and the head thrusts forward
- Hyperextension of the knees, allowing the client to slide to the foot of the bed
- Pressure on the posterior aspect of the knees, decreasing circulation to the feet
- External rotation of the hips
- Arms hanging unsupported at the client's sides
- Unsupported feet or pressure on the heels
- Unprotected pressure points at the sacrum and heels

Supine Position. The supine position is a back-lying position. In the supine position, the relationship of body parts is essentially the same as in good standing alignment except that the body is in the horizontal plane. Pillows, trochanter rolls, and hand rolls or arm splints are used to increase comfort and reduce injury to the skin or musculoskeletal system. The mattress should be firm enough to support the cervical, thoracic, and lumbar vertebrae. Shoulders are supported, and the elbows are slightly flexed to control shoulder rotation. A foot support is used to prevent footdrop and maintain proper alignment. The following are some common trouble areas for clients in the supine position (see Skill 42-1 for preventive measures):

- Excessive cervical flexion because the pillow at the head is too thick and the head thrusts forward
- Head flat on the mattress
- Shoulders unsupported and internally rotated

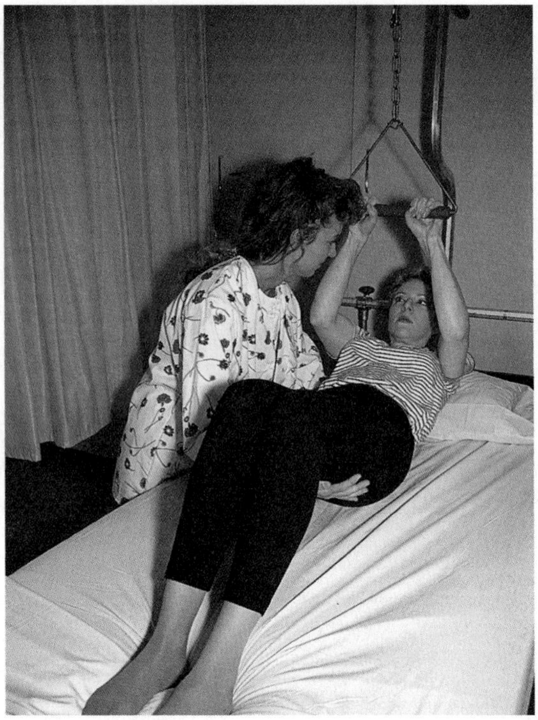

FIGURE **42–22** Client using a trapeze bar.

- Elbows extended
- Thumb not in opposition to the fingers
- Hips externally rotated
- Unsupported feet
- Unprotected pressure points at the occipital region of the head, vertebrae, coccyx, elbows, and heels

Prone Position. The client in the prone position is lying chest down. Often the head is turned to the side. If a pillow is under the head, it should be thin enough to prevent cervical flexion or extension and maintain alignment of the lumbar spine. Placing a pillow under the lower leg permits dorsiflexion of the ankles and some knee flexion, which promotes relaxation. If a pillow is unavailable, the ankles should be in dorsiflexion over the end of the mattress. The nurse should assess for and correct any of the following potential trouble points (see Skill 42-1 for preventive measures):

- Neck hyperextension
- Hyperextension of the lumbar spine
- Plantar flexion of the ankles
- Unprotected pressure points at the chin, elbows, hips, knees, and toes

Studies show the prone position reduces risk of pressure ulcers. Areas located over the body prominences have the highest interface pressures, which result in a greater likelihood of developing ulcers. Defloor (2000) found that the prone position resulted in the lowest interface pressures, reducing the risk of skin breakdown. Although the prone position is seldom used in practice, nurses should consider this as an alternative, especially in clients who normally sleep in this position.

Side-Lying Position. In the side-lying (or lateral) position, the client is resting on the side with the major portion of body weight on the dependent hip and shoulder. A 30-degree lateral position is recommended for clients at risk for pressure ulcers (see chapter 43). Trunk alignment should be the same as in standing. For example, the structural curves of the spine should be maintained, the head should be supported in line with the midline of the trunk, and rotation of the spine should be avoided. The following trouble points are common in the side-lying position (see Skill 42-1 for preventive measures):

- Lateral flexion of the neck
- Spinal curves out of normal alignment
- Shoulder and hip joints internally rotated, adducted, or unsupported
- Lack of support for the feet
- Lack of protection for pressure points at the ear, shoulder, anterior iliac spine, trochanter, and ankles
- Excessive lateral flexion of the spine if the client has large hips and a pillow is not placed superior to the hips at the waist

Sims' Position. Sims' position differs from the lateral position in the distribution of the client's weight. In Sims' position, the weight is placed on the anterior ilium, humerus, and clavicle. Trouble points common in Sims' position include the following (see Skill 42-1 for preventive measures):

- Lateral flexion of the neck
- Internal rotation, adduction, or lack of support to the shoulders and hips
- Lack of support for the feet
- Lack of protection for pressure points at the ilium, humerus, clavicle, knees, and ankles

Transfer Techniques. Nurses often provide care for immobilized clients whose position must be changed, who must be moved up in bed, or who must be transferred from a bed to a chair or from a bed to a stretcher. Use of proper body mechanics enables the nurse to position, move, or transfer clients safely and also protects the nurse from injury to the musculoskeletal system. Although nurses use many transfer techniques, the following general guidelines should be followed in any transfer procedure:

- Raise the side rail on the side of the bed opposite the nurse to prevent the client from falling out of bed
- Elevate the level of the bed to a comfortable working height
- Assess the client's mobility and strength to determine what assistance the client can offer during transfer
- Determine the need for assistance from other care providers or mechanical lifts
- Explain the procedure to the client and describe what is expected of the client
- Assess for correct body alignment and pressure areas after each transfer

Safety Alert. The nurse should recognize personal strength and limits. Moving a completely immobilized client alone is dangerous and not allowed in many agencies. The nurse who is attempting transfer or moving techniques for the first time should request help to reduce the risk of injury to self and client.

Moving Clients. Clients require various levels of assistance to move up in bed, move to the side-lying position, or sit up at the side of the bed. For example, a young, healthy woman may need only a little support as she sits at the side of the bed for the first time after childbirth, whereas an older person may need help from one or more nurses to do the same task 1 day after abdominal surgery.

The nurse should always enlist the client's help to the fullest extent possible. To determine what the client is able to do alone and how many people are needed to help move the client in bed, the nurse assesses the client to determine whether the illness contradicts exertion (e.g., cardiovascular disease). Next, the nurse determines whether the client comprehends what is expected. For example, a client recently medicated for post-operative pain may be too lethargic to understand instruction; thus, to ensure safety, two nurses are needed to move the client in bed. The nurse then determines the comfort level of the client. The nurse also evaluates personal strength and knowledge of the procedure. Finally, the nurse determines whether the client is too heavy or immobile for the nurse to complete the procedure alone (Nelson et al., 2003). If in doubt, the nurse should always request assistance from another person. The nurse collaborates with the physiotherapist, occupational therapist, and physician to plan for mobilizing the bariatric client; mechanical transfer devices may be warranted, and agency lifting and transferring policies must be followed. Skills 42-1 and 42-2 describe the steps commonly used in moving clients in bed and transferring them to a sitting position at the side of the bed.

Transferring a Client From a Bed to a Chair. Transfer of a client from a bed to a chair by one nurse requires assistance from the client and should not be attempted with a client who cannot help (see Skill 42-2). The nurse explains the procedure to the client before the transfer. Moving obstacles out of the way also prepares the environment. The chair is placed next to the bed with the chair back in the same plane as the head of the bed. Placement of the chair allows the nurse to pivot with the client and to transfer the client's weight quickly.

A safe transfer is the first priority. The nurse who is doubtful about personal strength or the client's ability to help should request assistance. A **transfer belt** should be used with all clients being transferred for the first time and thereafter as deemed necessary. A transfer belt (called a **gait belt** when used for walking with a client) helps prevent caregiver back injuries and promotes the safe transfer of the client. It is a leather belt that encircles the client's waist and has handles attached for the nurse to hold. It is applied over the client's clothing, never over bare skin. The belt is tightened so that it is snug but does not cause discomfort or impair breathing, and the buckle is placed off-centre in the front or in the back. The buckle should not be over the spine.

Often a hydraulic lift can be used to transfer clients (see Skill 42-2). The client should sit and dangle the feet at the side of the bed for a minute before standing. The client should then stand at the side of the bed for another minute so that he or she can quickly sit down on it in case of dizziness or fainting. When moving a client from a bed to a wheelchair, both nurses must use proper body

Text continued on p. 1481

Skill 42-1 Moving and Positioning Clients in Bed

Delegation Considerations

The skills of moving and positioning clients in bed can be delegated to unregulated care providers (UCPs). The nurse is responsible for assessing the client's level of comfort and for any hazards of immobility. It is important for the nurse to instruct the UCP on any limitations affecting movement and positioning of client in bed.

Equipment

- Pillows
- Drawsheet or pull sheet
- Positioning devices as required (e.g., trochanter roll, extra pillows, footboard, hand rolls, etc.)

Steps	Rationale
1. Assess client's body alignment and comfort level while client is lying down.	Provides baseline data for later comparisons. Determines ways to improve position and alignment.
2. Assess for risk factors that may contribute to complications of immobility:	Increased risk factors require client to be repositioned more frequently.
a. Paralysis: hemiparesis resulting from cerebrovascular accident; decreased sensation	Paralysis impairs movement, causes muscle tone changes; sensation can be affected. Because of difficulty in moving and poor awareness of involved body part, client is unable to protect and position body part for self.
b. Impaired mobility: traction or arthritis or other contributing disease processes	Traction or arthritic changes of affected extremity result in decreased range of motion (ROM).
c. Impaired circulation	Decreased circulation predisposes client to pressure sores.
d. Age: very young, older adults	Premature and young infants require frequent turning because their skin is fragile. Normal physiological changes associated with aging predispose older adults to greater risks for developing complications of immobility.
e. Level of consciousness and mental status.	Comatose or semicomatose clients are unable to verbalize areas of skin pressure, increasing the risk for skin breakdown.
3. Assess client's physical ability to help with moving and positioning:	Enables nurse to use client's mobility and strength. Determines need for additional help. Ensures client and nurse safety.
a. Age	Older adult client may move more slowly and with less strength.
b. Level of consciousness and mental status	Determines need for special aids or devices. Clients with altered levels of consciousness may not understand instructions and may be unable to help.
c. Disease process	Cardiopulmonary disease may require client to have head of bed elevated.
d. Strength, coordination	Determines amount of assistance provided by client during position change.
e. ROM	Limited ROM may contraindicate certain positions.
4. Assess physician's orders. Clarify whether any positions are contraindicated because of client's condition (e.g., spinal cord injury; respiratory difficulties; certain neurological conditions; presence of incisions, drain, or tubing).	Placing client in an inappropriate position could cause injury.
5. Perform hand hygiene.	Reduces transfer of micro-organisms.
6. Assess for the presence of tubes, incisions, and equipment (e.g., traction).	Will alter positioning procedure and may affect client's ability to independently change positions.
7. Assess ability and motivation of client, family members, and primary caregiver to participate in moving and positioning client in bed in anticipation of discharge to home.	Determines ability of client and caregivers to assist with positioning.
8. Raise level of bed to comfortable working height, and get extra help if needed.	Raises level of work to centre of gravity and provides for client's and nurse's safety.
9. Perform hand hygiene.	Reduces transfer of micro-organisms.

Steps	Rationale
10. Explain procedure to client.	Decreases anxiety and increases client co-operation.
11. Position client flat in bed if tolerated.	Repositioning from a flat position decreases friction and possible shear on client's skin.

Critical Decision Point: Before flattening bed, account for all tubing, drains, and equipment to prevent dislodgement or tipping if caught in mattress or bed frame as bed is lowered.

Steps	Rationale
12. Position client in bed.	
A. Assist client in moving up in bed (one or two nurses). NOTE: Only a young child or a lightweight client requiring minimal assistance can be safely moved by one nurse.	
(1) Remove pillow from under head and shoulders, and place pillow at head of bed. Ask client to cross arms across the chest.	Prevents striking client's head against head of bed. Reduces surface area and friction.
(2) Face head of bed.	Facing direction of movement prevents twisting of nurse's body while moving client.
(a) Each nurse should have one arm under client's shoulders and one arm under client's thighs.	
(b) Alternative position: position one nurse at client's upper body. Nurse's arm nearest head of bed should be under clients' head and opposite shoulder; other arm should be under client's closest arm and shoulder. Position other nurse at client's lower torso. The nurse's arms should be under client's lower back and torso.	Prevents trauma to client's musculoskeletal system by supporting shoulder and hip joints and evenly distributing weight.
(3) Place feet apart, with foot nearest head of bed behind other foot (forward-backward stance; see illustration).	Wide base of support increases balance. Stance enables nurse to shift body weight as client is moved up in bed, thereby reducing force needed to move load.
(4) Ask client to flex knees with feet flat on bed.	Decreases friction and enables client to use leg muscles during movement.
(5) Instruct client to flex neck, tilting chin toward chest.	Prevents hyperextension of neck when moving client up in bed.
(6) Instruct client to assist moving by pushing with feet on bed surface.	Reduces friction. Increases client mobility. Decreases workload.
(7) Flex knees and hips, bringing forearms closer to level of bed.	Increases balance and strength by bringing centre of gravity closer to client. Uses thighs instead of back muscles.
(8) Instruct client to push with heels and elevate trunk while breathing out, thus moving toward head of bed on count of three.	Prepares client for move. Reinforces assistance in moving up in bed. Increases client co-operation. Breathing out avoids Valsalva manoeuvre.

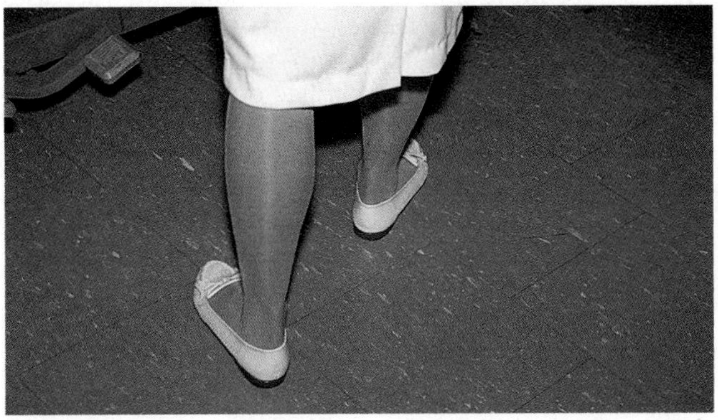

STEP **12A(3)** Position of feet: feet placed apart in a forward-to-backward stance.

Skill 42-1 Moving and Positioning Clients in Bed—cont'd

Steps	Rationale
(9) On count of three, rock and shift weight from front to back leg. At the same time, client pushes with heels and elevates trunk.	Rocking enables nurse to improve balance and overcome inertia. Shifting weight counteracts client's weight and reduces force needed to move load. Client's assistance reduces friction and workload.
B. Move immobile client up in bed with drawsheet or pull sheet (two nurses)	
(1) Place drawsheet or pull sheet under client by turning side to side. Have sheet extend from shoulders to thighs. Return client to supine position.	Supports client's body weight and reduces friction during movement.
(2) Position one nurse at each side of client.	Distributes weight equally between nurses.
(3) Grasp drawsheet or pull sheet firmly near the client.	
(4) Place feet apart with forward-backward stance. Flex knees and hips. Shift weight from front to back leg, and move client and drawsheet or pull sheet to desired position in bed.	Facing direction of movement ensures proper balance. Shifting weight reduces force needed to move load. Flexing knees lowers centre of gravity and uses thighs instead of back muscles.
(5) Realign client in correct body alignment.	Prevents injury to musculoskeletal system.
C. Position client in supported Fowler's position (see illustration)	
(1) Elevate head of bed 45 to 60 degrees.	Increases comfort, improves ventilation, and increases client's opportunity to socialize or relax.
(2) Rest client's head against mattress or on small pillow.	Prevents flexion contractures of cervical vertebrae.
(3) Use pillows to support arms and hands if client does not have voluntary control or use of hands and arms.	Prevents shoulder dislocation from effect of downward pull of unsupported arms, promotes circulation by preventing venous pooling, and prevents flexion contractures of arms and wrists.
(4) Position pillow at lower back.	Supports lumbar vertebrae and decreases flexion of vertebrae.
(5) Place small pillow or roll under thigh.	Prevents hyperextension of knee and occlusion of popliteal artery from pressure from body weight.
(6) Place small pillow or roll under ankles.	Prevents prolonged pressure of mattress on heels.

Critical Decision Point: To keep feet in proper alignment and prevent footdrop, place footboard at bottom of client's feet.

Steps	Rationale
D. Position hemiplegic client in supported Fowler's position	
(1) Elevate head of bed 45 to 60 degrees.	Increases comfort, improves ventilation, and increases client's opportunity to relax.
(2) Position client in sitting position as straight as possible.	Counteracts tendency to slump toward affected side. Improves ventilation and cardiac output; decreases intracranial pressure. Improves client's ability to swallow and helps to prevent aspiration of food, liquids, and gastric secretions.

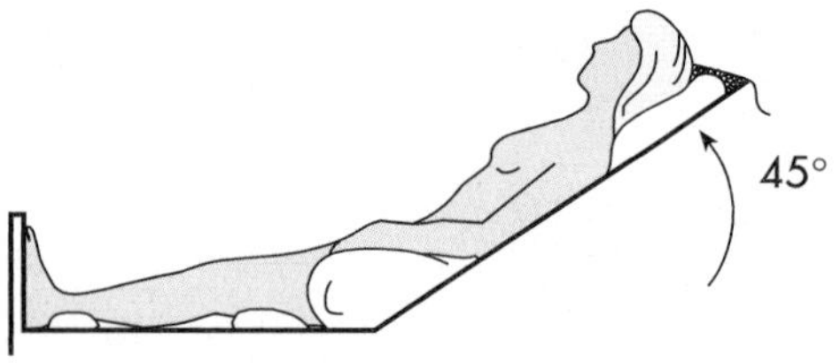

STEP **12C** Supported Fowler's position with footboard in place.

Steps	Rationale
(3) Position head on small pillow with chin slightly forward. If client is totally unable to control head movement, hyperextension of the neck must be avoided.	Prevents hyperextension of neck. Too many pillows under head may cause or worsen neck flexion contracture.

Critical Decision Point: If the client has a paralyzed extremity, provide support for involved arm and hand on overbed table in front of client. Place arm away from client's side and support elbow with pillow.
- Position *flaccid* hand in normal resting position with wrist slightly extended, arches of hand maintained, and fingers partially flexed; may use hand grip or section of rubber ball cut in half; clasp client's hands together.
- Position *spastic* hand with wrist in neutral position or slightly extended; fingers should be extended with palm down or may be left in relaxed position palm up. It may be difficult to position spastic hands without the use of specially made splints for the client.

Steps	Rationale
(4) Flex client's knees and hips by using pillow or folded blanket under knees.	Ensures proper alignment. Flexion prevents prolonged hyperextension, which could impair joint mobility.
(5) Support feet in dorsiflexion with firm pillow or footboard.	Prevents footdrop. Stimulation of ball of foot by hard surface has tendency to increase muscle tone in client with extensor spasticity of lower extremity.
E. Position client in supine position	
(1) Be sure client is comfortable on back with head of bed flat.	Some clients' physical conditions will not tolerate supine position.
(2) Place small rolled towel under lumbar area of back.	Provides support for lumbar spine.
(3) Place pillow under upper shoulders, neck, or head.	Maintains correct alignment and prevents flexion contractures of cervical vertebrae.
(4) Place trochanter rolls or sandbags parallel to lateral surface of client's thighs.	Reduces external rotation of hip.
(5) Place small pillow or roll under ankle to elevate heels (see illustration for Step 12C).	Reduces pressure on heels, helping to prevent pressure sores.
(6) Place footboard or firm pillows against bottom of client's feet.	Maintains dorsiflexion and prevents footdrop.
(7) Place footboots on client's feet, if necessary.	Maintains feet in dorsiflexion. Prevents footdrop.
(8) Place pillows under pronated forearms, keeping upper arms parallel to client's body (see illustrations).	Reduces internal rotation of shoulder and prevents extension of elbows. Maintains correct body alignment.
(9) Place hand rolls in client's hands. Consider physiotherapy referral for use of hand splints if necessary.	Reduces extension of fingers and abduction of thumb. Maintains thumb slightly adducted and in opposition to fingers.

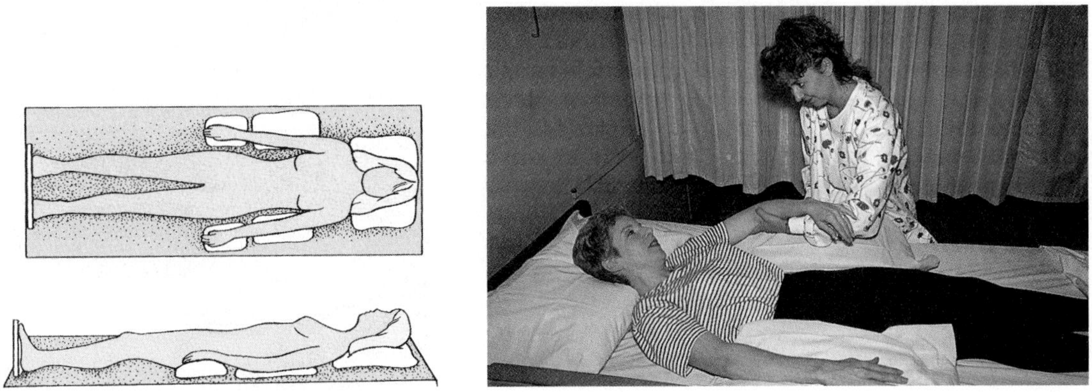

STEP **12E(8)** Supine position with pillows in place.

Skill 42-1 Moving and Positioning Clients in Bed—cont'd

Steps	Rationale
F. Position hemiplegic client in supine position	
(1) Place head of bed flat.	Necessary for positioning in supine position.
(2) Place folded towel or small pillow under shoulder or affected side.	Decreases possibility of pain, joint contracture, and subluxation. Maintains mobility in muscles around shoulder to permit normal movement patterns.
(3) Keep affected arm away from body with elbow extended and palm up. (Alternative is to place arm out to side, with elbow bent and hand toward head of bed.)	Maintains mobility in arm, joints, and shoulder to permit normal movement patterns. (Alternative position counteracts limitation of ability of arm to rotate outward at shoulder [external rotation]. External rotation must be present to raise arm overhead without pain.)

Critical Decision Point: Position the affected hand in one of the recommended positions for flaccid or spastic hand.

Steps	Rationale
(4) Place folded towel under hip of client's involved side.	Diminishes effect of spasticity in entire leg by controlling hip position.
(5) Flex affected knee 30 degrees by supporting it on pillow or folded blanket.	Slight flexion breaks up abnormal extension pattern of leg. Extensor spasticity is most severe when client is supine.
(6) Support feet with soft pillows at right angle to leg.	Maintains foot in dorsiflexion and prevents footdrop. Pillows prevent stimulation to ball of foot by hard surface, which has tendency to increase muscle tone in client with extensor spasticity of lower extremity.
G. Position client in prone position	
(1) With client supine, roll client over arm positioned close to body, with elbow straight and hand under hip. Position on abdomen in centre of bed.	Positions client correctly so that alignment can be maintained.
(2) Turn client's head to one side and support head with small pillow (see illustration).	Reduces flexion or hyperextension of cervical vertebrae.
(3) Place small pillow under client's abdomen below level of diaphragm (see illustration).	Reduces pressure on breasts of some female clients and decreases hyperextension of lumbar vertebrae and strain on lower back.
(4) Support arms in flexed position level at shoulders.	Maintains proper body alignment. Support reduces risk of joint dislocation.
(5) Support lower legs with pillows to elevate toes (see illustration).	Prevents footdrop. Reduces external rotation of hips. Reduces mattress pressure on toes.

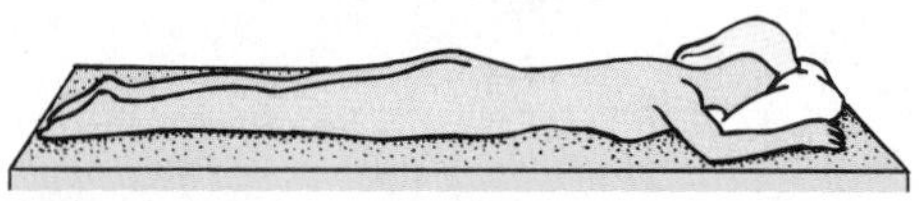

STEP **12G(2)** Prone position, head supported with pillow.

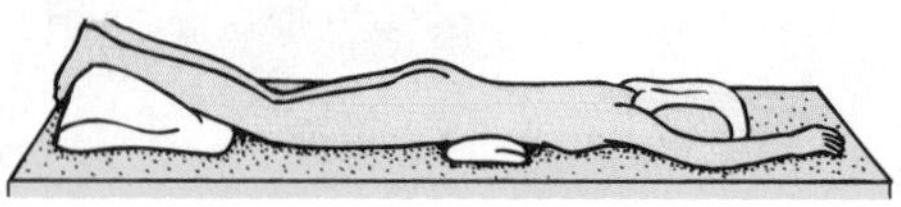

STEP **12G(3)** Prone position, pillow under client's abdomen and feet.

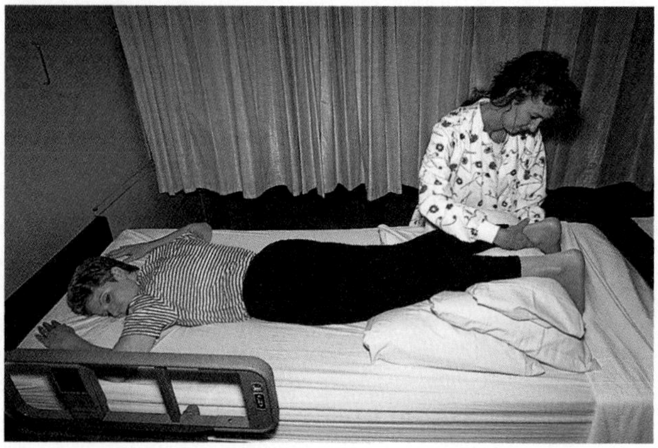

STEP **12G(5)** Prone position.

Steps	Rationale
H. Position hemiplegic client in prone position	

Critical Decision Point: Increase frequency of position if pressure areas begin to appear, joint mobility becomes impaired or worsened, or client complains of discomfort. Consult with physiotherapist and occupational therapist as needed. Use 30-degree lateral position (see Figure 43-18).

Steps	Rationale
(1) Move client toward unaffected side.	Creates room for proper client alignment in centre of bed when client is rolled onto abdomen.
(2) Roll client onto side.	
(3) Place pillow on client's abdomen.	Prevents sagging of abdomen when client is rolled over; decreases hyperextension of lumbar vertebrae and strain on lower back.
(4) Roll client onto abdomen by positioning involved arm close to client's body, with elbow straight and hand under hip. Roll client carefully over arm.	Prevents injury to affected side.
(5) Turn head toward involved side.	Promotes development of neck and trunk extension, which is necessary for standing and walking.
(6) Position involved arm out to side, with elbow bent, hand toward head of bed, and fingers extended (if possible).	Counteracts limitation of arm's ability to rotate outward at shoulder (external rotation). External rotation must be present to raise arm over head without pain.
(7) Flex knees slightly by placing pillow under legs from knees to ankles.	Flexion prevents prolonged hyperextension, which could impair joint mobility.
(8) Keep feet at right angle to legs by using pillow high enough to keep toes off mattress.	Maintains feet in dorsiflexion.
I. Position client in lateral (side-lying) position	
(1) Lower head of bed completely or as low as client can tolerate.	Provides position of comfort for client and removes pressure from bony prominences on back and buttocks.
(2) Position client to side of bed.	Provides room for client to turn to side.
(3) Prepare to turn client onto side. Flex client's knee that will not be next to mattress. Place one hand on client's hip and one hand on client's shoulder.	Positioning will set up leverage for easy turning.
(4) Roll client onto side toward you.	Rolling client toward nurse decreases trauma to tissues. In addition, client is positioned so that leverage on hip makes turning easy.
(5) Place pillow under client's head and neck.	Maintains alignment. Reduces lateral neck flexion. Decreases strain on sternocleidomastoid muscle.
(6) Bring shoulder blade forward.	Prevents client's weight from resting directly on shoulder joint.
(7) Position both arms in slightly flexed position. Upper arm is supported by pillow level with shoulder; other arm, by mattress.	Decreases internal rotation and adduction of shoulder. Supports both arms in slightly flexed position.
(8) Place tuck-back pillow behind client's back. (Make by folding pillow lengthwise. Smooth area is slightly tucked under client's back.)	Provides support to maintain client on side.
(9) Place pillow under semiflexed upper leg level at hip from groin to foot (see illustrations).	Maintains leg in correct alignment. Prevents pressure on bony prominence.
(10) Place sandbag parallel to plantar surface of dependent foot.	Maintains dorsiflexion of foot. Prevents footdrop.

Skill 42-1 *Moving and Positioning Clients in Bed—cont'd*

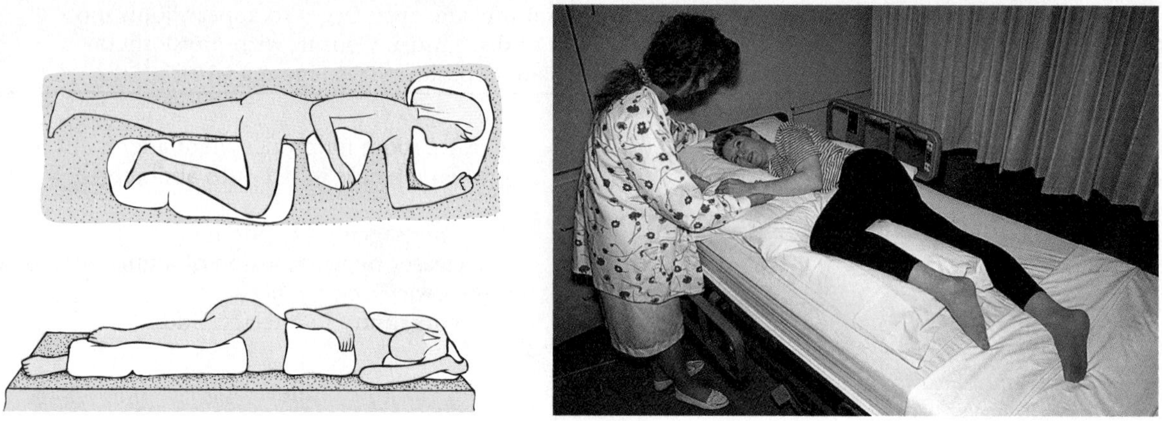

STEP **12I(9)** Side-lying position with pillows in place.

Steps	Rationale
J. Position client in Sims' (semiprone) position	
(1) Lower head of bed completely.	Provides for proper body alignment while client is lying down.
(2) Be sure client is comfortable in supine position.	Prepares client for position. Client is rolled partially onto abdomen.
(3) Position client in lateral position, with dependent arm straight along client's body and with client lying partially on abdomen.	
(4) Carefully lift client's dependent shoulder and bring arm back behind client.	
(5) Place small pillow under client's head.	
(6) Place pillow under flexed upper arm, supporting arm level with shoulder.	Maintains proper alignment and prevents lateral neck flexion. Prevents internal rotation of shoulder. Maintains alignment.
(7) Place pillow under flexed upper legs, supporting leg level with hip.	Prevents internal rotation of hip and adduction of leg. Flexion prevents hyperextension of leg. Reduces mattress pressure on knees and ankles.
(8) Place sandbags or pillows parallel to plantar surface of foot (see illustration).	Maintains foot in dorsiflexion. Prevents footdrop.

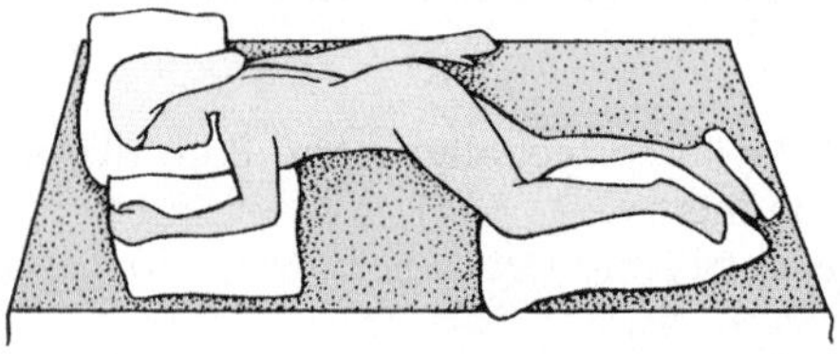

STEP **12J(8)** Sims' (semiprone) position with pillows in place.

Steps	Rationale

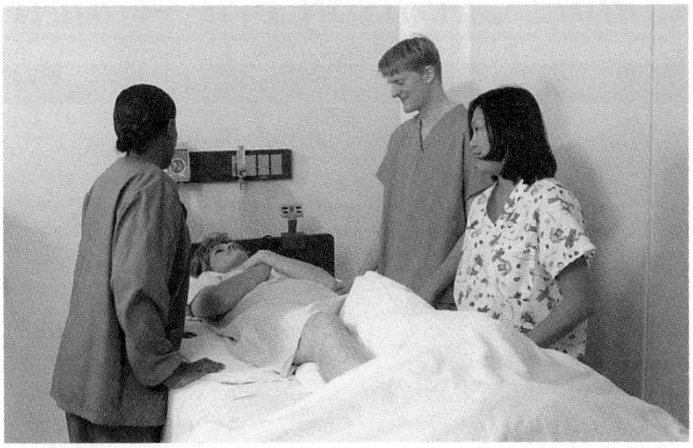

STEP **12K(3)** Position nurses on each side of client.

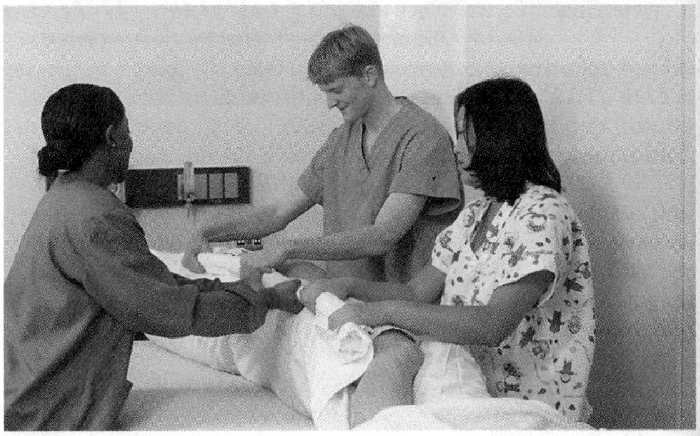

STEP **12K(5)** Move client as a unit, maintaining proper alignment.

K. Logrolling the client (three nurses)

Critical Decision Point: Supervise and aid UCPs when there is a physician's order to **logroll** a client. Clients who have suffered from spinal cord injury or are recovering from neck, back, or spinal surgery often need to keep the spinal column in straight alignment to prevent further injury.

Steps	Rationale
(1) Place pillow between client's knees.	Prevents tension on the spinal column and adduction of the hip.
(2) Cross client's arms on chest.	Prevents injury to arms.
(3) Position two nurses on side of bed to which the client will be turned. Position third nurse on the other side of bed (see illustration).	Distributes weight equally between nurses.
(4) Fanfold or roll the drawsheet or pull sheet.	Provides strong handles in order to grip the drawsheet or pull sheet without slipping.
(5) Move the client as one unit in a smooth, continuous motion on the count of three (see illustration).	This maintains proper alignment by moving all body parts at the same time, preventing tension or twisting of the spinal column.

Skill 42-1 Moving and Positioning Clients in Bed—cont'd

Steps	Rationale

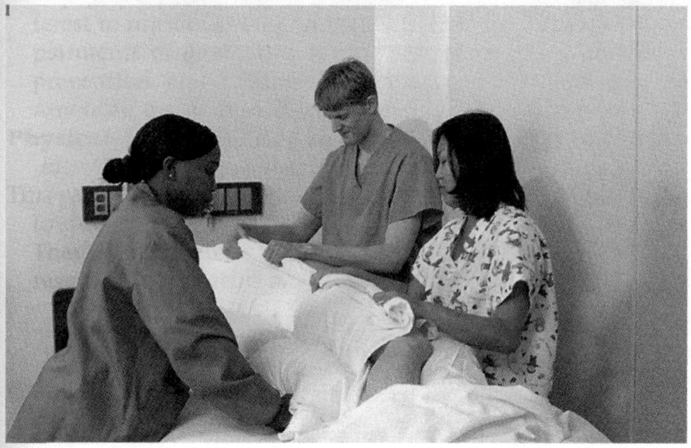

STEP **12K(6)** Place pillows along client's back for support.

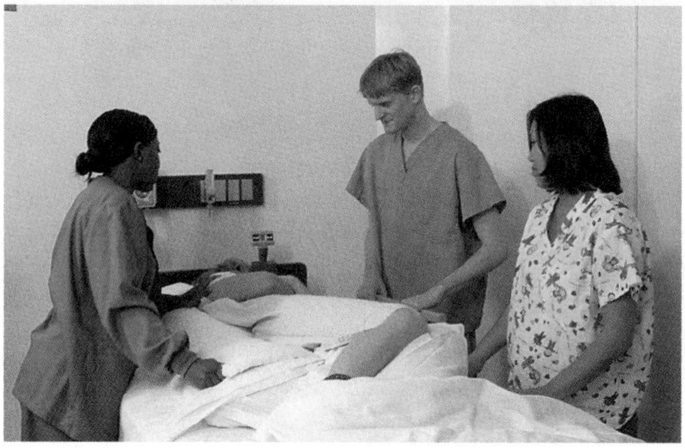

STEP **12K(7)** Gently lean client as a unit against pillows.

Steps	Rationale
(6) Nurse on the opposite side of the bed places pillows along the length of the client (see illustration).	Pillows keep client aligned.
(7) Gently lean the client as a unit back toward the pillows for support (see illustration).	Ensures continued straight alignment of spinal column, preventing injury.
13. Perform hand hygiene.	Reduces transmission of micro-organisms.
14. Evaluate client's level of comfort and ability to assist in position change.	Clients with reduced activity tolerance and increased levels of pain may find position changes very tiring and will need post-position change interventions to restore their level of comfort.
15. Following each position change, evaluate client's body alignment and presence of any pressure areas.	Prompt identification of poor alignment reduces risks to the client's skin and musculoskeletal systems.

Unexpected Outcomes and Related Interventions

- Joint contractures develop or worsen.
  - Improper positioning results in shortening of muscles.
- Skin shows areas of erythema and breakdown.
  - Frequency of repositioning is inadequate.
  - Place turning schedule above client's bed.
- Client avoids moving.
  - Indicates fear of pain.
  - Medicate as ordered by physician to ensure client's comfort before moving.
  - Allow pain medication to take effect before proceeding.

Recording and Reporting

- Record procedure and observations (e.g., condition of skin, joint movement, client's ability to assist with positioning).
- Report observations at change of shift and document in nurses' notes.

Home Care Considerations

- Teach family the importance of body mechanics for themselves and the client.
- Teach client and family about the signs of skin breakdown and the importance of safety during positioning for clients with decreased sensation.

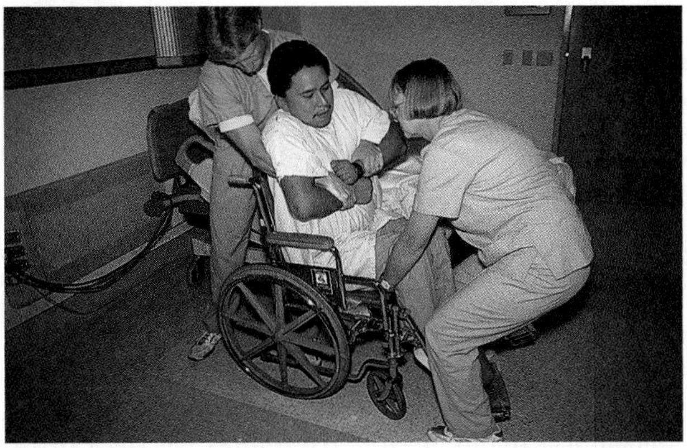

FIGURE **42–23** Transferring an immobile client from bed to wheelchair.

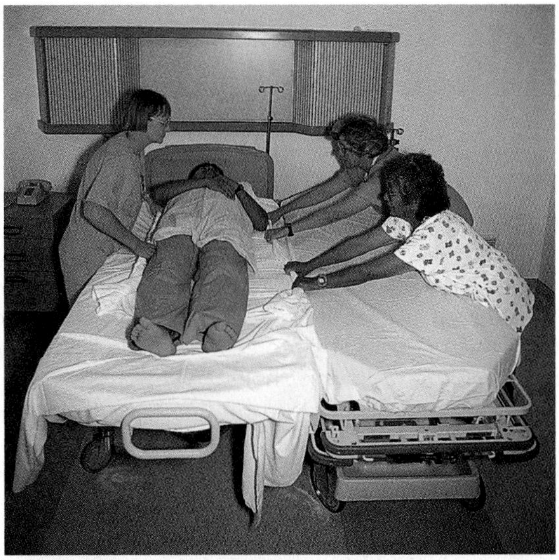

FIGURE **42–24** Use of a drawsheet to transfer a client from bed to stretcher.

mechanics (Figure 42–23). If a client has an immobile lower extremity from a cast or paralysis, the transfer should be toward the unaffected leg.

Transferring a Client From a Bed to a Stretcher. An immobilized client who must be transferred from a bed to a stretcher or from a bed to another bed often requires a three-person carry (see Skill 42-2). This technique is best implemented when personnel who are doing the lifting are similar in height. If their centres of gravity are within the same plane, they can lift as a team. Another way to transfer a client is by using a drawsheet (lift sheet) or a quilted transfer pad placed under the client (Figure 42–24). The drawsheet serves as a "cradle" while the client is being transferred to the stretcher. In this technique, nurses need to be on opposite sides of the bed and holding onto the drawsheet when transferring the client to the stretcher. The stretcher and the bed are placed side by side so that the client can be transferred quickly and easily using the lift sheet. As with all procedures, safety is the priority. Safety is increased in the three-person team if the lifters work together and one person assumes the leadership role.

Caution is used when the client has or is suspected of having spinal cord trauma. If the client must be moved, a transfer board should be placed under the client to maintain spinal alignment before transferring the client to a stretcher. The client should be prepared for the transfer and asked to help when possible (e.g., by folding the arms over the chest). The environment should be free from obstacles, and unnecessary equipment should be removed from the bed.

Restorative Care. The goal of restorative care for the client who is immobile is to maximize functional mobility and independence and reduce residual functional deficits such as impaired gait and decreased endurance. The focus in restorative care is not only on ADLs that relate to physical self-care, but also on **instrumental activities of daily living (IADLs).** IADLs are activities that are necessary to be independent in society beyond eating, grooming, transferring, and toileting and include such skills as shopping, preparing meals, banking, and taking medications.

The nurse uses many of the same interventions as described in the health promotion and acute care sections, but the emphasis is on working collaboratively with clients and their significant others and with other health care professionals. The goal is to enhance quality of life by helping the client return to maximal functional ability in both ADLs and IADLs.

Intensive specialized rehabilitation such as occupational or physiotherapy is common. The client, if in an institution, will likely go to the therapy department two to three times a day. The nurse's role is to work collaboratively with these professionals and reinforce exercises and teaching. For example, after a stroke or brain attack, a client will likely receive gait training from a physiotherapist, speech rehabilitation from a speech therapist, and training from an occupational therapist on food preparation or other household chores. Working with allied health professionals on an interdisciplinary plan of care, the nurse can reinforce and enhance mobilization. The therapy may not be able to restore total functional health but may help the client adapt to the mobility limitations or complications.

Common restorative interventions are focused on regaining mobility. There are evidenced-based protocols that demonstrate that performing exercises to maintain or regain joint mobility and teaching the use of assistive devices for walking are common restorative nursing interventions (Box 42-10). Items frequently used to help adapt to mobility limitations include walkers, canes, wheelchairs, and assistive devices such as toilet seat extenders, reaching sticks, special silverware, and clothing with Velcro closures.

Joint Mobility. To ensure adequate joint mobility, the nurse can teach the client about ROM exercises. When the client does not have voluntary motor control, the nurse institutes passive ROM exercises. Walking also increases

Text continued on p. 1490

Skill 42-2 Using Safe and Effective Transfer Techniques

View Video

Delegation Considerations

The skills of effective transfer techniques can be delegated to unregulated care providers (UCPs). Clients who are transferred for the first time after prolonged bed rest, extensive surgery, critical illness, or spinal cord trauma usually require supervision by professional nurses. When delegating this skill, the nurse should do the following:

- Instruct the UCP to seek assistance before moving or lifting a heavy client.
- Instruct the UCP on any client limitations that may affect safe transfer techniques.

Equipment

- Transfer belt, sling, or lapboard (as needed), non-skid shoes, bath blankets, pillows.
- Wheelchair: Position chair at 45-degree angle to bed, lock brakes, remove footrests, lock bed brakes.
- Stretcher: Position at right angle (90 degrees) to bed, lock brakes on stretcher, lock brakes on bed.
- Mechanical/hydraulic lift: Use frame, canvas strips or chains, and hammock or canvas strips.

Steps	Rationale
1. Assess the client for the following:	Provides information relative to the client's abilities, physical status, ability to comprehend, and the number of individuals needed to provide safe transferring.
a. Muscle strength (legs and upper arms)	Immobile clients have decreased muscle strength, tone, and mass. Affects ability to bear weight or raise body.
b. Joint mobility and contracture formation	Immobility or inflammatory processes (e.g., arthritis) may lead to contracture formation and impaired joint mobility.
c. Paralysis or paresis (spastic or flaccid)	Client with central nervous system damage may have bilateral paralysis (requiring transfer by swivel bar, sliding bar, or mechanical lift) or unilateral paralysis, which requires belt transfer to "best" (unaffected) side. Weakness (paresis) requires stabilization of knee while transferring. Flaccid arm must be supported with sling during transfer.
d. Orthostatic hypotension	Determines risk of fainting or falling during transfer. Immobile clients may have decreased ability for autonomic nervous system to equalize blood supply, resulting in drop of 20 mm Hg or more in systolic blood pressure or 10 mm Hg in diastolic blood pressure when rising from sitting position.
e. Activity tolerance	Determines ability of client to assist with transfer.
f. Presence of pain	Pain may reduce client's motivation and ability to be mobile. Pain relief before transfer enhances client participation.
g. Vital signs	Vital sign changes such as increased pulse and respiration may indicate activity intolerance (see chapter 27).
2. Assess client's sensory status: a. Adequacy of central and peripheral vision b. Adequacy of hearing c. Loss of peripheral sensation	Determines influence of sensory loss on ability to make transfer. Visual field loss decreases client's ability to see in direction of transfer. Peripheral sensation loss decreases proprioception. Clients with visual and hearing losses need transfer techniques adapted to deficits. Clients with cerebrovascular accident (CVA) may lose area of visual field, which profoundly affects vision and perception.

Critical Decision Point: Clients with hemiplegia also may "neglect" one side of the body (inattention to or unawareness of one side of body or environment), which distorts perception of the visual field.

Steps	Rationale
3. Assess client's cognitive status.	Determines client's ability to follow directions and learn transfer techniques.

Critical Decision Point: Clients with head trauma or CVA may have perceptual cognitive deficits that create safety risks. If client has difficulty in comprehension, simplify instructions and maintain consistency.

Steps	Rationale
4. Assess client's level of motivation: a. Client's eagerness versus unwillingness to be mobile b. Whether client avoids activity and offers excuses	Altered psychological states reduce client's desire to engage in activity.
5. Assess previous mode of transfer (if applicable).	Determines mode of transfer and assistance required to provide continuity. Transfer belts should be used with all clients being transferred for the first time and thereafter as deemed necessary.
6. Assess client's specific risk of falling when transferred.	Certain conditions increase client's risk of falling or potential for injury. Neuromuscular deficits, motor weakness, calcium loss from long bones, cognitive and visual dysfunction, and altered balance increase risk of falls.
7. Assess special transfer equipment needed for home setting. Assess home environment for hazards.	Transfer ability at home is greatly enhanced by prior teaching of family and support people, assessment of home for safety risks and functionality.
8. Perform hand hygiene.	Reduces transmission of micro-organisms.
9. Explain procedure to client.	Increases client participation.
10. Transfer client.	
A. Assist client to sitting position (bed at waist level)	
(1) Place client in supine position.	Enables nurse to assess client's body alignment continually and to administer additional care, such as suctioning or hygiene needs.
(2) Face head of bed at a 45-degree angle, and remove pillows.	Proper positioning reduces twisting of nurse's body when moving the client. Pillows may cause interference when the client is sitting up in bed.
(3) Place feet apart with foot nearer bed behind other foot, continuing at a 45-degree angle to the head of the bed.	Improves balance and allows transfer of body weight as client is sitting up in bed.
(4) Place hand farther from client under shoulders, supporting client's head and cervical vertebrae.	Maintains alignment of head and cervical vertebrae and allows for even lifting of client's upper trunk.
(5) Place other hand on bed surface.	Provides support and balance.
(6) Raise client to sitting position by shifting weight from front to back leg. Pivot feet as weight is shifted from front to back leg so that the upper body does not twist.	Improves balance, overcomes inertia, and transfers weight in direction in which client is moved.
(7) Push against bed using arm that is placed on bed surface.	Divides activity between arms and legs and protects back from strain. By bracing one hand against mattress and pushing against it as client is lifted, part of weight that would be lifted by the back muscles is transferred through the arm onto mattress.
B. Assist client to sitting position on side of bed with bed in low position	
(1) Turn client to side, facing you on side of bed on which client will be sitting (see illustration).	Decreases amount of work needed by client and nurse to raise client to sitting position.
(2) With client in supine position, raise head of bed 30 degrees.	Prepares client to move to side of bed and protects from falling.

Skill 42-2 Using Safe and Effective Transfer Techniques—cont'd

Steps	Rationale

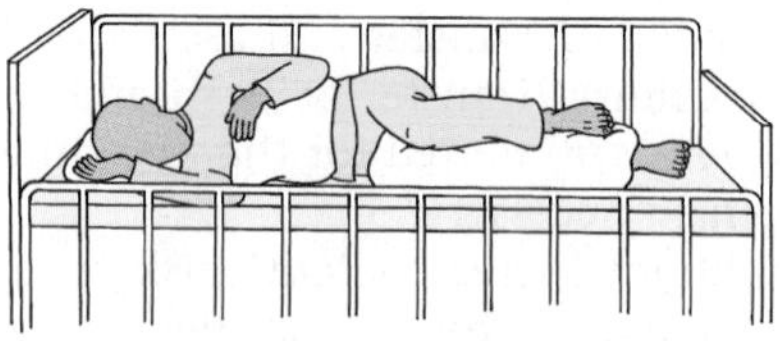

STEP **10B(1)** Side-lying position.

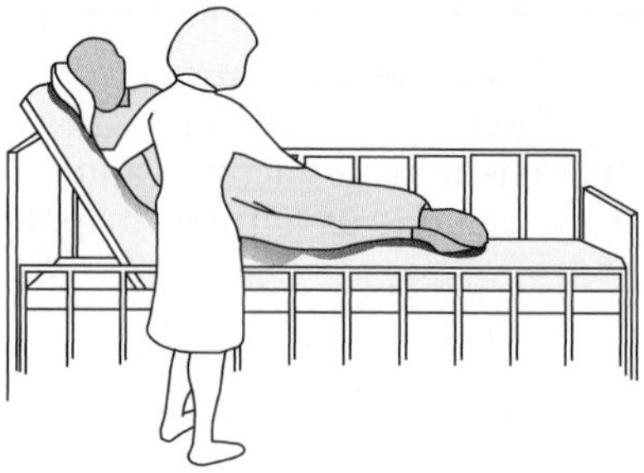

STEP **10B(6)** Nurse places arm over client's thighs.

Steps	Rationale
(3) Stand opposite client's hips. Turn diagonally so that you face client and far corner of foot of bed.	Places nurse's centre of gravity nearer client. Reduces twisting of nurse's body by facing direction of movement.
(4) Place feet apart with foot closer to head of bed in front of other foot.	Increases balance and allows nurse to transfer weight as client is brought to sitting position on side of bed.
(5) Place arm nearer head of bed under client's shoulders, supporting head and neck.	Maintains alignment of head and neck as nurse brings client to sitting position.
(6) Place other arm over client's thighs (see illustration).	Supports hip and prevents client from falling backward during procedure.
(7) Move client's lower legs and feet over side of bed. Pivot toward rear leg, allowing client's upper legs to swing downward.	Decreases friction and resistance. Weight of client's legs when off bed allows gravity to lower legs, and weight of legs assists in pulling upper body into sitting position.
(8) At same time, shift weight to rear leg and elevate client (see illustration). Pivot feet in the direction of movement to avoid twisting of upper body.	Reduces client risk for falling. Immobilized clients may experience light-headedness or dizziness when assuming a sitting position.
C. Transferring client from bed to chair with bed in low position	
(1) Assist client to sitting position on side of bed. Have chair in position at 45-degree angle to bed.	Positions chair within easy access for transfer.
(2) Apply transfer belt or other transfer aids.	Transfer belt maintains stability of client during transfer and reduces risk of falling (Owen, Welden, & Kane, 1999). Client's arm should be in sling if flaccid paralysis is present.
(3) Ensure that client has stable non-skid shoes. Weight-bearing or unaffected (strong) leg is placed forward, with affected (weak) leg back.	Non-skid soles decrease risk of slipping during transfer. Always have client wear shoes during transfer; bare feet increase risk of falls. Client will stand on unaffected (stronger, or weight-bearing) leg.

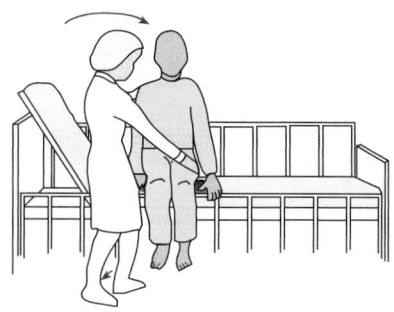

STEP **10B(8)** Nurse shifts weight to rear leg and elevates client.

Steps	Rationale

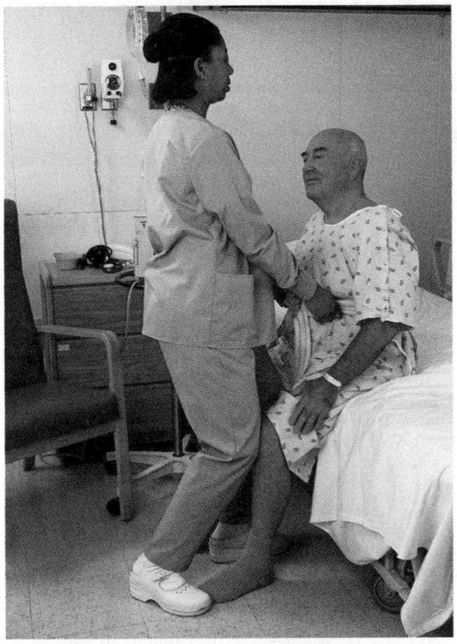

STEP **10C(5)** Nurse flexes hips and knees, aligning knees with client's knees.

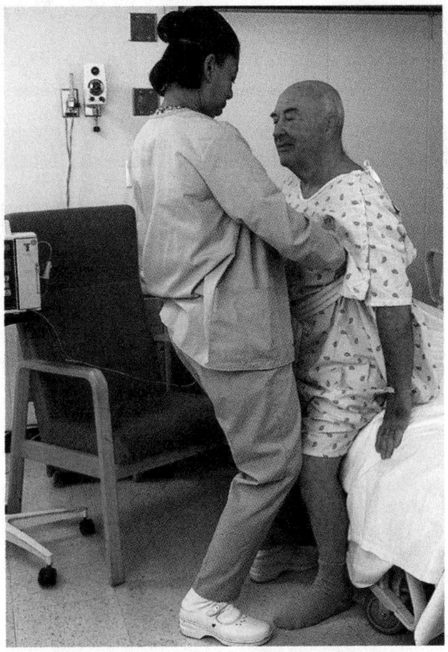

STEP **10C(7)** Nurse rocks client to standing position.

Steps	Rationale
(4) Spread feet apart.	Ensures balance with wide base of support.
(5) Flex hips and knees, aligning knees with client's knees (see illustration).	Flexion of knees and hips lowers the centre of gravity to object to be raised; aligning knees with client's allows for stabilization of knees when client stands.
(6) Grasp transfer belt from underneath.	Transfer belt is grasped at client's side to provide movement of client at centre of gravity. Clients with upper extremity paralysis or paresis should never be lifted by or under arms.

Critical Decision Point: A transfer belt or gait belt with handles should be used in place of the under-axilla technique. The under-axilla technique has been found to be physically stressful for nurses and uncomfortable for clients (Owen et al., 1999).

Steps	Rationale
(7) Rock client up to standing position on count of three while straightening hips and legs and keeping knees slightly flexed (see illustration). Unless contraindicated, client may be instructed to use hands to push up if applicable.	Rocking motion gives client's body momentum and requires less muscular effort to lift client.
(8) Maintain stability of client's weak or paralyzed leg with knee.	Ability to stand can often be maintained in paralyzed or weak limb with support of knee to stabilize.
(9) Pivot on foot farther from chair. Instruct client to stand straight. Pivot body in direction of chair, instructing client to take small steps toward chair. Ask client to tell you when the chair touches the back of his or her knees.	Maintains support of client while allowing adequate space for client to move.
(10) Instruct client to use armrests on chair for support and ease client into chair (see illustration).	Increases client stability.
(11) Flex hips and knees while lowering client into chair (see illustration).	Prevents injury to nurse from poor body mechanics.

Skill 42-2 Using Safe and Effective Transfer Techniques—cont'd

Steps	Rationale

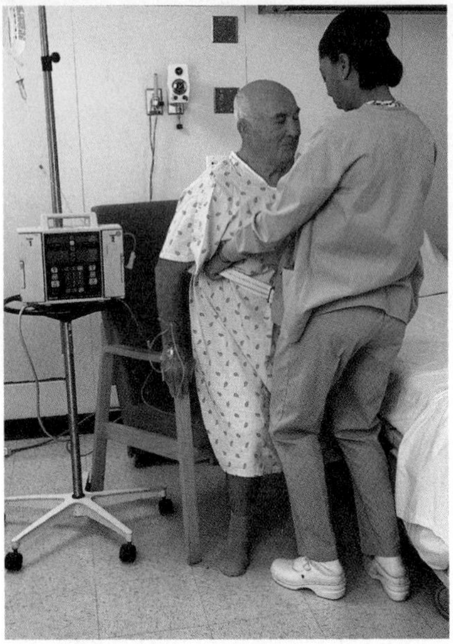

STEP **10C(10)** Client uses armrests for support.

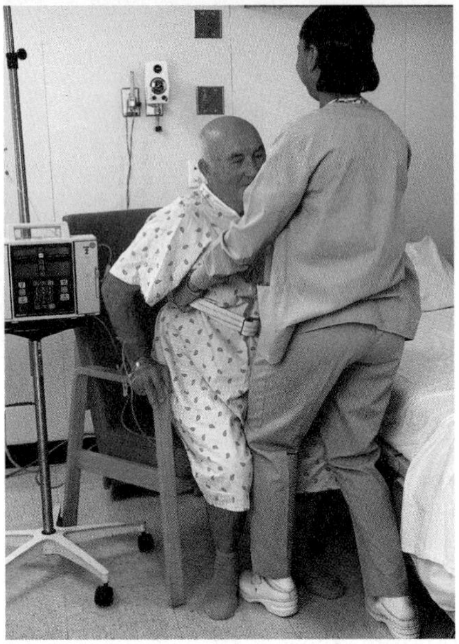

STEP **10C(11)** Nurse flexes hips and knees while easing client into chair.

Steps	Rationale
(12) Assess client for proper alignment for sitting position. Provide support for paralyzed extremities. Lapboard or sling will support flaccid arm. Stabilize leg with bath blanket or pillow.	Prevents injury to client from poor body alignment.
(13) Praise client's progress, effort, or performance.	Continued support and encouragement provide incentive for client perseverance.
D. Perform three-person carry from bed to stretcher (bed at stretcher level)	
(1) Three nurses stand side by side facing side of client's bed.	Prevents twisting of nurses' bodies. Client's alignment is maintained.
(2) Each person assumes responsibility for one of three areas: head and shoulders, hips and thighs, and ankles.	Distributes client's body weight evenly.
(3) Each person assumes wide base of support with foot closer to stretcher in front and knees slightly flexed.	Increases balance and lowers centre of gravity of person lifting.
(4) Arms of lifters are placed under client's head and shoulders, hips and thighs, and ankles, with fingers securely around other side of client's body (see illustration).	Distributes client's weight over forearms of lifters.

Critical Decision Point: Verify that clients with spinal cord injuries are stabilized before transfer. The inexperienced care provider should not attempt to move the spinal cord-injured client.

Steps	Rationale
(5) Lifters roll client toward their chests. On count of three, client is lifted and held against nurses.	Moves workload over lifters' base of support. Enables lifters to work together and safely lift client.

Steps	Rationale

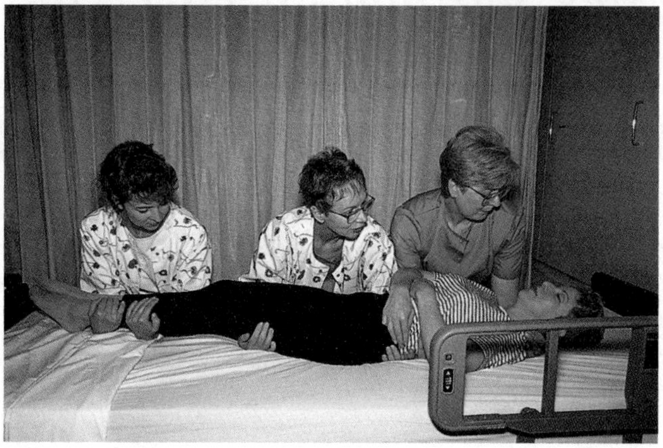

STEP **10D(4)** Proper positioning of lifters during three-person transfer.

Steps	Rationale
(6) On second count of three, nurses step back and pivot toward stretcher, moving forward if needed.	Transfers weight toward stretcher.
(7) Gently lower client onto centre of stretcher by flexing knees and hips until elbows are level with edge of stretcher.	Maintains nurses' alignment during transfer.
(8) Assess client's body alignment, place safety straps across body, and raise side rails.	Reduces risk of injury from poor alignment or falling.
E. Use mechanical/hydraulic lift to transfer client from bed to chair	
(1) Bring lift to bedside.	Ensures safe elevation of client off bed. (Before using lift, be thoroughly familiar with its operation.)
(2) Position chair near bed, and allow adequate space to manoeuvre lift.	Prepares environment for safe use of lift and subsequent transfer.
(3) Raise bed to high position with mattress flat. Lower side rail.	Maintains nurses' alignment during transfer.
(4) Keep bed side rail up on side opposite you.	Maintains client safety.
(5) Roll client on side away from you.	Completes positioning of client on mechanical/hydraulic sling.
(6) Place hammock or canvas strips under client to form sling. Place two canvas pieces so that lower edge fits under client's knees (wide piece), and upper edge fits under client's shoulders (narrow piece).	Two types of seat are supplied are supplied with mechanical/hydraulic lift: hammock style is better for clients who are flaccid, weak, and need support; canvas strips can be used for clients with normal muscle tone. Hooks should face away from client's skin. Place sling under client's centre of gravity and greatest portion of body weight.
(7) Raise bed rail.	Maintains client safety.
(8) Go to opposite side and lower side rail.	
(9) Roll client to opposite side and pull hammock (strips) through.	Completes positioning of client on mechanical/hydraulic sling.
(10) Roll client supine onto canvas seat.	Sling should extend from shoulders to knees (hammock) to support client's body weight equally.
(11) Remove client's glasses, if appropriate.	Swivel bar is close to client's head and could break eyeglasses.
(12) Place lift's horseshoe bar under side of bed (on side with chair).	Positions lift efficiently and promotes smooth transfer.
(13) Lower horizontal bar to sling level by releasing hydraulic valve. Lock valve.	Positions hydraulic lift close to client. Locking valve prevents injury to client.
(14) Attach hooks on strap (chain) to holes in sling. Short chains or straps hook to top holes of sling; longer chains hook to bottom of sling.	Secures hydraulic lift to sling.

Skill 42-2 Using Safe and Effective Transfer Techniques—cont'd

Steps	Rationale
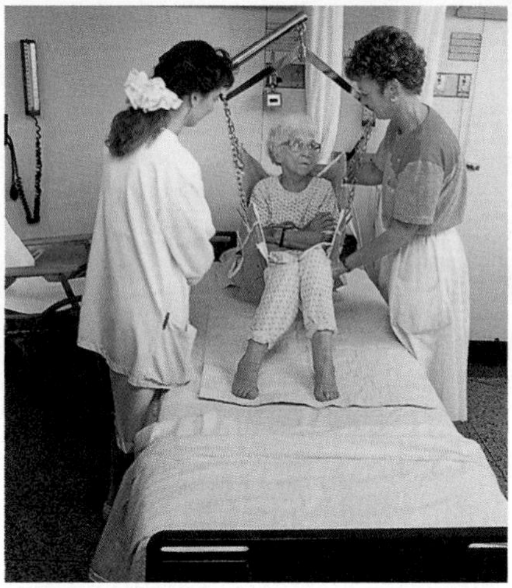 STEP **10E(17)** Proper placement of sling under client.	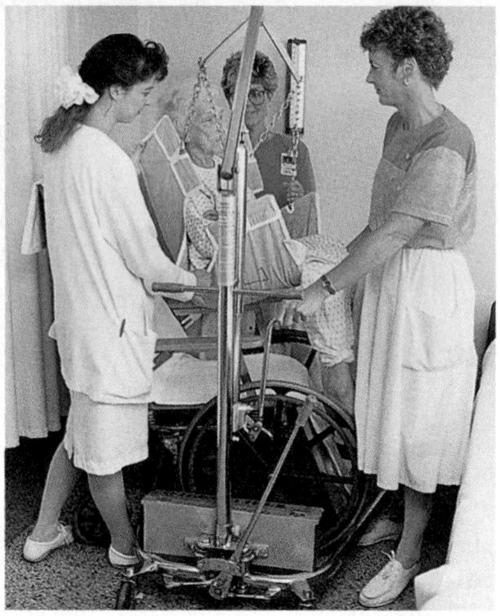 STEP **10E(20)** Use of hydraulic lift to lower client into chair.
(15) Elevate head of bed.	Positions client in sitting position.
(16) Fold client's arms over chest.	Prevents injury to paralyzed arms.
(17) Pump hydraulic handle using long, slow, even strokes until client is raised off bed (see illustration).	Positions client in sitting position.
(18) Use steering handle to pull lift from bed and manoeuvre to chair.	Moves client from bed to chair.
(19) Roll base around chair.	Positions lift in front of the chair in which client is to be transferred.
(20) Release check valve slowly (turn to left) and lower client into chair (see illustration).	Safely guides client into back of chair as seat descends.
(21) Close check valve as soon as client is down and straps can be released.	If valve is left open, boom may continue to lower and injure client.
(22) Remove straps and mechanical/hydraulic lift.	Prevents damage to skin and underlying tissues from canvas or hooks.
(23) Check client's sitting alignment and correct if necessary.	Prevents injury from poor posture.
11. Perform hand hygiene.	Reduces transmission of micro-organisms.
12. With each transfer, evaluate client's tolerance and level of fatigue and comfort.	Increased activity may result in symptoms associated with activity intolerance (e.g., increased pulse, changes in blood pressure, increased respirations, and decreased level of comfort). These clients may find transfer very tiring and will need post-transfer interventions to restore their level of comfort.
13. Following each transfer, evaluate client's body alignment.	Prompt identification of poor alignment reduces risks to the client's skin and musculoskeletal systems.

Unexpected Outcomes and Related Interventions

- Client unable to comprehend and follow directions for transfer.
  - Cognitive impairment affects learning and retention.
  - Reassess continuity and simplicity.
- Client sustains injury on transfer.
  - Indicates improper transfer technique was used.
  - Evaluate incident that caused injury (e.g., assessment inadequate, change in client status, improper use of equipment).
  - Complete incident report according to agency policy.
- Client's level of weakness does not permit active transfer.
  - Physical impairments require increased assistance from nursing personnel.
  - Increase bed activity and exercise to heighten tolerance.
- Client continues to bear weight on non-weight-bearing limb.
  - Certain conditions (e.g., hip fractures) need to be non-weight bearing through healing process.
  - Reassess client's understanding of weight-bearing status.
- Client transfers well on some occasions, poorly on others.
  - Transfers may be difficult when client is fatigued or in pain; assess before transfer (allow for a rest period before transferring, or medicate for pain if indicated).
  - Periodic confusion may also alter performance.
- Client is unable to stand for time required in transfer.
  - Results from increased fatigue, orthostatic hypotension, or pain.
  - Provide for adequate assistance during transfer.
- Localized areas of erythema develop that do not disappear quickly.
  - Complete pressure ulcer assessment and appropriate interventions (see chapter 43).

Recording and Reporting

- Record procedure, including pertinent observations: weakness, ability to follow directions, weight-bearing ability, balance, ability to pivot, number of personnel needed to assist, and amount of assistance (muscle strength) required.
- Report any unusual occurrence to nurse in charge. Report transfer ability and assistance needed to next shift or other caregivers. Report progress or remission to rehabilitation staff (physiotherapist or occupational therapist).

Home Care Considerations

- Teach family members about proper body mechanics for themselves and the client.
- Provide community resources for hospital equipment that can be used in the home setting (e.g., transfer belts, mechanical lifts) to assist in safe transfer techniques.

Evidence-Based Practice Guideline

Box 42-10

Exercise Promotion: Reinitiating Exercise in the Previously Immobile Client

- Assist client in contemplating change in activity level.
- Increase client's awareness of current activity.
- Provide information about the benefits of exercise.
- Determine any barriers to exercise.
- Provide choices of activities.
- Assist client in preparing for an activity program.
- Provide information about how to safely carry out the exercise (e.g., proper walking, safety considerations).
- Assist client in strengthening exercise tolerance and activity.
- Emphasize client's ability to become more active.
- Provide resources for social exercise groups (e.g., fitness groups, community walking programs, walking in local shopping malls).
- Assist client in establishing an activity program.
- Provide positive, constructive feedback.
- Increase activity as appropriate for client's mobility status.
- Assist client in developing a long-term exercise plan.
- Visit the client during an exercise program.
- Assist client in maintaining an activity program.
- Recognize each success.
- If relapse occurs, remind client that it is okay and to continue with the exercise program.
- Maintain a supportive environment.
- Encourage family and friends to participate in the exercise program.

Adapted from "Evidence-Based Protocol: Exercise Promotion: Walking in Elders," by N. Jitramontree, in *Series on Evidence-Based Practice for Older Adults,* edited by M. G. Titler (Series Ed.), 2001, Iowa City, IA: The University of Iowa College of Nursing Gerontological Nursing Interventions Research Center, Research Dissemination Core.

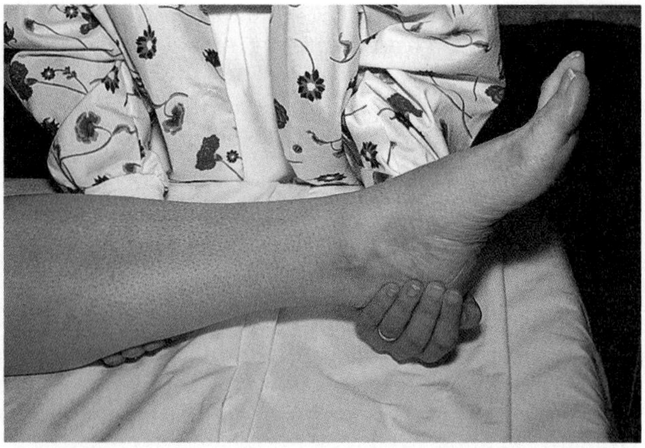

FIGURE **42–25** Using a cupped hand to support a joint.

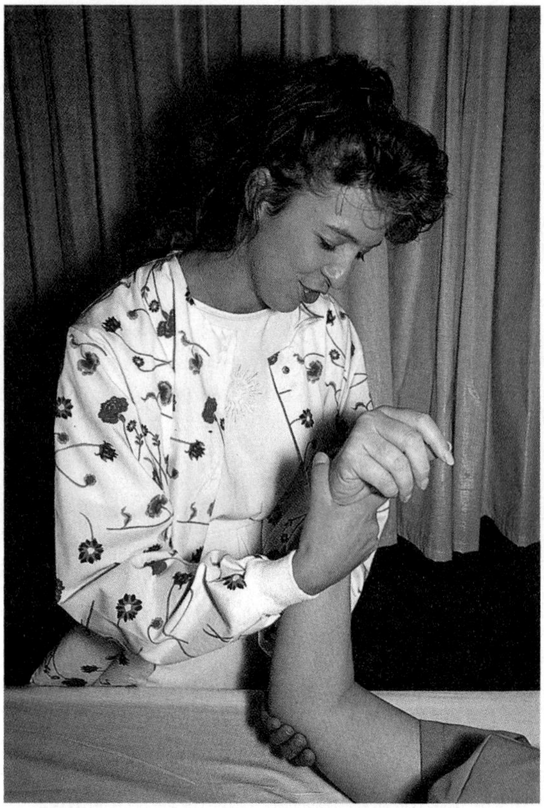

FIGURE **42–26** Supporting the joint by holding the distal and proximal areas adjacent to the joint.

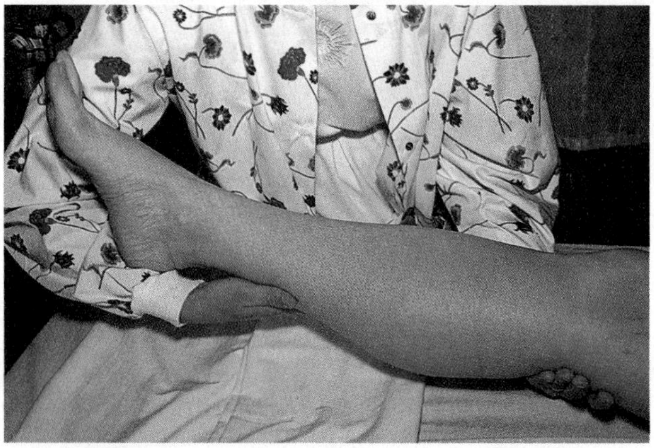

FIGURE **42–27** Cradling the distal portion of an extremity.

joint mobility. Occasionally clients need to use assistive devices such as crutches or walkers to help them walk (see chapter 32).

Range-of-Motion Exercises. Clients with restricted mobility are unable to perform some or all ROM exercises independently. This limitation can be identified in clients in whom one extremity has limited movement or in completely immobilized clients. The nurse provides ROM exercises to maintain maximum joint mobility.

To ensure that clients routinely receive ROM exercises, the nurse should schedule them at specific times, perhaps with another nursing activity, such as during the client's bath. This enables the nurse to systematically reassess mobility while improving the client's ROM. In addition, bathing usually requires that extremities and joints are put through complete ROM.

Unless contraindicated, the care plan should include moving the client's extremities through the fullest ROM possible. ROM exercises may be active, passive, or somewhere in-between. With a weak client, for example, the nurse may support an extremity while the client performs the movement, or the client may be able to move some joints actively while the nurse passively moves others. In general, exercises should be as active as health and mobility allow. Passive ROM exercises should begin as soon as the client's ability to move the extremity or joint is lost. Movements are carried out slowly and smoothly, just to the point of resistance, and should not cause pain. The nurse should never force a joint beyond its capacity. Each movement should be repeated five times during the session.

When performing passive ROM exercises, the nurse stands at the side of the bed closest to the joint being exercised. Passive ROM exercises are performed using a head-to-toe sequence and moving from larger to smaller joints. If an extremity is to be moved or lifted, the nurse places a cupped hand under the joint to support it (Figure 42–25), supports the joint by holding the adjacent distal and proximal areas (Figure 42–26), or supports the joint with one hand and cradles the distal portion of the extremity with the remaining arm (Figure 42–27). The following sections describe an overview of nursing considerations for ways to support major joints in the body. See Table 42-2 for detailed ROM exercises and illustrated motion for each joint.

Neck. A flexion contracture of the neck is a serious disability because the client's neck is permanently flexed with the chin close to or actually touching the chest. Ultimately, the client's body alignment is altered, the visual field is changed, and the level of independent functioning is decreased.

Shoulder. The shoulder is controlled by the deltoid muscle, which is the only muscle that exerts its full strength when in complete elongation. When caring for a client with limited shoulder mobility, the nurse may need to provide support devices for the shoulder, such as slings when the client is standing or sitting or pillows when the client is in bed. Correctly positioning the shoulder prevents pain, joint dislocation, and further changes in body alignment.

Elbow. The elbow functions optimally at an angle of about 90 degrees. An elbow fixed in full extension is disabling and limits the client's independence.

Forearm. Most functions of the hand are best carried out with the forearm in moderate pronation. When the forearm is fixed in a position of full supination, the client's use of the hand is limited.

Wrist. The primary function of the wrist is to place the hand in slight dorsiflexion, the position of functioning. Therefore, full ROM is not as great a priority as maintaining the wrist in a functional position. When the wrist is fixed in even a slightly flexed position, the grasp is weakened. In the immobilized client, the functional position of the wrist can be achieved by using splints.

Fingers and Thumb. The ROM in the fingers and thumb enables the client to perform ADLs and activities requiring fine motor skills, such as carpentry, needlework, drawing, and painting. The functional position of the fingers and thumb is slight flexion of the thumb in opposition to the fingers.

Hip. Because the lower extremities are involved chiefly with locomotion and weight bearing, stability of the hip joint may be more important than its mobility. For example, if the hip has no mobility but is fixed in a neutral position and fully extended, it is possible to walk without a significant limp.

Contractures often fix the hip in positions of deformity. Excessive abduction makes the affected leg appear too short, whereas excessive adduction makes the affected leg appear too long. In either case, the client has limited mobility and walks with an obvious limp. Internal and external rotation contractures cause an abnormal and unbalanced gait.

Knee. A primary function of the knee is stability, which is achieved by ROM, ligaments, and muscles. However, the knees cannot remain stable under weight-bearing conditions unless there is adequate quadriceps power to maintain the knee in full extension. ROM exercises should include pulling the knee into full extension.

An immobile knee joint can result in serious disability. The degree of disability depends on the position in which the knee is stiffened. If the knee is fixed in full extension, the person must sit with the leg thrust out in front. When the knee is flexed, the person limps while walking. The greater the flexion, the greater is the limp.

Ankle and Foot. Without full ROM of the ankle, there will be gait deviations. If the joint is not stable, the person will fall. If joint mobility is diminished, the nurse should maintain the joint in a position in which walking can be carried out with a forward rolling motion from the heel onto the forefoot.

When the person relaxes as in sleep or coma, the foot relaxes and assumes a position of plantar flexion. As a result, the foot may become fixed in plantar flexion (footdrop), which impairs the ability to walk. Inversion and eversion must also be avoided to allow the foot to rest flat on the floor.

Toes. Excessive flexion of the toes results in clawing. When this is a permanent deformity, the foot is unable to rest flat on the floor and the client is unable to walk properly. Flexion contractures are the most common foot deformity associated with reduced joint mobility.

Adequate ROM gives the necessary mobility to carry out ADLs and exercise. In addition, adequate ROM in the lower extremities allows walking.

Walking. In the normal walking posture, the head is erect; the cervical, thoracic, and lumbar vertebrae are aligned; the hips and knees have appropriate flexion; and the arms swing freely with the legs. Illness or trauma can reduce activity tolerance, so that assistance in walking is required. In addition, temporary or permanent damage to the musculoskeletal and nervous systems may necessitate use of an assistive device for walking.

Helping a Client to Walk. When a client's mobility has restricted the ability to walk, the nurse must assess the client's activity tolerance, tolerance to the upright position (orthostatic hypotension), strength, presence of pain, coordination, and balance to determine the amount of assistance needed.

The nurse explains how far the client should try to walk, who is going to help, when the walk will take place, and why walking is important. In addition, the nurse and client determine how much independence the client can assume.

The nurse also checks the environment to be sure that there are no obstacles in the client's path. Chairs, overbed tables, and wheelchairs are cleared out of the way so that the client has ample room to walk safely. Before starting, rest points should be established in case activity tolerance is less than estimated or the client becomes dizzy. For example, a chair might be placed in the hall for the client to rest if needed.

The nurse should provide support at the waist so that the client's centre of gravity remains midline. This can be achieved by placing both hands at the client's waist or using a gait belt. While walking, the client should not lean to one side because this alters the centre of gravity, distorts balance, and increases the risk of falling. The nurse walks to the side and slightly behind the client (Figure 42–28).

A client who at any point appears unsteady or complains of dizziness should be returned to a nearby bed or chair. If the client faints or begins to fall, the nurse should assume a wide base of support with one foot in front of the other, thus supporting the client's body weight. The nurse extends one leg and lets the client slide against the leg and gently lowers the client to the floor, protecting the head. Although lowering a client to the floor is not difficult, the student should practise this technique with a friend or classmate before attempting it in a clinical setting.

Clients with **hemiplegia** (one-sided paralysis) or **hemiparesis** (one-sided weakness) often need assistance to walk.

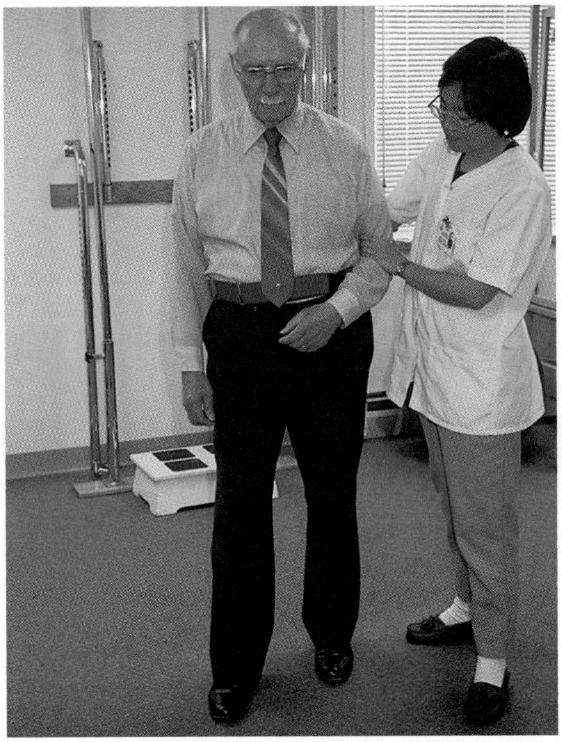

FIGURE **42–28** When helping a client walk, the nurse uses a gait belt and walks slightly behind the client's side. (From *Mosby's Canadian Textbook for the Support Worker,* by S. A. Sorrentino, 2004, Toronto, ON: Elsevier Canada.)

The nurse always stands on the client's affected side and supports the client by holding one arm around the client's waist (or uses a gait belt once the client's stability is ensured) and the other arm around the inferior aspect of the client's upper arm so that the nurse's hand is under the client's axilla. Providing support by holding the client's arm is incorrect because the nurse cannot easily support the weight to lower the client to the floor if the client faints or falls. In addition, if the client falls with the nurse holding an arm, a shoulder joint may be dislocated.

A nurse who does not have a lot of strength and who is unable to ambulate a client alone should request help. The two-nurse method helps distribute the client's weight evenly. The two nurses stand on either side of the client. Each nurse's near arm is around the client's waist, and the other arm is around the inferior aspect of the client's arm so that both nurses' hands are supporting the client's axillae.

Using Assistive Devices for Walking. Clients who are recovering from a lengthy illness that required bed rest and whose mobility is impaired frequently require assistive devices to assist in ambulation. These devices include canes, walkers, and crutches (see chapter 32). The client and family must be educated in the use of these devices.

NP Evaluation

Client Care. To evaluate outcomes and response to nursing care, the nurse measures the effectiveness of all interventions. The actual outcomes are compared with the outcomes selected during planning. The nurse evaluates specific interventions designed to promote body alignment, improve mobility, and protect the client from the hazards of immobility. Client and family teaching to prevent future risks to body alignment and hazards of immobility is also evaluated (Figure 42–29). The evaluation enables the nurse to determine whether new or revised therapies are required and if new nursing diagnoses have developed.

Client Expectations. Clients who are immobile and dependent on others for some or all of their needs can become overly dependent or try to do too much themselves too early. Finding the interdependent balance between independence and dependence is a difficult task. Clients will want control over their mobility that is personally satisfactory. In the client who is completely dependent on others for care, control over how and when things are done may be very important. Do clients feel they are treated with dignity? Do caregivers treat them as adults? Are they given opportunities to make meaningful choices?

Key Concepts

- Body mechanics are the coordinated efforts of the musculoskeletal and nervous systems as the person moves, lifts, bends, stands, sits, lies down, and completes daily activities.
- Coordinated body movement requires integrated functioning of the skeletal system, skeletal muscles, and nervous system.
- The skeletal system provides bony support structure for movement, attachment of ligaments and muscles, protection of vital organs, some of the regulation of calcium, and production of red blood cells.
- The nervous system provides initiation and voluntary control of movement.
- Coordination and regulation of muscle groups depend on muscle tone; activity of antagonistic, synergistic, and anti-gravity muscles; and neural input to muscles.
- Balance is assisted through nervous system control by the cerebellum and inner ear.
- Range-of-motion exercises include one or all of the body joints and can be active or passive.
- Body alignment is the condition of joints, tendons, ligaments, and muscles in various body positions.
- Balance is achieved when there is a wide base of support, the centre of gravity falls within the base of support, and a vertical line falls from the centre of gravity through the base of support.
- Developmental stages influence body alignment and mobility; the greatest impact of physiological changes on the musculoskeletal system is observed in children and older adults.
- The risk of disabilities related to immobilization depends on the extent and duration of immobilization and the client's overall level of health.

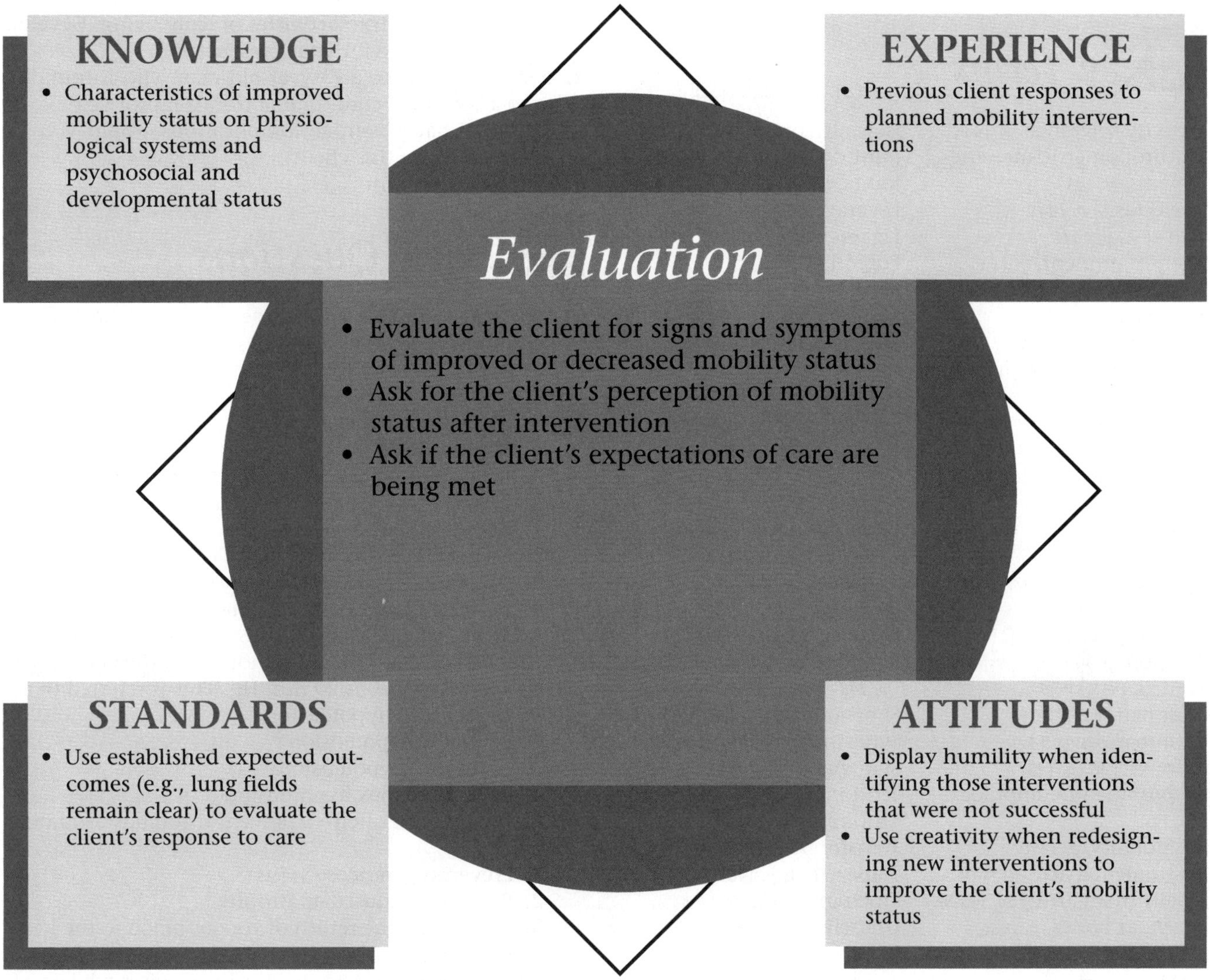
KNOWLEDGE
• Characteristics of improved mobility status on physiological systems and psychosocial and developmental status
EXPERIENCE
• Previous client responses to planned mobility interventions
Evaluation
• Evaluate the client for signs and symptoms of improved or decreased mobility status
• Ask for the client's perception of mobility status after intervention
• Ask if the client's expectations of care are being met
STANDARDS
• Use established expected outcomes (e.g., lung fields remain clear) to evaluate the client's response to care
ATTITUDES
• Display humility when identifying those interventions that were not successful
• Use creativity when redesigning new interventions to improve the client's mobility status

FIGURE **42–29** Critical thinking model for immobility evaluation.

- Immobility may result from illness or trauma or may be prescribed for therapeutic reasons (bed rest).
- Immobility presents hazards in the physiological, psychological, and developmental dimensions.
- The nurse uses the nursing process and critical thinking synthesis to provide care for clients who are experiencing or are at risk for the adverse effects of impaired body alignment and immobility.
- After identifying nursing diagnoses, the nurse plans and implements interventions to prevent or minimize the hazards and complications of impaired body alignment and immobilization.
- Clients with weakness and with impaired nervous, skeletal, or muscular system functioning often require nursing assistance to attain proper body alignment while in bed or sitting and to transfer from a bed to a chair.
- Positioning devices help clients maintain good body alignment while lying or sitting.
- Assistive devices to promote walking include canes, walkers, and crutches.

Key Terms

Activity tolerance, *p. 1448*
Anthropometric measurements, *p. 1454*
Atelectasis, *p. 1442*
Bed rest, *p. 1441*
Body alignment, *p. 1436*
Body mechanics, *p. 1435*
Cartilage, *p. 1437*
Cartilaginous joint, *p. 1437*
Chest physiotherapy (CPT), *p. 1464*
Concentric tension, *p. 1437*
Deconditioning, *p. 1436*
Disuse osteoporosis, *p. 1442*
Eccentric tension, *p. 1437*
Embolus, *p. 1455*
Exercise, *p. 1448*
Fibrous joint, *p. 1437*
Flat bones, *p. 1436*
Footdrop, *p. 1443*
Friction, *p. 1436*
Gait, *p. 1448*
Gait belt, *p. 1471*
Hemiparesis, *p. 1491*
Hemiplegia, *p. 1491*
Hypostatic pneumonia, *p. 1442*
Immobility, *p. 1440*
Instrumental activities of daily living (IADLs), *p. 1481*
Irregular bones, *p. 1436*
Isometric contraction, *p. 1437*
Isotonic contraction, *p. 1437*
Joint contracture, *p. 1443*
Joints, *p. 1437*
Leverage, *p. 1437*
Ligaments, *p. 1437*
Logroll, *p. 1479*
Long bones, *p. 1436*
Mobility, *p. 1440*
Muscle atrophy, *p. 1440*
Muscle tone, *p. 1438*
Negative nitrogen balance, *p. 1441*
Neurotransmitters, *p. 1439*
Orthostatic hypotension, *p. 1442*
Osteoporosis, *p. 1442*
Pathological fractures, *p. 1436*
Posture, *p. 1436*
Pressure ulcer, *p. 1444*
Range of motion (ROM), *p. 1437*
Short bones, *p. 1436*
Synarthrotic joint, *p. 1437*
Synovial joint, *p. 1437*
Tendons, *p. 1437*
Thrombus, *p. 1442*
Transfer belt, *p. 1471*
Trapeze bar, *p. 1469*
Trochanter roll, *p. 1468*
Unossified, *p. 1437*
Urinary stasis, *p. 1443*

Critical Thinking Exercises

1. You are caring for a 57-year-old man who has just had a bilateral total knee replacement for osteoarthritis. He is 2 days post-operative and beginning to transfer to a chair with help. He is 45 kg overweight and has a history of deep vein thrombosis. He has compression stockings, continuous passive range of motion, and a heparin/saline lock. Make a list of potential nursing diagnoses.
2. When you are doing a home visit for a 75-year-old woman, the client's granddaughter runs in and says, "Did you show the nurse the sore on your leg that you got from falling yesterday?" What questions about mobility are important to ask the client? How do you begin your assessment?
3. You are working in a long-term care facility. The nurse in charge asks you to help her with a program titled, "Lifestyle Choices: Living Life to Its Fullest." She asks you to participate and discuss how regular exercise can improve overall health and to show how exercise can be incorporated into activities of daily living. Develop a content outline for your presentation.
4. You are caring for a 75-year-old man who is immobilized after spinal cord trauma from a motor vehicle accident. What potential complications would you be assessing for in this client?

Review Questions

1. A client is unable to dorsiflex or invert her foot, a condition known as
   1. Kyphoscoliosis
   2. Footdrop
   3. Torticollis
   4. Kyphlordosis
2. A physiological risk associated with prolonged immobility is
   1. Decreased bone resorption
   2. Increased cardiac workload
   3. Decreased serum calcium levels
   4. Increased hemoglobin formation
3. A client has been on bed rest for several days. The client stands and the nurse notes that the client's systolic pressure drops 20 mm Hg. This is referred to as
   1. Orthostatic hypotension
   2. Rebound hypotension
   3. Positional hypotension
   4. Central venous hypotension
4. Elastic stockings help to prevent thrombus formation by
   1. Preventing varicose veins
   2. Preventing muscular atrophy
   3. Facilitating the return of venous blood to the heart
   4. Ensuring joint mobility
5. The client at greatest risk for developing adverse effects of immobility is a
   1. 3-year-old child with a fractured femur
   2. 48-year-old woman following a thyroidectomy
   3. 78-year-old man in traction for a broken hip
   4. 38-year-old woman undergoing a hysterectomy
6. A client has been immobilized for 5 days because of extensive abdominal surgery. When getting this client out of bed for the first time, a nursing diagnosis related to the safety of this client would be
   1. Pain
   2. Impaired skin integrity
   3. Altered tissue perfusion
   4. Risk for activity intolerance
7. Heparin and low-molecular-weight heparin are the most widely used drugs in the prophylaxis of deep vein thrombosis. Common dosage for heparin therapy is
   1. 5000 units given subcutaneously 2 hours before surgery and repeated every 8 to 12 hours
   2. 500 units given subcutaneously 2 hours before surgery and repeated every 8 to 12 hours
   3. 500 units given subcutaneously 8 hours before surgery and repeated every 8 to 12 hours
   4. 5000 units given subcutaneously 8 hours before surgery and repeated every 2 to 4 hours

8. The following device allows the client to pull with the upper extremities to raise the trunk off the bed, to assist in transfer from bed to wheelchair, or to perform upper arm exercises:
   1. Trapeze bar
   2. Trochanter roll
   3. Hand rolls
   4. Footboard
9. The client in this position is lying chest down:
   1. Supine
   2. Prone
   3. Fowler's
   4. Lateral
10. When positioning a client in the supported Fowler's position, the nurse places a small pillow under the client's thighs to
    1. Decrease intracranial pressure
    2. Support the lumbar vertebrae
    3. Prevent occlusion of popliteal artery
    4. Prevent pressure of mattress on heel

References

Ackley, B., & Ladwig, G. (2002). *Nursing diagnosis handbook: A guide to planning care* (5th ed.). St. Louis, MO: Mosby.

Agency for Healthcare Research and Quality. (2003). *Pressure ulcers in adults: Prediction and prevention.* Retrieved March 21, 2005, from *http://www.guideline.gov/summary/summary.aspx?ss=15&coc_id=2589&nbr=1815*

Andrews, M., & Boyle, J. (1999). *Transcultural concepts in nursing care* (3rd ed.). Philadelphia: Lippincott.

Association of Workers' Compensation Boards of Canada. (1999). *Work injuries and diseases, 1996–1998* (pp. 20—27). Ottawa, ON: Author.

Banks-Wallace, J. (2000). Staggering under the weight of responsibility: The impact of culture on physical activity among African American women. *The Journal of Multicultural Nursing and Health, 6*(3), 24–30.

Bergquist, S. (2001). Subscales, subscores, or summative score: Evaluating the contribution of Braden scale items for predicting pressure ulcer risk in older adults receiving home health care. *Journal of Wound, Ostomy, and Continence Nursing, 28,* 279–289.

Black, J., Hawks, J., & Keene, A. (2001). *Medical-surgical nursing: Clinical management for positive outcomes* (6th ed.). Philadelphia: Saunders.

Brown, J., & Josse, R. (2002). 2002 Clinical practice guidelines for the diagnosis and management of osteoporosis in Canada. *Canadian Medical Association Journal, 167*(Suppl. 10), S1–S34.

Byrne, B. (2001). Deep vein thrombosis prophylaxis: The effectiveness and implications of using below knee or thigh length graduated compression stockings. *Heart & Lung, 30*(4), 277–284.

Cooper, K., et al. (2001). Health barriers to walking for exercise in elderly primary care, *Geriatric Nursing, 22*(5), 258–262.

Defloor, T. (2000). The effect of position and mattress on interface pressure. *Applied Nursing Research, 13*(1), 2–11.

Deitrick, J. E., Whedon, G. D., & Shorr, E. (1948). Effects of immobilization upon various metabolic and physiological functions of normal men. *American Journal of Medicine, 4,* 3–36.

Dochterman, J. M., & Bulechek, G. M. (Eds.). (2004). *Nursing interventions classification (NIC)* (4th ed.). St. Louis, MO: Mosby.

Dumas, C. (2001). Rehab and the bariatric patient. *Rehab Management, 14(9),* 44–45.

Ebersole, P., & Hess, P. (2001). *Geriatric nursing and healthy aging.* St. Louis, MO: Mosby.

Grer, M. W., & Shekleton, M. E. (1989). *Basic pathophysiology: A holistic approach* (3rd ed.). St. Louis, MO: Mosby.

Im, E., & Choe, M. (2004). Korean women's attitudes toward physical activity. *Research in Nursing and Health, 27*(1), 4–18.

Jain, S., & Brown, D. R. (2001). Cultural dance: An opportunity to encourage physical activity and health in communities. *American Journal of Health Education, 32*(4), 216–222.

Jitramontree, N. (2001). Evidenced-based protocol: Exercise promotion: Walking in elders.In M. G. Titler (Series Ed.), *Series on evidence-based practice for older adults* (pp. 1–53). Iowa City, IA: The University of Iowa College of Nursing Gerontological Nursing Interventions Research Center, Research Dissemination Core.

Johnson, M. (2000). Perceptions of barriers to healthy physical activity among Asian communities. *Sport Education and Society, 5*(1), 51–70.

Lance, R., et al. (2000). Comparison of different methods of obtaining orthostatic vital signs. *Clinical Nursing Research, 9*(4), 479–491.

Ludwick, R. (1999). Clinical decision making: Recognition of confusion and application of restraints. *Orthopedic Nursing, 18,* 65–72.

Ludwick, R., Dieckman, B., & Snelson, C. (1999). Assessment of the geriatric orthopaedic trauma patient. *Orthopedic Nursing, 18,* 13–18.

Maher, A., Salmond, S., & Pellino, T. (2002). *Orthopaedic nursing* (3rd ed.). Philadelphia, PA: Saunders.

McCance, K. L., & Huether, S. E. (2002). *Pathophysiology: The biologic basis for disease in adults and children* (4th ed.). St. Louis, MO: Mosby.

Melillo, K., et al. (2001). Perceptions of older Latino adults regarding physical fitness, physical activity, and exercise. *Journal of Gerontological Nursing, 27*(9), 38–46.

Moorhead, S., Johnson, M., & Maas, M. (Eds.). (2004). *Nursing outcomes classification (NOC)* (3rd ed.). St. Louis, MO: Mosby.

Nelson, A., et al. (2003). Safe patient handling movement. *American Journal of Nursing, 103*(3), 32–43.

Nunnelee, J. (1997). Low molecular-weight heparin. *Journal of Vascular Nursing, 15*(3), 94–96.

Ontario Hospital Association. (2002). *Zero-lift policies: Are they for everyone?* Health Care Health & Safety Association of Ontario. Retrieved February 22, 2005, from Ontario Hospital Association Web site: *http://www.oha.com/client/OHA/OHA_LP4W_LND_WebStation.nsf/resources/Zero+Lifts/$file/ZeroLifts.pdf*

Owen, B., Welden, N., & Kane, J. (1999). What are we teaching about lifting and transferring patients? *Research in Nursing & Health, 22,* 3–13.

Registered Nurses Association of Ontario. (2002a). *Assessment and management of stage I to IV pressure ulcers.* Retrieved February 22, 2005, from *http://www.rnao.org/bestpractices/completed_guidelines/BPG_Guide_C2_pressure_ ulcer.asp*

Registered Nurses Association of Ontario. (2002b). *Prevention of falls and fall injuries in the older adult.* Retrieved February 22, 2005, from *http://www.rnao.org/bestpractices/completed_guidelines/BPG_Guide_C1_Prevent_Falls.asp*

Resnick, B. (2000). Functional performance and exercise of older adults in long-term care settings. *Journal of Gerontological Nursing, 26*(3), 7–16.

Sorrentino, S. A. (2004). *Mosby's Canadian textbook for the support worker.* Toronto, ON: Elsevier Canada.

Takata, S., & Yasui, N. (2001). Disuse osteoporosis. *Journal of Medical Investigation, 48,* 147–156.

Van Haastregt, J., et al. (2000). Preventing falls and mobility problems in community-dwelling elders: The process of creating a new intervention. *Geriatric Nursing, 21*(6), 309–314.

Recommended Web Sites

American Association of Rehabilitation Nurses: Related Sites:

http://www.rehabnurse.org/sites/index.html

This page provides an extensive list of links to Web pages of interest to nurses working with clients with actual/potential impairments or disabilities. It provides information about both prevention and treatment. Although the content has an American orientation, it is also useful to Canadian nurses.

Physical Activity Guide to Healthy Active Living:

http://www.hc-sc.gc.ca/hppb/paguide/index.html

This page is a general guide to physical activity and includes links to specific physical activity guides for older adults and children. These activity guides are a good source of consumer education regarding the benefits of activity.

The Osteoporosis Society of Canada: Health Professionals Resource Links:

http://www.osteoporosis.ca/english/For%20Health%20Professionals/Related%20Links/default.asp?s=1

The Osteoporosis Society of Canada is a national organization working toward educating and supporting individuals and communities in the prevention and treatment of osteoporosis. This site provides numerous links to Web pages featuring evidence-based information on osteoporosis.

43

Skin Integrity and Wound Care

Janice C. Colwell, RN, MS, CWOCN
Deborah Mings, RN, MHSc, ACNP, GNC(C) (Canadian author)

Objectives

Mastery of content in this chapter will enable the student to:

- Define the key terms listed.
- Describe how wounds are classified.
- List common causes of pressure ulcers.
- List the four stages of pressure ulcers.
- List factors that impair wound healing.
- Describe the differences between wounds healing by primary and secondary intention.
- Discuss the three phases of wound healing.
- Differentiate the types of wound drainage.
- Describe wound-related complications.
- Describe how to assess for a client's risk of developing pressure ulcers.
- Describe how to assess the skin for signs of a pressure ulcer.
- Explain how to assess wounds in emergency and stable settings.
- List nursing diagnoses associated with impaired skin integrity.
- Develop a nursing care plan for a client with impaired skin integrity.
- List nursing measures to prevent pressure ulcer formation.
- List appropriate nursing measures for a client with a wound.
- State evaluation criteria for a client with impaired skin integrity.

The skin is the body's largest organ, contributing to one sixth of the total body weight (Wysocki, 2000). It is a protective barrier against disease-causing organisms; it is a sensory organ for pain, temperature, and touch; and it can synthesize vitamin D. Injury to the skin poses risks to safety and triggers a complex healing response. One of the nurse's most important responsibilities is to monitor skin integrity and plan and implement interventions to maintain skin integrity. Knowing the normal healing pattern helps the nurse to recognize alterations that require intervention.

Scientific Knowledge Base

Skin Integrity

The skin is comprised of three layers: the epidermis, dermis, and subcutaneous fatty tissue (Figure 43–1). The **epidermis,** or the top layer, consists of several layers of epithelial cells. The stratum corneum is the thin, outermost layer of the epidermis. It consists of flattened, dead, keratinized cells. The cells originate from the innermost epidermal layer, commonly called the

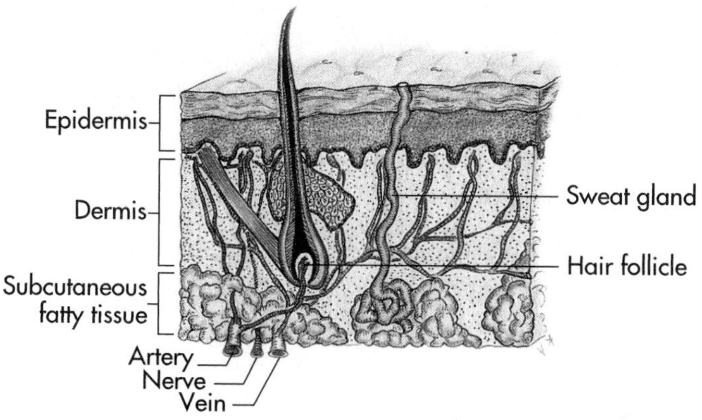

FIGURE **43–1** A cross section of the skin reveals three layers: epidermis, dermis, and subcutaneous fatty tissue.

basal layer. Cells in the basal layer divide, proliferate, and migrate toward the epidermal surface. After cells reach the stratum corneum, they flatten and die. This constant movement ensures replacement of surface cells sloughed during normal desquamation. The thin stratum corneum protects underlying cells and tissues from dehydration and prevents entrance of certain chemical agents. The stratum corneum allows evaporation of water from the skin and permits absorption of certain topical medications.

The **dermis,** the inner layer of the skin, provides tensile strength, mechanical support, and protection to the underlying muscles, bones, and organs. It differs from the epidermis in that it contains mostly connective tissue and few skin cells. **Collagen** (a tough, fibrous protein), blood vessels, and nerves are found in the dermal layer. Fibroblasts, which are responsible for collagen formation, are the only distinctive cell type within the dermis.

Subcutaneous tissue is mostly made up of fat, blood vessels, and connective tissue. This layer binds the skin to underlying structures, regulates body and skin temperature, and stores energy in the form of fat.

Understanding skin structure helps the nurse maintain skin integrity and promote wound healing. Intact skin protects the client from chemical and mechanical injury. When the skin is injured, the epidermis functions to resurface the wound and restore the barrier against invading organisms, and the dermis responds to restore the structural integrity (collagen) and the physical properties of the skin.

Wound Classifications

A **wound** is a disruption of normal anatomical structure and function that results from pathological processes beginning internally or externally to the involved organ(s) (Lazarus et al., 1994). Skin wounds are usually classified according to the following criteria:

- *Cause.* An *intentional wound* is created for therapy (e.g., surgical incisions, venipunctures for intravenous [IV] therapy). An *unintentional wound* occurs unexpectedly and is caused by trauma (e.g., falls, vehicle accidents, stabbings).
- *Intactness of the skin.* An *open wound* involves a break in skin, and loss of blood and body fluids occurs through the wound. A *closed wound* does not involve a break in the skin and can result in internal hemorrhage. Table 43-1 lists types of open and closed wounds.
- *Depth.* Wound depth refers to the tissue layers affected by the wound. *Partial-thickness wounds* are shallow wounds involving loss of the epidermis and possibly partial loss of the dermis. They heal by regeneration. *Full-thickness wounds* involve the dermis, epidermis, subcutaneous tissue, and possibly even muscle, bone, and supporting structures (e.g., tendon and joint capsules). These wounds generally heal by scar formation.
- *Cleanliness.* Cleanliness refers to risk of infection and includes the following:
  - *Clean wounds* contain no pathogenic organisms. Closed wounds are usually clean, as are closed surgical wounds created under sterile condition, provided they do not enter the alimentary, respiratory, or genital tracts.
  - *Clean-contaminated wounds* are intentional wounds made under aseptic conditions that involve a body cavity that normally harbours micro-organisms (i.e., surgical wounds that enter the alimentary, respiratory, or genital tracts). These wounds have a greater risk of infection than do clean wounds.
  - *Contaminated wounds* exist under conditions in which the presence of micro-organisms is likely. Contaminated wounds may show signs of inflammation and have a high risk of infection. Unintentional, open wounds are generally contaminated. Wound contamination also occurs in surgical wounds if there has been a break in surgical asepsis.
  - *Infected wounds* contain large amounts of bacteria (usually above 10^5 organisms per gram of tissue) and show signs of infection. Examples include any wound that does not properly heal and grows organisms, surgical incisions into infected areas, and traumatic injuries that rupture the bowel.
- *Duration of wound: acute versus chronic.* An *acute wound* follows the normal healing process in an orderly and timely way (Kane, 2001). Acute wounds usually have clean and intact edges and are easily cleaned. A *chronic wound* does not heal easily and the skin does not soon return to its normal appearance and function. Any wound that is continually exposed to friction, pressure, or moisture can become chronic. Chronic wounds are caused by various factors; for example, open wounds on the lower legs and feet may be caused by decreased blood flow (arterial ulcers) or poor blood return through the veins (stasis ulcers). When discussing chronic wounds, this chapter focuses on pressure ulcers because these wounds are very prevalent in health care facilities and can often be prevented with good nursing practice. Many strategies presented in this chapter for healing and prevention of pressure ulcers can be applied to other chronic wounds.

Pressure Ulcers

Pressure ulcer, pressure sore, decubitus ulcer, and *bedsore* are terms used to describe chronic wounds caused by unrelieved, prolonged pressure. A **pressure ulcer** is a localized area of tissue necrosis that develops when soft tissue is compressed between a bony prominence and an external

Table 43-1 Types of Wounds

Type	Description	Implications for Healing
Contusion (closed wound)	Bruising of the skin caused by a blow to the body by a blunt object. Skin appears swollen and discoloured.	Wound is more severe if internal organ is contused. Wound may cause temporary loss of function of body part. Localized bleeding into tissues may form hematoma (collection of blood).
Abrasion (open wound)	A scraping or rubbing of the skin's surface. May be unintentional (e.g., skinned knee from a fall) or intentional (e.g., a dermatological procedure for removing scar tissue)	Wound is painful from exposure of superficial nerves; deeper tissues are not involved. There is risk of infection from exposure to contaminated surface.
Incision (open wound)	A cut to the skin made by a sharp instrument (e.g., knife or scalpel), resulting in a wound with clean, straight edges. Usually intentionally produced.	The wound may be deep or shallow and is often painful.
Laceration (open wound)	Tearing of tissues resulting in irregular wound edges. Usually an unintentional injury caused by trauma (e.g., knife wound, accident involving machinery, tissues cut by broken glass).	Wound is usually created by contaminated object and is at risk for infection. Depth of wound determines other complications.
Puncture (open wound)	Entry of the skin and underlying tissues by a sharp object.	Risk of infection is high.
Penetrating (open wound)	Piercing of the skin and underlying tissues with a foreign object or instrument; usually unintentional (e.g., stab wound).	Risk of infection is high. Wound may cause internal and external hemorrhage; damage to organs possible.
Ulcer (open wound)	A break in skin or mucous membrane with loss of surface tissue and necrosis (decay) of epithelial tissue.	Risk of infection is high. A chronic wound.

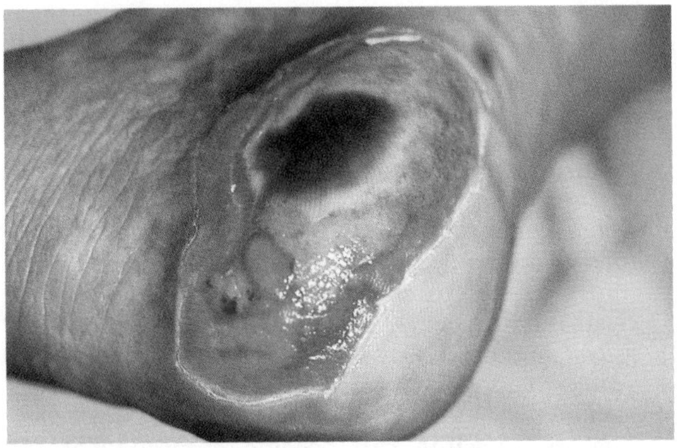

FIGURE **43–2** Pressure ulcer with tissue necrosis.

surface for a prolonged period of time (National Pressure Ulcer Advisory Panel [NPUAP], 1995b; Figure 43–2).

Pressure ulcers have a high prevalence rate in all health care settings. It is estimated that approximately 26% of clients in Canadian health care settings develop pressure ulcers (Houghton & Woodbury, 2004). Acute care settings have a prevalence rate of 25%; non-acute care settings (including long-term care facilities), 30%; and community care/home care settings, 15% (Houghton & Woodbury, 2004).

The impact of pressure ulcers on quality of life is significant, as normal activities may be restricted, healing time may be lengthy, and high costs are associated with pressure ulcer care. Although treatment of pressure ulcers is more costly than prevention (Richardson, Gardner, & Frantz, 1998), preventive measures are also expensive. Extra equipment, such as specialty beds and mattresses, and increased nursing time are needed to administer these measures. When an ulcer develops, mean hospital costs and length of stay increase (Allman et al., 1999).

Causes of Pressure Ulcers. Many factors contribute to the formation of a pressure ulcer. Pressure is the major cause. Tissues receive oxygen and nutrients and eliminate metabolic wastes via the blood. Unrelieved pressure restricts blood flow and therefore interferes with cellular metabolism and the function or survival of the cells. When blood supply to the tissues is deficient **(ischemia),** the tissue decays **(necrosis),** causing an ulcer.

Pressure occurs when the tissue is compressed between a bone and an external surface, usually the surface of a bed or chair. Therefore, pressure ulcers occur over a bony prominence. These bony prominences are called *pressure points* because they bear the weight of the body in certain positions and thus are at greatest risk for forming pressure ulcers (Figure 43–3). Pressure points include, for example, the elbows, hips, shoulder blades, ankle bones, sacrum, knees, and heels. Low pressures over a prolonged period of time can cause tissue damage, as can high-intensity pressure over a short period of time. Figure 43–4 shows a pressure ulcer that has developed on a client's heel from the pressure exerted by the heel on the mattress. A frequent repositioning schedule and the use of pressure-relieving devices (e.g., pillows, foam wedges, therapeutic mattresses) minimize the risk of pressure.

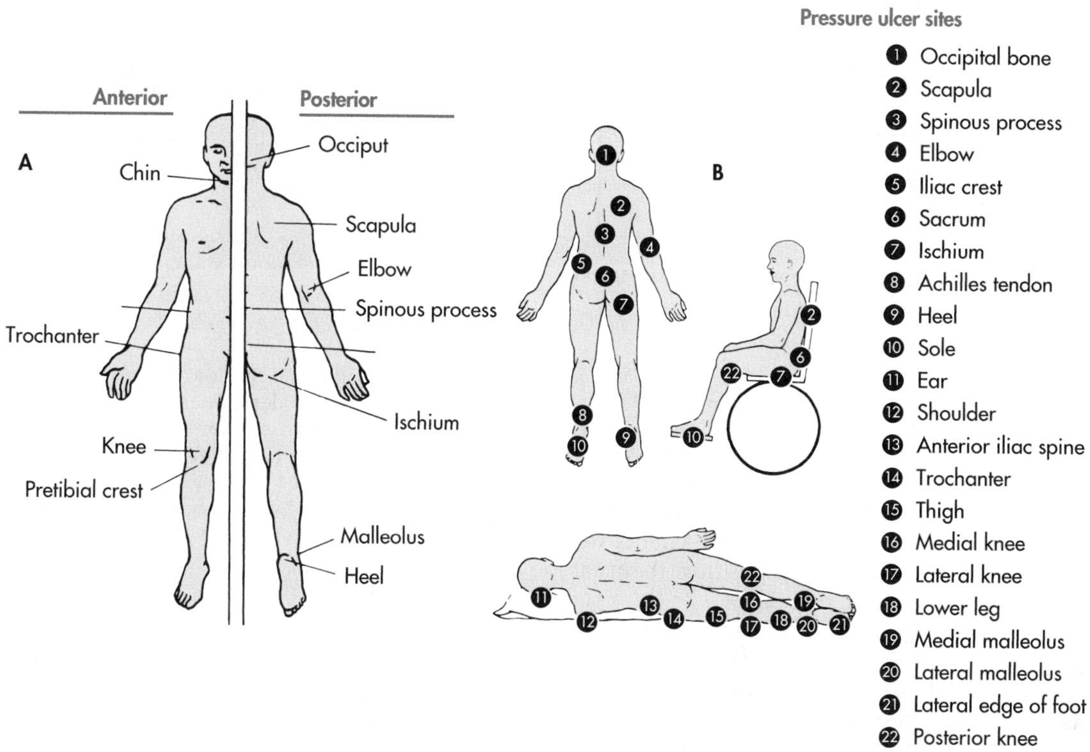

FIGURE **43–3** **A,** Bony prominences most frequently underlying pressure ulcer. **B,** Common pressure ulcer sites. (Adapted from "Developing Standards for Wound Care," by C. C. Trelease, 1988, *Ostomy/Wound Management, 20,* p. 46.)

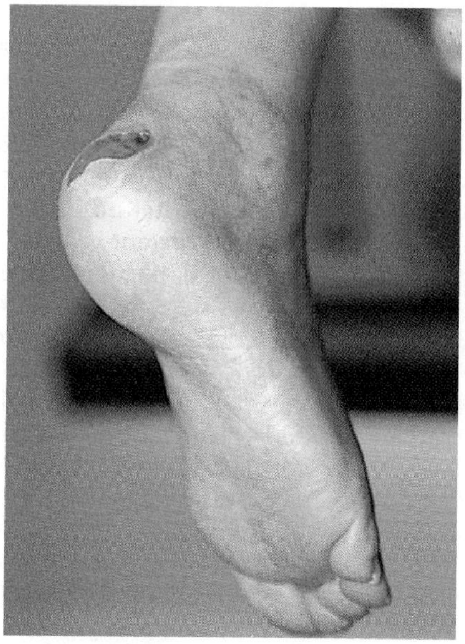

FIGURE **43–4** A pressure ulcer on the heel caused by pressure exerted by the mattress.

Although pressure is the greatest factor causing pressure ulcers, other factors work with pressure to damage the skin:

- *Friction.* **Friction** is the mechanical force of two surfaces rubbing across one another. Friction occurs when skin is dragged across a coarse surface such as bed linens, a cast, or a brace, often resulting in an abrasion and making the skin vulnerable to further breakdown. A friction injury can occur when a client is dragged rather than lifted from the bed surface during position changes. The use of turning sheets and trapeze bars will decrease the effects of friction (Dolynchuk et al., 2000).
- *Shearing force.* **Shearing** is the force that moves the layers of muscles and bones in a direction opposite to the skin. The underlying tissue capillaries are stretched and angulated by the shear force. As a result, necrosis occurs deep within the tissue layers. The tissue damage occurs deep in the tissues, causing undermining at the point of pressure. Shearing most often occurs when a client slides down or is dragged up in a bed or chair. The skin and subcutaneous layers adhere to the surface, but the layers of muscles and bones slide in the direction the body is moving (Figure 43–5). The risk of shearing can be minimized by keeping the head of the bed below 30 degrees and properly positioning clients in wheelchairs (Dolynchuk et al., 2000).
- *Moisture.* Prolonged moisture on the skin causes **maceration** (the softening of the skin), which can lead to skin breakdown. Moisture can be caused by wound drainage, excessive perspiration, and incontinence. Keeping the client's skin clean and dry is essential for preventing pressure ulcers (see chapters 34 and 40).

Clients are more vulnerable to pressure if they are unable to easily and independently change positions. The

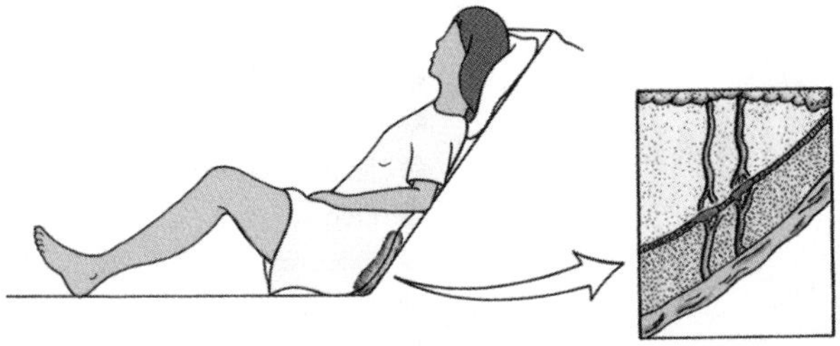

FIGURE **43–5** Sketch of shearing force exerted against sacral area.

following conditions therefore increase the risk of developing pressure ulcers:

- *Impaired mobility.* Clients who are restricted to a bed or wheelchair or who are unable to move certain parts of the body without assistance are less able to reposition themselves to relieve pressure. Immobile clients depend on the nurse to frequently reposition them (at least every 2 hours) to relieve pressure.
- *Altered level of awareness.* Clients who are confused, disoriented, or have changing levels of consciousness are unable to protect themselves from pressure ulcer development (e.g., clients in a coma or with Alzheimer's disease). They may be able to feel the pressure but may not understand how to relieve it or how to communicate their discomfort.
- *Impaired sensory perception.* Clients with altered pain perception (e.g., clients with paralysis or neurological disease) may not be able to respond to warning signs of increased pressure. They may not change position or ask assistance in changing positions. Sedative medications can also decrease sensory perception.

Finally, certain factors that are intrinsic to the client also affect tissue tolerance and increase the risk of pressure ulcer development, including the following:

- *Blood supply.* Chronic vascular diseases, such as diabetes, prevent areas of the body from having proper blood flow, thus increasing the risk of pressure ulcers.
- *Nutritional status.* Malnutrition is a serious risk factor for developing pressure ulcers. Poorly nourished skin is prone to injury. Inadequate intake of protein, calories, fluids, and nutrients—particularly zinc and vitamins A and C—is associated with greater risk of pressure ulcer development and poor wound healing (Dolynchuk et al., 2000).
- *Advanced age.* Changes to the skin that naturally occur with aging make older adults more prone to developing pressure ulcers (Box 43-1). Age can alter skin characteristics and make skin more vulnerable to damage.

Stages of Pressure Ulcer Formation. A pressure ulcer, like other chronic wounds, is classified in stages according to its severity. These stages range from redness of the skin to a deep, open wound with blackened tissue. There are several different staging systems that are used clinically (Agency for Health Care Policy and Research [AHCPR], 1994). The staging system devised by the National Pressure Ulcer Advisory Panel (NPUAP, 1989) is recommended by the Registered Nurses Association of Ontario (RNAO; 2002a, 2005) and the Canadian Association of Wound Care (CAWC). The NPUAP staging system is as follows:

- *Stage I.* A stage I pressure ulcer is an observable pressure-related alteration of intact skin whose indicators, as compared with an adjacent or opposite area on the body, may include changes in skin temperature (warmth or coolness), tissue consistency (firm or beefy feel), and/or sensation (pain, itching). The ulcer appears as a defined area of persistent redness in lightly pigmented skin, whereas in darker skin tones, the ulcer may appear with persistent red, blue, or purple hues (Figure 43–6, *A*). There are no open skin areas.
- *Stage II.* With a stage II ulcer, there is partial-thickness skin loss involving the epidermis, dermis, or both. The ulcer is superficial and presents clinically as an abrasion, blister, or shallow crater (Figure 43–6, *B*).
- *Stage III.* At stage III, there is full-thickness skin loss, involving damage to or necrosis of epidermis, dermis, and subcutaneous tissue. Tissue damage may extend down to, but not through, underlying fascia. The ulcer presents clinically as a deep crater, with or without undermining of adjacent tissue (Figure 43–6, *C*).
- *Stage IV.* A stage IV ulcer involves full-thickness skin loss with extensive destruction, tissue necrosis, or damage to muscle, bone, or supporting structures (e.g., tendon and joint capsules) (Figure 43–6, *D*).

Pressure ulcer staging is used to describe the pressure ulcer depth at the point of assessment. Thus, once the pressure ulcer is staged, this stage endures even as the pressure ulcer heals. Pressure ulcers do not progress from a stage III

Focus on Older Adults **Box 43-1**

Changes in Skin and Other Factors That Increase the Risk of Pressure Ulcers

- The attachment between the epidermis and dermis becomes flattened in older adults, allowing the skin to be easily torn in response to mechanical trauma (e.g., tape removal). This also increases the skin's susceptibility to shearing forces.
- The underlying muscle and tissues (hypodermis) thins with age; thus, older adults have little subcutaneous padding over bony prominences (Wysocki, 2000).
- The production of new skin cells slows down, meaning the epidermis does not replace itself as quickly as in younger adults and wound healing is slower.
- The normal age-related changes, such as reduced skin elasticity, increased skin dryness, and decreased collagen, cause the older adult's skin to be easily bruised and susceptible to injury, especially shearing forces (Wysocki, 2000).
- Concomitant medical conditions and medications prescribed to treat them may interfere with wound healing.
- Aging causes impaired immune function, which slows epithelialization and wound healing (Waldrop & Doughty, 2000).

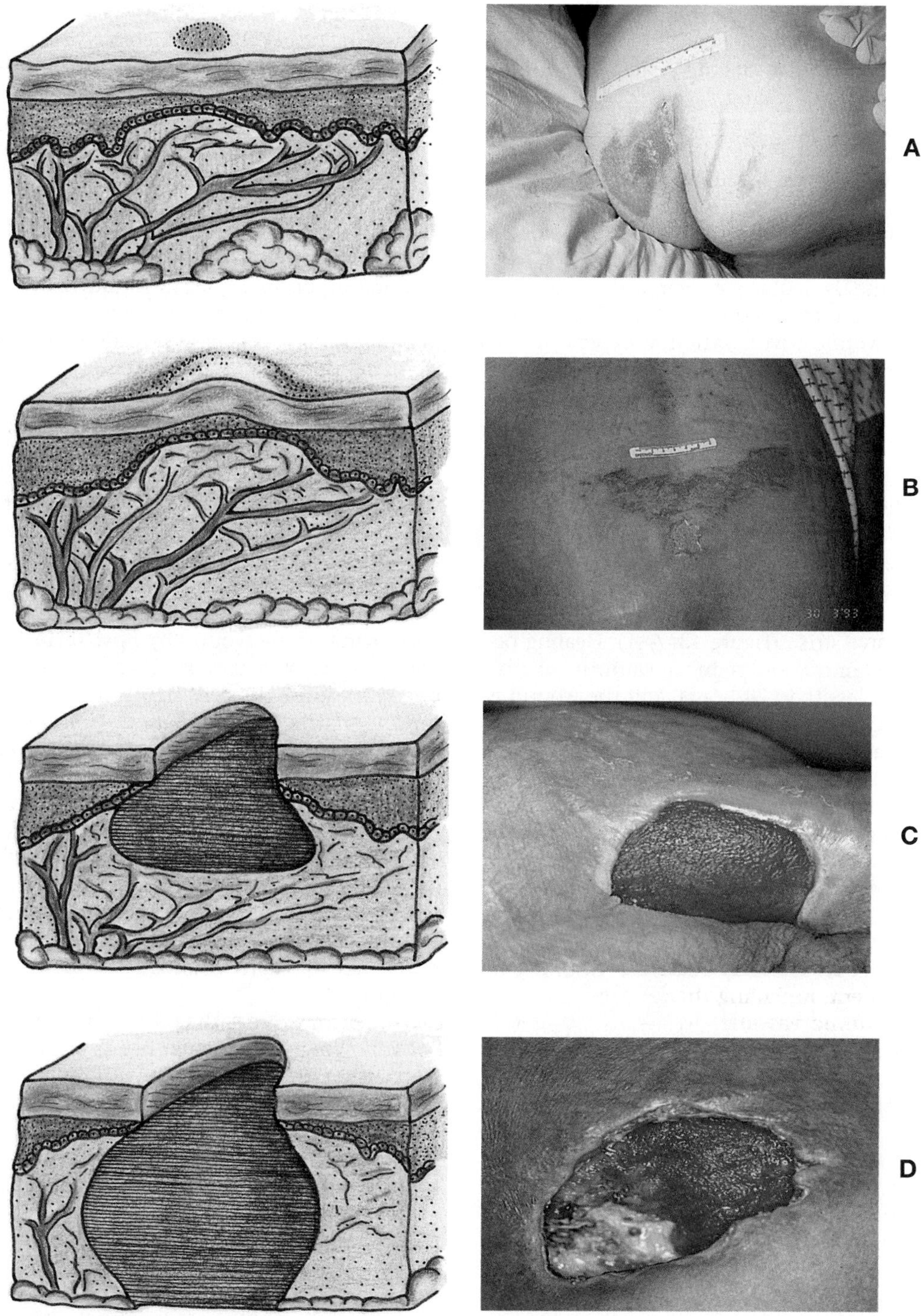

FIGURE 43–6 Diagram of stages of pressure ulcer formation. **A,** Stage I pressure ulcer. **B,** Stage II pressure ulcer. **C,** Stage III pressure ulcer. **D,** Stage IV pressure ulcer. (Courtesy Laurel Wiersma, RN, MSN, Clinical Nurse Specialist, Barnes-Jewish Hospital, St. Louis, MO.)

to a stage I; rather, a stage III ulcer demonstrating signs of healing is described as a healing stage III pressure ulcer (Cooper, 2000). Therefore, this staging system should not be used to measure wound healing.

Wound Healing

Wound healing is the process leading to total wound closure. Many factors can impair or prolong wound healing (Table 43-2), including poor nutrition. Normal wound healing requires adequate nutrition (Table 43-3).

Whether a wound is acute (e.g., surgical wound) or chronic (e.g., pressure ulcer), the wound healing process is the same for all wounds, with variation depending on the location, severity, and extent of injury. Wound healing is often described in terms of types of healing and phases of healing.

Types of Wound Healing. Depending on the nature of the wound, wounds heal by either primary intention or secondary intention. Wounds that have little or no tissue loss, such as a clean surgical incision, heal by **primary intention.** That is, the edges of the wound are brought together **(approximated)** and closed using sutures (stitches), staples, clips, or adhesive strips (Figure 43–7, *A*). Healing occurs quickly; the inflammation (redness, warmth, edema) typically subsides in less than 24 hours, and the wound is resurfaced between days 4 and 7 (Waldrop & Doughty, 2000). There is usually minimal scarring.

In contrast, a wound involving loss of tissue, such as a second- or third-degree burn or pressure ulcer, cannot have its edges approximated and therefore heals by **secondary intention** (Figure 43–7, *B*). The wound is left open until it becomes filled with tissue arising from its base. It takes longer for a wound to heal by secondary intention, and thus the chance of infection is greater. Scarring generally occurs and may be severe, resulting in permanent loss of tissue function.

Phases of Wound Healing. The wound healing process can be divided into three distinct but overlapping phases: inflammation, proliferation, and remodelling.

Inflammatory Phase. The inflammatory phase is the body's reaction to tissue damage and begins within minutes of injury and lasts up to 3 days, depending on the thickness of the wound. During this phase, the wound establishes **hemostasis** (cessation of bleeding) through constriction of injured blood vessels and clot formation. Clots contain platelets and a **fibrin** matrix that later provides a framework for cellular repair. Damaged tissue and mast cells secrete histamine, resulting in vasodilation of surrounding capillaries and exudation of serum and white blood cells into damaged tissues. This results in localized redness, edema, warmth, and throbbing. The inflammatory response is beneficial, and there is no value in attempting to cool the area or reduce the swelling unless the swelling occurs within a closed compartment (e.g., ankle or neck).

Leukocytes (white blood cells) reach the wound within a few hours. The primary acting white blood cell is the neutrophil, which begins to ingest bacteria and small debris. The second important leukocyte is the macrophage. Macrophages are the "garbage cells" that clean a wound of bacteria, dead cells, and debris by phagocytosis. Macrophages continue the process of clearing the wound of debris and release growth factors that attract **fibroblasts,** the cells that synthesize collagen (connective tissue). Collagen can be found at wound sites as early as the second day and is the main component of scar tissue.

In a clean wound, the inflammatory phase accomplishes control of bleeding and establishes a clean wound bed. The inflammatory phase is prolonged if too little inflammation occurs, as in debilitating disease such as cancer or after administration of corticosteroids. Too much inflammation also prolongs healing because arriving cells compete for available nutrients.

Proliferative Phase. The proliferative phase results in the filling and coverage of the wound bed. The proliferative phase begins with the appearance of new blood vessels and lasts from 3 to 24 days. The main activities during this phase are the filling of the wound with **granulation tissue** (a soft, pink form of connective tissue that forms on the surface of the wound), **contraction** (inward movement of edges) of the wound, and the resurfacing of the wound by **epithelialization** (the formation of epithelial cells). Fibroblasts are present in this phase; these are the cells that synthesize collagen, providing the matrix for granulation. Collagen mixes with the granulation tissue, and this matrix supports the epithelialization. Collagen provides strength and structural integrity to a wound. During this period, the wound begins to contract, reducing the area that requires healing. Last, the epithelial cells migrate from the wound edges to form a new surface. Epithelial cells can only migrate across a moist surface; therefore, a moist environment facilitates wound closure. Wounds that are kept moist resurface more quickly than wounds left open to air (Waldrop & Doughty, 2000).

In a clean wound, the proliferative phase accomplishes the following: the vascular bed is re-established (granulation tissue), the area is filled with replacement tissue (collagen and granulation tissue), and the surface is repaired (contraction and epithelialization). Impairment of healing during this stage usually results from systemic factors such as age, anemia, and poor nutritional status.

Remodelling Phase. The remodelling phase results in the maturation of the wound and may take place for more than a year, depending on the depth and extent of the wound. The collagen scar continues to reorganize and gain strength for several months. However, unless a wound is minor, the healed wound usually does not have the tensile strength of the tissue it replaces. Collagen fibres undergo remodelling or reorganization before assuming their normal appearance. Usually scar tissue contains fewer pigmented cells (melanocytes) and has a lighter colour than normal skin.

Wound Drainage

During the inflammatory phase of wound healing, **exudate** (liquid drainage) escapes from blood vessels and is deposited in tissue or on the wound surface. The amount of drainage varies depending on wound size and location.

Table 43-2 Factors That Impair Wound Healing

Physiological Effects	Nursing Implications
Infection	
Wound infection prolongs the inflammatory phase, delays collagen synthesis, prevents epithelialization, and may lead to additional tissue destruction (Waldrop & Doughty, 2000).	Observe for indications of wound infection: the presence of pus; change in odour, volume, or character of wound drainage; redness in the surrounding tissue; fever; or pain.
Malnutrition	
Deficiencies in any of the nutrients may impair all phases of healing (Stotts, 2000a; see Table 43-3). Stress from burns or severe trauma increases nutritional requirements.	A balanced intake of various nutrients is critical to support wound healing. Provide balanced diet rich in protein, carbohydrates, lipids, vitamins (especially A and C), and minerals (especially zinc). Assess ability to chew foods; if problem noted, provide with liquid supplements. Provide adequate amounts of calories and fluid.
Age	
Aging alters all phases of wound healing. Vascular changes impair circulation to wound site. Reduced liver function alters synthesis of clotting factors. Inflammatory response is slowed. Formation of antibodies and lymphocytes is reduced. Collagen tissue is less pliable. Scar tissue is less elastic.	Instruct client on safety precautions to avoid injuries. Be prepared to provide wound care for longer period. Teach support people in home wound care techniques.
Obesity	
Fatty tissue lacks adequate blood supply to resist bacterial infection and deliver nutrients and cellular elements for healing.	Observe obese client for signs of wound infection and dehiscence.
Impaired Oxygenation	
Low arterial oxygen tension alters synthesis of collagen and formation of epithelial cells. If local blood flow is poor, tissues fail to receive needed oxygen. Decreased hemoglobin in blood **(anemia)** reduces arterial oxygen levels in capillaries and interferes with tissue repair.	Provide diet adequate in iron, vitamin B_{12}, and folic acid. Monitor hemoglobin and oxygen saturation levels in clients with wounds.
Smoking	
Smoking reduces amount of functional hemoglobin in blood, thus decreasing tissue oxygenation. Smoking may increase platelet aggregation and cause hypercoagulability. Smoking interferes with normal cellular mechanisms that promote release of oxygen to tissues.	Discourage client from smoking by explaining its effects on wound healing.
Drugs	
Corticosteroids reduce inflammatory response and slow collagen synthesis. Anti-inflammatory drugs suppress protein synthesis, wound contraction, epithelialization, and inflammation. Prolonged antibiotic use may increase risk of superinfection. Chemotherapeutic drugs can depress bone marrow function, lower number of leukocytes, and impair inflammatory response.	Carefully observe clients receiving these drugs because signs of inflammation may not be obvious. Vitamin A can counteract effects of corticosteroids. Caution client to use only prescribed medications.
Vascular Diseases	
The ability to perfuse the tissues with adequate amounts of oxygenated blood is critical to wound healing (Waldrop & Doughty, 2000). Peripheral vascular disease (common in clients with diabetes) reduces circulation and impairs tissue perfusion.	Instruct clients with vascular diseases to take preventive measures to avoid cuts or breaks in skin. Provide preventive foot care.
Radiation	
Fibrosis and vascular scarring eventually develop in irradiated skin layers. Tissues become fragile and poorly oxygenated.	Observe closely for wound complications in clients who have had surgery after radiation.
Wound Stress	
Vomiting, abdominal distension, and respiratory effort may stress suture line and disrupt wound layer. Sudden, unexpected tension on incision inhibits formation of endothelial cell and collagen networks.	Control nausea with ordered anti-emetics. Keep nasogastric tubes patent and draining to avoid accumulation of secretions. Instruct and help client to splint abdominal wound during coughing.

Table 43-3 Role of Selected Nutrients in Wound Healing

Nutrient	Role in Healing	Recommendations	Sources
Calories	Fuel for cell energy "Protein protection"	30–35 kcal/kg/day	
Protein	Neogenesis, collagen formation, wound remodelling	1.20–1.50 g/kg/day, or enough to maintain positive nitrogen balance	Poultry, fish, eggs, beef
Vitamin C (ascorbic acid)	Collagen synthesis, capillary wall integrity, fibroblast function	*DRI: 75–90 mg/day Supplement if deficient 500 mg bid × 3 months Low toxicity	Citrus fruits, tomatoes, potatoes, fortified fruit juices
Vitamin A	Epithelialization, wound closure Can reverse corticosteroid effects	*DRI 700–900 mg/day Supplement if deficient 6700 mg (20 000 units × 10 days)	Green leafy vegetables (spinach), broccoli, carrots, sweet potatoes, liver
Zinc	Collagen formation and protein synthesis	*DRI 8–11 mg/day Supplement if deficient 25 mg elemental zinc bid with meals × 2 months Use with caution—large doses can be toxic May inhibit copper metabolism and impair immune function	Vegetables, meats, legumes
Fluid	Essential fluid environment for all cell functions	20–30 mL/kg/day Increase by another 10–15 mL/kg if client is on an air-fluidized bed	Use non-caffeine, non-alcoholic fluids without sugar Water is best—6 to 8 glasses/day

* DRI-Dietary reference intakes (see chapter 39).
Adapted from "Nutritional Aspects of Wound Healing," by E. A. Ayello, D. R. Thomas, and M. A. Litchford, 1999, *Home Healthcare Nurse, 17*(11), p. 719; and "Nutritional Assessment and Support," by N. A. Stotts, in *Acute and Chronic Wounds: Nursing Management* (2nd ed.), edited by R. A. Bryant, 2000, St. Louis, MO: Mosby.

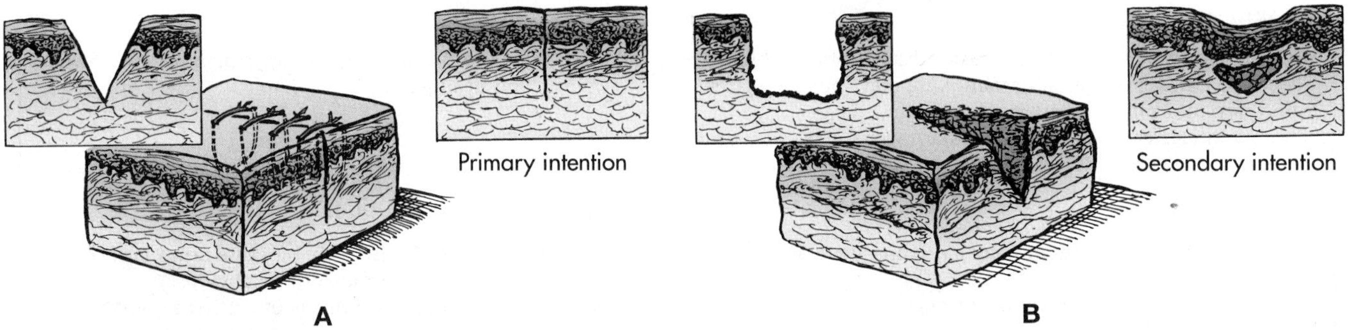

FIGURE **43–7** **A,** Wound healing by primary intention, such as with a surgical incision. Wound healing edges are approximated and closed with sutures, staples, or adhesive tapes, and healing occurs by connective tissue deposition. **B,** Wound healing by secondary intention. Wound edges are not approximated, and healing occurs by granulation tissue formation and contraction of the wound edges. (From *Acute and Chronic Wounds: Nursing Management,* 2nd ed., edited by R. A. Bryant, 2000, St. Louis, MO: Mosby. Used with permission.)

Bleeding and infection also affect the amount and character of drainage. The nurse observes and measures drainage.

There are four major types of wound drainage (Table 43-4):

- ***Serous drainage***—Clear, watery plasma. Serum does not contain blood cells or platelets. An example is the fluid in a blister.
- ***Purulent drainage***—Thick drainage that contains pus. Purulent drainage varies in colour depending partly on the organisms in the pus and may be green, yellow, or brown.
- ***Serosanguineous drainage***—Thin, watery drainage that is blood-tinged. This type of drainage is commonly seen in surgical incisions.
- ***Sanguineous drainage***—Bloody drainage. Large amounts of sanguineous drainage may indicate a hemorrhage; this type is frequently seen in open wounds. Bright drainage means fresh bleeding; darker drainage means older bleeding.

A wound that has excessive exudate may support bacterial growth, macerate the periwound skin, and slow the healing process. If excessive wound exudate is present,

Table 43-4 Types of Wound Drainage

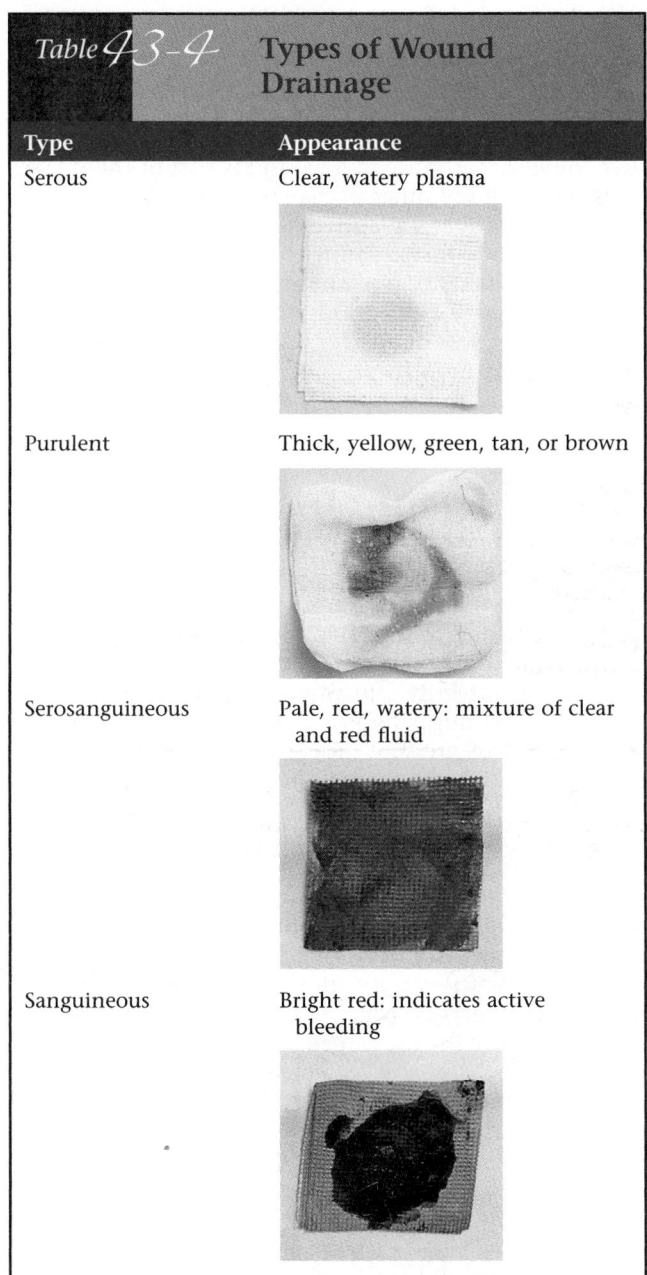

Type	Appearance
Serous	Clear, watery plasma 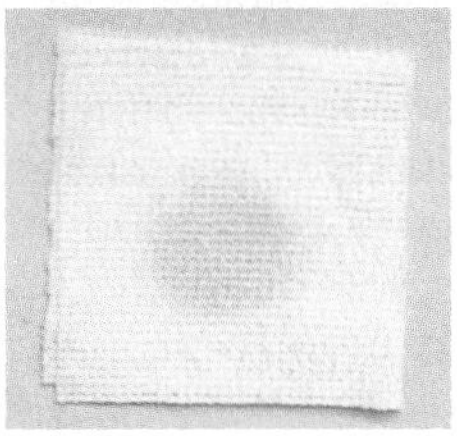
Purulent	Thick, yellow, green, tan, or brown 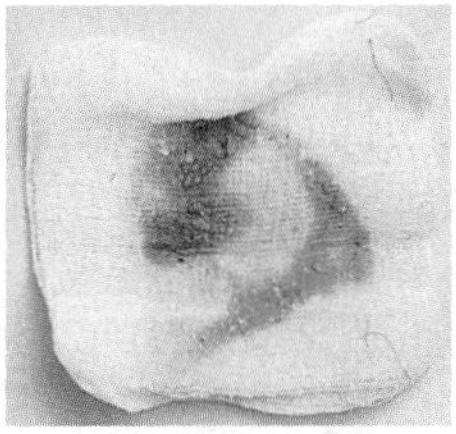
Serosanguineous	Pale, red, watery: mixture of clear and red fluid 
Sanguineous	Bright red: indicates active bleeding 

the nurse must evaluate the volume, consistency, and odour of the drainage to determine if signs of infection are present.

Nursing Knowledge Base

Complications Related to Wound Healing

Several complications can arise during the process of wound healing, including hemorrhage, wound infection, dehiscence, evisceration, and fistulas.

Hemorrhage. **Hemorrhage,** or bleeding from a wound site, is normal during and immediately after the initial trauma. Hemostasis occurs within several minutes unless large blood vessels are involved or the client has poor clotting function. Hemorrhage occurring after hemostasis may indicate a slipped surgical suture, a dislodged clot, infection, or erosion of a blood vessel by a foreign object (e.g., a drain). Hemorrhage may occur externally or internally. For example, if a deep surgical suture slips from a blood vessel, bleeding occurs internally within the tissues and there are no visible signs of blood unless a surgical drain is present at the site (a drain is inserted into tissues beneath a wound to remove fluid that collects in underlying tissues). The nurse can detect internal bleeding by looking for distension or swelling of the affected body part, a change in the type and amount of drainage from a surgical drain, or signs of hypovolemic shock. A **hematoma** is a localized collection of blood underneath the tissues. It appears as a swelling, change in colour or sensation, warmth, or mass that often takes on a bluish discoloration. A hematoma near a major artery or vein is dangerous because pressure from the expanding hematoma may obstruct blood flow.

External hemorrhaging is obvious. If bleeding is extensive, the dressing becomes saturated and blood may drain through the dressing and pool beneath the client. The nurse should closely observe all wounds for hemorrhage, particularly during the first 24 to 48 hours after surgery or injury.

Infection. Wound infection is the second most common nosocomial (hospital-related) infection (see chapter 29). According to the Centers for Disease Control and Prevention (CDC; 2001), a wound is infected if purulent material drains from it, even if a culture is not taken or has negative results. A sample of drainage from an infected wound may not reveal bacteria because of poor culture technique or administration of antibiotics. Positive culture findings do not always indicate an infection because many wounds contain colonies of non-infective resident bacteria. In fact, all chronic dermal wounds are considered contaminated with bacteria. It is generally agreed that wounds with more than 100 000 (10^5) organisms per gram of tissue are infected (Bowler, 2003; Robson, 1997). The types of micro-organism, their interactions with each other and with the wound environment, the local conditions, and host resistance are key factors that collectively influence infection and healing of a wound. The likelihood of wound infection is greater when the wound contains dead or necrotic tissue, there are foreign bodies in or near the wound, and the blood supply and local tissue defences are reduced. Bacterial wound infection inhibits wound healing.

A contaminated or traumatic wound may show signs of infection early, within 2 to 3 days. A surgical wound infection usually does not develop until the fourth or fifth post-operative day. Box 43-2 lists classic signs of wound infection.

Dehiscence. When a wound fails to heal properly, the layers of skin and tissue may separate. This most commonly occurs before collagen formation (3 to 11 days after injury). **Dehiscence** is the partial or total separation of wound layers. A client who is at risk for poor wound healing (e.g., is malnourished) or for a local infection is at risk for dehiscence (Candido, 2002). Obese clients also

Box 43-2 Classic Signs of Wound Infection

- Pain and tenderness at the wound site
- Erythema (reddening of the surrounding tissue)
- Edema (swelling), **induration** (increased firmness of tissue)
- Inflammation of wound edges
- Purulent discharge
- Warmth in surrounding tissue
- Fever, chills
- Foul odour
- Elevated white blood cell count
- Delayed healing

Chronic Wounds

The above signs and symptoms as well as the following:

- Increased exudates
- Bright red discoloration of granulation tissue
- New areas of slough or breakdown on the wound surface
- Undermining (dead space under the edges of the wound)

have higher risk because of the mechanical strain placed on their wounds and the poor healing qualities of fat tissue. Dehiscence most commonly involves abdominal surgical wounds and occurs after a sudden strain, such as coughing, vomiting, or sitting up in bed. Clients often report feeling as though something has given way. When there is an increase in serosanguineous drainage from a wound, the nurse should be alert for the potential for dehiscence. A strategy to prevent dehiscence is to place a folded blanket or pillow over the abdominal wound when the client is coughing. This provides a splint to the area, supporting the healing tissue when coughing increases the intra-abdominal pressure.

Evisceration. With total separation of wound layers, **evisceration** (protrusion of visceral organs through a wound opening) may occur. The condition is an emergency that requires surgical repair. When evisceration occurs, the nurse places sterile towels soaked in sterile saline over the extruding tissues to reduce chances of bacterial invasion and drying of the tissues. If the organs protrude through the wound, blood supply to the tissues is compromised. The client should be allowed nothing by mouth (NPO), observed for signs and symptoms of shock, and prepared for emergency surgery.

Fistulas. A **fistula** is an abnormal passage between two organs or between an organ and the outside of the body. Most fistulas form as a result of poor wound healing or as a complication of disease, such as Crohn's disease. Trauma, infection, radiation exposure, and diseases such as cancer can prevent tissue layers from closing properly and allow the fistula tract to form. Fistulas increase the risk of infection. Chronic drainage of fluids through a fistula can predispose a person to skin breakdown by increasing tissue moisture. Fluid loss also places the client at risk for fluid and electrolyte imbalances.

Psychosocial Impact of Wounds

Wounds affect clients physically and psychosocially. A wound can strip away dignity and the client's sense of independence. Psychological stress can impact on wound healing (Kiecolt-Glaser et al., 1995). The client's psychological response to a wound is part of the nurse's assessment. Body image changes may impose great stress on the client's adaptive mechanisms. In addition, changes in body image influence self-concept (see chapter 22) and sexuality (see chapter 23). Factors that may affect the client's perception of the wound include the presence of scars, drains (drains may be necessary for weeks or even months after certain procedures), odour from drainage, and temporary or permanent prosthetic devices.

Critical Thinking

When caring for clients who have impaired skin integrity and chronic wounds, the nurse must integrate knowledge from nursing and other disciplines, previous experiences, and information gathered from clients to understand the risks to skin integrity and wound healing (Figure 43–8). Knowledge of normal musculoskeletal physiology, the pathogenesis of pressure ulcers, normal wound healing, and the pathophysiology of underlying diseases enables the nurse to have a scientific basis for care. The AHCPR, the RNAO, and the CAWC have guidelines for assessment of risk for impaired skin integrity, prevention measures, and interventions to promote wound healing. These and other standards of practice should be applied. Past experience with clients at risk for impaired skin integrity or with clients with wounds increases the knowledge base from which the nurse can identify interventions. Finally, the nurse must be disciplined during assessment to obtain comprehensive and correct assessment data. Because chronic wounds are difficult to heal, the nurse must be diligent in evaluating nursing interventions and determining which interventions are effective and which need to be modified.

Nursing Process

NP Assessment

A major aspect of nursing care is the maintenance of skin integrity. Consistent, planned skin care interventions are critical to ensuring high quality in care (Box 43-3). Nurses constantly observe their clients' skin for breaks or impaired skin integrity.

Assessing for Risk of Pressure Ulcers. Prevention and treatment of pressure ulcers are nursing priorities. On admission to hospitals, long-term care facilities, other health facilities, and home care programs, clients should be assessed for risk of pressure ulcer development (AHCPR, 1992). Because pressure ulcers have multiple etiological factors, assessment for pressure ulcer risk includes several important factors (Skill 43-1).

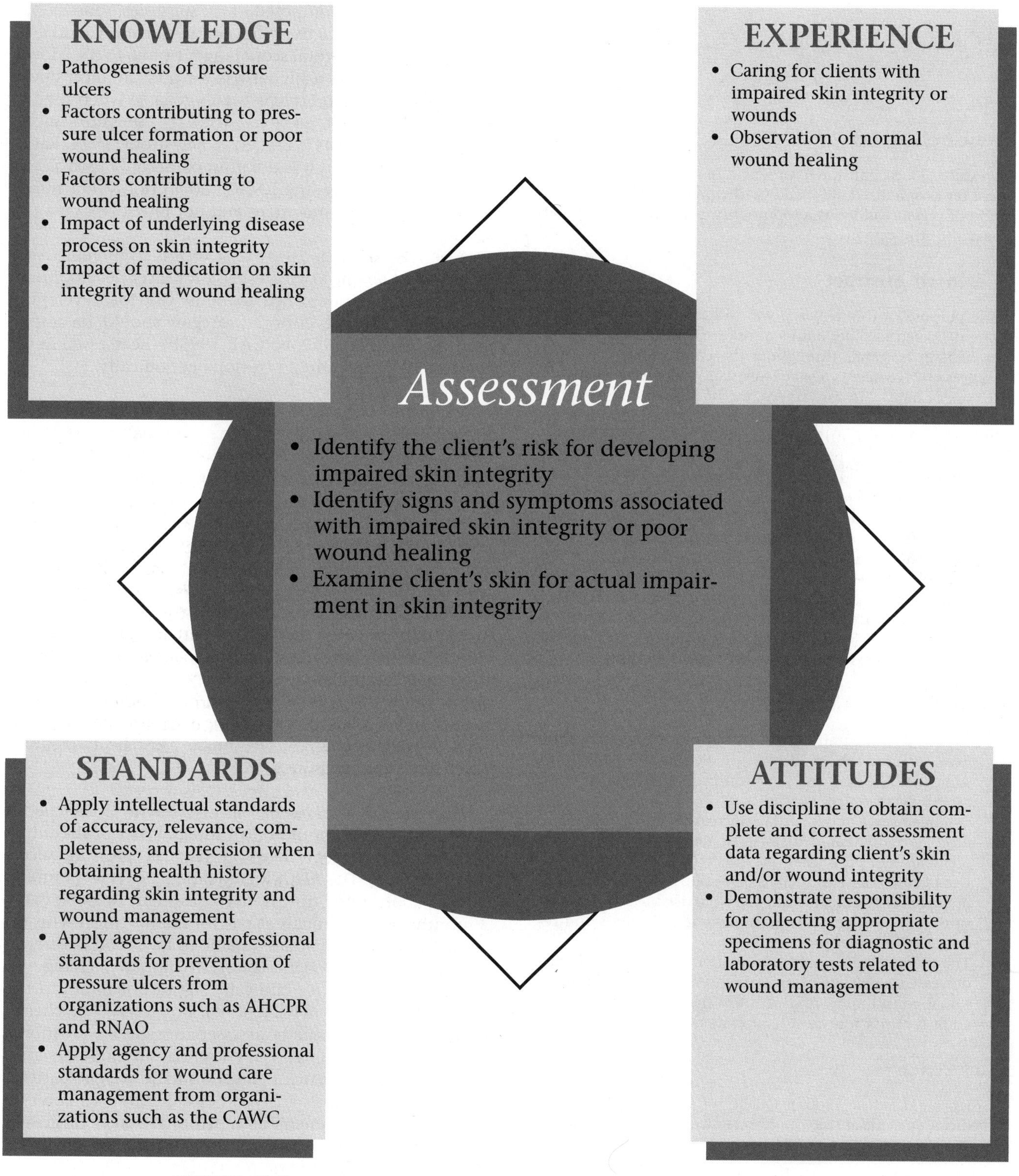
KNOWLEDGE
• Pathogenesis of pressure ulcers
• Factors contributing to pressure ulcer formation or poor wound healing
• Factors contributing to wound healing
• Impact of underlying disease process on skin integrity
• Impact of medication on skin integrity and wound healing
EXPERIENCE
• Caring for clients with impaired skin integrity or wounds
• Observation of normal wound healing
Assessment
• Identify the client's risk for developing impaired skin integrity
• Identify signs and symptoms associated with impaired skin integrity or poor wound healing
• Examine client's skin for actual impairment in skin integrity
STANDARDS
• Apply intellectual standards of accuracy, relevance, completeness, and precision when obtaining health history regarding skin integrity and wound management
• Apply agency and professional standards for prevention of pressure ulcers from organizations such as AHCPR and RNAO
• Apply agency and professional standards for wound care management from organizations such as the CAWC
ATTITUDES
• Use discipline to obtain complete and correct assessment data regarding client's skin and/or wound integrity
• Demonstrate responsibility for collecting appropriate specimens for diagnostic and laboratory tests related to wound management

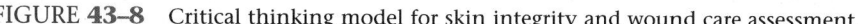

FIGURE **43–8** Critical thinking model for skin integrity and wound care assessment.

Research Highlight — Box 43-3

Quality Care and Pressure Ulcer Risk

Research Focus

Pressure ulcers continue to present a major health care problem for hospitalized older adults. The prediction and prevention of pressure ulcers is a top priority and must be included as part of the care plan.

Research Abstract

The purpose of this research was to examine the quality of care delivered to older adults at risk for pressure ulcer development in hospitals throughout the United States. Medical records of 2425 clients aged 65 years and older were evaluated for use of daily skin assessment, use of pressure-reducing device, documentation of being at risk, repositioning for a minimum of 2 hours, nutritional consultation for at-risk individuals, and staging of pressure ulcer. The associations between the previously noted process of care and the occurrence of pressure ulcer development were determined. Results showed compliance with the process of care: use of daily skin assessment, 94%; use of pressure-reducing device, 7.5%; documentation of being at risk, 22.6%; repositioning for a minimum of 2 hours, 66.2%; nutritional consultation, 43.3%; stage I pressure ulcer staged, 20.2%; and stage II or greater ulcer stage, 30.9%. The authors felt that the results suggest that caregivers in U.S. hospitals have numerous opportunities to improve care related to pressure ulcer prediction and prevention.

Evidence-Based Practice

- Lack of documentation of clients at risk demonstrates the need for hospitals to increase prediction and prevention strategies. Use of a risk scale can provide triggers to plan care to decrease risk factors.
- Extended stays of over 7 days increase the risk of pressure ulcer development. Nurses must remain vigilant in the prevention of pressure ulcers in clients with longer stays.
- Use of care practices such as daily skin assessment, use of pressure-relief surfaces, and objective risk assessment measures (e.g., Braden Scale) identified at-risk clients and reduced evidence of pressure ulcers.
- The use of a nutritional consultation was associated with decreased incidence of pressure ulcers, suggesting a nutritional consultation may sensitize the staff that the older adult is at risk for pressure ulcer development.

Reference

Lyder, C. H., et al. (2001). Quality of care for hospitalized medicare patients at risk for pressure ulcers. *Archives of Internal Medicine, 161*(12), 1549–1554.

Pressure ulcer risk assessment should be done systematically (AHCPR, 1992; NPUAP, 1989). Several risk assessment scales (Bergstrom, Demuth, & Braden, 1987; Norton, McLaren, & Exon-Smith, 1962) developed by nurses enable systematic risk assessment of clients. The **Braden Scale** is noted in the AHCPR (1992) and RNAO guidelines (2005) as being a valid tool for assessing pressure ulcer risk (Figure 43–9). It is composed of six subscales: sensory perception, moisture, activity, mobility, nutrition, and friction and shear. The total score ranges from 6 to 23; a lower total score indicates a higher risk for pressure ulcer development. The Braden Scale is highly reliable when used to identify clients at greatest risk for pressure ulcers (Bergstrom et al., 1987; Braden & Bergstrom, 1994; Ratliff & Bryant, 2003), and it is the most commonly used assessment tool. However, the RNAO (2005) notes that nurses must apply clinical judgment and not rely solely on a risk assessment tool.

A benefit of a risk assessment tool is to increase early detection of clients at greatest risk for ulcer development. Once a client is identified to be at risk for developing pressure ulcers, prevention strategies should be implemented (AHCPR, 1992; NPUAP, 1995b). Reassessment for pressure ulcer risk should be done periodically.

Mobility Assessment. Assessment includes documenting the level of mobility and the potential effects of impaired mobility on skin integrity. Assessment of mobility should also include data regarding the quality of muscle tone and strength. For example, the nurse determines whether the client can lift weight off of the sacral area and roll the body to a side-lying position. The client may have adequate range of motion to move independently into a more protective position. Finally, the nurse notes the client's activity tolerance (see chapter 32).

Mobility must be assessed as part of baseline data. If the client has some degree of independence in mobility, the nurse reinforces the frequency of position changes and measures to relieve pressure. The frequency of position changes is based on ongoing skin assessment and is revised as data change. The nurse must be meticulous when assessing pressure sites.

Nutritional Assessment. An assessment of the client's nutritional status should be an integral part of the initial assessment data for clients at risk for pressure ulcers (Stotts, 2000a). The AHCPR guidelines (1994) recommend that an abbreviated nutritional assessment be done every 3 months for individuals at risk for malnutrition. This includes individuals who are unable to take food by mouth or who have experienced an involuntary change in weight. Parameters for clinically significant malnutrition have been defined (AHCPR, 1994; Box 43-4). The client's mouth and skin should be assessed for signs of nutritional deficiencies (see chapter 39). The client's hydration status, especially the amount of fluids and the weight pattern, should also be assessed (Ayello et al., 1999). Chapter 39 discusses the assessment of nutritional status in greater detail. Nurses should always consult with dietitians to establish an appropriate treatment plan (RNAO, 2002a).

Albumin is a frequently measured variable used to evaluate the client's protein status. Serum albumin levels are good predictors of malnutrition in all age groups. Prealbumin is an excellent measure of nutritional status because it reflects what has been absorbed, digested, and metabolized (Stotts, 2000a). Clients with a potential for or actual decreased serum albumin levels or poor protein intake need a nutritional evaluation to ensure proper caloric intake (AHCPR, 1994; Ratliff & Bryant, 2003).

Skill 43-1 Assessment for Risk of Pressure Ulcer Development

Delegation Considerations

Assessment of clients for risk of pressure ulcers should not be delegated to unregulated care providers (UCPs). However, the UCP may have other aspects of client care delegated, and the nurse should instruct the UCP to do the following:

- Report to the nurse any changes, such as redness, blistering, abrasion, or cuts to the client's skin.
- Keep the client's skin dry and provide hygiene following incontinence of urine or stool or exposure to other body fluids.
- Reposition the client according to the frequency established on the nursing care plan or agency policy.
- Avoid trauma to the client's skin from tape, pressure, friction, or shear.

Equipment

- Risk assessment tool: Braden Scale (used in this skill) or other, according to agency policy
- Documentation record

Steps	Rationale
1. Identify at-risk individuals needing prevention and the specific factors placing them at risk.	Determines factors that increase the client's risk for developing pressure ulcers (Braden, 2001).
a. Use a validated risk assessment tool such as the Braden Scale.	Ensures consistent, reliable, comparable assessments (AHCPR, 1992; NPUAP, 1995b; RNAO, 2005).
b. Assess the client upon admission to hospitals, long-term care facilities, home care programs, and other health care facilities.	Provides a baseline assessment.
c. Inspect the condition of the client's skin at least once a day (see Box 43-6) and examine all bony prominences, noting skin integrity. (Check agency policy for reassessment and reassess at periodic intervals.) If redness or discoloration is noted, use thumb to gently palpate area of redness. The discoloration may vary from pink to deep red.	Routine skin assessments will identify changes in client's pressure ulcer risk. Non-blanchable erythema or discoloration in the client's skin may be an early indicator of skin injury (Pieper, 2000).

Critical Decision Point: In dark-skinned clients, the discoloration appears as a deepening of the normal ethnic colour (see Box 43-5). Darkly pigmented skin does not always show direct changes in colour (Bennett, 1995; NPUAP, 1998).

Steps	Rationale
d. Observe all assistive devices, such as braces or casts, and medical equipment, such as nasoenteral tubes and catheters, for pressure points.	Presence of medical equipment has the potential to cause pressure and skin breakdown to sensitive regions, such as the nares, ears, over bony prominences, and other pressure areas.
2. Determine the client's ability to respond meaningfully to pressure-related discomfort (sensory perception).	Clients with completely, very, or slightly limited ability to respond to pressure-related discomfort cannot communicate discomfort, will have a limitation in the ability to feel pain, and thus will have a risk for developing pressure ulcers.
3. Assess the degree to which the client's skin is exposed to moisture.	A person whose skin is exposed to excessive moisture has an increased risk of skin breakdown.
4. Evaluate the client's activity level.	The client who is bedfast, chairfast, or only walks occasionally will be at risk for developing pressure areas because of the degree of physical inactivity.
a. Determine the client's ability to change and control body position (mobility).	Potential for friction and shear increases when the client is completely dependent on others for position change.
b. Determine client's preferred positions.	Weight of body will be placed on certain bony prominences, and the client may resist repositioning off these areas.

Skill 43-1 Assessment for Risk of Pressure Ulcer Development—cont'd

Steps	Rationale
5. Assess the client's usual food intake pattern (nutrition).	A client who never eats a complete meal or rarely eats a complete meal is at risk for pressure ulcer formation.
a. Review weight pattern and nutritional laboratory values (see Box 43-4).	Decreased nutrition status is linked with pressure ulcer formation and poor pressure wound healing (AHCPR, 1994).
b. Complete fluid intake assessment.	Fluid imbalance, either dehydration or edema, can increase the client's risk for pressure ulcers.
6. Evaluate the presence of friction and/or shear.	The client who has a problem in moving, requires maximum assistance in moving, or slides against sheets when moved is at an increased risk of skin damage.
7. Document the risk assessment (Cooper, 2000).	The documentation will provide a baseline for comparison of increased or decreased risk for development of pressure ulcers and allow planning of interventions.
a. As the Braden Scale scores become lower, predicted risk becomes higher.	Scores: 15 to 16, mild risk 13 to 14, moderate risk 10 to 12, high risk 9 or below, very high risk
b. Link the risk assessment to preventive protocols.	Prevention protocols will target problem areas to assist in prevention of skin breakdown (Braden, 2001).
c. Institute mild-risk interventions (score of 15 to 16). Plan of care should include frequent turning; maximum remobilization; heel protection; use of pressure-reducing support surface; and managing moisture, nutrition, and friction and shear.	Decreases the risk of skin breakdown.
d. Institute moderate-risk interventions (score of 13 to 14). Plan of care should include interventions for mild risk (Step 7c), as well as using foam wedges to position the client in the 30-degree lateral position.	Decreases the increased risk of skin breakdown with appropriate interventions.
e. Institute high-risk interventions (score of 10 to 12). Plan of care should include interventions for moderate risk (Step 7d), as well as turning the client with small shifts in weight.	Addresses the factors that contribute to skin breakdown and plans for interventions to address the causative factors.
f. Institute very high-risk interventions (score of 9 or below). Plan of care should include interventions for high-risk (Step 7e) as well as using a pressure-relieving surface if the client has uncontrolled pain or severe pain exacerbated by turning.	Plan interventions to decrease the effects of immobility, decreased sensory perception, moisture, friction, shear, decreased activity, and nutritional issues in a high-risk individual.
8. Provide education to client and family regarding pressure ulcer risk and prevention.	Assists clients and family to understand the interventions designed to reduce pressure ulcer risk.
9. Evaluate measures to reduce pressure ulcer development	
a. Observe client's skin for areas at risk.	Determines over time client's response to risk-reduction interventions.
b. Observe tolerance of client for positioning.	Frequent change in position further reduces client's risk for pressure ulcer development.
c. Monitor the success of a toileting program or other measures to reduce the frequency of incontinence of urine or stool.	Determines timeliness of a toileting program or schedule to assist the client in meeting elimination needs.
d. Evaluate nutrition laboratory values.	Determines the success of nutritional supplements in improving nutritional status.

Unexpected Outcomes and Related Interventions

- Skin does not blanch (turn white or pale colour) when firmly pressed, has purple discoloration, or has significant colour change.
  - Reassess frequency of turning schedule.
  - Implement agency's skin care protocols.
  - Consider support surface to reduce pressure ulcer risk.

Recording and Reporting

- Record client's risk score.
- Record appearance of skin under pressure.
- Describe position, turning intervals, pressure-relieving devices, and other prevention strategies.
- Report any need for additional consultations for the high-risk client.

Home Care Considerations

- Instruct caregiver on the use of the 30-degree lateral position. This position reduces pressure over the trochanter.
- Pressure-relief manoeuvres need to be individualized for client need and home environment. Provide family with resources for hospital equipment.

Body Fluids. Continual exposure of the skin to body fluids also increases the client's risk for skin breakdown and pressure ulcer formation. Some body fluids, such as saliva and serosanguineous drainage, are not caustic to the skin and the risk of skin breakdown from exposure to these fluids is low. However, exposure to urine, bile, stool, acetic fluid, and purulent wound exudates carries a moderate risk for skin breakdown, especially in clients who have other risk factors, such as impaired mobility or poor nutrition. Exposure to gastric and pancreatic drainage has the highest risk for skin breakdown. It is important to prevent and reduce the client's exposure to body fluids, and when exposure occurs, meticulous hygiene and skin care must be provided.

Assessing the Skin for Signs of Pressure Ulcers. The nurse should assess the skin for signs of pressure ulcers at least once a day; however, high-risk clients will need more frequent skin assessments, such as at the beginning of each nursing shift. The neurologically impaired client; the chronically ill client in long-term care; the client with diminished mental status; and the intensive care unit, oncology, hospice, or orthopedic client have increased potential for developing pressure ulcers.

Assessment for signs of pressure ulcers requires visual inspection and palpation of the skin. Baseline assessment is performed to determine the client's normal skin characteristics and any actual or potential areas of breakdown. The nurse pays particular attention to areas located over bony prominences, under casts, traction, splints, braces, collars, or other orthopedic devices.

An early indicator of a pressure ulcer is persistent (nonblanching) reddened skin. When the skin is being compressed, blood flow is slowed and the skin becomes pale. After the pressure is relieved, the skin in the affected area turns red **(erythema),** a result of the blood vessels expanding (vasodilation) to allow more blood into the area to overcome the ischemic episode (Ratliff & Bryant, 2003). This process is called **normal reactive hyperemia.** The nurse assesses the reddened area by pressing a fingertip over it. If the area blanches (turns white or pale colour) and the erythema returns when the finger is removed, the reactive hyperemia is likely transient (Figure 43–10). If, however, the reddened area does not blanch when finger pressure is applied **(abnormal reactive hyperemia),** deep tissue damage should be suspected (Figure 43–11). Note, however, that reddening of the skin and **blanching** do not occur in clients with darkly pigmented skin. Box 43-5 lists characteristics of intact dark skin that might alert the nurse to the potential for pressure ulcers.

When hyperemia is noted, the nurse documents the location, size, and colour and reassesses the area after 1 hour. When abnormal reactive hyperemia is detected, the nurse can outline the affected area with a marker to make reassessment easier. In addition, the nurse palpates for induration, noting the size in millimetres or centimetres of the induration around the injured area. The nurse also uses palpation to note changes in temperature of the surrounding skin and tissues.

Box 43-6 lists the steps required to assess the skin for signs of pressure ulcers.

Assessing Wounds. The nurse often assesses wounds under two conditions: at the time of injury (emergency setting) and after therapy when the wound is relatively stable (stable setting). Each condition requires the nurse to make different observations and to take different actions. Regardless of the setting, it is important for the nurse to initially obtain information regarding the cause and history of the wound (Box 43-7).

Emergency Setting. The nurse may see wounds in any setting, including clinic, emergency department, youth camps, or the nurse's own backyard. The type of wound determines the criteria for inspection. For example, the nurse need not inspect for signs of internal bleeding after an abrasion but should do so in the event of a puncture wound.

After a client's condition has been judged to be stable based on the presence of spontaneous breathing, a clear airway, and a strong carotid pulse, the nurse inspects the wound for bleeding. An abrasion will have very little bleeding but may appear "weepy" because of plasma leakage from damaged capillaries. A laceration may bleed more profusely, depending on its depth and location. For example, minor scalp lacerations tend to bleed profusely because of the rich blood supply to the scalp. Lacerations greater than 5 cm long or 2.5 cm deep can cause serious bleeding. Puncture wounds bleed in relation to the depth and size of the wound; for example, a nail puncture does

Client's Name ____________ Evaluator's Name ____________ Date of Assessment

Sensory Perception Ability to respond meaningfully to pressure-related discomfort	1. Completely limited Unresponsive (does not moan, flinch, or grasp) to painful stimuli due to diminished level of consciousness or sedation. OR Limited ability to feel pain over most of body surface.	2. Very limited Responds only to painful stimuli. Cannot communicate discomfort except by moaning or restlessness. OR Has a sensory impairment that limits the ability to feel pain or discomfort over half of body.	3. Slightly limited Responds to verbal commands, but cannot always communicate discomfort or need to be turned. OR Has some sensory impairment that limits ability to feel pain or discomfort in one or two extremities.	4. No impairment Responds to verbal commands. Has no sensory deficit that would limit ability to feel or voice pain or discomfort.
Moisture Degree to which skin is exposed to moisture	1. Constantly moist Skin is kept moist almost constantly by perspiration, urine, etc. Dampness is detected every time client is moved or turned.	2. Very moist Skin is often, but not always, moist. Linen must be changed at least once a shift.	3. Occasionally moist Skin is occasionally moist, requiring an extra linen change approximately once a day.	4. Rarely moist Skin is usually dry. Linen only requires changing at routine intervals.
Activity Degree of physical activity	1. Bedfast Confined to bed.	2. Chairfast Ability to walk severely limited or non-existent. Cannot bear own weight and/or must be assisted into chair or wheelchair.	3. Walks occasionally Walks occasionally during day, but for very short distances, with or without assistance. Spends majority of each shift in bed or chair.	4. Walks frequently Walks outside the room at least twice a day and inside room at least once every 2 hours during waking hours.
Mobility Ability to change and control body position	1. Completely immobile Does not make even slight changes in body or extremity position without assistance.	2. Very limited Makes occasional slight changes in body or extremity position but unable to make frequent or significant changes independently.	3. Slightly limited Makes frequent though slight changes in body or extremity position independently.	4. No limitations Makes major and frequent changes in position without assistance.
Nutrition *Usual* food intake pattern	1. Very poor Never eats a complete meal. Rarely eats more than 1/3 of any food offered. Eats two servings or less of protein (meat or dairy products) per day. Takes fluids poorly. Does not take a liquid dietary supplement. OR Is NPO and/or maintained on clear liquids or IVs for more than 5 days.	2. Probably inadequate Rarely eats a complete meal and generally eats only about 1/2 of any food offered. Protein intake includes only three servings of meat or dairy products per day. Occasionally will take a dietary supplement. OR Receives less than optimum amount of liquid diet or tube feeding.	3. Adequate Eats over half of most meals. Eats a total of four servings of protein (meat, dairy products) each day. Occasionally will refuse a meal, but will usually take a supplement if offered. OR Is on a tube feeding or total parenteral nutrition regimen that probably meets most of nutritional needs.	4. Excellent Eats most of every meal. Never refuses a meal. Usually eats a total of four or more servings of meat and dairy products. Occasionally eats between meals. Does not require supplementation.
Friction and Shear	1. Problem Requires moderate to maximum assistance in moving. Complete lifting without sliding against sheets is impossible. Frequently slides down in bed or chair, requiring frequent repositioning with maximum assistance. Spasticity, contractures, or agitation leads to almost constant friction.	2. Potential problem Moves feebly or requires minimum assistance. During a move, skin probably slides to some extent against sheets, chair, restraints, or other devices. Maintains relatively good position in chair or bed most of the time but occasionally slides down.	3. No apparent problem Moves in bed and in chair independently and has sufficient muscle strength to lift up completely during move. Maintains good position in bed or chair at all times.	
				TOTAL SCORE

NOTE: Clients with a total score of 16 or less are considered to be at risk of developing pressure ulcers (15 to 16 = mild risk; 13 to 14 = moderate risk; 10 to 12 = high risk; 9 or less = very high risk).

FIGURE **43–9** Braden Scale for predicting pressure ulcer risk. (Courtesy Barbara Braden and Nancy Bergstrom.)

Box 43-4 Warning Signs of Significant Malnutrition

- Serum albumin is less than 35 g/L
- Total lymphocyte count is less than 1800/mm^3
- A loss of 5% of usual weight in 1 month, 7.5% in 3 months, or 10% in 6 months
- A body mass index of ≤18.5 (see chapter 39)
- Body weight that is less than 80% of usual weight.
- An intake consistently less than 60% of dietary reference intake
- A reduction in food intake to 50% of normal in the last week

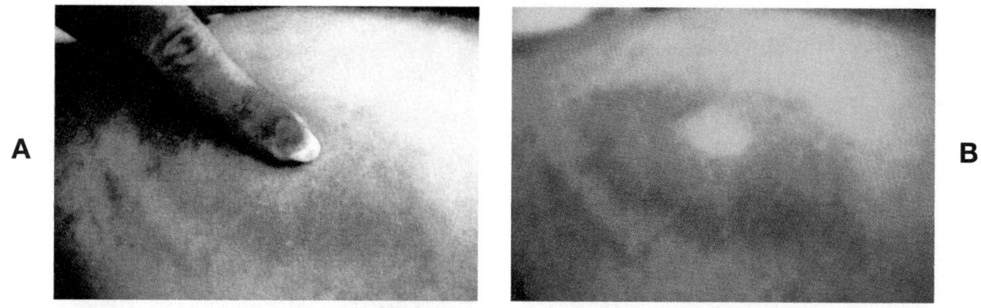

FIGURE **43–10** Normal reactive hyperemia. When a fingertip is pressed over the reddened area **(A),** the area turns white or pale colour (blanches) for a brief period of time **(B).** (From "Detection and Management of Early Tissue Pressure Indicators: A Pictorial Essay," by M. Pires and A. Muller, 1991, *Progressions, 3*[3], p. 3.)

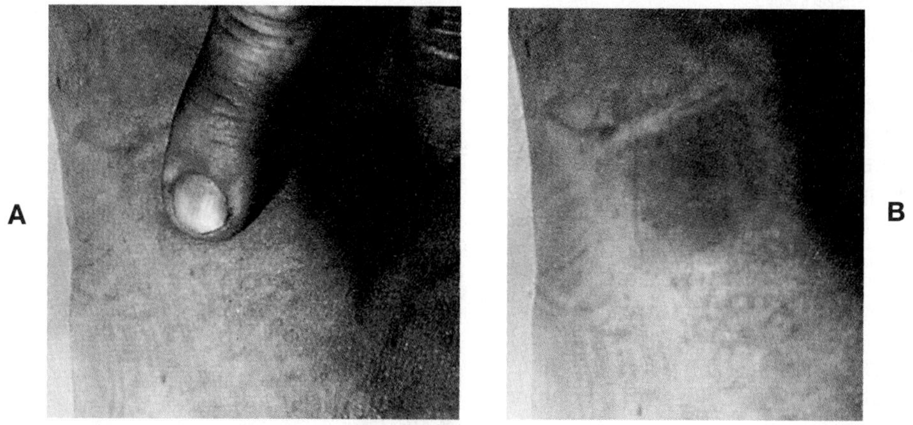

FIGURE **43–11** Abnormal reactive hyperemia. When a fingertip is pressed over the reddened area **(A),** the area does not blanch but remains consistently reddened, which is an indication of deep tissue injury. (From "Detection and Management of Early Tissue Pressure Indicators: A Pictorial Essay," by M. Pires and A. Muller, 1991, *Progressions, 3*[3], p. 3.)

not cause as much bleeding as a knife wound. The primary dangers of puncture wounds are internal bleeding and infection.

The nurse next inspects the wound for foreign bodies or contaminant material. Most traumatic wounds are dirty. Soil, broken glass, shreds of cloth, and foreign substances clinging to penetrating objects can become embedded in the wound.

The size of the wound is the next criterion for inspection. A deep laceration requires suturing. A large, open wound may expose bone or tissue that should be protected.

When the injury is a result of trauma from a dirty penetrating object, the nurse determines when the client last received a tetanus toxoid injection. Tetanus bacteria reside in soil and in the gut of humans and animals. A tetanus antitoxin injection is necessary if the client has not had one within the past 5 years.

Stable Setting. When the client's condition is stabilized (e.g., after surgery or treatment), the nurse assesses the wound to determine progress toward healing. If a dressing covers the wound and the physician has not ordered it

Box 43-5 Signs of Skin Breakdown in Dark Skin

Assessment Issues

Natural or halogen light sources are best for assessing skin.

Fluorescent light source should be avoided because it casts a bluish hue, making accurate assessment difficult.

Do not confuse the normal hyperpigmentation of Mongolian spots (seen on the sacrum of Black, Aboriginal, and Asian clients) with signs of skin breakdown.

The Gaskin's Nursing Assessment of Skin Color (GNASC) may be a useful took for identifying changes in dark skin colour (Gaskin, 1986).

Colour

Appears darker than surrounding skin

May have purplish/bluish hue in localized areas

Temperature

Initially, increased warmth when compared with surrounding skin

Later, coolness as tissue is devitalized

Touch	Appearance
Indurated	Blisters
Edema	Taut
Soft, boggy	Shiny
	Scaly

changed, the nurse should not directly inspect the wound unless serious complications are suspected. In such a situation, the nurse should inspect only the dressing and any external drains. If the physician prefers to change the dressing, the physician will assess the wound at least daily. When the nurse removes dressings, care is taken to avoid accidental removal or displacement of underlying drains. Because removal of dressings can be painful, it may help to give a prescribed analgesic at least 30 minutes before exposing a wound.

Acute wounds may require close monitoring (every 8 hours). Chronic wound assessment may be conducted less frequently. Depending upon the topical management system, the wound should be evaluated with every dressing change, usually not more than once per day.

Wound Appearance. The nurse measures the dimensions of the wound and notes its location and stage (if healing by secondary intention). Wound dimensions should include consistent measurements of depth, length, and width. The nurse uses a ruler to measure the longest and widest aspect of the wound surface in centimetres or millimetres (length × width). These measurements can provide overall gross changes in size as an indicator of healing.

The nurse also notes whether the wound edges are closed and the degree of approximation. A surgical incision healing by primary intention should have clean, well-approximated edges. Crusts often form along the wound edges from exudate. A puncture wound is usually a small, circular wound with the edges coming together toward the centre. If a wound is open (i.e., the wound edges are separated), the nurse inspects the condition of tissue at the wound base. The nurse also looks for complications such as dehiscence. The outer edges of a wound normally appear inflamed for the first 2 to 3 days, but this slowly disappears. Within 7 to 10 days, a normally healing wound resurfaces with epithelial cells, and the edges close.

The nurse assesses the amount (percentage) and appearance (colour) of tissue. Red, moist tissue is granulation tissue, and pink-purple tissue is newly formed epithelialization. Red and pink tissues indicate healing. Yellow tissue may be **slough** (stringy substance attached to wound bed), and black or brown tissue is generally **eschar** (necrotic, or dead tissue). Slough and eschar must

Box 43-6 Procedural Guidelines

Skin Assessment

Delegation considerations: Assessment for presence of skin breakdown is a nursing responsibility and should not be delegated to unregulated care providers (UCPs). However, it is important that the nurse instruct the UCP to immediately report the following:

- Any changes in the client's skin
- Client's exposure to body fluids (e.g., urine, feces, wound drainage, gastric secretions)

1. Obtain appropriate skin assessment documentation record (check agency policy).
2. Observe pressure points. Compression over bony prominences for prolonged periods of time can cause tissue ischemia and cell injury or death (AHCPR, 1992).
   a. Bony prominences—heels, ankles, knees, hips, sacral area, ischial area, spinal area, shoulders, and elbows (see Figure 43–3)
   b. Cast edges, area next to nasoenteral tubes, drainage tubes, or oxygen tubing
3. When reddened areas are found, gently press the area with a fingertip to assess the ability of the tissue to blanch. Normal reactive hyperemia is present when a reddened area blanches upon palpation. If the area does not blanch, suspect tissue injury.
4. Check perineal area for signs of reddened, irritated skin. Perineal skin is at high risk for skin breakdown in the client with fecal and/or urinary incontinence.
5. Observe areas where tape, tubing, casts, or splints are in contact with skin.
6. Note previous areas of skin breakdown, check for any breaks in the skin integrity, and note nonblanching erythema in these areas. Areas of previous skin breakdown do not heal to the same strength as intact non-injured skin; therefore, these areas are at higher risk of skin breakdown.
7. Determine if potential or actual skin breakdown is present and institute appropriate preventive or treatment protocols.
8. Record appearance of skin under pressure.
9. Record all preventive or treatment protocols that were initiated.

Box 43-7 Wound History Assessment Questions

What caused the wound?
When did the wound occur? What is its location and dimensions?
What happened to this wound since it occurred? What were the changes, and what caused them? What treatments, activities, or care have slowed or helped the wound-healing process? Are there special needs for this wound to heal?
Are there associated symptoms such as pain or itching with the wound? How are they being managed, and are they effective?
When did the client last receive a tetanus shot?
What is the goal for the client, wound, and healing?

Adapted from "Assessing the Patient With a Wound," by N. A. Stotts and C. E. Cavanaugh, 1999, *Home Healthcare Nurse, 17*(1), pp. 27–35.

Table 43-5 Assessment of Abnormal Healing in Primary and Secondary Intention Wounds

Primary Wounds	Secondary Wounds
Incision line poorly approximated	Pale or fragile granulation tissue; granulation tissue bed may be excessively dry or moist
Drainage present more than 3 days after closure	Exudate present
Inflammation increases in first 3–5 days after injury	Necrotic or slough tissue present in wound base
No epithelialization of wound edges by day 4	Epithelialization not continuous
No healing ridge by day 9	Fruity, earthy, or putrid odour present
	Presence of fistula(s), tunnelling, undermining

Adapted from "Assessing the Patient With a Wound," by N. A. Stotts and C. E. Cavanaugh, 1999, *Home Healthcare Nurse, 17*(1), p. 27.

be removed before the wound can heal. The condition of the skin surrounding the wound should be evaluated for redness, warmth, maceration (softening of the skin due to moisture), or **edema** (swelling). The presence of any of these factors on the skin surrounding the wound can indicate wound deterioration. If infection develops, the area directly surrounding the wound typically becomes brightly inflamed, swollen, warm, and tender (see Box 43-2). Table 43-5 lists assessment characteristics for abnormal wound healing in primary and secondary wounds.

Skin discoloration usually results from bruising of interstitial tissues or hematoma formation. Blood collecting beneath the skin first takes on a bluish or purplish appearance. Gradually, as the clotted blood is broken down, shades of brown and yellow appear.

Character of Wound Drainage. The nurse notes the amount, type (see Table 43-4), colour, odour, and consistency of drainage. The amount of drainage depends on the location and extent of the wound. For example, drainage is minimal after a simple appendectomy. In contrast, wound drainage is moderate for 1 to 2 days after drainage of a large abscess. Excessive exudates can indicate the presence of a wound infection.

If the nurse needs an accurate measurement of the amount of drainage within a dressing, the dressing can be weighed and compared with the weight of the same dressing when clean and dry. A rule of thumb is 1 g by weight of drainage equals 1 mL of volume of drainage. Another method of quantifying wound drainage would be to chart the number of dressings used and the frequency of change. An increase in the number or frequency of dressings will indicate a relative increase or decrease in wound drainage.

If the drainage has a pungent or strong odour, an infection should be suspected. The nurse should describe the wound's appearance according to characteristics observed. An example of accurate recording follows:

> Abdominal incision is 5 cm in width, in RLQ [right lower quadrant]; edges well approximated without inflammation or exudate. 1.2-cm diameter circle of serous drainage present on one 4 × 4 gauze changed every 8 hours.

Assessment Tools. The use and documentation of a systematic approach to wound assessment leads to better decision making and optimum outcomes (Ratliff & Bryant, 2003; Weir, 2001). Using a wound assessment tool enables the nurse to accurately compare the past and current state of the wound. It also provides a common language that can be used by all staff when discussing healing (Dolynchuk et al., 2000).

There are numerous tools available for assessing the healing wound. Many have been developed specifically for pressure ulcers, including, but not limited to, the Pressure Sore Status Test (PSST), the Pressure Ulcer Scale for Healing (PUSH), and the Bates-Jensen Wound Assessment Tool (BWAT; Figure 43–12). Several of these assessment tools are undergoing validity and reliability testing, and they are being used more frequently (Bates-Jensen, 1997; RNAO, 2002a). An agency may develop or adapt an assessment

BATES-JENSEN WOUND ASSESSMENT TOOL NAME________________________

Complete the rating sheet to assess wound status. Evaluate each item by picking the response that best describes the wound and entering the score in the item score column for the appropriate date.

Location: Anatomic site. Circle, identify right **(R)** or left **(L)** and use **"X"** to mark site on body diagrams:

___ Sacrum and coccyx ___ Lateral ankle
___ Trochanter ___ Medial ankle
___ Ischial tuberosity ___ Heel Other Site ___

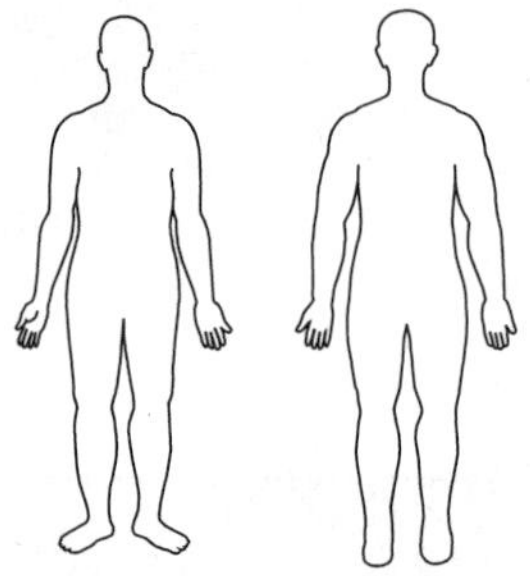

Shape: overall wound pattern; assess by observing perimeter and depth.

Circle and date appropriate description:

___ Irregular ___ Linear or elongated
___ Round/oval ___ Bowl/boat
___ Square/rectangle ___ Butterfly Other Shape ___

Item	Assessment	Date Score	Date Score	Date Score
1. Size	1 = Length × width <4 sq cm 2 = Length × width 4–<16 sq cm 3 = Length × width 16.1–<36 sq cm 4 = Length × width 36.1–<80 sq cm 5 = Length × width >80 sq cm			
2. Depth	1 = Non-blanchable erythema on intact skin 2 = Partial-thickness skin loss involving epidermis and/or dermis 3 = Full-thickness skin loss involving damage or necrosis of subcutaneous tissue; may extend down to but not through underlying fascia; and/or mixed partial and full thickness and/or tissue layers obscured by granulation tissue 4 = Obscured by necrosis 5 = Full-thickness skin loss with extensive destruction, tissue necrosis, or damage to muscle, bone or supporting structures			
3. Edges	1 = Indistinct, diffuse, none clearly visible 2 = Distinct, outline clearly visible, attached, even with wound base 3 = Well-defined, not attached to wound base 4 = Well-defined, not attached to base, rolled under, thickened 5 = Well-defined, fibrotic, scarred or hyperkeratotic			
4. Undermining	1 = None present 2 = Undermining <2 cm in any area 3 = Undermining 2-4 cm involving <50% wound margins 4 = Undermining 2-4 cm involving >50 % wound margins 5 = Undermining >4 cm or tunneling in any area			
5. Necrotic Tissue Type	1 = None visible 2 = White/gray non-viable tissue and/or non-adherent yellow slough 3 = Loosely adherent yellow slough 4 = Adherent, soft, black eschar 5 = Firmly adherent, hard, black eschar			
6. Necrotic Tissue Amount	1 = None visible 2 = <25% of wound bed covered 3 = 25% to 50% of wound covered 4 = >50% and <75% of wound covered 5 = 75 % to 100% of wound covered			

FIGURE **43–12** Bates-Jensen Wound Assessment Tool (BWAT). Based on Pressure Sore Status Tool (PSST). (Courtesy Barbara Bates-Jensen, Reseda, CA.)

Item	Assessment	Date Score	Date Score	Date Score
7. Exudate Type	1 = None 2 = Bloody 3 = Serosanguineous: thin, watery, pale red/pink 4 = Serous: thin, watery, clear 5 = Purulent: thin or thick, opaque, tan/yellow, with or without odor			
8. Exudate Amount	1 = None, dry wound 2 = Scant, wound moist but no observable exudate 3 = Small 4 = Moderate 5 = Large			
9. Skin Color Surrounding Wound	1 = Pink 2 = Bright red and/or blanches to touch 3 = White or grey pallor or hypopigmented 4 = Dark red or purple and/or non-blanchable 5 = Black or hyperpigmented			
10. Peripheral Tissue Edema	1 = No swelling or edema 2 = Non-pitting edema extends <4 cm around wound 3 = Non-pitting edema extends ≥4 cm around wound 4 = Pitting edema extends <4 cm around wound 5 = Crepitus and/or pitting edema extends ≥4 cm around wound			
11. Peripheral Tissue Induration	1 = None present 2 = Induration, <2 cm around wound 3 = Induration 2-4 cm extending <50% around wound 4 = Induration 2-4 cm extending ≥50% around wound 5 = Induration >4 cm in any area around wound			
12. Granulation Tissue	1 = Skin intact or partial-thickness wound 2 = Bright, beefy red; 75% to 100% of wound filled and/or tissue overgrowth 3 = Bright, beefy red; <75% and >25% of wound filled 4 = Pink, and/or dull, dusky red and/or fills ≤25% of wound 5 = No granulation tissue present			
13. Epithelialization	1 = 100% wound covered, surface intact 2 = 75% to <100% wound covered and/or epithelial tissue extends >0.5 cm into wound bed 3 = 50% to <75% wound covered and/or epithelial tissue extends to <0.5 cm into wound bed 4 = 25% to <50% wound covered 5 = <25% wound covered			
	TOTAL SCORE			
	SIGNATURE			

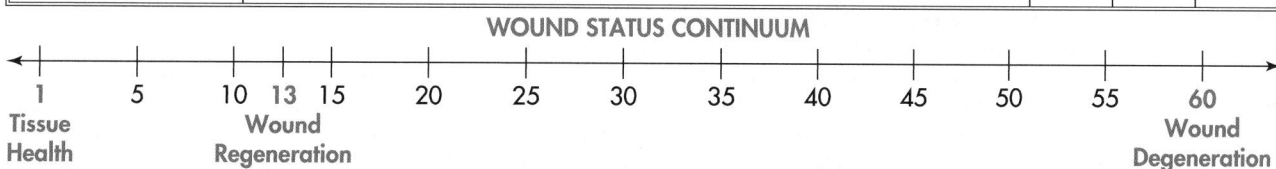

WOUND STATUS CONTINUUM

1 5 10 13 15 20 25 30 35 40 45 50 55 60

1 Tissue Health — 13 Wound Regeneration — 60 Wound Degeneration

Plot the total score on the Wound Status Continuum by putting an "X" on the line and the date beneath the line. Plot multiple scores with their dates to see-at-a-glance regeneration or degeneration of the wound.

FIGURE **43–12, cont'd** Bates-Jensen Wound Assessment Tool (BWAT). Based on Pressure Sore Status Tool (PSST). (Courtesy Barbara Bates-Jensen, Reseda, CA.)

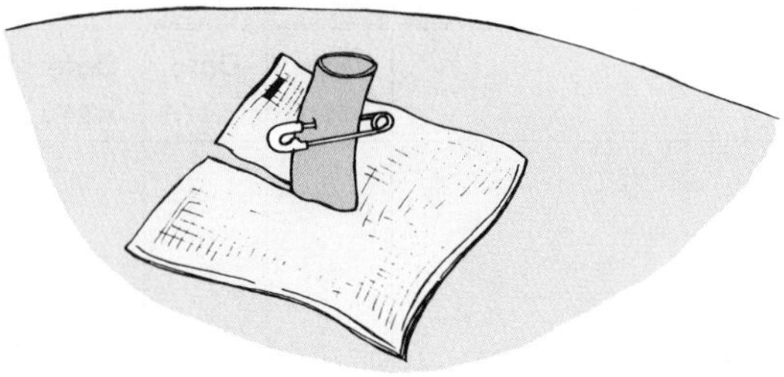

FIGURE **43–13** Penrose drain.

tool for its own setting. Check with agency policy for the use of wound assessment tools.

Drains. The physician inserts a drain into or near a surgical wound if a large amount of drainage is expected. Some drains are sutured in place. Caution should be exercised when changing the dressing around drains that are not sutured in place to prevent accidental removal. A Penrose drain may lie under a dressing; at the time of placement a pin or clip is placed through the drain to prevent it from slipping farther into the wound (Figure 43–13). It is usually the physician's responsibility to pull or advance the drain as drainage decreases to permit healing deep within the drain site.

The nurse assesses the number of drains, drain placement, character of drainage, and condition of collecting apparatus. First, the nurse observes the security of the drain and its location with respect to the wound. Next, the nurse notes the character of drainage. If there is a collecting device, the nurse measures the drainage volume. Because a drainage system must be patent, the nurse looks for drainage flow through the tubing and around the tubing. A sudden decrease in drainage through the tubing may indicate a blocked drain, and the physician should be notified. When a drain is connected to suction, the nurse assesses the system to be sure that the pressure ordered is being exerted. Evacuator units such as a Hemovac or Jackson-Pratt device (Figure 43–14) exert a constant low pressure as long as the suction device (bladder or bag) is fully compressed. These types of drainage devices are often referred to as self-suction. When the evacuator device is unable to maintain a vacuum on its own, the nurse notifies the surgeon, who can then order a secondary vacuum system (such as wall suction). If fluid is allowed to accumulate within the tissues, wound healing will not progress at an optimal rate and the risk of infection is increased.

Wound Closures. Surgical wounds are closed with staples, sutures, or wound closures. A frequent mode of skin closure is the stainless-steel staple. The staple provides more strength than nylon or silk sutures and tends to cause less irritation to tissue. The nurse looks for irritation around staple or suture sites and notes whether closures are intact. The nurse may choose to count sutures when the physician has removed a portion of them. Normally for the first 2 to 3 days after surgery, the skin around sutures or staples is edematous and reddened. Continued swelling may indicate that the closures are too tight. The skin can be cut by overly tight suture material, leading to wound separation. Sutures that are too

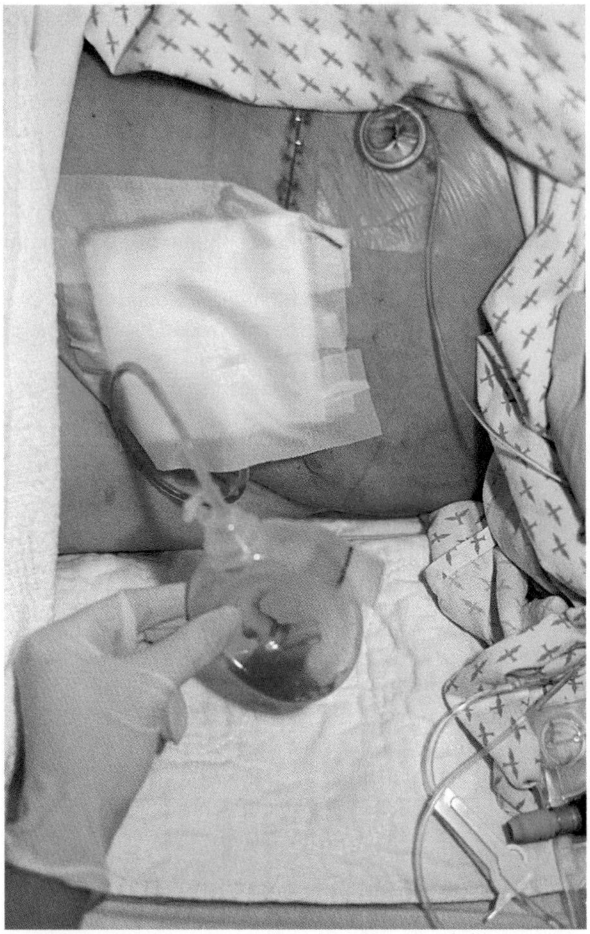

A

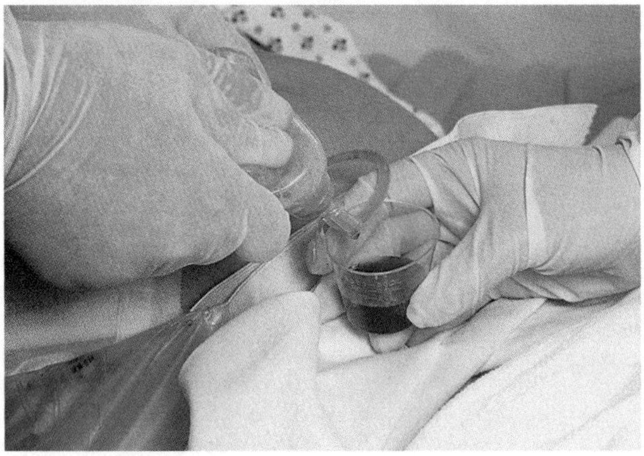

B

FIGURE **43–14** Jackson-Pratt drainage device. **A,** Drainage tubes and reservoir. **B,** Emptying drainage reservoir.

tight are a common cause of wound dehiscence. Early suture removal reduces formation of defects along the suture line and minimizes chances of scar formation.

Palpation of Wounds. When inspecting a wound, the nurse may observe swelling or separation of wound edges. While wearing gloves, the nurse lightly palpates wound edges, detecting localized areas of tenderness or drainage collection. The nurse gently applies the fingertips along

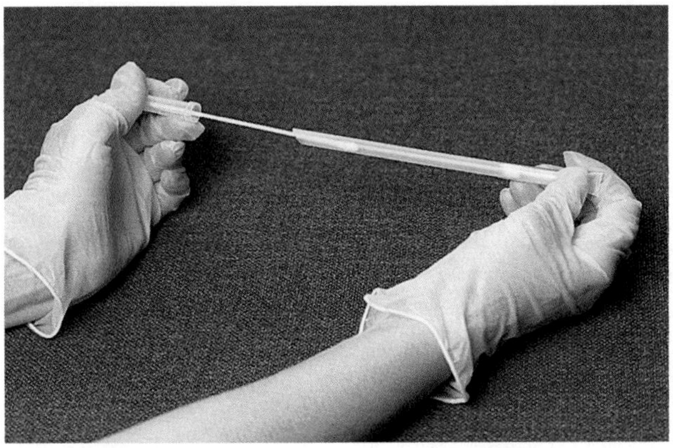

FIGURE **43–15** Wound culturette tube.

Box 43-8 Swab Procedure for Obtaining a Wound Culture*

- Clean the wound surface with a non-antiseptic solution.
- Moisten the swab with normal saline.
- Rotate the swab in 1 cm^2 of clean tissue in the open wound. The tip of the swab should be rolled from side to side in a zigzag pattern over the part of the wound with the most obvious signs of infection. Apply pressure to the swab to elicit tissue fluid.
- Insert the tip of the swab into the appropriate sterile container and transport to the laboratory immediately.

*Check agency policy to determine need to obtain physician order. Adapted from "Wound Infection: Diagnosis and Management," by N. A. Stotts, in *Acute and Chronic Wounds: Nursing Management* (2nd ed.), edited by R. A. Bryant, 2000b, St. Louis, MO: Mosby.

the wound edges. If pressure causes fluid to be expressed, the nurse notes the character of the drainage. It may be necessary to collect the drainage for culture. The client is normally sensitive to palpation of wound edges. Extreme tenderness may indicate infection.

Wound Cultures. If the nurse detects purulent or suspicious-looking wound drainage, or observes a change in a previously healing chronic wound, obtaining a specimen of the drainage for culture may be necessary (see chapter 29). The nurse never collects a wound culture sample from old drainage. Resident colonies of bacteria from the skin grow within exudate and may not be the true causative organisms of a wound infection. The nurse cleans a wound first with normal saline to remove skin flora. Aerobic organisms grow in superficial wounds exposed to the air, and anaerobic organisms tend to grow within body cavities. The nurse uses a different method of specimen collection for each type of organism.

To collect an aerobic specimen, the nurse uses a sterile swab from a culturette tube (Figure 43–15 and Box 43-8). If wound edges are separated, the nurse slowly and gently inserts the tip of the swab into the wound to collect deeper secretions. The nurse needs to apply sufficient pressure with the swab to cause some tissue fluid to be expressed in an area the size of 1 cm^2 and collected onto the tip of the swab (Stotts, 2000b). After collecting the specimen, the nurse returns the swab to the culturette tube, caps the tube, and crushes the inner ampule containing the medium for organism growth. The medium must moisten and coat the swab tip. The nurse immediately sends the labelled specimen to the laboratory for bacterial culture (AHCPR, 1994).

If drainage from a deep body cavity has a foul odour, there is a chance of anaerobic organism growth. The nurse uses a sterile syringe tip to aspirate drainage from the inner wound. Afterward, the nurse applies a sterile needle to the syringe and expels air from the syringe and needle. The nurse then removes the needle and replaces it with a sterile cap. In some institutions, the nurse may inject the specimen into a special vacuum tube containing culture medium.

Most microbiology laboratories routinely perform a direct gram stain on swab specimens submitted for culture. The results of this test often allow the physician to order appropriate treatment before culture results are available (normally within 24 to 72 hours). No additional specimens are usually required.

Pain. Wound pain influences the client's ability to function and quality of life. Pain, or any change in pain, is a key predictor of wound infection and inflammation. The AHCPR (1994) has recommended that the assessment and management of pain be included in the care of clients with wounds.

Wound pain can be divided into three categories (Krasner, 2001, as cited in Reddy et al., 2003):

1. *Non-cyclic acute wound pain*—occurs during manipulation of the wound, such as with debridement. Use of local anaesthetic and adequate preparation of the client can help reduce this pain.
2. *Cyclic acute wound pain*—accompanies regular procedures, such as dressing changes and client repositioning. In addition to the previous strategies, use of non-traumatic dressings, soaking dressings before removal, and allowing client control can minimize this type of pain.
3. *Chronic wound pain*—persistently felt by the client, even when the wound is not being manipulated. Medications and non-pharmacological treatment can be used (see chapter 38).

A thorough pain assessment includes noting the location, frequency, onset, duration, intensity, and exacerbating and relieving factors of the pain. Pain intensity can be measured by using a validated pain scale with each assessment (see chapter 38).

Client Expectations. When clients have an acute surgical or traumatic wound, the wound may heal promptly and without complications. However, when pressure ulcers or other chronic wounds are present, the course of treatment is lengthy and costly. Because the client and family must be involved with wound care management, it is important to know the client's expectations. A client who has realistic goals and is informed about the length

Nursing Diagnostic Process — Box 43-9

Assessment Activities	Defining Characteristics	Nursing Diagnosis
Inspect surface of skin.	Presence of wound, break in skin integrity Yellow, foul-smelling drainage from wound Edges of wound not approximated Sutures remain in place	Impaired skin integrity related to contaminated wound
Inspect wound for signs of healing.	Brown-red drainage 5 days after surgery Edges of wound not approximated	
Obtain client's temperature, heart rate, and white blood cell count	Client is febrile, heart rate is 125 beats per minute, leukocyte (white blood cell) count is 12 000/mm³	

of time required for wound healing is more likely to adhere to the specific therapies designed to promote wound healing and prevent further skin breakdown.

Nursing Diagnosis

Assessment reveals whether *impaired skin integrity* exists or whether the client is at risk. In addition, the assessment data may reveal more than one diagnosis. For example, suppose a post-operative client has purulent drainage from a surgical wound and reports tenderness around the area of the wound. These data would support a nursing diagnosis of *infection* (Box 43-9). After completing an assessment of the client's wound, the nurse identifies nursing diagnoses that will direct supportive and preventive care. There are multiple nursing diagnoses that may be associated with impaired skin integrity and wounds:

- Risk for infection
- Imbalanced nutrition: less than body requirements
- Acute or chronic pain
- Impaired physical mobility
- Impaired skin integrity
- Risk for impaired skin integrity
- Ineffective tissue perfusion

The client may be at risk for poor wound healing because of previously defined factors that impair healing (see Table 43-2). Thus, even though the client's wound may appear normal, the nurse identifies nursing diagnoses, such as *impaired nutrition* or *impaired tissue perfusion,* that direct nursing care toward support of wound repair.

The nature of a wound can cause problems unrelated to wound healing. Alteration in comfort and impaired mobility are problems that have implications for the client's eventual recovery. For example, a large abdominal incision can cause enough pain to interfere with the client's ability to turn in bed effectively.

Planning

After identifying nursing diagnoses, the nurse develops a plan of care for the client who has actual or is at risk for impaired skin integrity. During planning, the nurse again synthesizes information from multiple resources (Figure 43–16). Professional standards are especially important to consider when developing a plan of care.

Clients who have large or chronic wounds have multiple nursing care needs. For example, consider the following scenario:

> A nurse is caring for Mrs Martha Dobroskay. Mrs. Dobroskay is 65-years old and has a 30-year history of diabetes mellitus, for which she takes insulin. Her diabetes is poorly controlled due to her inability to adhere to a 1200-calorie diet. She is 30 kg overweight. For the last 10 years, she has reported decreased sensation to her lower extremities. She does not practise good foot care; she cuts her own toenails and goes barefoot. She was admitted to the hospital for elective repair of an abdominal aneurysm. The surgery went well, but post-operatively Mrs. Dobroskay had difficulty ambulating and performing coughing and deep-breathing exercises. On her second post-operative day, she developed a post-operative pneumonia, which required intravenous antibiotics. During the course of her pneumonia, Mrs. Dobroskay refused to walk, she became incontinent of urine and stool, and she complained about position changes. After her position was changed, she would reposition herself on her back. Two weeks after her surgery, Mrs. Dobroskay developed a large draining sacral wound, which is now 6 cm in diameter and is a stage IV pressure ulcer. In addition, she has a smaller, stage III ulcer on her left heel. Skin assessment also reveals areas of non-blanching redness over pressure points, especially on the right heel and over both hips.

When planning for care for Mrs. Dobroskay, a concept map can help to individualize care for her multiple health problems and related nursing diagnoses (Figure 43–17). This map assists the nurse in using critical thinking skills to organize complex client assessment data and related nursing diagnoses with the client's chief medical diagnosis. As the nurse identifies linkages between the nursing diagnoses and the chief medical diagnosis, the concept map also links potential interventions with the client's health care needs.

Goals and Outcomes. Nursing care is based on the client's identified needs and priorities. Goals and expected outcomes are established. From the goals, the nurse plans interventions according to the risk for pressure ulcers, the

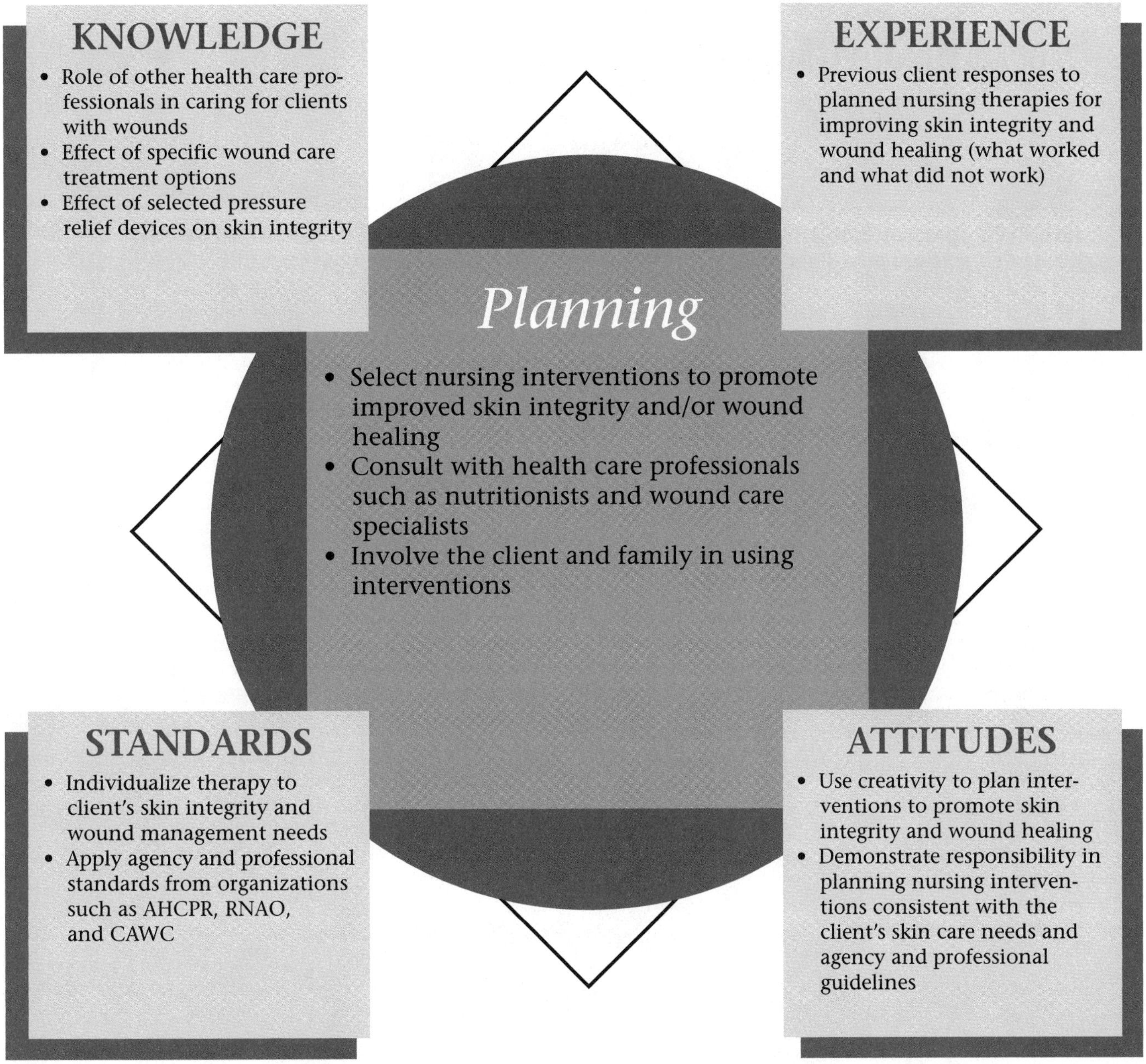
KNOWLEDGE
• Role of other health care professionals in caring for clients with wounds
• Effect of specific wound care treatment options
• Effect of selected pressure relief devices on skin integrity
EXPERIENCE
• Previous client responses to planned nursing therapies for improving skin integrity and wound healing (what worked and what did not work)
Planning
• Select nursing interventions to promote improved skin integrity and/or wound healing
• Consult with health care professionals such as nutritionists and wound care specialists
• Involve the client and family in using interventions
STANDARDS
• Individualize therapy to client's skin integrity and wound management needs
• Apply agency and professional standards from organizations such as AHCPR, RNAO, and CAWC
ATTITUDES
• Use creativity to plan interventions to promote skin integrity and wound healing
• Demonstrate responsibility in planning nursing interventions consistent with the client's skin care needs and agency and professional guidelines

FIGURE **43–16** Critical thinking model for skin integrity and wound care planning.

type and severity of the wound, or the presence of any complications that can affect wound healing (e.g., infection, poor nutrition, peripheral vascular diseases, or immunosuppression; see Care Plan).

A goal frequently identified when working with a client with a wound is to see wound improvement within a 2-week period. The outcomes of this goal might include the following:

- Higher percentage of granulation tissue in the wound base
- No further skin breakdown in any body location
- An increase in the caloric intake by 10%

These outcomes can be reasonable if the overall goal for the client is to heal the ulcer. Other goals of care for clients with wounds include the following: promoting wound hemostasis, preventing infection, promoting wound healing, maintaining skin integrity, gaining comfort, and health promotion.

Setting Priorities. The nursing care priorities in wound care are established from the comprehensive client assessment and goals and established outcomes. These priorities also depend on whether the client's condition is stable or emergent. An acute wound needs immediate intervention, whereas in the presence of a chronic, stable wound, the client's hygiene needs may have a greater priority. When there is a risk for pressure ulcer development, preventive interventions, such as skin care practices, elimination of shear, and frequent repositioning, are high priorities. Promotion of wound healing is a major nursing

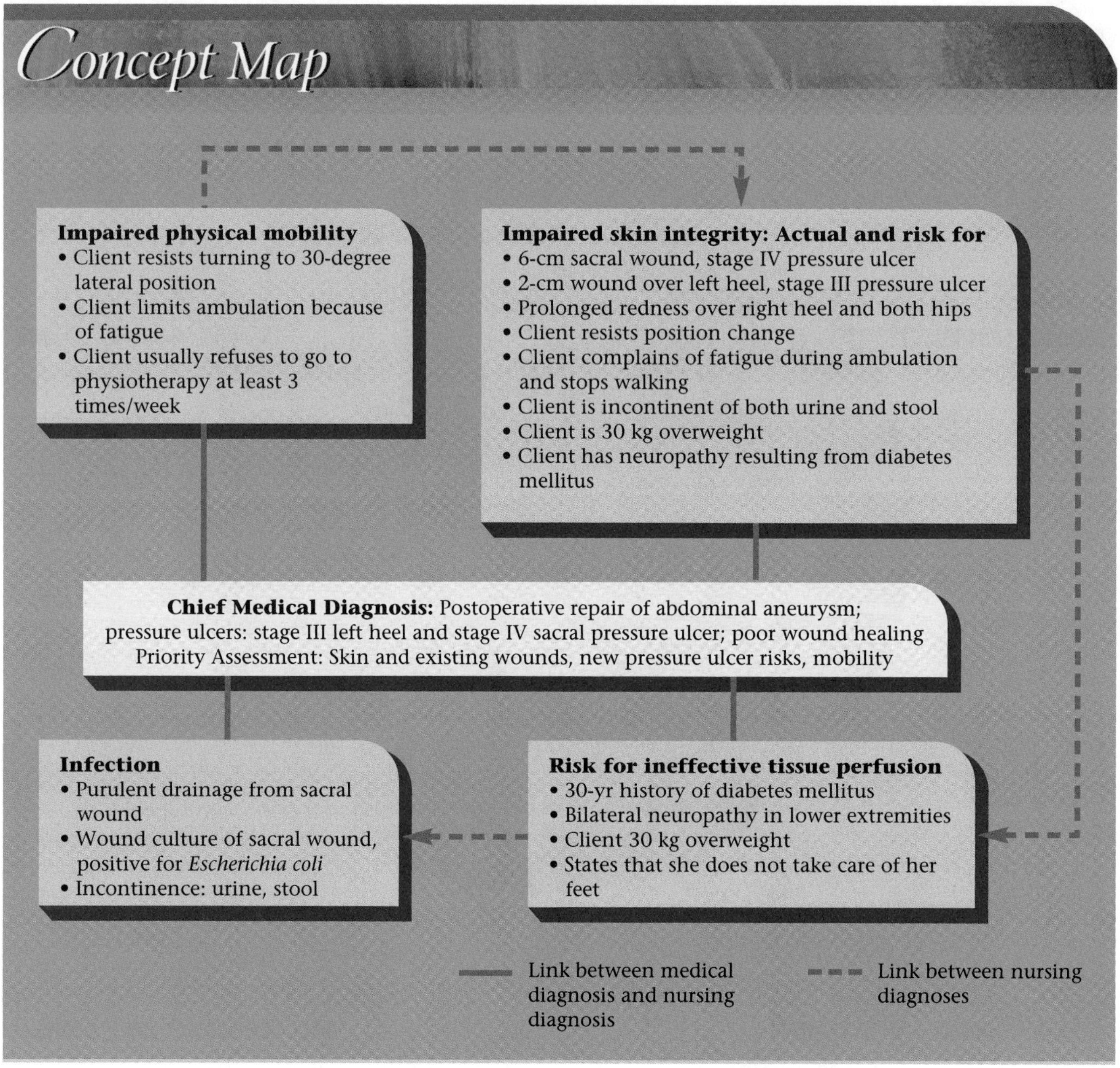
Concept Map
Impaired physical mobility
• Client resists turning to 30-degree lateral position
• Client limits ambulation because of fatigue
• Client usually refuses to go to physiotherapy at least 3 times/week
Impaired skin integrity: Actual and risk for
• 6-cm sacral wound, stage IV pressure ulcer
• 2-cm wound over left heel, stage III pressure ulcer
• Prolonged redness over right heel and both hips
• Client resists position change
• Client complains of fatigue during ambulation and stops walking
• Client is incontinent of both urine and stool
• Client is 30 kg overweight
• Client has neuropathy resulting from diabetes mellitus
Chief Medical Diagnosis: Postoperative repair of abdominal aneurysm; pressure ulcers: stage III left heel and stage IV sacral pressure ulcer; poor wound healing
Priority Assessment: Skin and existing wounds, new pressure ulcer risks, mobility
Infection
• Purulent drainage from sacral wound
• Wound culture of sacral wound, positive for Escherichia coli
• Incontinence: urine, stool
Risk for ineffective tissue perfusion
• 30-yr history of diabetes mellitus
• Bilateral neuropathy in lower extremities
• Client 30 kg overweight
• States that she does not take care of her feet
Link between medical diagnosis and nursing diagnosis
Link between nursing diagnoses

FIGURE **43–17** Concept map for client with a chronic wound.

priority, and the type of wound care administered depends on the type, size, and location of the wound, and overall treatment goals.

Other client factors to be considered when establishing priorities include client preferences, daily activities, and family factors. These factors are important regardless of the setting for health care. The priorities of care may not vary from outpatient, home, acute care, or restorative care settings.

Continuity of Care. Clients moving between care settings should have advanced notice in order to ensure a smooth transfer of care (RNAO, 2005). Consistency of pressure ulcer prevention and care between settings is essential. Ensuring that funding and equipment are in place is important to prevent interruption in the place of care. Communication of client information between settings, both in writing and verbally, will enhance the process. Specifically, the following information should be provided (RNAO, 2005):

- Risk factors
- Details of pressure points and skin condition prior to transfer
- Type of bed/mattress and seating required
- Stage, site, and size of existing ulcers
- History of ulcers, previous treatments, and dressings used
- Type of dressing currently used and frequency of change
- Any adverse reactions to dressing products

Nursing Care Plan

Impaired Skin Integrity

Assessment

Mrs. Stein is 3 weeks post-operative following a total hip replacement. She does not complain of discomfort at the operative site; however, she complains of a painful, burning sensation in the sacral region.

Assessment Activities	Findings/Defining Characteristics
Obtain an oral temperature.	Elevated temperature is noted.
Ask Ms. Stein how the surgical site limits her mobility.	She relates that her hip always aches and the pain is increased upon movement. She tells you that she prefers to keep the hip immobile to keep the pain level down. Position of comfort is supine, and Mrs. Stein resists position changes.
Perform a total body skin assessment, paying special attention to the sacral area.	Hyperemia is noted over the sacral area; this reddened area does not blanch upon palpation (Pieper, 2000). Skin over sacrum is blistered and has an abrasion (Braden, 2001). No other areas are noted to be open, with the exception of the surgical site.

Nursing Diagnosis: Impaired skin integrity related to pressure on the bony prominence in the sacral region.

Planning

Goal	Expected Outcomes*
	Tissue Integrity
Injury to client's skin and underlying tissue resulting from pressure on the bony prominence will be reduced within 2 to 4 weeks.	Client will have intact skin integrity in the area of non-blanching erythema. Mrs. Stein will maintain intact skin over other pressure points. Client's skin will remain clean and dry.
	Immobility Consequences: Physiological
Client's ability to tolerate position changes will improve within 2 to 4 weeks.	Reactive hyperemia will be within normal limits in all pressure points except sacral region. Reactive hyperemia in sacral region will have a decrease in non-blanchable pressure areas.

*Outcome classification labels from *Nursing Outcomes Classification (NOC)* (3rd ed.), edited by S. Moorhead, M. Johnson, and M. L. Maas, 2004, St. Louis, MO: Mosby.

Interventions†	Rationale
Pressure Management	
Reposition client every 90 minutes. Offer pain medication at least 20 minutes before position change.	Repositioning removes pressure and allows normal hyperemic response. Frequency of turning is based on initial assessment (AHCPR, 1994; Pieper, 2000; RNAO 2005).
Place client on a low-air-loss overlay.	Clients with pressure ulcer development are at greater risk for new ulcers and need preventive measures to prevent ulcer progression (AHCPR, 1994; NPUAP, 1995a, 1995b).
Site Care	
Keep area dry and clean; avoid rubbing the area.	Moisture can soften the skin and cause a break in the skin integrity. Rubbing an area of non-blanching erythema can cause further tissue damage (AHCPR, 1992; Ratliff & Bryant, 2003).

†Intervention classification labels from *Nursing Interventions Classification (NIC)* (4th ed.), edited by J. M. Dochterman and G. M. Bulecheck, 2004, St. Louis, MO: Mosby.

Continued

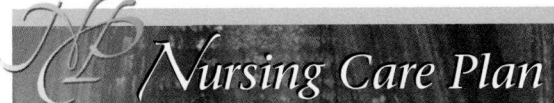

Nursing Care Plan

Impaired Skin Integrity—cont'd

Evaluation

Nursing Actions	Client Response/Findings	Achievement of Outcome
Perform a daily total body skin assessment. Chart results.	No new skin breakdown noted.	Client reports no other areas of pain or discomfort.
	Decreased redness at the sacral area.	Client reports decreased pain at the sacral site.
Palpate the reddened area over the sacrum.	Sacral area begins to show signs of normal reactive hyperemia and blanching following palpation.	Sacral region is improving; no break in epidermis.
	Other pressure points have normal reactive hyperemia and blanching.	Other pressure points remain intact.

Box 43-10 Home Care Recommendations

Ulcer/Wound Assessment

Assessment and documentation of the pressure ulcer should be carried out at least weekly, unless there is evidence of deterioration, in which case both the pressure ulcer and the client's overall management must be reassessed immediately. In the home setting, this may require the assistance of the client and family because weekly assessment by health care providers is not always feasible.

Psychosocial Assessment and Management

- Assess resources (e.g., availability and skill of caregivers, finances, equipment) of individuals being treated for pressure ulcers in the home. A successful treatment program requires adequate caregiver and equipment resources.
- Caregivers need to be evaluated for their ability to comprehend and implement the treatment requirements.
- Caregivers should also be evaluated for their level of strength and endurance.
- Economic factors should be considered, because they may limit the supply and availability of equipment, as well as opportunities to relieve caregivers.
- An approach is suggested that focuses upon the psychosocial and physical factors affecting wound care (Teare & Barrett, 2002).

Ulcer Care Dressings

- Consider caregiver time when selecting a dressing.
- In the home setting, caregivers may choose more expensive dressing materials to reduce the frequency of dressing changes.

Infection Control

- Clean dressings may also be used in the home setting.
- Clean dressings, as opposed to sterile dressings, are recommended for home use until research demonstrates otherwise. This recommendation is in keeping with principles regarding nosocomial infections and with past success of clean urinary catheterization in the home setting, and it takes into account the expense of sterile dressings and the dexterity required for application. The "no-touch" technique can be used for dressing changes. This technique is a method of changing surface dressings without touching the wound or the surface of any dressing that might be in contact with the wound. Adherent dressings should be grasped by the corner and removed slowly, whereas gauze dressings can be pinched in the centre and lifted off.
- Disposal of contaminated dressings in the home should be done in a manner consistent with local regulations and the policy and procedures of the home care provider.

Adapted from *Treatment of Pressure Ulcers* (Clinical Practice Guideline No. 15, AHCPR Publication No. 95-0653), Agency for Health Care Policy and Research, Panel for the Treatment of Pressure Ulcers in Adults, 1994, Rockville, MD: Author, U.S. Department of Health and Human Services.

- Need for ongoing nutritional support
- Summary of relevant laboratory results

Anticipating the client's discharge wound care needs and related equipment and resources, such as referral to a home care agency or outpatient wound care clinic, can assist in improving wound healing and the client's level of independence. Clients and their families may need to continue the objectives of wound management after discharge (Box 43-10). The nurse and client work together to establish ways of maintaining client involvement in nursing care and to promote wound healing whether the client is in the hospital or at home.

Implementation

Health Promotion. Prevention is perhaps the most effective intervention for problems with skin integrity and wound care. Prompt identification of at-risk clients and their risk factors aids in prevention of pressure ulcers.

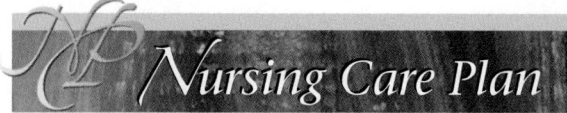

Box 43-11 RNAO Recommendations to Prevent Pressure Ulcers in At-Risk Clients

Equipment and Positioning

- Use pressure reducing/relieving equipment.
- Establish and post an individualized repositioning schedule.
- Use proper position, transferring, and turning techniques. Consult with occupational therapists or physiotherapists for advice.
- Replace standard mattress with one that has low interface pressure, such as a high-density foam.
- Do not use donut-type devices or products that localize pressure to a new area.
- For high risk clients experiencing surgical intervention, the use of pressure-relieving surfaces intraoperatively should be considered.

For clients restricted to bed:

- Use an interdisciplinary approach to plan care.
- Reposition the client at least every 2 hours, or sooner if high risk.
- Use pillows or foam wedges to avoid contact between bony prominences.
- Use devices (pillows, foam wedges) that totally relieve pressure on the heels and bony prominences of the feet.
- Avoid positioning directly on the trochanter. Position client at a 30-degree lateral position to either side (see Figure 43-18).
  To reduce shearing forces, maintain the head of the bed at the lowest elevation consistent with medical condition and restrictions. An elevation of 30 degrees or lower is recommended.
- Use lifting devices (e.g., manual or electric lifts, lifting sheets) to move rather than drag clients during transfer and position changes

For clients restricted to a chair:

- Use an interdisciplinary approach to plan care.
- Have the client shift weight every 15 minutes, if able.
- Reposition client at least every hour if client is unable to shift weight.
- Use pressure-reducing devices for seating surfaces (not donut type)
- Consider postural alignment, distribution of weight, balance and stability, and pressure reduction when positioning clients in chairs or wheelchairs.
- Refer to physiotherapy and occupational therapy for seating assessment and special adaptations.

Hygiene and Skin Care

- Do not massage over bony prominences.
- When bathing the client, avoid hot water and use a pH balanced, non-sensitizing cleansing agent. Apply minimal friction and force when cleansing the skin.
- Use lubricating moisturizers and creams with minimal alcohol content to rehydrate dry skin.
- Use protective dressings (e.g., liquid barrier films, transparent films, hydrocolloids) or protective padding to reduce friction injuries.
- If there is excessive moisture or incontinence:
  - Gently cleanse the skin at time of soiling. Avoid friction during care with the use of a spray perineal cleanser or soft wipe.
  - Assess and treat urinary incontinence (see chapter 40).
  - When moisture cannot be controlled, use absorbent pads, dressings, or briefs that wick moisture away from the skin. Replace pads and linens when damp.
  - Protect skin with a moisture barrier ointment.
  - If unresolved skin irritation exists in a moist area, consult with the physician for evaluation and topical treatment.
  - Establish a bowel and bladder program.

Nutrition

- Ensure hydration through adequate fluid intake.
- A nutritional assessment should be conducted on entry to a new health care environment and when the client's condition changes. If a nutritional deficit is suspected:
  - Consult with a dietitian.
  - Investigate factors that compromise dietary intake (especially protein or calories) and offer the client support with eating.
  - Plan and implement a nutritional support and/or supplementation program for nutritionally compromised clients.
  - Consider alternative nutritional interventions if dietary intake remains inadequate (see chapter 39).
  - Nutritional supplementation for critically ill older clients should be considered.

Mobility

- Consult with the care team regarding implementing a rehabilitation program to improve the client's mobility and activity status, if consistent with overall goals of care.

Adapted from *Risk Assessment and Prevention of Pressure Ulcers* (pp. 9–13), Registered Nurses Association of Ontario, 2005 (Revised). Retrieved March 29, 2005, from *http://www.rnao.org/bestpractices/completed_guidelines/BPG_Guide_C1_Pressure_Ulcers.asp*

Prevention of Pressure Ulcers. When the client is immobile, the major risk to the skin is the formation of pressure ulcers. Nursing interventions focus on prevention. The first step in prevention is to assess the client's risk factors for pressure ulcer development (see Assessing for Risk of Pressure Ulcers). The nurse then plans for the reduction or elimination of identified risk factors.

Box 43-11 is a summary of RNAO-recommended nursing interventions to prevent pressure ulcers in at-risk clients. Major areas of nursing interventions for prevention of pressure ulcers include the use of pressure-reducing and pressure-relieving equipment (including therapeutic mattresses), proper positioning of the client, hygiene and skin care, nutrition, and mobility. Client education on preventing pressure ulcers is also important. The following sections address issues that are related to some of these areas.

Topical Skin Care. The goal of bathing is to ensure that the moisture retention and barrier functions of the skin are not jeopardized. (See Box 43-11 for recommended interventions when bathing the client.) When the skin is cleansed, soaps and hot water must be avoided. Soaps and alcohol-based lotions cause drying and leave an alkaline residue. The alkaline residue discourages the growth of normal bacteria, thus promoting an overgrowth of opportunistic bacteria that can then enter an open wound

(AHCPR, 1992). There are many mild cleansing agents available for skin care, and their use needs to be matched to the specific needs of the client. Nurses should check that the product has a pH within the 4 to 7 range, ingredients are not contraindicated for the client, and the product has been tested for dermal irritation and antimicrobial efficacy.

Skin should be cleansed gently and then patted or air-dried. Once completely dried, moisturizer should be applied to keep the epidermis well lubricated but not oversaturated. Efforts should be make to control, contain, or correct incontinence, perspiration, and wound drainage (Ratliff & Bryant, 2003). When clients have an incontinent episode, the area should be gently cleansed and dried and a thick layer of moisture barrier applied to the exposed areas. A moisture barrier protects the skin from excessive moisture and bacteria found in the stool.

Urinary incontinence may be treated with behavioural techniques, medication, and surgery. Behavioural techniques are used to help clients learn ways to control their bladder and sphincter muscles. Two examples are bladder training and habit retraining (see chapter 40). The expertise of an advanced practice nurse with a focus on enterostomal therapy, wound care, or management of incontinence should be used in caring for at-risk clients.

Use of absorbent pads and garments should be considered only after other measures have been tried. The nurse should use only products that wick moisture away from the client's skin (AHCPR, 1992b; Ratliff & Bryant, 2003). Underpads should be chosen judiciously because some of these pads do not wick the drainage away from the client's skin and can cause skin damage.

Positioning. Turning and positioning the client to offload areas of increased pressure is one of the easiest ways to prevent pressure ulcers from developing. Positioning interventions are designed to reduce pressure and shearing force to the skin. Elevating the head of the bed to 30 degrees or less will decrease the chance of pressure ulcer development from shearing forces (AHCPR, 1992; RNAO 2005). The immobilized client's position should be changed at least every 2 hours; frequency of repositioning depends on the client's activity level, perceptual ability, and daily routines (Braden, 2001). The RNAO (2002a) recommends that a written turning and positioning schedule be used.

When repositioning, positioning devices (e.g., pillows, foam wedges) should be used to protect bony prominences (AHCPR, 1992, 1994; RNAO, 2005). Position the client in a 30-degree lateral position to either side in order to avoid lying the client over a bony prominence (AHCPR, 1992; RNAO, 2005; Figure 43–18). To prevent shear and friction injuries, the nurse should use a sheet or lifting device to lift rather than drag the client when changing positions.

> ***Safety Alert.*** Incorrect positioning of an immobile client can create a shearing injury. When repositioning the client, place a flat folded sheet under the client's body. Obtain assistance for repositioning and, with at least one other caregiver, lift the sheet up and toward the new position. Dragging the client on the sheets will place the client at high risk for shearing and friction injuries.

Clients able to sit in a chair should be limited to sitting in the same position for 1 hour or less. Again, the exact time is individualized, but the nurse should not allow the client to sit for a period longer than the recommended time that was calculated during assessment. Thus, if the interval is every 1 hour, the client should remain in a sitting position for less than 1 hour. In the sitting position, the pressure on the ischial tuberosities is greater than in the supine position. In addition, a client at risk for skin breakdown in a sitting position should be taught to shift weight every 15 minutes (AHCPR, 1992; Ratliff & Bryant, 2003). Shifting weight provides short-term relief on the ischial tuberosities. A client should also sit on foam, gel, or an air cushion to redistribute weight away from the ischial areas. Rigid and donut-shaped cushions are contraindicated because they reduce blood supply to the area, resulting in wider areas of ischemia (AHCPR, 1994).

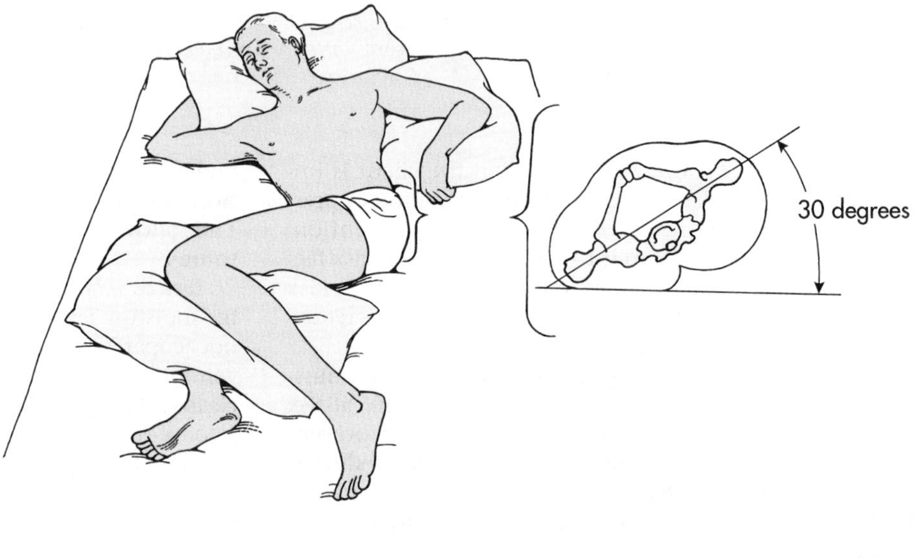

FIGURE **43–18** Thirty-degree lateral position in which pressure points are avoided. (From "Mechanical Forces: Pressure, Shear, and Friction," by B. Pieper, in *Acute and Chronic Wounds: Nursing Management,* 2nd ed., p. 244, edited by R. A. Bryant, 2000, St. Louis, MO: Mosby.)

After the client is repositioned, the nurse reassesses the skin (see Assessment of Skin for Signs of Pressure Ulcers).

Therapeutic Beds and Mattresses. Clients at risk for pressure ulcers should use a specialized mattress (RNAO, 2002a). A variety of support surfaces, including specialty beds and mattresses, have been designed to reduce the hazards of immobility to the skin and musculoskeletal system. However, no single device eliminates the effects of pressure on the skin, and none of these eliminates the need for meticulous nursing care.

It is important to understand the difference between a pressure-reducing and a pressure-relieving support surface. A mattress that is **pressure relieving** relieves the interface pressure (the pressure between the body and the support surface) below 32 mm Hg (capillary closing pressure). Mattresses that are **pressure reducing** reduce the interface pressure, but not necessarily below the capillary closing pressure (AHCPR, 1994). Table 43-6 lists some of the many available pressure-relieving and -reducing support surfaces. When used correctly, these therapeutic mattresses

Table 43-6 Pressure-Reduction and Pressure-Relief Mattresses

Product	Mechanism of Action	Advantages	Disadvantages
Pressure-Reduction Mattresses			
Foam (5- to 10-cm overlay or mattress)	Reduces pressure, friction, and shear	• Low cost • Lightweight • Provides comfort	• Thinner foams offer little pressure reduction • Retains moisture • Increases dermal temperature • Risk of bacterial contamination
Air-filled mattress (available in an overlay)	Interconnected air-filled cells, inflated to appropriate level	• Easy to clean • Lightweight • Versatile	• Over- or underinflation can increase pressure • Accidental puncture possible • Proper set-up and ongoing care difficult
Pressure-Relief Products			
Low-air-loss bed (full bed or overlay)	Bed: The entire surface is a powered, inflated surface with air loss Overlay: Powered surface, constant inflation and air loss at the surface; place over the bed mattress	• Prevents skin breakdown in clients who cannot be turned or have existing skin breakdown • Covering decreases moisture • Proper calibration results in interface pressures <25 mm Hg	• Expensive • No temperature control • Improper calibration possible • Client must be turned to decrease pulmonary complications
Air-fluidized high-air-loss bed	Bed frame with silicone-coated beads that become fluidized when air is pumped through the beads	• Appropriate for clients with burns or multiple stage III or IV pressure ulcers • Protects new grafts and flaps • Antishear, antifriction surface • Allows for ease of client movement • Minimizes maceration produced by incontinence or perspiration by drying the skin • Pressures <25 mm Hg	• Expensive • Significant fluid loss, up to 2400 mL/day • Contraindicated for clients on limited intake or with unstable neurological status • Can dry out wounds • Client transfers may be difficult • May cause motion sickness
Kinetic therapy low-air-loss bed	Provides continuous passive motion to promote mobilization of respiratory secretions; also provides low-air-loss therapy	• Appropriate for clients at risk for or who have developed atelectasis and/or pneumonia • Short-term use • Client turned automatically 200 times/day • Total pressure relief • Eliminates friction, shear, maceration	• Expensive • Small-framed clients at high risk of falls • No temperature control

Adapted from *Assessment and Management of Stage I to IV Pressure Ulcers* (pp. 82–83), Registered Nurses Association of Ontario, 2002a. Retrieved April 14, 2004, from *http://www.rnao.org/bestpractices/completed_guidelines/BPG_Guide_C2_pressure_ulcer.asp*

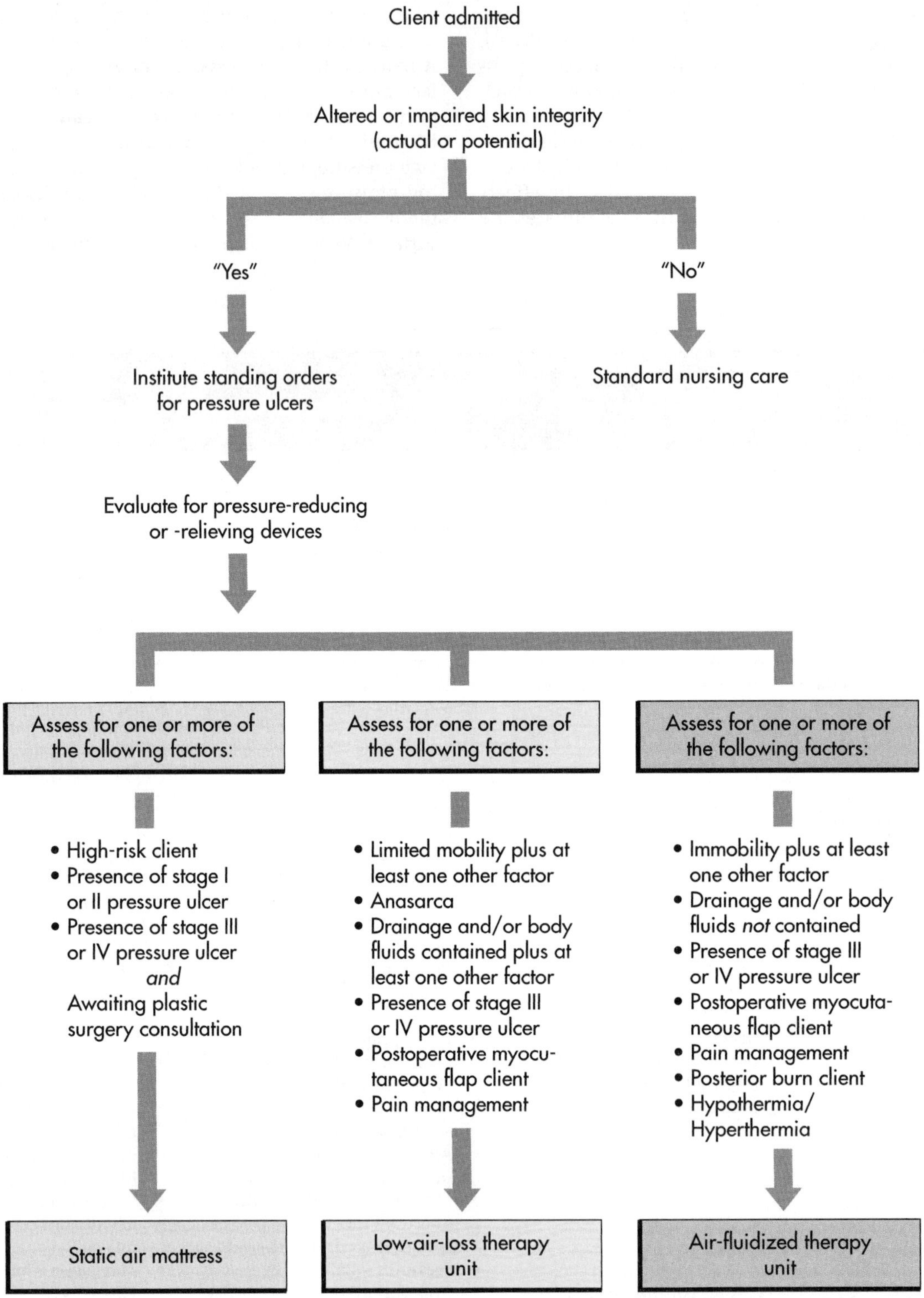

FIGURE **43–19** Flow diagram for ordering specialty beds. (From "Specialty Beds: Decision-Making Made Easy," by C. Thomas, 1989, *Ostomy/Wound Management, 23,* p. 51.)

and specialty beds assist in reducing pressure ulcers in clients at risk.

When selecting a support surface, the nurse should know the client's needs and risks and the purpose for the support surface; a flow chart may be helpful (Figure 43–19). The purposes of support surfaces are to provide comfort, postural control, and pressure management (Krouskop & van Rijswijk, 1995). Clients and families need to be taught the reason for and proper use of the beds or mattresses (Box 43-12). Some common errors with support surfaces are placing the wrong side of the support surface toward the client, not plugging support

Client Teaching Box 43-12

Therapeutic Beds and Mattresses

Objective

- Client and family will describe understanding of the purposes and basic operations of the therapeutic bed or mattress.

Teaching Strategies

- Explain to client and family the reasons for the therapeutic bed.
- Explain proper body mechanics while using the therapeutic bed.
- Educate family about the use and care of the therapeutic bed.
- Explain to client and family about additional pressure-relief measures.

Evaluation

- Client and family will state basic purposes for the therapeutic bed or mattress.
- Client and family will be able to describe the function of the therapeutic bed or mattress.
- Client and family will be able to demonstrate use of a therapeutic bed or mattress and other pressure-relief measures.

surfaces into the electrical source, not turning on the power source for powered support surfaces, failing to do "hand checks" for some support surfaces, and improperly inflating some support surfaces.

Education. Education of the client and caregivers is an important nursing function (Erwin-Toth & Stenger, 2001). There are a variety of educational tools—including videotapes and written materials—that can be used when teaching clients and caregivers or family to prevent and treat pressure ulcers. Written materials are available on a variety of topics, including dressing changes; there are also guides for measuring wounds and charts for positioning clients. AHCPR (1992, 1994) has booklets for clients on pressure ulcer prevention and treatment that can be helpful when teaching clients and their caregivers or family. The RNAO (2002b) has a fact sheet entitled, *Taking the Pressure Off: Preventing Pressure Ulcers,* that is available to clients and their caregivers.

Pressure ulcer treatment and prevention strategies and options should involve the client and caregiver whenever possible. Include information on pain, discomfort, and possible outcomes and duration of treatment if known. Teaching should be individualized, especially for older clients.

Emergency Care. In an emergency setting, the nurse uses first aid measures for wound care. For a traumatic wound, first aid interventions include stabilizing cardiopulmonary function, promoting hemostasis, cleansing the wound, and protecting the wound from further injury.

Hemostasis. After assessing the type and extent of the wound, the nurse controls bleeding of a laceration by applying direct pressure on the wound with a sterile or clean dressing, such as a washcloth. After bleeding subsides, an adhesive bandage or gauze dressing taped over the laceration allows skin edges to close and a blood clot to form. If a dressing becomes saturated with blood, the nurse adds another layer of dressing, continues to apply pressure, and elevates the affected part. Further disruption of skin layers should be avoided. A physician should suture serious lacerations. Pressure dressings used during the first 24 to 48 hours after trauma help maintain hemostasis.

A puncture wound is allowed to bleed to remove dirt and other contaminants, such as saliva from a dog bite. When a penetrating object, such as a knife blade, is present, it is not removed. Removal could cause massive, uncontrolled bleeding. Except for skull injuries, the nurse may apply pressure around the penetrating object, but not on it, and the client should be transported to an emergency facility.

Emergency Cleansing. The process of cleansing a wound involves selecting both an appropriate cleansing solution and using a mechanical means of delivering that solution without causing injury to the healing wound tissue (AHCPR, 1994). Gentle cleansing of a wound removes contaminants that might serve as sources of infection. However, vigorous cleaning by using a method with too much mechanical force can cause bleeding or further injury. For abrasions, minor lacerations, and small puncture wounds, the nurse first rinses the wound with normal saline and lightly covers the area with a dressing. When a laceration is bleeding profusely, the nurse should only brush away surface contaminants and concentrate on hemostasis until the client can be cared for in a clinic or hospital.

Protection. Regardless of whether bleeding has stopped, the nurse protects the wound from further injury by applying sterile or clean dressings and immobilizing the body part. A light dressing applied over minor wounds prevents entrance of micro-organisms. In the home, a clean towel may be the best secondary dressing. A bulky dressing applied with pressure minimizes movement of underlying tissues and helps immobilize the entire body part. A bandage or cloth wrapped around a penetrating object should immobilize it adequately.

Acute Care. Ongoing treatment of wounds requires a holistic team approach that uses the expertise of several multidisciplinary health care professionals (Dolynchuk et al., 2000). In addition to nurses, the team can include physicians, ostomal therapists, physiotherapists, occupational therapists, dietitians, social workers, pain specialists, rehabilitation specialists, and pharmacists.

Aspects of pressure ulcer treatment include local care of the wound and supportive measures such as adequate nutrients and relief of pressure (Skill 43-2). When treating a pressure ulcer, the wound should be reassessed for location, stage, size, tissue type and amount, exudate, and surrounding skin condition (Cooper, 2000).

Skill 43-2 Treating Pressure Ulcers

Delegation Considerations

Treatment of pressure ulcers should not be delegated to unregulated care providers (UCPs). In some practice settings, *non-sterile* dressing application may be delegated to UCPs for chronic, established wounds where the protocol has been evaluated and designated by a nurse. The *assessment* of the wound remains within the scope of the nurse even if the dressing change is delegated to a UCP. When aspects of client care or dressing change are delegated, the nurse should instruct the UCP to report the following immediately:

- Changes in skin integrity
- Pain, fever, or wound drainage
- Any potential contamination to existing dressing (e.g., client incontinence or other bodily fluids, dressing becomes dislodged)

Equipment

- Disposable (i.e., non-sterile) gloves
- Sterile gloves
- Plastic bag for dressing disposal
- Measuring device
- Cotton-tipped applicators
- Topical cleansing agent
- Dressing of choice (see Table 43-7)
- Hypoallergenic tape (if needed)
- Documentation record
- Scale for assessing wound healing

Steps	Rationale
1. Assess client's level of comfort and need for pain medication.	Dressing change procedure is better tolerated if pain is controlled.
2. Determine if client has allergies to topical agents.	Topical agents may cause localized skin reactions.
3. Review order for topical agent or dressing.	Ensures that proper medication and treatment are administered.
4. Close room door or bedside curtains. Position client to allow dressing removal.	Area should be accessible for dressing change.
5. Perform hand hygiene and apply clean gloves. Remove dressing and place in plastic bag.	Reduces transmission of micro-organisms and prevents accidental exposure to body fluids.
6. Assess pressure ulcer(s). All pressure ulcers should be individually assessed (see illustration).	Assessment of a pressure ulcer should be comprehensive.
a. Note colour, type, and percentage of tissue present in the wound base.	The tissue type will assist in the choice of dressing. Consistent assessment will provide the basis for evaluating wound progress (Cooper, 2000).
b. Measure width and length of the ulcer(s). Width is determined by measuring the dimension from left to right, and the length is from top to bottom (see illustration).	Ulcer size will change as healing progresses and therefore the longest and widest areas of the wound will change over time. Measuring the width and length by measuring consistent areas will provide a consistent measurement (Goldman & Salcido, 2002).
c. Measure depth of pressure ulcer using sterile cotton-tipped applicator or other device that will allow measurement of wound depth (see illustration).	Depth measure is important for determining wound volume. Although surface area adequately represents tissue loss in stage I and II ulcers, volume more adequately represents tissue loss in deeper stage III and IV wounds. Undermining represents the loss of the underlying tissue (subcutaneous and muscle) to a greater extent than the skin.
d. Measure depth undermining skin using a cotton-tipped applicator and gently probing under skin edges (see illustration).	Undermining may indicate progressive tissue necrosis and must be accommodated with an appropriate dressing.
7. Assess the periwound skin; check for maceration, redness, denuded area.	Deterioration of the skin around a wound may indicate infection, excessive wound exudate, or skin stripping from adhesive removal (Colwell, 2003).
8. Change to sterile gloves (check agency policy).	Aseptic technique must be maintained during cleansing and application of dressings. Refer to institutional policy regarding use of clean or sterile gloves.

Steps	Rationale

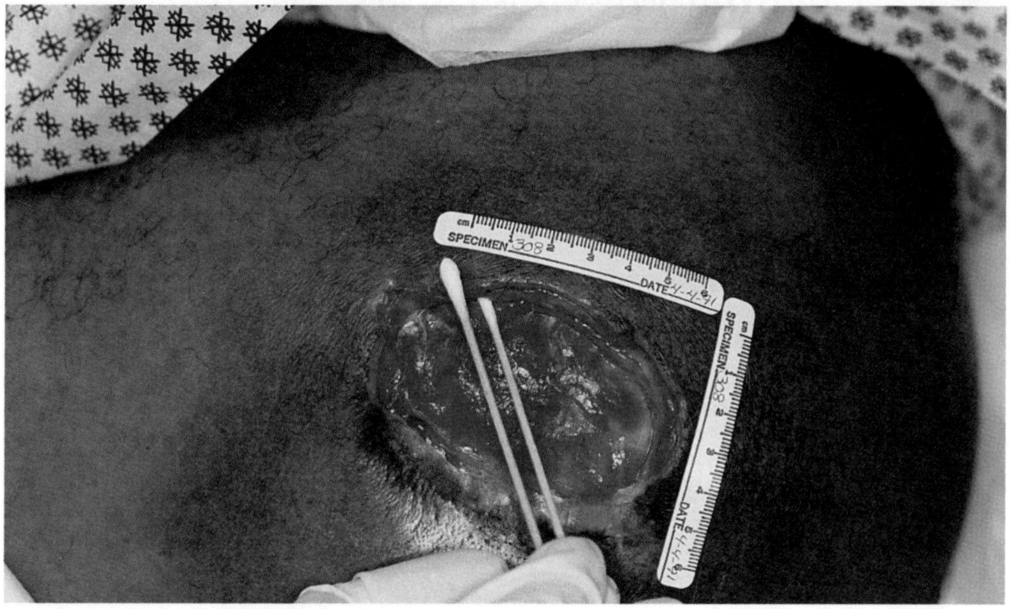

STEP **6** Measuring wound depth (Steps b, c, and d).

Steps	Rationale
9. Cleanse ulcer thoroughly with normal saline or cleansing agent. Use irrigating syringe for deep ulcers.	Removes wound debris.
10. Apply topical agents, as prescribed:	
A. Enzymes	
(1) Apply thin, even layer of ointment over necrotic areas of ulcer only. Do not apply enzyme to surrounding skin.	Thick layer of ointment is not necessary. Thin layer absorbs and acts more effectively. Excess medication can irritate surrounding skin (Rolstad et al., 2000). Some enzymes can cause burning, paresthesia, and dermatitis to surrounding skin. Check manufacturer's direction for frequency of application.
(2) Apply gauze dressing directly over ulcer.	Protects wound. Prevents bacteria from entering wound.
(3) Tape securely in place.	Keeps dressing in place.
B. Hydrogel	
(1) Cover surface of ulcer with hydrogel using applicator or gloved hand.	Provides maintenance of a moist wound environment.
(2) Apply dry gauze, hydrocolloid, or transparent film dressing over wound and adhere to intact skin.	Covers wound base, maintaining hydrogel wound interface.
C. Calcium alginate	
(1) Pack wound with alginate using applicator or gloved hand.	Provides maintenance of wound moisture while absorbing excess drainage.
(2) Apply dry gauze, foam, or hydrocolloid over alginate. Tape in place.	Holds alginate against wound surface.
11. Remove gloves and dispose of soiled supplies. Perform hand hygiene.	Reduces transmission of micro-organisms.
12. Complete ulcer information required for one of the wound-healing scales per agency's protocol.	Allows comparison of assessments over time to determine progress toward wound healing.

Critical Decision Point: A clean pressure ulcer should show evidence of some healing within 2 to 4 weeks.

Skill 43-2 Treating Pressure Ulcers—cont'd

Steps	Rationale
13. Compare subsequent ulcer measurements.	Wound assessment scales such as the BWAT (see Figure 43–12) can be used to quantify and measure pressure ulcer healing. Use agency-approved scale.
14. Do *not* use the pressure ulcer staging system to measure pressure ulcer healing.	System measures depth of wound, not healing (NPUAP, 1995a, 1995b).

Unexpected Outcomes and Related Interventions

- Skin surrounding ulcer becomes macerated.
  - Reduce exposure of surrounding skin to topical agents and moisture.
  - Consider the use of a liquid skin barrier on periwound skin.
- Ulcer becomes deeper with increased drainage.
  - Notify physician for possible change in pressure ulcer status.
  - Obtain necessary wound cultures.
  - Obtain additional consults (e.g., wound care specialist).

Recording and Reporting

- Record assessment of ulcer in client's record.
- Describe type of topical agent used, dressing applied, and client's response.
- Report any deterioration in ulcer appearance.

Home Care Considerations

- Cost can be a factor. Some clients have more time than financial resources. They may choose a less expensive treatment option such as dressing material.
- Disposal of contaminated dressings in the home should be done in a manner consistent with agency policy and local regulations (AHCPR, 1994).
- Discuss need for therapeutic mattress.

Whether the wound is chronic or acute, the goal of wound management is to maintain a healthy local wound environment (Rolstad, Ovington, & Harris, 2000). The wound care team implements measures to prevent infection (i.e., cleanse and debride the wound as appropriate) and protect the wound (i.e., apply dressings). The nurse may also be involved with caring for sutures, evacuating drainage, applying bandages and binders, and implementing heat and cold therapies.

An important factor not to overlook is that the wound will not heal unless contributing factors are controlled or eliminated. Therefore, it is critically important that the causative factors (e.g., shear, friction, pressure, and moisture) be addressed, or it is unlikely that the wound will heal despite therapy (Rolstad et al., 2000).

Preventing Infections. Infection is the result of entry and multiplication of micro-organisms in the tissues of a host (see chapter 29). The likelihood of a wound becoming infected is related to microbial load, the type of micro-organism, and the ability of the host to resist infection. Host resistance is often the critical factor in determining whether an infection will take place. Host resistance is lowered by poor tissue perfusion, poor nutritional status, local edema, immunocompromising medications or conditions, and other factors such as smoking and drug or alcohol abuse. The presence of foreign material such as necrotic debris, retained packing materials, or small fragments of gauze dressing will also decrease host resistance and thus increase the risk of infection. Prevention of wound infection includes wound cleansing and removal of non-viable tissue. In certain situations, such as with extensive burn wounds, a physician may order application of topical antimicrobial agents to prevent infection.

Cleansing. Although a moderate amount of wound exudate promotes epithelial cell growth, the physician may order cleansing of a wound or drain site if a dressing does not properly absorb drainage or if an open drain deposits drainage onto the skin. Wound cleansing requires good hand hygiene and aseptic techniques (see chapter 29).

Wounds are cleansed with normal saline or a commercial wound cleanser that is non-cytotoxic (will not damage or kill cells, such as fibroblasts and healing tissue; RNAO, 2002a; Rolstad et al., 2000). Commonly used solutions that are cytotoxic, and therefore should not normally be used to clean granulating wounds, are Dakin's solution (sodium hypochlorite solution), acetic acid, povidone-iodine, and hydrogen peroxide. Saline or non-cytotoxic solutions are applied with sterile gauze or by irrigation. The following three principles are important when cleansing a wound or the area surrounding a drain:

1. Cleanse in a direction from the least contaminated area, such as from the wound or incision to the surrounding skin (Figure 43–20) or from an isolated drain site to the surrounding skin (Figure 43–21).

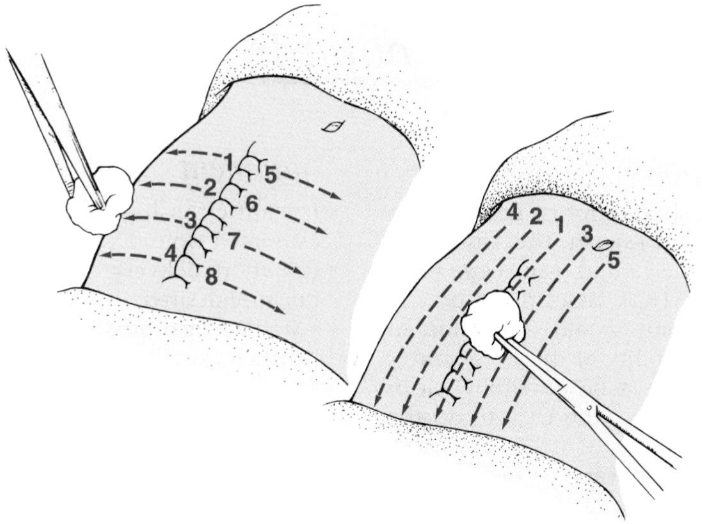

FIGURE **43–20** Methods for cleansing a wound site.

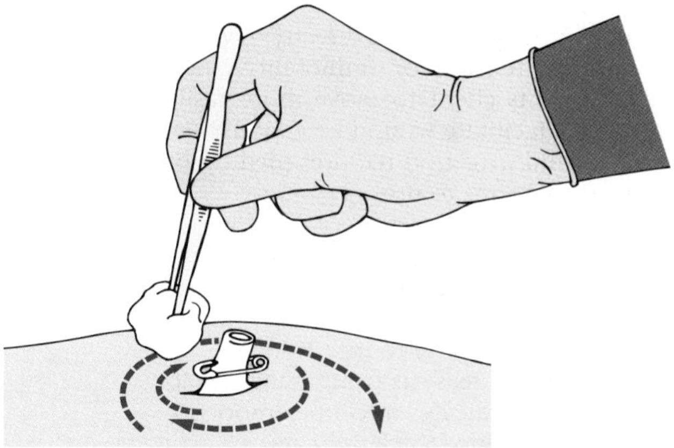

FIGURE **43–21** Cleansing a drain site.

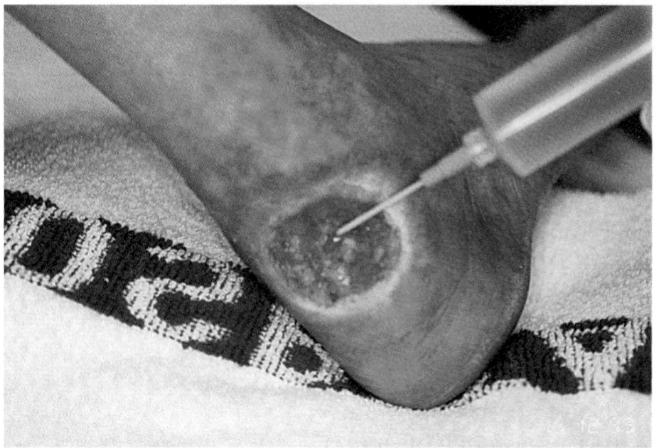

FIGURE **43–22** Wound irrigation.

2. Use gentle friction when applying solutions locally to the skin.
3. Never uses the same piece of gauze to cleanse across an incision or wound twice.

A drain site can be contaminated because moist drainage harbours micro-organisms. If a wound has a dry incisional area and a moist drain site, cleansing moves from the incisional area toward the drain. The nurse uses two separate swabs or gauze pads, one to cleanse from the top of the incision toward the drain and one to cleanse from the bottom of the incision toward the drain. To cleanse the area of an isolated drain site, the nurse cleans around the drain, moving in circular rotations outward from a point closest to the drain. In this situation, the skin near the site is more contaminated than the site itself. To cleanse circular wounds, the nurse uses the same technique as in cleansing around a drain.

Irrigation is a common method of delivering the wound-cleansing solution to the wound and removing debris. The nurse uses an irrigating syringe to flush the area with a constant low-pressure flow of solution. The gentle washing action of the irrigation cleanses a wound of exudate and debris. Irrigations are particularly useful for open, deep wounds.

Irrigation of an open wound requires sterile technique. The nurse uses a 35-mL syringe with a 19-gauge needle (AHCPR, 1994; Ratliff & Bryant, 2003) to deliver the solution, using an irrigation system that has a safe pressure and will not damage healing wound tissue (Figure 43–22). To reduce surface bacteria and tissue trauma, the nurse should use 100 to 150 mL of solution (RNAO, 2002a). It is important to never occlude a wound opening with a syringe, because this results in the introduction of irrigating fluid into a closed space. If this were to occur, the pressure of the fluid could cause tissue damage and discomfort. A wound should always be irrigated with the syringe tip over but not in the drainage site. Fluid should flow directly into the wound, from the least to most contaminated area. Skill 43-3 lists steps for wound irrigation.

Tissue Debridement. **Debridement** is the removal of non-viable, necrotic tissue. Removal of necrotic tissue is necessary to rid the ulcer of a source of infection, to enable

Skill 43-3 *Performing Wound Irrigation*

Delegation Considerations

The skill of wound irrigation should not be delegated to unregulated care providers (UCPs). In the case of a chronic wound, cleansing of the wound using *clean* technique can be delegated to a UCP. Assessment of any wound, care of acute new wounds, and evaluation of wound irrigation is the responsibility of the nurse and is never delegated. When a wound is stable or requires clean irrigation, the nurse should instruct the UCP to do the following:

- Report any change in wound appearance or increased wound drainage to the nurse.
- Use proper clean technique to avoid cross-contamination from irrigation syringes and equipment.

Equipment

- Irrigant/cleansing solution (volume 1.2 to 2 times the estimated wound volume)
- Irrigation delivery system depending on amount of pressure desired:
  - Sterile irrigation 35-mL syringe with sterile soft angiocatheter or 19-gauge needle (AHCPR, 1994) *or*
  - Hand-held shower or whirlpool
- Disposable gloves
- Sterile gloves
- Waterproof underpad, if needed
- Dressing supplies
- Disposable waterproof bag
- Gown, if risk of spray
- Goggles, if risk of spray

Steps	Rationale
1. Assess client's level of pain. Administer prescribed analgesic 30 to 45 minutes before starting wound irrigation procedure.	Discomfort may be related directly to wound or indirectly to muscle tension or immobility. Increased comfort level permits client to move more easily and be positioned to facilitate wound irrigation.
2. Review medical record for physician's prescription for irrigation of open wound and type of solution to be used.	Open wound irrigation requires medical order, including type of solutions to use.
3. Assess recent recording of signs and symptoms related to client's open wound.	Data are used as baseline to indicate change in condition of wound (Cooper, 2000).
a. Condition of skin and wound	
b. Elevation of body temperature	May indicate response to infection.
c. Drainage from wound (amount, colour)	Amount will decrease as healing takes place.
d. Odour	Strong odour indicates infectious process.
e. Consistency of drainage	Leukocytes produce thick drainage.
f. Size of wounds, including depth, length, and width	Determines stage of healing.
4. Explain procedure of wound irrigation and cleansing.	Information will reduce client's anxiety.
5. Perform hand hygiene.	Reduces transmission of micro-organisms.
6. Position client comfortably to permit gravitational flow of irrigating solution through wound and into collection receptacle. Position client so that wound is vertical to collection basin.	Directing solution from top to bottom of wound and from clean to contaminated area prevents further infection. Positioning client during planning stage provides bed surfaces for later preparation of equipment.
7. Warm irrigation solution to approximate body temperature.	Warmed solution increases comfort and reduces vascular constriction response in tissues.
8. Form cuff on waterproof bag and place it near bed.	Cuffing helps to maintain large opening, thereby permitting placement of contaminated dressing without touching refuse bag itself.
9. Close room door or bed curtains.	Maintains privacy.
10. Apply gown and goggles if needed.	Protects nurse from splashes or sprays of blood and body fluids.
11. Put on disposable gloves and remove soiled dressing and discard in waterproof bag. Discard gloves.	Reduces transmission of micro-organisms.
12. Prepare equipment; open sterile supplies.	
13. Put on sterile gloves.	

Steps	Rationale
14. To irrigate wound with wide opening:	
a. Fill 35-mL syringe with irrigation solution.	Flushing wound helps remove debris and facilitates healing by secondary intention.
b. Attach 19-gauge needle or angiocatheter (see Figure 43–22).	Provides ideal pressure for cleansing and removal of debris.
c. Hold syringe tip 2.5 cm above upper end of wound and over area being cleansed.	Prevents syringe contamination. Careful placement of the syringe prevents unsafe pressure of the flowing solution.
d. Using continuous pressure, flush wound; repeat steps 14a, b, and c until solution draining into basin is clear.	Clear solution indicates that all debris has been removed.
15. To irrigate deep wound with very small opening:	
a. Attach soft angiocatheter to filled irrigating syringe.	Catheter permits direct flow of irrigant into wound. Expect wound to take longer to empty when opening is small.
b. Lubricate tip of catheter with irrigating solution; then gently insert tip of catheter and pull out about 1 cm.	Removes tip from fragile inner wall of wound.
c. Using slow, continuous pressure, flush wound.	

Critical Decision Point: CAUTION: Splashing may occur during this step.

Steps	Rationale
d. Pinch off catheter just below syringe while keeping catheter in place.	Avoids contamination of sterile solution.
e. Remove and refill syringe. Reconnect to catheter and repeat until solution draining into basin is clear.	
16. To cleanse wound with hand-held shower:	Useful for clients able to shower with assistance or independently. May be accomplished at home. A shower table is helpful for bed-bound or acutely ill clients.
a. With client seated comfortably in shower chair, adjust spray to gentle flow; water temperature should be warm.	
b. Cover showerhead with clean washcloth if needed.	
c. Shower for 5 to 10 minutes with showerhead 30 cm from wound.	

Critical Decision Point: Consider culturing a wound if it has a foul and purulent odour, inflammation surrounds the wound, a non-draining wound begins to drain, or client is febrile.

Steps	Rationale
17. Obtain cultures, if needed, after cleansing with non-bacteriostatic saline.	Routine culturing of open wounds is not recommended in the AHCPR guidelines (1994). They recommend using quantitative bacterial cultures (tissue biopsy or wound fluid by needle aspiration) rather than swab cultures, which often detect only surface bacterial contaminants.
18. Dry wound edges with gauze; dry client if shower or whirlpool is used.	Prevents maceration of surrounding tissue caused by excess moisture.
19. Apply appropriate dressing (see Skill 43-2 and Skill 43-4).	Maintains protective barrier and healing environment for wound.
20. Remove gloves and, if worn, mask, goggles, and gown.	Prevents transfer of micro-organisms.
21. Dispose of equipment and soiled supplies. Perform hand hygiene.	Reduces transmission of micro-organisms.
22. Assist client to comfortable position.	
23. Assess type of tissue in the wound bed.	Identifies wound healing progress and determines type of wound cleansing needed.
24. Inspect dressing periodically.	Determines client's response to wound irrigation and need to modify plan of care.
25. Evaluate skin integrity.	Determines if extension of wound has occurred.
26. Observe client for signs of discomfort.	Client's pain should not increase as a result of wound irrigation.
27. Observe for presence of retained irrigant.	Retained irrigant is a medium for bacterial growth and subsequent infection.

Skill 43-3 Performing Wound Irrigation—cont'd

Unexpected Outcomes and Related Interventions

- Wound does not appear to heal.
  - Obtain wound culture.
  - Notify physician, who may change dressing and/or irrigation frequency.
- Wound drainage increases.
  - Apply more absorbent gauze.
  - Increase the frequency of irrigation.

Recording and Reporting

- Record wound irrigation and client response on progress notes.
- Immediately report any evidence of fresh bleeding, sharp increase in pain, retention of irrigant, or signs of shock to attending physician.
- At change of shift, report expected and unexpected outcomes that have actually occurred.

Home Care Considerations

- Teach client and caregiver how to make normal saline, especially if cost is an issue. Normal saline can be made by using 10 mL of salt in 1 L of boiling water (Barr, 1995).
- Tell client and caregiver that because normal saline has no preservatives, it should be discarded 24 to 48 hours after it is first opened or made (Barr, 1995).

visualization of the wound bed, and to provide a clean base necessary for healing. An exception to the rule that all eschar be debrided is a dry necrotic heel pressure ulcer. Heel ulcers with dry eschar need not be debrided if they do not have associated edema, erythema, fluctuance, or drainage (AHCPR, 1994).

The method of debridement will depend on which is most appropriate to the client's condition and care goals (AHCPR, 1994). It is important to remember that during the debridement process, some increase in wound exudate, odour, and size may occur. Pain that occurs with debridement needs to be assessed and prevented or effectively managed. Methods of debridement include mechanical, autolytic, enzymatic, and sharp/surgical.

One method of mechanical debridement is the use of wet-to-dry saline dressings. The nurse places a saline-moistened dressing into the wound to absorb necrotic tissue and debris. The dressing is allowed to dry thoroughly so that it adheres to the necrotic tissue. When the dry dressing is removed, the dead tissue is pulled away too (debridement). Because devitalized and viable tissue are both removed, this method is not used routinely. It should never be used in a clean, granulating wound. Other methods of mechanical debridement are wound irrigation (high-pressure irrigation and pulsatile high-pressure lavage) and whirlpool treatments (Ramundo & Wells, 2000).

Autolytic debridement uses synthetic dressings over the wound to allow the eschar to be self-digested by the action of enzymes that are present in wound fluids (AHCPR, 1994). It can be accomplished by using dressings that support moisture at the wound surface (e.g., hydrogel, hydrocolloid, transparent film dressings). If the wound base is dry, a dressing that will add moisture is used; if there is excessive exudate, a dressing that absorbs the excessive moisture while maintaining moisture at the wound bed is used. If tissue autolysis does not occur within 24 to 72 hours, another form of debridement should be used.

Enzymatic debridement is the most selective mode of debridement and relies on naturally occurring enzymes applied to the wound surface to degrade debris (Dolynchuk et al., 2000). The only licensed enzymatic product is collagenase. Its function is to degrade immature collagen in the wound matrix. It appears to be the most useful in the removal of eschar from large wounds where surgical techniques are not practical. Debridement can be facilitated by cross-hatching or scoring the hard eschar with scissors or a scalpel before applying the collagenase. However, this technique can cause excessive amounts of exudates with the breakdown of the necrotic tissue, and can create local irritation, maceration, and possibly infection.

Surgical debridement is the removal of devitalized tissue by using a scalpel, scissors, or other sharp instrument. Physicians usually perform surgical debridement of a pressure ulcer. Nurses should check their provincial or territorial nursing practice act to see if surgical debridement is covered as a nursing function in their jurisdiction. It is the quickest method of debridement. It is usually indicated when the client has signs of infection.

Dressings. The more extensive the wound, the larger the dressing required. The use of dressings requires an understanding of wound healing. A variety of dressing materials are commercially available. The correct dressing selection can facilitate wound healing (Currence, 2001;

Rolstad et al., 2000). The dressing type will depend on the assessment of the wound and the phase of wound healing. The objectives for the wound care must be identified and the dressing choice will become clear. A wound that requires infection management will require a different set of dressings than a wound that requires the removal of non-viable tissue.

For surgical wounds that heal by primary intention, it is common to remove dressings as soon as drainage stops. In contrast, when the nurse dresses a wound healing by secondary intention, the dressing material becomes a means for providing moisture to the wound or assisting in debridement.

Purposes of Dressings. A dressing may serve several purposes:

- Protecting a wound from micro-organism contamination
- Aiding hemostasis
- Promoting healing by absorbing drainage and debriding a wound
- Supporting or splinting the wound site
- Protecting the client from seeing the wound (if perceived as unpleasant)
- Promoting thermal insulation of the wound surface
- Providing a moist environment

When the skin becomes broken, a dressing helps reduce exposure to micro-organisms. However, when wound drainage is minimal, the healing process forms a natural fibrin seal that can eliminate the need for a dressing. A dressing is always needed for wounds with extensive tissue loss.

Pressure dressings promote hemostasis. Applied with elastic bandages, a pressure dressing exerts localized downward pressure over an actual or potential bleeding site. A pressure dressing eliminates dead space (a cavity within a wound) in underlying tissues so that wound healing progresses normally. The nurse checks pressure dressings to be sure they do not interfere with circulation to a body part. The nurse assesses skin colour, pulses in distal extremities, changes in sensation, and the client's comfort. Pressure dressings are not routinely removed.

A primary function of a dressing on a healing wound is to absorb drainage. Most traditional surgical dressings have three layers: a contact or primary layer, an absorbent layer, and an outer protective or secondary layer. The contact dressing covers the incision and part of the adjacent skin. Fibrin, blood products, and debris adhere to the contact dressing's surface. A problem can occur if the wound drainage dries, causing the dressing to stick to the suture line. Improper removal of the dressing can cause disruption of the healing epidermal surface. If the dressing is sticking to the surgical incision, the dressing should be lightly moistened with saline solution. This will cause the dressing to become saturated, thus loosening it from the incisional area and allowing removal without trauma to the incisional area.

The dressing technique will vary depending on the goal of the treatment plan for the wound. For example, if the goal is to maintain a moist environment for a clean granulating wound, it is important for the nurse to prevent the saline-moistened gauze dressing from drying and sticking to the healing wound. However, if the goal of care is to mechanically debride the wound, a saline wet-to-dry dressing technique is used (see Tissue Debridement).

Box 43-13 AHCPR Dressing Recommendations

- Use a dressing that will keep the ulcer bed continuously moist. Wet-to-dry dressings should be used only for debridement and are not considered continuously moist saline dressings.
- Use clinical judgment to select a type of moist wound dressing suitable for the ulcer. Studies of different types of moist wound dressings have shown no differences in healing outcomes.
- Choose a dressing that keeps the surrounding intact (periulcer) skin dry while keeping the ulcer bed moist.
- Choose a dressing that controls exudate but does not desiccate the ulcer bed.
- Consider caregiver time when selecting a dressing.
- Eliminate wound dead space by loosely filling all cavities with dressing material. Avoid overpacking the wound.
- Monitor dressings applied near the anus, because they are difficult to keep intact.

Adapted from *Treatment of Pressure Ulcers* (Clinical Practice Guideline No. 15, AHCPR Publication No. 95-0653), Agency for Health Care Policy and Research, Panel for the Treatment of Pressure Ulcers in Adults, 1994, Rockville, MD: Author, U.S. Department of Health and Human Services.

Dressings applied to a draining wound require frequent changing to prevent micro-organism growth and skin breakdown. Bacteria grow readily in the dark, warm, moist environment under a dressing. Skin surfaces become macerated and irritated. Periwound skin breakdown can be minimized by keeping the skin clean, dry, and reducing the use of tape.

The absorbent dressing layer serves as a reservoir for additional secretions. The wicking action of woven gauze dressings pulls excess drainage into the dressing and away from the wound.

The final outer layer of a dressing helps prevent bacteria and other external contaminants from reaching the wound surface. Usually, the outer dressing is made of a thicker dressing material. Adhesives can be applied to this layer, securing the dressings.

A dressing should support a moist wound environment if the wound is healing by secondary intention. A moist wound base facilitates epithelialization, thus allowing the wound to resurface as quickly as possible.

Types of Dressings. Dressings vary by type of material and mode of application (wet or dry; Skill 43-4). They should be easy to apply, comfortable, and made of materials that promote wound healing. The AHCPR guidelines (1994) are helpful when selecting dressings based on the goal of wound treatment (Box 43-13).

For pressure ulcers in particular, the type of dressing is usually based on the stage of the pressure ulcer and the objective of the dressing. Table 43-7 lists some of the many types of dressings appropriate for each stage. Before placing a dressing on a pressure ulcer, the nurse must

Text continued on p. 1545

Table 43-7 Dressing by Ulcer Stage

Dressing (example of two brand names)	Mechanism of Action	Comments
Stage 1		
Transparent film dressing (Tegaderm, Bioclusive)	Protects from friction injury Maintains moisture in wound Barrier against moisture and bacteria	Adhesive, semi-permeable polyurethane membrane Promotes formation of new granulation tissue Allows visualization of area May be left in place up to 7 days if occlusive seal remains Be careful when removing because skin can be torn; stretch away from the wound to lift; apply without stretching
Thin hydrocolloid dressing (X-thin DuoDerm, Restore X-Thin)	Provides protection of reddened area by decreasing surface injury	Flexible, occlusive dressing that can remain in place up to 5 days; translucent, allowing visualization of the area Maintains moisture within wound Can be used over all chronic ulcers
Stage II		
Hydrocolloid dressing (DuoDerm, Comfeel)	Interacts with the wound fluid to provide a moist environment	Can stay in place until the seal is broken, allowing for enhanced healing
Composite dressing (Viasorb, Alldress)	Traps wound moisture and provides surface protection	Provides absorbent, non-adherent layer over wound with occlusive cover
Hydrogel dressing (Curafil, Woun'Dres)	Provides moisture to a clean granular wound, supporting re-epithelialization	Requires secondary dressing
Foam dressing—non-adhesive (3M Foam, Sof-Foam)	Absorbs exudates and debris while maintaining moist environment*	Provides a non-linting, insulating layer over wound May or may not have film coating Is absorbent and non-adherent to wound base May be used with topical agents Do not use if wound is dry unless the goal is to suppress hypergranulation
Stage III		
Polyurethane foam adhesive (Allevyn, Curafoam)	Maintains moist wound environment*	Absorbs exudates For maximum absorption, needs direct contact with wound without additional taping Adhesive or safe-tac maintains placing of dressing Adhesive dressings may be difficult to remove without damaging skin
Hydrocolloid dressing (Duoderm, Comfeel)	Interacts with the wound fluid to provide a moist environment	Can cause slough tissue to soften by autolysis Effective with moderate amount of wound drainage
Hydrogel dressing (Curafil, Woun'Dres)	Provides moisture to a clean granular wound, supporting re-epithelialization	May be used to soften necrotic tissue, allowing for debridement Available in sheet dressing that can be packed into wound
Calcium alginate dressing (Kaltostat, AlgiSite)	Absorbs excessive moisture Exudates wounds	Soft, non-woven pads or rope that turn to a gel when moist Easy to apply and remove When a gel, may have a foul odour; do not mistake this for infection Conforms to the shape of the wound Can be left in wound bed until saturated, up to 72 hours
Stage IV		
Hydrocolloid dressing (DuoDerm, Comfeel)	Interacts with the wound fluid to provide a moist environment	Only indicated for a clean wound and generally used with a filler dressing
Hydrogel dressing (Curafil, Woun'Dres)	Provides moisture to a wound and can be used to loosen necrotic tissue	Used to fill tunnelled areas
Gauze roll dressing (Intersorb, Kerlix)	Provides moisture to wound when moistened with solution Wicks drainage away from wound	Gauze roll should be moistened with an appropriate solution, wrung out, unrolled, and packed lightly into wound Requires a secondary dressing Changed when soak through is noted on secondary dressing Generally requires dressing changes every 8 to 12 hours

*As with *all* occlusive dressings, wounds should *not* be clinically infected.
Adapted from "Wound management products by category," by Susan Russell, RN, ET, BScN, MN, CWON for Janssen-Ortho Inc©. Revised June 2004.

Skill 43-4 Applying Dry and Wet-to-Dry Dressings

View Video

Delegation Considerations

Controversy about delegating wound care to unregulated care providers (UCPs) exists. The care of acute new wounds and those that require sterile technique for dressing change should not be delegated to UCPs. In some settings, aspects of wound care such as dressing change can be delegated. This may include the changing of dressings using *clean* technique for chronic wounds. The assessment of the wound remains within the scope of the nurse even if the dressing change is delegated to a UCP. When aspects of client care or dressing change are delegated, the nurse should instruct the UCP to immediately report the following:

- Pain, fever, bleeding, or wound drainage.
- Any potential contamination to existing dressing (e.g., client incontinence or other bodily fluids, dressing becomes dislodged).

Equipment

- Sterile gloves
- Variety of gauze dressings and pads
- Irrigation kit
- Cleansing solution
- Sterile solution
- Disposable gloves
- Tape, ties, or bandage as needed
- Waterproof bag
- Extra gauze dressings or abdominal (ABD) pads

Steps	Rationale
1. Perform hand hygiene. Obtain information about size and location of wound to be dressed.	Reduces transmission of micro-organisms. Helps nurse to plan for proper type and amount of supplies needed. Alerts nurse when assistance is needed to hold dressings in place.
2. Assess client's level of comfort.	Removal of dry dressing can be painful; client may require pain medication.
3. Review orders for dressing change procedure.	Indicates type of dressing or applications to use.
4. Explain procedure to client and instruct client not to touch wound area or sterile supplies.	Decreases anxiety. Sudden, unexpected movement on client's part could result in contamination of wound and supplies.
5. Close room or cubicle curtains and windows.	Provides privacy and reduces airborne micro-organisms.
6. Position client comfortably and drape with bath blanket to expose only wound site.	Provides access to wound, yet minimizes unnecessary exposure.
7. Place disposable bag within reach of work area. Fold top of bag to make cuff (see illustration).	Ensures easy disposal of soiled dressings. Prevents soiling of bag's outer surface.
8. Apply face mask and protective eyewear, if splashing may occur, and perform hand hygiene	Reduces transmission of pathogens to exposed tissues. Protects nurse from splashes.
9. Put on clean, disposable gloves and remove tape, bandage, or ties.	Prevents transmission of infectious organisms from soiled dressings to nurse's hands.
10. Remove tape: pull parallel to skin; pull toward dressing; remove remaining adhesive from skin.	Pulling tape toward dressing reduces stress on suture line or wound edges.
11. With gloved hand, carefully remove gauze dressings one layer at a time, taking care not to dislodge drains or tubes.	Appearance of drainage may be upsetting to client. Removal of one layer at a time reduces the chance of accidental removal of underlying drains.
a. If dressing sticks on a wet-to-dry dressing, do not moisten it; instead, gently free dressing and alert client of potential discomfort.	Wet-to-dry dressing should debride wound. Do not wet the dressing to remove it. It is supposed to be dry so that as it is removed from the wound, it also removes necrotic tissue from the wound.

Critical Decision Point: Never use a wet-to-dry dressing in a clean granulating wound. Use only for debridement.

12. Observe character and amount of drainage on dressing and appearance of wound.	Provides estimate of drainage amount and assessment of wound's condition.

Skill 43-4 Applying Dry and Wet-to-Dry Dressings—cont'd

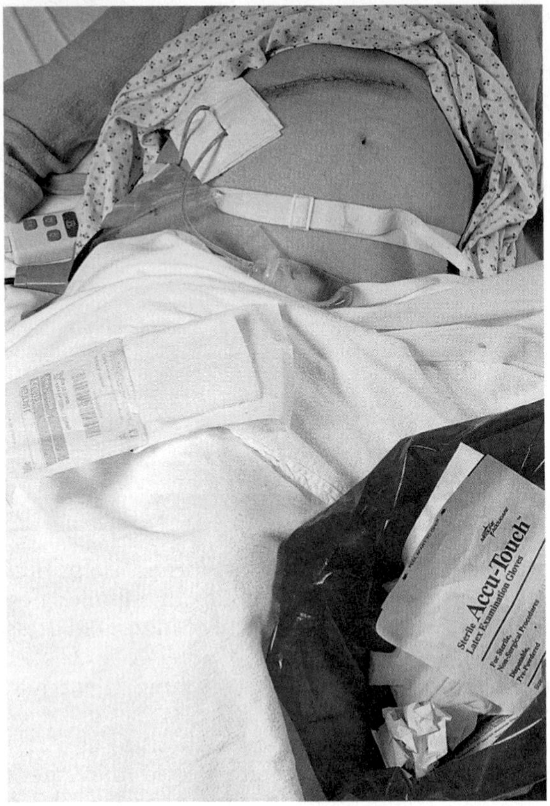

STEP **7** Disposable waterproof bag placed near the dressing site.

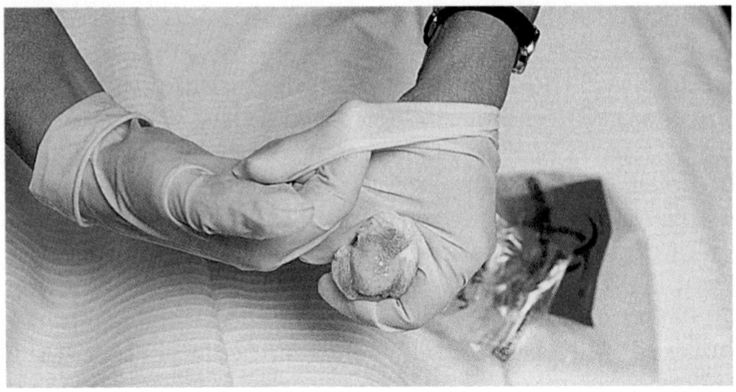

STEP **13** Removal of disposable glove over contaminated dressing.

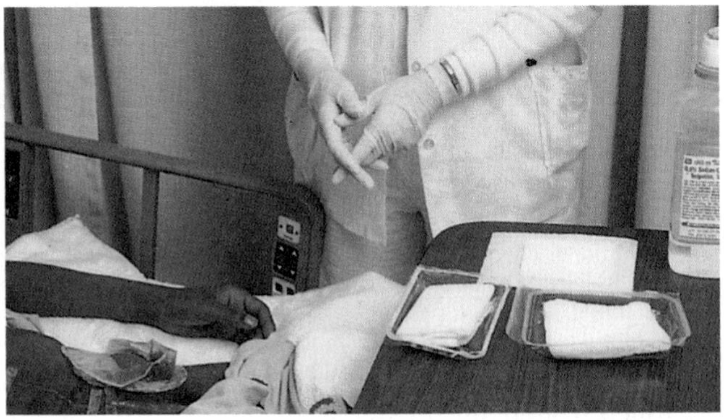

STEP **14** Sterile dressing equipment.

Steps	Rationale
13. Fold dressings with drainage contained inside, and remove gloves inside out. With small dressings, remove gloves inside out over dressing (see illustration). Dispose of gloves and soiled dressings in disposable bag. Perform hand hygiene.	Reduces transmission of micro-organisms. Prevents contact of nurse's hands with material on gloves.
14. Open sterile dressing tray or individually wrapped sterile supplies. Place on bedside table (see illustration).	Sterile dressings remain sterile while on or within sterile surface. Preparation of supplies prevents break in technique during dressing change.
15. Cleanse wound: a. Pour ordered solution into sterile irrigation container. b. Using syringe, gently allow solution to flow over wound. c. Continue until the irrigation flow is clear. d. Dry surrounding skin.	
16. Apply dressing: **A. Dry dressing**	
(1) Apply sterile gloves.	Allows handling of sterile supplies without contamination.
(2) Inspect wound for appearance, drains, drainage, and integrity.	Indicates status of wound healing.
(3) Cleanse wound with solution:	
(a) Clean from least-contaminated area to most-contaminated area.	Prevents contamination of previously cleaned area.
(4) Dry area.	Provides protection and absorption of wound drainage.

Steps	Rationale

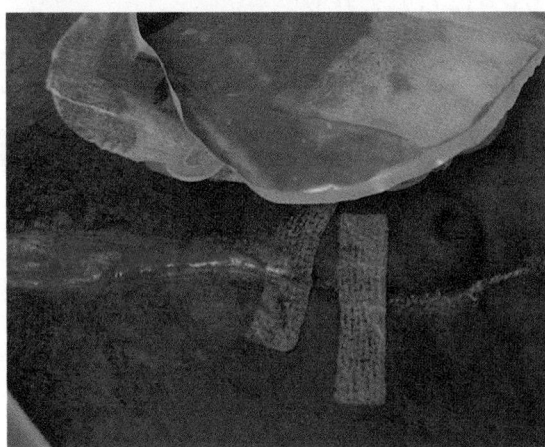

STEP **16B(3)** Exposure of wound facilitates assessment of wound and any drainage.

Steps	Rationale
(5) Apply sterile dry dressing covering wound	Protects wound from external environment.
(6) Apply topper dressing if indicated.	
B. Wet-to-dry dressing	
(1) Apply disposable gloves.	
(2) Remove old dressings, discard.	
(3) Assess surrounding skin (see illustration). Discard gloves.	Surrounding skin assessment provides an evaluation of wound management.
(4) Apply sterile gloves.	Allows handling of sterile supplies without contamination.
(5) Cleanse wound base with normal saline. Assess wound base.	Cleansing removes wound debris for adequate assessment.
(6) Moisten gauze with prescribed solution. Wring gauze out. Unfold.	Gauze should be moist to allow for absorption of wound debris.
(7) Apply moist, fine-mesh, open-weave gauze as a single layer directly onto the wound surface. If wound is deep, gently pack dressing into wound base with sterile gloves or forceps until all wound surfaces are in contact with the gauze. If tunnelling is present, use a cotton-tipped applicator to place gauze into tunnelled area. Be sure gauze does not touch the surrounding skin (see illustration).	Inner gauze should be moist, not dripping wet, to absorb drainage and adhere to debris. Wound should be loosely packed to facilitate wicking of drainage into absorbent outer layer of dressing. Having inner gauze too wet (so that it does not dry) is a common error in technique for this type of dressing (Barr, 1995).
(8) Cover with sterile dry gauze and topper dressing.	Topper dressing prevents strikethrough of wound drainage and provides a surface to tape the dressing in place.
17. Secure dressing.	
a. Tape: Apply non-allergenic tape to dressing.	The goal for securing a dressing is to keep the dressing in place and intact without causing damage to underlying and surrounding skin.
b. Montgomery ties (see Figure 43–27)	
(1) Expose adhesive surface of tape on end of each tie.	
(2) Place ties on opposite sides of dressing.	
(3) Place adhesive directly on skin or use skin barrier.	Skin barrier (Stomahesive) protects intact skin from stretch and tension of adhesive tape.
(4) Secure dressing by lacing ties across it	
c. For dressings on an extremity, secure dressing with roller gauze or Surgiflex elastic net (see illustration).	

Skill 43-4 Applying Dry and Wet-to-Dry Dressings—cont'd

Steps	Rationale

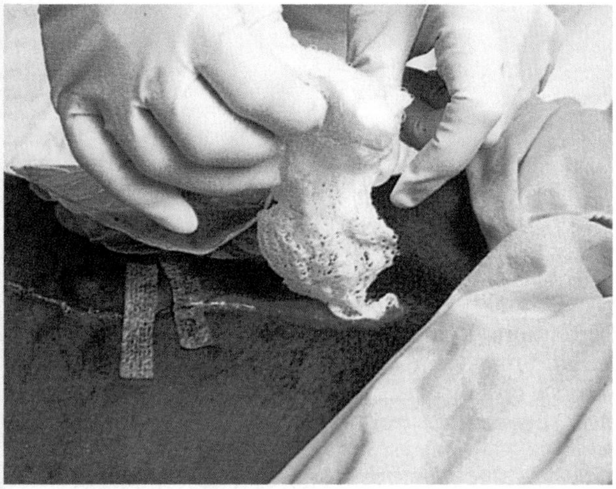
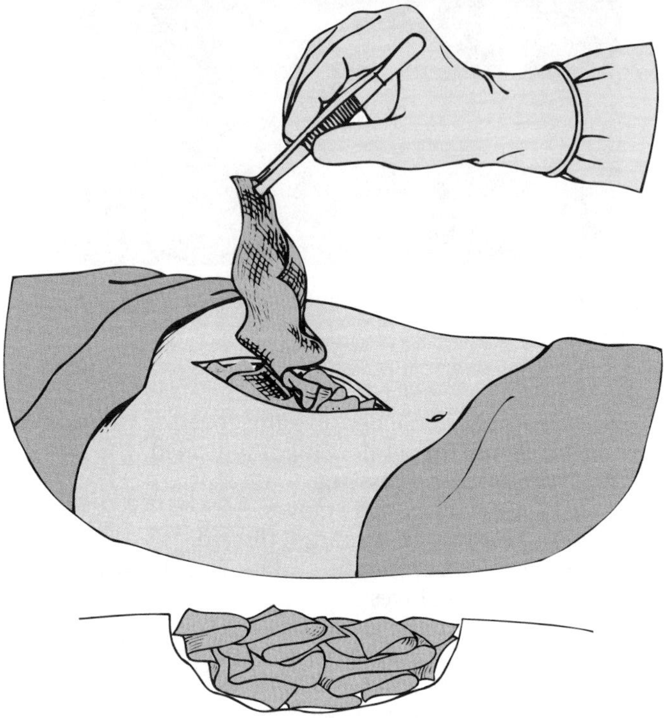

STEP **16B(7)** Packing wound with single layer of gauze.

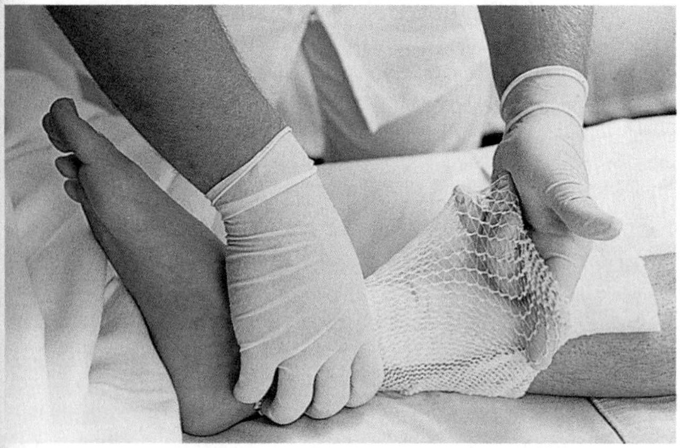

STEP **17c** Elastic net securing a lower extremity dressing.

Steps	Rationale
18. Remove gloves and dispose of in bag. Remove any mask or eyewear.	Reduces transmission of infection.
19. Dispose of supplies and perform hand hygiene.	Reduces transmission of infection.
20. Assist client to comfortable position.	Promotes client's sense of well being. Enhances comfort.

Unexpected Outcomes and Related Interventions

- Wound appears inflamed, tender, with or without drainage.
  - Monitor client for signs of infection (e.g., increased temperature, white blood cell count).
  - Obtain wound culture.
  - Notify physician.
- Wound drainage increases.
  - Increase frequency of dressing changes.
  - Notify physician, who may consider drain placement to facilitate wound drainage.
- Wound bleeds during dressing change.
  - Observe colour. If drainage is bright red and excessive, might need to apply pressure.
  - Inspect along dressing and underneath client to determine amount of bleeding.
  - Obtain vital signs as needed.
  - Notify physician.
- Client reports a sensation that "something has given way under the dressing."
  - Observe wound for increased drainage or separation of sutures.
  - Protect wound. Cover with sterile moist dressing.
  - Instruct client to lie still.
  - Notify physician.

Recording and Reporting

- Report brisk, bright red bleeding or evidence of wound dehiscence or evisceration to physician immediately.
- Report wound and periwound tissue appearance, colour, and tissue type and presence and characteristics of exudate, type and amount of dressings used, and tolerance of client to procedure.
- Record client's level of comfort.
- Write date and time dressing applied on tape in ink (not marker).

Home Care Considerations

- More expensive specialty dressings may be used because they decrease the frequency of dressing changes.
- Clean dressings may also be used in the home setting.
- Disposal of contaminated dressings in the home should be done in a manner consistent with agency policies and local regulations.

know the stage of the pressure ulcer, the goal of the dressing, and the principles of wound care.

Gauze sponges are the oldest and most common dressing. They are absorbent and are especially useful for wicking away the wound exudate. Gauze does not interact with wound tissue and thus causes little wound irritation. Gauze is available in different textures and in squares of 4 × 4 inches or 2 × 2 inches and rolls of various lengths. Gauze sponges can be saturated with solutions and used to cleanse and pack a wound. When used to pack a wound, the gauze is saturated with the solution (usually normal saline), wrung out, unfolded, and lightly packed into the wound. The purpose of this type of dressing is to provide moisture to the wound, yet to allow wound drainage to be wicked into the gauze pad. Unfolding the dressing allows a more efficient wicking action. For wounds that require debridement, the moistened contact dressing is allowed to dry to facilitate necrotic tissue removal when the gauze is pulled from the wound bed.

Non-adherent gauze dressings such as Telfa are used over clean wounds with little or no drainage. Telfa gauze has a shiny, non-adherent surface that does not stick to incisions or wound openings but allows drainage to pass through to the gauze.

Another type of dressing is a self-adhesive, transparent film. This type of dressing traps the wound's moisture, providing a moist environment (Figure 43–23). Transparent film dressings are ideal to protect high-risk skin or for small, superficial wounds such as partial-thickness wounds. A film dressing can also be used as a secondary dressing and for autolytic debridement of small wounds. It has the following advantages:

- Adheres to undamaged skin
- Serves as a barrier to external fluids and bacteria but still allows the wound surface to "breathe" because oxygen can pass through the transparent dressing
- Promotes a moist environment that speeds epithelial cell growth
- Can be removed without damaging underlying tissues
- Permits viewing of the wound
- Does not require a secondary dressing

Hydrocolloid dressings are dressings with complex formulations of colloids, elastomeric, and adhesive components. These dressings are adhesive and occlusive. The wound contact layer of this dressing forms a gel as fluid is absorbed and maintains a moist healing environment. Hydrocolloids can be used to support healing in clean granulating wounds as well as to autolytically debride necrotic wounds. These dressings come in a variety of sizes and shapes. This type of dressing has the following functions:

- It absorbs drainage through the use of exudate absorbers in the dressing.
- It maintains wound moisture.
- It slowly liquefies necrotic debris.
- It is impermeable to bacteria and other contaminants.
- It is self-adhesive and moulds well.
- It can be used as a preventive dressing for high-risk friction areas.
- It may be left in place for 3 to 5 days, minimizing skin trauma and disruption of healing.

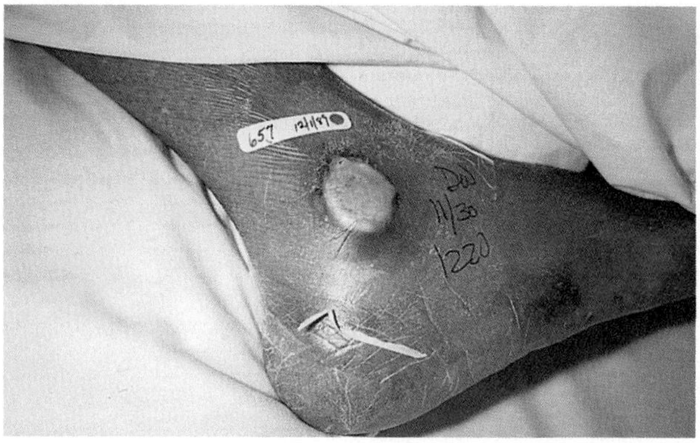

FIGURE **43–23** Transparent film dressing.

Hydrocolloid dressings are most useful on shallow to moderately deep dermal ulcers. A disadvantage of hydrocolloid dressings is that most cannot absorb sufficient drainage from heavily draining wounds, and some are contraindicated for use in full-thickness and infected wounds. Some hydrocolloids may leave a residue in the wound bed that can be confused with pus.

Hydrogel dressings are water- or glycerine-based amorphous gel-impregnated gauze or sheet dressings. Hydrogels also come in a tube, where the gel can be squirted onto the wound base. This type of dressing hydrates wounds and can absorb moderate amounts of exudate. Hydrogel dressings are used on partial-thickness and full-thickness wounds, deep wounds with some exudate, necrotic wounds, burns, and radiation-damaged skin. They are useful in painful wounds, because they are very soothing to the client and do not adhere to the wound bed, thus causing little trauma during dressing removal. A disadvantage is that some hydrogels require a secondary dressing and care must be taken to prevent periwound maceration.

Hydrogel preparations have the following advantages:

- They are soothing, reducing pain in the wound.
- They provide a moist environment.
- They can debride the wound (by softening the necrotic tissue).
- They do not adhere to the wound base.

There are many other types of dressings available. For example, foam dressings and calcium alginate dressings are used in wounds with large amounts of exudate and in wounds that need packing. Foam dressings are also used around drainage tubes to absorb drainage. Calcium alginate dressings are manufactured from seaweed and come in sheet and rope form. The alginate forms a soft gel when it comes in contact with wound fluid. These highly absorbent dressings can be used on infected wounds and do not cause trauma when removed from the wound. They should not be used on dry wounds and require a secondary dressing.

Several manufacturers produce composite dressings. These dressings combine two different dressing types into one dressing. Alternative dressings can also be used to cover and protect certain types of wounds. Examples are large wounds, wounds with drainage tubes or suction catheters in the wound, wounds that need frequent dressing changes, and fistulas. In these wounds, pouches or special wound collection systems are used to cover the wound and collect the wound drainage. Some of these devices have a plastic door on the front of the wound pouch, allowing the nurse to change the wound packing without removing the wound pouch from the skin.

The type of dressing used varies as the wound heals. Continued reassessment is essential (Colwell, 2003). For example, a transparent film dressing may be used initially to autolytically debride the wound. Once the wound is cleansed of necrotic tissue, a new dressing may be chosen.

Changing Dressings. To prepare for changing a dressing, the nurse must know the type of dressing, whether drains or tubing are present, and the type of supplies needed for wound care. Poor preparation may cause a break in aseptic technique or accidental dislodging of a drain. The nurse's judgment in modifying a dressing change procedure is important during wound care, particularly if the character of a wound changes. Notifying the physician of any change is essential.

The physician's order for changing a dressing should indicate the dressing type, the frequency of changing, and any solutions or ointments to be applied to the wound. An order to "reinforce dressing prn" (add dressings without removing the original one) is common right after surgery, when the physician does not want accidental disruption of the suture line or bleeding. The medical or operating room record usually indicates whether drains are present and from what body cavity they drain. After the first dressing change, the nurse describes the location of drains and the type of dressing materials and solutions to use in the client's care plan. The CDC (2001) recommends the following during the dressing change procedure:

- The skin beneath the tape is also assessed.
- The nurse should perform thorough hand hygiene before and after wound care.
- Personnel should not touch an open or fresh wound directly without wearing sterile gloves.
- Dressings over closed wounds should be removed or changed when they become wet or if the client has signs or symptoms of infection and as ordered.

There is a growing body of literature about sterile versus clean dressings. The AHCPR guidelines (1994) recommend that clean dressings be used on pressure ulcers and that the caregiver should wear disposable (clean) gloves when providing care.

To prepare a client for a dressing change, the nurse does the following:

- Administers required analgesics so that peak effects occur during the dressing change
- Describes steps of the procedure to lessen client anxiety
- Gathers all supplies required for the dressing change
- Recognizes normal signs of healing
- Answers questions about the procedure or the wound

Often it is necessary to teach clients how to change dressings in preparation for home care. The nurse must demonstrate dressing changes to the client and family and then provide an opportunity for the client or family member to practise. Usually in this situation, wound healing has progressed to the point that risks of complications such as dehiscence are minimal. The client

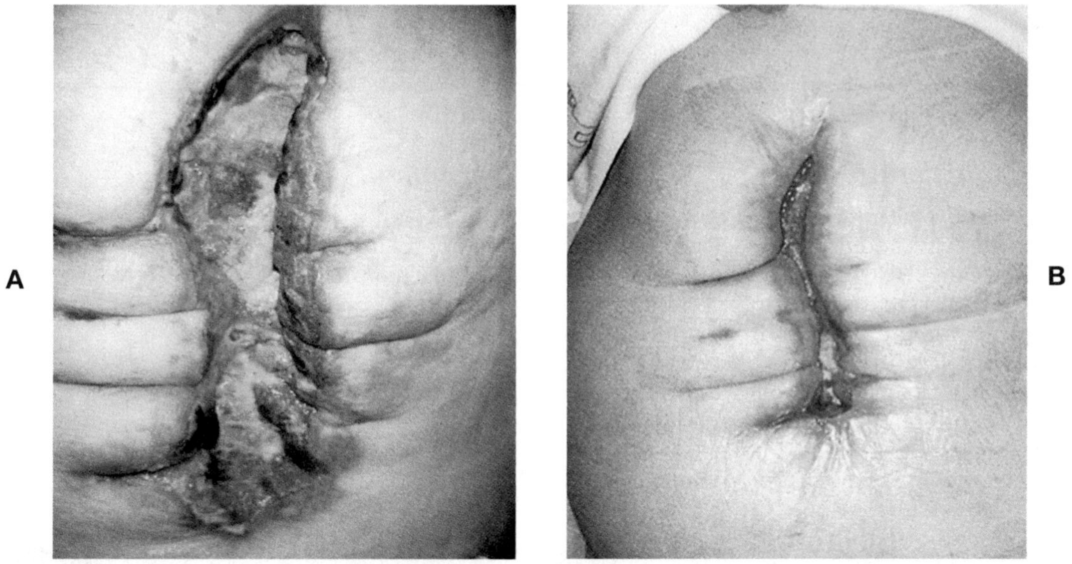

FIGURE **43–24** **A,** Dehisced wound before Wound V.A.C. therapy. **B,** Dehisced wound after Wound V.A.C. therapy. (Courtesy Kinetic Concepts, Inc., San Antonio, TX.)

should be able to change a dressing independently or with assistance from a family member before discharge. Clients without family help may require home care assistance for dressing changes. Skill 43-4 outlines the steps for changing dry and wet-to-dry dressings.

Packing a Wound. The first step in packing a wound is to assess the size, depth, and shape of the wound. These wound characteristics are important in determining the size and type of dressing used to pack a wound. The dressing should be flexible and must be able to be in contact with the entire wound surface. The nurse must make sure that the type of material used to pack the wound is appropriate. If gauze is the appropriate dressing material, the gauze is saturated with the ordered solution, wrung out, unfolded and lightly packed into the wound. The entire wound surface should be in contact with part of the moist gauze dressing (see Skill 43-4). The AHCPR guidelines (1994) recommend that wound dead space should be eliminated by loosely filling the entire wound cavity with the dressing material. It is important to remember that to prevent abscesses, the wound cavity needs to be filled so that areas are not "walled off" (AHCPR, 1994).

The wound should not be packed too tightly, as overpacking the wound may cause pressure on the tissue in the wound bed. The wound should be packed only until the packing material reaches the surface of the wound; there should never be so much packing material in the wound that it extends higher than the wound surface. Wound packing that overlaps onto the wound edges can cause maceration of the tissue surrounding the wound. It can also impede the proper healing and closing of the wound.

Vacuum-Assisted Closure. A new treatment modality for chronic wounds is **vacuum-assisted closure** (the brand name is **Wound V.A.C,** which is a device that assists in wound closure by applying localized negative pressure to draw the edges of a wound together; (Figure 43–24, *A, B*). Wound V.A.C. accelerates wound healing by promoting the formation of granulation tissue in order to completely close or improve the health of a wound in preparation for a skin graft. The use of negative pressure removes fluid from the area surrounding the wound, thus reducing local edema and improving circulation to the area (Chua et al., 2000; Figure 43–25). In addition, after 3 to 4 days of therapy, bacterial counts in the wound drop (Argenta & Morykwas, 1997; Evans & Land, 2001).

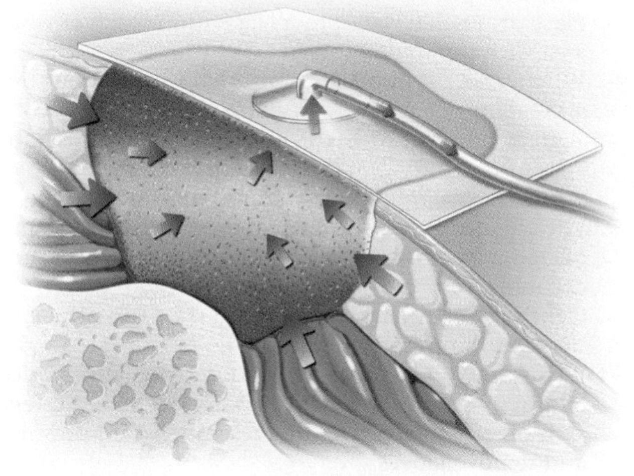

FIGURE **43–25** Wound V.A.C. system using negative pressure to remove fluid from area surrounding the wound, reducing edema and improving circulation to the area. (Courtesy Kinetic Concepts, Inc., San Antonio, TX.)

Wound V.A.C. may be used to treat acute and chronic wounds (Skill 43-5). The schedule for changing Wound V.A.C. dressings varies. An infected wound may need a dressing change every 24 hours, whereas a clean wound can be changed three times a week (Chua et al., 2000;

Text continued on p. 1552

Skill 43-5 *Implementation of Vacuum-Assisted Closure*

View Video

Delegation Considerations

Assessment for and placement of Wound Vacuum Assisted Closure (V.A.C.) should not be delegated to unregulated care providers (UCPs). Other aspects of the client care may be delegated, but the nurse is responsible for wound assessment and evaluation of wound care interventions. When delegating aspects of care the nurse must instruct the UCP to report the following:

- Any change in client's temperature or level of comfort
- Change in the pressure in the V.A.C. unit
- Any change in the integrity of the Wound V.A.C. dressing

Equipment

- V.A.C. unit (requires physician order; Figure 43–26)
- V.A.C. foam dressing
- Tubing for connection between V.A.C. unit and V.A.C. dressing
- Gloves, disposable and sterile
- Scissors (sterile)
- Skin prep/skin barrier
- Moist washcloth
- Plastic trash bag
- Linen bag

Steps	Rationale
1. Perform hand hygiene. Assemble supplies.	Reduces transmission of micro-organisms. Organizes procedure.
2. Position client comfortably and drape to expose only wound site. Instruct client not to touch wound or sterile supplies.	Maintaining client comfort assists in completing skill smoothly. Draping provides access to wound while minimizing unnecessary exposure.
3. Place disposable waterproof bag within reach of work area with top folded to make a cuff.	Facilitates safe disposal of soiled dressings.
4. When V.A.C. is in place, push therapy on/off button.	
a. Keeping tube connectors with V.A.C. unit, disconnect tubes from each other to drain fluids into canister.	Deactivates therapy and allows for proper drainage of fluid in drainage tubing.
b. Before lowering, tighten clamp on canister tube.	
5. With dressing tube unclamped, introduce 10 to 30 mL of normal saline, if ordered, into tubing to soak underneath foam.	Facilitates loosening of foam when tissue adheres to foam (Chua et al., 2000).
6. Gently stretch transparent film horizontally and slowly pull up from the skin.	Reduces stress on suture line or wound edges and reduces irritation and discomfort.
7. Remove old V.A.C. dressing, observing appearance and drainage on dressing. Use caution to avoid tension on any drains that are present. Discard dressing and remove gloves.	Determines dressings needed for replacement. Avoids accidental removal of drains because they may or may not be sutured in place.
8. Apply sterile or disposable gloves. Irrigate the wound with normal saline or other solution ordered by the physician. Gently blot to dry.	Irrigation removes wound debris.

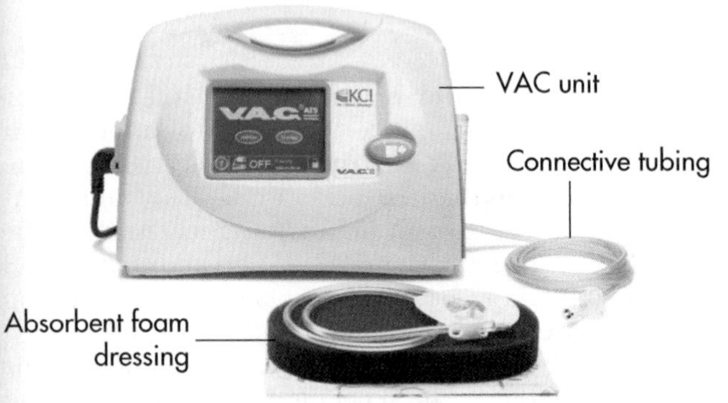

FIGURE **43–26** Wound V.A.C. unit. *Top to bottom:* V.A.C. unit itself, connective tubing to go between V.A.C. unit and V.A.C. dressing, absorbent foam dressing. (Courtesy Kinetic Concepts, Inc., San Antonio, TX.)

Steps	Rationale

Critical Decision Point: When drainage looks purulent, there is change in amount or colour, or it has a foul odour, wound cultures should be obtained even when they are not ordered for that particular dressing change (Chua et al., 2000).

Steps	Rationale
9. Measure wound as ordered: at baseline, first dressing change, weekly, and discharge from therapy. Remove and discard gloves.	Objectively documents wound healing process in response to negative pressure
10. Depending on the type of wound, apply sterile gloves or new disposable gloves.	Fresh sterile wounds require sterile gloves. Chronic wounds may require clean technique. However, do not use the same gloves worn to remove old dressing because cross contamination may occur (Stotts et al., 1997).
11. Prepare V.A.C. foam.	
a. Select appropriate foam.	Black, polyurethane (PU) foam has larger pores and is most effective in stimulating granulation tissue and wound contraction. White, polyvinyl alcohol (PVA) soft foam is denser with smaller pores and is used when the growth of granulation tissue needs to be restricted (Kinetic Concepts Inc. USA [KCI], 1999).
b. Using sterile scissors, cut foam to wound size. Dressing must be cut to fit the size and shape of the wound including tunnels and undermined areas.	

Critical Decision Point: Clients may experience more pain with the black foam because of excessive wound contraction. For this reason, they may need to be switched to the PVA soft foam.

Steps	Rationale
12. Gently place foam in wound; be sure that the foam is in contact with entire wound base and margins and tunnelled and undermined areas (see illustration Step 12, *A*).	Maintains negative pressure to entire wound. Edges of the foam dressing must be in direct contact with the client's skin (Broussard, Mendez-Eastman, & Frantz, 2000).
13. Apply wrinkle-free transparent dressing over foam and secure tubing to the unit (see illustration Step 12, *B* and *C*).	Connects the negative pressure from the V.A.C. unit to the wound foam.

Critical Decision Point: For deep wounds, regularly reposition tubing to minimize pressure on wound edges. In addition, clients with restricted mobility or sensation must be repositioned frequently to prevent client from lying on the tubing and causing skin damage (KCI, 1999).

Steps	Rationale
14. Apply skin protectant, such as skin prep or Stomahesive wafer, to skin around the wound.	Protects periwound skin from injury that may result from the occlusive dressing.
15. Apply Wound V.A.C. dressing. Secure tubing to transparent film, aligning drainage holes to ensure an occlusive seal (see illustration Step 12, *C*). Do not apply tension to drape and tubing.	Ensures that the wound is properly covered and a negative pressure seal can be achieved (Box 43-14). Excessive tension may compress foam dressing, produce a shear force on periwound area, and impede wound healing (KCI, 1999).
16. Secure tubing several centimetres away from the dressing.	Prevents pull on the primary dressing, which can cause leaks in the negative pressure system (Chua et al., 2000; KCI, 1999).

Skill 43-5 Implementation of Vacuum-Assisted Closure—cont'd

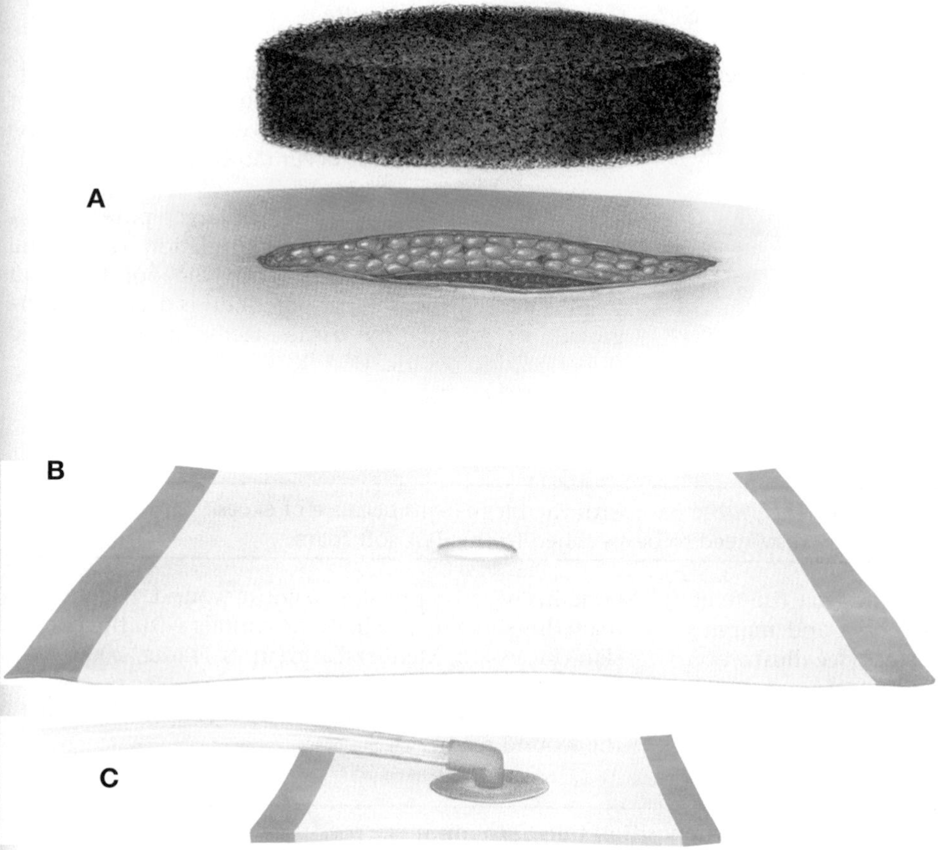

STEP **12** Dressing application. **A,** Properly sized foam to cover wound (Step 12). **B,** Wrinkle-free transparent dressing applied over foam (Step 13). **C,** Secure tubing to the foam and transparent dressing unit (Step 15). (Courtesy Kinetic Concepts, Inc., San Antonio, TX.)

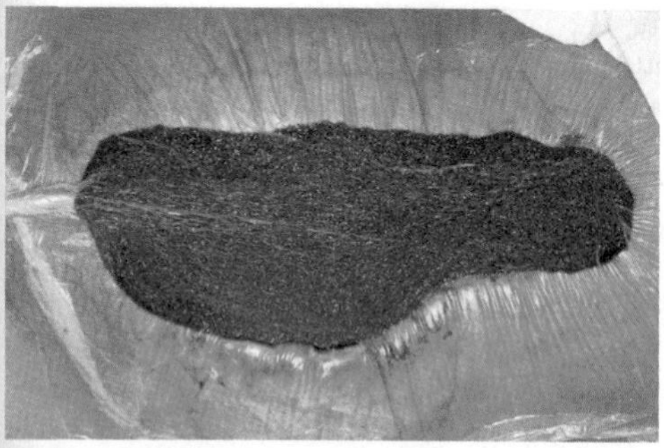

STEP **17** Foam dressing, transparent dressing, and Wound V.A.C. tubing secured over existing wound. (Courtesy Kinetic Concepts, Inc., San Antonio, TX.)

Steps	Rationale
17. Once wound is completely covered (see illustration), connect the tubing from the dressing to the tubing from the canister and V.A.C. unit. a. Remove canister from sterile packaging and push into V.A.C. unit until a click is heard. **NOTE: An alarm will sound if the canister is not properly engaged.**	Intermittent or continuous negative pressure can be administered at 50 to 200 mm Hg, according to physician order and client comfort. The average is 125 mm Hg (Baxandall, 1996; Chua et al., 2000).

Steps	Rationale
b. Connect the dressing tubing to the canister tubing. Make sure both clamps are open.	
c. Place V.A.C. unit on a level surface or hang from the foot of the bed. **NOTE: The V.A.C. unit will alarm and deactivate therapy if the unit is tilted beyond 45 degrees.**	
d. Press in green-lit power button and set pressure as ordered.	
18. Discard old dressing materials; remove gloves and perform hand hygiene.	Reduces transmission of micro-organisms.
19. Inspect Wound V.A.C. system to verify that negative pressure is achieved.	Negative pressure is achieved when an airtight seal is achieved.
a. Verify that display screen reads THERAPY ON.	
b. Be sure clamps are open and tubing is patent.	
c. Identify air leaks by listening with stethoscope or by moving hand around edges of wound while applying light pressure.	
d. If a leak is present, use strips of transparent film to patch areas.	
20. Compare wound with baseline wound assessment.	Provides objective documentation of wound healing.
21. Verify airtight dressing seal and proper negative pressure.	In order to achieve prescribed vacuum level, the wound must be covered with an airtight seal. This airtight seal and the negative pressure promote wound drainage, circulation, and healing.

Unexpected Outcomes and Related Interventions

- Wound appears inflamed and tender, drainage has increased, and an odour is present.
  - Notify physician.
  - Obtain wound culture.
  - Increase frequency of dressing changes.
- Client reports increase in pain.
  - If using black foam, switch to the PVA foam product.
  - Client may need more analgesic support when V.A.C. is initiated.
  - Negative pressure may need to be reduced.
- Negative pressure seal has broken.
  - Take preventive measures: Shave hair around wound, avoid wrinkles in transparent dressing, and avoid use of adhesive remover because it may leave residue that hinders film adherence.
  - Reinforce with transparent dressing strips.

Recording and Reporting

- Record appearance of wound, colour, characteristics of any drainage, and presence of wound healing augmentation.
- Record pressure setting of Wound V.A.C.
- Record date and time of dressing change.
- Report brisk, bright bleeding, evidence of poor wound healing, and possible wound infection.

Home Care Considerations

- Wound V.A.C. can be used in the home safely. Client may need clinic visits or home care nursing visits to monitor wound healing.
- Provide resources to client for supplies for Wound V.A.C.
- Instruct family and caregiver regarding proper disposal of contaminated product.

Box 43-14 Maintaining an Airtight Seal

To avoid wound desiccation, the wound must stay sealed once therapy is initiated. Problem seal areas include wounds around joints and near the sacrum. The following points may assist in maintaining an airtight seal:

- Shave hair around wound.
- Cut transparent film to extend 3 to 5 cm beyond wound parameter.
- Avoid wrinkles in transparent film.
- Patch leaks with transparent film.
- Use multiple small strips of transparent film to hold dressing in place before covering dressing with large piece of transparent film.
- Avoid adhesive remover because it leaves a residue that hinders film adherence.

From "Vacuum-Assisted Wound Closure," by P. C. Chua et al., 2000, *American Journal of Nursing, 100*(12), pp. 45–48.

Mendez-Eastman, 1998). As the wound heals, the wound base is redder and granulation tissue lines the surface of the wound. The wound has a stippled or granulated appearance. The surface area of the wound may increase or decrease depending on wound location and the amount of drainage removed by the Wound V.A.C. system. As the wound heals, paler areas in the wound may develop. This indicates an increase in fibrous tissue (Mendez-Eastman, 1998).

Securing Dressings. The nurse may use tape, ties, bandages, or a secondary dressing and cloth binders to secure a dressing over a wound site. The choice of anchoring depends on the wound size and location, the presence of drainage, the frequency of dressing changes, and the client's level of activity.

The nurse most often uses strips of tape to secure dressings if the client is not allergic to tape. Non-allergenic paper and plastic tapes minimize skin reactions. Common adhesive tape adheres well to the skin's surface, whereas elastic adhesive tape compresses closely around pressure bandages and permits more movement of a body part. Skin that is sensitive to adhesive tape can become severely inflamed and denuded and may even slough when the tape is removed. It is important to assess skin under tape at each dressing change.

Tape is available in various widths such as 1.5, 2.5, 5, and 7.5 cm. The nurse chooses the size that sufficiently secures the dressing. For example, a large abdominal wound dressing must remain secure over a large area despite frequent stress from movement, respiratory effort, and possibly abdominal distension. Strips of 7.3-cm adhesive better stabilize such a large dressing so that it does not continually slip off. When applying tape, the nurse ensures that it adheres to several centimetres of skin on both sides of the dressing and that it is placed across the middle of the dressing. When securing the dressing, the nurse presses the tape gently, exerting pressure away from the wound. This way, tension occurs in both directions away from the wound, minimizing skin distortion and irritation. Tape is never applied over irritated or broken skin. Some nurses protect the skin beneath the tape with a skin sealant product.

To remove tape safely, the nurse loosens the tape ends and gently pulls the outer end parallel with the skin surface toward the wound. The nurse applies light traction to the skin away from the wound as the tape is loosened and removed. Adhesive remover can also be used to loosen the tape from the skin. The traction minimizes pulling of the skin. If tape covers an area of hair growth, the client experiences less discomfort if the nurse pulls the tape in the direction of hair growth.

To avoid repeated removal of tape from sensitive skin, the nurse can secure dressings with pairs of reusable Montgomery ties (Figure 43–27). Each section consists of a long strip; half contains an adhesive backing to apply to the skin, and the other half folds back and contains a cloth tie or a safety pin and rubber band combination to be fastened across a dressing and untied at dressing changes. A large, bulky dressing may require two or more sets of Montgomery ties. Another method to protect the surrounding skin on wounds that need frequent dressing changes is to place strips of hydrocolloid dressings on either side of the wound edges, cover the wound with a dressing, and then apply the tape to the hydrocolloid dressing. To provide even support to a wound and immobilize a body part, the nurse may apply elastic gauze or cloth bandages and binders over a dressing.

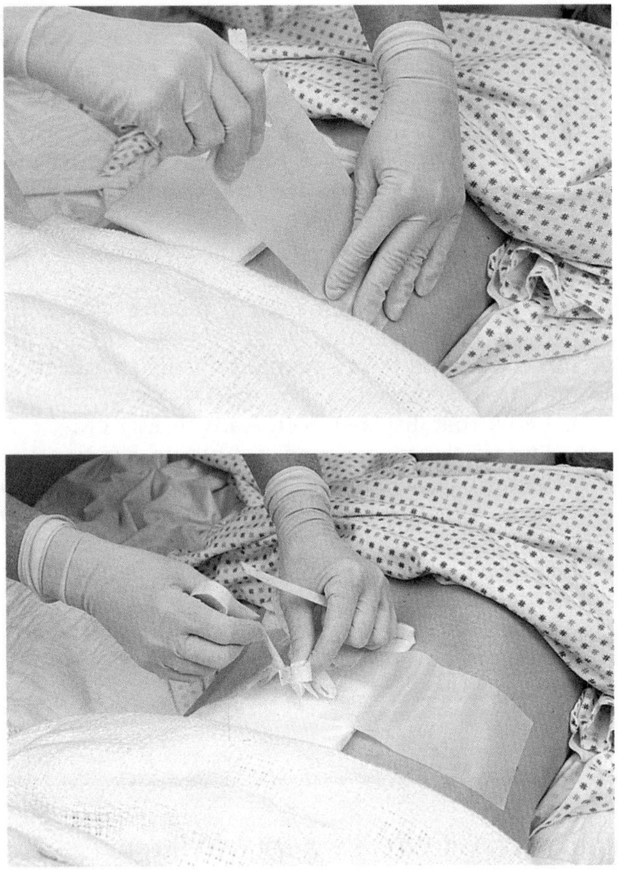

A

B

FIGURE **43–27** Montgomery ties. **A,** Each tie is placed at side of dressing. **B,** Securing ties encloses dressing.

Comfort Measures. A wound can be painful, depending on the extent of tissue injury. The nurse uses several techniques to minimize discomfort during wound care. Careful removal of tape, gentle cleansing of wound edges, and careful manipulation of dressings and drains minimize stress on sensitive tissues. Careful turning and positioning also reduce strain on a wound. Administration of analgesic medications 30 to 60 minutes before dressing changes (depending on a drug's time of peak action) also reduces discomfort.

Suture Care. A surgeon closes a wound by bringing the wound edges as close together as possible to reduce scar formation. Proper wound closure involves minimal trauma and tension to tissues with control of bleeding.

Sutures are threads used to sew body tissues together. Metal staples may also be used to close a wound (Figure 43–28). The client's history of wound healing, the site of surgery, the tissues involved, and the purpose of the sutures determine the suture material to be used. For example, if the client has had repeated surgery for an

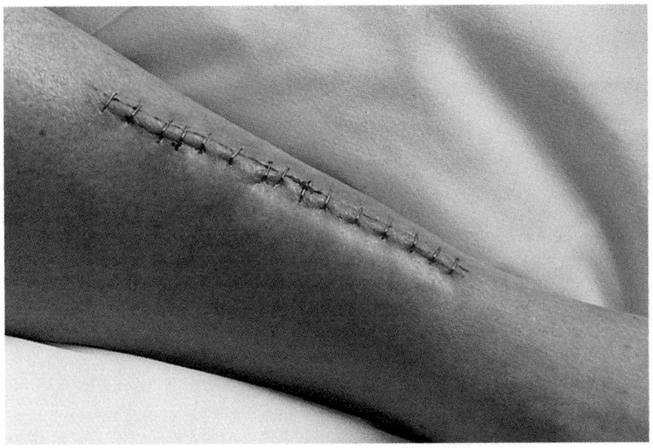

FIGURE **43–28** Incision closed with metal staples.

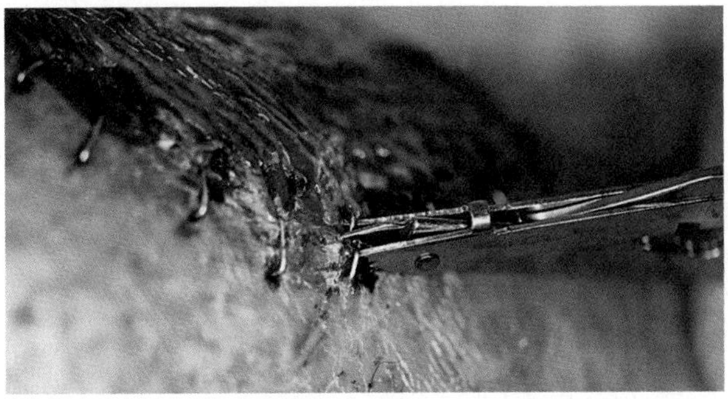

FIGURE **43–29** Staple remover.

abdominal hernia, the physician might choose wire sutures to provide greater strength for wound closure. In contrast, a small laceration of the face calls for the use of very fine Dacron (polyester) sutures to minimize scar formation.

Sutures are available in a variety of materials, including silk, steel, cotton, linen, wire, nylon, and Dacron. Sutures come with or without sharp surgical needles attached. Steel staples are commonly used. They cause less trauma to tissues than sutures, yet provide extra strength. Wounds are also often closed with tape closures such as Steri-Strips applied over the wound.

Sutures are placed within tissue layers in deep wounds and superficially as the final means for wound closure. Deep sutures are usually an absorbable material that will disappear over time. Sutures are foreign bodies and thus are capable of causing local inflammation. The surgeon can minimize tissue injury by using the finest suture possible and the smallest number necessary.

Policies vary within institutions as to who may remove sutures. If it is appropriate that the nurse remove them, a physician's order is required. An order for suture removal is not written until the physician believes that the wound has closed (usually in 7 days). Special scissors with curved cutting tips or special staple removers slide under the skin closures for suture removal (Figure 43–29). The physician usually signifies the number of sutures or staples to remove. If the suture line appears to be healing in certain locations better than in others, the physician may choose to have only some sutures removed (e.g., every other one).

To remove staples, the nurse simply inserts the tips of the staple remover under each wire staple. While slowly closing the ends of the staple remover together, the nurse squeezes the centre of the staple with the tips, freeing the staple from the skin.

To remove sutures, the nurse first checks the type of suturing used (Figure 43–30). With intermittent suturing, the surgeon ties each individual suture made in the skin. Continuous suturing, as the name implies, is a series of sutures with only two knots, one at the beginning and one at the end of the suture line. Retention sutures are placed more deeply than skin sutures and may or may not be removed by the nurse, depending on agency policy. The manner in which the suture crosses and penetrates the skin determines the method for removal. The most important principle in suture removal is to never pull the visible portion of a suture through underlying tissue. Sutures on the skin's surface harbour micro-organisms and debris. The portion of the suture beneath the skin is sterile. Pulling the contaminated portion of the suture through tissues may lead to infection. The nurse clips suture materials as close to the skin edge on one side as possible and pulls the suture through from the other side (Figure 43–31).

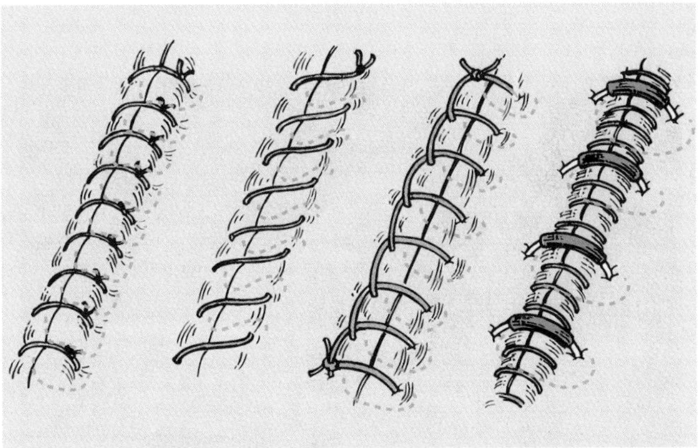

A B C D

FIGURE **43–30** Examples of suturing methods. **A,** Intermittent. **B,** Continuous. **C,** Blanket continuous. **D,** Retention.

Drainage Evacuation. When drainage interferes with healing, drainage evacuation can be achieved by using either a drain alone or a drainage tube with continuous suction. The nurse may apply special skin barriers, including hydrocolloid dressings, around drain sites, similar to those used with ostomies (see chapter 41). The skin barriers are soft materials applied to the skin with adhesive. Drainage flows on the barrier but not directly on the skin. **Drainage evacuators** (Figure 43–32) are convenient, portable units that connect to tubular drains lying within a wound bed and exert a safe, constant, low-pressure vacuum to remove and collect drainage. The nurse ensures

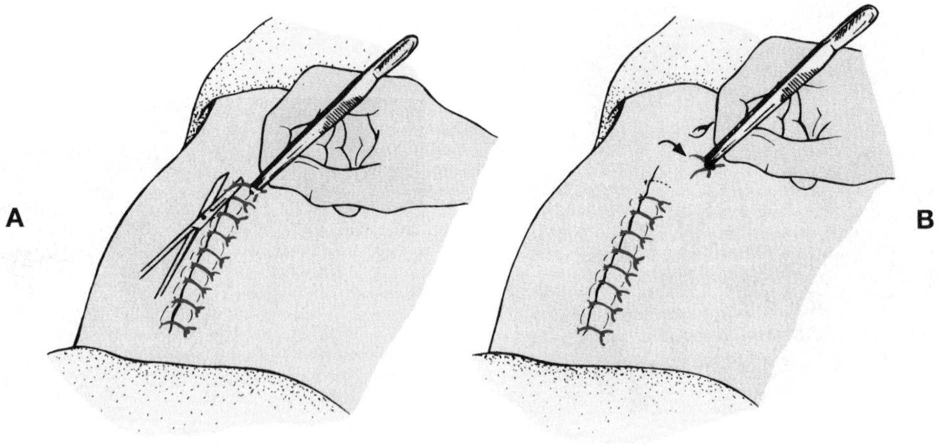

FIGURE **43–31** Removal of intermittent suture. **A,** The nurse cuts the suture as close to the skin as possible, away from the knot. **B,** The nurse removes the suture and never pulls the contaminated stitch through tissues.

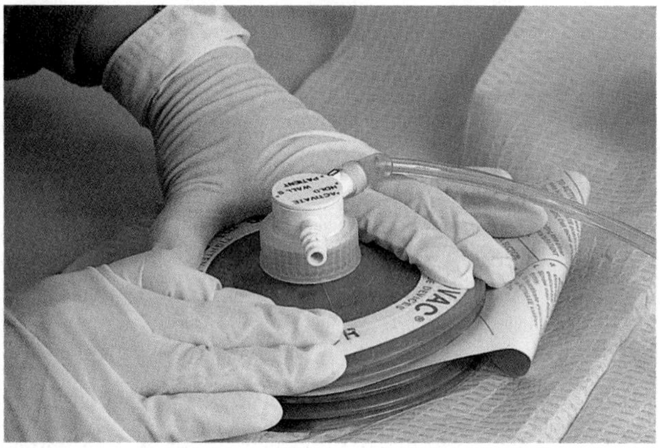

FIGURE **43–32** Setting the suction on a drainage evacuator. 1. With the drainage port open, the level on the diaphragm is raised. 2. The nurse pushes straight down on the lever to lower the diaphragm. 3. Closure of the port prevents escape of air and creates vacuum pressure.

that suction is exerted and that connection points between the evacuator and tubing are intact. The evacuator collects drainage that the nurse assesses for volume and character every shift and as needed. When the evacuator fills, the nurse measures output by emptying the contents into a graduated cylinder and immediately resets the evacuator to apply suction.

Bandages and Binders. A simple gauze dressing is often not enough to immobilize or provide support to a wound. Binders and bandages applied over or around dressings can provide extra protection and therapeutic benefits by doing the following:

- Creating pressure over a body part (e.g., an elastic pressure bandage applied over an arterial puncture site)
- Immobilizing a body part (e.g., an elastic bandage applied around a sprained ankle)
- Supporting a wound (e.g., an abdominal binder applied over a large abdominal incision and dressing)
- Reducing or preventing edema (e.g., a well-supporting bra to minimize breast discomfort after delivery of a baby)
- Securing a splint (e.g., a bandage applied around hand splints for correction of deformities)
- Securing dressings (e.g., elastic webbing applied around leg dressings after a vein stripping)

Bandages are available in rolls of various widths and materials, including gauze, elasticized knit, elastic webbing, flannel, and muslin. Gauze bandages are lightweight and inexpensive, mould easily around contours of the body, and permit air circulation to prevent skin maceration. Elastic bandages conform well to body parts but can also be used to exert pressure.

Binders are bandages that are made of large pieces of material to fit a specific body part. Most binders are made of elastic or cotton. An abdominal binder and a breast binder are examples.

Principles for Applying Bandages and Binders. Correctly applied bandages and binders do not cause injury to underlying and nearby body parts or create discomfort for the client. For example, a chest binder must not be so tight as to restrict chest wall expansion. Before a bandage or binder is applied, the nurse's responsibilities include the following:

- Inspecting the skin for abrasions, edema, discoloration, or exposed wound edges
- Covering exposed wounds or open abrasions with a sterile dressing
- Assessing the condition of underlying dressings and changing if soiled
- Assessing the skin of underlying areas that will be distal to the bandage for signs of circulatory impairment (coolness, pallor or cyanosis, diminished or absent pulses, swelling, numbness, and tingling) to provide a means for comparing changes in circulation after bandage application.

The nurse explains to the client that all bandages or binders feel relatively firm or tight. A bandage should be carefully assessed to be sure that it is properly applied and is providing therapeutic benefit. Soiled bandages should be replaced.

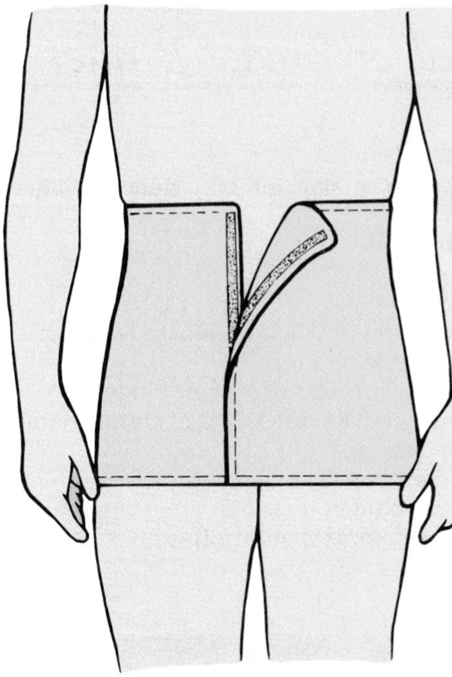

FIGURE **43–33** Securing an abdominal binder with Velcro.

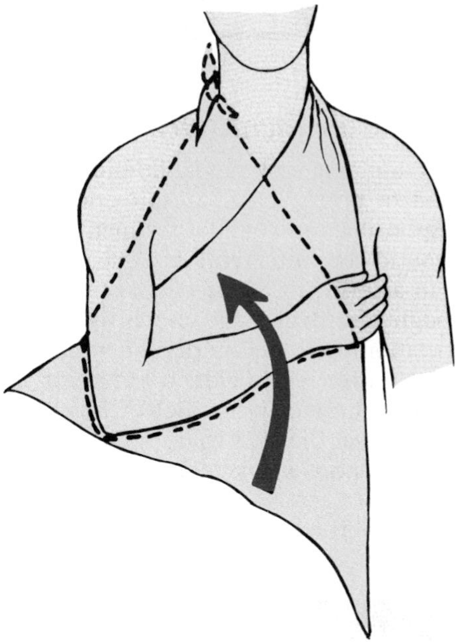

FIGURE **43–34** Application of a sling.

Binder Application. Binders are especially designed for the body part to be supported. The most common types of binders are the abdominal binder and breast binder (Skill 43-6). Breast binders, used to provide support after breast surgery or to exert pressure to reduce lactation in a woman after childbirth, are now being replaced with well-fitting bras.

An abdominal binder supports large abdominal incisions that are vulnerable to tension or stress as the client moves or coughs. The nurse secures an abdominal binder with safety pins, Velcro strips, or metal stays (Figure 43–33).

Slings. Slings support arms that have muscular sprains or fractures. A commercially manufactured sling consists of a long sleeve that extends above the elbow, with a strap that fits around the neck. In the home, a large triangular piece of cloth can be used. The client may sit or lie supine during sling application. The nurse instructs the client to bend the affected arm, bringing the forearm straight across the chest. The open sling fits under the client's arm and over the chest, with the base of the triangle under the wrist and the triangle's point at the client's elbow (Figure 43–34). One end of the sling fits around the back of the client's neck. The nurse brings the other end up and over the affected arm while supporting the extremity. The nurse ties the two ends at the side of the neck so that the knot does not press against the cervical spine. The loose material at the elbow can be folded evenly around the elbow and pinned. The lower arm and hand should always be supported at a level above the elbow to prevent the formation of dependent edema.

Bandage Application. Rolls of bandage can secure or support dressings over irregularly shaped body parts. Each roll has a free outer end and a terminal end at the centre of the roll. The rolled portion of the bandage is its body, and its outer surface is placed against the client's skin or dressing.

The nurse may use a variety of bandage turns, depending on the body part to be bandaged (Table 43-8). After a bandage is applied, the nurse assesses, documents, and immediately reports changes in circulation, skin integrity, comfort level, and body function (e.g., ventilation or movement). The nurse who applies a bandage can loosen or readjust it as necessary. The nurse should have a physician's order before loosening or removing a bandage applied by a physician. Skill 43-7 describes the steps for applying an elastic bandage.

Heat and Cold Therapy

Assessment for Temperature Tolerance. Before applying heat or cold therapies, the nurse assesses the client's physical condition for signs of potential intolerance to heat and cold. The nurse first observes the area to be treated. Alterations in skin integrity, such as abrasions, open wounds, edema, bruising, bleeding, or localized areas of inflammation, increase the client's risk of injury. Because the physician commonly orders heat and cold applications to be placed on traumatized areas, the baseline skin assessment provides a guide for evaluating skin changes that might occur during therapy.

Assessment includes identification of conditions that contraindicate heat or cold therapy. An active area of bleeding should not be covered by a warm application because bleeding will continue. Warm applications are contraindicated when the client has an acute, localized inflammation such as appendicitis because the heat could cause the appendix to rupture. If a client has cardiovascular problems, it is unwise to apply heat to large portions of

Skill 43-6 Applying an Abdominal or Breast Binder

Delegation Considerations

The skills of applying a binder (abdominal or breast) can be delegated to unregulated care providers (UCPs). The nurse is responsible for wound assessment and the evaluation of wound care interventions. The nurse must also complete an assessment of the client's ability to breathe deeply, cough effectively, and move independently; of skin for irritation/abrasion; of incision/wound and dressing; and of comfort level before a binder or sling is applied for the first time. When delegating this skill, the nurse must instruct the UCP to do the following:

- Immediately report any change in client's respiratory status.
- Report increase in wound drainage.
- Report changes in skin integrity under or adjacent to the binder.
- Remove the binder at prescribed intervals.

Equipment

- Disposable gloves, if wound drainage is present
- Abdominal binder:
  - Correct size cloth/elastic straight binder
  - Safety pins, (6 to 8), unless Velcro closure or metal fasteners are attached
- Breast binder:
  - Correct size binder
  - Safety pins (approximately 12), unless Velcro closure is attached

Steps	Rationale
1. Observe client with need for support of thorax or abdomen. Observe ability to breathe deeply and cough effectively.	Baseline assessment determines client's ability to breathe and cough. Impaired ventilation of lung can lead to alveolar atelectasis and inadequate arterial oxygenation.
2. Review medical record if medical prescription for particular binder is required and reasons for application.	Application of supportive binders may be used on nursing judgment. In some situations, physician input is required.
3. Inspect skin for actual or potential alterations in integrity. Observe for irritation, abrasion, skin surfaces that rub against each other, or allergic response to adhesive tape used to secure dressing.	Actual impairments in skin integrity can be worsened with application of a binder. Binder can cause pressure and excoriation.
4. Inspect any surgical dressing.	Dressing replacement or reinforcement precedes application of any binder.

Critical Decision Point: Dressing should be clean and dry, and incision/wound should be entirely covered by dressing.

Steps	Rationale
5. Assess client's comfort level, using analogue scale of 0 to 10 (see chapter 38) and noting any objective signs and symptoms of pain.	Data will determine effectiveness of binder placement.

Critical Decision Point: Expect client in moderate-to-severe pain to have diaphoresis, tachycardia, and elevated blood pressure.

Steps	Rationale
6. Gather necessary data regarding size of client and appropriate binder.	Ensures proper fit of binder.
7. Explain procedure to client.	Promotes client's understanding and co-operation.
8. Teach skill to client or significant other.	Reduces anxiety and ensures continuity of care after discharge.
9. Perform hand hygiene and apply gloves (if likely to contact wound drainage).	Reduces transmission of micro-organisms.
10. Close curtains or room door.	Maintains client's comfort and dignity.
11. Apply binder.	
A. Abdominal binder	
(1) Position client in supine position with head slightly elevated and knees slightly flexed.	Minimizes muscular tension on abdominal organs.
(2) Fanfold far side of binder toward midline of binder.	Reduces time client remains in uncomfortable position.

Steps	Rationale
(3) Instruct and help client to roll away from nurse toward raised side rail while firmly supporting abdominal incision and dressing with hands.	Reduces pain and discomfort.
(4) Place fanfolded ends of binder under client.	Permits placement and centring of binder with minimal discomfort.
(5) Instruct or assist client to roll over folded ends.	
(6) Unfold and stretch ends out smoothly on far side of bed.	Maintains skin integrity and comfort.
(7) Instruct client to roll back into supine position.	Facilitates chest expansion and adequate wound support when binder is closed.
(8) Adjust binder so that supine client is centred over binder using symphysis pubis and costal margins as lower and upper landmarks.	Centres support from binder over abdominal structures, which reduces incidence of decreased lung expansion.

Critical Decision Point: Cover any exposed areas of an incision or wound with sterile dressing.

Steps	Rationale
(9) Close binder. Pull one end of binder over centre of client's abdomen. While maintaining tension on that end of binder, pull opposite end of binder over centre and secure with Velcro closure tabs, metal fasteners, or horizontally placed safety pins (see Figure 43–33).	Provides continuous wound support and comfort.
B. Breast binder	
(1) Assist client in placing arms through binder's armholes.	Eases binder placement process.
(2) Assist client to supine position in bed.	Supine positioning facilitates normal anatomical position of breasts; facilitates healing and comfort.
(3) Pad area under breasts if necessary.	Prevents skin contact with undersurface.
(4) Using Velcro closure tabs or horizontally placed safety pins, secure binder at nipple level first. Continue closure process above and then below nipple line until entire binder is closed.	Horizontal placement of pins may reduce risk of uneven pressure or localized irritation.
(5) Make appropriate adjustments, including individualizing fit of shoulder straps and pinning waistline darts to reduce binder size.	Maintains support to client's breasts.
(6) Instruct and observe skill development in self-care related to reapplying breast binder.	Self-care is integral aspect of discharge planning. Skin integrity and comfort level goals are ensured.
12. Remove gloves and perform hand hygiene.	Prevents cross-infections.
13. Assess client's comfort level, using analogue scale of 0 to 10 and noting any objective signs and symptoms.	Helps determine effectiveness of binder placement. Binders should not increase discomfort.
14. Adjust binder as necessary.	Promotes comfort and chest expansion.
15. Observe site for skin integrity, circulation, and characteristics of the wound. (Periodically remove binder and surgical dressing to assess wound characteristics.)	Determines that binder has not resulted in complication to skin, wound, or underlying organs.
16. Assess client's ability to ventilate properly.	Identifies any impaired ventilation and potential pulmonary complications.
17. Identify client's need for assistance with activities such as hair combing.	Mobility of upper extremities may be limited, depending on severity and location of incision.

Skill 43-6 Applying an Abdominal or Breast Binder—cont'd

Unexpected Outcomes and Related Interventions

- Client's pain increases.
  - Remove binder and assess wound.
  - Reapply binder using less pressure.
- Client's respiratory rate decreases.
  - Remove binder.
  - Encourage client to cough and deep breathe.
  - Reapply binder using less pressure.
- Client develops impaired skin integrity under the binder.
  - Remove binder.
  - Initiate skin care measure to heal affected site.

Recording and Reporting

- Report any skin irritation to nurse at between-shift report.
- Record application of binder, condition of skin, circulation, integrity of dressing, and client's comfort level.
- Report ineffective lung expansion to physician immediately.

Home Care Considerations

- Abdominal and breast binders can be washed and hung to dry.
- Instruct caregiver to avoid excessive pressure with binder application.

the body because the resulting massive vasodilation may disrupt blood supply to vital organs.

Cold is contraindicated in the following situations:

- If the site of injury is already edematous—cold further retards circulation to the area and prevents absorption of the interstitial fluid.
- If the client has impaired circulation (e.g., arteriosclerosis)—cold further reduces blood supply to the affected area.
- If the client has neuropathy (which causes numbness and loss of feeling, especially in hands and feet)—the client is be unable to perceive temperature change and damage resulting from temperature extremes.
- If the client is shivering—cold applications may intensify shivering and dangerously increase body temperature.

The nurse also assesses the client's response to stimuli. Sensation to light touch, pinprick, and mild temperature variations (see chapter 28) reveals the ability of the client to recognize when heat or cold becomes excessive. If a client has peripheral vascular disease, the nurse pays particular attention to the integrity of extremities. For example, if the physician's order is to apply a cold compress to a lower extremity, the nurse should assess circulation to the leg by assessing for capillary refill, observing skin colour, and palpating skin temperatures, distal pulses, and edematous areas. If signs of circulatory inadequacy are present, the nurse should question the order.

Level of consciousness influences the ability to perceive heat, cold, and pain. If a client is confused or unresponsive, the nurse must make frequent observations of skin integrity after therapy begins.

The nurse must also assess the condition of equipment being used. Electrical equipment should be checked for cracked cords, frayed wires, damaged insulation, and exposed heating components. Equipment containing circulating fluids should not have leaks. The nurse also checks equipment for evenness of temperature distribution.

Local application of heat and cold to an injured body part can be therapeutic. Before using these therapies, however, the nurse must understand normal body responses to local temperature variations, assess the integrity of the body part, determine the client's ability to sense temperature variations, and ensure proper operation of equipment. The nurse is legally responsible for safe administration of heat and cold applications.

Bodily Responses to Heat and Cold. Exposure to heat and cold can cause systemic and local responses. Systemic responses occur through heat-loss mechanisms (sweating and vasodilation) or mechanisms promoting heat conservation (vasoconstriction and piloerection) and heat production (shivering; see chapter 28). Local responses to heat and cold occur through stimulation of temperature-sensitive nerve endings within the skin. This stimulation sends impulses from the periphery to the hypothalamus, which becomes aware of local temperature sensations and triggers adaptive responses for maintenance of normal body temperature. If alterations occur along temperature-sensation pathways, the reception and eventual perception of stimuli will be altered.

The body can tolerate wide variations in temperature. The normal temperature of the skin's surface is 34° C, but temperature receptors usually adapt quickly to local temperatures between 45° and 15° C. Pain develops when local temperatures exceed this range. Excessive heat causes a burning sensation. Cold produces a numbing sensation before pain.

The body's adaptive ability creates the major problem in protecting clients from injury resulting from temperature extremes. A person initially feels an extreme change in temperature but within a short time hardly notices it. This can be dangerous because a person insensitive to heat and cold extremes can suffer serious tissue injury. The nurse must recognize clients most at risk for injuries from heat and cold applications (Table 43-9).

Local Effects of Heat and Cold. Heat and cold stimuli create different physiological responses. The choice of heat or cold therapy depends on local responses desired for wound healing.

Effects of Heat Application. Heat generally is quite therapeutic, improving blood flow to an injured part

Table 43-8 Types of Bandage Turns

Type	Description	Purpose or Use
Circular	Bandage turn overlapping previous turn completely 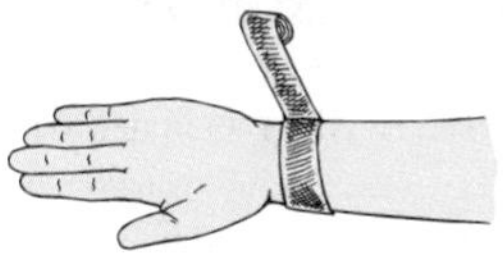	Anchors bandage at the first and final turn; covers small part (finger, toe)
Spiral	Bandage ascending body part, with each turn overlapping previous one by one-half or two-thirds width of bandage 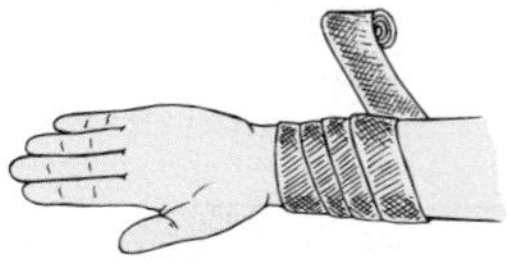	Covers cylindrical body parts such as wrist or upper arm.
Spiral-reverse	Turn requiring twist (reversal) of bandage halfway through each turn 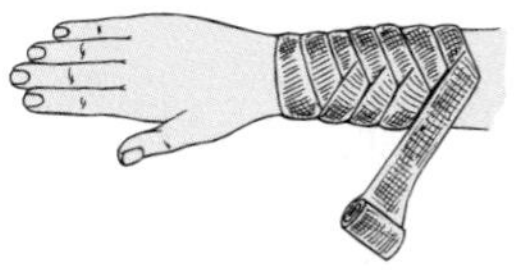	Covers cone-shaped body parts such as forearm, thigh, or calf; useful wth nonstretching bandages such as gauze or flannel
Figure eight	Oblique overlapping turns alternately ascending and descending over bandaged part; each turn crossing previous one to form figure eight 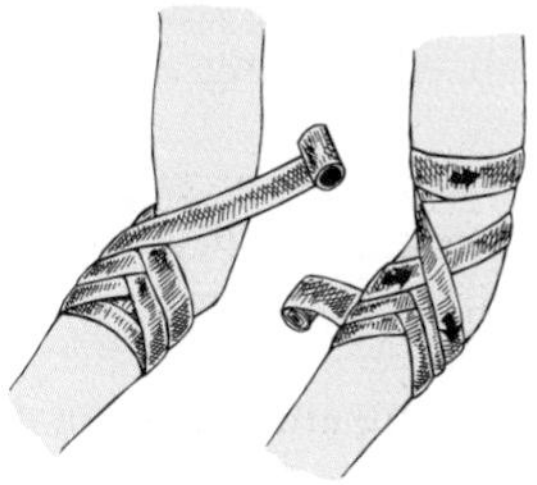	Covers joints; snug fit provides excellent immobilization
Recurrent	Bandage first secured with two circular turns around proximal end of body part; half turn made perpendicular up from bandage edge; body of bandage brought over distal end of body part to be covered with each turn folded back over on itself 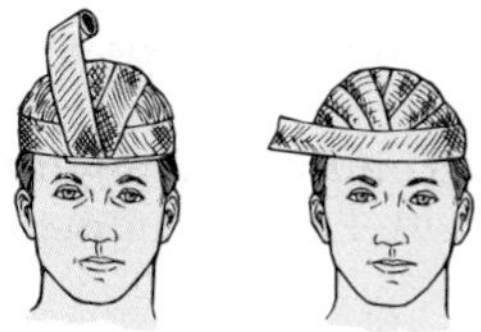	Covers uneven body parts such as head or stump

(Table 43-10). If heat is applied for 1 hour or more, however, blood flow is reduced by a reflex vasoconstriction as the body attempts to control heat loss from the area. Periodic removal and reapplication of local heat restores vasodilation. Continuous exposure to heat damages epithelial cells, causing redness, localized tenderness, and even blistering.

Effects of Cold Application. The application of cold can initially diminish swelling and pain (see Table 43-10). Prolonged exposure of the skin to cold results in a reflex vasodilation. The cell's inability to receive adequate blood flow and nutrients results in tissue ischemia. The skin initially takes on a reddened appearance, followed by a bluish purple mottling with numbness and a burning type of pain. The skin's tissues can freeze from exposure to extreme cold.

Factors Influencing Heat and Cold Tolerance. The body's response to heat and cold therapies varies depending on certain situations:

- A person is better able to tolerate short exposure to temperature extremes.
- Certain areas of the skin are more sensitive to temperature variations. These areas include the neck, inner aspect of the wrist and forearm, and perineal region. The foot and palm of the hand are less sensitive.

Skill 43-7 *Applying an Elastic Bandage*

Delegation Considerations

The application of an elastic bandage can be delegated to unregulated care providers (UCPs). The nurse is responsible for wound assessment and the evaluation of the wound. In addition, the nurse is responsible for assessing for adequate circulation to the extremity distal to the elastic bandage (e.g., pulse, skin temperature, capillary refill). When delegating this skill to a UCP, the nurse must instruct about any restrictions that the client might have (e.g., unable to independently raise leg or independently roll over). The nurse must also instruct the UCP to report the following:

- Any change in the skin colour of the client's injured extremity
- Any increases in client's pain

Equipment

- Correct width and number of bandages
- Safety pins, clips, or adhesive tape
- Disposable gloves, if wound drainage is present

Steps	Rationale
1. Perform hand hygiene and apply gloves if needed. Inspect skin for alterations in integrity as indicated by abrasions, discoloration, chafing, or edema. (Look carefully at bony prominences.)	Altered skin integrity contraindicates the use of elastic bandages.
2. Inspect surgical dressing. Remove gloves and perform hand hygiene.	Surgical dressing replacement or reinforcement precedes application of any bandage.
3. Observe adequacy of circulation (distal to bandage) by noting surface temperature, skin colour, and sensation of body parts to be wrapped.	Comparison of area before and after application of bandage is necessary to ensure continued adequate circulation. Impairment of circulation may result in coolness to touch when compared with opposite side of body, cyanosis or pallor of skin, diminished or absent pulses, edema or localized pooling, and numbness or tingling of part.
4. Review medical record for specific orders related to application of elastic bandage. Note area to be covered, type of bandage required, frequency of change, and previous response to treatment.	Specific prescription may direct procedure, including factors such as extent of application (e.g., toe to knee, toe to groin) and duration of treatment.
5. Identify client's and primary caregiver's present knowledge level of skill if bandaging will be continued at home.	Ensures that planning and teaching are individualized.
6. Explain procedure to client.	Increased knowledge promotes co-operation and reduces anxiety.
7. Teach skill to client or primary caregiver.	Reduces anxiety and ensures continuity of care after discharge.
8. Perform hand hygiene and apply gloves if drainage is present.	Reduces transmission of micro-organisms.
9. Close room door or curtains.	Maintains client's comfort and dignity.
10. Help client to assume comfortable, anatomically correct position.	Maintains alignment. Prevents musculoskeletal deformity.

Critical Decision Point: Bandages applied to lower extremities are applied before client sits or stands. Elevation of dependent extremities for 20 minutes before bandage application will enhance venous return.

Steps	Rationale
11. Hold roll of elastic bandage in dominant hand and use other hand to lightly hold beginning of bandage at distal body part. Continue transferring roll to dominant hand as bandage is wrapped.	Maintains appropriate and consistent bandage tension.

Critical Decision Point: Toes or fingertips should be visible for follow-up circulatory assessment.

Steps	Rationale
12. Apply bandage from distal point toward proximal boundary using variety of turns to cover various shapes of body parts (see Table 43-8).	Bandage is applied in manner that conforms evenly to body part and promotes venous return.
13. Unroll and very slightly stretch bandage.	Maintains uniform bandage tension.
14. Overlap turns by one-half to two-thirds width of bandage roll.	Prevents uneven bandage tension and circulatory impairment.
15. Secure first bandage with clip or tape before applying additional rolls.	
a. Apply additional rolls without leaving any uncovered skin surface. Secure last bandage applied.	Prevents wrinkling or loose ends.
16. Remove gloves if worn and perform hand hygiene	Reduces transmission of micro-organisms.
17. Assess distal circulation when bandage application is complete and at least twice during 8-hour period.	Early detection and management of circulatory impairment ensures healthy neurovascular status.
a. Observe skin colour for pallor or cyanosis.	
b. Palpate skin for warmth.	
c. Palpate pulses and compare bilaterally.	
d. Ask if client is aware of pain, numbness, tingling, or other discomfort.	Neurovascular changes indicate impaired venous return.
e. Observe mobility of extremity.	Determines whether joint immobility is attained and whether bandage is too tight, which would restrict movement.
18. Have client demonstrate bandage application.	Return demonstration documents learning.

Unexpected Outcomes and Related Interventions

- Impaired circulation distal to elastic bandage
  - Release bandage.
  - Palpate extremity and assess pulse, temperature, and capillary refill.
  - Reapply dressing with less pressure.
- Break in skin under elastic bandage
  - Remove bandage.
  - Reapply bandage with less pressure.
- Client unable to perform dressing change
  - Reinstruct client on bandage application.
  - Observe client apply bandage.

Recording and Reporting

- Document condition of wound, integrity of dressing, application of bandage, circulation, and client's comfort level.
- Report any changes in neurological or circulatory status to nurse in charge or physician.

Home Care Considerations

- Instruct client or caregiver not to make bandages too tight, which interferes with circulation.
- Elastic bandages that are used to reduce swelling are best applied to the feet in the morning, before getting out of bed.
- Always remove an elastic bandage daily and inspect

Table 43-9 Conditions That Increase Risk of Injury From Heat and Cold Application

Condition	Risk Factors
Very young clients or older clients	Thinner skin layers in children increase risk of burns. Older clients have reduced sensitivity to pain.
Open wounds, broken skin, stomas	Subcutaneous and visceral tissues are more sensitive to temperature variations. They also contain no temperature receptors and fewer pain receptors.
Areas of edema or scar formation	Reduced sensation to temperature stimuli occurs because of thickening of skin layers from fluid buildup or scar formation.
Peripheral vascular disease (e.g., diabetes, arteriosclerosis)	Body's extremities are less sensitive to temperature and pain stimuli because of circulatory impairment and local tissue injury. Cold application further compromises blood flow.
Confusion or unconsciousness	Perception of sensory or painful stimuli is reduced.
Spinal cord injury	Alterations in nerve pathways prevent reception of sensory or painful stimuli.
Abscessed body site (e.g., tooth or appendix)	Infection is highly localized. Application of heat may cause rupture with spread of micro-organisms systemically.

Table 43-10 Therapeutic Effects of Heat and Cold Applications

Physiological Response	Therapeutic Benefit	Examples of Conditions Treated
Heat		
Vasodilation	Improves blood flow to injured body part; promotes delivery of nutrients and removal of wastes; lessens venous congestion in injured tissues	Improves blood flow to injured body part; promotes delivery of nutrients and removal of wastes; lessens venous congestion in injured tissues
Reduced blood viscosity	Improves delivery of leukocytes and antibiotics to wound site	
Reduced muscle tension	Promotes muscle relaxation and reduces pain from spasm or stiffness	
Increased tissue metabolism	Increases blood flow; provides local warmth	
Increased capillary permeability	Promotes movement of waste products and nutrients	
Cold		
Vasoconstriction	Reduces blood flow to injured body part, preventing edema formation; reduces inflammation	Direct trauma (sprains, strains, fractures, muscle spasms); superficial laceration or puncture wound; minor burn; suspected malignancy in area of injury or pain; injections; arthritis and joint trauma
Local anaesthesia	Reduces localized pain	
Reduced cell metabolism	Reduces oxygen needs of tissues	
Increased blood viscosity	Promotes blood coagulation at injury site	
Decreased muscle tension	Relieves pain	

- Exposed skin layers are more sensitive to temperature variations.
- The body responds best to minor temperature adjustments. If a body part is cool and a hot stimulus touches the skin, the response is greater than if the skin were already warm.
- A person has less tolerance to temperature changes to which a large area of the body is exposed.
- Tolerance to temperature variations changes with age.
- Clients who are very young and old are most sensitive to heat and cold.
- If a client's physical condition reduces the reception or perception of sensory stimuli, tolerance to temperature extremes is high, but the risk of injury is also high.
- Uneven temperature distribution suggests that the equipment is functioning improperly.

> ***Safety Alert.*** Before application of heat or cold therapy, the client should understand its purpose, the symptoms of temperature exposure, and precautions taken to prevent injury. Box 43-15 provides methods for the safe application of heat and cold therapy.

Application of Heat and Cold Therapies. A prerequisite to using any heat or cold application is a physician's order, which should include the body site to be treated and the type, frequency, and duration of application. The nurse should consult the agency's procedure manual for correct temperatures to use.

Choice of Moist or Dry. Heat and cold applications can be administered in dry or moist forms. The type of wound or injury, the location of the body part, and the presence of drainage or inflammation are factors considered in selecting dry or moist applications. Box 43-16 summarizes advantages and disadvantages of both.

Warm, Moist Compresses. For open wounds, sterile, warm, moist compresses improve circulation, relieve edema, and promote consolidation of pus and drainage. A compress is a piece of gauze dressing moistened in a prescribed warmed solution. A pack is a larger cloth or dressing applied to a larger body area.

Heat from warm compresses dissipates quickly. To maintain a constant temperature, the nurse must change the compress often or apply a waterproof heating pad over the compress. Because moisture conducts heat, any device's temperature setting should be lower for a moist compress than for a dry application. A layer of plastic wrap or a dry towel can also be used to insulate the compress and retain heat. Moist heat promotes vasodilation and evaporation of heat from the skin's surface. For this reason, a client may feel chilly. The nurse controls drafts within the room and keeps the client covered with a blanket or robe. Skill 43-8 describes the steps for applying a warm, moist compress to an open wound.

Warm Soaks. Immersion of a body part in a warmed solution promotes circulation, lessens edema, increases muscle relaxation, and can provide a means to debride wounds and apply medicated solution. A soak can also be accompanied by wrapping the body part in dressings and saturating them with the warmed solution.

The nurse positions the client comfortably, places waterproof pads under the area to be treated, and heats the

Box 43-15 Safety Suggestions for Applying Heat or Cold Therapy

Explain to the client sensations to be felt during the procedure.
Instruct the client to report changes in sensation or discomfort immediately.
Provide a timer, clock, or watch so that the client can help the nurse time the application.
Keep the call light within the client's reach.
Refer to the agency's policy and procedure manual for safe temperatures.
Do not allow the client to adjust temperature settings.
Do not allow the client to move an application or place hands on the wound site.
Do not place the client in a position that prevents movement away from the temperature source.
Do not leave unattended a client who is unable to sense temperature changes or move from the temperature source.

Box 43-16 Choice of Dry or Moist Applications

Advantages

Moist Applications

Moist application reduces drying of skin and softens wound exudate.
Moist compresses conform well to body area being treated.
Moist heat penetrates deeply into tissue layers.
Warm moist heat does not promote sweating and insensible fluid loss.

Dry Applications

Dry heat has less risk of burns to skin than moist applications.
Dry application does not cause skin maceration.
Dry heat retains temperature longer because it is not influenced by evaporation.

Disadvantages

Moist Applications

Prolonged exposure can cause maceration of skin.
Moist heat will cool rapidly because of moisture evaporation.
Moist heat creates greater risk for burns to skin because moisture conducts heat.

Dry Applications

Dry heat increases body fluid loss through sweating.
Dry applications do not penetrate deep into tissues.
Dry heat causes increased drying of skin.

solution to about 40.5° to 43° C. After immersing the body part, the nurse covers the container and extremity with a towel to reduce heat loss. It is usually necessary to remove the cooled solution and add heated solution after about 10 minutes. The goal is to keep the solution at a constant temperature. The nurse never adds a hotter solution while the body part remains immersed. After any soak, the nurse dries the body part thoroughly to prevent maceration.

Sitz Baths. The client who has had rectal surgery, an episiotomy during childbirth, painful hemorrhoids, or vaginal inflammation may benefit from a **sitz bath,** a bath in which only the pelvic area is immersed in warm fluid. The client sits in a special tub or chair or in a basin that fits on the toilet seat so that the legs and feet remain out of the water. Immersing the entire body causes widespread vasodilation and nullifies the effect of local heat application to the pelvic area.

The desired temperature for a sitz bath depends on whether the purpose is to promote relaxation or to clean a wound. The procedure normally lasts 20 minutes. The nurse may need to add warm water during the procedure to maintain a constant temperature. Agency procedure manuals recommend safe water temperatures. A disposable sitz basin contains an attachment resembling an enema bag that allows gradual introduction of warmer water.

The nurse prevents overexposure of the client by controlling drafts and draping bath blankets around the client's shoulders and thighs. The client should be able to sit in the basin or tub with feet flat on the floor and without pressure on the sacrum or thighs. Because exposure of a large portion of the body to heat can cause extensive vasodilation, the nurse should assess the pulse and facial colour and ask whether the client feels light-headed or nauseated.

Commercial Hot Packs. Commercially prepared, disposable hot packs apply warm, dry heat to an injured area. By striking, kneading, or squeezing the pack, chemicals are mixed and release heat. Package directions recommend the time for heat application.

Cold, Moist, and Dry Compresses. The procedure for applying cold, moist compresses is the same as that for warm compresses. Cold compresses should be applied for 20 minutes at a temperature of 15° C to relieve inflammation and swelling. They may be clean or sterile.

There are commercially prepared cold packs that are similar to the disposable hot packs for dry applications. They come in various shapes and sizes to fit different body parts. When using cold compresses, the nurse observes for adverse reactions such as burning or numbness, mottling of the skin, redness, extreme paleness, and a bluish skin discoloration.

Skill 43-8 Applying a Warm, Moist Compress to an Open Wound

Delegation Considerations

This skill can be delegated to unregulated care providers (UCPs). The nurse is responsible for wound assessment and evaluation of wound care interventions. When delegating this skill to a UCP, the nurse must do the following:

- Caution caregiver to maintain proper temperature of application during duration of treatment.
- Caution caregiver to keep application in place for only the length of time specified in physician's orders.
- Have caregiver notify the nurse when treatment is complete so that an evaluation of client's response can be made.

Equipment

- Prescribed solution warmed to appropriate temperature
- Sterile gauze dressings or commercially prepared compresses
- Sterile container for solution
- Dry bath towel
- Disposable gloves
- Sterile gloves
- Waterproof pad
- Ties or tape
- Heating pad (optional)
- Bath blanket

Steps	Rationale
1. Refer to physician's order for type of compress, location and duration of application, desired temperature, and agency policies regarding temperature of compress.	Ensures safe and correct application.
2. Refer to medical record to identify any systemic contraindications to heat application.	Heat causes vasodilation, which aggravates active bleeding. Heat applied to localized area of acute inflammation or tumour may cause rupture or activate cell growth.
3. Perform hand hygiene.	Reduces transmission of micro-organisms.
4. Inspect condition of exposed skin and wound on which compress is to be applied.	Provides baseline to determine changes in skin during heat application.

Critical Decision Point: Very thin or damaged skin is more susceptible to injury from heat. Nonintact skin and drainage from wounds are indications to wear gloves.

Steps	Rationale
5. Assess client's extremities for sensitivity to temperature and pain by measuring light touch, pinprick, and temperature sensation.	Clients insensitive to heat or cold sensations must be monitored closely during treatment.
6. Assemble equipment and supplies.	Organization of supplies prevents unnecessary delays in the procedure.
7. Explain steps of procedure and purpose to client. Describe sensations to be felt, such as decreasing warmth and wetness. Explain precautions to prevent burning.	Minimizes client's anxiety and promotes co-operation during the procedure.
8. Close door and bedside curtains.	Decreases drafts, thus decreasing the transmission of micro-organisms. Provides for client privacy.
9. Assist client in assuming comfortable position in proper body alignment and place waterproof pad under area to be treated.	Compress remains in place for several minutes. Limited mobility in uncomfortable position causes muscular stress. Pad prevents soiling of bed linen.
10. Expose body part to be covered with compress and drape client with bath blanket.	Prevents unnecessary cooling and exposure of body part.
11. Prepare compress:	Ensures orderly procedure.
a. Pour solution into sterile container.	
b. If using portable heating source, warm solution. Commercially prepared compresses may remain under infrared lamp until just before use. Open sterile packages and drop gauze into container to become immersed in solution.	Compresses must retain warmth for therapeutic benefit.

Critical Decision Point: Diabetic clients, survivors of stroke, and clients with peripheral neuropathy are particularly at risk for thermal injury.

Steps	Rationale

Critical Decision Point: Temperature must be tested by applying sterile solution to nurse's forearm (without contaminating solution).

Steps	Rationale
12. Apply disposable gloves. Remove any existing dressing covering wound. Dispose of gloves and dressings in proper receptacle.	Reduces transmission of micro-organisms.
13. Assess condition of wound and surrounding skin. Inflamed wound appears reddened, but surrounding skin is less red in colour.	Provides baseline to determine skin changes following compress application.

Critical Decision Point: If skin surrounding wound is reddened, application may be contraindicated.

Steps	Rationale
14. Apply sterile gloves.	Allows nurse to manipulate sterile dressing and touch open wound.
15. Pick up one layer of immersed gauze, wring out any excess solution, and apply it lightly to open wound.	Excess moisture macerates skin and increases risks of burns and infection. Skin is sensitive to sudden change in temperature.
16. In a few seconds, lift edge of gauze to assess for redness.	Increased redness indicates burn.
17. If client tolerates compress, pack gauze snugly against the wound. Be sure all wound surfaces are covered by the warm compress.	Packing of compress prevents rapid cooling from underlying air currents.
18. Cover moist compress with dry sterile dressing and bath towel. If necessary, pin or tie in place. Remove sterile gloves.	Dry sterile dressing will prevent transfer of micro-organisms to wound via capillary action caused by moist compress. Towel insulates compress to prevent heat loss.
19. Apply waterproof heating pad over towel (optional). Keep it in place for desired duration of application.	Provides constant temperature to compress.
20. Change warm compress using sterile technique every 5 minutes or as ordered during duration of therapy.	Prevents cooling and maintains therapeutic benefit of compress.
21. Inspect affected area covered by compress and heating pad every 5 to 10 minutes.	Assists in determining effects of application.
22. Ask every 5 to 10 minutes if client notices any unusual burning sensation not felt before application.	It may be difficult to assess burn merely by colour changes if wound is inflamed or drainage is present.
23. After prescribed time, apply disposable gloves and remove pad, towel, and compress. Reassess wound and condition of skin, and replace dry sterile dressing as ordered.	Continued exposure to moisture will macerate skin. Prevents entrance of micro-organisms into wound site.
24. Assist client to preferred comfortable position.	Maintains client's comfort.
25. Dispose of equipment and soiled compress. Perform hand hygiene.	Reduces transmission of micro-organisms.
26. Have client explain and demonstrate application.	Evaluates client's understanding of and ability to perform procedure.

Skill 43-8 Applying a Warm, Moist Compress to an Open Wound—cont'd

Unexpected Outcomes and Related Interventions

- Client's wound remains the same.
  - Report to physician.
  - Evaluate the continued use of warm compress.
- Client's skin is broken, erythematous, and warm to the touch.
  - Verify that correct temperature of compress is maintained.
  - Institute skin care practices.

Recording and Reporting

- Record type, location, and duration of application.
- Note solution and temperature.
- Describe condition of wound and skin before and after treatment, as well as client's response to therapy.
- Describe any instructions given and client's ability to explain and perform procedure.
- Report unusual findings to nurse in charge or physician.

Home Care Considerations

- When necessary, assess availability of primary caregivers to assist clients in application of compress, their understanding of purpose of procedure, and their willingness to comply with procedure and not leave client with compress in place beyond prescribed time limit.
- Assess physical environment to determine existence of adequate facilities to prepare warm compress and provide for sterile technique.

Cold Soaks. The procedure for preparing cold soaks and immersing a body part is the same as for warm soaks. The desired temperature for a 20-minute cold soak is 15° C. The nurse controls drafts and uses outer coverings to protect the client from chilling. It may be necessary to add cold water during the procedure to maintain a constant temperature.

Ice Bags or Collars. For a client who has a muscle sprain, localized hemorrhage, or hematoma or who has undergone dental surgery, an ice bag is ideal to prevent edema formation, control bleeding, and anaesthetize the body part. Proper use of the bag requires the following steps:

1. Fill the bag with water, secure the cap, invert to check for leaks, and pour out the water.
2. Fill the bag two-thirds full with crushed ice so that the bag can mould easily over a body part.
3. Release any air from the bag by squeezing its sides before securing the cap, because excess air interferes with conduction of cold.
4. Wipe off excess moisture.
5. Cover the bag with a flannel cover, towel, or pillow case.
6. Apply the bag to the injury site for 30 minutes; the bag can be reapplied in an hour.

NP Evaluation

Client Care. Nursing interventions for wound care and reducing the risk of pressure ulcers are evaluated by determining the client's response to nursing therapies and by determining whether each goal was achieved. To evaluate outcomes and responses to care, the nurse measures the effectiveness of interventions. The optimal outcomes are to prevent injury to the skin and tissues, reduce injury to the skin and underlying tissues, and restore skin integrity.

Because each client has different risk factors for impaired skin integrity, nursing interventions must be individualized. Clients with minimal mobility impairments or relatively stable health status may need only a few measures. Nursing interventions for reducing and treating pressure ulcers are evaluated by determining the client's response to nursing therapies and by determining whether each goal was achieved (Figure 43–35).

To evaluate outcomes and responses to care, the nurse measures the effectiveness of interventions. This often occurs over an extended period of time, requiring the nurse to make careful ongoing assessments of the client with an ulcer. The nurse also evaluates specific interventions designed to promote skin integrity and to teach the client and family to reduce future threats to skin integrity.

The nurse evaluates the client's and family's need for additional support services (e.g., home care, physiotherapy, and counselling) and initiates the referral process. The nurse also evaluates the need for additional referrals to other experts in wound care when indicated, such as nurses certified in wound care. Care of the client with a pressure ulcer requires a multidisciplinary team approach.

Client Expectations. The client and caregiver need to understand how to prevent or treat pressure ulcers. Clients may enter into the wound-healing phase with unrealistic expectations with regard to the duration of care. The nurse needs to collect evaluation data about the

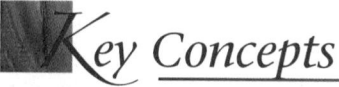

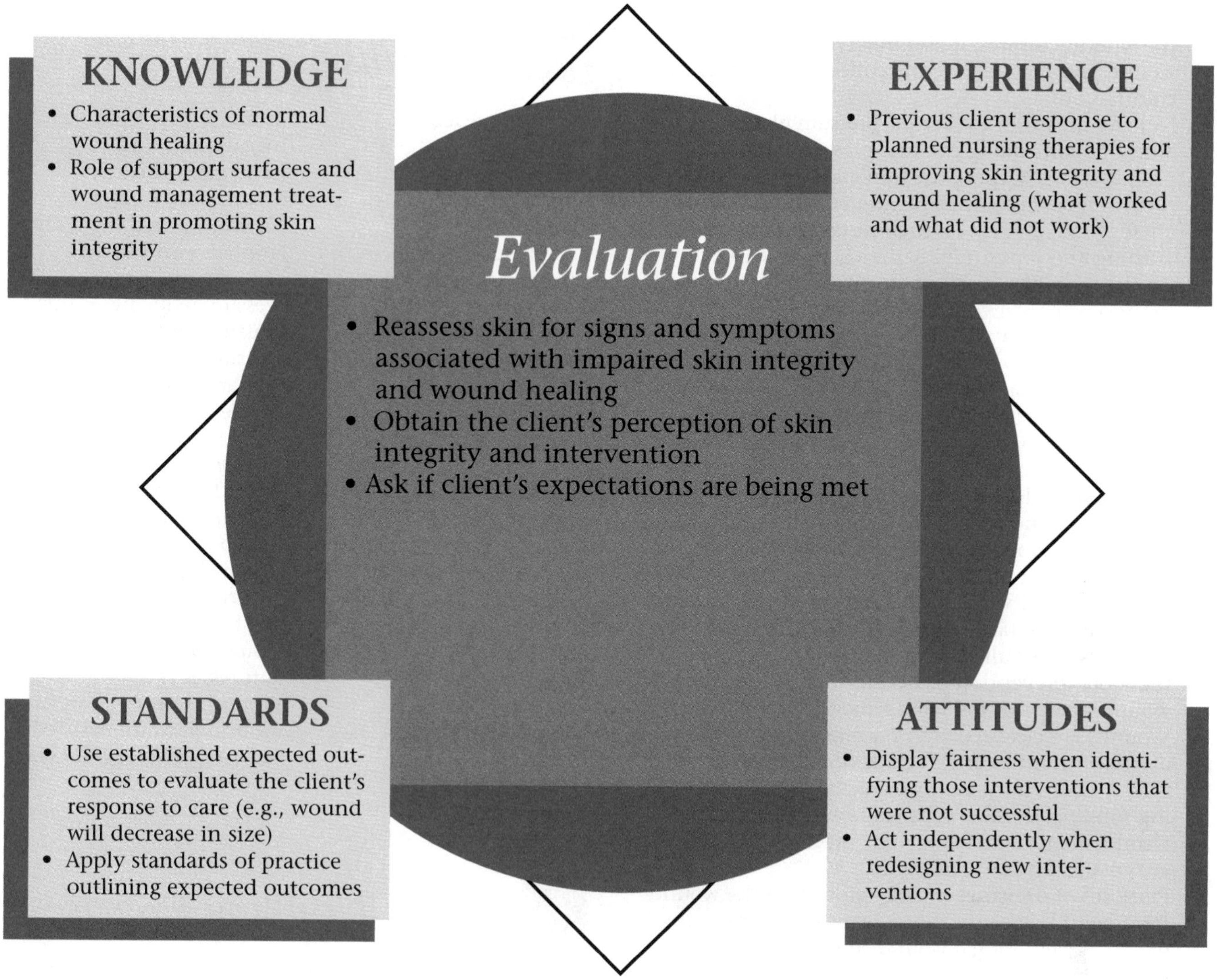
KNOWLEDGE
• Characteristics of normal wound healing
• Role of support surfaces and wound management treatment in promoting skin integrity
EXPERIENCE
• Previous client response to planned nursing therapies for improving skin integrity and wound healing (what worked and what did not work)
Evaluation
• Reassess skin for signs and symptoms associated with impaired skin integrity and wound healing
• Obtain the client's perception of skin integrity and intervention
• Ask if client's expectations are being met
STANDARDS
• Use established expected outcomes to evaluate the client's response to care (e.g., wound will decrease in size)
• Apply standards of practice outlining expected outcomes
ATTITUDES
• Display fairness when identifying those interventions that were not successful
• Act independently when redesigning new interventions

FIGURE **43–35** Critical thinking model for skin integrity and wound care evaluation.

client's perception of wound care management. Clients with chronic wounds are often cared for in their homes and have certain expectations about their level of comfort, lifestyle, independence, and privacy. Therefore, the nurse must determine from the client whether his or her expectations were respected and met.

Key Concepts

- Wounds can be classified according to cause, intactness of skin, depth, cleanliness, and whether they are acute or chronic.
- Pressure ulcers occur over bony prominences and are the result of reduced blood supply to the tissue caused by unrelieved pressure.
- Although external pressure is the primary cause of pressure ulcers, other contributing factors include friction; shearing force; moisture; impaired mobility, level of consciousness, and pain perception; poor nutritional status; vascular disease; and advanced age.
- According to the NPUAP staging system, a pressure ulcer is classified as being in one of four stages according to it severity; this staging system should not be used to measure wound healing.
- Wounds that have little or no tissue loss heal by primary intention; wounds with extensive tissue loss heal by secondary intention.
- Wound healing proceeds through three phases: inflammatory, proliferative, and remodelling.
- Assessing for risk of pressure ulcers is important in decreasing the opportunity for pressure ulcer development.
- The nurse must meticulously assess the skin for signs of pressure ulcers, including assessing for blanching and abnormal reactive hyperemia.
- Wound assessment includes observing the wound appearance (its size, location, stage, and periwound skin condition), the character of the wound

drainage, the condition of drains (if present), and the wound closures; it also involves palpating the wound and may require the collection of a wound culture sample.
- Nursing measures to prevent pressure ulcers are aimed at controlling external pressure on bony prominences; keeping the skin clean, free of moisture, well lubricated, and hydrated; and promoting an adequate diet that is high in protein and calories.
- Turning and repositioning the client at least every 2 hours to relieve pressure is one of the easiest ways to prevent pressure ulcers from developing.
- Therapeutic beds and mattresses reduce the effects of pressure; selection is based on assessment data to identify the best bed for individual needs.
- Principles of wound first aid include control of bleeding, cleansing, and protection.
- Ongoing treatment of wounds requires a team approach, including nurses, physicians, ostomal therapists, physiotherapists, occupational therapists, dietitians, social workers, pain specialists, rehabilitation specialists, and pharmacists.
- The chances of wound infection are greater when the wound contains necrotic tissue, retained packing materials, or small fragments of gauze dressing; therefore, prevention of wound infection includes wound cleansing and debridement.
- Wounds are cleansed with normal saline or a commercial wound cleanser that is not cytotoxic; irrigation is a common method of delivering the cleansing solution to the wound and removing debris.
- Debridement methods include mechanical, autolytic, enzymatic, and sharp/surgical.
- Purposes of dressings include protecting the wound from contamination, aiding hemostasis, absorbing drainage, debriding a wound, and promoting a moist environment.
- Suture removal requires a physician's order.
- A bandage or binder should be applied in a manner that does not impair circulation or irritate the skin.
- Heat and cold applications can be administered in dry or moist forms; the type of wound or injury, the body part being treated, and the presence of drainage or inflammation are factors to consider when selecting dry or moist applications.
- An acute sprain, closed fracture, or bruise responds best to cold applications.

Key Terms

Abnormal reactive hyperemia, *p. 1513*
Anemia, *p. 1505*
Approximated, *p. 1504*
Blanching, *p. 1513*
Braden Scale, *p. 1510*
Collagen, *p. 1499*
Contraction, *p. 1504*
Debridement, *p. 1535*
Dehiscence, *p. 1507*
Dermis, *p. 1499*
Drainage evacuators, *p. 1553*
Edema, *p. 1517*
Epidermis, *p. 1498*
Epithelialization, *p. 1504*
Erythema, *p. 1513*
Eschar, *p. 1516*
Evisceration, *p. 1508*
Exudate, *p. 1504*
Fibrin, *p. 1504*
Fibroblasts, *p. 1504*
Fistula, *p. 1508*
Friction, *p. 1501*
Granulation tissue, *p. 1504*
Hematoma, *p. 1507*
Hemorrhage, *p. 1507*
Hemostasis, *p. 1504*
Induration, *p. 1508*
Irrigation, *p. 1535*
Ischemia, *p. 1500*
Maceration, *p. 1501*
Necrosis, *p. 1500*
Normal reactive hyperemia, *p. 1513*
Pressure reducing, *p. 1529*
Pressure relieving, *p. 1529*
Pressure ulcer, *p. 1499*
Primary intention, *p. 1504*
Purulent drainage, *p. 1506*
Sanguineous drainage, *p. 1506*
Secondary intention, *p. 1504*
Serosanguineous drainage, *p. 1506*
Serous drainage, *p. 1506*
Shearing, *p. 1501*
Sitz bath, *p. 1563*
Slough, *p. 1516*
Sutures, *p. 1552*
Wound, *p. 1499*
Wound Vacuum Assisted Closure (Wound V.A.C.), *p. 1547*

Critical Thinking Exercises

1. When removing a saline-moistened dressing from a sacral pressure ulcer, you note that the gauze is dripping with beige-coloured fluid. What assessments should be made, and after the assessment, what should be done next? What could be the possible cause of this drainage?
2. After changing a client's position, you observe redness over the bony prominences. How should this area be assessed?
3. You have just admitted a client from a long-term care facility to your division. On initial assessment, you assess a stage III pressure ulcer. How do you determine the type of care and dressing to use with this particular pressure ulcer?
4. You are providing care to an older, incontinent, dark-skinned man who is bed-bound. How will you assess for pressure ulcers in this client? What measures can you take to prevent his skin from breaking down?

Review Questions

1. The following type of pressure ulcer has an observable pressure-related alteration of intact skin whose indicators, compared with an adjacent or opposite area on the body, may include changes in one or more of the following: skin temperature (warmth or coolness), tissue consistency (firm or beefy feel), and/or sensation (pain, itching):
   1. Stage I
   2. Stage II
   3. Stage III
   4. Stage IV
2. Serous drainage from a wound is defined as
   1. Fresh bleeding
   2. Clear, watery plasma
   3. Thick and yellow
   4. Beige to brown and foul smelling
3. Post-operatively, the client with a closed abdominal wound reports a sudden "pop" after coughing. When the nurse examines the surgical wound site, the sutures are open and pieces of small bowel are noted at the bottom of the now opened wound. The correct intervention would be to
   1. Allow the area to be exposed to air until all drainage has stopped
   2. Place several cold packs over the areas, protecting the skin around the wound
   3. Cover the areas with sterile saline-soaked towels and immediately notify the surgical team; this is likely to indicate a wound evisceration
   4. Cover the area with sterile gauze; place a tight binder over the areas. Ask the client to remain in bed for 30 minutes because this is a minor opening in the surgical wound and should reseal quickly
4. When repositioning an immobile client, the nurse notices redness over a bony prominence. When the area is assessed, the red spot blanches with fingertip touch, indicating:
   1. A local skin infection requiring antibiotics
   2. Abnormal reactive hyperemia
   3. Deep tissue damage
   4. The reactive hyperemia is likely transient
5. When obtaining a wound culture to determine the presence of a wound infection, the specimen should to be taken from the
   1. Necrotic tissue
   2. Drainage on the dressing
   3. Wound drainage
   4. Wound after it has first been cleansed with normal saline
6. One measure nurses use to prevent pressure ulcers is to
   1. Position the client in a 30-degree lateral position
   2. Use a donut-type device
   3. Reposition the client at least every 3 hours
   4. Elevate the head of the bed 30 degrees or more
7. The best description of a hydrocolloid dressing is
   1. A seaweed derivative that is highly absorptive
   2. Premoistened gauze placed over a granulating wound
   3. A debriding enzyme that is used to remove necrotic tissue
   4. A dressing that forms a gel that interacts with the wound surface
8. A binder placed around a surgical client with a new abdominal wound is indicated for
   1. Collection of wound drainage
   2. Reduction of abdominal swelling
   3. Reduction of stress on the abdominal incision
   4. Stimulation of peristalsis (return of bowel function) from direct pressure
9. For a client who has a muscle sprain, localized hemorrhage, or hematoma, the following helps prevent edema formation, control bleeding, and anaesthetize the body part:
   1. Binder
   2. Ice bag
   3. Sling
   4. Sitz bath
10. Application of a warm compress is indicated
    1. To relieve edema
    2. For a client who is shivering
    3. To promote healing by simulating blood flow
    4. To protect bony prominences from pressure ulcers

References

Agency for Health Care Policy and Research, Panel for the Prediction and Prevention of Pressure Ulcers in Adults. (1992). *Pressure ulcers in adults: Prediction and prevention* (Clinical Practice Guideline No. 3, AHCPR Publication No. 92-0047). Rockville, MD: Author, U.S. Department of Health and Human Services.

Agency for Health Care Policy and Research, Panel for Treatment of Pressure Ulcers in Adults. (1994). *Treatment of pressure ulcers* (Clinical Practice Guideline No. 15, AHCPR Publication No. 95-0653). Rockville, MD: Author, U.S. Department of Health and Human Services.

Allman, R. M., et al. (1999). Pressure ulcers, hospital complications, and disease severity: Impact on hospital costs and length of stay. *Advances in Wound Care, 12*(1), 22–30.

Argenta, L. C., & Morykwas, M. J. (1997). Vacuum-assisted closure: A new method for wound control and treatment: Clinical experience. *Annals of Plastic Surgery, 38*(6), 563–576.

Ayello, E. A., Thomas, D. R., & Litchford, M. A. (1999). Nutritional aspects of wound healing. *Home Healthcare Nurse, 17*(11), 719–729.

Barr, J. E. (1995). Principles of wound cleansing. *Ostomy/Wound Management, 41*(Suppl. 7A),15S–21S.

Bates-Jensen, B. (1997). The Pressure Sore Status Tool a few thousand assessments later. *Advances in Wound Care, 10*(5), 65–73.

Baxandall, T. (1996). Tissue viability: Healing cavity wounds with negative pressure. *Nursing Standard, 11*(6), 49–51.

Bennett, M. A. (1995). Report of the Task Force on the Implications for Darkly Pigmented Intact Skin in the Prediction and Prevention of Pressure Ulcers. *Advances in Wound Care, 8*(6), 34–35.

Bergstrom, N., Demuth, P. J., & Braden, B. J. (1987). A clinical trial of the Braden scale for predicting pressure sore risk. *Nursing Clinincs of North America, 22*(2), 417–428.

Bowler, P. G. (2003) Bacterial growth guideline: Reassessing its clinical relevance in wound healing. *Ostomy Wound Management, 49*(1), 44-53.

Braden, B. J. (2001). Risk assessment in pressure ulcer prevention. In D. L. Krasner, G. T. Rodeheaver, & R. G. Sibbald (Eds.), *Chronic wound care: A clinical source book for healthcare professionals* (pp. 641–652). Wayne, PA: HMP Communications.

Braden, B. J., & Bergstrom, N. (1994). Predictive validity of the Braden Scale for pressure sore risk in a nursing home population. *Research in Nursing & Health, 17*(6), 459–470.

Broussard, C. L., Mendez-Eastman, S., & Frantz, R. (2000). Adjuvant wound therapies. In R. A. Bryant (Ed.), *Acute and chronic wounds: Nursing management* (2nd ed., pp. 431–454). St. Louis, MO: Mosby.

Bryant, R. A. (Ed.). (2000). *Acute and chronic wounds: Nursing management* (2nd ed.). St. Louis, MO: Mosby.

Candido, L. C. (2002). Treatment of surgical wound dehiscence. *Dermatology Nursing, 14*(3), 177–178, 181.

Centers for Disease Control and Prevention. (2001). Feeding back surveillance data to prevent hospital acquired infections. *Emerging Infectious Diseases, 7*(2), 295–298.

Chua, P. C., et al. (2000). Vacuum-assisted wound closure. *American Journal of Nursing, 100*(12), 45–48.

Colwell, J. (2003). Skin integrity and wound care. In P. A. Potter & A. G. Perry (Eds.), *Basic nursing: essentials for practice* (5th ed.). St. Louis, MO: Mosby.

Cooper, D. M. (2000). Assessment, measurement, and evaluation: Their pivotal roles in wound healing. In R. A. Bryant (Ed.). *Acute and chronic wounds: Nursing management* (2nd ed., pp. 51–84). St. Louis, MO: Mosby.

Currence, S. (2001). Product selection in the new millennium. In D. L. Krasner, G. T. Rodeheaver, & R. G. Sibbald (Eds.), *Chronic wound care: A clinical source book for healthcare professionals* (pp. 321–328). Wayne, PA: HMP Communications.

Dochterman, J. M., & Bulechek, G. M. (Eds.). (2004). *Nursing interventions classification (NIC)* (4th ed.). St. Louis, MO: Mosby.

Dolynchuk, K., et al. (2000). Best practices for the prevention and treatment of pressure ulcers. *Ostomy/Wound Management, 46*(11), 38–52.

Erwin-Toth, P., & Stenger, B. (2001). Teaching wound care to patients, families and healthcare providers. In D. L. Krasner, G. T. Rodeheaver, & R. G. Sibbald (Eds.), *Chronic wound care: A clinical source book for healthcare professionals*. Wayne, PA: HMP Communications.

Evans, L., & Land, L. (2001). Topical negative pressure for treating chronic wounds: A systematic review. *British Journal of Plastic Surgery, 54*(3), 238–242.

Gaskin, F. C. (1986). Detection of cyanosis in the person with dark skin. *Journal of National Black Nurses' Association, 1,* 52–60.

Goldman, R. J., & Salcido, R. (2002). More than one way to measure a wound: An overview of tools and techniques. *Advances in Skin & Wound Care, 15*(5), 236–243.

Houghton, P. E, & Woodbury, M. G. (2004). The prevalence of pressure ulcers in Canadian Healthcare Settings. Ostotomy *Wound Management, 50*(10), 22–39.

Kane, D. P. (2001). Chronic wound healing and chronic wound management. In D. L. Krasner, G. T. Rodeheaver, & R. G. Sibbald (Eds.), *Chronic wound care: A clinical source book for healthcare professionals* (pp. 7–10). Wayne, PA: HMP Communications.

Kiecolt-Glaser, J. K., et al. (1995). Slowing of wound healing by psychological stress. *Lancet, 346,* 1194–1196

Kinetic Concepts Inc. USA. (1999). *The V.A.C.: Vacuum assisted closure—Guidelines for use, physician and caregiver reference manual.* San Antonio, TX: Author

Krouskop, T., & van Rijswijk, L. (1995). Standardizing performance-based criteria for support surfaces. *Ostomy/Wound Management, 41*(1), 34–36, 38, 40–45.

Lazarus, G. S., et al. (1994). Definitions and guidelines for assessment of wounds and evaluation of healing. *Archives of Dermatology, 130*(4), 489–493.

Mendez-Eastman, S. (1998). When wounds won't heal. *RN, 61*(10), 20–23.

Moorhead, S., Johnson, M., & Maas, M. (Eds.). (2004). *Nursing outcomes classification (NOC)* (3rd ed.). St. Louis, MO: Mosby.

National Pressure Ulcer Advisory Panel. (1989). Pressure ulcer prevalence, cost and risk assessment: Consensus development conference statement. *Decubitus, 2*(2), 24–28.

National Pressure Ulcer Advisory Panel. (1995a). *NPUAP proceedings of the Fourth National NPUAP Conference.* Washington, DC: Author.

National Pressure Ulcer Advisory Panel. (1995b). *Pressure ulcer research: Etiology, assessment, and early intervention.* Buffalo, NY: Author.

National Pressure Ulcer Advisory Panel. (1998). *Position statement on stage I assessment in darkly pigmented skin.* Retrieved March 1, 2005, from *www.npuap.org/archive/positn4.htm*

Norton, D., McLaren, R., & Exon-Smith, A. N. (1962). *An investigation of geriatric nursing problems in hospital.* Edinburgh, Scotland: Churchill Livingstone.

Pieper, B. (2000). Mechanical forces: Pressure, shear and friction. In R. A. Bryant (Ed.), *Acute and chronic wounds: Nursing management* (2nd ed., pp. 221–264). St. Louis, MO: Mosby.

Pires, M., & Muller, A. (1991). Detection and management of early tissue pressure indicators: A pictorial essay. *Progressions, 3*(3).

Ramundo, J., & Wells, J. (2000). Wound debridement. In R. A. Bryant (Ed.), *Acute and chronic wounds: Nursing management* (2nd ed.). St. Louis, MO: Mosby.

Ratliff, C. R., & Bryant, D. E. (2003). *Guidelines for the management of pressure ulcers.* Glenview, IL: Wound, Ostomy and Continence Nurses Society, Clinical Practice Guideline Series.

Reddy, M., et al. (2003). Practical treatment of wound pain and trauma: A patient-centered approach. An overview. *Ostomy/Wound Management, 49*(Suppl. 4A), 2–15.

Registered Nurses Association of Ontario. (2002a). *Assessment and management of stage I to IV pressure ulcers.* Retrieved April 14, 2004, from *http://www.rnao.org/bestpractices/completed_guidelines/BPG_Guide_C2_pressure_ulcer.asp*

Registered Nurses Association of Ontario. (2002b). *Health education fact sheet: Taking the pressure off: Preventing pressure ulcers.* Retrieved May 1, 2004, from *www.rnao.org/bestpractices/ PDF/Press_Ulcer_Fact_Sheet.pdf*

Registered Nurses Association of Ontario. (2005). *Risk assessment and prevention of pressure ulcers.* (Revised) Retrieved March 29, 2005, from *http://www.rnao.org/bestpractices/completed_guidelines/BPG_Guide_C1_Pressure_Ulcers.asp*

Richardson, G. M., Gardner, S., & Frantz, R. A. (1998). Nursing assessment: Impact on type and cost of interventions to prevent pressure ulcers. *Journal of Wound, Ostomy, and Continence Nursing, 25*(6), 273–280.

Robson, M. C. (1997). Wound infection: A failure of wound healing caused by an imbalance of bacteria. *Surgical Clinics of North America, 77*(3), 637–650.

Rolstad, B. S., Ovington, L., & Harris, A. (2000). Principles of wound management. In R. A. Bryant (Ed.), *Acute and chronic wounds: Nursing management* (2nd ed., pp. 85–124). St. Louis, MO: Mosby.

Russell, S. (2004). "Wound management products by category." Janssen-Ortho Inc©.

Stotts N. A. et al. (1997). Sterile versus clean technique in postoperative wound care of patients with open surgical wounds in the post-op period: pilot study. *Journal of Wound, Ostomy and Continence Nursing, 24*(1), 10–16.

Stotts, N. A. (2000a). Nutritional assessment and support. In R. A. Bryant (Ed.), *Acute and chronic wounds: Nursing management* (2nd ed., pp. 41–50). St. Louis, MO: Mosby.

Stotts, N. A. (2000b). Wound infection: Diagnosis and management. In R. A. Bryant (Ed.), *Acute and chronic wounds: Nursing management* (2nd ed., pp. 179–188). St. Louis, MO: Mosby.

Stotts, N. A., & Cavanaugh, C. E. (1999). Assessing the patient with a wound. *Home Healthcare Nurse, 17*(1), 27–35.

Teare, J., & Barrett, C. (2002). Using a quality of life assessment in wound care. *Nursing Standard, 17*(6), 59–60, 64, 67–68.

Thomas, C. (1989). Specialty beds: Decision-making made easy. *Ostomy/Wound Management, 23,* 51–53, 57–59.

Trelease, C. C. (1988). Developing standards for wound care. *Ostomy/Wound Management, 20.*

Waldrop, J., & Doughty, D. (2000). Wound-healing physiology. In R. A. Bryant (Ed.), *Acute and chronic wounds: Nursing management* (2nd ed., pp. 17–40). St. Louis, MO: Mosby.

Weir, D. (2001). Pressure ulcers: Assessment, classification, and management. In D. L. Krasner, G. T. Rodeheaver, & R. G. Sibbald (Eds.), *Chronic wound care: A clinical source book for healthcare professionals* (pp.619–628). Wayne, PA: HMP Communications.

Wysocki, A. B. (2000). Anatomy and physiology of skin and soft tissue. In R. A. Bryant (Ed.), *Acute and chronic wounds: Nursing management* (2nd ed., pp. 1–16). St. Louis, MO: Mosby.

Recommended Web Sites

Canadian Association for Enterostomal Therapy:
http://www.caet.ca

This professional association promotes education, research, and standards for enterostomal nursing practice. Enterostomal nurses are prepared at the post-graduate level to offer care to clients with the following conditions: abdominal stomata (opening), fistulae, draining wound, and selected disorders of the integumentary (skin), gastrointestinal, and genitourinary systems.

Canadian Association of Wound Care:
http://www.cawc.net

The Canadian Association of Wound Care (CAWC) Web site has quick reference guides and best practice articles available for downloading on all aspects of wound care practice.

National Pressure Ulcer Advisory Panel:
http://www.npuap.org

The National Pressure Ulcer Advisory Panel (NPUAP) provides multidisciplinary leadership for improved client outcomes in pressure ulcer prevention and management through education, public policy, and research.

Registered Nurses Association of Ontario Best Practice Guidelines:
http://www.rnao.org/bestpractices/index.asp

This Web site provides links to the Registered Nurses Association of Ontario (RNAO) Best Practice Guidelines, including *Risk Assessment and Prevention of Pressure Ulcers* and *Assessment and Management of Stage I to IV Pressure Ulcers.*

Wound, Ostomy, & Continence Nurses Society:
http://www.wocn.org

The Wound, Ostomy, & Continence Nurses (WOCN) Society is a professional nursing society that supports the practice and delivery of expert health care to individuals with wounds, ostomies, and incontinence.

44

Sensory Alterations

Janice Boundy, RN, PhD
Marion Allen, RN, PhD (Canadian author)

Objectives

Mastery of content in this chapter will enable the student to:

- Define the key terms listed.
- Differentiate among the processes of reception, perception, and reaction to sensory stimuli.
- Discuss the relationship of sensory function to an individual's level of wellness.
- Discuss common causes and effects of sensory alterations.
- Discuss common sensory changes that occur with aging.
- Describe how to assess a client's sensory status.
- Identify nursing diagnoses relevant to clients with sensory alterations.
- Develop a plan of care for clients with visual, auditory, tactile, speech, and olfactory deficits.
- List interventions for preventing sensory deprivation and controlling sensory overload.
- Describe conditions in the health care agency or client's home that can be adjusted to promote meaningful sensory stimulation.
- Discuss ways to maintain a safe environment for clients with sensory deficits.

Imagine the world without sight, hearing, or the ability to feel objects, taste foods, or smell aromas. People rely on a variety of sensory stimuli to give meaning and order to events occurring in their environment. The senses are tightly interwoven in forming the perceptual base of our world (Ebersole & Hess, 2001). Stimulation comes from many sources in and outside the body, particularly through the senses of sight **(visual),** hearing **(auditory),** touch **(tactile),** smell **(olfactory),** and taste **(gustatory).** The body also has a **kinesthetic** sense that enables a person to be aware of the position and movement of body parts without seeing them. **Stereognosis** is a sense that allows a person to recognize an object's size, shape, and texture. The ability to speak is not considered a sense, but it is similar to a sense in that without it, the client may lose the ability to interact meaningfully with others. When sensory function is altered, the person's ability to relate to and function within the environment changes drastically. Meaningful stimuli allow a person to learn about the environment and are necessary for healthy functioning and normal development.

Many clients seeking health care have pre-existing sensory alterations (e.g., cataracts). Others may develop sensory alterations as a result of medical treatment (e.g., hearing loss from antibiotic use). Clients who have partial or complete loss of a major sense may have developed or may need to find alternate ways to function safely within the environment. If sensory alterations occur early in life, clients may have developmental and socialization problems because of difficulty in interacting with people and the environment.

The environment of a health care setting (e.g., a noisy intensive care unit [ICU]) can cause sensory alterations. A health care setting is often a place of unfamiliar sights, sounds, and smells, as well as minimal contact with family and friends. The nurse must understand and help meet the needs of clients with sensory alterations, as well as recognize clients most at risk for developing sensory problems. The nurse helps clients learn to interact and react safely and effectively in their environment.

Scientific Knowledge Base

Normal Sensation

The nervous system continually receives thousands of bits of information from sensory nerve receptors, relays the information through appropriate channels, and integrates the information into a meaningful response. Sensory stimuli reach the sensory receptors and can elicit an immediate reaction or present information to the brain to be stored for future use. The nervous system must be intact for sensory stimuli to reach appropriate brain centres and for the individual to perceive the sensation. After interpreting the significance of a sensation, the person can then react to the stimulus. Table 44-1 summarizes normal hearing and vision.

Reception, perception, and reaction are the three components of any sensory experience. Reception begins with stimulation of a nerve cell called a receptor, which is usually designed for only one type of stimulus, such as light, touch, or sound. In the case of special senses, the receptors are grouped close together or located in specialized organs (McCance & Huether, 2002), such as the taste buds of the tongue or the retina of the eye. When a nerve impulse is created, it travels along pathways to the spinal cord or directly to the brain. For example, sound waves stimulate hair cell receptors within the organ of Corti, which causes impulses to travel along the eighth cranial nerve to the acoustic area of the temporal lobe. Sensory nerve pathways usually cross over to send stimuli to opposite sides of the brain. The actual perception or awareness of unique sensations depends on the receiving region of the cerebral cortex, where specialized brain cells interpret the quality and nature of sensory stimuli. When the person becomes conscious of the stimuli and receives the information, perception takes place. Perception includes integration and interpretation of the stimuli based on the person's experiences. A person's level of consciousness influences how well stimuli are perceived and interpreted. Any factors lowering consciousness impair sensory perception. If sensation is incomplete, such as blurred vision, or if past experience is inadequate for understanding stimuli such as pain, the person may react inappropriately to the sensory stimulus.

It is impossible to react to all of the multiple stimuli entering the nervous system. The brain prevents sensory bombardment by discarding or storing sensory information. A person will usually react to stimuli that are most meaningful or significant at the time. After continued reception of the same stimulus, however, a person stops responding and the sensory experience goes unnoticed. For example, a person concentrating on reading a good book may not be aware of music in the background. This adaptability phenomenon occurs with most sensory stimuli except for those of pain.

The balance between sensory stimuli entering the brain and those actually reaching a person's conscious awareness maintains a person's well-being. If an individual attempts to react to every stimulus within the environment

Table 44-1 Normal Hearing and Vision

Function	Anatomy and Physiology
The Ear	
Transmits to the brain an accurate pattern of all sounds received from the environment, the relative intensity of these sounds, and the direction from which they originate	Two ears provide stereophonic hearing to judge sound direction. The external ear canal shelters the eardrum and maintains relatively constant temperature and humidity to maintain elasticity. The middle ear is an air-containing space between the eardrum and oval window. It contains three small bones (malleus, incus, and stapes) called ossicles. The eardrum and ossicles transfer sound to the fluid-filled inner ear. Movement of the stapes in the oval window creates vibrations in the fluid that bathes the membranous labyrinth, which contains the end organs of hearing and balance. The union of the vestibular (balance) and cochlear (hearing) portions of the labyrinth explains the combination of hearing and balance symptoms that may occur with inner ear disorders. Vibration of the eardrum is transmitted through the bony ossicles. Vibrations at the oval window are transmitted in perilymph within the inner ear to stimulate hair cells that send impulses along the eighth cranial nerve to the brain.
The Eye	
Transmits to the brain an accurate pattern of light reflected from solid objects in the environment and transformed into colour and hue	Light rays enter the convex cornea and begin to converge. Fine adjustment of light rays occurs as they pass through the pupil and through the lens. Change in the shape of the lens focuses light on the retina. The retina has a pigmented layer of cells to enhance visual acuity. The sensory retina contains the rods and cones—photoreceptor cells sensitive to stimulation from light. Photoreceptor cells send electrical potentials by way of the optic nerve to the brain.

or if there is insufficient variety and quality of stimuli, sensory alterations will occur.

Sensory Alterations

The most common types of sensory alterations are sensory deficits, sensory deprivation, and sensory overload. When a client has more than one sensory alteration, the ability to function and relate effectively within the environment can be seriously impaired.

Sensory Deficits. A loss in the normal function of sensory reception and perception is a **sensory deficit.** In Canada, one in nine individuals will experience severe vision loss by the age of 65 years; this increases to one in four by age 85 (Canadian National Institute for the Blind, 2001). Approximately 4 of every 100 Canadians have impaired hearing, which establishes this sensory deficit as among the most prevalent in the country (Health Canada, 2002).

When senses are impaired, the sense of self is impaired. Initially, a person may withdraw by avoiding communication or socialization with others in an attempt to cope with the sensory loss. It becomes difficult for the person to interact safely with the environment until new skills relying on other existing functions are learned. When a deficit develops gradually or when considerable time has passed since the onset of an acute sensory loss, the person learns to rely on unaffected senses. Some senses may even become more acute to compensate for an alteration. For example, blind clients may rely more on their senses of hearing for information about the world.

Clients with sensory deficits may change behaviour in effective or ineffective ways. For example, one client with a hearing impairment may turn the unaffected ear toward the speaker to hear better, whereas another client may shun people to avoid the embarrassment of not being able to understand their speech.

Many conditions and diseases cause sensory deficits (Box 44-1). Certain sensory deficits occur more commonly in select ethnic groups. For example, the frequency and severity of glaucoma is higher among Black Canadians as compared with Whites (Elolia & Stokes, 1998). Certain types of glaucoma are more prevalent among the Inuit and Asian-Canadian populations and less prevalent among people of European and African descent (Elolia & Stokes, 1998). Other statistics have shown that otitis media is more prevalent among Inuit and First Nations populations (Stout & Kipling, 1999). As well, the prevalence of diabetes and diabetic retinopathy is higher in Aboriginal communities (Maberley, 2000).

Sensory Deprivation. The reticular activating system in the brain stem mediates all sensory stimuli to the cerebral cortex. Even in deep sleep, clients are able to receive stimuli. Sensory stimulation must be of sufficient quality and quantity to maintain a person's awareness. The sensory deprivation that clients experience may relate to the need for a comforting touch. Clients in ICUs are often exposed to physical touch, but it is usually associated with technical intervention rather than with a personal, comforting touch (Urden, Stacy, & Raugh, 2002). Decrease in stimuli can occur when clients are placed in isolation. This can reduce the number of people entering their room and contact with the outside world. As well, nurses are required to follow transmission-based precautions, which include the use of masks and gloves. Masks may prevent visualization of caregivers' faces and gloves will alter the sense of touch.

When a person experiences an inadequate quality or quantity of stimulation, such as monotonous or meaningless stimuli, **sensory deprivation** occurs. Three types of sensory deprivation are reduced sensory input (e.g., caused by sensory deficit from visual or hearing loss), elimination of order or meaning from input (e.g., exposure to strange environments), and restriction of the environment (e.g., bed rest or reduced environmental variation) that produces monotony and boredom (Ebersole & Hess, 2001).

There are many effects of sensory deprivation (Box 44-2). The symptoms can easily cause nurses and physicians to believe that a client is psychologically ill and confused, is suffering from severe electrolyte imbalance, or is under the influence of psychotropic drugs. Therefore, the nurse must always be aware of the client's existing sensory function and the quality of stimuli within the environment.

Sensory Overload. When a person receives multiple sensory stimuli and cannot perceptually disregard or selectively ignore some stimuli, **sensory overload** occurs. Excessive sensory stimulation prevents the brain from appropriately responding to or ignoring certain stimuli. Because of the multitude of stimuli leading to overload, the person no longer perceives the environment in a way that makes sense. Overload prevents meaningful response by the brain; the person's thoughts race, attention moves in many directions, and anxiety and restlessness may occur. As a result, overload causes a state similar to that produced by sensory deprivation. However, in contrast to deprivation, overload is individualized. The amount of stimuli needed for healthy function varies with each individual. A person's tolerance to sensory overload may vary by level of fatigue, attitude, and emotional and physical well-being.

The acutely ill client may easily be affected by sensory overload. The client in constant pain or who undergoes frequent monitoring of vital signs or who has irritation from drainage tubes is at risk. Multiple stimuli can combine to cause overload even if the nurse offers a comforting word or provides a gentle back rub. Clients may not benefit from nursing interventions because their attention and energy are focused on more stressful stimuli. Another example is the client who is hospitalized in an ICU, where the activity is constant. Lights are always on. Sounds can be heard from monitoring equipment, staff conversations, equipment alarms, and the activities of people entering the unit. Even at night, an ICU can be very noisy.

The behavioural changes associated with sensory overload can easily be confused with mood swings or simple disorientation. The nurse must look for symptoms such as racing thoughts, scattered attention, restlessness, and anxiety. Clients in ICUs sometimes resort to constantly fingering tubes and dressings. Constant reorientation and control of excessive stimuli become an important part of the ICU client's care.

Box 44-1 Common Diseases and Conditions Causing Sensory Deficits

Visual Deficits

Presbyopia: A gradual decline in the ability of the lens to accommodate or to focus on close objects. Individual is unable to see near objects clearly.

Cataract: Cloudy or opaque areas in part or the entire lens that interfere with passage of light through the lens. Cataracts usually develop gradually, without pain, redness, or tearing in the eye. Eventually leads to blurring and dimming of vision. Although associated with aging, cataracts can also be caused by diabetes, injury to the eye, or medications, especially steroids.

Dry eyes: Results when tear glands produce too few tears. Common in older adults and results in itching, burning, or blurred vision.

Glaucoma: A condition of increased fluid pressure inside the eye that can eventually damage the optic nerve. Left untreated, can result in visual field loss, decreased visual acuity, a halo effect seen around objects, and blindness. Can be idiopathic in origin or may be caused by eye injury, inflammation, tumours, diabetes, or medications such as steroids.

Diabetic retinopathy: Long-term or poorly managed diabetes can lead to progressive damage to the blood vessels of the retina, resulting in decreased vision or blindness.

Macular degeneration: Condition in which the macula (specialized portion of the retina responsible for central vision) loses its ability to function efficiently. First signs may include blurring of reading matter, distortion or loss of central vision, and distortion of vertical lines. Is a common cause of blindness in people over the age of 50 years, but may also affect younger adults and children.

Hearing Deficits

Presbycusis: A common progressive hearing disorder in older adults.

Cerumen accumulation: Buildup of cerumen (earwax) in the external auditory canal. Cerumen, which is normally absorbed in a younger person's ear, becomes hard and collects in the canal and causes a conduction deafness.

Otosclerosis: The hardening of the ossicles in the middle ear, resulting in gradual and progressive hearing loss that is usually accompanied by **tinnitus** (background noises in the ear, usually hissing or ringing sounds or discrete tones or pulses). Otosclerosis is a hereditary condition.

Meniere's disease: A disorder of the inner ear that is characterized by hearing loss, tinnitus, and **vertigo** (sudden loss of balance). It likely is caused by increased fluid in the inner ear. This disorder usually begins in people between the ages of 20 and 50 years.

Otitis media: Infection of the middle ear; common in infants and children. Recurrent or chronic otitis media can cause damage to the eardrum or middle ear, resulting in permanent hearing loss.

Balance Deficit

Benign positional vertigo: Common condition in older adulthood, usually resulting from vestibular dysfunction. Frequently an episode of vertigo or disequilibrium is precipitated by a change in position of the head.

Taste Deficit

Xerostomia: Decrease in salivary production that leads to thicker mucus and a dry mouth. Result of medications such as antihistamines. Can interfere with the ability to eat and leads to appetite and nutritional problems.

Taste alterations: Alterations, manifested by food aversions and decreased caloric intake, can occur frequently in clients with cancer (Sherry, 2002).

Neurological Deficits

Peripheral neuropathy: Disorder of the peripheral nervous system. Commonly caused by diabetes, carpal tunnel syndrome, and neoplasms (Ebersole & Hess, 2001). Symptoms include loss of sensation, numbness and tingling of the affected area, and stumbling gait.

Stroke: Cerebrovascular accident caused by clot, hemorrhage, or emboli disrupting blood flow to the brain. Creates altered proprioception with marked incoordination and imbalance. Loss of sensation and motor function in extremities controlled by the affected area of the brain also occurs. A stroke affecting the left hemisphere of the brain results in symptoms on the right side such as difficulty with speech. A stroke on the right hemisphere will have symptoms on the left side, which may include visuospatial alterations such as loss of half of a visual field or inattention and neglect.

Nursing Knowledge Base

Factors Affecting Sensory Function

When delivering care, the nurse can address many factors that affect sensory function, including the client's age, the quantity and quality of stimuli, social interaction, and family and environmental factors.

Age. Infants are unable to discriminate sensory stimuli because nerve pathways are immature. Visual changes during adulthood include presbyopia (inability to focus on near objects), which leads to the need for reading glasses. These changes usually occur from ages 40 to 50 years. Changes normally associated with aging include reduced visual fields, increased glare sensitivity, impaired night vision, reduced accommodation and depth perception, and reduced colour discrimination. Hearing changes include decreased hearing acuity, speech intelligibility, pitch discrimination, and hearing threshold. Older adults hear low-pitched sounds best but have difficulty hearing conversation over background noise. Speech sounds are garbled, and there is a delayed reception and reaction to speech. Older adults have difficulty discriminating the consonants (*z, t, f, g*) and high-frequency sounds (*s, sh, ph, k*). A problem with

Box 44-2 Effects of Sensory Deprivation

Cognitive

Reduced capacity to learn
Inability to think or problem solve
Poor task performance
Disorientation
Bizarre thinking
Regression
Increased need for socialization, altered mechanisms of attention

Affective

Boredom
Restlessness
Increased anxiety
Emotional lability (i.e., rapid mood swings)
Panic
Increased need for physical stimulation

Perceptual

Alterations in the following:
Visual/motor coordination
Colour perception
Apparent movement
Tactile accuracy
Ability to perceive size and shape
Spatial and time judgment

Adapted from *Toward Healthy Aging: Human Needs and Nursing Response* (5th ed.), by P. Ebersole and P. Hess, 2001b, St. Louis, MO: Mosby.

age-related hearing loss is that some individuals may not even be aware of their deficit (Tolson, 1997). A serious concern for those with a hearing deficit is that they may be inappropriately labelled as confused (Maas et al., 2001).

Gustatory and olfactory changes include a decrease in the number of taste buds in later years and a reduction of olfactory nerve fibres by the age of 50 years. Reduced taste discrimination and reduced sensitivity to odours are common.

Proprioceptive changes after the age of 60 years include increased difficulty with balance, spatial orientation, and coordination. Older adults experience tactile changes, including declining sensitivity to pain, pressure, and temperature.

Older adults are a high-risk group because of normal physiological changes involving sensory organs. However, the nurse must be careful to not automatically assume that a client's sensory problem is related to advancing age. For example, adult sensorineural hearing loss can be caused by metabolic, vascular, and other systemic alterations or by exposure to excess and prolonged noise. Hearing loss may also be a side effect of medications such as thiazide diuretics. A client may benefit from a referral to an **audiologist** or **otolaryngologist** if the assessment reveals serious hearing problems.

Quality of Stimuli. Meaningful stimuli reduce the incidence of sensory deprivation. In the home, meaningful stimuli may include pets, background music, television, family photos, and a calendar and clock. The same types of items should be present in a long-term care facility. In a health care setting, the nurse notes whether clients have roommates or visitors. The presence of others can offer positive stimulation. However, a roommate who constantly watches television, persistently tries to talk, or continuously keeps lights on can contribute to sensory overload. A client can become disoriented in a barren environment such as in an isolation room that gives few signals for normal sensory perception. The presence or absence of meaningful stimuli influences alertness and the ability to participate in care.

Quantity of Stimuli. Excessive stimuli in an environment can cause sensory overload. The frequency of observations and procedures performed in an acute care setting may be stressful. If the client is in pain, has many tubes and dressings, or is restricted by casts or traction, overstimulation can be a problem. A hospital environment is full of sensory stimuli that may contribute to sensory overload. The sounds of electrical monitors and equipment, bright lighting around-the-clock, and the odours of body fluids are just some examples. Also, a client's room may be near repetitive or loud noises (e.g., an elevator, stairwell, or nurses' station).

Conversely, not enough meaningful stimuli can cause sensory deprivation. Living in a confined environment, such as a long-term care facility, places people at risk for sensory deprivation. Although most quality long-term care facilities offer meaningful stimulation through group activities, environmental design, and mealtime gatherings, there are exceptions. The individual who is confined to a wheelchair, has poor hearing or vision, has decreased energy, or avoids contact with others is at significant risk for sensory deprivation. If the environment creates monotony, the individual has a reduced capacity to learn and to think.

Social Interaction. Clients with hearing loss tend to decrease the time spent with social activities and verbal communication (Resnick, Fries, & Verbrugge, 1997). Children with hearing deficits may be inattentive, uncooperative, or easily bored (Wong, Perry, & Hockenberry, 2002). Often a client is too embarrassed to continually ask another person to repeat what has been said; instead, the person avoids communication. Clients who find their lifestyles influenced by a hearing loss may experience loneliness and lowered self-esteem.

Family Factors. The amount and quality of contact with supportive family members and significant others can influence the degree of isolation the client feels. The absence of visitors during hospitalization or residency in a long-term care facility can also affect sensory status. This is a common problem in hospital intensive care settings, where visitation is often restricted. A pattern of social isolation can contribute to sensory changes. The ability to discuss fears or concerns with loved ones is an important coping mechanism for most people. Therefore, the absence of meaningful conversation can cause a person to become sensorially deprived, and the nurse may not be alerted until behavioural changes occur.

Environmental Factors. A person's work environment can also increase risk for sensory alterations. Individuals who are exposed to loud noises at work or who have occupations involving risk of exposure to chemicals or flying objects should be screened for hearing and visual problems. Clients who use their hands in a repetitive fashion (e.g., computer programmers) are at risk for carpal tunnel syndrome, a condition characterized by swelling or inflammation of the wrists. This inflammation creates pressure on the nerve as it passes through the narrow area in the wrist. The client experiences numbness, tingling, pain, and weakness in the hand while performing fine hand movements (Ruda, 2000).

A hospitalized client can be at risk for sensory alterations from exposure to environmental stimuli or a change in sensory input. Clients who are immobilized because of bed rest or physical encumbrances (e.g., casts or traction) are at risk, because they are unable to have free movement and seek out meaningful interactions. Clients placed in isolation because they have a communicable disease are also at risk (see chapter 29) because of lack of interactions with visitors.

As a result of illness or hospitalization, a client is often confined to an unfamiliar environment. This does not mean that all hospitalized clients have sensory alterations. However, the nurse must carefully assess clients who are subjected to continued sensory stimulation (e.g., clients in ICU settings and those requiring long-term hospitalization or multiple therapies). The nurse assesses the client's environment, both within the health care setting and the home, looking for factors that pose risks or that need adjustment to provide safety and more stimulation.

Critical Thinking

Critical thinking involves synthesizing knowledge and information gathered from clients, experience, and intellectual and professional standards. The nurse anticipates the information necessary, analyzes the data, and makes decisions regarding client care. During assessment (Figure 44–1), the nurse must consider all critical thinking elements that build toward making appropriate nursing diagnoses.

In the case of sensory alterations, the nurse must integrate knowledge of the normal anatomy and physiology of the sensory and nervous systems and the pathophysiology of sensory deficits, factors that affect sensory function, and therapeutic communication principles. This knowledge enables the nurse to conduct appropriate assessments, anticipate what to recognize when a client describes a sensory problem, and recognize abnormalities. For example, knowing the normal symptoms of a cataract helps the nurse recognize the pattern of visual changes in a client with a cataract.

Previous experiences in caring for clients with sensory deficits enable the nurse to recognize limitations in function in each new client and how limitations might affect the client's ability to carry out daily activities. For example, after caring for a client with a hearing impairment, the nurse will be able to conduct a more effective assessment of the next client.

Critical thinking attitudes and standards, when applied during assessment, ensure a thorough and accurate database from which to make decisions. For example, perseverance is needed to learn details as to how visual changes influence a client's ability to socialize. Standards of care and practice, such as those from the Canadian Ophthalmology Society, the Registered Nurses Association of Ontario, and the Canadian Gerontological Nurses Association, provide criteria for screening sensory problems and for establishing standards for competent, safe, effective care and practice. Using critical thinking, the nurse can conduct a thorough assessment and then plan, implement, and evaluate care that will enable the client to function safely and effectively.

Nursing Process

NP Assessment

When assessing clients with or at risk for sensory alterations, the nurse must have an understanding of how the client's particular illness may lead or has led to sensory changes. As well, all of the factors that may influence sensory function must be considered. For example, if the client has a hearing impairment, the nurse needs to adjust his or her communication style and then focus the assessment on relevant criteria related to hearing deficits. The nurse collects a history that also assesses the client's current sensory status and the degree to which a sensory deficit affects the client's lifestyle, psychosocial adjustment, developmental status, self-care ability, and safety. The assessment must also focus on the quality and quantity of environmental stimuli.

Sensory Alterations History. The nursing health history includes assessment of the nature and characteristics of sensory alterations or any problem related to an alteration (Goldblum, 2004). When taking the sensory alterations history, the nurse should consider the ethnic background of the client because certain alterations are higher in some ethnic groups (see Sensory Deficits). The nurse begins by asking the client to describe the sensory deficit, as in the following examples:

- Describe your hearing loss.
- Describe how your vision is affected.
- Explain how use of your hands has changed.

Knowledge about the onset and duration of the sensory alteration can be helpful. The nurse begins to learn how long the client has taken measures to adjust to the alteration:

- How long have you had a visual problem?
- When did you begin to feel numbness in your hands? In your legs?

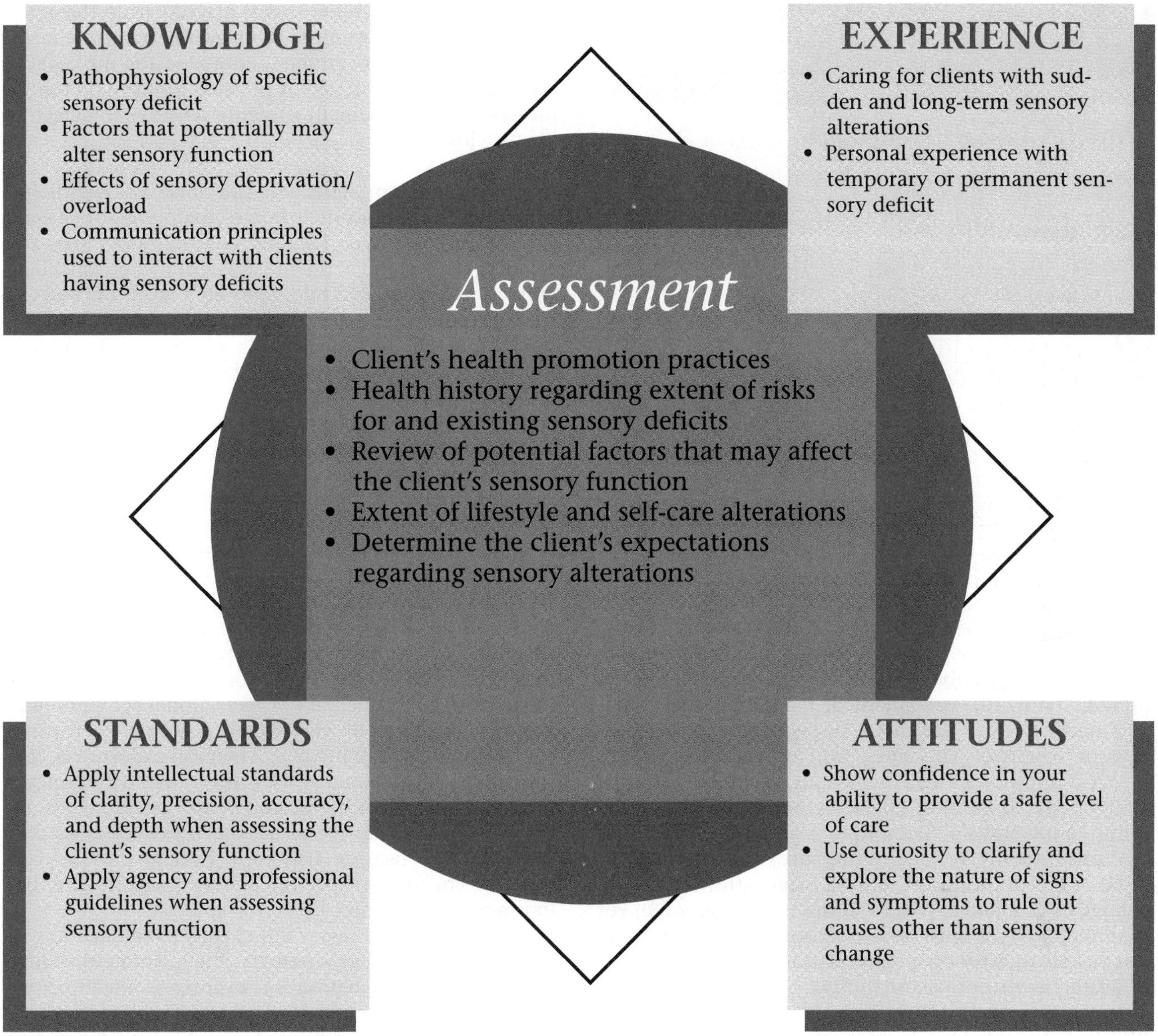
KNOWLEDGE
• Pathophysiology of specific sensory deficit
• Factors that potentially may alter sensory function
• Effects of sensory deprivation/ overload
• Communication principles used to interact with clients having sensory deficits
EXPERIENCE
• Caring for clients with sudden and long-term sensory alterations
• Personal experience with temporary or permanent sensory deficit
Assessment
• Client's health promotion practices
• Health history regarding extent of risks for and existing sensory deficits
• Review of potential factors that may affect the client's sensory function
• Extent of lifestyle and self-care alterations
• Determine the client's expectations regarding sensory alterations
STANDARDS
• Apply intellectual standards of clarity, precision, accuracy, and depth when assessing the client's sensory function
• Apply agency and professional guidelines when assessing sensory function
ATTITUDES
• Show confidence in your ability to provide a safe level of care
• Use curiosity to clarify and explore the nature of signs and symptoms to rule out causes other than sensory change

FIGURE **44–1** Critical thinking model for sensory alterations assessment.

- How long have you noticed being unable to hear conversations clearly?

It is also useful to assess the client's self-rating for a sensory deficit. Lewis-Cullinan and Janken (1990) found that a client's self-rating for hearing was one of the most important defining characteristics for the nursing diagnosis of *disturbed sensory perception (auditory)*. The nurse can simply say, "Rate your hearing as excellent, good, fair, poor, or bad." Then, from the client's self-rating, the nurse may explore more fully the client's perception of a sensory loss. This provides a more in-depth look at how the client's quality of life has been influenced. In the specific case of hearing problems, a screening tool developed by Ventry and Weinstein (Weinstein, 1994) has been found to be effective in identifying clients needing audiological intervention. The screening version of the Hearing Handicap Inventory for the Elderly (HHIE-S) is a 5-minute, 10-item questionnaire designed to assess how a client perceives the emotional and social effects of hearing loss (Weinstein, 1994). The greater the handicapping effect from the hearing loss, the higher the scores (Demers, 2001).

A health history can also reveal any recent changes in a client's behaviour. Often friends or family are the best resources for this information because the client may be unaware of any change. The nurse asks the following:

- Has the client shown any recent mood swings (e.g., outbursts of anger, nervousness, fear, or irritability)?
- Have you noticed the client avoiding social activities?

It is important to remember that many adults are sensitive about admitting losses and may hesitate to share information.

Mental Status. Mental status assessment is an important component of any evaluation of sensory function

Box 44-3 Assessment of Mental Status

Physical Appearance and Behaviour

Motor activity, posture, facial expression, hygiene

Cognitive Ability

Level of consciousness, abstract reasoning, calculation, attention, judgment
Ability to carry on conversation; ability to read, write, and copy figure
Recent and remote memory

Emotional Stability

Agitation, euphoria, irritability, hopelessness, or wide mood swings
Auditory, visual, or tactile hallucinations, illusions, delusions

(Box 44-3). Observing the client during history taking, during the physical examination, and during nursing care provides valuable data for evaluation of a client's mental status. An assessment of mental status is valuable particularly if the nurse suspects sensory deprivation or overload. The nurse will observe the client's physical appearance and behaviour, measure cognitive ability, and assess the client's emotional status. The Mini-Mental Status Examination is an example of a tool that can formally be used to measure disorientation, altered conceptualization and abstract thinking, and change in problem-solving abilities (see chapter 28). For example, a client with severe sensory deprivation may not be able to carry on a conversation, remain attentive, or display recent or past memory.

Physical Assessment. To identify sensory deficits and their severity, the nurse assesses vision, hearing, olfaction, taste, and the ability to discriminate light touch, temperature, pain, and position. Chapter 28 describes assessment techniques in detail. Table 44-2 summarizes assessment techniques for identifying sensory deficits. Data will be more accurate if the examination room is private, quiet, and comfortable for the client.

The nurse also relies on personal observation of the client to detect sensory alterations. Ebersole and Hess (2001) have identified some typical observations indicating hearing loss, which include the following: the client seems inattentive to others, responds with inappropriate anger when spoken to, believes people are talking about him or her, has trouble following clear directions, asks to have something repeated, has monotonous voice quality and speaks unusually loud or soft, has the television unusually loud, and answers questions inappropriately.

The typical physical tests used to screen for hearing impairment rely on an examiner's whispered voice or a tuning fork. The Welch-Allyn audioscope is very effective for measuring hearing acuity. The hand-held instrument includes an ear speculum that is placed within the external ear canal. The examiner can view the tympanic membrane to ensure that cerumen is not blocking the canal. A tonal sequence is initiated by pressing a button on the audioscope. The instrument is highly sensitive to detecting hearing loss.

Ability to Perform Self-Care. The nurse assesses clients' functional abilities in their home environment or health care setting, including feeding, dressing, grooming, and toileting. For example, the nurse assesses whether a client with altered vision can find items on a meal tray and can read directions on a prescription. The nurse also determines a visually impaired client's ability to perform daily routines such as reading bills, writing cheques, or driving a vehicle at night. If a client seems sensorially deprived, is concern shown for grooming? Does a client's loss of balance prevent rising from a toilet seat safely? Can the client with a stroke manipulate buttons or zippers for dressing? Any impairment in the ability to perform self-care has implications for planning discharge from a health care setting and in providing resources within the home.

Health Promotion Habits. The nurse must assess the daily routines that clients follow to maintain sensory function. What type of eye and ear care is incorporated into daily hygiene? For those individuals who participate in sports (e.g., racquetball) or recreational activities (e.g., motorcycle riding), or who work in a setting where ear or eye injury is a possibility (e.g., chemical exposure or constant exposure to loud noise), the nurse determines if safety glasses or hearing protective devices are worn. Do clients who use assistive devices such as eyeglasses, contact lenses, or hearing aids know how to provide daily care (see chapter 34)? Are the devices used, and are they in proper working order?

The nurse also assesses the client's adherence to routine health screening. When was the last time the client had an eye examination or hearing evaluation? For adults, routine screening of visual and hearing function is imperative to detect problems early. This is especially true in the case of glaucoma, which if undetected can lead to permanent visual loss. Recommended screening guidelines are usually structured according to age. When a client begins to show a hearing deficit, routine screening should be incorporated in regular examinations.

Hazards. A client with sensory alterations is at risk for injury if the living environment is unsafe. For example, a client with visual impairment cannot see potential hazards clearly. A client with proprioceptive problems may lose balance easily and fall. The condition of the home, the rooms, and the front and back entrances can be problematic to the client with sensory alterations. Some of the more common hazards include the following:

- Uneven, cracked walkways leading to front/back door
- Doormats with slippery backing
- Extension and phone cords in the main route of walking traffic
- Loose area rugs and runners placed over carpeting
- Bathrooms without shower or tub grab bars
- Water faucets unmarked to designate hot and cold

Table 44-2 Assessment of Sensory Function

Assessment	Behaviour Indicating Deficit (Children)	Behaviour Indicating Deficit (Adults)
Vision		
Ask client to read newspaper, magazine, or lettering on menu. Measure visual acuity with Snellen chart (see chapter 28). Assess visual fields and depth perception. Assess pupil size and accommodation to light. Ask client to identify colours on colour chart or crayons.	Self-stimulation, including eye rubbing, body rocking, sniffing or smelling, arm twirling; hitching (using legs to propel while in sitting position) instead of crawling	Poor coordination, squinting, underreaching or overreaching for objects, persistent repositioning of objects, impaired night vision, accidental falls
Hearing		
Perform conventional assessment, including whisper and tuning fork (see chapter 28). Perform audiometry, if indicated. Observe client conversing with others. Compare client's ability to recognize consonants with ability to distinguish vowels. Assess client's perception of hearing ability and history of tinnitus. Inspect ear canal for hardened cerumen.	Frightened when unfamiliar people approach, no reflex or purposeful response to sounds, failure to be awakened by loud noise, slow or absent development of speech, greater response to movement than to sound, avoidance of social interaction with other children	Blank looks, decreased attention span, lack of reaction to loud noises, increased volume of speech, positioning of head toward sound, smiling and nodding of head in approval when someone speaks, use of other means of communication such as lip-reading or writing, complaints of ringing in ears
Touch		
Assess client for sensitivity to light touch and temperature (see chapter 28). Check client's ability to discriminate between sharp and dull stimuli. Assess whether client can distinguish objects (coin or safety pin) in the hand with eyes closed. Ask whether client feels unusual sensations.	Inability to perform developmental tasks related to grasping objects or drawing, repeated injury from handling of harmful objects (e.g., hot stove, sharp knife)	Clumsiness, overreaction or underreaction to painful stimulus, failure to respond when touched, avoidance of touch, sensation of pins and needles, numbness
Smell		
Have client close eyes and identify several non-irritating odours (e.g., coffee, vanilla).	Difficult to assess until child is 6 or 7 years old, difficulty discriminating noxious odours	Failure to react to noxious or strong odour, increased body odour, increased sensitivity to odours
Taste		
Ask client to sample and distinguish different tastes (e.g., lemon, sugar, salt). (Have client drink or sip water and wait 1 minute between each taste.) Ask client if recent weight change has occurred.	Inability to tell whether food is salty or sweet, possible ingestion of strange-tasting things	Change in appetite, excessive use of seasoning and sugar, complaints about taste of food, weight change
Position sense		
Perform conventional tests for balance and position sense (see chapter 28).	Clumsiness, extraneous movement, excessive arm swinging in those with hyperactivity or learning difficulty	Poor balance and spatial orientation, shuffling gait, reduced response to brace self when falling, more precise and deliberate movements

- Bathroom floor with slippery surface
- Absence of smoke detectors in rooms
- Unlit stairways, lack of handrails
- Cluttered floors, furniture, including footstools
- Kitchen equipment (e.g., ranges, irons, toasters) with hard-to-read settings

In the hospital environment, caregivers often forget to rearrange furniture and equipment to keep paths from the bed and chair to the bathroom and entrance clear. Walking into a client's room and looking for safety hazards must be a routine part of every nurse's care. The nurse checks for the following:

- Is the call light within easy, safe reach?
- Are intravenous (IV) poles on wheels and easy to move?
- Are footstools in the middle of the room?
- Are suction machines, IV pumps, or drainage bags positioned so that a client can rise from a bed or chair easily?

Visually impaired clients may also be unable to read medication labels and syringe gauges. The nurse therefore must ask the client to read a label to determine whether the client can adequately see the dosage and frequency instructions. If a client has a hearing impairment, the nurse checks to see whether the sounds of a doorbell, telephone, smoke alarm, and alarm clock are easy to discriminate.

Communication Methods. Clients with existing sensory deficits often develop alternative ways of communicating. To interact with the client and to promote interaction with others, the nurse must understand the client's method of communication (Figure 44–2). A deaf or hearing-impaired client may read lips, use sign language, listen with the help of a hearing aid, or read and write notes.

Visually impaired clients are unable to observe facial expressions and other non-verbal behaviours that clarify the content of spoken communication. Instead, they rely on voice tones and inflections to detect the emotional tone of communication. Clients with visual deficits often learn to read Braille, although decreased tactile acuity of the fingers may make this more difficult in older people. Clients with **aphasia** may be unable to produce or understand language. **Expressive aphasia,** a motor type of aphasia, is the inability to name common objects or to express simple ideas in words or writing. For example, a client may understand a question but be unable to express an answer. Sensory or **receptive aphasia** is the inability to understand written or spoken language. The client may be able to express words but is unable to understand questions or comments of others. **Global aphasia** is the inability to understand language or communicate orally.

The temporary or permanent loss of the ability to speak is extremely traumatic to an individual. The nurse assesses a client's alternative communication method and whether it causes anxiety in the client. Clients who have undergone laryngectomies often write notes, use communication boards or laptop computers, speak with mechanical vibrators, or use esophageal speech. Clients with endotracheal or tracheostomy tubes have a temporary loss of speech. Most use a notepad to write their questions and requests. However, the client may become incapacitated and unable to write messages. The nurse needs to determine whether the client has developed a sign language or system of symbols to communicate needs. If not, the nurse may need to assist the client in developing a meaningful one during the temporary loss.

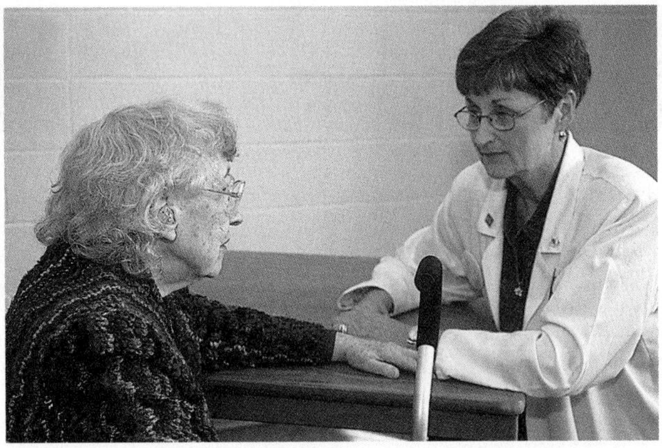

FIGURE **44–2** Nurse sits at eye level so that client with hearing impairment can communicate.

To understand the nature of a communication problem, the nurse must know whether a client has trouble speaking, understanding, naming, reading, or writing. Depending on the nature of the problem, the nurse selects the best way to interact with the client. For example, if the person has a visual deficit or is blind, the nurse speaks normally from a reasonably close distance and ensures that there is sufficient lighting. For someone who is hearing impaired, the nurse speaks clearly with a moderate rate of speech and pauses to determine understanding.

Social Support. It is important for the nurse to know the client's social skills and level of satisfaction with the support given by family and friends. Is the client satisfied with the support made available from friends? Is the client able to solve problems with family members? Does the family offer the support needed when the client requires assistance as a result of a sensory loss? The long-term effects of sensory alterations can influence family dynamics and a client's willingness to remain active in society.

Use of Assistive Devices. The nurse should assess the use of assistive devices (e.g., hearing aids or glasses) and the sensory effects for the client. This includes learning how often the devices are used daily, the client's or family caregiver's method for cleaning, and the client's knowledge of what to do when a problem develops. However, just because the client has an assistive device, the nurse should not assume that it works or that the client uses it or benefits from it (McConnell, 2002).

Other Factors Affecting Perception. Factors other than sensory deprivation or overload may cause impaired perception (e.g., medications or pain). The nurse assesses the client's medication history, which includes prescribed and over-the-counter medications, as well as herbal products. This history includes gaining information regarding the frequency, dose, method of administration, and last

Nursing Diagnostic Process — Box 44-4

Assessment Activities	Defining Characteristics	Nursing Diagnosis
Assess client's visual acuity.	Has reduced ability to see objects clearly. Needs brighter light to read. Has trouble distinguishing edges of stairs.	Risk for injury related to visual impairment from cataract formation
Visit home setting and inspect for any hazards that may pose risks to client.	Lighting in rooms, hallways, and stairwells is very dim. Carpet in living room is old, and edges are curled up. Steps lead up to front entrance of home.	
Review medical record from clinic visit.	Client has been diagnosed as having cataracts in both eyes.	

time these medications were taken. Some antibiotics (e.g., streptomycin, gentamicin, and tobramycin) are **ototoxic** and can permanently damage the auditory nerve; chloramphenicol can irritate the optic nerve. Narcotic analgesics, sedatives, and antidepressant medications can alter the perception of stimuli. The nurse also conducts a thorough pain assessment when pain is suspected to be causing perceptual problems (see chapter 38).

Client Expectations. Clients depend on their senses to provide them with information so as to respond or react to a specific situation or problem. Therefore, clients expect caregivers to recognize and appropriately manage and adjust their environment to meet their sensory needs. This would include assisting the client in adapting his or her lifestyle as a result of a sensory impairment. The nurse should determine from the client exactly what the client expects to achieve and what interventions have been helpful in the past in the management of the client's limitation. The nurse should remember that clients with sensory alterations may have strengthened their other senses and expect the caregivers to anticipate their needs (e.g., for safety and security).

Nursing Diagnosis

After assessment, the nurse reviews all available data and looks for patterns and trends suggestive of a health problem relating to sensory alterations (Box 44-4). For example, a client's advanced age, apathy, inattentiveness during conversations, and self-rating of hearing as "poor" are all defining characteristics for the nursing diagnosis of *disturbed sensory perception (auditory)*. The nurse validates findings to ensure accuracy of the diagnosis. For example, the diagnosis of *disturbed thought processes* could mistakenly be made if the nurse does not confirm the client's hearing deficit and perception of poor hearing.

The nurse determines the factor that likely causes the client's health problem. In the previous example, impacted cerumen is the cause of the client's hearing alteration. The etiology or related factor of a nursing diagnosis is a condition that can be affected by nursing interventions. The etiology must be accurate; otherwise, nursing therapies will be ineffective. For a client with impacted cerumen, regular irrigations of the ear canal have the potential for improving auditory perception (Wong et al., 2002). In contrast, if the client's auditory alteration were related to hearing loss from nerve deafness, nursing interventions for alternative communication methods would be necessary.

The client may also have health care problems for which sensory alteration is the etiology, such as with the diagnosis of *risk for injury*. For example, 25% of falls causing injury among older adults are attributed to vision problems (Health Canada, Division of Aging and Seniors, 2002). The nurse may also select nursing diagnoses by recognizing the way that sensory alterations affect a client's ability to function (e.g., self-care deficit). In addition, most clients present themselves to health care professionals with multiple diagnoses (Figure 44–3). In the example of the concept map, a client with retinal detachment has the nursing diagnosis of disturbed sensory perception, which can lead to risk for falls and fear. The nurse must recognize patterns of data that reveal health problems created by the client's sensory alteration. Examples of nursing diagnoses that might apply to clients with sensory alterations include the following:

- Impaired adjustment
- Impaired verbal communication
- Risk for injury
- Impaired physical mobility
- Self-care deficit, bathing/hygiene
- Self-care deficit, dressing/grooming
- Self-care deficit, toileting
- Situational low self-esteem
- Disturbed sensory perception
- Social isolation
- Disturbed thought processes
- Altered socialization

Planning

During planning, the nurse uses critical thinking skills to synthesize information from multiple resources (Figure 44–4), including knowledge gained from the assessment and knowledge of how sensory deficits affect normal functioning. In this way, the nurse can recognize the extent of

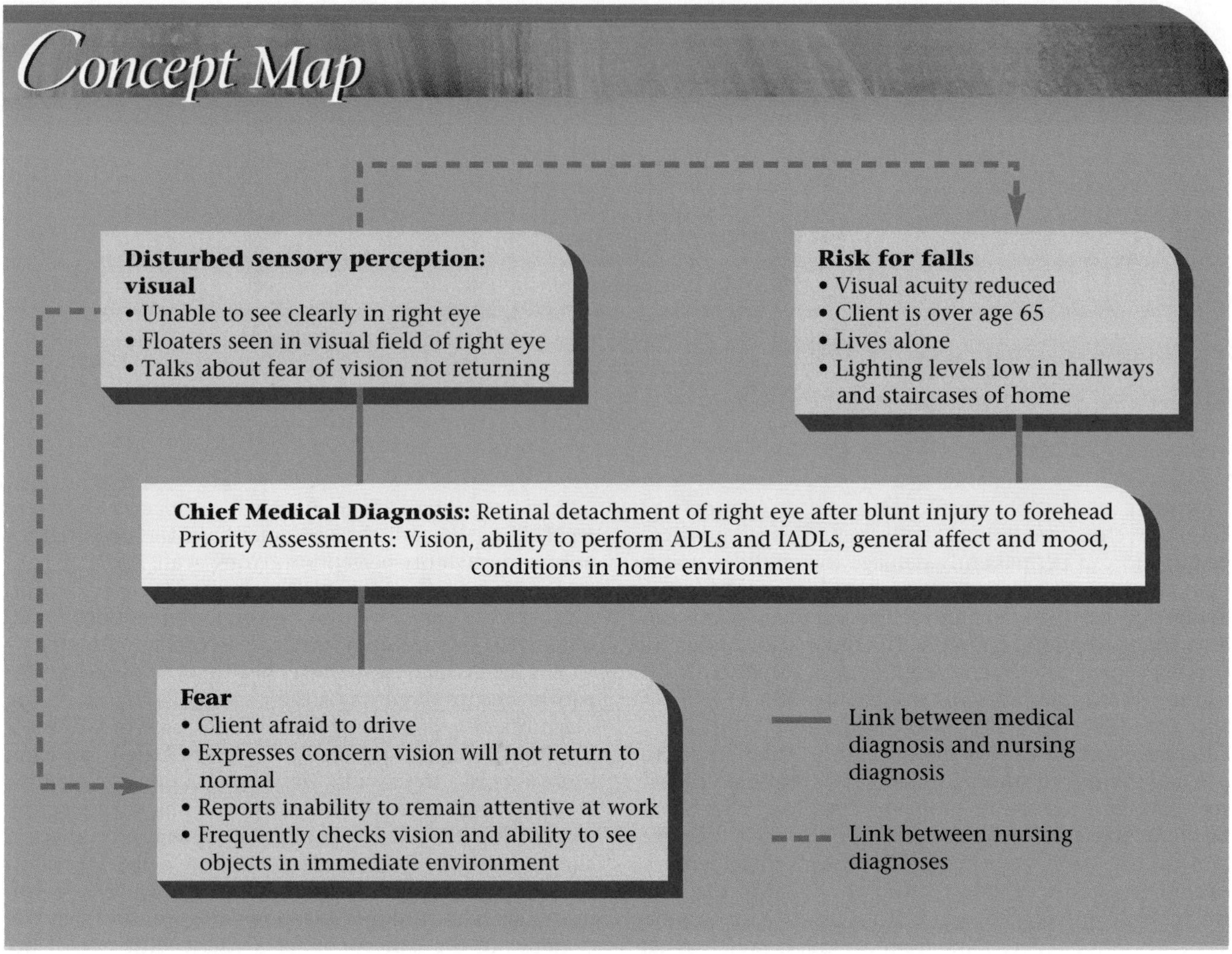
Concept Map
Disturbed sensory perception: visual
• Unable to see clearly in right eye
• Floaters seen in visual field of right eye
• Talks about fear of vision not returning
Risk for falls
• Visual acuity reduced
• Client is over age 65
• Lives alone
• Lighting levels low in hallways and staircases of home
Chief Medical Diagnosis: Retinal detachment of right eye after blunt injury to forehead
Priority Assessments: Vision, ability to perform ADLs and IADLs, general affect and mood, conditions in home environment
Fear
• Client afraid to drive
• Expresses concern vision will not return to normal
• Reports inability to remain attentive at work
• Frequently checks vision and ability to see objects in immediate environment
Link between medical diagnosis and nursing diagnosis
Link between nursing diagnoses

FIGURE **44–3** Concept map for client with retinal detachment of right eye after blunt injury to forehead.

the client's deficit and know the type of interventions most likely to be helpful. The nurse also considers the role that health professionals can play in planning care and the available community resources that may be useful. Previous experience in caring for clients with sensory alterations can be invaluable when planning nursing approaches.

When applying critical thinking to planning care, professional standards can be particularly useful. These standards, in the form of clinical pathways or clinical practice guidelines, often recommend scientifically proven interventions for the client's condition. For example, clients who have visual deficits and are hospitalized may be placed on a fall prevention protocol that will incorporate research-based precautions to ensure client safety.

Goals and Outcomes. During planning, the nurse develops an individualized plan of care for each nursing diagnosis (see Care Plan). The nurse and client partner together to develop a realistic plan that incorporates what the nurse knows about the client's sensory problems and the extent to which sensory function can be maintained or improved. If maintenance or improvement is not realistic, preventing injury and learning alternate ways of maintaining independence is key. Goals and outcomes should be realistic and measurable. A goal of care for a client with an actual or potential sensory alteration may include "The client will regain improvement in hearing acuity within 2 weeks." Associated outcomes for this goal might include the following:

- The client will report using communication techniques for improved reception of messages within 2 weeks.
- The client will successfully demonstrate the technique for cleansing the hearing aid within 1 week.
- The client and family will be observed using proper communication skills to send and receive messages.
- The client will self-report improved hearing acuity.

Setting Priorities. Priorities of care must be set with regard to the type and extent of sensory alteration that affects a client. For example, a client who enters the emergency department after experiencing eye trauma may have priorities of reducing anxiety and preventing further injury to the eye. In contrast, a client who is being discharged from an outpatient surgery department following

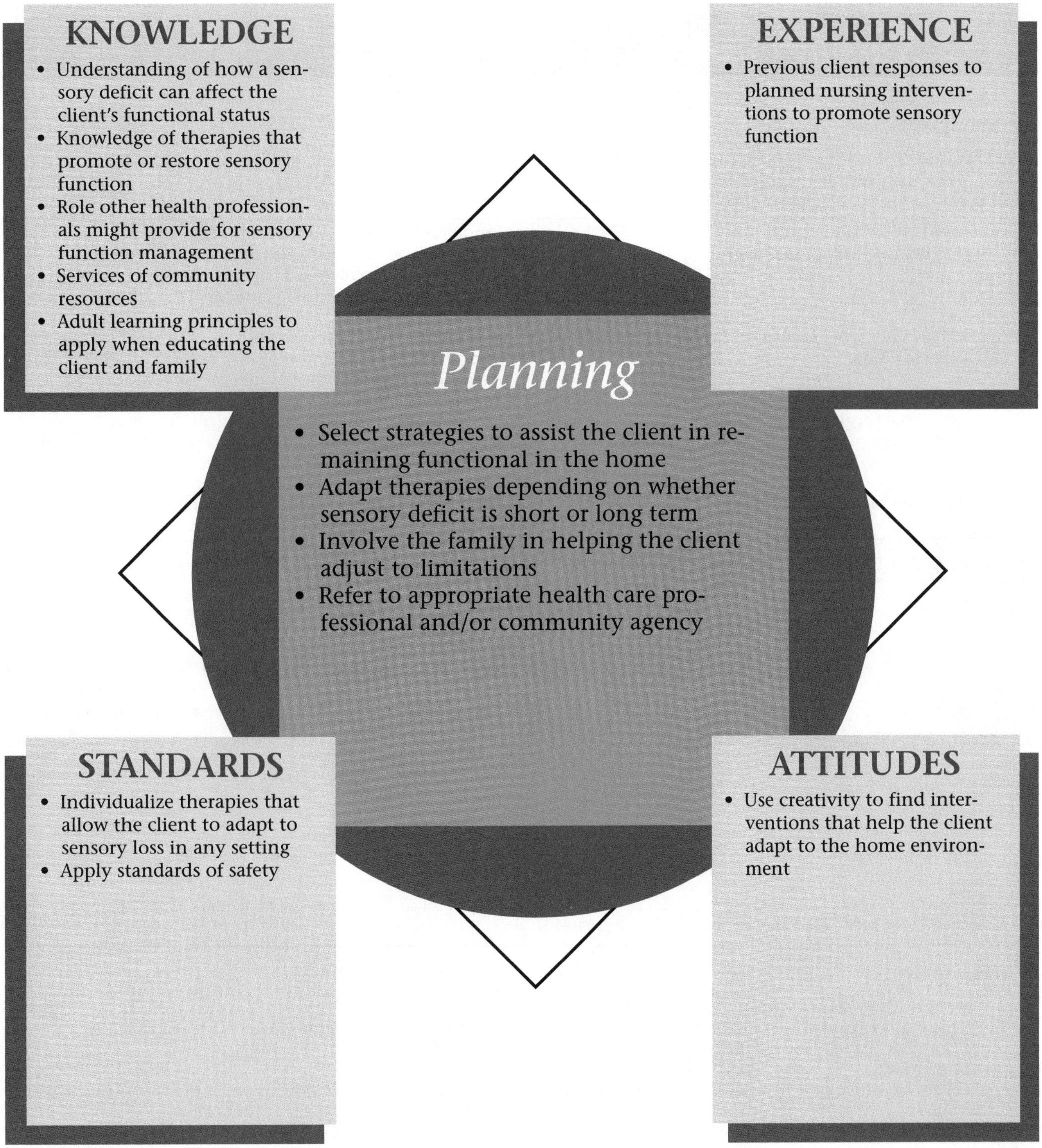
KNOWLEDGE
• Understanding of how a sensory deficit can affect the client's functional status
• Knowledge of therapies that promote or restore sensory function
• Role other health professionals might provide for sensory function management
• Services of community resources
• Adult learning principles to apply when educating the client and family
EXPERIENCE
• Previous client responses to planned nursing interventions to promote sensory function
Planning
• Select strategies to assist the client in remaining functional in the home
• Adapt therapies depending on whether sensory deficit is short or long term
• Involve the family in helping the client adjust to limitations
• Refer to appropriate health care professional and/or community agency
STANDARDS
• Individualize therapies that allow the client to adapt to sensory loss in any setting
• Apply standards of safety
ATTITUDES
• Use creativity to find interventions that help the client adapt to the home environment

FIGURE **44–4** Critical thinking model for sensory alterations planning.

cataract removal may have the priority of learning about any self-care requirements. However, safety is always a top priority. The client can also help prioritize aspects of care. For example, clients may wish to learn ways to communicate more effectively or to participate in favourite hobbies, given their sensory limitation.

Some sensory alterations are short term (e.g., a client suffering sensory/perceptual alterations as a result of sensory overload in an ICU). Appropriate interventions are thus likely to be temporary (e.g., frequent reorientation or introduction of intimate and pleasant stimuli such as a back rub). Sensory alterations such as permanent visual

Nursing Care Plan

Disturbed Sensory Perception

Assessment

Judy Long, a 70-year-old receptionist, tells the community health nurse that lately her vision is blurred. She comments that she is having her neighbour drive her places. Judy visited an ophthalmologist, and she is scheduled for surgery in 3 weeks.

Assessment Activities	Findings/Defining Characteristics
Ask Judy to describe her vision changes.	Judy states, "My left eye seems to have a film over it that makes my vision blurred. I am having difficulty reading. I also have difficulty with night driving; the headlights are large and blurred."
Ask Judy to describe any life changes that have occurred since the change in vision.	Judy indicated that she has always worked, managed her home, and done volunteering. She says she is losing her independence because she has to have someone drive her and she is now hesitant to use stairs at home.
Assess Judy's visual acuity.	Judy cannot read the Snellen chart with the left eye.
Ask Judy the results of the visit to the ophthalmologist.	Judy states that she was told she has a cataract in the left eye and a beginning one in her right eye; surgery is planned in 3 weeks on her left eye.
Conduct a home hazard assessment.	There is clutter in the home, dim lighting, and stairs without handrails going into the house.

Nursing Diagnosis: Disturbed sensory perception related to altered sensory reception of senile cataract.

Planning

Goals	Expected Outcomes*
	Safety behavior: Home Physical Environment
Client will maintain independence in a safe home environment.	Client will verbalize changes made to protect and maintain visual acuity for indoor and outdoor activities in 2 weeks. A safety check of the client's home will show removal of safety hazards in 1 week.
	Client will explain plans for alternate transportation to work and social activities in 1 week.
	Sensory Function: Vision
Client will maintain existing visual function.	Client will use visual aid devices in 1 week.

*Outcome classification labels from *Nursing Outcomes Classification (NOC)* (3rd ed.), edited by S. Moorhead, M. Johnson, and M. L. Maas, 2004, St. Louis, MO: Mosby.

Interventions†	Rationale
Environmental Management	
Instruct client to keep walking area in home and work area free of clutter, footstools, and electric cords and to avoid rearranging furniture.	Keeping the area clutter free reduces the risk of injury (Hensel, 2000).
Instruct client to reduce glare by wearing dark-coloured sunglasses outside.	Clients have better visual acuity when they protect their eyes from bright light (Ebersole & Hess, 2001).
Teach client to use a light over the shoulder for reading and writing.	People with cataracts see better with wider illumination (Ebersole & Hess, 2001).
Provide magnifier for client to use to read newspaper and mail.	Devices will provide magnification to improve visual acuity.
Emotional Support	
Encourage client to express feelings regarding loss of vision and lifestyle changes.	People who experience visual loss grieve over loss of independence (Vader, 1992).
Family Involvement	
Confer with client on selecting a family member, friend, or community resource person who can provide transportation until after the eye condition has been corrected.	An alternate means of transportation will foster safety (Hensel, 2000).

†Intervention classification labels from *Nursing Interventions Classification (NIC)* (4th ed.), edited by J. M. Dochterman and G. M. Bulecheck, 2004, St. Louis, MO: Mosby.

Nursing Care Plan

Disturbed Sensory Perception—cont'd

Evaluation

Nursing Actions	Client Response/Finding	Achievement of Outcome
Ask client to describe the changes that have made the home environment safer. During a home visit, observe the home environment for safety hazards.	Judy responds that the family has removed the clutter and handrails have been placed at the entryway. Lighting has been placed behind her chair, and there are 100-watt lights in the living room.	Judy reports feeling safer walking the stairs and moving about in her home. The home hazards have been reduced.
Observe client's verbal and non-verbal responses to the lifestyle adaptations.	Judy says, "I feel safer with walking in my home."	
As Judy uses magnifier, have her read a medication label.	Judy is able to read name of medication and dosage correctly.	Visual acuity has not been further compromised.
Ask if client is able to maintain a degree of independence with the environmental and lifestyle modifications.	Judy states, "I am more independent at home, and until surgery I do not mind someone driving for me."	Judy has attained some degree of independence.
Ask client to identify source of transportation.	Judy says a family member has agreed to drive her shopping and for surgery.	Judy has transportation through the weeks required for the surgical experience.

loss require long-term goals of care for clients to adapt. However, clients who have sensory alterations at the time of entering a health care setting are usually most informed about how to adapt interventions to their lifestyles. People with sensory impairment need to control whatever part of their care they can. Sometimes it becomes necessary for the client to make major changes in self-care activities, communication, or socialization.

Continuity of Care. When developing a plan of care, the nurse considers all resources available to clients. The family can play a key role in providing meaningful stimulation and learning ways to help the client adjust to any limitations. As part of a multidisciplinary health care team, the nurse may also refer the client to other health care professionals. Early referrals to occupational or speech therapists, for example, can speed a client's recovery. If a client has experienced a major loss of sensory function and is also unable to manage medical needs such as medication self-administration or dressing changes, referral to home care may be an option. There are also numerous community-based resources (e.g., Canadian National Institute for the Blind [CNIB], Canadian Association of Independent Living Centres, Canadian Hearing Society). The nurse may be able to arrange a volunteer to visit a client or have printed materials made available that describe ways to cope with sensory problems.

Implementation

Nursing interventions involve the client and family so that a safe, pleasant, and stimulating sensory environment can be maintained. The most effective interventions enable the client with sensory alterations to function safely with existing deficits and to continue a normal lifestyle. Learning to adjust to sensory impairments can occur at any age with the proper support and resources. The nurse uses measures to maintain a client's sensory function at the highest level possible.

Health Promotion. Good sensory function begins with prevention. Almost everyone becomes exposed to risks in the environment that may cause sensory alterations. When clients enter primary health care settings, the nurse can take the opportunity to review common-sense approaches for reducing risk of sensory loss (Box 44-5).

Screening. Preventable blindness is a worldwide health issue (Smith, 2003). Therefore, prevention of visual impairment begins with children and requires appropriate screening (Wong et al., 2002). There are three recommended interventions: (a) screening for rubella or syphilis in women who are considering pregnancy; (b) adequate prenatal care to prevent premature birth (with the danger of exposure of the infant to excessive oxygen); and (c) periodic screening of all children, especially newborns through preschoolers, for congenital blindness and visual impairment caused by refractive errors, ambylopia, and **strabismus** (the misalignment of the eyes).

Visual impairments are common during childhood. The most common visual problem is a **refractive error** such as nearsightedness. The nurse's role is one of detection and referral. Parents must know signs suggesting visual impairment (e.g., failure to react to light and reduced eye contact from the infant). The nurse instructs parents to report these signs to a physician immediately. Vision screening of school-age children and adolescents can detect problems early. The school nurse or public health nurse is usually responsible for vision testing.

Children at risk for hearing impairment include those with a family history of childhood hearing impairment,

Focus on Primary Health Care — Box 44-5

Sensory Alterations

Major goals in primary health care settings are health promotion, disease prevention, early detection, and referral. In the community, primary health care related to sensory alterations is delivered in doctors' offices, homes, community centres, schools, and industry. Public health nurses, for example, conduct newborn hearing screenings during well-baby clinics and reinforce the importance of parents following the Canadian Ophthalmology Society eye examination guidelines. In ophthalmologist's offices, the ophthalmic nurse can reinforce health-promoting practices as well as guide the client to find appropriate resources to assist in living with visual impairment. In school health programs, the nurse can stress the importance of maintaining the health of eyes and ears. Occupational health nurses play a key role in preventing injury. For example, the nurse can help ensure that safety standards are followed and that first aid stations (e.g., eyewash fountains in case the eye is splashed with a chemical) are appropriately placed.

Nurses are often consulted for guidance when changes in vision and hearing occur. Knowledge of screening techniques, such as the use of the Amsler grid for macular degeneration, is important. It is also important that the nurse know normal aging changes as well as signs and symptoms of common diseases so that appropriate suggestions for referral can be made.

Box 44-6 Tips for Preventing Eye Injury in Children

Infants and Toddlers

Avoid toys with long, pointed projections.
Do not allow child to walk or run with pointed object in hand.
Keep pointed instruments and tools out of reach.

Preschoolers

Supervise use of sharp or pointed objects such as scissors.
Teach child to walk carefully when carrying pointed objects.
Keep child away from projectile activities.
Begin to teach respect for firearms and fireworks.

School-Age Children and Adolescents

Teach proper use of potentially dangerous equipment such as power tools, fireworks, and sports equipment (hockey sticks or pool cues).
Stress use of eye protection when playing hockey, ball and racquet sports, shooting, using power tools, or riding motorcycles.
Warn children not to look directly at the sun even when wearing sunglasses.
Be sure corrective lenses are made of safety glass, which is shatterproof.

perinatal infection (rubella, herpes, cytomegalovirus), low birth weight, chronic ear infection, and Down syndrome. Nurses should advise pregnant women of the importance of early prenatal care, avoidance of ototoxic drugs, and testing for syphilis or rubella.

Children with chronic middle ear infections, a common cause of impaired hearing, should receive periodic auditory testing. Parents must be warned of the risks and should seek medical care when the child has symptoms of earache or respiratory infection.

Hearing loss from noise-induced environments was once thought to affect primarily older individuals; however, recent research has observed this loss in youth and young adults aged 20 to 30 years old. This loss is attributed to exposure to noise at constantly high levels, such as from portable music devices, automobile stereo systems, and concerts. This hearing impairment results in loss of sound quality. Sounds are barrel-like, and consonants are hard to hear. According to provincial occupational health and safety legislation, workers must use hearing protection devices to minimize or prevent hearing loss. As well, the various provincial jurisdictions mandate occupational noise exposure limits. Nurses should routinely teach parents and children to take precautions when involved in activities associated with high-intensity noise. The nurse should assess clients for noise exposure and participate in providing hearing conservation classes for teachers, students, and clients (Lusk, 2002; McCullagh, 2002).

In Canada, glaucoma is the second leading cause of blindness and affects 1 in 100 Canadians over the age of 40 years. The risk is eight times higher among Blacks. It is important to recommend that clients between the ages of 40 and 64 years have an eye examination every 2 to 4 years. Examinations should occur every 1 to 2 years if there is a family history of glaucoma or if the client is of African ancestry, has had a serious eye injury in the past, is taking steroid medications, or is over 65 years of age (Smith & Wilbur, 2004).

The guidelines for hearing screening for adults are less prescriptive. Generally, if a client works or lives in an environment where there is a high noise level, routine screening is highly recommended (Meadows, 2003) and may be mandated by occupational health and safety measures in the workplace. Nurses in occupational settings can assess for symptoms of tinnitus and make prompt referrals. Early detection may prevent hearing disabilities (Griest & Bishop, 1998; Lusk, 2002). Adults must not accept hearing loss as a natural part of aging. Once a client acknowledges his or her hearing loss, it is important to have regular hearing testing. Nurses should encourage clients to follow through with recommendations for hearing aids.

Preventive Safety. Trauma is a common cause of blindness in children. Penetrating injury from propulsive objects such as firecrackers, slingshots, rubber bands, or rocks or from penetrating wounds from sticks, scissors, or toys are just a few examples. Parents and children require counselling on ways to avoid eye trauma (Box 44-6). Safety equipment can easily be found in most sports shops and large department stores. In some Canadian jurisdictions, legislation or association bylaws may mandate the wearing of protective equipment (e.g., visors in minor hockey).

Adults are at risk for eye injury while playing sports and working in jobs involving exposure to chemicals or flying objects. Occupational Health and Safety has guidelines for safety in the workplace. Employers are required to have employees wear eye goggles or use equipment such as hearing protective devices (HPDs) to reduce the risk of injury. Nurses in occupational health settings can reinforce use of protective devices.

Preventing hearing loss requires individuals to avoid exposure to continuous high noise levels and brief loud impulse noise. HPDs should be worn by clients who must work around noise. Earplugs and earphones are useful in blocking high-decibel sounds (Box 44-7).

Another means of prevention involves regular immunization of children against diseases capable of causing hearing loss (e.g., rubella, mumps, and measles). Public health nurses, nurse practitioners, and nurses who work in physicians' offices, schools, and community clinics should reinforce the importance of early and timely immunization. When a child or an adult develops any type of health problem, caution should be used in prescribing drugs that are ototoxic.

Use of Assistive Devices. Health promotion requires appropriate use of assistive aids and good, routine hygiene measures. A client who wears corrective contact lenses, eyeglasses, or hearing aids should make sure that they are kept clean, accessible, and functional (see chapter 34). It is helpful to have a family member or friend also know how to clean an assistive aid (Box 44-8).

It is critical for contact lens wearers to frequently clean lenses and to use the appropriate solutions for cleaning and disinfection. With the rise in use of soft contact lenses, particularly extended-wear lenses, some clients have become casual with regard to both the care and wearing time of the contacts; as a result, there has been an increase in serious corneal infections. Infrequent lens disinfection, contamination of lens storage cases and contact lens solutions, and use of homemade saline add to a client's risk. Swimming while wearing lenses also creates a serious risk of infection.

Wearing a hearing aid no longer has to be a social stigma. There are a wide variety of aids that not only successfully enhance a person's hearing, but can also be cosmetically acceptable. Chapter 34 summarizes the types of hearing aids available and tips for proper care and use.

Smith and Wilbur (2004) identified factors that determine a person's likelihood for wearing a hearing aid: perceived need for improved hearing, attitude toward the hearing problem, and motivation to seek solutions. Acknowledging a need to improve hearing is a person's first step. The nurse can give clients useful information on the benefits of wearing a hearing aid. It is also important to have a significant other available to assist with hearing aid adjustment. If a client has any of the following ear conditions, a hearing aid cannot be used: visible congenital or traumatic deformity of the ear, active drainage in the last 90 days, sudden or progressive hearing loss within the last 90 days, acute or chronic dizziness, unilateral sudden hearing loss within the last 90 days, visible cerumen accumulation or a foreign body in the ear canal, pain or discomfort in the ear, or an audiometric air-bone gap of 15 decibels or greater. The nurse can detect all but the last of these on physical examination

Research Highlight — Box 44-7

Farmers' Use of Hearing Protection

Research Focus

Noise-induced hearing loss is a consequence of exposure to high noise levels and is preventable by the appropriate use of hearing protection devices (HPDs). The focus of this research was to identify factors affecting farmers' use of HPDs. Farmers use a variety of equipment that routinely exposes them to hazardous high-noise levels. Nurses need to focus assessment and interventions to promote effective use of HPDs among farmers and others. Additional research is needed to evaluate the impact of educational interventions for those exposed to high noise levels.

Research Abstract

Within the framework of Pender's Health Promotion Model, this study examined factors that influence farmers' use of HPDs. Pender's model of health-promoting behaviours shows a relationship between understanding and knowledge to explain and predict behaviour. A sample of 139 farmers was tested at a farm show in the midwest United States. The researchers found that interpersonal support (encouragement and praise from others), situational factors, and perceived barriers were significant predictors for whether farmers used HPDs. The study showed that 17% of the farmers used HPDs with high noise levels and the majority (56%) never used HPDs. The results of the study as compared with other studies of workers' use of hearing protection showed that construction workers have more encouragement and support for the use of HPDs than the farmers, who commonly work in isolation.

Evidence-Based Practice

- Assess farmers for noise-induced hearing loss.
- Design and evaluate teaching tools to educate health care providers regarding the use of HPDs to include farmers and others exposed to high noise levels (e.g., workers in natural resource-based industries such as mining and forestry).
- Teach the value of HPDs for prevention of hearing loss to all workers, including farmers.
- Educate professionals on the necessity of family support for use of HPDs.
- Refer clients with suspected hearing impairment to a hearing clinic or to an audiologist for testing.

Reference

McCullagh, M., Lusk, S. L., & Ronis, D. L. (2002). Factors influencing use of hearing protection among farmers: A test of the Pender Health Promotion Model. *Nursing Research, 51,* 33–39.

Client Teaching Box 44-8

Troubleshooting Hearing Aid Malfunction

Objectives

- Family member will identify source of malfunction in hearing aid.
- Family member will demonstrate hearing aid care.

Teaching Strategies

- Show family member locations on hearing aid device where damage (e.g., cracks, fraying) is likely to occur: ear mould or case, earphone, dials, cord, and connection plugs.
- Demonstrate battery replacement: Have extra set of unused batteries available.
- Review method to check volume: turn dial to maximum gain and then check. Is voice clear?
- Consult manufacturer's directions for specific care measures for cleaning battery case and ear mould.
- Review factors to report to hearing aid laboratory: static, distortion of sound, poor volume quality.

Evaluation

- Have family member describe types of common malfunctions with hearing aid.
- Have family demonstrate battery removal and cleaning.

and should refer to or recommend that the client see an otolaryngologist or audiologist for further counselling (Ebersole & Hess, 2001).

Promoting Meaningful Stimulation. Life becomes much more enriching and satisfying when meaningful and pleasant stimuli exist within the environment. There are many ways that the nurse can help clients make adjustments to their environment so that it becomes more stimulating. This is best done when the nurse considers the normal physiological changes that accompany sensory deficits.

Vision. As a result of the normal changes of aging, the pupil's ability to adjust to light is diminished. As a result, older adults can be very sensitive to glare. The nurse can suggest ways for the client to minimize glare by selecting satin and non-gloss finishes for walls and countertops in the home and choosing sheer curtains, tinted windows, or adjustable shades to reduce outdoor light. Wearing sunglasses outside can reduce the glare of direct sunlight.

The ability to read is important to everyone. Therefore clients should be encouraged to use their glasses whenever possible (e.g., during procedures and client instruction); it helps clients to remain oriented, maintain some control, and retain their dignity (Larsen, Hazen, & Martin, 1997). Clients with reduced visual acuity may need more than corrective lenses. A pocket magnifier can help a client read most printed material. Telescopic lens eyeglasses are smaller, easier to focus, and have a greater range. There are also books and other publications available in larger print. If a client has a legal or other important document he or she wishes to read, standard copying machines have enlarging capabilities. There are now closed-circuit television magnifying units or portable/desktop video magnifiers using solid state digital technology that enlarge written characters. Minimum and maximum magnification varies from 12 to 60 times the original, depending on screen size.

With aging, a person experiences a change in colour perception. Perception of the colours blue, violet, and green usually declines. Brighter colours such as red, orange, and yellow are easier to see. The nurse can offer suggestions of ways the client may decorate a room and paint hallways or stairwells so that differentiations can be made in surfaces and objects in a room.

Hearing. To maximize residual hearing function, the nurse works closely with the client to suggest ways to modify the environment. Telephones and televisions can be amplified. Alarm clocks that shake the bed or activate a flashing light are useful adaptive devices. An innovative way to enrich the lives of those with a hearing impairment is recorded music. Music recorded in the low-frequency sound cycles can be heard by clients with severe hearing loss.

One way to help an individual with a hearing loss is to ensure that the problem is not impacted cerumen. With aging, cerumen thickens and builds up in the ear canal. Excessive cerumen occluding the ear canal can cause a **conductive hearing loss.** Irrigation of the canal with tepid water in a 60-mL syringe (see chapter 34) will remove cerumen. Removal of cerumen can significantly improve the client's hearing ability. Lewis-Cullinan and Janken (1990) and Moore et al. (2002) conducted investigations to study the effect of cerumen impaction on hearing. Improvement in hearing test scores occurred in most subjects after cerumen removal, and in the Moore et al. study, mental status also improved.

Taste and Smell. The nurse can easily promote the sense of taste by using measures to enhance remaining taste perception. Good oral hygiene keeps the taste buds well hydrated. Taste perception is heightened if foods are well seasoned, differently textured, and eaten separately. Flavoured vinegar or lemon juice can add tartness to food. The nurse should always ask the client what foods are most taste appealing. If taste perception is improved, food intake and appetite will also improve.

Stimulation of the sense of smell with aromas such as brewing coffee, cooking garlic, and baking bread can heighten taste sensation. The client should avoid blending or mixing foods, because these actions make it difficult to identify tastes. Older adults should chew food thoroughly to allow more food to contact remaining taste buds.

Smell can be improved by strengthening pleasant olfactory stimulation. A client's environment can be made more pleasant with smells such as cologne, mild room deodorizers, fragrant flowers, and sachets, although the nurse must assess for allergies or sensitivities before using these items. The nurse should also encourage clients to sniff food before eating. When the nurse assists clients with eating or sets up a meal tray in a health care setting, naming the foods may help clients imagine the aromas.

The client is again an important resource. Certain aromas may actually cause clients to lose their appetites.

Removal of unpleasant odours improves the quality of a person's environment. The nurse should keep a client's room clean, empty bedpans or urinals, remove and dispose of soiled dressings, and keep bathroom doors closed.

Touch. Clients with reduced tactile sensation usually have the impairment over a limited portion of their bodies. The nurse can stimulate existing function by providing touch therapy. If the client is willing to be touched, hair brushing and combing, a back rub, and touching of the arms or shoulders are ways of increasing tactile contact. When sensation is reduced, a firm pressure may be necessary for the client to feel the nurse's hand. Turning and repositioning can also improve the quality of tactile sensation. When invasive procedures are being performed, it is important to use touch by holding the client's hands and keeping them warm and dry.

If a client is overly sensitive to tactile stimuli **(hyperesthesia),** the nurse must minimize irritating stimuli. Keeping bed linens wrinkle-free and protecting the skin from exposure to irritants are helpful measures. If the client has numbness and tingling or pain in the hands, as with carpal tunnel syndrome, special wrist splints may be worn to dorsiflex the wrist to relieve the nerve pressure. For those clients who use computers, there are special keyboards and wrist pads available to decrease the pressure on the median nerve and aid in relief of pain and promote healing.

Establishing Safe Environments. When sensory function becomes impaired, individuals become less secure and the world around them becomes smaller. Older adults in particular find it important to feel secure about their immediate environment. Feeling safe allows a person to function within the home and helps provide a sense of independence. The nurse can make recommendations to assist clients in making their living environment safer without restricting their independence. During a home visit or while completing an examination in the clinic, the nurse can offer several useful suggestions for home safety. The nature of the actual or potential sensory loss determines the safety precautions taken.

Adaptations for Visual Loss. Whether a visual alteration is a result of injury, eye disease, or the changes of aging, safety becomes a factor if visual acuity, peripheral vision, adaptation to the dark, and depth perception are permanently reduced. With reduced peripheral vision, a client cannot see panoramically because the outer visual field is less discrete. This creates a special hazard for driving or walking in crowded areas. Adults with reduced adaptation to the dark require three times as much light to see objects as they did as young adults. With reduced depth perception, a person cannot see how far away objects are located, making walking down stairs or over uneven surfaces dangerous.

> ***Safety Alert:*** To create a safe environment, the nurse begins by looking at the results of the home environment assessment (see chapter 33).

Driving is a particular safety hazard for anyone with visual alterations. Reduced peripheral vision may prevent a driver from seeing a car in an adjacent lane. Reduced adaptation to the dark and a sensitivity to glare makes driving at night a significant risk. Vision is a primary consideration for safety, but there are other factors as well. In the case of older adults, decreased reaction time, reduced hearing, and decreased strength in the legs and arms may further compromise driving skills. Safety tips for those who continue to drive include the following: drive in familiar areas, do not drive during rush hour, avoid major highways for local drives, use rear-view and side-view mirrors when changing lanes, avoid driving at dusk or night, go slow, but not too slow, keep the car in good working condition, and carry a cellular phone (but do not use while driving).

Visual alterations make conducting normal activities of daily living difficult for the person. Because of reduced depth perception, clients can trip on throw rugs, runners, or the edge of stairs. All flooring or carpeting should be kept in good repair. The nurse can advise the client to use low-pile carpeting. Thresholds between rooms should be level with the floor. Clutter should be removed to ensure clear pathways for walking. Furniture should be arranged so that a client can move about easily without fear of tripping or running into objects. Any stairwell should have a securely fastened handrail extending the full length of the stairs.

Front and back entrances to the home, work areas, and stairwells need to be properly lighted. The nurse encourages the client to have lights with higher wattage and wider illumination installed. Fluorescent lighting should be avoided. A light switch should be located at the top and bottom of stairwells. It is also important that lighting on the stairs does not cast shadows. The nurse should ensure that the client is able to clearly see the edge of each step, especially the first and last. When possible, steps inside and outside the home should be replaced with ramps.

When a client is unable to see visual contrasts, a number of interventions can be helpful. Sometimes settings on electrical appliances and equipment are only highlighted in black and white or shades of grey. Colour contrasts help to distinguish settings. Coloured tape, paint, nail enamel, or raised label dots can be used to colour-code appliance dials. Colour can also be useful to highlight the edge of stairs. Applying a broad strip of coloured tape at the stair edge can help a person better see the edges. The nurse can help the client tour the home to find opportunities for colour-coding. Telephones with large numbers may be helpful.

The nurse can also ensure that the client is able to self-administer medications safely. Labels on medication containers should be in large print. A friend or spouse should always be familiar with dosage schedules. People who are visually impaired may have some difficulty manipulating eyedroppers. Eye-drop dispensers are available and often allow older or visually impaired people to independently administer their own drops.

Adaptations for Reduced Hearing. Important environmental sounds (e.g., doorbells and alarm clocks) may best be heard if amplified or changed to a lower-pitched, buzzer-like sound. There are also sound lamps that respond with light to sounds such as doorbells, burglar alarms, smoke detectors, and babies crying. These lamps can be purchased from hearing aid dealers, telephone companies, and appliance stores. Signalling devices allow the deaf person greater independence. Family members or anyone who calls the client regularly should learn to let the phone ring for a longer period. Amplified receivers for telephones and telephone communications devices use a computer and printer to transfer words over the telephone for people who are hearing impaired. Both sender and receiver must have the special device to complete a call. A relay service also is available from most telephone companies. This is a phone operator service that translates voice to text and vice versa.

Adaptations for Reduced Olfaction. A reduced sensitivity to odours means that the client may be unable to smell leaking gas, a smouldering cigarette or fire, or tainted food. The client should use smoke and carbon monoxide detectors and other alternative precautions such as checking ashtrays or placing cigarette butts in water. A client can learn to check dates on food packages and the colour and texture of food. Leftovers should be kept in labelled containers with the preparation date. Pilot gas flames should be checked visually or professionally on a regular basis.

Adaptations for Reduced Tactile Sensation. When clients have reduced sensation in their extremities, they are at risk for injury from exposure to temperature extremes. The nurse should caution them on the use of water bottles or heating pads (see chapter 43). The temperature setting on the home water heater should be no higher than 48.8° C.

Promoting Communication. A sensory deficit can cause a person to feel isolated because of an inability to communicate with others. It is important for individuals to be able to interact with people whom they encounter. This problem can complicate a nurse's effectiveness in teaching clients information and skills. The nature of the sensory loss influences the methods and styles of communication that nurses can use (Box 44-9). Communication methods can also be taught to family members and significant others.

When beginning a conversation with a client who has a hearing deficit, it helps to reduce any background noise by turning off or lowering the volume of any TV, appliance, or radio. It is also helpful to have conversations in settings where there are better acoustics, which aid in controlling and muffling extraneous background noises. In a group setting, it is better to form a semicircle in front of the client so that the client can see who is speaking next; this helps foster group involvement. The client with a hearing impairment may be able to speak normally. However, the deaf client's inability to hear self-spoken words may cause serious speech alterations. Clients may use sign language (American Sign Language or Quebec Sign Language) or lip-reading, write with a pad and pencil, or learn to use a computer for communication. Special communication boards that contain common terms used in nursing care (e.g., *pain, bathroom, dizzy,* or *walk*) help clients express their needs.

Client instruction is one aspect of communication. There are teaching booklets available in large print for clients with visual loss. The client who is blind may require more frequent and detailed verbal descriptions of information. This is particularly true if there are no instructional booklets written in Braille. Visually impaired clients can learn by listening to audio tapes or the sound portion of a televised teaching session. Clients with hearing impairment may benefit from written instructional materials and visual teaching aids (e.g., posters and graphs). Demonstrations by the nurse are very useful. In a 1997 Supreme Court ruling, provinces must now pay for sign language interpreters for deaf clients when they receive medical treatment.

Acute Care. When clients enter acute care settings for therapeutic management of sensory deficits or as a result of traumatic injury, the nurse tries to maximize sensory function existing at the time. Safety is an obvious priority until the client's sensory status is either stabilized or improved. For example, clients with sensory deficits have a high risk for falls in the acute care environment. It also becomes very important to know the extent of any existing sensory impairment before the acute episode of illness so that the nurse can reinforce what the client already knows about self-care or plan for more instruction before and following discharge.

Clients in ICUs and those who are acutely ill are also at risk for developing sensory alterations. The constant activity within an ICU and the frequent monitoring of the acutely ill can easily cause clients to experience sensory overload. The nurse's main challenge becomes introducing regular, meaningful stimulation so that clients maintain a clearer perception of their immediate environment. Ongoing explanations help to orient the client to any new stimuli within the environment and reduce fear and disorientation.

Orientation to the Environment. The client with recent sensory impairment requires a complete orientation to the immediate environment. Reorientation to the institutional environment may be provided by ensuring that name tags on uniforms are visible, addressing the client by name, explaining where the client is (especially if clients are transported to different areas for treatment), and using conversational cues to time or location. The tendency for clients to become confused can be reduced by offering short and simple, repeated explanations and reassurance. Family members and visitors can also help orient clients to the hospital surroundings.

A client with serious visual impairment must feel comfortable in knowing the boundaries of the immediate environment. Normally, clients see physical boundaries within a room. The blind or severely visually impaired client must touch the boundaries or objects to gain a sense of their surroundings. The client needs to walk through a room and feel the walls to establish a sense of direction. The nurse can help by describing objects within the room, such as furniture or equipment. It takes time for the client to absorb a room's arrangement. The client may need to reorient again, with the nurse explaining the location of key items (e.g., call light, telephone, and chair). It also helps to always approach a blind client from the front to avoid startling him or her.

Box 44-9 Communication Methods

Clients With Aphasia

Listen to the client and wait for the client to communicate.
Do not shout or speak loudly (hearing loss is not the problem).
If the client has problems with comprehension, use simple, short questions and facial gestures to give additional clues.
Speak of things that are familiar to and of interest to the client.
If the client has problems speaking, ask questions that require simple yes or no answers or blinking of the eyes. Offer pictures or a communication board so that the client can point.
Give the client time to understand; be calm and patient.
Do not pressure or tire the client.
Avoid patronizing and childish phrases.

Clients With an Artificial Airway

Use pictures, objects, or word cards so that the client can point.
Offer a pad and pencil or Magic Slate for the client to write messages.
Do not shout or speak loudly.
Give the client time to write messages because these clients become easily fatigued.
Provide an artificial voice box (vibrator) for the client with a laryngectomy to use to speak words or phrases.

Clients With Hearing Impairment

Get the client's attention. Do not startle the client when entering the room. Do not approach a client from behind. Be sure the client knows you wish to speak.
Face the client and stand or sit on the same level. Be sure your face and lips are illuminated to promote lip-reading. Keep hands away from mouth.
If the client wears glasses, be sure they are clean so that your gestures and face can be seen.
If the client wears a hearing aid, make sure it is in place and working.
Speak slowly and articulate clearly. Older adults may take longer to process verbal messages.
Use a normal tone of voice and inflections of speech. Refrain from speaking with something in your mouth or with your hand in front of your mouth.
When you are not understood, rephrase rather than repeat the conversation.
Use visible expressions. Speak with your hands, your face, and your eyes.
Do not shout. Loud sounds are usually higher pitched and may impede hearing by accentuating vowel sounds and concealing consonants. If it is necessary to raise your voice, speak in lower tones.
Talk toward the client's best or unaffected ear. Use written information to enhance the spoken word.
Do not restrict a deaf client's hands. Never have IV lines in both of the client's hands if the preferred method of communication is sign language.
Avoid eating, chewing, or smoking while speaking.
Avoid speaking from another room or while walking away.

It is important to keep all objects in the same position and place. Simply moving a chair aside may create a dangerous safety hazard. The nurse should ask the client if any item should be arranged to make ambulation easier. Traffic patterns should be kept clear and use of furniture with sharp edges avoided. The client who is blind always needs extra time to perform tasks. The client needs a detailed description of how to perform an activity and will move slowly to remain safe.

Bedridden clients are at risk for sensory deprivation. Normally, movement gives an integrated awareness of the self through vestibular and tactile stimulation. A person's sensory perception is influenced by movement patterns. The limited movement of bed rest changes how a person interprets the environment; surroundings seem different, and objects seem to assume shapes different from normal. A person who is on bed rest requires routine stimulation through range-of-motion exercises, positioning, and participation in self-care activities (as appropriate). Comfort measures such as washing the face and hands and providing back rubs can help to improve the quality of stimulation and lessen the chance of sensory deprivation. Planning time to talk with clients is also essential. The nurse should explain unfamiliar environmental noises and sensations. A calm, unhurried approach during contact with a client gives the nurse quality time to help reorient and familiarize the client with care activities. The client who is well enough to read will benefit from a variety of reading materials.

Communication. The most common language disorder following a stroke is aphasia. As a result of a disruption in blood flow to the brain, the speech centre becomes damaged, altering a person's ability to use or understand spoken words. Depending on the type of aphasia, the inability to communicate can be frustrating and frightening. The nurse should initially establish very basic communication and recognize that aphasia does not indicate intellectual impairment or degeneration of personality. The nurse explains situations and treatments that are pertinent to the client because the client may be able to understand the spoken word (Ebersole & Hess, 2001). Because a stroke often causes partial or complete paralysis of one side of the client's body, an aphasic client may need special assistive devices. Communication boards have been developed for several levels of disability. Sensitive pressure switches, activated by the touch of an ear, nose, or chin, can control electronic communication boards (Ebersole & Hess, 2001). Clients who have had a stroke usually require referrals to speech therapists to develop appropriate rehabilitation plans.

In acute care hospitals or long-term care facilities, nurses often care for clients with artificial airways (see chapter 35). For example, an endotracheal tube is inserted into the oropharynx and down through the vocal cords of the larynx into the upper bronchus. The placement of the tube prevents a client from speaking. In this case, the nurse must use special communication methods to help the client express needs (see Box 44-9). The client may be completely alert and able to hear and see the nurse normally. Giving the client time to convey needs and requests is very important. Creative communication techniques (e.g., a communication board or a laptop computer) can be used.

Controlling Sensory Stimuli. The nurse controls excessive stimuli for clients at risk for sensory overload. Clients need time for rest and freedom from stress caused by frequent monitoring and repeated tests. The nurse can reduce sensory overload by organizing the care plan. Combining activities such as dressing changes, bathing, and vital sign measurement in one visit prevents the client from becoming overly fatigued. The client also needs scheduled time for rest and quiet. Planning for rest periods often requires co-operation from family, visitors, and health care colleagues. Coordination with laboratory and radiology departments may help minimize the number of procedures the client must undergo. The nurse may encourage a family member to sit quietly with a client or involve the client in an undemanding repetitive activity such as combing hair. Helping clients to become as mobile and independent as possible within prescribed limits provides meaningful stimulation.

When clients experience sensory overload or deprivation, the resultant behaviour can be difficult for family or friends to accept. The nurse encourages the family not to argue with or contradict the confused client, but to calmly explain location, identity, and time of day. Engaging the client in a normal discussion about familiar topics may assist in reorientation. Pre-arranging tests and procedures with departments reduces the amount of time needed for tests and examinations. Anticipating client needs such as voiding helps reduce uncomfortable stimuli.

The nurse can also try to control extraneous noise in and around the client's room. It may be necessary to ask a roommate to lower the volume on a television or to move the client to a quieter room. Equipment noise should be kept to a minimum. Bedside equipment not in use, such as suction and oxygen equipment, should be turned off. The nurse also avoids abrupt loud noises, such as dropping objects or causing the overbed table to adjust to the lowest level suddenly. Nursing staff should also try to control laughter or conversation at the nurses' station. Nurses should allow clients to close room doors.

When the client leaves an acute care setting for the home environment, nurses should communicate with colleagues in the home care setting about the interventions that helped the client adapt to sensory problems. Similarly, information describing the client's existing sensory deficits should be reported. Continuity of care is achieved when the client is required to make only minimal changes in the home setting.

Safety Measures. The client with recent visual impairment often requires help with walking. The presence of an eye patch, frequently instilled eye drops, or the swelling of eyelid structures following surgery are just a few factors that cause a client to need more assistance than usual. A sighted guide can give confidence to the visually impaired person and ensure safe mobility. Ebersole and Hess (2001) listed four suggestions for a sighted guide:

- Ask the blind client if he or she wants a "sighted guide."
- If assistance is accepted, offer an elbow or arm. Instruct the client to grasp your arm just above the elbow. If necessary, physically assist the person by guiding his or her hand to your arm or elbow.
- Go one-half step ahead and slightly to the side of the blind person. The shoulder of the person should be directly behind your shoulder. If the person is frail, place the hand on your forearm.
- Relax and walk at a comfortable pace. Warn the client when you approach doorways or narrow spaces.

While walking the client, describe the course of movement and ensure that obstacles have been removed. A client with visual impairment should never be left standing alone in an unfamiliar area. For clients who undergo eye surgery, it is important to teach family members techniques for assisting with ambulation.

A visually impaired client who spends considerable time in bed should have a call light nearby. Necessary objects should be placed in front of the client to prevent falls caused by reaching over the bedside. At night, a night light with a red bulb can help reduce falls. The red light reduces the time required for the eyes to adapt to the dark and allows the client to see well enough to function without keeping the regular light on (Matteson & McConnell, 1988).

Nurses may rely on clients in health care settings to report unusual sounds, such as a suction apparatus running improperly or an IV pump alarm. However, the client with a hearing loss may not hear such sounds and thus requires careful monitoring by the nurse. The client can also benefit from learning to use vision to discover sources of danger. The nurse should never restrict both arms of deaf or hearing-impaired clients (e.g., with restraints or IV lines), because they need their hands to communicate. The nurse should face the client when speaking, use simple sentences, and speak more slowly and in a normal volume (McConnell, 2002). It is wise to note on the intercom button and a client's chart if the client is deaf or blind. A client lacking the ability to speak cannot call out for assistance. Clients should have message boards or the call light easily available.

Clients with reduced tactile sensation risk injury when their conditions confine them to bed because they are unable to sense pressure on bony prominences or the need to change position. These clients rely on nurses for timely repositioning, moving tubes or devices the client may lie on, and turning to avoid skin breakdown. When the client cannot sense temperature normally, the nurse should be extra cautious when applying heat and cold therapies (see chapter 43) and preparing bathwater. The nurse must frequently check the condition of the client's skin.

Restorative and Continuing Care

Maintaining Healthy Lifestyles. After a client has experienced a sensory loss, it becomes important to understand the implications of the loss and to make the adjustments needed to continue a normal lifestyle. Sensory impairments need not prevent a person from leading an active, rewarding life. Many of the interventions applicable to health promotion, such as adapting the home environment, can be used after a client leaves an acute care setting.

Understanding Sensory Loss. Clients who have experienced a recent loss must understand how to adapt so that their living environments can be safe and appropriately stimulating. All family members should understand the way that a client's sensory impairment affects normal daily activities. Family and friends can be more supportive when they understand sensory deficits and the types of elements that worsen or lessen sensory problems. For example, family and friends need to learn how to communicate with the person with a hearing loss. There are resources within a community that provide information that assists clients with personal management needs. For example, the Canadian National Institute for the Blind, the Canadian Hearing Society, and the Canadian Association of the Deaf offer resource materials and product information.

Socialization. The ability to communicate is gratifying. It tests our intellect, opens opportunities, and allows us to exchange the feelings we have about others. When interactions are hindered by sensory alterations, a person can feel ineffective and lose self-esteem. If clients feel socially unaccepted, they will perceive sensory losses as seriously impairing the quality of life.

Interacting with others can become a burden for many clients with sensory alterations. Asking people to continuously repeat what they say is both embarrassing and exhausting for a client with hearing loss. Many clients lose the motivation to engage in social situations. As a person withdraws from interaction, a deep sense of loneliness can develop. The nurse can introduce therapies to reduce loneliness, particularly for older clients (Box 44-10). In addition, family members must learn to focus on a person's ability to interact rather than on the person's disability. It should not be assumed, for example, that a person who is hard of hearing does not wish to speak. A blind person can still enjoy a walk through a park with a companion describing the sights around them.

Promoting Self-Care. The ability to perform self-care is essential for self-esteem. Frequently, family members and nurses believe that sensorially impaired clients require assistance, when in fact they can help themselves. There are useful guidelines to assist clients with visual or tactile impairment so that they can help themselves with daily living activities. For example, a meal tray can be set up as though food on the tray and condiments and drinks around the tray are numbers on the face of a clock (Figure 44–5). The visually impaired client can easily become oriented to the items after the nurse or family member explains each item's location.

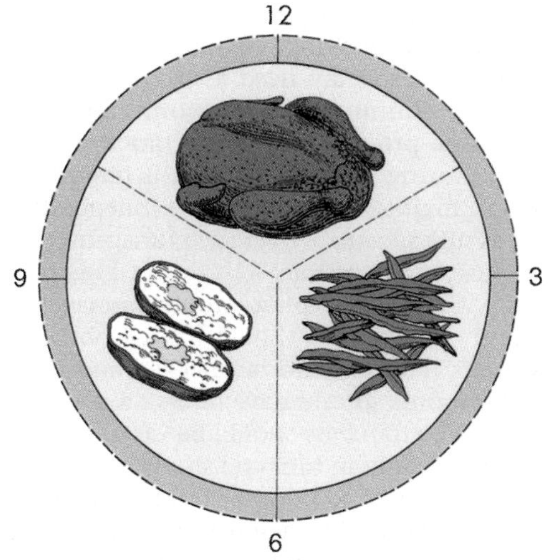

FIGURE 44–5 Location of food using the clock as a frame of reference.

Focus on Older Adults — Box 44-10

- Spend time with a person in silence or conversation.
- Use physical contact—holding a hand, embracing a shoulder—to convey caring.
- Recommend alterations in living arrangements if physical isolation is a factor.
- Assist older adults to keep in contact with people important to them.
- Obtain information about mutual help groups.
- Arrange for security escort services as needed.
- Suggest the client obtain a pet that is easy to care for.
- Link the client with religious organizations attuned to the social needs of older adults.

The client with visual problems needs assistance in reaching toilet facilities safely. Safety bars should be installed near the toilet. It may be helpful to have the bar a different colour than the wall for easier visibility. Towels should never be placed on safety bars, because they may interfere with a person's grasp. Toilet paper should be within easy reach. The use of colours, especially red, on drawers and other places helps promote functional independence (Swanson & Drury, 2001).

If tactile sense is diminished, the client can dress more easily with zippers or Velcro strips, pullover sweaters or blouses, and elasticized waists. If a client has partial paralysis and reduced sensation, the affected side should be dressed first. Family members responsible for selecting clothing for visually impaired clients should be encouraged to follow the client's preferences. Any sensory impairment has a significant influence on body image, and it is important for the client to feel well-groomed and attractive. A client may need assistance with basic grooming such as brushing, combing, and shampooing hair. The client also may need assistance with medication selection, clothing identification, and learning to manage routine procedures such as blood pressure and glucose monitoring (Cleary, 1995). It is important to assist clients in maintaining a degree of independence and in having as much control over the management of their care and lifestyle as possible.

Clients with proprioceptive problems may lose their balance easily. Floor mats should have rubberized, skid-proof bottoms. They should be checked and replaced as needed. Bathrooms should have non-skid surfaces in the tub and shower. Grab bars should be installed either vertically or horizontally in tubs and showers, depending on how the client is able to grasp or hold onto the bar. The nurse can instruct family members to supervise ambulation and sitting, make frequent checks to prevent falls, and caution the client against leaning forward.

NP Evaluation

Client Care. The client is the only one who will know if his or her sensory abilities are improved and which specific interventions or therapies are most successful (Figure 44–6). To evaluate the effectiveness of nursing interventions, the nurse uses critical thinking and makes comparisons with the baseline sensory assessment data to evaluate if sensory alterations have changed.

The nurse determines if the expected outcomes have been met. For example, the nurse uses evaluative data to determine whether care measures improve or at least maintain a client's ability to interact and function within the environment. The nature of a client's sensory alterations influences the way a nurse evaluates the outcome of care. For example, the nurse uses proper communication techniques with a client with a hearing deficit and then evaluates whether the client has gained the ability to hear or interact more effectively. When expected outcomes have not been achieved, there may be a need to change interventions or alter the client's environment. Family members may need to be involved in support of the client. The nurse may also consult with the multidisciplinary team (e.g., physician, occupation therapist, audiologist) for suggestions to achieve unmet needs. The client must be involved in all evaluation and planning activities.

If nursing care has been directed at improving sensory acuity, the nurse evaluates the integrity of the sensory organs and the client's ability to perceive stimuli. Any interventions designed to relieve problems associated with sensory alterations are evaluated on the basis of the client's ability to function normally without injury. When the nurse attempts to directly or indirectly (through education) alter the client's environment, evaluation is directed at observing whether the client makes environmental changes. When client teaching is designed to improve a client's sensory function, it is important to determine whether the client is following recommended therapies. Asking the client to explain or demonstrate self-care skills evaluates the level of learning that has occurred. It may be necessary to reinforce previous instruction if learning has not taken place.

Client Expectations. If the nurse has successfully developed a good relationship with a client and has a therapeutic plan of care, subtle behaviours often indicate the level of the client's satisfaction. The nurse may note that the client responds appropriately, such as by smiling. The nurse may observe that the client interacts more and is not asking to have information repeated. However, it is important for the nurse to ask the client if his or her sensory needs have been met. For example, the nurse may ask the client, "Can you tell me if you feel we have done all we can do to help improve your ability to hear?" If the client's expectations have not been met, then the nurse needs to spend more time understanding the client's needs and specific preferences. Working closely with the client and family will enable the nurse to redefine those expectations that can be realistically met within the limits of the client's condition and therapies. The interventions are effective when the client's goals and expectations have been met.

Key Concepts

- Sensory reception involves the stimulation of sensory nerve fibres and the transmission of impulses to higher centres within the brain.
- When sensory function is impaired, the sense of self is impaired and can affect the ability to socialize.
- Sensory deprivation results from an inadequate quality or quantity of sensory stimuli.
- Aging usually results in a gradual decline of acuity in all senses.
- Clients who are older, immobilized, or confined in isolated environments are at risk for sensory alterations.
- Assessment of a client's health promotion habits helps reveal risks for sensory impairment.
- An older adult often will not admit to a sensory loss.
- An assessment of hazards in the environment requires the nurse to tour living areas in the home and to look for conditions that increase the chances of accidents such as falls.
- The plan of care for clients with sensory alterations should include participation by family members. The extent of support from family members and significant others can influence the quality of sensory experiences.
- Clients with sensory deficits develop alternative ways of communicating that rely on other senses.
- Care of clients at risk for sensory deprivation includes introducing meaningful and pleasant stimuli for all senses.
- To prevent sensory overload, the nurse controls stimuli and orients the client to the environment.
- Clients with artificial airways can communicate effectively with communication boards, laptop computers, and written messages.

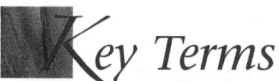

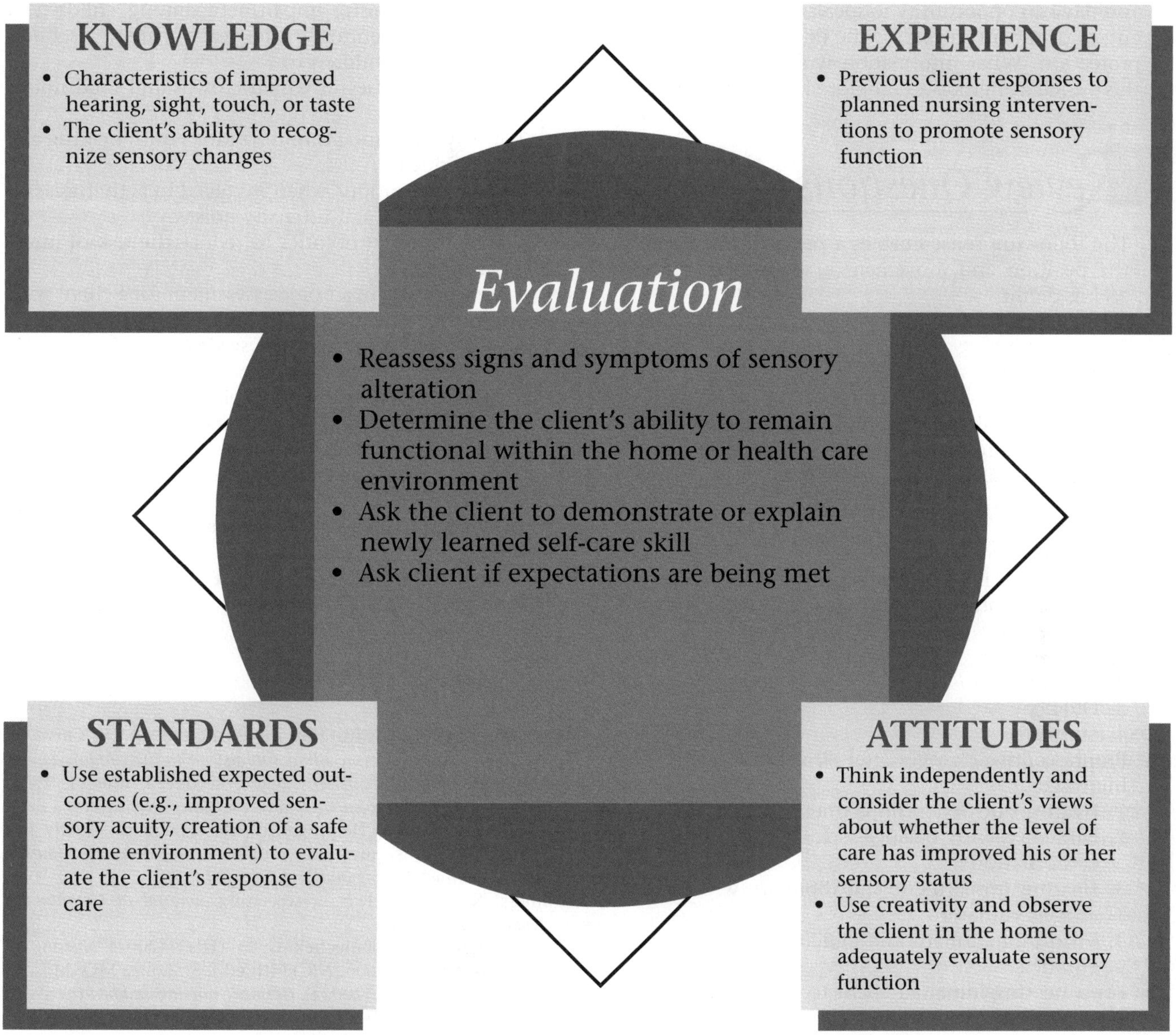
KNOWLEDGE
• Characteristics of improved hearing, sight, touch, or taste
• The client's ability to recognize sensory changes
EXPERIENCE
• Previous client responses to planned nursing interventions to promote sensory function
Evaluation
• Reassess signs and symptoms of sensory alteration
• Determine the client's ability to remain functional within the home or health care environment
• Ask the client to demonstrate or explain newly learned self-care skill
• Ask client if expectations are being met
STANDARDS
• Use established expected outcomes (e.g., improved sensory acuity, creation of a safe home environment) to evaluate the client's response to care
ATTITUDES
• Think independently and consider the client's views about whether the level of care has improved his or her sensory status
• Use creativity and observe the client in the home to adequately evaluate sensory function

FIGURE **44–6** Critical thinking model for sensory alterations evaluation.

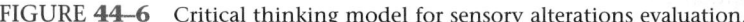

Key Terms

Aphasia, *p. 1582*
Audiologist, *p. 1577*
Auditory, *p. 1573*
Conductive hearing loss, *p. 1590*
Expressive aphasia, *p. 1582*
Global aphasia, *p. 1582*
Gustatory, *p. 1573*
Hyperesthesia, *p. 1591*
Kinesthetic, *p. 1573*
Olfactory, *p. 1573*
Otolaryngologist, *p. 1577*
Ototoxic, *p. 1583*
Proprioceptive, *p. 1577*
Receptive aphasia, *p. 1582*
Refractive error, *p. 1587*
Sensory deficit, *p. 1575*
Sensory deprivation, *p. 1575*
Stereognosis, *p. 1573*
Strabismus, *p. 1587*
Tactile, *p. 1573*
Tinnitus, *p. 1576*
Vertigo, *p. 1576*
Visual, *p. 1576*

Critical Thinking Exercises

1. Mr. Tully is a 54-year-old farmer who is having a physical examination. Overall, his health is good. His wife reports that over the past year, he has lost interest in being involved in social gatherings, is more irritable, and often has asked her to repeat what was said. Recently, he has complained of a constant buzzing in his ears. What assessment data are needed? What specific interventions may be needed?
2. Mrs. Marfell, 79 years old, is visiting the outpatient cardiac centre for a routine checkup. The nurse notices that the client needed help reading the physical forms. She also told the nurse she is having increased difficulty driving at night. What additional assessment data should the nurse gather from Mrs. Marfell?

3. You have an opportunity to speak with a group of parents and students regarding the importance of hearing protection. What information would you share with this varied age group to promote healthy hearing?

Review Questions

1. The following sense enables a person to be aware of the position and movement of body parts without seeing them:
   1. Auditory
   2. Kinesthetic
   3. Tactile
   4. Gustatory
2. A sense that allows a person to recognize an object's size, shape, and texture is
   1. Stereognosis
   2. Kinesthetic
   3. Tactile
   4. Gustatory
3. A client who is in constant pain and undergoes frequent monitoring of vital signs is at risk for experiencing sensory
   1. Deprivation
   2. Deficits
   3. Overload
   4. Stimuli
4. Proprioceptive changes after 60 years of age include increased
   1. Hearing and vision impairment
   2. Difficulty with balance, spatial orientation, and coordination
   3. Hearing impairment and difficulty with balance and coordination
   4. Vision impairment and difficulty with spatial orientation
5. For a hearing-impaired client to hear a spoken conversation, the nurse should
   1. Approach a client quietly from behind
   2. Face the client when speaking; use a louder-than-normal tone of voice
   3. Select a public area to have a spoken conversation
   4. Face the client when speaking; speak slower and in a normal volume
6. When obtaining a history of the client's hearing loss, the nurse should ask
   1. How long have you been deaf?
   2. Do you also have vision problems?
   3. Why don't you pay attention to me while I speak?
   4. How does your hearing now compare with your hearing a year ago?
7. A realistic goal for an older adult client who drives is to
   1. Drive very, very slowly all of the time
   2. Use rear-view and side-view mirrors when changing lanes
   3. Always drive at night to prevent sun glare
   4. Drive during rush hour when others are on the road
8. To prevent hearing impairment among children, a nursing intervention is to teach parents, schoolteachers, and children to
   1. Avoid activities in which crowds and loud noises occur
   2. Delay childhood immunizations until hearing can be verified
   3. Take precautions when involved in activities associated with high-intensity noises
   4. Administer antibiotics to reduce the risk of infections
9. A high-priority in a home assessment for a client with diminished olfaction is the inclusion of
   1. A low-temperature water setting
   2. Extra lighting in hallways
   3. Smoke detectors on all levels
   4. Amplified telephone receivers
10. Sensory deficits happen when a problem with sensory reception or perception occurs. As a result, clients may
    1. Withdraw socially to cope with the loss
    2. Rely solely on one sense
    3. Respond normally to stimuli
    4. Function safely within their environment

References

Canadian National Institute for the Blind. (2001). *The Canadian National Institute for the Blind submission to the commission on the future of health care in Canada.* Retrieved June 11, 2004, from *http://www.cnib.ca/eng/publications/health_care.htm*

Cleary, M. E. (1995). Helping the person who is visually impaired: Concerns, questions, remedies, and resources. *Journal of Ophthalmic Nursing and Technology, 14,* 205–211.

Demers, K. (2001). Hearing screening. *Journal of Gerontologic Nursing, 27*(11), 8–9.

Dochterman, J. M, & Bulechek, G. M. (Eds.). (2004). *Nursing interventions classification (NIC)* (4th ed.). St. Louis, MO: Mosby.

Ebersole, P., & Hess, P. (2001a). *Geriatric nursing and healthy aging.* St. Louis, MO: Mosby.

Ebersole, P., & Hess, P. (2001b). *Toward healthy aging: Human needs and nursing response* (5th ed.). St. Louis, MO: Mosby.

Elolia, R., & Stokes, J. (1998). Monograph series on aging-related diseases: XI. Glaucoma. *Chronic Diseases in Canada, 19*(4), 157–169.

Goldblum, K. (2004). Obtaining a complete and pertinent patient history. *Insight, 29*(2), 17–22.

Griest, S. E., & Bishop, P. M. (1998). Tinnitus as an early indicator of permanent hearing loss. *American Association of Occupational Health and Nursing Journal, 46,* 325–329.

Health Canada, Division of Aging and Seniors. (2002). *Barriers to senior's autonomy: Sensory loss—hearing. Aging Vignette #88.* Retrieved June 14, 2004, from *http://www.hc-sc.gc.ca/seniors-aines/pubs/vignette/vig88_e.htm*

Hensel, S. L. (2000). Sensory function. In A. G. Lueckenotte (Ed.), *Gerontologic nursing* (2nd ed., pp. 695–720). St. Louis, MO: Mosby.

Larsen, P. D., Hazen, S. E., & Martin, J. L. H. (1997). Assessment and management of sensory loss in elderly patients. *AORN Journal, 65,* 432–437.

Lewis-Cullinan, C., & Janken, J. K. (1990). Effect of cerumen removal on the hearing ability of geriatric patients. *Journal of Advanced Nursing, 15,* 594–600.

Lusk, S. L. (2002). Preventing noise-induced hearing loss. *Nursing Clinics of North America, 37,* 257–262.

Maas, M. L., et al. (Eds.). (2001). *Nursing care of older adults: Diagnoses, outcomes, & interventions.* St. Louis, MO: Mosby.

Maberley, D. (2000). *Diabetes and diabetic retinopathy in Canadian aboriginal peoples: A literature review.* British Columbia Centre for Epidemiologic and International Ophthalmology. Retrieved June 17, 2004, from *http://www.interchange.ubc.ca/bceio/DR_paper.html*

Matteson, M. A., & McConnell, E. S. (1988). *Gerontological nursing: Concepts and practice.* Philadelphia: W. B. Saunders.

McCance, K. L., & Huether, S. E. (2002). *Pathophysiology: The biologic basis for disease in adults and children* (4th ed.). St. Louis, MO: Mosby.

McConnell, E. A. (2002). How to converse with a hearing impaired patient. *Nursing, 32*(8), 20.

McCullagh, M. (2002). When hearing becomes a part of healing. *Orthopedic Nursing, 21*(4), 64–68.

Meadows, C. (2003). Assessment of the auditory system. In W. J. Phipps et al. (Eds.), *Medical-surgical nursing health and illness perspectives* (7th ed., pp. 1909–1918). St. Louis, MO: Mosby.

Moore, A. M., et al. (2002). Cerumen, hearing, and cognition in the elderly. *Journal of the American Medical Directors Association, 3,* 136–139.

Moorhead, S., Johnson, M., & Maas, M. (Eds.). (2004). *Nursing outcomes classification (NOC)* (3rd ed.). St. Louis, MO: Mosby.

Resnick, H. E., Fries, B. E., & Verbrugge, L. M. (1997). Windows to their world: The effects of sensory impairments on social engagement and activity time in nursing home residents. *Journal of Gerontology Series B-Psychological Sciences & Social Sciences, 52B*(3), S135–144.

Ruda, S. C. (2000). Nursing assessment: Musculoskeletal system. In S. M. Lewis, M. Heitkemper, & S. Dirksen (Eds.), *Medical-surgical nursing: Assessment and management of clinical problems* (5th ed., pp. 1745–1761). St. Louis, MO: Mosby.

Sherry, V. W. (2002). Taste alterations among patients with cancer. *Clinical Journal of Oncology Nursing, 6,* 105–106.

Smith, S. C. (2003). Problems of the eye. In W. J. Phipps et al. (Eds.), *Medical-surgical nursing health and illness perspectives* (7th ed., pp.1885–1908). St. Louis, MO: Mosby.

Smith, S. C., & Wilbur, M. E. (2004). Vision and hearing problems. In S. M. Lewis, M. Heitkemper, & S. Dirksen (Eds.), *Medical-surgical nursing: Assessment and management of clinical problems* (6th ed.), St. Louis, MO: Mosby.

Stout, D. & Kipling, G. D. (1999). *Emerging priorities for the health of First Nations and Inuit children and youth.* Retrieved June 22, 2004, from *http://www.hc-sc.gc.ca/fnihb-dgspni/fnihb/sppa/ppp/emerging_priorities_youth.htm*

Swanson, E. A., & Drury, J. (2001). Sensory/perceptual alterations. In M. L. Maas et al. (Eds.), *Nursing care of older adults: Diagnoses, outcomes and interventions.* St. Louis, MO: Mosby.

Tolson, D. (1997). Age-related hearing loss: A case for nursing intervention. *Journal of Advanced Nursing, 26,* 1150–1157.

Urden, L. A., Stacy, K. M., & Raugh, M. E. (2002). *Thelan's critical care nursing: Diagnosis and management* (4th ed.). St. Louis, MO: Mosby.

Vader, L. A. (1992). Vision and vision loss. *Nursing Clinics of North America, 27,* 705–714.

Weinstein, B. E. (1994). Age-related hearing loss: How to screen for it, and when to intervene. *Geriatrics, 49*(8), 40–47.

Wong, D. L., Perry, S. E., & Hockenberry, M. J. (2002). *Maternal child nursing care* (2nd ed.). St. Louis, MO: Mosby.

Recommended Web Sites

The Canadian Hearing Society:
http://www.chs.ca/

The Canadian Hearing Society provides services that prevent hearing loss and promote the independence of deaf and hearing-impaired people.

Canadian Helen Keller Centre:
http://www.chkc.org/main/index.htm

The Canadian Helen Keller Centre (CHKC) provides free training programs to individuals who are deaf-blind in order to help them increase and maintain their independence and autonomy, access services in the community, and decrease isolation. This Web site offers links relevant to deaf-blindness and communicating with people who are deaf-blind.

Canadian National Institution for the Blind:
http://www.cnib.ca/

The Canadian National Institution for the Blind (CNIB) is a national, voluntary organization that offers information and support to people with visual loss.

45

Care of Surgical Clients

Marilyn Schallom, RN, MSN, CCRN, CCNS
Frances Fothergill-Bourbonnais, RN, BScN, MN, PhD (Canadian author)

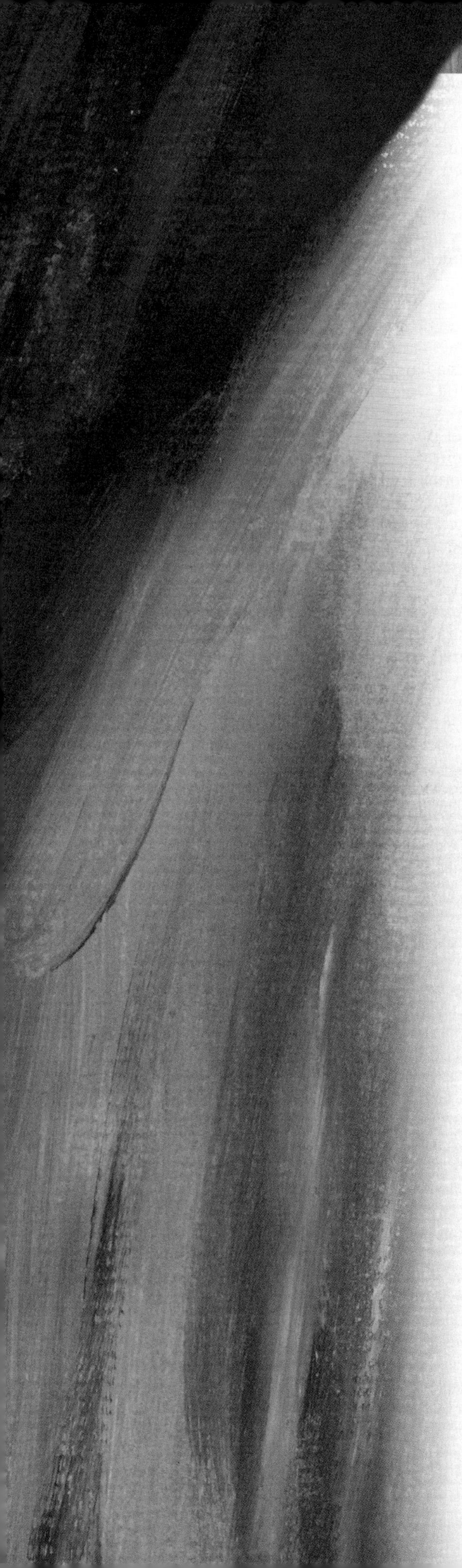

Objectives

Mastery of content in this chapter will enable the student to:

- Define the key terms listed.
- Understand the dimensions of perioperative nursing care.
- Differentiate between classifications of surgery and types of anaesthesia.
- List factors to include in the preoperative, intraoperative, and post-operative assessment of a surgical client.
- Demonstrate post-operative exercises: diaphragmatic breathing, coughing, incentive spirometer use, turning, and leg exercises.
- Design a preoperative teaching plan
- Prepare a client for surgery.
- Explain the nurse's role in the operating room.
- Describe the rationale for nursing interventions designed to prevent post-operative complications.
- Explain the difference and similarities in caring for ambulatory (outpatient) surgical clients versus inpatient surgical clients.

Perioperative nursing care includes nursing care given before (preoperative), during (intraoperative), and after surgery (post-operative). Surgical procedures take place in a hospital, although some minor surgical procedures can be done in a physician's office. Perioperative nursing is based on the nurse's understanding of several important principles, including the following:

- Excellence in perioperative practice
- Multidisciplinary teamwork
- Effective and therapeutic communication and collaboration with the client, the client's family, and the surgical team
- Effective and efficient client assessment and intervention in all phases
- Advocacy for the client and the client's family
- Understanding of cost containment

The nurse must practise surgical asepsis, thoroughly document care, and emphasize client safety in all phases of care. The nursing process provides a basis for perioperative nursing, with the nurse individualizing strategies so that the client has continuity of care from admission into the health care system through convalescence. Use of the nursing process can help the nurse anticipate needs and minimize complications.

The continuing care of the surgical client has shifted from hospital-based convalescence to home-based convalescence, with the client and family assuming increased responsibility. As the length of hospital stay decreases, the educational needs of the clients and their families increases. Clients are sent home with complex medical or surgical conditions that require education and follow-up. Effective teaching and early discharge planning are essential to ensure positive surgical outcomes (Gershenson et al., 1999).

History of Surgical Nursing

Surgery gave physicians the means to treat conditions that were difficult or impossible to manage purely by medicinal applications. Early surgeons had little knowledge of the principles of asepsis, and anaesthesia techniques were primitive and unsafe. Indeed, a surgeon's success was based on speed. The discovery of anaesthesia in the 1840s revolutionized surgery. Anaesthesia provided for the combination of analgesia, muscle relaxation, and amnesia, which allowed the surgical procedure time to be extended. The value of handwashing and the development of the germ theory in the 1860s (Pasteur) and 1870s (Koch) triggered the study of aseptic technique, which reduced post-operative infections and mortality. Joseph Lister (1827–1912) was associated with antisepsis or *listerism*. Initially, antisepsis was one way to protect clients from pathogens in the environment. Experimenting with carbolic acid dressings and continuous carbolic acid sprays during surgical operations, Lister described in 1867 a reduced incidence of gangrene and mortality. He eventually abandoned carbolic acid by 1890, when Koch demonstrated heat to be more effective than chemicals for sterilizing instruments (Porter, 1997). Therefore, Pasteur, Lister, and Koch helped provide a scientific basis to prevent infection in hospitals.

Asepsis and the techniques associated with it ensured that the client did not acquire in-hospital infections. The germ theory influenced nursing practice through the creation of carefully delineated steps in procedures in order to preserve asepsis (McPherson, 1996). Nurses working in the first operating rooms (ORs) cleaned the rooms and equipment, prepared the solutions and dressings, performed technical tasks such as obtaining supplies, administered anaesthetics as graduates, and occasionally accompanied the client to the surgical ward to deliver nursing care.

In Canada, OR nursing began to be part of training at the Montreal General Hospital in 1890 (Nurses life in the Montreal General Hospital, 1892). Toronto General Hospital, St Michael's Hospital in Toronto, and the Winnipeg General Hospital quickly followed. OR nursing in the early 20th century became organized around the therapeutic technology of surgery. Nurses ensured that the aseptic conditions of the surgical environment were maintained by all personnel and, along with physicians, became the first specialists in anaesthesia. As separate sterile ORs developed, OR nursing became a specialty separate from anaesthesia and surgical nursing. Two roles emerged: the sterile scrub nurse, who handled the instruments and passed them to the surgeon, and the circulating nurse, who ensured that all sponges used in operations were accounted for outside the client's body and that aseptic conditions were maintained. OR nursing was confined to activities in and around the OR. It became a well-established field of practice by the 1920s. During WW II, a proliferation of courses developed that focused on OR nursing. These post-diploma courses enabled nurses to then join the military, where they were highly valued to work with trauma clients (Toman, Heap, & Frize, in press).

The trend of including OR experience in training continued into the 1960s. However, during the 1970s, a change occurred in nursing education, whereby nurses were expected to acquire a broad knowledge base. As a result, many schools eliminated OR experience from the curriculum, believing that it only focused on manual skills (Sandelowski, 2000). What was not recognized was the role that OR nurses played in ensuring clients' comfort and safety and continuity of care before, during, and after surgery.

In 1956 in the United States, the Association of Operating Room Nurses (AORN) was formed. The organization developed standards of nursing practice that outlined the scope of responsibility of the perioperative nurse. AORN was the first nursing organization to develop structure, process, and outcome standards as defined by the American Nurses Association. Today, AORN has changed its name to the Association of Perioperative Registered Nurses; however, AORN is still used as their acronym. The organization continues to be a driving force for the practice of perioperative nursing and works closely with Canadian associations.

In Canada, the Operating Room Nurses Association of Canada (ORNAC) was founded in 1983. The mission of this professional nurses organization is to promote and advance excellence in preoperative client care and enhance professional and personal development of OR nurses. It sets the standards for Canadian perioperative nursing practice. Specifically, the ORNAC recommends that (a) perioperative nurses have a sound knowledge base in nursing, the sciences, and the humanities and use the nursing process for decision making; (b) administration and management provide direction, support, and resources as required; and (c) an assigned registered nurse (RN) is designated "in charge" and is responsible for direct supervision and provision of client care.

Opportunities exist in conjunction with the Canadian Nurses Association for RNs to obtain perioperative nursing certification. In addition to the National Association of Perianesthesia Nurses of Canada (NAPAN), there are provincial associations. For example, The Ontario Perianesthesia Nurses Association (OPANA) was founded in 1985 to represent all nurses involved in the care of a client in the post-anaesthetic phase. OPANA has developed standards of perianaesthesia nursing practice (2000) that are used by Ontario hospitals.

Ambulatory Surgery

A recent change in the surgery setting is the advent of **ambulatory surgery,** also referred to as outpatient surgery, short-stay surgery, or same-day surgery. These services are provided within a hospital setting. Over half of all surgical procedures are conducted on an outpatient basis and include ophthalmic, gastroenterological, gynecological, eye-ear-nose-throat, orthopedic, cosmetic/restorative, and general procedures. One-day surgery in which the client is admitted the day of surgery and observed overnight (23-hour admission) has also increased in popularity.

There are distinct benefits for the client who has ambulatory surgery. Anaesthesia drugs that metabolize rapidly with few after-effects allow shorter operative times. Nurses recognize the benefit of early post-operative ambulation and encourage clients to assume an active role in recovery. Ambulatory surgery also eliminates the need for hospital stays. This reduces the possibility of acquiring nosocomial infections, which occur when clients become colonized with bacteria found in the hospital setting. Procedures such as tumour biopsies and gallbladder removal **(cholecystectomy)** can now be done using laparoscopic procedures. Because of the small incision, a laparoscopic cholecystectomy involves only a few hours to a 24-hour hospital stay and a recovery period of a week. In contrast, a traditional open cholecystectomy involves a large abdominal incision. Clients require a 3- to 5-day hospitalization and at least a 4-week recovery period. Thus, many surgeons use laparoscopic procedures for a variety of surgical interventions, thereby decreasing the length of surgery, hospitalization, and associated costs.

Ambulatory surgery requires that nurses provide extensive pre- and post-operative teaching and assess the client's available support systems and readiness for self-care. As well, home care nurses must refer the client to appropriate community agencies. Discharge instructions and follow-up care are essential for preventing complications.

Scientific Knowledge Base

Classification of Surgery

The types of surgical procedures are classified according to seriousness, urgency, and purpose (Table 45-1). A procedure may fall into more than one classification. For example, surgical removal of a disfiguring scar is minor in seriousness, elective in urgency, and reconstructive in purpose. Frequently, the classes overlap. An urgent procedure is also considered major in seriousness. The same operation may be performed for different reasons on different clients. For example, a gastrectomy may be performed as an emergency procedure to resect a bleeding ulcer or as an urgent procedure to remove a cancerous growth. The classification indicates to the nurse the level of care a client might require. Hospitals have a system for prioritizing the booking of surgeries based on their classification.

The American Society of Anesthesiologists (ASA) assigns classification on the basis of a client's physiological condition independent of the proposed surgical procedure (Table 45-2). Intraoperative difficulties occur more frequently with clients who have a poor physical status classification (Rothrock, 2003). ASA physical status class I and class II clients are acceptable for ambulatory surgery. Clients in classes IV and V require inpatient surgery because they are at higher risk for complications (e.g., cardiac or pulmonary complications). The ASA classification system is used in Canadian hospitals.

Nursing Knowledge Base

Nursing knowledge offers important contributions for the care of the perioperative client. For example, nursing research has shown the benefit of preoperative education in promoting positive client outcomes following

Table 45-1 Classification for Surgical Procedures

Type	Description	Example
Seriousness		
Major	Involves extensive reconstruction or alteration in body parts; poses great risks to well-being	Coronary artery bypass, colon resection, removal of larynx, resection of lung lobe
Minor	Involves minimal alteration in body parts; often designed to correct deformities; involves minimal risks compared with major procedures	Cataract extraction, facial plastic surgery, tooth extraction
Urgency		
Elective	Is performed on basis of client's choice; is not essential and may not be necessary for health	Bunionectomy, facial plastic surgery, hernia repair, breast reconstruction
Urgent	Is necessary for client's health, may prevent additional problems from developing (e.g., tissue destruction or impaired organ function); not necessarily emergency	Excision of cancerous tumour, removal of gallbladder for stones, vascular repair for obstructed artery (e.g., coronary artery bypass)
Emergency	Must be done immediately to save life or preserve function of body part	Repair of perforated appendix, repair of traumatic amputation, control of internal hemorrhaging
Purpose		
Diagnostic	Is surgical exploration that allows physician to confirm diagnosis; may involve removal of tissue for further diagnostic testing	Exploratory laparotomy (incision into peritoneal cavity to inspect abdominal organs), breast mass biopsy
Ablative	Is excision or removal of diseased body part	Amputation, removal of appendix, cholecystectomy
Palliative	Relieves or reduces intensity of disease symptoms; will not produce cure	Colostomy, debridement of necrotic tissue, resection of nerve roots
Reconstructive/Restorative	Restores function or appearance to traumatized or malfunctioning tissues	Internal fixation of fractures, scar revision
Procurement for transplant	Removal of organs and/or tissues from a person pronounced brain dead for transplantation into another person	Kidney, heart, or liver transplant
Constructive	Restores function lost or reduced as result of congenital anomalies	Repair of cleft palate, closure of atrial septal defect in heart
Cosmetic	Performed to improve personal appearance	Blepharoplasty to correct eyelid deformities; rhinoplasty to reshape nose

Table 45-2 Physical Status (PS) Classification of the American Society of Anesthesiologists

Class	Description	Characteristics and Examples
PS-I	A normal healthy client	No physiological, biological, organic disturbance
PS-II	A client with a mild systemic disease	Disease imposes minimal restriction on activity; e.g., hypertension (HTN), obesity, diabetes mellitus
PS-III	A client with a severe systemic disease that limits activity but is not incapacitating	Disease limits activity; e.g., severe diabetes with systemic complications; history of myocardial infarction, angina pectoris, or poorly controlled HTN
PS-IV	A client with a severe systemic disease that is a constant threat to life	E.g., severe cardiac, pulmonary, renal, hepatic, or endocrine dysfunction
PS-V	A moribund client who is not expected to survive without the operation	Surgery is done as a last recourse or resuscitative effort; e.g., major multi-system or cerebral trauma, ruptured aneurysm, or large pulmonary embolus
PS-VI	A client declared brain dead whose organs are being removed for donor purpose	

Note: The addition of an "E" to the physical status class indicates emergency surgery, such as PS-IE, PS-IIE, and so on.

Data from *Alexander's Care of the Patient in Surgery* (12th ed., p. 223), by J. C. Rothrock, 2003, St. Louis, MO: Mosby; and *Surgery: Scientific Principles and Practice* (2nd ed., p. 446), by L. Greenfield et al., 1997, Philadelphia: Lippincott-Raven.

surgery. Structured preoperative teaching that includes the AORN standards (2004) and return demonstration of post-operative exercises has been shown to improve outcomes such as pain severity, pulmonary function, length of stay, and clients' level of anxiety.

There is also significant evidence-based knowledge available for proper wound care interventions. Nursing research has contributed to what is known about the characteristics of wound healing and the types of applications most likely to be beneficial (see chapter 43).

Within the OR setting, knowledge has improved the standards for infection control and client safety. For example, surgical hand scrubs (see chapter 29) can now be performed without the use of brushes as a result of research that has shown the efficacy of alcohol-based hand antiseptics in reducing bacteria on the skin (Hobson et al., 1998; Larson et al., 1990). Evidence-based practice changes within the OR improve the quality of care for surgical clients and ultimately improve client outcomes.

Critical Thinking

Successful critical thinking requires a synthesis of knowledge, information gathered from clients, experience, critical thinking attitudes, and intellectual and professional standards. Clinical judgments require the nurse to anticipate the information necessary, analyze the data, and make decisions regarding client care. A client's condition is always changing. During assessment (Figure 45–1), the nurse must consider all of the elements that build toward making appropriate nursing diagnoses.

In the case of caring for the perioperative client, the nurse makes clinical care decisions by integrating knowledge of anatomy, physiology, pathophysiology, and the surgical stress response with previous experiences in caring for surgical clients and information gathered from the client, such as medical and surgical history, potential for surgical risk, and coping resources. The use of critical thinking attitudes such as perseverance is needed to develop a plan of care that provides successful perioperative care (e.g., airway management, infection control, pain management, and discharge planning). Professional standards and guidelines developed by, for example, the AORN, NAPAN, and ORNAC, provide valuable information for perioperative management and evaluation of process and outcomes. However, the nurse should review guidelines within the context of new emerging evidence-based practice and agency policies.

The Nursing Process in the Preoperative Surgical Phase

Surgical clients enter the health care setting in different stages of health. A client may enter the hospital on a predetermined day feeling relatively healthy and prepared to face elective surgery. In contrast, a victim of a motor vehicle collision may face emergency surgery with no time to prepare. The ability to establish rapport and maintain a professional relationship with the client is an essential component of the preoperative phase. Nurses must do this quickly but compassionately and effectively.

The surgical client may undergo tests and procedures to confirm or rule out problems requiring surgery. Most testing is performed before the day of surgery. Usually clients scheduled for ambulatory surgery have tests done several days before surgery. Testing done the day of surgery is usually limited to such tests as glucose monitoring for the client with diabetes. Nurses must be familiar with the tests, their purpose, and how to monitor results.

The client meets many health care personnel, including surgeons, anaesthesiologists, physiotherapists, and

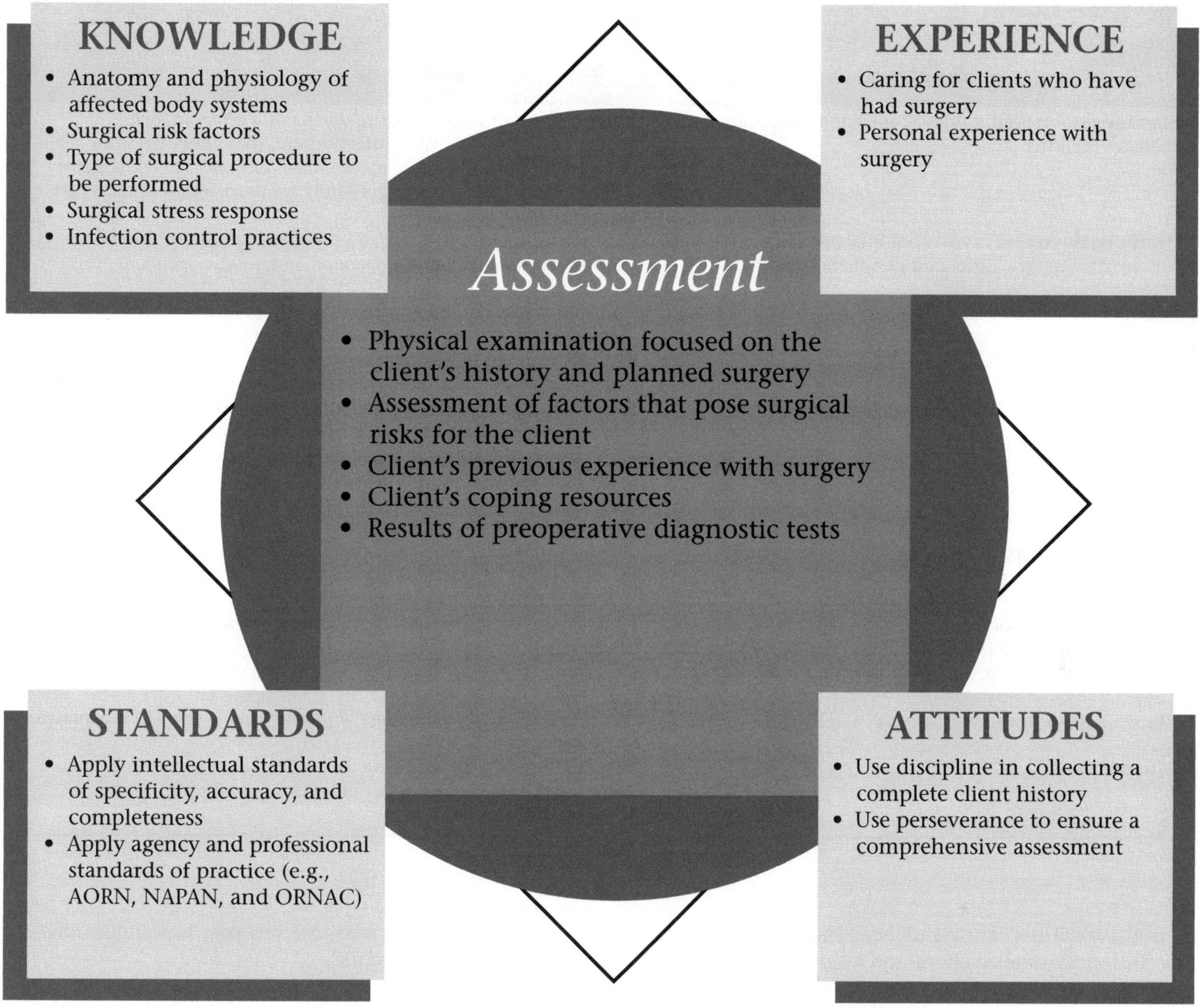
KNOWLEDGE
• Anatomy and physiology of affected body systems
• Surgical risk factors
• Type of surgical procedure to be performed
• Surgical stress response
• Infection control practices
EXPERIENCE
• Caring for clients who have had surgery
• Personal experience with surgery
Assessment
• Physical examination focused on the client's history and planned surgery
• Assessment of factors that pose surgical risks for the client
• Client's previous experience with surgery
• Client's coping resources
• Results of preoperative diagnostic tests
STANDARDS
• Apply intellectual standards of specificity, accuracy, and completeness
• Apply agency and professional standards of practice (e.g., AORN, NAPAN, and ORNAC)
ATTITUDES
• Use discipline in collecting a complete client history
• Use perseverance to ensure a comprehensive assessment

FIGURE **45–1** Critical thinking model for surgical client assessment.

nurses. All play a role in the client's care and recovery. Family members attempt to provide support through their presence but face many of the same stressors as the client. The nurse must effectively communicate with the client and family because the nurse-client relationship is the foundation of care (see chapter 14). The nurse assesses the client's physical, emotional, and spiritual well-being and cultural heritage; recognizes the degree of surgical risk; coordinates diagnostic tests; identifies nursing diagnoses and nursing interventions; and establishes outcomes in collaboration with the client and the client's family. Pertinent data and the plan of care are communicated among the surgical team.

NP Assessment

The aim of the assessment of the surgical client is to establish the client's baseline preoperative function to assist in preventing and recognizing possible post-operative complications. Assessment of the surgical client can be extensive. Ambulatory and same-day surgical programs require that client data be completed several days in advance. A multidisciplinary team approach is essential. Clients are admitted only hours before the surgical event; thus, nurses must organize and verify data obtained preoperatively to implement a perioperative plan of care. This occurs not only with the ambulatory care client, but also with the client who will require a more prolonged hospital stay. Increasingly, clients are admitted the day of surgery, even for such major procedures as open heart and bowel surgery.

The majority of assessments begin in the physician's office or a preadmission clinic before admission for surgery. Clients may answer a self-report inventory and a nurse may complete an initial physical examination, draw or complete laboratory tests, begin teaching, identify potential risks, answer questions, and initiate paperwork. This streamlines the care required by the client on the day of surgery. Nurses in the immediate preoperative

Table 45-3 Medical Conditions That Increase the Risks of Surgery

Type of Condition	Reason for Risk
Bleeding disorders (thrombocytopenia, hemophilia)	Increase risk of hemorrhaging during and after surgery.
Diabetes mellitus	Increases susceptibility to infection and may impair wound healing from altered glucose metabolism and associated circulatory impairment. Stress of surgery may cause increases in blood glucose levels.
Heart disease (recent myocardial infarction, dysrhythmias, congestive heart failure) and peripheral vascular disease	Stress of surgery causes increased demands on myocardium to maintain cardiac output. General anaesthetic agents depress cardiac function.
Obstructive sleep apnea	Administration of opioids increases risk of airway obstruction post-operatively. Clients will desaturate as revealed by drop in O_2 saturation by pulse oximetry.
Upper respiratory infection	Increases risk of respiratory complications during anaesthesia (e.g., pneumonia and spasm of laryngeal muscles).
Liver disease	Alters metabolism and elimination of drugs administered during surgery and impairs wound healing and clotting time because of alterations in protein metabolism.
Fever	Predisposes client to fluid and electrolyte imbalances and may indicate underlying infection.
Chronic respiratory disease (emphysema, bronchitis, asthma)	Reduces client's means to compensate for acid-base alterations (see chapter 36). Anaesthetic agents reduce respiratory function, increasing risk for severe hypoventilation.
Immunological disorders (leukemia, acquired immunodeficiency syndrome [AIDS], bone marrow depression, and use of chemotherapeutic drugs or immunosuppressive agents)	Increases risk of infection and delayed wound healing after surgery.
Abuse of street drugs	People abusing drugs may have underlying disease (HIV/hepatitis), which affects healing.
Chronic pain	Regular use of pain medications may result in higher tolerance. Increased doses of analgesics may be required to achieve post-operative pain control.

period assess the client's understanding of previous teaching and individualize client and family care.

The physician performs a comprehensive history and physical examination with follow-up by the preadmission nurse. In this case, the nurse needs to review assessments and testing already completed and to highlight significant information (e.g., the client being on diuretics). The nurse focuses on key measurements for all body systems to ensure that no obvious problems are overlooked and that the client has understood education previously provided. Even though the surgeon will screen the client before scheduling surgery, preoperative assessment occasionally reveals an abnormality that delays or cancels surgery. For example, the client may have a cough and low-grade fever on admission. This may indicate the onset of infection, and the surgeon will need to be notified immediately.

Nursing Health History. The nurse conducts an initial interview to collect a client history similar to that described in chapter 28. If a client is unable to relate all of the necessary information, the nurse relies on family members as resources.

Medical History. A review of the client's medical history should include past illnesses and the primary reason for currently seeking medical care. The client's current medical record and medical records from past hospitalizations are excellent sources of data.

Pre-existing illnesses can influence the choice of anaesthetic agents used and the client's ability to tolerate surgery and reach full recovery (Table 45-3). Candidates for ambulatory surgery must be carefully screened for medical conditions that may increase the risk for complications during or after surgery. For example, a client who has a history of congestive heart failure may experience a further decline in cardiac function both intraoperatively and post-operatively. Intravenous (IV) fluids may need to be administered at a slower rate, or a diuretic may need to be given if blood transfusions are required.

Risk Factors. Various conditions and factors increase a person's risk in surgery. Knowledge of risk factors enables the nurse to take necessary precautions in planning care.

Age. Very young clients are at risk during surgery because of immature physiological status. During surgery, nurses and physicians are especially concerned with maintaining an infant's normal body temperature. The infant's shivering reflex is underdeveloped, and often wide temperature variations occur. Anaesthesia adds to the risk because anaesthetics can cause vasodilation and heat loss.

During surgery, an infant has difficulty maintaining a normal circulatory blood volume. The total blood volume of an infant is considerably less than that of an older child or an adult. Even a small amount of blood loss can be serious. A reduced circulatory volume makes it difficult for the infant to respond to increased oxygen demands during surgery. In addition, the infant is highly susceptible to complications associated with dehydration. However, if blood or fluids are replaced too quickly, overhydration may occur. Other important and unique aspects of a child's surgical care include airway management, treatment of seizures, management of temperature alterations, identification and treatment of emergence delirium and delayed emergence from anaesthesia, treatment of pain and agitation, and availability of age-appropriate emergency equipment and medications.

Older clients are also at risk for complications. With advancing age, a client's physical capacity to adapt to the stress of surgery is hampered because of deterioration in certain body functions. Despite the risk, the majority of clients undergoing surgery are older adults. Table 45-4 summarizes physiological factors that place older clients at risk during surgery.

Nutrition. Normal tissue repair and resistance to infection depend on adequate nutrients. Surgery intensifies this need. After surgery, a client requires at least 1500 kcal/day to maintain energy reserves. Increased protein, vitamins A and C, and zinc facilitate wound healing (see chapters 39 and 43). A malnourished client is prone to poor tolerance to anaesthesia, negative nitrogen balance, delayed blood clotting mechanisms, infection, poor wound healing, and the potential for multiple organ failure. If a client has elective surgery, attempts to correct nutritional imbalances before surgery should be made. However, if a malnourished client must undergo an emergency procedure, efforts to restore nutrients occur after surgery.

Obesity. Obesity increases surgical risk by reducing respiratory and cardiac functions. Hypertension, coronary artery disease, diabetes mellitus, and congestive heart failure are common in the **bariatric** (obese) population. Embolus, **atelectasis** (partial or total collapse of the alveoli), and pneumonia are also more frequent post-operative complications in the obese client. The client may have difficulty resuming normal physical activity after surgery. The obese client is susceptible to poor wound healing and wound infection because of the structure of fatty tissue, which contains a poor blood supply. This slows delivery of essential nutrients, antibodies, and enzymes needed for wound healing (see chapter 43). It is often difficult to close the surgical wound of an obese client because of the thick adipose layer. An obese client is also at risk for **dehiscence** (opening of the suture line).

Immunocompetence. For the client with cancer, radiation therapy may be given preoperatively to reduce the size of the cancerous tumour so that it can be removed surgically. Radiation has some unavoidable effects on normal tissue, such as excess thinning of skin layers, destruction of collagen, and impaired vascularization of tissue. Ideally, the surgeon waits to perform surgery 4 to 6 weeks after completion of radiation treatments. Otherwise, the client may face serious wound-healing problems. In addition, chemotherapeutic drugs used for cancer treatment, immunosuppressive medications used to prevent rejection after organ transplantation, and steroids used to treat a variety of inflammatory conditions increase the risk for infection.

Fluid and Electrolyte Imbalance. The body responds to surgery as a form of trauma. As a result of the adrenocortical stress response, sodium and water are retained and potassium is lost within the first 2 to 5 days after surgery. The severity of the stress response influences the degree of fluid and electrolyte imbalance. The more extensive the surgery, the greater is the stress response. A client who is hypovolemic or who has serious preoperative electrolyte alterations is at significant risk during and after surgery. For example, an excess or depletion of potassium increases the chance of dysrhythmia during or after surgery. If the client has pre-existing renal, gastrointestinal, or cardiovascular abnormalities, the risk of fluid and electrolyte alterations is even greater.

Pregnancy. The perioperative plan of care must address the needs of the mother and the developing fetus. Surgery is performed on the pregnant client only on an emergency basis. All major systems of the mother are affected during pregnancy. For example, cardiac output significantly increases, as does respiratory tidal volume to accommodate the increase in metabolic rate. Gastrointestinal motility decreases, hormone levels increase, and energy levels decrease with advancing pregnancy. Laboratory and hemodynamic values change. Fibrinogen levels increase, making pregnant clients more susceptible to the development of deep vein thrombosis because of increased coagulability. Hemoglobin and hematocrit levels decrease, mostly as a result of the effects of hemodilution (increased circulating volume). The white blood cell (WBC) count is elevated when the woman is near term and postpartum without the presence of infection. However, infection must always be ruled out in the presence of an elevated WBC. General anaesthesia is administered with caution because of the increased risk of fetal death and preterm labour. Psychological considerations for mother and family are essential.

Previous Surgeries. A client's past experience with surgery can influence physical and psychological responses to a procedure. The previous type of surgery, level of discomfort, extent of disability, and overall level of care provided are factors the nurse asks the client to recall. The nurse addresses any complications that the client experienced. It is also important to assess clients for motion sickness, nausea, and vomiting with previous surgeries (Gan, 2002; Tramer, 2001). These factors increase the risk for aspiration. Prior anaesthesia records may be a useful source of information if other previous problems occurred. This information helps the nurse anticipate the client's preoperative and post-operative needs.

Previous surgery may also influence the level of physical care required after a surgical procedure. For example, a client who has had a previous thoracotomy for resection of a lung lobe has a greater risk for post-operative pulmonary complications than a client with intact normal lungs.

Table 45-4 Physiological Factors That Place the Older Adult at Risk During Surgery

Alterations	Risks	Nursing Implications
Cardiovascular System		
Degenerative change in myocardium and valves	Reduced cardiac reserve	Assess baseline vital signs. Recognize the longer time period required for heart rate to return to normal following stress on the heart and evaluate the occurrence of tachycardia accordingly (Eliopoulos, 2001).
Rigidity of arterial walls and reduction in sympathetic and parasympathetic innervation to heart	Alterations predispose client to post-operative hemorrhage and rise in systolic and diastolic blood pressure	Maintain adequate fluid balance to minimize stress to the heart. Ensure blood pressure level is adequate to meet circulatory demands.
Increase in calcium and cholesterol deposits within small arteries; thickened arterial walls	Predispose client to clot formation in lower extremities	Instruct client on techniques for performing leg exercises and proper turning. Apply elastic stockings, sequential compression devices.
Integumentary System		
Decreased subcutaneous tissue and increased fragility of skin	Prone to pressure ulcers and skin tears	Assess skin every 4 hours; pad all bony prominences during surgery. Turn or reposition at least every 2 hours (see chapter 43).
Pulmonary System		
Rib cage stiffened and reduced in size	Reduced vital capacity	Instruct client on proper technique for coughing, deep breathing, and use of spirometer.
Reduced range of movement in diaphragm	Residual capacity (volume of air left in lung after normal breath) increases, reducing amount of new air brought into lungs with each inspiration	When possible, have client ambulate and sit in chair frequently.
Stiffened lung tissue and enlarged air spaces	Alteration reduces blood oxygenation	Obtain baseline oxygen saturation; measure as indicated throughout perioperative period.
Renal System		
Reduced blood flow to kidneys	Increased risk of shock when blood loss occurs.	For clients hospitalized before surgery, determine baseline urinary output for 24 hours.
Reduced glomerular filtration rate and excretory times	Limits ability to eliminate drugs or toxic substances.	Assess for adverse response to drugs.
Reduced bladder capacity	Voiding frequency increases, and larger amount of urine stays in bladder after voiding. Sensation of need to void may not occur until bladder is filled.	Instruct client to notify nurse immediately when sensation of bladder fullness develops. Keep call light and bedpan within easy reach. Toilet every 2 hours or more frequently if indicated.
Neurological System		
Sensory losses, including reduced tactile sense	Decreased ability to respond to early warning signs of surgical complications.	Inspect bony prominences for signs of pressure that client may not sense. Orient client to surrounding environment. Observe for nonverbal signs of pain.
Decreased reaction time	Confusion after anaesthesia	Allow adequate time to respond, process information, and perform tasks. Institute fall precautions (RNAO, 2002b).
Metabolic System		
Lower basal metabolic rate	Reduced total oxygen consumption.	Ensure adequate nutritional intake when diet is resumed, but avoid intake of excess calories.
Reduced number of red blood cells and hemoglobin levels	Ability to carry adequate oxygen to tissues is reduced.	Administer necessary blood products. Monitor blood test results.
Change in total amounts of body potassium and water volume	Greater risk for fluid or electrolyte imbalance occurs.	Monitor electrolyte levels and supplement as necessary.
Impaired thermoregulatory mechanisms	Cold operating rooms; exposure of body parts during procedure, IV fluids, medications.	Ensure careful, close monitoring of client temperature; provide warm blankets; monitor cardiac function; warm IV fluids.

Table 45-5 Drugs With Special Implications for the Surgical Client

Drug Class	Effects During Surgery
Antibiotics	Antibiotics can potentiate action of anaesthetic agents. For example, if taken within 2 weeks before surgery, amino-glycosides (gentamicin, tobramycin, neomycin) may cause mild respiratory depression from depressed neuromuscular transmission.
Antidysrhythmics	Antidysrhythmics can reduce cardiac contractility and impair cardiac conduction during anaesthesia.
Anticoagulants	Anticoagulants alter normal clotting factors and thus increase risk of hemorrhaging. They should be discontinued at least 48 hours before surgery. Aspirin is a commonly used medication that can alter clotting mechanisms.
Anticonvulsants	Long-term use of certain anticonvulsants (e.g., phenytoin [Dilantin] and phenobarbital) can alter metabolism of anaesthetic agents.
Antihypertensives	Antihypertensives may interact with anaesthetic agents to cause bradycardia, hypotension, and impaired circulation. They may inhibit synthesis and storage of norepinephrine in sympathetic nerve endings.
Corticosteroids	With prolonged use, corticosteroids cause adrenal atrophy, which reduces the body's ability to withstand stress. Before and during surgery, dosages may be temporarily increased.
Insulin	Diabetic clients' need for insulin after surgery is altered. Stress response and IV administration of glucose solutions can increase dosage requirements after surgery. Decreased nutritional intake can decrease dosage requirements.
Diuretics	Diuretics potentiate electrolyte imbalances (particularly potassium) after surgery.
Nonsteroidal anti-inflammatory drugs (NSAIDs)	NSAIDs inhibit platelet aggregation and may prolong bleeding time, increasing susceptibility to post-operative bleeding.
Herbal therapies: ginger, gingko, ginseng	Some herbal therapies have the ability to affect platelet activity and increase susceptibility to post-operative bleeding. Ginseng may increase hypoglycemia with insulin therapy.

Perceptions and Understanding of Surgery. The surgical experience affects not only the client, but the entire family. The nurse therefore must prepare both the client and the family for the surgical experience. Identification of a client's and family's knowledge, expectations, and perceptions allows the nurse to plan teaching and to provide individualized emotional support measures.

Each client feels fearful when entering the surgical setting. Some fears are due to past hospital experiences, warnings from friends and family, or lack of knowledge. The nurse assesses the client's understanding of the planned surgery and its implications. The nurse might ask questions such as, "Tell me what you think will happen before and after surgery" or "Explain what you know about surgery." If a client is misinformed or unaware of the reason for surgery, the nurse must confer with the physician before the client is sent to the surgical suite. The nurse also determines if further explanations are needed related to routine preoperative and post-operative procedures. When a client is well prepared and knows what to expect, the nurse reinforces the client's knowledge and maintains accuracy and consistency.

Medication History. If a client regularly uses prescription or over-the-counter medications, the surgeon or anaesthesiologist may temporarily discontinue the drugs before surgery or adjust the dosages. Certain medications have special implications for the surgical client, creating greater risks for complications or interacting with anaesthetic agents (Table 45-5). For example, the nurse instructs clients in a preadmission unit to ask the physician if usual medications should be taken the morning of surgery. Clients should also be asked if any herbal preparations are used, because many clients do not view herbs as medications and may omit them from their medication history (see chapter 31). Certain herbs may interfere with the action of other medications (the pharmacist must be consulted). Nurses in the preadmission clinic determine if the client is taking any herbal medications. For hospitalized clients, prescription drugs taken preoperatively are automatically discontinued post-operatively unless the physician reorders them. It is important for the nurse to be aware of the client's previous medications that likely need to be resumed post-operatively (e.g., antihypertensives).

Allergies. The nurse must assess for allergies to drugs that may be given during a phase of the surgical experience. In addition, it is also critical to assess for latex, food, and contact allergies (e.g., to tape, ointments, or solutions). A client may be too young or have too few exposures to drugs to know if he or she has allergies. The type of allergic response is very important to assess. Allergies need to be delineated from unpleasant side effects. For example, the client may state that codeine causes nausea (a side effect), or it may cause hypotension and confusion (an allergy). When asking a client about allergies, realize that the term *allergy* can be confusing for some clients. Asking a client if he or she has ever "had a problem with a medication or substance" may be another helpful approach to questioning.

It is critical that the client specifically be asked about latex allergies because a latex-free environment must be provided for clients with latex allergies. The nurse ensures that a list of the client's allergies is noted appropriately in the client's chart and/or the hospital computer system, as well as any other places designated by institutional policy, such as an allergy band.

Smoking Habits. The client who smokes is at greater risk for post-operative pulmonary complications than a client who does not. The chronic smoker already has an increased amount and thickness of mucous secretions in the lungs. General anaesthetics increase airway irritation and stimulate pulmonary secretions, which are retained as a result of reduction in ciliary activity during anaesthesia. After surgery, the client who smokes has greater difficulty clearing the airways of mucous secretions and needs education on the importance of post-operative deep breathing and coughing (see chapter 35).

Alcohol Ingestion and Substance Use and Abuse. Habitual use of alcohol and illegal drugs predisposes the client to adverse reactions to anaesthetic agents. The client may also experience a cross-tolerance to anaesthetic agents, necessitating higher-than-normal doses. In addition, the physician may need to increase post-operative dosages of analgesics. Clients with a history of excessive alcohol ingestion may also be malnourished, which may contribute to delayed wound healing. These clients are also at risk for liver disease, portal hypertension, and esophageal varices (predisposing the client to bleeding disorders). The client who habitually uses alcohol and is required to remain in the hospital longer than 24 hours is also at risk for acute alcohol withdrawal and its more severe form, delirium tremens.

Family Support. It is important for the nurse to determine the extent of the client's support from family members or friends. Because blood relations do not always define family, it is best to have the client identify his or her source of support (see chapter 16). Surgery often results in temporary or permanent disability that requires added assistance during recovery. The client usually cannot immediately assume the same level of physical activity enjoyed prior to surgery. Often a client returns home with dressings to change or exercises to perform. With ambulatory surgery, clients and families assume responsibility for post-operative care. The family is an important resource for the client with physical limitations and provides the emotional support needed to motivate the client to return to a previous state of health. The family may better remember preoperative and post-operative teaching as well.

The nurse should ask if family members or friends could provide support. The client may want someone else present when the nurse provides instructions or explanations. Family presence should be encouraged when feasible, especially for clients in the ambulatory setting. Often a family member can become the client's coach, offering valuable support during the post-operative period, when the client's participation in care is vital.

Occupation. Surgery may result in physical alterations that hinder or prevent a person from returning to work. The nurse assesses the client's occupational history to anticipate the possible effects of surgery on recovery and eventual work performance. The nurse explains any restrictions before a client returns to work, such as lifting, use of the extremities, or climbing stairs. When a client is unable to return to a job, the nurse confers with a social worker or occupational therapist to refer the client to job-training programs or to help the client seek economic assistance.

Preoperative Pain Assessment. Surgical manipulation of tissues, treatments, and positioning on the OR table may result in post-operative pain for the client. Pain is a very personal experience and requires an individualized plan of care. Preoperatively, the nurse should conduct a comprehensive pain assessment (see chapter 38), including the client's and family's expectations for pain management following surgery. The nurse should begin education regarding pain management as soon as possible (Barnes, 2001). The preoperative assessment should introduce to the client the use of a pain instrument to rate the presence and severity of pain post-operatively (see chapter 38). Several instruments for both pediatric and adult clients have shown reliability and validity (Summers, 2001). Frequent pain assessments with the client are necessary to alert the nurse to treat the pain and assess the adequacy (outcome) of pain interventions.

Review of Emotional Health. Surgery is psychologically stressful. The client may be anxious about the surgery and its implications. Clients often feel that they are powerless over their situation. Family members may perceive the client's surgery as a disruption of their lifestyle. Hospitalization and the recovery period at home may be lengthy. The family is usually concerned about the client returning to a normal, productive life. When the client has chronic illness, the family may be fearful that surgery may result in further disability or hopeful that it may improve their lifestyle. To understand the impact of surgery on a client's and family's emotional health, the nurse assesses the client's feelings about surgery, self-concept, body image, and coping resources.

It is often difficult to assess feelings thoroughly when ambulatory surgery is scheduled. The nurse usually has less time to establish a relationship with the client. Box 45-1 describes a study that explored the needs of ambulatory surgery clients. In some outpatient surgical programs, the nurse may visit with a client in the home or on the telephone before surgery. In a hospital room, the nurse should choose a time for discussion after admitting procedures or diagnostic tests are completed. The nurse explains that it is normal to have fears and concerns. The client's ability to share feelings partially depends on the nurse's willingness to listen, be supportive, and clarify misconceptions.

If the client feels powerless, the nurse should attempt to determine the reason. The medical diagnosis may generate apprehension of increased dependence and loss of physical or mental function. The thought of being "put to sleep" under anaesthesia may create concern about loss of control. Many clients feel the need to retain the power to make decisions about treatment. The nurse must assure clients of their right to ask questions and seek information.

A client may be angry about the need for surgery. For example, a young person may feel that it is unfair to have a disorder that typically affects older people. Surgery may occur at a time when it is inconvenient or potentially disruptive. The client may occasionally express anger by verbally attacking the nurse or physician. Being argumentative or overly demanding, refusing to co-operate, and criticizing the nurse's efforts to provide care are manifestations of anger and anxiety.

Research Highlight Box 45-1

Perceptions of Ambulatory Care Surgical Clients

Research Focus

Over the past decade, the number of ambulatory surgical procedures has continually increased. Nursing care of the ambulatory surgery client must be condensed into shorter time periods in all phases of perioperative care. Ensuring that the needs of ambulatory surgery clients are met is imperative.

Research Abstract

The purpose of this study was to explore the perceptions and views of ambulatory surgery clients. A study of 16 clients who underwent abdominal surgical procedures in an ambulatory surgery setting was conducted. Data were collected by intensive semi-structured interviews conducted in the surgeon's office at the time of the 1-week post-operative appointment. Topics in the interviews included clients' recall of how they felt the night before surgery, experiences the day of surgery, whether the perioperative experience met their expectation, feelings regarding the discharge process, and the experience of recovering at home. The interviews were then analyzed. Three areas were identified: fear, knowing, and presence. This study supported the importance of the nurse's presence through the perioperative experience and provided the perioperative nurse with an understanding of the needs of the ambulatory surgery client.

Evidence-Based Practice

- Fear in general was expressed, and fear of anaesthesia was discussed most often. Frequently, clients discuss their fears indirectly. Nurses must listen to clients for cues and provide them an opportunity to express their fears.
- Clients often had insufficient knowledge about what to expect preoperatively and post-operatively despite a good understanding of the surgical procedure itself. Education and reinforcement of the education is important throughout all phases of the perioperative experience.
- Clients wanted to know they mattered as an individual. Nurses should address clients by name and listen to individual requests and concerns. Incorporate the individual and the support system into the plan of care.
- Clients wanted to know the nurse was truly there for them both physically and emotionally.
- Connection with family or significant others is important throughout the perioperative experience.

Reference

Costa, M. J. (2001). The lived perioperative experience of ambulatory surgery patients. *AORN Journal, 74*(6), 874–881.

Body Image. Surgical removal of any diseased body part often leaves permanent disfigurement, alteration in body function, or concern over mutilation. Loss of certain body functions (e.g., with a colostomy or ureterostomy) may compound a client's fears. The nurse assesses for the body image alterations that clients perceive will result from surgery. Individuals will respond differently depending on their culture, self-concept, and degree of self-esteem (see chapter 22).

Often surgery changes the physical or psychological aspects of clients' sexuality. Excision of breast tissue, colostomy, ureterostomies, hysterectomy, or removal of the prostate gland may affect the clients' perceptions of their sexuality. Some surgeries (e.g., hernia repairs) require the client to temporarily refrain from sexual intercourse until the return to normal physical activity.

The nurse should encourage clients to express concerns about sexuality. The client facing even temporary sexual dysfunction requires understanding and support. Discussions about the client's sexuality should be held with the client's sexual partner so that they can gain a shared understanding of how to cope with limitations in sexual function.

Coping Resources. Assessment of feelings and self-concept helps reveal whether the client can cope with the stress of surgery. The physiological effects of stress are well documented. Activation of the endocrine system results in the release of hormones and catecholamines (epinephrine, norepinephrine), which result in increases in blood pressure, heart rate, and respiration. Platelet aggregation also occurs, along with many other physiological responses. The nurse must be aware of these responses and assist with stress management (see chapter 26). The nurse asks the client about past stress management. If the client has had previous surgery, the nurse should determine behaviours that helped resolve any tension or nervousness. The nurse may instruct the client on relaxation exercises that can help control anxiety.

When reviewing the client's coping resources, the nurse asks the client about specific family members and friends who may provide support. Once they are identified, the nurse includes these individuals in any client teaching and interventions to manage stress and anxiety.

Culture. Culture is a system of beliefs that have developed over time and subsequently been passed on through many generations (Lipson, Dibble, & Minarik, 1996). Clients come from diverse cultural and religious backgrounds. These backgrounds affect the way each client perceives and reacts to the surgical experience. If cultural, ethnic, and religious differences are not acknowledged and planned for in the perioperative plan of care, desired surgical outcomes may not be achieved. Therefore, learning about a client's cultural and ethnic heritage helps the nurse provide effective perioperative care. Although it is important to recognize and plan for differences based on culture, it is also necessary to recognize that members of the same culture are individuals and may not hold these shared beliefs. Box 45-2 highlights cultural care aspects in the perioperative period.

Client Expectations. Clients rely on their caregivers for information, comfort, pain control, adequate monitoring, and performance of interventions that ensure their safety throughout the surgical experience. This requires the nurse to have a caring attitude, advocate for the client, be skilled in surgical assessment and interventions,

Cultural Aspects of Care Box 45-2

Providing individualized education and perioperative nursing care to clients of various cultural, religious, and ethnic groups can be challenging. Using a variety of resources within a health care agency, in the literature, and from the Internet will help the nurse to provide culturally sensitive care.

Implications for Practice

- Preoperative assessment should include a cultural assessment with questions such as primary language spoken, feelings regarding surgery and pain, pain management, expectations, support system, and feelings toward self-care with post-operative implications (e.g., Does client relate to concept of pain? Does client have feelings about gender of caregiver? Does client follow custom that gives family members control over decisions?).
- Use a professional interpreter to communicate with a client whose language is different than yours.
- Use pictures or phrase cards with various languages to communicate with a client whose language is different than yours; these cards can be used to assess pain, comfort, temperature, and so forth.
- Provide preoperative and post-operative educational materials in a variety of languages.

Adapted from "Developing a Transcultural Patient Care Web Site," by H. P. De Ruiter and K. E. Larsen, 2002, *Journal of Transcultural Nursing, 13*(1), pp. 61–70; and "Pain as the Fifth Vital Sign: Will Cultural Variations Be Considered?" by M. Douglas, 1999, *Journal of Transcultural Nursing, 10*(4), p. 285.

and anticipate the client's needs throughout the perioperative period. The nurse must understand the client's expectations in order to develop an individualized care plan. Does the client expect full pain relief or simply to have pain reduced? Does the client expect to be independent immediately after surgery, or does he or she expect to be fully dependent on the nurse or family? These are only a few of the questions that need to be asked of the surgical client to establish a care plan congruent with the client's needs and expectations.

Physical Examination. The nurse conducts a partial or complete physical examination, depending on the client's preoperative condition (see chapter 28). Assessment focuses on findings related to the client's medical history and on body systems that will likely be affected by the surgery. The nursing assessment should complement the surgeon's and anaesthesiologist's physical examination (Barnes, 2002).

General Survey. The nurse observes the client's general appearance. Gestures and body movements may reflect weakness caused by illness. The client may appear malnourished. Height, body weight, and history of recent weight loss are important indicators of nutritional status.

Preoperative vital signs, including blood pressure while sitting and standing, provide important baseline data with which to compare alterations that occur during and after surgery. Some institutions request that blood pressure be obtained in both arms for comparison. Anxiety and fear commonly cause elevations in heart rate and blood pressure. As the effects of the anaesthesia diminish after surgery, the nurse compares findings with the preoperative baseline. Preoperative assessment of vital signs is also important to rule out fluid and electrolyte abnormalities (see chapter 27).

An elevated temperature before surgery is a cause for concern. If the client has an underlying infection, the surgeon may choose to postpone surgery until the infection has been treated. An elevated body temperature increases the risk of fluid and electrolyte imbalance after surgery.

Head and Neck. The condition of oral mucous membranes is one indicator of the level of hydration. A dehydrated client is at risk for developing serious fluid and electrolyte imbalances during surgery. Inspection of the soft palate and nasal sinuses can reveal sinus drainage, indicative of respiratory or sinus infection. Cervical lymph node enlargement may reveal local or systemic infection.

The nurse inspects the jugular veins for distension. Excess fluid within the circulatory system or failure of the heart to contract efficiently may lead to jugular vein distension and reveal a risk for cardiovascular complications during surgery.

During the examination of the oral mucosa, loose or capped teeth must be identified because they could become dislodged during endotracheal intubation. Dentures must be noted so that they can be removed before surgery, especially if general anaesthesia is required.

Integument. The nurse carefully inspects the skin, especially over bony prominences, such as the heels, elbows, sacrum, and scapula. During surgery, a client must lie in a fixed position, often for several hours. As a result, the client may have an increased risk for pressure ulcers (see chapter 43), especially if the skin is thin and dry and has poor turgor (Schoonhoven, Defloor, & Grypdonck, 2002). Chronic use of steroids also increases the client's susceptibility to skin tears. The overall condition of the skin also reveals the client's level of hydration. An older adult is at high risk for alteration in skin integrity from positioning and sliding on the OR table, causing shearing and pressure.

Thorax and Lungs. Assessment of the client's breathing pattern and chest excursion aids in assessing ventilatory capacity. A decline in ventilatory function places the client at risk for respiratory complications. For example, a client who has high abdominal surgery will have difficulty breathing deeply because of a painful abdominal incision. Auscultation of breath sounds will indicate whether the client has pulmonary congestion or narrowing of airways.

Existing atelectasis or moisture in the airways will be aggravated during surgery. Serious pulmonary congestion may cause postponement of the surgery. Certain anaesthetics can cause laryngeal muscle spasm; thus, if the nurse auscultates wheezing in the airways preoperatively, the client is at risk for further airway narrowing during

Table 45-6 Common Diagnostic Tests Performed Preoperatively Based on Client History

History	Test
Hepatic disease	International Normalized Ratio, partial thromboplastin time (INR/PTT); liver enzymes, such as serum aspartate aminotransferase; alkaline phosphatase
Medications:	
Diuretics	Blood urea nitrogen (BUN), creatinine, electrolytes
Steroids	Electrolytes, glucose
Anticoagulants	INR/PTT
Cardiovascular disease	BUN, creatinine, complete blood count (CBC), chest X-ray study, electrocardiogram (ECG)
Pulmonary disease	CBC, chest X-ray study, ECG
Central nervous system disease	White blood cell (WBC) count, electrolytes, BUN, creatinine, glucose, and electroencephalography (EEG)

surgery and after extubation (removal of the endotracheal tube); therefore, the physician should be made aware of these findings.

Heart and Vascular System. The nurse assesses the character of the apical, radial, and peripheral pulses; the capillary refill; and the colour and temperature of extremities. If peripheral pulses are not palpable, a Doppler instrument should be used for assessment of their presence. Acceptable capillary refill occurs in less than 3 seconds. Measurement of capillary refill and assessment of peripheral pulses are particularly important for the client having vascular surgery or for a client who may have casts or constricting bandages applied to the extremities after surgery (see chapter 28).

Abdomen. The nurse assesses the abdomen for size, shape, symmetry, and presence of distension. Assessment of preoperative bowel sounds is useful as a baseline. The nurse should also ask whether the client has regular bowel movements and inquire about the colour and consistency of stools.

Neurological Status. Preoperative assessment of neurological status is imperative for all clients receiving general anaesthesia. The baseline neurological status assists with the assessment of ascent from anaesthesia. During the health history and physical assessment, the nurse observes the client's level of orientation, alertness, and mood, noting whether the client answers questions appropriately and can recall recent and past events. A client who will have surgery for neurological disease (e.g., brain tumour or aneurysm) may demonstrate an impaired level of consciousness or altered behaviour.

If the client is scheduled for spinal anaesthesia, preoperative assessment of gross motor function and strength is important. Spinal anaesthesia causes temporary paralysis of the lower extremities (see chapter 38). The nurse should be aware if a client enters surgery with weakness or impaired mobility of the lower extremities so that when the spinal anaesthetic wears off, the nurse will not expect full motor function to return.

Diagnostic Screening. Before a client has surgery, the surgeon may order diagnostic tests to screen for pre-existing abnormalities. Ordered tests are determined by the client's history and physical assessment. Table 45-6 contains common diagnostic tests performed preoperatively based on the client's medical history. Tests are also determined by the procedure itself. For procedures where blood loss is expected (e.g., hip and knee replacements), a type and cross-match would be indicated preoperatively. The surgeon will designate the number of blood units to have available during surgery. Table 45-7 gives the purpose and normal values for the more common blood tests. If diagnostic tests reveal severe problems, the surgeon may cancel surgery until the condition stabilizes. The nurse is responsible for the preparation of clients for diagnostic studies and for coordinating completion of the tests. The nurse also reviews diagnostic results as they become available, not only to alert physicians to these findings and to assist with planning appropriate therapy, but also to integrate these findings into decisions related to client care.

If a client is over the age of 65 years or has heart disease, an electrocardiogram (ECG) is mandatory. The ECG measures the electrical activity of the heart to assess the heart rate, rhythm, and other factors. A chest X-ray (an examination of the condition of the heart and lungs) is required for thoracic surgery or if the client has certain medical conditions.

Pulmonary function testing and arterial blood gas analysis may be performed on clients with pre-existing lung disease. Blood glucose levels are measured on diabetic clients.

Autologous infusions are an option for some clients who choose to donate their own blood before surgery to ease their anxiety over the risk of transfusion-related infections. Although Canadian Blood Services screens all blood donors and blood products for infections such as HIV and hepatitis, some clients are more comfortable donating their own blood. The donation usually must be made several weeks before the scheduled surgery. The client who does self-donation may exhibit a lower hemoglobin and hematocrit level on the day of surgery. Autotransfusion via the use of a cell-saver device in surgery may be possible if physicians are anticipating large blood loss (e.g., open heart surgery). The cell saver, although expensive, returns washed red blood cells to the client and has created positive outcomes in terms of

Table 45-7 Diagnostic Screening for Surgical Clients

Measurement and Normal Values	Interpretation
Complete blood count (CBC) *RBC:* Men: 4.7–5.14 × 10^{12}/L Women: 4.2–4.87 × 10^{12}/L *Hgb:* Men: 132–173 g/L Women: 117–155 g/L *Hct:* Men: 0.43–0.49; Women: 0.38–0.44 *WBC:* Adults and children >2 years: 4.5–11 × 10^9/L	Peripheral venous sample of blood measures red blood cells (RBCs), white blood cells (WBCs), hemoglobin (Hgb), and hematocrit (Hct). May reveal infection, low blood volume, and potential for oxygenation problems. Surgeon may order blood replacement.
Serum electrolytes *Sodium (Na):* 136–145 mmol/L *Potassium (K):* 3.5–5.0 mmol/L *Chloride (Cl):* 98–106 mmol/L *Bicarbonate (HCO_3):* 22–26 mmol/L	Peripheral venous sample of blood reveals significant fluid and electrolyte imbalances preoperatively. Attention is given to Na, K, and Cl levels. IV fluid replacement may be indicated preoperatively.
Coagulation studies *INR:* 0.76–1.27 *APTT:* 30–40 seconds *Platelets:* 150–400 × 10^9	International normalized ratio (INR), activated partial thromboplastin time (APTT), and platelet counts reveal clotting ability of blood. Reveals clients at risk for bleeding tendencies and thrombus formation.
Serum creatinine *Men:* 53–106 umol/L *Women:* 44–97 umol/L	Ability of kidneys to excrete creatinine, by-product of muscle metabolism, indicates renal function. Elevated level can indicate renal failure.
Blood urea nitrogen (BUN) 2.9–7.5 mmol/L	Ability of kidneys to excrete urea and nitrogen indicates renal function. BUN becomes elevated if client is dehydrated. Preoperative IV fluid replacement may be needed.
Glucose *Fasting:* 4.2–6.1 mmol/L	Finger stick or peripheral blood sample. Clients may require treatment of low or high levels preoperatively and post-operatively. Elevated blood sugar results from a deficiency in insulin secretion (Type 1 diabetes), insulin action, or combination of both (Type 2 diabetes).

Adapted from *Mosby's Diagnostic and Laboratory Test Reference* (7th ed.), by K. D. Pagana and T. J. Pagana, 2003, St. Louis, MO: Mosby; and *Davis's Comprehensive Handbook of Laboratory and Diagnostic Tests With Nursing Implications,* by Z. Burgess Schnell, A. M. Van Leeuwen, and T. R. Kranpitz, 2003, Philadelphia: F. A. Davis.

length of client stay (Rothrock, 2003). Autologous infusions are commonly used in orthopedic surgery.

NP Nursing Diagnosis

The nurse clusters patterns of defining characteristics gathered during assessment to identify nursing diagnoses for the surgical client (Box 45-3). The client with pre-existing health problems is likely to have a variety of risk diagnoses. For example, a client with pre-existing bronchitis who has abnormal breath sounds and a productive cough will be at risk for *ineffective airway clearance.* In addition, a client who undergoes a surgical procedure is at risk for developing infection at the surgical site, the IV site, or the bloodstream (sepsis). A diagnosis of *risk for infection* will require the nurse's attention from admission through convalescence.

The related factors for each diagnosis establish directions for nursing care that will be provided during one or all of the surgical phases. For example, the diagnosis of *risk for infection related to an invasive procedure* will require different interventions than if the related factor were *inadequate immune response.* Preoperative nursing diagnoses allow the nurse to take precautions and actions so that care provided during the intraoperative and post-operative phases is consistent with the client's needs.

Nursing diagnoses made preoperatively will also focus on the potential risks a client may face after surgery. Preventive care is essential so that the surgical client can be managed effectively. The following are common nursing diagnoses relevant to the surgical client:

- Ineffective airway clearance
- Risk for latex allergy response
- Anxiety
- Disturbed body image
- Risk for imbalanced body temperature
- Ineffective breathing pattern
- Ineffective coping
- Fear
- Risk for deficient fluid volume
- Risk for infection
- Risk for perioperative-positioning injury
- Deficient knowledge (specify)
- Impaired physical mobility
- Acute pain
- Powerlessness
- Impaired skin integrity
- Disturbed sleep pattern
- Delayed surgical recovery

NP Planning

During planning, the nurse again synthesizes information from multiple resources (Figure 45–2). For example, knowledge pertaining to adult learning principles, coupled with the client's unique needs, will ensure a well-designed

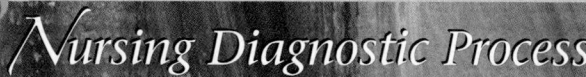

Nursing Diagnostic Process — Box 45-3

Assessment Activities	Defining Characteristics	Nursing Diagnosis
Ask client to describe previous surgical experiences.	Client mentions a traumatic prior experience with surgery	Fear related to knowledge deficit and previous surgical experience
Ask client about preoperative education/preparation before admission.	Unaware of preoperative testing	
Observe client's non-verbal behaviour.	Client's behaviour indicates fear and tension	
Assess vital signs.	Increased heart rate	

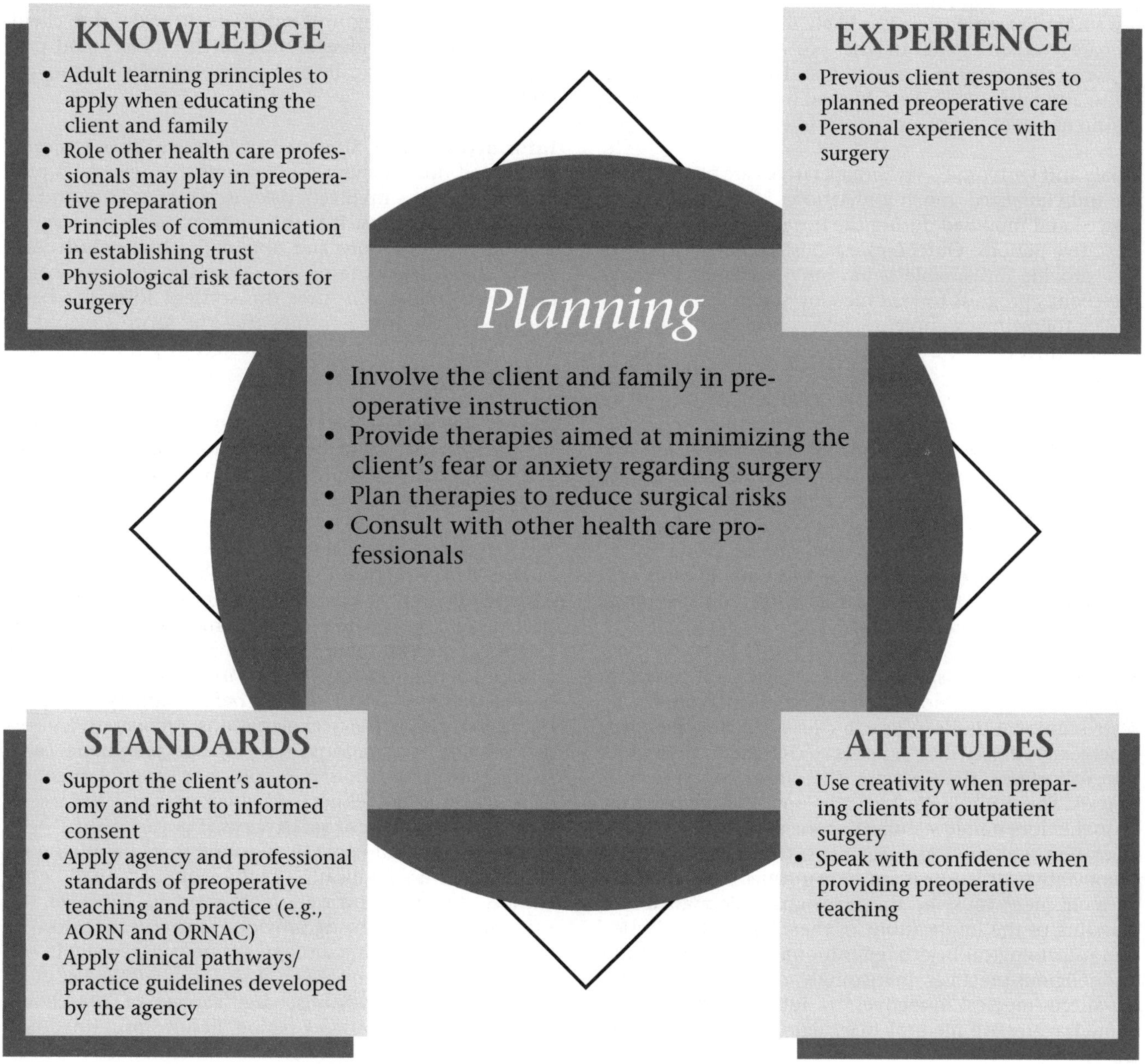
KNOWLEDGE
• Adult learning principles to apply when educating the client and family
• Role other health care professionals may play in preoperative preparation
• Principles of communication in establishing trust
• Physiological risk factors for surgery
EXPERIENCE
• Previous client responses to planned preoperative care
• Personal experience with surgery
Planning
• Involve the client and family in preoperative instruction
• Provide therapies aimed at minimizing the client's fear or anxiety regarding surgery
• Plan therapies to reduce surgical risks
• Consult with other health care professionals
STANDARDS
• Support the client's autonomy and right to informed consent
• Apply agency and professional standards of preoperative teaching and practice (e.g., AORN and ORNAC)
• Apply clinical pathways/practice guidelines developed by the agency
ATTITUDES
• Use creativity when preparing clients for outpatient surgery
• Speak with confidence when providing preoperative teaching

FIGURE **45–2** Critical thinking model for surgical client planning.

preoperative teaching plan. Critical thinking ensures that the client's plan of care integrates the nurse's knowledge, previous experience, and established standards of care. Previous experience in caring for surgical clients helps the nurse anticipate how to approach client care (e.g., complications to prevent and anticipate, and methods to reduce anxiety). Professional standards are especially important to consider when the nurse develops a plan of care. These standards often provide a scientific basis for selecting effective nursing interventions. The nurse develops an individualized plan of care for each nursing diagnosis (see Care Plan). The nurse and client set realistic expectations for care.

Successful planning requires the involvement of the surgical client and family in establishing the care plan. Early client involvement minimizes surgical risks and post-operative complications. A client informed about the surgical experience is less likely to be fearful and can prepare to participate in the post-operative recovery phase so that outcomes can be met. Diagnosis, interventions, and outcomes are established to ensure recovery or maintenance of the preoperative state.

Goals and Outcomes. The preoperative care plan is based on individualized nursing diagnoses. This plan is reviewed and modified during the intraoperative and post-operative periods. Outcomes established for each goal of care provide measurable behavioural evidence to gauge the client's progress toward meeting stated goals.

The following example provides a goal of care and expected outcomes relevant for the preoperative surgical client:

- Client is able to verbalize significance of post-operative exercises.
- Client verbalizes prevention of lung congestion and pneumonia as reasons for deep breathing and coughing exercises and incentive spirometer.
- Client verbalizes promotion of blood flow to prevent leg clots as reason for post-operative leg exercises.
- Client verbalizes rationale for early ambulation as it improves lung function, assists with return of bowel function, and promotes recovery.

Setting Priorities. Using clinical judgment, the nurse prioritizes nursing diagnoses and interventions from the assessed unique needs of each client. Clients requiring emergency surgery may experience changes in their physiological status that require the nurse to reprioritize quickly. For example, if a client's blood pressure begins to drop, hemodynamic stabilization becomes a priority over education and stress management. Generally, when the preoperative situation is more controlled, the approach to each client must be thorough and reflect an understanding of the implications of the client's age, physical and psychological health, educational level, and cultural and religious practices. Increasingly, clients are preparing advanced medical directives to indicate their wishes should aggressive medical treatment be required following surgery.

Continuity of Care. For ambulatory surgery clients and clients admitted the day of their scheduled surgery, preoperative planning occurs days before admission to the hospital. Frequently, preoperative education begins in the physician's office, continues during the scheduled preadmission testing visit, and is reinforced by the nurse the day of admission. Preoperative instruction gives the client time to think about the surgical experience, make necessary physical preparations (e.g., altering diet or discontinuing medications), and question post-operative procedures. The ambulatory surgical client usually returns home on the day of surgery. Thus, well-planned preoperative care ensures that the client is well informed and able to be an active participant during recovery. The family or spouse can also play an active supportive role for the client.

NP Implementation

Preoperative nursing interventions provide the client with a complete understanding of the surgery and prepare the client physically and psychologically for surgical intervention.

Informed Consent. Surgery cannot be legally or ethically performed until a client understands the need for a procedure, the steps involved, risks, expected results, and alternative treatments. It is the surgeon's responsibility to explain the procedure and obtain the **informed consent.** The nurse witnesses the client signing the consent form (see chapter 8). After the consent form has been completed, the nurse ensures that the form is placed in the client's medical record. The record goes to the OR with the client.

Health Promotion. Health promotion activities during the preoperative phase focus on health maintenance, prevention of complications, and support of possible rehabilitation needs post-operatively.

Preoperative Teaching. Education is an important aspect of the client's surgical experience. Preoperative teaching concerning a client's expected post-operative behaviour, provided in a systematic and structured format with teaching and learning principles, has a positive influence on the client's recovery. Nurses in preadmission clinics may call clients up to 1 week before surgery to clarify questions and reinforce explanations. Preoperative information and instructions may include telephone calls, mailings from the physician's office or hospital, preoperative teaching guidelines and checklists, and the use of videotapes or **clinical pathways** (Figure 45–3).

Lookinland and Pool (1998) found that clients who received structured education before admission had better clinical outcomes and were more satisfied. However, despite the education being provided to clients, retention of information following discharge is poor, especially in the older adult population (Bean & Waldron, 1995). Lee et al. (1998) conducted post-discharge surveys of 206 clients hospitalized over a 6-week period. Results from this study indicated that continuity of care was enhanced if education was provided before, during, and after discharge. They found that half of the clients who were contacted requested additional education. Therefore, it seems ideal to attempt perioperative education before admission,

Nursing Care Plan

Deficient Knowledge Regarding Preoperative and Post-operative Care Requirements

Assessment

Mrs. Campana is an 80-year-old woman scheduled to be admitted in 5 days for elective bowel resection. Joe Marrero is the nurse in the clinic surgery service assigned to prepare Mrs. Campana for surgery. During Joe's initial discussion with Mrs. Campana, he observes her to be alert and oriented. Mrs. Campana has severely reduced visual acuity but is able to hear Joe's questions clearly.

Assessment Activities	Findings/Defining Characteristics
Ask Mrs. Campana about previous surgeries and her experience with them.	She responds, "I had surgery over 20 years ago, and I was in the hospital for 10 days."
Ask Mrs. Campana what she has been told regarding her surgery.	She states her surgeon explained the procedure with a drawing of the bowel and the location of the part to be removed.
Ask Mrs. Campana what she has been told regarding preoperative preparation and what to expect post-operatively.	She states she received information from the surgeon's office regarding medicines to stop and those she should take the morning of surgery, her diet before surgery and when to stop eating, and who to call for questions. She does not recall receiving information regarding what to expect post-operatively.
Assess Mrs. Campana's ability to read typical font type.	She is unable to read the font on the newspaper; she can read the headlines with her glasses.
Assess Mrs. Campana's family/support system for preoperative and post-operative assistance.	She states her daughter will be coming in town the day of surgery to help her after surgery

Nursing Diagnosis:

Deficient knowledge regarding preoperative and post-operative care requirements related to lack of exposure to information.

Planning

Goals	Expected Outcomes*
	Knowledge: Treatment Procedures
Client will understand the post-operative routines of surgical care by day before surgery.	Client will discuss monitoring routines following surgery by morning of surgery in the preoperative period. Client will be able to describe importance of post-operative exercises by morning of surgery, including turn, cough, and deep breathing, incentive spirometer, leg exercise. Client will be able to describe schedule for activity and nutritional management following surgery by day 1 post-operatively.
Client will participate actively in post-operative recovery activities by day 1 following surgery.	Client will successfully perform post-operative exercises by morning of surgery in the preoperative period.

*Outcome classification labels from *Nursing Outcomes Classification (NOC)* (3rd ed.), edited by S. Moorhead, M. Johnson, and M. L. Maas, 2004, St. Louis, MO: Mosby.

Interventions†	Rationale
Teaching Preoperative	
Provide client with audio-tape program that explains preoperative and post-operative routines. Supply instruction booklet designed for visually impaired. Make a follow-up call to client and call the daughter to allow them the opportunity to ask questions and voice concerns. Document all phases of education provided to client in client's record, preoperative before admission, day of surgery, and post-operative.	Preadmission education can require less teaching time and better performance of exercises on admission. Education has a beneficial effect in reducing post-operative anxiety (Shuldham, 1999).
On admission to hospital, demonstrate to client and daughter the performance of post-operative exercises and how to get out of bed.	Demonstration is an effective method to reinforce didactic instruction.
Explain sensations to be expected post-operatively (e.g., incisional pain, IV, nasogastric tube, wound care).	Teaching about sensory aspects (what the client sees, feels, smells) should be structured (Shuldham, 1999).
Give client opportunity to return demonstrate post-operative exercises before surgery.	Return demonstration measures client learning and provides opportunity to reinforce instruction.
Correct any unrealistic expectations client or daughter may have regarding surgery.	Unrealistic expectations, when unmet, can contribute to client's anxiety. Psychological preparation for surgery reduces anxiety.

†Intervention classification labels from *Nursing Interventions Classification (NIC)* (4th ed.), edited by J. M. Dochterman and G. M. Bulecheck, 2004, St. Louis, MO: Mosby.

Continued

Nursing Care Plan

Deficient Knowledge Regarding Preoperative and Post-operative Care Requirements—cont'd

Evaluation

Nursing Actions	Client Response/Finding	Achievement of Outcome
Ask client to describe typical monitoring and care activities following surgery. Document evaluation of client's understanding and demonstration of learned activities in client's record.	She is able to verbalize typical monitoring and care following surgery. She states the booklet and audio tape were both helpful.	Mrs. Campana has a good understanding of the typical post-operative course.
Observe client's demonstration of post-operative exercises.	She is able to demonstrate leg exercises and deep breathing and coughing exercises but is having difficulty with incentive spirometer use.	Mrs. Campana is able to demonstrate most of post-operative exercises but needs further teaching and practise on incentive spirometer use.
Explore with client and daughter if they have any remaining fears or concerns.	Both Mrs. Campana and her daughter deny any fears or concerns at the present time.	Informational and psychological needs of Mrs. Campana and her daughter have been met.

during the hospital stay, and after discharge. Including family members in perioperative preparation is advised.

Often a family member is the coach for post-operative exercises when the client returns from surgery. The family may also recognize untoward events that may unfold once the client is home. Therefore, they need to be aware of what are normal expectations after discharge from hospital. If anxious relatives do not understand routine post-operative events, it is likely that their anxiety will heighten the client's fears and concerns. Preoperative preparation of family members before surgery can help to minimize anxiety and misunderstanding.

The nurse should provide clients with information about sensations typically experienced after surgery. Preparatory information helps clients anticipate the steps of a procedure and thus helps them form realistic images of the surgical experience. When events occur as predicted, clients are better able to cope and attend to the experiences. For example, in the OR, the anaesthesiologist may apply ointment to clients' eyes to prevent corneal damage. Warning clients about sensations of blurred vision will reduce their anxiety on awakening from surgery. Sensations that the nurse may describe include expected pain at the surgical site, tightness of dressings, dryness of the mouth, or the sensation of a sore throat resulting from an endotracheal tube.

Anxiety and fear are barriers to learning, and both emotions are heightened as surgery approaches. The nurse assesses the surgical client's readiness and ability to learn. If the client is capable of and receptive to learning, the nurse presents information in a logical sequence, beginning with preoperative events and advancing to intraoperative and post-operative routines. The following demonstrates client understanding of the surgical experience.

Client Cites Reasons for Preoperative Instructions and Exercises. If given a rationale for preoperative and post-operative procedures, the client is better prepared to participate in care. Every preoperative teaching program includes explanation and demonstration of post-operative exercises: diaphragmatic breathing, incentive spirometry, coughing, turning, and leg exercises. These exercises are designed to prevent post-operative complications (Skill 45-1).

If the client is measured for elastic stockings or **pneumatic compression devices,** teaching about the purposes and nursing care that will be required following application is necessary (see chapter 42).

After explaining each exercise, the nurse demonstrates it. The nurse acts as a coach, guiding the client through each exercise. For example, the nurse assesses whether the client is sitting properly and helps the client place the hands in the proper position during breathing. The nurse then allows the client time for independent practice and returns to evaluate effectiveness before surgery.

Client States the Time of Surgery. The client and family should be told the approximate time that surgery will begin. If the hospital has a busy OR schedule, it is best to let them know if other procedures are scheduled before the client's. The surgeon usually informs the client and family of the anticipated length of surgery. Unanticipated delays may occur for many reasons. The family needs to be aware that delays do not necessarily indicate a problem.

Client Knows Where the Post-operative Unit Is and Where the Family Will Be During Surgery and Recovery. The unit to which the client is admitted before surgery may be different from the post-operative unit. The family needs to know where the client will be taken after surgery. The nurse also explains where the family can wait and where the surgeon will attempt to find family members after surgery. Many institutions have implemented programs in which the circulating nurse gives periodic reports to the family in the waiting room for prolonged surgeries. If the client will be taken to a special unit, it helps to orient the client and family members to the unit's environment before surgery. Programs to connect with

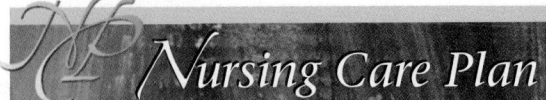

The Ottawa Hospital | L'Hôpital d'Ottawa

CLINICAL PATHWAY – PLAN CLINIQUE

Total Hip Replacement: Primary/Revision
Remplacement total de la hanche : primaire/réintervention

☐ Civic ☐ Gen.-Gén.

Addressograph/Plaque

PAU — Unité pré-admission

Date: yyaa ________ mm ______ dj ______

Critical Path

- **Assessment & teaching per PAU standards and procedure specific education material**

Tests
- PTT, INR
- CBC
- Type and screen to ensure minimum of 2 units pRBCs (including autologous blood)

Additional testing if required per PAU standards

✓ if done

☐ Na, K, Cl, Glucose, Creatinine
☐ Chest X-ray
☐ Pregnancy test
☐ ECG
☐ Urinalysis

Additional Orders
- Consult Physio
- Consult OT if patient has pre-existing medical issues / compounding medical complications / cognitive issues that impact on discharge planning
- X-rays: (Films required) AP pelvis (top of film @ ASIS) and lateral of affected hip

Discharge Planning
- Discuss expected length of stay
- Initiate Discharge Preparation Clinical Pathway

Patient Outcomes

Patient/Family Teaching
- Understands pre-op instructions and events
- Understands usual post-op course, plan for pain management, and usual self care measures to prevent post-op complications

Discharge Planning
- Understands usual lenth of stay
- Appropriate discharge plan in place or if not suitable discharge plan in place – social work has been consulted

Patient progress corresponds with clinical pathway

Physiotherapy:
☐ Yes ☐ No Signature: ____________________
Time: ________ NTV – circle above, VC ________

Nursing:
☐ Yes ☐ No Signature: ____________________
Time: ________ NTV – circle above, VC ________

Day of Surgery Pre-op — SDA/SDCU — Jour de la chirurgie pré-opératoire

Date: yyaa ________ mm ______ dj ______

Critical Path

- **Assessment and teaching per Same Day Admission standards and procedure specific education material.**

Tests ✓ if done

☐ Glucose meter: for diabetic patient
☐ PTT/INR: for patient normally taking warfarin (Coumadin) – Unless normal result obtained after warfarin discontinued per pre-op instructions
☐ Electrolytes: for dialysis dependant patient – Unless acceptable post-dialysis results obtained within 24 h of surgery
☐ CBC if autologous blood donor

Additional Orders
- IV NS at 50 mL/h (or D5W at 100 mL/hr if diabetic) if IV medications to be given in SDA/SDCU
- Naproxen E 500 mg with 30 mL water on arrival to SDCU (approx. 2 hrs pre-op unless contraindicated)

Antibiotics:

1. If No history of allergy to penicillin or to other beta-lactam antibiotics;
   or
   History of non-life threatening reaction to penicillin or other beta-lactam antibiotics (eg. rash, diarrhea, stomach upset)

   IV Cefazolin on chart for administration in OR:
   - 1g if BMI < 30 (or Weight < 90 kg & height info not available)
   - 2g if BMI ≥ 30 (or Weight ≥ 90 kg & height info not available)

Or

2. If patient has a history of life threatening reaction (hypotension, bronchospasm, urticaria, angioedema) to penicillin or other beta-lactam antibiotics

   IV Vancomycin:
   - If BMI < 30 (or Weight < 90 kg & height info not available) 1 g over 60 min pre-op
   - If BMI ≥ 30 (or Weight ≥ 90 kg & height info not available) 1.5 g over 90 min pre-op

Patient Outcomes

Patient Teaching
- Compliant with pre-op instructions
- Understands usual events/expectations of operative day
- Understands usual post-op course, plan for pain management, and usual self care measures to prevent post-op complications

Patient progress corresponds with clinical pathway

Nursing:
☐ Yes ☐ No Signature: ____________________
Time: ________ NTV – circle above, VC ________

Variance Codes (VC)

186	Activity variance
653	Consult not sent by Day 3
492	Not discharged by end of pathway – continued need for acute care
510	Not discharged by end of pathway – non-medical reason
NTV	Non-Tracked Variance
OFF	Ordered off clinical pathway

CP 4A ENGLISH (REV 02-2005) ID CHART – DOSSIER

FIGURE **45–3** Preoperative client instructions for a clinical pathway for a total hip replacement. The first day of a 6-day pathway highlights what the client can expect before surgery. (Courtesy of The Ottawa Hospital, Ottawa, ON.)

the family have also been developed in the same-day admit and day-surgery area. For example, the Queen Elizabeth II Health Sciences Centre in Halifax, Nova Scotia, has created the role of the surgical liaison nurse to provide communication and support for families of surgical clients (Fowlie, Frances, & Russell, 2000).

Client Discusses Anticipated Post-operative Monitoring and Therapies. The client and family need to know about post-operative events. If they understand the frequency of post-operative vital sign monitoring before surgery occurs, they will be less apprehensive when nurses measure vital signs. The nurse can also explain whether the client is likely to have IV lines, monitoring lines, dressings, or drainage tubes or will require ventilator support.

Client Describes Surgical Procedures and Post-operative Treatment. After the surgeon has explained the basic purpose of a surgical procedure, the client may ask the nurse additional questions to clarify misunderstandings. Preestablished teaching standards, such as those integrated in clinical pathways for preoperative and post-operative care (Figure 45–4), give the nurse an excellent guide for instruction. A good starting point is to ask what the client has been told. If the client has limited understanding about the surgery, the nurse can provide additional explanations. If necessary, the surgeon can be asked to reinform the client.

Client Describes Post-operative Activity Resumption. The type of surgery a client undergoes affects the speed with which normal physical activity and regular eating habits can be resumed. The nurse explains that it is normal to progress gradually in activity and eating. If the client tolerates activity and diet well, activity levels will progress more quickly.

Client Verbalizes Pain-Relief Measures. One of the surgical client's fears is pain. The family is also concerned for the client's comfort. Pain after surgery is expected. The nurse informs the client and family of interventions available for pain relief (e.g., analgesics, positioning, splinting, and relaxation exercises; see chapter 38). The client needs to know the schedule for analgesic drugs, the route of administration, and their effects.

Surgical clients may avoid taking pain-relief drugs for fear of becoming dependent. The nurse should encourage the client to use analgesics as needed and explain to the client that the risks of becoming dependent are almost negligible. Explain to the client that unless the pain is controlled, it will be difficult for the client to participate in post-operative therapy such as mobilization. The client should be encouraged to inform nurses before the pain becomes a constant discomfort. If a client waits until pain becomes excruciating, an analgesic may not provide relief at the dose ordered. Clients who will have patient-controlled analgesia (PCA) after surgery should know how to push the button when beginning to feel discomfort and understand that use of PCA will not cause overmedication (see chapter 38). The client should also know the length of time that it takes for the drug to begin working. Information from preoperative assessment will be helpful to the nurse when teaching about pain-relief measures. Pain reporting and expectations regarding pain management based on a client's cultural beliefs are areas that need to be explored individually and systematically through research (Douglas, 1999; Ramer et al., 1999).

Client Expresses Feelings Regarding Surgery. If the client is admitted to hospital during the preoperative surgical phase, frequent visits by staff, diagnostic testing, and physical preparation for surgery consume a lot of time, and the client has few opportunities to reflect on the surgical experience. The nurse must recognize the client as a unique individual. The client and family need time to express feelings about surgery. The client's level of anxiety influences the frequency of discussions. While delivering bedside care, the nurse can encourage expression of concerns. The family may wish to discuss concerns without the client present so that their fears will not frighten the client and vice versa. The establishment of a trusting and therapeutic relationship with the client and family allows this to happen.

Acute Care. Acute care activities in the preoperative phase focus on interventions to physically prepare the client for surgery.

Physical Preparation. The degree of preoperative physical preparation depends on the client's health status and the surgery to be performed. A seriously ill client receives more supportive care in the form of medications, IV fluid therapy, and monitoring than the client facing a minor elective procedure. The nurse explains the purpose of all procedures.

Maintenance of Normal Fluid and Electrolyte Balance. The surgical client is vulnerable to fluid and electrolyte imbalances as a result of inadequate preoperative intake, excessive fluid losses during surgery, and the physiological effect of third spacing of fluid in the initial post-operative period (see chapter 36). A client traditionally took nothing by mouth (NPO) after midnight on the morning of surgery to keep the stomach empty and thus reduce the risk of vomiting and aspiration. Recommendations for preoperative fasting have been published by a task force from the American Society of Anesthesiologists (ASA, 1999). They recommended fasting from intake of a light meal or non-human milk for 6 or more hours, breast milk for 4 or more hours, and clear liquids for 2 to 3 hours before elective procedures requiring general anaesthesia, regional anaesthesia, or sedation.

Agencies vary as to the extent these guidelines have been adopted. The nurse removes fluids and solid foods from the client's bedside and posts a sign over the bed to alert hospital personnel and family members about fasting restrictions. The client may be instructed to take specific medications (e.g., cardiovascular medications, anticonvulsants, or antibiotics) with a sip of water. Although the parameters of preoperative fasting have changed over the past 10 years, studies demonstrate that recent guidelines have not been fully implemented and multidisciplinary improvement processes may be required (O'Callaghan, 2002; Williams, 1999).

Text continued on p. 1626

Skill 45-1 Demonstrating Post-operative Exercises

View Video

Delegation Considerations

The skill of demonstrating post-operative exercises should not be delegated to unregulated care providers (UCPs). However, other aspects of client care may be delegated.

- Educate the UCP to encourage clients to practise exercises regularly following instruction.
- Instruct the UCP to inform the nurse if client is unwilling to perform these exercises.

Equipment

- Pillow or wrapped blanket (used to splint surgical incision during coughing)
- Incentive spirometer
- Positive expiratory pressure (PEP) device and nose clip

Steps	Rationale
1. Assess client's risk for post-operative respiratory complications. Review medical history to identify presence of chronic pulmonary conditions (e.g., emphysema, asthma), any condition that affects chest wall movement, history of smoking, and presence of reduced hemoglobin.	General anaesthesia predisposes client to respiratory problems because lungs are not fully inflated during surgery and cough reflex is suppressed, so that mucus collects within airway passages. After surgery, client may have reduced lung volume and require greater efforts to cough and deep breathe; inadequate lung expansion can lead to atelectasis and pneumonia. Client is at greater risk to develop respiratory complications if other chronic lung conditions are present. Smoking damages ciliary clearance and increases mucus secretion. Reduced hemoglobin level can lead to inadequate oxygenation.
2. Assess ability to cough and deep breathe by having client take deep breath and observing movement of shoulders and chest wall. Measure chest excursion during deep breath. Ask client to cough after taking deep breath.	Reveals maximum potential for chest expansion and ability to cough forcefully; serves as baseline to measure ability to perform exercises after surgery.
3. Assess risk for post-operative thrombus formation. (Older clients, those with active cancer, and clients immobilized for more than 3 days are most at risk.) Observe for localized tenderness along the distribution of the venous system, swollen calf or thigh, calf swelling more than 3 cm compared with asymptomatic leg, pitting edema in symptomatic leg, and collateral superficial veins. If any of these signs are present, notify the physician.	Venous stasis, hypercoagulability, and vein trauma exist simultaneously for thrombus formation to occur (Lewis et al., 2004). After general anaesthesia, circulation is slowed, thus increasing risk of clot formation. Immobilization results in decreased muscular contraction in lower extremities, which promotes venous stasis.

Critical Decision Point: A positive Homans' sign (calf pain when dorsiflexing client's foot with knee flexed) has been found to have a low specificity for deep vein thrombosis (DVT) diagnosis and often is not present or may be present when no DVT exists (Anand et al., 1998; Tick et al., 2002).

Steps	Rationale
4. Assess client's ability to move independently while in bed.	Determines existence of any mobility restrictions.
5. Explain post-operative exercises to client, including importance to recovery and physiological benefits.	Information allows client to understand significance of exercises and can motivate learning. People tend to learn new skills when benefits can be gained.
6. Demonstrate exercises.	
A. Diaphragmatic breathing	
(1) Assist client to comfortable sitting position on side of bed or in chair or standing position.	Upright position facilitates diaphragmatic excursion.
(2) Stand or sit facing client.	Allows client to observe breathing exercise.
(3) Instruct client to place palms of hands across from each other, down and along lower borders of anterior rib cage. Place tips of third fingers lightly together (see illustration). Demonstrate for client.	Position of hands allows client to feel movement of chest and abdomen as diaphragm descends and lungs expand.

Skill 45-1 Demonstrating Post-operative Exercises—cont'd

Steps	Rationale

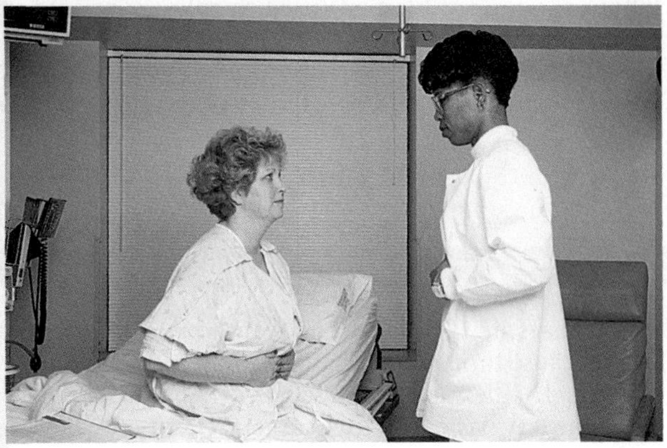

STEP **6A(3)** Client learns how to feel proper abdominal breathing.

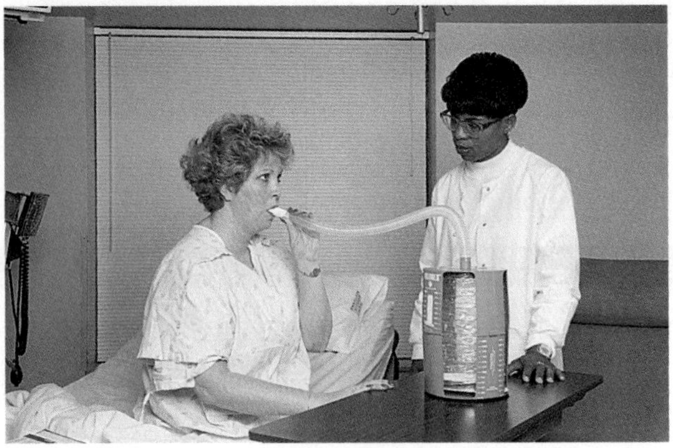

STEP **6B(4)** Client inhales using incentive spirometer.

Steps	Rationale
(4) Have client take slow, deep breaths, inhaling through nose and pushing abdomen against hands. Tell client to feel middle fingers separate during inhalation. Demonstrate.	Taking slow, deep breaths prevents panting or hyperventilation. Inhaling through nose warms, humidifies, and filters air.
(5) Explain that client will feel normal downward movement of diaphragm during inspiration. Explain that abdominal organs descend and chest wall expands.	Explanation and demonstration focus on normal ventilatory movement of chest wall. Client develops understanding of how diaphragmatic breathing feels.
(6) Avoid using auxiliary chest and shoulder muscles while inhaling and instruct client in same manner.	Using auxiliary chest and shoulder muscles increases useless energy expenditure.
(7) Have client hold slow, deep breath for count of three and then slowly exhale through mouth as if blowing out a candle (pursed lips). Tell client middle fingertips will touch as chest wall contracts.	Allows for gradual expulsion of all air.
(8) Repeat breathing exercise three to five times.	Allows client to observe slow, rhythmic breathing pattern.
(9) Have client practise exercise. Instruct client to take 10 slow, deep breaths every hour while awake during post-operative period until mobile.	Repetition of exercise reinforces learning. Regular deep breathing prevents post-operative complications.
B. Incentive spirometry	
(1) Perform hand hygiene.	Reduces transmission of micro-organisms.
(2) Instruct client to assume semi-Fowler's or high-Fowler's position.	Promotes optimal lung expansion during respiratory manoeuvre.
(3) Either set or indicate to client on the device scale, the volume level to be attained with each breath.	Establishes goal to volume level necessary for lung expansion.
(4) Demonstrate to client how to place mouthpiece of spirometer so that lips completely cover mouthpiece (see illustration).	Demonstration is reliable technique for teaching psychomotor skill and enables client to ask questions.
(5) Instruct client to inhale slowly and maintain constant flow through unit, attempting to reach goal volume. When maximal inspiration is reached, client should hold breath for 2 to 3 seconds (see illustration) and then exhale slowly. Number of breaths should not exceed 10 to 12/minute in each session.	Maintains maximal inspiration and reduces risk of progressive collapse of individual alveoli. Slow breath prevents or minimizes pain from sudden pressure changes in chest.

Steps	Rationale

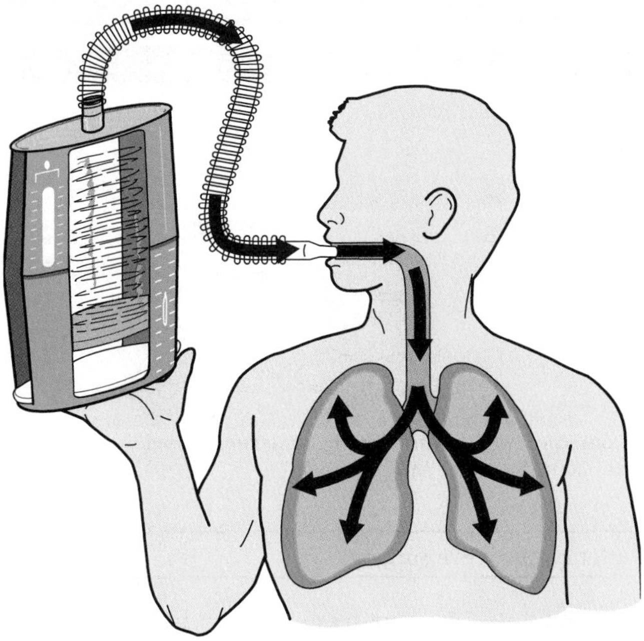

STEP **6B(5)** Incentive spirometer increases flow of air into lungs.

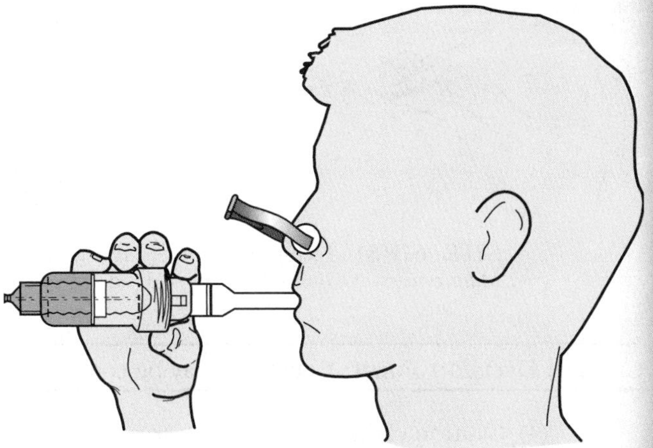

STEP **6C(3)** Positive expiratory pressure device.

Steps	Rationale
(6) Instruct client to breathe normally for short period.	Prevents hyperventilation and fatigue.
(7) Have client repeat manoeuvre until goals are achieved.	Ensures correct use of spirometer.
(8) Perform hand hygiene.	Reduces transmission of micro-organisms.
C. Positive expiratory pressure (PEP) therapy and "huff" coughing	
(1) Perform hand hygiene.	Reduces transmission of micro-organisms.
(2) Set PEP device for the setting ordered.	The higher the setting, the more effort will be required by the client. Ideally it should deliver 10 to 20 cm H_2O during passive expiration (American Association for Respiratory Care [AARC], 2002).
(3) Instruct client to assume semi-Fowler's or high-Fowler's position and place nose clip on client's nose (see illustration).	Promotes optimal lung expansion and expectoration of mucus (AARC, 2002).
(4) Have client place lips around mouthpiece. Client should take a full breath and then exhale two to three times longer than inhalation. Pattern should be repeated for 10 to 20 breaths.	Ensures that all breathing is done through the mouth and that the device is used properly.
(5) Remove device from mouth and have client take a slow, deep breath and hold for 3 seconds.	Promotes lung expansion before coughing.
(6) Instruct client to exhale in quick, short, forced exhalations or "huffs."	"Huff" coughing, or forced expiratory technique, promotes bronchial hygiene by increased expectoration of secretions.
D. Controlled coughing	
(1) Explain importance of maintaining upright position.	Position facilitates diaphragm excursion and enhances thorax expansion.
(2) Demonstrate coughing. Take two slow, deep breaths, inhaling through nose and exhaling through mouth.	Deep breaths expand lungs fully so that air moves behind mucus and facilitates effects of coughing.
(3) Inhale deeply third time and hold breath to count of three. Cough fully for two or three consecutive coughs without inhaling between coughs. (Tell client to push all air out of lungs.)	Consecutive coughs help remove mucus more effectively and completely than one forceful cough.

Skill 45-1 Demonstrating Post-operative Exercises—cont'd

Steps	Rationale

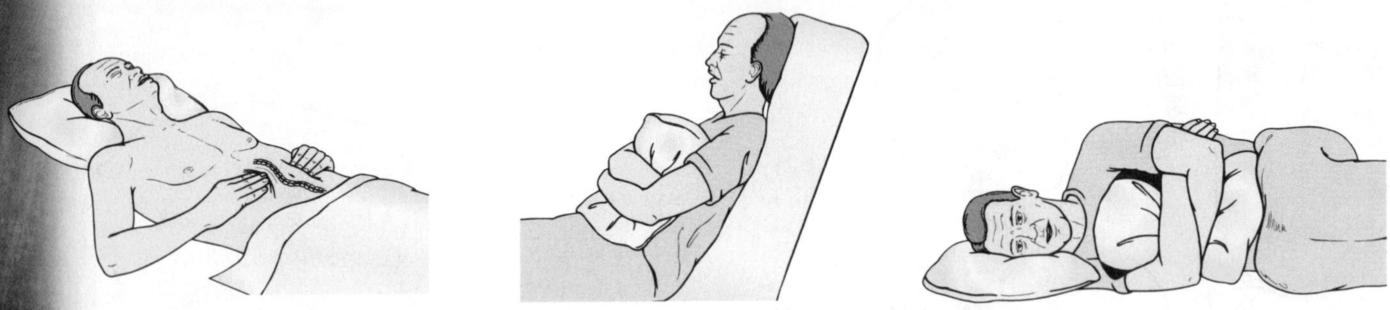

STEP **6D(5)** Techniques for splinting incision. (From *Medical-Surgical Nursing: Assessment and Management of Clinical Problems*, 6th ed., by S. Lewis, et al., 2004, St. Louis, MO: Mosby.)

Critical Decision Point: Coughing may be contraindicated after brain or eye surgery.

Steps	Rationale
(4) Caution client against just clearing throat instead of coughing. Explain that coughing will not cause injury to incision when done correctly.	Clearing throat does not remove mucus from deep in airways. Post-operative incisional pain makes it harder for the client to cough effectively.
(5) If surgical incision will be abdominal or thoracic, teach client to place one hand over incisional area and other hand on top of first. During breathing and coughing exercises, client presses gently against incisional area to splint or support it. Pillow over incision is optional (see illustration).	Surgical incision cuts through muscles, tissues, and nerve endings. Deep breathing and coughing exercises place additional stress on suture line and cause discomfort. Splinting incision with hands provides firm support and reduces incisional pulling. (Some clients prefer to have pillow to place over incision.)
(6) Client continues to practise coughing exercises, splinting imaginary incision. Instruct client to cough two to three times every 2 hours while awake.	Value of deep coughing with splinting is stressed to effectively expectorate mucus with minimal discomfort.
(7) Instruct client to examine sputum for consistency, odour, amount, and colour changes.	Sputum consistency, odour, amount, and colour changes may indicate presence of pulmonary complication, such as pneumonia.
E. Turning	
(1) Instruct client to assume supine position and move to side of bed if permitted by surgery. Have client move by bending knees and pressing heels against the mattress to raise and move buttocks (see illustration). Top side rails on both sides of bed should be in up position.	Positioning begins on side of bed so that turning to other side will not cause client to roll toward bed's edge.
(2) Instruct client to place right hand over incisional area to splint it.	Supports and minimizes pulling on suture line during turning.
(3) Instruct client to keep right leg straight and flex left knee up (see illustration). If back or vascular surgery was performed, client will need to logroll or will require assistance with turning.	Straight leg stabilizes client's position. Flexed left leg shifts weight for easier turning.

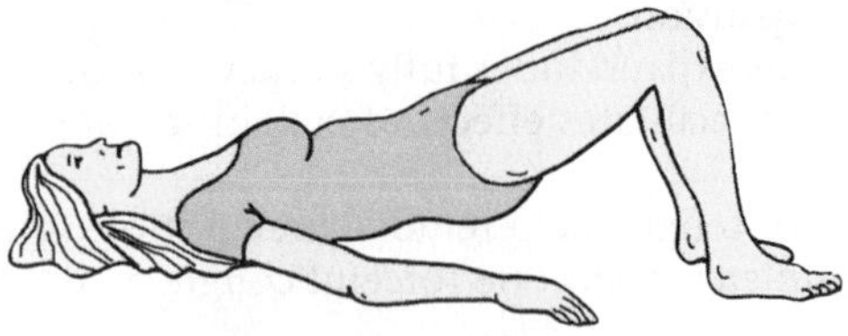

STEP **6E(1)** Buttocks lift.

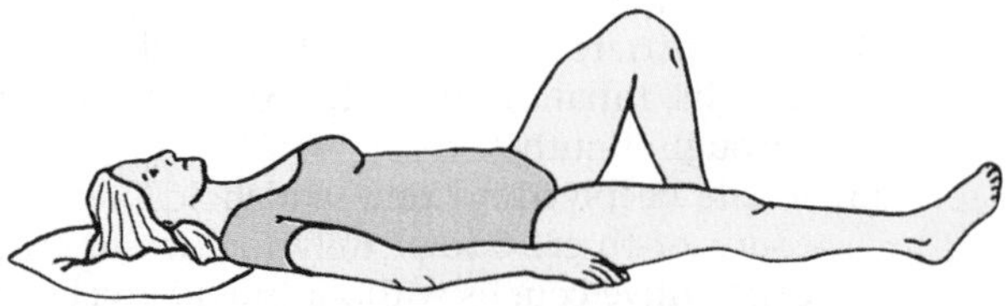

STEP **6E(3)** Leg position for turning.

Steps	Rationale
(4) Have client grab right side rail with left hand, pull toward right, and roll onto right side.	Pulling toward side rail reduces effort needed for turning.
(5) Instruct client to turn every 2 hours while awake.	Reduces risk of vascular and pulmonary complications.
F. **Leg exercises**	
(1) Have client assume supine position in bed. Demonstrate leg exercises by performing passive range-of-motion exercises and simultaneously explaining exercise.	Provides normal anatomical position of lower extremities.
(2) Rotate each ankle in complete circle. Instruct client to draw imaginary circles with big toe (see illustration). Repeat five times.	Leg exercises maintain joint mobility and promote venous return to prevent thrombi.
(3) Alternate dorsiflexion and plantar flexion of both feet. Direct client to feel calf muscles contract and relax alternately (see illustrations *A* and *B*). Repeat five times.	Stretches and contracts gastrocnemius muscles.
(4) Perform quadriceps setting by tightening thigh and bringing knee down toward mattress, then relaxing (see illustration). Repeat five times.	Contracts muscles of upper legs, maintains knee mobility, and enhances venous return.
(5) Have client alternately raise each leg straight up from bed surface, keeping legs straight and then have client bend leg at hip and knee (see illustration). Repeat five times.	Promotes contraction and relaxation of quadriceps muscles.
7. Have client practise exercises at least every 2 hours while awake. Instruct client to coordinate turning and leg exercises with diaphragmatic breathing, incentive spirometry, and coughing exercises.	Repetition of sequence reinforces learning. Establishes routine for exercises that develops habit for performance. Sequence of exercises should be leg exercises, turning, breathing, incentive spirometry, and coughing.
8. Observe client's ability to perform all five exercises independently.	Ensures that client has learned correct technique. Documents client's education and provides data for instructional follow-up.

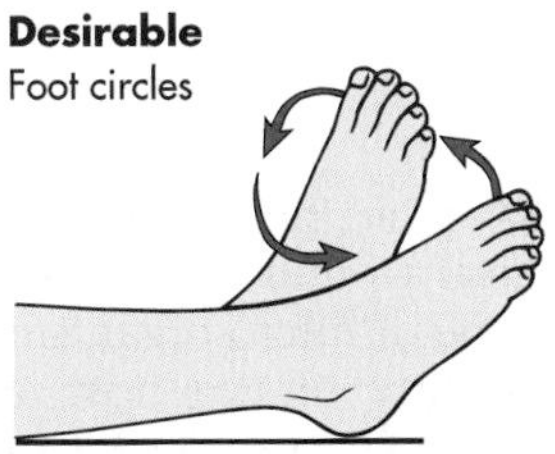

STEP **6F(2)** Foot circles. (From *Medical-Surgical Nursing: Assessment and Management of Clinical Problems,* 6th ed., p. 406, by S. Lewis, et al., 2004, St. Louis, MO: Mosby.)

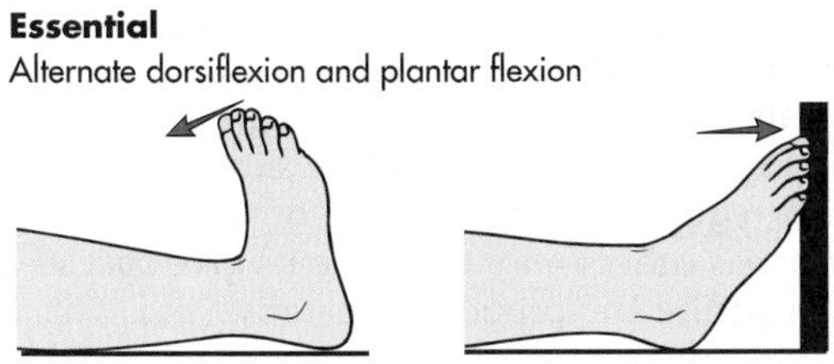

STEP **6F(3) A,** Alternate dorsiflexion and plantar flexion. (From *Medical-Surgical Nursing: Assessment and Management of Clinical Problems,* 6th ed., by S. Lewis, et al., 2004, St. Louis, MO: Mosby.)

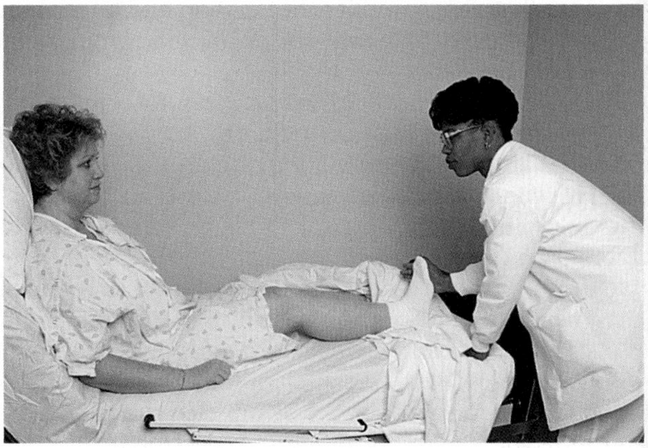

STEP **6F(3) B,** Client pushes feet to perform plantar flexion.

Skill 45-1 Demonstrating Post-operative Exercises—cont'd

Steps	Rationale

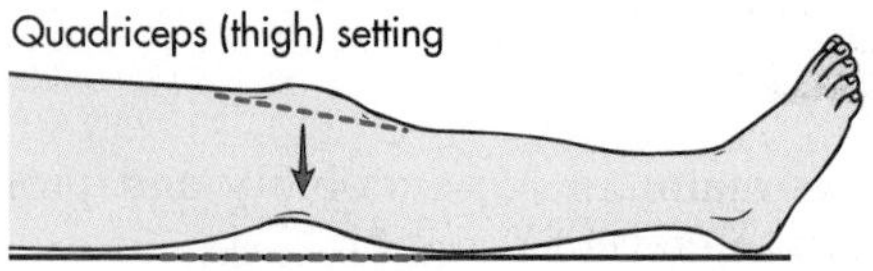

STEP **6F(4)** Quadriceps (thigh) setting. (From *Medical-Surgical Nursing: Assessment and Management of Clinical Problems,* 6th ed., by S. Lewis, et al., 2004, St. Louis, MO: Mosby.)

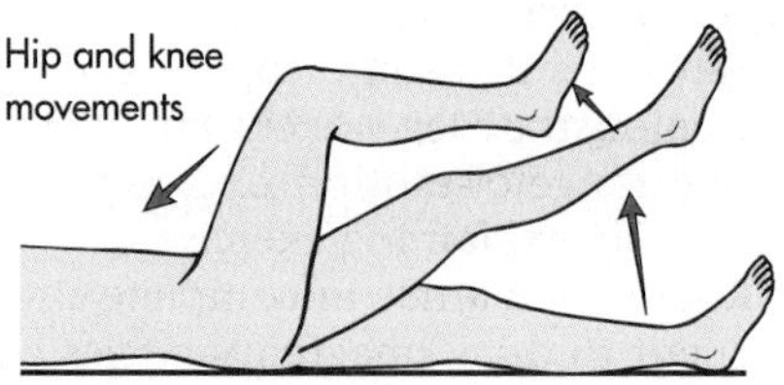

STEP **6F(5)** Hip and knee movements. (From *Medical-Surgical Nursing: Assessment and Management of Clinical Problems,* 6th ed., by S. Lewis, et al., 2004, St. Louis, MO: Mosby.)

Unexpected Outcomes and Related Interventions

- Client is unable to perform exercises correctly preoperatively.
  - Assess for the presence of anxiety, pain, and fatigue.
  - Teach client stress reduction techniques, pain management strategies, or both.
  - Repeat teaching using more demonstration or re-demonstration at time when family or friends are present.
- Client is unwilling to perform exercises post-operatively because of incisional pain of thorax or abdomen (deep breathing, coughing, and turning) or because of surgery involving lower abdomen, groin, buttocks, or legs (leg exercises, turning).
  - Instruct client to ask for pain medication 30 minutes before performing post-operative exercise or to use patient-controlled analgesia (PCA) immediately before exercising.
  - Report to surgeon inadequate pain relief and need to change analgesic or increase dose.

Recording and Reporting

- Record exercises demonstrated and whether client can perform them independently.
- Report any problems client has in practising exercises to nurse assigned to client on next shift for follow-up.

A client who is at home the evening before surgery must understand the importance of the specific fasting period that is ordered. The nurse can allow clients to rinse the mouth with water or mouthwash and brush the teeth immediately before surgery as long as they do not swallow water. The nurse notifies the surgeon and anaesthesiologist if the client has eaten or drunk fluids during the fasting period.

During surgery, normal mechanisms for controlling fluid and electrolyte balance, including respiration, digestion, circulation, and elimination, are disturbed. The surgical procedure may cause extensive losses of blood and other body fluids. The surgical stress response aggravates any fluid and electrolyte imbalance. The client's preoperative diet should include foods high in protein, with sufficient carbohydrates, fat, and vitamins. If a client cannot eat because of gastrointestinal alterations or impairments in consciousness, an IV route for fluid replacement is started. The physician assesses serum electrolyte levels to determine the type of IV fluids and electrolyte additives to administer. Clients with severe nutritional imbalances may require supplements with concentrated protein and glucose (see chapter 39).

Reduction of Risk of Surgical Wound Infection. The risk of developing a surgical wound infection is determined by the amount and type of micro-organisms contaminating a wound, susceptibility of the host, and the surgical wound itself. All three factors interact to cause infection. Antibiotics may be ordered in the preoperative period. Risk of wound infection decreases when an antibiotic is present in sufficient concentrations at the wound site before incision (Polk & Christmas, 2000). Antibiotics given before surgery may be administered orally or by IV. Increasingly, antibiotics are administered in the OR immediately before surgery (Dellinger et al., 1994).

Micro-organisms grow and multiply on the skin. Without proper skin preparation, the risk of post-operative wound infection is high. Many surgeons have clients bathe or shower the evening before surgery. Some physicians may request clients to bathe or shower more than once, whereas others may have clients give special attention to cleansing the proposed operative site. This attention could include use of an antibacterial soap. Depending on the surgical procedure, a client may also shower the morning of surgery. If the surgical procedure involves the head, neck, or upper chest area, the client

Patient(e) ______________________ Chart No. – Nº du dossier ______________________

Post-op Day 1 — Jour 1 post-opératoire

Date: yyaa ________ mm ______ dj ______

Critical Path	Patient Outcomes
Assessments/Treatments • VS, NVS, O_2 sat q4h → q shift • Check dressing • Monitor Intake & Output **Activity** • DB&C • Exercise program • Pivot transfer with walker • Comfirm weight bearing status • Up in chair x 2 ________ initial, ________ initial • Ambulate x 1 with assistance: ________ initial • Assistive devices, specify: ______________ **Nutrition** • Diet as ordered **Elimination** • Catheter as ordered **Patient Teaching** • Reinforce exercise program • Hip precautions • Ensure patient has Total Hip Replacement patient information booklet	**Pain Control** • Indicates adequate pain control **Activity** • Completes transfer with assistance • Performs exercises according to self directed exercise program **Prevention of DVT** • Demonstrates appropriate exercises & positioning for prevention of DVT • Verbalizes understanding of anticoagulant therapy **Patient Teaching** • Verbalizes understanding of "Total Hip Replacement" instructions and exercise program • Demonstrates: – Proper positioning – Understanding of mobility aids

Patient progress corresponds with clinical pathway

Physiotherapy:

☐ Yes ☐ No Signature: ______________ Time: ________ NTV – circle above, VC ________

Nursing:

D ☐ Yes ☐ No Signature: ______________, Initial ________ Time: ________ NTV – circle above, VC ________

E ☐ Yes ☐ No Signature: ______________, Initial ________ Time: ________ NTV – circle above, VC ________

N ☐ Yes ☐ No Signature: ______________, Initial ________ Time: ________ NTV – circle above, VC ________

D = 8-12 h day shift **E** = evening shift, if applicable **N** = 8-12 h night shift

Variance Codes (VC)

186	Activity variance	**510**	Not discharged by end of pathway – non-medical reason
653	Consult not sent by Day 3	**NTV**	Non-Tracked Variance
492	Not discharged by end of pathway – continued need for acute care	**OFF**	Ordered off clinical pathway

 CHART – DOSSIER CP 5A (3 – 7)

FIGURE **45–4** Post-operative client instructions for a clinical pathway for a total hip replacement. Highlights what the client can expect the first day after surgery. (Courtesy of The Ottawa Hospital, Ottawa, ON.)

may be required to shampoo the hair. Cleansing and trimming of fingernails and toenails may also be necessary.

The need for hair removal is less common now and depends on the amount of hair, location of the incision, and surgical procedure planned (AORN, 2002b). Hair removal can damage and cause breaks in the client's skin, which may allow for the entry of micro-organisms. If required, hair is removed with a clipper or shaver as close to the time of surgery as possible. Short hospital stays are known to reduce the chance of a nosocomial (hospital acquired) infection. Respiratory, urinary tract, and wound infections can all be acquired during hospitalization. This is one advantage to having ambulatory surgical procedures, because the client usually returns home when the surgery has been completed.

Prevention of Bowel and Bladder Incontinence. The client may receive a bowel preparation (e.g., a cathartic or enema) if the surgery involves the lower gastrointestinal system or lower abdominal organs. Manipulation of portions of the gastrointestinal tract during surgery results in absence of peristalsis for 24 hours or longer. Enemas and cathartics, such as GoLYTELY, cleanse the gastrointestinal tract to prevent intraoperative incontinence and postoperative constipation. An empty bowel reduces risk of injury to the intestines and minimizes contamination of the operative wound if a portion of the bowel is incised or opened accidentally, or if colon surgery is planned. The surgeon's plan may read "give enemas until clear." This means that the nurse is to administer enemas until the enema return contains no solid fecal material (see chapter 41). Too many enemas given over a short time, however, can cause serious fluid and electrolyte imbalances. Most agencies recommend a limit to the number of enemas (usually three) a nurse may administer successively.

The bladder is not prepared until the morning of surgery. The nurse instructs the client to void just before leaving for the OR and before giving preoperative medications. An empty bladder prevents a client from being incontinent during surgery. This is important during abdominal surgery, when it may become necessary for the surgeon to manipulate the bladder. An empty bladder also makes abdominal organs more accessible during surgery. The nurse in the OR often inserts a Foley catheter to maintain an empty bladder.

Promotion of Rest and Comfort. Rest is essential for normal healing. Anxiety about the impending surgery can easily interfere with the ability to relax or sleep. The underlying condition requiring surgery may be painful, further impairing rest.

If the client is admitted to hospital prior to the day of surgery, the nurse should attempt to make the client's environment quiet and comfortable. Sometimes the client is ordered a sedative-hypnotic or anxiolytic agent for the night before surgery. Sedative-hypnotics (e.g., temazepam [Restoril]) affect and promote sleep. Anxiolytic agents (e.g., alprazolam [Xanax]) act on the cerebral cortex and limbic system to relieve anxiety.

An advantage to ambulatory surgery or same-day surgical admissions is that the client is able to sleep at home the night before surgery. The client is likely to get more rest in a familiar environment. The non-hospitalized client may also have medication ordered by the physician if apprehension about surgery interferes with a good night's rest.

Preparation on the Day of Surgery. The nurse completes a number of routine procedures before releasing the client for surgery.

Hygiene. Basic hygiene measures provide additional comfort before surgery. The client may want to bathe before surgery. Because the client cannot wear personal nightwear to the OR, the nurse provides a clean hospital gown. If the client has been NPO the last several hours, the client's mouth may be very dry. The nurse may offer the client mouthwash and toothpaste, again cautioning the client not to swallow water.

Hair and Cosmetics. During surgery with the client under general anaesthesia, the client's head is positioned to introduce an endotracheal tube into the airway (see chapter 35). This procedure may involve manipulation of the client's hair and scalp. To avoid injury, the nurse asks the client to remove hairpins or clips before leaving for surgery. Hairpieces or wigs should also be removed. Long hair can be braided. The client will wear a disposable hat before entering the OR.

During and after surgery, the anaesthesiologist and nurses assess skin and mucous membranes to determine the client's level of oxygenation and circulation. Therefore, all makeup (lipstick, powder, blush, nail polish) should be removed to expose normal skin and nail colouring. Pulse oximetry is capable of recording accurate measurements through most nail polish colours, but removal is still considered good practice. Contact lenses, false eyelashes, and eye makeup must also be removed. The client's glasses can be stored or given to the family immediately before the client enters the OR.

Removal of Prostheses. It is easy for any type of prosthetic device to become lost or damaged during surgery. The client must remove all prostheses, including partial or complete dentures, artificial limbs, artificial eyes, and hearing aids. If a client has a brace or splint, the nurse checks with the physician to determine whether it should remain with the client.

For many clients, it is embarrassing to remove dentures, wigs, or other devices that enhance personal appearance. Privacy should be offered as the personal items are removed. Clients may be allowed to keep personal items until they reach the preoperative area. For safekeeping, dentures must be placed in special containers labelled with the client's name and other identification required by the agency. In many agencies, nurses must document an inventory of all prosthetic devices or personal items and have them locked away according to agency policy. It is also common practice for nurses to give prostheses to family members or to keep items like dentures at the client's bedside. Documentation in the nursing notes, surgical checklist, or per agency policy should reflect these actions.

Safeguarding Valuables. If a client has any valuables, the nurse should give them to family members or secure them for safekeeping. Many hospitals require clients to sign a release to free the institution of responsibility for lost valuables. Valuables can usually be stored and locked in a designated location. Often clients are reluctant to remove wedding rings or religious medals. A wedding band can be taped in place. However, if there is a risk that the client will experience swelling of the hand or fingers (related to mastectomy, hand surgery, fluid shifts), the band should be removed. Many hospitals allow clients to pin religious medals to their gowns, although the risk of loss increases. For safety, other metal items, such as for pierced areas, should also be removed. The location of valuables is documented per hospital policy.

Preparing the Bowel and Bladder. The client may require an enema or cathartic the morning of surgery to ensure that the colon is empty. If so, it should be given at least an hour before the client is scheduled to leave, allowing time for the client to defecate without rushing. The client should void before surgery. If the client is unable to void, it should be noted on the preoperative checklist. An indwelling urinary catheter may be placed if the surgery is long or the incision is in the lower abdomen.

Vital Signs. The nurse measures a final preoperative set of vital signs. The anaesthesiologist uses these values as a baseline during surgery. If preoperative vital signs are abnormal, surgery may need to be postponed. The nurse notifies the physician of abnormalities before sending the client to surgery.

Documentation. Before the client goes to the OR, the nurse checks the contents of the medical record to be sure that pertinent laboratory results are present. The nurse checks consent forms for accuracy of information. A preoperative checklist (Figure 45–5) provides the nurse with guidelines to ensure nursing interventions are completed. The nurse also checks the nurse's notes to be sure that documentation of care is current. This is especially important if the hospitalized client experienced unpredicted problems the night before surgery.

Performing Special Procedures. A client's condition may warrant special interventions before surgery. The client may need IV infusions started or a nasogastric tube inserted before leaving for surgery. These procedures may also be done once the client is in the preoperative area, but are usually done in the OR.

Administering Preoperative Medications. The advent of ambulatory surgery has reduced the use of preoperative medications. However, the anaesthesiologist or surgeon may order preanaesthetic drugs ("on-call medications," "preops") to reduce the client's anxiety, the amount of general anaesthesia required, the risk of nausea and vomiting and resultant aspiration, and respiratory tract secretions.

The nurse provides all nursing care measures before giving the client preoperative medications at the prescribed time. The consent form needs to be signed before the administration of these medications. In addition, the client should be helped to void. Because the drugs cause sedation, the client should not be allowed to leave the bed or stretcher until surgical personnel arrive to transport the client to the OR. The client should be warned to expect drowsiness and a dry mouth.

> ***Safety Alert:*** Explain to the client the effects of the preoperative medications. Remind the client to remain in bed or on the stretcher. The side rails should be raised and the bed or stretcher kept in the low position. The call light is placed within easy reach of the client.

Latex Sensitivity/Allergy. As the incidence and prevalence of **latex sensitivity** and allergy increases, the need for recognition of potential sources of latex is critical. The Canadian Society of Hospital Pharmacists (2001) released new guidelines recommending procedures to prevent and treat occupational latex allergy. Guidelines developed through Canadian and American health care organizations are also available for the management of latex allergies and safe latex use in health care facilities (Sussman & Gold, 2004).

The OR and post-anaesthesia care unit (PACU) contain innumerable products that contain latex. Some common sources include gloves, IV tubing, syringes, and rubber stoppers on bottles and vials. Latex is also present in objects that may be overlooked, including adhesive tape, disposable electrodes, endotracheal tube cuffs, protection sheets, and ventilator equipment. Those most at risk include people with genetic predisposition to latex allergy, children with spina bifida, clients with urogenital abnormalities or spinal cord injury (because of a long history of catheter use), clients with a history of multiple surgeries, health care professionals, and workers who manufacture rubber products (Paquet, 1998). Symptoms of a latex reaction can include local effects ranging from urticaria and flat or raised red patches to vesicular, scaling, or bleeding eruptions. Acute dermatitis may also be present. Rhinitis and rhinorrhea are other common reactions in both mild and severe latex reactions. Immediate hypersensitivity reactions can be life-threatening, with the client exhibiting focal or generalized urticaria, edema, bronchospasm, and mucous hypersecretion, which can compromise respiratory status. Vasodilatation compounded by increased capillary permeability can lead to circulatory collapse and eventual death. Because the client may be draped during surgery, any unexplained acute deterioration in a previously healthy client should be investigated for possible latex allergy (Shoup, 1998).

Protocols exist for clients with a latex allergy or sensitivity. Clients with this allergy are identified preoperatively. Latex kits are available. These kits include latex-free equipment (e.g., a latex-free ambu bag) and follow the clients throughout their hospitalization. A reference binder is kept that indicates supplies, medications, and appropriate care options for latex-sensitive clients. It is recommended that the client with a latex allergy be scheduled as the first case of the day in the OR. The room should be thoroughly cleaned, including all equipment, and all unnecessary items removed (Doepke, 1998). The client can then be safely accommodated by using appropriate latex-free items during the perioperative period and recovery. Box 45-4 lists precautions for clients with latex sensitivity or allergy.

Eliminating Wrong Site and Wrong Procedure Surgery. Whenever an invasive surgical procedure is to be performed, the nurse and surgeon must be sure the site has been marked by the surgeon (see agency policy). Indelible ink may be used to mark left and right distinction, multiple structures (e.g., fingers), and levels of the spine. The nurse also verifies the client and the procedure to be performed. In addition, once the client reaches the OR, the client is introduced to the surgical team. The client is asked to describe what procedure is being performed and to indicate the site. The consent form is verified.

The Ottawa Hospital | L'Hôpital d'Ottawa
❑ Civic ❑ General
❑ Riverside

PREOPERATIVE CHECKLIST
FEUILLE DE VÉRIFICATION PRÉOPÉRATOIRE

PART-PARTIE 1
To be completed prior to the patient leaving the Nursing Unit.
À être remplie avant le départ du patient de l'Unité des soins.

Patient is-Le(la) patient(e) est:
❑ **calm-calme** ❑ **anxious-anxieux(se)**
❑ **tearful-en larmes** ❑ **other-autre:**

CHART REVIEW-RÉVISION DU DOSSIER	Yes Oui	No Non	N/A S/O	CHART REVIEW-RÉVISION DU DOSSIER	Yes Oui	No Non	N/A S/O
❑ Allergies Allergies ❑ Allergy band Bracelet d'allergies ❑ Latex allergy Allergie au latex				Addressograph plate Plaque d'adressographe			
Caution sheet-Feuille de précaution Civic and Riverside only-seulement				Anesthesia record Fiche d'anesthésie			
Consent completed as per policy Consentement rempli d'après la politique				Medication record/MAR Fiche des médicaments/RAM			
Consult notes/Medical history Notes de consultation/Antécédents médicaux				Nursing History Histoire des soins infirmiers			
				Old chart if required Dossier antérieur si nécessaire			

ASSESSMENT-ÉVALUATION	Yes Oui	No Non	N/A S/O	ASSESSMENT-ÉVALUATION	Yes Oui	No Non	N/A S/O
Identity bracelet verified-Bracelet d'identité vérifié				Precautions - if yes, check-si oui, cocher: ❑ contact(es) ❑ total(es) ❑ airborne-aériennes ❑ droplet-gouttelettes			
Removed-Enlevé - Medic alert bracelet/necklace-collier				Communication barrier-Conflit de communication			
Teeth-Dents : ❑ capped-couronne ❑ loose-branlante				Interpreter present-Interprète présent			
Removed-Enlevé(s) : ❑ dentures-dentiers ❑ bridge-pont				Skin integrity problem-Problème de l'intégrité de la peau Site:			
❑ glasses-lunettes ❑ contacts-verres de contacts				Surgical implants-Implants chirurgicaux Site:			
❑ hearing aid-appareil auditif							
❑ jewellery/body piercing-bijoux/perçage corporel				Pacemaker/Internal defibrillator Stimulateur cardiaque/Défibrillateur interne			
Pregnancy possibility-Possibilité de grossesse							
If yes, physician notified: (Name) Si oui, médecin avisé : (Nom)				Antibiotics ordered-Antibiotiques ordonnés			
				Sent to OR with patient-Envoyés au bloc avec patient			

❑ Ate-Ingestion de nourriture last-dernière: ❑ Water-Ingestion d'eau last-dernière: ❑ Void-Miction last-dernière: ❑ Catheterized-Cathétérisé

DIAGNOSTIC TESTS ORDERED AND ON CHART EXAMENS DIAGNOSTIQUES DEMANDÉS ET AU DOSSIER	Yes Oui	N/A S/O	DIAGNOSTIC TESTS ORDERED AND ON CHART EXAMENS DIAGNOSTIQUES DEMANDÉS ET AU DOSSIER	Yes Oui	N/A S/O
ECG			Urinalysis-Analyse d'urine		
CBC			Type & Screen-Hémotypologie et dépistage		
PTT/INR			Autologus-Auto-transfusion-units-unités		
Electrolytes / BUN			Chest X-Ray-Radio pulmonaire		

CARE PLAN DE SOINS

SIGNATURE (Nurse-Infirmière) Init.

SIGNATURE (Nurse transferring patient to OR-Infirmière transférant patient au bloc) Init. DATE

PART-PARTIE 2 To be completed by OR nurse-À être remplie par l'infirmière du bloc opératoire

1. ❑ Patient identified-Patient identifié
2. ❑ Patient chart reviewed-Dossier du patient révisé
3. ❑ Consent checked-Consentement vérifié
4. ❑ Surgical site identified as per policy-Site chirurgical identifié d'après la politique ❑ N/A-S/O
5. Positional problems-Problèmes de position : ❑ N/A-S/O ❑ Yes-Oui :

Verbal lab report obtained, physician notified Médecin avisé après l'obtention du rapport de lab Name-Nom Time-Heure

CARE PLAN DE SOINS

Signature Date (yyaa-mm-dj) Time-Heure

ORA 06 (04/2004) Cat.: 412550 **CHART-DOSSIER**

FIGURE **45–5** Preoperative checklist. (Courtesy of The Ottawa Hospital, Ottawa, ON.)

Evidence-Based Practice Guideline — Box 45-4

Latex Precautions

1. Survey the client care area and remove products containing latex (e.g., exam gloves, rubber sheets, or blood pressure cuff).
2. Place a latex precautions label on the client's chart and latex precautions signs on the door to the client's room and/or transport cart.
3. Use only non-latex gloves. Order an adequate supply.
4. Review supplies to be used for the client, and substitute with latex-free supplies.
5. Review medications to be administered and verify that they are latex-free. Include the following steps:
   a. Notify pharmacy of need for latex precautions.
   b. Verify that all prescribed medications are latex-free.
   c. Place a sign in area where medications (including mixing solutions) are kept, indicating that the client is on latex precautions.
   d. Use latex-free syringes.
6. Review intravenous supplies to be used and verify that they are latex-free. Include the following steps:
   a. Use latex-free solutions.
   b. Use latex-free tubing, buretrols.
   c. Use latex-free syringes, including those for patient-controlled analgesia.
   d. Use latex-free tape.
7. Verify that bedding and support garments are latex-free (e.g., mattress protectors, antiembolism stockings, and binders).
8. Verify that dressings and tape are latex-free.
9. Notify family and visitors of the use of latex precautions.
10. Routinely survey the client care area and verify latex products are not present (e.g., examination gloves, balloons).
11. Before transfer to another area or agency, notify care providers of need for latex precautions.
12. Education programs about latex allergy should be provided to health care providers, clients, and family or caregivers. This education should include the following:
    a. Definition of latex allergy
    b. Exposures to latex
    c. Latex avoidance
    d. Signs and symptoms of a reaction to latex
    e. Emergency treatment of a reaction to latex

Adapted from "Evidence-Based Protocol: Latex Precautions," by V. M. Steelman and M. G. Titler, in *Series on Evidence-Based Practice for Older Adults*, edited by M. G. Titler (Series Ed.), 2001, Iowa City, IA: The University of Iowa College of Nursing Gerontological Nursing Interventions Research Center, Research Dissemination Core.

NP Evaluation

Client Care. The nurse in the preoperative area will be the source for evaluating outcomes in the preoperative period (Figure 45–6). With regard to the preoperative client's plan of care, limited time is available to evaluate the outcomes. The client's current status is compared with expected outcomes to determine whether new or revised interventions or nursing diagnoses need to be implemented.

Because interventions continue during and after surgery, evaluation of many goals and outcomes do not occur until after surgery. For example, the nurse will not be able to evaluate the success of preventing post-operative wound infection or promoting return of normal physiological function until a few days after surgery. If the client is having ambulatory surgery, the client will return home; therefore, the effectiveness of certain interventions may not be easily evaluated.

Client Expectations. Determining whether the client's expectations have been met regarding preoperative teaching may be difficult. The nurse is evaluating the client in a hurried atmosphere because there are many things that need to be accomplished in a short amount of time. The client's surgery may be an emergency, or performance of various procedures may make it difficult for the nurse to find time for evaluation. The client may feel somewhat depersonalized by the need to complete procedures. It is important that the nurse remember to attend to the emotional needs (privacy, fear, anxiety) of the client, as well as the physical needs. The client should be given an opportunity to state whether expectations have been met. If expectations are unmet, the nurse will need to work closely with the client to redefine expectations that can be realistically met within the time limits imposed by this particular setting.

Transport to the Operating Room

Personnel in the OR notify the nursing division or ambulatory surgery area when it is time for surgery. In many hospitals, a nursing orderly or transporter brings a stretcher for transporting the client. The transporter checks the client's identification bracelet against the client's chart to be sure that the right person is going to surgery. Because the client may have received preoperative drugs, the nurses and transporter assist the client in transferring from bed to stretcher to prevent falls. The ambulatory surgery client may ambulate to the OR if able and not medicated. Provide the family an opportunity to visit before the client is transported to the OR. Nurses then direct the family to a waiting area. In some hospitals, the family may be allowed to wait with the client in the OR holding area until he or she is transported into the OR.

After the client leaves the nursing division, the nurse prepares the bed and room for the client's return if the client is returning to the same nursing division. A postoperative bedside unit should include the following:

- Sphygmomanometer, stethoscope, and equipment to take a temperature
- Emesis basin
- Clean gown
- Washcloth, towel, and facial tissues
- IV pole
- Suction equipment (if needed)
- Oxygen equipment (if needed)
- Extra pillows for positioning the client comfortably

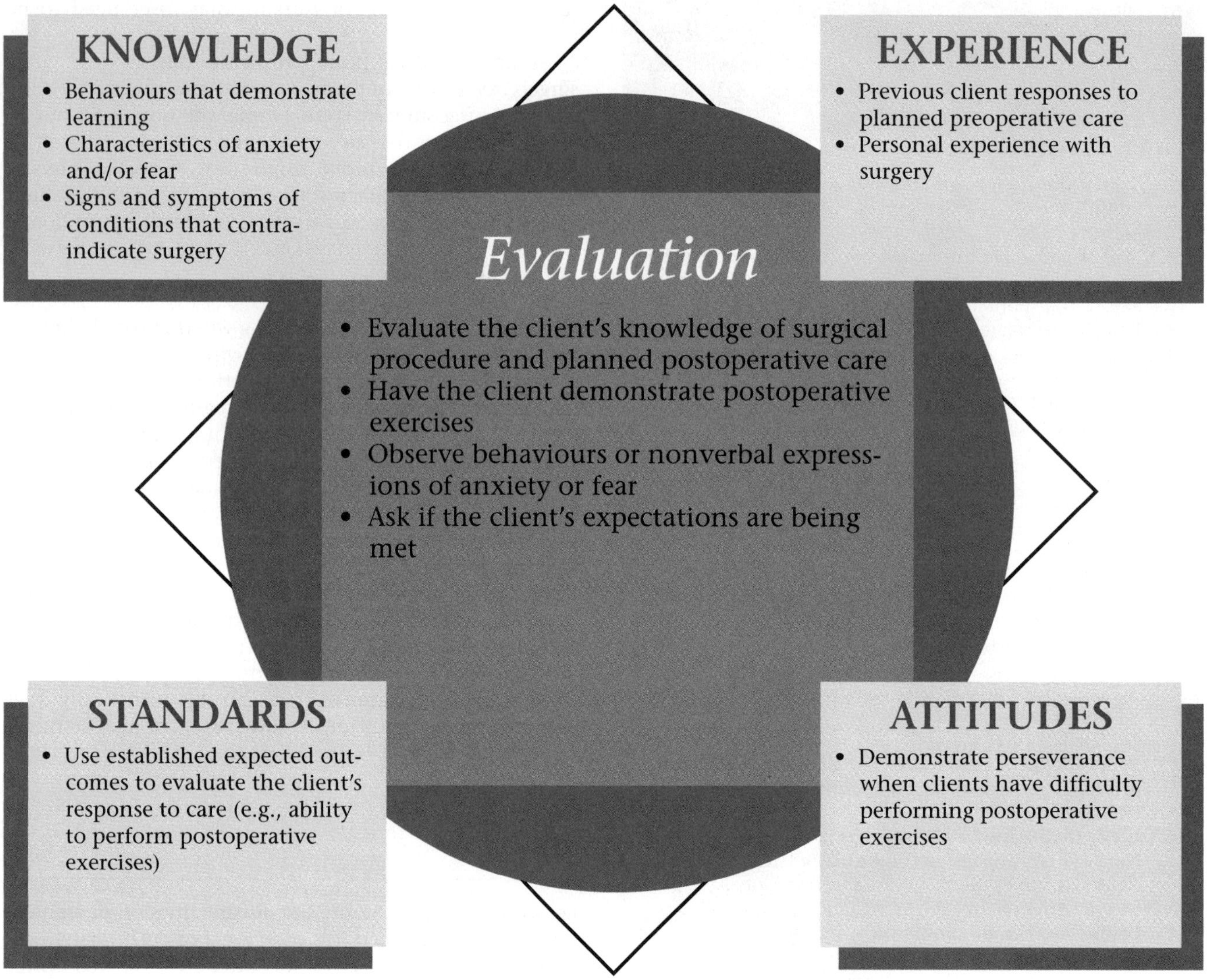
KNOWLEDGE
• Behaviours that demonstrate learning
• Characteristics of anxiety and/or fear
• Signs and symptoms of conditions that contra-indicate surgery
EXPERIENCE
• Previous client responses to planned preoperative care
• Personal experience with surgery
Evaluation
• Evaluate the client's knowledge of surgical procedure and planned postoperative care
• Have the client demonstrate postoperative exercises
• Observe behaviours or nonverbal express-ions of anxiety or fear
• Ask if the client's expectations are being met
STANDARDS
• Use established expected out-comes to evaluate the client's response to care (e.g., ability to perform postoperative exercises)
ATTITUDES
• Demonstrate perseverance when clients have difficulty performing postoperative exercises

FIGURE **45–6** Critical thinking model for surgical client evaluation.

- Bed pads to protect bed linen from drainage
- Bed raised to stretcher height with bed linens pulled back and furniture moved to accommodate the stretcher and equipment (such as IV lines)

Intraoperative Surgical Phase

Care of the client during surgery requires careful preparation and knowledge of the events that occur during the surgical procedure. The nurse usually functions in one of two roles in the OR: circulating nurse or scrub nurse. The **circulating nurse** must be an RN. Responsibilities of the circulating nurse include review of the preoperative assessment, establishing and implementing the intraoperative plan of care, evaluating the care, and providing for continuity of care post-operatively. The circulating nurse assists with procedures as needed such as endotracheal intubation and blood administration. In addition, this nurse monitors sterile technique and a safe OR environment, assists the surgeon and surgical team by operating non-sterile equipment, provides additional supplies, verifies sponge and instrument counts, and maintains accurate and complete written records.

The **scrub nurse** may be an RN or a registered practical nurse. This nurse maintains a sterile field during the surgical procedure, assists with applying sterile drapes, hands the surgeons the instruments and other sterile supplies, and counts the sponges and instruments.

Preoperative (Holding) Area

In most hospitals, the client enters a holding area outside the OR, also known as the preanaesthesia care unit. The nurse explains the steps to be taken in preparing the client for surgery, verifies that appropriate data has been obtained, assesses a client's readiness both physically and emotionally, and reinforces teaching (Sullivan, 2000). Nurses in the holding area are members of the OR staff and wear surgical scrub suits, hats, and footwear in accordance with infection-control policies. In some ambulatory surgical settings, a perioperative primary nurse admits the client, circulates for the operative procedure, and manages the client's recovery and discharge.

In the preoperative area, the nurse or anaesthesiologist may insert an IV catheter into the arm to establish a route for fluid replacement and IV drugs. A large-bore (18-gauge) IV catheter is used for easy infusion of fluids and blood products if necessary. The nurse also applies a blood pressure cuff. The cuff will remain in place throughout surgery so that the anaesthesiologist can assess blood pressure readings. The nurse usually reviews the preoperative checklist, and the anaesthesiologist may perform a client assessment at this time.

If any preoperative medications have been given, the client begins to feel drowsy. The temperature in the holding area and adjacent OR suites is usually cool, and the client should be offered an extra blanket. The client's stay in the holding area is usually brief.

Admission to the Operating Room

Nurses transfer the client to the OR via a stretcher. The client is usually still awake and will notice nurses and physicians wearing complete surgical masks, gowns, and eyewear. The staff carefully transfers the client to the OR table, being sure that the stretcher and table are locked in place. After the client is on the table, the nurse fastens a safety strap around the client. The nurse supports the client by explaining procedures and encouraging the client to ask questions. Sights and sounds in the surgical suite can seem frightening to clients.

The Nursing Process in the Intraoperative Surgical Phase

NP Assessment

In the holding area, the nurse conducts a focused preoperative assessment to verify that the client is ready for surgery and to plan intraoperative care. Because clients will not be able to speak for themselves while under general anaesthesia, this preoperative assessment in the OR is important for the client's safety.

> ***Safety Alert:*** Verification of client name by client response compared with chart and ID bracelet is done before sedation. The chart is reviewed for consent forms, allergies, medical history, physical assessment findings, test results, and verification of preoperative medications. The nurse verifies with the client the planned surgical procedure and the surgical site before anaesthesia is administered. Some agencies have the client mark the surgical site. The nurse ensures that prosthetic devices and valuables have been removed.

The nurse reviews the preoperative care plan to establish an intraoperative care plan and assesses the client's psychological comfort.

NP Nursing Diagnosis

The nurse reviews preoperative nursing diagnoses and modifies them to individualize the care plan in the OR.

NP Planning

Goals and Outcomes. Client-centred outcomes of preoperative care extend into the intraoperative phase. For example, a goal would be to maintain skin integrity. Expected outcomes include the following:

- Client will have intact skin and show no signs of redness.
- Client will be free of burns at the grounding pad.

NP Implementation

A primary focus of intraoperative care is to prevent injury and complications related to anaesthesia, surgery, positioning, and equipment used. The perioperative nurse serves as an advocate for the client during surgery and protects the client's dignity and rights at all times.

Acute Care

Physical Preparation. After safely securing the client on the OR table, the nurse applies monitoring devices to the client before surgery. Clients receiving general and regional anaesthesia undergo continuous ECG monitoring during surgery. Small plastic electrodes are placed on the chest and extremities to record electrical activity of the heart. A monitor in the OR displays the heart's electrical activity. Pulse oximetry will be used to monitor oxygen saturation. An electrical cautery grounding pad is applied to the skin. **Antiembolism stockings** may be applied intraoperatively (especially for long cases) or post-operatively according to agency policy (see chapter 42). The nurse documents device application and client tolerance to procedures.

Introduction of Anaesthesia. Clients undergoing surgical procedures receive one of four types of anaesthesia: general, regional, local, or conscious sedation.

General Anaesthesia. Modern anaesthetic agents are much easier to reverse and allow the client to recover with fewer untoward effects. **General anaesthesia** results in an immobile, quiet client who does not recall the surgical procedure. The client's amnesia acts as a protective measure from the unpleasant events of the procedure. An anaesthesiologist gives general anaesthetics by IV and inhalation routes through the three phases of anaesthesia: induction, maintenance, and emergence. Surgery requiring general anaesthesia involves major procedures with extensive tissue manipulation or during a procedure when analgesia, muscle relaxation, immobility, and control of the autonomic nervous system are desired.

Induction includes the administration of agents and endotracheal intubation. The maintenance phase includes positioning the client, preparation of the skin for incision, and the surgical procedure itself. Appropriate levels of anaesthesia are maintained during this phase. During emergence, anaesthetics are decreased and the client begins to awaken. Because of the short half-life of today's medications, emergence often occurs in the OR.

The duration of anaesthesia depends on the length of surgery. The greatest risks from general anaesthesia are the side effects of anaesthetic agents, including cardiovascular depression or irritability, respiratory depression, and liver and kidney damage.

Regional Anaesthesia. Induction of **regional anaesthesia** results in loss of sensation in an area of the body. The method of induction influences the portion of sensory pathways that are anaesthetized. No loss of consciousness occurs with regional anaesthesia, but the client may be sedated. The anaesthesiologist gives regional anaesthetics by infiltration and local application. Administration techniques include nerve blocks and spinal or epidural anaesthesia, and IV regional anaesthesia.

Risks are involved with infiltrative anaesthetics, particularly in the case of spinal anaesthesia. Because the level of anaesthesia may rise, which means that the anaesthetic agent moves upward in the spinal cord, breathing may be affected. This migration of anaesthetic depends on the drug type, amount, and client position. If the level of anaesthesia rises, respiratory paralysis may develop, requiring resuscitation. Elevation of the upper body prevents respiratory paralysis. The client may have a sudden fall in blood pressure, which results from extensive vasodilation caused by the anaesthetic block to sympathetic vasomotor nerves and pain and motor nerve fibres. The client requires careful monitoring during and immediately after surgery.

Because the client is responsive and capable of breathing voluntarily, it is unnecessary for the anaesthesiologist to use an endotracheal tube. OR personnel can gain a false sense of security because of the client's relative alertness. Nurses must remember that burns and other trauma can occur on the anaesthetized part of the body without the client being aware of the injury. It is therefore necessary to frequently observe the position of extremities and the condition of the skin.

Local Anaesthesia. **Local anaesthesia** involves loss of sensation at the desired site (e.g., a growth on the skin or the cornea of the eye). The anaesthetic agent (e.g., lidocaine) inhibits nerve conduction until the drug diffuses into the circulation. It may be injected locally or applied topically. The client experiences a loss in pain and touch sensation. Local anaesthesia is commonly used for minor procedures performed in ambulatory surgery. Physicians may infiltrate the operative area with local anaesthetics to promote post-operative pain relief.

Conscious Sedation. **Conscious sedation** is routinely used for procedures that do not require complete anaesthesia but rather a depressed level of consciousness. A client under conscious sedation must independently retain a patent airway and airway reflexes and must be able to respond appropriately to physical and verbal stimuli (Litwack, 1999). Short-acting IV sedatives, such as midazolam, are given.

Advantages of conscious sedation include adequate sedation and reduction of fear and anxiety with minimal risk, amnesia, relief of pain and noxious stimuli, mood alteration, elevation of pain threshold, enhanced client cooperation, stable vital signs, and rapid recovery. A variety of diagnostic and therapeutic procedures are appropriate for conscious sedation (burn dressing changes, some cosmetic surgery, pulmonary biopsy and bronchoscopy, colonoscopy, and many others; Litwack, 1999).

Nurses assisting with the administration of local anaesthesia and conscious sedation must demonstrate competency in the care of these clients. Knowledge of anatomy, physiology, cardiac dysrhythmias, procedural complications, and pharmacological principles related to the administration of individual agents is essential. Nurses must also be able to assess, diagnose, and intervene in the event of untoward reactions and demonstrate skill in airway management and oxygen delivery. Resuscitation equipment must be readily available when local anaesthesia or conscious sedation is used (AORN, 2002a).

Positioning the Client for Surgery. During general anaesthesia, the nursing personnel and surgeon often do not position the client until the stage of complete relaxation is achieved. The choice of position is usually determined by the surgical approach. Ideally the client's position provides good access to the operative site and sustains adequate circulatory and respiratory function. It should not impair neuromuscular structures. The client's comfort and safety must be considered.

Normal range of joint motion is maintained in an alert person by pain and pressure receptors. If a joint is extended too far, pain stimuli provide a warning that muscle and joint strain is too great. In a client who is anaesthetized, normal defence mechanisms cannot guard against joint damage, muscle stretch, and strain. The muscles are so relaxed that it is relatively easy to place the client in a position the individual normally could not assume while awake. The client often remains in a given position for several hours. Although it may be necessary to place a client in an unusual position, the nurse should attempt to maintain correct alignment and protect the client from pressure, abrasion, and other injuries. Attachments to the operating table allow protection and padding of extremities and bony prominences. Positioning should not impede normal movement of the diaphragm or interfere with circulation to body parts. If restraints are necessary, the nurse pads the area to be restrained to prevent skin trauma.

Documentation of Intraoperative Care. During the intraoperative phase, the nursing staff continues the preoperative care plan. For example, strict asepsis must be followed to minimize the risk of surgical wound infection. IV fluid infusion and monitoring of urinary and nasogastric output are examples of actions the nurse takes to maintain fluid balance. Throughout the surgical procedure, the nurse keeps an accurate record of client care activities and procedures performed by OR personnel. Documentation of intraoperative care provides useful data for the nurse who cares for the client post-operatively.

Evaluation

Interventions implemented during the intraoperative phase are evaluated throughout the surgical procedure.

Client Care. The nurse performs intraoperative evaluation of the client. Vital signs and intake and output are continuously monitored. The client's body temperature during the procedure and on completion of the surgical procedure is measured. The skin is inspected under the grounding pad and at areas where pressure from positioning may have been exerted. Schoonhoven et al. (2002) conducted research related to the development of pressure ulcers during surgery of more than 4 hours. Of the 208 clients in the study, 44 developed ulcers in the first 2 days following surgery. Therefore, careful monitoring and preventive measures must be taken during and following surgery.

Client Expectations. For clients not undergoing general anaesthesia, the nurse frequently questions them regarding pain, numbness, perceived room temperature, and overall comfort. The circulating nurse provides updates to family members in the waiting room.

Post-operative Surgical Phase

After surgery, a client's care can become complex as a result of physiological changes that may occur. Clients who have undergone general anaesthesia are more likely to face complications than those who have had only local anaesthesia or conscious sedation. The client who has had general anaesthesia usually has undergone extensive surgery as well. In contrast, an ambulatory surgical client who has had local anaesthesia with no sedation and has stable vital signs may be immediately discharged. A client who has undergone regional or general anaesthesia usually is transferred to the post-anaesthesia care unit (PACU) to be stabilized before discharge to the nursing unit or back to the ambulatory surgery area.

To assess a client's post-operative condition, the nurse applies critical thinking while relying on information from the preoperative nursing assessment, knowledge regarding the surgical procedure performed, and events occurring during surgery. This information helps the nurse to detect any change and make decisions about the client's care. A variation from the client's norm may indicate the onset of surgically related complications. Along with the anaesthesiologist, the circulating nurse may accompany the client to the PACU and report to the nurse to provide continuity of care.

A client's post-operative course involves two phases: the immediate recovery period and post-operative convalescence. For an ambulatory surgical client, recovery normally lasts only 1 to 2 hours, and **convalescence** occurs at home. For a hospitalized client, recovery may last a few hours, and convalescence occurs over 1 or more days, depending on the extent of surgery and the client's response.

Immediate Post-operative Recovery

Before the arrival of the client in the PACU, the PACU nurse obtains data from the surgical team in the OR regarding the client's general status and need for special equipment and nursing care. Careful planning allows the nursing staff to consider placement of clients in the PACU. For example, clients who undergo spinal anaesthesia are aware of their surroundings and may benefit from being in a quieter part of the PACU, away from clients needing frequent monitoring. The client with a serious infection such as tuberculosis should be isolated from other clients. Standard precautions/routine practices for infection control are used for all clients (see chapter 29). The nurse must be familiar with agency and professional protocols related to preventing respiratory infection transmission (Ontario Ministry of Health and Long-term Care, 2004)

When the client is admitted to the PACU, the personnel notify the client care area of the client's arrival. This allows the nursing staff to inform family members. The nurse usually advises family members to remain in the designated waiting area so that they can be found when the surgeon arrives to explain the client's condition. It is the surgeon's responsibility to describe the client's status, the results of surgery, and any complications that may have been encountered. The nurse can be a valuable resource to the family if complications have arisen in the operative phase.

When the client enters the PACU (Figure 45–7), the nurse and members of the surgical team confer about the client's status. The surgical team's report includes a review of anaesthetic agents administered so that the PACU nurse can anticipate how quickly a client should regain consciousness and can anticipate analgesic needs. A report on IV fluids or blood products administered during surgery alerts the nurse to the fluid and electrolyte balance. The surgeon often reports special concerns (e.g., whether the client is at risk for hemorrhaging or infection). The anaesthesiologist discusses whether there were complications during surgery, such as excessive blood loss or cardiac irregularities. Frequently this report takes place while PACU nurses are admitting the client. The

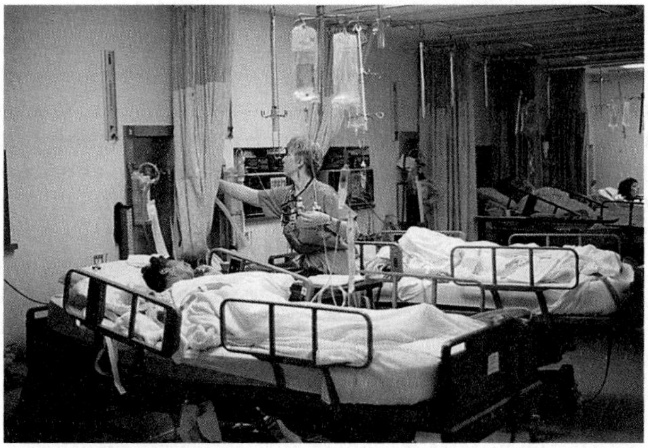

FIGURE **45–7** Post-anaesthesia care unit.

nurse will attach the client to monitoring equipment such as the non-invasive blood pressure monitor, ECG monitor, and pulse oximeter. Clients usually receive some form of oxygen in this immediate recovery period. The nurse in the PACU takes vital signs when the client arrives and confirms these with the surgical team.

After reviewing events in the OR, the PACU nurse makes a complete assessment of the client's status. The assessment should be performed rapidly and thoroughly and be targeted to the needs of the post-surgical client. Standards of perianaesthetic nursing practice, such as those of OPANA (2000), are a guide for agencies in outlining the urgent nature and components of the admission assessment as well as ongoing monitoring of client status. A systems approach to assessment is discussed in a later section outlining the nursing process in post-operative care. Nursing care in the PACU focuses on monitoring and maintaining respiratory, circulatory, neurological, and fluid and electrolyte status; assessing wound status; and assessing and managing pain (see The Nursing Process in Post-operative Care).

Discharge From the Post-Anaesthesia Care Unit

The nurse evaluates readiness for discharge from the PACU by comparing vital sign stability with the preoperative data. Other outcomes for discharge include body temperature control, good ventilatory function, orientation to surroundings, absence of complications, minimal pain and nausea, controlled wound drainage, adequate urine output, and fluid and electrolyte balance. Clients with more extensive surgery requiring anaesthesia of longer duration usually recover more slowly. Many PACU staff use an objective scoring system that helps delineate when clients may be discharged. The Aldrete score, or the **Post-Anesthesia Recovery Score (PARS),** is the most widely used scoring tool (Table 45-8). The client must receive a composite score of 8 to 10 before discharge from the PACU. Some agencies have modified this scoring system; for example, some remove extremity movement and add presence of pain, and some agencies require that the client have a composite score of 10 before discharge from the PACU. If the client's condition is still poor after 2 to 3 hours, the stay lengthens or the surgeon may transfer the client to an intensive care unit.

When the client is ready to be discharged from the PACU, the nurse calls the nursing unit to report the client's status, including vital signs, respiratory status, the type of surgery and anaesthesia performed, any complication occurring in surgery or the PACU, blood loss, level of consciousness, general physical condition, and presence of IV lines, drainage tubes, and dressings. The PACU nurse also reviews physician orders that require attention. The PACU nurse's report helps the nurse on the acute client care area to anticipate special client needs and obtain necessary equipment. Any outstanding family issues are also addressed.

Personnel, who may include nurses, return the client on a stretcher. Staff members assist in safely transferring the client to a bed (see chapter 32). The PACU nurse, if helping to transport the client, shows the acute care nurse the recovery room record and reviews the client's condition and course of care.

Table 45-8 Modified Aldrete Score

Parameter	Task	Score
Activity	Able to move four extremities voluntarily or on command	2
	Able to move two extremities voluntarily or on command	1
	Unable to move extremities voluntarily or on command	0
Respiration	Able to breathe deeply and cough freely	2
	Dyspnea or limited breathing	1
	Apneic	0
Blood pressure	±20% of preanaesthetic level	2
	±20%–49% of preanaesthetic level	1
	±50% of preanaesthetic level	0
Consciousness	Fully awake	2
	Arousable on calling	1
	Not responding	0
Oxygen saturation	SpO_2 >90% on room air	2
	Needs O_2 inhalation to maintain SpO_2 >90%	1
	SpO_2 <90% even with extra O_2	0
Totals		

Adapted from "A Post-Anesthetic Recovery Score," by J. A. Aldrete and D. Kroulik, 1970, *Anesthesia and Analgesia, 49,* pp. 924–934; and "Modifications to the Post-Anesthesia Score for Use in Ambulatory Surgery," by J. A. Aldrete, 1998, *Journal of Perianesthesia Nursing, 13*(3), p. 148.

Recovery in Ambulatory Surgery

The thoroughness and extent of post-operative recovery care depends on the ambulatory client's condition, type of surgery, and anaesthesia. There are two phases of post-anaesthesia recovery. During phase I, the nurse focuses on helping the client safely transition from a totally anaesthetized state to one requiring less acute interventions. After clients become stable and no longer require such intensive monitoring, the nurse transfers them to phase II recovery. During phase II, the nurse focuses on continuing the recovery process, addressing client needs, and preparing the client and family for discharge from phase II (OPANA, 2000).

With new anaesthetic agents and techniques, clients experience a more rapid awakening in the OR (Apfelbaum et al., 2002; Fredman et al., 2002; Saar, 2001). Therefore, some ambulatory surgery clients may bypass phase I. This is known as fast tracking (White et al., 2003). Phase II recovery may consist of a room equipped with medical recliner chairs, side tables, and footrests. Kitchen facilities for preparing light snacks and beverages are usually located in the area, along with bathrooms. Aldrete (1998) has added five more areas of functional assessment for the ambulatory surgery client, which constitute the **Post-Anesthesia Recovery Score for Ambulatory Patients (PARSAP;** Table 45-9). The phase II environment is designed to promote the client's and family's comfort and well-being

Table 45-9 **Expanded Post-Anesthetic Recovery Score for Ambulatory Patients**

Parameter	Task	Score
Activity	Able to move four extremities voluntarily or on command	2
	Able to move two extremities voluntarily or on command	1
	Unable to move extremities voluntarily or on command	0
Respiration	Able to breathe deeply and cough freely	2
	Dyspnea or limited breathing	1
	Apneic	0
Blood pressure	±20% of preanaesthetic level	2
	±20%–49% of preanaesthetic level	1
	±50% of preanaesthetic level	0
Consciousness	Fully awake	2
	Arousable on calling	1
	Not responding	0
Oxygen saturation	SpO_2 >90% on room air	2
	Needs O_2 inhalation to maintain SpO_2 >90%	1
	SpO_2 <90% even with extra O_2	0
Dressing	Dry and clean	2
	Wet but marked and not increasing	1
	Growing area of wetness	0
Pain	Pain free	2
	Mild pain handled by oral medication	1
	Severe pain requiring parenteral medication	0
Ambulation	Able to stand up and walk straight*	2
	Vertigo when erect	1
	Dizziness when supine	0
Fasting-feeding	Able to drink fluids	2
	Nauseated	1
	Nausea and vomiting	0
Urine output	Has voided	2
	Unable to void but comfortable	1
	Unable to void and uncomfortable	0
Totals		

NOTE: Total score must be at least 18 for client to be discharged to home.
*May be substituted by Romberg's test, or picking up 12 clips in one hand.
Adapted from "A Post-Anesthetic Recovery Score," by J. A. Aldrete and D. Kroulik, 1970, *Anesthesia and Analgesia, 49*, pp. 924–934; and "Modifications to the Post Anesthesia Score for Use in Ambulatory Surgery," by J. A. Aldrete, 1998, *Journal of Perianesthesia Nursing, 13*(3), p. 148.

Client Teaching Box 45-5

Post-operative Instructions for Ambulatory Surgical Clients

Objective

- Client will verbalize resources to contact for assistance.
- Client will describe signs and symptoms of post-operative problems.
- Client will list the name and dose of medications to self-administer.
- Client will describe guidelines related to specific surgery.

Teaching Strategies

- Give instruction sheet with physician's or nurse's telephone number, surgery centre's number, and follow-up appointment date and time. Allow client and family to ask questions.
- Explain to family member the signs and symptoms of infection for which to observe.
- Explain name, dose, schedule, and purpose of medications. Provide drug information leaflets.
- Explain activity restrictions, diet progression, and any special wound care related to specific surgery. Provide instruction sheet with clear, focused explanations.

Evaluation

- Have client describe signs indicating potential problems and normal convalescence
- Have client explain when and how to call health care professionals such as the home care nurse
- Have client recite date for follow-up appointment
- Have client and family member describe signs and symptoms of infection
- Have client verbalize name of drug, dose, and when to take
- Have client demonstrate proper activity/movement and wound care

until discharge. The nurse monitors clients but not at the same intensity as during phase I. In phase II recovery, nurses initiate post-operative teaching with clients and family members (Box 45-5).

Ambulatory surgical clients are discharged to home when they meet certain criteria. A client being monitored by the PARSAP must achieve a score of 18 or higher before being discharged. An exception may be allowed if the client was unable to walk or use extremities before surgery (Aldrete, 1998). Post-operative nausea and vomiting may occur once the client is home even if the symptoms were not present at the time of discharge. Options for therapy include the prophylactic use of the drug ondansetron (an orally disintegrating tablet), transcutaneous acupoint electrical stimulation, or a transdermal scopolamine patch (Gan, 2002).

Written post-operative instructions and prescriptions are reviewed with the client and family, and the nurse ensures that they verbalize understanding of these instructions. The client is discharged to a responsible adult.

Post-operative Convalescence

Inpatient clients are kept in the PACU until their condition stabilizes; they are then returned to the post-operative nursing unit. Ambulatory surgery clients will return home. Nursing care focuses on returning the client to a relatively functional level of wellness as soon as possible. The speed of convalescence depends on the type or extent of surgery, risk factors, and post-operative complications.

The Nursing Process in Post-operative Care

Nursing care in the PACU focuses on managing pain and monitoring and maintaining respiratory, circulatory, fluid and electrolyte, and neurological status. Other important factors to assess include temperature control, skin and incision/wound status, and genitourinary and gastrointestinal function. However, these factors are not unique to the PACU setting. The nurse on the acute care unit continues assessment of these critical factors on a less intensive basis until the client's discharge from the acute care facility.

NP Assessment

After the assessment on the client's arrival to PACU, the nurse repeats evaluation of vital signs and other key observations at least every 15 minutes or more frequently, depending on the client's condition and unit policy. This assessment usually continues until discharge from the PACU. Once the client is returned to the surgical unit, the nurse admitting the client takes vital signs immediately in order to compare them with the PACU findings. Vital sign monitoring on the post-operative nursing unit should initially be hourly for 4 hours and then every 4 hours, unless complications develop. Frequency of assessment should always be based on the client's current condition, which can change rapidly, especially during the post-operative period.

The nurse thoroughly documents the assessment, including vital signs, respiratory status, level of consciousness, condition of dressings and drains, comfort level, IV fluid status, and urinary output measurements. Client data can be entered on flow sheets, a computerized client record, or written progress notes. The initial findings are a baseline for comparing post-operative changes.

Once the client returns to the acute care area, the nurse focuses on completing the assessment, meeting the client's immediate needs, and providing opportunity for the family to be with the client. The nurse can explain the purpose of post-operative procedures or equipment and the client's status. The family should know that the client will fall in and out of sleep for most of the rest of the day from the effects of general anaesthesia and pain medication. The family should also be reminded that frequent assessments are to be expected and that limited sensation and movement in the extremities may remain for several hours if the client had spinal or epidural anaesthesia.

Respiration. Certain anaesthetic agents may cause respiratory depression. Thus, the nurse is especially alert for shallow, slow breathing and a weak cough. The nurse assesses airway patency, respiratory rate, rhythm, depth of ventilation, symmetry of chest wall movement, breath sounds, and colour of mucous membranes. If breathing is unusually shallow, placement of the hand near the client's nose or mouth allows the nurse to feel exhaled air. Pulse oximetry should reflect 92% to 100% saturation. Some agencies now have directives that allow the nurse to administer oxygen at 3 L/minute via nasal prongs if the client has a saturation of less than 92%.

The client often has an oral or nasal airway (see chapter 35) inserted in the OR after removal of the endotracheal tube to maintain a patent airway until the client can protect his or her airway. As the client awakens in the PACU, the client will spit out the airway or the nurse asks the client to spit out the airway. The ability to do so signifies the return of a normal gag reflex.

One of the nurse's greatest concerns is airway obstruction. A number of factors can contribute to obstruction, including weak pharyngeal/laryngeal muscle tone from anaesthetics; secretions in the pharynx, bronchial tree, or trachea; and laryngeal or subglottic edema (Litwack, 1999). In the post-anaesthetic client, the tongue causes the majority of airway obstructions. Ongoing assessment of airway patency is crucial. Clients are often kept in side-lying positions until airways are clear.

In the acute care area, the nurse continues to assess respiratory status and breath sounds. Older clients, smokers, and clients with a history of respiratory disease are prone to developing complications such as atelectasis or pneumonia. The client is also assessed for any signs of shortness of breath with activity.

Circulation. The client is at risk for cardiovascular complications resulting from actual or potential blood loss from the surgical site, side effects of anaesthesia, electrolyte imbalances, and depression of normal circulatory regulating mechanisms. Careful assessment of heart rate and rhythm, along with blood pressure, reveals the client's cardiovascular status. A rhythm strip is usually obtained post-operatively, compared with preoperative ECG tracings, and mounted on the PACU record. The vital signs are monitored at least every 15 minutes throughout the recovery phase. The nurse compares preoperative vital signs with post-operative values. The physician should be notified if the client's blood pressure drops progressively with each check or if the heart rate changes or becomes irregular.

The nurse assesses circulatory perfusion by noting capillary refill, pulses, and the colour and temperature of the nail beds and skin. If the client has had vascular surgery or has casts or constricting devices that may impair circulation, the nurse assesses peripheral pulses and capillary refill distal to the site of surgery. For example, after surgery to the femoral artery, the nurse assesses posterior tibial and dorsalis pedis pulses. The nurse also compares pulses in the affected extremity with those in the non-affected extremity.

A common early circulatory problem is hemorrhage. Blood loss may occur externally through a drain or incision, or internally. Either type of hemorrhage may result in a fall in blood pressure; elevated heart and respiratory rate; thready pulse; cool, clammy, pale skin; and restlessness. Often the first sign of hemorrhage is restlessness. However, signs such as thready pulse and clammy skin are noted much later, after significant blood loss has occurred. The surgeon must be notified if changes such as these are noted. The nurse maintains IV fluid infusion and may need to increase IV replacement fluids. The nurse monitors the client's vital signs every 15 minutes or more frequently until the client's condition stabilizes. Oxygen may need to be continued. Volume replacement and medications to promote perfusion to vital organs such as the brain may be considered. Blood counts and coagulation studies are drawn and sent to the laboratory. The potential for cardiovascular complications remains when the client is transferred to the acute care area. The nurse continues to assess the same factors that were identified in the PACU.

Temperature Control. The OR and recovery room environments are extremely cool. The client's anaesthetically depressed level of body function results in a lowering of metabolism and fall in body temperature. When clients begin to awaken, they complain of feeling cold and uncomfortable. The length of time spent in the OR and laminar flow rooms contributes to heat loss. Surgeries that require an open body cavity also contribute to heat loss. Older adults and pediatric clients are at higher risk for developing problems associated with hypothermia.

In rare instances, **malignant hyperthermia** develops, a genetically determined condition and a life-threatening complication of anaesthesia. Malignant hyperthermia causes tachypnea, tachycardia, premature ventricular contractions, unstable blood pressure, cyanosis, skin mottling, and muscular rigidity. An elevated temperature occurs late. Although it is often seen during the induction phase of anaesthesia, symptoms may recur 24 to 72 hours post-operatively (Karlet, 1998). Without prompt detection and treatment, it can be fatal.

Temperature is monitored closely in the acute care area. Because an elevated temperature may be the first indication of an infection, the nurse evaluates the client for a potential source of infection, including the IV site (if present), the surgical incision or wound, and the respiratory and urinary tracts. The physician must be notified, because a further evaluation, including blood, sputum, and urinary cultures, will likely be needed.

Fluid and Electrolyte Balance. Because of the surgical client's risk for fluid and electrolyte abnormalities, the nurse assesses the hydration status and monitors cardiac and neurological function for signs of electrolyte alterations (see chapter 36). Laboratory values will be monitored and compared with the client's baseline values.

An important responsibility of the nurse is maintaining patency of IV infusions. The client's only source of fluid intake immediately after surgery is through IV catheters. The nurse inspects the catheter insertion site to ensure that the catheter is properly positioned within a vein so that fluid flows freely. Accurate recording of intake and output helps assess renal and circulatory function. The nurse measures all sources of output, including urine, surgically placed drains, gastric drainage, and drainage from wounds, and notes any insensible loss from diaphoresis. Daily weights may be assessed post-operatively if the client has a known cardiac history (e.g., heart failure). It is important to compare pre- and post-operative weights and be consistent in the scale, amount of clothing, and time of day to obtain accurate weight measurement.

Neurological Functions. In the PACU, the client is often drowsy. As anaesthetic agents are metabolized, the client's reflexes return, muscle strength is regained, and a normal level of orientation returns. A client should at least be oriented to self and the hospital before discharge from the PACU. The nurse assesses gag reflexes (see chapter 28), hand grips, and movement of extremities. If a client has had surgery involving a portion of the neurological system, the nurse conducts a more thorough neurological assessment, including assessing pupil size and reaction.

Clients with regional anaesthesia begin to experience a return in motor function before tactile sensation. The nurse checks the client's sensation along **dermatomes** (segmental skin areas innervated by specific segments of the spinal cord). Knowing where anaesthesia was introduced, the nurse is able to check the distribution of the spinal nerves affected (see chapter 28). Typically, the nurse assesses the dermatome level by touching the client bilaterally and documenting where the client feels touch. The sense of touch can be tested using, for example, a paper clip. Assessment of extremity strength, movement, and sensation continues to be important if spinal or epidural anaesthesia has been given, although the client should remain in the PACU until sensation and voluntary movement of the lower extremities have been re-established.

Skin Integrity and Condition of the Wound. In the PACU, the nurse assesses the condition of the client's skin, noting rashes, petechiae, abrasions, or burns. A rash may indicate a drug sensitivity or allergy. Abrasions or petechiae may result from a clotting disorder or inappropriate positioning or restraining that injures skin layers. Burns may indicate that an electrical cautery grounding pad was incorrectly placed on the client's skin. Burns or serious injury to the skin should be documented by an incident report (see chapter 13). The nurse should also note if the client is complaining of any burning or pain in the eye that could indicate a corneal abrasion.

After surgery, most wounds are covered with a dressing that protects the site and collects drainage. The nurse observes the amount, colour, odour, and consistency of drainage on dressings. Serosanguineous drainage is the most common type of drainage occurring immediately after surgery. The nurse estimates the amount of drainage by noting the number of saturated gauze sponges. If drainage appears on the outer surface of a dressing, another way of assessing drainage is by drawing a circle around the outer perimeter of the drainage and dating it with the time noted. This way, the nurse can easily note if drainage is increasing (see chapter 43).

Many physicians prefer to change surgical dressings the first time so that they can inspect the incisional area. The nurse on the surgical nursing unit will usually have the first opportunity to view and thoroughly assess and document the status of the incision or wound. Initially, it is important to note if wound edges are approximated and no active bleeding or drainage is present. Wound assessment is especially important because it forms the baseline for continued monitoring during the client's hospital stay.

It is also important to assess the client's mobility level. If the client is unable or unwilling to turn, pressure ulcer development is a concern. The nurse should use the Braden Scale to determine the client's risk of developing pressure ulcers (RNAO, 2005). Preventive measures such as a turning schedule and pressure-reduction devices can be instituted (see chapter 43).

Genitourinary Function. Depending on the surgery, a client may not regain voluntary control over urinary function for 6 to 8 hours after anaesthesia. An epidural or spinal anaesthetic may prevent the client from feeling bladder fullness. The nurse palpates the lower abdomen just above the symphysis pubis for bladder distension. If the client has a urinary catheter, there should be a continuous flow of urine of 30 to 50 mL/hour in adults (Metheny, 2000). The nurse observes the colour and odour of urine. Surgery involving portions of the urinary tract normally causes bloody urine for at least 12 to 24 hours, depending on the type of surgery. The acute care nurse will provide ongoing assessment of genitourinary function.

Gastrointestinal Function. Anaesthetics slow gastrointestinal motility and may cause nausea. Normally during the immediate recovery phase, faint or absent bowel sounds are auscultated in all four quadrants. The nurse inspects the abdomen for distension that may be caused by accumulation of gas. In a client who has had abdominal surgery, distension will develop if internal bleeding occurs; however, this is a late sign of bleeding. Distension may also occur in the client who develops a **paralytic ileus** from handling of the bowel in surgery.

The acute care nurse closely monitors the client's initial oral intake for potential aspiration or the presence of nausea and vomiting. Assessment also includes checking for return of peristalsis every 4 to 8 hours. Routinely, the nurse auscultates the abdomen to detect return of normal bowel sounds; 5 to 30 loud gurgles per minute over each quadrant indicates that peristalsis has returned. High-pitched tinkling sounds accompanied by abdominal distension suggest that the bowel is not functioning properly. The nurse asks if the client is passing gas (flatus). This is an important sign indicating normal bowel function. If a nasogastric tube is in place, assess the patency of the tube (see chapter 41) and the colour and amount of any drainage.

Comfort. Pain management is included in the overall aim of ensuring client comfort. Comfort is also achieved through nursing measures such as bathing and providing clean bedding. As clients awaken from general anaesthesia, the sensation of pain becomes prominent. Pain can be perceived before full consciousness is regained. Acute incisional pain causes clients to become restless and may be responsible for temporary changes in vital signs. It is difficult for clients to begin coughing and deep breathing exercises when they experience pain. The client who had regional or local anaesthesia may not initially experience pain because the incisional area is still anaesthetized.

Assessment of the client's discomfort and evaluation of pain-relief therapies are essential nursing functions. Pain scales are an effective method for nurses to assess post-operative pain, evaluate response to analgesics, and objectively document pain severity (see chapter 38). By frequently assessing pain, the nurse can evaluate the effectiveness of interventions (e.g., positioning, analgesics) throughout the client's recovery.

Client Expectations. The nurse assesses the client's and family's expectations and perceived progress in the recovery and convalescence phases. Ongoing assessment of expectations regarding pain control, comfort level, dietary intake, activity level, and readiness for discharge are also performed. The nurse determines the client's and family's expectations regarding needs at home and these are incorporated into the plan of care.

Nursing Diagnosis

The nurse determines the status of problems identified from preoperative nursing diagnoses and clusters new relevant data to identify new diagnoses. Previously defined diagnoses, such as *impaired skin integrity,* may continue as a post-operative problem. The nurse may also identify new risk factors leading to identification of nursing diagnoses. For example, an older client who has undergone major abdominal surgery and who has a pre-existing problem of reduced hip mobility resulting from arthritis will likely have the diagnosis of *impaired physical mobility.* The surgery itself may add risk factors for the client. The nurse also considers the needs of a client's family when making diagnoses. For example, the inability of the family to cope with the client's condition requires the nurse's intervention. Dialogue early on with the family can identify any challenges.

Planning

Because of the critical nature of the immediate post-operative period, the plan of care in the PACU involves close monitoring of the client and frequent assessments to ensure return to stable physiological function. During the convalescent phase, the nurse uses current physical assessment data and analysis of the preoperative nursing health history for planning the client's care. The surgeon's post-operative plan also offers guidelines. Typical post-operative plans include the following:

- Frequency of vital sign monitoring and special assessments
- Types of IV fluids and rates of infusion
- Post-operative medications (especially those for pain and nausea)
- Resumption of preoperative medications as condition allows (some oral medications will be converted to the IV route with appropriate dose adjustment)
- Fluids and food allowed by mouth
- Level of activity that the client is allowed to resume
- Position that the client is to maintain while in bed
- Intake and output
- Laboratory tests and X-ray studies
- Special directions (e.g., surgical drains to suction, tube irrigations, dressing changes)

Goals and Outcomes. The nurse considers the effects of the stress of surgery and limitations it produces when establishing goals, expected outcomes, and interventions for the individual client. Measurable outcomes help to ensure timely and appropriate recovery from surgery. For example, the client at risk for impaired mobility should have specific outcomes selected that include targeted ambulation (e.g., steps to take and distance down hallway) and range of joint movement. After each outcome is met, the client will ultimately achieve the goal of independent mobility at a preoperative level or better. The nurse carefully considers all goals of care established during the preoperative surgical phase. The following is an example of goals and expected outcomes for the postoperative period:

- Client achieves a return of normal physiological function after surgery.
- Client's vital signs return to preoperative baseline.
- Client's airway is patent and respirations are even and unlaboured.
- Client's temperature returns to baseline. Client's fluid and electrolyte levels remain balanced.
- Client returns to previous level of activity.

Setting Priorities. In the PACU, priorities of care include the assessment and stability of the client's airway; intervention for an impaired airway; assessment of the client's respiratory, circulatory, neurological, and fluid and electrolyte status; and pain control. As the client progresses on the acute care unit, priorities should focus on advancement of client activity to return the client to preoperative functioning or better. The client will generally have multiple nursing diagnoses (Figure 45–8). The nurse may re-establish priorities several times as the status of the client's health problems change.

Continuity of Care. In the recovery phase, the nurse collaborates on the plan of care with staff from respiratory therapy, physiotherapy, occupational therapy, dietary, social work, home care, and other areas to meet the needs

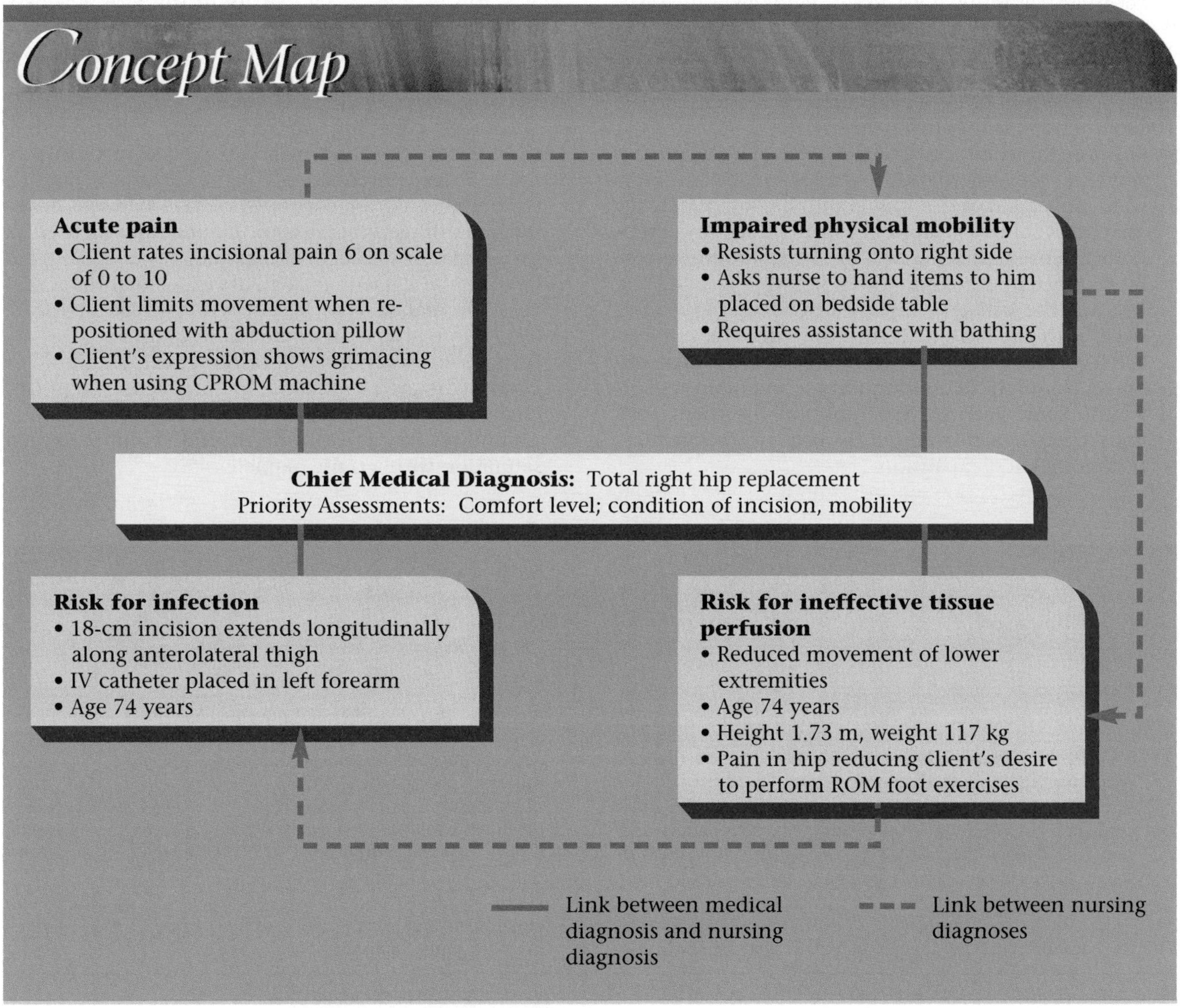
Concept Map
Acute pain
• Client rates incisional pain 6 on scale of 0 to 10
• Client limits movement when repositioned with abduction pillow
• Client's expression shows grimacing when using CPROM machine
Impaired physical mobility
• Resists turning onto right side
• Asks nurse to hand items to him placed on bedside table
• Requires assistance with bathing
Chief Medical Diagnosis: Total right hip replacement
Priority Assessments: Comfort level; condition of incision, mobility
Risk for infection
• 18-cm incision extends longitudinally along anterolateral thigh
• IV catheter placed in left forearm
• Age 74 years
Risk for ineffective tissue perfusion
• Reduced movement of lower extremities
• Age 74 years
• Height 1.73 m, weight 117 kg
• Pain in hip reducing client's desire to perform ROM foot exercises
Link between medical diagnosis and nursing diagnosis
Link between nursing diagnoses

FIGURE **45–8** Concept map for surgical client with total hip replacement.

of the client. The goal of all of these disciplines is to assist the client to return to the best possible level of functioning with a smooth transition to home. The family's role in the plan of care to foster recovery is also essential.

NP Implementation

Health Promotion. Primary causes of post-operative complications include the surgical wound, the effects of prolonged immobilization during surgery and convalescence, preoperative risks such as age (Box 45-6), and the influence of anaesthesia and analgesics. Nursing interventions in the post-operative period are directed at preventing complications so that the client returns to the highest level of functioning possible. Failure of the client to become actively involved in recovery adds to the risk of complications (Table 45-10). Virtually any body system can be affected. The nurse must consider the interrelationship of all systems and therapies provided.

Maintaining Respiratory Function. To prevent respiratory complications, the nurse begins pulmonary interventions early. The benefits of thorough preoperative teaching are realized when clients are able to participate actively. When the client awakens from anaesthesia, the nurse may need to assist him or her in maintaining a patent airway. The following measures maintain airway patency:

- Position the client on one side with the face downward and the neck slightly extended to facilitate a forward movement of the tongue and the flow of mucous secretions out of the mouth. A small folded towel supports the head. Another positioning technique to promote a patent airway involves slightly elevating the head of the bed and slightly extending the client's neck, with the head turned to the side. The nurse in the PACU may need to perform a jaw thrust manoeuvre and/or chin lift continuously to maintain the airway in some clients. Never position the client with arms over or across the chest because this reduces maximum chest expansion.
- Suction artificial airways and the oral cavity for mucous secretions (see chapter 35). Care must be taken to avoid eliciting the gag reflex, which might cause vomiting.

The following measures promote expansion of the lungs:

- Encourage diaphragmatic breathing exercises every hour while clients are awake. Maximal inspirations lasting 3 to 5 seconds open up alveoli.
- Instruct clients to use an incentive spirometer for maximum inspiration. The client should try to reach the inspiratory volume achieved preoperatively on the spirometer.
- Encourage early ambulation. Walking causes clients to assume a position that does not restrict chest wall expansion and stimulates an increased respiratory rate.
- Help clients who are restricted to bed to turn on their sides every 1 to 2 hours while awake and to sit when possible. Turning permits expansion of the lungs. Sitting causes lowering of abdominal organs, thus facilitating diaphragmatic movement and lung expansion.
- Keep the client comfortable. A client who is comfortable will be able to participate in the post-operative regimen. Assess, document, treat, and evaluate the client's pain on a regular basis.

The following measures promote removal of pulmonary secretions if they are present:

- Encourage coughing exercises every 2 hours while clients are awake and maintain pain control to promote a deep, productive cough. Coughing may be contraindicated for clients who have had eye or intracranial surgery because of the potential increase in intraocular or intracranial pressure.
- Provide oral hygiene to facilitate expectoration of mucus. The oral mucosa becomes dry when clients are NPO or are placed on limited fluid intake.
- Initiate orotracheal or nasotracheal suction for clients who are too weak or are unable to cough (see chapter 35).
- Administer oxygen as ordered and monitor oxygen saturation with a pulse oximeter.

Box 45-6

Focus on Older Adults

- Age alone is no longer a parameter for determining the benefit one can achieve from a surgical procedure. Consequently, nurses are caring for many more surgical clients of advanced age and are required to know the age-related factors that impact a surgical procedure (Eliopoulos, 2001).
- A smaller margin of physiologic reserve makes the older adult less able to compensate during the perioperative period for changes that can occur due to infection, hemorrhage, alterations in blood pressure, and fluid/electrolyte abnormalities.
- Older clients are at greater risk for post-operative delirium after procedures such as hip replacement. A rapid decline in cognitive function, fluctuations in awareness and orientation, disturbed sleep-wake cycle, and personality and mood changes characterize the typical presentation (Lueckenotte, 2000).
- Altered and unexpected drug responses are often related to different pharmacokinetics in the older adult. Thus, the nurse caring for the perioperative older client must be alert to the possibility of a high risk for adverse medication events with the administration of anaesthetic agents and post-operative analgesics, especially narcotics (Lueckenotte, 2000). "Start low and go slow" should be the guiding principle when medicating older adults because of their slower drug-clearance capability.

Data from *Gerontologic Nursing* (5th ed.), by C. Eliopoulos, 2001, Philadelphia: Lippincott; and *Gerontologic Nursing* (2nd ed.), by A. G. Lueckenotte, 2000, St. Louis, MO: Mosby; and Assessment and Management of Pain, RNAO, 2002. Retrieved September 1, 2004, from *http://www.rnao.org/bestpractices/index.asp*

Table 45-10 Post-operative Complications

Complication	Cause
Respiratory System	
Atelectasis: Collapse of alveoli with retained mucous secretions. Signs and symptoms include elevated respiratory rate, dyspnea, fever, crackles auscultated over involved lobes of lungs, and productive cough.	Inadequate lung expansion. Anaesthesia, analgesia, and immobilized position prevent full lung expansion. There is greater risk in clients with upper abdominal surgery who have pain during inspiration and repress deep breathing.
Pneumonia: Inflammation of alveoli. It may involve one or several lobes of lung. Development in lower dependent lobes of lung is common in immobilized surgical client. Signs and symptoms include fever, chills, productive cough, chest pain, purulent mucus, and dyspnea.	Poor lung expansion with retained secretions or aspirated secretions.
Hypoxemia: Inadequate concentration of oxygen in arterial blood. Signs and symptoms include restlessness, dyspnea, high or low blood pressure, tachycardia or bradycardia, diaphoresis, and cyanosis.	Respirations are depressed by anaesthetics or analgesics. Increased retention of mucus with impaired ventilation occurs because of pain or poor positioning.
Pulmonary embolism: Embolus blocking pulmonary arterial blood flow to one or more lobes of lung. Signs and symptoms include dyspnea, sudden chest pain, cyanosis, tachycardia, and drop in blood pressure.	Same factors lead to formation of thrombus or embolus. Immobilized surgical client with pre-existing circulatory or coagulation disorders is at risk.
Circulatory System	
Hemorrhage: Loss of large amount of blood externally or internally in short period of time. Signs and symptoms include hypotension, weak and rapid pulse, cool and clammy skin, rapid breathing, restlessness, and reduced urine output.	Slipping of suture or dislodged clot at incisional site. Clients with coagulation disorders are at greater risk.
Hypovolemic shock: Inadequate perfusion of tissues and cells from loss of circulatory fluid volume. Signs and symptoms are same as for hemorrhage.	In surgical client, hypovolemic shock is usually caused by hemorrhage.
Thrombophlebitis: Inflammation of vein often accompanied by clot formation. Veins in legs are most commonly affected. Signs and symptoms include swelling and inflammation of involved site and aching or cramping pain. Vein feels hard, cordlike, and sensitive to touch.	Venous stasis is aggravated by prolonged sitting or immobilization. Trauma to vessel wall and hypercoagulability of blood increase risk of vessel inflammation.
Thrombus: Formation of clot attached to interior wall of a vein or artery, which can occlude the vessel lumen. Signs and symptoms include localized tenderness along distribution of the venous system, swollen calf or thigh, calf swelling >3 cm compared with asymptomatic leg, pitting edema in symptomatic leg, collateral superficial veins, and decrease in pulse below location of thrombus (if arterial).	Venous stasis (see discussion of thrombophlebitis) and vessel trauma. Venous injury is common after surgery of legs, abdomen, pelvis, and major vessels. Clients with pelvic and abdominal cancer or traumatic injuries to the pelvis or lower extremities are at high risk for thrombus formation.
Embolus: Piece of thrombus that has dislodged and circulates in bloodstream until it lodges in another vessel, commonly lungs, heart, brain, or mesentery.	Thrombi form with increased coagulability of blood (e.g., polycythemia and use of birth control pills containing estrogen).
Gastrointestinal System	
Paralytic ileus: Non-mechanical obstruction of the bowel caused by physiological, neurogenic, or chemical imbalance associated with decreased peristalsis.	Handling of intestines during surgery can lead to loss of peristalsis for a few hours to several days.
Abdominal distension: Retention of air within intestines and abdominal cavity during gastrointestinal surgery. Signs and symptoms include increased abdominal girth, tympanic percussion over abdominal quadrants, client complaints of fullness and "gas pains."	Slowed peristalsis from anaesthesia, bowel manipulation, or immobilization. During laparoscopic surgeries, influx of air for procedure causes distension.
Nausea and vomiting: Symptoms of improper gastric emptying or chemical stimulation of vomiting centre. Client complains of gagging or feeling full or sick to stomach.	Abdominal distension, fear, severe pain, medications, eating or drinking before peristalsis returns, and initiation of gag reflex.
Genitourinary System	
Urinary retention: Involuntary accumulation of urine in bladder as result of loss of muscle tone. Signs and symptoms include inability to void, restlessness, and bladder distension. It appears 6–8 hours after surgery.	Effects of anaesthesia and narcotic analgesics. Local manipulation of tissues surrounding bladder and edema interfere with bladder tone. Poor positioning of client impairs voiding reflexes.
Urinary tract infection: An infection of the urinary tract as a result of bacterial or yeast contamination. Signs and symptoms include dysuria, itching, abdominal pain, possible fever, cloudy urine, white blood cells and leukocyte esterase positive on urinalysis.	Most frequently a result of catheterization of the bladder.

Continued

Table 45-10 Post-operative Complications—cont'd

Complication	Cause
Integumentary System	
Wound infection: An invasion of deep or superficial wound tissues by pathogenic micro-organisms; signs and symptoms include warm, red, and tender skin around incision; fever and chills; purulent material exiting from drains or from separated wound edges. Infection usually appears 3–6 days after surgery.	Infection is caused by poor aseptic technique or contaminated wound or surgical site before surgical exploration. For example, with a bowel perforation, the client is at increased risk for a wound infection because of bacterial contamination from the large intestine.
Wound dehiscence: Separation of wound edges at suture line. Signs and symptoms include increased drainage and appearance of underlying tissues. This usually occurs 6–8 days after surgery.	Malnutrition, obesity, preoperative radiation to surgical site, old age, poor circulation to tissues, and unusual strain on suture line from coughing or positioning cause dehiscence.
Wound evisceration: Protrusion of internal organs and tissues through incision. Incidence usually occurs 6–8 days after surgery.	See discussion of wound dehiscence. Client with dehiscence is at risk for developing evisceration.
Skin breakdown: Result of pressure or shearing forces. Surgical clients are at increased risk if alterations in nutrition and circulation are present, resulting in edema and delayed healing.	Prolonged periods on the operating room (OR) table and in the bed post-operatively can lead to pressure breakdown. Skin breakdown results from shearing during positioning on the OR table and improper pulling of the client up in bed.
Nervous System	
Complex pain situations: These might include situations in which pain is unresponsive to standard treatment or where there are multiple sources of pain (RNAO, 2002a).	The source may be related to, for example, surgical site or concomitant injuries or pathology.

Preventing Circulatory Complications. Measures directed at preventing circulatory complications avert circulatory stasis. Some clients are at greater risk of venous stasis because of the nature of their surgery or medical history. The following measures promote normal venous return and circulatory blood flow:

- Encourage clients to perform leg exercises at least every hour while awake. Exercise may be limited in an affected extremity involving vascular repair or realignment of fractured bones and torn cartilage.
- Apply elastic antiembolism stockings or pneumatic compression stockings as ordered by the physician (see chapter 42). The antiembolism stockings should be removed every 8 hours and left off for 1 hour; in some agencies, they are left off overnight. Perform a thorough assessment of the skin of the lower extremities at this time.
- Encourage early ambulation. Some clients are expected to ambulate the evening of surgery, depending on the severity of the surgery and their condition. Even if a client has an epidural catheter or PCA device, ambulation should be encouraged. The degree of activity allowed progresses as the condition improves. Before ambulation, the nurse assesses the client's vital signs. Abnormalities may contraindicate ambulation. If vital signs are at baseline, the nurse first helps the client to sit on the side of the bed. Client complaints of dizziness are a sign of postural hypotension. A recheck of the client's blood pressure determines whether ambulation is safe. The nurse assists with ambulation by standing at the client's side and making sure that the client can walk steadily. The first few times out of bed, clients may be able to walk only a few metres. This should improve each time. Evaluate tolerance to activity by periodically assessing the pulse rate as the client ambulates.
- Avoid positioning clients in a manner that interrupts blood flow to extremities. While in bed, clients should not have pillows or rolled blankets placed under the knees. Compression of the popliteal vessels can cause thrombi. When clients sit in chairs, their legs should be elevated on footstools. A client should never be allowed to sit with one leg crossed over the other.
- Administer anticoagulant drugs as required. Physicians often order prophylactic doses of anticoagulants, such as heparin or Fragmin (dalteparin) for clients at greatest risk for thrombus formation.
- Promote adequate fluid intake. Adequate hydration prevents concentrated buildup of formed blood elements, such as platelets and red blood cells. When the plasma volume is low, these elements may gather and form small clots within blood vessels.

Achieving Rest and Comfort. A surgical client's pain increases as anaesthesia effects diminish. The client becomes more aware of the surroundings and more perceptive of discomfort. The incisional area may be only one source of pain. Irritation from **abdominal gas,** drainage tubes, tight dressings or casts, and the muscular strains caused from positioning on the OR table can cause discomfort.

It is common to administer narcotic analgesics immediately after surgery. Initial analgesic doses are usually given by IV infusion in the PACU and titrated to client comfort. After an anaesthetized client is awake and aware, PCA may be used. This is given by IV or subcutaneous infusion or via an epidural, as with fentanyl or morphine. The PCA system allows clients to administer their own analgesics from a specially prepared pump (see chapter 38). If clients gain a sense of control over their pain, they usually have fewer post-operative problems. Gagliese et al. (2000) found that both young and older adult surgical clients were able to use a PCA to attain adequate levels of pain relief. The use of subcutaneous PCA was found in one research study to result in lower pain scores and less sleep disturbance from pain (Dawson et al., 1999). Many clients receive epidural analgesia that may be continued throughout the recovery period (see chapter 38).

The nurse in the acute care area continues pain assessment and determines the effectiveness of interventions. If the client has a PCA and is using it more frequently than the amount programmed, the nurse should contact the physician or the advanced practice nurse on the acute pain service to increase the amount of medication that the client can receive. The PCA gives the nurse a useful monitor of the effectiveness of pain medication. As oral intake is tolerated, the nurse facilitates changing the client's pain medication from IV to oral administration. It is important to ensure adequate coverage when the client is switched from an IV to an oral route of pain medication (Snell, Fothergill-Bourbonnais, & Durocher-Hendriks, 1997).

The importance of non-pharmacological interventions should not be overlooked. The nurse should assess which care measures may contribute to pain and use non-pharmacological measures to treat them. An example would be to lower the head of the bed and use a pillow for incisional splinting while turning a client with recent abdominal surgery. The nurse can also use other methods of promoting pain relief, such as positioning, back rubs, distraction, or imagery. Pain can significantly slow recovery. The client becomes reluctant to cough, breathe deeply, turn, ambulate, or perform necessary exercises. The nurse assesses the client's pain thoroughly (see chapter 38). It should not be assumed that the pain is incisional. When the client asks for pain medication, the nurse determines the location, intensity, and character of the pain. During the first 24 to 48 hours after surgery, the nurse should provide analgesics on a regular basis around the clock to improve pain control (AHCPR, 2002; RNAO, 2002a). If pain medications are not relieving discomfort, the nurse should notify the physician or the acute pain service after completing a thorough assessment. Recognizing potential complications of analgesics and what to do if they occur is an important role for the post-operative nurse.

Acute Care

Temperature Regulation. Temperature regulation is important in the post-operative period. Clients are often cool after surgery; the PACU nurse provides warmed blankets in the immediate post-operative period. If the temperature is 35.6° C or below, a warming device such as the Bair Hugger may be used. Increasing body warmth causes the client's metabolism to rise and circulatory and respiratory functions to improve.

Shivering may not be a sign of hypothermia but rather a side effect of certain anaesthetic agents. Meperidine (Demerol) may be given in small increments to decrease shivering. Deep breathing and coughing helps to expel retained anaesthetic gases.

Malignant hyperthermia is a potentially lethal condition that can occur in clients receiving general anaesthesia. It should be suspected when there is unexpected tachycardia and tachypnea; jaw muscle rigidity; body rigidity of limbs, abdomen, and chest; or hyperkalemia. Temperature elevation is a late sign. The nurse will immediately administer dantrolene sodium ordered by the physician.

Infection is another possible cause of temperature elevation. The following interventions decrease the risk of post-operative infections: encouraging deep breathing and coughing, assisting with early ambulation, promptly removing in-dwelling urinary catheters and IV catheters, and providing aseptic care of the surgical wound. Cultures will be obtained from clients suspected of having infections (see chapter 43).

Maintaining Neurological Function. Orientation to the environment is important in maintaining the client's mental status. The nurse reorients the client, explains that surgery is completed, and describes procedures and nursing measures. The client who was properly prepared before surgery is less likely to be anxious when nurses provide care. Any change in level of consciousness should be promptly reported to a physician.

Maintaining Fluid and Electrolyte Balance. An important nursing responsibility is maintaining patency and prescribed rate of IV infusions and monitoring fluid and electrolyte balance in the post-operative period. As the client begins to take and tolerate oral fluids, the IV rate will be decreased. When an ambulatory surgical client awakens and is able to tolerate fluids by mouth without gastrointestinal upset, the IV catheter is removed. When the client no longer needs a continuous IV infusion, the IV line may be saline locked to preserve the site for antibiotics or other use (see chapter 36). The client may also receive blood products depending on blood loss during and after surgery.

Promoting Normal Bowel Elimination and Adequate Nutrition. Normally a client who has had general anaesthesia does not receive fluids to drink in the PACU because of bowel sluggishness, the risk of nausea and vomiting, and grogginess from general anaesthesia. To minimize nausea, the client should avoid sudden movement. For clients identified to be at high risk for the development of nausea and vomiting or clients who must not vomit (e.g., eye surgery), a combination of antiemetics may be recommended (Gan, 2002; Tramer, 2001). If the client has a nasogastric tube, the nurse ensures it remains patent (see chapter 41). Occlusion of a nasogastric tube results in accumulation of gastric contents within the stomach.

The client will likely begin taking ice chips or sips of fluids once returned to the acute care unit. If these are tolerated, a clear liquid meal will usually be ordered. Interventions for preventing gastrointestinal complications promote return of normal elimination and faster return of normal nutritional intake. It takes several days for a client who has had surgery on gastrointestinal structures (e.g., a colon resection) to resume a normal diet.

Normal peristalsis may not return for 2 to 3 days. In contrast, the client whose gastrointestinal tract is unaffected directly by surgery can resume dietary intake after recovering from the effects of anaesthesia. The following measures promote return of normal elimination:

- Maintain a gradual progression in dietary intake. For the first few hours after surgery, a client receives only IV fluids. If bowel sounds are active and the physician orders a normal diet the first evening after surgery, first provide clear liquids, such as water, ginger ale, broth, or tea, after nausea subsides. Overloading with large amounts of fluids may lead to distension and vomiting. If the client tolerates liquids without nausea, advance the diet as ordered. Clients who have had abdominal surgery are usually NPO the first 24 to 48 hours. As peristalsis returns, provide clear liquids, followed by full liquids, a light diet of solid foods, and finally a client's usual diet. Encourage intake of foods high in protein and vitamin C.
- Promote ambulation and exercise. Physical activity stimulates a return of peristalsis. The client who suffers abdominal distension and "gas pain" may obtain relief while walking.
- Maintain an adequate fluid intake. Fluids keep fecal material soft for easy passage. Fruit juices and warm liquids are especially effective.
- Administer fibre supplements, stool softeners, and rectal suppositories as ordered. If constipation or distension develops, the physician may attempt to stimulate peristalsis with cathartics or enemas.
- Promote adequate food intake by stimulating the client's appetite:
  - Remove sources of noxious odours and provide small servings of non-spicy foods.
  - Assist the client to a comfortable position during mealtime. The client should sit if possible to minimize pressure on the abdomen.
  - Provide desired servings of food. For example, a client may be more willing to face the first meal when servings are not large.
  - Provide frequent oral hygiene. Adequate hydration and cleansing of the oral cavity eliminate dryness and bad tastes.
  - Provide meals when the client is rested and free from pain. Often a client loses interest in eating if mealtime has been preceded by exhausting activities, such as ambulation, coughing and deep breathing exercises, or extensive dressing changes. When a client has pain, the associated nausea often causes a loss of appetite.

Promoting Urinary Elimination. The depressant effects of anaesthetics and analgesics impair the sensation of bladder fullness. If bladder tone is reduced, the client has difficulty starting urination. However, clients should void within 8 to 12 hours after surgery. Because a full bladder can be painful and often causes restlessness in recovery, it may become necessary to insert a catheter. If the client has an in-dwelling urinary catheter, the goal should be to have it removed as soon as possible because of the high risk for the development of a nosocomial bladder or urinary tract infection.

Clients who undergo surgery of the urinary system frequently have an in-dwelling urinary catheter inserted to maintain free urinary flow until voluntary control of urination returns. The following measures promote normal urinary elimination (see chapter 40):

- Help the client to assume normal positions during voiding. The male client may need assistance to stand to void. Bedpans make voiding difficult. A female client will have better results if she is able to use a toilet or bedside commode.
- Check the client frequently for the need to void. A surgical client restricted to bed needs assistance in handling and using bedpans or urinals. Often the client acquires a sudden feeling of bladder fullness and urgency to void and will need help quickly.
- Assess for bladder distension. If a client does not void within 8 hours of surgery or if bladder distension is present, it may be necessary to insert a straight urinary catheter. A physician's order is needed. Continued difficulty in voiding may require an in-dwelling catheter, although the risk for a urinary tract infection increases.
- Monitor intake and output. Urine output should be at least 30 mL/hour for adults. If the urine is dark, concentrated, and low in volume, the physician should be notified. A client can easily become dehydrated as a result of fluid loss from the surgical wound. Measure intake and output for several days after surgery until normal fluid intake and urinary output are achieved.

Promoting Wound Healing. A surgical wound undergoes considerable stress during convalescence. The stress of inadequate nutrition, impaired circulation, and metabolic alterations increase the risk for delayed healing (see chapter 43). A wound may also undergo considerable physical stress. Strain on sutures from coughing, vomiting, distension, and movement of body parts can disrupt the wound layers. The nurse protects the wound and promotes healing. A critical time for wound healing is 24 to 72 hours after surgery, after which a seal is established. If a wound becomes infected, it usually occurs 3 to 6 days after surgery. A clean surgical wound usually does not regain strength against normal stress for 15 to 20 days after surgery. The nurse uses aseptic technique during dressing changes and wound care (see chapters 29 and 43). Surgical drains must remain patent so that accumulated secretions can escape from the wound bed. Ongoing observation of the wound identifies early signs and symptoms of infection.

Maintaining/Enhancing Self-Concept. The appearance of wounds, bulky dressings, and extruding drains and tubes threatens a client's self-concept. The effects of surgery, such as disfiguring scars, may create permanent changes in the client's body image. If surgery leads to impairment in body function, the client's role within the family can change significantly.

The nurse observes clients for alterations in self-concept. Clients may show revulsion toward their appearance by refusing to look at incisions, carefully covering dressings with bedclothes, or refusing to get out of bed because of tubes and devices. The fear of not being able to return to a functional role in their families may even cause clients to avoid participating in the care plan.

The family becomes an important part of the efforts to improve the client's self-concept. The nurse explains the client's appearance to the family and ways to avoid nonverbal expressions of revulsion or surprise. The family needs to be accepting of the client's concerns and encourage the client's independence. If the condition is permanent, the family and client go through a grieving process. Coping strategies develop over time to manage the situation. The following measures help to maintain the client's self-concept:

- Provide privacy during dressing changes or inspection of the wound. Keep room curtains closed around the bed, and drape the client so that only the dressing or incisional area is exposed.
- Maintain the client's hygiene. Wound drainage and antiseptic solutions from the surgical skin preparation dry on the skin's surface and cause irritation. When clients return to the unit, they should be given a post-operative bath and provided oral hygiene. In addition, a complete bath the first day after surgery can make the client feel renewed. When the gown becomes soiled by wound drainage, offer a clean gown and washcloth. Keep the client's hair clean and neatly combed. Offer frequent oral hygiene. Room deodorizers may be useful if the odour from drainage seems particularly troublesome to the client and family.
- Prevent drainage devices from overflowing. Contents of drainage collections are measured every 8 hours for output recording and are emptied as they become full. The client sometimes becomes preoccupied with observing the gradual collection of drainage, and some drainage devices can leak contents if they become too full.
- Maintain a pleasant environment. Self-concept is heightened by being in pleasant, comfortable surroundings. Store or remove unused supplies and keep the client's bedside orderly and clean.
- Offer opportunities for the client to discuss feelings about appearance. A client who avoids looking at an incision may need to discuss fears or concerns. A client having surgery for the first time is often more anxious than one who has had multiple surgeries. When the client chooses to look at an incision for the first time, the area should be clean. Eventually, the client should be able to care for the incision site by applying simple dressings or cleaning the affected area.
- Provide the family with opportunities to discuss ways to promote the client's self-concept. Encouraging independence can be difficult for a family member who has a strong desire to assist the client in any way. By knowing about the appearance of a wound or incision, family members can be supportive during dressing changes. The topic or tone of a conversation can also help family members support a client dwelling on fears and concerns. Family members should not avoid discussing the future. However, they need help to know when it is appropriate to discuss future plans. Then the client and family can work together to discuss realistic plans for the client's return home.

Box 45-7

Focus on Primary Health Care

Recovery at Home

Regardless of the length of time the client spends in hospital, it is essential that the nurse ensure that the client and family have the appropriate information and skills needed to continue a successful recovery at home. However, time is often very limited, with the move to preadmission units and short hospital stays. A comprehensive approach is needed to ensure continuity of care from hospital to home. A client often has to continue dressing care, follow activity restrictions, continue medication therapy, and observe for signs and symptoms of complications on returning home. In addition, the client needs someone to be present for the first 24 hours to ensure that there is no delayed reaction from the anaesthetic, such as difficulty breathing. A referral to home care assists clients unable to perform self-care activities. Close association with home care services is required for some clients if there is a need for dressing changes or physiotherapy. It is useful to have a case management nurse in attendance at discharge to know what a client can effectively perform.

Restorative and Continuing Care. The nurse, client, and family work to prepare the client for discharge. Education regarding wound care, activity level, diet, medications, and specifics related to the type of surgery is an ongoing process throughout hospitalization. After discharge, some clients will need assistance from home care with tasks such as wound care (Box 45-7). With ambulatory surgery clients, focused education within the limited time is essential. Including the family or significant other person provides a resource for the client once home (see Box 45-5). With both ambulatory and hospitalized surgical clients, nurses provide a wide variety of written educational materials. For example, educational materials with many pictures should be used with clients who do not speak the nurse's language or have limited reading ability. Materials should be sensitive to various cultures and religions. However, the provision of materials does not ensure understanding. Verification, return demonstration, and ongoing clarification are required.

NP Evaluation

Client Care. The nurse evaluates the effectiveness of care provided to the surgical client on the basis of expected outcomes following nursing interventions. In all surgical settings, the nurse consults with the client and family to gather evaluation data. The nurse can evaluate the ambulatory surgical client's outcomes via a telephone call to the client's home, asking specific questions to determine if complications have developed and if the client understands restrictions or medications. The call is usually placed 24 hours after surgery, which allows the nurse to evaluate the progress of recovery.

In an acute care setting, the evaluation of a surgical client is ongoing. If a client fails to progress as expected, the nurse revises the client's plan of care according to the priorities of the client's needs. Every effort is made to assist the client in returning to as healthy and functional a state as possible. The nurse's evaluation also includes determining the extent to which the client and family have learned self-care measures.

Client Expectations. With short hospital stays and ambulatory surgery, it is especially important to evaluate client expectations early in the post-operative process. Pain relief is usually a priority. Asking the client if everything possible has been done to alleviate pain, including non-pharmacological measures, can determine if the client's needs have been met. Timeliness of response to the client's needs, such as scheduled times for pain medication and prompt answering of a call light, may increase satisfaction. The client usually wants to be discharged from acute care as soon as possible and when indicated by the physician. Ensuring that discharge plans are in place facilitates that process and enhances the client's satisfaction with care.

Key Concepts

- Perioperative nursing is nursing care provided to the surgical client before, during, and after surgery.
- Surgery is classified by level of severity, urgency, and purpose.
- The preoperative period may be several days or only a few hours long.
- Preoperative assessment of vital signs and physical findings provides an important baseline with which to compare post-operative assessment data.
- Nursing diagnoses of the surgical client may pose implications for nursing care during one or all phases of surgery.
- Primary responsibility for obtaining informed consent rests with the client's surgeon.
- Structured preoperative teaching has a positive influence on a client's post-operative recovery.
- Basic to preoperative teaching is explanation of all preoperative and post-operative routines and demonstration of post-operative exercises.
- In ambulatory surgery, nurses must use the limited time available to educate clients, assess their health status, and prepare them for surgery.
- A routine preoperative checklist is a guide for final preparation of the client before surgery.
- Many responsibilities of nurses within the OR focus on protecting the client from potential harm.
- All medications taken before surgery are automatically discontinued after surgery unless a physician reorders the drugs.
- Family members are important in assisting clients with any physical limitations and in providing emotional support during post-operative recovery.
- Assessment of the post-operative client centres on the body systems most likely to be affected by anaesthesia, immobilization, and surgical trauma.
- Accurate pain assessment and intervention are necessary for healing.

Key Terms

Abdominal gas, *p. 1644*
Ambulatory surgery, *p. 1602*
Antiembolism stockings, *p. 1633*
Atelectasis, *p. 1607*
Bariatric, *p. 1607*
Cholecystectomy, *p. 1602*
Circulating nurse, *p. 1632*
Clinical pathways, *p. 1616*
Conscious sedation, *p. 1634*
Convalescence, *p. 1635*
Dehiscence, *p. 1607*
Dermatomes, *p. 1639*
General anaesthesia, *p. 1633*
Informed consent, *p. 1616*
Latex sensitivity, *p. 1629*
Local anaesthesia, *p. 1634*
Malignant hyperthermia, *p. 1639*
Paralytic ileus, *p. 1640*
Perioperative nursing, *p. 1601*
Pneumatic compression devices, *p. 1618*
Postanesthesia Recovery Score (PARS), *p. 1636*
Postanesthesia Recovery Score for Ambulatory Patients (PARSAP), *p. 1636*
Preoperative teaching plan, *p. 1616*
Regional anaesthesia, *p. 1634*
Scrub nurse, *p. 1632*

Critical Thinking Exercises

1. An 82-year-old client is admitted for surgery of a fractured hip caused by a fall. What post-operative complications are seen in the older client undergoing this type of surgery?
2. Mr. B. is a 52-year-old client who will have thoracic surgery. He has a 30-year history of smoking one pack of cigarettes per day. What type of pulmonary preventive measures would you expect Mr. B to need post-operatively?
3. Mrs. C. was admitted for ambulatory surgery for an inguinal hernia repair. What discharge criteria would be used for Mrs. C., and what discharge instructions would she require?
4. Your client is scheduled for abdominal hysterectomy at 2:00 PM. Based on NPO guidelines, what fasting schedule should you implement in collaboration with the surgeon and anaesthesiologist?

Review Questions

1. An obese client is at risk for poor wound healing post-operatively because
   1. Ventilatory capacity is reduced
   2. Fatty tissue has a poor blood supply
   3. Risk for dehiscence is increased
   4. Resuming normal physical activity is delayed
2. The nurse should ask each client preoperatively for the name and dose of all prescription and over-the-counter medications taken before surgery because they
   1. May cause allergies to develop
   2. Are automatically ordered post-operatively
   3. May create greater risks for complications or interact with anaesthetic agents
   4. Should be taken the morning of surgery with sips of water

3. A client who smokes two packs of cigarettes per day is most at risk post-operatively for
   1. Infection
   2. Pneumonia
   3. Hypotension
   4. Cardiac dysrhythmias
4. Family members should be included when the nurse teaches the client preoperative exercises to that they can
   1. Supervise the client at home
   2. Coach the client post-operatively
   3. Practise with the client while waiting to be taken to the operating room
   4. Relieve the nurse by getting the client to do exercise every 2 hours
5. In the post-operative period, measuring input and output helps assess
   1. Renal and circulatory function
   2. Client comfort
   3. Neurological function
   4. Gastrointestinal function
6. In the PACU, one measure to maintain airway patency is to
   1. Suction the pharynx and bronchial tree
   2. Give oxygen through a mask at 10 L/minute
   3. Position the client so that the tongue falls forward
   4. Ask the client to use an incentive spirometer
7. The following measure promotes normal venous return and circulatory blood flow
   1. Suctioning artificial airways and the oral cavity
   2. Monitoring fluid and electrolyte status every shift
   3. Having the client use incentive spirometry
   4. Encouraging the client to perform leg exercises at least every hour while awake
8. A client with an international normalized ratio (INR) or an activated partial thromboplastin time (APTT) greater than normal is at risk post-operatively for:
   1. Anemia
   2. Bleeding and formation of thrombi
   3. Infection
   4. Cardiac dysrhythmias
9. When the client is deep breathing and coughing, it is important to have the client sitting because this position
   1. Is more comfortable
   2. Facilitates expansion of the thorax
   3. Increases the client's view of the room and is more relaxing
   4. Helps the client to splint with a pillow
10. In the post-operative period, if a client has unexpected tachycardia and tachypnea, jaw muscle rigidity, body rigidity of limbs, abdomen and chest, or hyperkalemia, the nurse should suspect
    1. Infection
    2. Hypertension
    3. Pneumonia
    4. Malignant hyperthermia

References

Agency for Health Care Policy and Research. (2002). *Acute pain management: Operative or medical procedures and trauma.* (Clinical Practice Guideline No. 1, AHCPR Publication No. 92-0032). Rockville, MD: Public Health Service, U.S. Department of Health and Human Services.

Aldrete, J. A. (1998). Modifications to the post anesthesia score for use in ambulatory surgery. *Journal of Perianesthesia Nursing, 13*(3), 148–155.

Aldrete, J. A., & Kroulik, D. (1970). A post-anesthetic recovery score. *Anesthesia and Analgesia, 49*(6), 924–934.

American Association for Respiratory Care. (2002). *AARC Clinical Practice Guideline: Use of positive airway pressure adjuncts to bronchial hygiene therapy.* Retrieved September 1, 2004, from *http://www.rcjournal.com/online_resources/cpgs/papcpg.html*

American Society of Anesthesiologists Task Force on Preoperative Fasting. (1999). Practice guidelines for preoperative fasting and the use of pharmacologic agents to reduce the risk of pulmonary aspiration: Application to healthy patients undergoing elective procedures. *Anesthesiology, 90*(3), 896–905.

Anand, S. S., et al. (1998). Does this patient have deep vein thrombosis? *Journal of the American Medical Association, 279*(14), 1094–1099.

Apfelbaum, J. L., et al. (2002). Eliminating intensive postoperative care in same-day surgery patients using short-acting anesthetics. *Anesthesiology, 97*(1), 66–74.

Association of Operating Room Nurses. (2002a). Recommended practices for managing the patient receiving moderate sedation/analgesia. *AORN Journal, 75*(3), 642–651.

Association of Operating Room Nurses. (2002b). Recommended practices for skin preparation of patients. *AORN Journal, 75*(1), 184–187.

Association of Operating Room Nurses. (2002d). *Standards, recommended practices, and guidelines.* Denver, CO: Author.

Barnes, S. (2001). Pain management: What do patients need to know and when do they need to know it? *Journal of Perianesthesia Nursing, 16*(2), 107–108.

Barnes, S. (2002). Patient preparation: The physical assessment. *Journal of Perianesthesia Nursing, 17*(1), 46–47.

Bean, P., &Waldron, K. (1995). Readmission study leads to continuum of care. *Nursing Management, 26,* 65–68.

Burgess Schnell, Z., Van Leeuwen, A. M., & Kranpitz, T. R. (2003). *Davis's comprehensive handbook of laboratory and diagnostic tests with nursing implications.* Philadelphia: F. A. Davis.

Canadian Society of Hospital Pharmacists. (2001). *Guidelines for preparing medications for natural rubber latex (NRL) sensitive/allergic patients.* Ottawa, ON: Author.

Costa, M. J. (2001). The lived perioperative experience of ambulatory surgery patients. *AORN Journal 74*(6), 874–884.

Dawson, L., et al. (1999). Improving patients' postoperative sleep: A randomized control study comparing subcutaneous with intravenous patient-controlled analgesia. *Journal of Advanced Nursing, 30*(4), 875–881.

Dellinger, E. P, et al. (1994). Quality standard for antimicrobial prophylaxis in surgical procedures. *Clinical Infectious Diseases, 18,* 422–427.

De Ruiter, H. P., & Larsen, K. E. (2002) Developing a transcultural patient care web site. *Journal of Transcultural Nursing, 13*(1), 61–70.

Dochterman, J. M., & Bulechek, G. M. (Eds.). (2004). *Nursing interventions classification (NIC)* (4th ed.). St. Louis, MO: Mosby.

Doepke, S. (1998). Identifying the risk. *Seminars in Perioperative Nursing, 7*(4), 226–238.

Douglas, M. (1999). Pain as the fifth vital sign: Will cultural variations be considered? *Journal of Transcultural Nursing, 10*(4), 285.

Eliopoulos, C. (2001). *Gerontologic nursing* (5th ed.). Philadelphia: Lippincott.

Fowlie, P., Francis, H., & Russell, S. (2000). The surgical liason nurse: A perioperative communication with families. *The Canadian Nurse, 96*(8), 30–33.

Fredman, B., et al. (2002). Fast-track eligibility of geriatric patients undergoing short urologic procedures. *Anesthesia and Analgesia, 94*(3), 560–564.

Gagliese, L., et al. (2000). Age is not an impediment to effective use of patient-controlled analgesia by surgical patients. *Anesthesiology, 93*(3), 601–610.

Gan, T. J. (2002). Postoperative nausea and vomiting—Can it be eliminated? *Journal of the American Medical Association, 287*(10), 1233–1236.

Gershenson, T. A., et al. (1999). Tilling the soil: Nurturing the seeds of patient and family education. *Journal of Nursing Care Quality, 13*(6), 83–91.

Greenfield, L., et al. (1997). *Surgery: Scientific principles and practice* (2nd ed.). Philadelphia: Lippincott.

Hobson, D. W., et al. (1998). Development and evaluation of a new alcohol-based surgical hand scrub formulation with persistent antimicrobial characteristics and brushless application. *American Journal of Infection Control, 26,* 507–512.

Karlet, M. C. (1998). Malignant hyperthermia consideration for ambulatory surgery. *Journal of Perianesthesia Nursing, 13*(5), 304–312.

Larson, E. L., et al. (1990). Alcohol for surgical scrubbing? *Infection Control and Hospital Epidemiology, 11,* 139–143.

Lee, N. et al. (1998). A survey of patient education postdischarge. *Journal of Nursing Care Quality, 13*(1), 63–70.

Lewis, S., et al. (2004). *Medical-surgical nursing: Assessment and management of clinical problem* (6th ed.). St. Louis, MO: Mosby.

Lipson, J., Dibble, S., & Minarik, P. (1996). *Culture and nursing care: A pocket guide.* San Francisco: UCSF Nursing Press.

Litwack, K. (1999). *Core curriculum for perianesthesia nursing practice* (4th ed.). Philadelphia: Saunders.

Lookinland, S., & Pool, M. (1998). Study on effect of methods of preoperative education in women. *AORN Journal, 67*(1), 203–213.

Lueckenotte, A. G. (2000). *Gerontologic nursing* (2nd ed.). St. Louis, MO: Mosby.

McPherson, K. (1996). *Bedside matters: The transformation of Canadian nursing, 1900–1990.* Toronto, ON: Oxford University Press.

Metheny, N. M. (2000). *Fluid and electrolyte balance: Nursing considerations* (4th ed.). Philadelphia: Lippincott.

Moorhead, S., Johnson, M., & Maas, M. (Eds.). (2004). *Nursing outcomes classification (NOC)* (3rd ed.). St. Louis, MO: Mosby.

Nurse's life in the Montreal General Hospital. (1892, October). *Dominion Monthly Magazine,* pp. 541–550.

O'Callaghan, N. (2002). Pre-operative fasting. *Nursing Standard, 16*(36), 33–37.

Ontario Ministry of Health and Long-Term Care. (2004, April 15). *Standard for all Ontario health care facilities/settings for high-risk respiratory procedures under nonoutbreak conditions.* Toronto, ON: Author.

Ontario Perianesthesia Nurses Association. (2000). *Standards of perianesthetic nursing practice.* Toronto, ON: Author.

Pagana, K. D., & Pagana, T. J. (2005). *Mosby's diagnostic and laboratory test reference* (7th ed.). St. Louis, MO: Mosby.

Paquet, J. (1998). Latex hypersensitivity: The IgE response. *Seminars in Perioperative Nursing, 7*(4), 203–205.

Polk, H. C., & Christmas, A. B. (2000). Prophylactic antibiotics in surgery and surgical wound infections. *American Surgeon, 66*(2), 105–111.

Porter, R. (1997). *The greatest benefit to mankind: A medical history of humanity.* New York: W. W. Norton.

Ramer, L., et al. (1999). Multimeasure pain assessment in an ethnically diverse group of patients with cancer. *Journal of Transcultural Nursing, 10*(2), 94–101.

Registered Nurses Association of Ontario. (2002a). *Assessment and management of pain.* Retrieved September 1, 2004, from *http://www.rnao.org/bestpractices/index.asp*

Registered Nurses of Ontario. (2002b). *Prevention of falls and fall injury in the older adult population.* Retrieved September 1, 2004, from *http://www.rnao.org/ bestpractices/index.asp*

Registered Nurses of Ontario. (2005). *Risk assessment and prevention of pressure ulcers.* (Revised). Retrieved March 29, 2005, from *http://www.rnao.org/bestpractices/completed_guidelines/BPG_Guide_C1_Pressure_Ulcers.asp*

Rothrock, J. C. (2003). *Alexander's care of the patient in surgery* (12 ed.). St. Louis, MO: Mosby.

Saar, L. (2001). Use of a modified postanesthesia recovery score in phase II perianesthesia period of ambulatory surgery patients. *Journal of Perianesthesia Nursing, 16*(2), 82–89.

Sandelowski, M. (2000). *Devices and desires: Gender, technology and American nursing.* Chapel Hill: The University of North Carolina Press.

Schoonhoven, L., Defloor, T., & Grypdonck, M. (2002). Incidence of pressure ulcers due to surgery. *Journal of Clinical Nursing, 11,* 479–487.

Shoup, A. (1998). Why latex allergy now? *Seminars in Perioperative Nursing, 7*(4), 222–225.

Shuldham, C. (1999). A review of the impact of pre-operative education on recovery from surgery. *International Journal of Nursing Studies, 36,* 171–177.

Snell, C. C., Fothergill-Bourbonnais, F., & Durocher-Hendriks, S. (1997). Patient controlled analgesia and intramuscular injections: A comparison of patient pain experiences and postoperative outcomes. *Journal of Advanced Nursing, 25,* 681–690.

Steelman,V. M., & Titler, M. G. (2001). Evidence-based protocol: Latex precautions. In M. G. Titler (Series Ed.), *Series on evidence-based practice for older adults.* Iowa City, IA: The University of Iowa College of Nursing Gerontological Nursing Interventions Research Center, Research Dissemination Core.

Sullivan, E. E. (2000). Preoperative holding areas. *Journal of Perianesthesia Nursing, 15*(5), 353–354.

Summers, S. (2001). Evidence-based practice. II. Reliability and validity of selected acute pain instruments. *Journal of Perianesthesia Nursing, 16*(1), 35–40.

Sussman, G., & Gold, M. (2004). *Guidelines for the management of latex allergies and safe latex use in health care facilities.* Retrieved September 1, 2004, from *http://www.acaai.org/public/physicians/latex.htm*

Tick, L. W., et al. (2002). Practical diagnostic management of patients with clinically suspected deep vein thrombosis by clinical probability test, compression ultrasonography, and D-dimer test. *American Journal of Medicine, 113,* 630–635.

Toman, C., Heap, R., & Frize, M. (in press). *Canadian women in engineering and science: Historical and contemporary perspectives.* Ottawa, ON: University of Ottawa Press.

Tramer, M. R. (2001). A rational approach to the control of postoperative nausea and vomiting: Evidence from systematic reviews. II. Recommendations for prevention and treatment, and research agenda. *Acta Anaesthesiologica Scandinavica, 45,* 14–19.

White, P. F., et al. (2003). PACU fast-tracking: An alternative to 'bypassing' the PACU for facilitating the recovery process after ambulatory surgery. *Journal of Perianesthesia Nursing, 18*(4), 247–253.

Williams, J. R. (1999). Pre-operative fasting: Putting research into practice. *Nursing Standard, 13*(39), 33–35.

Recommended Web Sites

Canadian Anesthesiologists' Society:
http://www.cas.ca
This Web site offers client information and guidelines about anaesthesia.

National Association of PeriAnesthesia Nurses of Canada:
http://www.napanc.org/
Perianaesthesia nurses are registered nurses with advanced knowledge in the care of clients during all phases of perianaesthesia, including post-anaesthetic care units and same-day surgery.

Operating Room Nurses Association of Canada:
http://www.ornac.ca
This Web site provides practice standards for Canadian operating room nurses.

Appendix PRACTICAL NURSING IN CANADA

History of Practical Nursing in Canada

Practical nursing is the second largest regulated nursing group in Canada. It has a relatively short history, becoming a profession only in the late 1930s. Initially beginning as a hands-on hospital-based program with few common standards and little legislative control, practical nursing has evolved into a profession that requires a sound knowledge base and is publicly accountable under legislative control.

The Beginnings of Practical Nursing

In some respects, practical nursing has always existed. Whenever people have provided "hands-on" nursing care, they have been providing practical nursing care. It has only been in recent years, however, that practical nursing has been recognized as a distinct profession requiring formal education. Until about the mid-1970s, only minimal high school preparation was necessary for entry into a practical nursing program, and the program was most often a short apprenticeship in a hospital setting. No licensure exam was required. There was also no official registration, protected title, or professional body.

The Evolution of Practical Nursing

Practical nursing has evolved in a similar way in most provinces. It has also followed a similar pattern that other occupations have followed when establishing themselves as professions. Abbott (1988) studied 130 occupations, and noted that as they evolve into professions, they tend to establish the following:

1. A national professional association
2. Government-sponsored licensing legislation
3. Professional examinations
4. A professional school separate from other professions
5. A university-based professional education
6. A code of ethics
7. A national-level journal
8. An accreditation (USA) or certification (UK) program

Except for requiring a university-based education, practical nursing has established all the other steps. (And a university-based practical nursing education is now being offered in the USA.) Abbott, however, does not note the series of name and designation changes that seem to be unique to practical nursing, nor does his list highlight the increasing tendency to more and more education, which some have termed "creeping credentialism."

Canada

As early as 1914, the Canadian National Association for Trained Nurses (since 1924, called the Canadian Nurses Association [CNA]) recognized the value of practical nursing, especially for providing care to clients in the home (College of Licensed Practical Nurses of Alberta [CLPNA], 2001). The first practical nurses were usually called either a nursing aide (if female) or an orderly (if male). Their relatively short training period focused on hands-on care rather than knowledge (CLPNA, 2001).

In 1931, there were 4,698 practical nurses in Canada. By 1947, this figure had increased to 7,973, largely due to increased hospital service needs following the Second World War. The first formal education program specifically for practical nurses (as opposed to nursing aides or orderlies) began in Manitoba in 1945 (Canadian Institute for Health Information, 2002; College of Licensed Practical Nurses of BC, 2003). The first legislative acts controlling the education, testing, licensing, regulation, and practice of practical nursing were introduced in the 1940s.

Over the years, practical nurses in Canada have undergone many changes in designation as well as function. They have struggled to achieve self-regulation, rather than government-regulation, of their profession.

Many of the changes in the education of the practical nurse reflect the same changes that occurred earlier in the education of the registered nurse. Practical nurses have been required to obtain higher levels of education. Education programs became longer and more complex. They moved from hospital schools to postsecondary institutions, such as colleges. Rather than continuing to emphasize tasks and procedures, education programs began focusing more on holistic principles of nursing.

In the 1980s, most provinces developed regulations to govern practical nurses and were requiring graduates to write a licensing exam provided by what was then the Canadian Nurses' Association Testing Service (CNATS). Graduates of practical nursing programs across Canada (except in Quebec) now must pass a national registration exam before they can begin professional practice. (Quebec has its own practical nursing exam.)

Table A1.1 presents historical highlights in the evolution of practical nursing in selected provinces.

United States

In the USA, the first practical nurse program was started by the Ballard School in New York in 1893, with a three-month course to train women in simple nursing care, emphasizing care of infants and children, older adults, and the disabled in their own homes (McLennan Community College, 2004).

Table A1.1 History of Practical Nursing in Certain Provinces

Province	Year	Significant Developments, Comments
BC	1951	*Practical Nurse Act* passed
	1965	*Practical Nurses' Act* legally approved; Established Council of LPNs as the licensing body under auspices of Ministry of Health
	1977	BC practical nurses required to write Canada-wide licensing exam
	1989	Ministry of Advanced Education, Training, and Technology strongly supports future role of LPNs in health care
	1991	Publication of Closer to Home, a document endorsing laddering for nursing education from Aide to LPN to diploma RN to degree RN; Council of LPNs becomes an independent regulatory body
	1992–93	12-month college program piloted that differentiates LPN and RN roles based on client acuity and complexity of care required
	1996	Council becomes the College of LPNs of BC under HPA *(Health Professions Act)*
MB	1945	First official practical nurse education program in Canada
PEI	1952	*Licensed Nursing Assistants Act* proclaimed
	1960	Training for nursing assistants centralized in one place
	1963	Association of Licensed Nursing Assistants incorporated
	1994	Training program moves from hospital to college
	2002	*New Licensed Practical Nurse Act* affirms title of LPN
AB	1945	First school for nursing aides in Calgary, sponsored by Dept. of Veterans Affairs and Canadian Vocational Training
	1947	Nurses Aide Act passed, allowing licensing for certified nursing aide; training program is 40 weeks long
	1958	Dept. of Public Health takes over training of nurses aides
	1964	Entrance requirements for nurses aide program increased to Grade 10
	1967	Dept. of Education begins orderly program for male aides
	1972	Alberta Certified Nursing Aide Association becomes a founding member of the Canadian Association of Practical Nurses and Nursing Assistants
	1974	Certified nursing aides appeal to human rights commission about pay inequities between them and orderlies; nursing aides win
	1978	Nursing Assistant Registration Act combines aide and orderly in one category of RNA (Registered Nursing Assistant)
	1979	Health Occupation Act becomes HDA (Health Disciplines Act)
	1987	Professional Council of RNAs (PCRNA) becomes first health discipline under HDA (council is regulating body for RNAs); Nursing assistant graduates required to write CPNRE national licensing exam
	1990	RNAs change title to LPN; Council becomes PCLPN
	1998	Council changes its name to College of LPNs (CLPNA)
	1999	HDA becomes HPA (Health Professions Act), which will eventually include all regulated health professions under their separate provincial colleges
SK	1955	Professional affairs of the Certified Nursing Assistant/Licensed Practical Nurse controlled by RNs under SK RN Association Act
	1988	Certified Nursing Assistants Act passed
	1992	Above Act is amended to Licensed Practical Nurses Act; SALPN (SK Association of LPNs) has legal authority to regulate practice of LPNs
ON	1938	Centres begin offering 6-month courses for nursing assistants
	1941–45	With approval of ON Dept. of Health, RNAO (Registered Nurses Association of Ontario) sponsors eight 6-month training programs for nursing assistants
	1947	Nurses Act is amended to allow title of Certified Nursing Assistant (CNA)
	1953	Training is increased to 10 months
	1957	Part-time evening programs and high school programs (Grades 11 and 12) started
	1963	Title is changed to RNA (Registered Nursing Assistant)
	1990	RNA training programs moved to community colleges
	1993	Title is changed to RPN (Registered Practical Nurse)
	2002	CNO (College of Nurses of Ontario) passes a regulation to require all RPNs to obtain their basic diploma through an enhanced 2-year program in a provincial college (CAAT), beginning January 2005
	2003	Government asks CNO to revise regulation allowing for the education of RPNs by private colleges as well as by the CAATs

From Canadian Institute for Health Information, College of Licensed Practical Nurses of BC, College of Licensed Practical Nurses of Alberta, College of Nurses of Ontario, Saskatchewan Association of Licensed Practical Nurses, Prince Edward Island Licensed Practical Nurses, Registered Practical Nurses Association of Ontario

The Americans were the first to use the term LPN (Licensed Practical Nurse), setting a precedent that many Canadian provinces and territories have since followed.

United Kingdom and Australia

Prior to the early 1990s, nursing education in the United Kingdom was provided in nursing schools attached to hospitals. Project 2000, started in the early 1990s in the United Kingdom, aimed to increase the professional stature of nursing by removing it from its hospital service base and placing it in postsecondary educational institutions. Today, nursing education in the United Kingdom, as in Canada and the USA, takes place in the postsecondary school system at the college or technical school level (Nursing Courses UK, n.d.). Courses in enrolled nursing (the closest equivalent to practical nursing) no longer officially exist. Therefore, practical nurses from other countries cannot be certified in nursing in the United Kingdom. They must first undergo extensive theoretical and clinical upgrading.

In Australia, the practical nurse is referred to as an Enrolled Nurse (EN) and is legally considered to be "the second level nurse in a 2 tier qualified nursing framework of professional care workers. By legislation . . . an enrolled nurse must work under the direction and supervision of a registered nurse" (Enrolled Nurses Professional Association of New South Wales, 2000). This situation is very similar to many Canadian provinces in that it recognizes nursing as a profession carried out by two levels of practitioners.

The Demand for Practical Nursing

In the late 1940s and early 1950s, demand for practical nurses increased significantly in most jurisdictions. A number of factors were responsible for this increased demand, including political and economic pressures, changes within the nursing profession, and ecological and sociological factors.

Political and Economic Pressures

As roles for women expanded after the Second World War and more opportunities were available in a range of occupations and professions, the numbers of nurses decreased. This shortage of registered nurses came at a time when client acuity (i.e., their level of sickness) was increasing in institutions. As well, an increasingly aged population was requiring more supportive care in communities and long-term care facilities, and private enterprise began exerting a greater economic influence on health care.

Because of this increased public demand for safe and competent practice occurring at the same time as economic and manpower challenges, practical nursing became more important within the health care system. Practical nursing offered an economical but highly competent work force to meet the needs of hospital and long-term care clients.

Changes within Nursing

Nursing Education

The changing methods of educating nurses also contributed to the manpower and economic challenges in the health care sector. For many years, hospitals and other health care agencies depended on nursing students for the more or less free staffing of their institutions. When nursing education moved from a hospital base to a postsecondary base (beginning in the early 1970s), there was a sudden decrease in the numbers of staff available. Institutions responded by employing greater numbers of poorly trained health care assistants (i.e., unlicensed assistive personnel, unregulated health care workers) to provide basic care. This move to a lesser-trained work force has not always benefited the public, who now demand accountability and professionalism in health care. This increased public demand has resulted in higher standards and legal licensing requirements for all categories of nurse, including the practical nurse.

Registration Laws

The introduction of registration requirements for RNs also influenced the rise of the practical nurse. Nurse registration laws in the earlier part of the 20th century protected the title of "registered nurse"; however, they could not control other forms of non-registered nursing. As long as unregulated health care workers did not claim to be registered, they could still practise many nursing activities. This enabled agencies to save money by hiring these less expensive but less qualified workers.

Following the Second World War, the public began demanding more qualified practitioners. As a result, nurse registration laws were amended to allow the creation of a second-level nurse. Most provinces now have two levels, or categories, of nursing practitioners: (a) registered nurses, who are educated at a high level and are responsible for a complex client base, and (b) practical nurses, who have less education and are responsible for stable and predictable clients. In the four western provinces, a third category exists, that of Registered Psychiatric Nurses (RPNs).

Development of Levels within the Nursing Profession

As noted above, Canadian nursing has evolved into two levels of professional practitioners (and in the four western provinces, three): registered nurses and practical nurses. Compare nursing with the medical profession. Medicine essentially has one level of practitioner, a medical doctor and many subspecialties (e.g., pediatrics, ophthalmology, orthopedics, and so on). Medicine also ceded limited activities to other professions without danger of losing its own professional position. For example, ophthalmologists (MDs specializing in vision disorders) are authorized to measure vision and prescribe corrective lenses. However, their practice involves many more responsibilities than these two simple functions. Therefore, they cede these two functions to optometrists without any danger to their own professional position. Optometrists have a unique limited scope of practice and make no claims to be medical doctors. In the USA, doctors also have physician's assistants to perform limited tasks. Like optometrists, these workers do not claim to be MDs.

Between the medical profession and its various offshoots, it can thus be seen that the boundaries of practice are quite distinct. Medicine has retained to itself the central tasks of diagnosis and treatment of human disease states, functions that are clear in the public mind. Nursing, however, has developed a much less definitive practice, dividing the professional knowledge base and functions somewhat less clearly and neatly. The basic theory and practice is common to both levels of nurse practitioner; the two levels of nurses are divided only by depth of knowledge and complexity of care required. However, client complexity, predictability, and stability are hardly absolute. They are easily changeable and can be difficult to define. As a result, practitioners and the public are sometimes unsure about the boundaries between registered and practical nurses. This blurring of boundaries is well supported in the HPRAC (Health Professions Regulatory Advisory Council) report of June 1996, which states that "the distinction between nurses (RPNs, RNs, and NPs [nurse practitioners]) are not publicly understood, and they are not as great as distinctions between professions regulated by the OMA [Ontario Medical Association] for instance" (HPRAC, p. 10).

Exploring the theories of ecology and sociology as they apply to nursing can offer further insights into the development of two levels of nursing. These theories consider reactions to change and competition among groups for functions, power, rewards, and even professional survival.

Ecological and Sociological Factors

Ecology Theory Applied to Nursing

Ecology theory in general describes changes in populations resulting from environment and evolution. Ecology theory originally referred only to plants and animals, but has been expanded by some authorities to apply to social groups like companies and professions (Wilson, 1992).

In order to survive, groups must (a) compete for niches (places or functions in any system) and (b) evolve to cope effectively with environmental changes. Groups that have too narrow a function or who fail to compete successfully lose their niche to other groups. Niches may also change, so successful adaptation requires either competing for a new niche or getting into the niche first and establishing a solid place.

Two concepts in biological evolution that can be applied to practical nursing are the concepts of speciation and hybridization. In speciation, the species divides into one or more subspecies, each with its own particular function or niche. In hybridization, the new species adopts characteristics of one or more of the ancestor species (Van House & Sutton, 1996).

Applying the concept of speciation to nursing, one can see that the functions of the species of "nurse" have evolved. Out of the single species, two "subspecies" have arisen: the registered nurse—who usually has a university degree and is educated to cope with a wide variety of client (environmental) challenges, and the practical nurse—who has a college diploma and is educated to cope with a limited variety of client challenges. Some provinces also have a third subspecies, the registered psychiatric nurse, who is college educated to cope with the narrower niche of clients with mental illness. The niche for the registered nurse is wider than that of the practical nurse, and the niche for the registered psychiatric nurse is the narrowest of all.

The concept of hybridization can also be applied to nursing. Nursing has adopted characteristics of other species; in particular, it has adopted ideas and technology that have previously been exclusively medical functions. For example, taking blood pressure, starting IVs, and making certain types of diagnoses are now nursing functions but used to be medical functions.

It is interesting to note that while nursing has developed speciation, medicine has avoided speciation and instead developed specialization. Where nurses share functions, doctors cede specific unwanted functions to different sectors. It is this sharing of functions among practical and registered nurses that contributes to the public and professional confusion about the roles of the two levels of nurses.

Sociology Applied to Nursing

Sociology is the study of group roles, functions, and interactions. Abbott's unique theory about professions (1988) can be melded with ecology theory to provide more insight into the development of professions. According to Abbott, a profession attempts to keep certain tasks or problems for itself, and shares them with others only if it can do so without endangering its own niche.

Abbott also believed that a profession protects itself and its niche position by possessing a sound knowledge base. In other words, acquiring knowledge is central to developing a strong professional identity. Abbott believed that knowledge sets a true profession apart from a mere occupation:

> Practical skill grows out of an abstract system of knowledge and control of the occupation lies in control of the abstractions that generate the practical techniques.... Any occupation can obtain licensure (e.g., beauticians) or develop an ethics code (e.g., real estate). But only a knowledge system governed by abstractions can redefine its problems and tasks, defend them from interlopers, and seize new problems.... Abstraction enables survival in the competitive system of professions.

Professional tasks are either objective (knowledge and technology based), or subjective (culturally or legally based) in nature. Some objective tasks unique to nursing have been the development of the nursing process and nursing diagnoses. Subjective tasks are most clearly seen in the legal criteria for nursing defined in each province. For example, the *Ontario Regulated Health Professions Act* (RHPA) defines three authorized acts that may be performed by nurses in that province: performing a procedure below the dermis or mucus membrane; placing an instrument, hand, or finger into a body opening; and administering a substance by injection or inhalation. Of course, there is much overlap here. That is, the authorized nursing acts in Ontario are both knowledge and technology based and legally defined.

Objective tasks are more resistant to change than are subjective tasks. Environment often brings in new tasks, new knowledge, and new technology. The successful profession adopts the knowledge and new tasks it wants, strives to maintain current knowledge and tasks it considers worth keeping, and works to prevent other professions from intervening in its acquired knowledge and task base (its ecological niche). A successful profession is supported in this by subjective forces from the environment, such as legal sanctions, public opinion, and workplace practices and rules, all of which are reflective of the culture and the society.

Practical nursing has had mixed success in these areas. Most jurisdictions have enacted definitive legal supports (such as registration, licensing, and protected title) for a particular knowledge base and specified range of tasks. However, practical nursing is still striving to clarify its role for both the public and the government. Its knowledge and practice are very similar to that of the registered nurse (varying only in depth and skill level as noted previously). The workplace in many provinces is also challenged to make appropriate use of the practical nurse's skills in many areas, avoiding either under-use or exploitation of the practical nurse's knowledge and skill set.

> Abbott's analysis also casts light on the debate raging in most professional schools—what is the perfect balance between theory and practice? A student focusing solely on theory (or the abstract knowledge base) lacks the skills and tools to practice the profession; however, Abbott warns that practice-based knowledge lacks abstraction. An exclusive focus on the tools and service models leaves the student with no ability to extend the underlying knowledge base to new niches. In times of rapid change in niches, a thorough understanding of the knowledge base, not simply the tools and skills, is most likely to provide safe passage to the new environment. (Van House & Sutton, 1996, p. 8)

Practical nursing in Canada is striving to achieve a balance in both theory and practice. Basic education is increasing in complexity and promoting the concept of lifelong learning for the professional. In addition to basic education, many practical nurses complete credentialing in specialty areas after graduation, which enhances the individual's knowledge base and adaptive ability as well as increases professional credibility in the public mind.

Failure to adapt to changes can result in a loss of niche, role, and position. A profession could become like the panda, endangered because it has an extremely narrow niche in the ecosystem and is unable to adapt to the changing environment (Van House & Sutton, 1996). On the other hand, having a niche that is too broad could result in the profession losing political (public, governmental, and inter-professional) support. Too much knowledge or task sharing between specific niches (blurred boundaries) could also threaten survival of a professional species.

We have addressed some reasons for the development of practical nursing as a unique profession and provided some theoretical insights. However, why distinct levels (or species) have developed within nursing is still unanswered. It remains to be seen whether this division of professional nursing into two (and three) levels of practitioner will strengthen or weaken nursing as a profession and preserve its position in the health care system.

Practical Nursing Today: Issues and Trends

Like other evolving professions, practical nurses face many issues and trends pertaining to their educational requirements and clinical roles. Many of the same issues and trends are apparent across the country.

Educational Preparation

Client needs are becoming ever more complex. Practical nurses must respond to increased client acuity, wide cultural and social variations among clients, and a continuing trend toward home and community care. In response, practical nurse education is also becoming more demanding.

Entry to a Practical Nurse Program

There is a trend toward higher entry requirements for practical nursing programs. At one time, only a Grade 9 or 10 level of education was required for entry into a practical nursing school. Now, Canadian practical nursing programs require that applicants have a high school diploma. Most require that they also have high marks in language and in one or two sciences. Many postsecondary institutions also allow mature students without a high school diploma if they can demonstrate equivalent learning through other forms of education.

Location and Length of Program

In most Canadian jurisdictions, practical nursing programs are offered in postsecondary institutions, and they run for about two academic years (approximately four semesters). The programs require two years in order to address the complexity of the client base and the need for knowledgeable and flexible professional care. Also, in most provinces and territories, new graduates do not have a prolonged orientation to clinical practice. Therefore, educational programs prepare the student to face immediate responsibilities in the initial job placement (College of Nurses of Ontario, 2003).

Instructors in Practical Nurse Programs

Canadian nursing instructors are usually required to have clinical experience and educational preparation that is at least one level beyond that of their students. At one time, this meant that registered nurses taught aides and practical nurses. Today, almost without exception, registered nurses with baccalaureate degrees teach in practical nursing programs. Many have master's degrees or PhDs in nursing, education, or other related areas.

Practical nurses are most often involved with teaching students in the clinical area. Usually these practical nurse teachers are employees of the agency in which clinical practice takes place, and they serve a mentoring and occasionally supervisory role under the direction of the clinical instructor. However, some Ontario colleges have begun employing practical nurses as course instructors.

Student Clinical Practice

The practical nurse can work almost anywhere as long as the client's condition is predictable and stable. Why, then, are appropriate clinical placements for students not easily found? There are two main reasons.

First, many acute care areas (e.g., surgery, acute medicine, and pediatric wards, to name a few) either do not use or limit the use of practical nurses in client care. Even though documented professional standards indicate that practical nurses are qualified to work in such areas, many institutional bureaucracies and individual staff are either unfamiliar with new standards or feel personally and legally uncomfortable with them.

Second, many areas are inundated with students from various health care fields requesting clinical placements, often at the same time. This problem is especially prominent in the larger urban centres, with many university and college health care students competing for clinical placements. As a result, practical nursing schools may sometimes be required to take clinical placements for their students at inconvenient times and in inconvenient places.

Not having appropriate clinical placements is a serious issue for students. Practical nursing students need to be placed in clinical settings where they can work to their full scope of practice. If they do not have this opportunity, their educational experience will suffer.

Entry to Practice Requirements

The professional regulatory college is mandated by the government to set minimum entry to practice requirements in order to promote public safety and professional accountability. Usually, professional groups tell the regulatory college what these requirements should be.

In most Canadian jurisdictions, entry to practice requirements for practical nursing include the following:

- Graduation from an approved postsecondary program for practical nursing, with the appropriate number of hours of theory and practice and with the appropriate courses taken
- A clear police criminal record check
- A sound knowledge base in all aspects of the nursing process (assessment, planning, implementing, and evaluating nursing care) for clients throughout the life span
- Ability to function independently with clients in stable and predictable conditions and collaboratively under supervision of other health care professionals, especially registered nurses, with clients in more acute, unpredictable, or unstable conditions
- Ability to work in a variety of settings with individuals, groups, and families (Ontario specifies that the practical nurse does not work independently with communities and populations)
- Ability to apply ethical practice standards
- Ability to collaborate and communicate with others, including the client and other health care personnel (including health teaching)
- Ability to be accountable for own actions and to work within the scope of practice
- Ability to be a lifelong learner
- Ability to cope effectively with change

Credentialing is done by the professional registering body through its admission criteria, because the "government itself does not have the resources or expertise to ensure that professional competence, credibility and integrity are maintained in the numerous health professions" (May, 2003, p. 10).

It is important to note that these entry to practice standards measure minimal standards for practice (although that minimum appears to be increasing). They are not guarantees of safe practice.

Trend to More Education

For some time, there has been a trend toward more entry to practice requirements (also called "creeping credentialism"). A number of factors have been claimed as being responsible for this trend, including new and rapid developments in technology, increased public expectations, professional competitiveness and turf protection, increased postsecondary education trends, and expanded markets.

These increases in entry to practice requirements have both positive and negative aspects for the individual professional, the professions, the workplace, the government, and society in general. The positive effects may include maximizing employment opportunities, increasing national and international mobility, increasing the quality of service to the public, and enhancing research potential and development. The negative effects may include the following:

- Increasing educational costs for the individual and society
- Delaying the entry of the professional into the job market
- Causing problems in workplace collective agreements
- Exacerbating job shortages
- Creating economic burdens for employers because people with more credentials tend to expect a higher wage

Some authorities also think that increased credentialing may possibly ill serve rural, small, or isolated communities because professionals may be reluctant to take employment in these settings for economic and ongoing educational reasons (DuPerron, 2003; Lowi-Young, 2003; May, 2003).

Continuing Education Issues

Laddering

Should health care aides be allowed to become practical nurses? Should practical nurses be allowed to become diploma nurses? Should diploma nurses be allowed to become degree nurses? The concept of educational laddering acknowledges that knowledge and expertise are acquired in various ways, and it provides a means by which individuals can progress in their careers without being forbidden reasonable access to other levels or categories. The key phrase here is reasonable access. Because registered nursing and practical nursing aspire to different levels of practice, the applicant's previous experience must be carefully considered in order to protect the discipline of nursing.

Postgraduate Certification

It is not necessarily in the nursing profession's best interest to promote the concept that a practical nurse is less vital to health care than is a registered nurse. Practical nurses can further their education and their contribution to the profession by specializing, just as registered nurses can.

Practical nurses have endless opportunities to obtain certification in specialty areas after graduation from the basic program. These certificates may be offered to practical nurses or to both registered and practical nurses. Such examples include, but are not limited to, certification in operating room technique and management, foot care, gerontology and geriatric nursing, dialysis, women's health, and occupational nursing.

The Role of the Practical Nurse

Most jurisdictions recognize that practical nursing is a separate category within the broader field of professional nursing. Most jurisdictions also recognize that practical nurses follow the same nursing practice and theory as registered nurses, but have a more basic understanding of the theory and care for clients with more stable and predictable conditions.

Indeed, the CLPNA (2003) agrees, saying that the main difference between registered nurses and practical nurses is their knowledge base. Although they study the same material, registered nurses study it for a longer period of time and in more depth. They therefore have a stronger foundation in clinical practice, decision-making, critical thinking, leadership, research, and resource management. Practical nurses, on the other hand, have a strong foundation in clinical practice and decision-making and critical thinking skills.

Practical nurses are usually employed in chronic care settings and in gerontology and geriatrics. Increasingly, however, health care agencies and institutions are considering allowing practical nurses to care for more acutely ill clients. For example, British Columbia is considering allowing practical nurses in operating rooms. Some areas are beginning to employ practical nurses in acute care wards with a client base that is less stable. Consequently, practical nurse programs are often providing training for skills needed in acute care settings (e.g., dressing changes, IV therapy).

Many practical nurses are eager to assume these new roles and responsibilities in acute care settings, and they are legally entitled to do so. However, they have difficulty gaining employment in these settings because there are many barriers arising from institutional culture, personal prejudices, and past practices.

Registered nurses continue to act as gatekeepers for the nursing profession, restricting entry of practical nurses into certain aspects of the nursing niche. Most nursing managers are registered nurses with baccalaureate degrees or postgraduate degrees. They sometimes resist allowing practical nurses into certain clinical areas for a combination of reasons: unwillingness to give up some of their duties, belief that patient acuity is too high to be able to use practical nurses, lack of understanding about the latest changes in practical nursing education, fear of litigation, bureaucratic pressures, or union pressures to maintain RN positions. Practical nurses themselves may present barriers due to personal fears associated with role change.

Much has been made recently about studies claiming that client outcomes are better when registered nursing staff is used, and this no doubt has worked against the hiring of practical nurses. However, as Kazanjian (2000) notes, this research must be read carefully and critically. She questions its methodologies and emphasizes that because it is an American study, its conclusions may not be relevant to Canadian nurses: "Major differences exist between U.S. and Canada in the structure of the professions of nursing, rendering the relevance of such U.S. research less firm in Canada" (p. 10).

Workplace Issues

The nursing profession currently has a high rate of attrition and frequent occurrences of stress and burnout in the workplace. Many factors create this climate of unease in the workplace:

- The pay is relatively poor for the work provided.
- Full-time nursing positions are decreasing and part-time positions are increasing as employers try to retrench and save money. Consequently, many part-time nurses have to be employed in more than one job in order to receive an adequate income.
- Patients are entering hospitals with a higher level of acuity, and there are higher patient loads.
- Care requirements are becoming more complex.
- Practice settings are shifting to community and long-term care, but full-time nursing positions are actually declining in the community, teaching facilities, and small institutions.
- There is an actual or perceived lack of institutional support for nursing activities. Many practical nurses feel discouraged when the nursing system fails to recognize or fully use their abilities.
- Bed closures, downsizing, and increased use of unregulated health care workers seem to be the rule rather than the exception.

Work Force Issues

Practical nursing numbers are increasing slowly, but an actual shortage is forthcoming as nurses reach retirement age, are downsized, are replaced by other personnel, or leave nursing altogether.

The nursing work force is aging, and high retirement rates are pending. This will increase attrition rates and place extra strain on remaining personnel. For example, according to the Nursing Effectiveness, Utilization and Outcomes Research Unit (NRU) (2003), 75% of full-time practical nurses in Ontario are 40 years of age or older and only 3% are younger than 24. This means that by 2008, Ontario will lose 5,125 practical nurses, assuming they work until age 65. If they retire at age 55, the expected losses nearly double to 9,131. As the NRU points out, these losses will greatly affect the community and long-term care sectors because the need for practical nurses will increase as our population ages.

Canada is having problems recruiting practical nurses from other jurisdictions. Fewer practical nurses are immigrating to Canada, in large part due to actual or perceived diminished job opportunities. In addition, because of the concern about accountability and public safety—as well as a tendency to niche and turf protection—regulating authorities often are not quick in accepting the credentials of a practical nurse from another jurisdiction. The so-called "creeping credentialism" tendency may present significant blocks to the licensing of nursing professionals from other provinces or countries. According to some authorities, Canadian immigration policy often "fails to recognize the skills and qualifications that foreign-trained workers bring to Canada" (Access Issues for Regulators Workshop 2, 2001, p. 3).

Employment Trends

Practical nursing is one of the largest regulated health professions in Canada, second only to registered nursing. The Canadian Institute for Health Information (CIHI) (2002) estimates there are 230,957 registered nurses and 60,123 practical nurses working in Canada.

Table A2.1 summarizes the numbers of practical nurses per capita for each province and two of the territories. The table shows that the numbers of practical nurses per capita vary across the country, with British Columbia having the lowest number (10.3 practical nurses per 10,000 people) and Newfoundland and Labrador having the highest (51.9 practical nurses per 10,000 people).

Table A2.1 Practical Nursing Trends in Canada

Province or Territory*	Practical Nurses/ 10,000 People	Numbers Employed (and % of Total)	Percentage in Hospitals	Percentage in Nursing Homes	Percentage in Community Health	Percentage in Other Work Settings
All Canada	19.1	60,123 (100%)	47	35	8	10
BC	10.3	4,262 (7.1)	62	25	4	6
AB	14.2	4,435 (7.4)	63	23	7	6
SK	19.9	2,011 (3.3)	68	15	7	6
MB	19.6	2,250 (3.7)	42	42	7	9
ON	19.7	23,827 (39.6)	48	25	10	3
QC	19.5	14,560 (24.2)	38	54	2	3
NB	30.8	2,333 (3.9)	48	45	3	2
NS	31.2	2,950 (4.9)	47	35	10	4
PEI	42.3	593 (1.0)	45	43	4	8
NL	51.9	2,759 (4.6)	45	52	1	1
NWT	21.5	79 (0.1)	67	12	0	19
YT	19.1	64 (0.1)	28	44	1	19

*Information for Nunavut not available.
Adapted from Canadian Institute for Health Information: *Workforce trends of licensed practical nurses in Canada, 2002*. Retrieved January 25, 2004, from *http://secure.cihi.ca/cihiweb/dispPage.jsp?cw_page=AR_365_E*

Employment Status of Practical Nurses

In some provinces, most practical nurses work full-time. The highest percentage of full-time practical nurses is in the Northwest Territories, where over 70% of all practical nurses are employed full-time. The next highest percentage is in Newfoundland and Labrador, where 60% of practical nurses work full-time. In other provinces, most practical nurses work part-time, Manitoba having the highest percentage at about 56% of the practical nurse work force. Ontario and Quebec seem to be the most balanced of the provinces and territories, with the percentage of full-time and part-time workers clustering just at or slightly above the 40% mark in each case. Saskatchewan and Newfoundland and Labrador have the highest numbers of practical nurses classified as casual workers (CIHI, 2002, Table 13, p. 64).

Workplace Settings

Table A2.1 also summarizes the percentage of practical nurses working in the various settings. The public may think that practical nurses work exclusively in nursing homes. This is indeed a key area of employment for about 35% of practical nurses, but a greater number, about 47%, work in hospitals. Only about 8% work in the community, and the remaining approximately 10% work in other areas.

Practical nurses may find employment in a variety of settings. According to the CIHI (2002), "other" places of employment include business, industry, occupational health offices, private nursing agencies, private duty, physicians' offices, family practice units, self-employment, schools and other educational institutions, and voluntary associations like the Lung Association.

These trends in workplace settings raise some concerns. If clients requiring nursing care are increasingly found in the community and not in institutions like hospitals and nursing homes, then why is the practical nurse found in such low numbers in the community or the setting called "other"? Perhaps these statistics reflect reluctance on the part of other health care workers to permit practical nurses to function at the full scope of practice for which they are prepared.

Standards and Scope of Practice

Standards of Practice

As a regulated profession, practical nursing is responsible for establishing its own standards of practice. The professional regulatory body for practical nurses in each jurisdiction (e.g., the provincial college of practical nurses) has the authority to set standards of practice for its members. It also has the authority to ensure members meet these standards.

Standards of practice are written statements that detail the level of performance expected of nurses in a particular jurisdiction. They provide general guidelines about several aspects of professional practice and performance. In so doing, they provide a bar against which the practice of any nurse can be continually measured. They also demonstrate to the public that the profession of practical nursing is dedicated to protecting public safety and providing a high level of quality care.

Although they differ in details, most standards of practice for practical nurses in Canada offer performance guidelines for the following areas (among others): the nursing process (i.e., assessment, participation in nursing diagnoses, planning, implementation, evaluation), ethics, education, leadership, research, and collaborating with others.

Each individual nurse and the regulatory body are responsible for standards—the nurse for knowing and using them, and the regulatory body for publishing and enforcing them. As well, the professional association and employers must support these standards in practice as well as theory. Finally, members of the public are responsible for being good consumers of the professional health care they receive.

Ethics in Nursing

Ethics refers to the moral principles or values that guide us when deciding what is right and what is wrong. Ethics influence our behaviour and relationships with others. Providing ethical nursing care means the nurse forms a dynamic, caring, helping relationship with the client in order to help the client achieve and maintain optimal health.

Regulatory bodies for practical nursing are responsible for establishing and promoting codes of ethics. These codes of ethics guide practical nurses in ethical decision-making. They also uphold ethical standards for practical nurses. The following values are promoted in most codes of ethics for practical nurses:

- Being accountable for one's actions
- Upholding the client's rights to privacy and confidentiality
- Providing care that maintains the client's dignity
- Demonstrating respect for the client at all times
- Promoting integrity by providing safe, competent, and ethical nursing care
- Evaluating one's work and maintaining competency

Continuing Education and Expanded Competencies

The practical nurse is expected to continue to grow professionally and acquire a greater range of knowledge, skill, and judgment beyond that of the minimal entry to practice standards. Many educational opportunities are available to the nurse from postsecondary institutions, professional organizations, employers, and charitable agencies (e.g., the Canadian Diabetic Association). Increasingly, nurses are encouraged to attend educational events offered by other health care professionals, such as respiratory therapists, pharmacists, physiotherapists, and gerontologists. This cross-professional education is also immensely valuable in encouraging greater understanding and collaboration among members of the health care team.

Inevitably, nurses in various areas will develop different competencies. This presents individual and workplace challenges. As individual competencies are enhanced and scopes of practice are expanded, nurses and employers must continuously seek clarification of their roles. Nurses are accountable for their actions at all times. The employer needs to remain fully aware of the new competencies of nurses, both at entry level and beyond. Employers must also develop clear policies to address the expanded practices of all nursing staff.

Challenges to Working to Full Scope of Practice

Perhaps the best way to maintain competency is to continually use one's skills and training. Unfortunately, many employers do not allow practical nurses to work to their full scope of practice. As mentioned in Chapter One, the potential of practical nurses is often not recognized by the system, for both personal and political reasons. For example, the College of Licensed Practical Nurses of BC (CLPNBC) recognized in 2002 that practical nurses are often not permitted to administer medications, even though medication administration has been an entry-level competency for practical nurses in British Columbia since 1984.

When barriers are put in place [that] inappropriately restrict the practice of nursing by licensed practical nurses, the satisfaction and professional growth of the licensed practical nurse as well as their nursing colleagues may be eroded. The competencies of the licensed practical nurse are lost when they are unable to practice appropriately. (CLPNBC, 2003, p. 2)

Nevertheless, many areas make efforts to allow practical nurses to work to their full scope of practice, thus bringing them from a task orientation to a competency base—and in the process, improving client care and professional job satisfaction.

Collaboration

The practical nurse is a team member, so should always be working in a collaborative fashion with other health care personnel. Collaboration includes communicating with the client, the family, and other health care workers to define, implement, and evaluate the plan of care. Collaboration with the client and family includes focusing on real and perceived needs and wishes and how they intersect with medical and nursing plans. The practical nurse makes suggestions and referrals to individual members of the health care team and in team meetings where client care and concerns are discussed. Collaboration with the health care team includes clear and appropriate verbal and written communications.

Scope of Practice

Scope of practice refers to the legal limits of one's professional role. Three categories of care providers provide nursing care: unregulated care providers (e.g., nurse's aides, support workers), practical nurses, and registered nurses. Each category of care provider has its own scope of practice. These scopes of practice are different because each category of care provider has different education, legal authority, and performance requirements.

Table A3.1 compares the scopes of practice for practical and registered nurses in New Brunswick. (Each province

Table A3.1 Scope of Practice Requirements for Practical and Registered Nurses in New Brunswick

	Practical Nurse	Registered Nurse
Education for entry to practice	College diploma or certificate; Program length 1–2 years	University baccalaureate degree (BScN or BN); Program length 4 years
Legislated scope	Under RN supervision or direction and/or physician direction*; Has greater independence in care of stable and predictable clients; Under close direction of RN or assists RN in care of unstable or unpredictable clients	Independent practice of nursing for all clients; Collaborates with physicians and other health care personnel
Client	Individuals, families, and groups	Individuals, families, groups, communities, and populations
Application of nursing process	Participates in client assessment and developing a care plan; Implements interventions and evaluates effectiveness	Determines client status, integrates, analyzes, interprets, implements; Evaluates care and makes independent judgments

*Supervision and direction need not always be carried out in person, but may be accomplished by agency policies and procedures and by maintaining a collaborative consultative relationship between the practical and the registered nurse. For some functions, the practical nurse may function independently. For the sake of client and professional safety, collaboration must exist at all times in health care, no matter what the task or who is performing it.

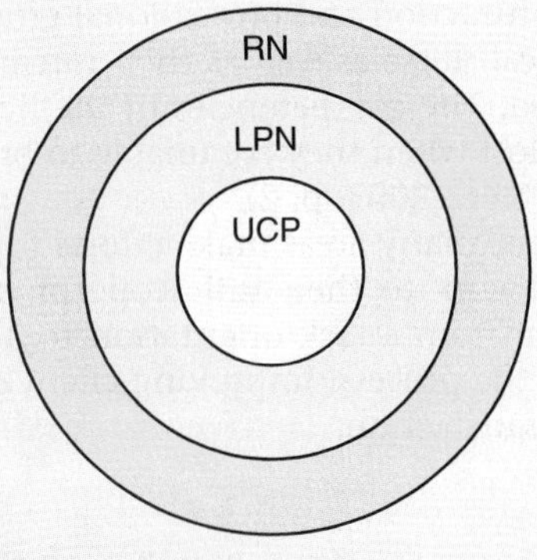

FIGURE **A3–1** Care Providers' Scope of Practice (Adapted from Nurses Association of New Brunswick and Association of New Brunswick Licensed Practical Nurses: Working together: A framework for the registered nurse and the licensed practical nurse, 2003, p. 4. Retrieved January 29, 2004, from *http://www.nanb.nb.ca/pdf_e/Publications/General_Publications/RN-LPN%20(e)1.pdf*)

and territory has similar scope of practice requirements for nursing in its jurisdiction.) In Table 3.1, notice that practical nurses have a more limited scope of practice in that they must assist an RN or be closely supervised by an RN when providing care for unstable patients. They may work independently only with clients in stable conditions. Registered nurses, however, may independently provide care for all clients.

Figure A3.1 illustrates the expanding scopes of practice among the three categories of nursing care providers. It shows that unregulated care providers have the most limited scope of practice, practical nurses have a more expanded scope of practice, and registered nurses have the largest scope of practice. Registered nurses are ultimately responsible for the direction of nursing care.

Notice that this figure uses a solid line to separate each scope of practice. In reality, the boundaries between the scopes of practice vary. Between registered and practical nurses, the scope of practice is much less definitive and the boundaries are sometimes blurred, because both levels of nurses share a base knowledge and practice and develop new competencies during clinical practice. However, the boundaries between practical nurses and unregulated care providers are more definite, because little of the basic knowledge or competencies are shared between the two roles. Indeed, the roles of practical and registered nurses are "separate and overlapping" (Nurses Association of New Brunswick and Association of New Brunswick Licensed Practical Nurses, 2003, p. 2). As the CLPNBC (2003) stated, "the accepted nursing competencies for [registered and practical nurses] have significant overlap with each other and therefore are accepted as shared competencies that provide the foundation of partnership" (p. 1).

Leadership: Supervising and Delegating

The practical nurse is often in a position to supervise or to delegate, as well as to be the recipient of supervision and delegation. In order to supervise and delegate, the practical nurse must have sufficient knowledge, skill, and judgment. Supervision and delegation, although different skills, both serve to protect the public and the profession by ensuring that a skill is performed safely and competently. The same principles of supervision and delegation are applicable to both levels of nurse.

Supervision

Supervision is usually required by individuals who are new to a skill or role, such as students of a profession, new members of a profession, and professionals or nonprofessionals (such as family members or unregulated health care workers). The person who is supervising is usually experienced in that knowledge and skill and may or may not be a member of the same profession or occupational group.

Supervision is an intervention and usually an ongoing relationship. The purposes of supervision are to (a) enhance competent functioning of an inexperienced person and (b) protect the public and the professional practice. Because supervision requires continual observation, monitoring, and evaluation, the supervisor must have a positive, collaborative relationship with the person being supervised. Both parties in the relationship must understand the roles each must play. The ongoing nature of most supervision allows the relationship to grow and develop. People should be supervised until they can safely perform the task alone. Supervision may occur in many forms, such as a one-on-one observation, an interview with the client who has received care, or an analysis of the written report of a task. The supervisor provides evaluative information about the task performed as soon as is feasible.

If supervision of a skill occurs in a more isolated instance, the development of a relationship and the analysis of progress are more difficult.

Delegation

In delegation, authority to perform a restricted task or function is transferred to another person or group. It is crucial for the nurse to make this decision carefully. The professional standards are quite clear in this matter. Before delegating a task to another, the nurse must ensure that the person has the required knowledge, skill, and judgment to perform that function. The nurse must consider numerous other factors before a function is delegated to someone else: the associated risks and benefits to the client, the need for another person to perform the task, the ability of the person to maintain competence in the procedure over time, and whether adequate supervision can be provided once the skill has been learned. A useful discussion of the Five Rights of Delegation is available from the Massachusetts Board of Registration in Nursing Web site (noted in references). The five rights include (a) the right task, (b) the right circumstances, (c) the right person, (d) the right direction or communication, and (e) the right supervision and evaluation. These rights are applicable to nurses working at all levels.

In addition, the nurse must know institutional policies and procedures about delegation and whether the particular function may be legally delegated. This is particularly crucial today when there has been a rapid increase in unregulated health care workers with varied skill sets and functions within the health care system. Responsibility does not stop once a task is delegated to another. The delegating nurse retains ultimate responsibility for the task being completed correctly. The College of Nurses of Ontario has provided a useful decision tree to help the nurse decide whether a function can be delegated to another (Figure A3.2).

Clinical Skills

Medication Administration

Medication administration is a specific knowledge-based clinical skill that is part of the practical nursing scope of practice in some jurisdictions but not in others. In most cases, it must be delegated to the practical nurse because it is a restricted activity requiring special education and competence to be performed safely. Even if it is part of the scope of practice, there may be reluctance to allow practical nurses to use this skill. Boundary issues with accompanying confusions about who may administer what medications, to whom, and when become evident in some areas. Medication administration competencies for practical nurses remain in continuous change between and even within jurisdictions. For instance, in some areas of Alberta, practical nurses are permitted to give injections (intradermal, subcutaneous, intramuscular), and in other areas, they are not (Canadian Practical Nurses Association, 2003). In some jurisdictions, practical nurses may monitor IV therapy, and in other jurisdictions, they may not. There is a tremendous variation in practice across the country, between institutions in a region, and even within an institution itself.

Other Clinical Skills

The same points about medication administration apply to many other skills for which a practical nurse may acquire the specific knowledge and competency. In most cases, practical nurses can and do acquire other clinical skills beyond those needed for entry to practice. The restrictions on these skills are the same as those for the RN; the practical nurse must usually take a specific course to acquire the needed knowledge and skill base, and must usually be employed in an area allowing frequent enough application of this skill to maintain continued competency levels. For example, courses are available to learn about various types of dialysis, but entry into these courses is usually confined to those employed or soon to be employed in this area, where they will require the skill and will be able to use the skill often enough to maintain competency.

Whether an added skill may be practised by a practical nurse is sometimes restricted by legislation and/or local institutional or health region policy. Theoretically, any health care skill a family member or lay person can be taught should be able to be acquired by a nurse, the parameters being the same: a proper knowledge base and demonstrated initial and continued competency and judgment in application of the skill. However, practical nurses need to be aware of the possible unique legal restrictions on their roles. Whether sensible or not, these legal restrictions do not apply in the same way to family members.

Because there is increasing complexity in the individuals and groups requiring nursing, there is a corresponding variation in functions that can be assigned to practical nurses and where and in what context these functions may be performed. Some of the more common added competencies for practical nurses in many jurisdictions include (but are not limited to) operating room techniques, special foot care, orthopedic care, gerontology, community care, and mental health care.

The only commonality in this modern day appears to be continued rapid change. The nurse must be careful never to assume that standards and scopes of practice are the same within or between institutions, between jurisdictions, or over time. One way to keep pace with change

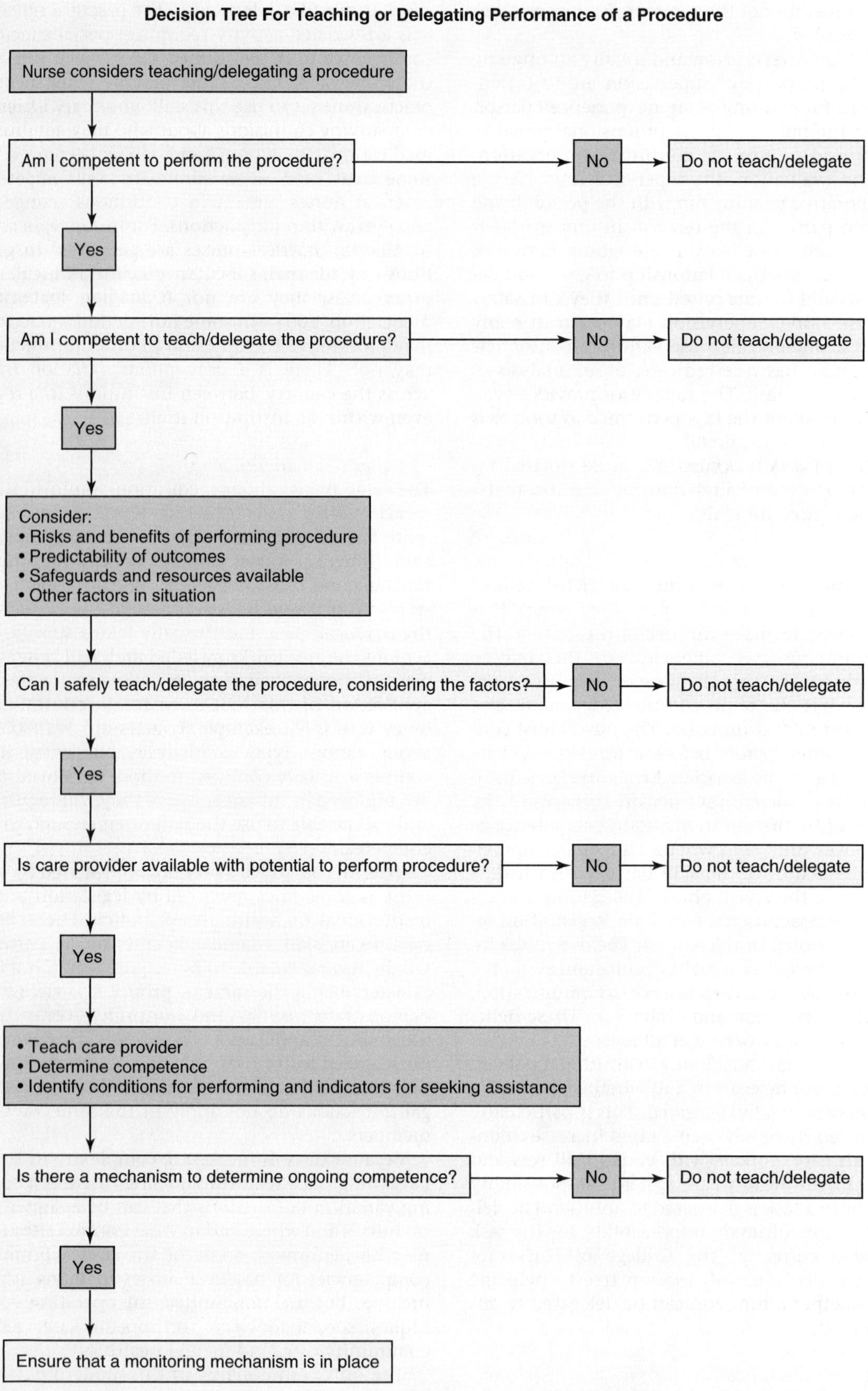

FIGURE **A3–2** Decision Tree for Teaching or Delegating Performance of a Procedure (From College of Nurses of Ontario: Working with unregulated care providers, 2004, p. 17. Retrieved March 28, 2004, from *http://www.cno.org/docs/prac/41014_workingucp.pdf*)

is to keep in close contact with a variety of sources: the professional association, the regulatory body, agency policies, and the ever-expanding body of health care knowledge.

Legislation, Regulatory Bodies, and Professional Associations

Legislation, regulatory bodies, and professional associations govern the practice of nursing. These have been created to protect public safety and promote ethical practice.

Legislation

In most provinces and territories, nursing practice has similar legal regulatory requirements (educational, registration, and complaints and disciplinary processes) and professional standards (scope and standards of practice, and competency issues). Laws that govern regulated health professions serve to protect the best interests of the public by regulating health care practitioners and determining how, what, and where they practise.

Acts That Govern Specific Health Care Professions

In all provinces and territories (except two), each profession has its own governing law, called an act. For example, medical doctors, registered nurses, practical nurses, chiropractors, and so forth each have a professional act. These acts list specific tasks that those professionals are allowed to perform because they have the required skills. However, the skills of one profession often overlap with those of another, causing confusion for public and professionals alike.

Acts That Govern Multiple Health Care Professions

Two provinces (Ontario and British Columbia) have removed or are in the process of removing separate acts for individual health professions and are replacing them with a single, generic act that applies to all health professions. In Ontario, this law is called the *Regulated Health Professions Act* (RHPA), and in British Columbia, it is called the *Health Professions Act* (HPA). This move has been made for several reasons:

- The public is demanding safe and accountable practice.
- New technology, which is increasingly complex and invasive, is potentially dangerous if improperly used. Trained professionals must administer with great care treatments such as radiation therapy, drugs for cancer, surgery, and even injections.
- People requiring health care have increasingly complex physical, emotional, and social needs.
- As many professions expand their scope of practice and acquire new knowledge and skill sets, significant overlap occurs between various groups. These general health care acts are an attempt to apply a regulatory structure common to all.
- Health care professionals are more mobile today (i.e., they move between jurisdictions) and may have wide variations in knowledge and competence.
- There is an increased number and variety of health care professions.
- It is fundamentally just to have set standards and expectations that are applicable to all groups wanting to be regulated by the health act. This also applies to foreign-trained professionals who apply to enter the profession in Canada (Registered Nurses Association of British Columbia [RNABC], 2003a).

These generic health care acts list (a) professions that are regulated by the law and (b) activities that only members of certain professions are authorized to perform. These restricted activities are called reserved acts (in British Columbia) and controlled acts (in Ontario); they refer to:

> clinical activities that may present a risk of harm and are therefore reserved for special professions only. Examples of reserved or controlled actions are diagnosing, prescribing medications, managing labour, ordering and applying hazardous forms of energy (including diagnostic ultrasound, electricity, laser and x-ray) and setting or casting a simple fracture. (RNABC, 2003a, p. 4)

Different health care professions are legally permitted to perform certain restricted activities. For instance, diagnosing a disease is a controlled act that is usually restricted to the medical profession. In Ontario, the RHPA lists 13 controlled acts, 3 of which can be performed by nurses.

All the laws governing the actions of health care professionals, whether they are profession-specific acts or generic health care acts, make statements about the type of educational background required to enter a professional school and the type and length of education the professional schools must offer. The laws also require the profession to set up a governing body to monitor and regulate professional practice in the public interest.

It may seem that these laws are excessively cumbersome and confusing. However, they are a reasonable attempt to establish uniform professional competencies and thereby protect the public. In addition, the laws encourage an increased uniformity between provincial education systems and registration policies, allowing health professionals a greater mobility between jurisdictions (College of Nurses of Ontario [CNO], 2003).

Regulatory Bodies

"Throughout North America, hundreds of organizations like the College of Nurses of Ontario evolve and grow along with the professions they regulate" (CNO, 2003, p. 9).

According to the professional and health care acts, each profession must have a regulatory body that governs it. Depending on the province or territory, this regulatory body may be called a college, council, association, or board. Its primary mandate is to protect the public by controlling the activities of the professionals. In order to practise or use their professional title, all professionals must be members of their regulatory body.

Functions of the Regulatory Body

Each regulatory body uses many methods to protect the public. It ensures that its members have been properly educated; meet the minimum entry standards; maintain continued competence; and have the required knowledge, skill, and judgment to practise the particular profession. Almost all regulatory bodies perform the following functions:

- Ensuring professionals have the necessary credentials to practise in that province or territory
- Determining whether qualifying exams are necessary
- Registering the professional as a member of the profession once all criteria for membership have been met
- Keeping a public register of the names, registration numbers, and business addresses of all members
- Defining scope of practice and competency standards, according to professional standards and the existing laws
- Ensuring that members renew or update registration and maintain competency criteria on a regular basis
- Receiving complaints from the public or other professionals about personal practices of members, investigating these complaints, and disciplining members as necessary
- Publishing disciplinary results regularly (i.e., name, registration number, offense, and disciplinary decision)

"The privilege of professional registration ensures that the registered members must meet the minimal education and competence requirements of the profession. For the public, registration also provides the expectation of professional service and ethical standards." (College of Licensed Practical Nurses of British Columbia [CLPNBC], n.d.)

Because the names, registration numbers, and business addresses of registered health care professionals are made public, some people have expressed concern that members' right to privacy is compromised. However, regulatory bodies and most provincial and territorial governments believe this information is necessary for public safety. Therefore, they consider that protecting the public safety supersedes the professional's right to privacy. In many areas, governments also permit the publication of disciplinary action against a health care professional, believing that doing so fulfills this mandate of serving the best interests of the public.

Protecting or Reserving Titles

Usually, regulatory bodies are also responsible for ensuring that the members' professional title (e.g., LPN, Dr.) is protected, or reserved. This means that only registered members are authorized to call themselves by the professional title. The protected title is usually related to the terms used in the jurisdiction, but protection is usually also extended to other, synonymous terms. For example, in Ontario, the following related terms are all protected: nurse, registered practical nurse, RPN, LPN, PN, and their variants.

The College of Licensed Practical Nurses is the provincial regulatory body responsible for superintending the profession of licensed practical nursing in the public interest. As such, the College sets the requirements for the privilege of using the professional titles related to Licensed Practical Nurses. The professional title assures the public and other care providers that the individual has met the minimal requirements for entry into the profession and maintains competence to practice as a professional licensed practical nurse. (CLPNBC, n.d.)

In all provinces and territories (except Ontario), the official designation of the practical nurse is LPN (Licensed Practical Nurse). In Ontario, the official designation is RPN (Registered Practical Nurse).

Obtaining Criminal Record Checks

Because professionals have positions of power, there are inevitable concerns that they could take advantage of vulnerable people, especially young children and older adults. In response, some provinces and territories require people registering with a regulatory body to undergo a criminal record check.

Self-Regulation

To what extent should governments be involved in the regulation of a health care profession? Surely professionals are capable of regulating themselves and do not require paternalistic interference from government bureaucrats. There has to be a balance between public good and individuality, between government laws and professional input. Professional self-regulation in nursing means that each nurse is expected to assume personal responsibility for maintaining competence and personal, physical, social, and emotional fitness to practice. Self-regulation also means that nurses establish standards of practice and an ethical framework for the nursing profession as a whole.

> Self regulation is a privilege that is entrusted by society to a college to regulate the profession in the public interest. . . . Self-regulation for nursing means that . . . nurses determine standards of practice and ethics for the profession and ensure that these are met. The alternative would be for someone else, such as government or a consumer board, to independently set such standards and ethics. (RNABC, 2003b, p. 4)

The Registration Process for the Practical Nurse (Credentialing)

In all territories and provinces of Canada, nurses wanting to register with the local regulatory body must go through a specific process. The regulatory body (also called a registering body) in each jurisdiction determines whether the applicant has sufficient educational background and competency for registration in the particular area. To be registered as practical nurses, applicants must prove that their education meets requirements for theoretical and clinical hours in specified topics and clinical areas. They also must provide evidence of competent practice by passing a licensing exam and/or providing evidence of recent competent work in the practical nursing field. As already noted, in many jurisdictions, applicants must also pass a criminal record check before registering to practice.

Registering Locally

Successful graduates of a practical nursing school submit their names to the local licensing authority for permission to write the national certification exams. As a general rule, students must write the certifying exam in the province or territory in which they received their education because they must be recommended to write the exam by their local registration body. The students are notified of where and when exams will be written. Once the exam is written, the student will be notified of the results by mail. Usually, the school receives a summary of the passes/fails in that class and information about their success relative to other schools in the jurisdiction. Privacy of exam marks is an issue in many areas. In Ontario, for instance, students must sign a waiver allowing their exam results to be included in the information sent to their educational institution. When the exam results are sent to the school, the student names are blacked out.

After passing the licensing exam and (if required) completing a criminal record check, the new graduate then applies to the regulatory body to be registered as a practical nurse.

Registering in Another Province or Territory

Just as they would in their own jurisdictions, applicants wanting to register in a province or territory in which they have not been educated must formally apply for registration. This generally means the applicants must submit official transcripts from their school, indicating both hours and topics of theory and practice they completed in the basic program. They must show competent practice by submitting a record of success in the national certification exam or its equivalent from another country. If they are not recent graduates, they must also provide evidence of a sufficient amount of recent (within the last three to five years) appropriate work in practical nursing. If they have not already done so, they may have to complete a criminal record check (at their own expense). If the certification exam, educational background, or recent nursing experience is not accepted by the regulatory body, then the applicant may be required to write the Canadian exam and take a theoretical or clinical nursing course to upgrade to Canadian standards.

Registering in Other Countries

The registration process for the USA, the United Kingdom, and Australia is very similar to the Canadian process. The applicants must prove to the foreign regulatory body that (a) they have successfully completed a basic nursing education program that includes a specified number and type of theoretical and clinical hours, and (b) they are capable of competent nursing practice (i.e., they have successfully written the exam and/or have recent practical experience). Countries vary in how they accept Canadian certification exams and basic nursing program clinical and theoretical hours. In the USA and Australia, the nurse is certified in the specific state or territory; in the United Kingdom, the nurse is certified nationally.

Practical nurses planning to relocate to another jurisdiction (country, state, or province) should contact the new registering/licensing body well in advance because they may have different requirements for professional practice. The procedure for attaining registration in a new jurisdiction can take up to three months if there are no complications or deficiencies, but it can take much longer if there are problems.

Professional Associations

In Prince Edward Island and Ontario, the professional association is separate from the regulatory body (e.g., the College of Nurses of Ontario is the regulatory body, and the Registered Practical Nurses Association of Ontario is the professional association). However, in all other provinces and territories, they are the same body. The purpose of most professional associations is to advocate for and promote the particular profession they serve. The LPN Association of Prince Edward Island (2003) states that its goals are to:

- Foster public recognition and awareness of the profession
- Encourage members to interact and take pride in their profession
- Promote proficiency, continuing education, and career development among members
- Represent members collectively in relations with other persons and organizations
- Provide for services to members such as group liability insurance
- Promote action and work for improvements in regard to health issues
- Pursue such other goals as the Association may consider necessary to advance the profession and further the interest of its members

The above highlights the fundamental differences between a regulatory body and a professional association. Protection of the public is the distinct mandate of the regulatory body, whereas promoting professional development is the mandate of the professional association. Many nurse leaders and politicians believe that regulatory bodies and professional associations should not be combined because doing so may lead to public confusion and conflict of interest issues. Of course, the professional association works closely with the regulatory body. It would not serve the profession well if its constituents did not cooperate with the regulators about issues of professional practice. In the interests of both professional issues and public accountability, the two separate groups (professional association and regulatory body) must remain in continuous, effective communication.

The provinces and territories that do not have a professional association separate from the regulatory body depend on the Canadian Practical Nurses Association (CPNA) for professional advocacy and promotion issues. The CPNA mission states in part that it promotes education, research, and excellent nursing practice and it collaborates in the development of national practical nursing standards. Unlike membership in the regulatory body, membership in the professional association is usually voluntary.

The Canadian Association of Practical Nurse Educators (CAPNE), an affinity group of the nationwide Association of Canadian Community Colleges (ACCC), offers educational and networking opportunities and holds yearly conferences for educators throughout Canada.

Benefits of Membership in the Professional Association

Members of professional associations enjoy the following benefits:

- Receiving emotional support from other professionals by sharing thoughts, feelings, and ideas.
- Enhancing personal and collective knowledge base, thus contributing to individual and group growth.
- Being part of a strong force for change. It is often easier for a group to effectively lobby for changes than it is for individuals.
- Achieving some economic advantages (e.g., better insurance rates through a group plan).
- Having opportunities to network.

In summary, nursing is a complex profession that exists in a challenging environment under constant legal and professional changes. No nurse works alone, but is always in an environment with the public and other professionals. Each nurse must understand how legislation, regulatory bodies, and professional associations work together to inform safe and competent practice.

The Future of Practical Nursing in Canada

It is not possible to know the future of practical nursing, but it is possible to make reasonable predictions based on current and projected trends. The health care system in Canada is continually changing, and these changes have an impact on practical nursing. In order to cope effectively, nurses must be proactive and view change as a challenge and opportunity rather than a threat. By doing so, nursing will maintain or advance its niche position in health care.

Both Abbott (1988) and Wilson (1992) believed that organisms and professions that do not respond to change will lose their niche positions and either fade to unimportant entities controlled by others or die out completely. According to Wilson, "homogeneity means vulnerability" (p. 301). The Romanow Report repeated this same idea when it stated the following: "In the face of uncertainty, the solution is not to sit back and wait for the outcomes of potential challenges" (Government of Canada, 2002, p. xxxiv).

General Health Care Trends

A number of current and projected changes can potentially impact practical nursing. The following issues are generally increasing in Canada, and they each have an impact on the delivery of health care services:

- Costs of health care; the individual consumer will have to pay more.
- Privatization of health care with less government funding.
- Use of technology, including robotics for treatment and computer technology for communications and teaching.
- Public access to information.
- Population diversity.
- Public demands for a voice in health care and competent health care services.
- Medico-legal litigation.
- Percentage of older adults in the population.
- Post-acute care, rehabilitation, palliative care, long-term care, and chronic care in the home rather than in hospitals or other institutions.
- Patient acuity; hospital patients are increasingly ill, so hospitals are becoming large intensive care units.

Specific Health Care Issues in Canada

The Romanow Report (Government of Canada, 2002) makes several suggestions about the unique needs of Canadians that will impact practical nursing:

- Government should increase strategies that promote physical activity and reduce obesity.
- Efforts to reduce smoking should be expanded.
- Immunization programs require closer attention, especially in response to new infectious diseases and increased population mobility between countries.
- Services to new Canadians, visible minorities, people with disabilities, Aboriginal people, and rural and isolated populations require more attention and funding.
- Home care is one of the fastest-growing sectors of the health care system; investing more in home care will improve services and quality of life for home care clients and will also save the system money by keeping people out of hospitals and long-term care facilities.
- Better services are required in mental health care, post-acute care, rehabilitation, and palliative care.
- Canada needs a national approach to health human resources planning, so one province does not "poach" scarce health professionals from other provinces.

Implications for Practical Nursing

Continuous rapid change requires professionals to respond appropriately in order to cope effectively. Practical nurses need to be lifelong learners and develop increasingly broad-based competencies to adapt to changing occupational demands. This is not the time to focus solely on one narrow skill set or cling stubbornly only to the knowledge base given in undergraduate school.

Modern technological treatment is increasingly expensive and time intensive. Nursing will need to focus more on issues of illness prevention and health promotion. The practical nurse will have to upgrade knowledge and skills in the areas of epidemiology and principles of teaching and learning for clients throughout the life span.

Because health care problems are often too complex to be addressed by any one person, practical nurses will have to focus more on working collaboratively in teams and networks of health care providers. This will require nurses to be increasingly aware of scope of practice and changes in scope of practice among all workers. Because of this emphasis on collaborative teamwork, there will probably be more emphasis on outcome-based care frameworks (called in the text "care maps," or critical pathways) rather than on more narrow frameworks unique to only one profession (such as the nursing care plan). Having all health care team members work from the same model would simplify care issues and reduce the chance of error.

As more health care services are offered by the private sector, nurses will encounter different and challenging ethical issues. Nurses will need to be more aware of conflict of interest situations. They may find that their professional values clash with corporate interests. In this respect, professional colleagues and the professional association will become increasingly important sources of information and support. Practical nurses will have to consider strengthening their national association and in some provinces and territories having a more direct and local input in the form of a provincial association.

As consumer demands for and awareness of available information sources increase, nurses will continue to need to focus on the client and empowering clients to be active participants in their own health care. For instance, nurses will need to actively participate in health promotion and disease prevention strategies, such as providing information to reduce infectious and chronic lifestyle-related diseases like cancer, diabetes, obesity, and heart–lung disorders. Health teaching for individuals and groups in the areas of diet, exercise, and reducing bad health habits like smoking will become increasingly important. To provide effective teaching, nurses will have to develop and maintain skills in the use of computers and the Internet.

Nurses work with an increasingly diverse and multicultural population base. The nurse will thus have to develop more knowledge and skill in applying concepts from the humanities and social sciences such as psychology, sociology, and anthropology.

Possible Evolution of the Practical Nurse Role

Changes in Educational Standards for Entry to Practice

In view of the likely expanding roles for the practical nurse, a high school diploma must be the minimal requirement for entry into a practical nursing program. The applicant must have a firm grounding in communication skills (written and oral) as well as two senior sciences to cope with the increased scientific base of nursing. Some knowledge of or fluency in a second language would be useful in this increasingly multicultural society. Perhaps practical nurse education programs should recruit more in second-language communities.

Practical nurse education programs need to be at least two academic years in length and must occur in a postsecondary institution that meets general program standards for preparing professionals to meet entry to practice requirements. This program must be academically sound and contain pure science, social science, and humanities components. Should the practical nurse decide to continue with studies in registered nursing, the practical nursing program should be accepted in whole or in part toward a university baccalaureate program. Private postsecondary schools may present some issues about control of program standards and conflict of interest between profit taking and the public interest, although this need not be so if regulating authorities closely monitor these schools.

As noted in earlier in this Appendix, "laddering" into registered nursing is not the only option for practical nurses to enhance their professional careers. Many opportunities exist for nurses to gain expertise in specific health care areas while retaining a practical nursing identity.

Should a university degree in practical nursing be available? Some places in the USA offer degrees in practical nursing, but this raises some questions. If university degrees become common, what would be the difference between practical nursing and registered nursing? Would the levels of nurses and their currently separate scopes of practices become even more blurred, or would they merge? Does the public need two very similar practitioners with the same education?

If practical nursing required a degree, this would mean registered nurses would be required to have master's degrees. A master's degree might even become a requirement for entry to practice for the RN. This is already happening in the USA and much of Canada, where a Master's in Nursing is required for almost all entry-level teaching or administrative positions and most nurse practitioner (RN extended class) positions. This scenario may appeal to health care agencies because they could employ more practical nurses, presumably for less cost than the same number of registered nurses. However, if university degrees in practical nursing were required, professionals educated at this level would demand higher pay. Thus, the health care system would not be much further ahead economically.

Will practical nursing remain a recognized health care profession, or will it be swallowed up by professions on either side of it: the RN/baccalaureate on one side, and the unregulated health care worker on the other? If practical nursing fails to maintain or expand the knowledge base, then unregulated care workers will chip away and perhaps absorb nursing competencies into their own skill set.

Scope of Practice and New Competencies

Currently, registered nursing claims a greater depth of knowledge and a broader practice base than practical nursing. Consequently, registered nurses act as gatekeepers for nursing practice. They are unlikely to share too many of their responsibilities with practical nurses because doing so would cause them to lose their niche position and possibly cause professional death. It is more likely that the scopes of practice for the two nursing levels will continue as they are.

Practical nursing will continue to be allowed to develop separate postgraduate competencies in specific areas because specific competencies do not directly threaten the separate scopes of practice. In the future, more of these competencies may involve community health, telephone consultations and advice ("Telehealth"), disease prevention (epidemiology), rehabilitation, palliative care, special needs populations, and health teaching opportunities for groups and individuals. Likely, practical nurses will also have many opportunities to work with multicultural groups, including new immigrants, Aboriginal people, and rural populations. The practical nurse will continue to work in long-term and chronic care settings.

If professionals in acute care increase their use of the critical pathway (care map) system, practical nurses could have expanded roles in areas like ICUs (intensive care units). They would be able to work with less stable patients because the critical pathway system allows for more interdependence and collaboration, technological and personnel help, and distinct instructions for care and consultation. The registered nurse would continue with the role of case manager.

What is the Final Answer?

What will happen to practical nursing in the future? No one knows for sure, but we do know from ecological and sociological studies of professions that individuals and groups—both animal and human—grow, develop, change, flourish, fade out, and disappear. According to Wilson (1992), "environment is the theatre and evolution is the play" (p. 82).

Practical nurses and registered nurses are likely to always maintain separate scopes of practice for survival reasons.

But practical nursing can strengthen its position by developing more diverse and specialized competencies in this changing society. It must develop those competencies that address the needs of the environment. It must change to meet health care demands. For nurses, health care—more specifically nursing—is the theatre, and constant change is the play. If practical nurses wish to maintain their particular niche in the health care system, it is essential that they respond effectively in this environment of continued rapid change.

Key Terms

Acuity Level of sickness.

Attrition The process of losing numbers from a group (such as people failing a course or retiring from or quitting jobs).

Competence "The integration and application of knowledge, skills, attitude, and judgment required for safe, ethical, and appropriate performance in an individual's nursing practice." (RNABC, 2003b, p. 26)

Controlled act (reserved act) A clinical skill that may present a danger to the public if not performed properly and therefore may be performed only by certain health professionals.

Credentialing The process of officially acknowledging that a person is competent in an occupation or profession. Licensure and certification are two forms of credentialing.

Creeping credentialism The trend toward higher entry to practice requirements.

Delegation The transfer of authority to perform certain restricted activities.

Educational Laddering A process whereby a person progresses from one level of practice to another as a result of acquiring extra formal and/or informal education.

Environmental scan An analysis of the external and internal issues that can affect a person or an organization.

Epidemiology The study of disease occurring in populations.

Gatekeeper One who monitors or oversees the actions of others.

Jurisdiction A particular legal or geographic area of practice, e.g., Ontario, Vancouver Island Health Authority, etc.

Paraprofessional A person who performs a particular skill that requires special training, but the skill level required is much less than that of a professional. (Para is a prefix from Greek with various meanings, including beside, near, like.)

Proactive To think or plan ahead and anticipate change.

Professionalization The process of developing into a profession.

Protected title A title that can be used only by a person officially licensed in a profession or occupation in a particular area. For example, in Alberta, only a practical nurse registered with the College of Licensed Practical Nurses of Alberta can use the abbreviation or title LPN. The person can use this title only in Alberta. The person cannot use the title in BC unless the person is also registered in BC as an LPN.

Registration Once a person is licensed to practise a particular profession in a specific area, that person's name goes on an official register of practitioners.

RPN In Ontario, refers to registered practical nurse; in the four western provinces, refers to registered psychiatric nurse.

Semi-professional A synonym of paraprofessional, meaning partly professional.

Specialization Developing expertise in a specific area of an occupation or profession (e.g., emergency nursing, mental health nursing, pediatric nursing).

Speciation In biology, refers to the development of a new species or subspecies from the original.

Reactive To react to an observed problem or change that has already occurred.

Scope of nursing practice The legal limits of nurses' professional role; the activities nurses are educated and authorized to perform.

Stakeholder An individual or group with a vested interest in the organization and/or function of another.

Standard of practice Written statements describing the desired level of performance against which actual performance will be compared.

Supervision The process of overseeing the performance of a person or group.

Unregulated health care worker (also called unlicensed care worker [UCW], unlicensed assistive personnel [UAP], unlicensed care personnel [UCP]). A person, paid or volunteer, whose practice is not licensed under the law in a jurisdiction—such as ward aide, orderly, home care worker, or family member.

References

Abbott, A. D. (1988). The system of professions: An essay on the division of expert labor. Chicago: University of Chicago Press.

Access Issues for Regulators Workshop 2. (2001). Panel discussion. Retrieved January 25, 2004, from *http://www.maytree.com/PDF_Files/AIRRisingStandards.pdf*

Canadian Institute for Health Information. (2002). Workforce trends of licensed practical nurses in Canada. Retrieved January 25, 2004, from *http://secure.cihi.ca/ cihiweb/dispPage.jsp?cw_page=AR_365_E*

Canadian Nurses Association. (1993). The scope of nursing practice: A review of issues and trends. Ottawa: Author.

Canadian Practical Nurses Association. (2003). CLPNA report to CPNA. Available from Canadian Practical Nurses Association Web site, *http://www.cpna.ca*, under "Member Reports."

College of Licensed Practical Nurses of Alberta. (2001). History of the licensed practical nurse in Alberta. Available from CLPNA Web site, *http://www.clpna.com*

College of Licensed Practical Nurses of Alberta. (2003). Collaborative nursing practice in Alberta. Retrieved January 15, 2004, from CLPNA Web site, *http://www.clpna.com/doc_collaborationdocument.pdf*

College of Licensed Practical Nurses of British Columbia. (n.d.). Position statement: Use of protected titles for licensed practical nurses in British Columbia. Retrieved February 15, 2004, from *http://www.clpnbc.org/pdf/UseOfTitle.pdf*

College of Licensed Practical Nurses of British Columbia. (2002). Position statement: Medication administration for licensed practical nurses in British Columbia [Revised]. Retrieved January 29, 2004, from *http://www.clpnbc.org/pdf/MedicationAdministrationRevisedOct2002.pdf*

College of Licensed Practical Nurses of British Columbia. (2003). History of LPNs in Canada. Available from CLPN of BC Web site, *http://www.clpnbc.org*

DuPerron, B. (2003). National forum on changing entry-to-practice requirements in allied health professions Panel 2—Workplace implications. Retrieved January 25, 2004, from *http://www.accc.ca/ftp/events/All_Health2003/DuPerron_summary.rtf*

College of Licensed Practical Nurses of British Columbia. (2003). Position statement: The appropriate utilization of licensed practical nurses. Retrieved January 29, 2004, from *http://www.clpnbc.org/pdf/AppropriateUtilizationMarch2003.pdf*

College of Nurses of Ontario. (2003, June) Fact sheet: What is nursing? Retrieved January 25, 2004, from *http://www.cno.org.docs/general/43060_fsPractisingnursing.pdf*

College of Nurses of Ontario. (2003, December). Pushing the boundaries at CLEAR. Communiqué, 28(4), 9–11.

College of Nurses of Ontario. (2004). Working with unregulated care providers. Retrieved January 28, 2004, from *http://www.cno.org/docs/prac/41014_workingucp.pdf*

Enrolled Nurses Professional Association of New South Wales. (2000). What is an enrolled nurse? Retrieved January 20, 2004, from *http://enpansw.org/whatis.htm*

Government of Canada. (2002). Building on values: The future of health care in Canada [Romanow Report]. Ottawa: Commission on the Future of Health Care in Canada. Retrieved February 20, 2004, from *http://www.hc-sc.gc.ca/english/care/romanow/hcc0086.html*

Health Professions Regulatory Advisory Council. (June, 1996). Advice to the Minister of Health: Separate College for Registered Practical Nurses. Retrieved April 22, 2004, from *http://www.hprac.org/downloads/rpn/rpc2.pdf*

Kazanjian, A. (2000). Nursing workforce study, Vol. V: Changes in the nursing workforce and policy implications. University of British Columbia: Centre for Health Services and Policy Research. Retrieved January 26, 2004, from *http://www.chspr.ubc.ca/hhru/pdf/hhru00-7NWPv5.pdf*

Licensed Practical Nurses Association of PEI. (2003). Mandate. Available from LPNAPEI Web site, *http://www.peilpn.com/1%20LPNAPEI%20mandate.htm*

Lowi-Young, M. (2003). Are degrees for entry-to-practice necessary? The employer perspective. Annual Meeting of the Michener Institute. Retrieved January 26, 2004, from *http://www.michener.on.ca/about/ness_degrees.php*

Massachusetts Board of Registration in Nursing. (2000). The five rights of delegation. Retrieved April 19, 2004, from *http://www.state.ma.us/reg/boards/rn/advrul/thefive.htm*

May, D. (2003). Changing entry level education requirements: Is the neo-classical model helpful? [Economics 6030, MER Program, Memorial University]. Retrieved January 26, 2004, from *http://www.nlhba.nf.ca/Web_Site_Files/LR/ETP.pdf*

McLennan Community College. (2004, Spring). Historical development of vocational nursing. Retrieved January 23, 2004, from *http://www.mclennan.edu/syllabi/VNSG/VNSG1119.html*

Nurses Association of New Brunswick and Association of New Brunswick Licensed Practical Nurses. (2003). Working together: A framework for the registered nurse and the licensed practical nurse. Retrieved January 29, 2004, from *http://www.nanb.nb.ca/pdf_e/Publications/General_Publications/RN-LPN%20(e)1.pdf*

Nursing Courses UK. (n.d.). About nursing-training. Retrieved January 23, 2004, from *http://www.nursingcourses.co.uk/about_nursing/training.html*

Nursing Effectiveness, Utilization and Outcomes Research Unit. (2003). Trends for registered practical nurses in Ontario: Fact sheet. Available from Nursing Effectiveness, Utilization and Outcomes Research Unit Web site, *http://www.fhs.mcmaster.ca/nru/publications/factsheets/factsheets.htm*

Practical nurses in Canada. Retrieved January 25, 2004, from *http://secure.cihi.ca/cihiweb/dispPage.jsp?cw_page=AR_365_E*

Registered Nurses Association of British Columbia. (2003a). In touch: Keeping you informed. Vancouver: Author.

Registered Nurses Association of British Columbia. (2003b). Standards for registered nursing practice in British Columbia. Publication No. 128. Vancouver: Author.

Van House, N. A., & Sutton, S. A. (1996). The panda syndrome: An ecology of LIS education [Electronic version]. Journal of Education for Library and Information Science, 37(2), 131–147.

Wilson, E. O. (1992). The diversity of life. Cambridge: Harvard University Press.

Review Question ANSWERS

For answers with rationales see answer key beginning on p. 1675.

Chapter 1
1. 1
2. 4
3. 1
4. 1
5. 2
6. 3
7. 2
8. 3
9. 2
10. 2

Chapter 2
1. 2
2. 2
3. 3
4. 1
5. 3
6. 1
7. 4
8. 1
9. 2
10. 4

Chapter 3
1. 2
2. 3
3. 4
4. 3
5. 1
6. 2
7. 2
8. 1
9. 2
10. 3

Chapter 4
1. 1
2. 2
3. 3
4. 4
5. 4
6. 2
7. 2
8. 3
9. 1
10. 1

Chapter 5
1. 4
2. 3
3. 1
4. 1
5. 3
6. 1
7. 1
8. 2
9. 2
10. 2
11. 2

Chapter 6
1. 4
2. 4
3. 1
4. 3
5. 2
6. 1
7. 2
8. 3
9. 3
10. 4

Chapter 7
1. 3
2. 4
3. 3
4. 1
5. 4
6. 2
7. 3
8. 4
9. 1
10. 2

Chapter 8
1. 1
2. 1
3. 2
4. 4
5. 2
6. 2
7. 4
8. 4
9. 4
10. 3

Chapter 9
1. 2
2. 2
3. 1
4. 2
5. 1
6. 1
7. 4
8. 3
9. 1
10. 4

Chapter 10
1. 4
2. 4
3. 1
4. 4
5. 3
6. 4
7. 2
8. 1
9. 4
10. 1

Chapter 11
1. 2
2. 4
3. 1
4. 2
5. 4
6. 2
7. 4
8. 3
9. 3
10. 1

Chapter 12
1. 1
2. 3
3. 1
4. 1
5. 1
6. 4
7. 1
8. 2
9. 3
10. 3

Chapter 13
1. 1
2. 1
3. 3
4. 3
5. 1
6. 3
7. 3
8. 2
9. 1
10. 4

Chapter 14
1. 4
2. 3
3. 2
4. 1
5. 1
6. 3
7. 4
8. 3
9. 2
10. 2

Chapter 15
1. 3
2. 4
3. 4
4. 1
5. 3
6. 1
7. 3
8. 1
9. 2
10. 1

Chapter 16
1. 4
2. 2
3. 4
4. 4
5. 3
6. 2
7. 1
8. 4
9. 1
10. 3

Chapter 17
1. 3
2. 2
3. 3
4. 4
5. 3
6. 1
7. 3
8. 1
9. 2
10. 1

Chapter 18
1. 4
2. 1
3. 1
4. 1
5. 4
6. 2
7. 1
8. 2
9. 3
10. 4

Review Question RATIONALES

Chapter 1

1. The correct answer is 1. The Lalonde Report shifted emphasis from a medical to a behavioural approach to health. It concluded that the traditional medical approach to health care was inadequate and that "further improvements in the environment, reductions in self-imposed risks, and a greater knowledge of human biology" are necessary to improve the health status of Canadians.

2. The correct answer is 4. The *Ottawa Charter for Health Promotion* supported a socio-environmental approach to health. It identified prerequisites for health as peace, shelter, education, food, income, a stable ecosystem, sustainable resources, social justice, and equity.

3. The correct answer is 1. Labonte (1993) categorized the major determinants of health in a socio-environmental approach as psychosocial risk factors and socio-environmental risk conditions. Political, social, and cultural forces affect health and well-being directly and indirectly through their influence on personal health behaviours. Socio-environmental risk conditions can lead to psychosocial risk factors, which then result in unhealthy behaviours

4. The correct answer is 1. Given that the determinants of health are broad, healthy public policy must extend beyond traditional health agencies and government health departments to other sectors such as agriculture, education, transportation, labour, social services, energy, and housing. Therefore, policy-makers in all government sectors and organizations should know the health consequences of their policies.

5. The correct answer is 2. Primary prevention includes activities that protect against a disease *before* signs and symptoms occur. Examples include immunization to prevent infectious diseases and reduction of risk factors such as inactivity, smoking, and air pollution.

6. The correct answer is 3. Rather than focusing only on helping people develop healthy behaviours, health promotion seeks to create healthy public policy, supportive environments, community action, and personal skill. Health promotion is committed to empowerment and community-based health planning and addresses health issues within the context of the social, economic, and political environment. It therefore is political.

7. The correct answer is 2. The belief that health is primarily an *individual* responsibility is most congruent with the behavioural approach to health. The behavioural approach places responsibility for health on the individual, thereby favouring health promotion strategies such as education, assuming that if people know the risk factors of disease they will engage in healthy behaviours.

8. The correct answer is 3. Rather than focusing primarily on interventions at the societal level, the population health promotion model advocates interventions be implemented toward individuals and families, communities, individual sectors of society (such as health or environmental sectors), and society as a whole.

9. The correct answer is 2. Income and social status are the greatest determinants of health. Canadians who live in poverty have poorer health and are more likely to die earlier and to suffer more illnesses than those with higher incomes, regardless of age, sex, race, culture, and place of residence.

10. The correct answer is 2. Health promotion is directed toward increasing the level of well-being and self-actualization.

Chapter 2

1. The correct answer is 2. Canada contributes 9.7% of its gross domestic product to health care; comparatively, the United States contributes 13.9%.

2. The correct answer is 2. The social safety net includes programs such as family allowance, welfare, and unemployment insurance. Medicare is also a key element of Canada's social safety net.

3. The correct answer is 3. The first universal social program in Canada was family allowance. The *Family Allowance Act* (1945) gave every family a monthly allowance, regardless of means.

4. The correct answer is 1. The five principles of the *Canada Health Act* include public administration, comprehensiveness, universality, portability, and accessibility.

5. The correct answer is 3. Community services are directed at primary and secondary care and should be easily accessible to clients in locations where they live, work, play, and attend school. An adult daycare centre is a community agency. It may be associated with a hospital or long-term care facility or exist as independent centres.

6. The correct answer is 1. The five levels of health care services are promotive, preventive, curative (diagnosis and treatment), rehabilitative, and supportive (including home care, long-term care, and palliative care).

7. The correct answer is 4. Hospitals and other institutions account for the largest share of total health care expenditures (39.4%), followed by drugs (16.2%) and remuneration for physicians (12.9%).

8. The correct answer is 1. Health care cost accelerators include new technology, new pharmaceuticals, an increase in chronic and new diseases, and changing demographics and expectations.

9. The correct answer is 2. Illness prevention services help clients, families, and communities reduce risk factors for disease and injury. Prevention strategies include clinical (screening, immunizing), behavioural (lifestyle change, support groups), or environmental (societal pressure for a healthy environment).

10. The correct answer is 4. Tertiary care is specialized and highly technical care in diagnosing and treating complicated or unusual health problems. Clients who require tertiary care present with an extensive, often complicated, pathological condition.

Chapter 3

1. The correct answer is 2. Florence Nightingale, who is considered the founder of modern nursing, spearheaded the movement to improve standards of nursing care in the mid-19th century.

2. The correct answer is 3. Marguerite d'Youville formed the Sisters of Charity of Montreal, a Canadian order of nuns, in 1737. They began as a small group of women who pooled their possessions to form a refuge for the poor and needy, and eventually became the first visiting nurses in Canada.

3. The correct answer is 4. The first doctoral nursing program was established at the University of Alberta Faculty of Nursing in 1991.

4. The correct answer is 3. An advanced practice nurse is a clinical nurse with graduate preparation who provides primary care, usually in partnership with a physician or group of physicians. The advanced practice nurse has authority to prescribe medications (with the exception of narcotics) and treat health problems within the scope of nursing practice.

5. The correct answer is 1. A code of ethics defines the principles by which nurses function. The first code of ethics for nursing was developed by the International Council of Nurses in 1953 and was adopted by the Canadian Nurses Association (CNA) in 1954. The most recent update to the CNA Code of Ethics was in 2002.

6. The correct answer is 2. Professional nursing organizations establish educational and practice standards for nurses, carry out the regulatory functions of registration and licensure, and discipline members who do not meet the standards. They also collaborate with other health professions' organizations on matters of mutual interest and help their members maintain competence through continuing education. They do not monitor unregulated care providers.

7. The correct answer is 2. In all provinces and territories, nursing practice acts regulate the licensure and practice of nursing. Each province or territory defines for itself the scope of nursing practice because constitutional responsibility for education and health care rests with individual provinces (i.e., the legal limits of nurses' professional role).

8. The correct answer is 1. Because health is a provincial responsibility, each professional nursing organization is responsible for developing the standards for nursing practice in its particular province. The standards provided by the CNO for nurses in Ontario include accountability, continuing competence, ethics, knowledge, knowledge application, leadership, and relationships.

9. The correct answer is 2. In all provinces except Ontario and Quebec, provincial nursing associations assume responsibility for defining and monitoring standards.

10. The correct answer is 3. Nursing unions are primary participants as the representatives of nurses in particular provinces/territories at the bargaining table when new contracts are negotiated.

Chapter 4

1. The correct answer is 1. The overall goals of a population health approach are to maintain and improve the health of the entire population and to eliminate health disparities. The population health approach provides a framework for thinking about health and for taking action to improve the health of populations. Action is primarily directed at community levels.

2. The correct answer is 2. Public health nursing merges knowledge from the public health sciences with professional nursing theories to safeguard and improve the health of populations in the community.

3. The correct answer is 3. Community-based nursing involves acute, chronic, and palliative care of clients and families that enhances their capacity for self-care and promotes autonomy in decision making.

4. The correct answer is 4. Vulnerable populations of clients are those who are likely to develop health problems as a result of excess risks, who have barriers to access to health care services, or who are dependent on others for care.

5. The correct answer is 4. Competent care of vulnerable populations does not include offering financial or legal advice.

6. The correct answer is 2. Physical, emotional, and sexual abuse, as well as neglect, are major public health problems affecting older adults, women, and children

7. The correct answer is 2. A successful community health nursing practice requires an ability to build relationships with the community and be responsive to changes within the community.

8. The correct answer is 3. Perinatal classes, infant care, child safety, and cancer screening are just some of the health education programs in which a nurse in community practice may participate as a nurse educator.

9. The correct answer is 1. The nurse as consultant provides information and supports participation in health activities. In this role, the nurse responds to inquiries about and makes referrals to community resources.

10. The correct answer is 1. The community can be viewed as having three components: structure or locale, the people, and the social systems.

Chapter 5

1. The correct answer is 4. A theory is a purposeful set of assumptions or propositions that show relationships between concepts. Theories are useful because they provide a systematic view of explaining, predicting and prescribing phenomenon.

2. The correct answer is 3. The drive for early nursing theorizing came from nursing educators, who noted that traditional ways of preparing professional nurses were becoming outdated.

3. The correct answer is 1. The nursing process originally involved four steps: assessment, planning, intervention, and evaluation.

4. The correct answer is 1. Each conceptual framework attempted to define nursing by creating a theoretical definition for the substance and structure of the key bodies of knowledge needed to understand clinical situations. This knowledge was called the metaparadigm concepts and included person, environment, health, and nursing.

5. The correct answer is 3. The problem confronting theorists remained: How does one organize and make sense of all possible bodies of knowledge that nursing might draw from and apply them intelligently to the challenges that arise in an individual clinical case?

6. The correct answer is 1. Kuhn challenged the traditional notion of science as a logical progression of discoveries. He argued that major scientific developments occurred when scientists thought about problems in radically new and different ways.

7. The correct answer is 1. The main features of the McGill model include a focus on health rather than illness and treatment, on all family members rather than the patient alone, on family goals, rather than on the nurse's, and on family strengths rather than their deficits.

8. The correct answer is 2. Peplau defined the core of nursing as the interpersonal relationship between the nurse and the client. He viewed this relationship as interactive and therapeutic, with a goal of having the client live independently away from the hospital.

9. The correct answer is 2. Canadian theorist Evelyn Adam articulated the essence of nursing as a helping process. From her perspective, the nurse played a complementary-supplementary role in supporting the client's strength, knowledge, and will.

10. The correct answer is 2. Systems theory accounted for the whole of an entity (the system) and its component parts (subsystems) as well as the interactions between the parts and the whole.

11. The correct answer is 2. Parse's nursing model does not articulate goals for nursing in the traditional sense of defining health; instead, it relies on the notion of people in a continuous process of making choices and changing health priorities.

Chapter 6

1. The correct answer is 4. The first provincially approved doctoral nursing program was established at the University of Alberta Faculty of Nursing in 1991.

2. The correct answer is 4. Carper (1978) described empirics as "knowledge that is systematically organized into general laws and theories for the purpose of describing, explaining and predicting phenomena of special concern to the discipline of nursing."

3. The correct answer is 1. The scientific method is characterized by systematic, orderly procedures that seek to limit the possibility for error and minimize the likelihood that any bias or opinion by the researcher might influence the results of research.

4. The correct answer is 3. Ethnography is chosen if the research question leads to the study of behaviour within a specific group or culture. Ethnography

involves the observation and description of behaviour in social settings. It comes from anthropology, where it provides the means to study the culture of groups of people.

5. The correct answer is 2. Subjectivity from the participants' perspective is sought in qualitative research. Because of the nature of the data, rich with personal experience and example, the research is usually reported in a literary style, similar to storytelling.

6. The correct answer is 1. The grounded theory is "discovered," developed, and verified through a rigorous process of data collection and analysis. Glaser and Strauss advocated that researchers not review the literature prior to carrying out the study, as they might be influenced by what others have found. The strength of the grounded theory approach comes from examining the situation afresh and opening up the possibility of a new perspective on an old problem.

7. The correct answer is 2. The sample in a survey design should be representative of the population so that generalizations can be made on the basis of the sample data.

8. The correct answer is 3. Naming other participants in not required for informed consent. The consent form must describe the purpose of the study, the role of the subjects, types of data that are to be obtained, how the data are obtained, the duration of the study, subject selection, procedures, risks to the subject, potential benefits, alternatives to participation, and contact information.

9. The correct answer is 3. A quasi-experimental research design is one in which groups are formed and the conditions are controlled, but the subjects are not randomly assigned to a control group or treatment conditions.

10. The correct answer is 4. As well as using knowledge based on systematic research studies, evidence-based practice also takes into account a nurse's clinical experience, practice trends, and client preferences.

Chapter 7

1. The correct answer is 3. By understanding their personal values, nurses better understand their clients' and colleagues' values. "Value conflict" is when personal values are at odds with those of a client, colleague, or institution. Values clarification plays a major role in resolving these dilemmas.

2. The correct answer is 4. Justice refers to fairness. The term often is used during discussions about resources. What constitutes a fair distribution of resources may not always be clear.

3. The correct answer is 3. Maleficence refers to harm or hurt; thus non-maleficence is the avoidance of harm or hurt. In health care ethics, ethical practice involves not only the will to do good, but also the equal commitment to do no harm.

4. The correct answer is 1. Beneficence refers to taking positive actions to help others. Commitment to beneficence helps to guide difficult decisions wherein the benefits of a treatment may be challenged by risks to the client's well-being or dignity.

5. The correct answer is 4. Autonomy refers to a person's independence. Autonomy represents an agreement to respect another's right to determine a course of action. Respect for another's autonomy is fundamental to the practice of health care. It is why clients are included in all aspects of decision making regarding their care.

6. The correct answer is 2. The Canadian Nurses Association (CNA) publishes a code of ethics (2002) that outlines nurses' professional values and ethical commitments to their clients.

7. The correct answer is 3. The nurse does not make decisions for the client. Advocating for the client includes protecting the client's right to choice by providing information, obtaining informed consent for all nursing care, and respecting clients' decisions.

8. The correct answer is 4. A utilitarian system of ethics proposes that the value of something is determined by its usefulness.

9. The correct answer is 1. The ethic of care explores the notion of care as a central activity of human behaviour. Those who write about ethic of care maintain that ethical theory based on principles is a male-biased theory. They advocate a more female-biased theory that is based on understanding relationships, especially personal narratives.

10. The correct answer is 2. Each step in the processing of an ethical dilemma resembles steps in critical thinking. The nurse begins by gathering information and moves through assessment, identification of the problem, planning, implementation, and evaluation.

Chapter 8

1. The correct answer is 1. Statute law is created by elective legislative bodies such as Parliament and provincial or territorial legislatures. Examples of provincial statutes are the nursing practice acts throughout the country, which describe and define nursing practice within each province.

2. The correct answer is 2. If a client denies understanding the consent form or the nurse suspects the client does not understand, the nurse must notify the physician or nursing supervisor.

3. The correct answer is 2. The inappropriate or unjustified use of restraints (e.g., by confining a person to an area, using physical or chemical restraints) may be viewed as false imprisonment.

4. The correct answer is 4. Negligence in nursing is conduct that falls below a standard of care established by law. No intent is needed for negligence to occur. It is characterized chiefly by inadvertence, thoughtlessness, or inattention. Therefore, failing to raise the side rails when they are ordered is negligence.

5. The correct answer is 2. Informed consent is part of the physician-client relationship. Because nurses do not perform surgery or direct medical procedures, obtaining clients' informed consent does not usually fall within the nursing duty.

6. The correct answer is 2. When nurses provide consent forms for clients to sign, the clients should be asked if they understand the procedures for which consent is being given. If they deny understanding or the nurse suspects they do not understand, the nurse must notify the physician or nursing supervisor.

7. The correct answer is 4. If a client is harmed as a direct result of a nursing student's actions or lack of action, the liability is generally shared by the student, instructor, hospital or health care facility, and university or educational institution.

8. The correct answer is 4. A nurse providing emergency assistance at an accident scene would not be covered by an employer's insurance policy because the care given would not be the responsibility of the employer. However, some provinces have passed "Good Samaritan" laws (e.g., Alberta's *Emergency Medical Aid Act*) that prevent voluntary rescuers from being sued for wrongdoing unless it can be proven that they displayed gross negligence.

9. The correct answer is 4. The physician is responsible for directing medical treatment. Nurses are obligated to follow physicians' orders unless they believe the orders are in error, violates hospital policy, or would harm clients.

10. The correct answer is 3. Whenever information is requested on a client by any third parties, including insurance companies or employers, nurses must obtain a signed release by the client before releasing confidential information.

Chapter 9

1. The correct answer is 2. The processes of enculturation and acculturation facilitate cultural learning. Socialization into one's primary culture as a child is known as enculturation. The process of adapting to and adopting characteristics of a new culture is acculturation.

2. The correct answer is 2. In Canada, rather than assimilation, the preferred outcome is multiculturalism, where immigrants and others maintain their culture and different people of diverse cultures interact peacefully within the nation. Canadians believe, as enshrined in the multiculturalism policy, that citizens should be able to retain their unique ethnic cultures and traditions within a Canadian context.

3. The correct answer is 1. Cultural awareness is being aware of one's own background, and involves an in-depth self-examination to recognize biases, prejudices, and assumptions about other people.

4. The correct answer is 2. Culturally competent care is a process whereby nursing care is delivered based on knowledge of the client's cultural heritage, beliefs, and attitudes. It requires the practitioner to bridge cultural gaps in caring, work with cultural differences, and enable clients and families to receive meaningful care.

5. The correct answer is 1. Ethnocentrism is the root of stereotypes, biases, and prejudices against others perceived to be different from the valued group.

6. The correct answer is 1. When action is taken on one's prejudices, discrimination occurs, which is treating people unfairly based on their group membership.

7. The correct answer is 4. The dominant value orientation in North American society is individualism and self-reliance in achieving and maintaining health. Caring approaches generally promote the client's independence and ability for self-care.

8. The correct answer is 3. Disparities in health outcomes between the rich and poor illustrate the influence of socio-economic factors in morbidity and mortality. Social factors such as poverty and lack of access to health resources compromise the health status of the poor and unemployed.

9. The correct answer is 1. Clients may suffer cultural pain when their valued way of life is disregarded by practitioners

10. The correct answer is 4. The high value that Western society places on individual autonomy and self-determination may be in direct conflict with diverse groups. Advance directives, informed consent, and consent for hospice are examples of mandates that may violate clients' values.

Chapter 10

1. The correct answer is 3. The functional nursing model of care delivery is task focused, not client focused. Tasks are divided, with one nurse assuming responsibility for certain tasks, for example, hygiene and dressing changes, and another nurse assuming responsibility for other tasks such as medication administration.

2. The correct answer is 4. The primary nursing model of care delivery aimed to place RNs at the bedside and improve nursing accountability for client outcomes and relationships among staff

3. The correct answer is 1. Case management is a care management approach that coordinates and links health care services to clients and their families while streamlining costs and maintaining quality

4. The correct answer is 4. Working in a decentralized structure has the potential for greater collaborative effort, increased staff competency, and a greater sense of professional accomplishment and satisfaction.

5. The correct answer is 3. Accountability means being answerable for one's actions. It involves follow-up and reflection on one's decisions to evaluate effectiveness

6. The correct answer is 4. Communication with staff is one of the manager's greatest challenges, especially in a large work group. A manager can use several approaches to communicate quickly and accurately with all staff. Examples are circulating newsletters, posting minutes of committee meetings, and using list servers and e-mail.

7. The correct answer is 2. Second-order priority needs are actual problems for which the client or family has requested immediate help, such as comfort measures.

8. The correct answer is 1. First-order priority needs are an immediate threat to a client's survival or safety, such as an obstructed airway, loss of consciousness, or an anxiety attack.

9. The correct answer is 4. Unregulated care provides (UCPs) should not be assigned sole responsibility for client care. The nurse in charge of client care decides which activities the UCP can perform independently and which activities must be performed by the nurse and UCP in partnership. UCP have been trained to bathe clients.

10. The correct answer is 1. An outcome reveals if interventions are effective, if clients progress, how well standards are being met, and if changes are necessary. A client outcome is a measure of the client's status after receiving care.

Chapter 11

1. The correct answer is 2. Critical thinking is an active, organized, cognitive process used to carefully examine one's thinking and the thinking of others. It involves forming conclusions, making decisions, drawing inferences, and reflecting.

2. The correct answer is 4. Core critical thinking skills, when applied to nursing, are useful in showing the complex nature of clinical decision making. Self-regulation involves self-examination and self-correction. The nurse reflects on his experiences and identifies ways he can improve his own performance.

3. The correct answer is 1. An important aspect of critical thinking is reflection, the process of purposefully thinking back or recalling a situation to discover its purpose or meaning. Nurses should think back on a client situation, make sense of the experience, and thus gain insight into the meaning of the situation.

4. The correct answer is 2. Intuition is the direct understanding of particulars in a situation without conscious deliberation. It is an inner sense that something is so. It occurs when an experienced nurse walks into a client's room, looks at the client's appearance without the benefit of a thorough assessment, and senses that the client is about to deteriorate physically.

5. The correct answer is 4. At the basic level of critical thinking, a learner trusts that experts have the right answers for every problem. Thinking is concrete and based on a set of rules or principles. For example, a nurse uses an institution's procedure manual to confirm how to insert a Foley catheter.

6. The correct answer is 2. The nursing process consists of five steps: assessment, nursing diagnosis, planning, implementation, and evaluation. During the planning phase, the nurse determines care priorities.

7. The correct answer is 4. The nursing process consists of five steps: assessment, nursing diagnosis, planning, implementation, and evaluation. During the evaluation phase, the nurse evaluates whether the nursing action has been effective.

8. The correct answer is 3. The first component of critical thinking is a nurse's knowledge base. This varies according to a nurse's educational experience, including basic nursing education, continuing education courses, and additional university degrees. In addition, it includes the initiative a nurse shows in reading the nursing literature to remain current in nursing science.

9. The correct answer is 3. A critical thinker does not usually accept or reject another person's ideas without question. To think independently, one questions others' ways of interpreting knowledge and looks for rational and logical answers to problems.

10. The correct answer is 1. A nurse is responsible for correctly performing nursing care activities based on standards of practice. Standards of practice are the minimum level of performance expected of nurses to provide safe, competent, and ethical care (Canadian Nurses Association, 2004). For example, the nurse does not take shortcuts (e.g., failing to identify a client) when administering medications.

Chapter 12

1. The correct answer is 1. The purpose of the assessment is to establish a database about the client's needs, health problems, and responses to these problems. The data contain information about health practices, family and social support, goals, values, and expectations about the health care system.

2. The correct answer is 3. During data clustering, nurses organize data and focus attention on client functions needing support and assistance for recovery. Focused data clustering using a systems approach or another health patterns approach assists the nurse to correctly classify and organize data.

3. The correct answer is 1. A nursing diagnosis is a clinical judgment about individual, family, or community responses to actual and potential health problems or life processes.

4. The correct answer is 1. *Family coping: potential for growth related to unexpected birth of twins* is a wellness nursing diagnosis. This type of nursing diagnosis describes responses to levels of wellness in a client that has a readiness for enhancement. In other words, the client wishes to achieve a higher level of wellness.

5. The correct answer is 1. Once a nurse assesses a client's condition and identifies appropriate nursing diagnoses, a plan is developed for the client's nursing care.

6. The correct answer is 4. Priorities are based on the urgency of the problem, the client's safety and desires, the nature of the treatment indicated, and the relationship among the diagnoses.

7. The correct answer is 1. Indirect care interventions are treatments performed away from the client but on behalf of the client or group of clients. Examples of indirect care include actions aimed at managing the client's environment (e.g., safety and infection control), documentation, and interdisciplinary collaboration.

8. The correct answer is 2. An out-of-date or incorrect care plan compromises the quality of nursing care, whereas review and modification enable the nurse to provide timely nursing interventions to best meet the client's needs.

9. The correct answer is 3. The evaluation process, which determines the effectiveness of nursing care, includes five elements: (a) identifying evaluative criteria and standards, (b) collecting data to determine whether the criteria or standards are met, (c) interpreting and summarizing findings, (d) documenting findings and any clinical judgment, and (e) terminating, continuing, or revising the care plan.

10. The correct answer is 3. As goals are evaluated, the nurse makes adjustments to the care plan as indicated. If a goal was successfully met, that portion of the care plan is discontinued. Unmet and partially met goals require the nurse to continue intervention. After a nurse reassesses a client, nursing diagnoses may be modified or added with appropriate goals and expected outcomes, and interventions are established.

Chapter 13

1. The correct answer is 1. Accrediting agencies such as the Canadian Council on Health Services Accreditation (CCHSA) offer guidelines for documentation.

2. The correct answer is 1. Use of an institution's accepted abbreviations, symbols, and system of measures (e.g., metric) ensures that all staff members use the same language in their reports and records.

3. The correct answer is 3. To limit nursing liability, nurses must clearly document the individualized, goal-directed nursing care that was provided to a client. The record must describe exactly what happened to a client.

4. The correct answer is 3. Data recorded, reported, or communicated to other health care professionals are confidential and must be protected.

5. The correct answer is 1. Clients frequently request copies of their health records, and they have the right to do so. Each institution has policies for controlling the manner in which records are shared. In most situations, clients are required to give written permission for release of medical information.

6. The correct answer is 3. Critical pathways or CareMaps are multidisciplinary care plans that include client health concerns, key interventions, and expected outcomes within an established time frame.

7. The correct answer is 3. Acuity records (also known as workload measurement systems) provide a method of determining the hours of care and staff required for a given group of clients. A client's acuity level is based on the type and number of nursing interventions required for providing care in a 24-hour period.

8. The correct answer is 2. Ideally, discharge planning begins at admission. Nurses revise the care plan as the client's condition changes. The client and family members are involved in the discharge planning process so that they have the information needed to return home.

9. The correct answer is 1. An increasing number of older adults require care in long-term care facilities. Because many individuals will live in this setting for the rest of their lives, they are referred to as residents rather than clients.

10. The correct answer is 4. A telephone order (TO) involves a physician stating a prescribed therapy over the phone to an RN. A verbal order (VO) may be accepted when there is no opportunity for a physician to write the order, as in emergency situations. Clarifying for accuracy is important when an RN accepts physician's orders over the telephone or verbally. The order needs to be verified by repeating it clearly and precisely. The RN is responsible for writing the order on the physician's order sheet in the client's permanent record and signing it.

Chapter 14

1. The correct answer is 4. Assessment of a client's ability to communicate includes gathering data about the many contextual factors that influence communication. These include the participants' internal factors and characteristics, the nature of their relationship, the situation prompting communication, the environment, and the socio-cultural elements present. Assessing these contextual factors helps the nurse make sound decisions during the communication process.

2. The correct answer is 3. Active listening means to be attentive to what the client is saying both verbally and non-verbally. Several non-verbal skills have been identified as facilitative skills for attentive listening. S—Sit facing the client. O—Observe an open posture (i.e., keep arms and legs uncrossed). L—Lean toward the client. E—Establish and maintain intermittent eye contact. R—Relax.

3. The correct answer is 2. A helping relationship between nurse and client does not just happen—it is created with care and skill and is built on the client's trust in the nurse. Statements reflecting empathy are highly effective because they tell the person that the nurse heard the feeling content, as well as the factual content, of the communication. It is used to establish trust.

4. The correct answer is 1. Gender influences how we think, act, feel, and communicate. Male and female communication patterns tend to differ, which can sometimes create barriers to effective communication. Males communicate to achieve goals, establish individual status and authority, and compete for attention and power. Females communicate to build connections with others, include others, and co-operate with, respond to, show interest in, and support others.

5. The correct answer is 1. Nurses function in roles that require interaction with multiple health team members. Many elements of the nurse-client helping relationship are also applied in these collegial relationships, which are focused on accomplishing the work and goals of the clinical setting. It is especially important to involve the client and family in decisions about the plan of care to determine whether suggested methods are acceptable.

6. The correct answer is 3. Clarifying: To check whether understanding is accurate, the nurse can restate an unclear or ambiguous message to clarify the sender's meaning. Instead of restating the message, the nurse can also ask the other person to rephrase it, explain further, or give an example of what the person means.

7. The correct answer is 4. Focusing is used to centre on key elements or concepts of a message. If conversation is vague or rambling or clients begin to repeat themselves, focusing is a useful technique.

8. The correct answer is 3. Giving personal opinions: When the nurse gives a personal opinion, it takes decision making away from the client. It inhibits spontaneity, stalls problem solving, and creates doubt.

9. The correct answer is 2. A tip for improved communication with older adults is to stick to one topic at a time.

10. The correct answer is 2. In the zones of personal space and touch, the personal zone (45 cm to 1 m) includes nursing activities such as sitting at a client's bedside and taking the client's nursing history.

Chapter 15

1. The correct answer is 3. Touch is one way to offer comfort and communicate concern and support. Touch leads to a connection between nurse and client. However, touch can convey many messages; it must be used with discretion.

2. The correct answer is 4. To know a client means that the nurse avoids assumptions, focuses on the client, and engages in a caring relationship with the client that reveals information and cues that facilitate critical thinking and clinical judgments. Knowing the client is at the core of the process by which nurses make clinical decisions.

3. The correct answer is 4. Spiritual health is achieved when people find a balance between their own life values, goals, and belief systems and those of others. Research has shown a link between spirit, mind, and body. An individual's beliefs and expectations can and do have effects on the person's physical well-being.

4. The correct answer is 1. The family is an important resource. Success with nursing interventions often depends on the family's willingness to share information about the client, their acceptance and understanding of therapies.

5. The correct answer is 3. Strategies to enable nurses to demonstrate more caring behaviours include introducing greater flexibility into the work environment structure, rewarding experienced nurse mentors, improving nurse staffing, and providing nurses with autonomy over their practice.

6. The correct answer is 1. Nurses make caring a part of the philosophy and environment in the workplace by incorporating care concepts into standards of nursing care, thus establishing the guidelines for professional conduct.

7. The correct answer is 3. A nurse demonstrates caring by helping family members become active participants in a client's care.

8. The correct answer is 1. Listening includes not only "taking in" what a client says, but also interpreting and understanding what is said and reflecting that understanding to the person talking.

9. The correct answer is 2. Presence involves a person-to-person encounter that conveys closeness and a sense of caring that involves "being there" and "being with" clients.

10. The correct answer is 1. Knowing the behaviours that clients perceive as caring helps nurses to understand what clients expect of them as caregivers. Establishing a reassuring presence, recognizing an individual as unique, and being attentive to the client are recurrent caring behaviours identified by researchers. All clients are unique; however, understanding common behaviours that clients associate with caring will help the beginning student learn to express caring in practice.

Chapter 16

1. The correct answer is 4. The nurse must think of family as defined by each individual. In other words, the nurse can think of the family as a set of relationships that the client identifies as family or as a network of individuals who influence each other's lives, whether or not there are actual biological or legal ties.

2. The correct answer is 2. The blended family is formed when both parents bring children from previous relationships into a new, joint living situation, or when there are children from the current union and children from previous unions living together.

3. The correct answer is 4. The rate of teenagers giving birth has been declining steadily over the last 25 years, probably due to increased sexual education, the availability of contraceptives, and the use of abortion.

4. The correct answer is 4. The family is the primary social context in which health promotion and disease prevention take place. The family's beliefs, values, and practices also strongly influence health-promoting behaviours of its members.

5. The correct answer is 3. Recently, health promotion research has started to focus on the stress-moderating effect of hardiness and resiliency as factors that contribute to long-term health. Family hardiness is the internal strengths and durability of the family unit. Family resiliency is the ability to cope with expected and unexpected stressors.

6. The correct answer is 2. When the family as client is the approach, the nurse focuses on the entire family—its processes and relationships (e.g., parenting or family caregiving).

7. The correct answer is 1. Internal structure: The people who are included in the family and how they are connected to each other. Specifically, this question assesses family composition, a subcategory of internal structure. Composition refers to the individual members who form the family. The family composition is not limited to the traditional, nuclear family, but may include any of the various family forms.

8. The correct answer is 4. Expressive functioning refers to the ways in which people communicate. Emotional communication is a subcategory of expressive functioning and refers to the range and types of feelings that are expressed by the family.

9. The correct answer is 1. Circular questions facilitate change by inviting the family to discover their own answers; they help explain a problem.

10. The correct answer is 3. In an effective family interview, the nurse can engage a family to assess, explore, and identify strengths and problems. The nurse can also decide to intervene or refer the family to another health professional.

Chapter 17

1. The correct answer is 3. Psychomotor learning involves acquiring skills that require the integration of mental and muscular activity. Teaching a client to use a walker requires the use of the psychomotor domain. The client masters skills by manipulating equipment and practicing manual skills.

2. The correct answer is 2. If a client's learning ability is impaired, the nurse should modify or postpone teaching activities. Any physical condition (e.g. pain, fatigue, or hunger) that depletes energy also impairs the ability to learn. Therefore, the nurse should teach the client when pain medications are working.

3. The correct answer is 3. Readiness to learn is related to the grieving stage. Clients cannot learn when they are unwilling or unable to accept the reality of illness. However, properly timed teaching can help a client to adjust to illness or disability. When a client is in denial or disbelief, teach in present tense (e.g., explain what client needs to know to be discharged).

4. The correct answer is 4. As a child matures, intellectual growth moves from concrete to abstract. By

developing topics for discussion that require problem solving, the nurse is considering the adolescents' level of development and will engage the students in learning about nutrition.

5. The correct answer is 3. Behavioural objectives are measurable and observable and indicate how learning will be evidenced. An objective is more precise when it describes the conditions or timing under which the behaviour occurs (e.g., the client will perform breast self-examination correctly before the end of the teaching session).

6. The correct answer is 1. The telling approach is useful when limited information must be taught (e.g., preparing a client for an emergency diagnostic procedure).

7. The correct answer is 3. Role-play helps teach new ideas and attitudes. During role-play, clients play themselves or someone else and rehearse a desired behaviour.

8. The correct answer is 1. Learning disabilities are disorders that may impair ability to acquire, organize, remember, understand, or apply information. When teaching clients with learning disabilities or other barriers to learning, a recommended technique is to demonstrate procedures such as measuring dosages and then ask for return demonstrations (provides opportunity to clarify instructions and time to review procedures).

9. The correct answer is 2. Generally, teaching and learning begin when a person identifies a need for knowing or acquiring an ability to do something.

10. The correct answer is 1. Demonstrations help teach psychomotor skills such as preparing a syringe. The client is able to observe a skill before practicing it.

Chapter 18

1. The correct answer is 4. Growth is the quantitative, or measurable, aspect of an individual's increase in physical measurements. Measurable growth indicators include changes in height, weight, teeth, skeletal structures, and sexual characteristics.

2. The correct answer is 1. Moral development is the ability of an individual to distinguish right from wrong and to develop ethical values on which to base his or her actions.

3. The correct answer is 1. Organicism refers to a theoretical focus on the organism itself. Theories in this tradition hold that development is a result of biologically driven behaviour and the person's adaptation to the environment.

4. The correct answer is 1. There are three major categories of factors that influence human growth and development: genetics, environment, and the interaction between these two. The family is an example of an environmental factor. Family influences through its values, beliefs, customs, and specific patterns of interaction and communication.

5. The correct answer is 4. Psychiatrist Roger Gould believes his research describes a sequential process that takes place between the internal life (personality) of adults and their outer world (culture, lifestyle).

6. The correct answer is 2. The fourth theme, identified in individuals in their 40s, "The die is cast," is indicative of resignation and the belief that possibilities are limited. The personality is set. Changes in career are believed to be less likely to be successful. Parents are blamed for their lack of choices. Regret is faced for mistakes made with children.

7. The correct answer is 1. During formal operations, the individual's thinking moves to abstract and theoretical subjects. Thinking can venture into such subjects as achieving world peace, finding justice, and seeking meaning in life. Adolescents can organize their thoughts in their minds. New cognitive powers allow the adolescent to do more far-reaching problem solving.

8. The correct answer is 2. The microsystem consists of the immediate settings, activities, and personal relationships of the individual. Examples of microsystems include family, classroom, workplace, or recreation group.

9. The correct answer is 3. Daniel Keating and Clyde Hertzman's population health approach (1999) maintains that human development is a population phenomenon. They refer to the strong association between the health of a population, developmental outcomes, and the social and economic forces affecting the larger society. Therefore, improving community housing would be an attempt to improve the health of the population.

10. The correct answer is 4. According to resilience theory, protective processes protect from adversity and include social supports, such as quality daycare.

Chapter 19

1. The correct answer is 1. Maternal risk factors associated with preterm labour include physiological stresses such as renal and cardiovascular disease, diabetes mellitus, or uterine and cervical abnormalities.

2. The correct answer is 1. The most extreme physiological change occurs when the newborn leaves the *in utero* circulation and develops independent respiratory functioning. Nursing care is directed at maintaining an open airway, stabilizing and maintaining body temperature, and protecting the newborn from infection.

3. The correct answer is 3. Infants who are breast-fed, especially those in more northerly areas, need to receive a vitamin D supplement.

4. The correct answer is 4. According to Piaget (1952), during the preoperational thought stage of cognitive development, toddlers recognize that they are separate beings from their mothers, but they are unable to assume the view of another. They use symbols to represent objects, places, and people. This function is demonstrated when children imitate the behaviour of another that they viewed earlier (e.g., pretend to shave like daddy).

5. The correct answer is 3. The play of preschool children becomes more social after the third birthday as it shifts from parallel to associative play. Most 3-year-old children are able to play with one other child in a co-operative manner in which they make something or play designated roles such as mother and baby. By the age of 4 years, children play in groups of two or three, and by 5 years, the group has a temporary leader for each activity.

6. The correct answer is 2. Preschoolers average 12 hours of sleep a night and take infrequent naps.

7. The correct answer is 1. Motor development in the school-age child: 8-10 years: Can learn to floss teeth effectively and be independent in tooth care.

8. The correct answer is 2. Infections account for the majority of all childhood illnesses; respiratory infections are the most prevalent. The common cold remains the chief illness of childhood.

9. The correct answer is 3. Good communication skills are critical for overcoming peer pressure and unhealthy behaviours. The following are some hints for communicating with adolescents: do not avoid discussing sensitive issues, ask open-ended questions, look for the meaning behind their words or actions, be alert to clues to their emotional state, and involve other individuals and resources when necessary.

10. The correct answer is 3. Injuries, including self-inflicted injuries and injuries caused by motor vehicle accidents and poisoning, are the leading cause of death in adolescents.

Chapter 20

1. The correct answer is 2. The young adult has usually completed physical growth by the age of 20 years.

2. The correct answer is 1. The nurse's role in health promotion is to identify lifestyle risk factors and provide education and support to reduce unhealthy behaviours.

3. The correct answer is 4. When determining what the amount of information the individual needs to make decisions about the prescribed course of therapy, the nurse should consider those factors that may affect the individual's compliance with the regimen, including educational level, socio-economic factors, and motivation and desire to learn.

4. The correct answer is 4. A common physiological change in the second trimester is the sensation of Braxton-Hicks contractions, which are caused by the expanding uterus and preparation of the uterus for labour.

5. The correct answer is 2. Motor vehicle accidents causing injuries and fatalities are double the rate in 20- to 24-year-olds than for the population as a whole. Motor vehicle accidents are the leading cause of accidental injury for young and middle adults.

6. The correct answer is 2. Close friends and associates of the single young adult may also be viewed as the individual's "family."

7. The correct answer is 3. A family history of a disease may put a young adult at risk for developing it in the middle or older adult years. For example, a young man whose father and paternal grandfather had myocardial infarctions (heart attacks) in their 50s has a risk for a future myocardial infarction.

8. The correct answer is 3. In the middle adult years, as children depart from the household, the family enters the post-parental family stage. Time and financial demands on the parents decrease, and the couple faces the task of redefining their relationship.

9. The correct answer is 3. Health teaching and health counselling are often directed at improving health habits.

10. The correct answer is 3. The physiological response to stress can be avoided. The nurse uses relaxation techniques, imagery, and biofeedback to recondition the client's response to stress.

Chapter 21

1. The correct answer is 4. Two factors contribute to the projected increase in the number of older adults: the aging of the baby boom generation and the growth of the population segment over 85 years. The baby boomers are the large cohort of adults born between 1946 and 1964.

2. The correct answer is 3. Various theorists have attempted to describe the complex biopsychosocial process of aging. Although many theories have been developed, there is no single universally accepted theory that predicts and explains the complexities of the aging process.

3. The correct answer is 3. The three common conditions affecting cognition are delirium, dementia, and depression. The nurse may find that distinguishing

among these three conditions is challenging but essential.

4. The correct answer is 2. Sexuality is increasingly recognized as an important factor in the care of older adults. All older adults, whether healthy or frail, need to express sexual feelings. Sexuality involves love, warmth, sharing, and touching, not just the act of intercourse.

5. The correct answer is 1. The older adult's libido does not decrease, although frequency of sexual activity may decline. An older woman who does not understand physical changes affecting sexual activity may be concerned that her sex life is nearly over with the onset of menopause. The older man may feel the same when he discovers a change in the firmness of his erection, a decreased need for ejaculation with each orgasm, or a longer recovery period between episodes of intercourse.

6. The correct answer is 3. Presbyopia is common in older adults and is the gradual decline in the ability to focus on near objects.

7. The correct answer is 1. Presbycusis, common in older adults, affects the ability to hear high-pitched sounds and sibilant consonants such as *s, sh,* and *ch.*

8. The correct answer is 1. Taste buds atrophy and lose sensitivity. The older adult is less able to discern among salty, sweet, sour, and bitter tastes.

9. The correct answer is 4. The antero-posterior diameter of the thorax increases. Because of the increased incidence of osteoporosis in older adults, vertebral changes due to osteoporosis lead to dorsal kyphosis, the curvature of the thoracic spine sometimes called "dowager's hump."

10. The correct answer is 1. Frontal-temporal dementia has an insidious onset and progresses slowly. Early symptoms include poor hygiene, lack of social tact, hyper-orality, and sexual disinhibition. Incontinence is an early symptom in frontal-temporal dementia, although it is a late symptom in the more common Alzheimer's disease.

Chapter 22

1. The correct answer is 2. Self-concept is how one thinks about oneself. It is a subjective sense of the self and a complex mixture of unconscious and conscious thoughts, attitudes, and perceptions. Mastectomy is a surgical procedure that alters the appearance and function of the body. Although the changes may not be apparent to others when the individual is dressed, these bodily changes have a significant impact on the individual.

2. The correct answer is 2. One of the self-concept developmental tasks of 1- to 3-year-olds is developing self through modeling, imitation, and socialization.

3. The correct answer is 4. Identity involves the internal sense of individuality, wholeness, and consistency of a person over time and in various circumstances.

4. The correct answer is 3. Body image depends only partly on the reality of the body. Body image involves attitudes related to the body, including physical appearance, structure, or function. Feelings about body image include those related to sexuality, femininity and masculinity, youthfulness, health, and strength. These mental images are not always consistent with a person's actual physical structure or appearance.

5. The correct answer is 1. Through the process of reinforcement-extinction, certain behaviours become common or are avoided, depending on whether they are approved and reinforced or discouraged and punished.

6. The correct answer is 4. Through the process of identification, an individual internalizes the beliefs, behaviour, and values of role models into a personal, unique expression of self.

7. The correct answer is 3. An individual's identity is affected by stressors throughout life but is particularly vulnerable during adolescence, a time marked by great change.

8. The correct answer is 1. Identity confusion results when people do not maintain a clear, consistent, and continuous consciousness of personal identity.

9. The correct answer is 3. Self-esteem: asking clients how they feel about themselves gives the nurse information about their self-esteem.

10. The correct answer is 1. Increasing the client's self-awareness is achieved through establishing a trusting relationship that allows the client to openly explore thoughts and feelings.

Chapter 23

1. The correct answer is 3. Gender identity refers to the degree to which a person identifies as male, female, or some combination. It begins in infancy as the child becomes aware of the differences of the sexes and perceives that he or she is male or female.

2. The correct answer is 2. Sexual health means a person has freedom from physical and psychological impairment, awareness of and positive attitudes toward sexual functioning, and accurate knowledge about sexuality.

3. The correct answer is 4. Sexual dysfunction is the absence of complete sexual functioning.

4. The correct answer is 1. A major problem in dealing with STIs is that symptoms are absent or go unnoticed. Finding and treating the people who have

them can be difficult. Some people may not even know that they are infected.

5. The correct answer is 2. The most common bacterial STI is genital chlamydia. (HIV/AIDS is a *viral* STI.) A chlamydial infection may cause an abnormal genital discharge and burning with urination. There are many serious complications of genital chlamydia in women, including chronic pelvic pain, infertility, and ectopic pregnancy.

6. The correct answer is 1. Contraceptive methods that require a health care provider's intervention include hormonal contraception, intrauterine devices (IUDs), the diaphragm, the vaginal contraceptive ring, the cervical cap, and surgical procedures (vasectomy and tubal ligation).

7. The correct answer is 2. Birth control pill: Effectiveness rates are as follows: birth control pills, 98% to 99%; contraceptive sponge, 80% to 91%; vaginal spermicide, 78% to 90%; female condom, 79% to 85%.

8. The correct answer is 2. The most valuable tool that the nurse can develop for providing care in areas of sexuality is effective, non-judgmental communication. A perceptive and educated approach to talking about sexuality can offer the support that many clients require. Effective communication about sexuality requires caring, sensitivity, tact, compassion, the use of appropriate language, and non-discriminatory attitudes.

9. The correct answer is 3. When caring for older adults, nurses may adjust their assessment approach. When gathering a sexual history from an older adult, it is important to keep in mind that the older adult may have difficulty discussing intimate details with health care providers. The nurse has the responsibility to help maintain the sexuality of older adults by offering the opportunity to discuss any concerns. Often, asking questions on the topic of sexuality in a comfortable, relaxed manner facilitates older adults' discussing their sexual needs.

10. The correct answer is 1. A useful framework to guide planning is the PLISSIT model developed by Annon (1976). The *P* stands for permission giving. During assessment, the nurse's questions can bring up the topic of sexuality and can give the individual permission to talk about sexual concerns. *LI* stands for limited information, which involves providing basic information regarding sexuality and sexual functioning. *SS* stands for specific suggestions, whereby the nurse provides specific suggestions regarding a sexual concern or issue. The concern expressed might be one that the nurse is not equipped to address. In this case, the nurse should refer to another health care provider. The *IT* stands for intensive therapy. At this level of intervention, the nurse's role would be to refer the client to a qualified practitioner, such as a social worker or sex counsellor for individualized therapy.

Chapter 24

1. The correct answer is 3. Caring for a client's spiritual needs means caring for the whole person, accepting his or her beliefs and experiences, and helping the client with issues surrounding meaning and hope.

2. The correct answer is 2. Atheist: There are individuals who either do not believe in the existence of God (atheist) or who believe that any ultimate reality is unknown (agnostic). This does not mean that spirituality is not an important concept for the atheist or agnostic. Atheists search for meaning in life through their work and their relationships with other individuals.

3. The correct answer is 4. When a person has the attitude of something to live for and look forward to, hope is present. Hope is a multi-dimensional concept that provides comfort while enduring life threats and personal challenges.

4. The correct answer is 4. Canadian Hutterites believe that it is not appropriate to pray for good health, but rather wisdom to live a healthy life or bear suffering without complaint.

5. The correct answer is 4. A ritual can provide the client with structure and support during difficult times. If rituals are important to the client, the nurse uses them as part of nursing intervention.

6. The correct answer is 1. The ability to establish presence is part of the art of nursing. It is not simply being in the same room with a client while performing procedures or sharing information. Presencing involves "being with" a client versus "doing for" a client. Presencing involves offering a closeness with the client, physically, psychologically, and spiritually.

7. The correct answer is 1. Some sects of Hinduism are vegetarians. The belief is not to kill any living creature.

8. The correct answer is 4. Some members of the Jehovah's Witnesses may avoid food prepared with or containing blood.

9. The correct answer is 2. Members of the Mormon faith abstain from alcohol, caffeine, and tobacco.

10. The correct answer is 1. Clients who experience terminal illness or who have been recently disabled by disease or injury will require the nurse's support in grieving over and coping with their loss. Supporting a client during times of grief can be enhanced by a spiritual relationship with the client.

Chapter 25

1. The correct answer is 1. An actual loss is any loss of a person or object that can no longer be felt, heard, known, or experienced by the individual. Lost objects that have been valued by a client include any possession that is worn out, misplaced, stolen, or ruined by disaster.

2. The correct answer is 2. A perceived loss is any loss that is uniquely defined by the grieving client. It may be less obvious to others.

3. The correct answer is 3. Situational loss includes any sudden, unpredictable external event.

4. The correct answer is 4. During Bowlby's phase of disorganization and despair, an individual may endlessly examine how and why the loss occurred.

5. The correct answer is 4. During Kübler-Ross's stage of depression, the person finally realizes the full impact and significance of the loss and may feel overwhelmingly lonely and withdraw from interpersonal interaction.

6. The correct answer is 2. Worden's Task III is to adjust to the environment in which the deceased is missing. According to Worden, a person does not realize the full impact of a loss for at least 3 months. At this point, many friends and associates stop calling and the person is left to ponder the full impact of loneliness.

7. The correct answer is 3. Loneliness and *problems associated with completing the tasks of daily living* are two of the most common and difficult adjustments for older bereaved spouses.

8. The correct answer is 1. General nursing care goals for clients with a loss include accommodating grief, accepting the reality of a loss, and renewing regular relationships.

9. The correct answer is 2. For transplantation of organs, the client must be maintained on ventilatory and circulatory support until vital organs are harvested. The family must clearly understand that the client is "brain dead," that the equipment (i.e., ventilator and vasopressor medications) is not keeping the client alive but keeping the physical body in a state so that the organs will not be damaged before harvesting.

10. The correct answer is 3. Palliative care allows clients to make more informed choices, achieve better alleviation of symptoms, and have more opportunity to work on issues of life closure.

Chapter 26

1. The correct answer is 1. The medulla oblongata controls vital functions necessary for survival, including heart rate, blood pressure, and respiration.

2. The correct answer is 4. The general adaptation syndrome (GAS) has a three-stage reaction to stress. During the alarm reaction, rising hormone levels result in increased blood volume, blood glucose levels, epinephrine and norepinephrine amounts, heart rate, blood flow to muscles, oxygen intake, and mental alertness.

3. The correct answer is 2. Ego-defence mechanisms are indirect methods of coping with stress. Denial is avoiding emotional conflicts by refusing to consciously acknowledge anything that might cause intolerable emotional pain.

4. The correct answer is 3. Post-traumatic stress disorder (PTSD) begins with an acute stress disorder.

5. The correct answer is 3. Situational stress can arise from the person's current circumstances, such as moving, changing jobs, and adjusting to a chronic illness or condition.

6. The correct answer is 2. The nurse uses the interview to determine the client's perception of the stressor by asking the client what is of the most concern at this time.

7. The correct answer is 4. Three primary modes of intervention for stress are to decrease stress-producing situations, increase resistance to stress, and learn skills that reduce physiological response to stress. A support group provides emotional support to a client experiencing stress.

8. The correct answer is 2. In the presence of anxiety-provoking thoughts and events, a common physiological symptom is muscle tension. Physiological tension will be diminished through a systematic approach to releasing tension in major muscle groups.

9. The correct answer is 4. Rapid changes in health care technology, diversity in the workforce, organizational restructuring, and changing work systems can place stress on nurses.

10. The correct answer is 1. A crisis creates a turning point in a person's life because it changes the direction of a person's life in some way. The precipitating event usually occurs from 1 to 2 weeks before the individual seeks help, but it may have occurred within the past 24 hours. Generally, a crisis is resolved in some way within approximately 6 weeks.

Chapter 27

1. The correct answer is 3. Bradycardia is a slow heart rate, below 60 beats per minute in adults. Bradypnea is an abnormally slow rate of breathing, less than 12 breaths per minute.

2. The correct answer is 1. An inefficient contraction of the heart that fails to transmit a pulse wave to the peripheral pulse site creates a pulse deficit. To assess

a pulse deficit, the nurse and a colleague assess radial and apical rates simultaneously and then compare rates. The difference between the apical and radial pulse rates is the pulse deficit.

3. The correct answer is 1. The normal temperature range gradually drops as individuals approach older adulthood. The older adult has a narrower range of body temperatures than the younger adult. Oral temperatures of 35° C are not unusual for older adults in cold weather. However, the average body temperature of older adults is approximately 36° C.

4. The correct answer is 2. Blood pressure measurements will not be accurate unless the correct size blood pressure cuff is applied appropriately.

5. The correct answer is 3. If cuff is too small, it tends to come loose as inflated and results in false high readings.

6. The correct answer is 1. The blood pressure measurements indicate that the client has orthostatic hypotension. If orthostatic hypotension is assessed, the client is assisted to a lying position and the physician or nurse in charge is notified. While obtaining orthostatic measurements, the nurse observes for other symptoms of hypotension such as fainting, weakness, or light-headedness.

7. The correct answer is 2. If the nurse detects an abnormal rate while palpating a peripheral pulse, the next step is to assess the apical rate. The apical rate requires auscultation of heart sounds, which provides a more accurate assessment of cardiac contraction.

8. The correct answer is 1. Conduction is the transfer of heat from one object to another with direct contact. Heat conducts through contact with solids, liquids, and gases. When the warm skin touches a cooler object, heat is lost. Conduction normally accounts for a small amount of heat loss. The nurse increases conductive heat loss when applying an ice pack or bathing a client with a cool cloth.

9. The correct answer is 3. Diseases causing poor oxygenation such as asthma or chronic obstructive pulmonary disease (COPD) cause an increase in pulse rate.

10. The correct answer is 1. The basic techniques of inspection, palpation, and auscultation are used to determine vital signs.

Chapter 28

1. The correct answer is 4. The nursing diagnosis is made after completion of both the health history and the physical examination, and any necessary diagnostic or laboratory tests. The quality, intensity, and location of the symptom or sign are three of the ten characteristics of a symptom/sign assessed by nurses. Information about the ten characteristics provides the nurse with comprehensive information about the symptom/sign.

2. The correct answer is 4. Recent memory involves the recall of events that occurred within the previous 24 hours, such as what was eaten for breakfast. Immediate recall is the ability to recall information such as a telephone number which has been learned within the last few minutes. Remote memory is the ability to recall significant information learned in the past such as birthdays or historical events.

3. The correct answer is 2. When the nurse conducts an otoscopic examination, the client is always asked to tilt the head away from the side being examined. For example, if examining the (R) ear, the nurse asks the client to tilt the head slightly toward the (L) shoulder. This positioning enhances the nurse's ability to see the ear structures. Straightening of the ear canal, using the largest ear speculum that fits the ear canal without touching the skin, and moving the otoscope slowly all permit the nurse to visualize the ear structures.

4. The correct answer is 3. Nurses assess the consistency of the nodes, the definition of the node borders, the mobility or fixation of a node, and the presence of node tenderness. These are four of the characteristics that nurses assess when palpating lymph nodes. They also assess enlargement, location, size, shape, and surface characteristics of the nodes. During palpation of lymph nodes, nurses do not assess turgor, moisture, temperature, or colour that are all characteristics of skin. Configuration is a characteristic of skin lesions.

5. The correct answer is 3. Adventitious breath sounds are unexpected. When nurses hear crackles, rhonchi, wheezes or friction rubs, they need to identify their location in the lungs, determine when they occur in inspiration and/or expiration, and confirm that they do not clear with coughing or after several deep inspirations. The ratio of inspiratory phase to expiratory phase is one way of determining the type of expected breath sound as vesicular, bronchovesicular, or bronchial.

6. The correct answer is 4. If the PMI is palpated 4 cm to the left of the left midclavicular line, the nurse suspects the presence of an enlarged left ventricle. The nurse expects the PMI to be palpated at about the 5th left interspace only, to be palpated during the first two thirds of systole, and to feel like a brisk tap against the palpating finger.

7. The correct answer is 2. To ensure accurate comparison for percussion of symmetric areas, nurses keep the force of the percussion blow consistent between sides. During percussion, nurses use a brisk, arc-like, but relaxed wrist motion, apply the pleximeter finger firmly to the skin surface, and use the lightest percussion blow to achieve clear percussion notes.

8. The correct answer is 3. Nurses palpate the paravertebral muscles bilaterally for symmetry of bulk and to detect tenderness or spasm, but do not assess the attachments of the paravertebral muscles to the 24 vertebrae. They assess curvatures, alignment, and range of motion of the spine when inspecting the spine.

9. The correct answer is 3. The testicles of a young adult male are smooth and slightly rubbery. An elderly male client is expected to demonstrate age-related changes that include diminished and grey pubic hair, a more pendulous scrotal sac because of dartos muscle relaxation, and a small penis, whether circumcised or uncircumcised.

10. The correct answer is 2. Clients should be able to perform point-to-point testing accurately whether eyes are closed or open. When a client can perform the test accurately with eyes open, but not with eyes closed, the client has lost position sense because of the lack of visual cues. Vision aids accuracy. Without visual cues, the test cannot be performed with accuracy when position sense is lost.

Chapter 29

1. The correct answer is 1. If an infection can be transmitted from one person to another, it is a communicable (infectious, contagious) disease.

2. The correct answer is 1. Hepatitis A is transmitted by direct contact. Direct contact involves physical skin-to-skin contact between an infected or colonized individual and a susceptible host.

3. The correct answer is 4. The interval when a client manifests signs and symptoms specific to type of infection (e.g., common cold manifested by sore throat, sinus congestion, rhinitis) is the illness stage.

4. The correct answer is 2. Hand hygiene is the most important and most basic technique in preventing transmission of infections. Hand hygiene includes using an instant alcohol hand antiseptic before and after providing client care, handwashing with soap and water when hands are visibly soiled, and performing a surgical scrub when necessary. The components of good handwashing include using an adequate amount of soap, rubbing the hands together to lather the soap and create friction, and rinsing under a stream of water.

5. The correct answer is 2. Washing times of at least 10 seconds are needed to remove most transient microorganisms from the skin. If the hands are visibly soiled, more time may be needed.

6. The correct answer is 2. Before isolation measures are instituted, the client must understand the nature of the disease or condition, the purposes of isolation, and steps for carrying out specific precautions. The nurse also takes measures to improve the client's sensory stimulation during isolation.

7. The correct answer is 4. Gowns or cover-ups protect health care workers and visitors from coming in contact with infected material, blood, or body fluid.

8. The correct answer is 2. Gloves should be removed promptly after use, before touching noncontaminated items and environmental surfaces, and before going to another client.

9. The correct answer is 3. An autoclave is used to sterilize surgical instruments, parenteral solutions, and surgical dressings.

10. The correct answer is 1. When a nurse is doing a surgical handwashing, he or she must keep hands above elbows.

Chapter 30

1. The correct answer is 1. Right documentation has been added to the traditional five rights of medication administration to enhance medication safety. Documentation is an important part of safe medication administration. Because medication errors may result from inaccurate documentation, nurses must ensure that the appropriate documentation exists before giving medications.

2. The correct answer is 2. A medication order is required for any medication to be administered by a nurse. Before any other interventions, the nurse ensures that the medication order contains all of the elements. If the medication order is incomplete, the nurse should inform the prescriber and ensure completeness before carrying out the medication order.

3. The correct answer is 1. The primary contraindications to giving oral medications include the presence of gastrointestinal (GI) alterations, the inability of a client to swallow food or fluids, and the use of gastric suction.

4. The correct answer is 1. A medication error is any event that could cause or lead to a client receiving inappropriate medication therapy or failing to receive appropriate medication therapy. Most medication errors occur when a nurse fails to follow routine procedures such as checking dose calculations, deciphering illegible handwriting, or administering medications with which the nurse is unfamiliar.

5. The correct answer is 4. This example demonstrates how the formula applies with solid dose forms. The physician orders 500 mg orally (PO) of Keflex. The medication is available in tablets containing 250 mg.

   500 mg/250 mg × 1 tablet = Number of tablets to administer

   The fraction 500/250 equals = 2. Therefore,

   2 × 1 tablet = 2 tablets to be administered.

6. The correct answer is 3. Subcutaneous injections involve placing medications into the loose connective tissue under the dermis. Because subcutaneous tissue is not as richly supplied with blood as the muscles, medication absorption is somewhat slower than with intramuscular injections.

7. The correct answer is 1. The nurse is responsible for following legal provisions when administering controlled substances (drugs that affect the mind or behaviour), which can be dispensed only with a prescription. Violations of the *Narcotic Control Act* are punishable by fines, imprisonment, and loss of nurse licensure or registration.

8. The correct answer is 2. Pharmacokinetics is the study of how medications enter the body, reach their site of action, are metabolized, and exit the body. The nurse uses knowledge of pharmacokinetics when timing medication administration, selecting the route of administration, judging the client's risk for alterations in medication action, and observing the client's response.

9. The correct answer is 4. Official publications, such as the *British Pharmacopoeia* and the *Canadian Formulary,* set standards for drug strength, quality, purity, packaging, safety, labelling, and dosage form. Physicians, nurses, and pharmacists depend on these standards to ensure that clients receive pure drugs in safe and effective dosages.

10. The correct answer is 1. Administration of the *Food and Drugs Act* and the *Controlled Drugs and Substances Act* is carried out by the Health Protection Branch (HPB) of the federal government. Before a new drug can be marketed in Canada, an application for approval must be made to the HPB. After intensive testing, the HPB reviews the application. When sufficient information has been accumulated to ensure its safety, the drug is released for general use.

Chapter 31

1. The correct answer is 3. Despite the success of allopathic medicine (traditional Western medicine), many conditions such as arthritis, chronic back pain, gastrointestinal problems, allergies, headaches, and insomnia are difficult to treat, and more clients are exploring alternative methods to relieve their symptoms.

2. The correct answer is 4. Many of the complementary therapies, such as acupuncture, contain diagnostic and therapeutic methods specific to their field, whereas others, such as guided imagery and breathwork, are generally easily learned and applied.

3. The correct answer is 1. One survey reported that half of Canadians had used alternative therapies in the previous year. Of these, 88% thought the care they received was either somewhat or very helpful. Most respondents (81%) reported using alternative therapies to prevent illness or to maintain wellness.

4. The correct answer is 1. Holistic nursing regards and treats the mind, body, and spirit of the client. Nurses can use holistic interventions such as relaxation therapy, guided imagery, music therapy, simple touch, massage, and prayer. Such interventions affect the whole person (mind-body-spirit) and are economical, non-invasive, non-pharmacological complements to medical care.

5. The correct answer is 1. Some CAM therapies and techniques use natural processes such as breathing, concentration, and simple touch to help clients feel better and cope with chronic conditions. Nurses can learn these kinds of techniques with minimum preparation, and many of these procedures can be used with clients as independent nursing practice (Dossey et al., 2000). Adequate assessment and the client's permission are prerequisite for implementation.

6. The correct answer is 1. One of the principles of these therapies is that the individual must be actively involved in the treatment. Clients achieve better responses if they practice the techniques or exercises daily. The client must commit to implementing and maintaining the therapy until a desired outcome is achieved.

7. The correct answer is 3. St. John's Wort is effective as a mild antidepressant and sedative, along with offering some protection against viruses. Clinical trials investigating the effectiveness of St. John's Wort against AIDS have begun.

8. The correct answer is 1. Meditation can augment the effects of certain drugs. For example, individuals taking anti-hypertensive, thyroid-regulating, antidepressant, or anti-anxiety medications should be monitored. Prolonged practice of meditation techniques may, in some cases, lead to the reduced need for certain medications, and some doses of medications may need to be adjusted.

9. The correct answer is 2. Biofeedback techniques are frequently used in addition to relaxation interventions to assist individuals in learning how to control specific autonomic nervous system responses.

10. The correct answer is 2. Therapeutic touch (TT) is a training-specific therapy that was developed in the 1970s by a nurse, Dr. Dolores Krieger. Although the philosophical and religious assumptions of TT are different from those of other Eastern healing modalities, they are similar in that both involve trained practitioners who attempt to direct their own balanced energies in an intentional and motivated manner toward those of the client.

Chapter 32

1. The correct answer is 3. To reduce the risk of injury to the client or nurse, the nurse must know and practise proper body mechanics. This includes knowledge of the actions of various muscle groups, understanding of the factors involved in the coordination of body movement, and familiarity with the integrated functioning of the skeletal, muscular, and nervous systems.

2. The correct answer is 1. Proprioception is the awareness of the position of the body and its parts. Proprioception is monitored by proprioceptors located on nerve endings in muscles, tendons, and joints. Posture is regulated by the nervous system and requires coordination of proprioception and balance.

3. The correct answer is 2. When standing, running, lifting, or performing activities of daily living (ADLs), a person must have adequate balance. Balance is controlled by the nervous system, specifically by the cerebellum and the inner ear. The major function of the cerebellum is to coordinate all voluntary movement, particularly highly skilled movements, such as those required in skiing.

4. The correct answer is 1. A client with a right-sided cerebral hemorrhage and damage to the right motor strip may have left-sided hemiplegia. However, a client with a right-sided head injury may only have cerebral edema (but not destruction) of the motor strip.

5. The correct answer is 1. Older adults may walk more slowly and appear less coordinated. They may also take smaller steps, keeping their feet closer together, which decreases the base of support. Thus, body balance may become unstable, and they are at greater risk for falls and injuries.

6. The correct answer is 4. Clients are more open to developing an exercise program if they are at the stage of readiness to change their behaviour. Information on the benefits of regular exercise may be helpful to the client who is not at the stage of readiness to act.

7. The correct answer is 2. It has become increasingly clear that children are becoming less active, resulting in an increase in childhood obesity. Children and adolescents spend a great deal of their time in school; however, in Canada today most children do not receive the recommended five periods of physical activity per week. Physical education has become an optional subject in most secondary schools, and only 18% of teenagers are accumulating enough daily activity to meet the international guidelines for optimal growth and development.

8. The correct answer is 2. Bending at the knees helps to maintain the nurse's centre of gravity and lets the strong muscles of the legs do the lifting.

9. The correct answer is 2. If the client has a syncopal episode or begins to fall, the nurse should assume a wide base of support with one foot in front of the other, thus supporting the client's body weight. The nurse then extends one leg and lets the client slide against the leg and gently lowers the client to the floor, protecting the client's head.

10. The correct answer is 3. In a three-point gait, weight is borne on both crutches and then on the uninvolved leg, and the sequence is repeated. The affected leg does not touch the ground during the early phase of the three-point gait.

Chapter 33

1. The correct answer is 3. Noise pollution occurs when the noise level in an environment becomes uncomfortable to the inhabitants of the environment. A health care facility can be polluted by noise. The sounds of machines, people talking, intercoms, and paging systems can create increased noise levels. It may produce a syndrome called *sensory overload,* which is a marked increase in the intensity of auditory and visual stimuli.

2. The correct answer is 2. In Canada, accidental injuries are the leading cause of death for people between the ages of 1 and 44 years.

3. The correct answer is 3. Motor vehicle accidents are the leading cause of accidental injury, followed by falls and fire.

4. The correct answer is 2. Adolescents are at risk for injury from motor vehicle accidents, suicide, and substance abuse.

5. The correct answer is 1. Advancing age and the concurrent physiological changes in vision, hearing, mobility, reflexes, circulation, and the ability to make quick judgments all predispose older adults to falls.

6. The correct answer is 2. WHMIS consists of three main elements: worker education programs, cautionary labelling of products, and provision of Material Safety Data Sheets (MSDSs).

7. The correct answer is 2. Procedure-related accidents occur during therapy. They include medication and fluid administration errors, improper application of external devices, and accidents related to improper performance of procedures (e.g., Foley catheter insertion).

8. The correct answer is 3. Restraints are NOT considered a long-term intervention. Restraints are used only after other alternatives have been tried, and the least restrictive method of restraint is used. The use of restraints must be part of the client's medical treatment. Restraints are considered a short-term intervention, and once they have been applied, regu-

lar assessments are needed to determine whether or not they should be continued.

9. The correct answer is 3. The poison control centre phone number should be visible on the telephone in homes with young children. In all cases of suspected poisoning, this number should be called immediately.

10. The correct answer is 4. When a client is having a seizure, the nurse should NOT insert a tongue depressor into the client's mouth. Significant injury to the client's oral cavity is rare, even during the most violent seizures. Injury may instead occur from a caregiver forcing an object into the client's mouth and from the teeth biting down on a hard object. Soft objects may break in the mouth during a seizure and be aspirated. Therefore, Epilepsy Canada recommends not inserting objects into the person's mouth during a seizure.

Chapter 34

1. The correct answer is 1. Because hygiene care requires close contact with the client, the nurse uses communication skills to promote a caring therapeutic relationship and to use the time with the client for teaching and counselling. The nurse can integrate other nursing activities during hygiene care, including client assessment and interventions such as range-of-motion exercises, application of dressings, or inspection and care of intravenous sites.

2. The correct answer is 3. A client's personal preferences for hygiene are influenced by a number of factors. No two individuals perform hygiene in the same manner, and it is important that the nurse individualize the client's care from knowledge about the client's unique hygiene practices and preferences. Hygiene care is never routine.

3. The correct answer is 4. Head lice require a source of human blood to survive. Transmission is by direct contact (i.e., head to head). The parasite is found on scalp attached to hair strands.

4. The correct answer is 1. Clients most in need of perineal care are those at greatest risk for acquiring an infection (e.g., clients who have in-dwelling urinary catheters, clients who are recovering from rectal or genital surgery or childbirth, or uncircumcised males).

5. The correct answer is 1. A back rub or back massage usually follows the client's bath. It promotes relaxation, relieves muscular tension, and stimulates skin circulation.

6. The correct answer is 2. Clients will experience conditions that threaten the integrity of oral mucosa. For example, mucosal changes associated with aging, use of chemotherapeutic drugs, or dehydration requires the nurse to adapt oral hygiene approaches. More frequent mouth care and use of anti-infective agents are examples of ways the nurse will revise approaches to meet client needs.

7. The correct answer is 3. Unconscious clients and those with artificial airways (e.g., endotracheal or tracheal tubes) need more frequent and specialized oral hygiene. These clients have an increased risk of aspiration and subsequently aspiration pneumonia, and they also have more problems with dry and inflamed oral mucosa.

8. The correct answer is 2. Depending on the client's age and physical condition, the room temperature should be maintained between 20° C and 23° C. Infants, older adults, and the acutely ill may need a warmer room. However, certain ill clients benefit from cooler room temperatures to lower the body's metabolic demands.

9. The correct answer is 2. File the toenails straight across and square; do not use scissors or clippers. Consult a podiatrist as needed.

10. The correct answer is 4. In an open bed, the top covers are folded back so that a client can easily get into bed.

Chapter 35

1. The correct answer is 1. Anemia, a lower than normal hemoglobin level, is a result of decreased hemoglobin production, increased red blood cell destruction, and/or blood loss. Clients will have complaints of fatigue, decreased activity tolerance, and increased breathlessness, as well as pallor (especially seen in the conjunctiva of the eye) and an increased heart rate.

2. The correct answer is 2. Carbon monoxide is the most common toxic inhalant that decreases the oxygen-carrying capacity of blood. The affinity for hemoglobin to bind with carbon monoxide is greater than 200 times its affinity to bind with oxygen, creating a functional anemia. Because of the bond's strength, carbon monoxide is not easily dissociated from hemoglobin, making the hemoglobin unavailable for oxygen transport.

3. The correct answer is 1. Hypovolemia is caused by conditions such as shock and severe dehydration resulting from extracellular fluid loss and reduced circulating blood volume. With a significant fluid loss, the body tries to adapt by increasing the heart rate and peripheral vasoconstriction to increase the volume of blood returned to the heart and, in turn, increase the cardiac output.

4. The correct answer is 3. Fever increases the tissues' need for oxygen, and as a result, carbon dioxide production also increases. If the febrile state persists, the metabolic rate remains high and the body begins to break down protein stores, resulting in

muscle wasting and decreased muscle mass. Respiratory muscles such as the diaphragm and intercostal muscles are also wasted.

5. The correct answer is 1. Left-sided heart failure is an abnormal condition characterized by impaired functioning of the left ventricle as a result of elevated pressures and pulmonary congestion. If left ventricular failure is significant, the amount of blood ejected from the left ventricle drops greatly, resulting in decreased cardiac output.

6. The correct answer is 1. Right-sided heart failure results from impaired functioning of the right ventricle characterized by venous congestion in the systemic circulation. Right-sided heart failure more commonly results from pulmonary disease or as a result of long-term left-sided failure. Right-sided heart failure results from impaired functioning of the right ventricle characterized by venous congestion in the systemic circulation. Right-sided heart failure more commonly results from pulmonary disease or as a result of long-term left-sided failure. As the failure continues, the amount of blood ejected from the right ventricle declines, and blood begins to "back up" in the systemic circulation. Clinically, the client has weight gain, distended neck veins, hepatomegaly and splenomegaly, and dependent peripheral edema.

7. The correct answer is 2. Cyanosis, blue discolouration of the skin and mucous membranes caused by the presence of desaturated hemoglobin in capillaries, is a late sign of hypoxia. The presence or absence of cyanosis is not a reliable measure of oxygenation status.

8. The correct answer is 1. A person who starts smoking in adolescence and continues to smoke into middle age has an increased risk for cardiopulmonary disease and lung cancer.

9. The correct answer is 3. Frequent changes of position are simple and cost-effective methods for reducing the risks of stasis of pulmonary secretions and decreased chest wall expansion.

10. The correct answer is 4. The most effective position for clients with cardiopulmonary diseases is the 45-degree semi-Fowler's position, using gravity to assist in lung expansion and reduce pressure from the abdomen on the diaphragm.

Chapter 36

1. The correct answer is 1. Hypokalemia is one of the most common electrolyte imbalances, in which an inadequate amount of potassium circulates in ECF. When severe, hypokalemia can affect cardiac conduction and function. Because the normal amount of serum potassium is so small, there is little tolerance for fluctuations. The most common cause of hypokalemia is the use of potassium-wasting diuretics such as thiazide and loop diuretics.

2. The correct answer is 4. An infant's proportion of total body water (70% to 80% total body weight) is greater that that of children or adults. Infants are not protected from fluid loss because they ingest and excrete a relatively greater daily water volume than do adults. Therefore, they are at a greater risk for fluid volume deficit (FVD) and hyperosmolar imbalance because body water loss is proportionately greater per kilogram of weight.

3. The correct answer is 2. Older adults experience a number of age-related changes that can affect fluid, electrolyte, and acid-base balances. They have a decreased thirst sensation, which may affect their oral intake of fluids. The kidneys have a decrease in glomerular filtration rate and in the number of filtering nephrons. These changes can mean that in the presence of sodium depletion or overload, the older adult may be unable to maintain homeostasis and the imbalance is instead worsened.

4. The correct answer is 4. For clients in health care settings, intake and output (I&O) measurement is a nursing intervention routinely used for clients following a procedure, clients who are febrile, clients with restricted fluids, or clients who receive diuretic or intravenous (IV) therapy. Output includes urine, diarrhea, vomitus, gastric suction, and drainage from post-surgical wounds or other tubes.

5. The correct answer is 1. Health promotion activities in the area of fluid, electrolyte, and acid-base imbalances focus primarily on client teaching. Clients and caregivers need to recognize risk factors for these imbalances and implement appropriate preventive measures.

6. The correct answer is 3. Total parenteral nutrition is a nutritionally adequate hypertonic solution consisting of glucose and other nutrients and electrolytes given through an in-dwelling or central IV catheter that may be inserted peripherally or percutaneously, implanted, or tunnelled. TPN is used as an intervention in severe cases of malnutrition.

7. The correct answer is 1. Under no circumstances should potassium chloride (KCl) be given IV push. A direct IV infusion of KCl may be fatal. If an IV is to have additives added, a physician's order must be obtained that includes the required additives.

8. The correct answer is 1. The client's microflora and contamination by insertion are initially controlled for in the procedure for IV insertion. However, the other factors are controlled through conscientious use of infection-control principles. This begins with thorough hand hygiene before and after the nurse handles any component of the IV system.

9. The correct answer is 3. An infiltration occurs when IV fluids enter the surrounding space around the venipuncture site. This is manifested as swelling

(from increased tissue fluid) and pallor and coolness (caused by decreased circulation) around the venipuncture site.

10. The correct answer is 1. Phlebitis may be prevented by the routine removal and rotation of IV sites. The Centers for Disease Control and Prevention (CDC) recommends replacing peripheral venous catheters and rotating sites at least every 72 to 96 hours.

Chapter 37

1. The correct answer is 4. Excessive daytime sleepiness (EDS) is the most common complaint of people with obstructive sleep apnea (OSA). People with severe OSA may report experiencing a disruption in their daily activities because of sleepiness.

2. The correct answer is 2. In hospitals and long-term care facilities, it is difficult to provide clients with the time needed to rest and sleep. However, the nurse plans care to avoid awakening clients for non-essential tasks. The nurse can schedule assessments, treatments, procedures, and routines for times when clients are awake. For example, a nurse should not wake a stable client to check vital signs.

3. The correct answer is 1. The use of non-prescription sleeping medications is not advisable. Clients should learn the risks of such drugs. Over the long term, these drugs can lead to further sleep disruption even when they initially seemed to be effective. Older adults should be cautioned about using over-the-counter antihistamines because of their long duration of action that can cause confusion, constipation, urinary retention, and increased risk of falls.

4. The correct answer is 1. Clients should be cautioned about the dosage and use of herbal compounds because active ingredients can vary from product to product. Herbal compounds may create interactions with prescribed medication, and concurrent use should be avoided.

5. The correct answer is 1. Although dreams occur during both non-rapid eye movement (NREM) and rapid eye movement (REM) sleep, the dreams of REM sleep are more vivid and elaborate and are believed to be functionally important to learning, memory processing, and adaptation to stress

6. The correct answer is 3. Beta-adrenergic agents can cause nightmares, insomnia, and awakenings from sleep.

7. The correct answer is 4. Limiting alcohol, caffeine, and nicotine and decreasing fluids 2 to 4 hours before sleep may promote sleep for older adults.

8. The correct answer is 4. The Canadian Paediatric Society recommends that apparently healthy infants be placed in the supine position during sleep because of an association between the prone position and the occurrence of sudden infant death syndrome (SIDS).

9. The correct answer is 4. Narcolepsy is a dysfunction of mechanisms that regulate the sleep and wake states. Excessive daytime sleepiness (EDS) is the most common complaint associated with this disorder. During the day, the person may suddenly feel an overwhelming wave of sleepiness and fall asleep; REM sleep can occur within 15 minutes of falling asleep.

10. The correct answer is 4. Sleep needed during the school years is individualized because of varying activity and health levels. Six-year-olds average 11 to 12 hours of sleep nightly, whereas 11-year-olds sleep 9 to 10 hours. The 6- or 7-year-old can usually be persuaded to go to bed by encouraging quiet activities.

Chapter 38

1. The correct answer is 1. Although traditionally pain has been viewed simply as a symptom of an illness or condition, pain itself is now considered to be a separate disease.

2. The correct answer is 2. Chronic pain is generally defined as pain that has been present for at least 6 months, persists beyond the normal time of healing, may not have an identifiable cause, serves no biological benefit, and leads to great personal suffering.

3. The correct answer is 3. One of the common misconceptions about pain management is that administering analgesics regularly will lead to drug addiction.

4. The correct answer is 1. Cognitively, toddlers and preschoolers are unable to recall explanations about pain or associate pain with experiences that can occur in various situations.

5. The correct answer is 4. An accurate diagnosis is made only after a complete assessment has been performed. In the diagnosis of pain, the nurse considers the client's withdrawal from communication, grimacing, moaning, and verbalizations of discomfort.

6. The correct answer is 3. Descriptive scales are used both to assess pain severity and evaluate changes in a client's condition. A rating of 7 or more on a 0 to 10 scale requires immediate attention. The dose was insufficient.

7. The correct answer is 2. Teaching clients about pain reduces anxiety and helps them achieve a sense of control. When a client is anticipating pain, the nurse needs to explain procedures and associated discomfort. A confident explanation of the procedure helps a client place trust in a nurse. When clients are informed about an upcoming painful experience, they often perceive the actual experience as less unpleasant.

8. The correct answer is 1. Non-pharmacological interventions include cognitive-behavioural and physical approaches. The goals of cognitive-behavioural interventions are to change pain perceptions, alter pain behaviour, and provide a greater sense of control. Relaxation and guided imagery are examples.

9. The correct answer is 3. One way to maximize pain relief while minimizing drug toxicity is to administer the medication on a regular around-the-clock (ATC) basis rather than on an as-needed (prn) basis. The Canadian Pain Society, the American Pain Society, and the AHCPR have stated that if pain is anticipated for the majority of the day, ATC administration should be considered. This is to prevent breakthrough pain, which is hard to control once it appears.

10. The correct answer is 3. A drug delivery system called patient-controlled analgesia (PCA) is a safe method for post-operative and cancer pain management that most clients prefer. The client gains control over pain, and pain relief does not depend on nurse availability. Small doses of medications are delivered at short intervals, stabilizing serum drug concentrations for sustained pain relief.

Chapter 39

1. The correct answer is 4. Carbohydrates are the main source of energy in the diet.

2. The correct answer is 2. Proteins are essential for synthesis (building) of body tissue in growth, maintenance, and repair.

3. The correct answer is 4. When the intake of nitrogen exceeds the output, the body is in positive nitrogen balance, which is required for growth, normal pregnancy, maintenance of lean muscle mass and vital organs, and wound healing.

4. The correct answer is 1. Water composes 60% to 70% of total body weight.

5. The correct answer is 2. The most reliable method for verification of placement of small-bore feeding tubes is X-ray examination.

6. The correct answer is 2. Parenteral nutrition (PN) is a form of specialized nutrition support in which nutrients are provided intravenously. Clients who are unable to digest or absorb enteral nutrition benefit from PN. Clients in highly stressed physiological states such as sepsis, head injury, or burns are also candidates for PN therapy.

7. The correct answer is 2. *Helicobacter pylori* is a bacterium that causes peptic ulcers.

8. The correct answer is 1. Inflammatory bowel disease includes Crohn's disease and idiopathic ulcerative colitis.

9. The correct answer is 3. Nutritional therapy for hypertension includes kilocalorie reduction to promote weight loss as appropriate, decreased sodium intake, and potassium-rich foods if potassium-wasting diuretics are part of the treatment.

10. The correct answer is 2. Home-bound older adults with chronic illness have an increased risk of poor nutrition.

Chapter 40

1. The correct answer is 2. The normal adult urine output is 1,500 to 1,600 mL/day.

2. The correct answer is 1. Renal alterations result from factors that cause injury directly to the glomeruli or renal tubule, interfering with their normal filtering, reabsorptive, and secretory functions. Selected causes include transfusion reactions, diseases of the glomeruli, and systemic diseases such as diabetes mellitus.

3. The correct answer is 2. Postrenal alterations result from obstruction to the flow of urine in the urinary collecting system anywhere between the renal pelvis and urethral meatus. Urine is formed by the urinary system but cannot be eliminated by normal means. Urinary obstruction can be caused by calculi (stones), blood clots, or tumours.

4. The correct answer is 3. Acidic urine inhibits bacterial growth and may prevent UTIs. Therefore, fluids that promote an acidic urine (e.g., cranberry juice) should be made available as part of the fluid intake for clients at risk for UTI.

5. The correct answer is 3. Hospital-acquired UTIs are often related to poor hand hygiene, improper catheter care, or faulty catheterization technique.

6. The correct answer is 1. The urine appears concentrated and cloudy because of the presence of white blood cells (WBCs) or bacteria.

7. The correct answer is 1. Prompted voiding is a useful strategy for clients with cognitive and/or physical impairment who rely on caregiver assistance.

8. The correct answer is 3. With stress incontinence, urine loss results from increased intra-abdominal pressure (e.g., coughing, sneezing, laughing, lifting). It usually involves a small volume of urine loss (less than 50 mL); it usually occurs in women or in men following radical prostatectomy. Pregnancy and delivery, weak pelvic floor muscles, heavy lifting, and obesity are sometimes contributing factors.

9. The correct answer is 1. The drainage bag should never be raised above the level of the client's bladder. The bag should hang on the bed frame or wheelchair without touching the floor. Urine in the bag and tubing can become a medium for bacteria,

and infection is likely to develop if urine flows back into the bladder.

10. The correct answer is 4. Care must be taken to ensure that whatever type or size of condom is used, blood supply to the penis is not impaired. Therefore the condom should be snug and secure but does not cause constriction to blood flow.

Chapter 41

1. The correct answer is 4. Most nutrients and electrolytes are absorbed in the small intestine, specifically by the duodenum and jejunum.

2. The correct answer is 3. Lactose intolerance is the inability to digest lactose, the predominant sugar in milk and milk products. It is caused by a shortage of the enzyme lactase, which is normally produced by the cells that line the small intestine and is needed to digest lactose. Lactase frequently disappears in adulthood, and as a result, lactose cannot be absorbed, resulting in diarrhea, gaseous distension, and cramping.

3. The correct answer is 4. A common laboratory test that can be done at home or at the client's bedside is the fecal occult blood testing (FOBT), or guaiac test, which measures microscopic amounts of blood in feces. It is useful as a diagnostic screening test for colon cancer.

4. The correct answer is 1. Antidiarrheal opiate agents decrease intestinal muscle tone to slow passage of feces. Opiates inhibit peristaltic waves that move feces forward, but they also increase segmental contractions that mix intestinal contents and expose the contents to the mucosal absorbing surface.

5. The correct answer is 3. An obvious sign of impaction is the inability to pass a stool for several days, despite the repeated urge to defecate. When a continuous oozing of diarrhea stool develops, impaction should be suspected. The liquid portion of feces located higher in the colon seeps around the impacted mass.

6. The correct answer is 4. Cleansing enemas promote the complete evacuation of feces from the colon. The maximum amount given to an adult is 750 to 1,000 mL.

7. The correct answer is 3. The specific signs and symptoms of a client not tolerating an enema include abdominal pain more than a pressure sensation, abdominal cramping, abdominal distension, or rectal bleeding. The enema must be stopped. Notify physician and obtain vital signs.

8. The correct answer is 2. One of the greatest problems in caring for a client with an NG tube is maintaining comfort. The tube is a constant irritation to nasal mucosa. The nurse must assess the condition of the nares and mucosa for inflammation and excoriation.

9. The correct answer is 1. The stool discharged from an ostomy is called effluent.

10. The correct answer is 1. A nurse trained to care for ostomy clients is an enterostomal therapist (ET).

Chapter 42

1. The correct answer is 2. Footdrop is the inability to dorsiflex and invert the foot because of peroneal nerve damage. The foot is permanently fixed in plantar flexion and the person is therefore unable to lift the toes off the ground.

2. The correct answer is 2. The effects of bed rest or immobilization on the cardiovascular system include orthostatic hypotension, increased cardiac workload, and thrombus formation.

3. The correct answer is 1. After bed rest, clients usually have increased pulse rate and decreased pulse pressure and blood pressure. A large decrease in blood pressure when arising to a sitting or standing position (a drop of 20 mm Hg or more in systolic blood pressure and of 10 mm Hg in diastolic blood pressure) is known as orthostatic hypotension, and can result in light-headedness and fainting.

4. The correct answer is 3. Elastic stockings (sometimes called thromboembolic device hose; TED) help to maintain external pressure on the muscles of the lower extremities and thus may promote venous return.

5. The correct answer is 3. Immobility can have a significant effect on the older adult's levels of health, independence, and functional status.

6. The correct answer is 4. Increased activity may result in symptoms associated with activity intolerance (e.g., increased pulse, changes in blood pressure, increased respirations, and decreased level of comfort). This can jeopardize the client's safety.

7. The correct answer is 1. Heparin and low-molecular-weight heparin (LMWH) are the most widely used drugs in the prophylaxis of deep vein thrombosis (DVT). Standard heparin is considered the gold standard for treatment because it has been well studied and validated. Common dosage for heparin therapy is 5,000 units given subcutaneously 2 hours before surgery and repeated every 8 to 12 hours until the client is fully mobile or discharged.

8. The correct answer is 1. The trapeze bar is a triangular device that descends from a securely fastened overhead bar attached to the bed frame. It allows the client to use the upper extremities to raise the trunk off the bed, to assist in transfer from bed to wheelchair, or to perform upper arm exercises.

9. The correct answer is 2. The client in the prone position is lying face or chest down.

10. The correct answer is 3. When a client is in supported Fowler's position, placing a small pillow or roll under the thigh prevents occlusion of popliteal artery from pressure from body weight. It also prevents hyperextension of the knee.

Chapter 43

1. The correct answer is 1. A stage I pressure ulcer is an observable pressure-related alteration of intact skin whose indicators, as compared with an adjacent or opposite area on the body, may include changes in skin temperature (warmth or coolness), tissue consistency (firm or beefy feel), and/or sensation (pain, itching).

2. The correct answer is 2. Serous drainage is clear, watery plasma.

3. The correct answer is 3. When evisceration occurs, the nurse places sterile towels soaked in sterile saline over the extruding tissues to reduce chances of bacterial invasion and drying of the tissues. If the organs protrude through the wound, blood supply to the tissues is compromised. The client should be allowed nothing by mouth (NPO), observed for signs and symptoms of shock, and prepared for emergency surgery.

4. The correct answer is 4. When the skin is being compressed, blood flow is slowed and the skin becomes pale. After the pressure is relieved, the skin in the affected area turns red (erythema), a result of the blood vessels expanding (vasodilation) to allow more blood into the area to overcome the ischemic episode. This process is called normal reactive hyperemia. The nurse assesses the reddened area by pressing a fingertip over it. If the area blanches (turns white or pale colour) and the erythema returns when the finger is removed, the reactive hyperemia is likely transient. If, however, the reddened area does not blanch when finger pressure is applied (abnormal reactive hyperemia), deep tissue damage should be suspected (Figure 43-11).

5. The correct answer is 4. If the nurse detects purulent or suspicious-looking wound drainage, or observes a change in a previously healing chronic wound, obtaining a specimen of the drainage for culture may be necessary. The nurse never collects a wound culture sample from old drainage. Resident colonies of bacteria from the skin grow within exudate and may not be the true causative organisms of a wound infection. The nurse cleans a wound first with normal saline to remove skin flora.

6. The correct answer is 1. To reduce the risk of pressure ulcers, the nurse should position the client alternately in the supine position and in a 30-degree lateral position to either side in order to avoid lying the client over a bony prominence.

7. The correct answer is 4. Hydrocolloid dressings are dressings with complex formulations of colloids, elastomeric, and adhesive components. These dressings are adhesive and occlusive. The wound contact layer of this dressing forms a gel as fluid is absorbed and maintains a moist healing environment.

8. The correct answer is 3. To provide even support to a wound and immobilize a body part, the nurse may apply elastic gauze or cloth bandages and binders over a dressing.

9. The correct answer is 2. For a client who has a muscle sprain, localized hemorrhage, or hematoma or who has undergone dental surgery, an ice bag is ideal to prevent edema formation, control bleeding, and anaesthetize the body part.

10. The correct answer is 1. For open wounds, sterile, warm, moist compresses improve circulation, relieve edema, and promote consolidation of pus and drainage.

Chapter 44

1. The correct answer is 2. A kinesthetic sense enables a person to be aware of the position and movement of body parts without seeing them.

2. The correct answer is 1. Stereognosis is a sense that allows a person to recognize an object's size, shape, and texture.

3. The correct answer is 3. When a person receives multiple sensory stimuli and cannot perceptually disregard or selectively ignore some stimuli, sensory overload occurs. The client in constant pain or who undergoes frequent monitoring of vital signs is at risk. Multiple stimuli can combine to cause overload.

4. The correct answer is 2. Proprioceptive changes after the age of 60 years include increased difficulty with balance, spatial orientation, and coordination.

5. The correct answer is 4. For a client with hearing impairment, the nurse should face the client when speaking, use simple sentences, and speak more slowly and in a normal volume.

6. The correct answer is 4. The nursing health history includes assessment of the nature and characteristics of sensory alterations or any problem related to an alteration. The nurse begins by asking the client to describe the sensory deficit. For example, "How does your hearing now compare with your hearing a year ago?"

7. The correct answer is 2. For older adults: Do not drive during rush hour. Use rear-view and side-view

mirrors when changing lanes. Avoid driving at dusk or night. Go slow, but not too slow. Keep the car in good working condition.

8. The correct answer is 3. Hearing loss from noise-induced environments was once thought to affect primarily older individuals; however, recent research has observed this loss in youth. Nurses should routinely teach parents and children to take precautions when involved in activities associated with high-intensity noise. The nurse should assess clients for noise exposure and participate in providing hearing conservation classes for teachers, students, and clients.

9. The correct answer is 3. Olfactory is the sense of smell. If a client cannot smell, the client may not smell smoke if there were a fire. A fire alarm would be essential.

10. The correct answer is 1. When senses are impaired, the sense of self is impaired. Initially, a person may withdraw by avoiding communication or socialization with others in an attempt to cope with the sensory loss.

Chapter 45

1. The correct answer is 2. The obese client is susceptible to poor wound healing and wound infection because of the structure of fatty tissue, which contains a poor blood supply. This slows delivery of essential nutrients, antibodies, and enzymes needed for wound healing.

2. The correct answer is 3. If a client regularly uses prescription or over-the-counter medications, the surgeon or anaesthesiologist may temporarily discontinue the drugs before surgery or adjust the dosages. Certain medications have special implications for the surgical client, creating greater risks for complications or interacting with anaesthetic agents.

3. The correct answer is 2. The client who smokes is at greater risk for post-operative pulmonary complications than a client who does not.

4. The correct answer is 2. The family is an important resource for the client with physical limitations and provides the emotional support needed to motivate the client to return to a previous state of health. Often a family member can become the client's coach, offering valuable support during the post-operative period.

5. The correct answer is 1. Accurate recording of intake and output helps assess renal and circulatory function. The nurse measures all sources of output, including urine, surgically placed drains, gastric drainage, and drainage from wounds, and notes any insensible loss from diaphoresis.

6. The correct answer is 3. Position the client on one side with the face downward and the neck slightly extended to facilitate a forward movement of the tongue and the flow of mucous secretions out of the mouth.

7. The correct answer is 4. To promote normal venous return and circulatory blood flow, encourage clients to perform leg exercises at least every hour while awake. Other measures include applying elastic stockings or pneumatic compression stockings as ordered, encouraging early ambulation, positioning the client so that blood flow is not interrupted, administering anticoagulant drugs as ordered, and promoting adequate fluid intake.

8. The correct answer is 2. International normalized ratio (INR), activated partial thromboplastin time (APTT), and platelet counts reveal clotting ability of blood, which reveals clients at risk for bleeding tendencies and thrombus formation.

9. The correct answer is 2. Maintaining an upright position facilitates diaphragm excursion and enhances thorax expansion.

10. The correct answer is 4. Malignant hyperthermia is a potentially lethal condition that can occur in clients receiving general anaesthesia. It should be suspected when there is unexpected tachycardia and tachypnea; jaw muscle rigidity; body rigidity of limbs, abdomen, and chest; or hyperkalemia. Temperature elevation is a late sign.

Index

C

D

M

O

P

T

U

V

W

Special Features

Client Teaching

Concept Maps

Special Features—cont'd

Research Highlights

Nursing Care Plans

Procedural Guideline

Skills and Procedures

Special Features—cont'd